Brief Table  of Contents

Continued

Davis Advantage
for MEDICAL-SURGICAL NURSING
SECOND EDITION

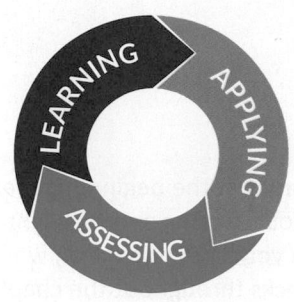

BUILDING **CONFIDENCE** & **KNOWLEDGE** for

- Class
- Exams
- NCLEX®

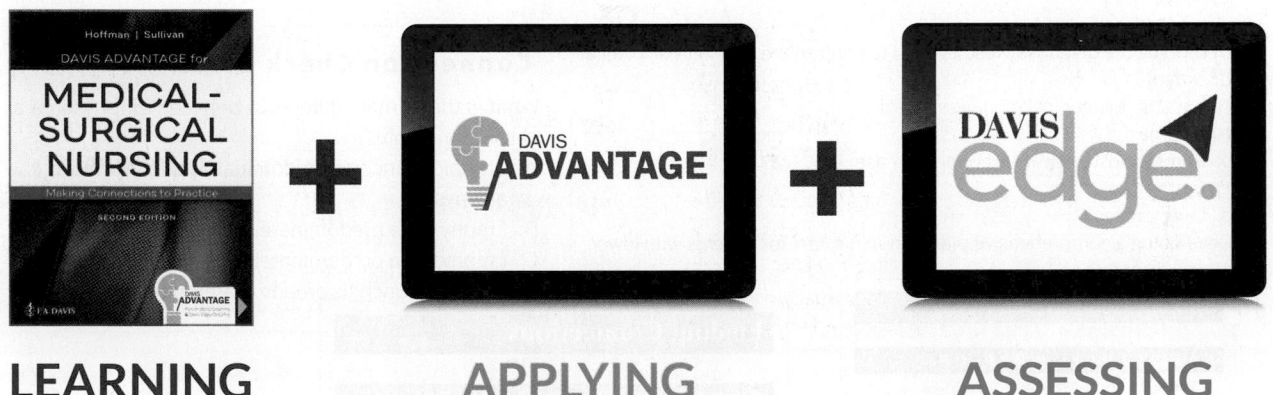

LEARNING + **APPLYING** + **ASSESSING**

Your journey to success begins here!

Davis Advantage for **Medical-Surgical Nursing** combines your textbook with an interactive, personalized learning and quizzing experience that makes this challenging, but must-know content easier to master.

Follow the instructions on the inside front cover.
UNLOCK YOUR RESOURCES TODAY!

Hoffman | Sullivan

DAVIS ADVANTAGE for

MEDICAL-SURGICAL NURSING

Making Connections to Practice

SECOND EDITION

F.A DAVIS

DAVIS ADVANTAGE
Personalized Learning
& Davis Edge Quizzing

LEARNING
APPLYING
ASSESSING
YOUR

LEARNING

Connecting concepts from the written word to the real world

Medical-Surgical Nursing, 2nd Edition helps you to make the connections between concepts and patient care to prepare you for real-world nursing practice.

STEP #1 Build a solid foundation.

LEARNING OUTCOMES

Content in this chapter is designed to assist in:

1. Describing the epidemiology of lower airway disorders
2. Correlating clinical manifestations to pathophysiological processes of:
   a. Asthma
   b. Chronic obstructive pulmonary disease
   c. Cystic fibrosis
   d. Lung cancer
3. Describing the diagnostic results used to confirm the diagnosis of lower airway disorders
4. Discussing the medical management of:
   a. Asthma
   b. Chronic obstructive pulmonary disease
   c. Cystic fibrosis
   d. Lung cancer
5. Developing a comprehensive plan of nursing care for patients with lower airway disorders
6. ~~rmacological, dietary, and lifes~~ ~~y diso~~

Learning Outcomes at the beginning of each chapter guide your reading and highlight the information you'll need to know, while **Connection Checks** throughout the chapters test how well you've mastered the material.

Connection Check 26.2

What is the primary difference between emphysema and chronic bronchitis?
A. Chronic bronchitis predominately affects the large airways.
B. Emphysema predominately affects the large airways.
C. Emphysema predominately affects the alveoli.
D. Chronic bronchitis predominately affects the alveoli.

Making Connections

CASE STUDY: WRAP-UP

Clifford continues to be short of breath and to wheeze. His SpO$_2$ remains acceptable while he receives oxygen via the nasal cannula. After the first three nebulizer treatments, his peak flow reading is repeated. It is slightly improved but not back to baseline. Clifford then receives Prednisone 60 mg intramuscularly (IM). The symptoms slowly begin to subside. A repeat of the peak flow reading reveals continued improvement. When Clifford's symptoms are fully resolved, he is discharged from the emergency department with a prescription for an oral prednisone taper. Before he leaves, hospital personnel ensure that he has an appointment with his primary care provider to review this hospital visit and update his asthma action plan.

Case Study Questions

1. What is the most important component of the medical management of Mr. Davis?
   A. Breathing techniques
   B. Disease management through education
   C. Use of "rescue" medications
   D. Use of a peak flow meter
2. If there are no wheezes and diminished breath sounds upon reassessment, what conclusion can the nurse make?
   A. Mr. Davis has resolved his respiratory condition.
   B. Mr. Davis has responded to the bronchodilator therapy.
   C. Mr. Davis has a partially obstructed airway.

Finding Connections

CASE STUDY: EPISODE 1

Follow this patient throughout the chapter.

Clifford Davis is a 39-year-old male with a history of asthma who presents to the emergency department with shortness of breath and inability to carry on a conversation. He is assuming a tripod position and exhibits pursed-lip breathing. He has a nonproductive cough. He woke up coughing, followed by chest tightness, which prompted a call to the rescue services. His vital signs are blood pressure (BP), 121/65 mm Hg; heart rate (HR), 150 bpm; respiratory rate (RR), 40. He has audible wheezes bilaterally. He has been a one-pack/day smoker for 15 years.

Finding Connections are case studies that illustrate key points and bring the content to life. Follow each case study as it unfolds throughout the chapter to see how the theory you're learning applies to practice. Then, answer the critical-thinking questions at the end of **Making Connections Case Study: Wrap-Up.**

Safety Alerts focus on potential hazardous or high-risk issues related to the specific chapter content.

Nursing Management provides clear and well-defined nursing care guidance to help you to understand the nurse's role. Begin with scientific explanations for presenting clinical manifestations, then follow the nursing process to prioritize care. For easy reference, **Nursing Interventions** are formatted into **Assessments**, **Actions**, and **Teaching** categories with bulleted rationales that explain the 'hows' and 'whys' of treatment.

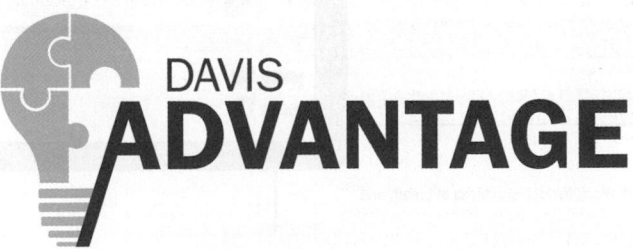
DAVIS ADVANTAGE

To explore learning resources for this chapter, go to **Davis Advantage** and find...

- Answers to in-text questions
- Chapter Resources and Activities
- NCLEX®-Style Chapter Review Questions
- Bibliography

Additional learning resources and activities are available for every chapter on **Davis Advantage**.

Nursing Management
Assessment and Analysis
The clinical manifestations presented by the patient are due to increased airway resistance, increased work of breathing, and increased sputum production. They include:

- Cough
- Increased sputum production
- Dyspnea
- Use of accessory muscles
- Tripod positioning
- Inability to talk in full sentences
- Pursed-lip breathing
- Changes in skin coloring
- Anxiety

Nursing Diagnoses
- **Impaired gas exchange** related to altered oxygen delivery and alveoli destruction
- **Ineffective airway clearance** related to decreased energy, dyspnea, ineffective cough
- **Activity intolerance** related to fatigue and dyspnea
- **Anxiety** related to breathlessness

Nursing Interventions
■ **Assessments**
- Oxygen saturation
  An SpO₂ of less than 90% indicates a significant oxygenation problem. The goal is to maintain the SpO₂ at 90% or above.
- Respiratory rate
  Monitor respiratory rate to avoid hypoventilation—the respiratory drive in COPD is hypoxemia, not hypercapnia. See Safety Alert.
- Breath sounds
  The presence of crackles and wheezes may indicate airway obstruction. Crackles indicate the premature closing of the airways.
- Pursed-lip breathing
  Patients with COPD display pursed-lip breathing to keep the airways open longer and prolong exhalation, allowing for increased time for oxygen and carbon dioxide exchange.
- Cough
  Cough is a cardinal sign of pulmonary disease. It is a protective mechanism for the tracheobronchial tree.
- Temperature
  Increased temperature is a sign of an infectious trigger.
- Dyspnea
  Use of the visual analog dyspnea scale allows the patient to identify his or her own level of dyspnea because dyspnea is a subjective experience.
- Weight
  Monitoring weight identifies nutritional deficiencies—with prolonged increased work of breathing and decreased energy, the ability to eat decreases.

■ **Actions**
- Administer bronchodilators as ordered.
  Bronchodilators are bronchial smooth muscle relaxants that help open the airway. Beta₂-agonists (short-acting beta-agonists [SABAs] and long-acting beta-agonists [LABAs]) relax the smooth muscles of the airway by stimulating beta-adrenergic receptors, resulting in antagonism to bronchoconstriction. Anticholinergics relax and enlarge the airways in the lungs, making breathing easier. Also, anticholinergics can also protect the airways from bronchospasm and may reduce the amount of mucus produced by the airways.
- Provide oxygen.
  Increase the SpO₂ to 90%. Patients may be placed on continuous oxygen therapy if the SpO₂ is less than or equal to 88% or the PaO₂ is less than or equal to 60 mm Hg.
- Position—semi-Fowler's
  The semi-Fowler's position increases oxygenation by allowing adequate lung expansion.
- Provide small, frequent meals with dietary supplements.
  Small, frequent meals take less energy to consume and avoid excessive pressure on the diaphragm that may be associated with a large meal.

■ **Teaching**
- Breathing techniques—pursed-lip breathing (Box 26.3)
  Pursed-lip breathing keeps the airways open longer and prolongs exhalation, allowing for increased time for oxygen and carbon dioxide exchange.
- Pacing of activities
  Pacing decreases the work of breathing and conserves energy.

LEARNING
APPLYING
ASSESSING

DAVIS
ADVANTAGE

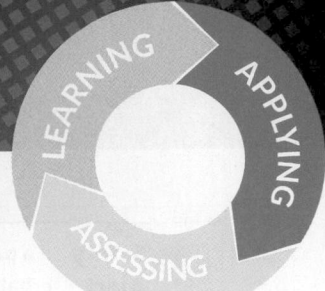

APPLYING

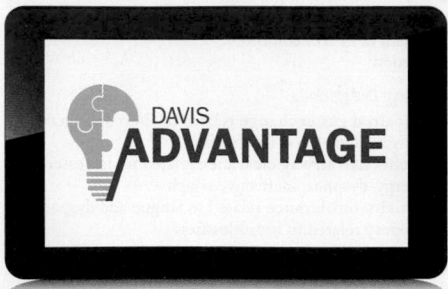

A personalized learning experience tailored to your needs

Put a study plan to work that's based on your strengths and weaknesses. Engaging, interactive content helps you make the connections and master key Med-Surg topics.

STEP #2 Make the connections and apply your knowledge.

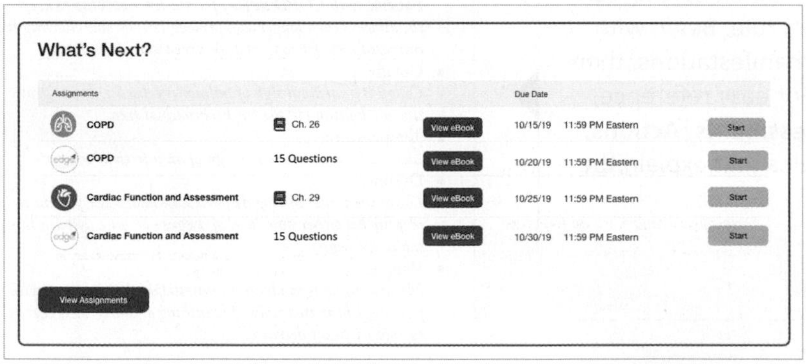
What's Next?
Assignments
Due Date
COPD
Ch. 26
View eBook
10/15/19 11:59 PM Eastern
Start
COPD
15 Questions
View eBook
10/20/19 11:59 PM Eastern
Start
Cardiac Function and Assessment
Ch. 29
View eBook
10/25/19 11:59 PM Eastern
Start
Cardiac Function and Assessment
15 Questions
View eBook
10/30/19 11:59 PM Eastern
Start
View Assignments

Assignments in Davis Advantage are mapped to a specific chapter in your book. Begin by reading from your printed text or click the ebook button to be taken to the chapter in your **FREE integrated ebook.**

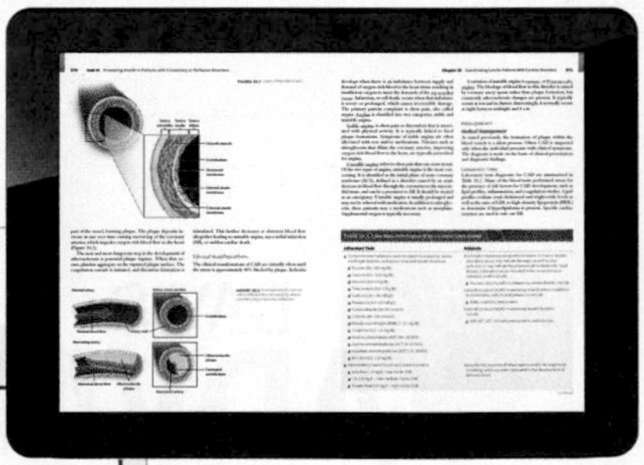

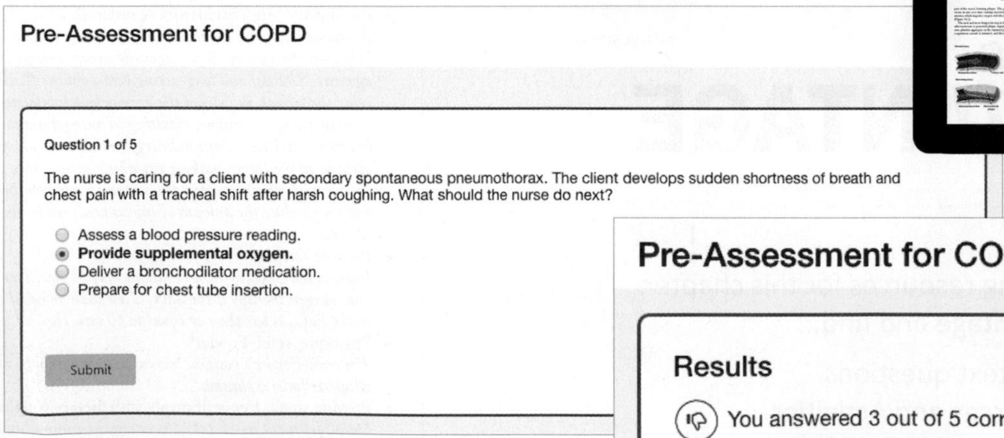
Pre-Assessment for COPD
Question 1 of 5
The nurse is caring for a client with secondary spontaneous pneumothorax. The client develops sudden shortness of breath and chest pain with a tracheal shift after harsh coughing. What should the nurse do next?
Assess a blood pressure reading.
Provide supplemental oxygen.
Deliver a bronchodilator medication.
Prepare for chest tube insertion.
Submit

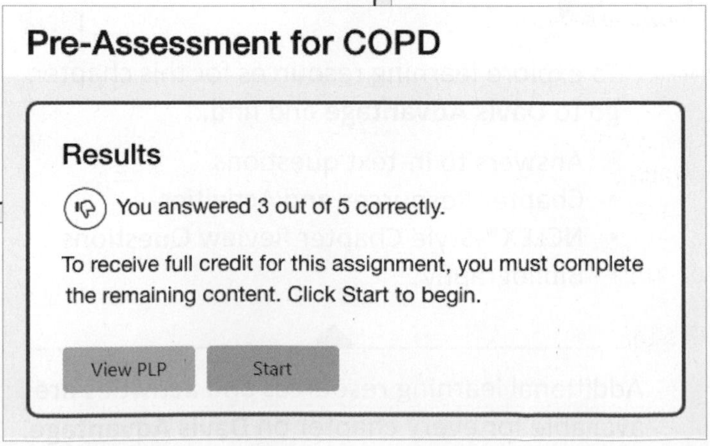
Pre-Assessment for COPD
Results
You answered 3 out of 5 correctly.
To receive full credit for this assignment, you must complete the remaining content. Click Start to begin.
View PLP
Start

Following your reading, take the **Pre-Assessment** quiz to evaluate your understanding of the content. You'll receive **immediate feedback** that identifies your strengths and weaknesses.

Don't miss the complete list of videos in the back of the book.

COPD

Video

Activity

Post-Assessment

Chronic Obstructive Pulmonary Disease (COPD)

alpha-1 antitrypsin

80%-90%

View Transcript   Next

Animated mini-lecture videos make key concepts easier to understand, while **interactive learning activities** allow you to apply your knowledge and make the connections.

COPD

Video

Activity

Post-Assessment

Question 1 of 8

This or That? For each topic, select the answer which best classifies the following vocabulary term or patient data.

Caused by the destruction of alveoli

Chronic Bronchitis   Emphysema   Both

INCORRECT. Hypoxemia refractory to the administration of oxygen therapy is common in patients who are diagnosed with ARDS; therefore, the priority nursing action is to monitor pulse oximetry readings. A decrease in pulse oximetry readings from the baseline occurs due to intrapulmonary shunting. While auscultating heart sounds may be required, it is more appropriate to auscultate lung sounds as crackles may be present due to fluid buildup or lung sounds may be diminished due to atelectasis and fibrotic changes in the lungs.

Next

After working through the video and activity, a **Post-Assessment** quiz tests your mastery. The results feed into your **Personalized Learning Plan**, where your instructor is able to view them.

Post-Assessment for COPD

Question 1 of 5

The client with emphysema comes to the emergency department with difficulty breathing. What assessment finding should the nurse anticipate?

○ Excess mucous production
● **Barrel shaped chest**
○ Hypoventilation
○ Blueish skin tones

Submit

Personalized Learning at a Glance

Advantage Assignments: Average

Average Score   Time Spent   Participation

18 mins   15 / 63

Edge Assignments

Average Score   Time Spent   Participation

15 mins   13 / 63

Performance Summary

Congratulations! You have demonstrated competency in Pulmonary Embolism & Asthma

The following topics could use further study and review. Focus study time on:

Fluid and Fluid Imbalances

Electrolyte Balance

View PLP

Your dashboard provides a snapshot of your **performance at a glance** as you work through your assignments.

Advantage Assignments

DISPLAY:

Assignments	Pre-Assessment	Video	Activity	Post-Assessment	Date Complete	
Pulmonary Embolism Chapter 27					10/05/19 10:10 AM Eastern	Review
Obstructive Sleep Apnea Chapter 25					10/10/19 10:30 PM Eastern	Review
Asthma Chapter 26					10/12/19 10:36 PM Eastern	Review
COPD Chapter 26					10/14/19 10:44 PM Eastern	Review
Cardiac Function & Assessment Chapter 28						Continue
The Electrical Conduction System Chapter 29						Continue

View All

Key: ≤ 69%   70% - 79%   80% - 100%

Your **Personalized Learning Plan** is mapped to your needs and tracks your progress by topic to identify the exact areas that require additional study.

Online content subject to change upon publication.

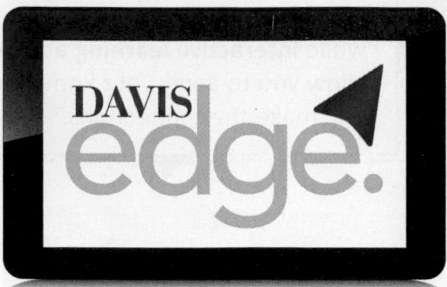

ASSESSING

Building mastery and improving test scores with Personalized Quizzing

NCLEX®-style Q&A provides the additional practice you need to master Med-Surg content and improve your scores on classroom exams.

LEARNING
APPLYING
ASSESSING

STEP #3 Study smarter, not harder with Davis Edge quizzing.

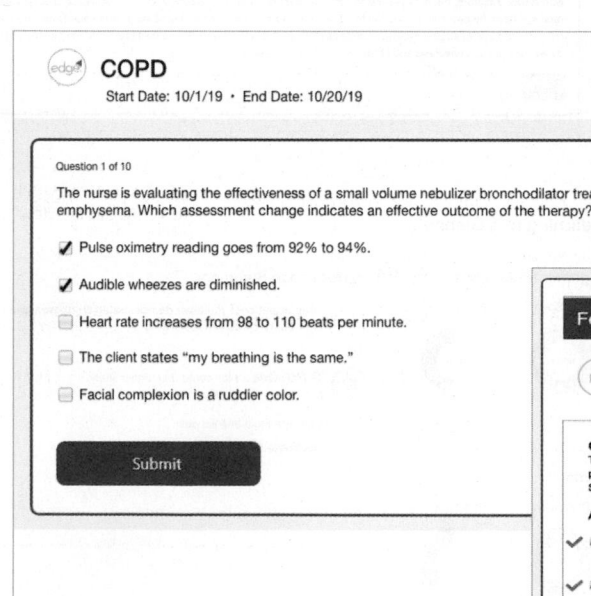

NCLEX®-style questions assess your understanding and challenge you to think critically. Practice with standard format questions like **multiple choice,** as well as more difficult format types such as **select all that apply.**

Immediate feedback with **comprehensive rationales** explains why your responses are **correct** or **incorrect**. Page-specific references direct you to the relevant content in your *Medical-Surgical Nursing* text, while **Test-Taking Tips** improve your test-taking skills.

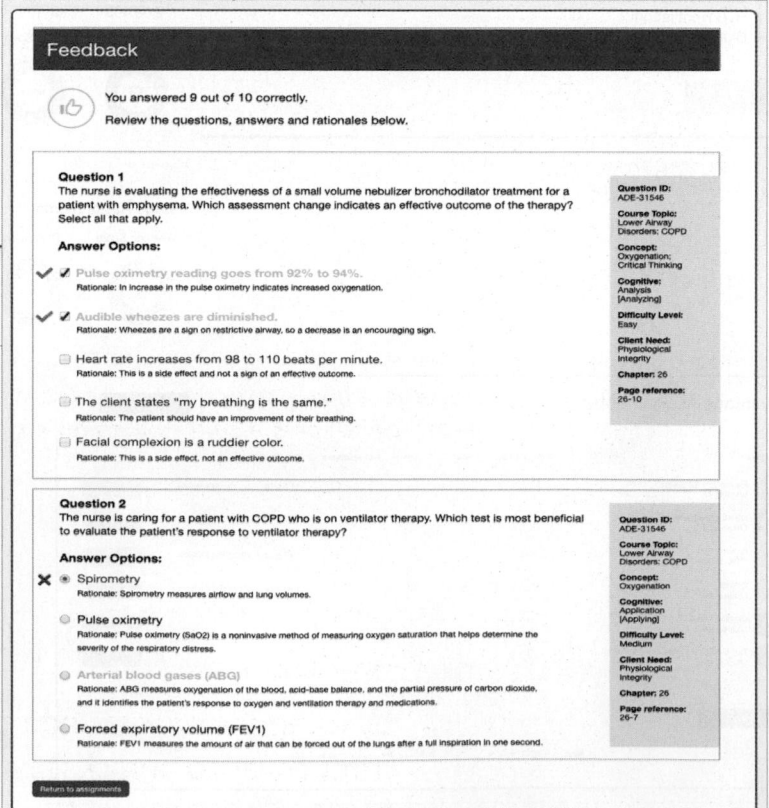

Online content subject to change upon publication.

As you complete the **Davis Edge assignments** created by your instructor, your
Personalized Learning Plan identifies your strengths and weaknesses topic by topic.

Edge Assignments

ACTIVE | ALL

Assignments are NCLEX-style assessments generated by your instructor.

Assignments		Competency	Percent Correct	Date Complete		
edge	Obstructive Sleep Apnea	15 Questions	👍	75%	10/10/19	10:30 PM Eastern	Review
edge	COPD	15 Questions	👍	90%	10/19/19	10:30 PM Eastern	Review
edge	Cardiac Function & Assessment	15 Questions	👎	68%	10/29/19	10:30 PM Eastern	Review

View All

Key: 👎 ≤ 69%   👍 70% - 79%   👍 80% - 100%

Practice Quizzes

Create Practice Quiz

Students may generate their own practice quizzes (NCLEX-style assessments to test or expand their understanding of topics).

Assignments		Competency	Percent Correct	Date Complete		
edge	Postoperative Care	15 Questions	👍	85%	9/11/19	10:40 PM Eastern	Review
edge	Shock	15 Questions	👍	79%	9/25/19	10:45 PM Eastern	Review

View All

Key: 👎 ≤ 69%   👍 70% - 79%   👍 80% - 100%

Create your own **practice quizzes** to focus on topic areas where you
are struggling, or as a study tool to review for an upcoming exam.

GET STARTED

by using the access code on the inside
front cover to unlock **Davis Advantage**
for **Medical-Surgical Nursing** today!

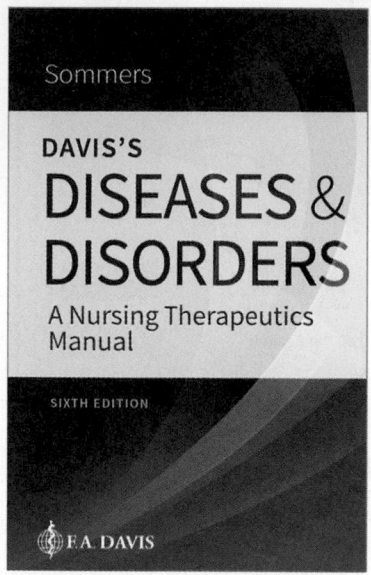
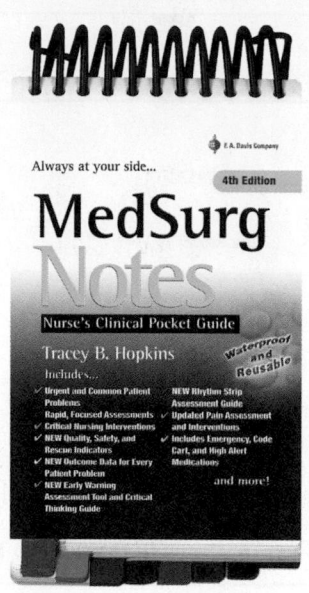
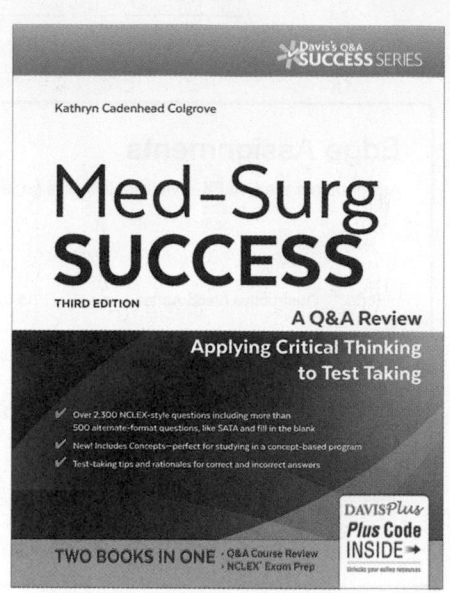
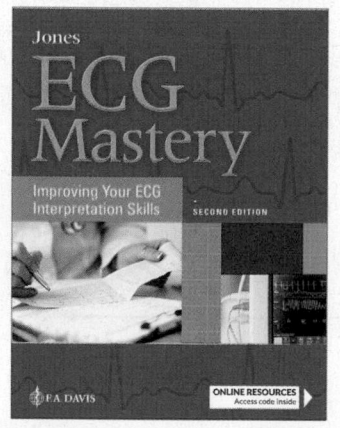

DAVIS ADVANTAGE for

MEDICAL-SURGICAL NURSING

Making Connections to Practice

SECOND EDITION

Janice J. Hoffman, PhD, RN, ANEF
Clinical Professor
Department of Nursing
Towson University
Towson, Maryland

Nancy J. Sullivan, DNP, RN
Assistant Professor/Simulation Director
Johns Hopkins University School of Nursing
Baltimore, Maryland

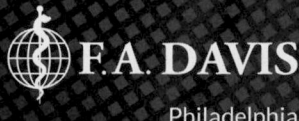

F.A. DAVIS

Philadelphia

F. A. Davis Company
1915 Arch Street
Philadelphia, PA 19103
www.fadavis.com

Printed in the United States of America

Last digit indicates print number: 10 9 8 7 6 5 4 3 2

Publisher, Nursing: Terri Wood Allen
Senior Content Project Manager: Adrienne D. Simon
Electronic Project Manager: Sandra Glennie and Eric Van Osten
Design and Illustrations Manager: Carolyn O'Brien
With Illustrations by Jeanne Robertson CMI and Lindsay Coulter, BFA, CMI

As new scientific information becomes available through basic and clinical research, recommended treatments and drug therapies undergo changes. The author(s) and publisher have done everything possible to
make this book accurate, up to date, and in accord with accepted standards at the time of publication. The
author(s), editors, and publisher are not responsible for errors or omissions or for consequences from application of the book, and make no warranty, expressed or implied, in regard to the contents of the book. Any
practice described in this book should be applied by the reader in accordance with professional standards of
care used in regard to the unique circumstances that may apply in each situation. The reader is advised
always to check product information (package inserts) for changes and new information regarding dose
and contraindications before administering any drug. Caution is especially urged when using new or
infrequently ordered drugs.

Library of Congress Cataloging-in-Publication Data

Library of Congress Control Number:2019946038

About the Authors

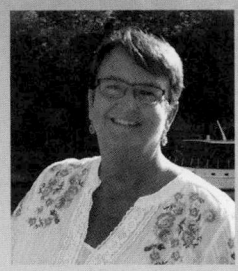

Janice J. Hoffman,
PhD, RN, ANEF

Dr. Hoffman began her nursing career on active duty as a United States Navy Nurse Corps Officer. She transitioned to the Navy Reserves after 7 years and retired in 2005 as a captain. Her experiences in the U.S. Navy were the start of her interest in and passion for teaching, as she served as a staff development officer involved in medical corps, nurse corps, and hospital corps training.

With a nursing career spanning over 40 years, she has taught in graduate, baccalaureate, associate, and diploma nursing programs, as well as serving in staff-development positions in acute care and military facilities. Dr. Hoffman's areas of expertise include clinical decision making, new graduate transition, preceptor development, curriculum development, and teaching strategies. She has presented nationally and internationally on effective teaching and learning strategies, curriculum development, and new graduate nurse transition. Dr. Hoffman is a member of the editorial board and a manuscript reviewer for *Nurse Educator* and also serves as a reviewer for the *Journal of Nursing Education* and *Journal of Professional Nursing*.

She completed her Bachelor of Science in Nursing from the University of North Carolina at Chapel Hill. While she was receiving her Master of Science in Nursing Education from California State University Fresno, her master's thesis investigated self-directed learning among registered nurses. She obtained her PhD in Nursing from the University of Maryland School of Nursing, Baltimore, where she studied critical thinking in undergraduate students. An expert in new graduate transition, she has developed and implemented nurse internship and residency programs in large academic health centers, military facilities, and community hospitals.

In addition to this textbook, Dr. Hoffman has been a contributing author to several nursing fundamentals, pathophysiology, pharmacology, and critical care nursing textbooks. She has published manuscripts on new graduate transition, teaching strategies, and nursing care of patients with neurological disorders. An expert in test development, she has served as an item writer and item reviewer for the National Council of State Boards of Nursing. Dr. Hoffman has received more than $1.8 million in grant funding to support seamless academic progression, particularly in RN-to-BSN programs.

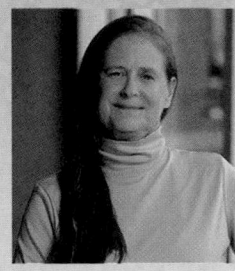

Nancy J. Sullivan,
DNP, RN

Dr. Sullivan's career has spanned over 40 years, which has allowed her the opportunity to experience a tremendous variety of nursing roles. She began her career in critical care/trauma nursing with both adult and pediatric patients. These experiences sparked an interest in critical care nursing that remains today. She also has nurse management experience and 11 years of experience in a nurse educator role working with new graduate nurses. Since 2005, she has held several faculty positions, such as clinical instructor, clinical course coordinator, and theory course coordinator for both critical care and medical-surgical nursing courses.

She received her Bachelor of Science in Nursing from the University of Maryland, Baltimore, in 1975 and her Master of Science in Trauma/Critical Care Nursing from the same school in 1992. In 2013, she received her DNP from the Johns Hopkins University School of Nursing after completing a project focusing on rapid-cycle deliberate practice simulation.

Dr. Sullivan has authored manuscripts and presented locally, nationally, and internationally on the topics of the use of simulation in nursing education and resuscitation. She was also a contributing author in a nursing pharmacology textbook, writing a chapter focusing on antiarrhythmic drugs.

Presently, Dr. Sullivan is an assistant professor and the clinical simulation director for the Johns Hopkins University School of Nursing. She has primary responsibility for the simulation program for the prelicensure program as well as overseeing the integration of simulation into the advanced practice DNP programs. She is also presently the theory course coordinator for the last in a series of three medical-surgical nursing courses. Her research interests include using simulation in nursing education and resuscitation training.

The Sigma Theta Tau International Honor Society of Nursing acknowledged the first edition of Dr. Hoffman's and Dr. Sullivan's text with the Capstone International Nursing Book Award.

ACKNOWLEDGMENTS

Both authors would like to acknowledge the many students and faculty who have provided feedback to the first edition of our book. It has been so gratifying and humbling to hear how you are using our book to facilitate your teaching and learning. To the students, a special thank you for your feedback, as this book was written with you, the students, in mind!

BOTH AUTHORS DEDICATE THIS BOOK TO:

The dedicated and resourceful people at F. A. Davis Company who have been instrumental in the development of the first and second editions of this medical-surgical textbook. It was through their guidance, support, patience, and expertise that this textbook has become a reality. Thank you to Terri, Adrienne, Beth, and all the other reviewers, editors, and others involved. We also would like to thank the many contributing authors who shared their expertise and time in the development of this book. It is only their sharing of their expertise and experience that this book is a reality.

JANICE HOFFMAN ALSO DEDICATES THIS BOOK TO:

My husband, Paul, who has unselfishly given up weekend activities and vacation days to allow me to devote time to this work! Hopefully, we will have more time to explore Virginia now!

My two sons, Bryan and Joshua, and their wives, Erika and Kaitlyn, who have been unconditionally supportive and patient as I worked on "THE BOOK." Their love and encouragement are a constant source of joy in my life, and their children (my grandchildren—Lilly, Benton, and Joey Rose) are such great diversions!

A special tribute to my parents, Wallace and Lorraine Joyce, who were always a great source of love, support, and encouragement.

A special acknowledgment to Dr. Anne Belcher and Dr. Marilyn Oermann, who have consistently supported my academic career over the years and provided valuable mentoring.

Finally, heartfelt thanks to my coauthor, Dr. Nancy Sullivan! We have been friends and colleagues for years, and there is no one with whom I would rather have shared this journey. I hope you and Mark now have more time to enjoy your spectacular home!

NANCY SULLIVAN ALSO DEDICATES THIS BOOK TO:

My wonderful husband, Mark, who has contributed steadfast support and invaluable advice during the hours spent in the writing and revising of this book. A true partner.

My parents, Charles and Lydia, whose love and support I will always cherish, and a special tribute to my mother, who inspired me to become a nurse. It was through her example that I realized from a very early age that I wanted to be a nurse—just like her!

Finally, warmest thanks to my coauthor, Dr. Janice Hoffman! In addition to her friendship, she has been a mentor guiding me through my career, providing support and opportunities that have helped move me forward. Thank you, Janice!

The title of this book is important because it describes the approach to the design and pedagogy of this nursing textbook. We believe that it is the connections that nurses make between the clinical presentation of the patient, the nursing actions, and *most importantly,* the rationales for those actions that promote clinical judgment and clinical decision making. *Medical-Surgical Nursing: Making Connections to Practice* is a concise, focused medical-surgical nursing text designed to prepare contemporary nursing students for adult health practice areas. This text is designed to teach associate degree (ADN), baccalaureate degree (BSN), and entry-level master's degree (MSN) nursing students. It is designed to serve as the primary text for medical-surgical and/or acute care courses.

According to the Nursing Executive Center of the Advisory Board (2008), there is a growing academic–practice gap demonstrated by recent nursing school graduates. In particular, nursing executives surveyed in these studies prioritized the following as areas in which new graduates lack expected knowledge and competency:

- Knowledge of pathophysiology of patient conditions (34%)*
- Knowledge of pharmacological implications of medications (28%)*
- Decision making based upon the nursing process (20%)*
- Interpretation of assessment data (18%)*

(The asterisks indicate the percentage of frontline nurse leaders' satisfaction with the specific new graduate nurses' proficiency.)

Medical-Surgical Nursing: Making Connections to Practice not only provides content related to pathophysiology and pharmacology but also presents it in a format that fosters an understanding of the relationships between the physiology, pathophysiology, clinical manifestations, and management of these disorders. This approach fosters a more accurate interpretation of data and better clinical judgment and decision making.

ORGANIZATION

Medical-Surgical Nursing: Making Connections to Practice introduces a contemporary, student-centered learning approach to nursing education. With its concise content and explicit correlations between pathophysiology, clinical presentation, medical management, and nursing management, learners' thinking will be focused on understanding and applying the underlying principles to the management of disorders seen in adult patients. The consistent structure and organization in each of the chapters support learning and mastery of content.

The beginning of the text presents current professional issues/content pertinent to the medical-surgical population (cultural considerations, ethical principles, interprofessional implications, etc.). The second unit provides the foundational clinical concepts that are woven throughout the text (geriatric considerations, pain management, oncology overview, fluid and electrolyte balance, etc.). Perioperative content is the focus of Unit III, which describes the management of patients in pre-, intra- and postoperative settings. This unit provides a broad overview of the operative experience that supports the specific discussions of surgical procedures presented in the disorder chapters.

The heart of the book is the chapters focusing on body system units. Consistent with the *Healthy People 2020* and *2030* recommendations, there is comprehensive content on decreasing the risk and managing the complications of diseases such as heart disease, stroke, diabetes mellitus, chronic kidney disease, and cancer. The *Healthy People 2020* and *2030* objectives are also used to guide content related to genomics and interprofessional care management. The final section of the book focuses on special populations and again incorporates those conditions outlined in *Healthy People 2020* and *2030*, including obesity and substance use disorders. There are also chapters related to environmental injuries and trauma as well as management of mass casualties. In this second edition, based on the opioid crises in the United States, we have expanded this content, particularly in the chapters on pain and substance use disorders.

With an emphasis on health and wellness, each body system unit includes an assessment chapter, which is an overview of normal function, followed by chapters detailing selected disorders. The pathophysiology discussed in the disorder chapters is presented with an emphasis on how the clinical manifestations are directly related to alterations in normal function. Again, the focus is on assisting the learner in transferring prior learning in order to better understand the disease process. This approach is also consistent with most nursing programs, which require anatomy and physiology as prerequisites to their programs. The disorder chapters consistently present the epidemiology, pathophysiology, clinical manifestations, and medical and nursing management of selected medical-surgical disorders. With a focus on "making connections," the rationales for medical, nursing, and interprofessional interventions are directly related to the underlying physiology and/or pathophysiology. Critical thinking and clinical judgment are facilitated with this approach because it requires the learner to consistently address the "whys" and "hows" of clinical presentation and treatment plans for patients with specific disease processes. The nursing care is presented with scientific explanations for the presenting clinical manifestations, and formatted as assessments, actions, and teaching interventions with rationales that correlate directly back to the physiological and/or pathophysiological content in the chapter—again, "making connections."

Critical care nursing content is integrated into most of the body system units, with a dedicated critical care chapter for the management of patients in cardiovascular, neurological and neurosurgical, respiratory, and burn intensive care units. Additionally, there is a chapter dedicated to the management of patients in various shock states, with guides to hemodynamic monitoring.

PEDAGOGICAL FEATURES

Numerous pedagogical features are incorporated into the book to facilitate student learning.

- **Learning Outcomes** guide the organization and content of each chapter. A consistent approach is used, with each assessment and disorder chapter having similar learning objectives to support the learner in developing a systematic approach to learning new content.
- **Essential Terms** are introduced at the beginning of each chapter and are highlighted and defined the first time they are used in the chapter.
- **Concepts** are used to guide the presentation of the content and are listed at the beginning of each chapter. These concepts are particularly relevant to nursing programs using a concept-based approach to their nursing curriculum.
- **Connection Checks** are multiple-choice questions incorporated throughout each chapter. Questions are integrated throughout the chapters and align with the chapter objectives. The successful completion of the Connection Checks helps ensure the student's understanding of the material as he or she moves through the chapter. An Answer Key for all of the Connection Check questions is at the end of the book for quick access; answers with rationales for each question are available online in the Davis Advantage Resources.
- **Case Studies** are used in each chapter. At the beginning of the chapter, the case study is titled "Finding Connections" and presents a patient case related to the chapter content. The case is introduced three times in each chapter and supports the learner in applying the chapter content. At the end of the chapter, "Making Connections" provides a wrap-up of the case study.
- **Case Study Questions** are presented at the end of the final "episode" of the case study and include five questions that require the application of the case study content to answer correctly. Answers with detailed rationales for these questions are available online in the Davis Advantage Resources.
- **Nursing Process Approach** is used to present the nursing management, including assessment, action, and teaching interventions and scientific rationales.
- **Evidence-Based Practice Boxes** are included in each chapter and present the latest evidence for a practice discussed in the respective chapter.
- **Safety Alerts** in chapters focus on potential hazardous or high-risk issues related to the specific chapter content.

- **Geriatric/Gerontological Considerations Boxes** present content focused on the special needs of older adults, including assessment findings associated with aging as well as special considerations in the care of this population.
- **Transitional Care Boxes** highlight the coordination required for patients with complex healthcare needs as they transition from different levels of healthcare settings on the basis of their care-coordination needs.
- **Genetic Connections Boxes** are included in chapters where there are genetic links related to the incidence, pathophysiology, or treatment modalities.
- **Figures and Graphics** are included to provide representative art to support student comprehension.

Online Chapter Resources

- **NCLEX®-Style Chapter Review Questions** are presented online for each chapter for review of the overall chapter content.
- **Finding Connections Assessment Questions** ask the learner to apply anatomy and physiology content. Again, this stresses the importance of understanding anatomy and physiology as the basis of understanding disorders and not merely memorizing signs and symptoms.
- **Prioritization Activities** are included in selected disorder chapters and provide at least two presentations/scenarios that allow the student to prioritize the care for these patients.
- **NANDA-NIC-NOC Tables** are available in selected case studies and support the learner in applying the nursing process to the care of the patient.
- **Concept Maps** are included in selected case studies and have a consistent approach that describes the connections/relationships between normal anatomy and physiology, pathophysiology, clinical manifestations, and management.
- **Community Resource Boxes** are available for selected disorders and other selected chapters and present a list of public and community resources to provide services and information pertaining to selected disorders.

THE TEXT IN RESPONSE TO STUDENT-CENTERED LEARNING

Medical-Surgical Nursing: Making Connections to Practice is a concise textbook that uses an integrated approach that reduces redundancies while at the same time making the important correlations more explicit. The textbook is based on the underlying physiology and pathophysiology of specific disorders generally seen in medical-surgical settings. The consistent focus on explicit correlations between pathophysiology, clinical presentation, and treatment plans facilitates critical thinking and provides the basis for better clinical decisions. Using this type of framework, which integrates clinical judgment to guide decision making, promotes consistency in approach and provides a more focused discussion. With an emphasis on student-centered learning and technology, this medical-surgical textbook provides nursing students and faculty with the most up-to-date resources and information available through Web/online references.

The consistent approach to each assessment and disorder chapter facilitates student comprehension and fosters a structured approach to learning this complex content. The writing style supports reading comprehension, and the frequent Connection Checks allow students to self-evaluate their progress. Consistent headings and features also support the student in developing a systematic approach to learning complex content. The concise, focused approach of each disorder chapter is presented in a straightforward manner, with all content presented in an organized format from epidemiology to the evaluation of nursing care.

THE TEACHING AND LEARNING PACKAGE

How students learn is evolving. In this digital age, we consume information in new ways. Online, we are spoon-fed information in bite-size, dynamic chunks.

In order to meet the needs of today's learners, how faculty teach is also evolving. Classroom time is valuable for active learning. This approach makes students responsible for the key concepts, allowing faculty to focus on clinical application. Relying on the textbook alone to support an active classroom leaves a gap. *Davis Advantage Med-Surg* fills that gap with the following resources:

- **A Strong Core Textbook** that provides the foundation of knowledge that today's nursing students need to pass the NCLEX® and enter practice prepared for success.

- **Online Student Tools** to learn and practice the content in an engaging, interactive format. **Pre-Assessment Quizzes** test students on their comprehension of a key topic and then give them a **Personalized Learning Plan** to work through that is based on their strengths and weaknesses. They are engaged in an interactive experience that uses multimedia content to help spark connections and bring concepts to life. Once students complete the interactive experience, **Post-Assessment Quizzes** assess their comprehension of the material.

- **Online Instructor Resources** are aimed at creating a dynamic classroom experience that relies heavily on interactive participation and is tailored to students' needs. Results from the post-assessments are available to faculty, in aggregate or by student, and inform a **Personalized Teaching Plan** that faculty can use to deliver a targeted classroom experience. Faculty will know students' strengths and weaknesses *before* they come to class and can spend class time focusing on where students are struggling. Suggested in-class activities are provided to help create an interactive, hands-on learning environment that helps students connect more deeply with the content. NCLEX-style questions from the **Instructor Test Bank** and **PowerPoint** slides that correspond to the textbook chapters are referenced in the Personalized Teaching Plans.

- **Davis Edge Med-Surg** online quizzing to promote assessment and remediation, using an adaptive format with NCLEX®-style questions. Faculty can set up a review and remediation system to take a constant pulse of classroom performance. The results are provided in real time and feed to a gradebook. Comprehensive rationales for all answer options are provided for students and explain why an answer is correct or incorrect.

Contributors

Valerie G. Bader, PhD, CNM
Assistant Teaching Professor
University of Missouri Sinclair School
of Nursing
Columbia, Missouri

Lourdes Carhuapoma, RN, MS, ACNP-BC, CCRN
Acute Care Nurse Practitioner
The Johns Hopkins Hospital
Baltimore, Maryland

JoAnn Fitzgerald Conroy, DNP, MSN, RN
Professorial Lecturer in Nursing
The George Washington University
School of Nursing
Ashburn, Virginia

Linda Cook, PhD, RN, CNS, ACNP
Assistant Professor
University of Maryland School of
Maryland
Baltimore, Maryland

Denise Cost, CHPN, C-RN, MSN, BSN
Professional Nurse and Nurse Educator
(Retired)
The Visiting Nurse Service of New York
New York, New York

Carrie Cox, MSN, RN
Community Outreach and Clinical
Education Coordinator, Clinical
Research Nurse
Johns Hopkins Bayview Medical Center,
Johns Hopkins Bum Center
Baltimore, Maryland

Mary K. Donnelly, DNP, MPH, ANP-BC, ACNP-BC, CNL
Assistant Professor; Chair, Graduate
Nursing
University of San Francisco School
of Nursing and Health Professions
San Francisco, California

Wanda E. R. Edwards, DNP, RN, PMHCNS, PMHNP-BC
Nurse Practitioner
Health and Business Consultants,
Psychological Institutes of Michigan
Southfield, Michigan

Deborah A. Ennis, MSN, RN, CNE
Senior Professor of Nursing
Harrisburg Area Community
Harrisburg, Pennsylvania

Kristen A. Farling, DNP, ANP-BC, CUNP
Nurse Practitioner
The Johns Hopkins Hospital Brady
Urological Institute
Baltimore, Maryland

Monica J. Filburn, MSN, RN, PNP
Interim Chair, Department of Nursing,
Professor of Nursing
Harrisburg Area Community College
Harrisburg, Pennsylvania

Barbara Fitzsimmons, MS, RN, CNRN
Nurse Educator, Department of
Neurosciences Nursing
The Johns Hopkins Hospital
Baltimore, Maryland

Eleni Flanagan, DNP, MBA, RN-BC
Assistant Director of Nursing
The Johns Hopkins Hospital
Baltimore, Maryland

Cynthia Fox, MS, RN, CORLN
Nursing Faculty
University of Maryland Medical Center
and University of Maryland School
of Nursing
Baltimore, Maryland

Trisha Fronczek, MS, RN-BC, CCRN
President
Trial Run, LLC
North Huntingdon, Pennsylvania

Adriana Glenn, PhD, MA, MN, RN, FNP-BC
Assistant Professor, Nursing
George Washington University
Ashburn, Virginia

Jana Goodwin, PhD, RN, CNE
Assistant Professor, Director BSN
Program
University of Maryland School of
Nursing
Baltimore, Maryland

Kristy Gorman, MS, RN, OCN
Clinical Nurse
Baltimore County Public Schools
and University of Maryland Medical
Center
Baltimore, Maryland

Thomasine D. Guberski, PhD, CRNP
Director, Health Program
Institute of Human Virology of the
University of Maryland School
of Medicine
Baltimore, Maryland

Dawn Hohl, PhD, RN
Senior Director of Transitions and Patient
Experience
John Hopkins Home Care Group
Baltimore, Maryland

Kelly Krout, DNP, MSN, RN
Director, Quality Management
Johns Hopkins Bayview Medical Center
Baltimore, Maryland

Susan Kulik, DNP, MBA, RN
Director, Accreditation and Regulatory
Activities
John Hopkins Medicine International
Baltimore, Maryland

Amy S. D. Lee, DNP, ARNP, WHNP-BC
Clinical Associate Professor
The University of Alabama, Capstone
College of Nursing
Tuscaloosa, Alabama

Sherrie Lessans, RN, PhD, CNL
Assistant Professor, Director Clinical
Nurse Leader Program
University of Maryland, Baltimore
School of Nursing
Baltimore, Maryland

Vickie M. Lester, MSN, RN-BC, CNE
Clinical Assistant Professor
University of North Carolina-Chapel Hill
Chapel Hill, North Carolina

Megan Lynn, PhD, MBA, RN
Nurse Manager
University of Maryland
Baltimore, Maryland

Shari J. Lynn, MSN, RN
Instructor
Johns Hopkins University School
of Nursing
Baltimore, Maryland

Jamelia Maher, BSN, RN, CNOR
OR Clinical Instructor
The Johns Hopkins Hospital
Baltimore, Maryland

Margaret McCormick, MS, RN, CNE
Clinical Associate Professor
Towson University
Baltimore, Maryland

Lynn McDonald, DNP, RN
Nurse Coordinator
The Johns Hopkins Hospital
Baltimore, Maryland

Alice M. Moore, MPA, MSN, NHA, CRNP
Simulation Educator
Johns Hopkins University Schools
    of Medicine and Nursing
Baltimore, Maryland

Diane J. Morey, PhD, MSN, RN, CNE
Campus Dean of Nursing
West Coast University
North Hollywood, California

Kathleen T. Ogle, PhD, RN, FNP-BC, CNE
Associate Professor and Graduate
    Program Director
Towson University, Department of Nursing
Towson, Maryland

Denise Owens, RN, MS, CCRN-K
Course Director
University of Maryland School of Nursing
Rockville, Maryland

Sharon Owens, ACNP-BC, PhD
Assistant Director of Nursing
The Johns Hopkins Hospital
Baltimore, Maryland

Vinciya Pandian, PhD, MBA, MSN, RN, ACNP-BC, FAAN
Assistant Professor
Johns Hopkins University School of Nursing
Baltimore, Maryland

Catherine R. Ratliff, PhD, GNP-BC, CWOCN, CFCN
Associate Professor/NP
University of Virginia Health System
Charlottesville, Virginia

Maren M. Reinholdt, PhD, MSN, RN
Clinical Faculty
Johns Hopkins University School of
    Nursing
Baltimore, Maryland

Susan Renda, DNP, ANP-BC, FNAP, FAAN
Assistant Professor, Associate Director
    DNP Advanced Practice Program
Johns Hopkins University School of
    Nursing
Baltimore, Maryland

Susan Sartorius-Mergenthaler, MA, RN
Oncology Clinical Trials Sr. Research
    Nurse Referral Coordinator
Johns Hopkins School of Medicine,
    Department of Oncology
Baltimore, Maryland

Brenda Shelton, DNP, APRN-CNS, RN, CCRN, AOCN
Clinical Nurse Specialist
Sidney Kimmel Cancer Center at
    The Johns Hopkins Hospital
Baltimore, Maryland

Diane Vail Skojec, DNP, MS, ANP-BC
Lead Nurse Practitioner
The Johns Hopkins Hospital
    Department of Surgery
Baltimore, Maryland

Sarah Smith, RN, MS
Nurse Educator
The Johns Hopkins Hospital Nurse
    Residency Program
Baltimore, Maryland

Sandra M. Swoboda, RN, MSN, FCCM
Research Program Coordinator,
    Simulation Educator
Johns Hopkins University Schools
    of Medicine and Nursing
Baltimore, Maryland

Laura Syron, MSA, MPH, RN
Nurse Manager
Johns Hopkins Home Care Group
Baltimore, Maryland

Sarah Tarr, MSN, RN
Full-Time Lecturer
Belmont University
Nashville, Tennessee

Gladdi Tomlinson, RN, MSN
Professor of Nursing
Harrisburg Area Community College
Harrisburg, Pennsylvania

Nina M. Trocky, DNP, RN, NE-BC, CNE
Associate Professor and Associate Dean
    Baccalaureate Nursing Program
University of Maryland School of Nursing
Baltimore, Maryland

Mallory Trosper, MSN, RN, CRNP-BC
Clinical Instructor, Johns Hopkins University
Acute Care Nurse Practitioner, Division
    of Neurosciences
The Johns Hopkins Hospital
Baltimore, Maryland

Regina Donovan Twigg, DNP, RN, CNE
Clinical Associate Professor and Assistant
    Chair, Department of Nursing
Towson University
Towson, Maryland

Marida Twilley, MSN, RN-BC
Nurse Educator
The Johns Hopkins Hospital
Baltimore, Maryland

Sherri Ulbrich, PhD, RN, CCRN, CNE
Associate Teaching Professor
University of Missouri Sinclair School
    of Nursing
Columbia, Missouri

Joanne M. Walker, MS, RN, CWOCN
Nurse, Wound and Ostomy (Retired)
The Johns Hopkins Hospital
Baltimore, Maryland

Stephanie Walter-Coleman, RN
ICU/ED Float Pool RN
Johns Hopkins Bayview Medical Center
Baltimore, Maryland

Jennifer Wenzel, PhD, RN, CCM, FA, AN
Associate Professor, Department of Acute
    and Chronic Care; Principal Faculty,
    Center for Innovative Care in Aging
Johns Hopkins University School
    of Nursing
Baltimore, Maryland

Dianne Whyne, RN, MS
Director of Operations (Retired)
Johns Hopkins CEPAR
Baltimore, Maryland

Kelley Miller Wilson, DNP, MSN, CMS, RN
Assistant Professor, Program Director
    BSN Program
Georgetown University School
    of Nursing and Health Studies
Washington, DC

Elizabeth K. Zink, MS, RN, CCNS, CNRN
Clinical Nurse Specialist
The Johns Hopkins Hospital
Baltimore, Maryland

Maya Zumstein-Shaha, PhD, MS, RN
Professor
Bern University of Applied Sciences,
    Department of Health, Division of
    Applied Research and Development,
    Master of Science in Nursing
Bern, Switzerland

Contributors to the First Edition

Laura Alberico-Klug, BA, BSN, RN, CWON
Annapolis, Maryland

Diana-Lyn Baptiste, DNP, MSN, RN
Baltimore, Maryland

Gail Biba, MSN, RN, CNRN
Baltimore, Maryland

Victoria Buechel, RN, MSN, CCNS, CCRN
Nashville, Tennessee

Margaret Clifton, RNC-BC, MS
Lincoln, Rhode Island

Linda K. Cook, PhD, RN, CCRN, CCNS, ACNP-BC
Baltimore, Maryland

Denise Cost, CHPN, C-RN, MSN, BSN
New York, New York

Carrie A. Cox, MS, RN
Baltimore, Maryland

Melissa C. Custer, BSN, RN, CCRN
Baltimore, Maryland

Mary K. Donnelly, DNP, MPH
Baltimore, Maryland

Dzifa Dordunoo, PhD, RN
Baltimore, Maryland

Wanda E. R. Edwards, DNP, RN, PMHCNS-BC, NP
Detroit, Michigan

Deborah Ennis, MSN, RN, CNE
Harrisburg, Pennsylvania

Kristen Ann Farling, DNP, CRNP, CUNP
Baltimore, Maryland

Monica J., Filburn RN, MSN, PNP, TNCC, PALS and ACLS Certifications
Harrisburg, Pennsylvania

Barbara Fitzsimmons, MS, RN, CNRN
Baltimore, Maryland

Eleni Flanagan, RN, MSN, MBA
Baltimore, Maryland

Dawn Foster, PhD, ACNP-BC, CCRN-K
Charlottesville, Virginia

Cindy Fox, MS, RN, CORLN
Baltimore, Maryland

Trisha C. Fronczek, MS, RN-BC, CCRN
North Huntingdon, Pennsylvania

Jana Goodwin, PhD, RN, CNE
Baltimore, Maryland

Conrad Gordon, RN, BSN, MS
Baltimore, Maryland

Kristy Gorman, MS, RN, OCN
Baltimore, Maryland

Thomasine D. Guberski, PhD, CRNP
Baltimore, Maryland

Gail Gustafson, CRNP, MSN
Harrisburg, Pennsylvania

Rita Herzog, MSN, RN, CNRN
Baltimore, Maryland

Vanessa K. Hill, MSN, BSN, NP-C
Birmingham, Alabama

Dawn Hohl, RN, PhD
Baltimore, Maryland

Susan L. Humphreys, PhD, RN, NE-BC
Baltimore, Maryland

Shannon Idzik, DNP, CRNP, FAANP
Baltimore, Maryland

Anela Kellogg, MSN, RN
Baltimore, Maryland

Bernice King, DNP, APRN
Washington, DC

Dina A. Krenzischek, PhD, RN, MAS, CPAN, CFRE, FAAN
Baltimore, Maryland

Kelly Krout, DNP, MSN, RN
Baltimore, Maryland

Susan Kulik, DNP, MBA, RN
Baltimore, Maryland

Amy S. D. Lee, DNP, ARNP, WHNP-BC
Baltimore, Maryland

Sherrie Lessans, PhD, RN
Baltimore, Maryland

Vickie M. Lester, MSN, RN-BC, CNE
Chapel Hill, North Carolina

Cathleen Lindauer, RN, MSN, CEN
Baltimore, Maryland

Megan Lynn, PhD, MBA, RN, FNE-A
Baltimore, Maryland

Shari Lynn, MSN, RN
Baltimore, Maryland

Jamelia S. Maher, RN, BSN, CNOR
Baltimore, Maryland

Anna Rose Martin, MS, RNC-OB, IBCLE
Baltimore, Maryland

Rita Moldovan, RN, DNP, ACHPN
Baltimore, Maryland

P. Lea Monahan, PhD, RN
Macomb, Illinois

Diane J. Morey, PhD, MSN, RN, CNE
Salem, Virginia

Jackie Newsome-Williams, PhD, RN, ANP-BC
Baltimore, Maryland

Denise Owens, RN, MS, CCRN
Rockville, Maryland

Sharon G. Owens, ACNP-BC, PhD
Baltimore, Maryland

Larry Purnell, PhD, RN, FAAN
Newark, Delaware

Catherine R. Ratliff, PhD, GNP-BC, CWOCN, CFCN
Charlottesville, Virginia

Lynn Richards-McDonald, DNP, RN
Baltimore, Maryland

Karen Ritchey, RN, MSN, CNOR
Baltimore, Maryland

Reviewers

Terri Astorino, DEd, MSN, RN
Associate Professor of Nursing
Edinboro University
Edinboro, Pennsylvania

**Andrietta Wright Barnett, DNP,
APRN, FNP-BC**
Visiting Professor
Chamberlain University
Walterboro, South Carolina

Tracy Blanc, RN, MSN
Associate Professor
Ivy Tech Community College, Terre
    Haute Campus
Terre Haute, Indiana

Tammy Clemens, MSN, RN, NP-C
Clinical Instructor/Course Manager
University of Alabama in Huntsville
Huntsville, Alabama

Lorraine S. Collins, MSN, RN, CNOR
Associate Professor of Nursing
Piedmont Virginia Community College
Charlottesville, Virginia

Lenore Cortez, MSN, RN-BC
Clinical Instructor of Nursing
Angelo State University
San Angelo, Texas

Stacy Flaten, MSN, RN
Nursing Instructor
Minot State University
Minot, North Dakota

Krysia Hudson, DNP, RN, BC
Assistant Professor
Johns Hopkins University School
    of Nursing
Baltimore, Maryland

Susan Irvine, MS, RN
Faculty Program Director
Excelsior College
Albany, New York

Neena Tresa John, RN, MSN
Assistant Professor
Ivy Tech Community College
Evansville, Indiana

Lynn Lagasse, MSN, RN, CNE
Assistant Clinical Professor of Nursing
Keene State College
Keene, New Hampshire

**Mary Jane Larmon, MBA, MSN,
RN-BC, CCRN, Alumnus**
Director
Sharon Regional School of Nursing
Sharon, Pennsylvania

Susan McCarthy, DNP, APRN
Professor of Nursing
Finger Lakes Community College
Canandaigua, New York

Janell McKethan, MSN, RN, CMSRN
Registered Nurse
Atlanta VA Medical Center
Atlanta, Georgia

Terri Peterson, RN, MSN Ed
Nursing Faculty
Atlanta Technical College
Atlanta, Georgia

Kimberlie Rippey, MSN, RNC
Instructor of Nursing
Finger Lakes Community College
Canandaigua, New York

Rebecca Rubin, MS
Instructor
South Piedmont Community College
Monroe, North Carolina

**Suzanne H. Tang, DNP, APRM,
FNP-BC, PHN**
Professor and Assistant Director
    of Nursing
Rio Hondo College
Whittier, California

**Regina Donovan Twigg, DNP,
RN, CNE**
Clinical Associate Professor & Nursing
    Program Coordinator
Towson-Hagerstown
Towson University, Department of
    Nursing
Towson, Maryland

Geraldine Tyrell, DNP, RN, CNE
Director & Associate Professor
Bethel College
North Newton, Kansas

**Julia Vincente, PhD, MSN,
RN, CCRN**
Clinical Education Consultant, Critical
    Care Residency Program
Martin Health System
Stuart, Florida

Karol Yundt, MSN, RN
Assistant Professor of Nursing
Northampton Community College
Bethlehem, Pennsylvania

SPECIAL THANKS TO OUR CULTURE ADVISORY BOARD REVIEWERS:

Victoria Haynes, DNP, APRN, FNP-C
Coordinator of Diversity & Cultural Competency/Associate
    Professor
School of Nursing
MidAmerica Nazarene University
Olathe, Kansas

**Marilyn A. Ray, RN, PhD, CTN-A, FSfAA, FAAN,
FESPCH (hon.), FNAP**
Colonel (Ret.), United States Air Force, Nurse Corps
Professor Emeritus
The Christine E. Lynn College of Nursing
Florida Atlantic University
Boca Raton, Florida

Contents

Chapter 5: Palliative Care and End-of-Life Issues 52

UNIT II
CLINICAL PRINCIPLES OF MEDICAL-SURGICAL NURSING 61

Chapter 6: Geriatric Implications for Medical-Surgical Nursing 61

Chapter 7: Oxygen Therapy Management 80

Chapter 24: Coordinating Care for Patients With Infectious Respiratory Disorders   459

Chapter 25: Coordinating Care for Patients With Upper Airway Disorders   476

Chapter 26: Coordinating Care for Patients With Lower Airway Disorders   495

Chapter 38: Coordinating Care for Patients With Peripheral Nervous System Disorders   844

Chapter 39: Coordinating Care for Critically Ill Patients With Neurological Dysfunction   862

UNIT IX
PROMOTING HEALTH IN PATIENTS WITH ENDOCRINE DISORDERS   903

Chapter 40: Assessment of Endocrine Function   903

UNIT XI
PROMOTING HEALTH IN PATIENTS WITH INTEGUMENTARY DISORDERS   1063

Chapter 49: Assessment of Integumentary Function   1063

Chapter 50: Coordinating Care for Patients With Skin Disorders   1094

Chapter 51: Coordinating Care for Patients With Burns   1148

Chapter 63: Coordinating Care for Patients With Urinary Disorders   1473

UNIT XV PROMOTING HEALTH IN PATIENTS WITH REPRODUCTIVE DISORDERS   1489

Chapter 64: Assessment of Reproductive Function   1489

Chapter 65: Coordinating Care for Female Patients With Reproductive and Breast Disorders   1506

Unit I

Professional Foundations of Medical-Surgical Nursing

Chapter 1

Foundations for Medical-Surgical Nursing

Janice Hoffman

INTRODUCTION

Medical-surgical nursing has historically been practiced in acute care facilities across the United States. However, with changes in healthcare delivery, legislation, and insurance coverage, medical-surgical nursing is now practiced in many different practice settings, including hospitals, same-day surgical centers, acute rehabilitation centers, ambulatory care settings, long-term care agencies, and patients' homes. No longer considered a "stepping-stone" to more complex patient care settings (intermediate care, critical care, etc.), medical-surgical nursing focuses on the management of acutely ill adult patients. Medical-surgical nurses are the largest group of practicing nursing professionals.

According to the **Academy of Medical-Surgical Nurses (AMSN)**, the only professional nursing organization dedicated to medical-surgical nursing, the foundation of all nursing practice has its roots in this practice area. The mission of the AMSN is to "promote excellence in medical-surgical nursing" (AMSN, 2018), and the AMSN has an average membership of over 11,000 registered nurses. The strategic plan of the AMSN is in Box 1.1. Over the years, medical-surgical nursing has developed into a specialty practice area, and registered nurses who meet specific requirements are eligible for certification in this practice area through the **Medical-Surgical Nursing Certification Board (MSNCB)**. These nurses earn the credential **Certified Medical-Surgical Registered Nurse® (CMSRN)**. Box 1.2 provides the domains of nursing tested by the MSNCB.

Certification in medical-surgical nursing is also available through the American Nurses Credentialing Center (ANCC); registered nurses with this certification are entitled to the credential of Registered Nurse-Board Certified (RN-BC).

COMPETENCIES IN MEDICAL-SURGICAL NURSING

Entry-level nursing programs, including associate, baccalaureate, master's (including Clinical Nurse Leader), and doctoral degrees, focus on the preparation of nurses to practice competently in the various medical-surgical settings. Competency in the management and coordination of adult medical-surgical patients requires a strong background in the sciences, including anatomy and physiology, chemistry, microbiology, pathophysiology, and pharmacology. Throughout this text, there is an emphasis on correlating the nursing care of this adult patient population to the physiological and pathophysiological bases of selected disease processes. Promoting an understanding of the relationships between the physiology, pathophysiology, clinical manifestations, and management of these disorders fosters more accurate interpretation of data, enhanced critical thinking, and better clinical decision making.

Box 1.1 Academy of Medical-Surgical Nurses Strategic Framework

Mission

The mission of the Academy of Medical-Surgical Nurses (AMSN) is to promote excellence in medical-surgical nursing.

Vision

Medical-surgical nurses use their powerful voice and focused action to continuously improve patient care.

Values

Medical-surgical nursing is a distinct specialty with its own body of knowledge. We believe patients receive better care when medical-surgical nurses:

- Engage in ongoing professional development
- Use evidence-based practices
- Speak with a unified voice
- Serve as leaders on healthcare teams
- Have the necessary resources to deliver excellent care
- Practice in a healthy work environment

Strategic Message

The AMSN is a vibrant community of medical-surgical nurses who care about

- Improving patient care
- Developing personally and professionally
- Advocating for the specialty of medical-surgical nursing
- Connecting with other nurses who share their compassion and commitment

Adapted from American Academy of Medical-Surgical Nurses. (2015). *Strategic plan and initiatives and outcome*. Retrieved from https://www.amsn.org/sites/default/files/documents/about-amsn/strategic-plan/AMSN-Strategic-Plan.pdf

Box 1.2 Domains of Nursing Practice for Medical-Surgical Nursing Certification

1. Helping Role
2. Teaching-Coaching Function
3. Diagnostic and Patient Monitoring
4. Effective Management of Rapidly Changing Situations
5. Administering and Monitoring Therapeutic Interventions and Regimens
6. Monitoring and Ensuring the Quality of Healthcare Practices
7. Organizational and Work Role Competencies

This focus on competency is particularly important because the **Nursing Executive Center of the Advisory Board** has reported that recent nursing school graduates have demonstrated an academic-practice gap. The Nursing Executive Center serves nursing administrators through data collection around best practices, strategic initiatives, and operational issues. In this specific study, nursing executives described that new graduates lacked the expected knowledge and competency in the following areas:

- Knowledge of pathophysiology of patient conditions (34%)*
- Knowledge of pharmacological implications of medications (28%)*
- Decision making based on the nursing process (20%)*
- Interpretation of assessment data (18%)*

*Percentage of front-line nurse leaders who were satisfied with the specific new graduate nurse proficiency.

Although this study was completed in 2008, the issue related to the readiness for practice of new graduate nurses continues, particularly in acute care settings. As a result, there is a growing body of knowledge related to addressing this academic-practice gap through the establishment of academic-practice partnerships. Suggested strategies to better prepare the nurse graduate for the realities of practice include the increased use of simulation in nursing education programs, extended transition to practice and residency programs, as well as the establishment of academic service partnerships.

Competencies Related to the Nursing Process

Equally important to the practice of medical-surgical nursing are competencies in the **nursing process**, clinical decision making, evidence-based care, **patient-centered care**, quality and safety, and interprofessional practice. The nursing process includes assessment, diagnosis, planning, implementation, and evaluation and ultimately guides patient care. Throughout this text, there is a strong emphasis on using the nursing process to guide the delivery of safe, effective, and patient-centered nursing care.

The nursing process is closely associated with the nurse's clinical decision making, and the role of the medical-surgical nurse in key decision making with patients and families is evident in the current healthcare environment. Higher patient acuity and increased complexity of patients' care needs, accompanied by shorter lengths of stay in acute care settings, place the nurse in the vital role of ensuring that patients are prepared for transitions to different levels of care. Facilitating the patient's and family's understanding of treatment plans and discharge teaching is a primary responsibility of the registered nurse.

Connection Check 1.1

Which factors have led to the expansion of medical-surgical nursing from traditional acute care facilities to other settings? *(Select all that apply.)*
A. Increases in healthcare complexity
B. Shortage of registered nurses
C. Changes in insurance coverage
D. Shortened hospital lengths of stay
E. Low salaries for registered nurses in hospitals

EVIDENCE-BASED NURSING CARE

Evidence-based nursing practice is the foundation of professional nursing practice. Based on a problem-solving approach to healthcare delivery, nursing care practices and protocols are based on the best evidence from research studies and the expertise of clinicians. Medical-surgical nursing incorporates evidence-based practice principles in order to provide the highest-quality and most cost-effective care to patients and families. Evidence-based care is characterized by clinical decisions that are based on the use of the best available evidence, clinical expertise, and patient preferences (see Evidence-Based Practice). The steps of the evidence-based process are listed in Box 1.3.

Evidence-Based Practice

Bedside Shift Reporting

Based on recommendations by The Joint Commission to more actively involve patients in their care, as well as to standardize hand-off communications during a change of care providers, hospitals have implemented nurse-to-nurse bedside shift reporting. In this research, focused on increasing patient involvement in their care and improving patient satisfaction, a quasi-experimental, between-group, pre-implementation and post-implementation study was conducted at a 149-bed hospital to examine compliance with bedside shift reporting. The intervention included a standardized approach to bedside reporting along with a change management strategy that included support from nursing leadership to consistently use this reporting approach. In addition to educating the nurses in the use of SBAR (situation, background, action, and response) to provide the bedside report, consistent monitoring of compliance and leadership support contributed to the effectiveness of this study. Five months after implementation, both patient satisfaction and compliance with nurse-to-nurse bedside reporting had increased.

Scheidenhelm, S., & Reitz, O. E. (2017). Hardwiring bedside shift report. *Journal of Nursing Administration, 47*(3), 147–153.

Box 1.3 Steps of Evidence-Based Practice

- Develop the question.
- Search and collate the best evidence.
- Evaluate the quality of the evidence.
- Integrate evidence into practice.
- Evaluate outcomes of practice change.
- Disseminate the evidence.

The utilization of the best evidence requires the registered nurse to possess competencies in locating and evaluating the quality of data. Typically, there is a clinical question or problem identified that guides the initiation of an evidence-based project. Once the question has been defined, a literature review is conducted to assess the current state of the science around the question. Skills in conducting effective literature searches and analyzing findings are crucial for the nurse in locating and evaluating the quality of evidence required to guide clinical practice. Increasingly, nursing programs incorporate these search strategies into their curriculum, often in collaboration with college/university libraries.

Once data have been located, the evaluation of the quality of the evidence is the next step in the process. Box 1.4 outlines one process for the evaluation of data and describes the types of data that are used to determine the quality, validity, and reliability of evidence. The lowest numerical rating of the level of evidence in this approach correlates with the highest level of evidence. For example, **systematic reviews** of randomized controlled studies (Level I) are the highest level of evidence because they include data from selected studies that randomly assigned participants to control and experimental groups. **Randomized controlled studies** are considered the gold standard of research, with their findings most valuable. Level II evidence is based on the results of a single randomized controlled study. **Quasi-experimental studies** (Level III) also use the control and experimental groups but lack the random assignment. Research that is designed as a **case-control study** includes two groups, those with a specific disorder and those without, and then comparisons are made between the two groups. **Cohort studies** use a group of people (cohort) who are initially free of disease and are then followed over a period of time to examine whether the development of new cases differs between those with and without exposure to some type of disease, environmental hazard, or other factor. Both case-control and cohort studies are often conducted in epidemiological research and are considered Level IV evidence. Descriptive and qualitative studies do not use an experimental design with control and experimental groups; they provide

findings based on observations of populations and phenomena. Systematic reviews of descriptive studies (Level V), because they include numerous studies as opposed to a single descriptive study (Level VI), provide a higher level of evidence. The lowest level of evidence (Level VII) is expert opinions from individuals and committees. Although higher levels of evidence are preferred, there are not always randomized controlled studies available to answer all questions posed in an evidence-based review of the literature.

The importance of evidence-based care is also reflected in the **American Nursing Credentialing Center (ANCC) Magnet® Recognition program**, in which Magnet status is awarded to healthcare facilities that demonstrate excellence in the recruitment, recognition, and retention of nursing staff as well as excellence in patient care and quality. Because quality patient care is associated with a foundation in evidence-based findings, the AMSN's *Scope of Medical-Surgical Nursing Practice* provides dissemination of evidence-based practice guidelines for medical-surgical nurses.

Connection Check 1.2

In designing an evidence-based practice guideline for a medical-surgical unit, which source provides the most reliable information?
A. Content from a textbook
B. Manuscript in a nursing journal
C. Results from research studies
D. Information from a professional activity

PATIENT-CENTERED CARE IN THE MEDICAL-SURGICAL SETTING

The importance of patient-centered care is highlighted in the **Institute of Medicine's (IOM) 2003 report** *Health Professions Education: A Bridge to Quality*. As acute care hospital lengths of stay shorten, the patient's interactions with members of the healthcare team and particularly one-on-one time with the primary healthcare provider are affected. Complicating these patient encounters are greater requirements for documentation and justification for care. From the patient's perspective, the requirements of the system often seem to overshadow the patient's concerns. The results of patient satisfaction surveys that evaluate hospital stays often report dissatisfaction regarding time spent with members of the healthcare team.

Patient-centered care is a benchmark that acute care facilities are evaluated against, and nursing care is an important component of this evaluation. Because nursing care is provided 24 hours a day in acute care settings, patients often base their evaluations of the quality of their care on interactions with nursing staff. Patient-centered care focuses on treating patients and families with dignity and respect and engaging patients and families in decision making about care decisions. Competencies of medical-surgical nurses that are closely associated with patient-centered care

---

Box 1.4 Evaluating Levels of Evidence

- **Level I** Evidence from systematic reviews of randomized controlled studies (RCTs)
- **Level II** Evidence from at least one RCT
- **Level III** Evidence from quasi-experimental studies
- **Level IV** Evidence from case-control and cohort studies
- **Level V** Evidence from systematic reviews of descriptive or qualitative studies
- **Level VI** Evidence from a single descriptive or qualitative study
- **Level VII** Evidence from expert individual authorities or committees

include effective communication skills, empathy, caring, and compassion. Equally important are the clinical competency and knowledge base of the registered nurse.

The relevance of patient-centered care is further underscored by the Hospital Consumer Assessment of Healthcare Providers and Systems (HCAHPS), a survey that provides a standardized approach to collecting data from patients about their experiences in hospitals. The nine essential topics included on the HCAHPS survey are listed in Box 1.5.

Patient-centered care and communication are also incorporated into **The Joint Commission (TJC)** Standards for Hospitals. The Joint Commission is an independent, not-for-profit organization that accredits and certifies approximately 77% of hospitals in the United States. Accreditation and certification by TJC are recognized as the standard of patient care, effectiveness, and safety and foster continuous process improvements. Aspects of patient-centered care are incorporated into the accreditation, including data related to patient participation in the plan of care and visitation rights. The vision statement of TJC focuses on promoting safe, high-quality, and best-value healthcare across all healthcare settings.

The Beryl Institute is also an organization that fosters patient-centered care through the "patient experience" that is influenced by all the interactions and experiences encountered, based on the organization's culture and practices. Results from a 2017 study by The Beryl Institute found that efforts focused on supporting patient experiences are expanding, are a top priority for healthcare agencies, and can be tied to positive healthcare outcomes. Consistent with TJC's mission, The Beryl Institute supports patients and families being well informed and actively involved in all healthcare decisions.

Connection Check 1.3

The medical-surgical nurse needs to be knowledgeable of which organization that scores patient-centered care via a telephone survey of selected patients after discharge?

A. The Joint Commission
B. The Beryl Institute
C. The Carnegie Institute
D. The Hospital Consumer Assessment of Healthcare Providers and Systems

---

PATIENT SAFETY OUTCOMES

Providing safe, quality care is a priority for medical-surgical nurses. The Joint Commission annually publishes **National Patient Safety Goals** aimed at improving patient safety through goals that focus on potential problems in the healthcare setting. The 2018 goals identified the following areas to improve patient safety:

- Identify patients correctly
- Improve staff communication

Box 1.5 Hospital Consumer Assessment of Healthcare Providers and Systems (HCAHPS) Topics

- Communication with providers
- Communication with nurses
- Responsiveness of hospital staff
- Pain management
- Communication about medications
- Discharge information
- Cleanliness of the hospital environment
- Quietness of the hospital environment
- Transition of care

- Use medicines safely
- Use alarms safely
- Prevent infection
- Identify patient safety risks
- Prevent mistakes in surgery

These patient safety goals are integral to safe, quality patient care in the medical-surgical setting.

Accurate patient identification is required throughout the patient experience, especially during assessments, while preparing patients for procedures and surgical procedures, and during medication administration. Effective staff communication is also integral to safe patient care, particularly during "hand-offs," such as change-of-shift reports, receiving patients, and transferring patients to other departments. The SBAR (Box 1.6) is one approach to decreasing communication barriers and focuses on a standard way to state the Situation, Background, Assessment, and Recommendation of patient events. Used to enhance communication with healthcare providers, nurses often use SBAR to report changes in patient conditions. SBAR enhances communication with

---

Box 1.6 The SBAR Approach for Effective Communication

SBAR is an acronym that correlates to:

   Situation: Brief statement of the problem or issue being addressed
   Background: Data related to the current situation
   Assessment: Summary of causes, significance, severity of situation
   Recommendation: Specific actions needed to address the situation

The SBAR method provides a consistent process for communication, particularly in high-risk situations. Of particular value is the focus on making a recommendation that focuses on a definitive approach to addressing the issue or clinical problem.

healthcare providers, and nurses often use SBAR to report changes in patient conditions. Box 1.7 provides an example of SBAR communication between the healthcare provider and nurse around a patient demonstrating difficulty voiding after a surgical procedure. Safety measures around medication administration have been implemented in medical-surgical settings and include practices that prevent interruptions during the preparation and administration of medications. Additionally, the nurse must follow the rights and responsibilities required for safe medication administration and ensure that the rationales for all medications are associated with the patient condition.

Medical-surgical nurses play an integral role in the prevention of infection and surgical errors. Hospital stays may be extended because of infection, particularly those associated with hospital-acquired infections. Many acute care facilities have implemented increased surveillance and evidence-based guidelines to prevent these types of infections, including catheter-associated urinary tract infections and central line infections. Additionally, surgical settings have implemented "time-outs" (requiring all personnel involved in the procedure to stop to make sure that the patient is identified, the correct anatomical site is identified, and all equipment is in working order) and special procedures for marking surgical sites. Better patient outcomes are associated with effective communication and collaboration in patient care settings. The proper use of alarm settings on equipment used for patient monitoring is also essential in the medical-surgical setting. The nurse must ensure that the alarm parameters are individualized to the patient as well as ensuring that the alarms are heard and responded to in a timely manner.

Because of the increased emphasis on quality and safety, in 2005 the Robert Wood Johnson Foundation funded a project focused on educating nursing students on patient safety and healthcare quality. These funds established the **Quality and Safety Education for Nurses (QSEN)** initiative designed to prepare nurses with the required knowledge, skills, and attitudes to foster continuous improvement of quality and safety in healthcare settings. Based on the Institute of Medicine's recommendations (Box 1.8), the QSEN initiative developed competencies for both prelicensure and graduate nursing students (Box 1.9).

Connection Check 1.4

The medical-surgical nurse implements SBAR to promote effectiveness in which aspect of quality and safety in patient care?

A. Surveillance
B. Communication
C. Organization
D. Cost-effectiveness

INTERPROFESSIONAL COLLABORATION AND COMMUNICATION

Because of the complexity and high acuity of most adult patients in medical-surgical settings, interprofessional collaboration is imperative to the promotion of effective patient outcomes. In 1999, the IOM reported in *To Err Is Human: Building a Safer Health System* that between 44,000 and 98,000 deaths occurred in U.S. hospitals because of preventable medical errors. In 2009, another report by the Institute of Healthcare Improvement estimated that there were approximately 40,000 incidences per day in U.S. hospitals that resulted in patient harm. In both of these studies, ineffective communication among the interprofessional healthcare team was identified in a root-cause analysis of

---

Box 1.7 SBAR Example

Situation:

Hello, Dr. Jones. This is Steve, the registered nurse caring for Ms. Sandra Williams in Room 732 on South Wing. I am contacting you because she arrived from the post-anesthesia care unit (PACU) and has not voided in more than 6 hours.

Background:

She was admitted to the hospital this morning, and you performed a lumbar laminectomy this morning for a herniated disc at L4–L5.

Assessment:

Ms. Williams is complaining of inability to void. According to her operative reports, she received 1,500 mL of IV fluid during the surgical procedure and in the PACU, and the indwelling catheter was removed prior to transfer from the PACU 6 hours ago; at the time, she had 800 mL of urine output. She has received an additional 250 mL of IV fluid since arriving on the unit.

Recommendation:

I recommend that an intermittent catheterization be performed at this time.

Box 1.8 Institute of Medicine's Competencies for Health Professionals

- Provide patient-centered care
- Work in interdisciplinary teams
- Employ evidence-based practice
- Apply quality improvement
- Utilize informatics

From Greiner, A., & Knebel, E. (Eds.). (2003). *Health professions education: A bridge to quality. Institute of Medicine (US) Committee on the Health Professions Education Summit.* Washington, DC: National Academies Press. Retrieved from http://www.ncbi.nlm.nih.gov/books/NBK221528/

Box 1.9 Quality and Safety Education for Nursing (QSEN) Competencies

- Patient-Centered Care
- Teamwork and Collaboration
- Evidence-Based Practice (EBP)
- Quality Improvement (QI)
- Safety
- Informatics

these medical errors. The Joint Commission includes an accreditation standard that addresses the importance of effective communication.

Medical-surgical nurses are members of interprofessional healthcare teams and in acute care settings are often in the role of care coordinator. The nurse participates in interprofessional rounds with the physicians, advanced practice registered nurses, pharmacists, discharge planners, social workers, and other members of the healthcare team. Additionally, because nurses are the primary direct provider in the acute care setting, they are often the key to communication between the various healthcare members as well as with specialists and consultants who may be episodically involved in the patient's care. Effective clinical reasoning and communication skills are crucial to this role of the medical-surgical nurse as a care coordinator. (The roles of care coordinator and interprofessional teams are discussed in Chapter 2.)

With the increased focus on interprofessional patient care teams, attention is also being given to the importance of educating future healthcare providers together. Faculty at schools of medicine, nursing, pharmacy, social work, and other healthcare professional educational settings are working collaboratively to design and implement interprofessional educational programs. The use of patient care simulations using high-fidelity mannequins provides safe environments for these future healthcare team members to practice interprofessional communication and teamwork. This increased focus on educating future healthcare providers together is based on findings of increased safety and quality in hospitals with effective interprofessional care teams.

Connection Check 1.5

Which outcome of interprofessional teams is associated with an increased focus on educating health professional students together?
A. Decreased hospital costs
B. Increased safety and quality
C. Decreased length of stay
D. Increased patient satisfaction

CHAPTER SUMMARY

Medical-surgical nursing is a specialty area characterized by competencies that are applicable for patients across the healthcare continuum, from acute care hospitals to home settings. As members of the largest subspecialty in nursing, medical-surgical nurses are eligible for certification in this practice area through the AMSN or the ANCC.

Foundational to medical-surgical nursing are evidenced-based practices that foster the delivery of safe, effective care that is based on research findings and clinical expertise and incorporates patient participation. Another growing focus of medical-surgical nursing is patient-centered care, which is also an important benchmark for acute care facilities. Patient-centered care focuses on treating patients and families with dignity and respect and engaging patients and families in decision making about care decisions. The importance of patient-centered care is demonstrated by its incorporation into TJC's Accreditation Standards for Hospitals. Interprofessional coordination and teamwork are also essential to effective patient outcomes in the complex health system in the United States. Medical-surgical nurses work closely in interprofessional teams including providers, social workers, pharmacists, and other disciplines to plan and implement the best evidence-based care.

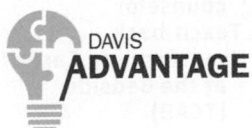

DAVIS ADVANTAGE | To explore learning resources for this chapter, go to **Davis Advantage** and find:
– Answers to in-text questions
– Chapter Resources and Activities
– NCLEX®-Style Chapter Review Questions
– Bibliography

Chapter 2

Interprofessional Collaboration and Care Coordination

Laura Syron and Dawn Hohl

LEARNING OUTCOMES

Content in this chapter is designed to assist in:

1. Discussing the importance of successful transitions for medical-surgical patients
2. Describing changes in the healthcare landscape
3. Describing models of transitional care
4. Exploring the role of the registered nurse in patient-centered transitional care programs
5. Defining interprofessional collaboration in the healthcare setting
6. Identifying the roles of healthcare professionals coordinating care for patients
7. Exploring unique patient situations requiring or enhanced by interprofessional collaboration

CONCEPTS

- Collaboration
- Communication
- Healthcare System
- Medication
- Nursing Roles
- Promoting Health
- Safety

ESSENTIAL TERMS

Affordable Care Act (ACA)
Care Transitions Program
Case manager (CM)
Certified registered nurse practitioner (CRNP)
Chaplain
Community health worker (CHW)
Comorbidity
Delegation
Goal-directed care
Guided Care Program
Home-care coordinator (HCC)
Interpreter
Interprofessional care team (ICT)
Interprofessional collaboration (IC)
Interprofessional education (IPE)
Legal counsel
Licensed practical nurse (LPN)
Licensed vocational nurse (LVN)
Multidisciplinary "rounds" (MDRs)
Occupational therapist (OT)
Palliative care coordinator
Patient and Family Advisory Council (PFAC)
Patient care coordinator
Patient-centered care
Patient-centered medical home (PCMH)
Pharmacist
Physical therapist (PT)
Physician
Post-discharge call nurse
Project BOOST (Better Outcomes for Older Adults Through Safe Transitions)
Project RED (Re-engineered Discharge)
Rapid response team
Registered dietitian/nutritionist (RD)
Registered nurse (RN)
Respiratory therapist (RT)
SBAR
Speech-language pathologist (SLP)
Social worker (SW)
Substance abuse counselor
Teach-back
Transforming Care at the Bedside (TCAB)
Transition guide (TG)
Transitional care
Transitional care model (TCM)
Transitional care nurse (TCN)
Unlicensed assistive personnel (UAP)

Finding Connections

CASE STUDY: EPISODE 1

Follow this patient throughout the chapter.

Mr. Frank Garfield is a 67-year-old gentleman admitted after an acute cerebrovascular accident (CVA). The patient has a history of well-managed hypertension and atrial fibrillation, lives with his wife of 46 years, and was functionally independent prior to admission. The patient now presents with right-sided weakness and aphasia and has been placed on four new medications, including an anticoagulant. He has been seen by various members of the interprofessional care team (ICT) including the unit-based nurse practitioner (NP). The patient and his wife are Spanish-speaking and are able to carry on simple conversations in English. The nurse recognizes the need to begin interprofessional collaboration (IC) to develop a safe discharge plan to return this patient to an optimal level of function and transition to the next level of care…

INTRODUCTION

The state of healthcare in the United States is dynamic and very complex. For a patient to safely and effectively navigate through our healthcare system requires coordination among all members of the ICT. However, access to care that is coordinated, safe, and focused on the patient's unique needs across all care settings has eluded many patients, particularly the elderly and chronically ill. The Institute of Medicine (IOM) released two important reports, *To Err Is Human: Building a Safer Health System* (2000) and *Crossing the Quality Chasm: A New Health System for the 21st Century* (2001) that address the quality and fragmentation of healthcare throughout the United States. These documents recommend the necessary transformations in healthcare needed to provide safe, effective, patient-centered, efficient, timely, and equitable care. Nursing practice, which has historically been setting defined rather than patient centered, is part of this transformation. There is an increasing focus on care coordination across settings, particularly for patients with chronic disease who experience frequent changes in health status and require multiple transitions among providers and settings. Vulnerable patients are put at greater risk during transitions if care is not coordinated, communication among professionals is inadequate, socioeconomic factors are inadequately addressed, and the needs of the patient and caregivers are not taken into consideration. Care coordination and managing patient transitions across care settings are integral parts of nursing care and an expanding role for the registered nurse (RN). Medical-surgical nursing quality and safety competencies and targeted knowledge, skills, and attitudes are necessary to prepare the RN to lead care management strategies and transitional care services across the care continuum.

Connection Check 2.1

Which phase of care is most critical for medical-surgical patients?

A. Acute hospital phase
B. Prehospital care phase
C. Transition phase
D. Discharge phase

OVERVIEW OF TRANSITIONAL CARE

The safety of the patient is at risk during transitions between care settings, particularly following an acute hospitalization. The patient's needs may go unmet, and there is the risk for medication errors and adverse clinical events. The readmission rates of hospitalized patients, particularly Medicare beneficiaries, are one driving factor in the call for improved **transitional care** services. Nearly one in five Medicare patients discharged from a hospital is readmitted within 30 days. Of these readmissions, 76% may be preventable. These readmission rates are often attributed to a lack of coordination of care as patients are discharged to rehabilitation facilities, long-term care agencies, or back to their homes. Without a plan to ensure continuous and coordinated care, these patients may be readmitted with complications. Although all hospital readmissions may not be related to the most recent hospitalization, insurance companies and other payers consider unplanned admissions as wasteful spending and, in some cases, may deny reimbursement or may charge penalties for readmissions within that 30-day window post-discharge. Data trending the numbers of unplanned readmissions after a recent hospital stay are used to measure the quality of hospital care. Focusing on more efficient and effective transitional practices and models should decrease the incidence of unplanned readmissions. The implementation of evidence-based practice to guide post-discharge calls, one important aspect of transitional care, is an example of how readmission rates can be lowered with care coordination (see Evidence-Based Practice).

Increasing access, improving quality and safety, and lowering costs are the basic principles of the Patient Protection and **Affordable Care Act (ACA)** signed in 2010. Transitional care programs have demonstrated that with the prevention of avoidable readmissions, patient safety and quality of care improve, and costs are lowered. For these reasons, transitional care is a high priority in the act. The Community-Based Care Transitions Program (Section 3026), Centers for Medicare and Medicaid Services (CMS) Innovation (Section 3021), Health Homes (Section 2703), and the Medicare Shared Savings Program (Section 3022) all support transitional care services.

Transitional care programs are patient centered and typically manage the transitions of patients from acute care to post–acute care settings. The goals are to avoid poor health outcomes, ensure continuity of care, and

Evidence-Based Practice

Improving Post-Hospital Discharge Telephone Reach Rates Through Pre–Hospital Discharge Face-to-Face Meetings

Calling a patient 24 to 48 hours after hospital discharge is an important component of care-coordination programs aimed at reducing readmission rates. The purpose of the call is to assess the patient's condition, ensure patient understanding of the post-discharge plan of care, and triage the patient as necessary to appropriate providers. A study recently published by Vergara et al (2017) demonstrated that the use of face-to-face meetings by a telephonic case manager with patients prior to discharge improved the rate of post-discharge call reach. The brief pre–hospital discharge meeting assisted patients in understanding the reasons for the call, identified the best times to call using accurate telephone numbers, and instructed patients how to prepare for the call by having their discharge instructions with them. Additionally, the telephonic case manager was no longer a stranger on the telephone but someone the patients had met. These factors combined may have significantly helped to increase post-discharge reach rates.

Vergara, F. H., Davis, J., Sheridan D. J., Sullivan, N. J., & Budhathoki, C. (2017). Improving post-hospital discharge telephone reach rates through pre-hospital discharge face-to-face meetings. Professional Case Management, 22(6), 275–283. http://dx.doi.org/10.1097/NCM.0000000000000243

Important strategies in managing the transition from acute to post-acute settings include:

- Initiating care coordination/transition planning at least 24 hours prior to discharge
- Organizing post-discharge follow-up services for patients requiring chronic disease management
- Providing specific discharge teaching related to symptoms requiring immediate treatment
- Coordinating with care providers responsible for management in discharge settings
- Providing a comprehensive medication review

Connection Check 2.2

What is considered the hospital's span of responsibility for the patient?

A. Admission to discharge
B. Admission to 30 days post-discharge
C. Admission to 15 days post-discharge
D. Admission to full recovery

EVIDENCE-BASED MODELS OF TRANSITIONAL CARE

Several models of transitional care have emerged in response to the call for improved coordination across the care continuum: the transitional care model (TCM), the Care Transitions Program, Project Red, and Project BOOST. Another transitional care plan is the patient-centered medical home (PCMH), a model for comprehensive, patient-centered primary care. A model that focuses on quality and safety in the hospital, Transforming Care at the Bedside (TCAB), was developed as an important first step in ensuring safe transitions across the continuum.

The Transitional Care Model

The transitional care model (TCM) is a nurse-led multidisciplinary program that was developed by Mary Naylor, an advanced practice nurse at the University of Pennsylvania. Transitional care nurses (TCNs) manage patients as they transition across the care continuum from inpatient settings to other settings, including skilled nursing facilities and home. Using evidence-based care-coordination methods, the TCN collaborates with other healthcare team members, including providers, nurses, social workers, discharge planners, and pharmacists, to plan care. The goal of this model is to prevent complications, provide continuity of care, and increase patients' and caregivers' abilities to manage their care. The TCM focuses on chronically ill, high-risk adults. Common medical and surgical conditions often included in this model are heart failure, diabetes mellitus, chronic kidney disease, and postsurgical hip surgery. Because many of these patients have multiple **comorbidities** (two or more coexisting medical conditions or disease processes), coordination

facilitate safe transitions between care settings. Unlike disease-management and case-management programs that are ongoing, transitional care is time limited. Emphasis is on the coordinating care, facilitating patient engagement and education, addressing the causes of poor outcomes, and avoiding preventable readmissions, focusing on the 30-day time period following discharge. A meaningful transition plan will include addressing those socioeconomic factors that affect the health of the individual. To support vulnerable patients and address these socioeconomic issues, the transitional care nurse will use a spectrum of community resources and programs. There are many organizations, Web sites, and providers who specifically address the immediate needs of patients out of the hospital and home in their communities. These resources answer questions, provide necessary medical equipment, and suggest community support groups of people who are dealing with similar disorders or issues. Go to **www.DavisAdvantage.com** for a listing of community resources specific to the disorders discussed in this book.

of care is critical to safe, quality care. In this model, the TCN visits the patient in the hospital and, following discharge, visits the patient weekly at home for a month. The TCN then conducts follow-up phone calls during the second month. The patient is followed for approximately 8 weeks. Specific TCN tasks include monitoring symptoms, education, and training and assisting with medication management. Results from National Institute of Health studies demonstrate that the TCM significantly improves patient safety and healthcare outcomes, enhances quality of life and satisfaction with care, and reduces overall healthcare costs.

The TCN can be an advanced practice nurse or a bachelor's level nurse. The typical caseload for most TCNs is 15 to 20 patients. The role of care coordinator or TCN is expected to grow as reimbursement is linked with decreasing admissions to acute care settings and cost-effective care management. Incorporating the competencies of a medical-surgical nurse with those of a care manager and patient advocate, this role requires knowledge of evidence-based care, working in interprofessional teams, quality improvement, and financial issues related to care delivery across multiple episodes of care.

The Care Transitions Program

Developed by Eric Coleman at the University of Colorado Health Sciences Center, the Care Transitions Program employs nurses as "transitions coaches" to manage chronically ill or seriously ill patients as they transition between healthcare settings. The transitions coach does not provide direct skilled care but, rather, uses effective communication to provide education and guidance to ensure a safe transition. In studies using a "coaching" approach, it has been demonstrated that patients who received education, encouragement, and coaching had lower rehospitalization rates. In the Coleman model, transition coaches visit the patient in the hospital and follow up with one home visit and phone calls for a 4-week time period. Patients receive tools to learn self-management skills that include recognizing and responding to "red flags" that indicate worsening of their condition, managing medications, managing their own personal health record, and completing follow-up care with their primary provider.

Project RED and Project BOOST

Project RED (Re-engineered Discharge) and Project BOOST (Better Outcomes for Older Adults Through Safe Transitions) are national programs that also seek to improve care as patients transition from acute care settings to post–acute care settings by improving the discharge processes. The objectives of Project BOOST, led by the Society of Hospital Medicine, are to identify patients at risk for readmission on admission, reduce 30-day readmission rates, decrease length of stay, and improve communication of patient care information during discharge. A risk-assessment tool developed by Project BOOST helps to identify patients at risk for adverse events after discharge. Called the *8P Scale,* this assessment tool is completed on admission and identifies

risk factors such as polypharmacy, problem medications, physiological issues, poor health literacy, principal diagnosis, patient support, prior hospitalizations, and palliative care. The 8P Scale is used by the ICT to determine appropriate post-discharge needs.

Project RED, or Re-Engineered Discharge, is a research group based at Boston University Medical Center that develops and tests strategies that improve hospital discharge processes. The RED is based on 12 interrelated components that promote patient safety and decrease readmissions. The 12 components are as follows:

- Ascertain need for and obtain language assistance.
- Make appointments for follow-up medical appointments and post-discharge tests/labs.
- Plan for the follow-up of results from laboratory tests or studies that are pending at discharge.
- Organize post-discharge outpatient services and medical equipment.
- Identify the correct medicines and a plan for the patient to obtain and take them.
- Reconcile the discharge plan with national guidelines.
- Develop and teach a written discharge plan the patient can understand.
- Educate the patient about his or her diagnosis.
- Assess the degree of the patient's understanding of the diagnosis and discharge plan.
- Review with the patient what to do if a problem arises.
- Expedite transmission of the discharge summary to clinicians accepting care of the patient.
- Provide telephone reinforcement of the discharge plan.

Both Project RED and Project BOOST offer tools, the 8P Scale and the comprehensive discharge instruction tool, that aid the ICT in safely and appropriately planning for the patient's discharge. These tools also complement the strategies of the TCM and the Care Transitions Program.

Patient-Centered Medical Home/Guided Care Program

Also included in the Affordable Care Act are programs and initiatives focusing on the patient-centered medical home (PCMH). An enhanced model of primary care, the PCMH engages ICTs to address and care for patients with multiple comorbidities. Specifically, the PCMH promotes care that is patient-centered, comprehensive, interprofessionally coordinated, and accessible on a long-term basis. The Guided Care Program is an example of a PCMH that has improved patient outcomes and quality and reduced costs through nursing interventions. Guided care nurses work closely with the interprofessional team to coordinate care for the patient with a chronic illness. They assist in coordinating the transition between sites providing care, assess the patient and caregiver in their home, create an evidence-based care plan, promote self-management, and facilitate access to community resources. As noted, unlike TCNs, the guided care nurse works with the patient on a long-term basis.

Transforming Care at the Bedside Model

Based on the 2001 IOM report, the **Transforming Care at the Bedside (TCAB)** project was implemented in 2003 to address the recommendations related to improving the quality and safety of patient care on medical-surgical units. Specific aims of this program also address the importance of retention of nurses at the bedside, participation of patients and family in their care experiences, and interprofessional team effectiveness.

The TCAB model focuses on the following themes: (1) safe and reliable care, (2) vitality and teamwork, (3) patient-centered care, (4) value-added processes, and (5) transformational leadership. In this project, front-line nurses and staff work on the development and implementation of action plans to address the overall quality and safety of care. Full participation of patients and families is integral to the project. Other priorities of TCAB include transformative change and continuous learning and discovery as changes in practice are implemented and evaluated. Hospitals participating in the initial phases of this model reported fewer codes, decreased patient injuries secondary to falls, lower readmission rates, reduced nurse turnover, and an increase in the time RNs spent in direct patient-care activities. The development of **rapid response teams** also grew as a result of TCAB efforts. These teams in acute care settings are composed of clinicians who provide critical care expertise at the patient's bedside or point of care and typically include a critical care provider or intensivist, critical care registered nurse, pharmacist, and respiratory therapist. They respond when a patient shows signs of deterioration in an effort to recognize and reverse the problem before a cardiac arrest occurs.

Patient Education

An essential component of IC and all care models striving for effective in-hospital and transitional care is patient education. Patient teaching can be conducted in any setting (hospital bedside, clinic, or home) by any member of the team. It is essential that the patient demonstrates an understanding of the diagnoses and plan of care in order to safely transition to home and avoid readmission. **Teach-back** is an effective teaching strategy used to enhance patient education (Box 2.1).

Connection Check 2.3

What is the focus of transitional care programs? *(Select all that apply.)*

A. Supporting the patient after hospital discharge
B. Coaching and teaching to enhance patient understanding
C. Providing patient-centered discharge instructions
D. Ensuring evidence-based medical therapy
E. Providing adequate pain control during hospitalization

Box 2.1 Teach-Back

Teach-back is a patient education strategy that involves imparting knowledge and then asking for the information to be restated to ensure patient understanding. This teaching should be accompanied by written material for the patient to use as an ongoing resource.

The components of teach-back include:

- Providing patient education in understandable, plain language, avoiding medical jargon
- Asking patients to repeat back what they understood in their own words in a nonshaming fashion—it is *not* a quiz!
- Avoiding the use of close-ended questions, such as "Do you understand?" or "Do you have any questions?"
- Reexplaining any areas of confusion
- Reassessing understanding by asking the patient to repeat back again
- Talking slowly and teaching in chunks, frequently assessing understanding

THE NURSE AS PATIENT CARE COORDINATOR

The RN providing direct care to patients is directly involved in the coordination and management of care in the acute care setting. Because of the increasing complexity of healthcare and the growing numbers of patients requiring chronic care management, the role of the RN as a **patient care coordinator** is evolving in acute care, rehabilitation, long-term, and home-care settings. Because patients are frequently discharged from acute care settings still in need of follow-up and nursing care, home health nursing is a growing practice area for acute care and medical-surgical nurses. The American Academy of Ambulatory Care Nursing (AACN) developed the Care Coordination and Transition Management (CCTM) Model to standardize the practice of ambulatory nurses as well as acute, subacute, and home health nurses in care-coordination and transition-management roles. The CCTM is grounded in care management and chronic disease management. The RN in care-coordination and transition-management roles practices across the care continuum, applying appropriate evidence-based interventions that focus on patient safety and quality of care during care transitions. To facilitate continuity of care across the care continuum, the RN must use interprofessional collaboration and coordinate healthcare services and community resources. The CCTM Model provides a core curriculum and dimensions or competencies necessary for the RN to be successful in care coordination and transition management roles. Expected knowledge, skills, and attitudes are identified for each dimension, which include advocacy, support for self-management, education and engagement of patient and family, cross-setting communication and transition, coaching and counseling of patients and families, nursing process, teamwork and collaboration, patient-centered care planning, and population health management. Developing the knowledge, skills, and attitudes needed for each dimension will help the RN meet the needs of patients and families with complex chronic illness and healthcare needs.

Connection Check 2.4

What roles does the nurse have in transitional care programs? *(Select all that apply.)*

A. Directing patient care in the inpatient setting
B. Coaching the patient after discharge
C. Managing chronic conditions after discharge
D. Directing patient care in the clinic setting
E. Assessing the patient's risk for readmission

CASE STUDY: EPISODE 2

Mr. Garfield is monitored as he slowly demonstrates signs of recovery. When the care manager meets with the patient's wife, she expresses concern that she is not sure she can care for him at home in his present condition but knows that he has expressed a desire to come home. She asks questions about what to do if his condition takes a turn for the worse because he has told her he "never wants to be on a machine." If she does take him home, she has no equipment in the home and does not know anything about his care or medications. During ICT rounds, the team discusses the need to engage therapists (physical, occupational, and speech), a pharmacist, and a nutritionist. Dual discharge-planning referrals are being made. A consult to the home-care coordinator (HCC) is made to develop a home-care plan. A second referral is made to the social worker for long-term planning should a skilled nursing facility be considered to assist with rehabilitation and advance life-planning decisions…

INTERPROFESSIONAL COLLABORATION

Interprofessional collaboration (IC) occurs when two or more professionals work together to solve problems or coordinate care. The concept that the "whole" is more than the sum of its parts is particularly meaningful when looking at the value of IC. Interprofessional collaboration is a partnership between a team of health professionals and a patient in a participatory and coordinated approach to shared decision making and communication. An important component is the inclusion of the patient and family in care and transition planning. This coordinated effort is ideally done in an atmosphere of mutual respect and shared responsibility for outcomes of care.

When the **interprofessional care team (ICT)** convenes, each individual's professional training and knowledge are used to optimize the patient's health outcomes. Team members are confident in their knowledge of each other's roles and how they contribute to the patient's care, can activate the team when needed, and hold each other accountable to meet goals. The purpose is to formulate and deliver a plan of care that is goal directed and team focused. **Goal-directed care** focuses on the overall aim for each patient. Daily care objectives remain focused on that overall goal, facilitating the efficient use of time and resources.

The evolving changes in healthcare financing and reimbursement are creating new imperatives for interprofessional teamwork. Well-coordinated collaboration allowing efficient and cost-effective care is not only good but is also essential in meeting contemporary healthcare financial challenges. As an example, a study that explored collaboration between the nurse and pharmacist when reconciling medications at admission and discharge found that preventing one discrepancy in every 290 patient encounters would offset the cost of the intervention. These findings demonstrate that investing in ICT collaboration may be an efficient and cost-effective way to ensure safe care.

Interprofessional Communication

Team members convene in a variety of ways with the purpose of providing a forum for team communication. This forum provides the opportunity to listen to other team members' assessments and recommendations, provide specific input, and make collaborative decisions. The ICT may convene in a regularly scheduled structure, such as daily rounds, or on an as-needed basis for highly complex patients or for patients who experience frequent readmissions. In a hospital setting, **multidisciplinary "rounds" (MDRs)** may be conducted on nursing units. The goal is to discuss each patient with all ICT members present in order to develop a comprehensive plan of care for both in-hospital and transitional care. This is done in an effort to improve hospital care, reduce unnecessary hospital days (decrease length of stay), and prevent readmissions. Rounds may be in a walking format where the group moves from patient to patient. This format facilitates the timely inclusion of the patient in the care-planning process. This is optimal to the process of **patient-centered care**; however, the length of rounds can be significant, necessitating the need to consider rounding in a conference room setting. Rounds conducted away from the bedside in a conference room can be structured to ensure maximum efficiency. The discussion should be limited to 2 to 5 minutes per patient. On a typical nursing unit, this results in rounds lasting about 1 hour. Included content is designed to cover daily care planning and discharge needs and includes the discussion of:

- Brief overview of the clinical situation
- The overall medical plan/plan for the day
- A risk screen that indicates a patient's potential need for post–acute care needs and complex discharge planning
- Caregiver involvement as applicable
- Patient engagement, teaching needs, and health literacy

- A discussion by each discipline that addresses the plan to prepare the patient for a safe transfer to home, including what needs to be completed prior to discharge (e.g., insulin administration return demonstration, transfer to chair independently, able to safely swallow without choking)
- Planned discharge date
- Specific actions that need to be completed in order for the discharge to occur (e.g., family needs to visit the skilled nursing facility, home infusion company needs to secure authorization, hospital bed and Hoyer lift need to be delivered to the home, provider follow-up appointment within 1 week). If a patient presents with frequent readmissions, the team may reach out to the previous level of care to assess the situation that is not supporting the patient (e.g., may confer with the home health nurse to assess what led to the readmission, such as not taking medications or lack of caregiver support)
- A discussion of required documents for discharge or transfer so that paperwork can be completed in a timely fashion

As discussed, the ideal is to have all team members present for the discussion, but that is not always possible. At these times, the team member facilitating the discussion may need to consult the missing ICT member prior to or after rounds to provide or receive a patient update or seek advice or information about patient plans. **SBAR** (Situation, Background, Assessment, Recommendation) is an effective communication technique used to facilitate concise and accurate communication between members of the team. It is especially useful when attempting to convey a message to a team member not present during rounds. See Box 2.2 for an example of SBAR.

Connection Check 2.5

Which statement by the nurse indicates an understanding of the benefits of multidisciplinary care? *(Select all that apply.)*

A. "I'm glad the social worker can focus on finding a placement for this patient."

B. "I don't have time for this teaching; the nutritionist can go over dietary plans."

C. "The occupational therapy evaluation made it clear there are more issues with activities of daily living (ADLs) to resolve before this patient can be discharged."

D. "I'm not worried about length of stay. The bean counters can deal with that."

E. "Discharge planning is much easier when we talk about it together as a team."

Interprofessional Education

Future generations of ICTs are being shaped, and interprofessional education (IPE) is a part of that development. Interprofessional education is necessary for effective

Box 2.2 SBAR

An effective form of communication that can be utilized to report changes and problems or provide a report on a patient is SBAR (situation, background, assessment, and recommendation). This is a structured method of communicating important information that needs attention and action. It is commonly used among interprofessional care team members as a standard of practice. This technique assists team members in being succinct, consistent, and thorough when sharing and handing off information or care updates.

Example of SBAR (Home-Care Coordinator [HCC] Calling Provider to Request Approval to Set Up Home Care):

S = Situation

Dr. XXX, this is XXX. I am the HCC on unit A and am calling you about your patient Mrs. XX. She has experienced two readmissions and expresses concern about her ability to manage her medications.

B = Background

She was admitted with dehydration following a prior admission for congestive heart failure (CHF). She reports confusion with her medications, and it is suspected that she double doses on her diuretics. She lives alone and plans to return home; she agrees that she needs more home support and has asked her daughter to more actively participate in her care.

A = Assessment

My assessment is that she meets the eligibility criteria for home care and would benefit from and is accepting of services.

R = Recommendation

If you are in agreement, I will make all the necessary arrangements. I will need three items from you: an order in the record, a completed face-to-face certification, and Medical Orders for Life-Sustaining Treatment (MOLST). Do you have any questions? Agree with this plan?

IC. It is defined as two or more disciplines learning how they work together in the hospital setting and outpatient settings. In the setting of IC, IPE is focused on each discipline understanding its respective skills, roles, and scope of practice. In doing this, each member can best engage the others appropriately for their expertise in patient care and together provide well-coordinated care. As an example, it is important that the inpatient team understands home-based services and available community services. This helps to ensure that all factors necessary to include in the transitions of care to improve safety are there. This process results in greater efficiency and confidence in managing the discharge process.

There is increasing recognition that IPE holds promise for preparing health professionals as collaborative-ready practitioners. Students who participate in an introductory

IPE course early in their professional preparation develop and maintain positive attitudes toward IC and learning.

The nurse should become knowledgeable about all members of the team and should educate the team as to the nursing role in each unique patient care setting. The nurse should also take responsibility, along with other members of the team, for the education of the patient as to the members of the ICT and their roles. Patients and family can easily become confused on whom to consult for specific questions. If they lack confidence or are hesitant, they may not clarify critically important care needs. Members of the ICT use their respective areas of expertise to educate patients; explain indications for contacting the provider; and coordinate posthospital care, including provider appointments and home care. As noted previously, patient participation in the ICT is essential to ensure that the patient's goals and preferences are integrated into the plan.

Connection Check 2.6

Which statement by the nurse about discharge planning indicates understanding about the role of the multidisciplinary team?

A. "This patient had a fairly uncomplicated hospital admission. There's no need to involve the team in this discharge plan."

B. "Our physical therapist is busy today. I'll take care of the physical therapy evaluation."

C. "Let's make sure we are all in agreement about the discharge plans for this patient in multidisciplinary rounds today."

D. "We need this bed for an emergency admission. I'm okay with discharging this patient before the occupational therapy evaluation."

COMPOSITION AND ROLES OF THE INTERPROFESSIONAL CARE TEAM

In the healthcare setting, a variety of professionals work directly or indirectly with the patient to help him or her return to optimal health. Each professional has unique training and addresses a particular aspect of patient care. Together, these various healthcare professionals form the ICT and contribute to the development and implementation of a plan of care for the patient throughout the continuum of care (Fig. 2.1). The ICT typically consists of but is not limited to the professionals discussed in the following subsections.

Registered Nurse

The **registered nurse (RN)** is the professional who utilizes the nursing process to care for the patient: to assess, plan, implement, and evaluate. The nurse performs the patient assessment and formulates the appropriate nursing diagnoses. The plan of care is formulated on the basis of the assessment and nursing diagnoses. The plan is implemented and evaluated; revisions are made on the basis of the evaluation. Because of the 24/7, around-the-clock responsibility of RNs, they are the eyes and ears of the healthcare team members. The RN provides feedback to the provider on the efficacy of medical interventions and reports normal and abnormal objective or subjective assessment findings. Most importantly, the RN is the patient advocate, intervening on the patient's behalf to ensure appropriate care and providing patient teaching to facilitate positive outcomes after discharge, including hand-offs to other levels of care. The RN may also function in a charge nurse role. In that role, the nurse's focus broadens from a specific patient assignment to the nursing unit as a whole. That focus includes staffing; patient movement such as discharge, transfer, or admissions; and oversight and support of all staff on the nursing unit, such as new nurses, **licensed practical nurses (LPNs)** or **licensed vocational nurses (LVNs)**, and unlicensed assistive personnel.

The LPN/LVN role functions under the direction of and **delegation** by the nurse. This list is not comprehensive, but as an example, LPNs/VPNs can provide direct patient care that includes helping with activities of daily living, such as bathing, toileting, and feeding. They can also obtain vital signs or laboratory specimens, complete wound care or dressing changes, and administer some medications. Unlike the RN, they do not have the same level of authority or responsibility and cannot make independent decisions.

Unlicensed assistive personnel (UAP) is a grouping of paraprofessionals who play a critical role in maintaining safe and accessible care. These paraprofessionals are responsible for the completion of patient care tasks, such as obtaining vital signs, and assisting patients with their personal care needs, such as activities of daily living (ADLs) and personal care. They must receive appropriate training and demonstrate competence before assuming new or expanded responsibilities within the clinical setting. Delegating and monitoring of the UAP is defined in policy and under the Nurse Practice Act. The UAP is accountable to and works under the supervision of the registered nurse when performing a delegated patient care activity and requires ongoing monitoring. With all patient care roles, it is important that communication during the planning and provision of care is maintained to ensure safe, effective care.

Delegation

Specifics regarding the "Five Rights of Delegation" are included in Table 2.1. It is important for team members to understand the authority of the RNs and the delegatee's scope of practice as it relates to patient care. Also important is understanding the rules within each specific setting because the rules may vary from institution to institution, such as from hospital to home care.

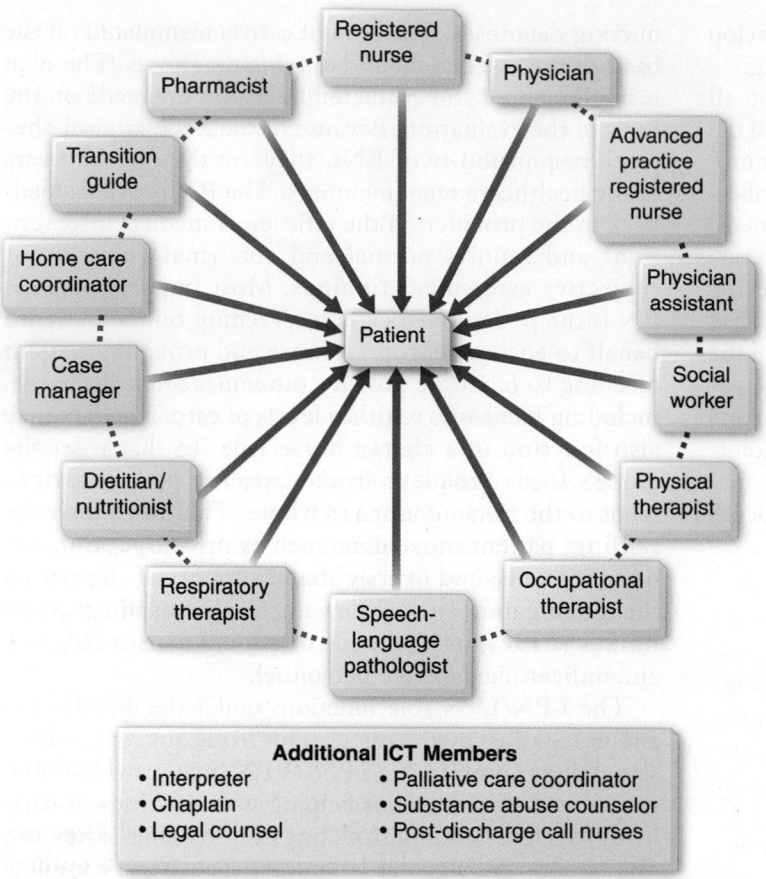

Additional ICT Members
- Interpreter
- Chaplain
- Legal counsel
- Palliative care coordinator
- Substance abuse counselor
- Post-discharge call nurses

FIGURE 2.1 The interprofessional care team (ICT).

Table 2.1 Five Rights of Delegation

Right Task	The activity falls within the delegatee's role or in policies of the nursing practice, including expectations and limits of the activity and provision of competency training.
Right Circumstance	The health condition of the patient must be stable. If there is a change, the delegatee must communicate this to the licensed nurse, who reassesses the situation and the appropriateness of the delegation.
Right Person	The licensed nurse, along with the employer and the delegatee, is responsible for ensuring that the delegatee possesses the appropriate skills and knowledge to perform the activity.
Right Directions and Communication	Each delegation situation should be specific to the patient, the licensed nurse, and the delegatee. The licensed nurse is expected to communicate specific instructions for the delegated activity to the delegatee; the delegatee, as part of two-way communication, should ask any clarifying questions. The delegatee must understand the terms of the delegation and must agree to accept the delegated activity. The licensed nurse should ensure that the delegatee understands that she or he cannot make any decisions or modifications in carrying out the activity without first consulting the licensed nurse.
Right Supervision and Evaluation	The licensed nurse is responsible for monitoring and evaluating the delegated activity. The delegatee is responsible for communicating patient information to the licensed nurse during the delegation situation. The licensed nurse should be ready and available to intervene as necessary. The licensed nurse should ensure appropriate documentation of the activity is completed.

From National Council of State Boards of Nursing. (2016). National guidelines for nursing delegation. *Journal of Nursing Regulation, 7*(1), 5–11. Retrieved from https://www.ncsbn.org/NCSBN_Delegation_Guidelines.pdf

Providers

Physician

The physician (MD) is the healthcare professional who, after reviewing the history and physical examination and results from laboratory and radiology findings, makes a diagnosis and plan for medical care. The physician typically leads the ICT with input from the entire team. Mid-level practitioners or advanced practice providers may also provide leadership of the team under the direction of the physician. They include certified registered nurse practitioners (CRNPs) and physician assistants (PAs).

Certified Registered Nurse Practitioner

Working with and under the direction of a physician, CRNPs can diagnose and manage most common and many chronic illnesses. They perform physical examinations, order and interpret diagnostic tests, provide counseling and education, and write prescriptions. The CRNP role in discharge planning varies by institution, but when involved, this role assists the attending physician in assessing the patient's post–acute care needs; coordinating necessary referrals; ordering important follow-up services; and most importantly, conveying this information to the patient, family, and ICT. The CRNP may attend rounds on behalf of the attending and liaise between the ICT and attending, which is particularly useful for surgeons who may be unavailable when in the operating room. For example, the CRNP may work with the HCC by ordering the home health services and medical equipment, ordering laboratory work, and writing prescriptions for discharge medications. The CRNP may also assist in completing required transition documents, such as those required by specific insurers in order to qualify for care, written orders needed at the next level of care, and discharge instructions forms. A transition call may also be placed to the community physician apprising this physician of the inpatient care experience and post-discharge plan. The CRNP, depending on the model of care within the institution, is typically available for post-discharge calls and possibly for clinic visits. Of note, because this role is a nursing role, the CRNP may be able to assist with making recommendations for specific nursing care as well.

Physician Assistant

Similar to the NP, PAs obtain medical histories, perform examinations and procedures, prescribe medications and treatments, order and interpret diagnostic tests, diagnose on the basis of those assessments and tests, and assist in the operating room. They typically work with specific physicians, may attend rounds on behalf of the attending, and may also assist with the discharge planning and transition-of-care plan as described previously for the CRNP.

Social Worker

The social workers (SWs) are the professionals who assess the psychosocial functioning of patients and families. They intervene as necessary, connecting patients and families to necessary supports and resources in the community. They can also provide supportive counseling and help the patient strengthen his or her network of social supports. The SW assists with specific transition care planning, such as guardianship for patients who cannot make sound decisions, facility transfers, and assistance with insurance or medical care provisions.

Rehabilitation Therapy

Physical Therapist

The physical therapist (PT) is the professional who assesses and provides training and education on physical strength, gait, and mobility for the patient. This professional may also provide wound care and teach transfer techniques, secretion clearance techniques (ways to cough and bring up secretions), and neuromuscular reeducation (relearning to walk or use an affected limb with maximum function). The PT evaluates and assists the patient in utilizing techniques to maximize his or her safety during and after the hospitalization.

Occupational Therapist

The occupational therapist (OT) is the professional who assesses and retrains the patient to perform ADLs, such as bathing, brushing teeth, dressing, cooking, and doing laundry, and performing skills necessary to return to optimal functions. This professional utilizes adaptive equipment to assist patients in performing these activities, such as a grabber or adaptive utensils. The OT also provides visual and spatial perceptual retraining, such as using a double-vision eye patch and teaching the art of scanning the environment (gathering information about the external environment as an aid in planning a course of action), as well as energy conservation for patients with poor endurance, such as those with chronic respiratory conditions.

Speech-Language Pathologist

The speech-language pathologist (SLP) is the professional who assesses, diagnoses, and treats patients with disorders relating to speech, language, swallowing, voice, and cognitive communication. The SLP develops specific exercises and recommends food consistencies for patients with dysphagia, dysarthria, and a tracheostomy to help prevent complications.

Respiratory Therapist

The respiratory therapist (RT) is the professional who specializes in airway management. As part of and in collaboration with the healthcare team, the RT is responsible for maintaining the airway through the administration of oxygen, nebulized medications, and assessment of respiratory status and lung function (through pulmonary function tests and other assessment methods). The RT cares for patients with all types of respiratory disorders: upper airway disorders such as sinusitis, nasal trauma and fractures, and laryngeal cancer and lower airway disorders such as chronic obstructive pulmonary disease, asthma, restrictive lung disease, and respiratory distress syndrome. The RT is able to perform arterial blood gases to monitor oxygenation, ventilation, and acid–base balance and also manages ventilators under the direction of the provider.

Registered Dietitian/Nutritionist

The **registered dietitian/nutritionist (RD)** is the professional who assesses the patient's nutritional needs, develops meal plans, and provides education about dietary modifications related to the individual's disease process. The RD promotes healthy eating habits and assists patients in adapting to acceptable diets according to their healthcare needs, such as recommending a low-sodium diet for patients with congestive heart failure, a low-carbohydrate diet for patients with diabetes, or a low-fat diet for patients with heart disease. The RD also assists in designing enteral and parenteral plans for patients who can no longer eat by mouth and require gastrostomy tubes and central line nutrition.

Case Manager

The **case manager (CM)** may come from a variety of backgrounds, typically an RN with an advanced nursing degree or a social worker. This team member utilizes the processes of assessing, planning, facilitating, advocating, and providing available resources to meet the individual's health needs with sound quality and cost-effective outcomes in mind. A CM incorporates the input of the ICT to plan in-hospital care and discharge transition care. This professional monitors services to ensure that the patient has the available resources to return to optimal health. This may include conferring with the provider to make a hospice referral for a patient with a terminal illness or assisting a patient in securing medications, which is difficult because of affordability, all while incorporating the patient and family's preference and requests into the plan.

Home-Care Coordinator

A **home-care coordinator (HCC)**, typically an RN, identifies home-care needs proactively while the patient is in the hospital/skilled nursing facility or emergency department, or in lieu of hospitalization, the HCC may coordinate care from a provider's office. The HCC facilitates the provision of services in the home, including nursing, therapy, infusion, and respiratory care and medical equipment (e.g., hospital bed), and establishes the necessary resources needed for home care prior to discharge.

Transition Guide

The **transition guide (TG)**, typically an RN with an advanced practice degree, assists patients during and after transitions (such as from hospital to home or a skilled nursing facility), with the goals of ensuring a smooth transition, identifying and managing readmission risks, and assisting with aligning possible resources to aid in the patient's plan of care. The TG may meet with the patient prior to discharge and reconnect by phone and/or via home visits and is typically accessed when other home-based services are not warranted or when the patient is not eligible. These roles are typically paid by the hospital in a cost-avoidance strategy to minimize readmissions.

Pharmacist

The **pharmacist** is actively involved in the management of the patient's medications, including:

- Reconciling the patient's medications between transitions of care (from home to the hospital and then from hospital to home)
- Reviewing medication orders for appropriateness and adjustment to the hospital formulary
- Monitoring of medication interactions
- Monitoring of adverse medication reactions
- Monitoring of therapeutic medication levels
- Providing medication counseling to the patient and family members
- Providing patient teaching on new or complex medications

The pharmacist oversees pharmacy technicians who assume responsibility for preparing medications. The pharmacist is an important ICT member because of his or her skills in identifying the best medication regimens for the patient, considering such factors as costs and caregiver skills (e.g., ability to inject medications long term).

> **(!) Safety Alert** A pharmacist should review all medication orders before administration to the patient to ensure that there are no medication interactions, allergies, or other safer alternatives that should be considered.

Ad Hoc Members

Ad hoc members of the ICT may include:

- Interpreter
- Chaplain
- Community health worker
- Legal counsel
- Palliative care coordinator
- Substance abuse counselor
- Post-discharge call nurses

The **interpreter** is the professional who facilitates the understanding of medical information by translating the information from English to the patient's native tongue, and vice versa. The interpreter needs to have command of the specific language that he or she translates and should also have the ability to translate the medical terms effectively. Specific competencies are required in order to interpret in the healthcare setting. Family members should not be relied on as interpreters because they may not accurately impart all of the information the patient needs to hear and understand.

The **chaplain** is the professional who has an educational background in religion. The chaplain provides spiritual comfort to patients and family members in need.

The **community health worker (CHW)** is an emerging role in the healthcare setting. CHWs serve as a point of connection between the patient's community and the rest of the health system. This role receives basic healthcare training and focuses on behavioral health concepts and important concepts related to patient engagement and motivational factors to promote health. It is important that the ICT understands the specifics of the CHW's role because there are many different types of CHWs. CHWs may address single health issues (e.g., diabetes) or multiple chronic issues, and they have differences in their levels of knowledge, training, and practice settings. Many focus on communities with which they have experience, or where they reside, to heighten credibility with and acceptance by patients.

The **legal counsel** is the professional who has judicial education, particularly in healthcare law, and provides legal perspective and support when resolving legal matters in the healthcare setting. This professional protects the rights of the patients and healthcare professionals in the healthcare system and works to identify safety risks and reduce them.

The **palliative care coordinator** is an advanced practice RN who provides information and support for the patient and family members when the patient needs disease, pain, or symptom management or is in need of hospice care when the patient has a terminal illness. This professional facilitates end-of-life discussions with the patient, family, and healthcare team and helps coordinate the care at home or in a facility.

The **substance abuse counselor** can be an SW, counselor, or RN but is typically a professional with a degree or certificate in addiction counseling. This team member provides counseling, support, and resources for patients who are addicted to substances, most commonly alcohol or prescription or illicit drugs such as heroin, cocaine, or marijuana. This counselor can help facilitate inpatient or outpatient detoxification programs for patients with substance abuse problems.

Post-discharge call nurses perform follow-up calls to patients after hospital discharge. They contact the patients who transition home with lower levels of support. Typically, this call is made in the first 24 to 48 hours after discharge to assess how the transition home is progressing. The calls are typically scripted and involve data collection for outcome measures or identification of missed discharge-planning opportunities and activities. The post-discharge call nurse hopes to identify potential challenges early in an attempt to prevent a readmission. Clinical symptom algorithms may be used to make a determination of a stable or unstable condition. An example is inquiring about weight gain, breathing, or fatigue in a patient

with congestive heart failure (CHF). Post-discharge calls can be very helpful in making necessary connections, such as home care for patients who thought they would be comfortable providing their own care at home but, once there, find it to be overwhelming and confusing. The post-discharge call nurse may also have the opportunity to answer questions for a caregiver who was not present during the discharge teaching process. Last, calls may assist with learning about the patient's experience with care in the hospital and give the patient the opportunity to voice complaints and/or compliments.

The patient is the center of the interprofessional effort; however, another important member of the care team is the **Patient and Family Advisory Council (PFAC)**. Most hospitals have PFACs that empower patients and their families and caregivers to participate in the improvement of patient care. PFACs are evolving across the continuum of care. Patients and family members on these councils provide feedback about their experiences of care, review care processes, and evaluate new programs, to name a few areas in which they are involved. The members may also be care mentors and advocates in specific care areas. The team may interact with specific members or access the PFAC through a request to provide input, evaluate a specific care matter, or provide general feedback.

Connection Check 2.7

The nurse is caring for a patient who has experienced a CVA. Which ICT members should be involved in this patient's care? *(Select all that apply.)*

A. Occupational therapist
B. Physical therapist
C. Physician
D. Case manager
E. Legal counsel

UNIQUE PATIENT SITUATIONS REQUIRING OR ENHANCED BY INTERPROFESSIONAL COLLABORATION

All patients benefit from IC, but there are several situations where effective collaboration clearly maximizes patient outcomes (Box 2.3). Complex patients with multisystem disease require the expertise of many disciplines. Examples include patients with transplants, those with a chronic disease such as CHF or chronic pulmonary obstructive disease, and patients with cancer. Another example is the patient with catastrophic traumatic injuries involving orthopedic, neurological, cardiovascular, and respiratory issues. These patients require providers from many disciplines working collaboratively with the nurse at the bedside, as well as input from the pharmacist, nutritionist, OT, and PT to design the plan of care. Elderly patients with limited resources or limited caregiver options and patients with impaired mental status are equally challenging. They require collaboration between all members of the team but especially home care, social work, and CMs to facilitate the availability of the necessary resources in the hospital and at home.

Discharge planning must begin the day of admission; especially with short lengths of stay, it is imperative to discover any issues that may affect a successful transition plan. Key to that is determining the details about the patient's social network, such as:

- Are there family members or friends available to help upon discharge?
- Does the patient have a home to return to, or should the patient return home?
- Can the patient afford the medications ordered? Does the patient have transportation to the provider's office?

An example of a patient who clearly needs and would benefit from effective IC is one going home with a new tracheostomy. There are many questions and issues to be considered. Examples (not an exhaustive list) of the care-planning process/questions for that patient include:

- Who is assuming primary responsibility for managing the tracheostomy? Backup? Third-level backup?
- Has teaching been completed prior to discharge? Can the primary and secondary caregivers successfully demonstrate at least three return demonstrations of tracheostomy care and suctioning?
- When will the patient get the tracheostomy changed? Have the supply sizes been specified so that the proper equipment is ordered?
- What emergency equipment is in place, such as an Ambu bag and suction equipment?
- Has oxygen been ordered? Has the household considered all the oxygen safety factors?
- What other equipment is needed? Hospital bed? Bedside commode? Wheelchair? Suction machine?
- Have home healthcare services been ordered?

Connection Check 2.8

Which statement by the nurse indicates an understanding of the benefits of interprofessional collaboration in providing care for patients with chronic illness? *(Select all that apply.)*

A. "Social work can be consulted to assist with long-term counseling."

B. "Family members need to be included, with the patient's approval, to assess their willingness to assist in the long-term care of the patient."

C. "Each member of the ICT participates in patient education and can use teach-back as a technique to determine synthesis of the information."

D. "The ICT is concerned about developing a solid discharge plan that produces positive outcomes for the patient and prevents readmissions."

E. "Direct care nurses are not involved in long-term care planning for patients with chronic illness."

Box 2.3 Advantages of Interprofessional Collaboration

- Enhanced communication between members of the team
- Improved understanding of all team members' roles and responsibilities
- More timely discharge and transition planning
- Greater safety in the discharge transition process
- Improved patient satisfaction with the discharge transition process
- Improved team member satisfaction
- Decreased unnecessary hospital days
- Decreased 30-day readmission rates

Making Connections

CASE STUDY: WRAP-UP

Mr. Garfield's discharge plan is discussed in rounds. He continues to be hypertensive during the hospitalization, so he will need to go home with a prescription for an antihypertensive and close monitoring. Social work will work on insurance support for his prescriptions. An interpreter is available to help the nurse, pharmacist, and RD with patient teaching related to his hypertension, diet, and the action/frequency/side effects of the medications. Teach-back is used to ensure that Mrs. Garfield is retaining the teaching provided. Mrs. Garfield decides to take the patient home. On day 3 of the hospitalization, she assists the nurses in delivering his care. On day 4, she provides care all on her own, with supervision, to gain confidence and skills prior to discharge. The HCC works to arrange equipment (hospital bed, bedside commode, and a wheelchair) and home-care services to including nursing, all three therapists (PT, OT, and speech), a SW, and a home health aide. A referral is made to a local skilled nursing facility just in case the plan fails at home. A follow-up provider appointment is made for the first week after discharge.

Case Study Questions

1. Which statement by Mr. Garfield indicates that teaching has been effective?
   A. "I don't need to get lab work when I feel well."
   B. "I'll take my pill when I don't feel good."
   C. "I have to take this pill even if I feel good."
   D. "My blood pressure isn't really that high; it won't cause a problem until it gets really high."

2. Which members of the interprofessional home-care team are necessary for Mr. Garfield's care? *(Select all that apply.)*
   A. Home-care nurse
   B. Home health aide
   C. Speech-language pathologist
   D. Primary care provider
   E. Palliative care provider

3. Which statement is true about the follow-up appointment?

    A. The appointment can be canceled if the patient is doing well.

    B. The appointment can be delayed if the patient is feeling well.

    C. It is important to follow up with the provider as planned.

    D. The appointment is unnecessary if the patient refuses to go.

4. Which statement is *incorrect* about working with a patient who primarily speaks a different language?

    A. An interpreter is always advised when imparting important information.

    B. Family members can be used to interpret when necessary.

    C. Written teaching materials should be in the patient's native language.

    D. Non-English-speaking patients require advance discharge planning.

5. Excellent interprofessional collaboration in Mr. Garfield's care is evidenced by which of the following statements?

    A. All members of the team worked according to their specialty to determine an appropriate discharge plan.

    B. Only the team members necessary were involved in designing Mr. Garfield's discharge plan.

    C. Only the inpatient team was necessary in developing the discharge plan.

    D. Only the outpatient team was necessary in developing the discharge plan.

CHAPTER SUMMARY

The need for better patient care coordination, particularly smoother transitions of care between different care facilities, is a growing concern in the U.S. healthcare system. Increased medical errors, often resulting in patient harm; increased length of stays in hospital settings; and increased healthcare costs are all driving factors for better care coordination and interprofessional team collaboration.

Patient-centered transitional care and other care-management initiatives are within the nursing scope of practice. Transitional care models and patient-centered medical homes put nurses in leadership positions to help coordinate care; engage patients, caregivers, and providers; and safely transition patients between care settings. Nurses in these positions easily transition with the patient and become a link to care. The transitional care model (TCM), Care Transitions Program, and guided care are evidence-based practices that utilize nurses in providing patient-centered care coordination across the care continuum. Increasing transitional care and care-management programs is part of the new healthcare landscape, and it will require well-prepared nurses to assist in further development and implementation.

Interprofessional collaboration (IC) is an equal partnership among the varied healthcare professionals and the patient, all working together to provide care to patients. While in the hospital, patients receive care from the IC. When preparing the patient for discharge, the role of the IC is to prepare to transition care to the patient and family. The essential components of this collaboration are coordination, communication, and shared responsibility. The purpose is to formulate and deliver a plan of care that is goal directed and team focused. Goal-directed care focuses on the overall aim for each patient. Daily care objectives remain focused on that overall goal, facilitating the efficient use of time and resources. Patient teaching and teach-back are integral parts of the interprofessional care team (ICT) process.

Members of the team include the registered nurse, physician, social worker, physical therapist, occupational therapist, respiratory therapy, nutritionist, case manager, pharmacist, and speech-language pathologist. Other members of the team include an interpreter, chaplain, legal counsel, home-care coordinator, palliative care coordinator, transition guide, and substance abuse counselor. The ICT may round and review patient care or speak informally but often uses a standardized communication. such as SBAR (see Box 2.2).

Interprofessional collaboration improves the care of the patient by increasing coordination between all healthcare disciplines. Time and resources are utilized more efficiently. Discharge issues are identified early, facilitating a return to home in a timely fashion. Interprofessional collaboration enhances the professional satisfaction of the members of the healthcare team. Ultimately, the outcomes of IC include improved communication, enhanced safety, decreased costs of care, prevention of unnecessary readmissions, and positive patient outcomes. The patient benefits from care delivered by an interprofessional approach, and the practice of the nurse is enhanced.

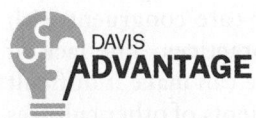
DAVIS ADVANTAGE

To explore learning resources for this chapter, go to **Davis Advantage** and find:
 – Answers to in-text questions
 – Chapter Resources and Activities
 – NCLEX®-Style Chapter Review Questions
 – Bibliography

Chapter 3

Cultural Considerations

Nina Trocky

LEARNING OUTCOMES

Content in this chapter is designed to assist in:

1. Differentiating between cultural competence, awareness, and sensitivity
2. Describing social factors that predispose patients to health disparities
3. Using a cultural competency model to assess knowledge, attitudes, and beliefs
4. Explaining how bias may influence nursing judgment
5. Explaining the social determinants of health

CONCEPTS

- Assessment
- Communication
- Diversity
- Nursing Roles
- Self

ESSENTIAL TERMS

Ageism
Bias
Conscious (explicit) bias
Cultural awareness
Cultural competence
Cultural sensitivity
Culture
Disparity
Diversity
Ethnicity
Ethnocentrism
Gender identity
Health disparity
Health literacy
Identify
Implicit bias
Literacy
Race
Social determinants of health
Stereotype
Transcultural nursing
Xenophobia

Finding Connections

CASE STUDY: EPISODE 1

Follow this patient throughout the chapter.

Liu Huìwén is a 79-year-old female born in Taiwan. She speaks Mandarin, with limited English. Mrs. Liu recently moved in with her daughter and son-in-law because she requires more assistance to complete activities of daily living. Mrs. Liu's daughter has found her crying during the day and is not sure if Mrs. Liu is taking her Coumadin and other medications prescribed by her primary care physician and cardiologist (Mrs. Liu has heart failure and atrial fibrillation). Mrs. Liu asks her daughter to take her to a Chinese medicine store...

INTRODUCTION

The ethnic and racial composition of the United States is continually evolving. In the past 25 years, the minority population has been increasing while the majority population has been on the decline. According to the U.S. Census Bureau, African American/black and Asian minority populations have increased, as has the number of Hispanics. Nursing care must be culturally competent in order to best serve the evolving diverse population. Cultural competence in healthcare is having the knowledge, abilities, and skills to deliver care congruent with the patient's cultural beliefs and practices. The lack of skills related to cultural competence can make it difficult for nurses to communicate with patients of other cultures and races; therefore, knowledge of other cultures is imperative. In addition to awareness of other cultures, nurses must avoid being ethnocentric and remain bias-free.

Ethnocentrism is the universal tendency of human beings to think that their individual ways of thinking, acting, and believing are the only right, proper, and natural ways. Nurses must remain nonjudgmental to optimize relationships and maximize quality care for all patients.

The concepts of ethnicity, culture, race, bias, identity, and inclusion are potential influences on nurses' judgment and behaviors, affecting the ability to deliver culturally competent and patient-centered care. Nurses have no way of knowing an individual's personal values and beliefs, national heritage, feelings about sexual identity, experiences within the healthcare system, or health literacy, based solely on appearance and demographic data. Nurses must develop essential skills in this area, enabling them to work with and care for a cross-cultural and ethnically diverse workforce and patient population. Becoming a competent healthcare professional requires each individual to evaluate and assess his or her knowledge of other cultures and also requires an understanding of personal biases and stereotypes (generalized beliefs about a particular category of people) that inhibit the ability to provide compassionate and patient-centered care to all. Moreover, elimination of racial and ethnic disparities in healthcare is needed, and nurses are instrumental in developing care congruent with the principles of a social justice and human rights orientation. The provision of culturally congruent care and sensitivity in developing care based on patients' beliefs and values are core competencies in nursing education.

ETHNICITY, RACE, IDENTITY, CULTURE, AND CULTURAL BELIEF SYSTEM

Race and ethnicity are related but different concepts. Both terms are associated with how individuals choose to self-identify (identify means how a person views him- or herself). Both race and ethnicity place individuals within a social category and begin to establish a personal and group identity.

The American Sociological Association defines race as the physical differences that groups and cultures consider socially significant, such as skin color, hair texture, and eye shape or color. The U.S. Office of Management and Budget defines the racial categories that are used in all aspects of our daily lives, including employment applications, official census data, and even Medicaid applications. Self-reporting is the primary method of racial identification, using the following five categories from the U.S. Census Bureau:

- White—a person having origins in any of the original peoples of Europe, the Middle East, or North Africa
- Black or African American—a person having origins in any of the black racial groups of Africa
- American Indian or Alaska Native—a person having origins in any of the original peoples of North and South America (including Central America) and who maintains tribal affiliation or community attachment

- Asian—a person having origins in any of the original peoples of the Far East, Southeast Asia, or the Indian subcontinent, including, for example, Cambodia, China, India, Japan, Korea, Malaysia, Pakistan, the Philippine Islands, Thailand, Taiwan, and Vietnam
- Native Hawaiian or other Pacific Islander—a person having origins in any of the original peoples of Hawaii, Guam, Samoa, or other Pacific Islands

In 2000, the U.S. census offered survey participants the option to select more than one race as the racial category to more accurately describe the changing demographics of the United States and account for the children born to parents of different races. The number of children of two or more races is expected to more than double between 2018 and 2060, from 5% to 11%.

Ethnicity is related to race, but the terms are not synonymous. Ethnicity is the perception of oneself as belonging to one or more ethnic groups, including a commitment to cultural customs and rituals. For demographic purposes, the U.S. Census Bureau makes the distinction between people of Hispanic and non-Hispanic origin, and this information may be included in healthcare data. On an admission intake form, for example, the patient may select "White, non-Hispanic," where "White" is the race and "non-Hispanic" is the ethnicity. However, all patients who self-identify as the same ethnicity may not share all of the same practices or preferences. For example, individuals of Hispanic ethnicity may share a common language (e.g., Spanish) and religion (e.g., Catholic), or they may share a language but not a religion. Another example is an individual who identifies as an Alaskan Native and may refer to him- or herself as a member of a particular tribal community and language group (e.g., Aleut or Eyak). Race and ethnicity are elements of a broader concept called culture. Culture is complex. At first, a person may simply explain that he or she is Irish or Jewish or African in relation to culture. However, that is a very limited view of culture. Culture relates to dynamic patterns of behaviors based upon beliefs and values, communication, customs, language, roles and relationships. These interrelated patterns influence expected behaviors associated with ethnic, racial, religious or social groups that are shared and transmitted to following generations.

When thinking about "culture," individuals consider how much of self is visible to others and how much is kept hidden, yet everything about self—visible or hidden—interacts to create the individual's cultural belief system. Cultural belief systems are personally defined and unique to each individual; they reflect what is valuable and true to that individual, based on ideas and stories individuals tell themselves from a social and personal context.

In healthcare, an individual's belief system influences information processing, including interactions with providers and the overall healthcare system. For example, food may be considered a medicine by certain individuals because food is used to restore health, whereas others may not see food and diet from such a holistic perspective. As caring professionals, nurses must develop their ability to provide culturally competent care—embracing a patient's belief system and preferences, ensuring that care is inclusive, just, and respectful.

CULTURAL COMPETENCE, AWARENESS, AND SENSITIVITY

Cultural competence, awareness, and sensitivity are similar yet different terms. Each term reflects critical knowledge, skills, and abilities that enable nurses to provide care that is appropriate for each patient's unique set of needs. Learning the differences between each term is the first step. Knowing that differences exist, having the ability to be open to and accepting of these differences, and choosing to avoid judging or assigning value to the differences is the goal.

Cultural Competence

The term *competence* is not new to nursing and healthcare. Competence refers to a person demonstrating proficiency, knowledge, and/or skill. Registered nurses learn how to take blood pressures and often must complete an annual validation to demonstrate competency for that essential skill, and they are then expected to complete that task correctly, every time. Cultural competence is the ability of healthcare providers and organizations to effectively deliver healthcare services that meet the social, cultural, and linguistic needs of patients. Culturally competent care means that nurses learn about each patient and tailor nursing actions to the individual patient and the patient's needs.

Culturally competent care is essential to all nursing interventions. In fact, it is a professional expectation set forth by the American Nurses Association (ANA) *Standards of Professional Practice*. Specifically, Standard 8 explains that "the registered nurse practices in a manner that is congruent with cultural diversity and inclusion principles," which is demonstrated in a number of ways. The elements of Standard 8 explain how nurses apply knowledge of culture and inclusion to develop care that is appropriate, sensitive, and reflective of current nursing practice (Box 3.1).

Total cultural competency requires the recognition that care must be equal, respect **diversity**, and be free of bias. Equal care means that every patient is treated the same, and as a result, patient care outcomes are similar. For example, a nurse provides two different patients information about heart failure. One patient is a college graduate who possesses a high level of literacy, whereas the other patient has less education and a lower level of literacy. The nurse confirms both patients fully understand the material and provides additional literacy support to either patient as necessary. This ensures that both patients receive equal access to the information.

Box 3.1 American Nurses Association Standards of Professional Practice: Standard 8

The registered nurse practices in a manner that is congruent with cultural diversity and inclusion principles.
 Competencies for the registered nurse:

1. Demonstrates respect, equity, and empathy in actions and interactions with all healthcare consumers.
2. Participates in life-long learning to understand cultural preferences, worldview, choices, and decision-making processes of diverse consumers.
3. Creates an inventory of one's own values, beliefs, and cultural heritage.
4. Applies knowledge of variations in health beliefs, practices, and communication patterns in all nursing practice activities.
5. Identifies the stage of the consumer's acculturation and oppression in practice within and among vulnerable cultural groups.
6. Considers the effects and impact of discrimination and oppression on practice within and among vulnerable cultural groups.
7. Uses skills and tools that are appropriately vetted for the culture, literacy, and language of the population served.
8. Communicates with appropriate language and behaviors, including the use of medical interpreters and translators in accordance with consumer preferences.
9. Identifies the cultural-specific meaning of interactions, terms, and content.
10. Respects consumer decisions based on age, tradition, beliefs and family influence, and stage of acculturation.
11. Advocates for policies that promote health and prevent harm among culturally diverse, underserved, or underrepresented consumers.
12. Promotes equal access to services, tests, interventions, health promotion programs, enrollment in research, education, and other opportunities.
13. Educates nurse colleagues and other professionals about cultural similarities and differences of healthcare consumers, families, groups, communities, and populations.

From American Nurses Association. (2015). *Nursing scope and standards of practice* (3rd ed.). Washington, DC: Author.

Cultural Awareness

Realizing that each patient sees and interprets things in his or her own way is the first step toward becoming culturally aware. Awareness may be defined as knowledge or understanding of a subject, issue, or situation, and cultural awareness is rooted in a desire to interact with the patient in a real and authentic fashion. **Cultural awareness**, therefore, is the realization and recognition that personal beliefs and values impact cultural health beliefs and potentially the view of those who are different. It is a critical starting point that nurses choose not to impose personal views on others. Awareness brings humility, further introspection, and empathy, which can help the nurse develop care that respects each patient's unique needs. To fully respect the differences of individual patients, nurses must actively create an environment and tone that are inclusive and without judgment. A nurse must be culturally aware to provide care that is appropriate for each patient and respectful of each patient's beliefs. For example, in some cultures, it might be appropriate and acceptable to physically stand very close to the person to whom you are speaking. In another cultural, physical space or distance between those in conversation is necessary, fostering comfort. Being culturally aware means that the nurse honors the patient's need for distance and does not force his or her own need to stand close to the patient. Awareness means the nurse is curious, wishing to know more, and choosing to act in a way that honors the patient's needs, not his or her own needs. Acknowledging and understanding the differences among patients and learning from them is the start of a nurse's cultural awareness.

Cultural Sensitivity

In order to provide culturally competent care, nurses must demonstrate **cultural sensitivity**: an understanding, thoughtfulness, and kindness that leads to inclusiveness and equity. Cultural sensitivity relates to an appreciation of one's personal needs and emotions, as well as to others' cultural practices, that lead to patient-centered care. This is especially important because, no matter the setting, nurses care for patients who come from diverse backgrounds. In fact, The Joint Commission (2017) developed an application, Cultural Sensitivity for Health Care Professionals, to help healthcare professionals improve their ability to deliver culturally sensitive care and strengthen communication skills with patients and families.

As nurses, caring is a hallmark behavior that promotes actions, attitudes, and behaviors that respect all cultures and all patients as individuals. Having a caring mindset and being open to considering and appreciating a patient's culture require time and desire. These are attributes of a professional registered nurse and reflect the ANA's commitment to respecting the human rights of all persons and avoiding personal biases and stereotypes that lead to inequity.

Connection Check 3.1

Select the statement that reflects a culturally sensitive response to a patient's question.

A. Can you try to decrease your smoking while you work?

B. How do your religious beliefs impact your healthcare decisions?

C. What is the biggest barrier to you making a lifestyle change?

D. When do you think it is possible for you to decrease your salt intake?

HEALTH DISPARITIES AND HEALTH EQUITY

Registered nurses must be committed to reducing health inequities and disparities by customizing patients' plans of care. Applying the *Standards of Professional Practice* ensures that the nurse's role is to fulfill a social contract, based on social justice, modifying care by responding to the needs of patients. Raising awareness is the first step in addressing barriers to health equity. As awareness is raised, nurses improve the ability to recognize actions that perpetuate unjust and unequal care and treatment that contribute to social injustice.

Health Disparities

A **disparity** is a difference, inequity, discrepancy, or gap. According to the Office of Disease Prevention and Health Promotion, a **health disparity** is a health difference that is closely linked with social, economic, or environmental disadvantages. Health disparities are real and preventable, and they exist in all age groups, cultures, races, ethnic groups, religions, and populations who are vulnerable by virtue of sexual identity.

Any difference in a health outcome that is related to bias, injustice, exclusion, marginalization, and social determinants of health may be viewed as a disparity. For example, in the U.S., infant mortality rates are 2.2 times higher in African Americans compared with non-Hispanic whites, and the rate of postneonatal mortality for non-Hispanic blacks and American Indian/Alaskan Natives is more than twice that of non-Hispanic whites. This may be the result of many social factors (Box 3.2) or may result from the biases and discriminatory behaviors of providers. For the patient, the degree of risk and vulnerability grows as the number of social factors increases.

Age

A patient's age is an important consideration in the provision of culturally competent care. Age is one of many factors that informs the nurse's actions when developing a plan

---

Box 3.2 Social Factors Affecting Healthcare Equity

- Age
- Differences in education
- Disabilities
- Economic instability
- Gender
- Income inequality
- Limited English proficiency
- Limited social support
- Mental illness
- Race
- Sexuality
- Social isolation

of care. However, assuming that patients of the same age, young or old, act and feel the same way is a misperception. **Ageism**, or stereotyping and discriminating based solely on the patient's age, marginalizes the patient and results in dehumanizing and inappropriate care. The following examples show how nurses exhibit ageism:

- When admitting a 79-year-old female for elective surgery, the nurse avoids asking a question about alcohol intake because the likelihood of alcoholism is "pretty low" in her age group. The nurse assumes the female patient does not drink alcohol and misses the opportunity to assess the patient for alcohol use disorder.
- During a health assessment, the nurse notices that the older adult male appears underweight and assumes the patient is malnourished. The nurse fails to ascertain that the patient is a long-distance runner whose weight has been stable for several years. Moreover, upon finding this out, the nurse questions the importance of physical activity in "someone his age." The nurse dismisses the importance of exercise to the patient's social and spiritual well-being.

Nurses must take steps to avoid judging and stereotyping patients based on age because these actions affect a patient's ability to receive the most appropriate care. These effects may be associated with health disparities because older adults may have limited access to healthcare, whereas in many older adults, the use of healthcare services increases. With the price of medications and other out-of-pocket costs, senior adults are faced with the financial burden of prescription medication use, which may result in delayed healthcare and unmet healthcare needs. Nurses have the opportunity to assess patients using an age-relevant lens that supports the identification of appropriate resources to address patient needs.

Race

To support a healthcare workforce empowered to address and embrace the diversity in the patient population, the U.S. Congress formed the Office of Minority Health (OMH) in 1986. The OMH supports research, projects, and other initiatives to promote a better understanding of health risk factors and successful prevention and intervention strategies for minority populations. Despite the work done by the OMH, there are still problems with health equity for minority populations. The 2010 census noted that although several health indicators (e.g., life expectancy, infant mortality) did improve for the general population, minority groups continued to have a greater incidence of preventable disease, death, and disability compared with nonminorities.

Gender and Sexuality

Gender is defined as the socially constructed characteristics of women and men, such as norms, roles, and relationships of and between groups of women and men. However, how one identifies oneself may be different from how others describe the person. **Gender identity** is how one defines and sees oneself. For example, a patient appears to be anatomically male, yet the patient identifies as female. This is gender identity and may lead to gender bias in the nurse. The nurse's actions can lead to inappropriate treatment of the patient, such as avoiding contact other than when it is necessary. Gender bias is the end result of negative stereotyping (e.g., assuming all males who are transitioning to a female act in a certain way) and can lead to gender discrimination or the unequal treatment of the patient. Nurses must be able to avoid gender bias and discrimination in order to establish a therapeutic relationship that is free from judgment, personal opinions, or the power to demoralize the patient and/or family. Nurses must develop care based on the acceptance of all patients for who they are, not how the nurse might think they should be, and that care should be both compassionate and equitable.

Sexuality or sexual orientation is linked with gender identity and refers to which individuals a person chooses for romantic and sexual encounters. Both gender identity and sexual orientation are individually and personally defined and may be different from how others may "see" them. A nurse might hold the opinion that men "look" a certain way and women might "act" a certain way; these ideas reflect a broad generalization that is unacceptable and harmful. Holding on to one's personal perceptions regarding sexuality leads to behavior that negatively impacts one's interactions with others, which is called gender stereotyping. The nurse's role is to ensure gender equality and facilitate care that respects all patients' rights and preferences.

In 2016, the National Institute on Minority Health and Health Disparities (NINHD), a part of the U.S. Department of Health and Human Services, designated sexual and gender minorities as a health disparity population. This designation allows the NINHD to specifically address the need for research among lesbian, gay, bisexual, and transgender populations, including those who may be questioning sexual orientation, identity, and expression. Subsequent studies have shown that the social stigma associated with transgender patients plays a role in the degree of patient engagement with medical care. For HIV-positive transgender youth and emerging adults, this was found to result in missed HIV care appointments. Because HIV is a chronic disease, missed HIV visits may lead to greater morbidity and a higher viral load for the individual, which can increase the chance of HIV transmission.

Economics

The possession of adequate financial resources for day-to-day living expenses and to pay for healthcare services greatly impacts an individual's ability to obtain healthcare. The high costs of healthcare services and health insurance create a financial barrier for patients with limited resources. Information related to both past and present financial resources is useful in determining gaps in healthcare or deterioration in health status and function that may be attributable to economic factors. Through a better understanding of the patient's financial needs, the nurse identifies the support services (e.g., patient assistance programs for prescription medications) that are appropriate for the patient.

When patients face economic and financial barriers to accessing healthcare, there may also be delays in receiving care and/or accessing primary care services that potentially prevent definitive care and hospitalization. Often, income level and employment are associated with health insurance access. Health insurance increases a patient's access to primary care and preventative care. Additionally, the Peterson Center on Healthcare noted that in 2016, an estimated 1 in 10 adults reported that healthcare costs resulted in a delay in seeking care or in avoiding care altogether. Other research, for example, has found that younger black men with healthcare insurance are more likely to participate in prostate cancer screening. As a nurse, understanding the financial barriers and supporting access to healthcare and services for all patients is a vital part of helping patients achieve the highest possible level of health.

Language and Literacy

Communication is a vital part of any patient encounter. The concepts of literacy and health literacy are essential components of providing patient-centered care. **Literacy** is the ability to read, write, speak, and compute and solve problems, and **health literacy** is the ability to appropriately locate, comprehend, and use health information and services. Patients must have an adequate understanding of their treatment plan, medications, and health status in order to make informed decisions. When given teaching materials, patients must be able to read and understand the content accurately, as well as to be able to read printed materials and contact the healthcare provider if experiencing unusual symptoms.

Patients with language barriers or poor levels of health literacy use healthcare services differently compared with patients with higher health literacy and may experience poorer outcomes. Patients with low health literacy are less likely to access preventative services, such as mammograms and influenza vaccinations; are less knowledgeable about their chronic conditions, making them less able to adequately manage disease; have higher hospital admissions and emergency room visits; and have lower medication management capacity (i.e., having the ability to identify, open, and describe the dose and timing of their medications).

Geography

According to the Robert Wood Johnson Foundation, each individual is affected by three interrelated environments either promoting or jeopardizing his or her health: physical, social, and service environments. The physical environment is the "built environment," which includes housing structures, retail shops, and commercial spaces, plus the natural environment, such as parks, trees, and walking trails. The social environment refers to the presence and quality of the relationships and connections individuals have with others, such as neighbors. Finally, the service environment includes the neighborhood resources associated with education, employment, transportation, healthcare, grocery shopping, recreation, and other services directly or indirectly tied to health.

Where a person lives may create health disparities because an individual's health is directly affected by elements that increase or decrease wellness; a person's immediate neighborhood influences his or her health. Consider the phrase "place matters." When a neighborhood has plenty of green space and parks, crime is low, and streets and sidewalks are in good working order, individuals might feel compelled to enjoy the outside space, embrace exercise, and spend time talking to neighbors. Compare that scenario to a neighborhood where crime is high, city services are marginal, and many homes are vacant and boarded up. Physical safety might be a concern that encourages an individual to stay inside, avoid public spaces, and limit outside hobbies. Consider a neighborhood that has limited public transportation and the ways to access a bus, subway, or train might inhibit one's ability to find work, shop for groceries, and access preventative healthcare services. Likewise, consider a neighborhood where elementary schools lack adequately prepared teachers and sufficient textbooks and do not have a school nurse. Children in this neighborhood may have a foundational education that is inferior compared with children living in a neighborhood where schools are exceptional and have superior teachers and state-of-the-art classroom resources.

Physical geography also influences what the individual breathes (e.g., clean air versus polluted air), the quality of the drinking water, and what diseases people living in that area may be exposed to (e.g., HIV, tuberculous, alcoholism). Geography and health arc very closely linked, and when considered together, they allow the nurse to consider patient risk factors and health needs from a broader perspective. The nurse's role is to identify the degree to which geography negatively impacts health and develop opportunities and provide resources that the patient may access to minimize the risk for disease.

Bias and Discrimination

Every individual has the potential for forming an opinion that is unfair or prejudicial in some way. This perception is termed **bias**. An individual, as well as groups of individuals, may hold multiple biases. There are two aspects to bias that are important to understand because both are associated with inferior, insensitive, and inappropriate healthcare. Implicit or unconscious bias is related to associations outside conscious awareness that foster a negative evaluation of a person on the basis of irrelevant characteristics such as race, gender, age, and so forth. Implicit bias may emanate from negative and positive stereotypes and impact one's judgment and is automatically activated and often unintentional.

Implicit bias is subconscious and may be visible through subtle behaviors, such as being more relaxed when addressing one patient while being distant or aloof with another.

Implicit bias explains the potential differences between explicit beliefs and actions to treat everyone equally and the influence of hidden *negative* implicit associations on beliefs and actions.

Conscious bias, or **explicit bias**, is blatant, purposeful, targeted, and intentional. For example, conscious bias results when an individual has deliberate thoughts and feelings about an individual, such as an obese male as well as groups of obese individuals. The intent of conscious bias is to demonstrate whether or not the negative aspects or evaluations of the individual or group are true. Bias can lead to stereotyping, which is grouping all individuals in a group together and forming a broad generalization (e.g., "all homeless individuals are illiterate"; "Native Americans are typically obese and live on reservations").

Bias and Healthcare Professionals

Healthcare professionals have personal belief systems, values, and attitudes. These personal attitudes, values, and beliefs can impede a provider's ability to understand and accept patients with different backgrounds or belief systems or patients who may not do things or act in a way that the professional "expects." This lack of understanding and acceptance can affect patient care and, ultimately, patient outcomes.

In 2002, the Institute of Medicine (now referred to as the National Academy of Medicine) reported that differences in patient care may be related to the behaviors of healthcare professionals, specifically bias, or prejudice directed toward certain groups; greater clinical uncertainty when interacting with minority patients; and beliefs, or stereotypes, held by the provider regarding the behavior or health of minorities. The report *Unequal Treatment: What Healthcare Providers Need to Know About Racial and Ethnic Disparities in Healthcare* explains that there are differences in the way patients respond to treatment and interventions as well as variations in their treatment-seeking behaviors. Despite this and other reports, unequal treatment and health inequity are still evident in the current healthcare environment. Providers must adjust practices to address patient behaviors, attitudes, and care responses, and they must not allow bias to enter into patient care practices.

It has also been found that healthcare providers who stereotype patients based on personal misperceptions and biases negatively influence patient outcomes and contribute to healthcare disparities. Research exploring the impact of the implicit racial and ethnic biases of healthcare professionals and the impact on health outcomes revealed low or moderate levels of implicit bias in healthcare professionals toward people of color. Several studies noted that healthcare professionals characterized African American patients as less cooperative and responsible. Surveys have found that healthcare providers in some Veterans Affairs Medical Centers display bias in relation to patients with mental illness. These findings are based on reports from each provider about the amount of contact with patients with mental illness, as well as with personally known individuals with mental illness. Stigmatizing attitudes were lower for providers who had more contact with patients and nonpatients with mental illness.

The provider–patient relationship can also create a power dynamic in which the provider has the bulk of the power. This can alter interactions between healthcare providers and patients if providers consider the patients to be "less than" themselves or "beneath" them. The power imbalance fueled by the negative impact of bias and stereotyping can result in actions that are aggressive toward the patient and can lead to unfair treatment by the provider.

When an individual is afraid and demonstrates hatred or exhibits "an attitudinal orientation of hostility against non-natives in a given population," this is called xenophobia (United Nations Educational and Scientific and Cultural Organization, 2017). **Xenophobia** is often expressed by fear, intolerance, dislike, and prejudice against individuals from other countries.

Biases, conscious or unconscious, are not limited to characteristics such as ethnicity and race; biases may exist toward any social group. Bias, discrimination, stereotyping, and hatred alter judgment, influence behavior, and create isolation and disassociation between nurses and patients and/or family members. The distortions in healthcare provider judgment and decision making are key contributors to patient safety events as well as health inequality and disparities.

Connection Check 3.2

Select the response that acknowledges that social factors place patients at risk for health disparities.
A. Anyone can be poor and have limited income; that does not impact access to healthcare.
B. Having faith and being religious help patients deal with health adversity.
C. Many patients speak another language, but translations services help them a lot.
D. Unemployment is a barrier that negatively impacts housing, food, and healthcare access.

Connection Check 3.3

Which thought by the nurse suggests that the nurse is considering whether unconscious bias is influencing his or her judgment?
A. "All obese patients just make bad nutritional decisions."
B. "I wonder if my feelings about abortion made me say that."
C. "Is cultural awareness as important as cultural competency?"
D. "Why do they all act that way?"

CASE STUDY: EPISODE 2

Mrs. Liu is admitted to the hospital for rectal bleeding. During the nursing assessment, the nurse learns about Mrs. Liu's recent move to live with her daughter and son-in-law and their visit to the Chinese medicine store. The nurse does not understand why Mrs. Liu went to the Chinese medicine store. Further discussions reveal that Mrs. Liu consulted the local deity (or spiritual leader) when her bleeding first began to ask for guidance. Mrs. Liu brings in her prescriptions, Coumadin and Digoxin, and a vial, without a label, containing blue pills.

The nurse becomes concerned when she learns that the bleeding started 5 days prior to admission and that Mrs. Lui did not contact her primary care physician. Mrs. Liu's daughter explains that her mother values traditional Chinese medicine over Western medicine. Despite that, the nurse recommends some tests to determine the cause of the bleeding. After testing, the nurse determines that Mrs. Liu's rectal bleeding was a consequence of an elevated international normalized ratio (INR). The Coumadin dose is decreased, Mrs. Liu's rectal bleeding resolves. However, the nurse now notices that Mrs. Liu appears withdrawn, avoiding eye contact whenever the nurse enters the room. The nurse considers that Mrs. Liu might feel socially isolated, unable to fully participate in her care management, perhaps because of a language barrier or unfamiliarity with the Western medical system. Mrs. Liu's daughter explains that Mrs. Liu feels fearful…

ELIMINATING DISPARITIES AND CREATING HEALTH EQUITY

Social Determinants of Health

The **social determinants of health** (SDOH) consist of a variety of circumstances and conditions "in the environments in which people are born, live, learn, work, play, worship, and age that affect a wide range of health, functioning, and quality-of-life outcomes and risks" (Office of Disease Prevention and Health Promotion, 2018c). The SDOH include specific factors, such as socioeconomic status; level of education; neighborhood and physical environment where one resides; employment, unemployment, or underemployment; presence of social support networks; and ability to access healthcare. Healthcare providers must consider the relevant SDOH for each patient and address those SDOH relevant to improving health and reducing disparities in health and healthcare.

The SDOH model (Fig. 3.1) serves as a visual representation framework for the *Healthy People 2020* and *2030* population health indicators. These indicators show high-priority issues that impact the health and well-being of all individuals

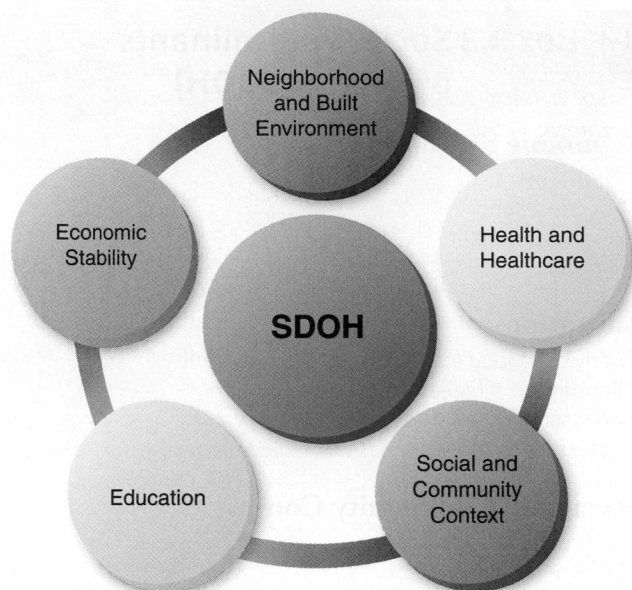

FIGURE 3.1 The social determinants of health (SDOH) model

but especially those who are vulnerable, marginalized, and burdened by social factors. Examples of leading health indicators are suicide, obesity, and substance abuse. Additionally, genetics plays an important role in one's ability to maintain health, and given that genetic makeup cannot be altered, nursing efforts must focus on modifiable elements contributing to the individual determinants of health (e.g., homelessness or low literacy).

The SDOH model has five key elements:

- Economic stability
- Education
- Social and community context
- Health and healthcare
- Neighborhood and built environment

Box 3.3 shows the social factors that are included in each of the five SDOH elements. The care provided to the patient must acknowledge the influence of each SDOH element on the current health situation as well as the role of each determinant in the patient's pathway to improved health. Failing to consider the SDOH when providing care is a barrier to providing patient-centered care.

Healthy People Initiative

The United States has a national initiative centered on creating health equity by focusing on health promotion, disease prevention, and quality of life. According to the Office of Disease Prevention and Health Promotion, the *Healthy People* initiative focuses on 10-year national objectives meant to improve the health of all Americans by utilizing science-based initiatives. Three key goals serve as the foundation:

- Encourage collaborations across communities and sectors.
- Empower individuals toward making informed health decisions.
- Measure the impact of prevention activities.

Box 3.3 Social Determinants of Health (SDOH)

Economic Stability

- Employment
- Food insecurity
- Housing instability
- Poverty

Education

- Early childhood education and development
- Enrollment in higher education
- High school graduation
- Language and literacy

Social and Community Context

- Civic participation
- Discrimination
- Incarceration
- Social cohesion

Health and Healthcare

- Access to healthcare
- Access to primary care
- Health literacy

Neighborhood and Built Environment

- Access to foods that support healthy eating patterns
- Crime and violence
- Environmental conditions
- Quality of housing

Based on Office of Disease Prevention and Health Promotion. (2018). *Determinants of health*. Retrieved from https://www.healthypeople.gov/2020/about/foundation-health-measures/Determinants-of-Health.

In each of the 10-year goals, the focus is on addressing health for all and reducing inequities and health disparities for some social groups over another. In *Healthy People 2000*, the goal was to reduce health disparities for Americans. In *Healthy People 2010*, the goal was to eliminate health disparities. In *Healthy People 2020*, the goal is more specific and direct: to achieve health equity, eliminate disparities, and improve the health of all groups. *Healthy People 2020* also covers more vulnerable groups, including LGBTQ populations, as well as those with special needs and considerations. *Healthy People 2030* objectives, published in 2020, include objectives specifically focused on eliminating health disparities by addressing the SDOH and improving access to quality healthcare.

When nurses develop culturally competent care, conscious decisions are made to minimize barriers to care, including all determinants of health conditions and factors. Although each patient presents unique needs, nurses may use the *Healthy People* framework and the learning health indicators to develop patient, family, and community interventions that contribute to the improved health of the nation.

Improving Health Literacy

There are several evidence-based interventions that may be incorporated into a healthcare provider's practice to improve health literacy, thereby minimizing the potential barrier of the patient's ability to understand the plan of care. These interventions include:

- Incorporating technology and Web sites with realistic pictures and clear captions to improve comprehension
- Integrating teach-back and plain language into instructions to improve knowledge retention
- Using simple language and photograph- and pictogram-based care plans to improve patients' disease management abilities
- Developing print materials to be at the seventh- to eighth-grade reading level

Language and Literacy

It is important to assess patients for individual language needs and for healthcare providers to adjust their communication style to meet these needs. Patients with limited ability to speak, write, or read English (individuals with limited English proficiency [LEP]) face additional barriers. Additional safeguards must be in place within healthcare organizations to prevent or minimize potential discrimination. Specifically, Title VI of the Civil Rights Act of 1964 states: "no person in the United States shall, on the ground of race, color, or national origin, be excluded from participation in, be denied the benefits of, or be subjected to discrimination under any program or activity receiving Federal financial assistance." Applicable to all facets of life in the United States, this law is also relevant to supportive services in healthcare, such as medical translators and language resources. Per the Civil Rights Act, printed materials in languages other than English must be available for patients based on the patient population being served. Patients deemed LEP must be provided with services that support their ability to access healthcare and services, communicate with healthcare providers, and receive information in a manner that facilities their understanding. These practices reflect the incorporation of cultural awareness principles in the provision of individualized care.

Culturally and Linguistically Appropriate Services (CLAS)

The Office of Minority Health (OMH) formed the Center for Linguistic and Cultural Competency in Health Care (CLCCHC) to address the unmet needs of patients seeking healthcare and to decrease barriers to healthcare literacy. The CLCCHC developed Culturally and Linguistically Appropriate Services (CLAS) as national standards for healthcare facilities to use when developing services, policies, and educational materials to mitigate health inequities and disparities related to individuals with LEP. The CLAS focus is respect and responsiveness, which translates into respecting the wholeness of each individual and responding to each individual's needs, preferences, and desires in order to provide services that reflect an individual's culture and language preferences. The goal of these services is to support healthcare professionals in facilitating positive health outcomes for diverse populations. The 15 CLAS standards are listed in Box 3.4.

Connection Check 3.4

What is the most accurate description of the social determinants of health?

A. Biological, socioeconomic, psychosocial, behavioral, or social factors influencing an individual's health

B. Factors that contribute to health inequity, discrimination, and healthcare professional bias

C. National standards that are used to develop culturally competent and linguistically appropriate patient care

D. Services used within healthcare facilities to identify which patients require culturally competent care

CULTURAL ASSESSMENT MODELS

Models of cultural competence serve as a framework to meet the increasing heterogeneity of patient populations. These theories and models exist to assist nurses in developing culturally and linguistically appropriate healthcare that is free of behaviors, attitudes, and judgments influenced by fear, discrimination, and bias. Each model offers healthcare professionals a means to understand personal uncertainties and knowledge gaps related to patients with different experiences, needs, beliefs systems, and cultures. All of the theories and models highlight the importance of developing an authentic connection based on acceptance, understanding, and respect for human life.

Box 3.4 National Standards for Culturally and Linguistically Appropriate Services (CLAS) in Health and Healthcare Standards

Principal Standard:

1. Provide effective, equitable, understandable, and respectful quality care and services that are responsive to diverse cultural health beliefs and practices, preferred languages, health literacy, and other communication needs.

Governance, Leadership, and Workforce Standards:

2. Advance and sustain organizational governance and leadership that promotes CLAS and health equity through policy, practices, and allocated resources.
3. Recruit, promote, and support a culturally and linguistically diverse governance, leadership, and workforce that are responsive to the population in the service area.
4. Educate and train governance, leadership, and workforce in culturally and linguistically appropriate policies and practices on an ongoing basis.

Communication and Language Assistance Standard:

5. Offer language assistance to individuals who have limited English proficiency and/or other communication needs, at no cost to them, to facilitate timely access to all healthcare and services.
6. Inform all individuals of the availability of language assistance services clearly and in their preferred language, verbally and in writing.
7. Ensure the competence of individuals providing language assistance, recognizing that the use of untrained individuals and/or minors as interpreters should be avoided.
8. Provide easy-to-understand print and multimedia materials and signage in the languages commonly used by the populations in the service area.

Engagement, Continuous Improvement, and Accountability:

9. Establish culturally and linguistically appropriate goals, policies, and management accountability, and infuse them throughout the organization's planning and operations.
10. Conduct ongoing assessments of the organization's CLAS and related activities, and integrate CLAS and related measures into measurement and continuous quality improvement activities.
11. Collect and maintain accurate and reliable demographic data to monitor and evaluate the impact of CLAS on health equity and outcomes and to inform service delivery.
12. Conduct regular assessments of community health assets and needs and use the results to plan and implement services that respond to the cultural and linguistic diversity of populations in the service area.
13. Partner with the community to design, implement, and evaluate policies, practices, and services to ensure cultural and linguistic appropriateness.
14. Create conflict and grievance resolution processes that are culturally and linguistically appropriate to identify, prevent, and resolve conflicts or complaints.
15. Communicate the organization's progress in implementing and sustaining CLAS to all stakeholders, constituents, and the general public.

Based on Office of Minority Health. (2018, June 11). *Center for Linguistic and Cultural Competency in Health Care.* Retrieved from https://minorityhealth.hhs.gov/omh/browse.aspx?lvl=2&lvlid=34; and Office of Minority Health. (n.d.). *What is CLAS?* Retrieved from https://www.thinkculturalhealth.hhs.gov/clas/what-is-clas

Transcultural Nursing

Transcultural nursing acknowledges that nurses meet and care for patients who are different from themselves, and these differences may present a challenge. Learning about patients' cultural backgrounds, experiences, and desires requires nurses to enter into meaningful conversations about how patients' cultures affect their lives, thereby decreasing discrimination and bias. The recognition by the nurse of how culture influences an individual's values, beliefs, and worldviews reflects cultural awareness. This also underscores the importance of nurses acknowledging that these differences exist and respecting these differences.

Transcultural Nursing Model

Nursing theorist Madeline Leininger based the Transcultural Nursing (TCN) cultural assessment model on a humanistic approach that broadly supports individuals, organizations, communities, and societies and linking caring within the context of culture. In her work, Leininger blended concepts from both nursing and anthropology to explain caring as the central link between the human being (the patient) and the nurse (provider of care). The concept of caring is considered as assisting, supporting, or enabling the patient's behaviors while also helping the patient improve health and performance. A nurse who practices humanistic care seeks to understand and know the person, the human being, in order to improve health and ameliorate suffering.

Culture Care Diversity and Universality Theory

Leininger's Culture Care Diversity and Universality Theory explains that nurses must first know the patients they are caring for—individual patterns, beliefs, practices, and personal expressions. The nurse is then informed and able to provide care that is congruent with the belief systems of the patients. The term *transcultural nursing* refers to the nurse's desire to cross the divide and meet the patient where he or she is, as an individual in a global and diverse patient population. Culturally competent care only occurs when culture care values are known and serve as the foundation for meaningful and just care, shifting from less aware to more aware. Moreover, Leininger explains that nurses must be educated and immersed in learning about the nuances of a patient's cultural beliefs and values so that the care provided does not harm or prevent the patient from attaining the highest degree of possible health. The Culture Care Diversity and Universality Theory focuses on examining and addressing the differences and similarities of global cultural care.

Sunrise Model

Leininger depicts the Culture Care Diversity and Universality Theory using the Sunrise Model (Fig. 3.2), which shows the factors and conditions that influence care. The concept of a sunrise is one that is most fitting to represent the process of cultural awakening; the rising sun begins first with a dim light but soon becomes bright. In a similar way, the professional nurse may begin with little cultural knowledge but strives to become aware and to expand knowledge and practice to better develop culturally focused interventions for the most vulnerable patients.

In the model, the outermost "ring" represents cultural care and the worldview, the way in which the nurse views the world. This worldview informs the nurse's knowledge about patients, families, and/or communities within the healthcare system. Nurses use their education to learn more about the next ring, which includes cultural and social dimensions that influence each patient: technological, religious/philosophical, kinship/social, cultural values and lifeways, political and legal, economic, and education. By addressing the language and environmental barriers, nurses create pathways that respect patients' experiences, patterns, and practices, leading each to a state of holistic health. Finally, the nurses integrate patients' folk or traditional health beliefs with the professional healthcare systems to devise care that is respectful, just, and patient centered.

ASSESSING CULTURAL COMPETENCE

Characteristics of Cultural Diversity

Cultural specifics affect individual health beliefs and behaviors. Knowledge of the cultural specifics of the groups in a community helps explain why patients from different cultures have different expectations of healthcare. The six cultural specifics that influence health are communication, space, time orientation, social organization, environmental control, and biological variations.

Communication

Communication is an exchange of information, ideas, and feelings, including verbal and nonverbal language (i.e., spoken language, gestures, eye contact, and even silences). Language differences present one of the most difficult obstacles to providing individualized, patient-centered care. Even when the nurse and the patient speak the same language, culture influences how feelings and thoughts are expressed and which verbal and nonverbal expressions are appropriate to use.

Assessment and Strategies

Ask the following questions:

- By what name do you prefer to be called?
- What language do you speak at home?
- Are you able to read and write in English?
- If not, what language is preferred?

Incorporate the following actions:

- Be an active listener, and become comfortable with silence.
- Avoid appearing rushed.
- Be formal with greetings until told to do otherwise.

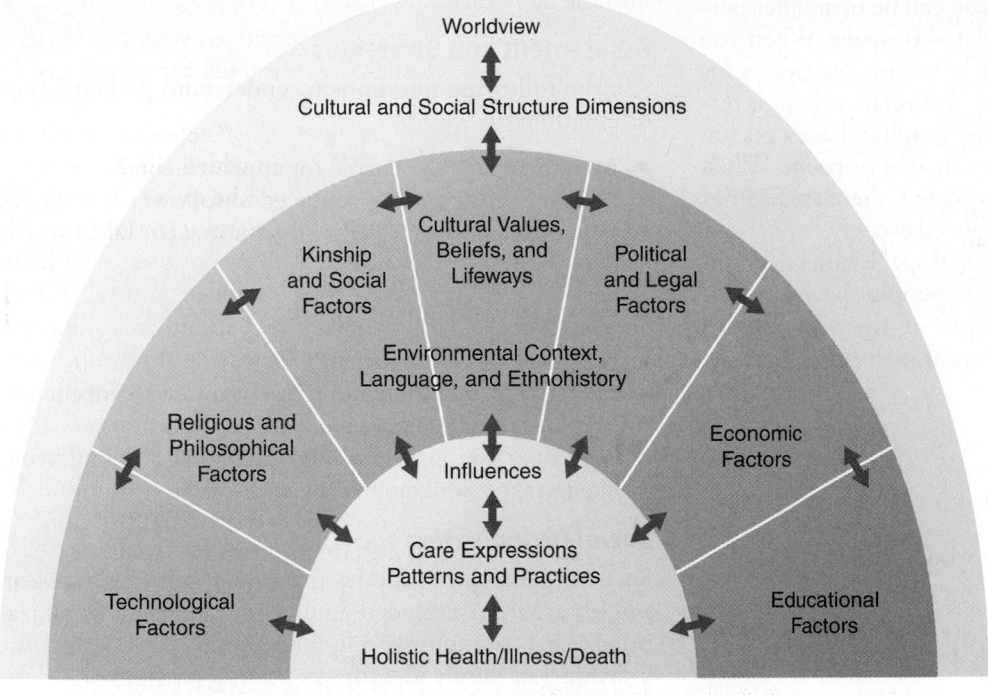

Leininger's Sunrise Enabler to Discover Culture Care
Culture Care

Worldview

Cultural and Social Structure Dimensions

Kinship and Social Factors

Cultural Values, Beliefs, and Lifeways

Political and Legal Factors

Environmental Context, Language, and Ethnohistory

Religious and Philosophical Factors

Influences

Economic Factors

Care Expressions Patterns and Practices

Technological Factors

Educational Factors

Holistic Health/Illness/Death

Focus: Individuals, Families, Groups, Communities, or Institutions in Diverse Health Contexts of

Influencers

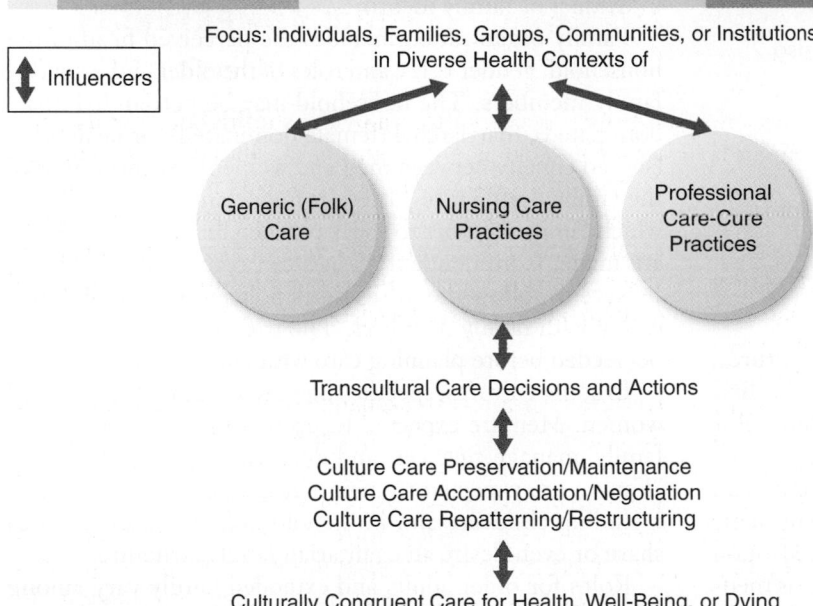

Generic (Folk) Care

Nursing Care Practices

Professional Care-Cure Practices

Transcultural Care Decisions and Actions

Culture Care Preservation/Maintenance
Culture Care Accommodation/Negotiation
Culture Care Repatterning/Restructuring

Culturally Congruent Care for Health, Well-Being, or Dying

FIGURE 3.2 Leininger's Culture Care Diversity and Universality Theory—The Sunrise Enabler Model.

- Take greeting cues from the patient.
- Speak slowly and clearly. Do not speak loudly or with exaggerated mouthing.
- Explain why you are asking specific questions.
- Give reasons for treatments.
- Repeat questions as needed.
- Provide written instructions in the patient's preferred language.
- Obtain an interpreter if needed.

Nurses should refrain from relying on untrained individuals to interpret, especially family members. Although it may seem logical that a patient's best advocate is a family member, it is risky to rely on family members to interpret medical or health information for the following reasons:

- Family members may not be proficient in medical terminology.
- They may not possess the skills needed to interpret.
- They may unintentionally or intentionally omit or alter important information.
- Using family members to interpret may raise privacy issues protected by the Health Insurance Portability and Accountability Act of 1996 (HIPAA).
- If children are used as translators, they may not be emotionally mature enough to handle the information being conveyed.

Space

Space refers to a person's personal space, or the boundaries that determine how close one person can be to another person. A person's comfort level is related to space. When you invade another's personal space, a common reaction is for the person to move away from you. A similar concept is territoriality, which is related to the geographic space a person views as owned or claimed, such as an area or room. When an individual's personal space is protected, there are feelings of safety, security, control, and reduced anxiety.

Within all cultural groups, personal space varies depending on the relationship between the people speaking: intimates versus acquaintances, people of the same versus opposite sex, and people of a different position within the social hierarchy.

Assessment and Strategies

Ask the following questions:

- Are you comfortable?
- Do you have any concerns you would like to discuss?

Incorporate the following actions:

- Ensure patients are comfortable before interviewing them.
- Maintain appropriate physical distances while also observing for cues.
- Be aware of cultural differences.
- Be aware of physical objects that may be a barrier to comfort.
- Make sure that the patient's physical environment is arranged to ensure safety, security, confidentiality, and familiarity.

Time Orientation

Time orientation varies among people of different cultures, and the perception of time has two dimensions. The first dimension is related to clock time versus social time. For example, some cultures have a flexible orientation to time and events, and appointments take place when the person arrives. For others, time is less flexible, and appointments and social events are expected to start at the agreed-upon time. For many, social events may be flexible, whereas medical appointments and business engagements start on time.

The second dimension of time relates to whether the culture is predominantly concerned with the past, present, or future. Past-oriented individuals maintain traditions that were meaningful in the past and may worship ancestors. Present-oriented people accept the day as it comes, with little regard for the past; the future is unpredictable. Future-oriented people anticipate a bigger and better future and place a high value on change. Some people balance all three views—they respect the past, enjoy living in the present, and plan for the future.

Differences in time orientation are important considerations when planning nursing interventions. It is important to understand patients' time orientation to best prepare them for the timing of appointments, tests, and treatments.

In addition, an assessment of the patient's usual routines is necessary in order to incorporate these as much as possible into the daily care.

Assessment and Strategies

Ask the following questions to understand patients' time orientation:

- Are you normally on time for appointments?
- Are there any routines you need to follow?
- What time do you usually eat your meals? Take your bath?

Incorporate the following actions:

- Have a clock in the patient's room.
- Assess for orientation and reorient to time as needed.
- Prepare patients before a procedure or test.
- Give time options when appropriate (e.g., "Would you like to take a walk now or in an hour?").

Social Organization

Social organization includes the family unit (e.g., nuclear, single parent, or extended family) and the wider organizations (e.g., community, religious, ethnic) with which the individual or family identifies.

Family organization includes the perceived head of the household, gender roles, and roles of the older and extended family members. The household may be patriarchal (male dominated), matriarchal (female dominated), or egalitarian (shared equally between men and women). An awareness of the family dominance pattern is important for determining which family member to speak to when healthcare decisions are made. Confidentiality issues can complicate this issue. Be sure to follow the institution's policies when communicating with family members. The patient's permission may be needed before planning care with family members.

In some cultures, specific roles are outlined for men and women. Men are expected to protect and provide for the family, manage finances, and deal with the outside world. Women are expected to maintain the home environment, including childcare and household tasks. Not all societies share or even desire an egalitarian family structure.

Roles for older adults and extended family vary among culturally diverse groups. In some cultures, adults are seen as being wise, are deferred to for making decisions, and are held in high esteem. Children are expected to provide for older family members when they are no longer able to care for themselves. In other cultures, although older people may be loved by family members, they may not be given such high regard and may be cared for outside the home when self-care or assistance with daily activities becomes a concern.

The extended family is very important in some groups, and a single household may include several generations living together out of desire rather than out of necessity. The extended family may include both blood-related and non-blood-related persons who are given family status. In other families, each generation lives in a separate home or living space.

Assessment and Strategies

Ask the following questions:

- Who makes the decisions in your household?
- Who takes care of money matters, does the cooking, or is responsible for childcare?
- Who decides when it is time to visit a healthcare provider?
- Who lives in your household?

Incorporate the following actions:

- Observe the use of touch between family members.
- Let family members decide where they want to stand or sit for comfort.

Environmental Control

Environmental control consists of three major concepts: people's perception of the ability to control what happens to them and their health, beliefs about health and illness, and beliefs in alternative healthcare therapies such as folk medicine. For example, if individuals do not believe they have control of their health, they may not be receptive to nursing interventions that require self-confidence, such as self-administration of insulin. Regarding health beliefs, if individuals believe that illness is due to a spiritual cause and not bacteria or believe in folk healing practices, they may not understand the need to take antibiotics. Nurses need to consider their patients' cultural values and beliefs, especially when they differ from those of the dominant Western healthcare view.

Distinctions are made between health and illness and what people do to promote or maintain health and to prevent and treat illnesses. Not all patients use a Western healthcare system or provider. Many people try some form of alternative therapy before seeking treatment. People also use alternative therapies and religious systems, such as prayer, in combination with the scientific medical system.

Assessment and Strategies

Ask the following questions:

- How do you define health? Illness?
- Do you have any special beliefs about health and illness?
- What do you do to keep well?
- When you feel ill, what is the first thing you do to get better?
- How do you deal with pain?
- How do you and your family express grief?
- Are there any cultural beliefs or practices that I need to know about to plan your care?

Incorporate the following actions:

- Be aware of possible cultural beliefs and practices.
- Never stereotype based on what you know about different cultures; always ask for specific information.
- Perform a cultural assessment on all of your patients.

- Ask if patients have received treatments of any kind for their illness.
- Ask about religious beliefs and practices.
- Encourage helpful practices and discourage those that are harmful.

Biological Variations

Biological variations include ways in which people are different genetically and physiologically, including body variations and medication metabolism. Biological variations create susceptibility to certain diseases and injuries and explain differences in response to treatment. Consequently, clinical trials (medication studies) now recommend incorporating biological variations.

Biological variations also refer to differences in nutritional practices, including the personal meaning of food, food choices and rituals, food taboos, and how food and food substances are used for health promotion and wellness. Cultural beliefs influence what people eat or avoid. In addition to being important for survival, food offers security and acceptance, plays a significant role in socialization, and can serve as an expression of love.

Culturally congruent dietary counseling, such as adapting preparation practices and including ethnic food choices, can reduce health risks. Whenever possible, determine a patient's current dietary practices. Counseling about food group requirements or dietary restrictions must respect an individual's cultural background. Most cultures have nutritional practices for health promotion and disease prevention. For many, a balance of different types of foods is important for maintaining health and preventing illness.

Assessment and Strategies

Ask the following questions:

- Are there any genetic disorders or diseases related to your cultural background?
- Are you satisfied with your weight?
- Are you active? What is your normal exercise pattern?
- Do you protect your eyes and skin from the sun? From possible injuries?
- Do you have any medication or food allergies?
- Has anyone in your family had any major illnesses?
- What do you eat to stay healthy?
- What do you eat when you are ill?
- Are there certain foods you do not eat? Why?
- Do certain foods cause you to become ill? What are they?
- Who purchases the food in your household?
- Who prepares the food in your household?

Incorporate the following actions:

- Teach about biological variations that may pertain to the patient.
- Determine and respect usual eating patterns whenever possible.
- Teach good nutrition habits, taking into account patient preferences. Refer to a dietitian if appropriate.

Connection Check 3.5

Which action by the nurse reflects the use of a cultural competency model to assess knowledge, beliefs, and attitudes?

A. Acknowledging that education level plays a role in the ability to buy a home

B. Believing that patients bring on their own illness by making poor choices

C. Considering how similar spiritual beliefs are to those of another nurse

D. Thinking about how one American Indian tribe member looks like another

Making Connections

CASE STUDY: WRAP-UP

The nurse requests an interprofessional team meeting to discuss and develop a discharge plan addressing Mrs. Liu's care needs. A medical interpreter is assigned to Mrs. Liu and will follow her as both an inpatient and outpatient. This consistency is important to establish trust and to give the interpreter the opportunity to assess Mrs. Liu's health literacy needs. Social workers will work with Mrs. Liu to identify a Taiwanese community center, helping her to build a social group of friends and peers. The nurse working in the Coumadin Clinic will contact Mrs. Liu, with the assistance of the interpreter, to perform medication reconciliation and symptom management and will also determine if Mrs. Liu has visited the Chinese medicine practitioner. If Mrs. Liu has visited the Chinese medicine practitioner, the nurses plan to gently probe her to determine if she began any new complementary therapies. All communications, assessments, and interventions will be documented in the electronic medical record, allowing the primary care physician and cardiologist to access critical patient information during Mrs. Liu's medical visits.

Case Study Questions

1. Mrs. Liu is challenged by a low level of health literacy; what interventions might the nurse suggest to the interprofessional care team?
   A. Ask if she wants to continue to see the Chinese medicine practitioner.
   B. Locate a family member who can translate all healthcare documents for her.
   C. Secure relevant patient teaching materials written in her native language.
   D. Talk only to her daughter and son-in-law to expedite all communications.

2. The nurse verbalizes annoyance and fear when learning about the visit to the Chinese medicine practitioner. This attitude best reflects which characteristic?
   A. Bigotry
   B. Discrimination
   C. Hatred
   D. Xenophobia

3. What resources might the nurse secure to improve the nurse's knowledge of the cultural beliefs and values of Taiwanese patients?
   A. Calling the nurse manager to discuss the situation
   B. Consulting with the care coordination manager to discuss CLAS standards
   C. Discussing the patients with other staff nurses during hourly rounds
   D. Managing all communications quickly through the patient's daughter

4. How might feelings of social isolation influence Mrs. Liu's ability to adapt to her new living environment?
   A. Attributing loneliness to food items she has never eaten
   B. Developing new hobbies and interests to fill up her day
   C. Fearing engagement with Western healthcare providers
   D. Making long-term plans with her daughter and son-in-law

5. Which strategy reflects a nurse's ability to apply communication to culturally specific influences in an encounter with Mrs. Liu?
   A. Actively listening following a question placed to Mrs. Liu
   B. Increasing the tone of voice after Mrs. Liu appears confused
   C. Nodding to Mrs. Liu when she is speaking
   D. Quickly calling in the interpreter, then walking out of the room

CHAPTER SUMMARY

Nurses care for patients who are diverse, different, and complex, and this is the reality of the world. It is of utmost importance that nurses are aware that differences exist while remaining open to assessing all factors contributing to each patient's ability to strive for the highest level of health. All this must be done without assigning judgment, stereotyping, and displaying bias.

Becoming a culturally competent healthcare provider means demonstrating care, compassion, and tolerance to all human beings. This process requires the nurse to acknowledge differences and similarities among patients, groups, and populations. Understanding key terminology and concepts helps to minimize barriers that prevent the nurse from providing care that is free of bias, judgment, stereotypes, and the cultural bias of the nurse and other members of the healthcare team to facilitate the provision of individualized and patient-centered care.

There are several cultural competence models to assist nurses in assessing their knowledge, skills, and abilities so that they may appropriately guide their actions, ensuring culturally competent and appropriate healthcare. Nurses may apply the Culture Care Diversity and Universality Theory and Sunrise Enabler Model of Leininger to help them assess their knowledge, skills, and attitudes toward becoming culturally competent professionals and to enhance care delivery for diverse populations. Additionally, consideration of the six cultural specifics that influence health ensures the nurse's actions are focused on minimizing health disparities and maximizing care based on the unique needs of each patient.

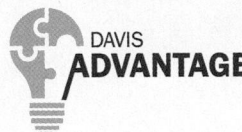

To explore learning resources for this chapter, go to **Davis Advantage** and find:
- Answers to in-text questions
- Chapter Resources and Activities
- NCLEX®-Style Chapter Review Questions
- Bibliography

Chapter 4

Ethical Concepts

JoAnn Conroy

LEARNING OUTCOMES

Content in this chapter is designed to assist in:

1. Identifying professional standards that guide ethical nursing practice
2. Defining ethical principles
3. Describing ethical theories
4. Addressing ethical dilemmas associated with the care of the acutely ill adult
5. Discussing how ethical principles guide decision making for the registered nurse

CONCEPTS

- Assessment
- Collaboration
- Communication
- Ethics
- Nursing Roles

ESSENTIAL TERMS

Advance directive
Autonomy
Beneficence
Casuistry
Common good
Confidentiality
Consequentialism
Deontology
Fidelity
Informed consent
Justice
Living will
Nonmaleficence
Paternalism
Respect
Sanctity of life
Self-determination
Veracity
Virtue

Finding Connections

CASE STUDY: EPISODE 1

Follow this patient throughout the chapter.

Joseph Michaels is a 45-year-old male who is attending a 4th of July picnic when he suddenly feels dizzy, with loss of balance, trouble speaking, and a sudden headache. Family members assist Mr. Michaels in lying down, blame the symptoms on the hot day, and wonder if he has consumed too much alcohol. After a short while, he feels better and returns to the party. On the way home that evening, he again experiences the dizziness and headache, and his wife decides to take him to the local emergency department. Because he also demonstrates right-sided hemiplegia, global aphasia, and dysphagia, he undergoes a diagnostic evaluation and is diagnosed with a cerebrovascular accident, admitted to the intensive care unit, and started on anticoagulant therapy...

THE ROLE OF ETHICS IN NURSING

As nurses gain autonomy in their professional roles, their responsibility and accountability for sound clinical judgment grow as well. Today's complex healthcare environment presents a myriad of ethical and bioethical challenges to all healthcare providers. Nurses spend a disproportionately large amount of time with patients and serve as their advocates, protectors, and trusted confidantes. In many instances, nurses must guide patients and families in making difficult choices, and in some cases, they must make decisions on their behalf, in consultation with other members of the interdisciplinary team. These decisions are often complex and sometimes controversial. Ethical theories and principles provide a moral framework for sound decision making. In many cases, there is no apparent *good* decision, only a list of the *best possible* options, which speaks to the challenging moral relativity that often accompanies ethical decision making. Ethical principles also guide the moral traditions, values, and behaviors of professional nursing, which are outlined in the *Code of Ethics for Nurses* ("the *Code*") we use today (Box 4.1).

Box 4.1 Guide to the *Code of Ethics for Nurses:* Interpretation and Application

Provision 1

The nurse practices with compassion and respect for the inherent dignity, worth, and unique attributes of every person.

Provision 2

The nurse's primary commitment is to the patient, whether an individual, family, group, community, or population.

Provision 3

The nurse promotes, advocates for, and protects the rights, health, and safety of the patient.

Provision 4

The nurse has authority, accountability, and responsibility for nursing practice; makes decisions; and takes action consistent with the obligation to promote health and to provide optimal care.

Provision 5

The nurse owes the same duties to self as to others, including the responsibility to promote health and safety, preserve wholeness of character and integrity, maintain competence, and continue personal and professional growth.

Provision 6

The nurse, through individual and collective effort, establishes, maintains, and improves the ethical environment of the work setting and conditions of employment that are conducive to safe, quality healthcare.

Provision 7

The nurse, in all roles and settings, advances the profession through research and scholarly inquiry, professional standards development, and the generation of both nursing and health policy.

Provision 8

The nurse collaborates with other health professionals and the public to protect human rights, promote health diplomacy, and reduce health disparities.

Provision 9

The profession of nursing, collectively through its professional organizations, must articulate nursing values, maintain the integrity of the profession, and integrate principles of social justice into nursing and health policy.

From American Nurses Association. (2015). *Code of ethics for nurses with interpretive statements.* Silver Spring, MD: Author.

BIOETHICS

The field of bioethics is similar to ethics but is broader in scope. It is both a concept and a movement that considers our past missteps as well as the breadth and consequences of our technological advances; just because we can, should we? It is an interdisciplinary shared consideration of moral philosophy as it relates to standards and methods of treatment of disease in individuals. Bioethics is an ongoing public conversation that manifests through the formation of health policy, through media coverage, at professional conferences, on the pages of professional journals, and in numerous other venues. It often considers questions engendered by the moral consequences of our technological advances, such as cloning and genetic testing (see Evidence-Based Practice). Its history stems from earlier events, both good, such as Watson and Crick's paper about DNA in 1953 and the first heart transplant in 1967, and bad, such as the syphilis research performed on African American males by the U.S. Public Health Service in Tuskegee, Alabama. All of these events, both positive and negative, signaled increasing complexity and the need for a new way of thinking and greater input from a more diverse body of knowledge and pool of disciplines.

Evidence-Based Practice

Ethics Related to Genetic Testing in Patients with Cancer

Genetic testing and genomics are rapidly expanding practices in the management of patients with cancer. Nurses working in oncology may face ethical issues, and this case study examined the impact of cancer genetics and ethics on patients and families with familial adenomatous polyposis (FAP). Because genetic testing can provide information about the impact of a hereditary cancer syndrome, like FAP, this case study considered ethical issues, particularly those related to an individual's rights. In this case study, there were differences in opinion among family members about whether they wanted to know the results related to their risk of future cancer development. The case study includes a discussion about the differences between legal obligations to share genetic information and the moral obligation to share genetic testing results. Nurses working in areas where genetic testing and genomics are growing need to consider how these advances affect their practice, as well as their responsibilities regarding the ethical issues of cancer genetics.

Beamer, L. C. (2017). Ethics and genetics: Examining a crossroads in nursing through a case study. *Clinical Journal of Oncology Nursing, 21*(6), 730–737.

THE BELMONT REPORT

Due to the past harm caused to individuals in the name of research in places like Tuskegee and Nuremberg, a commission was formed in 1976 to create a set of principles to govern the use of human subjects in research. The commission met at the Smithsonian Institute in the Belmont Conference Center. The resultant document, entitled the *Belmont Report*, is used to this day. The report describes three basic ethical principles to be applied to any research involving human subjects: respect for persons, beneficence, and justice. These are broad terms that need increased specificity when applied to a particular situation. For example, the principle of beneficence means to "do good," but does it also mean to "do no harm"? The *Belmont Report* outlines requirements for such situational specificity. Since the time of its publication, the *Belmont Report* has engendered the inclusion of additional ethical principles, such as **nonmaleficence** (do no harm) and autonomy (individual right to choose for oneself).

Two important developments came out of the report's publication, each with direct implications for current nursing practice. First, any research involving human subjects, which may be conducted on nursing units, must be approved by the organization's institutional review board (IRB) to ensure that the proposed research methodologies will not cause any harm to the research subjects.

In consideration of the principle of autonomy, which states that a mentally competent individual of legal age (therefore not a child) has the right to choose for him- or herself, the practice of informed consent was created. This practice protects patients' rights to decide what is best for themselves once they are provided with key information about the risks and benefits of a diagnostic test, treatment, surgical procedure, and other diagnostic or treatment modalities. The informed-consent process must contain all of the needed elements (information, voluntary participation, and mental competence) in order to be considered legal. It is imperative for nurses to know that the provider is responsible for obtaining patient consent. Nurses cannot obtain informed consent on behalf of a surgeon, anesthesiologist, or other direct-care provider performing a procedure, but they may witness the consent form.

PROFESSIONAL STANDARDS FOR ETHICAL PRACTICE: GUIDANCE DOCUMENTS FOR NURSES

The *Code of Ethics for Nurses* and *Nursing: Scope and Standards of Practice* are separate documents; however, both provide a framework for the practice of nursing where ethical decision making and care are the expected norm rather than the exception.

American Nurses Association Code of Ethics

One of the distinguishing characteristics of any profession is its code of ethics. The code of ethics for the profession is the social contract with the public concerning the moral behaviors of the members of the profession. Nursing first began to discuss a code of ethics in 1896, when a group of nursing leaders met to discuss the practice of nursing in the United States. The forerunners to the official code of ethics were generally based on the (Florence) Nightingale Pledge, which was and still is administered to graduating nurses. That first organization to address the code of ethics for nurses eventually became the American Nurses Association (ANA), and the first official code of ethics for nurses, the Code for Professional Nurses, was accepted by the ANA House of Delegates in 1950.

The Code for Professional Nurses has been updated and revised over the years to the *Code of Ethics for Nurses* ("the *Code*") we use today (see Box 4.1). It reflects the social contract that nursing has with the public, encompassing the moral traditions, values, and trust that the public has come to associate with nursing. The obligations that nurses have toward themselves, patients, and communities are all guided by ethical principles. There are no right or wrong behaviors identified in ethical principles, only guidelines for the moral practice of nursing.

Throughout the *Code*, the predominating principle is **justice**. Registered nurses have been voted the most trusted healthcare professionals again and again in public opinion polls. Nursing has a strong and long-standing commitment to social justice at every level, for both the individual as well as the community. Social justice relates to the equal treatment of all persons irrespective of race, ethnicity, gender, social status, or religion. Today's nurse must be culturally competent and attuned to the needs of vulnerable populations.

In order to practice sound ethical decision making, nurses must know and understand their own personal value systems. The value system of the nurse and the values of the organization in which the registered nurse is employed are fundamental to ethical behavior. However, these are not always compatible. What is considered ethical behavior in one situation may not apply in another. When a nurse is seeking employment, it is important that he or she examine the stated beliefs of the organization before accepting a position. Most organizations set forth a framework for ethical decision making. However, there may be moral conflicts encountered by a nurse involving certain reproductive services provided by the employer if these are not consistent with the nurse's personal moral position on birth control and abortion.

Many situations in healthcare are ambiguous, morally confronting, and have no clear-cut solution. The *Code* serves as a guide for the nurse; it does not tell the nurse what the *right* answer is in situations calling for ethical decision making. The first three provisions of the *Code* speak to the individual nurse and the responsibilities and commitment of the nurse in building a relationship with the patient. These provisions are based on equal **respect** for the patient and the need to advocate for the patient's rights regardless of race, gender, or culture. Provisions 4, 5, and 6 provide guidance for the nurse in the workplace environment, focusing on personal and professional accountability for the nursing care provided, professional behavior, and maintaining professional practice competency.

Connection Check 4.1

The initial nursing code of ethics was based on which work?
A. The Bill of Rights
B. The Nightingale Pledge
C. The Hippocratic Oath
D. The International Council of Nurses

ANA Scope and Standards of Practice

The ANA first published the *Standards of Nursing Practice* in 1973. This document defined a generic level of competency common to all practicing nurses and used the nursing process as the framework. Since that time, there have been revisions and updates. In 2015, *Nursing: Scope and Standards of Practice* (3rd ed.) was published to guide nursing practice.

The scope of nursing practice describes the who, what, when, where, why, and how of nursing practice. Nursing today is practiced in many different settings requiring knowledge and skill in the biological, physical, social, and behavioral sciences. Registered nurses are licensed by the state in which they practice and work collaboratively with other healthcare professionals.

Nursing is both an art and a science that includes caring, compassion, and respect for human dignity. The natural sciences are foundational to nursing practice. Through the use of critical thinking, nurses gather pertinent information, which is turned into action in the form of the nursing process. The nursing process is identified as the primary decision-making method for registered nurses and entails the collection of both subjective and objective data, analysis of the data to determine an appropriate nursing diagnosis, formulation of desired patient outcomes, creation of a plan to accomplish the outcomes, provision of care, and evaluation of the patient response.

There are 16 standards of professional nursing practice divided into two subsets: the 6 standards of practice and the 10 standards of professional performance, both of which are based on the nursing process. The first six standards define the practice of nursing for the registered nurse (RN) as well as the graduate-level-prepared advanced practice registered nurse (APRN). The remaining 10 standards define the roles and responsibilities of professional performance. Again, the registered nurse and the graduate-level advanced/specialty nurse roles and responsibilities are defined. Standard 7 addresses ethical nursing practice.

International Nursing Council Code of Ethics

The International Council of Nurses (ICN) is an organization that promotes ethical nursing practices throughout the world. The standards, guidelines, and policies of the ICN are accepted globally for the basis of nursing practice and policy. The ANA is the representative member for the United States.

The goals of the ICN are to (1) influence global health policy by (2) advancing nurses and nursing practice and (3) bring nursing together worldwide. The code of ethics of the ICN guides registered nurses worldwide in setting priorities, making ethical judgments, and taking action when faced with an ethical dilemma. The core values of the ICN promote ethical practice through (1) visionary leadership, (2) innovativeness, (3) solidarity, (4) accountability, and (5) social justice. The ICN code of ethics describes what nurses are held accountable for in terms of their core values, making nurses responsible for promoting health, preventing illness, and alleviating suffering on a global level.

ETHICAL PRINCIPLES AND THEORIES RELEVANT TO NURSING

The study of ethics is a branch of philosophy. Ethics assumes that individuals have choices for their decisions and behaviors. The choices are concerned with right and wrong; in other words, there are good choices and bad choices. The decision-making process for choosing a behavior or making a certain decision is complex and can be controversial. Although the ethical theories used in nursing are prescriptive and provide a framework for decision making, no single theory or principle is sufficient for every instance.

The most common ethical principles that provide the foundation of ethical practice and decision making for nurses:

1. **Beneficence** concerns people acting positively on behalf of the perceived well-being of others.
2. **Autonomy** involves the individual's personal right to make decisions concerning him- or herself. Nurses must provide support and advocacy for the individual patient's choices, regardless of whether they agree with them.
3. **Justice** requires fair and equal treatment for everyone regardless of race, religion, or gender. At the level of community, questions of equitability are taken

into account in decision making, such as the greatest good for the greatest number and the allocation of scarce resources during times of disasters or emergency.

4. **Fidelity** expects the nurse to be accountable for commitments made to others, to the self, and to the profession, based on the **virtue** of caring.

5. Nonmaleficence examines issues related to who may be harmed by actions and how any harm can be minimized or averted. This also relates to nurses' need to remain competent in their practice and exercise moral courage in reporting suspected/observed incidents of malpractice, abuse, or diversion.

6. **Veracity** is the requirement to tell the truth and to refrain from intentionally misleading or deceiving a patient to influence decisions (related to paternalism, described in item 8). Veracity or truth telling is also part of nonmaleficence, described in item 5.

7. **Confidentiality** requires that information is not shared beyond those who have a need to know. Nurses must remain vigilant regarding their use of social media, as outlined in later this chapter.

8. **Paternalism** is the inappropriate intention to protect individuals from their own involuntary actions or choices in the name of beneficence, which actually violates their right to self-determination (autonomy). Paternalism is often seen in the care of the older adult and in male-dominant cultures.

ETHICAL THEORIES TO SUPPORT NURSES IN DECISION MAKING

Ethical decision making can be highly complex and often ambiguous. The following ethical theories offer some foundational perspective and are provided as a guide to how individuals decide the relative moral "rightness or wrongness" of a decision or behavior. Because the human condition is so variable in both personal circumstance and situational elements, it is important to remain mindful of the term *relative* when engaging in ethical decision making. There are no absolutes; nurses must strive to make the *best possible* decision for a specific individual patient given the variables at hand while respecting and supporting the patient's autonomy.

An example of this is the concept of the **common good**, which considers what decision will be most beneficial for the greatest number of people and relates to the theory of utilitarianism. This theory is often associated with matters of social justice, the allocation of scarce resources, and emergency and disaster response. Another example is the concept of the **sanctity of life**. Healthcare providers are taught early and consistently that anything that will cause a patient to die is harmful. Although

the principle of nonmaleficence states that healthcare providers must do no harm, there are times when forcing life and enforcing lifesaving measures may be considered harmful. Respecting the wishes of the patients and their families can be difficult for healthcare providers if those wishes conflict with the basic value system of the provider. There are no right or wrong answers when working through ethical dilemmas, only the *best possible* solutions for the patient encountering a particular set of circumstances. In these situations, there are resources, such as hospital-based ethics committees (discussed later in this chapter), that can provide support, shared wisdom, and consultation to patients, family members, and providers.

Connection Check 4.2

Which ethical principle deals with ensuring truthfulness and commitment?
A. Autonomy
B. Beneficence
C. Justice
D. Veracity

Deontology

The deontological perspective of determining the rightness or wrongness of behavior is derived from the Greek term *deontos*, which means "a duty to obey." **Deontology** is most frequently associated with the philosopher Immanuel Kant, who felt that a moral individual, although self-determined, must base his or her actions on duty, which he saw as superior to actions based on love. Those who use deontology as their ethical framework inherently believe there is a right and a wrong for all acts based on fixed laws. Neither the situation in which the act occurs nor the consequences resulting from the act are considered. There are no exceptions, and any characteristics of the environment or situation are not considered when making decisions. Using purely this perspective, a patient in a vegetative state will not be removed from life support if the removal of the assistive device will hasten death. The healthcare team has a duty to do no harm, and removing life support would result in death.

This example considers the concept of the sanctity of life. Traditional healthcare education teaches providers that anything that will cause a patient to die is harmful. Although the principle of nonmaleficence states that healthcare providers must do no harm, there are times when forcing life and enforcing lifesaving measures may indeed be considered harmful. Respecting the wishes of the patients and their families can be difficult for healthcare providers if those wishes conflict with the deontological value system of the provider. In these situations, there are resources such as hospital-based ethics committees that can share the decision-making burden.

Consequentialism and Utilitarianism

In contrast to deontology, **consequentialism** determines the rightness or wrongness of a decision or behavior by the end result of the action. The utilitarian perspective is sometimes called the *greater-good perspective* and is based on the work of two British philosophers, Jeremy Bentham and John Stuart Mill. Utilitarianism aims at maximizing desired positive outcomes, such as lives saved, and minimizing harm, such as lives lost. The characteristics of the environment and the situation, as well as the consequences of the action, are an essential part of the decision-making process.

Using the utilitarian perspective, that same patient in a vegetative state on life support considered through the lens of deontology in the previous section can be removed from the ventilator and allowed to die. This is based on the decision meeting with the wishes of the patient and family, who view the death as a greater good than lingering and suffering in a vegetative state.

In addition, there are two similar theories to consider: act utilitarianism and rule utilitarianism. *Act utilitarianism* theory states that the consequences of an act are predictable and that the choice that yields the greatest benefit for the most people is the right and ethical choice. Act utilitarianism does not take into account personal feelings or societal constraints and is not concerned with justice, beneficence, or individual autonomy but with what will benefit the most individuals even if individual rights are infringed. Examples of act utilitarian-based actions include the potential enforcement of mandatory quarantine in times of epidemic and mandatory vaccination laws aimed to prevent such an epidemic. *Rule utilitarianism* theory is similar to act utilitarianism but takes into account any fairness laws that may exist, which sometimes come up in persons unable to receive certain vaccines due to allergies, for example. Therefore, justice and beneficence are valued. However, there can be the possibility of conflicting rules, resulting in no ethically correct answer. The theory itself poses potential dilemmas for both society and the individual.

CASE STUDY: EPISODE 2

Because of persistent swallowing problems, video fluoroscopy is conducted, and the findings indicate a severe swallowing disorder. Because of the danger of aspiration, the provider orders a nasogastric tube inserted for feeding purposes, with plans for possible gastrostomy tube placement if the dysphagia does not resolve. The family members tell the nurse they do not want any type of permanent feeding tube placed in the patient…

If the deontological perspective is used in the decision as to whether to place the device as described in the case study, the device will be placed because of the duty to do no harm.

Leaving the nasogastric tube in place may result in irritation to the nasal passages and oropharyngeal area, skin irritation from the tape and tube around the outside of the nares, and a potential for placement errors that result in fluid being introduced into the lungs. So the right action would be to place a more permanent feeding device directly into Mr. Michaels's stomach because it is safer for the patient. However, the patient's family does not want a permanent feeding tube.

Rights

The rights theory can be useful if it is used in conjunction with another ethical theory; it cannot stand alone. This theory states the rights set by society are to be afforded the highest priority and protected at all cost. Individuals can also give rights to others if they are in a position to do so. The primary issue with this theory is that society has to determine the rights it wishes to uphold; but in order to do this, society must determine its priorities and goals, and these priorities must be backed with laws or legislation. One example is the right for all citizens to be provided healthcare. Although a vehicle for this has been created in the form of the Affordable Care Act, it is at risk due to its associated costs to business, and there is no guarantee that society will continue to uphold and support it.

Casuistry

The term **casuistry** is derived from the Latin word for *case*. It examines the outcomes and lessons learned from earlier benchmark or *paradigm* cases to make ethical decisions. It uses inductive reasoning to examine significant facts and outcomes in past similar cases as a means to project possible future outcomes on which to base ethical decision making. Casuistry has a more holistic and personal focus than the more all-or-nothing approaches of deontology and utilitarianism. Although it is not considered to be flawless, it is a highly valued addition to the ethical toolbox in today's complex bioethical environment where healthcare providers are faced with coming to terms with the unintended consequences of technological advancements.

There are many other theories that have characteristics that are useful in ethical decision making. However, no single theory is applicable in all situations. By using a combination of theories, it is oftentimes possible to arrive at the *most ethical* decision. For nurses interested in further study, there are philosophy courses and continuing education opportunities that focus on ethical decision making.

Connection Check 4.3

Which ethical theory is based on obeying laws?
A. Autonomy
B. Deontology
C. Rights
D. Consequentialism

ETHICAL DILEMMAS

The complexity of today's nursing practice cannot be understated. Nursing ethics considers situations where there are no clear right or wrong answers; what may be right for one patient may be very wrong for another. Today's nursing practice takes place in many different settings, increasingly outside of the traditional acute care hospital, where there is an environment of support from other healthcare providers. Practice settings such as community health fairs, schools, private homes, shopping malls, homeless shelters, and soup kitchens are the new norm. Often, the nurse is the only healthcare provider at the site and has to independently work through an ethical dilemma.

As previously discussed, the predominating principle of the ANA's *Code* is justice, and although there are nine provisions to guide the nurse, there is no step-by-step process for nurses to use to solve ethical dilemmas. There is, however, a process that nurses use every day, the *nursing process*, that when applied to ethical decision making can assist the nurse in making a complex decision (Box 4.2).

Today, nursing is emerging in many states as an autonomous and independent profession by virtue of being a licensed profession. This is exemplified in the 2010 Institute of Medicine report *The Future of Nursing: Leading Change,* *Advancing Health*, which includes recommendations to increase the numbers of baccalaureate-prepared nurses to 80% by 2020, to double the number of nurses with a doctorate by 2020, and to remove scope-of-practice barriers for APRNs. In the past, practice within the hospital setting saw the typically male physician in charge of the patient's care and the typically female nurse following physician orders. There was an unspoken attitude that nurses were subservient members of the healthcare team due to sexist views of the place of females in society and the gaps in educational preparation between physicians and nurses. In today's practice environment, there are more male nurses, more APRNs functioning as providers, and improved interdisciplinary communication across healthcare teams. The nurse who chooses to practice within a hospital setting is no longer considered subservient. Each healthcare organization has a stated mission and vision that govern the roles and responsibilities of nurses and other healthcare team members. Nurses are expected to practice ethically within the scope and standards of practice and to be vocal and involved when ethical dilemmas present themselves.

Nurses are frequently placed in situations where decisions require an examination of ethical issues. They have a duty (fidelity) to the patient to provide care that is competent and respectful of each patient's individual situation. Sometimes this may be in conflict with the nurse's own beliefs, the organization's beliefs and protocols, or the provider's/practitioner's beliefs.

A *dilemma* can be defined as a problem with one or more alternative solutions where each of the alternative solutions presents ethical or practicality problems and where all solutions are equally unpleasant. Almost all ethical dilemmas in nursing involve the right to **self-determination** (autonomy) of the patient and relate to the patient's right to make his or her own decisions about treatment. Although nursing practice has many such dilemmas, the following discussion is limited to some of the more commonly seen scenarios related to healthcare.

Box 4.2 Suggested Ethical Decision-Making Process

Assess/Diagnose

Determine exactly what must be decided. Sometimes the issue is hidden within the emotional or cultural/ethnic/religious characteristics of the patient and family. The nurse must determine how these factors affect or define the issue.

Plan

Formulate at least three alternatives to solve the issue. Each alternative must be examined for practicality, legal issues, patient and family characteristics such as personal wants and desires, the social and environmental aspects of the alternative, financial considerations, and the long- and short-term viability and consequences of each alternative. Ideally, the alternative is chosen by the healthcare team (which includes the nurse) and the family. Sometimes ethics committees assist in choosing the alternative.

Implement

Once the alternative is chosen, actions to achieve the greatest benefit with the least amount of risk are carried out.

Evaluate

Determine if the desired effect has occurred or new information is available that might alter the plan and/or implementation.

Connection Check 4.4

In addressing an ethical dilemma, which principle guides decision making focused on minimizing harm to the patient?
A. Beneficence
B. Justice
C. Nonmaleficence
D. Fidelity

Informed Consent

As discussed earlier regarding the *Belmont Report*, **informed consent** simply means that the patient has been fully informed by the provider responsible for the treatment or procedure. This consent includes information related to necessity, what is physically involved in the treatment or procedure, and the associated risks and benefits. This allows the patient to make a knowledgeable determination as to whether to agree to have the proposed treatment or procedure. The patient who is giving consent for the procedure must be mentally competent to make this decision. For patients who are minors or deemed mentally incompetent, the parent(s) or appointed guardian must give consent following the same informed-consent procedure.

Informed consent is required for all invasive treatments/procedures. All information must be provided in a language or format that the patient understands, with an opportunity for the patient to ask questions. The information is provided by the person who will be performing the treatment/procedure. Neither the healthcare provider nor any member of the healthcare team is allowed to coerce the patient to give consent for the treatment/procedure. Although it is not the responsibility of the nurse to obtain informed consent on behalf of an absent or unwilling provider, the nurse may be asked to witness a consent process. In this case, the nurse is validating *only* that the patient, parent, or guardian/surrogate was observed signing the consent form.

The patient has the right to refuse a treatment/procedure, refuse receipt of the information about the treatment/procedure, or waive the informed consent and still have the procedure. Whenever a patient refuses any part of the informed consent, there must be comprehensive documentation of the refusal in the patient's medical record.

There are instances when informed consent by the patient, parent, or guardian is not required, and almost all of these are in emergency situations where withholding or delaying the treatment/procedure to seek consent would be deleterious to the patient. Healthcare organizations have policies that guide the actions of the provider performing an emergency treatment/procedure because it is necessary to "save life or limb." In addition, parental consent is not needed for minors seeking treatment for sexually transmitted infections. In some states, minors may be considered emancipated (those who are married, pregnant, or financially independent), allowing them to give consent. In other instances, the treatment/procedure can be ordered by the courts or other legal authority, and the patient, parent, or guardian does not need to give consent.

Registered nurses participating in research are often involved with human subjects. As outlined in the *Belmont Report*, any individual who takes part in a research study must be informed of the study's goals, any known benefits and risks associated with participation, what the individual can expect by being a participant, and that he or she has the right to refuse or withdraw at any time without consequences. All research studies using human subjects must be approved by the agency's institutional review board (IRB).

Do-Not-Resuscitate Directives

The customary definition of death is the absence of a heartbeat and respiration. However, with today's technological advances in healthcare, there are situations where patients may have significant and irreversible brain injuries, but because the brainstem is still intact, the patient still has a pulse and respirations. This damage to the brain may lead to an irreversible loss of consciousness or a persistent vegetative state, but there are unassisted heartbeats and respirations. Decisions regarding life-sustaining procedures raise many ethical questions, and these decisions require communication between the healthcare providers, the patient, and the family.

Patients have the right to refuse or accept life-sustaining treatment. The primary issue is to determine whether the patient is mentally competent to make that decision. Once competency is determined, the information needed by the patient to make this decision revolves around whether (1) by accepting treatment, the patient will return to an acceptable state of health; (2) by accepting treatment, the patient will continue in a compromised health state with no hope of returning to an acceptable state of health for an indefinite period; or (3) by accepting treatment for a terminal illness, the dying process will be prolonged. All of these situations bring up ethical issues. What is in the best interest of the patient is the question that must be posed.

Most healthcare organizations have policies related to do-not-resuscitate (DNR) orders, and it is up to the patient and the provider to follow the procedures set forth in the policy for the particular agency. A DNR order must be displayed in a visible spot in a patient's room because it is the exception to the rule in healthcare agencies that mandate that in the event of cardiac or respiratory arrest, cardiopulmonary resuscitation must be initiated by a competent person. Consultation between the patient (or patient's family in the case of an unconscious or incompetent patient) and the provider should precede any written DNR orders and usually revolves around issues of quality of life. A DNR order should be reviewed periodically and updated as the patient's condition changes. With the increased use of palliative care to maximize the quality of life, for some patients and families, prolonging life may not be a welcome option. Nurses who have personal belief systems related to DNR orders that would compromise their ability to enforce a DNR order should transfer the care of that patient to another nurse and consider changing their practice setting if this type of dilemma is frequently encountered.

A relatively new program called the physician order for life-sustaining treatment (POLST) is based on effective communication between patients with life-threatening illnesses and providers. Although similar to an advanced directive (discussed in the next section), which everyone should have, a POLST is created at the time a patient develops a condition that is seen as life-threatening. It contains documentation of agreed-upon orders and a promise by providers to honor the patient's wishes for treatment concerning procedures such as intubation, feeding tubes, and the use of specific medications. In essence, the program provides a DNR order that is independent of a specific healthcare organization. POLST programs have been implemented at some level in all 50 states and the District of

Columbia. However, levels of usage and incorporation as a standard of care vary widely from state to state. How the program is administered and what it is called (e.g., medical orders for life-sustaining treatment [MOLST], physician orders for scope of treatment [POST], and clinician orders for life-sustaining treatment [COLST]) varies from state to state as well. Decisions on determining resuscitation status are informed by documents optimally created by patients before they become seriously ill. They include the advance directive and living will.

Advance Directives

An **advance directive** is a document that is designed to communicate the final wishes of patients in the event they cannot speak for themselves and is created when the patient is competent and in open communication with the provider, family, and close friends. Sometimes religious leaders are also a part of these conversations. The directive is a set of precise instructions for the type and duration of care the patient wants. Different scenarios may be presented with the circumstances outlined regarding life-sustaining procedures and treatments.

Living Wills

A **living will** is a legal document created by a competent person that provides the person's desires for medical care in the event the person is unable to independently make decisions regarding care. The requirements for living wills vary by state and may also be referred to as a type of advance directive, healthcare directive, or a provider's directive. This document describes specifics about life-prolonging treatments the person will allow and those that will not be allowed and becomes effective only when the person becomes incapacitated to the point that he or she cannot make decisions for him- or herself.

Withdrawal of Fluids and Nutrition

The decision to withdraw fluids and nutrition is one of the most challenging ethical dilemmas that a nurse may confront. The patient, family, and provider ultimately make this decision collaboratively. Withdrawal of fluids and nutrition to patients is commonly referred to the healthcare agency's ethics committee for review and input. The decision to withdraw fluids and nutrition is not made lightly because it violates the responsibility of the provider and the nurse to promote comfort. It is often difficult for the family to understand and accept. Nurses exhibit beneficence and fidelity by explaining the rationale for withdrawing nutrition to anxious patient families and reassuring them of the comfort and benefit derived from these measures. Patients who are in the dying phase do not need fluid or nutrition in the amounts that are necessary to sustain life, and the addition or forcing of fluids or nutrition may be detrimental to the patient's comfort. The dying phase varies by individual patient and may take several days or a relatively short period. Often, there is a tendency for the family to request fluids and nutrition at levels the patient had in the past. However, as the body begins to shut down, the circulation becomes slower, so the addition of extra fluid may cause increased fluid in the lungs, causing difficulty breathing, peripheral edema, ascites, or vomiting. The addition of nutrition from either enteral feedings or IV sources may cause vomiting, constipation, or bowel obstruction from the reduced gastric emptying. In addition, there is the chance of aspiration because of the reduced gag reflex.

Pain Control

Pain is often referred to as the "fifth vital sign" and should be assessed by the nurse upon each patient encounter. The perception of pain is a personal experience for every individual, and only the patient can describe its location, duration, and intensity. Every report of pain, either by the patient or the family/significant other/surrogate on the patient's behalf, should be evaluated by the nurse, and what the patient reports about the pain, including intensity, characteristics, and past effective methods of relief, is to be accepted by the healthcare provider. Patients who are experiencing pain need to be shown empathy and respect and given choices for pain relief. The alternatives for pain relief should be explained, including the advantages and disadvantages, benefits, and risks. The nurse should accept the patient's decision for pain management regardless of personal beliefs. Once the patient has chosen the method of pain relief, it should be implemented and evaluated by the nurse. This evaluation includes a dialogue with the patient concerning the effectiveness of the measure and what the nurse has observed in relation to the relief of pain.

Nurses must be self-aware of and vigilant against any bias, organizational or social pressure regarding patients labeled as "drug-seeking" or "hypochondriacal," or any other factors that may inhibit sound clinical judgment and the provision of appropriate pain control. Further, nurses must display moral courage to advocate for proper pain management from providers who may be hesitant to provide the higher doses of medication required to properly control pain in the suffering patient.

Genetic Testing, Reproductive Technology, and Selective Abortion

New ethical dilemmas arise from advances in the knowledge and techniques of genetic testing and human reproduction. Mendelian laws of heredity state that there is a one in four chance of a child being affected with a disorder if both parents are carriers of an *autosomal-recessive* gene, a one in two chance the child will be a carrier, and a one in four chance the child will not have the disorder or be a carrier. For *autosomal-dominant* disorders, there is a one in two chance the child will inherit the gene. A child inheriting this gene will have the disorder.

The sex chromosomes also present the possibility of a child inheriting a disorder. X-linked disorders depend on the chromosome, X or Y, on which the mutant gene is attached. Females can contribute only X chromosomes to conception, whereas a male can contribute an X or a Y. If the male contributes an X, the result will be a female child, whereas if the male contributes a Y, the child will be a male. Mutant genes carried on the X chromosome result in the child being affected with the disorder if the child is a male but only a one in two chance of the child being affected if the child is a girl. It would take two X chromosomes with the mutant gene attached for a female to be affected.

There are techniques that detect the presence of genetic disorders in addition to a blood test for individual genetic mapping. Amniocentesis is a procedure that withdraws amniotic fluid from the pregnant uterus that allows testing for certain genetic disorders. This test is not performed before the 15th or 16th week of gestation, and results may not be available until the 20th week of gestation, when selective abortion is more problematic. Chorionic villi sampling, which can be completed in the first trimester, tests placental tissue for genetic disorders, and selective abortion can be done in the first trimester. However, there is a higher risk of spontaneous abortion with this procedure. Prenatal diagnosis of genetic disorders is completed, and then comes the ethical dilemma about whether to decide to abort (selective abortion) the fetus if a disorder is detected.

There are many ethical issues regarding abortion in general and selective abortion specifically. There is a group of disability rights advocates who claim that selective abortion is discrimination. There are also well-known religious and cultural objections to abortion for any reason. The nurse who practices in a setting where abortions are performed must define individual values in relation to abortion and selective abortion, but the nurse's individual values must not be allowed to impact the patient's right to self-determination (autonomy).

Genetic testing does not affect only pregnant women. Individuals who have a history of a disorder in their family may also be tested. There are some disorders that do not produce clinical manifestations until middle age. Huntington's disease is an adult-onset problem but is transmitted genetically. Clearly devastating disorders such as Huntington's, Tay-Sachs, sickle cell anemia, and cystic fibrosis can be detected through genetic testing before conception, thereby preventing transmission. It is considered wrong to coerce individuals to undergo genetic testing for social control over reproductive decisions. Coercive measures for selective abortion after testing are an invasion of rights and a form of paternalism.

Advances in reproduction technology are making it possible for women who have been diagnosed as infertile to become pregnant or to donate the ovum to a surrogate mother who will carry the fetus. Other options include artificial insemination of the ovum with sperm from a sperm bank and in vitro fertilization, in which the sperm fertilizes the ovum in a laboratory and then the embryo is inserted into the uterus of the woman. Couples can elect to have the woman's ovum fertilized with the man's sperm and frozen for later use. As reproductive technology continues to advance, there are ethical concerns that may arise for the nurse.

The ethical questions that arise in reproductive technology are complex and often revolve around religious values and legal issues. Many religious ethicists say that the use of reproductive technology for the purpose of producing a baby is morally wrong, and if a third party has donated either the ovum or sperm, adultery has been committed. On the other hand, if the wife donated the ovum and the husband donated the sperm, some of these same ethicists contend that this is within the bounds of a marital framework and is permissible. However, if more than one embryo is produced for implantation, or if unneeded or unsuitable embryos are discarded, this can create issues regarding the morality of discontinuing life. Nurses who practice in fertilization centers are frequently confronted with these matters.

In cases where there is a surrogate mother, there can be legal issues concerning who is the mother of the child: the genetic mother or the gestational mother? Where there have been ovum or sperm donors with no relation to the mother, in the case of a single woman or the couple in a husband/wife situation, who is the legal parent? Surrogacy contracts differ from state to state, with various approaches to the social policy aspects. There are no definitive answers for the nurse.

Experimental Therapies

As with genetics, knowledge and technology in treating disease are rapidly advancing and lead to issues related to research involving human beings. Human subjects research is divided into two categories: therapeutic and nontherapeutic research. Nontherapeutic research, primarily for the advancement of knowledge, results in outcomes not intended to be of benefit to the human subject. In therapeutic research, the human subject is expected to benefit from the treatment, vaccine, new medication, or diagnostic procedure that is being investigated. However, the distinctions between the two categories are often difficult to discern. Therapeutic research may not have the intended beneficial result, and there may be unintended consequences of nontherapeutic research that do benefit the subject. In any kind of research using human subjects, the concern for informed consent is an issue. The person who becomes a research subject must be fully informed of the risks and benefits of participating, consent must be voluntary, and the person must be allowed to withdraw from the study at any time with no repercussions. But in some research, the risks and benefits might not be known.

Biomedical research enhances the advancement of medical treatment by investigating various alternatives in medications, procedures, and treatments so that healthcare practices are evidence based. Ethical issues arise when the rights of the human subjects are examined. Do patients who have a certain disease have a duty to participate in a study even though they may not want to, even though the results may provide help for others? Is it ever ethical to give a participant a disease so that the effects of various treatments or medication can be studied? There are those who contend that the answer to the previous questions is yes, as long as only minimal risk is involved. But how does one define *minimal risk*? The nurse who practices in the field of research must define personal values that could be challenged by specific research studies.

Inability to Afford Prescribed Care

There is ongoing debate in the United States about whether access to healthcare is a fundamental human right. Healthcare in the United States is not available to all citizens on an equal basis. Those who have health insurance or can afford to pay healthcare costs enjoy a level of care that may lead to a longer life expectancy and increased quality of life. However, many people cannot afford healthcare because of a lack of health insurance or the inability to pay for care. The Affordable Care Act (ACA) of 2010 was initially designed to close the gap between those who can afford healthcare and those who cannot. Due to many complicating factors and the perceived inordinate cost of healthcare, it is unclear how long the ACA will remain in effect or in its current form.

Does society have an obligation to its citizens to provide healthcare for all? If so, does the individual person have an obligation to participate in behaviors that decrease health risks? The theories of justice give some insight into the issues involved in the ethics of care. The libertarian viewpoint is that citizens have a right to individual liberty, life, and property and that governments cannot take those away to give to someone else. A socialist viewpoint is that all individuals of a society are equal and that governments have an obligation to ensure that equality is maintained, so those who have more must provide for those who have less. The liberal point of view is that those who have more should help those who have less.

There are agencies in most communities that assist those who cannot afford healthcare or who cannot afford treatment. There is a difference in those who cannot afford healthcare and those who cannot afford treatment. Insurance may give the individual the ability to seek healthcare, but insurance may pay for only a portion of the prescribed treatment or none at all.

Organ and Tissue Donation

The issue of organ donation and transplantation has many considerations. Organ transplantation has been performed since 1954, when the first kidney was transplanted into the donor's twin. There have been many advances since then, but there is also a scarcity of donor organs, which creates an ethical dilemma concerning the allocation of scarce resources and "who" receives the organ or tissue. There is a great deal of fear about becoming an organ donor among people due to a general mistrust of the medical profession and how death is defined and determined. Public education programs are aimed at dispelling misconceptions and clarifying organ procurement criteria.

Organ donors are solicited in many ways. Many people indicate they are an organ donor through a special decal on their driver's license or by indicating the desire to donate in a will. Although this may be the wish of the individual, the family of the patient can overturn this decision at the time of death of the potential donor. Individuals who are victims of trauma may become donors when the physician determines that the patient is brain dead and requests a donation of unaffected organs from the family. The donor is placed or continued on mechanical ventilation, which keeps the organs oxygenated but also gives the appearance to the family of the donor still being alive, which can make an already difficult decision even more agonizing. Organ procurement teams are specially trained to work with families to encourage organ donation. Although some families are willing to share their loved one's organs with another, some have religious or cultural edicts against this. The nurse may be from a religious or cultural background that prohibits organ donation, but these beliefs cannot interfere with the patient's or family's decisions.

When a person needing a transplant is identified, he or she is added to a national list, created by the National Organ Transplant Act of 1984, to await an organ with the right specifications to become available. The severity of disease is a determinant in where the patient is placed on this list, leading to the sickest patients being placed higher on the list. Many people die before their desired organ or tissue becomes available. The ethical issue of justice arises when there is more than one person needing the same organ when it becomes available. The decision as to which patient gets which organ, or any organ, is based on criteria established by the Organ Procurement and Transplantation Network (OPTN), a division of the U.S. Department of Health and Human Services (HHS).

ETHICAL ISSUES IN PROFESSIONAL PRACTICE

Moral Courage

Truth telling has its costs and involves moral courage, and it takes moral courage for nurses to stay strong and resilient in the face of many forms of adversity in today's practice settings. Moral courage involves actions that stand up to wrongdoing. It requires the willingness to be honest in the face of personal risk. For many nurses, it is a fundamental part of their fabric and a key reason they sought out the profession. There is ample reason to celebrate the moral courage of nurses, for in many cases, they go to extremes and expose themselves to personal harm in order to advocate for and protect the rights of their patients. No wonder that nurses are consistently voted the most trustworthy professionals.

Discernment

Moral courage requires the practice of discernment. As nurses practice over time, they gain clinical and practical wisdom and the quality of discernment, which allows them to gather pertinent data in a given situation and create informed conclusions based on their accumulated practice-based wisdom. Although the role of bias and burnout, among other factors, must also be considered, experienced nurses know intuitively when they must speak up about certain conditions, behaviors, or situations that violate patient or professional ethical standards. Although there are clear-cut situations—for example, when a colleague is observed diverting medications or abusing a patient, or a surgeon refuses to honor a "time-out" in the operating room, or an informed consent was witnessed as being subtlety coerced—many situations requiring moral courage are murky and uncertain.

Nurse–Patient Communication

Nurses spend proportionately more time with their patients than do other healthcare providers and have more opportunities to connect and form trusting relationships with them. This is not to minimize the trusted relationship that many providers have with their patients. However, when patients receive difficult or complex information from their providers, questions evolve, often when the provider is no longer available, leaving the nurse to answer them. Nurses must learn to carefully navigate the line between what they can and cannot divulge to a patient, based on both scope-of-practice and professional and organizational guidelines. This can be an ethically challenging situation when a patient and/or family is desperate for information that the nurse cannot (but wishes to) divulge to the patient. It takes just as much moral courage and discernment to speak, or refrain from speaking, as it does to report an injustice. However, the nurse can advocate for the patient by discussing the patient's wishes for more information with the direct health-care provider.

Social Media, Computers, and HIPAA

There is a saying about the paradox of your best feature also being your worst. This has never been truer than at the intersection of social media and healthcare. Nurses can access and share knowledge with colleagues and create professional relationships and communities of interest with nurses in other cities and countries. Social media has also brought many patients into closer and more frequent contact with their providers via encrypted virtual private networks (VPNs). Patients can search for health information online, although not all of it is reliable. As consumers, potential patients having elective procedures can review

Medicare's Hospital Consumer Assessment of Healthcare Providers and Systems (HCAHPS) to decide which hospital best meets their care needs and expectations. These data, accessible via the Internet and disseminated through social media, have made hospitals more accountable for their patient outcomes.

However, a tragic number of nurses, physicians, and students have seen a promising career go by the wayside due to the indiscriminate use of social media sites, upon which they have, often unwittingly, posted information that proved to be sensitive and/or damaging to their patients and organizations. Some mistakenly think that by not mentioning the patient or organization's name, they are not violating anyone's privacy. This is not accurate. Social media users are savvy and clever and can piece together information nurses are unaware they are providing. The best practice is for nurses to refrain from even the smallest mention of patient- and workplace-related events in their social media use.

In other computer-related, career-ending events, nurses have violated Health Insurance Portability and Accountability Act (HIPAA) and organizational guidelines prohibiting them from seeking access to charts of patients they know from other aspects of their lives, such as neighbors or their children's teachers. In other words, they did not access the patient's medical record on a "need-to-know" basis but, rather, in a self-satisfying inquiry that does not reflect fidelity, veracity, or beneficence toward any patient.

A relatively new phenomenon called "patient-targeted Googling" (PTG), initially used by psychiatrists, citing the need to locate and reconnect with at-risk patients inconsistent in their appointments, has become a greater issue among nurses and providers. The ethical principle of fidelity, which encompasses confidentiality and the right to patient privacy, suggests that to "Google" someone with whom one is in a caregiver–patient or provider–patient relationship, where a power imbalance in favor of the provider already exists, is a violation of professional boundaries and of the patient's privacy, unless there is urgent concern over the patient's well-being. Nurses are all human and therefore possess a native inquisitiveness; however, as professionals, curiosity must be curtailed in the name of veracity and fidelity to patients, families, and their privacy.

Duty to Warn

Although Provision 3 of the ANA *Code* states that the nurse will promote and protect the right to patient confidentiality, there are exceptions to this rule. When a patient shares information with a nurse or provider that indicates that the patient is a danger to him- or herself or others, or contains disclosure of certain past crimes, such as rape or incest, or any other vital information that is critical to the well-being of another, the nurse may disclose the information to outside parties, optimally with the guidance and support of the institution's organizational leadership.

The exception for disclosure of this type of information came out of a landmark 1976 court case known as *Tarasoff v. Board of Regents of the University of California*. In the case, a psychiatric outpatient who was also enrolled as a student at the university and receiving counseling at the student health center told his therapist of plans to kill his girlfriend. The therapist reported this to the campus police, who did not take appropriate action and warn the victim of the threat, who was later killed by the student. Her parents sued the involved staff and the school's board of regents. This case fundamentally changed the practice and definition of confidentiality.

Workplace Incivility and Horizontal Violence

Although the phrase "Nurses eat their young" is both negative to the profession and widely known to many, it wasn't until 2015 that the ANA published a position statement on workplace incivility. Nurse-on-nurse aggression is not a new phenomenon. In some ways, there is an inherent setup for this condition by the widely disparate variation in professional preparation. No other profession has as many approved levels of "entry into practice" educational preparation as does nursing. This includes associate degree, diploma (hospital based), baccalaureate, as well as entry master's degree programs, including the clinical nurse leader, all leading to eligibility to seek the licensure to be a registered nurse. If one also considers age, race, and gender biases, by combining all of these "nurses" on a unit, under the pressures of understaffing or high-acuity patients, with good, bad, or uncertain leadership, it easy to see a prescription for conflict.

Connection Check 4.5

In managing care for competent patients, which interventions or activities require the patient's informed consent? *(Select all that apply.)*
A. Participation in a research study
B. Change in room/unit
C. Invasive diagnostic studies
D. Operative procedures
E. Discharge time and day

ETHICS COMMITTEES: SUPPORT FOR ETHICAL DECISION MAKING

Ethical decision making is not easy and usually involves conflicting beliefs and priorities. One of the primary roles for the nurse in a situation where there may be conflicting solutions is to recognize that there may be a question of ethics involved and to get the appropriate personnel involved.

Role of Interprofessional Care

Interprofessional teams include physicians, APRNs, clinical nurse specialists, staff nurses, social workers, pharmacists, dietitians, chaplains, and physical and occupational therapists and are responsible for addressing issues or concerns beyond a strictly medical focus. For instance, a treatment that may seem in the best interest of the patient could be examined by the team of professionals in relation to quality of life following the treatment, the time the treatment may take and any long-term consequences that may result, the cost of the treatment, or the recovery time associated with the treatment. The team must be able to present a wider range of options for the same problem.

Ethics Committees

An ethics committee consists of healthcare providers from many different disciplines. Ethics committees are similar to an interprofessional team, but an ethics committee examines ethical dilemmas as they arise in an agency and creates policies to assist with decision making. An ethics committee also provides guidelines for potential ethical problems, serves as a forum for open discussion of the problem, and acts as the patient's advocate, as needed. Ethics committees usually have one of three distinct structures but can blend these structures as needed:

1. The autonomy model facilitates decision making for the competent patient.
2. The patient benefit model uses substituted judgment and facilitates decision making for the incompetent patient.
3. The social justice model considers broad social issues and is accountable to the institution.

The ethics committee is responsible for creating the policies by which ethical decisions are made so that the rights of the patients are protected. The committee also describes the roles of each member of the healthcare team and the patients and families in making decisions.

Making Connections

CASE STUDY: WRAP-UP

The family has stated they do not want a gastrostomy tube placed. It is the responsibility of the nurse and the healthcare team in general to provide enough information about the entire issue of the feeding tubes, both nasogastric and a skin-level device. Informed consent or dissent can be made only when the family has as much information about the benefits of each feeding device and the consequences of each device. In the case of Mr. Michaels, part of the information needed is that his hemiplegia is improving, and he responds appropriately to commands and the surrounding environment. The decision is made to hold a conference to discuss whether a permanent tube should be placed. Additionally, a competency evaluation is scheduled for Mr. Michaels to determine his ability to make informed decisions based on his improving level of consciousness.

Case Study Questions

1. To begin to assist this patient and family with decision making concerning a gastrostomy tube, which action should the nurse do first?
   A. Report the family's decision to the prescriber.
   B. Inform the family that the provider will make the best decision.
   C. Offer to have another patient who has a gastrostomy tube talk with the family.
   D. Check the patient's chart for an advance directive or living will.

2. In checking for the presence of a living will for Mr. Michaels, the nurse is using which ethical principle?
   A. Autonomy
   B. Beneficence
   C. Justice
   D. Nonmaleficence

3. As Mr. Michaels's level of consciousness improves and he is following commands, what must be evaluated prior to making the decision about placement of the gastrostomy tube?
   A. Mental competency
   B. Swallowing
   C. Psychomotor abilities
   D. Vision and hearing screening

4. Mr. Michaels is found to be mentally competent, but the family still does not want the gastrostomy tube placed. In the event the tube is not placed, this could be considered a violation of which ethical principle?
   A. Veracity
   B. Beneficence
   C. Self-determination
   D. Confidentiality

5. As a result of the difference between the family members' and Mr. Michaels's wishes, the nurse should request which consultation?
   A. Ethics committee
   B. Interprofessional meeting
   C. Hospital chaplain
   D. Family lawyer

CHAPTER SUMMARY

Registered nurses in today's world face ethical challenges almost daily. Knowing the guidelines provided by professional organizations, understanding individual value systems, and enlisting the available support systems assist in helping the nurse to make choices that are in the best interest of the patients. Nurses must be familiar with essential ethical principles that guide decision making in the clinical setting. It is important that the nurse be knowledgeable of the role of autonomy, beneficence, confidentiality, fidelity, justice, nonmaleficence, veracity, and paternalism in providing care. These ethical principles are used in assisting patients and families in making difficult decisions related to advance directives, living wills, organ transplantation, life-prolonging procedures, and genetic testing. Ethics committees are available in most acute care settings to support the patient, family, and healthcare team in resolving potential ethical dilemmas.

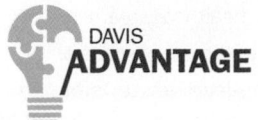

DAVIS ADVANTAGE | To explore learning resources for this chapter, go to **Davis Advantage** and find:
- Answers to in-text questions
- Chapter Resources and Activities
- NCLEX®-Style Chapter Review Questions
- Bibliography

Chapter 5

Palliative Care and End-of-Life Issues

Jennifer Wenzel and Maya Zumstein-Shaha

LEARNING OUTCOMES

Content in this chapter is designed to assist in:

1. Discussing the meaning of palliative care and hospice care
2. Listing the domains of palliative care
3. Analyzing the nursing care priorities for patients near the end of life
4. Developing communication and support strategies for family members
5. Explaining moral distress in end-of-life issues
6. Identifying nursing self-care strategies

ESSENTIAL TERMS

Advanced care planning (ACP)
Hospice care
Moral distress
Palliative care (PC)
Postmortem care

CONCEPTS

- Assessment
- Comfort
- Communication
- Ethics
- Grief and Loss
- Legal

Finding Connections

Follow this patient throughout the chapter.

Mrs. Kelso is a 79-year-old female with hypertension, past myocardial infarction, chronic obstructive pulmonary disease (COPD), congestive heart failure, and peptic ulcer disease. She had been living in her own home and was able to bathe and feed herself and perform light housework until she fell at home and suffered a subdural hematoma. The hematoma was surgically evacuated. Since the surgery, she has lost the ability to walk and has had ongoing changes in her mental status. She is not oriented to person, time, or place and does not interact with her caregivers. She sleeps most of the day, with only occasional periods of wakefulness. These changes in her mental status have resulted in the loss of full decisional capacity. Mrs. Kelso's daughter, Nancy, has become her surrogate decision maker with the input of other family members. They elect to continue fully aggressive care because their primary goal is Mrs. Kelso's survival. She is eventually discharged to a rehabilitation facility in an attempt to improve her mobility...

HISTORICAL BACKGROUND

Early in the last century, the focus of healthcare was on the provision of comfort, mostly at the time of death. With an average life expectancy of 47 years in the United States, patients usually died at home, surrounded by loved ones, following a sudden acute illness such as an infectious disease or an accident. As the century progressed, standard public health interventions such as water and sewage treatment and mass inoculation helped prevent and manage disease outbreaks. Injuries sustained during World Wars I and II brought about advances in preventing and treating infections and improved surgical techniques. Today, the United States has an average life expectancy of 78 years. Millions of Americans have benefited from innovations, including organ transplantation; advances in cardiac care involving pacemakers, vessel stents, coronary bypass surgery, and implanted defibrillators; gene therapy; cancer treatment; perinatal and neonatal care; laparoscopic surgery; imaging techniques; antibiotics; and immunotherapy.

Even though people are living longer with chronic illnesses that are better managed by scientific advances, they are also living longer with disability. There is ample evidence that patients with advanced disease have inadequate knowledge about illness progression, receive inappropriate or inadequate care, have poorly managed symptoms, and experience spiritual distress and financial worries. Disease progression and the aging process can result in treatment efforts that have marginal benefits, do not improve function, and can cause suffering. This results in death from a chronic illness that follows exacerbations over many years. Seventy percent of these deaths occur in hospitals and institutional settings. The economic consequences of this care are significant. The number of Americans aged 65 and older is expected to double to more than 71 million by 2030, and more than 25% of Medicare expenditures account for care provided at the end of life.

PALLIATIVE CARE

Palliative care (PC) is a specialized form of care that focuses on relief of pain and other symptoms and stress associated with a severe illness. It includes, but is not limited to, **hospice care**, which focuses on the care of a patient with a terminal illness who has less than 6 months to live. Palliative care was developed in response to the poorly met needs of an increasingly aging population. Many patients benefit from PC, which focuses on the relief of suffering and maximizing the quality of life for patients with a serious, life-threatening illness and their families. Provided by an interprofessional team, PC is given concurrently with curative treatment that meets the patient's goals (Fig. 5.1). This care serves patients in all situations, including those who depend on technology such as dialysis or artificial ventilation, as well as those with chronic progressive conditions; acute, serious, and life-threatening illness; and terminal illness. Having basic proficiency in PC skills is the responsibility of all professional healthcare providers. Specialty training and certification are available for nurses and providers.

Palliative care has been shown to improve symptom management and patient and family satisfaction. In a randomized study of patients with non–small cell lung cancer, those who received PC experienced a better quality of life. They were less depressed and received fewer aggressive interventions at the end of life. They also survived longer than those who received standard care. Palliative care is provided in hospital, outpatient, and community settings. It is also provided for patients under hospice care with a projected prognosis of 6 months or less. Palliative care provides continuity of care across healthcare settings, including the outpatient clinic, hospital, rehabilitation or nursing facility, home, and hospice.

Connection Check 5.1

Hospice care is *not* appropriate in which of these circumstances?

A. The patient decides to forego curative treatment.
B. The patient's prognosis is 3 to 6 months.
C. The patient is undergoing experimental chemotherapy.
D. The patient is receiving palliative chemotherapy.

Domains of Palliative Care

In 2004, the National Consensus Project published clinical practice guidelines to promote quality PC across all care settings. These guidelines, or domains of care, provide a useful structure for discussing nursing implications for PC.

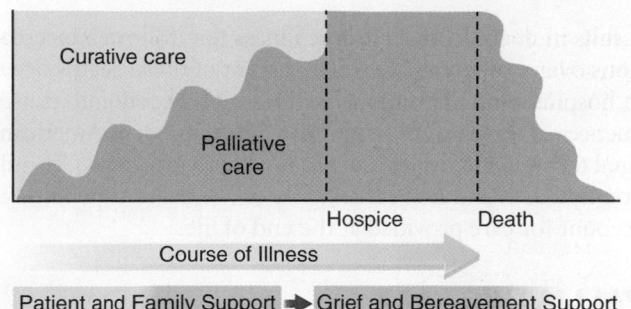

FIGURE 5.1 Integrated palliative care model.

Domain 1: Structure and Process of Care

The structure and process of care domain addresses the plan of care provided by nurses and providers with advanced PC training. The plan should incorporate the patient's goals, preferences, and values while recognizing that they may change over time. The plan of care should travel with the patient across healthcare settings. Patients and families should be educated about hospice care when death may occur within the year (Table 5.1). The topic should be reintroduced as the patient declines. The healthcare team should assess and improve, as necessary, patient and family knowledge about the disease course, prognosis, and benefits and risks/burdens of diagnostic evaluation and treatments.

Domain 2: Physical Aspects of Care

Physical aspects of care address the need to assess, treat, and document symptoms such as pain, dyspnea, constipation, and nausea using standardized scales to evaluate the effectiveness of the interventions. Patient outcomes should be documented. There should be follow-up with provider colleagues for continuing orders to provide effective symptom management.

Domain 3: Psychological and Psychiatric Aspects of Care

Psychological and psychiatric aspects of care state that the PC plan should assess and document the presence of anxiety, depression, and delirium using available standardized scales such as the Memorial Symptom Assessment Scale and the Edmonton Symptom Assessment Scale. The patient's symptoms should be managed in a safe and timely manner

Table 5.1 Hospice Care

Frequently Asked Question	Answer
Who can receive hospice?	Anyone, regardless of diagnosis, with a prognosis of 6 months or less who has decided not to pursue curative treatment (exceptions may be made for time-limited palliative treatment such as radiation or artificial nutrition; also, Affordable Care Act [ACA] pediatric patients are not required to forgo curative treatment)
What are the levels of care under hospice?	1. Routine home care 2. Continuous home care 3. Inpatient respite care 4. General inpatient care
How is hospice provided?	● In the home by a team of nurses, health aides, social workers, and others ● In an inpatient hospice unit with 24-hour nursing and other caregivers ● In a nursing home with intermittent visits provided by the home hospice team
Who can contact hospice?	The patient, the family, the attending provider, or any member of the team can contact hospice; the hospice will contact the patient's primary care provider to sign orders for hospice.
When should hospice be contacted?	When the patient does not want to pursue curative therapy; when life expectancy is 6 months or less
How long can a patient receive hospice care?	As long as the provider certifies the patient is terminally ill with a life expectancy of 6 months or less if the disease runs its expected course
What services are provided?	Intermittent nursing; home health aide; social work; pastoral care; physical therapy; nutrition services; provider visits; volunteers; bereavement services; medical equipment; medications to manage symptoms; short-term acute inpatient care, including respite care, counseling, and pain and symptom management
How is it paid for?	Medicare A, Medical Assistance, and most major health insurance plans provide hospice coverage.
What is not covered?	Treatment for the terminal illness that is not for symptom relief; care given by another provider that was not arranged for by the hospice; care from another provider that duplicates the care hospice is required to provide

that is acceptable to the patient and his or her family. The patient and family should be assisted with their emotional or psychological reactions to functional impairment and loss. They should be connected with coping resources such as grief and bereavement services.

Domain 4: Social Aspects of Care, Including Advanced Care Planning

Social aspects of care address the need to facilitate regularly scheduled patient and family conferences with the interprofessional team to discuss the goals of care, prognosis, and advance care planning and to offer support. It includes assessment of patient and family social networks; cultural, legal, and financial concerns; caregiver availability; and coping skills, as well as access to medications and equipment. These aspects should be incorporated into the plan of care.

Nurses are important in **advanced care planning (ACP)**, a process in which patients, with support from care providers, family, and important others, make decisions about future healthcare. The concept of ACP is based on the premise that persons with life-threatening chronic diseases or polymorbidity and their families need to be assisted by healthcare professionals to identify and determine preferences and wishes about end of life and respective decision making. As part of ACP, a person may elaborate an advance directive to indicate his or her preferences about the end of life. ACP can be employed for any illness but is specifically recommended in the context of chronic diseases or polymorbidity with a potentially fatal outcome; the recommendation is to initiate this early in the disease process, well before any issues of incompetency or incapacity may arise. ACP includes three main aspects: ensuring full comprehension about the disease and its treatment; clarifying expectations about proposed treatments; and determining therapeutic goals, preferences, and wishes.

Domain 5: Spiritual, Religious, and Existential Aspects of Care

Spiritual, religious, and existential aspects of care incorporate the patient's religious, spiritual, and existential concerns and practices into the plan of care. Spiritual care is based on the patient's preferences.

Domain 6: Cultural Aspects of Care

Caring for patients, families, and communities within increasingly diverse practice settings necessitates cultural sensitivity and cultural competency. This is especially true when issues arise that elicit cultural, philosophical, and personal views surrounding death and dying and how to appropriately intervene or manage care. Being confronted with the end of life is challenging in most cultures around the world, and healthcare providers need to be well prepared to manage cultural aspects of care.

Cultural humility may be an especially effective framework for navigating highly sensitive and emotionally charged discussions and interactions surrounding palliative care or end-of-life decisions. Awareness of power imbalances and an inclusive and open approach to incorporating a variety of perspectives and practices are important components of provider training, communication, and practice,

promoting mutual empowerment, respect, partnership, and optimal care outcomes.

Consideration of the cultural aspects of PC should address the patient and family's cultural beliefs about care, such as:

- How healthcare decisions are made
- Preferences for how and to whom information is disclosed
- Dietary preferences
- Family communication
- Perspectives on death, suffering, and grieving
- Funeral/burial preferences

Domain 7: Care of the Imminently Dying

Care of the imminently dying addresses the need to recognize, document, and inform family and other team members of the transition to the active dying phase. It addresses the need to educate the family about the signs and symptoms of dying (Table 5.2) and to appropriately treat

Table 5.2 Physical and Psychological Changes Prior to Death	
Stage	**Description**
1. Early stage: acceptance that death is approaching	The patient may begin to withdraw. There may be a loss of interest in social contacts. As the body slows, there may be a loss of appetite because the body has decreased needs; however, the patient does not experience hunger or thirst. The patient decreases participation in activities and begins to sleep more.
2. Middle stage: weeks before death	There is a decline in mental status; the patient will become confused and disoriented, sleeping most of the time. Physical changes include decreases in body temperature and blood pressure. The pulse rate may become irregular. Respirations become labored and rapid. Skin color begins to change as circulation is diminished. Speaking slows or ceases altogether.
3. Late stage: days or hours before death	The patient may experience a very brief and limited surge of energy in a last effort at physical exertion and expression. Afterward, previously noted symptoms worsen. Coma ensues, extremities become cool and mottled, and the respiratory pattern becomes more rapid and labored (Cheyne–Stokes respiration). There is a loss of ability to manage secretions because of loss of the swallow reflex. Congestion in the airways causes respirations to sound loud and wet. Death follows.
	Hearing is thought to be one of the last senses to lapse before death, so care should be taken to act as if the dying person is aware and able to hear even if he or she is unresponsive.

the patient. The family should be supported throughout this process.

Symptom Management

Symptom management in the dying patient includes being aware of and treating the typical signs of distress that occur during the dying process. Several of the most common symptoms include pain/general discomfort, respiratory distress, and delirium. If the patient is unable to express his or her pain, an observational pain scale will note the presence of facial grimacing, moaning/groaning, and restlessness. Opiates, such as morphine, and adjuvant medications are often the treatment of choice. However, nonpharmacologic ways to address pain or to manage symptoms should also be explored. These can include acupressure, essential oils, sea bands, the use of fans for dyspnea, and other emerging complementary and alternative therapies (see, for example, http://www.caresearch.com.au).

Respiratory signs/symptoms can include dyspnea, tachypnea, upper airway "gurgle," and the use of accessory muscles for breathing. Anticholinergic medications help dry the secretions, lessening the gurgle. Other treatment modalities for respiratory distress during the active dying phase include elevating the head of the bed and the use of opiates. Concomitant use of sedatives with opiates acts synergistically to relax the patient, calm the breathing, and alleviate pain. Nurses, at times, express the fear that administering opiates to a dying patient may hasten death. The ethical principle of double effect states that a nurse's conduct is moral and ethical if the primary intent is to ease pain and respiratory distress (Box 5.1).

Delirium can be managed by calm verbal reassurance. Surrounding the patient with familiar sights, sounds, and smells is also beneficial. Haloperidol or benzodiazepines (lorazepam, midazolam) can be used to manage hyperactive delirium in dying patients. Causes of delirium such as medications, constipation, or a full bladder should be ruled out before other measures are tried.

Connection Check 5.2

Mrs. Jones is receiving hospice care in the nursing home. During the assessment, the nurse observes the patient is unconscious and has wet, noisy respirations and cool, mottled extremities. The nurse understands which of the following actions are indicated? *(Select all that apply.)*

A. Notifying the patient's family
B. Requesting an order for an anticholinergic medication
C. Notifying the patient's provider
D. Performing a sternal rub to assess the patient's response
E. Performing a full systems assessment

Family Support

Family support (Box 5.2) includes offering the family an opportunity to participate in the patient's care. This may include providing mouth care and applying lip balm, bathing, massaging aching joints, or reading to the patient. Maintaining

Box 5.1 Principle of Double Effect

The principle of double effect, often invoked concerning the effect of opiates at the end of life, implies that an intended good effect such as pain management is ethically permissible even if it produces an unintended secondary effect, hastening death. There is no evidence to support this cause-and-effect relationship in pain management at the end of life. There is a wide margin of safety with the use of opiates and sedating medications to manage symptoms.

Box 5.2 Care of the Family

- Assess family understanding of the patient's diagnosis and dying.
- Inform family members that the patient is dying. Open a space for them to express grief.
- Invite family members to care for the patient as they feel comfortable: bathing, massaging bony prominences, applying lip balm, or reading to the patient.
- Bring in the patient's favorite music; use headphones.
- Bring in favorite quilts or family pictures.
- If young children cannot visit, have them write a note that can be shared with the patient. Alternatively, have them call on the phone.
- Have family members record stories from the past and share them with the patient. This can become a family legacy.
- If family members are unable to visit, have them call the patient's room. Other family members or nursing staff can hold the phone to the patient's ear. This can be done even if the patient is comatose.

communication with the family is of paramount importance. Nurses are not always sure of what to say to the family of a dying patient. Expressing concern and understanding of their distress is one simple way to begin to establish a bond. The use of reflective listening is a technique to help family members process their experience (Box 5.3). When possible, incorporate patient and family preferences for the site of dying: home or inpatient hospice. Assure everyone that effective pain and symptom management is being provided.

Encourage the family to communicate with the patient prior to death. Allow each family member, as desired, private time with the patient to express his or her final thoughts. Sometimes family members are unsure about what to say. Providing simple suggestions helps facilitate the process. Some feel that actually saying a final good-bye allows the patient to go on his or her final journey. See Box 5.4 for suggested communications with the dying patient.

Offering the family private time in the room to view the patient's body after death can help facilitate the grieving process. Some families may decline the viewing, preferring to remember the person as he or she was when still alive. Foot traffic near the patient's room should be monitored for noise so that a respectful presence is maintained. Incorporate a bereavement care plan that includes follow-up after the death.

Box 5.3 Communication With the Family

Use reflective listening to help the family process the dying experience:

- How are you doing?
- What are you worried or anxious about?
- What questions do you have?
- I can see this is difficult for you.
- How did you hear the news?
- How are other family members coping?
- What are some of your favorite memories of the patient?
- What will you miss most about the patient?
- Do you think the patient is comfortable?
- Do you need anything at this time?

Box 5.4 Communication With the Dying Patient

Talking with a loved one as death approaches is difficult. The following phrases may help guide the conversation and make it meaningful for both the patient and the family member or friend. These phrases may also be used by the dying patient to help express important thoughts and feelings before dying.

"Thank you for. . ."
"I forgive you for . . ."
"Please forgive me for . . ."
"I love you."
"Good-bye."

Connection Check 5.3

Mr. Smith's wife is in the terminal stage of chronic obstructive pulmonary disease (COPD). He is very anxious that his wife be comfortable during her last hours. The nurse finds him tearful in the hall outside the room. Which communication should the nurse use first?

A. "My aunt had COPD, and she died on a ventilator. Count your blessings that your wife is not on a machine."
B. "I can see you're upset, Mr. Smith. Would you like to talk about it?"
C. "Is your family here?"
D. "Do you think your wife would like a visit from pastoral care?"

Postmortem Care

Postmortem care involves preparing the body for eventual disposition to the funeral home. The body should be treated with respect, incorporating the family's religious and cultural practices. Practices vary by state and/or local jurisdiction, but if there is to be an autopsy, tubes and catheters

usually must remain in place. If no autopsy is planned, remove tubes and cleanse soiled areas of the body. Taking the time to involve other nurses in this care provides an opportunity for the staff to engage in a ritual of farewell. After completing the care, each nurse/staff member can pause for a moment to say good-bye to the patient before the body is transported to the morgue or funeral home.

Domain 8: Ethical and Legal Aspects of Care

Important to this domain is addressing the patient's decisional capacity (Box 5.5) and determining who the patient's surrogate decision maker is if the patient is unable to make decisions for himself or herself. This domain also addresses the nurse's role as patient advocate, assuring the patient or surrogate that preferences are known and will be honored and that ethical care will be provided. This includes the patient's right to full disclosure of information and refusal of treatment. The ethical principle of beneficence is demonstrated by providing care that benefits the patient, such as good symptom management. Addressing the patient's spiritual distress and respecting wishes for the use of life-sustaining treatment are examples of nonmaleficence, or not doing harm to the patient. Providing equitable access to hospice and PC for all patients is an example of the principle of justice.

After the goals of care are determined, the team translates them into medical orders. Usually, the attending provider recommends appropriate interventions that promote comfort. Decisions need to be made regarding the use of life-sustaining treatments, including cardiopulmonary resuscitation, artificial ventilation, dialysis, artificial hydration and nutrition, antibiotics, and vasopressors. Ongoing discussions of these interventions should consider the benefits and burdens or risks they pose in meeting the patient care goals (Box 5.6).

Connection Check 5.4

The nurse asks the patient and family members if they have any questions about the patient's diagnosis and plan of care. This is an example of which PC domain?
A. Physical aspects of care
B Psychological and emotional aspects of care
C. Ethical and legal aspects of care
D. Structure and process of care

Box 5.5 Decisional Capacity

The patient is deemed to have decisional capacity if these criteria are met:

- Ability to understand the nature and consequences of the proposed treatment
- Ability to rationally evaluate the burdens, benefits, and risks of treatment
- Ability to communicate a decision

Box 5.6 A Well-Managed Death

- Appropriate pain and symptom management
- Avoiding a prolonged dying process
- Clear communication about decisions by patient, family, and provider
- Adequate preparation for death for both the patient and loved ones
- Feeling a sense of control
- Finding a spiritual or emotional sense of completion
- Affirming the patient as a unique and worthy person
- Strengthening relationships with loved ones
- Not being alone

CASE STUDY: EPISODE 2

While in rehabilitation, Mrs. Kelso develops a urinary tract infection and sacral decubitus ulcers. Unable to participate in intensive physical therapy, she is discharged home bedbound after 10 days, with 24-hour caregivers. After 1 week at home, her home-care nurse notes that she is hypotensive and tachycardic. She is taken to the emergency department, where she is intubated and subsequently admitted to the intensive care unit with a diagnosis of sepsis. Cultures reveal an infected central line, pneumonia, and osteomyelitis related to the decubitus ulcers. Her respiratory status eventually stabilizes, and she is extubated. She is often delirious, calling out and speaking in a confused manner. Although she is unable to tell the staff she is in pain, her discomfort is clear as she moans when turned and screams when her sacral dressings are changed...

ETHICAL IMPLICATIONS AND MORAL DISTRESS

Nurses deliver highly technological and complex care, with an expectation that all of their actions will work toward enhancing the patient's well-being in all domains: physiological, psychological, relational, social, and spiritual. Nurses correctly feel they have an ethical obligation to advocate for the patient.

Unfortunately, sometimes the valuation of "doing well" and "the patient's best interest" can differ among the patient, his or her family members, and members of the healthcare team. Disagreements often occur over the choice of treatments, patient prognosis, and acknowledgment that the patient is dying. At times, the nurse may believe the patient's best interest is being violated. However, nurses often have difficulty acting according to their values and goals for the patient and difficulty voicing their concerns in practice. This may be due to working in a traditional power structure that lacks collaborative relationships with providers. Sometimes, nurses feel ignored or not respected as professionals. Thus, they often feel caught between the patient and the provider's decisions for patient care. In this context, nurses are regularly confronted with decisions they do not agree with but are expected to implement. This can lead to a sense of disintegration of the nurse's personal integrity.

Nurses who regularly face these situations can suffer **moral distress**, which involves the inability to do the morally correct thing because of situational factors. Factors that contribute to creating moral distress include high stress in the work environment; time and resource pressures; high-technology care situations; and differences in values, attitudes, and cultural or religious beliefs among patients, families, and staff.

Unaddressed moral distress has serious consequences. Nurses begin to feel disengaged from patients, resulting in poor patient care. Feelings of anger, frustration, powerlessness, dissatisfaction, and emotional and physical exhaustion can lead to burnout. There is no longer a sense of joy in working with patients and families. Moral distress also results in decreased job satisfaction, increased staff turnover, and ultimately, nurses choosing to leave the profession.

Nurses cope with moral distress by talking with other nurses about the situation and sharing their feelings and values with their peers. They also share with and receive support from nurse managers and chaplains. They share decisions with colleagues, sometimes acceding to the majority opinion. Such discussions enable the nurse to consider alternatives in the situation. Providing education in ethical decision making and instituting ethics rounds can help manage moral distress. Nurses who have developed expertise, experience, problem-solving skills, and an ability to take risks tend to take action in an ethical manner when confronted with moral dilemmas. These nurses may act as role models and are a valuable resource for new nurses.

Healthcare organizations must also be responsive by developing and implementing processes that help nurses recognize and name moral distress. Nurse leaders and administrators need to recognize factors that contribute to moral distress. Monitoring of mechanisms that produce moral distress allows the organization to address moral distress in a systematic fashion. Initiatives to promote open dialogue about ethical concerns among team members can transform the care environment so that nurses and others feel safe voicing their concerns and are empowered to act in an ethical manner. The organization's ethics committee may be helpful in addressing conflicts regarding the goals of care, healthcare decisions, and advance care planning. The ethics committee may also model behaviors of respectful listening that encourage dialogue.

Connection Check 5.5

The nurse understands that moral distress may result in which of the following? *(Select all that apply.)*
A. Physical exhaustion
B. Disagreements among staff
C. Anger at family
D. Anger at providers
E. Feelings of undeserved power

Nurse Self-Care

Nurses are in the privileged position of caring for patients when they are perhaps most vulnerable: the time preceding their death. While advocating for patients so that their values, goals, and preferences are heard and honored, nurses may also feel a sense of loss and grief over the impending death. When involved in stressful care situations, nurses may not take the time to process the experience with trusted friends or professionals. The end result may be a walling off of emotions in an effort to protect from feelings of distress. Nurses do not have to settle for this result.

As individuals, nurses can build self-care activities into their daily schedules. Talking with trusted friends or nursing colleagues, journaling, engaging in aerobic exercise, gardening, practicing yoga, meditating, and praying can help recharge emotional batteries.

As a team, nurses can employ stress-reducing strategies, such as:

- Performing postmortem care together
- Pausing for a moment of silence during the monthly staff meeting to remember those who have died in care
- Sending the family a bereavement card

Nursing management should plan regularly scheduled unit debriefings facilitated by crisis intervention staff, pastoral care, or social workers. Managers should take advantage of employer-provided counseling services to help staff process stressful care situations.

Again, as individuals, nurses should reflect on their role as the final caregivers who make a difference for patients at a crucial time in their lives. The nurse is sometimes the only person who attends a dying patient. It should be remembered that this is a privilege and an honor. Appropriating the experiences of death and loss deepens a sense of shared humanity and forms a sense of compassion and the ability to be more fully present for future patients and families in care.

Connection Check 5.6

The nurse understands that appropriate actions to take after a distressing discussion with a provider over end-of-life issues for a patient include which of the following?
A. Avoid communicating with the provider except through the electronic medical record
B. Having a drink after work to calm frazzled nerves
C. Arguing with colleagues who disagree
D. Soliciting support from a nurse manager or ethics consultation

Making Connections

CASE STUDY: WRAP-UP

As Mrs. Kelso's condition continues to deteriorate despite aggressive care, the need to discuss healthcare goals, expectations, and hopes for recovery becomes clear. The healthcare team believes that the patient is dying. As family members discuss their hopes and fears for the patient with the nurse, they become tearful. Using active listening, the nurse encourages the family to talk about the patient's past life, her relationships with her family, her love for gardening, and her involvement in church activities. The nurse asks the family if the patient ever expressed her wishes about end-of-life care. They state simply, "Our mother did not want to suffer." The healthcare team discusses Mrs. Kelso's potential and actual suffering—physically, emotionally, and spiritually—and, with the family, develops a plan that includes palliative and hospice care.

They develop a plan for the management of pain and respiratory distress. Morphine sulfate is ordered. The patient ceases moaning, her facial muscles relax, and her respiratory rate decreases to 18 per minute with no use of accessory muscles. The nurse documents her findings and incorporates symptom management into the care plan. Mrs. Kelso is transferred to inpatient hospice. She dies 2 days later.

Case Study Questions

1. The nurse caring for Mrs. Kelso understands that her first priority should be to do which of the following?
   A. Call the chaplain
   B. Ask family members for their understanding of the situation
   C. Address the patient's pain
   D. Call the ethics committee

2. Efforts to support family members include which of the following? *(Select all that apply.)*
   A. Assuring them that the end is near and that it is okay to go home
   B. Encouraging final private conversations with the patient
   C. Asking them to bring a few of the patient's favorite things to her room
   D. Telling them to encourage the patient to hold on for them
   E. Encouraging active discussions about favorite family memories

3. The nurse understands that the use of morphine sulfate to treat symptoms may result in which of the following? *(Select all that apply.)*
   A. Improved mobility
   B. Relief of pain
   C. Slowing of respirations
   D. Relief of nausea
   E. Improved appetite

4. As an experienced palliative care nurse, your response to Mrs. Kelso's nurse when expressing concern that giving pain medication and sedatives may hasten patient death is which of the following?
   A. "Don't worry—we do this all of the time."
   B. "We are covered ethically by the principle of double effect."
   C. "Don't worry—we have a doctor's order."
   D. "We are covered ethically by the principle of beneficence."

5. Mrs. Kelso's death can be described as a well-managed death for which reason?
   A. It allowed enough time for the family to accept it was coming.
   B. It occurred in the hospice unit.
   C. There was appropriate pain and symptom management.
   D. The family accepted the care team's decisions.

CHAPTER SUMMARY

The need for PC arose as advances in healthcare brought about not only longevity but also increased chances of surviving with long-term disability. Palliative care addresses the needs of patients with chronic illness and their families in order to alleviate and prevent suffering in all its forms and promote the best possible quality of life.

The domains of PC include the structure and process of care, physical aspects of care, psychological and psychiatric aspects of care, social aspects of care, spiritual and religious aspects of care, cultural aspects of care, care of the imminently dying, and ethical and legal issues. Ensuring that the patient and family have needed information about the diagnosis and prognosis is part of the structure and process of care. Symptom management and family support are also essential in the care of the imminently dying patient.

As care providers who spend the most time at the bedside, nurses play a pivotal role in providing PC by advocating for patient preferences, educating the patient and family about the disease process, and assisting them in processing the experience by engaging them in advanced care planning as well as reflective listening and by probing what is important to them. Often, the nurse provides a supportive presence, bearing silent witness in the midst of an experience that inspires awe: the death of the beloved. Nurses may experience moral distress as they try to advocate for the patient's best interest while being expected to carry out treatments they find morally distressing. Moral distress may result in staff turnover, anger, frustration, and extreme fatigue. Interventions at both the individual and organizational levels can help manage moral distress.

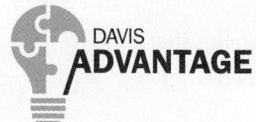
DAVIS ADVANTAGE

To explore learning resources for this chapter, go to **Davis Advantage** and find:
– Answers to in-text questions
– Chapter Resources and Activities
– NCLEX®-Style Chapter Review Questions
– Bibliography

Unit II

Clinical Principles of Medical-Surgical Nursing

Chapter 6

Geriatric Implications for Medical-Surgical Nursing

Denise Cost

LEARNING OUTCOMES

Content in this chapter is designed to assist in:

1. Defining the demographics of the aging population
2. Discussing age-related physiological changes
3. Identifying common healthcare issues of older adults
4. Analyzing care priorities for geriatric patients
5. Developing support strategies for older adults

CONCEPTS

- Assessment
- Cognition
- Fluids and Electrolytes
- Nutrition
- Perfusion
- Safety

ESSENTIAL TERMS

Activities of daily living (ADLs)
Adaptation
Advance directives
Ageism
Aging in place
Alzheimer's dementia
Atrophy
Cachexia
Calcification
Cognitive
Deconditioning
Delirium
Dementia
Depression
Homeostasis
Homeostenosis
Instrumental activities of daily living (IADLs)
Living will
Polypharmacy
Sarcopenia
Sclerosis
Senescence
Stenosis

Finding Connections

CASE STUDY: EPISODE 1

Follow this patient throughout the chapter.

Mrs. Gomez is an 87-year-old Hispanic woman with a history of hypertension and arthritis. She developed new-onset shortness of breath and was hospitalized. In the hospital, she was diagnosed as having heart failure and was discharged to home with six new medications, oxygen therapy, and a sodium-restricted diet. Mrs. Gomez is a widow and lives alone in her apartment. She has extended family members who live in the same apartment building. She speaks some English but mostly Spanish. She has been referred for home-care services and has been assigned a primary nurse…

OVERVIEW OF AGING

Demographics

The process of aging is universal and inevitable and affects all species. Interest in and study of aging is peaking as the number of people who are considered elderly has rapidly increased. Presently, *old age* is defined by three stages. The age range of 65 to 75 is considered "young-old," the range of 75 to 85 is "old," and from 85 upward is termed the "old-old" or "oldest old." As Americans live longer, the growth in the number of older adults is unprecedented. The dramatic growth is due in part to the so-called "baby boomer" population, those people born between the years 1946 and 1963, who have started to turn 65. Over the past 10 years, the population 65 and over increased from 36.6 million in 2005 to 47.8 million in 2015 (a 30% increase) and is projected to more than double to 98 million. In 2016, 23% of persons age 65 and over were members of racial or ethnic minority populations; 9% were African Americans (not Hispanic), 4% were Asian or Pacific Islander (not Hispanic), 0.5% were Native American (not Hispanic), 0.1% were Native Hawaiian/Pacific Islander (not Hispanic), and 0.7% of persons 65+ identified themselves as being of two or more races. Persons of Hispanic origin (who may be of any race) represented 8% of the older population (Box 6.1).

U.S. Census Bureau statistics show that women continue to live longer than men. Based on the 2012 census, there are approximately 22.9 million older women and 17.3 million older men. The overall life expectancy for the U.S. population is 77.2 years. Older men are much more likely to be married. Forty-two percent of older women are widows, and of women 75 and older, 49% live alone. The financial status of older persons reveals a median income of $25,877 for men and $15,282 for women. Their major sources of income are reported to be Social Security (reported by 87%), assets

Box 6.1 Health Disparities in the Geriatric Population

- *Healthy People 2020* defines a *health disparity* as "a particular type of health difference that is closely linked with social, economic, and/or environmental disadvantage." Minority populations are increasing overall in the United States. They are among the leading victims of hypertension and diabetes. Disparities occur when differences in outcomes are related to bias and a system of care that is not culturally sensitive.
- The Census Bureau predicts that racial and ethnic minority populations will grow to half of the U.S. population in 3 decades. The National Institutes of Health has a research agenda in place to address the increasing health needs of populations suffering from inequities. Some health disparities are demonstrated in the following facts:
  - A comparison of rates by race reveals that black women and men have much higher rates of death from coronary heart disease in the 45-to-74 age-group.
  - The same black–white difference was seen among women and men who died of stroke.
  - Older adults, non-Hispanic blacks, U.S.-born adults, and adults with lower family income, less education, public health insurance, diabetes, obesity, or a disability all have a higher prevalence of hypertension than their counterparts.
  - The disparity by race/ethnicity, socioeconomic status, disability status, and education level is still substantial. Non-Hispanic blacks have the highest percentage of householders living in inadequate, unhealthy housing, followed by Hispanics and American Indians/Alaska Natives.
  - As of 2015, whereas 20% of measures showed disparities getting smaller for blacks and Hispanics, most disparities have not changed significantly for any racial and ethnic groups.

From Agency for Healthcare Research and Quality. (2017). *2016 national healthcare quality and disparities report*. Retrieved from http://www.ahrq.gov/research/findings/nhqrdr/nhqdr16/summary.html

income (54%), private pensions (28%), government employee pensions (14%), and earnings (25%). Almost 8.9% of older adults live below the poverty line.

Connection Check 6.1

The nurse is preparing a discharge plan for a 78-year-old woman. Which likely scenario should the nurse anticipate?
A. The patient will drive herself home.
B. The patient lives in a homeless shelter.
C. The patient is a widow and lives alone.
D. The patient receives a government pension.

AGE-RELATED CHANGES AND COMMON HEALTH ISSUES

Death in advanced years is not caused by "old age" but by disease processes or infections. Older adults are at greater risk for illness because of the normal decline in **adaptation** that occurs in the body. Most of the changes of aging become apparent when the body is placed under stress. **Homeostasis** is the body's ability to adapt to or return to a normal state of balance after being subjected to a threat or stress. Such stressors include injury, exposure to pathogenic organisms, changes in fluid and nutritional intake, and the effects of medication. The failure of homeostasis is termed **homeostenosis**. This is defined as the characteristic progressive decrease in homeostatic reserve that occurs in every organ system with aging. The physiological reserves are present, but they are being used to maintain homeostasis. Therefore, when a challenge occurs, there is less reserve to call upon for compensation.

Senescence refers to normal age-related changes in the organ systems. Individual humans age differently, but there are changes that affect all people in a similar manner. In general, there are several processes that affect all body systems. **Sclerosis** is the hardening of tissue due to fibrous tissue overgrowth. **Stenosis** is the narrowing or constricting of a passage or orifice. **Atrophy** is defined as a wasting away or decrease in the size of an organ. **Calcification** occurs normally as part of bone formation. However, calcium and calcium salts can be deposited abnormally in other organs, including blood vessels. On a functional level, there is a general tendency for slowing, shrinking, and stiffening. Gait slows down, height is diminished, and range of motion decreases. Organ systems develop these changes at differing rates between individuals and within an individual. Mobility and strength in an 85-year-old man may be good while he suffers from cataracts and markedly diminished hearing. His 85-year-old neighbor may need to use a walker but has excellent vision and hearing.

These processes do not necessarily bring on disease, but they create limitations in normal activities. Healthy aging entails compensation for these limitations by way of healthy lifestyle choices and interventions in factors that can be controlled.

The following sections and accompanying tables describe the body systems and the physiological alterations that occur.

Common Cardiovascular Health Issues

Age-related cardiovascular changes are listed in Table 6.1. They include a decreased number of pacemaker cells, stenosis of the heart valves, and stiffening and narrowing of arterial walls.

Heart and Vascular Diseases

Heart and vascular diseases, such as *hypertension (HTN)*, *coronary artery disease (CAD)*, and *myocardial infarction (MI)*, occur as a result of sclerotic changes in blood vessels and heart wall muscle tissues, particularly coronary arteries. Systolic blood pressure rises because of the stiffening of systemic arteries. When blood flow is decreased to the heart muscle, death of the tissue (infarction) occurs.

Heart Failure

Heart failure (HF) is most often caused by MI or HTN. Damaged heart muscle results in weakened contractility. The pumping function of the heart becomes impaired, and fluid accumulation develops in the lungs and tissues. Pulmonary edema (fluid in the lungs) causes shortness of breath and the inability to breathe while lying flat and can be life threatening. Edema in dependent areas of the body, most often the feet and legs, can develop as well and is an early sign of heart failure. One in every 100 people over age 65 has heart failure, and 80% of those hospitalized with heart failure are over 65.

Atrial Fibrillation

Changes in the pacemaker cells in the atrium contribute to the development of atrial fibrillation (AF). The pacemaker cells fire sporadically, resulting in a rapid twitching of the atria. This produces inefficient filling of the ventricles and a backup of blood in the atria. The main danger of AF is the formation of blood clots in the right atrium, which puts the patient at risk for systemic embolization. Stroke is the

Table 6.1 Age-Related Cardiovascular Changes

Change	Consequence
• Reduced number of pacemaker cells in the sinoatrial (SA) node	• Decrease in maximum heart rate with age
• Decreased cardiac responsiveness to beta-adrenergic stimuli	• Increased tendency for arrhythmias, atrial fibrillation
	• Reduced heart-rate control that impairs ability to adapt to stressors
• Left atrial enlargement	• Fourth heart sound heard normally in older adults
	• Increased risks of hypertension and heart failure
• Stenosis (narrowing or constriction) of heart valves	• Rise in systolic blood pressure
• Increased fibrosis and calcification of heart chambers and valves	
• Stiffening of artery walls	
• Narrowed arteries and weakened venous valves	• Slowed venous return, resulting in edema
• Formation of atherosclerotic plaques that can block blood flow	• Increased risk of venous thrombosis and stroke
• Decline in baroreflex response to arterial pressure	• Diminished blood pressure responses
	• Orthostatic hypotension

most common complication of atrial fibrillation and the resultant embolization.

Heart Disease

Heart disease continues to be the number one cause of death in those over 65. Stroke is the fifth-leading cause of death. Risk factors that can be modified to prevent heart disease and stroke include HTN, high cholesterol levels, diabetes, smoking, obesity, poor diet, and physical inactivity. Consistent with *Healthy People 2020, Healthy People 2030* stresses addressing and improving these factors could substantially reduce the number of deaths from cardiovascular disease.

CASE STUDY: EPISODE 2

The goal is to have Ms. Gomez safely age in place: to remain living where she has lived for years, a familiar place in which she is comfortable (Box 6.2). The primary nurse from the home healthcare service will assess her needs and determine which services are necessary for Ms. Gomez to remain safely at home. Before the first home visit, the primary nurse needs to arrange for a Spanish interpreter and a family member to be present so that they can support and assist the patient during the assessment. An informed consent form for home-care services must also be obtained before the nurse can conduct an assessment. A complete physical and psychosocial assessment, a home safety assessment, and an assessment of the patient's medications are needed in order to develop nursing diagnoses and a plan of care to address Ms. Gomez's needs. In addition, the nurse will need to prioritize educating Ms. Gomez on home oxygen use and safety and assess her risk of falling as part of the home safety assessment. On the basis of the assessment findings, the nurse will determine what other support services are needed. The nurse will communicate with the primary health provider to obtain medical orders for all anticipated services and to confirm medications. A plan of care based on the problems identified and nursing interventions to address them will then be implemented...

⚠ Safety Alert   The Joint Commission identified five safety goals for home care for 2018:

1. **Correctly identifying the patient.** Use at least two ways of identifying the patient, such as the patient's name and date of birth, for example. Even in the home environment, it is possible to visit or examine the wrong person, especially if there are many other family members present. Verification of the patient's first and last name and having another family member present to confirm the identity will prevent misidentification.

2. **Using medications safely.** Record and communicate correct information about a patient's medications. Compare new medications with the medications being taken previously. In the home, the nurse must use communication, teaching, and organizational skills to educate the patient about his or her medications. This includes indications, side effects, and dosing intervals. The nurse helps the patient develop a system for organizing the medications, usually accomplished with a "mediplanner" pill container (Fig. 6.1). This is a major priority for home care in order to avoid dangerous medication interactions and side effects.

3. **Preventing infection.** The home-care nurse must follow accepted practices of hand washing and maintenance of the equipment carried into each visit in order to prevent the spread of pathogens into the home and outside to the community. Use the hand-cleaning guidelines from the Centers for Disease Control and Prevention (CDC) or the World Health Organization (WHO) when washing hands. Use accepted maintenance practices for equipment brought into the home in order to prevent the spread of pathogens in the home and outside to the community.

4. **Preventing falls.** Older adults are at increased risk for falls. A careful review of medications that may have side effects of dizziness, weakness, or sleepiness is a priority, as is education of the individual about fall prevention.

5. **Identifying safety risks.** These risks include environmental hazards such as loose carpeting, damaged electrical connections, or clutter and trash that pose a fire hazard. If there is oxygen in the home, safety measures to prevent the risk of fire must be taught, and the residence must be identified at the entrance as having oxygen on the premises.

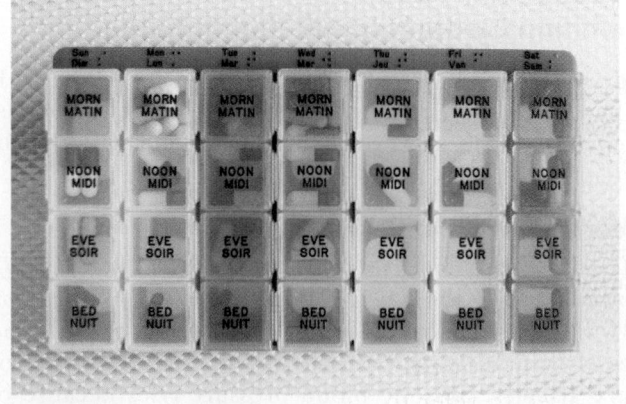

FIGURE 6.1 Typical mediplanner container.

Box 6.2 Aging at Home

The Centers for Disease Control and Prevention defines **aging in place** as independently and comfortably remaining in one's own home regardless of income, age, or disabilities. An assessment is completed to determine the resources necessary to safely remain at home. Occupational therapy, physical therapy, and home healthcare are resources to support aging in place. Overall, this process has been aided by legislation that supports older adults staying at home, assistive technologies such as telehealth for remote health and wellness monitoring, and technologies that support safety and home security. Also built into this model are communities and activities designed to decrease isolation and increase involvement with others. Group social activities and potluck dinners are examples. Volunteers or family members who can help with shopping and home maintenance are key ingredients for successful aging in place.

Table 6.2 Age-Related Respiratory Changes

Change	Consequence
• Ossification of laryngeal cartilage (becomes bony) • Less mobile vocal fold movement • Atrophy of vocalis muscle	• Voice becomes weak, breathy, rough, and hoarse.
• Costochondral cartilage calcification • Decreased chest wall compliance • Atrophy of intercostal muscles	• By age 65, inspiration becomes dependent on the abdominal muscles.
• Progressive loss of lung elastic recoil, decreasing lung compliance, and decreasing surface area for gas exchange	• Decline in PaO_2
• Diminished laryngeal and cough reflexes	• Increased risk of aspiration and aspiration pneumonia
• Reduced diaphragm strength • Decreased pulmonary reserves	• Increased risk of respiratory failure

Common Respiratory Health Issues

Age-related respiratory changes are listed in Table 6.2. They include stiffening and calcification of the cartilage that separates the bones within the rib cage (costochondral cartilage), atrophy of the intercostal muscles, and loss of lung elastic recoil. As a result of the homeostenotic changes previously discussed, there is an increased risk of respiratory failure from all causes. Combined, lower respiratory diseases are the fourth-leading cause of death in people aged 65 and over. Nonpulmonary conditions such as malnutrition, stroke, heart failure, Parkinson's disease, and **delirium** impact pulmonary issues. For example, gastrostomy tube feeding has a significant risk for aspiration. Tube feedings are commonly administered in older adult patients with dementia who can no longer eat or swallow safely.

Pneumonia

Pneumonias include bacterial, viral, and aspiration as well as diffuse aspiration bronchiolitis. A decrease in the lung's elastic recoil and diminished compliance cause decreased alveolar expansion. Weakened cough reflex and diaphragm strength allow secretions to pool in the lungs, contributing to infections. In addition, older adults tend to have impaired swallowing, which puts them at risk for aspiration and pneumonia. The use of thickening agents in liquids helps decrease the risk of aspiration by making liquids thicker and easier to swallow.

Chronic Obstructive Pulmonary Disease/Asthma

Chronic obstructive pulmonary disease (COPD) is a term used to refer to two conditions, emphysema and chronic bronchitis (Fig. 6.2). Smoking is the primary

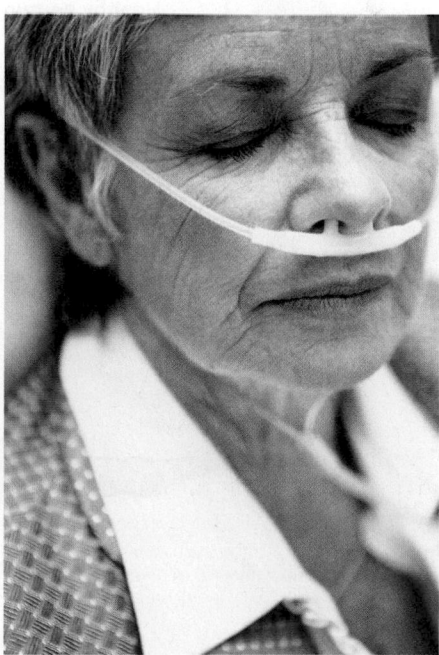

FIGURE 6.2 Older adult patients with chronic obstructive pulmonary disease often need continuous oxygen.

risk factor for COPD. Those aged 65 and over have the highest rate of chronic bronchitis. Asthma affects 5% to 7% of the over-65 population, and this age-group accounts for 60% of all asthma-related fatalities. Indoor allergens are more likely to be triggers for asthma because older adults spend more time in the home than outside.

Common Neurological Health Issues

Age-related neurological changes are noted in Table 6.3. They include atrophy of the brain, decreased numbers of neuronal cells, and reduced cerebral white matter and blood flow.

Dementia

Dementia is defined as a progressive **cognitive** decline that affects a person's social and occupational functioning (Fig. 6.4). Loss of the ability to think, reason, and remember interferes with communicating and relating to others. In addition, dementia prevents accomplishing **instrumental activities of daily living (IADLs),** such as paying bills, making appointments, shopping, and maintaining a household. It can become severe enough to affect the individual's ability to perform **activities of**

Table 6.3 Age-Related Neurological Changes	
Change	**Consequence**
• Atrophy of the brain, occurring mainly in the cerebrum	• These anatomic changes may not have direct clinical consequences; new synapses continue to form to compensate for neuronal losses.
• Decreased number of neuronal cells, which varies from one region to another	
• Reduced cerebral white-matter volume	• Decreases in information processing
• Decrease of 20% in cerebral blood flow	• Slower working memory
• Synaptic loss and decreased dendritic connections	• Increased response time
	• Decreased reaction time
• Slowed nerve conduction time in peripheral nervous system shows	• Decreased motor time is task specific; familiar tasks are not affected.
• Formation of neurofibrillary tangles (aggregates of "tau" protein; see Figure 6.3) and senile plaque (can be present without dementia)	• Development of Alzheimer's dementia

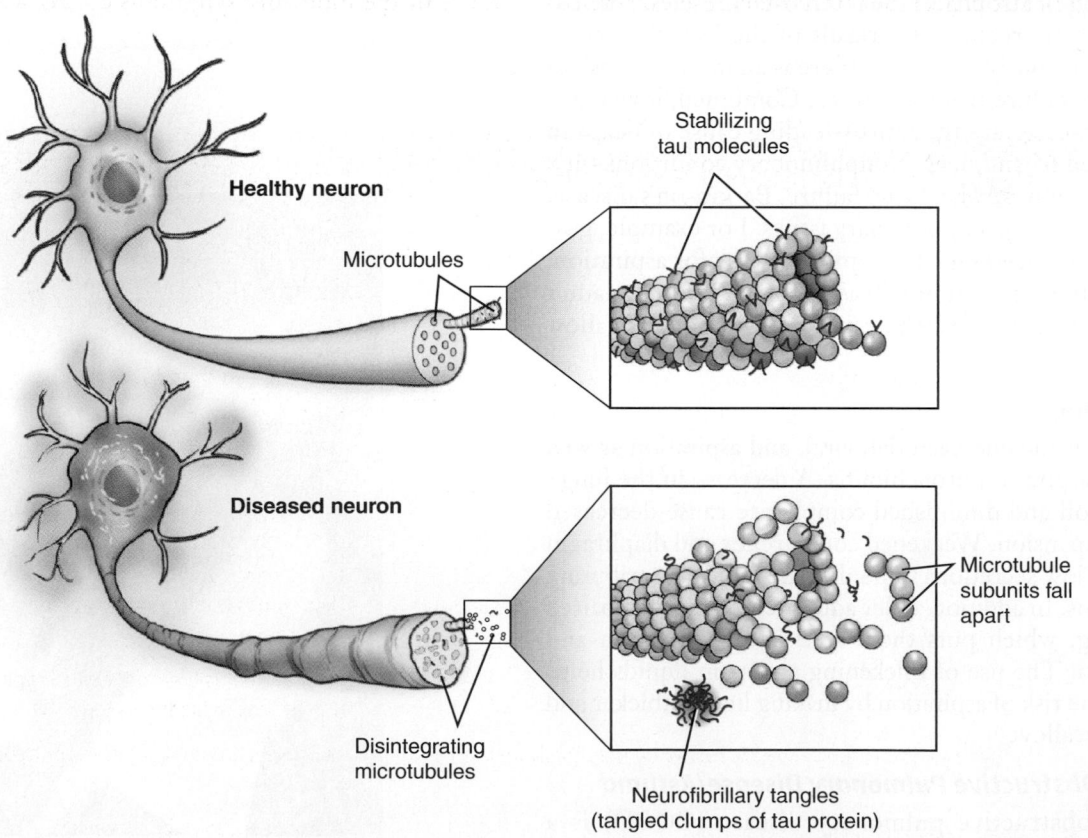

FIGURE 6.3 Neurofibrillary tangles.

Healthy neuron

Microtubules

Stabilizing tau molecules

Diseased neuron

Microtubule subunits fall apart

Disintegrating microtubules

Neurofibrillary tangles (tangled clumps of tau protein)

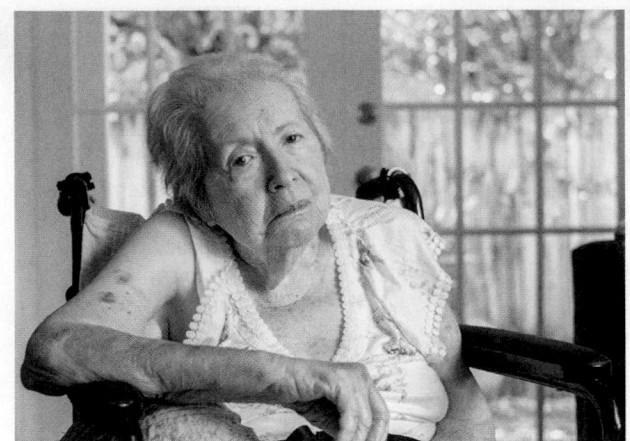

FIGURE 6.4 Older adult woman with dementia.

daily living (ADLs), such as dressing, bathing, eating, and walking.

Dementia stems from a variety of pathological conditions. The most common is **Alzheimer's dementia**, which occurs in 50% to 80% of cases. According to the Alzheimer's Association, 5.7 million Americans are living with Alzheimer's, and by 2020, this number will rise to nearly 14 million. It is the sixth-leading cause of death in the United States. One in three seniors dies with Alzheimer's or another form of dementia. It kills more people than breast cancer and prostate cancer combined.

Some other causes of dementia are Parkinson's disease, Lewy body dementia, multi-infarct dementia, and vascular dementia. Delirium is the short-term, acute loss of some cognitive abilities. Differentiating dementia from delirium is a major clinical challenge when caring for older adults. Table 6.4 notes the differences between dementia and delirium.

Depression

It is a myth that depression is a normal part of aging. However, it is a common problem for older adults, and it needs to be treated so that the individual can have the best quality of life. The normal emotional changes that accompany aging can develop into clinical depression. It has been found that older adults with depression are underdiagnosed and undertreated. The National Institutes of Health has reported that depression in people aged 65 and older is a major public health problem. The suicide rate of people 80 to 84 years of age is twice that of the general population.

Some symptoms of depression are similar to naturally occurring changes of aging and make diagnosis more challenging. For instance, lower energy levels, difficulty sleeping, less appetite, aches and pains, and difficulty remembering details are some of the symptoms shared by depression and the aging body. The symptoms of a major depressive episode are the same regardless of age—the presence of five or more of the following symptoms during a 2-week period

Table 6.4 Differentiating Dementia and Delirium

Feature	Dementia	Delirium
Course	Chronic, gradual onset	Acute; onset often in the evening
Progression	Slow but even	Abrupt
Duration	Months to years	Hours to less than 1 month
Awareness	Clear	Reduced
Alertness	Generally normal	Fluctuating, lethargic, or hypervigilant
Orientation	May be impaired	Generally impaired; fluctuates in severity
Memory	Recent and remote impairment	Recent and immediate impairment
Thinking	Impaired judgment; word finding and abstraction are difficult.	Disorganized, distorted, fragmented; speech is incoherent.
Perception	Misperceptions can be absent.	Illusions, delusions, and hallucinations are present; patient has difficulty distinguishing reality.
Psychomotor behavior	Normal; may have loss of some previously learned skills	Variable; can be hypokinetic or hyperkinetic
Sleep/wake cycle	Fragmented; frequent naps	Disturbed; day–night reversal

that represents a change from previous functioning *and* at least one of the symptoms is depressed mood or loss of pleasure or interest:

1. Depressed mood most of the day nearly every day
2. Markedly diminished interest or pleasure in all or most activities
3. Significant, unintentional weight loss or decreased appetite nearly every day
4. Insomnia or hypersomnia (sleeping too much)
5. Psychomotor agitation or retardation (slowness or speed of movement)
6. Fatigue or loss of energy
7. Feelings of worthlessness or excessive guilt feelings
8. Diminished ability to think or concentrate
9. Recurrent thoughts of death, recurrent suicidal ideation

Once depression is identified, treatment must be prompt and aggressive, using pharmacological and nonpharmacological measures. Most antidepressants are effective for older adults. Care must be taken with the older class of antidepressants, such as amitriptyline, because these medications can cause lowered blood pressure and sedation.

Most depressed people find that support from family and friends, involvement in self-help and support groups, and psychotherapy are helpful. Psychotherapy is especially beneficial for those who prefer not to take medicine. It also is helpful for older adults who cannot take medications because of side effects, interactions with other medicines, or other medical illnesses. Psychotherapy in older adults can address a broad range of functional and social consequences of depression. The nurse is in a key position to identify possible clinical depression and to place a psychiatric referral.

Parkinson's Disease

Parkinson's disease is a degenerative condition that primarily affects movement. It causes tremor, rigidity, and gait disturbances and can also adversely affect speech.

Cerebrovascular Accident

Cerebrovascular accident (stroke) is primarily a vascular disease with neurological consequences. Paralysis, weakness, and speech and vision impairments can range from minor to devastating. If treated immediately, neurological damage can be minimized or prevented.

Common Cognitive Issues

Age-related cognitive changes are noted in Table 6.5. They include mostly changes in memory and information processing. The Mini-Cog screening tool described in Box 6.3 can be used to assess cognitive impairment.

Cardiovascular health is the best physical predictor of intellectual ability in old age. In the absence of disease, older adults who keep mentally and physically active retain their mental and cognitive skills. When tasks do not require

Table 6.5 Age-Related Cognitive Changes

Change	Consequence
• Episodic memory diminishes with age. • Free recall diminishes. • Working memory ability decreases. • Semantic memory is maintained or may increase. • Processing speed decreases.	• Evident in tasks requiring learning and recall of items that are not meaningful, for example, phone numbers • The ability to recall unrelated words from a list decreases. • The ability to multitask successfully declines with aging, along with reduced ability to process complex incoming information. • Memory of facts and meanings and intellectual ability are unchanged. • If speed is not crucial, information is retrieved as well as in younger people.

Box 6.3 Mini-Cog Assessment for Cognitive Impairment

The Mini-Cog is a validated, quick, simple screening tool for assessing cognitive impairment. It can be administered in 3 minutes. The assessment is completed through evaluation of memory and the ability to accurately draw a specific time on a clock. Specifically, after the patient's attention has been gained, he or she is asked to remember three unrelated words. The patient is then asked to draw the face of a clock and then draw in the hands of the clock depicting a specific time, such as 11:10. Scoring is based on how many words the patient is able to remember and whether or not the clock and time are drawn correctly.

From Borson, S., Scanlan, J. M., Chen, P., & Ganguli, M. (2003). The Mini-Cog as a screen for dementia: Validation in a population-based sample. *JAGS, 51*(10), 1451–1454.t

speed, older people perform as well as younger people. The older adult's ability to solve practical problems is generally higher than that of young adults. New learning may be more difficult, and it takes more time to store new knowledge in accessible memory. This can impact health education for older adults.

Common Renal Issues

Age-related renal changes are noted in Table 6.6. In general, all of the changes in the renal system together result in the consequences noted.

Table 6.6 Age-Related Renal Changes

Change	Consequence
● Decrease in the size of the renovascular bed	● Impaired tubular reabsorption
● Decreased renal blood flow	● Reduced ability to conserve and excrete sodium
● Selective loss of cortical vasculature	● Impaired concentrating ability
● Sclerosis of glomeruli	● Reduced response to antidiuretic hormone
● Loss of glomeruli	● Inability to excrete an acid load
● Decrease in tubular size and number	● Greatly increased risk for fluid and electrolyte imbalances of many types
● Exaggerated renal vasoconstrictive response to sympathetic stimulation	● Decline in creatinine clearance

Table 6.7 Age-Related Genitourinary and Reproductive Changes

Change	Consequence
● Decline in bladder capacity, contractility, and control	● Incontinence of urine
● Decline in urethral length and sphincter strength	● Increased risk of urinary infection
● Prostate hypertrophy	● Narrowing of the urethral lumen with incomplete bladder emptying, incontinence
● Detrusor muscle instability	● Risk of uterine prolapse in females
● Pelvic floor muscle weakness	
● Atrophy of uterus and vagina	● Cessation of reproductive capacity
● Markedly reduced production of estrogen and ovarian fibrosis	● Decreased libido
● Decreased testosterone levels	● Erectile dysfunction

Common health issues include:

- Greatly increased risk of dehydration, not only from renal changes but also from a delayed and less-intense thirst response
- Decreased excretion of drugs and toxins, with an associated increase in side effects and morbidity
- Hyponatremia and hypernatremia related to impaired renal-diluting capacity and concentrating ability
- Both hypokalemia and hyperkalemia, which can occur from gastrointestinal losses and diuretic use. Hyperkalemia is more common in older adults

Common Genitourinary and Reproductive Changes

Age-related genitourinary and reproductive changes are noted in Table 6.7. Changes include a general decline in bladder function and capacity, uterine and vaginal atrophy, and decreased reproductive hormone levels.

Incontinence is a problem in both men and women. Stress incontinence is more common in women. Male urinary dysfunction is characterized by hesitancy, a weak urinary stream, and a feeling of incomplete bladder emptying as a result of benign prostatic hypertrophy. Sexual dysfunction occurs in both sexes as a result of hormone decreases, organ atrophy, and decreased sexual fluids.

Connection Check 6.2

The nurse is performing a cardiovascular assessment of an older adult patient. Which physical signs of normal aging can be expected?
A. Irregular pulse and diminished lung sounds
B. Heart rate of 88 bpm and a heart murmur
C. Systolic blood pressure of 150 mm Hg and a fourth heart sound
D. Productive cough and hoarseness

Common Gastrointestinal Changes

Age-related gastrointestinal changes are noted in Table 6.8. Typical changes include slowed gastric emptying, delayed transport through the colon, increases in acid secretion, and a decrease in the organ size of the liver and pancreas.

Common health issues include:

- Increased risk of gastric and duodenal ulcers and atrophic gastritis
- Gastroesophageal reflux disease
- Vitamin B_{12} deficiency and resultant anemia
- Increased feeling of fullness after a meal, with resultant reduced intake and possible nutritional deficiency
- Bone loss
- Constipation and fecal impaction. These are frequent and major problems for seniors. Delayed colon transit time and decreased strength of contraction, a tendency toward dehydration, and

Table 6.8 Age-Related Gastrointestinal Changes

Change	Consequence
• Slowed gastric emptying	• Gastric distention and anorexia
• Gastric mucosal atrophy	
• Increased secretion of gastrin (hormone that increases gastric acid secretion)	• Risk of ulcer formation
• Impaired gastric mucosal barrier function	
• Reduced secretion of intrinsic factor, a protein necessary for the absorption of vitamin B$_{12}$	• Impaired vitamin B$_{12}$ absorption
• Delayed colonic transit	• Constipation
• Decreased rectal wall sensitivity	
• Decreased colonic contraction strength	
• Decreased calcium absorption	• Contributes to bone loss
• Decrease in liver size and blood flow	• Impaired clearance of drugs
• Decrease in pancreas mass and enzyme reserves	• Reduced insulin secretion; increased insulin resistance

side effects from multiple medications all play a contributing role.

- Increased risk of adverse reactions and toxicity from medications as a result of liver changes
- Type 2 diabetes mellitus, also known as adult-onset diabetes, is considered epidemic among older adults. It accounts for 95% of all cases of diabetes in adults. Diagnosed and undiagnosed diabetes occurs in more than 26% of adults aged 65 and over. It can be prevented with a combination of weight loss, exercise, and dietary limitation of fats and calories.

Nutritional Issues

Related to gastrointestinal status, nutrition in older adults can be less than optimal for a variety of reasons. As part of the aging process, the senses of taste and smell diminish and can make food seem less appetizing. In addition to the previously mentioned changes in feelings of fullness and a tendency toward constipation, there can be problems with dentition and chewing that interfere with eating a well-balanced diet. A contributing factor in malnutrition is the presence of dysphasia, or difficulty swallowing, leading to loss of appetite, dehydration, and weight loss. Dysphasia also sometimes leads seniors to "pocket" food or medication in their cheeks, leading to an increased risk of aspiration.

Medications can have side effects affecting appetite and taste, which can lead to lowered intake of food. Seniors may have more difficulty shopping and cooking because of decreased mobility. Social isolation and having meals alone can decrease the enjoyment of eating and lead to decreased intake. Those with early-onset dementia and short-term memory impairment can simply forget to eat without assistance or reminders.

A comprehensive nutritional assessment is part of the nurse's responsibility when caring for seniors in any setting (Box 6.4). In addition, the nurse can collaborate with the nutritionist or registered dietitian because this health professional can conduct a detailed nutritional assessment.

Of particular concern is geriatric "failure to thrive," which is a condition of unintended weight loss in older adults. The term was borrowed from pediatrics in the 1970s. The Institute of Medicine defines *failure to thrive* as "weight loss of >5%, decreased appetite, poor nutrition, physical inactivity often associated with dehydration, depression, immune dysfunction and low cholesterol." It is a multidimensional problem with four chief characteristics: impaired physical functioning, malnutrition, depression, and cognitive impairment. In 25% to 35% of those affected, there is no identifiable medical cause.

Cachexia is the loss of weight and muscle mass and cannot be reversed nutritionally. It is generally associated with cancer, untreated or unsuccessfully treated AIDS, and COPD. This age-related wasting has multiple physical, psychological, and sociological causes. If not treated early, it can lead to rapid physical decline and has a poor prognosis.

Box 6.4 Mini Nutritional Assessment

The Mini Nutritional Assessment is a screening tool used to assess the nutritional status of those aged 65 and over. The purpose of the tool is to identify individuals who are malnourished or at risk for malnourishment.

It consists of six screening questions and 12 assessment questions that seek to correlate readily available data. Some of the data measured by this tool are appetite, typical foods and liquids consumed, mobility, living situation, number of medications taken, recently experienced psychological stress, midarm and midcalf circumferences, and body weight. One advantage of the tool is that it eliminates the need for blood testing.

The clinician can use this tool along with information regarding the individual's preferences, cultural influences, and usual mealtime desires to perform a comprehensive nutritional assessment.

The tool and more details on its background and application can be viewed online at the Hartford Institute for Geriatric Nursing Web site (http://consultgeri.org/try-this/general-assessment/issue-9).

Common Musculoskeletal Changes

Age-related musculoskeletal changes are noted in Table 6.9. Decreases in muscle mass, stiffening of tendons and ligaments, decreased bone density, and increased bone loss are common.

Common health issues include:

- Arthritis, with chronic joint and skeletal pain
- Osteoporosis, with risk of fractures caused by trauma and spontaneous fractures
- Limitations in movement and ability to perform tasks, resulting in increasing dependence on others for assistance with all activities
- Development of **sarcopenia**, which is the loss of muscle mass and increase in body fat that occurs with aging. In order to prevent a reduced quality of life due to loss of strength and function, interventions to address dietary needs and exercise are needed. These include increased protein intake and resistance training. Protein supplementation in combination with resistance-training exercises enhances muscle protein synthesis and improves body composition by increasing lean mass in relation to fat mass.

- Increased risk of falls as well as risk of sustaining injuries when falls occur (Boxes 6.5 and 6.6)

Fall prevention programs in the hospital should include strategies initiated before falls occur, not after a fall has been sustained. Age is a risk factor for falls because of the associated altered or ineffective gait and mobility. A more recent approach accepts that falls cannot be completely prevented. In light of this, emphasis is placed on exercise, strengthening muscles, and gait training and on teaching older adults how to fall safely without developing disabling fear.

Deconditioning, a rapid loss of strength, can occur when a patient is hospitalized or bedbound. In this process, bedrest or prolonged immobilization brings about

Box 6.5 Factors Associated With Increased Risk of Falls

- Confusion and disorientation
- Symptomatic depression
- Altered elimination
- Male gender
- Dizziness or vertigo
- Particular categories of medications: benzodiazepines and antiepileptics
- Higher score on "get-up-and-go test" (see Box 6.6)

From Hendrich, A. (n.d.). *Fall risk assessment for older adults: The Hendrich II Fall Risk Model.* Retrieved from http://consultgeri.org/try-this/general-assessment/issue-8

Box 6.6 Get-Up-and-Go Test

Assessment of poor balance and gait can be accomplished with a portion of the complete Tinetti get-up-and-go test. The assessment can be done by simply asking the patient to rise out of a chair and take several steps in a straight line. Patient steps are observed and should be purposeful and steady. To conduct the test, follow these steps:

- Ask the patient to rise.
- Remain close in case the patient begins to fall.
- Ask him or her to walk forward to a specified spot, turn, return to the chair, and sit back down.
- Look for shuffling gait, lack of arm swing, unequal shoulder or hip height, the ability to turn without support, and the ability to stand and sit in a controlled fashion.
  Score 0 = Patient can rise unassisted/hands-free.
  Score 1 = Patient rises using arms to push up in one attempt.
  Score 3 = Patient makes several attempts to push up and succeeds to stand.
  Score 4 = Patient is unable to stand without assistance.
  A total accumulative score of 5 or more indicates a higher risk of falls.

From Hendrich, A. (n.d.). *Fall risk assessment for older adults: The Hendrich II Fall Risk Model.* Retrieved from http://consultgeri.org/try-this/general-assessment/issue-8

Table 6.9 Age-Related Musculoskeletal Changes

Change	Consequence
Decrease of 30%–40% in muscle mass	Reduced strength of upper and lower extremities
Increased intramuscular and subcutaneous fat	Loss of muscle mass (sarcopenia)
Decline in tensile strength of ligaments and tendons	Increased risk of deconditioning; a rapid loss of strength
Stiffening of ligaments and tendons	Reduced joint range of motion
Stiffer collagen in cartilage	
Decreased bone density and bone remodeling	Osteopenia and osteoporosis
Increased bone loss	Increased risk for fractures
Decreased vitamin D absorption	
Decrease in hand and foot movement speed	Increased risk for falls
Significant decline in one-legged balance	Management of activities of daily living and instrumental activities of daily living becomes more challenging, including dressing, bathing, ambulating, doing household chores, shopping, and writing.
Gait changes, including reduced stride length and walking speed	
Decreased grip strength	
Presence of postural tremor	

pathological changes in muscles and bones that result in serious disability for older adults. It is estimated that 31% of older adults are discharged from a hospitalization with deconditioning and a significant decrease in ability to perform ADLs.

CASE STUDY: EPISODE 3

The home-care nurse completes the first visit with the assistance of the Spanish interpreter and the patient's daughter, who lives in the same building. The findings include some shortness of breath with activity, no lower extremity edema, and normal breath sounds. Initial vital signs are as follows:

Heart rate: 95 bpm

Blood pressure: 154/88 mm Hg

Respiratory rate: 22

Temperature: 98.8°F (37.1°C)

The patient's weight is obtained on a home scale. The nurse now has baseline measurements against which to gauge future changes. For patients with HF, weight changes of 2 pounds or greater in 24 hours or 5 pounds in a week require immediate intervention to prevent exacerbation of heart failure or pulmonary edema and rehospitalization. Education on the safe use of home oxygen is conducted by the nurse, and both the patient and her daughter are able to give a correct return demonstration. The home-care nurse sees that Ms. Gomez has come home from the hospital with a decreased ability to ambulate steadily and has suffered a loss of strength and muscle tone. On the basis of all of these findings, the nurse identifies several problems that need to be addressed in the plan of care: decreased activity tolerance, deconditioning, and potential for exacerbation of HF. Interventions to address these findings include directing the patient to maintain her daily weight and providing education on a low-salt diet. A referral for physical therapy is also indicated in order to develop a strength-building program and provide placement of assistive devices (cane, walker, wheelchair) as needed for the provision of safe ambulation. A home health aide is also requested to assist Ms. Gomez with her personal care and her ADLs while she builds her strength and activity tolerance.

The nurse encourages Ms. Gomez to express her concerns and fears related to increasing dependence on others and her changing role in the family. "I'm so tired and weak," she responds. "I'm a useless old lady now. I used to cook for everyone, and now I don't have the energy." It will be important for the nurse to reinforce progress as it develops and to help keep Ms. Gomez focused on her recovery. The nurse will utilize both family and outside social and community agencies to keep Ms. Gomez engaged and supported...

Common Immunological and Skin Changes

Age-related immunological and skin changes are noted in Table 6.10. There is a general diminishing of immune functioning. The skin's ability to function as a barrier is also diminished.

Common immunological and skin-related health issues include:

- Blunted responses to infection, making diagnosis more difficult. Older adults are less likely to have a fever or elevated white blood cell count or obvious manifestation of symptoms. When older adults develop infections, particularly urinary tract infections, the only sign that may be apparent is a change in their behavior. They may not have any pain or changes in their pattern of urination but will display sudden mood shifts, memory loss, inattention, confusion, or lethargy. These are beginning signs of delirium and need to be investigated immediately (see Table 6.4 on dementia and delirium).

Table 6.10 Age-Related Immunological and Skin Changes

Change	Consequence
• Decrease in phagocytic activity and bactericidal function	• Increased susceptibility to and mortality from infections
• Decrease in T-cell function	
• Decreased inflammatory responsiveness	• Altered clinical signs of acute infection; absence of fever
• Decreased antibody response to antigen stimulation of 90% by age 75	• Decreased allergic reactions
• Diminished antibody production in response to vaccination or infection	• Reactivation of infectious diseases
• Reduction in humoral immunity	
• Decreased melanocytes	• Increased skin cancer risk
• Decreased collagen	• Dry skin; rough skin
• Progressive loss of elastic tissue	• Low-grade skin infections
• Decreased elasticity	• Slow wound healing; weak scars
• Ineffective DNA repair	
• Loss of dermal thickness	• Decreased barrier function
• Smaller adjoining surface between dermis and epidermis	• "Paper-thin" skin
	• Less resistance to shearing forces
	• Increased potential for skin tears

- Increased risk of skin breakdown from pressure when older persons are sedentary, immobile, or bedbound. Four forces that contribute to skin breakdown are friction, pressure, shearing, and maceration. Prevention or moderation of these mechanisms is essential to avoid skin breakdown.

- Shingles that occurs with a history of herpes zoster (chickenpox). The significance of a shingles outbreak is the risk of developing chronic severe pain even after the shingles lesions have healed. This is termed *postherpetic neuralgia* (PHN) and is most common in older adults. A new shingles vaccine called Shingrix (recombinant zoster vaccine) was licensed by the U.S. Food and Drug Administration (FDA) in 2017. The CDC recommends that healthy adults 50 years and older get two doses of Shingrix, 2 to 6 months apart. Shingrix provides strong protection against shingles and PHN.

- Increased incidence of xeroderma (dry, rough skin) and associated itching

- Intrinsic and extrinsic factors that are responsible for skin problems in older adults. Intrinsic factors are controlled by cellular processes that are programmed by genetic inheritance. Extrinsic aging is the result of external factors such as environmental conditions, smoking, ultraviolet light, medications, and chronic illness. Intrinsic and extrinsic factors can affect the ability of the skin to regenerate and aid in wound healing.

Common Sensory Changes

Age-related sensory changes are noted in Table 6.11. Decreases in visual acuity and hearing are common. The prevalence of hearing loss doubles with every age decade, and nearly two-thirds of Americans older than 70 years have a clinically significant hearing impairment, according to the Institute of Medicine and the National Research Council. The hearing loss that occurs with age is usually caused by the intrinsic aging of the auditory system. It rarely develops into total deafness. It can most often be managed with a hearing aid. There are many types and varieties from which to choose, and they fit a range of budgets. Hearing loss can be partially prevented by protecting the ears and hearing from excessive noise. The damage from noise is cumulative over a lifetime.

Common health issues related to vision and hearing loss include:

- Safety concerns related to the older adult's ability to navigate his or her environment. Whether older adults are in their homes or outside of them, vision and hearing impairments prevent awareness of obstacles to walking, objects in pathways, oncoming pedestrians or vehicles, and changing traffic signals. Vision impairments can prevent safe medication administration if labels and directions are misread or are unreadable. Safe operation of devices and appliances can be affected as well. In particular, the

Table 6.11 Age-Related Sensory Changes	
Change	**Consequence**
• Gradual opacity of lens	• Decreased visual acuity
• Increased corneal thickening	• Decreased ability to discriminate between color intensities, particularly blues and greens
• Yellowing of lens	
• Impaired adaptation to darkness	• Decreased ability to focus in dim light; increased sensitivity to glare
• Increased rigidity of the pupil	• Reduced adaptation to changes in light intensity
• Decreased elasticity of lens capsule	• Presbyopia (failure to bring near objects into focus)
• Hardening of the lens	
• Loss of accommodation	
• Reduction in fine oculomotor control	• Decreased dynamic visual acuity
• Reduction depth perception	• Decreased ability to detect movement and judge distances, which can affect driving skills
• Decreased lacrimation	• Dry eyes; increased risk of eye infections
• Presbycusis (age-related hearing loss distinct from other causes of hearing loss) that occurs for unknown reasons	• Loss of high-frequency tones
	• Impaired discrimination in source of sound

question of how long safe driving can continue is a difficult issue. Often, older adults resist giving up the ability to drive because it signals a major loss of independence. The safety concerns of all are a priority in making the decision to stop driving.

- Hearing problems that contribute to miscommunication. Conversations and comments directed to the individual can be misinterpreted. Older adults may begin to avoid social contacts because they cannot really hear what others are saying. When healthcare practitioners are conducting assessments and interviews, incomplete or erroneous information may be collected as a result of the older adult not understanding what is being asked. Lower tones of voice are heard better than high-pitched tones.

- There are long-term and public health implications of sensory impairments, including the risk for costly health outcomes of disability, depression, cognitive impairment, and dementia. Sensory loss impedes self-care and independence and can therefore negatively affect caregivers.

SAFETY AND PSYCHOSOCIAL ISSUES

Care priorities can be broadly discussed as safety and psychosocial issues. Safety considerations are a priority and have been discussed throughout this chapter in relation to the physical changes that naturally occur with aging. They include physical safety and medication safety. Another safety concern is the potential for abuse and being protected from possible abusive situations involving strangers and caregivers alike. Complicating the maintenance of safety for older adults is the fact that they often do not perceive that they are at risk. Psychosocial priorities include successfully navigating the transition into an older adult, attending to the social isolation and loneliness that can accompany old age, attending to housing and financial issues that accompany that transition, and establishing a plan of care or advance directives if the older adult becomes critically ill. When older adults have a chronic illness, an important goal is to prevent hospitalization and maintain care for the individual in his or her home environment. This requires additional services to maintain a safe home environment, with modifications suited to increased needs and the provision of medical equipment needed to treat various conditions.

Safety Issues

Physical Safety

Naturally occurring changes in strength, flexibility, balance, and reflex time combine to put older adults at risk for accidents and falls. If the home environment is not upgraded to compensate for the frailties of age, there can be risks of falling in the bathtub or shower, tripping over rugs and electrical cords, and falling from stepladders and makeshift climbing devices. There is less room for compensation and less margin for safety when a fall does occur. There is a greater chance of serious injury, such as fracture, hemorrhage, or loss of consciousness. Older adults may have fewer social supports and family members available to help or check on them, so they may be injured and unable to move or summon help in a timely manner.

Another important safety issue is driving. Older adult drivers are at risk and put others at risk. Decreased speed of reflex responses and decision making as well as visual and hearing problems can prevent awareness of dangerous traffic situations. Early, unrecognized dementia can impair an older adult's ability to follow traffic lights, directions, and other drivers' signals.

In the hospital setting, older adult patients have safety issues due to the development of behavioral problems as a result of the illness for which they are hospitalized. Sudden severe illness, dehydration, infections, and dementia can result in delirium. Patients with delirium suffer from confusion, disorientation, and altered level of consciousness and sometimes have aggressive behavior. In the past, the use of restraints was common in these circumstances to keep older adults safe, but it is now recognized that the current standard of practice is the avoidance of either physical or chemical (medicating with sedatives or antipsychotics) restraints. The present approach combines investigating possible causes of the behavior; addressing unmet needs and physiological conditions; reducing fall risk by modifying the environment; and providing close, continual observation and assistance (Box 6.7). Included in the approach is the use of the least invasive treatments. The challenge is to balance the patient's rights with his or her safety.

Medication Safety

In addition to the dangers of physical trauma from falls and accidents, older persons are at risk of injury from their own medications. The average number of prescription medications taken by those over age 65 is six. The individual may also take a number of over-the-counter medications. Each medication has its own side effects, and the combination of drugs increases the chances for adverse or deleterious effects. Older adults often need education, guidance, and support in order to follow the medication regimens that their primary providers are prescribing. Some of the normal aging changes in visual acuity, memory, and strength can interfere with correct and successful medication management. Problems such as being able to read the prescription label, remembering to take the medication at the right time and the right number of times a day, being able to open the pill bottle or container, and being able to go to the drugstore for refills if the pharmacy does not deliver are all factors that increase the risk of errors in medication management.

Box 6.7 The 4 Ps

In an effort to increase patient safety and decrease patient falls, many hospitals have implemented the evidence-based practice of hourly rounding. The focus of the hourly rounding is on the 4 Ps: pain, potty, positioning, and possessions. Patients are checked to ensure that their pain needs are met and that their essential possessions (call bell, tissues, glasses) are close at hand. Patients are asked if they need to visit the bathroom or if they need a change of position. In addition to increased patient safety, improved skin integrity or decreased skin breakdown and increased patient satisfaction are outcomes of hourly rounding focusing on the 4 Ps.

Safety Alert **Treatment by Tic Tac**
A creative exercise for medical residents at the University of California, Irvine

Medication regimens can be confusing and difficult to follow. Patients often do not take their medications the way they are prescribed. Nonadherence to medication regimens can cause adverse events, sometimes leading to hospitalization, nursing home placement, and death.

A 1-week-long "Mock Medication Compliance Exercise" using different flavors of Tic Tacs was developed. Medical residents were asked to take five mock medications for 7 days:

- "Lisinopril 20 mg" bid
- "Metformin 500 mg" tid
- "Fosamax 70 mg" weekly
- "Coumadin 5 mg," 1 tablet on Monday, Wednesday, and Friday and 1/2 tablet on Tuesday, Thursday, Saturday, and Sunday
- "Pravastatin 40 mg" at bedtime

The regimen was designed very deliberately to address the multiple issues providers must consider and nurses must monitor before and after prescribing:

1. Five mock prescriptions were given because research indicates that most medication problems start when drug lists are at least five medications long.
2. All "medications" prescribed were given at various times during the day to illustrate the complexities of drug regimens.
3. Each "medication" was to be taken as if it were a real drug.
   A. "Fosamax," for example, was to be taken on an empty stomach with a glass of water while in an upright position.
   B. "Metformin" was to be taken with food to avoid potential gastrointestinal intolerance. Participants were forced to remember to take "metformin" with them to work so that they could take it at lunchtime.
   C. "Pravastatin" was deliberately prescribed because it is one of the statins less likely to interact with "Coumadin."
   D. "Lisinopril" was given because "the patient" was diabetic and would normally take an angiotensin-converting enzyme inhibitor to prevent nephropathy.

There was only one resident who was 100% compliant. He happened to have worked as a pharmacy technician before starting medical school. Most residents were not completely compliant with the medication regimen. The reasons residents did not take the Tic Tacs were very similar to the reasons patients usually give: forgot them at home, got too busy to take them at home, didn't like the way the Tic Tacs tasted, had difficulty opening a child-resistant prescription vial, or had difficulty cutting the "Coumadin" Tic Tac in half. All residents reported that it was a difficult and very eye-opening experience.

Polypharmacy has been identified as a major problem for older adults. Polypharmacy is generally defined as being prescribed six or more medications and/or using a potentially inappropriate medication. Tools containing criteria for medication evaluation are readily available for the nurse to use. One of the most commonly used tools is the Beers Criteria for Potentially Inappropriate Medication Use in Older Adults.

Safety Alert **Beers criteria**
The Beers criteria identify medications that have been determined by an expert consensus panel as having potential risks that outweigh their potential benefits. It was last updated in 2015. The criteria apply to adults aged 65 years and older. This tool helps nurses identify medications that may increase the risk of adverse drug reactions. The purpose is to increase safety in medication use and improve medication monitoring. Part 1 of the tool lists 48 individual medications or classes of medications to avoid in older adults. The following are some of the medications identified in Part 1:

Amitriptyline (Elavil)
Barbiturates except phenobarbital
Cyclobenzaprine (Flexeril)
Diazepam (Valium)
Diphenhydramine (Benadryl)
Hydroxyzine (Vistaril)
Hyoscyamine (Levsin, Anaspaz)
Meperidine (Demerol)
Naproxen (Aleve, Naprosyn)
Promethazine (Phenergan)

The successful treatment of disease depends on compliance with the ordered regimens. People who are in compliance with their medications reduce their risk of rehospitalization and emergency department visits. When seniors have self-care confidence and take the right medication at the right time in the right form and dose, the chances of increased effectiveness and successful treatment of their condition increase greatly (see Evidence-Based Practice).

Evidence-Based Practice

Beyond Social Support: Self-Care Confidence Is Key for Adherence in Patients With Heart Failure

A study from 2017 demonstrated that heart failure patients who have confidence in their ability to provide self-care had an improved ability to adhere to their plan of care. Interventions targeting self-care confidence are crucial.

Hammash, M. H., Crawford, T., Shawler, C., Schrader, M., Lin, C. Y., Shewekah, D., & Moser, D. K. (2017). Beyond social support: Self-care confidence is key for adherence in patients with heart failure. *European Journal of Cardiovascular Nursing, 16*(7), 632–637.

Potential for Abuse

The potential vulnerability of older adults due to increased physical weakness and possible cognitive impairment as well as the stress that they may place on their caregivers makes them unintended and intended targets for abuse. They may suffer physical and emotional abuse at the hands of their caregivers. They may be neglected or abandoned if, for example, the caregiver becomes overly stressed. Older adults can also become victims of scams and financial exploitation by strangers. Their bank accounts are sometimes depleted by the caregivers who have assumed responsibility for their finances. Although the true frequency of elder abuse is not entirely known, a 2010 study published in the *American Journal of Public Health* found that 10% of people over the age of 60 are subject to emotional, physical, or sexual abuse or to neglect. Other studies have determined that elder abuse is vastly underreported, indicating that for every reported case, there are 24 unknown cases. The CDC has released new uniform definitions for elder abuse. Releasing uniform definitions of elder abuse will help guide future research and provide a more accurate depiction of elder abuse cases across the country. This in turn can help increase elder abuse funding at the government level.

> **Safety Alert** ● The CDC defines elder abuse as "an intentional act or failure to act by a caregiver or another person in a relationship involving an expectation of trust that causes or creates a risk of harm to an older adult." In addition, the CDC has identified and defined five types of elder abuse:
> ● Physical abuse: Intentional use of physical force—including hitting, kicking, pushing, slapping, and burning—that causes illness, pain, or injury.
> ● Sexual: Forced or unwanted sexual interaction, including unwanted sexual contact or penetration or noncontact sexual harassment.
> ● Emotional or psychological: Verbal or nonverbal behaviors that inflict anguish, mental pain, fear, or distress, including name-calling, humiliating, destroying property, or preventing someone from seeing friends or family.
> ● Neglect: Failure to meet basic needs, such as food, water, shelter, clothing, hygiene, and essential medical care.
> ● Financial: Improperly using money, benefits, belongings, property, or assets. Examples of financial abuse include taking money from a bank account or changing a will.

Psychosocial Issues

Psychosocial Transition

Those aged 65 and over are entering a unique developmental stage. Becoming old is not only a biological process but also a social and cultural one. As people age, their roles and status in life change, and they acquire another social identity. In the United States, the social identity of older adults is often one of being less valued and less important. Older adults are often neglected, dismissed, or ignored. They can experience a form of discrimination termed **ageism**, where they are treated with less respect and consideration because of their advanced age.

One of the tasks this group faces is how to accept a different and more dependent role after an adult lifetime of independence. Older adults need to adjust to job loss or retirement from a career and physical losses that range from minor vision, hearing, and mobility impairments to major disabilities from the chronic diseases and illnesses of old age. Issues concerning the management of one's material and financial belongings are now evident. There are losses of friends, family, and spouses through death. There is an alteration in self-image as the aging body changes in sometimes drastic ways. Sexual identity and sexual activity are dramatically changed as well. Sometimes complicating this adjustment, older adults commonly live in senior communities, which are designed to provide for their special needs and activities but they also act to segregate this population from the rest of the community and the society around them. All of these changes can increase the potential for social isolation.

There is the also the realization of mortality and the associated spiritual, philosophical, and intellectual processes that people face toward the end of life. Eric Erikson described eight developmental stages in life, the last one being late adulthood from age 60 to death. In this stage, the strength of wisdom comes from accumulated experience. As one looks back on life, there is a sense of accomplishment and contentment that the individual has made a contribution to the world in his or her own way. One has acceptance of the life one has lived. Erikson called this *integrity*. There is also the possibility of despair, with the look back showing perceived failures and uncertainty about life's meaning. This can contribute to a fear of death. As with all developmental tasks, older adults learn through a process of awareness and realization, trial and error, adaptation, acceptance, and integration of the newly changed self and new roles into the personality. As a healthcare provider, the nurse needs to have an awareness of this stage and develop strategies to assist and educate older persons while maintaining their dignity and autonomy as much as possible (Box 6.8).

Advance Directives

Families are the first source of care and comfort that people look to in times of need. Those who cared for the young must now depend on the young to care for them. When older adults are planning for their future, an open discussion with family members should take place regarding what kind of care they would like to receive if they become incapacitated. These wishes can be delineated in legal documents referred to as **advance directives**. It is most important to have someone older adults trust acting on their behalf if they become unable to speak for themselves. A healthcare proxy is a legally recognized document that outlines who has the authority to act on the older adult's behalf in making medical decisions.

Another important document is a **living will**. The living will outlines acceptable healthcare choices and treatments as well the treatments that are not acceptable. As part of the living will, the person may decide to direct healthcare providers not to perform cardiopulmonary resuscitation (CPR) if he or she should suffer a cardiac arrest. This is termed a *do-not-resuscitate (DNR) order*. These important decisions should be made while the older adult is still able to clearly and accurately communicate his or her desires regarding medical treatment in the event of a serious or terminal illness.

Family members most often fill the role of healthcare proxy as well as serving as legal guardians of the older adult's finances, which is termed a *power of attorney*. When there are no family members alive or willing to assume these responsibilities, friends, neighbors, or any trusted, willing, and capable adult can fulfill these roles. In cases where there is no one available, a court-appointed guardian is necessary.

Box 6.8 Interventions to Help Decrease Social Isolation

The nurse advocates for and facilitates the following measures:

- Assessment of family and community resources for possible contacts
- Assessment of family members' proximity to the senior and their ability to visit/transport
- Identification of neighbors who are available to help
- Location of community senior centers, volunteer organizations/ YMCA, and faith-based organizations able to provide support
- Ensuring safe transport so that seniors can leave the home for activities:
  1. Arrange senior transportation vans.
  2. Locate other local organizations providing care service.
  3. Assist in arranging transportation and senior-discount fares.

The nurse is in an important position to facilitate and encourage these conversations and decisions.

Housing and Finances

Most people reaching retirement age and beyond hope to be able to live independently for as long as possible. Some of them have homes that are paid for and family members who are willing and able, both physically and geographically, to assist them. Some have retirement income and savings that will be used to supplement their Social Security income. A few will continue to work in some capacity either because they need to or because they want to work and stay active. For others, there will be obstacles if they do not have retirement benefits or have not saved enough money. There may be no family members willing or able to help them. They may not be physically able to live on their own and may have to relocate to a community where help is available or hire assistants to come into their home. Often, the first people who become aware of these circumstances are healthcare practitioners. When older adults are hospitalized and a discharge plan is formulated, it may be discovered that there is no one at home to assist the recovering older adult.

RESOURCES

With the growing population of aged individuals and the "oldest old" increasing in numbers, the caregivers themselves are advancing in years; a 90-year-old woman might have her 70-year-old daughter as a caregiver who has needs of her own. The "graying" of America is bringing about a crisis in the circumstances of living to old age without the necessary resources. In addition, the increasing numbers of Alzheimer's patients and those suffering from other forms of dementia are placing serious financial and emotional burdens on caregivers. There are growing numbers of agencies that provide information, education, support, and links to other agencies for caregiver assistance. There is very little availability of volunteer assistance in home care for older adults. Most of the agencies that provide aides and homemaker assistants charge an hourly fee for the services.

The first place to seek assistance is the local community or city of residence. Community and government agencies offer support by way of education, referrals to smaller groups, and links to Web sites. In addition, literature can be downloaded or received in the mail, and help with applying for financial assistance can be provided. Community groups often give free assistance on a limited basis and have volunteers available to provide transportation to senior centers, shopping centers, or doctor appointments. There are some groups that provide free meals and food delivery and transportation services. These are usually church- or religion-affiliated organizations.

The Social Security Office can provide information. State governments have a senior citizens department and an office of aging. The federal government also has an Office of Aging.

There are a growing number of geriatric care managers who are experts in knowing about and finding resources. These can include assistance in finding housing; assistance in the home for a range of activities; and management of financial resources, including filing Medicaid applications.

Medicare is the government health insurance program that covers medical expenses for people aged 65 and over. It provides for care in the hospital, provider visits, and limited home-care assistance. Many people are not aware that Medicare does not cover nursing home care and that the coverage for home care does not extend past a few months. After this period, patients and their families must develop a plan using a combination of family and privately hired help.

Medicaid is the government insurance program for those whose incomes are below a certain level at which they are unable to afford the healthcare they need. Medicaid provides for nursing home care or care at an assisted living facility. It also provides for a nursing attendant in the home for 8 or more hours a day if the patient has his or her own home and a caregiver who has assumed responsibility for super-vision of his or her affairs.

In order to manage the issues that present themselves in this stage of life, it is usually necessary to put together several strategies that combine the following: a private-pay, supplemental insurance plan; community agencies such as Meals on Wheels or senior centers; Social Secu-rity, Medicare, and/or Medicaid; and available family or neighbors. The most active community and government agencies serving as resources for older adults and their caregivers, with links to their Web sites, can be found on www.DavisAdvantage.com.

Connection Check 6.4

The nurse caring for an older adult patient with early signs of dementia incorporates which priority nursing diagnosis into the plan of care?
A. Altered nutrition, less than nutritional requirements
B. Altered nutrition, greater than nutritional requirements
C. Risk for injury
D. Activity intolerance

Connection Check 6.5

While assisting family members in finding resources to care for their father, the nurse is aware that which agency can provide assistance with nursing home costs?
A. Medicare
B. Social Security Administration
C. Medicaid
D. Department of Health and Human Services

Making Connections

CASE STUDY: WRAP-UP

The home-care nurse makes a follow-up visit to Ms. Gomez to evaluate the effectiveness of the plan of care and to continue assessing and monitoring the patient's physical and psychosocial status. Ms. Gomez has weighed herself and recorded the result with the assistance and guidance of her home health aide and her daughter. The nurse provides education to all three about the patient's medications and supervises the daughter in filling the mediplanner. A physical therapist has visited and has initiated a home exercise program with Ms. Gomez. The nurse reviews with the patient her dietary intake for the previous day and reinforces the need for strict salt restriction in order to avoid fluid retention. To promote incentive for maintaining this, the nurse reminds Ms. Gomez that the goal is to prevent rehospitalization. Ms. Gomez continues to express feelings of frustration and hopelessness about her diagnosis and the aging process. The nurse requests a social work referral to provide a more in-depth psychosocial assessment and emotional support. During subsequent visits, the nurse assesses the patient for the absence of symptoms, no weight gain, the absence of edema, reduction of salt intake, and adherence to the medication schedule. Ms. Gomez is evaluated for returning strength and gradual increase in activity tolerance. The goal of aging at home is accomplished through collaboration with a team of people that includes the patient and her family, the provider, the home health aide, the physical therapist, and the social worker.

Case Study Questions

1. Which statement by Ms. Gomez indicates that the teaching has been effective?
   A. "I'm not concerned with my weight as long as I take my pills."
   B. "Walking too much puts a strain on my heart."
   C. "I need to take my medications to stay out of the hospital."
   D. "As long as I take my meds, I can use salt."

2. The nurse monitors Ms. Gomez for the development of cognitive issues. Which clinical manifestations are early indications of the development of dementia? *(Select all that apply.)*
   A. Short-term memory impairment
   B. Acute onset of reduced awareness
   C. Gradual onset of impaired judgment
   D. Fluctuating levels of alertness
   E. Personality changes

3. The nurse caring for Ms. Gomez, who is suffering from deconditioning from the recent hospitalization, should add what to the plan of care? *(Select all that apply.)*

   A. Maintenance of bedrest to prevent a fall

   B. Range-of-motion exercises

   C. Limited dietary intake because of decreased activity

   D. Referral for physical therapy

   E. Education for safe ambulation and fall prevention

4. The nurse includes which information in the teaching plan about the management of heart failure? *(Select all that apply.)*

   A. Strict portion control at meals

   B. Daily weight and record

   C. Taking stairs instead of elevators

   D. Avoiding artificial sweeteners

   E. Salt restriction and salt substitutes

5. Which of these assessment findings will alert the nurse to possible worsening of heart failure? *(Select all that apply.)*

   A. Sudden inability to breathe while lying flat

   B. Blurred vision

   C. Craving for sweets

   D. Loose bowel movements

   F. A weight gain of 2.5 pounds in 1 day

CHAPTER SUMMARY

The demographics of older adults show that they are an increasingly larger percentage of the U.S. population and are growing rapidly. Older women outnumber older men and are more likely to be widows and live alone. Minority populations are steadily growing and require a culturally sensitive approach in order to achieve positive outcomes. One consequence of increased numbers of older adults is growing pressure on families, communities, and government agencies as they try to meet their care needs.

Age-related changes in each system come primarily as a result of slowing and stiffening processes and the atrophy of organs. Systolic hypertension and a fourth heart sound are examples of normal consequences of the aging process. Respiratory changes put older adults at higher risk of infection. Gastrointestinal changes can result in decreased appetite and constipation as well as nutritional deficiencies. Renal changes result in a decrease in effective functioning over time. Musculoskeletal changes are evident in the decreased muscle mass of older adults, which is one factor that puts them at an increased risk for falls.

The cognitive changes of aging and the rising incidence of dementia are particularly challenging care issues. Most older adults retain their intellectual abilities but experience decreases in the speed of processing and the amount of information that can be processed at one time. However, the incidence of dementia is growing, with Alzheimer's dementia being the most common form afflicting older adults. This presents an increasingly significant care burden on individuals and on society as a whole.

The safety of older adults is a priority because they are at greater risk of injury as a result of decreases in strength, balance, and reaction time. Fall prevention is a priority of care in all care settings where older adults are seen. Adherence to medication regimens is not only a safety concern, but evidence has also shown that it produces a greater likelihood of positive outcomes and decreased hospitalizations and emergency department visits for patients with heart failure. Another safety priority is protection from abuse, both unintentional and intentional.

Documenting end-of-life wishes with an advance directive and living will after conversations with family members is essential to ensure that the older adult's healthcare priorities are maintained.

Knowledge of how and where to find resources to assist older adults is essential to the nurses who care for older adults in greater numbers. The federal government and individual state governments have established departments of aging that provide extensive information and referral sources for patients, caregivers, and professionals alike. Medicare and Medicaid are government agencies that provide healthcare coverage for older adults. Medicaid is the government program that covers nursing home costs when individual finances have been depleted.

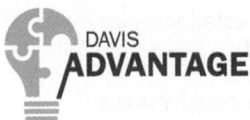

DAVIS **ADVANTAGE** | To explore learning resources for this chapter, go to **Davis Advantage** and find:
- Answers to in-text questions
- Chapter Resources and Activities
- NCLEX®-Style Chapter Review Questions
- Bibliography

Chapter 7

Oxygen Therapy Management

Denise Owens

Finding Connections

CASE STUDY: EPISODE 1

Follow this patient throughout the chapter.

Sarah Graham, a 70-year-old Caucasian female, presents to the emergency department with complaints of shortness of breath, chills, weakness, and having a productive cough with yellow/green secretions. At night, she sleeps with two pillows behind her back to make it easier to breathe. Mrs. Graham is having difficulty trying to finish a sentence without stopping to rest to catch her breath. It hurts when she tries to take a deep breath, and the cough gets worse.

History includes chronic obstructive pulmonary disease (COPD), hypertension (HTN), osteoarthritis, and hypothyroidism.

T	101°F (38°C)
Pulse	102 beats per minute
RR	32 breaths per minute
BP	142/84 mm Hg
PO	88% on room air

History: She has a history of COPD, HTN, osteoarthritis, and hypothyroidism.

Social History: Mrs. Graham states that she smokes one pack of cigarettes per day but has decreased the number of cigarettes because of her difficulty in breathing. She has smoked since she was 16 years old. She has not had much of an appetite the last several days and complains of being tired and weak all the time.

Home Medications:

Boniva IV every 3 months

Lisinopril 40 mg every day

Potassium 20 mEq every day

Vitamin D 1,000 units every day

Synthroid 0.1 mg every day

Fish oil every day

Colace 100 mg as needed

Spiriva 1 capsule inhalation daily...

OVERVIEW OF OXYGEN THERAPY

Physiology

The human body requires oxygen in order to sustain life. The inhaled air consists of 21% oxygen, 78% nitrogen, and 1% miscellaneous gases. Through ventilation, perfusion, and diffusion, oxygen is delivered to the cells and carbon dioxide (CO_2) is removed to maintain proper oxygenation and tissue perfusion. **Ventilation** is the movement of air in and out of the lungs. **Perfusion** is the gas exchange of oxygen and CO_2 at the alveoli-capillary membrane. **Diffusion** is the movement of solutes from an area of high concentration to an area of low concentration. **Oxygenation** is the process of oxygen passively diffusing from the alveoli to the blood, where the oxygen attaches to the hemoglobin or dissolves in the plasma. This process of the transport of oxygen from the inhaled air to the cells and the transport of CO_2 in the opposite direction is called **respiration**. The main function of the respiratory system is to deliver oxygen to the lungs (ventilation) where, through diffusion, oxygen is released into the blood at the alveolar-capillary membrane (perfusion); the oxygen is then transported to the tissues, and CO_2 is transported by the blood to the lungs and released at the alveolar-capillary membrane through diffusion and then released as a gas.

The respiratory system consists of the upper respiratory tract and the lower respiratory tract. As air enters the body through the upper airways (the nose, mouth, pharynx, nasopharynx, oropharynx, laryngopharynx, and larynx), the air is warmed, humidified, and filtered as it passes through these structures into the lower respiratory tract. As the air enters the lower respiratory tract (the trachea, bronchi, bronchioles, and into the alveoli), the air continues to be filtered by hairlike cilia that line the respiratory tract. In some patients who are unable to maintain a normal airway, a **tracheotomy** (surgical opening of the trachea) may be performed to create a **tracheostomy** (an opening/stoma directly into the trachea). The care of patients with tracheostomies is discussed throughout this chapter.

The alveoli surface area has two types of cells that make gas exchange possible. Type I cells (squamous) are thin, flat cells that allow for rapid gas exchange between the alveoli and the blood. Type II cells (pneumocytes) secrete **surfactant**, a phospholipid and protein substance that covers the alveoli to prevent the alveoli from collapsing by reducing surface tension in the alveoli, allowing for gas exchange to take place. Surface tension is the force present within the alveoli of the lungs that causes the alveoli to collapse. The surfactant reduces the surface tension, therefore reducing the tendency of the alveoli to collapse. When the lungs have improved **compliance** (ease of expansion of the lungs), less effort is needed to expand the lungs. Oxygen diffuses across the capillary bed that surrounds the alveoli from an area of higher concentration to the blood, the area of lower concentration. Oxygen is carried to the tissue in two ways: 97% of the oxygen is attached to hemoglobin, and 3% is dissolved in plasma. Carbon dioxide is carried by the circulatory system to the lungs, where it is removed from the blood through diffusion into the alveoli and is exhaled as gas.

The normal PaO_2 (partial pressure of oxygen in arterial blood) level, the part of total blood gas pressure exerted by oxygen gas, is 80 to 95 mm Hg, and the normal SaO_2 (percentage of oxygen saturation of arterial blood) level is 95% to 100%. When these levels are sustained, there is adequate oxygenation for the body.

The disruption in oxygenation can be either in ventilation or perfusion, causing **hypoxia** and **hypoxemia**. Hypoxia occurs secondary to insufficient oxygen to meet the metabolic demands of the cells, tissues, and organs. Hypoxemia develops when there are low levels of oxygen in the arterial blood. When there is a disruption in oxygenation, the cells may become hypoxic (decreased oxygen) because of an inadequate amount of oxygen in the system, causing a decrease in tissue oxygenation.

Hypoxemia is manifested when the PaO_2 level in the blood becomes less than 60 mm Hg or the SaO_2 level becomes less than 90% when breathing room air. Hypoxemia also occurs when the PaO_2 level and/or SaO_2 is less than a desirable amount for specific clinical situations, particularly when supplemental oxygen is administered. Trauma, acute myocardial infarction, and surgery are examples of acute care situations in which hypoxemia may develop.

The patient who does not have adequate oxygenation may experience early signs of hypoxia, including a change in mental status, anxiety, restlessness, and/or confusion, because the cells in the brain are not receiving an adequate supply of oxygen. Other clinical manifestations include increased respiratory and heart rates, as well as **dyspnea** (subjective feeling of difficulty breathing). On the basis of the clinical presentation, these patients may require supplemental oxygen to maintain proper oxygenation to the cells.

Oxygen therapy is initiated when an oxygenation concentration higher than room air (21%) is needed to treat or prevent the hypoxia. Oxygen is a medication and requires an order from a healthcare provider. When a patient is receiving oxygen therapy, the patient must be closely monitored to prevent complications associated with oxygen therapy. When evaluating the oxygen order, the nurse adheres to the six rights of medication administration and continuously monitors the concentration of oxygen that is prescribed by the healthcare provider.

Connection Check 7.1

The nurse includes which nursing diagnosis in the plan of care for the patient admitted with pneumonia?
A. Anxiety related to hypoxia
B. Deficient knowledge related to cause of disorder
C. Fear related to the threat of pain
D. Ineffective breathing pattern related to decreased surfactant

Age-Related Considerations

Through the aging process, the pulmonary function of the older adult undergoes changes, which are not the same in every aging adult and may vary in each individual person. These changes include the loss of lung elasticity, an enlargement and rigidity of the chest wall, a decrease in muscle strength, and a decrease in alveolar surface area. Elastin and collagen changes cause a loss of lung elasticity. Intercostal cartilage calcifies, causing the chest wall to enlarge and become rigid. Respiratory muscles weaken because of the increased loss of mobility of the chest wall. The decrease in alveolar surface area causes a decrease in the diffusion capacity for oxygen, causing lower oxygen levels in the older adult. These changes can lead to decreased expansion of the lungs, less depth with breathing, less effective cough, a decrease in gas exchange, and alveolar collapse, all of which affect ventilation and perfusion in the aging adult. Older adults who have a significant history of smoking, a sedentary lifestyle, obesity, and a diagnosis of chronic disease, along with the changes in pulmonary function associated with the aging process, are at greater risk for developing hypoxia and hypoxemia (see Geriatric/Gerontological Considerations).

Geriatric/Gerontological Considerations

The Older Population

Between 2010 and 2050, the United States is projected to experience rapid growth in the older population. In 2050, the number of Americans 65 and older is projected to be 88.5 million. The baby boomers are largely responsible for the increase in the older population.

With the aging population growing and people living longer, more of the aging population will have health problems. The older adult is at risk for aspiration and infection due to the aging process and other health issues, including pulmonary conditions and pulmonary diseases. Patient education is needed and should include adequate nutrition and leading a healthy lifestyle.

National Center for Health Statistics. (2016). *Chapter 1: Introduction. Healthy People 2020 midcourse review*. Retrieved from https://www.cdc.gov/nchs/healthy_people/index.htm

Indications for Supplemental Oxygen

Oxygen therapy is initiated with the intent of treating and preventing the clinical manifestations of hypoxia. Indications for oxygen therapy include PaO_2 less than 60 mm Hg or SaO_2 less than 90% in a patient breathing room air or a PaO_2 and/or SaO_2 below the indicated or prescribed range for the patient's clinical situation. Conditions that result in low PaO_2 or SaO_2 levels include respiratory, cardiac, and/or central nervous system disorders. Oxygen therapy may be indicated when there is an increased need for oxygen, such as a patient with a fever, infection, anxiety, and/or anemia, to meet the metabolic demands of these conditions. These conditions cause an increase in the work of breathing and an increased workload of the heart to meet the metabolic demands at the cellular level. The oxygen needs are unmet because of ventilation (intake) and/or perfusion (delivery) problems, and the cells become hypoxic, which can lead to the death of the cell. The body at this time requires an oxygen concentration greater than 21%. Through oxygen therapy, the patient can receive the higher concentration of oxygen that the body requires.

In order to prevent the cells, tissues, and organs from dying, supplemental oxygen may be required to meet the needs of the body and to sustain life. Oxygen therapy is ordered to maintain a PaO_2 level greater than 80 mm Hg and an SaO_2 level greater than 95%, to decrease the workload of the heart, and to decrease the work required by the patient to maintain optimal oxygen levels. Oxygen therapy is used for both acute and chronic medical conditions.

Contraindications to Oxygen Administration

Generally, there are no contraindications to oxygen therapy when appropriate assessment, including a history of respiratory disease, and indications are present. Use extreme caution with patients who are hypoxic and have chronic **hypercapnia** or **hypercarbia** (increased $PaCO_2$ levels in the blood), which is often observed in patients with COPD. In a patient with COPD, a low PaO_2 level (hypoxia) is the patient's primary drive for breathing. Oxygen therapy should be started with caution in patients with COPD because delivering too much oxygen may interfere with the hypoxic drive for breathing, leading to decreased respiratory effort and ultimately rate.

Oxygen Monitoring and Measurement

The need for and the effectiveness of oxygen therapy are assessed and monitored by physical assessment of the patient, pulse oximetry, and arterial blood gas (ABG) analysis. **Pulse oximetry** is a noninvasive method that can be used in any setting to obtain the oxygen saturation of hemoglobin (SpO_2) in the blood. The pulse oximeter is the device used to perform the measurement. It uses a light sensor that has two sources of light (red and infrared) that pass through the skin to measure the amount of hemoglobin saturated with oxygen. The light is absorbed by the hemoglobin in the blood; the more hemoglobin saturated with oxygen, the higher the oxygen saturation. The measurement is converted to a digital value representing the percentage of hemoglobin saturated with oxygen. Normal SpO_2 levels are 95% to 99%.

The pulse oximeter can be used as an intermittent assessment or as a continuous monitoring measurement. When used intermittently, the pulse oximeter can be used on an as-needed (prn) basis for patients who may be at risk for hypoxemia. Examples include patients on a medical-surgical floor who are admitted with pneumonia who may experience hypoxia or patients after surgery who may be at risk for hypoxia because of the depressant effects of anesthesia. The pulse oximeter can be used continuously on the patient who is being weaned from oxygen therapy or the patient who is intubated and requires a continuous display

of the oxygen saturation. In addition to the SpO_2 level, many pulse oximeters display the pulse rate. Many health-care facilities use the pulse oximeter when assessing the vital signs of the patient to monitor the patient's SpO_2 level.

The pulse oximeter is most often applied to the finger, but the earlobe, bridge of the nose, or the toe also can be used. The accuracy in the reading of the pulse oximetry depends on several variables, including the hemoglobin level of the patient, adequate perfusion to the area where the pulse oximeter is placed, the temperature of the area where the pulse oximeter is placed, and the patient's ability to oxygenate. The pulse oximeter does not have the ability to measure ventilation or the $PaCO_2$ and can lead to a potential delay in the detection of hypercapnia. Pulse oximetry is one part of a complete assessment of the patient's oxygenation status and is not a substitute for the need to obtain ABGs. When documenting the results of the patient's pulse oximetry, the nurse should include the SpO_2 level, the amount of oxygen the patient is receiving, and the patient's respiratory rate.

Arterial blood gas analysis is used to measure the pH, PaO_2, $PaCO_2$, HCO_3^- (bicarbonate), and SaO_2 levels of the blood. The ABG sample is obtained through an arterial puncture, usually via the radial or femoral artery, or through an indwelling arterial line or pulmonary artery catheter. Obtaining an ABG provides the most accurate measurement of cellular oxygenation, and the results guide the management and treatment for patients with oxygenation and acid–base disorders. See Table 7.1 for normal ABG values.

NONINVASIVE OXYGEN DELIVERY METHODS

There are a number of different noninvasive oxygen delivery devices available for the treatment of patients with oxygenation issues, and several factors are considered when ordering oxygen therapy. These factors include the patient's age, disease process (acute or chronic), degree of hypoxia, and the ability of the patient to tolerate the oxygen device that is ordered.

Table 7.1 Normal Arterial Blood Gas Values

Arterial Blood Gas	Normal Range
pH	7.35–7.45
PaO_2	80–95 mm Hg
$PaCO_2$	35–45 mm Hg
HCO_3^-	22–26 mEq/L
SaO_2	95%–100%

CASE STUDY: EPISODE 2

A physical examination reveals a frail woman who complains of shortness of breath, chills, and weakness, and she has a productive cough of yellow/green sputum. She states that at night she has to use two pillows to make her breathing easier. Now she has problems trying to finish a sentence without stopping to take a breath. It hurts when she tries to take a deep breath, and she notices the coughing gets worse. Mrs. Graham is alert and oriented times 3, crackles are noted in the lower bases of the lungs with an occasional expiratory wheeze, and her peripheral pulses are palpable but weak. Her abdomen is flat with bowel sounds present. An indwelling urinary (Foley) catheter is placed, with 80 mL of amber-colored urine noted in the urinary drainage bag. Her skin is warm to the touch and pink in color. She is placed on the cardiac monitor, which reveals a heart rate of 102 bpm with occasional premature ventricular contractions. A peripheral IV line is started with 0.9% normal saline at 80 mL an hour.

The following diagnostic results are received:

Chest x-ray indicates consolidation in the lower lobes of the lungs.

ABGs:

pH	7.32
PaO_2	56 mm Hg
$PaCO_2$	52 mm Hg
HCO_3^-	30 mEq/L
SaO_2	88%

Hematology results:

WBC	14,000 mm^3
RBC	6.2 g/dL
Hgb	18 g/dL
Hct	54%
Plt	380,000 mm^3

A **sputum culture** is sent to the laboratory.

Blood cultures ×2 are sent to the laboratory.

Because of these findings, Mrs. Graham is started on a Venturi mask at 28% oxygen…

Low-Flow Delivery Devices

Low-flow delivery devices include the nasal cannula, simple face mask, partial rebreather mask, and nonrebreather mask. These low-flow delivery systems provide oxygen in concentrations that vary with the patient's respiratory pattern. The supplemental oxygen is mixed with the room air, which lowers the oxygen level that is actually delivered to the patient. The true amount of oxygen that is delivered to the patient, known as the fraction of inspired oxygen (FiO_2), cannot be determined and can vary according to the patient's ability to breathe (see Table 7.2 for details on obtaining an oxygen saturation reading).

Nasal Cannula

The nasal cannula device delivers oxygen through tubing that has two soft prongs on one end that are placed into the patient's nares (Fig. 7.1); the other end of the tubing is connected to an oxygen source. This is the most commonly used delivery system because it is more comfortable, mobile, easy to use, and less expensive than other delivery systems. The nasal cannula is used for patients who require low levels of oxygen to maintain adequate oxygenation, and it works well for the patient who has adequate ventilation but requires a higher oxygen concentration than what is available in room air. This delivery device of supplemental oxygen is used most commonly with patients in the hospital, long-term care units, and home settings. The oxygen concentrations of 24% (1 L/min) to 44% (6 L/min) are administered via the nasal cannula. Patients with chronic lung disease or those who require long-term oxygen therapy find the nasal cannula easy to use and comfortable to wear. The patient who retains CO_2, such as the patient with COPD, will use the lower amount of oxygen (1–2 L/min) so that the patient does not lose the hypoxic drive to breathe. The oxygen can be humidified when it is passed through a bubbling humidifier of sterile water to decrease the risk of irritation to the nasal passage and drying of the mucous membranes. The area behind the ears where the oxygen tubing is placed, as well as the nasal septum, should be assessed for skin breakdown.

Face Masks

Face masks are used when a patient requires a higher oxygen concentration. There are several different types of masks used, including simple, partial rebreather, and nonrebreather masks. The mask should fit properly on the patient's face, covering the patient's mouth and nose, and is kept in place with elastic straps that go around the head. This delivery system is hard to use on a patient who is anxious or claustrophobic. Assess for skin breakdown under the mask and behind the ears. The disadvantage to the face mask is that it must be removed for the patient to eat. The patient is placed on a nasal cannula when eating, and the mask is replaced after eating.

Simple Face Mask

The simple face mask (Fig. 7.2) is used when the patient needs a moderate amount of oxygen to maintain an adequate PaO_2 level. This device uses oxygen flow rates between 5 and 10 L/min and can deliver oxygen concentrations from 40% to 60%. The amount of oxygen that the patient receives depends on the patient's respiratory pattern and proper fitting of the mask. The higher flow rate (5–10 L/min) assists the patient in preventing rebreathing of exhaled CO_2 that can be retained in the mask, thus delivering more oxygen. Rebreathing exhaled CO_2 may lead to complications such as hypoxemia because the patient does not receive an adequate supply of oxygen. This device is used for short-term oxygen therapy and is useful when transporting a patient.

Table 7.2 Obtaining an Oxygen Saturation Reading

Action	Rationale
Wash hands.	Decreases transmission of microorganisms
Explain the procedure to the patient and/or family members.	Informs patient and family of the purpose of procedure and decreases anxiety and apprehension about procedure
Select a sensor site; the finger is used most frequently. Remove nail polish.	Nail polish decreases light transmission and alters reading of the pulse oximeter.
Choose a site that has signs of adequate perfusion (warm skin, adequate capillary refill) and is free of moisture.	Peripheral vasoconstriction, edema, and moisture can interfere with the SpO_2 reading because of decreased circulation to these areas.
Apply the sensor to allow the light source to be directly opposite the light detector.	This allows for proper determination of the pulse oximetry reading.
Turn device on when sensor is in place.	Allows time for self-testing and detection of the waveforms before values are displayed
Determine accuracy of detected waveform by comparing the displayed pulse rate on the device to the simultaneously assessed heart rate of the patient.	If the pulse rate detected by the oximeter does not correlate with the patient's actual heart rate, the oximeter is not detecting sufficient arterial blood flow. Consider reapplying the sensor again or attaching the sensor to another area such as the earlobe.
Leave sensor in place until oximeter displays constant value and pulse display reaches full strength.	Reading usually takes 10–30 seconds depending on the site used.
Monitor for excessive movement.	Movement may result in a false reading; ask the patient to rest the hand on a flat surface.
If monitoring oxygen saturation continuously, assess the SpO_2 alarm limits that are set. The alarms are usually preset by the manufacturer.	Alarms should be set to alert the nurse of any changes in the patient's condition.
Assess skin integrity under the sensor every 4 hours and adjust pulse oximeter as needed.	The sensor can cause skin irritation or tissue ischemia.
If SpO_2 is assessed intermittently, remove probe and turn device off.	Allows for the patient to continue with activities. Batteries will not last if device is left on.
Wash hands.	Decreases transmission of microorganisms
Documentation includes the SpO_2 results, type and amount of oxygen therapy delivered, vital signs, and education provided to patient and/or family.	Readings are one segment of a complete evaluation of the patient. This allows for comparing of patient data and monitoring for any changes in the patient's condition.

Partial Rebreather Mask

A partial rebreather is a simple mask with a reservoir bag attached (Fig. 7.3). The patient breathes in the oxygen from the reservoir bag; on exhalation, the bag refills with oxygen, and the exhaled gases exit through small holes on both sides of the mask. This allows for a greater concentration of oxygen to be delivered to the patient than with the simple face mask. Oxygen flow must be maintained to keep the reservoir bag one-third to one-half full on inspiration. Maintaining a flow rate of 8 to 10 L/min to this device can provide 50% to 75% oxygen to the patient. This device is useful for short-term oxygen therapy.

Nonrebreather Mask

A nonrebreather mask is similar to the partial rebreather mask except this mask has one-way valves (Fig. 7.4). There is a one-way valve between the bag and the mask that prevents the exhaled air from entering the bag, thus ensuring a higher/more accurate oxygen concentration in the reservoir. This device also has one-way valves on both sides of the mask to prevent room air from entering the mask on inhalation. The reservoir bag must be kept inflated at one-third to one-half full on inspiration so that the patient receives the optimal amount of oxygen, and there should be a minimal flow rate of 10 L/min to maintain bag inflation. The nonrebreather mask can provide up to 90% oxygen to the patient.

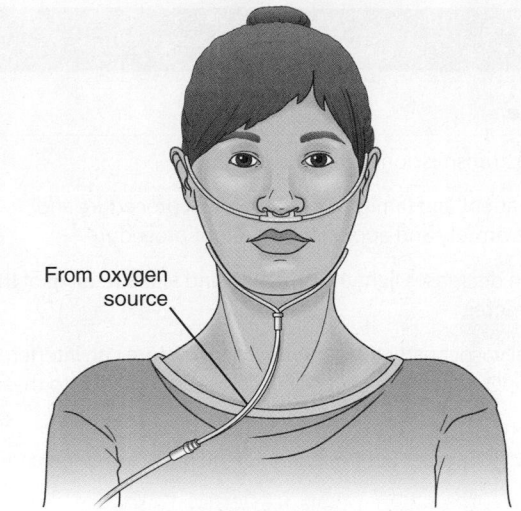

FIGURE 7.1 Nasal cannula.

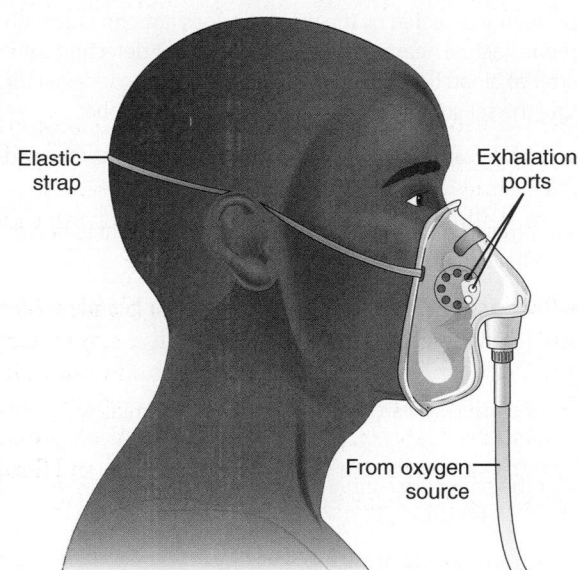

FIGURE 7.2 Simple face mask.

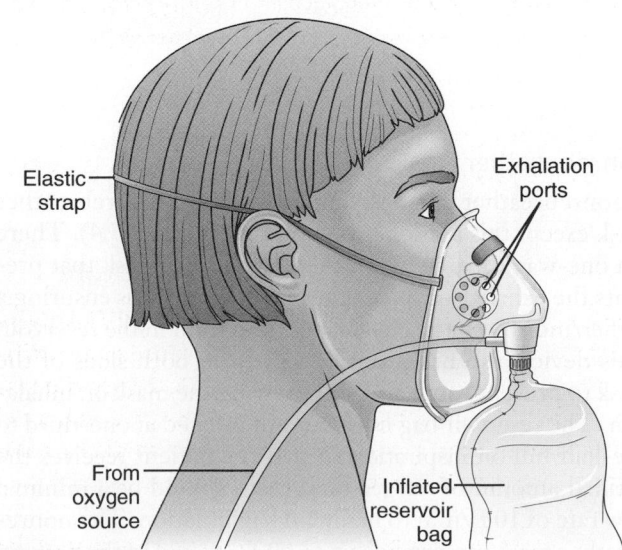

FIGURE 7.3 Partial rebreather.

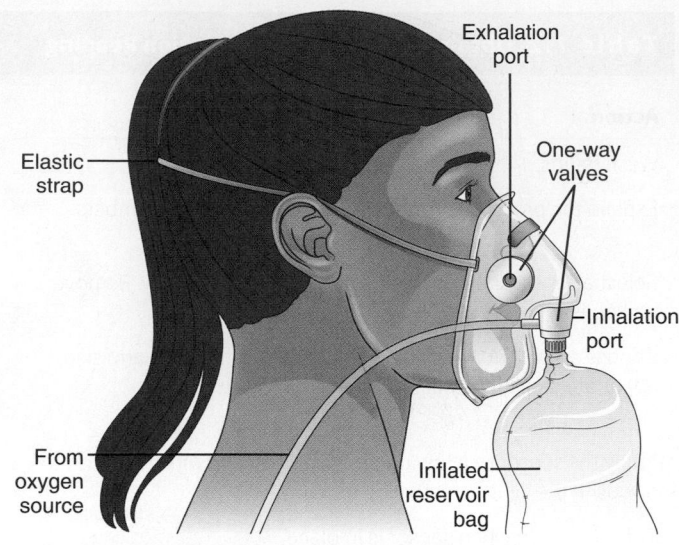

FIGURE 7.4 Nonrebreather mask.

High-Flow Delivery Devices

High-flow delivery devices include the Venturi mask, aerosol mask, tracheostomy collar, T-piece adapter, and face tent. These high-flow devices deliver set oxygen concentrations regardless of the patient's breathing pattern. Humidity is provided with the oxygen with specific devices. The oxygen source is passed through a humidifier that allows the oxygen concentration to be humidified before reaching the patient. The humidifier has a dial that is used to adjust the oxygen concentration being delivered to the patient. This provides the patient with oxygen concentrations of 24% to 100% with a minimal flow of 10 L/min.

Venturi Mask

The Venturi mask is the most commonly used high-flow delivery device because this device delivers the most accurate oxygen concentration (Fig. 7.5). This device can deliver oxygen concentrations of 24% to 60% by using different adapters and by adjusting the oxygen flow from 2 to 15 L/min. The adapter indicates the flow rate of oxygen that should be maintained to provide the prescribed percentage of oxygen to the patient. The mask is fitted to the face, and an adaptor is attached to the bottom of mask; the other end of the adapter is attached to the oxygen tubing, and then the tubing is connected to the oxygen source. There are Venturi masks that have an adapter with a dial to determine the oxygen concentration to be delivered to the patient. The patient with a chronic lung disorder benefits from this device because this device delivers a more accurate oxygen concentration to the patient on inspiration.

Aerosol Mask

The aerosol mask is indicated for the patient who requires high-humidity oxygen concentrations. The patients who benefit from aerosol masks are those who have been extubated (discontinuation of an endotracheal tube [ETT]), those who have had upper airway surgery, or those with thick secretions. This device delivers aerosol therapy that

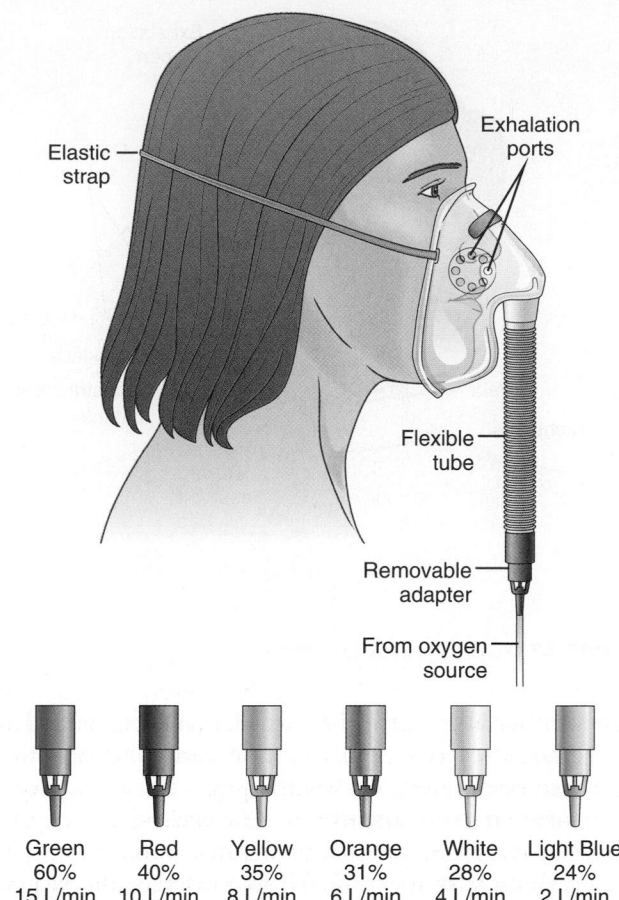

FIGURE 7.5 Venturi mask.

| Green 60% 15 L/min | Red 40% 10 L/min | Yellow 35% 8 L/min | Orange 31% 6 L/min | White 28% 4 L/min | Light Blue 24% 2 L/min |

Elastic strap — Exhalation ports — Flexible tube — Removable adapter — From oxygen source

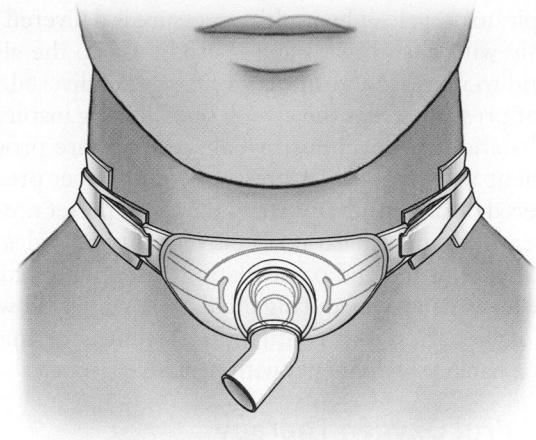

FIGURE 7.6 Tracheostomy collar.

includes humidification and/or medications in order to liquefy secretions for easier removal. It is also used to humidify the respiratory tract, relieve **bronchospasm** (contraction of the smooth muscles of the bronchioles), and reduce edema of the respiratory tract.

Tracheostomy Collar

The tracheostomy collar is used for patients with a tracheostomy. This device allows humidified oxygen to be delivered to the patient via the tracheostomy collar because the air is inhaled directly through the tracheostomy and bypasses the usual humidification and filtration processes provided by the nose and mouth. This collar fits over the tracheostomy site, and there are adjustable straps that fit around the patient's neck (Fig. 7.6). The device provides high humidity with the prescribed oxygen concentration.

T-Piece Adapter

The T-piece adapter, much like the tracheostomy collar, is a device that may be used when weaning a patient from the **mechanical ventilator** who still has an endotracheal, nasotracheal, or tracheostomy tube in place. This device connects an oxygen source with humidification to the ETT or tracheostomy tube. The T-piece adaptor provides high humidity with the desired oxygen concentration and allows a spontaneous breathing trial (SBT) to be performed prior to extubating the patient. The SBT requires the patient to

maintain spontaneous breathing through the T-piece adapter.

Face Tent

The face tent is a device used for patients who have facial trauma, have burns, or have had upper airway surgery. The device fits under the chin and extends just above the ears. This device allows the delivery of oxygen mixed with a mist.

High-Flow Nasal Cannula

High-flow nasal cannula uses an air-oxygen blender (blends O_2 with compressed air), active humidifier, single heated tube, and nasal cannula to deliver heated and humidified medical gas up to 60 L/min. The advantages include reduced anatomical dead space, positive end-expiratory pressure (PEEP), constant FIO_2, and humidification. Soft and flexible nasal prongs are used for the comfort of the patient.

Connection Check 7.2

The nurse is reviewing orders on the patient who is to receive supplemental oxygen. It is a priority for the nurse to follow up with the provider about which order?

A. Nasal cannula at 2 L/min
B. Venturi mask at 24% concentration
C. Nasal cannula at 8 L/min
D. Venturi mask at 50% concentration

Noninvasive Positive-Pressure Ventilation

Noninvasive positive-pressure ventilation (NPPV) delivers positive pressure to the airway without the use of an artificial airway to keep the alveoli open and decreases the risk of nosocomial infections. The positive pressure is delivered to the patient using a nasal mask, a full face mask, or nasal pillows. The patient can receive **continuous positive airway pressure (CPAP)** or **bi-level positive airway pressure (BIPAP)**. Continuous positive airway pressure provides the patient with a preset, continuous positive pressure throughout the respiratory cycle. The positive pressure is delivered continuously with each breath and is used to keep the alveoli open and to increase the amount of oxygen delivered. The constant pressure keeps the alveoli open during inspiration and exhalation. Bi-level positive airway pressure provides the patient with two preset pressures; one preset pressure is delivered during inspiration, and the other preset pressure is delivered during exhalation. This modality provides positive pressure at the end of exhalation along with a higher positive airway pressure during inhalation, which allows for better oxygenation and ventilation. A ventilator may be used as a backup for patients with periods of apnea.

Long-Term Oxygen Therapy

Long-term oxygen therapy may be indicated for the treatment of hypoxemia in patients with a diagnosis of COPD or with specific clinical conditions associated with hypoxemia, such as heart failure, cystic fibrosis, or sleep apnea. Indications for long-term oxygen therapy include a PaO_2 level less than or equal to 55 mm Hg or an SaO_2 level less than or equal to 88% in patients breathing room air or a PaO_2 of 55 to 59 mm Hg or SaO_2 less than or equal to 89% with specific clinical conditions such as cor pulmonale, heart failure, or polycythemia greater than 55%. Some of these patients may not meet the criteria for continuous home oxygen therapy but may develop hypoxemia during exercise, ambulation, or during sleep. The indication for oxygen therapy during specific activities, but not continuously, includes an SaO_2 level falling to levels less than or equal to 90%. The nasal cannula can be used for continuous or intermittent oxygen therapy in the home.

Transtracheal oxygen therapy (TTOT) is another option for long-term oxygen therapy for patients and delivers oxygen directly into the trachea using a small, flexible, plastic catheter (Fig. 7.7). Surgical placement can be done as an outpatient under local anesthesia (modified Seldinger technique), or placement can be done as an inpatient using conscious sedation anesthesia. Advantages to using TTOT over a nasal cannula include less nasal and ear irritation and the catheter being less visible. Some patients have been shown to have a reduction in oxygen flow requirements by 50% to 60% in resting oxygen flow rate and a 30% decrease with activity. The patient and caregiver must be educated on the TTOT procedure, care of the tracheal stoma (opening into the trachea created by the tracheostomy), replacement of the catheter, home oxygen use, and mucus problems that may develop when using TTOT. The TTOT team provides the education and support for the patient and caregiver.

Oxygen Delivery

The nurse instructs the patient and/or caregiver in oxygen safety and informs the patient and/or caregiver of the different ways oxygen is available. Oxygen is available in liquid oxygen, compressed oxygen, or as an oxygen concentrator. Liquid oxygen is made by cooling the oxygen gas, changing it to a liquid. Liquid oxygen is often used for people who are more active because large amounts of oxygen can be stored

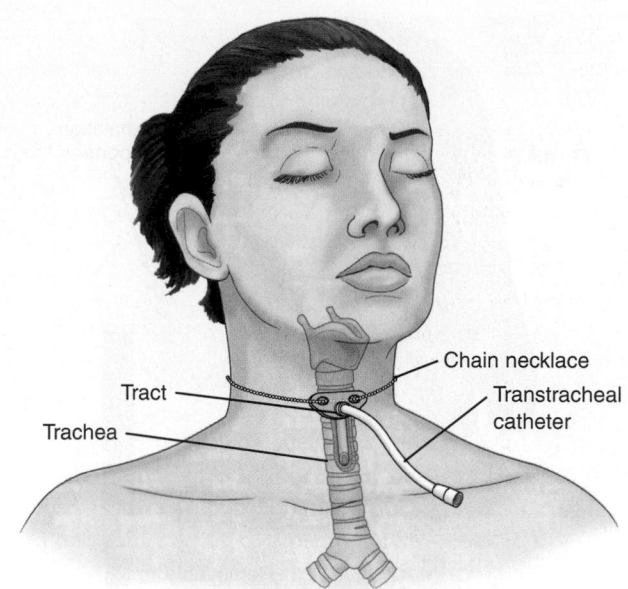

FIGURE 7.7 Transtracheal oxygen therapy.

in smaller portable units. These smaller units can be refilled from a large reservoir canister. The disadvantage is that there is an evaporation loss when the canisters are not used.

An **oxygen concentrator** is an electrical device that produces oxygen by removing nitrogen, water vapor, and hydrocarbons that are in the air and extracts the oxygen. The advantage of this system is that it does not need to be resupplied and is less expensive than liquid oxygen. Oxygen concentrators can deliver oxygen at concentrations of 85% or greater and include stationary devices, portable devices, and systems that can transfill oxygen cylinders. This method is less expensive and easy to maintain, and the concentrator runs on electricity or a battery. The disadvantages are that some devices are noisy, and people may need a backup source of oxygen in case of a power failure.

Compressed oxygen is stored under pressure and can be supplied in large cylinders to be used as stationary units in the home. The large tanks are heavy and can be used only in a stationary manner. Smaller units are available for portability and as backup units in case of a power failure or equipment malfunction. See Box 7.1 for instructions for in-home oxygen use.

A respiratory therapist is involved in the transition from the hospital to the use of long-term oxygen in the home. Respiratory therapists assess, treat, and evaluate patients with respiratory or cardiopulmonary disorders. They consult with other healthcare professionals and practice under the direction of the healthcare provider.

> **!** **Safety Alert** The Joint Commission's 2014 National Patient Safety Goals require a home safety risk assessment that includes a functional smoke detector, fire extinguisher, and home safety plan.

Box 7.1 Education for Patients Receiving Home Oxygen

- The referral agency for home oxygen equipment contacts the patient and/or caregiver to set a delivery time for oxygen equipment and supplies to the home.
- The agency sends a respiratory therapist or a home health nurse to demonstrate the use, care, and cleaning of the equipment.
- There are three types of oxygen sources that are available: liquid oxygen, compressed gas, and an oxygen concentrator.
- The education starts in the hospital and continues on discharge to home.
- Explain and educate the patient and caregiver.
- Oxygen is a fire hazard. Oxygen makes a flame burn hotter and faster.
- Never smoke or let anyone smoke while oxygen is in use.
- Place "No Smoking" signs within the home.
- Keep oxygen at least 6 feet away from flames or heat sources, such as gas stoves, space heaters, candles, and fireplaces.
- Check all electrical equipment that is within the same room as the oxygen for frayed cords.
- Keep a fire extinguisher in the home near the oxygen source.
- Store and keep oxygen tanks in an upright position.
- Do not change the settings of the oxygen without the healthcare provider's permission.
- Check the amount of oxygen in the tank and order more in advance so that it does not run out.
- Always have extra equipment and supplies in case of an emergency.
- Discuss an emergency plan; in case of power failure, call 9-1-1.
- Observe the tops of the ears and behind the ears for skin breakdown; the ears may be padded if irritation is noted.
- Assess oral and nasal passages for dryness and/or irritation; water-based gel may be used for protection.

COMPLICATIONS OF OXYGEN THERAPY

Oxygen Toxicity

Oxygen toxicity can develop as a result of the administration of an oxygen concentration equal to or greater than 50% over 24 to 48 hours. The high levels of oxygen can cause damage to the alveolar-capillary membrane and inactivate surfactant production in the lungs. Loss of surfactant production can result in the walls of the alveoli sticking together and collapsing. The collapse of the alveoli makes it very difficult to reinflate the alveoli, and they can become filled with fluid or blood if there is damage to the alveoli. This can lead to pulmonary edema, **atelectasis** (collapse of alveoli), and hemorrhage and can progress to acute respiratory distress syndrome (ARDS). Prevention of oxygen toxicity is essential for patients who are receiving oxygen therapy and can be facilitated by administering the lowest oxygen concentration to maintain the PaO_2 level within the patient's normal range.

Absorption Atelectasis

Absorption atelectasis occurs when high levels of oxygen are administered and cause the alveoli to collapse. The high levels of oxygen dilute the nitrogen that normally prevents the alveoli from collapsing and replace nitrogen with oxygen in the alveoli. The high level of oxygen causes the nitrogen to be "washed out" of the alveoli. The oxygen diffuses from the alveoli into the bloodstream faster than it is replaced by inhaled oxygen, causing the alveoli to collapse.

Mucous Membrane Dryness

Oxygen has a drying effect on the mucous membranes because the humidification of the inspired air is lessened for the patient who is receiving oxygen therapy. When oxygen therapy is prescribed at levels greater than 4 L/min via nasal cannula, humidification should be added. The humidification occurs when the oxygen is passed through sterile water, causing bubbling in the container, and then goes through the tubing to the patient's mask or cannula. This process restores the humidity that is normally present in the room air.

Infection

Oxygen therapy can be a potential cause of infection. The equipment used to deliver oxygen, such as the humidifier, nebulizer, nasal cannula, oxygen tubing, and/or masks, can be a source of bacteria causing infection due to moisture that may accumulate. Healthcare facilities have protocols and/or policies in place that state when the equipment is to be changed to prevent the cause of infection.

Precautions in Oxygen Therapy

Delivering oxygen to patients with COPD may inhibit their stimulus to breathe. In patients with chronic lung disease such as COPD, the stimulus for breathing is hypoxia rather than an increase in CO_2 levels. The central chemoreceptors located in the medulla are normally sensitive to the increased arterial carbon dioxide ($PaCO_2$) levels. These receptors stimulate breathing and increase the respiratory rate. Patients with chronic lung disease have a gradual increase in $PaCO_2$ levels; thus, the normal stimulus to breathe is diminished. The respiratory center becomes less sensitive to the elevated CO_2 levels that usually stimulate the respiratory center, and the stimulus to breathe becomes the low arterial oxygen (PaO_2) levels. The decreased oxygen levels are sensed by the peripheral chemoreceptors located in the aortic arch and the carotid sinuses. These oxygen receptors then take over as the primary drive to breathe in the patient with chronic lung disease; this is called the hypoxic drive. This physiological change requires the nurse to titrate the oxygen to meet the individual needs of the patient with COPD.

In the management of the patient with chronic lung disease receiving oxygen therapy, it is important to frequently assess the patient for any changes in oxygen saturation, level of consciousness, and rate and depth of respirations as well as to frequently monitor ABG results. Oxygen-induced hypoventilation may be a concern for patients with chronic lung disease, but not treating the hypoxia is a greater threat to the patient. Withholding oxygen therapy can lead to greater hypoxia and can threaten life. Oxygen therapy is ordered at the lowest level of oxygen needed to treat the hypoxemia.

Connection Check 7.3

What is the most important information for the nurse to include in the teaching plan about the management of home oxygen therapy? *(Select all that apply.)*

A. Do not change the settings of the oxygen without the healthcare provider's permission.
B. Place "No Smoking" signs within the home.
C. Oxygen is a fire hazard.
D. Others may smoke around you as long as you do not smoke.
E. Keep a fire extinguisher near the oxygen source.

Connection Check 7.4

The nurse is caring for a patient who is receiving oxygen therapy via the Venturi mask. Which complications are associated with oxygen therapy? *(Select all that apply.)*

A. Oxygen toxicity
B. Cachexia
C. Bradycardia
D. Absorption atelectasis
E. Increased dead space

INVASIVE OXYGEN DELIVERY

Artificial Airways

Airway management is the first priority for clinical care and involves maintaining a patent passage for the inhaled air to move through the upper airways to the lower airways to achieve adequate ventilation. The upper and lower airways can become narrowed or blocked as a result of secretions, a foreign object, or constriction of the airways. An airway that is not patent leads to oxygen deprivation. Without oxygen, cells begin to die, and death of the patient may result within minutes. Through the use of artificial airways, the patient can be ventilated and provided with adequate oxygen to maintain tissue perfusion.

Endotracheal Tube

An endotracheal tube (ETT) is an artificial airway used to maintain a patent airway when a patient is having respiratory distress. An ETT is a long tube made of polyvinyl chloride that is passed either nasally or orally through the vocal cords into the trachea and is placed just above the carina (the point where the trachea divides into the left and right

mainstem bronchi (Fig. 7.8). The cuff (an inflatable balloon that encircles the lower end of the ETT) is inflated to prevent air from leaking around the ETT, to minimize the risk for aspiration and to secure the ETT in place. Adult sizes range from 7.5 to 9.0 mm. Oral intubation is preferred over nasal intubation because it is quicker and allows visualization of the vocal cords during intubation, as opposed to nasal intubation, which is considered "blind" intubation because the vocal cords cannot be seen during the procedure. Nasal intubation is used when the patient has facial or oral trauma or when oral intubation is not possible. The patient may develop sinusitis after nasal intubation. A certified nurse anesthetist, anesthesiologist, pulmonologist,

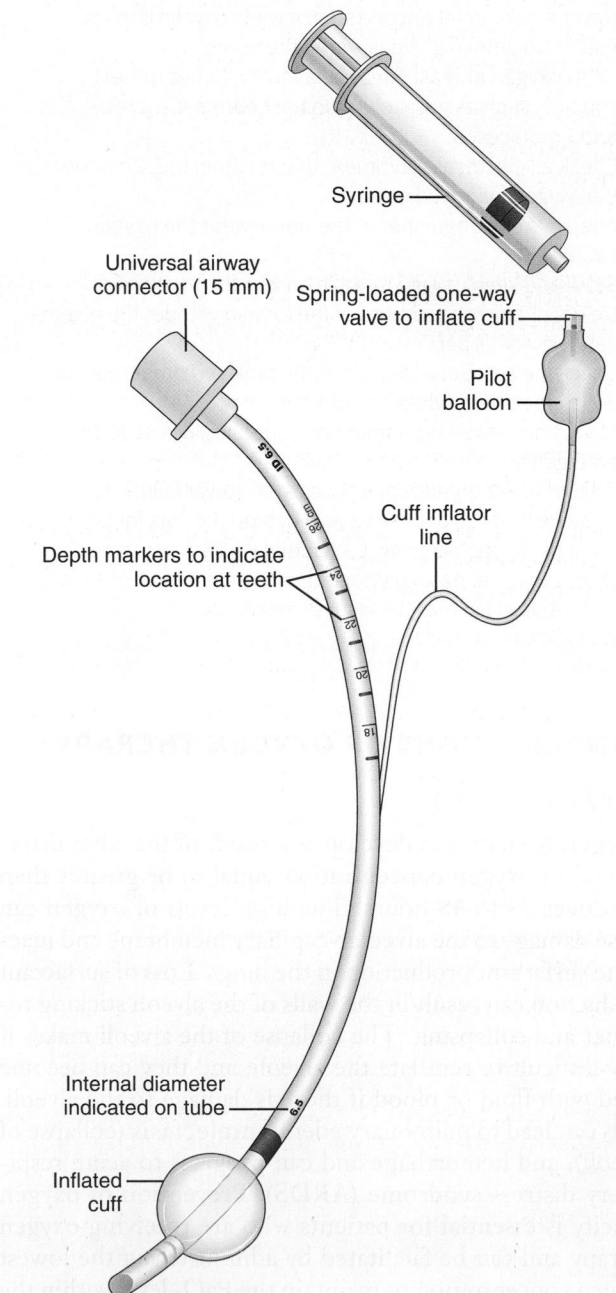

FIGURE 7.8 Endotracheal tube (ETT).

intensivist, or acute care nurse practitioner usually performs the intubation.

Indications

Endotracheal tubes are indicated when there is upper airway obstruction, apnea, high risk for aspiration, ineffective airway clearance, and/or respiratory distress. These tubes are also placed to deliver general anesthesia via an endotracheal tube and may be required after the surgical procedure to maintain the airway. In all of these situations, there is a need for assistance to maintain adequate ventilation and perfusion.

Nursing Considerations

An interprofessional team approach is used when a patient requires intubation. The nurse ensures all needed personnel are at the bedside, including anesthesia, the healthcare provider, the respiratory therapist, and other nurses to assist in the procedure. Considerations include the following:

- Explain the procedure and the reason for intubation to the patient (if patient is able to understand) and family members.

- Maintain proper airway management using a manual resuscitation bag with a face mask connected to 100% oxygen source throughout the intubation procedure.
- Position the intubation tray at the bedside.
- Ensure suction is available throughout the procedure to ensure a patent airway.

During intubation, the nurse coordinates the care of the patient. The nurse continuously monitors the patient, including vital signs; continuous pulse oximetry; and signs of hypoxia, dysrhythmias, and aspiration. If intubation takes longer than 15 to 30 seconds, the intubation needs to stop, the patient is manually ventilated to prevent hypoxia or cardiac arrest, and then a second attempt to place the ETT is initiated (Table 7.3). It is often the responsibility of the nurse to ensure that the procedure is stopped in the event that the attempted intubation exceeds 30 seconds.

Once the patient is intubated, endotracheal placement is verified by an end-tidal CO_2 device, indicating CO_2 is released in expired air from the lungs. If the tube is inadvertently placed in the esophagus, the end-tidal CO_2 is negative. The nurse also verifies proper placement by assessing

Table 7.3 Process for Endotracheal Intubation

Action	Rationale
Preparation	
Explain the procedure and the reason for intubation to the patient (if patient is able to understand) and family members.	Allows for cooperation by the patient and less anxiety and apprehension by the family and patient
Maintain proper airway management using a manual resuscitation bag with face mask connected to 100% oxygen source throughout the intubation procedure.	Proper oxygenation prevents hypoxia that can lead to decreased cerebral perfusion and possibly death.
The healthcare provider, nurse, anesthesia provider, and respiratory therapist will all assist in the intubation procedure.	An interprofessional team meets the needs of the patient.
The nurse ensures all equipment is at the bedside and properly functioning. An intubation tray is positioned at the bedside for use by the anesthesia provider during intubation. Respiratory therapy brings the ventilator to the bedside.	Functioning equipment is required for a successful intubation. Most intubation trays include laryngoscopes, endotracheal tubes (ETTs) of different sizes, lubricant, stylet, syringe for balloon inflation, oral airways, Magill forceps, and CO_2 detector; an ETT holder should be available once the ETT is in place. The nurse makes sure all materials are present and functioning.
Restraints may be required; assess need once patient is intubated.	Prevents accidental extubation by patient
Suction setup is ready to be used throughout the procedure to ensure a patent airway: Yankauer for oral secretions and in-line suction once the patient has been intubated.	Removes increased secretions to allow for proper oxygenation
Personal protective equipment is made available to all the staff members who will be assisting in the intubation procedure.	Decreases transmission of microorganisms and secretions
Wash hands.	Decreases transmission of microorganisms

Continued

Table 7.3 Process for Endotracheal Intubation—cont'd

Action	Rationale
Intubation Process	
Premedicate as required to promote patient compliance and decrease anxiety.	To facilitate endotracheal intubation, the provider will sedate the patient prior to the procedure. In some instances, a paralytic is also used, and in these cases a sedative must be administered.
The patient's head is placed in the "sniff" position.	This allows for easier access/visualization to the vocal cords for intubation.
Prior to intubation, the patient is hyperoxygenated with 100% O_2.	Provides protection from suction-induced hypoxia
The anesthesia provider inserts the laryngoscope into the patient's mouth until the vocal cords are seen; the ETT is inserted through the vocal cords and stops above the carina.	The ETT is placed above the carina where the trachea branches into the right and left bronchioles; this allows for adequate oxygenation.
The cuff of the ETT is inflated, and either respiratory therapy or the nurse assesses for bilateral lung sounds; a CO_2 detector is used to assist in verifying placement.	To ensure proper placement of the ETT
Secure the ETT with the ETT holder.	Assists in maintaining proper positioning of the ETT
The patient is attached to the ventilator, and settings are ordered by the healthcare provider.	A closed system between the patient and the ventilator allows for proper ventilation for the patient.
Placement of an orogastric tube (OGT) or nasogastric tube (NGT) can be performed at this time. Proper verification of placement can be done.	This allows for proper nutrition and for medication administration.
A portable chest x-ray is ordered, and then daily chest x-rays are ordered.	To ensure proper placement of ETT and OGT/NGT.
Note tube placement at the lip or teeth and chart/report at change of shift.	This information allows for monitoring tube placement. If the tube requires adjustment, the respiratory therapist or registered nurse will adjust.
Management	
Assess frequently for change in vital signs, pulse oximetry (or can place SpO_2), respiratory status, cardiac rhythm, and level of consciousness.	The information reflects the patient's status for ventilation and oxygenation.
Monitor ventilator settings and alarm settings.	The priority is proper ventilation and oxygenation of the patient. When alarms are not immediately corrected, disconnect the patient from the ventilator and manually ventilate the patient.
Assess for suctioning needs every 2 hours along with lung sounds bilaterally in all lobes.	Suctioning assists the patient in removing secretions from the airways; assessing lung sounds provides information for the need to suction and proper ETT placement.
Check the water level for proper humidification.	Humidification allows for increases in secretion movement.
Empty the water that collects in the tubing delivering oxygen to the patient into a separate container.	If water collects in the delivery tubing, it leads to increased work for the ventilator to maintain proper oxygen flow. This results in increases in the peak airway (inspiratory) pressure and an area for microorganism production. Water accumulation in the tubing may also make the high-pressure alarm sound.
Check cuff pressure every 4 hours to maintain proper cuff inflation (usually done by respiratory therapy).	Cuff pressure that is too high causes ischemia in surrounding tissue. Cuff pressure that is too low allows for possible accidental extubation and aspiration. Low pressures may also interfere with the delivery of the ordered tidal volume.
Keep HOB elevated at 30 degrees and provide mouth care every 2 hours, daily sedation vacations, GI prophylaxis, and DVT prophylaxis.	These are the ventilator bundles used to decrease ventilator-associated pneumonia (see Evidence-Based Practice: What Is the ABCDEF Bundle?).

DVT = Deep vein thrombosis; GI = gastrointestinal; HOB = head of bed.

Evidence-Based Practice

What Is the ABCDEF Bundle?

The ABCDEF bundle is an evidence-based approach to caring for critically ill patients at the bedside, designed to prevent oversedation, prolonged ventilation, delirium, and other complications associated with unwanted outcomes of critically ill patients.

A = Assess, prevent, and manage pain

B = Both spontaneous awakening trials and spontaneous breathing trials

C = Choice of analgesia and sedation

D = Delirium—assess, prevent, and manage

E = Early exercise/ambulation

F = Family engagement and empowerment

Marra, A., Ely, E. W., Pandharipande, P. P., & Patel, M. B. (2017). The ABCDEF bundle in critical care. *Critical Care Clinics, 33*(2), 225–243.

for symmetrical chest rise and fall with ventilation, equal and bilateral lung sounds, no sounds heard over the abdomen, and an order for a portable chest x-ray to confirm placement. If lung sounds and chest wall movement are present only on the right side of the chest, the ETT may have been placed in the right main bronchus. Right mainstem bronchus intubation occurs because the right bronchus has a lesser angle to the trachea and is often wider than the left bronchus. With right mainstem intubation, the ETT needs to be repositioned and reassessed for correct placement.

The ETT is stabilized by inflating the ETT cuff with 20 to 25 mm Hg of air. High cuff pressures can result in ischemia to the surrounding tissue, pressure necrosis, and tracheal bleeding. Low cuff pressures can result in aspiration of secretions, inability to deliver effective ventilations, and unwanted early intubation. An ETT holder device assists in maintaining proper placement of the ETT. The ETT has centimeter markings on the tube, and the nurse documents at what centimeter the ETT is placed at the level of the teeth or lip. If the patient bites the ETT, this will temporarily occlude the tube, and an oral airway may be needed to ensure the patient receives the needed ventilator support by preventing biting.

The administration of a sedative, a paralytic, and an analgesic medication during the intubation procedure of the patient must be considered. This will decrease the risk of aspiration and injury to the patient. The goals for sedation and analgesics in a patient being intubated and placed on a mechanical ventilator are focused on providing comfort for the patient and maintaining synchrony between the patient's breathing and the mechanical ventilator rate.

ETT Management

The nurse documents the intubation procedure, including a complete assessment of the patient, the ETT size, the ETT position, the location of the ETT (centimeter marking at the lip, teeth, or gum), the ventilator settings, and the patient's response to the procedure.

The role of the nurse is to ensure proper ETT management by maintaining a patent airway, monitoring the patient for complications, maintaining proper cuff inflation, providing oral care and suctioning as needed, maintaining correct tube placement, monitoring oxygenation and vital signs, and educating the patient and family members. This role is shared with the respiratory therapist, who works closely with the nurses in managing the patient who has an ETT and is also being mechanically ventilated. The respiratory therapist maintains the proper cuff pressure, assesses the patient frequently, adjusts the ETT on an as-needed basis, gives ordered respiratory treatments, and obtains the ABGs when ordered. In some settings, the nurse may be the person responsible for repositioning the ETT and obtaining ABG samples.

Communication is often difficult with a mechanically ventilated patient. Using different methods of communication is important to assist the patient in communicating with the interprofessional team and family members. There are various ways to communicate with the patient that can minimize feelings of isolation, frustration, and anxiety about the care and the surroundings. Despite the inability of the patient to speak, there are methods available to assist the patient. Intubated patients can communicate with their family members and the interprofessional team through letter and picture boards, writing paper, gestures, or lip reading. Explain the equipment and the patient's surroundings to the patient to help alleviate stress and anxiety.

Connection Check 7.5

The nurse is caring for a patient who has just been orally intubated. Which action should the nurse take first?

A. Assess for symmetrical chest rise and fall with ventilation.

B. Provide mouth care to ensure a clean oral cavity.

C. Assess the need for nutritional support through an oral nasogastric tube.

D. Provide a communication board for the patient and family.

Suctioning is required in a patient with an artificial airway to remove secretions and to maintain a patent airway, and it allows for optimal ventilation and oxygenation in the patient who is unable to clear secretions. Swallowing is impaired due to the placement of the ETT. An in-line suction system device may be used in a patient who has an artificial airway and is receiving mechanical ventilation. The in-line suction catheter prevents the interruption of ventilation and oxygenation that the patient is receiving by the ventilator. These devices are known to decrease infection rates and allow for suctioning of the lower airway.

Suctioning increases the risk for hypoxemia and bronchospasm, so suction only as needed. Assess the patient to determine if suctioning is necessary because some patients require suctioning every 1 to 2 hours, whereas other patients may require less suctioning. To determine if the patient requires suctioning, assess breath sounds for wheezes, crackles, and/or rhonchi; these sounds may indicate a need for suctioning (Table 7.4). Other indications may include coughing, audible secretions, increase in pulse or respirations, decreased SaO_2 level, visible secretions, and/or restlessness (Table 7.5).

Table 7.4 Characteristics of Breath Sounds

	Character	Indication
Wheezes	Musical High pitched Squeaking	Air squeezed through narrowed passages caused by secretions, bronchospasm, edema, inflammation
Crackles	Loud, low-pitched, bubbling, and gurgling sound	On inhalation, air comes in contact with secretions in the trachea and large bronchi.
Rhonchi	Musical Low pitched Snoring/moaning	Airflow obstruction from thick secretions or fluid in the large airways

Table 7.5 Suctioning Using In-Line or Closed Suction Catheters

Steps	Rationale
Wash hands and put on protective equipment.	Reduces transmission of microorganisms
Explain procedure to patient and family members if present at the time of the procedure; encourage patient to cough to assist in removing the secretions if patient is alert.	Explaining the procedure will reduce the likelihood of apprehension and anxiety.
Place patient in a semi-Fowler's position.	Elevating the HOB will allow for easier ventilation for the patient.
Continuously monitor patient's cardiac rhythm, BP, pulse, respiration, and SaO_2 level before, during, and after the procedure.	Monitoring the patient for changes in VS can alert the nurse to complications such as dysrhythmias, decreased oxygenation, and vagal response that may occur during this procedure.
Attach the in-line suction catheter or closed suction catheter system to suction.	Attaching the catheter to suction allows for removal of secretions from the airways.
Turn on suction and set suction vacuum up to 160 mm Hg.	This level of suction allows for adequate negative-pressure suctioning.
Hyperoxygenate the patient by activating the 100% oxygen button on the ventilator. The 100% oxygen button that is located on the ventilator provides 100% oxygen for approximately 2 minutes.	Hyperoxygenation assists in providing protection from suction-induced hypoxia.
Insert the catheter quickly without applying suction, far enough to stimulate the cough reflex.	Applying suction during catheter insertion increases the risk of hypoxia and trauma to tissue.
Apply suction and rotate catheter as the catheter is gently withdrawn, with each suctioning event lasting no longer than 10 seconds.	Suctioning for longer than 10 seconds can cause hypoxia, cardiopulmonary compromise, or vagal response.
Hyperoxygenate the patient again with 100% of FiO_2 via the ventilator 100% oxygen button.	Hyperoxygenation assists in providing protection from suction-induced hypoxia.
If secretions are still present, repeat the procedure with a maximum of three passes of catheter; provide a rest period of 10–20 seconds between suction procedures.	Suctioning can produce hypoxia, dysrhythmias, and bronchospasm. Repeated suctioning can remove excessive secretions.

Table 7.5 Suctioning Using In-Line or Closed Suction Catheters—cont'd

Steps	Rationale
Rinse the catheter with sterile saline solution while maintaining suction. This allows the saline to rinse the catheter without the saline going into the artificial airway. This is done between passes of the catheter and when the procedure is done.	Secretions that remain in the suction catheter can reduce the catheter's ability to remove excessive secretions.
Suction the patient's mouth and, if indicated, provide mouth care to the patient; use a separate suction line when providing mouth care.	Removes upper airway secretions and microorganisms that may introduce infection
Check the ventilator settings.	Assessing the ventilator settings ensures that the settings are correct.
Assess the patient's breath sounds, VS, cardiac monitor, and SaO_2 and document findings after procedure.	Suctioning can induce cardiac dysrhythmias, hypoxia, and bronchospasm.
If at any time during the suctioning procedure the patient's pulse oximeter decreases or if the patient's heart rate decreases, stop suctioning and give 100% oxygen.	Suctioning can induce hypoxia and stimulate the vagal response.
Document procedure, color, consistency, and amount of secretions noted and patient's response in the medical records.	Provides information about the procedure, information about the secretions that may indicate infection, or change in secretions

BP = Blood pressure; HOB = head of bed; VS = vital signs.

Complications

Complications of endotracheal intubation include unplanned extubation, aspiration, and infection. Unplanned extubation can be caused by the patient pulling out the ETT or by unwanted movement of the ETT during repositioning or transfer of the patient. To prevent unplanned extubation, provide the patient with adequate sedation and analgesics, use soft wrist restraints only if necessary, and explain the reason for the ETT to the patient and family members. The nurse is responsible for ensuring that the ETT is in the proper position and is secure at all times during repositioning and transferring of the patient. If an unplanned extubation does occur, the nurse calls for assistance, stays with the patient, and provides airway management until assistance arrives and the patient is reintubated as indicated. Airway management includes proper head positioning of the patient to allow an open airway and manually ventilating the patient using a 100% oxygen source, usually a manual resuscitation bag.

During and after placement of an ETT, there is the risk for aspiration of gastric contents or aspiration of secretions because the ETT passes through the epiglottis, and the patient loses the protection of the epiglottis to prevent aspiration. The ETT does have an inflatable cuff, but this does not totally prevent aspiration from occurring. Other ways to prevent aspiration include maintaining the head-of-the-bed elevation above 30 degrees unless contraindicated (this minimizes aspiration of gastric secretions), providing frequent mouth care (this decreases the risk of colonization of the oral secretions that, if aspirated, can lead to an infection), suctioning of the mouth and above the cuff of the ETT (this decreases the likelihood of oral secretions pooling around the ETT), and maintaining proper inflation of the ETT cuff at 20 to 25 mm Hg (this decreases the incidence of oral secretions and/or gastric secretions from being aspirated into the lungs).

An ETT provides an opportunity for infection to occur because it bypasses the natural defenses provided by the upper airway. Continuous or intermittent subglottic suction is available with some ETTs; these ETTs include a subglottic suction adaptor that suctions at the area above the cuff to prevent secretions from going into the lungs and causing infection and aspiration.

Tracheostomy

If a patient requires mechanical ventilation for longer than 7 to 14 days, a tracheotomy is usually performed to prevent the laryngeal and upper airway damage that is associated with the prolonged use of an ETT. A tracheostomy is indicated to provide a stable airway in patients who require long-term ventilator support, to allow access to the lower airway for suctioning, and to relieve upper airway obstructions. The tracheostomy tube replaces the ETT and provides the patient with improved comfort and patient safety.

Advantages of a tracheostomy include decreasing airway resistance; allowing air to enter directly into the trachea and the lungs; allowing for decreased workload of breathing compared with air traveling from the upper airways to the lower airways; and allowing for improved oral care over the ETT, which is passed through the mouth, making oral care more difficult. Other advantages include improved airway security due to the fact that an ETT is not as secure as a tracheostomy tube, improved access for the removal of pulmonary secretions, and improved patient comfort. The tracheostomy tube allows the oral cavity to be free of tubes, making it easier for reading lips, and in time, patients may be able to eat with a tracheostomy in place (Fig. 7.9).

Endotracheal Tube   **Tracheostomy**

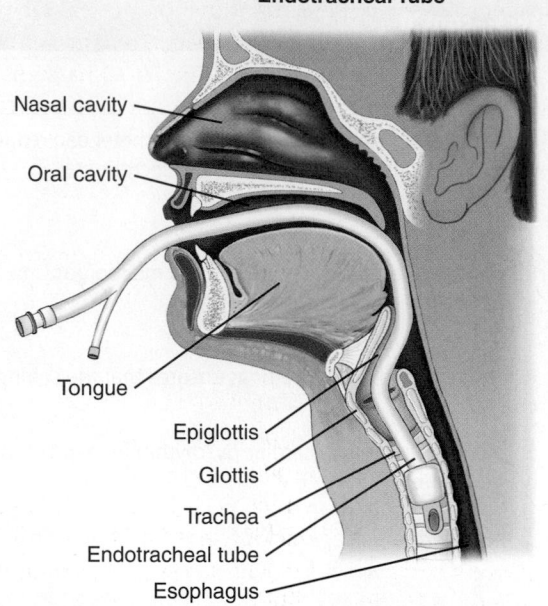

FIGURE 7.9 Endotracheal tube (ETT) versus tracheostomy.

Disadvantages of a tracheostomy are the inability to communicate verbally, similar to the patient with an ETT.

To perform a surgical tracheotomy, the patient's shoulders are elevated, and the head is extended. The skin over the second tracheal ring is identified, and a vertical incision of 2 to 3 cm in length is made (Fig. 7.10). A second incision is made entering the trachea. There are different techniques and incisions used, and they depend on the surgeon and the reason for the tracheostomy. Once the trachea has been entered, the tracheostomy tube is placed and secured with sutures and a tracheostomy tube holder, and a chest x-ray is ordered to ensure proper placement of the tracheostomy tube.

Tracheostomy tubes are permanent or temporary, and there are a number of different types and sizes of tracheostomy tubes. The type and size of the tracheostomy tube used depend on the patient's size and the rationale. Most tracheostomy tubes consist of an outer cannula with a neck plate, an inner cannula, and an obturator (Fig. 7.11). The outer cannula is the tube that holds the tracheostomy open. The neck plate extends from the sides of the outer tube. There are holes in the neck plate that attach the Velcro strap around the neck. The inner cannula locks inside of the outer cannula. The obturator is used to insert a tracheostomy tube. Most tracheostomy tubes are made of polyvinyl chloride, silicone, or polyurethane; a few are made of metal (silver or stainless steel).

Tracheostomy tubes may have an inner cannula that can be removed for cleaning or a disposable inner cannula. There are also cuffed and uncuffed tracheostomy tubes. A

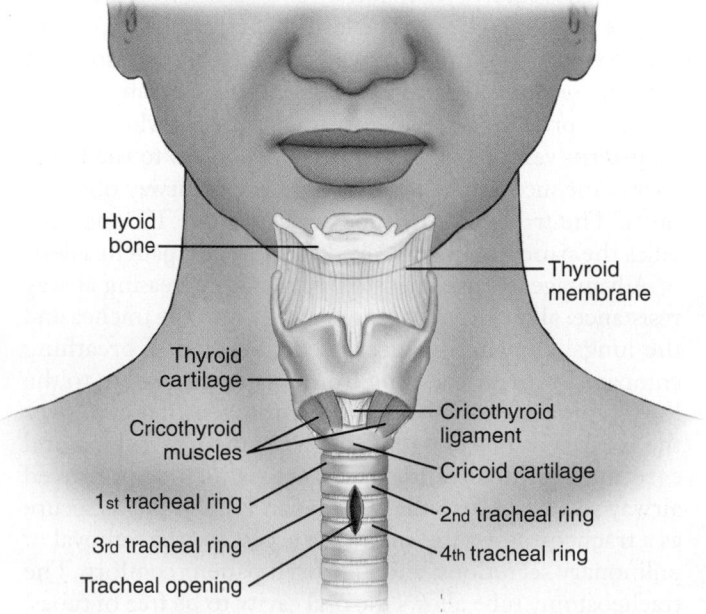

FIGURE 7.10 Tracheostomy.

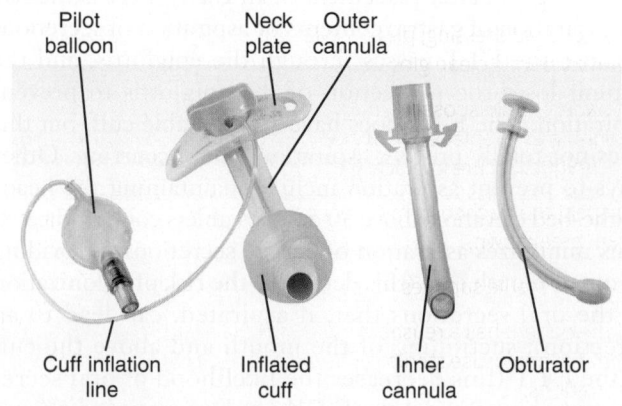

FIGURE 7.11 Parts of a tracheostomy tube.

cuffed tracheostomy tube is used for the patient who needs continuous mechanical ventilation or a patient who is at risk for aspiration. It is recommended that cuff pressure be maintained at 20 to 30 cm H_2O to decrease the risk of injury to esophageal tissue and aspiration. An uncuffed tracheostomy tube is used for patients who are ready for **decannulation** (the process of removing the tracheostomy tube) or are not receiving mechanical ventilation. The fenestrated tracheostomy tube is similar to the cuffed tube, with the exception that this tube has small openings above the cuff that allow the patient to speak. The fenestrated tracheostomy tube has a removable inner cannula and a plastic plug. If the inner cannula is removed, the cuff deflated, and the plastic plug in place, the patient is able to speak and breathe through the natural airways. This allows the healthcare provider to assess the patient's ability to breathe using the oral/nasal route in preparing for possible decannulation. The Passy-Muir speaking valve is an example of a one-way speaking valve that attaches to the hub of a nonfenestrated tracheostomy tube. The Passy-Muir valve opens on inhalation, allowing air to pass and enter into the lungs. Then on exhalation, the valve closes, and the air must exit and passes through the vocal cords to produce speech.

Indications

Indications for the creation of a tracheotomy include the need to provide long-term mechanical ventilation, to bypass upper airway obstruction, to allow removal of respiratory secretions, to allow for a more secure airway, and to allow oral intake and speech in a patient requiring a long-term tracheostomy tube. A long-term tracheostomy tube also allows for increased mobility for the patient and decreases the risk of aspiration compared with an ETT.

Tracheostomy Care

Tracheostomy care is provided each shift and as needed or as indicated by the facility's policy and protocol. This care is provided to maintain a patent airway and to prevent infection (Table 7.6).

Suctioning a Tracheostomy

Assess the patient to determine if suctioning is necessary. Some patients require suctioning every 1 to 2 hours, and other patients may require less suctioning. Assess breath sounds for wheezes, crackles, and/or rhonchi; these sounds may indicate a need for suctioning. Other indications may include coughing, audible secretions, an increase in pulse or respirations, or restlessness (Table 7.7).

 Safety Alert If at any time during the suctioning procedure the patient's oxygen saturation decreases or the heart rate drops, suctioning should be stopped and 100% oxygen administered.

Table 7.6 Best Practice for Tracheostomy Care

Actions	Rationale
Gather supplies and prepare for procedure.	Allows for an organized procedure
Provide patient and family, if present, the rationale for the procedure.	Decreases the patient's and family's level of anxiety and apprehension
Wash hands and apply personal protective equipment.	Decreases transmission of microorganisms
Suction the tracheostomy as needed.	Removal of secretions from inner cannula and lower airways allows for better oxygenation and reduces the need for coughing during the procedure.
Remove old dressing; place in biohazard bag along with soiled gloves; put on clean gloves.	Decreases transmission of microorganisms
If patient has disposable inner cannula, remove the old inner cannula and replace with a new inner cannula using aseptic technique. Secure in place. Remove soiled gloves.	Secures inner cannula and decreases transmission of microorganisms
Inspect the tracheostomy site for signs of infection, irritation, and skin breakdown.	Irritation or skin breakdown can lead to infection.
Prepare sterile supplies from tracheostomy cleaning kit.	Decreases transmission of microorganisms
If the patient has a reusable inner cannula, remove and clean the inner cannula; use sterile saline and a small brush to remove secretions.	Normal saline loosens and removes secretions from the inner cannula. Brushing the inner cannula removes the secretions that are not easily removed.

Continued

Table 7.6 Best Practice for Tracheostomy Care—cont'd

Actions	Rationale
Rinse with sterile saline and replace inner cannula after drying with sterile 4 × 4s.	Rinsing with normal saline cleans the inner cannula.
Replace inner cannula and secure in place.	Secures the inner cannula and reestablishes airway
Clean around the stoma site with sterile cotton-tipped applicators moistened with sterile saline. Cleanse the plate of the tracheostomy with sterile cotton-tipped applicators moistened with sterile saline. Do not allow any solution into the tracheostomy stoma. Using dry 4 × 4 gauze, dry the stoma area.	This removes secretions from stoma/plate site and cleans the area. Drying the area around the stoma/plate decreases microorganism growth and excoriation of the area.
Place a new sterile tracheostomy dressing under the tube plate.	Dry surfaces provide decreased growth of microorganisms and skin excoriation. Dressing absorbs any drainage and prevents pressure from the plate.
Replace the Velcro tracheostomy holder if soiled. The tracheostomy tube holder should be changed with two caregivers.	The use of two caregivers prevents accidental dislodgement of the tracheostomy tube.
Allow room for one to two fingers' width of space between the Velcro tube holder and the neck.	The two-finger method prevents the tube holder from being too tight.
Remove gloves and wash hands.	Decreases transmission of microorganisms
Document procedure, how patient tolerated procedure, education that was done with patient, and assessment of the stoma site.	Allows for interprofessional team to note any changes at the tracheostomy site. Excoriated skin can lead to infection; increased secretions indicate the need for increased tracheostomy site care.

Table 7.7 Suctioning the Tracheostomy Tube/Nasotracheal

Actions	Rationales
Wash hands and put on protective equipment.	Decreases transmission of microorganisms and secretions
Explain the procedure to patient and family members if present at the time of the procedure.	Decreases the patient's and family's level of anxiety and apprehension
Encourage the patient to cough to assist in removing the secretions if the patient is alert.	Assists with secretion removal
Place patient in a semi-Fowler's position.	Promotes secretion removal and prevents aspiration
Turn on suction and set suction vacuum up to 120 mm Hg.	This level of suction allows for adequate negative-pressure suctioning.
Open suction catheter kit and place sterile drape on bedside table. Do not allow sterile suction catheter to touch unsterile area.	Decreases transmission of microorganisms
Open sterile saline container and fill with sterile saline solution, approximately 100 mL. Do not touch the inside of the sterile container.	Saline is used to "flush" the tubing after each suction procedure.
Open lubricant and squeeze on sterile field. Lubricant is needed only when suctioning nasotracheal; it is not used for artificial airways.	Lubricant allows for easy passage of the nasotracheal suction catheter.
Apply sterile gloves, pick up suction catheter with dominant hand (keep sterile), and attach the catheter to the suction tubing. Use nondominant hand when touching the suction tubing (this hand will be nonsterile).	Decreases transmission of microorganisms and maintains sterility of suction catheter

Table 7.7 Suctioning the Tracheostomy Tube/Nasotracheal—cont'd

Actions	Rationales
Suction a small amount of saline to make sure the equipment is functioning correctly. Apply small amount of lubricant on catheter if performing nasotracheal suctioning.	Equipment must be functioning correctly to perform this procedure.
Remove oxygen device with nondominant hand and hyperoxygenate the patient by providing 100% oxygen via an Ambu bag that is connected to 100% oxygen. Hyperoxygenate with 4–6 breaths.	Hyperoxygenation assists in providing protection from suction-induced hypoxia and should provide approximately 2 minutes of 100% oxygen before the procedure.
Instruct the patient to take a deep breath.	Insert during inspiration when the epiglottis is open.
Insert the catheter quickly; do not apply suction on insertion of the catheter. Insert catheter far enough to stimulate the cough reflex.	Applying suction during catheter insertion increases the risk of hypoxia and trauma to the mucosa.
Apply suction and rotate catheter as the catheter is gently withdrawn over a maximum period of 10 seconds by placing thumb of nondominant hand over the catheter.	Suctioning longer than 10 seconds can cause hypoxia, cardiopulmonary compromise, or vagal response and damage to the mucosa.
Encourage patient to cough.	Allows for easier removal of secretions
Reoxygenate the patient again with 100% of FiO_2 via the Ambu bag for 2–3 breaths.	Hyperoxygenation assists in providing protection from suction-induced hypoxia.
Rinse the catheter with sterile saline solution while maintaining suction. This will allow the saline to rinse the catheter between suction attempts.	Secretions that remain in the suction catheter can reduce the catheter's ability to remove excessive secretions.
If secretions are still present, repeat procedure for a maximum of three passes of the catheter; provide a rest period of 20–30 seconds between passes of the catheter.	Suctioning can produce hypoxia, dysrhythmias, and bronchospasm. Repeated suctioning can remove excessive secretions.
When the procedure is complete, replace oxygen source to patient, clean area, and discard per hospital policy.	Allows proper patient oxygenation after the procedure
Suction patient's mouth and, if indicated, provide mouth care to the patient. Use a separate suction line when providing mouth care.	Removes upper airway secretions and microorganisms that may introduce infection
Assess the patient's breath sounds, vital signs, cardiac rhythm if the patient is on monitor, and SaO_2 level throughout the procedure and after the procedure.	Monitoring of the patient's vital signs allows for discontinuation of the procedure if the patient's heart rate or oxygen saturation drops because of hypoxia or vagal stimulation.
Document procedure, patient's response, and breath sounds; include color, consistency, and amount of secretions noted and patient's BP, pulse, respirations, and SaO_2 level before, during, and after the procedure.	Provides information about the procedure and information about the secretions that may indicate infection or change in secretions

BP = Blood pressure.

Immediate Post-Tracheostomy Complications

Accidental tracheostomy tube decannulation within the first 72 hours of the surgical procedure is considered a medical emergency because the tracheostomy is not mature, and during reinsertion, there is a greater risk for tissue damage and unsuccessful ventilation. If accidental decannulation occurs, the nurse must stay with the patient, call for assistance from respiratory therapy and a healthcare provider, and provide manual ventilation using a manual resuscitation bag with 100% oxygen. Because the patient will be anxious, offer assurances that help is on the way. When

the respiratory therapist or the healthcare provider arrives, insertion of a new tracheostomy tube will be attempted. Best practices require that replacement tracheostomy tubes are maintained at the bedside; this includes a tube equal in size and a tube that is one size smaller, along with an intubation tray.

Tube obstruction caused by secretions can be prevented by encouraging the patient to deep breathe and cough, suctioning, and providing humidification with the oxygen source. Humidification is often indicated even if the patient does not require supplemental oxygen because the inspired air is not warmed, filtered, and humidified through the nose and mouth as with normal breathing. The patient with a tracheostomy has less of an effective cough because of the inability to close the glottis. A small amount of bleeding from the tracheostomy site is expected for the first few days. Report moderate to large amounts of bleeding or a continuous oozing of blood to the healthcare provider.

A **pneumothorax** is a collection of air in the pleural cavity. This complication may occur during the tracheotomy procedure if the lung is pierced during the procedure, allowing air to enter the chest cavity. A chest x-ray is always ordered after the procedure to verify placement and to assess for a pneumothorax. **Subcutaneous emphysema** can occur if there is a puncture or tear in the trachea and air moves into the surrounding tissue. The air can move into the neck area, chest, or even the face. If this occurs, the skin becomes edematous with air and feels like a crackling sensation when palpated with the fingers and hand. Notify the healthcare provider immediately if this finding is observed.

Infection can occur early or late in a patient with a tracheostomy. While the patient is in the hospital, it is imperative to use aseptic techniques when providing tracheostomy care and when suctioning the patient. Teach the patient and/or caregiver about tracheostomy care before discharge, have the patient or family member return demonstrate the correct procedure, and ensure follow-up with home care once the patient has been discharged.

Long-term complications of a tracheostomy may include infection, tracheal stenosis, or tracheoesophageal fistula. Tracheal stenosis is a narrowing of the trachea due to scar tissue that forms from irritation of the mucosal lining of the trachea from the cuff. To prevent tracheal stenosis, maintain proper cuff pressures, prevent pulling of the tracheostomy tube, and maintain proper positioning of the tracheostomy tube. A tracheoesophageal fistula can develop as a result of overinflation of the tracheostomy cuff. The excessive pressure from the cuff causes a fistula (hole) to occur between the trachea and the esophagus. Prevention includes maintaining proper cuff pressures.

THERAPEUTIC MODALITIES

Incentive Spirometry

The **incentive spirometer** (Fig. 7.12) is a handheld respiratory device designed to assist the patient in deep-breathing exercises and encourage the patient to breathe slowly and deeply to allow lung expansion and to prevent or reverse atelectasis. When taking a slow, deep breath in and holding it, the alveoli expand, reducing the risk for collapse and assisting with oxygenation.

Indications

The incentive spirometer is ordered by the healthcare provider for patients who have had a surgical procedure and patients diagnosed with chronic breathing problems or

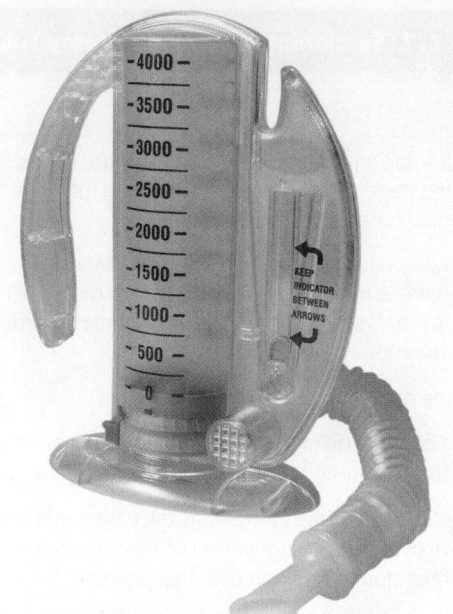

FIGURE 7.12 Incentive spirometer.

pulmonary issues. Patients ordered bedrest or patients with an extended hospital stay associated with decreased or limited mobility may benefit from the use of an incentive spirometer to reduce the possibility of developing atelectasis, which increases the risk for pneumonia.

Nursing Implications

Encourage the patient to use this device 5 to 10 times per hour while awake. Set the incentive spirometer goals on the basis of the patient's individual performance. For surgical patients, teaching and setting of incentive spirometer goals are best if completed preoperatively because postoperative pain or sedation may impair respiratory effort. Repeated use of the incentive spirometer can improve lung expansion and assist in removing secretions from the airways (Box 7.2).

Chest Physiotherapy

Chest physiotherapy (CPT) is ordered when the patient requires assistance in removing pulmonary secretions. Chest physiotherapy consists of percussion, vibration, and **postural drainage**. After CPT, the patient is encouraged to breathe deeply and cough to clear the airways. Some patients may require suctioning to assist in removing the secretions if they are unable to produce an effective cough to independently clear the airways. The goal is to move the secretions to the main airways so that the patient is able to produce an effective cough to clear the airways, thus allowing for improved ventilation. Chest physiotherapy is ordered 1 hour before meals or 3 hours after meals, and a bronchodilator may be ordered before CPT to allow for bronchial dilation. Percussion and vibration along with postural drainage assist the patient in removing pulmonary secretions.

Box 7.2 Use of the Incentive Spirometer

- Explain the correct use and indication for incentive spirometry.
- Assist the patient to a sitting position (semi-Fowler's) if no contraindications are noted. (This allows for optimal lung expansion during this breathing exercise.)
- Instruct the patient to exhale completely.
- Instruct the patient to place the mouthpiece in the mouth and place the lips tightly around the mouthpiece. (This allows for a good seal around the mouthpiece.)
- Instruct the patient to take in a slow, smooth, deep breath, like inhaling through a straw. When the patient has reached maximal inspiration and cannot inhale any more, instruct the patient to hold his or her breath for approximately 3 seconds. Then have the patient exhale smoothly and slowly. (This allows for good expansion of the alveoli to prevent or treat atelectasis.)
- Encourage the patient to use the device 5–10 times per hour while awake or as directed by the healthcare provider. Have the patient rest a few seconds between exercises and cough after each session. (This repeated exercise improves lung expansion and promotes airway clearance of the secretions.)
- Keep the incentive spirometer at the bedside within the patient's reach.
- Document exercises and effectiveness in the patient's medical record.

Postural drainage uses gravity to assist in removing pulmonary secretions. Through percussion and vibration, the secretions become loose and drain into the larger airways so that the patient can cough or the nurse can assist with suctioning the secretions if the patient is unable to independently clear secretions. Postural drainage consists of using different positions that use gravity to allow drainage of different segments of the lungs (Fig. 7.13). The head must be lower than the chest; this allows the secretions to drain toward the trachea, where they can be easily expectorated or suctioned if needed. The position of the patient depends on the segment of the lung that needs to be drained. Bronchodilators and mucolytic medications may be ordered before postural drainage to improve secretion removal. Pillows, a positional hospital bed, or a tilt table may be used to achieve the different positions. Each position should be held for 3 to 15 minutes or longer if ordered by the healthcare provider. Positions are modified if indicated by the patient's condition or tolerance to the treatment. Patients with chronic respiratory and cardiac conditions, for example, COPD or heart failure, may be unable to tolerate having the head lower than the chest.

Chest percussion is performed by lightly striking the chest wall over the area of the lung segment that is being drained. Use cupped hands so that the fingers and thumb are closed, and strike the chest wall while alternating cupped hands (Fig. 7.14). This percussion facilitates the secretions to move into the larger airways and allows the patient to cough and free the airways of secretions. Perform

percussion over the patient's gown or over a thin layer of clothing to protect the skin. Do not perform percussion over buttons, snaps, or zippers. Percussion is performed only to the area of the chest wall ordered by the healthcare provider and can be performed manually or by a mechanical device that is ordered by the healthcare provider.

Vibration is performed with the hands in a flat position. The hand moves repeatedly, causing a vibration to the area of the segment of the lung that needs to be drained. This is performed during exhalation to assist in loosening the secretions and inducing a cough.

Other airway clearance devices can be ordered to clear pulmonary secretions, including the Acapella and the high-frequency chest wall compression device. The Acapella is a handheld device that can be used in any setting to mobilize secretions. Acapella uses positive expiratory pressure and airway vibration and is easier to tolerate than CPT for some patients. The high-frequency chest wall compression device is a vibrating, air-filled vest that causes a continuous, gentle vibrating motion to assist the patient in removing pulmonary secretions. Devices such as the high-frequency chest wall compression device can be used in the home on patients who are discharged from the hospital and require assistance in mobilizing secretions. With proper patient education, the patient and/or caregiver can use the devices without assistance.

Connection Check 7.6

When the nurse is performing postural drainage for the patient, which factor promotes the movement of secretions to the upper airways?
A. Dilation of alveoli
B. Action of the cilia
C. Muscle contraction
D. Force of gravity

Nebulizer Treatments

Nebulizer treatments are prescribed by a healthcare provider and are usually administered by a respiratory therapist or another trained healthcare provider. Nebulizer treatments use bronchodilators, corticosteroids, and/or mucolytic agents to assist in thinning secretions, to reduce bronchospasm, and to reduce edema or inflammation of the bronchioles. Some medications that are prescribed may require saline to be added. The nebulizer changes the liquid medication into a mist; this is done either by a compressor machine that creates high air pressure that causes the liquid to become a mist or by an ultrasonic machine that uses high-speed vibration that causes the liquid to become a mist. The mist/medication that is produced is inhaled into the airways and lungs. Auscultation of the breath sounds and monitoring of vital signs are performed before and after each treatment. The breath sounds, vital signs, and patient response to the treatment are noted in the patient record.

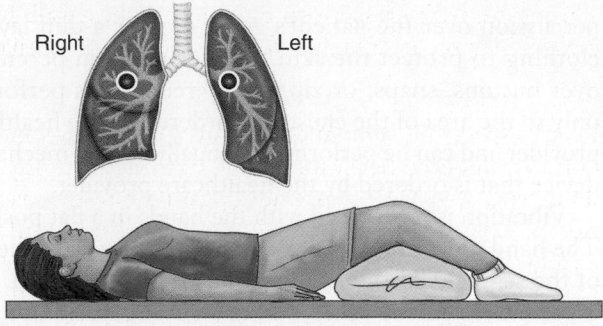

Anterior segments

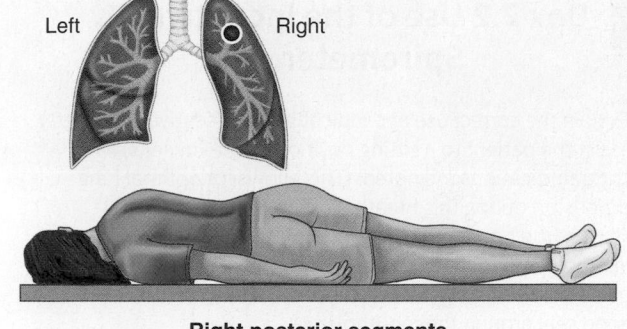

Right posterior segments

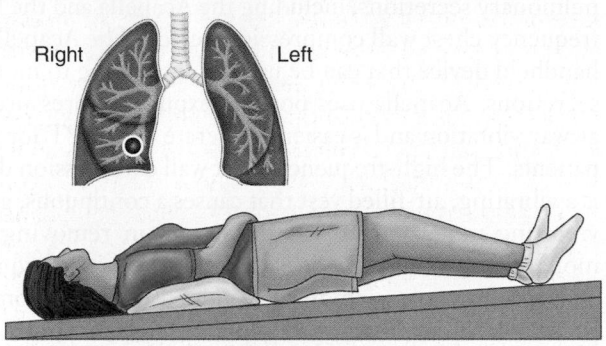

Right middle lobe

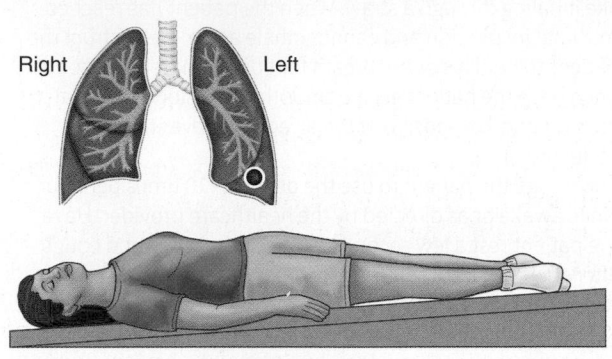

Left lingular

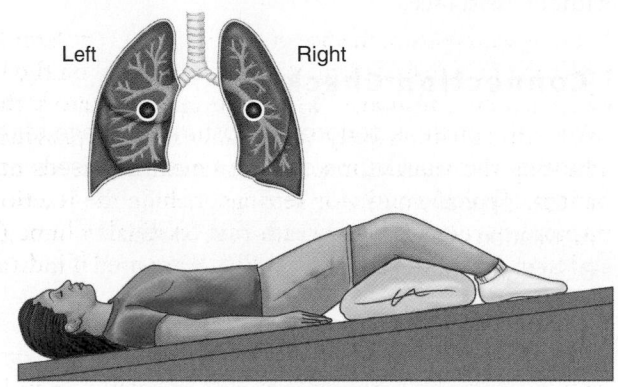

Anterior segments (lower lobes)

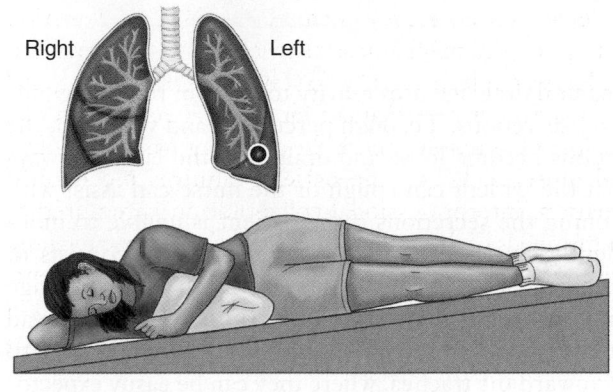

Left lateral segment

FIGURE 7.13 Common positions for postural drainage.

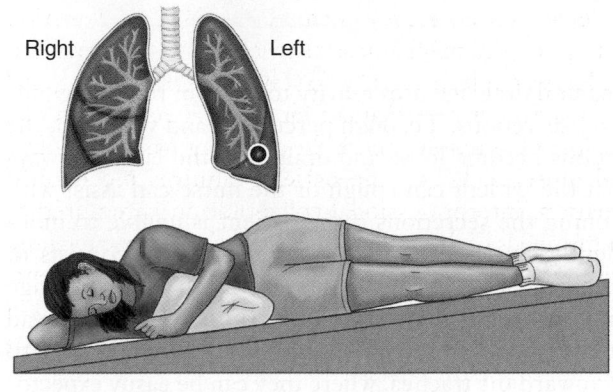

FIGURE 7.14 Cupped hand.

Intermittent Positive-Pressure Breathing

Intermittent positive-pressure breathing (IPPB) devices are prescribed by the healthcare provider to improve lung expansion, to deliver aerosol medications, or to assist the patient in ventilation. IPPB is indicated for patients who need to improve lung expansion, patients with pulmonary atelectasis when other therapies have been unsuccessful (incentive spirometry, CPT, and deep-breathing exercises), patients with an inability to clear secretions due to ineffective cough, and patients who require short-term ventilatory support. The patient receives intermittent positive pressure to the airways to maintain adequate gas exchange or to deliver aerosol treatments.

OVERVIEW OF MECHANICAL VENTILATION

Mechanical ventilation (Fig. 7.15) is required when a patient cannot maintain adequate ventilation and/or perfusion. Indications for mechanical ventilation include acute

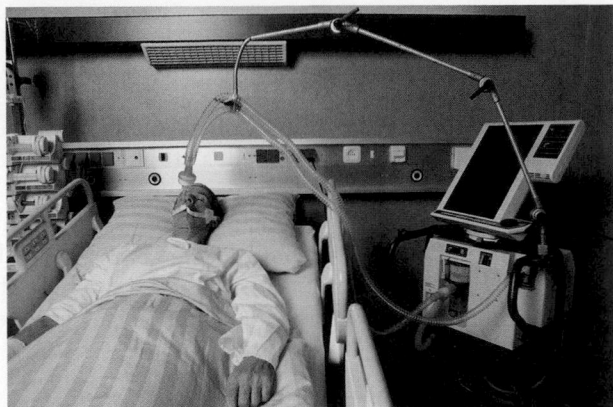

FIGURE 7.15 Mechanical ventilation.

respiratory failure; heart failure; exacerbation of COPD; protection of the airway due to cardiac arrest, drug overdose, or respiratory depression; and spinal cord or neurological trauma. The goal of mechanical ventilation is to support the patient until the underlying pathophysiological process is corrected. Mechanical ventilation is not a cure but is used to support the patient to improve ventilation and perfusion and to decrease the patient's work of breathing until the acute problem is managed. Once the underlying condition is corrected, mechanical ventilation may be discontinued. Patients who cannot support their own ventilatory needs or who cannot maintain optimal oxygenation may require the mechanical ventilation on a permanent basis. For example, patients who suffer a high cervical spinal injury may require permanent mechanical ventilation due to the loss of function of both the diaphragm and the intercostal muscles. When the patient requires mechanical ventilation, interprofessional collaboration is required to meet the needs of the patient. The role of the nurse includes providing continuous monitoring and assessment, preventing complications from mechanical ventilation, monitoring the equipment for any problems, and providing emotional support to the patient and family. Other members of the team may include the primary healthcare provider, respiratory therapist, dietitian, physical therapist, and social worker.

Types of Mechanical Ventilation

Negative-Pressure Ventilation

Negative-pressure ventilation is a noninvasive mechanical ventilation modality used for patients with respiratory disorders usually associated with neuromuscular disorders that impede the normal respiratory muscle function, such as muscular dystrophy. During spontaneous breathing, negative pressure is created when the thoracic cavity expands, causing intrapulmonary pressure to drop and air to flow into the lungs. This type of ventilation is similar to natural respiration. The negative-pressure ventilator provides a negative (pulling) pressure on the external chest wall, assisting in ventilation. The patient is fitted with a shell that connects to a ventilator. Through the use of the ventilator, the air is removed from the area between the patient and the shell,

causing negative pressure on the external chest wall. Examples include the iron lung and the chest cuirass ventilator.

Positive-Pressure Ventilation

Positive-pressure ventilation usually requires placement of either an endotracheal tube (ETT) or a tracheostomy tube. This type of ventilator provides positive-pressure ventilation to support the patient who has impaired ventilation, and it is provided by exerting positive pressure on the airways, pushing air into the lungs, causing the alveoli to participate in gas exchange. Exhalation occurs passively. Positive-pressure ventilation can be delivered by pressure-cycled or volume-cycled ventilators. Pressure-cycled ventilators deliver air into the lungs until a preset air pressure is reached. Exhalation remains passive. One issue with this type of ventilation is that the **tidal volume** (the amount of air delivered per breath) varies depending on lung compliance and resistance. Volume-cycled ventilators deliver air into the lungs until a preset volume is reached. A constant tidal volume is delivered regardless of lung compliance and resistance. The volume of air that is delivered is constant with each breath that is given by the ventilator. There is a preset pressure limit that prevents excessive pressure to the lungs with both pressure- and volume-cycled ventilators.

Mechanical Ventilator Settings

Patients who require the use of a mechanical ventilator have prescribed ventilator settings that are adjusted on the basis of the patient's response. The nurse and respiratory therapist work collaboratively with the healthcare provider in adjusting the ventilator settings to meet the needs of the patient. Typical ventilator settings include the fraction of inspired oxygen (FiO_2), breath rate (f), tidal volume (Vt), and flow. Pressure support and PEEP are used if indicated.

Fraction of Inspired Oxygen

The setting for FiO_2 indicates the amount of oxygen the patient receives via the mechanical ventilator. The FiO_2 may be started at 100% if the patient is extremely hypoxic and then decreased on the basis of ABG results. The ventilator can provide FiO_2 from 21% to 100% depending on the needs of the patient. The goal of this setting is to maintain a PaO_2 above 60% mm Hg and an SaO_2 above 90% to 92% at the lowest possible oxygen setting.

Rate

The rate is the number of respirations the patient receives per minute via the ventilator, and the usual setting is 8 to 12 breaths per minute. The setting depends on the mode selected and whether the patient can breathe spontaneously or whether the ventilator needs to provide mandatory ventilation for the patient. The rate may be gradually decreased in a patient who is breathing spontaneously until the patient is able to maintain adequate ventilation. When the respiratory rate of a patient on a mechanical ventilator is assessed, the number documented includes the numbers of both ventilator and spontaneous breaths.

Tidal Volume

Tidal volume (Vt) is the amount of preset air that is delivered with each breath. The usual setting is 8 to 10 mL/kg, and this setting is based on the patient's ideal body weight. Adjustments are made according to the ABG results. Large amounts of Vt may cause **barotrauma** (injury to the lungs caused by positive pressure) or increase the risk for ventilator-associated lung injury. Lower amounts of Vt may be ordered on patients with adult respiratory distress syndrome or acute lung injury. Using a lower Vt decreases the risk of further injury to the lungs.

Flow

The flow is the velocity of gas flow or volume of gas per minute.

Positive End-Expiratory Pressure

Positive end-expiratory pressure (PEEP) is positive pressure applied at the end of expiration to help prevent alveolar collapse, assist patent alveoli, and redistribute fluid from the alveoli. PEEP improves oxygenation, allowing the FiO_2 level to be lowered. This is important because prolonged use of high FiO_2 can cause lung injury. PEEP is often ordered at levels between 3 to 5 cm H_2O to minimize alveolar collapse and based on the patient's underlying pathophysiology. PEEP is generally indicated in patients who are being mechanically ventilated with ventilator modes such as assist-control ventilation, synchronized intermittent mandatory ventilation, or pressure-control ventilation. PEEP is referred to as CPAP when applied to spontaneously breathing patients.

Modes

There are different modes of mechanical ventilation available to meet the patient's breathing needs. The mode refers to how the breaths are delivered by the ventilator to the patient.

Assist-Control Ventilation

Assist-control (A/C) ventilation, also known as continuous mandatory ventilation (CMV), is the mode used for patients who have weak respiratory muscles and may be unable to maintain adequate ventilation. The respiratory rate and volume of breaths are preset. If the patient does not initiate a breath, the ventilator delivers the breaths at the preset rate and volume. If the patient does initiate a breath, the ventilator delivers the preset volume (assisted breath), allowing the patient to control the rate of breaths. The disadvantage of this mode is that in the hyperventilating patient, respiratory alkalosis can develop if the respiratory rate increases above a normal rate because the ventilator continues to deliver a preset volume with each initiated breath. Causes of hyperventilation can include pain, acid–base imbalance, and/or anxiety.

Intermittent Mandatory Ventilation

Intermittent mandatory ventilation provides a combination of ventilator-assisted breaths and spontaneous breaths of the patient. This mode is used for patients who can breathe spontaneously but at a volume and/or rate that does not meet adequate oxygenation. This mode makes sure that a preset volume and rate of breaths are given per minute regardless of the patient's efforts. This mode allows the patient to initiate a breath, but the volume is limited to what the patient is able to produce, decreasing the risk of barotrauma, but can lead to the patient breathing against the ventilator. As the patient exhales, the ventilator may be delivering a breath. This is called "bucking the ventilator."

Synchronized Intermittent Mandatory Ventilation

Synchronized intermittent mandatory ventilation (SIMV) is used for patients who are being weaned from the ventilator and those patients who require some assistance to maintain adequate ventilation. If the patient does not initiate a breath, the ventilator delivers the preset volume and rate per minute to the patient. This mode allows the patient to breathe spontaneously at his or her own volume and rate between the breaths given by the ventilator. This mode synchronizes with the patient's efforts to breathe. When used for weaning, the number of breaths given by the ventilator can be decreased so that the patient takes over and breathes spontaneously, without the assistance of the ventilator. This mode is sometimes used with **pressure support** (continuous positive pressure during inspiration) to decrease the workload of breathing for patients who are able to produce spontaneous breaths because there is increased respiratory effort required for the patient to breathe through the ETT.

Airway Pressure-Release Ventilation

Airway pressure-release ventilation is a mode designed for spontaneously breathing patients who require a high level of pressure to effectively recruit alveoli. The high level of pressure forces the alveoli open and contributes to gas exchange. The inflation period is long, and breaths may be initiated spontaneously as well as by the ventilator. This mode allows spontaneous breathing at a preset CPAP that is interrupted by pressure release to a lower pressure. This mode is believed to reduce the risk of ventilator-induced lung injuries such as barotrauma.

Pressure-Support Ventilation

Pressure-support ventilation (PSV) may be used as an independent mode or in conjunction with CPAP or SIMV. This mode gives a set positive pressure during spontaneous inspirations. The patient breathes spontaneously with the patient's own volume, rate, and inspiratory time but has continuous positive pressure that is maintained during inspiration. This continuous positive pressure assists in reducing the workload of breathing and keeping the alveoli open. When used for weaning, the pressure support helps the patient to overcome the dead space of the ETT.

CASE STUDY: EPISODE 3

Mrs. Graham becomes confused and combative, her SaO_2 drops to 82%, and she pulls off her Venturi mask. Her BP drops to 88/46, and her ABGs are as follows:

ABGs:

pH	7.24
PaO_2	58 mm Hg
$PaCO_2$	62 mm Hg
HCO_3^-	34 mEq/L
SaO_2	82%

Mrs. Graham is intubated and given a 1,000-mL bolus of 0.9% NS and is transferred to the medical intensive care unit. Upon arrival, she is given another 1,000-mL bolus of NS, vancomycin 1 g IV ordered STAT, and an order to continue the vancomycin 1 g IV every 12 hours.

Ventilator settings are as follows:

SIMV:

Vt	550
FiO_2	100%
SIMV	12
PEEP	5 cm H_2O

Admission orders:

VS every hour

Continuous ECG and PO monitoring

ABGs 2 hours after intubation

Daily labs: ABGs, CBC, chemical profile

Portable CXR and ECG daily

IV D5$^1/_2$ NS with 20 mEq of KCl at 84 mL/hr

Enoxaparin (Lovenox) 40 mg subcutaneous daily

Famotidine (Pepcid) 20 mg intravenous push (IVP) daily

Methylprednisolone (Solu-Medrol) 125 mg IVPB every
  8 hours

Nebulizer treatments with albuterol (Ventolin) 2.5 mg every
  4 hours and prn

Bedrest

Maintenance of ventilator settings

Strict I/O every hour

HOB elevated at 30 degrees

Mouth care every 4 hours and prn

Daily sedation vacation

Smoking cessation

Place orogastric tube and begin Pulmocare (enteral nutrition formula) @ 20 mL/hr; increase by 10 mL/hr until a goal of 40 mL/hr is established. Hold tube feedings for residual greater than 100 mL.

The following ABG results are obtained after 2 hours on the previously mentioned settings of the ventilator.

ABGs:

pH	7.36
PaO_2	90 mm Hg
$PaCO_2$	46 mm Hg
HCO_3^-	30 mEq/L
SaO_2	98%

Complications Associated With Mechanical Ventilation

The nurse is responsible for assessing the patient and the ventilator to maintain proper functioning. Complications that are associated with mechanical ventilation include hypotension, infection, barotrauma, aspiration, and ventilator-associated pneumonia (VAP). The ventilator has an alarm system that the nurse is required to monitor. The alarm indicates when there is a need for intervention. The nurse immediately assesses the patient and the ventilator to find out what is interfering with the ventilator and causing the alarm. The alarms that most often are activated are the high-pressure alarm and the low-pressure alarm (Table 7.8).

> **! Safety Alert** A ventilator alarm alerts the nurse that something is wrong with the pressure, volume, or rate of air being delivered to the patient. When an alarm is activated, it is the nurse's responsibility to immediately check the patient's ventilation and oxygenation; the priority assessment is the patient first, then the ventilator. If the nurse cannot immediately identify the problem, the nurse disconnects the patient from the ventilator and uses a manual resuscitation bag to ventilate the patient while calling for assistance. Failure to ensure adequate ventilation can result in injury to the patient, such as an anoxic brain injury or death.

Hypotension

Hypotension may develop secondary to changes in pressure in the chest cavity and is associated with positive-pressure modalities of mechanical ventilation. Because the delivered breaths are "pushed" into the lungs via positive-pressure ventilations, the pressure in the chest cavity increases. This increased intrathoracic pressure decreases venous return to the right side of the heart and ultimately decreases cardiac output. Fluids may be ordered by the healthcare provider to correct the hypotension; ventilator settings may also need to be adjusted. Sedatives or opioids may be a contributing factor to the hypotension and may need to be adjusted to elevate the blood pressure.

Table 7.8 Mechanical Ventilator Alarms

Cause	Intervention
High-Pressure Alarm	
Mucous plug or increased secretions	Suction as needed.
Patient biting the ETT	Insert an oral airway to prevent biting.
Pneumothorax	Assess for asymmetrical chest rise and decreased breath sounds over pneumothorax site; contact healthcare provider immediately.
Patient anxious and fighting the ventilator	Assess the patient, provide emotional support, and reevaluate sedation/analgesic need.
Kink in the tubing	Assess the tubing from ventilator to patient to ensure no kinking of the tube is present.
Water collected in the ventilator tubing	Empty water from the ventilator tubing.
Low-Pressure Alarm	
Cuff leak	Assess for cuff leak, check cuff pressure, and call for respiratory and healthcare provider.
Leak in the ventilator circuit	Assess all connections and tubing.
Patient stops breathing in the pressure support modes or SIMV.	Assess patient; notify the healthcare provider.

ETT = Endotracheal tube; SIMV = synchronized intermittent mandatory ventilation.

Infection

Infection is a potential complication because the normal defenses of the upper and lower respiratory systems are bypassed. The ETT or the tracheostomy tube can become a direct source to the lungs because both increase the risk of introduction of infectious substances. Normally, the upper and lower airways protect against infection by hair-like cilia that line the respiratory tract and filter the air before it reaches the lungs.

Barotrauma

Barotrauma is a complication of the mechanical ventilator due to the increased positive pressure applied to the lungs, which can cause alveolar rupture. Overdistention of the alveoli can lead to an excessive amount of air entering into the pleural space, causing a tension pneumothorax. This can be a life-threatening situation for the patient, and the nurse must notify the healthcare provider immediately and prepare for chest tube insertion to allow removal of trapped air in the pleural space.

Aspiration

Aspiration of gastric secretions and pulmonary secretions is a potential complication because the natural defense of the epiglottis is bypassed when an artificial airway is in place. Elevating the head of the bed (HOB) reduces the risk of aspiration. See the following section for additional nursing measures.

Ventilator-Associated Pneumonia

Ventilator-associated pneumonia (VAP) is a serious healthcare-associated infection resulting in high morbidity, high mortality, and high costs of treatment. Aspiration of oropharyngeal and/or gastric fluids is presumed to be an essential step in the development of VAP, and it typically develops 48 hours or more after endotracheal intubation.

Guidelines for preventing VAP include (1) minimizing sedation, including daily spontaneous breathing trials (SBTs) for patients without contraindications; (2) facilitating early exercise and mobilization; (3) using ETTs with subglottic secretion drainage ports for patients requiring greater than 48 to 72 hours of intubation; (4) elevating the HOB 30 to 45 degrees; and (5) changing the ventilator circuit only when visibly soiled or malfunctioning (Boxes 7.3 and 7.4).

Nursing Management for a Mechanically Ventilated Patient

Nursing Diagnoses

- **Ineffective airway clearance**
- **Ineffective breathing pattern**
- **Impaired gas exchange**
- **Risk for trauma**
- **Decreased cardiac output**
- **Impaired verbal communication**
- **Risk for infection**

Nursing Interventions

▨ Actions

- HOB elevation between 30 and 45 degrees unless contraindicated
  Reduces the risk for aspiration of gastric contents
- Clear airway secretions with suctioning, CPT, frequent position changes, and increasing activity.
  Reduces the risk of aspiration and clears the airways of secretions
- Daily "sedation vacation" and a readiness-to-wean assessment
  Holding sedation is necessary to determine the patient's potential for readiness to wean from the mechanical ventilator. Excessive sedation may decrease the respiratory rate and effort.
- Peptic ulcer disease prophylaxis
  Medications that reduce gastric acidity have been shown to protect patients from developing peptic ulcer disease and gastrointestinal bleeding.
- Deep vein thrombosis (DVT) prophylaxis
  Treatments with anticoagulants and sequential compression devices have been shown to reduce the risk for DVT that may develop in patients who require prolonged mechanical ventilation.

Box 7.3 The American Association of Critical-Care Nurses (AACN) Practice Alert: Prevention of Ventilator-Associated Pneumonia (VAP) in Adults

Alert Statements

Critically ill patients who are intubated are at risk for the development of ventilator-associated pneumonia (VAP). The reported incidence rate of VAP has been steadily declining. It is uncertain whether the decrease is related to prevention efforts, reporting definitions, or a combination of the two.

Expected Nursing Practice

Collaborate to identify patients for whom implementation of noninvasive positive-pressure ventilation (NIPPV) may be appropriate to prevent the need for intubation.

Assess readiness to extubate daily through combined spontaneous awakening trials (SATs; sedation interruption/minimization) and spontaneous breathing trials (SBTs), unless clinically contraindicated. Maintain and improve physical conditioning through early exercise and mobility. Elevate the head of the bed (HOB) to 30 to 45 degrees unless clinically contraindicated in patients receiving mechanical ventilation, as well as patients at high risk for aspiration. Minimize pooling of secretions above the endotracheal tube cuff by using an endotracheal tube with subglottic suction capability in patients with anticipated intubation greater than 48 to 72 hours. Change ventilator circuits only if visibly soiled; do not change ventilator circuits routinely. Perform oral care using chlorhexidine. Use ventilator bundles to reduce ventilator-associated events (VAEs) and VAP.

From American Association of Critical-Care Nurses. (2017). AACN practice alert: Prevention of ventilator-associated pneumonia in adults. *Critical Care Nurse, 37*(3), e22–e25.

- Daily oral care with chlorhexidine
  Oral care using chlorhexidine has been shown to decrease dental plaque that can cause bacterial growth.

Connection Check 7.7

The nurse is screening patients for their risk of developing VAP. The nurse considers which patient at greatest risk?

A. A patient who was extubated within 24 hours of being intubated

B. A patient intubated and placed on mechanical ventilation less than 72 hours ago

C. A patient with the head of the bed elevated 45 degrees

D. A patient who was placed on a nasal cannula after being extubated

Box 7.4 Healthcare-Associated Infections

Healthy People 2020 has indicated emerging issues in healthcare-associated infections (HAIs). Healthcare-associated infections are among the leading causes of preventable deaths in the United States and increase the healthcare costs each year. The goal of *Healthy People 2020* is to reduce, prevent, and eventually eliminate HAIs. Ventilator-associated pneumonia is one of the infections among the HAIs that *Healthy People 2020* is addressing. The group plans to target HAIs through evidence-based strategies that the Institute for Healthcare Improvement has adapted.

Weaning From Mechanical Ventilation

When a patient is intubated and placed on a mechanical ventilator, the primary goal is to frequently assess the need for continued intubation and mechanical ventilation. **Respiratory weaning** is a gradual process going from ventilator dependence to spontaneous breathing. The patient is assessed daily to determine readiness for the weaning process and discontinuation of the ventilator. The patient should demonstrate evidence that the underlying cause of respiratory failure has been reversed before the patient can be weaned from the ventilator. Indications that the patient may be ready for the weaning process include the ability to breathe spontaneously, support adequate oxygenation, and maintain hemodynamic stability.

Patient Criteria for Weaning

The patient is monitored for stable vital signs/ABGs, minimal secretions, adequate oxygenation, and spontaneous breathing and is free of sedation medications (Box 7.5).

Weaning Methods

Once the patient has met the weaning criteria, the patient is assessed with a spontaneous breathing trial (SBT). The

Box 7.5 Weaning Criteria

Criteria for Weaning

The criteria should be individualized for each patient.

Reversal of the underlying cause of respiratory failure
Ability to maintain:
pH greater than or equal to 7.25 during spontaneous ventilation
PEEP less than or equal to 5–8 cm H_2O
FiO_2 less than or equal to 0.4–0.5
PaO_2/FiO_2 ratio greater than 150–200
Hemodynamic stability, meaning no active myocardial ischemia or hypotension (patients receiving a low dose of vasopressors may be considered for weaning)
Ability to initiate an acceptable inspiratory effort

PEEP = positive end-expiratory pressure.

SBT is completed using a mode of partial support. The most common methods used in SBT are pressure support or CPAP or via a T-piece (see Evidence-Based Practice: T-Piece or Pressure Support Ventilation for Weaning From Mechanical Ventilation).

- Pressure support is used to assist the patient in overcoming the resistance of the ETT and assists the alveoli with perfusion support. The patient must have the ability to breathe spontaneously.
- CPAP is used to assist the patient in overcoming the ETT resistance because there is constant pressure maintained throughout the respiratory cycle. The patient must have spontaneous breathing because there is no additional inspiratory support.
- The T-piece is used when the ventilator is disconnected and the patient breathes through the ETT. Supplemental oxygen is provided, but there is no support provided by the ventilator. The patient must be monitored closely for an increased work of breathing because the small diameter of the ETT requires more patient effort for inspiration.

If the patient tolerates the SBT for 30 to 120 minutes without tachycardia, hypertension, hypotension, deteriorating ABG results, or arrhythmias, the patient is usually extubated. Following extubation, the patient is placed on oxygen via a face mask or nasal cannula for a period of time, and oxygenation and perfusion are continually assessed.

Evidence-Based Practice

T-Piece or Pressure-Support Ventilation for Weaning From Mechanical Ventilation

Two techniques used for spontaneous breathing trials (SBTs) for patients being weaned from mechanical ventilation are the use of a T-piece or pressure-support ventilation (PSV). Because there is no clearly preferable technique, a systematic review was conducted that included MEDLINE, Embase, SciELO, Google Scholar, CINAHL, ClinicalTrials.gov, and Cochrane CENTRAL databases through June 2015. The review included randomized controlled trials in adult patients being weaned from mechanical ventilation and compared outcomes of T-piece and PSV. The specific outcomes reviewed included weaning failure, reintubation rate, intensive care unit (ICU) mortality, and weaning duration. SBT technique was not found to be related to weaning success, ICU mortality, or reintubation. There were specific subgroup analyses that found that PSV might be superior to T-piece weaning in patients who were classified as "simple to wean." However, in patients found to require prolonged weaning, the T-piece was associated with shorter weaning duration. Because of the low level of evidence, the authors recommend further comparison studies related to SBT techniques, particularly in difficult-to-wean patients and those with COPD.

Pellegrini, J. A., Moraes, R. B., Maccari, J. G., de Oliveira, R. P., Savi, A., Burns, K. E., & Teixeira, C. (2016). Spontaneous breathing trials with T-piece or pressure support ventilation. *Respiratory Care, 61*(12), 1693–1703.

Weaning Complications

Reintubation is the major concern with patients after extubation. The team should be ready with an intubation tray at the bedside in case the patient becomes unstable and requires reintubation. Aspiration is another concern with a patient who is being extubated. As the tube is removed, the patient can breathe in and aspirate secretions in the respiratory tract. The patient is suctioned before extubation, and the patient is instructed to cough as the tube is being removed to reduce the incidence of aspiration. The healthcare provider orders oxygen either by nasal cannula or by face mask. The patient requires continuous monitoring after extubation. Monitor vital signs, continuous pulse oximetry, cardiac status, and respiratory status, including respiratory rate and effort. The patient may experience a sore throat and be hoarse after extubation because of the irritation to the vocal cords and throat from the ETT. Encourage deep-breathing and coughing exercises. The use of an incentive spirometer will assist the patient with lung expansion. Monitor the patient for any signs of airway obstruction, such as dyspnea, cyanosis, coughing, and stridor. **Stridor** is an abnormal, high-pitched, crowing sound heard on inspiration that is caused by edema of the glottis or laryngospasm. Notify the healthcare provider immediately for reintubation of the patient.

Connection Check 7.8

A nursing preceptor is observing a newly hired nurse prioritizing patient rounds. Correct prioritization of assigned patients is indicated if the new nurse assesses which patient first?

A. A patient with cellulitis of the right lower leg
B. A patient who was extubated 2 hours ago
C. A patient who was ordered nebulizer treatments prn
D. A patient with an IV of D51/2 NS at 125 mL/hr

Making Connections

CASE STUDY: WRAP-UP

Daily ABGs and chest x-rays are obtained. Mrs. Graham goes through daily sedation vacations, and on the third day, she successfully passes the weaning trial and is extubated and placed on 2LNC of oxygen and maintains a PO of 94%.

Mrs. Graham and her family are provided with teaching on the following to prevent further exacerbations:

Medication therapy, including reason, action, time, adverse effects

Importance of making follow-up appointments

Smoking cessation

Breathing exercises

Signs of respiratory infection

Avoiding exposure to people with infections

Need to balance rest and exercise

Discharge planning is begun to transfer Mrs. Graham to a short-term rehabilitation facility to focus on reconditioning and maximizing independence.

Case Study Questions

1. The nurse correlates which clinical manifestations observed in Mrs. Graham to hypoxia?

   A. Shortness of breath

   B. Chills

   C. Productive cough

   D. Fever

2. The nurse identifies which of the following as benefits to placing Mrs. Graham on a Venturi mask? *(Select all that apply.)*

   A. It delivers low levels of oxygen.

   B. It minimizes rebreathing of exhaled CO_2.

   C. It does not require high flow rates of oxygen.

   D. It provides a more precise concentration of oxygen.

   E. It provides higher concentrations of oxygen.

3. In observing Mrs. Graham for changes in respiratory status, which findings correlate with worsening hypoxia?

   A. Decreased $PaCO_2$

   B. Decreased respiratory rate

   C. Decreased heart rate

   D. Decreased PaO_2

4. What is the rationale for Mrs. Graham being ordered Pepcid (famotidine) 20 mg IV Push daily when intubated and placed on the mechanical ventilator?

   A. To decrease inflammation in the airways

   B. To reduce gastric acidity

   C. To minimize constipation

   D. To enhance gastric emptying

5. The nurse correlates which ventilator setting as most important in preventing alveolar collapse in Mrs. Graham while intubated?

   A. FiO_2 of 100%

   B. Vt of 550 mL

   C. PEEP of 5 cm H_2O

   D. SIMV with rate of 12

CHAPTER SUMMARY

The main function of the respiratory system is to deliver oxygen to the lungs, where, through diffusion, oxygen is released at the alveolar-capillary membrane into the blood and CO_2 is removed from the blood through diffusion and is released as a gas that is transported to the atmosphere. Oxygen therapy is initiated when patients require a higher concentration than is found in room air, with the goal of oxygen therapy being to treat or prevent hypoxia. The effectiveness of oxygen therapy can be assessed by monitoring the pulse oximeter and by obtaining arterial blood gases.

Endotracheal tubes are indicated when there is upper airway obstruction, apnea, high risk for aspiration, ineffective airway clearance, and/or respiratory distress. Therapeutic modalities include the use of incentive spirometry, chest physiotherapy, nebulizer treatments, and intermittent positive-pressure breathing.

Indications for the use of a mechanical ventilator include acute respiratory failure; heart failure; exacerbation of COPD; protection of the airway due to cardiac arrest, drug overdose, or respiratory depression; and spinal cord or neurological trauma. Complications associated with mechanical ventilation include hypotension, barotrauma, aspiration, and ventilator-assisted pneumonia (VAP).

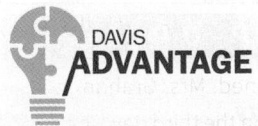

DAVIS **ADVANTAGE** To explore learning resources for this chapter, go to **Davis Advantage** and find:
- Answers to in-text questions
- Chapter Resources and Activities
- NCLEX®-Style Chapter Review Questions
- Bibliography

Chapter 8

Fluid and Electrolyte Management

Linda Cook

LEARNING OUTCOMES

Content in this chapter is designed to assist in:

1. Reviewing basic concepts related to fluid and electrolyte balance
2. Describing the role of the endocrine, renal, and respiratory systems in the regulation of fluid and electrolyte balance
3. Explaining the significance of osmolality, osmolarity, blood urea nitrogen (BUN), creatinine, and urine specific gravity in relation to fluid and electrolyte status
4. Discussing changes in fluid and electrolyte balance associated with aging
5. Describing the pathophysiology, clinical presentations, and management of dehydration, hypovolemia, and hypervolemia
6. Correlating laboratory data and clinical manifestations related to disorders in:
   a. Sodium balance
   b. Chloride balance
   c. Potassium balance
   d. Magnesium balance
   e. Calcium balance
   f. Phosphorus balance
7. Explaining nursing considerations related to patients with fluid and electrolyte disorders

CONCEPTS

- Assessment
- Fluid and Electrolyte Balance
- Medication
- Nutrition

ESSENTIAL TERMS

Active transport
Anions
Anuria
Blood urea nitrogen
Cations
Colloidal osmotic pressure (oncotic pressure)
Concentration gradient
Creatinine
Diffusion
Electrolytes
Extracellular fluid
Filtration
Fluid volume deficit
Fluid volume excess
Glomerulosclerosis
Homeostasis
Hydrostatic pressure
Hypertonic
Hypotonic
Interstitial space
Intracellular fluid
Isotonic
Lymph
Natriuretic peptide hormones
Oliguria
Orthostatic hypotension
Osmolality
Osmolarity
Osmosis
Osmotic diuresis
Osmotic pressure
Passive transport
Plasma
Pulmonary edema
Resorption
Rhabdomyolysis
Solute
Specific gravity
Third spacing
Tonicity
Transcellular fluid

Finding Connections

CASE STUDY: EPISODE 1

Follow this patient throughout the chapter.

Henrietta Morrison is an 80-year-old female admitted with a complaint of shortness of breath. She has a history of coronary artery disease, hypertension, and heart failure. She is complaining of a 2-week weight gain of 15 pounds, swollen ankles, and an inability to lie flat at night to sleep. Her current medications include furosemide (Lasix) 20 mg by mouth daily, K-Tabs 10 mEq by mouth twice daily, digoxin (Lanoxin) 0.25 mg by mouth daily, lisinopril (Prinivil) 10 mg by mouth twice daily, and spironolactone (Aldactone) 25 mg by mouth twice daily. She is waiting for the diagnostic tests to be completed, including a complete blood count (CBC), prothrombin time/international normalized ratio (PT/INR), activated partial thromboplastin time (aPTT), basic metabolic profile (BMP), brain natriuretic peptide (BNP), and a chest x-ray…

Table 8.1 Ion Concentration of the Intracellular and Extracellular Fluid Compartments

Ion	Intracellular	Extracellular
Sodium	10	140
Potassium	140	4
Chloride	4	104
Bicarbonate	10	24
Biphosphate	100	3
Calcium	1	5

Values are in milliequivalents per liter of water.

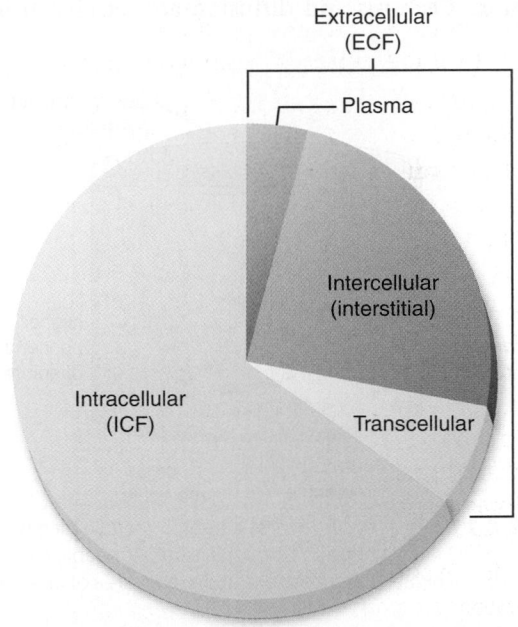

FIGURE 8.1 Compartments of total body water. The extracellular fluid (ECF) is composed of plasma, interstitial fluid, and transcellular fluid.

BASIC CONCEPTS OF FLUIDS

Disturbances in fluids and **electrolytes**, electrically charged particles in solution and active chemicals, are seen in patients for a variety of reasons and can have significant impacts on nursing care. Understanding the interactions of fluids and electrolytes is important for nurses as they provide care to patients in a variety of clinical settings.

Fluid Composition

Fluids and electrolytes exist within the body, are dynamic in nature, and are maintained in constant balance, or **homeostasis**, within the body. Electrolytes are responsible for many chemical reactions that produce energy. Energy generation occurs as **cations** (ions with net positive charge) and **anions** (ions with net negative charge) combine and split, resulting in energy creation for organ-level activity such as cardiac and skeletal muscle contractions. During the process of ionization, anions gain electrons, whereas cations lose electrons. Sodium (Na^+), potassium (K^+), calcium (Ca^{++}), magnesium (Mg^{++}), and hydrogen (H^+) ions are the major cations in body fluid. Chloride (Cl^-), bicarbonate (HCO_3^-), and phosphate (HPO_4^-) ions are the major anions in body fluids (Table 8.1).

Water is the primary constituent of cells and surrounds each cell. Water is distributed throughout the body, with 55% of the average female body and 65% of the average male body being composed of water. Total body water is distributed between four compartments, the intracellular, extracellular, intercellular, and plasma compartments (Fig. 8.1).

Intracellular fluid (ICF) includes all fluid present within the cells, with **extracellular fluid** (ECF) being found outside the cell. Sixty-five percent of total body water is found in ICF, and the remaining 35% is ECF. Extracellular fluid is further divided into intercellular, plasma, and transcellular. Intercellular, or interstitial, fluid is found between cells and is 25% of total body water. Intercellular fluid surrounds all cells, providing nutrients to the cell and facilitating waste removal. **Lymph** fluid is considered interstitial fluid, and as lymph enters the lymphatic system, it returns protein and excess interstitial fluid to the circulatory system. **Plasma** accounts for 8% of total body water and is located in the intravascular system. Total blood volume within the circulatory system is 6 L, of which 3 L is plasma. **Transcellular fluid** is only 2% of total body water and consists of fluids located in the gastrointestinal (GI), respiratory, and urinary tract and glandular, intraocular, and cerebrospinal fluids.

Extracellular and intracellular fluids are separated by the capillary wall and cell membrane. The capillary wall and cell membrane are permeable membranes allowing water to shift easily between the cells, **interstitial spaces** (area surrounding tissue cells), and plasma. Fluid is drawn back into the intracellular space from the blood through **osmosis**, which is the movement of water through a semipermeable membrane from an area of higher water concentration to an area of lower water concentration (Fig. 8.2). The goal of osmosis is to equalize water and **solute** (substance dissolved in a solution) concentrations on both sides of the membrane. In order to maintain equal distribution of solutes or particles between membranes, diffusion occurs. **Diffusion** moves solutes or particles from an area of higher concentration to an area of lower concentration (Fig. 8.3). The difference in the concentration of solutes or particles between membranes is the **concentration gradient**. A concentration gradient allows for particles to evenly distribute themselves throughout a solution. Osmosis and diffusion are **passive transport** processes because no energy is required for the movement of water or solute through a semipermeable membrane to occur. Larger molecules require energy to move into a cell. This process is called **active transport**. Active transport moves an ion or molecule against a concentration gradient.

Fluid Intake and Output

Fluid is kept in a balanced state through the intake and output (I&O) of fluid and is achieved through normal physiology. On average, 2,500 mL of fluid is processed daily by the body through gains and losses. Intake of fluid is through solid food, fluid, and cellular anaerobic respiration. Cellular anaerobic respiration uses glucose to create adenosine triphosphate (ATP) for energy, with a by-product being water. The primary loss of body water is in the urine. Additional fluid is lost in the stool, in exhaled air through the respiratory system, and from the skin as perspiration (Fig. 8.4).

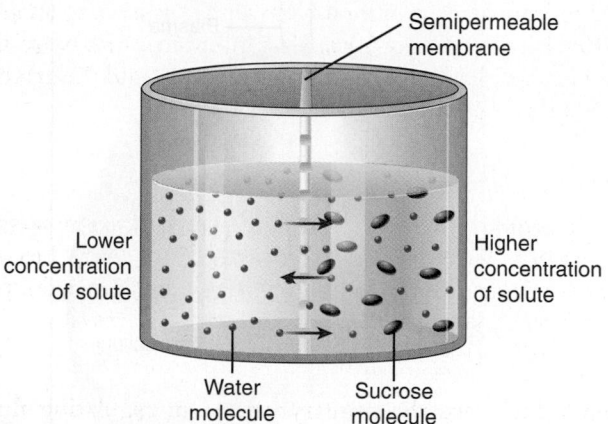

FIGURE 8.2 Osmosis occurs across a semipermeable membrane and reflects the movement of water through a semipermeable membrane from an area of higher water concentration to an area of lower water concentration.

Connection Check 8.1

The nurse understands that cerebrospinal fluid is considered which type of fluid?

A. Intracellular
B. Interstitial
C. Transcellular
D. Plasma

FLUID AND ELECTROLYTE REGULATION

Osmosis

Regulation of intracellular and extracellular fluids is based on fluid shifts from a higher concentration of solute to a lower concentration through the membrane separating them. A shift of water occurs until there is a balance in solute concentration and is dependent on the fluid concentration gradient. This process is called osmosis and is dependent on the number of particles in the solution; the number of particles or solutes per unit of solution determines **osmolality** and is measured as the total number of solute

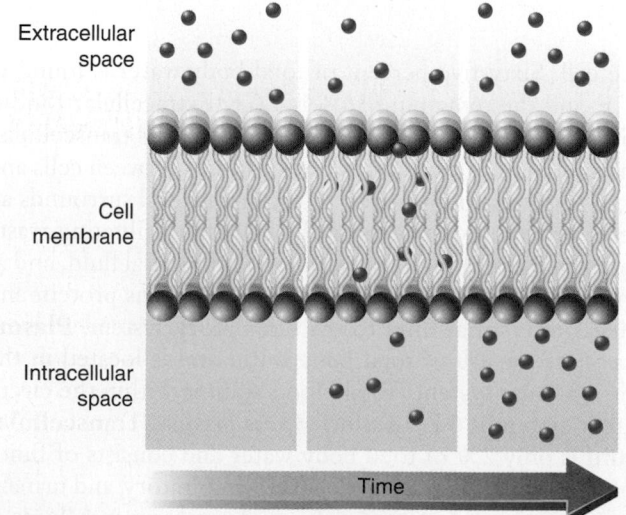

FIGURE 8.3 Diffusion moves solutes or particles from an area of higher concentration to an area of lower concentration. Solutes move from the extracellular fluid (ECF) through the cell membrane to the intracellular fluid (ICF) over time.

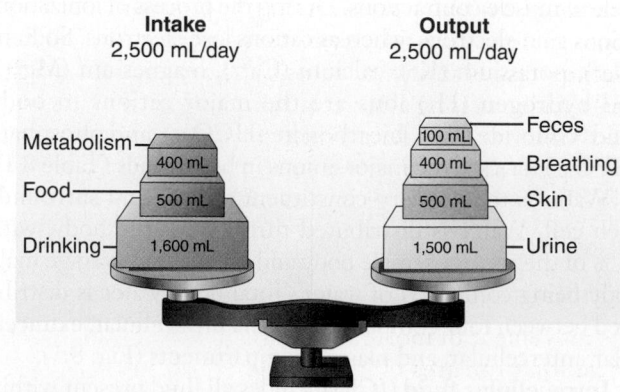

FIGURE 8.4 Daily intake and output are typically equal. Fluid intake includes fluids, food, and metabolic processes, and output includes urine and fluid loss through the skin, lungs, and bowel.

particles per kilogram. Additional terms associated with osmosis are *osmotic pressure*, *oncotic pressure*, and *osmotic diuresis*.

Osmotic pressure is the ability of a solution to draw water across a membrane, and it is affected by the **tonicity** of fluids. Tonicity is the ability of solutes to cause an osmotic driving force that promotes the movement of water across a membrane from one compartment to another. Fluids are classified as **isotonic**, **hypotonic**, or **hypertonic** on the basis of the particle concentration in body fluids. Milliequivalents per liter (mEq/L), milliosmoles per liter (mOsm/L), and millimoles per liter (mmol/L) are how particle concentrations in body fluids are measured. The number of milliosmoles in a kilogram (mOsm/kg) of solution is the osmolality of a solution, whereas **osmolarity** is the number of milliosmoles found in a liter of solution. The normal range for serum osmolality is 275 to 295 mOsm/kg. The normal range for the calculated osmolarity for body fluid and plasma is 270 to 300 mOsm/L, and osmolarity close to 300 mOsm/L is the value at which the body functions best. Isotonic fluids have the same osmolarity as plasma and body fluids, so no fluid is pulled across the cell membrane when these fluids are administered. Hypotonic solutions have a lower concentration of solutes than within the cell, causing fluid movement into cells. Hypertonic solutions have higher concentrations of solutes than within cells, causing fluids to shift out of the cell and into the ECF, causing cells to shrink.

The pressure created by solutes, nondiffusible plasma proteins (primarily albumin) dissolved in fluid, exerts oncotic pressure and pulls fluid toward the solute. **Colloidal osmotic pressure**, also known as oncotic pressure, is a form of osmotic pressure that pulls fluid from the interstitial space back into the intravascular space, increasing the circulating volume. The presence of albumin creates a higher concentration of protein in the intravascular plasma, which exerts colloidal osmotic pressure in the venous end of the capillary, returning fluid to the circulatory system. Plasma protein osmotic function maintains a fluid balance between the interstitial and intravascular spaces. If there is an increase in the intravascular volume from the shifting of fluids from the interstitial space to the intravascular space, there is also an increase in blood volume to the kidneys, leading to an increase in urine output. This resulting increase in urine output is **osmotic diuresis**. Osmotic diuresis also occurs as a result of the body's effort to remove high levels of glucose (hyperglycemia) and in response to mannitol or radiographic contrast media. Hyperglycemia results in increased osmotic pressure within the renal tubules, causing a decreased reabsorption of water back into the intravascular fluid. Mannitol and radiographic contrast media, both of which are administered intravenously, have a high osmolality, leading to osmotic diuresis.

Diffusion

The movement of molecules from an area of higher concentration to an area of lower concentration is **diffusion**. In any change in the concentration of electrolytes in either the interstitial fluid or plasma, the change is swiftly followed by a shift in electrolytes to restore balance in the concentration. Once balance is restored, diffusion continues without shifting of electrolytes.

Diffusion occurs as a result of the membrane transport system, which assists with the passage of a specific ion or molecule through the cell membrane. In some instances, the ion or molecule must be moved against a concentration gradient and requires the expenditure of energy. This use of energy is considered active transport and is accomplished through pumps. The sodium–potassium pump is an example of active transport. High concentrations of sodium and potassium are maintained in the ECF and ICF, respectively, because of the active transport of potassium.

Filtration

Filtration is the process by which water and dissolved substances (solutes) cross a membrane as a result of **hydrostatic pressure**, which is the pressure exerted on the walls of blood vessels by fluid, primarily water. Movement of solutes occurs from an area of high hydrostatic pressure to an area of low hydrostatic pressure. Examples of filtration are the glomerular filtration system of the kidneys and the arterial end of the capillary.

Regulatory Mechanisms

Balance, or homeostasis, of fluid is accomplished by several regulatory mechanisms and processes in the body. Homeostasis between fluids and regulation of I&O are achieved by the renal, endocrine, and respiratory systems.

Role of the Renal System

The kidneys are the primary organs in regulating fluid volume and electrolyte balance to maintain homeostasis. Through the glomeruli, the renal capillary network, the kidneys process approximately 170 L of plasma daily. Selective reabsorption of water and electrolytes occurs in the glomeruli, maintaining homeostasis of plasma osmolality and fluid (see Geriatric/Gerontological Considerations). Urine output is 1 to 2 L per day.

Geriatric/Gerontological Considerations

Renal Changes That Influence Fluid and Electrolyte Balance

With aging, there are renal changes that influence fluid and electrolyte balance. Renal blood flow decreases due to vascular changes, which can result in ischemia and the death of renal cells. Kidney size decreases with age due to cortical tissue loss from **glomerulosclerosis** (hardening of the glomeruli in the kidney). There is a decrease in glomerular filtration rate (GFR) due to reductions in the glomerular capillary plasma flow rate and reabsorption of water. A history of chronic hypertension, heart failure, and diabetes also predisposes the older adult to kidney failure.

Role of the Endocrine System

Control of fluid and electrolyte balances is maintained by the renin–angiotensin–aldosterone system (Fig. 8.5), antidiuretic hormone (ADH), and natriuretic peptides. The renin–angiotensin–aldosterone system also assists in maintaining blood pressure and intravascular fluid status. In response to a decrease in blood pressure or blood flow, renin is released from the juxtaglomerular cells of the kidneys and works on angiotensinogen (from the liver), converting it to angiotensin I. Angiotensin I is then converted to angiotensin II in the lungs by angiotensin-converting enzymes. Angiotensin II is a potent vasoconstrictor that also stimulates the release of aldosterone and stimulates the thirst mechanism, increasing fluid intake. Aldosterone release is also stimulated by an increase in urine sodium or a decrease in extracellular sodium and is secreted by the adrenal cortex. Aldosterone promotes the retention of sodium and water in the distal nephrons of the kidney, restoring blood volume.

Antidiuretic hormone is synthesized in the hypothalamus and released from the posterior pituitary gland and is released in response to changes in blood osmolality sensed by osmoreceptors located in the hypothalamus. These osmoreceptors are sensitive to blood plasma concentration and stimulate the release of ADH in response to increases in osmolality. In addition to osmoreceptors, there are baroreceptors, located in the aortic arch, carotid arches, and the left atrium, that also respond to changes in circulating blood volume and blood pressure. If there is a decrease in arterial blood pressure, baroreceptors stimulate the sympathetic nervous system, causing renal arteriole constriction that decreases glomerular filtration and increases the release of aldosterone and reabsorption of sodium and water. Antidiuretic hormone directly influences water reabsorption in the distal tubules and collecting ducts in the kidneys. The reabsorbed water is then returned into the vascular system, reducing serum osmolality and increasing circulating volume. Once serum osmolality returns to normal, 275 to 295 mOsm/kg, the release of ADH is inhibited (Fig. 8.6).

Natriuretic peptide hormones are released from specialized cells within the walls of the atrium (atrial natriuretic peptide [ANP]) and ventricles (brain natriuretic peptide [BNP]) in response to increased blood volume and blood pressure. As a result of the release of ANP and BNP, reabsorption of sodium by the kidney and the increase in glomerular filtration rate result in increased urine output that is high in sodium.

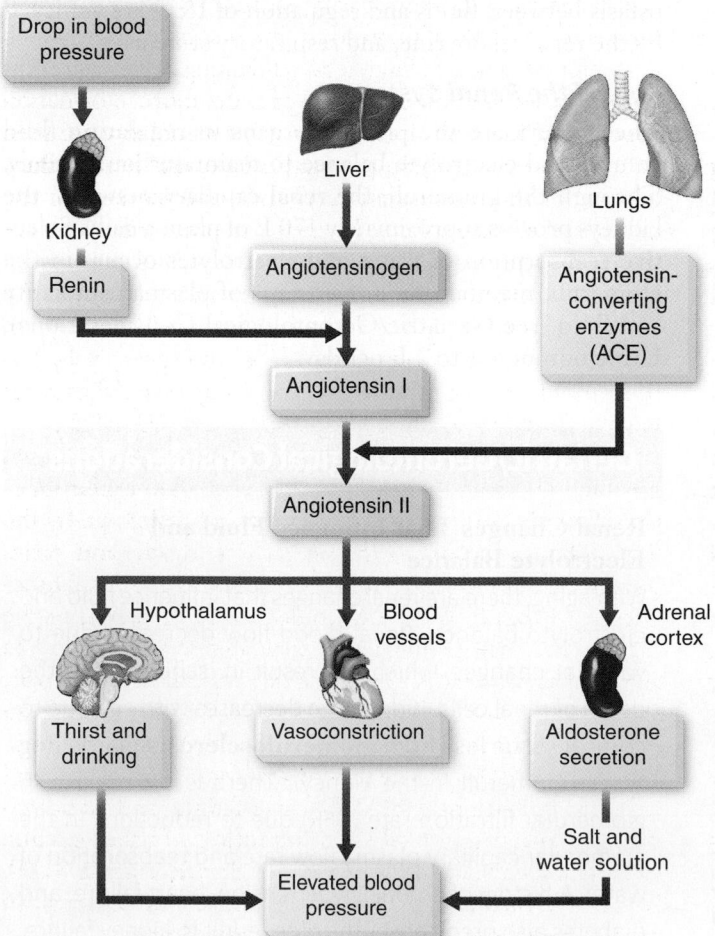

FIGURE 8.5 Fluid and electrolyte balance and blood pressure regulation through the renin–angiotensin system.

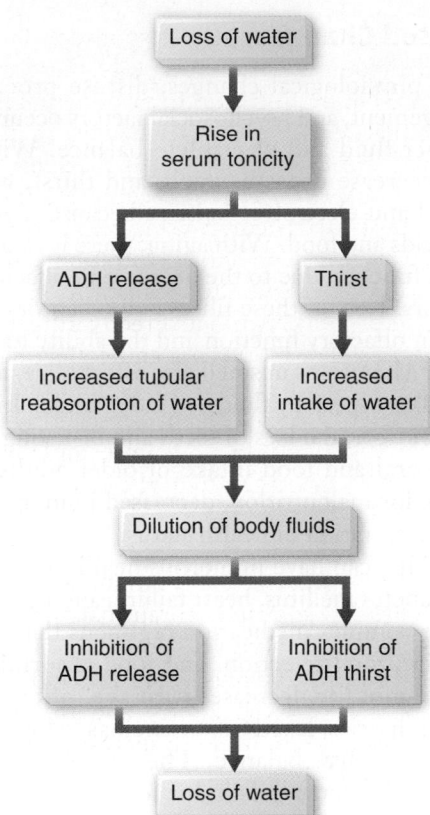

FIGURE 8.6 Role of antidiuretic hormone (ADH) in fluid regulation. ADH secretion increases with thirst and increased serum osmolality and decreases with decreased serum osmolality.

Role of the Respiratory System

Fluid loss occurs from the lungs through vaporization, which occurs as a result of inspired air being warmed and humidified by the body. With exhalation, the warmed, humidified air is released from the lungs. Approximately 300 mL of water is lost through the lungs daily, and that amount can be higher during hyperventilation or tachypnea or if the patient is receiving mechanical ventilation.

Insensible Losses

Insensible water loss occurs through the skin, lungs, and stool. Insensible water loss is not controllable and can be significant in the total amount because of the lack of awareness of this fluid loss. Increased insensible water losses can also be seen in hypermetabolic states such as trauma, burns, fever, and thyroid crisis because of fluid loss from impaired skin integrity, an increase in perspiration with fever, and hypermetabolism with thyroid crisis. In a hot, dry environment, insensible water loss increases because of evaporation of body water from the skin. Loss of water through perspiration is variable and is controlled by body temperature, vasodilation, and the autonomic nervous system. With increases in body temperature, the autonomic nervous system is stimulated by the hypothalamus to cause vasodilation. Vasodilation increases blood flow through the periphery, allowing conduction of heat into the environment. Insensible loss of water also increases via the GI tract in severe diarrhea or ulcerative colitis.

Connection Check 8.2

The nurse correlates which physiological response to the secretion of natriuretic peptide hormones?
A. Increase in urine output
B. Increase in blood pressure
C. Increase in blood volume
D. Increase in serum osmolality

Indicators of Fluid Status

The fluid status of patients is evaluated through a review of body weight, serum osmolality, blood urea nitrogen (BUN), creatinine, and urine specific gravity. Physical assessment findings also contribute to the evaluation of fluid status. Measurement of body weight and comparison to the patient's normal weight provides information regarding fluid loss or retention.

Osmolality is the concentration of a solution as determined by the number of solutes in a kilogram of water in blood and urine. Collection of a blood specimen and a random urine specimen at the same time is the most effective means to evaluate osmolality. The normal ratio between urine and blood osmolality is 3:1, with a normal range of serum osmolality of 275 to 295 mOsm/kg and a random urine specimen osmolality of 50 to 1,200 mOsm/kg of water. Evaluation of urine osmolality is a more exact measurement of urine concentration than specific gravity because it depends on the number of particles of solute found in a unit of solution, which is a better reflection of fluid status. Obtaining urine and serum osmolality levels at the same time provides more information about renal function. Increases in urine osmolality are seen in **fluid volume deficit**, prerenal failure, and heart failure because of the concentration of urine and increase in the number of particle solutes. Decreases in urine osmolality are seen in hyponatremia, **fluid volume excess**, and diabetes insipidus because of the dilution of urine and decrease in the number of particle solutes. Increases in serum osmolality are seen in hyperglycemia, hypernatremia, and severe dehydration, and decreases in serum osmolality are seen with renal failure, diuretic use, and fluid volume excess (Table 8.2).

Blood urea nitrogen (BUN) measures the nitrogen portion of urea and serves as a measure of glomerular function. Urea is the end product of protein breakdown by the liver. The normal BUN level is 8 to 21 mg/dL and varies with urine output, which reflects fluid status and renal function. Increases in BUN due to decreased perfusion of the kidneys are seen in impaired renal function secondary to sepsis, shock, stress, and congestive heart failure. In sepsis, shock states, and heart failure, blood is shunted away from the kidneys to maintain perfusion to the heart and brain. Decreases in BUN can be seen in syndrome of inappropriate antidiuretic hormone (SIADH), liver failure, and malnutrition. In patients with SIADH, retention of water occurs, diluting the circulating blood volume, thus decreasing BUN. In liver failure and malnutrition, there is a decrease in protein metabolism, resulting in decreased urea.

Table 8.2 Serum and Urine Osmolality

Conditions That Increase Osmolality

Serum	Urine
• Dehydration/sepsis/fever/ sweating/burns	• Dehydration
• Diabetes mellitus (hyperglycemia)	• SIADH
• Diabetes insipidus	• Adrenal insufficiency
• Uremia	• Glycosuria
• Hypernatremia	• Hypernatremia
• Ethanol, methanol, or ethylene glycol ingestion	• High-protein diet
• Mannitol therapy	

Conditions That Decrease Osmolality

Serum	Urine
• Excess hydration	• Diabetes insipidus
• Hyponatremia	• Excess fluid intake
• SIADH	• Acute renal insufficiency
	• Glomerulonephritis

SIADH, Syndrome of inappropriate antidiuretic hormone.
From RnCeus.com. (n.d.). *Serum and urine osmolality.* Retrieved from http://www.rnceus.com/renal/renalosmo.html

Creatinine is the by-product of muscle creatinine phosphate metabolism. Creatinine production is constant as long as muscle mass remains constant and serves as a better indicator of kidney function than BUN. Creatinine values range from 0.5 to 1.2 mg/dL depending on the muscle mass of the individual. The normal ratio of BUN to creatinine is 10:1 to 20:1.

Specific gravity is a measurement of dissolved chemicals in urine and reflects the ability of the kidneys to concentrate urine and is affected by the number and size of particles (minerals and salts) in urine. Hydration status, urine volume, and the number of particles impact the normal range of specific gravity. The normal range for specific gravity is 1.005 to 1.030. High values of specific gravity indicate concentrated urine and can be seen in patients with decreased renal perfusion or dehydration or in patients with SIADH. Lower values of specific gravity indicate dilute urine and are seen with diuretic use, diabetes insipidus, and increased fluid intake.

Connection Check 8.3

The nurse assesses for which clinical manifestations in the patient with dehydration? *(Select all that apply.)*
A. Increased urine specific gravity
B. Increased serum BUN
C. Increased serum osmolality
D. Decreased serum osmolality
E. Decreased BUN-to-creatinine ratio

Age-Related Changes

Numerous physiological changes, disease processes and their management, and psychosocial factors occurring with aging impact fluid and electrolyte balance. With aging, there is a decrease in taste, smell, and thirst, which can impact fluid and electrolyte balance because it affects the intake of fluids and food. With aging, there is also a decline in olfactory function due to the decrease in olfactory fibers and receptors. Loss of these fibers and receptors results in a decrease in olfactory function and the ability to discriminate smells. Alterations in smell also affect taste, impacting the oral intake, especially fluids, of older adults. In addition to the loss of taste, the loss of teeth and ill-fitting dentures impact the oral and food intake of older adults, placing them at risk for malnutrition, decreased immunity, weight loss, and deterioration of health status.

Older adults can have numerous health issues, such as arthritis, diabetes mellitus, heart failure, and hypertension, that require complex medication regimens that can influence appetite, food selection, and food absorption. Gastrointestinal motility decreases with age, often requiring the use of cathartics, laxatives, or enemas, which can alter fluid and electrolyte balance. The use of diuretics can result in a fluid volume deficit due to increased urine production. Fluid volume deficits can also occur when older adults limit fluid intake because of problems with bladder control and mobility. Ill-fitting dentures and the absence of teeth can affect food choices, which can result in electrolyte imbalances.

With aging, older adults are at risk for lack of financial resources to purchase and prepare nutritionally balanced meals. Lack of transportation, reduced income, healthcare expenses, and disabilities can limit the older adult's ability to maintain adequate dietary intake. Loneliness and depression can impact the older adult's interest in preparing foods and eating. Cognitive changes associated with dementia and Alzheimer's disease impact the ability to recognize the need for and ability to ingest adequate food and fluid and can result in confusion about the need to eat, swallowing difficulties, and forgetting how to use eating utensils.

Connection Check 8.4

In the aging adult, which of the following impacts food and fluid intake?
A. Increased sensitivity to smells
B. Increased sensitivity to texture in foods
C. Decreased manual dexterity
D. Decreased olfactory function

FLUID IMBALANCES

Alterations in fluid balance occur frequently in patients, and the nurse's role is to identify them, initiate interventions, and evaluate the effects of the intervention. Fluid volume deficit and excess often lead to the need for evaluation and treatment (Table 8.3).

Table 8.3 Comparison of Fluid Volume Deficit and Fluid Volume Excess

Assessment Parameters	Fluid Volume Deficit	Fluid Volume Excess
Weight	Decreased	Increased
Vital signs		
Heart rate	Increased	Increased
Blood pressure	Decreased (orthostatic hypotension)	Increased
Respirations	Clear	Crackles or wheezing
Skin turgor	Decreased	Increased
Edema	None	Dependent
Jugular vein	Flat	Possible distention
Urine output	Decreased	Normal or low
Urine specific gravity	Increased	Decreased

Hypovolemia: Fluid Volume Deficit

A fluid volume deficit is a decrease in fluid in the body and can occur in the interstitial, intravascular, or intracellular spaces. Fluid volume deficits are a common problem and may coexist with acid-base and/or electrolyte imbalances. A fluid volume deficit develops when fluid losses exceed fluid intake.

Causes

Fluid volume deficits occur as a result of excessive loss of fluids, insufficient intake of fluid, or fluid shifts. Gastrointestinal loss of fluid through vomiting, diarrhea, and nasogastric suction contributes to excessive loss of fluids. Increased perspiration during strenuous exercise or extreme heat without adequate fluid replacement can contribute to a fluid volume deficit. Additional causes of fluid losses include hemorrhage, diabetes insipidus, diabetic ketoacidosis, and adrenal insufficiency.

Insufficient intake of fluid can occur because of nausea; anorexia; or an inability to swallow as a result of an oral injury, neck trauma, or a cerebrovascular accident (stroke). Altered thirst mechanism can also decrease the recognition of the need to drink. Inability to communicate thirst and to access fluid also contributes to insufficient fluid intake. Aggressive treatment of fluid volume excess with diuretics can also result in a fluid volume deficit.

Fluid shifts into the interstitial space or **third spacing** occurs when fluid leaves the vascular space and enters the space between cells, becoming unavailable to support normal physiological activities. As fluid shifts into the interstitial space, circulating blood volume decreases, resulting in a decrease in blood flow to the organs of the body. Patients can become hypotensive, tachycardic, or restless and have decreased urine production. Third spacing can be seen in trauma, burns, cirrhosis, or right-sided heart failure and is often related to a decrease in oncotic pressure. Fluid can shift into the abdomen (ascites), pleural space (pleural effusion), or soft tissues (peripheral edema) or be lost through disrupted skin integrity as with burn injuries.

Laboratory Values

Routine laboratory studies to evaluate fluid volume status include electrolytes, specifically sodium and potassium; hemoglobin and hematocrit; serum osmolality; BUN in relationship to creatinine; urine specific gravity; and urine osmolality. In a fluid volume deficit, elevations of serum osmolality, urine specific gravity, and urine osmolality are observed as the kidneys work to conserve water. The kidneys conserve water as a result of the role of aldosterone through reabsorption of sodium, and ADH increases water reabsorption in the distal nephrons.

Hemoglobin and hematocrit also may be decreased if the fluid volume deficit is secondary to hemorrhage or elevated with the loss of fluid volume. Hemoglobin is the protein molecule within red blood cells that carries oxygen. Hematocrit is the percentage of red blood cells in the volume of whole blood and is dependent on the number and size of red blood cells. With decreased circulating volume, hematocrit is falsely elevated. Normal values for hemoglobin are 14 to 17.3 g/dL for adult males and 11.7 to 15.5 g/dL for adult females, and hematocrit is 42% to 52% for adult males and 36% to 48% for adult females.

Elevation of the BUN-to-creatinine ratio occurs as a result of decreased renal perfusion and function, which occur in shock states or dehydration. A BUN elevation is seen secondary to dehydration because of the retention of waste products. Serum sodium levels elevate with loss of water. Hypokalemia may occur in severe gastrointestinal (GI) fluid loss such as diarrhea because of the rapid passage of stool through the colon, resulting in the inability of the colon to reabsorb potassium. Gastrointestinal fluids contain sodium, potassium, bicarbonate, and chloride.

Clinical Manifestations

Depending on the cause, fluid volume deficits can develop quickly, and if the deficit is severe, patients may exhibit pronounced clinical manifestations. Weight loss, loss of skin turgor, concentrated urine output, **oliguria** (low urine output), thirst, and dry mucous membranes are indications of a fluid volume deficit. Severe, rapid fluid losses may be seen in hemorrhage, burns, or extensive losses from the GI tract. Additional clinical manifestations observed with significant fluid loss may include weak, rapid peripheral pulses; flattened neck veins; hypotension; anxiety; restlessness; and cool, clammy, pale skin.

Management
Medical Management
Identification of the etiology of the fluid losses and implementation of appropriate interventions are the first steps in correcting fluid volume deficits. Intake of oral fluids is the

preferred method of water replacement if the fluid deficit is not severe. In situations where the patient is unable or it is not feasible to replace fluid orally, or the loss is rapid and severe, alternative methods must be used. Provision of IV isotonic solutions, such as 0.9% normal saline (NaCl) or lactated Ringer's solution, expands plasma volume and corrects hypotension. The rate of infusion is dependent on the severity of fluid loss and patient symptoms. Once hypotension has been corrected, IV solutions and the infusion rate are adjusted to correct electrolyte disturbances and correct deficits in total body water. IV solutions of D5 0.45% NaCl or 0.45% NaCl can replace deficits in total body water and are used as maintenance fluids (Table 8.4).

Close monitoring of patient response to fluid replacement is essential. Assessment of vital signs, pulmonary and neurological function, and urine output identifies improvement in patient status and prevents the development of fluid volume overload. Improvement in neurological status includes a decrease in restlessness and improvement in mental status. Pulmonary clinical manifestations of fluid overload are increased respiratory rate, cough, development of crackles, and decreased oxygen saturation. If urine output continues to be low, further evaluation of fluid status and renal perfusion assists in determining if additional fluid is required.

Complications

Complications of fluid volume deficit occur with losses of large amounts of fluid volume. Hypovolemic shock can develop, as evidenced by hypotension, tachycardia, and signs of organ hypoperfusion, such as cool and clammy skin, oliguria progressing to **anuria** (lack of urine output), decreased level of consciousness, and tachypnea.

Nursing Management

Assessment of patients for fluid volume deficit includes collecting a health history, performing a physical assessment, reviewing diagnostic results, and calculating I&O. Collection of a health history focuses on the onset and duration of clinical manifestations, any recent illness, and medication use. Physical assessment findings may include dry mucous membranes, poor skin turgor, weak peripheral pulses, changes in vital signs, and weight loss. Changes in vital signs such as heart rate greater than 100 beats per minute and hypotension can indicate the presence of a significant fluid volume deficit. Hypotension, especially **orthostatic hypotension** (a decrease in blood pressure within 3 minutes of standing when compared with blood pressure from the sitting or supine position), and tachycardia with a weak, thready pulse indicate a fluid volume deficit. Monitoring of vital signs provides information regarding the patient's response to treatment. In addition to vital signs, assessment of mucous membranes; skin turgor; and urine specific gravity, color, and volume provides information about

fluid volume status. Laboratory data may include elevated hemoglobin and hematocrit, serum sodium levels, and BUN. The nurse continues the physical assessment for signs of correction of fluid deficit, such as moist mucous membranes, improved skin integrity, and an increase in urine output.

> **⚠ Safety Alert** Patients with significant hypovolemia are at risk for orthostatic or postural hypotension. The nurse needs to monitor the patient closely when changing the patient's position, particularly when sitting or standing, because the patient is at risk for dizziness and falls.

Early recognition of patients at risk for the inability to independently provide an adequate oral intake of fluid assists in preventing the development of fluid volume deficit and is identified through monitoring of output. Ensuring fluid replacement as prescribed assists in correcting a fluid volume deficit. Administering oral liquids or IV fluids as ordered assists in correcting fluid volume deficits. Monitoring I&O is one means to evaluate patient response to interventions to correct fluid volume deficits. Depending on patient status, assessment of I&O is completed in specified hourly increments. Monitoring laboratory results, especially serum electrolytes and osmolality, hemoglobin, and hematocrit, provides information about the patient response to treatment. Obtaining daily weights also provides information about the patient's response to interventions.

CASE STUDY: EPISODE 2

Henrietta continues to complain of shortness of breath. Physical assessment findings include an irregular heart rate of 124 beats per minute, 3-cm jugular vein distention, bilateral crackles to mid-level of both lungs, 3+ pitting edema to both lower extremities, and abdominal distention. Her chest x-ray shows bilateral pulmonary congestion. Her laboratory work shows hemoglobin 10 g/dL, hematocrit 30%, Na+ 130 mEq/L, K+ 4.9 mEq/L, BUN 29 mg/dL, creatinine 0.8 mg/dL, and albumin 3.2 g/dL. A saline lock is inserted, and furosemide (Lasix) 40 mg is administered by IV push...

Hypervolemia: Fluid Volume Excess

A fluid volume excess occurs as a result of increased water and sodium retention. An increase in sodium always results in an increase in water retention to maintain equilibrium. The presence of excess fluid can lead to increased intravascular fluid volume and interstitial fluid or edema.

Table 8.4 Common IV Fluids: Crystalloids and Colloids

	Action/Use	Nursing Considerations
Crystalloid		
Hypotonic: less than 250 mOsm/L	Shifts fluid out of vessels into cells	May worsen hypotension
	Hydrates cells	Can increase edema
0.25% NaCl		
0.45% NaCl	(D5W spares protein; provides calories and free water; treats hyperkalemia; is a diluent for IV medications)	May cause hyponatremia
5% D5W		(D5W may also irritate veins)
Isotonic: greater than 250 mOsm/L	No fluid shift	May cause fluid overload
	Vascular expansion	Generalized edema
0.9% NaCl	Electrolyte replacement	Dilutes hemoglobin
Lactated Ringer's (LR)		May cause hyperchloremic acidosis
		May cause electrolyte imbalance
		Pro-inflammatory in large doses
Hypertonic: greater than 375 mOsm/L	Shifts fluid back into circulation	Irritating to veins
	Vascular expansion	May cause fluid overload
D5 0.45% NaCl	Replaces electrolytes	May cause hypernatremia
D5 0.9% NaCl		May cause hyperchloremia
HS 3% or 5%		(HS slows inflammation and increases capillary permeability)
Colloid		
Albumin (plasma proteins)	Keeps fluid in vessels	May cause anaphylaxis (watch for hives, fever, chills, headache)
5% or 25%	Maintains volume	
	Used to replace protein and treat shock and erythroblastosis fetalis	May cause fluid overload and pulmonary edema
Dextran (polysaccharide)	Shifts fluids into vessels	May cause fluid overload and hypersensitivity
40 kDa or 70 kDa	Vascular expansion	Increased risk of bleeding
	Prolongs hemodynamic response when given with HS	Contraindicated in bleeding disorders, CHF, and renal failure
HES (synthetic starch)	Shifts fluid into vessels	May cause hypersensitivity and fluid overload
6% or 10%	Vascular expansion	Increased risk of bleeding
		Contraindicated in bleeding disorders, CHF, and renal failure
Mannitol (alcohol sugar)	Oliguric diuresis	May cause fluid overload
5% or 25%	Reduces cerebral edema	May cause electrolyte imbalances
	Eliminates toxins	Cellular dehydration
		Extravasation can cause tissue necrosis

CHF, Congestive heart failure; *D5W,* dextrose in water; *HES,* hetastarch; *HS,* hypertonic saline; *NaCl,* sodium chloride.

Causes

Disease processes or conditions that result in retention of sodium and water include cirrhosis, heart failure, stress conditions causing a release of ADH and aldosterone, adrenal gland disorders, and the use of corticosteroids. Patients receiving sodium-containing fluids in excessive amounts are also at risk for fluid volume excess. Ingestion of excessive amounts of salt in the diet also contributes to the development of fluid volume excess.

Laboratory Values

Laboratory tests that are assessed with suspected fluid volume excess include serum electrolytes, hematocrit, BUN, serum osmolality, and albumin. In fluid volume excess, hematocrit and BUN may be low secondary to dilution. Hypoalbuminemia presents in cirrhosis because of alterations in protein synthesis secondary to liver dysfunction. Hyponatremia and low serum osmolality may be present in chronic renal failure because of the dilution of blood volume.

Clinical Manifestations

Manifestations of fluid volume excess present in the form of weight gain, ascites, edema, and increased urinary output. Cardiac manifestations of fluid volume excess include hypertension, tachycardia, elevated central venous pressure, development of S_3 heart sounds, and jugular vein distention. In patients with heart failure, cardiac output is not able to meet the oxygen demands of the body. To meet these oxygen demands, the sympathetic nervous system is activated, increasing the heart rate and cardiac contractility, both of which increase blood pressure. As a result of decreased tissue perfusion, activation of the renin–angiotensin system occurs. Angiotensin II stimulates the release of aldosterone, which then promotes sodium and water reabsorption by the kidneys, further increasing the circulating blood volume. An extra heart tone, S_3, is present because of the large amount of blood volume entering the ventricles during diastole. Jugular vein distention develops as blood backs up in the right side of the heart. Respiratory symptoms develop as fluid leaks from the pulmonary capillaries into the alveoli because of the increased circulating blood volume and the inability of the left heart to pump the blood volume forward into the circulatory system. Respiratory symptoms include cough, tachypnea, adventitious breath sounds (i.e., crackles, wheezing), orthopnea, and decreased oxygen saturation.

Management

Medical Management

Management of fluid volume excess is aimed at prevention, correcting/managing the underlying cause, and treating the clinical manifestations. In patients at risk for fluid volume excess, limiting the daily intake of fluid and sodium and monitoring daily weight assist in preventing fluid retention and facilitating early recognition of fluid overload. Terminating or decreasing the infusion rate of sodium-containing IV fluids assists with fluid volume status. Use of diuretics may be required to promote excretion of excess fluid volume. In patients with renal compromise who do not respond sufficiently to diuretic therapy, renal dialysis may be required.

Complications

Worsening heart failure with progressive **pulmonary edema** is a complication of fluid volume excess. As left ventricular function continues to fail, fluid accumulates in the interstitial spaces of the lungs and in the alveoli. Pulmonary edema can occur as a result of an acute exacerbation of chronic heart failure, in the setting of an acute myocardial infarction and acute or chronic renal failure. Pulmonary edema is a potentially life-threatening condition due to progressive hypoxia that develops as oxygen exchange is compromised because of fluid in the alveoli. Emergent interventions include oxygen therapy, diuretics, morphine, and vasodilators.

Oxygen therapy may range from supplemental oxygen via nasal cannula to endotracheal intubation with mechanical ventilation. Mechanical ventilation provides positive end-expiratory pressure that decreases the movement of fluid from the pulmonary capillaries into the alveoli, improving oxygenation. The type of intervention is determined by the patient's arterial blood gas results, oxygen saturation, and signs of respiratory distress. (See Chapter 9 for more information on mechanical ventilation.)

Administration of morphine in small doses of 2 to 3 mg via IV push (IVP) promotes peripheral venous dilation, which reduces preload by redistributing blood volume in the periphery. In addition to peripheral vasodilation, morphine reduces anxiety. This reduction of preload secondary to decreased venous return can minimize the fluid overload of pulmonary edema.

Administration of IV diuretics such as furosemide (Lasix) promotes rapid diuresis, decreasing the circulating blood volume. Close monitoring of urine output to evaluate the patient's response is important. Electrolyte values, particularly potassium, must be monitored with diuretic administration because some of these medications are potassium wasting and others are potassium sparing. Patients with acute or chronic renal failure who develop fluid volume excess may require emergent renal dialysis. Vasodilators such as nitroglycerin or nitroprusside (Nipride) also may be administered intravenously to promote venous dilation and decrease preload. Both medications are titrated to patient response, and the blood pressure is closely monitored.

Nursing Management

Assessment of patients for fluid volume excess includes collecting a health history, performing a physical assessment, reviewing laboratory data, monitoring weight, and calculating I&O. Collection of a health history focuses on the onset and duration of symptoms, any recent illness, previous health issues, and current medication use and compliance. Physical assessment findings may include adventitious breath sounds (crackles), the presence of the extra heart sound S_3, abdominal distention or ascites, peripheral edema, a distended jugular vein, and altered mental status. If the patient status allows, obtain a weight upon admission to assist in evaluating patient response to treatment.

Nursing care is aimed at early recognition of clinical manifestations of fluid volume excess. Monitoring I&O, performing a physical assessment for signs of fluid overload, and evaluating patient response to interventions to resolve fluid volume excess are essential nursing interventions. Obtaining a daily weight provides additional information regarding fluid loss. Each kilogram of weight (2.2 pounds) is equivalent to 1 L of fluid. Providing patient education regarding medications such as diuretics, limiting intake of sodium and fluid, and the importance of daily weight assists patients in preventing the development of fluid volume excess. Patient education also needs to include specific criteria for the patient to contact the healthcare provider regarding clinical manifestations of fluid volume excess.

Connection Check 8.5

The nurse assesses for which clinical manifestations in the patient with hypervolemia?

A. Bradycardia

B. S_3 heart sound

C. Postural hypotension

D. Decreased skin turgor

CASE STUDY: EPISODE 3

Over the next 3 days, Henrietta has 6 L of urine output. Her breath sounds demonstrate crackles in the bases bilaterally and an SaO$_2$ of 97% on room air. Follow-up laboratory work shows hemoglobin 15 g/dL, hematocrit 43%, Na$^+$ 155 mEq/L, K$^+$ 2.9 mEq/L, BUN 49 mg/dL, creatinine 1.2 mg/dL, and albumin 3.2 g/dL. She is given 40 mEq of potassium chloride, and her diuretics are held for 2 days…

ELECTROLYTE DISORDERS

Alterations in electrolyte balances are common in patients for a variety of reasons, including acute illnesses or as a result of medication usage. Nurses play a vital role in recognizing these alterations in electrolyte balance and seeking corrective interventions. Electrolyte imbalances place patients at risk for serious negative health outcomes and are found in all healthcare settings (Tables 8.5–8.7).

Sodium

Sodium is the most prevalent electrolyte in ECF, with 95% of physiologically active sodium located in the ECF. Sodium levels are a key determinant of the osmolality of ECF and control the distribution of water within the body. The

Table 8.5 Electrolyte Values

Electrolyte	Normal Value Range
Serum sodium	135–145 mEq/L
Serum chloride	97–107 mEq/L
Serum potassium	3.5–5.0 mEq/L
Serum magnesium	1.6–2.2 mg/dL
Total serum calcium	8.2–10.2 mg/dL
Ionized calcium	4.6–5.3 mg/dL
Serum phosphorus	2.5–4.5 mg/dL
Serum osmolality	275–295 mOsm/kg
Urine osmolality	250–900 mOsm/kg

Table 8.6 Intracellular Versus Extracellular Electrolytes

Intracellular	Extracellular
Potassium	Sodium
Magnesium	Chloride
Phosphorus	Bicarbonate

normal range of sodium is 135 to 145 mEq/L. Sodium levels are controlled by thirst, ADH, and the renin–angiotensin–aldosterone system. The thirst mechanism is stimulated, and the release of ADH is seen in patients with elevated sodium levels. Increased oral intake and water reabsorption result in restoring normal serum sodium levels. Excessive free water intake and release of ADH can result in low serum sodium levels. The sodium–potassium pump facilitates transfer of sodium from the ECF to the ICF and transfer of potassium from the ICF to the ECF, creating an action potential. This action potential is responsible for cardiac and skeletal muscle contractions and nerve impulse transmission.

Sodium levels are maintained through the functioning of the kidneys under the influence of ADH, aldosterone, and natriuretic peptide. Sodium ions are positively charged, and chloride ions are negatively charged, and they maintain the balance of positive and negative charges. Sodium intake occurs as a result of the ingestion of food and fluids. The 2015 Dietary Guidelines for Americans report that the Institute of Medicine recommends a daily intake of sodium between 1,500 and 2,300 mg, with the goal to limit sodium intake as much as possible.

Table 8.7 Common Electrolyte Disturbances

Electrolyte	Clinical Manifestations	Treatment
Sodium (Na⁺) 135–145 mEq/L		
Hyponatremia Serum sodium level less than 135 mEq/L	Headache, lethargy, confusion, seizures, nausea/vomiting, coma	• Fluid restriction • In severe neurological symptoms, 3% NaCl • Oral sodium supplements • Loop diuretics
Hypernatremia Serum sodium level greater than 145 mEq/L	Disorientation, hallucinations, agitation, restlessness, neuromuscular irritability, confusion, seizures, lethargy, tachycardia, dry mucous membranes, skin flushed, agitation, thirst	• Fluid replacement 0.45% NaCl or D5W • Treatment of underlying cause
Chloride (Cl⁻) 97–107 mEq/L		
Hypochloremia Serum chloride levels less than 97 mEq/L	Irritability, hypotension, tetany, shallow respirations, and hyperexcitability of muscles and nerves	• 0.45% or 0.9% NaCl • Correction of underlying cause
Hyperchloremia Serum chloride levels greater than 107 mEq/L	Deep, rapid respirations, lethargy, tachypnea, decreased cognitive ability, and hypertension	• 0.45% NaCl • Correction of underlying cause
Potassium (K⁺) 3.5–5.0 mEq/L		
Hypokalemia Serum potassium level less than 3.5 mEq/L	Weakness, lethargy, generalized weakness, hyporeflexia, ECG changes (ST depression), PVCs, nausea/vomiting, constipation, abdominal cramping	• Increased dietary intake or supplementation • Slow-K, KCl liquid, powder or tablets • IV replacements (KCL runs, KCL aliquots): **Peripheral IV:** KCL 10 mEq in 100 mL NaCl or D5W over 1 hour **Central line** (PICC, triple-lumen catheter, or portacath): KCL 10 or 20 mEq in 100 mL NaCl or D5W to infuse over 1 hour *__Never__ administer as IVP
Hyperkalemia Serum potassium level greater than 5.0 mEq/L	Generalized weakness, muscle cramps, paresthesia to weakness, ECG changes (abnormal rhythms, widened QRS complex), bradycardia, sinus arrest, heart blocks, or ventricular dysrhythmias	• Sodium polystyrene sulfonate (Kayexalate), 50% dextrose, and IV regular insulin IVP bolus • Sodium bicarbonate 50 mEq IVP • Calcium gluconate • Albuterol nebulization for 1 hour • Loop diuretics
Magnesium 1.6–2.2 mg/dL		
Hypomagnesemia	Muscle weakness and cramping, paraesthesia, tetany, twitching, tremors, hyperactive reflexes, tachycardia, nausea/vomiting, seizures, anorexia, dysrhythmias such as tachycardia and PVCs, paroxysmal atrial tachycardia, ventricular fibrillation or tachycardia, emotional lability	• IV replacement • Magnesium 2 g in 100 mL NaCl or D5W over 1 hour • Magnesium tablets • IVP during Code Blue situation

Table 8.7 Common Electrolyte Disturbances—cont'd

Electrolyte	Clinical Manifestations	Treatment
Hypermagnesemia	ECG changes, widened QRS, hypotension, bradycardia, atrial fibrillation, intraventricular conduction delay, drowsiness, lethargy, decreased deep tendon reflexes, decreased platelet clumping, delayed formation of thrombin	Increased fluids
Calcium (Ca⁺) 8.2–10.2 mg/dL		
Ionized calcium 4.6–5.3 mg/dL		
Hypocalcemia	Anxiety, confusion, irritability, paresthesias, + Chvostek/Trousseau sign, tetany, twitching, tremors, focal numbness, muscle spasms, biliary colic, dysphagia, wheezing, and bronchospasm	• IV calcium • Oral supplementation (calcium tablets, Tums)
Hypercalcemia	Abdominal discomfort, constipation, nonspecific joint and bone aches, decreased deep tendon reflexes, hypertension, bradycardia thirst, lethargy, muscle weakness	• IV fluids • Loop diuretics • Bisphosphates
Phosphorus 2.5–4.5 mg/dL		
Hypophosphatemia	Confusion, apprehension, seizures, coma, skeletal or general smooth muscle weakness; respiratory insufficiency resulting from diaphragmatic dysfunction	• Phosphorous supplementation • Neutra-phos powder • K Phos IV replacement
Hyperphosphatemia	Positive Chvostek or Trousseau sign, hyperreflexia, soft tissue calcification, tetany bone and joint pain, muscle weakness, anorexia, paresthesias, delirium, convulsions, seizures, coma hypotension, heart failure and a prolonged QT interval on ECG	• PhosLo capsules • Oral phosphate-binding medications • If normal renal function, IV NS and loop diuretics

D5W, Dextrose in water; *DTR*, deep tendon reflex; *ECG*, electrocardiogram; *IVP*, intravenous push; *KCl,* potassium; *NaCl,* sodium chloride; *PICC,* peripherally inserted central catheter; *PVC,* premature ventricular contraction.

Sodium and water imbalances are common in a variety of patient populations. Changes in water balance, either by intake or loss through excretion, gastrointestinal losses, or illness, impact serum sodium levels and can result in hypernatremia. In patients with hypovolemia (fluid deficit), there is a loss of both water and sodium. Hyponatremia is seen in patients who are not able to eliminate water, resulting in dilution of the intravascular fluid. The presences of edema is primarily the result of the retention of water and sodium as seen in heart failure, liver disease, or renal failure.

Hyponatremia

Hyponatremia refers to serum sodium values that are less than 135 mEq/L and is the most common electrolyte disorder. Representing the amount of water in relationship to serum sodium, hyponatremia often results from disturbances in water. This disturbance in water balance can result in hypovolemic hyponatremia, euvolemic hyponatremia, or hypervolemic hyponatremia (Table 8.8).

In patients with hypovolemic hyponatremia, there is a decrease in the total body sodium and water in ECF as a result of the renal or extrarenal loss. The use of loop and thiazide diuretics is a cause of renal water loss, with thiazide diuretics being more likely to cause hyponatremia through renal loss of sodium. Sodium may also be lost secondary to diarrhea, vomiting, hyperglycemia with glycosuria, and perspiration. Clinical manifestations of hypovolemic hyponatremia include weight loss, orthostatic hypotension, tachycardia, abdominal cramping, and polydipsia (increased thirst).

Euvolemic hyponatremia occurs when there is an increase in total body water with no evidence of edema or hypovolemia. This can be seen in patients with SIADH and other endocrine disorders, such as severe hypothyroidism or adrenal insufficiency, both of which impair water excretion. Euvolemic hyponatremia also can be seen in psychotic polydipsia (excessive thirst) because antipsychotic medications have an anticholinergic effect, causing dry mouth and increased thirst.

Table 8.8 **Types of Hyponatremia**

	Hypervolemic	Euvolemic	Hypovolemic
Total body water	Increased—relative greater water retention	Increased—due to ingestion of large amounts of water	Decreased—loss of water
Total body sodium	Increased	Normal or unchanged value	Decreased—greater loss of sodium
Management	• Sodium and water restrictions • Treatment of underlying cause	• Limit free-water intake • Treatment of underlying cause	• Isotonic saline replacement • Treatment of underlying cause
Causes	Congestive heart failure Nephrotic syndrome Cirrhosis Advanced kidney disease Acute kidney injury	Hypothyroidism SIADH Medications • Carbamazepine • Opioids • Barbiturates • Vincristine • Phenytoin • Pantoprazole	Diuretic excess Salt-losing renal disease Severe diarrhea and vomiting Gastric suctioning Addison's disease Third spacing (burns or pancreatitis)

SIADH, Syndrome of inappropriate antidiuretic hormone.

Hypervolemic hyponatremia, causing an increase in ECF, occurs secondary to increases in total body water and is seen in patients with heart failure, cirrhosis, and nephrotic syndrome. Hypoperfusion in heart failure results in activation of the renin–angiotensin–aldosterone, norepinephrine, and ADH hormonal compensation mechanisms, leading to water and sodium retention. Hypoalbuminemia, from cirrhosis or nephritic syndrome, results in a decrease in the osmotic pressure of the intravascular volume, allowing fluid shifts to the interstitial space.

Clinical Manifestations

Clinical manifestations of hyponatremia are dependent on the severity, cause, and rapidity of onset. In the setting of acute hyponatremia, treatment needs to be started quickly to prevent cerebral edema and neurological decline, whereas slow onset should be treated more conservatively. In acute or severe hyponatremia, serum sodium levels of less than 120 mEq/L develop in less than 48 hours; these patients have the greatest risk for neurological complications. Cerebral edema and higher mortality rates are seen in patients with acute hyponatremia. Neurological clinical manifestations include lethargy, headache, confusion, gait disorders, nausea, and vomiting. Seizures, coma, permanent brain damage, and death may occur because of cerebral edema if severe hyponatremia is not recognized and treated. A slow decline in serum sodium levels may delay the onset of symptoms, and a chronic decrease in sodium can result in adaptation of brain cells to the new osmotic equilibrium, causing fewer symptoms.

> **Safety Alert** In the acute onset of sodium levels less than 120 mEq/L, the patient is at high risk for life-threatening neurological changes. These can occur due to brain swelling and intracranial hypertension that can result in brainstem herniation and respiratory arrest. If not treated quickly, this can result in permanent brain damage or death.

Management

Medical Management

Treatment of hyponatremia is based on the etiology of the sodium deficit, speed of development, and assessment for potential causes. Initially, the treatment of hyponatremia is the replacement of sodium via oral, enteral, or parenteral means and restriction of fluid intake. If the patient can tolerate food, intake of a regular diet can provide enough sodium to correct the deficit.

Replacement of volume in patients with hypovolemic hyponatremia with isotonic saline (0.9% NaCl) restores fluid volume and resolves symptoms. In patients with euvolemic hyponatremia, restriction of water intake to less than 1 L per day assists in restoring normal sodium levels but may be difficult to enforce. In patients with chronic hyponatremia, slow correction of sodium levels is important. A correction rate on the average of 0.5 mEq/L/hr for a total of 8 to 12 mEq/L/day is recommended to prevent osmotic demyelination. Osmotic demyelination or central pontine myelinolysis, leading to severe damage to the myelin sheath, can occur with aggressive or rapid replacement of sodium and can progress to worsening neurological function. Several patient populations, including those with a history of alcohol abuse, burns, or malnourishment and elderly women on thiazide diuretics, are at high risk for the development of osmotic demyelination during the correction of hyponatremia.

In patients exhibiting neurological symptoms, administration of hypertonic saline solution (3% or 5% sodium chloride) intravenously may be required at a rate of about 1 mL/kg/hr. If seizures are present or the patient is exhibiting signs of brain herniation, hypertonic saline may be infused at 2 to 3 mL/kg/hr for the first few hours. Hypertonic saline solution must be administered judiciously because of the potential for developing fluid volume overload. Administration of hypertonic saline solution should take place in a monitored unit with frequent assessments of the patient for indications of improvement in severe neurological symptoms and fluid volume overload. Infused through a central line via an IV pump, hypertonic saline is administered until the resolution of neurological symptoms, and then treatment focuses on management of the underlying disease process causing the hyponatremia. Infusion of hypertonic saline should be terminated prior to reaching normal serum sodium levels to prevent overcorrection of hyponatremia, which can lead to the development of excessive water diuresis, resulting in hypernatremia.

Decreasing circulating volume in hypervolemic hyponatremia is accomplished through the use of loop diuretics, fluid and sodium restriction, and treatment of the underlying fluid retention. In patients with cirrhosis, sodium and water restriction and the use of aldosterone antagonists such as spironolactone (Aldactone) can treat hyponatremia by causing the kidneys to eliminate unneeded water and sodium. With the progression of cirrhosis, liver transplant is the only effective treatment of hyponatremia secondary to hepatic failure (see Table 8.8).

Pharmacological interventions for hyponatremia include demeclocycline (Declomycin), lithium (Eskalith), and vasopressin-receptor antagonists such as conivaptan (Vaprisol) and tolvaptan (Samsca). Inhibition of the kidney's response to vasopressin is accomplished with the administration of demeclocycline (Declomycin) and lithium; both inhibit the reabsorption of water. Beneficial effects of demeclocycline may not be achieved for 1 to 2 weeks. Vasopressin receptor antagonists, referred to as "vaptans," block V2 receptors in the renal tubules, increasing the excretion of water. Tolvaptan (Samsca), lixivaptan (VPA-985), satavaptan (Aquilda), and conivaptan (Vaprisol) are examples of vasopressin-receptor antagonists.

Complications. Complications of hyponatremia include neurological symptoms such as lethargy, confusion, weakness, fatigue, muscle cramps, and postural hypotension. In severe acute hyponatremia, seizures, coma, and death can occur.

Nursing Management

Nursing management focuses on identifying patients at risk for the development of hyponatremia and monitoring sodium levels. Early recognition of hyponatremia can prevent the development of serious consequences such as seizures, decreased level of consciousness, coma, and death. Monitoring of fluid status through obtaining daily weights and measuring I&O can assist with early detection of water-balance issues. Observing the patient for signs of water losses or gain can serve as a warning sign of sodium imbalance. Neurological changes such as confusion, muscle twitching, lethargy, and seizures can indicate low sodium levels, especially in older adults. If hyponatremia is suspected, obtaining orders for urine osmolality and specific gravity can assist with monitoring sodium and water balance.

A key role that nurses play in managing hyponatremia is providing patient education. Goals of patient education include the importance of fluid and sodium intake and patient compliance. Sodium or salt intake increases the reabsorption of water, increasing the risk of redeveloping hyponatremia. Providing education to family members about clinical manifestations of hyponatremia can allow for earlier interventions. The nurse can include patient teaching related to sodium content in foods (Box 8.1).

Hypernatremia

Hypernatremia refers to serum sodium values greater than 145 mEq/L and often occurs as a direct result of water loss and/or the loss of sodium and water. Unavailability of water or inability to access water can result in water deficits. Changes in mental status, physical disabilities, dementia, or advanced age can limit the ability to verbalize thirst or physically consume water. Without adequate water intake, patients receiving hypertonic enteral feeding are at increased risk of developing hypernatremia. Water losses can also occur from diabetes insipidus, hyperglycemia, neoplasms, hypercalcemia, and hyperkalemia secondary to nephrogenic diabetes insipidus or medications such as lithium, demeclocycline, and amphotericin B. Neoplasms can also affect the hypothalamic osmoreceptors that regulate thirst. Increases in insensible loss of fluids through the respiratory system or skin can also result in water deficits. Losses of fluid

---

Box 8.1 Sodium Content of Common Foods

- Frozen pizza, plain cheese: 450–1,200 mg in 4 oz
- Soup (tomato), reconstituted: 700–1,260 mg in 8 oz
- Tomato juice: 340–1,040 mg in 8 oz (approximately 1 cup)
- Pretzels: 290–560 mg in 1 oz (28.4 g)
- Potato chips: 120–180 mg in 1 oz (28.4 g)
- Salsa: 150–240 mg in 2 Tbsp
- Salad dressing, regular fat, all types: 110–505 mg in 2 Tbsp
- Tortilla chips: 105–160 mg in 1 oz (28.4 g)
- Breads, all types: 95–210 mg in 1 oz
- Frozen vegetable, all types: 2–160 mg in $1/2$ cup

through the respiratory tract may be secondary to hyperventilation and tracheobronchitis. Burn injuries, febrile states, and exercise can result in loss of fluid through the skin.

Excessive ingestion of sodium also can result in hypernatremia. Use of sodium bicarbonate to correct metabolic acidosis and during cardiopulmonary resuscitation can result in an elevation of serum sodium levels. Close monitoring of sodium levels and prompt termination of sodium bicarbonate infusions after correction of metabolic acidosis minimize the risk of developing hypernatremia.

Clinical Manifestations

Clinical manifestations of hypernatremia include nonspecific neurological changes such as neuromuscular irritability, agitation, restlessness, lethargy, coma, and seizures. In the setting of severe hypernatremia, hallucinations, delusions, and disorientation may be present. Patients may complain of thirst and demonstrate signs of dehydration, including tachycardia, dry mucous membranes, flushed skin, decreased urine output, and orthostatic hypotension. In healthy persons, thirst serves as the mechanism to prevent the development of hypernatremia. In infants, a high-pitched cry and irritability are present because of brain damage secondary to subarachnoid hemorrhage that may result from hypernatremia.

Management

Medical Management

Medical management is aimed at limiting sodium intake or replacing water deficits through the infusion of hypotonic fluids such as 0.45% NaCl or 5% dextrose in water (D5W). Caution should be taken in order to prevent rapid correction of hypernatremia that may lead to fluid shifts into brain tissue, potentially resulting in cerebral edema. In an effort to correct hypernatremia, intracellular water shifts into the extracellular space, resulting in dehydration of brain cells. As water losses are replaced, water shifts back into brain cells. If rapid correction of water deficit occurs, this shift back into brain cells can result in cerebral edema, increasing the risk of seizures or permanent neurological damage. Termination of IV solutions with isotonic sodium or sodium bicarbonate should be the first step in the correction of hypernatremia. Correction of the water deficit should occur over 48 to 72 hours, preferably by use of enteral means if possible (see Evidence-Based Practice).

Evidence-Based Practice

Free Water Deficit Calculation and Replacement

In patients with hypernatremia, replacement of free water is required to return serum sodium levels to normal. The following formulas are used to calculate the free water deficit and the infusion rate and duration of D5W. In hypernatremia that has developed over days, correction of the

sodium level should occur at a rate not to exceed 0.5 mEq/L/hr and a total of 8 to 10 mEq/d. Rapid correction during this time can result in cerebral edema, which can cause permanent brain damage. If the hypernatremia is accompanied by a volume deficit, the intravascular volume needs to be replaced with isotonic sodium chloride prior to any free-water administration. Correction of a water deficit should occur over a 48- to 72-hour time frame.

Determine water deficit:

1. Total body water (TBW) = correction factor × weight in kilograms
   The correction factor is 0.6 for men, 0.5 for women and elderly men, and 0.45 for elderly women.
2. Water deficit (liter) = weight (kg) × correction factor
3. Change in serum Na^+ = (Infusate Na^+ – serum Na^+)/(TBW + 1)

As an example of the use of these calculations, consider an 80-year-old male who is admitted with severe dehydration. His weight is 70 kg. His serum sodium level is 165 mEq/L. To reduce his serum sodium, D5W is the infusate to be used (NA+ content = 0 in D5W). The calculations are as follows:

1. Total body water = 0.5 × 70 = 35L
2. Water deficit = 35 × 0.5 = 17.5 L
3. The retention of 1 L of D5W leads to a serum sodium reduction of –4.6: (0 – 165)/(35 + 1) = –4.6
4. Because the goal is to reduce the serum sodium by no more than 10 mEq/L in 24 hours, then 10/4.6 = 2.17 L of D5W is required. To compensate for natural water loss, and additional 1–1.5 L is added to total 3.67 (2.17 + 1.5) over 24 hours.
5. The infusion rate is 153 mL/hour.

D5W, dextrose in water.
Lukitsch, I., & Batuman, V. (2018). *Hypernatremia treatment & management.* Retrieved from https://emedicine.medscape.com/article/241094-treatment

 Safety Alert Correction of hypernatremia must be performed cautiously because of the risk of overcorrection that can lead to life-threatening complications such as cerebral edema secondary to fluid shifting into brain cells.

Complications. Complications of mild hypernatremia, sodium levels of 145 to 150 mEq/L, include the development of restlessness, weakness, disorientation, delusions, and hallucinations. With progression to severe hypernatremia, serum sodium levels greater than 152 mEq/L, seizures, stupor, coma, and potentially death can occur. If hypernatremia is due to fluid volume deficits, cardiac symptoms such as orthostatic hypotension and tachycardia may also be present.

Nursing Management

Nursing care is aimed at early recognition of patients at risk for hypernatremia through close monitoring of I&O. Close monitoring of patients, specifically those unable to access water independently, receiving enteral feedings, or demonstrating mental status changes or those with physical disabilities, dementia, or advanced age, enables early identification of the actual or potential development of hypernatremia.

Ensuring adequate intake of water in patients receiving enteral nutrition is accomplished by providing a water bolus several times throughout the day. In patients who are unable to access water, providing opportunities to ingest water throughout the day in sufficient quantities is an important role of nursing. If patients are unable to orally ingest adequate amounts of water, collaboration with the healthcare provider regarding alternative routes of fluid administration, such as parenteral or enteral methods (nasogastric or gastrostomy tube), may be required.

Monitoring of daily weights and serum sodium levels assists in providing baseline assessment data to guide interventions. Individuals engaging in strenuous activities are encouraged to ingest adequate amounts of water to prevent water loss and dehydration. Providing patient and family education regarding means to increase water intake can assist in the collaborative management of hypernatremia.

Patients with head injuries, postoperative neurological surgical procedures, or brain tumors are at risk for developing central diabetes insipidus related to decreased production of vasopressin, which promotes water reabsorption in the kidneys. Close monitoring of the hourly urine output volume, urine specific gravity, and serum sodium of patients at risk for the development of diabetes insipidus is an important nursing function.

Chloride

Chloride is found in the ECF and is the major anion as sodium chloride. The normal serum chloride value range is 97 to 107 mEq/L. Chloride is found in pancreatic and gastric juices as well as saliva, sweat, and bile. In addition to sodium, chloride is important in maintaining the osmotic pressure of ECF. The relationship between serum chloride and bicarbonate levels is an important indicator of the nature of acid-base disturbances because bicarbonate is the anion most often exchanged with chloride. Normal chloride levels are achieved through excretion and reabsorption of chloride in the kidneys.

Hypochloremia

Hypochloremia refers to serum chloride levels less than 97 mEq/L and occurs as a result of chloride loss. It is observed in patients with severe vomiting, burns, chronic respiratory acidosis, nasogastric suctioning, metabolic alkalosis, and Addison's disease (adrenal cortex insufficiency). In chronic respiratory acidosis, the buffer systems of the kidney retain bicarbonate and excrete chloride in order to re-establish acid-base balance. Hypochloremia in metabolic alkalosis occurs as a result of increases in plasma bicarbonate concentration due to the loss of hydrogen in the GI tract (nasogastric suctioning, vomiting, or diarrhea) or in the urine.

Administration of IV fluids low in chloride (D5W) or high in bicarbonate, hyponatremia, and decreased sodium intake can also lead to hypochloremia as a result of volume dilution and increases in urine output. Patients can develop hypochloremic metabolic alkalosis as serum chloride levels decrease and increases in sodium and bicarbonate reabsorption compensate for the loss of chloride through the GI tract. In patients with hypochloremia, hypokalemia and hyponatremia may also be present because of the renal loss of potassium and sodium.

Clinical Manifestations

Patients with hypochloremia may exhibit irritability, hypotension, tetany, shallow respirations, and hyperexcitability of muscles and nerves. If hypokalemia is also present, cardiac dysrhythmias may develop. Because of the relationship of sodium to chloride, hyponatremia may also be present with water excess and, if severe, can lead to seizures and death.

Management

Medical Management

Medical management is aimed at correcting the cause of hypochloremia and replacing chloride through the administration of 0.45% or 0.9% NaCl solution. If metabolic alkalosis is present, ammonium chloride may be prescribed. In metabolic alkalosis, there is an increase in sodium bicarbonate in the blood. Ammonium is used by the kidneys in place of sodium to maintain the acid-base balance. Correcting the metabolic alkalosis restores serum chloride levels.

Complications. Hypochloremia can develop as a result of hypokalemia, which can lead to cardiac dysrhythmias. Chloride levels parallel sodium levels, and in the presence of hypochloremia, hyponatremia and water excess can result in seizures and coma.

Nursing Management

Nursing care is aimed at early recognition of hypochloremia and implementing actions to assist in the correction of decreased serum chloride levels. Monitor patients for changes in the level of consciousness, respiratory effort, and muscle control, and promptly notify the provider of changes. The provision of patient education regarding foods high in chloride content and replacing fluid losses with electrolyte-containing fluids assists in preventing the reoccurrence of hypochloremia.

Hyperchloremia

Hyperchloremia is present if the serum chloride level is greater than 107 mEq/L and can result in bicarbonate loss, resulting in metabolic acidosis and hypernatremia. In hypernatremia, chloride is reabsorbed in the kidneys to maintain ion neutrality. Infusion of excessive levels of chloride relative to sodium can lead to hyperchloremia. Loss of bicarbonate ions through the GI and renal systems, combined with the use of 0.9% NaCl, 0.45% NaCl, and lactated Ringer's solution for fluid intake maintenance, can result in hyperchloremia. With the use of these IV solutions, chloride replaces bicarbonate to correct acidosis, leading to hyperchloremia.

Clinical Manifestations

Clinical manifestations of hyperchloremia are similar to those observed in fluid volume excess, metabolic acidosis, and hypernatremia. Comparable to hypernatremia, the clinical presentation of hyperchloremia includes deep and rapid respirations, lethargy, tachypnea, decreased cognitive ability, and elevated blood pressure.

Management

Medical Management

Identification and management of the underlying causes and correction of acid-base, fluid, and electrolyte disturbances guide the management of hyperchloremia. Administration of hypotonic IV solutions, such as 0.45% NaCl, to replace fluid losses assists in correcting serum chloride levels. A sodium bicarbonate infusion may be utilized to increase bicarbonate levels to increase the urinary excretion of chloride. In addition to sodium bicarbonate infusions, limiting the intake of fluids containing sodium and chloride and the use of diuretics assist in lowering chloride levels. If metabolic disturbances are present, correction of the underlying cause is essential to correcting hyperchloremia.

Complications. If left untreated, patients with hyperchloremia can develop cardiac dysrhythmias, decreased cardiac output, and coma.

Nursing Management

Nurses monitor patients for clinical manifestations, including changes in neurological, cardiac, and respiratory status that are typically seen in hyperchloremia, and promptly relay these changes to the healthcare provider. Neurological manifestations include decreases in cognitive ability and lethargy. Cardiac manifestations include hypertension and tachycardia from fluid overload. Deep, rapid respirations are also usually present. Provision of patient education regarding adequate hydration and how to manage hyperchloremia is required prior to discharge. Patient education includes the avoidance of foods high in chloride, such as processed meats, canned vegetables, eggs, bananas, cheese, and milk, and limited intake of free water (water without electrolytes).

Potassium

Potassium is the major intracellular electrolyte (cation) of the body, with 98% found within the cell. The remaining 2% is extracellular and is essential for neuromuscular function. The normal range of serum potassium is 3.5 to 5.0 mEq/L. The sodium–potassium pump (Fig. 8.7) controls the movement of potassium into and out of cells as needed for neuromuscular function and to maintain homeostasis. In conjunction with sodium, potassium produces action and resting membrane potentials of muscle and nerve cells. In the function of the sodium–potassium pump, potassium's role is just as important as sodium's for heat production (thermogenesis) and cotransport. Potassium is also important for the metabolic processes of the body and protein synthesis. Normal renal function is required to maintain normal levels of potassium, with 80% of the daily loss of potassium occurring through the kidneys. Daily replacement of potassium loss is easily achieved through daily food intake (Box 8.2).

Hypokalemia

Hypokalemia is associated with serum potassium levels less than 3.5 mEq/L and is further classified as mild (3.0–3.5 mEq/L), moderate (2.5–3.0 mEq/L), and severe (less than 2 mEq/L); it can reflect a real loss of potassium stores or a temporary shift of potassium into the cell. In the patient with respiratory or metabolic alkalosis, potassium ions shift intracellularly as hydrogen ions shift out of the cell in an effort to restore acid-base balance.

Potassium deficit can occur secondary to losses through the GI tract and renal system, actions of medications, transcellular shifts, and inadequate intake of potassium. Gastrointestinal losses of potassium occur as a result of diarrhea, vomiting, and gastric suctioning. Significant potassium loss can occur as a result of the loss of gastric secretions and then as a result of renal excretion of potassium to correct metabolic alkalosis from the gastric secretion loss associated with the loss of hydrochloric acid. Excessive use of enemas or laxatives contributes to potassium loss through the GI tract. Hypokalemia secondary to GI losses can also be seen in patients with anorexia, bulimia, or excessive use of laxatives.

Renal loss of potassium can occur as a result of hyperaldosteronism that leads to increased potassium excretion, resulting in severe potassium depletion. In the patient with hyperaldosteronism, aldosterone secreted from the adrenal cortex stimulates the reabsorption of sodium and the excretion of potassium. As sodium is reabsorbed, increased water is absorbed as well. Renal loss of potassium also occurs with the use of various medications, and diuretics are the most common medication related to hypokalemia. The use of loop diuretics, thiazide diuretics, and ethacrynic acid (Edecrin) with poor intake of potassium can result in hypokalemia. Additional medications that can cause hypokalemia include aminoglycosides, steroids, and beta-adrenergic agonists (albuterol or dobutamine).

Shifts of potassium intracellularly can occur for several reasons. In patients with hyperinsulin secretion, potassium shifts into hepatic and muscular cells are promoted because insulin makes cells more permeable to potassium. The release of catecholamines, such as epinephrine, during periods of

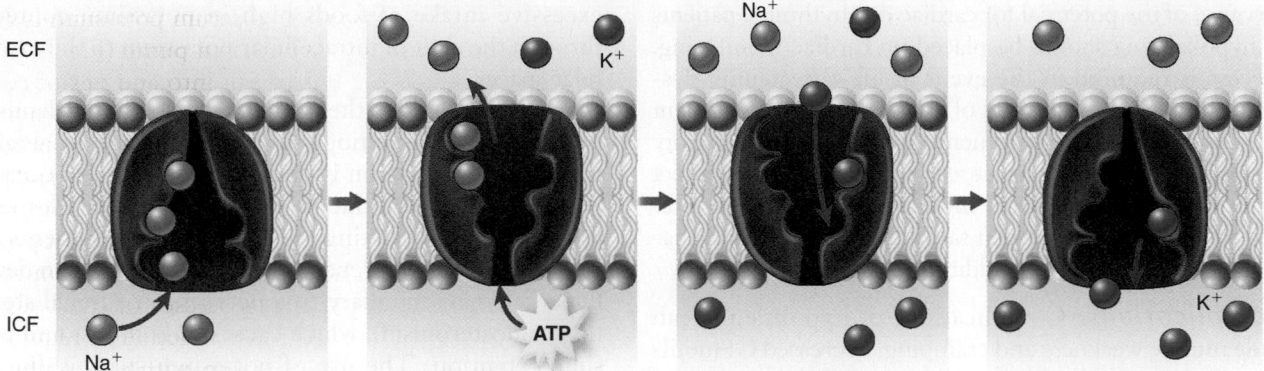

FIGURE 8.7 High concentrations of sodium and low concentrations of potassium are in the extracellular fluid (ECF), and diffusion occurs through ion channels in the cell membrane. The sodium–potassium pump maintains appropriate concentrations of these ions through active transport (adenosine triphosphate [ATP]).

Box 8.2 Potassium Content of Common Foods

- Spinach: 839 mg in 1 cup cooked
- Baked potato with skin: 738 mg in 1 small potato
- Tomato juice: 556 mg in 1 cup
- Mushrooms: 555 mg in 1 cup cooked
- Sweet potato: 475 mg in $1/2$ cup cooked
- Vegetable juice cocktail: 469 mg in 1 cup
- Banana: 422 mg in 1 medium-sized banana
- Cantaloupe: 417 mg in 1 cup
- Low-fat milk: 407 mg in 1 cup
- Kidney beans: 371 mg in $1/2$ cup cooked
- Avocado, California: 345 mg in $1/2$ avocado
- Tomato: 292 mg in 1 medium-sized tomato
- Kiwi: 284 mg in 1 kiwi
- Strawberries: 233 mg in 1 cup
- Orange: 232 mg in 1 medium-sized orange

---

stress, such as acute illness, post-cardiopulmonary resuscitation, and acute head injury, or during episodes of acute coronary ischemia can cause shifting of potassium intracellularly because of increased activity of sodium–potassium adenosine triphosphatase (ATPase).

Clinical Manifestations

Hypokalemia can result in a variety of physiological alterations, or patients may be asymptomatic if serum potassium levels remain greater than 3 mEq/L. Cardiac, pulmonary, neuromuscular, and GI symptoms can develop as a result of hypokalemia. Patients may experience weakness, lethargy, hyporeflexia, nausea/vomiting, constipation, abdominal cramping and electrocardiogram (ECG) changes (ST depression). In severe hypokalemia, cardiac or respiratory arrest can occur.

Cardiac symptoms in hypokalemia include the development of palpitations; premature atrial or ventricular complexes (PVCs), especially in patients with cardiovascular

disease; cardiac rate disturbances; and hypotension. In severe hypokalemia, sudden death can occur as a result of ventricular fibrillation. Respiratory complications can occur as a result of weakness of accessory muscles of the chest and abdomen, leading to hypoventilation, respiratory distress, and respiratory arrest. Neuromuscular symptoms include skeletal muscle weakness or cramping, paresthesias or paralysis, decreased muscle strength, and weakness of the GI tract. Anorexia, ileus, gaseous distention, abdominal cramping, prolonged gastric emptying, nausea, and vomiting can develop as a result of weakness of the GI muscles.

In the setting of prolonged potassium deficit, the inability of the kidneys to respond to ADH can result in polyuria, nocturia, and polydipsia. The resistance of the kidneys to ADH and increased stimulation of thirst results in polyuria, with potassium being lost with increased urine excretion. Nocturia occurs because of increased fluid intake during waking hours.

Management

Medical Management

Daily intake of potassium is essential for normal homeostasis. If adequate potassium levels are not achieved with dietary intake, supplemental potassium is required. Potassium replacement can be achieved using oral or parenteral routes, with oral being preferred because it is easy to administer, readily absorbed from the GI tract, and safe. In the setting of mild to moderate hypokalemia, oral replacement should suffice. In severe hypokalemia, administration of potassium both orally and parenterally may be required.

 Safety Alert   **Parenteral Potassium Administration**

Administration of IV potassium is considered a high-alert medication. Potassium is never to be administered as an IVP bolus. The total maximum 24-hour dose is 150 mEq. An infusion pump must be used when administering IV potassium.

Because of the potential for cardiac dysrhythmias, patients with hypokalemia should be placed on cardiac monitoring. IV access is required in the event of life-threatening dysrhythmias and IV replacement of potassium when the patient is not able to take oral replacement. Assessment of respiratory function is also a priority because low potassium levels affect the function of the respiratory muscles. Monitoring of respiratory rate, effort, and oxygen saturation provides information regarding the need for additional interventions.

Complications. Complications of hypokalemia can include muscle weakness and cramping, decreased GI motility, cardiac dysrhythmias, respiratory failure, cardiac or respiratory arrest, and death.

Nursing Management

Because of potentially life-threatening complications, monitoring patients at risk for developing hypokalemia is a key nursing role. This includes an assessment of serum potassium levels and physical assessment findings such as leg cramps and muscle weakness, as well as interpreting cardiac rhythm strips that can assist with early recognition of hypokalemia. Ventricular dysrhythmias are commonly seen in patients with hypokalemia and can progress to ventricular fibrillation, a life-threatening situation. In patients receiving digitalis, hypokalemia can potentiate the effects of digitalis by increasing blood levels of digoxin, leading to digoxin toxicity. Symptoms of digoxin toxicity include loss of appetite, nausea, vomiting, cardiac dysrhythmias, and visual disturbances.

Providing patient education regarding dietary sources of potassium, such as bananas, oranges, and raisins, to patients at risk for developing hypokalemia is an important nursing role. In addition, educating patients about clinical manifestations of hypokalemia can lead to early interventions to replace potassium.

Administration of a potassium replacement is another key nursing action. Oral replacement is the route of choice, with potassium supplements available in liquid, powder, caplet, and tablet forms. Parenteral replacement of potassium should be given slowly and never as an IVP medication because of the risk for cardiac dysrhythmias, cardiac arrest, and death. Potassium chloride can be administered parenterally in concentrated forms, 10 to 20 mEq in 100 mL of fluid over 1 to 2 hours, via an IV pump and preferably through a central access device. Potassium chloride is very irritating to small veins; high concentrations of potassium are not tolerated well by patients. Each institution has guidelines on concentrating and administering concentrated potassium solutions.

Hyperkalemia

Hyperkalemia is a serum potassium level greater than 5.0 mEq/L and is rarely seen in patients with normal renal function. Hyperkalemia is characterized as mild (5.0–6.0 mEq/L), moderate (6.1–7.0 mEq/L), and severe (greater than 7.0 mEq/L). Hyperkalemia can occur as a result of acute or chronic renal failure, medications, or excessive intake of foods high in potassium content or through the shift of intracellular potassium to the extracellular space.

Renal excretion is the primary regulation mechanism of potassium. In the setting of acute or chronic renal failure, excretion of potassium is diminished because of decreased potassium filtration due to a reduction in the glomerular filtration rate, resulting in hyperkalemia. Patients with Addison's disease (adrenal cortex insufficiency) can develop hyperkalemia secondary to a decrease in adrenal steroids (hypoaldosteronism), which causes sodium loss and potassium retention. The use of potassium-sparing diuretics, such as spironolactone (Aldactone), which inhibit the effects of aldosterone, allows excretion of water and sodium while retaining potassium. NSAIDs in the setting of renal insufficiency can result in hyperkalemia because these medications decrease renin secretion, which then decreases potassium excretion in the urine.

In addition to potassium-sparing diuretics and NSAIDs, potassium supplements, beta blockers, and digoxin/digitalis glycosides increase potassium levels because of decreased sodium–potassium ATPase activity. Combination medications, including potassium-sparing diuretics, place the patient at risk for hyperkalemia because of the inhibition of aldosterone binding to receptor sites. The use of potassium-based salt substitutes and intake of foods high in potassium, such as bananas, oranges, tomatoes, and high-protein diets, can result in hyperkalemia in patients with renal impairment.

Shifts of intracellular potassium to the ECF occur for several reasons. Metabolic acidosis, soft tissue injury (crush injury or burns), catabolism, and tissue lysis syndrome cause shifts or release of potassium from within the cell. In the setting of metabolic acidosis from acute renal failure, diabetic ketoacidosis, or lactic acidosis, hydrogen ions move into the cell in an attempt to correct acidotic pH levels, thus causing potassium to shift out of the cell. In the diuresis associated with diabetic ketoacidosis, there may be an increased loss of potassium in the urine, and potassium levels require vigilant monitoring as the hyperglycemia and metabolic acidosis resolve. In crush injuries or cellular breakdown, intracellular potassium is released into the bloodstream, leading to hyperkalemia.

In patients for whom hyperkalemia is unlikely, pseudohyperkalemia can occur because of hemolysis of blood samples, leukocytosis, thrombosis, and prolonged tourniquet use during phlebotomy. Pseudohyperkalemia occurs as a result of leakage of potassium from the cell, giving a false elevation of serum potassium levels. This disorder should be ruled out prior to intervening in patients with no risk of hyperkalemia.

Clinical Manifestations

Patients with hyperkalemia may complain of generalized fatigue, muscle cramps, palpitations, paresthesias, or weakness. The clinical presentation may not reflect the true extent of hyperkalemia, placing patients at high risk of cardiac arrest. The most important and potentially life-threatening consequence of hyperkalemia is its effect on the cardiac electrical conduction system. In patients with serum potassium levels greater than 6 mEq/L, ECG changes may be seen. Patients can develop bradycardia, sinus arrest, heart blocks, or ventricular dysrhythmias. Because of these cardiac rhythm abnormalities, patients can develop symptomatic hypotension. Initial ECG changes are narrow and peaked T waves, ST depression, and shortening of the QT interval (Fig. 8.8). If correction of serum potassium levels does not occur, progression in the severity of cardiac dysrhythmias and sudden cardiac death can occur. In potassium levels ranging from 6.5 to 7.5 mEq/L, there is a progression in the length of the PR, QRS, and QT intervals. In addition, there is a decrease in the amplitude of the R wave, with an increase in the depth of the S wave and depression of the elevation of the ST segment. In potassium levels greater than 7.5 mEq/L, there is a disappearance of the P wave with the development of junctional rhythms. The QRS complex widens and can proceed to the development of idioventricular rhythms. At potassium levels greater than 10 mEq/L, if immediate interventions are not undertaken, the QRS continues to widen to the development of a sine wave, which is preterminal. During assessment of the ECG, the sine wave is associated with the disappearance of the P wave and the merging of the QRS and T waves.

Management

Medical Management

Once the presence of hyperkalemia is recognized, an ECG should be obtained to assess for changes in cardiac rate and

rhythm. In situations where pseudohyperkalemia is suspected to be the cause of elevated potassium levels, repeated specimen collection and evaluation may be required. In patients with end-stage renal disease, prompt dialysis removes excessive serum potassium. In patients with hyperkalemia related to increased dietary or supplemental potassium intake, dietary modification and withholding of potassium supplements may be the only interventions required.

If ECG changes are present in the setting of hyperkalemia, the severity of the ECG changes will determine the priority of interventions. In severe hyperkalemia with widened QRS complexes and loss of P waves, parenteral administration of calcium is indicated. IV-administered calcium will not reduce serum potassium levels but will reverse ECG changes and decrease risks for ventricular dysrhythmias, and the effects from IV calcium are short-lived (30–60 minutes).

In the event of metabolic acidosis, correction of the underlying causes results in shifting of the potassium back into the cell. In diabetic ketoacidosis, correction of hyperglycemia through the use of short-acting IV insulin and volume replacement with normal saline (NS) solution corrects the acidosis, resulting in lowering of serum potassium levels. In metabolic acidosis from acute renal failure or lactic acidosis, the administration of sodium bicarbonate may be required. Sodium bicarbonate elevates the serum pH level by causing intracellular hydrogen to shift outside the cell, leading to potassium moving intracellularly. Sodium bicarbonate may be given as an IV bolus or continuous infusion until sufficient lowering of potassium is achieved.

IV administration of 25 to 40 g of 50% dextrose with 10 units of short-acting insulin promotes the movement of extracellular potassium into the cells. Use of regular insulin shifts glucose into the cell, and potassium follows glucose. The effects of IV 50% dextrose and short-acting insulin have an onset of 20 minutes and last 4 to 6 hours. The use of beta-adrenoceptor agonists such as albuterol (Proventil, Ventolin) in nebulized form can also result in a redistribution of the extracellular potassium intracellularly through activation of the sodium–potassium pump, sending potassium back into the cell. Dosing of albuterol is 4 times normal dosing, with onset of action in 30 minutes and benefits lasting 2 hours.

Elimination of potassium can also be achieved through the use of loop diuretics such as furosemide (Lasix) or bumetanide (Bumex). Loop diuretics inhibit the reabsorption of potassium, sodium, and chloride and the excretion of water. Caution is required with the use of loop diuretics because of the risk of development of a fluid volume deficit. The use of gastrointestinal cation exchangers such as sodium polystyrene sulfonate (Kayexalate) is another means to lower potassium levels. When administered, gastrointestinal cation exchangers cause an exchange of sodium for potassium in the gut, resulting in increased bowel elimination of potassium. Onset is slow, 2 hours, with the desired effect not seen for up to 6 hours.

K^+ Normal Range 3.5–5
Hyperkalemia Progression

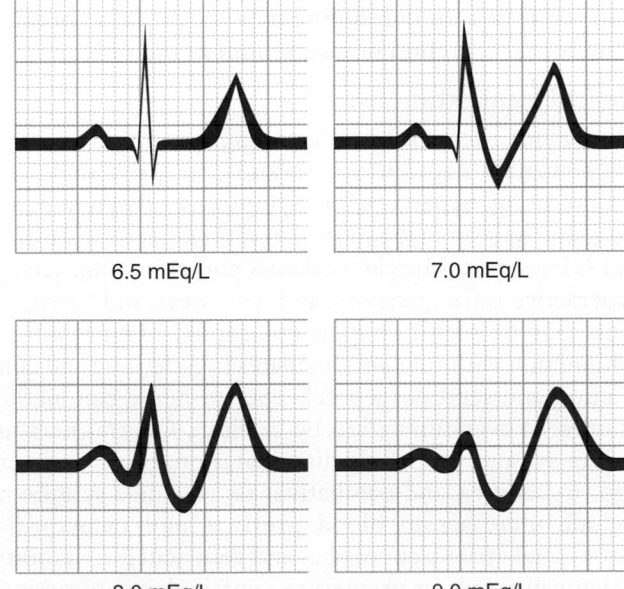

6.5 mEq/L 7.0 mEq/L

8.0 mEq/L 9.0 mEq/L

FIGURE 8.8 Initial electrocardiogram (ECG) changes are narrow and peaked T waves, ST depression, and shortening of the QT interval. In potassium levels ranging from 6.5 to 7.5 mEq/L, there is a progression in the length of the PR, QRS, and QT intervals. In potassium levels of greater than 7.5 mEq/L, there is a disappearance of the P wave with the development of junctional rhythms. As the potassium level exceeds 9.0 mEq/L, the QRS complex continues to widen.

Complications. Complications of hyperkalemia include cardiac dysrhythmias, which can progress to cardiac arrest and death. Muscular weakness with progression to paralysis can occur if hyperkalemia is not corrected. Gastrointestinal symptoms of nausea and diarrhea can also develop.

Nursing Management

Nurses must be alert to identify and monitor for clinical manifestations of hyperkalemia in high-risk patients, including those with cardiac dysrhythmias and muscle weakness. Monitoring and reporting elevations in BUN and creatinine (a reflection of renal function), serum glucose levels, and potassium and acid-base status also provide earlier identification of hyperkalemia. Elevations of BUN and creatinine indicate decreased renal function, which can result in decreased potassium excretion and hyperkalemia. Providing continuous cardiac monitoring with early recognition of the ECG changes associated with hyperkalemia enables early interventions. Resolution of the ECG changes can provide information about the effectiveness of interventions.

Administering medications as prescribed to lower elevated serum potassium levels and monitoring the results of measures used to lower potassium levels are important nursing roles. After administration of GI cation-exchange agents, it is important to monitor for the onset of GI effects. In patients treated with albuterol, monitor heart rate response for the potential development of tachycardia. The education provided to patients at risk of hyperkalemia should focus on limiting intake of foods high in potassium and potassium-based salt substitutes.

Magnesium

Magnesium, the fourth most abundant cation in the body, is needed for cellular functioning and has an interrelationship with the sodium–potassium–ATPase pump. Magnesium is also part of DNA and RNA transcription and is required for the production and function of adenosine triphosphate and protein synthesis. Needed for nucleic acid and protein synthesis, magnesium is also required for more than 300 biochemical reactions within the body. Magnesium alters the effects of calcium on smooth muscles, causing them to relax, and also antagonizes calcium ions at the presynaptic junction, reducing the release of acetylcholine. Acetylcholine is a major neurotransmitter of the autonomic nervous system and activates muscle function. Magnesium is needed for healthy bones and teeth, nerve and muscle function, and coagulation. It is also beneficial in preventing myocardial infarction, stroke, and osteoporosis. The normal reference range for magnesium is 1.6 to 2.2 mg/dL.

Hypomagnesemia

Hypomagnesemia is a serum magnesium level of less than 1.6 mg/dL and is seen in patients with malnutrition and excessive excretion of magnesium via the renal system. Hypokalemia and hypocalcemia may also be present in patients with hypomagnesemia. Calcium levels are affected by magnesium levels because of the dependence of the production of cyclic adenosine monophosphate on magnesium. Cyclic adenosine monophosphate controls the release of parathyroid hormone (PTH), which controls calcium levels. The relationship of hypomagnesemia and hypokalemia is not fully understood at present; it is thought that hypomagnesemia impairs sodium–potassium–ATPase, contributing to potassium wasting in urine.

People who chronically abuse alcohol are at risk for developing hypomagnesemia because of poor nutritional intake and GI malabsorption issues. Decreased absorption of magnesium in the GI tract can occur from inadequate dietary intake of food containing magnesium, diarrhea, damage to the small intestine resulting in poor absorption, and malnutrition. Malnutrition from low protein and calorie intake, high alcohol intake or chronic alcohol abuse, vomiting and diarrhea, laxative abuse, and dehydration can all result in hypomagnesemia.

Excess renal loss of magnesium in urine can be attributed to increased diuresis caused by loop diuretics, glycosuria, and chronic alcohol use. As urine output increases, increased magnesium loss occurs. In patients with elevated serum glucose levels, increased thirst (polydipsia) is present, resulting in increased urine output (polyuria). Alcohol is a diuretic, increasing urine output and losses of magnesium. Increased secretion of aldosterone, ADH, and administration of IV fluids all increase urine output, which may also lead to hypomagnesemia. Patients receiving certain diuretics (furosemide [Lasix], bumetanide [Bumex], and hydrochlorothiazide), chemotherapy agents (cisplatin), and antibiotics (amphotericin, cyclosporine, and gentamicin) are at risk for developing hypomagnesemia because of increased excretion of magnesium in the urine.

Clinical Manifestations

Clinical manifestations of hypomagnesemia, if present, are primarily neuromuscular and are associated with symptoms of hyperactivity. Symptoms of hypomagnesemia can be seen in the muscular, central nervous, cardiac, and GI systems. Muscle weakness and cramping, tetany, hyperactive reflex, tremors, and Trousseau and Chvostek signs may be seen in hypomagnesemia. Magnesium, in conjunction with calcium, regulates muscle tone and contraction and serves as a gatekeeper to nerve conduction to prevent overstimulation by calcium. Central nervous system symptoms include disorientation, psychosis, vertigo, irritability, and combativeness. Cardiac symptoms include increases in blood pressure and tachycardia, paroxysmal atrial tachycardia, and ventricular irritability, which can result in premature ventricular contractions (PVCs) and ventricular fibrillation or tachycardia. Anorexia, nausea, and vomiting may also be present. In patients with severe hypomagnesemia, seizures can develop because of alterations in electrical activity in the central nervous system (CNS). Seizures and emotional lability may occur.

Management

Medical Management

Because patients may not present with clinical manifestation of low serum magnesium levels, diagnostic laboratory results may be the first identification of hypomagnesemia. If hypomagnesemia is present, evaluation of potassium and calcium levels also needs to occur because magnesium is required to process potassium, and secondary to inhibited release of PTH, hypocalcemia can result. Replacement of magnesium is achieved through dietary increases in foods high in magnesium, such as whole grains and green leafy vegetables. Oral supplementation, such as magnesium oxide or magnesium gluconate, can also be given.

Replacement of magnesium IV may be required if patients are unable to tolerate oral intake or if clinical manifestations are present. IV administration of 2 to 4 grams of 50% magnesium sulfate diluted in D5W or 0.9% NaCl over 30 to 60 minutes is given to treat mild to severe magnesium deficits. In emergency treatment of ventricular fibrillation, 2 to 4 grams of 50% magnesium sulfate is administered as a bolus per Advanced Cardiac Life Support (ACLS) guidelines. During the administration of IV magnesium, monitoring of vital signs for early recognition of hypotension, changes in cardiac rate and rhythm, or the development of respiratory suppression is required.

Complications. Cardiac arrest from ventricular fibrillation and seizures can be life-threatening complications of hypomagnesemia. Prompt recognition of decreased serum magnesium, potassium, and calcium, all of which are important in the electrical stimulation and relaxation of smooth muscle, can assist in preventing these life-threatening complications.

Nursing Management

Recognition of and monitoring for clinical manifestations for patients at risk of hypomagnesemia is a nursing role. Providing safety interventions such as cardiac monitoring because of the risk of cardiac dysrhythmias, seizure precautions because of CNS hyperexcitability, and fall precautions because of muscle weakness and disorientation are examples of nursing interventions. With IV replacement, respiratory rate and effort are also monitored due to magnesium's respiratory-depression effects. Providing patient education regarding foods high in magnesium (Box 8.3) and the correct use of diuretics and laxatives also assists in preventing the reoccurrence of hypomagnesemia. In patients with chronic alcohol abuse–induced hypomagnesemia, nursing can provide counseling and referral to alcohol abstinence programs.

Hypermagnesemia

Hypermagnesemia is a serum magnesium level greater than 2.2 mg/dL, with the most common causes being over-replacement of magnesium deficits and renal insufficiency or renal failure. Because of the effective excretion of magnesium by the kidneys, hypermagnesemia is uncommon.

Box 8.3 Food Sources for Magnesium

- Halibut: 90 mg in 3 oz cooked
- Almonds, dry roasted: 80 mg in 1 oz
- Cashews, dry roasted: 75 mg in 1 oz
- Spinach, frozen: 75 mg in 1/2 cup cooked
- Nuts, mixed, dry roasted: 65 mg in 1 oz
- Cereal, shredded wheat: 55 mg in 2 rectangular biscuits
- Oatmeal, instant, fortified: 55 mg in 1 cup prepared with water
- Potato, baked w/skin: 50 mg in 1 medium-sized potato
- Peanuts, dry roasted: 50 mg in 1 oz
- Peanut butter, smooth: 50 mg in 2 Tbsp
- Wheat bran, crude: 45 mg in 2 Tbsp
- Black-eyed peas: 45 mg in 1/2 cup cooked
- Yogurt, plain, skim milk: 45 mg in 8 oz
- Bran flakes: 40 mg in 1/2 cup
- Rice, brown, long grain: 40 mg in 1/2 cup cooked
- Lentils: 35 mg in 1/2 cup cooked
- Avocado, California: 35 mg in 1/2 cup pureed
- Kidney beans: 35 mg in 1/2 cup canned
- Pinto beans: 35 mg in 1/2 cup cooked
- Wheat germ, crude: 35 mg in 2 Tbsp
- Chocolate milk: 33 mg in 1 cup
- Banana: 30 mg in 1 medium-sized banana
- Milk chocolate candy bar: 28 mg in 1.5-oz bar
- Milk, reduced fat (2%) or fat-free: 27 mg in 8 oz
- Bread, whole wheat, commercially prepared: 25 mg in 1 slice
- Raisins: 25 mg in 1/2 cup packed
- Whole milk: 24 mg in 1 cup
- Chocolate pudding: 24 mg in 4-oz ready-to-eat portion

Over-replacement of magnesium in the setting of hypomagnesemia or overuse of medications containing magnesium can lead to hypermagnesemia. Medications containing magnesium include milk of magnesia, magnesium citrate, aluminum-magnesium hydroxide (Maalox), and hydromagnesium aluminate. Older adults are at risk for hypermagnesemia because of decreased renal function and the use of magnesium-containing laxatives and antacids. Lithium toxicity can also result in hypermagnesemia because it decreases renal excretion of magnesium.

Because magnesium levels are affected by both renal and GI function, disorders of each may increase the risk of hypermagnesemia. Acute renal failure results in the inability of the kidneys to excrete magnesium in the urine, resulting in hypermagnesemia. In patients in whom destruction of soft tissue occurs, there is a release of intracellular magnesium. Soft tissue injuries include **rhabdomyolysis** (breakdown of muscle tissue that leads to the release of muscle fiber contents into the blood), burns, sepsis, trauma, and tissue lysis syndrome. Alternations in the GI tract can have an impact on serum magnesium levels. Intestinal hypomotility due to narcotics or anticholinergics and chronic constipation or bowel obstruction results in increased GI absorption and decreased elimination of magnesium through the GI tract.

Clinical Manifestations

Hypermagnesemia affects the cardiac, central nervous, respiratory, and hematologic systems. Cardiac symptoms in hypermagnesemia include hypotension due to vasodilation and dysrhythmias such as bradycardia, atrial fibrillation, and intraventricular conduction delays exhibited by widening of the QRS complexes. With serum levels greater than 10 mg/dL, heart blocks and asystole can occur. CNS clinical manifestations include drowsiness, lethargy, muscle weakness, loss of deep tendon reflexes, paralysis, and coma. Respiratory signs include a decrease in the respiratory rate that can lead to complete respiratory suppression. Hypermagnesemia is also associated with decreased platelet clumping and delayed formation of thrombin, increasing the risk of bleeding.

Management

Medical Management

Correction of hypermagnesemia is aimed at identifying the cause and intervening. If GI hypomotility is identified, the use of agents to promote GI motility, such as cathartics and enemas, stimulates GI loss of magnesium. Cessation of magnesium supplements, if present, and provision of IV hydration and loop diuretics to promote renal excretion of magnesium lower serum magnesium levels. Assessing the airway, breathing, and circulation and providing ventilatory support, treating cardiac dysrhythmias, and correcting hypotension with IV fluids are initial steps in the management of hypermagnesemia. In the setting of severe renal insufficiency or renal failure, hemodialysis with a low-magnesium dialysate may be required to lower serum magnesium levels. Administration of calcium gluconate 100 to 200 mg 10% solution in a continuous IV infusion (2–4 mg/kg/hr) may be required to antagonize the neuromuscular and cardiovascular effects of hypermagnesemia. Calcium reverses the effects of magnesium on smooth muscles, resolving clinical manifestations.

Complications. Serum magnesium levels of greater than 10 mg/dL can result in respiratory failure, stupor or coma, cardiac arrest, hypotension refractory to vasopressors, and death.

Nursing Management

Recognition of and monitoring for clinical manifestations of hypermagnesemia in patients at risk are a nursing priority. Nurses need to monitor vital signs for signs of hypotension, cardiac dysrhythmias, and respiratory depression. Neurological assessment includes monitoring for changes in the level of consciousness and deep tendon reflexes. Loss of deep tendon reflexes occurs because of the blockage of synaptic transmission of nerve impulses that occurs when magnesium levels reach 6 to 10. Older adults need to be provided with patient education focused on limiting the use of magnesium-containing laxatives and antacids. In patients at risk for developing hypermagnesemia due to renal insufficiency or renal failure, education regarding the identification of high-magnesium-content foods and over-the-counter medications is important.

Connection Check 8.6

The nurse identifies the patient with which electrolyte abnormality as having the greatest risk for ventricular fibrillation?

A. Hypochloremia
B. Hyponatremia
C. Hypocalcemia
D. Hypokalemia

Calcium

Calcium is utilized in processes such as cardiac contraction, blood coagulation, transmission of nerve impulses, and muscular contractions. Calcium is found primarily within bones (99%), with the remaining 1% found in the cells (0.7%) and the ECF (0.3%). The extracellular calcium is either ionized or free (50%); plasma-protein bound (40%); or complexed (10%) or chelated to citrate, phosphate, or sulfate. The ionized form of calcium is the active form of calcium that is involved with cellular functions. The plasma value of calcium is related to changes in plasma albumin, and low levels of albumin result in low levels of total calcium. In patients with low serum calcium levels, it is important for the nurse to also assess the serum albumin level. The ionized calcium levels are the most accurate measurements of active calcium. Normal values for ionized calcium are 4.6 to 5.3 mg/dL and for total calcium are 8.2 to 10.2 mg/dL. Calcium levels are tightly controlled by parathormone (PTH), calcitriol (vitamin D), and calcitonin (secreted by the thyroid gland).

Calcium is regulated on the basis of the functions of the parathyroid and thyroid glands. Parathyroid hormone (parathormone [PTH]) is secreted from the parathyroid glands that are located in the neck area, around the thyroid glands. There is a direct relationship between PTH and serum calcium levels; an increase in PTH leads to an increase in serum calcium. Parathyroid hormone leads to increases in reabsorption of calcium in the urine, in calcium reabsorption from the intestine (vitamin D required), and in osteoclastic (bone-breakdown) activity. Calcitonin, secreted by the thyroid gland, also has a role in calcium regulation. Serum calcium levels decrease as a result of calcitonin because it acts on the kidney to increase calcium excretion.

Hypocalcemia

Hypocalcemia is serum calcium levels less than 8.2 mg/dL with a normal albumin level or ionized calcium less than 4.6 mg/dL. Hypocalcemia also occurs as a result of vitamin D deficiency, hypoparathyroidism, diarrhea, malnutrition, lactation, pregnancy, chronic renal failure, bone disease, and chronic alcohol abuse. Vitamin D is required for calcium absorption from the GI tract. In patients with hypoparathyroidism, the PTH, which regulates calcium balance, is low, resulting in low serum calcium levels. Hypocalcemia develops from diarrhea, malnutrition, chronic alcohol abuse, inadequate absorption of calcium in the intestines, and inadequate vitamin D intake. During pregnancy, the fetus requires calcium for mineralization of the skeleton and for normal physiological functions, and lactation provides calcium for continued skeletal growth. In chronic renal failure, there is decreased absorption of calcium because of nonfunctioning kidneys and in response to hyperphosphatemia.

Clinical Manifestations

Clinical manifestations of hypocalcemia are dependent on the rapidity of onset and severity. There may be no symptoms in patients with chronic hypocalcemia. In acute moderate hypocalcemia, 6 to 7 mg/dL, signs include excitability of nerves and muscles, which can lead to focal numbness, muscle spasms, paresthesias, twitching, tremors, and tetany. Smooth muscle spasms can lead to biliary colic, dysphagia, wheezing, and bronchospasm. Cardiac effects of hypocalcemia include lengthening of the QT interval, which predisposes the patient to ventricular dysrhythmias. In addition, hypocalcemia can cause decreased myocardial contractility, which can lead to hypotension, angina, and congestive heart failure. Calcium is required by cardiac cells for contraction as part of the action potential, and it also prolongs the depolarization phase, making the heart less receptive to further stimulation. Patients may also experience anxiety, confusion, and irritability secondary to low calcium levels. Positive Trousseau (Fig. 8.9) and Chvostek (Fig. 8.10) signs are classic physical assessment findings in hypocalcemia. Depending on the level of hypocalcemia, twitching of the facial muscles is elicited along with carpal spasm. Clinical manifestations of chronic hypocalcemia also include coarse hair, brittle nails, cataracts, chronic pruritus, and dry skin.

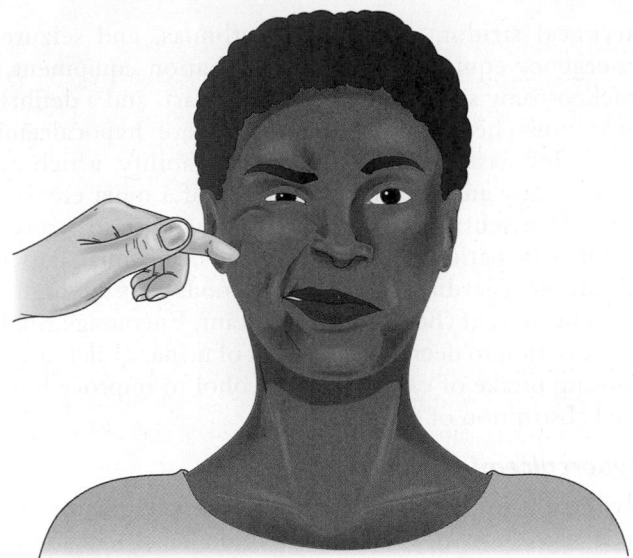

FIGURE 8.10 Chvostek sign. Tapping over the facial nerve leads to twitching of the face related to hyperexcitability at the neuromuscular junction due to hypocalcemia.

Management

Medical Management

Acute severe hypocalcemia, serum calcium levels less than 6.5 mg/dL, can produce life-threatening clinical manifestations and is often associated with other complex disease processes such as chronic renal failure, Crohn's disease, and pancreatitis. Initial care includes protection and maintenance of the airway and breathing, implementation of cardiac monitoring, and placement of an IV catheter. Evaluation of diagnostic results establishes the presence of hypocalcemia and other electrolyte abnormalities such as hypomagnesemia, hyperphosphatemia, or hypoalbuminemia. In severe symptomatic hypocalcemia, serum calcium levels less than 6.5 mg/dL, IV replacement of calcium is recommended. Calcium gluconate 0.5 mg/kg/hr IV in D5W over 10 to 15 minutes is administered and may be increased to 2 mg/kg/hr, not to exceed 3 to 4 g IV over 4 hours. The bolus is then followed by a continuous infusion until correction of the calcium deficit has occurred.

Re-evaluation of serum calcium levels should be done every 4 to 6 hours during replacement therapy to prevent hypercalcemia. If hypomagnesemia is present, it should be treated prior to treating hypocalcemia because correction of hypocalcemia is refractory until correction of hypomagnesemia has occurred. Magnesium resistance to PTH diminishes its secretion, affecting calcium concentration in the blood. In chronic hypocalcemia, oral calcium supplements and vitamin D are administered.

Complications. Cardiovascular collapse, refractory hypotension, laryngospasm, dysrhythmias, and decompensated heart failure can develop in acute severe hypocalcemia.

Nursing Management

Nursing care focuses on monitoring patients at risk for the development of hypocalcemia. Because of the potential for

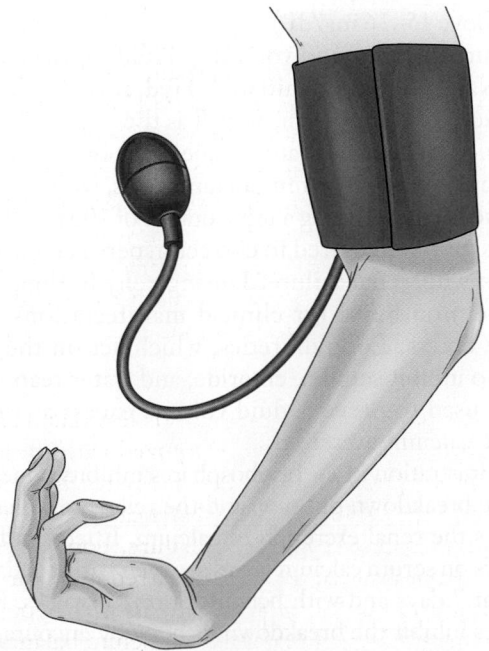

FIGURE 8.9 Positive Trousseau sign. With inflation of the blood pressure cuff, the fingers go into carpal spasm, indicating hypocalcemia.

laryngeal stridor, cardiac dysrhythmias, and seizures, emergency equipment such as intubation equipment, a tracheostomy set, a code/emergency cart, and a defibrillator must be readily available. Severe hypocalcemia causes increased neuromuscular excitability, which can cause tetany and seizures. Provision of a quiet environment is essential to decrease stimulation to prevent seizures in patients with severe hypocalcemia. Patient education regarding the intake of foods that are high in calcium content (Box 8.4) is important. Encourage smoking cessation to decrease excretion of urinary calcium and limiting intake of caffeine and alcohol to improve intestinal absorption of calcium.

Hypercalcemia

Hypercalcemia is a serum calcium level greater than 10.2 mg/dL with a normal albumin level and ionized calcium levels greater than 5.3 mg/dL. Malignancy and primary hyperparathyroidism are the principal causes of hypercalcemia. Bone metastasis secondary to breast carcinoma, lymphoma, multiple myeloma, and non–small-cell lung cancer can result in hypercalcemia. Humoral hypercalcemia of malignancy can occur as a result of cervical, ovarian, renal, bladder, or esophageal malignancies or head and neck and lung squamous-cell cancer because of increased osteoclastic activity within the bone. Osteoclastic activity results in bone destruction and the release of calcium into the ECF. In hyperparathyroidism, there is an increased release of PTH, resulting in increased release of calcium from bones, increased absorption of calcium in the intestine, and increased reabsorption in the renal system. Medications such as thiazide diuretics, lithium, and calcium carbonate, as well as theophylline toxicity and hypervitaminosis of vitamins A and D, can also cause hypercalcemia. Thiazide diuretics decrease the excretion of calcium in the urine. Lithium increases PTH, which increases serum calcium levels. Theophylline toxicity results in hypercalcemia due to stimulation of beta receptors in the bone, resulting in the release of calcium from the bone. Hypervitaminosis of vitamins A and D causes excessive bone **resorption** (the breakdown of bone resulting in the release of calcium), as well as increased calcium absorption in the intestines.

Box 8.4 Foods High in Calcium

- Milk: 290–300 mg in 8 oz milk
- Orange or grapefruit juice: 300 mg in 8 oz
- Canned salmon (with bones): 170–210 mg in 3 oz
- American cheese: 165–200 mg in 1-oz slice of cheese
- Broccoli: 160–180 mg in 1 cup
- Soybean curd (tofu): 145–155 mg in 4 oz
- Kale: 90–100 mg in 1/2 cup, cooked
- Ice cream or frozen dessert: 80–100 mg in 1/2 cup
- Egg: 55 mg in 1 medium-sized egg

Clinical Manifestations

As with hypocalcemia, clinical manifestations of hypercalcemia are related to the rapidity of onset and severity of elevation as well as the overall health status of the patient. The patient's clinical presentation may be nonspecific in hypercalcemia and include clinical manifestations such as bradycardia, hypertension, thirst, lethargy, muscle weakness, abdominal discomfort, constipation, and decreased deep tendon reflexes. Mild and chronic elevation of serum calcium levels may not produce any clinical manifestations. In acute moderate hypercalcemia, calcium levels of 11.5 to 18 mg/dL, anorexia, nausea, vomiting, lethargy, nonspecific joint and muscle aches, and confusion may be present.

Severe elevation in calcium levels can result in coma. Renal calculi, polyuria, dehydration, and, in the setting of calcium levels greater than 13 mg/dL, renal failure may develop. Renal calculi develop as calcium crystals combine to form stones. Renal calculi can obstruct urine flow, leading to renal failure. Calcium deposits within the kidney can impair renal function, resulting in renal failure. Skeletal fractures can occur from osteopenia secondary to calcium loss from the bone.

Management

Medical Management

Initial medical management is dependent on the severity of hypercalcemia and is aimed at stabilization and reduction of calcium levels. Reduction of serum calcium is achieved through increased calcium excretion and decreased resorption of calcium from bone. Discontinuation of medications associated with hypercalcemia and treatment of the underlying causes of hypercalcemia, such as malignancies, hyperparathyroidism, and renal failure, if possible, are additional initial interventions.

In patients with severe hypercalcemia (serum calcium levels above 15–16 mg/dL), hypovolemia is present because of polyuria, nausea, and vomiting. Fluid replacement with 0.9% NaCl should be initiated. Hydration facilitates the renal excretion of calcium, as well as the expansion of ECF. The fluid replacement rate is dependent on the severity of dehydration and the serum calcium levels, with the infusion rate aimed at maintaining a urine output of 100 to 150 mL/hr. Dialysis may be required to correct hypercalcemic states in patients with renal failure. During rehydration, patients must be monitored for clinical manifestations of fluid volume excess. Loop diuretics, which act on the loop of Henle to inhibit sodium, chloride, and water reabsorption, may be used to prevent fluid volume excess as well as to increase calcium excretion.

Administration of IV bisphosphates inhibits bone resorption, the breakdown of bone, and the release of calcium and increases the renal excretion of calcium. Effects of bisphosphonates on serum calcium levels are seen within 2 days, with a peak at 7 days and with benefits lasting 2 weeks. Bisphosphonates inhibit the breakdown of bone by encouraging osteoclasts (cells that destroy bone) to undergo cell death, preventing the release of calcium. Calcitonin also inhibits bone resorption and increases the renal excretion of calcium.

Calcitonin is administered intramuscularly or subcutaneously, with effects within several hours and lasting several days.

In hypercalcemia caused by malignancies, interventions are aimed at the treatment of the malignancies, which cause the release of calcium from the bone, through chemotherapy, surgical removal, or radiation therapy. The use of glucocorticoids in patients with multiple myeloma and hematological malignancies decreases intestinal absorption of calcium and increases renal excretion of calcium. Glucocorticoids inhibit vitamin D–mediated GI absorption of calcium and increase urinary calcium excretions, both of which lower serum calcium levels.

In hyperparathyroidism, treatment is aimed at controlling serum calcium levels and can be achieved through nonsurgical interventions or surgical removal of the parathyroid glands. Nonsurgical interventions include limiting intake of calcium-containing foods, maintaining good hydration, increasing mobilization, engaging in regular exercise activities, and avoiding medications that can impact calcium levels.

Complications. Hypercalcemic crisis occurs when serum calcium levels are greater than 14 mg/dL with the presence of clinical manifestations of acute hypercalcemia. Cardiac rhythm changes such as lengthening of PR and QRST intervals, T-wave changes such as flattening or inversion, and varying degrees of heart block can develop, progressing to cardiac arrest. Patients with acute hypercalcemia may have confusion and lethargy with potential progression to coma.

Nursing Management

Monitoring patients at risk for the development of hypercalcemia is the initial role of nursing. Because of cardiac and neurological clinical manifestations related to hypercalcemia, nurses assess for changes in cardiac rhythm and mental status. Encouraging early and frequent ambulation of patients at risk for hypercalcemia, as well as adequate hydration, assists in preventing elevated serum calcium in patients at risk. Monitor for clinical manifestations of fluid volume excess in patients receiving rehydration therapy in the setting of hypercalcemia. When encouraging oral hydration, provide patients with liquids of choice.

Connection Check 8.7

Which nursing action is the priority in the patient with a serum calcium of 6.0 mg/dL?

A. Prepare for placement of a nasogastric tube.

B. Place an intubation tray at the bedside.

C. Place an indwelling urinary catheter.

D. Prepare for emergency dialysis.

Phosphorus

Phosphorus is primarily found in combination with calcium in bones, with the remainder found inside cells. Phosphorus exists as phosphate in the body and is critical for numerous cellular processes, such as cellular energy metabolism, production of DNA and RNA, membrane structure, and regulation of enzyme and protein actions. Phosphorus levels are always evaluated in comparison to calcium because of their inverse relationship. Phosphorus levels are maintained with dietary intake and renal excretion. The normal value of serum phosphorus is 2.5 to 4.5 mg/dL.

Hypophosphatemia

Hypophosphatemia is a serum phosphorus level of less than 2.5 mg/dL, and clinical manifestations appear only when phosphorus levels are less than 1 mg/dL. Hypophosphatemia results from decreased dietary intake, decreased intestinal absorption of phosphorus, and increased renal excretion of phosphorus. Low phosphate levels may also be the result of shifts of phosphate from the intracellular space into the extracellular space, which leads to urinary loss. In respiratory alkalosis, phosphate shifts into the cell and is used for intracellular glycolysis, leading to phosphorus consumption. Hypophosphatemia can be seen in patients with extensive burns, diabetic ketoacidosis, critical illness, malnourishment, refeeding syndrome, alcoholism, and excessive antacid use. In extensive burns, the mechanism of development of hypophosphatemia is unclear, with salt and water diuresis that occurs after burn injury considered to be the cause. In diabetic ketoacidosis, insulin deficiency mobilizes intracellular phosphate, causing phosphate to shift to the extracellular space and leading to urinary loss. Phosphorus levels can also decrease in the treatment of DKA with insulin that moves glucose into the cell and phosphorus is consumed during phosphorylation. Critically ill patients may develop hypophosphatemia because of acid-base disturbances, acute kidney injury, or increased cellular uptake of phosphorus due to catecholamine release. In patients with malnourishment or refeeding syndrome, giving carbohydrates stimulates the release of insulin, which moves glucose and phosphate into the cell. Excessive antacid use results in binding of phosphate in the gut, preventing absorption. Hypophosphatemia may also be caused by hypercalcemia, lack of vitamin D, and hyperparathyroidism.

Clinical Manifestations

The clinical presentation of hypophosphatemia may include alterations in neurological, cardiac, and musculoskeletal function. Confusion, apprehension, seizures, and coma are neurological symptoms. The most commonly seen manifestation of hypophosphatemia is skeletal or smooth muscle weakness, including weakness in any muscle group. In addition to muscle weakness, respiratory insufficiency can develop from diaphragmatic dysfunction. Clinical manifestations of hypophosphatemia may also include tremors, paresthesias, joint stiffness, and bone pain.

Management

Medical Management

Determining and treating the cause of the intracellular-to-extracellular movement of phosphorus, known as transcellular shift, are the goals of treatment of acute moderate hypophosphatemia if no clinical manifestations are present. Correction of additional electrolyte disturbances (hypokalemia, hypomagnesemia, and hypocalcemia) facilitates the correction of serum phosphorus transcellular shifts. Hypokalemia and hypomagnesemia increase the renal loss of phosphorus. In the setting of acute severe hypophosphatemia or if the GI tract is nonfunctioning, IV replacement of phosphorus may be required until phosphorus levels are greater than 1.5 mg/dL. Caution must be given to prevent the development of hyperphosphatemia. Management of the phosphorus level focuses on ensuring adequate intake through foods, enteral feedings, and total parenteral nutrition, especially in patients at risk.

Complications. Patients with acute severe hypophosphatemia can develop widespread organ-system dysfunction due to depletion of ATP, which is responsible for intracellular energy transfer, and if phosphorus levels are low, energy production converts to glycolysis. Phosphorus is required for the delivery and release of oxygen to cells. In hypophosphatemia, cell dysfunction can occur, resulting in multiple-organ-system disorders. In critically ill patients, respiratory insufficiency and depressed cardiac contractility may be present. Cardiac dysrhythmias, impaired hepatic function, seizures, and depressed function of white blood cells can also occur because of intracellular ATP. Bleeding from platelet dysfunction and hemolysis are rare complications of severe hypophosphatemia.

Nursing Management

Monitoring and identifying patients at risk for developing hypophosphatemia are the roles of the nurse. Patients at greatest risk for hypophosphatemia are those with a history of chronic alcohol abuse, diabetic ketoacidosis treated with insulin, critical illness, or malnourishment or those with extensive burns. Patients with hypophosphatemia are monitored for clinical manifestations indicating changes in patient status, such as confusion, increased muscle weakness, and myocardial irritability. Nursing care is aimed at the treatment of emergent causes of hypophosphatemia and, with chronic disorders, at patient and family education regarding dietary sources for ensuring adequate intake of phosphorus.

Hyperphosphatemia

Hyperphosphatemia is defined as a serum phosphate level greater than 4.5 mg/dL. Renal failure is the most frequent cause of hyperphosphatemia and is secondary to decreased renal excretion of phosphorus. Additional causes include shifts from the intracellular to the extracellular space as a result of diabetic ketoacidosis (DKA) and increased ingestion with a decreased output of phosphorus. In DKA, phosphate levels increase secondary to intracellular phosphorus moving in to the extracellular fluid. Shifts of phosphorus can occur as a result of cellular breakdown, secondary to tumor lysis, acute hemolysis, or rhabdomyolysis. Increased intake of phosphorus can be seen in vitamin D intoxication, excessive use of oral saline laxatives, or phosphate replacement. Hyperphosphatemia may also be secondary to hyperthyroidism or hypoparathyroidism.

Clinical Manifestations

The clinical manifestations of hyperphosphatemia are similar to those seen in hypocalcemia because of the inverse relationship of phosphorus and calcium. Hypocalcemia is caused by phosphorous precipitating calcium and altering bone reabsorption of calcium through stimulation of the PTH, which may result in life-threatening hypocalcemia.

A positive Chvostek or Trousseau sign, hyperreflexia, soft tissue calcification, and tetany may occur with elevated phosphorus levels. Patients may complain of bone and joint pain, muscle weakness, anorexia, and paresthesias. Delirium, convulsions, seizures, and coma may also be noted. Cardiovascular symptoms such as hypotension, heart failure, and a prolonged QT interval on the ECG may be seen. Long-term effects of hyperphosphatemia include the development of calcifications found in soft tissue, the kidneys, the skin, the cornea, and blood vessels. Calcium calcifications play a key role in the development of cardiovascular disease and mitral and aortic stenosis and in the progression of renal disease, resulting in high morbidity and mortality of these patients.

Management
Medical Management

Identification of the underlying causes of hyperphosphatemia and treatment are the focus of medical management. Increasing renal excretion of phosphorus through volume replacement with IV normal saline and the use of loop diuretics facilitate the renal excretion of phosphorus. Because of the relationship of phosphorus and calcium, correction of hypocalcemia corrects hyperphosphatemia. In patients with severe renal insufficiency or renal failure, dialysis may be required if hypocalcemia is also present. Limiting the intake of phosphorus-containing foods may be adequate to control hyperphosphatemia. The use of phosphate binders in patients with renal failure is indicated because they inhibit absorption of phosphate through the GI tract.

Complications. Short-term complications of hyperphosphatemia include possible tetany from acute hypocalcemia. Long-term effects can be seen in any organ system and can result in vascular wall calcification and arteriosclerosis, kidney disease, bone and joint pain, and fractures.

Nursing Management

Monitoring and identifying patients at risk for developing hyperphosphatemia are the roles of the nurse. Nursing care is aimed at patient and family education regarding the dietary management of phosphorus intake. Dietary education focuses on foods to avoid, such as meats, nuts, high-protein foods, cheese, and other dairy products. Because of the inverse relationship between phosphorus and calcium, patient education needs to include the symptoms of hypocalcemia.

Making Connections

CASE STUDY: WRAP-UP

Henrietta is ready for discharge home. She continues to have fine crackles in her lung bases and trace peripheral edema in her lower extremities. Laboratory work collected today shows hemoglobin 11.7 g/dL, hematocrit 34%, Na⁺ 140 mEq/L, K⁺ 4.2 mEq/L, BUN 27 mg/dL, and creatinine 0.9 mg/dL. Her discharge medications include furosemide (Lasix) 40 mg by mouth daily, K-Tab 20 mEq by mouth daily, digoxin 0.125 mg by mouth daily, spironolactone (Aldactone) 25 mg by mouth twice daily, and carvedilol (Coreg) 6.25 mg by mouth twice daily. Discharge instructions include taking daily weights, calling her physician if a weight gain of 3 to 4 pounds over 3 days is noted, avoiding salt substitutes, and limiting fluid intake to 1,200 mL per day.

Case Study Questions

1. The charge nurse is reviewing the admission orders for Henrietta, who has been admitted with heart failure and renal insufficiency. It is a priority for the charge nurse to follow up with the provider about which order?
   A. Digoxin 0.125 mg by mouth daily
   B. Carvedilol (Coreg) 12.5 mg by mouth twice daily
   C. Bumetanide (Bumex) 1 mg by mouth twice daily
   D. Spironolactone (Aldactone) 25 mg by mouth three times a day

2. Which statement by Henrietta about potassium supplements indicates the need for further teaching?
   A. "In addition to the potassium supplement, I will eat a banana every day."
   B. "I can liberally use salt substitutes with my meals."
   C. "I should stop taking the K-Tab if I have no leg cramps."
   D. "Fruits and vegetables are a good source of potassium."

3. The nurse is providing discharge instructions to Henrietta regarding dietary sources of potassium. The nurse does not recommend which food as a source of high potassium content?
   A. Baked potato
   B. Apple
   C. Banana
   D. Cooked spinach

4. When providing discharge instructions for Henrietta, the nurse should include which of the following? *(Select all that apply.)*
   A. Weigh herself daily at the same time.
   B. Limit fluid intake to 3 L per day.
   C. Limit salt intake.
   D. Increase the intake of fresh fruits and vegetables.
   E. Report a 3-lb weight gain in 2 days to her primary care provider.

5. Which statement by Henrietta indicates the need for further teaching about hyperkalemia?
   A. "It is normal to have heart palpitations."
   B. "Fatigue and weakness are signs of low potassium."
   C. "Some of my medications make me at risk for high potassium."
   D. "I may have numbness and tingling when my potassium is high."

CHAPTER SUMMARY

Fluids are categorized as intracellular and extracellular, which includes plasma, intercellular (interstitial) and transcellular fluids. Patients at risk for fluid deficits are those who are unable to access fluids independently; have cognitive changes that diminish the thirst mechanism; or have increased fluid loss due to vomiting, diarrhea, or insensible fluid losses. Clinical manifestations of fluid volume deficits include tachycardia, hypotension, poor skin turgor, and weight loss. Patients at risk for fluid volume excess are older adults with compromised cardiac and renal functions. The clinical presentation of fluid volume excess includes crackles, tachycardia, hypertension, hypoxia, weight gain, and edema.

Sodium is the most prevalent electrolyte in the ECF and is required for many regulatory functions, including fluid and electrolyte balance and neuromuscular activity. The normal range of sodium is 135 to 145 mEq/L. Hyponatremia, a serum sodium level of less than 135 mEq/L, is the most common electrolyte disturbance seen in hospitalized patients. Hyponatremia occurs as a result of increased levels of ADH and aldosterone and fluid volume excess. Clinical manifestations often include neuromuscular manifestations, such as confusion, headache, and muscle cramps.

Hypernatremia, a serum sodium level of greater than 145 mEq/L, is seen in excess loss or decreased intake of water, decreased levels of ADH, and intake of excessive amounts of sodium. Treatment is aimed at the replacement of water. Clinical manifestations of hypernatremia include increased thirst, poor skin turgor, hypotension and tachycardia, confusion, and restlessness.

Chloride is the major ECF anion and works in conjunction with sodium to maintain osmotic pressure. The normal serum chloride value range is 97 to 107 mEq/L. Hypochloremia refers to serum chloride levels of less than 97 mEq/L and occurs as a result of chloride loss. Patients with hypochloremia may exhibit hypotension, tetany, shallow respirations, and hyperexcitability of muscles and nerves. Hyperchloremia is present if the serum chloride level is greater than 107 mEq/L and can result in bicarbonate loss, resulting in metabolic acidosis and hypernatremia. Clinical manifestations of hyperchloremia include deep and rapid respirations, lethargy, tachypnea, decreased cognitive ability, and increased blood pressure.

Potassium is the most abundant intracellular cation and is essential to neuromuscular function and metabolic processes. The normal range of serum potassium is 3.5 to 5.0 mEq/L. Hypokalemia, a serum potassium level of less than 3.5 mEq/L, is seen in patients with alkalosis, loss due to nasogastric suctioning, diuretic use, and increased renal loss. Treatment includes oral or IV replacement of potassium. Clinical manifestations of hypokalemia include muscle weakness, cardiac dysrhythmias, and altered carbohydrate metabolism. Hyperkalemia, a serum potassium level of greater than 5.0 mEq/L, is seen in patients with acidosis, cell trauma, and renal failure. Treatment is aimed at lowering potassium levels by causing a shift of potassium back into the cell, binding of potassium in the gut, and correction of acidosis. The clinical presentation of hyperkalemia includes muscle weakness and cardiac dysrhythmias.

Magnesium is the fourth most abundant cation in the body and is needed for cellular functioning, healthy bones and teeth, nerve and muscle function, and coagulation. The normal reference range for magnesium is 1.6 to 2.2 mg/dL. Hypomagnesemia is a serum magnesium level of less than 1.6 mg/dL and is seen in patients with malnutrition and excessive excretion of magnesium via the renal system. Clinical manifestations of hypomagnesemia include muscle weakness and cramping, tetany, hyperactive reflexes, and tremors. Hypermagnesemia is a serum magnesium level of greater than 2.2 mg/dL, with the most common causes being over-replacement of magnesium deficits and renal insufficiency or renal failure. Clinical manifestations of high serum magnesium levels include hypotension, dysrhythmias, muscle weakness, and loss of deep tendon reflexes.

Calcium is utilized in processes such as cardiac contraction, blood coagulation, transmission of nerve impulses, and muscular contractions. Normal values for ionized calcium are 4.6 to 5.3 mg/dL and for total calcium are 8.2 to 10.2 mg/dL. Hypocalcemia is serum calcium levels of less than 8.2 mg/dL with a normal albumin level or ionized calcium less than 4.6 mg/dL. Clinical manifestations of hypocalcemia include positive Trousseau and Chvostek signs, tetany, and laryngospasm. Cardiac signs including lengthening of the QT interval, ventricular dysrhythmias, and hypotension and angina secondary to decreased myocardial contractility. Hypercalcemia is a serum calcium level of greater than 10.2 mg/dL with a normal albumin level and ionized calcium levels greater than 5.3 mg/dL and is often associated with malignancies. Clinical manifestations include bradycardia, hypertension, abdominal discomfort, lethargy, and confusion.

Phosphorus exists as phosphate in the body and is critical for numerous cellular processes, such as cellular energy metabolism. The normal value of serum phosphorus is 2.5 to 4.5 mg/dL. Hypophosphatemia is a serum phosphorus level of less than 2.5 mg/dL. Confusion, apprehension, seizures, coma, and skeletal and smooth muscle weakness are clinical manifestations of hypophosphatemia. Hyperphosphatemia is a serum phosphate level of greater than 4.5 mg/dL, and renal failure is the most frequent cause. Clinical manifestations include positive Chvostek or Trousseau sign, hyperreflexia, soft tissue calcification, tetany, bone and joint pain, muscle weakness, anorexia, and paresthesias. Cardiovascular clinical manifestations may include hypotension, heart failure, and a prolonged QT interval on the ECG.

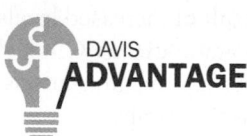

DAVIS
ADVANTAGE   To explore learning resources for this chapter, go to **Davis Advantage** and find:
- Answers to in-text questions
- Chapter Resources and Activities
- NCLEX®-Style Chapter Review Questions
- Bibliography

Chapter 9

Acid-Base Balance

Trisha Fronczek

LEARNING OUTCOMES

Content in this chapter is designed to assist in:

1. Describing the significance of acid-base balance for normal function
2. Stating the steps for arterial blood gas interpretation
3. Explaining the meaning of compensation
4. Comparing and contrasting major acid-base disorders
5. Describing the role of the respiratory and renal systems in acid-base balance
6. Explaining nursing considerations related to patients with acid-base disorders

CONCEPTS

- Assessment
- Fluid and Electrolyte Balance
- Oxygenation
- pH Regulation

ESSENTIAL TERMS

Acid
Acid-base balance
Acid-base imbalance
Anion gap
Base
Base excess
Bicarbonate
Bicarbonate buffers
Carbon dioxide
Chemical buffers
Compensation
Fully compensated
Hydrogen ion
Metabolic acidosis
Metabolic alkalosis
Oxygenation
PaO$_2$
Partially compensated
pH
Phosphate buffers
Protein buffers
Renal buffers
Respiratory acidosis
Respiratory alkalosis
Respiratory buffers
Uncompensated

Finding Connections

CASE STUDY: EPISODE 1

Follow this patient throughout the chapter.

Cory Nelson, 21 years old, presents via ambulance to the emergency department after a motor vehicle accident (MVA). When the car he was a passenger in struck a tree, Cory was wearing his seat belt. He sustained chest trauma due to the impact and has facial lacerations. The paramedic at the scene noted that Cory had alcohol present on his breath and slurred speech when questioned...

ACID-BASE BALANCE OVERVIEW

Acid-base balance refers to the homeostasis of the **hydrogen ion** (H+) concentration in body fluids. The body fluid's concentration of hydrogen ions is expressed as the body's **pH** level (Fig. 9.1). Body fluids are further classified as **acids** or **bases** according to their hydrogen ion concentration.

Hydrogen Ion Concentration

The hydrogen ion concentration of body fluids is vital to acid-base balance. The hydrogen ion concentration is measured in terms of the pH. The pH numerical value is inversely proportional to the number of hydrogen ions in the body fluid:

↑ Hydrogen ion concentration, ↓ pH (acid)
↓ Hydrogen ion concentration, ↑ pH (base)

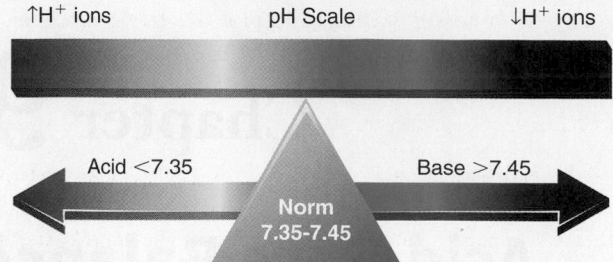

FIGURE 9.1 The relationship between hydrogen ions and the body's pH. As the hydrogen ion (acid) concentration increases, the pH level decreases, indicating acidosis. As the hydrogen ion concentration decreases, the pH level increases, indicating alkalosis.

The normal arterial blood pH range is 7.35 to 7.45. A pH level below 6.8 or above 7.8 is considered incompatible with life because cell function becomes seriously impaired.

 Safety Alert Fatal blood pH levels are less than 6.8 and greater than 7.8.

Acids

Acids are known as hydrogen ion donors. An acidic solution has more hydrogen ions and a pH of less than 7.35. The excess of hydrogen ions can be a result of overproduction of acids that causes the release of hydrogen ions or an under-elimination of acids that causes retention of hydrogen ions. Because hydrogen ions are positively charged ions, hydrogen ion excess in the blood causes imbalances in other electrolytes, such as calcium, potassium, and sodium. These imbalances can lead to disorders of the cardiac, central nervous, neuromuscular, and respiratory systems.

Bases

Bases are known as hydrogen ion acceptors. A base, or alkaline, solution has fewer hydrogen ions and a pH of greater than 7.45. Alkalosis can result from either an overproduction of base or an under-elimination of base. The most common base is **bicarbonate**, and the systems affected are the cardiovascular, muscular, and nervous systems.

Oxygenation

Oxygenation is measured using arterial blood gas (ABG) sampling. The **PaO₂** measures the partial pressure of oxygen in arterial blood and is the most important factor in determining how oxygen binds to hemoglobin. If the PaO_2 is high, then more oxygen is able to bind with hemoglobin; if the PaO_2 is low, then less oxygen is able to bind with hemoglobin. The SaO_2 measures the oxygen-carrying capacity of hemoglobin and can be assessed through the use of pulse oximetry. Primarily, SaO_2 is used to evaluate respiratory function and is not used to evaluate acid-base balance. Higher than normal PaO_2 and SaO_2 values are associated with unnecessarily high levels of supplemental oxygen administration. In contrast, lower than normal PaO_2 and SaO_2 values indicate hypoxemia (Table 9.1).

 Safety Alert Pulse oximetry is considered accurate for oxygen saturations of greater than 80%. Arterial blood gas analysis is recommended for oxygen saturations of less than 80%.

Carbon Dioxide

Carbon dioxide (CO_2) is the natural by-product of cellular metabolism. Carbon dioxide is measured by the $PaCO_2$ levels, which indicate the partial pressure of CO_2 in the arterial blood. The $PaCO_2$ is used to evaluate the respiratory component of acid-base balance. Primarily regulated by the ventilatory function of the lungs, normal arterial CO_2 levels are 35 to 45 mm Hg.

- $PaCO_2$ greater than 45 mm Hg is related to hypoventilation or excessive CO_2 retention, and therefore acidosis.

Table 9.1 Oxygenation Blood Gas Values		
Level	**Normal Value**	**Interpretation**
PaO₂	80–95 mm Hg	Measurement of partial pressure of oxygen in arterial blood
		PaO₂ less than 80 mm Hg = insufficient oxygen present; there is less chance of oxygen binding with hemoglobin
		PaO₂ greater than 95 mm Hg = there is more oxygen in the blood than necessary
SaO₂	>95%	The percentage of oxygen that is bound to hemoglobin
		SaO₂ less than 95% = oxygen saturation is insufficient to meet the body's needs
		SaO₂ greater than 95% = oxygen saturation is sufficient for the body's needs

- $PaCO_2$ less than 35 mm Hg is related to hyperventilation or excessive CO_2 exhalation, and therefore alkalosis.

Bicarbonate

Bicarbonate helps the body regulate pH and accomplishes this by its ability to accept a hydrogen ion (H^+). Regulated by the kidneys, bicarbonate is measured by the arterial blood HCO_3^- concentration and is used to evaluate the metabolic component of acid-base balance. Normal HCO_3^- values are between 22 and 26 mEq/L.

- HCO_3^- less than 22 mEq/L is acidosis.
- HCO_3^- greater than 26 mEq/L is alkalosis.

Connection Check 9.1

How does the nurse interpret an arterial pH of 7.47?
A. Acidosis
B. Alkalosis
C. Compensation
D. Homeostasis

REGULATION OF ACID-BASE BALANCE

To maintain the pH of the extracellular fluid within the narrow range, the body has three regulating mechanisms: chemical buffers, respiratory buffers, and renal buffers.

Chemical Buffers

The first line of defense against a change in the body's pH is **chemical buffers**. Chemical buffers include bicarbonate, phosphate, and proteins.

- **Bicarbonate buffers** are mainly responsible for buffering blood and interstitial fluid. They rely on a series of chemical reactions in which pairs of weak acids and bases combine with stronger acids and bases to weaken them. These chemical reactions are assisted by the kidneys and lungs.
- **Phosphate buffers** are found in the intracellular fluids as bicarbonates. They control small fluctuations in pH and respond quickly. They prove especially effective in the renal tubules, where phosphates exist in greater concentration.
- **Protein buffers** are the most abundant buffers in the body. They work both inside and outside of cells: hemoglobin inside the cell and albumin and globulins outside the cell. Protein buffers

work by binding with acids and bases to neutralize them.

Respiratory Buffers

Acid-base disturbances resulting from primary alterations in the $PaCO_2$ are regulated by **respiratory buffers**. Any retention of CO_2 or increase in the body's concentration of CO_2 produces an increase in hydrogen ions through the generation of carbonic acid (H_2CO_3). This lowers the pH and thus promotes the development of an acidotic state, which is observed in conditions such as chronic obstructive pulmonary disease (COPD). While in the acidotic state, chemoreceptors in the brain respond to the increased CO_2 levels by stimulating the respiratory system to increase the respiratory rate and depth in an effort to excrete CO_2 through the lungs (Table 9.2). Conversely, decreases in CO_2 concentration result in a decrease in hydrogen ions. This leads to a pH rise, and an alkalotic state results, as seen in conditions such as hyperventilation.

$$CO_2 + H_2O \Leftrightarrow H_2CO_3 \Leftrightarrow H^+ + HCO_3^-$$
Carbon dioxide + water $\Leftrightarrow$ carbonic acid $\Leftrightarrow$ hydrogen + bicarbonate

Renal Buffers

The **renal buffers** are the most effective, yet the slowest-acting buffering system and buffer by regulating bicarbonate levels. If the body is in a state of alkalosis, then the kidneys excrete HCO_3^- and reabsorb hydrogen ions (H^+). This results in urine becoming more alkaline, a drop in the blood bicarbonate levels, and a decrease in pH. If the body is in a state of acidosis, then the kidneys excrete hydrogen ions (H^+) and reabsorb HCO_3^-. This results in urine becoming more acidic, bicarbonate levels increasing, and the pH increasing (Table 9.3; Fig. 9.2).

This response to **acid-base imbalances** begins within hours but requires several days to be marginally effective. This is in comparison to the faster changes brought about through the increases or decreases in the respiratory rate.

Table 9.2 Respiratory System Role in Acid-Base Balance

CO_2	H^+ Ions	pH State	Body Response
Retention	↑	↓ pH (acid)	↑ Depth and rate of respirations
Excretion	↓	↑ pH (base)	↓ Rate of respirations

Table 9.3 Renal System Role in Acid-Base Balance

Body's State	HCO$_3^-$	H$^+$ Ions	pH State	Body Response
Alkalosis	Excrete	Reabsorb	Increase	Urine alkaline, ↓ blood HCO$_3^-$, ↓ pH
Acidosis	Absorb	Excrete	Decrease	Urine acidic, ↑ HCO$_3^-$, ↑ pH

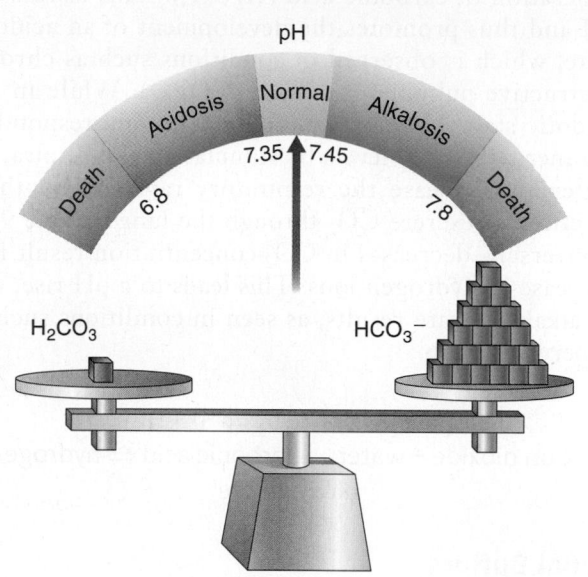

FIGURE 9.2 Normal pH results when the balance between carbonic acid (H$_2$CO$_3$) and bicarbonate (HCO$_3^-$) is maintained. Retention of CO$_2$ or an increase in the body's concentration of CO$_2$ produces an increase in hydrogen ions through the generation of carbonic acid (H$_2$CO$_3$). This lowers the pH and results in an acidotic state. If the body is in a state of alkalosis, then the kidneys excrete HCO$_3^-$ and reabsorb hydrogen ions (H$^+$). This results in urine becoming more alkaline, a drop in blood bicarbonate levels, and decreased pH. If the body is in a state of acidosis, then the kidneys excrete hydrogen ions (H$^+$) and reabsorb HCO$_3^-$. In all cases, a pH level below 6.8 or above 7.8 is considered incompatible with life, and death will likely ensue.

Connection Check 9.2

Which parameter of the ABG result correlates to the assessment of the base component?

A. pH
B. PaO$_2$
C. HCO$_3^-$
D. PaCO$_2$

RESPIRATORY AND RENAL COMPENSATION

Compensation describes physiological responses to an acid-base imbalance in an attempt to normalize pH. If the problem is of respiratory origin, then the kidneys work to correct. If the problem is of renal origin, then the lungs work to correct.

Respiratory Compensation

If the primary alteration in acid-base balance has resulted from a metabolic disorder, then the respiratory system may compensate by retaining or removing CO$_2$ while minimizing a change in the pH. The lungs may take as little as 5 to 15 minutes to begin compensation. The respiratory system responds to metabolic-based pH imbalances (Table 9.4) by

- **Metabolic acidosis**: increase in respiratory rate and depth
- **Metabolic alkalosis**: decrease in respiratory rate and depth

In older adults, respiratory compensation may be limited because of physiological changes associated with aging, including barrel chest and kyphosis (spinal curvature) that result in decreased lung compliance and recoil and increased work of breathing.

Renal Compensation

If the primary alteration in acid-base balance results from a respiratory disorder, then the renal system may compensate by excreting or retaining hydrogen and bicarbonate. The renal system may take as long as 24 hours to correct a respiratory-induced problem because there are three major renal mechanisms that work to compensate the disorder: tubular kidney movement of bicarbonate, kidney tubule formation of acids, and the formation of ammonium from

Table 9.4 Metabolic Acidosis and Metabolic Alkalosis

	Respiratory Compensation	Body Results
Metabolic acidosis: **Bicarbonate deficit**	↑ Rate and depth of respirations	Greater elimination of CO$_2$
Metabolic alkalosis: **Bicarbonate excess**	↓ Rate and depth of respirations	↑ CO$_2$ retention and ↑ carbonic acid accumulation

amino acid catabolism. The renal system responds to respiratory-based pH imbalances (Table 9.5) by

- **Respiratory acidosis**: increase in hydrogen excretion and bicarbonate reabsorption
- **Respiratory alkalosis**: decrease in hydrogen excretion and bicarbonate reabsorption

Renal function also changes with aging and includes atrophy of the kidney and decreased blood flow to the kidneys, leading to a decreased glomerular filtration rate. Renal compensation may be affected by these alterations in kidney function.

Arterial blood gases are further defined by their degree of compensation. An ABG can be **uncompensated, partially compensated,** or **fully compensated**. To determine the level of compensation, the pH, $PaCO_2$, and HCO_3^- are analyzed.

Steps to Determine Acid-Base Compensation

1. Does the pH range indicate acidosis or alkalosis? If pH is within the normal range, in which direction does it trend?
2. Has the $PaCO_2$ or HCO_3^- changed to account for the acidosis or alkalosis?
3. Has the opposite system worked to correct and shift back toward a normal pH?

Types of Compensation

The three types of compensation are:

Uncompensated: pH is abnormal, and either the $PaCO_2$ or the HCO_3^- is also abnormal. There is no indication that the opposite system has tried to correct the imbalance (Table 9.6).

Partially compensated: pH is abnormal, and both $PaCO_2$ and HCO_3^- are also abnormal (Table 9.7). This indicates that the opposite system has attempted to correct for the other but has not been completely successful.

Fully compensated: pH is normal, and both the $PaCO_2$ and HCO_3^- are abnormal (Table 9.8). The normal pH indicates that one system has been able to compensate for the other.

Table 9.6 Example of Blood Gas Results—Respiratory Alkalosis

Blood Gas 3 Results	Interpretation
pH: 7.51	Alkalosis
$PaCO_2$: 26 mm Hg	Alkalosis
HCO_3^-: 25 mEq/L	Normal
PaO_2: 90 mm Hg	Normal

Table 9.7 Example of Blood Gas Results—Partially Compensated Respiratory Alkalosis

Blood Gas 4 Results	Interpretation
pH: 7.49	Alkalosis
$PaCO_2$: 25 mm Hg	Alkalosis
HCO_3^-: 20 mEq/L	Acidosis
PaO_2: 95 mm Hg	Normal

Table 9.8 Example of Blood Gas Results—Fully Compensated Respiratory Alkalosis

Blood Gas 5 Results	Interpretation
pH: 7.44	Normal but greater than 7.4, so tends toward alkalosis
$PaCO_2$: 25 mm Hg	Alkalosis, primary problem
HCO_3^-: 19 mEq/L	Acidosis, compensatory response
PaO_2: 95 mm Hg	Normal

Table 9.5 Respiratory Acidosis and Respiratory Alkalosis

	Renal Compensation	Body Response
Respiratory acidosis: Carbonic acid excess	↓ H+ and ↑ HCO_3^-	Restore balance
Respiratory alkalosis: Carbonic acid deficit	↑ H+ and ↓ HCO_3^-	Restore balance

Maintaining a homeostatic pH environment is essential for normal body functioning. To achieve this goal, the body must constantly monitor its hydrogen ion concentration. When there is an increase or decrease in this balance, the body must use the blood bicarbonate, proteins, and phosphate buffer body fluids to compensate. There does come a time in the disease process when these buffers can no longer maintain adequate concentrations of hydrogen ions, and outside resources must be used to help the body compensate.

Connection Check 9.3

What acid-base imbalance does the nurse suspect on the basis of these results?

pH: 7.31
$PaCO_2$: 52 mm Hg
HCO_3^-: 28 mEq/L

A. Uncompensated respiratory acidosis
B. Partially compensated respiratory acidosis
C. Uncompensated metabolic acidosis
D. Partially compensated metabolic acidosis

ARTERIAL BLOOD GAS INTERPRETATION

Arterial blood gas analysis describes the set of values that are assessed to determine an individual's ability to maintain normal acid-base balance. Arterial blood gases are drawn from arteries such as the radial, brachial, or femoral and can also be obtained through an indwelling arterial line that may be present in one of these arteries. Arterial lines also provide continuous blood pressure (BP) monitoring and allow for arterial blood sampling. A patient with an arterial line must be cared for in the intensive care unit (ICU) or a monitored unit because of possible circulatory impairment to the affected limb, risk of hemorrhage, and the need for continuous arterial line monitoring.

Obtaining an Arterial Blood Gas

Most ABG samples are collected by a respiratory therapist or specially trained registered nurse (see institution's policy). Collection from the femoral artery, however, is usually performed only by a physician or advanced practice registered nurse (APRN). Before a radial puncture is performed, an Allen test should be conducted (Box 9.1). This test is conducted to ensure adequate collateral circulation in the event there is hemorrhage or thrombosis of the radial artery that is punctured.

Arterial Blood Gas Assessment

There are six parameters included in an ABG measurement:

1. pH
2. $PaCO_2$
3. HCO_3^-
4. Base excess
5. PaO_2
6. SaO_2

Blood acidity is reflected by pH levels, and the normal range is 7.35 to 7.45. A pH greater than 7.45 indicates alkalosis; a pH less than 7.35 indicates acidosis. If the level is normal or borderline, then the body may be attempting

Box 9.1 Performing an Allen Test

Rest the patient's arm on the mattress or bedside stand and support his wrist with a rolled towel. Tell him to clench his fist. Using your index and middle fingers, press on the radial and ulnar arteries. Hold this position for a few seconds.

Without removing your fingers from the patient's arteries, ask him to unclench his fist and hold his hand in a relaxed position. The palm will be blanched because pressure from your fingers has impaired the normal blood flow.

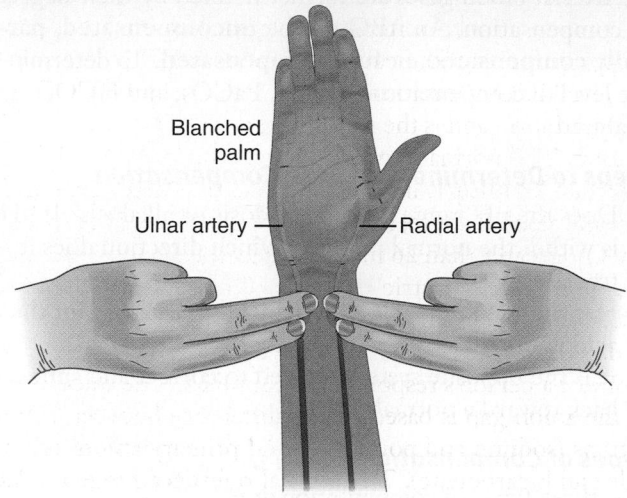

Release pressure on the patient's ulnar artery. If the hand becomes flushed, which indicates blood filling the vessels, you can safely proceed with the radial artery puncture. If the hand does not flush, select another site for the puncture.

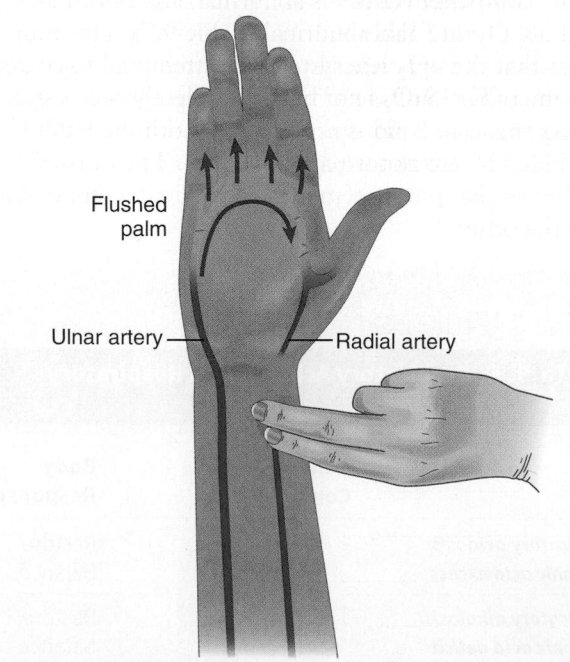

to compensate for a slightly abnormal or chronic acid-base imbalance. Compensation is the way in which the body responds to an acid-base imbalance in an attempt to normalize the pH of the blood.

The $PaCO_2$ level reflects the partial pressure of CO_2 in arterial blood and is adjusted by changes in the rate and depth of respiratory ventilation. The normal range is 35 to 45 mm Hg. A $PaCO_2$ greater than 45 mm Hg indicates hypoventilation or excessive CO_2 retention, as in COPD, drug overdose, or acute respiratory failure, and therefore respiratory acidosis. A $PaCO_2$ less than 35 mm Hg indicates hyperventilation or excessive CO_2 exhalation, and therefore respiratory alkalosis. Respiratory alkalosis may occur with an anxiety attack, pulmonary edema, hepatic failure, or inappropriate mechanical ventilator settings.

The HCO_3^- level reflects the arterial blood's HCO_3^- concentration and is the renal component of acid-base regulation. The normal range is 22 to 26 mEq/L. An HCO_3^- less than 22 mEq/L indicates acidosis and may occur with chronic alcohol abuse, starvation, or acute renal failure. An HCO_3^- greater than 26 mEq/L indicates alkalosis and may be the result of gastric drainage, diuretic use, or severe potassium depletion. An **anion gap** calculation may be used to determine the cause of metabolic acidosis and is a way to monitor a person's response to treatments. The calculation of the anion gap is based on the difference between major cations (sodium and potassium) and primary anions (chloride and bicarbonate). The normal reference range for the anion gap is 8 to 16 mEq/L. **Base excess** reflects the level of HCO_3^- and other bases such as proteins and hemoglobin, and the normal range is –2 to +2. A base excess less than –2 indicates an acid excess. A base excess greater than +2 indicates an acid deficit.

The PaO_2 level reflects the partial pressure of oxygen in arterial blood (Table 9.9). The normal range is 80 to 95 mm Hg. A PaO_2 level less than 80 mm Hg indicates hypoxemia. The SaO_2 level reflects hemoglobin's oxygen-carrying capacity. A normal value is anything greater than 95%. This value is not used to evaluate acid-base balance.

Steps for Interpreting Arterial Blood Gas

Step 1: Review the pH result. Is it normal (7.35–7.45), acidosis (<7.35), or alkalosis (>7.45)?

Step 2: Review the $PaCO_2$ result. Is it normal (35–45 mm Hg), acidosis (>45 mm Hg), or alkalosis (<35 mm Hg)?

Step 3: Review the HCO_3^- result. Is it normal (22–26 mEq/L), acidosis (<22 mEq/L), or alkalosis (>26 mEq/L; Tables 9.10 and 9.11)?

Step 4: Match either the $PaCO_2$ or HCO_3^- result with the pH result to determine the cause of the acid-base imbalance.

Step 5: Does either the $PaCO_2$ or HCO_3^- go in the opposite direction of the pH? This result indicates compensation by that system.

Step 6: Review the PaO_2 and SaO_2 results. If they are below normal limits, then the patient is hypoxic.

> **! Safety Alert** It is important to interpret blood gases as part of the complete patient assessment, which includes pertinent details such as past medical history, presenting complaint, and current patient status. Abnormal values need to be addressed quickly with the assistance of the healthcare team in order to establish a plan of care for the patient.

Table 9.9 Normal Arterial Blood Gas Values

ABG Value	Normal Range
pH	7.35–7.45
PaCO₂	35–45 mm Hg
HCO₃⁻	22–26 mEq/L
Base excess	–2 to +2
PaO₂	80–95 mm Hg
SaO₂	>95%

Table 9.10 Example of Blood Gas Results—Uncompensated Respiratory Acidosis

Blood Gas 1 Results	Interpretation
pH: 7.30	Acidosis
PaCO₂: 55 mm Hg	Acidosis
HCO₃⁻: 25 mEq/L	Normal
PaO₂: 85 mm Hg	Normal
SaO₂: 96%	Normal

Table 9.11 Example of Blood Gas Results—Uncompensated Metabolic Alkalosis

Blood Gas 2 Results	Interpretation
pH: 7.48	Alkalosis
PaCO₂: 41 mm Hg	Normal
HCO₃⁻: 28 mEq/L	Alkalosis
PaO₂: 86 mm Hg	Normal
SaO₂: 95%	Normal

Connection Check 9.4

Which acid-base imbalance should be suspected with these ABG results?

pH: 7.47
$PaCO_2$: 31 mm Hg
HCO_3^-: 24 mEq/L

A. Respiratory acidosis
B. Respiratory alkalosis
C. Metabolic acidosis
D. Metabolic alkalosis

Connection Check 9.5

When the body is in a state of alkalosis, what is the role of the renal buffers?

A. ↑ Excretion of water
B. ↓ Excretion of water
C. ↑ Excretion of HCO_3^-
D. ↓ Excretion of HCO_3^-

CASE STUDY: EPISODE 2

Cory presents to the emergency department with the following vital signs: afebrile, BP 100/62, respiratory rate (RR) 8, pH 7.30, PaO_2 80 mm Hg, $PaCO_2$ 65 mm Hg, HCO_3^- 24 mEq/L, blood alcohol level 0.24%. The clinical presentation upon arrival to the emergency department includes decreased responsiveness and respiratory distress. An emergent chest x-ray indicates a right-sided pneumothorax. Cory's treatment plan includes chest tube insertion for pneumothorax and artificial airway insertion for respiratory distress...

ACID-BASE DISORDERS

An individual's acid-base balance is essential to life. The two major categories of acid-base imbalances are acidosis and alkalosis. They are further classified according to respiratory and metabolic origin and degree of compensation. A thorough patient assessment, including ABG analysis, is vital for determining the type of imbalance and the treatment modality.

Respiratory Acidosis

Respiratory acidosis is the primary acid-base imbalance, resulting from altered ventilation leading to CO_2 retention. Characterized by a low pH and elevated CO_2 levels due to alveolar hypoventilation, respiratory acidosis may be acute or chronic, as in the case of COPD. The body attempts to

compensate by renal absorption of HCO_3^-. Box 9.2 lists the causes of respiratory acidosis, which are associated with suppressed ventilation leading to CO_2 retention. Box 9.3 presents the clinical manifestations of respiratory acidosis.

Arterial Blood Gas Results

The ABG results for respiratory acidosis are pH less than 7.35 and $PaCO_2$ greater than 45 mm Hg. With metabolic compensation, then the HCO_3^- is greater than 26 mEq/L.

Treatment

When the underlying cause is respiratory, the correction or improvement in ventilation is to lower the $PaCO_2$. When the underlying cause is nonrespiratory, then correction or improvement of the underlying cause must occur.

Possible Respiratory Treatments

- Bronchodilators to open constricted airways
- Supplemental oxygen
- Medications to treat hyperkalemia
- Antibiotics to treat infection
- Chest physiotherapy to remove secretions from the lungs
- Removal of a foreign body from the airway, if indicated
- Chest tube insertion to increase lung expansion or remove drainage
- Intubation to allow mechanical ventilation

Box 9.2 Causes of Respiratory Acidosis

- Central nervous system depression (head trauma, oversedation, anesthesia, high spinal cord injury)
- Pneumothorax
- Hypoventilation
- Bronchial obstruction and atelectasis
- Severe pulmonary infections
- Heart failure with pulmonary edema (congestive heart failure)
- Massive pulmonary embolus
- Myasthenia gravis
- Multiple sclerosis

Box 9.3 Clinical Manifestations of Respiratory Acidosis

- Dyspnea
- Restlessness
- Headache
- Tachycardia
- Confusion
- Lethargy
- Dysrhythmias
- Respiratory distress
- Drowsiness
- Decreased responsiveness

Possible Nonrespiratory Treatments

- Reversal of sedation to awaken the patient and increase the rate and depth of respirations
- Heart failure treatment such as diuretics to decrease fluid in the lungs

Nursing Management

Before a nursing diagnosis or intervention can occur, the nurse must obtain a comprehensive patient history, identify health problems associated with respiratory acidosis, check for clinical manifestations of respiratory acidosis, obtain vital signs for a baseline comparison with future vital signs, and assess ABG values, particularly the pH and $PaCO_2$.

Nursing Diagnoses

- **Impaired gas exchange** related to alveolar hypoventilation from underlying disease process
- **Acute confusion** related to disturbance in acid-base regulation
- **Impaired oral mucous membrane** related to abnormal breathing pattern
- **Disturbed sleep pattern** related to frequent treatments and procedures
- **Ineffective family coping** related to stress reaction from family member's illness

Nursing Interventions

Nursing interventions for patients with respiratory acidosis include maintaining the patient's airway; monitoring ABG levels; monitoring vital signs, especially respiratory rate and depth; administration of supplemental oxygen; assisting with intubation if necessary; monitoring potassium levels; administration of sedatives cautiously; and providing patient reassurance and teaching as needed.

Complications

Respiratory acidosis results from altered ventilation leading to CO_2 retention. In response to prolonged increased CO_2 levels, paralysis and coma may result from cerebral vasodilation.

Respiratory Alkalosis

Respiratory alkalosis is an acid-base imbalance caused by an increase in the rate of alveolar ventilation. Acute alveolar hyperventilation is frequently the result of anxiety and is commonly referred to as *hyperventilation syndrome*. Hyperventilation decreases serum CO_2 in the lungs and blood because CO_2 is eliminated by the increased rate of respirations. A decreased CO_2 concentration decreases the levels of carbonic acid and hydrogen ions circulating in the blood, therefore raising the arterial pH levels. The body tries to restore the pH to normal levels through renal compensation; in this process, renal excretion of bicarbonate is increased. Respiratory alkalosis may be acute, resulting from hyperventilation, or chronic, which can be difficult to identify because of the renal compensation. Patients in the early stage of pulmonary edema may present with a respiratory alkalosis due to the increased respiratory rate secondary to anxiety and hyperventilation associated with attempts to increase oxygenation. Causes of respiratory alkalosis are listed in Box 9.4 and are associated with increased ventilation leading to excessive CO_2 excretion. Box 9.5 provides an overview of the clinical manifestations of respiratory alkalosis.

Arterial Blood Gas Results

Arterial blood gas results for respiratory alkalosis are pH greater than 7.45 and $PaCO_2$ less than 35 mm Hg. With metabolic compensation, the HCO_3^- is less than 22 mEq/L.

Treatment

Several measures are indicated to correct the underlying cause:

- Discontinuation and possible removal of the causative agent (such as salicylates or other medications)
- Steps to reduce fever, including cooling measures and antibiotic therapy if the elevated temperature is secondary to an infectious process

Box 9.4 Causes of Respiratory Alkalosis

- Anxiety and nervousness
- Fear and pain
- Fever and gram-negative septicemia
- Hyperventilation
- Lung conditions such as pneumonia, pulmonary embolisms
- Thyrotoxicosis
- Central nervous system lesions
- Salicylate intoxication/overdose
- Hepatic failure
- Pregnancy
- Early pulmonary edema

Box 9.5 Clinical Manifestations of Respiratory Alkalosis

- Hyperventilation
- Light-headedness
- Confusion
- Decreased concentration
- Paresthesias
- Tetanic spasms in the extremities
- Cardiac dysrhythmias
- Palpitations
- Sweating
- Dry mouth
- Blurred vision

- Elimination of the source of sepsis by identifying the source
- Oxygen therapy to treat acute hypoxemia
- Sedative or anxiolytic therapy to treat anxiety
- Diuretics to treat pulmonary edema

Further measures taken to counteract hyperventilation include:

- Teaching the patient to breathe into a paper bag or cupped hands, which leads to "rebreathing" of exhaled carbon dioxide
- For intubated patients: adjusting mechanical ventilator settings as needed by decreasing the tidal volume (volume delivered with each mechanical breath) or rate (number of breaths per minutes)

Nursing Management

Before a nursing diagnosis or intervention can be developed, the nurse must obtain a patient history of clinical problems, identify health problems associated with respiratory alkalosis, assess clinical manifestations of respiratory alkalosis, obtain vital signs for a baseline comparison with future vital signs, and assess ABG results, particularly the pH and $PaCO_2$.

Nursing Diagnoses

- **Ineffective breathing pattern** related to hyperventilation secondary to anxiety
- **Anxiety** related to difficult situation
- **Risk for falls** related to light-headedness, confusion, and blurred vision

Nursing Interventions

Key nursing interventions for patients with respiratory alkalosis include assisting in achieving the goal of reducing the ventilation rate by encouraging slow, deep breathing; monitoring vital signs; providing emotional support and reassurance to the patient to reduce anxiety; assisting the patient with activities of daily living; and providing teaching as needed.

Complications

Respiratory alkalosis results from an increase in the rate of alveolar ventilation. Hyperventilation decreases serum CO_2 in the lungs and blood as CO_2 is eliminated by the excess respirations. Complications of respiratory alkalosis include seizures related to decreased oxygen-carrying capacity to cerebral cells and chest pain from cardiac and noncardiac causes related to anxiety and hyperventilation.

Metabolic Acidosis

Metabolic acidosis is an acid-base imbalance caused by an increased accumulation of metabolic acids that rise in proportion to a decrease in bicarbonate and result in decreased arterial pH. The decrease in serum bicarbonate is caused by one of the following mechanisms:

- Increase in the concentration of hydrogen ions in the form of nonvolatile acids, for example, ketoacidosis associated with diabetes mellitus or lactic acidosis

- Loss of alkali secondary to severe diarrhea or intestinal malabsorption
- Decreased acid excretion by the kidneys in acute or chronic renal failure

The decrease in arterial pH stimulates respirations. The body's attempt to compensate occurs rapidly and may reduce the $PaCO_2$ levels by as much as 10 to 15 mm Hg. The most important mechanism for ridding the body of excess hydrogen ions (H^+) is the increase in acid excretion by the kidneys. However, nonvolatile acids may accumulate more rapidly than they can be neutralized by the body's buffers. Another way to decrease excess hydrogen ions is for a cellular exchange to occur. The intracellular potassium is pumped outside the cell in exchange for the excess extracellular hydrogen ions. This increases the serum potassium levels while the intracellular potassium levels decrease, resulting in hyperkalemia. In Box 9.6, the causes of metabolic acidosis are listed. Box 9.7 lists the clinical manifestations of metabolic acidosis.

 Safety Alert In patients with metabolic acidosis related to hyperglycemia, potassium is moved outside the cell in exchange for hydrogen ions and may be excreted due to the osmotic diuresis associated with diabetic ketoacidosis. As the elevated blood glucose levels are normalized and acidosis resolves, potassium moves back into the cells, and the patient must be monitored for hypokalemia.

Arterial Blood Gas Results

Arterial blood gas results for metabolic acidosis are pH less than 7.35 and HCO_3^- less than 22 mEq/L. With respiratory compensation, the $PaCO_2$ is less than 35 mm Hg.

Treatment

Metabolic acidosis treatment depends on the underlying cause. Sodium bicarbonate replacement administered intravenously neutralizes blood acidity in patients with a pH lower than 7.1. As needed to maintain fluid balance,

Box 9.6 Causes of Metabolic Acidosis

Accumulation of Acid

- Renal failure
- Ketoacidosis
- Anaerobic metabolism
- Starvation
- Salicylate intoxication

Loss of Base

- Diarrhea
- Intestinal fistulas

Box 9.7 Clinical Manifestations of Metabolic Acidosis

- Headache
- Confusion
- Restlessness
- Lethargy
- Weakness
- Stupor/coma
- Kussmaul respirations
- Nausea and vomiting
- Dysrhythmias
- Warm, flushed skin
- Seizures
- Twitching
- Peripheral vasodilation

parenteral fluid replacement may be used. Rapid-acting insulin may be needed for patients with diabetes mellitus in order to reverse diabetic ketoacidosis and drive potassium back into the cells. Antidiarrheals may be used to treat diarrhea-induced bicarbonate loss. Dialysis may be needed for patients with renal failure or for metabolic acidosis caused by a toxic reaction to a medication. Lastly, mechanical ventilation may be initiated to assist respiratory compensation.

Nursing Management

Before a nursing diagnosis or intervention can occur, the nurse must obtain a patient history of clinical problems and identify health problems associated with metabolic acidosis, such as starvation, severe or chronic diarrhea, diabetic ketoacidosis, trauma and shock, and renal failure. Interventions include assessing the arterial bicarbonate, base excess, and serum CO_2 levels for metabolic acid-base imbalances, obtaining baseline vital signs for comparison with future vital signs, and checking laboratory results, especially blood glucose and serum electrolytes.

Nursing Diagnoses

- **Decreased cardiac output** related to severe metabolic acidotic state
- **Deficient fluid volume** related to nausea, vomiting, and increased urine output
- **Imbalanced nutrition, less than body requirements**, related to the body's inability to use nutrition
- **Acute confusion** related to the disturbance in acid-base regulation
- **Impaired oral mucous membranes** related to the increase in insensible fluid loss secondary to hyperventilation
- **Disturbed sleep pattern** related to frequent treatments and procedures
- **Ineffective family coping** related to the stress reaction

Nursing Interventions

Key nursing interventions for patients with metabolic acidosis are specific to the underlying cause and include

monitoring hemodynamic status through BP, pulse rate, respirations, and cardiac rhythm and assessing peripheral vascular status. Cautious administration of sodium bicarbonate may be indicated, along with providing patient reassurance and teaching as needed.

Complications

Metabolic acidosis results from an increased accumulation of metabolic acids that rise in proportion to bicarbonate and leads to a decreased arterial pH. If the pH falls below 7.0, cardiac dysrhythmia can occur. This happens as a result of changes in cardiac conduction, which occur in direct response to a decrease in pH and because of the effects of increased hydrogen ion concentration on plasma and intracellular potassium levels. If metabolic acidosis is caused by chronic renal failure, complications may include renal osteodystrophy (bone disease) and renal encephalopathy.

Metabolic Alkalosis

Metabolic alkalosis is an acid-base imbalance caused by an increased loss of acid. Most instances of this increased loss of acid are through the gastrointestinal tract, usually via vomiting or nasogastric suctioning, or through renal excretion. The loss in metabolic acid causes an increase in the arterial pH level, which in turn results in a reduction in the hydrogen ion concentration. The body's attempt to compensate occurs by creating a state of hypoventilation, which works to conserve $PaCO_2$ levels. Additionally, in order to increase serum hydrogen ion levels, serum potassium is pumped into the cell in exchange for the serum hydrogen ions. This decreases the serum potassium levels while the intracellular potassium levels increase, resulting in hypokalemia. In Box 9.8, the causes of metabolic alkalosis are listed. Box 9.9 lists the clinical manifestations of metabolic alkalosis.

Arterial Blood Gas Results

Arterial blood gas results for metabolic alkalosis are pH greater than 7.45 and HCO_3^- greater than 26 mEq/L. With respiratory compensation, the $PaCO_2$ is greater than 45 mm Hg.

Treatment

Metabolic alkalosis treatment depends on the underlying cause. Discontinuation of potassium-wasting diuretics and nasogastric suctioning may be necessary. Patients may be administered an antiemetic to treat underlying nausea and vomiting. Lastly, in order to increase renal excretion of bicarbonate, medications such as acetazolamide are administered if the patient is not volume compromised or hypokalemic.

Nursing Management

As with other acid-base imbalances, before nursing diagnosis or interventions can be proposed, the nurse must obtain a patient history and identify health problems associated with metabolic alkalosis, such as vomiting, gastric suction, and peptic ulcer disease. Additional interventions include assessing the arterial bicarbonate, base excess, and serum

Box 9.8 Causes of Metabolic Alkalosis

Accumulation of base

- Excess use of bicarbonate
- Lactate administration in dialysis
- Excess ingestion of antacids

Loss of acids

- Vomiting
- Nasogastric suctioning
- Hypokalemia
- Hypochloremia
- Administration of diuretics
- Increased levels of aldosterone

Box 9.9 Clinical Manifestations of Metabolic Alkalosis

- Muscle twitching and cramps
- Tetany
- Dizziness
- Lethargy
- Weakness
- Disorientation
- Convulsions
- Coma
- Nausea and vomiting
- Depressed respirations

CO_2 levels for metabolic acid-base imbalances, obtaining baseline vital signs for comparison with future vital signs, and checking laboratory results, especially blood glucose and serum electrolytes.

Nursing Diagnoses

- **Decreased cardiac output** related to electrolyte imbalances from metabolic alkalosis induced by gastric suctioning or potassium-wasting diuretics
- **Acute confusion** related to the disturbance in acid-base regulation
- **Ineffective family coping** related to stress or the diagnosis

Nursing Interventions

Key nursing interventions for patients with metabolic alkalosis are specific to the underlying cause but include monitoring hemodynamic status through respirations, pulse rate, and cardiac rhythm and assessing the patient's level of consciousness. Additional interventions include administering IV fluid (see Evidence-Based Practice) and electrolyte supplements as prescribed and providing patient reassurance and teaching as needed.

Evidence-Based Practice

0.9% Saline Infusions

Patients in acute care settings who receive 0.9% saline infusions are at greater risk of developing a hyperchloremic acidosis. Fluid resuscitation with 0.9% saline dilutes serum bicarbonate through plasma volume replacement with nonbicarbonate fluids. This evidence-based literature review included studies that related to potential complications associated with the use of 0.9% saline solutions in comparison to the infusion of lactated Ringer's or Plasma-Lyte. On the basis of the findings of this study, fluid replacement is better accomplished with chloride-restricted PlasmaLyte because of decreased acid-base disturbances.

Barker, M. E. (2015). 0.9% saline induced hyperchloremic acidosis. *Journal of Trauma Nursing, 22*(2), 111–116.

Complications

Metabolic alkalosis results from an increased loss of acid. The loss in metabolic acid causes an increase in the arterial pH level, which in turn results in a reduction of the hydrogen ion concentration. With a pH greater than 7.55, dysrhythmias and a coma may result from alterations in the depolarization of neuronal and cardiac muscle cells.

Connection Check 9.6

A patient has been diagnosed with an intestinal obstruction. The nurse inserts a nasogastric tube and attaches the tube to low intermittent suction. For which acid-base imbalance is the patient at greatest risk?
A. Respiratory acidosis
B. Respiratory alkalosis
C. Metabolic acidosis
D. Metabolic alkalosis

Connection Check 9.7

The patient's ABG results indicate worsening respiratory acidosis. He has rapid, shallow breaths and decreased bilateral breath sounds. Which intervention should be the nurse's first priority?
A. Administer an antibiotic for suspected pneumonia.
B. Administer diuretics for heart failure.
C. Encourage the patient to breathe into a brown paper bag.
D. Prepare the patient for intubation and mechanical ventilation.

Making Connections

CASE STUDY: WRAP-UP

Cory Nelson, 21 years old, presents via ambulance to the emergency department after a motor vehicle accident (MVA). When the car he was a passenger in struck a tree, Cory was wearing his seat belt. He sustained chest trauma due to the impact and has facial lacerations. The paramedic at the scene noted that Cory had alcohol present on his breath and slurred speech when questioned. Cory's vital signs in the emergency department are as follows:

Afebrile, BP 100/62 mm Hg, RR 8

Arterial blood gases are pH 7.30, PaO_2 80 mm Hg, $PaCO_2$ 65 mm Hg, HCO_3^- 24 mEq/L; and a blood alcohol level 0.24%

The patient's clinical presentation upon arrival to the emergency department includes a decreased level of consciousness, facial lacerations, and respiratory distress. An emergent chest x-ray reveals a right-sided pneumothorax. Cory undergoes oral intubation and is placed on a mechanical ventilator. A right-sided chest tube is inserted, and he is placed on continuous pain medication via infusion. An orogastric tube (OGT) is placed to provide gastric decompression as needed.

On day 2, the right-sided pneumothorax is resolving, and his respiratory status has stabilized. He is extubated and placed on oxygen 40% via face mask.

Case Study Questions

1. The clinical team immediately creates a plan for the patient on the basis of Cory's ABG results and current patient assessment. Cory is being treated for which acid-base disorder?
   A. Metabolic acidosis
   B. Metabolic alkalosis
   C. Respiratory acidosis
   D. Respiratory alkalosis
2. Cory's treatment plan includes chest tube insertion for pneumothorax and artificial airway insertion for respiratory distress. The clinical team also places immediate nursing orders for which of the following? *(Select all that apply.)*
   A. OGT insertion
   B. Electrocardiogram (ECG) monitoring
   C. Fleet enema
   D. Repeated ABGs
   E. Physical therapy and occupational therapy consults
3. Cory begins to regain consciousness and is extremely agitated. The clinical team wants to evaluate his neurological status before starting sedation to calm Cory. What nursing interventions should be used to calm Cory?
   A. Restrain Cory's wrists.
   B. Speak calmly with Cory when he is agitated.
   C. Remove Cory's parents from the room.
   D. Maintain a well-lit environment.

4. What is the highest-priority nursing diagnosis during the emergency phase of Cory's hospital course?
   A. Impaired oral mucous membrane related to abnormal breathing pattern
   B. Disturbed sleep pattern related to frequent treatments and procedures
   C. Ineffective family coping related to stress reaction
   D. Impaired gas exchange related to trauma and agitation
5. Cory successfully passes the neurological examination and is provided sedation. He is transferred to the ICU, where the new graduate nurse is having a difficult time managing Cory's nursing priorities. What are the top priorities that the new graduate nurse's preceptor emphasizes? *(Select all that apply.)*
   A. Provide patient and family teaching.
   B. Monitor vital signs.
   C. Monitor ABG levels.
   D. Monitor orogastric secretions.
   E. Maintain patient's artificial airway.

CHAPTER SUMMARY

Acid-base balance refers to the homeostasis of the hydrogen ion concentration in body fluids and is expressed as the body's pH level. The normal arterial blood pH range is 7.35 to 7.45. Acids are known as hydrogen ion donors and have a pH less than 7.35. Bases are known as hydrogen ion acceptors and have a pH greater than 7.45

An arterial blood gas (ABG) describes the set of values that permit the assessment of an individual's ability to maintain normal cell function. There are six parameters included in an ABG measurement: pH, $PaCO_2$, HCO_3^-, base excess, PaO_2, and SaO_2.

The two major categories of acid-base imbalances are acidosis and alkalosis. The categories are further classified according to respiratory and metabolic origin and levels of compensation. Nursing considerations related to patients with acid-base disorders are individualized and based on the imbalance origin and mode of compensation.

To maintain the pH of the extracellular fluid within the narrow range, the body has three regulating mechanisms: chemical buffers, respiratory buffers, and renal buffers. Compensation is the physiologic response to an acid-base imbalance in an attempt to normalize pH. If the imbalance is of respiratory origin, then the kidneys work to correct. If the imbalance is of renal origin, then the lungs work to correct. Arterial blood gases are further defined by their degree of compensation and can be uncompensated, partially compensated, or fully compensated.

Respiratory acidosis is the primary acid-base imbalance resulting from altered ventilation leading to CO_2 retention. Arterial blood gas results for respiratory acidosis are pH less than 7.35 and $PaCO_2$ greater than 45 mm Hg. If compensated, then the HCO_3^- is greater than 26 mEq/L.

Respiratory alkalosis is an acid-base imbalance caused by an increase in the rate of alveolar ventilation. Arterial blood gas results for respiratory alkalosis are pH greater than 7.45 and $PaCO_2$ less than 35 mm Hg. If compensated, then the HCO_3^- is less than 22 mEq/L.

Metabolic acidosis is an acid-base imbalance caused by an increased accumulation of metabolic acids that rise in proportion to bicarbonate and result in decreased arterial pH. Arterial blood gas results for metabolic acidosis are pH less than 7.35 and HCO_3^- less than 22 mEq/L. If compensated, then the $PaCO_2$ is less than 35 mm Hg.

Metabolic alkalosis is an acid-base imbalance caused by an increased loss of acid. Most instances of this increased loss of acid are from the stomach or the kidneys. Arterial blood gas results for metabolic alkalosis are pH greater than 7.45 and HCO_3^- greater than 26 mEq/L. If compensated, then the $PaCO_2$ is greater than 45 mm Hg.

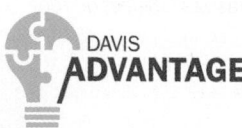

To explore learning resources for this chapter, go to **Davis Advantage** and find:
- Answers to in-text questions
- Chapter Resources and Activities
- NCLEX®-Style Chapter Review Questions
- Bibliography

Chapter 10

Overview of Infusion Therapies

Gladdi Tomlinson

LEARNING OUTCOMES

Content in this chapter is designed to assist in:

1. Discussing reasons patients require infusion therapy
2. Describing the characteristics of common IV solutions
3. Comparing peripheral and central venous access, including indications, access devices, and potential complications
4. Describing the equipment used to provide infusion therapy
5. Describing the potential complications of infusion therapy and strategies to prevent these complications
6. Explaining the procedure for safely administering blood products
7. Describing the special precautions required to safely administer parenteral nutrition
8. Developing a teaching plan for a patient receiving infusion therapy

CONCEPTS

- Assessment
- Fluid and Electrolyte Balance
- Medication
- Nutrition
- Skin Integrity

ESSENTIAL TERMS

Air embolism
Bolus
Central venous access (CVA)
Central venous access device (CVAD)
Central venous catheter (CVC)
Colloidal solutions
Crystalloid solutions
Electronic infusion device
Euvolemic
Extravasation
Flushing
Flushing and locking protocol
Hemolytic transfusion reaction
Implanted port
Incompatibility
Infiltration
Intraosseous
Intravenous access device (IVAD)
Keep vein open (KVO)
Locking
Midline catheter
Nonthrombotic
Normovolemic
Occlusion
Osmolarity
Peak and trough levels
Peripheral venous access
Peripherally inserted central catheter (PICC)
pH
Phlebitis
Priming
Vesicant

Finding Connections

CASE STUDY: EPISODE 1

Follow this patient throughout the chapter.

Jason Blair is a 21-year-old male who was involved in a motor vehicle accident and arrives in the emergency department with abdominal and lower extremity injuries. Upon arrival, he is tachycardic and hypotensive. He has one peripheral IV in his left forearm that is infusing 0.9% normal saline at 200 mL/hr. The emergency department provider and general surgeon are evaluating his injuries. Jason is a well-conditioned professional hockey player in excellent health…

INTRODUCTION

In today's healthcare environment, infusion therapy is delivered to patients across the continuum of care. Patients receive infusion therapy in hospitals, extended care facilities, outpatient clinics, infusion centers, and their own homes. Infusion therapy is undergoing rapid advancements as new evidence is constantly emerging to improve outcomes through improved techniques, equipment, and technologies. Research demonstrates that specialized "IV resource teams" result in better patient outcomes and reduced costs. However, generalist nurses in all practice settings are involved in the provision of infusion therapy and need to be knowledgeable in the most current evidence related to infusion therapy and competent in the care they provide to their patients.

The Infusion Nurses Society (INS) is a national organization that has established evidence-based practice standards of care to guide the delivery of infusion therapy. The standards were last revised in 2016 and are based on ranked evidence. A professional organization, the Infusion Nurses Certification Corporation, offers a national certification program that recognizes the expertise of nurses specializing in infusion therapy. The designation of Certified Registered Nurse of Infusion (CRNI©) is awarded after successfully passing a rigorous examination and completing the required hours of practice in infusion therapy.

Patients require infusion therapy for a variety of reasons, including fluid and electrolyte replacement, medication administration, blood product administration, and nutritional support. The duration of infusion therapy may be brief periods of hours or days to months or long-term therapy required for a lifetime.

Administration of IV fluids is initiated to both maintain and restore fluid and electrolyte balance when it is not possible to maintain this balance with the oral intake of fluids. To maintain fluid balance, adequate amounts of fluid need to be administered to account for sensible and insensible fluid losses. Fluid and electrolyte replacement may also be required because of losses related to hemorrhage, surgery, burns, vomiting, or diarrhea. IV administration of medications is indicated when the oral or other routes are not available or appropriate. Certain medications are administered only by the IV route because of their pharmacological composition or because of the need to be given intravenously to attain higher blood levels or faster action. When the gastrointestinal tract is unable to absorb sufficient amounts of nutrients, the IV route can be utilized. Solutions containing protein, lipids, and high concentrations of dextrose can provide the calories and nutrition needed to sustain life.

Blood products can be administered only intravenously and include packed red blood cells (RBCs), platelets, plasma, albumin, and clotting factors. They may be needed in acute situations or to correct deficits related to chronic conditions and require special precautions to ensure patient safety; they are presented later in the chapter.

Connection Check 10.1

The nurse recognizes that which patient may need infusion therapy? *(Select all that apply.)*
A. Patient who sustained trauma presenting to the emergency department
B. Patient with osteomyelitis receiving IV antibiotics at home
C. High school teacher during an annual health appraisal
D. Patient with cancer receiving parenteral chemotherapy
E. Patient with multiple sclerosis in remission

SOLUTIONS USED IN INFUSION THERAPY

Infusion therapy requires the specific IV fluid order by a licensed healthcare provider. The order needs to include the solution to be administered, any additives to the solution, and either the rate of infusion or the total dose or volume to be infused over a specific time frame.

The two major types of IV solutions are crystalloid solutions and colloidal solutions. **Crystalloid solutions** are composed of electrolytes dissolved in water and include dextrose solutions, sodium chloride solutions, balanced electrolyte solutions, and alkalizing and acidifying solutions. **Colloidal solutions** are composed of larger molecules, usually protein or starch, suspended in fluid and are not a true solution. Colloidal solutions are frequently referred to as *plasma volume expanders* because the larger molecules do not diffuse through cell membranes and draw fluid into the intravascular space. Colloidal solutions are used to maintain intravascular volume and prevent shock after major blood or fluid losses. Examples of colloidal solutions include albumin, dextran, and mannitol.

An important characteristic of IV solutions is **osmolarity**, a measure of the concentration of the solution that is expressed in terms of the number of particles (osmoles) per liter of solution. The concentration of the solution influences how water moves between the intracellular and extracellular compartments of the body. Normal blood and body solutions have a calculated osmolarity 270 to 300 mOsm/L. Solutions can be isotonic, hypotonic, or hypertonic (Table 10.1).

Isotonic solutions (Fig. 10.1A) have the same or nearly the same osmolarity as plasma and cause no movement of fluid into or out of cells. Isotonic solutions remain in the extracellular compartment in either the intravascular or interstitial compartments. The osmolarity of plasma varies from 270 to 300 mOsm/L, and solutions are considered to be isotonic if their osmolarity is between 250 and 375 mOsm/L. Isotonic solutions are administered to dehydrated patients with deficits in intravascular volume because they increase the amount of fluid circulating in the vascular system without causing movement of fluid in and out of cells.

Hypotonic solutions (Fig. 10.1B) have a lower solution concentration than plasma and cause fluid to move from the intravascular space into both the intracellular and interstitial spaces. Administration of hypotonic solutions hydrates cells but results in depletion of intravascular fluid volume. Hypotonic solutions are used in the management of hypernatremia, hyperosmolar conditions, hypertonic dehydration, and diabetic ketoacidosis after initial sodium chloride replacement. Extreme caution needs to be exercised when solutions that are not isotonic are administered because of resulting fluid shifts, and they should be administered only for brief periods.

Hypertonic solutions (Fig. 10.1C) have concentrations higher than plasma and cause fluid to move from the cells into the intravascular space. Because of the danger of circulatory overload, these solutions are given only in critical situations. Solutions with a concentration greater than 600 mOsm/L should be administered only via **central venous access (CVA)**, commonly referred to as a central line, where there is adequate blood flow to dilute the solution and prevent damage to the vein as the hypertonic solution infuses.

When administering any IV solution, the nurse needs to carefully monitor the fluid status of the patient regardless of the osmolarity of the solution being administered. This assessment includes respiratory status, vital signs, and skin turgor. Older adults and patients with compromised cardiovascular or renal function require even greater vigilance because of the risk of fluid overload.

The **pH** is a measure of the concentration of hydrogen ions in a solution and indicates the acidity or alkalinity of the solution. Most IV solutions are slightly acidic, which increases their stability and shelf life. Medications with a pH of less than 7 are acidic; those with a pH of greater than 7 are basic, or alkaline. Fluids or medications with a pH value of less than 5 or greater than 9 should be administered through a central line to avoid damage to the vein. (Acid-base disorders are discussed in more detail in Chapter 9.) The wrong diluent or incompatible solutions can alter the pH of a medication. Acidic medications are irritating to the walls of the vessels and can cause chemical **phlebitis**, which is irritation of the vein wall caused by the medication. Antibiotics are also a significant cause of phlebitis because of their low pH. Nurses need to be attentive to continually assessing peripheral IV sites where antibiotics are infusing to assess for signs of warmth and tenderness that may indicate phlebitis.

Table 10.1 Osmolarity of Intravenous Solutions

Isotonic	Hypotonic	Hypertonic
250–375 mOsm/L	Less than 250 mOsm/L	Greater than 375 mOsm/L
Examples:	Examples:	Examples:
• 0.9% sodium chloride (0.9% NaCl, normal saline [NS])	• 0.45% sodium chloride (0.45% NaCl, 1/2 NS)	• 3% sodium chloride
• 5% dextrose in water (D_5W)—becomes hypotonic in the body	• 2.5% dextrose in water	• 5% dextrose in lactated Ringer's
• Lactated Ringer's solution (LR)	• 0.33% sodium chloride	• 20% dextrose in water
		• 10% dextrose in water
		• Dextrose 5% in 1/2 NSS
		• Dextrose 5% NSS
		• Albumin 25%
Indications:	Indications:	Indications:
• Fluid deficits	• Diabetic ketoacidosis	• Severe dehydration
• Dehydration	• Hyperosmolar hyperglycemia	• Severe electrolyte imbalance
• Fluid challenges	• Hypertonic dehydration	• Hypotonic dehydration

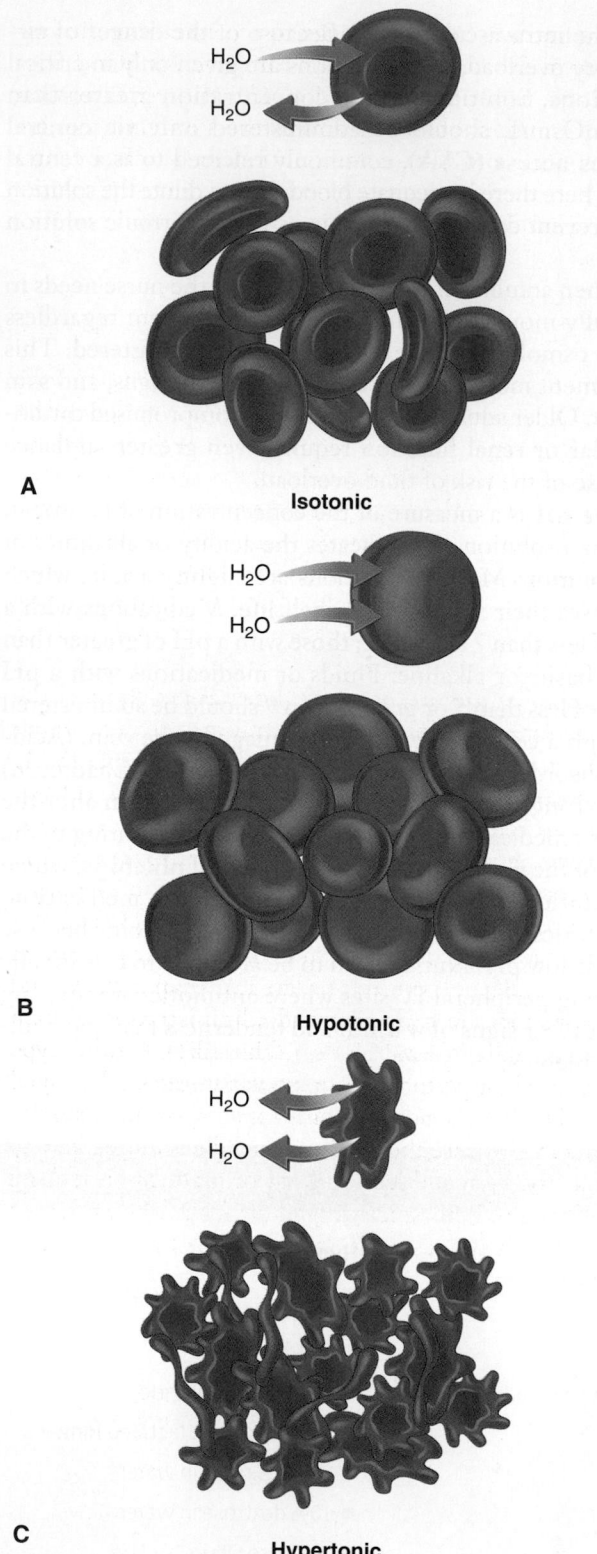

FIGURE 10.1 Effects of osmolality on fluid movement. *A,* Isotonic. The osmolality is the same in both the intracellular fluid (ICF) and extracellular fluid (ECF). There is typically no movement of fluid from cells when an isotonic solution is administered. If there is movement, it is equal between the two compartments due to the same osmolality. *B,* Hypotonic. With the administration of hypotonic solutions, fluid moves from the intravascular into the intracellular space. *C,* Hypertonic. With the administration of hypertonic solutions, fluids move from the cells into the intravascular space.

The use of the wrong diluents can also alter the pH of a medication, and incompatible solutions can greatly affect the medication's pH. **Incompatibility** is an undesirable reaction occurring between two medications or a medication and its diluent. There are three main types of medication incompatibility. Physical incompatibility is the reaction that causes a visible change. This change may be in the form of color, cloudiness, haziness, turbidity, the formation of precipitate, and even the formation of gas. Precipitate formation is the most common physical incompatibility. Calcium in medication or solution increases the risk for precipitate. Ringer's solution is an example of a solution with calcium. The second type is chemical incompatibility, which correlates to the breakdown of the medication. This reaction will most likely not be visible. The most common reaction is the acid-alkaline reaction that results in an unstable pH of one of the medications. The third type of incompatibility is therapeutic incompatibility that causes an increased or decreased therapeutic response. The incompatibility may be undetected until the patient shows no clinical response to the medication. Therapeutic incompatibility may occur with the use of two antibiotics. For example, aminoglycosides may be inactivated when given with penicillins or cephalosporins. Therefore, they must be given in separate sites, 1 hour apart. Also, if the medication requires **peak and trough levels** (measurements of medication levels before and after administration), the levels may show no therapeutic response. Nurses must be vigilant about checking compatibility when giving IV medications, whether it is two medications together or the administration of an IV medication by direct IV or IV piggyback with a primary solution. Compatibility charts are readily available in most facilities, and many healthcare facilities utilize IBM Micromedex® as the standard for checking the compatibility of medications. The pharmacist is also an additional resource for information about medication incompatibility.

Connection Check 10.2

The nurse anticipates which fluid movement when administering an isotonic IV fluid to a patient?
A. Causes fluid to move from the cells into the intravascular space
B. Causes fluid to move from the intravascular space into the intracellular space
C. Causes no or equal movement of fluid into or out of cells
D. Causes fluid to move from the intravascular space into the interstitial spaces

VEINS USED IN INFUSION THERAPY

Veins are the low-pressure blood vessels that return deoxygenated blood to the heart. Vein walls consist of three layers: the tunica intima (innermost layer), tunica media (middle layer), and tunica adventitia (outer layer) (Fig. 10.2A). The innermost layer consists of a single layer of endothelial cells lining the lumen of the vein. The middle layer contains smooth muscles that surround the vein, and the outer layer contains connective fibers that support the vein and nerve endings. Veins contain valves that aid the return of blood to the heart by preventing backflow of blood as veins are compressed by the surrounding skeletal muscles, thus facilitating blood return back to the central circulation.

The diameter of the veins and blood flow within the veins increase as the veins get closer to the heart. Larger veins with greater blood flow are appropriate when infusing larger volumes of fluid and when the osmolarity of the solution is high or the pH is outside the normal range. The vein also needs to be large enough to accommodate the vascular access device selected while allowing for blood flow around the device. Nurses need to take into consideration patient condition, characteristics of the solution to be infused, volume and rate of the solution to be infused, and type of **intravenous access device (IVAD)** available when planning infusion therapy.

TYPES OF INTRAVENOUS ACCESS DEVICES

Infusion therapy is divided into two general categories based on the location of the tip of the IVAD, peripheral or central. It is important to understand when peripheral infusion therapy is appropriate and when a CVA is preferred or required. The IVAD should be of the smallest gauge (size) and length with the fewest number of lumens and be the least invasive to provide the ordered infusion therapy.

Peripheral Venous Access

Peripheral venous access describes when the tip of the IVAD terminates outside of the central vasculature in a peripheral vein. The most common type of peripheral IVAD is the short over-the-needle catheter (Fig. 10.3). The flexible catheter is introduced into the vein over a metal needle that is then removed and discarded. The catheters range in length from 1 to 7.5 cm and in size from 14 to 27 gauge. Standardized catheter hub colors are used to identify catheter gauge (Table 10.2). Therapies utilizing a short peripheral catheter should be expected to last less than a week, and indications include hydration and administration of pain medications and some antibiotics (Table 10.3). Another type of IVAD used for peripheral venous access, the steel-winged device (Fig. 10.4), is indicated only for short-term or single-dose therapy because the rigid steel needle is more likely to puncture the vein and lead to fluid or medication leaking out of the vein. This steel-winged device is often referred to as a butterfly because of the appearance of wings on each side of the needle.

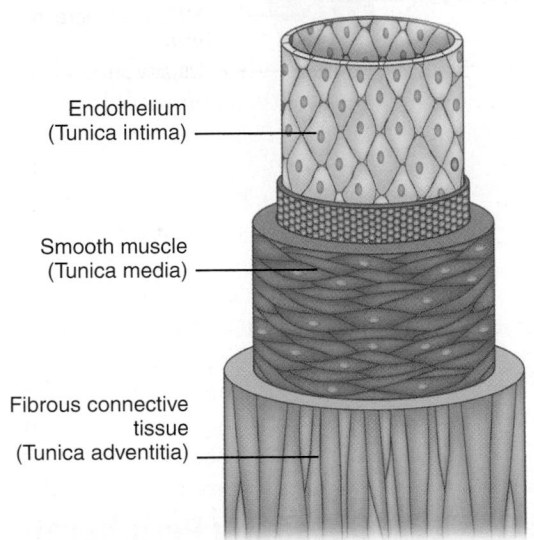

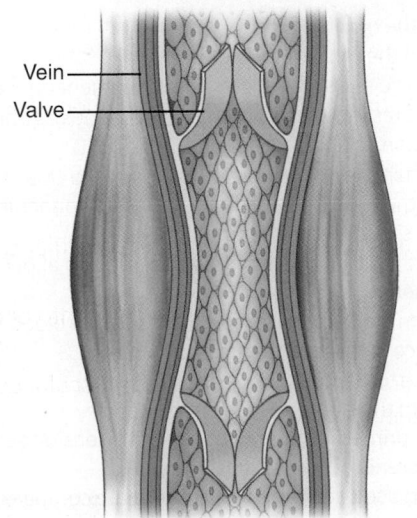

FIGURE 10.2 Layers of the vein. *A,* Vein walls consist of three layers: the tunica intima (innermost layer), tunica media (middle layer), and the tunica adventitia (outer layer). *B,* Valves in vein wall.

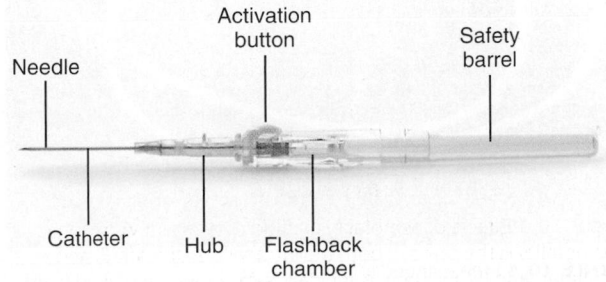

FIGURE 10.3 Over-the-needle peripheral catheter. The flexible catheter is introduced into the vein over a metal needle that is then removed and discarded. The Flashback chamber fills with blood when the vein is accessed, and the activation button progresses the catheter over the needle. The safety chamber protects the needle once the catheter is inserted to prevent inadvertent needle stick.

Table 10.2 Standard Colors Used to Identify Catheter Gauge

Gauge	Color
16	Gray
18	Green
20	Pink
22	Blue
24	Yellow

Table 10.3 Peripheral Catheter Gauge Selections

Catheter Gauge	Clinical Indications
14, 16, 18	Trauma, surgery, blood transfusion, need for rapid administration of large volumes
20	Continuous or intermittent infusions, blood transfusions
22	Continuous or intermittent infusions in small veins
24	Continuous or intermittent infusions in fragile veins

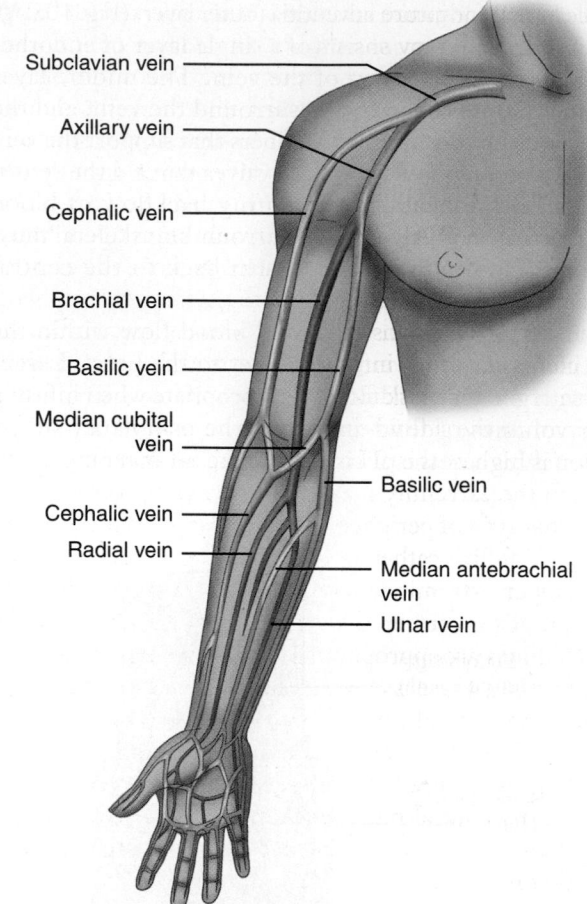

FIGURE 10.5 Veins of the upper extremities.

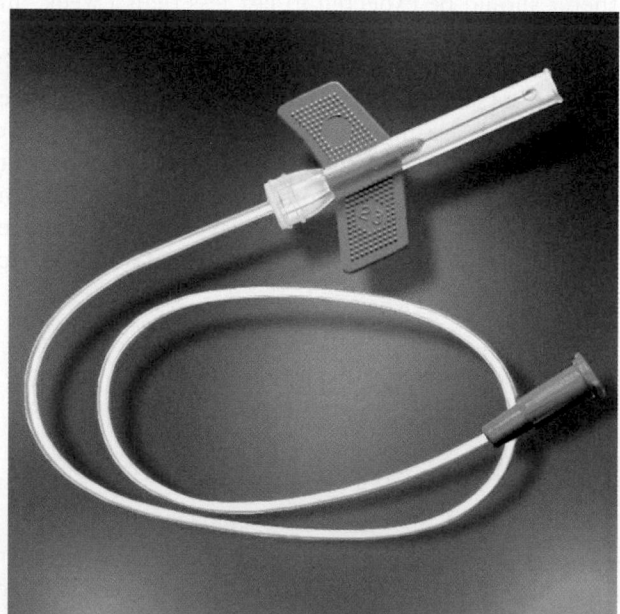

FIGURE 10.4 Steel-winged infusion set.

Short-term peripheral IV access is established in the superficial veins of the upper extremity (Fig. 10.5; Box 10.1). It is recommended to start therapy in the most distal available and appropriate vein and move upward with subsequent insertions. Using more distal sites first preserves

Box 10.1 Obtaining Peripheral IV Access

1. Verify the order.
2. Explain the procedure to the patient.
3. Select the needed catheter and equipment on the basis of the prescribed therapy and the patient's age and condition.
4. Wash hands and put on gloves.
5. Apply the tourniquet proximal to the venipuncture site.
6. Select site for venipuncture.
7. Clean the site with an antiseptic agent and allow it to dry completely.
8. Perform venipuncture and obtain positive blood return.
9. Advance catheter into vein.
10. Release tourniquet.
11. Activate the safety release for the needle.
12. Attach primed administration set or extension set.
13. Apply sterile occlusive dressing.
14. Discard used equipment in appropriate containers.
15. Remove gloves and wash hands.
16. Assess patient's tolerance of the procedure and the security of the catheter.
17. Document per institutional policy.

sites less distal for future insertions. Veins selected for short-term infusion therapy should be soft (nonsclerotic), non-tender, and not in an area where a previous infusion has infiltrated. Areas of the vein containing a valve should also be avoided. Veins in areas of flexion such as the wrist and antecubital fossa should be avoided if possible because it is more difficult to stabilize the IVAD in these areas. The movement of an IVAD that is not firmly secured can cause mechanical irritation of the vein. Recommended veins for peripheral infusion therapy include the metacarpal, cephalic, basilic, and median veins. Veins in the lower extremities are not recommended for infusion therapy in the adult patient because of the high risk for thrombophlebitis. Use of a vein in the arm on the side where a patient has had a mastectomy or has dialysis access is also contraindicated because venous return in the extremity may already be compromised.

Another type of peripheral infusion device is the **midline catheter**. Midline catheters are inserted in a peripheral vein in the upper extremities with tips that terminate distal to the shoulder in either the basilic, cephalic, or brachial vein. Midlines are appropriate for therapies expected to last between 1 and 4 weeks. The midline catheter is longer than the short peripheral catheter but is not a central catheter and should not be used to administer therapies when a central line is required, such as **vesicants** or other irritating solutions, parenteral nutrition solutions, or solutions with a pH of less than 5 or greater than 9 or osmolarity greater than 600 mOsm/L.

Connection Check 10.3

A patient is admitted with osteomyelitis and is going to require 3 to 4 weeks of IV antibiotics. Which IVAD is most appropriate for this patient?

A. 16-gauge central venous catheter
B. 18-gauge over-the-needle IVAD
C. 20-gauge midline catheter
D. 22-gauge steel-winged device

Central Venous Access

Central venous access (CVA) describes when the tip of the IVAD terminates in the central vasculature at the level of the superior vena cava or the inferior vena cava. Central venous catheters are made of silicone or polyurethane and come in many sizes and can have single or multiple lumens. Multiple-lumen catheters (Fig. 10.6) provide separate fluid pathways that make it possible to deliver two or more solutions at the same time. Each lumen, or fluid pathway, is totally separate from the other lumens. The fluid infused in each of the lumens leaves the **central venous access device (CVAD)** and enters the central venous system at different points along the catheter. These lumens are referred to as proximal, medial, or distal lumens depending on the location of the end of the fluid path on the catheter. Because the

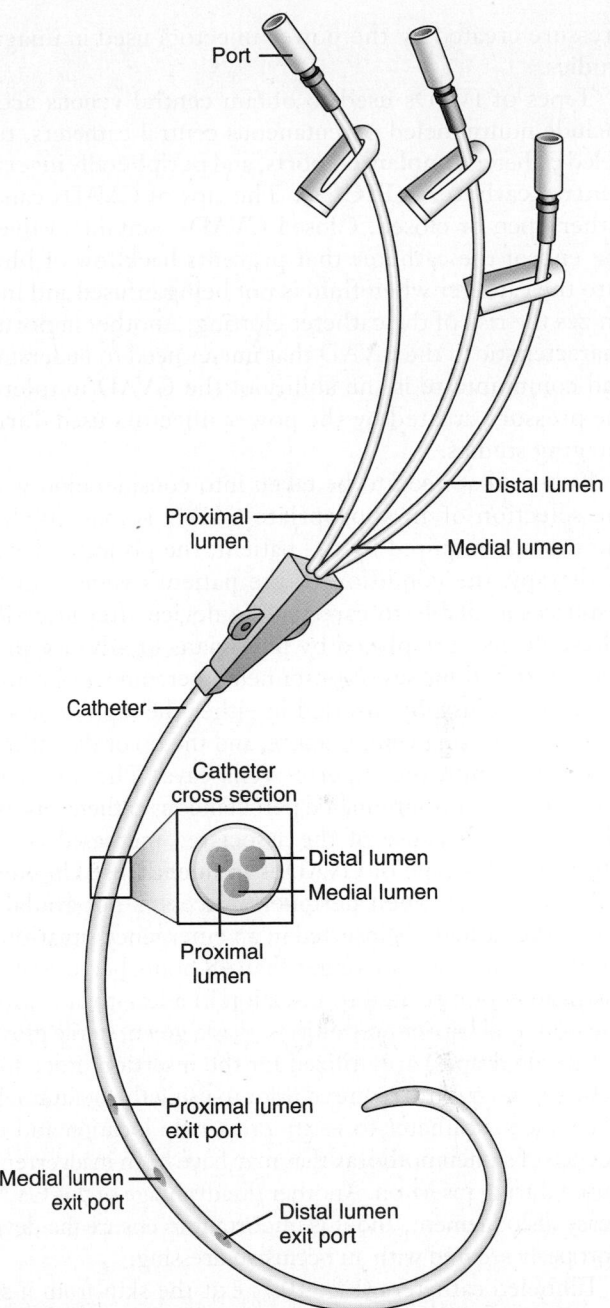

FIGURE 10.6 Multiple-lumen central venous catheter. Multiple-lumen catheters provide separate fluid pathways to deliver two or more solutions at the same time. The lumens are referred to as proximal, medial, or distal lumens depending on the location of the end of the fluid path on the catheter, and the corresponding exit ports are noted on the distal end of the catheter.

lumens are separate, incompatible solutions can be infused using the different ports attached to each of the lumens. Each port of the catheter is attached to a separate lumen that provides a distinct fluid pathway within the catheter. Each lumen requires initial flushing, which fills the catheter with the ordered IV solution, and flushing is also used to maintain the patency of the individual lumens if fluids are not being continuously administered. Manufacturers offer devices coated or impregnated with anti-infective agents and devices that can withstand the pressure created by the power injectors used in imaging studies.

Types of IVADs used to obtain central venous access include nontunneled percutaneous central catheters, tunneled catheters, **implanted ports**, and **peripherally inserted central catheters (PICCs)**. The tips of CVADs can be either open or closed. Closed CVADs contain a valve at the end of the catheter that prevents backflow of blood into the catheter when fluid is not being infused and minimizes the risk of the catheter clotting. Another important characteristic of the CVAD that nurses need to understand and communicate is the ability of the CVAD to tolerate the pressure created by the power injectors used during imaging studies.

Factors that need to be taken into consideration when the selection of an appropriate CVAD is made include the therapy required by the patient, the projected length of therapy, the condition of the patient's veins, and the resources available to care for the device after insertion. These devices are placed by physicians or advance practice registered nurses. Nontunneled percutaneous central catheters are usually inserted in either the jugular or subclavian veins using venipuncture, and the tip of the catheter is advanced into the superior vena cava. The use of the femoral vein for nontunneled percutaneous catheters is used with caution because of the associated increased risk of infection. This type of CVAD is frequently used in emergency situations when peripheral access is not available. When the catheter is inserted in an emergency situation, it should stay in place no longer than 48 hours because of the risk of infection related to insertion in a less-than-optimal situation. Full barrier precautions (mask, gown, sterile gloves, and sterile drapes) are utilized for the insertion procedure. A chest radiograph is required prior to using the nontunneled percutaneous catheter to verify proper tip location and the absence of a pneumothorax that may have been inadvertently caused during insertion. Another disadvantage of this CVAD is easy dislodgement, and it is important to ensure the device is properly secured with an occlusive dressing.

Tunneled catheters (Fig. 10.7) exit the skin from a site distal from the site where they enter the vein and are tunneled through the subcutaneous tissue between the exit and insertion site. The tip of the catheter is advanced from the insertion site to the central vascular. The tunneled portion of the catheter contains a Dacron cuff that tissue adheres to after insertion. The cuff stabilizes the catheter and provides a barrier to organisms, minimizing infection. This type of CVAD can be permanent and appropriate for patients requiring long-term therapy. The exit site is usually located on the chest and allows the patient easy access, promoting self-care. Tunneled catheters are inserted in nonemergency situations in sterile environments such as an operating or procedure room.

Implanted ports (Mediports) are also used for long-term therapy and offer the added advantage of requiring minimal care when not in use. An implanted port consists of a small reservoir with a septum and an attached catheter (Fig. 10.8).

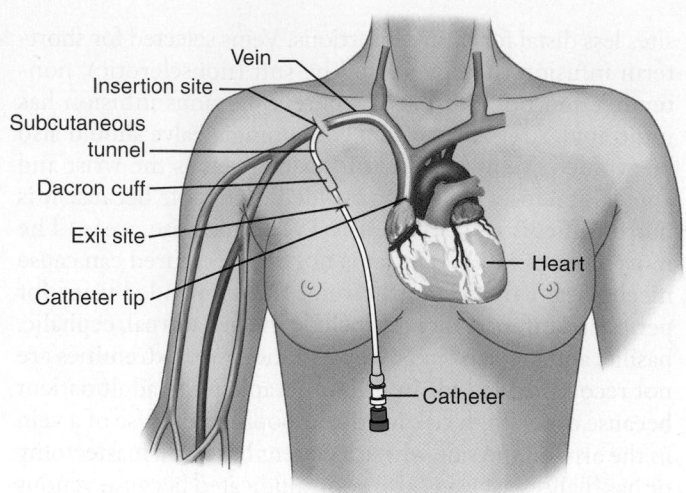

FIGURE 10.7 Tunneled central venous catheter. Tunneled catheters exit the skin from a site distal from the site where they enter the vein and are tunneled through the subcutaneous tissue between the exit and insertion site. The tip of the catheter is located in the central vasculature. The tunneled portion of the catheter contains a Dacron cuff that tissue adheres to after insertion.

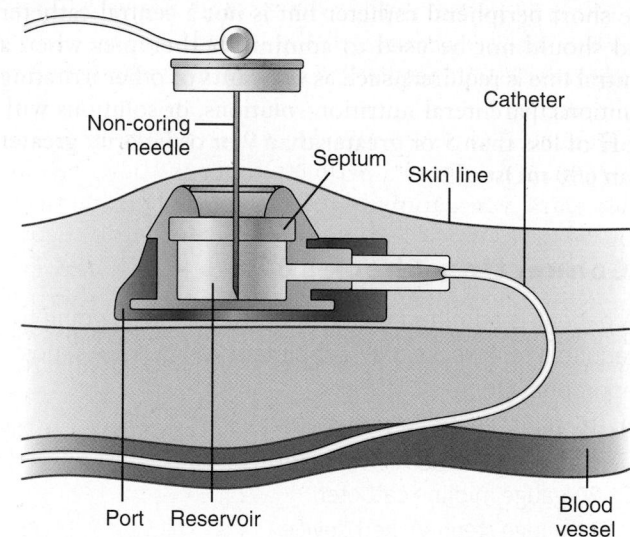

FIGURE 10.8 Implanted port. The implanted port consists of a small reservoir with a septum and an attached catheter. The reservoir is placed under the skin. The catheter is inserted in the vein near the reservoir, and the tip is advanced into the central vasculature. The entire device is located internally.

The reservoir is placed under the skin. The preferred site is the upper chest wall because it allows the patient to more easily care for the implanted port. These implanted ports can also be placed in the upper extremity, abdomen, and back. The catheter is inserted in the vein near the reservoir, and the tip is advanced into the central vasculature. The entire device is located internally. In order to use the device, it needs to be accessed with a specially designed noncoring needle that is inserted using sterile technique through the skin and into the septum of the reservoir. Noncoring needles (Fig. 10.9) have a different bevel angle, allowing the septum of the port to be punctured multiple times without

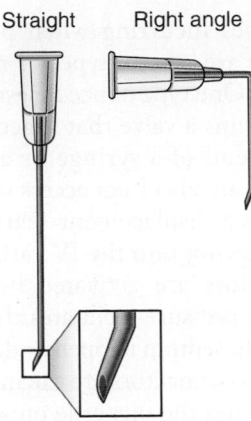

Straight   Right angle

FIGURE 10.9 Straight and right-angle noncoring needles. Noncoring needles have a different bevel angle, allowing the septum of the port to be punctured multiple times without damage.

damage. Once the implanted port is accessed with the noncoring needle, it needs to either have a continuous infusion maintained or be flushed periodically according to institutional policy. Implanted ports can have one or multiple ports, and each port communicates with a separate lumen in the catheter and needs to be flushed separately. When not accessed, the ports interfere minimally with the patient's daily activities and require only infrequent flushing to maintain patency.

Peripherally inserted central catheters (PICCs) are CVADs that are inserted into a peripheral vein and advanced into the central vasculature (Fig. 10.10). Peripherally inserted central catheters are frequently placed by registered nurses trained and competent in their insertion at the bedside with the assistance of ultrasound guidance. These catheters also have the advantage of being more cost-effective and easy to place and are appropriate for therapies of moderate to long-term duration. As with all CVADs, verification of tip placement is required with a chest radiograph prior to use. Ultrasound guidance can be used to confirm the placement

of PICCs. Recent studies show that the technique using electrocardiogram (ECG) guidance is more reliable and of lower cost compared with ultrasound guidance. The ECG-guided technique is accurate for the correct positioning in terms of catheter tip–carina distance and catheter tip–tracheobronchial angle.

The veins used for PICC insertion are usually the larger veins in the upper extremities. If infusion therapy using short peripheral therapy with repeated venipunctures has compromised these veins, PICC placement is much more difficult. Early placement of PICCs needs to be considered in patients who require therapies of longer than a few days to maximize the availability of veins that have not previously been accessed. The length of the fluid pathway in a PICC requires special attention to flushing to maintain patency because they need to be flushed before and after each use and periodically when not in use. Care needs to be taken when flushing a PICC so that excess pressure does not damage the thin walls of the catheter. Unless a PICC is specially designed to withstand higher pressures, only 10-mL or larger syringes, or flushing syringes especially designed to limit the amount of pressure they exert, should be used when flushing the PICC or administering medications through the PICC. If there is a possibility of the need for imaging studies requiring power injection, the power PICC is designed to withstand imaging contrast.

Access to the central venous system is also possible using the **intraosseous (IO)** (into bone marrow) route (Fig. 10.11). Using a handheld driver, the IO device is inserted into the vasculature of the bone marrow, allowing for infusion of fluids and medications. The insertion site is covered with a sterile occlusive dressing to decrease the risk of infection. Infusion rates of up to 1,800 mL per hour are possible, and the patient may require pain medications if experiencing discomfort and pressure during rapid infusions. The IO route is acceptable for any medication that requires a central venous route, and any medication

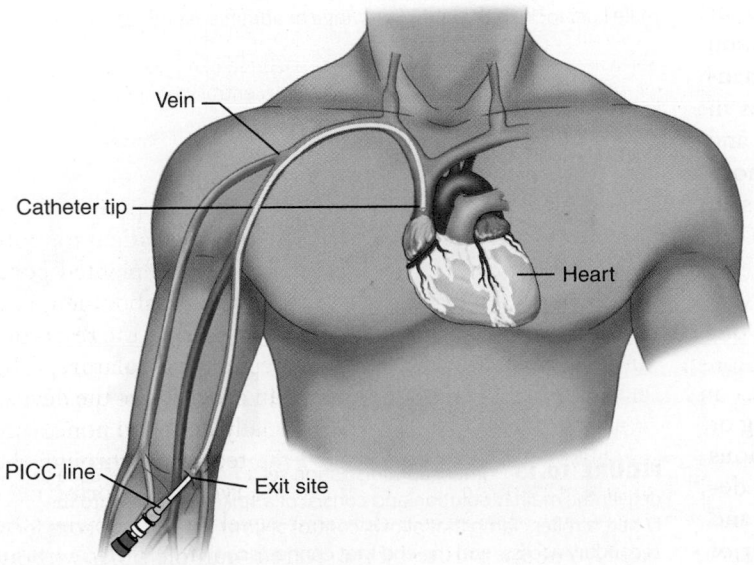

Vein

Catheter tip

Heart

PICC line — Exit site

FIGURE 10.10 Peripherally inserted central catheter. Peripherally inserted central catheters (PICCs) are central venous access devices (CVADs) that are inserted into a peripheral vein and advanced into the central vasculature.

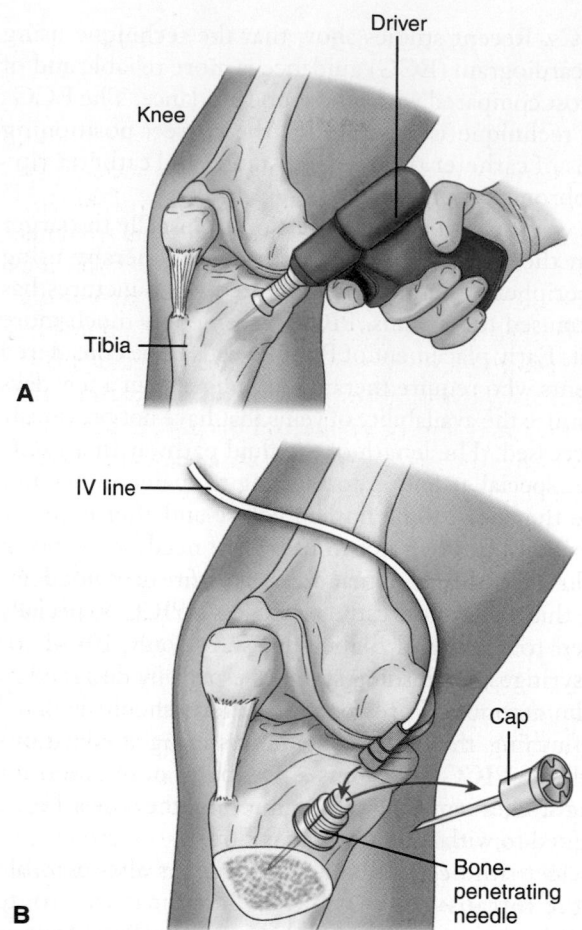

FIGURE 10.11 Obtaining intraosseous (IO) access. *A,* A handheld driver is used to access the bone marrow to place the IO device. *B,* The IO device is inserted into the vasculature of the bone marrow, allowing for infusion of fluids and medications.

or fluid that is administered by the IV route can be administered by this route.

Intraosseous access requires less skill than other types of venous access and can be accomplished in under 1 minute. It is especially useful in severely dehydrated patients and for prehospital vascular access. It is becoming more common for IO lines to be placed by emergency medical technicians prior to arrival to the hospital. Frequently used sites in the adult include the proximal humerus, proximal tibia, and distal tibia. The IO route provides rapid central venous access in emergency situations and is recommended as an alternative route in cardiopulmonary resuscitation by the American Heart Association.

EQUIPMENT USED IN INFUSION THERAPY

Infusion systems consist of the containers and the tubing or administration sets that deliver solutions and medications to the IV access device. Needleless systems have been developed and are mandated by the Occupational Safety and Health Administration (OSHA) to reduce the number of

needle-stick injuries incurring when providing infusion therapy, and there are several types of needleless systems available to nurses. One type of needleless system makes use of a port that contains a valve that is accessed with a male Luer lock on the end of a syringe or administration set (Fig. 10.12). There are also Luer access valve systems available with a positive displacement feature that prevents blood from backflowing into the IV catheter after use. All needleless connectors are activated by pressure in the syringe Luer. This pressure facilitates the syringe Luer to enter an already-split septum to open or depress the septum/plunger. Needleless connectors are the microbial gatekeepers between blood and the unsterile outside of the system. The needleless system aims to prevent microorganisms on the system surface from gaining access into the bloodstream. Disinfection of the needleless system surface is of primary importance prior to use. Disinfection/alcohol caps can be used for continuous disinfectant contact. Even with these caps, the needleless system must be cleaned with an alcohol wipe. The Joint Commission recommends a 10- to 15-second scrub. Allow the disinfectant to dry prior to accessing the system.

Administration sets are either primary or secondary sets (Fig. 10.13). Primary sets are used to deliver the main

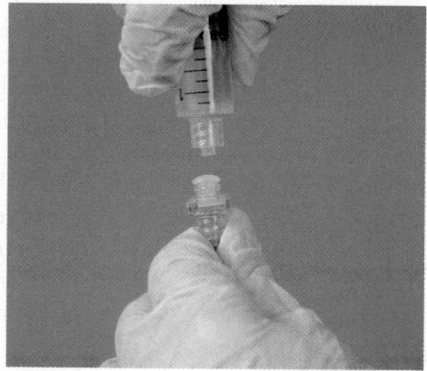

FIGURE 10.12 Luer-activated injection cap. This is a needleless system that uses a port that contains a valve that is accessed with a male Luer lock on the end of a syringe or administration set.

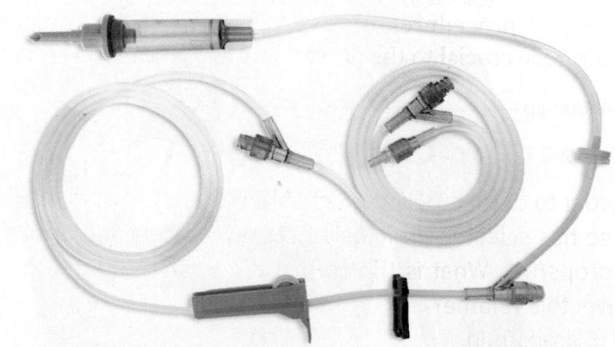

FIGURE 10.13 Primary administration set. Primary sets are used to deliver the main IV solution and consist of a spike that goes into the IV bag, a roller clamp that allows control of flow/infusion rate, ports for secondary access, and the end that connects to the IV catheter.

IV solution, and secondary sets are attached to the primary set to deliver additional solutions or intermittent medications into a y-site in the primary infusion set. These administration sets use gravity to deliver fluids into the vasculature. Administration sets allow for the control of delivery rates using a roller clamp. The infusion rate is determined by the drip factor of the infusion set. Macrodrop administration sets have drip factors of 10, 12, 15, or 20 drops/mL and are appropriate when delivering higher infusion rates. Microdrop administration sets have drip factors of 60 drops/mL and are appropriate when delivering rates of less than 100 mL/min. To determine the infusion rate:

milliliters per minute × drop factor = drops per minute

There are situations when more accurate rate control is needed than can be provided by gravity administration set roller clamps, and one possible solution is the use of an **electronic infusion device** or pump. These infusion pumps can deliver solutions and medications with a greater degree of accuracy and can alert the nurse to situations when the infusion has slowed or stopped because of kinked tubing or increased resistance that can indicate that the IV catheter is clotted or has infiltrated into the subcutaneous tissue. Some electronic infusion devices use standard administration sets, whereas others require administration sets specifically designed for use in the device. Electronic infusion devices assist the nurse in providing accurate infusion therapy, but the nurse is still responsible for monitoring the delivery of the therapy.

One of the most important safety features offered by many electronic infusion devices is the ability to enforce parameters for safe administration of medications through the use of a medication library that sets high and low limits for medication administration. These electronic infusion devices are called "smart pumps" and have been shown to greatly improve the safety of IV medication administration because they prevent the setting of infusion rates outside established safe parameters. However, recent studies have found that more than half of infusions contain errors. These errors are not technology related but, instead, deviations in hospital policies. Seventy-seven percent of hospitals use smart pump technology, but adherence to clinical practice policies and procedures and competence in smart pump operation are crucial to the prevention of medication errors.

Connection Check 10.4

In order to deliver 0.9% sodium chloride at 125 mL/hr, the nurse has selected an infusion set with a drop factor of 15 drops/mL. What is the correct drop rate required to deliver this volume?

A. 15 drops/min
B. 31 drops/min
C. 60 drops/min
D. 125 drops/min

NURSING MANAGEMENT OF INFUSION THERAPY

Monitoring and Preventing Complications

The fluid status of patients receiving IV fluids needs to be monitored to ensure that the intended outcome of therapy is being achieved; therapy should provide adequate amounts of fluid to maintain a **euvolemic** or **normovolemic** (having normal blood volume) state. Hypertonic and hypotonic fluids place the patient at the greatest risk for fluid imbalance and require more intense monitoring. Fluid status is monitored with physical assessment, periodic weights, and accurate measurement of intake and output. Laboratory values, particularly serum electrolytes, need to be monitored for further indications of fluid balance.

Phlebitis and Infiltration

Complications of peripheral infusion therapy include phlebitis and **infiltration**. Phlebitis, inflammation of the vein, is characterized by pain and erythema along the vein and is graded using a standardized scale according to signs, symptoms, and severity (Table 10.4). Peripheral sites that show signs of phlebitis should be removed and restarted in another location because phlebitis can progress to more serious conditions, including thrombus formation, cellulitis, and sepsis. The antecubital fossa site has been shown to have the lowest phlebitis rates, whereas hand veins have a high risk of phlebitis.

Causative factors of phlebitis are divided into three categories: chemical, mechanical, and bacterial. Chemical phlebitis is the result of the infusion of irritating solutions and medications that occurs when the peripheral vein does not allow for sufficient hemodilution of the IV fluid as it exits the catheter. Mechanical phlebitis is the result of the catheter irritating the vein wall and can be caused by introducing a catheter too large for the vein, inadequately securing the catheter, or movement of the catheter placed in an area of flexion such as the elbow or wrist. Bacterial phlebitis is the result of bacteria being introduced into the catheter

Table 10.4 Infusion Nurses Society Phlebitis Scale

Grade	Clinical Criteria
0	No clinical symptoms
1	Erythema at access site with or without pain
2	Pain at access site with erythema and/or edema
3	Pain at access site with erythema, streak formation, and/or palpable cord
4	Pain at access site with erythema, streak formation, palpable venous cord greater than 1 inch in length, and/or purulent drainage

Data from Infusion Nurses Society. (2016). *Infusion therapy standards of practice.* Norwood, MA: Author.

because of improper site cleaning prior to venipuncture, failure to clean ports prior to accessing the administration set, or failure to perform adequate hand hygiene (see Evidence-Based Practice: Use of Aloe Vera to Prevent and Treat Infusion Phlebitis). The insertion sites of peripheral vascular access devices need to be assessed at regular intervals for phlebitis, as defined by institutional policies. It is important to continue to assess the site after the peripheral catheter has been removed because phlebitis can develop after the infusion has been completed.

Evidence-Based Practice

Use of Aloe Vera to Prevent and Treat Infusion Phlebitis

Because of the risk of phlebitis associated with IV fluid administration, a systematic review was conducted in 2014 to examine the effects of the application of aloe vera to prevent and treat phlebitis. Inclusion criteria included randomized and quasi-randomized controlled studies of participants receiving topical aloe vera or aloe vera–derived products applied to the insertion site. There was a total of 43 reviews, with 35 of these being randomized controlled studies that represented 7,465 participants. The trials compared the application of aloe vera alone or with another non–aloe vera treatment, such as wet compresses of 75% alcohol or 33%, 50%, or 75% magnesium sulfate, with no treatment. The findings suggest that the application of fresh aloe vera alone or in combination with other non–aloe vera treatment may be effective in preventing and treating phlebitis secondary to placement of IV access devices. The authors recommend cautious interpretation of these results secondary to some issues with low methodologic quality.

Zheng, G. H., Chen, J. F., Chu, J. F., & Mei, L. (2014). Aloe vera for prevention and treatment of infusion phlebitis. *Cochrane Database of Systematic Reviews, 6,* CD009162. doi:10.1002/14651858.CD009162.pub2

Infiltration occurs when a solution or medication is inadvertently infused into the tissue surrounding the vein and is a complication that can occur with any IVAD, peripheral or central. When the solution or medication that infiltrates is a vesicant (able to cause blisters), an **extravasation** (leakage of IV fluid into subcutaneous tissue) has occurred. Medications that are classified as vesicants include specific antineoplastic agents, antibiotics, and vasoactive medications. Nurses administering vesicants require additional education to ensure competency, and infusion should be routinely assessed for possible infiltration at intervals established by institutional policy. Clinical manifestations of

infiltration include blanched skin, skin cool to the touch, edema, unexpected pain or burning at the insertion site or along the path of the vein, and leaking of fluid from the insertion site. Assessment intervals need to take into consideration the patient's condition, type of device, type of therapy, and risk factors. In the case of an extravasation, the infusion needs to be stopped immediately, and corrective action needs to be taken to minimize damage to the tissue.

Central Line Complications

Complications of central venous infusion therapy include infection, loss of patency, and air embolism. Strategies have been implemented in healthcare institutions to eliminate infections of **central venous catheters (CVCs)** because of their negative effects on patient outcomes and the high cost of treating central line–associated bloodstream infections. The use of maximal sterile barrier precautions, including mask, sterile gown and cap, sterile gloves, and large full-body drapes, while inserting a CVAD is now the standard of practice. Nurses play a key role in preventing these infections by following evidence-based best practices (see Safety Alert).

> **! Safety Alert** 2016 National Patient Safety Goal: Implement best practices or evidence-based guidelines to prevent central line–associated bloodstream infections.
> - Perform hand hygiene prior to line manipulation and dressing changes; use aseptic technique.
> - Disinfect catheter hub and injection port when accessing.
> - If assisting or supervising line insertion, maintain sterile technique, and speak up if sterile technique is broken; complete or collect line insertion checklist.
> - Educate patient and/or family prior to insertion regarding prevention of central line infection.

Loss of patency, or **occlusion**, of a CVC can delay the delivery of lifesaving therapies and may also mean the patient is subject to the risk and discomfort of insertion of another CVC. Occlusions can be the result of a thrombotic process when blood or fibrin in or around the catheter interferes with flow. Thrombotic occlusions can result in slowed infusion rate and resistance to flushing or the complete inability to infuse or flush the catheter. Proper flushing before and after use of the catheter and at intervals when the catheter is not in use decreases the occurrence of thrombotic occlusions. There are injection caps specially designed to prevent thrombotic occlusions; these caps create a positive pressure that prevents blood from refluxing into the catheter when not in use.

Occlusion can also be **nonthrombotic** (not resulting from a clot) and can result from medication precipitation. Medication precipitation occurs when incompatible medications are administered together or without adequate flushing between administrations of the incompatible medications. Nurses need to verify that medications being administered together by the IV route are compatible with the solution infusing and any other medications that may still be in the line or catheter.

An **air embolism** occurs when air is inadvertently introduced into the venous system. Air can be introduced if the catheter is damaged, during insertion and removal of CVCs, and if the connections in the IV delivery system (e.g., catheter hub, tubing, injection caps) are not tightly secured with Luer-locked connections. Nursing actions that can prevent air embolism include proper Trendelenburg positioning during CVC insertion (10–30 degrees), avoiding CVC insertion during inspiration, correcting hypovolemia prior to CVC insertion, ensuring all IV connections are intact and secure, and ensuring all lumens are capped and/or clamped. Additional actions include using Luer-locking connections, frequently checking the connections, and clamping catheters and injection sites when not in use. Other preventive measures include using infusion pumps, **priming** (flushing all the air out of the IV tubing with the ordered solution) all IV tubing prior to connecting to the CVC, expelling air out of all syringes prior to use, and inspecting all lines and connections. Ensure the central line dressing is intact, and use caution when prepositioning the patient. The CVC should be removed only by personnel competent to perform this procedure, and removal should be performed with the patient in a supine position. Prior to removal, the patient should be instructed to perform a Valsalva's maneuver or exhale during the removal to prevent the introduction of air into the line. The catheter should be removed slowly, and a sterile occlusive dressing should be placed over the insertion site immediately and left in place for 24 hours.

Connection Check 10.5

The nurse recognizes the presence of pain, redness, and streak formation at the site of a peripheral IV site as what grade of phlebitis?

A. 1
B. 2
C. 3
D. 4

Maintaining Intravenous Access

In order to maintain the patency of both peripheral and central IVADs, proper flushing is required, and all IVADs need to be flushed prior to use to establish that they have been placed properly and are functioning correctly. Single-use vials or prefilled syringes of preservative-free 0.9% saline are the preferred methods of delivering flushes because they require less manipulation and are less likely to be contaminated. Whenever manipulating an IVAD, it is imperative to perform hand hygiene and to clean the injection ports prior to every

entry. The injection port needs to be cleaned with alcohol or chlorhexidine and allowed to dry completely; the nurse follows institutional protocols regarding which agent is used to clean the port. Catheters are flushed with a volume twice that of the catheter and any attached extension tubing (Box 10.2). The INS recommends a **flushing and locking protocol**.

- "**Flushing**" is the act of moving fluids, medications, blood, blood products, and nutrients out of a vascular access device into the bloodstream, ensuring delivery of these components and verifying device patency.
- "**Locking**" is the instillation of a solution into a vascular access device to maintain device patency.

The patency of CVADs requires a continuous infusion or periodic flushing. As with peripheral catheters, CVADs need to be flushed after the administration of a medication or blood product when changing from a continuous infusion to an intermittent "locked" device and also after the withdrawal of blood and when not in use. The frequency of periodic flushing is determined by the type of CVAD and institutional policies. The volume used to flush the CVAD needs to be at least twice the volume of the catheter to be sure all contents of the IVAD are cleared with the flush. Institutional policy determines which CVADs used intermittently are "locked" with saline or with a heparin solution. Studies have shown that the patency of some catheters can be maintained without heparin, which decreases the bleeding complications associated with this anticoagulant.

All IVADs, with the exception of well-healed tunneled catheters, are dressed with a sterile occlusive dressing to prevent bacterial contamination of the site. Transparent semipermeable dressings offer the advantage of allowing a clear view of the insertion site for assessment, but gauze dressing occluded with tape is acceptable. Dressings should be changed immediately if they are no longer occlusive or become moist. Peripheral IVADs do not require routine dressing changes or site care. The frequency of CVAD

Box 10.2 Centers for Disease Control and Prevention (CDC) Protocol for Flushing Central Venous Lines

Positive-pressure technique (may not apply to neutral-displacement or positive-displacement needleless connectors):

- Flush the catheter, continue to hold the plunger of the syringe while closing the clamp on the catheter, and then disconnect the syringe.
- For catheters without a clamp, withdraw the syringe as the last 0.5 to 1 mL of fluid is flushed.

From Centers for Disease Control. (2011). *Guidelines for the prevention of intravascular catheter-related infections* [Updated 2017]. Retrieved from https://www.cdc.gov/infectioncontrol/guidelines/bsi/recommendations.html

dressing changes and site care is determined by institutional policy, type of CVAD, and type of dressing. Sterile gloves should be worn when changing a CVAD dressing to decrease the risk of infection.

A recent meta-analysis performed by the Cochrane Collaboration found no clear evidence for routine replacement of peripheral IV catheters. Rotating peripheral IV sites every 72 to 96 hours is unpleasant for the patient and expensive in terms of supplies and nursing time. The 2016 INS Infusion Nursing Standards of Care note that peripheral catheters should be replaced when clinically indicated, not at set intervals. Clinical indications for the removal of a peripheral catheter include whenever the patient reports discomfort or pain related to the infusion site and assessment findings indicating possible phlebitis, infiltration, or occlusion. IV tubing is changed according to institutional policy; there is no evidence that changing IV tubing more frequently than every 96 hours decreases the risk of infection (see Evidence-Based Practice: Peripheral IV Site Rotation Based on Assessment Findings).

Evidence-Based Practice

Peripheral IV Site Rotation Based on Assessment Findings

There are variations in practice related to the length of time that peripheral IV catheters may remain in place prior to changing sites. In many healthcare settings, agency policies require that sites be changed at specific time intervals (usually 72–96 hours), despite the absence of complications such as phlebitis and infiltration. A descriptive study, based on Duffy's Quality Caring Model and conducted in a 500-bed community hospital, included a convenience sample of 71 patients with 89 IV catheters. At the time of the study, the policy at this facility required that IV catheter sites be changed every 96 hours, despite the absence of complications. The findings of this study demonstrated that IV catheters could remain in place past the 96-hour time frame with routine assessment of the site. Thirty sites maintained patency for 96 to 200 hours, five sites maintained patency at 201 to 300 hours, and four sites were patent when assessed over 300 hours after initial placement. These findings also are consistent with 2011 recommendations from the Infusion Nurses Society stating that IV catheter site changes should be based on assessment data, including site, length and type of IV therapy, patency, and stabilization.

Helton, J., Hines, A., & Best, J. (2011). Peripheral IV site rotation based on clinical assessment vs. length of time since insertion. *MEDSURG Nursing, 25*(1), 44–49.

Routine replacements or exchanges of CVADs are not necessary if the catheter is functioning and there is no evidence of complications. The continued need for a short-term central catheter (PICCs and nontunneled percutaneous central catheters) needs to be evaluated daily by the interprofessional team to determine if the catheter is required. Consideration needs to be made to possibly administering infusion therapies by a less invasive peripheral approach or by other routes, such as oral.

CASE STUDY: EPISODE 2

Upon Jason's arrival in the emergency department, two large-bore (18-gauge) IV catheters are placed in his forearm, and the IV lines started in the field are discontinued. The nurse practitioner also inserts a nontunneled percutaneous central catheter. Blood samples are obtained for serum chemistries, complete blood count, and toxicology, and samples are also sent for type and crossmatch in the event Jason requires blood products. He is taken to the operating room for an emergency exploratory laparotomy, and in the post-anesthesia care unit (PACU), the nurse anesthetist places a triple-lumen CVC for the anticipated need for administration of blood products, IV fluids, and antibiotics. He is transferred to the surgical intensive care unit for postoperative management…

Administration of Intravenous Medications

Terms used to describe the method used to administer medications or solutions include *continuous infusion, intermittent infusion, bolus* (a specific amount of fluid over a short time period) *infusion,* and *IV push* (direct IV administration). The order of a licensed independent practitioner needs to indicate which method is to be used. Continuous infusion refers to the ongoing administration of a solution and can be ordered as a specific rate per hour (e.g., 125 mL/hr) or a volume over a time period (1,000 mL over 8 hours). Clarification needs to be obtained for orders indicating a "keep open rate" or "**keep vein open**" (KVO) to obtain a more clearly defined rate unless a "keep open rate" is defined in institutional protocols. Interpretation of such orders can vary greatly, particularly depending on the age and weight of the patient, and can lead to possible fluid overload. Veins should never be kept open with solutions containing medications such as potassium because insufficient amounts will be delivered to be therapeutic.

Intermittent infusions can be given through the injection port on the administration set of the continuous infusion ("piggyback") or infused into the injection port of the locked IVAD. Intermittent infusions concurrent with a continuous infusion need to be compatible with the continuous infusion. If not compatible, the continuous infusion needs to be stopped while the intermittent infusion infuses and the tubing of the infusion set is cleared or flushed with a compatible solution, usually 0.9% normal saline. Prior to administration of an intermittent infusion through a locked IVAD, the IVAD device needs to be flushed to ensure proper functioning of the device and clearing of any potentially incompatible solution. When the intermittent infusion is completed, the IVAD then needs to be flushed again and relocked. When intermittent infusions are administered either into a continuous infusion or into a locked IVAD, the IV system needs to remain closed, and the tubing should not be disconnected to prevent the introduction of microorganisms into the IV system. Flushing and administration of intermittent infusions are done through an injection port that has been cleaned with alcohol or chlorhexidine, per institutional protocol, and allowed to completely dry.

Bolus infusions are concentrated medications and/or solutions given over a short period of time. This is the method used when administering a "fluid bolus" or "fluid challenge" to a patient who may have a low urine output because of decreased fluid volume status. Boluses are usually administered with small-volume solution containers (250 or 500 mL) in a manner similar to an intermittent infusion but over a shorter time period. Patients receiving bolus infusions need to be monitored closely to ensure they are tolerating the volume infused.

IV push, or direct IV, is the manual administration of a medication using a syringe. Special attention needs to be given to the correct concentration and rate of administration of medications given with this method. Some medications need to be diluted prior to administration to ensure a safe concentration and to more accurately control the rate of administration. IV push medications can be given into a locked IVAD or into an IVAD with a continuous infusion. Prior to administration, the IVAD and any tubing between the injection port and the IVAD needs to be flushed to ensure proper functioning of the device and clearing of any potentially incompatible solution or medications. Flushing and administration of the IV push are done through an injection port that has been cleaned with alcohol or chlorhexidine and allowed to completely dry. After the IV push medication has been administered, the IVAD needs to be flushed again. Keep in mind that the rate of this flush needs to be at the same rate that is acceptable for the medication administration because the medication that is in the tubing and IVAD will be flushed through and administered to the patient at the flush rate.

Administration of Blood Products

Transfusion of blood components is a lifesaving therapy that includes risk and requires meticulous adherence to procedures and policies along with close monitoring of the patient. Modern practices for blood collection include multiple screening tests and volunteer donors, rendering the blood supply relatively free of the risk of transmissible diseases such as syphilis, hepatitis, and HIV. Transfusion of whole blood is rare because it is more efficient to administer only the portion of the blood, or component, required by the patient (Table 10.5). Also, one unit of donated blood can be separated into individual components that can benefit multiple recipients. Components commonly infused include RBCs, fresh frozen plasma (FFP), platelets, granulocytes, clotting factors, and albumin.

Prior to releasing a blood component for administration to a patient, the blood bank or laboratory carefully matches the intended component to the sample of the patient's blood to ensure that they are compatible using ABO, Rhesus (Rh), and human leukocyte antigen (HLA) testing. Antigens present on the surface of the RBC determine the ABO blood type of the patient. Antibodies to the ABO antigens are in the plasma, which means ABO antigens present on the transfused blood will be attacked by the antigens in the recipient's blood if they do not have the same ABO antigens. This causes a **hemolytic transfusion reaction**. The Rh antigen is another antigen on the RBC that is either present (Rh-positive) or absent (Rh-negative). Recipients who are Rh-negative should receive only Rh-negative blood, but recipients who are Rh-positive can receive either Rh-positive or Rh-negative blood (Table 10.6). Patient identification and specimen labeling of blood samples collected from the patient need to be done with extreme care and usually require independent identification by two separate

Table 10.5 Indications for Blood Component Transfusion	
Blood Component	**Indication**
Packed red blood cells (volume 225–350 mL)	Symptomatic anemia
	Acute and chronic blood loss
Plasma (fresh frozen plasma) (volume 200–250 mL)	Deficiency of plasma coagulation factors
	Massive transfusion in trauma
	Need for emergency reversal of elevated prothrombin time and international normalized ratio (PT/INR) that indicates increased risk of bleeding
	Disseminated intravascular coagulation (DIC)
Platelets (volume 40–70 mL)	Bleeding due to thrombocytopenia or platelet abnormalities
Granulocytes (volume 200–300 mL)	Neutropenia with infection, unresponsive to appropriate antibiotics
Albumin (volume varies)	Volume expansion when crystalloid solutions are not adequate

Table 10.6 ABO Compatibilities

Blood Component	Type-Specific Compatibilities	
Red blood cells (RBCs) and platelets	Donor	Recipient
	O	O, A, B, AB
	A	A, AB
	B	B, AB
	AB	AB
Fresh frozen plasma	Donor	Recipient
	O	O
	A	A, O
	B	B, O
	AB	AB, B, A, O

healthcare providers. The HLA system relates to proteins located on the surface of white blood cells and other tissues. Important to immune function, HLAs form in response to exposure to foreign substances. In blood transfusions and organ transplants, the immune system recognizes these cells or tissues as foreign substances, activating the HLA system and leading to transfusion reactions and organ rejection.

Because blood components are "living transplants," they need to be stored according to strict standards. Even though most blood components contain preservatives, they are stored in the laboratory until just prior to their transfusion. There are strict time limits placed on how long blood products can be outside of storage in the laboratory prior to administration and on the length of time over which they can be infused. Nurses must be knowledgeable of these timelines and follow the guidelines established by the institution where they practice. Compliance with these standards is monitored on the blood product administration forms required with the administration of each individual component. Each component or unit is accompanied by a unique form that provides information about the blood product.

Before the blood component is obtained from the laboratory, the patient's informed consent and an order for the administration of the blood component need to be confirmed. The order should indicate the type of blood component to be administered, the number of units or volume of the blood component to be infused, the flow rate or duration of the infusion, and other parameters for infusion. Because there is a limited amount of time allowed for the component to be outside the controlled storage conditions of the laboratory, the nurse needs to confirm adequate IV access and that all supplies and equipment needed for the transfusion are available prior to the blood component being released from the laboratory for administration. Once the component is obtained from the laboratory, there needs to be verification performed by two

licensed staff members, which includes matching the blood product to the order and matching the patient to the blood product. The blood product should agree with the type of component prescribed, the volume or number of units to be transfused, and the patient's full name and one other patient identifier. The ABO and Rh compatibility of the donor and recipient also needs to be confirmed prior to the initiation of the transfusion. The expiration date and the date and time the component was released from the laboratory need to be confirmed as acceptable.

> **Safety Alert**   The National Quality Forum has identified mismatched blood transfusions as an event that should never happen. Patient identification is the most important process in the safe administration of blood components. Fatal errors can occur because of mislabeled specimens or blood components and patient identification.

Immediately prior to starting the blood transfusion, a patient assessment needs to be completed, including baseline vital signs and respiratory status. The nurse needs to explain the procedure and confirm patient understanding, including clinical manifestations to immediately report. Blood transfusions can be an anxiety-producing situation, and adequate time for explanations and questions needs to be provided.

Close observation is required to detect any reaction the patient may have to the blood product (Table 10.7), especially during the first 15 minutes when reactions are most likely to occur. Assessments should continue at least every hour for the duration of the transfusion and should include respiratory status; vital sign status; and any complaints of discomfort, dyspnea, or itching.

The type of component ordered determines the method of administration and the type of equipment needed for the infusion. There are special filters and tubing for each type of blood component, but the only type of infusion solution used in flushing administration sets and IVADs, and in the administration of any of the blood components, is 0.9% sodium chloride. The rationale for this fluid is because it is isotonic and does not cause fluids to move into or out of the transfused RBCs. The gauge of the IVAD used for transfusion needs to be large enough to facilitate the required flow rates so that the blood is transfused within the prescribed time frame. An 18- to 20-gauge catheter is recommended for the infusion of packed RBCs in the adult population to prevent RBC lysis.

Packed RBCs consist of the cells that remain after the plasma portion of the whole blood is removed. Packed RBCs are the component that is used for most blood replacement therapy, including acute blood loss, and chronic symptomatic anemia that does not respond to pharmacological therapy. In certain situations, RBCs that have undergone

Table 10.7 Types of Transfusion Reactions

Transfusion Reaction	Cause	Clinical Manifestations	Interventions if Suspected
Acute hemolytic reaction	Infusion of ABO-incompatible blood	Fever Chills Hypotension Flank pain Vascular collapse	Stop the transfusion immediately. Notify the provider. Maintain blood pressure.
Febrile nonhemolytic reaction	Antibody reaction to granulocytes or platelets in infused blood component	Temp increase of 1°C or 2°F Chills Headache Chest pain	Stop transfusion; notify provider. Monitor vital signs. Possible administration of antipyretics Restart transfusion slowly.
Allergic reaction	Sensitivity to donor's plasma proteins	Itching Hives Facial flushing Anxiety Dyspnea	Stop transfusion; notify provider. Monitor vital signs. Possible administration of antihistamines Restart transfusion slowly.
Circulatory overload	Administration rate higher than patient tolerance	Headache Dyspnea JVD Edema Increased BP	Stop transfusion; notify provider. Monitor vital signs. Elevate HOB. Possible administration of diuretics and oxygen Restart transfusion slowly.

BP, Blood pressure; *HOB,* head of bed; *JVD,* jugular venous distention.

special processing are ordered to meet special patient needs. These types of packed RBCs include irradiated and leukocyte-reduced RBCs. Irradiating RBCs inactivates donor lymphocytes and reduces allergic and febrile reactions in some patients. Leukocyte-reduced RBCs decrease febrile reactions in recipients with high levels of leukocyte antibodies.

A single unit of packed RBCs has a volume between 225 and 300 mL and is usually infused over 1 1/2 to 2 hours but no longer than 4 hours. The integrity of blood products infused over periods greater than 4 hours is compromised, and any remaining product not infused in the 4-hour period needs to be returned to the laboratory. Administration sets used to infuse packed RBCs are either a straight or y-type set with a 170- to 260-micron filter. Filters of this size allow for the movement of the RBCs through the filter but stop any small clots or other debris. The tubing is primed with 0.9% sodium chloride prior to use.

Connection Check 10.6

A patient is ordered to receive a blood transfusion because of anemia. What is the recommended minimum gauge of the IV catheter to administer blood?

A. 16
B. 18
C. 20
D. 22

Administration of Total Parenteral Nutrition

The use of the intravenous route to provide nutrition is indicated only when it is not possible to provide adequate nutrition using the oral or enteral routes. Intravenous total parenteral nutrition (TPN) is associated with increased risks to the patient and greater costs. Parenteral nutrition solutions provide the major macronutrients (protein, carbohydrates, and lipids) along with required micronutrients (electrolytes, vitamins, and trace minerals) and water. The protein required by the body for growth, maintenance, and repair of tissues is provided in TPN in the form of amino acids in a combination that meets the body's needs. Carbohydrates used to generate energy for the body are supplied by dextrose in the TPN solution. Lipid emulsions may be included to provide an additional source of energy and serve as a source for essential fatty acids. Lipids can either be contained in the primary TPN solution or infused separately.

An interprofessional approach is required to design a TPN program that meets the needs of the individual patient, including the primary healthcare provider (physician, advanced practice registered nurse, physician's assistant), registered nurses, pharmacists, and dietitians. Total parenteral nutrition solutions are prepared in the pharmacy under special conditions to reduce the risk of bacterial contamination. Infusion of additional medications in the TPN solution is institution specific, and the risk of infection and medication incompatibilities needs to be carefully evaluated. Medications that are added in some institutions include insulin, heparin, and H_2-receptor antagonists.

Because of the high concentrations of dextrose, TPN therapy is initiated gradually, and the patient's glucose and fluid tolerance are evaluated as the infusion rate is gradually increased until the targeted rate is reached. Blood glucose levels may be monitored every 6 hours, and an insulin scale is used to control blood glucose levels. Similarly, when the therapy is being discontinued, the rate of infusion should be gradually decreased as the patient adjusts to decreased amounts of concentrated IV dextrose and fluids.

When TPN is infused, special precautions are implemented to prevent complications. Because of the high osmolarity of TPN solutions, they should be infused into a CVAD with the tip placement confirmed in the vena cava. This allows for hemodilution of the TPN solution, decreasing the risk of phlebitis, thrombosis, and pain. The infusion system used to administer TPN should remain a closed and dedicated line and should not be used to administer other medications or access the CVAD for any reason. The administration set used to infuse TPN should be changed every 24 hours to decrease the risk of contamination and infection.

Connection Check 10.7

The nurse recognizes the prevention of which complication as the primary rationale for initiating total parenteral nutrition at a slow rate?

A. Infection
B. Hyperglycemia
C. Discomfort
D. Air embolism

Patient Teaching

One of the most important roles of the professional nurse in infusion therapy is patient and family education because they have the right to be involved in their care. In order to be actively involved and make decisions about the care they receive, patients need to be educated on the alterations in their health that require infusion therapy, the infusion therapies prescribed, and the expected outcomes and possible complications of the therapies.

Prior to the insertion of any IVAD, peripheral or central, the patient needs to be educated and learning verified regarding the rationale for the IVAD, alternatives to the selected device, and expectations during the insertion of the device, including the level of expected discomfort. Patients are also educated on the measures used to decrease discomfort and possible complications. The practice of aseptic techniques needs to be explained to the patients, and return demonstration by the patient, family member, or significant other of aseptic technique in caring for the IV access is included in the education.

Patients are informed of the type of IV solution and/or medications to be administered, including the reasons they are being administered, expected outcomes, and possible complications. During therapy, the patient's understanding of the importance of reporting any unexpected outcomes and signs of possible complications is assessed. Patients are taught measures to prevent possible complications, including reporting any discomfort or redness at the insertion site, temperature elevation, and whenever the IVAD dressing is no longer occlusive or is wet. Patients are encouraged to monitor hand washing and proper cleaning of ports in the IV delivery system prior to entry by all healthcare personnel.

Connection Check 10.8

The nurse recognizes that education for patients receiving infusion therapy should include which information? (Select all that apply.)

A. Precautions for preventing infection
B. Signs and symptoms to report
C. Manufacturer of the IVAD
D. Purpose of infusion therapy
E. Calculation of infusion rates

It is the professional nurse's responsibility to administer IV solutions and medications as prescribed and know the expected outcomes and possible side effects of the solutions and medications administered. Additionally, it is an expectation that the nurse is competent in the techniques used to provide infusion therapy and in monitoring the patient for responses to therapy and the development of any undesired outcomes or complications. The need for continuous infusion therapy and IV access is evaluated periodically, and discontinuation is considered as soon as therapy can be delivered by other, less invasive routes.

Making Connections

CASE STUDY: WRAP-UP

Four days postoperatively, Jason develops a peritoneal abscess requiring IV antibiotics and analgesics, blood products, and TPN. He remains in the surgical intensive care unit for 3 days and receives four more units of packed RBCs. On day 4, he is transferred to the surgical intermediate care unit, and 10 days after admission, he is transferred to a short-term acute rehabilitation facility until he can be discharged home.

Case Study Questions

1. The nurse should be prepared to administer what IV solution to Jason as a result of the injuries he sustained in the motor vehicle accident?
   A. 5% dextrose in lactated Ringer's
   B. 5% dextrose in normal saline
   C. 0.45% normal saline
   D. 0.9% normal saline

2. What is the rationale for the placement of a nontunneled percutaneous central catheter for Jason?
   A. The catheter allows easy care of the catheter by Jason after discharge.
   B. There is a lower risk of infection and other complications.
   C. Jason prefers to not have an IV in his hand.
   D. There is an urgent need for fluid and medication administration.

3. The nurse recognizes that the multiple units of packed RBCs Jason received for blood loss after his motorcycle accident did not contain clotting factors and anticipates that which blood component may be required?
   A. Fresh frozen plasma
   B. Granulocytes
   C. Platelets
   D. Whole blood

4. Into which port of his triple-lumen CVAD can the nurse infuse the next dose of antibiotics? *(Select all that apply.)*
   A. Port with the parenteral nutrition infusion
   B. Port with the packed RBCs infusing
   C. Port where the patient-controlled analgesia is attached
   D. Port that is saline locked
   E. Port with 0.9% normal saline infusing

5. On assessing Jason's central line, the nurse notes that the Luer lock on one of the lumens is not tight and recognizes that this places him at risk for which complication?
   A. Air embolism
   B. Clotting of the catheter
   C. Infection
   D. Fluid loss

CHAPTER SUMMARY

Infusion therapy is an important part of the care provided to patients with a wide variety of conditions in many settings across the continuum of care. In order to provide safe and effective infusion therapy, nurses require specialized skills and knowledge of current evidence to guide their practice.

Infusion therapy is utilized to maintain fluid and electrolyte balances, administer medication and blood products, and provide nutritional support. In order to provide the safest care and prevent complications, nurses need to have knowledge of the anatomy and physiology of the vascular system, correct selection and care of various IV access devices, and the pharmacology of the medications and solutions administered intravenously. Nurses need to be alert to possible complications and perform interventions that minimize their occurrence and detect complications early when they do occur.

Intravascular devices selected to deliver infusion therapy should be the least invasive, with the smallest gauge and fewest number of lumens to provide the therapy prescribed. More invasive CVADs are indicated when larger volumes of fluid need to be delivered and for certain medications and solutions that require the greater hemodilution provided in the central vasculature. Specially designed CVADs are available to meet the needs of a variety of patients, including tunneled devices, ports, PICCs, and IO devices. CVADs are required for the administration of TPN due to the high osmolarity and glucose levels.

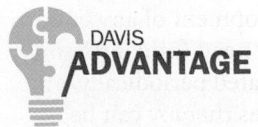

DAVIS
ADVANTAGE | To explore learning resources for this chapter, go to **Davis Advantage** and find:
| – Answers to in-text questions
| – Chapter Resources and Activities
| – NCLEX®-Style Chapter Review Questions
| – Bibliography

Chapter 11

Pain Management

Sherrie Lessans

LEARNING OUTCOMES

Content in this chapter is designed to assist in:

1. Explaining the pathophysiological processes that underlie the pain process
2. Defining types of pain
3. Describing components that comprise a comprehensive pain assessment
4. Examining pain management strategies
5. Developing a comprehensive plan of nursing care for patients with pain
6. Incorporating both pharmacological and nonpharmacological evidence-based interventions into a plan of care for patients with pain
7. Developing patient educational strategies to promote self-care and improved patient outcomes

CONCEPTS

- Assessment
- Comfort
- Communication
- Medication
- Safety

ESSENTIAL TERMS

Acupressure
Acute pain
Addiction
Adjuvant
Allodynia
Analgesia
Anesthesia
Biofeedback
Breakthrough pain
Chronic malignant pain
Chronic pain
Cutaneous pain
Dependence
Epigenetics
Expectancy
Gate control theory
Guided imagery
Hyperalgesia
Hypnosis
Meditation
Music therapy
Neuropathic pain
Nocebo
Nociceptive pain
Nociceptors
Opioid
Pain
Patient-controlled analgesia
Persistent pain
Placebo
Plasticity
Referred pain
Rubefacients
Somatic pain
Tolerance
Visceral pain

Finding Connections

CASE STUDY: EPISODE 1

Follow this patient throughout the chapter.

Martha Jessup is a 68-year-old African American female, 2 days following coronary bypass surgery. She has a medical history significant for hypertension, diabetes, and chronic renal insufficiency. At change of shift, Mrs. Jessup reports 6/10 pain at the surgical site. She further reports spasms in her lower back and "burning" pain that "shoots" down her right leg. She states that "I hurt my back when I was teaching" and has not taken her "usual back pain medications" for more than 3 days. Mrs. Jessup is grimacing; rubbing her right leg; guarding her incision site with a pillow; and taking short, shallow breaths.

Mrs. Jessup is demonstrating a mixed type of pain: acute postoperative pain related to the cardiac surgery and nonmalignant persistent pain in her lower back. In completing a comprehensive pain assessment, the nurse considers how Mrs. Jessup's age, gender, ethnicity, and prior pain experiences influence her pain experience. Her renal insufficiency with possible inherited genetic influences on pharmacokinetics and pharmacodynamics may influence how well she metabolizes her pain medications as well as her response to pain medications...

INTRODUCTION

Pain is the most universal and the most personal of symptoms, an emotional and sensory experience shaped by biological, sociocultural, and psychological factors, including genetics, gender, health status, and life experience. No one person experiences pain like any other. The same person may experience pain in different ways, at different times, and under different circumstances, challenging both assessment and treatment. Although pain is the number one reason patients consult a healthcare provider in the United States, pain remains poorly understood, with mixed treatment success. For most patients in pain, a thorough assessment leads to the identification of the source of pain, a diagnosis, and successful treatment. For other patients, the source of their pain is difficult to determine, and a diagnosis is difficult to make. Treatments for many pain problems may bring little in the way of sustained relief or may create challenging side effects to manage.

Pain disrupts lives and represents a significant public health problem. Even with new medications and treatments, most people experience at least one episode of sustained and unrelieved pain in their lifetime. One in three patients presenting to an emergency department identifies pain as the chief complaint, with more than 60% of patients reporting pain at primary care visits. For the hospitalized patient, pain accompanies surgical treatment, traumatic injury, childbirth, and invasive procedures. Often, the medications and treatments given to treat disorders such as cancer and cardiovascular disease cause pain and disability that linger beyond the treatment period. Pain interferes with sleep, activity, and nutrition patterns as well as relationships and social interactions. Pain contributes to a loss of independence and is frequently linked to the development of anxiety disorders and depression. One in every six adults in the United States reports **chronic pain**, a condition that is poorly managed or undertreated. Counting both the direct costs of provider visits and medications as well as the indirect costs of lost time from work or school and reduced productivity, the cost of pain is more than $100 billion each year according to the National Center for Health Statistics.

Nearly 9 of 10 American households have one or more pain relief therapies in their homes, including over-the-counter (OTC) oral medications, analgesic heat rubs, and heating pads. More than 50% of these same households also have prescription pain medications, usually an **opioid** (opium-based medication used for pain), sharing the medicine cabinet with OTC medications. However, thousands of patients each year fail to satisfactorily manage pain, and the search for pain relief often finds providers who are not knowledgeable about pain management or are unwilling to treat pain that lasts for more than a short acute episode. Relatively few pain specialists are in practice, and they are often concentrated in city centers not easily accessible to rural populations. Health insurance may cover only a portion of the costs associated with comprehensive pain care.

At the end of 2000, President William J. Clinton declared the 10-year period beginning January 1, 2001, the Decade of Pain Control and Research. During this time, funding for pain research nearly doubled, leading to new insights into the biology of pain and a greater appreciation for the pathology that is chronic pain. The American Pain Society, the American Nurses Association, and The Joint Commission all released standards of care requiring that patients be educated about their right to appropriate assessment and pain management, with a special emphasis on pain management in older adults and patients at the end of life. Health professional organizations reaffirmed ethical obligations to relieve pain and alleviate suffering, supporting the growth of an evidence-based intervention science with new approaches to assessment, pain management, and improved quality of life for pain sufferers. This emphasis on improved pain management did lead to innovations in pain treatment, including new classes of medications. By mid-decade however, these advances contributed to only a marginally more complete understanding of the bio-psycho-social complexity that is chronic pain, a tripling of the number of patients addicted to opioids, and an opioid overdose problem that has reached epidemic proportions. Significant challenges continue with pain management, with many gaps in translating research findings into evidence-based pain management practice. Most significant is a fundamental shift in the assessment and management of pain that is less focused on relieving all pain and more focused on improving comfort and functional engagement. This paradigm shift in pain care management will powerfully shape the next generation of health professionals.

DEFINITIONS OF PAIN

For most of the 20th century, the prevailing view was that pain reflexively followed tissue injury, with peripheral nerves rapidly generating and transmitting electrochemical pain messages to the spinal cord and brain, leading to an equally rapid pain response. This peripheral nervous system–centric view failed to explain how or why pain persists for many patients or why chronic pain often appears so disconnected from tissue injury and so difficult to treat. Attention refocused on the dynamic role of the brain and spinal cord in pain messaging in 1965 with the introduction of the seminal **gate control theory**. The impact of this theoretical rethinking and redefinition of pain cannot be overstated. Pain is now understood to be more than the simple transmission of incoming messages to the central nervous system; descending pathways are also widely distributed throughout the brain and spinal cord, which serve to boost or inhibit pain messaging. Many of these specialized pain-messaging and pain-processing pathways are associated with diverse brain structures, including those

shaping motivation, memory, and cognition. It is the job of the spinal cord to integrate input from peripheral tissues with this central descending input by gating "open" or "closed" pain messages to form a neurophysiological response. Although the spinal cord is largely in charge of pain message processing, pain perception is centered in the conscious brain. Pain represents the creative transformation of nerve impulses by the brain into a meaningful and emotion-filled perceptual experience (Fig. 11.1).

With this broader understanding of pain, however, comes confusion about definitions and terminology. Are there physiological differences between acute and chronic pain? Does all pain cause suffering? Is pain relief the same as having no pain? How do health professionals develop a consistent pain language while acknowledging that pain is "whatever the experiencing person says it is"? Second only to gate control theory, this assertion by Margo McCaffery has had the most profound effect on the way healthcare providers assess and manage pain. Although clinicians have largely accepted that pain is subjective, the subjectivity of the pain experience compels the need to prove that pain is present and challenges clinicians when observed pain behaviors are not consistent with other pain experiences. Reliance on self-reports has left clinicians wondering how best to distinguish pain that may signal a medical emergency from more benign pain or whether treatment has provided relief. In 2017 at the most recent consensus conference on

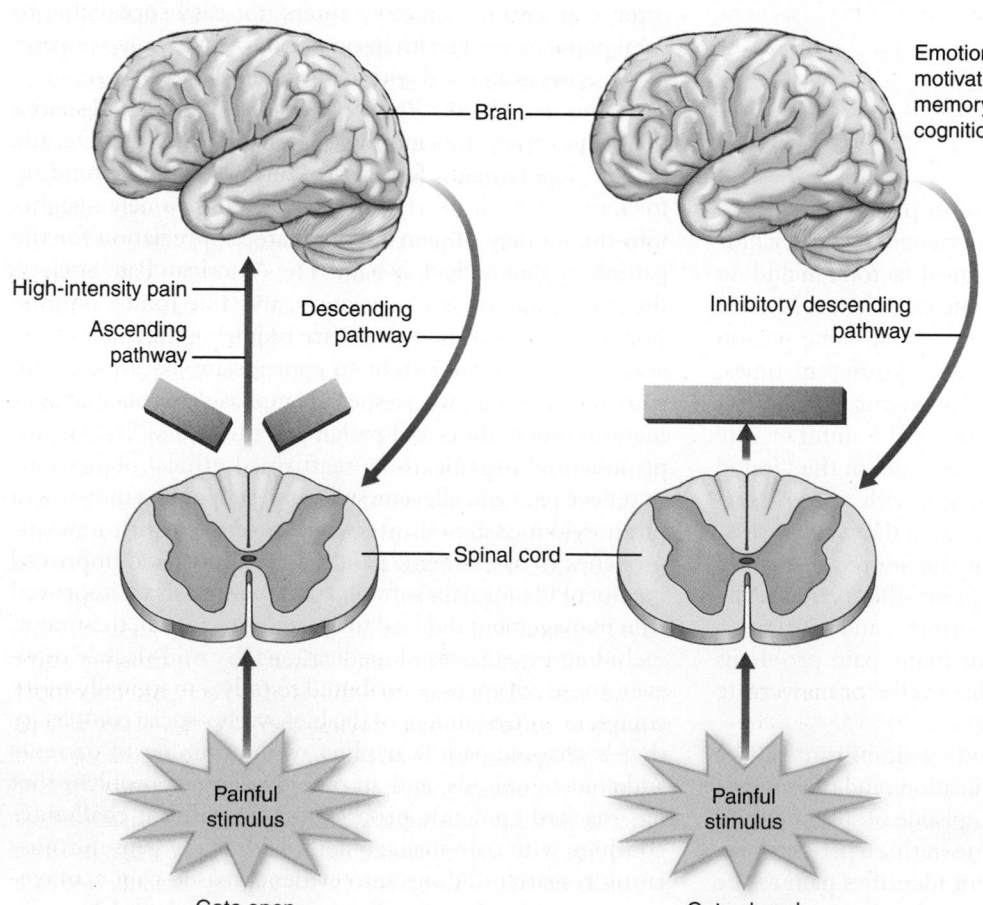

FIGURE 11.1 Pain perception (gate control theory). The spinal cord integrates painful stimuli from the periphery through descending input controlled by "open" or "closed" gates to form a neurophysiological response. The perception of pain is also influenced by the conscious brain that transforms these impulses into meaningful and emotion-filled experiences.

pain, experts reaffirmed the definition of pain as an unpleasant sensory and emotional experience associated with actual or potential tissue damage while acknowledging that much remains to be understood about the intersection of noxious conditions in the tissues and pain perception.

Distinguishing Acute and Chronic Pain

Of all the different ways to classify pain, the most common may be a distinction based on pain duration (Table 11.1). **Acute pain** is sudden in onset and usually of short duration, presenting immediately following noxious stimuli and tissue damage and continuing for several hours to several weeks. The close association between tissue injury and sudden onset of pain suggests acute pain serves a biological purpose, alerting us to actual or potential tissue damage and prompting withdrawal or avoidance behaviors. The quick pulling back of the hand, for example, following touching of a hot surface protects the hand from burns. Pain-induced guarding of an abdominal incision reduces tension at the surgical site, minimizing further trauma. Patients frequently describe acute pain as sharp or intense and can generally pinpoint the pain to a well-defined and specific body location. Acute pain is generally responsive to common pain management treatments and predictably resolves as tissue heals. Examples of acute pain include the pain that accompanies trauma such as fractures or wounds and procedure pain. One of the most common examples of acute pain for nurses is postoperative pain following surgical disruption of superficial skin and muscle. Because postoperative pain is common and predictable, it might be expected that it is well assessed and well managed. Evidence suggests, however, that nearly 70% of patients experience unrelieved pain at some point during their postoperative recovery. Patients themselves delay reporting postoperative pain, believing such pain is to be expected, whereas nurses frequently undermedicate, believing pain treatment may lead to respiratory depression and sleepiness, slowing recovery.

Pain that is present for more than 3 to 6 months, with or without an obvious link to tissue injury, is considered chronic pain. Chronic pain intensity can vary widely; patients describe pain that is achy, dull, stabbing, burning, and icy hot. Patients with chronic pain may also have difficulty localizing chronic pain with more precision than a general region of the body, such as the lower back or legs. Chronic pain is unpredictable in course and resistant to many common pain management approaches and, unlike acute pain, serves no apparent biological purpose. Examples of chronic pain include diabetic peripheral **neuropathic pain** (pain associated with damage or disease affecting the somatosensory nervous system), phantom limb pain following amputation, and fibromyalgia. Acute or chronic pain that responds to some therapeutic interventions but reoccurs when therapies reach the effective end of their dose is termed **persistent pain**. Examples of this type of pain include pain associated with wounds, arthritis, back pain, and some headaches. Although patients with persistent pain may have pain relief with medications, the application of heat, or the application of pressure at specific acupoints, these modalities have time-limited effectiveness, with pain returning as therapies "wear off." Persistent pain can be particularly frustrating for patients and caregivers because pain solutions appear to work, but there is not sustained pain relief. **Breakthrough pain** is a term used by pain experts without consensus to describe short-term bursts of acute pain that present against a background level of controlled or managed pain. Breakthrough pain can be caused by patient movements, by underlying or escalating pathology, or by being at or near the end of a medication dose. Frequently, breakthrough pain appears for unknown reasons but may be remedied by medication, dose, or schedule modification.

Although chronic pain cannot always be linked to a specific tissue injury, some forms of chronic pain coexist with other health problems with enough frequency that a comorbid relationship between other pathologies and chronic pain must be considered. In **chronic malignant pain**, for example, rapidly dividing cells associated with cancer growth invade and distort bone and other tissues, causing quite severe pain. More than two-thirds of cancer patients report moderate to severe pain during their illness, especially as cancer progresses or becomes unresponsive to therapy. So interconnected are pain and cancer in the minds of cancer patients that fear of pain and fear of addiction are almost as debilitating as fear of cancer and its consequences, in spite of evidence that fewer than 5% of cancer patients become addicted to aggressive and largely effective opioid therapy.

Table 11.1 Acute and Chronic Pain Characteristics

Acute Pain	Chronic Pain
Short duration—hours to weeks	Long duration—months to years
Sudden and fairly immediate onset—linked to tissue injury or damage	Sustained or spontaneously acute—cannot always be linked to identified tissue injury or damage
Alerts and prompts withdrawal, avoidance, and protective behavioral responses	Disrupts normal activities, limiting ability to work, sleep, eat, and socially interact
Predictable in course—intensity improves as tissue heals	Unpredictable in course—intensity waxes and wanes over time
Responsive to common pain management strategies	Inconsistently responsive to both common and adjuvant pain management strategies
Examples include traumatic pain, myalgia following exercise, and postoperative pain.	Examples include migraine headaches, low-back pain, peripheral neuropathy, arthritis, and fibromyalgia.

Cancer is not the only chronic illness in which pain is a regular and constant presence. Most patients with chronic illness report moderate to severe pain, including patients with arthritis, sickle cell anemia, irritable bowel syndrome, fibromyalgia, and lupus erythematosus. Some patients with chronic illness in fact report pain as their primary symptom, including patients with migraine or cluster headaches, chronic oral-facial pain, and postamputation pain. Referred to as *nonmalignant* or *noncancer chronic pain*, this type of pain inconsistently responds to common pain treatments, including anti-inflammatory medications and opioids, and is least likely to be adequately managed, according to patients and pain experts.

Connection Check 11.1

The nurse correlates which findings to the pathophysiology of chronic malignant pain?
A. Recent trauma
B. Rapidly dividing cells
C. Direct damage to nerve fibers
D. Persistent pain with no known etiology

Distinguishing Nociceptive and Neuropathic Pain

A second useful way to classify pain is by the point of origin. Pain originating in different tissues has unique biological features that shape both the presentation of pain and its responsiveness to therapy. **Nociceptive pain** results from stimulation of peripheral nerve fibers by noxious stimuli or conditions in superficial skin and tissues as well as bones, joints, and muscles or in organs. Specialized receptors on peripheral nerves sense and respond to noxious mechanical stimuli, including pressure and pinprick, as well as to a range of potentially tissue-injuring cold and hot temperatures. Other specialized peripheral neuron receptors sense and respond to noxious chemical stimuli, including acidic or basic substances, as well as many locally released chemicals, including enzymes and growth factors. Nociceptive pain, when originating in superficial tissues, is termed **cutaneous pain**. Pain originating deeper in the joints, bones, and muscles is called **somatic pain**, whereas pain that has its origins in the organs is termed **visceral pain** (Table 11.2). Cutaneous pain tends to be sharp, with intensity varying from mild to severe. It is easily located to a well-defined area. Examples of cutaneous pain include superficial cuts and minor burns and the pain that accompanies some procedures, such as phlebotomy. Somatic pain tends to be dull, achy, and difficult to localize, although the intensity can also vary from mild to severe. Examples of somatic pain include pain associated with inflammatory diseases of the joints such as arthritis, overuse injuries involving the muscle following exercise, trauma, and degenerative diseases of the bone. Visceral pain can be sharp or dull but is relatively difficult to localize. It can begin in any of the large organs in the thoracic or abdominal cavity, although the pain sensation is often present in a location some distance away from the source organ. This is known as **referred pain** and occurs when nerve fibers from normally high-sensory areas (superficial tissues) and input from normally low-sensory areas (visceral organs) all converge at a similar level of the spinal cord (Fig. 11.2). When visceral organs generate strong pain signals, the brain is not used to processing pain messages from these sites and interprets this input as coming from more superficial sites. Referred pain can be diagnostic for serious disorders and should be evaluated thoroughly.

The most challenging type of pain to assess and manage follows damage or injury to nervous system structures. This neuropathic pain presents with a mixture of both positive and negative symptoms. Patients report shooting, stinging, or "pins and needles" type of pain at the same time they describe areas where they lack feeling or sensation. *Peripherally generated neuropathic pain* presents in the peripheral tissues but may represent injury or dysfunction anywhere along the nerve pathway that supports that region of the body. Patients with phantom limb pain who, for example, have experienced a limb loss often continue to perceive pain, itching, and numbness in the absent limb. The loss of the limb involves a transection through the nerves supplying that limb. These damaged nerves continue to transmit nociceptive messages, often in hyperexcited bursts, that can permanently alter how the brain and spinal cord process incoming and descending pain messages. Even as the brain can visually recognize the loss of the limb, the perception of pain in the missing limb remains. Other examples of peripherally generated neuropathic pain syndromes include diabetic and alcohol-induced neuropathy, chemotherapy-induced neuropathy, and postherpetic neuralgia. *Centrally generated neuropathic pain* has its origins in injuries to the spinal cord and brain structures. Damage to the nerve roots that enter the spinal cord, the cord itself, or anywhere along ascending or descending central nociceptive pathways disrupts normal pain processing. Some parts of the pain-processing pathways can become hyperactive while others can lose function. New abnormal synaptic connections can form, contributing to sensations of pain that may be felt anywhere in the body. In some primary neurological conditions, such as stroke, Parkinson's disease, or multiple sclerosis, damage to neurons, their supporting myelin, or the nourishing glial cells that surround the brain and spinal tissue also disrupt pain processing. One condition that has features associated with both peripherally generated and centrally generated neuropathic pain is fibromyalgia. Patients complain of pain and stiffness in the muscle and joints that are often accompanied by cognitive dysfunction, fatigue, disturbed sleep, depression, and anxiety. Evidence suggests these symptoms are associated with abnormalities in the brain regions responsible for these body functions as well as altered neuroendocrine functioning and may follow either prolonged stress or emotional trauma.

Neuropathic pain can last for months to years. The vagueness of complaints, frequently in the absence of diagnosable injury, leads patients on an often-frustrating search for solutions, with many health providers wondering

Table 11.2 Cutaneous, Somatic, Visceral, and Neuropathic Pain Characteristics

Type of Pain	Origin	Patient Descriptors	Duration	Other Features	Patient Examples
Cutaneous	Superficial skin and tissues Easily localized	Tender, sharp, itchy	Short—hours to days	May be extra sensitive to touch in region around painful area; may have some numb areas next to very painful areas	Sunburn, minor cuts and scrapes, some types of procedural pain
Somatic	Deeper tissues, joints, and bones Can be more difficult to localize area of pain	Dull achy; can be described as cramping, crushing, stabbing, sore, spasm	Can be short to very long	Often presents with reflex muscle contractions and muscle tenderness	Arthritis fractures, exercise- or flu-induced myalgias, some types of procedural pain
Visceral	Mostly hollow organs in the abdominal or thoracic cavities, including heart, bladder, stomach, intestinal tract Difficult to localize area of pain; often referred to other body locations	Cramping, achy, dull, pressure, stabbing	Can be short or long; if long, can be intermittent or sustained	Often see autonomic nervous system effects, sweating, pallor, nausea, low heart rate and hypotension, syncope, restlessness	Myocardial pain, appendicitis, biliary and pancreatic obstructions, colitis
Neuropathic	Peripheral and central nervous system structures Difficult to localize; often represents area served by a nerve structure and not necessarily location of nerve injury or damage	Numbness, tingling, shooting, burning, pins and needles, electric shock, stabbing	Long—months to years	Pain often worse at night or at rest; can occur spontaneously without any overt stimuli	Postherpetic neuralgia, phantom limb pain, diabetic neuropathy, chemotherapy-induced neuropathy, carpal tunnel or spinal root compression

about the truthfulness of patient reports. Some patients with neuropathic pain feel dismissed by their healthcare providers as having mental health concerns and not actual pain. New insights into the biology of pain processing are leading to the broader understanding that neuropathic pain is pathological pain; whether arising out of injury to central or peripheral nervous structures, neuropathic pain represents true dysfunction and disorder in the nervous system.

PROCESSING PAIN MESSAGES

The Processing of Pain Messages in Acute Pain

The peripheral nerves that innervate peripheral tissues have several unique features that allow them to sense and transmit information rapidly across great distances on their way to the spinal cord and brain. Each nerve is composed of a bundle of single nerve fibers surrounded by connective tissue. Each nerve fiber is a long projecting axon for a single nerve cell or neuron leading to a cell body located near the entrance to the spinal cord. Some of these single projecting axons transmitting incoming sensory or afferent information, especially those innervating the distal extremities, can be several meters long. Along the dorsal side of the spinal cord, the cell bodies of these peripheral neurons are grouped in a nodular structure or ganglion called a *dorsal root* ganglion (DRG; Fig. 11.3A). Each DRG represents a large region of the body, and the chain of DRGs along the dorsal side of the spinal cord represents somatic regions, or dermatomes, on the body (Fig. 11.3B).

Dorsal root ganglion neurons are specialized at their terminal ends, all along their axons, and in their cell bodies to

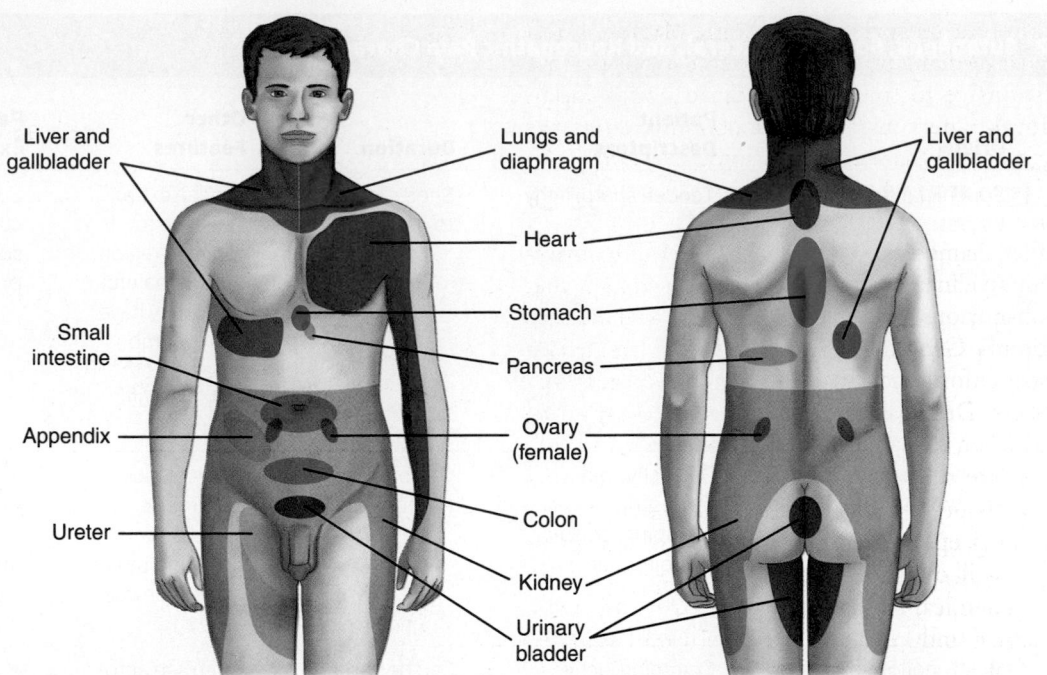

FIGURE 11.2 Common areas of referred pain. Referred pain occurs when nerve fibers from superficial tissues and visceral organs all converge to a similar level of the spinal cord. When visceral organs generate strong pain signals, the brain is not used to processing pain messages from these sites and interprets this input as coming from more superficial sites. Referred pain can be diagnostic for serious disorders and should be evaluated thoroughly.

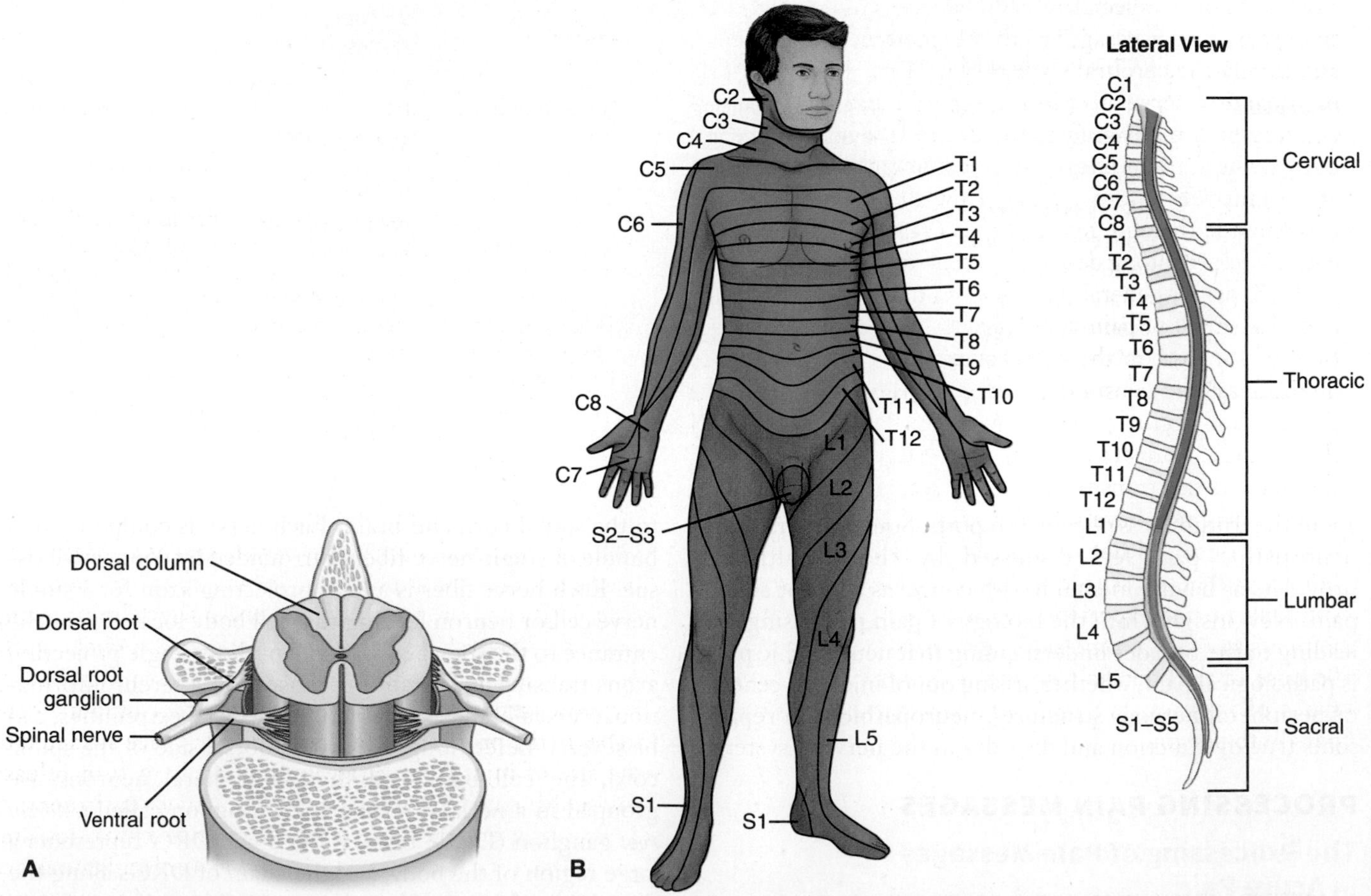

FIGURE 11.3 Dorsal root ganglion (DRG). *A,* Ganglion of nerve cell bodies entering the spinal cord. Cell bodies of peripheral neurons are grouped in a nodular structure or ganglion called a dorsal root ganglion. *B,* Dermatomes of the DRG ganglion chain along the body. Each DRG represents a large region of the body, and the chain of DRGs along the dorsal side of the spinal cord represents somatic regions, or dermatomes, on the body.

respond to different sensory stimuli. Some of these DRG neurons have large-diameter myelin-covered axons that are generally responsive to touch and proprioceptive input. Myelin is critical to nervous system functioning, serving as an insulating material that surrounds some nerve fibers to increase the speed at which electrical impulses move along the nerve fiber.

Some smaller-diameter DRG neurons have thinly myelinated axons, unmyelinated axons, or free nerve endings that respond to non-noxious temperatures as well as a wide range of noxious stimuli. Generally, nerve fibers with less myelin conduct sensory information more slowly than larger, fully myelinated fibers. Dorsal root ganglion neurons that selectively respond when stimuli become noxious or potentially injury inducing are called **nociceptors**. Some nociceptors are sensitive to tissue-injuring cold and hot temperatures, whereas other nociceptors are sensitive to mechanical pressure or pinprick. Still other nociceptors sense the presence of tissue-injuring chemical substances, including acids, bases, and specific injury-induced chemical substances released by the body.

Peripheral nociceptive neurons have the ability to convert a cellular response to noxious stimulation into an electrochemical message that is rapidly transmitted to the spinal cord along afferent (sensory) nerve pathways. Once in the spinal cord, peripheral sensory fibers make connections with other specialized pain-processing neurons that then relay pain messages to the brainstem, the forebrain, and finally the cerebral cortex (Fig. 11.4). This structural organization serves to filter, interpret, and influence ascending pain messaging to the brain. It is in the cerebral cortex where these electrochemical nociceptive messages are cognitively interpreted as pain. The pain response is coordinated through many of these same brain and spinal cord structures along descending pain-messaging pathways.

Acute pain is generally understood to be a product of this complex series of pain-processing steps. At every connection, or synapse, in the pain-processing system, there are important neurotransmitters that can either boost or inhibit the transmission of pain messages. In classic gate control theory, these neurotransmitters can either "open" or "close" the gate to the transmission of nociceptive information. Pain researchers have a better appreciation of how these neurochemicals either enhance or inhibit pain processing but are still at a loss to explain why patients experiencing similar injuries experience pain in very different ways. Patients may use a common language to describe their pain because of the specific pain pathways activated in specific types of injuries, but pain intensity varies widely from person to person.

Dysfunctional Pain Processing Is the Hallmark of Chronic Pain

Evidence suggests that what happens at the beginning of an injury may well shape the pain experience long term. In the earliest stages of an injury, damaged cells release a wide

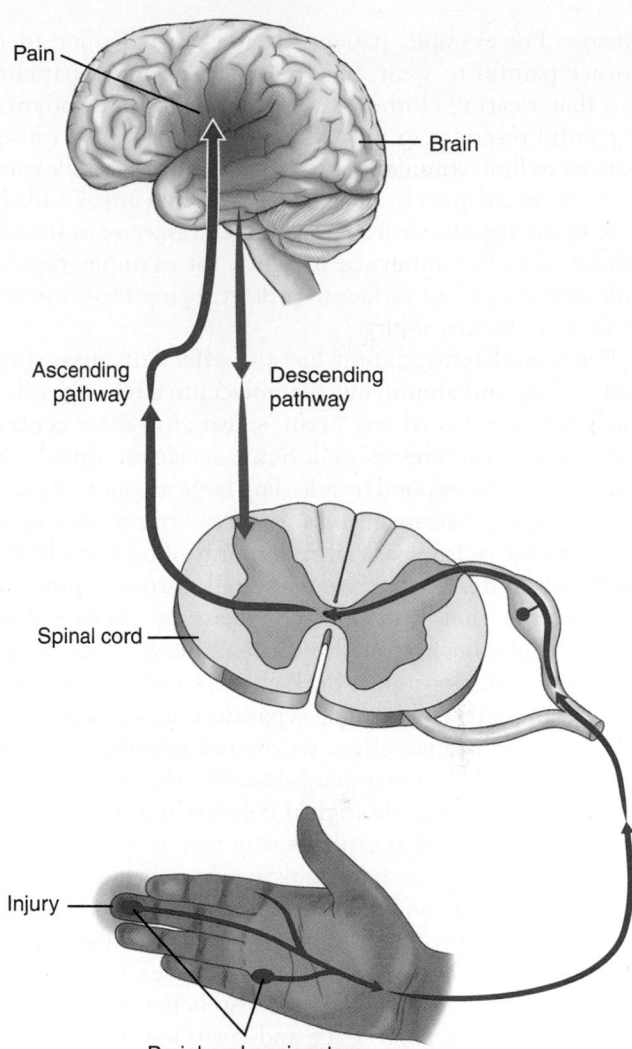

FIGURE 11.4 Peripheral sensory fibers make connections with other specialized pain-processing neurons. The noxious stimulation is converted into an electrochemical message that is rapidly transmitted to the spinal cord. Once in the spinal cord, peripheral sensory fibers make connections with other specialized pain-processing neurons that then relay pain messages to the brainstem, the forebrain, and the cerebral cortex, where the nociceptive messages are cognitively interpreted as pain. The pain response is coordinated through many of these same brain and spinal cord structures along descending pain-messaging pathways.

range of chemicals, including histamine, bradykinin, and prostaglandins. Some of these locally released chemicals specifically activate local nociceptors to begin transmitting pain messages to the brain and spinal cord. Other locally released chemicals serve to stimulate the inflammatory response, attracting macrophages and other immune cells to begin the process of local tissue repair. Once attracted to the site of injury, activated immune cells in turn release pain-enhancing chemicals into the local injury environment. These pain-enhancing chemicals include cytokines and growth factors. The net result of this local inflammatory response is to increase the sensitivity of injured tissue to any further stimuli. This sensitization of peripheral tissues serves a protective function to try to minimize further tissue damage. For example, patients do not normally find their clothes painful to wear, but following sunburn, patients find that wearing clothes is very painful. This **allodynia**, or painful response to normally innocuous stimuli, causes patients to limit stimulation to their injured tissue, allowing it to heal more quickly. These same patients are also likely to be **hyperalgesic**, with an exaggerated response to already painful stimuli. Sunburned patients, for example, rapidly withdraw from a hot surface to protect their already injured tissue from further injury.

Peripheral sensitization has the effect of increasing, prolonging, and amplifying the nociceptive messages that reach the spinal cord and brain, sensitizing these central nociceptive structures as well. Some sensitized spinal and brain nerve cells respond by releasing large amounts of pain-enhancing neurotransmitters, whereas other sensitized central nerve cells release large amounts of pain-inhibiting neurotransmitters. Sensitized nerve cells further respond to this increased neurotransmitter release by altering their synaptic relationships with adjacent nerve cells. Some synaptic connections quiet or die back, some new synapses appear, and some abnormal synaptic connections form, changing the balance of excitation and inhibition in pain processing. Some researchers describe the formation of these abnormal or pathological connections as a form of "cellular memory" that explains why pain may linger after all objective measures indicate tissues have healed.

This structural and functional reorganization of synapses is what allows nervous systems to respond to new experiences, including injury and disease; however, this synaptic flexibility feature, or **plasticity**, is also believed to be what contributes to the persistence and treatment resistance of many chronic pain conditions. There is still a great deal that is not known about how this synaptic reorganization occurs. Why, for example, do two people with similar injuries have different long-term pain experiences? One patient may have persistent pain that gradually resolves as the injury heals, whereas another patient goes on to develop debilitating chronic pain. Many chronic pain conditions have no clear-cut injury as a precipitating event, so it is not clear how or why chronic pain develops in such patients.

FACTORS SHAPING THE PAIN EXPERIENCE

Some people seem to have a lower threshold for pain, whereas others appear to tolerate a great deal of pain in spite of common anatomy and physiology. Evidence suggests many factors shape the pain experience, including prior experience with pain, expectations of pain, and anxiety, as well as attention to and the situational meaning of that pain for that particular patient. A woman in labor, for example, may be able to endure quite a bit of pain knowing that at the end of this painful experience will be a new life. This same woman in labor, however, may find labor more painful in a subsequent delivery if she had a difficult delivery with a previous birth. The expectation of pain

during phlebotomy is often enough to make this procedure quite painful for one person but not painful to another who is distracted and does not expect the procedure. Patients are naturally apprehensive before surgery, but evidence suggests that patients with higher anxiety use more pain medications in the postoperative period. Patients who receive preoperative education about what to expect and reassurances about postoperative pain medication report less preoperative anxiety and use less postoperative pain medications. Patients who normally describe themselves as having a high **tolerance** for pain find their tolerance influenced by fatigue, nausea, and their ability to cope in the moment. Environmental factors, such as ambient temperature, humidity, light, and noise, and the presence of other people shape the pain experience.

Sociocultural Determinants of Pain

One of the most powerful influences on the pain experience is the patient's cultural experience. Social mores and customs shape families, the communities of residence, and the larger culture, just as the larger culture, communities, and families shape biology and behavior. People learn how to respond to pain in subtle and obvious ways. In some families, stoicism is valued, whereas in other families, it is acceptable to more demonstrably display pain. Depending on how health and illness are defined within a community, pain may mean different things. A patient's cultural experience may lead to increased faith in Western medicine to diagnose and treat pain, whereas another patient's experiences may reinforce non-Western approaches to managing pain. Limited access to healthcare resources may inspire creative and folk solutions to pain that continue even when access to healthcare is ensured.

Evidence suggests that pain assessment and pain management are likely to qualitatively improve pain diagnosis and pain relief when patients and caregivers share a common ethnicity or cultural perspectives. When the cultural background of the caregiver differs from that of the patient, caregivers are more likely to misread or misjudge the intensity and severity of pain. Language barriers between patient and healthcare providers serve to exacerbate cultural differences. Although educational programs for health professionals attempt to infuse cultural sensitivity into standards and practice, most cultural effectiveness is often and inconsistently gained through trial-and-error learning in actual practice. Nurses need to be aware that language and culture shape the pain experience and should incorporate culturally specific and validated assessment tools and population- or pain-specific dosing guidelines into the standards of care.

The Influence of Gender and Genetics

Differences in pain sensitivities and the pain experience are both clinically and experimentally observed in humans. Inflammatory arthritis, irritable bowel syndrome, and neuropathic pain, for example, are among many pain conditions more prevalent among women. Cluster headaches, as well as some muscle and visceral pain syndromes, are more prevalent among men (Table 11.3). Prominent meta-analyses of human pain studies found gender differences in the majority of selected studies, with evidence suggesting women have lower thresholds for pain, rate noxious stimuli as more painful, and have a lower tolerance for intense pain than do men. Gender differences in both clinical and experimental pain generally do not present until after the age of puberty, suggesting a prominent role for sex-linked hormones. Women generally report more pain sensitivity to acute pain during all phases of their menstruating adult lives than do postpubescent men, although these gender differences in pain sensitivity seem to lessen after female menopause. Differences between men and women may represent clearly distinct molecular and neurohormonal pain mechanisms. Gender differences, however, may also reflect the influence of a wide range of cognitive, affective, and sociocultural factors. Many pain researchers use the terms *sex* and *gender* interchangeably, whereas others make critical distinctions between the two terms. When distinctions are made, the term *sex* refers to purely biological differences, whereas the term *gender* encompasses the larger psycho-social-cultural context associated with being masculine or feminine. Modeled and learned behaviors, life history, and factors other than biological differences may influence both pain processing and the pain experience. Gender-role expectations, for example, may discourage men from reporting pain or even seeking regular medical care. On the other hand, women are more likely to have an ongoing relationship with a healthcare professional and may feel freer to report painful symptoms, even as evidence suggests that healthcare professionals may not recognize gender differences in pain presentation or may not take female pain complaints as seriously as complaints presented by males. In children as young as 5 or 6, masculine and feminine stereotypes appear to manifest, with boys more likely

to say they do not pay attention to pain, whereas girls are more comfortable discussing their pain. The incidence of reported pain is higher in people, regardless of gender, when a history of physical or sexual abuse is present. There is also evidence to suggest that women in pain utilize a broader range of coping skills than do men, including how they self-medicate, employ palliative behaviors, and use social supports.

In addition to reported gender differences in pain sensitivities, men and women are noted to respond differently to analgesics. Several studies of hospitalized postoperative patients using **patient-controlled analgesia** (PCA) found that men required more opioid dosing to achieve pain relief than did females. PCA technology delivers a constant low level of background opioid dose that is supplemented by patients choosing to bolus deliver additional opioids, within preset dosing programming. It is not clear whether this difference in therapeutic response represents only sex-influenced differences in opioid metabolism or is a manifestation of a larger gender influence on threshold and self-management strategies. Nonopioid analgesia use differs between genders as well, with men reporting more analgesic relief with ibuprofen (Motrin), one of many NSAID compounds. That women can be simultaneously more sensitive to pain and more responsive to most analgesics suggests a number of mechanistic questions about pain that remain underexplored.

Few pain disorders feature true inherited dominant or recessive genes, although there are rare sensory and autonomic neuropathies that pass generation to generation as well as some familial migraine disorders. Case-controlled association studies of unrelated individuals, however, identify thousands of possible genetic variations between individuals that can influence pain thresholds, tolerance, and response to analgesics. Some of these genetic variants might cause a protein to be malformed or to be produced in excess quantities or even result in a critical protein not being produced at all. For example, genes that regulate the production of several inflammatory cytokines, including interleukin-6, interleukin-1, and interleukin-10, vary extensively between people, suggesting differences in how an inflammatory response can shape the pain experience. Genes that play a role in how nerve cells form connections or synapses with adjacent nerve cells also vary widely between people, suggesting that how a nervous system sensitized by injury structurally and functionally restructures synapses may influence who may develop chronic pain. Genes also shape the pharmacodynamics and pharmacokinetics of medication, increasing the likelihood of toxic effects or altering the body's ability to resolve pain. Gene differences in medication metabolism, for example, can vary across genders, across ethnic groups, and within ethnic groups depending on geography. Genes responsible for some enzymes in medication metabolism pathways, for example, appear in less than 5% of Caucasians of Northern European descent and in less than 1% of people from southern Asia but in more than 25% of people of African descent. Understanding

Table 11.3 Gender Differences in Prevalence of Human Pain Syndromes

Pain Syndromes More Prevalent in Females	Pain Syndromes More Prevalent in Males
• Inflammatory arthritis	• Cluster headaches
• Migraine headaches	• Back pain (slightly more prevalent)
• Irritable bowel syndrome	• Visceral pain from nonreproductive organs including the heart and pancreas
• Chronic orofacial pain	
• Temporomandibular pain	
• Neuropathic pain	
• Interstitial cystitis	

how individual genetic differences contribute to pain processing, pain perception, and pain relief is a major research goal, with the promise of targeted or individually designed pain treatments.

Epigenetics and Pain

Cells, particularly neurons, have evolved considerable ability to respond to both external and internal stressors. One critical evolutionary process involves how cells control access to DNA to shape a cellular response that is moment to moment and not dependent on any change in the basic nucleotide sequence of inherited DNA. **Epigenetics** refers to the cellular processes that allow access to the cell's DNA for transcription, regulation, and production of proteins critical to cell function. Compacting the nearly 2 meters of chromosomal DNA into the relatively small cell nucleus while allowing access for transcription and gene expression requires highly coordinated packaging processes that serve to temporally and functionally control access to DNA throughout the cell cycle. Histones are the chief compacting proteins within the nucleus, forming tight covalent bonds along the DNA backbone that essentially spool the DNA around the histone. The new histone–DNA spool, now called chromatin, organizes as repeating functional groupings of spooled DNA in a "bead on a string" formation, which can either open or restrict transcriptional access to the DNA as needed to shape a cell's response. It is this functionally relevant regulation of gene expression through dynamic remodeling and modification to chromatin that defines epigenetics. For example, the local changes around a cell that result from tissue injury release cellular contents such as histamine into the local tissue environment. This external stress to the cell alters signaling between and within cells that prompts chromatin to unspool a region of DNA, allowing transcription, replication, and the production of anti-inflammatory cytokines and glucocorticoids to respond to the local injury. This access to the DNA, however, is transient and often short-lived, with re-spooling of the DNA and tightening up of the chromatin access to DNA when no longer needed.

Chromatin remodeling processes result from the addition or removal of chemical groups, either to the histone molecule or the DNA molecule, within the chromatin complex. The addition of a methyl group, for example, is called methylation, and the addition of an acetyl group or phosphate group is called acetylation and phosphorylation, respectively. The orchestrated formation and disruption of chromatin that controls transcription also include ways to rapidly and dynamically demethylate and deacetylate protein structures, or remove phosphate groups, as well as recruit a wide range of other modifier proteins in the cell to shape a cellular response. These epigenetic processes have become increasingly important to the evolving science of pain management, representing new targets for pain medications and altering the way injury is managed from moment to moment.

Two of the most therapeutically intriguing insights arising from epigenetics research are suggestions that epigenetic mechanisms play a critical role in the transition from acute to chronic pain and that a wide range of environmental factors across the life span serve as epigenetic primers for individual pain and analgesic response. Evidence suggests that more than 1,000 genes in spinal cord neurons are epigenetically regulated within the first minutes to hours following a peripheral nerve injury. Often, these early modifications are followed by more sustained epigenetic processes shaping synaptic connectivity and are implicated in the formation of long-term pathological pain. Sustained DNA methylation, for example, has been linked to accelerated degeneration of vertebral disks in low-back pain in both animal models and human subjects. Sustained histone deacetylation has been identified as a factor driving long-lived neuropathic pain and decreased responsiveness to morphine analgesia. There is also compelling evidence that pain in the neonate, like that experienced by babies in the neonatal intensive care unit (NICU), epigenetically primes the nervous system, creating conditions that support the development of chronic pain later in life. New medications in development that target epigenetic processes include histone deacetylation inhibitors (HDAC inhibitors) that inhibit the removal of acetyl groups to stabilize DNA access and improve anti-inflammatory responses. Surgeons and anesthesiologists now recognize the pre-, intra-, and postoperative period as a very active period of epigenetic activity with the potential for shaping surgical outcomes. The promise in epigenetics lies in identifying the temporal ordering of chromatin remodeling changes linked to pathology, then therapeutically leveraging the transient and often reversible nature of epigenetic processes to interrupt or otherwise influence a health outcome.

Pain and Older Adults

As the proportion of the population over 65 years of age grows, healthcare providers are challenged to assess and manage pain in an increasingly older population of patients. The pain assessment tools used in most healthcare settings were developed and tested with younger adults and may lack reliability and validity as pain measures in older adults. For example, evidence suggests that verbal descriptor scales and numerical rating scales become more difficult to use as patients age, with a higher frequency of incomplete or unscored responses. The evidence further suggests that older patients who are not acculturated to visual analog scales or numerical rating scales in their formal education or who may have mild to moderate cognitive problems demonstrate problems reporting their pain using tools that require a level of abstract reasoning. Some older patients with pain reluctantly report pain, feeling as if pain is to be expected and normal or out of fear that pain signals pathology, leading to a diagnostic process that itself may be painful.

The evidence is mixed on the prevalence of pain and pain patterns in older patients. Some studies report that migraine headaches and low-back pain peak in middle age and decrease as patients age. Other studies report an increased incidence in all types of persistent pain, generalized musculoskeletal pain, and fibromyalgia in older patients. More than half of older patients report mild to moderate intermittent pain as they age, with the incidence of all types of pain more common in institutionalized elderly. Many of these studies date from the late 1980s and early 1990s, and relevant new research is needed to quantify pain experiences as patients age. There is no reason to expect that all types of pain will vary the same way as a function of age given that different pain mechanisms are responsible for different types of pain.

One type of pain in which differences between older and younger adults is most apparent is acute pain, especially acute pain associated with specific injuries or infections. Conditions that are painful in younger adults, such as urinary tract infections or duodenal ulcers, are likely to manifest as subtle behavioral changes in an older adult, including confusion, aggression, restlessness, or a loss of appetite.

The pathophysiological reason for this more subtle clinical presentation is not clear. It is theorized that age-related changes in these target organs or in pain-processing structures in the spinal cord and brain lead to an altered neurochemical response from sensitized nerve cells, changing the way nerve cells form synaptic connections. Instead of pain messages moving along established pain pathways, new synaptic connections are made that divert pain messages to other brain regions. Other types of visceral pain have an atypical presentation in older adults as well, with as many as 30% of adults reporting either no pain with myocardial infarction or referral patterns different from those of younger patients with myocardial pain. Similar atypical presentations are reported for older patients with pancreatitis and appendicitis. Older postoperative patients do, however, report more unrelieved pain, use analgesic agents longer than younger adults, and are more likely to have pain slow their surgical recovery. Inadequate pain control in older adults is associated with greater levels of postoperative confusion, depression of immune and respiratory systems, and increased mortality. Although evidence suggests that common pain treatments, including NSAIDs and opioids, are effective in managing pain in older adults, doses often need to be modified because of age-related changes in medication metabolism. Standard dosing may lead to more toxic side effects, whereas reduced dosages provide effective analgesia.

Connection Check 11.2

The nurse recognizes that the incidence of pain is greatest in which patient population?

A. Active teenagers
B. Unemployed adults regardless of age
C. Employed middle-aged and older adults
D. Older patients who are institutionalized

COMPREHENSIVE ASSESSMENT STRATEGIES FOR ACUTE AND CHRONIC PAIN

In early 1999, the Veterans Health Administration (VHA) began a system-wide initiative to improve pain management for the nearly 3.5 million veterans cared for nationwide. This VHA program, called "Pain as the 5th Vital Sign," requires measurement and documentation of patients' self-report of pain using a numeric rating scale for all clinical encounters. The American Pain Society soon championed this relatively straightforward way to improve pain management, believing the inclusion of pain assessment when assessing blood pressure, pulse, and respirations would give pain assessment clinical priority. This now familiar and widely accepted approach in most clinical settings asks patients to self-report their pain on a standardized 10-integer verbal or visual analog scale, with 0 representing no pain and 10 representing the worst possible pain. Visual scales are available for patients to use to assist in the communication of their pain score. Pain scores of 4 or higher require a clinician response, including a more comprehensive pain assessment and timely intervention. In the years since this initiative was launched, evidence suggests that the widespread use of numerical rating scales has improved awareness of the importance of pain assessment but has not always translated to improved pain management outcomes for patients. One of the big challenges in using a numeric rating scale is that this asks patients to measure their pain only on the single dimension of intensity and does not allow for a more nuanced self-report. A second challenge to using single-dimension tools such as numeric rating scales is that such tools are not designed to measure the mixed pain that most patients actually experience.

As this new decade in pain science is entered, there is a realization that this single-dimension pain scale has likely contributed to patients and caregivers believing the best pain score to have is 0. Pain specialists implicate the 0-to-10 pain-rating system as contributing to both the overprescribing of opioids and the larger opioid misuse epidemic. A new consensus is developing that measuring intensity is only one way to assess pain and analgesia response and that the most effective pain assessment approach is to assess across multiple dimensions of the pain experience.

Measuring Pain Intensity

The most commonly used pain assessment tools provide valuable and useful information to clinicians about pain intensity. When serially administered over the course of hours to days, these tools reliably measure pain levels in a single patient, allowing staff to implement pain management strategies and measure treatment response. Examples of unidimensional assessment tools include numeric rating scales, verbal rating scales, and visual analog scales. Verbal rating scales ask patients to rate their pain by looking at a list of descriptive words ordered from least to most intense (no pain, mild, moderate, and severe). Patients then select the one word that best describes their pain, with the evaluator assigning a point value that corresponds to the descriptor (no pain = 0, severe = 3). Visual analog scales are structured with a 10-cm horizontal or vertical line with labeled endpoints. One end of the scale is marked "no pain," and the other end is marked "worst pain ever" or uses a similar phrase to indicate intense pain. Patients place a mark on the line to indicate their level of current pain or indicate their pain by moving a sliding indicator, with the evaluator measuring the distance in centimeters from the low end of the scale as a numerical index of pain intensity. Often the patient is asked to evaluate the pain on not just one visual analog scale but several similarly constructed scales to assess different dimensions of pain besides intensity. Some of these other dimensions of pain include how disturbing or unpleasant the pain is, how close to the surface or how deep the pain is, and how disruptive the pain is to activities of daily living. These tools are reliable for measuring many types of acute pain, with evidence suggesting verbal rating scales are more effective with older people than the more common numeric rating scales (Fig. 11.5).

All of these unidimensional measures of pain are sensitive to measuring treatment response to both pharmacological and nonpharmacological interventions for many forms of acute pain, including burns, postoperative pain, and chronic noncancer pain. Although evidence suggests unidimensional scales may be less effective as measures of chronic pain or mixed acute and chronic pain, there is a clinical preference for numeric rating scales. Most clinicians find them easy to explain and relatively quick to administer; patients also find they are minimally intrusive and conceptually simple to understand. Visual analog scales can be more difficult to administer in many clinical settings, requiring preprinted forms and writing implements as well as

a patient whose vision and hearing are largely intact so that instructions are understood and followed. Patients with motor or physical impairments also have difficulty using visual analog scales. Some of these barriers to using visual analog scales were addressed with the introduction of the visual analog thermometer (Fig. 11.6).

Another useful approach to visual analog measures is to use cartoon faces expressing degrees of discomfort, unhappiness, and pain. Explanations are provided that direct the patient to choose the facial image that best describes how he or she is feeling, with each face associated with a specific score for quantification. Examples include the Wong-Baker FACES tool geared mostly to preverbal populations, such as children, and the FACES pain scale used with older adults with expressive aphasia. Such tools have not been found to be an effective assessment tool for patients with cognitive impairments or to bridge language and cultural differences. Patients from different ethnic backgrounds or who speak languages other than English may not understand or may not view the facial imagery in a qualitatively useful way for assessment.

Barriers to effective use of numerical rating scales, verbal rating scales, and visual analog scales include clinicians who doubt the accuracy of self-report. Some clinicians believe that including a subjective numerical assessment of pain at the same time objective data such as blood pressure and heart rate are collected overstates the qualitative usefulness of pain assessment information, especially because this measures only a single dimension of pain. Often these doubts about the accuracy of self-reports arise from the failure of unidimensional measures to support assessment and effective pain management in complex pain situations, such as in patients with chronic pain or addictions or at the end of life. Although pain intensity is an important aspect of the pain experience, it is not the only dimension of pain important to patients and therefore should not be the only dimension of pain important to clinicians.

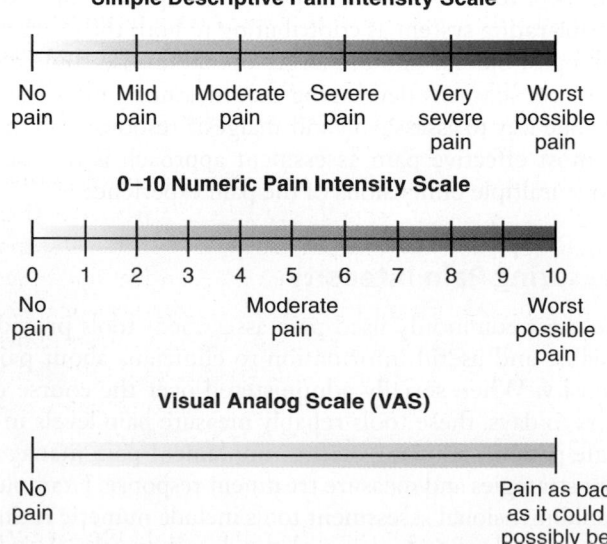

FIGURE 11.5 Pain scales. Pain scales allow patients to rate their pain, as well as responses to pain management modalities.

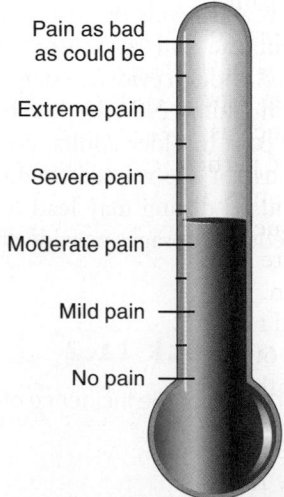

FIGURE 11.6 Pain thermometer. The visual analog thermometer is used with patients with motor or physical impairments who may have difficulty using visual analog scales.

The Focused Pain Assessment

OPQRST-AAA

One critical aspect of pain assessment that is underemphasized in most healthcare settings relying on unidimensional measures of pain is the follow-up required to make effective use of this screening measure. Although these tools often advise intervention at pain levels 4 and above, these tools are not designed to recommend specific pain measures. Clinicians have a range of therapeutic options available to them and require more information to appropriately evaluate clinical manifestations and choose an intervention. OPQRST-AAA is a useful mnemonic to use to evaluate pain symptoms, with each letter representing an important area of assessment.

- O: Onset of pain
  When the pain first begins is critical to understanding whether the pain is more acute or chronic in nature. Ask patients to describe what they were doing when the pain first started and whether the pain onset was sudden, gradual, or ongoing. Follow-up questions include "What do you believe is causing this pain?"
- P: Provocation
  External factors such as movement and clinician examination can elicit a pain response. Ask the patient whether any specific factor, such as turning in bed, sitting, or walking, makes the pain worse.
- Q: Quality of pain
  Descriptive words or phrases, such as *sharp, dull, stabbing, burning*, or *crushing*, can give clinicians insight into the pain experience for patients. Open-ended questions such as "Can you describe your pain to me?" can be particularly effective at drawing out pain descriptors. In an urgent situation, leading questions such as "Is your pain sharp or stabbing?" can generate specific and immediate assessment information.
- R: Region and radiation
  The location of the pain and whether it radiates or moves to other body areas can be diagnostically significant, especially for deep somatic and visceral pain. Ask patients to point to areas on their body where they feel the pain. Sometimes it can be helpful to ask patients if they can trace the borders of their pain to help localize the extent of the pain.

- S: Severity of pain
  The terms *severity* and *intensity* are often used interchangeably and generally mean the degree of discomfort associated with pain. Numerical rating scales are often used to gauge patient perception of pain intensity. Frequently, patients use this opportunity to compare this pain to a pain they experienced previously, as in "This is much worse than when I broke my arm" or "This is worse than childbirth." Patients also describe their pain in terms of how it limits their activities, such as "I cannot sleep" or "I cannot sit for long periods." These are important subjective comments that are worth noting in an assessment summary.
- T: Time and duration
  As with onset of pain, the length of time a patient reports pain is diagnostically significant. Ask patients how long the pain condition they are experiencing has been going on and whether it has happened before. Follow-up questions include whether the pain condition has changed for the better or worse since they first had the pain.
- AAA: Aggravating/Alleviating factors and Associated clinical manifestations
  Ask patients if there is anything they do that makes the pain better or worse. Sometimes focused questions will help them reflect, for example, "If you change your position, does this make the pain better?" or "Does sitting up help you feel better?" Follow-up questions include "Have you taken any medications that help you feel better?" or "Did you use a heating pad or put an ice pack on the area, and did it make it feel better or worse?" and "Do you have any other symptoms such as nausea, sweating, or odd sensations you can describe?"

A brief interview using the OPQRST-AAA mnemonic can be conducted in less than 5 minutes and can occur simultaneously with other assessment activities. The information gained through this structured questioning approach clarifies the nature of the pain experienced by the patient and informs the clinician's review and selection of effective therapeutic interventions.

Other approaches to more comprehensive pain assessment include using assessment tools that ask the patient to evaluate pain on several dimensions, including the functional impact of pain. Examples of this more comprehensive tool include the McGill Pain Inventory and the Multidimensional Pain Inventory. The use of such structured tools to assess dimensions of pain beyond intensity with structured OPQRST-AAA interviewing techniques yields more complete pain assessments to guide diagnoses and treatment decisions.

Physical Examination

There are many situations when a screening tool or serial measure, such as a numerical rating scale or the OPQRST-AAA mnemonic, yields insufficient information to support the diagnosis and management of pain. For example, some patients may not be verbal enough to describe or measure their pain. Other patients present with complex pain conditions that are not easily measured using unidimensional scales or qualified solely through subjective answers to structured interview questions. Selected physical assessment techniques tailored to the pain complaint can support bedside diagnosis to help clinicians choose appropriate therapeutic interventions. The most useful of these techniques for bedside clinicians may be palpation and assessment of range of motion (ROM). Muscle groups in the area of the pain should be palpated, and both verbal and nonverbal response to this palpation should be recorded. Clinicians should also record responses to any assessments of joint flexion, extension, side bending, and extremity lifting to determine whether pain is experienced with movement or whether there are any functional limitations. Consultation with members of the health team may lead to more extensive bedside testing, including a tailored neurological examination consisting of cranial nerve assessments and sensory testing of sensitivity to light touch, pressure, and pinprick, as well as reflexes. A more extensive assessment of motor function may include tests for motor weakness, coordination, balance, and loss of endurance. Many acute care settings provide comprehensive pain teams composed of physicians, nurse specialists, physical therapists, pharmacists, and social workers. These comprehensive pain teams should be consulted early in the presence of complex pain for the best clinical outcomes.

Connection Check 11.4

In assessing a patient's pain, the nurse asks the patient, "What makes the pain worse?" Which aspect of pain is the nurse determining?
A. Onset and duration
B. Intensity
C. Quality
D. Aggravating factors

NURSING MANAGEMENT OF PAIN

Patient and Nurse: The Therapeutic Partnership

Pain is so common to the patient experience that intervening to improve comfort and reduce suffering is central to the practice of nursing. When patients present with pain, it is frequently a nurse who first assesses the clinical presentation. It is also nurses who are often first to propose a remedy and to encourage self-management strategies. However, it is the critical role nurses play in understanding the larger context and impact of clinical manifestations, such as pain, that is at the core of what nurses are and what

nurses do. Although nurses, physicians, and other health team members work collaboratively to diagnose and treat health problems, it is nurses who are charged with recognizing the physiological and psychosocial responses to health problems that symptoms represent. Nurses are also charged with developing and implementing a comprehensive plan to address symptoms and the impact of those symptoms.

Effective interventions begin with comprehensive assessments of clinical manifestations of pain as well as functional health patterns. Specific tools or inventory forms are regularly used to collect initial or baseline data that establish physiological stability, the risk for physiological instability, and patient habits and routines. This data-collection step is critical to beginning to narrow down the range of risk for nursing diagnoses, identifying actual nursing diagnoses, and determining collaborative care problems with other disciplines. Although relatively few questions on most baseline assessment forms directly ask patients about their pain, in fact, most questions on comprehensive assessments are gathering pain-related information useful to planning effective interventions. Questions that ask patients how they perceive their health and well-being or that assess their knowledge of health practices add context to questions and answers about self-management of pain and adherence to prescribed treatment. Questions that determine usual patterns of food and fluid intake, as well as appetite and food preferences, add perspective to objective data gathered about weight lost or gained. In similar ways, questions that determine activity and exercise patterns, sleep–rest patterns, role and relationship patterns, and coping and stress tolerance patterns help nurses understand the larger impact of symptoms such as pain. This subjective portrait of a patient's health status is combined with physical assessment findings and other objective data to drive the identification of priority nursing diagnoses and a comprehensive plan of care.

The Care-Planning Process for Managing Acute and Chronic Pain

The reasoning process that guides the nurse from data collection to nursing diagnoses begins with listing individual signs, symptoms, and health needs. Next, the nurse evaluates the significance of individual pieces of data, sorting them into significance clusters or diagnostic cues. These diagnostic cues help nurses formulate diagnostic hypotheses. Diagnostic hypotheses represent inferences or tentative explanations for specific pieces or clusters of data cues that require further investigation. To confirm a diagnostic hypothesis, nurses may need to validate the accuracy and reliability of key pieces of data, distinguish normal from abnormal findings, and recognize inconsistencies and possible information gaps. Nurses, for example, may need to recheck a blood pressure or follow up a patient interview with a corroborative family interview.

CASE STUDY: EPISODE 2

On the third postoperative day after Mrs. Jessup's coronary bypass surgery, at change of shift, the night nurse reports that Mrs. Jessup is sleeping poorly at intervals. She was medicated for surgical-site pain twice with oral opioids and once with ketorolac (Toradol) IV. She got up twice with the assistance of two caregivers to use the bathroom but otherwise indicated she "was not up to walking in the hall." She remains on oxygen at 3 L via nasal cannula, with oxygen saturations in the low to mid-90s. She has a poor cough effort, and she is able to achieve only 450 mL with her incentive spirometer. She continues to report lower back spasms and shooting, burning pain down her right leg that is not relieved with pain medications.

The nurse quickly reviews the admission database to determine her functional health patterns at baseline, identifying long-standing sleep complaints and diminished activity patterns at home. The nurse completes the morning assessment: Mrs. Jessup's blood pressure is elevated at 165/84, her pulse rate is 104 bpm, and her respiratory rate is 22 and shallow. Diminished breath sounds at the bases are noted on auscultation. Mrs. Jessup reports pain that is 4/10 in the area of her incision, along with back and leg pain that "comes and goes" between 2/10 and 9/10. She is lying in bed, grimacing, and rarely opens her eyes. Her answers to questions are terse, short responses…

Nursing Diagnoses for Patients in Pain

The thinking language nurses use to organize and focus nursing care is the nursing process, organized around prioritized nursing diagnoses. A well-developed and well-constructed nursing diagnosis defines and shapes problem solving. When nurses identify a problem such as anxiety, insomnia, or delayed surgical recovery, they are choosing a diagnostic label that represents their reasoned conclusions arising out of data collection and data validation. This same process of reasoned evaluation of assessment data leads to the identification of related factors that have either caused or contributed to the identified health problem.

The value of diagnostic labels and the identification of related factors are often underappreciated. Not only do diagnostic labels focus nursing attention on prioritized care problems and define patient goals in the care-planning process, but the identification of related factors also guides critical interventions. It may seem self-evident that the grimacing postoperative patient reporting a variable 2/10 to 9/10 level in his or her pain should be diagnosed as being in acute pain, with the care goal being improved patient comfort. However, if this same patient is also breathing shallowly, guarding with incisional pain, and presenting with a decreased oxygen saturation level even on supplemental oxygen, the diagnostic label of ineffective respiratory function represents a more completely reasoned evaluation of a comprehensive assessment. Rather than being the primary problem, in this circumstance the acute pain the patient is experiencing is part of the related factors that are shaping the larger diagnosis of ineffective respiratory function. The nursing plan of care would include management of pain in either diagnosis. However, the nursing goal for this patient is not necessarily to improve comfort; rather, it is to improve respiratory functioning and gas exchange. Nurses who too narrowly diagnose either acute or chronic pain for their patients in pain run the risk of missing priority care problems by failing to acknowledge the significant life and health impacts of pain, as well as the risk of not choosing an intervention appropriate to meeting the larger care priority. A re-focus on understanding how to optimize and improve system functioning also has the benefit of increasing reliance on a broader range of pain management options, lessening overuse of pharmacological remedies, and reframing patient expectancy on improving comfort and not total pain relief.

For patients in pain, the impact is far ranging. The activation of pain-processing networks in the brain and spinal cord engages hormonal responses and stimulates sympathetic and parasympathetic nervous system responses. It is not uncommon to see elevations of heart rate and blood pressure as a result of pain, which can exacerbate preexisting health conditions such as heart failure or kidney impairment. Pain may limit the ability of someone to work or engage in previously enjoyable social situations. Pain may limit partner intimacy and alter interpersonal relationships. Pain may cause patients to question their beliefs, their values, and their self-worth. Pain may disrupt sleep or affect a patient's appetite. Pain medications may alter elimination patterns or compromise the physiological integrity of vital organs such as the liver or kidney. In order to develop a comprehensive plan of care for the patient in pain, it is critical to once again review how clinical manifestations impact functional health patterns. Many site-based comprehensive assessment forms use some organizing framework to understand the impact that the clinical presentation has on the well-being of the patient and the patient's family unit. This wide-ranging impact is reflected in the diversity of diagnostic labels that can focus nursing diagnoses for patients who are in pain (Box 11.1).

Identifying which diagnostic label best defines the patient's priority nursing problems rests with the reasoned interpretation of data cues, including the patient's subjective report of problem urgency as well as clinician interpretation of physiological stability. So not only must the diagnostic label be appropriately identified for each patient, but a focused nursing diagnosis must also identify the correct etiology (or "related to factors" that are part of the diagnostic statement), or nurses run the risk of not

Box 11.1 Nursing Diagnoses Relevant for Acute and Chronic Pain

- Acute pain; chronic pain
- Ineffective respiratory function
- Risk for aspiration
- Risk for injury: falls
- Ineffective management of therapeutic regimen
- Ineffective health maintenance
- Imbalanced nutrition greater or lesser than body requirements; deficit or excess fluid volume
- Constipation; risk for constipation
- Risk for impaired renal function
- Activity intolerance
- Impaired physical mobility
- Fatigue
- Insomnia; sleep deprivation; disturbed sleep pattern
- Anxiety; fear
- Acute confusion
- Disturbed body image
- Interrupted and dysfunctional family processes
- Impaired social interactions; social isolation
- Risk for loneliness
- Ineffective role performance
- Ineffective sexual patterns
- Compromised family coping; disabled family coping

intervening appropriately or wasting both nursing time and resources on ineffective interventions.

Measuring the Effectiveness of Care

Although data gathered through physical assessment, review of critical laboratory values, and structured questioning provide the evidence necessary to support the diagnostic labels that focus problem solving, this same evidence is used to measure both the success of nursing interventions and, ultimately, problem resolution. The nurse must provide both targeted pain medications and non–medication-based therapies designed to address the pain, such as thoughtful positioning and appropriately resourced assisted ambulation that promotes effective pulmonary hygiene. Organizing physical activity in the daytime combined with clustered nursing activities at night is an intervention designed to promote sleep and rest. When these care organizing strategies are combined with thoughtful use of massage and relaxation techniques, as well as pharmacologically appropriate medications to promote pain and sleep, nurses increase the likelihood that patients sleep more regularly and restfully. The success of nursing interventions and focused problem solving can be measured both by observational reports from night staff about the length of sleep periods overnight and by subjective reports from the patient about the quality of that sleep.

PAIN MANAGEMENT OPTIONS

Therapeutic Interventions to Promote Pain Relief

Pharmacological Treatment Options

The ready availability and general reliability of most pain medications mean that pharmacological treatments are among the first interventions used to bring pain relief. Since 2005, there has been tremendous growth in the variety of medications available, with strong evidence supporting the best pain practices. The nurse's role in intervening and advocating for effective pain management depends on understanding the broad range of treatment options.

Nonopioid Analgesics

Medications that reduce pain sensations without also inducing a loss of consciousness are called **analgesics**. The most common analgesics are nonnarcotic and nonopioid. This classification of pain medications includes three general categories of medications: salicylates (aspirin), acetaminophen (Tylenol), and NSAIDs. Medications such as ibuprofen or ketorolac exert their effect largely in the periphery, although some mechanisms of action have been identified in central nociceptive processing structures. Aspirin and NSAIDs are believed to reduce pain largely as a result of inhibiting local prostaglandin synthesis. Because prostaglandin is one of the chemicals released at the site of an acute injury that stimulates inflammation, the net effect of aspirin and NSAID administration is anti-inflammatory. Systemic effects of prostaglandin synthesis inhibition include a reduction in serotonin levels in the brain, lessening the effect of this critical pain-processing neurotransmitter. Acetaminophen has a similar analgesia effect as aspirin, although acetaminophen has few anti-inflammatory effects. Acetaminophen is believed to also activate one of the body's own natural pain-inhibiting neurochemical systems in the peripheral and central nervous systems, the cannabinoid system, to inhibit pain processing and minimize structural and functional reorganizing of central pain-processing synapses.

NSAIDs represent a broad category of anti-inflammatory medications. Originally developed to treat arthritis, they are also effective in treating a wide range of nonarthritic pain conditions. Because NSAIDs vary in both their potency and their elimination half-life (Table 11.4), different NSAIDs are recommended for specific pain complaints. Low-potency NSAIDs with a short elimination half-life, such as ibuprofen (Motrin, Advil), are particularly effective for patients with acute inflammatory pain, as well as visceral pain such as menstrual cramps. The rapid elimination of ibuprofen from the body means that it is safe to use for most patients, even those with severe liver or kidney impairments. NSAIDs with high potency and short elimination half-lives, including diclofenac (Voltaren) and ketorolac (Toradol), are effective in treating rheumatoid arthritis pain and acute gout. Because these NSAIDs also block the production of injury-induced proinflammatory molecules called *leukotrienes* in the upper

Table 11.4 Potency and Elimination Half-Life for Commonly Prescribed NSAIDs

Half-Life	Potency		
	Low	**Intermediate**	**High**
Short	Ibuprofen		Diclofenac (Voltaren)
	(Motrin, Advil)		Ketorolac (Toradol)
Intermediate		Diflunisal (Dolobid)	
		naproxen (Aleve, Naprosyn)	
Long			Oxicams (meloxicam, piroxicam)
			Selective COX-2 inhibitors
			Celecoxib (Celebrex)

respiratory tree, they are particularly effective at treating postoperative pain following lung and thoracic surgery. Intermediate- to high-potency NSAIDs with longer elimination half-lives, including diflunisal (Dolobid), naproxen (Aleve), and the oxicams (meloxicam), have proven effective at treating migraine headaches, activity-induced muscle aches, and even cancer pain, but they must be used cautiously with patients with renal impairment. Because the body depends on local prostaglandin release to support small vessel vasodilation, especially in the kidneys, blocking prostaglandin release impairs the ability of the kidney to cope with low renal blood flow. This prostaglandin-blocking effect is magnified in kidneys with preexisting blood flow–sensitive impairment. Nonopioid analgesics are very effective when combined with opioids, potentiating the opioid effects. Oxycodone has been combined with aspirin (Percodan), acetaminophen (Tylox, Percocet), and ibuprofen (Combunox) to treat acute dental pain, orthopedic pain, and cancer pain. Hydrocodone has also been successfully combined with acetaminophen (Lortab, Vicodin) as well as ibuprofen (Vicoprofen) to treat both acute and chronic pain.

Monitoring the Risks and Benefits of Nonopioid Analgesic Use

The broad benefits associated with nonopioid use need to be balanced with the risks associated with these therapies, including the risks associated with the mechanism of action and with the mechanisms of metabolic clearance. Aspirin, in addition to effects on prostaglandin synthesis, inhibits platelet aggregation, thus its secondary use for cardiovascular prophylaxis in patients at high risk for myocardial infarction or cerebrovascular accident (stroke). The reduced ability for platelets to aggregate following aspirin intake increases the risk for bleeding from wounds, incisions, and even minor cuts or scrapes. Patients taking aspirin as well as other anti-inflammatory medications, including most NSAIDs, are also at increased risk for thrombocytopenia (low platelet count).

This side effect is not well understood, but the relationship between medication intake and the onset of reduced platelet counts suggests that thrombocytopenia may result from an immune response to these medications in patients with a heightened systemic inflammatory response following injury. A drop in platelet counts can occur fairly quickly and is likely to reoccur with subsequent use of the medication.

Cyclooxygenase (COX) is an enzyme critical in the synthesis of prostaglandin. Aspirin and most NSAIDs interfere with prostaglandin synthesis by COX inhibition. There are two major COX isoenzyme variations, COX-1 and COX-2. These COX isoenzymes have similar functions, but inhibition of different COX isoenzymes has a different physiological effect and presents different side-effect risks. Cyclooxygenase-1 isoenzymes are present in every cell type throughout the body. Their role in producing nearly constant levels of prostaglandins and related molecules helps maintain physiological homeostasis in many organs, including the lungs, kidneys, and stomach. Inhibition of COX-1 by NSAIDs is particularly harmful to the gastrointestinal tract, disrupting the protective lining of the stomach and increasing the risk for gastrointestinal ulcers and bleeding even at recommended dosages and with short-term use. Inhibition of prostaglandin synthesis can also compromise uterine wall integrity, and for this reason, NSAIDs are discouraged in the third trimester of pregnancy to minimize the risk for premature labor. Cyclooxygenase-2 isoenzymes are produced only by activated immune cells, including macrophages. The anti-inflammatory and antipyretic effects of aspirin and NSAIDs are believed to be largely associated with COX-2 inhibition. To address the risk associated with COX inhibition, several NSAID compounds have been developed that leave COX-1 enzyme function intact but selectively block COX-2. These compounds, including celecoxib (Celebrex), have limited benefit for managing acute pain because of their slow absorption and slow elimination, but they are effective at managing chronic osteoarthritis pain.

> **⚠ Safety Alert**   Longitudinal studies of the selective COX-2 inhibitors revealed an increased risk of thrombotic events, including myocardial infarction and stroke, leading to rofecoxib (Vioxx) being pulled from the market in 2004. Other selective COX-2 inhibitors remain in use, with their risk for thrombotic events not fully quantified.

> **⚠ Safety Alert**
> - Be alert to combination medication preparations that contain acetaminophen, for example, Percocet, which includes acetaminophen and hydrocodone. Total acetaminophen doses should not exceed 3,000 mg in 24 hours because there is a risk for liver damage and failure.
> - Patients should also be instructed to read medication labels closely and avoid any that contain acetaminophen if they are taking prescription narcotics that also contain acetaminophen.
> - Recent studies link acetaminophen (Tylenol) taken during pregnancy to the development of attention deficit-hyperactivity disorders in children; because of the warnings and recommendations to limit the use of NSAIDs and acetaminophen during pregnancy, pregnant women should consult their providers for the best recommendations to manage pain and fever during pregnancy.

As with most high-potency NSAIDs with long elimination half-lives, selective COX-2 inhibitors should be used cautiously in patients with renal impairment.

Acetaminophen also inhibits COX, with specific selectivity for COX-2, but has few if any anti-inflammatory effects. Acetaminophen is metabolized in the liver and excreted in the kidneys. When used at therapeutic dose limits of 1,000 mg per single dose and 3,000 mg in 24 hours, acetaminophen is generally safe for use in patients with healthy livers. Doses need to be adjusted for patients with liver impairments or not used at all. Extra precautions need to be taken to educate patients about taking OTC acetaminophen with any other OTC or prescription products. Patients may not be aware, for example, that OTC cold preparations and prescription pain medications, such as Tylox and Vicodin, also contain acetaminophen. The risk of accidental overdose leading to liver failure has been associated with cumulative acetaminophen doses of greater than 3,000 mg per day.

Significant drug–drug interactions are also noted in patients taking nonopioid analgesics and prescription medications (Table 11.5). Because many of the nonopioids, including aspirin, acetaminophen, and NSAIDs, are OTC, patients may self-treat minor aches and pains but not appreciate the interaction effects with other common prescription medications, including insulins, antihypertensive medications, and diuretics.

Table 11.5 Drug–Drug Interactions With Common Over-the-Counter Nonopioid Analgesics

Nonopioid Medication	Decrease Effect of	Increase Effect of + Toxicity Risk	Monitor
Aspirin (acetylsalicylic acid)	Proton pump inhibitors, antacids, H₂-receptor blockers	Cyclosporine, tricyclic antidepressants, warfarin, calcium-channel blockers, oral contraceptives	Platelet counts Signs of bleeding
Ibuprofen (Advil/Motrin)	Thiazide diuretics	Digoxin, lithium, warfarin, cyclosporine, insulins	BUN, creatinine, AST, and ALT
Acetaminophen (Tylenol)		Increased hepatotoxicity with barbiturates, alcohol	AST, ALT, bilirubin, dark urine, BUN
Ketorolac (Toradol)	Thiazide diuretics	Lithium, cyclosporine Increased bleeding risk with anticoagulants and aspirin Increased renal impairment with ACE inhibitors	BUN, AST, ALT, dark urine, tinnitus may indicate toxicity
Celecoxib (Celebrex)	ACE inhibitors	Lithium, anticoagulants	Platelet counts, BUN

ACE, Angiotensin-converting-enzyme; *ALT,* alanine aminotransferase; *AST,* aminotransferase; *BUN,* blood urea nitrogen.

Corticosteroids

Corticosteroids are naturally occurring steroid hormones produced in the adrenal cortex. These steroids are involved with the body's stress response to illness and injury and play a role in the body's immune response and inflammation. Synthetic steroid hormones, such as prednisone (Deltasone) and hydrocortisone (Cortef), are used as anti-inflammatory agents to treat arthritis, bone pain, and painful dermatitis as well as visceral pain conditions, including lupus erythematosus, sarcoidosis, and inflammatory bowel disease. They are also successfully used to treat acute inflammation and pain following nerve and spinal cord injuries and are used as **adjuvant** (increasing effectiveness of other medications) therapy for pain control in cancer patients. Corticosteroids work by blocking the synthesis of proinflammatory molecules, such as prostaglandin and leukotrienes. Corticosteroids can be delivered at low doses in topical creams, ointments, and drops. Higher doses can be given orally, inhaled, directly injected in targeted regions such as joints, or delivered intravenously. Secondary effects of steroid use include improved appetite and mood, which can also shape the pain experience. High-dose or sustained corticosteroid use is associated with several side effects, including hyperglycemia, weight gain, myopathies, and Cushing's syndrome, as well as mental status changes, including delirium and psychosis. Dosage adjustments can minimize side effects; tapered discontinuation of corticosteroids is preferred over the sudden cessation of medication to prevent adrenal suppression and steroid withdrawal syndrome. Corticosteroids should not be used in combination with NSAIDs to minimize the risk of gastrointestinal bleeding.

Local Anesthetics

Local anesthetic agents are pharmacological substances, either topically applied or injected into nerves and tissue, that eliminate sensation and pain without the loss of consciousness associated with general **anesthesia**. Local anesthetics are generally used in a defined location to accommodate minor surgery or to regionally target pain. Lidocaine (Xylocaine) is the most commonly used local anesthetic medication. Lidocaine alters the excitability of neurons by blocking fast voltage-gated sodium (Na^+) channels in the cell membranes responsible for propagating pain messages along nociceptive pathways. It acts quickly, usually within 10 minutes, and can last as long as 2 hours. Bupivacaine (Marcaine) is more potent and longer lasting than lidocaine and is used often as an injection for nerve blocks and as an epidural anesthetic. Bupivacaine also carries a greater risk for central nervous system and cardiac toxicity, so doses must be carefully adjusted. It can take as long as 20 minutes for bupivacaine to achieve anesthesia, but the effects can last as long as 8 hours when given as an epidural. Bupivacaine can also be injected into the tissues around a surgical wound intraoperatively, providing pain relief for as long as 20 hours.

Local anesthetics relax vascular muscle walls, bringing increased blood flow into the region. This increased blood flow can increase systemic medication absorption, which shortens effective anesthesia times. To maximize local anesthetic effectiveness, these anesthetic agents are often combined with short-acting vasoconstricting agents such as epinephrine. This allows the anesthetic agent to stay regionally active for a longer period of time and limits potential systemic toxicity from too-rapid absorption. Local vasoconstriction also reduces bleeding in the area of injection. Epinephrine-lidocaine combinations, however, are not recommended for small, confined, vascular-rich areas, such as the penis, fingers, or toes, where local vascular constriction can cause inadequate blood flow and tissue necrosis.

> **Safety Alert** All medication labels should be read closely prior to administration. Vials containing lidocaine with epinephrine solutions look nearly identical to vials containing lidocaine without epinephrine, and using the wrong preparation can cause vascular injuries.

Local anesthetics are also diluted and compounded into sprays, pastes, and creams that can be applied to minor burns and abrasions. A commonly used mixture of local anesthetics (EMLA) is a combination ointment consisting of 2.5% lidocaine and 2.5% prilocaine and is applied to provide superficial dermal anesthesia for venipuncture, IV catheter insertion, and minor wound debridement. Applied 45 to 60 minutes before a procedure and covered with an occlusive dressing, EMLA provides up to 2 hours of local anesthesia once the occlusive dressing is removed. Dilute lidocaine anesthetic sprays and lozenges help soothe sore throats and aid in anesthetizing oral mucous membranes in preparation for tracheal or nasogastric intubation.

Topical Rubefacients

Rubefacients are topically applied substances that cause local dilation of blood vessels and reddening of the skin, producing local sensations of coolness and warmth that many people find soothing. Examples of rubefacients include rubbing alcohol, menthol-containing ointments and creams, salicylates (e.g., aspirin), and oil of wintergreen. Products such as Icy Hot and Bengay, which contain menthol, and aspirin-containing creams, such as Aspercreme and Myoflex, are used to treat low-back pain and general muscle aches associated with activity. Many homemade and folk recipes contain herbal rubefacients such as horseradish, nettle, garlic, cloves, rosemary oil, and turpentine. Rubefacients are believed to relieve pain by serving as a counterirritant. Rubefacients are often compounded to have a strong "medicinal" smell that is also believed to distract or offset the pain and are the most widely purchased OTC pain remedies after oral nonopioid analgesics. Rubefacients should not be used to treat painful dermatitis following radiation treatment because radiation damages epithelial cells and alters the permeability of the vascular bed, and the use of topical rubefacients can worsen radiation-induced dermatitis.

Capsaicin, the active ingredient in chili peppers, is frequently used in topical ointments and dermal patches to produce localized, soothing warm and hot sensations. Capsaicin is believed to activate specific temperature-sensitive receptors on peripheral neurons, causing a rapid propagation of warm and hot impulses to the spinal cord. At the level of the spinal cord, these heat impulses cause rapid release and emptying of stores of a pro-pain neurotransmitter called *substance P*. Until these neurotransmitter stores recover, which could be as long as 6 to 8 hours, these particular peripheral neurons cannot induce a pain response. In patient comparison studies, the evidence in support of capsaicin heat for providing effective pain relief is stronger than for the heat produced by other rubefacients. At low concentrations, capsaicin (Capzasin, Tiger Balm) is used to treat minor musculoskeletal aches and pains, including arthritis, backache, muscle strains, and sprains. At higher concentrations, capsaicin-containing ointments and patches have been used to treat the postherpetic neuralgia associated with shingles as well as other peripheral neuropathies. Gloves should be worn when applying capsaicin ointments and patches to avoid clinician exposure, and they should not be applied to open or broken skin. At higher doses, face masks, protective eyewear, and gloves are recommended for clinician safety. Capsaicin creams are not recommended immediately after hot baths or showers, nor are they recommended to be used with heating pads because the additional heat may allow for overabsorption of the medication.

Opioids

Considered primary in the treatment and management of acute pain, opioids are among the oldest known substances used for the treatment of pain. It is increasingly recognized that opioids are much less effective in managing the pathologies underlying most chronic pain conditions, and their use in chronic pain should be carefully evaluated. Opioids work by binding to opioid receptors that are located primarily in the brain, in the spinal cord, and along peripheral nerves

and the gastrointestinal tract. These opioid receptors are classified as delta-, kappa-, and mu-type receptors (Table 11.6), with the physiological effect of opioids dependent upon the location, type, and binding affinity between medication and receptor. Some opioid receptors located in ascending pain-transmission pathways are activated by opioid medications and block the effects of pro-pain neurotransmitters, including substance P and glutamate. Other opioid receptors located in descending pain pathways are activated by opioid medications and enhance naturally occurring pain-inhibiting processes. It is the action of opioids on receptors in other brain regions, such as the hypothalamus and pituitary gland, that produces the autonomic effects seen with opioids, including pupil constriction, dry mouth, lowered body temperature, and reduced sensitivity to cold. Opioid activation of receptors in the brainstem mutes the activity of the sympathetic nervous system and causes relaxation, sedation, slowed breathing, and reductions in anxiety. Other effects of opioids on brain receptors activate the chemoreceptor trigger zone, which can induce nausea and vomiting.

Opioids are used in the treatment of severe to moderate pain and are often administered to postoperative patients (Box 11.2). Although most often administered via the oral route, opioids may be given via the IV, subcutaneous, intraspinal, transdermal, rectal, and epidural routes. Oral dosages may provide the most consistent therapeutic levels of these medications, but they must be administered at appropriate intervals. Patients may not receive adequate pain

Table 11.6 Overview of Opioid Receptors and Physiological Effect of Opioid Binding		
Receptor	**Location**	**Opioid-Binding Effect**
Delta	Brain	Mild analgesia
	Peripheral sensory neurons	Antidepressant effects
		Stimulates respiration at low doses but slows respiration at high doses
Kappa	Brain	Analgesia
	Spinal cord	Sedation
	Peripheral sensory neurons	Miosis
		Dysphoria
Mu	Brain	Respiratory depression
	Spinal cord	Miosis
	Peripheral sensory neurons	Euphoria
	Intestinal tract	Reduced gastrointestinal motility

Box 11.2 Dsuvia—New Opioid Approved by the FDA

In 2018 a new opioid, Dsuvia, was approved by the U.S. Food and Drug Administration (FDA). However, in light of the opioid epidemic in the United States, the approval was met with controversy and some criticism. Dsuvia is a formulation of sufentanil that is administered sublingually through a 30-mg disposable, prefilled single-dose applicator. Restricted to use only in settings that provide direct supervision by healthcare providers, such as hospitals, surgical centers, and emergency departments, this medication is 10 times more potent than fentanyl. Proponents of the new medication describe some of the unique features of the medication, including the ability to quickly administer an opioid to patients who are unable to swallow oral medication or when IV access is unavailable. One of the primary target populations for this new medication is patients in military settings, where Dsuvia meets a specific but limited unmet medical need in treating military members on the battlefield. This medication is not intended to be used as a first-line choice for pain relief in the general population, and it is only indicated under direct supervision in patients whose pain has not been controlled by more conventional pain approaches.

Gottlieb, S. (2018). *Statement from Commissioner Scott Gottlieb, M.D., on agency's approval of Dsuvia and the FDA's future consideration of new opioids* (U.S. Food and Drug Administration Statement). Retrieved from https://www.fda.gov/NewsEvents/Newsroom/PressAnnouncements/ucm624968.htm

relief because of a fear of side effects or fear of addiction, which is not the same as tolerance. Tolerance is characterized by the need for increasing doses of medication to get the same pain results. **Addiction** is characterized by a compulsive behavioral pattern to take a medication for both its physiological and psychic effects without regard for the negative consequences associated with continued medication ingestion. The growth in addiction, particularly to new synthetic opioid formulations, over the last 5 years has reached epidemic proportions. The numbers of patients addicted to opioids tripled in the years between 2003 and 2014, with the number of opioid overdose deaths annually now exceeding those dying from gun violence and motor vehicle deaths combined. Although there has been a national initiative to limit opioid-prescribing patterns, opioid overdose deaths are cited as a significant contributing factor to the recent drop in life expectancy, the first such drop in more than 50 years.

Patients receiving opioids are at risk for several side effects, particularly related to actions at the mu receptor sites, and prevention and management of these effects are central to any plan of care for patients receiving opioids. Respiratory depression is the most critical adverse side effect of opioids and requires close patient monitoring, especially after IV administration. Nausea and vomiting, frequent side effects, usually develop shortly after the first doses. In the postoperative patient, assessment for nausea and vomiting is particularly important because it increases the risk of aspiration. Patients experiencing pain often have decreased physical activity and oral intake; these circumstances, along with the effects of opioids on the gastrointestinal system, increase constipation. Laxatives and stool softeners may be indicated to assist in the prevention or treatment of constipation. Other receptor-mediated adverse effects of opioids include urinary retention and pruritus. Opioids acting on opioid receptors in synaptically reorganized dysfunctional pain pathways can paradoxically increase pain in patients with chronic pain. This receptor response in patients who have taken opioids long term or who may also be addicted to opioids can confound the assessment and management of pain in this population, often leading to skepticism about pain severity and judgmental labeling of patients as "drug seeking." Consultation with pain management experts can assist providers in safe and appropriate pain management in this challenging pain circumstance (see Evidence-Based Practice: Opioid Use in Pain Management).

Evidence-Based Practice

Opioid Use in Pain Management

- Opioids are effective for managing acute pain such as postoperative or trauma-associated pain, with few therapeutic benefits in chronic pain conditions.
- Opioids are more effective when combined with NSAIDs as most acute pain has an inflammatory component.
- Opioids are most effective when combined with teaching and self-management instruction that shapes a realistic expectancy of the pain experience and pain relief. The goal should NOT be relief of all pain but improvement of functional engagement.

Chou, R., Gordon, D. B., de Leon-Casasola, O. A., Rosenberg, J. M., Bickler, S., Brennan, T., ... Wu, C. L. (2016). Management of postoperative pain: A clinical practice guideline from the American Pain Society, the American Society of Regional Anesthesia and Pain Medicine, and the American Society of Anesthesiologists' Committee on Regional Anesthesia, Executive Committee, and Administrative Council. *Journal of Pain, 17*(2), 131–157.

Morphine (Roxanol) is considered the gold standard of opioids and is used in the treatment of acute pain. Oral morphine agents are available in both short-acting and controlled-release (MS Contin) forms. In the acute setting, particularly with severe pain, and in the postoperative setting, IV morphine is common. Hydromorphone (Dilaudid) is another opioid used in the treatment of severe pain and is five times more potent than morphine (Fig. 11.7). Available only in short-release forms, this medication is frequently used in the treatment of acute pain, particularly via the IV route.

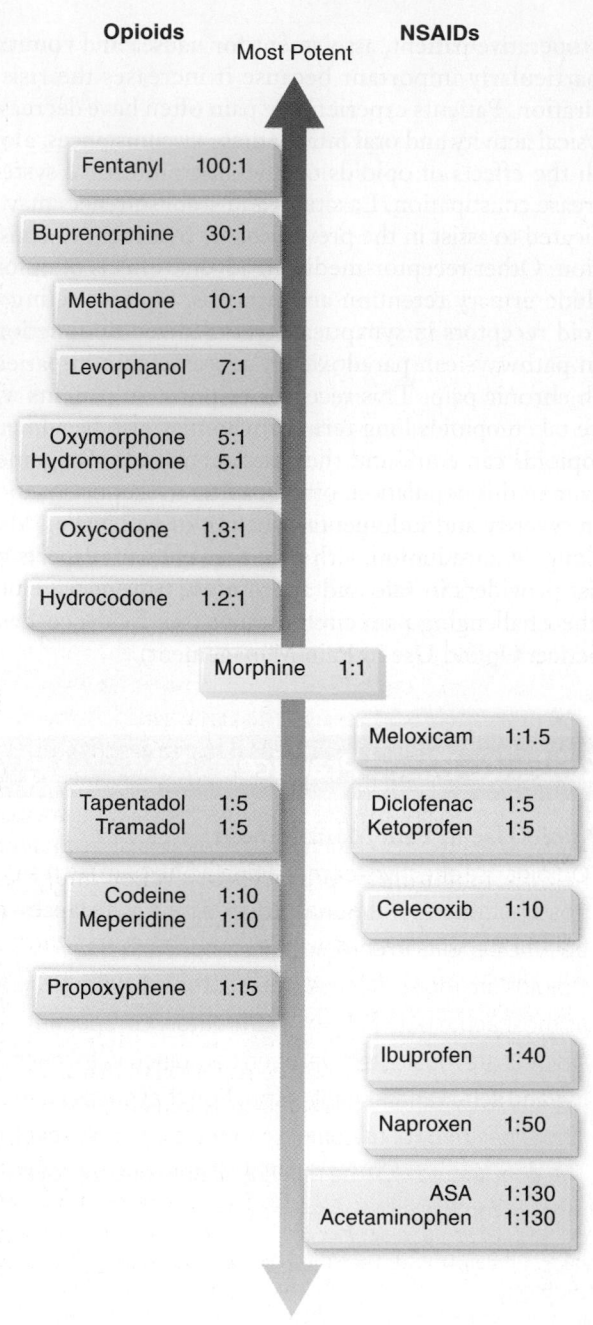

Opioids   NSAIDs
Most Potent

Fentanyl	100:1
Buprenorphine	30:1
Methadone	10:1
Levorphanol	7:1
Oxymorphone	5:1
Hydromorphone	5.1
Oxycodone	1.3:1
Hydrocodone	1.2:1

| Morphine | 1:1 |

| Meloxicam | 1:1.5 |

| Tapentadol | 1:5 |
| Tramadol | 1:5 |

| Diclofenac | 1:5 |
| Ketoprofen | 1:5 |

| Codeine | 1:10 |
| Meperidine | 1:10 |

| Celecoxib | 1:10 |

| Propoxyphene | 1:15 |

| Ibuprofen | 1:40 |

| Naproxen | 1:50 |

| ASA | 1:130 |
| Acetaminophen | 1:130 |

Least Potent

FIGURE 11.7 Not all opioids are created equal—understanding relative potency is a factor in pain management. New formulations are introduced all the time, and their potency should be considered in relation to the gold standard of morphine.

Newer synthetic opioids include different preparations of oxycodone, including the extended-release form branded as Oxycontin. This potent opioid, although marketed as having low addiction risk, is highly effective in relieving pain and is also highly addictive given its low cost and wide prescriptive availability. Until recently, this single agent was identified as being the most commonly abused opioid and responsible for a significant number of overdose deaths. Appropriately prescribed to manage short-term acute pain, this medication represents a significant treatment advantage over other commonly prescribed opioids; however, tighter prescription controls have not necessarily reduced opioid overdose deaths. Patients who previously have been taking oxycontin and find themselves addicted but without a ready source of that medication have switched their opioid of choice to cheaper and often illegally obtained heroin and fentanyl. Opioid overdose deaths remain a significant public health concern.

Connection Check 11.6

The nurse correlates respiratory depression and decreased gastrointestinal motility with the actions of which opioid receptor?
A. Delta
B. Kappa
C. Mu
D. Beta

Atypical Analgesics

Adrenergic Agonists

Clonidine (Catapres) is a direct-acting alpha-2 adrenergic agonist used to treat high blood pressure. Its side effects of analgesia and sedation prompted clinical trials to evaluate clonidine for pain relief. Oral dosing of clonidine for pain management has limited benefit for the treatment of acute and chronic pain because doses sufficient to produce pain relief create excessive sedation. Intrathecal and epidural infusions of clonidine, however, have been used to treat cancer pain and neuropathic pain as well as chronic pain in patients who have become tolerant to opioids. Clonidine activates alpha-2 receptors at the level of the spinal cord to reduce cellular excitability and has been demonstrated to potentiate the action of local anesthetics and opioids. A related compound, tizanidine (Zanaflex), used to treat muscle spasticity, has proven effective at treating some forms of myofascial pain and peripheral neuropathy.

Tricyclic Antidepressants

Tricyclic antidepressants (TCAs) comprise a large class of medications that modulate the effects of serotonin and the related neurotransmitter norepinephrine in the central nervous system. First used to treat mood disorders and major depression in the 1960s, TCAs became more widely used to treat pain with the discovery of the critical role of serotonin and norepinephrine in modulating naturally occurring opioids in descending pain pathways. Tricyclic antidepressants largely affect the reuptake of serotonin or norepinephrine at the level of the individual synapse in the brain, with the net effect being an increase in the amount of neurotransmitter available, enhancement of neurotransmission, and changes in the level of naturally occurring opioids in the central nervous system. The most commonly prescribed TCAs, amitriptyline (Elavil), clomipramine

(Anafranil), desipramine (Norpramin), imipramine (Tofranil), and nortriptyline (Pamelor), have proven effective at managing neuralgias, fibromyalgia, and migraine headaches as well as the pain associated with irritable bowel syndrome, posttraumatic stress disorders, and neuropathies. Although doses for pain relief are generally lower than those prescribed to treat depression, the stabilization of mood that accompanies TCA use is generally viewed as a positive outcome for patients with pain who also report depression.

⚠ Safety Alert Because older adults are sensitive to anticholinergic side effects, nortriptyline (Pamelor) and desipramine (Norpramin) are preferred agents over amitriptyline (Elavil) in this population. Dosage titration should begin at 10 to 25 mg per day and gradually adjusted until the patient reports pain relief. Ensure adequate time for a TCA trial. It may take as long as 8 weeks or more at maximal tolerated doses to determine the true effectiveness of TCAs in older adults. Baseline and periodic electrocardiograms should be routinely performed to assess for cardiac side effects in older adults taking TCAs. The selective serotonin uptake inhibitor paroxetine (Paxil) should also be used cautiously in older adults because of anticholinergic side effects.

Glutamate Receptor Antagonists and Gamma-Aminobutyric Acid Agonists

Glutamate is the principal excitatory neurotransmitter in the central nervous system. At the level of the spinal cord, glutamate interacts with several different receptors, including the N-ethyl-D-aspartic acid (NMDA) receptor. Calcium movement across NMDA receptors in spinal cord neurons is thought to influence how spinal neurons form synaptic connections with adjacent neurons, critically shaping "cellular memory" for pain. Blocking the activation of NMDA receptors is thought to limit the formation and permanency of abnormal synaptic connections. Ketamine (Ketalar) is the most commonly used medication to block glutamate activation of the NMDA receptor and has been successfully used to treat chronic pain resistant to most other analgesics. It is particularly useful at suppressing the central sensitization associated with surgical incisions and postherpetic neuralgia. Dose ranges for ketamine that produce analgesia are only slightly below dose ranges that produce pronounced hallucinations and ataxia; therefore, its use is largely restricted to anesthesia suites or emergency departments as part of pre-anesthesia induction or emergency sedation. Recent research has demonstrated that ketamine can be a life-saving therapy in depression that is nonresponsive to other antidepressant therapy. Although ketamine is an older and well-established analgesic, the overlap of brain regions shaping depression and chronic pain suggest that ketamine, and synthetic metabolites of ketamine in the body, may hold new and exciting promise in treating chronic pain.

Dilute topical preparations of ketamine in combination with other anesthetics and anti-inflammatory agents have been used to treat nerve pain and painful dermatitis following radiation for cancer treatment. The most common topical preparation includes 10% ketamine, 10% of the NSAID ketoprofen, and 5% lidocaine. Other topical ketamine preparations combine ketamine with clonidine, TCAs including amitriptyline and tramadol, and the local anesthetic mepivacaine. Medications closely related to ketamine are being evaluated in clinical trials to treat chronic pain syndromes. Amantadine (Symadine), commonly used to treat viral syndromes and the symptoms of Parkinson's disease, has demonstrated promising results in the treatment of neuropathic pain in cancer patients. Memantine (Namenda), used to treat the memory loss associated with Alzheimer's disease, is also in clinical trials, with significant reductions reported in diabetic neuropathic pain.

When pain messages originating in the periphery reach the spinal cord, both excitatory and inhibitory neurotransmitters are released at synaptic connections. *Gamma-aminobutyric acid* (GABA) is the principal inhibitory neurotransmitter in the central nervous system. When GABA interacts with specific receptors in the pain-processing systems, it changes the electrical conductivity from neuron to neuron, inhibiting pain processing. When injury leads to more permanent restructuring of pain synapses and dysfunctional cellular memory, it is often because there are fewer functional pain inhibition connections. Synthetic medications can be used to mimic the action of GABA by activating GABA receptors more widely, increasing pain inhibition. The most commonly prescribed GABA receptor agonist is baclofen (Lioresal). It is generally used to treat spastic movement disorders associated with spinal cord injury, multiple sclerosis, and amyotrophic lateral sclerosis. It has proven effective for the treatment of pain following nerve crush injuries, spinal cord injuries, and complex peripheral neuropathies in which the underlying cause may be difficult to determine.

Ion-Channel Blockers

Following the development of successful ion-channel–blocking agents, such as lidocaine, and the identification of other ion channels critical to pain processing, there has been great clinical interest in a broader ion-channel blockade to control pain. The anticonvulsant medications phenytoin (Dilantin), carbamazepine (Tegretol), and lamotrigine (Lamictal) are nonselective Na^+-channel blockers effective at treating neuropathic pain and trigeminal neuralgia. They must be used cautiously in patients also taking oral anticoagulants, including warfarin (Coumadin), because these can increase the therapeutic effect of anticoagulants (increasing the risk of bleeding) or cause toxicity. Tricyclic antidepressants, in addition to their effects on serotonin reuptake, block Na^+ channels as a secondary mechanism of action, limiting the propagation of pain messages, which may also help to explain their analgesic activity. Gabapentin (Neurontin) and pregabalin (Lyrica) are novel anticonvulsant medications with analgesic effects. Although gabapentin was initially synthesized to mimic the inhibitory neurotransmitter GABA, it is not believed to activate GABA receptors; instead, the analgesic mechanism of action is believed to be its binding to a subunit of ion channels that gate local calcium flow, limiting the propagation of pain messages. Both gabapentin and pregabalin, a more potent second-generation form of gabapentin, have proven effective at treating diabetic neuropathic pain and neuropathic pain following nerve injuries in the lower back. Other ion channels that influence calcium movement in pain-processing neurons and thus the propagation of pain messages have also been identified as potential analgesia targets. Blockers of L-type calcium channels, including nimodipine (Nimotop), verapamil (Calan), and diltiazem (Cardizem), allow for reduced doses of opioids when treating cancer patients, as well as a reduced need for postoperative analgesia following abdominal surgery (Table 11.7).

Decision Making for Effective Dose, Route, and Medication Choice

In spite of gains in pharmacology and a growing body of evidence to guide the best pain practices, too many patients wake each day in chronic pain, too many postoperative patients experience unrelieved pain that slows their recovery, and too many patients suffer at the end of life. Part of the challenge in balancing the risks and benefits of intervention is acknowledging that significant variability exists among individual patients in analgesia response. The therapeutic goal is to choose medications that provide the best pain relief with the fewest adverse effects for the individual. There are many factors to consider when making a therapeutic medication choice, including (1) the type, intensity, and duration of a patient's pain; (2) the patient's age, gender, and general health; (3) the potential for pain relief and side effects based on mechanism of action and analgesia potency; (4) the potential for drug–drug interactions with current medications; and (5) the potential to improve or worsen comorbid health conditions.

Effective pain management depends on understanding how the body releases medications from their formulation and how medications enter the circulation and are distributed throughout the body's tissues, as well as how medications are metabolized and excreted from the body. Identical medications can produce different results depending on the route of administration. Inhaled steroids, for example, provide more targeted treatment in the bronchial tree with fewer systemic effects than if the same steroid is delivered orally or intravenously. Although oral medications are preferred by most patients because they are more convenient and do not involve sterile procedures or potentially painful injections, many medications cannot be formulated for therapeutically effective gastrointestinal absorption into the bloodstream. Although many oral medications do have

Table 11.7 Dosing Guidelines for Common Atypical Analgesic Agents

Anticonvulsants–Ion-Channel Agonists	Route	Dose Range (mg/day)	Schedule	Practice Recommendations
Carbamazepine (Tegretol)	PO	600–1,200	q6–8 hours	
Clonazepam (Klonopin)	PO	0.5–3.0	q8 hours	
Phenytoin (Dilantin)	PO	1,500–3,000	q8 hours	Two loading doses of 500 mg each PO or IV at 4- to 6-hour intervals can establish a blood level for better long-term pain relief.
Gabapentin (Neurontin)	PO	300–3,600	q8 hours	
Tricyclic Antidepressants	**Route**	**Dose Range (mg/day)**	**Schedule**	**Practice Recommendations**
Amitriptyline (Elavil)	PO	50–150	Bedtime	Was first line; now desipramine is preferred with fewer side effects and equianalgesia
Desipramine (Norpramin)	PO	50–150	Bedtime	Preferred for elderly
Nortriptyline (Pamelor)	PO	50–150	Bedtime	
Doxepin (Sinequan)	PO	50–150	Bedtime	Can combine with nortriptyline for improved analgesia
Imipramine (Tofranil)	PO	50–150	Bedtime	

PO, by mouth.

the benefit of being able to be compounded for sustained release, many dosing errors have been associated with improper crushing of sustained-released medications, both by patients at home and by clinicians who may not be aware of sustained-release formulations. Oral medications are also frequently compounded with dyes and pharmacologically inert substances that are allergenic for many people. Over-the-counter oral analgesics, for example, should be used cautiously in patients with a significant allergy history or a documented allergy to red and yellow dyes.

In addition to the mouth serving as a convenient entry to the gastrointestinal tract, the mouth is also an area of very vascular-rich tissue, allowing medication access through the mucosa. Some opioids, such as buprenorphine (Buprenex) or methadone (Methadose), can be formulated for sublingual doses, compounded into a lozenge, or packaged as a lollipop. The Actiq lollipop contains the opioid fentanyl and is particularly effective at treating breakthrough pain between scheduled doses of other medications.

The rectal route can also be an effective route of administration for many patients, although it is associated with the most variable absorption and peak-onset effects. The rectal route also can stimulate bowel evacuation in patients with low levels of bowel continence, with a subsequent loss of unabsorbed medication, minimizing effective dosing. The IV route of administration is reliable in emergency situations or when a rapid therapeutic effect is desired, but its use is often more limited to care settings and not as readily available for home use. Intravenous medications have the advantage, however, of being able to deliver both a bolus dose of medication or continuous infusions. Bolus dosing provides for a relatively rapid onset of pain relief, usually within 5 to 7 minutes, whereas continuous infusions allow for a steady level of medication that keeps plasma concentrations of the medication more constant. Continuous infusions may allow for lower cumulative levels of medication to be delivered, which has the potential to reduce medication side effects. In addition to IV delivery of medications, other infusion devices can deliver pain medication via subcutaneous tissues. Small 25- to 30-gauge needles can be placed into the subcutaneous tissues and connected to a small refillable medication reservoir. Some patients can also have implanted subcutaneous medication reservoirs with tunneled infusion systems under the skin to continuously deliver small doses of medications. These infusion sites need to be continually monitored for redness, swelling, signs of medication leakage, and the formation of dependent edema in the affected extremity. Pain relief can be variable with these delivery systems, and sites generally need to be rotated every 6 to 7 days to minimize infection and tissue trauma.

Transdermal patches comfortably provide both targeted and systemic pain relief, although there are relatively few pain medications currently formulated for transdermal administration. The most common pain medication delivered by transdermal patch is fentanyl (Duragesic), a powerful opioid. Patients and families do appreciate the ability to self-medicate using this delivery system, with sustained medication delivery limiting the frequency of breakthrough pain; however, the risk of opioid-induced respiratory depression requires close monitoring of respiratory status. Transdermal patches may be applied to any clean, dry skin surface, although areas on the upper back and chest are recommended to minimize dislodging of the patch. It is important to remove old patches when new ones are applied so that patients are not overmedicated. New patches should be placed on rotating skin sites to minimize skin irritation. One important factor to consider with transdermal patches is that these sustained-release delivery devices can require up to 24 hours before effective pain relief is achieved, and often patients require a supplemental analgesic in the interim.

Intrathecal, epidural, or targeted injections into joints or nerve roots allow for regional analgesia with fewer systemic side effects but require specialist assessment and administration. Delivering medications directly into and around the spinal cord allows medications to act directly on specialized pain receptors and pain-processing networks of synapses to inhibit pain. The advantages of this targeted therapy include a generally longer duration of analgesia and at lower doses than can be achieved by other delivery methods. Often, targeted spinal analgesics combine an opioid with a local anesthetic to maximize pain relief by inhibiting several pain pathways. Side effects of targeted spinal analgesia and anesthesia include urinary retention and pruritus. Respiratory status must be closely monitored with targeted spinal opioid delivery and continued for several hours after discontinuation of therapy. Delayed respiratory depression has been noted, and patients should remain on continuous pulse oximeter monitoring for 8 to 12 hours after the medication has been discontinued. Frequent peripheral neurological and skin assessments should be performed with continuous targeted spinal analgesia, especially if opioids are combined with local anesthetic agents. Patients will have reduced sensation in the lower extremities and may not be able to readjust their position in response to pressure or other noxious stimulation. These patients should also have blood pressure monitored as well. Vascular tone can be affected by targeted spinal anesthesia, causing some pooling of blood in lower extremities, leading to lower systemic blood pressures and feelings of light-headedness. Epidural catheters are placed in the small space outside the dura mater of the spinal cord and are generally used for long-duration analgesia delivery, including pain relief in women in labor and some lower-extremity procedures. Implanted catheters connected to refillable reservoirs or pumps are used for days to months to provide long-lasting pain relief for patients with chronic pain. Intrathecal injections are usually single injections directly into the cerebrospinal fluid, bathing the spinal column with short-duration effects of 30 minutes to 8 hours.

Injections of corticosteroids and anesthetic agents directly into a muscle, joint, or nerve root are becoming increasingly common to treat such inflammatory complaints as osteoarthritis, bursitis, tendonitis, and rheumatoid arthritis.

Injection of anti-inflammatory agents is being used as a less invasive treatment for carpal tunnel and other entrapment syndromes as well as chronic myofascial pain. It is contraindicated in immune-suppressed patients and in the presence of bleeding disorders, as well as active joint or systemic infections. Although some clinicians prefer to use single agents, such as long-acting methylprednisolone, most clinicians inject a cocktail of lidocaine and both intermediate- and long-acting steroids. These injections can be painful and often require the sterility of a procedure or operating suite as well as ultrasound guidance for proper injection placement. Pretreatment with a local anesthetic can minimize injection discomfort, followed by icing of the injection site for long-term comfort. Patients should be educated to expect that swelling and increased pain may occur. Injections into an already painful joint or muscle are likely to cause short-term hyperalgesia (increased sensitivity to pain) of 1 to 2 days' duration. Muscle and joint injections, however, can produce analgesia for several months, allowing physical therapy and stretching to improve muscle tone and joint flexibility for sustained pain control. Although trained clinician delivery of anti-inflammatory medications directly into the muscle is proving effective at providing pain control, the delivery of other medications via intramuscular injections is becoming less common. Intramuscular injections do provide fairly rapid pain relief; however, effectiveness varies widely from person to person, and this method poses considerable risk to patients. Even with the careful identification of anatomical landmarks and proper injection technique, intramuscular injections can injure muscle, nerves, and soft tissues. Patients also find intramuscular injections painful and may delay seeking pain relief to avoid injection-induced pain.

Pain Management Guidelines

Principles established in 1987 by the World Health Organization (WHO) to guide pain management for cancer patients have been widely adapted to guide pain treatment for many different types of pain conditions. These principles suggest:

- Oral analgesics should be the first pharmacological treatment option used for most mild to moderate pain.
- Analgesics should be given at regular intervals rather than "on demand."
- Analgesics should be administered according to pain intensity as evaluated on a reliable measure of pain intensity.
- The goal of pain management is *not* to produce an absence of pain but to improve functional quality of life.
- Dosing should be adapted to the individual.
- Analgesics should be administered with attention to the details of dose and response.
- Evaluation of therapeutic response is critical to long-term pain management success.

The WHO developed a treatment ladder to guide analgesia prescribing in support of these treatment principles (Fig. 11.8). This three-step ladder recommends beginning

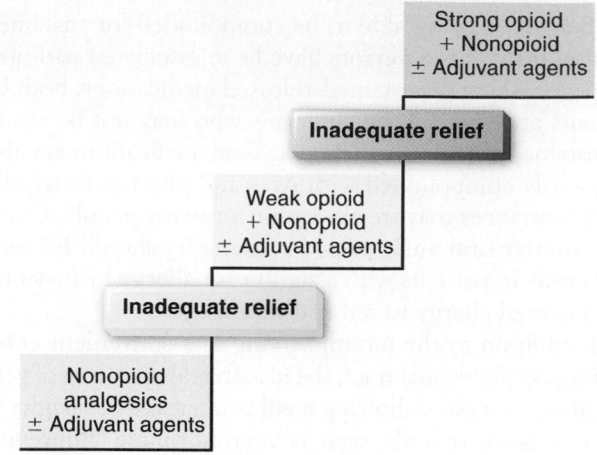

FIGURE 11.8 The World Health Organization three-step ladder. This three-step ladder begins with nonopioid analgesics (Step 1) and progresses to weak opioids (Step 2) and then stronger opioids (Step 3) as pain persists or becomes more severe.

with a nonopioid analgesic and progressing to weak opioids and then stronger opioids as pain persists or becomes more severe. Adjuvant therapies, including steroids, antidepressants, and anticonvulsant medications, can be added at any stage in the treatment ladder to maximize individual pain treatment success. The American Pain Society further endorses the use of nonopioid analgesics at each step in the pain treatment ladder even when opioids are prescribed, recognizing there are summative benefits of combining nonopioids and opioid analgesia agents that target both central and peripheral pain-processing pathways (Table 11.8).

Equianalgesia

Medications with different potencies and different mechanisms of action can often be used interchangeably to achieve similar levels of pain relief in cases of patient sensitivity or when tolerance to medication effects or addiction is a concern. A 25-mcg-per-hour fentanyl patch will gradually release pain medication, providing pain relief for up to 3 days. This dose provides an equivalent level of analgesia as that delivered by 30 to 40 mg of morphine delivered orally every 4 hours over a 24-hour period. Reference conversion charts list doses for common medications that can provide equal amounts of analgesia. Using the information in Table 11.9,

Table 11.8 Dose, Route, and Condition-Dependent Dosing for Common Nonopioid Analgesics

Common Nonopioid Analgesic	Route and Condition-Dependent Maximum Dose	Onset and Duration
Aspirin	PO/rectal 1–2 g in 24 hr	PO onset 15–30 min, peak 1–2 hr, duration 4–6 hr
	PO for arthritis 2–5 g in 24 hr	Rectal slow and variable onset, duration 4–6 hr
Acetaminophen	PO/rectal 1–4 g in 24 hr	PO onset 10–30 min, peak 1–2 hr, duration 4–6 hr
		Rectal slow and variable onset, duration 4–6 hr
Ibuprofen	PO 3.2 g in 24 hr	Onset 30 min, peak 1–2 hr, duration 6–8 hr
Ketorolac	PO/IM/IV 40 mg in 24 hr	PO onset 30–45 min, peak 2 hr, duration 4–6 hr
	IM 30-mg single dose	IM onset 15–30 min, peak 1–2 hr, duration 4–6 hr
	IV 15-mg single dose	IV onset 5–15 min, peak 1–2 hr, duration 4–6 hr
	PO/IM/IV dosing limited to 5 days and dosed no less frequently than every 4 hr	Should begin IV or IM dosing and transition to PO dosing
Celecoxib	One single loading PO dose of 400 mg followed by divided bid dosing 200 mg in 24 hr	PO onset in 45 min, peak onset 6–8 hr, duration 12 hr
	PO for arthritis up to 400 mg in 24 hr	

IM, Intramuscular; *IV*, intravenous; *PO*, by mouth.

Table 11.9 Equianalgesic Dosing for Management of Acute or Chronic Pain*

Medication	IM/SC/IV (mg)	PO/PR/SL (mg)	Hours of Pain Relief
Morphine	10	20–30	3–4
Codeine	120–130	200	3–4
Oxycodone	—	15–20	3–4
Hydromorphone	2	4	2–4
Meperidine	75–100	300	3–4
Acetaminophen with codeine (Tylenol #3)	—	Two tablets, each containing 300 of acetaminophen and codeine 30	3–4
Acetaminophen with oxycodone (Percocet)	—	Two tablets, each containing 325 of acetaminophen and oxycodone 2.5	3–6

IM, Intramuscular; *PO*, by mouth; *PR*, by rectum; *SC*, subcutaneous; *SL*, sublingual.
*Dose conversion recommendations are for treating chronic pain, and lower doses may be required for acute pain.

a patient receiving 75 to 100 mg of meperidine (Demerol) IV, for example, could instead receive 20 to 30 mg of morphine by mouth or sublingually, with similar pain control results.

Demand Dosing

Traditionally, pain medications have been administered by nurses either on an ordered frequency schedule or on an as-needed (prn) basis. This approach allows nurses to assess pain and to determine the most effective pain management treatment from a range of pain management options as well as to monitor for and prevent treatment-induced side effects. In spite of considerable professional education about the science of pain management, studies indicate that nurses routinely underestimate the amount of pain experienced by patients and significantly undertreat pain in a demand-dosing pain management model. There have been several theories put forth as to why demand-dosing models lead to poorer pain management outcomes. It has been suggested that nurses implicitly substitute their judgment as to how much pain the patient is experiencing over that subjectively reported by the patient. When asked to describe the key assessments and assumptions underlying their pain management decisions, nurses routinely report difficulties in validating subjective patient reports with objective clinical manifestations of pain. Although there are few well-studied or validated objective clinical manifestations of pain, when there are inconsistencies between a subjective report of patient pain and objective data, nurses tend to favor objective data. Nurses, for example, will question a patient self-report of pain of 10 on a scale of 1 to 10 when they bring pain medication to the bedside of a sleeping patient. This experience then tends to influence subsequent pain assessments such that nurses can become quite skeptical of patient self-reports if they do not conform to some preset image of what a patient in pain "should look like." Undertreatment is significantly more of a clinical issue when prn pain medications are part of the treatment plan. Rather than being seen as a direction to medicate a patient as needed, it is often interpreted as administrating a medication only on patient request. Nurses may administer pain medication at lower doses or at longer intervals than dosing guidelines suggest because of concerns about the development of respiratory depression or addiction.

Although evidence suggests that less than 1% of patients on long-term opioid treatment develop respiratory depression, **dependence**, and addiction, nurses report a belief that the risk of addition is as high as 60%, with the risk of respiratory depression nearly as high. They also report a belief that addiction to narcotics can develop in as few as 5 to 6 doses, contrary to evidence that suggests that true narcotic addiction requires weeks to months of medication consumption. These beliefs are particularly influential in emergency settings, where there is less opportunity to know patients and learn patient patterns. Both emergency department nurses and physicians are quicker to describe patients as "drug seeking" than clinicians in other acute settings, especially if the patient is a member of an ethnic group, younger, or from social groups that clinician bias defines as having an increased risk for addiction.

Demand dosing can have negative effects on patient outcomes in other ways. Waiting until a patient requests medications often means that patients are in more intense pain before receiving an analgesic. They may receive some temporary sedation and pain control only to rise again to peak levels of pain before being treated once again. This leads to peaks and troughs in pain control rather than achieving a more steady state of pain relief. Demand dosing puts authority and control in the hands of providers rather than in the hands of patients. Not only does this lack of control over pain management increase patient anxiety about when their next dose will be or whether they will find pain relief, but this anxiety can also actually exacerbate the pain experienced by patients. Strategies for improving the clinical effectiveness of demand-dosing models are outlined in Evidence-Based Practice: Maximizing the Effectiveness of Demand-Dosing Pain Management Models.

Evidence-Based Practice

Maximizing the Effectiveness of Demand-Dosing Pain Management Models

- Scheduling prn pain medications at regular intervals around the clock rather than waiting for patients to request medication maintains more constant blood levels and improves patient comfort.
- Analgesics used in combination are more effective than the use of single agents alone.
- The use of adjuvant therapies is *not* intended to replace analgesics or to be used to reduce the dose of primary analgesics.
- Dosages should be adjusted upward within an acceptable range and titrated to patient comfort, with the goal of total pain relief not a reduced level of pain.
- Side effects such as constipation, nausea, and pruritus are treatable and should not cause nurses to limit side-effect–inducing medications.
- Recognize that clinician beliefs and attitudes affect both the assessment and treatment of pain; patients who challenge beliefs and assumptions about pain management need effective pain management, not clinician judgment and skepticism.

American Pain Society. (2008). *Principles of analgesic use in the treatment of acute pain and cancer pain* (6th ed.). Glenview, IL: Author.
Pasero, C., & McCaffery, M. (2001). The undertreatment of pain. *American Journal of Nursing, 101*(11), 62–65.

Philosophically, patient-controlled analgesia (PCA) puts patients "back in charge" of their own analgesia. In practice, one of the few places patients can exercise much control over their dosing and scheduling of medications is in the home, and even then, prescriptive limits on how much pain medication may be dispensed and undereducated patients contribute to ineffective self-analgesia for most patients. In acute care settings, PCA is generally used to refer to self-control of medication delivery for the small subset of patients receiving medications via IV or subcutaneous infusions. Pumps have been designed to be programmable and responsive to interactive patient commands to administer medications. Often, these pumps are used first to deliver a bolus dose of medication, usually an opioid, and to provide a continuous low dose or background dose of analgesia. Patients who are experiencing pain can self-medicate by pressing a control button that delivers a preset additional dose above the background dose. Programming determines the maximum amount of medication that may be patient-delivered in a prescribed time frame; if the patient attempts to self-medicate beyond these dose and time limits, the patient is "locked out" of the system and cannot receive additional doses above the background dose.

The benefits of PCA are well documented. Patients report improved pain relief at lower doses of medication and with fewer side effects than with conventional approaches to pain management. Self-control over pain medication reduces anxiety about when a next dose might be delivered and about having to ask for medication. Patients are able to self-taper doses as their pain lessens and are generally able to discontinue pain medication earlier than with demand-dosing models of pain management. One of the challenges of PCA, however, is pain control during extended periods of daytime rest or night-time sleep. Basal levels of pain medications may be insufficient to provide sustained periods of pain control without waking to redose. Some pumps have more sophisticated programming algorithms that recognize patterns of self-medication and augment patient-delivered doses during periods of inactivity. Frequent patient assessments, which include patient education, ensure that the patient understands how to recognize when he or she needs additional doses and how to access the device.

Nonpharmacological Interventions

Nurses have long recognized the critical role of the healing environment in pain management. Bed linens that are clean and smoothed at intervals help bedbound patients feel more comfortable. Pillows and positioning devices that are soft and provide ergonomic support can minimize tension on incisions or reduce muscle spasms associated with deeper pain. Ambient light and temperatures, as well as odors and even color choices in the care environment, can stabilize and elevate mood, which can help moderate pain perception. Often used in more targeted ways for pediatric care areas, colors such as greens, yellows, and blues in more muted and balanced tones have been demonstrated to be therapeutic for adults as well. Yellows and greens have been used in postanesthesia recovery areas, for example, to promote a positive sense of wellness and security in patients emerging from anesthesia. Deeper blue tones have been suggested to promote relaxation and well-being in patients with nervous system dysfunction, including those with chronic neuropathic pain and those experiencing depression. In a similar way, specific odors have been therapeutically used to promote relaxation and pain relief. The smell of vanilla, for example, delivered via a diffuser or when applied as an essential oil to the skin, has been demonstrated to reduce anxiety and promote relaxation. The aroma of green apples has been used to reduce the pain associated with migraine headaches and arthritic joint pain. Colors used alone or in combination with aromatherapy are suggested to influence pain states by engaging the limbic system and contributing to the descending modulation of pain.

Nurses, however, are challenged to provide a calming and healing environment in most modern healthcare settings, which can be noisy and frenetic, with interruptions around the clock. Higher nurse-to-patient ratios or complex task lists often limit extended contact with patients. Evidence suggests, however, that successful care outcomes depend on how well nurses engage and meaningfully use the time they do spend with patients. The real value and power of nursing to affect care outcomes rest on the nurse's ability to mobilize a true and authentic presence in patient interactions. Forming a therapeutic alliance with a patient requires nurses to develop this ability to be present, being attentive, involved, and fully engaged in the moment of care. Presence communicates acceptance, empathy, and concern. This skill takes practice and patience to develop. The use of nonpharmacological interventions to full effect requires that nurses understand the mechanism of action, review supportive evidence, hold collaborative discussions with prescribing providers, and use themselves skillfully as therapeutic tools to effect positive outcomes.

Positioning

There is no one best position that promotes pain relief or comfort. Nursing efforts need to be focused on assisting a patient to find a position that the patient finds comfortable. Nurses can suggest side-lying positions or head elevations that may minimize stress on muscle groups or incisions. Nurses can also suggest upright sitting positions that encourage forward leaning. Such positions are often used to improve comfort for patients with dyspnea because they increase overall inspiratory muscle effort, allow for greater respiratory expansion, and decrease abdominal breathing as well as minimize the taking of guarded or shallow breaths. Many of these same respiratory issues affect patients in pain. Assuming respiratory-supportive positions can improve comfort for patients in pain. There are care guidelines that suggest position changes every 2 hours to promote skin integrity and minimize risks for skin breakdown. There are no similar guidelines, however, regarding the frequency of repositioning to aid in pain management. Nursing efforts again need to be focused on supporting patient choice in repositioning frequency. Evidence suggests that 45 minutes to 1 hour may be the comfort limit of most positioning strategies, although small adjustments in positions may allow for continued comfort between repositioning.

Heat and Cold Application

The application of heat and cold is situationally recommended to reduce pain associated with underlying muscle, skeletal, or neurological pathology. Cold is better than heat, for example, at reducing low-back pain with spasticity associated with nerve injuries and degenerative joint disease. Most patients, however, prefer heat to manage lower-back pain discomfort in the absence of spasm, although neither cold nor heat brings sustained or permanent pain relief. Activity-induced muscle pain such as that experienced in sports injuries, including acute strains and sprains, can be reduced with an early application of cold combined with pressure such as that provided by an elastic bandage. Local cooling of skin and underlying neuromuscular tissues reduces blood flow into the area, slowing the development of inflammation and inflammatory pain. Cooling-induced local vasoconstriction also limits bleeding into closed neuromuscular compartments around joints, slowing the development of painful tissue-deforming hematomas. Cooling also provides some local anesthesia effects by decreasing nerve conduction as well as increasing the threshold at which nociceptive receptors respond to several pain stimuli including pressure, pinprick, heat, and acidic conditions induced by local tissue injury. Cold has been used to provide a counterirritant effect, especially with dental pain. The application of cold combined with mentholated or alcohol spray has been used to increase the pain threshold for root canals and tooth extraction. This cold application works best when regionally applied to the skin web between the thumb and first finger on the same side of the body as the affected tooth, even as it is clearly some distance from the face and jaw region. This pain-relieving mechanism is not completely understood, but it is suggested that counterirritation activates sensory input into the spinal cord that engages natural inhibitory enkephalins and endorphins as well as influencing the descending modulation of naturally occurring opioids.

Both cold and heat have been used to provide relief from reflex muscle spasm associated with abdominal organ pain. Cold increases peristalsis and is preferred over heat application to the abdominal wall to address the pain associated with constipation, ileus, and mechanical bowel obstruction. Heat, on the other hand, reduces peristalsis and reduces acid production, helping to reduce the pain and discomfort associated with nausea, vomiting, and diarrhea. Heat has also been found to be superior to cold in reducing the reflex muscle spasms associated with menstrual cramps. Neither heat nor cold has been found effective in reducing the postoperative pain and discomfort associated with abdominal surgical approaches, although cold has been effective in reducing the postprocedural pain associated with gynecological surgery via vaginal approaches.

Heat can be delivered as wet or dry heat. Wet-heat technologies include paraffin wax and hydrotherapy baths, whereas dry-heat technologies include hot packs, heating pads, and radiant heat instruments such as heating lamps. Both wet- and dry-heat technologies allow for the sustained application of heat, with hydrotherapy having the additional benefits of allowing additional exercise or manipulation of painful joints with less resistance because of the buoyancy of being in the water. Hydrotherapy can also cleanse wounds less painfully because of the débriding action of whirlpool baths.

Cold can be delivered via ice packs, cold water baths, or commercially available cold-emitting chemical packs. Cloth layers are often placed between the skin and cold packs for patient comfort, but they can slow down cooling. The duration of cold application to achieve muscle cooling, relaxation of muscle spasm, and pain relief varies widely between patients and is somewhat dependent on the thickness of subcutaneous fat that insulates muscle. Even in a relatively slender patient with a thinner subcutaneous fat layer, effective cooling requires more than 10 continuous minutes of application. Heavier patients with localized thicker fat layers may require as long as 20 to 30 continuous minutes of cold application for effective pain relief. Heat applications are generally shorter in duration to achieve effective pain relief, lasting 5 to 15 minutes, although some patients require longer continuous heat applications for improved comfort.

Patient comfort can guide length of application, as can regular assessment of skin integrity at the site of heat or cold application. Skin must continue to blanch when pressed to ensure that there is sufficient regional blood flow to continue the application of cold. Cold application should be discontinued if the patient experiences shivering. Skin that reddens and is accompanied by acute stinging sensations signals the end of both heat and cold application. Any sudden onset of pain suggests that safe temperature limits have been exceeded and the application of heat or cold must be removed. There remains a significant research gap as to how frequently to apply heat and cold to achieve therapeutic benefits. It is not known, for example, if heat and cold should be applied hourly or whether outcomes are improved if heat or cold is applied at 2-, 4-, or 8-hour intervals. It is also not known whether heat and cold work best with concurrent use of any specific pharmacological options or dosing regimen.

Although heat and cold applications can provide tremendous benefits for patients, there are clinical situations in which heat or cold is contraindicated or where they should be used with caution. Heat is contraindicated if deep visceral infections or inflammatory conditions are present or suspected, such as with acute appendicitis. Heat increases vasodilation and regional blood flow, increasing the likelihood of endotoxin absorption and systemic distribution. Heat should also be used cautiously in anesthetized areas or with patients with decreased levels of consciousness. In both situations, natural protective mechanisms that allow a patient to withdraw from noxious or potentially tissue-injurious stimulation are diminished. Heat and cold applications should be used with caution in patients with impaired local circulation. Such patients will have more limited benefits because the affected vascular bed can neither therapeutically constrict nor dilate predictably, nor can safe limits on the duration of cold or heat application be determined. Patients with peripheral vascular disease or diabetes therefore are not likely to benefit from heat or cold applications to the extremities. Local temperature elevations increase local metabolic demands, but a reduced vascular bed cannot adapt, and the risk for tissue injury and necrosis increases. Heat should also not be applied to areas of hematoma or frank bleeding because the increased vascular flow to the heated area will increase hematoma formation and bleeding. Areas of malignancies, both superficial and visceral, should not have applications of heat. Without the ability to precisely control local temperature, heat may stimulate tumor growth. Heat should be used cautiously in the scrotal area because it affects sperm production and sperm health. If the whole body is submerged in heated water greater than 100°F

(38°C), body temperature must be monitored at 15-minute intervals. Whole-body immersion in heated water can override homeostatic temperature-regulation mechanisms and drive body temperatures up very quickly.

Cold applications have fewer contraindications or precautions. Rarely, patients become hypersensitive to cold, with local histamine release and the development of cold urticaria. Occasionally, large applications of cold can cause cold-sensitive patients to experience systemic effects of histamine release, including facial flushing, swelling around the eyes, and laryngeal edema. Other cold-sensitive patients produce hemolysins, agglutins, or cryoglobulins in response to cold that can cause tissue blanching, vascular compromise, and necrosis. These patients include those with Raynaud's syndrome. Pretesting a small area on the thigh to cold application is recommended to assess cold sensitivity. The presence of urticaria in response to cold should lead to limits on cold application.

Range of Motion and Exercise

Passive movement of a joint through its normal range of motion (ROM) is encouraged to prevent joint stiffness, promote motion, and prevent shortening of joint-supporting ligaments. Stiff or stiffening joints should be manually manipulated to the point of resistance but not pain. Patients can also be encouraged to actively move their joints through their normal ROM. More aggressive massage, targeted joint manipulation, progressive stretching, and vigorous exercise require specialized training and education for best outcomes. Evidence suggests that many inpatients, especially older adults, benefit from regular and targeted exercise or physical therapy. Even small increases in daily movement-focused exercise help improve balance, proprioception, gait, and muscle strength, shortening hospital lengths of stay and reducing readmissions associated with falls. Evidence further suggests that exercise improves mood as well as reduces symptoms of depression and anxiety, all of which shape the perception of pain. It is not completely understood why exercise has these wide-ranging effects. It is theorized that movement-focused exercise increases serotonin and norepinephrine levels throughout the central nervous system. These neurotransmitters activate the body's own opioid system, especially in descending pain pathways, with the net result being a reduction in pain. Studies are ongoing to evaluate the therapeutic benefits of movement-focused exercise on human neuropathic pain associated with traumatic nerve injuries, HIV and HIV treatment, and following chemotherapy. Nurses should work with other specialized disciplines to design and implement a comprehensive massage and exercise program that helps reduce pain and increase function.

Massage, Relaxation, Acupressure, and Energy-Based Therapies

Pain, even short-term pain, can be disabling, limiting movement, mobility, and function. Techniques that restore movement and soothe pain include massage, joint manipulation, and exercise. Massage involves the application of touch or force to muscles, tendons, and ligaments without changing the angle or position of joints. Specific massage techniques include effleurage or light stroking in a slow, repetitive, or rhythmic motion. Effleurage is particularly effective at reducing painful edema and can also be soothing when used to massage bony prominences or large body regions such as the back for bed-bound patients. Increasing applied pressure can influence deeper tissues and involves stroking in the direction of venous or lymph flow. Deeper stroking motions can improve blood flow, creating a sensation of warmth that many people find soothing. Muscle pain responds to kneading, where the skin and underlying tissues move with the hands. Kneading can be accomplished through a circular motion of the hands or moving the hands in a transverse fashion over the muscle.

A related technique uses pressure applied to specific body locations that correlate with specific healing areas or meridians in the body. These are the same locations that are used to place needles in acupuncture. Stimulation of these **acupressure** points produces both stress and pain relief. Similar to the specific application of cold to the skin web between the thumb and forefinger, firm pressure applied to this same area relieves same-side dental procedure pain, whereas firm pressure applied to the left lateral forehead can reduce discomfort associated with menstrual cramping. Tennis balls wrapped in socks can be used to stimulate several acupressure points along the lateral aspects of the spine. Patients can lie supine on and then move against the tennis balls to relieve the tension and discomfort associated with childbirth and low-back pain.

Many proponents of light and deep massage suggest that the benefits of massage go beyond the specific effects on muscle tension, lymph flow, and vascular beds. They argue that the laying on of hands and contact of skin to skin is uniquely healing. Physical proximity and physical interaction can be calming and reassuring when situationally and therapeutically used, communicating empathy and concern. Proponents of the healing power of touch further emphasize the essential energy or dynamic life force that is within each patient and each healer. It is working with and through this energy that shapes healing outcomes.

A number of noninvasive nonpharmacological interventions have been developed on the basis of this theoretical understanding, using physical proximity and touch to affect positive patient outcomes. These techniques include therapeutic touch, healing touch, and Reiki therapy. All of these therapies are based on the foundation that energy fields in the body need to be in harmony for there to be wellness. If energy fields are blocked or disturbed because of illness or pathology, this disharmony slows healing or leads to more illness. Those who use energy-based therapies consciously use their physical proximity with direct touch or near touch to influence the human energy field. What distinguishes these techniques from the more general use of touch in nursing practice is the training and mentored skill required to be a successful practitioner. Strong anecdotal evidence suggests that patients with specific pain conditions, including carpal tunnel, postoperative pain, and trauma, report significant pain relief following these energy-based therapies. When therapeutic touch, healing touch, and Reiki have been subjected to rigorous experimental studies using double-blind and placebo controls, pain relief is more mixed. Evidence suggests that energy-based therapies work best when combined with more traditional pharmacological interventions, allowing patients greater comfort and less anxiety at reduced analgesia doses than when pharmacological interventions are used alone.

Relaxation is defined as a deep level of rest that represents an integrated psychological and physiological response characterized by a decrease in sympathetic nervous system activation, decreased metabolic activity, and self-reported feelings of well-being. There is little consensus on what constitutes a relaxation intervention. Some clinicians use music, for example, to promote a relaxing, healing environment. Other clinicians suggest music has benefits on pain outcomes independent of relaxation and should not be considered strictly a relaxation intervention. Still other clinicians encourage specific breathing techniques or sequenced "tensing-relaxing" exercises of the extremity muscles to induce a state of relaxation.

In deep-breathing interventions, patients are asked to take a deep breath while simultaneously clenching their fists or staring at a focusing object. After a moment of breath holding, patients are instructed to slowly release their breath while relaxing their bodies to the point of being limp. In rhythmic breathing, patients are instructed to coordinate their breathing with more equal inhalation and exhalation cycles. Timing devices such as metronomes or patterned music can help establish rhythms. Deep breathing and rhythmic breathing techniques are commonly used with women in labor and in some procedure areas. Proponents of relaxation techniques suggest a range of theories as to why relaxation reduces pain. Advocates suggest that relaxation reduces muscle tension and spasm. Some suggest that having a patient focus on his or her breathing or "tensing-relaxing" specific muscle groups diverts attention in pain perception. Patient ability to relax varies, and it is important to remember that relaxation cannot be forced. It may be less effective during short hospital stays because it may take up to 3 weeks of practice using a selected relaxation technique before patients report positive results. One positive aspect of relaxation techniques is that patients report reduced levels of pain for as long as 6 to 8 hours even after relatively short relaxation sessions (10 to 15 minutes once a day).

In well-controlled studies using several different relaxation techniques, relaxation is usually combined with biofeedback. **Biofeedback** is the presentation of a sensory stimulus to a patient, usually visual or auditory, that changes in proportion to a self-reported or "fed-back" biological response. Examples of fed-back biological responses include electromyography (EMG) waveforms of muscle activity, skin temperature, electroencephalogram (EEG) waveforms of neurological activity, skin resistance, pulse rate, and blood pressure. Proponents suggest biofeedback enables the patient to objectively measure individual relaxation progress. Evidence suggests that biofeedback in conjunction with relaxation reduces the severity and frequency of muscle contraction or "tension" headaches, migraine headaches, and low-back pain. Unfortunately, poorly designed or underpowered studies outnumber more rigorous controlled studies, making it difficult to quantify the benefits of any particular relaxation technique.

Distraction Therapies

Any activity that cognitively refocuses attention to stimuli other than pain can serve as a therapeutic distraction. The most effective distractions are those that are interesting to and appropriate for the patient situation, as well as those that engage the widest range of senses. Large wall murals of nature scenes, for example, coupled with headphone-delivered nature sounds have been used to distract patients undergoing bronchoscopy and dental procedures, as well as during childbirth. Other techniques that can be used to cognitively refocus or distract patients in pain include many initiated by the patient, such as watching television, reading, doing puzzles or crafts, listening to music, and making phone calls or otherwise engaging in conversation. Nurses also use these same techniques to therapeutically distract patients. **Music therapy**, for example, is very versatile. Patients passively listen to music that they find enjoyable or relaxing; some patients use music to support meditation or use music to help them form distracting mental images. Some patients sing to distract, whereas others use music as a creative diversion for their pain by writing or performing music. Music is used to specifically manage the pain associated with headaches and childbirth and the pain associated with both cancer and cancer treatment. Humor is also used to distract patients in pain, whether it is watching a funny video of a favorite comedy routine, watching cartoons for children, or reading a funny story. Well-controlled studies of experimental pain demonstrate that humor increases the threshold and tolerance for both cold and pressure pain. Humor has a similar effect on pain threshold as on relaxation, so it is suggested that humor, or more critically, laughing, may be more of a relaxation technique than a distraction technique.

Guided imagery is a technique that therapeutically uses the patient's imagination to create mental pictures or situations that are soothing, relaxing, or pain relieving. Some practitioners describe guided imagery as helping patients to daydream in a very deliberative way, whereas others describe guided imagery as a form of self-hypnosis. Generally, patients being guided through the imagining process begin by closing their eyes and focusing on an image. This image is anything the patient finds useful, such as imagining a ball of healing energy or imagining their pain as electrical wires that can be cut. Other patients find that reliving a pleasant memory or imagining a visit to a favorite place distracts their attention from pain. **Meditation** is a related distraction technique in which patients focus their attention on a healing place or person. This healing place or person may have a religious or spiritual significance to the patient, and specific breathing or chanting phrases are used to achieve an altered state of peaceful contentment. Although some patients use meditation techniques to specifically divert attention away from painful or unpleasant situations, other patients practice meditation daily as a way of providing more consistent healing energy and a sense of peace in their lives, increasing the effectiveness of other pain management interventions. Evidence suggests that most distraction techniques work best for helping patients through an uncomfortable procedure or helping bridge the interval between receiving pain medication and when pain medicine takes full effect. Although distraction techniques are thought to be less effective for treating chronic or complex pain syndromes, some patients report sustained relief over several hours or as long as the techniques are in use. However, pain returns near or at previous levels when distraction techniques are no longer being used. Some patients also report feeling more tired and irritable after distraction sessions longer than 45 minutes to 1 hour.

Hypnosis is described as a special guided state of consciousness in which the focus of attention is therapeutically narrowed and the patient is believed to be more responsive to hypnotic suggestions. Proponents suggest that any patient can be placed in a state of altered or hypnotic consciousness, whereas others suggest that relatively few patients respond to hypnotic techniques, including specific relaxation exercises, the use of guided visualization imagery, and the shaping of expectations through hypnotic suggestion. There is considerable evidence from positron emission tomography that hypnosis may inhibit thalamic–somatosensory cortex pain pathways that are believed to be involved in the cognitive perception of pain. Hypnosis is used to treat the pain associated with burns and burn treatment, cancer, dental care, childbirth, and headache and following thoracic and abdominal surgery. Many of these nonpharmacological pain management techniques fall under the umbrella of complementary and alternative medicine (CAM), and the reader is referred to Chapter 12 for a broader discussion of CAM therapies.

Prayer

Prayer means different things to different people, and even patients who do not describe themselves as very religious often find a sense of peace and spiritual connection to all that is around them through the process of prayer. Patients may pray for improved health or a cure, or they may pray for the strength to endure suffering and limitations. For many patients, prayer is a way to feel less vulnerable, fearful, and isolated or to take back some of the control they feel they may have lost because of pain and illness. In many religions, prayer is used to establish a necessary connection with a higher power so that healing can happen. In this same way, patients pray for their caregivers to use their knowledge, skills, and technology for healing. For other patients, prayer and faith are not engaged with the expectation of a cure, but they do help to create positive energy to support healing. Prayer also has been used to relax the body, helping to create a more positive healing environment. Some religions use intercessory prayer, the prayer of strangers from a distance, to help channel healing energy toward someone who is ill in addition to private prayer.

Just as the importance of spirituality, prayer, and religion varies from patient to patient, health providers themselves have different spiritual and religious beliefs and differ among themselves as to how important spiritual beliefs are to healing. The intersection of religion and healthcare can be uncomfortable for healthcare professionals. Nurses are taught about different religions and cultures, with an emphasis on the importance of respecting beliefs and cultural traditions. However, nurses often find themselves in awkward patient care situations because they are unsure of how their own beliefs may support or conflict with those of their patients. Nurses may also find it challenging to support a patient's beliefs that are contradicted by provable science. Nurses or physicians may be asked to pray with patients or be asked if prayer can make a difference. Reflecting techniques can be helpful, with offers to provide support in any way patients find useful. Institutional resources such as chaplaincy services or outreach to spiritual contacts in the patient's home community can also help patients find prayer resources.

Invasive Treatment Options

Transcutaneous Electrical Nerve Stimulation

Transcutaneous electrical nerve stimulation (TENS) is an older nonpharmacological intervention used to treat postoperative pain, osteoarthritis, and chronic musculoskeletal pain. Transcutaneous electrical nerve stimulation is used under provider direction and by specially trained practitioners. Although the exact mechanism of action of TENS is not clearly understood, it is thought to interfere or compete with pain transmission or to stimulate nonpain receptors in the same location of the pain. Transcutaneous electrical nerve stimulation units (Fig. 11.9) are battery operated and have electrodes that are placed directly on the skin to produce tingling and vibratory sensations to decrease pain. Research continues to determine the exact mechanism of action of this therapy, as well as to determine the effectiveness of high- or low-intensity stimulation.

Deep Brain Stimulation

Used in the treatment of intractable pain for more than 50 years, deep brain stimulation (DBS) is often effective in selectively chosen patients. This nonpharmacological treatment for pain requires provider oversight, including the surgical implantation of brain pacemakers that send electrical impulses to specific parts of the brain. Consisting of three components, the DBS system includes an implanted pulse generator, the lead, and the extension, which are surgically placed. The lead is placed under local anesthesia through a hole that is drilled in the skull. The lead connects

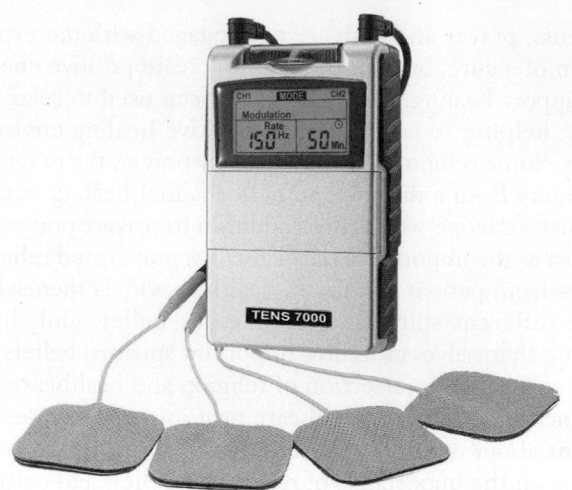

FIGURE 11.9 Transcutaneous electrical nerve stimulation (TENS) unit. The TENS unit is thought to work by interfering or competing with pain transmission or stimulating nonpain receptors in the same location as the pain. The units are battery operated, and electrodes are placed directly on the skin to produce tingling and vibratory sensations to decrease pain.

to the pulse generator by the extension that runs down the side of the head and neck, where it is placed subcutaneously below the clavicle. The patient must be awake during the procedure to test the electrical impulses for therapeutic effects. Deep brain stimulation is also used in the treatment of tremors in patients with Parkinson's disease.

Managing Pain and Pain Relief Expectancy

One of the more significant insights gained over the last decade in assessing and managing pain, including lessons learned through the overprescribing of opioids, is that clinicians have communicated to patients in ways both subtle and explicit that the goal of pain management is the relief of all pain. When patients rate their pain on a scale of 0 to 10, with 0 as the state of being in no pain and 10 being the worst pain they have experienced, the message patients receive is that a pain score of 0 is a desirable state to be attained. This **expectancy** of no pain often has antecedents in a preoperative visit where surgeons indicate that there will be some pain but that it can be relieved by pain medication, with encouragement to take pain medication as prescribed for their maximal comfort. Additionally, the no-pain message is reinforced by policies and procedures that include pain assessment with each vital sign assessment and follow up after medication is delivered to determine pain relief effectiveness. Mass-marketing messaging and advertising for pain medications also emphasize that pain is something to be extinguished as opposed to being managed as a part of life and work.

Recent research has identified the powerful role that reality-informed expectations of pain levels on analgesia can have in managing the pain experience. A profound change in pain management philosophy is the shift from an approach focused on the relief of all pain to an approach in which pain

is expected and in which the therapeutic goal of pain management is improved comfort. Much of this philosophical shift can be traced to a more complete understanding of both the **placebo** and **nocebo** effects. Aside from its use as a control in clinical trials, the placebo effect has often been narrowly and historically defined as the substitution of an inert substance for one that is pharmacologically active, with therapeutic effectiveness derived from convincing patients that they received the pharmacologically active agent. Any positive therapeutic benefit that was achieved was often taken as mistaken evidence that the underlying condition was not real. A more evidence-supported understanding defines the placebo effect as the positive cognitive modulation of behaviors and outcomes related to therapeutic treatment, with the nocebo effect referring to the negative modulation of behaviors and outcomes.

As early as the 1970s, evidence from studies in both animal and human subjects supported the role that opioid receptors play in the placebo effect. It was demonstrated that conditioning or training a subject to associate an external cue or tone with the delivery of analgesia and then the replacement of the analgesic with a saline solution paired with the same external cue would produce analgesia. That this analgesic effect could be blocked by pretreatment with an opioid-receptor blocker, like naloxone, implies that the saline, although not a pharmacological analgesic, was not inert. In this cueing-conditioning context, saline functioned as an analgesic based on how this substance worked with engaged brain regions to produce analgesia. More recent research has expanded the understanding of the involvement of more extensive brain regions in the placebo and nocebo effects, with broader receptor engagement throughout the brain.

There are many examples in clinical care where the placebo and nocebo effects shape an outcome, but the explicit connection between clinician cueing behavior and analgesic outcome has not been universally embraced as a therapeutic intervention. It is common, for example, to explain to patients that they will "feel a pinch" prior to phlebotomy, or to frame the resetting of a dislocated shoulder as a very painful, if temporary pain. In this way, clinicians communicate an expectancy of pain that has a link to a real-world experience. Pain expectancy, however, can also be shaped by forces outside the clinician. A patient, for example, who watches another patient have a smooth and relatively pain-free phlebotomy will be cued to expect a relatively low-pain phlebotomy experience, especially when reinforced through clinician cuing. Conversely, patients who enter the labor suite cued by family members and friends to expect labor to be painful may be less amenable to clinician cuing.

There is great potential in taking a more intentioned and collaborative approach to shaping pain expectancy and clinician cuing. Care providers across the continuum of care need to be consistent with shaping expectancy for pain experiences, including building new pain communication skill sets, with the goal being the communication of a more reality-based description of expected pain levels and a realistic outcome for analgesia interventions aimed at improving comfort and reducing but not eliminating pain.

MANAGING PAIN IN SPECIAL POPULATIONS

Managing Pain in Older Adults

Pain is such a common experience for older adults that it is often viewed and even dismissed as inevitable by both patients and caregivers alike (see Evidence-Based Practice: Educating Patients for Self-Management of Acute and Chronic Pain). Fear of addiction and oversedation and a misunderstanding of the mixed-pain conditions that most older adults experience lead to significant underdiagnosis, undertreatment, and needless suffering. Even experienced clinicians mistakenly assume older adults are more tolerant of or less sensitive to pain and that opioids should be the treatment of last resort. Ineffective pain management, however, is more likely to contribute to depression, anxiety, impaired mobility, social isolation, falls, sleep disturbances, reduced food and fluid intake, and malnutrition in older adults than in younger adults. This is often exacerbated by the costs of medications and insurer regulations that require high co-pays or limit prescriber treatment options. Older adult patients, however, are eight times as likely as the general adult population to live with a painful chronic health problem. Inflammatory conditions such as osteoarthritis affect up to 80% of older adults. Musculoskeletal pain commonly accompanies age-related changes in bone density, disk compression, and posture. Circulatory problems lead to fatigue, muscle cramps, aching vascular pain in the lower extremities, and sores that are slow to heal. Medication side effects and dental problems are also significant sources of orofacial pain.

Evidence-Based Practice

Educating Patients for Self-Management of Acute and Chronic Pain

- Patients need a realistic view of the type and intensity of pain they can anticipate with specific procedures or after traumatic injuries to better self-manage pain.
- Give patients multiple pain relief options to choose from and written guidelines on when each may be used to maximal effectiveness.
- Use more than single-dimension pain scales to help patients better qualify the impact of their pain; then help them define specific goals. Beyond reducing the level of pain, patients may find that improving the quality of their sleep is how they want to measure the success of their self-management.

- Provide written instructions on how to safely dose primary and adjuvant medications.
- Instruct patients on how to use nonpharmacological therapeutic options, including the application of heat/cold, relaxation techniques, and physical exercise.
- Provide patients with the Web addresses of reliable pain management information and resources; caution patients to evaluate "sure-fire" pain cures with a skeptical eye.
- Refer patients who are unable to achieve pain relief through self-management to reputable pain specialists who can recommend more aggressive therapeutic approaches.

American Pain Society. (2008). *Principles of analgesic use in the treatment of acute pain and cancer pain* (6th ed.). Glenview, IL: Author. Boyers, D., McNamee, P., Clark, A., Jones, D., Martin, D., Schofield, P., & Smith, B. (2013). Cost effectiveness of self-management methods for the treatment of chronic pain in an aging adult population: A systematic review of the literature. *Clinical Journal of Pain, 29*(4), 366–375.

There is a wide range of treatment options for managing pain in older adults, and often, utilizing multiple approaches leads to the best outcomes. Combining nonsteroidal anti-inflammatory medications and heat application to arthritic joints with a focused stretching and exercise regimen improves functional mobility, pain, and social engagement. Relaxation training combined with deep massage and antispasm medications is effective at relieving lower back pain. Acupressure, guided imagery, and music therapy have proved beneficial for older patients with severe orofacial pain. Although many of the same treatment options available to the wider populations of patients in pain can be used with older adults, adjustments in either dose or treatment intensity are often required to accommodate age-related changes in pharmacokinetics, pharmacodynamics, and general physiology. Doses of many medications, including NSAIDs, opioids, and steroids, need to be lowered or the frequency of administration adjusted to accommodate reduced kidney and liver function. Many older patients have comorbid health conditions and take other medications. The risk of potentially dangerous drug–drug interactions significantly increases with the addition of even one new medication, with NSAIDs particularly likely to interfere with common medications such as anticoagulants, thiazide diuretics, and both angiotensin-converting enzyme (ACE) inhibitors and calcium-channel blockers. An aging vascular system is less responsive to changes in temperature, and so applications of heat and cold, as well as therapeutic positioning, need to be shorter and very closely supervised to avoid the potential for injury.

Clinicians need to be vigilant to the development of adverse effects. Constipation, for example, is a more common response to opioids in older adults than in the general adult population but can be prevented or reduced in severity through adjustments in diet and exercise. Respiratory depression occurs at the same frequency in older adults as in the general population of adults; however, it may present at lower doses and last longer because of changes in the metabolism of medication. Confusion and delirium are much more common reactions to opioids in older adults than even respiratory depression, and keeping patients safe from injury and falls is critical.

Managing Pain in Adults With Cognitive or Communication Impairments

Although less than 20% of older Americans live in institutional settings such as assisted living or nursing homes, more than half of those who are in eldercare settings have cognitive impairments and dementia, challenging both assessment and treatment. This population more regularly interacts with nursing assistants and technicians who lack access to more effective assessment tools and adequate training to assess pain, leading to misconceptions that patients with dementia or patients with low cognitive skills do not experience pain. The blunted affect and nonexpressive facial expressions of many cognitively impaired patients lead caregivers to assume that the patient is not experiencing pain, especially if there is no clinical presentation that exhibits "typical" acute pain behaviors, such as groaning, grimacing, or muscle guarding. Given the prevalence of persistent and chronic pain in institutionalized older adults and the increasing presence of cognitively impaired patients in the general hospital population, there is no reason to assume that there is less pain in adults with cognitive impairment. Neurophysiological testing confirms that most cognitively impaired patients, including those with Alzheimer's, have an intact somatosensory cortex and can receive and process painful stimuli, although they may have difficulty understanding, interpreting, and communicating pain.

Assessing pain in the cognitively impaired adult requires a systematic approach and thorough documentation of assessment techniques and assessment results. Because attention and clarity of thought can vary by time of day and can be affected by medications, surroundings, and care routines, pain assessment should begin with an attempt at self-report. Tests of cognition such as the Mini-Mental State Examination, the Abbreviated Mental Test Score, or the St. Louis Mental Assessment can predict the ability to self-report. Patients who are verbal but cognitively impaired can reliably use more concrete visual analog scales to identify their pain, although they may have difficulty remembering previous self-reports and so may not be able to quantify whether they are feeling "better" or more comfortable following treatment.

If patients are not able to provide a verbal report, caregivers should systematically search for a potential cause for pain, beginning with a review of diagnoses, health issues, and procedure exposure. Cognitively impaired patients with wounds, arthritis, and cancer are as likely to have pain as cognitively intact elders, so the presence of pain should be assumed and treated accordingly. Similarly, cognitively impaired patients undergoing chemotherapy, rehabilitation activities, or diagnostic procedures should also be assumed to be in pain and appropriately proactively treated. If there are no known painful conditions or diagnostic activities, other physiologically distressful situations should be assessed and treated appropriately. For example, bed-bound patients should be repositioned, and all skin sites vulnerable to breakdown should be assessed. Ambulatory patients should have the fit of clothing assessed; belts or shoes that are too tight or the presence of clothing tags can cause unintentional distress. All patients should be toileted as part of the assessment process to be sure that undiagnosed continence issues or constipation are not causing pain or distress. A physical examination should survey each body area, moving each joint through passive and active ROM, with observations of differences in affect, mood, or nonverbal body signaling of discomfort. Special assessment attention should be focused on the most common sites of pain in older adults: the knee, hip, hands, and lower back. Hands-on assessments of joints and body regions are also likely to identify redness, heat, or other signs of inflammation or infection.

Observations of patient behavior, noting changes from baseline or routinely exhibited behaviors, can reliably indicate distress and pain in cognitively impaired patients, especially in settings where patients are regularly observed by the same caregivers or family members. Behavioral observations can be less reliable in hospitalized settings, where patients find themselves out of the structure of their normal routines, surrounded by unfamiliar noises and caregivers. Several dementias, including mid-stage Alzheimer's, are associated with "wandering" or "compelled walking" behaviors that hospital personnel worry will lead to falls or elopement. Physical or chemical restraints can exacerbate distress or mask pain, and clinicians must balance the need for patient safety with humane behavioral approaches to managing cognitive pathophysiology. Each cognitively impaired patient's behavioral responses to distress and pain are unique. Some patients may refuse food or withdraw from care and caregivers. Other patients may become belligerent, swear, or be physically violent. There is no set of behaviors that can reliably reflect pain intensity. These can be some of the most challenging patients for whom bedside hospital clinicians provide care.

Assessment skills that work with more cognitively intact patients are not reliably effective with cognitively impaired patients. Altered physiological parameters such as elevated blood pressure, heart rate, or respiratory patterns also do not reliably reflect pain in the presence of chronic or persistent pain; nervous systems have largely attenuated to painful input and do not fluctuate as predictably with pain. Patients with altered interaction patterns do not reliably respond to caring, nurturing caregiver behaviors. Nurses who are used to acknowledgments of their caring activities can be put off when cognitively impaired patients do not "give something back." It can be easy to become desensitized to the "yelling," plaintive calls for help, or quiet withdrawal of cognitively impaired patients and communicate to other caregivers this desensitization in reports with comments such as "He is a biter" or "She always yells like that."

Establishing a behavioral baseline is critical to pain assessment. Often, family members or caregivers from their regular care environment can provide behavioral details that provide this baseline to guide subsequent assessments. A comprehensive baseline should include behavioral patterns at rest and with activity. Behaviors that are more commonly associated with discomfort include guarding or bracing. Patients may be observed rubbing or massaging a body part. Some patients display escalating repetitive motions, such as clenching and unclenching a fist, tapping their hands or feet, or rocking. Facial expressions may change, with an increase in frowning, grimacing, brow furrowing, or clenching of teeth. Some patients may cry, yell, or become verbally abusive. Documentation of behavioral patterns helps subsequent clinicians understand the relationship between behavioral patterns and discomfort and be better prepared to intervene.

There are several instruments in development for use in both acute and long-term care. Most of these tools are measures of behavioral change suggesting pain or discomfort, but significantly, they do not measure pain intensity. The most widely used tools include the Pain Assessment in Advanced Dementia Scale, which summarizes behaviors into five pain indicators, and the Checklist of Nonverbal Pain Indicators, which sorts behaviors into six pain indicators (see Evidence-Based Practice: Assessing Pain in Cognitively Impaired Adults).

Evidence-Based Practice

Assessing Pain in Older Adults With Cognitive Impairments

Although pain assessment in older adults is sometimes challenging, individuals with moderate to severe dementia often self-report pain. This study evaluated self-reported, nurse-reported, and observational pain tools in a convenience sample of 156 older adults admitted to an acute geriatric ward. Observational pain was assessed through the Pain Assessment in Advanced Dementia (PAINAD) tool, and cognition and mood were evaluated with the Mini-Mental State Examination (MMSE) and the Geriatric Depression Scale (GDS015). Findings included statistically significant correlations between self-reported pain and the GDS-15 but not between self-reported pain and the MMSE. There was moderate agreement between self-reported pain and the PAINAD and fair agreement between self-reported pain and nurse-reported pain. The results of this study support the use of self-reported pain assessment data first in adults with cognitive impairment, with the use of an observational assessment tool when the individual is unable to self-report pain.

Ngu, S. S. C., Tan, M. P., Subramanian, P., Rahman, R. A., Kamaruzzaman, S., Chin, A., & Poi, P. J. H. (2015). Pain assessment using self-reported, nurse-reported, and observational pain assessment tools among older adults with cognitive impairment. *Pain Management in Nursing, 16*(4), 595–601.

If painful conditions are present or behavioral changes indicate that distress or pain is likely, nonpharmacological interventions and an analgesic trial are recommended. Nonopioid analgesics including NSAIDs should be considered first-line therapy, administered on a standing schedule rather than a prn schedule. Nonverbal or cognitively impaired patients may not be able to request pain medications. Psychotropic medications should be avoided if possible because they may blunt the behavioral evidence of pain without providing pain relief or may sedate the patient, making serial monitoring of behavior more challenging. Opioids can be safely administered to older and cognitively impaired patients but may require starting at lowered doses and titrating carefully to monitor for risks and side effects. Short-acting opioids are preferred if the patient's previous exposure to opioids is unknown because shorter half-lives allow for safer titration to manage pain. Hydromorphone and fentanyl are the preferred opioids in older adults with kidney or liver impairment, whereas meperidine should be avoided because of the adverse effects associated with a toxic metabolite, normeperidine. Similarly, propoxyphene (Darvon) has been associated with neuroexcitatory side effects, including dizziness and ataxia, in older patients. Carefully assess and document the behavioral response to interventions. Changes in behavior consistent with less discomfort and the reestablishment of baseline behaviors should be positive indicators that pain was present and that some measure of pain relief has been established.

Other therapies proven effective for managing pain in cognitively impaired adults include a tailored plan of physical activity and cognitive-behavioral therapy (CBT). Too often, cognitively impaired patients are restricted to their rooms or to their beds to ensure their safety, when safe outcomes are more likely if patients are out of their rooms and able to participate in regular physical activity. A physical therapist should be consulted to help design an activity schedule that exercises the full range of joints and promotes muscle strength and balance. Critical to the success of any activity plan of care is the incorporation of exercise into the daily routine. When administered by trained clinicians, CBT can help cognitively impaired patients replace ineffective behaviors with new behaviors that help focus their understanding of their situation and provide clinicians with new behavioral problem-solving strategies. Although this approach is more effective in outpatient or long-term settings, nurses in inpatient settings should avail themselves of nurse consultants who specialize in geriatric or cognitive impairments for care recommendations.

Making Connections

CASE STUDY: WRAP-UP

The assessment of Mrs. Jessup reveals that gas exchange and airway clearance are compromised, as is her quality of sleep. Her mobility is also compromised by persistent low-back pain following a preexisting back injury. Nursing diagnoses that focus the care Mrs. Jessup receives include:

1. **Ineffective respiratory function** related to positional guarding and shallow respiratory pattern secondary to surgically induced tissue trauma and reflex muscle spasm across thorax as evidenced by oxygen saturation values 92% to 94% on 3 L via nasal cannula, incentive spirometry volume at 450 mL, diminished breath sounds at the bases bilaterally to auscultation, and radiology reports of atelectasis in bases

2. **Disturbed sleep patterns** related to pain secondary to surgical incisions and lower-back injury exacerbated by frequent care interruptions associated with the hospital stay and medication side effects of diuretic use as evidenced by self-report of poor-quality sleep, nurse report of shortened sleep intervals of 1 to 2 hours overnight, and nurse report of total sleep hours less than 4 hours overnight

3. **Impaired mobility** related to chronic lower back pain secondary to preexisting traumatic injury exacerbated by neuropathic sensory dysfunction in feet and lower extremities as evidenced by observed inability to self-position to seated position with legs dangling; self-report of inability to bear weight on both feet simultaneously because of leg pain and weakness; and can ambulate no farther than 3 feet, requiring the assistance of two caregivers

Mrs. Jessup continues to rehabilitate from her coronary bypass surgery and is discharged to an inpatient rehabilitation facility that can address both her cardiac and chronic back pain issues. The plan is for her to be in the inpatient facility for 5 to 7 days and then be discharged to home. The goals are to increase her comfort and maximize her independence in activities of daily living.

Case Study Questions

1. What clinical manifestations can the nurse use to indicate the level of Mrs. Jessup's pain on a.m. assessment? *(Select all that apply.)*
   A. A subjective report of 6/10 pain level; shallow, guarded breathing; short, terse responses to questions
   B. Mrs. Jessup's report of poor overnight sleep and decreased supported ambulation
   C. Facial grimacing and observed rubbing of lower back and legs by patient
   D. Decrease in blood pressure
   E. Increased urinary frequency

2. The nurse correlates Ms. Jessup's clinical presentation with which type of pain?
   A. Acute pain
   B. Chronic pain
   C. Mixed acute and chronic pain
   D. Malignant chronic pain

3. Which pain management approach is best for Mrs. Jessup?
   A. NSAIDs and opioid medications, cold application to the back, supported ambulation, and distraction
   B. Aspirin and opioid medications, heat application to the chest and back, bedrest, and Reiki therapy
   C. Opioid medication, prayer, and music therapy
   D. TCA, TENS, and guided imagery

4. What is the best physiological explanation of why Mrs. Jessup may be experiencing chronic back pain?
   A. The injury she has in her back has just never healed.
   B. Non-nociceptive pain messaging has overtaken nociceptive pain messaging.
   C. Hyperexcited neurons at the time of injury created new pathological synaptic connections that persist.
   D. Chronic inflammation has reduced the effectiveness of descending inhibitory pathways.

5. What is the rationale for using ketorolac as the preferred NSAID to treat Mrs. Jessup?
   A. It is both high potency and has a long half-life for less breakthrough pain.
   B. It targets both prostaglandins and leukotrienes.
   C. It does not cause respiratory depression or constipation.
   D. It can be given every hour as needed to manage pain.

CHAPTER SUMMARY

Pain is a very individualized experience, and people with the same injuries or disease processes may exhibit very different clinical manifestations of pain. For many patients, the source of their pain can be readily identified, diagnosed, and treated. For other patients, the pathology underlying their pain is difficult to diagnose and to treat. Many factors shape the pain experience, including a patient's prior experience with pain as well as expectations for painful procedures and conditions. Other sociocultural and biological influences also shape the pain experience, including gender, genetics, ethnicity, and age. Females and males generally experience pain in different ways, with some pain conditions more prevalent in one as compared to another, whereas older patients generally present with more complex, mixed pain.

Acute pain serves a biological purpose, alerting to noxious and potentially tissue-injuring conditions and prompting tissue-protecting withdrawal and guarding behaviors. Chronic pain serves no similar biological function, representing true pathology and dysfunction in pain-processing structures. Painful sensations largely begin in peripheral tissues innervated by a fine network of nerves that transmit electrochemical messages to the spinal cord and brain. Some of these nerves carry proprioceptive and touch sensations. Specialized nerves that sense and transmit pain messages are called nociceptors. Some nociceptors respond to painful heat or cold, prick, or pressure, whereas others respond to noxious acidic and basic conditions in the tissues. With tissue injury comes a local release of pain-promoting substances, including prostaglandin and histamine. These substances sensitize peripheral tissues, amplifying the pain messages being sent to the central nervous system. Once in the spinal cord, incoming pain messages are processed and transmitted up the spinal cord and through serial regions of the brain, where pain is consciously perceived in the cerebral cortex. Descending pathways move through many of these same brain structures, returning to the spinal cord. It is in the spinal cord where incoming pain messages from the periphery are integrated with descending modulating pain messages to produce a neurophysiological pain response.

The peripheral sensitization that follows injury can lead to hyperexcited and sustained painful input into the spinal cord, sensitizing central neurons in the spinal cord and brain as well. Sensitized central neurons respond by producing more pro- and anti-nociceptive neurotransmitters. This hyperexcited nervous system alters nerve-to-nerve contact at the level of individual synapses. Some synapses die back while others newly form, altering the balance of excitation and inhibition in pain processing. This reorganization of synapses or plasticity at the level of the spinal cord is generally normal and adaptive in injury and illness. For some patients, however, this reorganization of synapses leads to dysfunctional synaptic connections forming, creating a long-lasting rerouting of pain messages, essentially a "cellular memory" for pain that can linger long after injuries heal and that can be very difficult to treat. Pain often accompanies many chronic illnesses such as arthritis and cancer. The most challenging pain conditions to manage follow injury to nociceptive structures, including the peripheral nerves, spinal cord, and brain.

Comprehensive pain assessments are essential to the nursing care of patients experiencing pain. There are many valid and reliable tools that have been developed to assess pain; these include relatively easy-to-administer numeric, verbal, and visual scales where patients can indicate pain intensity as well as their response to therapeutic interventions. For some populations with low verbal or abstract reasoning skills, such as children or cognitively impaired adults, cartoonlike scales display increasingly grimacing faces to represent different levels of pain intensity. Such tools can be helpful in measuring acute pain serially for one patient, although they can be less useful when measuring chronic pain or the mixed pain that most patients actually experience. In complex pain situations, it is often helpful to combine several scales to measure more than one dimension of pain, including how deep the pain is and how pain functionally disrupts lives. Pain assessments are culturally sensitive, and the use of any tools in pain assessment should be subject to rigorous review for use with special populations.

Nurses have the responsibility of recognizing the impact of clinical manifestations of pain on functioning and well-being. They are uniquely positioned in the healthcare system at the front lines of patient care to implement a tailored plan of care. Treatment options include a wide range of pharmacological and nonpharmacological interventions. For most patients in acute pain, NSAIDs or acetaminophen (Tylenol) is an effective first-line medication. These are easily accessible as over-the-counter (OTC) remedies and can be supplemented with OTC topical rubs, heating pads, or ice. Opioids are stronger medications available through provider prescription and are well suited to manage the pain associated with acute pain following traumatic injury, surgery, or dental pain. Opioids are also effective at managing the progressive chronic malignant pain that often accompanies cancer. The WHO advocates a stepwise approach to pain management that pairs nonsteroidal anti-inflammatory medications with progressively more potent narcotic medications as pain becomes more severe. Nurses should work collaboratively with the interdisciplinary team to integrate new classes of targeted pain medications, including sodium and calcium channel blockers as well as medications that act to alter neurotransmitter levels in the brain.

Nonpharmacological interventions include the selective use of heat and cold, positioning for comfort, and massage therapy. A team approach to pain management may include targeted physical therapy as well as a full range of CAM methods, including the skilled use of therapeutic touch or Reiki therapy, relaxation, hypnosis, acupressure, and aromatherapy. Special populations of patients challenge assessment and pain management, especially patients who are cognitively impaired. Family members and caregivers can aid in establishing a baseline and often provide context for atypical pain behaviors. A comprehensive use of stepwise

NSAID and opioids combined with CAM methods can reduce pain and improve quality of life for those with cognitive impairments or at the end of life. Effective pain management balances pain relief and functional improvement with the management of therapeutic side effects. Nurses need to monitor laboratory values, including kidney and liver function, and be alert to potentiated or reduced effectiveness of other medications because of drug–drug interactions. Although nurses do need to be alert to oversedation and the development of tolerance with some opioid medications, nurses also need to advocate for opioid use with patients and providers alike.

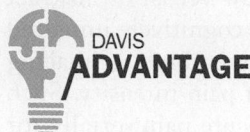

DAVIS ADVANTAGE

To explore learning resources for this chapter, go to **Davis Advantage** and find:
- Answers to in-text questions
- Chapter Resources and Activities
- NCLEX®-Style Chapter Review Questions
- Bibliography

Chapter 12

Complementary and Alternative Care Initiatives

Susan Sartorius-Mergenthaler

LEARNING OUTCOMES

Content in this chapter is designed to assist in:

1. Defining complementary and alternative medicine
2. Differentiating the classifications of complementary and alternative medicine
3. Discussing the nursing implications of complementary and alternative medicine

CONCEPTS

- Assessment
- Comfort
- Healthcare System
- Medication
- Nursing
- Nursing Role
- Promoting Health

ESSENTIAL TERMS

Acupuncture
Chiropractic medicine
Complementary and alternative medicine (CAM)
Conventional medicine
Holistic care
Integrative medicine
National Center for Complementary and Integrative Health (NCCIH)
Western medicine

Finding Connections

CASE STUDY: EPISODE 1

Follow this patient throughout the chapter.

Ms. E. Ellicott is a 52-year-old woman with a new diagnosis of hypertension. Her medical history is unremarkable except for occasional migraines. She states that her 82-year-old mother recently had a stroke and is recuperating at an inpatient rehabilitation center. Ms. Ellicott is an only child, and her mother lives 3 hours away. She is married and has two children, a 16-year-old girl and a 12-year-old boy. She is currently employed as a district attorney. Her husband owns a software company. Assessment: vital signs (VSs): temperature (T): 99.5°F (37.5°C), heart rate (HR): 80, respiratory rate (RR): 20, blood pressure (BP): 150/98. She is currently not taking medications. She states to the nurse that she is feeling overwhelmed with the new diagnosis of hypertension and the fact that her mother recently had a stroke…

INTRODUCTION

Conventional medicine, also known as **Western medicine**, is the dominant healthcare system in the United States, Canada, and most of Europe. Conventional medicine is a well-established, organized system that is rooted in scientifically proven theories. It is practiced by licensed providers, nurses, physical therapists and occupational therapists, social workers, and other allied healthcare professionals. **Complementary and alternative medicine (CAM)** is a collection of old-world traditions and healthcare practices that have been handed down through the generations. The therapies and products that are recognized as CAM are rooted in ancient wisdom traditions, folklore, and religious and spiritual practices. These traditional practices and doctrines are based on theoretical foundations and are performed by licensed and specially trained practitioners. The CAM model for delivery of care has three guiding principles, all described in Box 12.1.

The goals of CAM include the promotion of wellness, the prevention of illness, a reduction in treatment side effects, improvement of the immune system, and enhancement of quality of life. Although these goals of care are not unlike those of conventional medicine, CAM

Box 12.1 Guiding Principles of Complementary and Alternative Medicine

1. Recipient/Practitioner Partnership
   - Established relationship—builds trust, instills hope
   - Healing takes place in the context of the relationship
   - Treatment design is intrinsic to the holistic care model
2. Wellness Model of Care
   - Emphasizes healthy lifestyle—proactive approach to being well
   - Encourages self-awareness related to changes in the body and interconnectedness with lifestyle choices
   - Uses broad concepts for the promotion of health and wellness for the treatment of disease
3. Energy Paradigm
   - *Health* is defined as harmonious and balanced.
   - *Healing* is defined in the context of the whole person—mind, body, and spirit.
   - The basic theory involves a Life Force or Vital Force called *qi* that permeates and bonds all living things.
   - All living things have a universal spirit and wholeness.

Connection Check 12.1

The defining characteristics of CAM include which of the following? *(Select all that apply.)*
  A. Rooted in scientifically proven theories
  B. Rooted in ancient wisdom traditions
  C. A collection of old-world traditions
  D. A collection of old-world healthcare practices
  E. Works in isolation from conventional medicine

CLASSIFICATION OF CAM

The NCCIH classifies CAM according to specific techniques, methods, and applications. The five categories of CAM are:

1. Whole medical systems/alternative medicine systems
2. Mind/body therapies
3. Manipulative and body-based therapies
4. Energy healing therapies
5. Dietary supplements and botanical/herbal medicine

Whole Medical Systems/Alternative Medical Systems

Whole medical systems/alternative medical systems are time-honored ancient arts and practices with comprehensive methods of care that are used to nurture and promote the healing process. They are complete systems of theory and practice that are rooted in healing traditions. Treatments are personalized according to the physical, emotional, spiritual, religious, nutritional, and environmental needs of the patient. They are helpful in the management of emotional and psychological disorders such as chronic fatigue; stress, anxiety, and depression; symptoms related to menopause; and sleeping problems or insomnia. They are also helpful in the management of pain caused by arthritis, osteoarthritis, fibromyalgia, chronic back pain, carpal tunnel syndrome, migraines, sports injuries, and neuropathy. Examples include Ayurvedic medicine, traditional Chinese medicine, naturopathy, and Native American medicine.

Ayurvedic Medicine

Ayurvedic medicine is a 5,000-year-old integrated, natural medical system that originated in India. It uses a combination of herbs, yoga, massage, and diet to restore balance and wellness. The belief behind this treatment method is that there is an interconnection between the mind and the body. This distinctive connection, when encouraged, will facilitate, maintain, and restore health and well-being. It includes physical, mental, and spiritual practices to maintain inner harmony. The individual is evaluated on the basis of his or her unique, well-defined energy patterns, called *doshas*. According to the pattern of the *doshas*, various modalities are incorporated into a complex change in lifestyle.

healthcare practices are considered outside the sphere of conventional scientific methodologies, hence the terms *alternative* and *unconventional* as an approach to medical treatments. The term *complementary* refers to practices, treatments, or modalities that are stand-alone therapies or therapies that can be paired with conventional medicine to modify, restore, or renew balance; ease symptoms; or improve quality of life.

In 1992, the National Institutes of Health established the Office of Alternative Medicine (OAM) in response to the public's unforeseen and increasing interest in CAM. In 2014, the OAM name was changed to the **National Center for Complementary and Integrative Health (NCCIH)**. The NCCIH has identified pain, anxiety, depression, and headache as being among the top 10 reasons why adults seek CAM as an alternative and complement to managing healthcare needs.

Today, the NCCIH advocates for CAM through scientific, evidence-based research projects and provides a clearinghouse for safe and reliable information related to CAM. The NCCIH makes available academic research opportunities for investigators and offers a variety of educational formats for both healthcare providers and patients. The blending of conventional medicine and CAM is the nucleus of integrative medicine. As the term implies, **integrative medicine** joins together the best of Western medicine and the most effective CAM modalities. Philosophically, the foundation of integrative medicine is that of **holistic care**, treating the individual as a whole person—physically, mentally, and spiritually—to promote optimum health and well-being.

Traditional Chinese Medicine

Traditional Chinese medicine has been practiced for more than 5,000 years. This medical system (also referred to as **acupuncture**) is the oldest and most continuously practiced medicine in the world. The goal of treatment is to sustain the balance, or flow, of *qi*. *Qi* is defined as the universal Life Force or personal life force and is considered the connecting "energy" that influences all living and nonliving things. The flow of *qi* is facilitated by the acupuncturist's point placement of small needles, which are inserted just under the surface of the skin (Fig. 12.1). Each point represents a specific area and normalizes energetic function to stimulate the body's innate power to heal. The modern theory of acupuncture describes certain electrical properties stimulated by the needles, altering neurotransmitters in the body and resulting in changes associated with natural physiological chemicals.

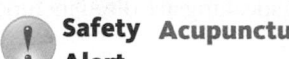

> **Safety Alert** **Acupuncture**
>
> Caution is advised for patients who are receiving chemotherapy and/or taking anticoagulants. Patients are at an increased risk for infection or bleeding under the following conditions:
>
> - Neutropenia (≤ 1,500/mm³)
> - Thrombocytopenia (≤ 50,000/mm³)
> - Elevated liver functions
> - Anticoagulation therapy
>
> Avoid inserting acupuncture needles in or around:
>
> - Radiation site areas
> - Burns
> - Direct tumor sites
> - Fractures
> - Varicose veins
> - Areas of lymphedema

Naturopathy

Naturopathy is a 100-year-old practice that integrates natural therapeutics such as acupuncture, hydrotherapy, manipulative therapy, homeopathy, and botanicals. The focus of care is on supporting health, not combating illness. Naturopathic providers integrate care according to the individual needs of the patient.

Native American Medicine

Native American medicine is a collection of indigenous customs, beliefs, and practices. It is believed that humans, community, and nature are interconnected and that healing must be restored to a state of wholeness to achieve optimal spiritual balance, well-being, and harmony. Native American healing traditions include shamanism, which represents a spiritual practice between the physical and spiritual worlds;

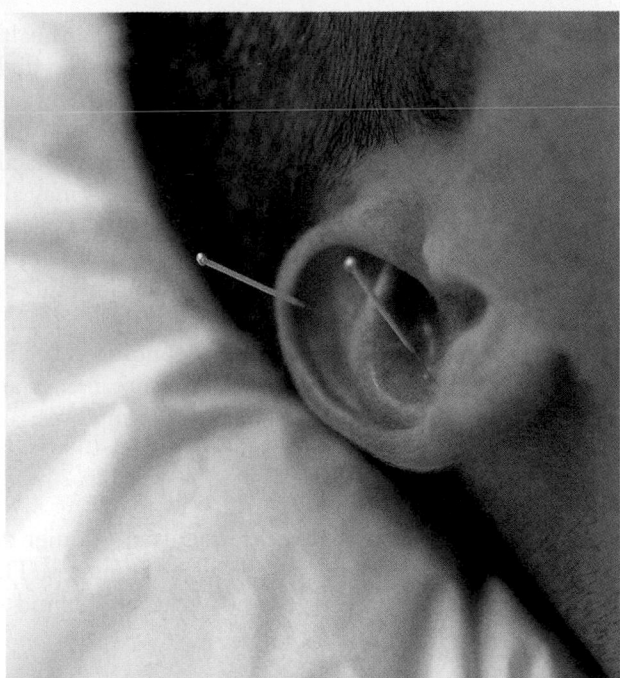

FIGURE 12.1 Auricular acupuncture. Considered microsystems of the body, the ears are used to treat conditions that are present anywhere in the body.

herbal medicine, defined by common practices such as the use of tinctures, salves, and teas; and ceremonial healing practices such as chanting, dancing, and singing to ask for spiritual help and guidance.

CASE STUDY: EPISODE 2

Ms. Ellicott is unsure what to do about her stress, which is related to her new diagnosis of hypertension and her worry for her mom after her stroke. She is so busy with her job and family that she is not sure which way to turn. Looking into acupuncture was recommended by a friend, but she is unsure if she is comfortable with that option. She is unfamiliar with CAM and is unaware of the many different modalities. After opening a discussion with the nurse, she finds she is interested in pursuing some form of alternative medicine as a way of relieving her stress…

Mind/Body Therapies

During the past 30 years, there has been scientific advancement in the field of neuroscience exploring the mind–body connection. It has been discovered that during mind/body treatment techniques, the limbic system and frontal cortex areas of the brain can have significant changes in patterns and functions. Research has shown that mental imagery can produce biochemical, immunological, and physiological changes in the body that have positive effects on health. Meditation, for example, can regulate the fight-or-flight response by slowing the heart, improving blood flow, and increasing the activity of the digestive tract. Many of the mind/body practices can be done in groups led by a facilitator or as a stand-alone practice. Many practices may also incorporate music, chanting, speaking, and reciting, such as prayer/spirituality, yoga, imagery, tai chi, and zero balancing (ZB). Mind/body therapies promote relaxation and are helpful in the management of emotional disorders such as stress, fatigue, and depression; physical conditions such as acute and chronic pain, elevated blood pressure, nausea and vomiting, and menopausal and menstrual symptoms; and nonverbal states by facilitating communication.

Meditation

Meditation is a self-directed technique used to quiet the mind and relax the body toward peace and calmness. This is achieved by closing the eyes and creating a sound or chanting. Methods include:

- Mindfulness meditation, or the practice of focusing on the present moment (Box 12.2)
- Transcendental meditation, or the repetition of a word or sound that has special meaning
- Breath meditation, which focuses on the process of inhaling and exhaling

Box 12.2 Mindfulness

Mindfulness is a practice of focusing active, open attention on the present moment.

A common technique to help engage in mindfulness is to focus on one's breathing, not controlling it but being aware of the natural breathing process. Another technique is focusing on areas of the body or body movements such as walking. While practicing mindfulness, it is not unusual for the mind to wander. When that happens, it is acknowledged in a nonjudgmental, accepting way, and then thoughts are returned to the present and whatever is the focus of the session. The practice of mindfulness can help ease feelings of tension and anxiety. It has been used to treat depression, insomnia, and pain, to name a few. A few practice tips include:

- Find a comfortable, safe place to sit or walk if the movement of the legs and feet is the focus.
- Set time limits when new to the practice (e.g., 5 or 10 minutes).
- Notice your breathing, body, or walking, again focusing on whatever is the emphasis of the session.
- Notice and be nonjudgmental when the mind wanders.
- Come back to the focus of the session.

Mindfulness does not require special equipment, and it can be practiced anywhere if it is safe to do so. If at work and having a stressful day, take a few minutes to be mindful to help ease the tension. Mindfulness can help build resilience in dealing with the everyday, common pressures in the workaday world.

Prayer/Spirituality

Prayer/spirituality is a commonly used practice that provides comfort for those who are ill or in distress and serves as a healing modality to promote empathy, love, and caring. Often used in religious and spiritually based communities, prayer may be done individually or in groups.

Yoga

Yoga is an example of a mind/body practice that incorporates breathing techniques, body movements, forms of exercise, diverse postures, meditation, and chanting. It is used to create a union of the mind, body, and spirit and to increase a sense of awareness and inner peace. Yoga is often used as a technique to quiet the mind and ease thought patterns.

Imagery/Guided Imagery

Another example is imagery, or guided imagery, which is used to promote relaxation and transform attitudes and behaviors. Music, chanting, and speaking are often included to enhance the meditative state.

Tai Chi

Tai chi is an ancient form of Chinese exercise that is considered a martial art; tai chi uses movement to balance the Life Force, or *qi*. It consists of low-impact body movements and breathing techniques that flow into each movement. The gentle, low-impact movements are helpful in reducing stress and alleviating the pain associated with osteoarthritis.

Zero Balancing

The final example in this classification is ZB. Zero balancing uses skilled touch to address the relationship between the energy and structures of the body. Zero balancing focuses primarily on specific skeletal joints that conduct and balance forces of gravity, posture, and movement. When the deepest and most dense tissues are addressed, the energy fields of the body and soft tissue clear or become unblocked, thereby contributing to an increase in vitality and better postural alignment. As with other mind/body therapies, ZB leaves the individual with feelings of calmness and inner peace.

> **! Safety Alert** Consult a provider for physical limitations or mobility restrictions before initiating any mind/body therapies if the following conditions are present:
> - Joint/back problems
> - Recent surgery or back injury
> - Uncontrolled hypertension
> - Glaucoma (some forms of physical activity may increase eye pressure)
> - Pregnancy

Manipulative and Body-Based Therapies

Manipulative and body-based therapies represent the largest, continuously organized complementary care profession. These methods have been used and respected for more than 1,000 years. At one time, a provider's hands were considered his or her greatest assets; Hippocrates discussed the benefits of touch and massage with his students. In the 1800s, Florence Nightingale valued massage as an essential nursing skill, and the first schools of nursing included massage therapy as a foundational skill in the nursing curriculum.

In the manipulative and body-based therapy classification system, practitioners are trained in various body manipulations and techniques, such as massaging or kneading of the body's soft tissues, muscles, tendons, and ligaments to realign the skeletal and lymphatic systems. There are more than 50 practices identified in this classification system, and all require specific training, certification, or state licensure for practice. Two examples of manipulative and body-based practices that are recognized around the world and require advanced degrees are chiropractic medicine and osteopathic medicine.

Manipulative and body-based techniques also incorporate strategies and techniques from mind/body medicine and energy medicine to enhance the overall effectiveness of treatment. In general, the most common use of body-based treatments is for musculoskeletal problems, which include back pain, neck pain, and arthritis. General benefits of manipulative and body-based therapies include enhancing the immune system; facilitating mental clarity and decreasing mental stress; relief of insomnia, asthma symptoms, and muscle tension; relief of nausea associated with chemotherapy; managing blood pressure and heart rate; and reduction of the pain caused by headaches, back and joint disorders, cancer, and surgery.

Massage Therapy

Massage therapy is defined as using one's hands to apply pressure and motion on the skin and underlying muscle of the recipient for the purposes of physical and psychological relaxation. Today, there are more than 30 types of massage therapy techniques, each requiring specific training and having a purpose that is uniquely its own. A few examples include Swedish massage, shiatsu, craniosacral massage, sports massage, and deep connective tissue massage.

Chiropractic Medicine

Chiropractic medicine uses the hands to manipulate the spine and body to restore spinal movement and overall body function. The general theory is that various forms of palpation and specific structural manipulation techniques can repair a dysfunctional relationship between the physical body and the nervous system and restore health. Research continues to sort out the effects of movement and manipulation and the relationship between the nervous system and improved physical functioning.

Osteopathic Medicine

Osteopathic medicine has been a continuous healing method since the late 1800s. It is the process of using one's hands to manipulate and palpate soft tissues, muscles, and bones, moving them in specific ways to bring the body back into optimal function and to restore health.

Reflexology

A unique form of body manipulation is reflexology. Within this specific discipline, it is believed that the body is divided into zones that are located in precise areas along the soles of the feet, the hands, and the ears (Fig. 12.2). Practitioners use various forms of pressure, touch, and manipulative

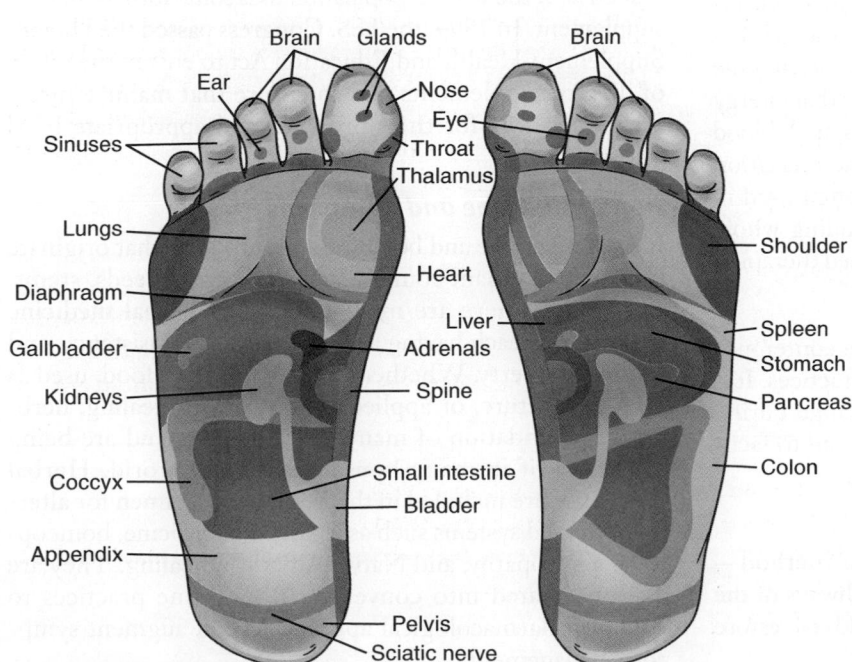

FIGURE 12.2 Reflexology. Reflex points on the soles of the feet that, when skillfully massaged, can relieve tension and treat illness.

techniques directed toward the zone or zones that need to effect physical change.

> **Safety Alert   Massage and body manipulation**
>
> Avoid massage under the following conditions or in the following areas:
>
> ● Radiation sites
> ● Burns
> ● Direct tumor sites
> ● Fractures
> ● Varicose veins
> ● Open wounds
> ● Areas with lymphedema
> ● Contraindicated in patients taking Coumadin (warfarin), Lovenox (enoxaparin injection), and heparin (heparin) products because of increased bleeding risk
> ● Caution during pregnancy—requires certification in pregnancy massage techniques

Energy Healing Therapy

Energy healing therapy is an ancient form of treatment. Energy healing therapy enables or reestablishes the balance or flow of energy, allowing the body to be restored to optimum health. *Energy* is a general term used to explain or describe the body's essence, or inner force. In this form of healing, the practitioner places his or her hands nearby or gently on the individual receiving the treatment to guide the flow of energy. In the 1970s, Dolores Krieger, a registered nurse (RN), introduced therapeutic touch (TT) as part of the nursing curriculum at New York University.

There is little scientific evidence to support the subtle effects of energy healing on the body. However, research has shown its effectiveness in decreasing anxiety and altering the perception of pain. Anecdotal evidence suggests that energy healing is beneficial for such imbalances as stress, high blood pressure, asthma, and pain. It can also promote relaxation and a sense of well-being. Energy healing is often used in combination with other forms of CAM, including whole medical systems and manipulative and body-based therapies.

Therapeutic Touch/Healing Touch

Therapeutic touch (TT), or healing touch, is a contemporary interpretation of several ancient healing practices. It is a consciously directed process of energy exchange during which the practitioner uses the hands to focus and to facilitate the healing process in someone who is ill.

Reiki

Much like TT, Reiki—an ancient Japanese method—disseminates energy along the centers and pathways of the body as a means of manipulating the energy fields to restore health and well-being.

Qi Gong

Breathing and movement add variety to the energy healing method known as *qi gong*, a 3,000-year-old Chinese healing modality. Often practiced in groups and with a skilled healer-facilitator, qi gong uses specific, gentle body movements with particular breathing techniques. This synergistic action allows the restoration of balance.

> **Safety Alert**   As with mind/body therapies, consult a provider for physical limitations or mobility restrictions before initiating any energy healing therapy if the following conditions are present:
>
> ● Joint/back problems
> ● Recent surgery or back injury
> ● Uncontrolled hypertension
> ● Glaucoma (some forms of physical activity may increase eye pressure)
> ● Pregnancy

Dietary Supplements, Herbal Medicine, and Botanicals

Dietary Supplements

Dietary supplements are the most common alternative modality in use today and are used to support the immune system, improve memory, aid digestion, decrease nausea, alleviate cold symptoms, reduce stress, reduce menopausal symptoms, decrease arthritic pain, support heart health, and enhance the condition of the skin and hair. Mineral, vitamin, hormone, and diet-based therapies are also included in this category. The World Health Organization has estimated that 80% of the world's population uses some form of dietary supplement. In 1994, the U.S. Congress passed the Dietary Supplement Health and Education Act to ensure the safety of dietary supplements and to ensure that manufacturers are responsible for their products and appropriate label information.

Herbal Medicine and Botanicals

Herbal medicine and botanicals are products that originate from natural plant sources such as flowers, seeds, stems, and fruits. There are more than 1,000 herbal medicine compounds, each having a unique quality, consistency, and healing property. Whether they are added to food, used as a tea or tincture, or applied to the skin for healing, herbs are the foundation of many CAM systems and are being made use of in many households in the world. Herbal medicines are included in the healthcare regimen for alternative-based systems such as Ayurvedic medicine, homeopathy, naturopathy, and Native American healing. They are also integrated into conventional medicine practices to support pharmacological approaches and augment symptom management.

Specifically, botanicals are used for their scent, flavoring, and healing properties. The term *natural* is often applied to this classification system. As nurses, we must be aware that although something may be a product from natural substances, it is not without potential risks. It is most important to consult an herbalist, naturopath, provider, or pharmacist before taking or applying an herbal or botanical product. Also, before combining herbal products and pharmaceutical products, check with the provider for potential risks of incompatibility and side effects that could cause harm. Benefits of herbal medicine include the management of gastrointestinal problems such as nausea, vomiting, constipation, and diarrhea. It can also help manage cough and congestion as well as pain, poor appetite, and insomnia.

⚠ Safety Alert Consult with a provider, pharmacist, or herbalist before taking, mixing, or combining herbs, botanicals, and vitamins with medications. Serious interactions and complications can occur when using these supplements in combination with pharmaceuticals. Read the label and instructions. Interactions or complications include:
- Allergy to plant content, causing:
  - Systemic effects
  - Local skin irritation
  - Asthma/respiratory distress
- Increased risk of bleeding
- Liver toxicity
- Decreased effectiveness of anesthesia

Connection Check 12.2

The classifications of CAM include which of the following? (*Select all that apply.*)

A. Hypertension prevention
B. Guided imagery
C. Recreational therapy
D. Massage therapy
E. Dietary supplementation

NURSING IMPLICATIONS: ASSESSMENT, EDUCATION, AND RESEARCH

As CAM continues to grow in popularity, it is vital that nurses be knowledgeable about the usefulness, safety, and appropriateness of CAM in order to guide patients through the labyrinth of Western medicine and complementary healthcare choices.

The NCCIH has identified dietary supplements and manipulative and body-based therapies, as well as yoga and mind/body therapies, as the most common CAM modalities

used by adults (Box 12.3). Additionally, 40% of adults use CAM for various illnesses and symptom relief, such as for pain relief, anxiety and depression, and insomnia. Most often, adults choose CAM for its natural characteristics and the quality of care that they receive. Individuals are seeking a value-driven partnership and rapport related to overall healthcare needs, and CAM supports that need as defined by the guiding principles of partnership, wellness, and energy models. A thorough assessment of the patient's attitudes related to CAM is an important first step in establishing a baseline holistic health assessment and building rapport with the patient and the family. Possessing an accepting and respectful communication style will enhance the effectiveness of the assessment and help build a trusting partnership.

Understanding the goals of care and how the patient will benefit from CAM is another component needed in building a foundation for competent, safe nursing care. Patients have constant access to CAM information via the Internet and popular press and through word of mouth. It is the responsibility of the nurse to ensure that patients have an understanding of the principles of CAM, the reasons for choosing CAM, and how the integration of therapies into their plan of care may benefit them. Providing and assisting individuals with finding accurate and reliable Web sites, well-written reading materials, and documented evidence-based research will help them and their family members make well-informed choices. Other information that is vital for patients is how to choose a CAM practitioner. Before treatment, patients may wish to interview CAM practitioners and review their qualifications and credentials. Box 12.4 is a guide to assist patients in finding a qualified and skilled CAM practitioner. Providing the patient with this list of provider questions will help to ensure that he or she receives treatment from a qualified therapist.

The use and acceptance of CAM in the conventional medical community are diverse and multifaceted. Some of the challenges of supporting an integrative healthcare approach are a shortage of qualified CAM practitioners; the

---

Box 12.3 Most Common Complementary and Alternative Medicine Modalities Used by Adults

1. Natural products
2. Deep breathing
3. Meditation
4. Chiropractic/osteopathy
5. Massage therapy
6. Yoga
7. Diet-based therapies
8. Progressive relaxation
9. Guided imagery
10. Homeopathic therapy

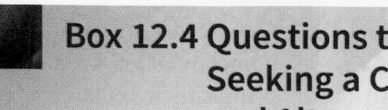

Box 12.4 Questions to Ask When Seeking a Complementary and Alternative Medicine Provider

1. What benefits can I expect from this therapy?
2. How will this therapy benefit my current condition?
3. Are there any risks associated with this therapy?
4. Should I expect any side effects from this therapy?
5. Will the therapy interfere with any of my daily activities?
6. How many sessions, and how often, will be needed for my condition?
7. How often will my progress or plan of treatment be assessed?
8. Will I need to buy any equipment or supplies?
9. Do you have any scientific articles or references about this particular treatment?
10. Can I use this therapy along with my conventional treatment plan and medications?
11. Could the therapy interact with conventional treatments?
12. Are there any conditions for which this treatment should not be used?
13. What type of education is required for this therapy?
14. Are you licensed for this type of therapy?
15. How long have you been in practice?
16. What are the costs for this form of therapy? Do you take insurance?

lack of knowledge related to CAM, which may deter open communication by conventional medicine healthcare providers; insufficient funding to support an integrated program; the lack of insurance reimbursement; and the need for more research to demonstrate and substantiate the effectiveness of treatment. Barriers to conducting research include limited funding, the lack of research infrastructure and standardization processes to interpret systemic reviews, and a limited number of patients to support trials. Most important is that the care is very nonstandard and personalized, so it is hard to evaluate on a large scale. Despite these challenges, CAM therapies are being sought out and used by the public with increasing frequency. This is an opportunity for nurses to consider evidence-based research projects related to CAM therapies to validate their clinical efficacy and ensure patient safety.

Connection Check 12.3

As a nurse who understands the guiding principles of CAM, your first step in guiding the patient is:
A. Referring the patient to a massage therapist to help manage stress
B. Explaining that the patient's *qi* is out of balance
C. Asking questions related to the presenting symptoms, work, and family to start building trust and rapport with the patient
D. Giving information related to a specific symptom the patient has reported to build a partnership with him or her

Making Connections

CASE STUDY: WRAP-UP

In a discussion with her nurse, Ms. Ellicott begins to explore CAM therapies in detail. In addition to acupuncture, there are other options to be considered. Manipulation and body-based therapies such as massage may be helpful. Mind/body therapies such as meditation or tai chi also seem promising. Ms. Ellicott and her nurse agree that a healthy diet that includes appropriate dietary supplements is a necessary foundation for any therapies considered.

Case Study Questions

1. Which of the following symptoms of Ms. Ellicott are listed among the NCCIH's top 10 reasons that adults seek CAM therapies? *(Select all that apply.)*
   A. Migraine headaches
   B. Depression
   C. Hypertension
   D. Anxiety
   E. Stress

2. Ms. Ellicott states to you that she is interested in CAM. You explain to her that the goals of CAM are: *(Select all that apply.)*
   A. To improve quality of life
   B. To repair and restore *qi,* the Life Force
   C. To promote wellness
   D. To treat hypertension
   E. To eliminate stress

3. Ms. Ellicott has decided that she would like to learn more about massage therapy, acupuncture, and guided imagery. She states, however, that she has concerns about the safety and efficacy of the treatments. Which of the following resources should you refer her to so that she can learn more about CAM?
   A. National Center for Complementary and Integrative Health (NCCIH)
   B. White House Commission on Complementary and Alternative Medicine
   C. Center for Integrated Medicine
   D. American Association of Acupuncture and Oriental Medicine
   E. All of the above

4. Ms. Ellicott is expressing concerns about being touched. You explain to her that there are CAM therapies that have a meditative and restful quality and do not involve touch. As the nurse, which of the following therapies do you suggest?
   A. Homeopathy
   B. Reflexology
   C. Yoga or prayer
   D. Massage therapy

5. Ms. Ellicott's provider is considering starting a hypertensive medication along with an anti-anxiety agent. Ms. Ellicott states that she has heard of herbal remedies that can help with depression and lower blood pressure. She states that she would like to take something more natural. As the nurse, your best response is:

   A. To discuss the use of herbal remedies with the provider

   B. To agree with Ms. Ellicott that because she is newly diagnosed with hypertension, trying an herb first is a good idea

   C. To explain to Ms. Ellicott that even though an herb is natural, there are contraindications when combining herbs with pharmaceutical medications

   D. To suggest further discussion with the provider along with a review of resources and collaboration with a pharmacist, naturopath, or herbalist

CHAPTER SUMMARY

The popularity of and growth in the field of CAM are expanding into hospital units, outpatient centers, and private provider offices, which are more commonly considered venues for conventional medicine. The National Health Interview Survey estimated that CAM is a multibillion-dollar industry and that those seeking CAM are paying more than a quarter billion dollars out of pocket annually for services. Although CAM systems are centuries old, CAM is a relatively new concept in the United States and other developed countries where conventional medicine is the dominant source for healthcare. The need for education is paramount, as are opportunities for CAM research to substantiate the effectiveness and best practices related to CAM therapies. Currently, 57 academic medical centers in the United States are part of the Consortium of Academic Health Centers for Integrative Medicine, whose mission is to advance the principles and practices of integrative medicine.

The NCCIH classifies CAM into five categories: old-world traditions, mind/body therapies, manipulative and body-based therapies, energy therapy, and dietary supplements and botanical/herbal medicine. Of these therapies, various forms of manipulative and body-based therapies, yoga, meditation, and breathing therapy are most commonly used by adults for symptoms such as pain, headache, anxiety, and depression. The goals of CAM include promotion of wellness, prevention of illness, reduction of treatment side effects, improvement of the immune system, and enhancement of quality of life—often reasons why 40% of adults seek CAM as an alternative for maintaining a healthy lifestyle. With 40% of the population using CAM, it is essential to include CAM in nursing education not only at the university level but also in hospital and outpatient settings so that the benefits and safety risks associated with CAM modalities are well understood. Along with advocating for educational opportunities, another fundamental need is for evidence-based research projects to ensure safe and competent care.

Bridging between the practices of Western medicine and CAM is a fundamental nursing role; being attuned to the guiding principles of CAM gives way to understanding the wisdom of integrative medicine, that is, treating an individual as a whole person—physically, mentally, and spiritually—to promote optimum health and well-being. Nurses are the channels for building collaborative partnerships so that all care, for all individuals, will be safe and best practices for individualized care will be considered.

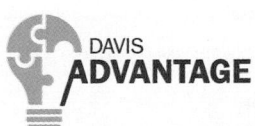

DAVIS ADVANTAGE | To explore learning resources for this chapter, go to **Davis Advantage** and find:
- Answers to in-text questions
- Chapter Resources and Activities
- NCLEX®-Style Chapter Review Questions
- Bibliography

Chapter 13

Overview of Cancer Care

Brenda Shelton

LEARNING OUTCOMES

Content in this chapter is designed to assist in:

1. Discussing the epidemiology of cancer
2. Explaining the pathophysiology of cancer cells
3. Describing vital diagnostic and preventive measures for the oncology patient
4. Identifying treatment options for oncology patients
5. Analyzing nursing care for the oncology patient
6. Developing teaching and support strategies for the oncology patient and family

CONCEPTS

- Assessment
- Cellular Regulation
- Fluid and Electrolyte Balance
- Infection
- Promoting Health

ESSENTIAL TERMS

Adjuvant therapy
Anaplasia
Anchorage dependence
Antineoplastic
Apoptosis
B symptoms/constitutional symptoms
Brachytherapy
Cancer
Carcinogen
Carcinogenesis
Carcinogenic
Chemoprevention
Chemotherapy
Contact inhibition
Dysplasia
Hematological malignancies
Malignant
Metastasis
Metastatic tumor
Neoadjuvant therapy
Neoplasia
Oncogene
Palliation
Primary tumor
Radiation therapy
Remission
Secondary tumor
Solid-tumor malignancies
Vesicants

Finding Connections

CASE STUDY: EPISODE 1

Follow this patient throughout the chapter.

Margaret Jones is a 49-year-old woman who has presented to her primary care provider with a new lump in her right upper, outer breast that was noted during showering. She reports no associated symptoms such as nipple discharge or breast pain. Mrs. Jones is premenopausal, stating she has noted no changes in her menstrual cycle. When the nursing medical history screening form is completed, the following are noted:

- Normal functional status, working as a schoolteacher
- Absence of smoking or substantial alcohol intake
- Family history of ovarian cancer in mother; maternal aunt dying of unknown abdominal cancer
- Past medical history of fibrocystic breasts, hypertension for 5 years, and moderate obesity

Physical examination shows:

- A palpable and immovable mass approximately 2 cm in size deep in the breast and near the axilla
- No other adenopathy is appreciable.
- Her abdominal organs are palpated as regular in size…

INTRODUCTION

Cancer is a constellation of diseases involving a **malignant** (unregulated) transformation of cells within a specific body system. Although there are many different types of cancers, all cancers are characterized by uncontrolled growth of malignant cells that compromises the integrity and function of normal, healthy cells. Cancer affects males and females of all ages, infants to adults. Its clinical presentation can vary from severe and acute clinical findings to a more chronic and indolent, or slowly developing, disease. Clinical features vary on the basis of cancer type, staging, and specific molecular characteristics.

EPIDEMIOLOGY

Cancer is the second leading cause of death worldwide, and rates are expected to increase over time. Globally, the most common types of cancer are lung, breast, colorectal, prostate, skin, and stomach cancer. However, cancer incidence (rate of new cases), prevalence (number of total cases), and mortality vary on the basis of gender, national socioeconomic indicators, and carcinogen exposure. Globally, women are more likely to develop breast, cervical, or colorectal cancer; men are more likely to develop lung, prostate, or colorectal cancer. Socioeconomic indicators are correlated with different cancer epidemiological patterns. In countries where life expectancy is beyond 70 years of age because of robust economic and healthcare systems, such as the United States, cancer is more common. This is because individuals are more likely to live longer in these countries, and older adults are simply more likely to develop cancer. It is well known that the competence of immune surveillance mechanisms weakens with aging, increasing the risk of missed mutations and the development of malignancy. Cancer is generally regarded as a disease of advanced age and is linked to mutations that occur over time. In developing countries where life expectancy is lower secondary to poor healthcare infrastructure and economic challenges, the risk of developing cancer is lower compared with the risk of contracting other diseases such as infectious disease. People simply do not live long enough to have high rates of cancer. Unfortunately, although there are fewer cases of cancer in developing countries, mortality is higher than in developed nations secondary to a healthcare infrastructure that is unable to effectively identify cancer early or provide treatment, accounting for 70% of worldwide deaths due to cancer. Cancer-causing infections such as hepatitis and human papillomavirus (HPV) are the attributable etiology for cancer in 25% of cases in developing countries. Finally, **carcinogen** (cancer trigger) exposure varies across nations for different reasons, leading to different cancer disease patterns. For example, rates of thyroid cancer and leukemia are higher in Ukraine than in other countries. This is believed to be associated with Ukrainian population exposure to **carcinogenic** levels of radiation after the 1986 explosion of the Chernobyl nuclear reactor. Food contaminants such as aflatoxins and water contaminants such as arsenic also contribute to cancers in specific populations.

Prevalence in the United States

Cancer is the second most common illness and cause of death in the United States. There were 1,735,350 cases projected for the United States in 2018. There is a high incidence of cancer in infants, children, and young adults, but it is primarily a disease more prevalent in elders. This is presumably because of increased rates of cell mutation with older age. Seventy-eight percent of all cancers are diagnosed in adults aged 55 years or older. Despite a general concept that cancer is typically a life-threatening disease, the majority of patients with cancer survive more than 5 years after diagnosis. The most current 5-year overall cancer survival rate based on data collected between 1975 and 2014 is estimated to be greater than 68%, up from 50% in the 1970s.

The most common cancers in adults in the United States in order of greatest incidence are prostate, breast, and lung. In men, prostate cancer is the most common, followed by lung and colorectal. In women, breast cancer is the most common, followed by lung and colorectal cancer. In children, leukemia is the most common, followed by brain tumors. Cancers that are detected at an early stage or with a slow proliferation rate are associated with longer survival. Prevalent cancers, such as breast and prostate cancers, are associated with excellent 5- to 10-year survival, but lung and colon cancers have a less promising prognosis unless detected when still surgically excisable. Cancers of highest risk are listed in Table 13.1.

Connection Check 13.1

Cancer is the _____ most common cause of death in the United States.
A. first
B. second
C. third
D. fourth

Risk Factors for Cancer

The most common risk factor for cancer is exposure to a carcinogen. Carcinogens are internal or external exposures that predispose individuals to DNA destruction, resulting in cellular mutation that may ultimately lead to malignant transformation of cells. Examples of some well-documented carcinogens are ionizing radiation, benzene, HPV, sun exposure, and tobacco. Carcinogen exposure alone is unlikely to trigger cancer. **Carcinogenesis**, the initiation and promotion of cancer, involves a series of other molecular changes that occur after exposure to carcinogens. For this reason, not all individuals with known risk factors or known exposure to a carcinogen develop the disease. Environmental, hormonal, and lifestyle factors; infectious disease; medications; immune status; and nutritional factors are all believed to influence the development of cancer.

In addition to carcinogens, there are other modifiable and nonmodifiable risk factors for cancer. Nonmodifiable cancer risk factors, or factors that the individual cannot alter to decrease the risk for cancer, include age and genetic predisposition. Advanced age increases the risk of cancer. This is believed to be related to greater exposure to carcinogens over time as well as changes in immune function. Another nonmodifiable risk factor is genetic predisposition.

Table 13.1 Cancer Statistics: Five Most Common Cancers by Gender

Males	Females
Prostate	Breast
Lung and bronchus	Lung and bronchus
Colon and rectum	Colon and rectum
Urinary bladder	Corpus and uterus
Melanoma of the skin	Thyroid

Data from Siegel, R. L., Miller, K. D., & Jemel, A. (2018). Cancer statistics, 2018. *CA: A Cancer Journal for Clinicians, 68*(1), 7–30. doi:10.3322/caac.21442

Approximately 5% to 10% of cancers are related to known genetic syndromes. Genetic counseling is a useful tool for identifying and screening individuals who have a family history of cancer or a known genetic syndrome associated with cancer. A generally recognized modifiable risk factor for cancer is lifestyle. Specifically, a sedentary lifestyle and poor diet and/or smoking put an individual at increased risk for cancer. Cancer associations with specific diseases, such as the relationship between colon cancer and inflammatory bowel disease or hepatic cancer resulting from hepatitis C infection, are modifiable but only as much as the management of the triggering disease. Regardless of whether a risk factor is modifiable or not, risk factors are believed to be cumulative, with multiple risks connoting additive cancer risk. Risk modification leading to primary prevention is possible in some circumstances, but when not preventable, frequent screening to detect cancer (secondary prevention) at its earliest stage is recommended.

PATHOPHYSIOLOGY

Carcinogenesis

Cancer initiation typically begins with carcinogen exposure, which subsequently triggers single- or multiple-gene mutations. An individual likely experiences multiple carcinogen exposures and genetic mutations over time; however, the immune system protects the individual by recognizing the mutation and initiating cell death. In carcinogenesis, the mutated cells are not detected by the immune system and are therefore able to proliferate and progress into cancer. The specific gene or multiple gene associations with different types of cancer is a growing field of study, and many cancers have identified mutations that can be abrogated with newer targeted antineoplastic therapies.

Cancer Characteristics

Cancer is characterized by two hallmark characteristics: uncontrolled cell growth and altered cell differentiation.

Uncontrolled Cell Growth

Normal cells grow in a structured pattern, and stimulation for cell growth is tightly controlled so that the number of cells produced by the body is roughly equivalent to the number of cells lost through cell death or shedding. Cancer cell growth and proliferation are unregulated by typical mechanisms. Normal cells are regulated by **contact inhibition** and stop growing and reproducing when they come into contact with other cells. Cancer cells lack contact inhibition. A regular cell cycle that ends with programmed cell death, **apoptosis**, is common with normal cells, but cancer cells do not undergo apoptosis. Normal cells typically need to anchor to either neighboring cells or basement cells so that they can plug into a nutrient-rich extracellular matrix to remain viable, but cancer cells do not have this type of **anchorage dependence** and can grow and flourish in atypical patterns and environments. This uncontrolled growth may result in **dysplasia** (Fig. 13.1),

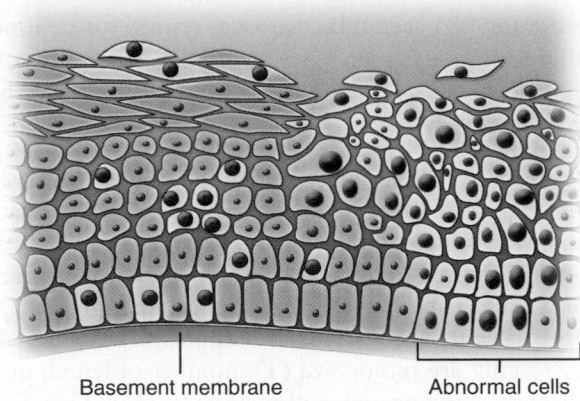

FIGURE 13.1 Mild dysplasia of cancer cells. Yellow cells indicate abnormal cells.

or deranged cell growth, in which cells vary in size, shape, and organization. In healthy tissue, dysplasia may be a risk for cancer, but it is not synonymous with cancer; it simply describes a cell-growth pattern but is often thought to be a precursor to malignant cell transformation. Another term often used to describe cell-growth patterns in cancer is **neoplasia**, which means uncontrolled cell proliferation. Like the term *dysplasia*, neoplasia is not synonymous with cancer because there are benign neoplasms; however, the term *neoplasia* describes a new cell-growth pattern that is characteristic of cancer. In summary, cancer cells are malignant neoplasms that grow uncontrollably and invade surrounding tissues and vessels. They have the capacity to destroy normal tissue, steal nutrition, create their own blood vessels, and survive even under anoxic or acidotic conditions.

Altered Cell Differentiation

Healthy, fully developed cells are well differentiated and have specific structural and functional characteristics. A malignant cell derives from a parent cell, such as a breast tissue cell, but no longer performs the expected functions of the parent cell, and the structure may be different as well. When a cell loses expected structure and function, it is called **anaplasia**. As cancer proliferation progresses, the cancer cell loses similarity to the parent cell. There is

a range in pathological presentation: Cancer cells may be well differentiated and look similar to the parent cell, undifferentiated and look nothing like the parent cell, or somewhere in between these extremes. Poorly differentiated cells are more difficult to treat. These cancers are often associated with more refractory and aggressive tumors, even if from the same tissue origin. The extent of differentiation is an important element in grading malignant neoplasms. Tumor grading is a mechanism to classify or describe tumors and is often used to plan treatment.

Metastasis

Cancer cells replicate and expand locally into masses of cells known as malignant tumors. The propensity for tumors to spread is called **metastasis** (Fig. 13.2). Cancer cells spread by cell-to-cell transfer, through the lymphatic system, or through the blood (hematogenous). Cell-to-cell transfer is characterized by direct invasion into adjacent cells. Lymphatic spread occurs when the tumor cells migrate into the lymphatic system using lymph channels that serve the organ where the cancer originated. Once in a lymph node, the cancer cell may be destroyed, grow into a mass, remain dormant, or spread to more distant lymph nodes and potentially into the vasculature. Hematological spread, or spread through the blood system, typically occurs when the cancer cell migrates into the venous system that drains the organ where the cancer originated.

Many cancers metastasize in a predictable pattern. For example, prostate cancer is notable for a tendency to spread by cell-to-cell transfer, so advanced disease is most likely to present with metastasis to nearby tissues, such as the rectum, pelvic floor, lower spine, or hip. Colorectal cancer commonly metastasizes hematogenously, and because the blood supply in closest proximity to the colon is the portal circulation, the liver is a common site of metastasis. When a tumor metastasizes, it often remains molecularly similar to the tumor of origin. That is to say, prostate cancer that has metastasized to the rectum has the same cellular and molecular qualities as prostate cancer; the prostate cancer cell has simply relocated

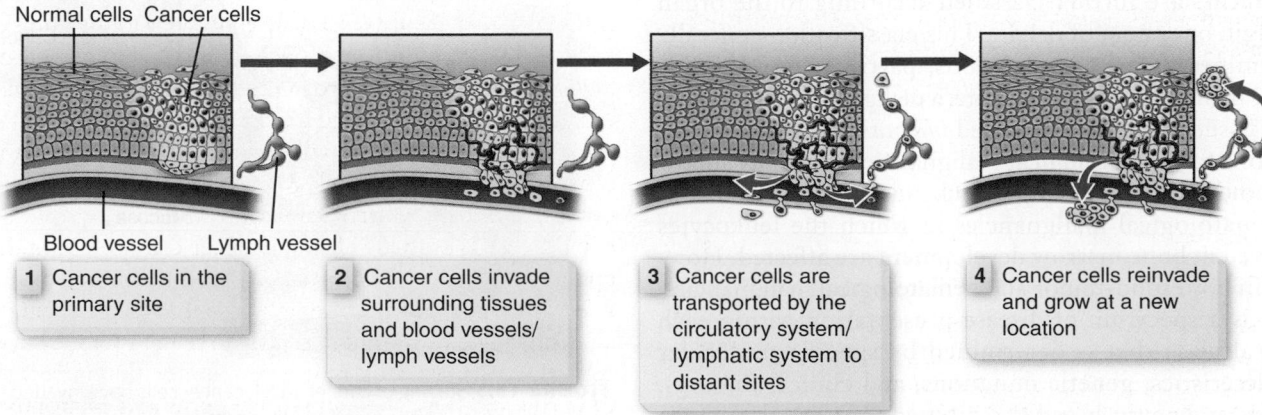

FIGURE 13.2 The stages of cancer metastasis.

to the rectum to create a prostate cancer tumor in the rectum. In other words, a rectal tumor originating from cancer of the rectum is different from a rectal tumor originating from cancer of the prostate. In the latter case, the tumor in the prostate is the **primary tumor**, and the tumor in the rectum is the **secondary tumor**, or **metastatic tumor**. Despite these similarities to the site of origin, metastatic lesions may also be molecularly unique and resistant to therapies that are effective for tumors in their primary site of origin.

Connection Check 13.2

What is the difference between the cells of a benign tumor and the cells of a malignant tumor?

A. The cells of benign tumors are typically aplastic.

B. The cells of malignant tumors are apoptotic.

C. The cells of malignant tumors lack contact inhibition.

D. The cells of benign tumors are characterized by uncontrolled cell growth.

TYPES OF CANCER

Cancers are generally divided into two main categories: solid tumors and hematological malignancies. **Solid-tumor malignancies** arise from specific body organs and grow into masses that invade and erode normal body tissue as they expand in size. An example of a solid-tumor malignancy is lung cancer. **Hematological malignancies** arise from cells of the hematopoietic cell line or from secondary immune organs such as the lymph nodes or spleen. The hematopoietic stem cell gives rise to all myeloid and lymphoid cells in the body, which later develop into cells of the blood system and immune system. A hematological malignancy can therefore affect any of the blood cells in the hematopoietic cell line, including red blood cells, white blood cells, and platelets. The three major subcategories of hematological malignancies are leukemia, cancers involving blood cells; lymphoma, cancers involving the lymphatic system; and multiple myeloma, cancers involving plasma cells and immunoglobulins.

Cancers are further classified according to the organ of origin or system of origin. This classification generally determines naming conventions, particularly for solid-tumor malignancies. To illustrate, a malignant tumor arising from tissue in the lung is called *lung cancer*. Naming conventions for hematological malignancies generally follow the same rules. For example, leukemia refers to a subclass of hematological malignancies in which the leukocytes involved in bone marrow development are affected. However, in both solid-tumor and hematological malignancies, there is a spectrum of disease presentation within each general class that is determined by specific molecular characteristics, genetic mutations, and clinical findings. Understanding the broad classification as well as the unique

presentation of a particular disease is critical for treatment planning.

STAGING

Once a cancer type has been diagnosed, the cancer is then further classified by stage. Staging is a classification system that considers the size of the tumor, burden of the disease, and extent of disease spread (Fig. 13.3). The stage of disease is used to plan patient assessment, clinical management, and treatment strategies. The basic components of solid malignancy staging are tumor size (T), number of lymph nodes involved (N), and presence of metastases (M). This TNM staging has differing combinations of tumor size or lymph nodes involved for each different kind of cancer. The American Joint Committee on Cancer (AJCC) has a book devoted to defining all staging systems. Cancer is generally staged along a continuum of one (I) through four (IV). A small tumor without obvious spread outside the organ is termed stage I, invasion of deeper tissues or involvement of local lymph nodes is stage II, large or locally invasive tumors are stage III, and cancers that have metastasized are considered stage IV. Some malignancies also include tumor-specific markers or molecular features in their staging system. All hematological malignancies are cancer stage IV at diagnosis because the disease is not well contained or localized because the hallmark clinical feature is that it is present in the hematological system at diagnosis.

CLINICAL PRESENTATION

Patients with cancer often initially present with three general types of symptoms:

- CAUTION symptoms
- Constitutional symptoms
- Malignancy-specific signs and symptoms

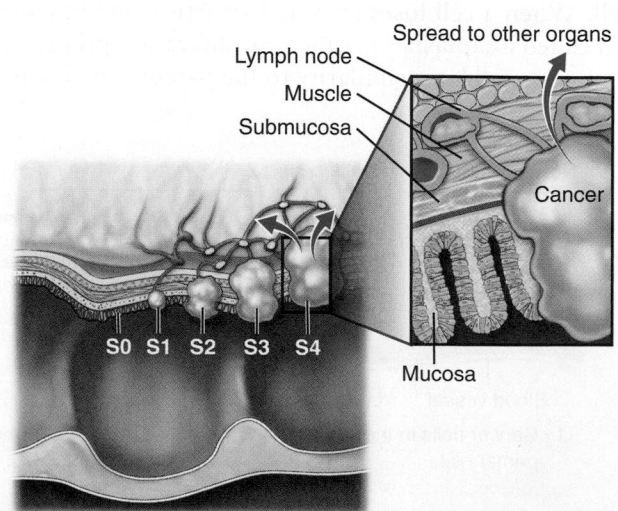

FIGURE 13.3 Staging of cancer. In S4, cancer cells have invaded surrounding tissue and spread to other organs.

CAUTION is an acronym used to describe common "warning signs" for cancer. Please see Box 13.1 for a full description. Often, patients experience a CAUTION symptom, and that serves as the impetus for visiting a doctor and therefore is a part of the initial clinical presentation. CAUTION symptoms occurring for more than 2 weeks warrant evaluation by a medical provider.

Cancer may also present with a constellation of vague symptoms, including fatigue, significant unexplained weight loss, fever of unknown etiology, and night sweats described as **constitutional symptoms**. This term is a formal classification in B-cell lymphoma. In B-cell lymphoma, constitutional symptoms are described as **B symptoms**, but fatigue is not an element of this formal classification system. B symptoms are considered an important prognostic indicator in B-cell lymphoma.

Finally, patients may present with symptoms characteristic of a specific malignancy; therefore, clinical presentation varies on the basis of the disease. These symptoms are related to the location of the primary cancer, the location of metastatic disease, metabolic changes associated with the malignancy, and the specific pathology of the disease. Symptoms and complications of solid tumors are often related to tumor-mass compression or erosion into normal anatomical structures. For example, individuals with primary brain cancer may present with pain secondary to tumor compression of nerves in the skull or signs of increased intracranial pressure from tumors that are occupying space within the cranium and minimizing room for functioning neurons, blood flow, and cerebrospinal fluid flow. This causes pain as well as other central nervous system changes. Please see Table 13.2 for key clinical features of specific cancers.

Box 13.1 CAUTION or Warning Signs of Cancer

C Change in bowel or bladder habits
A A sore that does not heal
U Unusual bleeding or discharge
T Thickening or lump in the breast or any other part of the body
I Indigestion or difficulty swallowing
O Obvious change in a wart or mole
N Nagging cough or hoarseness

Table 13.2 Common Cancers With Risk Factors and Defining Features

Cancer	Risk Factors	Clinical Signs and Symptoms	Common Sites of Metastases (in order of frequency)
Bladder cancer	Tobacco	Hematuria	Regional lymph nodes
	Cigarette smoking	Abdominal discomfort	Bone
		Distended abdomen	Lung
		Low-back pain	Skin
			Liver
Brain tumor	Alcohol, excessive	Headaches	Spinal cord
		Personality changes	
		Somnolence or hyperactivity	
		Memory deficits	
		Visual disturbances	
		Focal motor deficits	
Breast cancer	Endocrine disrupters: early menses, late menarche, nulliparity, late first child	Breast mass	Bone
		Axillary node enlargement	Lung
	Genetic propensity (*BRCA1*, *BRCA2*, *p53*)	Asynchrony of breasts	Lymph nodes
		Nipple discharge	Liver
	Obesity, high-fat diet		Brain

Continued

Table 13.2 Common Cancers With Risk Factors and Defining Features—cont'd

Cancer	Risk Factors	Clinical Signs and Symptoms	Common Sites of Metastases (in order of frequency)
Cervical cancer	Multiple sexual partners, early sexual contact Human papillomavirus Tobacco Oral contraceptives used over a long period of time	Vaginal bleeding, especially postcoital Vaginal discomfort Malodorous vaginal discharge Tumorous lesions on cervix Pain with sexual intercourse	Endometrium Vagina Extrapelvic wall Vulva
Colon cancer	Alcohol, excessive Beer consumption (rectal cancer only) Intestinal polyps, polyposis Obesity, high-fat diet Chronic bowel disease—Crohn's or ulcerative colitis	Altered bowel habit—may be constipation or diarrhea; thin, ribbonlike stools Blood in stool—overt or occult Abdominal fullness/distention Anorexia Weight loss Unexplained anemia	Liver Lung Muscle
Esophageal cancer	Alcohol, excessive Cigarette smoking	Dysphagia Indigestion/reflux Chest discomfort	Liver Lung Bones
Gastric cancer	Alcohol, excessive Gastric ulcers Asbestos Cigarette smoking *Helicobacter pylori* infection	Indigestion Loss of appetite Abdominal discomfort Postprandial fullness Nausea/vomiting	Lymph nodes Esophagus Periumbilical soft tissue Liver
Head and neck cancer	Alcohol, excessive Tobacco Wood dust Human papillomavirus infection	Oral lesions or bleeding Facial/oral/neck masses Pain in neck/jaw Lymph node enlargement of face/neck	Varies with each specific tumor region (e.g., soft tissue, oropharyngeal, nasopharyngeal) Lymph nodes Lung
Hepatic cancer	Alcohol, excessive Budd–Chiari syndrome Hepatitis A/B/C	Abdominal discomfort Nausea/vomiting Easy bruising Jaundice	Omentum/peritoneum Pleura

Table 13.2 Common Cancers With Risk Factors and Defining Features—cont'd

Cancer	Risk Factors	Clinical Signs and Symptoms	Common Sites of Metastases (in order of frequency)
Kidney cancer	Pesticides Solvent exposures Tobacco	Flank pain Hematuria Weight loss	Lymph nodes Lung Liver Bone Adrenal gland Brain Opposite kidney Subcutaneous skin nodules
Leukemia	Alkylating agents Genetic mutations Radiation exposure	Fatigue Anemia Chronic infection Bruising, petechiae, gum bleeding	Diffuse at diagnosis
Lung cancer, non-small cell and small cell	Asbestos Coal, soot, tar Pollution Tobacco Wood dust	Chronic cough Hemoptysis Dyspnea Chest discomfort Weight loss Paraneoplastic syndromes	Brain Bone Adrenal gland Contralateral lung
Lymphoma, Hodgkin's and non-Hodgkin's	Immunosuppression, chronic (e.g., long-term corticosteroids or after solid-organ transplant) Radiation Viruses—Epstein–Barr, HIV	Lymphadenopathy Palpable masses, subcutaneous tissue	Generally considered diffuse at diagnosis, but staging does allow for limited lower stage disease with limited lymph node groups involved
Melanoma	Sun exposure Ionizing radiation Family tendency	Skin lesions—varied color, irregular shape, raised or crusty texture Lesions that are new or growing Lesions on palms of hands, soles of feet	Lymph nodes Subcutaneous tissue Lung Brain Liver Bones
Multiple myeloma	Older age African American	Fatigue Dark, infrequent urine Bone pain	Not exactly metastatic, but bone and kidney infiltrations are signs of advanced disease

Continued

Table 13.2 Common Cancers With Risk Factors and Defining Features—cont'd

Cancer	Risk Factors	Clinical Signs and Symptoms	Common Sites of Metastases (in order of frequency)
Ovarian cancer	Genetic—*BRCA1*, *BRCA2* Endocrine disrupters—nulliparity, no breastfeeding, long-term oral contraceptive use	Abdominal fullness, bloating Fatigue	Peritoneum, omentum Pleura
Pancreatic cancer	Genetic—*BRCA2* Tobacco Diabetes Hereditary or chronic pancreatitis Hepatitis A/B/C Stomach ulcers Obesity	Nausea, vomiting Early satiety Vague abdominal discomfort Anemia Jaundice	Liver Peritoneum Lungs Bones
Prostate cancer	Age Family history Pesticides	Pelvic/rectal pain Dysuria Nocturia Erectile dysfunction	Bones Lymph nodes Rectum Bladder
Sarcoma	Arsenic Dioxins Herbicides Radiation, ionizing	Dependent upon location of mass—soft tissue masses or evidence of organ dysfunction that shows masses on radiological tests	Almost anywhere—extension of mass or recurrence at original site is common Lung (if not originating there) Abdominal-peritoneal (if not originating there)
Skin cancers	Radiation, ionizing UV/sun exposure	Dark, irregularly shaped skin lesions	Rare, soft tissues
Testicular cancer	Undescended testicles History of HIV Age (20–34)	Painless lump in scrotum Dull ache or heavy sensation in pelvis, anus, or scrotum	Lymph nodes Lung Liver Bones Brain
Thyroid cancer	Radiation, ionizing	Enlarged thyroid—diffuse and irregular Dysphagia	Lymph nodes Lung Bone
Uterine (endometrial) cancer	Early menarche, late menopause Estrogen replacement therapy Polycystic ovary disease Infertility Tamoxifen Diabetes mellitus Obesity	Abnormal menstrual cycles Vaginal bleeding, especially between cycles Lower abdominal pain/cramping	Lymph nodes Vagina Abdominal peritoneal cavity, omentum

GI, Gastrointestinal; *HIV,* human immunodeficiency virus; *UV,* ultraviolet.

Oncological Emergencies

Oncological emergencies are acute clinical complications that may occur in the presence of malignancy. They require urgent treatment to prevent long-term physiological deficits. Oncological emergencies may be secondary to the processes of tumor growth and invasion of body organs, metabolic changes from malignant cells, or a result of treatment. They are generally categorized as structural, metabolic, and hematological, but organ dysfunction may also be present. Probabilities of oncological emergencies vary with cancer type. The nurse should become familiar with oncological emergencies associated with specific cancers and when each emergency is more likely to be expected across the disease and treatment trajectory. This allows the nurse to anticipate the diagnosis and proactively manage symptoms. Management of oncological emergencies should be based on evidence-based practice as well as the patient's condition, prognosis, and preferences. If a patient is at the beginning of treatment and has the potential for recovery, the oncological emergency should be aggressively managed. On the other hand, if the emergence of an oncological emergency is an ominous sign of progressive disease, then the patient and the team may opt for a less aggressive, palliative approach to management. A summary of common oncological emergencies, important clinical features, and nursing implications is provided in Table 13.3.

Table 13.3 Selected Oncological Emergencies

Oncological Emergency	Pathophysiology	Clinical Presentation	Clinical Management	Nursing Implications
Bowel obstruction: most commonly found in tumors involving the bowel such as colon cancer and pancreatic cancer and abdominal masses such as ovarian, hepatic, and prostate cancers	Masses in bowel lumen obstruct normal flow of enteral contents, GI fluids, and wastes. External compression causes bowel obstruction. Obstructions can be partial or complete and involve the small or large bowel. The greatest danger of obstruction is rupture or perforation.	Obstruction causes reverse peristalsis with vomiting and abdominal distention. Bowel sounds are increased prior to the obstruction and diminished or absent after the obstruction. Stools may be thin or ribbonlike, or constipation with intermittent diarrhea may be present.	Best treated with surgery when resectable. Medical management: NPO/parenteral nutrition, peristaltic stimulants unless complete obstruction, when stimulants may cause intestinal rupture.	Detailed GI assessment: appetite; bowel movements; constipation; diarrhea; thin, ribbonlike stools; bowel sounds; presence of nausea, vomiting, distention, pain.
Hypercalcemia: most commonly found in cancers that metastasize to bone, such as breast, lung, and renal cancers, but can be related to paraneoplastic hormone production in lung and pancreatic cancers	Produced by bone demineralization (resorption) with release of calcium into systemic circulation. Bone invasion with tumor can activate osteoclasts; tumors may create their own parathormone-like substance, or renal dysfunction can contribute to this process.	Common symptoms include delirium symptoms, somnolence, muscle weakness, polyuria, bradycardia, nausea, and constipation. Symptoms vary depending on the calcium level and how quickly the hypercalcemia developed.	Hydration with normal saline dilutes calcium and enhances excretion of calcium. Bisphosphonates (e.g., pamidronate, zoledronate) are used as treatment or prevention of hypercalcemia in patients with bone metastases. Monoclonal antibody directed at the RANK ligand (denosumab) lowers calcium. Less-often-used agents that are still available in specific situations include calcitonin, corticosteroids, Mithracin, and strontium-98.	Monitoring of calcium, phosphorous, and renal function. Assessment for symptoms of hypercalcemia, such as: ● Delirium, somnolence, muscle weakness, fatigue, polyuria, bradycardia, nausea, constipation ● Provide hydration and medication as ordered.

Continued

Table 13.3 Selected Oncological Emergencies—cont'd

Oncological Emergency	Pathophysiology	Clinical Presentation	Clinical Management	Nursing Implications
Leukostasis: most commonly found in acute myelocytic leukemia with high white blood cell counts	Excessive immature white blood cells (most commonly myelocytes) cause capillary sludging, thrombosis, and rupture of vessels.	Congestion and dysfunction due to cell migration, inflammatory response, and hemorrhage within the organ; most commonly affect the kidney, lung, and brain	Emergency chemotherapy Leukopheresis Supportive interventions	Monitor white blood cell count. Assess for signs of occluded microcirculation, such as blurred vision, headache, transient ischemic attacks, cerebrovascular accidents, dyspnea, poor peripheral perfusion, and oliguria. Assess for signs of bleeding.
Pericardial effusions/ tamponade: most commonly found in cancers of the chest such as lung and breast cancers and also lymphoma; can also be found in any cancer that has metastasized to the chest	Small amounts of pericardial fluid (approximately 15–30 mL) exist in the pericardial space to allow for heart distention with blood filling the ventricles. When there is excess fluid accumulation in this space, it causes positive pressure in this space and impedes venous return of blood. This reduced blood inflow leads to impaired cardiac output.	Dyspnea is the most common although nonspecific symptom with which patients initially present. Acute signs of poor perfusion occur in most patients with pericardial effusion of noncardiac origin, but because it often progresses slowly in cases of neoplastic effusion, signs of progressive right heart failure may be more likely.	Immediate evacuation of excess fluid by needle or catheter pericardiocentesis or surgical placement of a pericardial window or shunt is recommended. Until expert clinicians can perform one of these procedures, large amounts of fluids are administered to increase the venous pressure above the pericardial pressure, permitting inflow of blood.	Assess vital signs, signs of dyspnea, poor perfusion, and signs of heart failure, such as respiratory distress, fatigue, and edema. Prepare for pericardiocentesis; administer IV fluids as ordered.
Pleural effusions: most commonly found when there are tumors in the chest, such as breast and lung tumors; also can be present in patients with leukemia, lymphoma, ovarian cancer, pancreatic cancer, and prostate cancer	Approximately 50–150 mL of fluid is normally in the pleural space to provide lubrication for lung expansion, but when excess fluid is in the space, it impedes breathing, increasing the work of breathing and compressing alveoli.	Dyspnea is the most common symptom. Increased work of breathing with use of accessory muscles, unequal chest excursion, and diminished breath sounds occur because of increased fluid in the pleural space. Resulting hypoxemia can cause confusion, anxiety, and agitation.	Intermittent therapeutic thoracenteses are commonly used until frequency is greater than weekly. Catheter drainage of pleural fluid (traditional chest tube or long-term silastic pleural catheter) used for palliation of symptoms unless a surgical talc pleurodesis can be performed. Bedside catheter pleurodesis with bleomycin, doxycycline, and talc may still be used when other therapies are unavailable.	Assess for dyspnea, shortness of breath, breath sounds, chest excursion equality, and signs of hypoxemia. Assess how frequently symptoms are appearing or progressively worsening.

Table 13.3 Selected Oncological Emergencies—cont'd

Oncological Emergency	Pathophysiology	Clinical Presentation	Clinical Management	Nursing Implications
Spinal cord compression: most commonly found when there are tumors near the spinal cord	Infectious or tumorous masses compress or invade the epidural space or its blood supply, leading to lack of communication from that level of the spine downward.	Symptoms are present in the dermatome affected. Pain and other sensory symptoms (numbness, tingling) precede motor weakness. Autonomic dysfunction is late.	Treatment based on etiology. Radiation therapy most common and produces rapid relief of symptoms if tumors are radiosensitive. If the cord is completely compressed, laminectomy (posterior approach preferred) can restore cord function. Rapid-onset corticosteroids provide immediate reduction of inflammation and symptoms. Vertebroplasty or kyphoplasty allows injection of cement between vertebrae for treatment of compression fractures.	Assess for back pain, weakness, numbness and tingling, unsteady gait, and loss of ability to distinguish hot and cold. Depending on level of compression, assess for constipation or incontinence.
Superior vena cava syndrome: most commonly found in chest tumors, lung cancer, and lymphoma	Tumor or tumor-involved lymph node compression of the soft-walled superior vena cava, causing reduced return of blood flow to the heart and venous congestion	Dyspnea is the most common clinical symptom, although venous congestion and edema of the upper body are common. Visual disturbances, headache, and altered mental status occur with cerebral edema. Prominent jugular veins, brachial veins, and chest vessels	Immediate chemotherapy or radiation, depending on the sensitivity of the tumor to specific therapy. Corticosteroids are administered to reduce inflammation. If a thrombus is present, systemic or catheter-directed thrombolytics are given. If vessel rupture is of concern, a superior vena cava stent with or without a graft may be performed.	Early assessment for dyspnea; edema of neck, face, and eyes (most severe in the morning); and prominent upper body vasculature. Later assess for signs of poor perfusion and decreased cardiac output, such as confusion, cyanosis, hypotension, and tachycardia.
Syndrome of inappropriate antidiuretic hormone (SIADH): most commonly found in patients who have primary or metastatic brain or lung cancer	Excess antidiuretic hormone (ADH) causes fluid volume retention and vasoconstriction; ADH receptors in the brain and lungs are stimulated and trigger ADH release. Some	Most clinical effects relate to the severity of hyponatremia, such as mental status changes or seizures. Fluid volume overload with effusions or edema and	Initial treatment is fluid restriction that causes increased sodium concentration and increased urine osmolarity. If ineffective, hypertonic saline may be administered, but sodium correction	Assess for signs of fluid overload, such as hypertension and hyponatremia, confusion, seizures, and coma. Restrict fluids and administer medication as ordered.

Continued

Table 13.3 Selected Oncological Emergencies—cont'd

Oncological Emergency	Pathophysiology	Clinical Presentation	Clinical Management	Nursing Implications
	tumors create their own ADH-like substance, producing the same effects.	dilutional reduced electrolytes and hematocrit are also common. Hypertension occurs even with mild SIADH but is more severe with fluid overload.	may not exceed 0.5 mEq/hr. For chronic SIADH, treatment may be lithium carbonate or demeclocycline.	
Tracheobronchial obstruction: most commonly found in patients who have lymphoma and lung cancer or centrally located metastatic lung lesions	Tumor-related obstruction or invasion of the major air-exchanging airways	Dyspnea with stridor is the most common finding. Wheezing may be present if the bronchi are involved. In severe and late-stage obstruction, breath sounds are absent, and chest excursion is reduced. Patients are more hypoxic than hypercarbic.	Immediate therapy with supportive interventions, such as bronchodilators or corticosteroids, provides immediate relief of symptoms to permit time for assessment for airway stent, laser therapy, cryotherapy, endobronchial brachytherapy, or photodynamic therapy. Definitive antineoplastic treatment is initiated simultaneously.	Assess for signs of respiratory distress, stridor, wheezing, and hypoxemia.
Tumor lysis syndrome (TLS): most commonly found in patients with rapidly proliferative tumors such as leukemia and lymphoma or therapy-sensitive tumors that respond quickly to treatment	Rapid cell lysis either with rapidly proliferative disease or after antineoplastic treatment. Lysing cells that cannot be cleared accumulate and cause electrolyte imbalance or renal dysfunction.	Primary clinical findings reflect the degree of electrolyte imbalance and renal dysfunction. Most patients are highly symptomatic with hypocalcemia and hyperkalemia. Acidosis may also produce unique features such as heart block and tachypnea. Hyperphosphatemia can cause renal dysfunction and worsening clinical symptoms.	Large-volume IV fluid administration with diuretics is immediately started to enhance excretion of electrolytes. Hyperuricemia is treated with rasburicase if the uric acid is already elevated, and allopurinol is given to prevent hyperuricemia for the patients at high risk for TLS. Electrolyte abnormalities are managed supportively. Patients are given Amphojel or other phosphate binders. If renal failure occurs, an initial hemodialysis treatment followed by continuous renal replacement therapy (CRRT) is recommended.	Assess for signs of hypocalcemia, such as paresthesias and numbness of the fingertips and perioral area, neuromuscular irritability, and severe signs such as laryngeal contraction. Assess for signs of renal dysfunction: elevated blood urea nitrogen (BUN), creatinine, decreased urine output. Assess for ECG changes such as heart block or peaked T waves indicative of dangerous hyperkalemia, and assess for hypotension.

GI, Gastrointestinal; *ECG,* electrocardiogram.

Other complications of cancer are common but are not classified as oncological emergencies. The presence of malignancy alters the microenvironment of the body, causing changes in hormonal balance, metabolic pathways, and cellular nutrition. Some of the complications of malignancy that are not clearly explainable but present in higher proportions of patients with cancer than those without it include anorexia/cachexia syndrome, hypercoagulation, effusions, fluid or electrolyte imbalances, glucose metabolism abnormalities, and clinical depression. Proactive prevention of deep vein thrombosis for patients with adenocarcinoma, large abdominal masses, or when clotting has been problematic is implemented in both inpatients and for patients being treated in the outpatient setting. Monitoring for these other complications and providing prompt interventions can minimize their associated negative outcomes.

Connection Check 13.3

The nurse understands that an important laboratory assessment parameter for a patient with cancer that has metastasized to bone is which of the following?

A. White blood cell count
B. Calcium level
C. Glucose level
D. Sodium/potassium level

PREVENTION

Cancer prevention initiatives fall into three levels: primary, secondary, and tertiary. Primary prevention is focused on identifying and modifying risk factors for cancer to reduce the probability that an individual will develop cancer. Secondary prevention is focused on early screening and detection of cancer in an effort to identify and control the disease early. Tertiary prevention is focused on reducing the complications of disease and improving the quality of life once an individual has been diagnosed with cancer. It is important to note that some cancers are not preventable because some risk factors are not easily modified or the risk factors and disease process are not well understood at this time. In these cases, general cancer prevention techniques and screening are recommended.

Primary Prevention

Primary prevention initiatives include:

- Risk factor modification
- Immunization
- Chemoprevention

Risk Factor Modification

There is increasing evidence that individuals can reduce their lifetime risk of developing certain types of cancers by avoiding known carcinogens. Primary cancer prevention initiatives are generally targeted at helping individuals identify their own cancer risk behaviors and modify their behavior in order to avoid exposure to carcinogens. An example of one such initiative is the multilevel approach to reducing tobacco use in the United States. There are system-level initiatives attempting to control national regulations and policy, as well as individual provider–patient initiatives to promote smoking cessation. Cancers linked to tobacco include cancers of the bladder, breast, lung, and pancreas. It has been shown that even after considerable exposure to tobacco, quitting smoking and remaining tobacco-free for 10 years can decrease the risk for lung cancer by 30% to 50%. A list of general cancer prevention guidelines is included in Box 13.2.

Immunization

Some cancers are believed to be triggered by viral exposure. An example of such a cancer is cervical cancer, believed to be triggered by HPV exposure. Exposure to HPV has also been linked to head and neck cancers of the oral, nasal, and pharyngeal regions. Other examples include hepatitis C, which is believed to trigger liver cancer, and Epstein–Barr virus (EBV), which has been associated with certain lymphomas. This does not mean that all individuals exposed to a potentially carcinogenic virus will develop viral disease and subsequently cancer, but the individual's lifetime cancer risk increases. Immunization against these viruses is recommended for susceptible individuals.

Chemoprevention

Chemoprevention is the administration of medications to reduce the risk of specific cancers in high-risk patients. Chemoprevention is a primary prevention strategy for some survivors of early-stage hormonal cancers such as breast and prostate cancers. High-risk patients who have been evaluated to be sensitive to chemoprevention are prescribed hormone stimulants or ablation agents that create hormonal environments that impede recurrence of the malignant cell

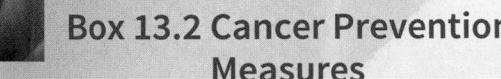

Box 13.2 Cancer Prevention Measures

- Avoid exposure to known carcinogens such as tobacco.
- Wear sunscreen every day.
- Prevent and/or treat infectious diseases known to be related to cancer: hepatitis B and C, human papillomavirus (HPV), HIV, *Helicobacter pylori (H. pylori)*.
- Maintain a healthy weight.
- Engage in regular moderate to vigorous physical activity.
- Eat a healthy, plant-based diet.
- Limit consumption of alcoholic beverages: no more than one drink a day for women and no more than two drinks per day for men.
- Recognize family risks, consider assessment or prophylactic interventions for genetic mutations, or alter screening practices.

clone. There are only a few chemoprevention agents available on the U.S. market, and providers must carefully evaluate the risks and benefits of therapy prior to the initiation of a chemoprophylaxis regimen. In addition to pharmaceutical chemopreventive agents, researchers are currently exploring the use of nutraceuticals, food and food products that may have medicinal properties, such as vitamins such as C and E and antioxidants, for cancer prevention. However, there is no conclusive evidence from high-quality clinical trials that supports the use of any nutraceuticals for chemoprevention at this time. In fact, some initial clinical trial results suggest that certain nutraceuticals may increase the risk of the development of specific cancers in certain populations.

Secondary Prevention

Secondary prevention is essentially cancer screening for early detection and management of the disease. Clinical outcomes are better for individuals diagnosed and treated for cancer earlier in the disease process compared with individuals diagnosed later in disease development. Ideally, individuals with cancer-related risk factors should have access to noninvasive screening tests that can identify cancer in its earliest stages, when it can be treated effectively with minimal risk of recurrence. Screening tests should be highly sensitive (able to detect in a low-risk population with few false negatives) and specific (able to accurately detect with few false positives). In order for a cancer screening test to provide the greatest benefit with the least harm, it must be cost-effective and easy to perform and have minimal adverse effects. Unfortunately, there are few cancer screening tests that meet these criteria. A summary of current cancer screening guidelines is included in Table 13.4.

For cancers that have no available standard screening test, clinician assessment is critical. Clinicians must become familiar with the individual patient's risk profile to determine high-risk cancers. Assessments may then be focused on organs or systems that present the highest cancer risk.

Table 13.4 Screening Guidelines

Type of Cancer	Screening Guidelines	Special Considerations for Health Disparities
General cancer checkup	Men and women aged 20 and older: • Discuss individual cancer risk factors and screening needs with your primary care provider during annual physical checkup. • Share family history of cancer—particularly first-degree relatives—with provider.	
Breast cancer	Women aged 40 and older: • Annual mammogram until age 55 years, then may switch to mammograms every 2 years • Annual clinical breast examination Women aged 20 to 39: • Clinical breast examination every 3 years	Caucasian women aged 40 and older have a higher risk of breast cancer than African American women aged 40 and older. African American women have higher breast cancer–associated mortality. Women from racial minority groups are: • More likely to be diagnosed with later stage and/or higher-grade cancer • At higher risk for breast cancer–related mortality • Less likely to have insurance Women with less than a high school education and of lower socioeconomic status are less likely to get mammograms. Medical assistance/financial assistance for screening is available through state-run Medicaid programs.
Cervical cancer	Women aged 21 to 29: • Screening every 3 years with regular Pap test Women aged 30 to 65: • Pap test plus HPV test every 5 years or • Pap tests every 3 years and HPV test every 5 years	Ethnic minorities and women of disadvantaged socioeconomic status are less likely to participate in screening.

Table 13.4 Screening Guidelines—cont'd

Type of Cancer	Screening Guidelines	Special Considerations for Health Disparities
Colon cancer	Men and women aged 45 and older (screening may be stopped over age 85): ● Stool assessment for low-risk individuals *or* ● Flexible sigmoidoscopy every 5 years *or* ● Colonoscopy every 10 years *or* ● Double-contrast barium enema every 5 years *or* ● CT colonography every 5 years	Incidence and mortality in African Americans are higher than in Caucasians; some suggest this is related to differences in socioeconomic status. In the United States, incidence and mortality among Asian/Pacific Islanders, American Indians/Alaskan Natives, and Hispanics/Latinos are lower than among Caucasians. Mortality of colon cancer is inversely associated with education. Globally, incidence and mortality are higher in the Western Hemisphere (United States, Canada, Europe) than the rest of the world. Individuals with lower socioeconomic status and/or no health insurance are less likely to participate in screening across all racial and ethnic groups.
Prostate cancer	Men aged 50 and older or men aged 45 and older with risk factors: ● Talk to your primary provider about the risks, benefits, and frequency of screening using: ● PSA level (blood test) ● Digital rectal examination	African Americans have highest incidence of prostate cancer among all racial groups in the United States. African Americans have higher mortality (two times) than Caucasians. Prostate cancer is common in the Western Hemisphere but rare in Asia and South America.
Lung cancer	No evidence-based consensus guidelines for the general population at this time ● American Cancer Society and National Comprehensive Cancer Network (NCCN) recommends yearly helical low-dose CT screening for high-risk patients (current smokers or those having quit within the past 15 years and have a 30-pack-year smoking history).	Incidence and mortality are higher in African American men than in Caucasian, Hispanic, and Native American/Alaskan Native men. Incidence and mortality in African American women and Caucasian women are similar; both are higher than in other races. Of individuals who smoke, African Americans and Native Hawaiians are at higher risk of developing lung cancer than are Caucasian Americans, Japanese Americans, or Latinos.
Melanoma	No evidence-based guidelines for the general population at this time ● American Cancer Society (ACS) recommends individuals monitor skin and skin changes (perform self-examination) annually to identify any concerning skin changes.	
Non-Hodgkin's lymphoma **Pancreatic cancer** **Multiple myeloma**	No evidence-based guidelines for the general population at this time	

CT, Computed tomography; *HPV,* human papillomavirus; *PSA,* prostate-specific antigen.
Source: American Cancer Society. (2019). *Cancer screening guidelines.* Retrieved from https://www.cancer.org/healthy/find-cancer-early/cancer-screening-guidelines.html

For example, if a patient has a significant family history of multiple myeloma, there is no consensus-driven standardized screening tool. The clinician may individualize the annual health examination to include a focused assessment for multiple myeloma, which may include urine analysis for Bence Jones protein—a characteristic sign of multiple myeloma. Although clinician-based, cancer-focused assessments vary across clinicians and may be imprecise secondary to limited guidance in the form of evidence-based practice, it is best to include cancer screening in primary care rather than not include it at all.

Evaluation of the family history for genetic cancer syndromes is an essential component of an optimal secondary cancer prevention program. The most well-known genetic cancer syndromes are related to *BRCA1*, *BRCA2*, *p53* (Li–Fraumeni syndrome), familial adenomatous polyposis, and retinoblastoma. The key assessment for familial cancer syndromes is the identification of two first- or second-generation relatives with one of the marker cancers. A family tree identifying specifics of the cancer and age at diagnosis can provide clues of familial cancers. Serum blood tests can detect the presence of the altered gene in an individual but may be imperfect in detecting the risk to future generations. Testing of family members experiencing cancer is the best method to determine if the cancer is potentially genetic in origin. A frequent misperception is that the genetic mutations place individuals at risk for a single cancer, but many of these known genetic syndromes confer a risk for several different cancers. For example, the *BRCA1* gene is associated with a higher risk for breast and ovarian cancer; however, the *BRCA2* gene is also known to convey increased risk for pancreatic or bile duct, prostate, or melanoma skin cancers and possible risk for bone, laryngeal/pharyngeal, esophageal, and gastric cancers.

Tertiary Prevention

Tertiary prevention focuses on reducing morbidity and mortality once a disease has been diagnosed. The treatment and management of the side effects of cancer or its treatment, which are discussed in subsequent sections, may be considered tertiary prevention.

CASE STUDY: EPISODE 2

After the history and physical examination are completed, Margaret is scheduled for a mammogram. The mammogram reveals a suspicious mass, so a biopsy is scheduled for the next week. A fine-needle aspiration biopsy reveals abnormal cells. Because of these findings, Ms. Jones's provider recommends that she see an oncologist for evaluation. An appointment is scheduled for the next week…

DIAGNOSING CANCER

The initial assessment for possible cancer is usually triggered when a patient presents to a provider with one of the seven CAUTION signs, constitutional symptoms, or other unexpected symptoms of unknown etiology. There are diagnostic tests designed to identify the specific cancer cells that uniquely define them as different from normal cells (cancer vs. nonmalignant tumors), tests that define the precise molecular makeup of the tumor (tumor markers, molecular or genetic profiling), and tests used to stage the disease (identify tumor size, lymph nodes involved, and spread). Tests from all three categories may be used to subsequently monitor the presence or absence of malignancy or the response to antineoplastic treatment. Nurses play a key role in translating essential information for patients, such as the intention of the diagnostic test, patient preparation and postprocedure care, what to expect during the test, and the anticipated time for results. Patients may require clarification when the same diagnostic tests are used for more than one purpose.

Diagnostic Evaluation

Diagnostic evaluation for cancer is dependent on the suspected cancer subtype, possible disease location, and expected extensiveness of the disease. It may include laboratory tests, radiological tests, ultrasound, invasive techniques, or combinations of these methods. Most initial diagnostic tests are performed to confirm the presence of masses associated with cancer. Radiological tests are most helpful for the detection of unusual masses, although ultrasound or even physical examination may also be valuable. Confirmation of malignant tissue requires a biopsy with cytopathological diagnosis, which is a diagnosis of disease based on the evaluation of cell pathology from cells obtained at biopsy.

Laboratory Tests

Laboratory diagnostic tests provide useful conjunctive information to validate some malignancies. Some laboratory tests can be performed on blood and serum, whereas others require a tissue sample. An example of a laboratory test is the prostate-specific antigen (PSA) test, obtained via a venous blood sample, used to validate the presence of prostate cancer. A high PSA level is associated with prostate cancer, although its presence is actually indicative of inflammation, and will reduce as the tumor shrinks in response to therapy. The PSA test has a high sensitivity (ability to accurately find cancer in patients who actually have cancer—true positive) but a low specificity (accurately identifying patients who do not have cancer—the test yields false positives), which means PSA elevations may not be cancer related. The PSA level is only one piece of information that can be considered in a definitive diagnosis of prostate cancer.

Laboratory diagnostic tests can also be used to track responses to therapy. These test results may be important for patients to adjust self-care. For instance, when patients are aware of their blood counts during chemotherapy, they are more able to understand when they are at risk for bleeding or infection and adjust their activities of daily living. Tumor markers may be assessed at initial diagnosis but also followed intermittently throughout and after treatment as one indicator of disease response.

Imaging

Imaging studies use radiographical, sonographical, or other technology to create images of the body for clinical evaluation. They are often used to assess the structure or function of body organs or systems. They are effective in identifying tissue masses, one of the most common presenting signs of cancer. Imaging studies allow for the detection of these tissue masses that are undetectable on physical examination. They are also used to detect metastasis, or tumor spread to other tissues. A computed tomography (CT) scan is indicated for general assessment of mass locations and involvement of vessels or body organs. In metabolically active tumors, positron emission tomography (PET) scans are preferred. Positron emission tomography scans typically involve the injection of radioactive material that, when imaged, appears to accumulate in areas of increased metabolic activity ("hot spots") that correspond to areas of disease. Magnetic resonance imaging (MRI) is preferred for evaluating changes in brain, joint, and breast tissues. Some of the imaging technologies use contrast, or the administration of dyes or radiosensitive markers, to enhance imaging details. Contrast is also helpful in identifying the involvement of blood and lymphatic vessels. Radiological imaging tests are useful in the diagnosis and assessment of solid tumor masses but may not be as useful for the diagnosis of hematological malignancies that are diffuse and do not present with masses (malignant lymphoma is the exception).

Biopsy

Biopsy is the primary method of obtaining samples required to determine the presence of malignancy. It is a surgical method of obtaining a tissue sample for evaluation, most commonly used in solid-tumor evaluation. Biopsies can be incisional (into the mass) or excisional (cut out the total mass and a margin around it). When an incisional biopsy, also known as a core biopsy, is performed, there is a danger of tracking malignant cells through the surrounding normal tissue. Excisional biopsy is preferred over incisional, and the standard margin of normal tissue to be removed (how much healthy tissue to remove around the suspected tumor) is dependent on the suspected malignancy. An alternative, less traumatic method of obtaining a tissue sample is via fine-needle aspiration (FNA) biopsy (Fig. 13.4). This method can be used when cells of interest are located close to the skin and can be extracted via a needle. This method yields fewer cells than traditional biopsy methods, but histological analysis is improved because cell structure is maintained. The limitation of FNA tissue sampling is that it may not be possible to conduct a thorough analysis of the tissue (DNA, molecular features, typing,

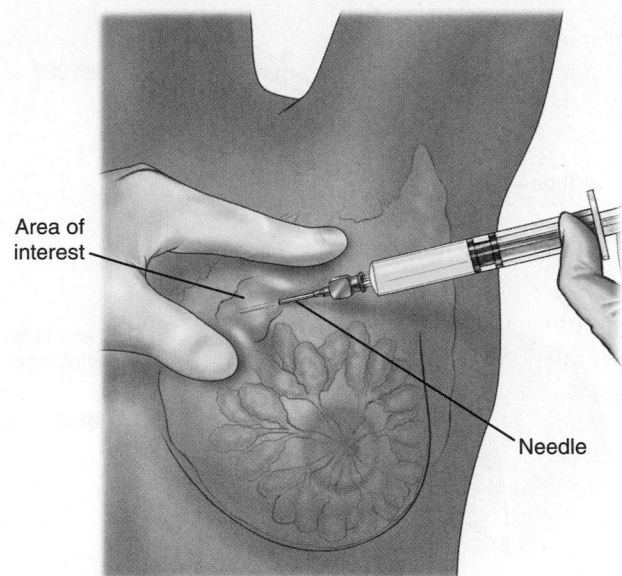

FIGURE 13.4 Fine-needle aspiration (FNA) breast biopsy.

etc.). Hematological malignancies are evaluated via bone marrow aspiration and biopsy, with cytopathological molecular testing for subtle cell differences.

Endoscopic Procedures

Endoscopic procedures, such as endoscopy and bronchoscopy, are performed with a rigid or flexible tube, light, and lens and allow visualization of hollow, tubelike structures in the body (e.g., the gastrointestinal tract) and may be necessary in order to access tissue for biopsy. An example is the use of bronchoscopy in the work-up for lung cancer. Bronchoscopy allows for visualization of the airways while also providing access to hard-to-reach tissue for sampling (Fig. 13.5).

Connection Check 13.4

What is the most specific method of diagnosing a malignancy?

A. Serum laboratory tests
B. MRI
C. CT scan
D. Biopsy

TREATMENT

The treatment of cancer varies according to the cell type and stage of disease and occasionally the markers that predict response to specific therapies. In addition, cancer treatment varies with the goal of care: cure, remission, maintenance/prevention of progression to extend life, or palliation. Whenever possible, the goal of cancer treatment is to cure the disease and maintain disease-free survival. Some resources define a disease cure as 5 years of disease-free survival; however, the interpretation of survivorship

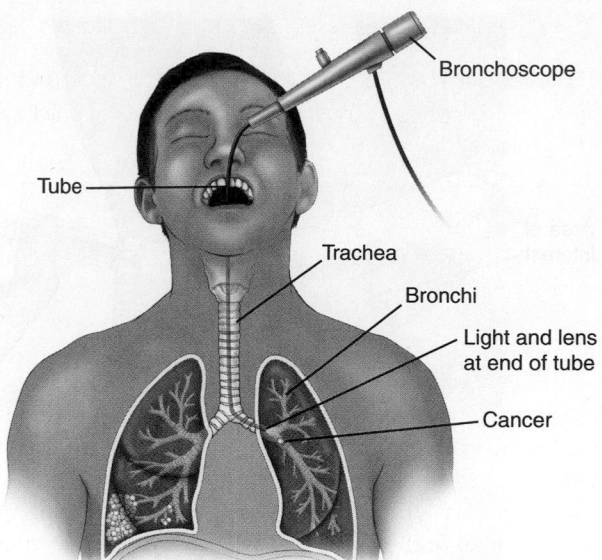

FIGURE 13.5 Bronchoscopy, a diagnostic procedure to look for evidence of cancer in the tracheobronchial tree.

and long-term disease-free status has been greatly debated. Many believe survivorship is a continuum that begins at the time of diagnosis and that disease-free survival is a more appropriate defining point than cure. Examples of cancers believed to be curable are early-stage, resectable cancers of the breast, cervix, colon, kidney, oropharynx, skin, testicles, and uterus.

If cancer is not curable, the goal may be simply to reduce tumor burden or prevent progression. Sometimes this may be referred to as **remission**, which is a disease-free state in which it is unclear if the disease has been eradicated or if this disease-free state will remain stable. Remission is often the goal of care in hematological malignancies. Long-term remissions based on suppression of the **oncogene** (the gene that has the potential to cause cancer) that produces cancers such as hairy cell leukemia and chronic myelogenous leukemia have reached a level of response that is relatively new to the oncology specialty. These patients remain disease-free as long as they consistently take their medications targeting the faulty cellular pathway, in much the same way as patients with hormonal disorders such as hypothyroidism can be free of clinical disease while maintained on hormonal replacement therapy. The hope is that scientific discovery leads to the identification of more targeted therapies that expand the number of patients who can experience this type of disease response. Although some diseases may have long periods of remission, such as many lymphomas, they are not considered curable because they will ultimately relapse.

Another goal of therapy may be to increase years of life—for example, to increase the projected life span from 2 years with untreated disease to 5 years with treatment. And finally, if the cancer is not curable or the harm from any treatment modality greatly exceeds the benefit, the primary goal may be **palliation**, the alleviation of the burdensome symptoms of cancer. Palliation is increasingly a consideration in all cancer treatments but typically not the primary consideration if a long-term disease-free status is possible. Patient-centered care reinforces that goals of treatment are mutually agreed on by patients, their significant others, and the healthcare team. Providing patient education regarding the language and meaning of these oncological treatment goals may be necessary to create a meaningful collaboration.

Treatment Modalities

Cancer treatment includes three broad modalities: surgical procedures, radiation therapies, and medical treatments. Treatment may be single therapy or may be multimodality. If a cancer treatment requires a multimodality approach, the definitive treatment is referred to as the primary therapy. A therapy that is used to shrink the tumor prior to definitive removal or destruction is called **neoadjuvant therapy**. Neoadjuvant strategies are used with many large solid tumors that are not resectable at diagnosis but may be after the initial treatment to shrink the size of the mass has been completed. **Adjuvant therapy** is defined as a treatment that is used in a patient who is currently disease-free or in remission but at high risk for relapse because of remaining microscopic malignant cells that will regrow at a later time. Evidence for the effectiveness of adjuvant treatment is currently limited to a handful of cancers, which includes breast, colon, head/neck, lung, and melanoma cancers. Ongoing trials using adjuvant therapy are in process for many other solid tumors, such as bladder, esophageal, pancreatic, renal, and testicular cancers and sarcoma. Patients with these cancers in moderate stages of disease who receive adjuvant therapy have a significantly increased disease-free survival rate. An example of a case in which all these terms may be relevant is a woman diagnosed with breast cancer who requires multimodality treatment: surgical, medical, and radiation interventions. The primary therapy is surgical because the main interest is to surgically remove the malignant tumor. Her oncology team determines she also needs neoadjuvant **chemotherapy** (medical therapy) to reduce the size of the tumor prior to surgery and adjuvant radiation therapy after surgery to decrease the risk of disease recurrence.

Surgical Treatment

Surgical resection of a tumor is the preferred cancer treatment modality because it offers the greatest probability of producing a cancer-free state. It is also the primary treatment modality for patients with solid-tumor malignancies. The primary goal of surgical oncology is total excision of malignant tumors and the local area of potential metastasis immediately surrounding the tumor. Surgical oncology also includes debulking of tumor masses (partially removing a tumor that cannot be completely excised). Redirection of vital functions after tumor removal and reconstructive procedures are also components of surgical oncology. Redirection and reconstructive procedures are necessary because surgical procedures for cancer usually involve the removal of the tumor as well as a margin of normal surrounding tissue, which may affect organs that perform vital functions. Surgery may often involve the reconstruction of normal blood vessels and nerves or the construction of drains. Removal of large masses may require the construction of diversions and ostomies, which are surgical openings to allow for the elimination of body waste. An example of a more extensive surgical procedure is the case of a patient with colon cancer who requires the removal of a section of the colon. If possible, the surgeon tries to connect the remaining pieces of the colon back together. If this is not possible, the patient will be unable to pass stool through an intact colon, requiring the creation of an opening (ostomy) through which the patient is able to pass stool. Another example of a more extensive surgical procedure is a mastectomy, or removal of a breast to remove a breast cancer tumor. Although this surgery does not necessarily impact vital body function, it does significantly impact the nervous and lymphatic systems. It also affects patient body image and quality of life. Because of these issues, a mastectomy is sometimes followed with reconstructive surgery. Advances in surgical oncology are allowing for surgical processes that are less invasive and that increasingly preserve vital organ structure and function. The impact of our enhanced knowledge of tumor biology has also provided greater opportunity to apply neoadjuvant therapy with successful later resection. This has led to higher numbers of patients with stage III locally advanced cancers realizing long-term remissions and cures.

Nursing considerations for the surgical oncology patient are similar to care for the general surgical patient. The patient may be at greater risk for infection and have increased morbidity compared with the noncancer patient, but this morbidity profile is secondary to the presence of remaining cancer and comorbidities. Nursing implications include a thorough understanding of the patient's goals of care, overall treatment plan, anticipated physical deficits, barriers to or facilitators of postoperative recovery, and self-care or education needs. It is not uncommon for patients with cancer to come to surgery with unique clinical problems that should be incorporated into the plan of care. Patients with cancer often have pain and are taking long-term medications for pain before surgery, requiring a modified postsurgical pain management plan. Patients may also have deconditioning, recent weight loss or malnutrition, altered skin integrity, and variable organ function. Rehabilitation and consultation with physical and occupational therapists are often required for optimal return to activities of daily living while adjusting to changes in body function. Anesthetic clearance may be impaired because of renal or hepatic dysfunction, and chronic infections may necessitate atypical antibiotic regimens. Nurses should thoroughly familiarize themselves with the recent medical history and consider the patient's physical and psychological status in planning care and education related to cancer surgery.

Connection Check 13.5

The nurse understands that the patient receiving chemotherapy prior to definitive surgical excision is receiving which type of treatment?

A. Secondary treatment
B. Adjuvant therapy
C. Neoadjuvant therapy
D. Primary treatment

Radiation Therapy

Radiation therapy is the localized delivery of ionizing radiation to intentionally destroy DNA structures within malignant cells and induce cell death. A radiation therapy treatment plan is designed with the goal of maximizing tumor exposure to radiation while minimizing injury to normal cells. Radiation therapy can be delivered externally via an external beam, internally via placement in a cavity or reservoir in the body (**brachytherapy**), or systemically via injection of a radioactive substance. These methods use different radioactive sources, chosen in part by the sensitivity of the defined tumors being treated. For external-beam radiation therapy, the radiation treatment plan is designed to deliver a planned total dose and is divided into "fractions." Fractions are the doses delivered in a single treatment. The normal fractionation cycle is a daily dose for 5 days followed by 2 days' rest. This cycle is repeated for 5 to 18 cycles. Radiation doses may be further divided into more than once per day, termed *hyperfractionation*, for the purposes of enhancing delivery to rapidly dividing tumor cells or to minimize some adverse effects. On occasions of severe tumor-related organ dysfunction or compression of major body organs (e.g., spinal cord compression, super vena cava syndrome, tracheobronchial obstruction), the daily dose may be higher for the initial 3 to 6 days in order to rapidly reduce the tumor size and its effects. The total radiation dose is determined by the amount of radiation needed to destroy the type and size of tumor. Available specialized techniques for the delivery of direct-beam radiation include intensity-modulated radiation therapy, conformal (three-dimensional) radiation therapy, invasive direct-beam therapy (e.g., intraoperative radiation or intrabronchial radiation), proton-beam therapy, and stereotactic radiation therapy. Stereotactic radiosurgery is a one-time treatment to a small, well-defined target in the body or brain. Cyberknife is the most common technique used. These techniques are designed to reduce injury to normal tissue while optimizing the radiation delivery to the tumor.

Brachytherapy, or internal delivery of low-dose or high-dose radiation, is an alternative method of delivering radiation therapy. Radioactive isotopes are placed in "seeds," which are then administered to the patient. These seeds may be infused via a catheter or surgically implanted. Low-dose brachytherapy allows for the continuous delivery of radiation in the body for as long as the source of active radiation remains in the body. This can be for a period of a few days or, in some cases, permanent. Low-dose brachytherapy is used in gynecological, prostate, head and neck, and brain cancers. High-dose radiation, such as radioactive isotopes, must be managed more closely than low-dose therapy. Radioactive isotopes are introduced into the body and allowed to dwell for a certain period and then removed in one treatment session. The patient may need multiple high-dose treatment sessions, but high-dose radiation therapy does not dwell within the patient unmonitored or for extended periods of time as may be the case for low-dose brachytherapy (Fig. 13.6).

Systemic radiation therapy typically involves the vascular administration of a radioactive substance. Radioactive iodine, for example, is sometimes used to treat thyroid cancer. The thyroid naturally attracts iodine, so the isotope concentrates in a local area after systemic delivery. Systemic radiation therapy may be administered with targeted therapy, such as a monoclonal antibody (see next section), to help the active isotope find the desired target. The monoclonal antibody targets a specific tissue or organ, and the radioactive isotope goes along for the ride. This technique is commonly used in the treatment of lymphoma that expresses a specific receptor so that the monoclonal antibody is able to carry radiation directly to the tumor.

Nursing considerations for the care of the patient receiving radiation therapy are related to symptom management and self-care. Because radiotherapy is delivered to a localized area, the adverse effects are usually a direct reflection of the body area treated. Common signs of local injury peak in the second to third week of treatment. Acute inflammatory effects are followed by fibrotic changes indicative of tissue injury. Inflammatory adverse effects and organ dysfunction

are possible outcomes. General patient education regarding skin care and management of treatment markings are provided to all patients.

Complications

Patients are evaluated before treatment and regularly throughout the radiation course for symptoms of inflammation, irritation, and altered mucosal integrity in the area receiving radiation. For some patients, this may be as minor as erythema of the skin, but assessment of radiation injury to internal structures such as the trachea may present as more subtle symptoms such as chest discomfort or cough. Fibrosis is a late effect of radiation, causing internal adhesions, fibrotic skin changes, and strictures (e.g., vaginal). Interventions may be routinely employed to reduce these effects (e.g., vaginal dilator) or implemented on an as-needed basis (e.g., feeding tubes for patients receiving neck or throat radiation).

Fatigue is a common adverse effect of both cancer and its treatment but is particularly prevalent in patients receiving radiation therapy. This symptom is thought to be related to the cumulative effect of cell damage and hence escalates throughout treatment, peaking at 3 to 6 weeks. It is important to provide patient education and support for activities of daily living such as transportation and self-care, realizing the prevalence and distress this symptom presents for patients. Evidence-based interventions include pacing of activities and mild to moderate exercise. Early patient education and reassurance can reduce the risk of misperceptions by patients and families or the fear that fatigue signals advancement of the cancer.

To minimize harmful exposure to radiation, the oncology nurse must be mindful of donning all appropriate personal protective equipment and following the self-care standards of the institution. This is particularly true for the nurse who handles potentially radioactive waste from patients receiving brachytherapy that may be eliminated in body fluids. Providing the same education to family members also prevents unintentional radiation exposure to individuals other than the patient.

Antineoplastic Medications

Antineoplastic medications are a broad class of chemicals and drugs used to treat cancer. Antineoplastic therapies are loosely divided into four different categories: (1) chemotherapy, (2) immunologic therapies, (3) targeted agents, and (4) hormonal agents. This type of therapy is indicated in patients with more advanced disease, diseases of the blood or bone marrow, or cancers that are not amenable to single-modality surgical or radiation therapy. Antineoplastic therapy is often administered systemically (IV), making it appropriate for more widespread advanced cancers. This route of administration is effective but also leads to a systemic side-effect profile. Some therapies act more specifically on tumor cell targets or receptors, whereas others are effective because they destroy *all* rapidly dividing cells, including most cancer cells. "Normal" rapidly dividing cells

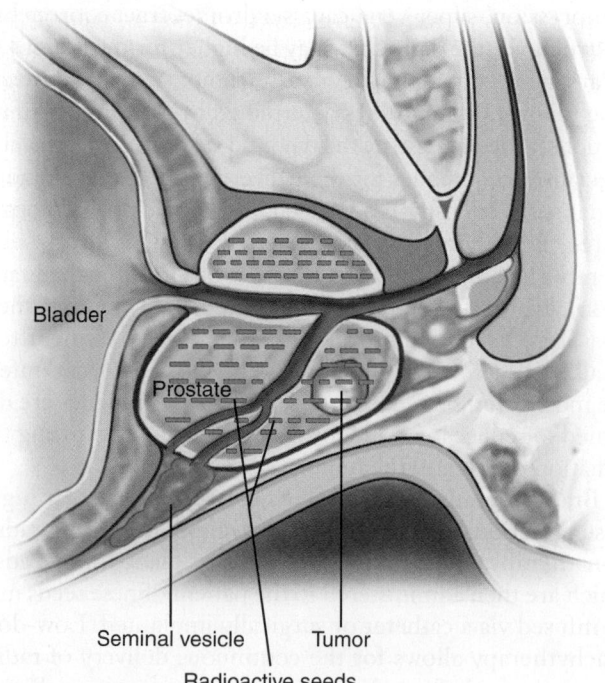

Bladder

Prostate

Seminal vesicle   Tumor

Radioactive seeds

FIGURE 13.6 Brachytherapy, radiation therapy delivered internally via placement in a cavity or reservoir in the body.

that are destroyed along with the cancer cells include hair, skin, intestinal tissues, and blood-forming cells. Additionally, a potential complication of the IV route is extravasation, or the infiltration of the medication out of the vessel and into the surrounding tissue. Many antineoplastic medications are **vesicants**, medications that can cause extensive damage to the tissue on direct contact. Great care must be taken by the nurse when administering these medications to avoid and prevent leakage of the medication into the tissue.

The selection of antineoplastic or targeted and immunologic agents is individualized according to the specific cancer type, molecular features, and location of the disease. Most antineoplastic medication therapies involve a combination of medications from different classes or categories that are able to destroy tumor cells at various phases of development. This ensures more effective destruction of the entire tumor cell population and balances the adverse effects common in a single class of medication. Each medication class has an adverse-effect profile that correlates to its mechanism of action, and common effects are seen with most medications within the class, termed "class effects." Chemotherapy regimens have been established through clinical trials evaluating the efficacy of single agents and then combined in specific doses and patterns of administration. They are often delivered every few weeks, with the plan to destroy a percentage of the tumor cells with each subsequent cycle until maximum control or cure is accomplished. The total dose of chemotherapy is carefully calculated according to the tumor type, growth rate, and total volume of the tumor mass. Any chemotherapy delays or dose reductions can compromise the potential for maximum response. Other considerations include the patient's baseline health status and comorbid conditions, the synergy of combination therapies, the adverse-effect profile, the social or financial circumstances of the patient, and previous therapies. Patients receiving antineoplastic medications require extensive education and support to understand the

treatment plan, monitoring, adverse-effect management, and self-care. Nurses often provide this education across several sessions and supplement verbal information with written reinforcement, multimedia information, and support networks. Given the complexity, physical symptoms, and possible associated anxiety, the involvement of the patient's family members is essential. Table 13.5 describes adverse effects associated with antineoplastic medications.

Stem Cell and Bone Marrow Transplants

Hematopoietic stem cell transplantation (HSCT) and bone marrow transplantation (BMT) are treatment methods for some cancers and hematological disorders. Hematopoietic stem cell transplantation/BMT involves two major steps: the administration of high-dose antineoplastic therapy (sometimes in combination with radiation therapy) followed by the infusion of hematopoietic stem cells (HSCT) or whole bone marrow (BMT). This method allows for the administration of high doses of antineoplastic/radiation therapy that would normally not be tolerated because high-dose chemotherapy and radiotherapy permanently damage bone marrow. The stem cell/bone marrow transplant essentially "rescues" the patient. If the stem cells are donated from another individual, the added benefit may be immunologic. The donated stem cells may work to fight the cancer in what is called a "graft-versus-tumor" effect. This therapy is normally administered to patients with nonmalignant hematological and immunologic disorders and hematological malignancies. The use of transplants for the treatment of refractory solid-tumor malignancies is not considered routine at this time. Variations within this therapy include variable levels of bone marrow destruction (fully myeloablative or nonmyeloablative); stem cells harvested from the periphery or bone marrow; and differing levels of genetic match (haploidentical or identical) and self (autologous; Fig. 13.7), related (allogeneic), or unrelated (matched unrelated) donors. Complications of HSCT/BMT may be related to the

---

Table 13.5 Common Adverse Effects Associated With Antineoplastic Medications and Nursing Implications

Common Adverse Effects	Nursing Implications
Alopecia—It is variable, but loss of hair typically begins soon after therapy begins. Again, variable, but hair begins to grow back several weeks after completion of therapy. Interestingly, when growing back, hair typically comes back different from pretherapy: curly, thicker, or a different color.	Loss of hair may cause a self-image disturbance, especially in women. They should be encouraged to investigate wigs or other head coverings to use during therapy. Patients should be reminded to cover their heads while outside to protect against sun damage.
Myelosuppression (bone marrow suppression)	Inform patients that a complete blood count will be assessed frequently during therapy.
	Instruct patients to call the provider immediately if a fever presents. Patients with myelosuppression and fever may be managed aggressively to prevent severe sepsis or shock.

Continued

Table 13.5 Common Adverse Effects Associated With Antineoplastic Medications and Nursing Implications

Common Adverse Effects	Nursing Implications
Nausea/vomiting	Administer prophylactic antiemetic therapy as ordered.
	Assess fluid and nutritional status frequently.
Hemorrhagic cystitis	Administer IV hydration before and after chemotherapy as ordered; prophylactic bladder protectant medication mesna (chemoprotectant medication to help prevent bladder toxicities) may be used.
Oral mucositis—inflammation and ulceration of the mucosal lining of the mouth, causing pain and difficulty with eating	Encourage frequent oral rinsing (every 2–4 hours) with toothbrushing to reduce severity of mucositis; encourage the use of 2% viscous lidocaine mouth rinse if ordered to help control pain. Oral saliva substitute may be recommended for comfort or to reduce severity of symptoms.
Hypersensitivity	Administer premedication for hypersensitivity as ordered.
	Emergency equipment should be readily available.
Infertility	Encourage patient to consider sperm or egg banking prior to therapy if desired.
Diarrhea	Administer antimotility agents for diarrhea as ordered.
	Assess fluid and nutritional status frequently.
Skin toxicities (palmar-plantar erythema)	Encourage the use of emollients to reduce skin toxicities.
	Teach patient to report severity of skin toxicities because it may require therapy break.
Cardiotoxicity	Teach patient that cardiac function will be monitored with echocardiograms or multi-gated acquisition scans (MUGAs). Many medications are held if decreased ejection fraction is found. Serum troponin levels may be drawn during curative therapy with doxorubicin to identify patients who may receive prophylactic treatment with cardioprotectant agents. Maintain fluid and electrolyte balance to reduce the risk of dysrhythmias.
Hepatic (liver) toxicity	Inform patient that hepatic function tests will be assessed regularly during therapy.
Pulmonary fibrosis	Inform patient that pulmonary function tests will be assessed periodically.
Clotting abnormalities—thromboses and/or bleeding	Some antineoplastic medications are never given within 6–8 weeks of major surgery because of bleeding risk.
	Prophylactic anticoagulation is common to prevent thromboses.
	The nurse and/or patient should frequently assess for bleeding.
	Teach patient about bleeding precautions; avoid falls or trauma, so no aggressive sports; avoid sharps such as razors, scissors, nail clippers; use stool softeners to avoid straining.
Peripheral neuropathy—weakness, numbness, and pain in hands or feet	Teach patient fall precautions; remove scatter rugs from home; remove any trip hazards such as electrical cords; use nonslip mats in your bathtub or shower.
Capillary permeability syndrome	Administer fluid replacement for hypovolemia as ordered. Weight assessment and management may be used to avoid fluid overload.
Menopausal symptoms	Teach patients possible effects regarding menopausal symptoms—hot flashes, insomnia, fatigue.

The Autologous Transplant Process

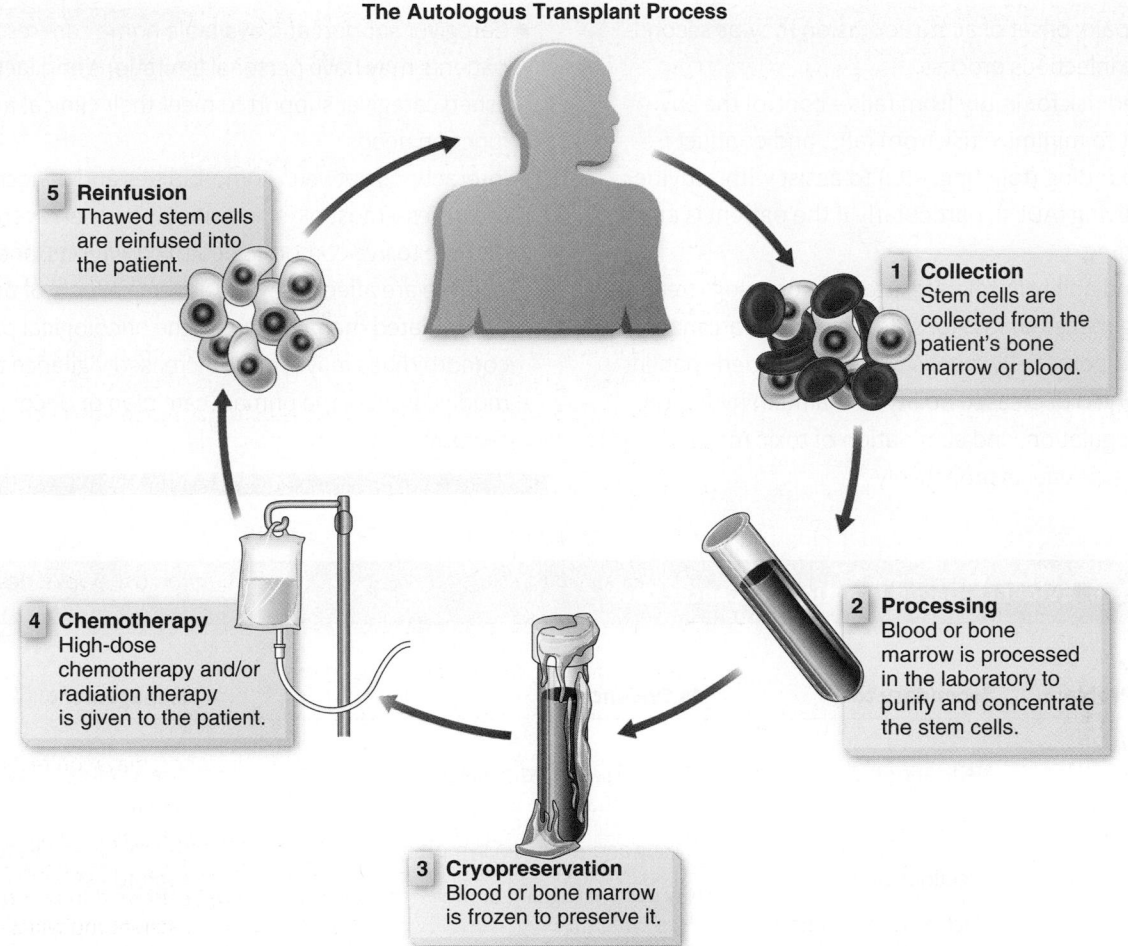

5 Reinfusion
Thawed stem cells are reinfused into the patient.

1 Collection
Stem cells are collected from the patient's bone marrow or blood.

4 Chemotherapy
High-dose chemotherapy and/or radiation therapy is given to the patient.

2 Processing
Blood or bone marrow is processed in the laboratory to purify and concentrate the stem cells.

3 Cryopreservation
Blood or bone marrow is frozen to preserve it.

FIGURE 13.7 An autologous bone marrow transplant.

chemotherapy/radiotherapy or linked to the transplant of foreign marrow.

NURSING MANAGEMENT

Nursing care of patients with cancer crosses all subspecialties of medical-surgical nursing and ambulatory primary care because the disease can affect any organ system and can be managed in a variety of clinical settings. Patient problems are based on the type of cancer, sites of metastases, stage of disease, comorbidities, and therapy plan. Nurses providing care to patients with cancer should have specialized training in the management of the specific antineoplastic therapy being delivered and the special needs of patients experiencing cancer.

Common medical-surgical problems may be managed differently in the patient with cancer on the basis of this specialized knowledge. For example, oncology patients may receive pain medications for both acute and chronic pain, yet the symptoms of constipation that may occur with opiates must also be considered as a symptom of tumor-related bowel obstruction. See Geriatric/Gerontological Considerations for care needs specific to the geriatric population. A list of common nursing diagnoses for the cancer patient with evidence-based care recommendations is provided in Table 13.6.

Geriatric/Gerontological Considerations

Older adults may have many comorbidities that require complex therapy or may already have some organ dysfunction, and their clinical presentation of disease sometimes differs from that of younger adults. Older individuals may also have unique reimbursement and treatment challenges, warranting a thorough socioeconomic evaluation for barriers to successful completion of the treatment plan. In order to provide safe care to older adults, nurses must be mindful of:

- Polypharmacy (multiple medications)—conduct medication reconciliation with patients; be mindful of potential medication interactions.
- Organ dysfunction—assess kidney and liver function in the physical assessment and via laboratory monitoring; be conscientious of the need for medication dose alterations, such as renal dosing, to minimize harm.
- Clinical presentation of infection—may not present with traditional signs and symptoms of infection, such as

fever or pain; onset of acute confusion may be secondary to an infectious process.

- Increased risk for injury from falls—control the environment to minimize risk from falls, and conduct frequent rounding (toileting, etc.) to assist with activities of daily living (ADLs), particularly if the patient is at risk for bleeding.
- Decreased ability to tolerate intensive oncology treatment regimens—assess for side effects that are more likely and potentially more severe in the elderly patient secondary to decreased ability to maintain hydration, thermoregulation, and elimination of toxic material; manage side effects proactively.

- Caregiver support and available home care resources—patients may have personal limitations and lack established caregiver support to meet their clinical and daily function needs.
- Interactions between comorbidities and cancer therapies—most older individuals have an average of three to five comorbid health conditions, and many of these are affected by the adverse effects of therapy. Coordinated management of the oncological plan and comorbidities may require increased vigilance and modification of the primary care plan or oncological therapy.

Table 13.6 Evidence-Based Practice for Cancer Care

Problem or Potential Problem	Secondary to	As Evidenced by	Management
Neurological			
Change in mental status	Medications (e.g., corticosteroids, voriconazole)	Patient disoriented to person, place, time, and/or situation	Use a delirium assessment tool routinely.
	Infectious disease	Waxing and waning of symptoms	Assess for associated symptoms.
	Electrolyte imbalance (calcium)	May be hypervigilant or more somnolent	Identify and correct underlying organic cause if possible (remove offending medication).
	Delirium (multifactorial)		Manage patient environment to reduce risk of harm.
			Reorient patient.
Cognitive impairment	Medication and hormonal therapy	Subjective self-report or clinician assessment of decreased attention; decreased concentration, executive function, information-processing skill; slowed psychomotor function, learning, and/or memory	Assess for cognitive changes.
	Disease		Evaluate for underlying organic disease and treat if possible.
	Delirium	(+) Change on Mini-Mental State Examination	Limited strong evidence-based recommendations exist for managing cognitive impairment; try supportive care and coping strategies based on symptoms.
		(+) Attentional Function Index	
		(+) Cognitive Failures Questionnaire	
Respiratory			
Ineffective breathing pattern	Pulmonary toxicity from chemotherapeutic agents (e.g., Bleomycin; targeted therapies)	Breathing rate outside expected normal range of 12–20 breaths/minute	Assess respiratory system, including oxygen saturation.
		Uneven breathing rhythm	Identify and correct underlying organic cause if possible.
		(+) Dyspnea on a numeric rating scale or dyspnea index	Pharmacotherapy for dyspnea: morphine
	Radiation therapy		Oxygen

Table 13.6 Evidence-Based Practice for Cancer Care—cont'd

Problem or Potential Problem	Secondary to	As Evidenced by	Management
	Decreased lung capacity (pneumectomy, lobectomy)		Pharmacology: benzodiazepines for dyspnea-induced anxiety
	Infection		Increase ambient airflow directed at the face (a fan).
	Sedation		Promote relaxation and stress reduction.
Impaired gas exchange	Anemia	Oxygen saturation less than 90%	Assess respiratory system, including oxygen saturation.
	Pulmonary tumor	Impaired chest excursion	ABG for assessment
	Radiation	Abnormal breath sounds assessment	Identify and correct underlying organic cause if possible.
	Pulmonary embolism	Evidence of decreased perfusion	
	Acute lung injury from treatment (chemotherapy, blood transfusion reaction)		Symptomatic support
			Oxygen therapy
	Pneumonia		Noninvasive ventilator support
	Pleural effusions		
	Fluid overload		
GI			
Anorexia	Disease-induced anorexia	Patient self-report	Assess GI system and nutritional and hydration status.
	Treatment-induced anorexia	(+) Patient-Generated Subjective Global Assessment (PG-SGA)	Pharmacotherapy: corticosteroids, progestins (megestrol acetate)
	Nausea and vomiting	Body mass index (BMI) less than baseline	Dietary counseling/diet diary
	Food intolerances	Decreased PO intake	
	Psychological distress	Cachexia	Monitor eating patterns, content, nutrient intake.
	Infection	Laboratory changes: decreased albumin or prealbumin	Evaluate need for/potential value of appetite stimulants.
Ineffective elimination pattern: diarrhea	Medication therapy (e.g., chemotherapy)	Increase of stools per day over baseline	Measure and document the frequency, volume, and character of stool output.
	Radiation therapy	(+) Diarrhea Assessment Scale	Assess for dehydration and electrolyte imbalances.
	Infection	(+) Per National Cancer Institute (NCI) Common Terminology Criteria for Adverse Events: diarrhea	Rule out infectious disease origin.
	Abnormal bowel integrity (e.g., bowel resections, ileostomy)	Establish baseline stool characteristics for comparison.	Consider dietary modifications.
	Graft-versus-host disease (GVHD) after hematopoietic stem cell transplant		Pharmacotherapy: PO loperamide, PO opiates, *or* IM/SQ octreotide

Continued

Table 13.6 Evidence-Based Practice for Cancer Care—cont'd

Problem or Potential Problem	Secondary to	As Evidenced by	Management
Ineffective elimination pattern: constipation	Medication therapy (e.g., opioids) Altered nutritional profile Altered fluid intake Altered mobility Altered daily routines	Decrease in stools per day; hard stools that are difficult to pass Subjective complaints of constipation (+) Constipation Assessment Scale Abdominal distention Abdominal/back pain Sensation of fullness	Measure and document the frequency, volume, and character of stool output. Pharmacotherapy: stool softeners and peristaltic stimulants; polyethylene glycol Establish fluid intake goals. Enhance normal routines and optimal mobility. Pharmacotherapy: prophylactic bowel regimen for patients on opioids *or* switch to less constipating opioids
Chemotherapy-induced nausea and vomiting (N/V)	Chemotherapy	Subjective complaints of nausea Emesis (+) Index of Nausea, Vomiting, and Retching (+) Per NCI Common Terminology Criteria for Adverse Events: nausea and vomiting	Assess and document cause of nausea and vomiting. Assess and document frequency, volume, and character of emesis. Benzodiazepine (lorazepam) for anticipatory N/V *or* combinations of 5-HT3, NK1 receptor antagonist, corticosteroids, benzodiazepine for acute and delayed nausea/vomiting Acupressure
Impaired oral mucous membrane (mucositis and stomatitis), xerostomia (dry mouth)	Disease Chemotherapy Hematopoietic stem cell therapy Oral infection Malnutrition	Subjective reports of oral discomfort and/or pain Redness, swelling of oral mucosae Sores or ulcerations on oral mucosae Dry mouth by self-report	Patient education on oral hygiene Oral care should include a soft toothbrush that is replaced regularly and frequent mouth rinsing. Cryotherapy for patients receiving rapid infusions of 5-FU or melphalan Pharmacotherapy: palifermin
Skin Radiodermatitis	Radiation therapy Intensity-modulated radiation therapy has decreased risk for radiodermatitis compared with conventional radiation therapy.	Rash on or near area exposed to radiation therapy characterized by mild to severe erythema, pruritus, desquamation (dry or moist), dryness, and/or pain Rash that may occur shortly after treatment to months after treatment	Encourage skin hygiene with mild, pH-neutral soaps.

Table 13.6 Evidence-Based Practice for Cancer Care—cont'd

Problem or Potential Problem	Secondary to	As Evidenced by	Management
			Pharmacology: prevent with calendula or hyaluronic acid cream
			Limited evidence-based recommendations for treatment
Rash and skin reactions other than radiodermatitis	Chemotherapy and targeted therapies	Rash or other dermatitis syndromes	Interventions as with radiodermatitis
	GVHD related to hematopoietic stem cell transplant	Hand–foot syndrome	Prepare patients for evaluations of potential treatable etiologies such as infections and GVHD and potential cultures or biopsies.
	Infection	Nail changes	
	Other medications		
Other			
Risk for bleeding	Thrombocytopenia (platelets less than 50,000)	Occult heme-positive excrement	Monitor complete blood count (CBC).
		Visible bleeding from soft tissue and mucous membranes	Assess for signs of bleeding.
		Bruising, ecchymoses	Maintain platelet threshold of at least 10,000–20,000 per mcL to reduce risk of spontaneous bleeding; consider higher thresholds prior to procedures or when receiving anticoagulant therapy.
			Platelet transfusion for patients below minimum platelet threshold.
			Manage environment and patient needs to reduce risk of injury and falls.
Risk for infection	Neutropenia (white blood cell [WBC] count less than 1,500/mm^3)	Fever	Monitor CBC.
		Constitutional symptoms	Assess for signs of infection, particularly temperature greater than or equal to 38°C (100.4°F).
	Impaired skin integrity	Purulent exudate	
	Mucositis	Organ-specific symptoms of infective secretions/excretions (e.g., cough and abnormal breath sounds with pneumonia)	Hand hygiene using soap and water
	Immune suppressive therapy		Strict adherence to standard precautions for general population and isolation precautions as needed
			Do not allow visitors with symptoms of respiratory infection.

Continued

Table 13.6 Evidence-Based Practice for Cancer Care—cont'd

Problem or Potential Problem	Secondary to	As Evidenced by	Management
			Pharmacology: influenza vaccine, prophylactic antibiotics, antivirals, and antifungals for patients at risk for severe neutropenia
Anxiety	Fears about disease	Patient self-report	Psychoeducational interventions: educate about disease, treatment, symptom management, and self-care.
	Concerns about treatment	(+) NCCN distress-thermometer	
	Concerns about symptoms		Psychosocial interventions: cognitive-behavioral therapy, individual or group counseling, support group
	Medication adverse effects		
			Pharmacotherapy: benzodiazepines
			Massage therapy
Fatigue	Disease	Patient self-report	Screen for organic causes that can be corrected (e.g., anemia, depression, sleep disturbances).
	Treatment	(+) Brief Fatigue Inventory	
	Infection	(+) Oncology Nursing Society Fatigue Scale	
	Specific complications (e.g., anemia)		Encourage exercise several times per week.
			Patient education on energy conservation and activity management
			Optimize sleep quality (good sleep hygiene).
			Relaxation training
			Massage and healing touch
Acute pain	Disease	Patient self-report	Assess pain.
	Treatment (surgery)	Reports pain on a numeric rating scale or a visual analog scale	Pharmacotherapy for nociceptive pain: acetaminophen, NSAIDs, opioids, fentanyl, methadone, corticosteroids
	Infection	(+) Brief Pain Inventory	
	Other medical-surgical conditions		
			Pharmacotherapy for neuropathic pain: antidepressants, gabapentin, pregabalin, topical lidocaine, opioids, tramadol
Chronic pain	Tumor infiltration	Patient self-report	Assess pain. See pharmacotherapy for acute pain.
	Postchemotherapy pain syndrome	Reports pain on a numeric scale or visual analog scale	
	Postradiation syndrome		
	Peripheral neuropathy		
	Phantom limb syndrome		

5-FU, Fluorouracil; *GI,* gastrointestinal; *IM,* intramuscular; *NCCN,* National Comprehensive Cancer Network; *PO,* per os; *SQ,* subcutaneous.

Connection Check 13.6

Which statement by the patient indicates that teaching about chemotherapy was effective?

A. "I know everyone loses their hair with chemo."
B. "I know it is important that I monitor my temperature."
C. "I know I should eat whatever I want so that I don't lose weight while on chemo."
D. "I understand that I can skip a chemo treatment if I don't feel well."

Making Connections

CASE STUDY: WRAP-UP

Mrs. Jones is diagnosed with stage III breast cancer. Her treatment plan includes chemotherapy followed by a mastectomy. The chemotherapy is done in an effort to decrease the size of the tumor prior to mastectomy. She is scheduled for a class that will provide information on chemotherapy: administration and side effects. After her mastectomy, she will be started on oral hormonal therapy and will start radiation therapy.

Case Study Questions

1. Mrs. Jones has stage III breast cancer. What does this mean?
   A. The tumor has spread to lymph nodes and other organs.
   B. The tumor is small and localized and has not invaded other organs.
   C. The tumor is large, locally advanced, and possibly in local lymph nodes.
   D. The tumor is large and has spread to the lymph and hematological systems but not to other solid organs.

2. Mrs. Jones's oral hormonal therapy is considered what type of treatment?
   A. Chemotherapy
   B. Adjuvant therapy
   C. Neoadjuvant therapy
   D. Primary treatment

3. The nurse is preparing to provide patient education to Mrs. Jones, who is about to start her first cycle of chemotherapy. In addition to self-management strategies and supplemental medications for persistent acute effects, the nurse will educate her on the importance of immediately calling her provider if she experiences what symptom?
   A. Hair loss
   B. Dry skin
   C. Fever
   D. Nausea

4. The nurse is about to start Mrs. Jones on her first dose of the taxane chemotherapy. This will be Mrs. Jones's first infusion of paclitaxel, a plant alkaloid which is a vesicant and can cause hypersensitivity reactions. What should be done as a part of the nurse's preparation for medication infusion? *(Select all that apply.)*
   A. Premedicate Mrs. Jones with vitamin K.
   B. Make sure emergency equipment (oxygen, medication) is working and easily accessible.
   C. Review Mrs. Jones's medical record to make sure she has had an electrocardiogram completed within the last 24 hours.
   D. Check Mrs. Jones's IV access by flushing the line and checking for good blood return.
   E. Check Mrs. Jones's blood glucose level.

5. Mrs. Jones is now presenting post-mastectomy for external-beam radiation therapy to her left breast and left chest wall. The nurse caring for Mrs. Jones pays particular attention to which of the following systems during the head-to-toe assessment? *(Select all that apply.)*
   A. Renal system
   B. Integumentary system
   C. Musculoskeletal system
   D. Cardiac system
   E. Respiratory system

CHAPTER SUMMARY

Cancer is a constellation of diseases involving a malignant transformation of cells within a specific body system. Cancer cells are characterized by uncontrolled cell growth and altered differentiation. Risk factors for cancer include exposure to a carcinogen (most common), age, and genetic predisposition. Advanced age increases the risk for cancer. Other factors include a sedentary lifestyle and poor diet. Risk factors are believed to be cumulative, with multiple risks connoting additive cancer risk.

Two broad classes of cancer are solid and hematological. Cancers are further classified according to the organ of origin or system of origin. Cancer is then further "staged" by evaluating the size of the tumor, the burden of the disease, and the extent of disease spread. The stage of disease is used to plan management and treatment strategies. Cancer presentation varies on the basis of tumor location and disease stage.

Diagnostic evaluation includes laboratory tests, imaging studies, biopsy, and endoscopic procedures. Three primary modes of cancer treatment are surgical, radiation, and medical antineoplastic therapy. Each treatment modality has unique side effects that must be managed to minimize morbidity and mortality.

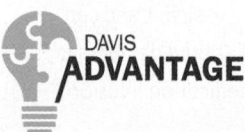

To explore learning resources for this chapter, go to **Davis Advantage** and find:
- Answers to in-text questions
- Chapter Resources and Activities
- NCLEX®-Style Chapter Review Questions
- Bibliography

Chapter 14

Overview of Shock and Sepsis

Nancy Sullivan

LEARNING OUTCOMES

Content in this chapter is designed to assist in:

1. Discussing the pathophysiology of shock
2. Identifying hypovolemic, cardiogenic, obstructive, and distributive shock
3. Describing the stages of shock
4. Describing the assessment of and monitoring techniques indicated for shock
5. Correlating clinical manifestations to pathophysiological processes of
   a. Hypovolemic shock
   b. Cardiogenic shock
   c. Obstructive shock
   d. Distributive shock
      • Neurogenic shock
      • Anaphylactic shock
      • Septic shock
6. Describing the medical management of selected shock states
7. Analyzing the nursing management of shock states
8. Discussing the complications associated with shock, including
   a. Disseminated intravascular coagulopathy
   b. Multiple-organ-dysfunction syndrome

CONCEPTS

- Assessment
- Fluid and Electrolyte Balance
- Infection
- Medication
- Oxygenation
- Perfusion
- pH Regulation

ESSENTIAL TERMS

Afterload
Anaphylactic shock
Anaphylaxis
Cardiac output (CO)
Cardiogenic shock
Central venous oxygen saturation (ScvO$_2$)
Compensatory stage
Contractility
Disseminated intravascular coagulopathy (DIC)
Distributive shock
Ejection fraction
Hemodynamic parameters
Hypovolemic shock
Initial stage
Lactate
Mixed venous oxygen saturation (SvO$_2$)
Multiple-organ-dysfunction syndrome (MODS)
Neurogenic shock
Obstructive shock
Oxygen consumption (VO$_2$)
Oxygen debt
Oxygen delivery (DO$_2$)
Preload
Progressive stage
Refractory stage
Sepsis
Septic shock
Systemic inflammatory response syndrome (SIRS)
Venous oxygen saturation

Finding Connections

CASE STUDY: EPISODE 1

Follow this patient throughout the chapter.

Mike Adams, a 42-year-old Caucasian male, is admitted to the emergency department from home with a complaint of shortness of breath. He has a history of hypertension and well-controlled diabetes. Upon presentation to the emergency department, his vital signs are as follows: temperature, 101.9°F (38.83°C); pulse, 120 bpm; respirations, 20; blood pressure, 90/54 mm Hg; and SpO$_2$, 91%. His chest radiograph reveals pneumonia. He is alert and oriented, but he complains of dizziness when changing positions. His weight is confirmed at 80 kg/176 lb.

The following orders are written for the patient:

Place two large-bore IV lines and infuse a 2.5-L (30-mL/kg) bolus of 0.9% normal saline and then begin 125 mL/hr.

Obtain complete blood cell count, serum electrolyte level, lactate level, and blood cultures.

Provide oxygen at 2 L/min via nasal cannula.

Begin administration of cefotaxime 2 g IV every 8 hours after blood cultures are drawn…

OVERVIEW OF SHOCK

The tissues of the body require a continuous supply of oxygen in order to maintain cellular functioning. Shock is a life-threatening syndrome that occurs when the circulatory system is unable to supply adequate amounts of oxygen to the tissues to meet basic metabolic requirements. This creates a state of tissue hypoxia, which is an imbalance of cellular oxygen supply and demand. Without immediate treatment to reverse this imbalance, organ system failure and death may result. Important concepts to understand when evaluating shock include cardiac output, oxygen delivery, oxygen consumption, and oxygen debt.

Cardiac Output

Cardiac output (CO) is the amount of blood ejected by the heart every minute. It is a function of stroke volume and heart rate (HR). The heart rate is simply the number of ventricular contractions per minute or heartbeats per minute. It can be affected by many variables. Stimulus from the autonomic nervous system or hormones from the adrenal medulla can adjust the HR up or down. Changes in blood pressure sensed by baroreceptors can also affect the HR.

Stroke volume is the amount of blood ejected with each ventricular contraction. It is influenced by three variables: preload, afterload, and contractility. **Preload** is the amount

of blood in the ventricles at the end of diastole. It is a reflection of a patient's fluid volume status. The values obtained to measure preload are sometimes referred to as *filling pressures*. An increase in preload may result in an increase in cardiac output. Conversely, a decrease in preload may decrease cardiac output. **Afterload** refers to the resistance to flow that the ventricle must overcome to eject its contents. Increasing afterload may make it harder for the heart to eject blood into the systemic circulation. **Contractility** refers to the force of the mechanical contraction. Poor contractility decreases stroke volume, thus decreasing cardiac output. These concepts related to cardiac output are discussed in depth in Chapter 28.

Oxygen delivery (DO$_2$) is the amount of oxygen delivered to the tissues. It is assessed through the evaluation of cardiac output and arterial oxygen content. Arterial oxygen content is a combination of hemoglobin levels, the percentage of hemoglobin saturated with oxygen, and the amount of oxygen dissolved in the plasma (the partial pressure of oxygen in arterial blood [PaO$_2$]). **Oxygen consumption (VO$_2$)** reflects the amount of oxygen extracted from the blood at the tissue level. It can be measured through evaluation of a blood sample, a **venous oxygen saturation**. The venous oxygen saturation level reflects the amount of oxygenated blood returned to the right heart. Oxygen consumption is typically stable at the tissue level. Normal SvO$_2$ values are between 60% and 75%. When that value falls below normal, it means the tissues are extracting more oxygen than normal. That results from a decreased DO$_2$, which may be a decrease in oxygen content, hemoglobin, or cardiac output. It may also reflect an inability to increase delivery in response to stressors such as pain or fever. **Oxygen debt** is the difference between normal VO$_2$ and VO$_2$ during the low-DO$_2$ state. The longer there is an imbalance between cellular oxygen supply and demand, the larger the oxygen debt becomes. This resulting oxygen debt must be repaid in order to maintain cellular function.

Connection Check 14.1

The nurse understands that which of these increase as the delivery of oxygen to the tissues falls below the tissues' requirements? *(Select all that apply.)*
A. VO$_2$
B. Oxygen debt
C. SvO$_2$
D. PaO$_2$
E. Preload

Classifications of Shock

Hypovolemic Shock

Hypovolemic shock results when there is a rapid fluid loss resulting in inadequate circulating volume. Most commonly, hypovolemic shock is secondary to blood loss from penetrating or blunt trauma or severe gastrointestinal (GI) bleeds. Examples of penetrating trauma include gunshot wounds and knife injuries. Blunt trauma examples include blood loss into the abdomen due to damage to the liver, trauma to the thoracic cavity resulting in a ruptured aorta, or long bone or femur fractures. Excessive fluid loss may be caused by severe vomiting or diarrhea. Extensive burns can also cause severe loss of fluids, resulting in hypovolemic shock.

Cardiogenic Shock

Cardiogenic shock is characterized as inadequate pumping ability of the heart muscle, most typically the result of an acute myocardial infarction (AMI). Independent of fluid volume status, the inadequate pumping of the heart results in decreased cardiac output and poor perfusion at the tissue level.

Distributive Shock

Distributive shock is the result of disease states such as sepsis, anaphylaxis, or neurogenic shock that cause poor vascular tone and vasodilation, resulting in increased vascular capacity and venous pooling. In this form of shock, a state of relative hypovolemia exists due to vasodilation without a concurrent increase in volume. Venous pooling results, causing a decreased venous return to the right heart.

Obstructive Shock

Obstructive shock is caused by a mechanical barrier to ventricular filling or ventricular emptying (increased afterload), causing decreased cardiac output. Examples of disorders resulting in impaired filling include cardiac tamponade and tension pneumothorax. An example of a disorder resulting in increased afterload is severe valvular disease.

See Table 14.1 for an overview of the classifications of shock.

Table 14.1 Classifications of Shock

Classification	Potential Cause
Hypovolemic shock	• External blood loss due to trauma, gastrointestinal bleeds, surgery
	• Internal bleeding due to fractures, dissecting aneurysms, hemothorax, retroperitoneal bleed
	• Fluid loss secondary to severe vomiting, diarrhea, excessive urination or burns
	• Third-space/transcellular fluid loss (pleural, peritoneal, joint spaces)
Cardiogenic shock	• Myocardial infarction
	• Severe valvular dysfunction
	• Severe heart failure
Distributive shock	• Sepsis
	• Anaphylaxis
	• Brain injury, spinal injury, or spinal anesthesia
Obstructive shock	• Tension pneumothorax
	• Cardiac tamponade
	• Severe valvular disease

Connection Check 14.2

The nurse understands that which patient is at risk of developing hypovolemic shock?

A. A patient with severe valvular disease
B. A patient receiving spinal anesthesia
C. A patient with severe diarrhea
D. A patient with a large pneumothorax

Stages of Shock

There are four distinct stages of shock: initial, compensatory, progressive, and refractory. Each stage is characterized by specific clinical manifestations, the initiation of compensatory mechanisms, and progressive indications of worsening hypoperfusion. Without effective treatment, shock progresses through the stages. The earlier the identification and treatment of shock take place, the better is the possible outcome.

Initial Stage

The **initial stage** of shock is marked by hypoxia due to decreased DO_2 to the cells. Clinical manifestations are subtle or subclinical, but cellular damage may be occurring. Invasive hemodynamic monitoring would note decreased cardiac output. Without identification and treatment at this stage, shock will progress to the next level.

Compensatory Stage

The **compensatory stage** is characterized by the initiation of compensatory mechanisms in an effort to maintain adequate volume, cardiac output, and blood flow to the tissues. These mechanisms include neural, endocrine, and chemical compensations.

Neural Compensation

Neural compensation is characterized by the detection of hypotension by baroreceptors in the carotid sinus and aortic arch that results in the stimulation of the sympathetic nervous system and the release of the catecholamines epinephrine and norepinephrine from the adrenal medulla. Heart rate and contractility increase, improving cardiac output. Also in response to this catecholamine release, systemic vasoconstriction occurs, resulting in increased blood pressure and redistribution of blood flow from nonessential organ systems, such as the kidneys, GI tract, and skin, to vital organs, such as the heart and brain.

Endocrine Compensation

Endocrine compensation or hormonal mechanisms that exert control over blood pressure include angiotensin II, epinephrine and norepinephrine, aldosterone, and antidiuretic hormone (ADH). Angiotensin II, created in response to low BP, is an end product of a series of events. After a drop in blood pressure, the kidneys respond by releasing the enzyme renin. Renin reacts with angiotensinogen to create angiotensin I. Angiotensin I is then converted in the lungs to angiotensin II via angiotensin-converting enzyme. Angiotensin II is a potent vasoconstrictor that increases blood pressure. Angiotensin II also acts on the adrenals to release aldosterone. The release of aldosterone promotes sodium and water reabsorption in the kidneys, which increases the circulating fluid volume. This is called the *renin–angiotensin–aldosterone system (RAAS)*. Aldosterone release is also stimulated by the release of adrenocorticotropic hormone in response to low blood pressure from the anterior pituitary, which then stimulates the adrenal cortex to release aldosterone. Also in an effort to increase the circulating volume, antidiuretic hormone is released by the posterior pituitary in response to decreased blood volume. It acts on the kidney to conserve water. Other compensatory mechanisms include the release of the catecholamines epinephrine and norepinephrine from the adrenal medulla, causing vasoconstriction as part of the fight-or-flight mechanism in the sympathetic nervous system. There is also a compensatory mechanism to increase glucose levels for energy. Circulating glucose levels are increased through the release of glucocorticoids from the adrenal cortex in response to decreased blood pressure.

Chemical Compensation

Chemical compensation is produced through the reaction of chemoreceptors in the aorta and carotid arteries that are stimulated by low oxygen levels. Low oxygen levels occur as a result of decreased blood flow through the alveoli. Tachypnea, or hyperventilation, occurs in an effort to increase circulating oxygen levels. The respiratory alkalosis that results causes a constriction of the carotid arteries. Although tachypnea is effective at improving oxygen levels, cerebral hypoxia and ischemia may result.

Progressive Stage

The **progressive stage** is marked by the failure of compensatory mechanisms to maintain adequate blood pressure and circulating fluid volumes. There is extensive shunting of blood to vital organs, which results in decreased blood flow to the periphery. Without effective treatment, profound hypoperfusion occurs, resulting in worsening metabolic acidosis, electrolyte imbalances due to the failure of the sodium–potassium pump, and respiratory acidosis.

Refractory Stage

The **refractory stage** is marked by prolonged inadequate blood supply to the cells, resulting in cell death and multisystem organ failure. There is a loss of aerobic metabolism, and only extremely inefficient anaerobic metabolism is available. Shock is irreversible at this stage.

Table 14.2 outlines the stages of shock and the clinical manifestations associated with each stage.

Connection Check 14.3

The nurse monitors for which clinical manifestations in the patient in compensatory shock?
A. Low but normal blood pressure, oliguria
B. Cold extremities, hyperglycemia
C. Weak pulses, hypoventilation
D. Hypotension, tachycardia

ASSESSMENT AND MONITORING OF SHOCK

The assessment and monitoring of shock are multifaceted. The first challenge is to quickly determine the presence and extent of shock. In some circumstances, such as obvious extensive external bleeding, a massive myocardial infarction, or rapid changes after spinal cord injury, shock may be evident quickly. Other times, it may be less obvious, such as bleeding that results in an internal sequestration or collection of blood that may occur with a femur fracture or retroperitoneal hemorrhage (i.e., blood accumulation in the abdominal cavity behind the peritoneum). Astute assessment and prompt response are essential to halt the progression of shock to the more advanced stages.

The second challenge is monitoring the progression of shock and resuscitation through physical assessment, hemodynamic monitoring, and laboratory analysis. Conventional parameters such as restoration of normal blood pressure are not adequate to gauge the extent of shock or the success of resuscitation strategies. The initiation of compensatory mechanisms in the second stage of shock may temporarily restore homeostasis without fully repaying the oxygen debt, allowing continuing hypoperfusion at the tissue level. Physical assessment parameters to assess perfusion at the tissue level, such as level of consciousness, urine output, respiratory status, pulse quality, skin color and/or mottling, and temperature, are important to monitor. Hemodynamic monitoring and laboratory analyses of endpoints, such as **lactate**, base deficit, venous oxygen saturation, and blood gas analysis, are also essential parameters to consider when evaluating the extent of shock and success of resuscitation.

Physical Assessment

Central Nervous System

Changes in central nervous system perfusion may be the initial indication of inadequate DO_2 to the tissues. As noted earlier, in addition to low DO_2, the respiratory alkalosis that results from tachypnea causes vasoconstriction of the

Table 14.2 Stages of Shock

Stage of Shock	System Response	Clinical Manifestations
Initial	• Decreased oxygen delivery to the tissues	• Subtle or no clinical manifestations
Compensatory	• Vasoconstriction • Increased sodium and water reabsorption • Shunting of blood away from nonessential organs • Increased glucose production	• Restlessness, confusion • Increased heart rate • Tachypnea • Respiratory alkalosis • Oliguria • Hyperglycemia • Decreased bowel sounds • Weak pulses • Cool, moist skin
Progressive	• Extensive shunting of blood away from nonessential organs • Failure of sodium–potassium pump	• Lethargy or coma • Hypotension • Dysrhythmias • Anuria • Absent bowel sounds • Severe metabolic acidosis • Respiratory acidosis • Cold extremities • Weak or absent pulses
Refractory	• Inefficient anaerobic metabolism • Extreme tissue hypoxia	• Coma • Severe hypotension • Severe metabolic and respiratory acidoses • Hepatic failure • Renal failure • Peripheral tissue ischemia and necrosis

carotid arteries, resulting in decreased cerebral blood flow. Restlessness, confusion, and irritability are several beginning indicators of poor cerebral perfusion. Without treatment, continued poor perfusion may progress to lethargy and coma.

Cardiovascular System

The cardiovascular system provides several parameters effective in the assessment of the presence or resolution of shock. Blood pressure is a valuable indicator of fluid status and cardiac output. A decreased blood pressure level can be indicative of a problem. In shock, blood pressure decreases because of inadequate venous return to the heart, vasodilation, or decreased contractility of the heart muscle. It is important to remember that a return to the baseline blood pressure level does not mean the resolution of the problem, but prolonged hypotension does indicate the continued presence of shock. A common finding indicative of the compensatory stage of shock is a narrow pulse pressure,

which results from compensatory vasoconstriction causing an increase in diastolic pressure with only a slight increase in systolic pressure.

Tachycardia is a typical finding due to stimulation of the sympathetic nervous system as a way to increase cardiac output. If shock is not resolved but is allowed to progress to later stages, the HR may slow. Skin color, temperature, quality of pulses, and capillary refill indicate perfusion in the extremities. Because of shunting of the blood to vital organs, the skin and periphery become cool, pale, mottled, or cyanotic, with thready pulses and sluggish capillary refill.

Respiratory System

The respiratory system also provides insight as to the presence and progression of shock. Early stages of shock are characterized by increased respirations done in an effort to increase oxygenation and decrease carbon dioxide (CO_2) levels due to the metabolic acidosis. Oxygenation can be measured through pulse oximetry, but poor peripheral circulation may cause inaccurate readings. Arterial blood gases (ABGs) may be necessary for more accurate assessment.

Renal System

The renal system provides a clear indication of poor perfusion if urine output decreases. Oliguria is a common finding in early shock because of decreased perfusion of the renal tubules, which stimulates the initiation of the renin–angiotensin–aldosterone system. If unresolved, later stages of shock will present with anuria, increased creatinine level, and other signs of acute renal failure.

Gastrointestinal System

The GI system indicates poor perfusion through sluggish, hypoactive bowel sounds that reflect a slowing of intestinal activity. Nausea and vomiting may also be present. The GI system is particularly vulnerable to poor perfusion and ischemia. Cell damage in the GI tract allows translocation of intestinal bacteria to the systemic circulation, increasing the risk of sepsis. Some have suggested that hypoperfusion in the GI system may initiate a systemic inflammatory response, which, if not resolved, may be the precursor to multiple organ dysfunction syndrome (MODS).

Hemodynamic Monitoring

Monitoring of blood pressure, cardiac output, and the variables that affect cardiac output provides valuable insights into the presence, stages, or resolution of shock. Invasive hemodynamic monitoring is done through an arterial line and a central venous catheter or pulmonary artery (PA) catheter.

Arterial Line

A critically ill patient in shock benefits from the placement of an arterial line. Blood pressure is continually displayed, and it provides easy access to blood for analysis, especially ABG samples. As mentioned previously, oxygenation is sometimes better measured through ABGs because of peripheral shunting and inaccurate pulse oximetry readings.

Pulmonary Artery Catheter

A pulmonary artery (PA) catheter is a flexible, balloon-tipped catheter that is guided through the right side of the heart and into the pulmonary artery. Pulmonary artery catheter monitoring allows the nurse to obtain detailed information about cardiac output and the variables that affect it: preload, also referred to as filling pressures; afterload; and contractility.

Although variable, the typical PA catheter has four lumens—proximal, distal, thermistor, and inflation—each of which leads to a specific port (Fig. 14.1). The proximal port, located approximately 30 cm from the tip of the catheter, typically resting just in the right atrium, is used to monitor right atrial pressure, a reflection of right heart preload, and *right ventricular end-diastolic volume*. It is also the port used to inject the solution to obtain a thermodilution cardiac output.

The distal lumen port is located at the tip of the PA catheter and rests within the pulmonary artery. Through this port, the nurse can monitor systolic, diastolic, and mean PA pressures and the pulmonary artery wedge pressure, also referred to as pulmonary artery occlusive pressure (PAOP). The PAOP is obtained when the balloon located at the

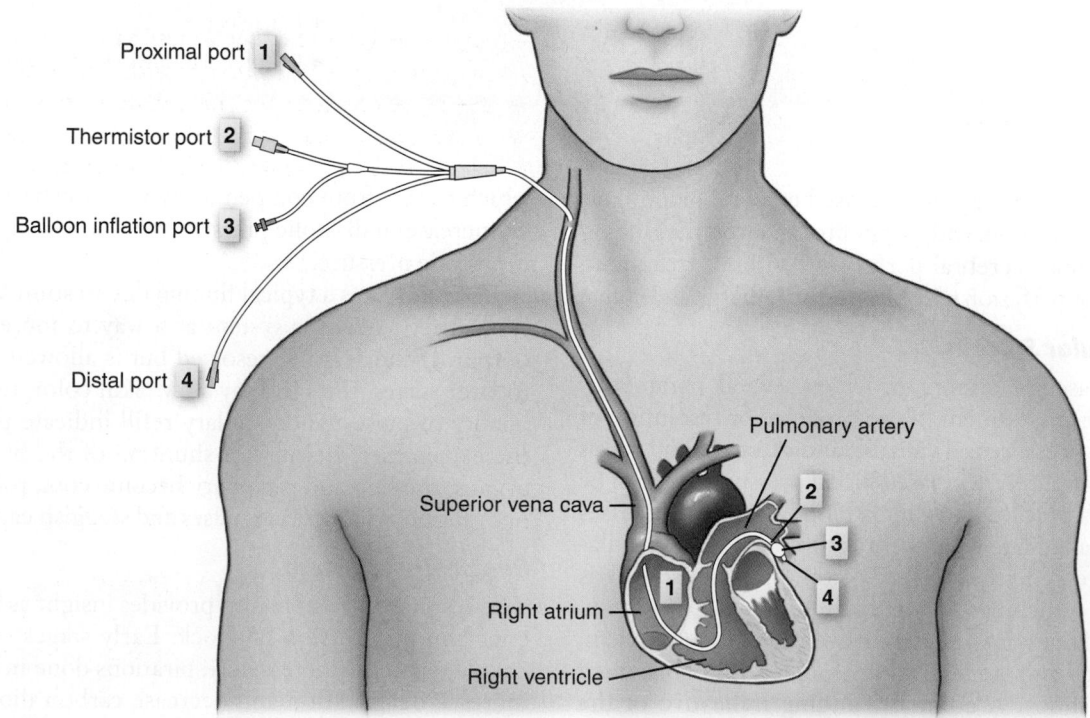

FIGURE 14.1 Pulmonary artery catheter.

end of the inflation lumen is inflated with 1.5 mL of air (Fig. 14.2). The balloon floats into a wedge position in the PA, which occludes that branch of the PA, obscuring data from the right heart. In this position, the values obtained reflect pressures proximal to the balloon or left heart pressures. Specifically, the PAOP reflects left heart preload or the amount of blood in the left ventricle at the end of diastole, also referred to as *left ventricular end-diastolic pressure*. The distal lumen port can also be used for drawing a venous oxygen saturation sample, specifically, a **mixed venous oxygen saturation (SvO$_2$)** sample. The SvO$_2$ obtained through a PA line provides a "mixed" sample of blood returned from both the superior and inferior vena cava, thus providing information on oxygen extraction throughout the entire body.

Cardiac output can be directly obtained through a PA catheter. There is a temperature sensor, or thermistor port, built into the tip of the PA catheter. It continuously measures the ambient blood temperature around it. To obtain a cardiac output, a small bolus of cooler saline is briskly injected into the PA catheter through the proximal port. As a result of the injection of cooler fluid, the temperature of the blood flowing by the sensor changes. The time it takes for the cold injectate to pass the sensor is measured in liters of blood pumped per minute. This is called the "thermodilution" method of obtaining cardiac output. Normal cardiac output is 4 to 6 L/min. Typically, cardiac output is indexed, meaning it is calculated on the basis of the patient's body surface area. A normal cardiac index is 2.5 to 4 L/min.

Other hemodynamic variables obtained through a PA catheter include afterload and contractility. Afterload, also known as *systemic vascular resistance*, is a calculated value obtained using mean arterial and mean right atrial pressure divided by cardiac output. Pulmonary vascular resistance, the afterload of the right heart, is obtained by substituting PA pressures into that calculation. Contractility is another value calculated through measurements obtained via the PA catheter. It is inferred by evaluating the right and left ventricular stroke work indexes, or calculations of work done by the heart with each contraction. As discussed, invasive hemodynamic monitoring with a PA catheter allows a more in-depth look at volume status and DO$_2$ but provides only a partial assessment of recovery.

The use of the PA catheter has not demonstrated a consistent benefit in the overall mortality of shock patients, so the decision to use this diagnostic monitoring tool should be based on individual case-based need by practitioners skilled in insertion and interpretation of the data. There are several less invasive tools for hemodynamic monitoring to help guide resuscitation in critically ill patients. One example presently in use is pulse contour analysis. This analysis estimates stroke volume through analysis of the systolic phase of the arterial waveform. Cardiac output is estimated through the calculation of HR × SV. There are several pulse contour systems; some require just an arterial line, some require the addition of a central line. They have limitations such as attempting to evaluate CO in a patient with an irregular heart rhythm. They continue to be evaluated for accuracy.

See Table 14.3 for a comparison of hemodynamic parameters in different types of shock and in early and late sepsis.

Central Venous Catheter

Central venous monitoring utilizes a long catheter threaded through the superior vena cava with the distal port resting in the superior vena cava immediately above the junction with the right atrium. This allows central venous pressure (CVP) monitoring. This value indicates a mean CVP, which,

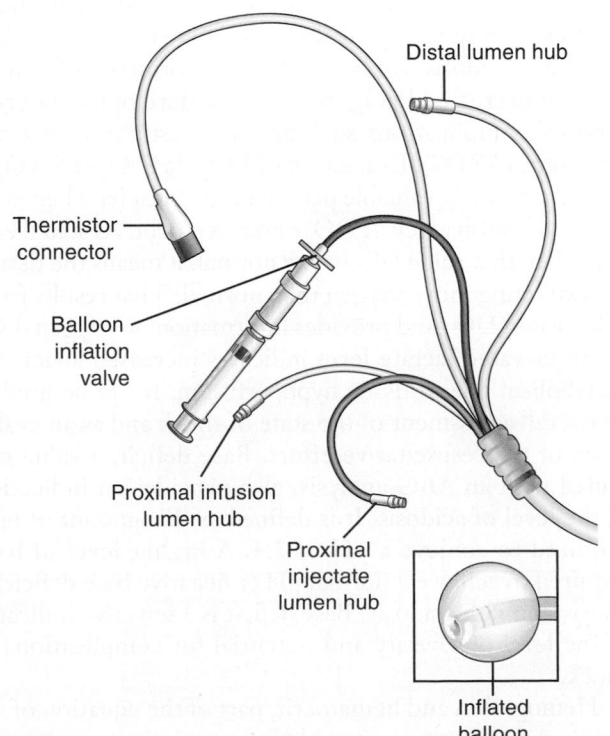

FIGURE 14.2 Pulmonary artery catheter with inflated balloon.

Labels: Distal lumen hub; Thermistor connector; Balloon inflation valve; Proximal infusion lumen hub; Proximal injectate lumen hub; Inflated balloon

Table 14.3 Comparison of Hemodynamic Parameters in Shock	
Classification of Shock	**Hemodynamic Parameters**
Hypovolemic shock	• Decreased cardiac output
	• Decreased central venous pressure (CVP) and pulmonary artery occlusive pressure (PAOP)
	• Increased systemic vascular resistance (SVR)
	• Decreased venous oxygen saturation (SvO$_2$ or ScvO$_2$)
	• Hypotension and tachycardia

Continued

Table 14.3   Comparison of Hemodynamic Parameters in Shock—cont'd

Classification of Shock	Hemodynamic Parameters
Cardiogenic shock	• Decreased cardiac output • Increased CVP and PAOP • Increased SVR • Decreased venous oxygen saturation (SvO$_2$ or ScvO$_2$) • Hypotension and tachycardia
Obstructive shock	• Decreased cardiac output • Variable CVP and PAOP • Increased SVR • Decreased venous oxygen saturation (SvO$_2$ or ScvO$_2$) • Hypotension and tachycardia
Distributive Shock	
Anaphylactic shock	• Decreased cardiac output • Decreased CVP and PAOP • Decreased SVR • Decreased venous oxygen saturation (SvO$_2$ or ScvO$_2$) • Hypotension and tachycardia
Neurogenic shock	• Decreased cardiac output • Decreased CVP and PAOP • Decreased SVR • Decreased venous oxygen saturation (SvO$_2$ or ScvO$_2$) • Hypotension and bradycardia
Early septic shock	• Increased cardiac output • Decreased CVP and PAOP • Decreased SVR • Increased venous oxygen saturation (SvO$_2$ or ScvO$_2$) • Normal or decreased blood pressure, tachycardia, and hyperthermia
Late septic shock	• Decreased cardiac output • Variable CVP and PAOP • Variable SVR • Decreased venous oxygen saturation (SvO$_2$ or ScvO$_2$) • Hypotension, tachycardia, and hypothermia

similar to the RAP, is used as an estimate of volume returning to the right heart or right heart preload, or the *right ventricular end-diastolic volume*. The CVP and RAP are typically the same or very similar unless there is a pressure differential between the SVC and the right atrium, and the terms are sometimes used interchangeably. For consistency purposes, this book will refer to the measure of right heart preload as CVP. A decreased CVP reading may be indicative of a low-volume state, such as hypovolemic shock or peripheral vasodilatation that occurs as a result of distributive shock. An elevated CVP may indicate increased volume that may occur with cardiogenic shock.

This line may also be used as a port to draw another type of venous oxygen saturation, specifically, a **central venous oxygen saturation (ScvO$_2$)**, if a PA line is not in place. Unlike the sample drawn through the PA line, the ScvO$_2$ provides information primarily on oxygen extraction in the brain and upper body (Fig. 14.3). Although ScvO$_2$ is not reflective of whole-body VO$_2$, good correlation has been found between SvO$_2$ and ScvO$_2$ for monitoring and treatment purposes.

Laboratory Analysis

Evaluation of laboratory studies provides valuable information regarding the presence, severity, or resolution of shock. Several very important indicators include ABG analysis, SvO$_2$ or ScvO$_2$, base deficit, and lactate level. Arterial blood gas analysis provides information on oxygenation, ventilation, and the presence of acidosis or alkalosis (metabolic or respiratory), which provides insight into the adequacy of treatment. Results will vary on the basis of early or late shock. As already stated, hyperventilation in early shock produces a respiratory alkalosis. In later stages of shock, a metabolic acidosis will be present. The presence of hypoxemia, or decreased PaO$_2$, indicates the development of respiratory complications such as acute respiratory distress syndrome (ARDS). Evaluation of VO$_2$ via SvO$_2$ or ScvO$_2$ is also an extremely valuable parameter to consider when evaluating the sufficiency of DO$_2$ or oxygen debt. As stated earlier, when that value falls below normal, it means the tissues are extracting more oxygen than normal. That results from a decreased DO$_2$ and provides information on oxygen debt.

An elevated lactate level indicates increased anaerobic metabolism due to tissue hypoperfusion. It can be used as an overall assessment of the state of shock and as an evaluation of the resuscitative effort. Base deficit, a value obtained with an ABG analysis, also provides an indication of the level of acidosis. It is defined as the amount of base required to achieve a pH of 7.4. A higher level of base required to achieve a normal pH (a negative base deficit) is consistent with acidosis. Base deficit is a sensitive indicator of the level of severity and potential for complications of shock.

Hemoglobin and hematocrit, part of the equation of arterial oxygen content, provide information about oxygen-carrying capacity and are valuable for determining the

Site of Measurement

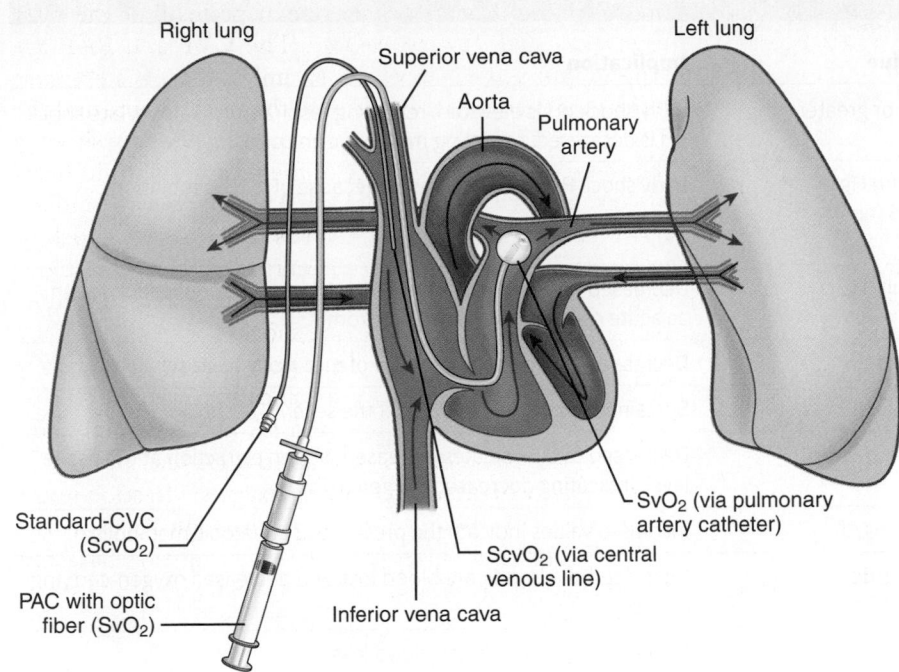

FIGURE 14.3 Measurement sites for ScvO₂ and SvO₂.

effectiveness of DO₂. Electrolytes, renal studies, liver studies, and glucose level are all valuable indicators of the state of shock. Unfortunately, by the time they are elevated, shock has progressed to later stages.

Table 14.4 lists laboratory tests that can aid in the evaluation of shock.

Connection Check 14.4

The nurse understands that which of the following are the best parameters for evaluating the severity of the shock state? *(Select all that apply.)*

A. SvO₂
B. Lactate level
C. Base excess
D. Glucose level
E. PaO₂

HYPOVOLEMIC SHOCK

Epidemiology

Hypovolemic shock is defined as inadequate intravascular volume producing decreased cardiac output that results when there is a severe loss of blood or fluids due to acute injury or illness. An acute bleed may be the result of penetrating or blunt trauma or massive GI bleeding. Rapid fluid loss may be due to severe vomiting and diarrhea, excessive urination, or loss of fluids due to burns. The most common cause of hypovolemia is blood loss. Incidence or prevalence data are unavailable because the data are reported for the causative mechanism rather than for the resultant hypovolemic shock.

Pathophysiology

Acute loss of circulating fluid volume results in decreased venous return to the right heart and decreased stroke volume and cardiac output, resulting in decreased perfusion at the tissue level. This decreased intravascular volume results in the initiation of several compensatory mechanisms. The initial response is the stimulation of the sympathetic nervous system, which increases the HR in an attempt to increase cardiac output. The sympathetic nervous system also stimulates the release of epinephrine and norepinephrine from the adrenal medulla, improving contractility and inducing systemic vasoconstriction. Blood pressure and cardiac output are increased. Blood flow is redirected from nonessential organs to vital organs such as the heart and brain.

The endocrine system, through the RAAS and the release of antidiuretic hormone from the posterior pituitary, increases sodium and water reabsorption in the renal tubules, effectively increasing venous return to the right heart. The end product of the renin–angiotensin–aldosterone system, angiotensin II, also produces potent systemic vasoconstriction that increases blood pressure and venous return.

Clinical Manifestations

Clinical manifestations vary depending on the stage of shock. Initially, the patient may be in a compensated state and have no outward symptoms. Without intervention, clinical manifestations appear because of the stimulation of compensatory mechanisms. In the early stages, blood pressure may remain within normal limits, but the HR is typically increased. The patient may present as restless or confused. Urine output decreases because of

Table 14.4 Laboratory Tests Valuable in the Evaluation of Shock

Laboratory Test	Abnormal Value	Implication
pH	Less than 7.35 or greater than 7.45	Early shock pH is elevated, reflecting respiratory alkalosis; late shock pH is decreased, reflecting metabolic acidosis.
Partial pressure of carbon dioxide in arterial blood (PaCO₂)	Less than 35 mm Hg or greater than 45 mm Hg	Early shock $PaCO_2$ is decreased because of hyperventilation.
Partial pressure of oxygen in arterial blood (PaO₂)	Less than 80 mm Hg	Decreased PaO_2 indicates the development of complications such as acute respiratory distress syndrome.
HCO₃	Less than 22 mEq/L	Decreased in late shock because of metabolic acidosis
Base deficit	Less than –2 mEq/L	Sustained negative levels reflect the severity of shock.
Mixed venous oxygen saturation (SvO₂)	Less than 60%	Decreased SvO_2 indicates increased oxygen extraction at the tissue level, indicating decreased oxygen delivery.
Lactate	Greater than 2 mg/dL	Increased values indicate the presence of anaerobic metabolism.
Hemoglobin	Less than 11.7 g/dL	Decreased levels indicate blood loss and decreased oxygen-carrying capacity.
Hematocrit	Less than 38%	Decreased values indicate blood loss.
Glucose	Less than 70 mg/dL or greater than 105 mg/dL	In the absence of diabetes, increased values indicate the initiation of fight-or-flight compensatory mechanisms.
Blood urea nitrogen	Greater than 21 mg/dL	Increased values indicate renal hypoperfusion.
Creatinine	Greater than 1.2 mg/dL	Increased values indicate acute renal failure.
Aspartate aminotransferase	Greater than 20 units/L	Increased values indicate hepatic injury.
Lactic dehydrogenase	Greater than 102 units/L	Increased values indicate hepatic injury.

the reabsorption of sodium and water. The skin becomes pale, cool, and clammy. Pulses are weak, with sluggish capillary refill. Hyperventilation is present, producing a respiratory alkalosis. Decreased or hypoactive bowel sounds are present because of the shunting of blood to vital organs. Hyperglycemia is evident because of the initiation of the fight-or-flight response in the initial compensatory phase.

Later stages of shock produce more pronounced clinical manifestations, such as lethargy; hypotension; metabolic and respiratory acidoses; anuria; cold, cyanotic skin with weak or absent pulses; and dysrhythmias. Without effective intervention, the patient enters the refractory stage of shock. Coma, severe hypotension, ischemic and necrotic cold extremities, renal failure, and hepatic failure follow.

Hemodynamic parameters that present in hypovolemic shock are a decreased central venous pressure and decreased PA occlusive pressure, which reflect decreased volume. Decreased venous oxygenation saturation, SvO_2 or $ScvO_2$, is present as a result of decreased cardiac output. An increased systemic vascular resistance reflects the initiation of compensatory mechanisms (see Table 14.3).

Management

Medical Management

Resuscitation priorities in hypovolemic shock include maximizing oxygenation, initiating fluid resuscitation, and identifying and treating the underlying cause. Maximizing oxygenation is essential in the treatment of the patient in shock. Assessing and stabilizing the patient's airway is the immediate first priority. High-flow oxygen via a 100% nonrebreather mask may be utilized if the patient is able to adequately maintain and protect his or her airway. Frequently spontaneous respiratory effort is inadequate requiring the need for intubation and positive-pressure mechanical ventilation. Positive-pressure mechanical ventilation should be used with caution because the associated increased intrathoracic pressures decrease cardiac output further, exacerbating poor DO_2 to the tissues.

Rapid fluid resuscitation is the mainstay of treatment for hypovolemic shock. The type of fluid used varies depending on the cause of hypovolemia. Nonhemorrhagic shock is typically treated with isotonic crystalloid fluids such as normal saline solution or lactated Ringer's solution. Fluid resuscitation strategies for trauma patients suffering large volumes of blood loss call for a balanced response that includes the minimization of crystalloids, 1:1:1 blood product replacement ratios with packed red blood cells (PRBCs), fresh frozen plasma (FFP) and platelets, and permissive hypotension. Whatever the cause of hypovolemia, it is important to continue resuscitation until the oxygen debt accumulated has been repaid. This is indicated by clinical signs such as stabilization of blood pressure, strong peripheral pulses, warm extremities, adequate urine output, no signs of a decreased level of consciousness, and lowering of lactate and base deficit to within normal limits. The patient with prolonged or unresponsive hypovolemia may need monitoring with a central venous monitor to evaluate filling pressures and cardiac output.

See Evidence-Based Practice: Fluid Resuscitation for a discussion of fluid resuscitation strategies in hemorrhagic shock.

Evidence-Based Practice

Fluid Resuscitation

Previous fluid replacement strategies in severe trauma began with the rapid infusion of crystalloid solutions, but increased morbidity and mortality are well documented with the use of excessive crystalloids. Resuscitation with normal saline solution, although initially producing an increase in blood pressure, ultimately results in a shift of fluid from the intravascular space into the interstitial and intracellular spaces. The most notable complication of this is adult respiratory distress syndrome. Crystalloid infusion also worsens coagulopathy through dilution and alters pH, resulting in acidosis, and excessive infusion of cold solution contributes to hypothermia, all of which result in the trauma triad of death: acidosis, hypothermia, and coagulopathy.

Recent research suggests a balanced resuscitation strategy for severe hemorrhagic shock: minimization of crystalloids, 1:1:1 blood product ratios for infusions, and permissive hypotension. Based on the significant experiential evidence in the military population, an approach utilizing equal amounts of packed red blood cells with fresh frozen plasma and platelets along with limited resuscitation with crystalloids may have a positive impact on overall survival. Additionally, maintaining a mean arterial pressure (MAP) of 50 rather than 65 or greater results in less bleeding and reduces the risk of dislodging a clot that may have formed to stop bleeding.

Cantle, P. M., & Cotton, B. A. (2017). Balanced resuscitation in trauma management. *Surgical Clinics*, 97(5), 999–1014.

Identifying and controlling further loss of blood or fluid is an obvious priority in this patient. If bleeding or fluid loss is not immediately apparent, diagnostic studies may be necessary to determine the cause of shock. An ultrasound and a focused assessment with sonography for trauma (FAST) may be necessary to determine if blunt trauma has caused thoracic or abdominal bleeding. Although obvious deformity may be evident, radiographs or computed tomography (CT) scans may be necessary to determine the presence of long bone or pelvic fractures, which can cause sequestration of large amounts of blood. Definitive treatment may include surgery to locate and control the source of bleeding, stabilization of fractures, and medications to control vomiting and diarrhea.

Nursing Management

Assessment and Analysis

The clinical manifestations of hypovolemic shock are related to the decrease in cardiac output and impaired blood flow to all vital organs. The manifestations vary depending on the stage of shock. Without adequate treatment, the results are hypotension; tachycardia with weak pulses; tachypnea; cold, cyanotic, and mottled skin; decreased or absent urine output; severely decreased level of consciousness; and severely decreased or absent bowel sounds. Continuing decompensation results in multiple organ system failures, as evidenced by increased renal studies such as blood urea nitrogen (BUN) and creatinine and increased liver function tests. The refractory stage is evidenced by coma, severe hypotension, bradycardia, and acute respiratory failure due to profound cellular hypoxia.

Hemodynamic parameters also vary according to the stage of shock. If a PA catheter is in place, decreased cardiac output will be noted beginning in the initial stage of shock. The compensatory stage is notable for an increase in systemic vascular resistance due to the sympathetic nervous system response. Central venous pressure and PAOP are decreased. Although initial compensation maintains a normal blood pressure, hypotension eventually results.

Nursing Diagnoses

- **Altered tissue perfusion** related to inadequate cardiac output
- **Inadequate oxygenation** related to poor gas exchange

Nursing Interventions
■ *Assessments*

- Neurological status
  A decreased level of consciousness occurs as a result of decreased cardiac output and carotid vasoconstriction that occurs as a result of hyperventilation and respiratory alkalosis.
- Vital signs
  Blood pressure may remain normal initially because of the stimulation of compensatory mechanisms. Tachycardia will be present as one of the compensatory mechanisms. Hypotension and bradycardia signal the end of effective compensation.

- Hemodynamic readings
  Decreased cardiac output occurs as a result of decreased filling pressures, as evidenced by decreased CVP and decreased PAOP. Increased systemic vascular resistance is evident as the sympathetic nervous system is stimulated, resulting in vasoconstriction to increase blood pressure and cardiac output.
- Urine output
  Decreased urine output occurs as a result of decreased cardiac output and stimulation of compensatory mechanisms that increase reabsorption of sodium and water.
- Skin color and temperature
  Cold and clammy skin may be a sign of decreasing peripheral perfusion and progressing shock.

  Laboratory Tests
- ABGs
  Initial ABGs may reflect a respiratory alkalosis due to hyperventilation. Later stages of shock reveal a metabolic acidosis due to anaerobic metabolism.
- Venous oxygen saturation; $SvO_2/ScvO_2$
  Decreased oxygen saturation is an indicator of inadequate oxygen delivery.
- Hemoglobin and hematocrit
  Hemoglobin and hematocrit values may be decreased if the cause of hypovolemic shock is bleeding.
- Metabolic profile
  Renal failure and liver failure, as evidenced by increased BUN and creatinine levels and liver function test results, may become evident as a result of decreased organ perfusion.
- Lactate/base deficit
  Increased lactate level and negative base deficit are evidence of poor perfusion at the cellular level. Decreasing lactate level is an endpoint demonstrating adequate resuscitation.

■ **Actions**

- Apply a 100% nonrebreather mask.
  Maximizing oxygenation is the number one priority.
- Anticipate and prepare for intubation.
  Intubation and mechanical ventilation may be required to improve oxygenation.
- Insert large-bore IV lines for fluid administration.
  Large-bore IV lines facilitate the rapid infusion of fluid necessary to reverse hypovolemic shock.
- Administer fluid replacement as prescribed:
  - Normal saline
  - Lactated Ringer's solution
  - Blood products
    Fluid replacement is the foundation of treatment in hypovolemic shock.

■ **Teaching**

- Instruct patient and family on the cause of hypovolemia.
  Depending on the cause of hypovolemia, patient and family understanding may help prevent a repeat occurrence.

- Allow family members visitation during hospital treatment; provide frequent updates on condition and treatment.
  Family visitation and information can help to decrease a patient's and family's anxiety.

Evaluating Care Outcomes

Rapid intervention with adequate oxygenation and fluid resuscitation may result in the restoration of hemodynamic stability. A well managed patient will be awake and alert with a stable blood pressure and have adequate urine output, warm extremities, strong peripheral pulses, and a normalizing lactate with the loss of fluid under control.

⚠ Safety Alert Permissive hypotension during resuscitation is a strategy that is recommended to reduce postresuscitation mortality and morbidity. One study compared patients who were resuscitated to a mean arterial pressure of 50 mm Hg with patients resuscitated to a mean arterial pressure of 65 mm Hg. The results were positive. Patients in the group with low mean arterial pressure required less fluid and blood administration and had decreased coagulopathy after treatment. It is thought that an increase in blood pressure may dislodge a newly formed clot, thus increasing the possibility of bleeding. Lower mean arterial pressures may decrease this risk.

Meticulous care must be taken to monitor the patient's hemodynamic status, including CVP, PAOP, blood pressure, SvO_2, and other endpoints of resuscitation, such as level of consciousness and urine output, to ensure the mean arterial pressure is adequate.

Connection Check 14.5

The nurse understands that which hemodynamic parameters are consistent with hypovolemic shock?

A. Decreased cardiac output, decreased systemic vascular resistance, decreased CVP

B. Decreased cardiac output, increased systemic vascular resistance, decreased CVP

C. Decreased cardiac output, increased systemic vascular resistance, increased CVP

D. Decreased cardiac output, decreased systemic vascular resistance, increased CVP

CARDIOGENIC SHOCK

Epidemiology

The prevalence of cardiogenic shock ranges from 5% to 10% in patients with AMI. The incidence is higher in men than in women because of the increased prevalence of coronary artery disease in males. The incidence of cardiogenic shock following AMI is higher in women. Cardiogenic shock has a mortality rate of approximately 50%, but the rate is higher in patients older than 75 and lower in younger patients.

Risk factors for cardiogenic shock include any disorder that results in the acute deterioration of myocardial mechanical contraction. Most commonly, cardiogenic shock results when more than 40% of the myocardium is damaged because of AMI. Other risk factors include end-stage congestive heart failure, cardiomyopathy, hypertension, diabetes, multiple-vessel coronary artery disease, and acute vascular disease.

Pathophysiology

Cardiogenic shock is defined as a state of hypoperfusion at the tissue level resulting from severe impairment of ventricular contraction in the presence of adequate vascular volume. As a result of damaged myocardium, there is a marked reduction in contractility, which reduces the **ejection fraction** (the percentage of blood ejected from the ventricle with each contraction) and cardiac output. The result is increased left and right ventricular filling pressures but decreased cardiac output. Venous oxygen saturation decreases with increased oxygen extraction at the tissue level because of low cardiac output. The ultimate result is univentricular or biventricular failure, profound hypotension, and pulmonary edema.

The decreased cardiac output leads to stimulation of compensatory mechanisms. In the case of cardiogenic shock, the sympathetic stimulation that increases HR and contractility also increases myocardial workload and myocardial oxygen demand, worsening the ischemia. Systemic vasoconstriction also increases the workload on an already-stressed heart by increasing afterload. Fluid retention induced by the renin–angiotensin–aldosterone system increases filling pressures, which ultimately contributes to the development of pulmonary edema and hypoxemia. The end result is a vicious cycle of increased cardiac workload and increased myocardial

oxygen demand combined with poor perfusion of myocardial tissue (Fig. 14.4). This worsens myocardial ischemia, which, if left untreated or unsuccessfully managed, ends in death.

Clinical Manifestations

Patients in cardiogenic shock frequently present with clinical symptoms similar to those of AMI, such as chest pain, diaphoresis, nausea, and vomiting. The decreased cardiac output, hypotension, and resulting compensatory mechanisms cause a decreased level of consciousness; decreased urine output; poor pulses; pale, cool skin; and decreased bowel sounds. Shortness of breath, crackles on auscultation, and decreased saturation of arterial blood with oxygen (SpO$_2$) are evident as a result of pulmonary edema. Decreased cardiac output greatly impairs tissue perfusion, leading to anaerobic metabolism that produces lactic acid, as evidenced by increased lactate levels. Arterial blood gases reveal a metabolic acidosis.

As shock progresses, clinical manifestations become more pronounced. Profound hypotension and bradycardia develop. Organ systems begin to fail. Laboratory analysis reveals increases in creatinine and liver enzymes, demonstrating renal and liver failure. Coma; cyanotic, mottled skin; absent bowel sounds; and anuria are present.

Hemodynamic parameters obtained through a PA catheter include increased CVP and PAOP. Systemic vascular resistance is high, and cardiac output is very low. Venous oxygen saturation is decreased.

Management

Medical Management

Laboratory and Diagnostic Tests

Laboratory and diagnostic tests related to cardiogenic shock include a 12-lead electrocardiogram (ECG), cardiac enzymes, and a chest radiograph. The initial diagnostic test

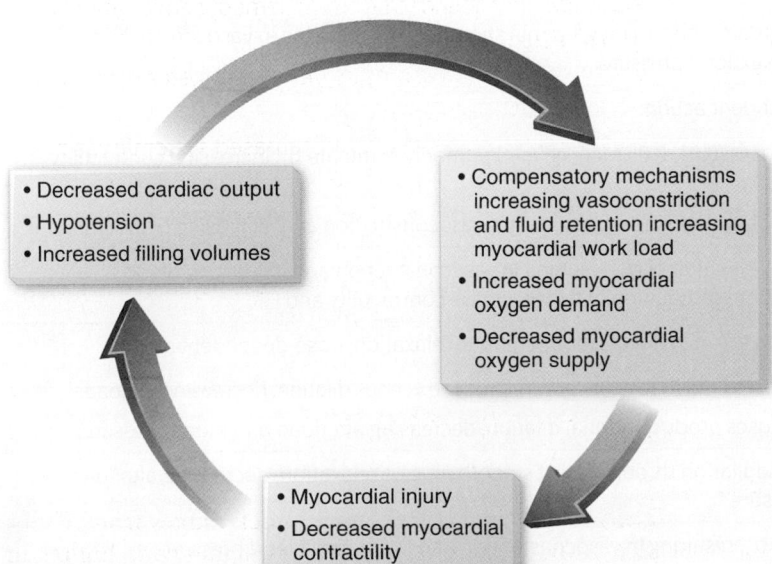

FIGURE 14.4 Vicious cycle of cardiogenic shock.

should be the 12-lead ECG, conducted to rule out or rule in myocardial infarction as the cause of shock. Cardiac enzymes will also help confirm the presence or absence of AMI. The chest radiograph is obtained to rule out other causes of hypotension and shock, such as tension pneumothorax or cardiac tamponade. A chest radiograph will also confirm the presence of pulmonary edema.

Treatment Priorities

Treatment priorities include stabilizing oxygenation and initiating drug therapy to increase blood pressure and cardiac output. Consideration of emergency revascularization, an attempt to restore blood flow through percutaneous coronary intervention, may be indicated. Intra-aortic balloon pump (IABP) therapy to increase myocardial oxygen supply and decrease myocardial oxygen demand may also be considered. If these treatments are not successful, a ventricular assist device (VAD) may be necessary.

Stabilizing Oxygenation

Providing 100% oxygen through a nonrebreather mask is a minimal first step to stabilize oxygenation. Intubation and mechanical ventilation are frequently necessary to support ventilation and maximize oxygenation. This may help decrease myocardial workload, increase myocardial oxygen supply, and preserve myocardial tissue.

Medications

Medications that support blood pressure through vasoconstriction (vasopressors), such as dopamine and norepinephrine, should be started to sustain blood pressure and help maintain adequate mean arterial pressure. Although there is no difference in mortality in most shock states with the use of dopamine or norepinephrine, there is some evidence that norepinephrine has a lower mortality rate in cardiogenic shock. Care should be taken when using vasopressors to increase blood pressure because they will also increase systemic vascular resistance, increasing myocardial workload. Inotropic support, medications such as dobutamine that increase myocardial contractility, should also be initiated to improve cardiac output. Nitroglycerin may be very carefully added in an attempt to decrease preload and afterload. It decreases preload through venous dilation and decreases afterload through arterial dilation. It will also decrease blood pressure, so it should be used with extreme caution. Nitroprusside may also be used with extreme caution to decrease afterload. Diuretics may also be used with caution in an attempt to decrease filling volumes. Morphine sulfate may also be administered. It is useful for several reasons. First, it helps relieve pain due to a myocardial infarction. Second, morphine is a vasodilator that decreases venous return and preload. Fentanyl may also be used for pain relief. See Table 14.5 for a list of medications commonly used in the

Table 14.5 Medications Commonly Used to Treat Shock States

Medication	Indication	Action
Dobutamine	Low cardiac output	Stimulates β_1 receptors; increases cardiac contractility and heart rate (HR)
Dopamine	Low cardiac output, hypotension, oliguria	Dose-dependent action: • A dose of 1–3 mcg/kg/min stimulates dopaminergic receptors on arteries in the heart, kidneys, brain, and abdomen, resulting in vasodilation; this will produce an increase in urine output (benefit of this diuresis is unclear). • A dose of 3–10 mcg/kg/min stimulates β_1, increasing contractility and HR. • A dose greater than 10 mcg/kg/min stimulates β_1, resulting in vasoconstriction and increasing blood pressure.
Epinephrine	Low cardiac output, hypotension	Dose-dependent action: • Lower doses (0.01–0.05 mcg/kg/min) primarily stimulate β_1, increasing contractility and HR. • Higher doses stimulate α_1, resulting in vasoconstriction and increasing blood pressure.
Norepinephrine	Hypotension, low cardiac output	Primarily stimulation of α_1, resulting in vasoconstriction and increasing blood pressure; some stimulation of β_1 to increase contractility and HR
Nitroglycerin	Preload and/or afterload reduction	Vasodilation through direct smooth muscle relaxation; dose-dependent action: • Lower doses (less than 40 mcg/min) produce venous dilation, decreasing preload. • Higher doses produce arterial dilation, decreasing afterload and blood pressure.
Nitroprusside	Preload and/or afterload reduction	Arterial vasodilation through direct smooth muscle relaxation, decreasing afterload and blood pressure
Phenylephrine	Hypotension	Stimulates α_1, resulting in vasoconstriction and increasing blood pressure
Vasopressin	Hypotension	Arterial vasoconstriction through smooth muscle contraction, increasing blood pressure

treatment of shock and Table 14.6 for information about adrenergic receptors affected by vasopressors.

Because many classes of medications are used in the treatment of cardiogenic shock, an arterial line is essential for continuous monitoring of blood pressure. Although not clearly beneficial in other forms of shock, a PA line has been shown to be helpful in the complex management of a patient in cardiogenic shock. The evaluation of cardiac output, preload, afterload, systemic vascular resistance, and SvO_2 is essential in order to gauge the response to treatment.

Emergency Revascularization

Early revascularization through percutaneous coronary intervention has been shown to increase short-term and long-term survival in most patients in cardiogenic shock. Percutaneous coronary intervention involves balloon angioplasty, or the insertion of a catheter through an artery up into the involved coronary artery and inflation of a balloon to break up the plaque causing the obstruction of flow. Typically, a stent is placed to maintain the patency of the vessel.

Intra-Aortic Balloon Pump Therapy

Intra-aortic balloon pump therapy may be considered when drug therapy does not improve cardiac output. The primary goal of IABP therapy is to increase myocardial oxygen supply and decrease myocardial oxygen demand. The IABP catheter is inserted into the aorta, usually via the femoral artery. Upon placement, the tip of the catheter should lie just below the aortic arch, about 2 cm from the left subclavian artery. There is a balloon at the tip of the catheter. It is timed to inflate at the start of diastole and deflate just before systole. When the balloon inflates, blood is displaced toward the coronary arteries and also into the systemic circulation, improving coronary and systemic perfusion. Deflating the balloon decreases afterload, thus decreasing the workload of the left ventricle (Fig. 14.5).

Ventricular Assist Device

A ventricular assist device (VAD) may be necessary if other treatments have not been successful. A VAD is a surgically inserted mechanical pump that assists the pumping of the left ventricle and decreases the workload of the heart. The pump works by displacing blood from the left ventricle into a receptor within the pump. The pump then works to eject blood into the aorta.

Nursing Management
Assessment and Analysis

The clinical manifestations of cardiogenic shock are related to a decrease in cardiac output and impaired tissue perfusion. They are similar to the presenting symptoms of AMI—chest pain, nausea, and diaphoresis—but also include hypotension, tachycardia, and tachypnea. Crackles on auscultation, shortness of breath (SOB), and decreased oxygenation may be present if the patient is in pulmonary edema. Systemically, the patient has a decreased level of consciousness and weak pulses with cold, cyanotic, and mottled skin. Urine output and bowel sounds are decreased or absent. Without successful intervention, profound hypotension, bradycardia, and hypoxia result.

Nursing Diagnosis

- **Altered tissue perfusion** related to inadequate cardiac output

Nursing Interventions
■ *Assessments*

- Neurological status
  Decreased level of consciousness occurs as a result of decreased cardiac output and carotid vasoconstriction that occurs as a result of hyperventilation and respiratory alkalosis.
- Vital signs
  Hypotension and tachycardia are present because of decreased cardiac output. Respiratory rate increases in an effort to increase tissue oxygenation and remove CO_2 to compensate for metabolic acidosis. Oxygenation may be decreased due to the presence of pulmonary edema
- Hemodynamic parameters
  Both right and left preloads are increased because of the impaired pumping ability of the heart, but cardiac output is low. As a result of compensation for low cardiac output, vasoconstriction occurs, increasing systemic vascular resistance.
- Breath sounds
  Crackles may be heard on auscultation due to the presence of pulmonary edema.
- Urine output
  Decreased urine output occurs as a result of decreased cardiac output and stimulation of compensatory mechanisms that increase reabsorption of sodium and water.
- Skin color and temperature
  Cold and clammy skin may be a sign of progressing shock.

Table 14.6 Adrenergic Receptors

Adrenergic Receptor	Locations	Response When Stimulated
α_1	Veins, arteries, arterioles	Vasoconstriction
α_2	Gastrointestinal tract	Decreased tone, secretions, and motility
β_1	Heart	Increased cardiac contractility and HR
β_2	Coronary arteries, bronchial smooth muscle, skeletal muscle vessels	Dilation of the coronary arteries and skeletal muscle vessels, relaxation of bronchial smooth muscle

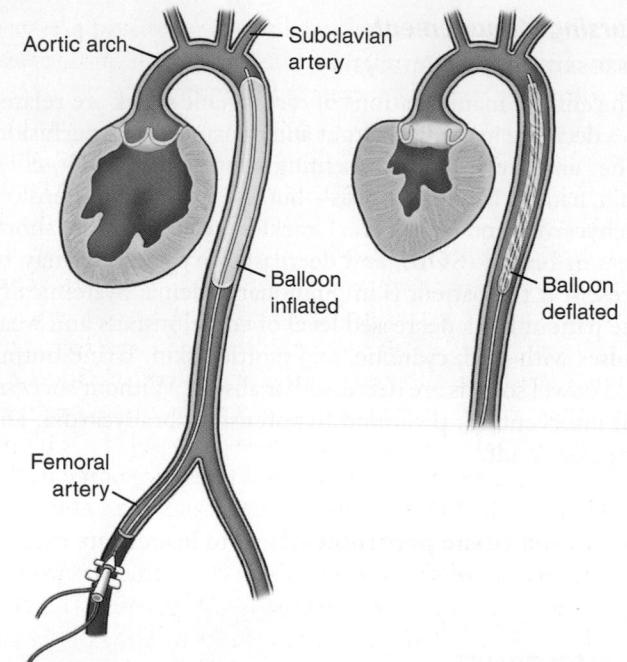

FIGURE 14.5 Intra-aortic balloon pump (IABP).

Laboratory Tests

- ABGs
  Initial ABGs may reflect a respiratory alkalosis due to tachypnea. Later stages of shock reveal a metabolic acidosis due to anaerobic metabolism.
- Venous oxygen saturation
  Decreased $SvO_2/ScvO_2$ is an indicator of inadequate DO_2.
- Metabolic profile
  Renal failure and liver failure as evidenced by increased BUN and creatinine levels and liver function test results may become evident because of decreased organ perfusion.
- Lactate/base deficit
  Increased lactate level and negative base deficit are evidence of poor perfusion at the cellular level. Decreasing lactate levels are an endpoint demonstrating adequate resuscitation.

▪ Actions

- Apply a 100% nonrebreather oxygen mask.
  Maximizing oxygenation is essential.
- Prepare for intubation and mechanical ventilation.
  Intubation and mechanical ventilation are frequently necessary with patients in cardiogenic shock in an effort to decrease VO_2 and increase oxygen availability.
- Administer medications as ordered:
  - Vasoactive medications such as norepinephrine or dopamine
    Vasoactive medications produce vasoconstriction, increasing blood pressure.
  - Inotropic medications such as dobutamine
    Inotropic medications increase contractility and cardiac output.
  - Diuretics
    Diuretics may be very cautiously utilized to decrease vascular volume if filling pressures are extremely elevated.

- Morphine sulfate
  Morphine will relieve pain, which can help to decrease myocardial VO_2. It will also decrease venous return through vasodilation.
- Administer fluids as prescribed.
  Fluids may be utilized cautiously to increase cardiac output if filling pressures are low and there are no signs of pulmonary edema.
- Restrict activity.
  Restricting activity will decrease cardiac workload and VO_2.

▪ Teaching

- Instruct patient and family about the importance of rest periods.
  Increased activity or stress levels cause increased myocardial VO_2 and can worsen the progression of shock.
- Teach patient and family about the causes of cardiogenic shock and myocardial infarction.
  Early recognition and treatment of myocardial infarction will help avoid a complication of cardiogenic shock.

Evaluating Care Outcomes

Rapid recognition of the presence of cardiogenic shock is essential in effective treatment. Swift intervention with inotropic and vasoactive support helps maintain adequate cardiac output and blood pressure to ensure sufficient oxygen supply to the tissues. Careful monitoring of clinical manifestations and hemodynamic status helps evaluate therapeutic interventions. Successful treatment is demonstrated by a satisfactory blood pressure level and cardiac output and adequate tissue perfusion. Cardiogenic shock is discussed in detail in Chapter 32.

Connection Check 14.6

The nurse correlates which of the following hemodynamic parameters to the patient with cardiogenic shock?

A. Decreased afterload
B. Increased contractility
C. Increased cardiac output
D. Increased right atrial pressure

OBSTRUCTIVE SHOCK

Epidemiology

As with hypovolemic shock, incidence and prevalence data are typically unavailable because the data are reported for the causative mechanism rather than the resultant obstructive shock.

Risk factors for obstructive shock include extracardiac disorders that impair ventricular filling or emptying. Impaired emptying is also referred to as *increased right or left afterload*. An example of a disorder resulting in increased right afterload is acute pulmonary embolism (PE). Examples of disorders resulting in impaired filling include cardiac tamponade and tension pneumothorax. These disorders are discussed in detail in Chapter 27.

Pathophysiology

Obstructive shock is caused by a mechanical barrier to ventricular filling or ventricular emptying (increased afterload) causing decreased cardiac output. As in cardiogenic shock, symptoms are independent of fluid volume status. The mechanical obstruction to the pumping action of the heart results in decreased cardiac output and poor perfusion at the tissue level. The specific pathophysiology varies depending on the cause of shock. For instance, a PE, typically the result of the mobilization of clot material to the lungs from a deep vein thrombosis (DVT), may result in obstructive shock. This results in extreme increases in right heart afterload due to an obstruction of blood flow into the lungs because of a clot or embolus in the PA. Alveoli are ventilated but not perfused, producing an extreme ventilation–perfusion mismatch.

Obstructive shock caused by cardiac tamponade is the result of excessive pressure on the heart muscle that occurs as fluid fills the pericardial sac. This may be the result of trauma to the cardiac muscle that results in bleeding and blood in the pericardial sac or a large, uncontrolled pericardial effusion. As the fluid accumulates around the heart, less blood enters the ventricles with each successive diastole, impairing ventricular filling.

Clinical Manifestations

As with other forms of shock, clinical manifestations are the result of decreased cardiac output and impaired peripheral perfusion: a decreased level of consciousness; decreased urine output; poor pulses; pale and cool skin; and decreased bowel sounds. Chest pain, nausea and vomiting, and shortness of breath are also common findings. Muffled heart sounds may be apparent with cardiac tamponade. Signs of right heart failure, such as jugular vein distention, may be noted with increased right heart afterload or impaired filling.

Hemodynamic parameters obtained through a PA catheter indicate variable CVP and PAOP depending on the problem, impaired filling or impaired emptying. Systemic vascular resistance is high, and cardiac output is very low. Venous oxygen saturation is decreased.

Management

Medical Management

As with other forms of shock, providing oxygen through a 100% nonrebreather mask is a minimal first step to stabilize oxygenation. Intubation and mechanical ventilation are frequently necessary to support ventilation and maximize oxygenation. Improving or enhancing oxygenation may help decrease myocardial workload, increase myocardial oxygen supply, and help preserve myocardial tissue. Vasoactive

medications may be utilized to help maintain blood pressure in the short term, but early definitive treatment of the cause of obstructive shock is necessary for survival.

If the cause of shock is impaired filling due to cardiac tamponade, the blood or fluid in the pericardial sac must be removed or drained as quickly as possible. This is a medical emergency. If the fluid is not promptly removed, death may ensue quickly. Removing the fluid or blood can be done through a procedure called pericardiocentesis. This procedure uses a large-bore needle inserted into the pericardial sac, guided by ultrasonography or echocardiography when possible, to remove the fluid. A pericardial window, a procedure to remove part of the pericardium to relieve pressure, may also be performed. After removal of the blood or fluid, it is essential to identify and treat the source of the problem. If the cause is left unknown and untreated, the cardiac tamponade may reoccur.

If the cause of shock is impaired ventricular emptying due to PE, the definitive treatment is to remove the clot through the use of thrombolytic therapy. Thrombolytics are medications capable of dissolving a clot. They are infused via a catheter directly into the clot. An alternative approach to minimize the dosage of thrombolytics is the combination of low-dose thrombolytics and targeted ultrasonic waves delivered through a catheter directly into the clot to aid in dissolution. If thrombolytics are contraindicated or unsuccessful, suction thrombectomy may be indicated. Suction thrombectomy is performed by inserting a catheter and guiding it toward the clot. The clot is essentially sucked through the catheter. Another option is a mechanical device at the tip of the catheter, such as a rotating head, that may be used to break up the clot. Infrequently, surgery (a pulmonary embolectomy) is required to remove the clot if other methods are unsuccessful. Depending on the cause of the PE, long-term anticoagulation therapy may be indicated to decrease the likelihood of a recurrent event.

Nursing Management
Assessment and Analysis

As in other forms of shock, the clinical manifestations of obstructive shock are related to a decrease in cardiac output and impaired tissue perfusion. Hypotension, tachycardia, and tachypnea are present. The patient has a decreased level of consciousness and weak pulses, with cold, cyanotic, and mottled skin. In addition, the patient may present with muffled heart sounds due to the presence of excessive fluid in the pericardial sac or signs of right heart failure due to elevated right heart afterload. As shock progresses, urine output and bowel sounds may become decreased or absent; typically, without definitive treatment of the cause, death occurs rapidly.

Nursing Interventions
- **Assessments**
- Neurological status
  Decreased level of consciousness occurs as a result of decreased cardiac output and carotid vasoconstriction that occurs as a result of hyperventilation and respiratory alkalosis.

Anxiety and restlessness may occur initially but will rapidly progress toward a further decreased level of consciousness without treatment.

- Vital signs
Hypotension and tachycardia are present because of decreased cardiac output. Respiratory rate increases in an effort to increase tissue oxygenation and remove CO_2 to compensate for metabolic acidosis.

- Hemodynamic parameters
Filling pressures are variable depending on the cause—elevated with impaired emptying; decreased with impaired filling. Both right and left afterloads may be increased as a result of mechanical resistance to ventricular emptying. Increased oxygen consumption is evidenced through a decreased venous oxygen saturation. Cardiac output is low.

- Urine output
Decreased urine output occurs as a result of decreased cardiac output and stimulation of compensatory mechanisms that increase reabsorption of sodium and water.

- Skin color and temperature
Cold and clammy skin is present as a result of poor peripheral perfusion.

Laboratory Tests

- ABGs
Initial ABGs may reflect a respiratory alkalosis due to hyperventilation.

- Venous oxygenation
Decreased $SvO_2/ScvO_2$ is an indicator of inadequate oxygen delivery.

■ Actions

- Apply a 100% nonrebreather oxygen mask.
Maximizing oxygenation is essential.

- Prepare for intubation and mechanical ventilation.
Intubation and mechanical ventilation are frequently necessary with patients in obstructive shock in an effort to decrease VO_2 and increase oxygen availability.

- Administer medications as ordered:
  - Vasoactive medications such as norepinephrine and dopamine
  Vasoactive medications produce vasoconstriction, increasing blood pressure and allowing the patient to stabilize until definitive treatment is implemented.
  - Anticoagulation via heparin administration if the cause of obstructive shock is PE
  Anticoagulation is used to decrease the formation of new clots and prevent the existing clot from increasing in size while the body is naturally dissolving it.
  - Thrombolytic therapy if the cause of obstructive shock is PE
  Thrombolytics are given to dissolve the clot.

- Prepare for definitive treatment of the cause, for example:
  - If cardiac tamponade:
    - Pericardiocentesis
    Pericardiocentesis is a procedure to drain fluid or blood from the pericardial sac, relieving pressure and allowing the ventricles to fill normally.

- Anticipate/prepare for emergency transport to the operating room for a pericardial window procedure
A pericardial window procedure will ease the pressure on the heart muscle, allowing the ventricles to fill.
- If PE:
  - Suction thrombectomy
  Suction thrombectomy is done to remove the obstruction to ventricular emptying.

■ Teaching

- Teach the patient and family about the causes of PE: avoid prolonged periods of inactivity, walk every hour, and drink plenty of fluids.
Mobilization helps reduce the likelihood of PE formation by decreasing the formation of a DVT, typically the initial source of the PE. Dehydration may increase the tendency to clot.

- Anticoagulation teaching:
  - Use electric razors, use soft toothbrushes, and avoid contact sports.
  Avoid potential causes of bleeding.
  - If on Coumadin:
    - Regular follow-up laboratory testing—international normalized ratio
    Determine effective dosing of anticoagulants.
    - Limit foods high in vitamin K, such as green leafy vegetables.
    These foods interfere with the efficacy of anticoagulants.

Evaluating Care Outcomes

Rapid recognition of the presence of obstructive shock is essential in effective treatment. Swift intervention with inotropic and vasoactive support helps maintain blood pressure, but definitive treatment of the cause is required to promote survival. Careful monitoring of clinical manifestations and hemodynamic status help evaluate therapeutic interventions. Successful treatment is demonstrated by satisfactory blood pressure and cardiac output and adequate tissue perfusion.

DISTRIBUTIVE SHOCK

Distributive shock is the result of disease states that cause poor vascular tone and vasodilation, resulting in increased vascular capacity and venous pooling. Even though blood volume is adequate, a state of relative hypovolemia exists because of decreased venous return to the right heart. Sepsis is the most common cause of widespread vasodilation and distributive shock. **Anaphylaxis**, another cause of distributive shock, is caused by the release of histamine, which results in vasodilation, decreased venous return, and hypotension. The least common form of distributive shock is neurogenic shock, which is due to a loss of vasomotor tone. There is a loss of stimulation from the sympathetic nervous system, resulting in the vessel walls relaxing and dilating. Venous return is decreased, and the patient is hypotensive, with a decreased cardiac output. Neurogenic shock can be caused by an injury to the brain, general or spinal anesthesia, or spinal cord injury.

Neurogenic shock (discussed in detail in Chapter 39) and anaphylaxis are discussed briefly here first. The major focus of this section is sepsis, which is discussed last.

Neurogenic Shock

Epidemiology and Pathophysiology

Neurogenic shock is caused by disruption of the sympathetic nervous system, typically as a result of spinal cord injury, regional spinal anesthesia, or an injury to the brain. The incidence of neurogenic shock is approximately 20% in patients with a cervical spinal cord injury. It is very uncommon in patients with lower spinal cord injuries. The sympathetic nervous system disruption causes several problems. First, vascular tone is significantly decreased, hampering vasoconstriction and leaving vessels relaxed and dilated. Vascular volume is increased in the peripheral vessels, but venous return to the right heart is decreased, resulting in decreased cardiac output. This is termed *relative hypovolemia*. This problem is made worse by the heart's inability to compensate through tachycardia. Also, unopposed parasympathetic activity may result in profound bradycardia. As with other types of shock, the decreased cardiac output of neurogenic shock causes systemic hypoperfusion, resulting in anaerobic metabolism and metabolic acidosis. These patients are especially susceptible to orthostatic hypotension.

Clinical Manifestations

Clinical manifestations include warm, dry skin and a flushed appearance due to systemic vasodilation. Hemodynamic parameters include decreased cardiac output, decreased right and left filling volumes, and decreased systemic vascular resistance.

Management

Medical Management

Treatment Priorities

The treatment focus is on providing cardiovascular support while attempting to resolve the primary cause of shock. Cardiovascular support is done through cautious fluid resuscitation and the use of vasoactive IV medications such as dopamine, epinephrine, norepinephrine, or phenylephrine (see Tables 14.5 and 14.6). If necessary, bradycardia is treated with atropine. Repeated episodes of bradycardia may require transcutaneous or transvenous pacing. Ventilatory support through intubation and mechanical ventilation may be required.

Nursing Management

Assessment and Analysis

The clinical manifestations of neurogenic shock are slightly different from the manifestations of other forms of shock. Similar to other forms of distributive shock, the patient has decreased cardiac output as a result of decreased vascular tone and reduced venous return; however, because of the disruption in the sympathetic nervous system, the patient may be bradycardic rather than tachycardic. The patient may appear pink and flushed as a result of vascular vasodilation.

Nursing Diagnosis
- **Altered tissue perfusion** related to decreased cardiac output

Nursing Interventions

Assessments
- Vital signs
  Hypotension may be present due to decreased venous return to the right heart secondary to systemic vasodilation. Bradycardia may be present because of the disruption of sympathetic nervous system activity.
- Hemodynamic parameters
  Cardiac output, CVP, and PAOP are low related to decreased venous return to the right heart secondary to systemic vasodilation. Systemic vascular resistance is low secondary to systemic vasodilation.
- Respiratory rate and SpO_2
  Respiratory rate may be low because of the injury causing neurogenic shock, such as cervical spinal cord injury, which may depress the respiratory rate and thus decrease oxygenation.

Actions
- Administer IV fluid as ordered.
  Cautious fluid resuscitation is provided to increase vascular volume to match the increase in the size of the vascular space due to the massive dilation.
- Administer IV medications as ordered:
  - Vasoactive drips
    Administration of vasoactive drips aids in increasing vasomotor tone and systemic vascular resistance.
  - Atropine
    Atropine is used for the treatment of bradycardia to block the action of the vagus nerve in the parasympathetic nervous system, increasing the HR.
- Prepare for transcutaneous pacing or transvenous pacing.
  Pacing may be necessary to treat recurrent episodes of bradycardia.
- Raise the head of the patient's bed slowly.
  Because of loss of systemic vasomotor tone, patients in neurogenic shock are particularly vulnerable to orthostatic hypotension.
- Apply venous thromboembolism prophylaxis, such as sequential compression devices or medication such as heparin.
  Patients in neurogenic shock are at high risk for venous thromboembolism, particularly in cases where the etiology of neurogenic shock is spinal cord injury.

Teaching
- If the cause of neurogenic shock is spinal cord injury, teaching related to the anticipated impact on the patient's immediate and future healthcare issues is vital. Psychosocial support from social workers, clergy, or a professional requested by the family is also essential in the care of the patient.
  A spinal cord injury has profound long-term healthcare and life implications. An understanding of treatment and outcomes is essential to maximize recovery.

Connection Check 14.7

The nurse understands that which of the following are clinical manifestations of neurogenic shock? *(Select all that apply.)*
A. Tachycardia
B. Vasoconstriction
C. Tachypnea
D. Decreased CVP
E. Bradycardia

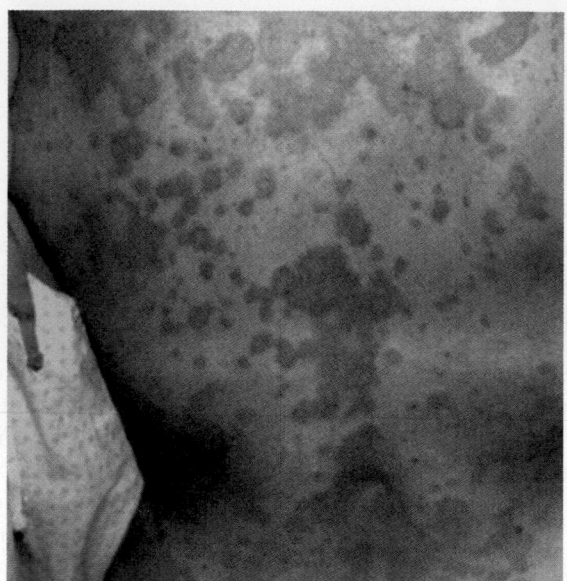

FIGURE 14.6 Urticaria.

Evaluating Care Outcomes

As with other forms of shock, prompt recognition and treatment of neurogenic shock are essential. Adding to the urgency is the patient's inability to compensate for the decreased cardiac output with tachycardia because of the disruption of the sympathetic nervous system. Pacing to maintain a normal HR may be required while the patient is treated and stabilized. A stabilized blood pressure, HR within normal limits, and adequate cardiac output are signs of a successful intervention.

Anaphylactic Shock

Epidemiology and Pathophysiology

Anaphylaxis, or **anaphylactic shock**, is a severe and life-threatening systemic hypersensitivity reaction. It is caused by an allergic reaction leading to a release of histamine and resulting in widespread venous dilation, increased capillary permeability, and smooth muscle contraction. The incidence of anaphylactic shock has been approximated at 30 to 950 per 100,000 people per year. Common triggers include food, such as seafood, and medications, such as antibiotics.

Common characteristics consist of sudden onset and rapid progression of symptoms that include airway compromise and circulatory collapse. Airway compromise is caused by airway muscle contraction and throat and/or tongue swelling. Circulatory collapse is caused by widespread vasodilation and capillary leak, resulting in decreased venous return and decreased cardiac output.

Clinical Manifestations

Clinical manifestations of airway compromise include shortness of breath, tachypnea, wheezing, stridor, cyanosis, and confusion due to hypoxia. Untreated, this will lead to respiratory arrest. Clinical manifestations of circulatory problems are tachycardia; hypotension; cool, pale, clammy skin; weak pulses; and edema. As in neurogenic shock, these patients are particularly vulnerable to orthostatic hypotension.

Also common are sudden onset and rapid progression of skin or mucosal changes. These changes include flushing, urticaria (an itchy, red, raised rash; Fig. 14.6), and angioedema, which is similar to the swelling of urticaria, only deeper. It is edema of the subcutaneous or submucosal tissues, usually occurring around the eyes and mouth. Hemodynamic changes include hypotension, tachycardia, decreased cardiac output, decreased filling pressures, and decreased systemic vascular resistance.

Management
Medical Management
Treatment Priorities

Treatment priorities include immediately removing the trigger if possible. If the trigger is the administration of antibiotics or blood, the infusion should be stopped immediately. If the trigger is a bee sting, the stinger should be removed. Sometimes the trigger is unknown or has been ingested, so removal is not possible. Maneuvers to induce vomiting are not recommended. Definitive treatment should not be delayed because cardiac arrest and death can ensue within minutes if treatment is delayed.

Treatment with intramuscular (IM) epinephrine is the immediate first treatment priority. Intramuscular is the preferred route of administration because it provides a consistent, rapid rise in therapeutic concentration and lowers the risk of cardiovascular complications that can be seen with IV administration. This dosing can be repeated two or three times. Most patients will respond, but if not, IV epinephrine may be administered. Epinephrine promotes bronchodilation, relieving respiratory distress, and vasoconstriction to aid in restoring blood pressure. Intravenous vasopressin has been found to be an effective alternative in refractory anaphylactic shock (see Table 14.5). The second priority is assessing the airway, maximizing oxygenation through the initiation of oxygen via a 100% nonrebreather, and preparing for intubation if the airway is compromised. Circulatory support via administration of IV fluid is essential. Other medications utilized to treat anaphylaxis include antihistamines, corticosteroids, and inhaled bronchodilators.

Nursing Management

Assessment and Analysis

Anaphylactic shock is characterized by a sudden and severe hypersensitivity reaction causing a release of histamine that results in smooth muscle contraction, widespread vasodilation, increased capillary permeability, and decreased venous return. This results in respiratory distress, circulatory collapse, and skin reactions. Airway compromise is manifested by wheezing, stridor, and shortness of breath. Skin reactions include itching, a raised red rash, and severe swelling, specifically around the eyes. Hemodynamically, the patient is hypotensive and tachycardic, with decreased filling pressures and decreased cardiac output.

Nursing Diagnoses

- **Impaired gas exchange** related to airway compromise
- **Impaired tissue perfusion** related to decreased cardiac output

Nursing Interventions

■ Assessments

- Vital signs/hemodynamic parameters
  Hypotension and decreased filling pressures are present because of widespread vasodilation, resulting in decreased venous return and cardiac output. Tachycardia results as a compensatory mechanism. Systemic vascular resistance remains low because of the vasodilation.
- Respiratory
  Shortness of breath, wheezing, and decreased oxygenation may be present because of airway smooth muscle contraction and edema of the throat and/or tongue.
- Skin/peripheral perfusion
  Urticaria and angioedema are indicators of an allergic reaction. Pale, cool, clammy skin is an indicator of poor peripheral perfusion related to decreased cardiac output.

■ Actions

- Remove trigger immediately.
  If possible, remove the trigger. If not possible, do not delay definitive treatment; the hallmark of anaphylaxis is sudden onset and rapid progression of symptoms.
- Administer IM epinephrine as ordered.
  Epinephrine promotes bronchodilation and vasoconstriction, helping to relieve respiratory distress and restore or maintain blood pressure.
- Apply oxygen via a 100% nonrebreather mask or prepare for intubation.
  Maximizing oxygenation is important in maintaining adequate delivery of oxygen to the tissues.
- Insert an IV line and administer IV fluid as ordered.
  Fluid shifts may occur with the increased vascular permeability. Infusion of IV fluids helps to increase and maintain vascular volume.
- Administer adjunctive medications as ordered:
  - Antihistamines
    Antihistamines may help counter histamine-mediated vasodilation and bronchoconstriction.
  - Corticosteroids
    The anti-inflammatory action of steroids may help shorten the anaphylactic reaction.
  - Inhaled bronchodilators
    Bronchodilators help relieve bronchoconstriction, relieving respiratory distress.

■ Teaching

- Teaching related to the cause of anaphylaxis
  Understanding the cause of the anaphylactic response is essential in avoiding a repeat occurrence.
- Administration of epinephrine via an EpiPen
  Typically, allergic reactions occur in the home or away from the hospital. Patients or family members must know how to use the EpiPen as a first-line treatment in an allergic reaction to avoid anaphylactic shock if possible.

Evaluating Care Outcomes

As with other forms of shock, prompt recognition and treatment of anaphylactic shock are essential. Without a rapid response, airway compromise and circulatory collapse can quickly lead to death. Successful treatment is demonstrated by stable hemodynamics; the resolution of airway compromise, as evidenced by a resolution of wheezing and shortness of breath; and the resolution of skin reactions, itching, and swelling.

CASE STUDY: EPISODE 2

Mike's condition deteriorates. He is admitted to the emergency department with a complaint of shortness of breath. His chest radiograph reveals pneumonia. Initially, he was alert and oriented, but he has since become confused and lethargic. He is admitted to the intensive care unit. Upon admission, his blood pressure is noted to be 80/50 mm Hg, with an HR of 130 bpm. His blood glucose level is 220 mg/dL. He is flushed, with bounding pulses and a temperature of 102.6°F (39.2°C).

Oxygen is maintained via a 100% nonrebreather mask. His SpO$_2$ is borderline at 90%. The staff anticipates intubation. Two liters of normal saline is given wide open. A Foley catheter is inserted to closely monitor urine output, and IV antibiotics are continued…

Sepsis/Septic Shock

Epidemiology

Accurately determining the incidence of sepsis is variable depending on sources and methods, but one international retrospective study indicated an incidence of 437 per 100,000 person-years between 1995 and 2015. Infection with gram-positive organisms is more commonly associated with the progression of sepsis, but infection with gram-negative organisms is still substantial. Fungal infections are increasing but are still fewer than bacterial infections. Mortality statistics vary also and range from 10% to 52% depending on disease severity, with older intensive care patients reporting the highest mortality. Most sources report that the incidence of sepsis is increasing. This may be attributed to innovations and changes in healthcare and our aging population. The use of invasive procedures and monitoring devices is much more common. This increases the patient's risk of infection. The use of chemotherapy and immunosuppressive medications is increasing, making patients more vulnerable to infection. A huge factor is the increase in antimicrobial resistance to antibiotics. Although the incidence is increasing, mortality is decreasing, which is thought to be due to increased sophistication in treatment.

There are ongoing efforts to more accurately define sepsis and septic shock. The Third International Consensus Definitions for Sepsis and Septic Shock (Sepsis 3) define **sepsis** as a life-threatening organ dysfunction caused by a deregulated host response to infection. **Septic shock** occurs when circulatory and metabolic abnormalities are profound, greatly increasing mortality. In the worst case, further complications such as **disseminated intravascular coagulopathy (DIC)**, a hematological disorder associated with enhanced coagulation, and secondary **multiple organ dysfunction syndrome (MODS)** may result. Figure 14.7 illustrates the defining characteristics and assessment criteria for sepsis.

Pathophysiology

The invasion of a pathogen initiates a series of complex responses by the host's immune system. The initial, immediate response is the activation of the innate immune response. This response is nonspecific to any antigen. It involves the mobilization of macrophages and neutrophils to the area; the activation of pro-inflammatory cytokines or signaling molecules; the activation of complement proteins, proteins that immobilize and break down pathogens; and the activation of the coagulation system. Activated coagulation produces a fibrin mesh to help localize the invading organism and activates bradykinin, which dilates vessels and increases capillary permeability. Local blood vessels dilate, increasing circulation to the involved area, which allows an influx of immune cells, causing local redness, warmth, and edema. This is done in an effort to kill the invading organism and keep the response localized. Sepsis occurs when the inflammatory response is no longer localized. The response becomes amplified and uncontrolled. The normal deactivation process, which decreases the production of pro-inflammatory cytokines and produces anti-inflammatory cytokines, is impaired. The excessive release of proinflammatory cytokines results in damage to the endothelial cells lining the blood vessels, producing vasodilation, decreased vasomotor tone, and increased capillary permeability. Ultimately, sepsis and septic shock result when proinflammatory cytokines overpower anti-inflammatory cytokines, resulting in overwhelming and excessive systemic inflammation, massive peripheral vasodilation, and increased

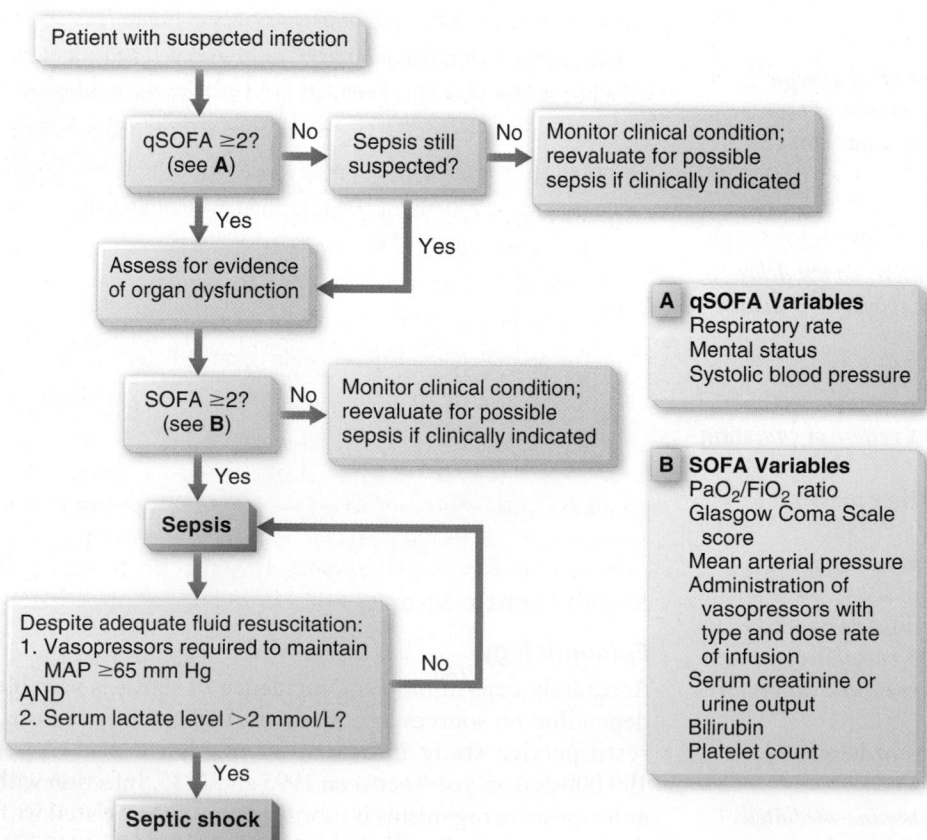

FIGURE 14.7 Algorithm to guide the identification of sepsis and septic shock.

capillary permeability. Other forces that contribute to widespread inflammation are substances produced by the invading organisms. Endotoxins released by gram-negative bacteria and exotoxins produced by gram-positive bacteria add to the pro-inflammatory effect.

A part of the excessive inflammation is activated and enhanced coagulation, resulting in widespread fibrin deposition and excessive clotting throughout the vascular system. It also results in decreased fibrinolysis (breakdown of clots). This occurs due to the decreased levels of activated protein C and antithrombin III seen in septic patients. The primary role of protein C is to modulate the production of thrombin and promote fibrinolysis. Antithrombin III deactivates thrombin. The role of thrombin in the coagulation cascade is to modulate the conversion of fibrinogen to fibrin clots. Decreased levels of both protein C and antithrombin III lead to enhanced formation of thrombin, resulting in clot formation and impaired fibrinolysis, which ultimately results in impaired blood flow due to microvascular clots and organ dysfunction.

Clinical Manifestations

The clinical manifestations of septic shock reflect the poor vascular tone and vasodilation that result in increased vascular capacity and blood pooling in the venous system. There is adequate blood volume, but a state of relative hypovolemia exists because of decreased venous return to the right heart. Septic shock is typically divided into early and late stages. Early stages of septic shock, sometimes termed *hyperdynamic* or *warm* sepsis, reflect the initial inflammatory response. The patient is tachycardic, with bounding pulses and warm, flushed skin, and is febrile. Blood pressure may be normal as a result of initial compensatory responses. Initial signs of decreased organ perfusion may be present, such as confusion and decreased urine output. Hemodynamic parameters indicate increased cardiac output that occurs as long as there is adequate fluid resuscitation. Filling pressures, CVP and PAOP, remain low. Systemic vascular resistance is low because of profound systemic vasodilation. Venous oxygen levels are temporarily increased due to the increase in cardiac output.

Late stages of septic shock, also referred to as *hypodynamic* or *cold* shock, are characterized by cool, pale skin; weak and thready pulses; and hypothermia. Tachycardia persists, but blood pressure remains low. Further signs of end-organ hypoperfusion, such as lethargy or coma and anuria, may be present. Hemodynamic parameters indicate decreased cardiac output with variable filling pressures depending on fluid resuscitation. Systemic vascular resistance may remain low but may increase as vasoconstriction occurs with compensation and drug therapy. Venous oxygen levels decrease, reflecting overall inadequate DO_2 to the tissues. Ultimately, venous oxygen levels may increase because of the maldistribution of blood flow in the microcirculation, resulting in decreased oxygen extraction at the tissue level.

See Table 14.3 for a comparison of hemodynamic parameters in different types of shock and in early and late sepsis.

Management

Diagnosis

Identification of infection is done through the evaluation of general non-specific indicators of infection such as fever, increased white blood cell count, changes in blood pressure, respiratory rate, and heart rate. There may also be signs of specific infections such as lung consolidation, frequent or painful urination, or peritonitis. Laboratory testing includes complete blood cell counts, metabolic profiles, urine testing, and cultures. Imaging procedures such as general radiographs, CT scans, or magnetic resonance images help identify and locate areas of abnormalities.

Assessment of the presence of sepsis is guided by the use of the Sequential Organ Failure Assessment (SOFA), with a higher score associated with higher mortality. Patient evaluation begins with a quick SOFA (qSOFA), which evaluates for an increased respiratory rate, decreased BP, and altered mentation. If indicated, evaluation continues with the SOFA. The SOFA rates patient deterioration through decreasing PaO_2/FiO_2 ratios, hypotension with or without vasopressor support, increased coagulopathies, decreased liver and renal function, and a decline in neurological status.

Medical Management

The European Society of Intensive Care Medicine, the Society of Critical Care Medicine, and the International Sepsis Forum initiated the Surviving Sepsis campaign in 2004. The goal of the campaign was to standardize care and reduce the high mortality associated with sepsis through the use of evidence-based practice. The guidelines were updated in 2018.

First-line therapy is prevention—hand washing, meticulous aseptic technique for invasive procedures, and elimination of invasive therapies when possible. Aggressive mouth care, including brushing the teeth with chlorhexidine products, in ventilated patients may help prevent ventilator-associated pneumonia.

Bundle of Care

Hour 1

The Surviving Sepsis campaign developed a bundle of care to help standardize the very complex treatment needed by patients in severe sepsis. They may vary hospital by hospital, but the basic elements should be adhered to in order to optimize treatment. The bundle includes activities that need to be completed within 1 hour after identifying sepsis. This recommendation is made with the understanding that treatment may not be completed in 1 hour, however, it clearly identifies that treatment should begin immediately (Table 14.7). The Surviving Sepsis Web site (http://www.survivingsepsis.org) is routinely updated and is an excellent source of information regarding treatment options.

Blood Work

Obtaining a serum lactate and two sets of blood cultures should be done immediately. Other recommended laboratory work includes: a complete blood count with differential,

Table 14.7 Surviving Sepsis Campaign Bundle of Care

Time Frame	Actions
Within 1 hour	• Measure lactate levels. Reassess if initial lactate is >2 mmol/L.
	• Obtain blood cultures (prior to administering antibiotics).
	• Administer broad-spectrum antibiotic.
	• Administer 30 mL/kg of crystalloid if patient hypotensive or lactate level at least 4 mg/dL.
	• Administer vasopressors if blood pressure is unresponsive during or after fluid resuscitation; maintain mean arterial pressure (MAP) at 65 mm Hg or above.

Adapted from Society of Critical Care Medicine. (n.d.). *Surviving Sepsis campaign.* Retrieved from http://www.survivingsepsis.org

coagulation studies, chemistries, liver function tests, and arterial blood gasses, as well as the culturing of any other potential sources of infection.

Antibiotics

Evidence suggests that prompt identification and treatment of the offending microorganism with antibiotics can decrease mortality in sepsis. It is recommended that antibiotics be administered within 1 hour of arrival at the hospital. Cultures should be done before antibiotics are administered to ensure appropriate antibiotic coverage.

Fluid Resuscitation

Fluid resuscitation is essential to restore hemodynamic stability, maximize DO_2, and begin repaying oxygen debt. A crystalloid solution such as normal saline or lactated Ringer's is commonly used to improve and maintain filling pressures. Evidence suggests that aggressive resuscitation in early sepsis has been shown to decrease mortality. Fluid resuscitation should be tapered as the patient demonstrates improvement. If fluid resuscitation is not successful at restoring blood pressure during or after administration, initiation of vasopressors to maintain a mean arterial pressure greater than 65 mm Hg may become necessary (see Table 14.5). The Surviving Sepsis campaign suggests the use of norepinephrine as the first-line vasopressor.

Corticosteroid Therapy

Adrenal insufficiency is sometimes a feature of sepsis, but the use of steroids in treatment is not routinely recommended. Studies have been inconclusive as to the benefits of low-dose steroids in septic shock. They have not been shown to decrease mortality in sepsis. The Surviving Sepsis guidelines recommend low-dose steroids only if the patient has not been responsive to fluid and vasopressor therapy.

Ongoing Monitoring

Frequent assessment of vital signs, peripheral perfusion, mental status, cultures, and laboratory analyses, including white blood cell count and differential and lactate, are essential. Hemodynamic parameters such as CVP or PAOP and SvO_2 or $ScvO_2$ help monitor responsiveness to therapy, but the use of a PA catheter, and thus PAOP and SvO_2, is

not recommended because the PA catheter has not been shown to have an improved impact on outcomes. Instead, monitoring of responsiveness to therapy can be done through evaluation of CVP and $ScvO_2$ in combination with dynamic measures such as monitoring cardiac output through echocardiology after a passive leg raise (PLR) maneuver. An increase in cardiac output demonstrates a good response to fluid resuscitation.

Connection Check 14.8

An older adult patient was admitted to the hospital 1 hour ago with a urinary tract infection, fever, tachycardia, hypotension, and confusion. The nurse anticipates which of the following interventions?

A. Assess fluid status; insert arterial line; insert central venous line.

B. Initiate a vasoactive drip; obtain lactate level and blood cultures.

C. Obtain blood and urine culture; initiate broad-spectrum antibiotics; fluid resuscitation.

D. Assess fluid status; obtain lactate level; insert central venous catheter.

Complications

Disseminated Intravascular Coagulopathy

Disseminated intravascular coagulopathy (DIC) is a hematological disorder most commonly caused by sepsis. It occurs because of enhanced coagulation that results from the release of procoagulant factors as part of the inflammatory response associated with sepsis. Disseminated intravascular coagulopathy is typically described in two phases: a clotting, or thrombotic, phase and a bleeding phase, but in some cases they may occur simultaneously. The initial thrombotic stage may last hours or several days. Once initiated, large amounts of thrombin are produced in response to decreased levels of protein C and antithrombin III, resulting in the excessive production of fibrin clots and consumption of clotting factors. As a result of the excessive coagulation, clots lodge in the microvasculature, causing ischemia and necrosis (Fig. 14.8). Patients present with cyanosis and ischemia in the fingers and toes and the tip of the nose. Organ ischemia may also be present. Patients are at risk for thrombophlebitis, PE, and stroke.

The second stage starts with the initiation of fibrinolysis. Although impaired in sepsis, the process of fibrinolysis occurs in an attempt to break down and remove the clots. The breakdown of the clot results in increased circulating fibrin degradation products, which are powerful anticoagulants. They impair the activity of thrombin, resulting in a decreased ability to form a fibrin clot. The combination of lack of available clotting factors and the anticoagulant properties of the fibrin degradation products results in excessive bleeding due to the inability to form clots. Diagnosis is based on the clinical picture in combination with laboratory results: decreased levels of fibrinogen, increased fibrin degradation products, increased D-dimer levels (an indicator of clot breakdown), decreased platelets, prolonged prothrombin and activated partial thromboplastin times, and decreased antithrombin III levels.

Management of DIC involves the vigorous treatment of the underlying disorder as well as treating other disorders caused by the excessive clotting and bleeding, such as hypotension, hypoxemia and respiratory distress, and the metabolic acidosis associated with poor tissue perfusion. Additional supportive treatment consists of volume replacement with crystalloids such as normal saline, blood replacement, and replacement of clotting factors with fresh frozen plasma and platelets. Identifying and correcting the cause are essential. The use of anticoagulation is not routinely recommended.

Multiple Organ Dysfunction Syndrome

Multiple organ dysfunction syndrome (MODS) is another complication that occurs as a result of the excessive inflammation associated with severe injury or sepsis. The cause of MODS is multifaceted. Several factors lead to decreased DO_2 to the organ systems, causing impaired tissue perfusion:

- Evidence suggests that apoptosis, or programmed cell death that occurs in all cells, is accelerated in sepsis.
- Widespread damage to the vascular endothelium, which occurs as a result of inflammation and causes the increased capillary permeability and vasodilation of sepsis, continues as a result of the excessive production of inflammatory mediators.
- The microvascular dysfunction that causes maldistribution of blood flow in the capillary beds continues, resulting in uneven flow to different organ systems.
- Enhanced coagulation leads to clots in the microcirculation, mechanically obstructing flow.

Additional factors include the following:

- The accelerated production of glucose as initial compensation eventually becomes harmful. This hypermetabolism causes increased cellular oxygen demand.
- The direct toxicity of mitochondrial cells that occurs with excessive inflammation affects the ability to use oxygen even when present.

Eventually, poor DO_2 coupled with increased oxygen demand and poor oxygen utilization results in profoundly impaired cellular functioning, metabolic acidosis, and organ failure.

The initial organ system to become symptomatic is typically the lungs, with the development of acute respiratory distress syndrome (ARDS). Sequential failure frequently includes the renal system, the hepatic system, and then the GI system. The mortality rate for ARDS averages 40%. Mortality increases as organ systems fail. Three or more systems are associated with an 80% to 90% mortality rate. There can be a 100% mortality rate if the cardiovascular and neurological systems are involved.

The focus of medical management of MODS is supportive in the form of controlling infection, maximizing oxygenation, and restoring and maintaining intravascular volume. Antibiotics are given as appropriate. Fluid is administered to maintain intravascular volume. Blood products are administered as necessary to maintain adequate hemoglobin levels. Mechanical ventilation is usually necessary to protect the airway and support oxygenation.

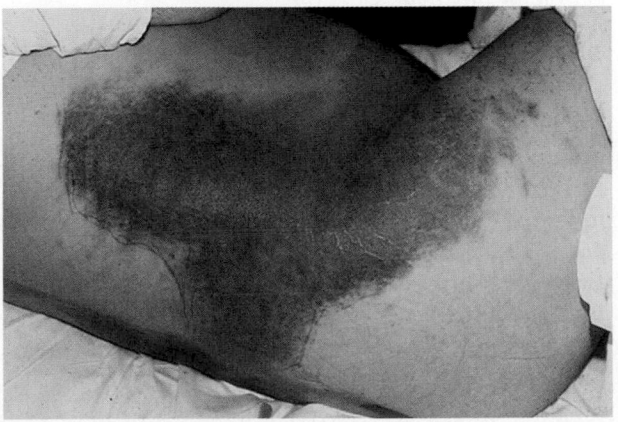

FIGURE 14.8 Disseminated intravascular coagulopathy.

Connection Check 14.9

The nurse understands that which of the following indicates the initial phase of DIC?

A. Bleeding from all puncture sites
B. Cold, mottled extremities
C. Increased antithrombin III levels
D. Increased fibrin degradation products

Nursing Management

Assessment and Analysis

Unlike other forms of shock, the early clinical manifestations of septic shock are related to the initial increase in cardiac output that occurs due to the tachycardia and decreased SVR associated with sepsis. The patient presents as warm and flushed, with bounding pulses. Later manifestations reflect the prolonged poor tissue perfusion. Hypotension, tachycardia, and hyperventilation are present. Systemically, the patient has a decreased level of consciousness and weak pulses, with cold, cyanotic, and mottled skin. Urine output and bowel sounds are decreased or absent. Without successful intervention, the clinical manifestations of enhanced coagulation, such as necrotic tissue in the extremities, begin to appear. In later stages, excessive bleeding from any puncture wounds, IV sites, or wounds begins.

Nursing Diagnosis

- **Altered tissue perfusion** related to inadequate cardiac output

Nursing Interventions

▪ Assessments

- Neurological status
  Decreased level of consciousness occurs as a result of decreased cardiac output and hyperventilation causing a decrease in cerebral blood flow.
- Vital signs
  Hypotension is present because of vasodilation, producing relative hypovolemia and decreased venous return. Tachycardia will be present as one of the compensatory mechanisms. Initially, the patient will be febrile as an adaptive response. In later stages, the patient will be hypothermic, potentially signaling the body's inability to continue the adaptive response.
- Hemodynamic readings
  Initially, cardiac output is increased; however, as sepsis progresses, cardiac output decreases as a result of continued decreases in filling pressures, such as CVP and pulmonary artery occlusion pressures. Initially, systemic vascular resistance is decreased as a result of widespread vasodilation. Later, it may increase due to compensation and vasopressor therapy.
- Urine output
  Decreased urine output occurs as a result of decreased cardiac output and the initiation of compensatory mechanisms.
- Skin color and temperature
  Initially, the patient's skin is flushed and warm because of increased cardiac output. Later, the skin becomes cold and clammy, signaling the progression of shock. Tissue necrosis in the extremities may indicate the enhanced coagulation of DIC.
- Bleeding
  Excessive bleeding from wounds and puncture sites may be present because of consumption of clotting factors in DIC.
  Laboratory Tests
- ABGs
  Initial ABGs may reflect a respiratory alkalosis due to hyperventilation. Hypercapnia and hypoxia are present as

respiratory failure worsens. Later stages of shock reveal a metabolic acidosis due to anaerobic metabolism.
- Venous oxygen saturation
  Decreased SvO_2 and $ScvO_2$ are typically indicators of inadequate oxygen delivery. In later sepsis, values may be elevated because of maldistribution of blood flow and are not indicative of recovery.
- Metabolic profile
  Renal failure and liver failure, as evidenced by increased BUN and creatinine levels and liver function test results, may become evident as a result of decreased organ perfusion.
- Lactate/base deficit
  Increased lactate level and negative base deficit are evidence of poor perfusion at the cellular level. Normalizing levels are an endpoint demonstrating adequate resuscitation. Sustained abnormal levels are indicators of increased risk of mortality.
- Clotting studies
  Decreased levels of fibrinogen, increased fibrin degradation products, increased D-dimer levels (an indicator of clot breakdown), decreased platelets, prolonged prothrombin and activated partial thromboplastin times, and decreased antithrombin III levels indicate the progression to DIC.

▪ Actions

- Meticulous hand washing and aseptic technique with all procedures
  Hand washing and aseptic techniques are basic interventions to help prevent and control infection.
- Administer oxygen as ordered.
  Maximizing oxygenation is essential.
- Anticipate and prepare for intubation.
  Intubation and mechanical ventilation may be required to improve oxygenation or if respiratory failure ensues.
- Obtain lactate level.
  Lactate levels are an indicator of adequacy of perfusion; increased levels signal the presence of anaerobic metabolism.
- Obtain two blood cultures from two different sites, obtain urine, sputum, and wound cultures.
  Cultures are obtained to identify the offending organism.
- Administer antibiotics as ordered after cultures are obtained.
  Antibiotics are the first-line treatment in an attempt to control the infection.
- Administer fluid replacement as ordered.
  Aggressive fluid replacement is the initial treatment to restore filling volumes and blood pressure in septic shock.
- Administer vasoactive drips such as norepinephrine as ordered.
  Vasoactive drips may be necessary to restore vascular tone if fluid replacement therapy is not effective at increasing blood pressure and cardiac output.
- Provide mouth care every 4 hours and when needed.
  Oral care is effective at reducing the occurrence of ventilator-associated pneumonia.
- Supportive care: nutrition, turning, DVT prophylaxis, range of motion exercises, mobilize as tolerated.
  These actions provide a supportive healing environment while active treatment of the underlying problem is provided.

Teaching

- Instruct the patient and family on the cause of sepsis and the importance of meticulous hand washing.
  Patient and family understanding of factors important in preventing, minimizing, and controlling infection are essential in the treatment.
- Allow family member visitation during hospital treatment.
  Family visitation can help decrease a patient's and family's anxiety.

Evaluating Care Outcomes

Rapid recognition of the presence of sepsis is essential in preventing progression along the continuum. Swift intervention with antibiotics and fluids is essential in maintaining cardiac output. Vasoactive support may be necessary if fluid replacement is not effective at maintaining blood pressure. Hemodynamic monitoring and frequent laboratory assessments are necessary to monitor the effectiveness of treatment. Supportive care, such as mouth care, frequent turning, nutrition, and DVT prophylaxis, is essential to prevent complications. Timely, aggressive medical care combined with meticulous monitoring and supportive care help ensure recovery. Successful treatment is demonstrated by a satisfactory blood pressure level and cardiac output and adequate tissue perfusion.

Making Connections

CASE STUDY: WRAP-UP

Mike's condition worsens. After admission to the intensive care unit and administration of several liters of normal saline, his blood pressure continues to deteriorate. He becomes increasingly lethargic and tachypneic, with a respiratory alkalosis. His urine output is noted to be decreasing, and laboratory values indicate the beginning of acute renal failure.

His deteriorating respiratory rate status requires intubation and mechanical ventilation. A central line is inserted to monitor CVP and $ScvO_2$. Aggressive fluid replacement is continued, and norepinephrine is started at 1.0 mcg/kg per minute. Antibiotics are continued.

After several days of frequent monitoring and meticulous care involving fluids and antibiotics, Mike begins to improve. His CVP normalizes, and his blood pressure finally begins to stabilize. The norepinephrine is decreased and then discontinued. His $ScvO_2$ returns to normal. After several days, Mike's respiratory status improves, and weaning parameters demonstrate that he is ready for extubation. His urine output improves, and his BUN and creatinine values return to normal.

Case Study Questions

1. Mike's nurse monitors him for which clinical manifestations in the early stages of septic shock?
   A. Decreased cardiac output
   B. Increased systemic vascular resistance
   C. Increased PA wedge pressure
   D. Increased cardiac output

2. It is a priority for Mike's nurse to follow up with the provider about which order?
   A. Start antibiotics.
   B. Prepare a norepinephrine drip.
   C. Take hourly vital signs.
   D. Send one set of blood cultures.

3. Mike's nurse incorporates which nursing diagnosis into the plan of care?
   A. Decreased cardiac output related to impaired contractility
   B. Decreased cardiac output related to increased afterload
   C. Impaired tissue perfusion related to vasodilation
   D. Impaired tissue perfusion related to loss of sympathetic tone

4. Mike's nurse evaluates which parameter as an indication of adequacy of treatment?
   A. CVP
   B. PAOP
   C. SpO_2
   D. SvO_2

5. Mike's nurse understands that which laboratory results indicate his condition is improving? *(Select all that apply.)*
   A. Increasing lactate level
   B. Decreasing base excess level
   C. Increasing $ScvO_2$ level
   D. Decreasing lactate level
   E. Increasing BUN and creatinine

CHAPTER SUMMARY

Shock is a syndrome that results from inadequate delivery of oxygen (DO_2) and nutrients to the tissues, resulting in poor tissue perfusion and impaired cellular metabolism. Without immediate treatment, organ system failure and death may result. Delivery of oxygen is assessed through the evaluation of cardiac output and arterial oxygen content. When DO_2 falls below the tissue requirements, also called *oxygen consumption* (VO_2), an oxygen debt results. Oxygen consumption can be indirectly measured through the evaluation of venous oxygen saturation, which reflects the amount of oxygenated blood returned to the right heart. Normal values are between 60% and 75%. When that value falls below normal, it signals that an oxygen debt is occurring because of a decrease in oxygen content, hemoglobin, or cardiac output. The longer the imbalance between oxygen supply and demand, the larger the debt becomes.

There are four distinct stages of shock:

- The initial stage is subtle or subclinical, but cellular damage may be occurring.
- The compensatory stage is characterized by the initiation of neural, endocrine, and chemical compensatory mechanisms to maintain adequate volumes and cardiac output.
- The progressive stage is marked by the failure of compensatory mechanisms.
- The refractory stage is marked by prolonged inadequate blood supply to the cells, resulting in irreversible multisystem organ failure.

The assessment and monitoring of shock involve the assessment of physical parameters such as level of consciousness, urine output, respiratory status, pulse quality, and skin color and temperature. It also requires invasive hemodynamic monitoring done through arterial lines or central venous or PA catheters. Laboratory analyses of endpoints such as lactate, blood gas analysis including base deficit, and SvO_2 are essential parameters to consider when evaluating the extent of shock and success of resuscitation.

Hypovolemic shock is defined as an acute loss of circulating fluid volume that results in a decreased venous return to the right heart, decreased stroke volume and cardiac output, and ultimately, decreased perfusion at the tissue level. Identifying and controlling further loss of blood or fluid is an obvious priority in this patient. Fluid replacement with normal saline or lactated Ringer's solution is the mainstay of initial resuscitation. Blood product replacement is necessary in the case of acute blood loss.

Cardiogenic shock is defined as a severe impairment of ventricular contraction in the presence of adequate vascular volume, resulting in decreased cardiac output. Treatment priorities include stabilizing oxygenation and drug therapy to increase blood pressure and cardiac output. Also considered is emergency revascularization, intra-aortic balloon pump therapy, or when other treatment fails, ventricular assist devices.

Distributive shock is the result of disease states that cause poor vascular tone and vasodilation, resulting in increased vascular capacity and venous pooling. This can be caused by sepsis, anaphylaxis, or neurogenic shock. Treatment priorities in anaphylactic shock include removing the trigger when possible, initiating drug therapy with IM epinephrine, and providing ventilatory support when necessary. Treatment priorities for neurogenic shock include cardiovascular support through fluid resuscitation and drug therapy and ventilatory support when necessary.

Sepsis and septic shock are two clinical conditions on a continuum that starts with infection and ends with septic shock and multiple organ dysfunction syndrome (MODS). Characteristically, the invasion of the host with a microorganism is the first step in the continuum, resulting in an inflammatory response. Identification of the offending microorganism and prompt treatment with antibiotics have been shown to decrease mortality in sepsis. Fluid resuscitation is essential to restore fluid deficits and maximize oxygen delivery. The initiation of vasopressors may become necessary if fluid resuscitation is not successful at restoring blood pressure.

Disseminated intravascular coagulopathy (DIC) and MODS are complications of shock and sepsis. Disseminated intravascular coagulopathy occurs because of the enhanced coagulation that results from the release of procoagulant factors as part of the inflammatory response associated with sepsis. Multiple organ dysfunction syndrome occurs as a result of the excessive inflammation associated with severe injury or sepsis. Factors such as widespread damage to the vascular endothelium cause increased capillary permeability, vasodilation, and microvascular dysfunction that result in maldistribution of blood flow in the capillary beds and enhanced coagulation, leading to clots in the microcirculation that mechanically obstruct flow to the organs.

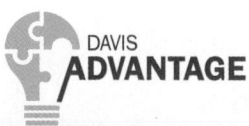

To explore learning resources for this chapter, go to **Davis Advantage** and find:
- Answers to in-text questions
- Chapter Resources and Activities
- NCLEX®-Style Chapter Review Questions
- Review Questions – Bibliography

Unit III

Managing the Surgical Experience

Chapter 15

Priorities for the Preoperative Patient

Deborah Ennis

LEARNING OUTCOMES

Content in this chapter is designed to assist in:

1. Discussing the essentials of the surgical experience
2. Explaining the priority assessments for the surgical patient
3. Identifying the vital preoperative preparation for the patient
4. Analyzing the nursing role in the preoperative process
5. Developing teaching and support strategies for the surgical patient and his or her family

CONCEPTS

- Assessment
- Fluid and Electrolyte Balance
- Legal
- Medication

- Nursing Roles
- Perioperative
- Safety

ESSENTIAL TERMS

Ablative surgery
Advance directive
Ambulatory (outpatient) surgery
Cosmetic surgery
Elective surgery
Emergency surgery
Exploratory (diagnostic) surgery
Informed consent
Intraoperative
Last oral intake
Minimally invasive surgery
NPO (nothing by mouth)
Palliative surgery
Post-anesthesia care unit (PACU)
Postoperative
Preoperative
Preoperative checklist
Reconstructive surgery
Robotic surgery
Telesurgery
Time-out
Urgent surgery

Finding Connections

CASE STUDY: EPISODE 1

Follow this patient throughout the chapter.

Maria Gonzalez is admitted to your facility for preparations for her total abdominal hysterectomy. She is 40 y.o. with two children aged 4 and 6 years. She has a history of fibroid tumors and deep vein thrombosis (DVT) with her most recent pregnancy. During your initial assessment, Maria informs you of her allergies to penicillin and latex. She has smoked 10 cigarettes a day for the past 20 years. Vital signs are noted as follows:

- Blood pressure (BP): 140/88 mm Hg
- Heart rate (HR): 80 bpm
- Respirations: 20/min
- Temperature: 98.7°F (37°C)
- Pain score: 0 out of 10...

INTRODUCTION

There are many different purposes and types of surgical procedures. Some common terms associated with the surgical process are:

- **Emergency surgery**—surgery that must be done immediately to save a patient's life, limb, or ability to function
- **Urgent surgery**—surgery that must be done within 24 to 48 hours to prevent permanent injury to the patient or death
- **Elective surgery**—surgery that may be necessary but can be planned around the patient's and surgeon's schedule
- **Ambulatory (outpatient) surgery**—surgery usually performed in 1 day, with the patient being admitted to the ambulatory surgical center (ASC) in the morning and discharged after acceptable recovery criteria have been met
- **Exploratory (diagnostic) surgery**—surgery performed to obtain a diagnosis and possible resolution
- **Ablative surgery**—surgery to remove tissue from an organ or area of the body
- **Palliative surgery**—surgery performed to decrease pain or symptoms in patients suffering from incurable illnesses
- **Reconstructive surgery**—surgery to restore function or a defect in an area of the body
- **Cosmetic surgery**—surgery to change or revise an area or structure of the body
- **Minimally invasive surgery**—surgery performed through very small openings in the skin, using instruments through with the surgeon can visualize the area such as a laparoscope
- **Telesurgery** or **robotic surgery**—surgery performed from a location other than the surgical suite, by use of robotic equipment

The operative experience is broken up into three phases: **preoperative**, **intraoperative**, and **postoperative**. Although each of these phases possesses unique nursing needs, the preoperative phase is a patient's first impression of the surgical setting. The preoperative phase commences when the decision for surgery is made and ends when the patient is transferred to the surgical suite. During this time, the preoperative nurse takes on a multitude of roles, including educator, advocator, and admittance nurse. It is crucial for the nurse to identify any potential needs the patient may have while in his or her care. The nurse's main priority is to complete a **preoperative checklist** (Fig. 15.1). Each facility's unique checklist ensures that the necessary documentation, admission assessment, physical preparation, and educational needs have been completed prior to the patient entering the surgical suite. This includes but is not limited to:

- A full medical history (including prescription, over-the-counter, herbal, and other alternative therapies)
- Assessment of the patient's health status
- Collection of information and paperwork necessary for intraoperative and postoperative care
- Completion of preoperative orders (IV antibiotics, thromboembolic-deterrent [TED] hose, etc.)
- Patient education regarding the entire surgical process
- Verifying the patient and a witness signed the informed consent
- The initial time-out—"pause for cause"—when the patient verifies:
  - All information on the identification band as correct
  - The name of the surgeon
  - The procedure that will be completed by the surgeon
  - The correct side of the body on which the surgery will occur if this is a unilateral procedure

These interventions not only identify potential issues prior to surgery but also ensure that all procedures are performed in a timely and safe manner.

INFORMED CONSENT

Informed consent is when a patient autonomously and cognitively grants permission to a provider to perform a surgical procedure after considering all alternatives, benefits, and risks of the procedure. Although obtaining consent is *not* the role of the nurse but that of the provider, it is the nurse's responsibility to ensure that the patient has all the

Preoperative/Preprocedure Checklist (Page 1 of 2)

MRN _____

DOB _____   PATCOM _____

RACE _____   SEX _____

Patient Identification Information

Name of Procedure/Surgery:	Sending Unit:		Phone Number:			
	Recent Weight: kg		Height: cm/in			
	Time of Vital Signs: _____ *(within 1 hour of transport)*		T	P	R	BP

DNR order? ☐ Yes ☐ No	**INTAKE**	**DATE**	**TIME**
	Last solid p.o. intake/tube feeding/breast milk: *(circle as appropriate)*		
	Last clear liquid p.o. intake:		

SECTION A: Required Pre-Op/ Preprocedure Elements	**Directions** If not done, please specify reason.	**Initials** Initial in appropriate box.		
1) The following are present:		Yes	No	N/A
• Isolation precautions: Type _____	*Note on front of chart. Call area before sending patient if on Airborne/Maximum Precautions*	_____		_____
• Nursing flowsheet and TPR	*For Non Clin Doc (Sunrise) units, place the past 24 hours in the chart*	_____		
• "Home" Medication List	*Provide printed copy in chart*	_____		
• Current day MAR	*Place last 24 hours in chart*	_____		
• If allergy, wristband applied		_____		
• If difficult airway is known, wristband applied		_____		
• Addressograph plate/label *(matches patient ID band)*	*Send only one plate*	_____		
• Correct ID band on patient *(matches addressograph)*		_____		
• Confirm second wristband is present in the chart	*For patients being sent to the OR (except L&D OR)*	_____		
2) Oxygen _____ L/min O₂ tank: _____ PSI	*Do not send tank with < 1000 PSI*	_____		
3) Pre-op/preprocedure prep *Do not give preoperative sedation if consent not obtained. If no to any below, please comment.*				
• Pre-op/preprocedure medications given if ordered		_____		
• Pre-op scrubs completed if ordered		_____		
• Bowel prep administered if ordered		_____		
• IV access present and patent	*(if no, notify procedure area)*	_____	_____	
4) Presence of any of the following items? *Check applicable policies for handoff/special equipment/transport needs*				
• External/internal insulin pump		_____		
• PCA (IV/SQ/epidural/intrathecal, peripheral nerve catheter) pump (circle appropriate)		_____		
• Pacemaker (external/internal) ventricular assist device, ICD (circle appropriate)	*Note: If nonmonitored unit and implantable cardioverter defibrillator (ICD) is off, patient must be transported on monitor*	_____		
• Circle appropriate: prostacyclin (Flolan®), tracheostomy, chest tube (indicate water seal or suction) Other: _____	*Send appropriate backup/emergency equipment/supplies as needed*	_____		
5) Continuous cardiac monitoring implemented if required	*Transport on a monitor*	_____		
6) Patient safety precautions implemented (e.g., lockable transport equipment; BP cuff sent; SCD sleeve left on for OR only; side-rails up; transport monitor charged)	*Assure transport monitor cord and/or extra battery sent with transport monitor*	_____		

Signature/Title	**Initials**	**Signature/Title**	**Initials**

FIGURE 15.1 Preoperative checklist.

Continued

Preoperative/Preprocedure Checklist (Page 2 of 2)

MRN _____

DOB _____ PATCOM _____

RACE _____ SEX _____

Patient Identification Information

7) Initial appropriate column for each item below. *Secure essential items/patient belongings per policy. Only send essential items with the patient (e.g., glasses/hearing aids) if they are needed to assist with the informed consent process.*

Items	Removed	N/A	Secured with: F = Family S = Security U = Unit P = Sent with patient	Items	Removed	N/A	Secured with: F = Family S = Security U = Unit P = Sent with patient
Jewelry (includes wedding ring)				Hearing aid			
Dentures/partial plates (no dentures for endoscopy, ECT or TEE)				False eyelashes/wig/hairpiece/hair pins			
Contact lenses/glasses				Face makeup/nail polish			
Artificial limb				Other:			

8) Location (or phone number) of family _____ ☐ N/A
   Relationship _____

9) Consent form for the procedure/surgery completed:
   DO NOT SEND to Operating Room without a signed, witnessed and dated consent. If consent is not present in the chart, notify the attending physician.

   ☐ Yes *Complete section B below and sign "Sending RN Validation" area.*

   ☐ No *If patient consentable, patient may be sent to procedure without consent; Skip section B below and send essential items such as glasses and hearing aid if applicable. Sign "Sending RN Validation" area.*

10) For OR cases, immediately post patient leaving the unit, transfer the patient's location to the appropriate OR holding area in Electronic Bed Board (EBB). For procedural areas, follow departmental guidelines for EBB transfers.

SECTION B: Complete this Preverification Section for all Consented Patients: For consents obtained in the procedural area, verification will be documented on procedural critical pathway.	Completed	Initials	Follow Instructions as Noted
1. Operative/procedural consent is present with the following information:			
a. Planned Procedure	☐ Yes ☐ No		
b. Operative side/site	☐ Yes ☐ No ☐ N/A		
c. Provider signature	☐ Yes ☐ No		
d. Patient/decision maker signature	☐ Yes ☐ No		
e. Witness Signature	☐ Yes ☐ No		If NO to 1–4: • OR Case—requires resolution per discussion with attending surgeon. • Non-OR case—notify procedure area (exceptions for site marking noted under #4).
f. Date/time for each signature	☐ Yes ☐ No		
2. Patient/decision maker agrees with planned procedure as documented on the consent.	☐ Yes ☐ No ☐ Parent/guardian/decision maker not available		
3. Patient/decision maker agrees with planned operative side/site as documented on the consent.	☐ Yes ☐ No ☐ N/A ☐ Parent/guardian/decision maker not available		
4. Site marking is visible; surgeon/provider initials on the planned operative side/site as documented on the consent. *Non-OR areas: site marking may be done in procedural area if applicable*	☐ Yes ☐ No ☐ N/A		

Section C: Sending RN Validation: _____ Date: _____ Time: _____
Signature

FIGURE 15.1–cont'd

information needed to make an informed decision about the procedure being offered. Working with the patient to identify and correct educational deficits not only makes the patient more comfortable about consenting to the surgical experience but also ensures the safest and most successful outcome. An informed patient is more likely to follow instructions preoperatively for preparation and postoperatively for recovery. It is important for the preoperative nurse to understand that every patient has the right to refuse a surgical intervention even when death is a risk of refusal of treatment. In the eyes of the law, treatment without consent is not allowed even at the risk of death.

Components of an Informed Consent

Surgical consent forms are similar in most institutions. Some may be preprinted; others must be completed to describe each procedure. Whichever form or forms are used, the required components are universal (Fig. 15.2).

Components of consents include:

- Consent for the procedure itself, which should include the following information:
  - Name of surgery, type of surgery, and reason for the surgery
  - Name of the surgeon to perform the surgery
  - Reason that intervention will benefit the patient

- All alternative options to surgery
- Potential outcomes if surgery is not performed
- Consent for anesthesia
- Consent to administer blood products

Anesthesia

Anesthesia consent is an additional consent the patient must sign. At this time, the anesthesiologist informs the patient of the type of anesthesia, the medications to be used, and the risks associated with the type of anesthesia planned. The anesthesiologist or nurse anesthetist may also describe how the medication is administered, such as epidural anesthesia or regional block. The role of the preoperative nurse remains

---

Consent for Performance of Procedures/Treatment/Operations or Other Procedures
Page 1 of 2

MRN _____

DOB _____ PATCOM _____

RACE _____ SEX _____

Patient Identification Information

Date: _____ PATIENT NAME (Print) _____

1) I hereby give my consent and authorize _____ and the Memorial General treatment team,
First name / Last name

to perform the following operation(s), treatment(s), or procedure(s) _____
(Identify operative site and side, use no abbreviations, and explain in nonmedical terms)

2) The indications, benefits, and probability of success of the operation(s), treatment(s), or procedure(s) have been explained to me in a manner that I understand. These include:

_____

3) The major risks and complications of the operation, treatment, or procedure have been explained to me in a manner that I understand. These may include such items as failure to obtain the desired result, discomfort, injury, need for additional treatment(s), and death. Additional risks include: _____

(Include common, infrequent, and local anesthesia risks)

4) I understand that the reasonable alternatives to the proposed operation(s), treatment(s), or procedure(s), including the major risks, benefits, and side effects of those alternatives are:

Alternatives: **Major Risks, Benefits, and Side Effects of Each Alternative:**

5) During the procedure, the provider may become aware of conditions which were not apparent before the start of the procedure. I consent to additional or different operations or procedures the provider considers necessary or appropriate to diagnose, treat, or cure such conditions.

6) Memorial General may dispose of any tissue or parts which are removed during the procedure. Memorial General may retain, preserve, and use these tissues or parts for internal educational and quality-improvement purposes without my permission, even if these tissues or parts identify me. However, Memorial General may only use or disclose tissues or parts that identify me for research with my permission or with the approval of a review board governed by federal laws protecting these activities. If the tissues or parts do not identify me, Memorial General may use them for scientific (research) purposes without my permission or action by a review board.

FIGURE 15.2 Informed consent form.

Continued

Consent for Performance of Procedures/Treatment/ Operations or Other Procedures
Page 2 of 2

MRN _____

DOB _____ PATCOM _____

RACE _____ SEX _____

Patient Identification Information

7) By signing below, I agree:
- That a provider has explained and answered all of my questions related to: _____
_____

(Operation/treatment/procedure as listed above)

- If I have further questions, I have the right to have those questions answered.
- That no guarantees were made concerning the outcome, as the practice of medicine and surgery is not an exact science.
- To have the operation(s), treatment(s), or procedure(s).
- That I have identified to a provider any restrictions on the sharing of information learned from the operation(s) or procedure(s).
- I have not given up my right to refuse treatment at any time.
- That I am entitled to a signed copy of this consent form.

For the following statement, if the patient does not agree, cross it out with a single line. The patient and provider shall initial, date, and time the cross-out:

- To allow observers or technical advisors to be present during the operation(s) or procedure(s).

_____
Patient Signature   Date   Time

_____
Signature (full name) of Provider Obtaining Consent   Title   Date   Time

First Name: _____ Last Name: _____ ID No. ☐ ☐ ☐ ☐ ☐
Provider's Name (PRINT)

_____
Witness Signature   Date   Time

☐ In-person   ☐ By phone/computer _____
Interpreter's Printed Name   Interpreter's Signature   Date   Time
(if in-person)

PATIENT IS UNABLE TO CONSENT BECAUSE: ☐ Patient is a minor   ☐ Patient lacks capacity
☐ Other (describe)_____

_____
Signature of Authorized Representative   Relationship   Date   Time

_____
Witness Signature   Date   Time

DO NOT COMPLETE THE SECTION BELOW UNTIL THE FINAL TIME-OUT IS CONDUCTED

Time-Out Verification

This documents that a final verification (time-out) was performed prior to starting the procedure. Documentation of time-out may be completed elsewhere in the patient's medical record (e.g., procedure/progress note, procedure flowsheet, checklist, ORMIS). I verify that the treatment team (for OR, minimum of provider, anesthesiologist/CRNA, circulating RN) participated in the time-out using active communication and that we verified the following:

- Correct patient identity
- Agreement on procedure to be done (as stated on the informed consent)
- Correct side and site procedure

_____
Signature and Title of Person Verifying Time-Out Was Performed   Printed First and Last Name

Document date and time that the time-out was performed: _____ _____ a.m./p.m.
Date   Time

FIGURE 15.2–cont'd

the same, one of patient advocate, ensuring that the patient understands the information being presented.

Blood Products

Consent to administer blood products may be a component of the general surgical consent or a separate form. The surgeon describes what situations will warrant the need for blood products and requests consent from the patient for their use. The nurse must be aware of cultural and religious obligations that prevent the patient from consenting to receive blood products. For example, because of religious beliefs, patients who are Jehovah's Witnesses will not consent to the use of blood products. In that case, the surgeon documents that the patient has refused blood products in the patient's chart. The preoperative nurse is responsible for identifying the patient as "no blood products" with a bracelet and sign on the patient's chart. Facilities have blood refusal forms that a patient is asked to sign if this situation presents. Providers can give blood without consent only in an emergency situation where the patient lacks the capacity to consent.

Inability to Consent

Special considerations occur when the patient is not able to consent for care. These situations include patients who are cognitively impaired or who are cognitively aware but unable to physically sign, a deaf patient or one who speaks another language, minors, or emergency situations. In situations where the patient is impaired, a medical power of attorney may be established for consent purposes. Patients who cannot physically sign but are able to make their own care decisions may sign with an "x." This consent needs to be witnessed by two people instead of just one as normally required. If the patient speaks another language or is deaf, a hospital interpreter may be used. For purposes of consent, this is desirable over a family member. The hospital interpreter is familiar with the medical terms being used. Also, the use of an anonymous interpreter avoids any bias that may occur with a family member during translation. Surgical consent for minors may be signed by the legal guardian of the child. However, if the child is old enough to understand the care, the procedure should still be explained.

In emergency situations, a verbal consent is acceptable. Written consent should be obtained in a timely manner following the surgery. If the patient is incapable of giving consent, two providers document the need for surgery. This is acceptable only if the patient's medical power of attorney or next of kin is unreachable or the surgery is emergent and the patient has no support present. Other situations require special permits done well before the procedure. An example of this is sterilization procedures. The patient must sign a unique consent 6 weeks prior to the surgery.

Advance Directives

The Patient Self-Determination Act of 1991 grants all patients the right to determine and direct their care in times of medical emergency: the right to create an **advance directive**. An advance directive defines a patient's wishes should he or she be deemed incompetent to express his or her wishes in a medical emergency. Facilities are required by law to provide the means and guidance to complete an advance directive if desired prior to surgery. Within the advance directive, the patient may name a durable medical power of attorney, usually a spouse or adult child, who is designated to make all medical decisions should the patient become incompetent. The advance directive also allows the patient to express desires related to organ donation and end-of-life issues.

As part of the advance directive, a living will defines care in the case of cardiac or respiratory failure or when the likelihood of recovery to a quality level of functioning is deemed unlikely. Patients may elect to have all necessary measures taken or may elect to stop life-sustaining procedures in the event of a cardiac arrest. The phrases "do not intubate," DNI, or "do not resuscitate," DNR, are recorded in the patient's chart. The patient also has the opportunity to express wishes in regard to feeding tubes or long-term ventilator-assisted breathing. The patient may select any combination of treatments he or she feels best matches his or her values and beliefs. It is imperative that if a patient has advance directives and/or a living will at the time of surgery, the nurse notes that on the chart and places a copy of these documents on the chart if the patient has brought them to the hospital.

Obtaining Informed Consent

Surgeon

The surgeon is solely responsible for obtaining consent in the presence of the patient and one witness. Family members or support persons may be present at this time. Informed consent for a scheduled procedure must be obtained prior to the administration of pain medications and sedatives or the induction of anesthesia because these medications may alter the patient's ability to make an informed decision. In addition to obtaining informed consent, the surgeon uses this uninterrupted time to ensure that all of the patient's and family member's questions are answered.

Preoperative Nurse

Many patients admit to not reading the entire consent before signing (Box 15.1). The role of the preoperative nurse is to clarify information and ensure patient understanding. Nurses correct common misconceptions and ease concerns of the patient, family members, or support persons.

In addition to reviewing the consent form and validating patient understanding, nurses often serve as the witness to the consent. The nurse is witnessing the physical signature, not the information provided. It is essential that the witness be with the patient as the consent is being signed. The nurse or other witness should never sign the consent form if the patient has not signed in his or her presence. As part of preoperative procedures, the nurse is also responsible for documenting that a signed consent has been placed in the patient's chart.

Box 15.1 Why Patients Do Not Read the Full Consent

The most common reasons patient do not read the form are:

- It is too long.
- There is too much information.
- It is too intimidating.
- It is typed in small print.
- The terms used are too medical or legal.

TIME-OUTS/PAUSE FOR CAUSE

Surgical errors and wrong-site procedures are a documented occurrence and have been identified by hospital accreditation organizations as an area for improvement. A **time-out** is a formal process of identification performed by the patient and the healthcare team to identify the correct patient, correct procedure, and correct surgical site. The preoperative nurse is a part of the time-out process.

The time-out, or "pause for cause," starts when the patient enters the surgical facility. On admission, the patient receives a wristband (Fig. 15.3) containing his or her identifying information.

After reviewing the wristband, the patient confirms that all the information is correct; it is essential that the wristband note accurate information before the patient is moved into the surgical suite. The first responsibility of the preoperative nurse is to review the information on the wristband with the patient and have the patient name the procedure and site. This time-out is performed again by the circulating nurse upon transfer to the surgical suite and once more immediately preceding incision by the entire team (Fig. 15.4). The surgeon marks the surgical site with his or her signature using a permanent marker. Some surgeons may require that, if possible, the patient marks the site him- or herself.

Components of a Time-Out

Although the process may vary in different facilities, the components of a time-out are consistent. The patient is asked to state his or her full name as printed on the identification bracelet and at least one other identifier, which is typically the patient's date of birth, although there are other acceptable identifiers (see Safety Alert). The patient is next asked to state the correct site and the procedure he or she is receiving. The surgeon then marks the correct site. As stated earlier, the process of identifying the patient, procedure, and site is completed again by the team immediately

prior to incision. Performing a time-out immediately prior to incision makes an irreversible mistake less likely.

 Safety Alert **Acceptable Patient Identifiers**

- Name
- Date of birth
- Social Security number
- Photo printed on band
- Address
- Telephone number

Connection Check 15.1

You are preparing a patient for surgery and have asked her to verify her information on her patient identification band. She tells you that the birth date is incorrect on her identification band. The most appropriate action by the nurse at this time is which of the following?

A. Cross out the birth date and put the correct one in its place with the nurse's initials.
B. Ask the family members to validate the patient's birth date.
C. Call the surgeon's office to validate the birth date.
D. Ask the admissions office to please send a corrected identification band.

PATIENT ASSESSMENT

The surgical patient requires a detailed medical history and assessment to ensure a safe and successful surgery. The preoperative nurse is responsible for obtaining and documenting this history on admission. If a patient has already been admitted to an inpatient unit and has a history on record, the information should be reviewed and documented on the preoperative record. This allows the preoperative nurse and surgeon to identify any patient learning and medical needs that are unique to his or her surgical experience.

Patient History

Completed patient medical, social, and surgical histories are the key to a successful surgical experience. These questions may be asked during a preoperative work-up or upon admission to the surgical facility. As the nurse prepares the patient for surgery, he or she asks a series of detailed questions. Some of the questions may be very personal and, at times, uncomfortable for the patient to answer. The nurse should remind the patient that this information is important in providing a safe outcome. It is also important to assure the patient that no judgment will be made on his or her responses and that the information will be used only for medical purposes. Box 15.2 lists the components of a complete patient history.

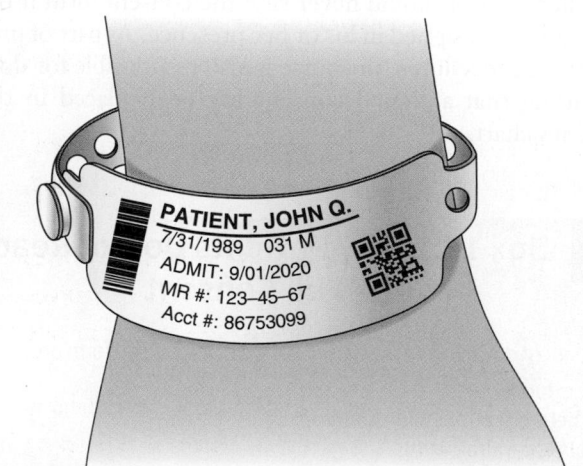

FIGURE 15.3 Patient armband.

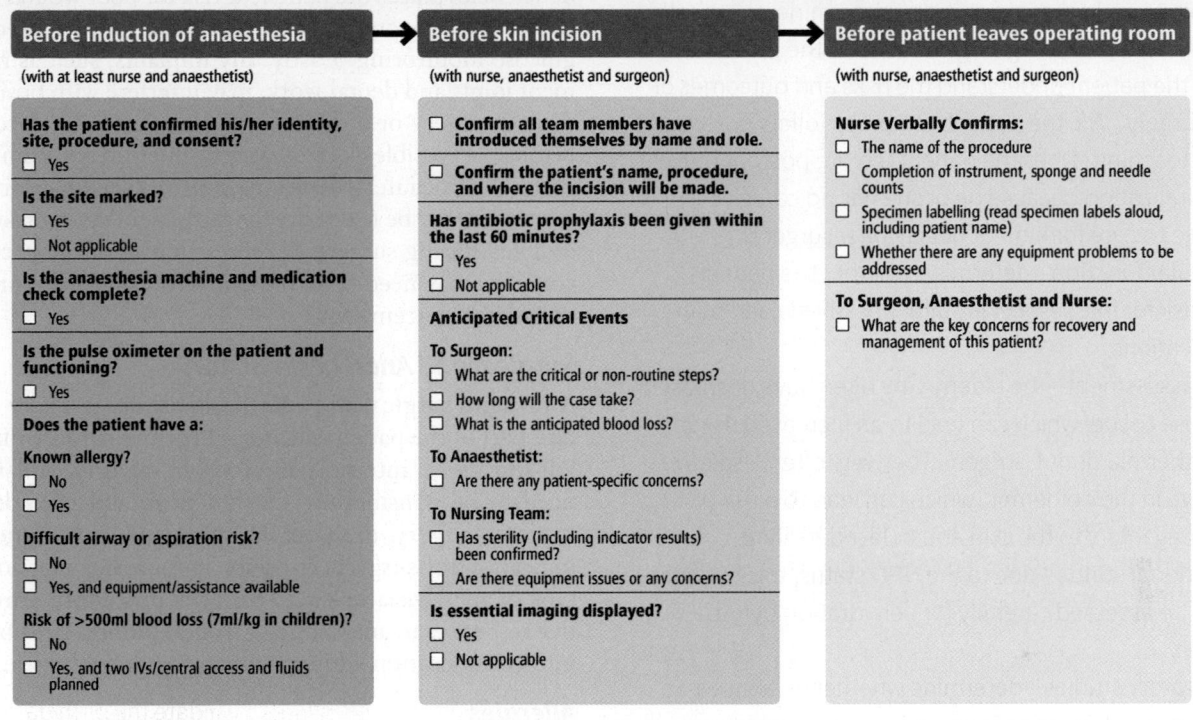

FIGURE 15.4 World Health Organization (WHO) surgical safety checklist.

Box 15.2 Components of a Complete Preoperative History

- Age (see Geriatric/Gerontological Considerations)
- Allergies and sensitivities to latex
- Current medications, including over-the-counter medications, vitamins, and herbal supplements
- Medical history and treatment plans
- Surgical history
- Previous anesthesia and responses to anesthesia
- Last oral intake
- Any medical implants or devices
- Any piercings
- Dental implants
- Nutrition deficiencies
- Family history
- Social history, including smoking and drug and alcohol habits
- History of mental illness or abuse
- Support system and living conditions
- Advance directives

Geriatric/Gerontological Considerations

Age and Preoperative History

The patient's age is important for a multitude of reasons; specifically, the elderly patient (65 or older) may have many issues that can interfere with a positive surgical outcome.

This patient must be assessed carefully for the following issues:

- Polypharmacy—the use of multiple medications, from multiple providers, purchased at multiple pharmacies. This can lead to medication interactions, which can also affect medications given during the perioperative period.
- Cardiac status—verify the presence of a preoperative electrocardiogram (ECG); place on the cardiac monitor and establish a baseline cardiac rhythm.
- Respiratory status—determine whether the patient is having any breathing difficulties. Establish a baseline

oxygen saturation on room air if the patient is not on oxygen at home or on the patient's normal administered oxygen level.

- Cognitive and sensory function—determine whether the patient is capable of giving consent for the procedure; does the patient understand the risks and outcomes of the surgery? Will the patient be able to follow postoperative teaching? Does the patient require postoperative hospitalization because he or she has no caregivers or is unable to care for him- or herself after surgery?
- Muscular function—determine whether the patient is at risk for falls, especially after anesthesia and pain medications.
- Skin assessment—the elderly very often have decreased adipose tissue, which can lead to an increased risk of hypothermia during surgery. They very often also have a change in the epidermis, which can lead to a risk of shearing injury to the skin and delayed healing.
- Nutritional status—due to the NPO status, this patient must be assessed carefully for dehydration before surgery.
- Laboratory studies—determine whether decreased renal/hepatic function is noted in the preoperative laboratory studies. Are all laboratory studies within normal range? The elderly patient typically has a decreased number of kidney nephrons and a decrease in the size of the liver, both which can affect how medications are metabolized.
- Chronic conditions—document all chronic conditions for which the patient is being treated.
- Support—it is important to ensure that the elderly patient has a strong support system and identify who will be responsible for helping the patient with any care needs he or she has when returning home.

Medical History

As the nurse asks questions pertaining to the patient's medical history, he or she should be taking special note of any conditions that will pose a risk during the surgical experience. For example, a patient with a history of DVT should be receiving coagulation studies prior to surgery. A patient with a cardiac condition may have an untoward response to anesthesia or may experience harmful hemodynamic changes during the surgical procedure and may require enhanced cardiac monitoring with a cardiologist's input before surgery. Chronic pulmonary conditions such as asthma, emphysema, and chronic bronchitis may complicate the removal of ventilatory support postoperatively and should be monitored with pulse oximetry and arterial blood gas (ABG) testing. These patients

may require extended intubation, and admission to the intensive care unit (ICU) postoperatively should be anticipated. The presence of chronic illness such as diabetes or immune deficiencies places the patient at risk for poor wound healing postoperatively and indicates the need for increased blood glucose monitoring. Lastly, any implants, such as replacement joints and dental work, may interfere with positioning during surgery or intubation. If a patient has a pacemaker, because of possible electromagnetic interference from the use of an electrocautery device to control bleeding during the surgery, it may be necessary for the patient's pacemaker to be disabled during surgery. A representative of the pacemaker company may need to be present before and after surgery to manage the pacemaker.

Surgical and Anesthesia History

A patient's surgical and anesthesia history is a very important part of the patient's history. Previous surgery may have left scar tissue, internal adhesions, or medical implants that need to be considered. The nurse should inquire about types of surgery, the year the surgery was performed, the indication for surgery, any poor incision healing, and what type of anesthesia was used for each procedure. Any negative responses to anesthesia or wound healing must be taken into consideration while planning the patient's care.

Allergies

All patient allergies must be documented to ensure patient safety. Allergies to medications, food, medical dyes, latex, medical adhesive, and environmental conditions must be documented along with the patient's physical response to exposure to these products. An alert bracelet is placed on the patient, and the surgical team is made aware. Allergies to antibiotics determine what pre- and postoperative prophylaxis medications are used. If a patient is allergic to antiseptic solutions such as Betadine or chlorhexidine, an alternative skin preparation must be selected. Latex allergies are a serious concern. Each facility must have adequate latex-free equipment available for these cases. In some outpatient settings, patients with latex allergies are scheduled as first cases of the day to ensure that the surgical suite is free of latex contamination. Many hospitals are choosing to create latex-free environments for all surgical suites for this reason.

Medications

Current medications are an extremely important part of the preoperative history (Table 15.1). The use of antihypertensives, anticoagulants, and antiarrhythmics, to name a few, can have a tremendous impact on the care provided in the operating room (OR). Herbal remedies and over-the-counter medications also may have potential interactions with medications used during the procedure and postoperatively or may increase the risk of bleeding.

Last Oral Intake

Last oral intake is an essential assessment parameter prior to anesthesia. The guidelines may be modified for different populations, but typically, all patients requiring

Table 15.1 Current Medications and Possible Implications

Medication Class	Potential Implications	Nursing Interventions	Rationale
Antiarrhythmic: ● Amiodarone ● Sotalol ● Ibutilide ● Dofetilide ● Dronedarone	Affect tolerance of anesthesia and potentiate neuromuscular blockers; depress cardiac function, output, and pulse	Obtain baseline electrocardiogram, vital signs. Monitor vital signs during the procedure. Communicate all medications to anesthesia team.	Continuous monitoring provides early detection of deviations.
Antihypertensives ● Captopril ● Clonidine HCl ● Metoprolol ● Atenolol ● Losartan ● Olmesartan ● Telmisartan ● Valsartan	Alter response to muscle relaxants and opioids May cause hypotensive crisis during and after the procedure	Monitor blood pressures. Communicate all medications to anesthesia team.	Hypotensive crisis can be prevented through monitoring and early detection.
Corticosteroids ● Dexamethasone ● Hydrocortisone ● Prednisone	Surgery increases need for higher doses in patients who use steroids for replacement therapy. May increase healing time because of blockage of collagen formation Increase risk of hemorrhage and may mask signs of infection	Assess for hyperglycemia, infection, bleeding, and wound healing. Splint incisions to promote healing. Continue therapy during the procedure.	Continuing therapy avoids withdrawal and adrenal crisis.
Anticoagulants ● Warfarin ● Heparin ● Aspirin	Increase risk of hemorrhage	Obtain baseline coagulation studies. Taper medication at least 48 hours prior to the procedure. Have vitamin K and protamine sulfate available as antidotes if excessive bleeding occurs during the procedure.	Obtaining coagulation studies at intervals during care can detect trends and potentially prevent hemorrhage. Vitamin K is the antidote for Coumadin; protamine sulfate is the antidote for heparin.
Nonsteroidal Anti-Inflammatory Drugs (NSAIDs) ● Ibuprofen, aspirin, naproxen	May prolong bleeding time and may cause intraoperative or postoperative bleeding	Inform physicians if the medication has not been withheld before surgery.	Bleeding risk must be assessed by the physicians.
Anticonvulsants ● Phenobarbital, phenytoin	These medications may alter the metabolism of anesthesia.	Must be alert for the potential of seizures because they can cause injury during a procedure. Maintain medication schedule Have suction and oral airway available.	Maintaining medication prevents seizures and injury.

Continued

Table 15.1 Current Medications and Possible Implications—cont'd

Medication Class	Potential Implications	Nursing Interventions	Rationale
Insulin	The patient will have a decreased need for insulin during the preoperative period due to decreased oral intake. Increased need postoperatively due to the stress of the surgery increasing glucose release Needs may fluctuate postoperatively because of decreased oral intake.	Closely monitor blood glucose levels pre-/intra-/postoperatively.	Essential to monitor glucose levels so that treatment can be quickly administered with abnormal glucose levels

surgical intervention should have had nothing to eat or drink (**NPO**) for at least 8 hours prior to the procedure. A patient who has eaten within 8 hours is at risk of aspiration, the introduction of food particles into the lungs through emesis. The preoperative nurse is responsible for documenting the last oral intake. Patients who have special needs, such as those with diabetes mellitus, may have altered NPO orders before surgery. Exceptions are sometimes made that allow patients to take essential medications with sips of water prior to the procedure. According to recent guidelines for elective procedures, the patient may be advised to be NPO 6 to 8 hours for solid foods and 2 hours for clear fluids (see Evidence-Based Practice).

Evidence-Based Practice

Preoperative NPO Status

General anesthesia depresses many of the body's protective reflexes, including the gag reflex that prevents stomach contents from entering the lungs. Preoperative fasting decreases stomach acid and volume to help prevent aspiration. In the past, it was accepted practice to instruct the patient to be NPO after midnight the night prior to his or her procedure. After review in 2012 and updates in 2017, the recommendation has changed to NPO for 8 hours for solid foods and 2 hours for clear fluids. These recommendations may vary based on pre-morbid conditions such as diabetes and age.

Practice guidelines for preoperative fasting and the use of pharmacologic agents to reduce the risk of pulmonary aspiration: Application to healthy patients undergoing elective procedures: An updated report by the American Society of Anesthesiologists Task Force on Preoperative Fasting and the Use of Pharmacologic Agents to Reduce the Risk of Pulmonary Aspiration. (2017). *Anesthesiology, 126*(3), 376–393.

There are different preoperative NPO parameters for children and infants:

- No solid food is allowed for 8 hours before surgery.
- Infant formula can be given up to 6 hours before surgery.
- Breast milk can be given up to 4 hours before surgery.
- Clear liquids can be given up to 2 hours before surgery.

Alcohol, Smoking, and Drug Use

Alcohol, smoking, and drug use are sometimes uncomfortable but important questions to ask of all patients. Smoking puts patients at risk for respiratory depression during the procedure and DVT during postoperative care. Because of changes in the pulmonary system, intubation and ventilation may also be compromised. Smoking may also increase the healing time for surgical wounds. Alcohol and drug use may compromise the patient's response to anesthesia. Additionally, postoperative pain management is complicated with recreational drug use, and such use must be taken into consideration when making discharge plans.

Special Considerations

When a patient history is obtained, some questions require privacy because of their sensitive nature. All psychosocial questions, such as questions about abuse at home and gynecological and mental illness, must be asked with no other family or support persons present. Any conflicting medical information from the patient's chart and the patient's responses should also be addressed at this time.

Connection Check 15.2

The nurse should report which of the following findings from a patient's history as increasing the risk for DVTs postoperatively? *(Select all that apply.)*

A. History of smoking
B. Age
C. History of DVTs with previous pregnancy
D. Borderline hypertension
E. Allergies

Physical Assessment

The physical assessment of the surgical patient is another component of the preoperative admission work-up. Assessment parameters include:

- Height and weight
- Vital signs
- Systems assessment

Height and Weight

Height and weight help the anesthesia provider determine fluid needs and medication dosages for anesthesia or antibiotics during the procedure. A patient with a high body mass index (BMI) may also require a larger operating table and recovery bed. Most operating tables have extensions that can meet increased weight requirements. In addition, the OR team may adjust diligence equipment used to transfer the patient.

Vital Signs

Vital signs are obtained by the nurse during the initial assessment. This includes blood pressure, respirations, pulse, temperature, and pulse oximetry. If available, the nurse should compare the admission vital signs with any previously recorded vital signs to note trends or major changes. If the initial set varies significantly from the patient's normal, a second set of vital signs may be taken 10 to 15 minutes later because many patients may be nervous, which may alter their vital signs. The presence of fever may be an indication of infection. That may necessitate a postponement of the surgical procedure. If the patient is held in the preoperative room for longer than 2 hours, a second set of vital signs may be required before transfer to the surgical suite.

Assessment of vital signs must include the fifth vital sign, pain. The patient is asked to rate pain in one of several ways. Examples of pain scales include:

- A scale of 0 to 10, with 10 being the worst pain the patient has ever experienced
- A series of faces ranging from a smile to a frown for pediatric patients

Another required admission question is the documentation of the patient's acceptable pain score. Each patient handles pain differently, and therefore a subjective pain scale is interpreted differently. This score is used by the post-anesthesia nurse and surgeon as a guide for adequate pain management.

Systems Assessment

During the initial assessment, the nurse performs a head-to-toe physical assessment of the preoperative patient. Key elements for the preoperative assessment are presented in the following subsections.

Cardiovascular Assessment

In addition to pulse and blood pressure, the nurse further assesses the patient's cardiovascular health. Peripheral pulses, color, skin turgor, capillary refill, temperature, and edema are important parameters to assess. The nurse also auscultates the heart for rhythm, rate, and murmurs.

Respiratory Assessment

The nurse assesses the patient's breathing for rate, depth, rhythm, and adventitious breath sounds such as crackles, rhonchi, or wheezing. Pulse oximetry is used to assess the patient's oxygen saturation on room air. In addition, the nurse should report any clubbing in the fingers, which could indicate long-term oxygen deprivation. The nurse must also ensure that the patient has a clear airway. The patient is asked to stick out his or her tongue, breathe with the head tilted up and with the chin down, and swallow. This ensures that an airway and any intubation may be safely maintained during the procedure. The anesthesiologist assesses the patient as well during his or her consultation.

Neurological Assessment

Prior to the induction of anesthesia, it is important for the nurse to obtain a baseline neurological evaluation. Assessment of general cognition and the ability to understand commands is important prior to the induction of general anesthesia. The nurse also assesses the movement, strength, and sensation of the extremities. This is especially important in a patient who will receive some type of regional block for the procedure. The presence of preoperative delirium or confusion may delay or postpone the procedure or necessitate admission to the hospital postoperatively.

Liver/Renal Assessment

It is important to note potential renal or liver disease in the surgical patient. The effects of anesthesia and other medications used before, during, and after an operation may be altered if the patient has decreased hepatic or renal clearance. A complete metabolic panel helps the team to identify any signs of dysfunction.

Integumentary Assessment

A general assessment of the patient includes assessing appearance, such as skin integrity and hygiene. Patients with poor skin turgor or fragile skin may heal more slowly than a healthy individual. Also, the team may want to be careful as to the type of dressings that are used to protect the skin from further damage beyond the incision. For example, in an older patient or a patient with fragile skin, the nurse may want to use a leg strap instead of an adhesive to secure a urinary catheter. If hygiene is an issue, the nurse may need to give extra instruction on wound care in an effort to decrease the risk for infection.

Gastrointestinal Assessment

It is important for the nurse to note typical bowel habits of the patient, especially if the patient will be admitted to the hospital after surgery. The nurse should also document the presence of normal bowel sounds and any areas of tenderness on the abdomen.

Genitourinary Assessment

The nurse should document any devices noted for urinary elimination, such as an indwelling urinary catheter. The nurse should have the patient void before entering the operating suite and note any unusual odor or color of the urine. The patient may wish to discuss any concerns about urination postoperatively; some patients worry about being able to get into the bathroom without assistance. The nurse should also document any perineal abnormalities on the chart.

Connection Check 15.3

Which of the following patients presents the greatest risk for a negative response to anesthesia?

A. A 40-y.o. male with high blood pressure

B. A 20-y.o. female with no prior surgical history

C. A 29-y.o. female with a history of stage II acute renal failure

D. An 85-y.o. male who drinks one glass of scotch every night

---

CASE STUDY: EPISODE 2

While Maria is interviewed, she expresses concern for her stay at the hospital and her upcoming procedure. Maria states that other than the birth of her children, this is the first time she has been in a hospital, and this is her first surgical procedure. She expresses anxiety over "being put under" and worries about how she will take care of her children after discharge…

PATIENT PREPARATION FOR THE SURGICAL EXPERIENCE

Laboratory Assessment

Preoperative laboratory work is essential in determining the patient's readiness for surgery. This can be done at an appointment prior to surgery or the morning of surgery. If done on the day of surgery, labs will be drawn as the nurse places an IV line to be used for venous access during surgery.

A type and screen to determine blood type and the presence of antibodies is drawn. This sample is used to cross-match blood in the event the patient needs blood during the surgical procedure. Often, facilities have the patient wear a blood identification bracelet with unique numbers that match the drawn sample for the purpose of easy and safe identification.

A complete metabolic panel provides baseline information on renal and liver functions, including liver enzymes,

albumin, electrolytes, blood urea nitrogen, and creatinine. This information helps in the selection of medications and dosages for the surgical procedure. Coagulation studies show how quickly the patient's blood clots after injury, determining any bleeding abnormalities. The CBC, or complete blood count, measures hemoglobin/hematocrit (blood volume and oxygen-carrying capability) and the white blood cell count for indications of infection. Any deviation from the facility's defined ranges should be reported to the surgeon or anesthesiologist, as appropriate, to be corrected to avoid complications. For example, a low platelet count or hemoglobin/hematocrit will be further decreased by surgery. The surgeon may ask for blood to be typed and cross-matched prior to the procedure, or the provider may ask for platelet administration before surgery. Clotting abnormalities may also require the administration of fresh frozen plasma before the procedure can begin.

Lastly, urine is measured for the presence of glucose, blood, protein, and specific gravity and the presence of ketones. These measures help determine the presence of infection or the hydration status of the patient. Women of childbearing age may be tested immediately prior to surgery for pregnancy.

Radiological Assessment

Radiological imaging is sometimes required prior to surgery. Common preoperative images are magnetic resonance imaging (MRI), computerized axial tomography (CAT scans), ultrasonography, or x-ray imaging. Imaging studies may also be required immediately before and during the surgery to monitor progress. An electrocardiogram (ECG) may also be performed prior to or on admission to the surgical facility, and cardiac monitoring may be ongoing.

Patient Teaching

It is important at this time to complete any necessary patient teaching. Patient teaching helps decrease anxiety, which has been shown to improve patient outcomes. Anxiety has been shown to increase postoperative pain medication requirements, necessitating more pain medication. This can affect the postoperative recovery by decreasing activity and mobility, which puts the patient at risk for complications such as DVT, pneumonia, and constipation. Anxiety also plays a role in increasing the risk of infection by decreasing the immune system response. Most facilities have a patient teaching record where teaching is documented.

The patient's family should be included in the preoperative teaching. At this time, the nurse should take the opportunity to have a discussion with the patient and his or her family support regarding what to expect during the patient's surgical and postoperative experience. For example, the nurse should discuss how long the procedure will be, how long the patient will be in the **post-anesthesia care unit (PACU)**, and how soon the family will receive an update on the patient's status and be able to see the patient. Discharge care may be covered at this time because the patient may be fatigued or drowsy after the procedure. The nurse can address any family concerns at that time as well. Lastly, the nurse should ensure that the family is guided to the appropriate waiting area where the staff will be able to locate them for updates. See Box 15.3 for a checklist of preoperative learning needs.

Physical Preparations

Intravenous Line (IV Line)

An IV line is inserted during the preoperative admission, typically for the purpose of the administration of anesthesia and fluids during the surgery. An 18-gauge catheter is preferred because this size is required for the administration of all blood products. Factors to consider when placing the IV line include the location of the procedure and if multiple sites are required. The IV should be labeled with gauge, time and date of placement, and the nurse's initials. The nurse may also administer any preoperative antibiotics at this time.

Bowel and Bladder Preparation

Patients receiving abdominal, intestinal, gynecological, or rectal surgery may be asked to perform a bowel preparation. This may be done by use of an enema or gentle laxatives that the patient self-administers at home the night before the procedure. The nurse should confirm and document that this preparation has been performed.

Patients scheduled for abdominal, gynecological, or long procedures may also require the insertion of an indwelling catheter to drain urine. This will keep the bladder empty during a procedure, preventing injury to the bladder. It also allows the surgical team to monitor output in the operating room and PACU.

Connection Check 15.4

During the initial assessment and admission questions, the nurse asks Maria for the time of her last oral intake. The patient replies, "I had dinner last night at 8 p.m., but I took a few sips of water this morning with my vitamins. The nurse's best response is which of the following?

A. Explain to the patient that just a sip of water should not be a problem for anesthesia but that the vitamins may be a problem. That information will be passed on to the anesthesiologist.

B. Tell the patient that the sip of water is not an issue because it was only a sip.

C. Inform the patient that her surgery will not be performed today because the risk is too high for a negative outcome.

D. Inform the patient that taking her vitamins before surgery was a good plan.

Box 15.3 Checklist of Preoperative Learning Needs

- Reason for procedure
- Nature of procedure
- Members of the surgical team
- Length of the procedure
- Location of the procedure
- Components and use of the pain scale
- Anesthesia plan
- Postoperative pain management plan
- Location of the incisions
- Presence of postoperative drains and dressings
- Surgical site preparation
- Ambulation guidelines after surgery
- Coughing and deep breathing exercises expectations
- Splinting incisional area when coughing to decrease the pain
- Family instructions—the patient should not be alone for the first 24 to 48 hours.

Skin Preparation

Prior to surgery, skin preparation is done to help prevent infection at the surgical site. Patients may be instructed to shower and wash with Betadine or hexachlorophene soap prior to admission. A surgical shave may be necessary depending on the patient's skin type and the location of the incision. If a shave is appropriate, the nurse uses a sterile electric clipper. A razor is not recommended because of the risk of infection caused by small nicks in the skin that may occur with a razor. Shaving may be done in the OR after the induction of anesthesia. In addition, the nurse should confirm that all body piercings have been removed and that nails are clear of polish.

Medications

Preoperative medications may be required. Patients with preoperative anxiety may be prescribed a benzodiazepine such as midazolam HCl, diazepam, or lorazepam. Antiemetics such as metoclopramide HCl or ondansetron HCl may be used preoperatively if a patient has a history of nausea and vomiting due to anesthesia.

Transfer

Preparing the patient for transfer to the OR suite is the final responsibility of the preoperative nurse. Before transport, the nurse should make sure that all consents have been signed; the history and assessment have been completed and documented, including vital signs; learning needs have been met; skin and bowel preparation are complete; and preoperative medication has been administered. The intraoperative nurse may accompany the patient to the surgical suite, or the anesthesia team may be responsible for this transport depending on the surgical suite's policies. Once transferred, the patient is now considered to be receiving intraoperative care.

> ⚠️ **Safety Alert** **Transfer of Patient to Surgical Suite**
>
> *The preoperative nurse must ensure that the following have been completed before transfer to intraoperative care:*
>
> - Patient identification
> - Physical preparations
> - Confirmation of NPO status
> - Documentation of complete medical history and admission vital signs and laboratory work
> - Allergy bracelet visible
> - Documentation of initial time-out
> - Copies of all appropriate documentation are in patient's file
> - Patient education with verbalized return of information
> - Family and patient questions answered

Connection Check 15.5

Maria's surgeon has asked that thromboembolic-deterrent (TED) stockings be placed on the patient before surgery as well as sequential compression devices on both legs to the knees. Maria asks the nurse what these devices will do for her. Which response by the nurse is most appropriate?

A. "They work together to make sure that you do not have a decrease in arterial blood flow in your legs during the surgery."

B. "They complement each other to prevent blood from backing up in your legs and causing a deep vein thrombosis due to your immobility during the surgery."

C. "They prevent deep tissue clotting during the surgery."

D. "The two devices do the same thing, but one is better during the surgery, and the other is better postoperatively."

NURSING MANAGEMENT

Nursing Diagnoses

- **Fear and anxiety** related to loss of control and the unknown
- **Knowledge deficit:** treatment procedure

Nursing Interventions

▪ *Assessments*

- Vital signs/oxygen saturation
  Initial vital signs provide a base to determine the patient's condition during and after the procedure. Increased or

decreased heart rate, increased or decreased blood pressure, increased temperature, and decreased oxygen saturation may necessitate a postponement of the procedure, if elective.

- Physical examination/laboratory analysis
  Evaluation of the physical exam and laboratory values determines readiness for the procedure, indicates necessary adjustments to be made prior to the procedure, and provides a baseline for comparison in the OR and postoperatively.

- Last oral intake
  NPO prior to the procedure is essential to guard against aspiration during intubation and extubation due to decreased gag reflexes.

- Confirm appropriate skin prep and bowel prep have been completed.
  Prepping the skin with a special soap prior to surgery helps reduce the risk of infection; a bowel prep prior to some abdominal, gynecological, or rectal surgeries is necessary to clear the bowel, which prevents the risk of peritoneal contamination if the bowel is compromised during surgery.

▪ *Actions*

- Ensure removal of jewelry and prosthetics.
  An electrocautery unit is used during operative procedures to decrease bleeding. Electricity may travel to any metal on the body, causing a burn. There is also a risk during positioning that the patient's ring may get caught in a piece of equipment, causing injury to the finger.

- Inform anesthesia and surgical personnel of the presence of any implants.
  A patient with a pacemaker may need to have the pacemaker disabled; the pacemaker company or a representative of the hospital needs to assume responsibility for this action. Personnel must also be aware of items such as central intravenous lines or Mediports, typically used for long-term medication therapy.

- Time-out
  Establishing the right patient, procedure, and site is essential to avoid operative errors.

- IV insertion
  An IV is necessary for fluid and medication administration.

▪ *Teaching*

- What to expect of the OR experience
  An understanding of what to expect of the OR experience helps control anxiety and increase patient comfort.

- How to prevent postoperative complications
  Knowledge of postoperative teaching, such as coughing, deep breathing, early ambulation, and leg and ankle exercises, significantly reduces the risk of postoperative complications.

Connection Check 15.6

When planning discharge education for a 65-y.o. male who is having a hip replacement, it is appropriate for the nurse to consider which of the following? *(Select all that apply.)*

A. The patient's resources at home for completing activities of daily living

B. The number of stairs in the patient's home

C. Transportation to follow-up appointments

D. Pre-existing medical conditions

E. The number of bathrooms in the home

Making Connections

CASE STUDY: WRAP-UP

Maria's nurse completes the preoperative preparation. An IV line is inserted, and normal saline is started. The anesthesia provider is reminded of Maria's allergies to penicillin and latex and her smoking history. Once completed, the nurse spends time with Maria, attempting to allay her fears by explaining what to expect in the OR and when she wakes up. They review potential plans for childcare postoperatively.

Case Study Questions

1. Maria expresses her anxiety about the procedure and anesthesia to her nurse. Which is the most appropriate response?

   A. Tell her, "It's okay; we do this every day."

   B. Assure her that her fears are normal and encourage her to use her consultation time with the surgeon and anesthesiologist to address her concerns.

   C. Share a story about your friend who had similar fears prior to her surgery.

   D. Document her concerns in the chart so that the PACU nurse will expect her to be anxious during recovery.

2. Maria is allergic to latex. What is the appropriate action to prevent an allergic reaction in the patient who is having surgery?

   A. Terminally clean the OR before her case and remove all latex products.

   B. Maria should be the first case of the day, and only nonlatex items should be used.

   C. All surgical suites are latex-free, so this is not a concern.

   D. Anesthesia should be prepared to intubate and treat her if a reaction occurs because there is no way to ensure a latex-free environment.

3. Because of Maria's smoking history, the nurse understands she is at great risk for which of the following? *(Select all that apply.)*

   A. Increased postoperative pain

   B. Difficulty with anesthesia

   C. Respiratory depression during the procedure

   D. Increased healing time after the procedure

   E. Deep vein thrombosis after the procedure

4. The nurse recognizes teaching has been effective by which of the following statements?

   A. "My neighbor was able to eat right up to the time of her procedure."

   B. "I know there is nothing you can do about nausea after the procedure."

   C. "So that IV line will stay in throughout the procedure?"

   D. "I know I will need blood during this procedure."

5. What is the priority responsibility of Maria's nurse before the procedure?

   A. Explaining the procedure and having Maria sign the consent form

   B. Reviewing the risks of anesthesia

   C. Marking the surgical site with the patient

   D. Ensuring completion of the preoperative assessment

CHAPTER SUMMARY

The preoperative phase of the surgical experience begins when the decision for surgery is made and ends when the patient is transferred to the surgical suite. During this time, the preoperative nurse takes on a multitude of roles, including educator, advocator, and admittance nurse.

Priority assessments include patient history and medications (prescribed and over the counter [OTC]), physical assessment, allergies, alcohol and drug use, and advance directives. The nurse must assess the elderly for specific concerns that may affect their surgical experience. It is essential to get a baseline for comparison in the intraoperative and postoperative periods, specifically with vital signs, cardiac rhythm, and oxygen saturation. Also, the assessment may identify a patient who requires additional monitoring to avoid complications associated with the procedure or anesthesia. Patient preparation includes education about the operative experience, IV insertion, labs, postoperative teaching, and family support. The patient should be aware of the potential for IV lines or drains that may be present postoperatively.

The nurse is involved in all aspects of preoperative care: patient education, time-outs, and confirmation of informed consent and family support. Education must include the many facets of the surgical experience, including postoperative care that will be vital to preventing complications, specifically coughing, deep breathing, and early mobility after surgery. The nurse must also be sure the patient is clear about postoperative medications and the regime for taking these medications. Teaching is a vital aspect of the preoperative nurse's care, to ensure that the transition to the operative suite and subsequent post-anesthesia care unit (PACU) is seamless and without adverse outcomes.

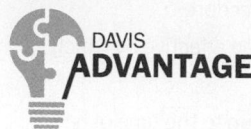

DAVIS
ADVANTAGE | To explore learning resources for this chapter, go to **Davis Advantage** and find:
- Answers to in-text questions
- Chapter Resources and Activities
- NCLEX®-Style Chapter Review Questions
- Bibliography

Chapter 16

Priorities for the Intraoperative Patient

Jamie Maher

Finding Connections

OVERVIEW OF THE SURGICAL EXPERIENCE

Surgical Settings

Surgical technology is changing every day. As new equipment is developed and evidence-based practice is integrated into surgical protocols, the setting of surgery also changes. Surgical procedures are not only performed in the traditional inpatient hospital setting but also in **outpatient surgical centers** that offer the same amenities.

Inpatient surgical settings perform surgical procedures that require admittance to a hospital unit postoperatively. Inpatient procedures are often very invasive and long. Patients require close monitoring and recovery for more than 24 hours after completion. Examples include procedures such as cardiac surgeries, which may require intensive care unit (ICU) care postoperatively with continuous monitoring. Joint replacements may require complex pain management. Inpatient surgery may also be indicated if admittance to the hospital after the procedure for rehabilitation is required.

Ambulatory or outpatient surgery is performed without admittance to a hospital unit before or after the procedure. The surgery center may be freestanding or located in a hospital. Also known as "same-day surgery," outpatient surgery is often less invasive, shorter in operating time, and requires less than 24 hours of monitored recovery time. Patients are often admitted 2 hours prior to surgery and discharged directly to their homes. Candidates for outpatient procedures typically have no other comorbidities, such as substantial medical histories. They do not need additional recovery care beyond post-anesthesia. Successful recovery at home requires the patient to be receptive to teaching prior to discharge from the surgical center and to have a caregiver who will be present with the patient at all times for at least 24 hours. Advances in surgical science have greatly increased the number of procedures that are done on an outpatient basis. Outpatient surgical examples include some ear, nose, and throat (ENT) procedures and oral and orthopedic surgeries. More complex procedures such as mastectomies can also be performed in an outpatient setting. Ambulatory surgery centers follow the same safety and clinical guidelines as an inpatient setting. These include the presence of an anesthesiologist, a sterile operating environment, and a **post-anesthesia care unit (PACU)**. Before a patient is discharged from the outpatient settings, goals are met regarding pain control and recovery education.

Freestanding outpatient surgery is a rapidly expanding option for many patients. Freestanding surgical centers tend to be located in a more convenient setting, away from the intimidating hospital setting. They allow more flexibility in scheduling for the patient. Family members are only separated from the patient during the actual procedure and are able to participate in the postoperative care and education. Freestanding surgical centers are less expensive than inpatient settings and often provide more face-to-face time with the nurse during the patient's stay.

Outpatient operative nursing poses unique challenges. The nurse needs to quickly identify and prioritize the patient's learning needs because there is a shorter recovery time and therefore less time to complete postoperative education. Also, some education may need to be completed during the preoperative time when the patient is more alert rather than sleepy after undergoing anesthesia.

Surgical Categories

Types of surgery can be divided into six subcategories. Diagnostic surgeries, such as biopsies, exploratory procedures, and laparotomies/arthroscopies, are performed to determine sources of disorders. Curative surgeries repair or remove causes of disorders. Restorative surgeries are those that repair disorders, such as a total hip replacement. They improve patient function by reconstructing mechanical parts of the body. Palliative procedures are for comfort and help relieve pain or symptoms of a disease process. Cosmetic surgeries restore or improve personal appearance, and lastly, transplant surgery is done to replace nonfunctioning or poorly functioning organs to improve or sustain life. Examples of this include kidney or heart transplants. Often the name of the surgery describes the nature of the procedure (Table 16.1).

Surgical procedures may be further classified as *elective*, *urgent*, or *emergency*.

- **Elective surgery** is surgery that the patient chooses to have. It is performed for his or her well-being but is not absolutely necessary. Most elective surgeries are scheduled at the patient's convenience, and many are performed in the outpatient setting. These often include plastic surgeries, oral surgeries, and orthopedic surgeries.
- **Urgent surgery**, although necessary, may be scheduled rather than done immediately. Examples include

Table 16.1 Suffixes for Surgical Procedures

Suffix	Meaning	Examples
-centesis	Puncture	Amniocentesis, thoracentesis
-ectomy	Removal	Cholecystectomy, hysterectomy
-lysis	Destruction	Electrolysis
-oscopsy	View with scope	Arthroscopy, endoscopy
-ostomy	Create an opening	Colostomy, ileostomy
-otomy	Incision	Episiotomy, tracheotomy
-plasty	To reshape or repair	Abdominoplasty, mammoplasty

hysterectomies, laminectomies, and hip or knee replacements.

- **Emergency surgery** is unscheduled and is done immediately to save a patient's life or limb. The need for this type of surgery is always unanticipated. Gunshot wounds, stabbings, and auto accidents often require emergency surgery.

Procedures can have a minor or major degree of risk. Minor procedures such as oral surgeries and dilations and curettage (D&C) are often performed under **local anesthesia**, hold less surgical risk for the patient's well-being, and require minimal post-anesthesia recovery. Major procedures are longer, more complex, and have a higher degree of risk. They are performed under general anesthesia and require overnight stays in the hospital, sometimes in the ICU setting. Cardiac procedures, neurological procedures, or thoracic procedures typically fall into this category.

Finally, surgical procedures are defined as simple or radical in extent. A simple procedure means that the surgeon is working within a small defined affected area. A radical procedure involves not only the small defined affected area but also the surrounding tissue. For example, a surgeon may only need to perform a simple tumor removal. Alternatively, a radical procedure involves removing the tumor and the surrounding tissues. A gynecologist may perform a simple hysterectomy where only the uterus is removed or may remove the fallopian tubes and ovaries in what is known as a radical total hysterectomy.

OVERVIEW OF THE SURGICAL TEAM MEMBERS

Each day, several million individuals worldwide face a surgical procedure of some kind. Surgical patients must depend on the knowledge and skills of surgical team members

who work in the OR. As in other healthcare settings, an efficiently functioning team in the surgical environment is of extreme importance to the patient. Respect for others' expertise, the ability to work harmoniously, and the art of communicating effectively are necessary ingredients for a well-functioning OR team.

The surgical procedure dictates the number and type of members on the surgical team. Normally, this team includes a surgeon; an anesthesia provider; a **perioperative registered nurse** (RN who works in the OR); and perhaps a variety of unlicensed assistive personnel, such as surgical technologists, OR associates, and critical care technicians. Team members are categorized as sterile, individuals who perform a surgical scrub and don a gown and gloves to work inside the **sterile field** (the identified surgical area considered free from microorganisms), and/or nonsterile, individuals who function outside the identified sterile field.

Sterile Team Members

Sterile team members are those who work within the sterile field and have the responsibility of maintaining **asepsis** (controlling the sterile field to avoid contamination by microorganisms) throughout the surgical procedure. The sterile field includes the OR table and the area closely surrounding it, an equipment stand called the **Mayo stand** that is conveniently positioned close to the patient, and the instrument table. The team members scrub their hands and arms with special disinfecting soaps and wear surgical gowns, caps, eyewear, gloves, and sturdy footwear (with or without optional shoe covers). Sterile team members include:

- The surgeon
- Surgical assistants
- The scrub nurse or surgical technologist

Surgeon

The **surgeon** is considered the leader of the surgical team and has the ultimate responsibility for performing the surgery in an effective and safe manner. Depending on the complexity of the surgical procedure, the surgeon may have one or more providers assisting. These providers may be interns or hospital residents who are participating in the surgery as part of their advanced training. There may also be other surgeons who are specialists in a particular field and part of the interprofessional team caring for the patient.

Surgical Assistants

Surgical assistants are practitioners with specialized training that allows them to assist with surgical procedures. These roles include physician assistants (PAs), surgical first assistants (SFAs), nurse practitioners (NPs), and RN first assistants (RNFAs).

The PA's primary role is to assist licensed providers. In addition to helping in the OR, the PA provides both preoperative and postoperative care for patients, freeing the surgeon to perform the more specialized care appropriate to his or her training and expertise. The PA's duties may include ensuring the acquisition of patient diagnostic films, records, laboratory studies, and history and physical examinations (also known as an H&P) and reporting any issues or concerns to the appropriate parties.

The SFA is typically a certified surgical technologist with additional specialized education or training. Under the surgeon's direction, the SFA provides aid in exposing of the surgical site, **hemostasis** (controlling blood flow and stopping or preventing hemorrhage), and other technical intraoperative functions as directed by the provider.

The RNFA or NP is an RN who has gone through extensive education beyond the traditional nursing preparation. The actual scope of the RNFA's/NP's practice in the perioperative environment is dependent on specific state regulations. In most instances, similar to the PA, the RNFA/NP functions interdependently with the surgeon during the procedure to assist in performing the operation.

Scrub Nurse, Surgical Technologist, and Operating Room Technician

The scrub nurse, surgical technologist, or operating room (OR) technician is also known as the **scrub**. This individual works directly with the surgeon within the sterile field by passing instruments, sponges, and other items needed during the surgical procedure. Before an operation, scrubs help prepare the OR by setting up surgical instruments and equipment, sterile drapes, and sterile solutions. They assemble both sterile and nonsterile equipment, checking to ensure that it is working properly. The scrub is also responsible for helping the surgical team don sterile gowns and gloves in preparation for the surgical procedure. Scrubs help count sponges, needles, instruments, and other miscellaneous supplies and help prepare, care for, and dispose of specimens taken for laboratory study. Depending on the institution's policies, scrubs may hold retractors, cut sutures, and assist with the application of surgical dressings. After an operation, scrubs assist with readying the room for the next procedure by restocking and cleaning.

Nonsterile Team Members

Nonsterile team members perform their duties outside the sterile field. These team members include but are not limited to:

- The anesthesia provider
- The circulating RN
- Unlicensed assistive personnel
- The OR director/coordinator/manager

Anesthesia Provider

The **anesthesia provider** is responsible for maintaining and sustaining the physiological status of the patient throughout the surgical process. This person may be an anesthesiologist or certified registered nurse anesthetist (CRNA). An anesthesiologist is a physician. CRNAs are advanced practice RNs trained to administer anesthetics. They can work independently or in collaboration with an anesthesiologist.

The anesthesia provider must be constantly aware of the surgeon's actions, doing everything possible to ensure the safety of the patient and reduce the stress of the operation. Specific responsibilities include providing smooth induction of the patient's **anesthesia** (temporary induced loss of sensation or awareness) in order to prevent pain; maintaining satisfactory degrees of relaxation of the patient; providing continuous monitoring of the patient's life functions, including oxygen exchange, circulatory functions, systemic circulation, and vital signs; and advising the surgeon of impending complications and independently intervening as necessary.

The anesthesia provider has contact with the patient during all phases of the surgical process: preoperative, intraoperative, and postoperative. During the **preoperative phase**, the anesthesia provider meets with the patient and conducts a preoperative interview. At this time, the patient's medical history and medications are reviewed, facilitating the development of a plan for managing these conditions during surgery. The upcoming surgery and options for anesthesia are also discussed.

During the **intraoperative phase**, the anesthesia provider administers anesthetic agents and carefully monitors the patient's vital signs, including heart rate and rhythm, blood pressure, and respiratory status. As the surgical procedure progresses, adjustments in anesthesia agents may be made to compensate for changes in the patient's physical condition. At the completion of surgery, the recovery phase begins. If a general anesthetic has been used, the anesthesia provider gradually stops the anesthesia administration to allow for the metabolism of the medications, thereby allowing the patient to regain consciousness.

The **postoperative phase** begins when the patient is transported from the operative suite to a PACU or ICU. If to the ICU, responsibility for patient care is assumed by the ICU medical team after a thorough hand-off from the surgical team. If to a PACU, the anesthesia care provider maintains the oversight of patient management. This includes but is not limited to airway management; pain, nausea, and vomiting management; and monitoring of physiological outliers, such as changes in vital signs. When PACU discharge criteria are met, the anesthesia provider approves the movement of the patient to the predetermined post-surgical destination (i.e., home, floor bed, or unit bed).

Circulating Registered Nurse

The circulating registered nurse (RN) observes the surgical procedure from a broad perspective, assisting the team in creating and maintaining a safe and comfortable environment for the surgical patient. The scope of the nurse's responsibilities includes:

- Initial assessment of the patient in the preoperative area. During this time, an essential role of the perioperative nurse is to establish a therapeutic relationship with the patient, attempting to calm fears and establish trust.

- Initial assessment upon admission to the OR
- Assisting the anesthesia provider with positioning, monitor placement, line placement, and patient monitoring
- Assisting the surgeon and scrub nurse/technologist with donning of sterile gowns, gloves, and other protective gear
- Anticipating the need for equipment, instruments, and medications
- Assisting the scrub nurse or technician by opening packages of sterile supplies necessary for the procedure
- Ensuring samples are appropriately labeled and sent to the laboratory for analysis
- Counting the number of sponges, needles, instruments, and other miscellaneous supplies used during the operation to prevent accidental retention or loss of an item in the surgical wound
- Documenting information pertinent to the surgery and the surgical patient

Unlicensed Assistive Personnel

Unlicensed assistive personnel are accountable to and work under the supervision of perioperative RNs. Their duties include patient transport to the OR and helping with the positioning and securing of patients on the operating table in preparation for their procedures. They may also be assigned other tasks, such as delivery of specimens to the laboratory, blood pickup, and equipment retrieval and housekeeping duties.

Operating Room Director/Coordinator/Manager

The OR director/coordinator/manager is responsible for oversight of the business aspect of the OR. This individual is accountable for budgets, staffing, and other areas critical in ensuring the efficient running of the OR.

Connection Check 16.1

Which of the following is the identified leader of the surgical team?

A. The circulating registered nurse
B. The anesthesia provider
C. The scrub nurse
D. The surgeon

PRIORITY ASSESSMENTS AND PROCEDURES

There are several priority assessments and procedures that are essential in ensuring a safe operative experience for the patient. These include:

- The preoperative assessment
- The surgical pause
- The surgical scrub
- The donning of surgical attire

Preoperative Assessment

The **preoperative assessment** is done by the perioperative nurses, typically in the preoperative area, and must accomplish, at a minimum, four goals:

1. Determine the patient's level of knowledge related to the planned surgery, potential complications, and interventions, such as insertion of an indwelling catheter, and provide education as appropriate. This time also allows the patient to voice specific concerns or questions regarding the procedure.
2. Confirm that informed consent for the proposed surgical procedure has been obtained. Informed consent discussions are intended to explain the proposed procedure in terms the patient can understand and is able to articulate.
3. Determine the patient's level of anxiety in order to support his or her management of preoperative fears and postoperative concerns. This is done by openly discussing the causes of anxiety, such as fear of death or disability, fear of pain, fear of poor prognosis, and fear of rejection if a transplant is the planned procedure.
4. Obtain relevant information about the patient, which may include:
   - Verification of the patient's name and date of birth, such as verifying that the medical record numbers match the patient's name band and paperwork
   - Verification of NPO status prior to surgery
   - Determination of medications taken in the morning prior to surgery
   - Assessment of skin color, temperature, and integrity (i.e., tattoos, bruises)
   - Verification of health history, including current medications
   - Verification of allergy status and specific allergic reactions the patient experiences, such as a rash or itching
   - Verification of placement of any metal implants, especially automatic implanted cardioverter defibrillators and pacemakers
   - Assessment of family support

Surgical Pause

The **surgical pause**, or **time-out**, is done prior to the start of the procedure to verify correct patient, correct procedure, correct surgeon, correct position, correct equipment, and correct imaging studies (radiography, etc.). The presence of implants, such as a pacemaker, is confirmed. If antibiotics were indicated, their administration is verified. If the surgical site involves laterality, the correct site is verified and clearly marked with the operating surgeon's initials.

This universal protocol developed by The Joint Commission also includes the introduction of all team members in the room; thus, it involves active communication among all members of the interprofessional team (see Evidence-Based Practice). It is consistently initiated by a designated member of the team and is conducted in a "fail-safe" mode, which means the surgical procedure does not commence until every question or concern has been resolved.

Evidence-Based Practice

Guideline Implementation: Team Communication

Communication is best defined as the meaningful exchange of information between individuals or groups. The need for effective communication in the perioperative setting is well recognized and vital to safe surgical practice. Studies aimed at exploring failures in communication and information transfer across the surgical care pathway indicate that poor communication contributes to an unsafe operating room culture and affects patient safety and employee engagement, decision making, efficiency, morale, and retention. More specifically, The Joint Commission cites communication failure as the leading root cause for medication errors, delays in treatment, and wrong-site surgeries as well as the second most frequently cited root cause for operative and postoperative events. The new Association of periOperative Registered Nurses (AORN) "Guideline for Team Communication" provides guidelines for using standardized processes to improve team communication. Key points include handovers between phases of care, pre-, intra-, and postoperative; a brief discussion on the surgical plan; a time-out or pause to verify the correct patient, procedure, site, and side; and a debriefing after the procedure to discuss what was done and what was learned or could be done better in the future.

Link, T. (2018). Guideline implementation: Team communication. *AORN Journal, 108*(2), 165-177.

Surgical Scrub

The **surgical scrub** is another key element of patient care in the OR that is done to prevent surgical site infections. Although the human hand represents a vital tool in the care of a patient, it also may act as a portal and transmitter of infection. The warm, moist conditions inside surgical gloves are an ideal environment for the rapid growth of microorganisms. To minimize the risk of infection to the patient, it is essential that OR personnel who will be directly involved in invasive surgical procedures follow appropriate hand-hygiene and hand-scrub procedures.

A systematic approach to this procedure is an efficient way to ensure proper technique is completed. The traditional surgical scrub starts with washing the hands thoroughly. This is followed by washing with a disposable scrub sponge from a clean area (the hand) to a less clean

area (the arm). Scrubbing with a long-acting, powerful antimicrobial sponge for at least 3 to 5 minutes allows adequate time to remove, inhibit, or kill as many microorganisms as possible and protect against infection if gloves develop holes, tears, or nicks during the operative procedure (Fig. 16.1). An alternative hand rub using a waterless alcohol-based preparation may be used, especially if surgical staff members are allergic to available antiseptic scrub solutions. Prior to performing the scrub, all jewelry must be removed. Nails should be clean and short. Nail acrylics and gels are not allowed.

Surgical Attire

Wearing of appropriate surgical attire is another important step in reducing the risk of postoperative infections. There are several levels of surgical attire. The first level is worn by everyone working in the OR. This apparel is popularly referred to as *scrubs* because it is usually worn in a scrubbed or sterile environment. Scrubs are the shirts and pants or dresses worn as uniforms by surgeons, nurses, and other support staff in the OR. The next level of attire, which is typically referred to as *surgical attire*, consists of the sterile gown and gloves worn by staff working directly within the sterile field. This attire includes gloves, caps, masks, gowns, protective eyewear, and sturdy footwear (Fig. 16.2; Box 16.1).

Connection Check 16.2

The OR nurse is completing a perioperative assessment for a patient who is scheduled for exploratory surgery. Which of the following interventions must be completed prior to this patient going into the OR? *(Select all that apply.)*

A. Verify operative consent has been signed.
B. Ensure allergy and ID bands are in place.
C. Remove the patient's personal clothing.
D. Determine evidence of advance directive.
E. Validate completed patient history and physical examination.
F. Determine NPO status (last food/fluid consumed).

ANESTHESIA

The term *anesthesia* is derived from the ancient Greek word *an-aisthesis*, meaning "lack of or no sensation." Without anesthesia, most surgical procedures performed today would not be possible. The goals of anesthesia are amnesia, analgesia, depression of reflexes, muscle relaxation, and manipulation of physiological systems and functions. These are accomplished through the use of balanced anesthesia, which consists of one to several agents, each with a different action. The agents used depend on the patient, the procedure, and the anesthesia provider's preference.

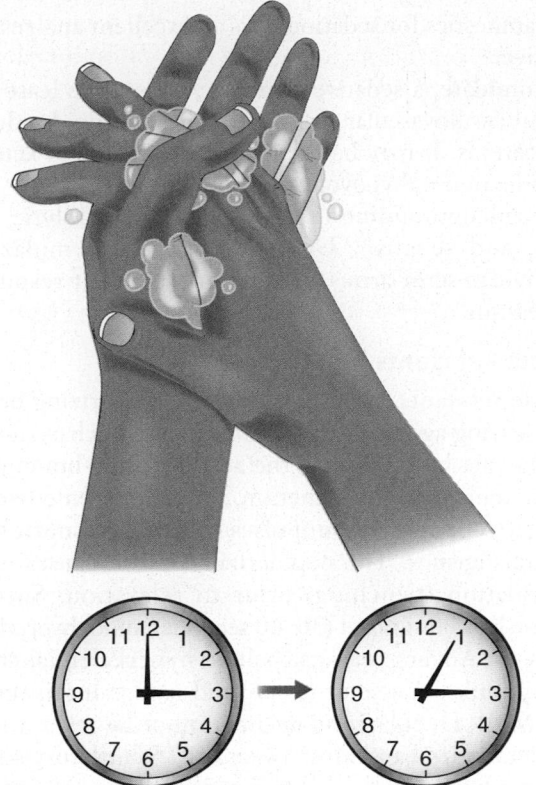

FIGURE 16.1 The surgical scrub.

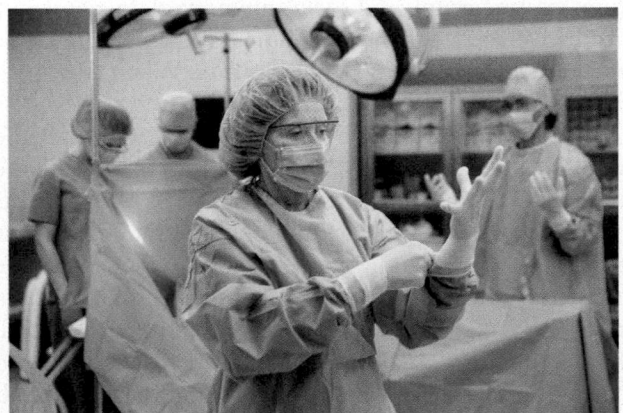

FIGURE 16.2 Surgical attire.

Box 16.1 Surgical Attire

- **Caps and masks** are made from paper and should never be reused because there is no way to properly clean them.
- **Gloves** protect the hands from infectious materials and protect patients from microorganisms on staff members' hands. The use of gloves *is not* a substitute for proper hand-washing techniques.
- **Masks** are worn to help contain moisture droplets expelled as staff members speak, cough, or sneeze. A mask is also a protective barrier against accidental splashes of blood or other contaminated body fluids. Masks should be changed between each patient contact.
- **Eyewear** protects staff in the event of an accidental splash of blood or other body fluid. Eyewear must always be worn when there is a potential for splash exposure.
- **Surgical gowns** are worn to reduce the transmission of microorganisms from the skin and clothing of members of the surgical team to the patient. They are made of fluid-resistant materials to also protect the surgical team against blood and other fluid exposures.
- **Sturdy footwear** is worn to protect the feet from injury by sharps or heavy items that may accidentally fall on them. Shoe covers are unnecessary if clean, sturdy shoes are available for use only in the surgical area.

Box 16.2 American Society of Anesthesiologists' Classification System

1. A normal healthy patient
2. A patient with mild systemic disease
3. A patient with severe systemic disease
4. A patient with severe systemic disease that is a constant threat to life
5. A moribund patient who is not expected to survive without the operation
6. A patient who is declared brain-dead and whose organs are being removed for donor purposes

Prior to surgery, each patient is given a preoperative physical examination and evaluation by the anesthesia team. On the basis of that evaluation, the patient is assigned a physical (P) status from the scale developed by American Society of Anesthesiologists (ASA) providers to assess and assign a perioperative risk, which helps in determining the anesthesia to be administered. This may also be called the *ASA status* using the same numbering system (Box 16.2).

Types of Anesthesia

There are four major types of anesthesia. They are general, regional, and local anesthetics and monitored anesthesia care (MAC).

General Anesthesia

General anesthesia is what the layperson calls "being put to sleep." Under general anesthesia, a patient is in a reversible unconscious state. General anesthesia provides all of the goals stated previously, including manipulation of physiological systems and functions. It is achieved using a variety of methodologies, either alone or together. These include inhalation of volatile agents (gases), IV agents, and muscle relaxants. The patient receiving a general anesthetic that includes the administration of a muscle relaxant requires ventilatory support in the form of an endotracheal tube (ETT). General anesthetics can also be administered without the use of muscle relaxants. In such instances the airway is frequently supported with supraglottic airways, such as a laryngeal mask airway (LMA), oral airway, or nasal airway. Airway management is discussed later in this chapter.

Volatile Agents

Volatile (inhalation or gas) anesthetic agents used in the United States include isoflurane, sevoflurane, desflurane, and nitrous oxide. The potency of the gases is identified as the minimum alveolar concentration needed to achieve the desired effect (the lower the minimum alveolar concentration, the more potent the gas). For example, sevoflurane has a minimum alveolar concentration of 2, whereas nitrous oxide has a minimum alveolar concentration of 105. Although these gases have been used for more than 100 years, their exact mechanism of action is not yet clearly understood. Some studies indicate that the synaptic transmission of nerve impulses is reversibly inhibited in areas of the central nervous system.

Intravenous Agents

Current IV anesthetics include:

- Barbiturates
- Benzodiazepines
- Opioids
- Propofol
- Ketamine
- Sedative-hypnotics

Barbiturates are central nervous system depressants. Examples include thiopental sodium, sodium methohexital, thiamylal, and Nembutal. They are excellent anesthetics and amnestics with a short onset and duration of action.

Benzodiazepines increase receptor availability for the inhibitory neurotransmitter gamma-aminobutyric acid. Examples include midazolam, diazepam, and lorazepam. They have a longer time to onset but have a longer duration than barbiturates. They are excellent amnestics but provide no analgesia.

Opioids bind to G-protein receptors as ligands or signaling molecules, producing analgesia. They also decrease the perception of pain. Examples include morphine, fentanyl, hydromorphone (Dilaudid), sufentanil, and remifentanil. They are excellent analgesics, but adverse effects include respiratory depression.

Propofol, sometimes referred to as "milk of anesthesia" because of its white color, is a hypnotic agent. It has a fast onset of action. The effects wear off quickly when the medication is discontinued. The patient is awake more quickly than with other sedatives. It is a good amnestic but provides no analgesia. For this reason, it is typically used in conjunction with analgesics.

Ketamine is a phencyclidine hydrochloride (PCP) derivative. It causes a dissociative state, which means the patient appears to be "dissociated" from the external environment but not necessarily asleep. Patients may experience hallucinations, so it is generally used in conjunction with amnestics for sedation. It is an excellent analgesic and sedative.

Etomidate, a sedative-hypnotic, causes the least detrimental cardiovascular changes of all nonopioid induction medications. It may be used as an alternative to ketamine for induction in hypovolemic patients.

Dexmedetomidine (Precedex) is an anxiolytic, analgesic, and sedative. Unlike fentanyl and midazolam, it provides semi-arousable sedation without respiratory depression.

Muscle Relaxants

Muscle relaxants are categorized as depolarizing or nondepolarizing agents. Depolarizing agents, such as succinylcholine, act by occupying the acetylcholine-binding sites at the neuromuscular junction. The membrane becomes depolarized; thus, no impulses can be transmitted, and paralysis ensues. The depolarizing action causes muscle fasciculation (twitching) prior to relaxation. Succinylcholine has a fast onset (30–40 seconds), quickly producing paralysis. Adverse effects include hyperkalemia, cardiac dysrhythmias, masseter spasm, and malignant hyperthermia (MH). Depolarizing agents cannot be reversed; they are metabolized and must "wear off." Ventilatory support is not withdrawn until the medication effects are no longer apparent.

Nondepolarizing agents, such as pancuronium, vecuronium, cisatracurium, and rocuronium, work by competing with native acetylcholine for binding at the neuromuscular junction without causing depolarization. When these medications are administered, progressive paralysis results as a chemical response. The reaction starts in the smaller muscles of the eyelids and face, then moves to the larger muscle groups, including the tongue, neck, and shoulder, and finally to the respiratory muscles: the intercostals, larynx, and diaphragm. The onset of action is longer, minutes compared to seconds. Nondepolarizing agents do not cause muscle fasciculation. Different agents have differing lengths of onset, duration, and hemodynamic effects. All nondepolarizing muscle relaxants can be reversed, which must be done before ventilatory support and airway protection are withdrawn. Some reversal agents are called *cholinergic agents*. They increase the amount of acetylcholine at the neuromuscular junction and reverse the relaxation. Examples include neostigmine, pyridostigmine edrophonium, and sugammadex. Because of cholinergic side effects such as bradycardia and increased secretions, anticholinergic medications are usually given concurrently. Examples of these are atropine and glycopyrrolates. See Table 16.2 for a list of anesthetic medications and Table 16.3 for the sequencing of anesthesia.

Complications of General Anesthesia

Untoward effects or complications of general anesthesia include:

- Hypoxia
- Respiratory and cardiovascular dysfunction

Table 16.2 Commonly Used Anesthetics

Medication	Use	Advantages	Disadvantages	Comments
IV Anesthetics				
Thiopental sodium (Pentothal)	Induction of anesthesia	Induction; short-acting barbiturate	May cause laryngospasm; large doses may cause apnea and cardiovascular depression	Can be administered rectally as well as intravenously
Sodium methohexital (Brevital)	Induction of anesthesia	Ultra short–acting barbiturate	May cause hiccups	Can be administered rectally as well as intravenously
Diazepam (Valium, Dizac)	Amnestic, hypnotic preoperative medication	Good sedation	Prolonged duration of effects	Residual effects for 20–90 hr
Midazolam (Versed)	Hypnotic, anxiolytic sedation; adjunct to induction	Excellent amnestic; water soluble (no pain with IV injection); short acting	Slower induction than thiopental	Often used for monitored anesthesia care and regional anesthesia or insertion of invasive monitors
Propofol (Diprivan)	Induction and maintenance of anesthesia; sedation with regional anesthesia or monitored anesthesia care	Rapid onset; rapid awakening after infusion discontinued	May have pain on injection	Short elimination half-life (34–64 min)
Ketamine (Ketalar)	Induction and occasionally maintenance of anesthesia (IV or intramuscular)	Short acting; patient maintains airway; good for small children and patients with burns or trauma	In large doses, may cause hallucinations and respiratory depression	Needs darkened, quiet room for recovery to prevent hallucinations
Etomidate (Amidate)	Induction of anesthesia	Least cardiovascular changes	May have pain on injection	
Dexmedetomidine (Precedex)	Anxiolytic, analgesic, and sedative	Provides semi-arousable sedation without respiratory depression	May cause bradycardia and hypotension	
Opioid Analgesics				
Morphine sulfate	Premedication; perioperative pain	Inexpensive; excellent analgesia; duration of 4–5 hr; euphoria; good cardiovascular stability	Nausea and vomiting; may be sedating in high doses	Used intrathecally and epidurally for postoperative pain
Fentanyl (Sublimaze)	Surgical analgesia; epidural infusion for postoperative analgesia	Good cardiovascular stability; duration of action 0.5 hr	May be sedating in high doses	Most commonly used opioid
Remifentanil (Ultiva)	Infused for surgical analgesia; small boluses given for brief, intense pain	Easily titratable; short duration; good cardiovascular stability	Expensive; requires mixing	

Continued

Table 16.2 Commonly Used Anesthetics—cont'd

Medication	Use	Advantages	Disadvantages	Comments
Sufentanil (Sufenta)	Surgical analgesia	Short duration of 0.5 hr; prolonged analgesia; good cardiovascular stability	Prolonged respiratory depression	
Depolarizing Muscle Relaxants				
Succinylcholine (Anectine, Quelicin)	Airway intubation; short cases	Rapid onset (30–40 sec); short duration	May cause fasciculations, postoperative myalgia; a trigger for malignant hyperthermia	Prolonged muscle relaxation with certain antibiotics
Nondepolarizing Muscle Relaxants				
Cisatracurium (Nimbex)	Intubation of the airway; maintenance of relaxation	No significant cardiovascular or cumulative effects	No histamine release	Good for renal failure patients
Rocuronium (Zemuron)	Intubation of the airway; maintenance of relaxation	Rapid onset (dose dependent)	Vagolytic that may increase heart rate	
Vecuronium (Norcuron)	Intubation of the airway; maintenance of relaxation	No significant cardiovascular or cumulative effects	Requires mixing	Mostly eliminated in bile
Pancuronium (Pavulon)	Maintenance of relaxation	Onset 2–3 minutes after administration	May cause tachycardia and increased heart rate	Mostly renal elimination
Cholinergic Agent				
Neostigmine (Prostigmin)	Reverses effects of nondepolarizing neuromuscular blocking agents	Prevents acetylcholine breakdown by inhibiting acetyl-cholinesterase		Given with either atropine or glycopyrrolate
Anticholinergics				
Atropine	Blocks the effects of acetylcholine; reverses muscle relaxants; treats sinus bradycardia	Increases heart rate; suppresses salivation and bronchial and gastric secretions	Depresses sweating; may cause dry mouth, flushing, dizziness	Selective at muscarinic receptor in smooth and cardiac muscles and exocrine glands
Glycopyrrolate (Robinul)	Similar to atropine	Slightly increases heart rate; does not cross blood–brain barrier	Prolonged duration of effects	Lower incidence of dysrhythmias than with atropine
Sugammadex	Reverse nondepolarizing neuromuscular-blocking agents	Fewer adverse effects than older reversal agents; does not inhibit acetylcholinesterase, so no cholinergic effects	Significantly interferes with oral contraceptives for 2 weeks after receiving it (inform women of childbearing age if used); may cause bradycardia	Approved December 2015. Rocuronium and Vecuronium are the most reliably reversed muscle relaxants with this agent

Table 16.3 Sequence of General Anesthesia

Stages	Actions
Induction	• Gain IV access and place monitors (blood pressure cuff, electrocardiogram leads, pulse oximeter); preoxygenate with oxygen via face mask. • Infusion of narcotics and/or muscle relaxants • Induction with sodium pentothal (propofol, ketamine, or etomidate) • Adequate sedation (indicated when patient becomes apneic and eyelid reflex disappears)
Intubation	• Place and secure airway.
Maintenance	• Maintain patient using balanced anesthesia.
Emergence	• Suction patient to decrease the chance of laryngospasm and aspiration. • Reverse residual muscle relaxant. • Provide oxygen to wash out inhalation agents. • Remove airway when patient is breathing on his or her own and follows commands.
Recovery	• Patient transported to post-anesthesia care unit (recovery room) or intensive care unit; vital signs monitored and oxygenation continued until patient is stable

- Hypotension
- Hypertension
- Fluid and electrolyte imbalances
- Residual muscle paralysis
- Neurological problems such as dementia, prolonged awakening, paresthesias
- Malignant hyperthermia

Malignant hyperthermia (MH) is a hypermetabolic state that can be caused by exposure to a triggering agent, such as a volatile gas anesthetic (except nitrous oxide) and/or succinylcholine. The triggering agent causes sustained muscular contractions related to an increase in intracellular calcium ion concentration. The sustained contractions result in signs of hypermetabolism. These include acidosis, tachycardia, hypercarbia, glycolysis, hypoxemia, and hyperthermia. The reaction usually begins to occur soon after the exposure, but it has been known to be delayed until the patient is in the recovery area.

The most specific sign of MH is skeletal muscle rigidity. However, the first sign noted by the anesthesia or nursing staff is an unexplained tachycardia. For the anesthesia provider, hypercarbia is the most sensitive indicator of potential MH. Myoglobinuria is another early sign. The patient's urine turns from dark amber to brown. Hyperthermia, the classic sign of MH, is usually a late sign.

> ⚠ **Safety Alert** Malignant hyperthermia is a medical emergency. Without quick and appropriate treatment, the patient will die. It is treated with dantrolene, a muscle relaxant that depresses the coupling mechanism in

skeletal muscles. Important nursing interventions include administering dantrolene and cooling the patient. This can be done by removing blankets and drapes, IV infusion of cold normal saline, ice bags around the body, and cold nasogastric lavage. If MH occurs during the intraoperative period, cold body cavity lavage can be done. When MH is diagnosed early and treated promptly, the mortality rate for the condition should be near zero. The incidence of MH in children is 1 in 30,000, and in adults, it is 1 in 100,000. About 1 in 2,000 may harbor the genetic change that makes an individual susceptible to MH. It can be found in all ethnic groups.

All patients should be asked preoperatively if they or any family members have had problems with anesthesia. Patients should be cautioned to wear an alert bracelet that indicates they are susceptible to MH when exposed to anesthesia.

Regional Anesthesia

Regional anesthesia is a local anesthetic used to block or anesthetize a nerve or nerve fibers. Types of regional anesthesia or blocks include spinal, epidural, caudal, and nerve blocks.

Spinal medication is injected into the spinal canal or intrathecal space surrounding the spinal cord, typically in the lower back or lumbar region (Fig. 16.3A). The injection lasts for several hours. It may also be given as continuous **spinal anesthesia** via a catheter. It is important to keep the head of the patient's bed flat after spinal anesthesia to avoid a headache.

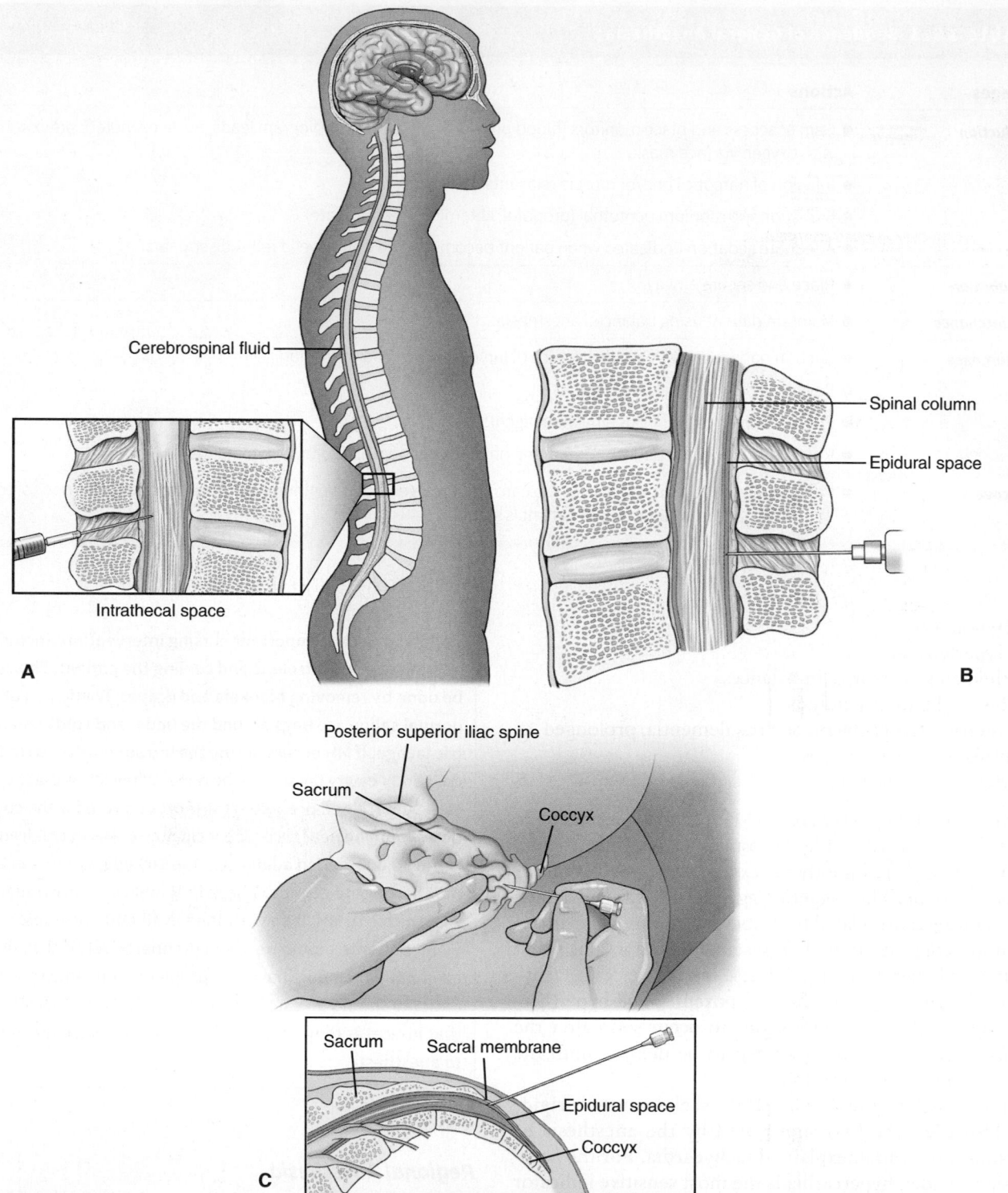

FIGURE 16.3 *A*, Intrathecal anesthesia injected into the spinal canal or intrathecal space surrounding the spinal cord. *B*, Epidural anesthesia injected into the epidural space. *C*, Caudal anesthesia injected into the epidural space through the caudal canal in the sacrum.

Epidural medication is injected into the epidural space into the lumbar region or thoracic region (Fig. 16.3B). A catheter is inserted for periodic or continuous injection. Spinal headache is avoided because the intrathecal space is not entered. Caudal is a form of epidural anesthetic where the medication is injected into the epidural space through the caudal canal in the sacrum (Fig. 16.3C).

A nerve block, anesthetizing of a nerve in an extremity, is done to allow surgery in a specific area (e.g., performing a block on the axillary nerve to allow surgery in the arm).

Untoward effects of epidural or spinal anesthesia may include the following:

- A rapid decrease in blood pressure due to vasodilation of the sympathetic nerves that control vasomotor tone, causing peripheral pooling and decreasing venous return. A vasopressor may be used to counteract this effect.
- Spinal headache is a risk with intrathecal anesthesia because of potential leakage of cerebrospinal fluid. It usually resolves in 1 to 3 days.
- Respiratory paralysis is a risk with a high intrathecal injection.
- Seizure is a risk if medication is injected intravascularly.
- Finally, nerve damage and epidural hematoma/abscess occur rarely.

Local Anesthetics

Local anesthetics cause a reversible conduction blockade of nerve impulses when they are placed in proximity to nerve membranes. The anesthetic diffuses into the nerves and inhibits the propagation of signals for pain and muscle contractions. Pain fibers are affected first, then sensory fibers and motor fibers. High concentrations inhibit all qualities of sensation as well as muscle control. Lower concentrations selectively inhibit pain sensation, with minimal effect on muscle power. Adverse reactions are due to overdosage, rapid absorption, and hypersensitivity. Reactions vary from mild (hives, itching, and rash) to severe (acute anaphylactic reaction). Examples include amides and esters, which are defined by their chemical composition.

Amides

- Lidocaine has a rapid onset and a short to intermediate duration of 60 to 120 minutes. The maximum dose is 4.5 mg/kg (30 mL in an average 70-kg adult). It has excellent spreading ability and is the main local anesthetic.
- Bupivacaine has a slow onset and a long duration of 4 to 8 hours. The maximum dose is 2 mg/kg (50 mL in an average 70-kg adult). It provides excellent postoperative analgesia.

Both medications may be mixed with epinephrine for its vasoconstrictive effects to help control bleeding at the procedure site. It also prolongs the action of the medications.

Esters

- Cocaine has a slow onset and medium duration. It is used in nasal surgery more for its vasoconstrictive effects than as an analgesic. It can cause hypertension and tachycardia as a result of increased catecholamine release.

Monitored Anesthesia Care

Monitored anesthesia care (MAC) provides anesthesia without unconsciousness. The patient has a decreased level of consciousness but maintains a patent airway and responds appropriately to verbal commands and physical stimulation. Objectives for the patient receiving MAC are:

- Maintenance of consciousness
- Elevation of pain threshold
- Enhanced cooperation
- Some degree of amnesia
- Minimal variation in vital signs
- Quick and safe return to activities of daily living

MAC couples sedation/analgesia with local anesthetics. The usual medications utilized are benzodiazepines such as diazepam and midazolam and narcotics such as fentanyl and meperidine. During the administration of both local anesthesia and MAC, signs are posted outside the OR alerting staff that the patient is awake. It is important that OR staff are mindful of conversations in the room and keep them to the minimum needed to communicate needs or to comfort the patient.

Connection Check 16.3

Which of the following is an example of a local anesthetic?

A. Diazepam
B. Lidocaine
C. Pavulon
D. Morphine

AIRWAY MANAGEMENT

Airway management is the process of protecting and ensuring adequate oxygenation and ventilation during an operative procedure. This is not only an essential component of care for patients receiving general anesthesia but also an important consideration with any kind of anesthesia that can potentially compromise the airway. Airway compromise can be caused by relaxation of the soft tissues of the oropharynx. This relaxed effect may create an occlusion of the trachea or trigger a **laryngospasm**, where the larynx constricts and cannot easily be re-expanded. The airway may also be compromised in patients who present with anatomical abnormalities such as a small mouth, short neck, inability to open the mouth fully, obesity, or facial or cervical injuries. See Table 16.4 for the different methods of managing airway patency in the OR.

Airway complications include:

- *Laryngospasm:* A reflexive and prolonged closure of the vocal folds in response to a trigger. It is most common during anesthesia induction/intubation or extubation. It is caused by stimulation of the airway by airway devices, secretions, or gastric contents.
- *Bronchial intubation*: This occurs when an ETT is passed below the carina into one of the mainstem bronchi, resulting in hyperinflation of the intubated lung and collapse (deflation) of the opposite lung.

Table 16.4 Types of Airway Devices

Name	Application	Indication	Comments
Face mask	Placed externally, covering patient's nose and mouth	To maintain the patient with spontaneous breathing	Use is dependent on factors such as the type and duration of the procedure and the patency of the airway.
Laryngeal mask airway	Inserted into the pharynx above the glottis, forming a low-pressure seal that allows positive pressure into the airway without entering the trachea (Fig. 16.4)	Used for patients undergoing anesthesia for brief and superficial surgeries	Less irritating than the standard endotracheal tube (ETT) and does not require muscle relaxants or laryngoscopy for placement
ETT	A tube inserted into the trachea just above the carina; may have a cuff that is inflated just enough to occlude the airway, preventing aspiration (Fig. 16.5)	Best method for managing the airway	Depending on the procedure and the patient's anatomy and physical condition, there are assorted variations of ETTs that can be used.
		Protects the airway, and the patient is able to breathe by spontaneous respirations with assistance as needed. Muscle relaxants can be given, and mechanical ventilation can be initiated.	

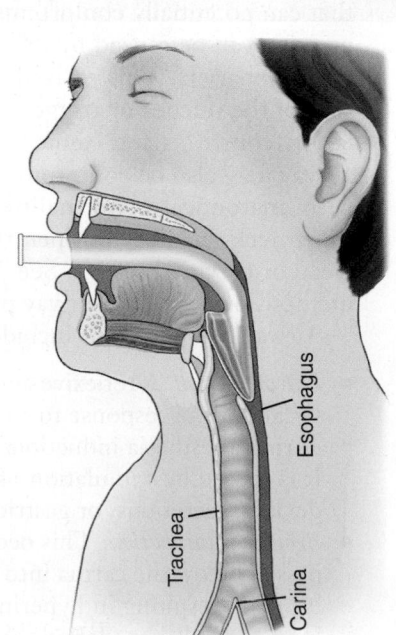

FIGURE 16.4 Laryngeal mask airway for airway protection during anesthesia.

Trachea

Esophagus

Carina

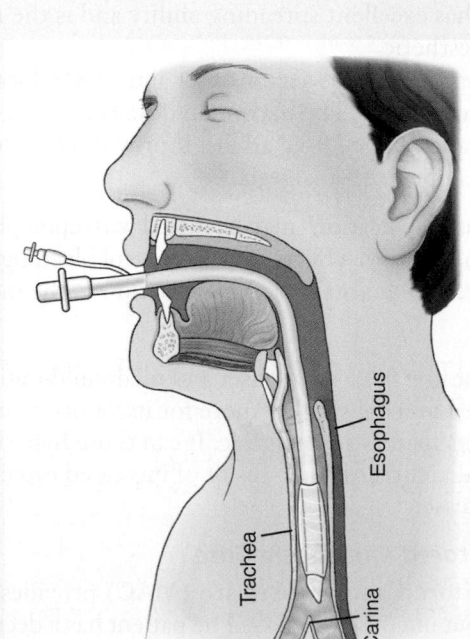

FIGURE 16.5 Endotracheal tube for airway protection during anesthesia.

Trachea

Esophagus

Carina

- *Tracheal and esophageal perforation*: This may occur during intubation if excessive force is applied or as a complication of the use of a stylet or other stiff intubation-assisting device.
- *Aspiration*: The patient regurgitates, and stomach contents or other secretions go into the lungs, resulting in pneumonia or airway obstruction.

Connection Check 16.4

Which of the following is an airway used to support airway management? *(Select all that apply.)*

A. MAC
B. MH
C. LMA
D. ETT
E. PCP

CASE STUDY: EPISODE 2

Review of Ms. Doe's laboratory and diagnostic studies reveals the following: white blood cell leukocytosis, 12,500/mm³; neutrophil count, 80%; and abdominal radiograph revealing hardened fecal material in the appendix. Findings from her physical examination include moderate abdominal distention and rebound pain on abdominal palpation. The attending surgeon schedules Ms. Doe for an emergency **exploratory laparotomy** (diagnostic surgery that allows providers to examine the abdominal organs) with possible **appendectomy** (removal of her appendix). Ms. Doe is transported emergently to the OR holding area from the ED. She was accompanied by her eldest daughter (the patient-identified spokesperson), who has since been escorted to the family lounge to await further information from the surgeon. As Ms. Doe arrives in the holding area of the OR, you observe that she is demonstrating nonverbal expressions of pain and is outwardly combative because she has previously expressed that she feels she will die on the operating table…

POSITIONING THE PATIENT IN THE OPERATING ROOM

Patient positioning for surgical procedures is done to provide for optimal anatomical exposure and patient safety. There are a variety of **positioning devices** utilized to ensure safe alignment of anatomical structures while contributing to surgical outcomes. The use of these devices may place the patient at risk for temporary or permanent injury. The challenge in positioning is to provide the exposure the surgeon needs in order to perform the procedure and allow for access to IV lines and monitoring equipment while also ensuring a safe, comfortable position for the patient.

Patient positioning is a collaborative activity involving all surgical team members. The surgeon determines the position that is appropriate for a specific procedure, and after consultation with the surgical team, the patient is placed in the appropriate position. The RN documents all positioning aids used and the team members assisting with patient positioning. The RN ensures that the patient is treated in a dignified manner throughout the positioning activity. The patient's dignity and right to privacy cannot be overlooked before, during, and after positioning activities.

Common Intraoperative Positions

There are four standard positions commonly used for surgical procedures. These positions are often modified according to the surgeon's preferences and surgical approaches and the patient's physiological requirements (Fig. 16.6). These positions are:

- Supine (Trendelenburg, reverse Trendelenburg, and Fowler's are modifications)
- Prone (jackknife is a modification)
- Lateral
- Lithotomy

Supine

The **supine** position (Fig. 16.6A) is the most frequently used patient position and is the most natural position for the body at rest. This position is used for procedures on the anterior surface of the body, including abdominal, abdominothoracic, vascular, orthopedic, head/neck, and ophthalmic operations. The patient is placed on his or her back with the legs extended and uncrossed and the arms on arm boards or at the sides with the palms down. Proper arm placement with extension at less than a 90-degree angle is necessary to avoid brachial plexus stretching and compression. The arms must not be positioned lower than the spinal column, and the spinal column should be in a straight line, with the legs parallel to the OR bed. The patient's head is in line with the spine, and the face is upward. The hips are parallel with the spine.

Trendelenburg

In the **Trendelenburg position** (Fig. 16.6B), the patient is placed in the supine position, and the OR bed is modified to a head-down tilt of 35 to 45 degrees. This position is used for procedures in the lower abdomen or pelvis when it is desirable to move the abdominal viscera away from the pelvic area for better exposure. Although exposure is increased, lung volume is decreased, and the pressure of the organs against the diaphragm mechanically compresses the heart.

Reverse Trendelenburg

In the **reverse Trendelenburg position** (Fig. 16.6C), the entire OR bed is tilted so that the patient's head is higher than his or her feet. This position is used for procedures on the head and neck to facilitate exposure, aid breathing, and

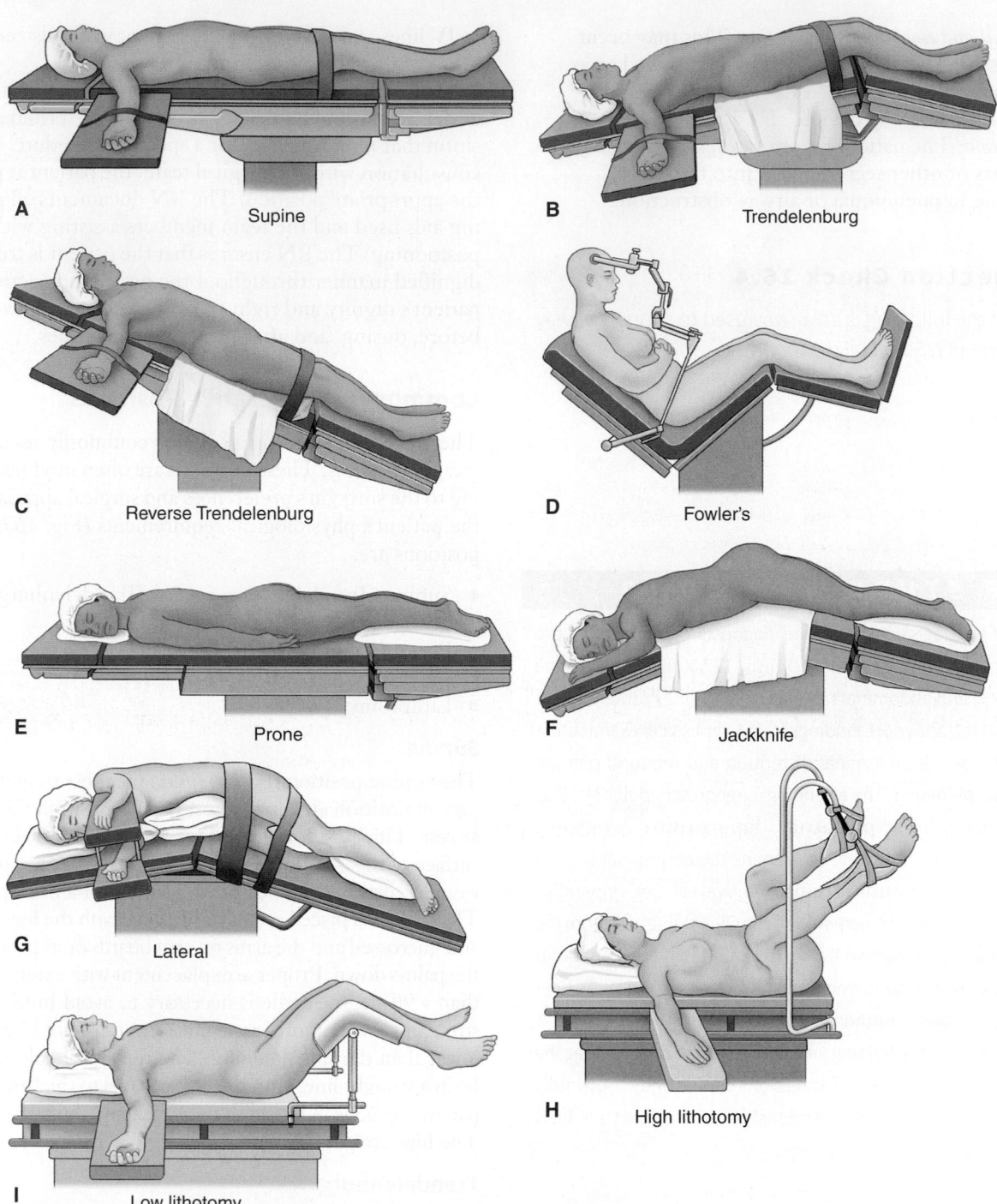

FIGURE 16.6 Common intraoperative positions: *A*, Supine position. *B*, Trendelenburg position. *C*, Reverse Trendelenburg position. *D*, Fowler's, or sitting, position. *E*, Prone position. *F*, Jackknife position. *G*, Lateral position. *H*, High lithotomy position. *I*, Low lithotomy position.

decrease blood supply to the operative area. A padded footboard is used to prevent the patient from sliding toward the foot of the bed.

Fowler's

For the **Fowler's position** (Fig. 16.6D), also called the sitting, lawn-chair, or beach-chair position, the patient is first placed in the supine position. The foot of the OR bed is lowered slightly, flexing the patient's knees. The body section is raised to 35 to 45 degrees, thereby becoming the backrest. The entire OR bed is tilted slightly, with the head end downward to prevent the patient from sliding. The patient's feet rest on a padded footboard. For cranial procedures, the head is supported in a headrest. This position can be used for shoulder or breast reconstruction procedures.

Prone

In the **prone** position (Fig. 16.6E), also known as the ventral recumbent or ventral decubitus position, the patient is placed facedown, resting on his or her abdomen and chest.

Chest rolls under the clavicles to the iliac crests raise the weight of the body from the abdomen and thorax. The arms may be supported along the sides of the body. The head is turned to one side, resting on a padded donut to prevent pressure on the ears, eyes, and face. Female breasts should be moved laterally to reduce pressure on them, and male genitalia must be positioned to be free from pressure.

Jackknife

The **jackknife position**, or Kraske position (Fig. 16.6F), is a modification of the prone position in which the patient is placed in the prone position on the OR bed and then inverted in a V position. The hips are over the center break of the OR bed between the body and leg sections. This position is used for gluteal and anorectal procedures.

Lateral

The **lateral** (lateral decubitus) position (Fig. 16.6G) is used primarily for thoracic, renal, and orthopedic (hip) procedures. The patient is placed in the supine position for anesthetizing and then turned to the unaffected side.

Lithotomy

In the **lithotomy** position, the patient is in the supine position, with the legs raised and abducted to expose the perineal region. The legs and feet are placed in stirrups that support the lower extremities. The lithotomy position is used for vaginal, obstetrical, urological, and rectal procedures and for radical resections of the groin, the vulva, and the rectal areas. There are two variations of the lithotomy position.

High Lithotomy

The high lithotomy position (Fig. 16.6H) is frequently used for procedures that require a vaginal or perineal approach.

Low Lithotomy

The low lithotomy position (Fig. 16.6I) is used in vaginal procedures and routinely for most laparoscopic surgeries. See Table 16.5 for risks and interventions related to surgical positions.

Table 16.5 Risks and Interventions for Surgical Positions

Position	Risks	Interventions
Supine	Pressure points: occiput, scapulae, thoracic vertebrae, olecranon process, sacrum, coccyx, knees, and heels	Pressure-reducing operating room (OR) mattress with additional padding as needed
	Pressure to peripheral vessels and nerves, primarily brachial plexus and ulnar nerves	Arm boards level with OR mattress, less than 90-degree extensions and palms up; ankles uncrossed
	Venous pooling of blood in the legs	Application of sequential compression devices
Trendelenburg	In addition to supine risks:	Close respiratory monitoring
	Diminished lung capacity	Slow, smooth postural transitions to diminish cardiovascular effects
	Shift in venous pooling toward heels	
	Sliding and shearing	Flex knees slightly; limit time in position.
Reverse Trendelenburg	In addition to supine risks:	Antiembolic or sequential compression stockings
	Deep vein thrombosis (DVT) in lower extremities	Padded footboard
	Sliding and shearing	
Fowler's	Pressure to scapulae, sacrum, coccyx, ischium, back of knees, and heels	Pressure-reducing OR mattress with additional padding as needed
	Air embolism if venous sinus is opened	Doppler probe over chest wall; insertion of central venous catheter
	Shearing	Momentary tilting of torso slightly away from the OR bed to allow skin to realign with skeletal structures
	DVT in lower extremities	
	Venous pooling that shifts toward lower body	Sequential compression stockings
		Slow, smooth postural transitions to diminish cardiovascular effects

Continued

Table 16.5 Risks and Interventions for Surgical Positions—cont'd

Position	Risks	Interventions
Prone	Pressure to cheeks, eyes, ears, breasts, genitalia, patellae, and toes	Use a pressure-reducing OR mattress with additional padding as needed; check ears, cheeks, eyes, and genitalia for pressure; tape eyes closed.
	Falls and dislodgment of airway, monitoring cords, and IV lines	Lock both beds; use a minimum of four people for turning patient; secure airway and all cords and lines.
	Diminished lung capacity	Chest rolls and close respiratory monitoring
	Injury to shoulders, arms, and upper extremity nerves	Arms on arm boards are flexed and pronated, with upper arms at less than 90-degree angle to the OR bed; pads placed above and below elbows to free ulnar nerve.
Jackknife	In addition to prone risks:	Check distal pulses before, during, and after positioning; if position maintained for extended time, use antiembolic or sequential compression stockings.
	DVT in lower extremities	
Lateral	Pressure to structures on dependent side: ear, shoulder, ribs, hip, greater femoral head, knee, and ankle	Use a pressure-reducing OR mattress with additional padding as needed; check that earlobes are not folded over; place pillow between knees and under ankles; be sure neck is in alignment.
	Risk of tilting and falling during procedure	Flex dependent leg for support; may require additional straps or wide tape to secure patient.
	Brachial plexus injury	Place padded roll under lower armpit.
	Venous pooling that shifts toward dependent side	Slow, smooth postural transitions to diminish cardiovascular effects
	Diminished capacity of dependent lung	Ventilator support includes positive end-expiratory pressure; anesthesia team inserts double-lumen ETT to ventilate dependent lung if a thoracotomy is performed.
	DVT in lower extremities	Check distal pulses before, during, and after positioning; use antiembolic or sequential compression stockings.
Lithotomy	Hip dislocations, fractures, and muscle and nerve injuries	Securely fasten stirrups to OR bed; avoid hyperabduction of hips and leaning against inner thighs.
	Pressure injuries to feet, ankles, and knees	Use stirrups that disperse support and pressure over wide areas; check distal pulses before and after positioning.
	Back strain	
	Diminished lung capacity	The buttocks should not hang off the edge of the torso section of the bed.
	Venous pooling that shifts toward head	Close respiratory monitoring
	DVT in lower extremities	Slow, smooth postural transitions to diminish cardiovascular effects
	Crushed fingers	Antiembolic or sequential compression stockings if patient in position for more than 2 hours
		Ensure fingers are away from the break in the OR bed when leg section is elevated.

Safety Alert Fourteen basic safety rules apply to all patients:

1. The side rails of the transport stretcher/bed are always up while the patient is on the vehicle.
2. At a minimum, two people are needed to assist the patient from the stretcher to the OR table.
3. The OR bed and stretcher are locked while the patient is being transferred.
4. Both side rails of the stretcher are down during transfer.
5. The safety strap is applied across the patient's thighs once he or she is on the OR table.
6. Body parts should not extend over the table.
7. The patient's legs should never be crossed.
8. Body parts should not come in contact with metal or an unpadded surface.
9. Always consult with the anesthesiologist before touching or moving an anesthetized patient.
10. Move the anesthetized patient slowly and gently.
11. Always check the pressure points and cautery pad if a patient is moved during the procedure.
12. Document baseline skin condition, position, and positioning devices/equipment.
13. Perioperative personnel should use proper body mechanics when transporting, moving, lifting, or positioning patients.
14. Positioning equipment should be used in a safe manner and according to the manufacturer's written instructions.

Positioning Devices

The choice of a particular positioning device for a surgical procedure depends on many variables. Patient variables such as height, weight, age, and physiological condition and the position required for the procedure influence which devices are used. The surgeon's preference affects the selection of a positioning device as well. Routine positioning devices used for most surgical procedures include but are not limited to the following: OR bed, headrest, arm boards, arm restraints, padding for bony prominences, blankets, pillows, safety straps, sandbags, bean bags, towels and sheets, foam pads, and gel-type devices.

Positioning Complications

Preoperative assessment of the patient is crucial in providing information about the patient's individual risk factors that may influence the selection of **positioning devices** and any alterations to a proposed position. Patients at high risk for complications due to positioning include:

- Geriatric patients, whose thin skin layer and impaired circulation make them susceptible to skin breakdown due to pressure and moisture

- Pediatric patients (immature systems)
- Extremely thin patients who may be malnourished, anemic, or hypovolemic
- Obese patients with an overabundance of fat tissue
- Paralyzed patients
- Diabetic patients who are already prone to skin breakdown
- Patients with prosthetic or arthritic joints
- Patients with edema and circulatory limitations
- Patients with medical conditions such as cancer that can alter cardiac, respiratory, or immune reserves
- Patients with infections
- Patients who have existing or previous trauma

Improper positioning may contribute to the development of a **pressure injury**. Also referred to as a decubitus ulcer, pressure injury is localized damage to the skin and/or underlying tissue, generally over a bony prominence. Pressure due to prolonged contact causes constriction of the blood vessels feeding the area and consequent damage to the skin and possibly underlying areas. High-risk situations include but are not limited to:

- Long surgical procedures
- Vascular surgery in which blood perfusion may be already compromised
- Demineralizing bone conditions (e.g., malignant metastasis or osteoporosis)
- Excessive sustained pressure on body parts due to surgical procedures or retraction

Connection Check 16.5

The nurse caring for a patient in the supine position on the OR table incorporates which nursing diagnosis into the plan of care?

A. Risk for fluid volume deficit
B. Risk for knowledge deficit
C. Risk for aspiration
D. Risk for potential alteration in skin integrity

NURSING MANAGEMENT

Nursing Diagnoses

- **Risk for impaired tissue and skin integrity**
- **Risk for infection**
- **Risk for injury** related to the surgical environment
- **Risk for knowledge deficit**
- **Risk for potential unplanned hypothermia** related to ambient room temperature and/or exposed body cavities
- **Risk for potential thrombus** related to prolonged immobility

Nursing Interventions

■ *Assessments*

- Ensure OR consent has been signed.
  Signed consent indicates the patient has had all risks, benefits, and alternatives to the procedure explained and is required before surgery can begin.
- Ensure the patient is correctly positioned and the appropriate patient positioning devices are used.
  Avoid unnecessary pressure points, thus skin breakdown or injury.
- Monitor staff in the use of a proper scrub and donning of OR attire, and validate that OR room and equipment have been thoroughly cleaned.
  Maintain sterility in the OR to prevent infection.
- Ensure readiness of the OR suite.
  Ensure a smooth procedure without unnecessary delays and or/complications.
  - Check that all necessary equipment/supplies are available.
    Having all equipment/supplies at the ready helps ensure a smooth procedure without unnecessary delays.
  - Ensure irrigation fluid and instruments are at the appropriate temperature.
    Fluid or instruments at inappropriate temperatures can cause skin irritation, breakdown, or burns or unwanted changes in patient temperature
  - Confirm flashed instruments are cool.
    Insufficiently cooled instruments can cause skin or tissue burns.

■ *Actions*

- Perform time-out.
  Time-out is a safety factor essential in preventing "preventable errors."
- Perform equipment safety check.
  Properly functioning equipment can prevent patient injury.
- Utilize **sterile technique** (avoiding the chances of exogenous items coming in contact with the catheter) while inserting a Foley catheter and setting up the sterile field.
  Proper sterile technique prevents patient infection.
- Assist the anesthesia care provider during intubation by applying cricoid pressure as indicated.
  Cricoid pressure can help prevent patient aspiration.
- Properly ground the patient as indicated.
  Proper grounding can prevent the patient from electrical injury and burns.
- Keep the patient safety belt in place while the patient is on the OR bed.
  Patient falls can be avoided through the proper use of a safety belt and side rails.
- Apply support hose and sequential compression devices (SCDs) as indicated.
  Deep vein thrombus can be prevented by the use of support hose and SCDs.

- Keep the patient warm with blankets, and use warm irrigation.
  Hypothermia can be avoided by using blankets and warm irrigation.
- Maintain a sterile field.
  Maintain sterility in the OR to prevent infection.
- Accurately record the number of sponges and sharps used on the count board.
  Accurate counting prevents retained foreign bodies.
- Accurately measure irrigation fluids and communicate the amount to the anesthesia care providers.
  Accounting for blood and fluid loss helps avoid a fluid deficit.
- Keep OR doors closed during the procedure.
  Maintain sterility in the OR to prevent infection.
- Keep hallways clear of extra equipment.
  An unobstructed path is necessary to ensure quick access to the patient in an emergency.

■ *Teaching*

- Explain to the patient your actions and what to expect when entering the OR.
  Decrease and manage the patient's fear of the operative experience.
- Keep the family updated during the procedure (at the time when surgery begins and then every 2 hours).
  Decrease and manage the family's fear of the operative experience.

Connection Check 16.6

The nurse understands that which actions are essential when providing support to the intraoperative patient and family during the OR experience? *(Select all that apply.)*

A. Introduce the patient and family to the surgical team members.
B. Give family members updates every 2 hours as possible during the procedure.
C. Explain what to expect from the operative experience.
D. Alert the family to mealtimes.
E. Explain that once the procedure is complete, the surgeon will discuss surgery outcomes.

Making Connections

CASE STUDY: WRAP-UP

The nurse caring for Ms. Doe alerts both the surgeon and anesthesiologist that she appears to be in pain and is combative. Her preoperative check is completed quickly, and she is provided with IV pain medication and a benzodiazepine for her anxiety. Her daughter is brought to her bedside to provide support while she waits to enter the OR. Soon after, Ms. Doe is transported into the

OR and transferred to the OR bed. Her daughter is escorted to the waiting area and is told she will be updated on a regular basis. After proper positioning and safety checks are completed, the time-out is performed and surgery is started. Ms. Doe has her appendix removed without complication.

Case Study Questions

1. If Ms. Doe indicates there is a family history of problems with anesthesia, it is important to discuss this with the anesthesia provider in order to avoid the use of which MH-triggering agent?

   A. Nitrous oxide

   B. Morphine

   C. Succinylcholine

   D. Ketamine

2. The nurse understands that surgical attire is worn for what purpose? *(Select all that apply.)*

   A. Prevent transmission of microorganisms between the patient and the team

   B. Promote cleanliness in the OR suite

   C. Prevent the spill of blood and body fluids to the surgical team's apparel

   D. Promote confidentiality of patient and staff identity

   E. Facilitate the surgical team working together collaboratively

3. Prior to the start of Ms. Doe's surgical procedure, all members of the surgical team participate in a time-out. Which of the following are components of the time-out? *(Select all that apply.)*

   A. Correct procedure

   B. Correct site

   C. Correct equipment

   D. Laterality

   E. Correct OR

4. While Ms. Doe is in the OR, what considerations will be taken to ensure her safety and positive outcome? *(Select all that apply.)*

   A. Time-out

   B. Maintenance of sterile technique

   C. Continuous patient monitoring

   D. Instrument count/sponge count

   E. Breaks for personnel

5. Potential adverse effects of the supine position for Ms. Doe's surgery include which of the following? *(Select all that apply.)*

   A. Skin breakdown in the heels and elbows

   B. Venous pooling in the legs

   C. Ulnar nerve injury

   D. Retinal detachment

   E. Cerebral edema

CHAPTER SUMMARY

Surgical procedures are classified as elective, which indicates they can be scheduled at the patient and surgeon's convenience; urgent, which means they should be performed within 48 hours; and emergent, which means the procedure needs to be performed immediately to prevent loss of life or bodily function. There are six types of surgery: palliative (to relieve symptoms or improve life quality), restorative (to restore bodily function), curative (removing disease through surgery), diagnostic (or exploratory—to diagnose disease), cosmetic (to improve or change the look of a patient), and transplant (to replace a poorly or nonfunctioning organ).

The surgical team includes the surgeon; an anesthesia provider; a perioperative RN; and a variety of unlicensed assistive personnel, such as surgical technologists and OR associates and/or critical care technicians. Team members who have a key function in a surgical procedure are usually categorized according to their roles and responsibilities in preparing for the operation—nonsterile team members and sterile team members. The surgeon is the identified team leader.

As the patient's advocate, the perioperative nurse has a vital responsibility to ensure patient safety during all surgical procedures. Procedures the OR nurse may perform to accomplish these goals include patient assessment, time-out or "surgical pause," planning, interventions during surgery, and postoperative evaluation. An essential component of safety is hand washing whenever necessary during the operative procedure.

An important part of the perioperative nurse's role is to quickly develop a therapeutic and trusting relationship with the patient and family to help with decreasing fear and managing anxiety regarding the operative experience. Ensuring that the patient is introduced to the anesthesia provider and talks with the surgeon is vital. Making sure the patient knows what to expect from the procedure helps decrease fear. Regular updates, ideally every 2 hours, should be given to the family during the procedure.

Anesthesia is the process of allowing the patient to be pain-free and comfortable during surgery. It also provides optimal operating conditions for the surgeon. There are four major types of anesthesia: general, regional, monitored anesthesia care (MAC), and local. An example of local anesthesia is lidocaine.

Malignant hyperthermia is a rare but potentially fatal complication of anesthesia, typically due to a genetic disorder making the patient more susceptible. When these patients are exposed to any of the volatile gases except nitrous oxide or succinylcholine, they exhibit signs of hypermetabolism. Left undetected and/or untreated, circulatory collapse and possibly death can occur in a short amount of time.

Airway management is the process of protecting the airway and ensuring adequate oxygenation and ventilation during the operative procedure. Oxygen delivery devices include the face mask, LMA, and ETT.

Patient positioning for surgical procedures requires the collaboration of the entire surgical team to provide for optimum anatomical exposure and patient safety. A variety of positioning devices may be used depending on the position necessary to perform the surgery. Positions include supine, Trendelenburg, reverse Trendelenburg, prone, lateral, and lithotomy. Skin breakdown is a risk when positioning the patient for surgery.

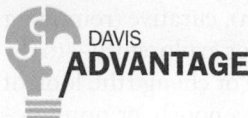

DAVIS ADVANTAGE

To explore learning resources for this chapter, go to **Davis Advantage** and find:
- Answers to in-text questions
- Chapter Resources and Activities
- NCLEX®-Style Chapter Review Questions
- Bibliography

Chapter 17

Priorities for the Postoperative Patient

Maren Reinholdt

Content in this chapter is designed to assist in:

1. Discussing the significance of the postoperative period
2. Explaining the priority assessments for the post-surgical patient
3. Developing support strategies for the surgical patient's family in the immediate postoperative period
4. Applying the vital postoperative interventions for the patient in the immediate postoperative period
5. Evaluating postoperative interventions on the inpatient unit

ESSENTIAL TERMS

Anesthesia
Hand-off
Patient-controlled analgesia (PCA)
Phase I
Phase II
Phase III
Post-anesthesia care unit (PACU)
Sedation

CONCEPTS

- Assessment
- Comfort
- Fluid and Electrolyte Balance
- Medication
- Perioperative
- Safety
- Skin Integrity

Finding Connections

CASE STUDY: EPISODE 1

Follow this patient throughout the chapter.

Howard Wells is a 70-year-old African American man. He is widowed and lives with his daughter, a nurse. Mr. Wells's daughter brought him to the hospital today for surgery. Mr. Wells has colon cancer and is scheduled to have a partial colectomy in the operating room. His additional significant medical history includes coronary artery disease and myocardial infarction 3 years ago; he is in chronic atrial fibrillation, has obstructive sleep apnea, and has type 2 diabetes. His regular medications include metoprolol, Coumadin, and omeprazole. Mr. Wells is scheduled to have general anesthesia and is to be admitted to the hospital for a few days after surgery. Mr. Wells's daughter will wait in the family waiting room during the procedure. She is eager to visit him in the post-anesthesia care unit...

INTRODUCTION

The postoperative period begins immediately after surgery and continues until the first follow-up postoperative physician visit. During this time, it is vital that the patient be closely monitored to ensure recovery and avoid serious complications that may occur related to the surgical experience. Postoperative care is delivered on a continuum. It begins in the post-anesthesia care unit immediately after surgery and continues either in a hospital setting or at home. The focus of this chapter is the specialized care delivered in the post-anesthesia care unit and important nursing assessments and interventions delivered on the general inpatient surgical unit.

THE POST-ANESTHESIA CARE UNIT

The **post-anesthesia care unit (PACU)** is the special critical care unit where patients are transferred immediately following **sedation** or **anesthesia** for surgical, diagnostic, or therapeutic procedures. Because of anesthesia, there is a temporary decrease in or loss of consciousness and loss of motor and reflexive control of respiration. The transition from anesthesia to recovery carries risks for potentially life-threatening complications as well as discomforts such as nausea and vomiting and pain. During this transition, patients need assistance to maintain a safe internal physiological balance.

The goal of care in the PACU is to safely allow the patient who has had anesthesia/sedation to awaken and resume normal bodily functions while controlling/minimizing pain and preventing complications of surgery and anesthesia. The PACU is generally located adjacent to the operating room (OR) or procedure area to decrease the time needed for transportation immediately following procedures and to ensure proximity to anesthesia providers if needed. The role of the nurse in the PACU is to frequently assess and monitor the patient's recovery from anesthesia and support and manage pain relief, maintaining and assessing the patient carefully. In addition, the nurse is responsible for educating the patient and family about the care following the PACU (next level of care), whether it be in the patient's home or in an acute care unit in the hospital.

Coordination of care with the staff and providers in the OR and the preoperative area as well as the availability of preoperative records defining all aspects of the patient's history are essential for the PACU nurse to adequately and completely assess the patient's condition, understand the potential risks or complications, and individualize care for each patient and family.

Post-Anesthesia Care Unit Phases of Care

The American Society of PeriAnesthesia Nurses has defined three levels of PACU care: phase I, phase II, and phase III. **Phase I** involves the nursing care provided in the immediate post-anesthesia period. This phase is generally in the PACU or intensive care unit (ICU). There is intensive, close monitoring of all vital signs with continuous electrocardiogram monitoring. There is a focus on cardiac, respiratory, and neurological functions, surgical-site monitoring, and pain and temperature control. The goals of care in this phase are to stabilize the patient's vital signs, allow the patient to awaken from anesthesia, and achieve adequate pain control. After meeting specific criteria, the patient is transferred to phase II care or to an inpatient unit. The specific discharge criteria vary by institution but generally include:

- An awake patient with a stable airway
- Adequate oxygen saturation
- Stable vital signs

In **phase II**, the monitoring is less intensive because the patient has met the criteria allowing transfer from phase I. The focus of nursing care is on preparing the patient to be discharged to an extended-care environment or home. Again, the patient needs to meet specific criteria for discharge home (Box 17.1).

Phase III, or extended observation of post-anesthesia care, focuses on providing ongoing care for those patients remaining in the postoperative care area after discharge criteria have been met. Extended observation starts after phase II

Box 17.1 Home Discharge Criteria

- The patient is awake and alert.
- Vital signs have returned to preoperative values.
- Tolerating liquids without nausea or vomiting
- Pain relief and comfort are provided with oral pain medications and nonpharmacological measures (e.g., positioning, pillow, cold and heat therapy).
- The patient is stable and able to walk safely.
- The patient is able to void (urinate) before discharge—voiding prior to discharge is typically required when urinary retention is a risk of the surgical procedure or the patient has a history of urine retention. The patient may go home without voiding if there is no risk per provider order.
- There are no signs of bleeding from the surgical site.
- Skin is intact, and the surgical wound is clean and dry.
- There are no adverse reactions or complications from surgery and nonsurgical procedures related to the surgery (e.g., radiology procedure).
- The patient demonstrates understanding of teaching, including medications and activities. It is critical that an interpreter is available if the patient does not speak or understand the English language.

critical elements have been met, but additional care is needed because a transfer bed is not ready or transportation home is unavailable. When this occurs, the nurse continues to monitor and provide care to this patient. A delay in discharge home when anticipated after a same-day surgery is most often caused by uncontrolled postoperative nausea and vomiting or pain, delays in the surgery schedule and OR availability, and social factors, such as a responsible adult not being present to take the patient home. The goal is to prepare the patient for transfer to an inpatient unit when a transfer bed is made ready or self-care and discharge home.

Connection Check 17.1

The nurse understands PACUs are designed for which of the following?

A. Managing the transition from anesthesia to long-term care
B. Managing the transition from anesthesia through phase III of recovery
C. Managing the transition from anesthesia through phase II of recovery
D. Managing the transition from anesthesia through rehabilitation

Post-Anesthesia Care Unit Settings

Post-anesthesia care is provided in a variety of settings. They include but are not limited to:

- Inpatient PACU
- ICU

- Outpatient PACU
- Procedure areas

Inpatient Post-Anesthesia Care Unit

The inpatient PACU is typically one big room, but recent PACUs are being designed with individual rooms for patient privacy. Patients are managed by anesthesia and nursing staff. Inpatient PACUs care for patients recovering from major or minor surgical procedures on a continuum from low to high risk of complications. Examples of surgical procedures requiring recovery in an inpatient PACU include radical retropubic prostatectomy, lung lobectomy, ileostomy reversal, nephrectomy, exploratory laparotomy, and open reduction and internal fixation of fractures.

The staffing varies according to the acuity level of the patients. The nurse–patient ratio can be 1:1 or 1:2. The extended-stay patients, patients meeting transfer or discharge criteria but requiring extended monitoring, may be in 1:3 ratios. The length of stay is generally short, 1 to 2 hours, except for the extended-stay patients, so patient flow is fast, with high volumes.

Intensive Care Unit

Postoperative care in the ICU is indicated for critically ill patients who require extensive and complex monitoring because of the high risk of complications. These patients are transferred directly to the ICU immediately following the operative procedure. They are managed by the ICU team and nursing staff. Examples of patients who undergo recovery in the ICU setting include patients undergoing transplant surgery, craniotomy, and coronary artery bypass procedures and trauma patients undergoing multiple procedures.

Outpatient Post-Anesthesia Care Unit

Outpatient post-anesthesia care is provided for patients going home after the procedure. The post-anesthesia care is delivered in the same outpatient setting where the procedure is performed. These settings include an outpatient area in the hospital setting, freestanding ambulatory surgery centers, providers' offices, urgent-care centers, and rural health clinics.

Examples of procedures done on an outpatient basis include orthopedic arthroscopic procedures and cholecystectomies. Outpatient procedures can also include more complex procedures such as mastectomy. Other procedures commonly performed in surgery centers or provider offices include diagnostic procedures, dental procedures, some plastic surgery, and ophthalmological procedures.

Procedure Areas

Patients undergoing procedures in a "procedure area" such as endoscopy or cardiac vascular interventional laboratories require postoperative monitoring and care in the procedural area if IV sedation or anesthesia is required for the procedure before return to the inpatient setting or being discharged home.

Connection Check 17.2

The nurse understands that a patient undergoing right upper lobe lobectomy requiring general anesthesia will receive recovery care in which of the following settings?
A. Outpatient PACU
B. Procedure area PACU
C. Surgical center PACU
D. Inpatient PACU

PATIENT CARE IN THE POST-ANESTHESIA CARE UNIT

Patients are all individuals and react differently to the different types of medications, treatments, surgery, procedures, or anesthesia. Therefore, postoperative nursing management should be individualized and should include:

- Assessment and monitoring of the patient's response to surgery and anesthesia
- Timely interventions to resolve the problems, concerns, and needs of patients (physical, psychological, emotional, spiritual)
- Evaluation of these interventions, including effects or adverse effects of medications (e.g., opioids)
- Reassessment of the patient's condition
- Evaluation of achievement of discharge criteria

Priority Assessments

The patient is brought into the PACU immediately following surgery accompanied by the anesthesia provider who provided care for the patient during the surgical procedure, a member of the surgical team, and an OR nurse. Good OR–PACU coordination is necessary to ensure a good transition of care. In addition to all of the priority needs, good communication is necessary during the initial transfer from the OR table to the correct stretcher or bed before transfer to the PACU; some patients may require a special bed to best meet their recovery needs.

On admission to the PACU, the patient is simultaneously connected to cardiac and other monitoring devices while an immediate assessment is performed. Critical areas of assessment on admission to the PACU include the following:

- Airway patency
- Respiratory status, including oxygen saturation (and capnography, if indicated) and auscultation of lung sounds
- Vital signs:
  - Blood pressure
  - Pulse: apical and peripheral
  - Cardiac monitor rhythm
  - Hemodynamic pressure readings if indicated
  - Temperature
- Neurological function, including level of consciousness, motor function, and sensation
- Temperature and color of skin

- Pain level/comfort level
- Condition of dressings; assessing for bleeding or drainage
- Condition of visible incisions
- Presence and patency of IV catheters, drains, and other catheters
- Hydration status and fluid therapy

Diagnostic Tests

Laboratory tests done postoperatively assess for bleeding, fluid loss, electrolyte imbalance, renal function, and clotting abnormalities. Table 17.1 outlines common laboratory tests done postoperatively. Depending on the patient and comorbidities, some of these tests are done in the initial recovery stage, such as a glucose test if it is a patient with diabetes, but most are done the next day, on postoperative day 1 (POD 1), as routine screening for postoperative complications.

Other studies done postoperatively may include:

- Chest radiograph
- Electrocardiogram (ECG)

A chest radiograph is done postoperatively if any complications from surgery due to central line placement, intubation, or anesthesia are suspected. An ECG is always done as a preoperative assessment. It is ordered postoperatively if any ECG changes were identified during surgery or after. Measurement of the ST segment among post-anesthesia patients will detect perioperative acute myocardial ischemia, and cardiac rhythm analysis may detect postoperative atrial fibrillation.

Table 17.1 Common Laboratory Tests in the PACU

Category	Significance
Prothrombin time/activated partial thromboplastin time (PT/aPTT); international normalized ratio (INR)/platelet count	These tests are done to evaluate clotting abnormalities. This is significant because of the possibility of bleeding postoperatively. It is also important to monitor if patients were on anticoagulants preoperatively. Normal values: PT: 10–13 seconds aPTT: 25–35 seconds INR: 0.9–1.1
Renal function: blood urea nitrogen (BUN), creatinine	Renal function may be decreased because of dehydration from blood or fluid loss. Consider age and renal disease. Normal values: BUN: 8–21 mg/dL Creatinine: 0.5–1.2 mg/dL
Glucose	Decreased glucose levels should be ruled out in cases of decreases in level of consciousness or inability to arouse postoperatively. Normal value: Glucose: 65–99 mg/dL fasting blood glucose level
Electrolytes: serum potassium (K), serum sodium (Na)	Values may be abnormal because of fluid loss, blood loss, or overhydration. Normal values: Potassium: 3.5–5.0 mEq/L Sodium: 135–145 mEq/L
White blood cell (WBC) count	An increase in the WBC count may indicate infection. Normal value: WBC count: 4.5–11.1 10^3/mm^3
Hematocrit/hemoglobin	Low values may indicate excessive blood loss. Normal values: Hematocrit: females, 36%–48%; males, 42%–52% Hemoglobin: females: 11.7–15.5 g/dL; males, 14–17.3 g/dL

PACU, Post-anesthesia care unit.

Pain Management

Pain management is an essential component of patient management in the PACU and beyond. In the preoperative area, the nurse assesses and documents the patient's physical and emotional status and discusses pain management following surgery. It is important that the nurse understands each patient's perception of pain, teaches him or her about postoperative pain management expectations, and engages the patient and family in developing a postoperative pain management plan. Important discussion and education points include:

- The importance of pain control and treating pain before it becomes severe
- The importance of reporting pain; terminology; pain scale that will be used in the PACU; patient's terminology regarding pain location and intensity
- Goals of treatment for pain, understanding that on a scale of 0 to 10, a goal of zero pain is often not realistic
- Pharmacological and nonpharmacological options available to manage pain in the PACU
- Fears about pain medication, such as addiction
- Chronic, current, or past use of opioids
- Nonpharmacological methods that the patient currently uses to reduce anxiety and improve comfort (e.g., music, deep breathing, prayer)
- Whether having family at the bedside is helpful or if the patient prefers to be alone

Pain Management Strategies

Although postoperative pain is expected in all patients, behavioral responses to pain vary widely from patient to patient. During the immediate postoperative period, anesthetic effects may mask or prevent the patient from reporting pain. The PACU nurse should use an appropriate method of pain assessment for the patient, such as a numerical scale, the Wong–Baker FACES scale, or a behavioral scale. The PACU nurse must know that there are physiological signs that indicate pain even if the patient is unable or unwilling to describe what he or she is feeling. These include restlessness; sweating; dilation of pupils; increase in respiration, blood pressure, and heart rate; and piloerection. Additionally, the patient may be frowning, opening his or her eyes widely, making facial grimaces, clenching the teeth, or moaning—all indications of pain. It is recommended that the nurse assume that pain is present, with or without overt symptoms, and provide treatment based on the knowledge that surgery is painful (see Evidence-Based Practice: Postoperative Pain Management Strategies).

Evidence-Based Practice

Postoperative Pain Management Strategies

In 2016, the American Pain Society, in conjunction with other professional organizations, published a clinical practice guideline on treating postoperative pain. The report states that although most patients experience pain postoperatively, less than half of the patients say that their pain is adequately controlled. The clinical practice guideline comprises 32 recommendations made by an expert panel after a systematic review of the evidence. The recommendations include preoperative evaluation for current opioid use and education about pain control expectations, tailoring of pain control plans to the individual patient and surgery, and the use of different pharmacological and nonpharmacological modalities (e.g., combining analgesics like ketamine, lidocaine, gabapentin, and pregabalin with opioids and the use of transcutaneous electrical nerve stimulation). The panel also recommends that clinicians provide education to all patients and primary caregivers on how to taper off pain medications.

Chou, R., Gordon, C. B., de Leon-Casasola, O. A., Rosenberg, J. M., Bickler, S., Brenan, T., ...Wu, C. L. (2016). Guidelines on the management of postoperative pain. *Journal of Pain, 17*(2), 131–157. doi:10.1016/j.pain.2015.12.008

The best results in postoperative pain management involve multimodal pharmacological therapy or synchronous administration of NSAIDs, acetaminophen, opioids, and local anesthetics. In addition to pain medication, studies demonstrate that a variety of nonpharmacological methods decrease pain (and the need for medication) postoperatively, such as music therapy, massage, prayer, and meditation; however, few PACUs offer these options to all patients as a part of their pain management programs.

Many postoperative patients are given a **patient-controlled analgesia (PCA)** pump for the delivery of opioid medications (Fig. 17.1). A PCA pump is an infusion of a prescribed amount of analgesia through an IV route when the patient pushes a button. This requires the patient to be able to understand and communicate effectively with the

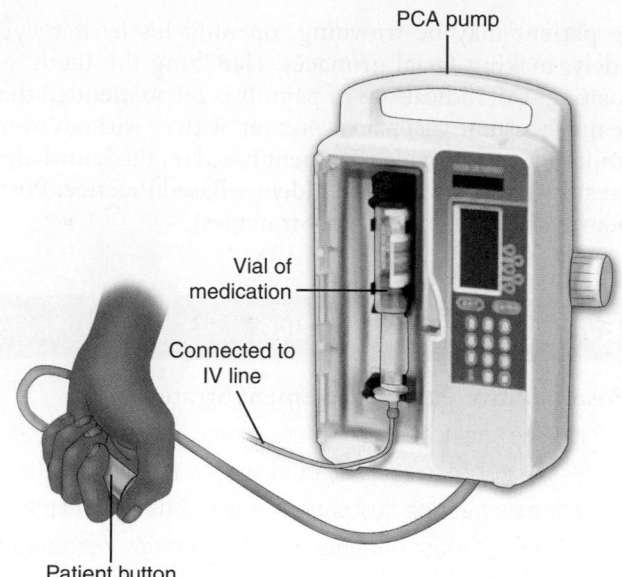

PCA pump

Vial of medication

Connected to IV line

Patient button

FIGURE 17.1 Patient-controlled analgesia (PCA) pump. The patient pushes a button when pain medication is required, resulting in the delivery of a preset dose of pain medication through the IV line.

nurse and might not be appropriate therapy if cognitive or communication problems exist. Assessment of the patient in the preoperative area prior to initiating PCA is essential to the safe implementation of this type of pain control. Also important is education that only the patient (not family members, the nurse, or other healthcare providers) should push the button to deliver a dose of the pain medication.

Management of Postoperative Nausea and Vomiting (PONV)

Postoperative nausea and vomiting (PONV) is often more anticipated and feared by patients than postoperative pain. In the immediate postoperative period, PONV can cause dehydration, electrolyte imbalance, wound dehiscence, and aspiration. Postoperative nausea and vomiting has been associated with an increased length of stay, a decreased ability to perform activities of daily living and return to school/work after discharge, and emergency department visits and hospital readmissions. Risk factors for PONV include being a young, nonsmoking female and having a history of PONV or motion sickness. Certain types of surgeries are more likely to cause PONV, such as cholecystectomies and laparoscopic, intra-abdominal, gynecological, and neurological surgeries. General anesthesia causes more PONV than regional anesthesia. The longer the patient is under general anesthesia, the more likely the patient is to experience PONV. High doses of the neuromuscular blockade reversing agent neostigmine also increase the likelihood of PONV.

In order to treat PONV, postoperative opioid use should be minimized, and hydration should be optimized. It is suggested that nausea be measured on a numerical scale, much

like pain, or a descriptor scale (mild, moderate, severe) so that providers can decide which antiemetic approach to use. This method of rating nausea gives nurses the ability to determine the effectiveness of different pharmacological agents. Multimodal pain management strategies should be taken to avoid relying on opioids alone, which increase PONV. Prophylactic treatment by using a combination of antiemetic medications in high-risk patients before surgery can help reduce PONV.

Connection Check 17.4

Which statement is true about the complicated nature of managing pain medication in the immediate post-anesthesia patient?

A. All patients respond to pain in the same way but have different medications ordered.

B. All patients respond to pain in different ways, potentially requiring different medications.

C. The synergy of all multimodal pain management is unpredictable.

D. Nonpharmacological methods of pain control do not work in the PACU setting.

CASE STUDY: EPISODE 2

Mr. Wells is transferred from the OR to the PACU. He is drowsy but responds to his name. He has on an oxygen mask, and a nasogastric tube is in place. He has a urinary catheter and is on the cardiac monitor, which shows atrial fibrillation with a rate of 85 beats per minute (bpm) and a respiratory rate of 12. His oxygen saturation is 97%. His breath sounds are clear and equal bilaterally. He has a dry abdominal dressing and two drains draining a small amount of sanguineous liquid. On his legs, he has intermittent pneumatic compression boots that are connected to the small pump on the bed. In addition to IV fluid that is running, Mr. Wells has a PCA pump, and he received IV doses of fentanyl and morphine before leaving the OR. He responds to his name and shakes his head "no" when asked if he has any pain. He says the pain is 1 on a scale of 0 to 10…

Potential Complications

Immediately following surgery and anesthesia, all patients are at risk for respiratory depression from anesthesia and pain medication and bleeding from the surgical procedure itself, requiring careful and frequent nursing assessment. In addition to these major complications, Table 17.2 includes additional serious complications that require either prevention or treatment in the PACU (see Geriatric/Gerontological Considerations).

Geriatric/Gerontological Considerations

The normal physiological decline associated with aging (see Chapter 6) can be exacerbated by the effects of stress of surgery, anesthesia, and immobility. Older adults are at higher risk for postoperative complications, delayed recovery, and an increased length of stay. The postoperative nurse should anticipate the following:

- Respiratory: decreased rib-cage expansion, increasing the risk for atelectasis; hypoxia; hypercarbia; increased work of breathing
- Cardiac: reduced cardiac output; hypotension, which can develop quickly; higher risk for postoperative atrial fibrillation; greater risk for orthostatic hypotension related to dehydration
- Renal: greater risk for postoperative volume overload and electrolyte imbalances; greater risk of medication toxicity—requires careful evaluation of dosage of medications excreted by the kidney
- Skin: more susceptible to friction, sheer, pressure, and moisture
- Delirium: higher risk postoperatively. Free from tethering devices as soon as possible, avoid physical restraint, use nonpharmacological interventions (e.g., reorientation, fall risk precautions, involve family in care), and consider administering antipsychotics.
- Immobility/decreased mobility: increased risk of deep vein thrombosis (DVT), pneumonia, pressure injuries, respiratory failure, delirium, orthostatic hypotension, and fatigue
- Nutrition: the older adult is more likely to have inadequate nutrients for wound healing and strength.

NURSING MANAGEMENT

Nursing Interventions

Assessment

- Neurological: level of consciousness/motor and sensation
  Anesthesia produces a decreased level of consciousness or a reversible loss of consciousness. A continued decrease in level of consciousness, restlessness, agitation, and confusion may indicate inadequate reversal of anesthesia or complications of anesthesia or could also be a result of hypoxia. Motor and sensation abilities must also be monitored to assess for the reversal of any nerve blocks administered during surgery for patient safety.

- Vital signs
  Any deviation from the normal range of values for blood pressure, heart rate, oxygenation saturation, respiratory rate, or temperature could indicate a postoperative complication.
  Excessive blood or fluid loss may cause hypotension and tachycardia.
  Excess catecholamine production from the physical and emotional stress of surgery may cause hypertension and tachycardia.
  Increased or decreased respiratory rate, use of accessory muscles, and decreased oxygen saturation may indicate inadequate reversal of or recovery from anesthesia. Increased temperature may be an indication of malignant hyperthermia, which can be triggered by anesthesia; hypothermia, not unusual postoperatively because of cool OR temperatures, prolonged skin exposure, and anesthesia that interferes with normal temperature control, may require warming measures.

- Peripheral pulses/skin temperature/skin color
  Weak peripheral pulses, cool skin temperature, and/or pale skin color could signify inadequate perfusion resulting from blood loss and decreased cardiac output.

- Urine output
  Decreased urine output, less than 30 mL/hr, may indicate dehydration due to fluid or blood loss or urinary retention.

- Pain
  Pain is an expected outcome of a surgical procedure but should be managed appropriately. Regular assessment of pain is necessary for the evaluation of pain management. Uncontrolled pain may be an indication of a complication.

- Skin/surgical incisions/wounds
  Extended time in intraoperative positioning may cause excessive pressure and skin breakdown. Excessive blood or drainage on wound dressings may indicate inadequate wound closure or bleeding and requires follow-up by the provider.

Actions

- Connect to continuous cardiac monitor immediately upon admission to the PACU.
  Changes in vital signs or dysrhythmias may indicate complications associated with anesthesia or the operative procedure.
- Start admission assessment immediately upon admission to the PACU.
  It is essential to get a baseline to understand the patient's presenting status.
- Document vital signs.
  Vital signs are often documented every 15 minutes to allow prompt response to changes as necessary.

Table 17.2 Potential Complications in the PACU

System	Complication	Intervention
Neurological	<ul><li>Drowsy and hard to arouse</li><li>Restless</li><li>Not following commands</li><li>Confusion</li></ul>	<ul><li>Check glucose level.</li><li>Hold pain medication.</li><li>Consider naloxone (Narcan).</li><li>Restrain as ordered.</li><li>Reorient/provide explanation/reassurance.</li><li>Have family present as possible.</li><li>Evaluate oxygenation; evaluate for alcohol withdrawal.</li></ul>
Respiratory	<ul><li>Airway obstruction/stridor</li><li>Inadequate oxygenation</li><li>Ineffective ventilation</li><li>Aspiration</li></ul>	<ul><li>Check airway and O_2 saturation.</li><li>Check breath sounds (auscultate).</li><li>Supplement oxygen as per provider's orders.</li><li>Consider ventilatory support.</li><li>Chest radiograph</li></ul>
Cardiovascular	<ul><li>Hypotension</li><li>Tachycardia</li><li>Bleeding</li><li>Venous thromboembolism (VTE)/pulmonary embolism (PE)</li><li>Dysrhythmias</li><li>Myocardial infarction</li><li>Fluid imbalance; dehydration/retention</li></ul>	<ul><li>Monitor vital signs.</li><li>Fluid and blood replacement as ordered.</li><li>For prevention of VTE: compression stockings, intermittent pneumatic compression boots</li><li>For treatment of VTE: anticoagulation</li><li>Monitor intake and output.</li><li>Monitor electrolytes.</li></ul>
Thermoregulation	<ul><li>Hyperthermia</li></ul>	<ul><li>Monitor for malignant hyperthermia.</li></ul> Initiate emergency treatment as necessary, including administration of dantrolene (see Chapter 16 for discussion of malignant hyperthermia).
	<ul><li>Hypothermia</li></ul>	<ul><li>Provide warm blankets or warming devices for hypothermia. Provide supplemental oxygen as shivering increases demand.</li></ul>
Gastrointestinal	<ul><li>Postoperative nausea and vomiting (PONV)</li></ul>	<ul><li>Administer antiemetics.</li><li>Anticipate and prevent aspiration if vomiting—head of bed elevated and/or side-lying position as possible.</li></ul>
Genitourinary	<ul><li>Urinary retention</li></ul>	<ul><li>Bladder scan</li><li>Consider Foley catheter.</li><li>Suggest standing (men) when attempting to void when possible.</li></ul>
Skin integrity	<ul><li>Skin breakdown or redness at pressure sites</li><li>Abnormal wound drainage; yellow/cloudy, bloody, foul-smelling</li><li>Severe wound complications such as dehiscence (wound rupture along surgical suture) or evisceration (extrusion of viscera outside the body through the surgical incision; Fig. 17.2)</li></ul>	<ul><li>Relieve pressure as possible through positioning and support with blankets and pillows.</li><li>Check amount of drainage, color, and frequency of dressing change; reinforce dressing and report to provider.</li><li>Dehiscence/evisceration requires immediate notification and intervention by the surgeon; maintain low Fowler's position, minimize movement, and cover wound with sterile saline dressing.</li></ul>

Table 17.2 Potential Complications in the PACU—cont'd

System	Complication	Intervention
Pain (see Chapter 11 for more information on pain control)	• Persistent pain may lead to deconditioning and respiratory comprise, such as atelectasis, through decreased mobility; hormonal response, such as excess catecholamine production resulting in hypertension and tachycardia; and neuropsychiatric effects, such as insomnia.	• Mild pain—nonopioid (e.g., acetaminophen, NSAIDs) • Moderate to severe pain—multimodal therapy: nonopioids, μ opioid agonists (e.g., morphine, hydromorphone, fentanyl), and adjuvants (e.g., anticonvulsants, local anesthesia, antidepressants) • Other pain modalities provided by the providers and supported by the nurses: preemptive analgesia (given preoperatively by anesthesia) and rescue analgesia (given postoperatively to supplement pain medication) • Other considerations: multimodal therapy (opioid and nonopioid analgesia to avoid unwanted sedation, regional blocks by anesthesia providers, and systemic or epidural patient-controlled anesthesia (PCA). Systemic PCA (IV) is used more often than epidural PCA for surgery below the waist or specific area that needs an analgesia block (e.g., thoracic block). • Comfort measures: physical/psychological (e.g., positioning, heat and cold therapies, sensory aids), sociocultural (e.g., family, caregiver, interpreter), psychospiritual (e.g., chaplain, religious objects), and environmental (e.g., reasonably quiet room, privacy)

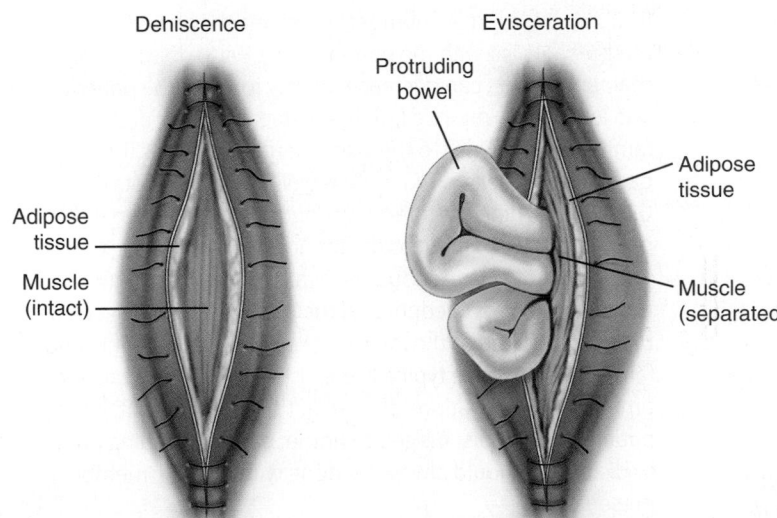

FIGURE 17.2 Surgical wound-healing complications include wound dehiscence; wound rupture along the surgical suture line; and wound evisceration, the extrusion of viscera outside the body through the surgical incision.

• Participation in hand-off from the OR
Good communication is essential for a smooth transition of care between the OR and PACU to ensure the patient's needs are met and complications are avoided as much as possible (Box 17.2).
• Continuous monitoring of patient's status
The initial PACU assessment is compared with the preoperative assessment. The assessment is monitored continuously to track the patient's recovery or to identify problems.
• Medicate as ordered for pain and nausea.
Nausea centers may be triggered by anesthesia; pain is a result of tissue trauma from surgery.

• Hand-off to inpatient unit if necessary (Box 17.3)
A clear, concise hand-off to the inpatient unit is essential for safe patient care.

▪ **Teaching**
• Family care (Box 17.4)
  • Inform family when the patient arrives in the PACU, and make contact every hour.
  • Communicate plan of care (i.e., time of transfer to bed or discharge home).
  • Allow visiting per hospital guidelines.

Box 17.2 Hand-Off of Care—OR to PACU

Transferring patient care, especially immediately after surgery, requires effective multidisciplinary communication. Without effective hand-off communication, there is an added risk of error due to lack of information and/or misinformation.

Following the admission assessment confirming the patient's stability, the PACU nurse participates in the **hand-off** communication with the three OR team members who have accompanied the patient in transfer (anesthesia, surgical team member, and OR nurse). This hand-off communication includes:

- Patient identification using two identifiers
- Significant medical history
  - Details about the surgical procedure/significant events that occurred in the OR
  - Significant laboratory results
  - Anesthesia and reversal agents administered intraoperatively
- Medications administered intraoperatively, including last dose of pain medication
- Fluid intake and estimated blood loss
- Placement of IV lines and drains
- Important home medications
- Discussion of actual and/or potential clinical issues (e.g., pain, changes in vital signs)
- Nonclinical information, such as family or placement issues
- Overall plan of care
- Team members' names and contact information

Both providers and the OR nurse give their own report. Prior to handing off care to the PACU nurse, the surgical provider and PACU nurse should discuss orders that have been written, the plan for pain management, and any potential complications that can be anticipated.

OR, Operating room; *PACU,* post-anesthesia care unit.

- If the patient is being discharged, provide discharge instructions with family members present. *Communicating and maintaining contact with a family member, as well as allowing visitation, is essential to help relieve anxiety and stress.*
  Because of the effects of anesthesia, the patient may not remember discharge instructions. Having a family member present is essential.

Connection Check 17.5

Upon patient admission to the PACU, the nurse understands that the priority intervention is which of the following?
A. Administer antiemetics.
B. Administer pain medication.
C. Connect patient to the monitor.
D. Start IV fluid.

Box 17.3 Hand-Off of Care—PACU to Inpatient Unit

The clear and concise hand-off of care from the PACU nurse to the inpatient unit nurse is crucial to a smooth and safe transition of care. Important components to include are:

- Surgical procedure
- Perioperative treatment course, including medications and fluids received intraoperatively
- Surgical complications, if any
- Past medical history
- Current vital signs
- Current assessment status
- Surgical incision and drain information
- Medications received for pain and/or nausea
- Plan for pain management
- Time for the receiving nurse to ask any clarifying questions to adequately prepare for accepting the patient into the nurse's care.

PACU, Post-anesthesia care unit.

Box 17.4 Family Visitation

Following the comprehensive admission assessment by the PACU nurse, a family member/loved one may be invited to have a brief visit with the patient in the PACU. It is believed that family visits can decrease anxiety for both the patient and loved one, improve family satisfaction, and encourage family support. Prior to the visit, the nurse ensures that the patient is awake and that pain is well controlled, sets expectations regarding the intended length of the visit, and explains the environment to the family member. During the visit, the PACU nurse should be available to answer questions about the procedure and the next level of care, such as being transferred to the inpatient surgical unit. Patients and family members are typically eager to know about transfer timing and expectations of care on the receiving unit. If the patient is being discharged to home, patient teaching prior to discharge should always be done with a family member present.

Many family members feel it is their right to be able to visit in the PACU; however, the nurse is empowered to terminate the visit depending on the patient, visitor, and unit circumstances. Protecting the safety, privacy, and confidentiality of all patients (and other family members) in the unit is a priority.

PACU, Post-anesthesia care unit.

PATIENT CARE ON THE INPATIENT UNIT

After receiving the hand-off from the PACU nurse, the inpatient nurse must review the new orders written by the provider on the postoperative inpatient unit to prepare to care for the patient in this new setting. Orders will contain information about vital sign parameters; activity and diet (see Evidence-Based Practice: Diet After Surgery); medications for postoperative pain, nausea, and vomiting; thromboembolism prophylaxis; postoperative imaging and laboratory studies; any special precautions related to the surgery; and the continuation of the patient's routine, preoperative medications. The nurse and staff of the inpatient unit can then begin setting up the room with the supplies necessary to support the patient.

Once the patient has arrived, taking vital signs and completing a thorough assessment should begin immediately to establish a baseline. This baseline can be compared to presurgical status and can be used to evaluate the patient's postoperative progress. Patients who are transferred to an inpatient unit are susceptible to many complications, so it is imperative that assessments identify any changes that need intervention.

Evidence-Based Practice

Diet After Surgery

Diet orders after surgery depend greatly on the type of surgery performed. The traditional idea of a patient progressing from ice chips or a clear liquid diet up to a regular diet is not supported by current evidence. For example, those who have had neurosurgery may not be able to eat until an evaluation of their swallowing ability has occurred because of possible cranial nerve disruption resulting in swallowing impairment. Patients who have had gastrointestinal surgery may have volume intolerance because of a risk for a leak at anastomosis sites in the postoperative period. Otolaryngology patients may not be able to eat a regular diet because they cannot chew or are at an increased risk for infection if foods pocket in surgical sites in the oral cavity. Some patients complain of very sore throats following intubation and benefit from choosing softer foods. Early feeding after surgery is generally safe, speeds recovery, shortens length of stay, and is more in line with patient preferences. Interestingly, some studies suggest gum chewing to recover bowel function more quickly when treating an ileus.

Boarin, M., Villa, G., Di Monte, V., Abbadessa, F., & Manara, D. F. (2017). The use of chewing gum for postoperative ileus prevention in patients undergoing radical cystectomy. *International Journal of Urology Nursing*, 11(3), 129–135. doi:10.111/ijun.12141

Short, V., Herbert, G., Perry, R., Atkison, C., Ness, A. R., Penfold, C., ... Lewis, S. J. (2015). Chewing gum for postoperative recovery of gastrointestinal function. *Cochrane Database of Systematic Reviews, 2015*(2), CD006506. doi:10.1002/14651858.CD006506.pub3

Willcutts, K. (2013). *Post-operative feeding: Time to move on.* [PowerPoint Slides]. Retrieved from https://www.cnmdpg.org/docs/Symposium/2013/Handouts/Willcutts,%20Kate%20Handout%20PostopFeeding CNM2013handout.pdf

Potential Postoperative Complications

Respiratory System

Some potential complications in the respiratory system include atelectasis, pneumonia, and pulmonary embolus, all potentially resulting in inadequate gas exchange, hypoxemia, and hypoxia. All are related to hypoventilation, venous stasis, and an ineffective cough secondary to immobility and pain. Immobility can cause an accumulation of mucus in the lungs, resulting in atelectasis and pneumonia. Immobility can also result in venous stasis and clot formation or deep vein thrombosis (DVT) formation, which can ultimately result in a pulmonary embolus. Pain can cause hypoventilation, which results in poor gas exchange and a weakened cough, further compromising the removal of secretions and oxygenation.

Cardiovascular System

The body's natural stress response to the surgical procedure may result in fluid and electrolyte complications. Acute stress and surgical fluid losses lead to a sympathetic response of tachycardia and vasoconstriction. There is increased secretion of adrenocorticotropic hormone (ACTH), stimulating the adrenals to release cortisol, hydrocortisone, and aldosterone. The pituitary is stimulated to release antidiuretic hormone (ADH), and the renin–angiotensin–aldosterone system (RAAS) is stimulated. All result in fluid retention, sodium retention, and urinary loss of potassium. This may result in fluid overload and hypokalemia. Hypokalemia affects cardiac contractility and may lead to lethal dysrhythmias. Conversely, fluid losses secondary to untreated or poorly treated preoperative dehydration, surgical fluid losses, bleeding, wound drainage, and/or vomiting may result in decreased cardiac output and poor tissue perfusion.

Neurological System

There are several severe neurological complications related to surgery and, more specifically, anesthesia. Delirium, defined as inattention and disorganized thinking, is a common complication affecting up to 70% of patients over 60 years of age. It is associated with persistent cognitive decline, prolonged ICU and hospital length of stay, and increased mortality. Treatment is mostly based on recognition of populations at risk and prevention. Preventative measures include decreasing the irritation of invasive lines, tubes, and drains that increase agitation as quickly as possible. Antipsychotic medications, such as low-dose haloperidol (Haldol), may be used as a treatment, along with reorientation and reassurance. Another complication common in the older patient is postoperative cognitive decline (POCD), which can be subtle and temporary or may last for weeks or months, causing delays in return to normal functioning such as work.

For both delirium and POCD, measures such as maintaining stable hemodynamic parameters, normal bowel and bladder functioning, early mobility, and frequent reorientation are helpful in preventing or limiting cognitive issues

Gastrointestinal System

Postoperative ileus (POI), a slowing of gastric and bowel mobility, is a complication largely associated with gastrointestinal (GI) surgery when there is manipulation of the bowel. It can also occur with other procedures due to anesthesia, immobility, opioid pain medication, and previous abdominal surgery. Patients present with nausea and abdominal pain. Interventions include insertion of a nasogastric tube to decompress the stomach to ease nausea and prevent vomiting and aspiration. Patients are kept nothing by mouth, NPO, until bowel motility returns.

Urinary System

Urinary retention can occur due to complications from anesthesia, opioids, and immobility. Anesthesia depresses the nervous system, which can affect the nervous system's control of micturition. This can result in a decreased sensation of a full bladder and urinary retention. Opioids may interfere with the patient's ability to fully empty the bladder. Immobility and bedrest impact the ability to fully relax the perineal structures to allow voiding and complete emptying of the bladder.

Integumentary System

A surgical procedure typically involves an incision through the skin and tissues, disrupting the first barrier to infection, the skin. Surgical-site infection is a risk in the perioperative period more commonly seen in older, immunosuppressed, or malnourished patients and those with longer hospital length of stays. The surgical site will appear red, warm, and edematous, with purulent drainage, and the patient will complain of increased pain—the cardinal signs of inflammation. In the worst-case scenario, the wound may dehisce; the sutures or staples fail, and the wound opens up. The wound must be cleaned and drained. Sterile saline dressings must be maintained until the wound is healthy enough to be reapproximated or resutured. Adequate nutrition is imperative for wound healing.

NURSING MANAGEMENT

Although postoperative needs are specific to the patient and surgical procedure, there are assessments and interventions that are common to all surgical patients. Case-specific needs are covered in the chapters where specific surgical procedures are discussed. This chapter focuses on common postsurgical needs. These patient assessments and interventions are crucial for safe patient care.

Nursing Interventions

▪ Assessment

- Respiratory status
  Low oxygen saturation and/or increased respiratory rate and work of breathing could signify a pulmonary embolism (PE), atelectasis, aspiration, or pneumonia. Adventitious lung sounds such as rhonci or diminished or absent sounds could
  also reveal atelectasis, aspiration, or pneumonia. Rales may indicate fluid overload.
- Vital signs—blood pressure (BP), heart rate (HR), and temperature: Monitor for trends in values.
  Deviations from normal vital signs could signify complications. The most common postoperative complication is hypotension and tachycardia due to blood or fluid loss. Hypertension and tachycardia may occur due to the stress response to surgery and pain. Increases in temperature may indicate infection due to pulmonary issues or surgical-site infection.
- Peripheral perfusion
  Cool, pale skin with weak pulses and delayed capillary refill may indicate decreased volume and cardiac output.
- Neurological
  Decreases in level of consciousness, confusion, agitation, or disorientation may indicate the onset of delirium or POCD. It may also be due to excessive pain medication or respiratory dysfunction. Irregularities in pupillary size and reaction or Glasgow Coma Scale (GCS) score may be due to increased intracranial pressure.
- GI
  Bowel sounds, flatus, and bowel movements reflect the return of GI motility. Postoperative nausea and vomiting may be associated with anesthesia. Absent or hypoactive bowel sounds, nausea, and vomiting may indicate paralytic ileus.
- Genitourinary (GU)
  Increased urine output in the initial postoperative period may be due to excessive IV fluids given intraoperatively. Decreased urination can result from dehydration or the release of antidiuretic hormone (ADH) and initiation of the RAAS due to stress and surgical fluid losses. Monitor for urinary retention that may be caused by complications from anesthesia, opioids, and immobility. Cloudy urine, tea- or cola-colored urine, and urine with a foul odor are signs of urinary tract infection.
- Skin/drains
  Assess surgical incisions and dressings for proximity of closed edges, presence and quality of drainage, and intactness of surrounding skin. Red, warm, edematous tissue with purulent drainage, along with complaints of increased pain, indicates infection. Assess for the presence and staging of any skin breakdown or pressure injuries that may be associated with prolonged positioning in the OR or immobility postoperatively.
- Drains
  Assess for excess, bloody, or cloudy drainage. Excessive or bloody drainage may indicate surgical-site bleeding. Cloudy drainage may indicate infection. Absent drainage may indicate a clogged drain.
- Pain
  Pain should be monitored and treated. Poorly controlled pain may indicate surgical complications or the need for alternate pain control treatment.
- Fluid and electrolyte balance; monitoring of glucose levels
  Fluid retention may occur due to activation of the RAAS and release of ADH in response to stress and dehydration.

Hypokalemia, a risk factor for lethal dysrhythmias, and hypernatremias may occur with the activation of the RAAS. Hyperglycemia may occur related to the stress of the surgical experience and is a risk factor for infection because high blood glucose fuels bacterial growth.

Actions

- Respiratory care
  Encourage patient to cough and breathe deeply to facilitate full lung expansion and airway clearance (see Evidence-Based Practice: Incentive Spirometry).
- Fluid management
  Maintain IV fluids as ordered to maintain intravascular volume. Start PO fluid as ordered with the return of bowel sounds. Maintain as tolerated/no nausea.
- Mobility: change position frequently; encourage ambulation as soon as possible.
  Mobility encourages lung expansion, requires muscle use to prevent atrophy, aids in DVT prevention, helps relieve constipation, aids in pain and fatigue relief, improves mood, reduces anxiety, increases comfort, instills a greater quality of life and independence, and is a factor in decreased length of stay.
- DVT/venous thromboembolism (VTE) prophylaxis
  DVTs, when they occur, commonly occur in the posterior calf, with noticeable redness, swelling, heat, and pain. A combination of administering anticoagulants as ordered, encouraging activity, and using compression devices is the most effective means of prevention.
- Diet management
  Provide diet as ordered. Nutrition is essential for healing. The progression and type of diet are unique to each type of surgical procedure but, in general, PO fluids and diet are started when bowel sounds return and are maintained as tolerated by the patient.
- Surgical site and wound management
  Change dressing as ordered, utilizing proper hand hygiene before and after care and correct use of clean and sterile gloves to prevent surgical-site infections. Provide complete documentation of wound assessment and care.
- Pressure-injury prevention
  Prolonged pressure deprives tissues of oxygen and nutrients, causing ulceration. Pressure injuries are most often found over bony prominences. To prevent pressure-injury development, patients should be encouraged to mobilize and adjust their position frequently. Those who are not able to do so should be assisted to turn and reposition every 2 hours. Encourage proper nutrition to promote skin integrity and wound healing.
- Fall prevention
  Encourage patients to call for assistance. Most falls happen when patients are trying to do something unassisted and/or without supervision, such as transferring from the chair to the bed or ambulating to the bathroom. Use bed alarms as necessary. Preoperative falls put patients at higher risk for postoperative falls.
- Managing constipation: administer stool softeners and laxatives as ordered.
  Constipation in the postoperative patient is a common occurrence due to the effects of anesthesia or other medications (particularly opioids), immobility, or improper hydration. Encourage the patient to ambulate, drink plenty of fluids, and eat a nutritious diet high in fiber. Medications other than or in conjunction with opioids to treat pain should be explored. Stool softeners add water into the bowel; laxatives improve bowel mobility to aid in defecation.
- Remove the Foley catheter as ordered.
  Removal of the indwelling Foley catheter helps prevent catheter-associated urinary tract infections (CAUTIs) and reduces the risk of falls by removing a tripping hazard.

Teaching

- Unit education
  Educate the patient on unit routines (e.g., frequency of vital signs and assessments, visitation hours, staff members on the unit), and orient the patient to his or her room (how to work the call bell, how to order food).
- Safety
  Topics include standard or isolation precautions, patient identification methods, fall precautions, activity or diet restrictions, and bleeding risk precautions.
- Discharge education (Box 17.5)
  Education is essential to ensure that the patient safely transitions to home and avoids readmission to the hospital. Teaching should be done in the presence of a family member or significant other who will help the patient upon returning home.

Evidence-Based Practice

Incentive Spirometry

Incentive spirometers are designed to give the patient visual feedback for deep breathing and lung expansion. The use of incentive spirometry has traditionally been a part of postoperative care, but the American Association of Respiratory Therapists no longer recommends routine, prophylactic use in postoperative patients. The guidelines state that "the use of Airway Clearance Therapy in the setting of atelectasis without retained airway secretions does not seem to be effective." The guidelines suggest early ambulation instead to expand the lungs and promote airway clearance.

Armstrong, C. O. (2017). Post-op incentive spirometry: Why, when, & how. *Nursing, 47*(6), 54–57. doi:10.1097/01.NURSE.0000516223.16649.02

Box 17.5 Home Discharge Instructions

- Signs and symptoms that need to be reported to the provider immediately
- When and how to take any prescriptions
- Signs and symptoms of infection
- Care of incision and dressings, bathing restrictions
- Activities allowed and prohibited (e.g., driving, exercising, sex, swimming, and weight restrictions)
- Dietary restrictions
- When and where to return for follow-up
- When to return to work/school

*More topics may be necessary to include based on the individual patient needs and the type of surgery performed (e.g., smoking cessation, signs and symptoms of hormonal imbalances, spinal precautions, signs and symptoms of a cerebrospinal fluid leak, or sternal precautions).

Making Connections

CASE STUDY: WRAP-UP

Mr. Wells's daughter has come in to visit at his bedside. She is happy that his surgery is over but is very worried about his post-surgical pain. The PACU nurse discusses the PCA pump with her and explains that her father has been resting comfortably and using the pump when needed. His vital signs are stable, and urine output has been good. Because Mr. Wells had bowel surgery, his nasogastric tube has been connected to low continuous suction as ordered by the surgeon. The nurse assesses his abdomen and hears no bowel sounds, but the incision is clean and dry. Soon Mr. Wells meets discharge criteria and is transferred to his inpatient bed.

Case Study Questions

1. The PACU nurse understands that the first priority for Mr. Wells upon admission to the PACU is which of the following?
   A. Informing the family of his status
   B. Checking vital signs and neurological status
   C. Providing pain medication
   D. Assessing the nasogastric tube

2. Initially upon admission, Mr. Wells remains sleepy and hard to arouse. The PACU nurse anticipates an order for which laboratory test?
   A. Glucose level
   B. Arterial blood gas
   C. Lactate level
   D. Liver function test

3. Shortly later, Mr. Wells becomes restless, and his heart rate goes up to 100 bpm. As the nurse assesses him, the priority assessment should include which interventions? *(Select all that apply.)*
   A. Check his dressing and drains for bleeding.
   B. Check his breathing and oxygen saturation.
   C. Check his pain and comfort level.
   D. Check to see if he has to have a bowel movement.
   E. Check his blood pressure and fluid volume status.

4. Before administering pain medication to Mr. Wells, the nurse's assessments include which of the following? *(Select all that apply.)*
   A. Sedation level
   B. Self-report of pain
   C. Vital signs
   D. Bowel sounds
   E. Urine output

5. The PACU nurse supports Mr. Wells's family by doing which of the following? *(Select all that apply.)*
   A. Informing family when the patient arrives in the PACU
   B. Allowing visitation immediately prior to transfer to his inpatient room
   C. Allowing visitation as safety and privacy allow
   D. Providing frequent updates
   E. Providing a visitation policy that allows visitation after discharge from the PACU

CHAPTER SUMMARY

The transition from anesthesia to recovery carries risks for potentially life-threatening complications. One of the most critical risk factors is that there is a temporary decrease in or loss of consciousness and loss of motor and reflexive control of respiration after anesthesia in the OR, so intense monitoring of respiratory status must occur. Also, the postoperative transition period is the time when many patients experience discomforts such as nausea, vomiting, and pain. During the transition from the OR, patients need assistance to maintain a safe internal physiological balance. Post-anesthesia care units (PACUs) specialize in managing both the potential life-threatening complications and the inevitable discomforts related to recovery from a surgical procedure.

Post-anesthesia care is provided in a variety of settings. They include but are not limited to the inpatient hospital PACU, intensive care unit (ICU), outpatient PACU, and procedure areas such as endoscopy. Examples of surgical procedures for which patients recover in an inpatient PACU include lung lobectomy, nephrectomy, exploratory laparotomy, and open reduction and internal fixation of fractures. Recovery from complex procedures with a high risk for complication, such as open-heart procedures, craniotomy, and transplantations, is done in an ICU setting. Patients who receive recovery care in an outpatient setting are able to go home the same day as the procedure, as are patients who receive recovery care in a procedure area.

Effective post-anesthesia care nursing requires knowledge of preoperative status, completion of an immediate postoperative assessment, and evaluation of pertinent laboratory and diagnostic studies. Priority assessments include vital signs and temperature; respiratory adequacy; postoperative cardiac status, including peripheral circulation; postoperative neurological status; IV patency; motor abilities and return of sensory and motor control in areas affected by local or regional anesthetics; and skin integrity. Priority interventions include connecting the patient to the monitor, completing the assessment, pain management, and management of nausea and vomiting. The post-anesthesia care nurse should inform the family of the patient's arrival into the PACU setting and allow visiting as soon as the assessment has been completed and the patient has been stabilized. Supporting the patient's family members and involving them in the discharge instructions is essential to recovery in the hospital or at home.

Patients who are transferred to an inpatient unit for continued monitoring and recovery from surgery are susceptible to many of the same complications as patients in the PACU, such as deep vein thrombosis (DVT) or pulmonary embolism (PE), wound infection, atelectasis, or pneumonia, or problems with gastrointestinal motility. The longer length of stay expands on the assessments and interventions done in the PACU, many of which are standard, but many are patient and surgery specific. Standard postoperative care includes assessment, monitoring, facilitating mobility, wound care, and very importantly, patient and family education.

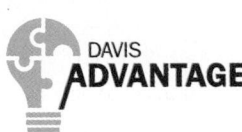
DAVIS ADVANTAGE

To explore learning resources for this chapter, go to **Davis Advantage** and find:
- Answers to in-text questions
- Chapter Resources and Activities
- NCLEX®-Style Chapter Review Questions
- Bibliography

Unit IV

Promoting Health in Patients With Immune Disorders

Chapter **18**

Assessment of Immune Function

Diane Vail Skojec

LEARNING OUTCOMES

Content in this chapter is designed to assist in:

1. Identifying key anatomical components of the immune system
2. Discussing the function of the immune system
3. Describing the procedure for completing a history and physical assessment of a patient with impaired immune function
4. Correlating relevant diagnostic examinations to immune function
5. Explaining nursing considerations for diagnostic studies relevant to immune function
6. Discussing changes in immune function associated with aging

CONCEPTS

- Assessment
- Immunity
- Infection
- Inflammation

ESSENTIAL TERMS

Adaptive (acquired) immunity
Antibodies
Antigen–antibody response
Antigen-presenting cells (APCs)
B lymphocyte (B cell)
Basophil
Cell-mediated immune response
Complement
Cytokines
Cytotoxic T cell
Dendritic cell
Eosinophil
Helper T cell
Humoral immune response
Immunoglobulin
Inflammation
Inflammatory response
Innate (natural) immunity
Leukocyte
Lymphocyte
Macrophage
Major histocompatibility complex (MHC)
Mast cell
Monocyte
Natural killer (NK) cell
Neutrophil
Phagocytosis
Plasma cell
Suppressor T cell
T lymphocyte (T cell)

Finding Connections

Follow this patient throughout the chapter.

Grace Hall is a 60-year-old female who presents to an urgent care clinic with a 4-day history of low-grade fever, malaise, headache, and an itching and painful sensation on the right side of her chest. She states that she has stopped exercising due to the discomfort and finds tight clothing to be irritating. Her maximum oral temperature has been 100.4°F (38°C). Ms. Hall denies weakness, dizziness, confusion, difficulty swallowing or breathing, cough, nausea, vomiting, diarrhea, and weight loss. She also denies exposure to ill individuals or recent travel...

INTRODUCTION

Immunity refers to the body's ability to resist infection and disease. Innate and adaptive immune responses provide three lines of defense against unwanted antigens (Fig. 18.1). **Innate (natural) immunity** provides the first and second lines. The first line consists of physical, biochemical, and mechanical barriers that offer surface protection to prevent

the invasion of microbes. When those barriers are breached, the second line of defense, the **inflammatory response**, is initiated to prevent and/or limit infection, clean out the debris of dead cells, and initiate tissue healing. The first and second lines are nonspecific, responding the same way for any invasion. The third line, **adaptive (acquired) immunity**, occurs by natural exposure; infection, transfer of maternal antibodies, or artificial exposure; vaccination; or infusion of immune serum globulin. This type of immunity is specific and protects by way of cellular-mediated and humoral-mediated mechanisms.

When competent, the immune system wards off the penetration of foreign microbes and the proliferation of abnormal or malignant cells. When the system is incompetent, the failure can lead to allergies, infection, cancer, and autoimmune and immunodeficiency disorders. Age, medications, nutrition, genetics, physical or emotional stress, and illness can all impact immunity and how the immune system functions.

OVERVIEW OF ANATOMY AND PHYSIOLOGY

Anatomy of the Immune System

Components of the immune system include the lymphatic system, primary and secondary lymphoid organs, and the cells and proteins involved in the immune response. The lymphatic system consists of lymphatic vessels and collecting ducts. Primary lymphoid, or central, organs include the thymus and bone marrow. Secondary lymphoid,

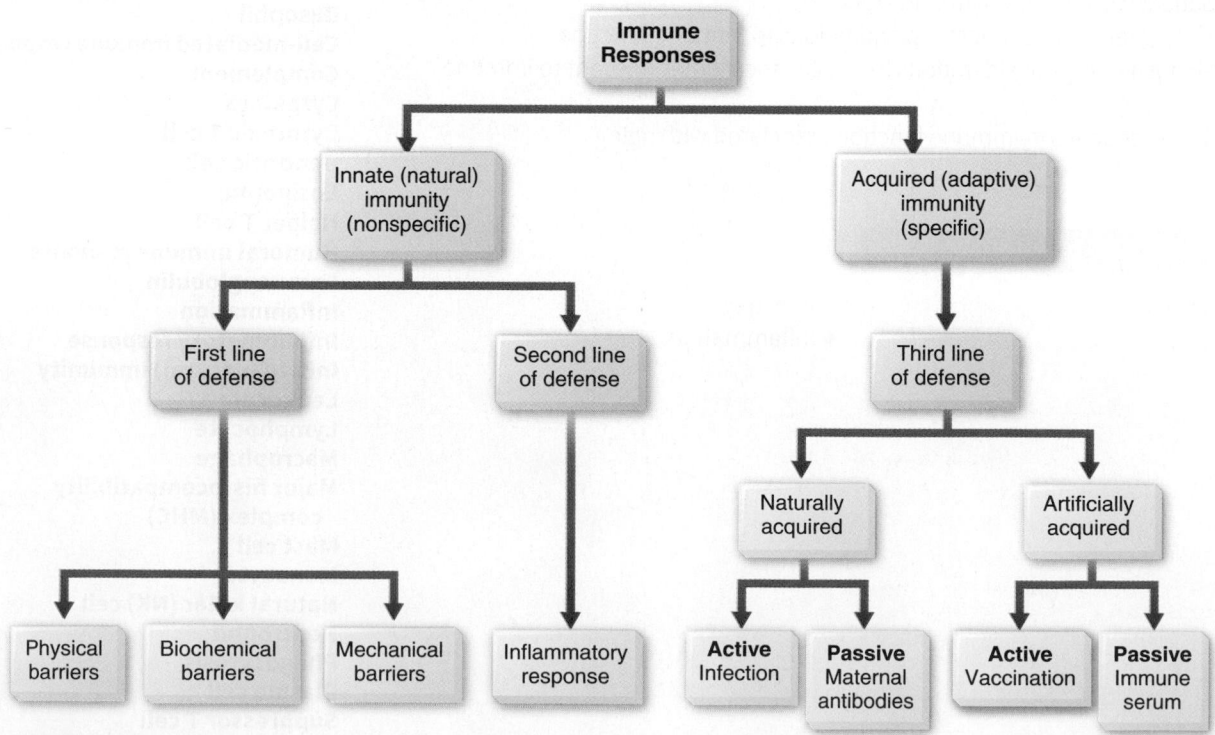

FIGURE 18.1 The immune response: innate (natural) immunity and acquired (adaptive) immunity.

or peripheral, organs include the spleen, lymph nodes, tonsils, adenoids, and Peyer's patches (Fig. 18.2). The cells and proteins include leukocytes (white blood cells [WBCs]), T and B lymphocytes (T cells and B cells), cells involved in the inflammatory response, antibodies, signaling proteins (cytokines), and other protein systems (complement system) that support the immune response. See Table 18.1 for an overview of the cells involved in the immune response.

Lymph Nodes and the Lymphatic System

Fluid continually filters out of the blood and into the interstitial space, the majority of which is reabsorbed back into the bloodstream. The lymphatic system is a network of vessels that transports excess interstitial fluid that has not been reabsorbed (lymph fluid) back to the bloodstream, helping to maintain fluid balance. This system contains thousands of lymph nodes strategically located superficially and deep within the tissues near the lymphatic vessels (Figs. 18.3, 18.4, and 18.5). The nodes are small glandular structures that house macrophages, **lymphocytes**, and **monocytes** that actively filter and phagocytize microorganisms and other invading particles from circulating lymphatic fluid. The lymph fluid moves through the lymphatic vessels, eventually emptying into the lymphatic ducts, the right lymphatic or thoracic duct, and returning to the general circulation through the subclavian veins. This filtering process prevents unwanted substances from reentering the bloodstream.

Thymus

The thymus is a soft organ located within the chest cavity near the heart. It is large in children and decreases in size into adulthood. It is the central lymphoid organ that produces thymosin (a hormone that stimulates T-cell production) and is where T-cell development takes place.

Bone Marrow

Within the cavities of bone resides bone marrow, or myeloid tissue, consisting of red (active) marrow and yellow (inactive) marrow. This is where B- and T-lymphocyte formation and differentiation of B cells and T cells occur. B cells stay within the bone marrow to mature. T cells migrate to the thymus to mature and become active as regulatory T cells (suppressor T cells) or effector T cells (helper T cells and cytotoxic T cells; Fig. 18.6).

Spleen

Approximately the size of a fist, the spleen is located in the left upper quadrant of the abdominal cavity. As a part of the lymphatic system, it serves as a blood filter. It is divided into compartments that contain red and white splenic pulp. The red pulp serves as the filtering site for old or damaged red blood cells. It can also store blood. The white pulp of

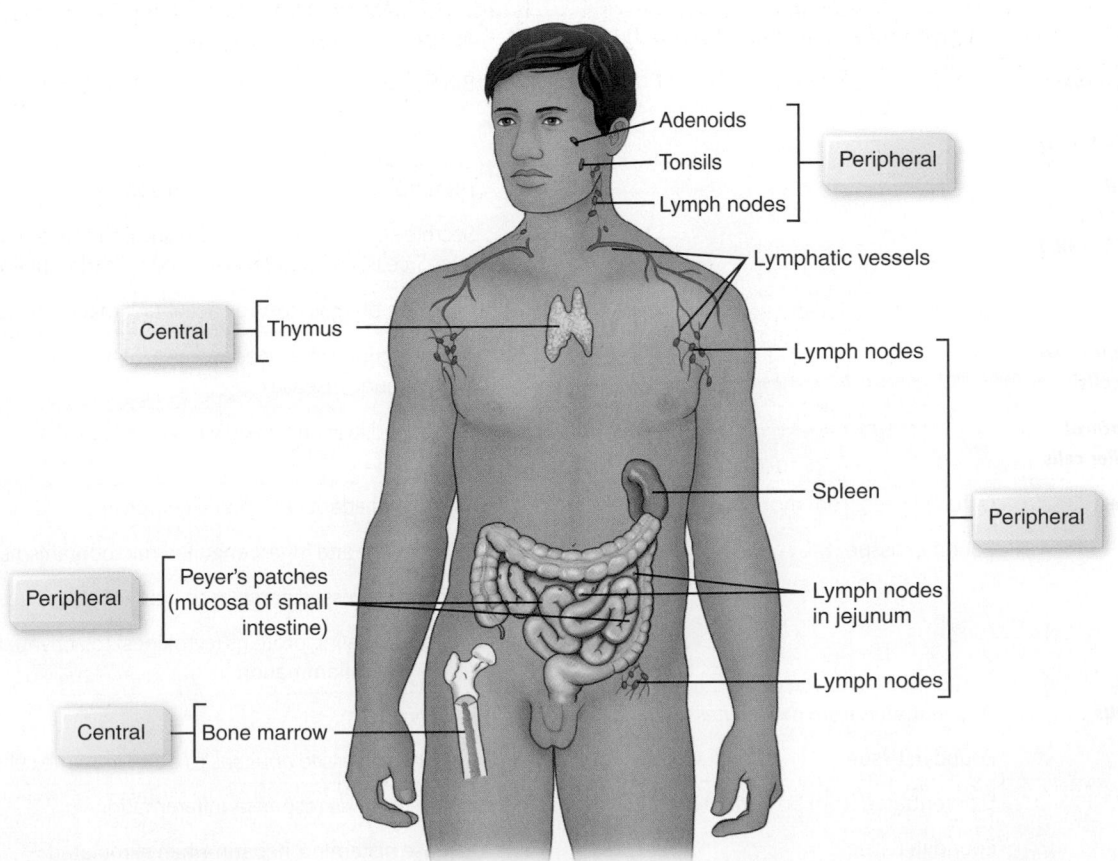

FIGURE 18.2 Central and peripheral organs of the immune system.

Table 18.1 Cells of the Immune System

Name	Site Produced/Found	Function
Leukocytes (**white blood cells**)	Formed in bone marrow and lymph tissue Found in the blood, lymphatic system, spleen, and body tissues	Innate and adaptive immune function
Neutrophils	Found in bone marrow, blood, and tissues	Innate immune response/inflammation Phagocytosis
Basophils	Found in circulation	Innate immune response/inflammation Release histamine, heparin when stimulated Associated with allergic reactions
Eosinophils	Found in tissue	Phagocytosis in parasitic infections, allergens Associated with allergic reactions
Monocytes	Found in circulation When they migrate to tissue, they differentiate into macrophages or dendritic cells.	Innate and adaptive immune response In the circulation: present pathogens to T cells to aid in recognition and destruction
Lymphocytes	Found in bone marrow, thymus, spleen, lymph nodes, and circulation	Coordinate adaptive immune responses
B cells	Formed and mature in the bone marrow	Adaptive/humoral immune response Responsible for antibody-mediated response: on activation, convert to plasma cells and produce antibodies or immunoglobins
T cells	Formed in bone marrow; mature in the thymus	Adaptive/cellular-mediated response
Cytotoxic T cells (**CD8 cells**)		Bind to and destroy invading viruses and cancer cells
Helper T cells (**CD4 cells**)		Humoral and cellular immune response Secrete signaling proteins (cytokines) to activate B cells, cytotoxic T cells, and natural killer (NK) cells (described below) Facilitate phagocytosis by activating macrophages
Suppressor T cells		Down-regulate immune response/prevent overactivity and autoimmune disease
Natural killer cells		Target and kill cancer and virus-infected cells
Macrophages	Differentiated from monocytes Found in tissue	Innate and adaptive immune response Phagocytize and ingest engulfed microorganisms Present processed antigens to helper T cells Secrete signaling proteins (cytokines) to activate helper T cells and inflammation
Dendritic cells	Differentiated from monocytes Found in tissue	Phagocytosis Present processed antigens to other immune cells
Mast cells	Differentiated from bone marrow cells Found in tissue	Innate immune response/inflammation Release histamine, heparin when stimulated Associated with allergic reactions Similar to basophils

A

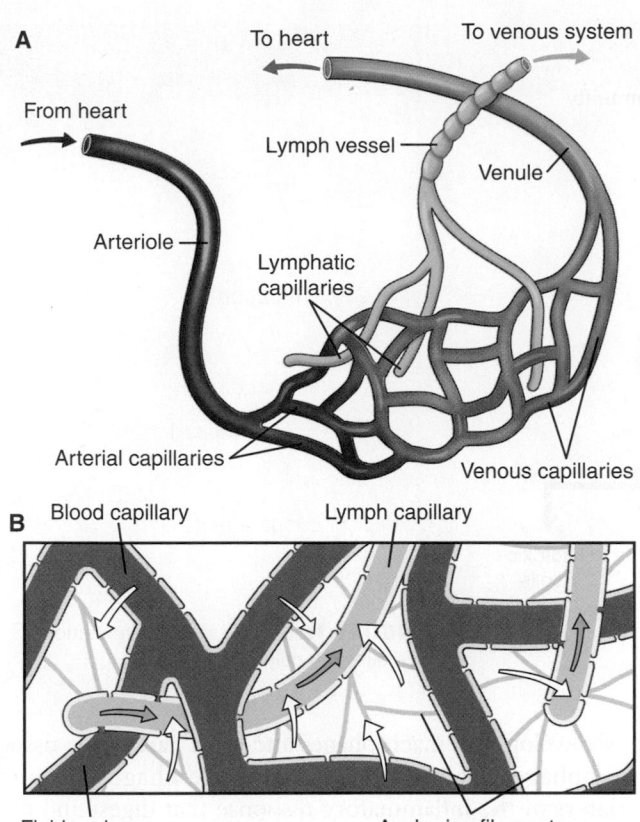

To heart

To venous system

From heart

Lymph vessel

Venule

Arteriole

Lymphatic capillaries

Arterial capillaries

Venous capillaries

B

Blood capillary

Lymph capillary

Fluid exchange

Anchoring filaments

FIGURE 18.3 Lymphatic capillary circulation. *A,* Representation of the interaction of lymphatic capillaries with the arterial and venous vascular system. *B,* Representation of the interaction of the vascular system and lymphatic system microcirculation.

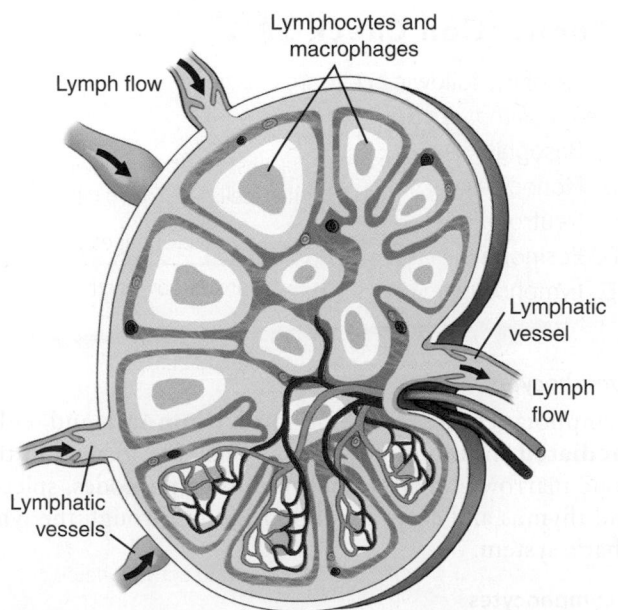

Lymphocytes and macrophages

Lymph flow

Lymphatic vessel

Lymph flow

Lymphatic vessels

FIGURE 18.4 Lymph node.

lymphoid tissue houses lymphocytes and macrophages, filtering unwanted debris like a lymph node. Although it is a redundant organ in the immune system, if it is removed due to accident or disease, the patient may become immunocompromised, with high-risk patients requiring lifetime antibiotics.

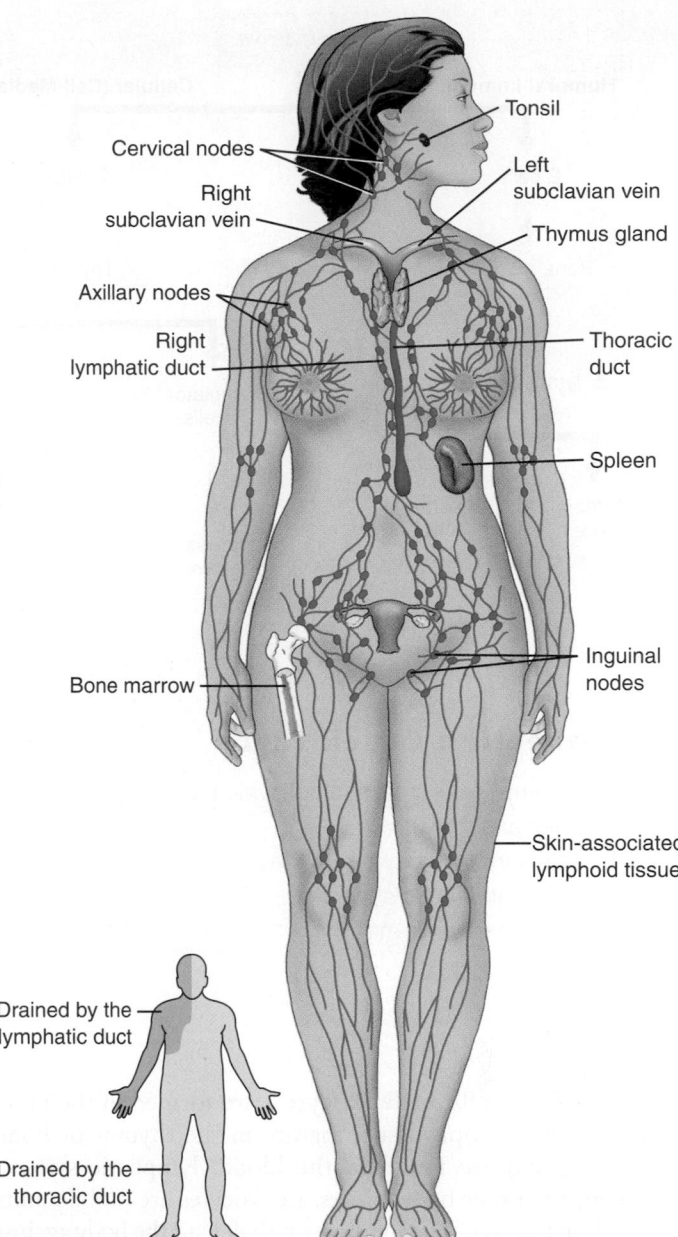

Tonsil

Cervical nodes

Left subclavian vein

Right subclavian vein

Thymus gland

Axillary nodes

Right lymphatic duct

Thoracic duct

Spleen

Bone marrow

Inguinal nodes

Skin-associated lymphoid tissue

Drained by the lymphatic duct

Drained by the thoracic duct

FIGURE 18.5 The nodes and vessels of the lymphatic system.

Tonsils, Adenoids, and Peyer's Patches

Additional lymphoid tissues, such as the tonsils, the adenoids, and Peyer's patches, are located in close proximity to mucosal surfaces within the body and provide another means of protection against invading microorganisms. The tonsils are located between the palatine arches on either side of the pharynx. They function as traps to protect against bacteria and viruses that are inhaled. Located at the nasopharyngeal border, the adenoids also defend against inhaled bacteria and viruses. Peyer's patches are lymphoid follicles located on the mucosa of the small intestine. They are known as intestinal immune sensors and defend against pathogens that gain entry to the intestinal tract. See Figures 18.2 and 18.5 for an overview of the structures of the immune system.

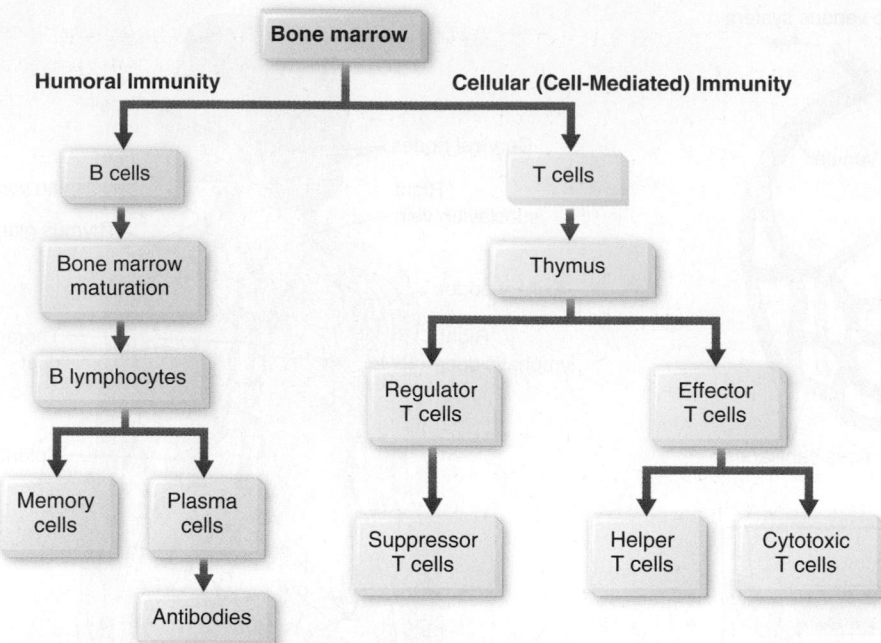

FIGURE 18.6 Process of differentiation of T-cell and B-cell lymphocytes.

Connection Check 18.1

Central lymphoid organs include which of the following?
A. Spleen and tonsils
B. Bone marrow and lymph nodes
C. Thymus and Peyer's patches
D. Thymus and bone marrow

Cells

Leukocytes

White blood cells, or **leukocytes**, are formed in the bone marrow and lymph tissue; mature in the thymus or bone marrow; and are found in the blood, lymphatic system, spleen, and other body tissues. Leukocytes are mobile units traveling through the bloodstream to defend the body against infection. There are five types of leukocytes: neutrophils, monocytes, eosinophils, basophils, and lymphocytes (B and T cells). They are further classified as granulocytes or agranulocytes depending on their function.

Granulocytes have granules in the cytoplasm and release histamines and other substances to defend the body against foreign materials by increasing capillary permeability through vasodilatory effects and mediating the inflammatory response. Neutrophils, basophils, and eosinophils are all phagocytic (cells that engulf bacteria and debris) granulocytes. **Neutrophils** are phagocytes of early inflammation that destroy bacteria. **Basophils** release heparin as an anticoagulant and histamine during the early inflammatory response. **Eosinophils** are phagocytes that destroy allergens and combat parasitic infections.

Agranulocytes (without granules in the cytoplasm) include monocytes and lymphocytes. In the bloodstream, monocytes are a part of the adaptive immune response, presenting pathogens to T cells for destruction. In the tissue, they develop into macrophages and are a part of the tissue macrophage system. **Macrophages** are phagocytes and initiators of the inflammatory response that digest and destroy, or phagocytize, microorganisms and other debris. They also activate helper T cells by secreting signaling proteins, called cytokines, and presenting processed antigens for destruction by the T cell.

Connection Check 18.2

Which of the following cells are classified as granulocytes? *(Select all that apply.)*
A. Basophils
B. Monocytes
C. Neutrophils
D. Eosinophils
E. Lymphocytes

Lymphocytes

Lymphocytes are active in both **humoral** and **cell-mediated immune responses**. They are formed in the bone marrow and are found in the lymph nodes, spleen, and thymus and enter the bloodstream through the lymphatic system.

B Lymphocytes

B lymphocytes (B cells) are the cells involved in humoral immune responses. They are a subset of lymphocytes that mature in the bone marrow and produce **antibodies**, or **immunoglobulins**. Antibodies bind with specific antigens, marking them for destruction by other components of the immune system, or directly neutralize the antigen by inhibiting an essential function necessary for its survival. Once B cells are exposed to a specific antigen for the first time, they proliferate and differentiate into **plasma cells** and memory cells. Plasma cells secrete antibodies after the first exposure to the antigen. Memory cells, restimulated by the same antigen, mount a specific **antigen–antibody response**, sometimes long after the initial exposure. B cells can function independently but typically require the help of T lymphocytes.

Immunoglobulins

The immunoglobulins (Igs), or antibodies, that B cells produce include the following five classes: IgA, IgD, IgE, IgG, and IgM. Immunoglobulin A is found in exocrine-gland secretions such as breast milk and tears. Immunoglobulin D plays a role in B-cell activation, and IgE is associated with allergic reactions and parasitic infections. Immunoglobulin G is effective against bacteria, viruses, and other toxins, and lastly, IgM is the initial antibody produced after an infection (Table 18.2).

T Lymphocytes

T lymphocytes (T cells) are participants in cellular-mediated immune responses. T-cell activation occurs when macrophages present the T cell with a phagocytized antigen. Their main functions include the elimination of cells infected by pathogens, continued activation of the inflammatory response against persistent infections, and regulation of innate and adaptive immune responses. T cells include **cytotoxic T cells**, **suppressor T cells**, and **helper T cells**. Cytotoxic T cells respond to foreign cells, including tumors,

non-self cells, and virus-laden cells. Helper T cells are important cells in both adaptive and innate immunity. They augment the effectiveness of the innate immune response by activating macrophages. They augment both humoral and cellular immunity through the activation of B cells to produce antibodies. They also activate cytotoxic T cells and natural killer cells. Suppressor T cells are activated by helper T cells when the immune response is no longer needed. **Natural killer (NK) cells**, another form of T cell, targets virus-infected and tumor cells. As individuals age, the number of NK cells increases. This increase helps to control infections in the elderly and is important for successful aging.

Dendritic and Mast Cells

Dendritic cells are a type of macrophage that reside in lymphoid tissue and are the most potent of the **antigen-presenting cells (APCs)**. APCs capture and engulf antigens, producing a molecule, the major histocompatibility complex (MHC), that identifies the antigen to aid in T-cell and B-cell recognition and response. The MHC process is discussed later in this chapter. When APCs attack an antigen, such as bacteria or a virus, they secrete signaling proteins (cytokines) that stimulate both the innate and adaptive immune response. **Mast cells** are heavily granulated and are found in the skin and lining of the respiratory and gastrointestinal tracts. Similar to basophils, they release heparin and histamine during the early inflammatory response. Mast-cell degranulation is responsible for many allergic reactions, including anaphylaxis, a severe systemic allergic reaction that is rapid in onset and can be fatal.

Proteins
Cytokines

Cytokines, which include interleukins (ILs), interferon (IFN), and tumor necrosis factor alpha (TNFα) are small proteins that act to regulate immune responses. They are produced in response to specific antigens by cells of the acquired immune system. They have systemic and local signaling effects that enable them to signal cells of the immune system. The production of ILs occurs predominantly by macrophages and lymphocytes in response to the initiation of the inflammatory response. They are responsible for the general enhancement or suppression of inflammation and the stimulation of leukocyte production and maturation. Interferons are proteins that protect against viral infections and tumor growth. They do not destroy a virus directly; rather, they prevent the virus from infecting the surrounding healthy cells and interfere with its ability to replicate. Tumor necrosis factor alpha, produced primarily by macrophages, enhances inflammation and is involved in the regulation and production of immune cells. Interleukins and IFNs rely on TNFα to mount an effective inflammatory response.

Complement System

Complement, a complex system of proteins, provides cell-killing effects for both innate and acquired immunity. Initiation of the complement can activate every component

Table 18.2 Immunoglobulins	
Immunoglobulin	**Function**
IgA	Dominant Ig found in secretory-gland secretions such as breast milk, sweat, saliva, mucus, and tears
IgD	Located primarily on the surface of developing B lymphocytes
	Plays a role in B-cell activation
IgE	The least concentrated Ig that acts as a mediator of many common allergic responses
	Also acts as a defender against parasitic infections
IgG	Most abundant of the immunoglobulins. Transported across the placenta and effective against bacteria, viruses, and other toxins.
IgM	Largest of the Igs
	First antibody produced during the primary response to an antigen
	Expressed by competent B cells

Ig, Immunoglobulin.

of the inflammatory response as well as "complement" the antibacterial function of antibodies. Complement proteins are synthesized primarily in the liver and circulate in the bloodstream in an inactive form until activated by bacteria, viruses, fungi, tumor cells, antigen–antibody complexes, or endotoxins. The complement system is activated through classic, lectin, and alternative pathways. The classic pathway is activated by antibodies of the acquired immune system bound to their specific antigens to form an antigen–antibody complex. The lectin pathway is activated through exposure to bacteria rather than antibodies. The alternative pathway is activated by polysaccharides in gram-negative bacterial and fungal cell walls.

Physiology of the Immune Function

Innate Immune Response

Innate immunity provides protective barriers and an inflammatory response that is immediate, nonspecific, and without memory as first and second lines of defense against threats that are foreign. An important first step in the immune response is to differentiate whether an invader is self (a self-antigen on the host's cells) or non-self (a foreign antigen). If recognized as non-self (i.e., from antigens such as a pathogen, pollen, or foreign tissue or blood product), an attack is mounted to stop and destroy the invading microorganism or toxin. To aid in the identification of self versus non-self, and to identify antigens to allow for a specific adaptive immune response, a group of proteins, the **major histocompatibility complex (MHC)**, codes for the antigens on APC cell surfaces to aid in recognition by the immune cells. That coding occurs when an APC cell, most commonly a dendritic cell, encounters an antigen, consumes it, and "presents" it on its surface to allow recognition by the immune cells. In humans, this process is called the *human leukocyte antigen* (HLA) system.

Physical, Mechanical, and Biochemical Barriers

The first line of defense relies on anatomical and biochemical barriers for protection. These all work in concert to mount a passive defense against pathogens. The epithelial cells of the skin, mucous membranes, and protective linings of the organs provide protection through the mechanisms of sloughing, coughing, sneezing, vomiting, and urination. Working with the physical and mechanical barriers, biochemical surface and glandular secretions such as tears, saliva, perspiration, and earwax provide additional means of protection.

Inflammatory Response

The second line is the inflammatory response that occurs due to tissue damage, such as a break in the skin, that introduces microorganisms. Inflammation may also be initiated through noninfectious processes, such as trauma or exposure to noxious compounds. The goal of **inflammation** is to prevent and/or limit infection and further damage to the involved area, remove debris, and prepare the area of injury for healing. Cellular mediators involved in the inflammatory response include those in the circulation (neutrophils, eosinophils, basophils, platelets, monocytes, and lymphocytes) and those in tissue (macrophage and mast cells). The proteins involved include complement, clotting factors, kinins (inflammatory mediators generated after tissue injury), and cytokines.

Initiation of the inflammatory response includes vasodilation and increased permeability of the capillaries stimulated by histamine released by mast cells, kinins, and other inflammatory mediators, such as prostaglandins and leukotrienes. Vasodilation increases blood flow to the inflamed area, facilitating leukocyte movement (chemotaxis) to the affected site. Increases in permeability allow the leukocytes to move into the tissues. Once in the tissue, invading organisms are engulfed and phagocytized. In order to limit infection and further damage, an area of margination or a border is created through the formation of fibrinogen clots around the area. The action of the inflammatory cells creates excess fluid and debris that are then removed by lymphatic vessels. Moving through the lymphatics, offending antigens identified through this process come in contact with lymphocytes residing in the lymph nodes, initiating the adaptive immune response with the production of antibodies. Lastly, a promotion of fibrous scarring to facilitate tissue repair and healing is seen. Clinical evidence that can be observed as a result of this response includes the cardinal signs of inflammation: redness and heat due to the increased blood flow and increased metabolic activity, edema due to the accumulation of fluid in the affected area, and pain due to the injury and swelling. Drainage, serous exudate or pus (a combination of dead immune cells and digested bacteria), may also be seen. Systemically, fever, chills, malaise, and an elevated WBC count (leukocytosis) may also occur as a result of the inflammatory response (Fig. 18.7).

Adaptive Immune Response

The adaptive immune response to foreign antigens consists of cellular and humoral responses. The cellular response is mediated by the T lymphocytes, and the humoral response is mediated by the B lymphocytes. For an immune response to be initiated, the foreign antigen must be recognized as non-self upon presentation by APCs via the MHC molecule on its surface. Each T or B cell recognizes only one antigen, but together as a group, they can recognize a host of foreign antigens (Fig. 18.8).

Acquired after birth, the adaptive immune response develops through active or passive immunity. In active immunity, antibodies or T cells are produced either after natural exposure to an antigen during illness or infection or after immunization. Passive immunity happens when preformed antibodies or T lymphocytes are transferred from one individual to another. For example, a newborn

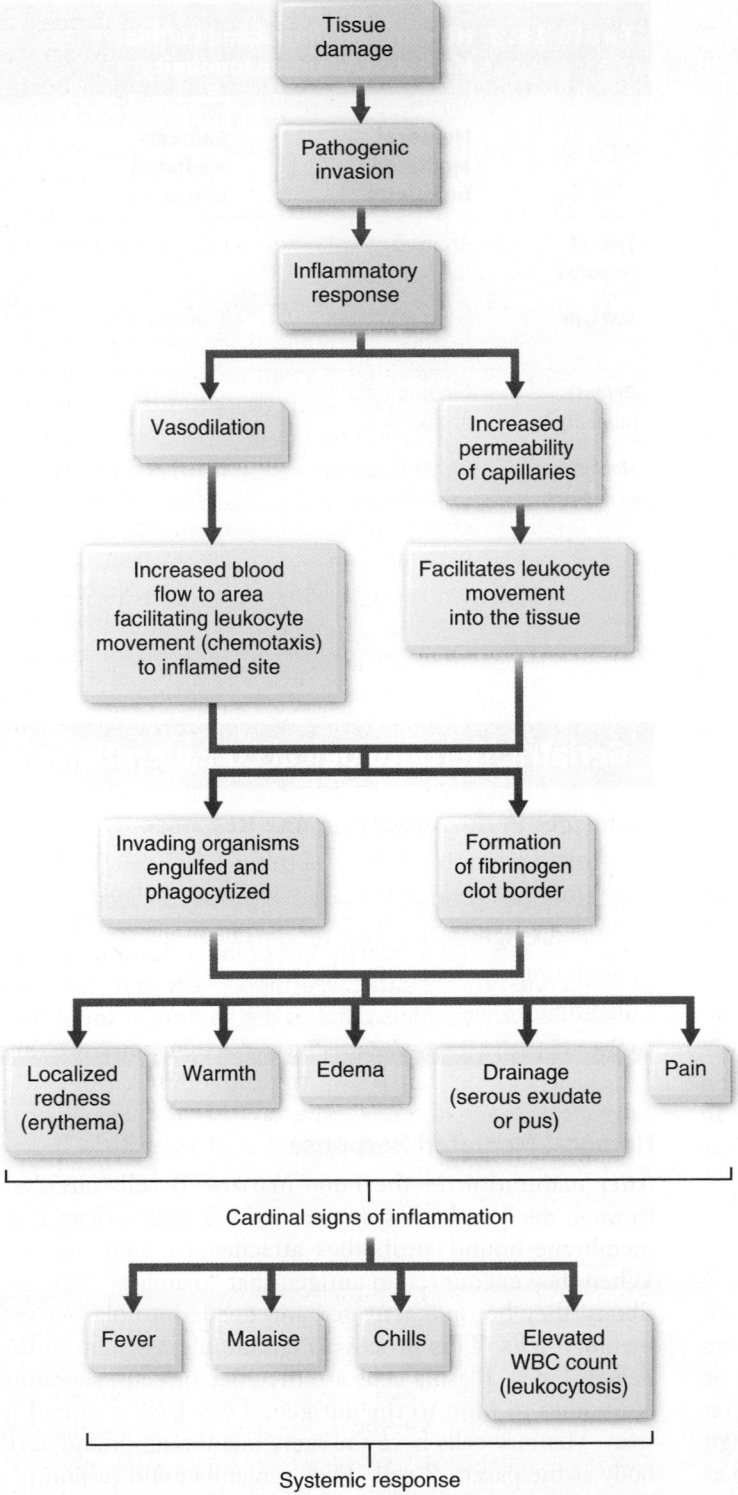

FIGURE 18.7 Acute inflammatory responses.

acquires immunity from his or her mother through the placenta, or an individual can acquire immunity through transfusion of antibody-laden blood products. Different from the immediate and nonspecific innate response, the adaptive immune response is delayed and very specific. It also has memory, which confers long-term protection (Table 18.3). Adaptive immunity works in tandem with innate immunity and relies on antigen-specific receptors on

T and B cells to mount a response against exposure to a threat or disease (see Fig. 18.8).

Cellular-Mediated Response

After formation in the bone marrow, undifferentiated T cells move to the thymus and develop specific surface antigen receptors in the process of maturation. *Naive* effector T cells (helper and cytotoxic T cells) leave the thymus and move to

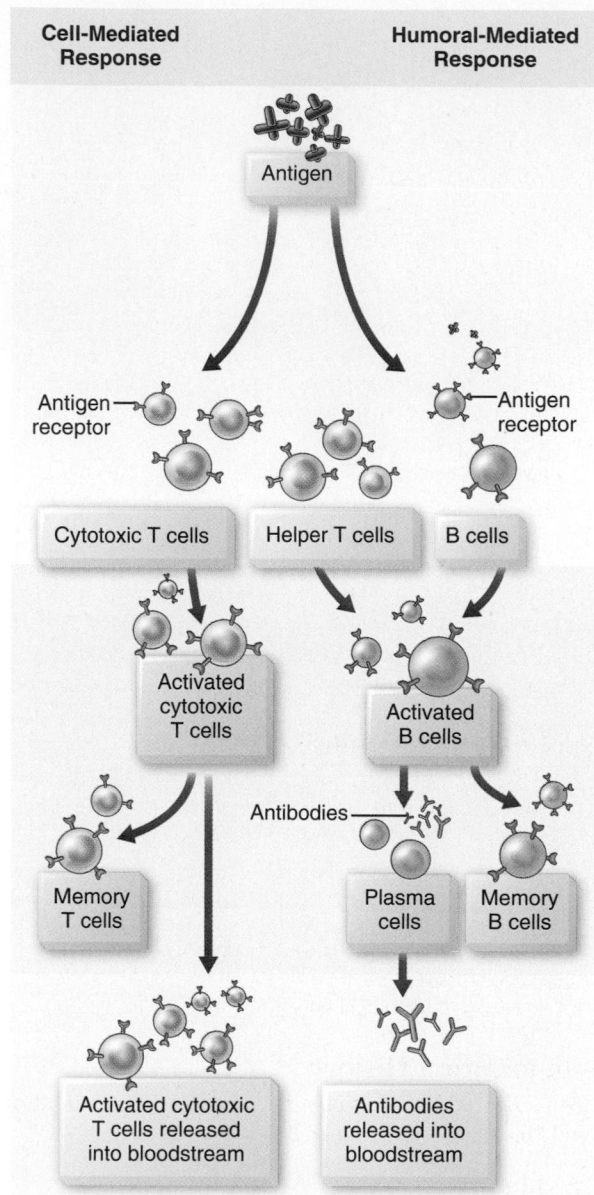

FIGURE 18.8 Adaptive immune response.

Table 18.3 Humoral-Mediated and Cellular-Mediated Adaptive Immunity

	Humoral-Mediated Immunity	Cellular-Mediated Immunity
Type of response	Antibody mediated	Cellular mediated
Cell type	B lymphocytes (B cells)	T lymphocytes (T cells)
Defense modality	Circulating antibodies	Cell-to-cell contact
Mechanism of defense	Defends against extracellular microorganisms: bacteria, viruses	Defends against intracellular microorganisms: viruses, fungi, bacteria, tumor and transplant antigens

Geriatric/Gerontological Considerations

Changes in the Aging Immune Response

The aged are noted to have a decline in T-cell function and antibody production when exposed to specific antigen challenges. They also tend to have an increase in circulating antibody levels, leading to autoimmune disorders.

Humoral-Mediated Response

After maturation in the bone marrow, B cells circulate through the lymphatic system as *naive* B cells with specific membrane-bound antibodies attached to their surface. When they encounter an antigen that "matches" their antibody, they become activated and divide into plasma and memory cells. This process is commonly assisted by the helper T cell. Plasma cells are the effector cells, secreting antibodies to bind to the antigen. They have a short life span. Memory cells have the same membrane-bound antibody as the parent B cell. They remember and respond to the same antigen if there is repeated exposure. They have a longer life span.

Antibodies defend against foreign substances in several ways. They can react between two antigens, causing them to clump, which is termed *agglutination*. Agglutination facilitates **phagocytosis** and enables the body to clear itself of the invading organism. Opsonization, a process in which the antigen–antibody binding is coated with a pasty substance, also facilitates phagocytosis and assists in the clearing of the invading organism.

lymphatic tissue throughout the body, ready for activation. This activation, followed by subsequent proliferation, occurs when there is binding of an antigen to a T-cell receptor following recognition through the MHC after presentation by the APCs. This allows direct destruction of foreign or abnormal cells and activation of other cells such as macrophages. This function is carried out by cytotoxic T cells. Activated T helper cells release signaling cytokines to other activated cells, B cells and cytotoxic T cells. This facilitates the process of proliferation and direct binding of the helper T cells to the B cells, which facilitates B-cell division to plasma cells and memory cells. T memory cells are also produced during this process to stimulate secondary cell-mediated immune responses. These memory cells have the ability to respond rapidly to additional exposures to the same antigen (see Geriatric/Gerontological Considerations).

CASE STUDY: EPISODE 2

CASE STUDY: EPISODE 2

The nurse practitioner at the clinic obtains a comprehensive health history and performs a physical examination on Ms. Hall. Her vital signs show her to have a low-grade fever, with a temperature of 100.2°F (37.8°C), a heart rate of 88 bpm, and a blood pressure reading of 128/82 mm Hg. Her examination is significant for an erythematous maculopapular rash with several vesicles on the right upper chest...

ASSESSMENT OF THE IMMUNE SYSTEM

Obtaining a comprehensive history and performing a thorough physical examination will assist the nurse in assessing a patient's immune function. Laboratory and other diagnostic tests are also helpful in the assessment of immune function.

History

Pertinent information to obtain from the patient or significant other includes the patient's age, current medications, allergies, and the current problem he or she is experiencing. Medications that have immune system side effects include antibiotics, anti-inflammatory and immunosuppressive agents, antimetabolites, antineoplastic agents, and thyroid-suppressive therapy. The medical and surgical history is also important to obtain in addition to the family and social history because some immunological problems are genetic or chemically induced. Also included should be nutritional status, infection history, prior immunizations, chronic illnesses, autoimmune disorders, and cancers.

Nutritional status is important to assess because suboptimal nutrition can negatively impact the immune system. Adequate vitamins and minerals are vital for the maturation of immune cells and their function. A fatty acid imbalance can have suppressive effects. Illness leading to inadequate oral intake may negatively alter nutritional status and the body's ability to fight off infection and disease. Childhood and adult immunizations should be assessed to make sure adequate protection is present. Tuberculin test administration and results and recent exposure to infections, including sexually transmitted diseases, are also important to assess. Box 18.1 details a comprehensive patient history. Table 18.4 details risk factors for immune system malfunction.

Physical Examination

Physical assessment includes the taking of vital signs; an inspection of the skin and mucous membranes; palpation of lymph nodes; and an examination of the neurological,

Box 18.1 Comprehensive Patient History

Current Problem
- Constitutional: fevers, chills, night sweats, weight loss, fatigue, malaise, rashes
- Dizziness; changes in mental status, memory, gait
- Shortness of breath, cough, wheezing
- Chest pain, palpitations, presyncope, syncope
- Loss of appetite, nausea, vomiting, diarrhea, abdominal pain
- Bleeding: site, characteristic, associated symptoms
- Enlarged nodes: site, characteristic, associated symptoms, predisposing factors
- Joint pain, stiffness, swelling, muscle weakness, myalgias, arthralgias
- Extremity swelling: unilateral/bilateral, characteristic, predisposing factors, associated symptoms, treatment
- Medications: chemotherapy, immunosuppression, antibiotics/antivirals, interferon, leukotriene antagonists
- Allergies and severity of reactions
- Physical activity and tolerance

Past Medical and Surgical History
- Childhood illnesses
- Medications: chemotherapy, antibiotics, immunosuppression, steroids
- Malignancy
- Recurrent infections
- Surgery or trauma (splenectomy)
- Chronic illnesses with or without risk factors
- Blood transfusions
- Tuberculosis (TB) or other infectious history

Immunization History
- Immunizations based on current Centers for Disease Control and Prevention (CDC) immunization guidelines

Family History
- Malignancy
- Anemia
- Recent infections
- TB history
- Immune disorders
- Hemophilia

Social History
- Lifestyle factors
- Smoking status
- Alcohol intake
- Illicit drug use
- Recent foreign travel
- Employment history
- Environmental exposure history

Table 18.4 Immune System Infection Risk Factors

Problem	Impact
Hepatic disease	Decreased neutrophil count
	Decreased phagocyte action
	Diminished immunoglobulin production
Malnutrition	Decrease in white blood cell count
	Diminished neutrophil activity
Pulmonary disease	Decreased neutrophil activity
Radiation therapy	Decreased white blood cell production
	Damage to first-line barrier defenses
Renal disease	Decreased neutrophil action
	Decreased immunoglobulin activity
Splenectomy	Loss of recognition and encapsulation of bacteria
Surgery	Disruption of normal flora
	Disruption of barrier defenses
	Reduced neutrophil action
Trauma	Disruption of barrier defenses
	Contamination from soil, water, objects

respiratory, cardiovascular, gastrointestinal, genitourinary, and musculoskeletal systems. In a patient with immune dysfunction, the normal inflammatory responses may be blunted, and subtle changes may be present.

Inspection

The nurse should perform a thorough assessment, inspecting each area of the patient's body for evidence of an immune disorder. Look for hypothermia or hyperthermia, enlarged lymph nodes, or edema. Also important to inspect are changes in skin color and skin integrity, rashes, dermatitis-type lesions, hematomas, petechiae, or purpura. Changes in level of consciousness, cognition, gait, and vision and hearing are important to note. Also important are changes in the respiratory system, such as tachypnea, air hunger, retractions, coughing, and nasal flaring. Collect and examine the urine for sediment, odor, and blood. Stool samples should be assessed for blood, smell, and the presence of diarrhea.

Auscultation

Listen to the lungs for adventitious (abnormal) breath sounds such as crackles, wheezing, rubs, or rhonchi. Also note if there is any decrease in or absence of breath sounds. Listen to heart sounds; note if tachycardia, rubs, or irregularity of heart rhythm is present. Check for bowel sounds and note if they are hyperactive, hypoactive, or absent.

Palpation and Percussion

Palpate the skin to check the temperature and whether clamminess is present. Also examine the lymph nodes for evidence of enlargement or tenderness. With light palpation, move the skin over the areas where nodes may be palpable. Nodes are not easily palpable in a healthy adult. If nodes are noted to be enlarged, tender, or fixed in position, this is cause for concern. Explore the adjacent area and regions that are drained by the enlarged node for signs of infection or malignancy. Cancerous nodes are not usually as tender as those from an infection or inflammatory process.

To assess the abdomen, perform light and deep palpations with percussion to assess for hepatosplenomegaly (enlargement of the liver or spleen), palpable masses, and the presence of abdominal fluid or abdominal pain. The liver and spleen may be enlarged because of infections, primary or metastatic cancer, or diseases of the blood or lymph system. Joints should be examined for mobility, pain, swelling, warmth, and erythema.

DIAGNOSTIC STUDIES

Diagnostic studies, including blood tests, skin tests, bone marrow aspiration and biopsy, and radiological imaging, may be necessary to evaluate the state of an individual's immune competence. Immune deficiencies that may occur can be primary (due to aberrant development of immune cells or tissues) or secondary (due to outside interference of the normal immune system) in nature. The disorders that follow may be due to infection, autoimmunity, hypersensitivity, or gammopathies (caused by abnormal protein produced by plasma cells). AIDS, which is caused by HIV, is an example of a secondary immune deficiency caused by a viral infection. Autoimmunity refers to the body's attack against tissue that is self, causing organ or tissue dysfunction. Hypersensitivity occurs when an exaggerated response to an antigen is present, and gammopathies are caused by an overproduction of Igs from the plasma cell.

Tests to evaluate immune disorders are obtained to identify antibody deficiencies, T-lymphocyte and neutrophil defects, and complement abnormalities. Specific tests to evaluate problems are based on the assessment and are related to the suspected deficiency or disorder. For example, if the patient has a history of chronic bacterial infections, a complete blood count (CBC) with differential to evaluate individual leukocyte counts may be ordered. If the patient is fighting an infection, a CBC to evaluate the WBC count and inflammatory markers such as C-reactive protein may be drawn to evaluate responsiveness to a prescribed antibiotic. If neutropenia (low neutrophil count) with a low absolute neutrophil count (ANC) is present, reverse isolation may be necessary to protect the patient from infections. Immune system deficiencies and disorders are more thoroughly discussed in additional chapters of this textbook.

The patient undergoing an immunological workup requires adequate preparation, education, and counseling regarding the studies that are ordered. Teaching will allow the patient to be prepared for the procedure. Ideally, the patient should repeat what he or she has been taught to evaluate comprehension of the material and should be encouraged to ask questions if clarification is needed. Patients may feel anxious or frightened about the pain and discomfort they might experience while undergoing testing. They may also experience anxiety and distress over a diagnosis based on test results. The nurse and health-care team should be ready to provide information and support. A summary of diagnostic studies can be found in Table 18.5.

Table 18.5 Diagnostic Tests for Immune Function

Function Evaluated	Diagnostic Test	Test Interpretation	Nursing Considerations
Leukocytes	Complete blood count with differential	Measures total leukocytes, with a breakdown of leukocyte types and percentage present	For all testing, provide patient teaching on what to expect, what the test is, and why it is being done.
		Increases in leukocytes with an increase in immature neutrophils, also know as band neutrophils, indicates infection or inflammation; referred to as a left shift	
	Leukocyte (white blood cell) total	Normal values: 4.5–11.1 10^3/mm^3	
	Differential:	Normal values: Number (%)	
	● Neutrophils	6,300 (40–70)	
	● Lymphocytes	4,100 (20–40)	
	● Monocytes	1,800 (2–8)	
	● Eosinophils	250 (1–3)	
	● Basophils	60 (less than 1)	
	● Absolute neutrophil count (ANC)	ANC calculates number of neutrophils available for fighting bacterial infections	
	● Absolute lymphocyte count (ALC)	ALC calculates number of lymphocytes available to fight viral and opportunistic infections	
Inflammation	Erythrocyte sedimentation rate	Screening for presence of inflammatory process	
	C-reactive protein	Detected if inflammatory process or tissue destruction is present	
Humoral immunity	Antibody production:		
	● Total immunoglobulin (Ig) levels: IgA, IgG, and IgM	Presence of antibody-producing B cells	
	● Levels of antibodies against vaccines	Ability to produce IgM, IgG antibodies	
	B-cell numbers:		
	● Lymphocytes with surface Ig	Presence of circulating B cells	
	● Flow cytometry		
Cellular immunity	Delayed hypersensitivity skin test:		
	● Skin test to measure reaction to exposed antigens	Presence of antigen-responsive T cells	

Continued

Table 18.5 Diagnostic Tests for Immune Function—cont'd

Function Evaluated	Diagnostic Test	Test Interpretation	Nursing Considerations
	T-cell numbers: • Numbers of T cells reacting to sheep erythrocytes or CD3 or CD11 antigen	Presence of circulating T cells	
	T-cell proliferation: • Proliferation response to mitogens (substances that stimulate mitosis)	Ability of T cells to divide with nonspecific stimulation	
	• Proliferation response to antigens	Ability of antigen-reactive T cells to respond to antigens	
Leukocyte and lymphocyte evaluation	Bone marrow evaluation: • Bone marrow aspiration	Status of blood-forming tissue	Prepare the patient for procedural specifics, including positioning and technique, pain or discomfort, and risk of bleeding or infection.
	• Bone marrow biopsy	Presence of hematological malignancies or primary bone marrow disorders	
Hypersensitivity	Tissue allergy panel	Ability to mount an antibody response to an injected antigen	Prepare the patient for possible discomfort at injection site and positive wheal reaction.
Phagocytic cell function	Nitroblue tetrazolium test	Status of phagocytic cell function to evaluate for chronic granulomatous disease	
Complement	Complement component: • Complement CH50 • Complement C3 level	Decreased if secondary deficiencies or autoimmune disorders	
	• Complement C4 level	Decrease can increase risk for pulmonary infections	
	• Complement fixation ratio	Decrease present with immune complex disease	
		Immunofluorescence to detect antigen–antibody reactions	
Specific antigen–antibody panels	Hepatitis A or B, cytomegalovirus, or respiratory syncytial virus	Immunofluorescence to detect antibodies or core antigens to specific viral antigens	
Organs and structures	Radiologic imaging: computed tomography scan, magnetic resonance imaging, ultrasound, positron emission tomography (PET) scan	Imaging to detect presence of lymphadenopathy, tumor formation, or metastatic disease	If contrast necessary, confirm absence of iodine allergy or previous contrast intolerance. Patient may be NPO for a period of time prior to the scheduled test. If patient claustrophobic, sedation may be necessary. For PET scan, blood sugar must be under 200 mg/dL.

AGE-RELATED CHANGES

Immune competence may decrease as the immune system changes and weakens with age. Aging has been noted to negatively affect both the innate and adaptive immune responses. *Immunosenescence* refers to those changes that occur with aging and their consequences—increased infection risk, increased risk of malignancy, and increased autoimmune disorders. Pneumonia and influenza are seen at much higher rates and are included in the top 10 causes of death for individuals aged 65 years and older. Atrophy of the thymus gland enhances with age, increasing the risk of viral infections. A greater incidence of shingles (herpes zoster virus) is seen in the older population; therefore, the shingles vaccine (Shingrix or Zostavax) is recommended for those 50 years of age and older.

Innate and adaptive immune responses actively provide defense against tumor cells. These responses decline with aging, creating an increased incidence of cancers. Older adults are also noted to have a decline in T-cell production and function and in antibody production when exposed to specific antigen challenges. They also tend to have an increase in the production of autoantibodies, leading to autoimmune disorders. Autoimmune disorders such as polymyalgia rheumatica, rheumatoid arthritis, and systemic lupus erythematosus are examples of problems due to increased autoantibody production.

A decrease in B-cell production and function and antigen-specific Ig activity may also be seen, creating a diminished immune memory and delayed hypersensitivity reactions. Malnutrition, which is associated with immune system defects, is sometimes seen in the older individual as a result of chewing and swallowing problems, blunted taste sensations, and chronic conditions that interfere with the absorption of food and nutrients. Additionally, economic factors, medication side effects, depressive moods, and decreased social interaction may all negatively impact oral intake and nutritional status in the aging population negatively impacting the immune response. Figure 18.9 and Table 18.6 detail age-related changes in the immune system.

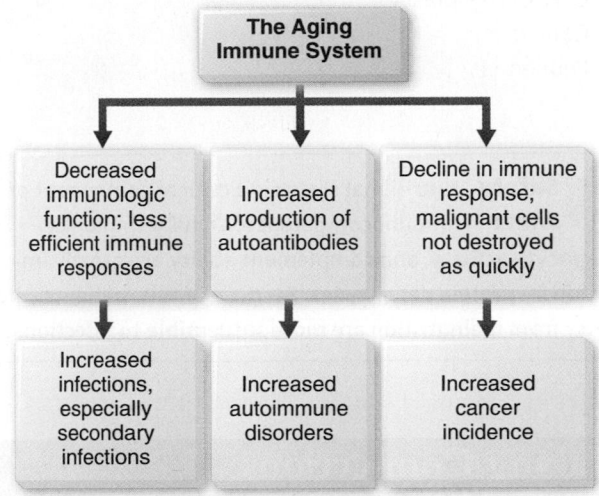

FIGURE 18.9 Age-related changes in the immune system.

Table 18.6 Age-Related Changes in the Immune System	
Innate Immune Response Changes	**Adaptive Immune Response Changes**
Hematopoietic cells	Thymic precursors
• Decreased number in bone marrow	• Decreased thymic size
• Decreased proliferation ability	• Decreased number of thymic precursors
Macrophages	T lymphocytes
• Decreased precursors in bone marrow	• Decreased number of immature T cells
• Decreased phagocytic capacity	• Decreased T-cell diversity
Neutrophils	• Decreased proliferation ability
• Decreased phagocytic capacity	• Decreased signaling ability
	• Decreased regulatory T-cell function
Natural killer cells	B lymphocytes
• Decreased number and percentage	• Decreased precursors in bone marrow
Dendritic cells	• Decreased peripheral B cells
• Increased number of myeloid dendritic cells	• Decreased antibody response
	• Increased autoreactive antibodies in the circulation

Connection Check 18.5

The nurse associates which of the following findings with immunosenescence in a 68-year old woman? *(Select all that apply.)*

A. Pneumonia

B. Shingles

C. Cervical dysplasia

D. Cancer

E. Leukemia

> **⚠ Safety Alert** Nutritional status is a critical component of immunocompetence. Cellular immunity, phagocyte activity, and complement ability are greatly impacted by protein deficiencies. Because of this, patients who suffer from malnutrition are more susceptible to infections.

Making Connections

CASE STUDY: WRAP-UP

Based on Ms. Hall's history of presenting symptoms and physical examination, she was diagnosed with herpes zoster (shingles). Herpes zoster is a reactivation of the chickenpox or varicella-zoster virus (VZV) that can result in post-herpetic neuralgia.

The nurse practitioner instructs Ms. Hall to increase her fluid intake and avoid exposure to individuals who may be immunosuppressed. She is instructed to immediately report if she develops increasing fever or pain. She will follow up every 1 to 2 weeks until resolution of her symptoms.

Case Study Questions

1. The nurse caring for a patient with herpes zoster incorporates which nursing diagnosis into the plan of care?
   A. Risk for bleeding
   B. Persistent fatigue
   C. Pain
   D. Inadequate nutrition

2. The nurse monitors for which advancing clinical manifestations in a patient diagnosed with shingles? *(Select all that apply.)*
   A. Worsening pain
   B. High fever
   C. Malaise
   D. Nausea
   E. Headache

3. A nurse providing care for a patient with shingles understands that the illness is caused by reactivation of which of the following viruses?
   A. Cytomegalovirus
   B. Epstein–Barr virus (EBV)
   C. Varicella-zoster virus (VZV)
   D. Human immunodeficiency virus (HIV)

4. The nurse includes which information in the teaching plan about the management of shingles?
   A. Limit fluid intake
   B. Encourage bed rest
   C. Post-herpetic neuralgia can develop
   D. Take antibiotics as directed

5. Which statement by Ms. Hall indicates that teaching has been effective?
   A. "I'm so glad I can continue my exercise schedule."
   B. "I need to stay away from my aunt who had a kidney transplant."
   C. "So I should contact you if I have more blisters appear?"
   D. "I don't drink a lot of fluids, so it shouldn't be hard for me to limit my fluid intake."

CHAPTER SUMMARY

The immune system is a network that remains in a continual mode of surveillance and on constant alert to defend the body against infection and disease. Lymphoid organs work in collaboration with specialized immunity and immune responses to afford this protection. Innate and adaptive immunity involve first-, second-, and third-line defenses that include physical and chemical barriers and inflammatory, cell-mediated, and antibody-mediated responses. Multiple bodily structures, including the circulatory, respiratory, and gastrointestinal systems, are involved in these protective mechanisms and work in concert to protect the host against infection and invasion by microorganisms.

Components of the immune system include the lymphatic system, the primary and secondary lymphoid organs, and the cells and proteins involved in the immune response. The lymphatic system defends the body against the invasion of microorganisms and consists of lymphatic vessels, lymph fluid, and collecting ducts. Primary lymphoid, or central, organs include the thymus and bone marrow. Secondary lymphoid, or peripheral, organs include the spleen, lymph nodes, tonsils, adenoids, and Peyer's patches.

Innate immunity provides the first two lines of defense. The first line is through anatomical, biochemical, genetic, or physiological barriers that include the skin and mucous membranes. Inflammatory responses provide the second line of defense with the assistance of IFN, complement, and phagocytosis. This response is rapid, nonspecific, and void of memory cells. Neutrophils are phagocytes and early responders to inflammation. Monocytes and macrophages respond later and stay longer to clean up debris at the site of inflammation. Eosinophils defend against parasitic infiltration, whereas NK cells eliminate viruses and cancer cells. Cytokines, including INF, IL, and TNF, are regulators of the inflammatory response. Local manifestations of inflammation include redness, heat, swelling, and pain.

The third line of defense is through adaptive immunity, which is acquired through natural or artificial exposure to an infection, antigen, or vaccine. This type of immunity protects through cell-mediated and antibody-mediated mechanisms by providing a specific antigen–antibody response with B- and T-cell activation. It can be active or passive immunity depending on whether the immune response originated in the host or in a donor.

When immune competence is present, the immune system prevents the penetration of foreign microbes or antigens and the proliferation of abnormal or malignant cells. Conversely, immune incompetence can lead to allergies, infection, cancer, and autoimmune and immunodeficiency disorders. Age, medications, nutrition, genetics, physical or emotional stress, and illness can all impact immunity and immune responses, thereby influencing the overall function of the immune system.

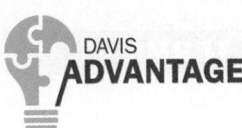

To explore learning resources for this chapter, go to **Davis Advantage** and find:
- Answers to in-text questions
- Chapter Resources and Activities
- NCLEX®-Style Chapter Review Questions
- Bibliography

Chapter 19

Coordinating Care for Patients With Immune Disorders

Diane J. Morey

LEARNING OUTCOMES

Content in this chapter is designed to assist in:

1. Describing the epidemiology of immune dysfunction
2. Describing pathophysiological processes of immune dysfunction
3. Correlating clinical manifestations to pathophysiological processes of
   a. B-cell deficiencies
   b. T-cell deficiencies
   c. Secondary immune deficiencies—therapy based
   d. Excessive immune response
4. Describing the diagnostic results used to confirm the diagnoses of selected immune dysfunctions
5. Discussing the medical management of:
   a. B-cell deficiencies
   b. T-cell deficiencies
   c. Secondary immune deficiencies—therapy based
   d. Excessive immune response
6. Describing complications associated with selected immune dysfunctions
7. Developing a comprehensive plan of nursing care for patients with immune dysfunction
8. Designing a teaching plan for a patient with immune dysfunction

ESSENTIAL TERMS

Allergen
Anaphylaxis
Angioedema
Antibody
Antigen
Atopic
Autoimmunity
Autosomal dominant
B-cell deficiencies
B lymphocytes
Complement
Cytotoxic
Histamine
Hypersensitivity reactions
Immunoglobulin E (IgE)
Immunoglobulin G (IgG)
Immunoglobulin M (IgM)
Immunosuppression
IV immune globulin (IVIG)
Primary immune dysfunction
Secondary immune dysfunction
T-cell deficiencies
Thymus gland
T lymphocytes
X-linked recessive

CONCEPTS

- Assessment
- Immunity
- Infection
- Inflammation
- Medication

Finding Connections

Follow this patient throughout the chapter.

Samuel Smith is a 50-year-old male patient who presents in the emergency department with a temperature of 101°F (38.3°C), a productive cough, fatigue, and difficulty breathing. He has a history of seasonal allergic rhinitis and mild asthma but no other significant health history. He does not report any known medication allergies. Initial orders include:

- Chest radiography
- Complete blood count
- Complete metabolic profile
- Pulse oximetry
- Sputum for culture and sensitivity...

Table 19.1 Warning Signs of Primary Immune Deficiency

Frequent Infections, Unusual Infections, or Unusual Complications of Usual Infections Are the Most Frequent Presentation of Immune Deficiency

- Eight or more new infections within 1 year
- Two or more serious sinus infections within 1 year
- Two or more months on antibiotics with little or no effect
- Two or more pneumonias within 1 year
- Failure of an infant to gain weight or grow normally
- Recurrent deep skin or organ abscesses
- Persistent thrush in the mouth or elsewhere on skin after age 1
- Need for IV antibiotics to clear infections
- Two or more deep-seated infections
- A family history of immune deficiency

INTRODUCTION

The immune system provides defense against microorganisms through first-line barriers to infection and the inflammatory and immune response. Additionally, it prevents the proliferation of cancer cells and initiates the healing of damaged tissue. Immune disorders may be due either to a deficiency or to overactivity and may involve one or more components of the immune system. Deficiency can result in disease processes; overactivation results in reactions that include **anaphylaxis** and autoimmune disorders.

OVERVIEW OF PRIMARY AND SECONDARY IMMUNE DYSFUNCTION

Primary immune dysfunction occurs in persons born with an immune system that is deficient or is limited in its ability to function. In this case, there is an intrinsic (inborn), congenital, or genetic cause. Most are inherited diseases, but some are the result of the interaction of predisposing genetic factors and environmental factors. These primary immunodeficiencies result from defects in **T lymphocytes**, B lymphocytes, natural killer cells, phagocytic cells, or the complement system. The majority are diagnosed in childhood. Table 19.1 lists warning signs that a primary immune dysfunction is present.

    Secondary immune dysfunction, or acquired immune deficiency, occurs when there is damage caused by an extrinsic or external environmental factor or agent. This arises secondary to some other disease process or exposure to medications or chemicals. Examples of secondary immune dysfunction include immune deficiency caused by HIV disease, irradiation, chemotherapy, malnutrition, or burns.

Secondary immune dysfunction comprises the majority of deficiencies presented in the clinical setting.

PRIMARY IMMUNE DYSFUNCTION: B-CELL DEFICIENCIES

One classification of primary immune dysfunction involves **B-cell deficiencies**. B cells are involved in producing a humoral immune response, which is the **antibody** response. An antibody, or immunoglobulin, is produced in response to a foreign substance known as an **antigen**. B-cell deficiencies involve a lack of differentiation of B-cell precursors into mature B cells or a lack of differentiation of B cells into plasma cells. One example of a B-cell deficiency is X-linked agammaglobulinemia (XLA).

X-Linked Agammaglobulinemia

Epidemiology

Agammaglobulinemia is an **X-linked recessive** inherited or congenital primary immune deficiency. It is the most common of the primary immune deficiencies and accounts for approximately 50% of cases. The term *X-linked recessive* means that the gene that causes this disease is located on the X chromosome. Humans have 46 pairs of chromosomes. One pairing identifies sex. Females have two X chromosomes; males have an X and a Y. X-linked agammaglobulinemia primarily affects males because it is unlikely that females will inherit two X chromosomes carrying the altered gene. Males get only one X chromosome. If their one X chromosome carries an altered or disease-carrying gene, they will have symptoms of the disease. Females may inherit one altered gene, which makes them a carrier of the disease. Figure 19.1 illustrates the genetic inheritance of XLA. An individual with a family history has the potential of

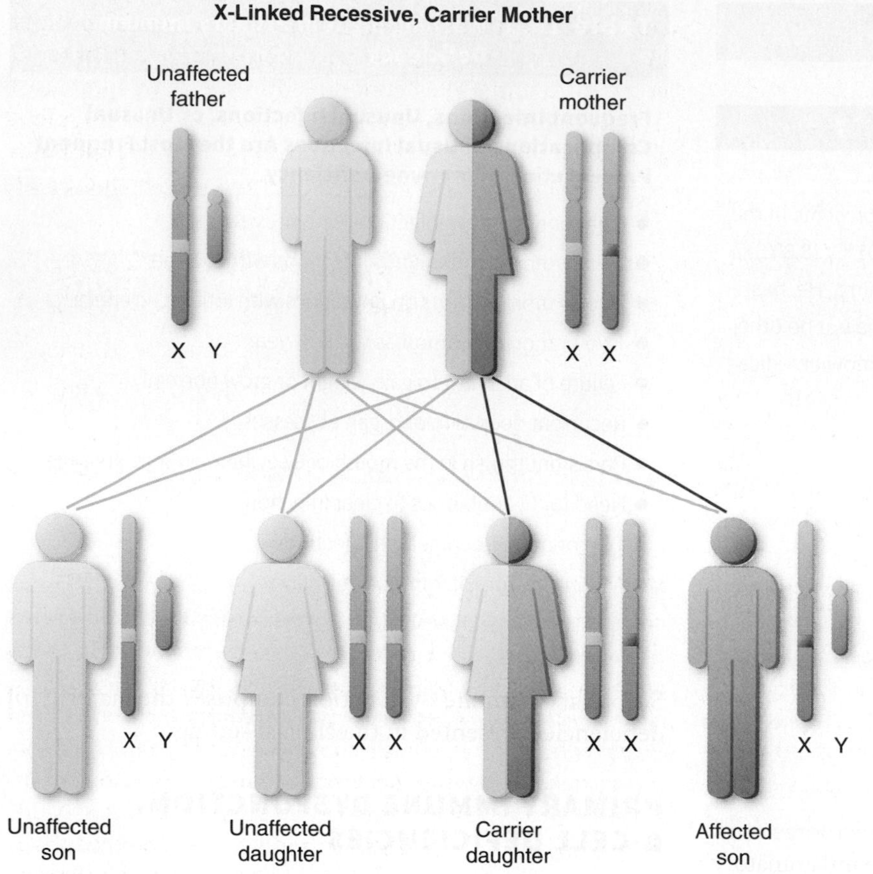

X-Linked Recessive, Carrier Mother

FIGURE 19.1 X-linked recessive genetic inheritance of disease. Males get only one X chromosome. The son who receives an altered gene on the X chromosome from his carrier mother will have symptoms of the disease. Females have two X chromosomes. The daughter who receives an altered gene on one X chromosome from her carrier mother will not manifest the disease but will be a carrier of the disease.

inheriting the disorder. It occurs at a frequency of about 1 in 250,000 male newborns. There is no ethnic predisposition. Prevalence is three to six per million males in all racial and ethnic groups. Symptoms do not appear until between 6 and 12 months of age because there is initial protection from the mother's antibodies. Many children die before their sixth birthday because of infection if the disorder is not identified and treated.

Connection Check 19.1

The nurse is screening patients for the risk of developing agammaglobulinemia. The nurse should consider which patient at greatest risk?

A. A 6-year-old female without any family history
B. A 35-year-old female with a respiratory infection
C. A 7-month-old male with recurrent infections
D. A 40-year-old male with a family history

Pathophysiology

X-linked agammaglobulinemia, also known as Bruton's agammaglobulinemia, is the result of a mutation of the *BTK* gene. The *BTK* gene is present on the long arm of the X chromosome, and its defect results in a deficiency of

Bruton's tyrosine kinase, which is essential for the development of the B lymphocyte. B cells are specialized white blood cells (WBCs) that, when mature, produce special proteins called antibodies or immunoglobulins. The BTK protein transmits chemicals that alert B cells to mature and produce antibodies. This type of B-cell deficiency is one in which immature B cells are present in normal numbers but are unable to mature. The inability to produce antibodies in response to the invasion of an antigen leaves the patient prone to severe bacterial infections.

Clinical Manifestations

Clinical manifestations include infections of the ears, lungs, skin, conjunctiva, and central nervous system. The presence of recurrent bacterial infections of the respiratory tract in childhood is the first indicator of the possibility of this disease. Chronic respiratory infections such as sinus infections and pulmonary disease are common clinical manifestations. Serious infections can develop in the bloodstream and internal organs. Patients can have recurrent pneumonia, meningitis, and septicemia with organisms such as *Streptococcus pneumoniae* and *Haemophilus influenzae*. They may also develop autoimmune disease, leukemia, or lymphoma. Patients tend to cope well with most short-term viral infections but are very susceptible to chronic viral infections such as hepatitis, polio, and enterovirus viruses.

Management

Medical Management

Diagnosis

Obtaining a detailed family history and history of infections is an important first step in a patient suspected to have an abnormal immune response. Frequent infections such as otitis media, more severe infections requiring hospitalizations, or atypical infections can be indicators. Diagnostics include B-lymphocyte surface marker assays, which identify specific cells involved in the immune response. These are general tests that can aid in the diagnosis of primary immunodeficiency disorders. They diagnose disorders by identifying abnormal numbers and percentages of B lymphocytes and help to evaluate immunodeficiencies. In X-linked agammaglobulinemia (XLA), blood tests indicate a lack of circulating B cells as well as low levels of immunoglobulins. A Western blot test can be done to determine if the BTK protein is being expressed—determining if the effects of the gene are appropriately manifested in a person. BTK expression is reported as present, absent, partial deficiency, or mosaic. Mosaic BTK expression indicates a carrier. Genetic testing can confirm the diagnosis. Women with a family member with XLA should seek genetic counseling. Periodic radiographs of the chest or sinuses in a child at risk are utilized to detect any signs of infection in its early stages.

Connection Check 19.2

The nurse monitors for which clinical manifestations in the patient diagnosed with XLA?
A. Low temperature
B. Recurrent respiratory infection
C. Low blood pressure
D. Diarrhea

Treatment

Treatment includes giving **IV immune globulin (IVIG)** to provide short-term passive immunity (see Geriatric/Gerontological Considerations). IV immune globulin is a sterilized solution made from human plasma. It contains the antibodies, mostly **immunoglobulin G (IgG)** or gamma globulin, to help protect against infection from various diseases. The dosage and the schedule are individualized, but typically IV immune globulin is given every 3 or 4 weeks. Gamma globulin can also be given by weekly subcutaneous injections. Both routes provide therapeutic concentrations of serum IgG.

Patients take a low dose of prophylactic antibiotics regularly, even when feeling well, if the episodes of infection are frequent. The aim of prophylactic antibiotics is to prevent an infection from starting. Aggressive treatment with specific antibiotics is initiated when the patient exhibits overt signs of infection. Patients should have an antibiotic

course at least twice as long as that used in normal, healthy individuals. Immunization with killed viral and bacterial vaccines is sometimes done to aid in the development of T-cell-mediated immune response, which may augment the protection that is obtained through immunoglobulin replacement. Vaccination with live viruses is contraindicated.

Geriatric/Gerontological Considerations

Geriatric patients have an elevated risk of acute renal failure, arterial or venous thrombosis, hemolysis, and allergic/hypersensitivity reactions during IVIG treatment.

Complications

Children with this disorder are prone to many different complications. Approximately 60% of individuals with XLA develop a severe, life-threatening bacterial infection, such as pneumonia, empyema, meningitis, sepsis, cellulitis, or septic arthritis. They may also develop a chronic viral enterovirus. When IV gamma globulin became available in the mid-1980s, the incidence of chronic enteroviral infection markedly decreased in individuals with XLA. However, some patients still develop enteroviral encephalitis, and some have neurological deterioration of unknown etiology.

> **! Safety Alert** Of patients with X-linked agammaglobulinemia (XLA), 5% to 10% developed vaccine-associated polio after vaccination with the live attenuated oral polio vaccine. For that reason, children with XLA and their siblings should be given inactivated polio vaccine rather than oral polio vaccine.

Nursing Management

Assessment and Analysis

Many of the clinical manifestations observed in the patient with XLA are directly related to infection of the respiratory tract, skin, conjunctiva, or ears. Common findings include:

General:
- Fever
- Changes in behavior (inconsolable crying), eating patterns, irritability, decreased activity

Respiratory:
- Increased respiratory rate
- Absent or decreased lung sounds

Skin:
- Rash
- Lesions

Conjunctiva:

- Redness or drainage

Ear:

- Pulling at the ears

Nursing Diagnosis

- **Risk for infection** related to compromised host defenses secondary to B-cell immunodeficiency

Nursing Interventions

■ Assessments

- Vital signs
  Increased temperature may indicate the presence of infection; respiratory rate may increase with respiratory infections in an effort to increase oxygenation.
- Assess lung sounds.
  Decreased or absent breath sounds or adventitious breath sounds may be present, with excessive secretions being common with respiratory infections.
- Inspect eyes and ears, skin and nails, rashes and lesions.
  Red, inflamed ears indicate an ear infection. Recurrent ear infections are the most common infection prior to diagnosis. Red conjunctiva with drainage indicates conjunctivitis, a common manifestation. Skin rashes and infections are frequently seen.
- Evaluate the infant or child's behavior and eating patterns.
  Irritability, decreases in activity, and poor appetite are signs of infection and illness.

■ Actions

- Administer IV gamma globulin as ordered.
  IV immune globulin contains antibodies to protect against infection, providing short-term immunity.
- Administer prophylactic antibiotic therapy as ordered.
  Prophylactic antibiotics may prevent infections.
- Anticipate prompt treatment with antibiotics when infection is present.
  Aggressive organism-specific treatment with antibiotics should begin as quickly as possible to prevent the development of extensive and more severe infections.

■ Teaching

- Teach parents of at-risk children about the 10 warning signs of primary immunodeficiency, and instruct them to speak to their provider if there are more than one of the conditions listed in Table 19.1.
  Prompt detection of XLA is essential to manage infections and initiate proper treatment with IVIG to avoid life-threatening complications.
- Institute precautions to prevent infection and minimize any source of infection in the environment at home related to foods (particularly raw foods) and water, domestic animals, or unsanitary conditions. Additionally, sites that accumulate stagnant water—such as sinks, toilets,

waste pipes, cleaning tools, and facecloths—readily support microbial growth and can become secondary reservoirs of infection.
Potential sources of infection should be identified and controlled as much as possible.

- Protect the patient from any direct contact with anyone with a contagious illness.
  To prevent infection from others
- Safe food handling and storage practices
  Food-based microorganisms can be a source of infection.
- Signs and symptoms of infection and when to seek medical attention, particularly any temperature of 100.5°F (38°C) or more
  Infection requires immediate treatment, and the family should not wait to report fever or symptoms of infection in an immunocompromised infant or child.
- Good hand washing
  To prevent infection
- Information regarding genetic disorders and community support groups
  Support for the family regarding understanding of genetic disorders and peer support are useful to cope with the disorder and manage the care of the patient.

Evaluating Care Outcomes

Appropriate antibiotic therapy and treatment with IVIG can help patients with XLA lead normal, active lives. The family and patient should be provided with information regarding the importance of preventing infection and when to contact their healthcare provider. Most patients have a good prognosis if they start the antibody replacement early.

Other B-Cell Deficiencies

Common Variable Immune Deficiency

Common variable immune deficiency (CVID) is the second category of B-cell deficiency. It is due to a lack of differentiation of B cells into plasma cells. This results in low levels of circulating antibodies. There are normal levels of B cells, but they fail to differentiate into antibody-secreting cells. The genetic basis is unknown, but it occurs in first-degree relatives of persons with IgA deficiency. It is similar to XLA in that it manifests with recurrent bacterial infections, but the infections tend to be less severe. This deficiency differs from XLA in that it appears in adolescents or in young adults between 15 and 35 years of age. It occurs equally in men and women. Patients with CVID have a tendency to develop autoimmune disorders, interstitial lung disease, hepatitis, non-Hodgkin's B-cell lymphoma, gastric cancer, hepatitis, and intestinal malabsorption. Treatment is similar to that of XLA.

Selective Immunoglobulin A

Selective IgA is the most common type of immunoglobulin deficiency. It affects 1 in 400 to 1 in 1,000 persons. The pattern of occurrence in families suggests an autosomal inheritance, but there is variability in its expression. As another example of the second type of B-cell deficiency, the cause of this deficiency is likely due to a block in the pathway that provides for the final differentiation of mature B cells to IgA-secreting plasma cells. Two-thirds of persons have no symptoms because normal IgG and IgM levels compensate for the deficiency. Fifty percent of those affected overcome the deficiency by the age of 14. Persons with IgA deficiency may develop anaphylactic reactions when IgA immunoglobulin is administered because of antibodies against IgA. Thus, this treatment is not utilized routinely. If blood is necessary, specially washed erythrocytes or IgA-deficient donors are used.

Immunoglobulin G Subclass Deficiency

Immunoglobulin G subclass deficiency affects one or more of the IgG subtypes but does not affect the overall levels of IgG. Because antibodies directed against carbohydrate and polysaccharide antigens are primarily IgG2, those with IgG2 deficiency are at greater risk for the development of sinusitis, otitis media, and pneumonia that is caused by polysaccharide-encapsulated microorganisms such as *S. pneumoniae*, *H. influenzae* type B, and *Neisseria meningitides*. Those with mild forms can be treated with prophylactic antibiotics. Those with more severe symptoms can be treated with IVIG.

PRIMARY IMMUNE DYSFUNCTION: T-CELL DEFICIENCIES

T lymphocytes include subtypes CD4 helper and CD8 **cytotoxic** T cells. They are responsible for the cell-mediated immune response that protects against fungal, protozoan, viral, and intracellular bacterial infections. They are also responsible for controlling malignant cell proliferation and coordination of the immune response. **T-cell deficiencies** lead to infections and other problems that are more severe than B-cell deficiencies. An example of a T-cell deficiency is DiGeorge's syndrome.

DiGeorge's Syndrome

Epidemiology

DiGeorge's syndrome, or congenital thymic hypoplasia, is an **autosomal-dominant** genetic condition that arises from the 22nd chromosome. Autosomal dominant means that the presence of only one altered gene is required for the disease to be present. Figure 19.2 illustrates the genetic inheritance of DiGeorge's syndrome. This disorder arises spontaneously and is present at birth. It is hard to identify anyone at risk for this disorder, but gestational diabetes is implicated in increasing risk. A population-based study conducted by the Centers for Disease Control and Prevention (CDC) found a prevalence of

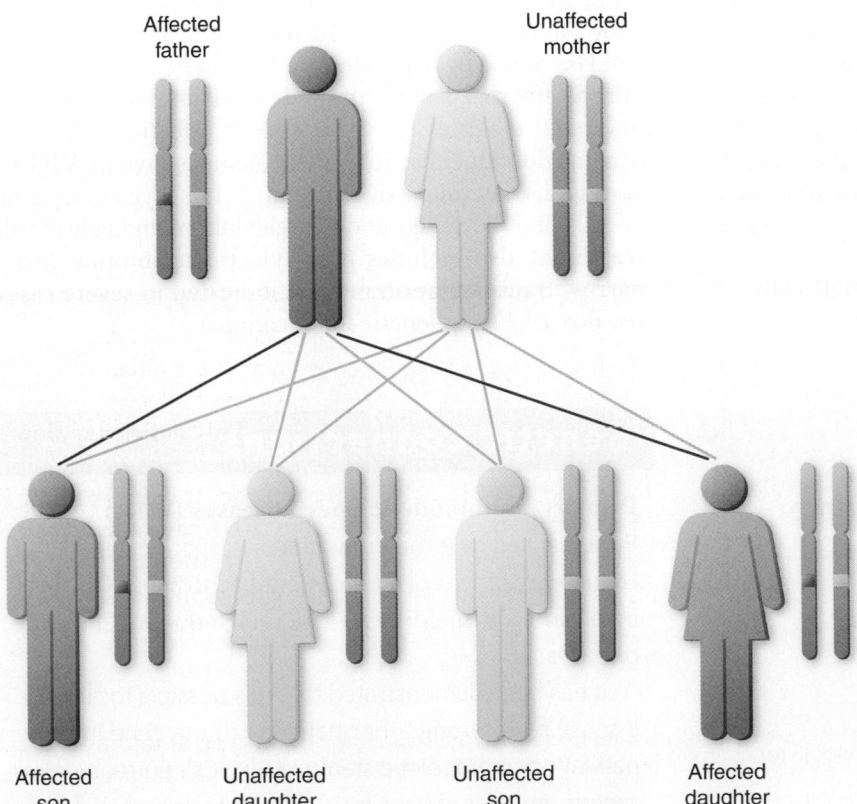

Autosomal Dominant

Affected father

Unaffected mother

Affected son

Unaffected daughter

Unaffected son

Affected daughter

FIGURE 19.2 Autosomal-dominant genetic inheritance of DiGeorge's syndrome. The child who receives the altered gene from an affected parent will manifest symptoms of the disease.

about 1 in 6,000 in whites, blacks, and Asians and 1 in 3,800 in Hispanics.

Pathophysiology

DiGeorge's syndrome arises from a disturbance of the normal embryological development of the pharyngeal pouches occurring between the 6th and 10th weeks of gestation. Pharyngeal pouches are the embryonic precursors to specific organ systems in the head, neck, and chest. For example, the third and fourth pharyngeal pouches develop into the thymus, parathyroid gland, and aorta. The pulmonary artery arises from the sixth pharyngeal pouch. The effects of DiGeorge's syndrome are dependent on which pharyngeal pouch is affected but typically involve dysfunction of the **thymus gland** and parathyroid, facial deformities such as cleft palate, and heart anomalies.

The thymus gland is responsible for T-cell production and differentiation. Thymus dysfunction results in T-cell deficiencies. The deficiencies vary depending on the amount of thymus that is affected. Because T cells help B cells mature, the lack of T cells usually affects B-cell activity also. T-cell function may improve with age depending on the severity of involvement.

Clinical Manifestations

Immune dysfunction caused by T-cell deficiencies results in recurrent infections. There are variations in the type and severity of dysfunction as a result of the extent of the body systems affected. If the patient has some limited thymic function, infections may be frequent but not necessarily severe. Infections include yeast, fungal, protozoan, and viral, such as chickenpox, measles, and rubella, which may be fatal. *Candida albicans* is almost always seen in patients with T-cell deficiencies. Frequent colds and ear infections are common. Other disorders are related to the specific body systems affected (Box 19.1). The acronym CATCH is formed by the first letter of each of these disorders. Because the disorder is caused by the deletion of a small piece of chromosome 22, the healthcare community sometimes refers to DiGeorge's syndrome as CATCH-22.

Other clinical manifestations include the following:

General

- Weakness or tiring easily
- Failure to thrive

- Failure to gain weight
- Difficulty feeding

Respiratory

- Frequent infections
- Shortness of breath
- Bluish skin due to low oxygen-rich blood

Other

- Twitching or spasms around the mouth, hands, arms, or throat
- Poor muscle tone
- Delayed development of infant milestones
- Delayed speech development
- Learning delays or difficulties, emotional and behavior problems
- Cleft palate or other problems with the palate
- Certain facial features, such as low-set ears, wide-set eyes, or a narrow groove in the upper lip

Management

Medical Management

Diagnosis

Diagnosis of the disorder is primarily done by genetic testing. DiGeorge's syndrome is determined with a finding of submicroscopic deletion of chromosome 22 detected by fluorescence in situ hybridization. Fluorescence in situ hybridization uses fluorescence microscopy to find specific features in DNA.

Treatment

Treatment includes pharmacological therapy, such as calcium supplements to prevent tetany and seizures, which could be caused by hypocalcemia from hypoparathyroidism if the parathyroid gland is affected. T-cell immune deficiency may require aggressive treatment of infections. As with agammaglobulinemia, treatment includes giving IVIG to provide short-term passive immunity. It is given every 3 or 4 weeks, and the dosage and the schedule are individualized. Treatment also includes prophylactic antibiotics. Bone marrow transplantation may be indicated in severe cases (see Box 19.2 and Genetic Connections).

Box 19.1 DiGeorge's Syndrome

The acronym CATCH summarizes the possible clinical manifestations of DiGeorge's syndrome:

- **C**ardiac abnormality (especially tetralogy of Fallot)
- **A**bnormal faces
- **T**hymic aplasia
- **C**left palate
- **H**ypocalcemia–hypoparathyroidism (See Chapter 43 for details.)

Genetic Connections

Primary Immunodeficiency Diseases (PIDs)

PID is caused by errors (mutations) in specific genes. The Human Genome Project has identified the specific genes involved in a majority of primary immunodeficiency diseases.

It has been demonstrated that it is possible to cure the disease by inserting a normal copy of the gene into the patient's hematopoietic stem cells (HSCs). Currently, viral vectors are tools utilized by molecular biologists to deliver genetic material into cells through a process known as insertional mutagenesis. This process is associated with risks and adverse effects, such as the development of leukemia-like disorders. Overcoming risks and determining safer vectors for gene therapy will allow for this process to become a more common and successful treatment. Gene therapy is still regarded as an experimental therapy. New and improved self-inactivating retroviral and lentiviral vectors that incorporate additional safety features are now in clinical trials.

Surgical Management

Surgery such as thymus tissue transplantation is an option if the thymus is absent. In that case, the child is extremely vulnerable to a number of severe infections. Ideally, the procedure is performed within 3 to 6 months of birth, prior to the onset of multiple infections. The tissue for this transplantation is obtained from infants having cardiac surgery. In cardiac surgery, in order to successfully visualize the heart, portions of the thymus gland are excised. With parental consent, that tissue can be saved for use in thymus transplantation for children with DiGeorge's syndrome. Surgery may also be an option to correct the cardiac defects of DiGeorge's syndrome, such as tetralogy of Fallot.

Box 19.2 Hematopoietic Stem Cell Transplantation

The process of taking hematopoietic stem cells (HSCs) from one person and transfusing them into another is called hematopoietic stem cell transplantation, or HSCT. Transplantation of HSCs represents the main treatment for several severe forms of primary immunodeficiency diseases. Traditionally, HSCs were obtained from the bone marrow but can now be obtained from peripheral blood or blood taken from the placenta at birth (umbilical cord blood). Transplantation of HSCs has the potential to replace the deficient immune system of the patient with a normal immune system and, thereby, effect a cure. The primary immunodeficiency diseases for which HSCT is most commonly performed include severe combined immune deficiency (SCID), Wiskott–Aldrich syndrome (WAS), and many other severe primary immunodeficiency diseases. Current challenges in HSCT include:

- Identifying candidates before significant damage from infection occurs
- If damage has occurred, determining the extent of tissue and organ involvement
- Recruiting donors with a match to the patient

Complications

DiGeorge's syndrome may cause problems with the development and function of the brain, resulting in learning, social, developmental, or behavioral problems. Delays in speech development and learning difficulties are common. Others develop disorders such as attention deficit-hyperactivity disorder, autism, or autism-related disorders. In later life, the patient is at increased risk of mental health problems, including depression, anxiety disorders, schizophrenia, and other psychiatric disorders.

Additionally, with a poor immune system due to the small thymus, patients may have an increased risk of autoimmune disorders, such as rheumatoid arthritis and Graves' disease. Patients with T-cell dysfunction are at risk for graft-versus-host disease. This is manifested when T cells in grafted tissue such as transfused blood attack and destroy the host's tissues.

Connection Check 19.3

The nurse is caring for a patient with DiGeorge's syndrome. Precautions are taken for decreased levels of which of the following?
A. B cells
B. Thyroid hormone
C. Serum calcium
D. Serum iodine

Nursing Management
Assessment and Analysis

The clinical manifestations of DiGeorge's syndrome are related to the disturbance of normal embryonic development of the pharyngeal pouches that leads to the eventual development of the thymus and parathyroid gland, facial structures, and cardiac structures. Table 19.2 summarizes the assessment data for DiGeorge's syndrome.

Nursing Diagnoses

- **Risk for complications** of opportunistic infections
- **Risk for infection** related to compromised host defenses secondary to T-cell immunodeficiency (inadequate function of B cells secondary to T-cell deficiencies)
- **High risk for ineffective airway clearance** related to laryngospasm secondary to hypocalcemia

Nursing Interventions
■ **Assessments**

- Vital signs
  Increased temperature may indicate infection; respiratory rate may increase with respiratory infections in an effort to increase oxygenation.
- Lung sounds
  Decreased or adventitious breath sounds may be present with a respiratory infection.
- Calcium levels
  Calcium levels may be decreased because of hypoparathyroidism.

Table 19.2 Assessment Data for DiGeorge's Syndrome

The Portions of Chromosome 22 Deleted in DiGeorge's Syndrome Play a Role in the Development of a Number of Body Systems and Result in Several Errors During Fetal Development

Assessment Data	Analysis/Explanation
● Recurrent infections	● Immunodeficiency occurs as a result of thymic hypoplasia, resulting in impaired T-cell production.
● Cardiac abnormality (especially tetralogy of Fallot) causes cyanosis, heart murmur, difficulty in feeding, failure to gain weight, retarded growth and physical development, dyspnea on exertion, clubbing of the fingers and toes, and polycythemia.	● Cardiac anomalies such as tetralogy of Fallot are a result of a disturbance of normal embryological development of the pharyngeal pouches—embryonic precursors to specific organ systems in the head, neck, and chest.
● Abnormal faces and craniofacial findings include auricular abnormalities, nasal abnormalities, "hooded eyelids," increased distance between the eyes (ocular hypertelorism), cleft lip and palate, asymmetric crying faces, and premature fusing of the cranial sutures.	● Deletion of the portion of chromosome 22 leads to abnormal development of the structures of the face.
● Cleft palate—velopharyngeal incompetence (VPI), which is the most common facial abnormality, may be a structural problem (short palate), a functional problem (hypotonia of the velopharyngeal musculature), or a combination of both.	● Because of the chromosome deletion, development of the palate is affected in utero. Sixty-nine percent of individuals with this syndrome have a palatal abnormality.
● Hypocalcemia	● Due to decreased functioning of the parathyroid gland, hypocalcemia is present in 17%–60% of patients and is most serious in the neonatal period.
● Assessment for possible feeding problems, such as significant gastroesophageal reflux; difficulty with sucking/swallowing, advancing feeds, addition of textured foods; and vomiting and constipation.	● About 30% of children have feeding difficulties: severe dysphagia requiring nasogastric tube feedings and/or gastrostomy tube placement related to nasopharyngeal reflux; prominence of the cricopharyngeal muscle, abnormal cricopharyngeal closure, and/or diverticulum; dysmotility in the pharyngoesophageal area.

● Tetany
Lack of plasma calcium due to hypoparathyroidism leads to increased neuromuscular activity such as sustained contractions.
● Monitor WBCs.
An increased WBC count is an indication of infection. Trending these values helps determine the presence of infection and evaluate the response to treatment.

▪ Actions

● Administer calcium supplements as ordered.
A low serum calcium concentration requires calcium supplementation to prevent complications such as tetany or bronchospasm.
● Infection control precautions and standard precautions, including thorough hand hygiene
Prevent infection: Implementation of hygiene practices is the best infection-preventive measure.
● Strategies for addressing feeding difficulties include modification of spoon placement when eating; treatment for gastroesophageal reflux with acid blockade, prokinetic agents, and postural therapy; and medication

to treat gastrointestinal dysmotility and facilitate bowel evacuation.
Feeding difficulties can occur with this syndrome in 30% of patients.
● Coordinate care for cardiac, infectious disease specialists, and speech pathologists.
An interprofessional evaluation involving healthcare providers from the following specialties is often necessary: genetics, plastic surgery, speech pathology, otolaryngology, audiology, dentistry, cardiology, immunology, child development, child psychology, and neurology.

▪ Teaching

● Overview of the disease process
It is important that the patient and family are able to both detect early signs of infection and prevent infection. Additionally, they need to understand the genetic disease.
● Growth and development milestones, need for early assessment for learning disabilities, need for ongoing medical care and evaluation
The family needs to know the normal developmental milestones in order to evaluate their child's development.

- Information and emotional support from networking with other parents of children with similar problems
The family needs to have community resources to provide support with their child's diagnosis.

Connection Check 19.4

What is the desired therapeutic effect of calcium supplements for the patient with DiGeorge's syndrome?
A. Improved muscular contractions
B. Prevention of tetany
C. Decreased heart rate
D. Increased bowel sounds

Evaluating Care Outcomes

The well-managed child has limited infections, no seizures, and growth and development within normal limits. This is accomplished through appropriate treatment with an interprofessional team, adequate monitoring for complications, and support for the caregivers of the child.

Other T-Cell Immune Deficiencies

DiGeorge's syndrome provides one example of a T-cell deficiency. Other T-cell deficiencies include chronic mucocutaneous candidiasis and hyper-IgM (HIGM) syndrome.

Chronic Mucocutaneous Candidiasis

Chronic mucocutaneous candidiasis is a T-cell disorder that is autosomal recessive. It involves the thymus and other endocrine glands, resulting in an autoimmune disorder. There is a combination of endocrine failure and immunodeficiency. Problems include hypocalcemia and tetany due to hypofunction of the parathyroid glands. There are recurrent *Candida* infections of the skin, nails, and mucous membranes. Morbidity is high because of endocrine dysfunction. Hypofunction of the adrenal cortex is the major cause of death.

Hyper-IgM Syndrome

Hyper-IgM (HIGM) syndrome is an X-linked immunodeficiency with low IgG and IgA serum levels, normal or high IgM and IgD levels, and absent IgG-specific antibodies. This was previously designated as a B-cell defect but is now known to be a T-cell defect. In this disorder, T cells do not have the ability to signal B cells to undergo switching to IgG and IgA and can produce only IgM. Although it is identified by the levels of antibodies, its cause is a defect in cell-mediated immunity. The estimated prevalence of HIGM is 2:1,000,000 males in families of European, African, and Asian descent. The diagnosis of HIGM is based on a combination of clinical findings, family history, and molecular genetic testing of CD40LG,

the only gene known to be associated with HIGM. As with XLA, clinical manifestations in boys are seen in the first 2 years of life. Recurrent infections include sinusitis, otitis media, tonsillitis, and pneumonia. Patients are also susceptible to opportunistic infections, especially *Pneumocystis jiroveci*, because of the cell-mediated immunity defect. Complications include the development of an autoimmune disease of the blood, such as hemolytic anemia, thrombocytopenia, and neutropenia.

Connection Check 19.5

The nurse correlates low levels of IgG with which disorder?
A. Selective IgA deficiency
B. CVID
C. HIGM syndrome
D. IgG subclass deficiency

PRIMARY IMMUNE DEFICIENCY OF BOTH T CELLS AND B CELLS

Severe combined immune deficiency (SCID) is a potentially fatal primary immunodeficiency. This disease involves a combined absence of T-lymphocyte and B-lymphocyte function. There are at least 13 different genetic defects that can cause SCID.

David Vetter, who was born with SCID, was known as the boy in the bubble. When he was born in 1971, a bone marrow transplant from an exactly matched donor was the only cure, and no one in his family was a match. For 12 years, David lived in a protected, germ-free environment at Texas Children's Hospital. In 1984, after receiving a bone marrow transfusion, David died from lymphoma, a cancer that was introduced into his system by the Epstein–Barr virus.

Another primary immunodeficiency disorder is Wiskott–Aldrich syndrome, which results from a combined B- and T-cell defect; its characteristics include recurrent infection, eczema, and thrombocytopenia. The bleeding problems are unique to this primary immunodeficiency disorder and are the result of unusually small, dysfunctional platelets. The inheritance is X-linked recessive.

Transitional Care

Primary Immune Dysfunction (PID) Adolescent and Adult Care

Pediatric patients are usually treated from an early age by the same physicians, nurses, and healthcare providers. The transition from adolescence to adulthood involves managing changes related to physical, social, psychological, and educational aspects of life. A defined and coordinated pathway guiding them toward adult services is necessary to avoid poor compliance with treatment, potential irreversible organ damage related to complications, reduced quality of life, and, very important, lower life expectancy as well as managing costs. A variety of disciplines related to PID services are required to coordinate adult care. They include:

- Access to essential providers:
  - Histopathologists familiar with lymphoid and infectious pathologies in PIDs
  - Respiratory medicine
  - Clinical hematology and hematological oncology
  - Gastroenterology (adult and pediatric)
  - Hepatology
  - Dermatology
  - Clinical genetics
- Access to:
  - Radiology services
  - Intensive care services
  - Other tertiary services may also be needed, for example, otorhinolaryngology (ENT), ophthalmology, neurology, and neurosurgery, as well as social services and psychiatric support

SECONDARY IMMUNE DYSFUNCTION: THERAPY-INDUCED DEFICIENCIES

Epidemiology

Secondary immune deficiencies are caused by a variety of factors, such as medication-induced **immunosuppression**, radiation, and surgery. The most common is medication-induced immunosuppression. Immunosuppressive therapy is prescribed to treat autoimmune disorders as well as to prevent transplant rejection. Immunosuppression is also a side effect of chemotherapy in the treatment of cancer. Chemotherapy can lead to leukopenia. This in turn results in decreased cell-mediated and humoral responses. Other medications that suppress the immune system are corticosteroids. Radiation therapy can also cause secondary immunodeficiency. Radiation destroys dividing and resting cells. With increased radiation, there is increased pancytopenia, which is a decreased number of all types of blood cells—red blood cells (RBCs), WBCs, and platelets. This causes a further suppression of the immune system function. Surgical removal of organs of the immune system, such as the lymph nodes, thymus, or spleen, also suppresses the immune response.

Pathophysiology

Chemotherapeutic medications used to treat cancer are cytotoxic, which means they target rapidly dividing cancer cells. Cells of the immune system are also naturally rapidly dividing and so are inadvertent targets of chemotherapeutic therapy. Cells such as WBCs, including lymphocytes and phagocytes, are destroyed by these medications. The result is a decrease in the number of circulating lymphocytes and phagocytes. Additionally, the medications cause general immunosuppression because remaining lymphocytes are unable to release antibodies and lymphokines, which are substances that bind to receptors on target cells, facilitating a directed immune response.

Immunosuppressive therapy, such as corticosteroid administration, is used to treat autoimmune disorders (discussed later in this chapter) or prevent transplant rejection by specifically targeting the immune system. The immunosuppressive medications interfere with cell-mediated immunity or the production of antibodies. Corticosteroids have anti-inflammatory effects in addition to immunosuppressive effects. The anti-inflammatory effects include stabilizing blood vessel membranes, decreasing permeability, and blocking the movements of neutrophils and monocytes. Immunosuppressive effects include decreased T cells because corticosteroids keep T cells in the bone marrow. This results in the suppression of cell-mediated immunity and lymphopenia as well as a decrease in the inflammatory response. There is also decreased IgG production and decreased antibody–antigen binding.

Management

Medical Management

Management of patients with secondary immune dysfunction is primarily preventive. Good hand washing is the first step. Avoiding contact with people who have obvious infections, such as a cough or cold, is recommended. Regular follow-up with the provider is necessary. Prompt action with any signs of infection, such as fever, chills, or cough, is essential. Any signs of urinary tract infection, such as difficulty with urination, bloody urine, or lower back pain, should be reported immediately.

Nursing Management
Assessment and Analysis

The goal of managing secondary immune deficiency is to protect the patient from infection. The nurse assesses for signs of infection, such as a fever over 100°F (37.8°C), chills, or cloudy and foul-smelling urine.

Nursing Diagnoses

- **Risk for complications** of opportunistic infections
- **Risk for infection** related to compromised host defenses secondary to therapy-induced immunodeficiency

Nursing Interventions
- **Assessments**
- Vital signs
  Increased temperature, hypotension, and tachycardia all indicate infection. The temperature increases in an attempt to kill organisms. Hypotension results because of

increased permeability causing fluid shifts and dehydration. Tachycardia occurs in an attempt to compensate for the hypotension.

- Signs of infection:
  - Monitor WBC and differential.
  Increased WBCs and leukocytes are part of the body's natural response to infection.
  - Breath sounds
  Decreased or adventitious breath sounds may be present with a respiratory infection.
  - Urine
  Cloudy or foul-smelling urine may indicate a urinary tract infection.
  - Skin
  Skin rashes or lesions indicate skin infections, which may occur with immunodeficiency.

■ Actions

- Practice good hand washing.
  Hand washing is the first step in preventing infections.
- Treat infection with antibiotics or antivirals as ordered.
  Antibiotics or antivirals specifically targeting the organism help control the infection.
- Anticipate changing or discontinuing the immunosuppressive medication if possible.
  With a change in medication, the cause of the secondary immune deficiency is removed. This is considered only if the infection is deemed a greater risk than the primary problem being treated with the immunosuppressive medications.

■ Teaching

- Avoid crowds or large gatherings, and avoid exposure to anyone with an obvious illness.
  To avoid exposure to infections
- Do not change cat litter boxes.
  Litter boxes expose the patient to toxoplasmosis.
- Avoid turtles and reptiles as pets.
  Turtles and reptiles carry diseases and bacteria such as Salmonella.
- Eat a low-bacteria diet. Avoid salads; raw fruit and vegetables; and undercooked meat, fish, and eggs.
  These foods can carry bacteria that can cause infection.
- Report any of the following:
  - Temperature greater than 100°F (37.8°C)
  - Cough
  - Cloudy urine
  - Any drainage from a wound
  Knowing the signs of infections and reporting them early to the healthcare provider can minimize infections and complications.

Evaluating Care Outcomes

A well-managed patient has a good understanding of the immune disorder and accompanying risks. This patient takes all appropriate precautions, practices good hand washing,

and knows when to contact the provider. If an infection does occur, it is treated promptly with the appropriate antibiotic or antiviral therapy.

EXCESSIVE IMMUNE RESPONSE

In contrast to the immune deficiencies, when the immune system is initiated inappropriately or when it overreacts, autoimmunity and hypersensitivity disorders occur. **Autoimmunity** is when the body initiates an immune response against self; antibodies are formed that respond to normal healthy cells and tissue. The body fails to recognize these normal cells as self, which causes an immune reaction to occur against the perceived antigen, the healthy cell. The cause of autoimmune diseases is still not completely known. Theories of causation include the inheritance of susceptible genes that may contribute to the failure of self-tolerance. Much research is being conducted in this area. Even with a genetic predisposition, some trigger is required for the initiation of autoreactivity. This may include an infectious agent such as a virus. Medications and hormones may be a trigger as well.

Autoimmune diseases are often classified as systemic or organ specific, as listed in Table 19.3. Some of these diseases are discussed in other chapters of the book. For example, lupus, rheumatoid arthritis, and scleroderma are discussed in Chapter 20 with connective tissue disorders. Graves' disease and diabetes are discussed in Unit IX with endocrine disorders. Myasthenia gravis and Guillain–Barré are discussed in Chapter 38 with peripheral nervous system disorders. Hematological disorders are discussed in Chapter 34.

A **hypersensitivity reaction** is when the immune response is overreactive to a foreign antigen. An antigen is a foreign protein that stimulates an immune response in a susceptible individual. Hypersensitivity reactions can be damaging to the body, may cause discomfort, and may also be fatal, as in anaphylaxis.

There are several categories of hypersensitivity reactions. They can be divided into five types—type I, type II, type III, type IV, and type V—as illustrated in Table 19.4. These types are based on the specific mechanisms and mediators that are involved in the process, the source of the antigen, and the length of time for the reaction to occur. This chapter discusses all of these hypersensitivity reactions but focuses on type I and type IV.

Hypersensitivity reactions and autoimmunity overlap. Many autoimmune diseases have hypersensitivity as part of their pathogenesis. Graves' disease is an autoimmune disorder that is a result of a type V hypersensitivity reaction. Systemic lupus erythematosus (SLE) is the result of a type III hypersensitivity reaction. Goodpasture's syndrome is an example of a type II hypersensitivity reaction. Similarly, most but not all hypersensitivity reactions are manifested in autoimmune disorders, but one that does not manifest as autoimmune is a type I hypersensitivity reaction—a typical allergic reaction.

Table 19.3   Examples of Known or Probable Autoimmune Diseases

Systemic Diseases or Non-Organ-Specific	Autoantigen	Organ-Specific Diseases	Autoantigen
Systemic lupus erythematosus*	DNA proteins	Blood:	
		Autoimmune hemolytic anemia	Erythrocytes
		Immune thrombocytopenic purpura	Platelets
Rheumatoid arthritis*	IgG, possibly cartilage	Central nervous system:	Unknown but suspected:
		Multiple sclerosis	Myelin basic protein
		Guillain–Barré syndrome	Antiganglioside antibodies
Scleroderma (progressive systemic sclerosis)	DNA proteins	Muscle:	
		Myasthenia gravis*	Acetylcholine receptor, acetylcholine
Mixed connective tissue disease	DNA proteins	Heart:	
		Rheumatic fever	Antibodies developed against group A streptococcus (GAS)
Sjogren's syndrome	Salivary gland cells, vaginal mucous cells, lacrimal gland cells	Eye:	
		Uveitis	Uveal tract cells (eyes)
Polymyositis-dermatomyositis	Unknown	Endocrine system:	
		Addison's disease	Adrenal cell
		Thyroiditis	Thyroid cell surface
		Type 1 diabetes mellitus	Islet cells, insulin, insulin receptor
		Graves' disease*	Thyroid-stimulating hormone receptor
		Gastrointestinal system:	
		Pernicious anemia	
		Ulcerative colitis	Intrinsic factor, parietal cell, B_{12} complexes
		Kidney:	
		Goodpasture's syndrome*	
		Glomerulonephritis	Glomerular basement membranes, pulmonary basement membranes
		Liver:	Unknown
		Primary biliary cirrhosis	
		Autoimmune hepatitis	
		Skin:	
		Psoriasis	Stratum corneum

*Hypersensitivity reaction.
DNA, Deoxyribonucleic acid; *Ig,* immunoglobulin

Table 19.4 Types of Hypersensitivity Reactions

Type of Hypersensitivity	Mechanism	Antigen	Antibody Involved	Mediators of Injury	Example
Type I: Immediate rapid allergic reaction	Reaction of IgE antibody with antigen-releasing mediators especially histamine	Pollen, dust, food, medications	IgE	Histamine, mast cells, leukotrienes, prostaglandins	• Allergic rhinitis • Asthma • Anaphylaxis
Type II: Cytotoxic reactions	Reaction of IgG with host cell membrane or antigen absorbed by host cell membrane	Cell surface of RBCs	IgG, IgM	Complement lysis Macrophages in tissues	• Transfusion reaction • Goodpasture's syndrome • Autoimmune thrombocy-topenic purpura • Myasthenia gravis
Type III: Immune complex reactions	Formation of immune complex of antigen and antibody that is deposited in walls of blood vessels, resulting in complement release and inflammation	Extracellular fungal, viral, bacterial	IgG, IgM	Neutrophils	• Systemic lupus erythematosus • Rheumatoid arthritis • Serum sickness
Type IV: Delayed hypersensitivity reactions; T-cell mediated	Reaction of sensitized T cells with antigen and release of lymphokines, which activate macrophages and cause inflammation	Intracellular or extracellular	None	Cytokines cytotoxic T cells, monocytes, macrophages, lysosomal enzymes	• Contact dermatitis to poison ivy • Positive TB skin tests • Latex allergy
Type V: Stimulated	Reaction of auto-antibodies with normal cell surface receptors, which stimulates continual overreaction of the target cell			Autoantibodies	• Graves' disease • B-cell gammopathies (increased levels of gamma globulins)

Ig, Immunoglobulin; *RBCs,* red blood cells; *TB,* tuberculosis.

Hypersensitivities

Type I Hypersensitivity Reaction: Immediate

Epidemiology

Type I hypersensitivity reaction is a rapid or immediate allergic reaction. There can be a local (**atopic**) reaction or a systemic reaction. The most common is allergic rhinitis or hay fever, a local reaction. The most severe form is anaphylaxis, a systemic reaction. A genetic predisposition exists for the development of allergic diseases. If both parents have allergies, there is an 80% chance the child will have allergies. If the mother is allergic, the child is likely to also have allergies. Approximately 20% of the population is atopic, which means having an inherited tendency to become sensitive to environmental **allergens,** the substances that cause an allergic response. Potential allergens include food, medications,

insect bites (e.g., bees, fire ants, hornets, yellow jackets, and wasps) and biting insects (e.g., mosquitoes), diagnostic testing substances (e.g., radiocontrast media), and blood.

In Western countries, between 10% and 25% of people annually are affected by allergic rhinitis. Allergic rhinitis affects 35.9 million individuals, which is about 11% of the population in the United States. It can be perennial or seasonal. Perennial rhinitis is caused by dust, molds, and animal dander. Seasonal rhinitis is caused by pollens from trees, weeds, or grasses. The person's immune system responds to the harmless material as though it were a real threat.

An accurate incidence of anaphylaxis is not known because of the differentiation between a full-blown anaphylactic response and milder cases. Milder forms are more common. There are up to 1,500 fatal cases of anaphylaxis annually. There are at least 40 deaths per year due to insect venom, about 400 deaths due to penicillin anaphylaxis, approximately 220 cases of anaphylaxis and 3 deaths per year due to latex allergy, and an estimated 150 people die annually from anaphylaxis due to food allergy. A recent review concluded that the lifetime prevalence of anaphylaxis is 1% to 2% of the population as a whole. The incidence of anaphylaxis appears to be increasing, especially cases in children attributed to food allergy.

Pathophysiology

The primary mediator of type I hypersensitivity reactions is **immunoglobulin E (IgE)**. The first time a patient is exposed to an allergen, IgE is produced. The IgE antibodies attach to mast cells. The next time the patient is exposed to that specific allergen, it binds to the IgE antibodies that are attached to the mast cells. This causes the mast cell to degranulate, releasing **histamine** and other chemicals such as leukotrienes and prostaglandins that cause smooth muscle contraction, vasodilation, increased vascular permeability, bronchoconstriction, and edema. This results in the symptoms associated with the allergy. The allergic reaction is illustrated in Figure 19.3.

Anaphylaxis is the most severe form of type I hypersensitivity reaction that exhibits the extremes of the symptoms. Table 19.5 indicates the specific mediator of a type I hypersensitivity reaction, its pathophysiological activity, and the symptoms it produces. Anaphylaxis can occur when these mediators are released systemically.

Clinical Manifestations

The various clinical manifestations may be local or systemic. Clinical manifestations of allergic rhinitis include nasal discharge, sneezing, and pruritus of the upper airways. The patient may complain of headache or sinus pressure. Typically, the patient has itchy, watery eyes. In anaphylaxis, a systemic response, there is an immediate response to an allergen. The patient complains of dyspnea and shortness of breath. Audible wheezes and/or crackles are present. A skin reaction or rash may appear. Patients may experience nausea, vomiting, or diarrhea. They complain of anxiety and often state they feel a flush of heat. **Angioedema**, swelling just below the surface of the skin, typically around the mouth and eyes, may also be present.

In an extreme anaphylactic reaction, there is a severe and rapid onset of symptoms. They include bronchospasm with extreme dyspnea and shortness of breath and wheezing. The patient may have hoarseness and stridor, a high-pitched crowing sound, which indicates narrowing of the airways. Severe or untreated reactions result in anaphylactic shock with hypotension and tachycardia due to the vasodilation and capillary leak.

Connection Check 19.6

The nurse monitors for which clinical manifestation in the patient diagnosed with a severe anaphylactic reaction?

A. Hypotension
B. Bradycardia
C. Diuresis
D. Hypertension

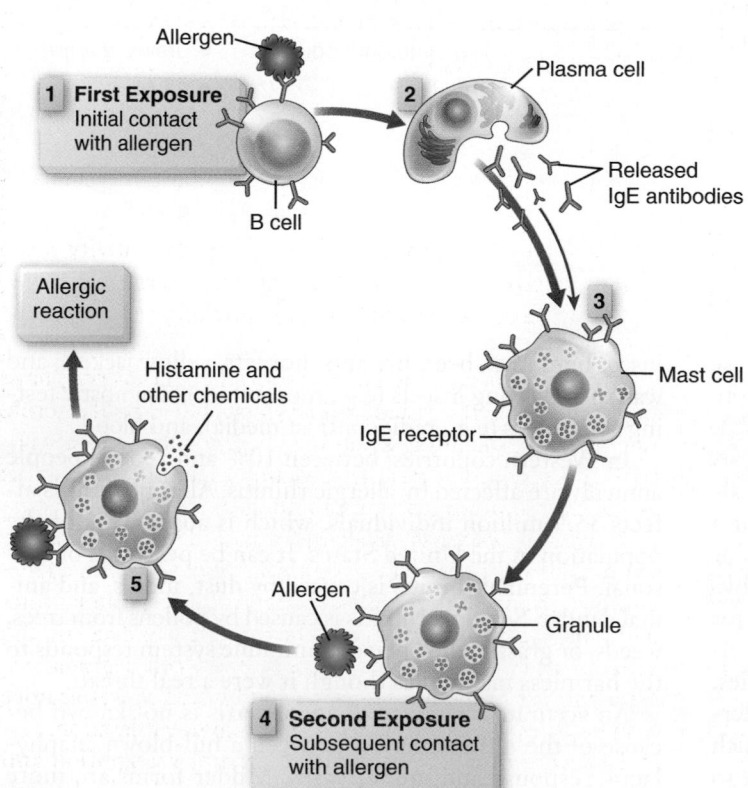

FIGURE 19.3 Steps in an allergic reaction. The first exposure to the allergen results in the formation of IgE antibodies, which attach to mast cells. On the second exposure, the allergen binds to the IgE antibodies that are attached to the mast cells, causing degranulation and the release of histamine and other chemicals.

Table 19.5 Mediators of Hypersensitivity Reactions, Pathophysiology, and Symptoms

Mediator	Pathophysiological Activity	Symptoms Produced
Histamine	Increases vascular permeability, constricts smooth muscle, increases gastric acid secretion	Edema of the airways and larynx, bronchial constriction, urticaria, angioedema, pruritus, nausea, vomiting, diarrhea, shock
Leukotrienes	Enhance the effect of histamine on the smooth muscle, constrict smooth muscle of the bronchi, increase vascular permeability	Bronchial constriction: wheezing
Platelet-activating factor	Platelet aggregation, stimulates vasodilation	Systemic hypotension, increase in pulmonary artery pressure
Kinins	Stimulate mucus secretion, increase vascular permeability	Bronchial constriction: wheezing, angioedema with painful swelling
Serotonin	Increases vascular permeability, stimulates smooth muscle contraction	Mucosal edema, bronchial constriction: wheezing
Prostaglandin	Stimulates smooth muscle contraction, increases capillary permeability, stimulates the inflammatory response, increases platelet aggregation, increases gastric acid creations	Bronchial constriction: wheezing, edema, nausea, and vomiting
Anaphylatoxins	Stimulate histamine release	Edema of the airways and larynx, bronchial constriction, urticaria, angioedema, pruritus, nausea, vomiting, diarrhea, shock

Management

Medical Management

Diagnosis. Diagnostics include a WBC count and differential. This test reveals an increase in eosinophils, which indicates the presence of an allergic response. Eosinophils are the key inflammatory cells seen in allergic rhinitis. As eosinophils increase, the symptom severity increases. A normal count is 1% to 2%. Someone with severe seasonal allergic rhinitis may have an eosinophil count as high as 12%.

Skin testing is performed to determine the specific allergen. Various allergens are introduced via a scratch test to determine which produce a positive reaction that indicates an allergy. The results are used to determine the causes of allergic rhinitis, urticaria or hives, and asthma. A localized reaction or wheal indicates a positive result within 15 to 20 minutes. Glucocorticoids and antihistamines are discontinued 5 days prior to testing. NSAIDs may also be discontinued before allergy testing. The forearm and the back are used as sites for scratch testing.

CASE STUDY: EPISODE 2

Mr. Smith's chest radiograph reveals pneumonia. He is placed on IV penicillin. The nurse returns to check on the patient and finds he is short of breath and extremely anxious about his symptoms and states that his skin is "itching" and he feels dizzy. Upon initial assessment, his pulse is rapid, his lips are blue tinged, a rash is apparent on his chest and arms, and wheezing is heard on auscultation of his lungs. The patient expresses a sense of impending doom. Vital signs at this time are:

- Blood pressure—85/50 mm Hg
- Heart rate—130 bpm
- Pulse oximetry—89%...

Treatment. Treatment of type I hypersensitivity reactions depends on the severity. Allergy management includes the identification, treatment, and prevention of allergic responses.

Avoidance therapy can be successful when the allergies have been identified. If a reaction does occur but is mild, merely removing the offending agent may be the only necessary action. If symptoms persist, antihistamines and decongestants are utilized. Decongestants can be used to decrease edema and secretions, especially in allergic rhinitis. Diphenhydramine hydrochloride (Benadryl), an antihistamine, decreases edema and constriction of smooth muscle in the respiratory tract and blood vessels. Steroids may be indicated to decrease the inflammatory response and decrease mast-cell degradation. Beta-agonist bronchodilators may aid in easing respiratory distress by causing respiratory smooth muscle relaxation.

In severe cases of anaphylaxis, prompt recognition and treatment are necessary to avoid a potentially fatal result (see Evidence-Based Practice). Emergency intervention and cardiopulmonary resuscitation may be necessary.

Evidence-Based Practice

Treatment of Anaphylaxis

Prompt recognition and treatment of an anaphylactic reaction are essential for a positive outcome. The most common clinical manifestations are skin reactions such as urticaria and angioedema, occurring in 90% of patients. Respiratory distress is seen in 50% of patients. First-line treatment includes the administration of intramuscular (IM) epinephrine. Epinephrine is effective as a respiratory smooth muscle relaxant and vasoactive medication to open airways to ease respiratory distress and constrict blood vessels to maintain the patient's blood pressure. It may be repeated every 5 to 15 minutes. Intravenous epinephrine is indicated in patients unresponsive to the IM doses. Glucagon is indicated in patients on beta blockers who are unresponsive to epinephrine. Second-line treatment includes antihistamines and corticosteroids, but importantly, they should not be given before or as first-line therapy.

Lee, S. E. (2017). Management of anaphylaxis. *Otolaryngologic Clinics of North America*, 50(6), 1175–1184.

Connection Check 19.7

The nurse understands that which actions of epinephrine help alleviate symptoms of anaphylaxis?

A. Dilates bronchioles, constricts blood vessels, improves cardiac contraction

B. Dilates blood vessels, constricts bronchioles, and slows cardiac conduction

C. Blocks histamine and decreases inflammation

D. Inhibits mast cells and decreases inflammation

Nursing Management

Assessment and Analysis. The clinical manifestations associated with a type I hypersensitivity reaction are caused by the release of histamine and other chemical mediators from mast cells upon exposure to the antigen. Typical results from histamine release include bronchoconstriction and increased capillary permeability. A runny nose, itching, red eyes, and rash are common. In extreme cases, the patient complains of shortness of breath and dyspnea. Wheezes are evident on auscultation.

Nursing Diagnosis

- **Risk for complications** of allergic reaction: wheals, itching, light-headedness, hypotension, wheezing, dyspnea, chest tightness, decreased level of consciousness, respiratory distress, and shock

Nursing Interventions

▪ Assessments

- Monitor respiratory rate, depth, and lung sounds; pulse oximetry; and arterial blood gases (ABGs).
  Because of bronchoconstriction produced by the histamine release, the respiratory rate may be increased. and wheezing, dyspnea and chest tightness, and throat or palate tightness may be present. Because of decreased oxygenation, the SpO_2 is decreased and the ABGs demonstrate hypoxemia.

- Blood pressure/pulse
  If anaphylaxis occurs, hypotension may be present because of vasodilation and capillary leak. Tachycardia is present as a compensatory response to the hypotension. Irregular and increased pulse and decreased blood pressure are also due to leukotriene release, which constricts airways and coronary vessels.

- General systems assessment
  Initial symptoms caused by the histamine release may be a rash and itching followed by watery red eyes, runny nose, and sneezing. Angioedema may be present. The patient may complain of feeling faint and diaphoretic. Diarrhea, stomach cramps, and abdominal pain may be present because of increased acid production due to histamine release.

▪ Actions

- Discontinue offending agent ASAP; if the offending agent is in an IV infusion, stop the IV medication, change the IV tubing, and hang normal saline.
  The medication causing the allergic reaction needs to be stopped to prevent any further reaction. The tubing has to be changed to prevent any further medication being infused.

- Administer oxygen as ordered via 100% nonrebreather.
  The vasodilation, capillary leak, and other shock responses are interfering with oxygenation and tissue perfusion. Starting oxygen enhances oxygen delivery to the tissues, especially the brain cells and cardiac muscle cells.

- Elevate the head of the bed as able; care is taken if hypotension is present.
  To improve ventilation, elevate the head of the bed, but do not compromise blood pressure if low.

- Medication administration as ordered
  - Administer diphenhydramine hydrochloride (Benadryl) as ordered.
    Diphenhydramine hydrochloride (Benadryl) is a histamine-receptor blocker; histamine is the main mediator in type I hypersensitivity reaction.
  - Administer corticosteroids as ordered.
    To inhibit the inflammatory response exacerbating the allergic response

- Administer bronchodilators as ordered.
  Beta agonists or bronchodilators facilitating bronchial smooth muscle relaxation may be indicated to ease bronchoconstriction.
- Anticipate order for STAT dose of intramuscular (IM) epinephrine if the reaction is severe.
  Epinephrine is the medication of choice to counteract anaphylactic shock by causing blood vessel constriction, raising blood pressure, and improving cardiac output through inotropic and chronotropic activity. It also acts as a beta-2 agonist to promote bronchial smooth muscle relaxation.
- Administer vasopressors as needed.
  If anaphylaxis occurs, vasoactive medications may be indicated to constrict blood vessels and increase blood pressure.
- Have emergency resuscitation equipment available (endotracheal intubation or tracheostomy) for possible progression to anaphylactic shock.
  As anaphylaxis progresses, there may be complete circulatory and ventilatory collapse requiring resuscitation.
- Stay with the patient and provide reassurance.
  Provide support to the patient who is anxious and fearful.

■ Teaching

- Educate patient regarding potential causes in the environment and ways to avoid exposure to the allergen.
  Minimizing any potential allergen exposure can prevent any future allergic or anaphylactic reaction.
- Educate the patient regarding the signs and symptoms of an initial reaction: rash and itching.
  The patient should know the possible signs and symptoms of a reaction to be able to react in a timely manner and prevent a more serious reaction.
- Educate the patient on the use of EpiPen.
  The EpiPen can inject a small dose of epinephrine when the patient has been exposed to an allergen and is at risk for anaphylaxis.
- Advise patient to obtain a Medic Alert bracelet or pendant and ensure that healthcare professionals are aware of any potential allergies.
  A Medic Alert bracelet alerts others to a patient's allergies. Healthcare professionals should be aware of any potential reactions to guard against potentially dangerous food or medication exposure.

Evaluating Care Outcomes

A well-managed patient is free of symptoms of the allergic reaction and has a normal oxygen level. With the removal of the offending agent and appropriate treatment of the allergic reaction with diphenhydramine hydrochloride (Benadryl), steroids, bronchodilators, and epinephrine if necessary, there is no further evidence of a rash, itching, or difficulty breathing. The patient is discharged when respiratory and cardiovascular assessment criteria have returned to baseline. After a severe allergic reaction for which the cause is not known, a trigger should be identified if possible. An allergist/immunologist should perform an evaluation, which may include a detailed history, physical examination, skin testing, in vitro testing, and

challenges when indicated. Future avoidance of the identified triggers should prevent subsequent anaphylactic episodes.

Connection Check 19.8

The nurse understands that information related to which of the following is a priority in the teaching plan about the management of an anaphylactic response to a bee sting?
A. Avoiding allergens
B. Wearing a Medic Alert bracelet
C. The use of an EpiPen
D. Immunotherapy through allergy shots

Type II Hypersensitivity Reaction: Cytotoxic

Type II antibody-mediated hypersensitivity reactions include three subtypes:

1. Complement and antibody-mediated cell destruction
2. Complement and antibody receptor-mediated inflammation
3. Antibody-mediated cellular dysfunction

Epidemiology

One example of a type II hypersensitivity reaction that causes cell destruction is erythroblastosis fetalis, which is due to Rh sensitization (Fig. 19.4). Rh sensitization occurs in approximately 1 in 1,000 births to Rh-negative women. The incidence of Rh-negative blood type is approximately 15% to 20% of Caucasians, 5% to 10% of African Americans, and less than 5% of individuals of Chinese and American Indian descent.

An example of type II hypersensitivity that causes inflammation is Goodpasture's syndrome, which is rare. It is more common in European populations, in which there is approximately one case present per million people per year. This syndrome is most common between ages 18 and 30 and again between 50 and 65. It is more common in males by a 6:1 ratio.

An example of type II hypersensitivity that causes cell dysfunction is myasthenia gravis. This disease affects approximately 2 out of 100,000 people. It can occur at any age but is most common in females 18 to 25 years of age and males 60 to 80 years of age.

Pathophysiology and Clinical Manifestations

The pathophysiology for each of the three subtypes of type II hypersensitivity has a basic component of complement and antibody-mediated cell involvement.

Subtype 1: Complement- and Antibody-Mediated Cell Destruction Hypersensitivity

Complement and antibody-mediated cell destruction hypersensitivity reaction is cytotoxic and antibody dependent. **Complement** is a series of proteins that distinguishes the individual's own cells from foreign substances: self-tolerance or self-recognition. When this function is not working, the individual is susceptible to autoimmune diseases as a result of the hypersensitivity reaction. The antibodies

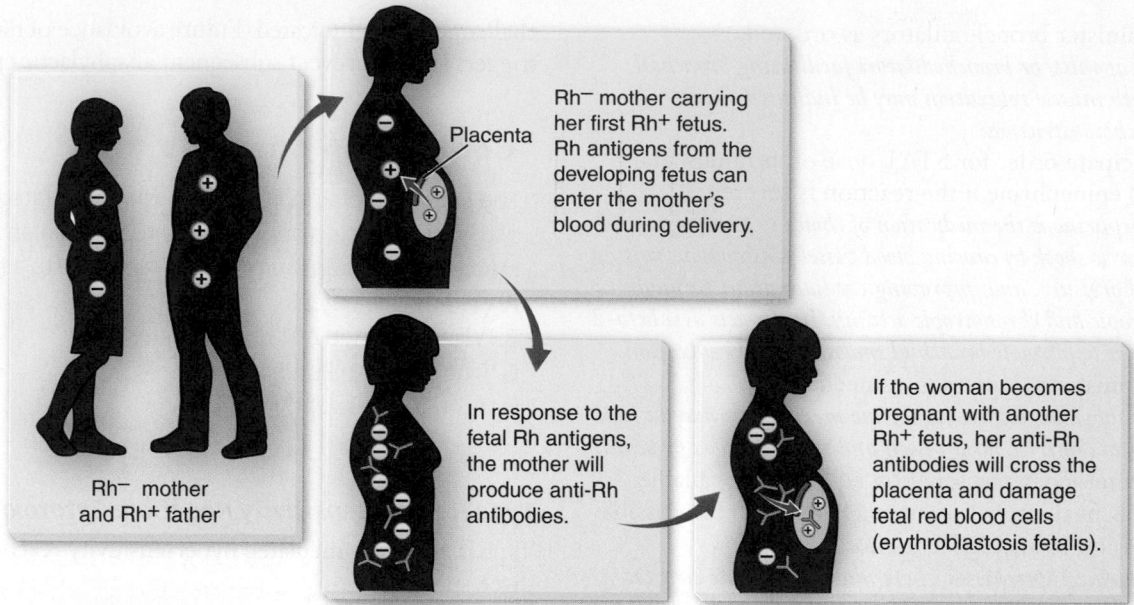

Rh⁻ mother carrying her first Rh⁺ fetus. Rh antigens from the developing fetus can enter the mother's blood during delivery.

Placenta

In response to the fetal Rh antigens, the mother will produce anti-Rh antibodies.

If the woman becomes pregnant with another Rh⁺ fetus, her anti-Rh antibodies will cross the placenta and damage fetal red blood cells (erythroblastosis fetalis).

Rh⁻ mother and Rh⁺ father

FIGURE 19.4 Rh sensitization. The Rh-negative mother develops anti-Rh antibodies during her first pregnancy in response to fetal Rh antigens entering her bloodstream. When pregnant again, the anti-Rh antibodies cross the placenta and damage fetal red blood cells.

involved in this hypersensitivity reaction are **immunoglobulin M (IgM)** and immunoglobulin G (IgG).

In subtype 1, the targeting of cells for deletion by antibodies is mediated by the complement system or by antibody-dependent cell-mediated cytotoxicity (ADCC). Destruction of cells by the complement-mediated system involves opsonization of cells or coating them with molecules that attract the phagocytes. Antibody-dependent cell-mediated cytotoxicity does not require complement. With ADCC, cells are coated with IgG antibody and are killed by various effector cells that bind to their target by the receptors for IgG; cell lysis results without phagocytosis. Examples of subtype 1 are blood transfusion reactions that occur when incompatible blood is transfused (Fig. 19.5; see Safety Alert), hemolytic disease of the newborn due to blood type (ABO) or Rh incompatibility, and certain medication reactions. In the example of medication reactions, medications or metabolites of medications bind to the surface of either red or white blood cells. This action causes an antibody response that lyses the medication-coated cell.

To avoid potentially fatal blood reactions, patients should receive only matching blood types, but in an *emergency,* there are some options (Table 19.6). Type AB blood is called a *universal recipient* because it lacks both anti-A and anti-B antibodies. Type O blood is called the *universal donor* because it lacks antigens.

If a patient receives incompatible blood, the patient will complain of chills, fever, pain, and a heat sensation at the transfusion site. A rash may develop. Antibodies coat the foreign erythrocytes, causing agglutination or clumping. The clumping blocks small blood vessels, resulting in ischemia. Neutrophils and macrophages phagocytize the clumped cells, causing the release of hemoglobin into the urine and plasma. This reaction causes vascular spasms in the kidney that can cause blockage of the renal tubules. The result can be acute renal failure from the hemoglobinuria. Coagulation is stimulated, which depletes clotting factors, resulting in massive bleeding.

Safety Alert Blood Transfusions and Hemolytic Transfusion Reactions

A person with type A blood has A antigens and anti-B antibodies.
A person with type B blood has B antigens and anti-A antibodies.
A person with AB blood has both A and B antigens and no antibodies.
A person with type O has no antigens and both anti-A and anti-B antibodies.

Subtype 2: Complement- and Antibody-Mediated Inflammation

Complement- and antibody-mediated inflammation causes inflammation rather than destruction. An example of this type is Goodpasture's syndrome, also known as antiglomerular basement antibody disease. Goodpasture's syndrome is an autoimmune disease triggered when the patient's immune system attacks the Goodpasture's antigen, an antigen in the glomerular basement membrane. The exact cause and trigger agent are not known. The antibody-mediated autoimmune reaction involves the glomerular and alveolar basement

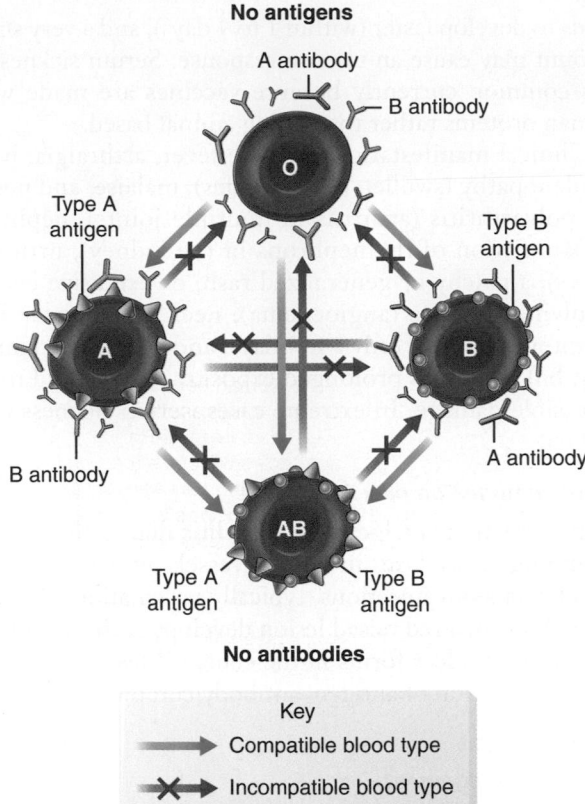

No antigens

A antibody

B antibody

O

Type A antigen

Type B antigen

A

B

B antibody

A antibody

Type A antigen

Type B antigen

AB

No antibodies

Key	
→	Compatible blood type
✕→	Incompatible blood type

FIGURE 19.5 Compatibility of blood types. AB is the universal recipient because it carries no antibodies. Type O is the universal donor because it carries no antigens. In addition to type O, type B can receive type B blood but not type A or AB. In addition to type O, type A can receive type A blood, but not type B or AB. Type O patients can only receive type O blood.

Table 19.6 Blood Types and Related Antigens

It Is Imperative to Check Blood Prior to Administration to Avoid a Potentially Fatal Reaction

Patient Blood Type	Antibodies	Antigens	Cannot Receive
Type A	Anti-B antibodies	A antigen	Type B or AB
Type B	Anti-A antibodies	B antigen	Type A or AB
Type AB	No antibodies	A and B antigens	Can have any blood type in an emergency
Type O	Anti-A and Anti-B	None	Type A, B, or AB

membranes. The antibodies combine with tissue antigen to activate complement. This causes deposits of IgG to form along the basement membranes of the lungs or kidneys. This disease is characterized by glomerulonephritis and hemorrhaging of the lungs and results in damage to the kidney and lungs. This is a rapidly progressing disorder.

Subtype 3: Antibody-Mediated Cellular Dysfunction

Antibody-mediated cellular dysfunction is a hypersensitivity reaction where the antibodies bind to cell-surface receptors. An example is myasthenia gravis. In myasthenia gravis, autoantibodies to acetylcholine receptors on the neuromuscular endplates are formed. The autoantibodies either block the action of acetylcholine or mediate the destruction of receptors. Either of these situations leads to decreased neuromuscular function and weakness. See Chapter 38 for more information on myasthenia gravis.

Management

Medical Management

As in type I hypersensitivity reactions, treatment of type II reactions requires removal of the medication or blood product that is causing the reaction. In addition, there are procedures to remove the offending blood components from the plasma. Plasmapheresis involves filtering the plasma to remove substances that precipitated the cytotoxic reaction. In this procedure, blood is removed via a catheter, RBCs and plasma are separated, and the RBCs are returned to the patient. In traditional plasmapheresis, the plasma is treated and returned to the patient. In plasma exchange, the patient's plasma is discarded and replaced by donor plasma. Plasmapheresis is covered in more detail in Chapter 20.

Goodpasture's syndrome is treated with corticosteroids and immunosuppressive medications in addition to plasmapheresis to slow the progression. Some patients require IVIG, a solution made from human plasma containing mostly IgG antibodies, to maintain antibody protection. Depending on the amount of renal involvement, dialysis may be necessary. Renal transplantation is an option for some patients.

Complications. Complications such as renal failure or hemolytic reaction may be life threatening. Renal function may be completely lost in a matter of days, a condition known as rapidly progressive glomerulonephritis. Lung damage, occurring as rapidly as the renal damage, may cause severe impairment of oxygenation requiring artificial ventilation. The patient may be anemic because of loss of blood through lung hemorrhaging over a long period. In Goodpasture's syndrome, lung hemorrhaging most often occurs in smokers and those with damage from lung infection or exposure to fumes. Medication reactions causing hemolytic reactions that cause cell lysis can produce transient anemia, leukopenia, or thrombocytopenia. Once the medication has been removed, these effects are corrected.

Type III Hypersensitivity Reaction: Immune Complex

Type III hypersensitivity reactions are immune complex–mediated reactions. These immune complex allergic disorders are mediated by the formation of antigen–antibody complexes. Similar to type I hypersensitivity reactions, there are two categories of type III reactions: systemic and local immune complex reactions. Examples of systemic immune complex reactions are systemic lupus erythematosus (SLE), rheumatoid arthritis, and serum sickness. A local immune complex reaction is Arthus reaction.

Epidemiology

Systemic lupus erythematosus may be caused by genetic, environmental, or unknown factors. In the United States, the prevalence of SLE is estimated to be about 53 per 100,000. Systemic lupus erythematosus occurs more frequently and with greater severity among those of non-European descent and is higher in those of Afro-Caribbean descent. Systemic lupus erythematosus is more common in females than males, 9 to 1, which is similar to other autoimmune diseases. Rheumatoid arthritis affects all ethnic groups, and women are affected 2.5 times more often than men. Arthus reaction is considered to be rare, and no specific prevalence is known.

Pathophysiology and Clinical Manifestations

A type III hypersensitivity reaction involves the formation of an antigen–antibody immune complex. Immunoglobulin G is the immunoglobulin involved. These immune complexes are large molecules of antibody combined with antigen and, due to their size, are difficult for the body to remove. Disease results when they are not removed but lodge in the tissues.

Systemic Immune Complex Disorders

Manifestations of rheumatoid arthritis are caused by the immune complexes that are lodged in joint spaces. When there are too many immune complexes, too much complement is activated, and an acute inflammatory response develops. Complement attracts neutrophils to the area of inflammation and stimulates the release of lysosomal enzymes. This release causes tissue damage, especially in small blood vessels where the immune complexes tend to lodge and the lack of blood supply causes tissue necrosis. This is followed by destruction of tissue, scarring, and fibrous changes.

Systemic lupus erthematosus produces antibodies against virtually any organ or tissue in the body. It forms immune complexes that lodge in the vessels, causing vasculitis; in the glomeruli, causing nephritis; and in the joints, causing arthralgia (joint pain) and arthritis. It affects the connective tissues and multiple organs, resulting in cardiovascular, renal, or neurological complications.

Serum sickness is an immune system reaction to certain kinds of medications, most commonly penicillin and other antibiotics or injected proteins (antiserum) used to treat immune conditions. Antiserum is given to enhance immunity, most commonly after a snake bite. Serum sickness occurs when the body mistakenly identifies a protein from the antiserum or medication as harmful and activates the immune system to fight it off. This results in the collection of immune complexes in blood vessel walls of the skin, joints, and kidney. The deposited complexes activate complement. This then increases vascular permeability, and phagocytic cells are recruited to the area that cause tissue damage and edema.

It usually develops within 7 to 12 days after initial exposure but sometimes can take as long as 3 weeks. If the patient is exposed to the substance a second time, serum sickness tends to develop faster (within 1 to 4 days), and a very small amount may cause an intense response. Serum sickness is less common currently because vaccines are made with human proteins rather than being animal based.

Clinical manifestations include fever, arthralgia, lymphadenopathy (swollen lymph nodes), malaise, and possibly polyarthritis (arthritis in multiple joints), nephritis (inflammation of the nephrons in the kidney), urticaria (hives), a patchy or generalized rash, or extensive edema involving the face (angioedema), neck, and joints. The symptoms may last only a few days, and damage is temporary, but if there is prolonged exposure, it may lead to irreversible damage. In extreme cases, serum sickness may be fatal.

Local Immune Complex Reactions

Arthus reaction is a localized vasculitis due to the deposit of immune complexes in dermal vessels after intradermal or subcutaneous injections, typically vaccinations. Within 4 to 10 hours, a red raised lesion develops at the site of the injection. An ulcer forms in the center. This is due to the in situ formation of antigen–antibody complexes.

Management

Medical Management

Removal of the offending agent is the first treatment. Symptom treatment for systemic immune complex reactions includes aspirin for joint pain and antihistamines for the pruritus. For the severe reactions, epinephrine or systemic corticosteroids may be utilized. Epinephrine is used for symptomatic relief of serum sickness, urticaria, and angioedema. Corticosteroids such as prednisone have been used to reduce the inflammation associated with serum sickness.

Type IV Hypersensitivity Reactions

Epidemiology

Type IV is a delayed-type hypersensitivity. Examples are poison ivy, the Mantoux test for tuberculosis, and latex allergy. Some patients may experience a mixed type I and type IV reaction. Latex allergy may be an immediate, rapid type I hypersensitivity reaction or a type IV delayed hypersensitivity reaction. The prevalence of latex allergy in the general population is approximately 2%. People at high risk for developing a latex allergy include healthcare workers who are routinely exposed to latex; patients who have undergone multiple surgical procedures, especially spina bifida patients; people with a previous history of atopic dermatitis or pre-existing hand dermatitis; and females.

Pathophysiology and Clinical Manifestations

Type IV cell-mediated/delayed-type hypersensitivity is also known as cell-mediated immune memory response or antibody independent. This reaction is different from the previous reactions in that it is mediated by cells rather than antibodies. This type of hypersensitivity reaction is delayed and is regulated by T lymphocytes that are damaging to cells or cytotoxic. The reaction usually occurs 24 to 72 hours after exposure to the antigen. Sensitized T lymphocytes are the cells that attack the antigens and release cytokines and thus mediate the reaction. The macrophages and enzymes released by macrophages are responsible for most of the tissue destruction. In the delayed hypersensitivity reaction, it takes 24 to 48 hours for a response to occur.

Clinical manifestations of a local reaction typical of a positive TB test include a wheal and flare reaction. This reaction is a raised area containing edematous fluid surrounded by red flare. The clinical manifestations of a latex allergy may range from local contact dermatitis, rhinitis, and conjunctivitis to pharyngeal edema and severe systemic reaction such as anaphylactic shock. The following Medical and Nursing Management section focuses on latex allergy.

Management

Medical Management

As in other hypersensitivity reactions, treatment is based on prevention, such as avoiding products that contain latex. If exposure does occur, antihistamines may help with a less severe reaction. Skin creams containing steroids help with the contact dermatitis. More severe reactions that occur with repeated exposure may require a trip to the hospital to receive oxygen, epinephrine, and IV corticosteroids to reduce the inflammatory response.

Nursing Management

Assessment and Analysis. The clinical manifestations seen with type IV hypersensitivity latex reaction are typically due to the tissue damage caused by the inflammatory response mediated by sensitized T cells. Mild reactions include:

- Local skin reactions, typically on the hands in relation to latex gloves
- Conjunctivitis
- Rhinitis

More severe reactions can include severe respiratory distress related to pharyngeal edema and anaphylactic shock as described previously under type I hypersensitivity reactions.

Nursing Diagnoses

- **Risk for localized tissue damage** related to hypersensitivity reaction secondary to latex allergy
- **Risk for impaired oxygenation** related to pharyngeal edema secondary to hypersensitivity reaction

Nursing Interventions

▪ Assessments

- Assess vital signs.
  A severe latex allergy reaction may produce clinical manifestations of anaphylaxis: respiratory distress with decreased oxygenation, hypotension, and tachycardia.
- Assess the skin.
  Mild reactions may include rashes, especially on the hands from latex gloves.

- Assess for previous history of latex allergy.
  A secondary exposure to latex after an allergic reaction may cause a more severe anaphylactic response because of already sensitized T cells.
- Assess for allergies for any of the following: avocado, chestnut, mango, papaya, passion fruit, tomato, raw potato, peach, banana, kiwi.
  Allergies to these substances may also indicate a sensitivity to latex.
- Assess for history of repeated surgical procedures or adverse reaction or complication related to surgery.
  Patients having repeated surgical procedures resulting in multiple exposures to latex are more likely to become sensitized and suffer an allergic response to latex.

▪ Actions

- Administer medications as ordered.
  Steroid skin creams and/or IV corticosteroids may be necessary to decrease inflammation. IM epinephrine may be necessary to relieve respiratory distress and increase blood pressure in a severe reaction.
- Eliminate exposure to latex products by using nonlatex alternatives: vinyl or neoprene gloves.
  The best treatment is prevention. A secondary exposure may lead to anaphylaxis.
- Protect patients from exposure to latex by:
  - Covering skin with cloth before applying the blood pressure cuff
  - Not allowing rubber stethoscope tubing to touch the patient
  - Not injecting through rubber ports on IV tubing
    As stated, overexposure to latex can exacerbate the hypersensitivity reaction. Avoidance of exposure is the best treatment.

▪ Teaching

- Teach the patient to avoid exposure to products that are commonly made of latex:
  - Healthcare equipment: wheelchair cushions, tourniquets, airways, endotracheal tubes, masks for anesthesia, electrode pads
  - Office/household products: erasers, rubber balls, tires, shoe soles, rubber bands, hot water bottles, cycle grips, baby bottle nipples, carpeting
    Any exposure can result in an anaphylactic reaction.
- Instruct the patient to wear a Medic Alert bracelet and inform healthcare providers of allergy.
  It is essential that the patient identify latex allergies to avoid exposure as much as possible and aid in the response should a reaction occur and the patient is unable to articulate the problem.
- Instruct the patient on the use and necessity of an EpiPen.
  The EpiPen delivers a small dose of epinephrine to counteract an allergic response, decreasing respiratory distress and increasing blood pressure.

Evaluating Care Outcomes. Patients can avoid the complications related to latex allergy by maintaining a heightened awareness of products in the environment that contain latex. Carrying an EpiPen and wearing a Medic Alert bracelet are necessary in the case of an inadvertent exposure to latex.

Type V Hypersensitivity: Stimulated

The type V designation can be noted as a distinct subcategory but is sometimes included in type II hypersensitivity reactions. This is an antibody-mediated cellular dysfunction that leads to a change in cell function but does not lead to cell death as in type II hypersensitivity reactions. This reaction is also called a *stimulatory reaction*. There is an excessive stimulation of a normal cell-surface receptor by an autoantibody. This stimulation results in a continuous turned-on state for the cell. An example of this is Graves' disease, which is a form of hyperthyroidism. An autoantibody binds to the thyroid-stimulating hormone receptor sites on the thyroid gland. The action of the binding results in a continual stimulation of thyroid cells to produce thyroid hormone. The normal feedback system is no longer working to stop the overproduction of thyroid hormones. The thyroid gland is normal, but the manifestations that are exhibited are those of hyperthyroidism. Graves' disease is discussed in detail in Chapter 43.

Making Connections

CASE STUDY: WRAP-UP

On auscultation, audible wheezing with decreased breath sounds in the lower lobes is noted. Mr. Smith complains of severe dyspnea and shortness of breath. Hoarseness is evident. Itchy skin wheals or hives have spread over his body, forming large, red blotches. Angioedema of his lips and mouth is visible. The nurse immediately discontinues the IV penicillin. The IV tubing is changed, and normal saline is initiated. Epinephrine 0.5 mg is administered IM stat. Oxygen therapy is provided via a 100% high-flow nonrebreather face mask. Oxygen saturation is monitored via pulse oximetry.

Mr. Smith is placed on a cardiac monitor, which reveals a heart rate of 130 bpm with occasional premature ventricular contractions (PVCs). His blood pressure (BP) is 85/50 mm Hg. His oxygen saturation improves to 90% after the initiation of oxygen. Diphenhydramine 50 mg is administered via IV push, and IV fluids are initiated. Albuterol, a beta agonist, is administered via nebulizer to relieve the bronchospasm. Emergency equipment for endotracheal intubation and possible tracheotomy is readied.

Mr. Smith's condition begins to improve. His shortness of breath lessens, and pulse oximetry indicates improved oxygenation at 95%. Vital signs reveal:

Blood pressure—110/60

Heart rate—90

Case Study Questions

1. The nurse caring for Mr. Smith, who is having an anaphylactic response to penicillin, incorporates which nursing diagnosis into the plan of care?
   A. Risk for ineffective gas exchange
   B. Risk for hyperventilation related to anxiety
   C. Pain related to bronchospasm
   D. Knowledge deficit: Prevention and treatment of anaphylaxis
2. Which is the priority nursing assessment for the nurse caring for Mr. Smith?
   A. Assessing bowel sounds
   B. A full head-to-toe assessment
   C. Monitoring respiratory status
   D. Assessing skin for a rash
3. The nurse caring for Mr. Smith understands that which of the following is the priority intervention when noting he is having a reaction to the penicillin infusion?
   A. Contact provider for orders.
   B. Ready emergency medications.
   C. Discontinue IV penicillin.
   D. Discontinue IV completely.
4. The nurse understands that Mr. Smith is having a potential allergic reaction by which of the following symptoms?
   A. Generalized fatigue
   B. Tachycardia and hypertension
   C. Abdominal pain and nausea
   D. Hypotension and tachycardia
5. The nurse monitors for which complication in the patient with progressing anaphylaxis?
   A. Circulatory failure
   B. Seizures
   C. Bradycardia
   D. Hypertension

CHAPTER SUMMARY

Primary immune dysfunction occurs in persons born with an immune system that is deficient or is limited in its ability to function. In this case, there is an intrinsic (inborn), congenital, or genetic cause. These primary immunodeficiencies result from defects in T lymphocytes, B lymphocytes, natural killer cells, phagocytic cells, or the complement system. The majority are diagnosed in childhood.

Secondary immune dysfunction, or acquired immune deficiency, arises secondary to some other disease process or exposure to medications or chemicals. Examples of secondary immune dysfunction include immune deficiency caused by HIV disease, irradiation, chemotherapy, malnutrition, or burns. Secondary immune dysfunctions comprise the majority of deficiencies presented in the clinical setting.

X-linked agammaglobulinemia is an X-linked recessive inherited or congenital primary immune deficiency. Clinical manifestations include infections of the ears, lungs, skin, conjunctiva, and central nervous system. The presence of recurrent bacterial infections of the respiratory tract in childhood is the first indicator of the possibility of this disease. Diagnostics include blood tests that show a lack of circulating B cells as well as low levels of immunoglobulins (Igs). Treatment includes giving IV gamma globulin (IVIG) to provide short-term passive immunity and aggressive treatment with specific antibiotics if the patient exhibits overt signs of infection.

T-cell deficiencies lead to infections and other problems that are more severe than B-cell deficiencies. An example of a T-cell deficiency is DiGeorge's syndrome. It typically involves the thymus gland and parathyroid dysfunction, causing hypocalcemia, facial deformities such as cleft palate, and heart anomalies. Treatment includes calcium supplements to prevent tetany and seizures, aggressive treatment of infections, prophylactic antibiotics, IVIG therapy, or thymic transplantation. Bone marrow transplantation may be indicated in severe cases.

Secondary immune deficiencies are caused by a variety of factors, such as medication-induced immunosuppression and chemotherapy, radiation, and surgery. Management of patients with secondary immune dysfunction is primarily preventive. The focus of nursing care priorities is assessing for signs of infection and prevention of infection. Teaching priorities are primarily avoiding exposure to infections, such as avoiding large crowds.

Hypersensitivity reactions and autoimmunity are examples of excessive immune responses. Autoimmunity is when the body initiates an immune response against self; antibodies respond to normal, healthy cells and tissue. Hypersensitivity is when the immune system responds inappropriately or overresponds to the presence of an antigen.

Type I hypersensitivity reaction is a rapid or immediate allergic reaction. There can be a local (atopic) reaction or a systemic reaction. The most common is allergic rhinitis, or hay fever, a local reaction. The most severe form is anaphylaxis, a systemic reaction. The primary mediator of type I hypersensitivity reactions is IgE. IgE causes mast cells to degranulate, releasing histamine and other chemicals, such as leukotrienes and prostaglandins, that cause smooth muscle contraction, vasodilation, increased vascular permeability, bronchoconstriction, and edema. In anaphylaxis, the primary mediator is histamine. The patient complains of extreme dyspnea and shortness of breath. Additional symptoms include hypotension, tachycardia, and in the extreme or untreated, anaphylactic shock. Treatment of type I hypersensitivity reactions depends on the severity. Nursing care priorities include discontinuing the offending agent as soon as possible, administering epinephrine IM, administering oxygen, and having emergency resuscitation equipment available. Other medications utilized include methylprednisolone, a glucocorticoid to decrease the inflammation, diphenhydramine, an antihistamine, and albuterol to help relieve respiratory distress. Patient teaching includes educating the patient regarding the signs and symptoms of an anaphylactic reaction and the use of an EpiPen.

Type II antibody-mediated hypersensitivity reactions include three subtypes: (1) complement and antibody-mediated cell destruction, (2) complement and antibody receptor-mediated inflammation, and (3) antibody-mediated cellular dysfunction. Subtype 1 involves cell destruction, subtype 2 involves inflammation, and subtype 3 involves cell dysfunction. One example of subtype 1 is the blood transfusion reaction that occurs when incompatible blood is transfused.

Type III hypersensitivity reactions are immune complex–mediated reactions. These immune complex allergic disorders are mediated by the formation of antigen–antibody complexes. Examples of systemic immune complex reactions are systemic lupus erythematosus, rheumatoid arthritis, and serum sickness.

Type IV cell-mediated/delayed-type hypersensitivity is also known as cell-mediated immune memory response or antibody independent. This reaction is different from the other reactions in that it is mediated by cells rather than antibodies. Examples are poison ivy, the Mantoux test for TB, and a latex allergy. Latex allergy may be an immediate, rapid type I hypersensitivity reaction or a type IV delayed hypersensitivity reaction. Nursing care priorities are to eliminate patient exposure to latex products by using nonlatex alternatives, such as vinyl or neoprene gloves. Teaching priorities include providing information about products commonly made of latex and emergency procedures if an immediate anaphylactic response should occur.

Type V hypersensitivity is an antibody-mediated cellular dysfunction that leads to a change in cell function. This reaction is also called a *stimulatory reaction*. There is an excessive stimulation of a normal cell-surface receptor by an autoantibody. This stimulation results in a continuous turned-on state for the cell. An example of this is Graves' disease, which is a form of hyperthyroidism.

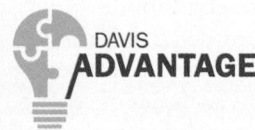

To explore learning resources for this chapter, go to **Davis Advantage** and find:
- Answers to in-text questions
- Chapter Resources and Activities
- NCLEX®-Style Chapter Review Questions
- Bibliography

Chapter 20

Coordinating Care for Patients With Connective Tissue Disorders

Kathleen Ogle

LEARNING OUTCOMES

Content in this chapter is designed to assist in:

1. Describing the epidemiology of connective tissue disorders
2. Correlating clinical manifestations to pathophysiological processes of:
   a. Osteoarthritis
   b. Rheumatoid arthritis
   c. Scleroderma
   d. Lupus erythematosus
   e. Gout
   f. Fibromyalgia
3. Describing the diagnostic results used to confirm the diagnosis of connective tissue disorders
4. Discussing the medical management of:
   a. Osteoarthritis
   b. Rheumatoid arthritis
   c. Scleroderma
   d. Lupus erythematosus
   e. Gout
   f. Fibromyalgia
5. Developing a comprehensive plan of nursing care for patients with connective tissue disorders
6. Designing a teaching plan that includes pharmacological, dietary, and lifestyle considerations for patients with connective tissue disorders

ESSENTIAL TERMS

Bouchard's node
Cartilage
Collagen
Connective tissue
Cytopenia
Disease-modifying antirheumatic drugs (DMARDs)
Effusion
Episcleritis
Heberden's node
Osteopenia
Osteophyte
Pericarditis
Pleural effusion
Pleuritis
Podagra
Raynaud's phenomenon
Rheumatoid nodule
Scleritis
Synovitis
Synovium
Tophi

CONCEPTS

- Assessment
- Comfort
- Immunity
- Inflammation
- Medication
- Mobility

Finding Connections

CASE STUDY: EPISODE 1

Follow this patient throughout the chapter.

Shannon Logan is a 32-year-old female patient who is referred to a rheumatology clinic by her primary care provider with complaints of multiple joint pain and swelling, fatigue, and morning stiffness. She is an elementary school teacher and has noticed that holding a marker has become progressively more difficult over the last 7 to 8 months. Because of morning stiffness lasting for more than 1 hour, she has to get up earlier to get ready for work. She complains of bilateral hand and wrist pain as well as pain and swelling in the second and third fingers bilaterally. By the end of the work day, she is extremely tired and is unable to carry on with her usual evening activities. She has a history of mild hypertension, which is treated with hydrochlorothiazide, but is otherwise in excellent health…

INTRODUCTION

Connective tissue, the most widely distributed and abundant tissue in the body, is an extracellular matrix made up of ground substance (a clear viscous fluid that aids in cellular adhesion to the matrix and facilitates the movement of substances between capillaries and cells), **collagen**, and elastic and reticular fibers. Cells, principally fibroblasts, participate in the synthesis of the matrix. Connective tissue provides support, structure, insulation, and cushion to tissues and organs of the body as well as fills space. In connective tissue disease, the collagen and elastin are typically damaged through inflammation or immune system dysfunction. Bone, cartilage, tendons, ligaments, lymphatic tissue, and blood are all examples of connective tissue.

OSTEOARTHRITIS

Epidemiology

Osteoarthritis is the most common form of arthritis in the United States. Affecting almost 27 million people in the United States, it is the leading cause of chronic disability in the country. It involves weight-bearing joints such as the knees, hips, feet, and lumbar spine, but it also affects the cervical spine, proximal interphalangeal joints, and distal interphalangeal joints of the hands (Fig. 20.1). Osteoarthritic involvement of the shoulders and elbows usually occurs after trauma, inflammation, or overuse.

There are multiple risk factors associated with osteoarthritis, including age, female sex, obesity, occupations that involve repetitive motions, sports activities, previous injury, muscle weakness, genetics, history of inflammatory arthritis, and other bone and joint disorders. Obesity is the single most modifiable risk factor contributing to osteoarthritis.

Obesity correlates most closely to the development of knee osteoarthritis; however, it has also been shown to correlate with the development of hand osteoarthritis, indicating that obesity itself, not only increased stress on weight-bearing joints and decreased exercise, may contribute to osteoarthritis. There have been links made between certain occupations and osteoarthritis. Individuals whose job entails repetitive knee bending are prone to develop knee osteoarthritis, and individuals who perform physical labor are at an increased risk for developing hand and hip osteoarthritis.

Aging is one of the most prevalent risk factors for developing osteoarthritis; only 0.1% of those aged 25 to 34 years are affected compared with 80% of individuals over age 55; however, osteoarthritis is not considered a normal process of aging. In general, women are more commonly affected by osteoarthritis than men. Osteoarthritis of the knees is more common in African American women than in Caucasian women. Osteoarthritis of the hands is most prevalent in women.

Connection Check 20.1

The nurse recognizes which patient to be at greatest risk for developing osteoarthritis?
A. A 70-year-old African American male
B. A 45-year-old Caucasian female
C. A 65-year-old obese African American female
D. A 30-year-old Caucasian male

Pathophysiology

Osteoarthritis is a disease that affects the joint as a whole because of biological, chemical, and viscoelastic changes within the joint. Tendons and ligaments are viscoelastic, meaning they lengthen while under tension but return to normal shape at rest. Cartilage, synovium, subchondral bone, synovial fluid, ligaments, periarticular muscle, and sensory nerves are altered by osteoarthritis. **Cartilage** is a material made primarily of water, collagen, proteoglycans, and elastin. Cartilage serves to provide joint protection by providing a smooth surface on which bones glide and disperses loads across the joint. When the cartilage is damaged from major trauma or repetitive microtrauma, osteophytes are formed by the body in an attempt to repair the damage. **Osteophytes** are projections of new cartilage and bone growth that form along joint lines, contributing to pain in the joint and decreased range of motion. Osteophyte formations on the proximal interphalangeal joints and distal interphalangeal joints are referred to as **Bouchard's nodes** and **Heberden's nodes**, respectively (Figs. 20.2A and B). Some of the new bone growth may break off as bone spurs and contribute to further cartilage loss. Cartilage loss is a clinical feature of osteoarthritis, causing the bone to be unprotected, which leads to the deterioration of joint function.

The **synovium** is a membrane that lines the noncartilaginous surfaces of highly mobile joints. It produces synovial fluid, serving to lubricate the joints. In osteoarthritis, the synovial membrane may become thickened and overproduce synovial fluid, causing more pain and even greater

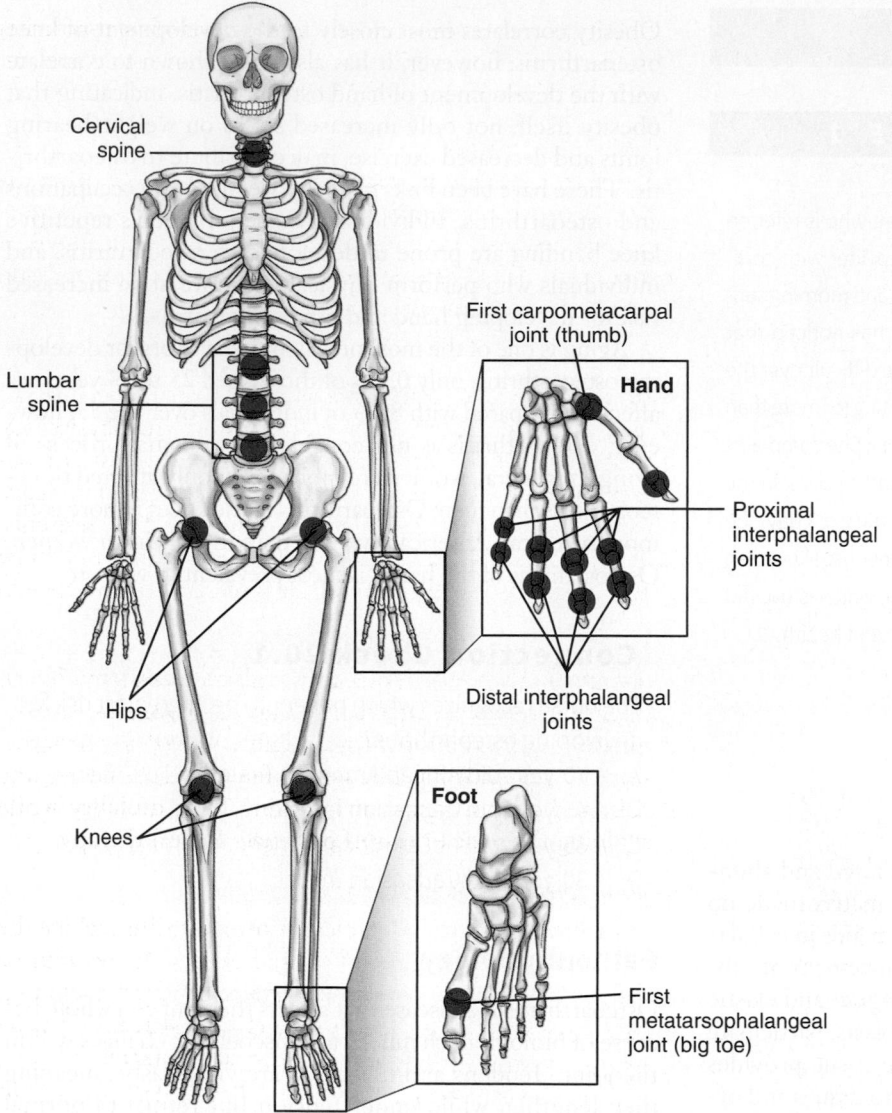

FIGURE 20.1 Common joints affected by osteoarthritis.

restriction on joint movement. Chronic **effusions**, an over-production of synovial fluid, may cause collateral ligaments to stretch, leading to joint laxity, or looseness, and mechanical instability, compounding joint damage. Muscles around the joints tend to atrophy as a consequence of decreased use of the joint. Radiographs may reveal sclerosis or cyst formation in the subchondral bone, which lies just below the cartilage. Ligaments, elastic band–type structures that connect bones to bones, may experience edema and fibrosis, also contributing to pain and decreased joint function (Fig. 20.3).

Clinical Manifestations

Clinical manifestations of osteoarthritis include progressive pain over time, decreased range of motion, tenderness to touch over the joint line or around the joint, bony swelling, soft tissue swelling, deformity, and instability. Crepitus, a crackling, grating sound or feeling due to air or gas under the skin, may also be present. This is due to cartilage breakdown in the joint. Patients typically experience more pain with activity, which improves with rest.

Connection Check 20.2

The nurse monitors for which clinical manifestations in the patient diagnosed with osteoarthritis? *(Select all that apply.)*
A. Pain that improves with activity
B. Joint pain
C. Joint swelling
D. Unsteady gait
E. Increased temperature

Management

Medical Management

Diagnosis

Diagnosis can be made based on clinical manifestations without laboratory testing or radiographs when the patient is 45 or older and presents with persistent usage-related pain in several joints and morning stiffness that lasts less than 30 minutes. The American College of Rheumatology

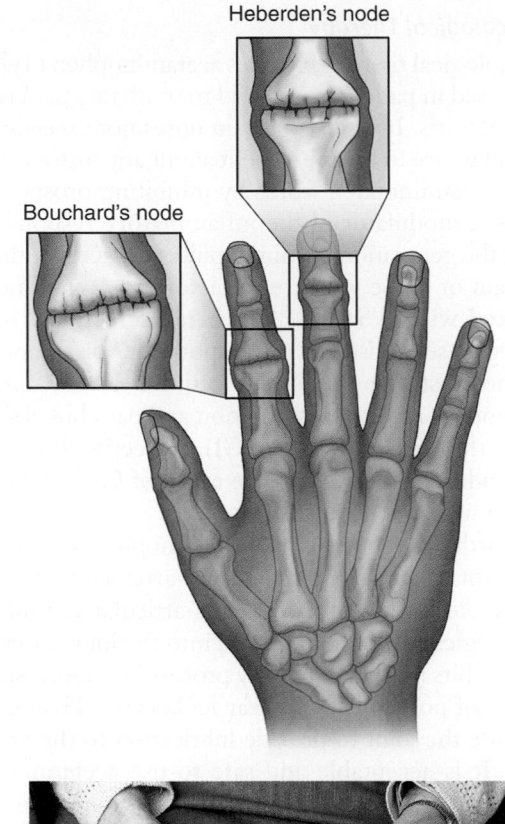

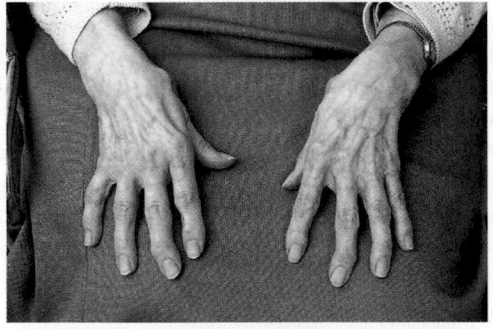

FIGURE 20.2 Osteoarthritis of the hand. *A,* Heberden's nodes and Bouchard's nodes. *B,* Clinical presentation of Heberden's and Bouchard's nodes.

(ACR) developed criteria for the diagnosis of osteoarthritis of the hand, hip, and knee initially in 1986. They are still current today (Boxes 20.1, 20.2, and 20.3).

Laboratory Testing

Laboratory testing may be performed to rule out other diagnoses, such as rheumatoid arthritis (RA). Laboratory testing should also be conducted as a part of the medical management of osteoarthritis in order to monitor for side effects related to medication use.

Radiographs

Plain radiographs of the affected joints, such as the hands, hips, knees, and spine, along with a history and physical examination can be used to confirm the diagnosis of osteoarthritis. Evidence of osteoarthritis includes joint-space narrowing, subchondral sclerosis or cysts, and the presence of osteophytes. Plain radiographs, however, may not show evidence of osteoarthritis until the disease is well advanced.

Treatment

Ideally, both pharmacological and nonpharmacological therapies should be utilized to treat osteoarthritis. Unfortunately, there is no therapy available to stop the progression of osteoarthritis. The goals of care include decreasing pain and improving or maintaining joint mobility while avoiding the toxic effects of pharmacological therapy.

Nonpharmacological Therapies

Nonpharmacological therapies for osteoarthritis include the following: weight loss if indicated; heat and cold compress applications; aerobic exercise; physical therapy, including range of motion and muscle-strengthening exercises; the use of ambulatory assistive devices; appropriate footwear, such as lateral-wedged insoles; occupational therapy; joint protection; energy conservation; and assistive devices for activities of daily living. Also important is patient education about self-management programs and social support.

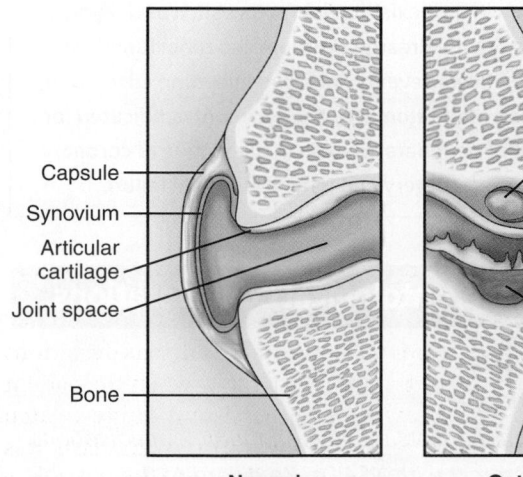

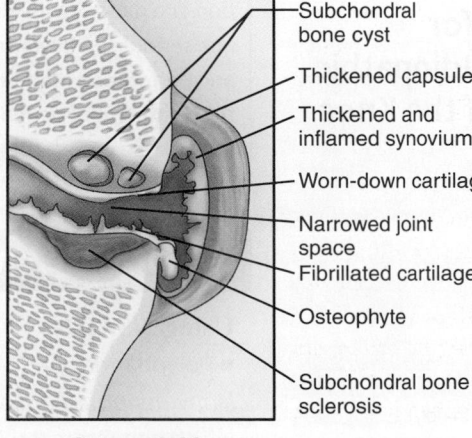

FIGURE 20.3 Osteoarthritis of the knee.

Box 20.1 Classification Criteria for Osteoarthritis of the Hand

Hand pain, aching, or stiffness and three or four of the following features:

- Hard tissue enlargement of 2 or more of 10 selected joints
- Hard tissue enlargement of two or more distal interphalangeal (DIP) joints
- Fewer than three swollen metacarpophalangeal (MCP) joints
- Deformity of at least 1 of 10 selected joints

    The 10 selected joints are the second and third DIP joints, the second and third proximal interphalangeal (PIP) joints, and the first carpometacarpal joints of both hands.

This classification method yields a sensitivity of 94% and a specificity of 87%. From Altman, R., Alarcón, G., Appelrouth, D., Bloch, D., Borenstein, D., Brandt, K., ... Wolfe, F. (1990). The American College of Rheumatology criteria for the classification and reporting of osteoarthritis of the hand. *Arthritis & Rheumatism, 33,* 1601–1610.

Box 20.2 Combined Clinical and Radiographical Classification Criteria for Osteoarthritis of the Hip

Hip pain and at least two of the following three features:

- Erythrocyte sedimentation rate less than 20 mm/hr
- Radiographical femoral or acetabular osteophytes
- Radiographical joint space narrowing

This classification method yields a sensitivity of 89% and a specificity of 91%. From Altman, R., Alarcón, G., Appelrouth, D., Bloch, D., Borenstein, D., Brandt, K., ... Wolfe, F. (1991). The American College of Rheumatology criteria for the classification and reporting of osteoarthritis of the hip. *Arthritis & Rheumatism, 34,* 505–514.

Box 20.3 Clinical Criteria for Classification of Idiopathic Osteoarthritis of the Knee

Knee pain plus three of the following criteria:

- Age greater than 50 years
- Stiffness less than 30 minutes
- Crepitus
- Bony tenderness
- Bony enlargement
- No palpable warmth

From Altman, R., Asch, E., Bloch, D., Bole, G., Borenstein, D., Brandt, K., ... Wolfe, F. (1986). Development of criteria for the classification and reporting of osteoarthritis: Classification of osteoarthritis of the knee. *Arthritis & Rheumatism, 29,* 1039–1049.

Pharmacological Therapy

Pharmacological therapy includes acetaminophen (Tylenol), which is used in patients with mild to moderate pain related to osteoarthritis. It is safe to use in doses not exceeding 4 g daily, but be sure to ask the patient about any history of liver disease. Acetaminophen works by inhibiting prostaglandin synthesis, a modulator of the inflammatory response, and blocking the generation of pain impulses. Patients with more severe pain or those who are refractory to acetaminophen are treated with NSAIDs, which nonselectively inhibit cyclooxygenase, an isoenzyme responsible for the production of the prostaglandins. Nonselective means inhibition of prostaglandin's role in inflammation and pain but also inhibition of the gastrointestinal (GI) protective function of prostaglandin, hence the adverse effect of GI bleeding and ulceration with NSAID use.

Osteoarthritis refractory to acetaminophen and NSAIDs may warrant treatment by using intra-articular injections of corticosteroids or hyaluronans. Intra-articular steroid injections strategically place the steroid into the joint space. The steroid inhibits the inflammatory process by suppressing the migration of polymorphonuclear leukocytes. Hyaluronans work inside the joint to provide lubrication to the articular surfaces. It is acceptable and safe to use acetaminophen, NSAIDs, and intra-articular medications in conjunction with each other; however, patients should not use more than one NSAID concomitantly because of increased risk of bleeding, development of gastric ulcers, and risk of renal damage (see Safety Alert and Geriatric/Gerontological Considerations). Opioid analgesics are an option but should be used sparingly because they may be habit forming. They bind to opioid receptors in the central and peripheral nervous systems, which decreases pain perception. See Table 20.1 for an overview of pharmacological treatment options.

> **Safety Alert** **NSAID Warning**
> NSAIDs may cause an increased risk of serous cardiovascular thrombotic events, myocardial infarction, stroke, renal insufficiency (especially in a "stressed" kidney, e.g., a patient with pre-existing risk factors such as dehydration or a patient with already compromised renal function), and serious GI adverse events, including bleeding, ulceration, and perforation of the stomach. They are contraindicated for the treatment of perioperative pain in the setting of coronary artery bypass graft surgery and patients in renal failure.

Geriatric/Gerontological Considerations

Using NSAIDs

- Polypharmacy

Many geriatric patients may be on multiple medications, which can interact with NSAIDs. Be aware of the possible medication interactions.

● Multiple comorbidities

Older patients may have multiple disorders. Confirm that NSAIDs are an appropriate treatment.

● Possible renal insufficiency

Use of NSAIDs carries an increased risk of renal complications and can exacerbate renal problems that are common in older patients.

● Use of current antiplatelet or anticoagulant therapy

NSAIDs can increase the risk of bleeding disorders and should not be used with antiplatelet or anticoagulant therapy.

Complications

Possible complications of osteoarthritis include chronic pain, decreased function, and toxic effects of medications.

Osteoarthritis can also negatively affect comorbid conditions such as diabetes and heart failure related to a decreased ability to exercise.

Surgical Management

Surgical interventions may be necessary for some patients suffering from disability and severe pain related to osteoarthritis. These procedures include arthroscopic irrigation and/or débridement, arthroscopic synovectomy, surgical fusion, and total joint replacement. Arthroscopic irrigation and/or débridement is a procedure in which the joint is irrigated and expanded in order to visualize the joint and remove debris that could be promoting joint inflammation. Synovectomy is a surgical procedure used to remove excessive growth of the synovial membrane in order to reduce joint inflammation. Surgical fusion is a procedure performed to fuse together the joint surfaces to eliminate any movement of the joint. Total joint replacement involves surgically replacing the joint surface with a prosthesis.

Table 20.1 Pharmacological Therapy for the Treatment of Osteoarthritis

Oral, Systemic Medications	Uses	Possible Side Effects
Acetaminophen	Mild to moderate pain	● Hepatic toxicity especially in those who use alcohol regularly ● Potentiation of warfarin
NSAIDs	Mild to moderate pain unresponsive to acetaminophen or severe pain	● Nephrotic toxicity ● Gastrointestinal bleeding ● Anticoagulation
Nonacetylated salicylates	Use as an alternative to NSAIDs for high-risk patients	● Ototoxicity
Opioid analgesics	Moderate to severe pain	● Nausea ● Constipation ● Confusion ● Drowsiness ● Respiratory depression ● Addiction
Topical, Local Medications		
Intra-articular corticosteroids	Use in conjunction with oral medications	● Local discomfort ● Temporary increase in blood glucose level
Intra-articular hyaluronans	Use in conjunction with oral medications	● Local discomfort ● Temporary increase in synovitis
Topical NSAIDs	Use as alternative to oral medications	● Local skin irritation
Topical capsaicin	Use as alternative to oral medications	● Local skin irritation

Nursing Management
Assessment and Analysis

Clinical manifestations of osteoarthritis are related to pain and decreased function of the affected joints. In addition, there may be clinical manifestations related to pharmacological therapy. The nurse may identify the following:

- Unsteady gait
- Bony enlargement or swelling of affected joints
- Fatigue
- Painful range of motion of affected joints
- Elevated serum creatinine secondary to NSAID use
- Elevated liver enzymes related to multiple medication use
- Constipation secondary to decreased physical activity and/or use of narcotic analgesics

Nursing Diagnoses

- **Pain** related to the disease process
- **Ineffective sleep patterns** related to pain
- **Self-care deficit** related to decreased range of motion

Nursing Interventions

▪ *Assessments*

- Vital signs
  Hypertension may occur related to chronic NSAID therapy that alters renal function, reducing sodium excretion and enhancing fluid retention.
- Weight
  The use of NSAIDs may alter renal function as noted previously, leading to weight gain.
- Skin integrity
  Skin breakdown may occur in bony prominences because of decreased physical mobility.
- Serum creatinine
  The use of NSAIDs may lead to renal impairment by inadvertently blocking essential prostaglandins, which maintain blood flow to the kidneys, resulting in an increase in serum creatinine, while blocking the targeted prostaglandins, which are necessary for pain control.

▪ *Actions*

- Administer analgesic and anti-inflammatory medications as ordered.
  Acetaminophen and NSAIDs reduce pain by inhibiting prostaglandin production, thus blocking the generation of pain impulses and inhibiting the inflammatory response. Opioids alter the perception of pain.
- Provide cold packs for painful joints.
  Cold reduces inflammation.
- Provide a heat pad for painful muscles.
  Heat relaxes muscles and causes vasodilation, which improves blood flow and promotes healing.

▪ *Teaching*

- Take medications only as prescribed.
  Misuse or overuse of analgesics and anti-inflammatories may lead to side effects and can be dangerous; NSAID therapy may increase the risk of myocardial infarction (MI), GI bleeding, stomach ulcers, renal insufficiency, and abnormal platelet function. See Safety Alert.
- Report chest pain, abdominal pain, abnormal bleeding, and blood in the stool or emesis.
  Signs of NSAID toxicity or MI
- Participate in regular physical activity.
  Physical activity promotes good health, weight management, joint mobility, muscle strength, cardiac health, and self-efficacy. It also can reduce stress, anxiety, and depression.
- Assist with referring the patient to occupational and physical activities.
  Fitting for assistive devices, splints, and other assistive devices should be done by physical and occupational therapists. Physical and occupational therapies should be utilized to improve or maintain joint function.
- Assist with referring the patient to orthopedic surgery when necessary.
  Surgery may be necessary for end-stage osteoarthritis once other treatments have failed.
- Assist with home healthcare referral.
  Home care may be utilized for a number of reasons, including assessing patients' homes for safety hazards and teaching patients and their families about the management of osteoarthritis.

Evaluating Care Outcomes

It is important for patients with osteoarthritis to maintain function. A well-managed patient has pain under control and has good, unrestricted movement. This may be achieved by utilizing both pharmacological and nonpharmacological modalities. Patient compliance with therapy is best achieved when they and their support system are well educated and understand why therapies are prescribed and the possible negative outcomes related to nonadherence.

RHEUMATOID ARTHRITIS

Epidemiology

Rheumatoid arthritis (RA) affects approximately 1% of the population. Females are three times more likely to be affected than males, and it is more prevalent in certain ethnic groups, such as Pima and Chippewa Indians. The onset of RA may occur at any age but is most common in the third through fifth decades, and the incidence increases after the sixth decade. The exact etiology of RA is unclear; however, it is well understood that genetics and environmental factors play a key role in the development of the disease. First-degree relatives of patients with RA are at a 1.5-fold higher risk than the general population. Environmental factors such as cigarette smoke, bacteria, and viruses have been implicated as initiating factors for the development of RA in the genetically predisposed population. Some patients initially diagnosed with RA may experience long-term remission within 1 year of onset. For those patients who do not enter remission, about 60% will be disabled within 10 years.

Pathophysiology

Rheumatoid arthritis is a chronic, systemic, autoimmune inflammatory disease characterized by an inflammatory process that affects diarthrodial, or freely moving, joints, causing pain and swelling. The involved joints are usually distributed in a symmetrical fashion, meaning bilateral wrists, ankles, or knees (Fig. 20.4). Rheumatoid arthritis primarily targets the synovial membrane. The exact pathophysiology is unclear; however, it is known that an unknown antigen triggers an immune response, leading to synovial tissue damage. The immune system essentially fails to

distinguish "self" from "non-self" and causes destruction to the synovium of joints. Inflammation of the synovium may lead to a dramatic increase in synovial fluid, impairing movement and causing pain. The synovial membrane becomes thickened and promotes the destruction of the joint (Fig. 20.5). In this process, antigens (substances that trigger an immune response in order to rid the body of that substance) activate monocytes and T lymphocytes; then immunoglobulin antibodies form immune complexes with antigens. Phagocytosis of the immune complexes generates an inflammatory reaction. Leukotrienes and prostaglandins are produced as a result of phagocytosis. Leukotrienes attract additional white blood cells, and prostaglandins modify inflammation. Collagenase, an enzyme that breaks down collagen, is also produced by leukotrienes and prostaglandins, leading to edema, proliferation of synovial membrane and pannus formation (a layer of vascular fibrous tissue), destruction of cartilage, and erosion of bone.

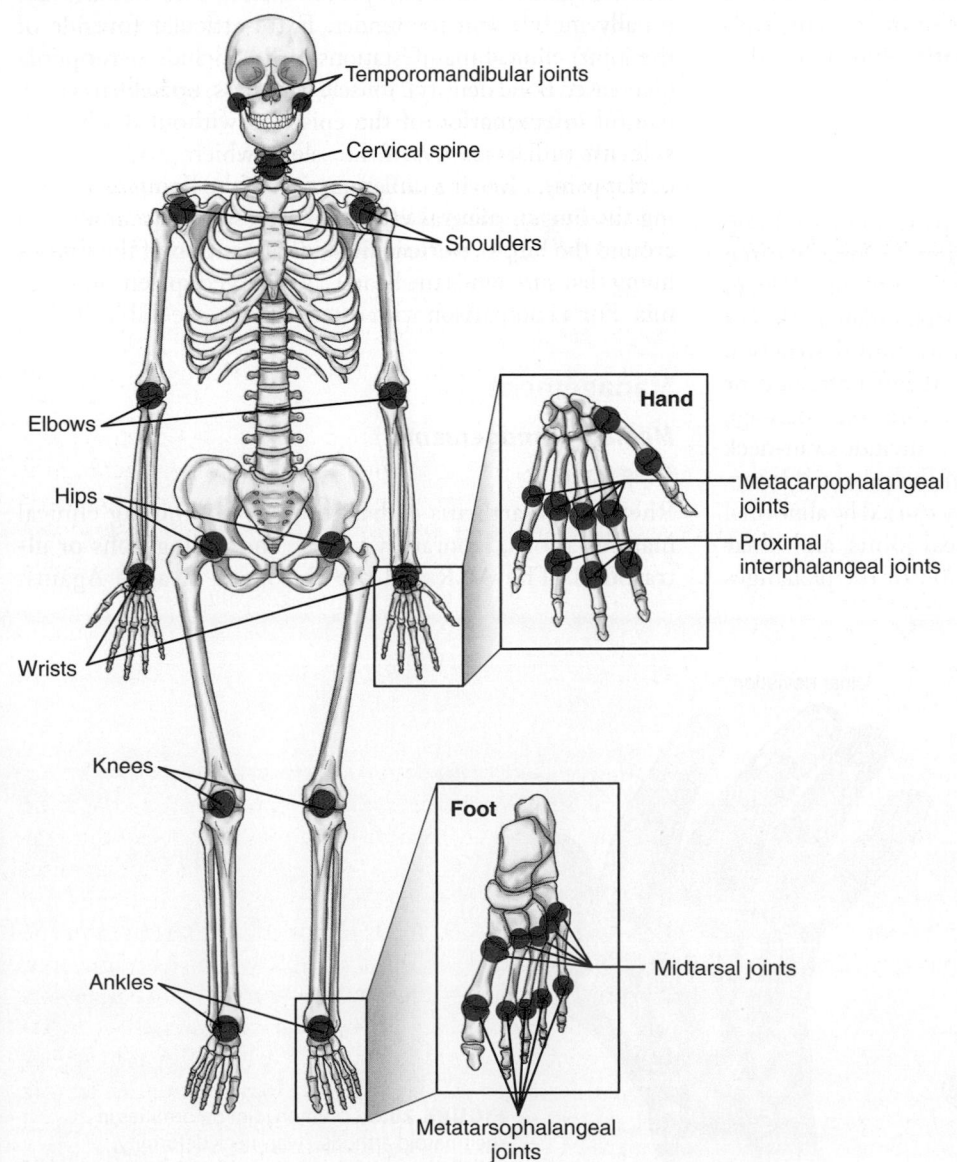

FIGURE 20.4 Common joints affected by rheumatoid arthritis.

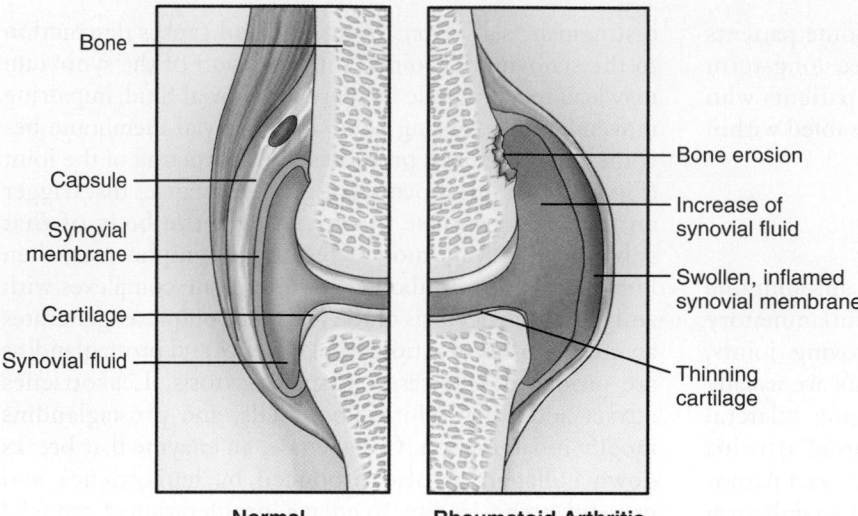

Normal   **Rheumatoid Arthritis**

Bone

Capsule

Synovial membrane

Cartilage

Synovial fluid

Bone erosion

Increase of synovial fluid

Swollen, inflamed synovial membrane

Thinning cartilage

FIGURE 20.5 Rheumatoid arthritis of the hand.

Less commonly, there is inflammation in other organs, including the lungs, heart, skin, kidneys, blood vessels, salivary glands, bone marrow, and the nervous system, leading to vasculitis, lung fibrosis, neuropathy, and kidney disease, to name a few.

Clinical Manifestations

Clinical manifestations include joint pain, joint swelling, erythema, morning stiffness, and fatigue. Onset is often insidious, with vague complaints of joint and muscle pain that evolves into joint pain with **synovitis**, inflammation of the synovial membrane, and can lead to joint destruction and deformity. Rheumatoid arthritis, if left untreated or inadequately treated, leads to irreversible joint damage and disability. Common joint deformities include swan-neck deformity caused by hyperextension of the proximal interphalangeal joints, boutonnière deformity caused by abnormal flexion of the proximal interphalangeal joints, and ulnar deviation caused by the lateral deviation of the phalanges

(Fig. 20.6). **Rheumatoid nodules** may be formed in subcutaneous tissue over bony prominences. The nodules are usually mobile and nontender. Extra-articular (outside of the joint) clinical manifestations of RA include **osteopenia** (decreased bone density), muscle weakness, **episcleritis** (red, painful inflammation of the episclera without discharge), **scleritis** (inflammation of the sclera, which produces deep ocular pain), **pleuritis** (inflammation of the lining surrounding the lungs), **pleural effusion** (excess fluid accumulation around the lungs), **pericarditis** (inflammation of the fibrous lining that surrounds the heart), an enlarged spleen, and anemia. For a comparison with osteoarthritis, see Table 20.2.

Management

Medical Management

Diagnosis

Rheumatoid arthritis is diagnosed by combining clinical manifestations, laboratory values, and radiographs or ultrasound. The ACR and the European League Against

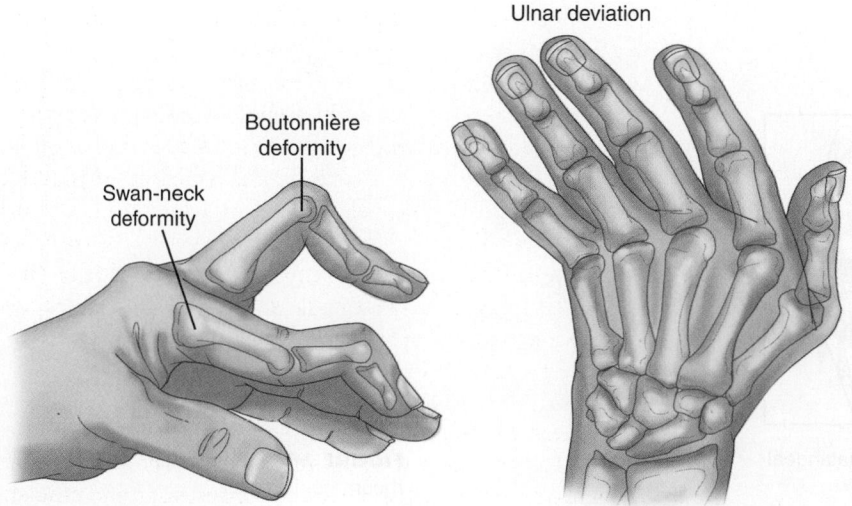

Ulnar deviation

Boutonnière deformity

Swan-neck deformity

FIGURE 20.6 Common joint deformities in rheumatoid arthritis: swan-neck deformity, boutonnière deformity, and ulnar deviation.

Table 20.2 Comparing Osteoarthritis to Rheumatoid Arthritis

	Osteoarthritis	Rheumatoid Arthritis
Morning stiffness	Less than 30 minutes	More than 30 minutes
Immune mediated	No	Yes
Typical joint involvement	• Large weight-bearing joints such as hips and knees • PIPs • DIPs • CMC • First MTP • Previously injured joints	• MCPs • PIPs • MTPs • Wrists • Elbows • Ankles • Knees
Symmetrical joint involvement	Not typical	Very typical
Systemic organ involvement	No	Yes

DIP, Distal interphalangeal; *CMC*, carpometacarpal; *MTP*, metatarsophalangeal; *MCP*, metacarpophalangeal; *PIP*, proximal interphalangeal

Rheumatism have worked together to update criteria for diagnosing RA in order to diagnose the disease at an early stage. The criteria assign point values to joint involvement, laboratory values, and duration of symptoms. When evaluating clinical manifestations, patients typically present with peripheral joint pain, which is usually symmetrical, and complain of morning stiffness lasting greater than 30 minutes. Symptoms persisting 6 weeks or longer are consistent with RA. Another important finding of RA is synovitis. Tenderness and synovitis are assessed by palpating each joint individually. Tenderness is subjective, whereas synovitis is objective. The clinician is usually able to detect the synovitis on examination via palpation or, if not detected by palpation, through ultrasonography.

Connection Check 20.3

When comparing osteoarthritis to RA, the nurse recognizes which of the following statements to be true? *(Select all that apply.)*

A. Osteoarthritic pain tends to get worse with activity, but RA gets better with activity.

B. Both RA and osteoarthritis are autoimmune diseases.

C. Patients with RA are at risk for developing extra-articular manifestations such as eye inflammation and lung disease, whereas osteoarthritis affects only joints and surrounding structures.

D. Patients with osteoarthritis typically have morning stiffness lasting less than 30 minutes hour, whereas RA patients typically complain of morning stiffness lasting greater than 30 minutes

E. Both RA and osteoarthritis affect joints in a symmetrical pattern.

Laboratory Testing

Laboratory testing is not conclusive but is done to help with diagnosis and to monitor for side effects related to medication use. The presence of the antibodies, rheumatoid factor, and anticyclic citrullinated peptides may assist in the confirmation of the diagnosis, but the absence of these does not exclude the diagnosis because approximately 25% to 30% of patients are negative for antibodies. Also, a positive rheumatoid factor does not always indicate the presence of RA. Other autoimmune diseases may have a positive rheumatoid factor. Acute-phase reactants such as C-reactive protein (CRP) and erythrocyte sedimentation rate (ESR) may be used to detect inflammation but are not specific for RA. Elevated CRP and/or ESR is an indicator that can be useful in distinguishing inflammatory from noninflammatory arthritis.

Obtaining information regarding renal and hepatic functions is necessary before initiating therapy because many medications used to treat RA can be toxic to the kidneys and liver. Baseline complete blood counts are necessary because antirheumatic medications may cause **cytopenia,** a reduced amount of blood cells. Common cytopenias include thrombocytopenia, a reduced number of platelets; leukocytopenia, a reduced number of white blood cells; and anemia, a reduced number of red blood cells. An elevated platelet count may indicate the presence of inflammation. Before the initiation of most biological therapies, an option for treatment of RA, a tuberculin skin test and hepatitis testing should also be performed because some biological therapies have the potential to reactivate dormant infections.

Radiographs

Conventional radiographs are used to assess for bony erosions and joint-space narrowing. Radiographs may be repeated during treatment to assess for disease progression and efficacy of pharmalogical therapy. Magnetic resonance imaging (MRI) may detect erosions not detected by conventional radiographs. Ultrasonography may also be used to assess for synovitis and erosions not detectable by plain radiographs and is a good option for patients who decline MRI because of cost or claustrophobia.

Treatment

Nonpharmacological Therapy

Education is very important in the management of RA. Patients must understand their disease and the measures they can take to help manage the disease. Range-of-motion exercises promote joint mobility, reduce stiffness, and improve muscle strength. Aerobic exercise promotes cardiac health. Physical and occupational therapies may be necessary to teach patients appropriate exercises, teach patients how to protect their joints, evaluate the need for assistive devices, and teach proper use of the devices. Proper nutrition is important to maintain good health, prevent obesity, and decrease the risk of heart disease. It is important for patients to take rest periods to manage fatigue and joint pain.

Pharmacological Therapy

The goal of pharmacological treatment is to control the inflammation that leads to joint and tissue destruction, decreasing joint pain, synovitis, and stiffness as well as maintaining joint function and preventing joint destruction. Treatment decisions are based on disease severity and response to medications. Initial treatments include analgesics, NSAIDs, and glucocorticoids. Analgesics, including acetaminophen and narcotic agents, provide only pain relief with no alteration in the disease process. Anti-inflammatory medications provide pain relief and some reduction in inflammation but do not alter the disease process. Glucocorticoids such as prednisone may be given orally, intramuscularly, intra-articularly, or IV and can actually suppress inflammation and alter the disease process but are not safe at high doses over long periods of time. Patients with RA whose disease does not respond very well to a combination of analgesics, anti-inflammatory agents, and low-dose prednisone are treated with **disease-modifying antirheumatic drugs (DMARDs)**.

Synthetic DMARDs include but are not limited to methotrexate (Rheumatrex), leflunomide (Arava), hydroxychloroquine (Plaquenil), sulfasalazine (Azulfidine), and tofacitinib (Xeljanz). Each alters the immune system in various ways, altering the inflammatory response to decrease inflammation and slow disease progression. These medications may be used alone as monotherapy or in conjunction with one another. Remember, before starting DMARD medications, patients should inform their healthcare provider of a history of or exposure to active tuberculosis. Fortunately, many patients respond well to methotrexate, which has been accepted as a first-line DMARD of choice to treat RA. Methotrexate is taken once weekly orally, subcutaneously, or intramuscularly (see Safety Alert). Traditionally, patients move on to additional or alternative medications if methotrexate alone does not control the disease (Table 20.3).

Table 20.3 Disease-Modifying Antirheumatic Medication Therapy	
Medication	**Mechanism of Action (MOA)**
• Methotrexate (Rheumatrex)	• Exact MOA is unknown, but it is thought to affect immune function
• Sulfasalazine (Azulfidine)	• Systemically interferes with prostaglandin synthesis
• Hydroxychloroquine (Plaquenil)	• Impairs complement-dependent antigen–antibody reaction
• Leflunomide (Arava)	• Inhibits pyrimidine synthesis, resulting in antiproliferative and anti-inflammatory effects
• Tofacitinib (Xeljanz)	• Inhibits Janus kinase; an inflammation mediator

Over the last decade, several medications, known as *biologics*, genetically engineered medications made from living organisms and their products, such as proteins, have obtained approval by the U.S. Food and Drug Administration to treat RA. These medications have proven to be beneficial in slowing or even halting the progression of RA. To date, the approved biological therapies must be infused IV or injected subcutaneously. Biologics target specific entities of the inflammatory cascade, thus interrupting the immune response and decreasing inflammation. See Table 20.4 for an overview of biological therapy.

 Safety Alert **Methotrexate Safety Warning**

- Patients on methotrexate must be monitored closely for hepatic toxicity while the dose is being escalated and periodically while on a maintenance dose.
- Take folic acid daily to prevent side effects such as oral ulcers.
- Avoid alcohol while taking this medication because of the risk of hepatotoxicity.
- Counsel female patients on proper birth control methods because of significant risk of teratogenicity, the capability of producing fetal malformation.
- Patients with renal insufficiency require lower doses of methotrexate.

Surgical Management

Surgical interventions including joint replacement or fusion may be necessary to help alleviate pain but may not actually improve function. Patients may choose to have surgical removal of rheumatoid nodules, but they may return over time.

Table 20.4   Biological Therapy Approved to Treat Rheumatoid Arthritis

Medication	Mechanism	Route
Infliximab (Remicade)	Binds to TNF	Intravenous
Etanercept (Enbrel)	Binds to TNF	Subcutaneous
Adalimumab (Humira)	Binds to TNF	Subcutaneous
Rituximab (Rituxan)	Targets B lymphocytes	Intravenous
Certolizumab (Cimzia)	Binds to TNF	Subcutaneous
Golimumab (Simponi)	Binds to TNF	Subcutaneous
Tocilizumab (Actemra)	Binds to IL-6 receptors	Intravenous
Abatacept (Orencia)	Modulates T-lymphocyte activation	Intravenous or subcutaneous

IL, Interleukin; *TNF,* tumor necrosis factor.

Complications

Many complications may be associated with RA, which may be caused by uncontrolled disease or as a result of pharmacological therapy. Patients can develop decreased function of joints and permanent joint deformities, which may lead to permanent disability if the disease is not well controlled. Extra-articular complications include increased risk of infection and increased risk of developing cancer.

Nursing Management

Assessment and Analysis

As with osteoarthritis, clinical manifestations of RA are related to pain and decreased function of the affected joints. In addition, there may be clinical manifestations related to pharmacological therapy. The nurse may identify the following:

- Unsteady gait
- Bony enlargement or swelling of affected joints
- Warmth and redness of joints
- Painful range of motion of affected joints
- Increased incidence of infection
- Elevated serum creatinine secondary to NSAID use
- Elevated liver enzymes secondary to methotrexate or leflunomide
- Constipation secondary to decreased physical activity and/or use of narcotic analgesics
- Nausea and oral ulcers related to methotrexate use
- Cough and/or shortness of breath due to interstitial lung disease, which can be caused by RA or by methotrexate therapy

- Self-care deficit
- Fatigue

Nursing Diagnoses

- **Pain** related to disease process
- **Ineffective sleep patterns** related to pain
- **Self-care deficit** related to decreased range of motion

Nursing Interventions

Assessments

- Joint pain and mobility
  Joint pain and mobility are indicators of treatment efficacy and disease progression.
- Temperature
  An increase in temperature is an indicator of infection.
- Laboratory testing
  - CRP and ESR
    Elevated values are indicative of inflammation.
  - Hemoglobin
    May be less than normal in patients with active RA, but a decreased value may also indicate a GI bleed, which can be caused by NSAID use.
  - Serum albumin
    Decreased value is correlated with increased disease severity because it is a negative acute-phase reactant and decreases in response to acute inflammation.
  - Platelet count
    May be elevated in very active disease because inflammation causes elevated platelet count.
  - Liver and renal function
    Elevated levels may be due to medications used to treat RA.
- Assess for pleural effusion, pericarditis, pleuritic, scleritis, episcleritis, and osteopenia.
  Extra-articular clinical manifestations of RA may be present due to the inflammatory changes outside of the joints.

Actions

- Administer analgesics and anti-inflammatories as ordered.
  Analgesics and anti-inflammatories provide pain relief by reducing inflammation but do not alter the disease process.
- Administer glucocorticoids as ordered.
  Glucocorticoids decrease pain by suppressing the inflammatory process and may alter the course of the disease.
- Administer DMARD therapy as ordered.
  DMARD therapy is very important in slowing disease progression by modulating the immune system and decreasing the inflammatory process.
- Administer biologics as ordered.
  Biologics have been shown to slow or halt the progression of RA through inhibition of tumor necrosis factor (TNF) or interleukins (ILs).

Teaching

- Importance of adherence to treatment plan
  It is essential to maintain the treatment plan to control disease progression.

- Report signs and symptoms of infection.
  Because of treatment with anti-inflammatories and immunosuppressive therapy, patients must be aware of signs and symptoms of infection and the importance of reporting these to their rheumatologist.
- Immunosuppressive therapy should be discontinued while patients have an active infection.
  Immunosuppressive therapy puts patients at a higher risk for developing infections and complications from infections.
- Assist with referral to an infectious disease specialist for patients with chronic or atypical infections.
  Patients with rheumatoid arthritis who are on immunosuppressive therapy are at risk for developing infections.
- Keep current with vaccinations.
  Patients with rheumatoid arthritis are at risk for infections due to treatment but should not receive live vaccines if on immunosuppressive therapy.
- Refer to physical and occupational therapies as needed.
  Therapy may preserve joint function and improve patients' quality of life.

Connection Check 20.4

The nurse knows that which of the following statements regarding laboratory values and RA are true? *(Select all that apply.)*

A. Patients with a positive rheumatoid factor definitely have RA.

B. An elevated CRP is indicative of inflammation but is not specific only for RA.

C. Certain DMARD therapies may cause laboratory abnormalities such as elevated liver enzymes, thrombocytopenia, and leukocytopenia.

D. Approximately 25% to 30% of patients who have RA do not have a positive rheumatoid factor.

E. Patients with RA have elevated cardiac enzymes due to pharmacological therapy.

Evaluating Care Outcomes

Important assessments of the efficacy of pharmacological therapy are the amount of joint tenderness and synovitis the patient is experiencing and the duration of morning stiffness.

It is possible to achieve remission by using effective medications. Having active patient involvement aids in that process (see Evidence-Based Practice). Teaching the importance of using antirheumatic medications properly and consistently is key in treating RA patients. Patients should understand that full efficacy cannot be achieved if the medication is not used consistently and that the medications can be dangerous if used more than directed. Ideally, the patient with well-controlled RA will have very few or no tender or swollen joints with minimal morning stiffness while experiencing little or no adverse effects from pharmacological therapy.

Evidence-Based Practice

PROMIS: Patient-Reported Outcomes Measurement Information System

The DREAM Remission Induction Cohort Study published in 2012 was designed to identify patients with early rheumatoid arthritis (RA) and evaluate the treatment strategies best able to achieve remission. The study developed the treat to target (T2T) strategy to guide care and determine treatment goals. Treat to target included the goal of clinical remission by adjusting medication therapy frequently and documenting the disease process frequently. The study suggested that clinical disease remission through use of effective medications is a realistic goal and should be the goal for every patient with RA. An important component of the success of the treatment program is active patient involvement. Standardizing and personalizing the T2T approach for RA using the Patient-Reported Outcomes Measurement Information System (PROMIS) was initiated as a way to increase patients' involvement in their plan of care. Patients were asked to complete a survey quarterly to identify the treatment domains most important to them. Options included pain management, fatigue, depression, physical function, and social function. The incorporation of the quarterly PROMIS questionnaires into clinic visits was found to be a viable process for incorporating patient preferences into a T2T approach to the management of RA.

Bacalao, E. J., Greene, G. J., Beaumont, J. L., Eisenstein, A., Muftic, A., Mandelin, A. M., . . . Ruderman, E. M. (2017). Standardizing and personalizing the treat to target (T2T) approach for rheumatoid arthritis using the Patient-Reported Outcomes Measurement Information System (PROMIS): Baseline findings on patient-centered treatment priorities. *Clinical Rheumatology, 36*(8), 1729–1736.

CASE STUDY: EPISODE 2

Ms. Logan presents with bilateral hand and wrist pain and pain and swelling in the second and third fingers. She also describes morning stiffness lasting longer than 1 hour and increased fatigue, which are symptoms consistent with RA. Initial laboratory testing reveals elevated rheumatoid factor, ESR, CRP, and anticyclic citrullinated peptide levels. Ultrasound reveals synovitis located in each wrist and bilateral second and third proximal interphalangeal joints...

SCLERODERMA

Epidemiology

The incidence of scleroderma is estimated to be 9 to 19 cases per million per year. The usual age of onset is 30 to 50 years; however, the age of onset for women ranges from 15 to 40 years, and the risk for developing scleroderma declines after menopause. The prevalence of scleroderma in women exceeds the prevalence in men by a ratio of 3:1 to 5:1. The disease affects all races, but African Americans are affected at a higher rate than Caucasians. African Americans tend to develop the disease earlier in life and are likely to have more diffuse disease with a worse prognosis. Scleroderma is not considered a hereditary disease, but patients who have a first-degree relative with scleroderma are more susceptible to developing the disease than the general population. It has also been suggested that, as in other autoimmune connective tissue diseases, environmental exposures such as infectious agents and occupational toxins may play a role in triggering the disease.

Pathophysiology

Scleroderma is a very complex disease that not only affects the skin but also may involve internal organs. The exact cause of scleroderma is unknown, but it is believed to be an autoimmune disease caused by many external triggers. Small-vessel vasculopathy (disease affecting blood vessels), pathological accumulation of collagen, and autoimmunity cause the disease manifestations. Tissue damage occurs when mononuclear cells cluster in tissues such as the skin, blood vessels, and organs, stimulating lymphokines that stimulate procollagen, causing insoluble collagen formation in excess. The inflammatory response causes edema, which leads to fibrotic changes, causing loss of elasticity and movement. Eventually, the tissue degenerates and becomes nonfunctional.

Clinical Manifestations

Scleroderma is divided into two main categories: localized and systemic. Localized scleroderma leads to morphea (isolated patches of hardened skin), linear scleroderma (lines of thickened skin affecting the tissues beneath), and scleroderma en coup de saber (thickened skin on the head). Localized scleroderma typically does not affect the internal organs. Systemic sclerosis is divided into the categories of diffuse and limited (Table 20.5).

Clinical manifestations of diffuse or limited systemic sclerosis may involve the skin, lungs, heart, kidneys, and musculoskeletal system. Skin manifestations include patches of thickened skin sometimes accompanied by itching, especially in the early stages. Patients with pulmonary involvement may experience dyspnea, nonproductive cough, and pulmonary fibrosis and have an increased risk of lung cancer. Conditions related to cardiac involvement include pericarditis, pericardial effusion, myocardial fibrosis, heart failure, and arrhythmia. Proteinuria and impaired renal function are common with renal involvement. Musculoskeletal complaints include swelling of the hands, joint pain, muscle pain, and fatigue. Three important manifestations of systemic sclerosis include Raynaud's phenomenon, scleroderma renal crisis, and pulmonary artery hypertension, all of which are due to abnormal vasoconstriction of

small vessels as a result of functional changes in the arteries. **Raynaud's phenomenon** results from vasospasm of the small vessels in the hands caused by exposure to cold. Vasospasm of the small vessels causes the fingers to blanch white, become blue from cyanosis, and then become red from reactive hyperemia. Raynaud's phenomenon is secondary to scleroderma and should not be confused with primary Raynaud's disease. Primary Raynaud's disease is common in the general population and does not result in permanent tissue damage, whereas Raynaud's phenomenon frequently causes permanent tissue damage and loss of digits due to chronic ischemia. Although mild renal dysfunction is common in scleroderma patients, scleroderma renal crisis occurs in approximately 10% to 20% of patients with diffuse systemic scleroderma but rarely in those with the limited cutaneous form. Scleroderma renal crisis is characterized by a sudden onset of severe hypertension, proteinuria, and progressive renal failure. Even with aggressive treatment, morbidity and mortality are high. Pulmonary artery hypertension symptoms develop insidiously, usually with a feeling of generalized weakness on exertion, then later dyspnea. Pulmonary disease is the leading cause of death in patients with systemic scleroderma. See Table 20.6 for clinical manifestations according to organ system.

| Table 20.5 Systemic Scleroderma: Limited Versus Diffuse ||
Limited	**Diffuse**
● Insidious onset	● Rapid onset
● Involves the skin of extremities distal to the elbows and knees	● Involves skin of extremities and trunk
● Internal organ involvement less likely and with late onset	● Most likely affects internal organs, typically within 2 years of onset
● Raynaud's phenomenon may precede disease diagnosis by years	● Raynaud's phenomenon may occur concurrently or after diagnosis

Connection Check 20.5

The nurse recognizes which patient with scleroderma to be at the highest risk for morbidity and mortality?

A. An 18-year-old Caucasian female with linear skin lesions noted on her face

B. A 20-year-old Hispanic male with patches of skin on the distal portions of his arms and legs

C. A 32-year-old Caucasian female presenting with thickened skin on her trunk

D. A 45-year-old African American male with Raynaud's disease

Table 20.6 Common Clinical Manifestations of Systemic Scleroderma

Organ System	Manifestations
Skin	• Thickened skin • Digital ulcers • Puffy hands • Pruritus • Superficial skin tenderness • Diffuse hyperpigmentation
Gastrointestinal	• Frequent heartburn • Dysphagia • Esophageal stricture • Erosive esophagitis • Postprandial bloating • Constipation • Malabsorptive diarrhea
Pulmonary	• Generalized fatigue • Shortness of breath • Dry cough • Lung fibrosis
Cardiac	• Arrhythmias • Heart failure • Pericarditis
Renal	• Renal insufficiency • Renal failure
Musculoskeletal	• Joint contractures • Tendon friction rubs • Muscle pain and weakness • Synovitis

Management

Medical Management

Diagnosis

The diagnosis of scleroderma is supported by the presence of clinical manifestations and serum antibodies. Laboratory testing may confirm a diagnosis of scleroderma but is not beneficial in excluding the diagnosis. Common laboratory tests include antinuclear antibody (ANA) screening, then testing for specific antibodies such as antitopoisomerase I (anti-scl-70), anticentromere, anti-RNA polymerase III, and anti-beta2-glycoprotein I. More than 95% of scleroderma patients have at least one of these antibodies present.

Radiographical testing may reveal subcutaneous calcification, distal esophageal hypomotility, and pulmonary fibrosis. Pulmonary function tests are important to assess the vital lung capacity and lung compliance. Echocardiograms should be done routinely to assess for pulmonary artery hypertension and myocardial involvement. Before treatment is initiated, more invasive tests such as bronchoalveolar lavage and right heart catheterization may be required for a definitive diagnosis of interstitial lung disease and pulmonary hypertension, respectively. Kidney biopsies are required to accurately diagnose renal disease.

Treatment

There is no single treatment to manage scleroderma. Treatment is focused on specific organ involvement and clinical manifestations. Systemic steroids such as prednisone suppress the immune response by reducing the migration of leukocytes and reducing the activity of the lymphatic system. Immunosuppressants, such as methotrexate, work by modulating the immune response to decrease inflammation. Antihistamines, such as loratadine (Claritin) and cetirizine (Zyrtec), may alleviate pruritus by blocking H_1 receptors on effector cells. Topical ointments and moisturizers are used to help soften the skin and relieve itching. Vasodilators such as amlodipine (Norvasc) or nifedipine (Procardia) are used to improve circulation and treat Raynaud's phenomenon, pulmonary hypertension, and renal impairment. See Table 20.7 for an overview of treatment options.

Complications

There are many possible complications related to systemic diffuse scleroderma, including infection, renal failure, heart failure, pulmonary fibrosis, and death. Complications should be addressed by healthcare providers based on the system affected and the degree of involvement.

Nursing Management

Assessment and Analysis

Clinical manifestations of scleroderma are related to multiple factors according to the extent of organ involvement as well as side effects of pharmacological therapy. The nurse may identify the following:

- Fatigue
- Thickened or hardened skin
- Digital ulcers
- Dyspnea
- Hypertension
- Decreased range of motion of joints
- Poor nutrition
- Frequent heartburn
- Dysphagia
- Cough

Nursing Diagnoses

- **Altered tissue perfusion** related to chronic ischemia
- **Fatigue** related to the disease process
- **Altered self-image** related to disfiguring skin lesions

Table 20.7 Overview of Treatment Options for Scleroderma

Organ System Involved	Manifestations	Treatment
Skin	• Localized skin thickening such as morphea	• Phototherapy and topical glucocorticoids (prednisone)
	• Pruritus	• Antihistamines and topical lubricants
	• Telangiectasia (vascular lesions formed near the surface of the skin)	• Green-tinted foundation makeup to disguise lesions; laser therapy for large lesions
	• Widespread skin involvement	• Immunosuppressive agents (methotrexate)
		• Physical therapy to limit contractures if skin involvement is over joints
Vascular	• Raynaud's phenomenon	• Avoidance of cold temperatures, stress, nicotine, caffeine, and vasoconstrictive medications (such as cold medications containing pseudoephedrine); wearing gloves and dressing warmly
		• Antiplatelet therapy using low-dose aspirin should be considered in patients with digital ulcers in order to reduce the risk of blood clots.
	• Pulmonary artery hypertension	• Surgical amputation of affected digit may be necessary in severe cases.
		• Vasodilators such as calcium channel blockers (amlodipine [Norvasc])
		• Endothelin-receptor antagonist (bosentan [Tracleer]) that blocks endothelin receptors in smooth muscle in order to inhibit vasoconstriction
		• Phosphodiesterase-5 inhibitor (sildenafil [Revatio]) that inhibits phosphodiesterase type 5 in smooth muscle of pulmonary vasculature to promote vasculature relaxation
	• Scleroderma renal crisis	• Angiotensin-converting enzyme inhibitors are used to help prevent and to treat scleroderma-related renal disease because they promote vasodilation of renal arteries, therefore improving blood flow through the kidneys.
Pulmonary	• Interstitial lung disease	• Immunosuppressive agents: cyclophosphamide is the primary immunosuppressive agent used to treat interstitial lung disease related to scleroderma.
		• Severe cases should be referred for lung transplantation.
Musculoskeletal	• Arthralgia and arthritis	• Analgesics (acetaminophen)
	• Decreased joint mobility	• NSAIDs (ibuprofen)
		• Low-dose glucocorticoids (prednisone)
		• Physical therapy to prevent or limit contractures
Gastrointestinal	• Gastroesophageal reflux disease	• Proton pump inhibitors (omeprazole) that suppress gastric acid secretion should be used even if patients are asymptomatic in order to prevent esophageal strictures.
	• Malabsorption and malnutrition	• Severe cases may require parenteral nutrition.
Cardiac	• Pericarditis	• NSAID therapy or glucocorticoids if NSAIDs are contraindicated

Nursing Interventions

▣ Assessments

- Vital signs at every assessment: blood pressure, heart rate and rhythm, respiratory rate
  Elevated blood pressure may be a sign of renal crisis. Elevated heart rate and ventricular arrhythmias may be present due to heart failure. Increased respiratory rate and effort may indicate interstitial lung disease, pulmonary vascular disease, or pulmonary artery hypertension.
- Auscultate lung sounds.
  The presence of crackles may be indicative of interstitial lung disease.
- Assess skin integrity and document skin thickening.
  Maintaining adequate records of skin involvement is important in monitoring disease progression.
- Assess the musculoskeletal system.
  Swelling of the hands, joint pain, muscle pain, and fatigue are common symptoms of scleroderma. Fibrosis around tendons and joint structures may lead to joint immobility.
- Auscultate bowel sounds and gather information regarding gastroesophageal motility.
  Chronic gastric reflux, difficulty swallowing, choking, cough, bloating, and alternating constipation and diarrhea are manifestations of GI involvement.
- Monitor serum creatinine and blood urea nitrogen (BUN).
  Monitor routinely to assess renal function and possible renal failure.

▣ Actions

- Administer medications as ordered: steroids, immunosuppressants, antihistamines, vasodilators, steroids, topical ointment.
  Steroids reduce the inflammatory response; immunosuppressants modulate the immune response to decrease inflammation; antihistamines alleviate pruritus by blocking H_1 receptors on effector cells; vasodilators dilate arterial vessels, improving circulation; and ointments soften skin and relieve itching.
- Perform range-of-motion exercises.
  Range-of-motion exercises improve joint mobility and help prevent contractures.
- Assist in referring the patient to pulmonologist, gastroenterologist, plastic surgeons, and physical therapy as needed.
  Diffuse scleroderma may lead to decreased pulmonary function, GI dysfunction, disfiguring skin lesions, and decreased joint mobility.
- Refer patients to counseling as needed.
  Many patients suffer from depression as a result of the diagnosis and clinical manifestations.

▣ Teaching

- Scleroderma disease process.
  Scleroderma is a very complicated disease that varies from one patient to another. Patients should understand and monitor for possible complications but realize that they may not experience all possible complications.

- Protect skin from trauma.
  Patients are at higher risk for infection and prolonged healing time related to decreased tissue perfusion.

Connection Check 20.6

In assessing the patient with scleroderma for pending renal crisis, which findings require an intervention by the nurse? *(Select all that apply.)*
A. Significant weight gain
B. Blood pressure 174/100 mm Hg
C. Creatinine 1.9 mg/dL
D. Clear urine output
E. BUN 15 mg/dL

Evaluating Care Outcomes

Diffuse systemic sclerosis is a very complicated and serious condition that is very difficult to treat and usually results in disability and shortened life span; there is no cure. Maintaining stable cardiac, pulmonary, and renal functions is the goal of treatment. Care is focused on monitoring, preventing, and managing complications. The maintenance of skin integrity may help minimize tissue loss, infection, and contractures. A well-controlled scleroderma patient maintains skin integrity and pulmonary, cardiac, GI, and renal functions.

LUPUS

Epidemiology

Systemic lupus erythematosus (SLE) affects fewer than 25 people per 100,000 in North America, South America, Europe, and Asia. Prevalence rates vary depending on gender, ethnicity, geographic location, and age. The female-to-male ratio in children affected by SLE is 3:1 but is as high as 15:1 for women during childbearing years. Statistically, African American women are almost four times more likely to develop the disease than Caucasian Americans; however, SLE occurs infrequently in blacks in Africa, Asians, and African Caribbeans. Hispanic Americans have a higher prevalence rate when compared to Americans of European descent in the United States. The age of onset varies according to gender and ethnicity, but overall, 65% of patients are diagnosed between the ages of 16 and 55. Many factors play a role in disease outcome. African Americans and Mexican Hispanics have a poorer prognosis related to renal disease than do Caucasians. Less-educated patients and those with low socioeconomic status are also more likely to have poorer disease control. Men are more likely than women to have renal disease, skin manifestations, laboratory abnormalities, neurological involvement, thrombosis, cardiovascular disease, and vasculitis, whereas women are more likely to suffer from Raynaud's phenomenon, photosensitivity, and mucosal ulceration. People who have relatives with SLE are at a higher risk than the general population for developing the disease. There have been genes identified that predispose humans to SLE.

Connection Check 20.7

The nurse recognizes which patient to be at the highest risk for developing SLE?
A. A 10-year-old Hispanic female
B. An 18-year-old African American male
C. A 30-year-old African American female
D. A 50-year-old Caucasian male

Pathophysiology

Systemic lupus erythematosus is a chronic inflammatory disease that can affect virtually any organ system. The exact etiology is unknown, as is the case with other autoimmune diseases, but the disease is triggered by multiple factors. Triggering factors include pregnancy, exposure to sunlight, illness, major surgery, silica dust, and medication allergies. Most clinical manifestations of SLE are attributed to antibodies and the creation of immune complexes that are deposited into tissues.

Clinical Manifestations

Clinical manifestations of SLE are diverse, do not follow a clinical pattern, and vary greatly from one person to another. The clinical course of SLE usually involves periods of remission and acute disease flares. See Table 20.8 for a description of clinical manifestations according to organ system.

Management

Medical Management

Diagnosis

Diagnosing lupus may be a complicated and frustrating process for most patients. There is no specific test used to diagnose SLE; rather, laboratory findings are used to support or confirm the diagnosis when combined with patient history and physical examination findings.

The ACR developed guidelines to help in the diagnosis of lupus. The Systemic Lupus International Collaborating Clinics revised and validated the classification criteria to aid in diagnosis. They identified 17 broad criteria that align with the clinical manifestations with specific definitions—some clinical, some immunologic. The clinical criteria include skin rashes such as the lupus malar rash, oral ulcers, thinning hair, joint tenderness, pleural or pericardial effusions, renal (urine protein) and neurological (seizures/confusion) disorders, and haematological disorders such as thrombocytopenia, leukopenia, or anemia. The immunological criteria include positive antinuclear antibody (ANA), low complement, positive anti-Sm, antiphospholipid antibodies, and positive anti–double-stranded DNA (anti-dsDNA). Four of the 17 criteria must present in order to support a

Table 20.8 Clinical Manifestations of Systemic Lupus Erythematosus

Organ System	Manifestations
Constitutional	• Fatigue
	• Fever
	• Difficulty concentrating
Mucocutaneous	• Rash
	Malar, also known as "butterfly rash" across the cheeks
	Discoid lesions, erythematous plaques covered by scale that typically appear on sun-exposed areas
	• Photosensitivity
	• Alopecia
	• Urticaria, palpable purpura, erythematous papules of fingers and palms, splinter hemorrhages, and digital ulcers caused by vasculitis
	• Oral, nasal, and anogenital ulcers
Musculoskeletal	• Joint pain with or without synovitis
	• Muscle pain and weakness
Renal	• Lupus nephritis
	• Proteinuria
	• Hematuria
Neurological	• Stroke
	• Seizures
	• Neuropathy
	• Psychosis
	• Organic brain syndrome
	• Depression
	• Anxiety
Cardiovascular	• Pericarditis
	• Endocarditis
	• Increased risk of cardiovascular disease
Pulmonary	• Pleurisy
	• Pleural effusion
	• Pneumonitis
	• Interstitial lung disease
	• Pulmonary hypertension
Ocular	• Retinal lesions
	• Rarely scleritis or uveitis
	• Dry eyes
Hematological	• Leukopenia
	• Anemia of chronic disease
	• Thrombocytopenia
	• Thromboembolism

diagnosis of SLE—at least one clinical and one immunologic. In clinical practice, however, patients may not have four criteria present to be diagnosed if there is sufficient evidence otherwise.

Laboratory Testing

Laboratory testing is used to confirm some of the clinical and immunological criteria. First, testing is done to confirm the presence of autoantibodies. Patients with SLE produce antinuclear antibody (ANA), confirming the existence of an autoimmune disease. The presence of ANAs does not in itself confirm the diagnosis of SLE because approximately 2% of healthy individuals are positive. Anti-dsDNA and anti-Sm antibodies are most specific for SLE because these autoantibodies are rarely found in other conditions. Antiphospholipid antibodies should also be assessed because the presence of these antibodies may lead to the formation of blood clots. Laboratory values to evaluate the clinical criteria include a complete blood count (CBC) to check for leukopenia (decreased white blood cell count), thrombocytopenia (decreased platelet count), and anemia (decreased red blood cells). Urinalysis with random protein and creatinine along with serum creatinine and BUN should be evaluated and monitored closely in order to detect kidney disease early. C-reactive protein and ESR are markers used to identify inflammation but are not specific for SLE. C-reactive protein and ESR may be monitored to assess for level of disease activity and response to treatment.

Radiographical Imaging

Radiographical imaging is beneficial to detect or assess some of the clinical criteria or to eliminate other causes of symptoms. See Table 20.9 for common radiographical diagnostic tools used to assess patients with SLE.

Treatment

Nonpharmacological Therapy

Nonpharmacological interventions include avoiding prolonged sun exposure and using sunscreen (SPF 50 or higher) on a daily basis. A well-balanced diet is recommended for proper nutrition. Frequent rest periods and a regular sleep schedule help combat fatigue. Regular exercise improves strength and maintains range of motion as well as a healthy weight.

Pharmacological Therapy

Pharmacological interventions for patients with SLE are typically based on disease manifestations. Antimalarial medications such as hydroxychloroquine (Plaquenil) are frequently used to treat patients with SLE. The exact mechanism of action of hydroxychloroquine is not fully understood; however, it is believed to impair complement-dependent antigen–antibody reactions. Hydroxychloroquine is also useful in treating constitutional symptoms such as fatigue as well as skin and joint manifestations. It also helps to prevent disease flares and serious organ disease such as lupus nephritis. The most common side effects related to hydroxychloroquine use are abdominal pain and nausea, which may improve over time (see Safety Alert).

Nonsteroidal anti-inflammatory medications such as ibuprofen are useful in treating arthralgias, myalgias, headaches, and fever. Glucocorticoids may be necessary to suppress inflammation in joints, kidneys, and other organ systems. Immunosuppressive agents such as methotrexate may be necessary to treat joint inflammation, which does not respond to NSAIDs or steroids. Glucocorticoids and immunosuppressive agents may be used in combination with hydroxychloroquine in order to treat more serious clinical manifestations. Belimumab (Benlysta) is a biological response modifier that was approved in 2011 for the treatment of SLE. It is the first new treatment to be approved for the treatment of SLE in more than 40 years. Belimumab is made of monoclonal antibodies that bind to proteins known as BLyS and interferes with the inflammatory cascade, decreasing the immune response that is responsible for causing clinical manifestations of SLE. See Table 20.10 for medications used to treat specific manifestations.

Table 20.9 Common Diagnostic Tools for Complications of Systemic Lupus Erythematosus

Diagnostic Tool	Implication
Plain radiograph	• Painful, swollen joints—assess for joint damage. • Chest—assess for lung disease and cardiomegaly.
Ultrasound	• Kidneys—assess size and rule out obstruction if there is evidence of renal impairment.
Echocardiogram	• Assess for pericardial involvement and elevated pulmonary artery pressure (SLE patients are at risk for developing pulmonary artery hypertension).
Computed tomography	• Abdominal pain—assess for pancreatitis. • Chest—assess for interstitial lung disease.
Magnetic resonance imaging	• Brain—assess neurological defects and cognitive dysfunction.

SLE, Systemic lupus erythematosus.

Table 20.10   Medications Used to Treat Clinical Manifestations of Systemic Lupus Erythematosus

Medication	Use
NSAIDs	• Musculoskeletal complaints • Fever • Headaches • Mild pleuritis or pericarditis
Low-dose oral glucocorticoids	• Joint pain with active synovitis • Rash
High-dose oral glucocorticoids	• Nephritis • Pneumonitis • Hematological abnormalities such as thrombocytopenia • Central nervous system disease • Systemic vasculitis
Topical glucocorticoids (clobetasol)	• Skin rash and oral/nasal ulcers
Immunosuppressive agents Methotrexate Azathioprine Cyclophosphamide Mycophenolate mofetil Thalidomide	• Joint pain and synovitis • Treatment of mild to moderate disease activity and as an alternative to long-term use of glucocorticoids; used to treat lupus nephritis and other organ-threatening manifestations • Treatment of severe SLE: lupus nephritis, central nervous system disease, pulmonary hemorrhage, and systemic vasculitis • Prevention of renal allograft rejection • Chronic cutaneous lupus
Biological response modifier Belimumab (Benlysta)	• Used in conjunction with traditional medications in SLE patients with serologically active disease

SLE, Systemic lupus erythematosus.

 Safety Alert   Common Lupus Medications

Plaquenil

Patients taking Plaquenil are required to have a baseline eye examination and then biannual or annual eye examinations to assess for retinal toxicity, which may be caused by long-term use.

Nonsteroidal Anti-inflammatory Medications

Nonsteroidal anti-inflammatory medications should be avoided in patients with renal impairment because of the inhibition of the prostaglandins responsible for preserving renal blood flow.

Surgical Management

Surgical interventions may include renal transplant for patients with severe lupus nephritis and joint replacement for patients at risk for avascular necrosis of large joints.

Complications

Lupus is a chronic disease with many possible complications, including renal failure, premature heart disease, interstitial lung disease, hypercoagulation, stroke, avascular necrosis of joints, and increased risk for infection. Complications may also arise from toxicities related to pharmacological therapy.

Nursing Management
Assessment and Analysis

There are many clinical manifestations related to SLE. The etiology is unknown, but it is thought to be attributed to antibodies and the creation of immune complexes, which are deposited into tissues. The nurse may identify the following:

• Fatigue
• Difficulty concentrating
• Joint pain
• Rash
• Photosensitivity
• Oral or nasal ulcers
• Dry eyes
• Dry mouth
• Hypertension
• Leukopenia
• Thrombocytopenia

- Alopecia
- Chest pain

Nursing Diagnoses

- **Fatigue** related to chronic inflammation and altered immunity
- **Altered skin integrity** related to rash
- **Altered self-image** related to manifestations such as rash and alopecia

Nursing Interventions

◼ Assessments

- Vital signs
  Hypertension may occur as a renal or cardiac complication of SLE, fever may be present due to infection that is a complication of treatment with immunosuppressants, and decreased oxygen saturation may be present because of the complication of interstitial lung disease.
- Past health history/head-to-toe physical assessment
  The diagnosis of SLE is based on the presence of 4 of 17 clinical manifestations in the patient's history and physical assessment, such as butterfly rash, oral or nasal ulcers, alopecia, musculoskeletal complaints, joint swelling, weight loss, and blood abnormalities.
- Monitor laboratory values: BUN and creatinine, urinalysis, CBC, CRP/ESR, coagulation studies.
  Elevated BUN and creatinine along with the presence of proteinuria may indicate decreased renal function and is one of the clinical criteria for SLE. Decreased white blood cells, platelets, and red blood cells are common in patients with SLE and may require intervention. Elevated CRP and/or ESR indicates inflammation and may require intervention. Coagulopathies are a complication of SLE.

◼ Actions

- Administer analgesics and anti-inflammatory medications as ordered.
  Most patients require analgesics and anti-inflammatory medications to manage the pain caused by inflammation.
- Administer medications as ordered to treat specific clinical manifestations.
  Managing clinical manifestations is imperative in the treatment of patients with SLE to help prevent complications. See Table 20.10 for medications used to treat clinical manifestations.

◼ Teaching

- Disease process
  It is very important for patients to understand the disease process in order to manage the disease and help prevent complications.
- Use sunscreen daily.
  Photosensitivity is common. Daily use of sunscreen helps prevent rash related to photosensitivity.
- Energy conservation and activity prioritization
  Fatigue is a common complaint and can be better managed by ensuring frequent rest periods and prioritizing activities.

- Keep up to date on immunizations, but avoid live vaccines.
  Patients at risk for infections due to treatment should not receive live vaccines if on immunosuppressive therapy.
- Avoid oral contraceptives in patients with SLE who have migraine headaches, Raynaud's phenomenon, a history of phlebitis, or antiphospholipid antibodies.
  Patients with SLE, specifically patients with the manifestations noted, have an increased risk of hypercoagulability, which may be heightened by the use of oral contraceptives.
- Assist in referrals to a pulmonologist, nephrologist, neurologist, cardiologist, and dermatologist as needed.
  Complicated clinical manifestations require the care of specialists to provide optimal care.

Evaluating Care Outcomes

Systemic lupus erythematosus is a complicated disease that can be very difficult to manage. Medication compliance plays a major role in controlling the disease. Disease flares are not unexpected and may consist of increased fatigue, fever, rash, arthritis, and mucosal ulcers as well as other common clinical manifestations. Frequent evaluations should be performed on a regular basis by a rheumatologist who monitors disease progression and treats new clinical manifestations as they arise. Patients with well-controlled SLE are high-functioning individuals who are able to carry out the usual activities of daily living.

GOUT

Epidemiology

Gout affects approximately 2% of people in the United States and is most commonly found in men aged 40 to 60 years and women aged 55 to 70. Risk factors for developing gout include obesity, hypertension, eating large amounts of meat and seafood, using thiazide diuretics, and consuming large quantities of alcohol. When metabolized, purine-rich foods such as seafood, meat, and alcohol increase uric acid production. Thiazide diuretics, such as hydrochlorothiazide, increase the net urate reabsorption in the renal tubules, therefore increasing the serum uric acid level.

Pathophysiology

Gout is a disease in which monosodium urate crystals are deposited in joints, bone, and soft tissues, accompanied by inflammation (Fig. 20.7). Hyperuricemia, an elevated uric acid level in the blood, must be present prior to the evolution of gout, but the presence of hyperuricemia is not indicative of gout. Hyperuricemia results from the overproduction of or diminished renal excretion of uric acid. Urate crystals are the result of an oversaturation of uric acid in the blood. The uric acid settles out of solution into soft tissues and joints. The body's attempt to rid itself of the crystal deposits results in an inflammatory process causing swelling, warmth, and intense pain in the affected joint. Gout attacks typically resolve after several days or weeks even if left untreated; however,

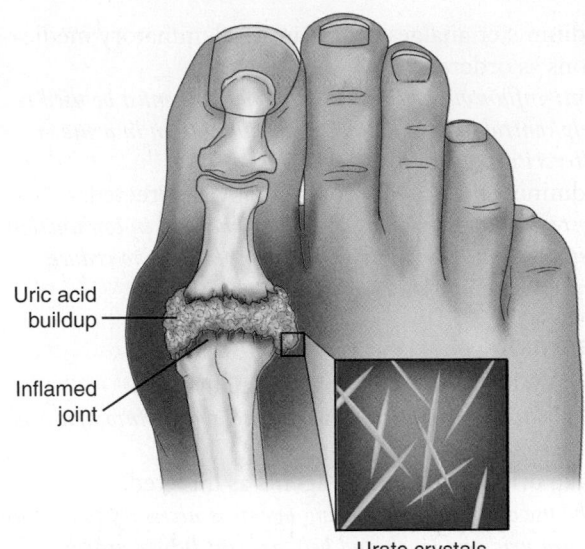

Uric acid buildup

Inflamed joint

Urate crystals

FIGURE 20.7 Urate crystal buildup in the great toe, a common presentation of gout.

gout can become a chronic inflammatory destructive arthritis. There are three phases of gout, which are termed *acute*, *intercritical*, and *chronic*. Acute gout usually involves one joint and is characterized by acute onset of pain, redness, and swelling. Intercritical gout is the asymptomatic period between gout attacks. If gout is left untreated, the attacks may come more often, with a shortened intercritical period. Chronic tophaceous gout is characterized by repeated attacks of many years, leading to the production of **tophi** (uric acid deposits or nodules in the joint) and joint destruction. About 80% of patients present with the first attack of gout affecting a lower extremity joint, typically the first metatarsophalangeal (MTP) joint. **Podagra** is the term used to identify gout in the first MTP. The severity of the attack typically peaks at 12 to 24 hours after onset.

Management

Medical Management

Diagnosis

A presumptive diagnosis of gout may be achieved by combining objective, subjective, and laboratory data, but the definitive diagnosis can be made only by observing crystals in synovial fluid or tophaceous material. Radiographical evidence is not necessary to diagnose gout; however, joint erosions and soft tissue nodules are radiographically consistent with chronic gouty arthritis. See Table 20.11 for the typical presentation of gout patients. Other diagnoses such as septic arthritis, trauma, and pseudogout should be ruled out. The presentation of septic arthritis and pseudogout may mimic acute gout and may not be differentiated by clinical examination alone. In some cases, it is necessary to examine joint fluid for uric acid crystals to make a definitive gout diagnosis.

Connection Check 20.8

The nurse assesses for which *initial* clinical manifestation in the patient diagnosed with gout?
A. Pain and inflammation in the shoulder
B. Pain and inflammation in the wrist
C. Pain and inflammation in the knee
D. Pain and inflammation in the great toe

Treatment

Nonpharmacological Therapy

Nonpharmacological treatment consists of weight management because obesity is a modifiable risk factor for gout. Alcoholic beverages, specifically beer, should be avoided because they increase uric acid production. Splinting of the affected joint may also be useful in protecting the joint and alleviating pain.

Pharmacological Therapy

Pharmacological treatment of gout depends on which stage the patient is in when requesting treatment. Acute gout management is focused on pain relief and reduction of inflammation. Common medications used include NSAIDs such as indomethacin (Indocin) and colchicine (Colcrys), which decrease the buildup of uric acid crystals in the joint. Glucocorticoids are used to reduce inflammation and provide pain relief. Management of intercritical gout consists of the use of NSAIDs and colchicine, whereas managing chronic gout focuses on the use of uric acid–lowering agents.

Table 20.11 Typical Presentation of Gout Patients

Subjective	Objective	Laboratory	Radiographical
• I have severe joint pain (usually great toe or knee). • I think my joint is swollen. • I cannot move my joint. • My joint feels hot when I touch it.	• Tenderness on palpation • Soft tissue swelling on examination accompanied by warmth and redness • Presence of tophi in the chronic gout patient	• Elevated serum uric acid level • Visualization of urate crystals found in synovial fluid on microscopic examination	• Plain radiographical findings are usually normal in early gout. • Erosions and soft tissue nodules may be present in chronic gout.

Uric acid–lowering agents such as allopurinol (Zyloprim) or febuxostat (Uloric) reduce serum uric acid by inhibiting the production of uric acid. One very important fact to remember is that acute gout is never treated with uric acid–lowering agents such as allopurinol. For unknown reasons, a rapid change in serum uric acid levels may provoke or worsen a gout attack.

> **(!) Safety Alert** Although aspirin is an NSAID, it should be avoided in the treatment of gout because it can increase uric acid levels by causing retention of uric acid.

Complications

Urate crystals can aggregate to form a stone, making gout patients more likely to experience kidney stones than the general population.

Nursing Management

Assessment and Analysis

Clinical manifestations of gout are related to pain and decreased function due to the accumulation of urate crystals and tophi nodules in the affected joints. The nurse may identify the following:

- Intense joint pain
- Tenderness on palpation of affected joint
- Swelling of affected joint
- Redness of affected joint
- Warmth over affected joint
- Decreased range of motion
- Presence of tophi

Nursing Diagnoses

- **Pain** related to the disease process
- **Knowledge deficit** related to the disease process and treatment

Nursing Interventions

■ Assessments

- Monitor uric acid level.
  Hyperuricemia promotes crystal formation.
- Assess for presence of tophi—lumps or hard nodules under the skin around joints.
  The presence of tophi is indicative of advanced gout.
- Assess for red, swollen, and painful joints.
  Red, swollen, and painful joints indicate an acute gout flare.
- Assess pain levels.
  Evaluating pain helps determine the occurrence of a flare and also evaluates the efficacy of treatment.

■ Actions

- Administer uric acid–lowering agents as directed.
  Uric acid–lowering agents are necessary to decrease serum uric acid and decrease the incidence of gout flares in chronic gout.

- Administer analgesics and anti-inflammatory medications as ordered.
  Anti-inflammatory agents and analgesics must be used to help control pain and decrease inflammation in acute or intercritical gout.
- Administer glucocorticoid therapy as directed.
  Systemic glucocorticoid therapy may be used in conjunction with or as an alternative to NSAID therapy to reduce inflammation in acute gout.

■ Teaching

- Avoid alcoholic beverages, especially beer.
  Alcohol is high in purines, which metabolize into uric acid, increasing serum uric acid levels.
- Take uric acid–lowering agents as directed.
  The use of uric acid–lowering agents is necessary to decrease serum uric acid levels and help prevent future attacks.
- Report gout flares promptly.
  Prompt treatment decreases the pain and the severity of gout flares.
- Proper nutrition
  Avoid high-purine foods, such as red meat, liver, and fish.

Connection Check 20.9

Which statement by the patient with gout indicates that further teaching is needed?

A. "Losing weight will help to reduce further gout attacks."
B. "I should report my diagnosis of gout to my cardiologist because taking some forms of diuretics may increase gout flares."
C. "Avoiding foods containing purines, such as red meats, seafood, and alcoholic beverages, will help to reduce the incidence of gout flares."
D. "I can drink alcohol if I limit the number of beers I drink."

Evaluating Care Outcomes

The goal of treating gout patients is to eliminate gout flares and prevent joint destruction. This is done by controlling the uric acid level. A well-managed patient takes gout-lowering agents appropriately; avoids foods containing purines, such as seafood and red meat; and limits alcohol consumption.

FIBROMYALGIA

Epidemiology

Fibromyalgia is the most common cause of chronic musculoskeletal pain in women between the ages of 20 and 55. The disorder affects approximately 4% of the U.S. population, with a greater prevalence in women. Fibromyalgia is commonly found in patients with rheumatic conditions such as RA, SLE, and Sjogren's syndrome. The onset of fibromyalgia usually occurs in middle adulthood but may occur in adolescence or later in life. Genetic factors may play a role in predisposing patients to the development of fibromyalgia.

Pathophysiology and Clinical Manifestations

Fibromyalgia is a chronic pain disorder of soft connective tissues that is characterized by widespread pain and other symptoms such as insomnia, fatigue, stiffness, and cognitive dysfunction (e.g., inability to focus or concentrate on tasks). The etiology and pathophysiology of this disorder are unclear, but current theories include the abnormal processing of stimuli by the central nervous system, causing normal pain signals to be amplified. The amplification of stimuli causes fibromyalgia patients to feel pain, whereas those without fibromyalgia would not feel pain. Fibromyalgia may be triggered by an infection or physical or emotional trauma. In females, the menstrual cycle can affect sensitivity to pain. Normal daily stress combined with common fibromyalgia symptoms can create a cycle that builds one on another (Fig. 20.8).

Management

Medical Management

Diagnosis

Laboratory testing is not necessary to diagnose fibromyalgia but may be necessary to rule out other diagnoses. History and physical assessment are used to diagnose fibromyalgia. Patients often report hurting all over or feeling as if they have the flu. Other complaints include fatigue, headaches, cognitive impairments, and abdominal pain. Physical examination of the patient is essentially normal, with no evidence of joint or muscle inflammation. In 1990, the ACR criteria for the diagnosis of fibromyalgia required that the patient experience pain at 11 or more of 18 specified locations (tender points) and have widespread pain. The assessment of tender points is done by applying approximately 4 kg of pressure (this is comparable to the pressure it would take to blanch your nail bed) to specific points on the patient's body (Fig. 20.9). Widespread pain involves pain on both sides of the body and above and below the waist.

Treatment

Nonpharmacological Therapy

Nonpharmacological therapy includes physical therapy, strength training, aerobic exercise, cognitive behavioral therapy, education, and self-management. Physical therapy is helpful in maintaining strength and function. Cognitive-behavioral therapy may be used to help understand the illness and change patients' behavioral response to pain. Self-management skills include utilizing relaxation techniques to minimize stress, establishing regular sleep patterns, and exercising regularly.

Pharmacological Therapy

Pharmacological therapy includes medications that alter chemicals in the brain, such as serotonin and norepinephrine, or block overactivity of nerve cells. Other medications that may prove useful are those that improve sleep and treat pain. The use of opioid analgesics is not recommended because they may be habit forming and usually are ineffective. Table 20.12 provides an overview of medications used for the treatment of fibromyalgia.

Nursing Management

Assessment and Analysis

The nurse may identify the following clinical manifestations in fibromyalgia patients due to enhanced pain perception and stress related to that enhanced pain:

- Fatigue
- Arthralgia and myalgia
- Headache
- Abdominal pain

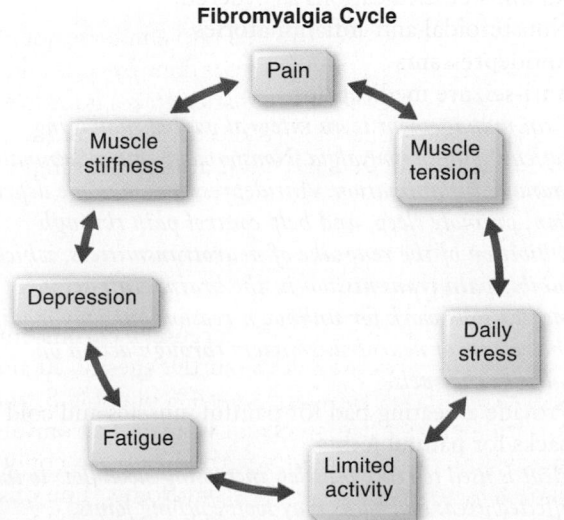

FIGURE 20.8 Fibromyalgia cycle.

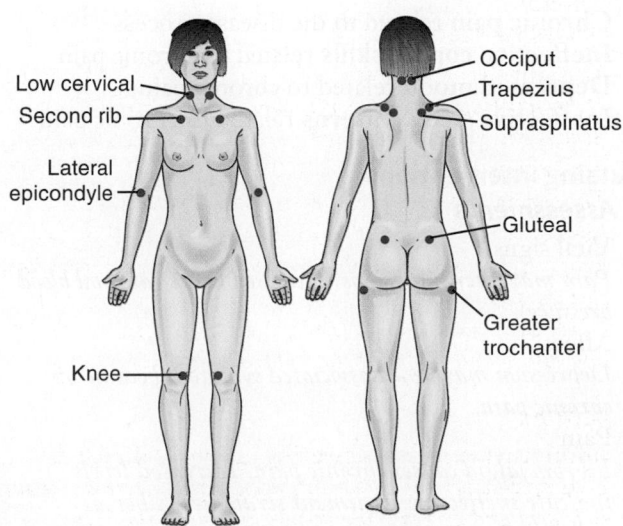

FIGURE 20.9 The 18 fibromyalgia tender points.

Table 20.12 Pharmacological Treatments for Fibromyalgia

	Medication	Action	Common Side Effects
Antidepressants to help with pain and promote sleep	Duloxetine (Cymbalta)	Inhibits norepinephrine and serotonin reuptake	Nausea
			Dry mouth
			Constipation
			Somnolence
	Milnacipran (Savella)	Inhibits norepinephrine and serotonin reuptake	Nausea
			Vomiting
			Constipation
			Insomnia
	Amitriptyline (Elavil)	Inhibits norepinephrine and serotonin reuptake	Drowsiness
			Dry mouth
			Dizziness
			Constipation
	Fluoxetine (Prozac)	Selectively inhibits serotonin reuptake	Nausea
			Headache
			Insomnia
			Nervousness
Anti-seizure medications to reduce pain	Pregabalin (Lyrica)	Binds alpha-2-delta subunit of calcium channels, reducing neurotransmitter release	Dizziness
			Weight gain

- Decreased desire to participate in activity
- Nonrestorative sleep
- Anxiety

Nursing Diagnoses

- **Chronic pain** related to the disease process
- **Ineffective coping skills** related to chronic pain
- **Depressed mood** related to chronic pain
- **Ineffective sleep patterns** related to chronic pain

Nursing Interventions

■ Assessments

- Vital signs
  Pain may alter vital signs (increased heart rate and blood pressure).
- Affect
  Depression may be an associated symptom because of chronic pain.
- Pain
  Fibromyalgia causes chronic pain. Increased levels indicate ineffective treatment strategies, whereas

decreased pain levels indicate effective treatment and self-management.

■ Actions

- Administer medications as ordered:
  Nonsteroidal anti-inflammatories
  Antidepressants
  Anti-seizure medications
  Pain management is an integral part of managing patients with fibromyalgia. Nonsteroidal anti-inflammatories manage inflammation. Antidepressants manage depression, promote sleep, and help control pain through inhibition of the reuptake of neurotransmitters, which inhibit pain transmission in the brain. Anti-seizure medications work for unknown reasons but may modify the release of neurotransmitters through action on calcium channels.
- Provide a heating pad for painful muscles and cold packs for painful joints.
  Heat is used to relax muscles, increasing blood flow to the affected area; cold packs may soothe aching joints.

■ *Teaching*

- Take medications only as prescribed.
  Improper use of medications can be very harmful. Proper use of medications is required in order to receive the desired effect.
- Participate in regular physical activity.
  Physical activity is necessary to maintain or improve strength and function.
- Teach effective coping skills.
  Effective coping skills are important to maintain a positive attitude and improve self-concept.
- Assist with referring the patient for a sleep study.
  Ineffective sleep may increase pain and fatigue.
- Assist with referring the patient to a mental health facility if necessary.
  Fibromyalgia patients may benefit from therapy to help deal with depression related to chronic pain.
- Assist with referral to occupational and physical therapies as needed.
  Occupational and physical therapists may formulate an exercise plan appropriate for the patient.

Evaluating Care Outcomes

Compliance with a healthy diet and exercise regimen and getting adequate rest are essential in managing fibromyalgia. Taking medications as prescribed helps to control the enhanced sensation of pain and the depression associated with the disease process. A well-managed patient has decreased pain and fatigue, healthy sleep patterns, and maintenance or improvement of strength and function (see Transitional Care).

Transitional Care

Connective Tissue Disorders

Considerations for all connective tissue diseases include:

- Evaluating the effects of medications due to declining renal function

May require more frequent follow-up to monitor medication levels and renal function

- Inadequate nutrition and exercise/ineffective or no support system

May require home-care follow-up to ensure proper nutrition and exercise

- Risk for falls

May require home safety evaluation; potential installation of grab bars in bathroom and shower

- Increased risk of depression

May require psychosocial follow-up

Connection Check 20.10

Which statement by the patient with fibromyalgia indicates that teaching has been effective?

A. "Because of my fibromyalgia, I may get inflammatory arthritis, which may lead to joint damage."

B. "I won't know for sure about my diagnosis until I have diagnostic tests such as x-rays and blood tests done."

C. "My only option to treat my pain is narcotic analgesics."

D. "It's frustrating, but I understand that fibromyalgia typically presents with a normal physical examination with no evidence of joint or muscle inflammation."

Making Connections

CASE STUDY: WRAP-UP

On the basis of the laboratory results indicating elevated rheumatoid factor, elevated ESR and CRP, and anticyclic citrullinated peptide, as well as synovitis on ultrasound in the affected joints, RA is diagnosed. Ms. Logan is started on ibuprofen and short-term low-dose prednisone. The rheumatologist discusses treatment options that are available to help control disease progression. Ms. Logan will most likely begin to use methotrexate to decrease the disease progression. She will follow up with the rheumatologist frequently until her disease is well controlled.

Case Study Questions

1. The nurse is reviewing the treatment plan for Ms. Logan. It is a priority for the nurse to follow up with the provider about which part of the plan?

   A. Ibuprofen 600 mg PO tid

   B. Prednisone 5 mg PO every day

   C. Oxycodone 5 mg PO every 6 hours prn

   D. Consid methotrexate if other options are unsuccessful in controlling pain

2. Which statement made by Ms. Logan regarding methotrexate indicates that teaching has been effective?

   A. "I guess I'll have to cut back to drinking only one beer a day."

   B. "Since the doctor ordered me to take six methotrexate pills a week, I can take one a day Sunday through Friday and skip taking a pill on Saturday."

   C. "My husband and I will use two effective means of birth control to prevent pregnancy if I start methotrexate."

   D. "If my joint pain and swelling get worse, I'll take more methotrexate then notify the doctor at my next appointment."

3. The nurse caring for Ms. Logan incorporates which nursing diagnosis into the plan of care?

   A. Impaired perfusion related to vasoconstriction secondary to RA

   B. Impaired oxygenation related to decreased respiratory effort secondary to RA

   C. Risk of injury related to unstable gait secondary to RA

   D. Imbalanced nutrition related to dietary limitations secondary to treatment of RA

4. The nurse caring for Ms. Logan after the initiation of methotrexate therapy monitors for which clinical manifestation?

   A. Weight gain

   B. Elevated liver enzymes

   C. Weight loss

   D. Decreased ESR

5. The nurse providing care for Ms. Logan should include which lifestyle modifications into the plan of care? *(Select all that apply.)*

   A. Limit range-of-motion exercise to reduce stress on joints.

   B. Begin high-carbohydrate, low-protein diet.

   C. Begin range-of-motion exercises to increase the flexibility of joints.

   D. Limit aerobic exercise to reduce stress on joints.

   E. Begin aerobic exercise for weight control.

CHAPTER SUMMARY

Connective tissues are made of collagen, elastin, and reticular fibers. Examples of connective tissues include bone, bone marrow, cartilage, tendons, ligaments, vasculature, and lymphatic tissue. Connective tissue diseases may affect any of these connective tissues.

Osteoarthritis is primarily a noninflammatory type of arthritis that results from weight bearing, trauma, infection, and overuse. Damage occurs within the joint, which leads to the deterioration of joint function. Osteoarthritis presents as joint pain, swelling, possible decreased range of motion, and at times, unsteady gait due to joint damage. Morning stiffness typically lasts less than 30 minutes, and pain tends to become worse with movement. The diagnosis of osteoarthritis is commonly made on the basis of symptoms and conventional radiographs. There is no cure for osteoarthritis, and there are no medications to greatly inhibit disease progression. Pain is treated with nonsteroidal anti-inflammatory medications, and in some cases narcotic medications are necessary. Nursing management consists of assessing for pain, swelling, redness, range of motion, and effectiveness of pain medications, as well as assessing for side effects related to medication management.

Rheumatoid arthritis, scleroderma, and lupus are autoimmune diseases that may affect multiple organ systems. These diseases may be difficult to diagnose and are not diagnosed solely by using laboratory data. Elevated CRP and ESR rates indicate inflammation but are not specific for RA. Patients may or may not present with a positive RA factor. A complete history and physical examination are extremely important in making these diagnoses. All of these diseases are more prevalent in women.

Rheumatoid arthritis is completely different from osteoarthritis. It affects only about 1% of the population. Rheumatoid arthritis is an autoimmune inflammatory disease that not only affects joints but may also affect other organ systems. Inflammation within each organ system is what causes organ or tissue damage. Morning stiffness usually lasts for greater than 30 minutes, and pain generally gets better with movement. Joint involvement is typically symmetrical. Lung disease related to RA is a common clinical manifestation that may be present even in the absence of joint inflammation. There are many good treatment options available to treat patients with RA, and it is possible to achieve clinical remission by using DMARDs. Nursing management includes assessing for pain, redness, and decreased mobility as well as assessment for organ involvement outside the musculoskeletal system.

Scleroderma is an autoimmune connective tissue disease characterized by secondary Raynaud's phenomenon, thickened and hardened skin, and multiple other internal organ manifestations. Localized scleroderma affects the skin but does not affect the visceral organs, whereas systemic scleroderma is more likely to involve the internal organs. Limited systemic scleroderma has a slower onset and involves the skin of the extremities; internal involvement occurs late in the disease. Diffuse systemic scleroderma, which has a rapid onset, involves the skin of the trunk and involves internal organs early in the disease. Disease-modifying antirheumatic medication therapy is used to treat scleroderma, but specific medications must also be used to treat specific organ involvement (i.e., vasodilators to treat pulmonary hypertension). Nursing management includes assessing for the symptoms of scleroderma and other organ system involvement. It also includes teaching appropriate skin care, assessing skin integrity, and monitoring for digital ulcers.

Systemic lupus erythematosus is an autoimmune disease mostly characterized by fatigue, fever, rash, photosensitivity, oral and nasal ulcers, alopecia, arthralgia, and myalgia. More serious manifestations include pericarditis, endocarditis, arthritis, interstitial lung disease, and lupus nephritis. Lupus primarily affects women of childbearing age. Nursing management includes educating the patient about the disease, the treatments, and what to report to the rheumatologist.

Treatment for RA, scleroderma, and lupus must be individualized for each patient but typically includes anti-inflammatories, analgesics, DMARDs, and biological agents.

Gout is a disease in which a state of serum hyperuricemia causes monosodium urate crystals to deposit in and around joints, which causes inflammation and leads to debilitating pain in the joint, with swelling and redness. It initially presents in a lower extremity joint, such as the great toe. Gout has three phases, acute, intercritical, and chronic, which are treated differently. Nursing management includes teaching about the disease, treatment options, and lifestyle modifications, including foods or drinks to avoid that increase in uric acid levels.

Fibromyalgia is a chronic pain syndrome characterized by widespread pain along with other symptoms, such as insomnia, fatigue, stiffness, and cognitive dysfunction. Patients typically present with a normal examination. Diagnosis is made through the evaluation of physical complaints. Nursing management focuses on the assessment of symptoms and includes teaching effective pain management and self-management.

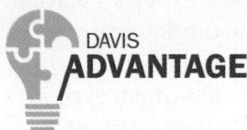

To explore learning resources for this chapter, go to **Davis Advantage** and find:
– Answers to in-text questions
– Chapter Resources and Activities
– NCLEX®-Style Chapter Review Questions
– Bibliography

Chapter 21

Coordinating Care for Patients With Multidrug-Resistant Organism Infectious Disorders

Gladdi Tomlinson

LEARNING OUTCOMES

Content in this chapter is designed to assist in:

1. Describing the epidemiology of multidrug-resistant organism infectious disorders
2. Correlating clinical manifestations to pathophysiological processes of:
   a. Methicillin-resistant *Staphylococcus aureus*
   b. Vancomycin-resistant *Enterococci*
   c. *Clostridioides difficile*
   d. *Acinetobacter baumannii*
   e. Carbapenem-resistant Enterobacteriaceae
3. Describing the diagnostic results used to confirm the diagnosis of infectious disorders
4. Discussing the medical management of:
   a. Methicillin-resistant *Staphylococcus aureus*
   b. Vancomycin-resistant *Enterococci*
   c. *Clostridioides difficile*
   d. *Acinetobacter baumannii*
   e. Carbapenem-resistant Enterobacteriaceae
5. Developing a comprehensive plan of nursing care for patients with multidrug-resistant-organism infectious disorders
6. Designing a teaching plan that includes pharmacological, dietary, and lifestyle considerations for patients with multidrug-resistant organism infectious disorders

ESSENTIAL TERMS

Acinetobacter baumannii
Airborne transmission
Bactericidal
Bacteriostatic
Carbapenem-resistant Enterobacteriaceae (CRE)
Coagulase-positive bacterium
Clostridioides difficile (*C. diff*)
Colonized
Contact isolation
Contact transmission
Endogenous pathogen
Exogenous
Facultatively anaerobic
Hand hygiene
Methicillin-resistant *Staphylococcus aureus* (MRSA)
Multidrug-resistant (MDR) organisms
Nonsporulating
Nosocomial infections
Peak levels
Probiotics
Trough level
Vancomycin-resistant *Enterococci* (VRE)
Vector-borne transmission
Vehicle transmission

CONCEPTS

- Assessment
- Fluid and Electrolyte Balance
- Immunity
- Infection
- Medication
- Safety

Finding Connections

CASE STUDY: EPISODE 1

Follow this patient throughout the chapter.

Joe Brown is a 76-year-old male who presents to his healthcare provider from his nursing home residence with a painful, red, swollen abdominal surgical wound that is warm to the touch and is draining pus. Joe had a cholecystectomy last week and is returning to his healthcare provider to get the staples removed. Joe has just finished his antibiotics. He takes metformin for his diabetes mellitus type 2 and is on Coumadin for atrial fibrillation...

INTRODUCTION

Infectious diseases have been plaguing the world for centuries. They are caused by pathogens—microorganisms that are capable of causing disease. For a pathogen to cause a disease, a susceptible host and a mode of transmission are required. A susceptible host usually has a weakened immune system or has had a breakdown in the body's defense mechanism. For an infection to be transmitted, a transport mechanism is required. Routes of transmission are contact, airborne, vehicle, and vector borne. **Contact transmission** occurs when a person or object comes in contact with a pathogen. **Airborne transmission** occurs when pathogens are carried through the air. **Vehicle transmission** is an indirect mode of transmission that occurs when a disease-carrying agent touches a person's body or is ingested. Similarly, **vector-borne transmission** is also an indirect mode of transmission that occurs when a vector, an organism that transmits a pathogen, bites or infects a person.

Contact transmission is the most common mode of transmission. In this mode, pathogens are introduced into the body by direct or indirect contact. When an infectious disease is spread by direct contact, the microorganisms are transferred directly from person to person. In indirect-contact transmission, microorganisms are spread from a source to a susceptible host by passive transfer from an inanimate object or fomite, an object or substance capable of carrying an infectious organism. Often in healthcare settings, patients acquire infectious diseases through indirect contact via the unclean hands of healthcare workers, from contaminated equipment, or from the contaminated environment. Infections that are acquired in the hospital and were not present on admission are called **nosocomial infections**. In 2016, the Centers for Disease Control and Prevention (CDC) reported the findings from the 2014 Healthcare Associated Infection (HAI) progress report. The survey results concluded that 1 in 25 inpatients in U.S. acute care hospitals had at least one healthcare-associated infection. The survey also revealed a 50% decrease in central line–associated bloodstream infections, a 17% decrease in surgical infections, an 8% decrease in *Clostridioides difficile* infections, a 13% decrease in methicillin-resistant *Staphylococcus aureus*, and no change in urinary tract infections. The Health and Human Services Department has implemented an *Action Plan to Prevent Healthcare-Associated Infections* goal of decreasing healthcare-associated infections by 25% by the year 2020.

Multidrug-resistant (MDR) organisms are common causes of nosocomial infections. **Methicillin-resistant *Staphylococcus aureus* (MRSA)**, vancomycin-resistant *Enterococci* **(VRE)**, *Clostridioides difficile* **(C. diff)**, *Acinetobacter baumannii*, and **carbapenem-resistant Enterobacteriaceae** are all examples of MDR organisms that cause nosocomial infections.

MULTIDRUG-RESISTANT ORGANISMS

Methicillin-Resistant *Staphylococcus Aureus*

Epidemiology

Staphylococcus aureus (S. aureus) is a common asymptomatic pathogen and is considered normal bacterial flora of humans. Two in 100 carry it, and approximately 30% of healthy individuals are **colonized** (the host carries the bacteria without active infection) with this pathogen in the nose, throat, axillae, toe webs, or perineum. The most common site of colonization is the anterior nares. Although 30% of people are colonized with *S. aureus*, fewer than 2% are infected with it.

The first case of MRSA was described in 1961, and the first documented outbreak occurred in the United States in 1968. In 2007, the Association for Professionals in Infection Control and Epidemiology reported that an estimated 1.2 million hospitalized patients acquire MRSA each year in the United States. Today, it is estimated that approximately 80% of *S. aureus* isolates from clinical cultures are MRSA. Methicillin-resistant *S. aureus* is the result of decades of unnecessary antibiotic use and is currently resistant to all beta-lactam antibiotics, including penicillins, cephalosporins, and carbapenems. It is also the most commonly identified MDR pathogen in North America, South America, Europe, Asia, Africa, and the Middle East.

A CDC study found that healthcare-initiated MRSA declined 54% between 2005 and 2011 and was down 13% in 2014. The CDC goal was a decrease of 25% by 2011. Data from the CDC and Healthcare-Associated Infections Progress Report continue to show progress; from 2011 to 2013, there were an estimated 8% fewer hospital-onset MRSA infections. Also, it is reported that there were 9,000 fewer deaths from MRSA in hospital patients in 2011 versus 2005. The National Healthcare Safety Network reported that the incidence of MRSA central line–associated bloodstream infections decreased in recent years in most intensive care units (ICUs), except in pediatric units. The decline in MRSA infection rates is attributed to general infection control efforts such as the use of alcohol-based hand rubs, improved **hand hygiene**, efforts targeted at eliminating bloodstream infections, and enhanced antimicrobial stewardship programs.

Historically, MRSA has been associated with healthcare; however, recently, a newer strain has been identified. The first case of community-acquired MRSA (CAMRSA) was reported in the United States in 1980. Community-acquired MRSA has become the most frequent cause of skin and soft tissue infections presenting to emergency departments in the United States. Hospital-acquired MRSA (HAMRSA) tends to lead to more invasive diseases such as bloodstream infections, surgical-site infections, and pneumonia.

Epidemiologically, HAMRSA and CAMRSA have different molecular characteristics. Community-acquired MRSA strains are resistant to beta-lactam and macrolide antimicrobials; however, they remain susceptible to many non–beta-lactam antimicrobials. Hospital-acquired MRSA strains are resistant to many other classes of antibiotics in addition to beta-lactam and macrolide antibiotics. Recent studies suggest that HAMRSA and CAMRSA should be treated on the basis of the type of infection and antibiotic susceptibility rather than the strain of bacteria.

Risk factors for HAMRSA include hospitalization in the past 12 months, soft tissue infection on hospital admission, hospitalization in intensive care, and residing in a long-term care facility, thus increasing the risk of exposure; invasive procedures or medical devices such as urinary catheters or IV lines that create a portal for the entry, including hemodialysis; and recent or long-term broad-spectrum antibiotic therapy allowing bacteria to become resistant to a specific antibiotic. Other risk factors include people with an immature or weakened immune system, such as young children, older adults, or people with HIV or AIDS as well as other comorbid conditions such as diabetes, cancer, chronic obstructive pulmonary disease, congestive heart failure, and immunosuppression.

Risk factors for CAMRSA include children younger than 2 years of age, athletes, IV drug users, men who have sex with men, military personnel, and persons living in correctional facilities or shelters. These risk factors are associated with close skin-to-skin contact, crowded living conditions, and poor hygiene (Table 21.1).

Pathophysiology

Staphylococcus aureus is an aerobic, gram-positive, **non-sporulating** (does not make spores capable of reproduction), **coagulase-positive bacterium** (produces the enzyme coagulase, which helps convert fibrinogen to fibrin). Because it is a coagulase bacterium, MRSA is coated with a fibrin wall that resists phagocytosis, making the bacterium more virulent, thus enabling it to protect itself from host defense mechanisms. Also, *S. aureus* has developed the ability to destroy the active lactam ring in the penicillin molecule by secreting an enzyme called beta-lactamase. This genetic mutation prevents the beta-lactam ring from binding to the bacterial cell; thus, the agent cannot exert its antimicrobial effects.

Methicillin-resistant *S. aureus* is not naturally found in the environment, but it is found on humans. *Staphylococcus aureus* and MRSA can live on surfaces and humans for days to weeks; it has a varying life span. When a person is colonized with MRSA, the **endogenous pathogen** (the pathogen residing on the body) can easily be transferred to the skin and other body areas, increasing the risk for infection (Fig. 21.1). For example, if a person is colonized with MRSA in the nose and he or she wipes the nose with the hand and then touches an open wound, the bacteria can then be transferred to the wound and cause an infection.

Methicillin-resistant *S. aureus* infections are also caused by **exogenous** (meaning "outside the body") sources. The mode of transmission from an exogenous source is contaminated surfaces. Methicillin-resistant *S. aureus* can be spread if an infected person touches the source of infection and then touches an object or surface. To prevent transmission from a contaminated surface, the CDC recommends covering cuts and open wounds with bandages and maintaining good hygiene, including bathing or showering regularly. The more common mode of transmission for MRSA is direct contact. Methicillin-resistant *S aureus* is easily spread, especially in hospitals and healthcare settings, from patient to patient or from body part to body part on the unclean hands of healthcare personnel or through improperly cleaned equipment. Thus, proper hand hygiene is essential when caring for patients with MRSA. A study done by Duke University found that the most commonly transmitted pathogen was *S. aureus*, including MRSA and methicillin-susceptible *S. aureus*. Contamination was from side rails, beds, supply carts, nurses' sleeves, and the pockets of nurses' uniforms.

Clinical Manifestations

Clinical manifestations of *S. aureus* commonly include minor skin infections, including pimples, abscesses, sties, and impetigo. Methicillin-resistant *S. aureus*, on the other hand, causes more serious infections, including pneumonia, skin and soft tissue infections, surgical-site infections, and bloodstream infections.

Complications

Because MRSA is resistant to numerous antibiotics, infections can often be difficult to treat and can cause serious complications as well as widespread infection. Infections with MRSA are associated with increased morbidity and mortality rates. The MRSA mortality rate overall is 20% to 50%. The highest mortality rates of 55.6% were observed among patients with MRSA-related septic shock. Patients with MRSA pneumonia had the next highest mortality rate at 32.4%, followed by MRSA endocarditis at 19.3%. Methicillin-resistant *S. aureus* bacteremia has a mortality rate of 10.2%, and the mortality of MRSA cellulitis is 6.1%. Patients with MRSA bacteremia have significantly longer lengths of stay, averaging 9.1 days, and the average hospital cost is significantly higher. The costs of MRSA average $20,000 per patient, with a total burden of $2.5 billion yearly. Patients who develop MRSA surgical-site infections have a 3.4-times-higher risk of death than a non-MRSA patient, and hospital costs are twice as much as the average hospital stay. Patients colonized with MRSA from a previous hospital stay have a 29% greater risk for developing bacteremia, pneumonia, or soft tissue infection within 18 months of colonization. Methicillin-resistant

Table 21.1 Risk Factors for Multidrug-Resistant (MDR) Organisms

Hospital-Acquired MRSA	Community-Acquired MRSA	VRE	Clostridioides Difficile	Acinetobacter Baumannii	CRE
Current/recent hospitalization	Less than 2 years of age	Prolonged hospitalization	Recent antibiotic use	Recent surgery	Weakened immune system
Residing in long-term care facility	Athletes	Weakened immune system	Greater than 64 years old	Invasive procedures/ medical devices	Disruption in the body's natural flora
Invasive procedures/ medical devices	IV drug abusers	Prolonged anti-biotic exposure	NGT or feeding tubes	Tracheostomy	Mechanical ventilation
Recent antibiotic use	Men who have sex with men	Invasive procedures/ medical devices	Prolonged hospitalization	Mechanical ventilation	Indwelling devices such as Foley catheters, central venous catheters, and feeding tubes
Weakened immune system	Military personnel	Comorbid conditions	Chemotherapy	Enteral feedings	
Comorbid conditions	Prison inmates		Gastrointestinal surgery	Recent antibiotic use	
Dialysis devices	People living in shelters		Acid-suppressing medications	Prolonged hospitalization	Patients in hospitals and long-term care facilities
Gastrointestinal disorders			Comorbid conditions	Intensive care unit admission	Older adults
				Prior hospitalization	Comorbid conditions: Heart disease Diabetes Renal disease
				Residing in long-term care facility	

CRE, Carbapenem-resistant Enterobacteriaceae; MRSA, methicillin-resistant *Staphylococcus aureus*; NGT, nasogastric tube; VRE, vancomycin-resistant *Enterococci*.

S. aureus infections can also lead to osteomyelitis and toxic shock syndrome, and ultimately, untreated infections can lead to multisystem organ failure and death.

Connection Check 21.1

Which are risk factors for MRSA infection? *(Select all that apply.)*

A. Surgery
B. Urinary catheters
C. Antibiotic use
D. Feeding tubes
E. Recent hospitalization

Vancomycin-Resistant *Enterococci*

Epidemiology

Enterococci are bacteria that normally live in the gastrointestinal tract and the female genital tract and are also found in the environment in soil, water, and food.

They are the third most common organisms seen in nosocomial infections. Traditionally, *Enterococci* have been considered low-grade pathogens; however, in the 1990s, they surfaced as an increasingly important cause of nosocomial infections. *Enterococci* are **facultatively anaerobic** (organisms that use aerobic metabolism if oxygen is present but can switch to anaerobic metabolism if oxygen is absent) gram-positive cocci.

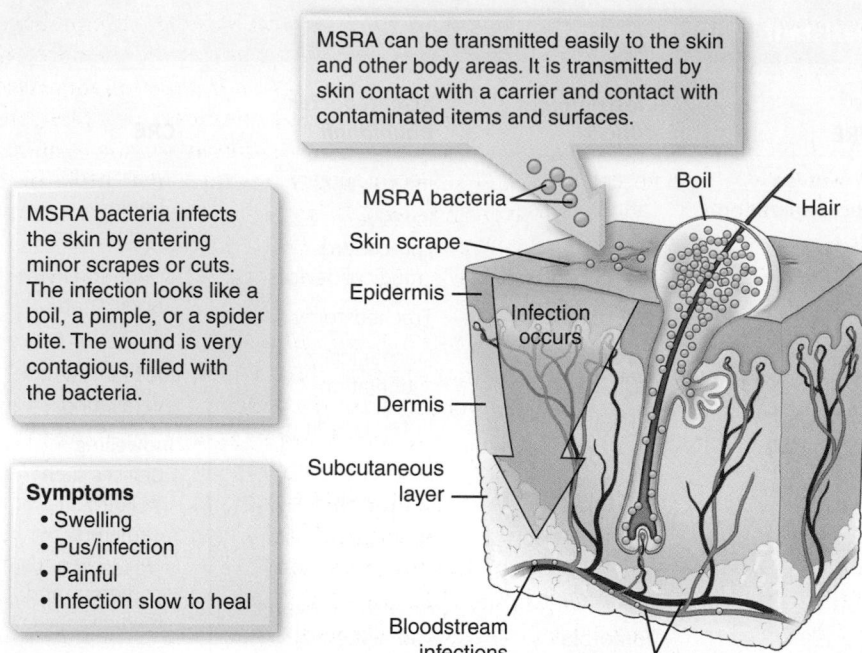

MSRA can be transmitted easily to the skin and other body areas. It is transmitted by skin contact with a carrier and contact with contaminated items and surfaces.

MSRA bacteria infects the skin by entering minor scrapes or cuts. The infection looks like a boil, a pimple, or a spider bite. The wound is very contagious, filled with the bacteria.

Symptoms
- Swelling
- Pus/infection
- Painful
- Infection slow to heal

MSRA bacteria
Skin scrape
Epidermis
Infection occurs
Dermis
Subcutaneous layer
Bloodstream infections
Blood vessels
Boil
Hair

FIGURE 21.1 Methicillin-resistant *Staphylococcus aureus* mode of infection; transmitted via skin contact with a carrier and entering through breaks in the skin.

In the late 1980s, the increasing prevalence of MRSA, as well as the discovery of antibiotic-associated diarrhea, resulted in an increased use of vancomycin and the emergence of VRE. Vancomycin-resistant *Enterococci* (VRE) were first reported in 1986 in Europe. The first case of VRE was reported in the United States in 1987. The exact origin of the vancomycin-resistant genes is unknown. Both *Enterococcus faecalis* and *Enterococcus faecium* are vancomycin-resistant species of *Enterococci. Enterococcus faecium* exhibits natural resistance to antimicrobial agents, including beta-lactams and aminoglycosides, and more than 95% of the VRE strains isolated in the United States are *E. faecium.* The majority of the remaining isolates are *E. faecalis,* which is a more pathogenic strain.

Since the emergence of VRE in the 1980s, the rates of VRE colonization and infection have risen steadily. In the United States, VRE infections mostly occur in hospitals and are not associated with community acquisition. They are associated with higher morbidity and mortality rates, higher healthcare costs, and prolonged lengths of hospital stay. The prevalence of VRE is highest among patients who are critically ill in ICUs. High VRE rates are also seen in hematology patients and organ-transplant recipients secondary to immunosuppression. Rates of VRE are significantly lower in western regions of the United States than in hospitals located in the eastern region. Larger hospitals or teaching centers also have significantly higher rates of VRE than smaller hospitals with fewer beds, secondary to increased severity of illness. Hand-hygiene compliance also affects the prevalence of VRE. Hospitals with observed hand-hygiene compliance rates at 59% or greater had significantly lower rates of VRE. Antibiotic stewardship is associated with lower rates of VRE. Efforts to reduce the use of vancomycin and cephalosporins have decreased the prevalence of VRE in the United States.

The risk factors for VRE are very similar to those for MRSA. They include prolonged hospital stays, people with weakened immune systems (such as patients in ICUs, transplant patients, and cancer patients, especially hematological malignancies), prolonged exposure to antibiotics (especially exposure to vancomycin and cephalosporins), and invasive procedures and devices. Severe comorbidities also are a risk factor for the acquisition of VRE (see Table 21.1).

Pathophysiology

Vancomycin-resistant *Enterococci* are hardy organisms and can remain viable on environmental surfaces for 7 days to 2 months. Patients can remain colonized with VRE for prolonged periods of time ranging from 7 weeks to 3 years. Although VRE are less virulent than MRSA, they can still cause many therapeutic problems because of their resistance to many antibiotics. They are spread by direct patient-to-patient contact or indirectly on the hands of healthcare personnel or on unclean patient care equipment. Colonization with VRE is associated with progression to VRE infection. Accordingly, there is a large emphasis on prevention because VRE outbreaks are very difficult to control owing to the fact that antibiotic use increases the microbial load of VRE and facilitates nosocomial transmission. They are also difficult to control because treatment options may be limited. A polypharmacological approach may be necessary.

Clinical Manifestations

Enterococci commonly cause urinary tract infections (UTIs), peritonitis (intra-abdominal and pelvic wound infections), and bacteremias; thus, clinical manifestations vary depending on the site of infection. Classic signs of UTI are back pain, pain on urination, the sensation of needing to urinate, and fever. Wound infections typically present as red and hot and, at times, with purulent drainage. Bacteremias present with signs of sepsis: tachycardia, hypotension, and fever.

Complications

One of the many complications of VRE is the growing list of resistance to antimicrobial agents as well as the emergence of vancomycin-resistant *S. aureus*. The vancomycin-resistant gene from VRE has been transferred to *S. aureus* isolates. This is quite disturbing because IV vancomycin is the medication of choice in the treatment of MRSA. Additional complications of VRE infections include prolonged hospital stays, prolonged antimicrobial therapy, higher attributable mortality rates, and increased cost of hospitalization. Vancomycin-resistant *Enterococci* bacteremia is associated with higher mortality rates than other *Enterococci* bacteremias because of antibiotic resistance. Another complication of VRE is endocarditis. *Enterococci* are the third most common cause of infective endocarditis. This is a problem because no agent has been approved by the U.S. Food and Drug Administration (FDA) for the treatment of VRE endocarditis.

Connection Check 21.2

The nurse is screening patients for their risk of developing VRE. The nurse should consider which patient at greatest risk?

A. The patient cared for at home
B. The patient with prolonged antibiotic exposure
C. The patient in a small community hospital setting
D. The patient hospitalized for an uncomplicated procedure

Clostridioides Difficile

Epidemiology

Clostridioides difficile (C. diff) was first detected in 1978. Increased use of antibiotics and the increased incidence of *S. aureus* infections are implicated in the emergence of *C. diff*. *Clostridioides difficile* is the most common cause of antibiotic-associated diarrhea in the United States, responsible for 12% of all hospital-acquired infections. The CDC identifies *C. diff* as one of the three most "urgent" threats to the public health system. In the mid-1990s, the incidence of *C. diff* in acute care hospitals was 30 to 40 cases per 100,000 patients. In 2001, the incidence had increased to almost 50 cases per 100,000 patients, and in 2005, it rose to 84 cases per 100,000. U.S. hospitals had a significant increase in *C. diff* infections between 2013 and 2014. Fifty percent or more of hospitalized patients are colonized with *C. diff* without showing symptoms of the disease. The risk of colonization increases steadily each day during hospitalization secondary to the daily risk of exposure to *C. diff* spores in a healthcare setting. The prevalence of *C. diff* in the stool of asymptomatic adults without recent hospitalizations is less than 2%. Ninety-six percent of patients infected with *C. diff* have received antimicrobial therapy

within the previous 3 months, and 85% of patients have received antimicrobials within 28 days prior to the onset of symptoms. The risk of recurrent *C. diff* infection increases in patients who have already had one infection. The rate increases from about 20% after the initial episode to about 40% after the first recurrence and to more than 60% after two or more recurrences. It is not known whether recurrence results from reinfection with a different strain or if it is the persistence of the strain responsible for the initial episode.

The risk factors for *C. diff* infections include the use of antimicrobials, particularly clindamycin, cephalosporins, and fluoroquinolones. Other risk factors include age greater than 64 years old; duration of hospitalization; immunocompromising conditions; chemotherapy; nasogastric (NG) tubes, including feeding tubes; gastrointestinal surgery; severe underlying illness; and the use of acid-suppressing medications such as histamine-2 (H$_2$) blockers and proton-pump inhibitors. The use of antimicrobial agents is a risk factor for *C. diff* infections because antimicrobials suppress the normal bowel flora and create an environment for *C. diff* to flourish. The greater the number of antimicrobials, the greater the number of doses, and the greater the duration of administration, the higher the risk of a *C. diff* infection. The prevalence of *C. diff* infections increases with age. People more than 85 years old are two times more likely to become infected compared with people aged 65 to 84 years old. Ironically, newborns and children in the first year of life have some of the highest rates of colonization but not infection. The use of acid-suppressing medications is a risk factor because these medications prevent the protective effect of stomach acid, which usually kills *C. diff* bacteria. Nasogastric tubes and gastrointestinal surgery increase the risk for *C. diff* infections because NG tubes are usually inserted in patients who have had gastrointestinal surgery who then undergo prolonged periods of no oral caloric intake and who are prescribed prolonged courses of postoperative systemic antibiotics. These patients also suffer from impaired bowel motility, which increases the risk for *C. diff* infections (see Table 21.1).

Pathophysiology

Clostridioides difficile is a spore-forming, gram-positive anaerobic bacillus. *Clostridioides difficile* spores are resistant to many types of disinfectants, heat, and dryness. They also can live for months on surfaces, in skin folds, and on the hands of healthcare workers. They are transmitted through the oral-fecal route. This occurs when a pathogen from feces is introduced into the oral cavity of a host. *Clostridioides difficile* is almost exclusively found in healthcare settings. The hands of healthcare workers are the primary source by which *C. diff* is spread during outbreaks. Environmental contamination is also a means by which the organism is spread secondary to its ability to survive in the environment for long periods of time. It can also be spread by direct person-to-person contact; thus, a patient with *C. diff* must be put on contact-isolation precautions.

Once a person becomes a susceptible host for *C. diff* by having one or more risk factors and has lost the protective normal flora in the colon secondary to antimicrobial therapy or decreased stomach acidity, its growth goes undetected and proliferates. The organism produces two toxins that cause the detrimental effects of the disease. One of the toxins produced is an enterotoxin, or toxin A, and the other toxin produced is a more potent cytotoxin, toxin B. Toxin A activates macrophages and mast cells, which release inflammatory mediators. The inflammatory mediators then cause disruption of the cell-wall junction, which results in increased permeability of the intestinal wall. Toxin B causes an increase in leukocytes and cytokines. Toxin B also causes degradation of the epithelial cells in the colon. Both toxins illicit a colonic inflammatory response that causes massive fluid secretions to move into the colon, resulting in diarrhea. As the *C. diff* infection worsens, purulent and necrotic debris accumulates and forms pseudomembranes (thin tissue layer covering the surface of the epithelium).

Clinical Manifestations

People who develop *C. diff* infections test positive for *C. diff* toxins in their stool. Although patients may be asymptomatic, the most common clinical manifestation is mild to moderate diarrhea.

Complications

Clostridioides difficile infections increase lengths of stay in healthcare facilities by 2.6 to 4.5 days, and costs nationally per infection range from $6,000 to $9,000. Unlike with MRSA and VRE, the attributable mortality of *C. diff* is low. The mortality rate has been reported as 6.9% at 30 days after diagnosis and 16.7% at 1 year. The rising incidence of the disease is causing higher mortality rates related to the increasing virulence of *C. diff* strains and the increasing host vulnerability. Severe *C. diff* infections lead to complications such as:

- Volume depletion (hypovolemia) and hypotension (low blood pressure)
- Renal insufficiency
- Electrolyte imbalances (hypo-/hyperkalemia, hypo-/hypernatremia)
- Hypoalbuminemia (low serum albumin levels)
- Peritonitis (inflammation of the peritoneum)
- Paralytic ileus (intestinal obstruction)
- Toxic megacolon (rapid dilation of the large intestines)
- Fulminant pseudomembranous colitis
- Sepsis
- Death

Complications are more common in patients with a white blood cell (WBC) count of 15.0 $10^3/mm^3$ or higher, and catastrophic complications occur in patients with a WBC count of 50.0 $10^3/mm^3$. Patients who are severely ill may require a subtotal colectomy (part of the colon is removed) with preservation of the rectum or colectomy (removal of the entire colon) for treatments for severe *C. diff*

infections that progress to fulminant pseudomembranous colitis, paralytic ileus, toxic megacolon, or sepsis.

Skin breakdown is also a complication of the disease. Excessive moisture, alkaline pH, colonization with microorganisms, and friction contribute to skin breakdown in patients with *C. diff*. Proper perineal cleansing is imperative. Creams and ointments that serve as a moisture barrier should be applied after cleaning to prevent skin breakdown. Fecal management systems can also be used in stool-incontinent patients to maintain skin integrity.

Acinetobacter Baumannii

Epidemiology

Acinetobacter has emerged as an important healthcare–associated pathogen. It was first identified in 1911 and was named *Micrococcus calcoaceticus*. In the 1950s, it became known as *Acinetobacter*. *Acinetobacter* is identified as an MDR organism because it is resistant to more than three classes of antibiotics. The CDC reported that the rates of *A. baumannii* resistance against the class of carbapenems increased from 9% in 1995 to 40% in 2004. The emergence of MDR *Acinetobacter* is due to the use of broad-spectrum antimicrobials and the transmission of strains among patients. The incidence of hospital-acquired *Acinetobacter* infections is continually increasing. Studies demonstrate that 17% to 26% of patients colonized with *Acinetobacter* in one or more sites may develop a clinical infection. The prevalence and resistance of *Acinetobacter* are also increasing in the community. Research has shown that increasingly resistant strains of *Acinetobacter* are being introduced into nursing homes and long-term care facilities, which is concerning because there are fewer resources for infection surveillance and prevention in these settings.

Acinetobacter baumannii outbreaks have been experienced throughout the world. They rarely occur outside of healthcare settings, and healthy people rarely get serious infections from this organism; however, outbreaks have been reported among U.S. military personnel dating back as far as the Korean War in 1955. The incidence of *Acinetobacter* infections is highest in ICUs. Within the past two decades, *Acinetobacter* has been responsible for increasing infections in ICUs globally. It causes an increase in morbidity and mortality as well as an increased length of stay in that setting. Studies suggest that there is a very low prevalence of *Acinetobacter* in the non–critically ill medical-surgical patient population.

Risk factors for MDR *A. baumannii* infections and colonization include recent surgery, central venous catheters, tracheostomy, mechanical ventilation, enteral feedings, exposure to antimicrobial agents, and underlying severity of illness. Vascular catheters and the respiratory tract have been identified as the most frequent source of *Acinetobacter* bacteremia. Other risk factors include prolonged hospitalization, ICU admissions, prior hospitalizations, and nursing home residence (see Table 21.1).

Pathophysiology

Multidrug-resistant *Acinetobacter* is a nonfermentative, aerobic, gram-negative coccobacillus that naturally inhabits water, soil, animals, and humans. It grows at varying temperatures and pH environments. More than 25 species within the *Acinetobacter* genus have been described. The most important species of this genus in human pathology is *A. baumannii*. It accounts for nearly 80% of *Acinetobacter* infections. It has been recovered from the skin, throat, and rectum of humans. It also colonizes the respiratory tract. This organism has the ability to survive for weeks to months on both dry and moist surfaces, which promotes transmission via contamination in hospital settings. Since 1974, higher rates of nosocomial *Acinetobacter* infections have been noted in the summer than in other seasons. Infection rates were approximately 50% higher from July to October than other times of the year. This is possibly due to the warmer, more humid air that favors the growth of *Acinetobacter* in its natural environment.

The mechanism by which the *Acinetobacter* species become resistant to antimicrobials is an impermeable outer membrane, antimicrobial-inactivating enzymes, reduced access to bacterial targets, and mutations that change targets or cellular function. This organism is spread by direct or indirect contact. Direct transmission occurs when *Acinetobacter* is transferred from patient to patient without a contaminated intermediate object or person. This usually occurs when an infected *Acinetobacter* patient and noninfected patient share the same room. Indirect transmission occurs when *Acinetobacter* is transferred through a contaminated object or person. The most common mode of transmission is through the unclean hands of healthcare workers who have cared for infected or colonized patients. Transmission commonly occurs through contaminated skin, body fluids, equipment, or the environment. Multidrug-resistant *Acinetobacter* outbreaks are often traced back to common-source contamination. Respiratory care equipment, wound care procedures, humidifiers, and patient care items have been named as sources of contamination in recent outbreaks.

Clinical Manifestations

Acinetobacter can infect or colonize many body sites. Typical sites of colonization and infection are the respiratory tract, blood, pleural fluid, peritoneum, urinary tract, surgical wounds, central nervous system (CNS), skin, and eyes. The most frequent clinical manifestations of *A. baumannii* infections are ventilator-associated pneumonia and bloodstream infections.

Complications

Many complications are associated with MDR *Acinetobacter* infections. They increase mortality, morbidity, length of hospitalization, and length of ventilator days. Patients with *Acinetobacter* bacteremia have a 5-day excess length of mechanical ventilation compared with patients without *Acinetobacter* infections. These infections also prolong an ICU stay by 6 days, with the median duration of hospitalization being 18 days.

Although difficult to prove secondary to the patient's severe underlying illnesses, the associated crude mortality rates range from 26% to 68% for MDR *Acinetobacter* infections. Other sources estimate the attributable mortality at 21.8%.

Carbapenem-Resistant Enterobacteriaceae (CRE)

Epidemiology

In 2018 the CDC reported about 9,300 CRE healthcare-associated infections in the United States. The CDC also reported that 50% of hospital patients who develop bloodstream infections from CRE bacteria die from them. Due to this, the CDC has labeled CRE an "urgent" concern, the CDC's highest level of concern. Enterobacteriaceae can cause infections in people in both the hospital and community setting. Healthy people are typically not at risk. Risk factors are similar to those for other MDR organism. They include any disorder or treatment that disturbs the body's natural flora. There is an increased frequency in older individuals, patients in hospitals and long-term care facilities, and a slight increase in women. Common comorbidities include diabetes, heart disease, and renal disease. Indwelling devices such as Foley catheters, central venous catheters, and feeding tubes increase risk.

Pathophysiology

Enterobacteriaceae include *Klebsiella* species and *Escherichia coli (E. coli)*. These organisms are normally found in the intestines, where they are typically harmless if contained, but if spread outside the intestine, they can cause serious infections, such as UTIs, bloodstream infections, wound infections, and pneumonia. Infections with CRE are usually spread through direct contact with infected or colonized people, particularly contact with wounds or stool. The resistance of CRE to carbapenems is caused by two main mechanisms: (1) the activity of β-lactamase enzymes that results in resistance to β-lactam antibiotics and (2) the production of carbapenemases, enzymes that hydrolyze (break down compounds in a reaction with water) carbapenem antibiotics.

Clinical Manifestations

Manifestations vary depending on the location of the infection—bloodstream, pneumonia, wound infections, or UTIs. Common manifestations include fever, chills, and signs of sepsis if the infection has not been successfully controlled.

Complications

Carbapenem-resistant Enterobacteriaceae are strains of bacteria that are resistant to carbapenem, a class of antibiotics typically used as a last resort for treating severe infections when other antibiotics have failed. These organisms are particularly dangerous and difficult because they have become resistant to nearly all available antibiotics. Because of this, mortality is high, especially in hospitalized patients.

CASE STUDY: EPISODE 2

Mr. Brown's abdominal wound is cultured. It is determined that he has an MRSA infection. His vital signs are:

BP: 110/66

HR: 110; atrial fibrillation noted on ECG

RR: 18

T: 100.5°F (38°C)

Bedside blood glucose monitoring: 140

Complicated by his history of diabetes and the presence of atrial fibrillation, it is essential that Mr. Brown receives prompt attention for his wound infection to avoid a systemic infection. He is admitted to the hospital for a course of IV vancomycin to be given every 12 hours...

MANAGEMENT OF MULTIDRUG-RESISTANT ORGANISMS

Medical Management

Diagnosis

Diagnosis of MDR organisms begins with detection. In an effort to contain outbreaks of VRE and MRSA, hospitals have initiated surveillance programs. A recent study suggests that lower rates of MRSA were found in healthcare settings where surveillance for antimicrobial-resistant organisms occurred. There is an MRSA risk assessment tool that is used to identify baseline data on MRSA incidence, prevalence, and transmission. The risk assessment helps to identify patient populations that are likely to be colonized or infected with MRSA. The purpose of the MRSA risk assessment is to prevent transmission through the development of a plan that is based on facility data and conditions. Thus, MRSA patient screening or active surveillance testing (AST) is individualized for each institution. With AST, MRSA cultures are obtained from patient populations identified as being at risk through the MRSA risk assessment. The most commonly cultured site is the anterior nares. Other sites that are typically screened for MRSA are areas of skin breakdown and draining wounds.

Tracking VRE colonization is done through active surveillance in high-risk populations. Some institutions perform VRE screening on any patient admitted to the intensive care environment. The screening is done through the collection of perianal specimens. These specimens are obtained by swabbing back and forth across the perianal region using culture swabs; if stool is present, the culture swab should be immersed in the stool.

There is no current surveillance for *C. diff* or *Acinetobacter*. If a patient is suspected of having *C. diff* secondary to watery diarrhea, a stool sample should be obtained. It is not recommended to test the stool of asymptomatic patients because infection is not likely. Once collected, the stool sample must be promptly sent to the laboratory. The *C. diff* toxins are unstable at room temperature, and false-negative results may occur in samples that are not tested within 2 hours of collection. *Clostridioides difficile* can also be diagnosed through direct visualization of the pseudomembranes via sigmoidoscopy or colonoscopy because it is nearly the exclusive cause of pseudomembranous colitis.

Currently, there are no specific recommendations regarding best practice for surveillance cultures for *Acinetobacter* because of the lack of verified effectiveness of screening cultures. However, in an outbreak situation, screening cultures may be a part of an enhanced intervention when rates are increasing. Suggested body sites for screening cultures include the nose, throat, skin sites such as the axilla or groin, the rectum, open wounds, and endotracheal aspirates. When environmental contaminants are suspected of playing a role in an outbreak, environmental or equipment culturing may be used. At present, there is no active screening for CRE. Infections are typically identified through blood, wound, sputum, or urine cultures.

Treatment

Hand Hygiene

The best treatment of MDR organisms begins with prevention—hand hygiene. The declining rates of some MDR infections have been attributed to the use of alcohol-based hand rubs and improved hand-hygiene programs. It is important to remember that alcohol-based hand rubs are not effective against *C. diff*.

 Safety Alert *Clostridioides difficile* **and Hand Washing**

- Alcohol-based hand sanitizers do not kill *C. diff* but just displace the spores.
- Healthcare workers, patients, and visitors must use soap and water and mechanical hand washing to perform hand hygiene when coming in contact with a patient who has *C. diff*.

Isolation

Patients in healthcare settings who are either colonized or infected with MDR organisms are placed on **contact-isolation** precautions (see Safety Alert: Isolation Precautions) to help reduce patient-to-patient spread of the organism within the hospital. Contact-isolation precautions include wearing gowns and gloves on entry to a patient's room, removing both the gown and gloves just prior to exiting, and performing proper hand hygiene before exiting. Past studies have shown that organisms remained on healthcare workers' isolation gowns, gloves, and hands before hand washing after caring for an infected or colonized patient. As noted previously, proper hand hygiene is essential with all MDR organisms. Patients colonized or infected with MDR organisms are placed in private rooms when available or placed in a room with other patients colonized or infected with the same organism. Contact-isolation precautions are typically continued throughout the duration of the hospital stay or, as in the case of *C. diff*, until the diarrhea has stopped. Discontinuation of contact precautions for MRSA patients may occur when clearance of the organism has been documented with three or more surveillance tests. Retesting patients to document clearance is commonly done 3 to 4 months after the last positive test result. However, some institutions consider MRSA-colonized patients to be colonized indefinitely.

During large MDR *Acinetobacter* outbreaks, patients are usually placed in a specific area or unit. Sometimes, the closure of an entire ICU is warranted to halt transmission. Dedicated nursing and respiratory staff, as well as dedicated equipment, is used to prevent further transmission.

 Safety Isolation Precautions Alert

- Isolation precautions *MUST* be used for patients with MRSA, VRE, *C. diff*, *Acinetobacter,* and CRE.
- Hand hygiene *MUST* be performed before healthcare workers put on isolation gowns and gloves.
- Isolation gowns *MUST* be secured at the neck and waist to effectively prevent bacteria transmission.
- Isolation gowns and gloves *MUST* be removed before the healthcare worker leaves the isolation patient's room.
- Hand hygiene *MUST* be performed before the healthcare worker leaves the isolation patient's room.

Medications

Methicillin-Resistant Staphylococcus Aureus

The most commonly used medication for the treatment of infections caused by MRSA is vancomycin (Vancocin), administered either IV or orally. The **trough level** (blood sample drawn after a dose is given but immediately before the next dose) should be monitored at least weekly to avoid toxic doses and maintain therapeutic levels. If trough levels are too high, vancomycin can cause nephrotoxicity as well as ototoxicity. Weekly blood urea nitrogen (BUN) and serum creatinine tests are recommended to assess kidney function because of the nephrotoxicity. Linezolid (Zyvox) given IV or orally is another antibiotic commonly used to treat skin and soft tissue infections caused by MRSA. Linezolid is a synthetic antibiotic of the oxazolidinone class and is **bacteriostatic** (stops organism reproduction) against *Enterococci* and *Staphylococci*. Recent studies have demonstrated that linezolid is equally as effective as vancomycin (Vancocin) for patients with skin and soft tissue infections.

Linezolid is given for 7 to 21 days depending on the infection. If it is given for more than 10 days, the patient should be monitored through evaluation of a complete blood count for myelosuppression, including anemia, leukopenia, pancytopenia, and thrombocytopenia. Linezolid may also cause diarrhea, nausea, and vomiting. Serious CNS reactions can occur when Linezolid is used together with serotonergic psychiatric medications. Patients taking Linezolid should avoid foods with high tyramine content (such as aged cheeses, dried/processed meats, alcohol, soy sauce) and should report any vision changes to their healthcare provider.

IV daptomycin (Cubicin) and IV tigecycline (Tygacil) are used for the treatment of complicated skin and soft tissue infections caused by MRSA. Daptomycin is a cyclic lipopeptide that has an antimicrobial spectrum similar to that of linezolid and exhibits **bactericidal** activity (kills the organism) against gram-positive organisms. Patients receiving daptomycin should be monitored for muscle pain and weakness and should have weekly creatine phosphokinase (CPK) levels drawn to assess for rhabdomyolysis (the breakdown of muscle tissue–releasing proteins into the blood). Patients with renal insufficiency need to have more frequent CPK level monitoring. Tigecycline is in the glycylcycline antibiotic class that has extended-spectrum activity against gram-positive, gram-negative, and anaerobic microorganisms. Tigecycline may cause diarrhea, nausea, and vomiting. It also decreases the effectiveness of oral contraceptives, so female patients should be instructed to use an alternative method of contraception while receiving this therapy.

Clindamycin (Cleocin) given IV or orally is one of the more commonly used antibiotics used to treat CAMRSA infections. Clindamycin has activity against aerobic and anaerobic gram-positive organisms including MRSA. The most common side effects of Clindamycin are diarrhea, and it can cause *C. diff*.

Sulfamethoxazole-trimethoprim (Bactrim) given IV or orally is also used to treat CAMRSA skin and soft tissue infections. Dosing must be adjusted for patients with impaired renal function. The most common side effects are gastrointestinal (nausea, vomiting, loss of appetite). Sulfamethoxazole-trimethoprim can cause sun sensitivity, so instruct patients to use sunscreen when going out into the sun. Patients should also report signs of jaundice, somnolence, and confusion to their healthcare provider because sulfamethoxazole-trimethoprim can cause fulminant hepatic necrosis. It is also important to instruct patients to stay hydrated to prevent the formation of renal stones while taking this medication.

Because MRSA has started to become resistant to many antibiotics, antibiotic stewardship must be practiced when prescribing medications. The CDC suggests that minor to moderate skin infections be treated with incision and drainage of abscesses without the use of antibiotics.

Currently, there are no recommendations to treat MRSA colonization; however, some institutions provide decolonization therapy. Decolonization therapy is the administration of local antimicrobial or antiseptic agents alone or in conjunction with antimicrobial therapy (Table 21.2). A typical therapy used to decolonize patients is 2% mupirocin (Bactroban) ointment administered intranasally; mupirocin ointment is often used along with chlorhexidine bathing to complete the decolonization process. Mupirocin ointment should not be used with other intranasal products, and contact with mupirocin ointment should be avoided with open wounds, burns, and eyes. It can also cause headaches, pharyngitis, and rhinitis.

Vancomycin-Resistant Enterococci

Vancomycin-resistant *Enterococci* infections are often difficult to treat and may require multiple antibiotics for treatment because most VRE isolates are resistant to penicillin and ampicillin. Susceptibility testing is recommended to verify the activity of the antimicrobial agent being used. Quinupristin-dalfopristin (Synercid) given via IV was the first antimicrobial agent available to treat VRE infections caused by *E. faecium*. Quinupristin-dalfopristin is a streptogramin and targets bacterial ribosomes, thereby inhibiting protein synthesis. This medication can be caustic to veins; thus, peripherally inserted central catheter (PICC) placement is recommended if long-term use is required. Dosages may need to be adjusted in patients with liver insufficiency or cirrhosis. The length of therapy depends on the type of infection. Common side effects of quinupristin-dalfopristin are joint pain, mild diarrhea, nausea and vomiting, and muscle pain.

Linezolid, daptomycin, and tigecycline are also used to treat VRE infections. Linezolid has activity against both *E. faecium* and non–*E. faecium* species. It is the only oral agent approved by the FDA for the treatment of infections caused by VRE. Daptomycin has been reported to be effective against more than 99.5% of VRE isolates. Tigecycline has in vitro activity against VRE, but clinical data are lacking for the treatment of VRE infections. Treatment for VRE colonization is not recommended because there is currently no antimicrobial agent available to eradicate VRE colonization. See Table 21.2 for a list of antibiotics used in the treatment of VRE.

Clostridioides Difficile

Before treatment for *C. diff* can begin, the suspected causative antibiotic must be stopped. In about 20% of patients, *C. diff* infection will resolve within 2 to 3 days of discontinuing the antibiotic to which the patient was previously exposed. Additionally, the use of antiperistaltic agents should be avoided because they may delay clearance of toxins from the colon and exacerbate toxin-induced colonic injury or precipitate ileus (an intestinal obstruction that results in the failure of intestinal contents to pass through) and toxic megacolon (a life-threatening complication of inflammatory bowel disease that causes rapid dilation of the large intestines, which results in septic shock).

Oral vancomycin is considered the first-line agent for the treatment of an initial episode of severe *C. diff* because

Table 21.2 Antibiotic Treatments for Infections With Multidrug-Resistant (MDR) Organisms

MRSA	VRE	Clostridioides Difficile	Acinetobacter	CRE
Vancomycin	Quinupristin-dalfopristin	Vancomycin	Ampicillin-sulbactam	Ceftazidime-avibactam
Linezolid	Linezolid	Fidaxomicin	Imipenem/Cilastatin	Meropenem-vaborbactam
Daptomycin	Daptomycin	Metronidazole	Meropenem	Polymyxin-based, combination such as polymyxin (colistin or polymyxin B) and meropenem
Tigecycline	Tigecycline		Tobramycin	
Clindamycin			Amikacin	
Sulfamethoxazole-trimethoprim			Tigecycline	Plazomicin
			Polymyxin B	
			Polymyxin E	
			Colistin	
			Minocycline	
			Doxycycline	

CRE, Carbapenem-resistant Enterobacteriaceae; *MRSA,* methicillin-resistant *Staphylococcus aureus*; *VRE,* vancomycin-resistant *Enterococci.*

it causes prompt symptom resolution and there is a significantly lower risk of treatment failure. It is effective because it is not absorbed in the intestines and kills the bacteria at the site of the infection in the colon. When oral vancomycin is not appropriate for the treatment of severe *C. diff* because of a coexisting ileus or toxic megacolon, IV metronidazole is used.

Fidaxomicin (Dificid) is also used to treat *C. diff* infections. It is a bactericidal agent against *C. diff* that inhibits RNA synthesis by RNA polymerases. Common side effects include vomiting and other gastrointestinal disorders. This medication is reserved for patients who have recurrent infections and probable vancomycin resistance. Oral metronidazole, once the treatment of choice, is an alternative if vancomycin or fidaxomicin is not available.

Recurrence of *C. diff* infections is seen in 20% to 30% of cases. Recurrence typically occurs 4 weeks after therapy has been completed. The recurrence rate for patients treated with metronidazole is 20.2%, and the recurrence rate for patients treated with vancomycin is 18.4%. Subsequent occurrences should be treated with vancomycin using a tapered regimen. In 2016, the FDA approved bezlotoxumab (Zinplava). It is indicated in the reduction of the recurrence of *C. diff* in patients who are receiving antibacterial medication treatment for *C. diff* infection and are at high risk for *C. diff* recurrence. Bezlotoxumab is a monoclonal antibody that binds to *C. diff* toxin B and neutralizes its effects. It is given as a single dose of 10 mg/kg and is administered by IV intermittent infusion over 60 minutes. The half-life is 10 days. Bezlotoxumab does not replace antibacterial treatment. See Table 21.2 for a list of antibiotics used in the treatment of *C. diff*.

Probiotics (live bacteria and yeasts) are another treatment that is used supplementally. Probiotics have effectively reduced the incidence of simple antibiotic-associated diarrhea and are sometimes used to treat recurrent *C. diff*; however, their efficacy is inconsistent. Another potential treatment option for recurrent *C. diff* is immunoglobulin therapy, but there is limited evidence supporting the efficacy of its use. Because of the inadequacies of current therapies as reflected by the high recurrence rate, the search is on for new antibiotics that inhibit vegetative cells of *C. diff* while preserving colonic flora during treatment.

Emerging as a treatment for recurring *C. diff* is fecal microbiota transplantation (FMT). The success rate of FMT in *C. diff* symptom resolution has been reported to be 81% to 94% in patients with recurrent disease. Fecal microbiota transplantation may restore the gut microbiota to create an environment resistant to *C. diff*. The treatment of FMT is indicated for patients who have had three or more occurrences of *C. diff* or who have had unsuccessful treatment with 6 to 8 weeks of vancomycin. Relatives who share similar microbiota are thought to be the most effective donors. The donor is screened for ova and parasites; HIV; and hepatitis A, B, and C. A stool culture and sensitivity may also be done. The fecal sample from the donor is combined with normal saline or water. Methods of administering the sample to the patient are nasogastric (25–50 mL) or colonoscopic (250–500 mL). Although frozen FMT oral capsules appear to be a viable delivery method, their clinical availability is limited, and their cost-effectiveness is still to be determined.

Connection Check 21.3

The nurse is reviewing orders for a newly admitted patient with *C. diff*. The nurse will follow up with the provider about which order?
A. PO Flagyl
B. Probiotics
C. Encouraging fluid intake
D. Imodium

Acinetobacter

Many different antimicrobial classes are used to treat MDR *Acinetobacter*; however, before treatment begins, susceptibility testing must occur because antibiotic resistance has increased over the last decade. Beta-lactamase inhibitors, especially sulbactams, possess the greatest intrinsic bactericidal activity against *A. baumannii*. Sulbactams, which in the United States are combined with ampicillin-sulbactam (Unasyn) given intravenously or intramuscularly, can be used for mild to severe cases of *A. baumannii* infections; however, the cure rate is only 67%. Better patient outcomes are associated with lower severity of illness. Ampicillin-sulbactam commonly causes diarrhea or a rash. It also decreases the effectiveness of oral contraceptives, so female patients should be instructed to use another form of contraception. Carbapenems given intravenously, such as imipenem/cilastatin (Primaxin IM) and meropenem (Merrem I.V.), are some of the most important therapeutic options for serious infections caused by MDR *Acinetobacter*. They have excellent bactericidal activity; however, the increasing carbapenem resistance is creating therapeutic challenges. It still remains the treatment of choice if the isolates retain susceptibility. Dosages need to be adjusted for patients with renal impairment. Carbapenems commonly cause nausea and headaches. They are also implicated in the development of Stevens-Johnson syndrome, a very rare toxic epidermal necrosis that causes the epidermis to separate from the dermis, typically because of a severe medication sensitivity.

Aminoglycoside agents such as IV tobramycin and IV amikacin are options for MDR isolates that retain susceptibility. Tobramycin maintains the highest susceptibility rates, and amikacin susceptibility has been reported at 53%. Tobramycin **peak levels** (medication levels obtained 30 minutes after administration) and trough levels should be obtained every 3 to 4 days to maintain a therapeutic dose. Amikacin may cause nephrotoxicity and ototoxicity; thus, peak and trough levels should also be monitored to maintain a therapeutic dose. Tigecycline, a glycylcycline agent, also has bacteriostatic activity against MDR *Acinetobacter*. However, the development of resistance to tigecycline has been reported recently.

Polymyxin agents are the most active agents in vitro against MDR *Acinetobacter*. They are cationic detergents that disrupt bacterial cell membranes, causing leakage of the cell contents, thus increasing permeability and leading to cell death. Polymyxin agents include Polymyxin B and Polymyxin E, which is also known as colistimethate sodium (Colistin). This class of medication has demonstrated its effectiveness as a treatment for highly drug-resistant gram-negative bacteria. The efficacy ranges from approximately 55% to more than 80%. Cure or improvement rates with colistin are 57% to 77% among severely ill patients. Resistance rates of MDR *Acinetobacter* for polymyxin agents are currently low. Polymyxin agents can be administered orally, intravenously, ophthalmically, intrathecally, or by inhalation. In the past, polymyxin agents could be administered intramuscularly, but the route was discontinued when Aminoglycosides became available. Polymyxins are poorly absorbed in the gastrointestinal tract, and gastrointestinal side effects are rarely reported with oral agents. Renal dose adjustment is required for patients with renal impairment.

Tetracycline agents, such as minocycline (Dynacin) and doxycycline (Doryx), are also used to treat MDR *Acinetobacter* infections. These agents can be given both intravenously and orally. Dosage and length of therapy vary depending on the type and severity of the infection. These agents decrease the effectiveness of oral contraceptives, so female patients should be instructed to use an alternative form of contraception. Tetracyclines also cause sun sensitivity, and patients should be instructed to use sunscreen when out in the sun for prolonged periods of time. It is recommended that tetracycline agents be taken, if prescribed orally, 1 hour before meals or 2 hours after meals to help with absorption. Adequate fluid hydration is also recommended to prevent esophageal irritation or ulcer. They may also cause gastrointestinal disturbances. Complete blood count (CBC) and liver and kidney function tests should be monitored if the patient is receiving chronic tetracycline therapy. See Table 21.2 for a list of medications used to treat *Acinetobacter* infections.

Connection Check 21.4

The nurse is screening patients for their risk of developing *Acinetobacter* infections. The nurse should consider which patient(s) at greatest risk? *(Select all that apply.)*

A. The patient on mechanical ventilation
B. The patient with a high-acuity illness
C. The patient recovering in the ICU overnight after surgery
D. The patient with prolonged antibiotic exposure
E. The patient with a wound infection

Carbapenem-Resistant Enterobacteriaceae

Treatment options are limited because no one antibiotic regimen has been shown to be better than another. As with other infections, treatment is based on the susceptibility of the organism. What follows is an overview because treatment is tailored to meet individual needs based on type of infection, comorbidities, and possible medication interactions. For serious infections caused by *Klebsiella*, ceftazidime-avibactam and meropenem-vaborbactam are acceptable options. These medications are given intravenously. They both work through the inhibition of bacterial cell-wall synthesis. They have reliable dosing and greater susceptibility, but data are limited. Options when neither of these is used are polymyxin-based combinations such as polymyxin (colistin or polymyxin B) and meropenem. These medications are also given intravenously and work through the disruption of the organism's outer cell membrane. These medications are associated with renal toxicity and neurotoxicity. Renal function should be carefully monitored, and the patient should be assessed for signs of neurological dysfunction. Some signs are mild, such as dizziness, diplopia, and weakness, but some adverse effects can be very serious, such as ataxia, dysphagia, dysphonia, psychosis, coma, and neuromuscular blockade leading to apnea. Polymyxin-based combinations and plazomicin are also options for other types of CRE. Plazomicin is given intravenously. It is associated with nephrotoxicity and ototoxicity, including hearing loss, tinnitus, and vertigo. Neuromuscular blockade is also associated with plazomicin.

Nursing Management

Assessment and Analysis

The clinical manifestations seen with MDR-organism infections are consistent with typical signs of infection: fever, tachycardia, tachypnea, and hypovolemia. Diarrhea is the prominent manifestation of *C. diff*, and MRSA wound infections can be red and warm with purulent drainage.

Nursing Diagnoses

- **Risk for deficient fluid volume** related to *C. diff* infection
- **Ineffective airway clearance** related to MDR pneumonia
- **Alteration in comfort** related to diarrhea and abdominal pain
- **Risk for perineal skin breakdown** related to frequent stools
- **Impaired tissue integrity** related to MDR wound infection
- **Impaired urinary elimination**: frequency related to urinary tract infection secondary to an MDR organism
- **Acute pain** related to wound infection secondary to an MDR organism

Nursing Interventions
Assessments

- Vital signs

  Increased body temperature is an immune response to an infection. A person's body temperature rises to try to kill the bacteria or virus that is causing the infection.

  Increased heart rate can occur due to fever and metabolic rate increases or hypovolemia.

  Tachypnea can occur secondary to pneumonia from infection with an MDR organism. Tachypnea is also caused secondary to a fever, which increases the metabolic rate, which then increases the work of breathing. Low blood pressure may indicate vasodilation due to systemic infection and hypovolemia. Hypovolemia can also occur secondary to fluid loss as a result of C. diff *diarrhea.*

- Oxygen saturation

  Monitor the patient's oxygen saturation. Decreased oxygen saturation can be a symptom of pneumonia caused by an MDR organism.

- Pain

  Pain is the fifth vital sign. Monitor patients for increased pain. Increased pain can be a sign of infection caused by an MDR organism; pain may also result from a fever.

- Skin turgor and mucous membranes

  Decreased skin turgor and dry mucous membranes can result from dehydration secondary to a C. diff *infection.*

- Urine output

  Decreased urine output is a sign of dehydration and can occur secondary to C. diff *diarrhea or may indicate the presence of a systemic infection with an MDR organism. It can also occur as an adverse side effect of antibiotics used to treat the infection.*

- Wound or surgical sites

  An infected wound or surgical site caused by an MDR organism may be red, swollen, painful, and warm to the touch and may have purulent drainage.

- Bowel movement frequency and consistency

  Increased bowel movement frequency can result in dehydration. When a person has a C. diff *infection, the bacteria proliferate and cause the release of toxins, resulting in an inflammatory response in the colon, which causes fluid to be secreted into the colon, resulting in diarrhea.*

- Skin integrity

  Monitor skin integrity to assess for skin breakdown or incontinence-associated dermatitis (IAD) secondary to C. diff *diarrhea.*

- Laboratory tests

  - White blood cell (WBC) count

    An increased WBC count is seen as part of the immune response; a large increase in WBCs may occur in C. diff *infections.*

  - Serum creatinine level

    Increased creatinine levels can occur when a patient is dehydrated or has an adverse reaction to antibiotic treatment, signaling decreased renal function.

  - Electrolyte and albumin levels

    Electrolyte and albumin levels may be decreased or increased secondary to dehydration from a C. diff *infection or any MDR-organism infection.*

Actions

- Hand hygiene

  To prevent the spread of MDR organisms: (1) alcohol-based cleansers are effective against nearly all MDR organisms, except C. diff; *(2) physical hand washing with soap and water is necessary to remove* C. diff.

- Place the patient on contact-isolation precautions.

  To prevent the spread of MDR organisms

- Administer medications as ordered:

  - Administer antibiotics.

    To treat infection of an MDR organism

  - Administer fever reducers.

    To decrease fever and complications associated with increased metabolic rate; also increases comfort

  - Administer pain medications.

    To decrease pain from wound or surgical-site infection

- Administer IV fluids or encourage the patient to drink fluids.

  To rehydrate from loss of fluid secondary to diarrhea from C. diff *infection or from infections with MDR organisms*

- Administer supplemental oxygen.

  To increase oxygen saturation secondary to MDR pneumonia

- Administer chest physiotherapy.

  To mobilize secretions in patients with MDR pneumonia and to increase oxygen saturation

- Encourage early mobilization.

  To decrease the risk of atelectasis secondary to MDR pneumonia and promote overall patient conditioning

- Stop administration of causative antimicrobial agent with a* C. diff *infection.

  To stop/decrease C. diff–*associated diarrhea*

- Perform wound care as ordered.

  To treat wound or surgical-site infection and promote wound healing

- Cleanse perineum and apply moisture barriers.

  To prevent skin breakdown or IAD secondary to C. diff–*associated diarrhea*

- Use fecal diversion or containment systems in the stool-incontinent patient.

  To prevent skin breakdown and increase comfort in C. diff *patients*

- Encourage family visits and the use of the telephone and television.

  To prevent depression in a patient in isolation with an MDR-organism infection

Teaching

- Contact-isolation precautions and hand washing (see Evidence-Based Practice)

  Teach patient and visitors the importance of wearing gowns and gloves when entering the room and removing the gowns and gloves when exiting the patient's room; also teach them the importance of performing hand hygiene after removing the gown and gloves.

- Take antibiotics as prescribed.

  Antibiotics should be taken as prescribed, and the patient should finish the course of antibiotics to prevent the reoccurrence of MDR infections.

- Clinical manifestations of infection
  It is important that the patient and family are able to recognize the signs and symptoms of infection.
- Sun protection
  Be aware of antibiotics such as tetracyclines that create sun sensitivities. Avoid prolonged sun exposure, wear sunscreen and appropriate covering clothing

Evidence-Based Practice

BUGG Study

A clinical trial was conducted to investigate the benefits of universal gowning and gloving (BUGG) in reducing the acquisition of methicillin-resistant *Staphylococcus aureus* (MRSA). The BUGG Study was sponsored by the Yale New Haven Health System Center for Healthcare Solutions in collaboration with the Agency for Healthcare Research and Quality (AHRQ), Centers for Disease Control and Prevention, University of Maryland, University of Iowa, and The Joint Commission. This observational study tested if doctors, nurses, and others wearing gloves and a gown while caring for all patients in an intensive care unit (ICU) would:

- Decrease the chance of patients getting an infection while in the hospital
- Decrease the chance of patients picking up bacteria as a result of being in the hospital
- Decrease the time a patient spends in the ICU or in the hospital
- Decrease the frequency of adverse events

A study by Harris et al. examined the results of that study. They found the following percentage decreases in MRSA acquisition:

- A reduction of 44% was due to universal gown and glove use.
- A reduction of 38% was due to improved hand hygiene.
- A reduction of 14.5% was due to decreased contact between healthcare workers and patients.

For more information on this clinical trial, go to the Web site ClinicalTrials.gov; the ClinicalTrials.gov Identifier is NCT01318213.

U.S. National Institutes of Health. (2015). *Benefits of universal glove and gowning* (BUGG). Retrieved from http://clinicaltrials.gov/ct2/show/NCT01318213
Harris, A. D., Morgan, D. J., Pineles, L., Perencevich, E. N., & Barnes, S. L. (2017). Deconstructing the relative benefits of a universal glove and gown intervention on MRSA acquisition. *Journal of Hospital Infection, 96*(1), 49–53.

Evaluating Care Outcomes

Infections due to MDR organisms can usually be successfully treated with antimicrobial therapy. Once the infection has been treated, the patient's vital signs and laboratory values should return to within normal limits. Patients should know the importance of finishing their antibiotic regimen to prevent the reoccurrence of infection. Patients and families should also know the clinical manifestations of a reoccurring infection in order to know when to seek healthcare advice.

Connection Check 21.5

What is the priority intervention to prevent the spread of MDR organisms?
A. Hand washing
B. Diagnostic cultures
C. Isolation precautions
D. Antibiotic administration

Making Connections

CASE STUDY: WRAP-UP

Upon his admission to the hospital, Mr. Brown's abdominal sutures are removed. The wound is irrigated; a sterile dressing is applied. The wound is left unsutured to facilitate drainage and allow for wound care. After 2 days and four doses of 1 g of IV vancomycin administration, Mr. Brown's wound infection is clearing. He remains in the hospital for 1 more day and two more doses of IV vancomycin. A vital sign check reveals:

BP: 130/80

HR: 80; atrial fibrillation still present

RR: 18

T: 98°F (37°C)

Bedside glucose monitoring: 98

At discharge, Mr. Brown receives instructions that include how to monitor his wound and change the dressing. Follow-up with the nursing home staff is arranged to help with dressing-change management. A follow-up appointment with his provider is set up for 2 weeks post-discharge. Mr. Brown is counseled to report any changes in the wound to his healthcare provider.

Case Study Questions

1. The nurse understands that Mr. Brown is at increased risk for a MRSA infection because of which factor(s)? *(Select all that apply.)*

   A. His recent hospitalization

   B. His history of atrial fibrillation

   C. His recent surgical procedure

   D. His residence in a long-term care facility

   E. His current use of the medication Coumadin

2. The nurse monitors for which clinical manifestations of MRSA in Mr. Brown's wound infection?

   A. Hyperglycemia

   B. Tachycardia

   C. Tachypnea

   D. Red, edematous, draining wound

3. The nurse should intervene immediately if Mr. Brown is noted to have which of the following symptoms?

   A. Depression

   B. Oliguria

   C. Decreased appetite

   D. Pain at the incision site

4. Which statement by Mr. Brown indicates the need for further teaching?

   A. "I need to be careful about the antibiotics I take."

   B. "I'll stop taking my antibiotics when I'm feeling better."

   C. "I never want to go to the hospital again."

   D. "I'll call my doctor if my blood sugar goes up."

5. Important transitional care plans for Mr. Brown include which of the following? *(Select all that apply.)*

   A. Follow-up with a home-care nurse

   B. Follow-up with a physical therapist

   C. Follow-up with his healthcare provider

   D. Follow-up with the emergency department

   E. Follow-up with a nutritionist

CHAPTER SUMMARY

Methicillin-resistant *S. aureus*, VRE, *C. diff*, *Acinetobacter*, and carbapenem-resistant Enterobacteriaceae are MDR organisms that plague healthcare settings because of their resistance to antimicrobial therapies. All of these organisms are easily spread within the healthcare setting by direct or indirect contact. Unclean hands of healthcare workers are one of the major causes of transmission of these organisms.

Proper hand hygiene is essential when caring for all patients and is especially vital for patients with MDR organisms. Alcohol-based hand rubs can be used for hand hygiene in patients with MRSA, VRE, and *Acinetobacter*, as well as hand washing with soap and water. However, hand washing with soap and water must be used to disinfect hands after contact with a patient with *C. diff*. Patients who are colonized or infected with MDR organisms are placed on contact-isolation precautions. Contact-isolation precautions are used to prevent the spread of the organisms in the healthcare setting. If private rooms are not available for patients with MDR organisms, they should be roomed with patients who are either colonized or infected with the same organism.

Methicillin-resistant *S. aureus* is the most well-known MDR organism, and it is the only MDR organism discussed in this chapter that is readily seen in the community as well as the healthcare setting. The most common MRSA infections seen in the community are skin and soft tissue infections. Vancomycin-resistant *Enterococci*, *C. diff*, and *Acinetobacter* infections are not seen in the community and are almost exclusively found in healthcare settings, particularly in the ICUs. Of the MDR organisms discussed in this chapter, *A. baumannii* is transmitted the most easily and is the most virulent. Carbapenem-resistant Enterobacteriaceae is an emerging "urgent" crisis because it is so difficult to treat.

All of the MDR organisms discussed in this chapter can both colonize and cause active infections in patients. Methicillin-resistant *S. aureus* causes common bacterial infections, including pneumonia, skin and soft tissue infections, surgical-site infections, and bacteremias. Vancomycin-resistant *Enterococci* commonly cause UTIs, peritonitis, and bacteremias. *Clostridioides difficile* is the cause of most antibiotic-associated diarrhea and can also cause pseudomembranous colitis, toxic megacolon, perforation of the colon, and sepsis. *Acinetobacter* causes bacteremias, pneumonia, meningitis, UTIs, and wound infections. Additionally, *Acinetobacter* is typically found in the more acute care setting or ICUs with intubated patients because of their increased susceptibility.

The risk factors associated with all of these MDR organisms are very similar. Hospitalizations, antibiotic use, invasive procedures, and residing in a long-term care facility are all common risk factors among MRSA, VRE, *C. diff*, *Acinetobacter*, and CRE. Similarly, they also have common complications. These MDR organisms all cause increased morbidity, mortality, and length of hospital stay. The use of proton-pump inhibitors or H_2 blockers is an additional risk factor for *C. diff* because they decrease the stomach's acid concentration, which helps destroy the organism.

Each MDR organism discussed in this chapter is extremely difficult to treat and has a set of specific antibiotic therapies. Antibiotic stewardship must be practiced when prescribing antimicrobial therapies for MDR organisms to prevent increased antibiotic resistance and the emergence of new MDR organisms. Additionally, once a patient has been diagnosed with *C. diff*, antiperistaltic agents should be avoided because they may delay the clearance of toxins from the colon.

Nursing implications when caring for patients with MDR-organism infections include impeccable hand hygiene, maintenance of isolation, administration of antibiotics as ordered, continual monitoring for resolution of infection or signs of systemic infection, and patient teaching. The single most important implication for nursing and the whole healthcare team is hand hygiene.

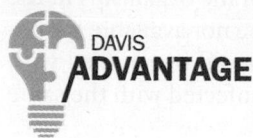

To explore learning resources for this chapter, go to **Davis Advantage** and find:
- Answers to in-text questions
- Chapter Resources and Activities
- NCLEX®-Style Chapter Review Questions
- Bibliography

Chapter 22

Coordinating Care for Patients With HIV

Thomasine Guberski

LEARNING OUTCOMES

Content in this chapter is designed to assist in:

1. Describing the etiology of human immunodeficiency virus (HIV) disorders
2. Discussing the epidemiology of HIV
3. Comparing and contrasting clinical presentations of the disease spectrum of HIV
4. Describing diagnostic results used to confirm the diagnosis of HIV
5. Developing a comprehensive plan of nursing care, including pharmacological, dietary, and lifestyle considerations, for patients with HIV disease

CONCEPTS

- Assessment
- Immunity
- Infection
- Medication
- Nursing Roles
- Safety

ESSENTIAL TERMS

Acquired immune deficiency syndrome (AIDS)
AIDS-defining condition
Antiretroviral therapy (ART)
CD4+ lymphocyte count
Human immunodeficiency virus (HIV)
Immune reconstruction inflammatory syndrome (IRIS)
Opportunistic infection (OI)
Pneumocystis carinii **pneumonia (PCP)**
Seroconversion
Serodiscordant
Viral load
Viral set point

Finding Connections

CASE STUDY: EPISODE 1

Follow this patient throughout the chapter.

Margo Castillo is a 45-year-old woman who presents to the emergency department with mild difficulty breathing for the past 2 days when walking a city block. She has had increasing fatigue for the past week. Prior to this, she had been relatively well except for several outbreaks of genital herpes in the past 6 months. The last outbreak was 2 months ago. She is currently on no medications. Her husband died of a blood infection 4 years ago…

OVERVIEW OF THE HIV/AIDS CONTINUUM

Like many chronic illnesses, HIV disease, caused by the human immunodeficiency virus (HIV), is comprised of several stages, ranging from acute infection to death. In an HIV-infected individual who does not receive treatment, the length of time from infection to death is approximately 12 years. In resource-limited countries, the time from infection to death is approximately 5 years. Malnutrition, tuberculosis (TB), and malaria are comorbidities that shorten the time the untreated patient survives.

June 2016 marked the 35th anniversary of the first reported cases of acquired immune deficiency syndrome (AIDS) in the United States. In June 1981, the Centers for Disease Control and Prevention (CDC) reported confirmed cases of *Pneumocystis carinii* pneumonia (PCP) in five previously healthy gay men. Because this disease occurs only in individuals with severely compromised immune systems, their new illness was called *acquired immune deficiency syndrome*. In 1985, when the antibody test for the HIV virus first became available, positive antibody tests confirming the presence of HIV antibodies were found in individuals who did not have signs or symptoms of AIDS. As a result of these findings, in 1986 the CDC published a disease classification system for individuals with a positive HIV test. Individuals were categorized into one of four mutually exclusive hierarchical groups on the basis of the presence or absence of signs or symptoms commonly associated with AIDS. This was the first recognition of the continuum of HIV/AIDS as a disease that progresses through stages, from acute HIV infection, asymptomatic HIV infection, and symptomatic HIV infection to the most advanced stage, AIDS.

Currently, anyone infected with HIV, regardless of the stage of his or her disease, is considered to have an HIV infection. In adults, the illness is then categorized into one of three different stages on the basis of the individual's **CD4+ lymphocyte count**, CD4+ percentage of total lymphocytes, or the presence or absence of certain infections commonly found in individuals with compromised immune systems, an **AIDS-defining condition**. If the person has an AIDS-defining condition, that person is considered to have AIDS regardless of CD4+ count (Table 22.1). Criteria for the stages of HIV infection in infants and children under the age of 13 are different from those for adults. Disease progression is from less severe to more severe. Once individuals are classified in a more severe stage, they cannot be reclassified into a less severe surveillance stage.

Outside the United States, a classification of HIV infection in adults and children developed by the World Health Organization (WHO) is used. The stages of HIV infection and criteria for classification are slightly different from those of the CDC classification. In addition, the WHO has a classification system for HIV based on response to treatment that allows individuals to move from severe to less severe stages.

According to the Joint United Nations Program on HIV/AIDS (UNAIDS), in 2010 approximately 33.3 million adults and children were living with HIV. Unlike many other infectious diseases, a vaccine to prevent the illness is not available. The constant change in the structure of the virus makes the development of a vaccine challenging. Until a vaccine is available, eliminating risky behaviors such as unprotected sex and IV drug use provides the major intervention to reduce transmission.

HUMAN IMMUNODEFICIENCY VIRUS (HIV)

Epidemiology

In 2016 UNAIDS estimated that approximately 1.8 million people were newly infected with HIV. This reflects a slow decline since the peak in 1997 due to an emphasis on prevention. With increased access to care and treatment for HIV, UNAIDS stated that in 2016 there was a decrease in the number of deaths to 1 million and an increase in the number of people living with HIV.

The picture in the United States is similar to that in the rest of the world. In 2016, the CDC estimated that since the beginning of the epidemic in the United States, approximately 2 million adults and children had been infected, and 600,000 had died. Currently, approximately 1.1 million individuals are living with HIV in the United States, and 15% are unaware of their infection. The latest statistics from the CDC indicate that in 2016, the new infection rate among gay men was 67% of new HIV infections, the highest of any group. This is a change from the early 2000s, when the highest new infection rates were via IV drug use and heterosexual transmission. African Americans are the racial and ethnic group most affected by HIV. The CDC states that in 2016, the highest rate of new infections among different racial and ethnic groups was in African American men, especially men who were having sex with men. HIV affects different populations in different ways. The highest incidence of HIV infections in the United States is found in Georgia, Louisiana, and Nevada, whereas the lowest is in Vermont.

HIV disease is most commonly a sexually transmitted disease, although a significant number of individuals contract the disease via IV drug use. Blood containing the HIV virus is injected into the bloodstream of an uninfected individual from an infected individual when needles or syringes are shared. A very small number of individuals are still infected with blood transfusions; the CDC notes one

Table 22.1 Classification of HIV Infection in Adults

Classification	CD4+ Count	CD4+ Percentage of Total Lymphocytes	AIDS-Defining Condition
HIV infection, stage 1	At least 500 cells/μL	At least 29%	None
HIV infection, stage 2	200–499 cells/μL	14%–28%	None
HIV infection, stage 3 (AIDS)	Less than 200 cells/μL	Less than 14%	Yes

Source: Centers for Disease Control and Prevention. (2008). Revised surveillance case definitions for HIV infection among adults, adolescents, and children aged <18 months and for HIV infection and AIDS among children aged 18 months to <13 years—United States, 2008. *MMWR, 57*(RR10), 1–8. Retrieved from http://www.cdc.gov/mmwr/preview/mmwrhtml/rr5710a1.htm

reported case since 2002. A smaller number of people, 0.36%, have gotten HIV through occupational exposure. Pregnant women or breastfeeding women infected with HIV can transmit the disease to their child. The latest figures available in the United States indicate that 99 children were born with HIV infection in 2016.

Connection Check 22.1

A nurse is screening patients for their risk of developing HIV. The nurse should consider which patient at greatest risk?
A. African American man
B. Asian woman
C. Caucasian man
D. Latino woman

Pathophysiology

The immune system protects the body by recognizing and destroying:

- Infectious agents such as bacteria, viruses, and parasites
- Abnormal cells
- Foreign objects—anything from splinters to transplanted organs

When an individual becomes infected with HIV, immune system functions are compromised, and the individual becomes more susceptible to a variety of infections. There is a chronic, persistent destruction of infection-fighting cells, the CD4+ cells, by the replication of HIV. The CD4+ cell is a type of T lymphocyte with CD4+ receptors on the cell surface, also called a *T helper cell*. Normally, when stimulated by a recognized antigen from a virus-infected cell, the CD4+ cell releases cytokines. This in turn activates B lymphocytes and killer T lymphocytes in an effort to destroy the invading organism. The HIV targets the CD4+ cell. The infected individual manifests various stages of HIV disease over the course of time. If the HIV infection is untreated, the individual eventually dies, usually from an **opportunistic infection (OI)**.

Viral Transmission, Acute Viral Infection, and Seroconversion

When a person is first infected with HIV, the virus causes an inflammatory reaction, bringing white blood cells and macrophages to the site of the inoculation with the virus. A virus particle attaches to specific receptors on the CD4+ cell, CD4+ receptors and co-receptors, and enters the cell. Once inside the cell, viral RNA is changed to viral DNA using the enzyme reverse transcriptase. The viral DNA is then integrated with the CD4+ lymphocyte cellular DNA in the nucleus of the lymphocyte. The HIV DNA is now in charge of cell reproduction and produces new viral proteins.

The viral proteins are assembled, and new HIV viruses are released, able to infect other CD4+ lymphocytes. The CD4+ lymphocyte is destroyed as the result of new viruses being produced (Fig. 22.1).

The result is a rapid decrease in the CD4+ lymphocyte count and a rapid increase in the **viral load**, the amount of HIV virus in the blood. During this time of acute viral infection, the individual may manifest symptoms of a flu-like viral illness: low-grade fever, generalized aches and pains, swollen lymph nodes, and generally feeling ill. After several weeks, the person's immune system develops antibodies to HIV, **seroconversion** occurs (the interval when HIV antibodies are first produced and rise to detectable levels), and the person tests positive for HIV.

Asymptomatic Chronic Infection

The immune system begins to exert control but is not able to eliminate viral replication. The CD4+ count increases to near normal, and the viral load drops to a set-point level. The **viral set point** occurs when viral replication is still taking place but the immune system is able to destroy the virus in equal amounts as is being produced. Over the years, the CD4+ count slowly falls, with the individual losing approximately 50 to 100 CD4+ cells per year, and the viral load slowly increases. This may take as long as 10 years.

Symptomatic Chronic Infection

As the HIV-infected individual's CD4+ count continues to fall, control over viral replication is slowly lost. The immune system becomes less able to fight off infections. Individuals begin to develop nonspecific symptoms, such as more frequent respiratory tract infections, skin problems, lymphadenopathy (enlarged lymph nodes), and weight loss. The CD4+ count falls more rapidly, and there is a rapid increase in viral replication. Once a person becomes symptomatic, the average time to the development of AIDS is 2 years.

Acquired Immune Deficiency Syndrome (AIDS)

As the CD4+ count continues to fall, the immune system is less and less able to fight off infections. Infections can use the "opportunity" of a nonfunctioning immune system to infect the body, or the immune system loses the ability to control infections that are in a dormant phase, allowing the infection to become reactivated. An HIV-infected individual has AIDS when the CD4+ count is less than 200 cells/μL or when he or she is diagnosed with one or more AIDS-defining illnesses.

Commonly occurring AIDS-defining illnesses in the United States are *Pneumocystis (carinii) jiroveci* pneumonia, *Mycobacterium avium* complex, toxoplasmosis, esophageal candidiasis, and recurrent bacterial pneumonia. Target organs for damage secondary to HIV are the kidneys, the peripheral and central nervous systems, and the cardiovascular system. The progression from viral transmission to AIDS is summarized in Box 22.1.

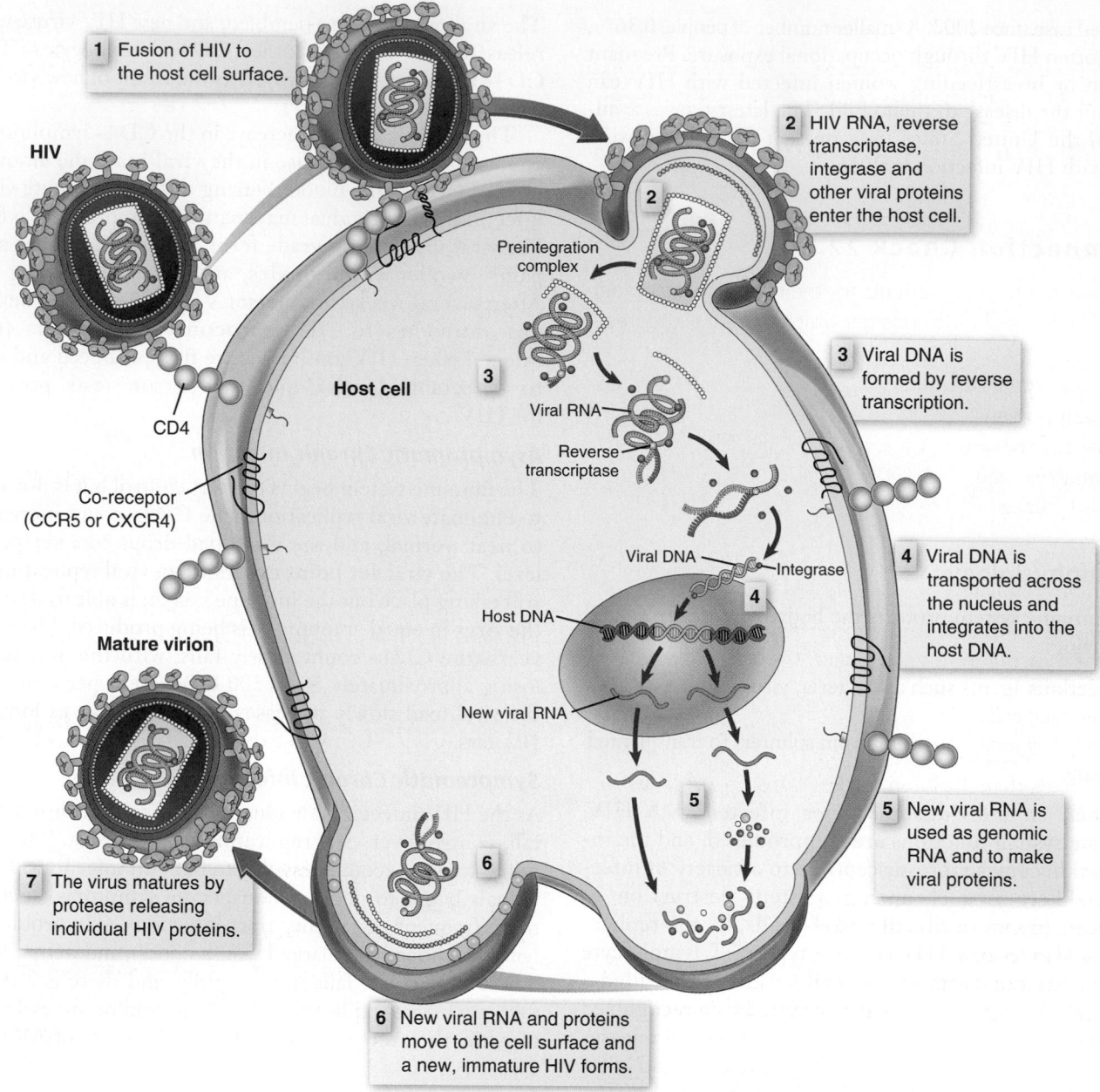

1 Fusion of HIV to the host cell surface.

HIV

CD4

Co-receptor (CCR5 or CXCR4)

Host cell

2 HIV RNA, reverse transcriptase, integrase and other viral proteins enter the host cell.

Preintegration complex

3

Viral RNA

Reverse transcriptase

3 Viral DNA is formed by reverse transcription.

Viral DNA — Integrase

Host DNA

4

4 Viral DNA is transported across the nucleus and integrates into the host DNA.

New viral RNA

5

5 New viral RNA is used as genomic RNA and to make viral proteins.

Mature virion

7 The virus matures by protease releasing individual HIV proteins.

6

6 New viral RNA and proteins move to the cell surface and a new, immature HIV forms.

FIGURE 22.1 HIV replication.

Box 22.1 Progression Through HIV/AIDS Stages

- Viral transmission
- Acute viral infection, 1 to 2 weeks
- Seroconversion
- Asymptomatic chronic infection, average = 3 to 10 years
- Symptomatic/AIDS, average = 2 years
- Death

Connection Check 22.2

Which of the following statements regarding viral replication is correct?

A. Endotoxin and/or exotoxin is required for viral proliferation.

B. The virus must use host white blood cells for viral proliferation.

C. Pathogenic replication is facilitated by the administration of antivirals.

D. The virus replicates by preventing phagocytosis by white blood cells.

Clinical Manifestations

Clinical manifestations observed in the patient with HIV/AIDS are most often related to impaired immune function and are typically a reflection of the OIs that occur as a result of HIV disease. The common signs and symptoms are:

- Fever
- Cough
- Weakness
- Nausea/vomiting
- Diarrhea
- Dysphagia, or difficulty swallowing
- Forgetfulness
- Skin lesions (Fig. 22.2)
- Shortness of breath, or dyspnea, on exertion
- Headache
- Vision changes
- Pain
- Night sweats
- Lymphadenopathy

Clinical manifestations indicating a deterioration in status requiring immediate attention by a healthcare provider are:

- New cough
- Increased fatigue
- Fever less than 97°F (36°C) or greater than 102°F (39°C)
- Night sweats
- New onset of headache
- New onset of visual blurring
- Recent change in mental status
- New skin lesions
- New onset of diarrhea
- Weight loss greater than 10% of previously recorded weight

See Table 22.2 for a list of the common clinical manifestations and their probable causes.

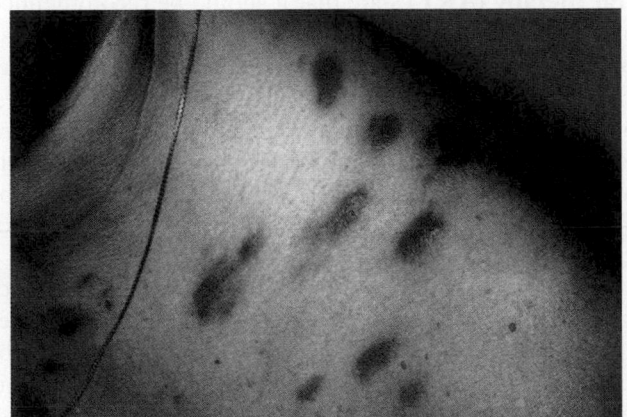

FIGURE 22.2 Kaposi's sarcoma lesions.

Table 22.2 Clinical Manifestations of HIV and Probable Cause

Clinical Manifestation	Probable Cause
Weight loss	Worsening disease
Fever	Infection
Night sweats	Mycobacterial infection
Cough	Pneumonia, tuberculosis
Dyspnea on exertion but not at rest	*Pneumocystis carinii* pneumonia
Unable to do usual activities	Neurological infections, anemia
Severe headache	Meningitis
Pain when swallowing	Oral or esophageal candidiasis, aphthous ulcers
Mental status changes	Central nervous system infection/tumor
Fatigue	Anemia, infection

CASE STUDY: EPISODE 2

Vital signs for Ms. Castillo are:

Temperature: 98°F (36.8°C)

Pulse: 104 bpm

Blood pressure: 100/50 mm Hg

Respirations: 28

Pulse oximetry: 92% on room air

She is put on 2 liters of oxygen via a nasal cannula. A peripheral IV is started, blood is drawn for a complete blood count and metabolic profile, and she is started on 0.9 normal saline 100 mL/hr...

Management

Medical Management

Diagnostic Testing

Diagnostic or screening tests assess for antibodies to the HIV virus. Rapid tests or point-of-care tests utilizing blood or oral fluids can be used in settings where a quick answer for the presence or absence of HIV antibodies is required, such as in health screening, occupational exposure, or labor and delivery. Rapid tests do not require a laboratory to perform the test. The results from the rapid tests are available in 5 to 30 minutes depending on the test used. Point-of-care positive tests are confirmed by an HIV-1/2 antibody assay performed by a laboratory.

A negative screening test does not require confirmation but should be repeated in 3 to 6 months, allowing time for antibodies to develop and be detected if they are present. HIV infection can also be confirmed by the presence of the HIV virus in the blood, the viral load. Although not contraindicated in adults, the viral load is most often used to confirm the presence of HIV infection in infants less than 12 months of age.

Although common comorbidities are not diagnostic of HIV, newly diagnosed HIV+ individuals are screened for these conditions. The common comorbidities are chronic hepatitis B and/or C. If there is a decrease in CD4+ count to less than 200 cells/µL, individuals testing positive for HIV are also screened for the presence of antibodies that could indicate a higher risk of developing certain OIs. These OIs include toxoplasmosis, TB, and syphilis. In addition, testing is done for anemia, kidney disease, liver disease, diabetes mellitus, and cholesterol. HIV+ women are screened for cervical cancer.

At the time of diagnosis, the patient's viral load and CD4+ count are obtained. The CD4+ count is obtained routinely every 3 to 6 months for the first 2 years on therapy and then every year. The viral load is also obtained every 3 months for the first 2 years on therapy for adherent patients, then is obtained every 6 to 12 months. Viral load is used as the primary indicator of treatment success or failure, but it is not recommended as an indicator for hospitalized patients. The viral load can be affected by other viral illnesses, resulting in a falsely high level. In U.S. cities with a high prevalence of HIV infection, newly infected individuals may be infected with a medication-resistant virus. A genotype assay, which determines changes in the viral gene sequence that make the virus resistant to antiretroviral therapy (ART) medications, is part of the initial evaluation. A genotype assay of viral tropism, a test to determine if there is a CCR5 coreceptor on the CD4+ cells, may also be done to help determine the cause of treatment failure and assist in the selection of ART.

Ongoing screening for TB should be routinely done every 6 months. In a person with a history of a positive purified protein derivative (PPD), an interferon gamma release assay (IGRA) such as the blood test QuantiFERON-TB Gold can be used to screen for TB. A positive test requires further evaluation for a current TB infection.

Connection Check 22.3

A nurse is caring for a patient in the emergency department. The patient asks for an HIV test. The nurse explains that a screening test can provide quick results and determine whether more testing is necessary. That test is a(n)

A. CD4+ count.
B. ELISA.
C. rapid test.
D. viral load.

Medications

Prophylaxis

If an HIV+ individual has a CD4+ count of 200 cells/µL or less, prophylaxis to reduce the risk of OIs, such as toxoplasmosis and PCP, is initiated prior to starting antiretrovirals. Individuals with a CD4+ count of 50 cells/µL or less are at risk for *M. avium* complex, a disseminated infection affecting multiple organs. As the immune system reconstitutes, patients will have a lower risk of developing opportunistic infections, and prophylaxis can be discontinued. Specifically, prophylaxis for toxoplasmosis and PCP can be discontinued in individuals when their CD4+ count has been greater than 200 cells/µL for at least 3 months. Prophylaxis for *M. avium* complex can be discontinued when the CD4+ count is greater than 100 cells/µL for 3 months.

> **⚠ Safety Alert** Individuals who have an allergic reaction to the sulfa component in Bactrim, a medication that is used for prophylaxis, may have a delayed manifestation of their allergy. The rash associated with an allergic reaction to Bactrim may not occur for 7 to 14 days after starting the medication. When assessing the patient who presents with a new rash, the nurse should ask about starting Bactrim within the past 2 weeks.
>
> The sudden onset of anemia in an individual who has recently started Bactrim may be a sign of another serious manifestation of an adverse reaction to the sulfa component. Hemolytic anemia caused by glucose-6-phosphate dehydrogenase (G6PD) deficiency (an enzyme that supports the functions of red blood cells) can be precipitated by an allergic reaction to sulfa. This is more common in African Americans.

Antiretroviral Therapy (ART)

Current Department of Health and Human Services (DHHS) 2017 recommendations for initiating **antiretroviral therapy (ART)** state that it should be recommended to all HIV+ individuals. Antiretrovirals interfere with the ability of HIV to reproduce itself (Fig. 22.3). Six classes of medications are currently available in the United States. Individuals are prescribed a minimum of three medications from at least two different classes. Most individuals are able to take a combination medication, one pill that contains three medications. The classes and their mechanism of action are described in Table 22.3.

Prior to the initiation of ART, hepatic and renal functions are evaluated. Significant physiological abnormalities influence the medication choice because medication metabolism takes place in the liver and kidneys. Once ART is begun, the CD4+ count will increase, and the HIV viral load will decrease to nondetectable levels. This is generally achieved in 6 to 8 weeks. The CD4+ counts and viral loads

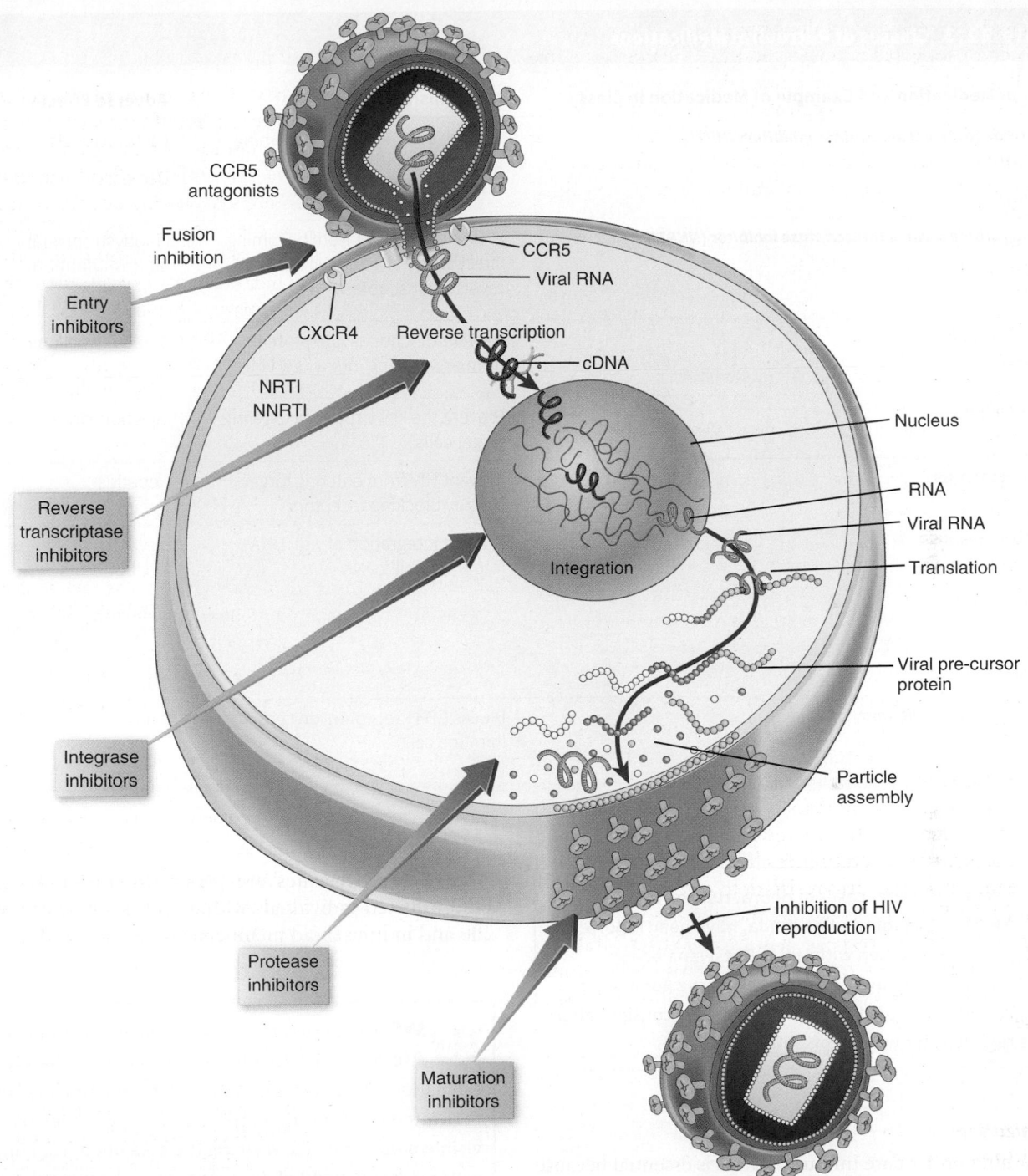

FIGURE 22.3 Targets for antiretroviral therapy (ART).

are followed at regular intervals, as recommended in the DHHS guidelines. For stable patients, the viral load may be obtained every 6 months and the CD4+ count yearly. Adherence to therapy is evaluated at each encounter to maintain a 95% adherence rate. One of the earliest signs of treatment failure is missing doses of medication or missing scheduled appointments.

Starting antiretrovirals is rarely an emergency. Critical to starting is a commitment to 100% adherence to therapy for a lifetime to reduce the possibility of viral resistance developing to therapy. Treatment preparation prior to starting

therapy is critical to success. Treatment preparation includes explaining:

- The advantages and disadvantages of therapy
- That taking ART is a lifetime commitment
- Why a certain medication combination was selected for that individual
- How and when to take the medications
- Side effects of the medications
- How to reduce potential side effects
- The effect of the medications on the immune system

Table 22.3 Classes of Retroviral Medications

Class of Medication and Example of Medication in Class	Mechanism of Action	Adverse Effects
Nucleoside reverse transcriptase inhibitors (NRTI) *Tenofovir* *Abacavir*	Prevent viral RNA from becoming viral DNA by inhibiting the enzyme reverse transcriptase	Lactic acidosis Decrease in bone density
Non-nucleoside reverse transcriptase inhibitor (NNRTI) *Etravirine*	Prevents viral RNA from becoming viral DNA by altering the enzyme reverse transcriptase	Lipodystrophy (abnormal fat redistribution)
Protease inhibitors *Darunavir*	Prevent functional viral proteins from assembling into a new virus	Diabetes mellitus Hyperlipidemia
Fusion inhibitors *Enfuvirtide*	Prevent the HIV virus from entering target cells	Injection-site reaction
CCR5 antagonists *Maraviroc*	Prevent HIV from entering target cells by blocking receptors	Hepatitis
Integrase inhibitors *Raltegravir* *Dolutegravir*	Prevent integration of viral DNA into the T cell's DNA	Elevated amylase or liver function tests Dolutegravir may increase the incidence of neural tube defects in the fetus.
Post-attachment inhibitors *Ibalizumab*	Blocks CD4+ receptors on certain immune cells	Diarrhea Rash

> **Safety Alert** Several cases of neural tube birth defects, including spina bifida, have been reported in babies born to women with HIV in Botswana being treated with dolutegravir. The Food and Drug Administration (FDA) recommends that clinicians should consider alternative regimens for women of childbearing age.

Immunizations

Maintaining up-to-date immunizations is essential because HIV+ individuals are more at risk for infections owing to their compromised immune systems. HIV+ patients with a CD4+ count of 200 cells/µL or greater should receive Pneumovax every 5 years to reduce the risk of pneumococcal pneumonia. PCV13 (Prevnar) should be given once. The influenza vaccine should be offered yearly, and patients are encouraged to receive it early in the season so that they can develop antibodies. The diphtheria, pertussis, and tetanus vaccine should be given every 10 years. The herpes zoster live-attenuated vaccine (ZVL) is recommended at age 60 for individuals with a CD4+ count of greater than 200.

Live-virus vaccines are generally contraindicated in HIV-infected individuals with a CD4+ count of less than 200 and in household members.

> **Safety Alert** Occupational exposure to blood or bodily fluids should be reported immediately. If the patient's HIV status is unknown, permission may be requested to do the appropriate screening. If there is visible blood or fluids, washing the area under running water is recommended. Do not squeeze the injured area because that may increase the possibility of infection. An HIV test to ascertain seropositivity is offered. If positive, a referral for care is initiated. If negative, antiretroviral medications are prescribed. The exact medications depend on the risk of the exposure and the patient's HIV treatment status if HIV+. Generally, two or three medications are prescribed to be taken for 28 days. HIV testing is done at 6 weeks, 12 weeks, and 4 to 6 months after exposure. Nursing mothers are encouraged to stop breastfeeding.

Connection Check 22.4

The nurse understands that which of the following are correct statements about HIV disease? *(Select all that apply.)*

A. HIV disease progresses in stages; HIV disease is diagnosed by determining viral load.

B. A CD4+ count of 500 cells/μL or more indicates HIV, not AIDS.

C. The Western blot test is diagnostic for HIV disease.

D. A CD4+ count of 200 cells/μL or less increases the chances for opportunistic infections.

E. ART is started immediately after diagnosis if the CD4+ count is less than 200 cells/μL.

Prevention

Prevention is a critical component of HIV care. Inadequate testing and compliance with the treatment plan or remaining in care remain barriers to the prevention of the initial HIV infection or progression through the continuum to AIDS. The HIV care continuum, or cascade of care, is used to estimate the percentage of HIV-infected individuals in each step of care from the acquisition of an HIV infection through engagement in care, including receiving ART and achievement of complete viral suppression. Approximately 85% of HIV+ individuals know their status, and only about 25% of HIV-infected individuals have a nondetectable viral load, potentially indicating patients not remaining in care.

A critical part of prevention is testing for HIV. Current recommendations state that all providers should offer routine opt-out screening for all individuals between the ages of 15 and 65. In HIV-negative individuals, yearly testing is recommended for those at high risk. *High risk* is defined as being in a community with an HIV prevalence of greater than 1%. Examples of high-risk communities include sexually transmitted infection clinic attendees and incarcerated individuals.

Antiretroviral therapy for HIV+ individuals is a cornerstone of prevention of the spread of the disease. When HIV+ individuals have a nondetectable HIV viral load, the risk of transmitting HIV to an HIV-negative partner is less than 3%. Another cornerstone of prevention is Truvada, a combination of the medications tenofovir and emtricitabine, also referred to as *preexposure prophylaxis* (PrEP). This medication has been approved for daily use to reduce the risk of acquiring HIV. Guidelines from the U.S. Public Health Service recommend its use by HIV-negative individuals who are part of an HIV **serodiscordant** couple (one partner is HIV positive, and one partner is HIV negative) and by those who engage in risky behaviors. Follow-up with a health-care provider every 3 months to assess medication adherence and provide reinforcement for additional risk-reduction behaviors is highly recommended. Prior to initiation of PrEP, acute and chronic hepatitis B must be ruled out (see Evidence-Based Practice).

Evidence-Based Practice

Preexposure Prophylaxis

Preexposure prophylaxis (PrEP) with Truvada is taken prior to exposure to reduce the likelihood of infection with HIV from an HIV+ partner. Except for the HIV-negative partner in long-term serodiscordant couples, PrEP is controversial because of the lifestyles associated with the practice of high-risk behaviors. It is well documented that exposure to blood and body fluids is the mode of transmission for HIV and that the risk of transmission is related to the viral load of the HIV+ individual. When taken with greater than 95% adherence, antiretroviral therapy reduces the HIV viral load to nondetectable levels in most persons. This reduces the risk of transmission to HIV-negative partners. However, only 25% of individuals infected with HIV in the United States have a nondetectable viral load.

A Cochrane Database systematic review of six clinical trials in both the United States and sub-Saharan Africa found that both the HIV-negative partner in serodiscordant couples and those individuals who practiced high-risk behaviors (such as commercial sex workers, sexually active young adults engaging in casual sex, men who have sex with men, and IV drug users) who were treated with daily Truvada showed significantly fewer new infections with HIV than those in the placebo groups. Efficacy ranged from 44% to 75% and was related to adherence in taking the medication. In one study of heterosexual women in sub-Saharan Africa, there was no significant difference in new HIV infections between the placebo and control groups. Adherence to the medication was low.

The availability of PrEP is not well known outside of individuals who have participated in clinical trials. When the availability and efficacy of treatment were made known to individuals practicing high-risk behaviors, more than 50% were interested in participating, provided the medication could be obtained at low or no cost.

Public health concerns include the cost of PrEP for a large number of individuals and the possibility of decreasing adherence over time. Another concern is the probability of the individual developing medication resistance to Truvada if he or she contracts HIV because Truvada alone has not been shown to suppress viral load.

Individuals who are at risk for HIV and are interested in taking PrEP need accessible and acceptable therapy. They need to understand the medical and social benefits of PrEP in order to make an informed decision. Other risk-reduction behaviors, such as the use of condoms in all sexual encounters, must be incorporated into the individual's treatment plan.

Balthazar, C., & Harris, L. A. (2014). A community perspective on PrEP [Abstract 63]. *Topics in Antiviral Medicine, 22*(e-1), 32.

Corneli, A. L., McKenna, K., Perry, B., Ahmed, K., Agot, K., Malamatsho, F., . . . Van Damme, L. (2014). FEM-PrEP: Participant explanations for non-adherence [Abstract 959LB]. *Topics in Antiviral Medicine, 22*(e-1), 503.

Hosek, S., Martinez, J., Santos, K., Mehrotra, M., Balthazar, C., Serrano, P., . . . Grant, R. (2014.) PrEP interest, uptake, and adherence among young men who have sex with men (YMSM) in the United States [Abstract 951]. *Topics in Antiviral Medicine, 22*(e-1), 498–499.

Kuo, I., Phillips, G., III, Magnus, M., Opoku, J., Rawls, A., Peterson, J., . . . Greenberg, A. (2014). Willingness to use pre-exposure prophylaxis among community-recruited injection drug users. *Topics in Antiviral Medicine, 22*(e-1), 501.

Okwundu, C. I., Uthman, O. A., & Okoromah, C. A. N. (2012). Antiretroviral pre-exposure prophylaxis (PrEP) for preventing HIV in high-risk individuals. *Cochrane Database of Systematic Reviews, 7*. doi:10.1002/14651858. CD007189.pub3

U.S. Public Health Service. (2014). *Preexposure prophylaxis for the prevention of HIV infection in the United States—2014: A clinical practice guideline.* Retrieved from http://www.cdc.gov/hiv/pdf/guidelines/ PrEPguidelines2014.pdf

Connection Check 22.5

A patient states that she has recently been treated for gonorrhea. Her last HIV test was 18 months ago. When you review the orders, you notice that an HIV test has been ordered. What do you do?

A. Explain that the test has been ordered and that she can opt out.

B. No discussion is necessary; just do the test.

C. Obtain her written consent for the test.

D. Provide pretest counseling before getting consent.

Complications

Complications of HIV disease are related to the decrease in immune function and consist of opportunistic infections and malignancies. When the CD4+ count is greater than 500 cells/μL, the individual often has no signs or symptoms related to HIV infection, although women may have an increased incidence of vaginal candidiasis unrelated to antibiotic use or diabetes. When the CD4+ count is between 500 and 350 cells/μL, individuals may have increased respiratory illnesses or dermatological manifestations such as herpes zoster. As the CD4+ count falls to between 350 and 200 cells/μL, the individual may notice an increase in infections mediated by the adaptive immune system and may develop symptoms of fever, fatigue, or severe bacterial infections. As the CD4+ cells continue to fall to below 200 cells/μL, the individual is considered to have AIDS. Individuals with AIDS are likely to develop specific OIs that are new infections or reactivations of dormant infections.

Examples of OIs associated with AIDS are PCP, cryptococcal meningitis, cryptosporidiosis *Candida* esophagitis, toxoplasmosis, cytomegalovirus (CMV), *M. avium-intracellulare* (MAC), and progressive multifocal leukoencephalopathy (PML) infections (Fig. 22.4).

Another complication of HIV disease is **immune reconstruction inflammatory syndrome (IRIS)**. This syndrome occurs as the CD4+ count increases and the immune system is able to respond to the presence of previously acquired OIs, such as cryptococcal meningitis. Paradoxically, the response is an overwhelming inflammatory response, making the symptoms of the infection worse.

Nursing Management

Assessment and Analysis

As stated earlier, clinical manifestations are most often a reflection of the OIs associated with HIV, such as frequent respiratory illnesses, pneumonia, meningitis, or *Candida* esophagitis. Common signs and symptoms are:

- Fever
- Cough
- Weakness
- Nausea/vomiting
- Diarrhea
- Dysphagia, or difficulty swallowing
- Forgetfulness
- Skin lesions
- Shortness of breath, or dyspnea, on exertion
- Headache
- Vision changes
- Pain
- Night sweats
- Lymphadenopathy

Nursing Diagnoses

- **Risk for infection** related to decreased immune function
- **Imbalanced nutrition**; less than body requirements
- **Risk for fluid volume deficit** related to gastrointestinal manifestations
- **Anxiety** related to disease diagnosis or progression of the disease
- **Knowledge deficit** related to self-care and the disease process

Nursing Interventions

◼ *Assessments*

- Temperature, pulse, respirations, oxygen saturation
  Fever is often the first indicator of an infection. In individuals with low CD4+ lymphocytes, there is an inability to release pyrogens, resulting in a low-grade fever even in the face of a significant infection. A drop in body temperature in the presence of infection is a sign of compensatory failure. An indirect measure of fever is an increase in the pulse rate above baseline. The respiratory rate may also increase in an effort to reduce the core body temperature.

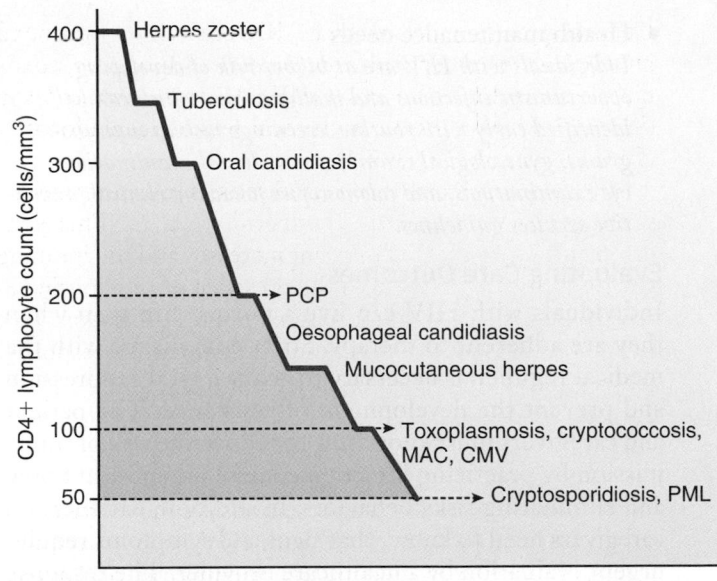

FIGURE 22.4 Association between opportunistic infections and CD4+ count.

Hypoxemia, or decreased oxygen-carrying capacity, may occur as a result of a decreased number of functional alveoli secondary to a respiratory infection such as PCP or from anemia secondary to a side effect of medication or pancytopenia from the invasion of the bone marrow by HIV.

- Weight trends
  Weight loss results from caloric expenditure exceeding caloric intake and can affect cellular metabolism. Weight loss of 10% or more can indicate worsening disease, treatment failure if the patient is on ART, or depression. It can lead to decreased albumin levels, impairing medication transport and utilization.

- CD4+ count
  There is a correlation between CD4+ count and the risk of developing certain OIs. The lower the CD4+ count, the more suppressed the individual's immune system is. Individuals with a low CD4+ count are more likely to have serious complications of HIV and non–HIV-related infections and a potentially blunted response to therapy.

- Viral load
  The viral load reflects the amount of viral replication. Viral load is an indicator of disease progression; the higher the viral load, the more quickly the disease progresses from HIV infection to AIDS.

- Adherence to ART
  An adherence rate of 95% or greater is essential to achieve viral suppression and prevent the development of resistance to one or more ART medications. If an individual misses one dose of even one medication during a day, the adherence rate for that day is 0%.

- TB status
  Although the incidence of TB has decreased overall, there has been an increase in TB in HIV-infected individuals, probably related to reactivation of a prior exposure.

- Immunization status
  Immunocompromised individuals should maintain up-to-date immunization status. They should not receive live-virus vaccines because of the risk of developing the disease. Immunizations in individuals with a CD4+ count less than 200 cells/μL may not be as effective because of the compromised ability to produce antibodies in response to the immunization.

- Depression
  HIV is often a stigmatizing illness requiring the infected individual, family members, and friends to confront behaviors or lifestyles that put the infected individual at risk for contracting the disease. Stigma may put distance between the HIV-infected individual and his or her support system.

■ Actions

- Utilize universal precautions consistently.
  Universal precautions are designed to prevent the spread of infections between individuals. In addition to HAND WASHING for a minimum of 15 to 30 seconds, which is the MOST IMPORTANT precaution, personal protective equipment may be required. The selection of personal protective equipment, such as gloves, goggles, and gowns, is related to the risk of exposure.

- Administer ART as prescribed and on time.
  Maintaining medication levels is critical to preventing medication resistance. Several medications that are commonly used have low resistance thresholds when subtherapeutic levels are present. Administering doses more than 1 or 2 hours after the usual time can increase the risk of the development of viral resistance.

- Provide nutritionally dense foods and small, frequent meals.
  Anorexia, nausea, and vomiting are commonly seen in individuals with HIV/AIDS as a result of medications or HIV infection. Persistent anorexia, nausea, or vomiting

can lead to dehydration, weight loss, and electrolyte imbalances. Small, frequent meals/snacks, incorporating foods such as nuts or nutritional supplements, will increase caloric intake and provide protein and essential micronutrients.

- Provide emotional support.
Complex emotional issues, such as sexuality, shame, and anger, may be associated with HIV/AIDS. Listening and being nonjudgmental can assist the patient in developing effective coping behaviors. Referral to a mental health professional may be needed. The focus is on living with HIV, not dying with HIV.

- Refer for social services evaluation.
Many patients need assistance with the cost of HIV medications, which can cost more than $12,000 a year and up. Individuals may be eligible for other programs and support services available through community organizations and the local, state, or federal government.

■ *Teaching*

- Avoidance of high-risk behaviors that increase the risk of transmission
Consistent use of condoms with every sexual encounter and avoiding the use of street drugs or alcohol or other situations that might impair judgment reduce the risk of transmitting HIV. These behaviors also reduce the risk of reinfection with a medication-resistant or more virulent strain of HIV.

- Adherence to treatment regimen
Adherence is essential in managing the progression of the disease. Taking medications as ordered and at the same time each day (plan administration times around activities of daily living) helps maintain therapeutic medication levels and decreases the risk of viral resistance developing. Understanding the name, purpose, and dosage of the medication and how to take the medication, potential side effects, and how to manage them contribute to maintaining greater than 95% adherence.

- Implementing infection-control precautions at home
Fear of transmission to other household members is a cause of stigma. Discussing specific methods of infection control will result in less stigma and enhance the protection of others from infection. Blood spills should be cleaned with a bleach solution. Avoid raw or undercooked eggs, meat, poultry, or fish to reduce the risk of diarrheal illnesses. Animal excrement should be taken care of by a non–HIV-infected, nonpregnant individual to avoid exposure to toxoplasmosis and other animal-borne illnesses.

- Signs and symptoms to report to the healthcare provider urgently
Early evaluation and intervention can reduce the morbidity and mortality associated with opportunistic infections or side effects of medications. Explain how to utilize a self-care symptom management manual.

- Health maintenance needs
Individuals with HIV are at higher risk of developing opportunistic infections and malignancies, which can be identified early with routine screenings such as mammograms, gynecological examinations, dental examinations, eye examinations, and colonoscopies following clinical preventive services guidelines.

Evaluating Care Outcomes

Individuals with HIV can live a normal life span when they are adherent to therapy. Strict compliance with the medical regimen is necessary to achieve viral suppression and prevent the development of resistance. The patient and caregivers must know how to reduce the risk of transmission by practicing infection control practices at home and eliminating risky behaviors. In addition, patients and caregivers need to know what signs and symptoms require urgent evaluation by a healthcare provider. The response to ART is determined by measuring the CD4+ count and the viral load. Within 6 to 8 weeks of therapy initiation, there is an increase in the CD4+ count and a decrease in the viral load. Over several months following the initiation of therapy, the viral load should reach nondetectable levels.

Transitional Care

HIV/AIDS has evolved into a chronic condition, with individuals experiencing symptoms related to aging, treatment side effects, and the disease process associated with HIV. In addition, those patients who are diagnosed late in the disease process may not recover immune function and are more likely to have disease-related symptoms, even with treatment. There is a need for palliative care for better symptom management. This should be incorporated into patient care from the time of diagnosis to death. Introducing the concept of palliative care as one intervention to improve quality of life is critical and, over time, may lead to other discussions, such as advanced directives and the need for hospice care.

Connection Check 22.6

A patient newly diagnosed with HIV asks about community support groups. What should the nurse do?

A. Contact psychiatry for an evaluation for depression.
B. Provide a list of groups in a neighboring community.
C. Request a referral to the social work department.
D. Suggest the patient contact the physician.

Finding Connections

CASE STUDY: WRAP-UP

Initial diagnostic results for Ms. Castillo are "confirmed HIV+": low white blood cell count, CD4+ count of 125 cells/μL, mild anemia, and normal renal and liver functions. She is experiencing symptoms of PCP. The common symptoms are a dry, persistent cough and mild shortness of breath with activity that occurs over several weeks. Patients often experience weight loss, fatigue, a low-grade fever, and hypoxia. Her healthcare provider orders PML *Cryptosporidiosis* antibiotic prophylaxis to treat her PCP. Consideration is given to preparing her to start ART.

Case Study Questions

1. Ms. Castillo is briefly admitted to the hospital for an evaluation. The charge nurse is reviewing her orders. It is a priority for the charge nurse to follow up with the provider about which order?
   A. Stopping antibiotic prophylaxis
   B. CD4+ count in the morning
   C. Applying PPD
   D. Dietary referral

2. The nurse caring for Ms. Castillo incorporates which nursing diagnosis into the plan of care?
   A. Imbalanced nutrition; more than body requirements
   B. Ineffective denial related to refusal to acknowledge diagnosis
   C. Risk for infection
   D. Risk for other-directed violence

3. When the nurse teaches Ms. Castillo about the ART she will soon start, which of the following will be helpful in increasing patient adherence?
   A. Centering medication taking on a daily activity
   B. Direct observation for negative side effects
   C. Increased frequency of medication administration
   D. Using multiple medications whenever possible

4. Which of the following would you include in your teaching plan for Ms. Castillo?
   A. Decreasing risky behaviors
   B. Emphasizing exploration of experimental treatments
   C. Implementing universal precautions at home
   D. Evaluating measures to decrease exposure to others

5. Which statement by Ms. Castillo indicates that teaching has been effective?
   A. "Anyone who touches me needs to wear gloves."
   B. "I can use alcohol in moderation with my medications."
   C. "I can take my medications late if I am out for the day."
   D. "I need to use condoms with every sexual encounter."

CHAPTER SUMMARY

When an individual becomes infected with HIV, immune system functions are compromised, and the individual becomes more susceptible to a variety of infections because of the chronic, persistent destruction of infection-fighting cells, the CD4+ cells, by the replication of HIV. The CD4+ cell is a type of T lymphocyte with a CD4+ receptor on the cell surface: a T helper cell. When stimulated by a recognized antigen from a virus-infected cell, cytokines are released. This in turn activates B lymphocytes and killer T lymphocytes. The HIV virus targets the CD4+ cell.

Approximately 1.7 million people are newly infected with HIV yearly. HIV disease is most commonly a sexually transmitted disease, although a significant number of individuals contract the disease via IV drug use. African Americans now have the highest new infection rate (45%), followed by Latinos (17%).

The individual manifests various stages of HIV disease over the course of time. If the HIV infection is untreated, the individual eventually dies, usually from an opportunistic infection (OI). Individuals infected with HIV are categorized into one of four mutually exclusive, hierarchical groups according to the presence or absence of signs or symptoms commonly associated with AIDS. This is the first recognition of the continuum of HIV/AIDS as a disease that progresses through stages from acute HIV infection, asymptomatic HIV infection, and symptomatic HIV infection to the most advanced stage, AIDS. Clinical manifestations are typically a reflection of the OIs that occur as a result of HIV disease. *P. carinii* pneumonia is the most common OI seen in HIV+ individuals.

Diagnostic or screening tests assess for antibodies to the HIV virus. Rapid tests utilizing blood or oral fluids can be used in settings where a quick answer for the presence or absence of HIV antibodies is necessary. A negative screening test does not require confirmation. A positive screening test requires confirmation by additional laboratory testing.

Medication therapy for an HIV+ individual who has a CD4+ count of 200 cells/μL or less starts with prophylaxis to reduce the risk of OIs and is initiated prior to starting antiretroviral therapy (ART). Antiretrovirals interfere with the ability of HIV to reproduce itself. Everyone infected with HIV should start ART as soon as possible after diagnosis.

Nursing management includes comprehensive assessment to assess response to therapy and the presence of OIs. Teaching is extremely important to help the patient understand the necessity of compliance with the medication regimen and the importance of avoidance of risky behaviors.

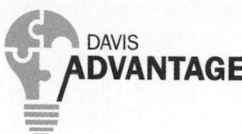

To explore learning resources for this chapter, go to **Davis Advantage** and find:
- Answers to in-text questions
- Chapter Resources and Activities
- NCLEX®-Style Chapter Review Questions
- Bibliography

Unit V

Promoting Health in Patients With Oxygenation Disorders

Chapter 23

Assessment of Respiratory Function

Megan Lynn

Finding Connections

CASE STUDY: EPISODE 1

Follow this patient throughout the chapter.

Mr. Larry Thomas is a 66-year-old male complaining of shortness of breath for the past 2 weeks. He has come to his provider's office for evaluation of his symptoms.

History of Present Illness:

Mr. Thomas reports chest pain that increases with coughing. He reports thick green/yellow sputum for the past week. His current weight is stable at 100 kg from his previous visit 6 months ago. He admits to occasionally smoking cigarettes...

INTRODUCTION

The respiratory system is a complex system that is divided into the upper and lower respiratory tracts. Air enters the respiratory system through the nose or mouth and travels to the lungs, where **respiration**; the exchange of oxygen and carbon dioxide between the outside air and the lungs occurs at the alveoli level. The major function of the respiratory system is to supply oxygen to and remove carbon dioxide from the body. Because of the complexity of the respiratory system, a thorough assessment should be completed by the nurse, including inspection, auscultation, percussion, and palpation to identify dysfunction. This chapter discusses the anatomy, physiology, assessment steps, and diagnostic tests specific to the respiratory system.

OVERVIEW OF ANATOMY AND PHYSIOLOGY

Functions of the Respiratory System

The major functions of the respiratory system are to perform the functions of **ventilation** and respiration. Ventilation occurs as air moves into and out of the respiratory system through the process of inspiration and exhalation. During ventilation, the structures of the respiratory system filter and humidify the air entering the system. The process of respiration occurs as oxygen and carbon dioxide are exchanged at the level of the alveoli. After respiration occurs, the circulatory system is responsible for transporting the oxygenated blood to the tissues of the body. This movement of oxygenated blood into the tissues is known as *perfusion*. The circulatory system provides the body with oxygenated blood and then returns deoxygenated blood back to the lungs to allow for re-oxygenation through the process of respiration. In addition to the processes of respiration and ventilation, the respiratory system is responsible for the following:

- *Acid-base balance*: The exchange of carbon dioxide for oxygen in the lungs and the renal secretion of bicarbonate maintain the body's pH between 7.35 and 7.45. If carbon dioxide levels rise within the body, this results in a decrease in the pH level: acidosis. If carbon dioxide levels decrease, this results in an increase in the pH level: alkalosis.
- *Speech*: The movement of air through the vocal cords allows vocalization of words.
- *Sense of smell*: The movement of air through the nose allows an individual to smell odors in the environment.
- *Fluid balance*: Water is excreted as water vapor through the exhalation process. This helps to maintain the body's fluid balance.

Connection Check 23.1

Which of the following is *not* a function of the respiratory system?
A. Acid-base balance
B. Temperature regulation
C. Fluid balance
D. Tissue perfusion

Anatomy of the Respiratory System

The easiest way to understand the structures of the respiratory system is to follow the path of air through the system. Air travels through the upper respiratory system to the lower respiratory system. The upper respiratory system consists of the nose, mouth, sinuses, pharynx (throat), and larynx. The lower respiratory system consists of the trachea and lungs. Figure 23.1 displays the major structures of the respiratory system.

Oxygen enters the respiratory system through the nose or mouth. The nose consists of two nares that are separated by a septum. The interior of each naris is lined with hair, which acts as a filter to prevent the entrance of microorganisms and/or foreign particulates into the respiratory system. Once oxygen passes through the nares, it encounters the three turbinates located within the nasal cavity. The turbinates are made of bone and are covered with cilia. Turbinates filter the air, and any foreign matter is filtered out through the cilia. In addition to filtering the air entering the nostril, turbinates are responsible for humidifying and warming the air. Around the nose are the paranasal sinuses—the ethmoid, frontal, sphenoid, and maxillary sinuses, named for the bones in which they are located. The sinuses are empty, air-filled cavities that humidify and warm inspired air; absorb shock, providing protection from facial trauma; provide voice resonance; and decrease the weight of the skull (Fig. 23.2).

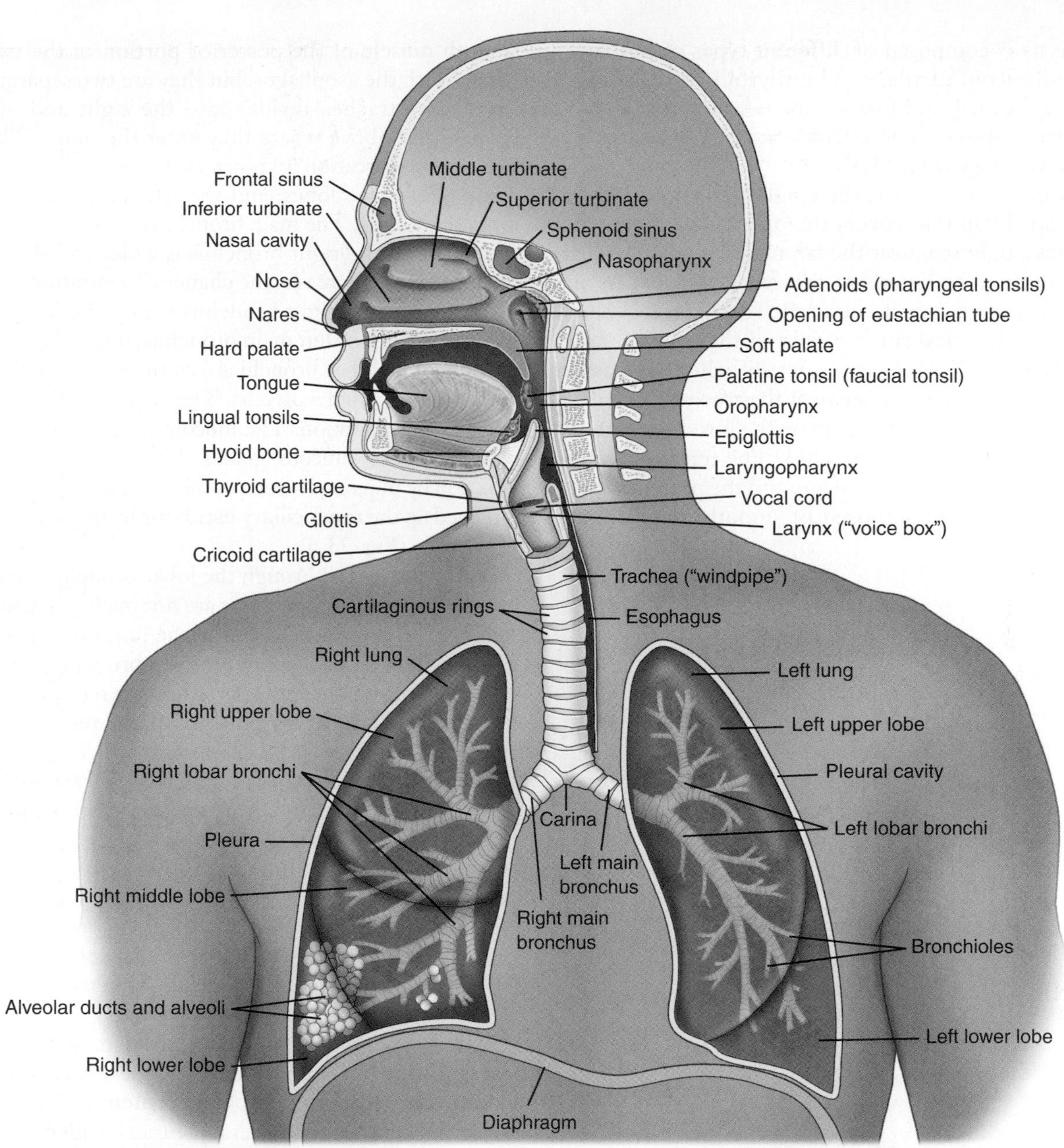

FIGURE 23.1 Major structures of the upper and lower respiratory system.

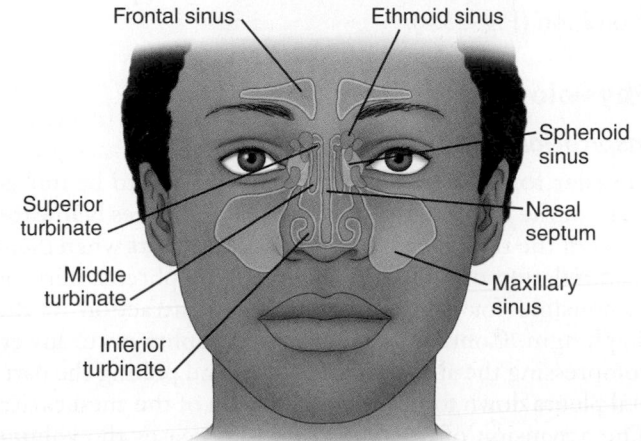

FIGURE 23.2 Frontal, ethmoid, and sphenoid sinuses: superior, middle, and inferior turbinates.

Once the air passes through the turbinates, it enters the pharynx. The pharynx is divided into the nasopharynx, oropharynx, and laryngopharynx. The area behind the nose is a mucous membrane called the *nasopharynx*. The ends of the eustachian tubes are located in the nasopharynx and connect the nasopharynx to the middle ear. Below the eustachian tubes are the adenoids. The adenoids filter out any foreign objects or microorganisms.

Once air passes the soft palate at the back of the mouth, it enters the oropharynx. The oropharynx is the mucous membrane located directly behind the mouth. Within the oropharynx are the palatine tonsils. The palatine tonsils, like the adenoids, are responsible for filtering out any foreign objects or microorganisms. Once the air moves past the oropharynx, it moves into the laryngopharynx. The laryngopharynx starts at the base of the tongue and continues to the larynx.

The larynx is composed of different types of cartilage: thyroid and cricoid cartilage. The thyroid cartilage protrudes from the neck and forms what is commonly known as the "Adam's apple." The cricoid cartilage is just below the thyroid cartilage (Fig. 23.3).

At the top of the larynx is the epiglottis. The epiglottis is a leaf-shaped flap that covers the opening of the larynx and provides a tight seal over the larynx when an individual is swallowing food or liquids to prevent aspiration. As air moves past the epiglottis, it enters the vocal cords, located in the larynx. The vocal cords consist of the true and false vocal cords (Fig. 23.4). Speech occurs when air passes through the glottis (located between the true vocal cords).

Once air leaves the larynx, it enters the lower respiratory system (see Fig. 23.1) via the trachea. The trachea is composed of C-shaped rings of cartilage, and the posterior portion of the trachea is composed of smooth muscle. The smooth muscle of the posterior portion of the trachea is shared with the esophagus, but they are two separate structures. The trachea divides into the right and left main bronchi just above where they enter the lungs. The point of trachea bifurcation is known as the *carina*. The right lung consists of three lobes, and the left lung consists of two lobes (Fig. 23.5). The main bronchi are composed primarily of cartilage. The right bronchus is wider and shorter than the left, which increases the chance of aspiration of foreign material into the right bronchus versus the left. Once air enters the right or left main bronchus, it travels to the lobar bronchi. The lobar bronchi are composed of cartilage, and the interior is lined with cilia. The cilia assist the lungs with mucous expectoration. The mucous, produced by epithelial goblet cells or mucous glands, functions as a barrier to infection by trapping bacteria or microorganisms. The mucous is moved up the **mucociliary escalator** by the beating motion of the cilia (Fig. 23.6).

Once air travels through the lobar bronchi, it enters the bronchioles. The bronchioles are not made of cartilage and thus rely on the elastic recoil of the lungs to remain open. The bronchioles divide into terminal bronchioles, and each terminal bronchiole branches to form two or more respiratory bronchioles. Air travels through the respiratory bronchioles to the alveolar ducts, both of which are lined with **alveoli**, to the alveolar sacs, which are clusters of alveoli. Gas exchange occurs from the respiratory bronchioles down (Fig. 23.7). The alveolar membrane is very thin, which enhances the transfer of oxygen and carbon dioxide across the alveolar membrane. Alveoli secrete a substance called **surfactant** that prevents collapse, or atelectasis, from occurring. If atelectasis occurs, the alveoli are unable to participate in gas exchange, thus limiting the gas-exchange capacity of the lungs.

The lungs are covered in a thin membrane called the **visceral pleura**. The inside of the chest cavity is covered in a membrane called the **parietal pleura**. The space between the parietal and visceral pleurae is called the **pleural space**. Pleural fluid, secreted by the pleural cells, is secreted between the two layers and acts as a lubricant. This allows the lungs to move freely during inspiration and expiration (Fig. 23.8).

Physiology of the Respiratory System

Inspiration

In order for ventilation to occur, there has to be movement of the diaphragm. The diaphragm resides below the lungs in the thoracic cavity. Inspiration occurs when there is stimulation of the phrenic nerve. The phrenic nerve is responsible for the movement and contraction of the diaphragm. Contraction causes the diaphragm to lower, compressing the abdominal contents and pulling the parietal pleura down to allow for expansion of the chest cavity. The expansion of the chest cavity increases the volume capacity of the lungs and decreases the pressure within the lungs to below atmospheric pressure. The decrease in

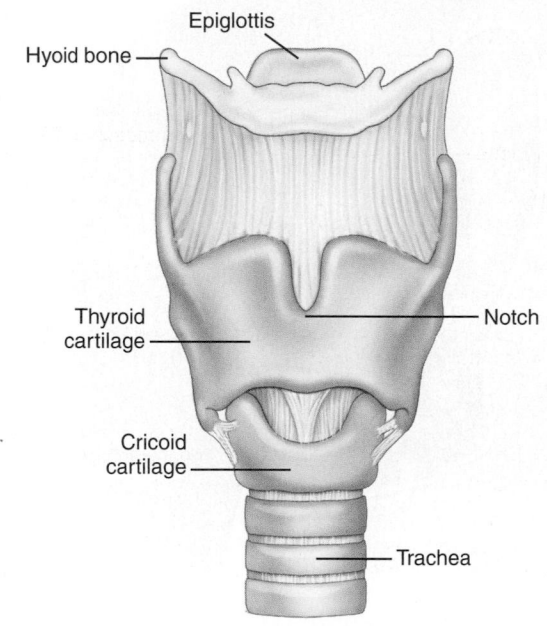

FIGURE 23.3 Thyroid and cricoid cartilages of the larynx.

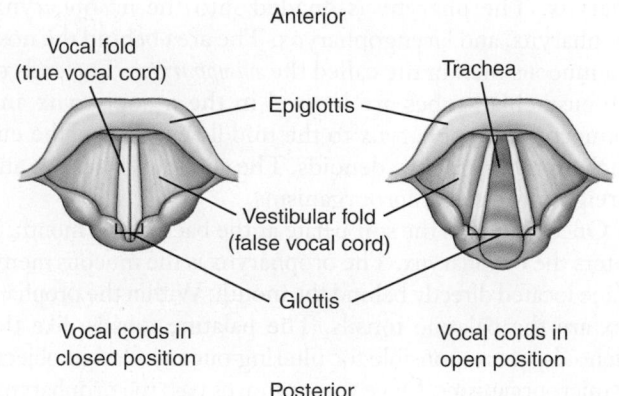

FIGURE 23.4 True and false vocal cords; sound is produced as air moves past the open true vocal cords.

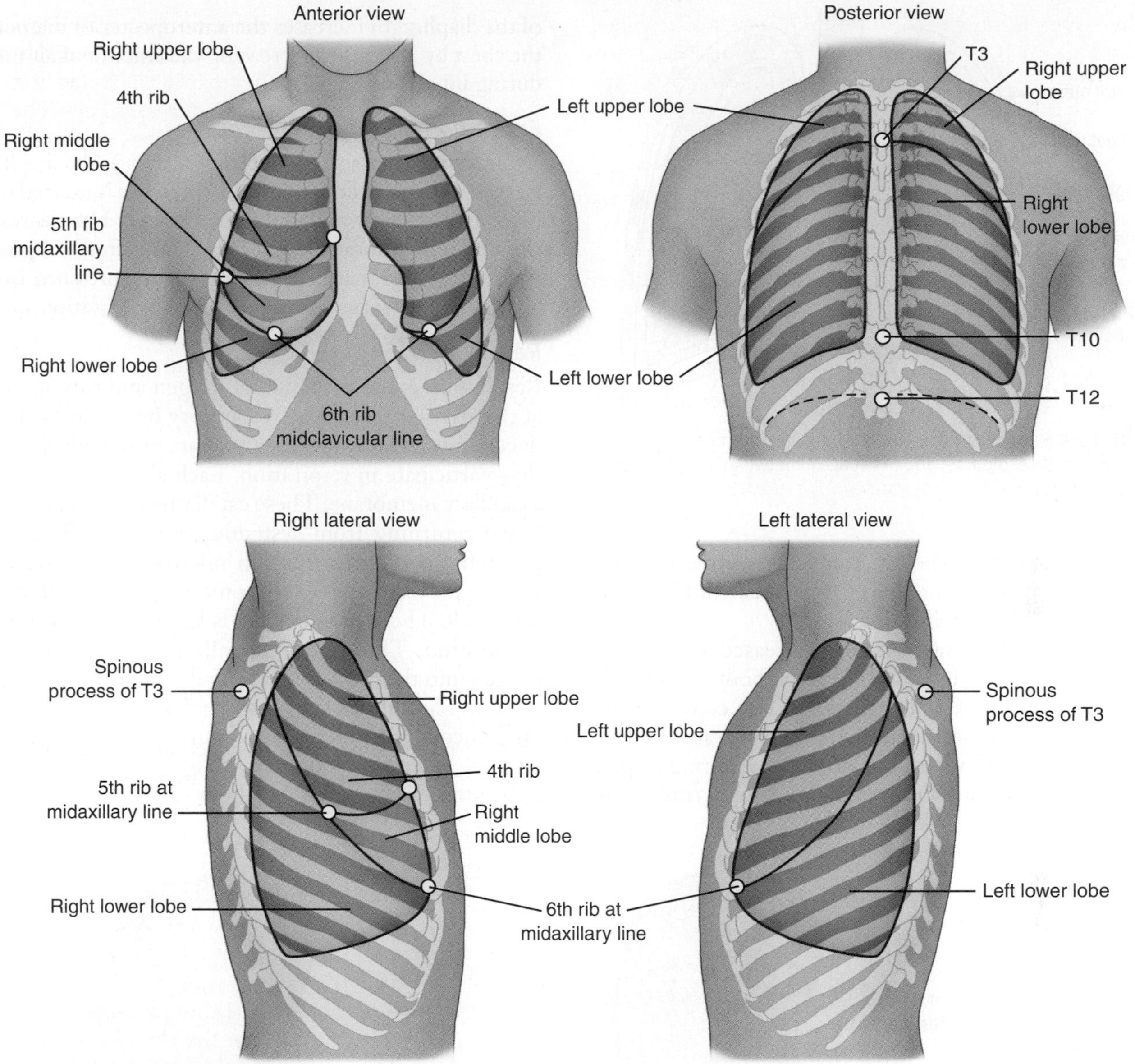

Anterior view

Right upper lobe
4th rib
Right middle lobe
5th rib midaxillary line
Right lower lobe
6th rib midclavicular line
Left upper lobe
Left lower lobe

Posterior view

T3
Right upper lobe
Right lower lobe
T10
T12

Right lateral view

Spinous process of T3
5th rib at midaxillary line
Right lower lobe
Right upper lobe
4th rib
Right middle lobe
6th rib at midaxillary line

Left lateral view

Left upper lobe
Spinous process of T3
Left lower lobe

FIGURE 23.5 Lobes of the lungs: upper, middle lower on the right; upper and lower on the left.

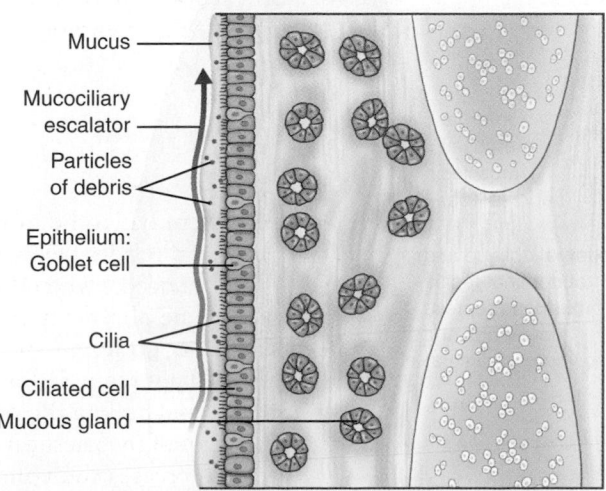

Mucus
Mucociliary escalator
Particles of debris
Epithelium: Goblet cell
Cilia
Ciliated cell
Mucous gland

FIGURE 23.6 The movement of mucus and bacteria or debris up the mucociliary escalator via the movement of the cilia.

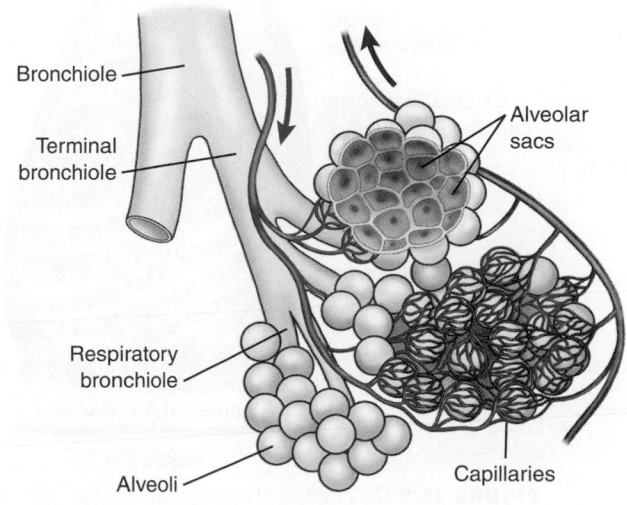

Bronchiole
Terminal bronchiole
Respiratory bronchiole
Alveoli
Alveolar sacs
Capillaries

FIGURE 23.7 Terminal airways; gas exchange takes place from the respiratory bronchiole down to the alveolar sac.

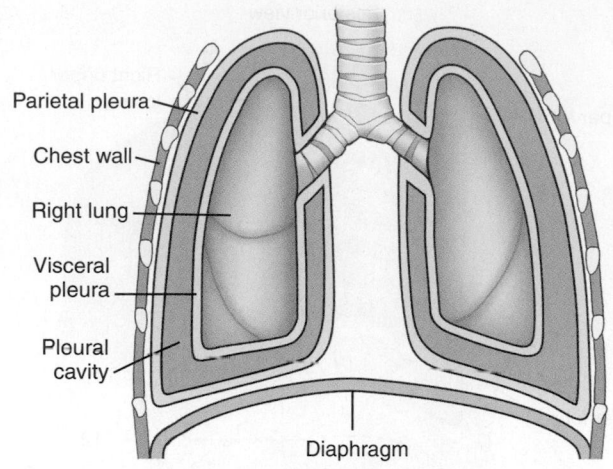

FIGURE 23.8 Membranes covering the lung and chest cavity, the parietal and visceral pleurae, and the space in between, the pleural space.

pressure of the lungs to below atmospheric pressure causes air to rush in because air moves from areas of high pressure to areas of low pressure.

During periods when there is increased demand for oxygen, such as periods of exercise, the body engages the muscles responsible for inspiration. They consist of the external intercostals, sternocleido mastoid, serratus anterior, and scalene muscles, which lift the rib cage during inspiration. The lifting of the rib cage combined with contraction

of the diaphragm increases the anteroposterior diameter of the chest by 20%, thus increasing the amount of air inhaled during inhalation (Fig. 23.9).

Expiration

Expiration is a passive process that occurs as the diaphragm relaxes. As the diaphragm relaxes, pressure is exerted on the lungs by the chest and abdominal cavity. The decrease in the size of the thoracic cavity causes an increase in pressure within the lungs that exceeds atmospheric pressure, causing air to passively leave the lungs through expiration.

Respiration

Respiration is the exchange of oxygen and carbon dioxide at the alveolar level. The respiratory bronchioles, alveolar ducts, and alveolar sacs contain or are lined with alveoli and thus participate in respiration. Each alveolus is covered in a capillary membrane. These capillaries carry deoxygenated blood returning from systemic circulation. The deoxygenated blood flows through microscopic capillary beds to allow the red blood cells to come into contact with the capillary wall. The area of contact is known as the **respiratory membrane**. This membrane allows for the diffusion of oxygen into the red blood cells and carbon dioxide into the alveoli. The diffusion of these gases occurs because of a difference in the concentrations and thus pressures exerted by these gases between the red blood cell and alveoli. The concentration of oxygen is higher within the alveoli, causing

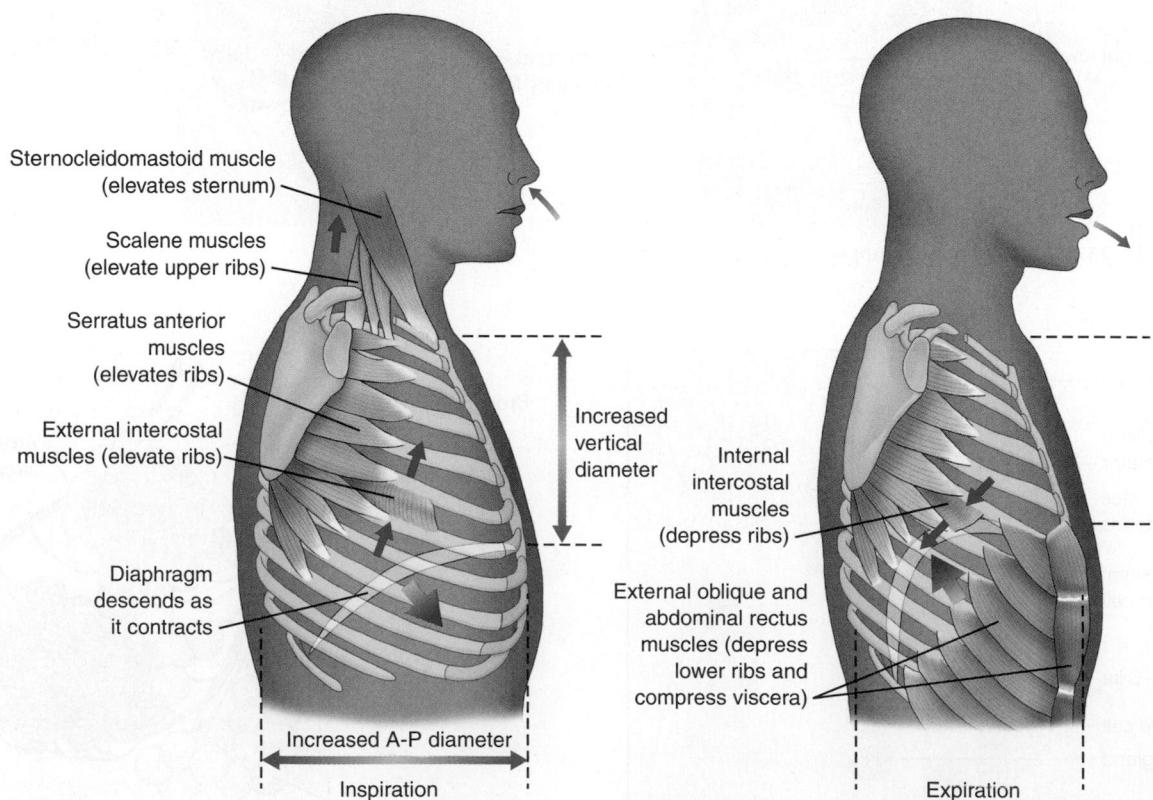

FIGURE 23.9 The muscles of respiration. The movement of the diaphragm and muscles of respiration during inspiration decrease the pressure within the lungs to below atmospheric pressure, allowing an influx of air. On expiration, the diaphragm relaxes and ascends, increasing pressure within the lungs and allowing air to passively exhale.

oxygen to diffuse across the respiratory membrane into the red blood cell. The concentration of carbon dioxide is higher within the red blood cell, causing the diffusion of carbon dioxide into the alveoli.

Dead Space/Shunt

Areas of the tracheobronchial tree that do not participate in gas exchange or respiration are referred to as **dead space**. There are two types of dead space within the respiratory system, anatomical and alveolar. All of the structures from the nose or mouth to the level of the respiratory bronchioles are filled with air but do not participate in gas exchange, so they are considered **anatomical dead space**. **Alveolar dead space** occurs when there is impaired or absent respiration at the level of the alveoli. This can occur when there is a lack of perfusion of the alveoli by the pulmonary capillaries. **Physiological dead space** is the sum of both anatomical and alveolar dead space. In patients with normal or healthy respiratory function, physiological dead space is typically equal to anatomical dead space.

Whereas dead space refers to alveoli that do not participate in gas exchange, **shunt** refers to blood that does not participate in gas exchange, or blood that returns to the left heart without being oxygenated. The two types of shunts are anatomical and physiological. Anatomical shunt refers to blood moving from the right to the left heart without traveling through the lungs. This can be caused by congenital heart defects. Physiological shunt occurs when alveoli are not functioning even though there is perfusion by the pulmonary capillaries. As a result, a portion of the blood returns to the left side of the heart deoxygenated. A shunt unit can occur as a result of atelectasis or collapse of the alveoli.

Ventilation–Perfusion Mismatch

Both dead space and shunt may result in a **ventilation–perfusion (V/Q) mismatch**. As noted previously, when there is no perfusion of functioning alveoli by the pulmonary capillaries (dead space) because of an obstruction of blood flow through the pulmonary capillaries, there is a high ventilation–perfusion mismatch, or adequate ventilation with poor perfusion. This can occur when there is a pulmonary embolism obstructing flow through the pulmonary artery. When there is adequate perfusion through poorly functioning alveoli (shunt), there is a low ventilation–perfusion mismatch, or poor ventilation with adequate perfusion (Fig. 23.10). A low V/Q mismatch can occur when a patient has pneumonia.

Connection Check 23.2

Which of the following structures actively participates in gas exchange?

A. Bronchi
B. Visceral pleura
C. Respiratory bronchioles
D. Terminal bronchioles

CASE STUDY: EPISODE 2

The evaluation of Mr. Thomas's complaint of shortness of breath continues with a medical history.

Past medical history: chronic obstructive pulmonary disease (COPD) and hypertension. He is unsure of his immunization status and does not remember receiving a PPD, or purified protein derivative skin test (most commonly a Mantoux test) to assess for TB, and he denies receiving a flu shot.

Past surgical history: Denies

Allergies: No known medication, food, or environmental allergies

Medications:

Amlodipine (Norvasc), 10 mg PO daily

Hydrochlorothiazide (HydroDIURIL), 25 mg PO bid

Salmeterol (Serevent), 50 mcg inhaled bid

Budesonide powder (Pulmicort), 90 mcg inhaled bid

Albuterol (Proventil), 2 puffs inhaled prn

Multivitamin, 1 tablet PO daily…

ASSESSMENT

History

History of present illness (HPI) is an important component of the assessment process. Information that should be obtained during the HPI includes:

- Factors that exacerbate or improve symptoms
- Pain
- Cough
- Change in weight
- Dyspnea

Factors That Exacerbate or Improve Symptoms

Factors that exacerbate or improve symptoms should be assessed to help determine the cause and degree of the illness. Factors such as walking, climbing stairs, or remaining at rest can indicate the level of strain on the respiratory and cardiac systems. If symptoms do not improve at rest, it may indicate a greater degree of dysfunction than for a patient whose symptoms are present only with activity but improve at rest.

Pain

Pain assessments should include quality, location, radiation, severity, and precipitating factors. Patients reporting pain in the thorax may have dysfunction of the cardiac, gastrointestinal, and/or respiratory system. Patients with a respiratory disease process may not experience any symptoms of pain because of the lack of sensory nerves in the lungs and visceral pleura. Conversely, the parietal pleura is able to generate a pain response. The parietal pleura may become inflamed (pleurisy) and cause pain that can be described as

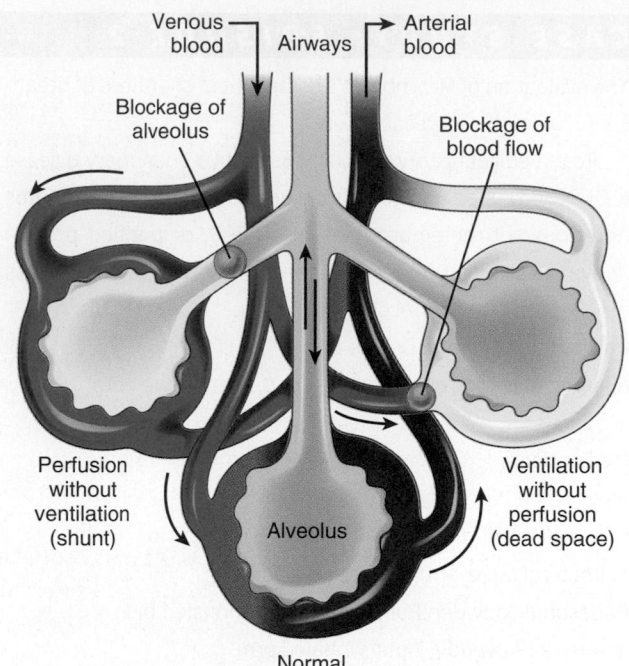

FIGURE 23.10 Ventilation–perfusion mismatch. On the left, perfusion without ventilation = shunt. On the right, ventilation without perfusion = dead space.

rubbing, sharp, or stabbing. It occurs because of the movement of the pleura during ventilation. In addition, pain caused by the respiratory system is normally increased with inspiration, deep breathing, and coughing because all of these cause movement of the parietal pleura.

Cough

Patients with a cough may have a productive or nonproductive cough. The frequency, duration, and presence of sputum production should be noted. The nurse should assess the color, volume, odor, consistency, and characteristics of the sputum. The assessment of the sputum will be helpful in understanding the possible causes of the cough. For example, pneumonia causes the production of thick sputum. A dry cough may be from asthma, a viral infection, or seasonal allergies.

 Safety Alert Patients reporting a productive cough with the following symptoms should be screened for tuberculosis (TB):

- Hemoptysis (bloody sputum)
- Low-grade fevers
- Weight loss
- Night sweats

Tuberculosis is a highly contagious illness that is transmitted via the air. Any patients with the previously listed symptoms should be placed in respiratory isolation until TB is ruled out to ensure the safety of the patient and providers.

Changes in Weight

Patients with recent weight changes need to be evaluated to determine if the changes in weight occurred with the onset of respiratory symptoms. Patients who have had recent weight gains and respiratory complaints will have an increased risk for sleep apnea or pauses in breathing during sleep. For patients with weight loss, the nurse needs to assess if the loss is due to lack of food intake. Many patients with respiratory complaints may have weight loss due to fatigue and shortness of breath with eating. Weight loss is common in chronic respiratory conditions such as COPD. A 24-hour food recall is a helpful tool to assess the dietary intake of a patient. The food recall will help the nurse understand the amount and the nutritional value of the patient's diet, providing insight into weight loss or gain.

Dyspnea

During assessment, **dyspnea**, the patient's perception of being short of breath, should be assessed for patients with respiratory complaints. It is important to note that dyspnea is based on the patient's perception; therefore, it is a subjective finding. Because dyspnea is a subjective finding, objective data are needed to identify the cause; dyspnea may be caused by nonrespiratory disease processes such as anxiety.

Health History

Once the nurse has evaluated the HPI, a detailed health history should be obtained. The nurse needs to assess the patient's current medications; allergies; past medical history; previous surgeries; family history; occupation/area of residence; and smoking, social, and recent travel histories.

Current Medications

Prescribed medications, herbal supplements, vitamins, and over-the-counter medications need to be documented. Patients with chronic respiratory disease processes should be asked about recent changes in medications, dosage, and/or frequency of administration. Changes in medication may account for the noted change in a patient's respiratory status. For example, a patient who starts a new respiratory medication but discontinues his or her previous therapy may experience improvement, worsening, or no change in symptoms. If the patient experiences a worsening in symptoms, it may indicate that the new medication regimen is not sufficient. In addition, many nonrespiratory medications have respiratory side effects. For example, angiotensin-converting enzyme (ACE) inhibitors used to treat hypertension may cause patients to develop a dry, nonproductive cough.

Allergies

The environment, food, and medications can all cause allergies. Environmental allergens may be found within or outside the home. Examples include fumes, chemicals, pollen, pets, and dust. Food allergies may be from food preservatives/additives or may be due to actual food items. Any allergy may cause shortness of breath, wheezing, or cough.

Past Medical History

Past medical history includes any previous acute illness, previous respiratory infections, and chronic disease processes. The current status of chronic disease processes should be noted (improving, worsening, or no change). The patient's immunization status should be evaluated, with particular attention to pertussis, pneumonia, and flu (novel and seasonal) vaccinations. In addition, patients should be asked for previous PPD results. Patients with a positive PPD need to have the date of the last chest x-ray documented.

Previous Surgeries

The patient's complete surgical history is important to note. Particularly relevant are surgical procedures impacting the respiratory system. For example, patients who have had a lobectomy have absent lung sounds over the affected area. A patient with a history of laryngectomy does not breathe through the mouth or nose; instead, the opening to the respiratory system is through the neck. Also important is that the nurse should assess if there is a history of respiratory complications following surgery (i.e., pulmonary embolism or atelectasis).

Family History

A family history of respiratory illnesses may increase the patient's genetic predisposition for illnesses (i.e., cystic fibrosis). Also, close contact with family members with infectious respiratory illnesses or respiratory irritants may be the cause of noted respiratory dysfunction. For example, patients who live in close contact with an individual diagnosed with TB need to be evaluated for the disease.

Occupation and Area of Residence

Certain occupations and areas of residence may contribute to or worsen respiratory disease processes. For example, patients who work in dusty environments may have respiratory symptoms in response to dust or other environmental allergens. Patients may be exposed to carcinogenic substances such as asbestos in their work environment. Patients who report occupational hazards or exposure to toxic substances need to be educated regarding the risks of their occupation and the importance of safety equipment to prevent complications.

Smoking History

Tobacco can be inhaled in the form of cigarettes or cigars or chewed in the form of chewing tobacco. Patients who report current or previous use of tobacco should be asked the type of tobacco used, amount or packs per day, number of years of use, and the quit date, if relevant.

Social History

The patient's social history, including alcohol and illicit drug use, should be evaluated for frequency of use, amount, route (for drug use), and number of years of use. Many illicit drugs can be smoked or inhaled, making the patient susceptible to respiratory illnesses.

Recent Travel History

Recent travel out of the country, especially to impoverished areas, may put the patient in contact with infectious respiratory disease processes such as TB. Symptoms that started after travel may assist in the diagnosis of the respiratory condition.

Physical Assessment

Inspection

Inspection is the first step in the assessment of the respiratory system. Abnormalities in the patient's level of consciousness and orientation status may indicate hypoxia. During inspection, the nurse should also assess the patient's speech. Patients should be able to speak freely and in full and complete sentences. Patients in respiratory distress may have difficulty speaking because of shortness of breath. The characteristics of the patient's fingernails may also indicate chronic respiratory dysfunction. Clubbing of the fingernails (Fig. 23.11) is a sign of chronic hypoxia and is a common assessment finding in patients with COPD.

The nose should be inspected to assess for symmetry and size. Each naris should be inspected for discharge, bleeding, masses, and/or swelling. The mucous membranes of the nares should be inspected for color. Pale or cyanotic mucous membranes may indicate tissue hypoxia.

The mouth should be inspected for open sores, bleeding, and/or masses. During inspection, the nurse should note the color and consistency of the mouth. The mucosa of the mouth should be pink and moist. Dry, cracked, or sticky mucous membranes may indicate dehydration. Mucous membranes that are pale or cyanotic may indicate tissue hypoxia.

The neck should be inspected for symmetry, skin discoloration, masses, cyanosis, and swelling. The position of the trachea (midline or any deviation to the right or left) should also be visualized during inspection of the neck.

The thorax should be inspected for skin integrity while identifying any scars, masses, lesions, or skin discoloration. The nurse should check for **retractions** on inspiration. Retractions occur when muscles pull inward during inspiration, sometimes causing the skin to pull in around ribs. This signifies increased work of breathing and respiratory distress. The nurse should also check for chest symmetry on inspiration and compare the thorax left to right and anterior to posterior (AP). Normally, the AP diameter when compared to the lateral diameter should be 1:2, whereas patients with chronic respiratory diseases such as COPD will have a ratio of 1:1. The nurse should inspect the spine while evaluating

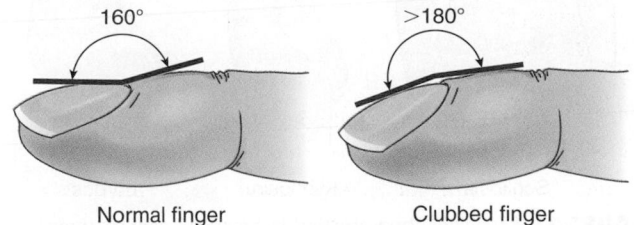

160°   >180°

Normal finger   Clubbed finger

FIGURE 23.11 Clubbing of the fingernails indicating chronic hypoxia.

the posterior thorax. Spinal deformities such as kyphosis, scoliosis, or lordosis can have an impact on the respiratory system (Fig. 23.12).

Vital signs, specifically the patient's respiratory pattern, rate, depth, and effort, should be assessed. The patient should be unaware that the nurse is obtaining the respiratory rate because patients tend to increase their respiratory rate if they know they are being observed. In order to take the respiratory rate, the nurse can count respirations and observe the chest wall while obtaining the patient's radial pulse. Respiratory rates greater than 20 are defined as **tachypnea**, whereas respiratory rates less than 12 are described as **bradypnea**. **Apnea** is defined as absent respirations. While the respiratory rate is obtained, signs of retractions, nasal flaring, and the use of accessory muscles can be observed. In addition, the **pulse oximetry** reading should be obtained. Pulse oximetry is discussed later in the chapter.

Palpation

The nurse should lightly palpate the trachea to ensure that it is midline and nontender. Following palpation of the trachea, the nurse can palpate the anterior and posterior thorax to assess for pain, crepitus, masses, and deformities. **Crepitus** occurs when air is trapped under the skin and is best described as a crackling feeling. Crepitus can be caused by a pneumothorax or trauma to the chest.

During palpation of the thorax, the nurse can assess for equal expansion of the lungs by placing both hands on the posterior thorax and having the patient inhale and exhale. As the patient breaths, both hands should rise equally during inspiration and return at the same rate during expiration. The nurse should also assess for tactile fremitus (vibration intensity) by placing hands on the patient's posterior thorax and having the patient say "ninety-nine." As the patient is speaking, the nurse should assess the vibration felt. Differences in vibrations between the right and left sides of the thorax may indicate conditions such as pneumonia or pleural effusions.

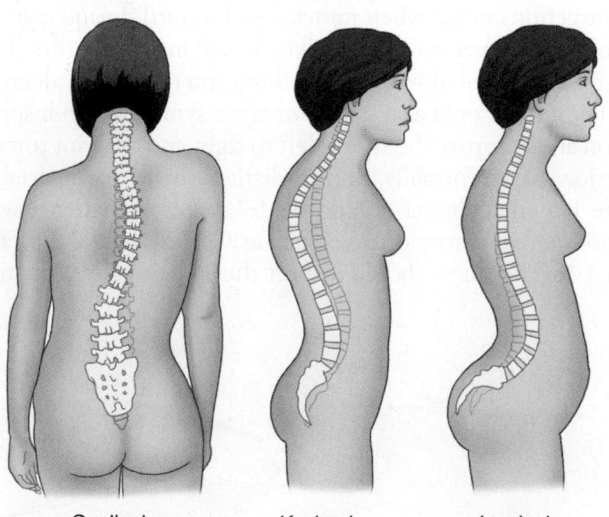

FIGURE 23.12 Spinal abnormalities that may impact breathing: scoliosis, kyphosis, and lordosis.

Scoliosis   Kyphosis   Lordosis

Percussion

Assessment of percussion between the ribs should be performed following palpation. The normal percussion sound heard over lung tissue is resonance. Table 23.1 describes the characteristics of each percussion sound and where it is heard normally. Table 23.2 details the respiratory conditions associated with each percussive sound when heard over lung tissue. Figure 23.13 demonstrates the appropriate sequence for percussion of the lungs.

Auscultation

The diaphragm of the stethoscope is used during auscultation of the respiratory system. The nurse should compare the sounds auscultated between the right and left lungs during inspiration and expiration. Careful attention should be given to ensure that the patient does not become dizzy or lightheaded during the assessment. See Figure 23.13 for the appropriate sequencing for auscultation.

Normal lung sounds can be divided into three types: bronchial, bronchovesicular, and vesicular lung sounds. Table 23.3 details the characteristics of each lung sound and the normal location for each sound.

Abnormal or adventitious lung sounds are crackles (rales), wheezes, rhonchi, and pleural friction rubs. Table 23.4 details the characteristics of adventitious lung sounds and the possible respiratory conditions associated with each adventitious sound.

⚠ Safety Alert Dyspnea is a subjective finding and, as such, will vary between patients. Patients who are reporting dyspnea and have any of the following assessment findings should be referred for immediate medical intervention:

- Unable to speak or able to speak only a few words
- Use of accessory muscles
- Retractions
- Adventitious lung sounds
- Tachypnea
- Pulse oximetry readings below baseline
- Abnormal percussion sounds
- Cyanosis
- Change in level of consciousness

Connection Check 23.3

Which of the following indicates an abnormal assessment finding of the respiratory system?

A. Symmetrical chest expansion
B. Muscle retractions with inhalation
C. The sound of resonance with percussion of lung tissue
D. Pink mucosa of the mouth and nares

Table 23.1 Percussion Sounds

Percussion Sound	Duration	Quality	Pitch	Normal Body Location for Percussion Sound
Resonance	Long	Hollow	Loud	Lung tissue
Flat	Short	Dull	High	Bone
Dull	Medium	Thud	Medium	Liver, heart, kidney, diaphragm
Tympany	—	Drumlike	Loud	Stomach
Hyperresonance	Longer than for resonance	Boom	Louder than for resonance	Sound not normally heard during assessment

Table 23.2 Percussion Sounds and Associated Respiratory Conditions

Percussion Sound	Potential Respiratory Conditions
Flat	Pleural effusion
Dull	Pneumonia, atelectasis, mass
Tympany	Large pneumothorax
Hyperresonance	Emphysema, chronic asthma, pneumothorax

Table 23.3 Normal Lung Sounds

Sound	Characteristic	Normal Auscultation Location
Bronchial	• Described as hollow • Loud intensity • Longer during expiration than inspiration	• Neck/trachea
Bronchovesicular	• Described as tubular • Moderate intensity • Sound heard equally during inspiration and expiration	• From first to second intercostal spaces
Vesicular	• Described as a gentle breeze • Soft intensity • Longer during inspiration than expiration	• Below the second intercostal space and peripheral lung fields

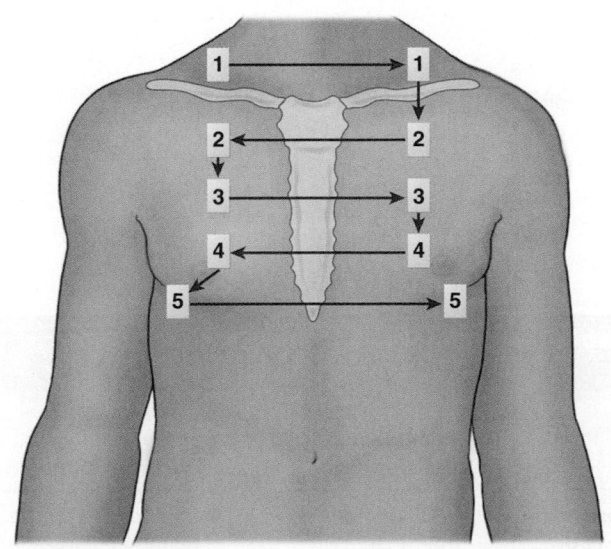

FIGURE 23.13 Sequencing for auscultation and percussion of the anterior chest.

DIAGNOSTIC STUDIES

Arterial Blood Gases

Description and Rationale

Arterial blood gas values include the partial pressure of carbon dioxide ($PaCO_2$), pH, bicarbonate (HCO_3^-), and partial pressure of oxygen (PaO_2) levels. Blood gases are used to assess acid-base balance. They can be used to determine oxygenation status because PaO_2 is the most accurate assessment, but pulse oximetry (discussed later in the chapter) is an easier, noninvasive way to assess oxygenation. Abnormal or low PaO_2 levels indicate hypoxemia. This does not indicate an acid-base imbalance; however, the body's compensatory mechanism of increasing the respiratory rate in response to hypoxemia decreases the $PaCO_2$ value, impacting the acid-base balance. An arterial blood gas sample is

Table 23.4 Abnormal or Adventitious Lung Sounds

Adventitious Sound	Characteristic	Respiratory Condition
Fine crackles (fine rales)	• Described as rubbing of hair follicles together • Cause: inflation of previously deflated lung tissue • Present during inspiration (early or late)	• Fibrosis • Bronchitis • Pneumonia • Chronic obstructive pulmonary disease (COPD)
Coarse crackles (coarse rales)	• Described as a popping/coarse sound • Cause: fluid or secretions in lower airways • Auscultated during early inspiration or expiration	• COPD • Sputum in airway • Pneumonia • Pulmonary edema • Congestive heart failure
Rhonchi	• Described as snoring • Cause: obstruction, sputum, or secretions typically in upper airways • Present during inspiration and expiration • May clear with coughing/suctioning	• Pneumonia/bronchitis • Masses (malignant or nonmalignant) • Foreign body
Wheezing	• Described as a squeaky musical instrument • Cause: bronchoconstriction and inflammation • Present during inspiration, expiration, or both	• Asthma • COPD
Stridor	• Described as a high-pitched sound during inspiration • Cause: airway obstruction of the throat or upper airway or spasms of the airway	• Allergic reaction • Epiglottis • Laryngitis
Pleural friction rub	• Described as grating or squeaking • Cause: inflammation of pleural space • Typically present during inspiration and expiration	• Pneumonia • Lung malignancy • Pleurisy

obtained directly from an artery through an arterial line or peripheral needle puncture.

Significance of Abnormal Values

The following are normal values for an arterial blood gas analysis:

PaO_2, 80 to 95 mm Hg
$PaCO_2$, 35 to 45 mm Hg
pH, 7.35 to 7.45
HCO_3^-, 22 to 26 mEq/L

Table 23.5 lists some respiratory conditions that cause acid-base abnormalities.

Patient Preparation

If the arterial blood gas specimen is being obtained through a peripheral needle puncture, the patient should be prepared for pain during the insertion of the needle. Because of the difficulty in puncturing the artery, the patient should be advised to remain still; any movement may cause difficulty in

Table 23.5 Respiratory Conditions That Cause Acid-Base Abnormalities

	Arterial Blood Gas Results	Associated With
Respiratory acidosis	$PaCO_2$: greater than 45 mm Hg pH: less than 7.35	• Chronic obstructive pulmonary disease • Pneumonia • Respiratory failure
Respiratory alkalosis	$PaCO_2$: less than 35 mm Hg pH: greater than 7.45	• Hyperventilation • May be associated with early asthma or pneumonia • Anxiety

obtaining a specimen. The patient may notice bruising and tenderness at the puncture site after specimen collection.

Nursing Implications

Prior to obtaining the specimen, the nurse should assess the patient's pulses and select a site that has a palpable pulse. The radial arteries are the most common site for obtaining peripheral arterial blood gas specimens. If the nurse elects to utilize the radial artery, assessment of the ulnar circulation needs to be evaluated utilizing the Allen test. The Allen test is done by asking the patient to clench his or her fist while compressing both the ulnar and radial arteries. Upon unclenching the fist, the hand should appear pale. Adequate ulnar circulation is indicated by the return to normal color after releasing pressure on the ulnar artery.

See Figure 23.14 for the appropriate technique for performing the Allen test.

After ulnar circulation is assessed, the nurse should confirm that all supplies are at the bedside, including a syringe designed for blood gas analysis and a cup of ice. Prior to insertion of the needle, the nurse preps the site with alcohol. If the patient's blood pressure is within normal limits, blood should enter the syringe immediately upon insertion of the needle into the artery. Once the specimen has been obtained, it should be promptly placed on ice. Direct pressure should be applied to the puncture site for several minutes, and then a pressure dressing is applied. The nurse should assess the puncture site to ensure that no bleeding is noted. Perfusion of tissue distal to the puncture site should also be assessed.

Pulse Oximetry

Description and Rationale

Pulse oximetry utilizes wavelengths of light to measure the saturation of hemoglobin with oxygen. It is a noninvasive way to monitor changes in the patient's oxygenation status.

Typically, pulse oximetry is obtained by placing a probe on a patient's finger, although some devices may be applied to the ear, toes, or forehead. Normal pulse oximetry readings are between 95% and 99%. Patients with chronic respiratory diseases may have baseline pulse oximetry readings below 95%. Pulse oximetry readings may be inaccurate if there is poor perfusion in the extremity being monitored. Poor perfusion can be caused by hypothermia, shock, cardiac arrhythmias, carbon monoxide poisoning, edema, peripheral vasoconstriction, tourniquets, and inflated blood pressure cuffs.

Significance of Abnormal Values

Pulse oximetry readings below 95% indicate that a patient may be experiencing hypoxemia. Abnormal pulse oximetry readings should be confirmed with arterial blood gases, especially when the patient's symptoms and pulse oximetry reading do not correlate. Pulse oximetry readings between 91% and 94% indicate mild hypoxemia, readings between 86% and 90% indicate moderate hypoxemia, and pulse oximetry readings of less than 85% indicate severe hypoxemia.

Patient Preparation

In order for a patient to have an accurate pulse oximetry reading, the fingernails need to be warm and free of nail polish. The patient should be asked to limit the movement of the finger the probe is placed on to ensure an accurate reading.

Nursing Implications

The nurse must confirm the accuracy of oximetry readings by evaluating the waveform (Fig. 23.15) and ensuring the pulse obtained through pulse oximetry correlates with the patient's heart rate. Without correlation, the accuracy of the reading should be questioned. It is also important to recognize that other conditions can affect the meaningfulness of the pulse oximetry reading. For example, the patient experiencing

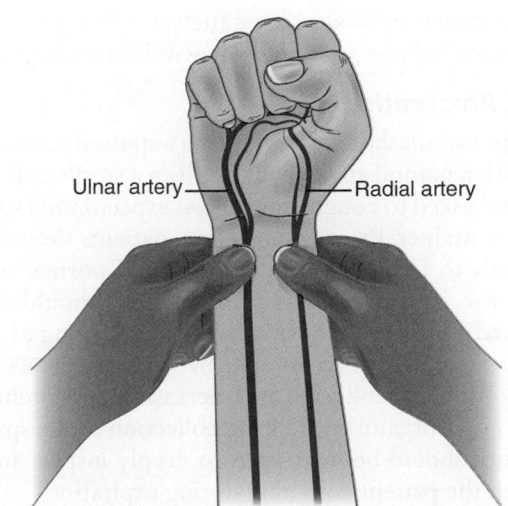

FIGURE 23.14 The Allen test to assess for adequacy of ulnar artery circulation.

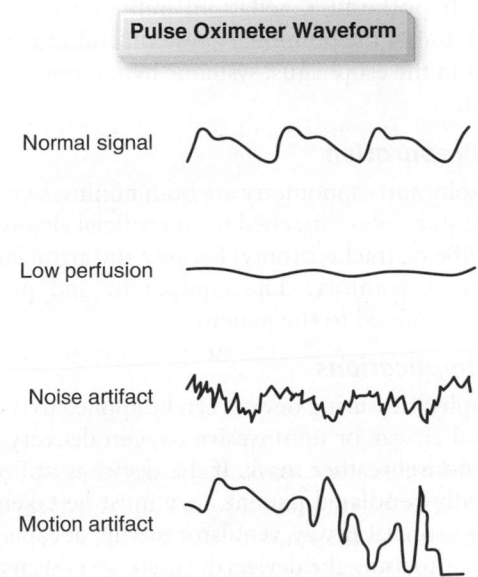

FIGURE 23.15 Pulse oximetry waveforms.

carbon monoxide poisoning may have a pulse oximetry reading of 100%, but the hemoglobin is saturated with carbon dioxide, not oxygen. Also, a patient with a pulse oximetry reading of 100% with a decreased hemoglobin level will still not have adequate tissue oxygenation.

Capnography and Capnometry

Description and Rationale

Capnography continuously monitors the $PaCO_2$ in the airway during inhalation and exhalation and provides a written tracing. **Capnometry** measures the amount of CO_2 exhaled without continuous tracing. Devices typically used for capnometry are sensor devices that provide a one-time reading of CO_2 levels. The most valuable CO_2 reading is the end-tidal CO_2 level. End-tidal CO_2 measures the maximal partial pressure of CO_2 obtained at the end of an exhaled breath. Normal end-tidal CO_2 readings are 2 to 5 mm Hg less than $PaCO_2$ readings for healthy patients.

Significance of Abnormal Values

Abnormal capnography and capnometry values indicate dysfunction of the respiratory system in expelling CO_2. Increases in end-tidal CO_2 levels may be from an increase in cellular metabolism, resulting in an increase in CO_2 production or hyperventilation that causes an increase in the excretion of CO_2 from the lungs. Disease processes that result in increased CO_2 levels are hyperthermia, trauma, burns, and sepsis. Decreases in the end-tidal CO_2 levels result from inadequate ventilation, respiration, or pulmonary perfusion. Conditions that cause this are slow cellular metabolism, resulting in less CO_2 production; hypoventilation, resulting in a decrease in the excretion of CO_2 from the lungs; and finally, conditions that cause an increase in alveolar dead space and shunt, which causes inadequate pulmonary capillary perfusion. This limits the diffusion of CO_2 into the alveoli, resulting in lower end-tidal CO_2 levels. Disease processes that result in lower end-tidal CO_2 levels are hypothermia, sedation, pulmonary embolism, hypoperfusion of the pulmonary system, endotracheal tube placement in the esophagus, systemic hypotension, and cardiac arrest.

Patient Preparation

Capnography and capnometry are both noninvasive and not uncomfortable unless attached to an artificial airway (endotracheal tube or tracheostomy) because the artificial airway may cause discomfort. The equipment and procedure should be explained to the patient.

Nursing Implications

Capnography measuring devices can be applied to the end of an artificial airway or noninvasive oxygen delivery devices such as a nonrebreather mask. If the device is utilized on a mechanically ventilated patient, care must be taken not to disrupt the artificial airway, ventilator tubing, or capnography device. Prior to using the device, the nurse should ensure that the capnography equipment is calibrated and zeroed.

Capnometry is typically utilized to confirm endotracheal tube placement after intubation. It is applied to the end of the endotracheal tube. The device will show a color change to blue, indicating the presence of CO_2 and intubation of the trachea. Endotracheal tube placement should also be confirmed by auscultation and chest x-ray. Continuous capnometry or monitoring of the end-tidal CO_2 level is also recommended for use during cardiopulmonary resuscitation (CPR) to evaluate the effectiveness of compressions. The American Heart Association states end-tidal CO_2 values between 10-20 mm Hg indicate adequate compressions.

Connection Check 23.4

You are caring for a patient who is currently receiving continuous pulse oximetry. Which of the following findings might indicate inaccurate readings?

A. The patient has a core body temperature of 94°F (34.5 °C).
B. The heart rate obtained through pulse oximetry correlates with the electrocardiogram heart rate.
C. The patient has the probe attached to her earlobe.
D. The patient's pulse oximetry is 95%, and the patient denies shortness of breath.

Sputum Analysis

Description and Rationale

A sputum analysis is done to check for microorganisms and/or abnormal cell growth. If microorganisms are identified, then a sensitivity test is performed to determine an effective antibiotic therapy. If abnormal cells are identified, analysis to determine if the cells are malignant or nonmalignant is indicated.

Significance of Abnormal Values

A sputum analysis positive for microorganisms indicates the presence of an infectious process such as TB or pneumonia. The presence of abnormal cells may indicate malignancy.

Patient Preparation

There are two methods for collecting a sputum culture. Patients with a natural airway will be given a sterile collection device and asked to cough and deposit expectorated sputum into the container. Prior to collection, patients should rinse the mouth to limit the contamination of normal mouth flora in the culture. In addition, patients should be instructed to collect sputum as early in the morning as possible because secretions accumulate overnight, increasing the volume of sputum collected and increasing the potential to identify microorganisms. During collection of the sputum, the patient should be instructed to deeply inspire and expire, with the patient coughing during expiration.

Patients with an endotracheal tube or tracheostomy will have the sputum culture collected by suctioning the airway and placing the contents into a sterile collection device. Suctioning may cause some discomfort to the patient, although the discomfort will be temporary.

Nursing Implications

Patients who require suctioning for the collection of a sputum sample will require hyperoxygenation prior to suctioning. Once the patient is hyperoxygenated, the nurse inserts the suction catheter connected to suction into the tracheostomy or endotracheal tube utilizing sterile technique. During the procedure, the nurse monitors the patient's respiratory rate and heart rate. If vital sign abnormalities are noted, the procedure is stopped, and the patient is hyperoxygenated until the vitals return to baseline.

Chest X-rays

Description and Rationale

Chest x-rays are diagnostic studies of the thorax that may identify problems with the lungs, heart, and pleural space. Chest x-rays are normally a first-line diagnostic test for patients with respiratory complaints because they are widely available and relatively inexpensive.

Significance of Abnormal Values

Chest x-rays will show if there are abnormalities of the heart or lungs. For the heart, chest x-rays are able to identify only abnormalities involving the size, shape, or placement of the heart. If abnormalities of the heart are noted during a chest x-ray, additional diagnostic tests are indicated. For the lungs, chest x-rays can identify masses, air or fluid in the pleural space, pneumonia, atelectasis, and possible TB infections. Many times, additional diagnostic tests are needed to confirm chest x-ray results. For example, a chest x-ray may identify possible TB, which is confirmed with a positive sputum culture.

Patient Preparation

Patients should remove any necklaces or jewelry that covers the neck or thorax prior to radiography. Female patients should remove their bra prior to having a chest x-ray. Any metal objects will obscure the view of the chest and thus the x-ray image.

Nursing Implications

The nurse or x-ray technician should drape all body areas not being x-rayed in a lead shield to minimize radiation exposure. For women of childbearing age, pregnancy status should be confirmed prior to the test. Women who are pregnant should receive education regarding the risk to the fetus prior to undergoing x-ray, and the test should be performed only if the benefits of the x-ray exceed the risks to the fetus.

Pulmonary Function Test

Description and Rationale

Pulmonary function tests evaluate lung volumes to determine the functioning of the lungs. The patient is asked to inspire and exhale into a mouthpiece. During the test, the patient is given instructions to alter his or her breathing patterns, allowing for different tests to be obtained. Before the test is started, normal values based on gender, weight, height, and smoking history are calculated to ensure the accuracy of the readings. See Table 23.6 and Figure 23.16 for a summary of normal pulmonary function results for a healthy adult male.

Significance of Abnormal Values

Pulmonary function values aid in the diagnosis of respiratory conditions. Table 23.7 discusses some possible causes of abnormalities related to the results of pulmonary function tests.

Patient Preparation

Prior to a pulmonary function test, the patient needs to refrain from smoking and eating for 8 hours. Also, the patient should abstain from bronchodilators (beta-2 agonists) for 4 to 6 hours prior to the test. The person administering the test should provide clear instructions to avoid unnecessary repetition.

Nursing Implications

The patient should be carefully monitored during the test to avoid any complications such as shortness of breath or bronchospasm.

Bronchoscopy

Description and Rationale

A bronchoscopy allows for direct visualization of the respiratory tract down to the level of the secondary bronchi. The two types of bronchoscopy are flexible and rigid. Flexible bronchoscopies are used to take tissue specimens or replace an endotracheal tube. Rigid bronchoscopy is used to remove obstructions or large amounts of secretions from the respiratory tract.

Significance of Abnormal Values

Abnormal findings on bronchoscopy assist in the diagnosis of respiratory conditions. Tissue specimens are analyzed to determine the presence of infectious processes or cellular abnormalities.

Patient Preparation

Because of the invasive nature of the procedure, patient consent should be obtained. Because of the need for sedation and the risk for aspiration, patients should not eat (should remain NPO) for at least 8 hours prior to the procedure.

Nursing Implications

Prior to beginning the procedure, the nurse should ensure that the appropriate consents have been signed and that a time-out procedure has been completed. The time-out should confirm the patient's identity and the procedure being performed. Flexible bronchoscopy can be performed at the bedside with the patient receiving moderate sedation. Rigid bronchoscopy typically requires general anesthesia and is performed in the operating room (OR).

Table 23.6 Summary of Normal Pulmonary Function Tests

Measurement	Typical Value	Definition
Respiratory volumes		
Tidal volume (TV)	500 mL	Amount of air inhaled and exhaled in one cycle during quiet breathing
Inspiratory reserve volume (IRV)	3,000 mL	Amount of air in excess of TV that can be inhaled with maximum effort
Expiratory reserve volume (ERV)	1,200 mL	Amount of air in excess of TV that can be exhaled with maximum effort
Residual volume (RV)	1,300 mL	Amount of air remaining in the lungs after maximum expiration; the amount that can never voluntarily be exhaled
Respiratory capacities		
Vital capacity (VC)	4,700 mL	The amount of air that can be inhaled and then exhaled with maximum effort; the deepest breath possible (VC = ERV + TV + IRV)
Inspiratory capacity (IC)	3,500 mL	Maximum amount of air that can be inhaled after a normal tidal expiration (IC = TV + IRV)
Functional residual capacity (FRC)	2,500 mL	Amount of air remaining in the lungs after a normal tidal expiration (FRC = RV + ERV)
Total lung capacity (TLC)	6,000 mL	Maximum amount of air the lungs can contain (TLC = RV + VC)
Forced vital capacity (FVC)	5,000 mL	Amount of air an individual can forcefully exhale after maximum inspiration
Forced expiratory volume (FEV1) (over 1 second or over 1 minute)	Depends upon the FVC	Amount of air an individual can forcefully exhale within a set time frame (1 second or 1 minute)
Forced expiratory flow (FEF)	Depends upon the FVC	Expiratory flow during different portions of the FVC. The flow readings are obtained during the beginning, middle, and last portion of the FVC.

Adapted from Saladin, K. S. (2018). *Anatomy & physiology* (8th ed.). New York, NY: McGraw-Hill

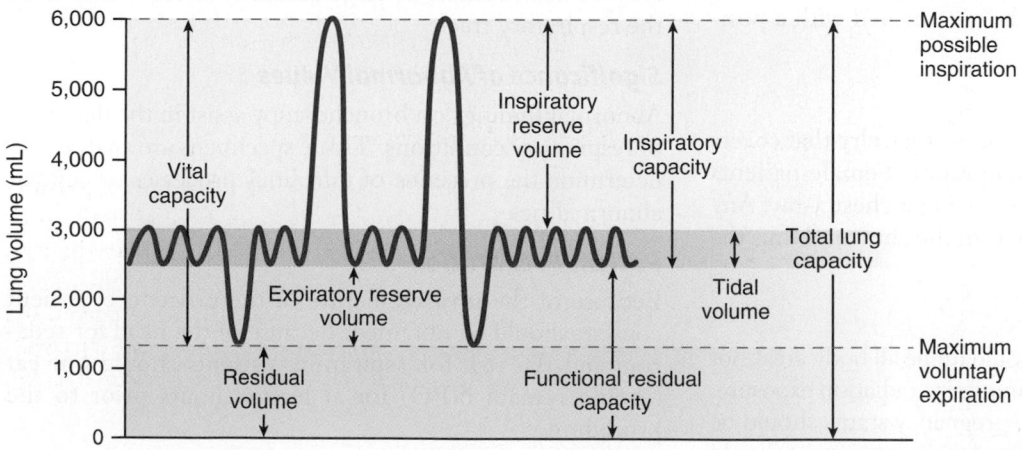

FIGURE 23.16 Respiratory volumes and capacities.

Moderate sedation involves giving the patient an IV pain medication and sedative. Depending on state and hospital protocols, this sedation may be administered by a nurse who has received specialized training in moderate sedation or an advanced practice nurse (i.e., a certified registered nurse anesthetist [CRNA]). Patients who receive moderate sedation are typically able to respond to verbal stimuli or gentle touch.

For flexible and rigid bronchoscopies, patients will need IV access and continuous cardiac monitoring, pulse oximetry, and blood pressure monitoring. Because patients are receiving moderate sedation or general anesthesia for the procedure, prior to starting the procedure, the nurse or OR staff needs to ensure that all of the emergency equipment is available at the bedside, including oxygen and suction. Nurses who are monitoring patients receiving moderate

Table 23.7 Disease Processes and Pulmonary Function Test Results

Pulmonary Function Test Result	Possible Disease Process
Increase in total lung capacity	Chronic obstructive pulmonary disease (COPD)
Decreases in total lung capacity	Sarcoidosis or pulmonary fibrosis
Decreases in forced vital capacity	COPD, sarcoidosis, pulmonary fibrosis, or neuromuscular diseases such as myasthenia gravis
Decreases in forced expiratory volume	COPD or may be caused by age-related changes
Decreases in forced expiratory flow	Disease processes related to obstructions such as asthma or COPD

sedation need to constantly evaluate the patient's condition and vital signs. If a patient receiving moderate sedation experiences respiratory depression, bradycardia, or hypotension, immediate action is needed on the part of the nurse. At the conclusion of the test, the patient should be monitored (vital signs, lung sounds, and mental status) every 15 minutes until his or her level of consciousness returns to baseline. During the recovery process, the nurse should assess for complications of the procedure, such as bleeding or hypoxia. The patient should remain on NPO status until the patient is alert and the gag reflex is intact.

Thoracentesis

Description and Rationale

A **thoracentesis** can be used as a diagnostic test or treatment depending on the disease process. During a thoracentesis, a needle is inserted into the pleural space to remove excess fluid/air.

Significance of Abnormal Values

If fluid is aspirated from the pleural space, it can be analyzed to determine if microorganisms or abnormal cells are present. If air is aspirated from the pleural space, this is consistent with a pneumothorax diagnosis. Thoracentesis can be used as a treatment option to remove fluid and/or air from the pleural space.

Patient Preparation

As with a bronchoscopy, the patient needs to sign a consent form and be informed of the benefits and risks of the procedure. This procedure is normally completed under local anesthesia, so the patient is fully awake during the procedure. Because patients are awake, they need to be instructed not to move but to remain as still as possible. In order to assist the provider with the procedure, the patient is placed in a sitting position. A bedside table is placed in front of the patient, and the patient leans against the table during the procedure. The patient should be informed that it is normal to feel the need to cough during the procedure and should be advised to try to deep breathe to avoid coughing.

Nursing Implications

Prior to starting the procedure, the nurse should ensure that the patient has signed the appropriate consent forms and that a time-out procedure has been completed. The nurse should assist the patient into a seated position on the side of the bed with a bedside table in front of the patient. The patient should then be instructed to lean on the table during the procedure. The nurse should assess for potential complications that may arise during the procedure by monitoring vital signs and pulse oximetry. Any changes in the patient's vital signs may indicate complications and the need for the procedure to be discontinued. The output from the site of the thoracentesis should be monitored because excess drainage (more than 500 mL) may cause hypotension. Most patients who report shortness of breath prior to the procedure report immediate relief of symptoms once the fluid or air is removed from the pleural space.

At the conclusion of the procedure, the nurse needs to reevaluate the patient's vital signs and lung sounds to assess for possible complications such as pneumothorax. A chest x-ray should also be obtained because of the high risk of pneumothorax. The patient should be encouraged to cough and deep breathe following the procedure to decrease the risk of atelectasis and promote good lung expansion.

Patients may be discharged home following a thoracentesis with education as to signs and symptoms of complications. Patients should be told to immediately report any of the following symptoms to their provider:

- Elevated heart rate/heart palpitations
- Dyspnea/shortness of breath (SOB)
- Chest pain
- Hemoptysis (bloody secretions)

The patient should also receive education regarding wound care following the thoracentesis. Following the procedure, a dry sterile dressing is typically applied to the site. The area should be assessed for drainage and bleeding immediately following the procedure and prior to discharge if the patient is having the procedure completed as an outpatient. A minimal amount of blood noted on the dressing is normal.

Lung Biopsy

Description and Rationale

A lung biopsy allows for a small piece of lung tissue to be removed and analyzed under a microscope. Lung biopsies can be performed percutaneously or through an open procedure. The type of biopsy performed is based on the location and size of the tissue requiring biopsy. A biopsy is typically ordered to confirm lung cancer, sarcoidosis, or pulmonary fibrosis.

Significance of Abnormal Values

Abnormal values may indicate an infectious process or malignancy.

Patient Preparation

Patients who are receiving a percutaneous lung biopsy will need the same preparation pre-procedure as patients receiving a bronchoscopy. Patients who are receiving an open biopsy will need to be NPO for at least 8 hours prior to the procedure because they will be receiving general anesthesia. Prior to the procedure, the patient will need to be educated about the postoperative period (i.e., open biopsies require the use of a chest tube in the postoperative period). Depending on the type of open biopsy performed and the patient's respiratory function, the patient may require intubation and mechanical ventilation in the postoperative period.

Nursing Implications

For percutaneous and open lung biopsies, there must be consent from the patient, and a time-out should be performed. During percutaneous biopsies, the nurse will assist the patient into the position that is utilized for a thoracentesis. Patients will receive a local anesthetic, injected at the site of the biopsy. During the procedure, the nurse will monitor the patient's vital signs, including pulse oximetry, for any complications that may arise. The nurse needs to remind the patient not to move or cough during the procedure.

Patients who are having an open biopsy will receive general anesthesia and will be monitored by an anesthesiologist or CRNA during the procedure. During an open biopsy, a thoracotomy will be performed, which will require a chest tube to allow for reexpansion of the lungs. The nurse will need to monitor the patient during the postoperative period to assess for complications arising from the surgery and anesthesia.

Connection Check 23.5

Which of the following is included in an arterial blood gas analysis?
A. End-tidal CO_2
B. Hemoglobin
C. $PaCO_2$
D. Sodium

AGE-RELATED CHANGES OF THE RESPIRATORY SYSTEM

There are anatomical, physiological, and immunological changes that occur in the respiratory system as age increases. Table 23.8 details each of these changes.

Connection Check 23.6

Which of the following is a finding attributable to age-related changes?
A. Kyphosis
B. AP-to-lateral diameter of 1:1
C. $PaCO_2$ of 47 on an arterial blood gas
D. $PaCO_2$ of 60 on an arterial blood gas

Table 23.8 Age-Related Changes of the Respiratory System

	Changes to Respiratory System	Impact
Structural changes	1. Stiffening of the thoracic cage 2. Decrease in height of thoracic vertebrae from osteoporosis 3. Kyphosis 4. Decrease in chest-wall compliance	Kyphosis and osteoporosis of the thoracic vertebrae cause a decrease in chest-wall compliance. The decrease in chest-wall compliance increases the residual volume, which decreases the function of the diaphragm. Therefore, elderly patients have increased residual volumes and respiratory effort during inspiration.
Changes related to muscle function	1. Decrease in strength of diaphragm 2. Decrease in strength of intercostals	The decrease in function/strength of the intercostals and diaphragm increases inspiratory effort to maintain adequate ventilation.
Tissue changes	1. Decrease in elasticity of tissue	The decrease in the elasticity of lung tissue increases the residual volume while decreasing vital capacity.
Reactivity of airway	1. Increase in potential for bronchoconstriction	The airways of older adults are more reactive than those of younger adults. Older adults have a delayed response to bronchodilators, increasing the possibility of hypoxia and hypercapnia from bronchoconstriction.

Table 23.8 Age-Related Changes of the Respiratory System—cont'd

	Changes to Respiratory System	Impact
Gas exchange	1. Depressed cough reflex and ventilatory response to hypoxia and hypercapnia 2. Delays in gas exchange across the alveolar membrane	Increased potential for episodes of hypercapnia and hypoxia
Immunological changes	1. Increase in the neutrophils in respiratory tissue 2. Decrease in the macrophages in respiratory tissue	The increase in neutrophils and decrease in macrophages create chronic inflammation of the lung tissue, which hinders gas exchange.

Data from Taffet, G. E. (2017). *Normal aging.* Retrieved from http://www.uptodate.com/contents/normal-aging

Making Connections

CASE STUDY: WRAP-UP

In addition to Mr. Thomas's complaint of shortness of breath, he reports chest pain that increases with coughing and thick yellow/green sputum for several days. His assessment is as follows:

Inspection upper respiratory system: Nasal and mouth mucosa are pink; no bleeding, masses, or deformities are noted in the upper respiratory system.

Inspection lower respiratory system: Patient has a respiratory rate of 20, with even and unlabored respirations. During the history, the patient is speaking freely and does not report any shortness of breath while talking. The patient has skin that is appropriate for his ethnic background, with no skin integrity issues noted during inspection.

Palpation: No masses, deformities, or crepitus are noted. Trachea is midline and nontender. The patient has equal lung expansion anterior and posterior; the patient reports pain that increases with inspiration.

Percussion: Dullness over right lower lobe, otherwise hyperresonance

Auscultation: Fine crackles in right lower lobe with inspiration and expiratory wheezes and diminished breath sounds noted throughout.

Vital signs:
Temperature: 100°F (38°C)
Respiratory rate: 22
Pulse oximetry on room air: 91% to 93%
Heart rate: 90 bpm
Blood pressure: 130/80 mm Hg

The chest x-ray notes pneumonia on the right lower lobe of the lung. On the basis of the diagnostic studies and assessment findings, the provider diagnoses Mr. Thomas with pneumonia and exacerbation of his COPD. Oral antibiotics are prescribed, and Mr. Thomas is advised to stay home from work until the symptoms subside.

Case Study Questions

1. Which of the following nursing diagnoses is the priority for Mr. Thomas on the basis of his diagnosis and symptoms?
   A. Impaired gas exchange
   B. Deficient knowledge
   C. Risk for infection
   D. Fluid volume deficit

2. Which of the following instructions should the nurse include in Mr. Thomas's teaching plan about the management of his pneumonia? *(Select all that apply.)*
   A. Begin a robust exercise program.
   B. Stop taking the antibiotics once his cough resolves.
   C. Smoking will exacerbate symptoms and should be avoided during recovery.
   D. To cough and deep breathe at least 10 times per hour to assist with airway clearance.
   E. Stay in bed to rest as much as possible.

3. Which statement by the patient with pneumonia indicates that teaching has been effective?
   A. "I will return to my provider's office if my symptoms are not improved 5 days after starting the antibiotics."
   B. "I can continue to smoke following my illness, and it will not have any impact on my respiratory status."
   C. "I will stop taking my blood pressure medication because it will increase my risk for developing pneumonia."
   D. "A fever is expected until I am finished with my course of antibiotics."

4. Which of the following indicates a worsening of Mr. Thomas's respiratory condition?
   A. Mr. Thomas is having difficulty speaking during the assessment.
   B. Mr. Thomas has wheezes bilaterally.
   C. Mr. Thomas's blood pressure has increased to 140/85 mm Hg.
   D. Mr. Thomas's pulse oximetry is 93% on room air.

5. On the basis of Mr. Thomas's past medical history, which of the following assessment findings will the nurse expect as a result?
   A. Clubbing of fingernails
   B. Wheezes upon auscultation
   C. Retractions on inspiration
   D. Poor skin turgor

CHAPTER SUMMARY

The respiratory system is a complex system that is divided into the upper and lower airways. Air enters the respiratory system through the nose or mouth and travels to the lungs, where respiration occurs at the alveoli level. The major functions of the respiratory system are ventilation and respiration. Ventilation occurs as air moves into the respiratory system through the process of inspiration. During ventilation, the structures of the respiratory system filter and humidify the air entering the system. The process of respiration occurs as oxygen and carbon dioxide are exchanged. Respiration, or air exchange, takes place in the respiratory bronchioles, which contain alveoli. Other functions of the respiratory system include acid-base regulation, temperature regulation, and fluid balance.

Because of the complexity of the respiratory system, a thorough assessment must be completed, including inspection, auscultation, percussion, and palpation, to identify dysfunction. If dysfunction of the system is noted, diagnostic tests can be ordered to determine the source of the dysfunction and assist in diagnosis. A finding of muscle retractions with inhalation is an abnormal finding indicating respiratory distress. Normal findings include symmetrical chest expansion, resonance with percussion, and pink mucosa.

Arterial blood gases and pulse oximetry are two tests to assess the adequacy of ventilation and respiration. Pulse oximetry is a less invasive means to determine oxygenation, but ensuring accuracy is essential. Arterial blood gases monitor $PaCO_2$, HCO_3^-, pH, and PaO_2. Other diagnostic tests include pulmonary function tests, chest radiography, bronchoscopy, biopsy, and thoracentesis.

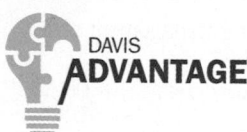
DAVIS
ADVANTAGE

To explore learning resources for this chapter, go to **Davis Advantage** and find:
- Answers to in-text questions
- Chapter Resources and Activities
- NCLEX®-Style Chapter Review Questions
- Bibliography

Chapter 24

Coordinating Care for Patients With Infectious Respiratory Disorders

Stephanie Walter Coleman

Finding Connections

CASE STUDY: EPISODE 1

Follow this patient throughout the chapter.

Mr. Harold Markham is a 70-year-old man who presents to the emergency department with fatigue, weight loss, and night sweats. He complains of a cough that produces rusty-colored or blood-streaked sputum. His vital signs are:

Blood pressure (BP) = 145/85 mm Hg

Heart rate (HR) = 95 bpm

Respiratory rate (RR) = 22

Pulse oximetry (SpO$_2$) = 92%

Temperature (T) = 100.3°F (38°C)

Mr. Markham works as a volunteer in the food service department of an HIV community support center. His past history consists of coronary heart disease with two cardiac stents (placed last year), mild emphysema, long-term type 2 diabetes, and arthritis. His current home medications are aspirin, 81 mg daily; ipratropium (Atrovent), 2 puffs three times daily; celecoxib, 100 mg twice daily; metformin, 500 mg twice daily; and an over-the-counter daily multivitamin…

INTRODUCTION

All body functions require a constant supply of oxygen to support their many metabolic activities. As a consequence of supplying continual oxygen, the respiratory tract maintains a persistent interface with the external physical environment, resulting in a high degree of direct exposure to microorganisms. It is for this reason that the respiratory tract is a common site of infection by pathogens. Fortunately, there is a series of complex, comprehensive, and efficient protective and defense mechanisms against harmful pathogens for both the upper and lower respiratory tracts.

The Upper Respiratory Tract

A wide variety of pathogens can produce infection within the respiratory tract, including bacteria, viruses, and fungi. As environmental air is inhaled, the first line of defense lies within the upper respiratory tract, which consists of the nasal cavities, the pharynx, and the larynx.

The nares and nasal cavities are equipped with coarse hairs (vibrissae) and a mucous layer that filter out and trap macroparticulates (large particles). In addition, the nasal cavities are lined with epithelial tissues and blood vessels that filter and warm the inspired air. The surface epithelium secretes antimicrobial peptides that exert a **bactericidal** effect on a variety of pathogens. The endothelial lining of the nasal cavities contains hairlike projections, called cilia, that,

through their wavelike motion, transport any particles trapped by the mucous lining back into the nasopharynx and oropharynx. This mechanism is called the **mucociliary escalator**. Here, the particulate matter is expelled from the respiratory tract by the protective sneezing and coughing reflexes. After inhaled air moves through the nasal cavities, the anatomy of the upper airway changes direction, causing any remaining large particles to come in contact with the back of the throat. The tonsils and adenoids (lymphoid organs) play an integral role in the development of an immune response to pathogens remaining in contact with the mucoid surfaces of the throat through trapping and filtering. Next, the larynx (voice box), which houses the epiglottis, provides mechanical protection of the airways. During breathing, the epiglottis remains open to allow air to pass into the trachea. While food and fluids are swallowed, the epiglottis closes, directing solid material into the esophagus and preventing **aspiration**, or movement of gastric contents into the airways.

Additional protective mechanisms of the upper respiratory tract are provided by the **colonization** (a collection of a number of bacteria small enough not to cause infection) of resident bacteria and some viruses. Examples of resident bacteria and viruses include but are not limited to forms of *Staphylococcus*, *Streptococcus*, spirochetes, mycobacteria, *Pseudomonas*, *Proteus*, and *Enterococcus*. This "normal flora" functions to maintain a healthy respiratory status by competing with pathogens for attachment sites in the respiratory mucous lining and producing bactericidal substances that destroy harmful microorganisms.

The Lower Respiratory Tract

The trachea marks the beginning of the lower respiratory tract, along with the bronchi, bronchioles, and alveoli. A layer of ciliated cells and the mucous-secreting cells within the trachea, bronchi, and bronchioles protect the lower respiratory tract via the mucociliary escalator from smaller-size particles that have avoided the upper airway defenses. Any pathogens that reach this area are trapped in an additional ciliated mucous layer and are driven upward via ciliary motion to the larynx and oropharynx, where they are swallowed and eventually destroyed by digestive enzymes in the stomach.

The lower respiratory tract houses no resident flora and is considered a "sterile site." This is in part due to the efficiency of the upper respiratory tract's ciliated epithelial lining in eliminating the majority of inhaled pathogens. Should pathogens gain access to the lowest portion of the respiratory tract (the alveoli), **alveolar** macrophages are the most important means of eliminating microorganisms from this area by phagocytosis. It is of the utmost importance that the alveoli remain free of pathogens because it is here that the vital exchange of gases occurs (Fig. 24.1). It is only when the respiratory epithelium becomes damaged or the sheer numbers of inhaled pathogens exceed the ability of these protective mechanisms to function that a respiratory infection occurs.

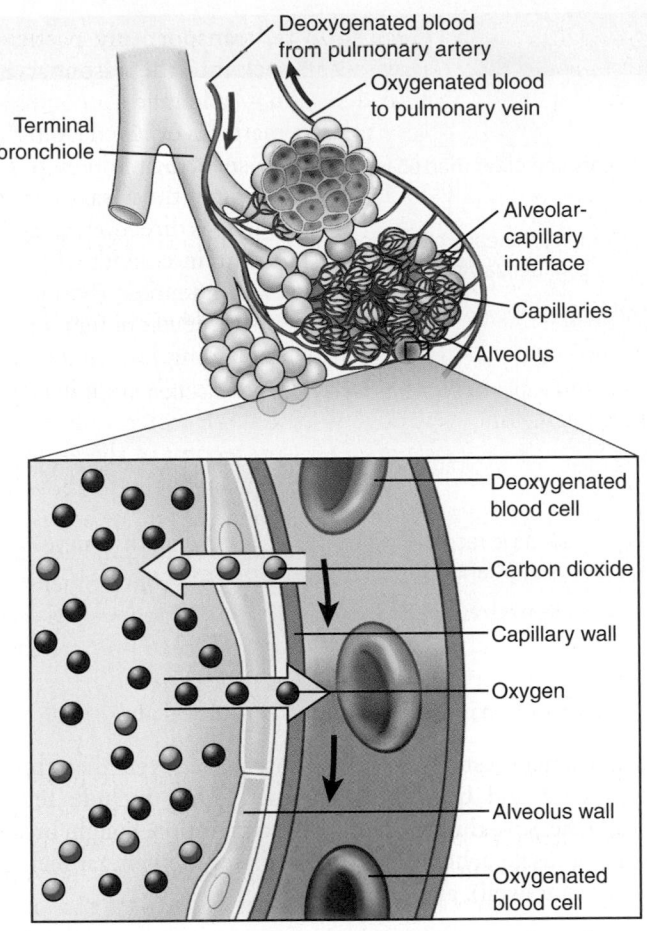

FIGURE 24.1 Gas exchange at the alveolar level: gases moving from areas of higher to lower concentration. Oxygen moves into the blood; carbon dioxide moves out of the blood.

Establishment of a Respiratory Tract Infection

In order for a respiratory infection to be fully established in the lower respiratory tract, the following barriers must be avoided and conditions met:

1. Avoidance of trapping in the mucociliary layer of the upper respiratory tract
2. Avoidance of the phagocytic action of the alveolar macrophages in the lower respiratory tract
3. Infectious organisms must be **airborne** (particles less than 5 μm that remain suspended in the air for a prolonged period of time) and have the ability to remain **virulent** (toxic) while in the air.
4. There must be sufficient numbers of infectious organisms inhaled and deposited on susceptible tissues within both the upper and lower respiratory tracts, preventing innate protective mechanisms from functioning effectively.

The Inflammatory Response of the Respiratory Tract

Once pathogens have been established in the respiratory tract, an inflammatory response is initiated. Direct stimulation by infecting organisms leads to the secretion of pro-inflammatory cytokines (interleukin [IL] and tumor necrosis factor [TNF]) by airway epithelial cells. Neutrophils (a type of white blood cell [WBC]) are recruited to the infected alveoli along with other immune cells and serum components (see Chapter 18). Capillary permeability increases, and the alveoli fill with fluid and plasma proteins. This accumulation of exudate (a mass of cells and fluid) provides the perfect medium for the proliferation of the infecting organism(s) and assists with movement to other nearby alveoli. The fluid- and exudate-filled alveoli are prevented from effective gas exchange at the alveolar-capillary level. This produces varying degrees of hypoxia depending on the severity of the infection.

INFLUENZA

Epidemiology

Influenza is a highly contagious infection that is rapidly spread from one individual to another. Outbreaks of influenza are tracked, recorded annually, and reported by the Centers for Disease Control and Prevention (CDC). The extent and severity vary widely among geographical areas throughout the United States. Localized outbreaks that affect more than the expected population (e.g., when the disease is expected to affect 15% of the population, but 40% become infected) are called *epidemics*. They occur at varying intervals, usually every 1 to 3 years. Epidemics typically begin abruptly, peak at 2 to 3 weeks, last approximately 2 to 3 months, and then rapidly subside. Global outbreaks (outbreaks that spread across a large geographical area) or outbreaks that are limited to a smaller geographical area but affect more people than expected (again using the example of an expected outbreak of 15%, but 70% of the population is affected) are referred to as *pandemics*. They also occur at variable intervals but less frequently than local outbreaks. The last influenza pandemic was the H1N1 pandemic in 2009, where estimates of the number of deaths ranged from 151,700 to 575,400. Morbidity and mortality rates were high, predominantly among those with underlying comorbid medical conditions or those of very young or advanced age. Other predominant risk factors for influenza are outlined in Table 24.1.

The CDC reported the highest influenza burden in the 2017–2018 season since the 2009 pandemic. Estimates for reported illnesses were 48 million, with 22 million doctors' visits, 959,000 hospitalizations, and 79,400 deaths.

Pathophysiology

Human influenza viruses are divided into three types, designated as A, B, and C. Influenza A viruses are divided into subtypes based on differences in two viral proteins—hemagglutinin (H) and neuraminidase (N). Influenza B is not broken down into subtypes but can be categorized by different strains. Influenza types A and B are responsible for epidemics of respiratory illness that occur mostly during the winter months and are often associated with increased

Table 24.1 **Risk Factors for Influenza Infection**

Risk Factor	Description
1. Age	Young children and older adults (younger than 2 years and older than 65 years) as a result of immature or less active immune systems
2. Occupation	Healthcare workers, family caregivers, daycare providers, and early childhood educators are more likely to be in frequent contact with those who are infected with the influenza virus.
3. Environmental	People living in dormitories, military quarters, and long-term care facilities who remain in close proximity for lengthy periods of time
4. Immune system compromise	Those with malignancies treated with chemotherapy, transplant recipients receiving anti-rejection medications, individuals with HIV/AIDS with CD4+ counts less than 200 cells/(L
5. Chronic illness	People with diabetes, renal failure, asthma, and cardiac and respiratory diseases are at higher risk for developing serious complications.
6. Pregnancy	Females who are considering pregnancy, are pregnant, or have recently given birth are at greater risk for developing severe viral pneumonia and have a four-fold overall mortality rate, even if they are otherwise healthy.

hospitalizations and deaths. The most extensive and severe outbreaks are from influenza A because of the tendency of the H and N antigens to mutate. Seasonal mutations of the viruses cause the emergence of a new and very different influenza virus and can contribute to a new pandemic. These mutations allow the viruses to escape the immune system surveillance of its host, making individuals susceptible to mutated influenza infections throughout their lives. Several pathogens that have been newly identified are hantavirus, metapneumoviruses, and coronavirus (SARS). Efforts to control the impact of influenza are focused on types A and B. Influenza C typically causes either no symptoms at all or a very mild respiratory illness. It is not associated with the occurrence of epidemics and does not have the serious public health concerns associated with influenza A and B.

The primary event that initiates an influenza infection is the aerosolization of small **droplets** (particles less than 5 μm that settle within 3–6 feet from point of release) from an infected individual's sneezing or coughing or by direct contact with fomites. **Fomites** are inanimate objects that can carry organisms and facilitate their transfer from one person to another, such as stethoscopes, scissors, or pens. The infectious agents are inhaled and become deposited on the epithelial cells of the upper respiratory tract. Over a period of approximately 4 to 6 hours, these infected cells reproduce and spread the virus to other respiratory cells, extending the infection throughout the respiratory tract. The incubation period (from the time of initial droplet inhalation to symptom development) lasts approximately 18 to 72 hours. The severity of the symptoms and subsequent illness are dependent on the amount of viruses shed during the replication phase and the number of respiratory cells affected. Virus shedding usually ends 2 to 5 days after symptoms first appear; therefore, it is important to remember that individuals are infectious for up to 7 to 10 days.

Clinical Manifestations

Clinical manifestations of the flu are more severe than those of a cold and have a rapid onset. They include fever, headache, sore throat, severe nasal congestion, cough, myalgia or muscle aches and pains, malaise (the general feeling of being unwell), and fatigue.

Management

Medical Management
Diagnosis

The diagnostic gold standard for identifying an influenza infection is a sampling of respiratory secretions for viral culture. The most significant drawback to this method is that viral cultures can take up to 10 days to provide confirmation. In emergency departments and outpatient clinics, the most commonly utilized tests for influenza are called **rapid influenza diagnostic tests (RIDTs)**. The identification of an influenza virus infection can be made in less than 30 minutes via nasopharyngeal/throat swab or nasal washings/aspirate. The sensitivity and specificity of RIDTs can be variable depending on the manufacturer's test used and the type of influenza virus circulating during a specific outbreak. Therefore, a negative RIDT does not necessarily mean that there is no influenza infection (a false-negative test). When utilizing an RIDT, clinicians should not make a diagnosis solely on the basis of the test result but should also consider the patient's symptoms and history and rely on their clinical judgment. Accepted influenza testing methods for types A and B are outlined in Table 24.2.

Circulating antibodies can be detected in the blood of individuals with an influenza infection within 2 weeks after initial infection. Specific laboratory tests conducted are hemagglutination inhibition, complement-fixation, and enzyme-linked immunosorbent assay.

Table 24.2 Approved Influenza Testing Methods for Types A and B

Method	Acceptable Specimens	Test Time
Viral cell culture (conventional)	Nasopharyngeal swab/bronchial wash, throat swab, nasal or endotracheal aspirate, sputum	3–10 days
Rapid cell culture	As above	1–3 days
Immunofluorescence, direct or indirect antibody staining	As above	1–4 hours
RT-PCR	As above	Varied; generally 1–6 hours
Rapid influenza diagnostic tests	Nasopharyngeal swab, throat swab, nasal wash, nasal aspirate	Less than 30 minutes

RT-PCR, Reverse transcription polymerase chain reaction.

Treatment

Treatment for influenza illness is directed primarily toward prevention by annual **vaccination**. Inoculation by inactivated influenza viruses that were identified as causing outbreaks the preceding year can provide up to 80% protection from the projected upcoming year's virus. Side effects from vaccinations occur infrequently and consist of low-grade fever and soreness at the injection site. Individuals who have an allergy to eggs should not receive this form of the vaccine because it contains an inactive ingredient of an egg protein. Alternative forms of vaccine (without this protein) are available. The most appropriate time of year for vaccination is in the early fall before the "flu season" begins.

Medications

Medications for the treatment of mild influenza illness are directed toward the relief of symptoms. Antipyretics/analgesics for fever and aches, adequate fluid intake to avoid dehydration, and rest are typically prescribed. For more serious forms of influenza or widespread local outbreaks, several antiviral medications are available for prophylaxis or treatment. The decision to treat flu symptoms utilizing antiviral medications is made on the basis of the severity of the presenting symptoms, such as an illness requiring hospitalization or a severe, complicated illness; the presence of any significant underlying comorbid risk factors; age greater than 65; and pregnancy or recent postpartum. The administration of antiviral medications does not "cure" the flu; however, further viral replication within the respiratory tract is impaired. This reduces the severity and duration of symptoms and plays a key role in preventing the risk of flu-related complications. The best results are achieved when antiviral medications are initiated within 24 to 48 hours of symptom onset. Antiviral medications are described in Table 24.3. Antibiotic preparations should be reserved for documented bacterial infections.

Complications

Primary influenza viral pneumonia is the least common but severest complication of influenza infection and occurs

Table 24.3 Antiviral Medications for the Treatment of Influenza

Antiviral Agent Generic (brand name)	Route	Treatment
Zanamivir (Relenza)	Inhaled	Influenza A and B
Oseltamivir (Tamiflu)	Oral	Influenza A and B
Peramivir (Rapivab)	IV	Influenza A and B
Baloxavir (Xofluza)	Oral	Influenza A and B
Rimantadine (Flumadine)	Oral	Influenza A

more frequently in individuals over the age of 65 years with or without chronic underlying illness. This complication is marked by progressive shortness of breath, persistent fever, and cardiovascular compromise. Dyspnea with negligible sputum production that may be visibly blood-streaked is also associated with the onset of a secondary bacterial pneumonia. Frequent bacterial organisms linked to secondary pneumonia are *Streptococcus pneumoniae*, *Staphylococcus aureus*, and *Haemophilus influenzae*. These organisms are resident "normal flora" within the nasopharynx that become pathologic when the respiratory defenses are altered. Secondary bacterial pneumonia classically presents as improvement in viral symptoms followed by an acute recurrence of symptoms and purulent nasal and tracheal secretions. Sinus and middle ear secondary bacterial infections may also accompany an influenza viral illness.

Nursing Management
Assessment and Analysis

The clinical manifestations observed in the patient with influenza—cough, headache, nasal congestion, sore throat, and fever—are typically the result of the inflammatory response once the virus has invaded the respiratory epithelium.

Nursing Diagnoses

- **Ineffective breathing pattern** related to infection of the lung
- **Decreased activity tolerance** related to hypoxia
- **Alteration in gas exchange—decreased** related to impaired alveolar-capillary interface
- **Fluid volume deficit** related to insensible losses from fever and tachypnea

Nursing Interventions

■ *Assessments*

- Vital signs
  Tachypnea: The body's first compensatory mechanism to a decreased oxygen delivery is increased respiratory rate and depth.
  Tachycardia: The body's second compensatory mechanism for a continued impairment of oxygen delivery is to raise the heart rate.
  Decreased oxygen saturation: Impaired gas exchange at the alveolar level results in hypoxia. Tachypnea and tachycardia decrease cardiac output, reducing perfusion and peripheral oxygen saturation.
  Fever occurs as a part of the inflammatory response.
- Neurological function
  Agitation, restlessness, anxiety, lethargy, and fatigue are the result of decreased tissue perfusion from altered alveolar gas exchange.
- Breath sounds
  Adventitious breath sounds such as rhonchi, crackles, and rales may be audible on lung assessment from fluid and exudates filling the alveoli. Audible wheezing is a result of airway reactivity due to inflammation and/or bronchospasm.
- General appearance
  Sudden onset of fever, chills, muscle aches, and fatigue in a generally ill-appearing patient
- Cough, nasal congestion, sneezing, rhinorrhea
  Primary viral pneumonia from influenza can cause coughing that lasts up to 2 weeks. Secretions that are white in color are consistent with viral infection. Purulent nasal discharge/sputum indicates a secondary bacterial infection.
- Peripheral pulses and skin temperature and color
  Diminished tissue perfusion causes blood to be shunted away from peripheral areas to the main core body organs. Peripheral pulses diminish, and skin becomes moist and pale. Peripheral cyanosis (bluish color to the nailbeds) is a late sign of tissue hypoxia.
- Laboratory values
  Arterial blood gases (ABGs): Primary respiratory infections may initially cause a respiratory alkalosis (increased pH, decreased carbon dioxide [CO_2]) in response to tachypnea. As the condition progresses, a respiratory acidosis (decreased pH, increased carbon dioxide [CO_2]) will develop.
  Positive RIDTs: These tests are sensitive, so a positive test is indicative of the presence of flu, but a negative test needs to be evaluated taking into account the patient's clinical presentation—a potential false negative.

■ *Actions*

- Initiate appropriate **isolation precautions** (Table 24.4).
  *Place patient on **droplet precautions** to avoid viral transmission. Personal protective equipment required includes a mask, gown, gloves, and eye protection if there is a risk of splashing of bodily fluids. The patient should wear a mask when outside the room. Visitors should wear a mask while in the room. A private room is desirable unless patients with similar infections are cohorted.*
- Administer humidified supplemental oxygen
  Improving oxygen delivery, reversing hypoxia, and maintaining moist respiratory mucosa are essential to avoid complications.
- Position patient in semi- to high Fowler's (head of bed raised to 30 degrees)
  Sitting up or elevating the head can provide for the relief of nasal drainage, promoting optimal lung expansion, preventing atelectasis, and preventing aspiration that can lead to secondary bacterial pneumonia.
- Medication administration
  - Administer antipyretics as ordered/indicated.
    Fever reduction can help reduce hyperdynamic effects on the respiratory and cardiovascular systems and increase patient comfort.
  - Administer antiviral medications if ordered/indicated.
    Early administration of antiviral medications (within 24–48 hours of symptom onset) offers the most favorable outcome for shortening the severity and duration of symptoms and decreasing the incidence of respiratory complications in high-risk patient populations.
  - Administer analgesics as ordered/indicated.
    Pain relief can increase comfort and allow for mobilization and effective coughing/expectoration of respiratory secretions.
- Provide adequate fluid intake.
  Replacing insensible losses from fever and tachypnea allows for optimal cardiovascular performance and liquefaction of respiratory secretions.
- Provide adequate nutritional intake.
  Adequate caloric intake is essential for cell recovery. Frequent small meals high in protein are recommended.
- Obtain cultures (nasal swabs, throat swabs, sputum, blood, and urine) before the administration of antiviral medications.
  To assess for the presence of bacterial infection before presence is masked by medication administration

■ *Teaching*

- Practice good hand hygiene.
  Hand washing is essential to prevent the spread of the virus to others.
- Disinfect frequently used objects and surfaces.
  Household cleaning products or soap and warm water are sufficient. Hospital-approved cleaners are to be used to disinfect horizontal surfaces during inpatient care.
- Limit contact with others for up to 10 days after the first symptoms appear or for at least 24 hours after fever has gone.
  Viral shedding continues from 10 days up to several weeks.

Table 24.4 CDC Isolation Precautions

Transmission-Based Precautions	Recommendation
General Principles	
	In addition to standard precautions, use transmission-based precautions for patients with documented or suspected infection or colonization with highly transmissible or epidemiologically important pathogens for which additional precautions are needed to prevent transmission.
Contact Precautions	
Patient placement	In acute care hospitals, place patients who require contact precautions in a single-patient room when available. When single-patient rooms are in short supply: ● Prioritize patients with conditions that may facilitate transmission (e.g., uncontained drainage, stool incontinence) for single-patient room placement. ● Place together in the same room (cohort) patients who are infected or colonized with the same pathogen and are suitable roommates.
Use of personal protective equipment (PPE)	Gloves, Gowns Discontinue contact precautions after signs and symptoms of the infection have resolved or according to pathogen-specific recommendations.
Droplet Precautions	Use droplet precautions as recommended for patients known or suspected to be infected with pathogens transmitted by respiratory droplets (i.e., large-particle droplets >5μ in size) that are generated by a patient who is coughing, sneezing, or talking.
Patient placement	In *acute care hospitals,* place patients who require droplet precautions in a single-patient room when available. When single-patient rooms are in short supply: Prioritize patients who have excessive cough and sputum production for single-patient room placement. Place together in the same room (cohort) patients who are infected with the same pathogen and are suitable roommates.
Use of PPE	Don a mask upon entry into the patient room or cubicle If transport is necessary, instruct patient to wear a mask. No mask is required for persons transporting patients on droplet precautions. Discontinue droplet precautions after signs and symptoms have resolved or according to pathogen-specific recommendations.
Airborne Precautions	Use airborne precautions as recommended for patients known or suspected to be infected with infectious agents transmitted from person to person by the airborne route.
Patient placement	In *acute care hospitals* and *long-term care settings,* place patients who require airborne precautions in an airborne infection isolation room (AIIR) that has direct exhaust of air to the outside or where the air is directed through high-efficiency particulate air (HEPA) filters.
Use of PPE	Wear a fit-tested N95 or higher-level respirator for respiratory protection. If transport or movement outside an AIIR is necessary, instruct patients to wear a surgical mask. Discontinue airborne precautions according to pathogen-specific recommendations.

From Centers for Disease Control and Prevention. (2007). *Isolation precautions.* Retrieved from https://www.cdc.gov/infectioncontrol/guidelines/isolation/index.html#5

- Report worsening shortness of breath; change in amount, color, and viscosity of pulmonary secretions; and recurrent fever.

  Viral infections can be mild at first, rapidly progressing to primary viral pneumonia or secondary bacterial pneumonia.

- Maintain adequate fluid intake.

  Insensible losses from tachypnea and fever can lead to dehydration and thickening of pulmonary secretions with difficult expectoration.

- Perform medication teaching for expected/desired effects, potential side effects, and expected duration of treatment.

  Take antiviral medications if they are prescribed for you. Make sure to take all of the medication—even if you begin to feel better. Explain that the addition of antibiotics may become necessary for the occurrence of a secondary bacterial infection.

  Antiviral medications do not "cure" the flu; they just shorten the duration and severity of symptoms and may prevent serious complications. The antiviral choice should be based on local community patterns and susceptibility.

- Be sure to get a flu vaccination every year.

  Vaccination is the best method of preventing the flu. As part of the national hospital performance measures, the Centers for Medicare and Medicaid Services (CMS) and The Joint Commission require all inpatients to be screened for the influenza vaccine and offered the vaccine prior to discharge if appropriate.

Evaluating Care Outcomes

Influenza may be avoided with flu vaccination. Mild cases of influenza usually resolve without complications. Indicators of resolving viral influenza infection are vital signs within the patient's normal limits, absence of fever for 24 hours after completion of antiviral medications (if prescribed), even and unlabored respirations, oxygen saturation above 92% or return to patient's baseline without oxygen administration, absence of nasal drainage, no sputum production, and a clear chest x-ray.

Connection Check 24.1

The nurse understands adequate teaching has been done by which of the following statements?

A. "I got a flu shot last year; I'm covered for a while."

B. "I don't need a flu shot; I never get sick."

C. "I guess it's important to get a flu shot every year."

D. "I don't get a flu shot, but I make sure my kids get one."

PNEUMONIA

Epidemiology

Infectious pneumonia can occur at any time and in individuals of any age. According to the CDC, in the United States, there are approximately 3 to 4 million cases reported annually. One-third of these cases occur in persons over 65 years of age. The National Center for Health Statistics reports that older individuals (over 65 years) are at higher risk of death from respiratory infections. Nearly 90% of deaths are in this age group, but pneumonia is also responsible for 16% of deaths in children under age 5. Overall, approximately 60,000 deaths are attributable to pneumonia each year. Pneumonia remains among the most frequent conditions for which the death rate has not significantly declined over the past decade.

Key risk factors for the development of pneumonia among the adult population include but are not limited to advanced age; long-term care residence; smoking; chronic respiratory disease (asthma, emphysema); immune system dysfunction (malignancy, transplantation, HIV/AIDS); altered mental status; prolonged immobility; aspiration of stomach contents or foreign material; prolonged nothing-by-mouth (NPO) status; diminished cough, gag, and/or swallow reflexes; exposure to air pollutants, gases, or noxious inhalants; and hospitalization for longer than 48 hours.

Pneumonia can be classified into several types: community-acquired pneumonia (CAP), methicillin-resistant *Staphylococcus aureus* (MRSA) community-acquired pneumonia (MRSA CAP), hospital-acquired pneumonia (HAP), and healthcare-associated pneumonia (HCAP). Table 24.5 describes the classifications and common causative organisms.

Community-acquired pneumonia occurs in individuals who have not been recently hospitalized or are living outside of a healthcare/long-term care facility. *Streptococcus pneumoniae* is the most common causative organism. Few clinical studies have been able to confirm MRSA as a frequent cause of CAP; however, the data to date may indicate that incidence is escalating. Methicillin-resistant CAP results from colonization of MRSA within the upper respiratory tract. This can produce mild, virtually asymptomatic illness that is customarily treated on an outpatient basis with oral antibiotics. Healthy individuals with no existing risk

Table 24.5	**Pneumonia Classifications and Common Causative Organisms**	
Community Acquired	**Hospital Acquired**	**Healthcare Associated**
Streptococcus pneumoniae	*Pseudomonas aeruginosa*	*Staphylococcus aureus*
Mycoplasma pneumoniae	*S. aureus*	Methicillin-resistant *S. aureus*
Haemophilus influenzae	*Klebsiella pneumoniae*	
Legionella	*Escherichia coli*	*P. aeruginosa*
Methicillin-resistant *S. aureus*	*Enterobacter* sp.	*H. influenzae*
Chlamydia pneumoniae		

factors for MRSA colonization are most frequently diagnosed with MRSA CAP after experiencing a viral illness.

Hospital-acquired pneumonia develops in patients after 48 hours of hospital admission. The diagnosis of healthcare-associated pneumonia is made 48 to 72 hours after admission and is accompanied by the following risk factors:

- Recent antibiotic therapy
- Receiving immunosuppressive therapy
- Diagnosed with a chronic disease
- Treated within healthcare facilities, such as dialysis clinics, adult daycare centers, and rehabilitation facilities, where they are in frequent, close contact with healthcare personnel and other patients who may be colonized with various infection-causing organisms

Pneumonia caused by atypical organisms is often associated with mild respiratory illness. The inability to identify them by culture or Gram staining is what makes them atypical. Examples of atypical organisms are *Mycoplasma*, *Chlamydophila* (from handling birds), *Legionella* (present in intricate water delivery systems), and *Bordetella pertussis* (responsible for whooping cough).

Connection Check 24.2

The correct statement about the prevalence of pneumonia is which of the following?
A. Pneumonia is no longer a major health problem.
B. The prevalence of pneumonia is increasing dramatically.
C. The prevalence and mortality are highest in persons older than 65 years.
D. The frequency has not declined, but mortality has declined.

Pathophysiology

Pneumonia is an inflammation of the lung **parenchyma** (functional lung tissue) resulting from a bacterial, viral, or fungal infection. Organisms enter the respiratory tract through inhalation of infected droplets or aspiration from the oropharynx. They evade the protective mechanisms of the respiratory tract and initiate the inflammatory process. The respiratory protective mechanisms become either ineffective or overwhelmed. An inflammatory cascade of events is initiated in response to the offending pathogen. Inflammatory mediators stimulate the production and release of neutrophils and macrophages that travel to the site of infection. Organisms continue to proliferate at the alveolar level. As the inflammatory response unfolds, protein-rich fluid and exudates fill the alveoli, impairing the exchange of oxygen and CO_2. A ventilation–perfusion mismatch results from adequate blood flow to a nonfunctioning, fluid-filled alveolar unit.

Organisms can localize to one or more lobes (**lobar** or multilobar pneumonia) or spread throughout the lung

parenchyma, resulting in the diffuse location of organisms (Figs. 24.2A and B). Bacteria causing pneumococcal pneumonia (*S. pneumoniae*) can gain access to the bloodstream, leading to septicemia and septic shock. Elderly individuals over the age of 65 years or those with chronic illness are at high risk for mortality from contracting this bacterial organism.

Clinical Manifestations

The clinical manifestations produced by the inflammatory response can vary from mild to severe and include:

- Fever
- Tachypnea/dyspnea
- Tachycardia
- Chills
- Cough, productive or nonproductive
- Pleuritic chest pain
- Fatigue
- Myalgia/arthralgia

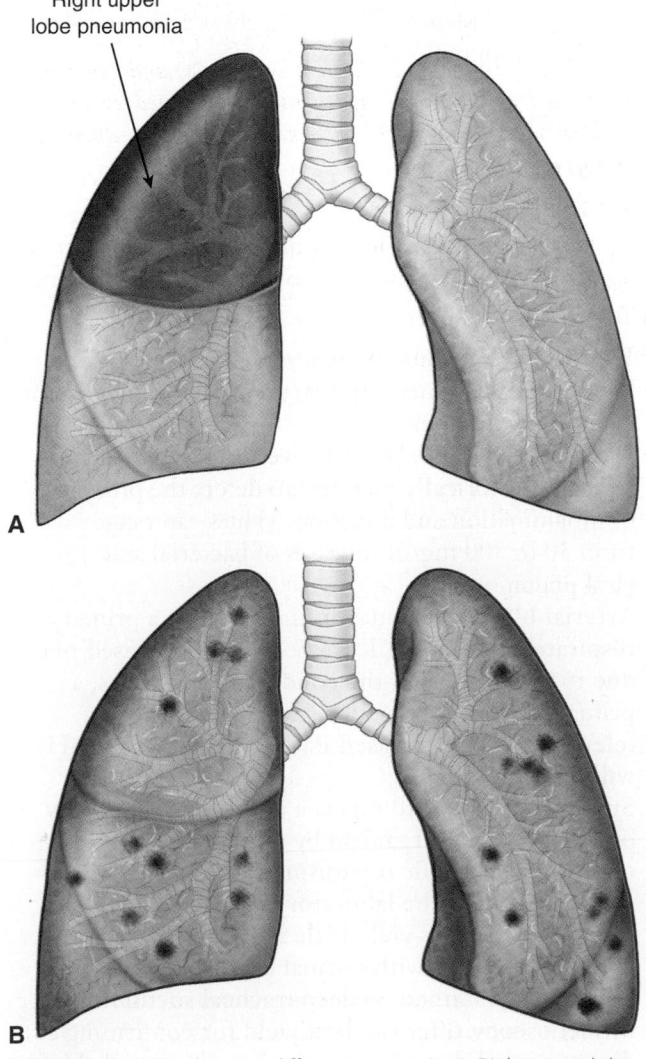

Right upper lobe pneumonia

FIGURE 24.2 Localizing or diffuse pneumonia. A, Right upper lobe lobar pneumonia. B, Diffuse pneumonia.

In more severe forms, additional manifestations can be:

- Purulent or blood-streaked sputum
- Hypotension
- Dysrhythmias

Awareness of the clinical manifestations and predictors of increased mortality is essential to help ensure the speedy identification and treatment of pneumonia. Validated clinical predictors of increased mortality and morbidity from severe infectious pneumonia include:

1. Altered mental status
2. Respiratory rate greater than 30 breaths per minute
3. Hypotension (systolic blood pressure less than 90 mm Hg)
4. Heart rate greater than 125 beats per minute
5. Body temperature less than 95°F (35°C) or greater than 104°F (40°C)
6. Arterial blood pH less than 7.35
7. Serum sodium level less than 130 mg/dL
8. Hematocrit less than 30%
9. PaO_2 less than 60 mm Hg on supplemental oxygen greater than or equal to 40%
10. Presence of pleural effusion on chest x-ray or computed tomography (CT) scan

Management

Medical Management

Diagnosis

Diagnosis is based on laboratory and imaging studies. Laboratory findings consistent with the diagnosis of pneumonia include:

- Elevated WBC count (leukocytosis) with elevated bands (immature neutrophils) on differential indicating acute inflammation
- Elevated C-reactive protein level, an accurate, sensitive, and historically used test to detect the presence of inflammation and infection. Values can range from 30 to 300 mg/dL in cases of bacterial and viral pneumonia.
- Arterial blood gases may initially reflect a primary respiratory alkalosis (decreased CO_2, increased pH) due to tachypnea. As the condition progresses, a primary respiratory acidosis with hypoxemia (elevated CO_2, decreased PaO_2, and decreased pH) will occur.
- Sputum cultures will reveal a preliminary category of the offending organism by Gram stain and confirm the specific organism after 24 to 48 hours of incubation in the laboratory. Expectorated sputum specimens yield little information because of contamination with normal oral bacteria. Specimens obtained by deep tracheal suctioning or bronchoscopy offer the best yield for confirming a diagnosis and directing the choice of antimicrobial management.

Imaging studies reveal:

- Chest x-rays may or may not show infiltrates and can be up to 72 hours behind in their ability to reveal an infectious process.
- Computed tomography scans of the chest may better demonstrate **consolidation** (solidification of lung tissue) and the presence of pleural effusions.

As noted previously with clinical manifestations, prompt diagnosis is essential in providing timely and effective treatment.

Treatment

The treatment of pneumonia is dependent on the type of pneumonia, an early diagnosis, and the overall health of the patient. Uncomplicated pneumonias can be effectively treated in the outpatient setting. More severe cases require hospitalization and supportive care. Because pneumonia may result in hypoxia, administration of oxygen to reverse or prevent hypoxia is an essential first step. In the case of patients with chronic lung pathology, high concentrations of oxygen can depress the drive to breathe. Those patients require careful monitoring while receiving oxygen. Ensuring adequate hydration is also an important intervention to support the patient's cardiovascular status and assist in thinning respiratory secretions for easy expectoration.

Medications

Bronchodilator therapy with albuterol (short-acting selective beta-2 adrenoceptor agonist) or Combivent (slow-onset anticholinergic agent) delivered either by aerosol nebulization or by metered-dose inhaler will open swollen and narrowed airways and promote ease of breathing.

Antibiotic therapy, the definitive treatment, is based on the offending organism, and initially, broad-spectrum antibiotics are initiated promptly. For HAP, antibiotic treatment is empiric—treatment based on clinical experience before the exact offending organism is identified. Because *Pseudomonas aeruginosa* is the major pathogen associated with HAP, initial treatment is focused on that organism. Specific antibiotic recommendations for the treatment of CAP, HCAP, and HAP are outlined in Table 24.6.

Complications

Severe MRSA CAP can lead to a necrotizing bacterial pneumonia requiring hospitalization. In aspiration pneumonia, the acidity of stomach contents is caustic to the delicate lung tissue. A necrotizing pneumonia may develop, resulting in fibrosis and scarring of the lung tissue. Pulmonary fibrosis and pulmonary hypertension from severe pulmonary infections can impair lung function after the respiratory infection resolves. Most antibiotics do not cross the blood–brain barrier, making the central nervous system a potential site of bacterial spread via the bloodstream. Acute meningitis can occur as a complication of a pneumococcal pneumonia.

Table 24.6 Recommended Antimicrobial Treatment for Community-Acquired Pneumonia

Patient Assessment	Recommended Antimicrobials
Outpatients	
● Previously healthy	
● No antibiotics within the past 3 months	Macrolides or doxycycline
● Comorbidities	Respiratory fluoroquinolones OR
● Have received antibiotics within the past 3 months	β-Lactam antibiotics and a macrolide
Inpatients (all)	Respiratory fluoroquinolones OR β-Lactam and a macrolide If CAMRSA: add vancomycin or linezolid

An empyema, a collection of purulent material in the pleural space, another possible complication, should be drained by the insertion of a chest tube. Pleurodesis, the injection of a sclerosing or scarring agent into the pleural space, causing the visceral and parietal pleura to "stick together," may be performed after the empyema has been resolved to prevent recurrence.

Other significant complications that can develop as a result of pneumonia include bacteremia (bacteria in the bloodstream); atelectasis, a complete or partial collapse of the lung more typically seen in the postoperative or immobile patient; septic shock; and acute respiratory failure with multiple organ failure. Evidence of organ impairment/failure due to decreased tissue perfusion includes:

- Agitation/confusion: It is important to stress that this may be the only presenting sign/symptom in those over 65 years of age.
- Peripheral cyanosis
- Central cyanosis
- Decreased urinary output/elevated creatinine level
- Hypoactive bowel sounds
- Increased liver function laboratory values (aspartate aminotransferase/alanine aminotransferase)

Nursing Management
Assessment and Analysis

The clinical manifestations in the patient with pneumonia result from the initiation of the inflammatory response and the buildup of fluid and exudate in the alveoli. They include fever; the deterioration of oxygenation, resulting in tachypnea and tachycardia; and the resultant decreases in cardiac output. This decrease in oxygen delivery results in shunting blood away from the periphery, producing weak and thready pulses. Exudate and excess secretions in the lungs and alveoli result in adventitious breath sounds such as wheezing, rhonchi, and rales.

Nursing Diagnoses

- Ineffective peripheral tissue perfusion related to decreased gas exchange
- Ineffective breathing pattern
- Impaired gas exchange
- Risk for acute confusion

Nursing Interventions

■ **Assessments**

- Vital signs
  Tachypnea: The body's first compensatory mechanism to a decreased oxygen delivery is increased respiratory rate and depth.
  Tachycardia: The body's second compensatory mechanism for a continued impairment of oxygen delivery is to raise the heart rate.
  Decreased oxygen saturation: Impaired gas exchange at the alveolar level results in hypoxia. Tachypnea and tachycardia decrease cardiac output, reducing perfusion and peripheral oxygen saturation.
  Fever occurs as a part of the inflammatory response.
- Neurological function
  Agitation, restlessness, anxiety, lethargy, and fatigue are the result of decreased tissue perfusion from altered alveolar gas exchange.
  Diminished cough, gag, and swallow reflexes resulting from altered levels of consciousness can contribute to aspiration risk.
- Breath sounds
  Adventitious breath sounds such as wheezing, rhonchi, crackles, and rales may be audible on lung assessment as a result of bronchospasm and/or fluid and exudates filling the alveoli.
- Peripheral pulses and skin temperature and color
  Diminished tissue perfusion causes blood to be shunted away from peripheral areas to the main core body organs. Peripheral pulses diminish, and skin becomes moist and pale. Peripheral cyanosis (bluish color to the nailbeds) is a late sign of tissue hypoxia.
- Respiratory secretions
  Purulent and/or bloody secretions may result from a buildup of exudate in the alveoli.
- Laboratory testing
  - Sputum microbiology
    Culture and sensitivity reports indicate the offending organism and list the antibiotics to which the organism is sensitive.
  - Arterial blood gases
    Bacterial respiratory infections may initially cause primary respiratory alkalosis (increased pH, decreased CO_2) due to increased respiratory rate. As the condition progresses, a primary respiratory acidosis will occur (decreased pH, increased CO_2).
- Intake and Output
  Insensible losses from fever and tachypnea along with decreased intake from malaise and increased work of breathing can lead to more serious tachycardia and dehydration.

▪ Actions

- Administer humidified oxygen as ordered.
  Oxygen administration helps maintain adequate oxygen levels. Humidification of respiratory tract mucous membranes helps liquefy secretions to facilitate expectoration. Careful administration should be given to the patient with chronic lung pathology in whom the drive to breathe comes from decreased oxygen levels.
- Administer antibiotics as ordered.
  Prompt administration of antibiotics to defeat the offending organism is the definitive treatment of choice.
- Pulmonary hygiene:
  - Incentive spirometry
  - Coughing and deep breathing
  - Postural drainage
  - Vibration/percussion
  - Early mobility
    Pulmonary hygiene is done in an effort to mobilize respiratory secretions and allow expectoration. This reduces the incidence of atelectasis and worsening pneumonia in hospitalized patients.
- Patient positioning
  Elevating the head of the bed to 30 degrees prevents aspiration of colonized nasopharyngeal secretions and gastric contents and facilitates lung expansion. Side-to-side turning assists with alveolar recruitment strategies to ensure maximum ventilation–perfusion.
  For infiltrates of only one lung, when turning, preferentially position patient with the good lung down to maximize perfusion to the functional alveolar units.
- Monitor intake and output.
  Optimal fluid balance assists with thinning respiratory secretions for ease of expectoration and maintains adequate tissue perfusion/oxygenation.
- Ensure adequate nutritional support.
  Adequate caloric intake is necessary for cellular recovery. Small, frequent meals that are high in protein and vitamins are recommended. Assess cough, gag, and swallow reflexes prior to offering food and drink. If reflexes are impaired, maintaining NPO status or initiating enteral feedings via feeding tube may be required until a formal swallow evaluation can be obtained and the degree of aspiration risk can be determined.
- Activity grouping
  Approach activities of care with intervals of rest. Fatigue and decreased tissue oxygen delivery limit activity tolerance.

▪ Teaching

- Hand hygiene and respiratory etiquette
  Frequent and effective hand washing is the most effective method for minimizing the spread of infectious organisms. Proper use and disposal of tissues for sneezing and coughing are also important.
- Encourage adequate rest.
  Introduce strategies to combat fatigue and conserve energy.

- Take antibiotics as prescribed; stress the importance of finishing all medication even if patients begin to feel better.
  Antibiotics offer a "cure" for bacterial infections. Incomplete treatment can lead to a recurrence of symptoms and the emergence of drug-resistant organisms.
- Encourage proper nutrition and fluid intake.
  Adequate nutrition is essential for healing and recovery from respiratory infections. Sufficient fluid intake can thin secretions for easy expectoration.
- Understanding of signs and symptoms indicating worsening respiratory status; how and where to seek medical attention
  Patients and families should be able to verbalize a clear understanding of which signs and symptoms indicate the need to seek medical attention.
- Encourage "at-risk" patients to get a pneumonia vaccine annually.
  Vaccination affords the best protection against future illness from pneumonia. As part of the national hospital performance measures, the CMS and The Joint Commission require all inpatients to be screened for the pneumonia vaccine and offered the vaccine prior to discharge if appropriate.

Evaluating Care Outcomes

Patients with mild cases of bacterial pneumonia are successfully managed as outpatients on oral antibiotic regimens. Most patients with pneumonia requiring hospitalization fully recover from their illness and are discharged without complications. A well-managed patient recovering from bacterial pneumonia will demonstrate stable vital signs, absence of fever for 24 hours after completion of antibiotic therapy, unlabored breathing, oxygen saturation above 92% (or return to patient's baseline) without the use of oxygen therapy, absence of cough/sputum production, and clear chest x-ray with increased energy levels and activity tolerance.

CASE STUDY: EPISODE 2

Mr. Markham's chest x-ray shows suspicious cavitating lesions. He is admitted to the medical unit with suspicion of TB. He is immediately put in isolation on airborne precautions. His temperature, heart rate, and respiratory rate remain elevated at 38°C (100.5°F), 100 bpm, and 24, respectively. His oxygen saturation decreases to 90%. He is started on oxygen via a face mask. An IV line is inserted, and IV fluids are started. Sputum and blood cultures are sent to the laboratory…

TUBERCULOSIS

Epidemiology

Tuberculosis (TB) is a significant and potentially life-threatening respiratory infection caused by the organism

Mycobacterium tuberculosis, an aerobic acid-fast bacillus (AFB). Tuberculosis infects one-third of the world's population. The CDC monitors the prevalence of TB in the United States and reported 9,093 new cases of TB (2.8/100,000 persons) in the United States in 2017, which represents a 1.8% decline from 2016, the smallest decline in 10 years. The majority of these new cases occurring in the United States were caused by reactivated latent tuberculosis infection (LTBI). Populations living outside of the United States, low socioeconomic groups that have obstacles in accessing healthcare, and racial and ethnic minorities have the highest incidence. Tuberculosis disproportionately affects blacks, Hispanics, and Asians. Tuberculosis is also a persistent problem in the homeless and incarcerated populations. Persons infected with HIV or who have AIDS are at exceptional risk of contracting TB or reactivating latent TB. This population poses a particular concern because of the extent of immunosuppression and the risk of contracting and spreading new strains of drug-resistant TB (MDR TB). An estimated 11 million people with HIV (one-third of the HIV population) are infected with *M. tuberculosis*. Tuberculosis is the leading killer of people with HIV infection.

Pathophysiology and Clinical Manifestations

Mycobacterium tuberculosis is typically transmitted by aerosolized droplets inhaled from the coughing or sneezing of an infected individual. Droplets of *M. tuberculosis* are tiny and can remain suspended in the air for several hours. Focused studies documenting transmission of active **tubercule** bacilli have shown that in close-contact situations, those whose sputum is infected with AFB are most likely to transmit the infection. It is estimated that up to 3,000 infectious nucleated droplets can be released in one cough. After the small infected droplets are inhaled, most of the bacilli remain within the upper airway and rarely cause active disease. Bacilli that manage to evade the mucociliary escalator defense are deposited within the alveoli and are quickly engulfed by phagocytic pulmonary macrophages. Once they are ingested by the macrophages, there is a slow but continued multiplication of the *Mycobacterium*. Tuberculosis is classified as follows:

- Latent tuberculosis infection (LTBI)
- Primary tuberculosis infection (PTBI)
- Primary progressive TB infection (PPTBI)
- Drug-resistant *M. tuberculosis* (MDR TB)

Latent Tuberculosis Infection

In those individuals with an intact immune system, a granuloma forms and limits further proliferation and spread of the *Mycobacterium*. Necrosis at the center of the granuloma leads to fibrosis and calcification. A calcified granuloma evident on chest x-ray is a classic sign of the type of TB termed **latent tuberculosis infection (LTBI)**. The inactive bacilli remain dormant within the

healed granuloma. Patients with LTBI have no symptoms, do not feel ill, and are not contagious. As long as the immune system remains intact, the bacilli remain in the healed tissue of the granuloma for the individual's lifetime and do not progress to TB infection. It is only when the immune system becomes compromised that the disease can become reactivated. The most common factors associated with reactivation are HIV infection, long-term diabetes, chronic renal disease, long-term steroid administration, sepsis, and malnutrition.

Primary Tuberculosis Infection

Individuals with a weakened immune response are unable to control the multiplication of *Mycobacterium*. Granuloma formation is initiated but is unable to progress to calcification and results in a **primary tuberculosis infection (PTBI)**. Primary TB infection is often asymptomatic and is confirmed only by positive sputum cultures and a positive skin test. This person is not infectious.

Symptomatic TB Infection

Symptomatic TB infection, referred to as **primary progressive TB infection (PPTBI)**, develops in a very small percentage of individuals who have been exposed to the bacterium. Initial symptoms are relatively nonspecific and consist of fatigue, weight loss, and night sweats. A cough develops eventually and produces a rusty-colored or blood-streaked sputum. As the disease progresses, dyspnea, orthopnea, and rales become evident.

Drug-Resistant Mycobacterium Tuberculosis

Drug-resistant *M. tuberculosis* (MDR TB) can be mono-drug or poly-drug resistant. This means that one or more of the first-line medications used for the treatment of TB are not effective. Drug-resistant TB can be caused by primary or secondary means. Primary resistance is caused by person-to-person transmission of the resistant organism. Secondary (acquired) resistant TB develops during treatment and results from an ineffective treatment regimen or an incomplete treatment regimen.

Management

Medical Management

Diagnosis

The diagnosis of TB infection is made by laboratory testing, a skin test, and chest x-ray. Laboratory testing consists of a sputum test for culture and acid-fast staining. Suspicious cavitating lesions (resulting from pathologic processes leading to necrosis and formation of a "gas-filled" space within the lung tissue) are seen on chest x-rays. The skin test is a positive purified protein derivative (PPD) screen skin test, also called a **Mantoux test**. The Mantoux tuberculin skin test is the standard method for determining if an individual is infected with the TB-causing organism. The test is administered by injecting 0.1 mL of PPD intradermally into the tissue of the forearm. Within 48 to 72 hours after injection, the administration site should be observed for any reaction (Table 24.7).

Individuals who have received a bacille Calmette–Guérin (BCG) immunization may show a false-positive PPD when not infected with the TB bacteria. Further testing in these individuals is required, such as a chest x-ray and/or blood testing using an interferon gamma release assay (IGRA). There are currently two IRGAs approved for use by the U.S. Food and Drug Administration (FDA): QuantiFERON®-TB Gold In-Tube (QTF-GIT) and T-SPOT® TB test (T-SPOT). These blood tests can determine if an individual has been infected with TB bacteria. A negative result indicates unlikely TB infection. A positive test confirms TB infection, and further work-up is necessary to establish whether the infection is latent TB or TB disease.

Treatment

According to the American Thoracic Society, the CDC, and the Infectious Diseases Society of America, the goals of treatment for TB infection are (1) to cure the patient and (2) to minimize the transmission of *M. tuberculosis* to other persons. A basic four-drug combination is recommended for the treatment of TB and should continue for 9 to 12 months (Table 24.8). The basic recommended treatment for TB is broadly applicable, but modifications may be necessary in special circumstances, such as HIV+, pregnancy, drug resistance, and children.

⚠ Safety Alert Immediate isolation of the patient with suspected or confirmed TB infection in a private room with negative airflow capabilities is a priority. Negative airflow occurs when air moves into the contaminated area or into the patient's room from bordering areas. The institution of **airborne precautions**, the use of an N95 mask respirator for healthcare personnel entering the patient's room (requires fit-testing), and a snug-fitting surgical mask for visitors are essential interventions. The patient's movement and transportation to other departments should be limited to essential needs only. Patients who must leave the negative-pressure room should also wear a surgical mask.

Complications

Extensive respiratory tissue destruction by *M. tuberculosis* can lead to respiratory failure, bronchopleural fistula formation (an abnormal pathway or sinus tract that develops between the bronchus and pleural space), and pleural effusions (collections of fluid in the pleural space). Untreated active TB can spread to parts of the body outside the respiratory system via the bloodstream and lymph circulation. Extrapulmonary TB can present as meningitis, lymphadenopathy, bone disease, and liver and kidney failure.

Connection Check 24.3

The nurse understands that the priority intervention with the patient with TB is which of the following?
A. Antibiotic administration
B. Initiation of isolation
C. TB test
D. Chest x-ray

Nursing Management

Assessment and Analysis

Unexplained weight loss, night sweats, fever, and chills are seen as a result of the inflammatory response, specifically the body's attempt to interact with the *Mycobacterium*. The *Mycobacterium* itself may also release fever-causing signals. Rusty-colored sputum occurs as a result of the destruction of lung tissue during granuloma formation. Tissue fragility and microbleeds result. The collection of WBCs presents in an attempt to wall off the infection, resulting in the production of sputum. Pleuritic chest pain is a result of chronic coughing.

Nursing Diagnoses

- **Ineffective airway clearance**
- **Alteration in gas exchange** related to necrosis of lung tissue
- **Alteration in comfort**: pain related to pleurisy
- **Ineffective coping** related to isolation and long-term therapy

Nursing Interventions

■ Assessments

- Oxygen saturation
  Decreased oxygen saturation occurs with the destruction of lung tissue, lessening the available surface area for air exchange.
- Temperature
  Fever is a result of the inflammatory process.
- Sputum
  Blood-tinged or rusty-colored sputum is present as a result of the destruction of lung parenchyma tissue.
- Breath sounds
  Wheezing from irritated airways; rales and rhonchi from fluid/exudates

■ Actions

- Humidified oxygen
  Humidified oxygen helps ensure adequate oxygen delivery to the tissues and maintains the integrity of the mucous membranes.
- Institute airborne isolation (see Table 24.4).
  Tuberculosis is an extremely contagious disease. Care must be taken to avoid transmission to other individuals, especially other hospitalized individuals with an increased risk for infection.

Table 24.7 Classification of Tuberculin Skin Test Reactions

5 mm or Greater	10 mm or Greater	15 mm or Greater
An **induration of 5 mm or greater** is considered positive in: • HIV-infected persons • A person having recent contact with a person with TB • Persons with fibrotic changes on chest radiography consistent with prior TB • Persons who are immunosuppressed including those with organ transplants	An **induration of 10 mm or greater** is considered positive in: • Recent immigrants from high-prevalence countries • IV drug abusers • Residents and employees of high-risk settings • Mycobacteriology laboratory personnel • Persons with clinical conditions that place them at high risk • Children younger than 4 years • Infants, children, and adolescents exposed to adults in high-risk categories	An **induration of 15 mm or greater** is considered positive in any person, including persons with no known risk factors for TB.

Adapted from Centers for Disease Control and Prevention. (2016). *Tuberculosis (TB) fact sheet.* Retrieved from http://www.cdc.gov/tb/publications/factsheets/testing/skintesting.htm

TB, tuberculosis.

Table 24.8 Recommended Tuberculosis Treatment Regimens

Initial Daily Treatment	Isoniazid	Rifampin	Pyrazinamide	Ethambutol
New infection/culture +	Daily dose × 2 months, then 4 additional months	Daily dose × 2 months, then 4 additional months	Daily dose × 2 months	Daily dose × 2 months
New infection/culture –	Daily dose × 2 months, then 2 additional months	Daily dose × 2 months, then 2 additional months	Daily dose × 2 months	Daily dose × 2 months
Isoniazid resistance	—	Daily dose × 6 months	Daily dose × 6 months	Daily dose × 6 months

• Administer antibiotics as ordered.
  Antibiotics are the definitive treatment for TB and are essential in controlling the spread of the disease.
• Ensure adequate nutrition.
  Adequate caloric intake to maintain optimum body weight is necessary for recovery. Often, patients report substantial weight loss during the time prior to diagnosis.

▪ Teaching

• Stress the importance of skin/blood testing for individuals living with or exposed to the infected person.
  Skin/blood testing helps monitor the spread of TB and ensures prompt treatment if necessary. TB is a reportable disease and is tracked by local, state, and federal health authorities. Healthcare providers are obligated to notify local health departments of an identified TB infection so that an investigation of contacts can be initiated and any positive TB infections can be identified and treated.

• Ensure that the patient and family understand the importance of completing all medications.
  Treatment for those who have become infected is necessary to prevent the spread of the disease and prevent complications that can occur from nontreatment. Incomplete treatment or interruptions in treatment can cause the emergence of drug-resistant forms of the bacterium. Directly observed therapy (DOT) may be necessary to ensure adherence.
• Assess the patient's support systems and community resources that will ensure successful adherence to the treatment plan after discharge.
  Early involvement of family, the medical team, and case management will provide the best support for the patient to comply with the established long-term treatment plan.

Evaluating Care Outcomes

The successful treatment of the patient with TB requires early detection and a comprehensive, interprofessional structure that addresses the clinical, psychosocial, environmental, and financial issues. Because of the long treatment period, patients need to be encouraged to follow the prescribed plan of care after discharge into the community (see Transitional Care). Indicators of resolving TB infection are the ability of the patient to gain and maintain a stable body weight, improved skin turgor and muscle tone, absence of cough and sputum production, even and unlabored breathing, and the cessation of fevers and night sweats.

Transitional Care

Tuberculosis

Once the patient with tuberculosis (TB) has been stabilized and has started therapy, treatment can continue at home. National TB treatment guidelines strongly recommend using **directly observed therapy (DOT)** when treating persons with active TB disease. Directly observed therapy is in place when a trained healthcare worker, home healthcare nurse, aide, or designated and trained individual provides the prescribed TB medications and watches the patient swallow every dose. Family members are typically excluded from this role. A recent study indicates that the use of mobile applications for "video" DOT is showing promise. The patient remains on home isolation, receiving periodic sputum cultures to determine the effectiveness of treatment. The need for home isolation may last up to 6 weeks depending on the patient's response to therapy.

Making Connections

CASE STUDY: WRAP-UP

Mr. Harold Markham is admitted to the medical unit with the diagnosis of TB. He remains in a private negative airflow room on strict isolation and airborne precautions. He is started on the four-drug combination therapy recommended for treatment of TB. He will stay on this drug therapy for 9 to 12 months. It is suspected that he was exposed to TB at the HIV clinic where he volunteers. Centers for Disease Control and Prevention personnel are alerted and sent to screen patients and staff at the clinic.

Case Study Questions

1. Which statement is correct related to isolation and airborne precautions for Mr. Markham?
   A. Mr. Markham should wear a mask at all times.
   B. Staff entering the room should wear a surgical mask.
   C. Visitors entering the room should wear an N95 mask respirator.
   D. Staff entering the room should wear an N95 mask respirator.

2. The nurse should question which order concerning Mr. Markham's care?
   A. Humidified oxygen via nasal cannula
   B. NPO
   C. Vital signs with oxygen saturation every 4 hours
   D. Activity as tolerated

3. Mr. Markham's TB can be characterized as which type of infection?
   A. An LTBI
   B. A PTBI
   C. A symptomatic, noncontagious TB infection
   D. A symptomatic TB infection

4. Which statement demonstrates adequate teaching has been done?
   A. "Wow! I'm going to be on these drugs for a long time!"
   B. "I can stop taking the drugs when I feel better."
   C. "My family doesn't need to wear a mask when they come to visit."
   D. "I'm looking forward to going down to the cafeteria to get something to eat."

5. What symptoms indicate a resolving TB infection? *(Select all that apply.)*
   A. Decreased sputum production
   B. Productive cough
   C. Stable body weight
   D. Fevers only at night
   E. Cessation of night sweats

CHAPTER SUMMARY

The human respiratory system has its own innate protective mechanisms to prevent infectious respiratory illness. When these mechanisms become overwhelmed or are impaired, viral, bacterial, and fungal infections occur. The patients at greatest risk for infectious airway disorders are the very young and those over 65 years of age, most often as a result of underlying chronic illnesses of the respiratory, cardiovascular, endocrine, and immune systems.

Clinical manifestations of infectious airway disorders can cause mild to severe symptoms, can occur suddenly or over a period of days to weeks, and can be highly contagious.

Influenza presents with a sudden onset of symptoms that includes fever with respiratory symptoms. Clear respiratory secretions indicate an influenza viral infection. Treatment is symptom based but may include antivirals with severe symptoms. The administration of antiviral medications does not cure a viral infection but does reduce the severity and duration of symptoms so that individuals can return to their daily activities sooner.

Pneumonia remains among the most frequent conditions for which the death rate has not significantly declined over the past decade. It can be viral or bacterial. Clinical manifestations include fevers, tachypnea, tachycardia, decreased SpO_2, fatigue, and a productive cough. Purulent respiratory secretions indicate a primary or secondary bacterial infection. Primary treatment options include bronchodilator therapy to open up inflamed airways and antibiotic therapy.

Tuberculosis is an extremely contagious disease that is most prevalent in at-risk populations. Night sweats with bloody or rusty sputum are common manifestations of TB infection. Treatment is long-term antibiotic therapy.

Vaccination with inactivated virus or bacterium is the best method for preventing the onset of respiratory illness due to influenza. Regular monitoring for TB is done through the Mantoux TB skin test. It is required in all healthcare workers. Blood testing using IRGAs for any positive skin test will confirm or rule out the presence of TB infection.

Any patient presenting with respiratory symptoms who is suspected of having a contagious respiratory illness should be placed in a private room or should be cohorted with patients with similar symptoms. Patients who present with unexplained weight loss, fever, and night sweats should be placed in an AFB negative airflow room immediately to prevent transmission within the healthcare facility.

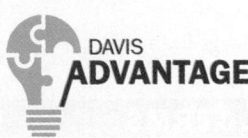

DAVIS
ADVANTAGE | To explore learning resources for this chapter, go to **Davis Advantage** and find:
– Answers to in-text questions
– Chapter Resources and Activities
– NCLEX®-Style Chapter Review Questions
– Bibliography

Chapter 25

Coordinating Care for Patients With Upper Airway Disorders

Linda Cook

LEARNING OUTCOMES

Content in this chapter is designed to assist in:

1. Describing the epidemiology of upper airway disorders
2. Explaining the pathophysiological processes of upper airway disorders
3. Correlating clinical manifestations to pathophysiological processes of
   a. Rhinitis
   b. Rhinosinusitis
   c. Obstructive sleep apnea
   d. Laryngitis
   e. Laryngeal cancer
   f. Laryngeal trauma
4. Describing the diagnostic results used to confirm the diagnoses of selected upper airway disorders
5. Discussing the medical management of:
   a. Rhinitis
   b. Rhinosinusitis
   c. Obstructive sleep apnea
   d. Laryngitis
   e. Laryngeal cancer
   f. Laryngeal trauma
6. Describing complications associated with selected upper airway disorders
7. Developing a comprehensive plan of nursing care for patients with upper airway disorders
8. Developing a teaching plan for patients with upper airway disorders

CONCEPTS

- Assessment
- Cellular Regulation
- Infection
- Inflammation
- Medication
- Nursing Roles
- Nutrition
- Oxygenation
- Promoting Heath

ESSENTIAL TERMS

Acute bacterial rhinosinusitis (ABRS)
Acute rhinosinusitis
Antihistamines
Apnea
Bronchoscopy
Continuous positive airway pressure (CPAP)
Decongestants
Dysphagia
Dyspnea
Electrolarynges
Esophageal speech
Fiberoptic laryngoscopy
Hemoptysis
Hypercapnia
Hypoxemia
Laryngeal cancer
Laryngeal mirror
Laryngeal trauma
Laryngectomy
Laryngitis
Obstructive sleep apnea (OSA)
Osteomeatal complex
Polysomnography
Rhinitis
Rhinorrhea
Rhinosinusitis
Stridor
Tracheostomy
Tracheotomy
Viral rhinosinusitis

Finding Connections

CASE STUDY: EPISODE 1

Follow this patient throughout the chapter.

Henry Comstock is a 56-year-old male who reports a history of snoring and frequently waking during the night. He works as a business manager. He weighs 260 pounds and is 5 ft 10 in. tall. His wife insisted that he see his primary care provider (PCP) because he frequently falls asleep when he sits for short periods of time. He is constantly irritable as a result of his lack of sleep...

RHINITIS

Epidemiology

Rhinitis is the most common problem with the nose and sinuses, affecting 20% of the population. Although not life threatening, rhinitis can impact quality of life by causing headaches, fatigue, sleep disturbances, and cognitive impairment. Rhinitis can result in widespread morbidity with significant financial impact from medical treatment costs, lost workdays with resulting reduced work productivity, and lost school days. Thirty to 60 million American adults and children experience allergic rhinitis.

Pathophysiology

Rhinitis is classified as allergic or nonallergic and acute or chronic. It is an inflammation and irritation of mucous membranes lining the nose (Fig. 25.1). It can also affect the eyes, throat, and ears. Allergic rhinitis is categorized as perennial (occurring throughout the year) or seasonal.

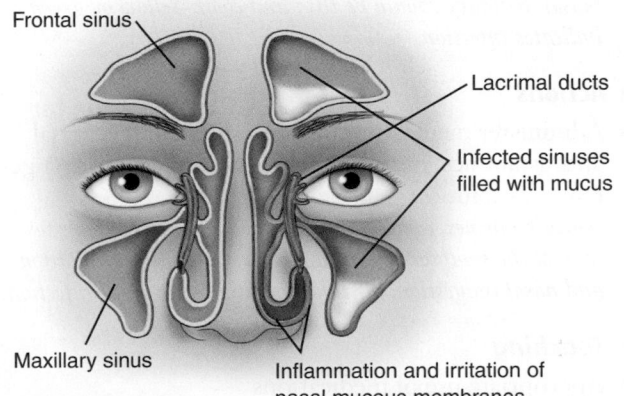

FIGURE 25.1 Rhinitis: inflammation of the mucous membranes and sinuses filled with mucus.

It occurs in response to exposure to allergens found in the environment, medications, foods, or occupational irritants. Common environmental allergens include mold, dust mites, cockroach droppings, weeds, trees, and animal dander. Foods that may induce allergic rhinitis include peanuts, cow's milk, nuts, eggs, and wheat. Medications such as angiotensin-converting enzyme (ACE) inhibitors, phosphodiesterase-5–selective inhibitors such as Viagra, penicillin-based medications, and aspirin and other NSAIDs may also induce symptoms. In response to the offending allergens, the lining of the nasal mucosa becomes inflamed, congested, and edematous. Mechanical obstructions within the nose or sinuses, such as polyps, nasal septal deviation, and hypertrophy of the nasal turbinate or sinus tumors, may also result in the development of rhinitis.

Nonallergic rhinitis presents similarly to allergic rhinitis but does not involve the immune system. The most common example of nonallergic rhinitis is the common cold, which is caused by a variety of viruses and is usually self-limiting unless a bacterial infection occurs simultaneously. Acute rhinitis can last 1 to 3 weeks; chronic rhinitis may last up to 12 weeks.

Clinical Manifestations

Symptoms of rhinitis include nasal itching, sneezing, nasal congestion, and **rhinorrhea** (runny nose, which is excessive nasal drainage). In chronic rhinitis, symptoms last 12 weeks or longer, with discolored nasal discharge and radiographical evidence of fluid levels within the sinuses.

Management

Medical Management
Diagnosis/Treatment

Treatment and management of rhinitis are dependent on the cause. Diagnosis is based on history and symptoms. Obtaining a history of the onset of symptoms that focuses on the pattern, seasonal aspects, environmental exposures to allergens in the home or work, and precipitating factors serves as the basis of determining treatment. If rhinitis is the result of a viral cause, medication to relieve symptoms may be prescribed. In patients with allergic rhinitis, allergy testing may be indicated, followed by a desensitizing regimen. Referral to an ear, nose, and throat specialist for assessment of nasal polyps, nasal septal deviation, and hypertrophy of the nasal turbinate or sinus tumors may be indicated. Avoidance of exposure to known allergens at home, at work, or in the environment will assist in limiting symptoms.

Effective management of asthma and obstructive sleep apnea (OSA), which can coexist or be complicating respiratory conditions, is often dependent on adequate and appropriate management of rhinitis. Asthma and rhinitis can both be triggered in response to allergens. Nasal inflammation as seen in rhinitis increases upper airway resistance, leading to OSA.

Medications

Pharmacological management in allergic and nonallergic rhinitis is aimed at symptom relief. The use of oral **antihistamines**, nasal spray antihistamines and corticosteroids, and decongestant medications can assist in the relief of symptoms (Table 25.1). Prescription and over-the-counter (OTC) antihistamines are the most common treatment of rhinitis symptoms of sneezing, rhinorrhea, and pruritus. Sedation, performance impairment, and anticholinergic effects such as dry mouth and eyes, constipation, and increased heart rate are common side effects of first-generation antihistamines. Second-generation OTC antihistamines such as loratadine (Alavert, Claritin) have less or no tendency to cause sedation. Long-term use of nonsedating antihistamines in rare cases results in mild acute liver injury.

Intranasal corticosteroid is the most effective treatment of allergic rhinitis and related symptoms when used on a regular basis. As-needed use of these nasal sprays can also be effective in relieving symptoms. There is no systemic effect from the use of intranasal corticosteroid medication. Intranasal sprays that contain antihistamines are effective at symptom relief and can work within minutes, whereas an intranasal corticosteroid may take days or weeks to provide full symptom relief. Antihistamine nasal sprays can result in systemic effects. These sprays are sometimes used in combination. Saline nasal sprays can be effective in relieving symptoms such as nasal congestion and sinus pressure–related effects. They moisten dry nasal mucous membranes to remove or reduce nasal plugs. Saline nasal sprays have no negative effects as can be seen with antihistamine or decongestants.

Decongestant medications can reduce nasal congestion and obstruction. Oral **decongestants** contain pseudoephedrine and phenylephrine, which reduce nasal congestion. Side effects of these medications include insomnia, irritability, and palpitations. The use of these medications should be avoided unless nasal antihistamines and a corticosteroid have been ineffective. They should also be avoided in patients with a history of cardiac disease, hypertension, glaucoma, cerebrovascular disease, and cardiac dysrhythmias because of the vasoconstriction caused by these medications. Decongestant nasal sprays such as oxymetazoline (Afrin) should only be used for a few days at a time because overuse may cause rebound congestion (severe congestion).

If infectious rhinitis is present, the administration of antibiotics is required, with the selection of the antibiotic based on patient history, allergies, and the severity of the infection.

Nursing Management

Assessment and Analysis

Symptoms of rhinitis are due to irritation and inflammation of the mucous membranes of the nose, resulting in sneezing, excessive nasal congestion, and nasal drainage.

Nursing Diagnoses

- **Alteration in comfort** related to sinus inflammation
- **Knowledge deficit** related to medication regimen
- **Risk for infection** related to inadequate primary defenses

Nursing Interventions

Assessments

- Vital signs
  Temperature elevation may indicate the presence of infection. Elevations in heart rate and blood pressure may be related to the medication used to treat symptoms.
- Peak flow rate and spirometry (if acute asthma exacerbation also present)
  Assessment of peak flow rate and spirometry may indicate the severity of exacerbation and response to therapy.
- Nasal drainage
  Nasal drainage should be thin and clear. Yellow or green indicates infection.

Actions

- Administer medications as prescribed: oral or nasal antihistamines, oral or nasal corticosteroids, decongestants, antibiotics.
  Antihistamines, corticosteroids, and decongestants are used to control the symptoms of excessive drainage, inflammation, and nasal congestion. Antibiotics are used to treat infection.

Teaching

- Appropriate use of medications
  Instruct patients to utilize medications as prescribed for best results. Avoid nasal decongestant use for greater

Table 25.1 Medications Used in the Treatment of Rhinitis

Symptom	Medication
Congestion, rhinorrhea	First-generation antihistamines such as diphenhydramine (Benadryl Allergy)
	Second-generation antihistamines such as loratadine (Alavert, Claritin)
	Decongestants such as guaifenesin (Robitussin, Mucinex)
	Nasal sprays:
	Corticosteroids sprays such as fluticasone (Flonase)
	Antihistamine sprays such as azelastine (Astelin)
	Saline nasal sprays
	Decongestant such as oxymetazoline (Afrin)

than 2 to 3 days at a time due to the risk of rebound congestion. Instruct the patient to complete antibiotic therapy as prescribed to avoid superinfection or the creation of antibiotic medication resistance.

- Avoidance of known allergens or triggers
  Reduced exposure to triggers is the first-line treatment to avoid symptoms.
- Preventing the spread of infection
  Instruct patients about the importance of hand hygiene and covering the mouth when coughing or sneezing. Dispose of facial tissues containing nasal drainage.

Evaluating Care Outcomes

Relief of symptoms is the expected outcome for the patient with rhinitis. A decrease in nasal drainage and congestion and the relief of headache can be achieved with the avoidance of allergens and the use of appropriate medications.

Connection Check 25.1

The nurse is caring for a patient with seasonal allergy-related rhinitis. The nurse correlates which of the following symptoms with rhinitis?

A. Productive cough
B. Earache
C. Rhinorrhea
D. Headache

RHINOSINUSITIS

Epidemiology

Rhinosinusitis is the symptomatic inflammation of the nasal cavity and the paranasal cavity. Rhinosinusitis is the preferred term when referring to sinusitis because it is a more comprehensive term. According to the American Academy of Otolaryngology–Head and Neck Surgery Foundation, one in eight Americans is affected by rhinosinusitis, resulting in 30 million people diagnosed each year. Healthcare-related costs are estimated at $11 billion annually. These costs are related to acute care and emergency department visits and surgical procedures on the paranasal sinuses.

Classification of rhinosinusitis is based on the duration of symptoms and includes acute, subacute, and chronic. Acute rhinosinusitis is defined as lasting less than 4 weeks; subacute is 4 to 12 weeks' duration. Chronic is more than 12 weeks and may include acute exacerbations of symptoms. **Acute rhinosinusitis** is further classified by etiology as either **acute bacterial rhinosinusitis (ABRS)** or **viral rhinosinusitis**. Viral upper respiratory infections that spread to the paranasal sinuses are the cause of most acute rhinosinusitis, which then can lead to bacterial infections. A deviated nasal septum, trauma to the nose, or tumors can interfere with nasal drainage and contribute to the development of acute rhinosinusitis. Annually in the United States, there are about 20 million cases of ABRS, with a

resulting healthcare cost of $3 billion. Healthcare needs for the treatment of ABRS include primary care office visits, diagnostic testing, antibiotics, and additional prescription medications for symptom management. The socioeconomic impact of ABRS through indirect costs is also significant because of the loss of workdays and decreased productivity.

Acute rhinosinusitis can progress to chronic rhinosinusitis (CRS), which is one of the most common chronic diseases. Fourteen percent to 16% of the U.S. population is affected by CRS. Chronic rhinosinusitis is more common in females, and the presence of nasal polyps is seen in 19% to 36% of patients. Chronic rhinosinusitis results in significant healthcare costs because of repeated visits to PCPs and the use of prescription medications. Chronic rhinosinusitis also has an impact on quality of life due to symptoms and impaired physical functioning.

Pathophysiology

Rhinosinusitis is infection and inflammation of the paranasal sinuses, the four paired air-filled spaces that surround the nasal cavity. They include the maxillary, frontal, sphenoid, and ethmoid sinuses. Inflammation of the nasal passages causes vasodilation, increased blood flow, and vascular permeability, reducing the size of the nasal passages. Nasal congestion occurs as a result of swelling of the nasal turbinates, bony structures along the nasal passages that aid in maintaining moisture and trapping airborne particles. This results in obstruction of nasal airflow (Fig. 25.2). Additional conditions that obstruct the flow of nasal secretions include a deviated nasal septum, trauma to the nose, and tumors. Lack of nasal airflow and increased drainage of nasal secretions provide the medium for bacterial growth. *Streptococcus pneumoniae*, *Haemophilus influenzae*, and *Moraxella catarrhalis* are the most common bacterial species in the culture results of patients with acute rhinosinusitis. Additional bacteria that cause rhinosinusitis include *Staphylococcus aureus* and anaerobes.

Clinical Manifestations

Acute rhinosinusitis is diagnosed by the presence of three symptoms: purulent nasal discharge; nasal obstruction; and facial pain, pressure, and fullness. Normal nasal secretions are clear. In acute rhinosinusitis, nasal secretions are colored or cloudy in nature. Nasal obstruction may be reported as congestion, stuffiness, or blockage of the nasal passages. Facial pain, pressure, and fullness may be located in the anterior face, in the periorbital areas, or as a diffuse or localized headache. The onset of these symptoms in relation to the development of upper respiratory symptoms indicates ABRS.

Additional symptoms may include fatigue, fever, maxillary dental pain, cough, and ear fullness or pressure. Nasal or purulent drainage may also be noted in the posterior pharynx. Indications of extra sinus involvement include signs of neck stiffness (due to the development of meningitis),

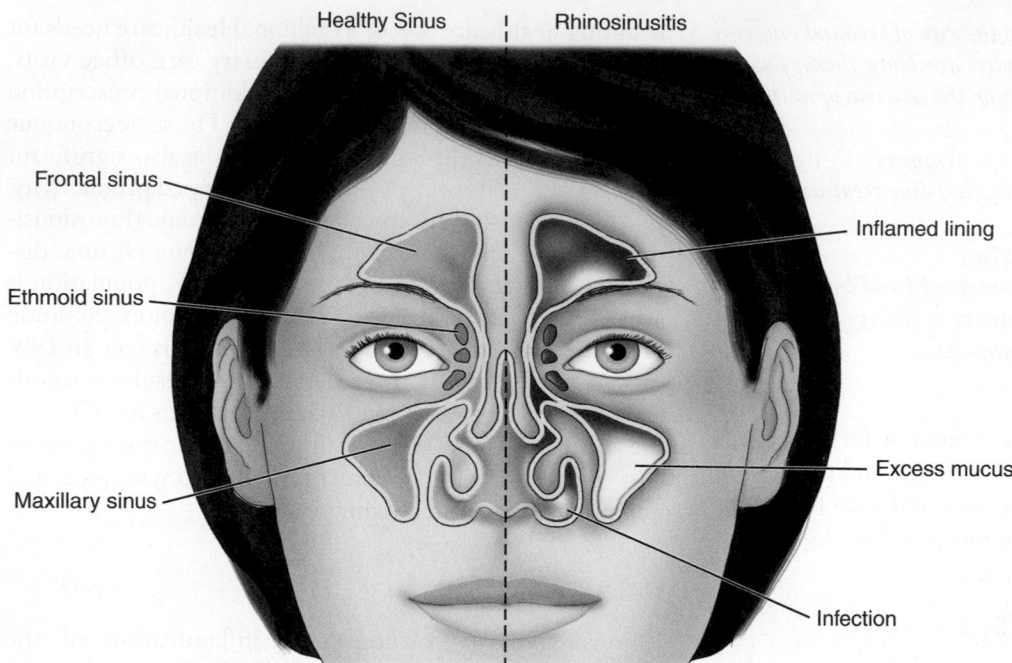

FIGURE 25.2 Rhinosinusitis: inflamed sinuses filled with excess mucus.

orbital protrusion, cellulitis of the face or orbit, and abnormal eye movement.

Management

Medical Management

Diagnosis

Diagnosis is primarily based on a physical examination and starts with the completion of a history and physical examination focusing on the ears, nose, throat, teeth, sinuses, and chest. During the physical examination, the provider is looking for signs of inflammation, tenderness, firmness, or redness. Light palpation or percussion of the sinuses using the index finger is done to evaluate the presence of pain. A vital sign assessment also needs to be completed to identify temperature elevation. Diagnostic testing may include radiographical imaging of the sinuses, computed tomography (CT), and magnetic resonance imaging (MRI) if patients do not meet clinical diagnosis criteria. On radiographical studies, fluid; thickening of the mucous lining of the sinuses; and the presence of polyps, opacities, or foreign objects may be found, indicating rhinosinusitis.

Treatment

The focus of treatment in acute rhinosinusitis is based on the etiology. Treatment goals include pain relief, reduction of nasal mucosal inflammation, and treating infection if present. Normal saline irrigation has local effects that reduce symptoms in acute rhinosinusitis. In this procedure, the patient pours or sprays normal saline into one nostril; it flows through the nasal cavity and pours out the other nostril. Irrigation is beneficial in the removal of infectious

debris, bacteria, allergens, and inflammatory mediators. It also decreases edema of the nasal mucosa and the viscosity of nasal secretions.

Caution must be taken to prevent antibiotic use in nonbacterial illnesses such as viral rhinosinusitis to prevent the development of antibiotic resistance, but in bacterial infections, antibiotic therapy is required. A delay in initiating antibiotic therapy may be indicated if the patient presents with symptoms of nonsevere illness (temperature less than 101°F [38.3°C] or with mild pain). If after 7 days the patient fails to improve or worsens at any time, antibiotics are prescribed. Amoxicillin or amoxicillin-clavulanate is the first-line therapy for most patients with ABRS because of its efficacy, safety, narrow microbiological spectrum, and low cost. In patients with penicillin allergies, doxycycline or a respiratory fluoroquinolone such as moxifloxacin or Levofloxacin is used. In patients who fail to respond within 48 to 72 hours of treatment or who have persistent symptoms, second-line antibiotics may be required. Second-line antibiotics most commonly used include second- or third-generation cephalosporins (cefuroxime [Ceftin], cefpodoxime [Vantin]), macrolides (clarithromycin [Biaxin]), fluoroquinolones (ciprofloxacin [Cipro], levofloxacin [Levaquin], moxifloxacin [Avelox]), and clindamycin (Cleocin).

Antipyretics and analgesics are used as needed to control temperature elevation and pain. The use of intranasal corticosteroids is recommended in patients with a history of allergic rhinitis.

The use of decongestants can be helpful in reducing obstruction of the **osteomeatal complex** (the bony structures around the drainage openings of the sinuses), facilitating drainage of the sinuses. Patients with hypertension should use caution when taking oral decongestants due to their action of vasoconstriction to reduce stuffiness, which can increase blood pressure. Medications typically used for symptomatic relief that should be used with caution include antihistamines that may cause drying of secretions, thus impairing mucus drainage, and topical decongestant sprays that, if used for more than 3 days, may result in rebound nasal congestion when discontinued. This is also referred to as rhinitis medicamentosa. Rhinitis medicamentosa results in nasal congestion without rhinorrhea or sneezing and is known as *rebound rhinitis* or *chemical rhinitis*. Treatment of rhinitis medicamentosa is the cessation of topical nasal decongestants.

Complications

Acute rhinosinusitis, if left untreated or inadequately treated, can lead to several potentially serious although rare complications that include orbital cellulitis, orbital abscess, osteomyelitis, meningitis, sepsis, and subdural abscess. Orbital cellulitis and orbital abscess occur from the transfer of a sinus infection to the area surrounding the eye. In the setting of chronic sinus infection, bacteria can infect the facial bones, resulting in osteomyelitis. Meningitis and subdural abscess occur when bacteria pass through the meninges. Mucoceles, collections of fluid, can develop within the sinuses, primarily the frontal or ethmoid sinuses, because of obstruction and can result in bony erosion.

Nursing Management
Assessment and Analysis

Symptoms of rhinosinusitis are due to obstruction in the flow of nasal drainage from inflammation of the sinus lining. Symptoms include a combination of facial pressure, sense of fullness or pain or nasal obstruction, and the presence of purulent (yellow-green) nasal discharge.

Nursing Diagnoses
- **Risk for infection** related to obstruction and inflammation of the sinus lining
- **Acute pain** related to nasal congestion

Nursing Interventions
■ *Assessments*
- Vital signs
  Temperature elevation may indicate the presence of infection. Increased blood pressure may be a side effect of the decongestants.
- Physical examination of the mouth, nose, and face
  Facial pressure, a sense of fullness or pain or nasal obstruction, and the presence of purulent (yellow-green) nasal discharge indicate impaired nasal drainage.
  Swelling, redness, and pain around the eyes may indicate an abscess or cellulitis.
- Percussion of sinuses
  Identifies presence of fluid within the sinus cavity, which results in pain

■ *Actions*
- Administer medications as prescribed: normal saline irrigation, decongestants, and antibiotics.
  Irrigation, decongestants, and antibiotics are used to control the symptoms of nasal congestion, excessive drainage, and inflammation. Antibiotics are used to treat bacterial infection.

Teaching
- Symptoms to report to provider
  Temperature, increase in pain, change in level of consciousness, redness, or edema around the face and eyes can indicate complications of rhinosinusitis.
- Instruct patients on correct medication usage.
  Instruct patients to read the content of the active ingredients and utilize medications as prescribed to prevent overdosing. Start taking decongestants at the onset of symptoms. Complete all antibiotics as prescribed. Limit use of decongestant nasal sprays to less than 4 days to avoid rebound congestion.
- Teach proper use of normal saline nasal rinse.
  - Lean over the sink with head tilted to one side.
  - Insert the spout of the neti pot or other irrigating device into the upper nostril.
  - Slowly pour the normal saline into the upper nostril while continuing to breathe through the mouth.
  - Allow fluid to drain out the lower nostril.
    Facilitates removal of debris and excess mucus

Evaluating Care Outcomes

With treatment, patients experience a decrease in and resolution of symptoms, such as relief of nasal congestion and drainage, headache, and facial pressure or sense of fullness. The resolution of a bacterial infection is managed through antibiotics. It is important that the patient completes antibiotic therapy as prescribed and reports unresolved symptoms to avoid the serious complications of orbital cellulitis, osteomyelitis, or chronic sinus infection.

Connection Check 25.2

Potential complications of rhinosinusitis include which of the following? *(Select all that apply.)*
A. Orbital cellulitis
B. Osteomyelitis
C. Meningitis
D. Pharyngitis
E. Orbital abscess

OBSTRUCTIVE SLEEP APNEA
Epidemiology

Obstructive sleep apnea (OSA) is a condition where the upper airway is obstructed during sleep, causing a narrowing of one or more sites of the upper airway, resulting in intermittent breathing patterns. It is estimated that 10% to

15% of females and 20% to 30% of males have OSA. Increased awareness and recognition, and thus testing, have resulted in an increased prevalence. A history of atrial fibrillation, nocturnal dysrhythmias, type 2 diabetes mellitus, heart failure, and pulmonary hypertension places patients at higher risk of OSA. Other risk factors for developing OSA include male gender, obesity, cigarette smoking, alcohol use, age between 40 and 65, craniofacial or upper airway soft tissue abnormalities, and menopause. Insulin resistance is seen in patients with OSA and is associated with increased severity. Increases in the prevalence of the risk factors have resulted in an increase in OSA.

Pathophysiology

Obstructive sleep apnea occurs during sleep as the upper airways narrow or collapse, increasing resistance to airflow (Fig. 25.3). Narrowing can occur in the retropalatal region, retroglossal region, or nose (Fig. 25.4).

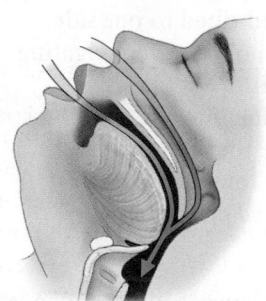 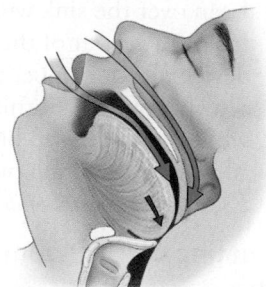

Normal breathing
• Airway is open.
• Air flows freely to lungs.

Obstructive sleep apnea
• Airway collapses.
• Air flow blocked to lungs.

FIGURE 25.3 Obstructive sleep apnea due to the collapse of the upper airways.

With the onset of sleep, the body muscle tone relaxes, which includes the muscles of the upper airway. With OSA, the normal work of breathing is unable to overcome the increased resistance in the upper airway, causing airway collapse. Narrowing of the upper airways increases inspiratory pressure and intrathoracic pressure, resulting in decreased minute ventilation and gas exchange. Ultimately, there are periods of **apnea**. During apnea, there is no tidal volume, or movement of air in or out; thus, no gas exchange occurs in the alveoli.

Hypoxemia (decreased concentration of oxygen in the blood), **hypercapnia** (increased concentration of carbon dioxide in the blood), acidosis, and increased sympathetic vasoconstrictive activity occur as a result of the decreased tidal volume and apnea.

Clinical Manifestations

Obstructive sleep apnea is characterized by the following symptoms: loud snoring, snorting, witnessed apnea, gasping during sleep, recurrent waking during sleep, or choking. Spouses often report that patients have disruptive snoring and have witnessed periods of apnea. Fifteen or more obstructive sleep events per hour are sufficient to diagnose the presence of OSA. Because of these frequent sleep disruptions, patients complain of excessive daytime sleepiness, falling asleep during quiet times, short and repetitive attention lapses, and taking intentional naps. Daytime sleepiness has been linked to workplace and motor vehicle accidents and cognitive complaints of poor motor performance, executive performance, and visuospatial learning; storage and recall of visual information about the spatial relationship of objects, and constructional ability.

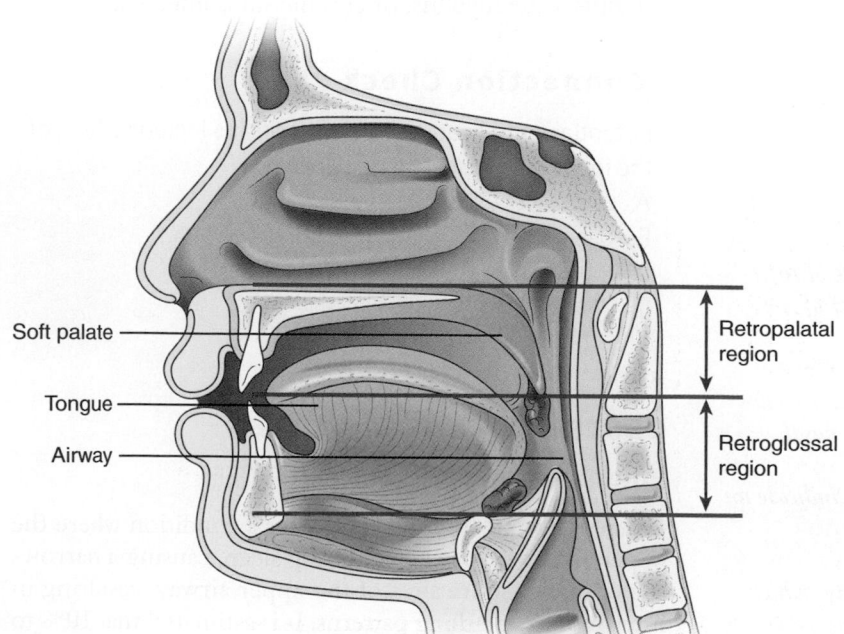

Soft palate

Tongue

Airway

Retropalatal region

Retroglossal region

FIGURE 25.4 Retropalatal region, retroglossal region of the upper airway.

Management

Medical Management

Diagnosis

Diagnostic testing begins with a sleep history, which includes gathering information on sleep patterns, a history of snoring, and daytime sleepiness. **Polysomnography** (a sleep study) is performed to diagnose OSA and can be conducted in an overnight sleep laboratory or using home portable monitoring. Numerous biophysiological measurements are obtained during sleep, including an electrocardiogram, pulse oximetry, respiratory airflow, eye and skeletal muscle movement, and an electroencephalogram. A key value obtained during the sleep study is the apnea-hypopnea index value, the number of apneic events each hour. It can be used to characterize the severity of OSA.

Treatment

Treatment of OSA requires multiple interventions and the active participation of the patient. The use of **continuous positive airway pressure (CPAP)** is the treatment of choice (Fig. 25.5). Continuous positive airway pressure prevents collapse of the upper airway through the use of pressure delivered through the use of a nasal, oral, or oronasal mask during sleep (Fig. 25.6). A CPAP machine delivers a continuous stream of positive pressure, keeping the airway open and providing an unobstructed airway. Patients are taught about the operation, care, and maintenance of the CPAP machine. Follow-up care is conducted for problem solving and to evaluate the effectiveness of therapy.

Weight management and loss are encouraged as a first-line intervention in conjunction with the use of CPAP. Positioning during sleep in a nonsupine position by using pillows is an effective secondary intervention. The avoidance of alcohol and sedatives before bedtime is an additional intervention.

Oral appliances that are custom-made for the patient may be used to maintain airway patency. Oral appliances assist with mandibular repositioning to hold the mandible in a forward position to keep the airway open. Forward positioning of the tongue is accomplished with tongue-retaining devices.

Surgical Management

Surgical procedures for OSA are classified as primary or secondary interventions. Surgical procedures are considered primary interventions for patients with severe obstructing anatomy that surgery can correct. Surgery is considered a secondary intervention in patients who are intolerant of CPAP or oral appliances. Surgical procedures that involve the airway include tonsillectomy and/or adenoidectomy, uvulopalatopharyngoplasty, septoplasty, nasal polypectomy, tongue reduction, and epiglottoplasty. These procedures remove excess tissue in the airway that interferes with maintaining adequate airflow. Bariatric surgery to facilitate weight reduction is also a consideration.

Complications

Obstructive sleep apnea is recognized as a mediator of cardiovascular disease because of recurrent hypoxemia, the release of inflammatory mediators such as endothelins (proteins that constrict blood vessels), and insulin resistance. In response to hypoxia, inflammatory mediators are released, which leads to the adherence of white blood cells to the endothelium, causing endothelial damage and atherosclerosis. The release of endothelin, a potent vasoconstrictor, results in endothelial dysfunction and damage. Severe nocturnal hypoxemia can result in cardiac ischemia, myocardial infarction, erectile dysfunction, stroke, atrial fibrillation, heart failure, and sudden cardiac death.

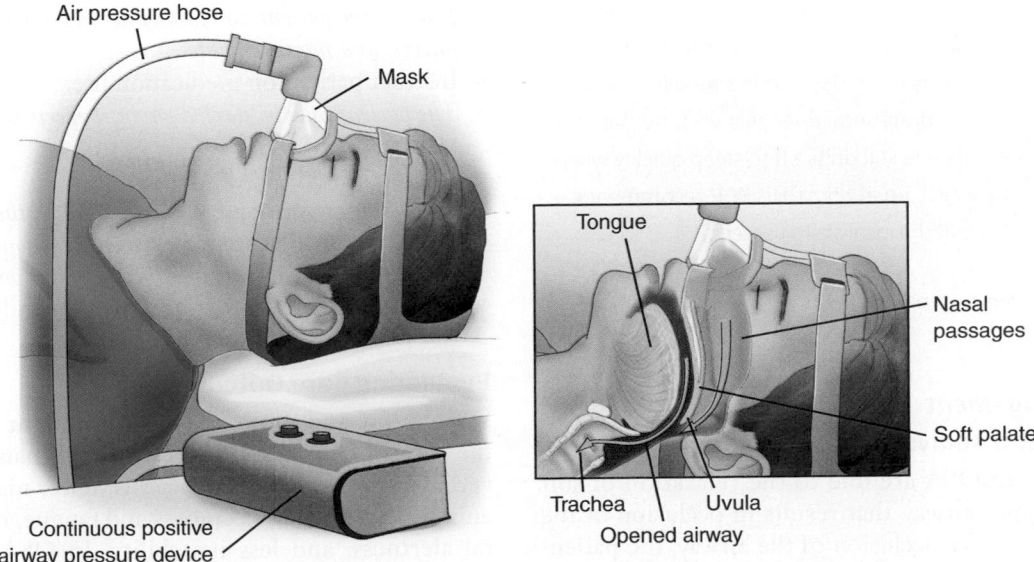

FIGURE 25.5 Continuous positive airway pressure (CPAP) machine with compressor and mask. The CPAP machine provides continuous positive airway pressure, keeping the upper airways patent.

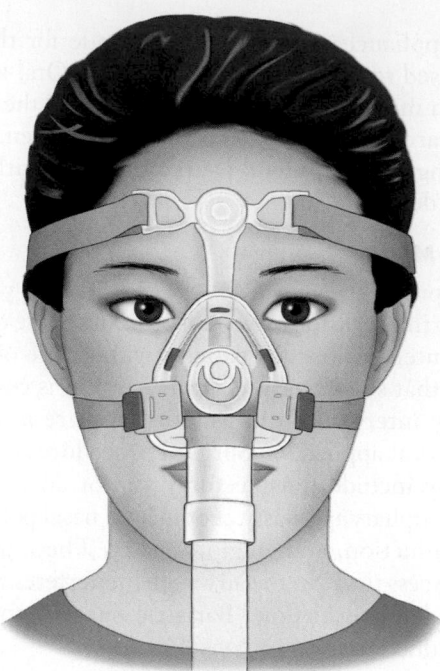

FIGURE 25.6 Continuous positive airway pressure mask.

Connection Check 25.3

Monitoring of which of the following biophysiological parameters occurs during a sleep study? *(Select all that apply.)*

A. Cardiac rhythm
B. Electroencephalogram
C. Eye movement
D. Blood pressure
E. Oxygen saturation

CASE STUDY: EPISODE 2

Henry returns to his PCP 6 weeks after his initial visit regarding his sleep patterns. He has increased his activity by walking 2 miles at the local school track every other day and has modified his diet by reducing his carbohydrate intake. At this visit, he has lost 8 pounds. His wife states he still drifts off to sleep quickly when sitting and abruptly wakes up at night. His PCP recommends a sleep study to be done at the local sleep center…

Nursing Management

Assessment and Analysis

The symptoms of OSA are due to the relaxation of soft tissue in the upper airway that results in occlusion of the airway. Because of the occlusion of the airway, the patient snores, and periods of apnea occur. During apnea, there is no oxygen exchange, resulting in hypoxia and hypercapnia.

As hypoxia and hypercapnia progress, the patient wakes and resumes breathing.

Nursing Diagnoses

- **Sleep deprivation** related to inability to breathe during sleep
- **Risk for decreased cardiac tissue perfusion** related to hypoxia during sleep
- **Ineffective sleeping pattern** related to cessation of breathing during sleep

Nursing Interventions

Assessments

- Vital signs
  Hypertension and dysrhythmias are common findings in OSA due to the hypoxia and release of inflammatory mediators as a result of the apneic episodes.
- Height and weight
  Obesity is a risk factor for OSA.
- Sleep, rest, and activity history
  Disruptive sleep patterns, daytime fatigue, increased sleepiness, and the presence of snoring indicate OSA.
- Assess for edema, bleeding, and respiratory distress postoperatively if a surgical option is pursued.
  Surgical procedures put the patient at risk for bleeding. Additionally, procedures in that area may cause respiratory distress if swelling occurs.

Actions

- Administer medications as ordered.
  Patients with OSA may have uncontrolled hypertension or cardiac dysrhythmias.
- Diagnostic testing
  Patient may undergo a sleep study, electrocardiogram, and echocardiogram.

Teaching

- Disease process
  Instruct the patient and family members about OSA, risk factors, and management.
- Instruct patient on medication use.
  The patient may be started on antihypertensive medications to control blood pressure.
- Instruction on CPAP
  Depending on the results of the sleep study, the patient may be started on CPAP therapy. Provide instruction on the use and maintenance of equipment and the application of the mask.
- Instruct patient on weight reduction and management
  Obesity is a risk factor for OSA.

Evaluating Care Outcomes

Weight loss and the use of CPAP at night may help with the control of OSA. Patients with well-managed OSA will verbalize improved sleep patterns, fewer night-time awakenings, less daytime sleepiness and fatigue, improved mental alertness, and less irritability. In OSA patients with hypertension, control of blood pressure values will be achieved.

LARYNGITIS

Epidemiology

Acute **laryngitis** is the most common disorder of the larynx. Causes of acute laryngitis include upper respiratory infection, environmental pollutants, gastroesophageal reflux disease (GERD), and the use of asthma inhalers. Vocal misuse or strain can also result in acute laryngitis. Vocal strain can occur from prolonged periods of talking, which may be seen in teachers or lawyers, for example; screaming or having to talk loudly as a result of environmental noise; or in attempts to communicate with someone with hearing loss. Attempts to maintain speech in the presence of laryngitis can further strain the vocal cords. Endotracheal intubation may also cause laryngeal edema resulting in acute laryngitis. Lung or throat cancer may manifest as laryngitis.

Pathophysiology and Clinical Manifestations

Laryngitis is an inflammation of the mucous membranes of the larynx. The predominant symptom is hoarseness, but symptoms similar to those of an upper respiratory infection may also be present, such as cough, postnasal drip, fatigue, and malaise. The symptoms of acute laryngitis typically last 7 to 10 days. Extreme airway obstruction and **stridor**, a high-pitched, wheezing breath sound caused by turbulent airflow in the partially obstructed larynx, may occur in patients after endotracheal intubation.

Management

Medical Management

Diagnosis

The diagnosis of laryngitis is based on patient complaint of hoarseness related to a current or recent upper respiratory infection. In patients with risk factors for developing cancers of the throat and lungs, further diagnostic evaluation may be warranted. Patients may require visual examination of the larynx by an ear, nose, and throat specialist through the use of a **laryngeal mirror** or **fiberoptic laryngoscopy**. A flexible fiberoptic laryngoscopy involves inserting a thin, flexible scope into the mouth or nose to the larynx to allow direct visualization. If polyps, inflammation, or tumors are present, x-rays or CT may be required.

Treatment

Treatment consists of voice rest, adding moisture to the air in the home with a humidifier or vaporizer, and drinking plenty of fluids. Avoidance of smoking and exposure to second-hand smoke is also important. The use of antibiotics is indicated in the setting of bacterial infection. If laryngitis lasts greater than 5 days after appropriate treatment and voice rest, evaluation for the presence of malignancy should be considered.

Nursing Management

Assessment and Analysis

Symptoms of laryngitis are due to inflammation of the larynx resulting in vocal hoarseness or the absence of voice. Additional symptoms may include dry throat, difficulty swallowing and eating, fever, and cough.

Nursing Diagnoses

- **Impaired verbal communication** related to the inflammatory process
- **Risk for infection** related to the inflammatory process
- **Risk for aspiration** related to the inflammatory process

Nursing Interventions

▣ **Assessments**

- Vital signs
  Temperature elevation may indicate an infection.
- Assessment of throat structures
  Increased edema of the throat structures could compromise the patency of the airway.
- Assess for the presence of stridor after extubation.
  Stridor indicates acute obstruction of the airway and is a medical emergency that may require reintubation.

▣ **Actions**

- Administer humidification as prescribed.
  Humidification may be ordered to reduce inflammation.
- Administer antibiotics as ordered.
  Antibiotics may be ordered to treat infection if present.
- Have emergency airway equipment readily available, especially if laryngitis occurs after extubation.
  Hoarseness and stridor after extubation indicate acute obstruction of the airway and are a medical emergency.
- Provide alternatives for communication (pen and paper or a communication board with pictures).
  Patients should be encouraged to rest the voice to prevent further trauma.

▣ **Teaching**

- Instruct on medication use.
  Complete all medications as prescribed.

- Instruct patient on voice rest and the need to use alternative modes of communication.
  Continued use of the voice will cause strain and delay the resolution of laryngitis.
- Increase intake of fluids.
  Fluids help soothe a sore throat.
- Smoking cessation
  Smoking irritates the larynx and can exacerbate symptoms.

Evaluating Care Outcomes

Voice rest, humidity, and increased oral intake help resolve laryngitis. Return of the patient's normal voice and resolution of accompanying symptoms reflect resolution of laryngitis and the effectiveness of treatment. Patients are encouraged to avoid activities that strain the larynx. If the laryngitis is a result of bacterial infection, the patient should take prescribed antibiotics as directed and use expectorant medication to manage secretions. In patients who develop acute laryngitis after extubation, resolution of stridor, ease of breathing, and adequate oxygenation levels indicate decreased obstruction and resolution of laryngitis.

Connection Check 25.5

The nurse is aware that there are several causes of laryngitis. Which of the following can cause laryngitis? *(Select all that apply.)*

A. Food allergies
B. Upper respiratory infection
C. Environmental pollutants
D. Gastroesophageal reflux
E. Obstructive sleep apnea

LARYNGEAL CANCER

Epidemiology

In 2018, the American Cancer Society reported an expected 13,150 new diagnoses of **laryngeal cancer**, with the diagnosis split into 10,490 cases in men and 2,660 cases in women. The number of deaths was estimated at 3,710. This reflects a decrease in the number of people diagnosed with laryngeal cancer because of the decrease in smoking.

Risk factors for the development of laryngeal cancer include tobacco and alcohol use, poor dietary habits, a compromised immune system, genetic syndromes, occupational hazards, gender, age, race, and GERD. In addition to being at higher risk for laryngeal cancer, patients with GERD are also at higher risk for cancer of the esophagus.

The use of tobacco in any form is the most important risk factor for the development of cancers of the head and neck, including the larynx. Cigarettes, pipes, cigars, and all forms of chewing tobacco raise the risk of laryngeal cancers because of the chemicals contained in tobacco products. Alcohol ingestion combined with tobacco use increases the risk of developing laryngeal cancer up to 100 times as compared with people do not use either product. In patients with a history of alcohol abuse, poor dietary habits are also often present, resulting in a lack of fiber intake and foods containing vitamins. Laryngeal cancers are more common in people who have compromised immune status as a result of immunosuppressant medications after organ transplant, hereditary diseases, or AIDS. People with genetic mutations resulting in syndromes such as *Fanconi anemia* and *dyskeratosis congenita* have an increased risk of developing cancer of the mouth and throat at an early age. Occupations where workers have intense and long exposure to certain chemicals; wood, coal or steel dust; paint fumes; and asbestos are at higher risk of laryngeal cancer. Laryngeal cancer is about four times more common in men than in women, although these statistics are changing as more women are smoking and using alcohol. Laryngeal cancer is slow growing, so more than half of the people with laryngeal cancer are over 65 years of age. It is more common in African Americans and Caucasians than among Latinos and Asians.

Pathophysiology

The larynx is divided into three main parts. The supraglottis is the uppermost part of the larynx above the vocal cords and includes the epiglottis. The middle part is the glottis and is where the vocal cords are located. The lower part of the larynx is the subglottis and is the area located between the vocal cords and the trachea. Laryngeal cancer usually originates from the squamous cells that line the larynx and hypopharynx, the part of the pharynx behind the larynx, the entrance to the esophagus. Changes in the squamous cells from irritation, usually from heavy alcohol drinking and smoking, result in the squamous cells becoming precancerous. According to the American Cancer Society, most precancerous cells do not become cancers, especially if the irritant is removed, but some advance into cancer cells. See Figures 25.7A and B for an illustration of the normal structures of the larynx; Figure 25.7C illustrates laryngeal cancer.

Clinical Manifestations

Clinical manifestations include hoarseness or a change in the voice that does not resolve in 2 weeks. Voice changes include lower-than-usual pitch and raspy and hoarse sounds. Additional symptoms include a persistent sore throat, constant cough, pain with swallowing, ear pain that does not go away, difficulty swallowing, trouble breathing, a lump or mass in the neck, and weight loss due to difficulty eating.

Management

Medical Management
Diagnosis

Diagnosis starts with the completion of a thorough health history, including general health information, other medical conditions, onset of symptoms, risk factors, and family

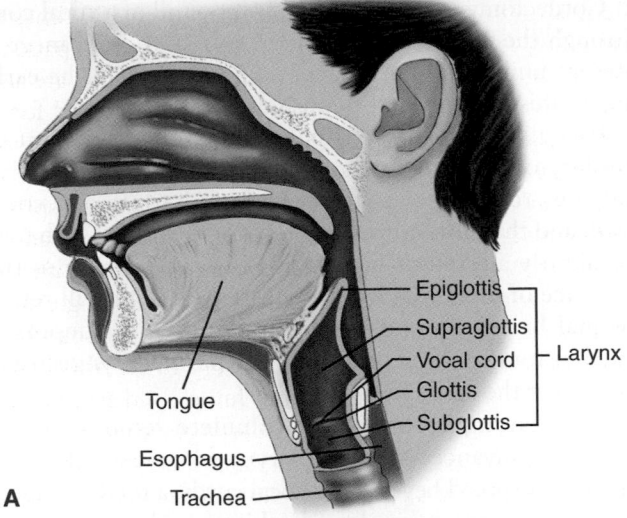

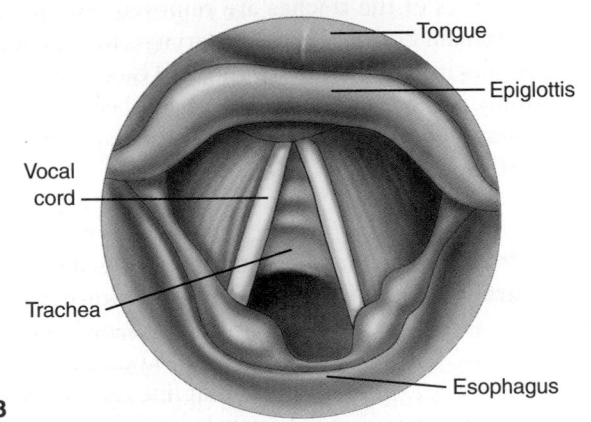

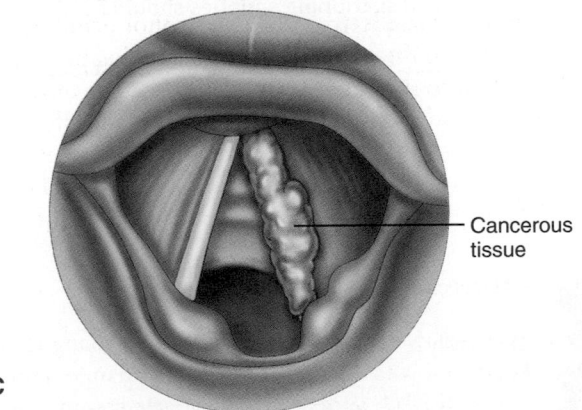

FIGURE 25.7 *A* and *B,* Normal structures of the larynx. *C,* Laryngeal cancer of the vocal cord.

and larynx are performed by an otolaryngologist with the use of a direct laryngoscopy with a flexible endoscope. Laryngoscopy allows for assessment of the vocal folds and glottis for the presence of ulcerations, nodules, polyps, strictures, bleeding, or tumors. Laryngoscopy may also be performed under general anesthesia, at which time samples or biopsies of suspicious tissue are obtained for evaluation (Fig. 25.8).

Diagnostic imaging includes a barium swallow, chest x-ray, CT, MRI, and positron emission tomography (PET). A barium swallow evaluates the throat and the ability to swallow. Chest x-rays are obtained to evaluate the lungs for the presence of lung cancer. The CT, MRI, and PET scans are completed to determine the presence of metastasis into the surrounding and distant soft tissues and for regional adenopathy, or lymph node involvement. The information obtained through biopsy and diagnostic imaging is used to determine the stage of the tumor and disease progression. Stages of laryngeal cancer are based on the size of the tumor, the involvement of the lymph nodes, and whether the cancer has spread to other sites within the body.

Diagnostic laboratory testing is also done to provide information about the overall health status of the patient. A complete blood count, blood chemistry profile, coagulation studies, and urinalysis provide vital information about the potential spread of laryngeal cancer, nutritional status, and organ function, such as the kidneys and liver. At present, there is no specific blood test or marker to assist in diagnosing laryngeal cancer.

Treatment

Treatment of laryngeal cancer is based on factors such as the stage of the disease, the location and size of the

history. Physical assessment of the neck, thyroid, lymph nodes, and muscle movement of the neck can indicate if tumor growth has invaded these structures. If these initial findings are suspicious for laryngeal cancer, a referral to an otolaryngologist (ear, nose, and throat specialist) or a head and neck surgeon is made.

Further diagnostic procedures include endoscopy and imaging. Visualization and examination of the pharynx

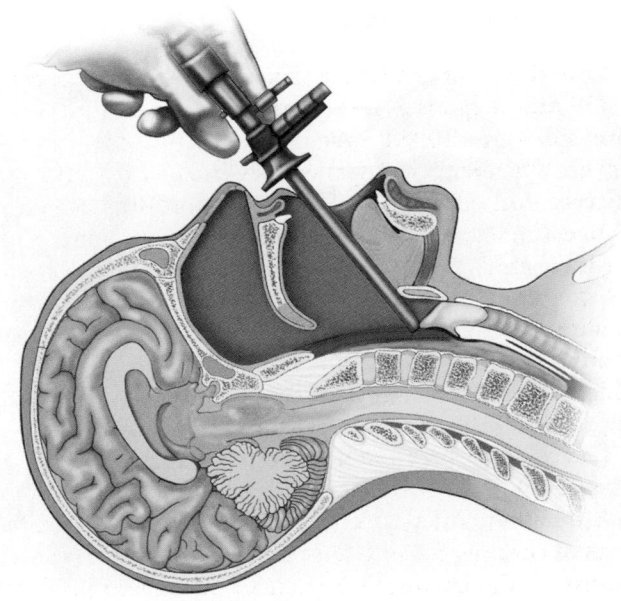

FIGURE 25.8 Laryngoscopy: direct visualization of the larynx.

tumor, and whether the current tumor is a reoccurrence. Treatment includes radiation therapy, surgery, and chemotherapy.

Radiation therapy is used to eliminate cancer cells and maintain the structure and function of the larynx. It is used to treat small tumors, to reduce tumor size prior to surgery, or in patients who are unable to undergo surgery. Radiation therapy is usually given 5 days a week for 6 to 8 weeks. Side effects of radiation include increased hoarseness; prolonged tissue healing; sore throat; difficulty swallowing; and if the salivary glands are involved, dry mouth (xerostomia).

Chemotherapy can be used in several different ways. It can be given at the same time as radiation therapy (chemoradiation) to improve the effectiveness of the radiation therapy. It can be given before radiation therapy to shrink larger tumors and make radiation therapy more effective. It can also be given prior to surgery to shrink larger tumors that are not easily excised. Finally, it can be used palliatively to help to control the cancer and relieve symptoms (palliative chemotherapy).

Surgical Management

Surgical procedures used to treat laryngeal cancer include laser surgery, cordectomy, partial **laryngectomy**, and total laryngectomy. The goal of surgical treatment is to remove the tumor and maintain the function of the larynx, speech, swallowing ability, and breathing.

Laser microsurgery is used to treat early forms of glottic cancers and is now considered the standard approach at many institutions. It utilizes a beam of light to remove the tumor. A cost-effective alternative to an open surgical procedure, laser microsurgery results in good functional outcomes and causes minimal morbidity.

Cordectomy is the removal of part or all of a vocal cord through the use of a transoral laser. If laryngeal cancer is present unilaterally on the vocal cords and is in the early stages, this option may be considered.

Partial laryngectomy is performed to remove part of the larynx in the early stages of laryngeal cancer. This includes removal of part of the larynx, only one vocal cord, and the tumor. Preservation of the voice, which may be slightly altered or hoarse, is achieved because of the presence of the remaining structures. Patients will retain normal breathing and swallowing ability. A temporary tracheostomy may be required after partial laryngectomy to protect the airway.

Total laryngectomy is the complete removal of the larynx. In advanced stages of laryngeal cancer where the cancer has spread beyond the vocal cords, a total laryngectomy is a curative procedure. In this procedure, the larynx and several rings of the trachea are removed. Swallowing ability will remain normal after total laryngectomy, but the surgery results in the inability to speak. The creation of a tracheostomy is required for breathing and because of the risk of aspiration of fluids and food after the removal of the epiglottis (Fig. 25.9).

⚠️ **Safety Alert** In patients with a tracheostomy, an obturator and a replacement tracheostomy tube should be kept at the bedside in the event of unexpected dislodgement of the tracheostomy tube. Ensure that the tube is secured in place with cloth tracheostomy ties or a Velcro tracheostomy tube holder. In addition, a suctioning unit and suctioning supplies should be at the bedside.

Before Laryngectomy

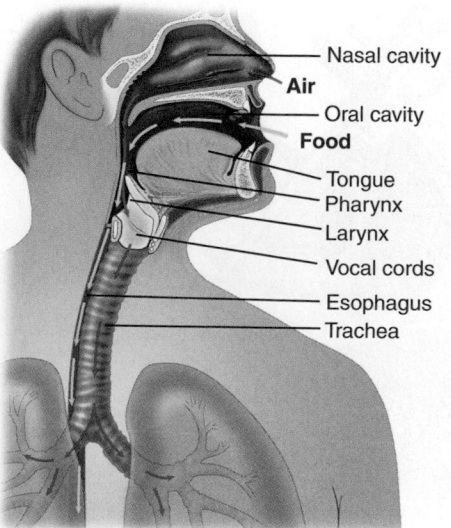

- Nasal cavity
- **Air**
- Oral cavity
- **Food**
- Tongue
- Pharynx
- Larynx
- Vocal cords
- Esophagus
- Trachea

After Laryngectomy

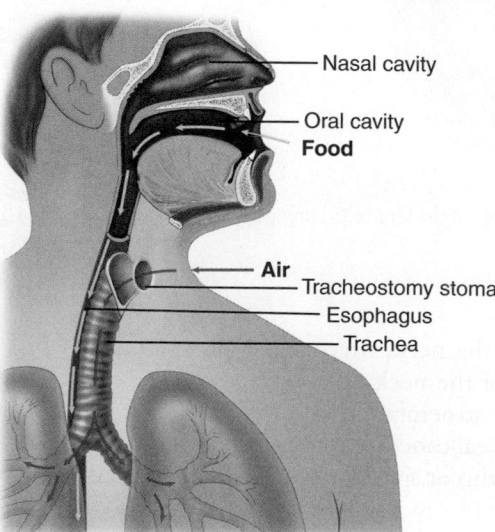

- Nasal cavity
- Oral cavity
- **Food**
- **Air**
- Tracheostomy stoma
- Esophagus
- Trachea

FIGURE 25.9 Surgical removal of the larynx and the creation of a tracheostomy to protect the airway.

Laryngeal cancer prognosis is dependent on the stage of the disease; the size, location, and grade of the tumor; the presence of metastasis; and the general health status, immune function, and age. Early diagnosis of laryngeal cancer has a high cure rate, with a 5-year survival rate of 80% to 95%. Advanced staging at diagnosis has a 5-year survival rate of 25% to 50%. The presence of comorbidities such as diabetes, heart disease, or hypertension also has an impact on survival. Smoking cessation is another factor increasing survival (see Evidence-Based Practice: Smoking Cessation). Because of the age of patients diagnosed with laryngeal cancer, usually in the 60- to 70-year-old age group, the cause of death may be related to other factors.

Evidence-Based Practice

Smoking Cessation
Medication therapy
First line

- Nicotine replacement therapies (nicotine gum, patches, or lozenges)
- Non-nicotinic medications (Varenicline [Chantix] or bupropion [Zyban])

Second line

- Clonidine* and nortriptyline*

Behavioral/counseling therapy

- Providing support increases the likelihood of success and can be in the form of group or individual counseling or telephone conversations.

Physical activity

- Increasing physical activity decreases the cravings and symptoms of anxiety, depression, and stress that may be experienced during smoking cessation.
- Increasing physical activity and exercise also can reduce weight gain after smoking cessation.

*Not approved by the U.S. Food and Drug Administration (FDA) for smoking cessation.
Rigotti, N. A. (2018). Patient education: Quitting smoking (beyond the basics). In J. K. Stoller & M. D. Aronson (Eds.), *UpToDate*. Retrieved from https://www.uptodate.com/contents/quitting-smoking-beyond-the-basics#H16

Nursing Management
Assessment and Analysis

The symptoms of laryngeal cancer are dependent on the location of the cancer. Laryngeal cancer affecting the vocal cords results in changes in voice quality and character or hoarseness. A lump in the neck, earache, or sore throat can be seen in tumors above the vocal cords.

Nursing Diagnoses
- **Ineffective airway clearance** related to surgical removal of the glottis
- **Impaired swallowing** related to laryngectomy/tracheostomy tube
- **Impaired verbal communication** related to removal of the larynx
- **Impaired body image** related to the surgical procedure
- **Risk for infection** related to the surgical procedure
- **Grieving** related to the change in body image, role performance, and potential death
- **Risk for nutritional imbalance, less than body requirement**, related to impaired swallowing, poor appetite

Nursing Interventions
Assessments
- Complete a review of risk factors
  Focus on risk factors for laryngeal cancer, such as smoking, alcohol use, and occupational exposure to chemicals.
- Review of symptoms/complaints
  Hoarseness, earache, and sore throat lasting several weeks need further evaluation.
- Skin/vocal/swallowing assessment
  Red, tender, peeling skin may result from radiation therapy. Radiation therapy may also cause worsening hoarseness and difficulty swallowing.
- Laboratory assessments: electrolytes, white blood cell (WBC) and platelet count
  Patients on chemotherapy may have alterations in their electrolyte balance. Also, they can become immunosuppressed, resulting in neutropenia, making them more susceptible to infection. Platelet counts may decrease, resulting in bleeding risk.

Postoperative
- Vital signs
  Decreased blood pressure may occur with blood loss; increased heart rate may be due to hypovolemia or pain.
- Oxygenation status
  Edema and increased secretions postoperatively may cause shortness of breath and decreased oxygenation.
- Patency of tracheostomy
  Bleeding or edema may occur postoperatively, impairing the patency of the tracheostomy.
- Weight, nutritional intake, calorie count
  Swallowing impairments postoperatively may impact adequate nutritional intake.

Actions
- Administer chemotherapy as ordered.
  Chemotherapy is used in combination with radiation and/or surgery in an effort to destroy cancer cells and reduce tumor size.
- Institute bleeding precautions as necessary.
  Chemotherapy may increase bleeding risk due to decreased platelet count.

Postoperative

- Tracheostomy care: use of humidified oxygen via a trach collar; pulmonary hygiene such as turning, coughing, deep breathing, and mobility; suctioning equipment, replacement tracheostomy tube (same size and one smaller), and obturator at bedside; tracheostomy care twice daily and as needed; management of oral secretions with a Yankauer suction tip (Fig. 25.10)

  Post-laryngectomy patients will have a permanent tracheostomy tube placed (Figs. 25.11 and 25.12). Good care is essential to maintain patency and decrease infection. Humidity, which will assist in moistening respiratory secretions, and pulmonary hygiene will facilitate secretion removal. Replacement equipment is necessary in case of unintended dislodgement of the tracheostomy. See Chapter 7 for more detailed information on tracheostomies.

- Institute aspiration precautions.

  Postoperatively, the patient is at risk for aspiration because of the removal of upper airway structures/epiglottis.

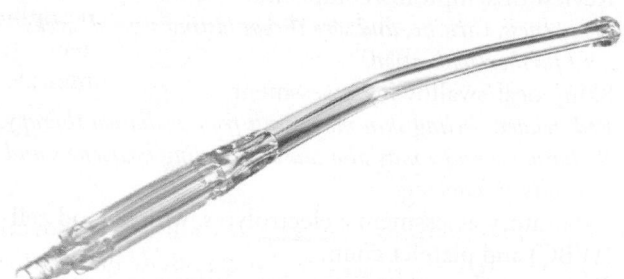

FIGURE 25.10 Yankauer suction tip.

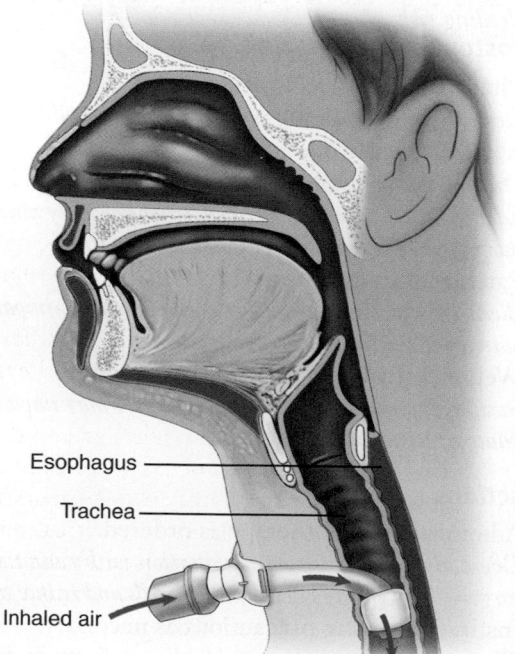

Esophagus

Trachea

Inhaled air

FIGURE 25.11 Tracheostomy: artificial airway created in the neck to allow for ventilation.

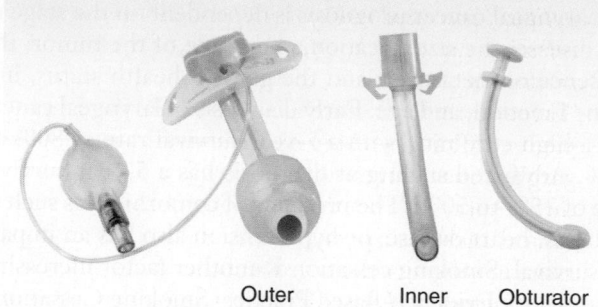

Outer cannula   Inner cannula   Obturator

FIGURE 25.12 Essential components of the tracheostomy tube.

- Provide means for communication.

  Post-laryngectomy, the patient will not be able to speak due to the removal of the larynx. Provide pen and paper and a picture board.

- Nutritional consultation

  Swallowing impairments may result in inadequate nutritional intake. Placement of a gastric or percutaneous esophageal gastrostomy tube may be required if the patient cannot maintain adequate nutritional intake.

■ Teaching

- Diagnostic testing and interventions such as direct laryngoscopy

  Understanding the testing and interventions may ease anxiety and increase compliance.

- Disease management

  *Depending on the location of the laryngeal cancer, the patient may undergo various interventions (laser surgery, laryngectomy, **tracheotomy**). Understanding the outcomes, such as loss of speech and creation of a **tracheostomy**, is essential.*

- Tracheostomy management: suctioning and tracheostomy care with return demonstration

  Skillful performance of suctioning and trach and stoma care is essential to keep the airway free from secretions and avoid infection.

- Radiation therapy care:
  - Skin care: avoid heating pad, ice pack, lotions or powders, sun exposure, extremes of temperature, and abrasive activities such as shaving at the radiation site; do not rub, scratch, or scrub the radiation treatment site; wear loose-fitting, soft clothing site; use a mild soap to clean the area.

    During radiation therapy, the skin can become red and tender and may peel. Radiation delays healing, so care must be taken to limit the additional potential for skin breakdown.

  - Oral care: use a soft-bristle toothbrush and brush and floss after each meal and at bedtime; suck on hard candy or chewing gum; examine the oral cavity for signs of infection, ulcerations, or bleeding.

    A decrease in the production of saliva, which may be permanent, can occur with radiation therapy, resulting in dry mouth or xerostomia. Changes in taste sensation, halitosis, increased risk of dental cavities, and oral infections can occur as a result of decreased saliva production.

- Throat care: limit voice use; eat soft foods, drink plenty of fluids; sucking on ice chips or use of saline gargling may decrease the discomfort. The use of throat sprays or mouthwashes that contain a local topical anesthetic prescribed by the provider may assist in relieving the sore throat.
  With radiation therapy, vocal hoarseness may worsen, and difficulty in swallowing or a sore throat may develop.
- Nutrition management: easy-to-eat, soft, nonspicy, non–acid-containing foods; small, frequent feedings; liquid nutritional supplements may be added.
  Swallowing impairments may result in inadequate nutritional intake.
- Chemotherapy management: take antiemetics prior to receiving chemotherapy and as needed; avoid crowds and persons with infections, and report any signs of infection immediately; report increases in bruising, presence of blood in the urine or stool, or increased fatigue.
  Chemotherapy may cause nausea and vomiting, immuno-suppression, and decreased platelets.
- Communication management: writing or picture boards, esophageal speech, electrolarynges
  Because of the loss of vocal cords with a laryngectomy, the ability to speak will be gone. Alternative forms of communication will be necessary. **Esophageal speech** *occurs through the use of swallowed air to create words in the mouth.* **Electrolarynges** *are mechanical devices that are placed against the neck and use vibrated air to create words.*

Evaluating Care Outcomes

The location, the treatment required (chemotherapy, radiation, surgery), and the presence of metastasis will determine the outcome of the patient with laryngeal cancer. In patients where early detection of laryngeal cancer has occurred, a complete recovery can be expected. If metastasis has occurred, the outcome is dependent on the metastasis site and the patient response to treatment. After laryngectomy, patients can return to normal activities using alternative means for communication. Patients are at risk for reoccurrence of laryngeal cancer if they continue to smoke and use alcohol.

Connection Check 25.6

The nurse is aware that the greatest risk factor for laryngeal cancer is

A. age.
B. alcohol use.
C. tobacco use.
D. occupational hazards.

LARYNGEAL TRAUMA

Epidemiology

Laryngeal trauma is rare. One form of trauma, the laryngeal fracture, occurs in approximately 1 patient per 14,000 to 42,000 emergency department visits and accounts for less than 1% of all blunt traumas. This is partially due to the protected location of the larynx, with the hard, bony structure of the cervical spine posterior and the mandible in a superior and anterior position. Laryngeal trauma is sometimes seen in females because of their slimmer, longer necks, but overall, males present with the highest percentage of laryngeal trauma because of a greater participation in body-contact sports such as fighting.

Pathophysiology

Laryngeal trauma occurs as a result of blunt or penetrating injuries, ingestion or inhalation of caustic agents to the neck, or pressure from prolonged endotracheal intubation. Blunt trauma can occur as a result of assaults, crush injuries, falls, motor vehicle crashes, sports, or strangulation. Penetrating injuries can occur from gunshots or stabbings. Patient outcomes are dependent on early recognition and maintenance of an adequate airway.

Clinical Manifestations

Clinical manifestations of laryngeal trauma are dependent on the extent of the injury. They include hoarseness, pain, stridor, **dyspnea** (difficulty breathing), **dysphagia** (difficulty swallowing), and **hemoptysis** (bloody sputum). The airway can become obstructed from edema or fracture of the laryngeal structures or hematoma development.

Management

Diagnosis and Medical/Surgical Management

Diagnosis is completed by conducting a physical inspection of the neck for signs of swelling, discoloration, subcutaneous emphysema, tracheal deviation, and open wounds. Diagnostic studies include cervical CT, fiberoptic laryngoscopy, or flexible **bronchoscopy**. During a laryngoscopy or flexible bronchoscopy, the provider uses a flexible tube with a fiberoptic system to view structures in the upper and lower airways (Fig. 25.13).

The priority of care in patients with laryngeal trauma is to ensure and maintain a patent airway. Maintenance of the airway may include endotracheal intubation or tracheostomy. Because of the potential of cervical spine injury in addition to laryngeal trauma, stabilization of the cervical spine is vital. Diagnostics wait until the airway is protected and the cervical spine is stabilized.

Surgical interventions, if necessary, include evacuation of hematoma, repair of lacerations, and stabilization/repair of fractures.

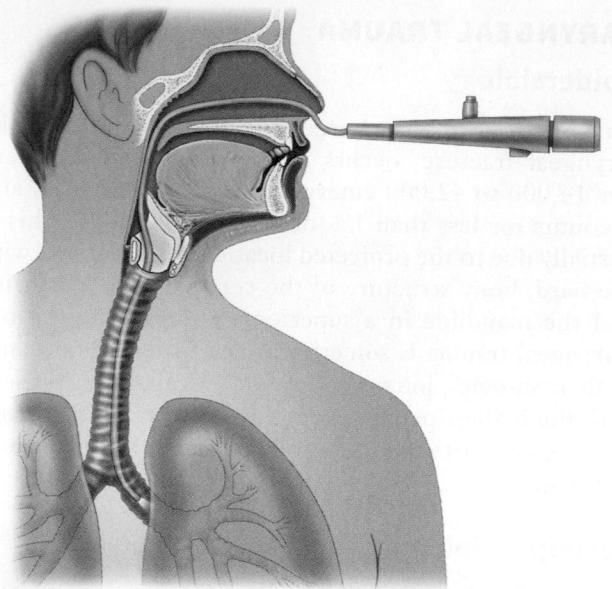

FIGURE 25.13 Flexible bronchoscopy allows for direct visualization of the upper and lower airways.

> **(!) Safety Alert** Patients who have experienced neck trauma are at high risk for airway occlusion or obstruction. Have an emergency tracheostomy insertion set at the bedside, and closely observe the patient for changes in respiratory rate, respiratory effort, and the development of adventitious breath sounds.

Nursing Management

Assessment and Analysis

Symptoms of laryngeal trauma are due to injury to the vocal cords and edema of the soft tissue of the neck. The patient may have a change in the quality and character of the voice or hoarseness, difficulty swallowing, or difficulty breathing. Discoloration and edema of the neck increase the suspicion of laryngeal trauma.

Nursing Diagnoses

- **Ineffective airway clearance** related to edema
- **Impaired gas exchange** related to laryngeal trauma
- **Impaired swallowing** related to edema

Nursing Interventions

■ Assessments

- Vital signs
  Increases in respiratory and heart rates, decreased oxygen saturation, and tachypnea indicate respiratory distress.
- Physical assessment of the neck and upper airway
  Identify risk for laryngeal trauma if discoloration, change in voice, stridor, use of accessory muscles for breathing, or restlessness indicating hypoxia are present.

■ Actions

- Have tracheostomy insertion tray and emergency equipment at the bedside.
  The patient may have a sudden loss of the airway requiring emergency tracheostomy.
- Provide humidified air via a face mask or face tent.
  Cool humidified air will help decrease airway edema.
- Keep the head of the bed elevated at 45 degrees or greater.
  Elevation of the head of the bed will assist in decreasing edema and maintaining a patent airway.
- Aspiration precautions
  Maintain nothing-per-os (NPO) status to protect the airway in the presence of edema and/or bleeding. Also, maintain NPO status until the need for surgery has been evaluated.

■ Teaching

- Symptoms to report to the healthcare provider and when to seek emergency medical care
  A compromise in airway patency can quickly progress to airway occlusion and death.
- Maintenance of voice rest
  Limit talking to prevent an increase in trauma to the larynx and to prevent edema.

Evaluating Care Outcomes

In patients with laryngeal trauma, early recognition of airway compromise is key. The nurse provides close monitoring of respiratory rate, effort, breath sounds, and oxygen saturation. Keeping the head of the bed elevated and providing adequate humidification will assist in decreasing edema to the area. Encouraging the patient to observe voice rest helps minimize additional irritation and avoid airway compromise.

Connection Check 25.7

In providing care for a patient with potential laryngeal trauma, a priority of care is
A. monitoring oxygen saturation every 2 hours.
B. having an emergency tracheostomy tray at the bedside.
C. continuous cardiac monitoring.
D. ensuring adequate oral intake of food.

Making Connections

CASE STUDY: WRAP-UP

Henry is found to have hypertension, with his blood pressure ranging from 150 to 170/90 to 100 mm Hg. His electrocardiogram shows sinus rhythm with frequent multifocal premature ventricular contractions. He is scheduled for a polysomnography (sleep study).

Henry's polysomnography study shows he has OSA. He is provided with a CPAP device with a nasal mask. He is started on hydrochlorothiazide 25 mg daily for his hypertension. Several months after diagnosis, he has lost 25 pounds. He reports that he is not as sleepy during the day and is more rested upon waking in the morning. His blood pressure currently is 130/82 mm Hg. His wife reports that he is less irritable and more energetic.

Case Study Questions

1. Henry is started on an antihypertensive after his diagnosis of hypertension. Which statement indicates Harry understands his education regarding the new medication?
   A. "I can stop taking this medication when I start sleeping better."
   B. "Sleeping through the night is the most important thing to consider."
   C. "I'm glad we found out I had high blood pressure so that I can treat it!"
   D. "This medication will help me sleep better."

2. The nurse provided patient education regarding the sleep study. Which statement made by the patient indicates he understands the procedure?
   A. "The study will occur in the cardiology department and will last 2 hours."
   B. "The sleep study will help determine the amount of sleep I need each night."
   C. "I will receive some sedation for the procedure and will need to have a ride home."
   D. "The test determines how deeply and what type of sleep I have."

3. After a sleep study confirms that Henry has OSA, the nurse is preparing to provide patient education regarding home management. The nurse includes which of the following instructions for Henry?
   A. The use of albuterol nebulization treatments to promote bronchodilation
   B. Use of nasal cannula oxygen delivery during sleep
   C. Use of a CPAP machine during sleep
   D. Keeping the head of the bed flat during sleep

4. The nurse is providing patient education regarding the use of the CPAP machine to Henry and his wife. Which of the following statements regarding CPAP are correct? *(Select all that apply.)*
   A. The machine utilizes a small compressor.
   B. CPAP provides extra oxygen at night.
   C. The face mask should snugly fit over the nose and mouth.
   D. There is an adjustment period to using the CPAP machine.
   E. You should use it only on nights you need to get up early in the morning.

5. After 4 months of using the CPAP machine, Henry determines that he would like to try to sleep without it. He feels slightly claustrophobic and thinks the weight loss may have improved his OSA. What does the nurse ask Henry and his wife to monitor if he stops using the CPAP machine? *(Select all that apply.)*
   A. Increased belching
   B. Irritability
   C. Snoring
   D. Voice quality
   E. Blood pressure

CHAPTER SUMMARY

Rhinitis is caused by irritation and inflammation of the mucous membranes of the nose. Symptoms of rhinitis include nasal congestion; rhinorrhea; sneezing; and itching of the nose, eyes, and ears. Causes of rhinitis include allergies, temperature or humidity changes, and the common cold. Treatment is aimed at symptom relief through the use of a decongestant.

Rhinosinusitis is the current terminology for sinusitis. Rhinosinusitis can be bacterial or viral in nature. A deviated nasal septum, trauma to the nose, or tumors can interfere with nasal drainage and contribute to the development of acute rhinosinusitis. Symptoms of rhinosinusitis include purulent nasal drainage, a sense of pressure, and facial pain. Treatment is dependent on whether a bacterial infection is present. Antibiotics, corticosteroids, pain medications, and saline nasal irrigation are treatment modalities for rhinosinusitis. Complications of rhinosinusitis include orbital cellulitis, osteomyelitis, subdural abscess, meningitis, and sepsis.

Obstructive sleep apnea (OSA) occurs as the soft tissue and muscles of the upper airway relax during sleep, occluding the airway. This results in apnea, hypoxia, and hypercapnia. The patient awakens frequently during the night. Signs and symptoms of OSA are excessive daytime sleepiness, insomnia, loud snoring, personality changes, impotence, hypertension, and cardiac dysrhythmias. Because of the increased prevalence of obesity, the incidence of OSA has increased. Obstructive sleep apnea results in the cardiovascular consequences of hypertension, cardiac dysrhythmias, and myocardial infarction. Treatment of OSA is weight reduction and the use of continuous positive airway pressure (CPAP).

Laryngitis occurs as a result of inflammation of the mucous membranes of the larynx. Acute laryngitis is the most common disorder of the larynx. Causes of acute laryngitis include upper respiratory infection, environmental pollutants, gastroesophageal reflux disease (GERD), and the use of asthma inhalers. Lung or throat cancer may manifest as laryngitis. If laryngitis is a result of infection, antibiotics are used. The patient is encouraged to rest her or his voice and increase oral fluid intake.

Risk factors for the development of laryngeal cancer include tobacco and alcohol use, poor dietary habits, a compromised immune system, genetic syndromes, occupational hazards, gender, age, race, and GERD. The use of tobacco in any form is the most important risk factor for the development of cancers of the head and neck, including the larynx. Diagnostic studies include flexible bronchoscopy, computed tomography, and laboratory studies. The treatment modalities required will be determined on the basis of the site and whether the cancer has metastasized. Surgery, radiation, and chemotherapy may be used to treat laryngeal cancers.

Laryngeal trauma occurs as a result of blunt or penetrating injuries to the neck, cervical spine injuries, and esophageal injuries. Symptoms of laryngeal trauma are dependent on the extent of the injury and include hoarseness, pain, stridor, dyspnea, dysphagia, and hemoptysis. Patients are at risk for loss of a patent airway, so emergency tracheostomy or intubation equipment should be at the bedside.

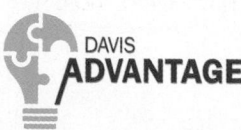

To explore learning resources for this chapter, go to **Davis Advantage** and find:
- Answers to in-text questions
- Chapter Resources and Activities
- NCLEX®-Style Chapter Review Questions
- Bibliography

Chapter 26

Coordinating Care for Patients With Lower Airway Disorders

Adriana Glenn

LEARNING OUTCOMES

Content in this chapter is designed to assist in:

1. Describing the epidemiology of lower airway disorders
2. Correlating clinical manifestations to pathophysiological processes of:
   a. Asthma
   b. Chronic obstructive pulmonary disease
   c. Cystic fibrosis
   d. Lung cancer
3. Describing the diagnostic results used to confirm the diagnosis of lower airway disorders
4. Discussing the medical management of:
   a. Asthma
   b. Chronic obstructive pulmonary disease
   c. Cystic fibrosis
   d. Lung cancer
5. Developing a comprehensive plan of nursing care for patients with lower airway disorders
6. Designing a teaching plan that includes pharmacological, dietary, and lifestyle considerations for patients with lower airway disorders

ESSENTIAL TERMS

Adjuvant therapy
Asthma
Bronchiectasis
Chronic bronchitis
Chronic obstructive pulmonary disease (COPD)
Cystic fibrosis
Emphysema
Exacerbation
Forced expiratory volume (FEV)
Forced vital capacity (FVC)
Neoadjuvant therapy
Peak expiratory flow
Pursed-lip breathing
Spirometry
Steatorrhea
Tripod position
Visual analog dyspnea scale

CONCEPTS

- Assessment
- Inflammation
- Medication
- Nursing Roles
- Oxygenation
- pH Regulation

Finding Connections

CASE STUDY: EPISODE 1

Follow this patient throughout the chapter.

Clifford Davis is a 39-year-old male with a history of asthma who presents to the emergency department with shortness of breath and inability to carry on a conversation. He is assuming a tripod position and exhibits pursed-lip breathing. He has a nonproductive cough. He woke up coughing, followed by chest tightness, which prompted a call to the rescue services. His vital signs are blood pressure (BP), 121/65 mm Hg; heart rate (HR), 150 bpm; respiratory rate (RR), 40. He has audible wheezes bilaterally. He has been a one-pack/day smoker for 15 years.

His medications include:

Hycodan cough elixir 1 to 2 tsp at bedtime (HS)

Zyrtec 5 mg bid

Advair 500/50 1 inhalation bid

Pulmicort Flexhaler 180 mcg bid

Tessalon Perles 200 mg tid

Ventolin 2 puffs prn…

INTRODUCTION

All lower airway disorders negatively impact oxygenation, ventilation, and gas exchange, thus affecting tissue perfusion. Some lower airway disorders can be chronic and progressive such as asthma, chronic obstructive pulmonary disease (COPD), and cystic fibrosis. Chronic and progressive lower airway disorders require meticulous management and lifestyle adjustments to achieve maximum wellness. Conversely, lung cancer can occur acutely and more often has a very poor 5-year survival rate. Lung cancer requires early detection and aggressive management to achieve maximum wellness. All patients attempting to optimally manage their lower airway disorders require thoughtful nursing care, support, and education.

ASTHMA

Epidemiology

Statistics updated in 2017 indicate asthma affects over 18 million Americans, including 6 million children. Approximately 8% of children and 8% of adults have asthma. In adults, it is more common in women than in men. In children, asthma is more common in boys. The rate of asthma among blacks is higher than in other racial or ethnic groups. Multiple-race, American Indian, or Native Alaskan people also have higher rates of asthma. Internationally, estimates of those who suffer from asthma are approximately 300 million people worldwide. This number is expected to increase by more than 100 million by 2025. The risk of death from asthma increases with age. Risk factors include a family history, frequent respiratory infections, eczema, and the presence of allergies such as rhinitis.

Pathophysiology

Asthma is a chronic lung disease characterized by an intermittent, reversible airway obstruction resulting from inflammation of the lung's airways and a tightening of the muscles that surround the airways. The condition affects the bronchial airways, not the alveoli. There is airway obstruction and bronchial hyperresponsiveness. The state of bronchial hyperresponsiveness and underlying inflammation of the small airways is easily triggered by exposure to irritants, exercise, cold weather, or risk factors. Irrritants include cigarette smoke, mold, pollen, dust, animal dander, air pollutants, and occupational irritants. Risk factors include viral infections, nasal polyps, allergic rhinitis, food and medication allergies, and emotional stress.

Exposure to triggers produces an inflammatory response. As a part of that immune activation, IgE antibodies bind to receptors on mast cells, causing degranulation and the release of inflammatory mediators, such as histamine and leukotrienes, which cause vasodilation and increase capillary permeability. There is edema of the airways and an increase in basophils, eosinophils, and neutrophils, which stimulate the production of mucus. The resulting thick, tenacious mucus causes a thickening of the airways and bronchial hyperresponsiveness. The release of histamine also causes constriction and spasm of the smooth muscles surrounding the bronchial tubes, causing bronchospasm of the bronchial tubes. The bronchospasms cause further narrowing of the airways. The bronchospasms, mucus production, and edema produce obstruction to the flow of air into and out of the lungs.

Clinical Manifestations

After exposure to a trigger, the patient exhibits clinical manifestations such as wheezing, dyspnea, coughing, increased sputum, and increased respiratory rate. The patient may also experience chest tightness and tachycardia, which may be secondary to decreased oxygenation or anxiety or a side effect of treatment with bronchodilators. A classic sign of an asthma attack is the inability to speak in full sentences.

Connection Check 26.1

A patient with asthma presents with which symptoms?

A. Cough, elevated blood pressure

B. Decreased respirations, fatigue

C. Increased respirations, wheezes

D. Increased sputum, decreased respirations

Management

Medical Management

Diagnosis

The diagnosis and assessment of asthma include a detailed patient history, pulmonary function tests, chest x-ray, and pulse oximetry and possibly arterial blood gases (ABGs). The detailed patient history should include childhood illnesses, family history of allergies or asthma, eczema, smoking history, occupational history, and exposure to environmental triggers. Additionally, the patient history should include the frequency of symptoms, whether they are triggered by any specific activity or time (day, evening, spring, or fall), how long the symptoms last, and mechanisms the patient uses to relieve the symptoms. The chest x-ray is needed to rule out any other respiratory conditions and to monitor progressive changes in the chest.

Pulmonary function tests (PFTs) are a predominant feature in evaluating asthma. PFTs are a group of tests used to evaluate the functioning of the respiratory system. Some of the more commonly used PFTs are spirometry, peak expiratory volume, and pulse oximetry. There are other PFTs available for use in confirming a diagnosis of asthma when routinely used tests or exams do not provide a clear diagnosis of asthma.

Spirometry is a test that measures airflow and lung volumes, such as the **forced expiratory volume (FEV)**. One of the major tests of pulmonary function is the forced expiratory volume in 1 second (FEV_1). The FEV_1 measures the amount of air forced out of the lungs after a full inspiration. The volume is measured at 1 second. The measurement is compared to a normal person's predicted volume based on age and gender. A decrease in this test of 15% to 20% below the predicted value for age and gender is diagnostic of asthma. An increase of 12% after administration of a bronchodilator is also diagnostic of asthma.

Peak expiratory flow readings measure the maximum airflow expired during a forced expiration. The patient's peak flow readings are compared to the personal best reading with a reading obtained during an **exacerbation** or "asthma attack." Patients are encouraged to monitor their peak flow values. The reading done during an exacerbation as compared to a personal best allows the patient to recognize the severity of the respiratory distress. The patient's asthma action plan (discussed later) is based on the peak flow readings (Box 26.1).

Both noninvasive and invasive methods can be used to obtain oxygen saturation levels in the blood. Pulse oximetry is a noninvasive method of measuring oxygen saturation (SpO_2). It can be used to help determine the severity of the respiratory distress. The normal pulse oximetry value is 95% to 100%. Pulse oximetry monitoring detects desaturation of the hemoglobin before the patient exhibits symptoms. Arterial blood gas monitoring is an invasive sampling of arterial blood to measure the oxygenation of the blood (PaO_2), acid-base balance, and the partial pressure of carbon dioxide ($PaCO_2$).

PaO_2 is an important term and component of ABGs. PaO_2 is the partial pressure of oxygen in arterial blood. PaO_2 reflects a more accurate measure of oxygen in the arterial

---

Box 26.1 Patient Education: Peak Flow Meter

Use of the Peak Flow Meter

- Before each use, make sure the sliding marker or arrow on the peak flow meter is at the bottom of the numbered scale (zero or the lowest number on the scale).
- Stand up straight. Remove gum or any food from your mouth. Take a deep breath (as deep as you can). Put the mouthpiece of the peak flow meter into your mouth. Close your lips tightly around the mouthpiece. Be sure to keep your tongue away from the mouthpiece. In one breath, blow out as hard and as quickly as possible. Blow a "fast hard blast" rather than "slowly blowing" until you have emptied out nearly all of the air from your lungs.
- The force of the air coming out of your lungs causes the marker to move along the numbered scale. Note the number on a piece of paper.
- Repeat the entire routine three times. (You know you have done the routine correctly when the numbers from all three tries are very close together.)
- Record the highest of the three ratings. Do not calculate the average. This is very important. You cannot breathe out too much when using your peak flow meter, but you can breathe out too little.
- Measure your peak flow at close to the same time each day. You and your healthcare provider can determine the best times. One suggestion is to measure your peak flow rate twice daily between 7 and 9 a.m. and 6 and 8 p.m. You may want to measure your peak flow rate before or after using your medicine. Some people measure peak flow both before and after taking medication. Try to do it the same way each time.
- Keep a chart of your peak flow rates. Discuss the readings with your healthcare provider.

---

blood than SpO_2. Once the PaO_2 in arterial blood falls below the threshold of 60 mm Hg, there is a steep reduction in SpO_2. Although a PaO_2 of 60 mm Hg is considered acceptable, a more acceptable range for PaO_2 is 80 to 95 mm Hg. Arterial blood gases provide the best information with regard to identifying the patient's response to oxygen and ventilation therapy and medications. Once asthma is diagnosed, the disease is classified based on the frequency and severity of the symptoms. One approach through the Global Initiative for Asthma guidelines identifies the level of control and the treatment recommended for asthma. Asthma is classified as "mild asthma," "moderate asthma," "severe asthma," and "uncontrolled asthma." Asthma severity may be assessed retrospectively through close evaluation of the treatment required to manage symptoms.

Treatment

The patient and healthcare provider develop an asthma action plan, which assists with decision making. The plan provides information and instructions on how the patient can manage his or her asthma based on peak expiratory flow readings, medications, an awareness or recognition of worsening symptoms and when to seek emergency care. The treatment of asthma includes assessment, monitoring, control of environmental factors, pharmacological treatment, and education. The patient's frequency of symptoms and triggers should be noted. Pulmonary function tests should be conducted regularly to track the patient's response to therapy. During an acute exacerbation, peak flow readings, pulse oximetry, and ABGs (in a very severe attack) are used to determine the severity of the attack. Control of environmental factors is a necessary part of the education program for the patient with asthma. Irritant exposure should be reduced once the irritant has been identified. Patient history or sensitivity testing will often reveal the likely irritant. Environmental smoke is associated with increased symptoms and decreased lung function. Patients should be advised not to smoke and to avoid "second-hand" smoke exposure. The patient should be counseled on the importance of being aware of the levels of air pollution and to avoid outside activities if the level is high. There are many air-monitoring apps available to assist patients in becoming more informed about the air quality in their area. Patients should avoid fumes from wood-burning stoves, fireplaces, aerosol sprays, and strong perfumes. They should also remove animals and/or birds from their home if they are sensitive to the dander. Stress and depression may also be factors that can precipitate an asthma attack.

Medications

Pharmacological treatment of the patient with asthma is based on the patient's response to previous treatment(s) and the level of engagement in the self-management plan. Patients are seen frequently when they begin a new medication (1–3 months) and when they experience an acute exacerbation (within a week). There are several classifications of medications that are used to treat asthma: anti-inflammatories, bronchodilators, anticholinergics, and leukotriene modifiers.

Anti-inflammatories, typically inhaled corticosteroids, reduce mucus production and swelling, making the airways less sensitive and less likely to react to asthma triggers that cause asthma symptoms. Bronchodilators such as beta$_2$-adrenergic agonists relax the bronchial smooth muscle, helping to open the airway and decreasing obstruction. Anticholinergics are another group of bronchodilators. Different from beta$_2$-adrenergic agonists, which relax the bronchioles or small airways, anticholinergics relax the muscles around the larger airways or bronchi. Leukotriene receptor antagonists are another class of medications that may be used to enhance asthma control if the usual medications are not effective. They are not steroids; they inhibit the leukotriene-mediated inflammatory process.

Medications also fall into two categories: long-term control medications and "rescue" medications. Long-term control medications are used daily regardless of the symptoms a patient is experiencing to achieve and maintain control of the asthma. The most effective long-term control medications for asthma are inhaled anti-inflammatories. Another long term control medication option for poorly controlled asthma or when inhaled gluccocorticoids are difficult to manage, such as in young children, is oral theophylline, a bronchodilator with anti-inflammatory

effects. "Rescue" medications are those medications used once an asthma attack has started; these are usually short-acting bronchodilators. Short-acting beta$_2$-adrenergic agonists are the gold standard because they are most effective. Short-acting beta$_2$-adrenergic agonists should be used for acute exacerbations of asthma only. Studies have shown that regular use of short-acting beta$_2$-adrenergic agonists results in more frequent and earlier exacerbations, tolerance, decreased baseline pulmonary function, and increased hyperresponsiveness. Oral anti-inflammatories such as prednisone may also be used in an acute exacerbation. As the attack subsides, oral anti-inflammatory medications are not abruptly stopped but decreased in dosage until they are discontinued.

New medications for poorly controlled asthma include anti-interleukin 5 (anti-IL5) and anti-immunoglobulin-E (anti-IgE) therapy. Anti-IL5 medications reduce the production and survival of eosinophils involved in the asthma attack. Anti-IgE medications help prevent the inflammatory response in allergic asthma. Figure 26.1 illustrates a stepwise approach to the treatment of asthma.

Complications

Status asthmaticus is an acute exacerbation of asthma that is unresponsive to repeated doses or treatment with the typical rescue medications (bronchodilators). It can vary from mild to severe with bronchospasm, inflammation, and excessive mucus production with mucus plugging. Patients report chest tightness, wheezing, dry cough, shortness of breath, and severe respiratory distress. This results in carbon dioxide retention, hypoxemia, and ultimately respiratory failure. Typical triggers include the recent onset of a viral respiratory illness, exposure to a potent irritant or allergen, or exercising in the cold.

Status asthmaticus is a life-threatening emergency requiring a prompt medical response. Treatment includes oxygen, IV fluids, systemic bronchodilators, and steroids to open the airways and decrease inflammation. Endotracheal intubation may be necessary in severe cases until symptoms are under control.

 Safety Alert • Absent or diminished breath sounds signify a decrease in the movement of air due to increased obstruction or respiratory exhaustion.
• If a patient's wheezing decreases and he or she has little or no breath sounds, this indicates the patient is not able to move air throughout the system. This is a medical emergency! It indicates respiratory failure. The patient may require mechanical ventilation.

Nursing Management
Assessment and Analysis

The symptoms the patient exhibits during an asthmatic attack are related to airway obstruction. These symptoms include:

• Dyspnea
• Use of accessory muscles of respiration

	STEP 1	STEP 2	STEP 3	STEP 4	STEP 5
Preferred Controller Choice		Low dose ICS	Low dose ICS/LABA**	Med/high ICS/LABA	Refer for add-on treatment, e.g., tiotropium,*† anti-IgE, anti-IL5*
Other controller options	*Consider low dose ICS*	*Leukotriene receptor antagonists (LTRA) Low dose theophylline**	*Med/high dose ICS Low dose ICS + LTRA (or + theoph*)*	*Add tiotropium*† Med/high dose ICS + LTRA (or 1 theoph*)*	*Add low dose OCS*
Reliever	As-needed short-acting beta²-agonist (SABA)		As-needed SABA or low dose ICS/formoterol#		

*Not for children <12 years
**For children 6–11 years, the preferred Step 3 treatment is medium dose ICS
#For patients prescribed BDP/formoterol or BUD/formoterol maintenance and reliever therapy
†Tiotropium by mist inhaler is an add-on treatment for patients ≥12 years with a history of exacerbations

FIGURE 26.1 Stepwise approach for asthma treatment.
Key: ICS, inhaled corticosteroid; LABA, long acting inhaled beta2 agonist; SABA, short acting inhaled beta2 agonist; LTRA, leukotriene receptor antagonist; OCS, systemic oral corticosteroid; anti-IgE , anti-immunoglobulin E; anti-IL5, anti-interluekin 5; tiotropium = anticholinergic drug; theophylline = broncodilator; BDP/formoterol = combined LABA and ICS

- Wheezes
- Elevated pulse
- Elevated blood pressure
- Increased anxiety
- Inability to lie flat
- Inability to talk in complete sentences
- Decreased peak flow readings

Nursing Diagnoses

- **Ineffective airway clearance** related to increased mucus production, bronchospasm, fatigue
- **Impaired gas exchange** related to dyspnea, fatigue
- **Ineffective breathing pattern** related to anxiety

Nursing Interventions

▪ Assessments

- Vital signs—pulse rate, temperature, respiratory rate, peak flow measurement
  Increased pulse rate may be a sign of poor oxygenation or anxiety or a side effect of treatment with bronchodilators; increased temperature is a sign of infection; a respiratory rate greater than 30 breaths per minute is due to increased anxiety and increased work of breathing due to bronchial constriction; peak flow values indicate the severity of the asthma attack and help monitor recovery.
- Oxygen saturation
  Oxygen saturation of less than 90% indicates significant oxygenation problems. The goal is to maintain the SpO_2 at 90% or above. Hypoxemia causes restlessness, anxiety, and increased blood pressure and pulse rate.
- Arterial blood gas
  The patient initially exhibits respiratory alkalosis caused by hyperventilation (decreased $PaCO_2$). As respiratory

difficulty increases, respiratory acidosis develops (increased $PaCO_2$).
- Breath sounds
  The presence of wheezing indicates narrowing of the airway—expiratory first, then inspiratory. Absent or diminished breath sounds signify a decrease in the movement of air due to increased obstruction or respiratory exhaustion.
- Level of consciousness
  Changes in level of consciousness are indicators of hypoxemia.
- Ability to speak in full sentences
  This demonstrates the ability to move air throughout the tracheobronchial tree; inability to speak in full sentences is an indicator of respiratory distress.
- Cough
  Irritation causes stimulation of the cough receptors.
- Use of accessory muscles
  Use of accessory muscles demonstrates respiratory fatigue.
- Position—**tripod position** (sitting upright with arms propped on a table) or semi-Fowler's position
  The patient may assume the tripod position in an attempt to decrease the work of breathing.
- Monitor dyspnea
  *Use of the **visual analog dyspnea scale** allows the patient to identify his or her own level of dyspnea because dyspnea is a subjective experience (Fig. 26.2).*
- Previous intubation
  The need for intubation in past asthma attacks is an indicator of severity.

▪ Actions

- Provide oxygen.
  Increase SpO_2 to 90% or greater.

Visual Analog Dyspnea Scale

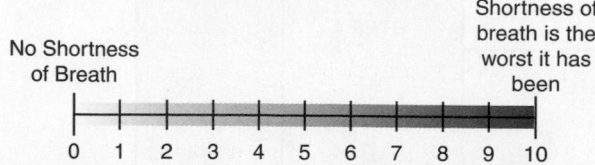

FIGURE 26.2 The visual analog dyspnea scale is a line that assesses the patient's degree of dyspnea. It is a 100-mm line that starts with "No shortness of breath" at one end and "Shortness of Breath is the worst it has been" on the opposite end. Only the patient can identify his or her perception of the dyspnea because dyspnea is a subjective experience. The patient identifies his or her dyspnea on the scale verbally by holding up his or her fingers or pointing to a point on the line. After treatment, the patient is reassessed using the same visual analog dyspnea scale.

- Administer bronchodilators as ordered.
  Bronchial smooth muscle relaxants help open the airway.
- Administer anti-inflammatory medication/steroids as ordered.
  Anti-inflammatory medication decreases the inflammation causing the airway obstruction.
- Administer anticholinergics as ordered.
  Anticholinergics relax the muscles around the larger airways or bronchi.

▪ Teaching

- Provide the patient with an individualized written asthma action plan (Fig. 26.3) that includes daily management of asthma and how to recognize symptoms of exacerbations.
  Control of asthma over time requires regular assessment and consistent management.
- Avoidance of risk factors
  Identify factors that trigger an attack.
- Pursed-lip breathing
  Pursed-lip breathing *keeps the airways open longer and prolongs exhalation, allowing increased time for oxygen and carbon dioxide exchange.*
- Medication education
  Control symptoms and manage disease. Oral steroids used during an exacerbation should be tapered, not abruptly discontinued, to avoid adrenal insufficiency.
- Peak flow meter (see Box 26.1)
  Monitor pulmonary status—establish a baseline and reassess during an acute exacerbation to determine the severity of respiratory distress.
- Smoking cessation
  Smoking is the leading cause of pulmonary disease.
- Proper inhaler technique (Box 26.2)
  Proper technique ensures maximum effectiveness of the inhaled medication. If the patient has trouble coordinating the inhalation and exhalation necessary for proper inhaler technique, recommend the use of an aerochamber.
- Cleaning of respiratory equipment
  Peak flow meters, nebulizers, metered-dose inhalers (MDIs), and aerochambers must be kept clean to prevent infections.

Evaluating Care Outcomes

A well-managed patient with asthma has decreased visits to the emergency department and relies on the use of "rescue" medications less often. The patient has minimal symptoms during the day and night. Supporting positive patient outcomes requires the patient to have adequate knowledge to manage his or her disease. The patient uses control medications as ordered and limits or avoids exposure to the irritants triggering asthma exacerbation. The patient ceases smoking, makes the home and environment as "allergy-free" as possible, monitors peak flow readings twice a day, and adheres to the asthma management plan. When the patient follows the treatment plan, the patient delays the progression of the asthma, experiences fewer exacerbations, and enjoys longer durations of being asymptomatic.

CASE STUDY: EPISODE 2

Clifford's SpO_2 reading upon arrival in the emergency department is 88%. He is started on nasal oxygen, which improves his saturation up to 96%. He is given prednisone by mouth after determining he has not taken his daily dose of anti-inflammatory medication. His peak flow reading is lower than his normal baseline. He is started on the first of three albuterol nebulizer treatments. His SpO_2 level maintains at 96%. He remains short of breath and tachycardic, with a heart rate of 135 bpm…

CHRONIC OBSTRUCTIVE PULMONARY DISEASE

Epidemiology

Chronic obstructive pulmonary disease (COPD) is composed of two diseases: emphysema and chronic bronchitis. It is the fourth-leading cause of chronic morbidity and mortality in the United States. COPD is projected to be the third-leading cause of death by 2020. Additionally, it is projected to rank fifth in 2020 in diseases worldwide. In 2014, almost 16 million people in the United States 18 years and older were diagnosed with COPD, and another 12 million adults are thought to have undiagnosed COPD based on low pulmonary function tests. The prevalence of COPD is higher among women and Caucasians. The Centers for Disease Control and Prevention (CDC) reports that American Indians/Alaskan Natives and multiracial non-Hispanics, those with less than a high school education, current or former smokers, and people with a history of asthma have an increased incidence of COPD. The highest rates of COPD are found in the Southeast and Midwest regions of the United States (Kentucky, Tennessee, Mississippi, and Alabama) and Puerto Rico.

Cigarette smoking is the primary cause of COPD. Approximately 80% to 90% of COPD deaths are caused by smoking. Other risk factors include occupational dust and chemicals, outdoor air pollution, and second-hand smoke.

Asthma Action Plan

For:_____ Doctor:_____ Date:_____

Doctor's Phone Number:_____ Hospital/Emergency Department Phone Number:_____

GREEN ZONE

Doing Well

- No cough, wheeze, chest tightness, or shortness of breath during the day or night
- Can do usual activities

And, if a peak flow meter is used,

Peak flow: more than _____ (80 percent or more of my best peak flow)

My best peak flow is:_____

Take these long-term control medicines each day (include an anti-inflammatory).

Medicine ➡	How much to take ➡	When to take it
_____	_____	_____
_____	_____	_____
_____	_____	_____
_____	_____	_____
_____	_____	_____
_____	_____	_____
_____	_____	_____
_____	_____	_____
_____	_____	_____

Before exercise   ☐ _____ ☐ 2 or ☐ 4 puffs_____ 5 minutes before exercise

YELLOW ZONE

Asthma is Getting Worse

- Cough, wheeze, chest tightness, or shortness of breath, or
- Waking at night due to asthma, or
- Can do some, but not all, usual activities

-Or-

Peak flow: _____ to _____ (50 to 79 percent of my best peak flow)

First ➡ Add: quick-relief medicine—and keep taking your GREEN ZONE medicine.

_____ ☐ 2 or ☐ 4 puffs, every 20 minutes for up to 1 hour
(short-acting beta$_2$-agonist) ☐ Nebulizer, once

Second ➡ If your symptoms (and peak flow, if used) return to GREEN ZONE after 1 hour of above treatment:

☐ Continue monitoring to be sure you stay in the green zone.

-OR-

If your symptoms (and peak flow, if used) do not return to GREEN ZONE after 1 hour of above treatment:

☐ Take:_____ ☐ 2 or ☐ 4 puffs or ☐ Nebulizer
(short-acting beta$_2$-agonist)

☐ Add:_____ mg per day For _____ (3–10) days
(oral steroid)

☐ Call the doctor ☐ before/ ☐ within _____ hours after taking the oral steroid.

RED ZONE

Medical Alert!

- Very short of breath, or shortness of breath, or
- Quick-relief medicines have not helped, or
- Cannot do usual activities, or
- Symptoms are same or get worse after 24 hours in yellow zone

-Or-

Peak flow: less than _____ (50 percent of my best peak flow)

Take this medicine:

☐ _____ ☐ 4 or ☐ 6 puffs or ☐ Nebulizer
(short-acting beta$_2$-agonist)

☐ _____ mg
(oral steroid)

Then call your doctor NOW. Go to the hospital or call an ambulance if:
- You are still in the red zone after 15 minutes AND
- You have not reached your doctor.

DANGER SIGNS
- **Trouble walking and talking due to shortness of breath**
- **Lips or fingernails are blue**

➡ • Take ☐ 4 or ☐ 6 puffs of your quick-relief medicine AND
• Go to the hospital or call for an ambulance _____ NOW!
(phone)

FIGURE 26.3 Sample asthma control plan.

Fewer than 5% of all COPD cases are caused by a deficiency of an enzyme called alpha-1 antitrypsin (AAT). AAT is produced in the liver and is present in the lungs. When present, it has lung-protectant properties. When deficient, there is an increased risk of developing emphysema. Both parents must carry the defective gene to increase the risk of deficient AAT. About 100,000 Americans have the AAT deficiency. Alpha-1 antitrypsin deficiency should be considered if a young person develops emphysema and has no history of smoking or exposure to smoke.

Box 26.2 Patient Education: Use of Metered-Dose Inhaler and Aerochamber

Use of the Metered-Dose Inhaler (MDI)

1. Remove the cap and shake the inhaler.
2. Breathe out gently.
3. Put the mouthpiece in your mouth, and at the start of inspiration, which should be slow and deep, press the canister down and continue to inhale deeply.

4. Hold the breath for 10 seconds or as long as possible, then breathe out slowly.
5. Wait for about a minute or as directed by your healthcare provider before repeating steps 2 through 4; if using a corticosteroid MDI, rinse mouth upon completion of doses.
6. Replace the cap on the MDI.

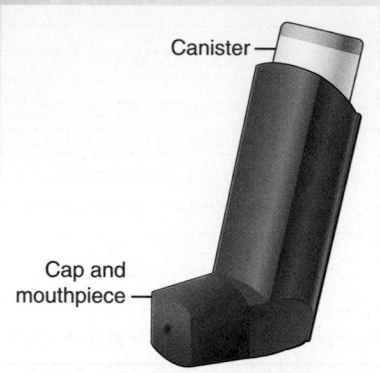

Canister

Cap and mouthpiece

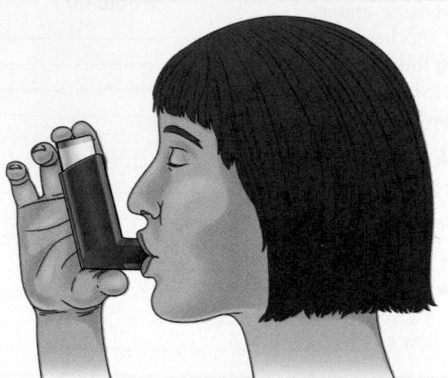

Use of the Aerochamber

1. Remove cap from the MDI.
2. Shake inhaler and insert in back of aerochamber (opposite of the mouthpiece).
3. Breath out completely and place mouthpiece of the chamber in your mouth and seal lips tightly around it.
4. Press canister once to release a dose of the medication.
5. Take a deep, slow breath in. (If you hear a whistling sound, you are breathing in too quickly.)

6. Hold breath for about 10 seconds (count slowly), and then breathe out through the mouthpiece.
7. Breathe in again but do not press canister.
8. Remove mouthpiece from mouth and breathe out.
9. Wait for about a minute or as directed by your healthcare provider before repeating steps 2 through 8; if using a corticosteroid MDI, rinse mouth upon completion of doses.
10. Replace the cap on the MDI.

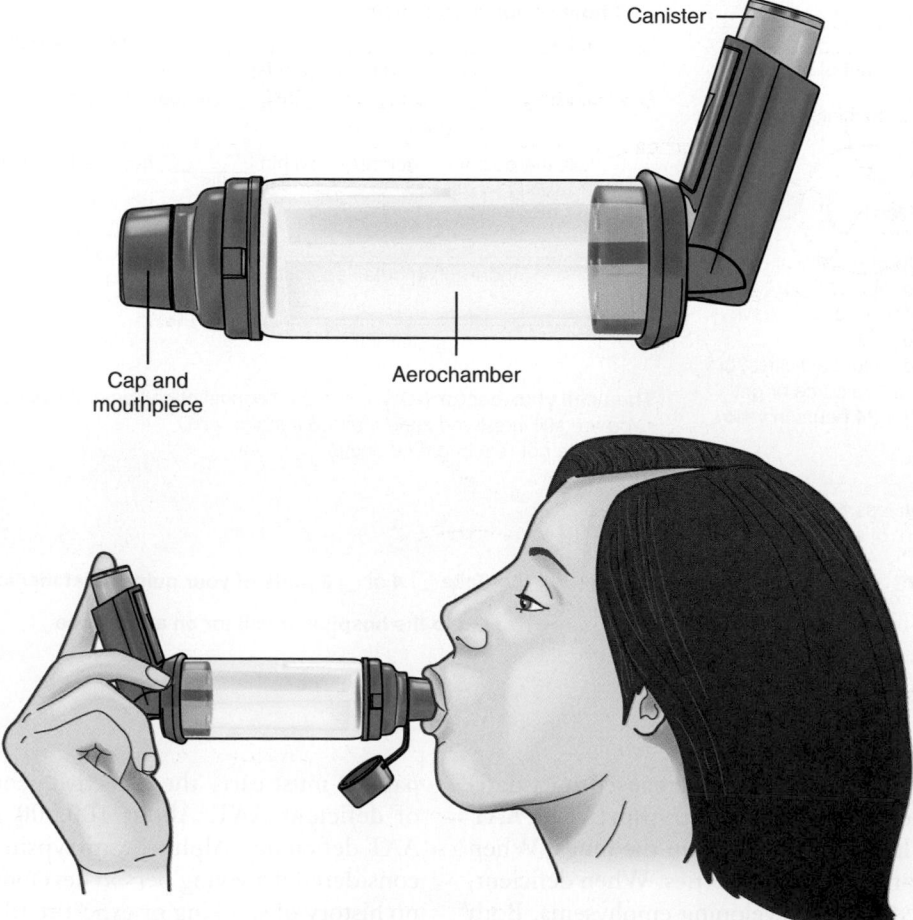

Canister

Cap and mouthpiece

Aerochamber

Pathophysiology

Chronic obstructive pulmonary disease is characterized by airflow limitations. The airflow limitation is progressive and is associated with an abnormal inflammatory response of the lung to noxious particles or gases. Both diseases in COPD cause obstruction to the airflow but in different ways (Fig. 26.4). **Emphysema** is a disease caused by the destruction of the alveoli. **Chronic bronchitis** affects the small airways and is defined as the presence of cough and sputum production for at least 3 months in each of 2 consecutive years. Thus, the chronic airflow limitation is caused by a mixture of small-airway disease and destruction of the lung tissue.

The patient with emphysema loses lung elasticity and develops hyperinflation of the alveoli. Inhaled pollutants (smoke, dust, chemicals, air pollution) result in the breakdown of elastin, which causes the alveoli to lose their elasticity and thus effective elastic recoil after exhalation. The small airways collapse prematurely, causing trapping of air in the alveoli and subsequent distention. Carbon dioxide cannot leave the alveoli, and oxygen cannot enter, resulting in an ineffective exchange of oxygen and carbon dioxide. The patient is hypoxemic, as evidenced by a low SpO_2 and PaO_2 (partial pressure of oxygen), and has carbon dioxide retention and chronic respiratory acidosis.

Chronic bronchitis is caused by inflammation of the bronchi and bronchioles by chronic exposure to smoke and environmental irritants. The inflammation causes an increase in the production of mucus cells, which produce a large amount of thick mucus. The walls of the bronchus thicken, causing airway obstruction. The smaller airways are usually affected before the larger airways. Also identified is an asthma-COPD overlap syndrome (ACOS) which significantly impacts disease trajectory and quality of life (see Evidence-Based Practice).

Clinical Manifestations

Clinical manifestations of the disease include increased work of breathing and shortness of breath. COPD is evidenced by the use of accessory muscles and the patient assuming the tripod position to help ease the work of breathing. The patient with emphysema often appears thin and has a "barrel chest," in which the ratio of the anteroposterior (AP) diameter to the transverse diameter of the chest is 2:2 rather than the normal ratio of 1:2. Patients with emphysema sometimes have a reddish complexion and appear to be puffing when breathing; hence, they may be referred to as a "pink puffer." Conversely, patients with chronic bronchitis are typically obese, have hypoxemia, and appear cyanotic and thus may be referred to as a "blue bloater"; they also have excessive mucus production with a productive cough. Additionally, patients with COPD are at risk for right heart failure due to chronic pulmonary hypertension resulting in right ventricular enlargement. This is referred to as cor pulmonale. Table 26.1 shows a comparison of chronic bronchitis, emphysema, and asthma.

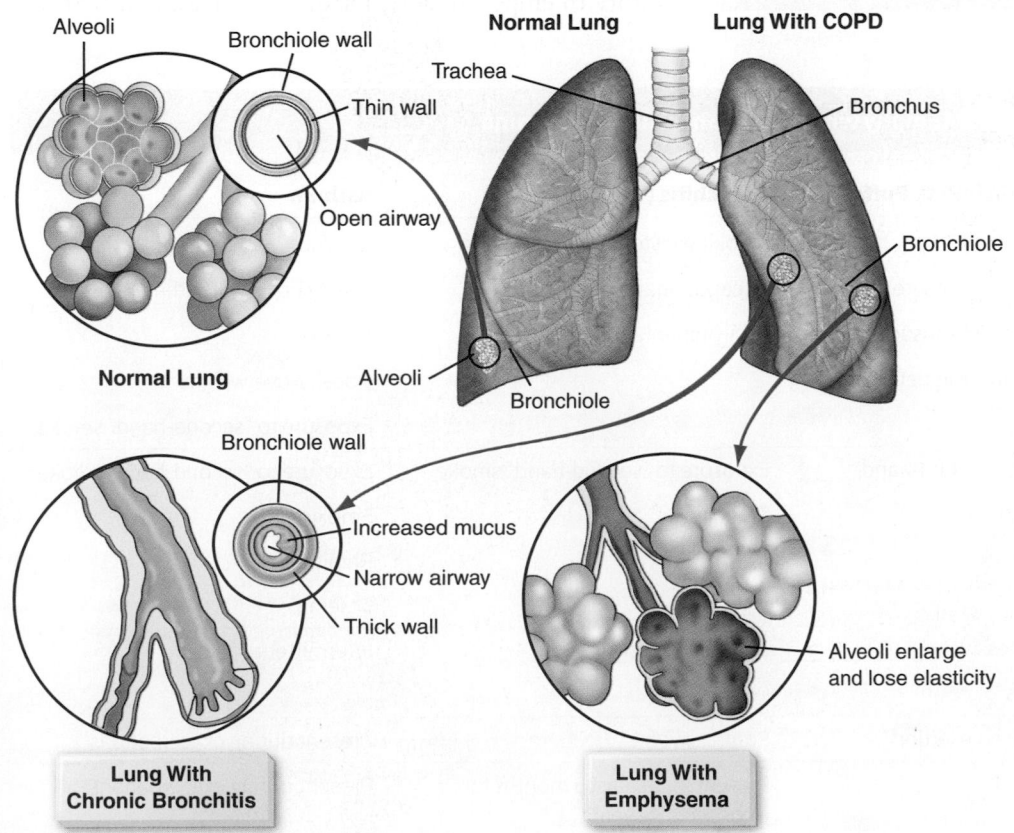

FIGURE 26.4 A normal lung versus a lung with COPD.

Evidence-Based Practice

ACOS

The term *asthma–COPD overlap syndrome (ACOS)* has been used to describe adults presenting with symptoms of both asthma and COPD. The prevalence rate is highly variable, from 15% to 55% depending on age and gender. These patients experience frequent exacerbations and a more rapid decline in lung function, with a correspondingly high mortality rate. They also consume a higher volume of healthcare resources than patients with COPD or asthma alone. There is a self-reported poor quality of life. Recognition of this diagnosis is key to successful management. The goals of treatment are similar to the goals for asthma and COPD: reduce exposure to risk factors, maintain lung function while reducing symptoms, prevent exacerbations, and maintain normal activity. Mainstays of treatment include anti-inflammatory medications and long-acting and short-acting rescue bronchodilators. Smoking cessation is essential.

Ding, B., & Small, M. (2017). Treatment trends in patients with asthma–COPD overlap syndrome in a COPD cohort: Findings from a real-world survey. *International Journal of Chronic Obstructive Pulmonary Disease, 12,* 1753–1763. doi:10.2147/COPD.S136314
Global Initiative for Chronic Obstructive Lung Disease. (2015). *Asthma-COPD overlap syndrome.* Retrieved from http://www.goldcopd.org/uploads/users/files/AsthmaCOPDOverlap.pdf

COPD is characterized by exacerbations occurring after exposure to pollutants such as smoke or respiratory infections such as a cold or flu. An exacerbation is a change in the natural course of the disease evidenced by a variation from the patient's daily baseline symptoms of dyspnea, cough, and/or sputum production. Exacerbations are typically acute in onset and may indicate the need for a change in usual patient management. Warning signs of an exacerbation include increasing shortness of breath, wheezing, more frequent or severe cough, anxiety, problems with sleep, and decreased appetite.

Management

Medical Management

Diagnosis

The diagnosis of COPD is based on patient history, physical assessment, and spirometry. Generally, a chest x-ray is obtained to rule out other causes of respiratory distress. A computed tomography (CT) scan may be considered when the lungs need to be viewed in more detail. Pulmonary function tests also aid in diagnosis. The most commonly performed pulmonary function test (PFT) is spirometry. Spirometry is the measurement of lung volumes and airflow. The two tests done by spirometry are **forced vital capacity (FVC)** and forced expiratory volume in 1 second (FEV_1). Forced vital capacity is the maximum volume of air exhaled during a forced expiration; FEV_1 is the volume of air expired in the first second of maximal expiration after a maximal inspiration. It is a measurement of the lung's ability to empty quickly. Diagnosis is based on both the

Table 26.1 Comparison of COPD (Emphysema and Bronchitis) and Asthma

	Emphysema ("Pink Puffer")	Bronchitis ("Blue Bloater")	Asthma
Risk factors	Smoking history	Smoking history	Smoking
	Occupational exposure	Occupational exposure	Family history of asthma
	Environmental exposure	Environmental exposure	Allergies
	Alpha-1 antitrypsin deficiency		Obesity/overweight
			Exposure to "second-hand" smoke
Health history	Exposure to "second-hand" smoke	Exposure to "second-hand" smoke	Exposure to "second-hand" smoke
	Smoking	Smoking	Smoking
			Rhinitis
			Eczema
Symptoms	Slow, progressive	Slow, progressive	Intermittent
	Continuous	Continuous	
Dyspnea	Progressive on exertion	Progressive	Present during exacerbations
Sputum production	Often present	Present for at least 3 months for 2 consecutive years	Present during exacerbations

Table 26.1 Comparison of COPD (Emphysema and Bronchitis) and Asthma—cont'd

	Emphysema ("Pink Puffer")	Bronchitis ("Blue Bloater")	Asthma
Bronchospasms	Premature closing of the airways with "air trapping"	Obstruction by thick, tenacious mucus	Airflow obstruction by inflammation and mucus
Reversible	Nonreversible	Nonreversible	Reversible
Airway affected	Alveoli are affected	Airways are affected	Airways are affected

value of FEV_1 and FEV_1/FVC. Using normal values for the sex, age, and height of the patient, the FEV_1 is measured, then calculated as a percentage of a normal value. The FEV_1/FVC is computed as a percentage of normal. Patients with COPD show a decrease in both the FEV_1 and the FEV_1/FVC.

Chronic obstructive pulmonary disease is a progressive disease. As the disease progresses, FEV_1 and FEV_1/FVC deteriorate, and exacerbations become more frequent and life threatening. The severity and progression of the disease correlate to the degree of abnormality of the tests. The Global Initiative for Obstructive Lung Disease has identified stages or grades of the disease: Grade I, mild; Grade II, moderate; Grade III, severe; and Grade IV, very severe. Table 26.2 describes the grades of COPD.

Treatment

The management plan for COPD has four goals: assess and monitor the disease, reduce modifiable risk factors, manage stable COPD, and manage exacerbations. Assessment includes regular pulmonary function tests and chest x-rays with an exacerbation to identify other thoracic abnormalities or progressive changes within the structure of the lungs. Additional important biological measurements in the COPD management plan include pulse oximetry (SpO_2) to determine the severity of hypoxemia during an exacerbation and

ABGs to measure the lungs' ability to clear carbon dioxide, as evidenced by $PaCO_2$ and acid-base balance. The ABGs also evaluate oxygenation through PaO_2 values and help identify the patient's response to oxygen therapy and medications. Finally, sputum cultures are assessed to identify organisms causing an infectious trigger to an exacerbation.

Reducing modifiable risk factors includes, if possible, decreasing or eliminating exposure to chemicals, dust, and air pollutants, especially smoke. The single most important modifiable risk factor is smoking cessation. Managing stable COPD includes health education regarding the risks and the warning signs of an exacerbation, oxygen therapy, moderate exercise as tolerated, and the mainstay of medical management: medications.

The cornerstone of pharmacological management is bronchodilators: beta$_2$-adrenergic agonists and anticholinergics used individually or in combination on an as-needed or regular basis to control symptoms. A way to evaluate the effectiveness of treatment and determine a course of therapy is to administer a bronchodilator treatment after the initial spirometry and then repeat the test. This approach helps determine how the lungs respond to the bronchodilator or how the pulmonary obstruction is reversed with the medication. Medication management progresses as the disease progresses and begins with inhaled bronchodilators on an as-needed basis. As the disease

Table 26.2 Gold Criteria for COPD Severity

In patients with FEV_1/FVC less than 0.70:

COPD Grade	Spirometry Values	Clinical Manifestations
Gold I Mild	FEV_1 greater than or equal to 80% of predicted normal value	Patient usually unaware of presence of disease
Gold II Moderate	FEV_1 50% to 79% of predicted normal value	Progressive shortness of breath with exertion
GOLD III Severe	FEV_1 30% to 49% of predicted normal value	Worsening shortness of breath Frequent COPD exacerbations
GOLD IV Very Severe	FEV_1 less than 30% of predicted normal value	Shortness of breath extreme, impairing quality of life COPD exacerbations life threatening

COPD = Chronic obstructive pulmonary disease; FEV_1, = forced expiratory volume at 1 second; FVC = forced vital capacity.

worsens, long-term bronchodilators are added. Inhaled glucocorticoids are added when and if the patient experiences frequent exacerbations.

Identifying and quickly managing exacerbations is essential because they can dramatically impair pulmonary function and accelerate disease progression. Inhaled bronchodilators and oral glucocorticoids are used, as well as antibiotics if the cause of the exacerbation is infection. Noninvasive positive-pressure ventilation can be used to improve oxygenation and ventilation as well as reduce the need for endotracheal intubation and ventilation.

Complications

A complication of COPD is secondary spontaneous pneumothorax (SSP). SSP is a spontaneous pneumothorax that occurs in patients with underlying lung disease. Of all cases of SSP, 50% to 70% are attributed to COPD. It is typically caused by the rupture of the hyperinflated alveoli or blebs. Patients present with dyspnea and chest pain. The presentation is more severe than in primary spontaneous pneumothorax—spontaneous pneumothorax without underlying lung disease—due to the already-existing pulmonary dysfunction. Treatment priorities include supplemental oxygenation and chest tube placement to remove air from the pleural space to allow re-expansion of the affected lung. Care of the patient with a chest tube is discussed in Chapter 27.

Nursing Management

Assessment and Analysis

The clinical manifestations presented by the patient are due to increased airway resistance, increased work of breathing, and increased sputum production. They include:

- Cough
- Increased sputum production
- Dyspnea
- Use of accessory muscles
- Tripod positioning
- Inability to talk in full sentences
- Pursed-lip breathing
- Changes in skin coloring
- Anxiety

Nursing Diagnoses

- **Impaired gas exchange** related to altered oxygen delivery and alveoli destruction
- **Ineffective airway clearance** related to decreased energy, dyspnea, ineffective cough
- **Activity intolerance** related to fatigue and dyspnea
- **Anxiety** related to breathlessness

Nursing Interventions

▪ Assessments

- Oxygen saturation
  An SpO$_2$ of less than 90% indicates a significant oxygenation problem. The goal is to maintain the SpO$_2$ at 90% or above.

- Respiratory rate
  Monitor respiratory rate to avoid hypoventilation—the respiratory drive in COPD is hypoxemia, not hypercapnia. See Safety Alert.
- Breath sounds
  The presence of crackles and wheezes may indicate airway obstruction. Crackles indicate the premature closing of the airways.
- Pursed-lip breathing
  Patients with COPD display pursed-lip breathing to keep the airways open longer and prolong exhalation, allowing for increased time for oxygen and carbon dioxide exchange.
- Cough
  Cough is a cardinal sign of pulmonary disease. It is a protective mechanism for the tracheobronchial tree.
- Temperature
  Increased temperature is a sign of an infectious trigger.
- Dyspnea
  Use of the visual analog dyspnea scale allows the patient to identify his or her own level of dyspnea because dyspnea is a subjective experience.
- Weight
  Monitoring weight identifies nutritional deficiencies—with prolonged increased work of breathing and decreased energy, the ability to eat decreases.

▪ Actions

- Administer bronchodilators as ordered.
  Bronchodilators are bronchial smooth muscle relaxants that help open the airway. Beta$_2$-agonists (short-acting beta-agonists [SABAs] and long-acting beta-agonists [LABAs]) relax the smooth muscles of the airway by stimulating beta-adrenergic receptors, resulting in antagonism to bronchoconstriction. Anticholinergics relax and enlarge the airways in the lungs, making breathing easier. Anticholinergics can also protect the airways from bronchospasm and may reduce the amount of mucus produced by the airways.
- Provide oxygen.
  Increase the SpO$_2$ to 90%. Patients may be placed on continuous oxygen therapy if the SpO$_2$ is less than or equal to 88% or the PaO$_2$ is less than or equal to 60 mm Hg.
- Position—semi-Fowler's
  The semi-Fowler's position increases oxygenation by allowing adequate lung expansion.
- Provide small, frequent meals with dietary supplements.
  Small, frequent meals take less energy to consume and avoid excessive pressure on the diaphragm that may be associated with a large meal.

▪ Teaching

- Breathing techniques—pursed-lip breathing (Box 26.3)
  Pursed-lip breathing keeps the airways open longer and prolongs exhalation, allowing for increased time for oxygen and carbon dioxide exchange.
- Pacing of activities
  Pacing decreases the work of breathing and conserves energy.

Box 26.3 Pursed-Lip Breathing (PLB)

- Sit upright with neck and shoulders relaxed.
- Inhale through the nose slowly, counting "one, two."
- Exhale through pursed lips as if you were blowing out a candle, slowly counting "one, two, three, four."
- Exhalation should be twice as long as inhalation.
- Continue PLB until shortness of breath is controlled.

- Smoking cessation program
  Smoking cessation is key to managing COPD and can change the course of the disease process.
- Nutritional needs
  Small, frequent meals decrease the work of breathing with less impact on the diaphragm.
- Medication regimen
  Knowledge regarding medications and their use; proper use of inhalers
- Vaccine prophylaxis
  Pneumococcal vaccination and an annual flu vaccine decrease the risk of disease exacerbations due to respiratory infections.
- Recognition of symptoms of exacerbation
  The patient and family should be aware of signs that signify the patient's respiratory system is more impaired.
- Coping strategies
  The patient and family should be aware of the lifestyle changes that may occur because of COPD. These include an inability to maintain an active lifestyle, an inability to care for oneself, depression, denial, and social isolation. Strong support and effective coping strategies are essential to managing the life changes.

> **⚠ Safety Alert** If a patient with COPD experiencing an exacerbation is on oxygen therapy, SpO$_2$ and respiratory rate must be monitored continuously until the condition is stabilized. If the patient is receiving too much oxygen, it may "blunt" the respiratory drive. The respiratory effort in a patient with COPD is triggered by the decrease in oxygen, not an increase in carbon dioxide, which is different from the patient with healthy lungs. Therefore, too much oxygen and high PaO$_2$ and SpO$_2$ may cause a decreased respiratory effort.

Evaluating Care Outcomes

A well-managed patient with COPD has decreased visits to the emergency department and fewer hospitalizations. A critical aspect of supporting patients in managing the disease is making sure the patient has adequate knowledge regarding COPD management. Medications should be taken as ordered, and avoiding or reducing exposure to people with colds or flu that may increase the risk of exacerbations

is key. The patient should cease smoking and maintain healthy dietary habits by eating small, frequent meals.

Connection Check 26.2

What is the primary difference between emphysema and chronic bronchitis?

A. Chronic bronchitis predominately affects the large airways.
B. Emphysema predominately affects the large airways.
C. Emphysema predominately affects the alveoli.
D. Chronic bronchitis predominately affects the alveoli.

CYSTIC FIBROSIS

Epidemiology

Cystic fibrosis is an inherited chronic disease that affects the lungs and digestive system. About 30,000 children and adults in the United States are affected with cystic fibrosis, with an estimated 1,000 new cases annually. There are approximately 70,000 affected individuals worldwide. Seventy percent of patients with cystic fibrosis are diagnosed by their second year of life. The disease most commonly affects Caucasians of North European descent. Males and females are equally affected. Blacks, Hispanics, Latinos, Asian Americans, and American Indians have lower incidence rates of cystic fibrosis. More than 10 million Americans are carriers of the defective cystic fibrosis gene.

Cystic fibrosis is the second most common life-shortening disorder occurring in childhood in the United States. The survival rate has increased since the 1950s and 1960s, when children were not expected to live into their teenage years. In the 1950s, children diagnosed with cystic fibrosis usually did not live long enough to attend school. Presently, more than 45% of patients with cystic fibrosis are over 18 years of age. The predicted median age of survival is the mid-30s. Due to the increased survival rate, more adults present with cystic fibrosis complications. Although other organs are affected, respiratory failure accounts for about 85% of the mortalities.

Pathophysiology

Cystic fibrosis is a genetic disease of the exocrine glands (glands that secrete hormones into ducts, also called duct glands), such as the sweat, salivary, and pancreas glands. Cystic fibrosis is caused by a defective gene, the cystic fibrosis transmembrane conductance regulator, or *CFTR*, gene that is carried by both parents (see Genetic Connections). The *CFTR* gene is linked to the production of a protein called the cystic fibrosis transmembrane conductance regulator. This protein functions as a channel to facilitate the transport of negatively charged chloride ions into and out of the cell. It also inhibits sodium transport channels, inhibiting sodium transport into the cell. Due to the extracellular ion concentration, water moves outside of the cell by osmosis, which maintains a thin layer of mucus on the epithelial cells. The genetic mutation disrupts the transport of chloride ions, sodium ions, and water, resulting in the production of a thick mucus that builds up on the epithelial cells (Fig. 26.5).

Genetic Connections

Cystic Fibrosis

Cystic fibrosis is a hereditary disease caused by a recessive defective gene. More than 10 million Americans are symptomless carriers of the defective cystic fibrosis gene. Genetic testing is performed to detect carriers. Each time two carriers of the defective gene have a child, the chances are:

- 25% (1 in 4) their child will have cystic fibrosis
- 50% (1 in 2) their child will carry the defective gene and not have cystic fibrosis
- 25% (1 in 4) their child will not carry the defective gene and not have cystic fibrosis

Genetic counseling is important for couples who might be at risk of carrying the gene as well as for all couples who are planning to become pregnant.

Cystic fibrosis is a multisystem disease that produces increased amounts of thick mucus in the respiratory, gastrointestinal (GI), and reproductive systems. The disease is characterized by thick, viscous mucus that clogs the lungs and obstructs the pancreas. Other organs that are affected include the liver, salivary glands, and testes. The mucus build-up in the GI system and pancreas leads to an exocrine insufficiency, blocking the transport of pancreatic enzymes and resulting in decreased breakdown and absorption of food. The patient may also develop a pancreatic endocrine insufficiency (insufficient secretion of the hormone insulin into the bloodstream to target organs), which results in cystic fibrosis–related diabetes.

The increase in thick, sticky mucus production in the lungs leads to mucus plugging of the airways, inflammation, and **bronchiectasis** (chronic dilation of the bronchioles). Initially, the upper lobes are affected by the disease. Stasis of the mucus leads to chronic respiratory infections. The organisms that cause the infection are often *Staphylococcus aureus* and *Haemophilus influenzae* in childhood and *Pseudomonas aeruginosa* in adults. Pulmonary disease is the most challenging aspect of managing cystic fibrosis and is the leading cause of mortality.

There are often reproductive problems with males who have cystic fibrosis. The thick mucus production results in plugging and deterioration of the vas deferens before birth. The vas deferens transports sperm from the testes to join the semen. This deterioration results in sterility, but modern reproductive technology may allow these patients to reproduce.

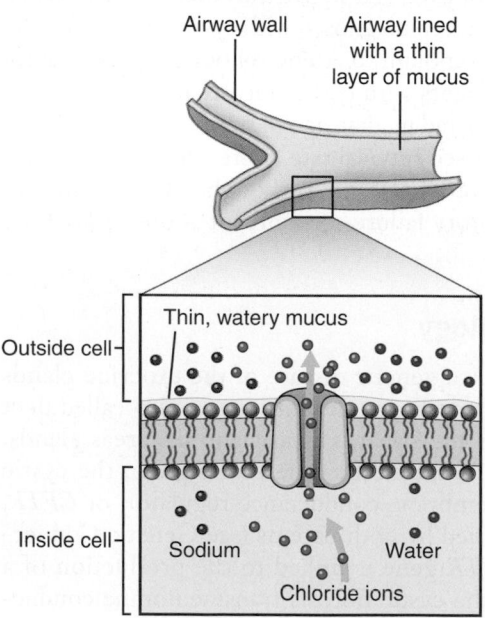

Cross Section of Normal Airway

Airway wall — Airway lined with a thin layer of mucus

Thin, watery mucus

Outside cell

Inside cell

Sodium — Water
Chloride ions

Normal CFTR Channel
Chloride ions freely move through the channel; Sodium and water transport is facilitated

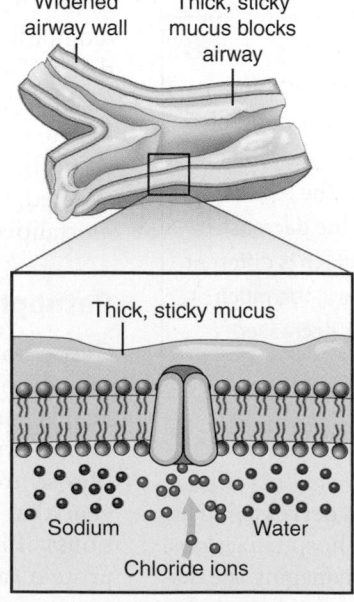

Cross Section of Airway with Cystic Fibrosis

Widened airway wall — Thick, sticky mucus blocks airway

Thick, sticky mucus

Sodium — Water
Chloride ions

Mutant CFTR Channel
Chloride, sodium and water transport is impaired causing thick, sticky mucus

FIGURE 26.5 A genetic mutation of the *CFTR* gene disrupts the transport of chloride and sodium ions and water in cystic fibrosis, resulting in thick mucus deposits on the epithelial cells.

Clinical Manifestations

The clinical manifestations are related to the organ systems affected and can vary significantly among patients. Respiratory symptoms include increased work of breathing, as evidenced by tachypnea and irregular breathing patterns. The patient presents with diaphoresis, nasal flaring, pursed-lip breathing, intercostal muscle retractions, and the use of accessory muscles. Other signs include a persistent cough that produces thick sputum, wheezing, a decreased ability to exercise, repeated lung infections, and inflamed nasal passages.

The GI effects are largely due to the accumulation of mucus in the pancreas, which hinders the release of pancreatic enzymes that help with the breakdown of food. Clinical manifestations of this include:

- Foul-smelling, greasy stools
- Poor weight gain and growth
- Intestinal blockage, particularly in newborns (meconium ileus)
- Severe constipation

Management

Medical Management

Diagnosis

Cystic fibrosis is primarily diagnosed through laboratory testing. The *CFTR* gene mutation in the sweat glands results in increased levels of chloride noted in the sweat because of the impairment of sodium chloride reabsorption. The sweat chloride test measures the concentration of chloride in the patient's sweat. A high level of chloride is an indication of cystic fibrosis. The normal value is less than 30 mEq/L. The test is positive for cystic fibrosis when the chloride level is greater than or equal to 60 mEq/L. Cystic fibrosis screening in newborns has been mandated throughout the United States since 2010. Newborn screening allows treatment to begin before symptoms develop.

Medications

The patient with cystic fibrosis takes the same medications as other patients with lower airway disorders, such as bronchodilators. In addition, the patient may take mucolytics to thin the mucus. Mucomyst (a mucolytic) and inhaled hypertonic saline increase the hydration of the airway to improve mucociliary clearance. The patient also takes anti-inflammatories such as ibuprofen to diminish the inflammatory response and slow the rate of decline in lung function.

Antibiotics are used for chronic pulmonary infections. The antibiotic most often used is tobramycin; its aerosolized form allows for minimal systemic effects. Azithromycin is another antibiotic frequently used. Fat-soluble vitamins (A, D, E, and K) are given as supplements because the long-term antibiotic therapy eradicates the normal flora of the GI tract. Pancreatic replacement enzymes are given to help with digestion and absorption of food. Patients, especially children and teenagers, may also need supplemental calories to maintain their weight and improve energy levels.

The most recent addition to pharmacological management of cystic fibrosis is the use of CFTR modulators. CFTR modulators are medications targeting specific defects caused by mutations in the *CFTR* gene. These treatments do not correct errors in the *CFTR* gene but attempt to correct the malfunctioning protein made by the *CFTR* gene. There are many different mutations causing defects in the protein. The currently developed CFTR therapies are effective only in people with specific mutations.

Surgical Management

Surgical management is an option for patients with cystic fibrosis. A lung or pancreas transplant or both may be considered. The transplant may extend the patient's life, but cystic fibrosis patients often have problems with other organs, which makes them a poor risk for the surgery. Also, transplantation does not cure the disease; the defective gene is still present. The patient may experience a reduction of symptoms initially but will then experience a gradual redevelopment of the disease.

Nursing Management

Assessment and Analysis

The patient with cystic fibrosis usually presents with a variety of symptoms related to the issues with blocked ducts in the sweat and pancreatic glands and the respiratory system. They include:

- Thick, sticky mucus
- Persistent coughing
- Tachypnea
- Frequent lung infections
- Wheezing or shortness of breath
- Poor growth or slow weight gain
- **Steatorrhea** (frequent greasy, bulky, fatty stools) or difficult bowel movements
- Very salty-tasting skin

Nursing Diagnoses

- **Ineffective airway clearance** related to increased sputum production
- **Impaired gas exchange** related to increased sputum
- **Fatigue** related to dyspnea
- **Risk for infection** related to stasis of mucus
- **Imbalanced nutrition**: less than body requirements related to impaired digestive process and absorption of nutrients, increased work of breathing

Nursing Interventions

■ *Assessments*

- Oxygen saturation
  Mucus plugging leads to decreased airflow and impaired gas exchange.
- Temperature
  Increased temperature is indicative of an infection.

- Respiratory rate
  Increased work of breathing causes an increase in the respiratory rate.
- Breath sounds
  Mucus plugging causes wheezing and crackles because of blockage of the airways and air trapping of the bronchioles.
- Weight
  Weight loss occurs because of the impaired pancreatic enzyme absorption disrupting the breakdown and absorption of food.
- Sputum for culture and sensitivities
  These tests identify the organism and appropriate antibiotic to ensure adequate therapy.

■ Actions

- Airway clearance techniques such as postural drainage and percussion
  The airway must be clear of secretions to maintain patency.
- Administer medications as ordered:
  - Bronchodilators
    Bronchial smooth muscle relaxants help open the airway and ease the work of breathing.
  - Antibiotics
    Manage respiratory infections
  - Mucolytics
    Thin secretions, facilitating airway clearance
  - CFTR modulators
    The medications correct the function of the defective protein made by the cystic fibrosis gene (they do not correct the gene itself).
  - Pancreatic enzymes
    Pancreatic enzymes aid in the breakdown and absorption of food.
  - Nutritional supplements
    Increase caloric and vitamin intake to increase energy and increase weight

■ Teaching

- Airway clearance techniques, the use of supplements to meet nutritional needs, taking medications as prescribed, and being aware of and avoiding risk factors of an exacerbation
  Most therapy for cystic fibrosis is performed on a daily basis in the home. In order to manage the disease, the patient and family need a strong understanding of the disease and effective treatment.
- Genetic screening
  The American College of Obstetricians and Gynecologists (ACOG) suggests all couples should be offered screening to identify if they are cystic fibrosis carriers (not just people considered "at risk" like Caucasians and individuals with a family history of cystic fibrosis) because the increasing diversity of the population makes it harder to assign a person to just one ethnicity.
- Genetic counseling
  Counseling should be offered to all couples who are planning to become pregnant.

Evaluating Care Outcomes

Well-managed patients with cystic fibrosis and their caregivers have adequate knowledge to manage the disease through airway clearance techniques and reduced exposure to risk factors for pulmonary infections; they are active participants in the plan of care. The patient presents with a well-controlled respiratory status and free from infection. The patient maintains adequate nutritional status by utilizing pancreatic enzymes, adequate diet, and nutritional supplements. The patient and/or the caregivers can identify changes that suggest an exacerbation of the condition in order to intervene as quickly as possible. These patients and their families use community resources that are available for information and support.

Connection Check 26.3

What is the priority treatment for a patient with cystic fibrosis?

A. Nutritional counseling
B. Airway clearance
C. Medication administration
D. Patient education

LUNG CANCER

Epidemiology

American Cancer Society (ACS) statistics for 2018 indicate that lung cancer remains the second most common cancer in both men and women. It is also the number one cancer killer in the United States for both men and women (about 154,050 deaths; 83,550 in men and 70,500 in women). The ACS estimated approximately 234,030 new cases of lung cancer for 2018.

Black men have a higher incidence of lung cancer than white men, whereas white women have a higher incidence than black women. Women have an overall lower incidence than men. Survival rates vary based the stage of disease at diagnosis. If diagnosed with stage 1A lung cancer, the survival rate is 49%; if diagnosed with stage IV lung cancer, the survival rate is 1%. When diagnosed with stage IV lung cancer, the disease has already spread to lymph nodes and other organs.

Lung cancer is most prevalent in persons over age 65. The major cause (90%) of lung cancer (and the most preventable) is smoking. The risk of developing lung cancer increases as the number of cigarettes smoked and the length of time spent smoking increase. Other risk factors include "second-hand" smoke, radon, occupational pollutants, and asbestos.

Pathophysiology

The uncontrolled growth of abnormal cells in the lungs causes lung cancer. There are two major types of lung cancer: non–small cell and small cell. Non–small-cell cancer represents 85% of lung cancers and consists of three different types of cells. They are squamous-cell carcinoma, adenocarcinoma, and large-cell carcinoma. The 5-year survival rate for those diagnosed with non–small-cell cancer if diagnosed in the early stages is good.

Small-cell cancer, also called oat-cell cancer, represents 15% of lung cancers. It grows quickly and metastasizes to other organs in the body. Independent of the stage at diagnosis, survival statistics are poor. Only 5% to 10% of those developing small-cell cancers survive for 5 years.

Clinical Manifestations

The symptoms of lung cancer are not typically evident early in the disease but become apparent as the disease advances. Symptoms include a new cough that does not go away or changes in a chronic cough, hemoptysis, shortness of breath, wheezing, hoarseness, and chest pain. Headache and bone pain may also be present. Weight loss is common. As the disease progresses, the symptoms worsen.

Management

Medical Management

Diagnosis

Diagnosis is made through several methods:

- Chest x-ray
- Computed tomography (CT) scan of the chest
- Sputum for cytology
- Bronchoscopy
- Positron emission tomography (PET) scans
- Bone scans and abdominal scans
- Mediastinoscopy

A chest x-ray or a CT scan of the chest may identify a pulmonary lesion. A cytology test on sputum may identify specific tumor cells. Bronchoscopy or mediastinoscopy allows direct visualization of the tissues to aid in the diagnosis of lung cancer. Bronchoscopy is the assessment of the larger airways, the trachea and bronchi, through a scope inserted through the mouth or nose. Mediastinoscopy is a surgical procedure that allows for direct visualization of the mediastinum. A scope is inserted through an incision in the chest that allows direct examination and collection of samples for biopsy. Bone scans and abdominal scans are performed to look for metastatic lesions. The PET scan is used to identify changes in the body's metabolism and function rather than structure. A PET scan can detect areas of increased metabolic activity as occurs with rapidly dividing cancer cells.

Nonsurgical Management

The treatment for lung cancer is interprofessional and is dependent on the type, size, location, and stage of the tumor. The components of nonsurgical treatment typically consist of a combination of radiation and chemotherapy. Pain management is also an important focus in treatment.

The chemotherapeutic agent used to treat lung cancer is dependent on the type and/or size of the tumor. It may be used in conjunction with surgery (discussed in the following section), or it may be the primary treatment option for more advanced cancers or if the patient is too ill for surgery.

Radiation therapy used in lung cancer treatment has great versatility. In situations where surgery is not an option, radiation can be used. Radiation can also be used palliatively to relieve symptoms or for pain control.

Pain control is a major component in lung cancer management. A pain relief ladder developed by the World Health Organization is helpful as a guideline for pain control (see Chapter 11, Fig. 11.7). Step 1 involves the use of nonopioid analgesics (acetaminophen or NSAIDs) for mild to moderate pain. Step 2 consists of a moderately potent opioid (codeine, hydrocodone, and oxycodone) plus a nonopioid for persistent pain or pain not controlled by Step 1. Step 3 includes the use of stronger opioids (morphine, fentanyl) plus a nonopioid for uncontrolled or severe pain. The use of adjuvant or additional medications is important to consider at all levels of treatment to relieve patient anxiety. Pain medication needs to be administered around the clock rather than on demand to avoid peaks of pain.

Palliative care services are appropriate to consider with the diagnosis of a life-threatening illness like lung cancer. Palliative care improves the quality of life of patients and their families. In addition to providing pain relief, palliative care can also help in the management of other distressing and debilitating symptoms, such as shortness of breath, nausea, and vomiting.

Surgical Management

Surgery is the preferred treatment if there is no metastasis. Surgery is primarily used for non–small-cell tumors. There are several types of pulmonary surgery depending on the tumor site and size (Fig. 26.6):

- Lobectomy is the removal of an entire lobe of the lung.
- Pneumonectomy is the removal of the entire lung.
- Wedge resection is the removal of a small section of a lobe of the lung.

Chemotherapy may be administered prior to surgery to reduce the size of the tumor to aid in resection. The administration of a chemotherapeutic agent in an effort to shrink the tumor prior to surgery is a type of **neoadjuvant therapy**. Additionally, chemotherapy can be used as **adjuvant therapy** after surgery to kill any remaining cancer cells. Similar to chemotherapy, radiation is also used to shrink the tumor prior to surgery or after surgery to kill any remaining cancer cells.

Connection Check 26.4

When should palliative care be initiated for patients diagnosed with lung cancer?

A. Upon diagnosis
B. After chemotherapy
C. After surgery
D. Upon patient request

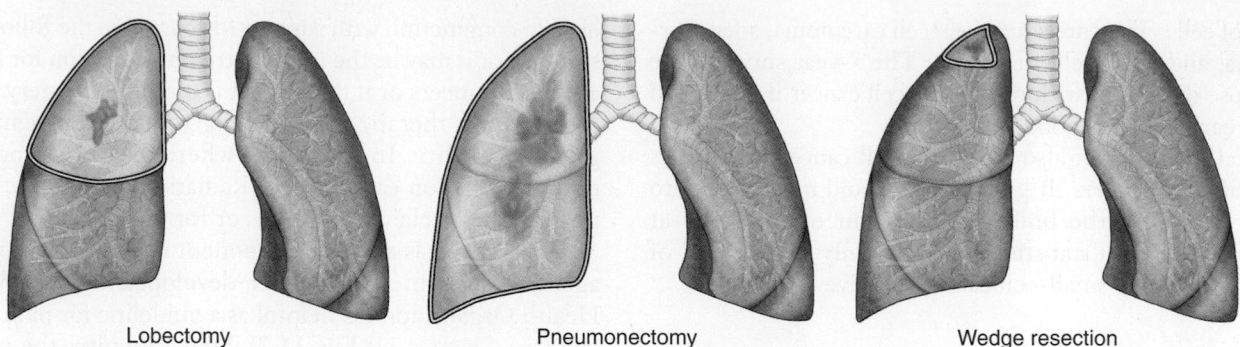

Lobectomy   Pneumonectomy   Wedge resection

FIGURE 26.6 Types of surgeries for lung cancer: lobectomy to remove cancer cells localized in one lobe, a wedge resection for cancer localized in one small area of the lung, and a pneumonectomy for cancer cells spread diffusely in the lung.

Nursing Management

Assessment and Analysis

The patient with lung cancer presents with the following characteristics as a result of abnormal cell growth and tumors in the lungs causing impaired chest movement and air exchange; they usually occur in the late stages of the disease:

- Persistent cough
- Dyspnea
- Wheezing
- Hemoptysis
- Chest pain
- Frequent episodes of pneumonia or bronchitis

Nursing Diagnoses

- **Ineffective gas exchange** related to disruption of pulmonary cells secondary to lung cancer
- **Anxiety** related to the inability to breathe effectively
- **Activity intolerance** related to fatigue and dyspnea

Nursing Interventions

Assessments

- Oxygen saturation
  Decreased SpO_2 is due to poor gas exchange. An SpO_2 of less than 90% indicates significant oxygenation problems.
- Temperature
  Increased temperature is a sign of infection.
- Breath sounds
  The presence of wheezes may indicate airway obstruction. Rhonchi indicate increased secretions in the upper airways.
- Cough
  Cough indicates an irritation of the tracheobronchial tree. The presence of hemoptysis indicates the rupture of small blood vessels.
- Pain
  Pain increases respiratory rate; anxiety decreases quality of life.
- Appetite/weight
  Appetite may be decreased because of the side effects of chemotherapy or loss of energy due to increased work of breathing. Monitoring the weight helps to identify nutritional deficiencies.

- Focused postoperative assessment:
  - Vital signs
    Hypotension and/or tachycardia may indicate excessive blood or fluid loss.
  - Breath sounds
    Diminished or absent breath sounds may indicate postoperative atelectasis.
  - Suture line
    A suture line that is reddened, warm to touch, and/or draining thick, yellow drainage indicates infection.
  - Chest tube
    - Monitor amount and color of chest tube drainage.
      Excessive bloody drainage may indicate a bleed within the chest. Cloudy drainage may indicate infection.
    - Monitor water-seal chamber.
      Persistent bubbling in the water-seal chamber indicates an air leak in the chest tube system.
    See Chapter 27 for a detailed description of chest tube care.

Actions

- Provide oxygen.
  Increase the SpO_2 to 90%.
- Administer medications as ordered.
  - Pain medications/Anti-anxiety medications
    Pain and anti-anxiety medications provide relief from both pain and anxiety, allowing better relaxation, increased expansion of the lungs to improve oxygenation, and improved quality of life.
  - Bronchodilators
    Bronchodilators, bronchial smooth muscle relaxants, open the airway and decrease the work of breathing.
- Provide small, frequent meals with dietary supplements.
  Small, frequent meals avoid excessive pressure on the diaphragm associated with a large meal. Dietary supplements increase nutritional caloric intake, providing energy for the work of breathing.
- Position—semi-Fowler's
  The semi-Fowler's position increases oxygenation by allowing full lung expansion.

- Focused postoperative actions
  - Maintain a closed chest tube system.
    A closed system prevents any inadvertent air leaks.
  - Never clamp the chest tube.
    Clamping the chest tube may result in increased air or fluid in the pleural space, worsening the pneumothorax, and may lead to a tension pneumothorax.
    See Chapter 27 for a detailed description of chest tube care.

Teaching

- Breathing techniques
  Controlled breathing techniques help to increase the clearance of sputum and reduce the sense of breathlessness. Pursed-lip breathing encourages the exchange of oxygen and carbon dioxide.
- Pacing activities
  Pacing conserves energy and decreases the work of breathing.
- Smoking cessation program
  Smoking cessation can change the course of the disease process.
- Nutritional needs
  Small, frequent meals decrease the work of breathing with less impact on the diaphragm.
- Medication regimen
  Knowledge regarding medications and their use, such as proper use of inhalers, increases the ability to manage the disease.
- Use of pain medications around the clock
  Improves patient comfort and quality of life by maintaining a level of pain control rather than suffering peaks of discomfort

Evaluating Care Outcomes

A well-managed patient with lung cancer has the pain under control, sufficient appetite and weight, and adequate oxygenation. Positive outcomes are achieved through around-the-clock pain medication; small, frequent meals; and appropriate use of oxygen and bronchodilators. Regular provider follow-up and palliative care referrals are essential to maintaining an optimal quality of life.

Connection Check 26.5

The nursing plan of care for a patient diagnosed with lung cancer includes which of the following? *(Select all that apply.)*
A. Education about disease management
B. Frequent assessment of pain levels
C. Reminders that recovery is coming soon
D. Frequent assessment of oxygenation
E. Weaning from oxygen because the disease is terminal

Making Connections

CASE STUDY: WRAP-UP

Clifford continues to be short of breath and to wheeze. His SpO_2 remains acceptable while he receives oxygen via the nasal cannula. After the first three nebulizer treatments, his peak flow reading is repeated. It is slightly improved but not back to baseline. Clifford then receives Prednisone 60 mg intramuscularly (IM). The symptoms slowly begin to subside. A repeat of the peak flow reading reveals continued improvement. When Clifford's symptoms are fully resolved, he is discharged from the emergency department with a prescription for an oral prednisone taper. Before he leaves, hospital personnel ensure that he has an appointment with his primary care provider to review this hospital visit and update his asthma action plan.

Case Study Questions

1. What is the most important component of the medical management of Mr. Davis?
   A. Breathing techniques
   B. Disease management through education
   C. Use of "rescue" medications
   D. Use of a peak flow meter

2. If there are no wheezes and diminished breath sounds upon reassessment, what conclusion can the nurse make?
   A. Mr. Davis has resolved his respiratory condition.
   B. Mr. Davis has responded to the bronchodilator therapy.
   C. Mr. Davis has a partially obstructed airway.
   D. Mr. Davis needs another nebulizer treatment.

3. What does the nurse recognize as the priority for Mr. Davis when a partially obstructed airway is suspected?
   A. Airway management
   B. Medication administration
   C. IV line insertion
   D. Patient education

4. What is a major component of the treatment program for Mr. Davis?
   A. A smoking cessation program
   B. A physical exercise program
   C. Genetic counseling
   D. Dietary counseling

5. Which statement about Mr. Davis's medications indicates the need for further teaching?
   A. "I use my albuterol (Proventil) when I am having difficulty breathing."
   B. "I wait 5 minutes between my inhalation puffs."
   C. "I will be able to discontinue all of my medications when my asthma is under control."
   D. "I should not suddenly stop taking the prednisone."

CHAPTER SUMMARY

Asthma is a chronic lung disease characterized by intermittent, reversible airway obstruction resulting from inflammation of the lung's airways and a tightening of the muscles that surround the airways. The patient with asthma presents with the symptoms of increased sputum, increased respirations, and wheezes. Effective treatment of asthma involves assessment and control of environmental triggers, monitoring of symptoms, pharmacological treatment, and education. Pharmacological management typically falls into two categories: long-term control medications and "rescue" medications. Long-term control medications are used daily to maintain control of the asthma. "Rescue" medications are those medications used once an asthma attack has started.

Chronic obstructive pulmonary disease is composed of two pulmonary diseases: emphysema and chronic bronchitis. Both diseases cause obstruction to the airflow but in different ways. The patient with emphysema has airway obstruction due to overdistention and air trapping of the alveoli. Chronic bronchitis results when there is inflammation of the bronchi and bronchioles. The inflammation causes an increase in the production of thick mucus. The walls of the bronchus thicken and cause airway obstruction. The management plan for COPD has four goals: monitor the disease, reduce exposure to risk factors, manage stable COPD, and manage exacerbations. The major components of pharmacological management are bronchodilators: beta$_2$-adrenergic agonists and anticholinergics used individually or in combination on an as-needed or regular basis to control symptoms.

The major diagnostic test for both asthma and COPD as well as other lower airway disorders is the pulmonary function test (FEV_1), which measures the amount of air that is moved in and out of the tracheobronchial tree. The FEV_1 is the amount of air forcefully exhaled within 1 second after a forced inhalation.

Cystic fibrosis is a genetic disease of the exocrine glands, such as the sweat, salivary, or pancreas glands. It is a multisystem disease that produces increased amounts of thick mucus in the respiratory, GI, and reproductive systems. The increase in thick, sticky mucus production leads to mucus plugging of the airways. It also blocks the pancreatic enzymes from breaking down and absorbing food. Medication management includes bronchodilators, mucolytics to thin the mucus, anti-inflammatories to diminish the inflammatory response, CFTR modulators, and antibiotics in the case of infection. Patients also require pancreatic replacement enzymes to help with digestion and absorption of food as well as supplemental calories to maintain weight.

Lung cancer is caused by the uncontrolled growth of abnormal cells in the lungs. There are two major types of lung cancer: non–small cell and small cell. The survival rate for those diagnosed with non–small-cell cancer is good at 5 years. Small-cell cancer grows quickly and metastasizes to other organs in the body. Only 5% to 10% of those developing small-cell cancers survive for 5 years. Treatment is multidisciplinary and is dependent on the type, size, location, and stage of the tumor. Medical management of lung cancer typically consists of a combination of surgery, radiation, chemotherapy, and pain management. Palliative care services are appropriate to consider from diagnosis through the course of the illness because they can improve the quality of life of patients and their families.

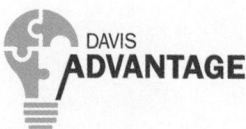
DAVIS
ADVANTAGE

To explore learning resources for this chapter, go to **Davis Advantage** and find:
- Answers to in-text questions
- Chapter Resources and Activities
- NCLEX®-Style Chapter Review Questions
- Bibliography

Chapter 27

Coordinating Care for Critically Ill Patients With Respiratory Dysfunction

Deborah Ennis

Finding Connections

CASE STUDY: EPISODE 1

Follow this patient throughout the chapter.

J.T. Winters is a 19-year-old male admitted to the emergency department after sustaining injuries in a motor vehicle collision (MVC). He was traveling at a high rate of speed when he lost control and went off the road. It is estimated that his car struck a tree at 35 miles per hour. He was not wearing a seat belt, but his air bag did deploy. He was conscious at the scene.

Upon his arrival to the emergency department, J.T.'s vital signs are as follows:

HR—115 bpm

SpO$_2$—93% (on 2 L N/C)

Temp—99.3°F (37.4°C)

BP—106/54 mm Hg

RR—32 breaths/minute

Pain—10/10

J.T. is complaining of pain across his sternum and on his left side. Inspection reveals a broad ecchymotic area across the front of his chest and a deformity along his left side in the region of his fifth through eighth ribs. With each inhalation, this part of his thorax moves inward. Someone uses the phrase "paradoxical movement" to describe what is observed. Upon auscultation, no breath sounds are heard on the left side. A chest tube is inserted, and 400 mL of blood is rapidly drained…

PULMONARY EMBOLISM

A **pulmonary embolism (PE)** is defined as the obstruction of one or more of the branches of the pulmonary artery by particulate matter that has an origin elsewhere in the body. A pulmonary embolus is most commonly caused by a thrombus. A pulmonary embolus can also be caused by a piece of tumor, amniotic fluid, air, or fat, referred to as a nonthrombotic pulmonary embolus (NTPE; Table 27.1). It is important to note that an amniotic fluid pulmonary embolus is fatal to the mother in two-thirds of the cases, with 70% of newborns surviving.

Epidemiology

There are many risk factors for PE, but by far, the greatest risk factor is the presence of a **deep vein thrombosis (DVT)**. **Virchow's triad** of venous stasis, vessel wall damage, and hypercoagulability is the major predisposing factor for the development of a DVT. The most common cause of DVT is prolonged immobility (Table 27.2).

Table 27.1 Sources of Pulmonary Emboli

Type	Source
Deep vein thrombus	Clot breaks loose from site of origin, most often from the deep veins of the leg or pelvis, then travels to the pulmonary vasculature.
Fat	Long-bone fracture
	Osteomyelitis
	Liposuction
Air	Central venous catheter (CVC) insertion—negative intrathoracic pressure can allow air to enter a CVC on insertion or if disconnected from a fluid source.
	Cardiopulmonary bypass
	Hemodialysis
Amniotic fluid	Amniotic fluid can move into the vascular space during delivery through placental vessels.
Tumor	Tumor sloughs off, and tumor particles travel to the pulmonary vasculature.

Table 27.2 Virchow's Triad

Predisposing Factor	Causes
Hypercoagulability	• Cancer
	• Oral contraceptives
	• Dehydration/hemoconcentration
	1. Sickle cell anemia
	2. Polycythemia vera
	3. Abrupt discontinuation of anticoagulants
Venous stasis	• Prolonged bedrest/immobility
	• Obesity
	• Burns
	• Pregnancy
	• Vasculitis/thrombophlebitis
	• Bacterial endocarditis
	• Any postoperative patient
Intimal damage of vessels	• Trauma
	• IV drug use
	• Atherosclerosis

Other risk factors for DVT include:

• Obesity
• Smoking
• Chronic heart disease

- Fracture (hip or leg)
- Hip or knee replacement
- Major surgery
- Major trauma
- Spinal cord injury
- History of previous venous thromboembolism
- Malignancy

The incidence of PE is approximately 1 to 2 per 1,000 persons in the United States. Annually, 50,000 to 100,000 patients die from PE. More than 40% of patients diagnosed with PE also have diagnosed DVT. Pulmonary embolism is the third most common cause of death in patients who are hospitalized for other reasons.

> (!) **Safety Alert** Elderly patients are the most likely recipients of knee or hip replacement surgery. Due to the fact that many of these patients experience limited mobility due to the pain from their disease and have a higher risk for DVT due to aging changes, these patients are at high risk for PE. The nursing assessment must be aimed at early identification of PE as a possible postoperative complication.

Pathophysiology

When a blood clot or other particulate matter travels to the lungs, it lodges in the pulmonary artery and blocks blood flow (Fig. 27.1). This obstruction results in an impaired ventilation-to-perfusion ratio (V/Q ratio) described as decreased or blocked blood flow or perfusion to functioning alveoli. This is called a **ventilation–perfusion mismatch (V/Q mismatch)**, a decreased blood flow to functioning alveoli or areas of the lung where gas exchange can take place if perfusion is adequate. A PE results in a high-ventilation/low-perfusion scenario—a high V/Q mismatch. This prevents gas exchange at the alveolar level, leading to **hypoxemia** (low blood oxygen levels) and local vasoconstriction in the affected pulmonary vascular bed. The PE also results in an increase in pulmonary vascular resistance (PVR) because blood flow cannot move past the venous obstruction. If the right ventricle cannot overcome this increased PVR, then left ventricular preload (blood flow to the left ventricle) is reduced. This leads to decreased oxygenation, decreased cardiac output, and hypotension. The combination of decreased oxygenation and reduced cardiac output results in inadequate tissue perfusion and **hypoxia** (inadequate oxygenation at the cellular level). The increased PVR also leads to pulmonary hypertension (high pressures in the pulmonary vasculature), causing a backflow of blood into the right ventricle and right heart failure. This can exacerbate if the vascular obstruction continues to grow.

Acute pulmonary emboli are classified as massive, submassive, or low risk (Table 27.3). Massive pulmonary emboli occur abruptly, with a sudden onset of symptoms

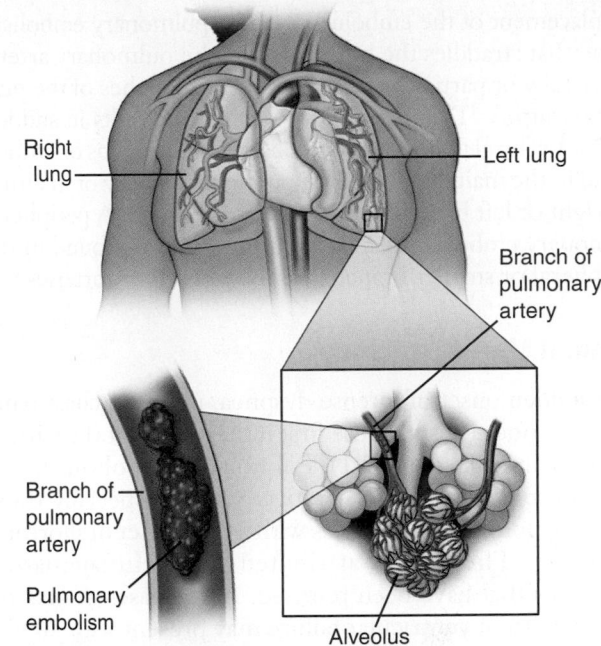

FIGURE 27.1 Pulmonary embolism.

Table 27.3 Pulmonary Embolism Classification	
Type	**Manifestations**
Massive	Acute pulmonary embolism with: • Prolonged hypotension requiring pharmacological support • Right and left ventricular dysfunction • Shock and/or cardiac arrest
Submassive	Acute pulmonary embolism with: • Normal blood pressure • Right ventricular dysfunction—evidenced by echocardiogram • Myocardial necrosis, indicated by elevated troponin I and elevated brain natriuretic peptide (BNP)
Low risk	Acute pulmonary embolism with: • Normal blood pressure • No right ventricular dysfunction • No elevated biomarkers (troponin or BNP)

following obstruction. An acute massive PE can cause rapidly developing right ventricular heart failure and death. A massive PE is present if more than 50% of the blood flow through the pulmonary artery is obstructed. A submassive PE is present when there is right heart dysfunction but no hemodynamic instability. A low-risk PE presents with no indications of heart dysfunction, elevated biomarkers, or hypotension. Pulmonary emboli are further categorized by the placement of the embolus. A saddle pulmonary embolism is one that straddles the bifurcation of the pulmonary artery, either fully or partially obstructing both branches of the pulmonary artery. This type of PE very often results in sudden death. A central pulmonary embolism is an embolus or emboli found in the main branch of the pulmonary artery or in either the right or left branch of the pulmonary artery. A peripheral pulmonary embolism is an embolism or emboli found in the peripheral or smaller branches of the pulmonary arteries.

Clinical Manifestations

The sudden onset of intense dyspnea, pleuritic chest pain, and tachypnea is usually the first indication that the patient has an acute PE (Box 27.1). Pulmonary embolism should be suspected in any postoperative patient, especially those following long-bone surgeries with a new onset of shortness of breath. The pain is attributed to the inflammatory mediators that have been released. In the cases of massive PE, acute right ventricular failure may present with jugular venous distention (JVD). Because of the decreased cardiac output, the patient may become hypotensive and tachycardic. The patient may also become tachycardic because of the hypoxemia caused by the increase in **dead-space ventilation** (nonperfused functioning alveoli). Cerebral perfusion may become compromised, making the patient anxious, restless, and/or confused. If pulmonary infarction has occurred because of hypoxia of pulmonary tissue, the patient may have hemoptysis (bloody sputum).

Management

Medical Management
Diagnosis
Imaging Studies
The diagnosis of PE is done through imaging studies and laboratory studies. The initial study for any patient presenting with chest pain is an electrocardiogram (ECG) to rule

---

out a myocardial infarction. There may be ECG changes in the case of massive PE, but they are nonspecific and not sensitive. Ischemic changes may be seen as inverted T waves and ST changes. Damage to the myocardium is represented by new Q waves and right bundle branch blocks. The predominant value of the ECG is to rule out myocardial infarction (MI).

An initial chest x-ray is done preliminarily to rule out other causes of the respiratory distress. It may show atelectatic changes similar to those of pneumonia and infiltrates at the area of the embolism.

The chest, spiral computed tomography (CT) scan with contrast is the most commonly ordered test to diagnose a PE. The scan can effectively identify central as well as peripheral emboli.

The ventilation–perfusion scan (V/Q scan) can be utilized if a CT scan is not available. A V/Q scan can identify areas of the lungs that are ventilated but not perfusing effectively. This is an indication of obstruction of the pulmonary vasculature or PE. The phrase "high probability" indicates that there is a V/Q mismatch.

The most definitive study for the diagnosis of PE is pulmonary angiography. This test allows for visualization of the pulmonary vasculature and therefore the detection of any obstruction. The invasive nature of this examination, coupled with the time it takes to perform the examination, limits its use when the patient is unstable. It also exposes the patient to more radiation than CT. This test is completed only if other studies are not conclusive and only in a stable patient.

Once the patient with an acute PE has been stabilized, a lower extremity venous ultrasound is usually conducted to determine the presence and extent of any DVT. Recurrent PE is a major cause of mortality for patients who have endured an acute PE. Discovery of a DVT helps guide inpatient and post-discharge therapy and education.

Laboratory Studies
A plasma D-dimer level is a very specific indicator of the possibility of the presence of a thrombus in the body. This level increases as the body removes clots through lysis as part of the normal clot-removal process. The D-dimer is the fibrin left behind from that lysis. A negative D-dimer rules out the possibility of a clot. A positive D-dimer indicates the presence of a clot but requires further testing. This test may be one of the first blood studies done for a patient with acute symptoms of a PE.

Laboratory studies very often include arterial blood gases (ABGs). Evaluation of ABGs in the presence of a PE will most likely reveal hypoxemia (PaO_2 less than 80 mm Hg) and respiratory alkalosis ($PaCO_2$ less than 35) due to the patient's increased respiratory rate. The hypoxemia is more profound in direct relation to the amount of pulmonary vessel obstruction the patient is experiencing. The ABGs may later reveal metabolic acidosis due to the hypoxemia because the body switches to anaerobic metabolism in the face of hypoxemia in the later stages of a PE.

Box 27.1 Common Signs and Symptoms of Pulmonary Embolism

- Dyspnea
- Accessory muscle use
- Pleuritic chest pain
- Tachycardia
- Tachypnea
- Crackles upon auscultation
- Cough
- Hemoptysis
- Unilateral lower extremity edema due to the presence of a deep vein thrombus (DVT); pain in extremity, with redness and warmth

As discussed previously, an acute PE may have cardiac manifestations. Because of the strain on the ventricles brought on by the PE, B-type natriuretic peptide (BNP) may be elevated. This peptide is released by overstretched ventricles under physiological stress. Levels above 100 pg/mL indicate heart failure. B-type natriuretic peptide is an insensitive test because not all patients with an acute PE have heart failure. Troponin I and troponin T may also rise, but this elevation is transient when compared with MI.

Treatment

Medication therapy when treating a patient with acute PE is primarily anticoagulation. Anticoagulation does not reduce the clot; it keeps the clot from getting larger and also helps to reduce the formation of other clots. In nonsymptomatic patients with a low-risk clot, anticoagulation usually consists of initiation of an oral factor Xa inhibitor that inhibits the conversion of prothrombin to thrombin. These medications require no laboratory monitoring as in the case of coumadin, but there is no reversal agent available. These patients do not require hospitalization. Intravenous heparin therapy is initiated with a symptomatic patient with any type of PE—blood clot, air, fat, or other particulate matter—because blood clots will adhere to any of those substances, making them larger and able to obstruct more blood flow. Typically, patients are started on IV heparin with a bolus followed by a continuous drip. The dosages are based on the patient's weight. Heparin therapy is monitored through the activated partial thromboplastin time (aPTT). Prior to the initiation of therapy, an aPTT is drawn and then repeated every 4 to 6 hours to monitor therapy. The therapeutic goal is 1.5 to 2.5 times the normal value, or 40 to 90 seconds. If the initial aPTT is below the designated therapeutic level, an additional heparin bolus may be given along with an increase in the rate of the infusion. If the aPTT is above therapeutic, the rate of the infusion will be reduced. In the cases of very high aPTT levels, the infusion may be held for a specified period of time before restarting the infusion at a lower rate. Once the aPTT is in the therapeutic range for two consecutive iterations, it is evaluated once every 12 or 24 hours. Each facility has established protocols for the assessment of aPTT for a patient receiving heparin. Reaching a therapeutic aPTT level within 24 hours has been shown to have better outcomes. Protamine sulfate is the reversal agent to heparin and must be readily available if active bleeding occurs. Subcutaneous low-molecular-weight heparin, fondaparinux, or unfractionated heparin may be prescribed in lieu of instituting a weight-based heparin protocol.

Anticoagulation continues after discharge with warfarin. Warfarin (Coumadin) therapy is monitored through the international normalized ratio (INR). The therapeutic anticoagulation goal is an INR of 2.0 to 3.0. It takes approximately 3 to 5 days to reach a therapeutic level, so initially, the two medications, heparin and warfarin, are prescribed concurrently. Warfarin may be continued following a PE, depending on severity, for 3 to 6 months. A factor Xa inhibitor could also be used on discharge rather than warfarin depending on patient and provider preference.

If a patient is hemodynamically compromised, thrombolytic therapy (alteplase) should be considered. Contrary to anticoagulation, systemic thrombolysis is responsible for lysis or removal of the clot from the pulmonary artery. The adverse effects of systemic thrombolytic agents may preclude their use. The risk of bleeding is of paramount concern. The main concern in the elderly patient is cerebral hemorrhage. Patients typically have IV heparin administration discontinued during the alteplase infusion. It is restarted after the infusion is complete. Absolute and relative contraindications must be taken into account before initiating this therapy (Table 27.4). Patients who are hemodynamically unstable may be candidates for catheter-directed thrombolysis (CDT) using a low-dose hourly infusion of tissue plasminogen activator (tPA) or urokinase. This therapy will administer the medication directly to the clot at the site, resulting in lysis of the clot and reducing the risk of bleeding complications. This therapy is considered safe and beneficial for patients with massive PE and those with submassive PE.

Intravenous isotonic fluid is used to decrease the viscosity of the blood. Caution must be exercised to ensure that the patient is not fluid-overloaded. In cases of recognized right ventricular compromise, IV fluid may be held, and an inotropic pharmacological agent that increases cardiac contractility, such as dobutamine, may be administered in order to overcome PVR and allow the left ventricle to maximize cardiac output. Hypotension can be managed with norepinephrine and vasopressin if it is not resolved with single-medication therapy.

Surgical Management

Surgical management is considered for acute massive PE resulting in hemodynamic instability where thrombolytic agents are contraindicated. The procedure is an

Table 27.4 Contraindications to Thrombolytic Therapy	
Absolute	**Relative**
History of hemorrhagic stroke	Severe hypertension (SBP greater than 200 mm Hg or DBP greater than 110 mm Hg)
Active intracranial neoplasm	Nonhemorrhagic stroke (within 2 months)
Recent surgery	Surgery in past 10 days
Recent trauma (less than or equal to 2 months)	Thrombocytopenia (platelets less than 100,000)
Active or recent internal bleeding (6 months)	History of bleeding tendencies

DBP, Diastolic blood pressure; *SBP*, systolic blood pressure.

embolectomy, or physical removal of the clot. There are two types of embolectomy, catheter or surgical. In addition to the CDT discussed above, rheolytic or rotational catheter embolectomy may be an option. In a rheolytic catheter embolectomy, pressurized saline is used to erode the clot. It requires a large venous catheter or sheath, so bleeding is a major risk. Another type of catheter embolectomy is the rotational embolectomy. A rotating tool is used to break down the clot. A standard cardiac catheter is used, so there is less risk to the patient. In general, catheter embolectomy is used for clots in the main and segmented or lobar pulmonary artery branches. The efficacy of catheter embolectomy is still being studied, but each method has a mortality rate of approximately 20%.

The more common type of embolectomy is the surgical embolectomy. This is a complex thoracic surgical procedure that requires cardiopulmonary bypass. Again, this procedure is usually performed when the patient has systemic hypotension and the use of thrombolytics is contraindicated. New studies indicate that the use of CDT could be an appropriate choice in lieu of a surgical approach, especially in the face of severe hemodynamic instability. The major determinant of the success of these procedures is when they can be performed prior to the onset of cardiogenic shock or cardiac arrest.

Inferior vena cava (IVC) filters are placed to prevent recurrent PEs (Fig. 27.2). The indications for IVC filter placement are active bleeding that disqualifies anticoagulation therapy, recurrent PE despite adequate anticoagulation

therapy, or evidence that hemodynamic or respiratory dysfunction is severe enough that another PE could be fatal. The filter allows for blood passage but is designed to trap any further emboli originating in the lower extremities. Complications of IVC filter placement are rare but include filter migration, erosion of the vena cava wall, obstruction due to filter thrombosis, and procedural complications. Retrievable IVC filters are now available, with the goal being the removal of the IVC when anticoagulation is again advisable.

Nursing Management

Assessment and Analysis

Assessment of a patient at risk for an acute PE requires astute monitoring. The clinical manifestations are nonspecific. Sudden onset of pleuritic chest pain, dyspnea, and tachypnea are the most common initial assessment findings. The presence of a PE has two distinct cardiac manifestations. If PVR is elevated, the early signs of right ventricular failure, such as JVD, may be seen. With a massive PE, preload to the left side of the heart may be dramatically reduced, causing a decrease in cardiac output and hypotension. A sudden change in mental status may occur if cerebral perfusion pressure is compromised. The patient may become anxious or express feelings of impending doom.

Nursing Diagnoses

- **Impaired gas exchange** related to interruption of pulmonary blood flow
- **Ineffective breathing pattern:** tachypnea related to pain and hypoxemia
- **Decreased cardiac output** related to increased PVR
- **Risk for bleeding** related to anticoagulant/thrombolytic therapy

Nursing Interventions

▪ *Assessments*

- Airway
  Is breathing effective to maintain oxygenation? Is the patient breathing comfortably or in respiratory distress? Mechanical ventilation may be required.
- Oxygenation
  The pulse oximetry reading decreases from baseline as a result of increased dead-space ventilation; blood is not properly oxygenated in the lungs.
- Frequent vital signs
  The pulse increases because of hypoxemia; blood pressure may decrease from baseline in cases of massive PE because of decreased left heart preload; tachypnea may occur due to decreased oxygenation and pain; fever may develop because of the inflammatory response.
- Chest pain
  Sudden-onset chest (pleuritic) pain with dyspnea and tachypnea is usually the first sign of acute PE, resulting from the release of inflammatory mediators.
- Laboratory values
  - ABGs (onset)
    Tachypnea causes respiratory alkalosis; PaO₂ is reduced because of increased dead-space ventilation.

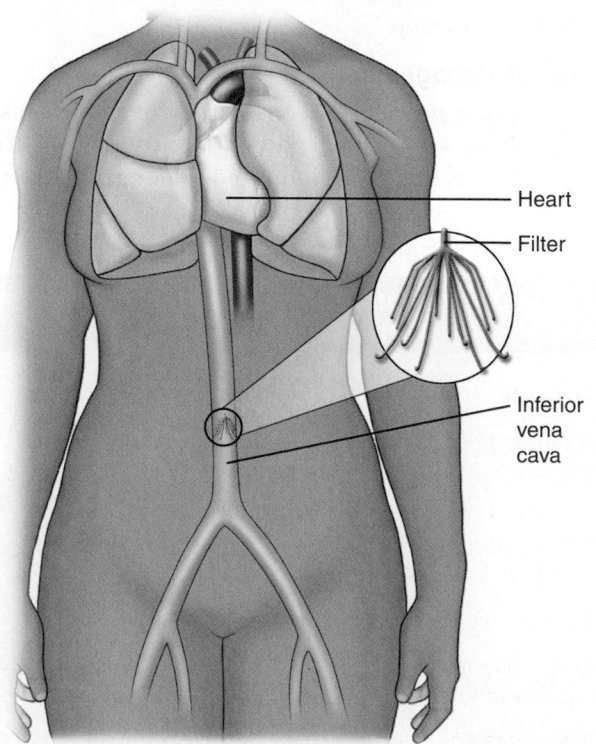

FIGURE 27.2 Inferior vena cava (IVC) filter placement. The filter allows for blood passage but traps emboli originating in the lower extremities, preventing travel to the heart and lungs.

Heart

Filter

Inferior vena cava

- ABGs (as disease progresses)
  Metabolic acidosis results from hypoxia and the subsequent transition to anaerobic metabolism.
- Lactic acid levels
  An increase confirms anaerobic metabolism.
- Coagulation studies
  APTT levels are monitored if the patient is on heparin; the prothrombin time (PT)/INR is followed if the patient is on warfarin.
- Monitor urine output.
  Urine output less than 0.5 mL/kg/hr is an early sign of shock.

■ Actions

- Elevate the head of the bed.
  Allows the diaphragm to drop, facilitating less work of breathing and better oxygenation
- Administer IV fluids.
  Decrease viscosity of blood; caution must be used in cases of right ventricular overload.
- Administer anticoagulation medications as ordered.
  Heparin infusion, warfarin, and factor Xa inhibitors limit the growth of PE and DVT and decrease the formation of new clots.
- Administer thrombolytic medications if ordered.
  Thrombolytics degrade the clot; if not contraindicated, they are used when patients are hemodynamically compromised.
- Administer inotropic agents if ordered.
  Inotropic agents increase cardiac contractility in an effort to augment cardiac output if the patient is hemodynamically unstable.
- Administer norepinephrine or vasopressin as ordered.
  These vasoconstrictive medications are given, if necessary, to maintain a systolic BP of at least 80 mm Hg.
- Institute bleeding precautions.
  The use of anticoagulants and/or thrombolytics can result in bleeding; minimize venipunctures; watch for blood in urine, stool, and sputum; watch for unusual bruising.
- Be prepared for intubation and resuscitation.
  Massive PE may result in cardiogenic shock and sudden death.

■ Teaching

- Disease process/lifestyle modifications
  The patient should understand the risks of PE and how to avoid future occurrences via lifestyle modifications.
  - Exercise regimen that includes aerobic exercise
    Exercise strengthens the patient's heart and cardiovascular system, improves venous return to the heart, and assists in the loss of weight.
  - Cardiac-prudent diet that minimizes saturated fats
    Heart-healthy diet to reduce damage to vasculature
  - Adequate fluid intake; at least eight 8-ounce glasses of water spread across each day
    Maintains hydration; decreases blood viscosity
  - Smoking cessation
    Reduces intimal damage to vasculature; decreases vasoconstriction caused by smoking, which decreases risk of clot formation in vasoconstricted vessels; improves overall health

- Medications
  Explain the mechanism of action of anticoagulants and thrombolytics; the patient will be required to have follow-up laboratory samples drawn if on warfarin to determine effective dosing of outpatient anticoagulants. Regular laboratory testing not necessary for patients on factor Xa inhibitors.
- Bleeding precautions
  Encourage the use of electric razors; use soft toothbrushes, no flossing. Avoid activities with a risk of bleeding, such as football.
- Diet
  Limit foods high in vitamin K; these foods interfere with the efficacy of warfarin.
- Signs and symptoms of a recurrent PE/DVT
  Be aware of the occurrence of unilateral lower extremity edema and pain in the extremity, with redness and warmth, which may be due to the presence of a DVT. Pleuritic chest pain and dyspnea may indicate recurrent PE.

Evaluating Care Outcomes

Patients who have suffered from a PE have an increased incidence of recurrent PE. By adhering to a medication regimen, improving diet, beginning an exercise program, staying adequately hydrated, and quitting smoking, the patient should remain free of a recurrence of a PE as well as reducing the most common cause, DVT of the lower extremities.

Connection Check 27.1

After oxygen has been administered, the next priority intervention the nurse would initiate for a patient with a pulmonary embolus is the administration of which of these therapies?

A. Normal saline IV fluid
B. IV heparin
C. Platelet administration
D. Antibiotics for inflammatory fever

ACUTE RESPIRATORY FAILURE

Epidemiology

Acute respiratory failure is when one or both of the gas-exchange functions of the lungs are compromised. The gas-exchange functions of the lungs are oxygenation and ventilation or carbon dioxide (CO_2) removal. Compromise of these functions leads to hypoxemia and/or **hypercapnia**, also referred to as hypercarbia (increased $PaCO_2$). There are two types of respiratory failure: type I, or **hypoxemic respiratory failure**, and type II, or **hypercapnic respiratory failure**.

Hypoxemic respiratory failure (type I) is characterized by a PaO_2 of less than 60 mm Hg despite increased inspired oxygen with a normal or low $PaCO_2$. Hypercapnic respiratory failure (type II) is characterized by a respiratory acidosis, a $PaCO_2$ greater than 50 mm Hg and pH less than 7.35. Hypoxemia may or may not be present.

The prevalence of acute respiratory failure varies depending on the definition, but it is a life-threatening disorder with a high mortality rate. Risk factors for hypoxemic respiratory failure include disease processes that produce a V/Q mismatch or impair oxygen diffusion at the alveolar level, such as pulmonary edema, pneumonia, or pulmonary embolus. Risk factors for hypercapnic respiratory failure include diseases that impair ventilation or cause hypoventilation. This type of respiratory failure is seen in patients with impaired chest-wall movement and thus impaired ventilation, such as acute asthma and narcotic overdose, or in patients with peripheral nervous system disorders that impair chest-wall movement, such as myasthenia gravis. This may also be seen in patients with chest-wall injury due to trauma that results in ventilatory impairment. Typically, these patients also present with hypoxemia if the cause is not quickly reversed. Risk factors are noted in Table 27.5.

Pathophysiology

In hypoxemic respiratory failure, gas exchange and oxygenation do not occur because of a V/Q mismatch, a shunt, or impaired diffusion. In the case of V/Q mismatch, one scenario is that the lungs are adequately ventilated but not perfused (dead-space ventilation), as in the case of a patient suffering from a PE (high V/Q); air is entering the lung, but the blood is blocked from reaching the alveoli due to the embolism, and thus no gas exchange occurs. The second scenario is when the lungs are perfused but inadequately ventilated (shunt), as in the case of the patient with atelectasis or pneumonia (low V/Q; Fig. 27.3). Blood is perfusing the lungs, but air cannot get to the alveoli due to fluid or exudate in the air spaces. An extreme V/Q mismatch is an **intrapulmonary shunt**, where there is no gas exchange at all because of a shunting of blood past collapsed alveoli, as in the case of atelectasis. Impaired diffusion occurs at the alveolar level. Either the distance for diffusion (gas exchange) is increased or the permeability of the **alveolar-capillary membrane** (ACM) is reduced. This is due to either collapsed alveoli; fluid in the alveoli or small airways, such as in pulmonary edema; or exudate in the small airways and/or alveoli, such as in pneumonia. The primary result is hypoxemia.

In hypercapnic respiratory failure, impaired ventilation occurs when there is a reduced ability of the lungs and respiratory apparatus to adequately expand (hypoventilation). The amount of air moved by the lungs is suboptimal. This means that the elimination of CO_2 does not take place adequately. Hypercarbia is the initial result, but hypoxemia eventually occurs without adequate treatment.

Clinical Manifestations

Acute respiratory failure results in hypercapnia and hypoxemia. Hypercapnia can produce headache, confusion, and a decreased level of consciousness or increased somnolence. The patient may be tachycardic and tachypneic and may also appear dizzy and flushed, with a pink coloring to the skin. In hypoxemia, clinical manifestations include increases in heart rate, respiratory rate, and blood pressure in an effort to increase oxygenation and perfusion. As the patient becomes more hypoxemic, there is less cerebral perfusion. This may manifest as restlessness, confusion, and/or anxiety. Eventually, without adequate treatment, the patient will present cyanotic with a greatly decreased level of consciousness or coma. It is important to remember that the patient will present not only with the clinical manifestations of respiratory failure but also with the clinical manifestations of the underlying cause or disease process (Table 27.6).

Connection Check 27.2

A patient with a diagnosis of pneumonia complains of a new onset of slight shortness of breath. For which of the following assessment findings would the nurse call the primary care provider immediately? *(Select all that apply.)*

A. The patient is voiding, but the amounts are decreasing.
B. The patient is sleeping more than usual.
C. There is a pink coloration to the skin.
D. The patient's secretions are thin and milky colored.
E. The patient thought it was the 3rd instead of the 5th of the month.

Table 27.5 Risk Factors for Acute Respiratory Failure

Impaired Ventilation (Hypoventilation)	Ventilation–Perfusion Mismatch	Impaired Diffusion (Alveolar)
• Airway obstruction	• COPD	• Pulmonary edema
• Respiratory muscle weakness/paralysis that can occur with neuromuscular disease such as myasthenia gravis	• Restrictive lung diseases (sarcoidosis, pulmonary fibrosis)	• ARDS
• Chest-wall injury	• Atelectasis	
• Anesthesia	• Pulmonary embolus	
• Opioid administration	• Pneumothorax	
	• ARDS	

ARDS, Acute respiratory distress syndrome; *COPD,* chronic obstructive pulmonary disease

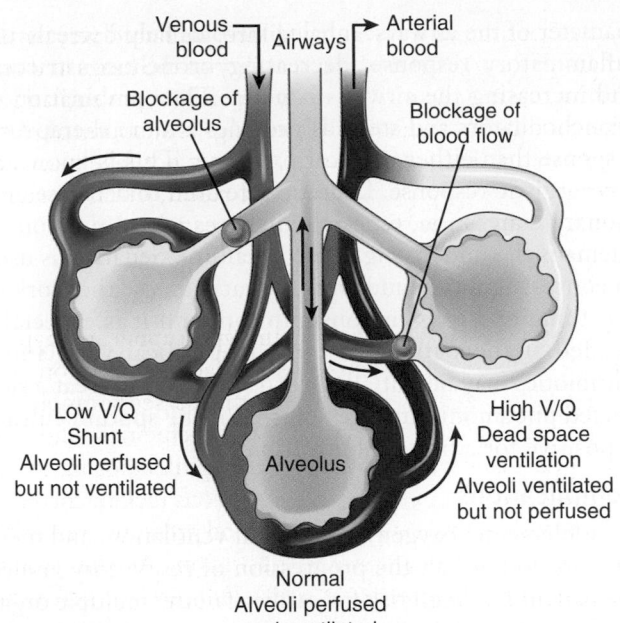

FIGURE 27.3 Ventilation–perfusion mismatch.

Table 27.6 **Clinical Manifestations of Respiratory Failure**		
Early	**Intermediate**	**Late**
• Dyspnea	• Confusion	• Cyanosis
• Restlessness	• Lethargy (due to increased CO$_2$)	• Coma
• Anxiety		
• Fatigue	• Pink skin coloration (due to increased CO$_2$)	
• Increased blood pressure (from baseline)		
• Tachycardia		

Management

Medical Management

Diagnosis

Laboratory and diagnostic tests include ABGs, venous oxygen saturation, hemoglobin and hematocrit, chest x-ray, and sputum cultures. Arterial blood gases are an excellent tool to assess the adequacy of both oxygenation and ventilation in the lungs. Hypoxemic respiratory failure has an initial period of respiratory alkalosis due to hyperventilation along with hypoxemia. Once the initial blood gases have been analyzed and treatment has been initiated, pulse oximetry can be used to monitor oxygenation. The goal is to have an SpO$_2$ greater than 94% (which correlates to a PaO$_2$ of approximately 80 mm Hg). Special care is taken for the patient with chronic obstructive pulmonary disease (COPD) because of the hypoxic drive to breathe (see Safety Alert).

Hypercarbic respiratory failure results in ABGs with a pH of less than 7.35 and a PaCO$_2$ of greater than 45 mm Hg. The PaO$_2$ may or may not be decreased initially but will eventually decrease without adequate treatment.

Venous oxygen saturation measures the amount of oxygenated blood returning to the heart to determine the adequacy of perfusion at the tissue level. It is correlated with perfusion failure or increased tissue oxygen demands. A normal venous oxygen saturation is 60% to 80%. A decreased venous oxygen saturation indicates inadequate cardiac output; the tissues are extracting more oxygen than normal because of the decreased oxygen delivery. A more detailed description of venous oxygen saturation and hemodynamic monitoring is given in Chapter 32.

The patient's hemoglobin and hematocrit should be analyzed to make certain that there are enough binding sites for oxygen to ensure adequate oxygen-carrying capacity. Red blood cells carry oxygen to the cells for cellular oxygenation. If there are not sufficient red blood cells, the oxygen-carrying capacity of the blood is diminished.

A chest x-ray may show an underlying pathology, such as heart failure, pulmonary congestion, pneumonia, or pneumothorax, that can explain the respiratory failure. As discussed earlier, PE as a cause of respiratory failure is diagnosed through laboratory testing and a CT scan. A sputum culture should be obtained to rule out a pathogenic (i.e., bacterial or viral) cause of the failure.

Treatment

Respiratory failure is not a disease—it is a condition caused by another disease or disorder. It is vital to treat not only the respiratory failure but also the underlying cause. If the cause is pulmonary edema, then that issue must be addressed as well as the oxygenation issues associated with the resulting respiratory failure. Careful attention to nutrition is also imperative to provide calories and energy for the increased work of breathing, as well as adequate hydration to keep secretions thin.

The treatment of respiratory failure begins with oxygen. In many cases of respiratory distress, minimal supplemental oxygen may help the patient's hypoxemic status. The use of a nasal cannula or Venturi mask may provide adequate support. This is not the case when a patient is suffering from respiratory failure. The patient in acute respiratory failure who has not responded to traditional methods of oxygen administration may be placed on a nonrebreather mask with 100% FIO_2. The mask is placed over the patient's nose and mouth and then secured to the patient using the elastic band. The oxygen flow meter is then turned on to its maximum setting. The reservoir bag of the mask should be inflated to ensure that the patient is receiving 100% oxygen.

In cases of severe V/Q mismatches where shunting of blood is occurring past nonfunctioning alveoli, supplemental oxygenation may not be sufficient to improve the patient's oxygenation status. In these cases, noninvasive or invasive positive-pressure ventilation may be necessary to open the alveoli to allow gas exchange. **Noninvasive positive-pressure ventilation (NPPV)**, such as bilevel positive airway pressure (BiPAP) or continuous positive airway pressure (CPAP), administered via a tight-fitting face mask, can be used to help increase oxygenation. In BiPAP, the patient receives two different pressures. A higher pressure during inhalation assists with the opening of the alveoli, and a lower pressure during exhalation keeps the alveoli from collapsing during/at the end of exhalation but also allows ease of exhalation. In contrast, CPAP maintains one continuous pressure throughout the respiratory cycle to help keep the alveoli open through inspiration and expiration.

Invasive positive-pressure ventilation requires an advanced airway, such as an endotracheal tube (ETT) or a tracheostomy tube, and mechanical ventilation. As with CPAP, during mechanical ventilation, positive pressure is maintained throughout the ventilatory cycle in the form of positive end-expiratory pressure (PEEP). The pressure is measured at the end of expiration, thus the name, but as stated, the positive pressure is maintained throughout the cycle. Mechanical ventilation is discussed in detail in Chapter 7.

Connection Check 27.3

The nurse understands that oxygen therapy for a patient with COPD requires close monitoring because of which of the following?

A. Hypoxic respiratory drive
B. Hypercapnic respiratory drive
C. Acidotic respiratory drive
D. Alkalotic respiratory drive

Medications

Medications such as inhaled bronchodilators, inhaled steroids, diuretics, sedation, and antibiotics are used in cases of acute respiratory failure. Bronchodilators open the airways by stimulating beta-2 receptors within the lungs. This helps to improve airflow because of an increase in the diameter of the airways. Inhaled steroids help decrease the inflammatory response, decreasing bronchoconstriction and increasing the airway diameter. The combination of bronchodilators and steroids provides a more therapeutic response than either medication alone. This is known as a synergistic response. Diuretics are used to decrease pulmonary congestion, especially in cases where pulmonary edema is the underlying cause of failure. Sedation is used to control agitation and anxiety that increase the work of breathing and oxygen consumption, and it is especially needed if the patient requires mechanical ventilation. Antibiotics may be initially broad spectrum to treat a suspected pneumonia and are adjusted if the sputum culture is positive for a bacterial infection.

Complications

If supplemental oxygen, mechanical ventilation, and medications do not halt the progression of respiratory failure, the patient is at high risk for cardiac failure, multiple organ dysfunction, and death.

Nursing Management

Assessment and Analysis

The clinical manifestations are due to the hypoxemia and hypercapnia of acute respiratory failure. Arterial blood gas analysis reveals a decreasing oxygenation status and/or increased CO_2 levels due to impaired oxygenation or ventilation. Changes in mental status may indicate a decrease in cerebral perfusion. Agitation indicates hypoxia; somnolence indicates hypercarbia. New-onset dyspnea, increased work of breathing, and tachypnea are early indicators of impending respiratory compromise. Tachycardia and hypertension are present initially as a compensatory response.

Nursing Diagnoses

- **Impaired gas exchange** related to **alveolar hypoventilation**, V/Q mismatching, and/or intrapulmonary shunting
- **Ineffective breathing pattern** related to muscular fatigue and/or neurological impairment

Nursing Interventions

Assessments

- Airway
  Is the airway patent? Is the patient breathing comfortably, or is there increased work of breathing? Does the patient require suctioning or assistance with airway secretions?
- Vital signs and oxygen saturation
  Blood pressure, pulse, and respiratory rate increase as a compensatory mechanism in an attempt to increase oxygenation in the presence of hypoxemia; fever may develop because of inflammation and/or infection. The pulse oximetry reading decreases from baseline because of the V/Q mismatch, impaired diffusion, and/or **alveolar hypoventilation***.*
- ABGs
  Hypoventilation of type II failure results in CO_2 retention, acidosis, and ultimately, decreased PaO_2; V/Q mismatch or diffusion defects of type 1 failure result in a decreased PaO_2.

- Cardiac monitoring
  Hypoxia and increased oxygen demand due to tachycardia may lead to dysrhythmias.
- Neurological assessment
  A change in mental status may be an early indication of impending respiratory failure.
  - Agitation
    Agitation is caused by hypoxemia.
  - Somnolence
    Somnolence is caused by hypercapnia.
- Breath sounds
  The underlying cause of respiratory failure may result in crackles (pulmonary edema) or rhonchi (pneumonia, COPD) or diminished or absent breath sounds (hypoventilation).
- Skin coloration
  Careful monitoring of skin coloration can be helpful in identifying changes in the patient.
  Cyanosis may be visible in the nail beds and around the mouth in the initial stages of hypoxemia; as central cyanosis sets in, the body may take on a blue or gray tinge.
  A deep pink coloration to the skin is highly indicative of increased CO_2 levels.

◾ Actions

- Administer oxygen (with humidity) as ordered.
  Supplemental oxygen is necessary to treat hypoxemia. Humidity helps to prevent mucosal drying and helps keep secretions thin so that they can be more easily coughed or suctioned up.
- Medication administration
  - Administer bronchodilating medications as ordered.
    Bronchial smooth muscle relaxants help open the airways.
  - Administer steroids as ordered.
    Reduce inflammation; synergistic effect with bronchodilating agents (administer bronchodilator medications first, then inhaled steroids to allow the steroids to be inhaled more easily into the bronchial tree)
  - Administer diuretics as ordered.
    Diuretics help decrease the pulmonary congestion that impairs ventilation.
  - Administer sedation as ordered (typically only in mechanically ventilated patients).
    Sedation helps decrease anxiety and agitation, helping to decrease the work of breathing and oxygen consumption.
- Elevate the head of the bed; sit the patient up in a chair.
  Positioning with the head elevated optimizes gas exchange, aids in the work of breathing, and decreases the risk of aspiration
- Position patient with the "good lung down."
  If the underlying disease is unilateral, positioning with the good lung down improves gas exchange by optimizing the V/Q ratio; gravity ensures the healthy lung maintains adequate blood flow to optimize ventilation to perfusion.

- Chest physical therapy and suctioning; ambulate as able.
  If excessive sputum is part of the underlying cause, positioning, postural therapy, percussion, vibration, and ambulation combined with assisted coughing or suctioning help mobilize and clear secretions.
- Administer IV fluids/hydration.
  Decreases viscosity of secretions; helps maintain intravascular volume.
- Administer nutritional support.
  The patient's metabolic needs must be met to promote healing.
- Be prepared for noninvasive or invasive positive-pressure ventilatory support.
  A severe V/Q mismatch may require the addition of positive pressure to adequately promote gas exchange.

◾ Teaching

- Disease process
  The patient should understand the risk factors and causes of acute respiratory failure and how to avoid future occurrences.
- Medications
  Explain the mechanism of action and the rationale for each medication. Dosing instructions, missed dosing, and the treatment regimen must be addressed.
- Pulmonary rehabilitation
  - Breathing techniques
    Techniques such as pursed-lip breathing and diaphragmatic breathing allow for better alveolar ventilation and improve gas exchange.
  - Energy conservation
    Work with the patient to determine priorities in daily living.
  - Exercise
    Aerobic exercise helps improve respiratory status.
- Infection prevention
  Hand washing and pneumococcal and influenza vaccinations help decrease the likelihood of infection.
- Diet and adequate hydration
  Adequate caloric intake is necessary for healing; adequate hydration helps ensure thin secretions.
- Smoking cessation
  Improves overall health and respiratory functioning; reduces incidences of pulmonary disease and cancer

Evaluating Care Outcomes

The initial goal of treatment for the patient with acute respiratory failure is to improve gas exchange. Pulmonary rehabilitation in the form of exercise training, nutritional counseling, and breathing strategies should be implemented to assist in the recovery from respiratory failure. The patient successfully treated is able to return to baseline respiratory function. Except in cases where the use of supplemental oxygen is the patient's underlying norm, a well-managed patient should not require supplemental oxygenation upon discharge. The patient should be able to return to baseline activities of daily living, work, and social commitments.

CASE STUDY: EPISODE 2

After stabilization of his injuries, J.T. is admitted to the intensive care unit (ICU). The bleeding into the thoracic cavity has stopped, but the lung has not fully expanded. On the second day in the unit, it is noted that his pulse oximetry readings continue to decline in spite of increased FIO_2 via 100% nonrebreather. He is tachypneic and tachycardic. A chest x-ray shows diffuse infiltrates bilaterally. An ABG shows the following: pH 7.50, $PaCO_2$ of 32, PaO_2 of 50, and HCO_3 of 28 while on 70% FIO_2. It is determined that J.T. has developed ARDS. J.T. is intubated, and mechanical ventilation is initiated...

Table 27.7 Direct and Indirect Causes of ARDS

Direct Injury	Indirect Injury
Aspiration	Sepsis, shock
Chest trauma	Pancreatitis
Pneumonia (infectious or aspiration)	Burns
Pulmonary contusion	Multiple blood transfusions; transfusion-related acute lung injury (TRALI)
Inhalation injury (smoke; toxins)	
Pulmonary embolus	Cardiopulmonary bypass
	Drug/alcohol overdose

ARDS, Acute respiratory distress syndrome.

ACUTE RESPIRATORY DISTRESS SYNDROME

Epidemiology

There are approximately 190,000 new cases of **acute respiratory distress syndrome (ARDS)** annually. Research shows that the prevalence of ARDS is between 15% and 18% of all mechanically ventilated patients. Despite the most modern technology and after numerous studies, mortality rates for ARDS remain high. Death is not usually due to respiratory failure but due to multiple organ dysfunction brought on by hypoxia and/or infection.

There are more than 50 causes for the development of ARDS. The most common cause is sepsis. Other causes include pneumonia, severe trauma, aspiration, massive transfusions, cigarette smoking, cardiopulmonary bypass, pneumonectomy, PE, and drug/alcohol overdose. A way of classifying ARDS is to determine if the cause is due to direct or indirect injury. Direct injury refers to damage or disruption of the respiratory system. Indirect causes are those processes or disorders that occur outside the respiratory system but have a deleterious effect on the lungs. Table 27.7 outlines a partial list of causes of ARDS; it is not meant to be a complete list.

Pathophysiology and Clinical Manifestations

Acute respiratory distress syndrome is defined by the following characteristics: acute onset of less than 7 days, refractory hypoxemia, and bilateral infiltrates ruling out cardiac pulmonary edema as the cause. It is further classified in terms of severity through evaluation of the **PaO_2/FIO_2 ratio**, the ratio of the partial pressure of oxygen over the fraction of inspired oxygen. To determine this ratio, divide PaO_2 by FIO_2. In a healthy individual, the PaO_2 averages 90 mm Hg (normal is 80 to 100). Breathing room air, the FIO_2 is 21% (or 0.21), so the equation is 90/.21 or a PaO_2/FIO_2 ratio of approximately 428. If a patient has a PaO_2 of 70 mm Hg while receiving 70% (0.7) FIO_2, the ratio is 100, which is diagnostic for severe ARDS (Table 27.8).

There are three phases of ARDS: exudative, proliferative, and fibrotic. The **exudative phase** typically occurs within 24 to 48 hours after injury. In this phase, as a result of the activation and release of inflammatory mediators, there is a disruption of the alveolar-capillary membrane (ACM). The ACM becomes dilated due to the inflammatory mediators, and this disturbance allows fluid to move from the capillaries into the interstitial space and into the alveoli. The disruption of the ACM also allows protein to move from the vascular space.

The presence of protein in the vascular space helps to maintain the colloid oncotic pressure. Loss of protein from the vascular space lessens the oncotic forces, worsening the movement of fluid into the alveoli. The alveolar and interstitial edema results in a severe V/Q mismatch, inadequate ventilation occurring in the face of adequate perfusion or blood flow, which results in hypoxemia; blood is shunted past the fluid-filled alveoli without being oxygenated.

In addition to the alveolar and interstitial edema, there is damage to the alveolar cells that produce surfactant. Surfactant is responsible for maintaining alveolar surface tension. Alveolar surface tension keeps the alveoli from fully collapsing at the end of expiration. If alveolar surface tension is lost, then the alveoli collapse. This is referred to as *atelectasis.*

Clinical manifestations in this phase include hyperventilation and tachycardia as a compensatory response to hypoxemia. Arterial blood gases reveal a respiratory alkalosis due to the hyperventilation. Cardiac output increases in an attempt to increase blood flow through the lungs. The chest x-ray reveals the increased alveolar fluid as bilateral infiltrates and is referred to as *pulmonary edema.* Unlike the pulmonary edema associated with a heart failure exacerbation (see Chapter 30), there is no evidence of increased left atrial or ventricular pressure, which would indicate left heart failure. This is referred to as *noncardiogenic pulmonary edema.*

Table 27.8 ARDS Severity

Level of ARDS	PaO$_2$/FIO$_2$ Ratio	Mortality Rate
Mild ARDS	200–300 on ventilator settings that include positive end-expiratory pressure (PEEP) or continuous positive airway pressure (CPAP) ≥5 cm H$_2$O	27%
Moderate ARDS	100–200 on ventilator settings that include PEEP ≥5 cm H$_2$O	32%
Severe ARDS	Less than 100 on ventilator settings that include PEEP ≥5 cm H$_2$O	45%

ARDS, Acute respiratory distress syndrome.

In the **proliferative phase**, neutrophils and other inflammatory mediators cross the damaged ACM and release toxic mediators that further damage both the alveolar and capillary epithelium. Diffusion defects result. The V/Q mismatch worsens, and pulmonary hypertension occurs because of locally occurring vasoconstriction in the lung caused by the hypoxemia. This results in right-sided heart failure due to the increase in PVR or high vascular pressures in the lung. Widespread fibrotic changes occur throughout the diseased lung tissue. The lungs become stiff and noncompliant, increasing the work of breathing.

Clinical manifestations in this phase include hypercarbia and worsening hypoxemia. As the process continues, PaCO$_2$ begins to rise despite hyperventilation. Increases in delivered oxygen do not alleviate the dropping PaO$_2$ caused by the increasingly impaired oxygen exchange across the fluid-filled and damaged ACM. This is refractory hypoxemia, meaning that in spite of increasing oxygen delivery to the patient, the hypoxemia does not improve and will eventually worsen. Lung compliance continues to deteriorate, continuing to increase the work of breathing. If the patient is on a ventilator, peak inspiratory pressures rise because of decreased compliance within the lung, requiring more pressure to deliver ventilatory volume.

In the **fibrotic phase**, there is diffuse fibrosis and scarring, resulting in greatly impaired gas exchange and compliance. Pulmonary hypertension worsens, as does the accompanying right-sided heart failure.

Clinical manifestations in this phase include a decreased left-heart preload due to the right heart failure and reduced capacity of the right ventricle to deliver blood to the lungs and on to the left side of the heart. This results in decreased blood pressure and cardiac output. The severe V/Q mismatch, diffusion defects, and intrapulmonary shunting result in refractory hypoxemia. The overall result is severe tissue hypoxia and lactic acidosis.

Connection Check 27.4

The pulmonary edema associated with ARDS is caused by
A. increased permeability of the ACM.
B. right ventricular failure with pulmonary hypertension.
C. left ventricular failure due to poor oxygenation.
D. fluid overload related to resuscitation in the first phase.

Management

Medical Management
Diagnosis
Imaging Studies
The key imaging procedure to help identify and guide treatment for ARDS is the chest x-ray. During the early phases of ARDS, serial chest x-rays can be used to identify the bilateral infiltrates that are the hallmark sign of this disease process. This is sometimes described as a "ground-glass appearance" and is also characterized as a "snow-screen effect" or whiteout effect on the chest x-ray.

Laboratory Testing
Laboratory testing includes ABGs; complete blood count (CBC) with differential; sputum, blood, and urine cultures; coagulation studies; electrolyte panels; and liver function tests. Arterial blood gases initially show hypoxemia and hypocapnia as alveolar compromise develops. A CBC with differential is done to determine if the cause is infection. An abnormally high white blood cell count (above 10,000) is indicative of an infectious process. Sputum, blood, and urine cultures are used to determine the source of any infection. Comprehensive metabolic panels, coagulation studies, and liver and renal function tests may be used to determine the cause of ARDS but are also used to determine if the hypoxia from the disease process is affecting other body systems. In some cases of ARDS, there is a disruption of the normal clotting cascade, resulting in impaired fibrinolysis. This can result in disseminated intravascular coagulopathy, discussed in Chapter 14.

Treatment
Mechanical Ventilation
Mechanical ventilation is the primary treatment for the refractory hypoxemia of ARDS. It is initiated as lung compliance decreases, work of breathing increases, and oxygenation continues to be refractory regardless of interventions such as NPPV and other oxygen therapies. There are several modes of ventilation used in ARDS. The most common is conventional ventilation using reduced tidal volumes and PEEP. Because of the loss of lung compliance, research has demonstrated that using lower **tidal volumes**—the volume of air moved with one breath, one

inhalation and exhalation—with mechanical ventilation can help improve oxygenation while also reducing the occurrence of **ventilator-induced lung injury (VILI)**, lung damage due to mechanical ventilation such as inflammatory-cell infiltrates, increased vascular permeability, pulmonary edema, and **barotrauma** such as alveolar rupture. The reduced tidal volumes result in hypercapnia, which is accepted as a side effect. Permissive hypercapnia, although not fully understood, has been demonstrated to have some protective effects for the lungs. Hypercapnia should be carefully monitored or avoided in a patient with increased intracranial pressure because it results in vasodilation, which increases cerebral blood flow. The use of a low tidal volume is combined with higher PEEP. This allows the alveoli to open and remain open while at the same time keeping peak airway pressures low. As discussed earlier, PEEP keeps the alveoli from collapsing, allowing maximum gas exchange to continue throughout the respiratory cycle.

Other ventilatory modes sometimes used in the treatment of ARDS are high-frequency oscillating ventilation and airway pressure-release ventilation (APRV). High-frequency oscillating ventilation delivers very small tidal volumes at high frequencies. It avoids lung overdistention and VILI while facilitating alveoli recruitment. Airway pressure-release ventilation utilizes an inverse inspiratory/expiratory ratio (longer inspiration than expiration) to facilitate oxygenation and gas exchange. It is a form of elevated or higher-than-baseline CPAP that has timed, regular, brief reductions in the set airway pressure or CPAP level. Oxygenation is supported during the timed, higher pressure. Removal of CO_2 is facilitated during the timed reduction in pressure. This mode of ventilation allows for spontaneous breathing, reduces the need for sedation or neuromuscular blockade, and reduces VILI.

Partial liquid ventilation is another form of ventilatory support where the lungs are filled with perfluorocarbon liquid to a volume less than or equivalent to functional residual capacity and then ventilated using a standard conventional mechanical ventilator. Perfluorocarbon has surfactant-like properties and good oxygen-carrying capacity. This mode of ventilation has been shown to decrease the shunt associated with ARDS and redistribute blood flow from dependent areas of the lung to nondependent areas. This form of ventilation has promise; research is ongoing to evaluate its safety and efficacy.

Another mode of oxygenation showing some promise is high-flow nasal cannulas (HFNCs). There is much research testing this treatment in the early phase of ARDS and in mild ARDS as a form of noninvasive ventilation (NIV). In this form of oxygenation, high-flow oxygen is humified, warmed, and delivered through soft, wide-bore nasal prongs. The high flow rate results in a "washout" of nasopharyngeal dead space, optimizing alveolar ventilation, and also increases nasopharyngeal airway pressure, producing a CPAP effect. The use of HFNC can improve oxygenation, decrease the work of breathing, and decrease the risk of nosocomial infection associated with invasive ventilation modes. As with other forms of NIV, some studies have shown a failure rate as high as 40%, requiring intubation and mechanical ventilation, indicating more research is required.

Another treatment to support gas exchange in severe ARDS is extracorporeal membrane oxygenation (ECMO). This technique uses a pump to circulate blood through an artificial lung outside of the body (extracorporeal), where oxygenation and CO_2 removal takes place. Blood is then returned into the bloodstream. This is a very invasive form of therapy with many inherent risks and complications, but recent technological improvements have made it safer, increasing its use. More research is needed to determine more clearly what subset of patients will benefit from this therapy.

Positioning

Patient positioning can be utilized as an adjunctive therapy in ARDS—specifically, placing the patient in a prone position. The proning of a patient while on mechanical ventilation may improve oxygenation through increased recruitment of collapsed posterior alveolar units and reduction in the V/Q mismatch. Via gravity, blood flow is directed to the better-aerated anterior portion of the lungs. It is best used in patients with severe ARDS if other ventilator strategies have not been successful. Careful, well-planned teamwork is required to successfully and safely put a critically ill patient with many IV lines and tubes in a prone position (see Evidence-Based Practice: The Use of Prone Positioning in the Patient with ARDS).

Evidence-Based Practice

The Use of Prone Positioning in the Patient With ARDS

Benefits:

- Dorsal lung reexpansion with improved oxygenation
- Aiding in secretion and extravascular water distribution, which decreases stress on the soft tissues of the lung
- Improved lung recruitment—opens more alveoli, improving oxygenation
- Reducing the need for higher PEEP and FIO_2, decreasing ventilator-induced lung injury (VILI)
- Overall effects reduce mortality in the ARDS patient.

Implementation:

- Should be implemented within 72 hours of diagnosis
- Up to 20 hours per day in the prone position is recommended for the best results.
- Can be accomplished by manually turning the patient in bed or by using a mechanical device that can turn

the patient as needed and place the patient in the Trendelenburg or reverse Trendelenburg position as needed

Contraindications:

- Spine instability
- Conditions that increase intracranial pressure
- Pregnancy—possible concerns
- Abdominal wounds—possible concerns
- Unstable peripheral fractures or rib fractures—possible concerns
- Need for frequent airway access—possible concerns

Nursing Considerations:

- Any change in baseline oxygenation parameters after proning should be cause for a new ABG determination.
- Eye and facial skin care must be an integral part of the patient's ongoing care, including eye lubricant and padding of areas of the face as required.
- Sedation may be required due to patient anxiety during the process.
- Enteral feedings should be stopped at least 1 hour before proning, and parenteral feeding may need to be considered.
- Ensure all tubes are free of compromise during the proning procedure and evaluated frequently during the process.
- Have a plan in place for a rapid return to the supine position in the case of hemodynamic compromise or cardiac arrest.
- Educate the family members on this process—including the pros and the cons—and answer all questions related to this treatment modality

ABG, Arterial blood gas; *ARDS,* acute respiratory distress syndrome; *PEEP,* positive end-expiratory pressure.

Drahnak, D. M. (2015). Prone positioning of patients with acute respiratory distress syndrome. *Critical Care Nurse, 35*(6), 29–37. doi:10.4037/ccn2015753

Munshi, L., Del Sorbo, L., Adhikari, N. K., Hodgson, C. L., Wunsch, H., Meade, M. O., . . . Fan, E. (2017). Prone position for acute respiratory distress syndrome. A systematic review and meta-analysis. *Annals of the American Thoracic Society, 14*(Suppl. 4), S280–S288.

Medications

If the cause of ARDS is infection, antibiotics are administered, broad spectrum initially, then narrow spectrum after the causative pathogen is identified. Corticosteroids are also used to decrease the inflammatory response, but their use for the treatment of a patient with ARDS is controversial. There is no evidence that the use of steroids improves

mortality and morbidity, but the anti-inflammatory properties are thought to reduce the migration of white blood cells to the affected areas of the lung. There is also some research that shows that there are less fibrotic changes in the lung during the fibrotic phase of the process. On the negative side, the use of corticosteroids can blunt the body's inflammatory response, making the patient more susceptible to secondary infections. Research regarding steroid use in ARDS is ongoing.

Neuromuscular blocking agents or paralytics are sometimes used when patients are mechanically ventilated. Neuromuscular blocking agents reduce the risk of barotrauma because of controlled patient–ventilator synchrony; the patient cannot take a breath out of sync with the ventilator. They also reduce oxygen demand by limiting muscle movement. If neuromuscular blocking agents are used, the patient must also receive pain and sedative medication to ensure optimum comfort during treatment. As stated earlier, the patient can be managed with the judicious use of sedatives without the use of paralyzing medications if on APRV mechanical ventilation. Paralytic agents are most often used for patients with severe ARDS, and their use must be reevaluated daily for each patient.

Hydration

Fluid management is an important component in the care of a patient with ARDS. Adequate hydration is necessary to maintain circulatory volume and also avoid issues with thick, dry secretions that may be difficult to clear and potentially cause plugged airways. Complicating the management of fluid balance is a decrease in venous return to the right side of the heart because of the increased intrathoracic pressure associated with the use of PEEP. This results in a decrease in cardiac output and systemic blood pressure, potentially requiring fluid resuscitation. If too much fluid is given, ARDS can worsen because of the increased permeability of the ACM. If an insufficient amount of fluid is administered, preload and blood pressure may decrease, resulting in decreased perfusion to the brain and other vital organs. The patient's urine output and hemodynamic volume status should be carefully monitored via a central venous or pulmonary artery (PA) catheter. Hemodynamic monitoring is discussed in detail in Chapter 32.

Nutrition

Adequate nutrition is a very important component of care for a critically ill patient with ARDS. Acute respiratory distress syndrome is associated with a proinflammatory, hypermetabolic state. Without adequate nutrition, malnutrition, loss of body mass, and reduced respiratory muscle strength can result. Enteral (nasogastric tube feedings through the gastrointestinal tract [GI]) or parenteral (IV nutrition via a peripheral or central venous catheter) nutrition should be initiated within 48 to 72 hours of the initiation of mechanical ventilation. Enteral nutrition is the preferred method unless contraindicated because of GI issues. Both have risks associated with them. Tube feedings are associated with aspiration, so care must be given to ensure that the feeding tube is properly placed, the head of the bed is elevated, and the tube feeding is turned off during those times when the patient is completely supine. Parenteral nutrition is associated with increased infections via the venous catheter.

Complications

Barotrauma

Acute respiratory distress syndrome results in a stiffening of the lungs and a loss of compliance (elasticity), requiring careful application of tidal volume and PEEP to maximize oxygenation without causing barotrauma. The patient is at risk for alveolar or lung rupture, resulting in **pneumomediastinum** (air in the mediastinal space) or **pneumothorax** (air in the pleural space), causing further hypoxemia.

Renal Failure/Multisystem Organ-Dysfunction Syndrome

Renal failure is a frequent complication of ARDS due to hypotension and the use of nephrotoxic medications to treat infection. It also may indicate the progression of ARDS to multisystem organ-dysfunction syndrome (MODS). Multisystem organ-dysfunction syndrome results from prolonged refractory hypoxemia, hemodynamic instability, and the inflammation associated with sepsis. Multisystem organ-dysfunction syndrome is discussed in detail in Chapter 14.

Ventilator-Associated Pneumonia

Any patient on mechanical ventilation is at risk for ventilator-associated pneumonia (VAP). When a patient has an artificial airway in place, normal mechanisms to protect the patient from pneumonia are compromised. The primary risks for pneumonia include the inability of the epiglottis to close and the potential drying out of the trachea and upper airways. Ventilator-associated pneumonia is difficult to detect when a patient is already ventilated because of ARDS, but there are some assessment findings that indicate its occurrence. Development of fever, leukocytosis, increased respiratory effort, and purulent secretions are hallmark signs of VAP. Sputum cultures will indicate infection. The earlier VAP is diagnosed, the earlier it can be treated.

Ventilator-associated pneumonia can be prevented by instituting some basic preventive techniques, such as regular mouth care (see Evidence-Based Practice: Preventing Ventilator-Associated Pneumonia). Suctioning of the ETT must be performed routinely as needed, as well as oropharyngeal suctioning to remove secretions from the mouth and throat. The ventilator circuit should be changed per hospital protocol, and care must be taken to avoid water buildup in the circuit. Sterile water should be used for the humidification of the air being delivered to the patient.

Evidence-Based Practice

Preventing Ventilator-Associated Pneumonia (VAP)

Important interventions to prevent VAP:

- Perform mouth care every 2 hours.
- Brush teeth every 12 hours with chlorhexidine.
- Keep the head of the bed elevated at all times at 30 degrees to prevent gastric aspiration.
- Conventional endotracheal tubes (ETTs) should be replaced with ETTs with subglottic secretion drainage. These are ETTs that have an extra port above the inflated cuff that is connected to low continuous suctioning. This prevents secretions that sit above the cuff from becoming infected with bacteria and then oozing down around the cuff into the airway, infecting the airway.

Prevention of ventilator-associated pneumonia in adults. (2017). *Critical Care Nurse, 37*(3), e22–e25. doi:10.4037/ccn2017460

Nursing Management

Assessment and Analysis

The clinical manifestations of ARDS are due to the refractory hypoxemia, pulmonary edema, and lung parenchymal changes of ARDS. The patient's increased work of breathing, evidenced by dyspnea, tachypnea, and accessory muscle use, may be the first indication present. Auscultation of breath sounds reveals crackles associated with pulmonary edema. Later, breath sounds may be diminished or absent because of the fibrotic lung changes and atelectasis. Anxiety and agitation may result from hypoxemia. The SpO_2 continues to decrease despite increasing FIO_2 levels. Initially, the ABGs demonstrate respiratory alkalosis due to the hyperventilation. Later, respiratory acidosis develops.

Nursing Diagnoses

- **Impaired gas exchange** related to disrupted pulmonary function as evidenced by increased work of breathing, refractory hypoxemia, and increased oxygen demand
- **Anxiety** related to hypoxemia, lack of cerebral perfusion, and loss of personal control
- **Imbalanced nutrition, less than body requirements**, related to increased metabolic demand

Nursing Interventions

Assessments

- Hemodynamic monitoring
  - Vital signs
    The pulse increases because of hypoxemia; this is a compensatory mechanism of the sympathetic nervous system in an attempt to increase oxygenation. The respiratory rate increases also in an attempt to increase oxygenation. Blood pressure may be decreased because of right-side heart failure and the increased intrathoracic pressure, thus the decreased venous return associated with PEEP.

- SpO$_2$/pulse oximetry
  The pulse oximetry reading may be low because of the V/Q mismatch and intrapulmonary shunting.
- Central venous pressure (CVP) or pulmonary artery (PA) pressure monitoring
  The CVP or PA pressure may be variable. They may be decreased because of the decreased venous return related to increased intrathoracic pressure. They may also be increased due to increased vasoconstriction in the lung.
- Neurologic assessment: level of consciousness (LOC) and pupillary assessment must be done at least every 1 to 2 hours.
  The patient with ARDS is at risk for neurological compromise due to the refractory hypoxemia and potential increase in PaCO$_2$ that can result in cerebral vasodilation. Frequent checks are necessary, especially if the patient is heavily sedated and chemically paralyzed or has a decreased ability to communicate due to intubation and mechanical ventilation.
- Respiratory assessment
  Crackles may be auscultated because of fluid buildup in the alveoli due to increased capillary permeability. Later, they may be diminished because of atelectasis and fibrotic changes in the lungs.
- Monitor urine output.
  A decreased urine output is an early sign of poor oxygen delivery to the tissues and shock.
- Monitor mechanical ventilation.
  Frequent monitoring of airway pressure on the ventilator is vital. Increases in airway pressure may indicate the presence of secretions or worsening lung compliance. Decreases in airway pressure may indicate a leak in the system.
- Monitor the ECG.
  Hypoxemia can lead to cardiac dysrhythmias.
- Laboratory tests
  - ABGs
    Initially, hypoxemia and respiratory alkalosis secondary to poor gas exchange and hyperventilation are present. Later, respiratory acidosis may occur because of increased PaCO$_2$ levels and the permissive hypercapnia of low-tidal-volume ventilation. Later, metabolic acidosis may be present because of worsening hypoxemia and decreased oxygen delivery to the tissues, signaling the transition to anaerobic metabolism.
  - Serum lactate level
    Increased serum lactate confirms anaerobic metabolism.
  - Liver/renal function blood tests
    Abnormal renal and liver values indicate the progression of ARDS to MODS.
  - Blood/sputum cultures/CBC
    Positive cultures may indicate the cause of ARDS. Later, positive cultures may be present because of complications associated with critical illness, such as indwelling lines and catheters or VAP. A CBC indicating an increased white blood cell count is another indicator of infection.
- Skin assessment
  Patients are at increased risk for skin breakdown due to immobility and hypoxemia/hypoxia.
- Chest x-ray
  Daily chest x-rays are done to monitor the progression or improvement of ARDS.

Actions

- Airway suctioning when indicated by the presence of secretions to ensure that the ETT is clear
  The ETT must remain clear of secretions to facilitate the delivery of ventilatory volume; increased secretions require increased pressure to deliver the preset volume or may actually block the ETT. Secretions are also a source of infection.
- Medication administration
  - Administer paralytic agents, analgesics, and sedative medications as ordered.
    Allows for maximum patient comfort during mechanical ventilation. Respiratory effort and patient–ventilator synchrony must be optimized to avoid barotrauma.
  - Administer inotropic/vasoactive agents as ordered.
    Inotropic medications are used to augment cardiac output; vasoactive medications may be necessary to support blood pressure.
  - Administer antibiotics as ordered.
    Antibiotics are necessary to treat infection if that is the cause or a complication of the critical illness.
- Patient positioning/activity
  - Placing the patient in the prone position—proning
    Proning allows for better oxygenation and alveolar recruitment by having the "good" side down. Proning increases the recruitment of collapsed posterior alveolar units and reduces the V/Q mismatch via gravity as blood flow is directed to the better-aerated anterior portion of the lungs.
  - Elevate the head of the bed.
    Elevating the head of the bed allows for better lung expansion and reduces the risk of aspiration.
  - Frequent position changes
    Frequent changes of position (as tolerated) help prevent skin breakdown.
  - Range-of-motion (ROM) exercises
    Range-of-motion exercises are necessary in the sedated or medically paralyzed bed-bound patient to preserve limb functioning and decrease contracture (severe joint stiffness).
- Infection protection/prevention
  - Hand washing
    Hand washing is the number one intervention in the effort to prevent infection.
  - Monitoring and care of central IV lines
    Central lines are a significant source of infection. Maintenance of strict sterile technique on insertion is key to infection prevention. Routine monitoring for redness or drainage at the insertion site, dressing changes per hospital protocol, IV tubing changes per hospital protocol, and evaluation of the continued need for many invasive lines are also key to preventing central line infection.
  - Foley catheter care
    Increased risk for iatrogenic infections such as urinary tract infection (due to Foley catheter) requires routine Foley catheter care and evaluation of necessity of continued use.

- Diligent mouth care
  Increased risk for VAP due to intubation requires mouth care every 2 hours.

■ *Teaching*

- Disease process
  The patient and the patient's support system should understand the pathophysiology of ARDS, the severity of the disease, and the treatment required. Understanding the medications, invasive lines, and mechanical ventilation may help decrease anxiety and provide some sense of control. Providing time for visiting as possible may help the family stay engaged and involved in the family member's care. Visiting also provides tremendous support for the patient.

Evaluating Care Outcomes

Successful treatment of a patient with ARDS should be considered a victory because of the high mortality rate. The optimal outcome for a patient with ARDS is to return to baseline respiratory function and a return to a lifestyle similar to that prior to the illness. Ideally, there are no long-term respiratory issues, but in reality, ARDS can do significant damage to the lungs and thereby impacts the patient's life post-discharge. The physical weakness, early fatigue, and change in lifestyle can take a tremendous toll on the patient. Helping the patient mentally adjust to any residual physical limitations is something that should be stressed for both family members and the healthcare team. Counseling may be required. Consistent medical follow-up and a realistic rehabilitation regimen maximize the patient's recovery.

CHEST TRAUMA

Epidemiology

Thoracic (chest) trauma accounts for approximately 16,000 deaths annually. Thoracic trauma is the direct cause in 20% to 25% of all trauma-related deaths and is a contributory cause for an additional 20% to 25% of deaths. Motor vehicle collisions (MVCs) are the most prevalent cause of thoracic injuries seen in emergency departments and trauma centers. In 2016, there were 34,439 MVCs resulting in fatality, with an overall number of 37,461 fatalities. These numbers have been decreasing over the past few years, most likely because of the increase in air bags in new cars and the improvement in car manufacturing to decrease crash fatalities. Older drivers (greater than 60 years of age) are more susceptible to injury. Other risk factors for injury include rate of speed, size of the vehicle, and seat-belt use or lack thereof. At speeds greater than 25 miles per hour, the vehicle's occupants are more likely to be injured. At greater speeds, driver reaction time is increased, meaning it takes longer to process and react to danger; there is a greater collision impact and a higher chance that objects may enter the passenger compartment on impact. This is called *intrusion* and can cause injury secondary to the collision. In a vehicle-to-vehicle collision, a smaller car provides limited protection, especially if struck by a larger vehicle. Finally, not wearing a seat belt puts drivers and passengers at risk of injury because of the collision with hard surfaces in the car, such as the dash, steering wheel, or windshield.

Pathophysiology

Chest trauma is divided into two types: blunt-force and penetrating trauma. Blunt chest trauma is the result of a blunt object hitting the chest or the chest striking a blunt surface such as a steering wheel. Blunt-force injuries can be further characterized as acceleration or deceleration injuries. Deceleration is when the movement of the body is suddenly stopped but the internal organs remain in motion and collide with the chest wall. Acceleration injury occurs when the body is abruptly set in motion (rear-end collisions) or when the body is hit by a rapidly moving object. When either occurs, chest organs and tissues are subject to impact and shearing forces. Blunt-force trauma is more diffuse than penetrating trauma and may cause injuries that may not be obvious at the time of initial assessment. Penetrating trauma is the result of sharp objects such as knives or bullets entering the chest and causing damage to internal structures or organs. Other causes of penetrating injury are objects that enter a motor vehicle during a collision (intrusion) or shrapnel from explosions. The depth, angle, and location of the penetration can differentiate whether the penetrating trauma is a superficial wound or is potentially life threatening. A gunshot wound into the lateral right chest, missing all major vessels, may be superficial. A gunshot wound to the middle of the left chest is life threatening.

Common injuries occurring as a result of chest trauma include fractured ribs, pneumothorax, and hemothorax. Fractured ribs are the most common injury associated with chest trauma. Normal chest wall movement—the diaphragm moving downward and the external intercostal muscles moving the rib cage up and outward—assists in generating the negative pressure required for inspiration and effective ventilation. When ribs are fractured, the integrity of the entire thorax and chest-wall movement are compromised. The patient cannot take deep, effective breaths, largely because of pain, effectively limiting the ability to maintain normal tidal volumes with each breath. Also, depending on the location of the rib fractures, there may be collateral penetrating damage to organs and vessels located near the site of injury, such as the liver.

A **flail chest** is defined as three or more adjacent ribs that have been fractured in two or more places as a result of blunt or crush chest trauma, resulting in a "free" segment of the ribs. "Paradoxical" chest-wall movement is the hallmark sign associated with a flail chest. With each inhalation, the damaged area moves inward; on exhalation, this section of the chest wall moves outward (Fig. 27.4). As with rib fractures as described previously, chest-wall movement is compromised largely because of pain and may result in respiratory insufficiency. The severity of the injury and the treatment are determined by the extent of the underlying lung injury or contusion more so than by the fractures themselves.

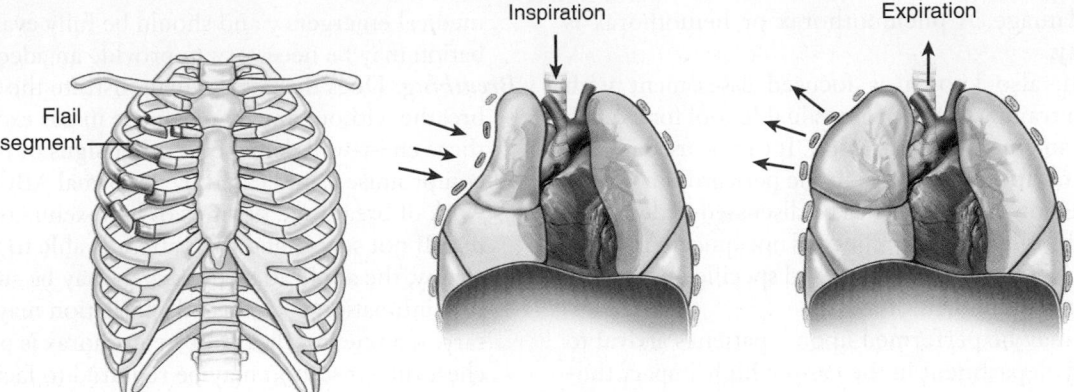

FIGURE 27.4 Flail chest. Paradoxical chest wall movement; on inhalation, the damaged area moves inward; on exhalation, the damaged area moves outward.

A pneumothorax may result from severe blunt or penetrating chest trauma where there is a disruption of the integrity of the lung parenchyma (Fig. 27.5). Pneumothorax is defined as the collection of air in the pleural space. A normal lung inflates during inspiration because of negative thoracic pressure in relationship to atmospheric pressure. As the diaphragm descends, the lung expands; air enters the airways and eventually fills the alveoli via the terminal bronchioles. When a pneumothorax occurs, there is a reduction in the negative thoracic pressure because of the presence of air in the pleural space. This makes inspiration more difficult, and the lung cannot adequately expand. This results in a reduction of gas exchange at the alveolar level, resulting in hypoxemia.

Different from a pneumothorax, a **hemothorax** is the presence of blood in the pleural space. It occurs if there has been a laceration of a pulmonary vessel with blunt or penetrating trauma. A hemothorax may result in two problems for the patient. As with pneumothorax, as blood fills the pleural space, the negative pressure is lost, limiting the lung's ability to expand. Second, the loss of blood from the

vascular space may result in hemodynamic compromise. Drainage greater than 1,500 mL is considered massive, and the patient may become hemodynamically unstable.

Clinical Manifestations

With all chest trauma, clinical manifestations may include decreased oxygenation and ventilation. Because of the inability to fully inflate the lungs, gas exchange is compromised, resulting in decreased oxygenation. Initially, hyperventilation occurs in an effort to increase oxygen availability to the tissues, but eventually, as the patient tires, CO_2 will begin to rise. Initial ABGs may indicate respiratory alkalosis due to hyperventilation, but respiratory acidosis will develop rapidly as CO_2 is not exchanged. An early sign of hypoxemia is agitation and anxiety, then a decreased level of consciousness. The patient typically reports shortness of breath. Subcutaneous emphysema, or air in the tissues under the skin, may occur with blunt trauma and pneumothorax. Pain is also a common clinical manifestation, further compromising chest-wall expansion and thus oxygenation and ventilation. The patient may exhibit splinting, assuming a protective posture around the site of injury. The arm on the affected side is held tightly against the body, and the patient bends to that side. This position further compromises lung expansion on the side of injury, and pneumonia may ultimately result.

Management

Medical Management

Diagnosis

Imaging Studies

Diagnostic evaluation following chest trauma includes several imaging studies, such as:

- Chest x-ray
- Ultrasonography
- Chest CT

A chest x-ray is done to evaluate the skeletal features of the chest and to evaluate the integrity of the lungs. The x-ray is viewed to look for fractures, lung expansion, or

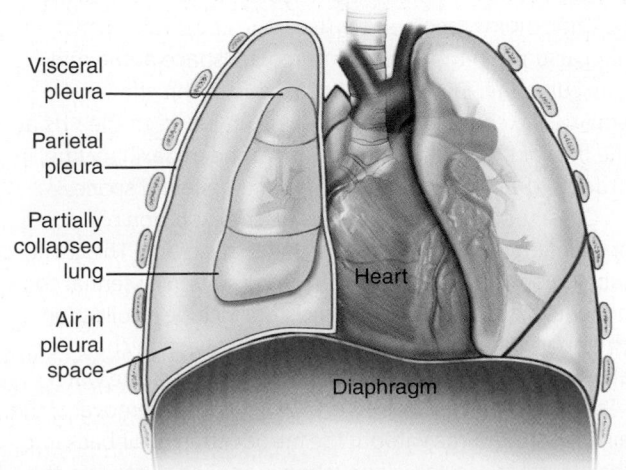

FIGURE 27.5 Pneumothorax. There is a reduction in the negative thoracic pressure because of air in the pleural space, resulting in an inability of the lung to fully expand.

mediastinal damage. A pneumothorax or hemothorax is visible on x-ray.

Ultrasound, also known as focused assessment with sonography in trauma (FAST), is a valuable tool for a quick assessment in an emergency situation. It can be used to rule out a **cardiac tamponade** (blood in the pericardium resulting in compression of the heart, to be discussed under complications), a life-threatening injury if not quickly treated. In addition, FAST is more sensitive and specific in diagnosing pneumothorax and hemothorax.

Chest CT may be performed upon a patient's arrival to the emergency department in the case of high-impact thoracic trauma. High-impact trauma involves rapid deceleration and may result in chest-wall deformities, multiple rib fractures, pneumothorax, or hemothorax. An abnormal chest x-ray indicating any of these conditions requires subsequent evaluation using CT. It is extremely useful in determining damage to the mediastinum or the aorta.

Laboratory Studies

Laboratory analysis includes:

- ABGs
- Serum lactate
- Hemoglobin/hematocrit
- CBC and complete metabolic profile, coagulation studies, and a type and crossmatch in the event that the patient needs a blood transfusion

Arterial blood gases are used to determine whether hypoxemia and abnormalities in the acid-base balance exist. As noted earlier, initial ABGs may indicate respiratory alkalosis due to hyperventilation, but the patient will quickly develop respiratory acidosis because of ineffective gas exchange and tiring.

A serum lactate level may be drawn to determine the adequacy of oxygen delivery to the tissues. If the respiratory system is significantly compromised, resulting in insufficient oxygen for cellular metabolism, anaerobic metabolism results. This causes the production of lactic acids, resulting in a rise in lactate levels within hours.

The hematocrit and hemoglobin may be reduced if there is any bleeding. This is important because the bleeding may be internal and not readily observable. Diagnostic imaging assists in identifying any bleeding within the chest.

Routine laboratories are drawn in any trauma situation. They include electrolyte panels, CBC, and coagulation studies as well as patient-specific tests. For example, if the patient is known to have heart failure, a B-type natriuretic peptide (BNP) and cardiac enzymes (myoglobin, troponin, and creatine kinase-muscle/brain [CK-MB]) may also be drawn.

Treatment

Treatment is guided by the common acronym ABC (airway, breathing, and circulation).

Airway: Evaluate the airway—Is the airway patent? Does the patient show any sign of respiratory compromise or obstruction? Partial or complete obstruction is a medical emergency and should be fully evaluated. Intubation may be necessary to provide an adequate airway.

Breathing: Does the patient demonstrate the ability to breathe without any compromise in gas exchange? Is there chest-wall damage or other signs of respiratory compromise as indicated by abnormal ABGs, increased work of breathing, or signs of hypoxemia or hypercapnia? If not severe and the patient is able to protect the airway, the application of oxygen may be sufficient. If not, intubation and assisted ventilation may be necessary. If a pneumothorax or hemothorax is present, chest tube insertion may be required to facilitate breathing and adequate oxygenation (Box 27.2).

Circulation: Is circulation sufficient? Does the patient have adequate pulses and skin color? Is the blood pressure within normal limits? If not, IV fluid resuscitation may be required to maintain hemodynamic stability. If the injury has resulted in blood loss, as in the case of a hemothorax, blood transfusions may be indicated.

 Safety Alert If the chest tube becomes disconnected from the drainage system, immediately submerge the end of the chest tube in sterile water to preserve the water seal. This prevents air from entering through the disconnected chest tube and reaccumulating in the pleural space. As quickly as possible, reconnect to a new chest tube system. Be aware of hospital policy. Some hospitals have protocols that allow the immediate reconnection to the original system.

If the chest tube becomes dislodged from the chest, apply a Vaseline gauze dressing and notify the provider immediately. Prepare for insertion of a new chest tube.

Box 27.2 Chest Tube Placement

Chest tube placement is indicated if a pneumo- or hemothorax occurs as the result of chest trauma. In the case of a pneumothorax, because air rises, the chest tube is placed high, usually in the second intercostal space at the midclavicular line. For a hemothorax, due to the effects of gravity, the chest tube is placed lower, between the ribs at the fifth or sixth intercostal space at the midaxillary line, in order to drain blood and fluid from the pleural space.

Chest tube placement allows for the expulsion of air and/or fluid while allowing the lung to reexpand. The chest tube is connected to a chest-drainage system. Essential components of the chest-drainage system include a collection chamber, water seal, and suction. The collection chamber allows for the accumulation of blood and fluid. The water seal acts like a one-way valve, allowing for the removal of the air/blood over time without the introduction of air back into the pleural space. Initially, suction is applied to assist in the reexpansion of the lung. The suction is discontinued as the lung reexpands.

Medications

Medications used for the patient suffering from chest trauma are primarily analgesic. A patient in extreme pain may not breathe deeply enough to avoid atelectasis. Initially, IV narcotic analgesia such as morphine is prescribed. A regional block or epidural analgesia may be administered to reduce pain without the narcotic side effects. This allows the patient to breathe more effectively. If there has been penetrating trauma, the patient is at an increased risk for an infection, so prophylactic broad-spectrum antibiotics may be prescribed.

Connection Check 27.5

The nurse understands that the priority action for a patient with a chest tube that has come disconnected from the chest-drainage system is which of the following?

A. Immediately cover the end of the chest tube with a sterile dressing.
B. Immediately submerge the end of the chest tube in sterile water.
C. Immediately reconnect the end of the chest tube with the drainage system.
D. Immediately page the provider to insert a new chest tube.

Complications

Tension pneumothorax (Fig. 27.6) may occur if air or blood collects in the pleural space and is not removed. If this is left untreated, the positive pressure in the pleural cavity increases, and the affected lung collapses. As the positive pressure increases, it may cause a mediastinal shift toward the unaffected side. This can result in compression of the heart, vena cava, aorta, and contralateral (unaffected) lung. Tracheal deviation toward the unaffected side is a hallmark sign of tension pneumothorax. This is a life-threatening emergency because left ventricular heart failure and reduced cardiac output can occur. In emergent cases of tension pneumothorax, a needle decompression, performed to remove the air from the pleural space, may be required. A large-bore needle (14- or 16-gauge) is inserted between the ribs at the second intercostal space at the midclavicular line to allow for rapid evacuation of air or blood. This is immediately followed by chest tube insertion.

Cardiac tamponade is caused by excessive air, fluid, or blood collecting in the pericardial sac (Fig. 27.7). When this occurs, the heart cannot adequately fill or contract because of the compression of the ventricles. It can manifest as hypotension, muffled heart sounds, and distended neck veins, which are known collectively as Beck's triad. Cardiac tamponade due to fluid accumulation in the pericardial sac is treated with a pericardiocentesis, the insertion of a large-bore needle into the pericardial space to drain the fluid. A small pericardial catheter (similar to a small chest

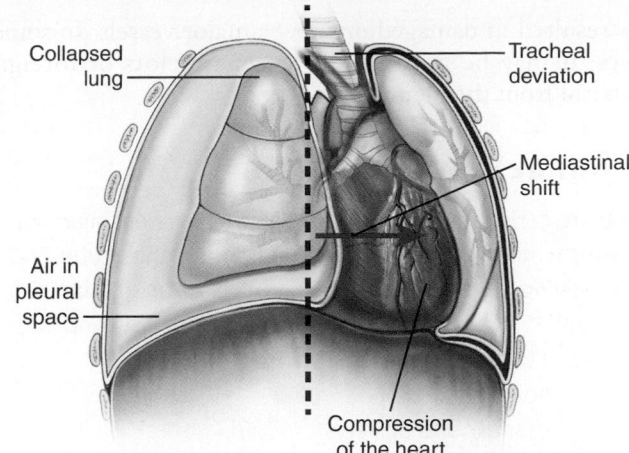

FIGURE 27.6 Tension pneumothorax. Accumulation of air or blood in the pleural space may result in a mediastinal shift and tracheal deviation toward the unaffected side, causing compression of the heart, vena cava, aorta, and unaffected lung.

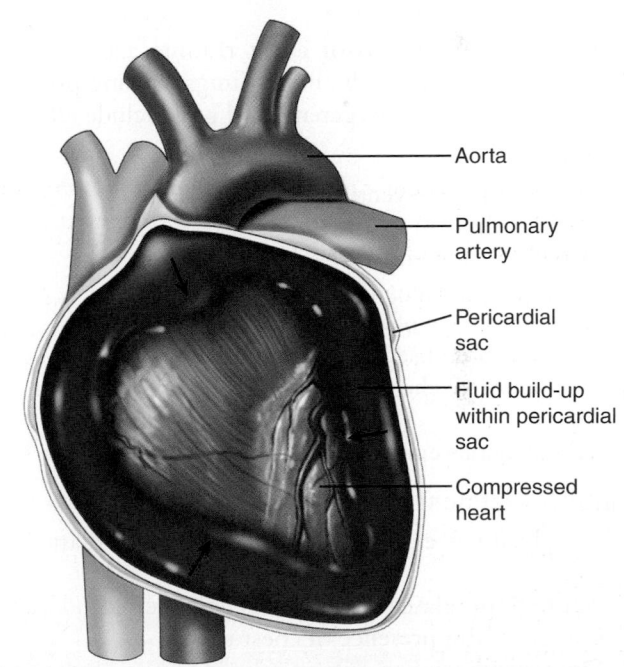

FIGURE 27.7 Cardiac tamponade.

tube but more flexible) may be placed to allow for continued drainage of the fluid until the cause can be determined and managed. A tension pneumothorax can create the same set of symptoms: compression of the heart due to the mediastinal shift, resulting in inadequate filling and contraction of the ventricles. Cardiac tamponade due to tension pneumothorax from excessive pleural effusion fluid collection is treated with an emergent thoracentesis; a needle insertion between the ribs for fluid removal.

Surgical Management

Surgical management may be indicated for patients with an unstable chest wall. In severe cases of flail chest, operative stabilization may be required. Thoracotomy, a surgical excision to the chest wall, is an option if the chest trauma has resulted in damaged organs or major vessels. In some cases, it may be necessary to evacuate clots or foreign material from the pleural space.

Connection Check 27.6

You are caring for a client who sustained a chest injury following a motor vehicle collision, requiring a chest tube, and is receiving morphine via patient-controlled analgesia (PCA) for pain. Which of the following would alarm you and initiate a call to the primary care provider?

A. Somnolence
B. Restlessness and anxiety
C. Itching at the IV site
D. Minimal amounts of bloody chest tube drainage

Nursing Management

Assessment and Analysis

Clinical manifestations of chest trauma are caused by damage to the chest wall and/or lungs causing problems with ventilation and oxygenation. They include all of the following:

- Tachypnea/hyperventilation
- Tachycardia
- Shortness of breath
- Decreased oxygenation
- Decreased level of consciousness
- Decreased or absent lung sounds
- Asymmetrical chest excursion (in the case of a flail chest)
- Subcutaneous emphysema (air under a layer of the skin)

Nursing Diagnoses

- **Impaired gas exchange** related to hypoventilation and pain
- **Acute pain** related to structural damage secondary to fractured ribs; presence of chest tube
- **Decreased cardiac output** related to hemorrhage and decreased circulating volume (hemothorax)

Nursing Interventions

Assessments

- Respiratory effort
  Increased work of breathing such as shortness of breath, accessory muscle use, or nasal flaring may indicate a need for further evaluation and treatment of chest trauma or pneumothorax and/or a need for an advanced airway
- Vital signs and pulse oximetry (SpO_2)
  Tachypnea and tachycardia may occur in response to decreased oxygen levels and increased oxygen demands and/or pain. Hypotension can indicate tension pneumothorax or cardiac tamponade due to compression of the heart, vena cava, and aorta. Hypotension can also indicate excessive blood loss with a hemothorax. Decreased SpO_2 may be present if there is ineffective respiration due to pain or

injury. Continuous readings help evaluate the response to treatment.

- Pain
  Severe pain due to fractures may limit the patient's ability to breathe deeply, which may result in decreased gas exchange.
- Level of consciousness
  Agitation, anxiety, and eventually, a decreased LOC may result from hypoxemia.
- ABGs
  Initial ABGs note a respiratory alkalosis due to tachypnea and hyperventilation. A decreased PaO_2 may be present because of the impaired ventilatory effort and decreased surface area available for gas exchange in a collapsed lung.
- Chest tube
  - Amount and color of drainage
    Red, free-flowing drainage in excess of 70 mL per hour (or the amount indicated by the provider) indicates hemorrhage; cloudiness may indicate an infection.
  - Water-seal chamber
    Initially, there is bubbling on expiration, indicating air removal from the pleural space. Later, after the air has escaped from the pleural space, the water level fluctuates with respiratory effort. When the pleural-wall disruption is healed, the water fluctuation may no longer be present. At that point, the patient should be evaluated for chest-tube removal. Continuous bubbling in the water-seal chamber is an indication of an air leak.
- Subcutaneous emphysema
  Subcutaneous emphysema produces a crackling feeling under the skin. It is not painful to the patient but may become uncomfortable if excessive. It is indicative of air from a chest injury escaping into the subcutaneous space, indicating potential chest trauma. Subcutaneous emphysema of the head and neck could be life threatening because the airway could be compromised.

Actions

- Apply oxygen as ordered.
  The patient with a chest injury is at risk for ineffective oxygenation and ventilation. Supplemental oxygen may be necessary.
- Anticipate and prepare for intubation.
  The patient with a severe chest injury may require an advanced airway to optimize ventilation and perfusion.
- Elevate the head of the bed.
  Allows for greater lung expansion; assists with work of breathing
- Encourage deep breathing and coughing, every 1 to 2 hours.
  Prevents atelectasis and assists in keeping airways clear
- Encourage ambulation as soon as possible.
  Prevents hazards of immobility; assists in returning respiratory function to normal
- Chest tube management
  - Maintain a closed system. Tape all connections, and secure the chest tube to the chest wall.
    These measures are important to prevent inadvertent tube removal or disruption of the system's integrity.

- Keep the collection apparatus below the level of the chest; keep tubing free from kinks or loops.
  Pleural fluid drains into the collection apparatus by gravity flow as well as low-level suction. Kinks or loops can interfere with drainage.
- **NEVER CLAMP THE CHEST TUBE!**
  Clamping the chest tube may result in increased air or fluid collection in the pleural space, worsening the pneumo- or hemothorax, and may result in a tension pneumothorax.
- When the chest tube is removed, immediately apply a sterile occlusive petroleum jelly dressing.
  An occlusive dressing prevents air from reentering the pleural space through the chest wound.
- Administer pain medications; encourage the use of patient-controlled analgesia before ambulation and pulmonary toileting.
  Control of the patient's pain allows for more effective pulmonary toileting and assists the patient in being able to tolerate ambulation/physical therapy.

■ *Teaching*

- Use of pain medications
  Pain medications should be used to ensure that pain from breathing post-injury does not reduce respiratory effort, which may result in ineffective gas exchange and a worsening of pulmonary status.
- Importance of:
  - Coughing and deep breathing
  - Ambulation
  - Splinting with pillow while coughing
    These actions help prevent complications such as atelectasis and pneumonia; splinting aids in patient comfort, allowing better effort.
- Motor vehicle safety: use seat belts; avoid distracted driving.
  Seat belts are proven to reduce injury. Distracted driving (e.g., talking on the phone or texting) has been shown to increase the occurrence of MVCs. Never drink and drive!

Evaluating Care Outcomes

A well-managed patient following chest trauma has unlabored respiratory effort, and ABGs within normal ranges. Lungs sounds are clear in all fields, and pain is under control. If the patient had a chest tube, skin integrity is intact.

Connection Check 27.7

The nurse anticipates which of the following in the initial care of a patient with ARDS?

A. Inotropic agents
B. Fresh frozen plasma (FFP)
C. Anticoagulants
D. Positive-pressure ventilation

Making Connections

CASE STUDY: WRAP-UP

J.T. remains in the intensive care unit (ICU), sedated on the ventilator. His is managed with conventional mechanical ventilation with low tidal volumes to protect his lungs from injury. His fluid balance is managed judiciously. He is started on enteral feeding to support his nutrition. Initially prone positioning is utilized to improve gas exchange. He has frequent position changes and ROM exercises. After 5 days of careful monitoring and meticulous care, J.T. begins to improve. His oxygenation status stabilizes, and he is able to be slowly weaned from the ventilator. By day 7 in the ICU, J.T. is extubated and out of bed to the chair.

Case Study Questions

1. The nurse is aware that J.T.'s hemothorax caused ineffective gas exchange due to which of the following mechanisms?
   A. Anxiety due to the need for a chest tube
   B. Blood collection in the pleural space reducing negative intrathoracic pressure
   C. Pain related to chest tube placement
   D. Blood collection in the pleural space increasing negative intrathoracic pressure

2. The nurse expects to see what oxygenation and ABG changes for J.T. when his ARDS begins to resolve?
   A. New-onset respiratory alkalosis
   B. An increasing PaO_2/FIO_2 ratio
   C. Resolving metabolic alkalosis
   D. A decreasing PaO_2/FIO_2 ratio

3. The nurse understands that J.T.'s initial "refractory hypoxemia" indicates what about the adequacy of his supplemental oxygen support?
   A. It is sufficient, and the FIO_2 can be reduced.
   B. It fails to maintain adequate oxygen saturation.
   C. It has caused signs of oxygen toxicity.
   D. It has caused alveolar collapse.

4. Which of the following are priorities in J.T.'s care? *(Select all that apply.)*
   A. Adequate nutritional supplementation
   B. Positioning with the good lung down
   C. Adequate hydration
   D. Maintain NPO status to prevent aspiration
   E. Elevate the head of the bed

5. The nurse understands that the rationale for the administration of sedative and analgesic medications to J.T. while on mechanical ventilation is which of the following? *(Select all that apply.)*

   A. Improve respiratory effort

   B. Reduce the pain

   C. Decrease oxygen consumption

   D. Increase patient–ventilator synchrony

   E. Increase mobilization

CHAPTER SUMMARY

A pulmonary embolism (PE) is defined as the obstruction of the pulmonary artery (or one of its branches) by particulate matter that has an origin elsewhere in the body. When a PE travels to the lungs, it lodges in the pulmonary artery and blocks blood flow. The biggest risk factor is the presence of a deep vein thrombosis (DVT). The most common cause of DVT is prolonged immobility. Medication therapy when treating a patient with acute PE is primarily anticoagulation.

Acute respiratory failure is when one or both of the gas-exchange functions of the lungs are compromised, leading to hypoxemia and/or hypercapnia (hypercarbia). There are two types of acute respiratory failure. Type I is known as acute hypoxemic respiratory failure. Type II is known as acute hypercapnic respiratory failure. Risk factors for hypercapnic failure include disease processes that impair ventilation or cause hypoventilation. Risk factors for hypoxemic failure include disorders that produce a ventilation–perfusion mismatch or that impair diffusion at the alveolar level. Treatment begins with oxygen. The patient in acute respiratory failure should be placed on a nonrebreather mask with 100% FIO_2. If the patient's oxygenation status does not improve, noninvasive positive-pressure ventilation (NIPPV) measures may need to be implemented.

Acute respiratory distress syndrome (ARDS) has the following characteristics: acute onset, refractory hypoxemia, and bilateral infiltrates consistent with pulmonary edema. Severity is characterized by the PaO_2/FIO_2 ratio. In the exudative phase, there is a disruption of the alveolar-capillary membrane (ACM). This disturbance allows fluid to move from the capillaries into the alveoli. In the proliferative phase, surfactant is compromised, alveolar surface tension is lost, and alveoli collapse. In the fibrotic phase, there is the development of fibrotic tissue within the ACM. As the disease progresses, lung compliance decreases, and the work of breathing increases. Mechanical ventilation is initiated for patients with ARDS because of refractory hypoxemia regardless of interventions such as NIPPV and other oxygen therapies.

Chest trauma is divided into two types: blunt force and penetrating. Blunt chest trauma is the result of a blunt object hitting the chest or the chest striking a blunt surface. Blunt-force injuries can also be classified as acceleration or deceleration injuries. Penetrating trauma is the result of sharp objects entering the chest and causing damage to internal structures or organs. In both cases, normal functioning of the respiratory system may be compromised. Examples include rib fractures and flail chest, both of which cause pain that diminishes the respiratory effort. Pneumothorax (air in the pleural space) and hemothorax (blood in the pleural space) result in a loss of the negative intrathoracic pressure necessary for inspiration. Chest tube insertion is required to restore negative pressure. Treatment is guided by the common acronym ABC: airway, breathing, circulation. Life-threatening complications include tension pneumothorax and cardiac tamponade. Both are medical emergencies and require immediate intervention.

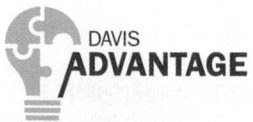

DAVIS **ADVANTAGE**

To explore learning resources for this chapter, go to **Davis Advantage** and find:
- Answers to in-text questions
- Chapter Resources and Activities
- NCLEX®-Style Chapter Review Questions
- Bibliography

Unit VI

Promoting Health in Patients With Circulatory or Perfusion Disorders

Chapter 28

Assessment of Cardiovascular Function

Nancy Sullivan

Finding Connections

CASE STUDY: EPISODE 1

Follow this patient throughout the chapter.

John Smith, a 57-year-old Caucasian male, has an appointment for his first physical in 4 years. He is in excellent health, with no particular complaints except "aches and pains after a hard day's work." He has no significant past medical history (PMH), takes no medications, and has no allergies. He is about 30 pounds overweight and drinks about five evenings a week. He quit smoking 2 years ago after smoking off and on for about 10 years. He does not exercise but does do heavy-lifting work around the house. Family history includes paternal death at 60 due to myocardial infarction; his mother is still alive and well …

OVERVIEW OF THE CARDIOVASCULAR SYSTEM

The primary function of the cardiovascular system is to deliver oxygenated blood to the tissues and return deoxygenated blood to the heart. This is accomplished through the interaction of a muscular pump, the heart (Fig. 28.1), and a large complex of **arteries** and **veins** (Fig. 28.2). The primary job of the heart is to propel blood from its left side into the aorta and the systemic circulation to provide oxygen and nutrients to the tissues. The amount of blood ejected from the left heart, the **cardiac output (CO)**, varies depending on the body's metabolic demands, increasing with exercise and decreasing when at rest. After circulating throughout the body, the blood returns to the right heart through the great veins, the superior and inferior vena cavae, to be delivered to the lungs to receive oxygen and remove carbon dioxide.

Vascular System

The arterial and venous vascular systems consist of a combination of arteries, veins, and **capillaries**. With the exception of the pulmonary artery, arteries carry oxygenated blood. Veins convey deoxygenated blood. The vascular system provides for:

- The delivery of oxygenated blood to the tissues
- The removal and transportation of cellular waste for excretion
- The return of circulatory volume to the right heart
- The return of lymph fluid back into the general circulation

Arterial System

The high-pressure arterial system consists of thick-walled muscular vessels whose function is to carry oxygenated blood from the heart to the tissues. This is accomplished through a series of vessels gradually decreasing in size, eventually entering the smallest vessels, the capillaries, where the actual oxygen and nutrient exchange takes place

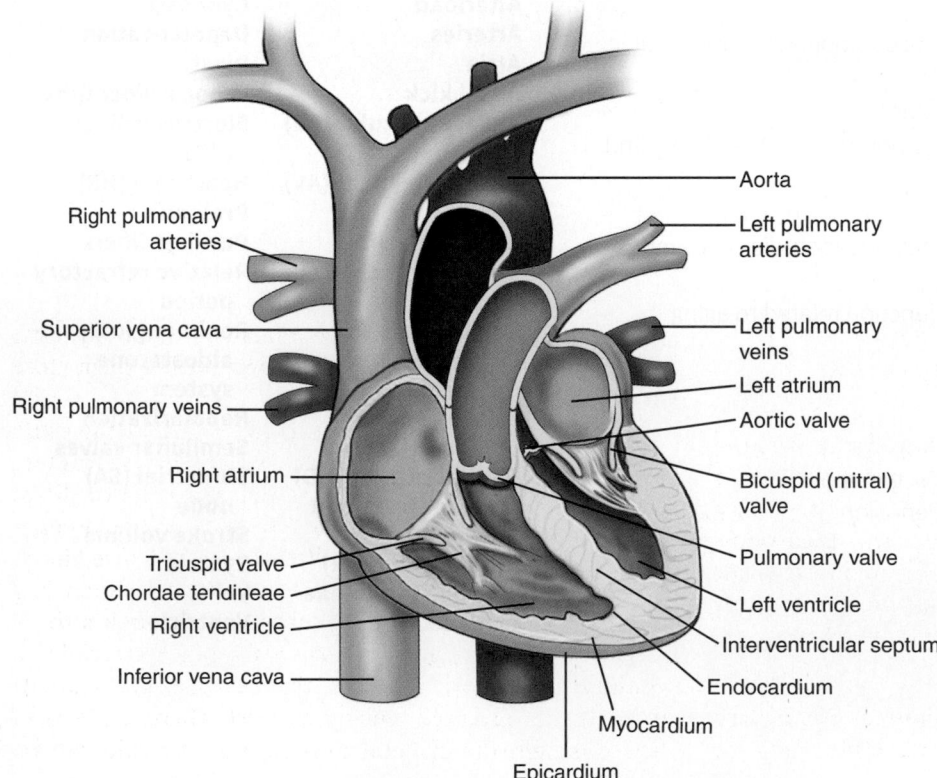

Right pulmonary arteries

Superior vena cava

Right pulmonary veins

Right atrium

Tricuspid valve
Chordae tendineae
Right ventricle

Inferior vena cava

Myocardium

Epicardium

Aorta

Left pulmonary arteries

Left pulmonary veins

Left atrium

Aortic valve

Bicuspid (mitral) valve

Pulmonary valve

Left ventricle

Interventricular septum

Endocardium

FIGURE 28.1 Major anatomical structures of the heart.

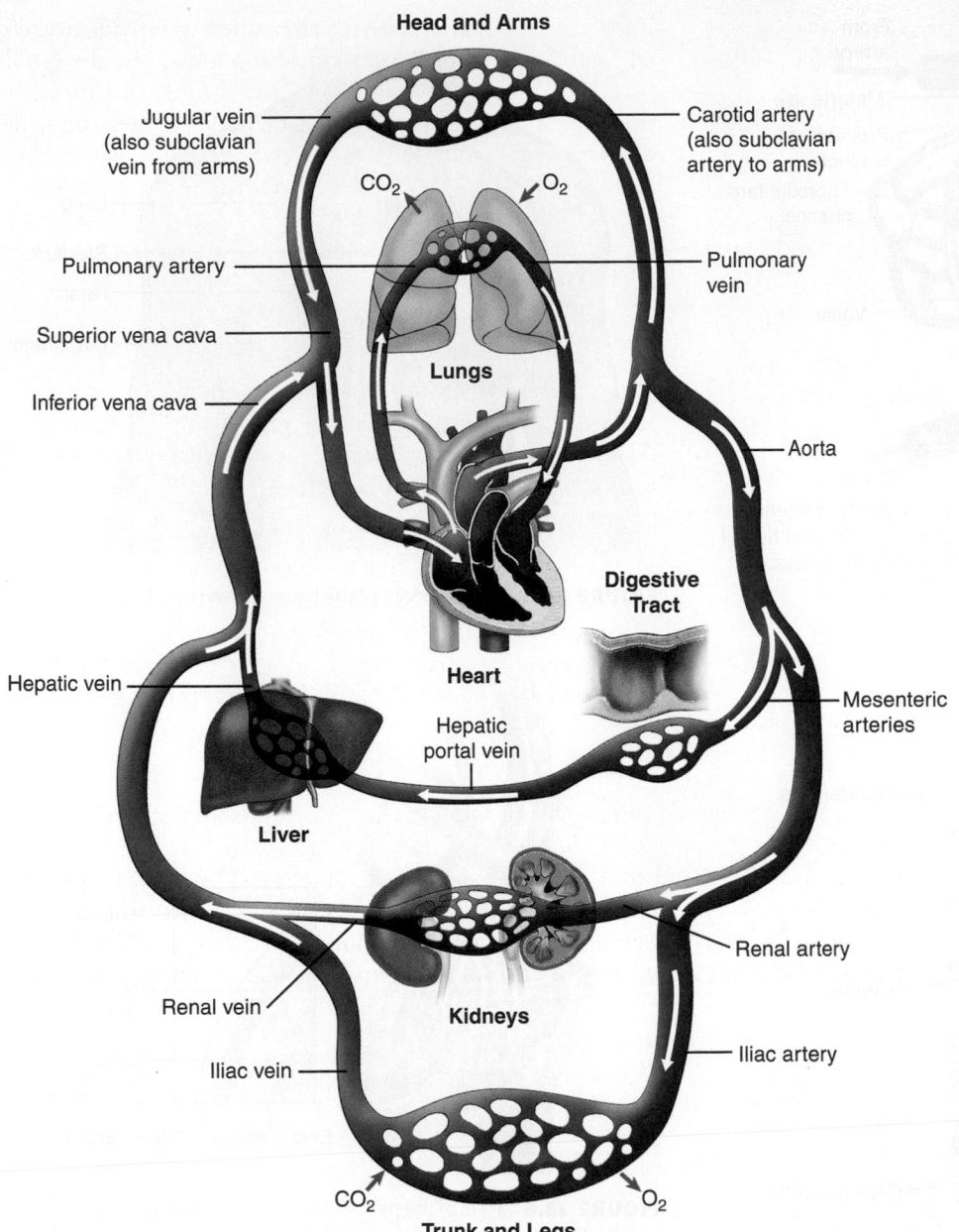

Head and Arms

Jugular vein
(also subclavian
vein from arms)

Carotid artery
(also subclavian
artery to arms)

CO_2 O_2

Pulmonary artery

Pulmonary
vein

Superior vena cava

Lungs

Inferior vena cava

Aorta

**Digestive
Tract**

Heart

Hepatic vein

Mesenteric
arteries

Hepatic
portal vein

Liver

Renal artery

Renal vein

Kidneys

Iliac artery

Iliac vein

CO_2 O_2

Trunk and Legs

FIGURE 28.2 Arterial and venous blood
flow through the systemic circulation.

(Fig. 28.3). The sequence of vessels is as follows: arteries to
arterioles to metarterioles to capillaries.

Venous System

In contrast to the arterial system, the venous system is a low-
pressure vascular circuit with vessels that contain valves to
prevent retrograde, or backward, flow. These vessels carry
blood from the capillary bed through venules, then veins,
back to the right heart. Veins also have the flexibility to adapt
to changes in volume without large changes in pressure.
This allows for the infusion of IV fluids and blood products.

Capillary Bed

The real work of the vascular system is done at the capillary
bed (Fig. 28.4). It is here where oxygen and nutrients are
delivered to the tissues and cellular waste is removed.

Capillaries are tremendously abundant in the body, estimated in the billions. Their abundance makes them close
to virtually every cell in the body.

The entire capillary system is never full at the same
time. There are muscle cells or precapillary sphincters
at the entrance of each capillary that constrict or dilate
to deliver or divert blood to areas of need. When precapillary sphincters are open, capillaries are filled with blood.
When a precapillary sphincter closes, that corresponding
capillary shuts down, and blood travels through a thoroughfare channel, going directly from metarteriole to
venule. In this way, blood is diverted to organ systems
in need. For example, during exercise, there is plentiful
flow through the skeletal muscle, but the skin can be
bypassed.

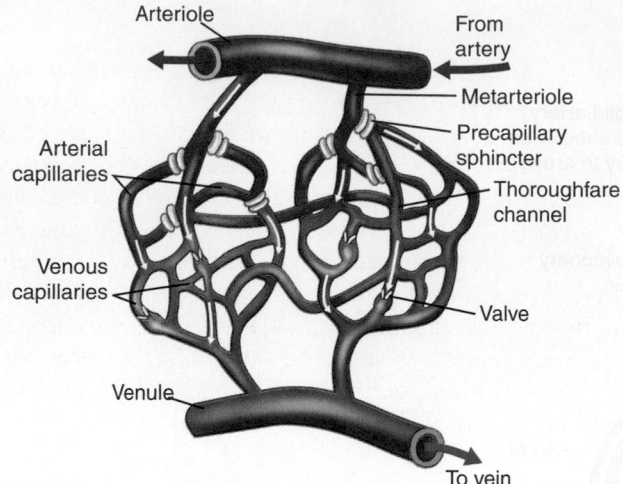

FIGURE 28.3 Blood flow through a capillary bed: artery to arteriole to metarteriole into the capillary. Flow is controlled through the action of the precapillary sphincter diverting flow to areas of need through a thoroughfare channel.

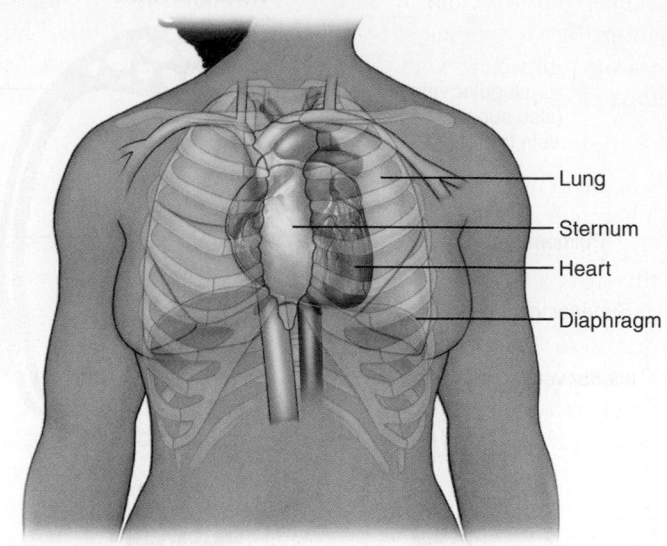

FIGURE 28.5 The placement of the heart within the chest.

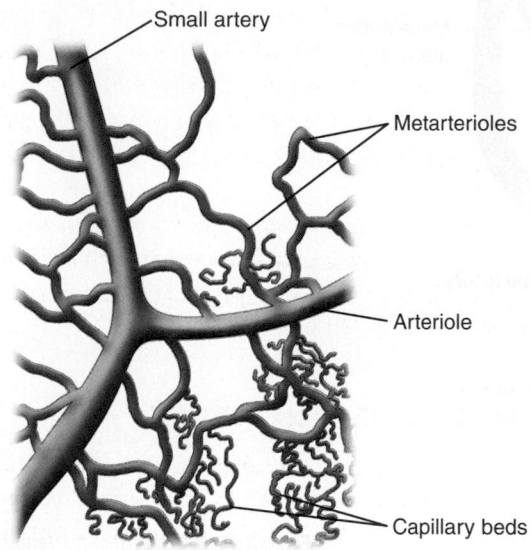

FIGURE 28.4 The capillary bed; capillaries are abundant in the body. Capillary beds are where oxygen and nutrients are delivered to the tissues and cellular waste is removed.

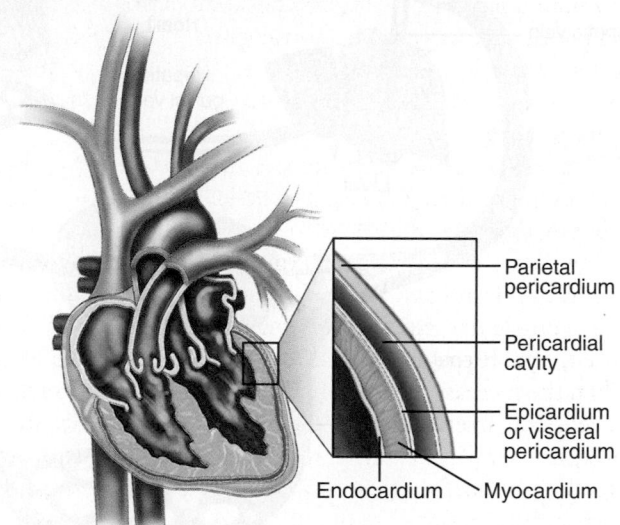

FIGURE 28.6 Layers of the pericardium; parietal and visceral pericardium and the three layers of the heart: epicardium, myocardium, and endocardium.

Anatomy of the Heart

The heart is a hollow, fist-sized organ located in the thoracic cavity between the lungs in a space called the *mediastinum*. It lies behind the sternum and rests on the diaphragm (Fig. 28.5). It is contained in a protective sac called the *pericardium*. The pericardium consists of two layers (Fig. 28.6). The outer layer, the pericardial sac or parietal pericardium, is a tough fibrous layer that turns inward at the base of the heart, forming the inner layer, the epicardium or visceral pericardium, which covers the heart surface. Between the two layers is a pericardial cavity containing serous fluid that provides a lubricant that allows the heart to beat without friction.

Layers

The heart muscle wall is composed of three layers (see Fig. 28.6). The thin outer layer of the heart is the epicardium, continuous with the inner layer of the pericardial sac. The thick middle layer, or myocardium, is the muscular layer responsible for the mechanical, contractile function of the heart. The thin inner layer is the endocardium. It lines the interior of the heart and the heart valves and is continuous with the inner layer, or endothelium, of the blood vessels.

Chambers

There are four chambers within the heart, the right and left **atria** and right and left **ventricles**. The right atrium receives deoxygenated blood from the systemic circulation through the great veins, the inferior and superior vena cava. Blood flows from the right atrium to the right ventricle. It is then delivered to the pulmonary circuit through the pulmonary artery. Newly oxygenated blood is returned to the left atrium via the pulmonary vein. It flows to the left ventricle and is then ejected into the aorta to the systemic circulation.

Valves

The heart needs valves (Fig. 28.7) to facilitate one-way flow. There are **atrioventricular (AV) valves** between the atria and ventricles on the right and left. The AV valve between the right atrium and ventricle is the tricuspid valve. The valve between the left atrium and ventricle is the bicuspid, or mitral, valve. When open, the valves allow flow from the atria into the ventricle. When the ventricles fill and the pressure within increases, the valves close to prevent retrograde flow back into the atria. The valves are connected to the muscle in the ventricle by fibrous cords, **chordae tendineae** (see Fig. 28.1), that prevent the valves from budging or turning inside out during ventricular contraction.

There are also **semilunar valves** between the ventricles and their respective arteries (pulmonary and aortic valves). The pulmonary valve is located between the right ventricle and pulmonary artery. The aortic valve is located between the left ventricle and aorta. Like the AV valves, they control the flow of blood between the ventricles and the pulmonary artery or aorta.

The valves in the heart open and close in response to changes in pressure. When the ventricles are relaxed during filling or **diastole**, the AV valves are open, allowing blood to flow into the ventricles. As the ventricles fill, the valves are forced upward and begin to close. The pressure increase from ventricular contraction forces the AV valves fully closed, which prevents backflow of blood into the atria. When the increase in pressure from ventricular contraction exceeds the arterial pressure in the pulmonary circuit or aorta, the semilunar valves open, allowing blood to flow into the pulmonary or systemic circulation. Figure 28.8 illustrates the pathway of blood flow through the chambers and valves.

Blood Supply to the Heart

In order for the heart to perform its work, it needs an adequate amount of oxygen and nutrients. The major vessels that supply blood to the heart are the left and right coronary arteries. They are the first arteries branching off of the aorta as it leaves the left ventricle, actually originating in the cusps of the aortic valve. The arteries branch off into arterioles and capillaries, then eventually merge into capillary veins that drain the blood into a coronary sinus, which eventually empties into the right atrium. Table 28.1 lists the coronaries, their primary branches, and the areas of the heart that they supply with oxygenated blood. Figure 28.9 illustrates the blood supply to the heart.

Connection Check 28.1

What is the composition of the heart?
A. Four chambers with four valves that control flow through the heart and lungs through changes in pressure
B. Four chambers and four valves that control flow through the heart and lungs through changes in oxygen levels
C. Two chambers on the right receiving blood from the high-pressure venous system and two chambers on the left sending blood into the low-pressure arterial system
D. Two chambers on the right receiving oxygenated blood from the venous system and two chambers on the left receiving deoxygenated blood from the pulmonary circuit

PHYSIOLOGY OF THE HEART

There needs to be both an electrical impulse conducted across the structures of the heart and a corresponding muscular contraction to facilitate the filling of the chambers of

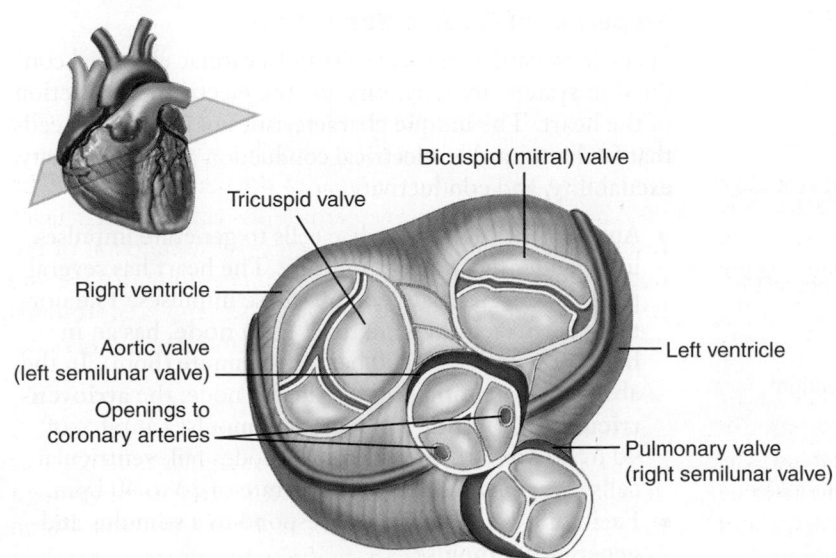

FIGURE 28.7 Cross-sectional view illustrating the valves of the heart. Note the openings to the coronary arteries in the aortic valve.

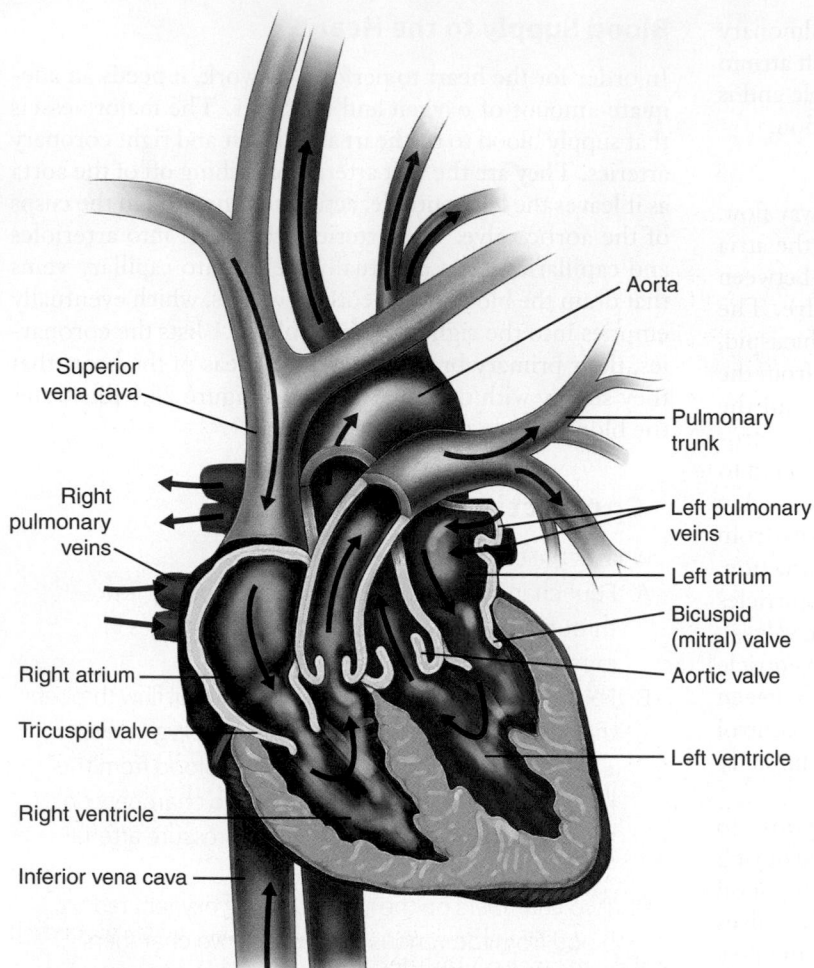

FIGURE 28.8 Pathway of blood flow through the heart.

Table 28.1	Coronary Arteries, Primary Branches, and the Areas of the Heart They Supply With Blood

Left Coronary Artery

Branches	Supplies
Left anterior descending (LAD) branch	Both ventricles
	Anterior interventricular septum
Circumflex branch	Anterior wall of the heart
	Left atrium
	Posterior wall of the left ventricle

Right Coronary Artery

Supplies the right atrium and sinoatrial node then branches off to:

Branches	Supplies
Right marginal branch	Lateral aspect of right atrium and ventricle
Posterior interventricular branch	Posterior aspect of both ventricles and interventricular septum

the heart and expulsion of blood into the systemic circulation. The next two sections will discuss each process and describe how they work together to produce sufficient cardiac output to deliver oxygenated blood to the tissues.

Cardiac Conduction System

Properties of Cardiac Muscle Cells

Specialized cardiac muscle cells and a cardiac electrical conduction system are necessary for the electrical conduction of the heart. The unique characteristics of the cardiac cells that facilitate cardiac electrical conduction are automaticity, excitability, and conductivity.

- Automaticity allows cardiac cells to generate impulses independently and rhythmically. The heart has several pacemaker cells that generate these impulses. The normal pacemaker, the **sinoatrial (SA) node**, has an inherent rate of 60 to 100 beats per minute (bpm). In the absence of an impulse from the SA node, the **atrioventricular (AV) node** can generate impulses at rates of 40 to 60 bpm. If the SA and AV nodes fail, ventricular cells can generate impulses at a rate of 20 to 40 bpm.
- Excitability is the ability to respond to a stimulus and generate an impulse.

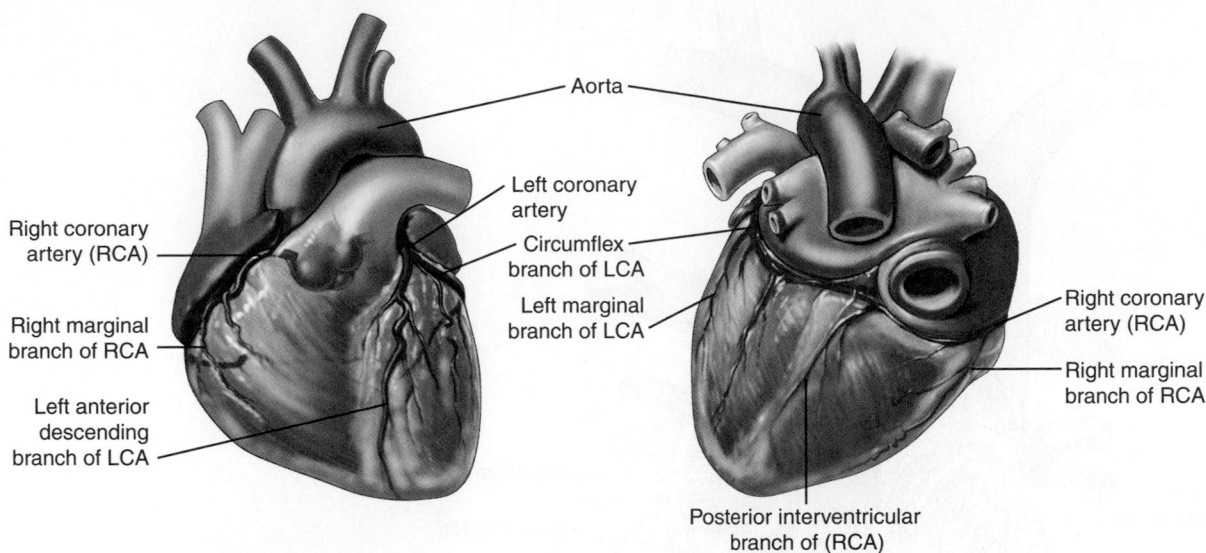

FIGURE 28.9 Blood supply to the heart.

- Conductivity allows cardiac tissue to transmit the impulses to neighboring connected cells.

Together, these properties allow cardiac tissue to act as a unit to propagate an impulse through the tissue and produce the muscular contraction necessary for the expulsion of blood during the cardiac cycle. Other properties unique to cardiac muscle cells include:

- Cardiac cells rely almost exclusively on aerobic metabolism for adenosine triphosphate production. Without the production of lactic acid that occurs with anaerobic metabolism, cardiac muscle can maintain its regular lifelong rhythm without tiring.
- Cardiac muscle relies on extracellular calcium to facilitate calcium release from the sarcoplasmic reticulum to produce its muscular contraction. This is referred to as calcium-induced calcium release. It is regulated by the slow inward flow of positively charged calcium ions during the action potential. Ion flow during the action potential is discussed in detail in this section of the chapter.
- Cardiac cells sustain a longer contraction, allowing ejection of blood from the atria and ventricles.
- Cardiac cells have a longer absolute refractory period, decreasing the possibility of repetitive, uncontrolled muscular contractions called *tetany*.

Cells of the Electrical Conduction System

The cells of cardiac electrical conduction system that generate and conduct the action potential follow this pathway:

1. The impulse originates in the SA node. The SA node has an inherent rate of 60 to 100 bpm.
2. The impulse spreads through the atria through the *internodal pathways* to the …
3. Atrioventricular node, where the impulse is delayed to allow for atrial contraction and complete ventricular filling.

4. It leaves the AV node through the **bundle of His** and branches off into the …
5. Right and left **bundle branches**, which travel down the interventricular septum to end in the …
6. **Purkinje fibers**, which extend the impulse into the ventricular tissue, facilitating ventricular contraction.

See Figure 28.10 for an illustration of the electrical conduction through the heart.

Action Potential of the Cardiac Conduction System

Electrical cardiac conduction is facilitated by the movement of ions across the cell membrane that is unique to cardiac cells. A stimulus begins the movement that produces the **cardiac action potential**, a process in which the membrane potential, the difference in charge between the interior and exterior of the cell, changes or goes up and down in a consistent pattern. **Depolarization** is the movement of ions preceding and facilitating cardiac mechanical contraction. **Repolarization** is the movement of ions back to the resting state, the cardiac resting membrane potential of −90 mV, to allow for the initiation of another action potential. There are five phases of the action potential (Fig. 28.11):

Phase 0: Rapid depolarization caused by the opening of sodium (Na^+) channels, allowing rapid Na^+ influx, moving the membrane potential to +30

Phase 1: Decrease in Na^+ influx, causing a slight movement toward negative of the membrane potential, producing an initial repolarization

Phase 2: Plateau state caused by an influx of calcium (Ca^{++}) through the opening of Ca^{++} channels balanced by a slight outflow of potassium (K^+)

Phase 3: Final repolarization caused by the closing of the Ca^{++} channels and the rapid outflow of K^+

Phase 4: Return to resting membrane potential

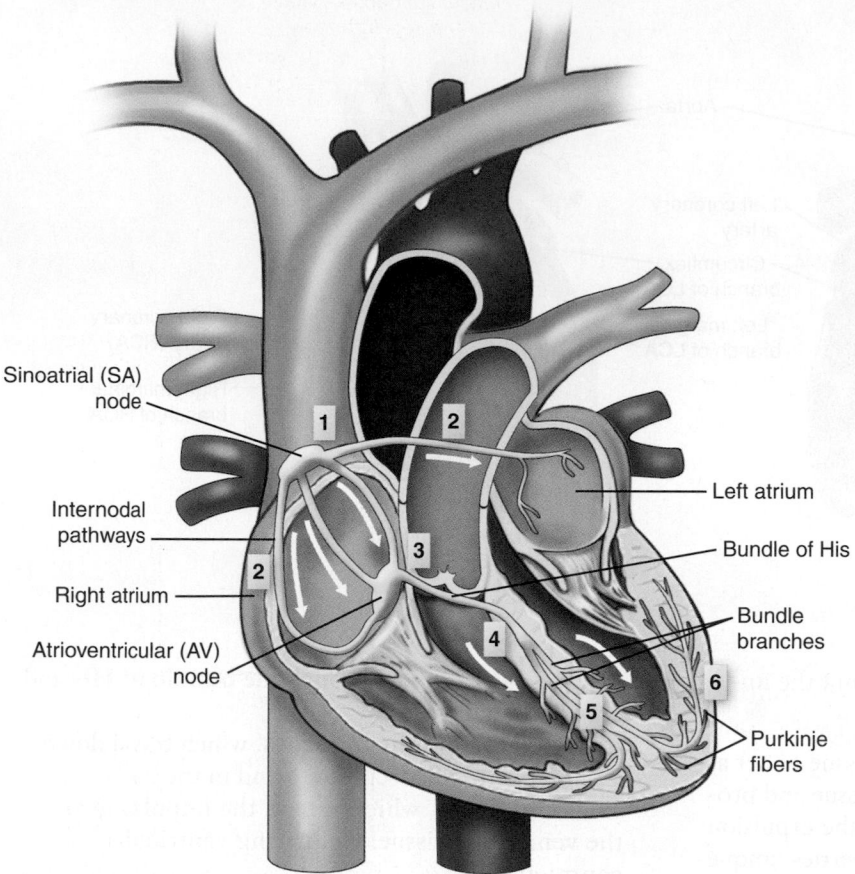

1 SA node fires.
2 Impulse spreads through atrial myocardium.
3 Impulse travels to the AV node.
4 Impulse leaves the AV node through the bundle of His.
5 Impulse travels through the bundle branches.
6 Impulse extends into the ventricular tissue through the Purkinje fibers.

FIGURE 28.10 Electrical conduction system of the heart: sinoatrial (SA) node, atrioventricular (AV) node, bundle branches and Purkinje fibers, and the impulse pathway.

An **absolute refractory period** occurs during and immediately following depolarization. During this time, the cell is unresponsive to any stimulus. This corresponds to phase 0 through the middle of phase 3. Immediately following the absolute refractory period is the **relative refractory period**. This represents a time when a greater-than-normal stimulus may initiate an impulse. This corresponds to the end of phase 3. Medications utilized to control irregular heart rhythms or dysrhythmias typically manipulate the movement of ions in some way.

Electrocardiogram

The electrical activity described previously produces waveforms, which can be amplified and viewed on a paper tracing called an **electrocardiogram (ECG)**. Electrodes placed on the wrists, ankles, and six locations around the chest produce a comprehensive picture of the cardiac electrical activity. Details on obtaining an ECG are discussed later in the chapter under diagnostic imaging tests.

The principal waveforms produced are the P wave, QRS complex, and T wave. The principal segments include

the PR segment and the ST segment. The intervals include the PR interval, QRS interval, and QT interval (Fig. 28.12).

- The *P wave* corresponds to atrial depolarization produced by the propagation of the impulse from the SA node through the atria. Atrial contraction takes place milliseconds after depolarization.
- The *PR interval* from the beginning of the P wave to the beginning of the QRS complex reflects the time required for atrial depolarization and the delay of the impulse at the AV node.
- The *PR segment*—the time immediately following the P wave to the beginning of the QRS complex—reflects the delay at the AV node.
- The *QRS complex* corresponds to ventricular depolarization. Ventricular contraction occurs after the QRS complex in the *ST segment*.
- The *QRS interval* reflects the time required for ventricular depolarization.
- The *T wave* corresponds to ventricular repolarization. Atrial repolarization occurs during ventricular

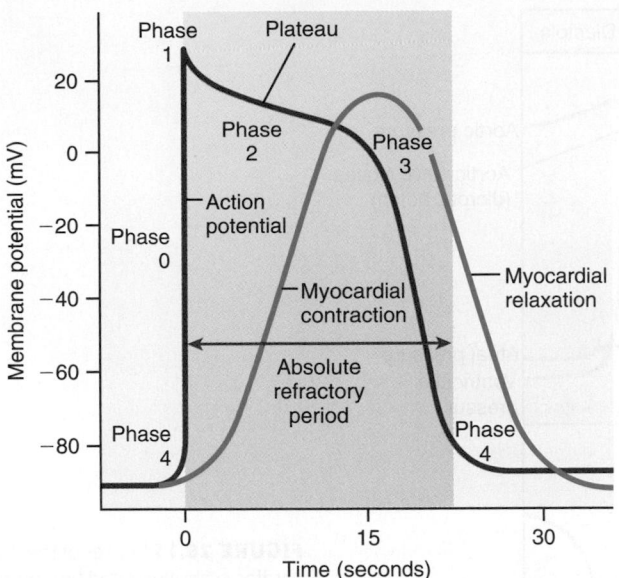

FIGURE 28.11 Phases of the cardiac action potential. Phase 0: Rapid depolarization caused by rapid Na⁺ influx, moving the membrane potential to +30. Phase 1: Deceases in Na⁺ influx, producing an initial repolarization. Phase 2: Plateau state caused by an influx of calcium (Ca⁺⁺) balanced by a slight outflow of potassium (K⁺). Phase 3: Final repolarization caused by the closing of the Ca⁺⁺ channels and the rapid outflow of K⁺. Phase 4: Return to resting membrane potential. The purple curve represents the action potential. The green curve represents the changes in cardiac muscle tension.

contraction. That waveform is not visible but is buried in the QRS complex.
- The *QT interval* reflects the time required for ventricular depolarization and repolarization.

Connection Check 28.2

Which is true of the electrical conduction system of the heart?
A. It is primarily controlled by the movement of uncharged ions.
B. It has a positive resting membrane potential.
C. It is reflected in the waveforms on the electrocardiogram.
D. It requires cells that respond only to a stimulus from the autonomic nervous system.

Cardiac Cycle

The cardiac cycle is defined as the circular sequence of events that produces the eventual muscular contraction that causes the ejection of blood from the right ventricle into the pulmonary circulation or from the left ventricle into the systemic circulation. This cycle works in coordination with the electrical cardiac conduction system, which is illustrated in Figure 28.13.

There are two parts to the cardiac cycle: **systole**, or contraction, and diastole, or relaxation. Diastole is when filling

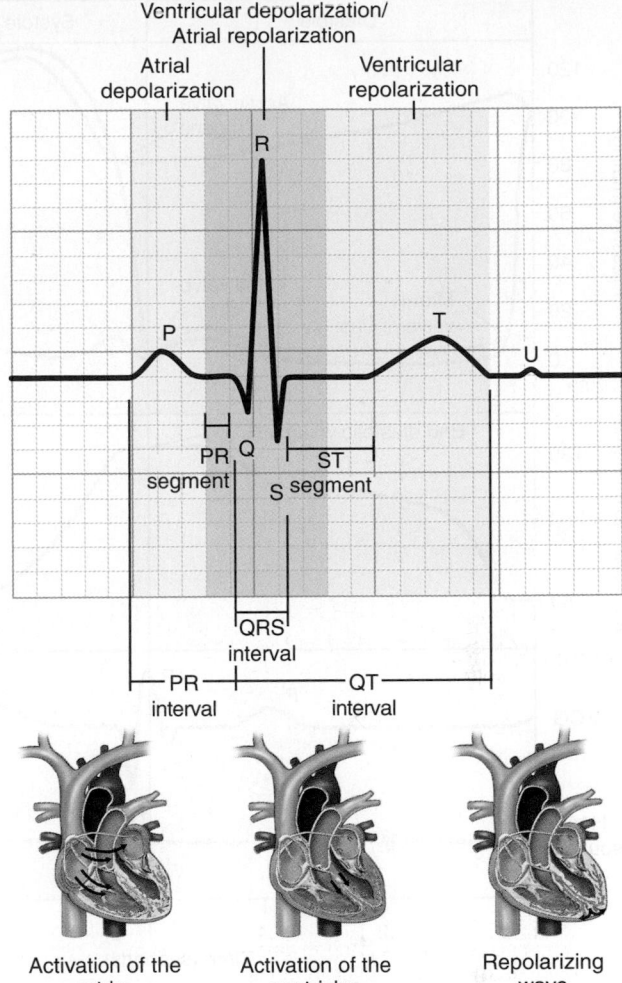

FIGURE 28.12 Cardiac waveforms and intervals. The *P wave* corresponds to atrial depolarization; atrial contraction occurs a millisecond after depolarization. The *PR interval* reflects the time required for atrial depolarization and the delay of the impulse at the atrioventricular (AV) node. The *PR segment* is the time immediately following the P wave to the beginning of the QRS complex and reflects the delay at the AV node. The *QRS complex* corresponds to ventricular depolarization; the *QRS interval* reflects the time required for ventricular depolarization. Atrial repolarization occurs during ventricular depolarization. That waveform is not visible but is buried in the QRS complex. The *ST segment* is where ventricular contraction occurs. The *T wave* corresponds to ventricular repolarization. The *QT interval* reflects the time required for ventricular depolarization and repolarization.

of the ventricles occurs and accounts for the first two-thirds of the cycle. Myocardial tissue perfusion occurs during diastole. Systole facilitates the ejection of blood from the ventricles and occurs during the last one-third of the cycle. This cycle is occurring simultaneously on the left and right sides of the heart.

Diastole

During diastole, the ventricles are relaxed, with a lower pressure than that of the atria, allowing the AV valves to open. Blood flows into the atria from the superior and inferior vena cava or from the pulmonary veins and then quickly flows into the ventricles. As blood flows into the ventricles,

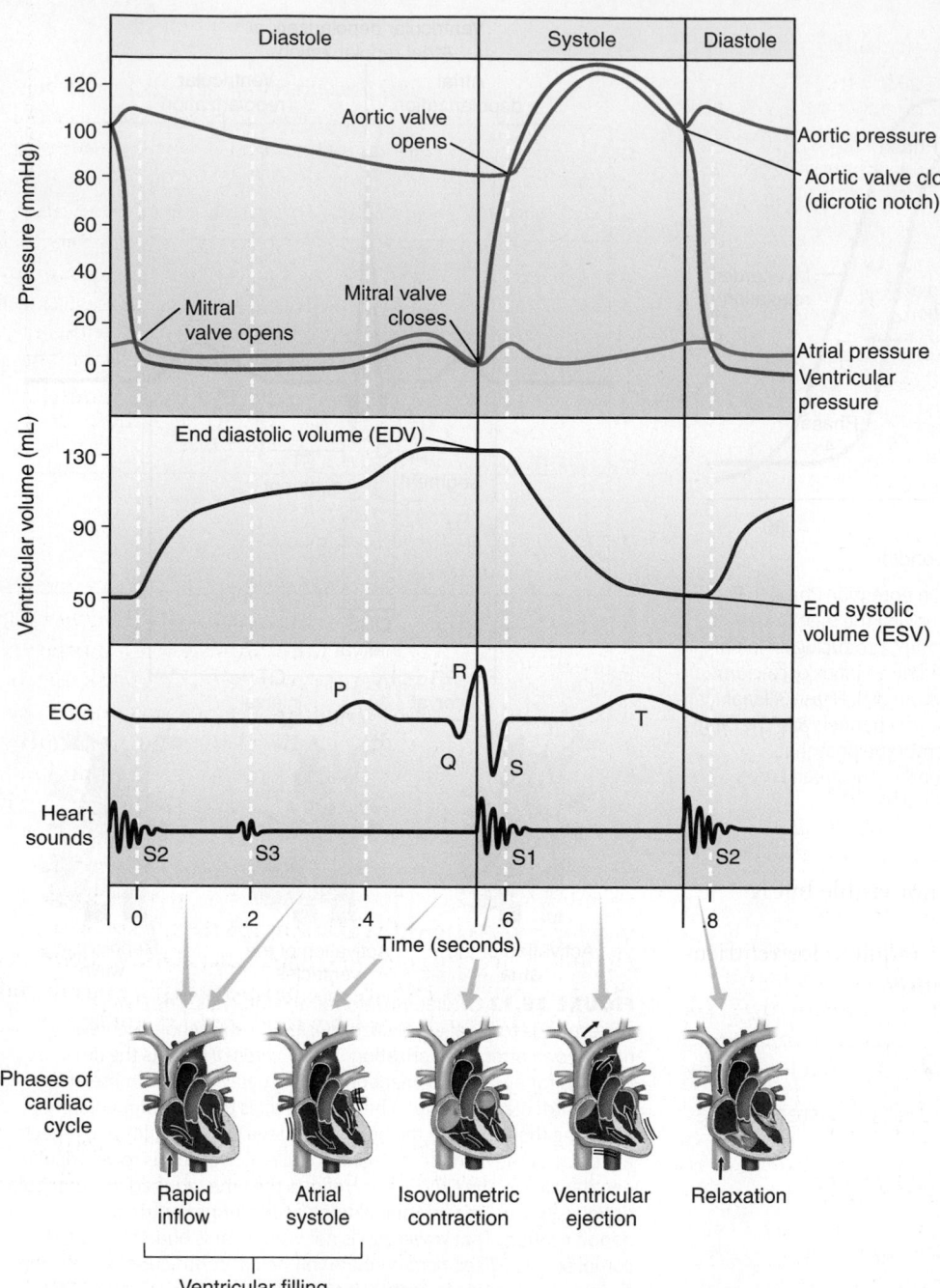

FIGURE 28.13 Phases of the cardiac cycle illustrated by volume and pressure changes in the left heart and corresponding electrocardiogram (ECG) changes and heart sounds. At time zero, the left ventricle (dark blue waveform) has a lower pressure than that of the left atrium (green waveform). The mitral valve opens, allowing blood to flow into the ventricle and quickly increasing the ventricular volume. The atria contract, completing ventricular filling to the end diastolic volume (red waveform). At time 0.6 seconds, pressure increases within the ventricle without any volume changes, an isovolumetric contraction, closing the mitral valve. Ventricular pressure eventually exceeds aortic pressure (purple line), opening the aortic valve and allowing a rapid ejection of blood into the systemic circulation. Note how atrial and ventricular systole occur milliseconds after depolarization, as illustrated by the P wave and QRS complex.

pressure drops in the atria and rises in the ventricles. The final phase of ventricular filling occurs when the atria contract, known as atrial systole, which accounts for the final 30% of ventricular filling. This is referred to as the **atrial kick**. The final volume in the ventricle at the end of diastole is the end diastolic volume. This is also referred to as **preload**.

Systole

At the completion of filling, the ventricles contact. During the initial phase of contraction, pressure increases, but there are no volume changes; thus, this is an isovolumetric contraction. The increased pressure in the ventricle causes the AV valves to close, preventing retrograde flow into the atria.

As ventricular pressure continues to increase during contraction, it eventually exceeds that of the aortic and pulmonic circuits. When this occurs, the semilunar valves are forced open, allowing a rapid ejection of blood into the pulmonary and systemic circulation.

Blood Pressure

Blood pressure (BP) is a reflection of the pressures generated during the cardiac cycle. It represents the force exerted against the vessel wall by blood flow. Factors that influence BP are the amount of blood ejected during systole, or CO, and the resistance to flow in the peripheral vessels, or peripheral vascular resistance.

Blood pressure is reported in two pressures, systolic and diastolic. Systolic is the peak pressure generated when blood is expelled from the left ventricle during ventricular contraction. Diastolic pressure is the minimal pressure maintained on the vessel walls during relaxation. Mean arterial pressure is the average pressure maintained throughout the cardiac cycle.

Regulation of BP is primarily controlled through changes in the factors that influence pressure: blood flow, or volume, and resistance to flow. Increases or decreases in blood volume or CO increase or decrease BP. Resistance, defined as opposition to flow, is chiefly a function of vessel diameter. Changes in flow and resistance are principally controlled by the autonomic nervous system (ANS) and hormones.

The ANS responds to messages sent by various sensory tissues in the body, **baroreceptors** and **chemoreceptors**. Baroreceptors, located in the aortic and carotid arches, are sensitive to changes in pressure. An increase in pressure stimulates the parasympathetic nervous system to dilate vessels and reduce the **heart rate (HR)** to reduce BP. The decrease in pressure stimulates the sympathetic nervous system to constrict vessels and increase the HR, which increases BP.

Chemoreceptors contained in collections of cells called *carotid bodies* and *aortic bodies* are located in the aortic arch and in the carotid arteries. They respond to changes in oxygen and CO_2 concentrations. Decreased levels of oxygen with increased levels of CO_2 produce acidosis. The chemoreceptors respond to decreased oxygen levels and acidosis by inducing vasoconstriction to increase BP and increase blood flow to the lungs, facilitating oxygen and CO_2 exchange. The respiratory rate (RR) is also increased.

Hormonal mechanisms that exert control over BP include angiotensin II, epinephrine and norepinephrine, aldosterone, and antidiuretic hormone. Angiotensin II, created in response to low BP, is an end product of a series of events. After a drop in BP, the kidneys respond by releasing the enzyme renin. Renin reacts with angiotensinogen to create angiotensin I. Angiotensin I is then converted in the lungs to angiotensin II via angiotensin-converting enzyme. Angiotensin II is a potent vasoconstrictor that increases BP. Angiotensin II also acts on the adrenals to release aldosterone. The release of aldosterone promotes sodium and water reabsorption in the kidneys, which increases circulating fluid volume. This is called the **renin-angiotensin-aldosterone system**. Epinephrine and norepinephrine, catecholamines released by the adrenal medulla, cause vasoconstriction, leading to increases in BP as part of the fight-or-flight mechanism in the sympathetic nervous system. Antidiuretic hormone is released by the posterior pituitary in response to the decreased blood volume. It acts on the kidney to conserve water. These concepts are discussed in more detail in Chapter 40.

Several other hormones, atrial natriuretic peptide (ANP) and brain natriuretic peptide (BNP), are released from heart tissue when fluid volumes are high. They stimulate vasodilation and diuresis. This is discussed in more detail in Chapter 30.

CARDIAC OUTPUT

Together, the electrical and muscular actions of the heart muscle fulfill the primary function of the cardiovascular system: the delivery of oxygenated blood into the systemic arterial circulation. The blood ejected from the left heart each minute to facilitate the delivery of oxygen and nutrients to the tissues is called the cardiac output (CO). Normal CO in an adult is 4 to 8 L/min. This value does not remain constant but is increased by exercise or activity and decreased in times of rest. Cardiac output is calculated by the formula HR × **stroke volume** (the amount of blood ejected with each ventricular contraction). That value can be indexed by dividing by the body surface area (height × weight) to reflect the different requirements related to body size.

Heart Rate

Heart rate (HR) is simply the number of cardiac contractions per minute. Heart rate can be affected by many variables. Stimulus from the ANS, although not initiating the heartbeat, does adjust it up or down. The HR can be increased or decreased depending on pressure. For instance, when BP is low, the HR is increased to maintain adequate CO. Stimulus from the sympathetic nervous system initiated by information from baroreceptors in the aortic arch and the carotids that are sensitive to changes in BP increase the HR through the release of norepinephrine. This is called a *positive chronotropic effect*. The parasympathetic nervous system slows the HR through the release of acetylcholine, a negative chronotropic effect. Other chemicals that can increase HR are the hormones epinephrine and norepinephrine released from the adrenal medulla.

Stroke Volume

Stroke volume is the amount of blood ejected with each ventricular contraction. It is influenced by three variables: preload, afterload, and contractility.

- **Preload** is the amount of blood in the ventricles at the end of diastole. It also refers to the amount of stretch of the muscle tissue at the end of filling. Increased volume produces increased stretch, which produces an increased contraction (Starling's law). This is true up to a point. Extreme overfilling decreases the effectiveness of the contraction, thus decreasing CO.
- **Afterload** refers to the resistance to flow the ventricle must overcome to open the semilunar valves and eject its contents. This is related to BP, vessel lumen diameter, and/or vessel compliance. The valves can meet resistance on both the right and left through the pulmonary artery or aorta. Hypertension on the right or left is implicated in the negative effects of increased afterload.
- **Contractility** refers to the force of the mechanical contraction. Contractile force can be increased with sympathetic stimulation or calcium release. It can be decreased in the face of hypoxia or acidosis.

Preload and afterload are reflected by measurements obtained through a centrally located IV line: preload = the central venous pressure; afterload = the systemic vascular resistance or pulmonary vascular resistance. The concept of cardiac output is discussed in more detail in Chapter 32.

Connection Check 28.3

A patient with hypertension has which physical symptom?
A. Decreased resistance, which may increase CO
B. Increased resistance, which may decrease CO
C. Increased resistance, which may increase CO
D. Decreased resistance, which may decrease CO

CASE STUDY: EPISODE 2

During the initial assessment, Mr. Smith offers no specific complaints. His PMH is negative for any significant disease. He does state he has aches and pains after a hard day at work; he does a lot of heavy lifting. He has no known allergies and is not taking any medication. His examination reveals:

BP—145/90 mm Hg

HR—84 bpm and regular

RR—16

His physical examination is unremarkable except for his stage 2 hypertension and excessive weight. His neurological, respiratory, and cardiovascular examinations are within normal limits ...

ASSESSMENT

History

Major risk factors for cardiovascular disease (CVD) include a family history of CVD, diabetes mellitus, chronic renal disease, hypertension, and dyslipidemia. A complete and thorough history that includes demographic data, family history, and personal history, including present health problems, is essential in the patient cardiovascular assessment. The patient is the primary source of information, but family members and medical records can also be very informative. Demographic data include age, sex, and ethnic background. These are all nonmodifiable risk factors. The family history can reveal significant information regarding the age, health status, and cause of death of immediate family members. Information regarding socioeconomic status is also important. Occupation, economic status, marital status, children, insurance, and support systems are important and can hint at a patient's ability to respond in times of need.

Modifiable risk factors in a patient's personal history include such things as weight, dietary habits, alcohol consumption, and smoking history. Excess consumption of fats

and sodium is a dietary habit that puts a patient at risk for heart disease. Smoking and excessive drinking are also implicated in heart disease. Activity level should be assessed. A sedentary lifestyle is a risk factor for cardiovascular disease; exercise promotes cardiovascular health.

Current Health Problems

After the patient's past history has been established, current health problems should be identified. The existence of diabetes, hypertension, and high cholesterol indicates a risk for heart disease. Significant complaints pertinent to heart disease include the presence of chest pain, difficulty breathing (dyspnea), cough, palpitations, edema, fatigue, and/or syncope.

Chest pain should be evaluated for its location, intensity, radiation, duration, and quality. Information related to the treatment that provides relief is also significant. Dyspnea and fatigue at rest or dyspnea on exertion are important to note. Palpitations are an indication of abnormal heart rhythms: dysrhythmias. Syncope is an indication of decreased CO resulting from problems with either the mechanical or electrical properties of the heart. Weight gain associated with edema indicates a weakened heart and potentially the presence of heart failure, discussed in more detail in Chapter 30.

Physical Assessment

General Assessment

The components of a cardiac physical assessment include an initial general assessment of the patient, inspection, palpation, and auscultation. The initial assessment starts with evaluating the patient's overall appearance, including color, diaphoresis, edema, and demeanor and restlessness, agitation, or confusion. The nurse's initial conversation can reveal information pertinent to the patient's orientation. Through observation, you can quickly determine weight and build, symptoms such as shortness of breath (SOB), and mobility. A patient with cardiac disease may appear pale, fatigued, or short of breath. Patients with late-stage heart failure will present with edema and appear frail and fatigued.

Other basic components of an initial cardiac assessment include an evaluation of HR and BP. The HR or pulse rate provides information on the efficiency and strength of the heart. A normal HR is 60 to 100 bpm. The HR can be determined in several ways, such as palpating the pulse over an artery close to the skin, typically the radial artery, and auscultating an apical HR. An apical rate can be auscultated by placing a stethoscope at the junction of the fifth intercostal space and the midclavicular line, the point of maximal impulse (PMI). A lower HR can indicate good physical conditioning, and thus an efficient heart, but it may also be an indicator of inadequate CO. If a low HR is associated with symptoms such as dizziness, SOB, or chest pain, further evaluation is required. Increases in HR naturally occur with exercise and exertion but are abnormal when occurring at rest. This may be due to many factors, some of which include a weak heart muscle, pain, fever, or inadequate fluid volume, all of which require further evaluation. A pulse deficit is occurring when, if performed at the same time, the radial pulse rate is less than the apical HR. A pulse deficit can indicate arrhythmias such as atrial fibrillation or premature ectopic beats.

Blood pressure provides information on the force of the heart's contraction and volume of CO as well as the resistance offered by the arterial vascular system. High BP indicates more resistance in the vessels, requiring higher pressures to produce an adequate CO. High BP increases the risk of heart failure, myocardial infarction, and stroke. The American Heart Association guidelines for BP levels were updated in 2017 (see Evidence-Based Practice). Hypertension is discussed in detail in Chapter 31. Low BP should be assessed for clinical significance. The presence of postural hypotension, a decrease of 20 mm Hg in BP when moving from a lying or seated position to a standing position accompanied by a 10% increase in HR, dizziness, SOB, and/or syncope, could indicate inadequate CO or blood volume and requires further evaluation.

Evidence-Based Practice

Guidelines for the Detection and Evaluation of High Blood Pressure in Adults

Based on evidence published by the American Heart Association in 2017, blood pressure in adults is categorized as normal, elevated, or hypertension; hypertension is further classified as stage 1 or stage 2. Categorization should be based on an average of two or more readings found two or more times on examination. If the systolic blood pressure (SBP) and diastolic blood pressure (DBP) fall into two different categories, the higher category should be assigned.

BP category	SBP		DBP
Normal	<120 mm Hg	and	<80 mm Hg
Elevated	120–129 mm Hg	and	<80 mm Hg
Hypertension			
• Stage 1	• 130–139 mm Hg	or	• 80–89 mm Hg
• Stage 2	• >140 mm Hg	or	• >90 mm Hg

Whelton, P. K., Carey, R. M., Aronow, W. S., Casey, D. E., Collins, K. J., Himmelfarb, C. D., ... & MacLaughlin, E. J. (2017). 2017 ACC/AHA/AAPA/ABC/ACPM/AGS/APhA/ASH/ASPC/NMA/PCNA guideline for the prevention, detection, evaluation, and management of high blood pressure in adults: A report of the American College of Cardiology/American Heart Association Task Force on Clinical Practice Guidelines. *Journal of the American College of Cardiology*, 71, e127–e248.

Inspection

Visual inspection is done to assess color, capillary refill time, edema, the presence or absence of jugular vein distention, and clubbing of the fingers or toes. Skin color and nailbed color in light-skinned people with adequate perfusion are pink. Poor perfusion produces a pale gray or bluish color. This is called **cyanosis**. In dark-skinned people, adequate perfusion produces the same pink coloring of the nailbeds. Cyanosis appears gray.

Cyanosis can be central or peripheral. Central cyanosis appears as blue coloring in the mucous membranes, lips, and tongue. It is usually caused by impaired heart or lung function. Peripheral cyanosis, or blue discoloration of the extremities, can be caused by heart or lung failure but may also indicate peripheral vasoconstriction or obstruction.

Capillary refill time is tested by compressing a finger or toe momentarily to stop the blood flow, producing a whitening effect, then releasing pressure and timing the return to the normal pink color. A return to color within 3 seconds indicates adequate peripheral circulation. Sluggish return may indicate arterial spasm or insufficiency.

Edema may be a sign of cardiac or liver issues. Bilateral lower extremity edema, if not associated with a local injury, generally indicates venous insufficiency or heart failure. Unilateral extremity edema, again if not associated with injury, can indicate a venous or lymphatic obstruction. Edema is identified as pitting or nonpitting. Pitting edema is characterized by an indenting of the skin that remains after pressure has been applied then released.

Distention of the jugular veins may be present in a patient with a constrictive disease such as pericarditis or cardiac tamponade. It is also seen in patients with right ventricular failure, valvular disease, or hypervolemia. It is often associated with poor contractile function of the heart that is present in heart failure (discussed in more detail in Chapter 30).

Clubbing of the fingers and/or toes indicates long-term perfusion problems produced by a decrease in oxygenated blood flow to the affected extremities. This is typically caused by congenital heart defects or chronic pulmonary disease. It can also be seen in patients with lung cancer.

Palpation

Assessment of skin temperature and pulses is done by palpation. Adequate CO produces warm skin temperatures. Cool or cold temperatures may indicate vasoconstriction, heart failure, or shock. Variations in temperature between different parts of the body may indicate vasoconstriction or vascular disease in the affected extremities.

Pulses typically palpated include the radial and dorsalis pedis pulses. A more extensive examination includes femoral, popliteal, and posterior tibial pulses. Strong, palpable pulses indicate adequate CO and good flow through the peripheral vessels.

Auscultation

Assessment of heart and lung sounds is done through auscultation.

Heart Sounds

The heart sounds ("lubb" and "dubb") that are heard during auscultation are produced by the closing of the valves during the cardiac cycle (Table 28.2). The first heart sound, S_1,

Table 28.2 Summary of Heart Sounds

Heart Sound	Cause	Description	Timing
S₁	Closure of AV valves	"Lubb"	
S₂	Closure of semilunar valves	"Dubb"	
S₃: Ventricular gallop	Ventricular dysfunction when heard in adults	Galloplike sounds	Early diastole
S₄: Atrial gallop	Decreased ventricular compliance	Galloplike sounds	Late diastole after atrial systole
Systolic murmur	Valvular disease such as aortic stenosis	Turbulent flow heard	Systole between S₁ and S₂
Diastolic murmur	Valvular disease such as aortic or pulmonic regurgitation	Turbulent flow heard	Diastole after S₂
Click	Mitral valve stenosis	High-pitched sound	Early diastole
Friction rub	Pericarditis	Harsh, scratching sound	Anywhere during the cardiac cycle

AV, Arterioventricular.

is the closing of the AV valves. It signifies the beginning of ventricular systole. The second heart sound, S₂, is the closing of the semilunar valves. It signifies the beginning of diastole. S₁ sounds longer and louder when compared with S₂, which is short and soft. Figure 28.13 illustrates where heart sounds are heard in the cardiac cycle.

Heart sounds vary with age. A third heart sound, S₃, can be heard in children and young adults. It is caused by vibration in the ventricular walls during filling or early diastole. If heard in an adult, it may indicate decreased ventricular compliance. The combined sounds of S₁, S₂, and S₃ resemble a gallop, thus the name *ventricular gallop*. A fourth heart sound, S₄, is heard in late diastole and occurs after atrial contraction. It also can indicate decreased ventricular compliance. It is known as an atrial gallop.

Fever, inflammation, excess fluid, and narrowed or incompetent valves are a few clinical situations that produce extra sounds, such as clicks, rubs, or murmurs. A click is a high-pitched sound heard early in diastole and is typically caused by mitral valve stenosis. Murmurs are usually caused by turbulent flow through the valves. That turbulence can be caused by regurgitation of blood through an incompetent valve, flow through a narrowed valve, or an increase in flow in hypermetabolic states such as hyperthyroidism or fever. A friction rub is described as a scratching or grating sound heard during both systole and diastole. The sound is produced by inflammation of the pericardium. It is diagnostic for pericarditis and is referred to as the pericardial friction rub.

When describing heart sounds, it is important to note:

- Pitch: high, medium, or low
- Quality, such as blowing or harsh
- Intensity, such as faint, quiet, or loud
- Timing during systole or diastole
- Location where heard best on the chest wall

Lung Sounds

Lung sounds give an indication of both lung and cardiac health. Clear breath sounds signify a healthy heart and lungs. Auscultation of rales, rhonchi, or rubs in the lung fields indicates the presence of fluid. These findings may be a result of pulmonary disease or congestive heart failure and decreased cardiac function. Heart failure is discussed in more detail in Chapter 30.

Connection Check 28.4

A nurse is providing care for a patient newly diagnosed with heart disease. Which dietary, activity, or lifestyle modification(s) should be included in the plan of care? *(Select all that apply.)*

A. Stopping smoking
B. Drinking lots of water
C. Limiting sedentary lifestyle
D. Eating a diet rich in red meat and protein
E. Limiting alcohol intake

DIAGNOSTIC STUDIES

Laboratory Markers as Predictors of Heart Disease

A lipid panel includes total cholesterol, low-density lipoproteins (LDLs), high-density lipoproteins (HDLs), and triglycerides. Cholesterol is a lipid necessary for the synthesis of hormones and cell walls. It is available through the ingestion of animal products (e.g., meat) and through synthesis in the liver. It is not soluble in blood, so it combines with proteins to form lipoproteins, LDLs and HDLs, to facilitate transport through the vascular system. Low-density lipoproteins primarily transport cholesterol into the cell but can also deposit it on the walls of arterial vessels. Elevated levels, greater than 100 mg/dL, are associated with an increased risk of heart disease. High-density lipoproteins, protective lipoproteins, transport cholesterol away from the cells to the liver for excretion. Therefore, opposite of LDLs, decreased levels of HDLs, less than 40 to 60 mg/dL, are a risk factor for heart disease. A total cholesterol level includes both LDLs and HDLs. Normal levels are 200 mg/dL or less. Increased levels are a risk factor for atherosclerotic vessel disease. Triglycerides, another lipid, store unused ingested calories in fat cells, which may be later released as an energy source between meals. Elevated levels, greater than 150 mg/dL, are another risk factor for heart disease.

Nonspecific Markers

Because diabetes and hyperglycemia are major risk factors for CVD, blood glucose levels are an essential laboratory value for evaluation. Increased homocysteine, an amino acid, is also a risk factor for heart disease. It can damage the lining of arterial walls, causing clot formation. Decreased dietary intake of folic acid and B vitamins is associated with increased levels of homocysteine. C-reactive protein is not specific for cardiac disease but is used in conjunction with other laboratory tests. Elevated levels reflect increased production of C-reactive protein in the liver secondary to systemic inflammation. Inflammation is implicated in the development of atherosclerosis. Coagulation studies such as platelets and fibrinogen levels, although not specific markers of cardiac disease, are commonly obtained for screening purposes. Increased platelets and fibrinogen levels are correlated with an increased risk of atherosclerotic heart disease. Prothrombin time, partial thromboplastin time, and international normalized ratio are measured in patients with increased risk of clot formation, such as patients with atrial fibrillation. They are also utilized to monitor anticoagulation therapy. Table 28.3 lists laboratory tests and normal values.

Nursing Implications

The nurse's responsibilities are primarily associated with patient education. Most of the laboratory tests mentioned previously do not require any specific patient preparation, but a lipid panel requires the patient to fast for approximately 8 to 12 hours prior to the test.

Laboratory Markers of Acute Cardiac Damage or Injury

Laboratory markers of acute cardiac damage or injury include enzymes or proteins that are elevated in response to cellular injury. Some are specific to cardiac tissue; others are more general and must be evaluated in conjunction with the specific tests.

Creatine kinase (CK) is a general marker of cellular injury. It is released from cells in the brain, skeletal muscle,

Table 28.3 Laboratory Predictors and Markers of Heart Disease

Laboratory Test	Normal Value*
Predictors of Heart Disease	
Lipid panel: Cholesterol	Less than 200 mg/dL
Low-density lipoproteins (LDLs)	Less than 100 mg/dL
High-density lipoproteins (HDLs)	Greater than 40–60 mg/dL
Triglycerides	Less than 150 mg/dL
Glucose	65–99 mg/dL
Homocysteine	4.4–10.8 mm/L
C-reactive protein	0 (only present when inflammation is present)
Coagulation studies: Platelets	150,000–400,000 mc/L
Fibrinogen levels	200–400 mg/dL
Prothrombin time (PT)	10–13 seconds
Partial thromboplastin time (PTT)	25–35 seconds
International normalized ratio (INR)	<2.0
Markers of Heart Disease	
Creatine kinase myocardial bands (CK-MB)	0–3 ng/mL
Troponin	Less than 0.4 ng/mL
Myoglobin	0–85 ng/mL
Brain natriuretic peptide (BPN)	Less than 100 pg/mL

*Values are a reference range and may vary by institution—they are just a guide.

and cardiac tissue after muscle damage has occurred. One isoenzyme of CK, creatine kinase myocardial bands (CK-MB) is the marker specific to cardiac tissue. When myocardial damage occurs, CK-MB is released from the cells. Increased levels can be seen at 3 hours after myocardial damage and can remain elevated for up to 36 hours before returning to normal.

Troponin is another specific marker of cardiac muscle damage and is the preferred method for diagnosing cardiac injury. It is a protein released from damaged tissue and, as with CK-MB, can elevate within 4 hours of injury. It can stay elevated for up to 10 days. Because it stays elevated longer than CK-MB, it is a valuable marker when attempting to diagnosis injury in the recent past.

Myoglobin, another protein, is released and elevated in muscle damage but is not specific for cardiac tissue. It can be used in conjunction with the other values to help rule out or rule in a myocardial infarction.

Brain natriuretic peptide (BNP) is released from over-stretched ventricular tissue. Physiological responses to increased levels of BNP include venous dilation, which decreases preload; arterial dilation, which decreases after-load; and diuresis. Elevations are an indicator of heart failure. Table 28.3 lists laboratory tests and normal values.

Nursing Implications

Nursing care related to obtaining CK, CK-MB, and troponin is primarily associated with the timing of the blood draws. When a patient is evaluated for acute injury, laboratory tests are obtained at baseline and then at regular intervals (typically 3 to 4 hours) for approximately 12 hours. It is important to obtain samples in a timely fashion and accurately note the time each blood sample is obtained.

Diagnostic Imaging Studies

Electrocardiography

The ECG is a basic diagnostic assessment that is completed routinely on patients to assess the electrical conduction system of the heart. It is a graphic recording of the heart's electrical activity. It can identify the presence of dysrhythmias, new or old heart muscle damage, electrolyte abnormalities, and/or cardiac hypertrophy. It is done by placing 10 electrodes on specific positions of the body (Fig. 28.14A), the bilateral upper and lower extremities (limb leads) and six positions around the left chest (chest or V leads). The chest positions are (see Fig. 28.14B):

V1: 4th intercostal space, just to the right of the sternum
V2: 4th intercostal space, just to the left of the sternum
V4: On the midclavicular line and 5th intercostal space

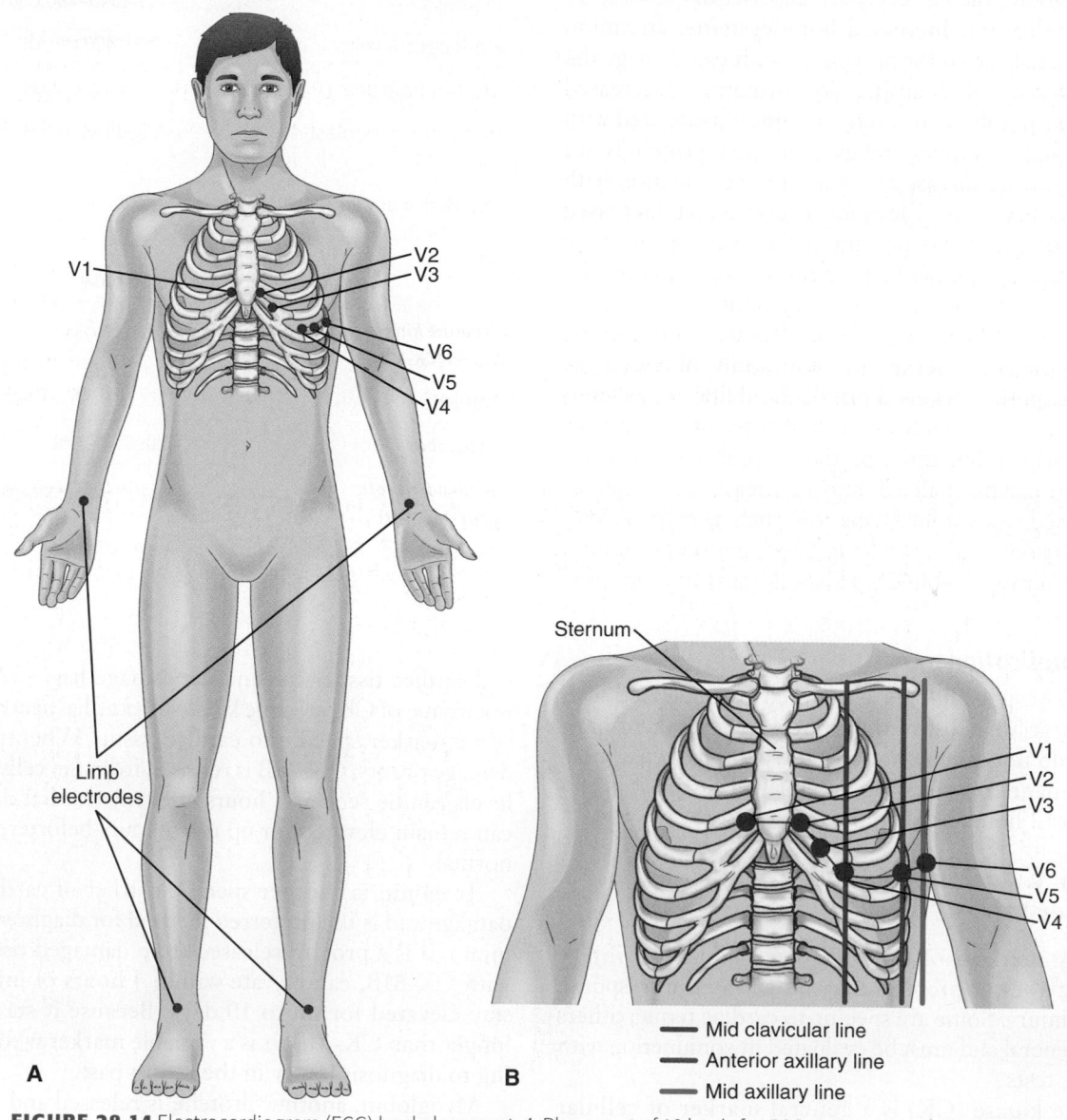

FIGURE 28.14 Electrocardiogram (ECG) lead placement. *A,* Placement of 10 leads for ECG. *B,* Location of six chest leads.

V6: On the midaxillary line, horizontal with V4
V5: Between V6 and V4 on the anterior axillary line
V3: Between V4 and V2

Nursing Implications

Electrocardiograms can be done with the patient resting or ambulatory. A resting examination is done with the patient supine and quiet. It is completed within several minutes. The skin must be clean, dry, and as free from hair as possible to ensure good electrode contact with the skin. If the patient has excessive chest hair, some hair may need to be shaved to ensure good contact.

An ambulatory examination (Holter monitoring) can be done continuously over several days while the patient maintains normal activities. In this way, symptoms such as chest pain, SOB, or syncope may be correlated with rhythm changes. The patient is instructed to keep a log of activities, especially noting the time and activity corresponding to adverse symptoms.

Radiology

The **chest x-ray (CXR)** is a general screening tool that provides information about the size, shape, and position of the heart. By itself, a CXR cannot diagnose heart disease but can highlight complications such as cardiac enlargement (Fig. 28.15) or pulmonary congestion. Pneumonia, pneumothorax, and other primary lung disorders are diagnosed via CXR. It is also used to confirm the placement of central venous catheters, endotracheal tubes, and chest tubes.

Nursing Implications

Preparation for a CXR is minimal. A hospital gown typically replaces any clothing worn on the upper body, especially a bra. The patient is instructed to hold his or her breath for several seconds while the film is obtained, minimizing movement and improving the quality and sharpness of the x-ray.

Echocardiography

Echocardiography uses ultrasound to provide information on the size and pumping function of the heart, blood-volume status, and valve function and integrity. Two common types of echocardiography are the transthoracic echocardiogram (TTE) and the transesophageal echocardiogram (TEE). The standard TTE is performed by placing a transducer on the patient's chest. The ultrasound waves are converted to a picture, which can be evaluated.

A TEE is obtained by placing the ultrasound transducer in the patient's esophagus. This provides information from the posterior of the heart. It is used when complications such as obesity or lung disease may obscure the standard TTE by interfering with the transmission of the ultrasound sound waves anteriorly. It also provides valuable information about the posterior aspect of the heart such as the left atrium (Fig. 28.16). Additionally, information about the presence of clots in the atrium, a risk factor for stroke, is more easily viewed through TEE.

Nursing Implications

Patients require education about the purpose and potential findings associated with echocardiography. When scheduled for a TEE, patients are instructed not to eat or drink for at least 8 hours prior to the procedure. Small sips of water with medications are the exception. Patients are given sedation for the test, so they should be

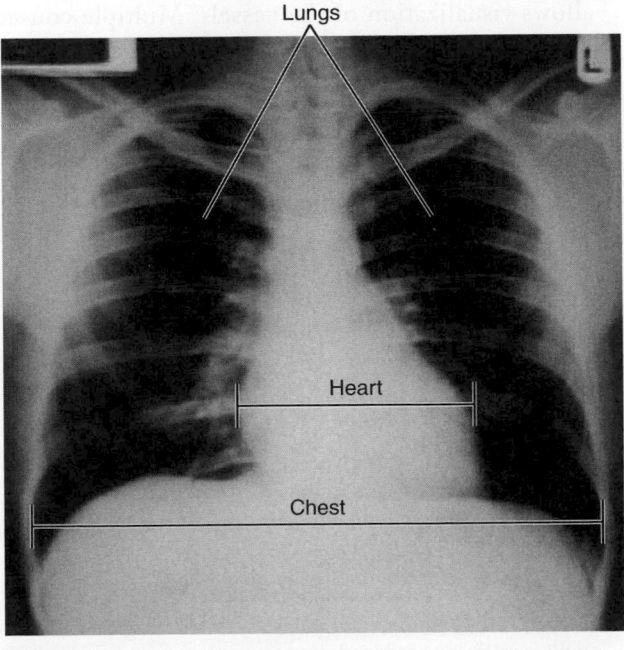

Normal heart

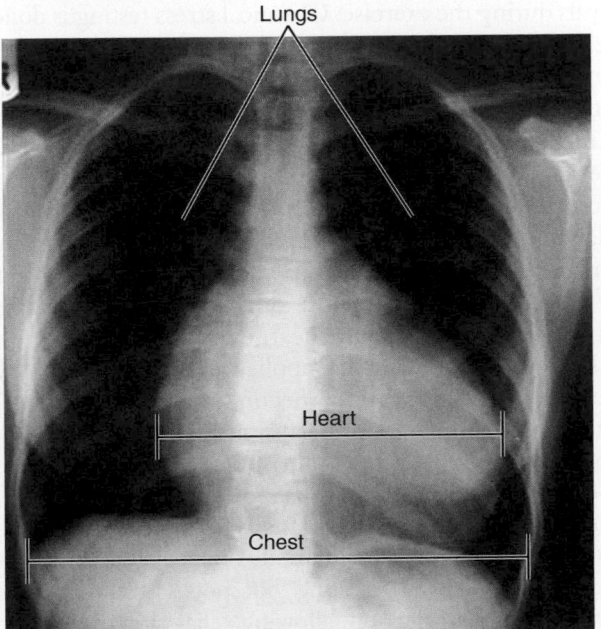

Enlarged heart

FIGURE 28.15 Chest x-ray (CXR) of normal heart and enlarged heart.

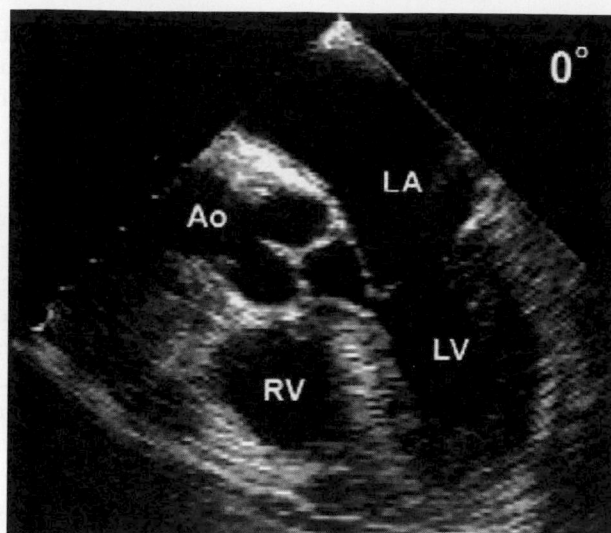

FIGURE 28.16 Transesophageal echocardiogram (TEE) demonstrating the chambers of the heart. *LA,* left atrium; *LV,* left ventricle; *RV,* right ventricle; *Ao,* aorta.

instructed to have someone with them who can drive them home.

Cardiac Stress Testing

A **cardiac stress test** is done to evaluate heart functioning during times of increased workload. It is a way to evaluate the functional ability of the heart. It is also a screening tool for symptoms of cardiovascular disease that may become apparent only when the heart is stressed. In that circumstance, symptoms such as chest pain, dizziness, dysrhythmias, or SOB may occur during the test.

Regular stress testing is typically done on a treadmill or stationary bike. The patient is attached to a monitoring system. Heart rate, rhythm, and BP are monitored at regular intervals during the exercise. Chemical stress testing is done if the patient is unable to exercise because of physical limitations. Cardiac stress is induced with IV administration of a medication such as dobutamine, a medication that stimulates the heart similar to exercise. The patient is monitored in the same fashion as the treadmill test.

Isotope or nuclear stress testing is a combination of a regular stress test and a chemical stress test. In this case, the chemical is an intravenously injected nuclear isotope tracer such as thallium. The purpose of this test is to visualize areas of poor perfusion in the heart due to blocked arteries. The isotope is more readily supplied to and picked up by tissues that have adequate perfusion, creating "hot spots" when imaged. Areas of poor perfusion get a lesser supply of the isotope, thus creating "cold spots." Imaging is done after exercise and at rest.

Another form of nuclear imaging is done with the isotope technetium. Opposite to thallium, this radioisotope becomes bound to damaged tissue, creating "hot spots." Imaging is done several hours after injection, allowing renal clearance of the medication not accumulated in the damaged cardiac tissue.

Nursing Implications

Patients are instructed to:

- Not eat or drink for 4 hours prior to the procedure to avoid any nausea that might be associated with heavy exercise
- Avoid smoking prior to the test
- Avoid caffeine prior to the test

During the procedure, the patient is closely monitored for the appearance of symptoms such as chest pain and/or dysrhythmias as noted previously. The nurse must be prepared to respond if patient decompensation occurs.

Catheterization and Angiography

Cardiac catheterization is an invasive x-ray procedure during which a radiopaque catheter is advanced through an artery or vein to the heart under fluoroscopy in order to evaluate cardiac filling pressures, CO, and valvular function. Both right and left heart studies can be conducted. A right heart catheterization can be done through a suitable vein (femoral, brachial, subclavian). The catheter is advanced to the right heart via the inferior or superior vena cava. A left heart catheterization is done through a suitable artery (femoral, brachial, radial). The catheter is advanced up through the aorta and into the left heart.

Coronary angiography is the primary reason cardiac catheterization is performed. It is a left-sided cardiac catheterization with the purpose of inspecting the coronary arteries for blockage and determining the necessity of revascularization procedures such as percutaneous coronary intervention or coronary bypass surgery. It is done through a technique called cineangiography. Once the catheter is in place, contrast dye is injected that allows visualization of the vessels. Multiple consecutive images (15 frames per second) are obtained, allowing visualization of the dye flowing through the specific arteries being studied, noting any areas of stenosis or blockage (Fig. 28.17).

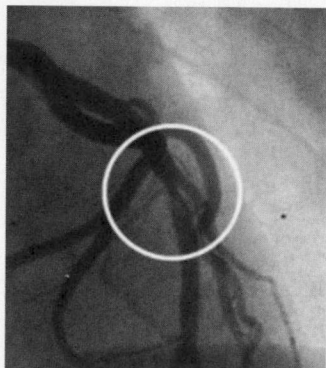

FIGURE 28.17 Coronary angiography. The circle indicates an area of stenosis in the left anterior descending coronary artery.

depolarization, and the T wave represents ventricular repolarization.

The blood ejected from the left heart is referred to as the *cardiac output (CO)*. The CO is calculated by the formula heart rate (HR) × stroke volume. Stroke volume is controlled by three variables: preload, afterload, and contractility. Cardiac output does not remain constant but is increased by exercise or activity as a result of an increase in the HR; it is decreased at times of rest.

The overall assessment of cardiovascular health includes the evaluation of many variables. The patient's history reveals modifiable and nonmodifiable risk factors, personal health history, and family history. Family history is an example of a nonmodifiable risk factor. When the patient is interviewed, current health problems are discussed as well as future goals. The physical examination of the patient will include a head-to-toe assessment and a laboratory assessment, which includes cardiac risk factors as well as a general laboratory evaluation. Laboratory tests specific for acute events such a myocardial infarction (CK-MB and troponin) are performed as necessary. An ECG is performed routinely at a physical examination. Other radiographical examinations, such as cardiac stress testing and echocardiograms, are performed as indicated by patient presentation. Cardiac angiography is indicated if coronary artery disease is suspected. Patient preparation prior to any examination includes patient teaching regarding the procedure, dietary restrictions and activity restrictions before and after procedures, and information about medications. During procedures that stress the heart, the nurse must be alert and ready to respond to any patient decompensation. Meticulous nursing care is necessary after cardiac catheterization to reduce strain and prevent bleeding from the cannula insertion site.

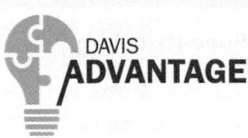

DAVIS
ADVANTAGE

To explore learning resources for this chapter, go to **Davis Advantage** and find:
- Answers to in-text questions
- Chapter Resources and Activities
- NCLEX®-Style Chapter Review Questions
- Bibliography

Chapter 29

Coordinating Care for Patients With Cardiac Dysrhythmia

Marida Twilley

LEARNING OUTCOMES

Content in this chapter is designed to assist in:

1. Defining the pathophysiology of rhythm disorders
2. Identifying a method to interpret electrocardiograms (ECGs)
3. Recognizing sinus, atrial, junctional, and ventricular dysrhythmias
4. Classifying first-, second-, and third-degree blocks
5. Explaining the types of pacing used in the treatment of certain dysrhythmias
6. Employing the appropriate intervention for each dysrhythmia reviewed
7. Differentiating the use of cardioversion from defibrillation
8. Analyzing the appropriate nursing interventions for patients with cardiac dysrhythmias
9. Designing an effective patient teaching plan for a patient experiencing atrial fibrillation

CONCEPTS

- Assessment
- Clotting
- Medication
- Perfusion

ESSENTIAL TERMS

Accelerated idioventricular rhythm (AIVR)
Agonal
Asystole
Atrial fibrillation (AF)
Atrial flutter (AFL)
Atrial tachycardia (AT)
Atrioventricular (AV) node
Complete heart block (CHB)
Dysrhythmia
First-degree AV block
Idioventricular rhythm (IVR)
Mobitz I
Mobitz II
Normal sinus rhythm (NSR)
Premature atrial contraction (PAC)
Premature junctional contraction (PJC)
Premature ventricular contraction (PVC)
Pulseless electrical activity (PEA)
Second-degree AV block type I
Second-degree AV block type II
Sinoatrial (SA) node
Sinus bradycardia (SB)
Sinus tachycardia (ST)
Supraventricular tachycardia (SVT)
Third-degree AV block
Ventricular fibrillation (VF)
Ventricular tachycardia (VT)
Wenckebach

Finding Connections

CASE STUDY: EPISODE 1

Follow this patient throughout the chapter.

Ms. Danielle Fletcher is a 68-year-old female who presents to the emergency department (ED) with complaints of acute lightheadedness and palpitations. She reports that she is becoming progressively more dyspneic (short of breath). Her medical history includes hypertension (HTN) and type 2 diabetes that is diet controlled. Ms. Fletcher is currently taking hydrochlorothiazide 12.5 mg daily and lisinopril 20 mg daily. On admission to the ED, Ms. Fletcher is triaged quickly to obtain baseline vital signs, such as blood pressure, heart rate (HR), respirations, and temperature, and a 12-lead electrocardiogram (ECG). A thorough history is obtained to determine onset and triggers of symptoms for this event. Ms. Fletcher's ECG reveals atrial fibrillation (AF)…

INTRODUCTION

An electrical conduction system with specialized muscle cells is necessary for the cardiac action potential that generates a heartbeat and thus cardiac output (CO). There is a designated pathway that the heart's normal electrical conduction travels. This pathway begins with the **sinoatrial (SA) node**, the heart's primary pacemaker, which can generate impulses at a rate of 60 to 100 beats per minute (bpm). The SA node is located in the upper wall of the right atrium near the superior vena cava. Once the SA node fires, the impulse travels through the atrial pathways and heads toward the **atrioventricular (AV) node**. This node can also be considered the gatekeeper of the heart's electrical conduction system. The AV node is responsible for allowing impulses to travel between the atria and the ventricles. Also, if for some reason the SA node fails to fire, the AV node can generate impulses at a rate of 40 to 60 bpm. Once the impulse has passed through the AV node into the ventricles, the impulse travels quickly through the ventricular pathways; the bundle branches and Purkinje fibers. Again, if the SA and AV nodes fail to

generate an impulse to stimulate the ventricles, then the ventricular pacer cells can generate impulses at a rate of 40 bpm or less. In a worst-case scenario, the Purkinje fibers can generate a ventricular rate of 20 bpm or less. The electrical conduction system is one of two components of the generation of heartbeat and cardiac output. The other component is the actual muscular contraction (squeeze). The electrical conduction system will stimulate the heart's muscle so that the chambers can contract/squeeze to force blood out of the heart. A fully functioning heart requires electrical conduction and mechanical contraction to produce CO.

When the impulse travels along the normal conduction pathway generated by the SA, it is called **normal sinus rhythm (NSR)**. It generates waveforms that indicate the firing of the SA node, the *P wave*, followed by a *QRS* complex indicating ventricular depolarization, and a *T wave*, indicating ventricular repolarization, all within the correct timing intervals (Fig. 29.1). These waveforms and intervals are discussed in detail later.

> ⓘ **Safety Alert**   **Pulseless Electrical Activity**
>
> There are occasions when the electrical conduction system is functional, but the heart muscle is not responding with a contraction. This is called **pulseless electrical activity (PEA)**. If not treated quickly, the electrical conduction system will eventually stop working because of the lack of oxygen to the heart's pacemaker cells. Causes of this in patients include hypoxia (lack of oxygen), hypovolemia (low blood/fluid volume in the circulatory system), hyper- or hypokalemia (high or low blood potassium levels), acidosis (excessive acid in the body), hypoglycemia (low blood glucose level), hypothermia (low body temperature), medication toxicities (overdose), pericardial tamponade (excessive blood/fluid around the heart), pneumothorax (collapsed lung), myocardial infarction, and pulmonary embolism (blood clot in the lung), to name just a few. The treatment for PEA is chest compressions, epinephrine, and treating the possible causes. With this in mind, it should not be assumed that a patient will have a pulse because you see a rhythm on a cardiac/heart monitor; make sure that you palpate for a pulse to confirm that the heart is pumping and circulating blood.

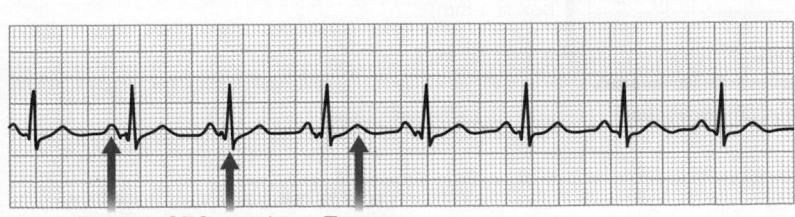

P wave   QRS complex   T wave

FIGURE 29.1 Normal sinus rhythm (NSR) with a P wave, QRS complex, and T wave.

EPIDEMIOLOGY

When there is a disruption in the electrical conduction system, an irregular rhythm or dysrhythmias can occur. Age is a primary risk factor for dysrhythmias. Older adults have fewer pacemaker cells in the SA node, and there may be fat deposits around SA node, causing a delay in the propagation of the action potential. Also, slowed impulse transmission may be related to calcification around the AV node and valves. Other risk factors that can put a patient at higher risk for developing a dysrhythmia include:

- Myocardial infarction (MI)
- Hypertension (HTN)
- Heart valve disease
- Heart failure (HF)
- Cardiomyopathy (CM)
- Infections
- Diabetes mellitus
- Sleep apnea
- Heart surgery (and procedures)
- Electrolyte disturbances
- Recreational drug use such as cocaine, alcohol, or tobacco
- Medication toxicities such as digoxin toxicity

PATHOPHYSIOLOGY

Dysrhythmias are disruptions in the cardiac conduction pathway or disorders of the electrical impulse conduction within the heart. They can result in deviations from a normal HR and/or rhythm, causing decreases in cardiac output (CO). Some dysrhythmias are lethal, causing a complete loss of CO, which results in cardiopulmonary arrest. Other dysrhythmias are apparent on ECGs but are symptomless. In between are symptomatic dysrhythmias that may require treatment. Symptoms of cardiac instability include:

- Palpitations (fast fluttering or beating in the chest or skipping beats)
- Hypotension
- Diaphoresis (sweating)
- Shortness of breath (SOB)
- Syncope (fainting)

- Lightheadedness
- Weakness and fatigue
- Dizziness
- Anxiety

Connection Check 29.1

As the nurse, you know that the following can cause rhythm disorders: *(Select all that apply.)*

A. Exercise
B. Electrolyte imbalances
C. Myocardial hypertrophy
D. Myocardial damage
E. Eating red meat

ECG REVIEW

Electrocardiogram

An ECG provides a graphic representation of the heart's electrical activity. When electrodes are placed on the patient's skin, they can monitor the flow of the electrical charges and transmit the corresponding waveforms to an ECG machine or cardiac monitor. The standard ECG has 12 leads or views of the electrical activity in the heart. Each lead has a negative and positive electrode or pole. The electrical impulse is measured as it moves between two poles or points. When the electrical impulse is moving toward a positive pole, the waveforms will be upright on the ECG. If the electrical impulse is moving away from the positive pole, it will produce a downward or negative deflection on the ECG. Waveforms vary in shape and size depending on which lead the monitor is set to read. The best lead to identify or interpret the heart's rhythm is lead II. Lead II mimics the heart's natural electrical direction in a healthy, normally positioned heart.

ECG Paper

When a patient receives an ECG or is placed on a cardiac monitor, the heart's electrical activity will be printed on specialized graph paper for interpretation. The ECG graph paper can measure both amplitude and time (Fig. 29.2).

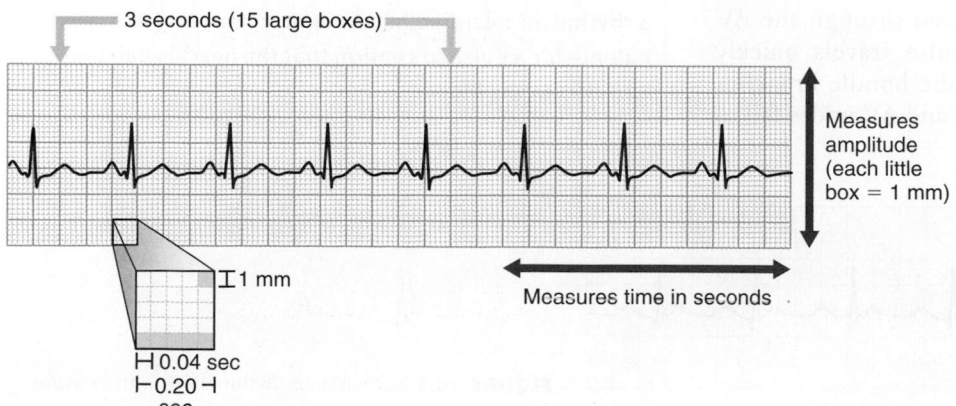

FIGURE 29.2 Electrocardiogram graph paper measures both amplitude and time.

The amplitude is measured on the vertical axis in millimeters (mm), whereas time is measured in seconds (sec) along the horizontal axis. The standard paper speed for ECGs is 25 mm per second. The graph paper is segmented into small and large boxes. Each small box is 1 mm in height (amplitude) and 0.04 sec in length. When looking at the graph paper, you will notice that there are darker lines that create a larger box. The larger boxes are divided into areas five small boxes high and five small boxes long. One large box equals 0.20 sec long (0.04 sec × five small boxes = 0.20 sec). This creates a quick reference when measuring the time intervals of the various waveforms discussed next.

Waveforms

The normal conduction pathway produces waveforms on an ECG that show the current as it travels across the heart tissue (Fig. 29.3). They are listed as follows in the order they normally appear on the ECG:

1. P wave
2. QRS complex
3. T wave
4. U wave

The *P wave* is the first waveform that is normally seen (Fig. 29.4). The P wave represents the SA node sending out an electrical impulse and represents atrial depolarization. This wave should be upright (positive deflection) with a rounded top in lead II. The P wave itself should not be longer than 0.10 sec in length and no higher than 2.5 mm.

The *QRS wave* (or *QRS complex*) is the next waveform that is normally seen (Fig. 29.5A). This complex represents ventricular depolarization. The ventricles depolarize from the endocardial layer (inside of the heart) to the epicardial layer (outermost layer of the heart). The QRS complex can take on many different forms (Fig. 29.5B). Normal QRS

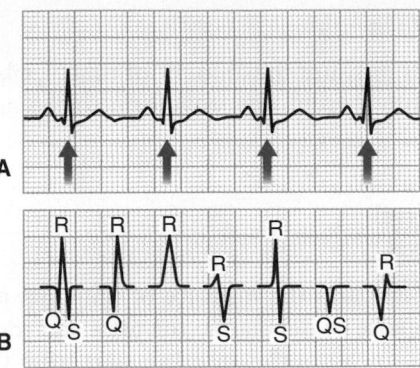

FIGURE 29.5 *A,* The QRS wave (or QRS complex): ventricular depolarization. *B,* The QRS complex can take many different forms.

complexes are usually pointy and skinny in width. As a rule of thumb, a wide QRS (greater than 0.10 sec or two and a half small boxes wide) means that there is something occurring in the ventricles causing the QRS to widen. For example, it may indicate that the impulse originated in the ventricles or that there is a block in the ventricles delaying the impulse from traveling through the ventricles to allow for a normal depolarization.

The *T wave* occurs after the QRS and represents ventricular repolarization (Fig. 29.6). This wave should be upright and rounded in lead II. Even though the T wave is not used for rhythm interpretation, it can be helpful in monitoring extreme electrolyte imbalances such as hypokalemia or hyperkalemia, disturbances with the myocardial oxygen supply, or other cardiac disorders such as pericarditis or ventricular aneurysm. There is no visible waveform that represents atrial repolarization. That is typically "buried" in the QRS complex.

The *U wave* represents Purkinje fiber repolarization and is rarely seen (Fig. 29.7). However, this waveform can be seen in patients with certain medication toxicities (e.g., digoxin toxicity) and electrolyte imbalances (e.g., hypokalemia). When a U wave is seen, it should be a small rounded wave in lead II. Be careful not to confuse it with the P wave.

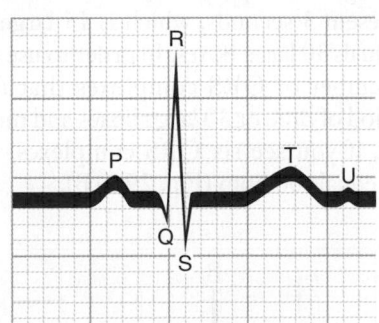

FIGURE 29.3 Waveforms seen on an electrocardiogram (ECG) that show the heart's electrical current as it travels.

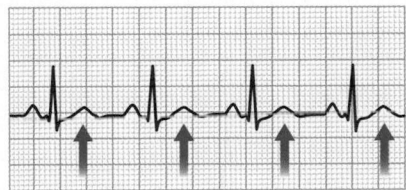

FIGURE 29.6 The T wave: ventricular repolarization.

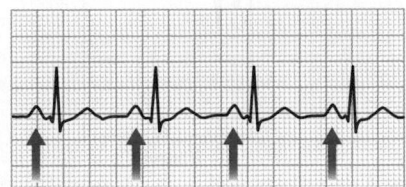

FIGURE 29.4 The P wave: atrial depolarization.

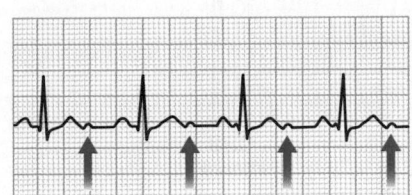

FIGURE 29.7 The U wave: Purkinje fiber repolarization.

Intervals

The intervals measure the amount of time it takes for the impulse to travel from one waveform to the next. They are the:

- PR interval
- QRS interval
- QT interval

The *PR interval* is the measure of time that it takes an electrical impulse to depolarize the atria and travel to the ventricles. To measure this interval, start from the beginning of the P wave (where it starts to leave the baseline) and count the number of small boxes to the beginning of the QRS complex (not the R wave; Fig. 29.8). The normal PR interval is from 0.12 sec (three small boxes) to 0.20 sec (five small boxes) in length.

The *QRS interval* is the measure of time to depolarize the ventricles. It is measured from where the QRS waveform leaves the baseline to where the QRS returns to the baseline (Fig. 29.9). The normal interval is 0.06 to 0.10 sec in length. As discussed previously, if the QRS is prolonged (more than 0.10 sec; equal to or more than three small boxes), it may be a sign of a disturbance within the ventricle itself (i.e., that the impulse originated in the ventricles or that there is a block in the ventricles delaying impulse travel time through the ventricles).

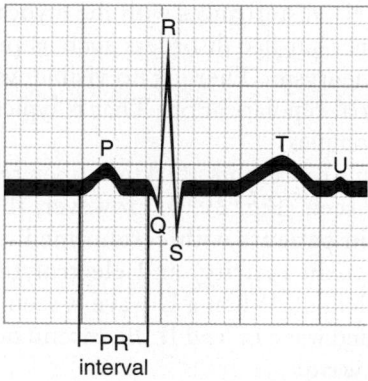

FIGURE 29.8 The PR interval: measure of time to depolarize the atria and travel to the ventricles.

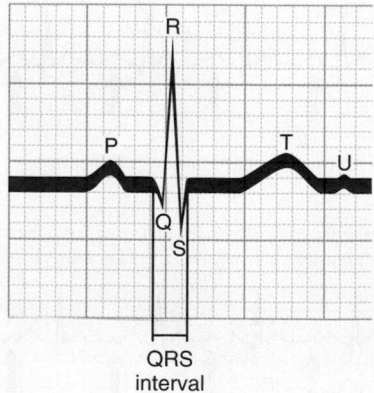

FIGURE 29.9 The QRS interval: the measure of time to depolarize the ventricles.

The *QT interval* is the measure of time that it takes the ventricle to depolarize and then repolarize. To measure a QT interval, start where the QRS leaves baseline and measure to where the T wave returns to baseline (Fig. 29.10). This interval is heart-rate dependent and should never be more than half the distance from one QRS to the next. A normal QT is usually less than or equal to 0.52 sec in length.

Steps in ECG Interpretation

When evaluating a cardiac rhythm, ask the following questions to help identify the rhythm seen on the ECG:

- Is the rate fast, slow, or normal?
- Is the rhythm regular; are complexes an equal distance from one to the next?
  - Are the distances from P wave to P wave equal throughout the strip? This is referred to as the *P–P interval.*
  - Are the distances from QRS wave to QRS wave equal throughout the strip? This is referred to as the *R–R interval.*
- Are there P waves present?
- Are there QRS complexes present?
- Are there T waves present?
- Are the intervals within normal limits (e.g., PR interval, QRS interval)?
- Is there a P wave before every QRS?
- Is there a QRS after every P wave?

Calculating Heart Rate

Establishing the heart rate (HR) is the first step in ECG evaluation. A *6-second strip* is a quick way to calculate an average HR, but it is not completely reliable if the rhythm is irregular. Electrocardiograph or monitor paper will print time markers, which may be vertical lines or arrows on the top or bottom of the strip (Fig. 29.11A). Most ECG/monitor paper time markers represent 3 seconds, which is 15 large boxes long; six seconds equals 30 large boxes. In order to use this method, count the number of QRS complexes that fall within a 6-second period of time or 30 large boxes and multiply by 10. For example, if you see six QRS complexes, multiply six by 10, which equals 60 bpm (Fig. 29.11B).

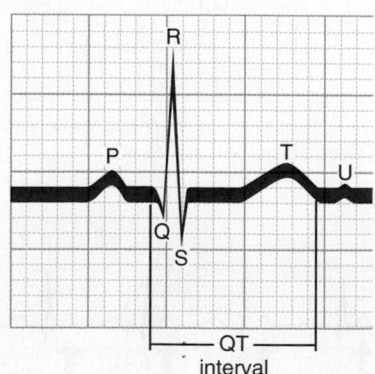

FIGURE 29.10 The QT interval: the measure of time that it takes the ventricle to depolarize and then repolarize.

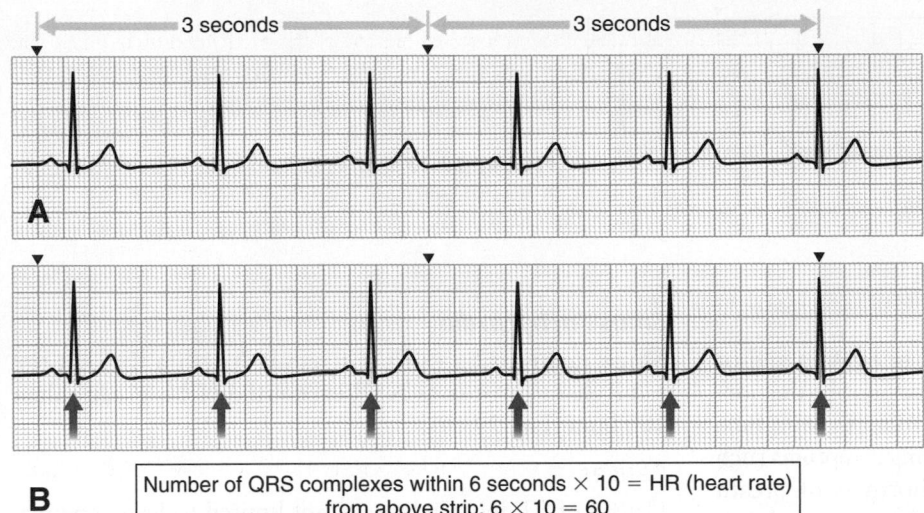

FIGURE 29.11 *A,* A 6-second strip. *B,* Calculating a heart rate using a 6-second strip.

Another method to calculate HR is to count the number of **small** boxes between two R waves and divide that number into 1,500. As an example, if there are 19 small boxes between two R waves, the calculation is 1,500/19 = HR of 79. One last method is to count the number of **large** boxes between two R waves and divide that number into 300; for example, for five large boxes, the calculation is 300/5 = HR of 60.

Calculating Regularity

An important step in evaluating an ECG is determining regularity. Regularity can be determined by counting the boxes between the waveforms being measured, such as P wave to P wave (P to P) or QRS complex to QRS complex (R to R). A regular rhythm will have the same number of boxes or equal space between waveforms or complexes (Fig. 29.12A). This is also called *marching out* the rhythm. *Marching out* the waveforms can help demonstrate if waves are falling early or late or are even hiding within another waveform. If the spaces are not equal, then it is considered irregular (Fig. 29.12B).

Connection Check 29.2

As the nurse caring for a patient on a cardiac monitor, you understand that which of the following steps are necessary to correctly identify the rhythm? *(Select all that apply.)*

A. Determine the rate
B. Determine the regularity
C. Determine if there is a QRS for every P wave
D. Determine if there is a P wave for every QRS
E. Determine if there is a U wave for every QRS

CARDIAC DYSRHYTHMIAS

Sinus Dysrhythmias

Sinus Bradycardia

Sinus bradycardia (SB) is a regular rhythm that has the same characteristics as NSR except the HR is less than 60 bpm (Fig. 29.13).

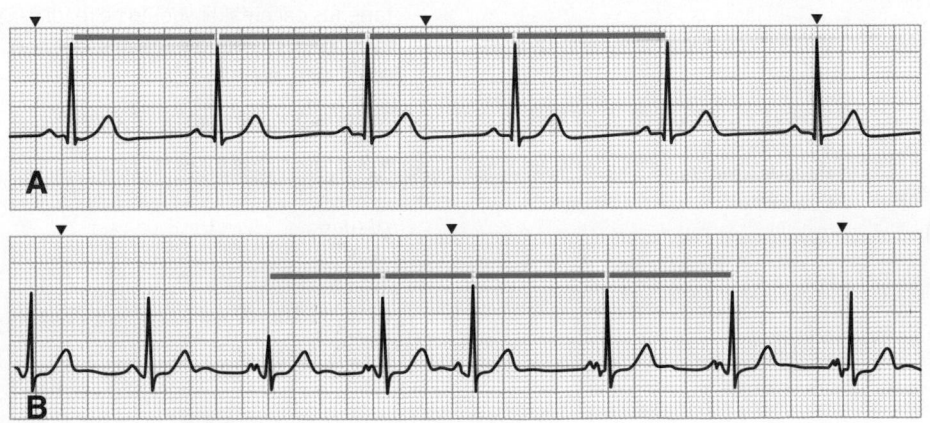

FIGURE 29.12 Marching out the waveforms. *A,* Example of a regular rhythm; equal distance R to R. *B,* Example of an irregular rhythm. Notice the difference in distance between R waves.

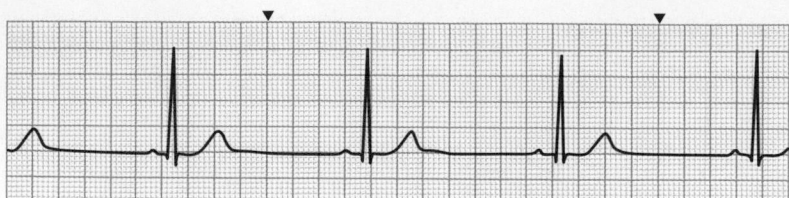

FIGURE 29.13 Sinus bradycardia (SB): sinus rhythm with a rate less than 60; in this strip, the rate is 40.

Causes

Causes of SB include but are not limited to hypoxia and/or hypothermia. It can occur during sleep, or it may be the normal rate in well-trained athletes. It is important to determine if the patient is symptomatic or experiencing symptoms such as syncope, chest pain, hypotension, shortness of breath (SOB), or diaphoresis while bradycardic. A symptomatic patient will require treatment. It may be normal in a nonsymptomatic patient, or that patient may just require observation.

Treatment

Treatment of symptomatic SB is atropine 0.5 mg IV push (IVP) (see Table 29.1).

Sinus Tachycardia

Sinus tachycardia (ST) is a regular rhythm that has the same characteristics as NSR except the HR is greater than 100 bpm (Fig. 29.14).

Causes

Causes of ST include but are not limited to fever, anemia, hypovolemia, hypotension, pulmonary embolism (PE), and myocardial infarction (MI).

Treatment

The treatment for ST is based on patient symptoms and possible causes. For example, if the patient is anemic and volume depleted, the treatment may be as simple as

Table 29.1 Overview of Medications for Cardiac Dysrhythmias

Medication Class	Medication Name(s)	Action	Indicated Rhythm	Special Considerations
Diagnostic/ Antiarrhythmic	Adenosine (Adenocard)	Slows down the heart rate temporarily to allow for better visualization of the rhythm	SVT	Dosing is rapid IV push of 6 mg followed by a 20-mL normal saline bolus; may repeat in 1–2 min with a dose of 12 mg followed by the normal saline bolus.
				If the patient has central venous access, the dose can be halved (e.g., 3 mg followed by 6 mg).
				Maximum dose: no more than two doses
				May result in asystole—The patient should be monitored, and a transcutaneous pacemaker should be readily available if the patient remains in prolonged asystole.
Antiarrhythmic	Amiodarone (Cordarone, Pacerone) Dronedarone (Multaq) Dofetilide (Tikosyn)	Slows the cardiac action potential, thus slowing the heart rate	VT VF AF	Amiodarone (Cordarone, Pacerone): ● IV preparation for continuous infusion must be in a glass bottle. Monitor: ● Pulmonary function test ● Thyroid function ● Liver function

Table 29.1 Overview of Medications for Cardiac Dysrhythmias—cont'd

Medication Class	Medication Name(s)	Action	Indicated Rhythm	Special Considerations
Anticholinergic	Atropine sulfate	Increases SA node stimulus and increases conduction through the AV node	Sinus bradycardia	Use cautiously with MI patients
Anticoagulant	Warfarin (Coumadin) Dabigatran (Pradaxa) Rivaroxaban (Xarelto) Apixaban (Eliquis) Edoxaban (Savaysa) Heparin	Inhibits clot formation	AF AFL	Monitor signs and symptoms of bleeding. Warfarin: ● Monitor INR or PT. Dabigatran, rivaroxaban, apixaban, and edoxaban: ● Monitor renal function. Heparin ● Monitor aPTT. ● Monitor platelets.
Beta blocker	Atenolol (Tenormin) Metoprolol (Lopressor) Carvedilol (Coreg) Sotalol (Betapace)	Negative chronotropic effects to help slow down the heart rate; decreases cardiac workload and oxygen demand	ST AF with RVR	Use cautiously in patients with: ● Heart failure ● Asthma Carvedilol is used in patients with heart failure for rate and rhythm control. Sotalol is used in AF rate and rhythm control.
Calcium channel blocker	Diltiazem (Cardizem)	Slows conduction through the AV node	AF AFL	Use cautiously in patients with heart failure.
Cardiac glycoside	Digoxin (Lanoxin)	Slows conduction through the AV node; improves cardiac contractility	ST AF AFL	Monitor: ● Digoxin levels ● Renal function Use cautiously in combination with amiodarone (Cordarone, Pacerone).
Vasopressor	Epinephrine	Produces vasoconstriction	VT VF	Ensure free-flowing IV. Use in combination with CPR.

AF, Atrial fibrillation; *AFL,* atrial flutter; *AV,* atrioventricular; *CPR,* cardiopulmonary resuscitation; *IV,* intravenous; *RVR,* rapid ventricular response; *SA,* sinoatrial node, *ST,* sinus tachycardia; *SVT,* supraventricular tachycardia; *VF,* ventricular fibrillation; *VT,* ventricular tachycardia.

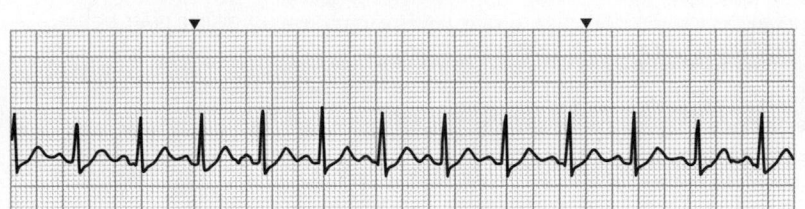

FIGURE 29.14 Sinus tachycardia (ST): sinus rhythm with a rate greater than 100; in this strip, the rate is 130.

administering red blood cells and IV fluids. Medications such as beta blockers or calcium channel blockers may be used to control or reduce the HR.

See Table 29.2 for a summary of sinus dysrhythmias.

Atrial Dysrhythmias

Atrial dysrhythmias are caused by pacemaker cells firing not from the SA node but from somewhere else within the atria. They include premature atrial contractions (PACs), atrial fibrillation (AF), and atrial flutter (AFL). Supraventricular dysrhythmias also arise from the atria with the exception of junctional tachycardias.

Premature Atrial Contractions

Premature atrial contractions (PACs) are non–life-threatening dysrhythmias that can be seen in NSR. In this dysrhythmia, a pacemaker cell close to the SA node fires earlier than expected (Fig. 29.15). This is an irregular rhythm due to the early impulse or beat. The PAC has a pause at the end of the complex called a *compensatory pause* allowing the conduction system to reset and resume the regular rhythm.

Causes

Causes of PAC include hypoxia, excessive stimulant ingestion (e.g., caffeine), infections, digoxin toxicity, and coronary artery disease.

Table 29.2 Summary of Sinus Dysrhythmias

Dysrhythmia	Signs and Symptoms	Medical Interventions	Nursing Interventions	Patient Teaching
Sinus bradycardia, asymptomatic	None	Assess and treat the causes as necessary: • Hypoxia • Ischemia • Electrolyte imbalance • Medication toxicities such as digoxin or calcium-channel-blocker overdose	*All asymptomatic sinus dysrhythmias:* Notify provider. Assess the patient for: • LOC • Palpable pulses • BP Obtain a 12-lead ECG.	*All asymptomatic sinus dysrhythmias:* Educate patient/family about signs and symptoms that can occur. Discuss signs and symptoms that warrant the patient or family contacting the primary care provider or healthcare provider or calling 911 for emergency help.
Sinus tachycardia, asymptomatic	None	Depends on the rate and cause of ST HR less than 150 bpm: Observe patient for possible signs of decompensation. Treat the causes: • Infection • Fever • Hypovolemia • Hypoxia • Ischemia • Electrolyte imbalance • Stimulants HR greater than 150 bpm (the patient can decompensate quickly): consider beta blockers to slow down the HR.		

Table 29.2 Summary of Sinus Dysrhythmias—cont'd

Dysrhythmia	Signs and Symptoms	Medical Interventions	Nursing Interventions	Patient Teaching

Sinus bradycardia, symptomatic	• Hypotension
	• Dizziness
	• Lightheadedness
	• Fainting
	• SOB
	• Sweating
	• Anxiety
		• Oxygen
		• Atropine IVP
		• Pacing
		
		Treat the causes:
		• Hypoxia
		• Ischemia
		• Electrolyte imbalance
		• Medication toxicities
			All symptomatic sinus dysrhythmias:
			
			Give oxygen per order.
			
			Assess the patient (initially and more frequently, e.g., every 5 min) for:
			• LOC
			• Palpable pulses
			• BP and HR
			
			Contact the authorized prescriber or medical emergency team.
			
			Obtain a 12-lead ECG.
			
			Ensure IV access is available and patent.
			
			Administer medication(s) as ordered.
			
			Prepare for transcutaneous pacing/cardioversion (if ordered).
			
			• Place defibrillator/pacing pads in an anterior/posterior (front/back) approach (see Fig. 29.30B).
			• Anticipate administration of a sedative such as midazolam (Versed) prior to the procedure if the patient has a stable BP.
			
			Stay with the patient (do not leave patient alone until he or she stabilizes or care is transferred to another healthcare provider).
				All symptomatic sinus dysrhythmias:
				
				Real-time education on problem at hand and treatment:
				• Medications: atropine
				• Intervention:
				  • 12-lead ECG
				  • Pacing
				
				After the patient stabilizes, a basic debriefing session should occur with the patient and/or family member(s) to allow them to ask questions that could not be asked during the emergency; this should help the patient/family to better understand what to do if this happens again.

Sinus tachycardia, symptomatic	• Hypotension • Dizziness • Lightheadedness • Fainting • SOB • Sweating • Anxiety • Palpitations	• Vagal maneuvers such as carotid massage • Beta blockers Treat the causes: • Hypoxia • Ischemia • Electrolyte imbalance • Medication toxicities • Stimulants		

BP, Blood pressure; *ECG,* electrocardiogram; *HR,* heart rate; *IVP,* intravenous push; *LOC,* level of consciousness; *SOB,* shortness of breath; *ST,* sinus tachycardia.

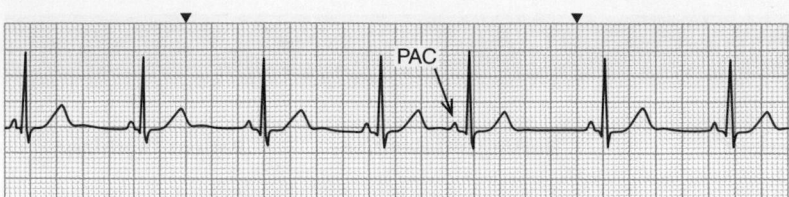

FIGURE 29.15 Premature atrial contractions (PACs); notice how the PAC occurs early or prematurely compared with the four previous complexes.

Treatment

The treatment for PACs is to monitor the frequency and eliminate the cause. This is especially important if the patient is symptomatic. If the patient gets PACs after drinking a pot of coffee in the morning, the "treatment" will be to eliminate or limit the coffee intake. This will help decrease the stimulus to the SA node and hopefully resolve the PACs.

Atrial Fibrillation

Atrial fibrillation (AF) is one of the most commonly seen dysrhythmias in the United States. The National Institutes of Health estimates that 2.2 million Americans are diagnosed with this dysrhythmia, and the American Heart Association (AHA) estimates that upward of 6.1 million Americans have been affected by AF, which often leads to other heart-related complications as well as increased risk of stroke. It accounts for roughly one-third of all hospital admissions due to dysrhythmias. The general classifications of AF are as follows: paroxysmal or spontaneously self-limiting, persistent or continuing beyond 7 days, long-standing or lasting more than 12 months, and permanent or persistent AF that is resistant to rhythm control therapies.

Atrial fibrillation has no *P waves*. It is best described as multiple pacemaker cells generating independent electrical impulses and causing chaos within the atria (see Figs. 29.16A, B, and C). It is characterized as irregularly irregular. The QRS complexes are usually narrow with irregular R–R intervals. Although the naked eye cannot measure an atrial rate in this rhythm, it can range from 300 to 600 bpm. The HR or ventricular response is determined by the AV node's ability to accept and transmit the impulses to the ventricle. When the AV node maintains the HR at less than 100 bpm, the AF is considered controlled (Fig. 29.16A). If the HR is greater than 100, the AF is considered uncontrolled and is called AF with rapid ventricular response (RVR; Fig. 29.16B).

Causes

The risk for AF increases with age. Causes include but are not limited to cardiomyopathy, pericarditis, hyperthyroidism, HTN, valvular disease, obesity, diabetes, chronic kidney disease, patients undergoing cardiac procedures or surgery, and coronary artery disease.

Complications

Loss of Cardiac Output

Because the atrial pacemaker cells are firing and competing against one another at such a rapid rate, the atria can only quiver instead of beating or contracting/squeezing normally. Without a normal atrial contraction, the heart can lose approximately 30% of its CO. This is referred to as *loss of atrial kick*, the filling force contributed by atrial contraction immediately before ventricular systole to maximize ventricular preload. This decrease in CO can cause significant symptoms for some patients, such as syncope, palpitations, and SOB.

Clots

Because the atria are not squeezing or contracting efficiently, blood pools in the atria, which can predispose the patient to clot formation. Blood clots moving through the circulation put the patient at risk for embolic events such as strokes. Care

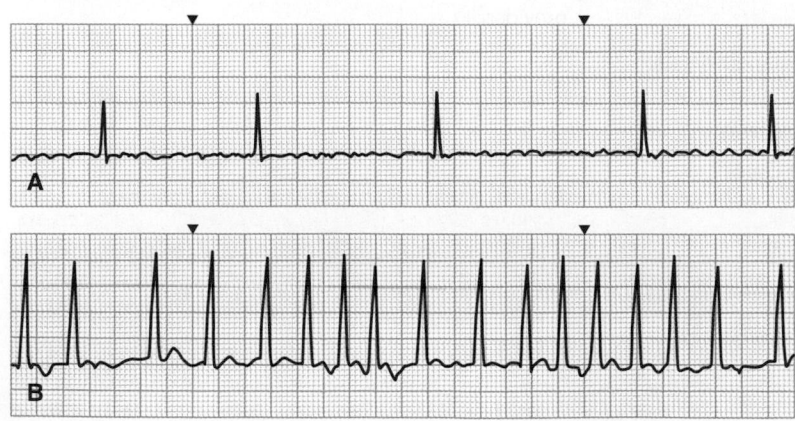

FIGURE 29.16 Atrial fibrillation (AF). *A,* Controlled AF with a ventricular rate of 50. *B,* Uncontrolled AF with rapid ventricular response (RVR).

should be taken when administering any treatments that could convert AF to NSR because of the increased risk of an embolus (blood clot) being forced out into the circulatory system.

Treatment

The treatment plan for AF is, in general, based on whether it is new onset or an established diagnosis in a patient. Other factors include ventricular response or HR and patient clinical manifestations. Anticoagulation should be considered in all patients with AF to prevent clot formation (see Table 29.1). Initial rate control is typically necessary in new-onset AF. Medications to control the HR, such as digoxin, beta blockers, and calcium channel blockers, are considered. Once the heart rate is managed, rhythm control is considered either through antiarrhythmic medications, cardiac ablation (scarring/destroying the tissue in the heart responsible for the irregular rhythm), or cardioversion. Typically, cardioversion (Table 29.3) is considered for AF after adequate anticoagulation is attained. Sometimes the atrium is evaluated for the presence of clots by transesophageal echocardiogram (TEE) prior to the procedure because it is not recommended if clots are present due to the risk of embolic events. If the patient is symptomatic (e.g., hypotensive, short of breath, having pain), urgent cardioversion may be required before adequate anticoagulation is attained. In that case, the patient should receive intravenous heparin as soon as possible with a loading dose before the procedure. Once initial stabilization has been attained or with established AF care, further treatment considerations include deciding on long-term rhythm or rate control, again with digoxin, beta blockers, and calcium channel blockers or antiarrhythmic medications (see Evidence-Based Practice).

Evidence-Based Practice

Follow Up From the AFFIRM Trial

In 2011, the AFFIRM trial, which investigated the mortality and morbidity of patients with AF and the relationship to rate and rhythm control, was published. The trial enrolled 4,060 patients with AF, with ages ranging from 46 to 80 years (mean age, 65 years).

The results showed the following:

- Increased mortality rates were associated with myocardial infarctions, coronary artery bypass graft, and digoxin therapy.
- Amiodarone was associated with increased intensive care unit stays and death.
- Rhythm control (converting the AF to sinus rhythm) and rate control in conjunction with anticoagulation therapy were equally effective in preventing strokes.

A follow-up study published in 2017 found that many patients turned to "crossover" treatment strategies to manage their symptoms. Of the study participants, 29% switched to rate from rhythm control, largely due to a failure to maintain rhythm control (45%) or intolerable side effects (20%). In addition, 12% switched to rhythm from rate control for similar reasons—failure to control the symptoms of AF (64%) and, again, intolerable side effects (3.6%). An interesting finding is that there was a significant difference in mortality in the subgroup of patients who switched to rate control compared with those who did not switch and maintained rhythm control. There was not a significant difference in the other subgroup, switch from rate to rhythm control, compared with the group that maintained rate control.

Maan, A., Zhang, Z., Qin, Z., Wang, Y., Dudley, S., Dabhadakar, K., … Heist, E. K. (2017). Impact of treatment crossovers on clinical outcomes in the rate and rhythm control strategies for atrial fibrillation: Insights from the AFFIRM (Atrial Fibrillation Follow_Up Investigation of Rhythm Management) trial. *Pacing and Clinical Electrophysiology, 40*(7), 770-778.

CASE STUDY: EPISODE 2

The patient history reveals that Ms. Fletcher has not been feeling well for several days. Her symptoms are related to a decrease in CO resulting from AF. She is seeking treatment in the ED because she became more short of breath and dizzy this morning. Anticoagulation therapy is indicated initially to prevent thrombus formation. She is placed on a heparin drip. Laboratory clotting studies are performed to evaluate the effectiveness of the heparin drip. She is placed on bleeding and fall precautions. Ms. Fletcher is given patient education on the risk of increased bleeding caused by the anticoagulation medication…

Atrial Flutter

Atrial flutter (AFL) is a dysrhythmia produced by a pacemaker cell other than the SA node. Because the SA node is not the primary pacemaker in this rhythm, there are no P waves. Flutter waves *(F waves)*, however, are present. F waves resemble a sawtooth pattern between narrow QRS complexes (Fig. 29.17). The atrial rate can range from 250 to 350 bpm. The number of F waves to a QRS complex can vary depending on the AV node's ability to accept and transmit impulses through to the ventricles which could produce a normal HR (60–100 bpm) or have an RVR response

Table 29.3 Summary of Cardioversion and Defibrillation

	Cardioversion	Defibrillation
Definition	Controlled electrical discharge of energy at the peak of the R wave	Uncontrolled electrical discharge of energy anywhere during the cardiac cycle
Indications	Symptomatic tachy dysrhythmias *with a pulse*: • Supraventricular (SVT) rhythms • AF with RVR (with caution) • AFL with RVR • VT with a pulse	Tachy dysrhythmias *without a pulse*: • VT • VF
Pad placement	Anterior/posterior (sometimes called *sandwiching the patient*; see Fig. 29.30B)	Anterior position (apex/sternum) used most often because of ease of application, but anterior/posterior approved (see Fig. 29.30A)
Energy level (joules; J)	SVT and AFL start between 50 and 100 J, then slowly increase to 200 J. AF starts between 120 and 200 J, then increases until maximum energy of 200 J. VT with a pulse starts at 120–200 J.	VT/VF = 200 J

AF, Atrial fibrillation; *AFL,* atrial flutter; *RVR,* rapid ventricular response; *SVT,* supraventricular tachycardia; *VF,* ventricular fibrillation; *VT,* ventricular tachycardia.
Based on American Heart Association (AHA) Advanced Cardiac Life Support (ACLS) guidelines: ACLS 2015 guidelines using biphasic defibrillator.

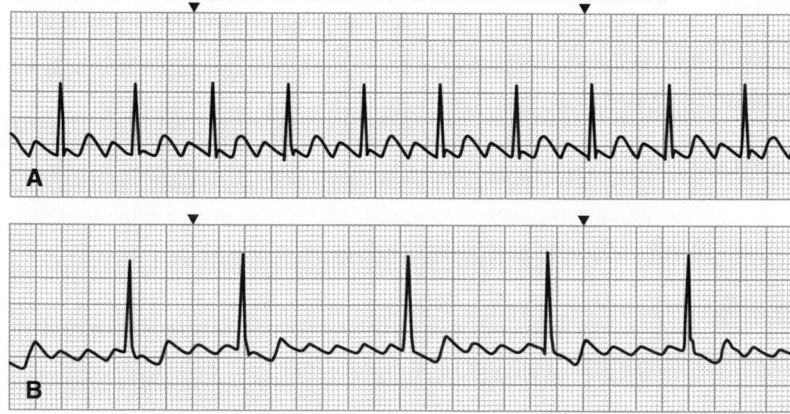

FIGURE 29.17 F waves. *A,* Atrial flutter (AFL; 2-to-1 conduction rate). *B,* AFL with a variable conduction rate.

(HR >150 bpm). Like AF, AFL can be a chronic or short-term dysrhythmia.

Causes

Causes of AFL in adult patients include acute MI, severe mitral valve disease, thyrotoxicosis (high thyroid hormone levels), and chronic obstructive pulmonary disease. Patients who have had surgical procedures within the chest, such as coronary artery bypass graft or pneumonectomy (removal of a portion of the lung), are prone to AFL. Atrial flutter can also be seen with digoxin toxicity.

Treatment

Treatment options for AFL are similar to those for AF. The goal of treatment is to control the ventricular rate

until the SA node takes over again, producing a normal rhythm. Beta blockers, calcium channel blockers, and digoxin can be used to control the ventricular rate (see Table 29.1). Some of these agents should be used cautiously because they can exacerbate HF symptoms and cause bradycardia. If a patient is still in AFL after the rate is controlled or is less than 100 bpm, then an antiarrhythmic may be ordered to chemically convert the rhythm back to an NSR.

Cardioversion (see Table 29.3) can be used to terminate the AFL but is not the first-line treatment unless the patient is severely symptomatic, and it may not be successful. Some of the symptoms that could warrant cardioversion include but are not limited to chest pain, hypotension, and SOB.

Supraventricular Tachycardia

Supraventricular tachycardia (SVT) is a rapid heart rhythm that originates above the ventricles. It most commonly appears as a regular, narrow QRS complex tachycardia. By definition, SVT is any narrow complex rhythm greater than 100 bpm, but can have HRs from 150 to 250 bpm (Fig. 29.18A). The rate may be slower depending on the patient's condition and the underlying cause of SVT. Another presentation is paroxysmal supraventricular tachycardia (PSVT), which is intermittent, coming on quickly and ending quickly (Fig. 29.18B).

Supraventricular tachycardia can be considered an umbrella term to capture one of five narrow complex tachycardia rhythms:

- Sinus tachycardia (ST; see Fig. 29.14), previously discussed in the sinus dysrhythmia section
- **Atrial tachycardia (AT)**, which is similar to ST except the electrical impulse is not generated from the sinus node. The electrical impulse is generated somewhere in the atria and can have unifocal (uniform appearance—originating from a single source; Fig. 29.19A) or multifocal (nonuniform appearance—originating from multiple sources; Fig. 29.19B) presentation.

- Atrial fibrillation with RVR (see Fig. 29.16C)
- Atrial flutter with RVR (see Fig. 29.17)
- Junctional tachycardia (JT), which is discussed in the junctional section later in the chapter (see Fig. 29.20C)

Treatment

The treatment for SVT is based on the symptoms and underlying rhythm. The key for treating SVT is to figure out the underlying rhythm while slowing down the HR. If the patient is symptomatic, medications (see Table 29.1) can be used, and electrical cardioversion can be considered; however, careful consideration should be taken if the underlying rhythm is not known.

See Table 29.4 for a summary of atrial dysrhythmias.

> **⚠ Safety Alert** Patients receiving adenosine (Adenocard) may experience prolonged periods of asystole after administration. Prior to administration of the medication, the patient should be on a monitor, and a transcutaneous pacemaker should be readily available should pacing of the patient be necessary.

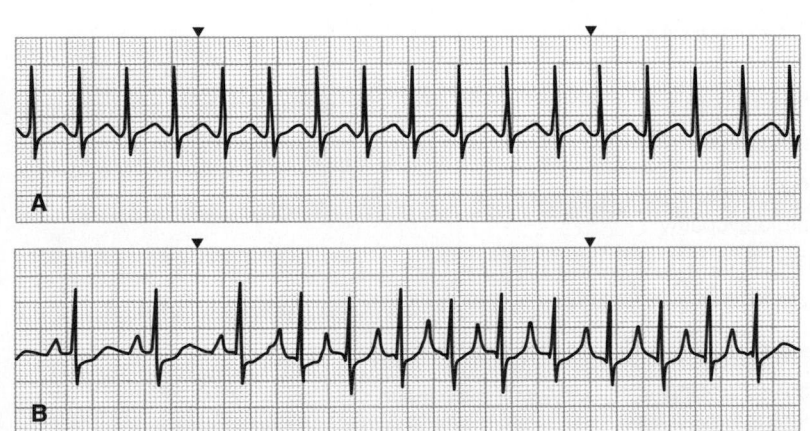

FIGURE 29.18 Supraventricular tachycardia (SVT). *A,* Continuous SVT with a heart rate of 170. *B,* Paroxysmal supraventricular tachycardia (PSVT).

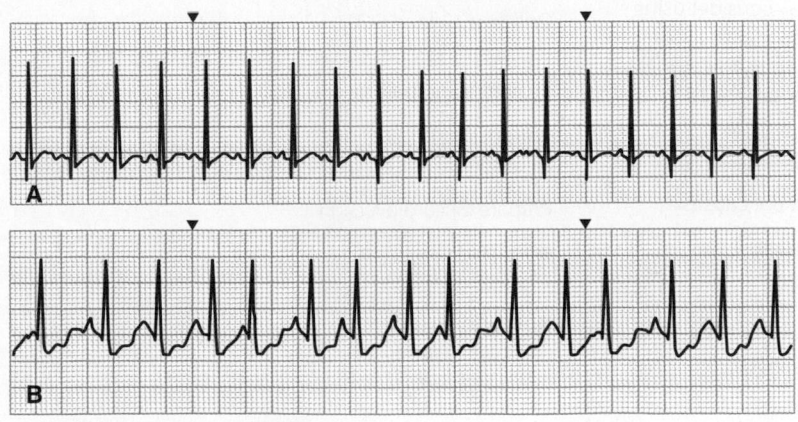

FIGURE 29.19 Atrial tachycardia (AT). *A,* Unifocal AT originating from the one pacemaker in the atria. *B,* Multifocal AT originating from many pacemakers in the atria.

Table 29.4 Summary of Atrial Dysrhythmias

Dysrhythmia	Signs and Symptoms	Medical Interventions	Nursing Interventions	Patient Teaching
Premature atrial contractions (PACs), asymptomatic	None	*All PACs:* Treat the causes if necessary: • Hypoxia • Ischemia • Electrolyte imbalance • Medication toxicities • Stimulants	*All PACs:* Assess the patient for: • LOC • Palpable pulses • BP and HR • Symptoms	*All PACs:* Educate patient/family about: • Causes • Signs and symptoms that need immediate attention • Appropriate actions if those symptoms occur
PACs, symptomatic	• Feeling of palpitations (skipping beats) • SOB • Sweating • Anxiety			
Atrial fibrillation (AF)/ atrial flutter (AFL), asymptomatic	• May feel palpitations	Depends on the rate and the patient's left ventricular function (LVF) Medication to: • Maintain rate control • Anticoagulate Treat underlying causes: • Acute MI • Severe mitral valve disease • Thyrotoxicosis • COPD • Pericarditis • Cardiomyopathy • HTN • CAD	Assess the patient for: • LOC • Palpable pulse • BP and HR Obtain a 12-lead ECG. Assess for other underlying causes.	Discuss clinical manifestations that indicate a need to contact a healthcare provider.
AF/AFL, symptomatic	• Hypotension • Dizziness • Lightheadedness • Fainting • SOB • Sweating • Anxiety • Palpitations	• Oxygen • Rate-controlling medications such as calcium channel blockers or beta blockers • May consider using amiodarone (Cordarone, Pacerone) to control the HR • Consider cardioversion. Treat the causes: • Infection • Fever • Hypovolemia • Hypoxia	Stay with the patient. Assess the patient: • LOC • Palpable pulse • BP and HR Obtain a 12-lead ECG. Ensure the IV access is available and patent. Administer medications as ordered. Prepare for cardioversion: • Place defibrillator pads. • Anticipate order for anti-anxiety medication.	Real-time education regarding the event, treatment, and ways to avoid it in the future

Table 29.4 Summary of Atrial Dysrhythmias—cont'd

Dysrhythmia	Signs and Symptoms	Medical Interventions	Nursing Interventions	Patient Teaching
		• Ischemia • Electrolyte imbalance • Stimulants		
Supraventricular tachycardia (SVT), asymptomatic • ST • AT • AF with RVR • AFL with RVR • JT	None	*All SVTs:* Treat the causes if necessary: • Hypoxia • Ischemia • Electrolyte imbalance • Medication toxicities • Stimulants	*All SVTs:* Assess the patient for: • LOC • Palpable pulses • BP and HR • Evolving symptoms	*All SVTs:* Educate patient/family about: • Causes • Signs and symptoms that need immediate attention • Appropriate actions if these symptoms occur
SVT, symptomatic • ST • AT • AF with RVR • AFL with RVR • JT	• Hypotension • Dizziness • Lightheadedness • Fainting • SOB • Sweating • Anxiety • Palpitations	• Oxygen • Adenosine to assist with determination of underlying rhythm • Rate-controlling medications such as calcium channel blockers or beta blockers • May consider using amiodarone (Cordarone, Pacerone) to control the HR • Consider cardioversion. Treat the causes: • Infection • Fever • Hypovolemia • Hypoxia • Ischemia • Electrolyte imbalance • Stimulants • MI • Medication toxicity	Stay with the patient. Assess the patient: • LOC • Palpable pulse • BP and HR Obtain a 12-lead ECG. Ensure IV access is available and patent. Administer medications as ordered. Prepare for cardioversion: • Place defibrillator pads. • Anticipate order for antianxiety medication.	Real-time education regarding the event, treatment, and ways to avoid it in the future

AT, Atrial tachycardia; *BP*, blood pressure; *CAD*, coronary artery disease; *COPD*, chronic obstructive pulmonary disease; *ECG*, electrocardiogram; *HR*, heart rate; *HTN*, hypertension; *JT*, junctional tachycardia; *LOC*, level of consciousness; *MI*, myocardial infarction; *RVR*, rapid ventricular response; *SOB*, shortness of breath; *ST*, sinus tachycardia.

Junctional Rhythms

Junctional rhythms begin within the AV node. The AV node is a cluster of pacemaker cells positioned between the atria and the ventricles. The AV node generates impulses at a rate between 40 and 60 bpm (Fig. 29.20A). If the rate increases to 61 to 100 bpm, it is identified as an accelerated junctional rhythm (Fig. 29.20B). If the HR is greater than 100 bpm, it is identified as a junctional tachycardia (Fig. 29.20C). In order for both the atria and the ventricles to depolarize during a junctional rhythm, the electrical impulse from the AV node must split and travel in different directions. The ventricular conduction pathway will accept the electrical impulse as usual. However, in order for the atria to depolarize, the electrical impulse must travel backward (the opposite direction of the normal conduction), producing a retrograde P wave. This will display as an inverted or upside-down P wave, an absent P wave that is buried in the QRS complex, or a retrograde P wave at the end of the QRS wave.

Premature Junctional Contractions

Premature junctional contractions (PJCs) are junctional impulses generated early by the AV node (Fig. 29.21). As with PACs, PJCs are not life threatening. They can present with an inverted P wave prior to, buried in, or after the QRS wave and will have a compensatory pause immediately following the PJC. Patients with PJCs are rarely symptomatic and typically do not require treatment.

Causes

Causes of junctional dysrhythmias include digoxin toxicity, acute MI, and heart surgery.

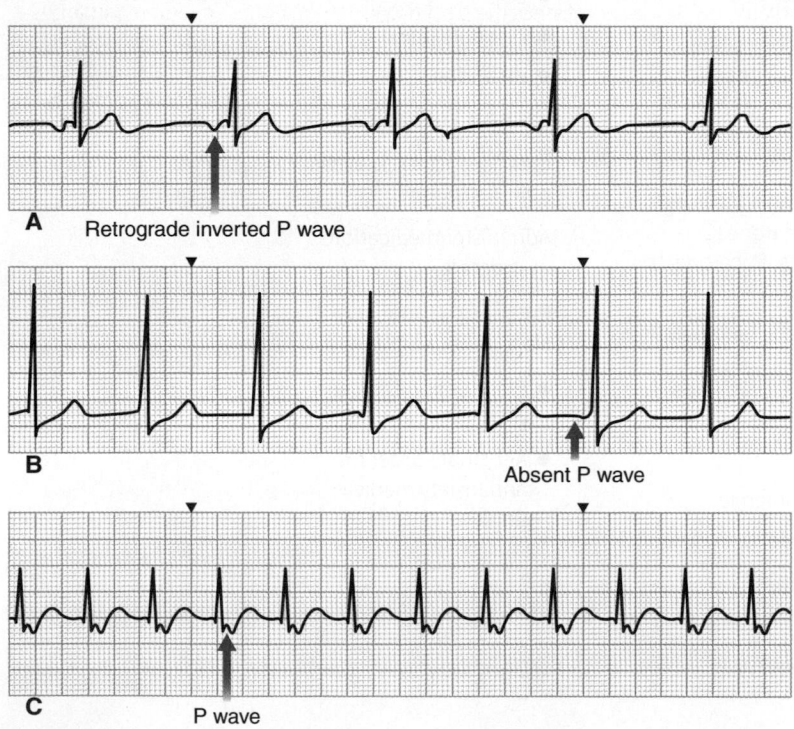

A Retrograde inverted P wave

B Absent P wave

C P wave

FIGURE 29.20 Junctional rhythms. *A,* Junctional rhythm with a ventricular rate of 50. *B,* Accelerated junctional rhythm with a ventricular rate of 70. *C,* Junctional tachycardia with a ventricular rate of 120.

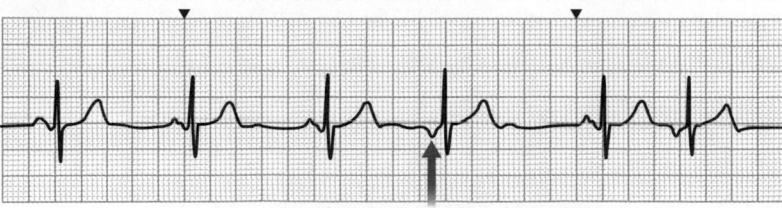

Premature junctional contraction with inverted P wave

FIGURE 29.21 Premature junctional contractions (PJCs); notice the inverted P wave.

Treatment

Treatment of junctional dysrhythmias is based solely on the patient's symptoms and possible causes. For example, if medication toxicity is the cause, then the medication should be stopped and reversed using an antidote if needed and if available.

See Table 29.5 for a summary of junctional dysrhythmias.

Connection Check 29.4

Which of the following is *not* an appropriate intervention for all atrial dysrhythmias?
A. An ECG
B. A pulse check
C. Blood pressure
D. Cardioversion

Ventricular Rhythms

Ventricular rhythms are those rhythms that originate somewhere within the ventricles. When an impulse starts in the ventricle, there is no P wave, and the QRS is usually wide (≥ 0.12 sec or three small boxes). The normal rate for pacemaker cells within the ventricles is 40 bpm or less. Types of ventricular rhythms include premature ventricular contractions (PVCs), ventricular tachycardia (VT), ventricular fibrillation (VF), and idioventricular rhythms (IVRs).

Premature Ventricular Contractions

Premature ventricular contractions (PVCs) are wide and atypical (or bizarre-looking) QRS complexes that fire earlier than expected from within the ventricles (Fig. 29.22). As with other premature contractions, there is a compensatory pause at the end to allow the heart's conduction system to

Table 29.5 Summary of Junctional Dysrhythmias

Dysrhythmia	Signs and Symptoms	Medical Interventions	Nursing Interventions	Patient Teaching
Junctional, asymptomatic	None	Treat the causes: • Ischemia • Medication toxicities (e.g., digoxin) • Hypoxia	Assess the patient for: • LOC • Palpable pulses • BP and HR Obtain a 12-lead ECG. Assess for other causes.	Education regarding signs and symptoms that warrant contacting a healthcare provider
Junctional, symptomatic	• Dizziness • Lightheadedness • Fainting • SOB • Sweating • Anxiety • Hypotension	• Oxygen • Atropine IVP • Pacing Treat the causes: • Infection • Fever • Hypovolemia • Hypoxia • Ischemia • Electrolyte imbalance • Stimulants • Medication toxicities (e.g., digoxin)	Get help and stay with the patient. Assess the patient for: • LOC • Palpable pulses • BP and HR Obtain a 12-lead ECG. Give oxygen per order. Ensure IV access is available and patent. Administer medication(s) as ordered. Prepare for TCP: • Place defibrillator/pacing pads in an anterior/posterior position. • Anticipate antianxiety medication.	Education regarding the event, treatment, and ways to recognize and avoid future occurrences

BP, Blood pressure; *ECG,* electrocardiogram; *HR,* heart rate; *IVP,* intravenous push; *LOC,* level of consciousness; *SOB,* shortness of breath; *TCP,* transcutaneous pacing.

reset. There are no P waves visible prior to the QRS because the impulse originated in the ventricle. Premature ventricular contractions coming from one ventricular pacemaker cell are called *unifocal PVCs* (Fig. 29.22A). If they come from multiple ventricular pacemaker cells, they are called *multifocal PVCs* (Fig. 29.22B). Two PVCs in a row is called a *couplet* (Fig. 29.22C). Three PVCs in a row is called a *triplet* or a *three-beat run of VT* (Fig. 29.22D). A PVC that occurs every other beat is called *bigeminy* (Fig. 29.22E). A PVC falling every third beat is called *trigeminy* (Fig. 29.22F).

Causes

Causes of PVCs include hypoxia, MI, CM, electrolyte imbalance, excessive stimulant ingestion (such as caffeine), hypertension, and recreational drug use.

Treatment

Treatment of PVCs is based on the patient's symptoms. If the patient is symptomatic, treatment includes correcting the cause and, rarely, antiarrhythmic therapy.

Ventricular Tachycardia

Ventricular tachycardia (VT) is defined as three or more PVCs (wide and fast impulses originating from the ventricles) in a row. The ventricular rate is usually greater than 150 bpm. It can be monomorphic (originating from one pacemaker cell; Fig. 29.23A) or polymorphic (originating from multiple pacemaker cells; Fig. 29.23B).

VT can be a life-threatening dysrhythmia as a result of the significant reduction in CO that can occur. A patient in VT might be able to maintain a pulse and a blood pressure

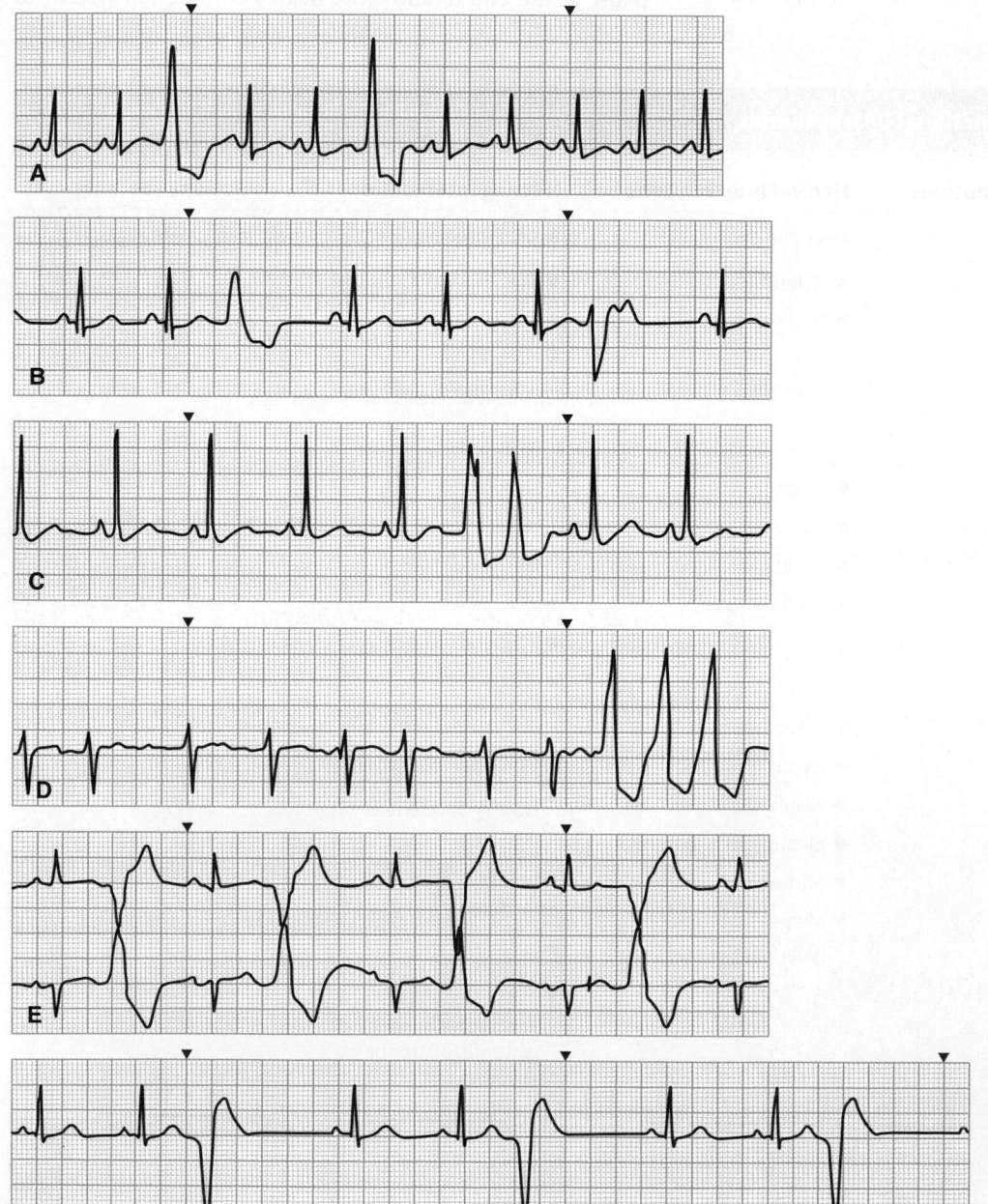

FIGURE 29.22 Premature ventricular contractions. *A,* Unifocal PVCs: notice how the PVCs present the same. *B,* Multifocal PVCs: notice how the PVCs present differently. *C,* Couplet. *D,* Triplet or a three-beat run of ventricular tachycardia (VT). *E,* Bigeminy. *F,* Trigeminy.

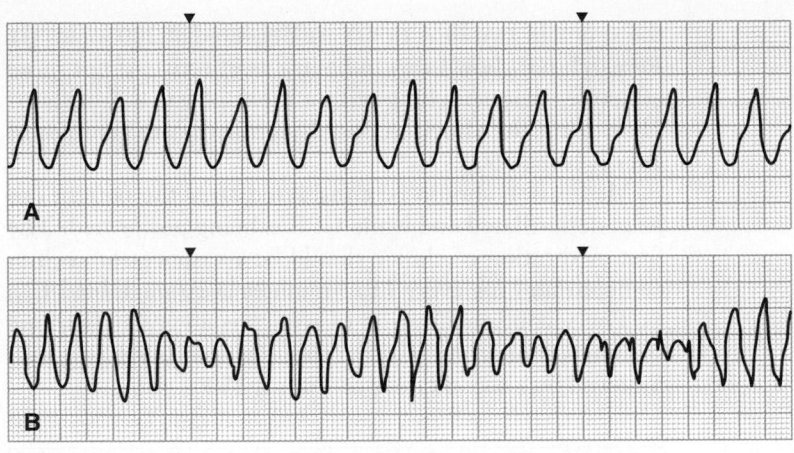

FIGURE 29.23 Ventricular tachycardia (VT).
A, Monomorphic: originating from one pacemaker cell.
B, Polymorphic: originating from multiple pacemaker cells.

for a limited time, but VT will cause death if prolonged or untreated.

Causes

Causes of VT include:

- Hypovolemia
- Hypoxia
- Acidosis
- Hypokalemia
- Hyperkalemia
- Hypoglycemia
- Hypothermia
- Toxins
- Cardiac tamponade
- MI
- PE

Treatment

Treatment for VT is based on the patient's presentation, which is either:

- VT with a pulse
- Pulseless VT

VT with a pulse describes a patient in VT who is maintaining a blood pressure and pulse with or without symptoms. The treatment options are antiarrhythmic medications such as amiodarone (Cordarone, Pacerone; see Table 29.1), electrolyte replacements such as potassium or magnesium, and/or cardioversion. Cardioversion is an electrical shock given to the patient at the time of ventricular depolarization (see Table 29.3). Cardioversion is typically reserved for a patient who is symptomatic such as hypotensive, SOB or complaining of chest pain.

Pulseless VT describes a patient who is in cardiac arrest. The first-line treatment is cardiopulmonary resuscitation (CPR) and defibrillation. In contrast to cardioversion, defibrillation is an electrical shock delivered anytime during the cardiac cycle (see Table 29.3). Other treatments include medications such as epinephrine and antiarrhythmics (e.g., amiodarone [Cordarone, Pacerone]).

Ventricular Fibrillation

Ventricular fibrillation (VF) is a lethal dysrhythmia requiring immediate treatment. It is the most frequently seen rhythm in cardiac arrests occurring outside of the hospital. Ventricular fibrillation occurs when the ventricle has multiple chaotic impulses rapidly firing (Fig. 29.24). This chaotic firing prevents the ventricles from pushing blood out of the heart, stopping CO and causing death. There are absolutely no identifiable P waves or QRS waves. The rhythm displayed on the ECG is a shaky or quivering line that can be very coarse (Fig. 29.24A) or fine (Fig. 29.24B).

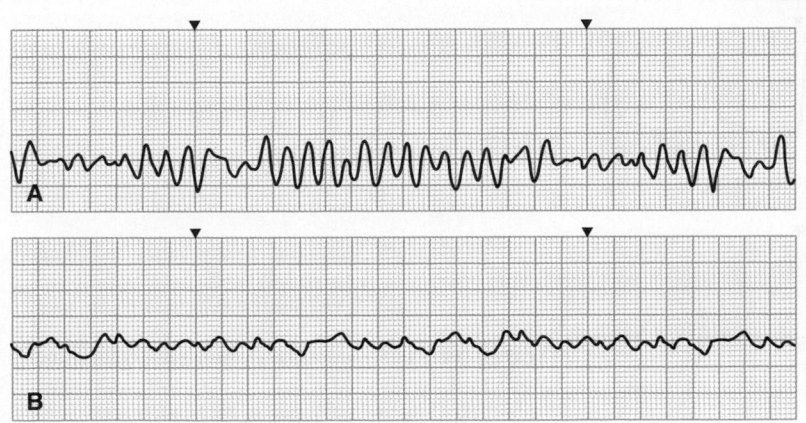

FIGURE 29.24 Ventricular fibrillation (VF). *A,* Coarse VF.
B, Fine VF.

Causes

Causes of VF include:

- Hypovolemia
- Hypoxia
- Acidosis
- Hypokalemia
- Hyperkalemia
- Hypoglycemia
- Hypothermia
- Toxins
- Cardiac tamponade
- MI
- PE

Treatment

Treatment requirements for VF start with chest compressions and include defibrillation and medication. Chest compressions and defibrillation are the most important interventions that can be done for a patient in VF. Chest compressions should be initiated immediately and maintained as continuously as possible. Compressions should not be paused/stopped longer than 10 seconds and should be paused only when applying external defibrillation pads and when discharging the electrical impulse from the defibrillator. To be effective, chest compressions need to be deep (2–2.4 inches in an adult) and fast (a rate of 100–120 bpm). Compressors need to switch every 2 minutes to limit fatigue and maintain continuous high-quality CPR.

Defibrillation (see Table 29.3) should be performed within 2 to 3 minutes (180 seconds) of the onset of VF for the best survival outcome. Studies have shown that for every minute a patient remains in VF without defibrillation, the survival rate decreases by 7% to 10%. When chest compressions are initiated prior to defibrillation, the effectiveness of the shock is increased. Shocks from biphasic defibrillators (delivering the shock in two directions) are delivered at 200 joules (J). Research has shown this to be just as effective, if not more effective, than shocking with a monophasic defibrillator (delivering the shock in one direction) set to its highest energy level, 360 J.

Medication should be considered after the patient has been defibrillated and while CPR is being performed. The first medication of choice should be a vasopressor such as epinephrine 1 mg every 3 to 5 minutes IVP (see Table 29.1).

The second medication of choice is an antiarrhythmic such as amiodarone (Cordarone, Pacerone) 300 mg IVP followed by a second dose of 150 mg IVP.

> **Safety Alert** When using the defibrillator to cardiovert or defibrillate a patient, be sure to look around the patient to confirm that no one is touching the patient while you loudly say, *"I am clear, you are clear, we are all clear"* prior to pushing the *SHOCK* button. This is to prevent electricity from traveling from the patient to another person accidentally.

Idioventricular Rhythm

Idioventricular rhythm (IVR) occurs when the SA and AV nodes fail to function and the rhythm is generated from the ventricle. The rate is usually less than 40 bpm (Fig. 29.25A) but could be between 40 and 100 bpm, which is called **accelerated idioventricular rhythm (AIVR;** Fig. 29.25B). The HR could also be less than 20 bpm, which is often called an **agonal** rhythm or *dying heart* (Fig. 29.25C).

Causes

Causes of IVR include MI, postcardiac arrest, medication and drug toxicities (e.g., cocaine, digoxin, anesthetics), electrolyte imbalances, myocarditis, CM, and congenital heart disease.

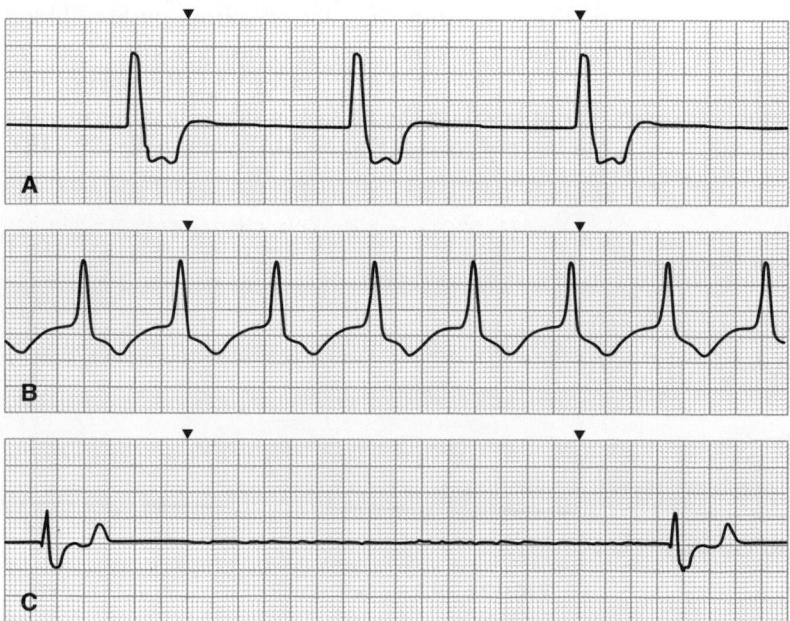

FIGURE 29.25 Idioventricular rhythm (IVR). *A,* IVR with a rate of 30. *B,* Accelerated idioventricular rhythm (AIVR) with a rate of 80. *C,* Agonal rhythm or dying heart.

Treatment

Treatment of IVR is based on the patient's symptoms. If the patient is symptomatic, the treatment includes correcting the cause, pacing, and atropine.

Connection Check 29.5

The nurse understands that rhythms originating in the ventricle have which of the following characteristics? *(Select all that apply.)*

A. Wide QRS complexes
B. Narrow QRS complexes
C. Only QRS complexes
D. Only fast rates
E. Only slow rates

Asystole

Asystole is a condition in which there is no measurable electrical activity originating from the heart. A straight or *flat line* is produced on the cardiac monitor (Fig. 29.26). Without an electrical stimulus, the cardiac muscles cannot squeeze or contract to force blood in or out of the heart's chambers. It is important to assess the patient to be sure that it is a true asystolic event. Occasionally, a loose ECG patch or wire from the monitor will cause a false reading. However, if it is a true asystolic event, the patient will be pulseless.

Compressions should be started immediately. The patient should be assessed with a second monitor lead, pausing compressions only briefly (< 10 seconds) to rule out a fine VF. If VF is confirmed, the patient should be defibrillated. If the second lead continues to show a *flat line*, asystole is confirmed, and defibrillation is not indicated. The treatment for asystole is CPR, epinephrine, and treating the cause, which is the same as that for VF addressed previously.

See Table 29.6 for a summary of ventricular dysrhythmias.

Connection Check 29.6

Which of the following dysrhythmias requires defibrillation?

A. Atrial tachycardia
B. Atrial fibrillation
C. Ventricular tachycardia with a pulse
D. Ventricular fibrillation

Heart Blocks

Heart blocks are caused by the delay or blockage of electrical conduction at the AV node. The AV node's blood supply comes from the right coronary artery (RCA). If the RCA becomes partially or completely blocked, the AV node is deprived of oxygen, which causes ischemia. If the AV node tissue becomes ischemic or dies, the electrical impulses originating in the atria will have difficulty traveling through the AV node to the ventricles along the usual pathway. The electrical impulses will need to find an alternative pathway, which could cause conduction delays or even an electrical disassociation of the atria and the ventricles. There are four types of heart blocks: first degree, second-degree type I, second-degree type II, and third degree.

Causes

The primary cause of most AV heart blocks is acute coronary syndrome. Acute coronary syndrome (ACS) is an umbrella term used to describe unstable angina, acute non–ST elevation MI (NSTEMI), and acute ST elevation MI (STEMI). Other causes of heart blocks include but are not limited to electrolyte imbalances and medication toxicities.

First-Degree AV Block

First-degree AV block looks very similar to an NSR except the PR interval is prolonged (> 0.20 sec or five blocks long; Fig. 29.27). This is due to the atrial depolarization being delayed in the AV node. Every atrial impulse gets through the AV node; it just takes longer. It is the same time interval each time.

Treatment

Treatment is not typically required for first-degree AV block unless the patient is having symptoms, which is very rare. If the patient is symptomatic, then the underlying causes are treated to alleviate the symptoms.

Second-Degree AV Block Type I

Second-degree AV block type I (also known as **Wenckebach** or **Mobitz I**) occurs when not all atrial impulses get through the AV node to the ventricles. There are more P waves than QRS complexes, and the PR interval gets progressively longer until a QRS is dropped (also referred to as dropping QRSs; Fig. 29.28). After the dropped QRS, the PR interval resets, and the process starts over. A helpful mnemonic is *longer, longer, longer, dropped; then you have a Wenckebach.* When identifying a heart block, look at the PR interval pattern after the dropped QRS complex. This is not considered a life-threatening dysrhythmia, and it is typically

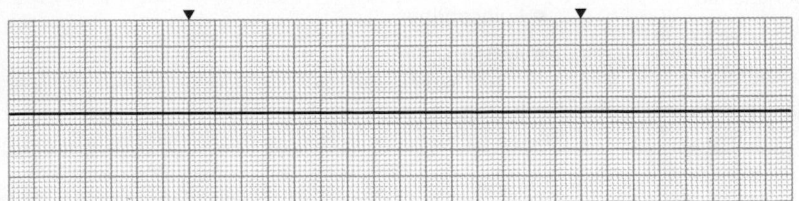

FIGURE 29.26 Asystole; no electrical activity.

Table 29.6 Summary of Ventricular Dysrhythmias

Dysrhythmia	Signs and Symptoms	Medical Interventions	Nursing Interventions	Patient Teaching
Premature ventricular contractions (PVCs), asymptomatic	None	*All PVCs:* Treat the causes if necessary: • Hypoxia • Ischemia • Electrolyte imbalance • Medication toxicities • Stimulants	*All PVCs:* Assess the patient for: • LOC • Palpable pulses • BP and HR • Symptoms	*All PVCs:* Educate patient/family about: • Causes • Signs and symptoms that need immediate attention • Appropriate actions if those symptoms occur
PVCs, symptomatic	• Dizziness • Lightheadedness • Fainting • SOB • Sweating • Anxiety • Palpitations • Hypotension			
Ventricular tachycardia with a pulse	• Dizziness • Lightheadedness • Fainting • SOB • Sweating • Anxiety • Palpitations • Hypotension	Follow AHA/ACLS guidelines: • Vagal maneuvers • Antiarrhythmic medications • Consider cardioversion. Treat the causes: • Hypovolemia • Hypoxia • Ischemia • Electrolyte imbalance • Toxins • Stimulants	Call for help. Stay with the patient. Frequent assessment for symptoms Frequent vital signs Obtain a 12-lead ECG. Ensure IV access is available and patent. Administer medication(s) as ordered. Prepare for cardioversion.	Education regarding dysrhythmia medications, treatment, signs and symptoms that require seeking treatment, and how to avoid future occurrences
Ventricular tachycardia without a pulse *Ventricular fibrillation*	• Unresponsive • No pulse • No BP	Follow AHA/ACLS guidelines: • CPR • Defibrillate • Medications–epinephrine, antiarrhythmics Treat possible causes: • Hypovolemia • Hypoxia • Acidosis • Hypokalemia • Hyperkalemia • Hypoglycemia • Hypothermia • Toxins • Cardiac tamponade • MI • PE	Activate medical emergency team. Start and maintain compressions. Defibrillate per ACLS guidelines. Ensure IV access is available and patent. Hang free-flowing IV fluids such as 0.9 NS. Administer emergency medications as ordered, such as: • Epinephrine • Antiarrhythmic (e.g., amiodarone [Cordarone, Pacerone])	Education regarding disease management to avoid future occurrences if patient has return of circulation and survives the event

Table 29.6 Summary of Ventricular Dysrhythmias—cont'd

Dysrhythmia	Signs and Symptoms	Medical Interventions	Nursing Interventions	Patient Teaching
Idioventricular rhythm, asymptomatic	None	Treat the causes if necessary: • Hypoxia • Ischemia • Electrolyte imbalance • Medication toxicities • Stimulants	Assess the patient for: • LOC • Palpable pulses • BP and HR	Educate patient/family about: • Causes • Signs and symptoms that need immediate attention • Appropriate actions if those symptoms occur
Idioventricular rhythm, symptomatic	• Dizziness • Lightheadedness • Fainting • SOB • Sweating • Anxiety • Palpitations • Hypotension • Decrease in level of consciousness	Treat the causes: • Hypovolemia • Hypoxia • Ischemia • Electrolyte imbalance • Toxins • Stimulants	Call for help. Stay with the patient. Frequent assessment for symptoms Frequent vital signs Obtain a 12-lead ECG. Ensure IV access is available and patent. Administer medication(s) as ordered. Prepare for TCP: • Place defibrillator/pacing pads in an anterior/posterior position (see Fig. 29.30B). Anticipate antianxiety medication.	Education regarding dysrhythmia medications, treatment, signs and symptoms that require seeking treatment, and how to avoid future occurrences
Asystole	• Unresponsive • No pulse • No BP	Follow AHA/ACLS guidelines: • CPR • Epinephrine Treat possible causes: • Hypovolemia • Hypoxia • Acidosis • Hypokalemia • Hyperkalemia • Hypoglycemia • Hypothermia • Toxins • Cardiac tamponade • MI • PE	Activate medical emergency team. Start CPR. Ensure IV access is available and patent. Hang free-flowing IV fluids such as 0.9 NS. Administer emergency medications as ordered, such as: • Epinephrine	Education regarding disease management to avoid future occurrences if patient has return of circulation and survives the event

AHA/ACLS, American Heart Association/Advanced Cardiac Life Support; *BP,* blood pressure; *CPR,* cardiopulmonary resuscitation; *HR,* heart rate; *LOC,* level of consciousness; *MI,* myocardial infarction; *NS,* normal saline; *PE,* pulmonary embolus; *SOB,* shortness of breath; *TCP,* transcutaneous pacing.

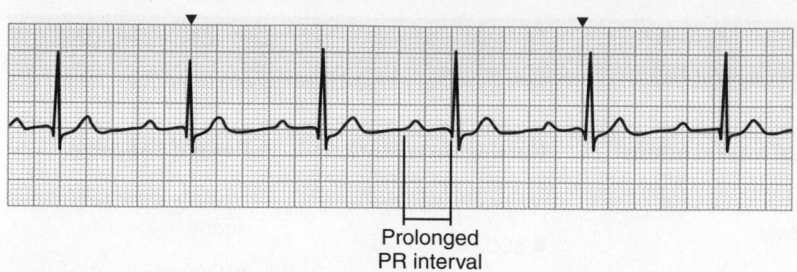

FIGURE 29.27 First-degree atrioventricular block: the PR interval is prolonged (> 0.20 sec); in this strip, the PR interval is 24.

Prolonged PR interval

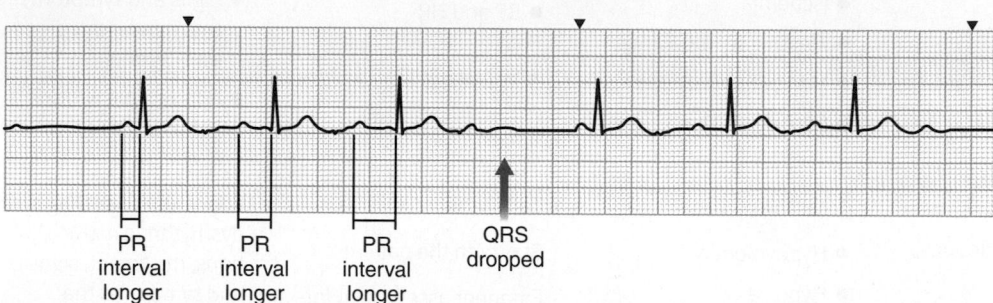

PR interval longer   PR interval longer   PR interval longer   QRS dropped

FIGURE 29.28 Second-degree atrioventricular block type I (Mobitz I or Wenckebach).

an intermittent rhythm; however, on rare occasions, it can be continuous.

Treatment

Treatment of second-degree AV block type I is considered only if the patient is symptomatic. Patients who cannot tolerate the loss of CO may experience symptoms such as dizziness, lightheadedness, and SOB. The treatment includes atropine 0.5 mg IVP to stimulate the heart to beat faster and, in extreme cases, temporary pacing.

Second-Degree AV Block Type II

Second-degree AV block type II (also known as **Mobitz II**) also drops QRS complexes, but unlike second-degree type I, the PR intervals are exactly the same length with each complex (see Fig. 29.29). This dysrhythmia is more alarming and is considered a potentially life-threatening dysrhythmia because it can quickly progress to a third-degree AV block.

Treatment

Treatment of second-degree AV block type II is dependent on the patient's symptoms. If the patient is symptomatic, then temporary pacing is the treatment of choice (see Table 29.7). Transcutaneous pacing (TCP) is the fastest pacing option, which is done by placing defibrillator pads on the patient's chest and back in the anterior-posterior

positions to externally pace the heart (see Fig. 29.30B). If time permits, other pacemaker options could be considered, such as a temporary transvenous pacemaker (TVP) or a permanent pacemaker.

Third-Degree AV Block

Third-degree AV block or **complete heart block (CHB)** occurs when the AV node is completely blocked and prevents any impulses from entering or exiting. There is no communication between the atria and the ventricles. The ECG records more P waves than QRS complexes (Fig. 29.31). The atrial rate is usually between 60 and 100 bpm, whereas the ventricular rate is usually less than or equal to 40 bpm.

In CHB, QRS complexes march out regularly and are independent of the P waves. Similarly, the P waves march throughout the rhythm strip at a regular rate. Sometimes the P waves are hidden within a QRS complex or the T wave, making it very important to march out the P waves to see where they fall.

Treatment

Treatment of CHB is initially based on treating the patient's symptoms, such as hypotension or SOB. Attempts are made to reverse the cause(s) if possible. Transcutaneous pacing is indicated in symptomatic CHB. Long-term treatment is typically the insertion of a permanent pacemaker (see Table 29.7; Fig. 29.32).

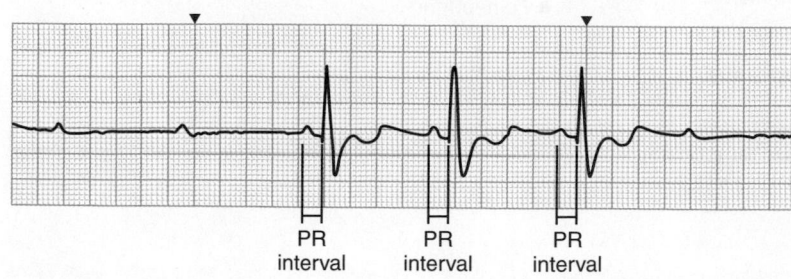

PR interval   PR interval   PR interval

FIGURE 29.29 Second-degree atrioventricular block type II (Mobitz II).

Table 29.7 Pacemaker Overview

Pacemaker Type	Placement or Location	Monitor	Nursing Care
External Pacemakers			
Transcutaneous (TCP)	Electro-pads (defibrillator pads) are placed on the patient's torso using an anterior/posterior position (see Fig. 29.30B).	Pacer spike prior to QRS	Place pads on the patient's chest and back. Medicate with sedative as ordered. Monitor patient: • HR • BP • Rhythm Stay with patient until stable. Maintain continuous cardiac monitoring to ensure detection of rhythm change or pacer failure.
Transvenous (TVP)	A pacer wire is inserted into the right ventricle (so that it touches the wall) through central venous access. The wire is attached to an external pacemaker. Usually done via internal jugular (IJ) vein	Pacer spike prior to QRS	Monitor patient: • HR • BP • Rhythm Maintain continuous cardiac monitoring to ensure detection of rhythm change or pacer failure. Monitor central venous access for signs of infection.
Transthoracic (TTP) (or epicardial pacer)	A pacer wire is surgically placed in the atrium or the ventricle and fed out through the skin. The externalized wire is attached to an external pacemaker.	Atria = pacer spike prior to P wave Ventricle = pacer spike prior to QRS (see Fig. 29.32A)	Monitor patient: • HR • BP • Rhythm Maintain continuous cardiac monitoring to ensure detection of rhythm change or pacer failure. Monitor incision site for signs of infection.
Internal Pacemakers			
Atrial	*For all internal pacemakers:* Pacer wires are placed in the atrium, ventricle, or both and attached to a small pacemaker generator placed under the skin near the clavicle (see Fig. 29.32B).	Atria = pacer spike prior to P wave	*For all internal pacemakers:* Monitor patient: • HR • BP • Rhythm Maintain continuous cardiac monitoring to ensure detection of rhythm change or pacer failure.
Ventricular		Ventricle = pacer spike prior to QRS	
Biventricular		Biventricle = double pacer spikes prior to QRS (due to having a pacer lead in each ventricle)	
Dual chamber		Pacer spike prior to P wave and QRS	Do not place medication patches or defibrillation pads over pacemaker. Monitor incision site for infection.

BP, Blood pressure; *HR,* heart rate.

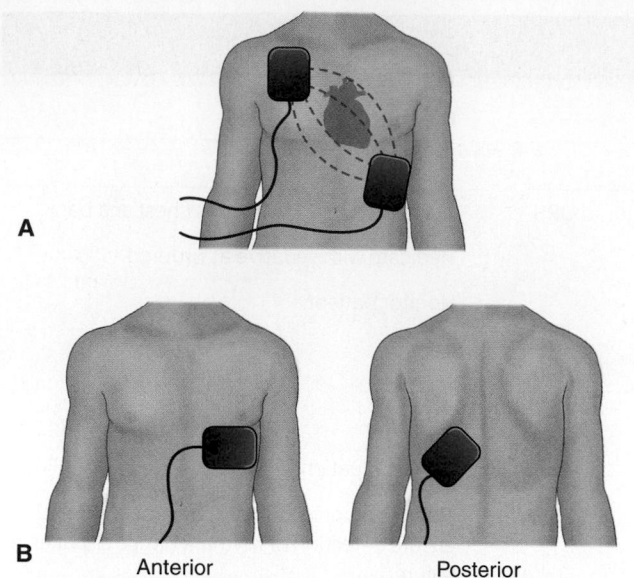

FIGURE 29.30 *A*, Apex/sternum pad placement. *B*, Anterior/posterior pad placement.

See Table 29.8 for a summary of heart blocks.

Connection Check 29.7

What do second-degree and third-degree heart blocks have in common?
A. Wide QRS complexes
B. Narrow QRS complexes
C. Dropped QRS complexes
D. No commonalities

Connection Check 29.8

Transcutaneous pacing should be considered for which of the following dysrhythmias?
A. VF
B. VT
C. Symptomatic heart block
D. AF

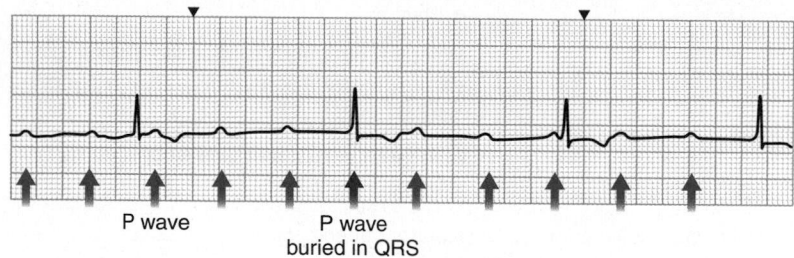

P wave

P wave buried in QRS

FIGURE 29.31 Third-degree heart block or complete heart block (CHB). R to R is regular, and P to P is regular, but there is no communication between the atria and the ventricles.

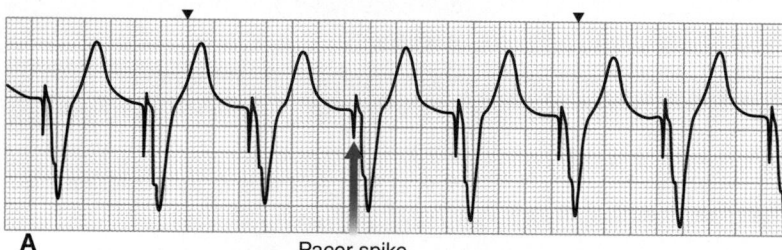

Pacer spike

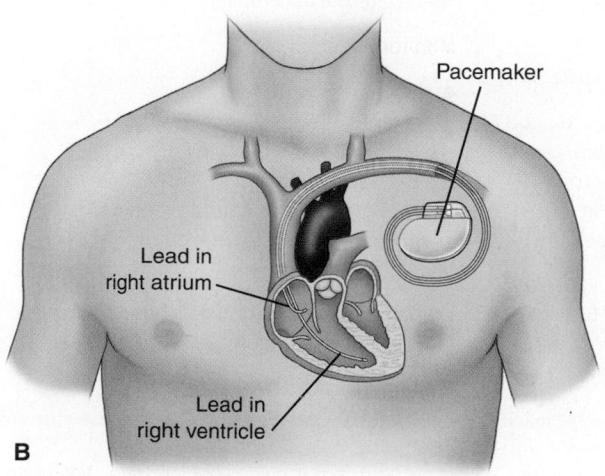

Pacemaker

Lead in right atrium

Lead in right ventricle

FIGURE 29.32 *A*, Example of ventricular paced rhythm with pacer spikes. *B*, Pacemaker implantation; there may be a lead in the atrium, ventricle, or both.

Table 29.8 Summary of Heart Blocks

Dysrhythmia	Signs and Symptoms	Medical Interventions	Nursing Interventions	Patient Teaching
First-degree AVB	None	No specific treatment is indicated for isolated first-degree block. Treat underlying cause if necessary.	Obtain vital signs. Assess patient for symptoms. Obtain a 12-lead ECG. Assess for causes.	Educate patient about dysrhythmia, underlying causes, and when to seek treatment.
Second-degree type I AVB, asymptomatic **Second-degree type II AVB, asymptomatic** **Third-degree complete heart block, asymptomatic**	None	Treat the causes if necessary: ● Hypoxia ● Ischemia ● Medication toxicities (e.g., digoxin) ● Electrolyte imbalance	Obtain vital signs. Assess patient for symptoms. Obtain a 12-lead ECG. Assess for other causes.	Educate patient about dysrhythmia, underlying causes, and when to seek treatment.
Second-degree type I AVB, symptomatic **Second-degree type II AVB, symptomatic** **Third-degree complete heart block, symptomatic**	● Dizziness ● Lightheadedness ● Fainting ● SOB ● Sweating ● Anxiety ● Hypotension	● Oxygen ● Atropine IVP ● Pacing Treat the causes: ● Hypoxia ● Ischemia ● Medication toxicities (e.g., digoxin) ● Electrolyte imbalance	Call for help. Stay with the patient. Frequent assessment for symptoms Frequent vital signs Obtain a 12-lead ECG. Give oxygen per order. Ensure IV access is available and patent. Administer medication(s) as ordered. Prepare for TCP. Anticipate administration of antianxiety medication.	Educate patient regarding dysrhythmia medications, treatment, signs and symptoms that require seeking treatment, and how to avoid future occurrences.

AVB, atrioventricular block; *ECG,* electrocardiogram; *IVP,* intravenous push; *SOB,* shortness of breath; *TCP,* transcutaneous pacing.

Nursing Management

Assessment and Analysis

Clinical manifestations for dysrhythmias are dependent on their impact on the patient's cardiac output. Some dysrhythmias have little impact on cardiac output and so have few manifestations. The more dangerous dysrhythmias, such as atrial fibrillation and ventricular rhythms or blocks, can greatly reduce cardiac output, causing SOB, pain, hypotension, fatigue, and if severe enough, death.

Nursing Diagnosis

● **Risk for decreased cardiac output** related to alteration in heart rhythm

Nursing Interventions

▪ Assessments

● Evaluate ECG and identify the rhythm.
   Recognizing the rhythm helps the nurse anticipate and respond appropriately.
● Determine if the patient is symptomatic versus asymptomatic.
   Symptomatic patients require immediate response and evaluation of causes; asymptomatic patients require observation and evaluation of causes.
● To assess if symptomatic, evaluate:
   ● Vital signs
      The lack of efficient contractile function of a heart experiencing dysrhythmias results in a decrease in CO and hypotension.

In an attempt to increase oxygenation in the face of decreased CO, SOB and tachypnea may occur. The HR may be faster, slower, regular rhythm, or irregular rhythm depending on the type of dysrhythmia.

- Change in level of consciousness
  Decreased blood pressure and thus CO may cause a decrease in blood flow to the brain, resulting in dizziness or syncope.
- Diaphoresis
  Diaphoresis is the result of the stimulation of the sympathetic nervous system in response to low CO.
- Chest pain
  Dysrhythmias may cause an imbalance in myocardial oxygen demand and supply, potentially resulting in chest pain.
- Poor peripheral circulation
  Decreased CO may cause weak peripheral pulses, cool extremities, and sluggish capillary refill. Poor contractile function may cause peripheral edema.
- Nausea and vomiting
  Shunting of blood away from nonessential organ systems during low-flow states may cause nausea and vomiting.
- Electrolyte levels and cardiac enzymes
  Dysrhythmias may indicate acute cardiac injury, which may be demonstrated by elevated cardiac enzymes.
  Elevated potassium levels can cause changes in the shape of the T wave.
  Electrolyte imbalances are sometimes the cause of dysrhythmias.

■ Actions

- Administer antiarrhythmic therapy as ordered.
  Antiarrhythmic medications limit the occurrence of dysrhythmias, helping to maintain an adequate CO and decrease the risk of life-threatening events associated with lethal dysrhythmias.
- Perform an ECG/maintain continuous ECG monitoring as ordered.
  Monitoring facilitates immediate recognition of dysrhythmias, which allows for prompt treatment as necessary.

- Be prepared to administer advanced cardiac life support in the event of a lethal dysrhythmia
  Cardiopulmonary resuscitation, defibrillation if indicated, and administration of emergency medications may restore adequate CO in a patient experiencing lethal dysrhythmias.
- Document the occurrence of dysrhythmias.
  Documentation helps evaluate the need for and/or the effectiveness of therapy.

■ Teaching

- Immediately report chest pain or chest discomfort.
  Prompt treatment is one way to help maximize positive outcomes when a patient is experiencing dangerous or lethal dysrhythmias.
- Take antiarrhythmic medications as prescribed.
  Maintaining adequate medication levels helps decrease the occurrence of adverse effects of dysrhythmias.
- Recognize signs of possible complications of dysrhythmias, such as strokes due to clot formation in AF.
  It is important that the patient (and family) is able to detect early signs of complications to ensure prompt treatment and reduce adverse effects.

See Table 29.9 for a quick dysrhythmia interpretation chart.

Connection Check 29.9

Signs or symptoms of symptomatic ventricular dysrhythmias include which of the following? *(Select all that apply.)*

A. Hypotension
B. Dizziness
C. Fever
D. Shortness of breath
E. Hypertension

Table 29.9 Quick Dysrhythmia Interpretation Table

Rhythm	Heart Rate	P Wave	QRS Complex	T Wave	P–P Regular	R–R Regular	PR Interval	QRS Interval
SR	Normal (60–100 bpm)	Yes	Narrow	Yes	Yes	Yes	Normal (0.12–0.2 sec)	Normal (0.04–0.1 sec)
SB	Slow (less than 60 bpm)	Yes	Narrow	Yes	Yes	Yes	Normal (0.12–0.2 sec)	Normal (0.04–0.1 sec)
ST	Fast (greater than 100 bpm)	Yes	Narrow	Yes	Yes	Yes	Normal (0.12–0.2 sec)	Normal (0.04–0.1 sec)
AF	Varies	No	Narrow	Yes (but may be hard to identify)	n/a	Irregular	n/a	Normal (0.04–0.1 sec)
AFL	Varies	F wave	Narrow	Yes (but may be hard to identify)	n/a	Usually regular but can vary on the basis of conduction rate	n/a	Normal (0.04–0.1 sec)
Junctional	Slower (usually) 40–60 bpm	Inverted when seen	Narrow	Yes	n/a	Yes	Less than or equal to 0.12 sec (when it can be measured)	Normal (0.04–0.1 sec)
SVT	Fast (greater than 100 but usually 150–250 bpm)	Sometimes seen inverted after QRS	Narrow	Yes	n/a	Yes	n/a	Normal (0.04–0.1 sec)
First-degree AVB	Normal	Yes	Narrow	Yes	Yes	Yes	Greater than 0.20 sec (measurement is consistent)	Normal (0.04–0.1 sec)
Second-degree AVB type I	Varies	Yes More P waves than QRS complexes	Narrow–wide Missing QRS complexes	Yes	Yes	Irregular	Starts normal then gets longer and longer until a QRS is dropped	Normal to wider
Second-degree AVB type II	Normal to slow	Yes More P waves than QRS complexes	Narrow–wide Missing QRS complexes	Yes	Yes	Yes	Normal to wide (but measurement is consistent)	Normal to wider
Third-degree AVB	Normal to slow	Yes More P waves than QRS complexes	Narrow–wide Missing QRS complexes	Yes	Yes	Yes	Vary because the P waves do not correlate to the QRS complex	Narrow–wide

AF, Atrial fibrillation; AFL, atrial flutter; AVB, AV block; SB, sinus bradycardia; SR, sinus rhythm; ST, sinus tachycardia; SVT, supraventricular tachycardia.

Making Connections

CASE STUDY: WRAP-UP

After being started on heparin, Ms. Fletcher is prepared for a TEE to determine if clots are present in her atria. If there are no clots, she may be a candidate for cardioversion. If clots are visualized, anticoagulation therapy will be continued. Ms. Fletcher's TEE reveals no clots. She is electively cardioverted because of her increasing instability. Her rhythm returns to NSR. She is admitted to a cardiac telemetry bed for observation overnight. She will need further education on the signs and symptoms of AF and her new medications. She is referred for follow-up to an appropriate dysrhythmia specialist.

Case Study Questions

1. What is the priority nursing action for Ms. Fletcher upon admission to the unit?
   A. Orientation to the room
   B. Initiating ECG monitoring
   C. Calculating intake and output
   D. Assessing pain level

2. The nurse monitors for which clinical manifestations in Ms. Fletcher? (*Select all that apply.*)
   A. Complaints of palpitations
   B. Complaints of shortness of breath
   C. Diaphoresis
   D. Fever
   E. Hyperglycemia

3. The charge nurse is reviewing new admission orders for Ms. Fletcher. It is a priority for the charge nurse to follow up with the provider about which order?
   A. Regular diet
   B. Discontinuing monitor
   C. Vital signs every 4 hours
   D. Saline lock

4. The nurse caring for Ms. Fletcher incorporates which nursing diagnoses into the plan of care? (*Select all that apply.*)
   A. Risk for decreased cardiac output
   B. Risk for embolic event
   C. Knowledge deficit
   D. Risk for poor nutrition
   E. Risk for bleeding

5. Which statement by Ms. Fletcher indicates that teaching has been effective?
   A. "I'm just glad the problem was fixed, and I don't need to go back to the doctor."
   B. "I'm glad I don't have to worry about having a stroke anymore."
   C. "I guess I need to follow up with a heart doctor."
   D. "I guess things will go back to normal now."

CHAPTER SUMMARY

Electrocardiogram interpretation is a useful tool to help identify dysrhythmias that affect efficient heart function. Key points to consider when interpreting dysrhythmias include the appearance and presence of P waves and QRS complexes, rate, and regularity.

Sinus rhythms originate in the sinoatrial (SA) node. Normal sinus rhythm is a rate of 60 to 100 bpm. Sinus tachycardia is a sinus rhythm with a rate of greater than 100 bpm. Sinus bradycardia is a sinus rhythm with a rate of less than 60 bpm.

Atrial rhythms are caused by pacemaker cells other than the SA node firing somewhere within the atria. Atrial dysrhythmias include premature atrial contractions (PACs), atrial fibrillation (AF), and atrial flutter (AFL).

Supraventricular tachycardia (SVT) is an umbrella term to capture narrow-complex tachycardias, such as sinus tachycardia, atrial tachycardia, junctional tachycardia, atrial fibrillation greater than 100 bpm, and AFL greater than 100 bpm.

Junctional rhythms begin within the atrioventricular (AV) node. Examples of junctional rhythms include premature junctional contractions, junctional rhythm, accelerated junctional rhythm, and junctional tachycardia.

Ventricular rhythms are those rhythms that originate somewhere within the ventricles. Examples include premature ventricular contractions (PVCs), ventricular tachycardia (VT) with a pulse, pulseless VT, and ventricular fibrillation (VF). Both pulseless VT and VF are lethal rhythms that require immediate treatment—immediate initiation of compressions and defibrillation within 2 to 3 minutes. Idioventricular rhythm occurs when the SA and AV nodes fail to function, which triggers the ventricles to generate an electrical impulse.

Asystole occurs when there is no electrical impulse from the heart, producing a flat line on the monitor. Treat immediately with chest compressions and epinephrine and determine the cause. Heart blocks are caused by delaying or blocking electrical conduction at the AV node. There are four types of blocks: first-degree AV block, second-degree type I (or Wenckebach or Mobitz I), second-degree type II (or Mobitz II), and third-degree heart blocks or complete heart block.

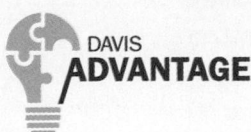

DAVIS
ADVANTAGE | To explore learning resources for this chapter, go to **Davis Advantage** and find:
– Answers to in-text questions
– Chapter Resources and Activities
– NCLEX®-Style Chapter Review Questions
– Bibliography

Chapter 30

Coordinating Care for Patients With Cardiac Disorders

Sherri Ulbrich

LEARNING OUTCOMES

Content in this chapter is designed to assist in:

1. Describing the epidemiology of cardiac disorders
2. Correlating clinical manifestations to pathophysiological processes of:
   a. Coronary artery disease
   b. Infectious endocarditis
   c. Myocarditis
   d. Pericarditis
   e. Valvular disease
   f. Heart failure
3. Describing the diagnostic results used to confirm the diagnosis of cardiac disorders
4. Discussing the medical management of:
   a. Coronary artery disease
   b. Infectious endocarditis
   c. Myocarditis
   d. Pericarditis
   e. Valvular disease
   f. Heart failure
5. Developing a comprehensive plan of nursing care for patients with cardiac disorders
6. Designing a teaching plan that includes pharmacological, dietary, and lifestyle considerations for patients with cardiac disorders

CONCEPTS

- Assessment
- Infection
- Inflammation
- Oxygenation
- Perfusion

ESSENTIAL TERMS

Acute coronary syndrome
Angina
Aortic stenosis
Atherosclerosis
Cardiac rehabilitation
Compensatory mechanism
Coronary artery bypass graft (CABG)
Coronary artery disease (CAD)
Ejection fraction
Embolization
Exercise stress test
Friction rub
Heart failure
Infective endocarditis
Ischemia
Murmur
Myocardial tissue
Myocarditis
Percutaneous transluminal coronary angioplasty (PTCA)
Pericardial effusion
Pericardiocentesis
Pericarditis
Prinzmetal's/variant angina
Pulmonary edema
Orthopnea
Regurgitation
Stable angina
Stenosis
Tamponade
Transcatheter aortic valve replacement
Unstable angina

Finding Connections

CASE STUDY: EPISODE 1

Follow this patient throughout the chapter.

Mr. Walter Thompson is a 57-year-old man with no significant past medical history except high blood pressure. He admits to being nonadherent with his meds because "I feel okay." He reports he was in his usual state of health until about 3 weeks ago. At that point, he reports feeling short of breath and fatigued unrelated to physical activity. Over the past 3 weeks, his symptoms have progressed to the point where he sleeps in his recliner every night. He is admitted to the step-down unit for further management…

CORONARY ARTERY DISEASE

Epidemiology

Coronary artery disease (CAD) affects an estimated 16.5 million people over the age of 20 and occurs when the blood vessels that deliver oxygen-rich blood to the heart muscle become obstructed or dysfunctional. It is also known as coronary heart disease or ischemic heart disease. The incidence increases with age for all people; however, there are racial and gender differences. According to the American Heart Association (AHA), the prevalence of CAD was higher in Caucasian males than in African and Hispanic American males (7.7%, 7.1%, and 5.9%, respectively). Among females, Hispanic women had the highest prevalence rate of 6.1%, followed by African American females at 5.7% and Caucasian females at 5.3%. The prevalence in American Indians and Native Alaskans is estimated to be highest of all groups at 9.3%. Studies have shown that postmenopausal women are three times more likely to have clinical symptoms of CAD than women of the same age who are premenopausal. This evidence suggests estrogen may be cardioprotective.

A newer diagnosis of nonobstructive coronary artery disease is becoming better understood and more frequently identified in patients. Although both diseases, obstructive and nonobstructive, can occur in both genders, men tend to have more obstructive disease, and women have nearly double the incidence of nonobstructive disease.

Risk factors are classified as modifiable or nonmodifiable. Modifiable risk factors are amenable to intervention. Nonmodifiable factors are inherent risk factors that are not amenable to intervention. Nonmodifiable risk factors include gender, race, heredity, and age. Men of all ages have a higher risk of heart disease than women. Risk increases with a family history of CAD and aging. Modifiable risk factors include increased total cholesterol, hypertension, diabetes, obesity, smoking, and physical inactivity. Stress and excessive alcohol consumption can also contribute to CAD risk. The risk factors for CAD are summarized in Table 30.1.

Pathophysiology

Traditionally, coronary artery disease is characterized by the obstruction of blood flow within the coronary arteries. **Atherosclerosis**, or plaque within the lumen of the vessels, is the principal cause of obstruction to blood flow. The arterial wall is made up of three layers: the tunica intima, tunica media, and tunica adventitia (Fig. 30.1).

The tunica intima is composed of endothelium and basement membrane. It has been suggested that atherosclerosis begins with an injury to the endothelium that causes an inflammatory response. That inflammatory response initiates a series of specific cellular and molecular reactions that lead to the accumulation of atherosclerotic plaque. Low-density lipoprotein (LDL) enters the tunica intima layer of the arterial wall and becomes trapped. Inside the tunica intima, the trapped LDL is modified through the process of oxidation. Once modified, the LDL attracts macrophages, which absorb the LDL to become foam cells. Fatty streaks within the tunica intima are an accumulation of foam cells. As the process continues, various components in the blood, such as macrophages, calcium, and cholesterol, adhere to the injured part of the vessel, forming plaque. The plaque deposits increase in size over time, causing narrowing of the coronary arteries, which impedes oxygen-rich blood flow to the heart (Fig. 30.2). When the heart muscle does not get enough oxygen and nutrients to meet its demands, myocardial **ischemia** results. This pathology is known as obstructive coronary artery disease.

The next and most dangerous step in the development of atherosclerosis is potential plaque rupture. When that occurs, platelets aggregate on the ruptured plaque surface.

Table 30.1 Risk Factors for the Development of Coronary Artery Disease	
Modifiable	**Nonmodifiable**
• Cigarette smoking	• Gender
• High total cholesterol, high LDL level, low HDL levels, and high triglycerides	• Race
• Hypertension	• Age older than 45 for men
• Diabetes	• Genetics/family history
• Obesity, particularly central obesity	• Being postmenopausal
• Sedentary lifestyle/physical inactivity	
• Stress	
• Excessive alcohol consumption	

HDL, High-density lipoprotein; *LDL,* low-density lipoprotein.

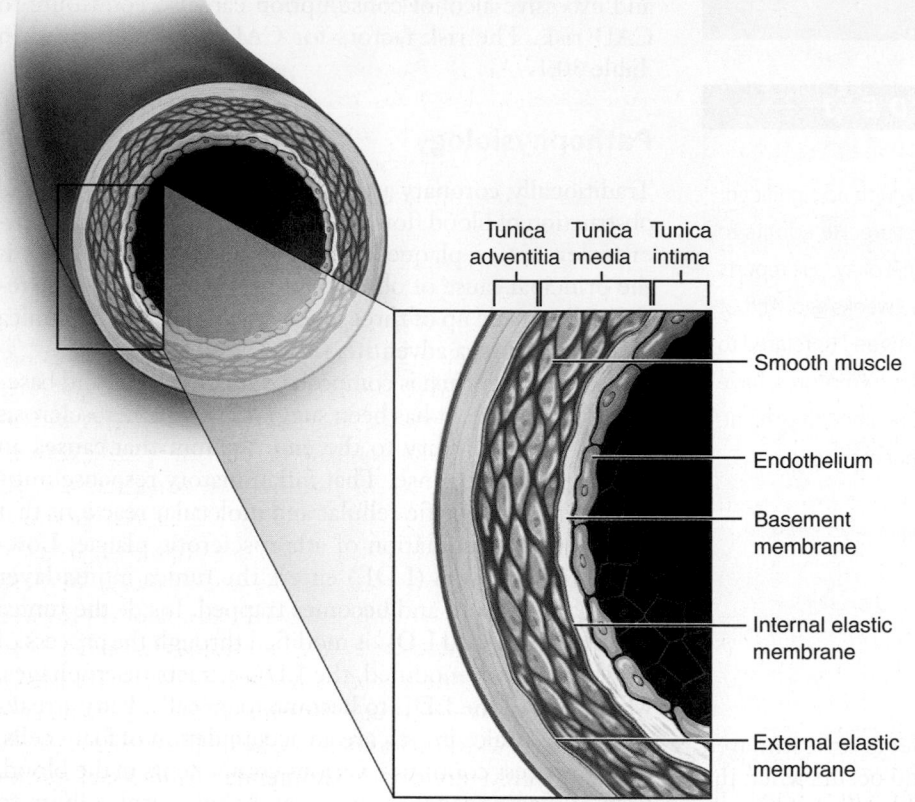

Tunica adventitia | Tunica media | Tunica intima

Smooth muscle

Endothelium

Basement membrane

Internal elastic membrane

External elastic membrane

FIGURE 30.1 Layers of the arterial wall.

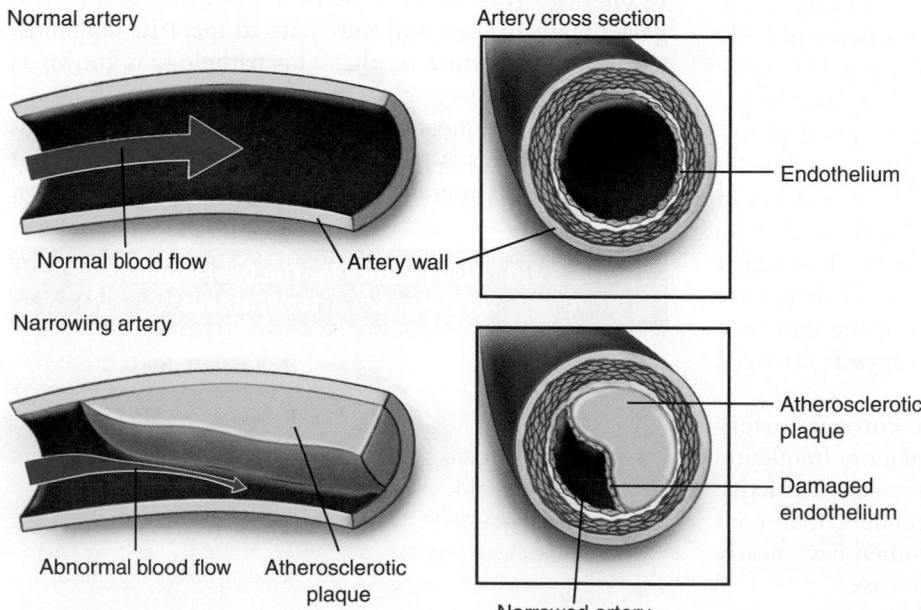

Normal artery

Normal blood flow | Artery wall

Narrowing artery

Abnormal blood flow | Atherosclerotic plaque

Artery cross section

Endothelium

Atherosclerotic plaque

Damaged endothelium

Narrowed artery

FIGURE 30.2 A comparison of a normal artery with an artery narrowed by atherosclerotic plaque deposits on the wall.

The coagulation cascade is initiated, and thrombus formation is stimulated. This clotting further decreases or obstructs blood flow altogether, leading to unstable angina, myocardial infarction (MI), or sudden cardiac death.

In nonobstructive coronary artery disease, patients have symptoms similar to obstructive coronary artery disease, but they do not have significant plaque that occludes the coronary arteries. Rather, ischemic symptoms are caused by reduced blood flow through the coronary microvascular system. In such cases, the microvascular system is not able to dilate in response to the myocardial demand for oxygen or may have stenosis.

Clinical Manifestations

The clinical manifestations of CAD are virtually silent until the artery is approximately 40% blocked by plaque in obstructive disease. Ischemia develops when there is an imbalance between supply and demand of oxygen-rich blood to the heart tissue, resulting in insufficient oxygen to meet the demands of the **myocardial tissue**. Infarction, or cell death, occurs when that imbalance is severe or prolonged, which causes irreversible damage. The primary patient complaint is chest pain, also called **angina**. Angina is classified into two categories, stable and unstable angina.

Stable angina is chest pain or discomfort that is associated with physical activity. It is typically linked to fixed plaque formations and is predictable. Symptoms of stable angina are often alleviated with rest and/or medications. Nitrates such as nitroglycerin that dilate the coronary arteries, improving oxygen-rich blood flow to the heart, are typically prescribed for angina.

Unstable angina refers to chest pain that can occur at rest. Of the two types of angina, unstable angina is the most concerning. It is identified as the initial phase of **acute coronary syndrome** (ACS) and is defined as a disorder caused by an acute decrease in blood flow through the coronaries to the myocardial tissue. It can be a precursor to MI and should be treated as an emergency. Unstable angina is usually prolonged and may not be relieved with rest or medication.

A variation of unstable angina is **Prinzmetal's, or variant, angina**. The blockage of blood flow in this disorder is caused by coronary artery spasm rather than plaque formation, but atherosclerotic changes are commonly present. It typically occurs at rest and in clusters. Interestingly, it normally occurs at night between midnight and 8 a.m.

Angina may radiate to the left arm, back, neck and jaw. Additional symptoms may accompany angina such as chest pressure, shortness of breath or dyspnea, fatigue, nausea, vomiting, diaphoresis, weakness, syncope, and epigastric discomfort. Men are more likely to present with classic exertional chest pain, whereas women are more likely to complain of atypical chest pain not associated with exertion. Women are also more likely to report fatigue, weakness, nausea, and dyspnea. Patients with diabetes also do not consistently present with chest pain, often having no signs and symptoms of CAD.

It is important to note that not all chest pain is caused by cardiac ischemia. Nonischemic causes can be aortic dissection, pericarditis, gallbladder disease, pleuritic pain, pulmonary embolism, pneumonia, and gastroesophageal reflux disease.

Management

Medical Management
Diagnosis

As stated previously, the formation of plaque within the blood vessels is a silent process. Often CAD is suspected only when the individual presents with clinical symptoms. The diagnosis is made on the basis of clinical presentation and diagnostic findings. Timely recognition of ischemia related to CAD is essential for prompt treatment and improved patient outcomes, particularly in cases where CAD has progressed to acute coronary syndrome or myocardial infarction. Delays in diagnosis can result in more myocardial damage from ischemia. When time is muscle, every minute counts.

Diagnostic Tests

Many of the blood tests performed assess for the presence of risk factors for CAD development, such as lipid profiles, inflammation, and coagulation studies. Lipid profiles evaluate total cholesterol and triglyceride levels as well as LDL and high-density lipoprotein (HDL). Specific cardiac biomarkers are used to rule out MI. Creatine kinase (CK) or creatine kinase–muscle/brain (CK-MB) and troponin (I or T) levels rise when myocardial injury occurs and are used to identify when ischemia has led to tissue damage. Because these biomarkers do not immediately rise with chest pain, they are measured every 6 hours after admission to the hospital to evaluate chest pain. This is known as serial cardiac enzyme or biomarker testing. Although most acute care facilities use both biomarkers, hospitals are increasingly using troponin alone as recommended in national guidelines. Recent evidence suggests that women may have a lower troponin threshold, which may be contributing to underdiagnosis of MI and worse outcomes. Laboratory tests diagnostic for CAD are summarized in Table 28.3 in Chapter 28.

An electrocardiogram (ECG) is often the initial test when CAD is suspected. During anginal episodes or symptoms of ACS, the ECG may show ST segment depression of greater than 0.5 mm or flat or inverted T waves that are indicative of ischemia. These changes return to normal when chest pain is relieved. It is important to note that ischemia in some patients may be electrically silent, with an ECG that appears normal. Serial ECGs may be done with cardiac biomarkers to rule out an infarction. If cardiac biomarkers and ECGs are normal, a patient may then undergo an **exercise stress test**. This is done to assess the function of the heart during exercise. Alternatively, for those who are unable to use a treadmill or stationary bicycle, pharmacological agents such as dobutamine can be used to increase heart rate, mimicking the effects of exercise on the heart. Stress echocardiograms are another option. Stress testing can be combined with nuclear imaging, such as thallium or technetium studies, to further evaluate perfusion to the heart. The goals of the stress test are (a) to determine whether there is reduced oxygen-rich blood flow to the heart tissue during physical activity and (b) to determine what parts of the heart are affected by the decreased blood flow. Descriptions of these tests can be found in Chapter 28.

The gold standard for diagnosing CAD is coronary angiography, a left-sided cardiac catheterization with the purpose of evaluating the coronary arteries for blockage.

This is performed to determine the location of the plaque within the coronary circulation, the degree of occlusion, and whether the area can be treated with percutaneous transluminal coronary angioplasty. The lack of major plaque limits the diagnostic value of this test in patients with nonobstructive CAD. Coronary computed tomography (CT) angiography, magnetic resonance angiography, and stress imaging techniques can be useful instead.

Treatment

Medications for patients with CAD are often prescribed with the goals of (a) stopping the aggregation of blood components to the injured endothelium, (b) controlling factors that led to damage of the endothelium, and (c) relieving symptoms (Table 30.2). Patients with stable angina at low risk for ACS are often prescribed aspirin and nitroglycerin along with medications to reduce risk factors, such as antihypertensives, antidiabetic agents, and cholesterol-lowering

Table 30.2 Medication Management for Patients With Coronary Artery Disease

Class of Medication	Mechanism of Action
Statins Examples: atorvastatin (Lipitor), simvastatin (Zocor)	Statins reduce total cholesterol when used for an extended period. Statins reduce cholesterol synthesis in the liver and increase clearance of LDL from the blood.
	This group of medications is contraindicated in patients with active liver disease or during pregnancy because of the possibility of causing muscle myopathies and marked decreases in liver function.
PCSK9 inhibitors Example: evolocumab (Repatha)	Increases LDL breakdown to reduce cholesterol level
	Available only as an injectable
Cholesterol absorption inhibitors Example: ezetimibe (Zetia)	Inhibits the absorption of cholesterol through the small intestine
Fibric acids Examples: gemfibrozil (Lopid)	Reduces cholesterol production and removes LDL cholesterol by reducing the liver's production of VLDLs and by speeding the clearance of triglycerides from the blood
	Should not be initiated in patients on statin therapy because of an increased risk for muscle symptoms or rhabdomyolysis
Nicotinic acid Example: niacin (Niaspan)	Reduces the production of triglycerides and VLDL and increases HDL levels
	Baseline hepatic transaminases, fasting blood glucose, and uric acid should be obtained before initiation and again during up-titration. Repeat labs every 6 months.
Bile acid sequestrants Example: cholestyramine (Questran)	Converts more cholesterol into bile acids, which are excreted in stool, thereby lowering cholesterol
	Usually used in combination with statin therapy, resulting in a further 10%–25% decrease in LDL levels
	Should not be used in individuals with baseline fasting triglyceride levels ≥300 mg/dL because severe triglyceride elevations can occur
Anticoagulants Examples: enoxaparin (Lovenox), heparin, bivalirudin (Angiomax), ticagrelor (Brilinta)	Prevents intracoronary thrombosis in patients who are hospitalized with ACS
Antiplatelet agents Examples: aspirin (Bayer aspirin, Ecotrin), clopidogrel (Plavix)	Inhibits platelet aggregation to prevent clot development

Table 30.2 Medication Management for Patients With Coronary Artery Disease—cont'd

Class of Medication	Mechanism of Action
Beta blockers Example: metoprolol (Lopressor, Toprol XL)	Inhibits the sympathetic nervous system response to physical activity, which decreases cardiac workload and oxygen consumption
ACE inhibitors and ARBs Examples: lisinopril (Zestril), losartan (Cozaar)	Reduces blood pressure, which decreases workload and oxygen demands Particularly beneficial in patient with HTN, diabetes, renal disease, and heart failure
Calcium channel blockers Examples: nifedipine (Adalat, Procardia), amlodipine (Norvasc)	Used when patients cannot tolerate beta blockers or in patients with HF Lowers blood pressure and increases blood flow through the coronaries Also prevents coronary artery spasms in Prinzmetal's/variant angina
Vasodilators Example: nitroglycerin (Tridil, Nitrostat)	Dilates coronary arteries to improve blood flow and oxygen supply to the myocardial cells Can also be given to reduce afterload See Medication Safety Alert for additional information on administration of nitroglycerin for chest pain and contraindications.

ACE, Angiotensin-converting enzyme; *ACS,* acute coronary syndrome; *ARB,* angiotensin II receptor blocker; *HDL,* high-density lipoprotein; *HF,* heart failure; *HTN,* hypertension; *LDL,* low-density lipoprotein; *VLDL,* very low-density lipoprotein.

medications. Aspirin prevents thrombus formation in the coronary artery. Nitroglycerin, a vasodilator, is used to manage anginal episodes, both at home and in the hospital. Nitroglycerin can be administered as sublingual tabs, as a spray or powder, intravenously, through transdermal patches, as an ointment, and by mouth with extended-release capsules. During anginal episodes, the sublingual and IV routes are preferred to restore blood flow promptly. Blood pressure should be monitored carefully due to the adverse effect of hypotension. Headaches can also occur and are best treated with nonopioid analgesics such as acetaminophen. Treatment of ACS in the acute care setting includes aspirin, supplemental oxygen, nitroglycerin, and morphine and can be referred to by the acronym MONA. Morphine can be given for angina pain in patients not responsive to nitroglycerin, but its use can be associated with hypotension, nausea, and vomiting. Beta blockers, additional anticoagulants, and possibly calcium channel blockers are also prescribed in ACS management. Treatment for nonobstructive CAD is being studied. Statins, angiotensin-converting enzyme (ACE) inhibitors, and beta blockers may be beneficial.

> ⓘ **Safety Alert** **Medication Safety Alert: Nitroglycerin**
>
> Nitroglycerin is an effective treatment for angina. Patients should be instructed to take this medication as prescribed,
>
> typically one tablet or spray under the tongue not to exceed three doses taken 5 minutes apart. If the symptom of angina (chest pain) is not relieved with three doses or if the pain worsens, they should be instructed to call emergency personnel. In addition, patients using medications such as sildenafil citrate (i.e., Revatio, Viagra) should be educated on the increased risk of hypotension with coadministration with nitroglycerin.

Percutaneous transluminal coronary angioplasty (PTCA) is the procedure most commonly performed to relieve symptoms caused by atherosclerotic changes in the coronary vessels. During this procedure, after the patient receives monitored anesthesia care (MAC), a catheter with a small balloon on its tip is advanced under fluoroscopy through a suitable artery, commonly the femoral or radial, to the area with atherosclerotic plaque. The balloon is inflated and deflated to open the lumen of the artery. During this time, patients may experience chest pain due to vessel occlusion. Once the lumen is open, a stent may be advanced to the location to hold the artery open and maintain adequate blood flow. Stent options include bare metal stents (BMS), drug-eluting stents (DES) to prevent clots, or the newer bioabsorbable stents. Patients frequently return from the procedure with a vascular closure device, such as an angioseal, applied to the access site to maintain hemostasis. This allows early ambulation. If no closure device is applied, strict bedrest for 6 to 8 hours is required until hemostasis is achieved. Figure 30.3 illustrates stent placement within the artery. Bleeding at the insertion site, abrupt vessel closure, dysrhythmias, and ruptured arteries are uncommon but potential complications from PTCA (see Genetic Connections: Pharmacogenetics and Anticoagulants). Care of the patient receiving a PTCA is outlined in Chapter 28.

Genetic Connections

Pharmacogenetics and Anticoagulants

Anticoagulants such as warfarin or clopidogrel are prescribed after percutaneous transluminal coronary angioplasty (PTCA). Patient responses to standard doses can vary greatly. Some patients need very low doses to reach therapeutic levels, whereas others require very high doses. Pharmacogenetics is the study of how a person's genes affect responses to medications. With scientific advances, genetic testing can now be used to determine responsiveness. In the case of warfarin, some patients are genetically fast metabolizers, which can result in an increased risk of clotting and the need for higher or more frequent doses. In contrast, slow metabolizers have an increased risk of bleeding and require lower or less frequent doses. Patients who are fast or slow metabolizers may also respond similarly to other types of medications. Pharmacogenetic testing is not widely used due to availability, clinician knowledge, and regulatory and reimbursement issues but may be valuable.

A more invasive surgical treatment is **coronary artery bypass grafting** (CABG). With CABG, blockages in coronary arteries are bypassed using other arteries from the chest or arm or veins from the legs. In the traditional CABG, patients undergo general anesthesia. A large incision through the sternum is made, and a cardiopulmonary bypass (CPB) is begun through large catheters in the vena cava or right atrium and aorta. A CPB provides continuous gas exchange and perfusion while the heart is stopped to provide a still, bloodless field for surgery. Then arteries or veins being used as bypasses are surgically attached to the diseased coronary artery, creating an alternate path for blood to flow around the blockage. Common vessels used are the internal thoracic (mammary) and saphenous vein. Bypasses made from arteries have greater longevity, but more bypasses can be made with saphenous veins, which require an additional incision in the leg. Multiple blockages may be bypassed in the same surgery. For example, a patient

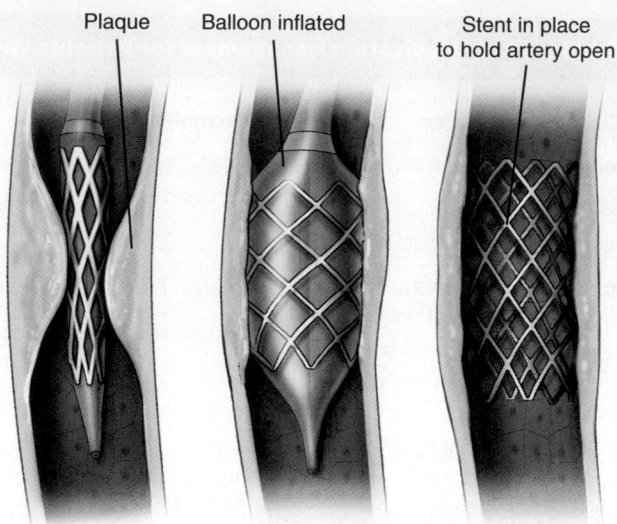

FIGURE 30.3 Stent placement within the artery. Step 1: A catheter with a small balloon on its tip is advanced to the area with atherosclerotic plaque. Step 2: The balloon is inflated and deflated to open the lumen of the artery. Step 3: The stent is advanced to hold the artery open and maintain adequate blood flow.

with four large coronary artery blockages would undergo a quadruple bypass.

Minimally invasive coronary surgery (MICS CABG) may be an alternative to CABG. MICS CABG involves a left chest incision and multiple smaller incisions that act as ports for instruments. A CBP is used, and multiple vessels can be bypassed. Minimally invasive direct coronary artery bypass (MIDCAB) is an option for some patients, in which incisions similar to those in MICS CABG are made. A pressor device placed through the chest incision immobilizes a part of the heart while the internal thoracic artery is used to bypass a single blockage. A similar procedure through a sternotomy incision allows for additional vessels to be bypassed. Because both procedures do not require a CPB, they are called off-pump or "beating heart surgery." Potential advantages of all these procedures include faster recovery times and fewer complications.

Patients who undergo CABG are sent to a critical care unit for intensive monitoring and care. Multiple hemodynamic monitoring catheters, chest tubes, an endotracheal tube, mechanical ventilation, a nasogastric tube, an indwelling bladder catheter, and a temporary pacemaker wire may all be needed postoperatively. Nursing care of the patient undergoing CABG is described in Chapter 32.

The decision between PTCA and CABG is made by the healthcare team and patient based on degree of disease, surgical risk, hemodynamic stability, and symptom severity. Other, less common invasive treatment strategies, such as atherectomy and transmyocardial laser revascularization (TMLR), may be performed in patients meeting limited criteria. During an atherectomy, plaque within the coronary artery is shaved and removed through a specialized catheter during cardiac catheterization. In TMLR, a patient's heart is surgically exposed, and a laser is used to create 20 to 40 tiny channels from the outside of the left ventricle to the chamber within. The outside openings are closed by clots, but the channels stay open on the inside. The procedure is also thought to stimulate angiogenesis; the formation of new blood vessels from pre-existing vessels.

Lifestyle Management

Diet and physical activity play an important role in the treatment of CAD and its risk factors of hypertension, hyperlipidemia, diabetes, and obesity (see Genetic Connections: Healthy Lifestyle Counters Genetic Risk). Maintaining a healthy body weight or a body-mass index (BMI) of less than 30 kg/m² is critical in the management of CAD. A diet that is low in saturated fat and sodium as well as high in fruits, whole grains, and vegetables and considers personal and cultural preferences should be discussed. Engaging in regular moderate-intensity physical activity at least 30 minutes a day, 5 days a week is recommended. Smoking cessation and avoiding exposure to smoking should be encouraged. Screening and treatment for depression can reduce ischemic events and improve quality of life in patients with CAD. Refraining from excessive alcohol use may reduce CAD risk. Patients with ACS, especially after PCI or CABG, should be referred and encouraged to participate in a comprehensive cardiac rehabilitation program. **Cardiac rehabilitation** is a supervised program of education, counseling, and supervised physical activity. Ideally, cardiac rehab begins before discharge and continues in the outpatient setting. Participation can improve morbidity and mortality, reduce angina episodes, and decrease rehospitalizations.

Genetic Connections

Healthy Lifestyle Counters Genetic Risk

Genetic and lifestyle factors are independent risks for coronary artery disease (CAD). However, in a study of over 55,000 participants, those persons at highest genetic risk for CAD reduced this risk by nearly 50% with healthy lifestyles. Healthy lifestyles included not smoking, not being obese, regular physical activity, and a healthy diet.

Complications

The primary complication of CAD is ACS, which includes unstable angina and MI. Myocardial infarction is discussed in detail in Chapter 32. Coronary artery disease may also result in dysrhythmias and heart failure. Women tend to have higher rates of adverse outcomes from CAD in general. These outcome differences have been attributed to limits in the diagnosis and treatment in nonobstructive CAD, particularly because most major diagnostic tests and treatments are focused on obstructive CAD. Gender bias in treatment has also been implicated in the higher number of adverse events in women.

Connection Check 30.1

After a percutaneous coronary angioplasty, what assessment should most concern the nurse?
A. Back discomfort
B. Chest pain
C. Capillary refill of less than 3 seconds
D. Hypoactive bowel sounds

Nursing Management
Assessment and Analysis

Careful assessment of chest pain and other manifestations of CAD is required to identify those patients with CAD and those patients who have stable angina that may be progressing to ACS. The clinical manifestations of CAD are the result of the imbalance of oxygen supply and demand to the myocardial tissue. The most common symptom is chest pain. Other, more nonspecific symptoms include:

- Epigastric discomfort
- Nausea and vomiting
- Diaphoresis
- Syncope
- Shortness of breath (SOB)
- Pain between shoulders/jawline

Nursing Diagnosis

- **Decreased tissue perfusion** related to inadequate blood flow secondary to the presence of plaque within the coronary arteries or microvascular dysfunction

Nursing Interventions
■ *Assessments*

- Vital signs
  Tachycardia and tachypnea can be manifestations of cardiac ischemia. Hypertension is a CAD risk factor. Nitroglycerin and morphine administration can result in hypotension.
- Pain assessment utilizing provoking factors, quality, region/radiation, severity, time (PQRST)
  Angina can be nonspecific in some patients; establishing location and quality can aid in the diagnosis of cardiac chest pain and disease progression. Headache can result from nitroglycerin administration.
- Electrocardiogram and continuous cardiac monitoring
  Depressed ST segment or flat or inverted T waves are indicative of ischemia; ST elevations are indicative of acute injury. Cardiac dysrhythmias may result from ischemia or infarction.
- Physical assessment
  Pallor, clamminess, nausea, vomiting, shortness of breath, and diaphoresis may indicate cardiac ischemia. Xanthomas are associated with hypercholesterolemia.
- Patient history
  Evaluate CAD risk factors and anginal patterns. Fatigue and weakness may be indicative of CAD. Identify potential noncardiac causes of chest pain, such as gastroesophageal reflux or respiratory disorders.

- Recreational drug use
  Illicit drug use (i.e., cocaine) can cause vasospasm, obstructing blood flow and causing symptoms that resemble CAD.
- Depression screening
  Depression may increase morbidity and mortality.
- Laboratory values
  - Cardiac biomarkers: troponin, CK/CK-MB
    Cardiac enzymes and troponin levels rise when the heart sustains an acute injury—can help differentiate between angina and MI pain.
  - Creatinine, blood urea nitrogen
    Assess renal function. The contrast dye used during heart catheterization is nephrotoxic.
  - Glycosylated hemoglobin (HgbA1c)
    Hyperglycemia occurs with diabetes and is a risk factor for CAD.
  - Lipid profiles: cholesterol, triglycerides, LDL, HDL
    Assess for hyperlipidemia, a risk factor for CAD development.

▪ Actions

- Administer oxygen to keep oxygen saturation greater than 93%.
  Supplemental oxygen optimizes oxygen delivery to the myocardium. Cardiac dysrhythmias, especially tachycardia, and anxiety increase myocardial oxygen consumption.
- Obtain ECG with the occurrence of chest pain.
  Evaluates new anginal episode for evidence of ischemia or injury. In cases of acute chest pain, an ECG within 10 minutes is recommended.
- Administer nitroglycerin as ordered.
  Dilates the coronary arteries to improve flow to the heart and relieve pain
- Administer aspirin as ordered.
  Prevents platelet aggregation
- Administer morphine as ordered if nitroglycerin does not relieve pain.
  Minimizes pain and decreases the workload on the heart. Monitor for adverse effects of hypotension, nausea, vomiting, and respiratory depression.
- Administer beta blockers/calcium channel blockers as ordered.
  Inhibit cardiac response to physical activity, decrease oxygen consumption; may consider holding prior to exercise test
- Administer statin medications as ordered.
  Reduce cholesterol level and decrease the risk of increased plaque formation

▪ Actions After PCI

- Perform cardiac catheterization care as described in Chapter 28.
- Report and treat chest pain immediately.
  Reocclusion, vasospasm, or stenosis can result in ischemia and requires prompt intervention.
- Administer additional anticoagulants.
  Prevents vessel occlusion by thrombus

- Maintain fluids through catheterization sheaths if left in place.
  Allows for immediate coronary access if return to catheterization lab is needed
- Maintaining bedrest and compression devices at the catheter insertion site.
  Promotes hemostasis and prevents bleeding

▪ Teaching

- Medication regimen
  Medication adherence lowers mortality and risk of hospitalization and MI.
- Angina management
  If angina occurs during activity, stop activity and rest. Take dose of nitroglycerin. Tabs can cause tingling or taste bitter when placed under the tongue. Not to exceed three doses 5 minutes apart. Caution patient about the use of the medication in the setting of light-headedness or dizziness because this can be indicative of hypotension. See Medication Safety Alert for more information.
- Bleeding precautions if on anticoagulants
  Avoiding activities that have high injury or fall risk, using a soft toothbrush and electric razor, and using caution with sharp objects reduces bleeding risk.
- Risk factor reduction strategies: physical activity, blood pressure management, healthy diet/weight loss, smoking cessation, decreased alcohol consumption, control of glucose
  Risk factor reduction can prevent primary disease and limits the progression of CAD.
- When to call providers or emergency services
  Unrelieved chest pain—chest pain at rest requires early intervention.
  For PCI patients: uncontrolled bleeding, swelling, redness, purulent discharge, and pain at insertion site or fever need prompt treatment.
- Encourage participation in cardiac rehabilitation for ACS patients after PCI or CABG.
  Reduces morbidity and mortality

Evaluating Care Outcomes

Patients with CAD can achieve optimal functional status by complying with prescribed medical therapy, maintaining a healthy diet, limiting alcohol, and engaging in regular exercise. Achieving desired activity levels and meeting self-care needs with minimal or no pain indicate achievement of care goals in this patient population. It is important that the patient understands the disease process, the medications used to treat it, and when to call 911.

INFECTIVE ENDOCARDITIS

Epidemiology

The exact prevalence of **infective endocarditis** (IE) is unknown; however, it is estimated that approximately 47,000 cases occur each year, and the number of cases has steadily risen since 2000. Infective endocarditis can be classified as native or prosthetic or as right or left sided. It most frequently affects the native mitral or aortic valves. The pulmonic valve is the least frequently affected. Individuals who abuse IV drugs tend to have right-sided or tricuspid valve infections.

Risk factors for IE include age (greater than 60), immunodeficiency, IV drug use, diabetes mellitus, the presence of prosthetic heart valves, prior history of endocarditis, congenital or structural heart disease, and the presence of an intravascular access or an implanted cardiac device. Recent studies have indicated others at risk of developing IE are persons with poor oral hygiene or periodontal disease, patients on hemodialysis, and patients with frequent exposures to the healthcare system or invasive procedures. Rheumatic heart disease is also considered a risk factor, but a sharp decline in the incidence in developed countries has lessened its impact. Mortality from IE is high, ranging from 20% to 40% of cases.

Connection Check 30.2

The nurse determines which patient is at greatest risk for developing IE?

A. A 22-year-old student undergoing a dental procedure

B. A 35-year-old man with a past medical history of IV drug use

C. A 65-year-old male heart transplant patient on immunosuppressive therapy undergoing a colonoscopy

D. A 70-year-old female with heart failure with an intravascular access device for home infusion

Pathophysiology

Infective endocarditis is defined as an infection of the innermost layer of the heart, the endocardium, most typically affecting the heart valves. Infective endocarditis begins with damage to the endocardial lining of the heart, which can occur as a result of turbulent blood flow. Turbulent blood flow is often caused by valve dysfunction. Platelet and fibrin deposit onto the injured area, forming what is known as a *nonbacterial thrombotic endocardial lesion*. Microorganisms introduced into the bloodstream through patient exposures circulate and can become trapped under the layers of platelet and fibrin deposits. These microorganisms and deposits grow into clumps known as *vegetation*. This vegetation can severely damage the valves of the heart (Fig. 30.4).

The etiology of IE is generally of bacterial origin, although other pathogens have been reported. The most common causative microorganisms are *Staphylococcus aureus* and *Streptococcus*. Infective endocarditis can also be caused by other bacteria, viruses, and fungi. The source of exposure to microorganisms in the blood has been historically linked to dental and other invasive procedures. However, it has been suggested that repeated exposures to microorganisms are more likely to cause IE than random exposure during a single dental or other invasive procedure.

Clinical Manifestations

Clinical manifestations of IE include red, painful nodes in the pads of the fingers and toes—Osler's nodes—and red, painless spots on the palms and soles, called *Janeway lesions*. *Splinter hemorrhages*, tiny blood clots that run vertically under nails, may also be present. Most patients have a heart **murmur**, the sound heard when there is

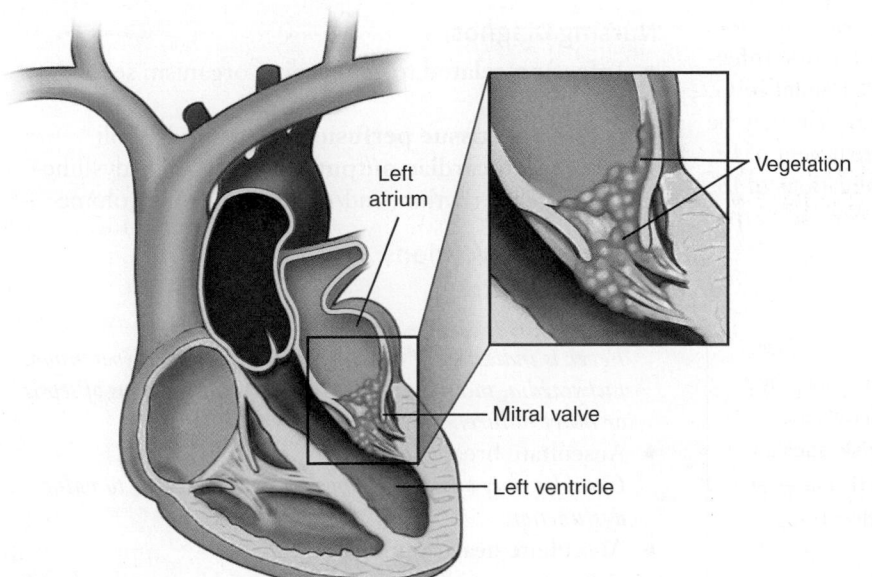

Left atrium

Vegetation

Mitral valve

Left ventricle

FIGURE 30.4 Mitral valve vegetation in infective endocarditis.

turbulent blood flow across a heart valve. They can also experience heart failure (HF), arrhythmias, weight loss, or night sweats. Other symptoms are similar to those of any infectious process, which include:

- Fever
- Fatigue
- Confusion (in older adults)

Management

Medical Management

Diagnosis

Diagnostic Tests

Tests used to confirm the diagnosis of IE are blood cultures, two sets from different sites, and transthoracic echocardiogram (TTE) or transesophageal echocardiogram (TEE). Echocardiography can identify valve dysfunction, vegetative growth, abscesses, and changes in heart size and pumping ability that can occur with IE. Echocardiography is described in more detail in Chapter 28. An elevated white blood cell count may also be indicative of infection.

Medications

Medication management consists primarily of IV antibiotic therapy. The increasing trend of microbial resistance has led to the use of combination therapy. The standard duration of treatment is 4 to 6 weeks but may be longer for prosthetic valves. Patients are often discharged to home on IV antimicrobial therapy. Shorter duration is recommended for some combination therapies. Oral antimicrobial agents are rarely used as initial treatment. Repeated blood cultures may be obtained until results are negative, indicative of adequate bactericidal effects. Prophylactic use of oral antibiotics is not routinely recommended but is used for patients at high risk (see Safety Alert).

The choice of antimicrobial agents is complex and based on the organism cultured and the sensitivity report, right-sided versus left-sided IE, native versus prosthetic valve involvement, patient comorbidity, and other factors. Infectious disease specialists are often consulted. Penicillin G, ceftriaxone, vancomycin, nafcillin, and gentamicin may be considered in various combinations for the treatment of IE. Supportive treatment for the common complications of IE, especially HF, is also indicated to optimize cardiac output and tissue perfusion.

> **⚠ Safety Alert** To prevent IE and reduce valvular disease, prophylactic antibiotics are recommended before dental procedures, and meticulous oral hygiene should be encouraged for patients at highest risk, such as those with a history of IE, intracardiac prosthetic material such as valves and defect closure devices, cardiac transplant, and congenital heart disease.

Surgical Management

The surgical treatment options for IE include valve repair or replacement. Surgery can remove infected tissue and reduce mortality and complications, but it also has significant risk. The timing of surgery is controversial, due to a lack of definitive evidence but early surgery is recommended for cases in which antimicrobial therapy has been ineffective in controlling the infection or when complications such as embolic events or heart failure are observed.

Complications

Embolic events are the major complication of IE and occur in 22% to 50% of cases. **Embolization** occurs when fragments of vegetation break free from the valve and travel to other parts of the body through the bloodstream. Embolic events are often a complication of left-sided IE and are rarely seen in right-sided IE. The emboli can travel randomly to any organ or tissue, resulting in obstructed blood flow and potential spreading of infection. Emboli from left-sided IE typically travel to the central nervous system (65%) but can also affect the kidneys, spleen, bowel, and extremities. Emboli traveling to the central nervous system (CNS) cause transient ischemic attacks or strokes. Right-sided IE is associated with pulmonary emboli.

Heart failure and dysrhythmias can also occur due to valvular dysfunction and abscesses in the conduction system. Strokes, heart failure, and dysrhythmias can be a part of the presenting symptoms of IE because they compel patients to seek treatment.

Nursing Management

Assessment and Analysis

The clinical manifestations of IE, such as positive blood cultures combined with fever, fatigue, and the lesions typically seen in the hands and feet, are due to infection. Sepsis can occur in conjunction with IE. Septic emboli can alter CNS and systemic perfusion. The damage to the heart valves can cause a new murmur and heart failure.

Nursing Diagnoses

- **Infection related** to an invading organism secondary to IE
- **Ineffective tissue perfusion** related to emboli
- **Decreased cardiac output** related to valve dysfunction, altered rhythm, and/or altered stroke volume

Nursing Interventions

▪ *Assessments*

- Vital signs
  Fever is indicative of ongoing acute infection. Hypotension, tachycardia, tachypnea, and low SpO_2 can be signs of sepsis or heart failure.
- Auscultate breath sounds.
  Crackles may be a sign of heart failure related to valve dysfunction.
- Auscultate heart sounds.
  A new or worsening murmur may occur due to valve damage.

- Assess neurological function.
  Neurological changes or deficits in pupils, grips, foot pushes, facial droop, and speech may be signs of CNS embolization.
- Assess extremities.
  Cyanosis or pallor, delayed capillary refill, and decreased peripheral pulses may indicate peripheral embolization. Edema could be a sign of heart failure related to valve dysfunction.
- Skin assessment
  Osler's nodes, Janeway lesions, and splinter hemorrhages are indicative of IE.
- Monitor diagnostic test results.
  Repeated culture reports are used to evaluate the effective treatment of IE. White blood cell (WBC) counts can indicate responsiveness to infection. Echocardiograms can evaluate the size of vegetation and valve function and can be used to predict the risk of complications.
- History of drug use, invasive procedures, implanted vascular or cardiac devices, or valve replacement surgery
  Common risk factors for IE

■ Actions

- Administer antibiotics as prescribed.
  Treatment for IE is long-term IV antibiotic treatment.
- Maintain IV access for antibiotic administrations.
  Intravenous access is essential for antibiotic administration. Long-term venous access, such as a peripherally inserted central catheter (PICC), may be considered.
- Administer heart failure medications as needed.
  Heart failure treatment optimizes cardiac output and tissue perfusion.
- Provide social support during prolonged hospitalization.
  Social isolation due to hospitalization may contribute to depression, anxiety, and anger.
- Refer patient to addiction counseling services if drug use has caused the disease.
  Stopping recreational IV drug use may help limit the reoccurrence of IE and lead to a better quality of life.

■ Teaching

- Good oral hygiene utilizing a soft toothbrush
  Bleeding gums provide a portal of entry for bacteria into the bloodstream. Poor dental hygiene may increase the recurrence of IE.
- Inform healthcare provider about IE history prior to any dental or invasive procedure.
  Prophylactic antibiotics may be prescribed to decrease the risk of IE.
- Completion of prolonged antibiotic regimen
  Completing the full course of antibiotics is critical to eradicating the infection and preventing recurrence and complications.

Evaluating Care Outcomes

Goals of care for patients with IE are control of the infectious process through antibiotic administration and minimizing complications. Patient education should focus on risk control, early detection, and prevention. A well-managed patient is free from infection and understands the signs of IE and when the healthcare provider should be contacted. (See Geriatric/Gerontological Considerations: Infective Endocarditis.)

Geriatric/Gerontological Considerations

Infective Endocarditis

Older people are at higher risk for infective endocarditis (IE) due to comorbidities, increasing numbers of invasive procedures, and greater use of implanted cardiac devices such as pacemakers and artificial valves. The required prolonged hospitalization and treatment can contribute to rapid functional decline. Evaluation for early discharge and home infusion therapy should be considered to maintain functional capabilities. An increase in fat mass, reduced renal function, and lower albumin levels require careful antimicrobial adjustments to optimize outcomes and reduce adverse effects. Serum medication levels, renal function, and culture reports should be routinely monitored. Confusion and agitation can challenge the maintenance of continuous IV access. Alternate medication routes may need to be considered. Aging is not a contraindication for surgery, but comorbidities and clinical status should be evaluated.

MYOCARDITIS

Epidemiology

Myocarditis is an inflammatory disease of the myocardium that is most commonly triggered by viral infection or autoimmune diseases. Men and young persons are most affected. It is a leading cause of dilated cardiomyopathy (discussed in Chapter 32) and the third leading cause of cardiac death in young athletes. About 1% to 5% of persons with viral illnesses may exhibit a form of myocarditis.

Pathophysiology

Viruses are the infectious agent in most cases of myocarditis. Coxsackie virus, adenovirus, parvovirus, and herpesvirus are frequent pathogens. Bacteria, parasites, and fungi can be the etiology. Autoimmune hypersensitivity reactions and toxin exposure can also cause myocarditis. Viral infection can directly damage the myocardium, and the patient's own immune responses can cause secondary damage. Myocardial inflammation and injury result, affecting the entire myocardium or localized areas of tissue.

Clinical Manifestations

Myocarditis can be classified as acute, subacute, or chronic. Symptoms vary widely from asymptomatic and mild cases to acute heart failure and cardiogenic shock. Common presenting symptoms are chest pain, dysrhythmias, dyspnea, palpitations, syncope, and heart failure. In the case of viral illness, sequelae such fever, fatigue, loss of appetite, and myalgia may also be experienced.

Management

Medical Management

Diagnosis

Diagnostic Tests

Patient history, C-reactive protein, troponin, brain natriuretic peptide (BNP), ECG, echocardiography, and magnetic resonance imaging (MRI) are used in the diagnostic process. Myocardial biopsy, also called endomyocardial biopsy, is the definitive test but is reserved for more acute cases.

Treatment

Some cases of myocarditis resolve within days, whereas others progress to heart failure and acute dilated cardiomyopathy that require significant intervention, which may include heart transplantation, implanted cardiac defibrillators, or mechanical circulatory support (see Chapter 32). Medical treatment focuses on the management of heart failure, dysrhythmias, and dilated cardiomyopathy. Antiviral immunosuppressants (prednisone and azathioprine) and immunotherapies such as immunoglobulin IgG may be used but have limited evidence of effectiveness.

Complications

Myocarditis is the most frequent cause of dilated cardiomyopathy. Heart failure and dysrhythmias, including sudden cardiac death, especially in young athletes, are also complications.

Nursing Management

Assessment and Analysis

Clinical manifestations of myocarditis, such as SOB, chest pain, fatigue, and dysrhythmias typical of the manifestations of heart failure are due to the weakened or damaged heart muscle.

Nursing Diagnosis

- **Risk for decreased cardiac output** related to myocardial dysfunction

Nursing Interventions

■ *Assessments*

- Vital signs
  Hypotension, hypertension, tachycardia, tachypnea, and hypoxia are signs of heart failure. Fever is indicative of infection.
- Cardiac rhythm
  Dysrhythmias are a common and dangerous clinical manifestation and must be identified and treated promptly.
- Assess for crackles, edema, jugular vein distention (JVD), weight gain, and decreased urine output.
  These are evidence of the weakened heart muscle seen with heart failure.

■ *Actions*

- Administer antivirals, antimicrobials, immunosuppressives, and immunoglobulins as ordered.
  Medications are administered depending on the cause of myocarditis.
- Administer heart failure medications as needed.
  Heart failure is a common manifestation and must be treated to optimize cardiac output and tissue perfusion.
- Provide emotional support.
  The diagnosis of myocarditis can cause fear and anxiety.

■ *Teaching*

- Complete the full medication treatment regime.
  Patients should continue to take medications as directed even if feeling better to ensure an effective/positive result.
- Avoid strenuous activities. Athletes should not participate in competitive sports while inflammation is present and need to be reevaluated in no less than 3 to 6 months before resuming sport.
  Activity restrictions may reduce the risk of sudden cardiac death.

Evaluating Care Outcomes

The primary goal is resolution of the underlying cause and reducing the symptoms of heart failure and risks of cardiomyopathy and sudden cardiac death. A well-managed patient is free of signs of infection and heart failure and is able to tolerate normal activity levels.

PERICARDITIS

Epidemiology

Pericarditis, inflammation of the pericardium, is diagnosed in about 5% of emergency room patients with chest pain not related to ischemia. About 80% of cases are idiopathic (unknown etiology) or are presumed to occur after a viral infection. Acute pericarditis is common following MI, occurring in about 15% to 20% of post-MI patients. The true prevalence of pericarditis is difficult to determine because persons with mild cases (subclinical) do not seek treatment. Some studies show that pericarditis occurs more in men and young and middle-aged persons. Recurrence is common, with 20% to 30% of persons having an additional episode. Pericarditis can be categorized as infectious (viral, bacterial, fungal, or parasitic), noninfectious (autoimmune, neoplastic, metabolic, trauma, and drug related), and idiopathic. Pericarditis can also be described as acute, chronic, or recurrent. The prognosis is generally good, with an in-hospital mortality rate of 1.1%.

Pathophysiology

The heart is surrounded by the two-layered pericardium, which protects the heart, reduces friction with surrounding structures, and helps to determine chamber size and pressure. The tough, fibrous outer wall is the parietal pericardium; the inner is the visceral pericardium, or epicardium. The space between contains approximately 20 to 60 mL of pericardial fluid. This fluid acts as a lubricant to prevent friction between the two layers. When the pericardium becomes inflamed, it is termed *pericarditis* (Fig. 30.5).

Clinical Manifestations

The most common clinical manifestation of pericarditis is pleuritic chest pain. This occurs in 85% to 90% of cases and can be differentiated from MI chest pain because it tends to be relieved by sitting up and leaning forward. **Friction rubs**, scratchy sounds that occur with each heartbeat, may be auscultated in 30% of cases. Box 30.1 describes how to assess for a friction rub. Other clinical manifestations include:

- New or worsening pericardial effusion (60%)
- ECG changes: diffuse ST-segment elevations or PR depression (60%)
- Fever

Management

Medical Management

Diagnosis

Diagnostic Tests

Tests used to diagnose pericarditis include ECG, chest x-ray, echocardiogram (transthoracic or transesophageal), cardiac CT scan, and MRI. The hallmark ECG changes include widespread ST-segment elevation or PR-segment depression (Fig. 30.6).

The finding of cardiomegaly and clear lung fields on chest x-ray may indicate a **pericardial effusion** (fluid buildup in the pericardial sac) and might be supportive of the pericarditis diagnosis. Pericardial effusion might also be evident on an echocardiogram, CT scan, or MRI.

Laboratory tests include serial cardiac biomarkers to rule out MI. Positive blood cultures, a complete blood count with a high WBC count, and positive inflammatory markers such as C-reactive protein or sedimentation rates may indicate the presence of infection or inflammation, leading to the diagnosis of pericarditis when combined with the associated clinical manifestations.

Medications

Medication management goals are to alleviate pain and stop the inflammatory process. Aspirin and other NSAIDs are indicated. Colchicine may be used as an additional anti-inflammatory medication with acetylsalicylic acid (ASA) or NSAIDS. If pain or inflammation is not relieved by ASA or NSAIDs, corticosteroids may be used. Additional treatment may be warranted depending on the etiology of the disease. For example, in addition to the use of anti-inflammatory agents, antimicrobial therapy may be instituted for bacterial pericarditis.

Complications

A complication of pericarditis is pericardial effusion. This is an accumulation of fluid in the pericardial space exceeding the typical 20 to 60 mL. Pericardial effusion is diagnosed by the use of chest x-ray, echocardiography, and ECG. Depending on the volume and clinical presentation, draining of the excess fluid, also known as **pericardiocentesis**, may be indicated. In a pericardiocentesis procedure, ultrasound guides needle insertion through the chest wall to aspirate the excess fluid.

Depending on the etiology, pericardial fluid may accumulate slowly (i.e., neoplastic), allowing the pericardium to stretch to accommodate the increased volume. Clinical symptoms in these cases gradually progress. In contrast, rapidly growing effusions overwhelm the stretching capacity of the

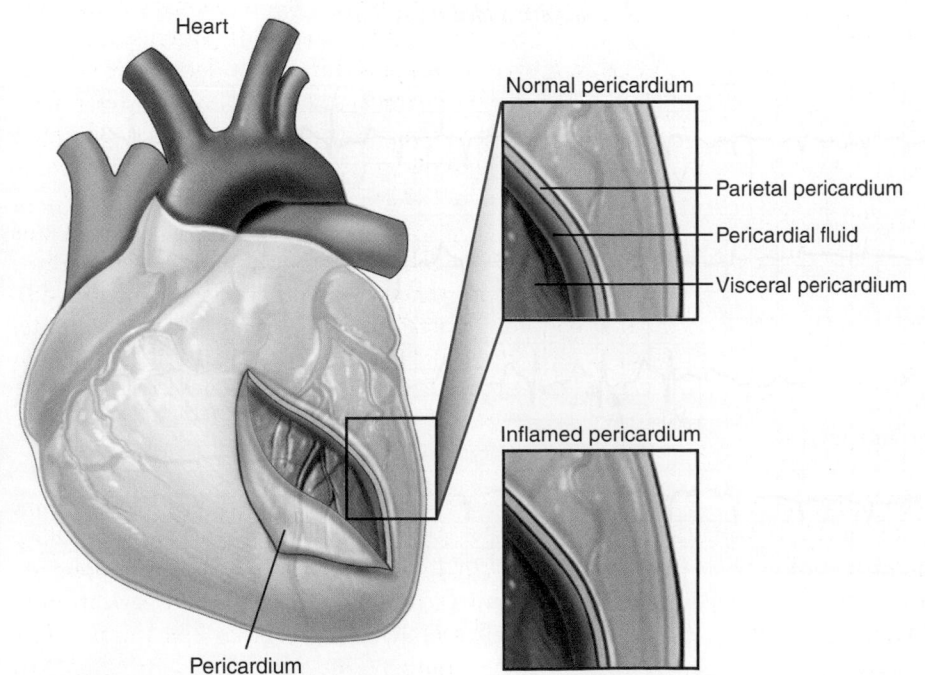

Heart

Normal pericardium

Parietal pericardium

Pericardial fluid

Visceral pericardium

Inflamed pericardium

Pericardium

FIGURE 30.5 Inflammation of the pericardium in pericarditis.

Box 30.1 How to Assess Pericardial Friction Rub

The sound of a pericardial friction rub is a result of the friction between the inflamed layers of the pericardium when the heart moves within the pericardial sac. It is best heard over the left sternal border at the end of expiration with the patient leaning forward. It produces a high-pitched, scratchy noise and is muffled when excessive fluid is present.

pericardium, resulting in an acute decompensation. If not treated emergently, the increased volume of fluid within the pericardial space can exert pressure on the heart, resulting in cardiac tamponade. In cardiac **tamponade**, the excessive fluid in the pericardial sac compresses the cardiac structures and dramatically decreases cardiac output. Common signs of pericardial tamponade include dyspnea, tachycardia, pulsus paradoxus, JVD, an enlarged heart, and muffled heart tones. Pulsus paradoxus is an abnormal drop in systolic blood pressure during inspiration. Beck's triad is the classic finding of hypotension, muffled heart sounds, and JVD but is only present in 10% to 40% of cases of tamponade. Emergent pericardiocentesis is indicated in this clinical presentation. Surgical management of pericardial effusions and cardiac tamponade may include a pericardial window, in which a window or fistula is created to drain excess fluid from the pericardial space.

Nursing Management

Assessment and Analysis

The major clinical manifestation of pericarditis is pain due to friction between the inflamed layers of the heart that occurs with movement. Excessive accumulation of fluid, or pericardial effusion, can result in acute decompensation due to the increased pressure around the heart limiting ventricular filling and contraction, resulting in decreased cardiac output.

Nursing Diagnoses

- **Chest pain** related to swelling and inflammation secondary to pericarditis
- **Risk for decreased cardiac output** related to cardiac structure compression

Nursing Interventions

■ Assessments

- Vital signs
  Hypotension, tachycardia, tachypnea, and pulsus paradoxus are indicative of cardiac tamponade, which is due to an excessive or sudden buildup of pericardial effusion. Fever is indicative of an ongoing infection.
- Pain
  Chest pain that is relieved by sitting up and leaning forward distinguishes pericarditis pain from the pain associated with MI.
- Auscultate heart sounds.
  A friction rub is a common finding in pericarditis. Muffled heart tones may indicate pericardial effusion or cardiac tamponade.
- ECG
  ST elevation or PR depression in all or most leads can be associated with pericarditis.

■ Actions

- Keep the head of the bed elevated.
  Pericardial effusion exerts pressure on surrounding organs, resulting in orthopnea (shortness of breath when lying down) and dyspnea. Raising the head of the bed relieves shortness of breath. Pain is also relieved by sitting in the upright position.
- Administer NSAIDs or ASA and colchicine medications as prescribed.
  Pain relating to pericarditis is associated with inflammation, so control is largely managed with anti-inflammatories. Steroids are added if necessary.

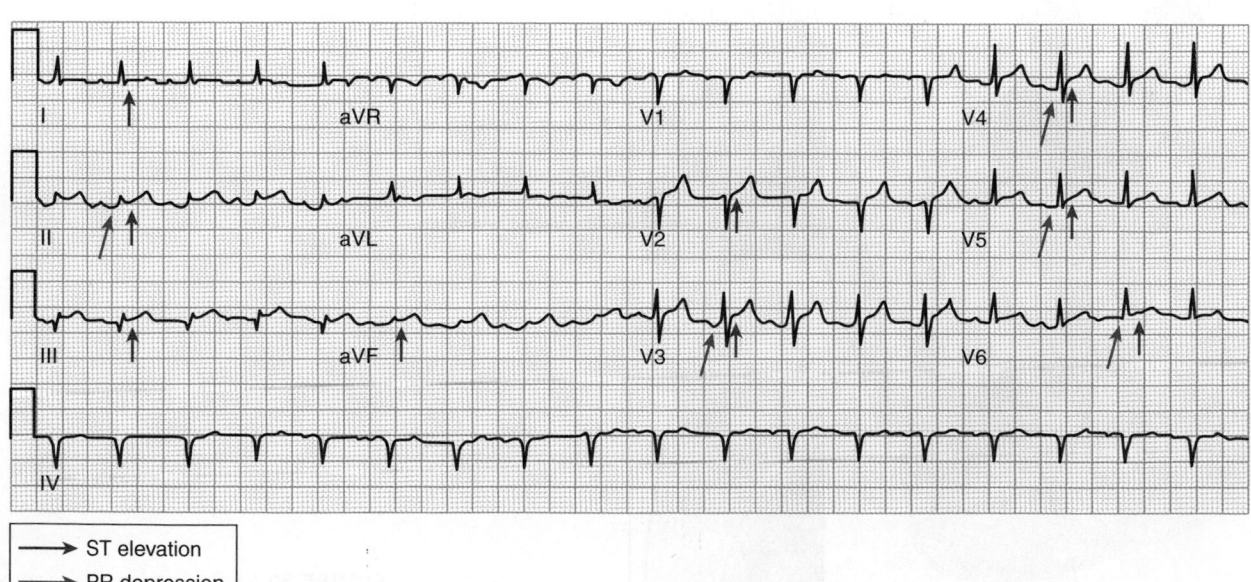

→ ST elevation
→ PR depression

FIGURE 30.6 Electrocardiogram illustrating ST elevation and PR depression associated with pericarditis.

- Provide emotional support.
  Anxiety can occur because of the fear that the pain is from a heart attack.

▧ *Teaching*

- Avoid strenuous activities until symptoms resolve or laboratory values return to normal.
  Activity restrictions may reduce the risk of sudden cardiac death, which is rare but has been reported.
- Distinguish between the pain of pericarditis and heart attack.
  Ensures patient will seek emergency help appropriately.

Evaluating Care Outcomes

The primary goal of care for a patient with pericarditis is pain relief. Early recognition and management of pericardial effusion are also important factors in the care of these patients. A well-managed patient is free from pain, shortness of breath, and indicators of cardiac tamponade. Ensuring that the patient and family are knowledgeable about the signs and treatment of the disease as well as the indicators of pericardial effusion is necessary to avoid the negative consequences associated with cardiac tamponade.

Connection Check 30.3

Which order would the nurse question in the initial management of acute pericarditis?
A. Aspirin
B. Colchicine
C. Prednisone
D. NSAIDs

VALVULAR DISEASE

Epidemiology

The prevalence of valvular disease in the general population is approximately 2.5%; it increases with age and occurs equally in men and women. The risk factors include infectious diseases such as IE and rheumatic fever, myocardial infarction, heart failure, congenital defects, and degenerative changes. Pregnancy has been shown to increase the risk of valvular disease because of the increased workload on the heart. Patients with risk factors for coronary artery disease are also at risk for valvular disease. The most common valvular diseases are **aortic stenosis** (Fig. 30.7) and mitral regurgitation. The least commonly affected valves are the tricuspid and pulmonic valves because of the low-pressure system in the right heart. Valvular disease can affect one or more valves at the same time.

Pathophysiology

There are several types of valvular disease: stenosis, insufficiency or regurgitation, and prolapse (Table 30.3). The pathophysiology of all valvular diseases is similar. Generally, in response to backward flow through the valve, referred to as **regurgitation**, or resistance to forward flow through the constricted or stenosed valve, signs of right- or left-sided HF develop. For instance, mitral valve regurgitation causes backward flow of blood into the left atrium. The increased blood volume raises the pressure in the atrium and pulmonary vessels and results in pulmonary edema and left-sided HF. Aortic valve stenosis obstructs the flow of blood from the left ventricle (LV), causing increased LV pressures. Left ventricle hypertrophy occurs to generate adequate force to open the valve. Over time, the LV fails, also resulting

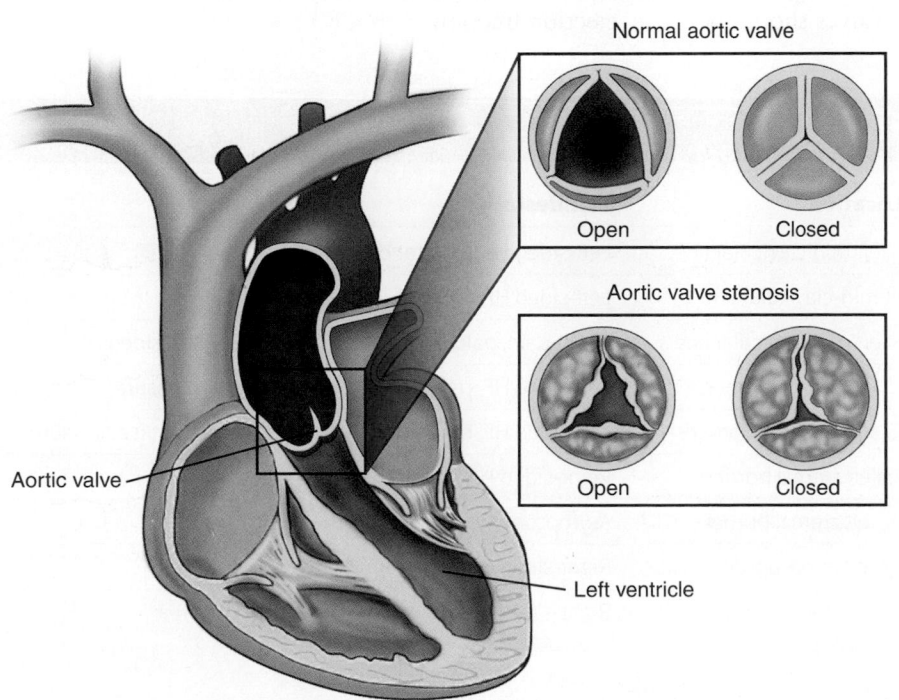

Normal aortic valve

Open   Closed

Aortic valve stenosis

Open   Closed

Aortic valve

Left ventricle

FIGURE 30.7 A comparison of a normal aortic valve with a valve narrowed in aortic stenosis.

Table 30.3 Types of Valvular Disease

Type	Description
Stenosis	Stiffening and thickening of the valve leaflets, caused by calcium deposits or scarring, narrow the opening and obstruct flow.
Regurgitation or insufficiency	Blood flows or leaks backward—ventricle to atria, aorta to the left ventricle, pulmonic circulation to the right ventricle—because of incomplete closing of the valve.
Prolapse	Valve leaflets bulge backward and do not close, causing regurgitation.

in the signs of left-sided HF. Insufficiency of the tricuspid valve causes backward flow and increased pressure in the right atrium, which results in signs of right-sided HF, such as JVD, generalized edema, and ascites.

Clinical Manifestations

Often, the first clinical sign of valvular disease is the auscultation of a murmur. A murmur can be the result of a high rate of blood flow through a valve, forward blood flow through a narrowed valve (**stenosis**), or backward blood flow through an incompetent valve (regurgitation). A cardiac murmur can be classified as systolic, diastolic, or continuous on the basis of where in the cardiac cycle it is best heard. Systolic murmurs can be heard during S_1 or *lub* when the ventricles are contracting. During this time, the aortic and pulmonic valves should be open, and the mitral and tricuspid valves should be closed. Diastolic murmurs can be heard during S_2 or *dub* when the ventricles are relaxing and the heart is filling. The mitral and tricuspid valves should be

open to allow for ventricular filling, and the aortic and pulmonic valves should be closed. Therefore, a systolic murmur can be heard with aortic or pulmonic stenosis or mitral or tricuspid regurgitation. In contrast, a diastolic murmur can be heard with aortic or pulmonic valve regurgitation or mitral or tricuspid stenosis. Another factor used to identify murmurs is the location of where the murmur is best heard based on the heart's auscultatory sites. Mitral valve murmurs are best heard at the apex of the heart. Table 30.4 identifies valve murmurs and their defining characteristics. Murmurs can be described in terms of sound qualities, but practice is needed to develop this skill. For instance, although it is not true in all cases, aortic stenosis typically produces a systolic murmur described as turbulent or harsh.

Most clinical manifestations of valvular disease resemble those of HF due to decreased cardiac output. They include:

- SOB, dyspnea, orthopnea
- Crackles
- Angina
- Syncope, dizziness
- Dysrhythmias
- Palpitations
- Fatigue
- Weight gain
- Edema
- Cool, pale extremities with weak pulses

Management

Medical Management

Diagnosis

Diagnostic Tests

Diagnostic tests used to diagnose valvular disease include:

- Echocardiogram to identify valve abnormalities and ejection fraction

Table 30.4 Valvular Disease Characteristics

Valve Disease	Auscultation Location	Manifestations
Mitral regurgitation	Systolic, 5th ICS left mid-clavicular line	Left-sided HF, palpitations
Mitral stenosis	Diastolic, ICS left mid-clavicular line	Left-sided HF
Mitral prolapse	Systolic, 5th ICS left mid-clavicular line	Chest pain, palpitations, syncope, anxiety, left-sided HF
Aortic regurgitation	Diastolic, 3rd ICS left sternal border	Left-sided HF, palpitations, widened pulse pressure
Aortic stenosis	Systolic, 2nd ICS, right sternal border	Left-sided HF, chest pain, syncope, narrowed pulse pressure
Pulmonary regurgitation	Diastolic, 3rd ICS left sternal border	Right-sided HF
Pulmonary stenosis	Systolic, 2nd ICS, left sternal border	Asymptomatic until severe, then right-sided HF
Tricuspid regurgitation	Systolic, 4th ICS left sternal border	Right-sided HF, atrial fibrillation
Tricuspid stenosis	Diastolic, 4th ICS left sternal border	Right-sided HF

HF, Heart failure; *ICS,* intercostal space.

- Chest x-ray to identify left or right heart hypertrophy and pulmonary edema
- Stress testing to identify functional capacity
- Heart catheterization as a definitive test for stenosis done prior to corrective surgery
- CT or MRI

Medications

Medication management for valvular disease is dependent on the etiology and degree of the disease. Valvular diseases with infectious etiology require antimicrobial therapy, whereas advanced valvular diseases require general HF management. That includes:

- Angiotensin-converting enzyme (ACE) inhibitors, angiotensin II receptor blockers (ARBs), or angiotensin receptor–neprilysin inhibitors (ARNIs) with beta blockers to reduce heart rate and blood pressure
- Diuretics to decrease preload and pulmonary congestion (see Safety Alert)

Medication management is also determined by the type of valve utilized in valve replacement, if necessary. Replacement valves are generally categorized as mechanical or tissue/bioprosthetic. Patients who undergo valve replacement with a mechanical prosthetic valve will need to be anticoagulated for life to prevent thrombotic events such as strokes. Tissue valves have recommended anticoagulation for only 6 months after placement but have less longevity. They are typically considered in patients who are older or cannot be anticoagulated.

 Safety Alert Care must be taken when managing blood pressure for patients with aortic stenosis. These patients require higher preload in order to generate adequate pressure for blood flow through the stenosed valve. Decreasing preload can lead to decreased cardiac output and hypotension.

Surgical Management

Surgical intervention to repair or replace diseased valves is often indicated and is based on the degree of valve dysfunction, symptom severity, and surgical risk. For patients needing valve replacement, open-heart surgery with a mechanical or bioprosthetic valve remains the standard approach. In these surgeries, patients undergo general anesthesia and are placed on cardiopulmonary bypass, and the diseased valves are replaced through a sternal incision or multiple smaller chest incisions. For patients with comorbidities, this comes with an increased risk of operative mortality; thus, fewer of these patients undergo surgical intervention. A more recent treatment option for aortic valve replacement is prosthetic valves that allow a transcatheter approach to valve replacement. In this procedure, called a **transcatheter aortic valve**

replacement (TAVR), a new valve is deployed through a catheter that is peripherally inserted and guided to the heart. The TAVR procedure is recommended particularly for intermediate- and high-operative-risk patients with aortic stenosis. Transcatheter mitral valve replacement is an emerging technology that is being studied and may be considered for patients who have severe regurgitation and symptoms with high surgical risk.

Overall, there is growing evidence that when possible, valvular repair yields better outcomes than replacement. Reparative surgery includes balloon valvuloplasty, commissurotomy, and mitral valve annuloplasty. Balloon valvuloplasty is a transcatheter procedure to repair stenosed valves. It involves inserting a balloon catheter through an appropriate vessel and advancing it to the heart. The balloon is inflated in the affected valve to enlarge the opening. Commissurotomy is a surgical procedure done to incise fused leaflets, widening the valve opening. Valve annuloplasty is a reconstructive procedure to repair the ring (annulus) that attaches and supports the valve leaflets. For patients with severe mitral valve regurgitation, a new procedure that partially clips the bulging leaflets together to reduce regurgitation and improve symptoms is being evaluated.

Complications

Valvular disorders can result in heart failure; cardiogenic shock; thromboembolism, including stroke; bleeding from anticoagulation; endocarditis; and dysrhythmias.

Connection Check 30.4

The nurse hears a loud systolic murmur at the second intercostal space right sternal border. What valve problem is the patient likely experiencing?
A. Aortic regurgitation
B. Aortic stenosis
C. Pulmonic regurgitation
D. Pulmonic stenosis

Nursing Management

Assessment and Analysis

Murmurs resulting from turbulent blood flow through diseased valves are heard with valve disease. Patients may be asymptomatic until valve function becomes significantly impaired, at which time clinical manifestations of HF related to decreased cardiac output and pulmonary congestion become prevalent.

They include:

- SOB
- Angina
- Syncope
- Dysrhythmia
- Palpitation
- Dizziness

- Fatigue
- Weight gain
- Poor color, cool extremities, weak peripheral pulses

Nursing Diagnoses

- **Decrease cardiac output** related to decreased stroke volume secondary to valve disease
- **Activity intolerance** related to decreased cardiac output secondary to HF due to valve disease

Nursing Interventions

■ Assessments

- Vital signs
  Hypertension, tachycardia, and tachypnea are indicative of HF due to increased resistance to flow and backflow of blood to the pulmonary system. Tachycardia occurs as a compensatory mechanism to increase cardiac output and oxygenation. Fever is indicative of infection and increases metabolic demands. Decreased SpO_2 occurs with pulmonary congestion.
- Pain assessment
  Chest pain and palpitations may occur with some murmurs.
- Monitoring for irregular heart rhythm
  Dysrhythmias, specifically atrial fibrillation, are common in valve disease.
- Peripheral vascular assessment
  Poor color, cool extremities, weak peripheral pulses, delayed capillary refill, and edema can indicate inadequate cardiac output.
- Breath sounds
  Crackles and orthopnea indicate pulmonary congestion.
- Activity tolerance
  Dyspnea on exertion, weakness, and fatigue indicate worsening HF.
- Auscultate heart sounds.
  Murmurs are typically the initial manifestation of valvular disease.
- Daily weights, intake and output
  Weight increases and intake greater than output can be indicative of HF.
- Monitor international normalized ratio (INR).
  Patients with valve replacements on warfarin need to maintain an INR that is two to three times normal.

■ Actions

- Provide supplemental oxygen and elevate the head of the bed.
  Oxygen and positioning increase oxygenation and ventilation.
- Administer medications as ordered: diuretics, ACE inhibitors, ARBs, ARNIs, beta blockers, antibiotics, anticoagulants.
  Medications are indicated for the relief of symptoms, not as a curative measure. Diuretics help decrease fluid overload; ACE inhibitors, ARBs, ARNIs, and beta blockers decrease heart rate and blood pressure, thus decreasing myocardial workload. Antibiotics are indicated if the valvular disease is caused by an infection such as IE. Anticoagulation decreases the risk of thrombus formation in patients with a prosthetic valve or patients in atrial fibrillation.

- Restrict sodium and fluids.
  To decrease fluid overload and reduce HF symptoms

■ Teaching

- Medication teaching
  Understanding and adhering to the medication treatment plan are essential for effective medication treatment.
- Consider prophylactic antimicrobials for dental procedures only for patients at high risk.
  Prevent (re)occurrence of infectious valvular disease
- Strict adherence to anticoagulation regimen if prosthetic valve
  Prevent thrombotic/embolic events (i.e., stroke)
- Anticoagulation precautions: avoid activities/sports that have a high risk for injury, report any injuries or falls to your provider, report anticoagulant use prior to any procedure, take care with shaving (electric razor preferred), take care with flossing to avoid bleeding, and limit alcohol consumption.
  Avoid activities/actions that increase bleeding risk.
- Maintain consistent intake of green leafy vegetables if taking warfarin.
  Green leafy vegetables impair the effectiveness of the anticoagulant warfarin.

Evaluating Care Outcomes

Successful management of patients with valvular disease requires maximizing cardiac output through repair or replacement of the damaged valve and controlling the symptoms of HF. Patients with valvular disease can achieve a high functional status by complying with the prescribed medical therapy, maintaining a healthy diet, and engaging in regular exercise. Vital signs within normal limits, increased energy, and an ability to actively participate in work and activities of daily living are indicative of disease control. The patient and family should be knowledgeable about the signs of decreased cardiac output and when they should report to their healthcare provider.

! Safety Alert **Orthostatic Hypotension**

Moving from a supine to an upright position is normally associated with a slight decrease in blood pressure. This is due to the pooling of blood in the lower extremities when the upright position is assumed, reducing the amount of blood returning to the heart and perfusion to the brain. In most people, the autonomic nervous system sends signals to the blood vessels in the lower extremities to constrict. Signals are also sent to the heart to increase rate. Both mechanisms increase cardiac output. In cardiac patients on many antihypertensive medications, the autonomic response can be impaired. Thus, moving to an upright position results in a feeling of dizziness and syncope, which puts the patient at risk for falls.

To measure orthostatic hypotension, have the patient assume a supine position for at least 2 minutes and record the blood pressure and heart rate. Then have the patient assume an upright position and record the blood pressure and heart rate. Generally, a reduction of 20 mm Hg or more in the systolic reading and/or 15 mm Hg in the diastolic value denotes the presence of orthostatic hypotension, also known as *postural hypotension*. In the patient who is highly symptomatic or with a history of syncope, this procedure can be performed in three stages: supine, sitting, and standing. The patient with orthostatic hypotension should be cautioned to transition from the supine or sitting to the standing position slowly by sitting briefly before standing. Some antihypertensive medications should be given with caution, starting with a lower dose and evaluating the patient's response, especially in older adults, to reduce the incidence of orthostatic hypotension.

CASE STUDY: EPISODE 2

Mr. Thompson is admitted to the step-down unit for further management. On physical examination, he is lying in bed with the head of the bed in a semi-Fowler's position. He is afebrile, with a temperature of 97.7°F (36.6°C). His blood pressure is 185/102 mm Hg. His heart rate is 124 beats per minute and appears to be irregular on the monitor. His respirations are 40 per minute and labored. Auscultation of his lung fields reveals crackles throughout. At a 30° angle, his jugular vein is distended and measures at 5 cm above the sternal border. He is on oxygen at 4 L/min via nasal cannula with an oxygen saturation of 95%. He has significant pitting edema of the lower extremities. Capillary refill is decreased to the fingers, and his extremities are cool to the touch…

HEART FAILURE

Epidemiology

The prevalence of heart failure (HF) is estimated at 6.5 million people aged 20 years or older in the United States, with about a million new cases each year. The lifetime risk of developing HF at age 40 is at least one in five for both men and women. The number of persons with heart failure is expected to continue rising. Heart failure is more common in people who are 65 years old or older, African Americans, people who are overweight, and people who have had a heart attack. Men have a higher rate of heart failure than women. The risk factors associated with the development of HF include:

- CAD
- Hypertension
- Diabetes mellitus
- Metabolic syndrome
- Obesity
- Smoking
- High sodium dietary intake

Other conditions that can cause heart failure include valvular dysfunction; cardiomyopathies; infectious and inflammatory heart disorders, such as pericarditis and endocarditis; dysrhythmias; and cardiotoxic substance exposure, such as alcohol, chemotherapy, and illicit drugs. With advances in management, mortality rates are declining but remain high at about 40% after 5 years from the time of diagnosis. Heart failure is a leading cause of hospitalizations among persons older than 65. The large number of persons with HF and hospitalizations related to HF contribute to an estimated annual cost of $39.2 billion.

Pathophysiology

Heart failure is a progressive disease characterized by myocardial cell dysfunction, resulting in the inability of the heart to pump enough cardiac output to meet the demands of the body. The normal physiology of the heart is governed by the Frank–Starling law, which states that the contractility of the myocardial muscle is influenced by the amount of blood within the ventricle prior to systole. In other words, high end diastolic volume stretches the myocardium, increasing the force of each contraction. However, in people with risk factors for HF, such as hypertension, the constant demands on the myocardial muscles over time cause them to become weakened and unable to pump effectively.

Compensatory mechanisms are activated in response to decreased stroke volume and cardiac output. These responses are actions that enable the body to maintain function. The sympathetic nervous system releases epinephrine and norepinephrine, resulting in an increased heart rate, increased myocardial contractility, and increased vasoconstriction in an effort to increase cardiac output. This additional workload stimulates ventricular remodeling, which results in hypertrophy or stiffening of the ventricular walls. Although sympathetic nervous system responses and ventricular remodeling may be successful in the short term, the long-term effects are damaging. They produce an increase in cardiac workload and cardiac oxygen consumption, worsening the failure.

The neurohormonal compensatory response leads to the activation of the renin-angiotensin-aldosterone system (RAAS). This is done in reaction to decreased blood flow to the kidneys. The kidneys interpret this as decreased volume and release an enzyme, renin. Renin converts angiotensinogen, an inactive peptide released by the liver, to angiotensin I. Angiotensin I is enzymatically converted to angiotensin II by angiotensin-converting enzyme released by the lungs. Angiotensin II produces peripheral vasoconstriction, which helps increase blood pressure and venous return to the heart. Angiotensin II also stimulates the release of aldosterone from the adrenal cortex, which results in sodium and water retention. As with the sympathetic nervous system, these changes are effective in the short term, but in the long term, they overtax an already weak heart with increased volume and workload.

Another neurohormonal compensatory response is the release of natriuretic peptides. Brain natriuretic peptide, or B-type natriuretic peptide (BNP), is a hormone produced by the ventricular cardiac muscle. It is released in reaction to "overstretching" of the ventricle in response to increased pressure and volume. The result is a natural diuresis as well as arterial and venous dilation. This action decreases both preload and afterload, which decreases the workload on the heart.

Heart failure is classified based on **ejection fraction** (EF), which is the percentage of blood that is ejected from the ventricle with each contraction. Normal values range from 55% to 70% of the total volume. Patients with low EF are diagnosed with heart failure with reduced ejection fraction (HFrEF), formerly called systolic heart failure. Patients with HFrEF have a weakened contraction, with an EF of 45% or less. Those patients with clinical manifestations of heart failure but an EF of greater than 45% are diagnosed with heart failure with preserved ejection fraction (HFpEF), formerly called diastolic heart failure. HFpEF is characterized by the inability of the ventricles to fill. These patients tend to be older and female. Traditionally, heart failure treatment focused on HFrEF, but there is a growing body of evidence to support HFpEF treatment. It is estimated that about half of HF patients have HFpEF, and half have HFrEF.

Heart failure is also described according to anatomical dysfunction, disease progression, and severity of symptoms. Heart failure can affect one or both sides of the heart. When both sides of the heart are affected, this is known as *biventricular failure*. Left-sided HF refers to the dysfunction of the left ventricle. Right-sided HF refers to the inability of the right side of the heart to effectively pump blood to the pulmonary vasculature.

Clinical Manifestations

Clinical manifestations of heart failure vary depending on the type, onset, and severity of the failure. The timing of onset and severity of symptoms can be used to determine if heart failure is acute or chronic. Acute heart failure has a sudden onset of symptoms and requires immediate intervention. Chronic heart failure describes the baseline set of symptoms and limitations that are relatively stable with treatment and self-management.

Some common signs include fatigue, weight gain, faster heart rates, and hypo- or hypertension. Heart murmurs may be present if the cause of HF is valve dysfunction. When auscultating heart tones, a third heart sound, S_3, may be a warning sign of worsening heart failure. An S_4 is common in chronic heart failure. The point of maximal intensity may be enlarged or displaced when ventricles enlarge. The clinical presentation of HF can depend on the side of the heart most affected (Table 30.5).

Table 30.5 Clinical Manifestations of Right- and Left-Sided Heart Failure

Right-Sided Heart Failure	Left-Sided Heart Failure
• Jugular vein distention • Dependent edema • Hepatomegaly • Ascites	• Shortness of breath or dyspnea or orthopnea • Crackles on auscultation • Pale color, weak pulses, cool temperature in extremities, delayed capillary refill • Fatigue, weakness

In left-sided HF, the weakened contraction results in poor peripheral perfusion and backflow of blood that causes fluid accumulation in the lungs. This produces classic symptoms such as SOB (dyspnea), orthopnea, fatigue, and crackles heard on auscultation. Other symptoms of left-sided failure include fatigue, poor color, weak pulses, and cool temperature in the extremities. The weakened contraction of the right ventricle, right-sided HF, results in a backflow of blood into the right atrium and venous circulation and is characterized by JVD, generalized dependent edema, hepatomegaly, and ascites. Left-sided HF can eventually cause right-sided HF, or the entire heart may be initially affected. If that happens, the symptom classification becomes less clear. In severe HF exacerbations, the patient may present with hypotension, cool extremities, decreased or no urine output, and poor or decreasing mentation. In such cases, both S_3 and S_4 may be heard.

There are several classifications of HF. The AHA and American College of Cardiology (ACC) classify the stages of HF development from A through D. The New York Heart Association (NYHA) classifies functional status as I through IV according to the clinical manifestations of HF (Table 30.6). It is important to note that a patient can fluctuate between NYHA classes I and IV with interventions such as diuresis; however, patients do not regress back to a previous stage in the AHA/ACC classification.

Management

Medical Management
Diagnosis

The diagnosis of HF is heavily dependent on history and physical assessment. The symptoms are fairly nonspecific, so diagnostic tests are done to rule out other disorders and determine the underlying cause. Diagnostic tools include chest x-ray, echocardiogram, and ECG to assess the presence of structural disease, ejection fraction, heart size, pulmonary congestion, or dysrhythmias. Multigated acquisition (MUGA) scans can also determine EF. Nuclear imaging studies, stress testing, and coronary angiography

Table 30.6 Comparison of Stages of Heart Failure Development and New York Heart Association Functional Classes

American Heart Association/American College of Cardiology Stages of Heart Failure Development	New York Heart Association Classification of Functional Status
A: Patient with risk factors but no LV impairment	I: No symptoms with physical activity, such as dyspnea or chest pain
B: Asymptomatic with LV hypertrophy and/or impaired LV function	II: Mild symptoms with ordinary activities
C: Current or past symptoms of HF	III: Marked limitation with physical activity but comfortable at rest
D: Refractory HF eligible for heart transplant, inotropic and/or mechanical support	IV: Severe limitation and distress with physical activity or at rest

HF, Heart failure; *LV,* left ventricle.

to evaluate blood flow to the heart are performed when coronary artery disease is suspected. In severe acute heart failure, hemodynamic monitoring with a pulmonary artery catheter can be useful.

Diagnostic Tests

Laboratory testing includes cardiac biomarkers, serum electrolytes, a complete blood count, urinalysis, glucose level, fasting lipid profile, liver function testing, and renal function tests. Electrolytes can be outside the normal range as a result of decreased kidney perfusion or medication. For example, potassium might be low because of diuretic therapy. Also, inadequate flow to the kidneys may impair renal function, resulting in elevated creatinine and blood urea nitrogen (BUN) levels. Decreased hemoglobin and hematocrit levels may indicate anemia, which may be a result of decreased blood flow to the kidneys that reduces the production and function of erythropoietin in the kidneys. Cardiac biomarkers such as troponin I or T are used to rule out an acute ischemic event. Other biomarkers, BNP and N-terminal pro-B-type natriuretic peptide (NT-proBNP), are increased because of the overstretching of the ventricles. Increased values in these tests can be used to diagnose HF; BNP and NT-proBNP can also guide clinical decision making and track a patient's response to therapy as well as indicate disease progression.

Medications

The medical management described here is predominantly for patients with HFrEF. These strategies have not been efficacious for patients with HFpEF. Management of patients with HFpEF focuses on the treatment of the underlying cause, blood pressure control, diuretics for fluid volume overload, and symptom management.

The goals of HFrEF management are the reduction of risk factors, manipulation of the critical components of cardiac output (preload, afterload, and contractility), and control of the compensatory mechanisms. Successful management slows disease progression, prevents complications, reduces morbidity and mortality, and improves quality of life. Risk-factor management may include blood pressure and glucose control, weight loss, optimizing serum lipids, and smoking cessation. Beta blockers are used to control the sympathetic nervous system compensatory response in HF, such as tachycardia, in order to decrease cardiac workload. Ivabradine, a new medication that slows sinus-node firing, can be added for greater control of heart rate in patients taking maximal doses of beta blockers or who do not tolerate beta blockers.

Preload is the amount of stretch in the heart at the end of diastole and is affected by the amount and pressure of blood returning to the heart. Aldosterone antagonist diuretics such as spironolactone (Aldactone) as well as loop diuretics such as furosemide (Lasix) are essential medications to decrease preload in patients with fluid retention. The use of spironolactone should be cautioned in patients with renal insufficiency because of the potential complication of hyperkalemia. In contrast, furosemide can cause hypokalemia and is often paired with a potassium replacement medication.

Afterload refers to the resistance within the vasculature. Increased afterload intensifies the workload on the heart, further impairing cardiac output. Afterload reduction is a main goal of medical management. Angiotensin-converting enzyme (ACE) inhibitors are usually the first line of medications used to control the RAAS compensatory response and reduce afterload. Angiotensin receptor blockers (ARBs) have a similar effect and can be used in patients who are intolerant of ACE inhibitors. Angiotensin receptor–neprilysin inhibitors (ARNIs) are a new class of medications that combine an ARB with a neprilysin inhibitor (valsartan with sacubitril) and can be used in place of an ACE inhibitor or ARB. Neprilysin is an enzyme that breaks down natriuretic peptides (BNP), which produces natural diuresis and vasodilation. By blocking neprilysin, natriuretic peptides remain active in increasing urine output and dilating blood vessels. Other medications that may be prescribed to reduce afterload include vasodilators such as hydralazine and isosorbide dinitrate. Calcium channel blockers, with the exception of amlodipine, should be avoided in HF due to their myocardial depressant effect and lack of demonstrated efficacy.

> **(!) Safety Alert** **Medication Safety Alert: ARNIs**
> Like ACE inhibitors, the neprilysin inhibitor in an ARNI prevents the breakdown of bradykinin as well as natriuretic peptides. Bradykinin is a cause of angioedema. The combination of an ACE inhibitor and ARNI significantly increases the risk of angioedema. An ARNI should not be given at the same time or within 36 hours of an ACE inhibitor. An ARNI should not be given to patients who had angioedema in the past.

Contractility is the force of the myocardial muscle contraction. A past mainstay of HF management has been digoxin (Lanoxin), an oral positive inotropic medication used to increase cardiac contractility and reduce heart rate. Its use is being questioned. Although patients realize a reduction in symptoms, overall mortality is not decreased. Patients on digoxin (Lanoxin) are prone to toxicities, with symptoms such as nausea and vomiting and visual disturbances (e.g., yellow halos around lights). Care must be taken to monitor patients closely to avoid the later signs of toxicity, such as bradycardia and dysrhythmias. See Table 30.7 for a summary of medications used in the treatment of HF.

Medical management of heart failure often requires multiple medications from different classes to achieve optimal results. For instance, patients can be prescribed spironolactone, furosemide, and carvedilol to manage their HF along with their other routine medications. In combination, these medications have been shown to improve survival in patients with HF by slowing or stopping the progression of ventricular remodeling and dysfunction.

An acute exacerbation of HF is typically treated with IV medications that can more quickly and effectively decrease preload and afterload and increase contractility. Nitroglycerin and nitroprusside (Nitropress), potent vasodilators, are commonly used. Intravenous inotropic agents (e.g., dopamine) can be used to increase contractility, whereas inodilators, agents with both positive inotropic and vasodilator effects (e.g., dobutamine and milrinone), provide positive inotropic effects and reduce afterload. All these medications require careful monitoring of blood pressure, heart rate, and cardiac rhythm and frequent assessments to guide therapy and avoid adverse effects.

Device and Surgical Intervention

As HF progresses, more invasive treatments are needed to support cardiac function and control the complications that result. Implantation of an automatic internal cardiac defibrillator (ICD) and a pacemaker may be considered for dysrhythmia control and ventricular resynchronization also

Table 30.7 Medications Used in the Management of Heart Failure

Medication	Indication
Angiotensin-converting enzyme inhibitors (captopril, enalapril)	Afterload reduction
Angiotensin receptor blockers (valsartan)	Afterload reduction
Angiotensin receptor–neprilysin inhibitor (valsartan/sacubitril)	Afterload and preload reduction
Arterial vasodilators (hydralazine, isosorbide dinitrate, nitroprusside)	Afterload reduction
Venous vasodilator (isosorbide dinitrate)	Preload reduction
Diuretics: *Loop diuretics (furosemide)* *Aldosterone receptor antagonists (spironolactone)*	Preload reduction
Beta blockers (carvedilol)	Decrease heart rate and myocardial workload
Inodilators (milrinone, dobutamine)	Increase contractility and reduce afterload
Inotropes (dopamine)	Increase contractility
I(f) current inhibitor (ivabradine)	Myocardial workload reduction by decreasing heart rate
Cardiac glycosides (digoxin/Lanoxin)	Enhance contractility (positive inotrope)

referred to as cardiac resynchronization therapy (CRT). Continuous IV inotrope therapy, an intra-aortic balloon pump, and other mechanical circulatory support (MCS) devices such as a ventricular assist device (VAD) can be used to support the failing heart. Depending on the cause of HF, valve replacement or heart transplantation may be considered. In addition to treatment, symptom management to improve healthcare-related quality of life (HRQOL) should always be considered. Palliative care is often indicated for patients with end-stage HF (NYHA class IV or AHA/ACC stage D).

Self-Management

Self-management is a critical component of HF treatment. Patients must assume responsibilities for symptom monitoring, medication adherence, and lifestyle changes. Daily weights taken at about the same time each day monitor fluid retention. Weight gain indicates fluid retention. A gain of 1 kg is the equivalent of 1,000 mL of fluid retention. A gain of more than 1 kg (2 lb) in a day or 2 kg (5 lb) in a week may be significant. Lifestyle changes typically include a sodium-restricted diet, maintaining optimal weight, and preventing cardiac cachexia. Sodium restriction to 1,500 mg/day is recommended in the early stages of HF, with a less restrictive recommendation of up to 4,000 mg/day in later stages. A high BMI is associated with a higher mortality and, although a lower BMI is generally positive, weight loss in a patient with HF may reflect cardiac cachexia which may also contribute to higher mortality.

Management interventions by the interprofessional healthcare team may have a beneficial effect on self management and thus on HF-related hospitalization and quality of life. Critical interventions by the healthcare team include teaching related to medications, sodium restriction, and weight management; symptom monitoring; screening for depression and mental health comorbidities; evaluating social support structures; planning and encouraging participation in cardiac rehabilitation; and implementing behavior-change strategies, such as motivational interviewing (see Evidence-Based Practice). Intensive intervention programs can combine in-patient interventions with home care and follow-up contacts. Self-management is affected by the patient perceptions of interactions with healthcare team members. Improved self-management occurs when patients perceive that their healthcare team members are responsive, interested in their individual needs, and share information. Poor communication and lack of continuity can be barriers to self-management.

Evidence-Based Practice

Cardiac Rehabilitation for Heart Failure

Persons with heart failure experience reduced capacity for physical activity, which can have detrimental effects on their quality of life and contribute to hospitalizations and mortality. The American Heart Association and American College of Cardiology recommend cardiac rehabilitation in the management of heart failure. A 2015 systematic review and meta-analysis that included 33 studies and 4,740 patients found that patients who participated in exercise-based cardiac rehabilitation programs had significantly fewer hospitalizations and improved quality of life. Long-term mortality may also be improved. Despite evidence from this study and many others, as well as reimbursement by the Centers for Medicare and Medicaid Services, referral to and attendance in such programs remain low. More patients with heart failure need to be referred to and encouraged to participate in cardiac rehabilitation.

Sagar, V., Davies, E., Briscoe, S., Coats, A., Dalal, H., Lough, F., . . . Taylor, R. (2015). Exercise-based rehabilitation for heart failure: Systematic review and meta-analysis. *Open Heart, 2*(1), e000163. doi:10.11356/openhrt-2014-000163

Geriatric/Gerontological Considerations

Heart Failure and Older Adults

Heart failure (HF) is more common with aging. Older patients are more likely to have heart failure with preserved ejection fraction (HFpEF), for which few evidence-based treatment guidelines exist. They often have five or six additional comorbidities, which create complexities in care and a greater potential for medication interactions. Depression, anxiety, and cognitive impairment, which often go undiagnosed, can reduce self-management abilities and medication adherence, warranting careful screening for these conditions. Few studies of HF focus exclusively on the older adult. Some studies show HF medications are underused in older adults, whereas others show that more intensive medication therapy is not associated with additional benefits. Many HF medications have hypotensive effects or cause nocturia, which may increase fall risk. A careful risk–benefit analysis of interventions is required, particularly when medication changes occur. Due to declining renal function, potential poor nutritional status, and greater risk for dehydration, older patients need to be monitored more carefully for adverse effects. Telephone and telemonitoring may be useful strategies after discharge.

Complications

Pulmonary edema is an acute complication of HF characterized by the accumulation of fluid in the interstitial and alveolar spaces of the lung, resulting from elevated filling pressures within the heart. The symptoms of pulmonary edema include SOB, low oxygen saturation, pink and frothy sputum, orthopnea, tachycardia, chest pain, and anxiety/fear. Treatments include supplementary oxygen administration and initiation of higher-dose or IV diuretics. Depending on the severity of the edema, the patient may need more aggressive respiratory support with continuous positive airway pressure (CPAP), bilevel positive airway pressure (BiPAP), or intubation with mechanical ventilation. Dysrhythmias can also occur as the heart enlarges and catecholamine levels increase.

Renal failure is another common complication seen in HF patients. This is due to the decrease in blood flow to the kidneys. Renal failure is discussed in more detail in Chapter 62.

Nursing Management
Assessment and Analysis

The clinical manifestations of HF are due to the weakened myocardial contraction resulting in decreased cardiac output, a backup of blood, and poor peripheral perfusion. Common findings include:

- Poor mentation
- Anorexia
- Exercise intolerance
- SOB, orthopnea
- JVD
- Dependent peripheral edema
- Weak peripheral pulses, cool extremities, delayed capillary refill
- Cardiac cachexia or generalized body wasting

Nursing Diagnoses

- **Impaired oxygenation** related to accumulation of fluid in the lungs secondary to HF
- **Decreased cardiac output** related to altered preload, afterload, and contractility
- **Ineffective peripheral perfusion** related to decreased cardiac output secondary to HF

Nursing Interventions

▪ *Assessments*

- Vital signs
  Hypertension is present because of the increased afterload. Hypotension may be caused by acute heart failure or be an adverse effect of medications. Tachycardia can be present as the heart attempts to compensate for decreased cardiac output. Tachypnea and decreased oxygen saturation may be present when fluid accumulates in the lungs because of left-sided HF.
- Breath sounds
  Crackles indicate pulmonary congestion.
- Monitoring for irregular heart rhythm or dysrhythmias
  Dysrhythmias are a common adverse effect of HF and medications used to treat HF.
- Skin color, temperature, peripheral pulses, and capillary refill time
  Pale or cyanotic color, cool extremities, weak peripheral pulses, and sluggish refill time result from inadequate cardiac output.
- Dry, persistent cough
  Common complication of ACE inhibitors
- Activity tolerance
  Dyspnea on exertion, weakness, and fatigue indicate decreased cardiac output and worsening heart failure.
- Urine output
  Output may be reduced with decreased renal perfusion. It can also be used to assess the effectiveness of diuretic therapy. Less than 30 mL/hr should be reported to the provider.
- Daily weight
  To evaluate fluid retention and effectiveness of diuresis
- Laboratory data
  Elevated BNP and NT-proBNP indicate overstretching of heart tissue. Elevated creatinine and BUN may be indicative of prerenal failure due to decreased cardiac output or overdiuresis. Elevated hepatic enzymes can be indicative of hepatomegaly; hypokalemia is a common complication of

diuretic administration. Anemia can be caused by reduced kidney perfusion resulting in decreased erythropoietin production and function
- Depression screening
  High rates of depression and anxiety are noted in the HF population. These can impact self-management.
- Social support
  Social isolation has been shown to be an independent predictor of mortality among HF patients.

▪ *Actions*

- Oxygen therapy
  To maintain adequate oxygenation
- Elevate the head of the bed and provide a fan for dyspnea.
  Maximize oxygenation and promote comfort
- Medication administration as ordered:
  - Administer diuretics.
    Diuretics decrease volume, thus preload.
  - Administer ACE inhibitors, ARBs, ARNIs, and vasodilators.
    Angiotensin-converting enzyme inhibitors, ARBs, ARNIs, and vasodilators decrease afterload, which helps to decrease the workload on the heart and decrease myocardial oxygen consumption.
  - Administer beta blockers.
    Beta blockers decrease the sympathetic response (heart rate), thus reducing myocardial oxygen consumption.
  - Administer inotropic agents.
    Enhance contractility
- Fluid and sodium restriction
  To prevent fluid overload

▪ *Teaching*

- Medication management
  Understanding and adhering to the medication treatment plan are essential for effective medication treatment.
- Maintain activity as tolerated. Alternate rest and activity periods.
  To reduce muscle wasting and functional losses; to decrease workload on the heart
- Low-salt diet
  To prevent fluid retention and exacerbation of HF
- Daily weight at home at the same time each day, preferably in the morning after voiding
  Evaluate fluid retention and need to call provider
- Cardiac rehabilitation
  Cardiac rehabilitation reduces mortality, improves functional status, reduces hospitalization, and improves quality of life.
- Signs and symptoms of worsening HF checklist (edema, SOB, fatigue, and orthopnea)
  Knowing the symptoms can expedite treatment and reduce hospitalizations.

Connection Check 30.5

What assessment would the nurse identify as a hallmark finding of left-sided heart failure?

A. Ascites
B. Bradycardia
C. Crackles
D. Edema

Evaluating Care Outcomes

Heart failure patients are at risk for frequent exacerbations due to even small changes in fluid status, salt intake, or being exposed to common ailments such as a cold. Reducing stressors that can lead to exacerbations is key. Successful management requires collaboration with the patient and family and the interprofessional team (physician, pharmacist, respiratory care therapist, dietitian, diagnostic technicians, social workers, and palliative care) to develop and implement a treatment plan. That plan should include frequent assessment, comprehensive patient education, and self-management. A well-managed patient has reduced dyspnea and fatigue, is able to actively participate in activities of daily living, and has reduced hospitalizations.

Making Connections

CASE STUDY: WRAP-UP

Mr. Thompson's ECG reveals atrial fibrillation with a heart rate of 130 to 140 bpm. His blood pressure continues to be high at 185/102 mm Hg. His respirations are still slightly labored and fast at 40 per minute. He continues on oxygen at 4 L/min via nasal cannula, with an oxygen saturation of 95%. The results of Mr. Thompson's diagnostic tests reveal:

- A chest x-ray indicates LV hypertrophy.
- A transthoracic echocardiogram indicates an EF of 30%.
- Cardiac biomarkers are negative for ischemia, with troponin I less than 0.1 ng/ml.
- Renal function tests reveal borderline failure, with a creatinine of 1.5 mg/dL and a BUN of 30 mg/dL.
- His BNP value is elevated to 500 pg/mL.
- Serum electrolytes reveal elevated potassium at 6.0 mEq/L.

It is determined that Mr. Thompson is in HF, and he begins treatment. A diuretic is administered; an ACE inhibitor and a beta blocker are ordered. His SOB and color begin to improve. His transient chest pain resolves with treatment.

Case Study Questions

1. The nurse has received the following orders for Mr. Thompson. Which order should the nurse implement first?
   A. Furosemide (Lasix) 40 mg IV
   B. Insert a Foley catheter
   C. Low-sodium, low-fat diet
   D. Apply sequential compression device

2. The nurse correlates which finding with Mr. Thompson's atrial fibrillation with a heart rate of 120 to 140 beats per minute?
   A. Acute decompensation requiring immediate cardioversion
   B. Loss of atrial kick requiring fluid resuscitation
   C. Increased workload of the heart requiring beta blockers
   D. Cardiac ischemia requiring immediate cardiac catheterization

3. The nurse understands that Mr. Thompson's sublingual nitroglycerin decreases chest pain through which mechanism of action?
   A. Dilating the coronary arteries to improve blood flow
   B. Decreasing preload to relieve symptoms of dyspnea
   C. Decreasing heart rate to decrease cardiac workload
   D. Converting atrial fibrillation into sinus rhythm

4. Which statement by Mr. Thompson indicates that teaching about hyperkalemia has been effective?
   A. "The water pill makes my potassium level high."
   B. "I should eat bananas because they make my potassium go down."
   C. "My liver is not working, so it holds on to the potassium."
   D. "My kidneys are not working which makes my potassium high."

5. The nurse providing care for Mr. Thompson should include which of the following in the discharge teaching plan? *(Select all that apply.)*
   A. Sodium restriction
   B. Daily weight
   C. Medication teaching
   D. Vigorous daily exercise
   E. Carbohydrate counting

CHAPTER SUMMARY

Atherosclerosis marks the beginning of coronary artery disease (CAD). The progression of plaque buildup is usually silent until occlusion of the vessel is significant enough to cause angina. Long-term effects include stable and unstable angina, myocardial infarction (MI), and sudden cardiac death due to extreme obstruction of blood flow in the coronary arteries. Many of the diagnostic blood tests performed, such as lipid profiles, assess for the presence of risk factors for CAD development. Specific cardiac enzymes are used to rule out MI. The gold standard for diagnosing CAD is a coronary angiogram. Medication for patients with CAD is often prescribed with the goals of (a) stopping the aggregation of blood components to the injured endothelium, (b) controlling factors that lead to damage of the endothelium, and (c) relieving symptoms. Percutaneous transluminal coronary angioplasty is the procedure most commonly performed to relieve symptoms. Nursing care priorities include vital signs and physical assessment and administering medication as ordered to manage risk factors and relieve symptoms. The teaching plan includes understanding the signs of an exacerbation and managing lifestyle to limit and control risk factors.

Infective endocarditis (IE) is the result of an infection of the innermost layer of the heart, the endocardium. The heart valves are the usual location for this lesion. The transthoracic echocardiogram (TTE) is the best at detecting the presence of vegetation. The primary treatment is IV antibiotics. Infective endocarditis unresponsive to antibiotic therapy can be treated with valve repair or replacement. Nursing assessment includes monitoring vital signs, especially for the presence of fever, which can be indicative of ongoing acute infection. Teaching includes the maintenance of good oral hygiene and informing the healthcare provider about IE history prior to any dental or invasive procedure.

Myocarditis is an inflammatory disease of the myocardium most commonly caused by viral infection or autoimmune diseases. Clinical manifestations include chest pain, dysrhythmias, dyspnea, palpitations, syncope, and heart failure. Medical treatment focuses on the management of heart failure, dysrhythmias, and dilated cardiomyopathy that may occur due to the inflammation. Treatment also includes medications to treat the cause.

Pericarditis is an inflammation of the membrane surrounding the heart, the pericardium. The chief clinical manifestation is pain. Tests used to diagnose pericarditis include an electrocardiogram (ECG), chest x-ray, TTE, cardiac computed tomography (CT) scan, and magnetic resonance imaging (MRI). The primary treatment is pain control with anti-inflammatories. Nursing priorities include pain assessment to evaluate the effectiveness of treatment and close monitoring for the complications of pericardial effusion and cardiac tamponade. Teaching priorities include distinguishing between pericarditis and heart attack to ensure the patient will seek emergency help appropriately when necessary.

Valvular disease refers to either narrowing or incomplete closure of the heart valves. In response to backward flow through the valve due to incomplete closure or resistance to forward flow through the stenosed valve, signs of right-sided or left-sided heart failure (HF) develop. Tests used to diagnose valvular disease include ECG, echocardiogram, and chest x-ray. The goals of medical therapy are to manage the manifestations of HF and prevent thrombus formation. Surgical intervention can include repair or replacement of valves. Nursing care priorities include assessment for signs of HF, which helps evaluate the effectiveness of treatment, and administration of medications as ordered to control the symptoms of HF. Medication management and anticoagulation precaution teaching are essential.

Heart failure is present when the heart loses its ability to pump blood effectively and is unable to produce enough cardiac output to meet the body's metabolic demands. Clinical manifestations of left-sided HF include shortness of breath (SOB), crackles, and poor peripheral perfusion. Symptoms of right-sided HF include jugular vein distention (JVD), hepatomegaly, ascites, and dependent edema. Treatment focuses on decreasing the workload of the heart by decreasing preload and afterload. Diuretics, angiotensin-converting enzyme (ACE) inhibitors, angiotensin receptor blockers (ARBs), angiotensin receptor–neprilysin inhibitors (ARNIs), and beta blockers are commonly prescribed. Nursing care priorities include assessment for signs of HF, which helps evaluate the effectiveness of treatment, and administration of medications as ordered to control the symptoms of HF. Medication and diet management and the manifestations of worsening HF are essential components of the teaching plan.

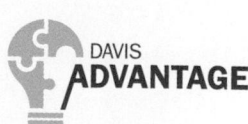

To explore learning resources for this chapter, go to **Davis Advantage** and find:
- Answers to in-text questions
- Chapter Resources and Activities
- NCLEX®-Style Chapter Review Questions
- Bibliography

Chapter 31

Coordinating Care for Patients With Vascular Disorders

Eleni Flanagan and Sarah Smith

LEARNING OUTCOMES

Content in this chapter is designed to assist in:

1. Describing the epidemiology of vascular disorders
2. Correlating clinical manifestations to pathophysiological processes of:
   a. Atherosclerosis/Arteriosclerosis
   b. Hypertension
   c. Peripheral arterial disease
   d. Carotid artery disease
   e. Aortic artery disease (aneurysms)
   f. Deep vein thrombosis
3. Describing the diagnostic results used to confirm the diagnoses of vascular disorders
4. Discussing the medical management of:
   a. Atherosclerosis/Arteriosclerosis
   b. Hypertension
   c. Peripheral arterial disease
   d. Carotid artery disease
   e. Aortic artery disease (aneurysms)
   f. Deep vein thrombosis
5. Developing a comprehensive plan of nursing care for patients with vascular disorders
6. Designing a teaching plan of care that includes pharmacological, dietary, and lifestyle considerations for patients with vascular disorders

ESSENTIAL TERMS

Abdominal aortic aneurysm (AAA)
Aneurysm
Ankle-brachial index (ABI)
Aortic dissection
Arteriosclerosis
Atherosclerosis
Carotid artery disease
Carotid artery stenting
Carotid endarterectomy (CEA)
Claudication
Deep vein thrombosis (DVT)
Essential (primary) hypertension
Hypertension
Hypertensive crisis
Hypertensive urgency
Peripheral arterial disease (PAD)
Plethysmography
Pulmonary embolism
Secondary hypertension
Stroke
Thoracic aortic aneurysm (TAA)
Venous thromboembolism (VTE)
Virchow's triad

CONCEPTS

- Assessment
- Inflammation
- Medication
- Nursing Roles
- Nutrition
- Perfusion
- Promoting Health

Finding Connections

CASE STUDY: EPISODE 1

Follow this patient throughout the chapter.

Mr. Brian More is a 62-year-old African American male who is brought into the emergency department by his daughter for occasional headaches, dizziness, and nocturia over the last 2 months. His past medical history includes hypercholesterolemia, diabetes mellitus type 2, obesity, and deep vein thrombosis (DVT). When a medical and family history is obtained, it is noted that Mr. More has smoked at least one pack of cigarettes per day for the last 40 years and that both of his parents died of stroke when they were in their mid-60s. He is currently on 40 mg PO Lipitor for his high cholesterol but denies use of any other medications...

INTRODUCTION

The overall function of the vascular system is to ensure adequate circulation of blood to all body tissues and capillary exchange between blood plasma, interstitial fluid, and tissue cells. Each tissue requires a minimum amount of blood per minute to sustain its metabolic activities and remove waste. The distribution of the cardiac output (CO) to various tissues depends on the interplay of (1) the pressure differences that drive the flow of blood and (2) the resistance to blood flow through specific blood vessels. See Chapter 28 for a more detailed overview of the anatomy and physiology of the vasculature. This chapter discusses disorders in the vasculature that impair or interfere with adequate delivery of oxygen and nutrients to the tissues.

ATHEROSCLEROSIS/ARTERIOSCLEROSIS

The primary culprits in many vascular disorders are arteriosclerosis and atherosclerosis. The terms are frequently used interchangeably. Although both conditions are types of vascular disease and may lead to the need for intervention or surgery, they are not the same.

Arteriosclerosis is a generic term describing the thickening or hardening of the arterial wall that is often associated with aging. This condition not only thickens the wall of the artery but also causes stiffness and a loss of elasticity. Arteriosclerosis includes three possible pathological processes. One, medial calcific sclerosis, occurs when calcium is deposited in the arterial wall. A second process, arteriolar sclerosis, involves the thickening of the smaller arterioles. The third process, atherosclerosis, occurs when low-density lipoprotein (LDL) particles build up in the arterial wall. Atherosclerosis is described in detail in the Pathophysiology section. To clarify, a patient with arteriosclerosis or hardened

arteries may not have atherosclerosis or plaque, but a patient with atherosclerosis does have arteriosclerosis. Patients often have both conditions. The focus of this chapter is atherosclerosis.

Epidemiology

The emerging epidemic of atherosclerotic disease in developing countries is thought to start in childhood and increase in prevalence with age. Changes occur in the arterial walls over time, which predisposes the older population to the development of atherosclerosis. Acquiring accurate data on the prevalence of the disease in the total population is difficult to obtain. It is more helpful to look at the prevalence of the disorders caused by atherosclerosis such as coronary artery disease, carotid artery disease, hypertension, abdominal aortic aneurysm (AAA), and peripheral arterial disease (PAD). This chapter reviews carotid artery disease, hypertension, AAA, and PAD. Coronary artery disease is discussed in depth in Chapter 30.

Risk factors that potentially stimulate atherosclerotic changes, causing damage to the arterial wall, include:

- Elevated cholesterol levels
- Elevated triglycerides
- Elevated low-density lipoprotein cholesterol (LDL-C)
- Low high-density lipoprotein cholesterol (HDLC)

Other risk factors of atherosclerosis include hypertension, diabetes, smoking, family history, obesity, and a sedentary lifestyle. Hypertension acts synergistically with other risk factors in the development of atherosclerosis. It causes a mechanical injury to the arterial walls that, over time, makes them harder and less elastic.

Diabetes is linked to atherosclerosis partially because of the increased LDLs and hyperglycemia associated with the disease. Hyperglycemia is thought to damage the intimal layer of the arterial wall.

Although tobacco use has declined in the United States, it remains the second leading cause of total deaths and disability. Tobacco smoke greatly worsens atherosclerosis and accelerates its growth in the coronary arteries, aorta, and arteries in the legs. Although cigarette smoke does not directly cause atherosclerosis, cigarette smoke and the by-products of tobacco cause vasoconstriction, hypertension, endothelial cell, and platelet dysfunction and increase circulating cholesterol. Second-hand smoke has also been shown to manifest these harmful effects. Smoking increases the risk of coronary artery disease two to four times above normal levels. Even smoking a few cigarettes a day or being exposed to cigarette smoke is correlated with an increased risk.

Some individuals have a family history of hyperlipidemia and increased cholesterol levels. Obesity and a sedentary lifestyle are linked to atherosclerosis because of their link to poor diet and increased cholesterol levels. Men have a higher incidence of atherosclerosis earlier in life than women; however, after menopause, the incidence of the disease is relatively equal in men and women. Degree of risk differs among Caucasians, African Americans, and Hispanics. There is an increased incidence of atherosclerosis among African Americans and Hispanics compared with Caucasians. This is partially because of an increased prevalence of smoking, diabetes, and hypertension in these races as compared with Caucasian Americans. Caucasians are more likely, however, to have abnormal serum lipid levels.

Connection Check 31.1

A patient teaching plan should focus on which risk factors for atherosclerosis? *(Select all that apply.)*
A. Obesity
B. Hyperlipidemia
C. Smoking
D. Age
E. Race

Pathophysiology

Atherosclerosis comes from the Greek words "athero," meaning "gruel" or "paste," and "sklerosis," meaning "hardness." Well documented in the literature, **atherosclerosis** is a disease in which LDL-C particles build up in the arterial wall.

Atherosclerosis is a slow, complex disease that typically starts in childhood and progresses while people grow older. In some people, it progresses rapidly, with symptoms becoming evident as young as 30 years of age. The lesions of atherosclerosis accumulate in large and medium-sized arteries. The exact pathophysiology remains under intense investigation, but the condition is thought to begin from vessel damage that causes an inflammatory response. After the vessel becomes inflamed, a fatty streak appears on the intimal surface, or inner lining, of the artery. Researchers believe that high circulating cholesterol levels promote the deposit of lipids into the arterial wall. In the presence of inflammatory mediators, they are oxidized by macrophages and perpetuate the inflammatory condition. It is best described as an inflammatory process comprising a series of highly specific cellular and molecular reactions that lead to the accumulation of atherosclerotic plaque. The presence of plaque thickens the inner layer of the artery significantly. The inner diameter of the artery shrinks, causing a decrease in blood flow, ultimately reducing oxygen supply to the affected tissues (Fig.31.1). Plaques can grow large enough to significantly reduce blood flow through an artery, but a more serious problem is when they become unstable and rupture. Plaques that rupture may cause blood clots to form that can block blood flow entirely. Ruptured plaques also have the potential to travel to another part of the body.

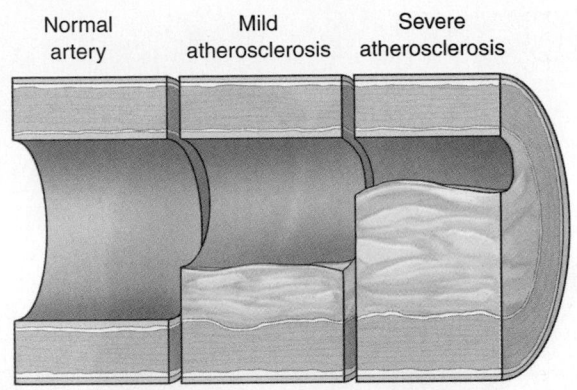

FIGURE 31.1 Atherosclerosis. The accumulation of atherosclerotic plaque shrinks the vessel diameter, decreasing blood flow.

Clinical Manifestations

There may be no symptoms of atherosclerosis until there is a critical narrowing of the artery that results in an emergency. Depending on the artery involved, the coronary or carotid arteries, plaque formation and/or rupture can lead to myocardial infarction, unstable angina, sudden cardiac death, or stroke. Specifically, atherosclerotic disease in the coronaries can result in chest pain or angina, shortness of breath, fatigue, and arrhythmias. As noted, it may also result in sudden cardiac death. Atherosclerotic disease in the carotids may result in a stroke. Manifestations of a **stroke** include sudden weakness (sometimes noted more on one side than the other), dizziness and loss of coordination, difficulty talking, facial droop, sudden vision problems, and sudden and severe headache. If blood supply to the arms or legs is reduced in a similar manner, it can cause significant pain and difficulty walking. If blood supply is completely occluded peripherally to the affected body part, it can eventually lead to gangrene. *Gangrene* is a medical term used to describe the death of tissues of the body. Gangrene can affect any part of the body; the most common sites include the toes, fingers, hands, and feet (Fig. 31.2).

Management

Medical Management

Identifying and controlling risk factors for the development of atherosclerosis are the basis of medical management. A decrease in serum LDL-C levels leads to a reduction in the risk of atherosclerotic cardiovascular disease. Medications used to lower lipid levels are the primary treatment modality. Anticoagulation is also used to decrease clot formation. Medication therapy is similar to that for coronary artery disease and is outlined in Table 30.2 in Chapter 30. Other options include modification in dietary habits, smoking cessation, and lifestyle modifications including an exercise and stress reduction plan. Proper management of diabetes is essential. Medical management for the disorders caused by atherosclerosis is discussed in detail throughout this chapter.

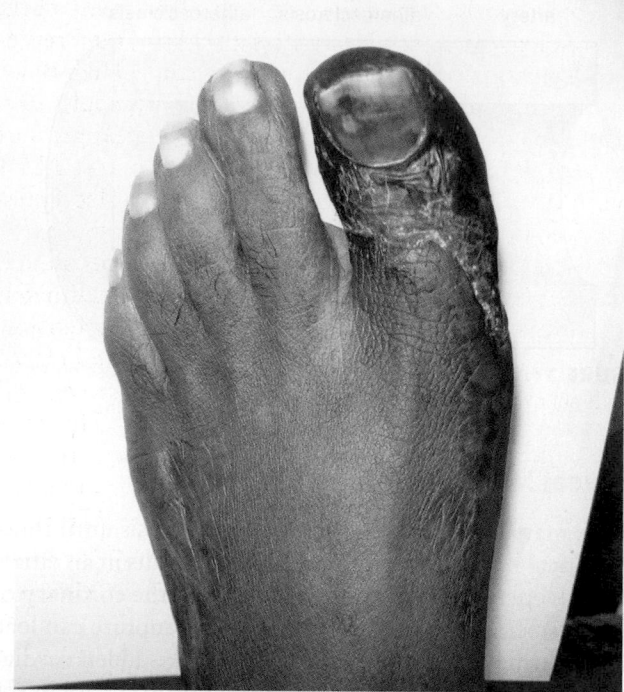

FIGURE 31.2 Patient foot with gangrene secondary to inadequate tissue perfusion.

Surgical Management

Surgical intervention is reserved for the irreversible manifestations of atherosclerosis such as chest pain or gangrene. Intractable chest pain caused by coronary artery disease requires coronary revascularization which can be done percutaneously or by surgical coronary artery bypass surgery. These management options for coronary artery disease are discussed in Chapter 30. Gangrene caused by atherosclerosis may require amputation. The use of surgical interventions must always be balanced against the risks of the procedure.

Nursing Management

Assessment and Analysis

The clinical manifestations of atherosclerotic disease vary according to the arteries involved. Disease in the coronary arteries results in chest pain, shortness of breath, and fatigue. Critical disease in the carotid arteries results in signs of stroke. Disease in the peripheral vascular system results in severe pain and difficulty walking. General nursing interventions for arteriosclerosis/atherosclerosis are outlined here.

Specific nursing management for disorders caused by arteriosclerosis/atherosclerosis—hypertension, carotid artery disease, and peripheral vascular disease—are discussed in detail throughout the chapter. Coronary artery disease is discussed in detail in Chapter 30, and stroke is discussed in detail in Chapter 39.

Nursing Diagnoses

- **Risk for ineffective tissue perfusion**: cerebral, related to interruption of carotid blood flow
- **Pain** related to decreased blood flow

Nursing Interventions

■ *Assessments*

- Complete patient history and cardiovascular assessment
  There is a genetic and environmental link to cardiovascular disease. Patients with a family history of cardiovascular disease have a higher prevalence of the traditional cardiovascular risk factors highlighting opportunities for prevention.
- Assess blood pressure (BP) in both arms
  Hypertension is a strong risk factor for atherosclerotic disease.
- Palpate pulses at all the major sites on the body and note any differences. Carotid arteries are palpated one at a time.
  Weak pulses may suggest poor flow through the artery. Palpate the carotids one at a time so as not to risk blocking flow to the brain.
- Auscultate for bruits
  A bruit is a turbulent, swishing sound that can be soft or loud in pitch. It is heard as a result of blood trying to pass through a narrowed artery.
  Bruits often occur in the carotid, aortic, femoral, and popliteal arteries. A bruit is considered abnormal, but it does not indicate the severity of the disease.
- Fasting lipid profile
  Low-density lipoprotein cholesterol (LDL-C)
  High LDL-C levels indicate an increased risk for atherosclerosis. Target LDL-C level is less than 100 mg/dL for healthy adults.
  High-density lipoprotein cholesterol (HDL-C)
  Low HDL-C levels indicate an increased risk for atherosclerosis.
  The target HDL-C level is greater than 40 mg/dL.
- Triglyceride levels
  Triglyceride levels may be elevated with atherosclerosis. Elevated triglycerides are considered a marker for other lipoproteins.
  A level of 150 mg/dL or above indicates hypertriglyceridemia.
- Homocysteine
  Homocysteine is a sulfur-containing amino acid derived from dietary protein. High serum levels of homocysteine may block production of nitric oxide on the vascular endothelium, making the cell walls less elastic and permitting plaque to build up.
- Glycosylated hemoglobin A1c (HgbA1c)
  Hyperglycemia is a risk for the development of atherosclerosis. An HgbA1c of greater than 7% may indicate poor glycemic control.

■ *Actions*

- Administer medications as ordered such as:
  - Antihypertensive medication
  - Lipid-lowering therapy including statin therapy
    There is a direct relationship between hypertension and increased cholesterol levels and atherosclerosis.

■ *Teaching*

- Blood pressure management—take medications as ordered
  Hypertension puts patients at risk for heart disease and stroke.
- Lifestyle changes such as:
  - Healthy diet
    A low-fat, low-cholesterol diet helps manage risk factors and slows the progression of atherosclerosis. Elevated homocysteine levels may be lowered by a diet enriched with B-complex vitamins, particularly folic acid.
  - Smoking cessation
    Toxins in tobacco smoke lower a person's HDL-C while raising levels of LDL-C.
    The nicotine and carbon monoxide in cigarette smoke damage the endothelium, which sets the stage for the build-up of plaque.
    If a smoker has hypertension, smoking can increase the risk of malignant hypertension.
  - Exercise
    Exercise can help to lower LDL-C and increase HDL-C.
    Exercise can also help reduce other risk factors of atherosclerosis such as high BP, diabetes, obesity, and stress.

Evaluating Care Outcomes

Arteriosclerosis/atherosclerotic disease and the related disorders can be well managed through adherence to a healthy diet, exercise, stress management, and very importantly, smoking cessation.

HYPERTENSION

Hypertension is a common and manageable chronic condition that is a major risk factor for atherosclerotic cardiovascular disease, heart failure (HF), stroke, kidney failure, vision loss, dementia, and circulation problems such as peripheral artery disease. Hypertension carries the risk for premature morbidity or mortality, which increases as systolic and diastolic pressures rise.

Epidemiology

The prevalence of hypertension is approximately 78 million individuals in the United States. Seventy million other Americans have prehypertension now referred to as elevated blood pressure. The overall prevalence of hypertension has not changed appreciably since 2009–2010. Among hypertensive Americans, 82% are aware of their condition. Approximately 75% are using antihypertensive medication; however, target BP control is attained only 53% of the time for individuals with diagnosed hypertension. Based on national data from 2011–2012, treatment of hypertension exceeded the Healthy People 2020 target goal of 69.5%. However, the control of hypertension has not met the goal of Healthy People 2020 (61.2% by 2020). Additionally, data from the

latest blood pressure guidelines from the American College of Cardiology/American Heart (ACC/AHA) for the Prevention, Detection, Evaluation, and Management of High Blood Pressure in Adults indicates that 45.6% of US adults have hypertension; death rates attributed to high blood pressure increased 10.5%, and the actual number of deaths rose 37.5% from 2005 to 2015. The total direct cost of high blood pressure could increase to an estimated $220.9 billion by 2035.

Risk factors include age, gender, race, and socioeconomic status. Blood pressure tends to rise with age. Approximately 65% of Americans aged 65 or older have hypertension. People with a normal BP at age 55 have a 90% lifetime risk of developing hypertension. Men and women are equally likely to develop high BP during their lifetimes. However, before age 45, men are more likely to have high BP than women. After age 65, the condition is more likely to affect more women than men. Race also plays a major factor in risk associated with hypertension. African American adults continue to have the highest prevalence of hypertension in the United States, and morbidity and mortality are highest in African Americans. It is also more prevalent in those of low socioeconomic status. Other major risk factors are outlined in Box 31.1.

Essential or **primary hypertension** accounts for 90% to 95% of the cases of hypertension in the adult population. Essential hypertension has no identifiable medical cause. It appears to be a multifactorial, polygenic condition. Heredity is a predisposing factor, but the exact mechanism is unclear (see Genetic Connections). It tends to be familial and is likely to be the consequence of an interaction between environmental and genetic factors. The risk for this type of hypertension can increase when heredity is combined with unhealthy lifestyle choices such as smoking or a poor diet. Essential hypertension is four times more common

Box 31.1 Major Risk Factors for the Development of Hypertension

Cigarette smoking
Obesity (body mass index ≥30 kg/m^2)
Physical inactivity
Excessive Alcohol use (more than two drinks per day for men and more than one drink per day for women)
Diet
Stress
Dyslipidemia*
Diabetes mellitus*
Microalbuminuria or estimated glomerular filtration rate of less than 60 mL/min
Age (older than 55 years for men, 65 years for women)
Family history of premature cardiovascular disease (men younger than age 55 years, women younger than age 65 years)

*Component of the metabolic syndrome

Genetic Connections

Genetic Factors Related to Essential Hypertension

More than 50 genes have been examined in association with hypertension. One of these genes, the angiotensinogen (*AGT*) gene, has been studied extensively. The results have shown that increasing the number of *AGT* genes increases blood pressure and hence may be a cause of hypertension. In general, these studies indicate essential hypertension has a large genetic component, but more research is indicated because the genetic influence upon hypertension is still not fully understood.

in African Americans than Caucasians. It accelerates more rapidly and is often more severe with higher mortality in African Americans.

Other notable risk factors associated with primary hypertension include obesity, salt sensitivity, renin elevation, insulin resistance, vitamin D deficiency, and cigarette smoking. Recent studies claim that obesity is a risk factor for hypertension because of the activation of the renin-angiotensin system and the sympathetic nervous system in adipose tissue. Other studies have linked insulin resistance with similar effects on the renin-angiotensin system and increased sympathetic nervous system activity. Salt sensitivity is an environmental factor that has received great attention. Approximately one-third of the population with essential hypertension is responsive to sodium intake. When sodium intake exceeds the body's capacity to excrete it through the kidneys, vascular volume expands secondary to movement of fluids into the intravascular compartment. This causes the arterial pressure to rise while the fluid volume and cardiac output (CO) increase. Local autoregulatory mechanisms attempt to counteract this by decreasing vascular resistance to maintain normotension.

Secondary hypertension is characterized by elevations in blood pressure due to a specific cause. Renal parenchymal disease affecting the renal medulla and renal cortex, where the "work" of the kidney is done, is the most common cause of secondary hypertension excluding obesity and alcohol abuse. It is responsible for 2% to 5% of all cases of secondary hypertension. Examples of renal parenchymal disease include chronic glomerulonephritis or pyelonephritis, polycystic renal disease, connective tissue disorders, and obstructive uropathy. Other causes of secondary hypertension include renovascular disease, pheochromocytoma, Cushing's syndrome, primary aldosteronism, congenital adrenal hyperplasia, hyperthyroidism, myxedema, and coarctation of the aorta. Excessive alcohol intake and use of oral contraceptives are also common causes of secondary hypertension, as is the use of sympathomimetics, NSAIDs, corticosteroids, cocaine, or licorice.

Pathophysiology

The mechanisms that cause hypertension are complex. Because BP is the result of CO × total peripheral vascular resistance (PVR), pathogenic mechanisms must involve increased CO, increased PVR, or both. Cardiac output is a function of heart rate (HR) and stroke volume (SV). Peripheral vascular resistance is a function of the autonomic nervous system and circulating hormones such as epinephrine. Any factor that increases HR, such as overactivity of the sympathetic nervous system, or increases circulating volume, such as fluid retention with increased sodium intake, increases BP. Any factor that increase PVR, such as angiotensin II, increases BP. In very-early hypertension or in younger people CO is increased and PVR is normal. Later or in older adults, increased PVR is predominant. Table 31.1 describes several mechanisms that may result in hypertension.

Table 31.1 Mechanisms That Result in Hypertension	
Increased sodium intake	● Increased sodium causes fluid retention, increasing stroke volume and blood pressure.
Renin-angiotensin-aldosterone system (RAAS)	● Excess angiotensin II results in vasoconstriction and increased blood pressure.
	● Excess angiotensin also results in increased aldosterone release (see below).
Aldosterone	● Excess aldosterone release results in sodium and water retention, which results in increased stroke volume and blood pressure.
	● Enhanced potassium (K) excretion also occurs, resulting in low plasma K.
	● Low plasma K increases vasoconstriction through closure of K channels.
Sympathetic nervous system	● Increased sympathetic activity is a primary precursor to hypertension. It can cause vasoconstriction, resulting in increased peripheral vascular resistance and increased blood pressure. It may also increase heart rate.
	● Overactivity of the sympathetic nervous system may result from either inappropriately elevated sympathetic drive from brain centers, an increase in synaptically released neurotransmitters in the periphery, or amplification of the neurotransmitter signal at the target tissue.

Connection Check 31.2

The nurse is screening patients for their risk of developing hypertension. The nurse should consider which patients at greatest risk? *(Select all that apply.)*

A. A 40-year-old Latino male who is obese and smokes two packs of cigarettes per day

B. A 35-year-old Asian female who has a familial history of diabetes mellitus type 1

C. A 78-year-old African American male with chronic renal insufficiency

D. A 25-year-old African American female track athlete with a healthy body mass index (BMI) who takes oral contraceptives

E. A 60-year-old Caucasian male with vitamin D deficiency and a history of cocaine use

Clinical Manifestations

Clinical manifestations of primary hypertension are typically evident only after long-term increased BP has resulted in target organ damage (TOD), to be discussed under Complications. Some symptoms of chronic uncontrolled hypertension are headaches, chest pain, vision changes, shortness of breath, renal dysfunction, dizziness, fatigue, or nosebleeds. Clinical manifestations related to secondary hypertension are the result of the disease processes that cause hypertension.

Management

Medical Management

Diagnosis

The diagnosis of hypertension is made on the basis of the average of two or more properly measured BP readings on two or more office visits. Treatment is indicated at that time but may begin immediately if two consecutive readings during a single visit indicate an extreme elevation. New (2017) ACC and AHA guidelines for the detection, prevention, management and treatment of high blood pressure lower the definition of high blood pressure to account for complications that can occur at lower numbers and to allow for earlier intervention. See Table 31.2 for the classifications of hypertension for adults aged 18 and older.

Once the diagnosis of hypertension has been made, providers attempt to identify the underlying cause on the basis of risk factors and other symptoms. Laboratory tests are performed to identify possible causes of secondary hypertension. Additional tests for diabetes and high cholesterol levels are performed because they are risk factors for the development of heart disease that require treatment. Tests typically performed in a hypertension work-up are classified in Table 31.3.

A thorough history and physical examination are done to detect TOD. The search for the presence of subclinical target organ damage (TOD) is strongly recommended because it allows a better stratification of cardiovascular

Table 31.2 Classification of Blood Pressure for Adults

Blood Pressure Classification	Systolic BP	Diastolic BP
Normal	Less than 120 mm Hg	and less than 80 mm Hg
Elevated	120–129 mm Hg	and less than 80 mm Hg
Stage 1 hypertension	130-139 mm Hg	or 80-89 mm Hg
Stage 2 hypertension	140 mm Hg or higher	or 90 mm Hg or higher
Hypertensive Crisis (consult doctor immediately)	Higher than 180 mm Hg	and/or higher than 120 mm Hg

Hypertensive Crisis

Hypertensive urgency: DBP greater than or equal to 120 mm Hg with no obvious target organ damage (TOD)*

Hypertensive emergency: DBP greater than or equal to 120 mm Hg with evidence of TOD*

*TOD is damage to the heart, eyes, or kidneys caused by hypertension.

DBP, Diastolic blood pressure; *SBP,* systolic blood pressure.

Table 31.3 Hypertension Laboratory Diagnostic Testing

System	Tests	Expected Findings If TOD Present
Renal	Microscopic urinalysis, proteinuria, serum BUN (blood urea nitrogen), and/or creatinine	Proteinuria Elevated BUN and creatinine
Endocrine	Serum sodium, potassium, calcium, TSH (thyroid-stimulating hormone)	↑Sodium ↑Potassium ↑TSH
Metabolic	Fasting blood glucose, total cholesterol, HDL and LDL cholesterol, triglycerides	Fasting glucose greater than 100 mg/dL ↑LDL, triglycerides ↓HDL
Other	Hematocrit, electrocardiogram, and chest x-ray	Left ventricular hypertrophy ↓Hematocrit

HDL, High-density lipoprotein; *LDL,* low-density lipoprotein
Source: Jameson, J. L., Fauci, A. S., Kasper, D. L., Hauser, S. L., Hauser, S. L., Longo, D. L., & Loscalzo, J. (2018). *Harrison's principles of internal medicine* (20th ed.). New York, NY: McGraw-Hill Medical

risk, encourages the achievement of a lower BP target than usual, and helps with the selection of the most appropriate medication regimen. To that end, testing is done to determine if hypertension has caused damage to the heart, eyes, or kidneys.

Treatment

An increase in recent years of illness and death due to hypertension has prompted experts to urge more effective BP control. To bring high blood pressure down to a healthy level, treatment guidelines recommend healthy lifestyle changes, medication, or both. Lifestyle changes alone may be the first step in patients with mildly elevated (systolic between 120-129 and diastolic < 80) blood pressure readings.

Medications

The new guidelines recommend only prescribing medication beginning at Stage I hypertension if a patient has already had a cardiovascular event such as a heart attack or stroke or is at high risk of heart attack or stroke based on age, the presence of diabetes mellitus, chronic kidney disease or calculation of atherosclerotic risk. If medications are necessary, there are a variety of medications used to treat high BP. Which medications are initially prescribed to a patient depends on numerous factors including ease of use, side effects, and coexisting medical conditions that may necessitate use of one agent versus another. Diuretics are commonly included in the treatment plan. Clinical trials have shown they enhance the antihypertensive efficacy of multiple medication regimens, are useful in achieving BP

control, and are more affordable than other antihypertensive medications. Combination therapy regimens can facilitate achievement of BP goals. Table 31.4 gives an overview of the antihypertensive medications that may be used individually or in combination with one another. When a treatment plan is considered for the patient, socioeconomic status and psychosocial stress as risk factors for high blood pressure should be considered in a patient's plan of care.

Connection Check 31.3

Which statement by the patient about the need for antihypertensive medication indicates the need for further teaching?
A. "I'm worried about a stroke if my BP is not controlled."
B. "Can my kidneys fail if I don't control my BP?"
C. "My BP is only slightly elevated, so I am ok."
D. "I guess I need to take this medication even if I feel OK."

Lifestyle Management

Lifestyle changes are an important component of hypertension management. These lifestyle changes include weight control, diet modification including reduced salt intake, lowering alcohol use, and regular exercise and relaxation.

Weight

Obesity is associated with severe hypertension and the need for multiple medications to control BP. Thus, weight loss

Table 31.4 Antihypertensive Medications

Medication	Description
Diuretics	Act on the kidneys to help the body eliminate sodium and water, reducing blood volume. Diuretics are often the first but not the only choice in high blood pressure medications.
Calcium channel blockers Amlodipine besylate (Norvasc) Diltiazem (Cardizem) Nifedipine (Adalat CC, Procardia XL)	Help relax/dilate the muscles of the blood vessels. Some slow the heart rate. In African American adults with hypertension but without heart failure or chronic kidney disease, including those with diabetes mellitus, initial antihypertensive treatment should include a thiazide-type diuretic or a calcium channel blocker. Two or more antihypertensive medications are recommended to achieve a blood pressure target of greater than 130/80 mm Hg in most adults, especially in African American adults, with hypertension.
Angiotensin-converting enzyme inhibitors	Help relax/dilate blood vessels by blocking the formation of angiotensin II, a vasoconstrictor, thus reducing blood pressure
Angiotensin II receptor blockers (ARBs)	Help relax/dilate blood vessels by blocking the action not the formation of angiotensin II, a vasoconstrictor; sometimes used in patients intolerant of ACE inhibitors
Beta blockers	Reduce the afterload on the heart and dilate blood vessels, causing the heart to beat more slowly and with less force
Combined alpha and beta blockers	Reduce nerve impulses that promote vasoconstriction and at the same time slow the heart rate and reduce afterload
Vasodilators	Relax the muscle tissue in the blood vessel walls and, in turn, lower the blood pressure
Central agonists	Decrease blood vessels' ability to contract and cause vasoconstriction

has clear benefits in reducing BP and the number of medications required to control it. Excess weight, especially excess fat stored in your abdomen, can raise blood pressure by increasing your blood volume and by changing the balance of pressure-regulating hormones. Even modest weight loss can have a positive impact. Research shows that losing just 7.7 pounds could reduce your risk for high blood pressure by 50% or more. The 2013 European Society of Hypertension and European Society of Cardiology guidelines recommend reducing BMI to 25 kg/m² and waist circumference to less than 102 cm in men and less than 88 cm in women.

Diet

High dietary salt intake is commonly associated with patients with resistant hypertension (hypertension resistant to treatment). High amounts of sodium found in many processed foods raise BP by facilitating water retention (which boosts blood volume) and even tightening small blood vessels. The association is more pronounced in salt-sensitive patients including older adults, African Americans, and patients with chronic kidney disease. Reducing dietary salt intake can reduce systolic BP and diastolic BP by 5 to 10 mm Hg and 2 to 6 mm Hg, respectively. African American and older adult patients tend to show greater benefits from reducing salt intake. Other dietary considerations include the minerals calcium, magnesium and potassium (found in low-fat and fat-free dairy products, such as milk and yogurt, as well as in produce and dried beans). They help the body regulate blood pressure; too little can raise blood pressure. Saturated fat (found in meat, cheese, butter, full-fat dairy products and many processed foods) may also raise blood pressure. A DASH (Dietary Approaches to Stop Hypertension) diet high in fruits, vegetables, and low-fat dairy products has been shown to lower elevated pressures (Table 31.5).

Table 31.5 DASH Diet Table

Type of Food	Servings on a 2,000-Calorie Diet
Grains and grain products (include at least three whole-grain foods each day)	6–8/day
Fruits	4–5/day
Vegetables	4–5/day
Low-fat or nonfat dairy foods	2–3/day
Lean meats, fish, poultry	6 or fewer/day
Nuts, seeds, and legumes	4–5 per week
Fats and oils	2–3/day
Sweets	5 or fewer/week

Alcohol Consumption

Heavy alcohol intake is associated with higher BP and with treatment-resistant hypertension. In one study, a small group of patients who quit heavy alcohol drinking reduced their systolic BP by 7.2 mm Hg and their diastolic BP by 6.6 mm Hg. Their prevalence of hypertension decreased from 42% to 12%. Moderating alcohol is very important. Although a small amount of alcohol may relax arteries, too much seems to have the opposite effect. Men should have no more than two drinks per day and women should have no more than one drink per day.

Exercise

Regular physical activity makes the heart stronger and may reduce weight if combined with a healthy diet. A stronger heart can pump more blood with less effort, reducing the force on the arteries, lowering BP. Becoming more active can lower systolic BP by an average of 5 to 10 mm Hg, which is as good as some BP medications. The ACC/AHA guidelines recommend at least 90 to 150 minutes per week of aerobic activity. Dynamic and isometric resistance exercise is also recommended.

Stress Management

The body's stress response releases hormones that temporarily raise blood pressure. To date, it is not clear whether mind-body therapies have a lasting effect on blood pressure or reduce the risk of hypertension. It is well researched that regularly practicing stress-soothing techniques such as breathing exercises, progressive relaxation, and fitness activities helps the recipient feel better, finding it easier to make other healthy changes. One technique, meditation, has been shown to reduce the risk for heart attacks and strokes in people with high blood pressure.

Connection Check 31.4

A nurse providing care for a patient whose BP readings are consistently 130/85 mm Hg should anticipate which medical plan of care? *(Select all that apply.)*
A. Diagnostic testing for TOD
B. Initiation of diuretics
C. Modifications of diet and exercise
D. Echocardiogram
E. A stress test

Complications

High BP is known as the "silent killer" because it can cause considerable damage to the heart, brain, and kidneys (target organs) before symptoms are apparent. The heart is most commonly affected by hypertension. When arterial pressure is high, the heart uses more energy to pump against the increased afterload caused by the elevated pressure in the aorta. Because of the increased afterload, the left ventricle gradually hypertrophies, causing diastolic dysfunction. The ventricle eventually dilates, causing dilated cardiomyopathy and HF due to systolic dysfunction. Heart failure is discussed in detail in Chapter 30.

Hypertension also compromises kidney function. The principal site of damage is in the arterioles leading to the renal system. The continual high pressures exerting force against the walls cause them to thicken, which narrows the lumen. The blood supply to the kidneys is gradually reduced. In response to the reduction in blood supply, the kidneys secrete more renin, which elevates the BP even more, complicating the problem. Eventually, the reduced blood flow may lead to the death of the kidney cells.

Stroke is a very serious complication of hypertension. Prolonged increases in BP may cause vessel rupture, which leads to hemorrhage and a sudden loss of function, resulting from a disruption of the blood supply to a part of the brain. It is the fourth-leading cause of death in the United States and the leading cause of disability. Hypertension is the most important but modifiable risk factor related to stroke. In clinical trials, antihypertensive therapy has been associated with reductions in stroke incidence averaging 35% to 40%. Please refer to Chapter 39 for a more detailed discussion of stroke. An **aneurysm** is another very serious complication of hypertension. An intracranial aneurysm is a dilation of the walls of the cerebral artery that develops as a result of weakness in the arterial wall. The aneurysm presses on nearby cranial nerves or brain tissue causing damage or ruptures causing subarachnoid hemorrhage and stroke.

Hypertensive crisis is an umbrella term for acute, severe elevations in BP. It comprises two conditions on a continuum: **hypertensive urgency** and hypertensive emergency. Hypertensive urgency is severely elevated BP (diastolic BP ≥120 mm Hg) with no obvious, acute TOD. Hypertensive emergency is differentiated from hypertensive urgency by evidence of TOD, which may include signs of stroke, papilledema, HF, or aortic dissection. Hypertensive emergency is the most serious but least common form of hypertensive crisis, representing only 5% of cases. It requires emergent attention. Blood pressure must be lowered immediately to halt TOD. The incidence is higher in older adults, African Americans, and men. Most patients seen in hypertensive crisis have a prior history of hypertension and have been prescribed antihypertensive medications at some point. Sudden escalation of essential, chronic hypertension is a common precipitant of hypertensive crisis. Medication interactions and/or withdrawal of treatment are also frequently precipitating factors.

Nursing Management

Assessment and Analysis

Hypertension is a silent disease. There are typically no symptoms until the disease is advanced and the damage to organs has been done. A physical examination may reveal no abnormality other than high BP.

Nursing Diagnoses

- **Risk for ineffective therapeutic regimen management** related to nonadherence to treatment
- **Risk for decreased CO** related to left ventricular hypertrophy and eventual left ventricle dilation secondary to increased afterload

Nursing Interventions

■ *Assessments*

- Neurological assessment
  It is important to assess signs and symptoms that could indicate TOD and cerebrovascular disease leading to possible complications such as stroke and aneurysm.
- Blood pressure
  Early detection and treatment of hypertension can prevent or minimize TOD. Measurements determine the treatment regimen prescribed.
- Heart rate
  Increased PVR can lead to increased HR or increased SV to compensate for the increased PVR.
- Examination of the optic fundi
  Hypertension may lead to retinal damage and eventually retinal hemorrhage because of the vascular changes caused by hypertension.
- Auscultation for carotid, abdominal, and femoral bruits
  Bruits are sounds created by blood flow through a stenosed or narrow vessel.
- Palpation of the lower extremities for edema and pulses
  Weak pulses and peripheral edema can indicate kidney disease and/or HF.
- Serum creatinine, blood urea nitrogen (BUN), estimated glomerular filtration rate, and 24-hour urine collection for creatinine clearance
  Abnormal levels indicate renal disease, which may develop in patients with hypertension.
- Albumin excretion rate
  Microalbuminuria is a significant marker of early cardiac, renal, and retinal structural and functional changes in essential hypertension.
- Calculation of BMI and waist circumference
  Obesity and diet are major risk factors in hypertension.

■ *Actions*

- Administer antihypertensive medications as ordered
  Clinical outcome trial data prove that lowering BP with a combination of one or several classes of medications reduces the complications of hypertension.
- Provide patient with DASH diet for meals
  A 1,600-mg sodium DASH eating plan has effects similar to those of antihypertensive single-medication therapy.

■ *Teaching*

- Adherence to antihypertensive medication regimen and lifestyle changes such as:
  - DASH diet and sodium restriction (diet rich in fruits, vegetables, and low-fat dairy products, and

reduced in saturated fat and cholesterol) greater than or equal to 1,600 mg sodium per day is recommended.

- Moderate exercise (at least 150 minutes of moderate aerobic activity per week, primarily aerobic exercise, which helps raise the heart rate to 70% to 85% of an individual's maximal heart rate, or endurance exercise supplemented by resistance exercise).
- Limit alcohol (no more than one drink per day for women, two drinks per day for men).
- Stress reduction
- Smoking cessation
  It is important that the patient and family are aware of the critical nature of adhering to the medication regimen and lifestyle changes. Long-term effects of TOD should be stressed as a risk factor with noncompliance. Expected side effects should be explained thoroughly so the patient knows what to expect and how to cope with the side effects.
- Monitoring blood pressure at home
  Teach and coach patients and family members to monitor BP consistently at home to improve BP management. Automatic BP cuffs can be purchased at local pharmacies.
- Signs and symptoms of TOD, stroke, and aneurysm
  Detecting signs and symptoms early can help prevent or stabilize renal, cardiovascular, cerebrovascular, and retinal disease.

Evaluating Care Outcomes

Patients need to understand and comply with the treatment regimen of antihypertensive medications and necessary lifestyle changes to achieve optimum health. A patient with well-controlled hypertension has a BP and HR within normal limits. Other indicators of well-controlled BP are increased energy and no headache, dizziness, or vision changes or other signs of TOD. The electrocardiogram (ECG) and echocardiogram remain normal or unchanged. Blood chemistries and urinalysis are within normal limits.

CASE STUDY: EPISODE 2

Mr. More demonstrates classic signs of chronic uncontrolled hypertension—headaches, dizziness, and nocturia. Initial diagnostic results show a BP reading of 180/122 mm Hg, HR 100 bpm, O_2 saturation of 96%, elevated fasting blood glucose (250), an elevated BUN (28 mg/dL) and creatinine (2.2 mg/dL), protein in his urine, elevated LDL (180 mg/dL), decreased HDL (30 mg/dL), and elevated triglycerides (300 mg/dL). The results are consistent with possible kidney and heart damage. Diagnostic testing continues in order to determine the level of damage. If one more BP reading confirms hypertension, Mr. More will be admitted to the hospital for observation and started on an antihypertensive medication regimen...

PERIPHERAL ARTERIAL DISEASE

Epidemiology

According to data from the AHA and the ACC from 2016, approximately 8.5 million people in the United States older than 40 years have **peripheral arterial disease (PAD)**. It is estimated that PAD affects 202 million people worldwide. PAD is associated with significant morbidly, mortality, and quality-of-life impairment.

Atherosclerosis is the main contributor to PAD. Therefore, the risk factors for atherosclerosis apply to PAD as well. They include key modifiable risk factors such as smoking, hypertension, diabetes, dyslipidemia, sedentary lifestyle, obesity, and ineffective stress management. Nonmodifiable risk factors include age, gender, ethnicity, and family history. A strong family history of coronary artery disease or PAD is an important predictor of its occurrence and subsequent prognosis.

Pathophysiology

PAD is a progressive and chronic condition where the obstruction of blood flow through the large peripheral arteries causes a partial or total arterial occlusion. This obstruction can be caused by a combination of atherosclerosis, inflammation, stenosis, embolus, and thrombus. Peripheral arterial disease deprives the lower extremities of oxygen and nutrients. The result of this inadequate tissue perfusion can be ischemia and necrosis, or cell death (Table 31.6).

Clinical Manifestations

The disease may be asymptomatic, identified only by a reduced BP in the ankle, or it may manifest symptoms of intermittent claudication or, in most patients, atypical lower extremity pain. Intermittent **claudication** is defined as muscle pain—ache, cramp, numbness, or sense of fatigue, classically in the calf muscle, that occurs during exercise and is relieved by a short period of rest. Atypical leg pain is described as limited or painful joints, cold and/or ulcerated extremities, or painful stretching to name a few. Both intermittent claudication and atypical leg pain have a cycle of exercise induced and rest relief. The typical patient with PAD experiences a profound limitation in exercise capacity and quality of life. In addition to affecting the limbs, PAD is a manifestation of systemic atherosclerosis which could be affecting other major vascular systems such as the cerebral and coronary circulations. Chronic PAD can be divided into four stages (Table 31.7).

Management

Medical Management

Diagnosis

The vascular assessment for PAD includes pulse palpation, auscultation for femoral bruits, and inspection of the legs and feet. To confirm the diagnosis of PAD, abnormal physical examinations findings must be confirmed with

Table 31.6 Buerger's Disease/Raynaud's Disease: Disorders Related to Poor Peripheral Circulation

	Buerger's Disease	Raynaud's Disease (Phenomenon)
Description	Acute inflammation and thrombosis in arteries and veins in the hands and feet	Temporary, severe vasoconstriction in the arteries of the fingers and/or toes in response to cold
Causes	Unknown but maybe autoimmune reaction triggered by smoking	Unknown
Risk Factors	Cigarette smoking	Cigarette smoking Alcohol use Connective tissue or autoimmune disorder
Clinical Manifestations	Claudication (exercise-induced pain) in hands/feet Numbness/tingling Raynaud's phenomenon Ulceration/gangrene of the digits	In response to cold: ● Distal extremities (finger tips, toes) turn white, then blue, then red as circulation returns ● Numbness ● Pain ● Severe: Ulceration/development of gangrene in finger pads
Treatment	Smoking cessation	Smoking cessation Use mittens rather than gloves Avoid stress Avoid sudden changes in temperature

Table 31.7 Stages of Peripheral Arterial Disease

Stage	Presentation
Stage I: Asymptomatic PAD	● No claudication/pain is experienced by patient. ● Bruit may be heard. ● Pedal pulses are decreased or absent.
Stage II: Claudication	● Muscle pain, burning, and cramping are experienced with exercise and are relieved by rest. ● Pain is reproducible with the same amount of exercise.
Stage III: Rest pain	● Pain is experienced at rest. ● Pain often awakens patient at night. ● Pain is described as numbness and burning and usually occurs in the distal portion of the extremity. ● Pain is often relieved by putting the extremity in the dependent position.
Stage IV: Necrosis or gangrene	● Ulcers and blackened tissue occur on the toes, the forefoot, or the heel of the foot. ● Gangrenous odor may be present.

diagnostic testing. Specifically, other comorbid causes of atypical leg pain should be ruled out before diagnosing PAD. Noninvasive testing for arterial disease has become a common method of diagnosis. This includes the ankle-brachial index (ABI), plethysmography, and graded-exercise treadmill test. These tests provide information about the arterial system with minimal risk. Anatomical imaging studies, including duplex ultrasound, computed tomography angiography, magnetic resonance angiography, and invasive angiography, are other diagnostic tools but are sometimes reserved for highly symptomatic patients who are being considered for revascularization.

Ankle-Brachial Index

The **ankle-brachial index (ABI)** uses a Doppler probe to compare the BP obtained at the ankle with the pressure obtained at the brachial artery. This is an inexpensive, noninvasive method of assessing PAD. Normally, BP readings in the ankle are higher than those in the upper extremities. This test provides a ratio known as the ABI. The value can be derived by dividing the ankle BP by the brachial BP (Fig. 31.3). An ABI of less than 0.9 in either leg is diagnostic of PAD (Box 31.2). An increased ABI is indicative of poorly compressible arteries which indicates calcification of the arteries; another indicator of vessel disease. As an alternative, particularly for diabetics, a toe-brachial index may be performed in a certified vascular laboratory.

Plethysmography

Plethysmography is another noninvasive test used to evaluate arterial flow in the lower extremities. Pulse volume recordings are plethysmographical tracings that detect changes in the volume of blood flowing through a limb. Pressure cuffs are placed on the thigh, calf, ankle, or foot. The pressure cuffs are inflated to 65 mm Hg, and a plethysmographical tracing is recorded at the various areas where the cuffs are placed. A normal pulse volume recording is similar to a normal arterial pulse wave tracing and consists of a rapid systolic upstroke and a rapid downstroke with a prominent dicrotic notch. With increasing severity of PAD, the waveforms are decreased or flattened depending on the degree of occlusion (Fig. 31.4).

Treadmill Test

A graded exercise treadmill test may give valuable information about the degree of peripheral arterial narrowing in patients who experience intermittent claudication. Once the resting pressures and pulse volume recordings are obtained, the patient is asked to walk on a treadmill at a constant speed, either at a constant grade (2 mph, 12% incline) or with a variable incline (0% at start, increased by 3.5% every 2–3 minutes). The former method exercises patients to a maximum of 5 minutes, whereas the latter continues for a maximum of an 18% incline. The graded exercise treadmill test:

1. Confirms the diagnosis of intermittent claudication and PAD
2. Demonstrates the objective functional limitation of PAD
3. Documents the effect of therapy on initial and absolute claudicating distances
4. Uncovers previously unrecognized coronary artery disease

Duplex Ultrasound

Duplex ultrasound uses the detection of sound waves to measure the velocity of blood flow. It is used to detect and localize vascular lesions and quantify the amount and severity of damage through blood flow velocity criteria.

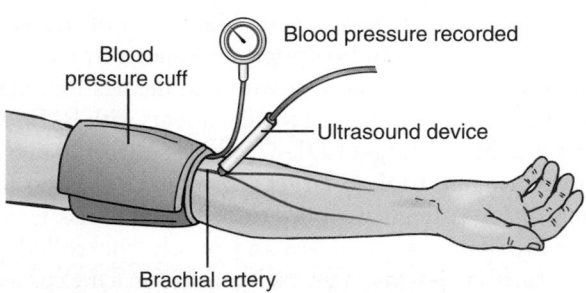

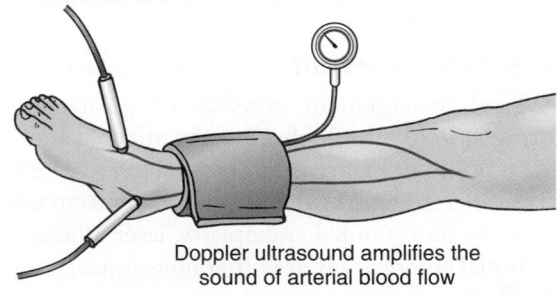

$$\text{ABI} \text{ (Ankle brachial index)} = \frac{\text{Ankle blood pressure}}{\text{Brachial blood pressure}}$$

FIGURE 31.3 Obtaining an ankle-brachial index (ABI). An ABI of less than 0.9 in either leg is diagnostic of peripheral arterial disease.

Box 31.2 Interpreting Ankle-Brachial Index Values

- Greater than 1.30 = Noncompressible arteries (stiff arteries)
- 1 to 1.29 = Normal
- 0.91 to 0.99 = Borderline PAD
- 0.41 to 0.9 = Mild to moderate PAD
- 0 to 0.4 = Severe PAD

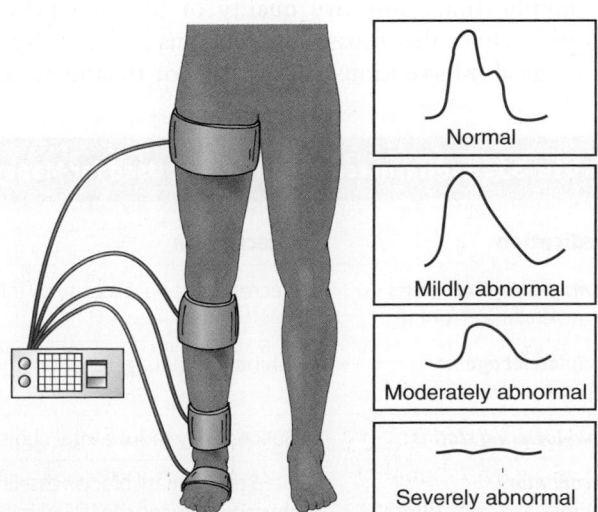

FIGURE 31.4 Plethysmography; damping of the wave form is indicative of peripheral arterial disease.

Computed Tomography Angiography

Computed tomography angiography (CTA) imaging is a CT scan that requires contract material to visualize blood vessels. It displays a roadmap of the vasculature which identifies the issues and is sometimes essential for determining interventional strategies. Advantages of CTA include quick noninvasive testing, wide availability, high resolution, and 3D imaging. The disadvantages of CTA include the lack of hemodynamic data, exposure to radiation, and use of contrast agents.

Magnetic Resonance Angiography

Magnetic resonance angiography (MRA) is a magnetic resonance test that focuses on the study of the vasculature. It uses contrast and noncontrast techniques when imaging the peripheral arteries. Noncontrast MRA has inferior resolution and may contain artefacts that limit the interpretation, but it is a valuable alternative for use in patients with mild to moderate chronic kidney disease for whom the use of contrast agents is not recommended. Vascular calcification can be underestimated by using MRA and this may affect revascularization procedures.

Angiography

Angiography imaging assessment consists of arteriography of the lower extremities. This is done to quantify the narrowing of the occluded vessels. Arteriography involves injecting contrast medium into the arterial circulation through a small sheath in the groin. Treatment options can be derived and refined via arteriography. One treatment option is balloon angioplasty for the occluded vessel with stent placement. Angiography can also provide a better visual for refinements for planned peripheral bypass surgery. Balloon angioplasty and peripheral bypass surgery are described in detail later.

Treatment

The primary goals of medical treatment and nursing care for patients with PAD are to provide relief of symptoms, prevent the progression of arterial disease and cardiovascular complications, improve quality of life, and provide education about the disease. Medications and nonsurgical and surgical interventions are options for treatment. The majority of patients with PAD are elderly with a significantly increased risk of myocardial infarction, stroke, and cardiovascular death. Nonpharmacological interventions such as weight reduction, smoking cessation, exercise, and adherence to a low-fat diet are first-line actions.

Medications

Medication therapies target the risk factors driving the progression of atherosclerosis in PAD. They include antihypertensive, antiplatelet, and statin agents. All of these medications have been associated with significant reductions in mortality in patients with PAD. Beta blockers can be used for BP control. They were previously thought to exacerbate intermittent claudication but are now currently recommended to achieve BP goals in PAD.

Antiplatelet agents such as acetylsalicylic acid (aspirin) and clopidogrel (Plavix) are commonly prescribed in patients with chronic PAD. Another antiplatelet agent, cilostazol, is an effective medical therapy for treatment of leg symptoms and walking impairment due to claudication. In addition to antiplatelet aggregation properties, it is also a vasodilator which can help improve blood flow through affected extremities. Unfortunately, significant side effects of headache, diarrhea, dizziness, and palpitations cause some patients to discontinue their treatment with that medication. Statin therapy is also recommended for all patients with PAD. The goal is to achieve a target LDL-C level less than 100 mg/dL. A more stringent LDL-C target is recommended (less than 70 mg/dL) in patients with PAD with multiple risk factors, especially diabetes, or severe and poorly controlled risk factors such as smoking, high triglycerides, or acute coronary syndrome. See Table 31.8 for pharmacological agents used for managing PAD.

Nonsurgical Management

Nonsurgical management consists of positioning or promoting vasodilation by having the affected limb in a dependent position. Exercise may be used to increase blood flow to the affected limb by increasing collateral circulation. Percutaneous transluminal angioplasty, laser atherectomy, and rotational atherectomy are other nonsurgical interventions for PAD.

Table 31.8 Pharmacological Agents Used for Managing Peripheral Arterial Disease (PAD)

Medication	Description
Hemorheological agents pentoxifylline (Trental)	Decrease blood viscosity by inhibiting platelet aggregation; increase blood flow to the affected extremity
Antiplatelet agents Aspirin or clopidogrel	Inhibit platelet aggregation, therefore decreasing the probability of vascular events
Lipid-lowering statins	Successfully reduce total cholesterol in most patients when used for extended period
Vasodilators angiotensin converting enzyme (ACE) inhibitors	Help relax/dilate blood vessels by blocking the formation of angiotensin II, a vasoconstrictor. ACE inhibitor therapy reduced the risk of myocardial infarction, stroke, or vascular morbidity in patients with peripheral arterial disease by approximately 25%.

Percutaneous Transluminal Angioplasty

Percutaneous transluminal angioplasty (PTA) is a nonsurgical, minimally invasive method of improving arterial blood flow. During this procedure, a cannula is inserted into or above an occluded or stenosed artery. The occluded artery is then dilated with a balloon catheter (Fig. 31.5). Success of the procedure is proven when it opens the vessel and restores or improves arterial blood flow. Stents may be used during this procedure to keep the vessel open. The transfemoral approach is the safest, most widely used, and most effective route for arteriography. If the femoral artery is not an option for catheterization secondary to surgery, arterial stenosis, or occlusion, alternative routes for arteriography include the brachial or axillary approach. Reocclusion may occur after percutaneous angioplasty. If this occurs, the procedure may be repeated. Some patients remain occlusion-free for up to 3 to 5 years, whereas other patients may experience reocclusion much sooner. The experience is patient specific. Patients must be educated on the importance of medication compliance and continued risk factor modifications. They are also educated on the signs and symptoms of reocclusion.

Laser-Assisted Angioplasty

Laser-assisted angioplasty is another minimally invasive intervention that can be done for patients with PAD. During this procedure, a laser probe is advanced through a cannula that is inserted into or above an occluded artery. This procedure is usually indicated for smaller occlusions in the distal superficial femoral, proximal popliteal, and common iliac arteries. Heat from the laser probe vaporizes the arteriosclerotic plaque to open the occluded or stenosed vessel. A PTA is often needed to further open the occlusion.

Rotational Atherectomy

Rotational atherectomy is another technique used to improve blood flow to the ischemic limbs of people with PAD. Rotational atherectomy is more commonly used for very hard, calcified stenotic lesions that are not amenable to balloon angioplasty. Rather than compressing plaque and stretching an artery narrowed by atherosclerotic plaque, the goal of atherectomy is removal of the plaque by breaking it into microfragments.

The occlusion is accessed the same way as for PTA and laser atherectomy. The rotational atherectomy device (rotoblader) is a high-speed rotary metal burr. The distal end of the burr is coated with fine abrasive bits that reach speeds of 100,000 to 120,000 rotations per minute. When the burr comes in contact with the calcific plaque, it breaks up the blockages into very small fragments (smaller than red blood cells), which can pass harmlessly into the circulation. Often, balloon angioplasty with stent placement is performed after rotational atherectomy to improve results.

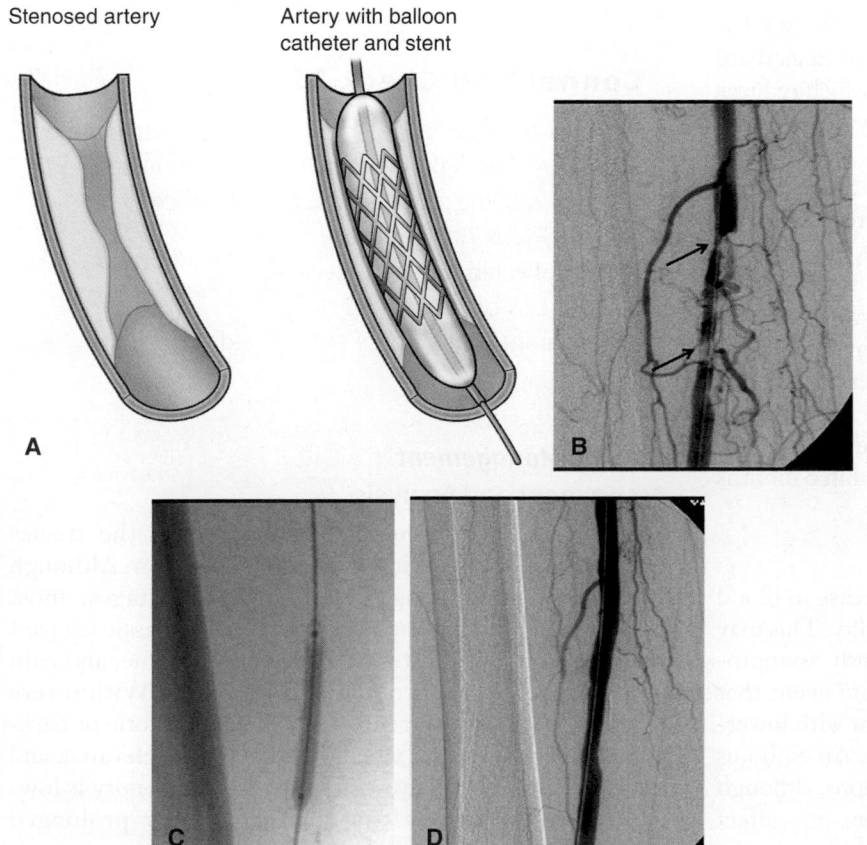

FIGURE 31.5 Percutaneous transluminal angioplasty (PTA). A, Plaque limiting flow in an artery, the artery is dilated with a balloon catheter and a stent is placed to keep the vessel open; B, Angiogram demonstrating a severe femoral artery stenosis (arrows) amenable to PTA; C, Balloon catheter dilation; D, Blood flow restored.

Surgical Management

Surgical or revascularization procedures are indicated when patients have severe pain at rest or claudication that interferes with the ability to perform activities of daily living (ADLs) or threatens loss of a limb.

Arterial revascularization is the surgical procedure most commonly used to increase arterial blood flow to the affected limb. Revascularization is accomplished through bypass grafting. Surgical bypass treats narrowed arteries by creating a bypass around a section of the artery that is blocked. Grafts used for bypasses are selected on an individual basis. Autogenous grafts, such as the patient's own saphenous vein, are most commonly used. If the saphenous vein is not suitable, then the cephalic or basilic arm veins may be used. Autogenous veins are often not long enough for use in vessels distal to the popliteal vessels, so composite grafts are constructed from multiple vein segments.

Synthetic grafts can be used if the patient's own vessels are not available for grafting. Synthetic grafts have been shown to be very effective in achieving patency in arteries above the knee. They have not been shown to be effective in occlusions distal to the popliteal vessels, hence the value of the autogenous composite grafts.

Complications

Critical Limb Ischemia

Critical limb ischemia (CLI) is the sustained, severe decrease of arterial blood flow to the affected extremity, which leads to chronic ischemia, rest pain, ulceration, gangrene, and, ultimately, limb loss if left untreated. Obstructive atherosclerotic arterial disease is the most common cause of CLI. Other contributing factors that lead to CLI or exacerbate the situation include diabetes and/or low CO, which reduces the blood flow to the microvasculature. Typically, CLI presents after an extended course of PAD.

Once PAD progresses to chronic CLI, the patient's prognosis is generally poor. Infection, cellulitis, and tissue breakdown can occur. All of these conditions increase the requirement for oxygenated blood, which is decreased because of the disease process. Without adequate tissue perfusion, tissue breakdown and ulcers worsen, and gangrene then becomes apparent. Almost half of patients with this level of CLI need revascularization to save the affected limb. Of the patients whose limbs cannot be revascularized, approximately 40% need major amputation within 6 months of initial diagnosis.

Acute Limb Ischemia

Acute limb ischemia (ALI) is the sudden decrease in blood flow to an extremity that threatens tissue viability. This may be the first manifestation of PAD in a previously asymptomatic patient, or it may be caused by an acute event that leads to symptomatic deterioration in a patient with lower-extremity PAD and intermittent claudication. An embolus is the most common cause of peripheral occlusions, although a local thrombus may be the cause. Occlusions may affect the upper extremities, but they are more common in the lower extremities. Emboli originating from the heart are the most common cause of acute arterial occlusions. Most patients with embolic occlusions have had an acute myocardial infarction (MI) or atrial fibrillation within the past few weeks.

Patients with ALI describe severe pain distal to the level of the occlusion that occurs at rest. The affected extremity is cool or cold, pulseless, and mottled. The toes may be blackened or present with gangrene. The following are the "six Ps" of ischemia:

- Pain
- Pallor
- Pulselessness
- Paresthesia
- Paralysis
- Poikilothermia (cool)

This patient requires immediate intervention. The goal of treatment is to preserve tissue and save the limb. Initiation of anticoagulation therapy with IV heparin is usually the first intervention to prevent further clot formation. Subsequent treatment for ALI includes interventions to restore blood flow, which relieves pain, helps heal ulcers, and possibly prevents amputation of the affected limb. Revascularization interventions include percutaneous transluminal angioplasty (PTA), bypass surgery, or surgical thrombectomy or embolectomy. Pain management and systemic antibiotics for infected skin or wounds are also indicated. If ALI is identified early and reperfusion interventions are promptly initiated, tissue may be salvaged.

Connection Check 31.5

The nurse is reviewing orders for a newly admitted patient with PAD in the right lower extremity. The nurse should follow up with the provider about which order?

A. Begin Plavix 75 mg PO daily
B. Keep affected extremity elevated
C. Begin Lisinopril 10 mg PO daily
D. Encourage light exercise as tolerated

Nursing Management

Assessment and Analysis

Clinical manifestations of PAD vary with the tissues involved and the severity of altered blood flow. Although PAD is often unrecognized in its early stages, most patients initially seek medical attention for classic leg pain referred to as intermittent claudication, fatigue, and pain in a specific muscle group during exertion. With severe arterial disease, the extremity is cold and cyanotic or darkened. Pallor may occur when the extremity is elevated, and dependent redness may occur when the extremity is lowered. Muscle atrophy can also accompany prolonged chronic PAD.

Nursing Diagnoses

- **Ineffective peripheral tissue perfusion** related to interruption of arterial blood flow to the peripheral tissue
- **Risk for impaired skin integrity** related to altered circulation or sensation
- **Chronic pain** related to decreased peripheral perfusion evidenced by the inability to walk for prolonged periods of time or having pain at rest

Nursing Interventions

Assessments

- Bilateral blood pressures
  Patients with diagnosed PAD have an increased risk of subclavian artery stenosis. Upper arm blood pressure difference of greater than 15 to 20 mm Hg is abnormal and suggestive of subclavian stenosis. Use the higher blood pressure measurement when calculating ABI and titrating blood pressure medications.
- Palpate all pulses in both legs
  Weak or absent pulses indicate poor blood flow through the extremity. The most sensitive indicator of arterial function is the quality of the posterior tibial pulse.
- Visual assessment of feet and limbs
  Signs of ulcer formation: sluggish capillary refill; dry, scaly, dusky, pale, or mottled skin; thickened toenails. Loss of hair on the lower calf, ankle, and foot indicate poor peripheral blood flow.
- Temperature
  Cool or cold temperature in the extremities indicates poor flow.
- Assess bilateral muscle tone
  Muscle atrophy can accompany prolonged chronic arterial disease.
- Assess pain
  Pain in the affected extremity with activity that is relieved with rest is indicative of PAD.

Actions

- Administer medications as ordered
  - Antihypertensives
    Controlling hypertension is necessary to help manage comorbidities, and it can improve tissue perfusion by maintaining pressures that are adequate to perfuse the periphery but not constrict the blood vessels.
  - Antiplatelet agents
    Patients with PAD and no contraindications to antiplatelet therapy should receive either aspirin or clopidogrel to inhibit clot formation.
  - Cilostazol
    Cilostazol has antiplatelet and vasodilation properties that can improve PAD symptoms.
- Proper positioning
  Keep the affected extremity dependent to facilitate blood flow.

Teaching

- Positioning
  Avoid crossing legs, which can further obstruct flow.
- Inspect feet daily
  Patients with PAD may develop ulcers on the bottom of their feet and between their toes. This should be monitored daily.
- Report chest discomfort or neurological changes immediately
  Patients with PAD have an increased risk for developing chronic angina, MI, or stroke.
- Lifestyle changes consistent with the management of atherosclerosis
  - DASH diet
  - Limit alcohol
  - Smoking cessation
  - Moderate exercise
    Atherosclerosis is the most common risk factor for PAD.

Evaluating Care Outcomes

The primary goals of medical treatment and nursing care for patients with PAD are to provide relief of symptoms, improve quality of life, provide education about the disease, and prevent the progression of arterial disease and cardiovascular complications. A well-managed patient is pain free and able to participate in normal physical activities without limitations.

CAROTID ARTERY DISEASE

Epidemiology

Carotid artery disease is a common atherosclerotic vascular disease. It can begin to develop in patients in their 40s, with the prevalence increasing with age, with as many as 11% of men 80 years of age or older presenting with the disease. It is thought that an occlusion of at least 50% will be present in 3% to 4% of the population. Men have a higher prevalence than women, and Caucasians and native Americans have a higher risk.

Risk factors associated with carotid artery disease are similar to those that cause atherosclerotic occlusive disease in other vessels: smoking, hypertension, diabetes, dyslipidemia, sedentary lifestyle, obesity, and ineffective stress management. Nonmodifiable risk factors include age, gender, ethnicity, and family history. Younger than 75 years, men have a greater risk than women. Older than 75 years, women have a greater risk. People with coronary artery disease have a greater risk of developing carotid artery disease.

Pathophysiology

Similar to atherosclerotic changes in other arteries, carotid artery disease is characterized by vessel wall thickening, plaque formation, and a progressive narrowing of the carotid artery. Plaque disruption and thrombus formation contribute to progressive narrowing of the lumen of the artery, which can cause adverse clinical events. Stenosis is most significant at the carotid bifurcation. This area is known as the carotid bulb, where the common carotid artery branches into the internal and external carotid arteries (Fig.31.6). The carotid bifurcation is an area of low-flow

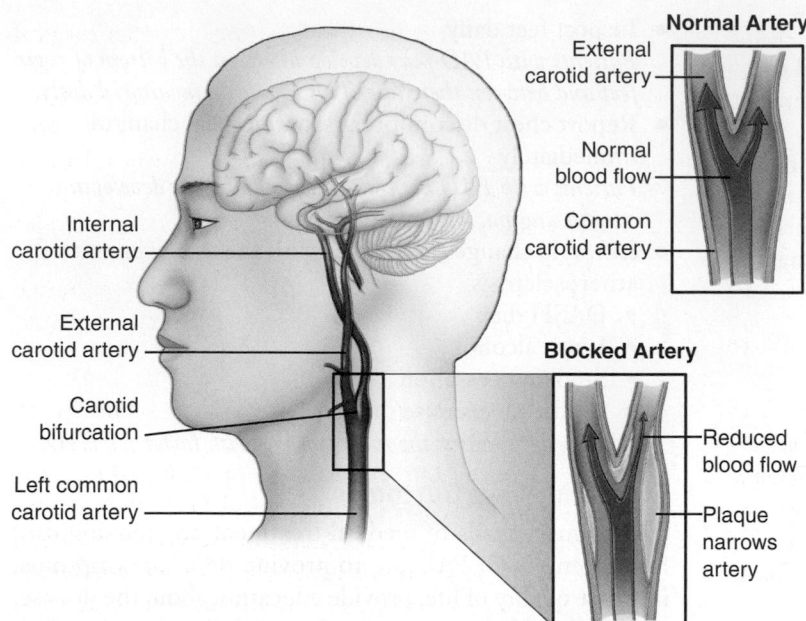

FIGURE 31.6 Plaque formation in the carotid arteries around the carotid bifurcation.

velocity and low-shear stress. While the blood circulates through the carotid bifurcation, there is a separation of flow into the low-resistance internal carotid artery and the high-resistance external carotid artery. With increasing degrees of stenosis in the internal carotid artery, flow becomes more turbulent, increasing the risk of atheroembolization: an embolism from atherosclerotic plaque. The severity of stenosis is commonly divided into three categories according to the luminal diameter reduction:

- Mild (<50%)
- Moderate (50%–69%)
- Severe (70%–99%)

Clinical Manifestations

Carotid artery disease is asymptomatic until the lumen of the vessel is obstructed to the point that cerebral perfusion is impaired. A bruit resulting from turbulent flow past the obstruction at the carotid bifurcation may be heard with a stethoscope.

The clinical manifestations of complications resulting from impaired cerebral perfusion such as stroke or transient ischemic attack (TIA) are discussed in Chapter 39. They include sudden weakness, sometimes noted more on one side than the other, dizziness and loss of coordination, difficulty talking, facial droop, sudden vision problems, and sudden and severe headache.

Management

Medical Management

Diagnosis

Diagnostic testing involves physical assessment and noninvasive and/or invasive procedures. Physical assessment of carotid artery disease includes auscultation over the blood

vessels in the neck. When the bell of the stethoscope is placed over the side of the neck anterior to the sternocleidomastoid muscle, a carotid bruit may be heard. This sound occurs when blood flow becomes turbulent while it hits an obstruction at the carotid bifurcation.

Noninvasive tests include carotid duplex scanning, computed tomography angiography (CTA), and magnetic resonance angiography (MRA). Duplex ultrasound is the most commonly used screening tool to evaluate for atherosclerotic plaque and stenosis of the external carotid artery (Fig. 31.7).

An invasive test, conventional carotid angiography, is the gold standard for diagnosis of the severity of carotid artery disease. This test involves inserting a catheter into an artery, typically the femoral artery, and guiding it up to the carotids. Contrast dye is injected through the catheter that allows visualization of the carotid arteries via radiographical

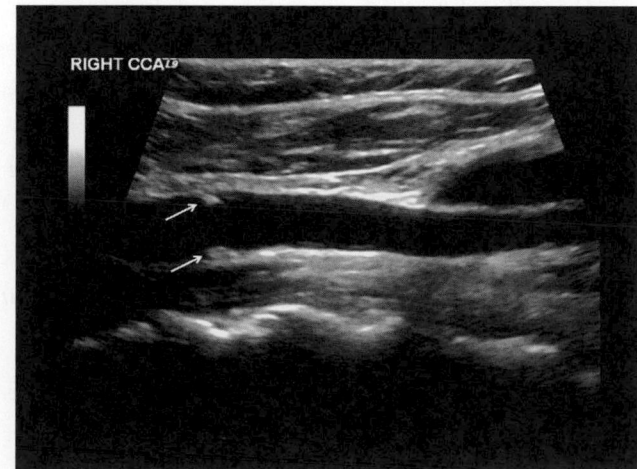

FIGURE 31.7 Doppler ultrasound of an atherosclerotic carotid artery showing plaque obscuring a portion of the vessel (arrows).

imaging. Because of the invasive nature of the test and the risks associated with it, noninvasive tests are more commonly used for diagnosis. See Table 31.9 for information on noninvasive diagnostic tests.

Treatment

Treatment for patients with carotid artery stenosis depends on the severity of the occlusion and whether the individual is symptomatic or asymptomatic. An **asymptomatic** patient is without a prior history of stroke or TIA. A **symptomatic** patient is one who presents with TIA, stroke in evolution, or completed stroke.

The management of asymptomatic patients starts with optimal medical therapy (OMT) which includes a combination of healthy lifestyle changes such as weight management, smoking cessation, limited alcohol consumption, and control of comorbidities such as diabetes and hypertension, and use of medications to manage the cause of atherosclerotic vascular disease. Medication management includes antiplatelet therapy with aspirin. Clopidogrel is an option if aspirin in contraindicated. Antihypertensive therapy for blood pressure control is essential. The AHA recommends maintaining blood pressure below 140/90 mm Hg. Many classes of medications, such as calcium channel blockers, angiotensin-converting enzyme inhibiters, and angiotensin receptor blockers, are effective in blood pressure control. Lipid-lowering therapy with statins is also recommended. Without stating an LDL-C target level as evidence, current guidelines suggest that the use of high-intensity statins shows a 50% reduction in LDL-C levels. Somewhat controversial is the use of invasive procedures to treat the obstruction itself. Patients would benefit from either surgical or endovascular revascularization but are at risk for the complications of the procedures, which include stroke. Current guidelines suggest revascularization in medically stable patients with carotid endarterectomy (CEA) or carotid artery stenting (CAS). Both procedures will be discussed below in detail. The management of symptomatic patients includes OMT but requires revascularization with CEA or CAS due to the presence of stroke or stroke symptoms unless excessive comorbidities put the patient at unreasonable risk of death.

Surgical Management

Revascularization options include carotid endarterectomy (CEA) or carotid artery stenting (CAS). CEA is a more invasive approach. There have been several studies comparing the efficacy of two procedures. A large multicenter randomized control trial, Carotid Revascularization Endarterectomy vs. Stenting Trial (CREST), was conducted in 2010 comparing outcomes for carotid-artery stenting with carotid endarterectomy. In 2016, a 10-year follow-up to CREST found no significant difference between patients who underwent carotid artery stenting and those who underwent carotid endarterectomy with respect to the risk of periprocedural stroke, myocardial infarction, or death and subsequent stroke. However, it appeared that in older patients (older than 70 years) adverse events were more common with stenting where younger patients had better results with stenting versus endarterectomy. The decision about which procedure to have requires careful consideration in regard to symptomatic versus asymptomatic, patient age, comorbid conditions, and severity of stroke symptoms.

Table 31.9 Noninvasive Diagnostic Tests for Assessing Carotid Artery Disease

Noninvasive Diagnostic Test	Rationale
Carotid duplex ultrasonography: a noninvasive test that uses high-frequency sound waves to measure real-time blood flow and detect blockages or other abnormalities in the carotids	This is the most widely used screening tool to evaluate for atherosclerotic plaque and stenosis. Ultrasonography is an accurate method for measuring the severity of stenosis.
Magnetic resonance angiography (MRA): utilizing IV contrast dye, the MRA uses magnetic fields and radio waves to show blockages inside the arteries	MRA is increasingly used to evaluate for atherosclerotic carotid occlusive disease. MRA can generate high-resolution noninvasive images of the carotid arteries. The radiofrequency signal characteristics of flowing blood are sufficiently distinct from surrounding soft tissue to allow imaging of the arterial lumen.
Magnetic resonance imaging (MRI): a test that uses a magnetic field and pulses of radio wave energy to make pictures of organs and structures inside the body without contrast dye	MRI of the brain is essential in the assessment of acute stroke patients. MRI can differentiate areas of acute ischemia, areas still at risk for ischemia, and chronic cerebral ischemic changes.
Computed tomography angiogram (CTA): utilizing IV contrast dye to highlight the carotid arteries, the CTA highlights any areas of blockage or stenosis using an ultrafast CT scanner	CTA has gained increasing popularity in the evaluation of carotid disease. The advantages of CTA over MRA include faster data acquisition time and better spatial resolution even in very tortuous vessels.

Carotid Endarterectomy

Carotid endarterectomy (CEA) is surgery to remove the plaque causing the occlusion in the carotid arteries. During the procedure, the plaque and arterial intima, along with portions of the media of the artery, are removed. A patch of autogenous vein or prosthetic material is then put in place (Fig. 31.8). The goal of the surgery is to improve blood flow through the carotid artery and prevent stroke. Wide fluctuations in the patient's BP are common, and excessive hypertension or hypotension may produce stroke. Perioperatively, the patient should have an intra-arterial catheter inserted to monitor BP so that cerebral perfusion can be maximized.

Following CEA, the patient is monitored in a postanesthesia care unit or an intensive care setting. Postoperative priorities include tight control of BP, frequent neurological reassessments (Table 31.10), and prevention of bleeding and incision site complications. Hospital lengths of stays vary, but usually patients are discharged within 48 hours postoperatively.

Medications post-CEA include antiplatelet aggregates, antihypertensives, and statins. Aspirin is recommended before CEA and may continue indefinitely postoperatively. Beyond the first month after CEA, aspirin, clopidogrel, or the combination of low-dose aspirin plus extended-release dipyridamole (inhibits clot formation) should be administered for long-term prophylaxis against reocclusion of the carotids.

Carotid Artery Stenting

Carotid artery stenting is a procedure performed in combination with carotid angioplasty. During carotid angioplasty, the common carotid artery is accessed with a guiding catheter or a long sheath. A balloon catheter is then guided to the area of the blockage or narrowing. Once in place, the balloon is inflated, and the fatty plaque is compressed against the arterial wall to increase the lumen of the vessel and improve blood flow. During the angioplasty procedure, a carotid stent (a small, metal mesh tube) is placed inside the carotid artery at the site of the blockage to provide support to keep the artery open. Prior to stent insertion, an emboli protection device (EPD) is deployed to capture distal emboli to prevent clots from traveling to the brain. Following EPD deployment, the stent is placed (Fig. 31.9). After placement, a post inflation of the stent with a balloon catheter is performed to achieve good stent expansion and adherence to the arterial wall. After stent placement, the EPD is removed.

The patient's neurological status, particularly level of consciousness, speech, and motor function, should be monitored throughout the stent procedure by the provider or the circulating nurse. It is important to avoid excessive sedation to facilitate this ongoing assessment. Intraprocedural management also includes adequate anticoagulation and hemodynamic monitoring.

Patients undergoing CAS are commonly pretreated with aspirin and clopidogrel prior to the procedure. Aspirin is continued life long, and clopidogrel is given for at least 1-month postprocedure. Administration of antihypertensive medication is recommended to control BP before and after CAS.

Nursing assessments postprocedure include frequent monitoring of vital signs, complete neurological assessment, and frequent access site monitoring. As with CEA, the focus is on recognizing and preventing the complications associated with carotid stenting.

Nursing Management

Assessment and Analysis

Carotid artery disease is asymptomatic until the lumen of the vessel is obstructed to the point that cerebral perfusion is impaired. A bruit resulting from turbulent flow past the obstruction at the carotid bifurcation may be heard with a stethoscope. Symptoms of a stroke—slurring of words, weakness, severe headache, sudden vision loss, facial droop, or dizziness—are secondary to impaired perfusion to the cerebral tissues.

Nursing Diagnoses

- **Risk for ineffective tissue perfusion: cerebral**, related to interruption of carotid blood flow
- **Risk for injury** related to loss of motor, sensory, or visual function

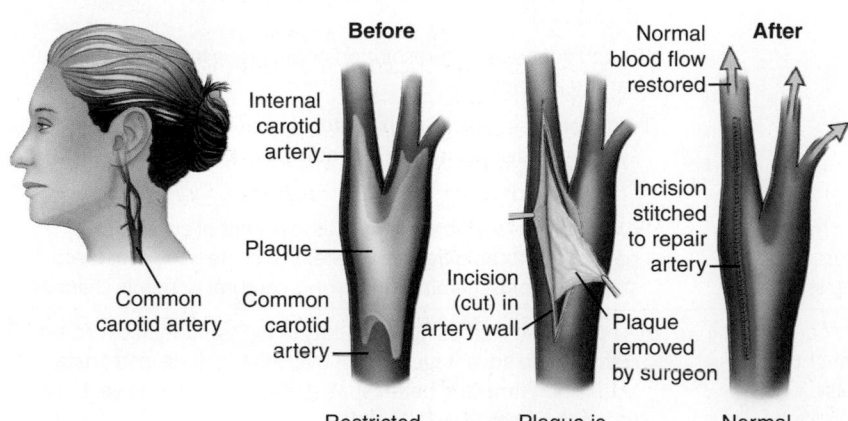

FIGURE 31.8 Removal of plaque from the carotid artery.

Table 31.10 Cranial Nerve Assessment Post-Carotid Endarterectomy (CEA)

The incidence of cranial nerve injury during carotid endarterectomy ranges from 3% to 23%. Lesions on the lower cranial nerves are mainly due to surgical maneuvers. Nurses must assess the function of these nerves after surgery. The damage can be temporary or permanent.

Cranial Nerve Name	Assessment
VII: Facial	Symmetry of face when smiling and showing teeth
X: Vagus	Swallowing, gag reflex, ask the patient to say "Ah"
XI: Spinal accessory	Shrug shoulders, rotate head side to side
XII: Hypoglossal	Tongue control and movement, ask patient to stick out tongue

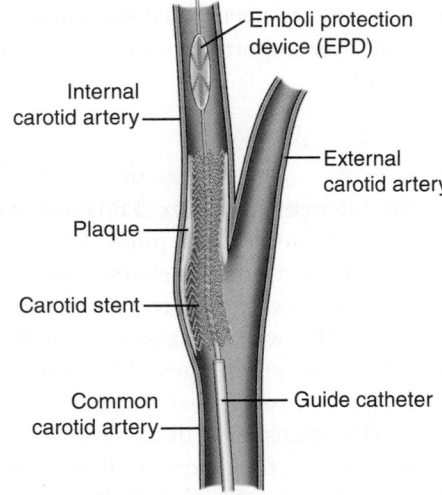

FIGURE 31.9 Carotid stenting with distal emboli protection device filter.

- **Anxiety** related to the invasive procedure or surgery, uncertainty of the outcome of the procedure

Nursing Interventions

Assessments

- Vital signs
  Hypertension is a risk factor for carotid artery disease. Fluctuations in blood pressure and bradycardia may be complications of treatment.
- Neurological assessment
  Difficulty speaking, weakness, facial droop, acute vision problems, and acute headache may be signs of stroke.
- Auscultation of the carotid arteries
  Asymptomatic carotid artery stenosis may be identified by the presence of carotid bruits, sounds created by blood flow through a stenosed vessel, on auscultation.

- Stroke history/signs of stroke
  Determines if patient is symptomatic or asymptomatic which impacts treatment

Postprocedure CEA/CAS

- Respiratory rate, SpO$_2$, stridor, tracheal deviation
  In CEA—Hematoma formation at the incision site can cause tracheal pressure resulting in respiratory distress, which can escalate rapidly as the hematoma enlarges.
- Vital signs: HR, BP
  In CEA—Prior to treatment, the carotid baroreceptor sensed a low pressure in the stenotic carotid artery. Following CEA, a new "normal" pressure may be sensed as a high pressure signalling the vagus nerve to respond, resulting in vasodilation, bradycardia, and hypotension. Prolonged hypertension may result in damage to the arterial graft, causing hemorrhage as well as placing the patient at risk of intracerebral haemorrhage.
  In CAS—Bradycardia, related to manipulation of the carotid sinus baroreceptors located in the carotid bulb, may occur during the procedure just after the stent implantation; Persistent hypotension can be caused by the effect of the stent on the carotid sinus baroreceptors.
- Post-CEA—Cranial nerves, specifically VII, X, XI, and XII (see Table 31.10)
  Retraction on the lower cranial nerves during surgery can result in temporary or permanent nerve damage due to trauma or edema.
- Post-CAS - Renal function
  Angiogram dye is nephrotoxic, especially in those patients who already have kidney disease.

Actions

- Administer antihypertensive medication as ordered to maintain BP below 140/90 mm Hg
  Prolonged increases in BP may cause vessel rupture, which leads to hemorrhage and stroke.
- Administer lipid-lowering medication as ordered
  Reducing LDL-C helps reduce plaque formation in the carotid vessels.
- Administer antiplatelet aggregates as ordered
  Antiplatelet therapy helps reduce platelet aggregation, resulting in decreased risk of obstruction in the vessel.
- Manage diabetes mellitus/maintain blood glucose within normal levels
  Poorly controlled diabetes mellitus results in increased plaque formation in the vessels due to the breakdown of fats for energy, increasing the risk for ischemic stroke.

Postprocedure CEA/CAS

- Keep systolic blood pressure strictly within ordered parameters
  To maintain integrity of the graft and/or flow through carotids
- If patient is hypotensive:
  - Reposition patient flat
    Increase blood flow to increase cerebral perfusion

- Anticipate orders for vasoactive drips or intravenous fluid bolus
  Vasoactive drips cause vasoconstriction to increase blood pressure. Fluid bolus increases circulating volume, increasing BP.
- If patient is hypertensive:
  - Maintain head of the bed at 30 degrees
    Facilitates venous drainage and avoids excessive increases in cerebral blood volume.
- Post-CEA—Keep head in neutral position
  Decreases strain on incision site and carotid artery.
- Post-CAS - Encourage fluid intake/Maintain IV fluids
  Flush the contrast dye through the kidneys

■ *Teaching*

- Clinical manifestations of a stroke: severe headache, facial drooping, loss of strength on one side, change in gag reflex, slurred speech, inability to stick out tongue and shrug shoulders equally; instruct patient and family to report neurological changes immediately.
  The best outcomes occur with rapid treatment.
- Lifestyle changes consistent with the management of atherosclerosis
  - DASH diet
  - Exercise
  - Smoking cessation
  - Limit alcohol
    Atherosclerosis is implicated in the development and progression of carotid artery disease.

Connection Check 31.6

A nurse is performing the immediate postoperative assessment of a patient who has just undergone CEA. What is the most important assessment to be reported immediately?

A. A complaint of 7/10 pain
B. Falling back to sleep after assessment
C. An asymmetric smile
D. Complaint of a sore throat

Evaluating Care Outcomes

A patient effectively managing carotid artery disease articulates awareness of risk factor modification such as compliance with the medication regimen and necessary lifestyle changes to limit complications. Adequate outcomes of care are demonstrated when the patient has no clinical manifestations of stroke or procedural complications such as pain, swelling, or bleeding.

AORTIC ARTERY DISEASE (ANEURYSMS)

Epidemiology

Approximately 15,000 people in the United States die each year of **abdominal aortic aneurysms (AAAs)**. Men develop AAAs four to five times more often than women. Caucasians develop AAAs more commonly than other racial groups. **Thoracic aortic aneurysms (TAAs),** the most common site for a dissecting aneurysm, occur most often in men between the ages of 40 and 70 years and have a high mortality rate even with surgical intervention.

Risk factors include family history, advanced age, male gender, smoking, atherosclerosis, treated and untreated hypertension, high total serum cholesterol, known coronary artery disease, and genetic and/or metabolic abnormalities. Atherosclerosis accounts for 75% of all AAAs, but of these risk factors, smoking is one of the most important. It is a risk factor that the patient can control, thus modifying the risk.

Genetics are a major factor in aortic aneurysms. Familial clustering of aortic aneurysms has been observed, with an estimated 15% to 20% incidence occurring in first-degree relatives of the individual with an aneurysm. Marfan's syndrome is the hereditary disease most closely linked to aneurysm. This syndrome results in the degeneration of the elastic fibers of the aortic media. Syphilis, patients born with bicuspid aortic valve, and Ehlers-Danlos syndrome, a rare genetic disorder, are other causes of AAAs. Chronic inflammation (aortitis) is implicated in the development of aneurysms. Blunt trauma, usually from motor vehicle crashes, can cause aneurysms in the descending thoracic or abdominal aorta. More importantly, blunt trauma can cause rupture of the aorta.

Pathophysiology

An aneurysm is a permanent localized dilation of an artery that forms when the middle layer (media) of the artery is weakened, producing a stretching effect in the inner layer (intima) and outer layers of the artery. While the artery widens, tension in the wall increases, further widening occurs, and the aneurysm enlarges. The diameter of the artery can be enlarged to at least two times the normal circumference. Hypertension is one cause of that tension and enlargement within the artery. Other causes include congenital problems such as Marfan's syndrome or acquired problems such as atherosclerosis.

Aneurysmal degeneration of the aorta and iliac arteries is referred to as aortic aneurysm. Aneurysms can occur in three different areas of the aorta. Ascending aortic aneurysms are located in the arch of the aorta, descending aortic aneurysms or thoracic aneurysms are located above the diaphragm, and abdominal aortic aneurysms (AAAs) are located below the diaphragm in the abdomen. The abdomen is the most common location (Fig. 31.10).

Aneurysms are classified as true or false. In true aneurysms, all three layers of the arterial wall are weakened. True aneurysms are further classified by their shape or form (Fig. 31.11). The most common forms are saccular and fusiform. A saccular aneurysm projects from only one side of the vessel. If an entire arterial segment becomes dilated, a fusiform aneurysm develops.

A false or pseudoaneurysm is not a distortion of the vessel wall but rather a leak from the artery. The leak is confined by the surrounding tissues, and eventually a blood clot forms. Pseudoaneurysms are typically caused by iatrogenic trauma

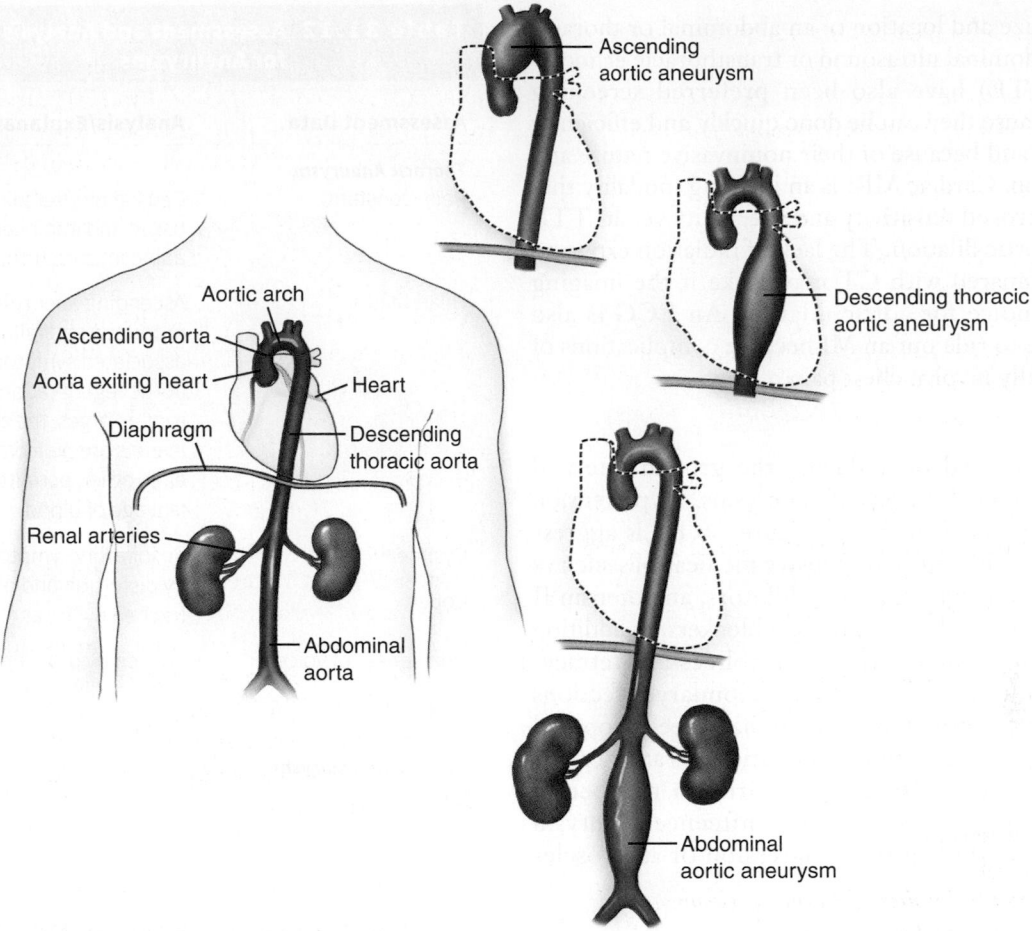

FIGURE 31.10 Thoracic and abdominal aneurysms; ascending aortic, descending aortic and abdominal aortic aneurysms.

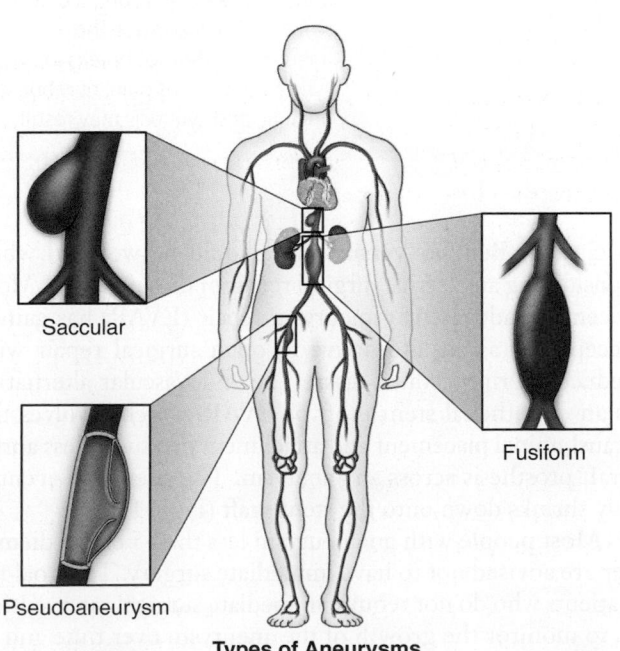

FIGURE 31.11 Types of aneurysms; saccular aneurysms project from only one side, a fusiform aneurysm is present when the entire arterial segment becomes dilated, a false or pseudoaneurysm is a leak from the artery typically caused by iatrogenic trauma that punctures the artery.

that punctures the artery. They are a known complication of percutaneous arterial procedures such as arteriography.

Clinical Manifestations

In most cases, aortic aneurysms cause no symptoms and are found when the patient is evaluated for another medical condition.

Clinical manifestations typically occur when a complication such as dissection or rupture occurs. There may be a palpable pulsatile mass in the abdomen with the AAA. Sometimes the patient presents with chest, back, or flank pain depending on the location of the aneurysm. The pain is typically not related to any activity and occurs spontaneously. Pain generally reflects a change in the aneurysm that needs immediate attention.

Management

Medical Management

Diagnosis

A number of imaging modalities can be used to detect and diagnose aortic dilation. Computed tomography scanning with IV contrast is considered the gold standard for assessing the size and location of an abdominal or thoracic aneurysm. Abdominal ultrasound or transthoracic echocardiography (TTE) have also been preferred screening modalities because they can be done quickly and efficiently at the bedside and because of their noninvasive nature and lack of radiation. Cardiac MRI is an imaging modality that has shown improved sensitivity and specificity versus TTE in detecting aortic dilation. The lack of radiation exposure with MRI compared with CT may make it the imaging modality of choice for aortic dilation. An ECG is also routinely done to rule out an MI because complications of aneurysm usually involve chest pain.

Medications

Treatment is focused on reducing the growth rate and preventing the complications of aneurysms. Hypertension is an important risk factor for rupture, so BP is aggressively managed with antihypertensive medications such as angiotensin-converting enzyme inhibitors, angiotensin II receptor blockers (ARBs), and/or beta blockers. In addition to antihypertensive medications, macrolides and tetracyclines, antibiotics that may inhibit secondary infections implicated in aneurysm development, have been proposed as a treatment for AAA with varying rationales and degrees of success. There is also evidence from a number of studies suggesting that statins may influence aneurysm growth rate by reducing the progression of atherosclerosis (Table 31.11).

Surgical Management

The size and location of the aneurysm along with the presence of symptoms are the determining factors for patient management (Table 31.12).

Currently, surgical intervention is shown to be the only treatment effective in preventing AAA rupture and aneurysm-related death. The most common surgical procedure for AAA has traditionally been a resection and repair (aneurysmectomy). In this procedure, the aneurysm is excised, and a graft is applied. Surgical repair is associated with risks that include bleeding, infection, MI, renal failure, and graft

Table 31.12 Assessment and Analysis for Aneurysms

Assessment Data	Analysis/Explanation
Thoracic Aneurysm	
Pain (constant)	Caused by stretching of the aortic tissue and impingement on adjacent structures
Heart failure	Ascending aneurysms may produce heart failure and its associated symptoms by causing aortic regurgitation. As the aortic root enlarges, the aortic valve leaflets are pulled away from each other, permitting backward leakage of blood.
Dyspnea Cough	Respiratory symptoms caused by distortion and obstruction of trachea by the aneurysm
Hoarseness of voice Dysphagia	Caused by distortion of the phrenic nerve or direct impingement on the esophagus by the aneurysm
Abdominal Aneurysm	
Pain	Pain occurs in the back and abdomen because of impingement on adjacent structures and stretching of aortic tissue
Abdominal throbbing	Noticeable, small pulsating mass near the navel due to increased aortic pressure
Cyanosis Blood clots	Blood can pool in the part of the aorta that is bulging, and a blood clot can develop inside the aneurysm. If the clot breaks loose, symptoms such as pain, numbness, tingling, and cyanosis may result.

Table 31.11 Medications Used in Aneurysm Management

Medication	Description
Macrolides	(Antibiotics) Inhibit abdominal aortic aneurysm (AAA) progression by reducing secondary infection within aortic wall
Tetracyclines	(Antibiotics) Inhibit matrix metalloproteinase (MMP), which is involved in aneurysm formation; decrease the rate of aneurysm expansion
Statins	Reducing the progression of atherosclerosis may influence aneurysm growth.

occlusion. Benefits versus risks should be weighed when considering an elective surgical repair of the aneurysm. More recently, endovascular aneurysm repair (EVAR) has gained acceptance as an alternative to open surgical repair with reduced periprocedural risks. The endovascular alternative is an endothelial stent graft or EVAR, which involves the transluminal placement and attachment of a sutureless aortic graft prosthesis across an aneurysm. The aneurysm eventually shrinks down onto the stent graft (Fig. 31.12).

Most people with an aneurysm less than 5 cm in diameter are advised not to have immediate surgery. The goal for patients who do not require immediate surgical intervention is to monitor the growth of the aneurysm over time and to maintain the BP at a normal level to decrease the risk of rupture. For those with small or asymptomatic aneurysms, regular ultrasounds or CT scans are necessary to monitor the growth of the aneurysm.

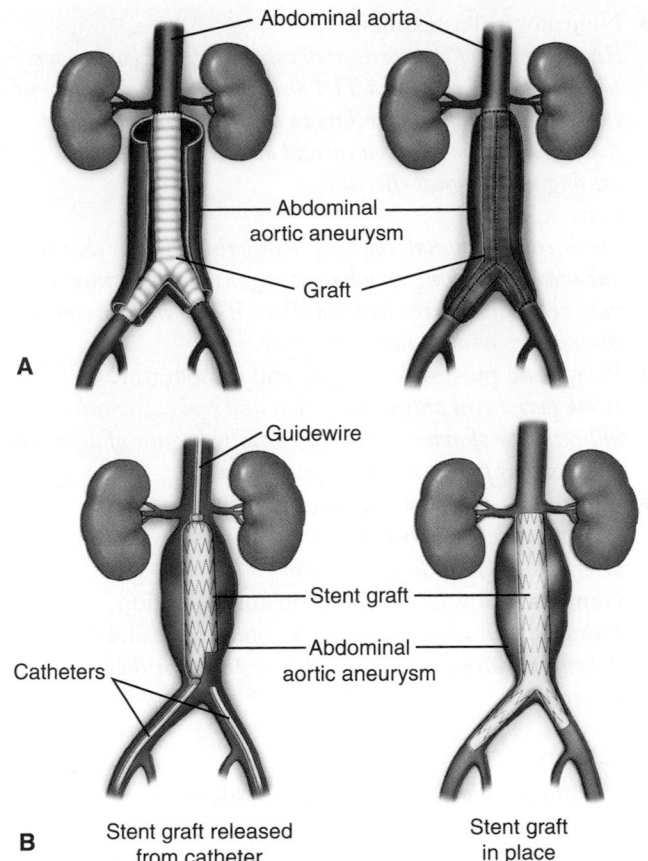

FIGURE 31.12 Aneurysm repair with surgery compared with stent placement. *A,* Aneurysmectomy; the aneurysm is excised, and a graft is applied. *B,* Endovascular aortic repair; placement and attachment of a sutureless aortic graft prosthesis across an aneurysm.

Patients with TAAs measuring 2.8 in. (7 cm) in diameter or with AAAs measuring 2 in. (5 cm) in diameter or those with smaller aneurysms that are producing symptoms are advised to have elective surgery (see Geriatric/Gerontological Considerations). A small aneurysm that expands more than 0.5 cm over a 6-month period of time should also be repaired surgically.

Geriatric/Gerontological Considerations

Elective Surgery

Most abdominal aortic aneurysms occur in patients between 60 and 90 years of age. Rupture is likely with coexisting hypertension and with aneurysms more than 6 cm wide. At this point, the risk of rupture is greater than the risk of death during surgical repair. Therefore, elective surgical repair should be considered carefully if the patient is able to withstand surgery and anesthesia. It is important that the healthcare team provides the patient and family with all the facts regarding the risk and benefit in order for the patient and family to make the most informed decision.

Complications

Aortic dissection (dissecting aneurysm) is thought to be caused by a sudden tear in the aortic intima creating a false lumen in the artery opening the way for blood to enter the aortic wall. Degeneration of the aortic media may be the primary cause for this condition, with hypertension being an important contributing factor. Dissection is also frequently linked with Marfan's syndrome. This is a life-threatening emergency because of the loss of circulation to any major artery arising distal to the dissection. The ascending and descending thoracic aortae are the most common sites, but dissections can also occur in the abdominal aorta (Fig. 31.13).

Classic signs and symptoms of aortic dissection are sudden onset of severe and persistent pain described as "tearing" or "ripping" in the anterior chest or back and extending to the shoulders, epigastric area, or abdomen. Diaphoresis, nausea, vomiting, faintness, and tachycardia are also common. Blood pressure is often markedly different from one extremity to another and often decreases because of loss of blood.

Rupture of the aortic aneurysm is the most life-threatening complication (Fig. 31.14). Rupture causes sudden and

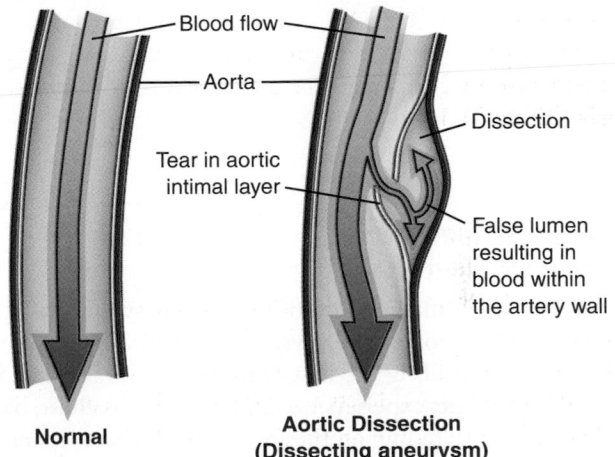

FIGURE 31.13 Aortic dissection (dissecting aneurysm).

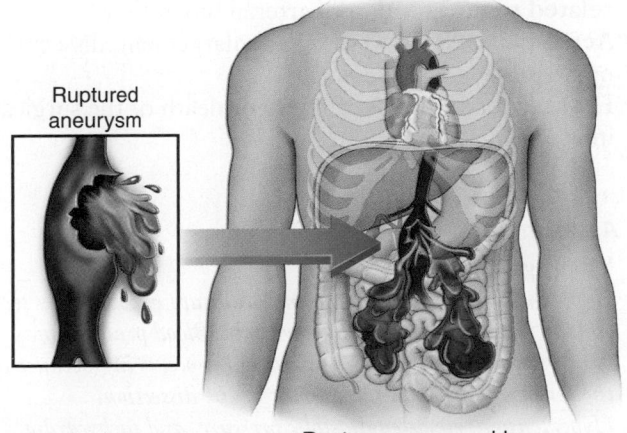

FIGURE 31.14 Ruptured aneurysm.

extreme loss of blood. Patients may present similar to those with a dissection with symptoms such as pain, tachycardia, and differing BPs between extremities, but in extreme cases, pain occurs then loss of consciousness due to hypovolemic shock from massive blood loss. The death rate in all patients with a ruptured abdominal aortic aneurysm (RAAA) or dissection is around 80%. One-third of all patients with an RAAA do not reach the hospital alive, and one-third do not have an intervention. Of the patients having an intervention, only half survive the intervention and admission.

Emergency surgical procedures are indicated for patients with a ruptured or dissecting abdominal aortic or thoracic aneurysm. Mortality rates increase dramatically once dissection or rupture has occurred as compared to the mortality rate if surgery is performed electively.

Connection Check 31.7

A nurse is assessing a patient in the emergency department with the complaint of sudden onset of severe back pain, tachycardia, and hypotension. Which interventions should the nurse anticipate? *(Select all that apply.)*

A. Electrocardiogram
B. Aortic arteriography
C. Ultrasonography
D. Chest x-ray
E. Computed tomography scan

Nursing Management
Assessment and Analysis

Most AAAs are small and do not cause any symptoms. The vast majority of thoracic aneurysms are silent, with rupture or dissection constituting the first symptoms. Overall, only 5% to 10% of patients experience symptoms such as chest, back, or flank pain depending on the location of the aneurysms.

Nursing Diagnoses

- **Risk for ineffective peripheral tissue perfusion related to** interruption of arterial blood flow
- **Acute pain** related to vascular enlargement, dissection or rupture
- **Fear** related to threat of injury or death or the surgical intervention

Nursing Interventions
▪ Assessments

- Vital signs
  Hypotension and tachycardia may indicate hypovolemia secondary to a loss of circulating volume. Blood pressure may vary between extremities if dissection is occurring because of the lessening of blood flow distal to the dissection. Hypertension, elevated diastolic pressure, and tachycardia can further weaken the vessel wall, increasing the risk that the aneurysm will enlarge, dissect, or rupture.

- Neurological assessment
  An aneurysm of the aortic arch can cause neurological symptoms similar to those of a TIA or stroke. The bulging aorta exerts pressure on the subclavian artery, decreasing blood flow through the common carotid arteries to the brain, causing neurological effects.

- Pain
  Persistent abdominal, chest, or back pain indicates that the aneurysm is pushing on adjacent organs and structures and may help pinpoint the location. Pain is also an indicator of a change such as dissection or rupture.

- Peripheral pulses, skin color, and temperature
  Weak peripheral pulses, poor color, and cool extremities indicate lack of arterial flow, potentially because of dissection or thrombus formation in the aneurysm.

- Peripheral sensation and motor response
  Paresthesias or paralysis may indicate pressure against the arteries supplying the spinal cord.

- Gentle abdominal auscultation and palpation
  Pulsatile abdominal masses may indicate an AAA. A bruit is caused by turbulent flow through the aneurysm.

▪ Actions

- Administer antihypertensives as ordered
  Antihypertensives control high BP, which is a major risk factor for aneurysm rupture.

- Administer statins as ordered
  Statins lower cholesterol and therefore reduce the risk of atherosclerosis, which may reduce the aneurysm growth rate.

- Administer tetracyclines and macrolides as ordered
  These types of antibiotics may inhibit AAA progression by reducing secondary infections within the aortic wall.

- Administer stool softeners as ordered
  Prevent strain on the aneurysm during defecation

- Create calm environment to reduce stress
  Reduction in stress has been shown to reduce BP and therefore lessen stress on the aneurysm.

▪ Teaching

- Signs and symptoms of aortic aneurysm and aortic dissection such as any new chest, abdominal, or flank pain, especially new pain not associated with increased activity
  It is important that the patient is able to detect signs and symptoms of an aortic aneurysm and aortic dissection to allow prompt intervention.

- Patients with Marfan's syndrome should be encouraged to do regular screening and call their provider with any new chest, abdominal, or flank pain.
  Patients with Marfan's syndrome are at increased risk for aneurysms due to the degeneration of the elastic fibers of the aortic media that occurs with that disease. Because of the emergent nature of aortic dissection, immediate recognition is essential to allow emergent repair.

- Following a strict treatment regimen which includes
  - Compliance with medications
  - Smoking cessation program if the patient is a smoker
  - Maintaining a healthy weight
  - Regular exercise
  - Avoid crossing or elevating legs to decrease pressure on the aorta and iliac arteries
  - Stress reduction
  - Following diagnostic testing and screening recommendations (includes regular blood pressure and cholesterol checks).
  - Obtaining regular ultrasounds to measure the aneurysm's growth
    Compliance with the treatment regimen is essential in successful management of aortic disease.

Connection Check 31.8

Which statements by a patient with a AAA indicate that teaching has been effective? *(Select all that apply.)*

A. "I need to quit smoking."

B. "I need to go to the emergency department immediately if I have new severe abdominal pain."

C. "The doctor may put me on blood thinners."

D. "I need to stay on my blood pressure medication."

E. "I should keep my legs elevated whenever possible."

Evaluating Care Outcomes

Patients with aortic aneurysms can achieve a good outcome by complying with the prescribed therapy. Blood pressure and HR within normal limits, strong peripheral pulses, normal skin color and texture, no complaints of abdominal, back, or chest pain, no complaints of wheezing and shortness of breath, no complaints of dysphagia or hoarseness, and a normal neurological assessment indicate a stable aneurysm.

DEEP VEIN THROMBOSIS

Epidemiology

Deep vein thrombosis (DVT) is a blood clot in a large vein, usually in the leg or pelvis. The prevalence of DVT is about 1 per 1,000 persons per year. Sometimes a DVT detaches from the site of formation and becomes mobile in the bloodstream. If the circulating clot moves through the heart to the lungs, it can block an artery supplying blood to the lungs. This condition is called **pulmonary embolism (PE)**. It is estimated that approximately 350,000 to 900,000 Americans each year suffer from DVT and PE. The disease process that includes DVT and/or PE is called **venous thromboembolism (VTE)**. At least 100,000 deaths may be directly or indirectly related to these diseases. Also, of note, approximately 10% to 30% of persons who survive the first occurrence of VTE develop another VTE within 5 years.

VTE is receiving increased attention from patient safety experts. A specific focus is on hospitalization as a risk factor as injury and surgery are causes of vascular injury and the prolonged bedrest often associated with hospitalization can cause venous stasis leading to clot formation. Approximately half of new VTE cases occur during a hospital stay or within 90 days of an inpatient admission or surgical procedure, and many are not diagnosed until after discharge.

Deep vein thrombosis is much less common in the pediatric population. Approximately 1 in 100,000 children younger than 18 years experience a DVT. This is possibly because of a child's higher heart rate, relatively active lifestyle, and fewer comorbidities when compared with adults. In pregnant women, it has an incidence of 0.5 to 7 per 1,000 pregnancies. It is the second-most common cause of maternal death in developed countries after bleeding.

Risk factors include increasing patient age, active cancer with or without concurrent chemotherapy, varicose veins, prior venous thrombosis, pregnancy, postpartum period, and oral contraceptive and hormone therapy. Surgery, trauma, hospital or nursing home confinement resulting in immobility, and procedures such as central vein catheterization or transvenous pacemaker insertion also increase the risk.

Pathophysiology

Virchow's triad describes the factors implicated in the formation of a venous thrombosis; decreased flow rate of the blood or stasis of blood flow, damage to the blood vessel wall; endothelial injury, and an increased tendency of the blood to clot (hypercoagulability).

Deep vein thrombosis, more common in the veins of the lower extremity, develop in the deep veins of the calf muscles or, less frequently, in the proximal deep veins of the lower extremity or upper arm. The deep veins that lie near the center of the leg are surrounded by powerful muscles that contract and force deoxygenated blood back to the lungs and heart. One-way valves prevent the backflow of blood between the contractions. Blood is squeezed up the leg against gravity, and the valves prevent it from flowing back to the feet. When the circulation of the blood slows down because of illness, injury, or inactivity, blood can accumulate or "pool," which provides an ideal setting for clot formation.

See Figure 31.15 for an illustration of DVT formation.

Clinical Manifestations

People with DVT may or may not have symptoms. The clot(s) can cause partial or complete blockage of circulation in the vein, which can lead to pain, swelling, tenderness, discoloration, or redness and warmth in the affected area. The clinical manifestations vary depending on the size, location, degree of vessel occlusion, and adequacy of collateral circulation. Table 31.13 describes common clinical manifestations associated with calf, femoral, iliofemoral, and upper extremity thrombosis. The presence of Homans' sign, calf pain elicited on dorsiflexion of the foot, may

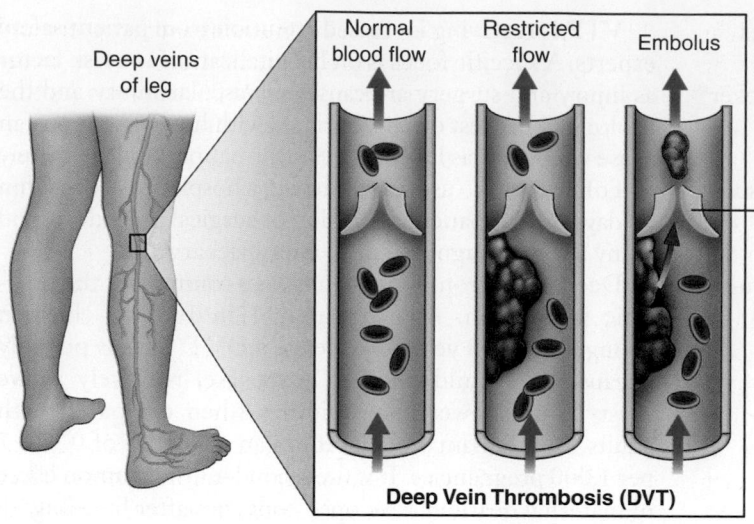

Deep Vein Thrombosis (DVT)

FIGURE 31.15 Deep vein thrombosis with the possibility of an embolus breaking off and traveling to the lungs.

indicate the presence of a DVT but its routine use in evaluation is not recommended as it is frequently misinterpreted and is not a reliable predictor.

Management

Medical Management

Diagnosis

Diagnostics include a combination of pre-test probability (PTP) testing, D-dimer testing, and compression ultrasonography (CUS). These have proven to be the most accurate, safe, and effective diagnostic tools for DVT. The evaluation of a patient with a suspected DVT begins with

an assessment of a set of clinical prediction rules, pre-risk probability, for DVT. The Wells score is a PTP scoring system that categorizes patients as high, moderate, or low probability. This is based on the presence of clinical features commonly associated with DVT and identification of an alternative diagnosis. Box 31.3 outlines both the PTP and DVT risk classification.

In patients with a low or moderate probability the next step is D-dimer testing. The D-dimer test is a global

Table 31.13 Common Signs and Symptoms Associated With Deep Vein Thrombosis	
Site	**Clinical Manifestations**
Calf thrombosis	Calf tenderness
	Distal swelling of affected extremity
Femoral thrombosis	Tenderness and pain in distal thigh and popliteal regions
	Swelling more prominent than with calf vein thrombosis alone
	Swelling may extend to knee
Iliofemoral thrombosis	Massive swelling in affected extremity
	Tenderness and pain involving entire extremity
Upper-extremity thrombosis	Swelling of affected extremity
	Dilated superficial veins
	Tenderness and pain
	Impaired mobility of extremity

Box 31.3 DVT Prerisk Probability Testing

Wells Score or Criteria: (Possible Score -2 to 8)

PRETEST – One point is given for each positive finding in the pretest, and 2 points are subtracted if an alternative diagnosis as likely as DVT is identified.

1. Active cancer (treatment within last 6 months or palliative) = 1 point
2. Calf swelling greater than 3 cm compared to other calf (measured 10 cm below tibial tuberosity) = 1 point
3. Collateral superficial veins (nonvaricose) = 1 point
4. Pitting edema (confined to symptomatic leg) = 1 point
5. Previously documented DVT = 1 point
6. Swelling of entire leg = 1 point
7. Localized pain along distribution of deep venous system = 1 point
8. Paralysis, paresis, or recent cast immobilization of lower extremities = 1 point
9. Recently bedridden greater than 3 days, or major surgery requiring regional or general anesthetic in past 4 weeks = 1 point
10. Alternative diagnosis at least as likely – subtract 2 points

    DVT RISK CLASSIFICATION
    High probability = 3 points
    Moderate probability = 1–2 points
    Low probability = 0 points

marker of coagulation activation by measuring fibrin degradation products produced from fibrinolysis (clot breakdown). A negative D-dimer test can exclude DVT without an ultrasound. Conversely, an elevated D-dimer suggests DVT but requires further testing to confirm the diagnosis because of the low specificity of the test. This low specificity is caused by the increase of the D-dimer level in other conditions, including infection, inflammation, cancer, surgery and trauma, extensive burns or bruises, ischemic heart disease, stroke, PAD, ruptured aneurysm or aortic dissection, or pregnancy. In the presence of a positive D-dimer or high probability PTP the next step is compression ultrasonography (CUS). It allows rapid and clear visualization of thrombi, including identification of unstable or floating thrombi, which may cause emboli.

Contrast venography, CT venography and MRI venography are other diagnostic tools but are rarely needed or utilized. These alternatives to ultrasound may be beneficial in selective cases, such as in the morbidly obese or when pelvic or abdominal thrombosis is suspected.

Prevention

The first step in treatment is prevention. In low risk patients, early ambulation may be all that is necessary. Venous thromboembolism (VTE) prophylaxis is indicated in at-risk hospitalized populations. In patients with a low bleeding risk pharmacological prevention is recommended. Preferred medications include low molecular weight heparin (LMWH), unfractionated heparin, or, in patients with heparin-induced thrombocytopenia (HIT), fondaparinux can be used. In patients with a higher risk of bleeding mechanical VTE prophylaxis is indicated. This includes the use of graduated compression stockings, venous foot pumps, and active external intermittent compression devices. The benefits of these methods include their effectiveness, ease of application, and safety especially in respect to bleeding. Intermittent compression devices apply external pressure to the limb which promotes blood flow velocity, reduces venous stasis, and increases levels of systemic fibrinolysis. Despite widespread use, there is limited evidence regarding the use of graduated compression stockings, venous foot pumps, or combined medical and mechanical prophylaxis.

Medications

Medication therapy typically consists of anticoagulation with unfractionated heparin or low molecular weight heparin (LMWH) followed by long-term oral anticoagulation with warfarin. These conventional anticoagulant therapies are widely used but have limitations. They require regular monitoring to maintain safe levels (see safety alert). Newer oral anticoagulant agents, including direct thrombin inhibitors (e.g., dabigatran etexilate) and direct factor Xa inhibitors (e.g., rivaroxaban, apixaban, and edoxaban) have been developed to overcome some of the limitations of conventional anticoagulant therapy.

These new oral agents have been evaluated for safety and efficacy in large, randomized clinical trials in the treatment and secondary prevention of VTE with results that are comparable to conventional therapy. These medications are important new treatment options for patients with VTE because they are effective and do not require regular monitoring.

The use of thrombolytic therapy such as tissue plasminogen activator (tPA) is not routinely administered in patients with DVT. These thrombolytic agents have a more rapid and complete thrombolysis, thus potentially preventing PE and decreasing the incidence of reoccurring DVT but are not associated with decreased mortality and are associated with increased risks for bleeding. Because of this, thrombolytics are only used under certain circumstances. They include patients who have failed conventional therapy with a clot that has been present for fewer than 14 days and have a low bleeding risk. Further assessment is made based on individual patient circumstances such as size and location of the clot and preexisting conditions. See Table 31.14 for a comparison of anticoagulant therapies.

 Safety Alert Essential teaching points for patients on warfarin:

1. Immediately report blood in sputum, emesis, stool, or urine.
2. Take the medication at the same time every day.
3. Never skip a dose of the medication.
4. Have laboratory values (international normalized ratio [INR]) checked on a regular basis.
5. Ensure that laboratory levels are safe to continue current dosage or change dosage.
6. Limit intake or maintain a consistent intake of green leafy vegetables that contain vitamin K (kale, spinach, collard greens, broccoli, okra, cabbage) that may counteract the action of warfarin.
7. Consult with your care provider before taking aspirin or Plavix in addition to warfarin.
8. Limit any physical activities that will increase bleeding risk such as contact sports.
9. Use an electric razor when shaving.
10. Use a soft toothbrush.

Surgical Management

Surgical management is rarely utilized to remove a DVT unless there is a massive occlusion that does not respond to medical treatment and the thrombus is of recent (1–2 days) onset. Thrombectomy is the most common surgical procedure for removing a clot.

Other less-invasive surgical procedures include balloon angioplasty, stent placement, and vena cava interruption. Balloon angioplasty widens the vein after a blood clot has been dissolved. As with other balloon angioplasty procedures, expanding the balloon in the vein causes the vein to widen and improves blood flow. Stent insertion can be utilized for DVT patients who have a vein that is prone to collapse. The stent expands once inserted and acts as a support for vein walls.

The purpose of vena cava interruption is to prevent PE. In this procedure, a provider surgically positions a filter inside the inferior or, not routinely, the superior vena cava between the DVT and the heart. Blood flows normally through the umbrellalike filter, but emboli are trapped, ensuring that they do not reach the lungs.

Table 31.14 Anticoagulant Therapy

Anticoagulant	Action	Possible Complications	Nursing Implications
Unfractionated heparin (UFH)	Inhibits clot formation by inhibiting clotting factors IIa (thrombin) and Xa, which in turn inhibits fibrin formation. Over a long period, the existing clot is slowly absorbed by the body.	Heparin-induced thrombocytopenia (HIT) – platelet aggregation caused by heparin-induced antiplatelet antibodies leads to thrombocytopenia	• Baseline laboratory determinants; *aPTT, **PT with ***international normalized ratio (INR), platelet count, and stool for occult blood are required before initiation • Dosage is weight based and nomograms typically using aPTT are used to measure therapeutic blood levels • Heparin should be continued 5–10 days • Oral anticoagulation should overlap • Protamine sulfate is an antidote for excessive bleeding
Low molecular weight heparin (LMWH) Enoxaparin (Lovenox) Dalteparin (Fragmin) Ardeparin (Normiflo)	Inhibits clot formation by inhibiting thrombin formation due to reduced factor IIa; has less of an effect on thrombin compared to heparin but maintains the same effect on factor Xa	Bleeding and thrombocytopenia (less bleeding risk than with UFH)	• Growing trend of using LMWH as replacement for UFH • Benefit is no laboratory monitoring unless treatment exceeds 7 days • Oral anticoagulation therapy should overlap • Home administration is a benefit
Xa inhibitors Rivaroxaban (Xarelto) Apixaban (Eliquis) Edoxaban (Savaysa) Dabigatran (Pradaxa)	Exert anticoagulant effect via direct inhibition of a single factor within the coagulation cascade (such as Factor Xa or thrombin), thereby prolonging clotting times	Bleeding	• Advantages include: rapid onset and offset of action which reduces having to use additional anticoagulants to bridge treatment, do not require frequent monitoring or redosing, have few medication interactions, and little to no food interactions. • No antidote available in the event of a major bleed • Diet and lifestyle teaching regarding bleeding risk are essential • Contraindicated in patients with severe renal impairment
Warfarin (Coumadin)	Works in the liver to inhibit synthesis of four vitamin K–dependent clotting factors	Bleeding	• Close monitoring required with laboratory values; PT/INR • Therapeutic levels monitored by INR • Takes 3–4 days to achieve therapeutic anticoagulation • Medication usually taken 3–6 months after deep vein thrombosis (DVT) • Vitamin K is the antidote for warfarin • Diet and lifestyle teaching are essential

Table 31.14 Anticoagulant Therapy—cont'd

Anticoagulant	Action	Possible Complications	Nursing Implications
Thrombolytics (streptokinase, urokinase, recombinant tissue plasminogen activators)	Dissolve existing thrombi and impair coagulation by increasing fibrinolytic activity through the conversion of circulating plasminogen to plasmin	Significant risk of hemorrhage, intracranial bleeding	• Nurse should watch for signs of bleeding and alert provider of fibrinogen level less than 100 mg/dL because of high bleeding risk • May prevent valvular damage and venous insufficiency • Contraindicated after surgery, trauma, strokes, or spinal injuries (increased bleeding risk)

*APTT or aPTT = Activated partial thromboplastin time evaluates the intrinsic and common coagulation pathways. It is used to evaluate the effectiveness of heparin

**PT = Prothrombin time evaluates the extrinsic coagulation pathway

***INR = International normalized ratio (a standardized measure of PT) evaluates the extrinsic coagulation pathway. It is used to evaluate the effectiveness of warfarin

Complications

The most serious life-threatening complication that can arise from DVT is a PE, which occurs in more than one-third of DVT patients. A PE occurs when a dislodged blood clot travels first to the heart and then to the lungs, where it can partially or completely block a pulmonary artery or one of its branches. The hemodynamic response to PE depends on the size of the embolus, coexistent cardiopulmonary disease, and neurohormonal effects. Clinical manifestations include:

- Shortness of breath
- Decreased oxygen saturation
- Tachycardia, hypotension
- Sweating
- Sharp chest pain (especially during deep breathing)
- Hemoptysis (bloody sputum)

These clinical manifestations are due to the clot in the pulmonary vasculature blocking flow through the lungs preventing oxygenation and ventilation, increasing pulmonary vascular resistance (PVR), increasing the workload on the right heart, and decreasing oxygen supply to the lung tissue itself. Hemodynamic decompensation occurs not only because of physical obstruction of blood flow but also because of the release of humoral factors such as serotonin from platelets, thrombin from plasma, and histamine from tissue. Pulmonary embolism can frequently cause death, particularly when one or more of the vessels that supply the lungs with blood is completely obstructed. For almost one-quarter of PE patients, the initial clinical presentation is sudden death.

Another complication that develops in 25% to 50% of patients after a DVT is post thrombotic syndrome (PTS). It is a chronic disorder with clinical features that range from minor limb swelling and discomfort to severe leg pain, intractable edema, irreversible skin changes, and leg ulceration. Prevention of PTS with the use of thromboprophylaxis is important because treatments are not very effective. Elastic compression stockings (ECSs) have the potential to prevent PTS by reducing venous hypertension and reflux, which are thought to be principal factors in the pathophysiology of PTS. However, a survey of thrombosis providers showed a lack of agreement on the benefits of ECSs or the optimum timing, indication, and duration of their use.

Connection Check 31.9

A patient has been admitted to the hospital for a PE. What is the priority nursing intervention?
A. Insert an IV line
B. Begin heparin drip as ordered
C. Check oxygen saturation
D. Determine patient allergies

Nursing Management

Assessment and Analysis

The clinical manifestations of DVT vary depending on the size, location, degree of vessel occlusion, and adequacy of collateral circulation. Patients may complain of pain, and there may be redness, swelling, and warmth due to obstruction of flow in the affected extremity.

Nursing Diagnoses

- **Ineffective peripheral tissue perfusion** related to interruption of venous blood flow
- **Acute pain** related to vascular inflammation and irritation and edema formation
- **Risk for impaired physical mobility** related to pain and discomfort of the affected extremities

Nursing Interventions

Assessments

- Vital signs with oxygen saturation
  Hypotension, tachycardia, and decreased oxygen saturation could indicate the presence of a PE or bleeding, especially if the patient is anticoagulated.

- Assess extremity for pain, tenderness, warmth, redness, or swelling
  Common symptoms of DVT that occur because of obstruction of blood flow and may indicate location of the clot
- Compare right and left calf, thigh, or arm circumferences
  Localized edema due to obstruction to blood flow in one extremity may suggest a DVT.
- Gentle palpation to inspect for induration
  Induration (hardening) helps to locate the placement of the clot in the blood vessel.
- D-dimer test
  Measures fibrin degradation products produced from clot breakdown. A positive result stratifies the patient into a high-risk category for DVT.
- Laboratory values: INR, PT/aPTT, hemoglobin, and hematocrit
  - The INR and PT/aPTT should be prolonged.
  - The hemoglobin and hematocrit should be within normal limits.
  The PT/INR evaluates the extrinsic coagulation cascade and is used to evaluate the effectiveness of warfarin.
  The aPTT evaluates the intrinsic coagulation cascade and is used to evaluate the effectiveness of heparin.
- Assess for signs of bleeding such as bruising, petechiae, hematuria, bloody stools
  Signs of bleeding may indicate a need to modify or decrease anticoagulation therapy.

■ Actions

- Early ambulation
  Bedrest has been recommended in the past, but recent studies show early ambulation does not result in more complications (see Evidence-Based Practice) and is key to prevention.
- Leg elevation
  When at rest, the affected extremity should be elevated at least 10 to 20 degrees above heart level to enhance venous return and reduce swelling.
- Compression stockings
  Should be worn at all times. Compression promotes venous return and decreases leg swelling.
- Avoid use of sequential compression devices (SCDs) in affected extremity
  An SCD may cause the thrombus to break away, resulting in an embolus.
- Encourage adequate fluid intake
  Prevents dehydration and sluggish blood flow, which exacerbates DVT growth
- Administer anticoagulation medications as ordered
  Anticoagulation with unfractionated heparin followed by long-term oral anticoagulation prevents the formation of new thrombi and inhibits the growth of the existing thrombi.
- Administer thrombolytic agent as ordered
  Thrombolytic agents dissolve existing thrombi and decrease the instance of vascular damage.

■ Teaching

- Prevention of reoccurrence with activities such as:
  - Early ambulation and active leg exercises
  - Monitor for adequate fluid intake to prevent dehydration and changes in blood flow
  - Avoid constricting clothing on the legs that might decrease venous flow, sitting with knees bent or crossed for long periods, standing for long periods
  - Remind patients that long car or airplane trips can increase the risk of DVT, so they should stay well hydrated and move around whenever possible or do leg exercises while sitting
  Encourage patients to engage in activity that decreases the incidence of DVT by maintaining adequate blood flow through the extremity and avoid activities or actions that constrict or limit blood flow.
- Signs and symptoms of bleeding such as bruising, bloody stools, petechiae
  It is important when taking anticoagulants that the patient (and family) is able to detect signs and symptoms of bleeding.
- Compliance with regular laboratory monitoring
  It is important that the patient (and family) understand the importance of compliance with laboratory draws and the medication regimen to reduce bleeding risk.
- Safety precautions when taking anticoagulants (see Safety Alert)

Evidence-Based Practice

Early Ambulation for Deep Vein Thrombosis (DVT): Bedrest versus early ambulation and standard anticoagulation in DVT management

Although it is not evidence-based, bedrest has been considered the cornerstone of management of deep vein thrombosis (DVT). A meta-analysis published in 2015 demonstrated that early ambulation combined with anticoagulation did not result in a higher incidence of complications such as pulmonary embolism (PE), progression of DVT, or death related to DVT.

Liu, Z., Tao, X., Chen, Y., Fan, Z., & Li, Y. (2015). Bed rest versus early ambulation with standard anticoagulation in the management of deep vein thrombosis: A meta-analysis. *PloS One, 10*(4), e0121388. https://doi: 10.1371/journal.pone.0121388

Connection Check 31.10

The nurse is caring for a patient on a heparin drip who was admitted for DVT 2 days ago. Which laboratory value is most important to report to the provider immediately?

A. A normal INR
B. An increased hematocrit
C. An increased platelet count
D. A normal aPTT

Evaluating Care Outcomes

Patients with a DVT can be safely managed by complying with prescribed anticoagulation therapy in combination with ambulation, compression stockings, and extremity elevation when resting. Stable vital signs and oxygen saturation along with decreased pain, swelling, and tenderness indicate a resolving DVT. Adjustments in anticoagulation therapy may be needed to maintain target laboratory values or prevent bleeding. Preventive patient teaching for high-risk individuals is essential to prevent initial and reoccurring DVT and PE. Patients should be able to maintain a healthy, active lifestyle by making adjustments in daily life that decrease DVT risk and by maintaining compliance with the treatment regimen.

Making Connections

CASE STUDY: WRAP-UP

Mr. More's BP readings continue to be elevated at 180/100 mm Hg with a high HR in the 100s. He is in a sinus rhythm. He is started on 40 mg Lasix, 400 mg PO labetalol, and 25 mg lisinopril and continued on his Lipitor 40 mg PO every day. An hour after his diuretic and antihypertensives are administered, his BP decreases to 150/90 mm Hg. After the next four doses over the next 2 days, his blood pressure normalizes to 125/80 mm Hg, and his HR is 72 bpm. After further diagnostic testing, Mr. More is diagnosed with left ventricular hypertrophy on echocardiogram and retinal damage to both of his eyes. Both can be prevented from progressing further with a combination of medication and heart-healthy lifestyle. His kidneys are responding well to the antihypertensive treatment, and his BUN and creatinine have normalized. A diabetic teaching consult and a nutritional assessment as well as an assessment of his lifestyle are completed by the nurse. It is determined that his diabetes will be managed through diet control; insulin will not be necessary at this time. He will be followed weekly for at least 3 months to ensure that his HgbA1c and blood glucose are normalized with diet control. Intensive teaching about the DASH diet, exercise regimen, and medication adherence is presented to Mr. More and his daughter. At the end of his admission, he is able to verbalize and demonstrate understanding of his treatment regimen and goal of care. Mr. More understands that he must follow up with outpatient care providers frequently for support with his disease.

Case Study Questions

1. Prior to admission to the unit, Mr. More's BP is 180/122 mm Hg and he is complaining of a headache and blurry vision. These signs and symptoms combined with his laboratory results suggest a concern for which of the following?
   A. Hypertensive emergency
   B. Stroke
   C. Hypertension urgency
   D. Diabetes

2. Upon admission, Mr. More's BP continues to be elevated at 188/122 mm Hg. Which order is most important for the nurse to implement first?
   A. Administer labetalol 400 mg PO
   B. Obtain a finger stick glucose reading
   C. Begin oxygen via nasal cannula at 2 L
   D. Administer Lipitor 40 mg PO

3. On the basis of patient history and the results of diagnostic tests, what are the priority assessments for Mr. More? *(Select all that apply.)*
   A. Strict intake and output
   B. Vital signs
   C. Finger stick blood glucose
   D. Cranial nerve assessment
   E. Swallowing evaluation

4. Priority teaching needs for Mr. More include which of the following? *(Select all that apply.)*
   A. Anticoagulation therapy
   B. Smoking cessation
   C. DASH diet
   D. Slow posture changes
   E. Eat a banana a day

5. Which statement by the patient about his medication regimen indicates the need for further teaching?
   A. "I will call my doctor if I am dizzy and short of breath."
   B. "I will take my BP medication only if my blood pressure is up."
   C. "One of my medications, Lasix, will make me urinate a lot."
   D. "I am able to take my labetalol and lisinopril at the same time."

CHAPTER SUMMARY

Atherosclerosis is a progressive inflammatory process that causes plaque formation within the artery. Plaque rupture can lead to myocardial infarction, unstable angina, or sudden death. Risk factors for atherosclerosis include elevated cholesterol levels, hypertension, smoking, diabetes, obesity, sedentary lifestyle, and family history. Risk factor modification is the initial action for patients who are at risk or evidenced to have atherosclerosis. Medication management is aimed at reducing lipid levels.

Hypertension is known as the "silent killer" because it can cause considerable damage to the heart, brain, and kidneys (target organs) before symptoms become evident. Early detection, prevention, and treatment are essential. The patient with the greatest risk of hypertension is a male over the age of 65 who is African American and of poor socioeconomic status. Definitive treatment is through antihypertensive medications, but diet and lifestyle modifications are essential. Nurses play a major role in effective prevention and treatment through education and follow-up regarding the importance of medication compliance, weight loss, diet, exercise, smoking cessation, and alcohol modification.

Peripheral arterial disease (PAD) is a progressive and chronic condition where the obstruction of blood flow through the large peripheral arteries causes a partial or total arterial occlusion leading to inadequate tissue perfusion and tissue ischemia. Patients with PAD often have atherosclerosis in the medium to large arteries including the aorta, the coronary arteries, and the carotid arteries. The treatment goals for patients with PAD are directed at providing symptom relief, education on risk factor modification, and reducing the risk of systemic cardiovascular morbidity and mortality.

Carotid artery disease is characterized by vessel wall thickening, plaque formation, and a progressive narrowing of the carotid artery. Treatment for patients with severe carotid stenosis includes antiplatelet aggregation medications combined with carotid revascularization such as carotid endarterectomy (CEA) or carotid artery stenting. Patients with carotid artery disease are at great risk for stroke. The risk of stroke is dependent upon the severity of the stenosis and the previous appearance of symptoms. Regular nursing assessment of neurological status is essential to detect signs of stroke. Patients need education on lifestyle modifications, adherence to the medication regimen, and reportable conditions such as neurological changes.

An aortic aneurysm is a permanent localized dilation of the ascending, descending, or abdominal aortic artery. Patients with greatest risk of aortic aneurysms are white males between the ages of 40 and 70. Atherosclerosis, family history, genetic diseases such as Marfan's syndrome, and smoking are the most frequent risk factors for AAA. Atherosclerosis accounts for 75% of aortic aneurysms. Aortic aneurysms may be asymptomatic. Following a strict regimen of medication compliance, healthy lifestyle, and regular screening is essential to successful management of aortic disease. A critical life-threatening complication of aortic aneurysm is rupture or dissection. Emergency surgery is the only treatment option. Symptoms of a ruptured or dissected aneurysm are severe back, chest, or flank pain; decreased BP; decreased red blood cell count; nausea; diaphoresis; pallor; and tachycardia.

Deep vein thromboses, or DVTs, typically form in the large vessels of the lower extremities. Risk factors include increasing patient age, surgery, trauma, hospital or nursing home confinement, active cancer with or without concurrent chemotherapy, pregnancy, postpartum period, oral contraceptives, and hormone therapy. Medical treatment with anticoagulants is indicated. Patient monitoring and teaching on the bleeding risk associated with anti_coagulation are imperative. Pulmonary embolism is a serious, life-threatening complication of DVT with clinical manifestations that include shortness of breath, tachycardia, sweating, and/or sharp chest pain especially during deep breathing.

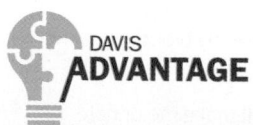
DAVIS ADVANTAGE

To explore learning resources for this chapter, go to **Davis Advantage** and find:
- Answers to in-text questions
- Chapter Resources and Activities
- NCLEX®-Style Chapter Review Questions
- Bibliography

Chapter 32

Coordinating Care for Critically Ill Patients With Cardiovascular Dysfunction

Sharon Owens

LEARNING OUTCOMES

Content in this chapter is designed to assist in:

1. Describing the indications and nursing implications for hemodynamic monitoring in the critically ill patient
2. Explaining the physiological relationship of hemodynamic parameters (preload, afterload, and contractility) to cardiac function
3. Correlating the clinical manifestations to the underlying pathophysiology of:
   a. Myocardial infarction
   b. Cardiomyopathy
   c. Cardiogenic shock
4. Explaining the rationales for relevant medical interventions in the treatment of patients with myocardial infarction, cardiomyopathy, and cardiogenic shock
5. Analyzing the nursing management of patients with myocardial infarction, cardiomyopathy, and cardiogenic shock
6. Developing a teaching plan for patients who have had a myocardial infarction or cardiogenic shock or who have cardiomyopathy

CONCEPTS

- Assessment
- Infection
- Medication
- Nursing Roles
- Nutrition
- pH Regulation
- Perfusion
- Safety

ESSENTIAL TERMS

Acute coronary syndrome (ACS)
Afterload
Angina
Arterial blood gas (ABG)
Arterial line
Cardiac index (CI)
Cardiac output (CO)
Cardiogenic shock
Cardiomyopathy
Central venous pressure (CVP)
Central venous oxygen saturation (ScvO$_2$)
Contractility
Mechanical Circulatory Support (MCS)
Mixed venous oxygen saturation (SvO$_2$)
Myocardial infarction (MI)
Oxygen delivery (DO$_2$)
Oxygen consumption (VO$_2$)
Oxygen utilization
Phlebostatic axis
Preload
Pulmonary artery wedge pressure (pulmonary artery occlusive pressure) (PAWP/PAOP)
ST elevation myocardial infarction (STEMI)
Non-ST elevation myocardial infarction (NSTEMI)
Stroke volume (SV)
Sympathetic nervous system
Unstable angina (UA)
Venous oxygen saturation

Finding Connections

CASE STUDY: EPISODE 1

Follow this patient throughout the chapter.

Mr. Martin King is a 68-year-old male who presents to the emergency department with complaints of crushing chest pain that starts in the center of his chest and radiates to the left shoulder. He is pale and diaphoretic and is complaining of nausea. His blood pressure (BP) is 105/60 with a heart rate of 110 bpm. Oxygen saturation is 90%. An electrocardiogram (ECG) is performed immediately. Admission orders include two liters of oxygen via nasal cannula, 1 tablet sublingual (SL) nitroglycerin to be repeated every 5 minutes for a total of 3 tablets as necessary, 325 mg of aspirin, and 2 mg of morphine sulfate IV if nitroglycerin does not relieve the pain. Two large-bore IVs are started. Blood work including a cardiac panel: troponin, creatine kinase (CK), creatine kinase–MB bands (CK-MB), complete metabolic panel (CMP), complete blood count (CBC), arterial blood gas (ABG), and coagulation studies is obtained. Metoprolol 5 mg IV is given cautiously. A chest x-ray is performed…

OVERVIEW OF HEMODYNAMIC MONITORING

Invasive hemodynamic monitoring is important to allow early identification and treatment of the complex medical problems of the critically ill patient. Physical examination can provide only a limited assessment of the patient's hemodynamic status. Advanced hemodynamic monitoring enables the nurse to assess for the presence of shock and cardiac and pulmonary abnormalities, as well as complications following myocardial infarction (MI). With the use of advanced monitoring systems, the nurse can evaluate the patient's immediate response to treatments including inotropic medications and mechanical support. Important concepts to understand when discussing hemodynamic monitoring include cardiac output, oxygen delivery, oxygen utilization and oxygen consumption.

Cardiac Output

Cardiac output (CO) is the volume of blood pumped by the heart each minute. It is dependent on stroke volume (SV) and heart rate (HR). Heart rate is the number of ventricular contractions per minute. It can be affected by many variables such as stimulus from the autonomic nervous system or hormones from the adrenal medulla. Changes in blood pressure (BP) can also affect HR.

Stroke volume is the volume of blood pumped by the left ventricle with each heartbeat. Stroke volume is dependent on three important factors: preload, afterload, and contractility.

Preload is the end diastolic pressure or volume that stretches the right or left ventricle. It reflects a patient's fluid volume status. The values obtained to measure preload are sometimes referred to as *filling pressures*. Factors affecting preload include blood volume, heart rate, body position, intrathoracic pressure from respirations, venous return of blood, atrial contraction, and valvular regurgitation.

Afterload is the force or resistance the ventricles must overcome to eject blood into the pulmonary circuit or aorta. Right heart afterload is reflected in the pulmonary vascular resistance (PVR). Left heart afterload is reflected in the systemic vascular resistance (SVR) and is representative of the force that the left heart must pump against to deliver the SV into the periphery.

Contractility is the inherent ability of the heart muscle to contract independent of preload and afterload. Effective contractility is a component of SV, helping to produce an adequate CO. Poor contractility directly affects CO and decreases SV.

Oxygen delivery (DO_2) is the amount of oxygen delivered to the tissues. It is determined through the evaluation of cardiac output and arterial oxygen content; hemoglobin levels, haemoglobin oxygen saturation, and the amount of oxygen dissolved in the plasma. **Oxygen utilization and oxygen consumption (VO_2)** reflects the relationship between oxygen delivery and oxygen extraction at the tissue level. It can be measured through a blood sample, a **venous oxygen saturation** that reflects the amount of oxygenated blood returned to the right heart. Oxygen consumption is typically stable at the tissue level. Normal VO_2 values are between 60% and 75%. When that value falls below normal it means the tissues are extracting more oxygen than normal. That results from a decreased DO_2 which may be a decrease in oxygen content, hemoglobin, or cardiac output. It may also reflect an inability to increase delivery in response to stressors such as pain or fever.

Hemodynamic Monitoring Systems

Hemodynamic monitoring systems include arterial, central venous, and pulmonary artery (PA or Swan-Ganz) catheters. When correctly assembled and attached to a monitor, these systems provide pressure readings that correspond to BP, right atrial (RA) or **central venous pressure (CVP)**, and pulmonary artery pressures. The readings are displayed as waveforms on the monitor. The system consists of transduced catheters attached to noncompressible pressure tubing and a pressurized normal saline flush bag to prevent backup of blood. The bag is pressurized to 300 mm Hg for the arterial catheter and 150 mm Hg for the central venous and PA catheters. Evidence has demonstrated flush bags only need to be pressurized, not heparinized; therefore, most institutions have changed their policies to reflect this standard (Fig. 32.1).

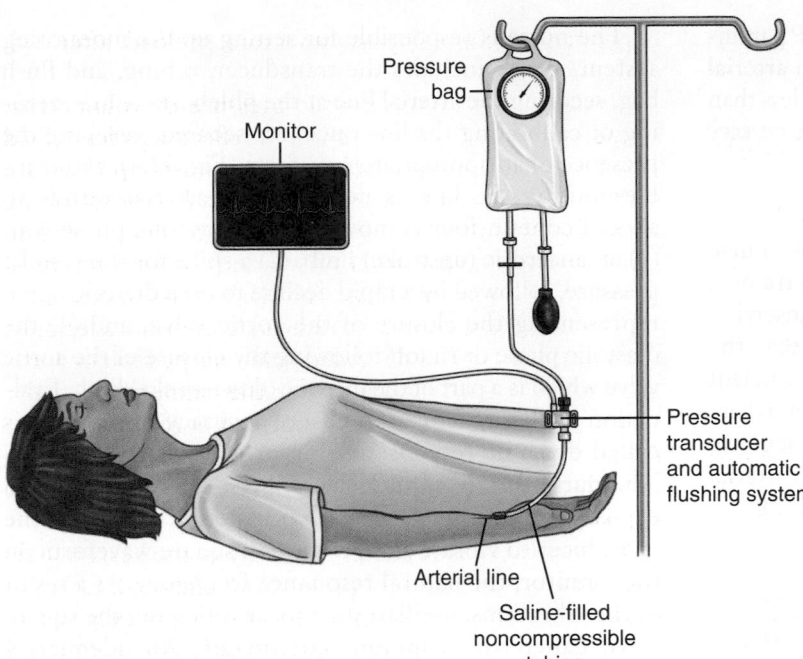

FIGURE 32.1 Pressure bag and transducer setup for invasive hemodynamic monitoring.

In order to obtain accurate readings, several conditions need to be present. First, the transducer should be secured at the **phlebostatic axis** (Fig. 32.2). This is the external reference point for the anatomical position of the right and left atria and the pulmonary artery. It is the midpoint of the left atrium, estimated as the fourth intercostal space in the midaxillary line with the patient in the supine position. If placed lower than the phlebostatic axis, the readings will be inaccurately high. If placed higher, the readings will be falsely low. Second, the tubing between the transducer and the cannula must be stiff, nonpliant, and less than 120 cm in length. Third, the transducer must be routinely calibrated, commonly referred to as "zeroing," to offset the atmospheric and hydrostatic pressures that may alter the reading. Finally, the transducer and tubing need to be free from blood and air to ensure accurate readings and waveform. This also helps avoid the introduction of emboli into the systemic circulation. The transducer includes a port for flushing blood and air bubbles from the system and obtaining blood samples. Many hospitals use an in-line closed system for blood sampling to reduce catheter-associated blood stream infections and reduce blood loss. The Venous

Arterial blood Management Protection (VAMP) system (Edwards Lifesciences, Irvine, CA, USA) is one type of closed in-line system. It is crucial that the nurse be aware of these implications when caring for the patient with invasive monitoring. Inaccurate readings could result in inappropriate and potentially harmful interventions to the patient.

Arterial Line

An **arterial line** is a small catheter inserted into an artery used to display a constant systemic BP. This allows for continual evaluation of interventions for the critically ill patient, especially those patients with a labile BP on vasoactive medications. This catheter can also be used to obtain **arterial blood gas (ABG)** samples, which are used to monitor a patient's acid-base and oxygenation status.

An arterial line is usually inserted into the radial artery (Fig. 32.3) but can also be inserted into the axillary, brachial,

FIGURE 32.2 The phlebostatic axis; midpoint of the left atrium, at the fourth intercostal space in the midaxillary line.

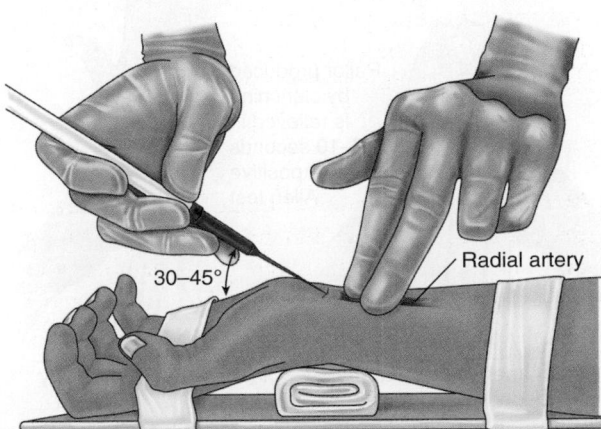

FIGURE 32.3 Arterial line insertion.

femoral, or dorsalis pedis artery. Normal systemic BP parameters are systolic BP less than 120 mm Hg, mean arterial pressure (MAP) 70 to 105 mm Hg, and diastolic BP less than 80 mm Hg. A MAP of 65 mm Hg is considered necessary for end-organ perfusion (Box 32.1).

Nursing Implications for Use of an Arterial Line

Providers, including physicians, physician assistants, nurse practitioners, and nurse anesthetists who have been trained, are responsible for arterial line insertion. Prior to insertion of a radial arterial line, the nurse must ensure that the provider performs an Allen test to confirm there is sufficient blood supply through the ulnar artery should the radial artery be damaged as a result of the cannulation. A negative Allen test indicates that it is not safe to place a radial arterial line; therefore, another site should be used (Box 32.2).

Box 32.1 Formula for Calculating Mean Arterial Pressure

Formula for calculating mean arterial pressure (MAP)

$$MAP = [(2 \times diastolic) + systolic]/3$$

Box 32.2 Performing an Allen Test

Ask the patient to elevate the hand and make a fist for approximately 30 seconds. While the hand is elevated in a fist, the ulnar and radial arteries are occluded via pressure. While still elevated, the hand is opened and should appear pale/whitish. While pressure over the radial artery is maintained, pressure over the ulnar artery is released. Normal color returns in 7 to 10 seconds in a positive test. A negative test, in which color does not return in 7 to 10 seconds, indicates insufficient blood supply through the ulnar artery.

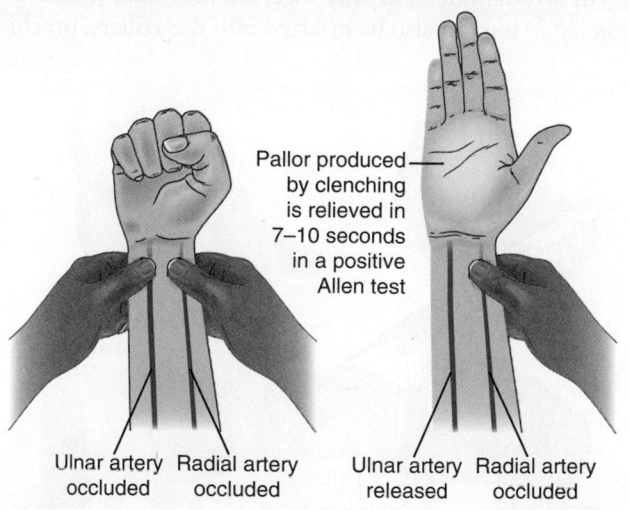

Pallor produced by clenching is relieved in 7–10 seconds in a positive Allen test

Ulnar artery occluded — Radial artery occluded   Ulnar artery released — Radial artery occluded

The nurse is responsible for setting up the monitoring system, which includes the transducer, tubing, and flush bag, securing the arterial line at the phlebostatic axis, zeroing or calibrating the line once it is secured, verifying the presence of an appropriate waveform (Fig. 32.4), and troubleshooting the line as needed. The arterial waveform should contain four components: the systolic phase with (1) an anacrotic (upstroke) limb, (2) a spike for the systolic pressure, followed by a rapid decline to (3) a dicrotic notch representing the closure of the aortic valve, and (4) the diastolic phase or runoff following the closure of the aortic valve which is a part of the dicrotic (downstroke) limb. Evaluation of the waveform to ensure accuracy of readings is called dynamic response testing or the square wave test. The nurse can do a quick flush of the arterial line which exposes the transducer to high pressure. This causes the transducer to vibrate and produces a square waveform on the monitor; the natural resonance frequency. As a result of the vibrations, oscillations appear following the square wave called the damping coefficient. An adequately damped waveform (normal) has two oscillations. An over-damped waveform has only one oscillation (little transducer vibration) and the tracing will lose its dicrotic notch. This may be caused by a clot in the catheter tip, or an air bubble in the tubing. When over-dampening occurs, the systolic BP may be under estimated and the diastolic BP may be overestimated. The underdamped trace will show numerous amplified oscillations, overestimate the systolic BP, and underestimate the diastolic BP. This may be caused by catheter artifact, noncompliant tubing, hypothermia, or tachycardia. The MAP remains the same in spite of damping.

The arterial site should be kept in view to prevent risk of catheter dislodgment and hemorrhage. The insertion site and area distal to the site must be monitored for adequate perfusion by checking color, warmth, capillary return, and movement. Observing the pulse oximetry waveform, with the probe placed distal to the insertion site, is an additional way that the nurse may continually observe for adequate perfusion. Additionally, appropriate alarms levels should be set on the monitor to alert the nurse with any change in pressure to allow prompt recognition and response.

When the arterial line is being discontinued, the dressing and sutures are first removed. The catheter is then removed, and pressure is applied over and above the insertion site for 3 to 5 minutes or until hemostasis is achieved. If the patient is at risk for bleeding, such as when receiving systemic anticoagulation, pressure should be applied for 10 minutes or longer to ensure hemostasis is achieved. A pressure dressing is then applied. The insertion site should be monitored to assure that hemostasis is maintained.

Complications

Complications from the use of arterial lines include blood loss that may occur if tubing becomes disconnected or

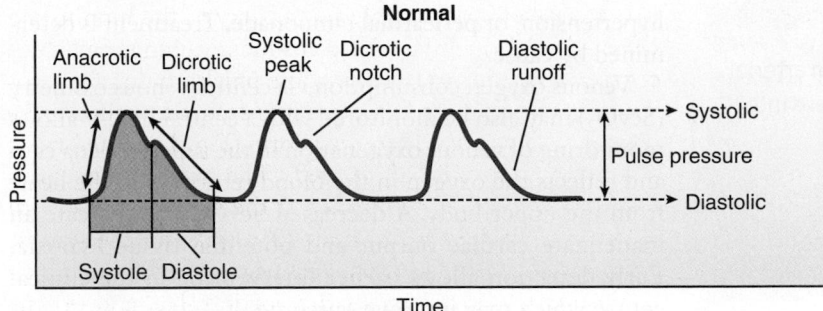

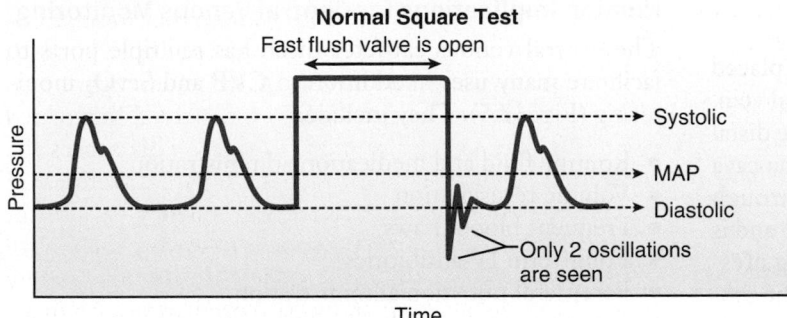

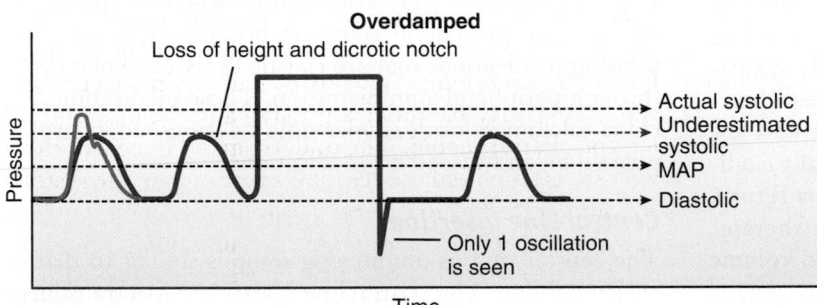

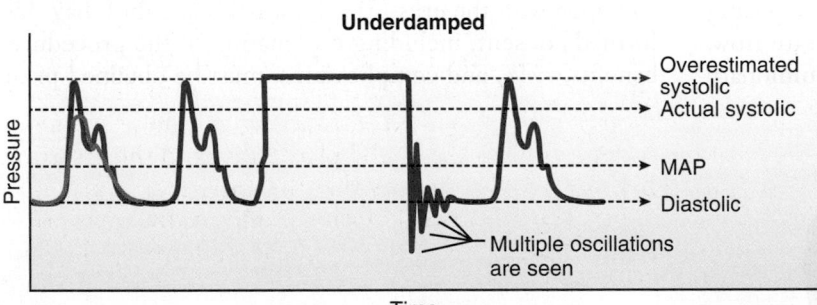

FIGURE 32.4 Arterial waveform. *A*, Normal arterial waveform. *B*, Normal square test. *C*, Overdamped waveform. *D*, Underdamped waveform.

the arterial line is accidentally displaced. There can be damage to the artery or occlusion of the artery, resulting in decreased flow distal to the site. As with any invasive device, infection is a risk (Box 32.3).

 Safety Alert   Arterial lines should be clearly marked so that IV medications are not given via this route. Inadvertent intra-arterial IV infusion can lead to tissue necrosis, gangrene, and loss of limb.

Box 32.3 Potential Arterial Line Complications

- Infection
- Occlusion of artery
- Hemorrhage due to tubing disconnection or line dislodgment
- Air emboli
- User error (inaccurate readings)
- Damage to artery

Connection Check 32.1

The nurse is managing the care of a patient with an arterial line. Which assessment finding warrants immediate intervention by the nurse?

A. An overdamped waveform on the monitor
B. Tubing disconnected from the arterial line
C. IV medications being infused into an arterial line
D. Redness at the arterial line insertion site

Central Venous Monitoring

Central venous monitoring utilizes a long catheter placed in the internal jugular (IJ), subclavian (SC), or femoral vein. It is threaded through the superior vena cava with the distal port or tip resting at the junction of the superior vena cava and right atrium. CVP monitoring can be done through this line. The CVP level indicates mean RA pressure and is typically used as an estimate of right ventricular filling pressures or volume returning to the right heart from the systemic circulation (**preload**). It is also used as an indication of right ventricular function. Normal CVP is 2 to 6 mm Hg. The CVP value may be influenced by many factors including intravascular volume, venous return, venous tone, sympathetic response, intrathoracic pressure, and right heart function. A decreased CVP reading may be indicative of a low volume state caused by hypovolemia or peripheral vasodilation which occurs in sepsis and reduces venous return. The treatment may be a fluid bolus, vasopressor therapy, or both. An elevated CVP may indicate increased volume that may occur with right heart failure. Central venous pressure may also be elevated when intrathoracic pressures or pressures in the pulmonary circuit are increased, requiring pressure in the right heart to increase to facilitate flow. This can occur with tension pneumothorax, pulmonary hypertension, or pericardial tamponade. Treatment is determined by cause.

Venous oxygen consumption via central venous oximetry ($ScvO_2$) may also be monitored with a central line. It allows monitoring of venous oxygenation in the superior vena cava and reflects the oxygen in the blood returning to the heart from the upper body. A decreased $ScvO_2$ may indicate an inadequate cardiac output and potential tissue hypoxia. Early detection allows earlier intervention in the clinical course which may improve outcomes.

Nursing Implications for Central Venous Monitoring

The central venous catheter often has multiple ports to facilitate many uses in addition to CVP and $ScvO_2$ monitoring (Fig. 32.5). They include:

- Routine fluid and medication administration
- Volume resuscitation
- Frequent blood draws
- Long-term IV antibiotics
- Parenteral nutrition administration
- Transvenous pacemaker insertion

These catheters may also be used when IV therapy is needed, and peripheral veins are not accessible or when infusing medications that are caustic to tissues when given through peripheral administration. These medications include calcium chloride, hypertonic solutions, amiodarone, potassium, and vasoactive medications.

Central Line Insertion

The central venous monitoring setup is similar to that of an arterial line. The central line is attached to a transducer via stiff, noncompressible tubing. The tubing is kept flushed and open with the pressurized normal saline flush bag. Informed consent, including explanation of the procedure, benefits, risks, and complications, must be obtained prior

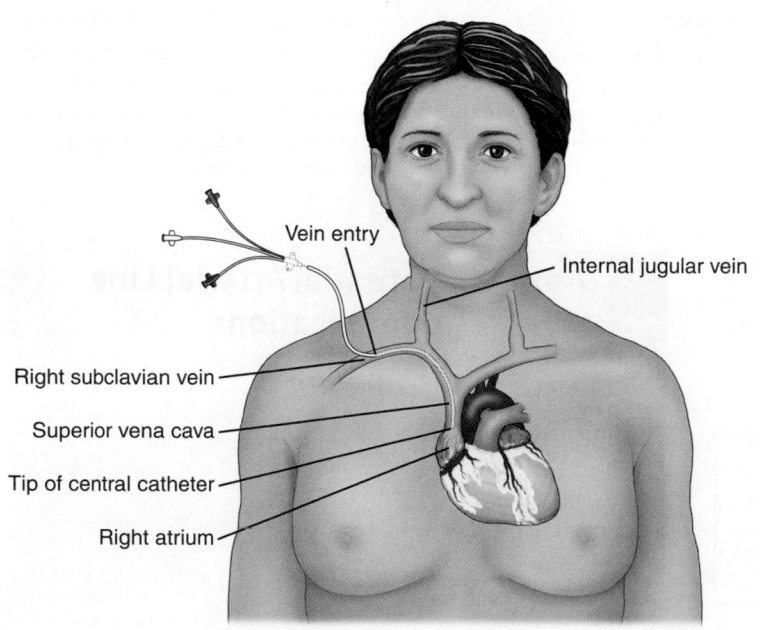

Vein entry

Internal jugular vein

Right subclavian vein

Superior vena cava

Tip of central catheter

Right atrium

FIGURE 32.5 The central venous pressure catheter with multiple ports inserted in the right subclavian vein with the tip resting at the junction of the superior vena cava and right atrium.

to line placement. Positioning the patient for an SC or IJ site may include placing a towel under the scapula to make the insertion site and landmarks more prominent. The patient should be placed in a Trendelenburg position (patient flat on back with feet 15 to 30 degrees higher than the head) unless the femoral vein approach is used, to reduce the risk of air embolism. Additionally, for the IJ approach, the Trendelenburg position will improve vessel distention, increasing the target size. Postprocedure, the catheter is secured by a suture, and an occlusive dressing is applied. The central line position must be verified by chest x-ray prior to its use.

The nurse plays a very important role during catheter insertion. Studies have demonstrated that using a checklist to assure adherence to evidence-based catheter insertion guidelines can significantly reduce catheter-related bloodstream infections. The nurse is empowered and obligated to stop the procedure if a violation of these guidelines is observed (Box 32.4).

Nursing Implications for Central Line Maintenance

The patient with a central line should be closely monitored, and maintenance of the catheter site and system should be closely observed. The central line must be well secured to the patient to avoid accidental removal or displacement. Patency of the central line can be maintained by normal saline or heparin flush, continuous IV fluids, or pressurized flush solution. Monitored lines must have appropriate alarm limits set. The transducer location reference point is the phlebostatic axis (see Fig. 32.2). Waveforms should be monitored with appropriate scale and assessed for dampened waveforms, which could be a sign of line malfunction or complications such as air or blood in the transducer. Invasive lines disrupt the integrity of the skin, increasing a patient's risk for infection. Infection may spread to the bloodstream,

leading to hemodynamic instability and sepsis. It is the nurse's responsibility to assess the insertion site for bleeding and signs of infection. To minimize risk of infection the nurse must use aseptic technique with any line care, minimize line handling, and maintain an occlusive dressing. Daily evaluation of line necessity and prompt removal when not necessary decreases infection risk. Conditions that should be reported to the provider include pressures outside ordered parameters, inability to correct a dampened waveform, impaired circulation, catheter dislodgement, bleeding or swelling at the insertion site, and signs of infection such as presence of swelling, redness, or discharge.

Nursing Implications for Central Line Removal

Prior to discontinuing the line, the nurse should prepare the patient by explaining the procedure. The dressing is removed, and the patient is placed in the Trendelenburg or supine position to prevent air embolism. The suture holding the central venous catheter are removed while ensuring it does not accidentally migrate out. Make sure all suture material has been removed. Ask the patient to hold his breath as the catheter is removed, again to prevent air embolism, and immediately cover the area with sterile gauze and apply pressure until hemostasis is achieved. Observe the patient after line removal for signs and symptoms of bleeding, air embolism, or infection of the site.

Complications

More than 5 million central venous catheters are placed each year in the United States, with an associated complication risk of greater than 15%. They include but are not limited to infection, air embolism, arrhythmias, and bleeding (Box 32.5).

Pulmonary Artery Catheter Monitoring

A PA (Swan-Ganz) catheter is a flexible, balloon-tipped catheter that is guided through the right side of the heart and into the pulmonary artery. The PA catheter may be inserted through the SC, internal or external jugular, or femoral vein. The typical catheter is 110 cm long and has four lumens, the distal, proximal, thermistor, and inflation lumens, each of which leads to a specific port. Some PA catheters have a second proximal lumen used for IV medication infusion (Fig. 32.6).

Box 32.4 Central Line Insertion Guidelines

Central line insertion guidelines shown to reduce bloodstream infections

1. Experienced provider inserting a line or providing supervision
2. Perform a time-out
3. Use proper hand hygiene
4. Don appropriate attire during insertion to include cap, mask, a sterile gown and gloves, and eye protection
5. Prep site with chlorhexidine antiseptic skin prep and let air dry
6. Drape patient utilizing sterile technique
7. Insert line; maintain sterile technique
8. Clean site with chlorhexidine and cover with sterile occlusive dressing
9. Optimal catheter site selection (attempting to avoid use of the femoral vein)
10. Daily review of the necessity of the line and prompt removal when unnecessary

---

Box 32.5 Potential Central Venous Line Complications

- Accidental arterial insertion
- Pneumothorax
- Nerve injury
- Vessel perforation
- Guidewire-induced arrhythmias
- Air embolism
- Venous thrombosis
- Bleeding
- Infection

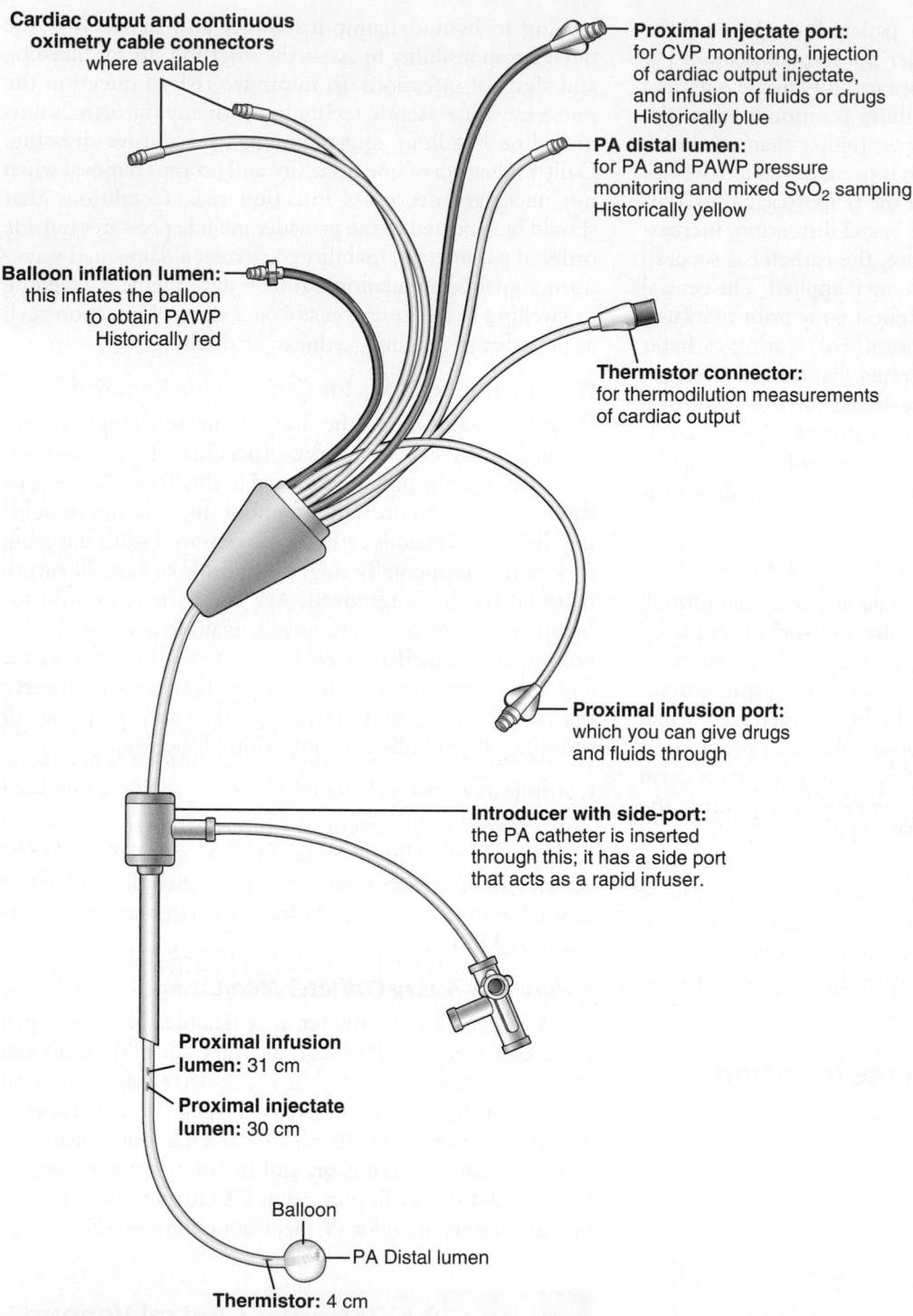

Cardiac output and continuous oximetry cable connectors
where available

Proximal injectate port:
for CVP monitoring, injection of cardiac output injectate, and infusion of fluids or drugs
Historically blue

PA distal lumen:
for PA and PAWP pressure monitoring and mixed SvO$_2$ sampling
Historically yellow

Balloon inflation lumen:
this inflates the balloon to obtain PAWP
Historically red

Thermistor connector:
for thermodilution measurements of cardiac output

Proximal infusion port:
which you can give drugs and fluids through

Introducer with side-port:
the PA catheter is inserted through this; it has a side port that acts as a rapid infuser.

Proximal infusion lumen: 31 cm

Proximal injectate lumen: 30 cm

Balloon

PA Distal lumen

Thermistor: 4 cm

FIGURE 32.6 Pulmonary artery catheter.

The distal lumen port is located at the tip, or end, of the PA catheter. Through this port, systolic, diastolic, and mean pulmonary artery pressures can be measured providing information about the left heart. Pulmonary artery pressures reflect the BP in the pulmonary artery. It is generated by the right ventricle ejecting blood into the pulmonary circulation. The pulmonary vascular system acts as resistance to the output from the right ventricle. The values are used to assess for pulmonary hypertension and right heart function. Normal parameters are pulmonary

artery (PA) systolic 15 to 30 mm Hg, and PA diastolic 4 to 12 mm Hg.

This port can also be used for drawing venous oxygen saturation via a mixed venous hemoglobin saturation (SvO$_2$). This value reflects the oxygen saturation of blood returned to the heart from both the superior and inferior vena cava therefore reflecting total body venous oxygen saturation.

The proximal port, located approximately 30 cm from the tip of the catheter in the right atrium, is used to monitor RA pressure (CVP). Central venous pressure is a reflection of right heart preload or right ventricular end-diastolic volume. The proximal port is also used to inject the solution used to obtain a thermodilution cardiac output (CO). There is a temperature sensor built into the thermistor lumen at the tip of the PA catheter. It measures the ambient blood temperature around it continuously. To obtain a CO, a small bolus of cooler normal saline is briskly injected through the proximal injectate port. Because of the injection of cooler fluid, the temperature of the blood flowing by the sensor changes. The time it takes for the cold injectate to pass the sensor is measured in liters of blood pumped per minute. This is called the "thermodilution" method of obtaining the CO. Normal CO is 4 to 8 L/min. Typically, CO is indexed, meaning it is calculated on the basis of the patient's body surface area (BSA). A normal **cardiac index (CI)** is 2.5 to 4 L/min/m^2.

The inflation lumen leads to the balloon, located less than 1 cm from the catheter tip. The **pulmonary artery wedge pressure** or **pulmonary artery occlusive pressure** (PAWP/PAOP) is obtained by inflating the balloon with a syringe included in the PA catheter kit and specifically designed for use with the balloon (1.5 mL of air). The PAOP reflects left heart preload or left ventricular end diastolic pressure. This pressure is obtained when the balloon is inflated and floats into a wedge position in the pulmonary artery which occludes that branch of the pulmonary artery obscuring data from the right heart. In this position, the values obtained reflect pressures proximal to the balloon in the left side of the heart. Normal values are 4 to 12 mm Hg. This value assumes normal pulmonary conditions. The use of PAOP is decreasing

because its use is associated with complications. In its place, the PA diastolic pressure may be used again, assuming a normal pulmonary vasculature and mitral valve.

The PA catheter also allows for indirect measurement of *afterload* via systemic vascular resistance (SVR) and pulmonary vascular resistance (PVR), and *contractility* via left ventricular stroke work index (LVSWI), and right ventricular stroke work index (RVSWI). Left heart afterload or the systemic vascular resistance is calculated using mean arterial pressure-central venous pressure/cardiac output (MAP-CVP/CO). Pulmonary vascular resistance is calculated as SVR, substituting pulmonary artery pressure for MAP and PAOP for CVP; PAP-PAOP/CP. The SVR and PVR can be indexed to a patient's body size by dividing by body surface area (BSA) to yield the systemic vascular resistance index (SVRI) and pulmonary vascular resistance index (PVRI). The normal SVR value ranges from 800 to 1,200 dynes*sec/cm^5, and the PVR value is less than 250 dynes*sec/cm^5. The normal SVRI is 1,900 to 2,400 dynes*sec/cm^5/m^2, and the PVRI is 200 to 400 dynes*sec/cm^5/m^2. Increasing afterload in an unhealthy ventricle increases cardiac workload, thus increasing myocardial oxygen consumption. It also decreases SV and CO.

Contractility can be inferred by evaluating stroke work indexes of the right and left ventricles. Stroke work indexes are measurements of work done by the heart with each contraction. They are calculated via measurements obtained through the PA catheter.

Table 32.1 describes normal cardiac values, causes of abnormal values, and treatment possibilities for CO disorders.

Table 32.1 Assessment of Cardiac Output

Value	Normal	Abnormal Low	Abnormal High	Intervention Low	Intervention High
Central venous pressure	5–10 cm H$_2$O	● Hypovolemia or peripheral vasodilation	● Right heart failure, tension pneumothorax, pulmonary hypertension, or pericardial tamponade	● Fluid bolus ● Vasopressor therapy	● Inotropic and vasodilator therapy; treatment of cause, i.e., chest tube for pneumothorax
Pulmonary artery (PA) ● Systolic (PAS) ● Diastolic (PAD)	 PAS, 15–30 mm Hg PAD, 4–12 mm Hg	● May be normal state or signs of hypovolemia and vasodilation	● Pulmonary hypertension, right heart failure	● Would treat only if other concerns present	● Inotropic and vasodilator therapy, diuresis
Pulmonary capillary wedge pressure	4–12 mm Hg	● May be normal state or signs of hypovolemia and vasodilation	● Pulmonary hypertension, cardiogenic shock, hypoxia, and acute respiratory distress syndrome	● Would treat only if other concerns present	● Inotropic and vasodilator therapy, diuresis

Table 32.1 Assessment of Cardiac Output—cont'd

Value	Normal	Abnormal Low	Abnormal High	Intervention Low	Intervention High
Cardiac output/ cardiac index	4–8 L/min 2.5–4 L/min/m²	• Myocardial infarction, all forms of shock except early septic shock	• Septic shock (early), hypervolemia, hyperthermia	• Fluid bolus, inotropic therapy, treatment of cause, i.e., MI	• Would treat only if other concerns present
Systemic vascular resistance/ systemic vascular resistance index	800–1,200 dynes*sec/cm⁵ 1,900–2,400 dynes*sec/cm⁵/m²	• Causes of vasodilation such as distributive shock	• Causes of vasoconstriction such as hypovolemia, hypotension, cardiogenic shock	• Fluid bolus • Vasopressor therapy	• Vasodilator therapy
Pulmonary vascular resistance/ pulmonary vascular resistance index	Less than 250 dynes*sec/cm⁵ 200–400 dynes*sec/cm⁵/m²	• May be normal state or signs of hypovolemia and vasodilation	• Pulmonary hypertension	• Would treat only if other concerns present	• Vasodilator therapy
Mixed venous oxygen saturation	60%–75%	• Increased oxygen needs of tissues • Low cardiac output • Low hemoglobin • Low oxygenation	• Later stages of sepsis and DIC with shunting of blood and/or microvascular clotting	• Increase cardiac output • Increase oxygen • Increase hemoglobin	• Treat the cause

Nursing Implications for the Pulmonary Artery Catheter

To ensure patient safety, it is essential that the nurse understand the mechanics of the PA catheter and the proper technique for assisting in catheter insertion and obtaining data. Providers, including physicians, nurse practitioners, and physician assistants, receive education and training to insert PA catheters, measure parameters, and interpret data. Nurses receive education and training to assist with the insertion, measure parameters, and interpret data.

As with the CVP line, the patient should be placed in the Trendelenburg position before insertion. During catheter insertion, the nurse monitors the waveforms while the catheter passes through the different chambers of the heart and into the pulmonary artery (Fig. 32.7).

Once the catheter is advanced into the right atrium, and as directed by the provider, the nurse must inflate the balloon before any further catheter advancement. Balloon inflation during catheter insertion helps the PA catheter float into the pulmonary artery and prevents trauma to the cardiac structures as it moves through the heart chambers and valves. When a PAOP is obtained, the balloon must be inflated no more than 1.5 mL. After the value is obtained,

it is essential that the nurse ensure the balloon is immediately deflated. The balloon will deflate passively and should not be manually deflated or forced to deflate. A PA catheter should never be inflated and remain in the wedge position for more than 10 to 15 seconds. If the balloon remains

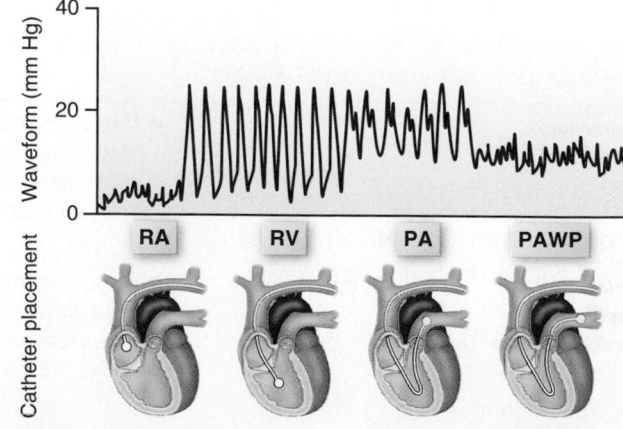

FIGURE 32.7 Pressure waveforms visible on the cardiac monitor during passage of the pulmonary artery line through the heart during catheter insertion.

inflated or in the wedge position there is the risk of accidental PA occlusion, hemorrhage, or PA infarction. If the waveform on the monitor indicates the catheter has remained in that wedge position, the nurse must verify that the balloon is not inflated and notify the provider for immediate intervention.

Care and risks of the PA catheter are the same as those with a central venous catheter; any handling of the line should be kept to a minimum to decrease infection risk, and an occlusive transparent dressing should be maintained and changed per hospital policy.

As with placement, the patient must be placed in a Trendelenburg position before removal. Remove any sutures holding the catheter in place, taking care not to cut the catheter. If possible, have the patient take a deep breath in and hold it during the withdrawal of the catheter. After removal, apply pressure for 3 to 5 minutes or until hemostasis is achieved. Observe the insertion site for potential bleeding. Subclavian veins are not compressible and are therefore more prone to bleeding if the coagulation studies are not within normal limits.

Complications

The data obtained through pulmonary artery (PA) catheters can be extremely useful in the management of a complex critically ill patient, but the use of PA catheters is in question. New methods of obtaining hemodynamic data are under development (see Evidence-Based Practice) because there is a significant degree of complications and risk with a PA catheter. Complications may be related to insertion, maintenance and use, or to interpretation of data. As with any invasive intervention, there is a risk of infection and bleeding. The PA catheter also carries the risk of PA rupture, infarction, or air embolism as a result of balloon rupture during inflation to measure the wedge pressure (Box 32.6). Questions have been raised about the precise indications, cost-effectiveness, and effect on clinical outcomes. Large observational studies, small randomized studies, and meta-analyses have confirmed no benefit (survival or days in hospital) from PA catheters in any medical or surgical population of critically ill patients. The decision to use a PA catheter should be done on an individual basis, according to the specific clinical presentation, weighing the risk versus the benefit for the individual patient.

Connection Check 32.2

The charge nurse is monitoring the care of several critically ill patients in the ICU. Which patient requires immediate intervention by the provider?

A. The patient with a PA catheter remaining in the wedge position

B. The patient with an SvO_2 of 55%

C. The patient with an SVR of 1,300

D. The patient with a CO of 3.2

Evidence-Based Practice

Newer Methods of Cardiac Output Monitoring

Noninvasive methods of measuring cardiac output are being developed because of the inherent risks associated with the pulmonary artery catheter. Several new methods include pulse contour analysis and transesophageal echocardiography (TEE). Pulse contour analysis provides information through the evaluation of the arterial pulse wave. Examples of pulse contour technologies are the FloTrac(tm)/Vigileo™ (Edwards Lifesciences, Irvine, CA) and PiCCO (PULSION medical system, Munich, Germany). Pulse contour analysis is based on the principle that stroke volume can be estimated through evaluation of the systolic portion of the arterial waveform. Cardiac output is then derived through analysis of stroke volume (SV) and heart rate. PiCCO requires an arterial line, and a central venous catheter. Similar to the PA catheter thermodilution method, cold solution is injected into the central line and is detected by a thermistor in the arterial line tip. FloTrac requires only an arterial line. Stroke volume is estimated via a calculation that evaluates the arterial waveform and specific patient demographics. Pulse contour technology has a number of limitations including inaccuracy in patients with irregular heart rhythms, right heart failure, and patients requiring low tidal volume mechanical ventilation.

Cardiac ultrasound via transesophageal echocardiography (TEE) may be used to provide real-time images of the cardiac structures and blood flow. Transthoracic echocardiography may help define pathophysiological abnormalities such as wall motion abnormalities, pericardial effusions, pulmonary hypertension, and valve abnormalities, in conjunction with other invasive or less-invasive monitoring. Although it cannot provide continuous monitoring, it can easily be repeated to quickly evaluate the response to an intervention. A TEE is obtained by placing a transducer in the esophagus next to the heart to produce images. TEE is used in the operating suites and in critical care units. There is, however, a significant learning curve for the provider, TEE is expensive, and continuous monitoring is not an option. There is a (low) risk of oropharyngeal bleeding and dislocation of the endotracheal tube.

Booker, K. J. (2015). Hemodynamic monitoring in critical care. *Critical Care Nursing: Monitoring and Treatment for Advanced Nursing Practice*, 73-86.

Mehta, Y., & Arora, D. (2014). Newer methods of cardiac output monitoring. *World Journal of Cardiology*, 6(9), 1022.

Box 32.6 Potential Pulmonary Artery Catheter Complications

Insertion
- Arrhythmias
- Misplacement
- Knotting of the long flexible catheter
- Myocardial, vessel, or valve rupture
- Pneumothorax during catheter insertion

Use and Maintenance
- Pulmonary infarction from lack of blood supply if balloon left in wedge position
- Pulmonary artery rupture from balloon inflation
- Air embolism from balloon rupture
- Thrombosis from catheter acting as a conduit for thrombus formation
- Bleeding
- Central line bloodstream infections
- Right heart/valve trauma

Data Misinterpretation
- Improperly calibrated monitors
- Over or underestimation of PAOP
- Lung zone misplacement

CASE STUDY: EPISODE 2

Mr. King's 12-lead ECG reveals the presence of ST-segment elevation in leads *II*, *III*, and *aVF*, which indicates an inferior wall myocardial infarction (MI). His troponin level is 12. The patient is diagnosed with acute inferior wall MI. After gastrointestinal bleeding is ruled out with a quick rectal examination, a heparin bolus is given IV and a heparin drip is started. His condition begins to deteriorate. Mr. King now has a BP of 75/50 mm Hg and a heart rate of 115 bpm. He is getting agitated, and his extremities are cool and pale. His ABG results, pH 7.23, PaCO$_2$ 34, PaO$_2$ 48, HCO$_3^-$ 20, reveal hypoxemia and metabolic acidosis. It is determined that he may be in cardiogenic shock. He is started on a norepinephrine IV drip to support his BP and a dobutamine IV drip to help improve cardiac contractility. He is intubated and immediately transported to the cardiac catheterization laboratory for coronary angiography and percutaneous coronary intervention (PCI)...

MYOCARDIAL INFARCTION

Epidemiology

Heart disease, which leads to MI, is the leading cause of death for men and women in the United States and not only results in serious illness and disability but also costs hundreds of billions of dollars per year. Approximately 630,000 people die of heart disease each year— one in every four deaths. Coronary heart disease was responsible for the death of 366,000 people in 2015. Currently, more than one in three adults lives with one or more types of cardiovascular disease.

Contributing risk factors for heart disease and MI include cigarette smoking, high low-density lipoprotein (LDL), type 2 diabetes, elevated adrenaline (catecholamines), obesity, inactivity, and hypertension. These risk factors are modifiable and significant because they can accelerate the development of heart disease and lead to earlier onset of symptoms. Additional nonmodifiable risk factors include male gender, postmenopausal female, and family history of heart disease.

An MI can occur at any time of day, but the most dangerous time for all types of cardiovascular emergencies is in the early morning hours. This includes not only MI but also sudden cardiac death, rupture of an aortic aneurysm, pulmonary embolism (PE), and stroke. A group from Harvard estimates that the increased risk of MI between 6 a.m. and noon is approximately 40%. The exact cause is unknown but may be due to higher levels of circulating adrenaline released during this time. Increased adrenaline may also contribute to feelings of acute loss or stress that occur during an evolving MI.

Pathophysiology

The term **myocardial infarction (MI)** refers to the destruction of heart muscle from lack of oxygenated blood supply. The most common cause of this obstruction is atherosclerosis. Atherosclerosis is the gradual buildup of plaque inside the wall of the artery. Rupture of this plaque results in thrombus formation and obstruction of coronary artery flow. Ischemia and death of heart muscle are the eventual outcomes. Heart muscle damaged by inadequate blood supply cannot maintain normal cardiac function, which results in decreased CO and the systemic symptoms associated with MI such as chest pain and poor tissue perfusion.

Stable angina is defined as episodes of intermittent chest pain present when the artery is narrowed 60% to 70%. It is typically associated with activity or exercise and is relieved by rest. Stable angina is not associated with damage to the heart muscle but is a warning sign for potential heart muscle damage. **Acute coronary syndrome** is an umbrella term used when there is concern for myocardial ischemia, and it encompasses unstable angina (UA), non-ST elevation MI (NSTEMI), and ST elevation MI (STEMI). Unstable angina is pain that is not associated with exercise and is not relieved by rest. It may present with ECG changes but no elevation in cardiac markers. It is an emergency requiring immediate treatment.

A NSTEMI is a partial occlusion of a major coronary vessel or complete occlusion of a minor coronary vessel causing reversible partial thickness heart muscle damage. In contrast, a STEMI is a complete occlusion of a major coronary vessel resulting in irreversible full thickness heart muscle damage (Fig. 32.8). Table 32.2 describes the characteristics of UA, NSTEMI, and STEMI.

The extent of damage is dependent upon the location of the blockage. The heart's blood supply originates from two major vessels, the left coronary artery and the right coronary artery. Severe occlusion of the right coronary artery results in symptoms of right heart failure. In addition, the forward delivery of blood to the left ventricle may be insufficient, resulting in symptoms of left heart failure.

The left coronary artery is referred to as the *left main* (LM). This branches off into the left anterior descending (LAD) and the circumflex (CIRC) coronary arteries. In some individuals, a third branch, the ramus coronary artery, arises between the LAD and the CIRC. An occlusion of the LM coronary artery is often referred to as the *widow maker* because interruption of its extensive coverage is associated with sudden death. A left coronary artery occlusion is most likely to produce extensive cardiac injury, with impairment of heart function, pulmonary congestion, and low CO. Table 32.3 lists different locations of myocardial damage with associated implicated vessels and lead changes seen on ECG.

Clinical Manifestations

The classic clinical manifestation of obstructed blood flow to the heart muscle is chest pain. As noted earlier, chest pain or angina, can be classified as stable or unstable. Stable, or exertional, angina typically occurs during activity, has a predictable pattern, and goes away with rest. Unstable, or rest, angina (UA) is much more serious because it can occur while at rest with no specific pattern and is not relieved by change in activity. Angina is a warning sign of impending MI. Unstable angina is a medical emergency requiring immediate intervention.

Symptoms in addition to chest pain when there is a complete occlusion of the vessel resulting in an MI and significant muscle damage include shoulder and arm pain (more often on the left), jaw and tooth pain, shoulder blade pain, upper back pain, shortness of breath, nausea and vomiting, sweating, and generalized fatigue. A right coronary artery MI, or right ventricle infarction, has very distinct characteristics. The patient may present with jugular vein distention (JVD), hypotension, bradycardia; due to damage to the sinoatrial (SA) node, nausea, and vomiting. An MI that involves the left coronary artery, or left ventricle infarction, has a worse prognosis with the highest risk of sudden death and congestive heart failure. Signs of a left ventricle infarct include dyspnea, tachycardia, and hypertension. The tachycardia and hypertension result from the loss of CO because of damage to the left ventricle and subsequent stimulation of sympathetic compensatory mechanisms. Hypotension will quickly evolve.

Clinical manifestations of MI can vary significantly from person to person, with gender one prominent distinction. Women are more likely to present with atypical MI symptoms including neck, shoulder blade, and jaw pain, as well as abdominal pain. The geriatric population

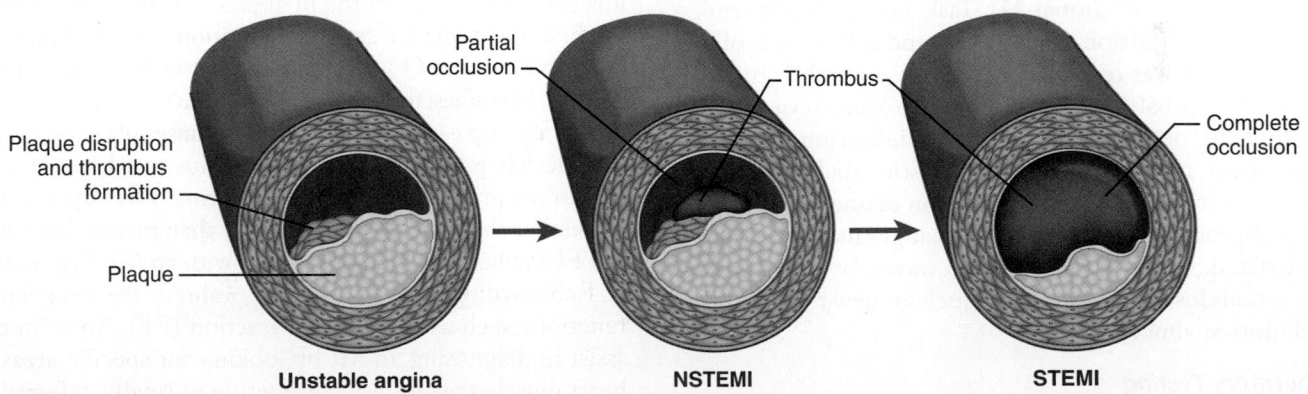

FIGURE 32.8 Acute coronary syndrome: Unstable angina, non-ST elevation myocardial infarction, and ST elevation myocardial infarction.

Table 32.2 Characteristics of Unstable Angina, Non-ST Elevation Myocardial Infarction and ST Elevation Myocardial Infarction

Unstable Angina	Non-ST Elevation Myocardial Infarction	ST Elevation Myocardial Infarction
May present with nonspecific or transient ST segment depressions or elevations	ST depressions (0.5 mm at least) or T wave inversions (1.0 mm at least) without Q waves in 2 contiguous leads with prominent R wave or R/S ratio >1	ST elevations
No elevation in cardiac markers	Elevated cardiac markers	Elevated cardiac markers

Table 32.3 Myocardial Infarction With Associated Electrocardiogram Leads and Coronary Artery Location

Type of MI	Associated ECG Lead Changes	Associated Coronary Artery
Anterior wall	Leads V1–V4	LAD
Posterior wall	Possibly leads V1–V4	CIRC or RCA
Lateral wall	Leads I, aVL, V5, V6	CIRC
Inferior wall	Leads II, III, aVF	RCA

CIRC, Circumflex; ECG, electrocardiogram; LAD, left anterior descending artery; MI, myocardial infarction; RCA, right coronary artery

may not exhibit classic angina symptoms or may have coexisting conditions which mimic angina. They may experience dyspnea, syncope, weakness, or confusion. Many patients, especially patients with diabetes, never have the typical symptoms but may present with symptoms of shortness of breath or fatigue. Cardiovascular etiologies should be considered for patients exhibiting these atypical symptoms.

Management

Medical Management

Diagnosis

In 2000, the First Global MI Task Force recommended a universal definition of MI to standardize care of MI patients. This was reviewed and updated in 2007. In 2012, the Third Global MI Task Force once again reviewed and updated the definition of MI. This definition states that there must be presence of diagnostic cardiac markers, preferably troponin, with the addition of one of the following: symptoms of ischemia, ECG changes indicative of new ischemia, development of ECG Q waves, or image testing that reveals loss of viable heart muscle or new regional heart wall motion abnormalities.

Laboratory Testing

Laboratory tests used to diagnose an MI include troponin, creatine kinase (CK), and CK-MB. Creatine kinase is a general marker of cellular injury. It is released from cells in the brain, skeletal muscle, and cardiac tissue after muscle damage has occurred. Creatine kinase–MB is the CK isoenzyme marker specific to cardiac tissue. When myocardial damage occurs, CK-MB is released from the cells. Increased levels can be seen at 3 hours and remain elevated for up to 36 hours before returning to normal. Cardiac troponin (I and T) are proteins expressed almost exclusively in the heart and are a specific marker of cardiac muscle damage. Troponin levels can elevate within 4 hours of injury and

can stay elevated for as long as 10 days. Because it stays elevated longer than CK-MB, it is a valuable marker when attempting to diagnose injury in the recent past. Troponin is the blood test of choice to diagnose acute MI (AMI).

While infarction progresses, cardiac function decreases. End-organ compromise should be assessed and monitored with routine blood work such as:

- A complete metabolic profile (CMP), which includes electrolytes and tests of organ system functioning such as renal values; BUN and creatinine
- Complete blood count (CBC), which includes hemoglobin, hematocrit, and white blood cell count
- Coagulation studies (prothrombin time, activated partial thromboplastin time, platelets)
- Arterial blood gas (ABG)

Diagnostic Testing

Diagnostic testing for MI can be performed through invasive and noninvasive tests. These tests include ECG, echocardiogram (echo), stress testing, and coronary angiography. An ECG has become the gold standard for diagnosis of MI. It is inexpensive, easy to perform, safe, and painless. Typical electrocardiogram changes diagnostic of AMI includes ST-segment elevation and the presence of Q waves. Electrocardiogram changes can occur in phases. The first observable ECG change is the presence of ST-segment depression indicating ischemia; NSTEMI. Although the changes may vary, typically if untreated, changes indicating the evolution from ischemia to infarction include tall narrow T waves, then ST-segment elevation, STEMI with T-wave inversion appearing. In the final phase, which can occur in the first hours, the ST-segment elevation is accompanied by development of a Q wave. Some patients do not develop a Q wave. In studies, the presence of a Q wave predicted a larger infarct and increased mortality. Other causes of Q waves may include left pneumothorax, myocarditis, cardiomyopathy, or chronic processes such as scleroderma. It is important to remember that women are less likely than men to have typical ECG changes when presenting with an MI (Fig. 32.9).

Echocardiography is used to evaluate the ventricular functions such as the ejection fraction (EF). An echo can assist in diagnosing an MI by looking for specific areas of heart muscle that are not contracting normally, referred to as *wall motion abnormalities*.

Although not done during the time an MI is evolving, stress testing is another way to evaluate heart function. Stress testing includes the exercise stress test, dobutamine/adenosine test, stress echo, and nuclear stress test. These tests are discussed in detail in Chapter 28. Testing is dependent upon the patient's needs and condition. These tests look at coronary blood flow as well as left ventricular function and wall motion abnormalities. A nuclear stress test is the best stress test for diagnosing myocardial ischemia. It reveals the amount of viable heart muscle, which helps to determine treatment.

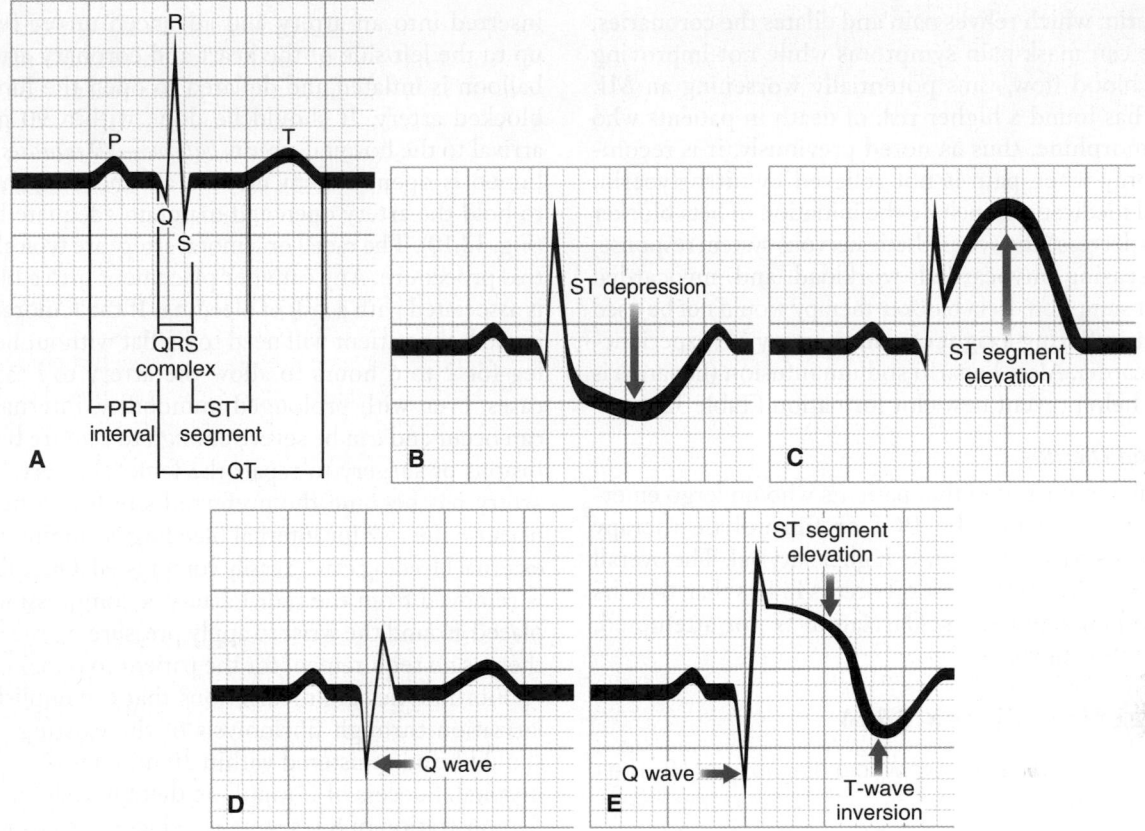

FIGURE 32.9 Electrocardiogram (ECG) waveforms illustrating the evolution of an MI. *A*, Normal ECG waveform. *B*, ECG waveform with ST depression indicating ischemia. *C*, ST elevation in acute myocardial infarction (AMI). *D*, Q waves after AMI. *E*, ECG waveform illustrating changes that occur with AMI.

Connection Check 32.3

The nurse is reviewing the laboratory results of her patient and notes that a cardiac troponin level was drawn. This test was drawn to determine which diagnosis?

A. Atrial fibrillation
B. Ventricular tachycardia
C. Myocardial infarction
D. Congestive heart failure

Coronary angiography is the gold standard for the diagnosis of flow-limiting coronary artery disease. During coronary angiography, a catheter is inserted into the radial or femoral, and advanced up to the heart. A radiopaque dye is injected through the catheter into the coronary artery while sequences of x-rays (fluoroscopy) are obtained. This allows visualization of any obstruction or narrowing of the coronary arteries. At the same time, a ventriculogram may be obtained. This involves positioning the catheter to allow injected dye to enter the left ventricle. The ventriculogram demonstrates how efficiently the left ventricle fills and pumps blood, how well blood flows through the aortic and mitral valves, and the size of the left ventricle.

Treatment

Once the diagnosis of MI is made, immediate patient management involves maximizing oxygenation and administering medications to control pain, dilate the coronaries, prevent clots, and decrease myocardial workload. Care then involves therapies to increase blood flow to cardiac tissue, or reperfusion therapy.

Medications

Immediately upon arrival to the hospital, the patient should receive oxygen, sublingual (SL) nitroglycerin, aspirin, and then pain medication such as morphine sulfate if pain is not relieved by the SL nitroglycerin. Oxygen is recommended for all patients with a suspected MI and specifically for patients in respiratory distress if the arterial saturation is less than 90% or for patients with a high risk of hypoxia. Nitroglycerin dilates the coronary arteries, increasing blood flow to the heart in an attempt to limit myocardial muscle damage and control pain. One tablet may be given sublingually every 5 minutes for a maximum of three doses as long as the patient maintains an adequate BP. If pain is not controlled with three doses, IV nitroglycerin will be started. Aspirin is given to help prevent platelets from enlarging the existing clot or new clots from forming. Morphine sulfate can be given to control pain; however, in contrast to nitroglycerin, which relives pain and dilates the coronaries, morphine can mask pain symptoms while not improving coronary blood flow, thus potentially worsening an MI. Research has found a higher risk of death in patients who received morphine, thus as noted previously, it is recommended only when pain is not relieved by nitroglycerin. Additional medications include the initiation of beta blocker therapy to decrease the sympathetic nervous system response, thus decreasing myocardial workload and myocardial oxygen consumption. Beta blocker therapy would not be used in a patient suffering a right coronary artery MI experiencing bradycardia. Also, heparin sodium infusion (heparin) is started to help prevent new clot formation (Table 32.4).

Reperfusion Therapy

It has been demonstrated that patients who undergo emergency revascularization by PCI or fibrinolytic therapy within 6 hours have significantly higher survival. The overall mortality when revascularization occurs in less than 6 hours is 38%. When rapid revascularization is not attempted, mortality rates approach 70%.

Connection Check 32.4

A nurse is caring for a patient with a diagnosis of MI. The patient calls the nurse because he is experiencing chest pain. The nurse administers an SL nitroglycerin tablet as prescribed. After 5 minutes, the chest pain is unrelieved by the nitroglycerin. The next nursing action is which of the following?

A. Administer another nitroglycerin tablet
B. Increase the flow rate of the oxygen
C. Contact the provider
D. Call the charge nurse

Percutaneous coronary intervention is the most preferred method for opening blocked blood vessels that cause MI. During PCI, a catheter with a small balloon on its tip is inserted into an artery and advanced under fluoroscopy up to the left side of the heart and coronary arteries. The balloon is inflated and deflated to open the lumen of the blocked artery. It should be done within 90 minutes of arrival to the hospital: *door to balloon—90 minutes*. Once the lumen is open, a stent may be advanced to the location to hold the artery open and maintain adequate blood flow (Fig. 32.10). The radial or femoral artery are typically used for this procedure. Any catheter placement into a blood vessel is associated with a risk of bleeding. If the femoral approach is used, the patient will need to lie flat without bending the leg for 2 to 6 hours to allow the artery to heal. In some cases, even with prolonged immobility, internal bleeding can occur and can be severe enough to require blood transfusions or surgery to repair the femoral artery. The radial artery has become the preferred site for catheterization because the risk for internal bleeding is eliminated and any external bleeding can be easily compressed. Once the catheter is removed from the radial artery, a compression device is placed around the wrist to apply pressure on the artery, and there is no requirement for the patient to remain immobile.

Fibrinolytics are medications that accomplish revascularization through fibrinolysis of the existing clot. They should be administered within 30 minutes of arrival to the hospital. Success of fibrinolytic therapy is defined as ECG demonstration of ST-segment reduction greater than 50% at 90 minutes. Fibrinolytics should be considered if not contraindicated and immediate PCI is not available. Contraindications include recent surgery or bleeding, presence of a peptic ulcer, uncontrolled hypertension, pregnancy, and noncompressible vascular punctures. The major complication of fibrinolytic therapy is bleeding, specifically an increased risk for intracranial hemorrhage.

Surgical Management

Coronary artery bypass grafting (CABG) is a surgical revascularization intervention that bypasses blockages in the coronary arteries causing the myocardial muscle damage. It

Table 32.4 Commonly Prescribed Medications for Myocardial Infarction

Classification	Medication	Action
Antiplatelet	Aspirin, clopidogrel (Plavix), eptifibatide (Integrilin)	Prevents platelets from forming new clots or increasing the size of the present clot
Anticoagulant	Heparin, enoxaparin (Lovenox), Factor XA inhibitors	Prevents formation of new clots
Narcotic	Morphine sulfate, hydromorphone (Dilaudid)	Relieves chest pain
Beta blocker	Metoprolol (Lopressor), Atenolol (Tenormin)	Decreases myocardial workload thus myocardial oxygen demand, limiting extension of injury
Nitrates	Nitroglycerin (Nitro-BID)	Dilate coronary arteries to increase blood flow to the heart muscle and relieve chest pain
Thrombolytics	Alteplase (Activase), reteplase (Retavase)	Revascularization of the heart muscle by dissolving clots in arteries

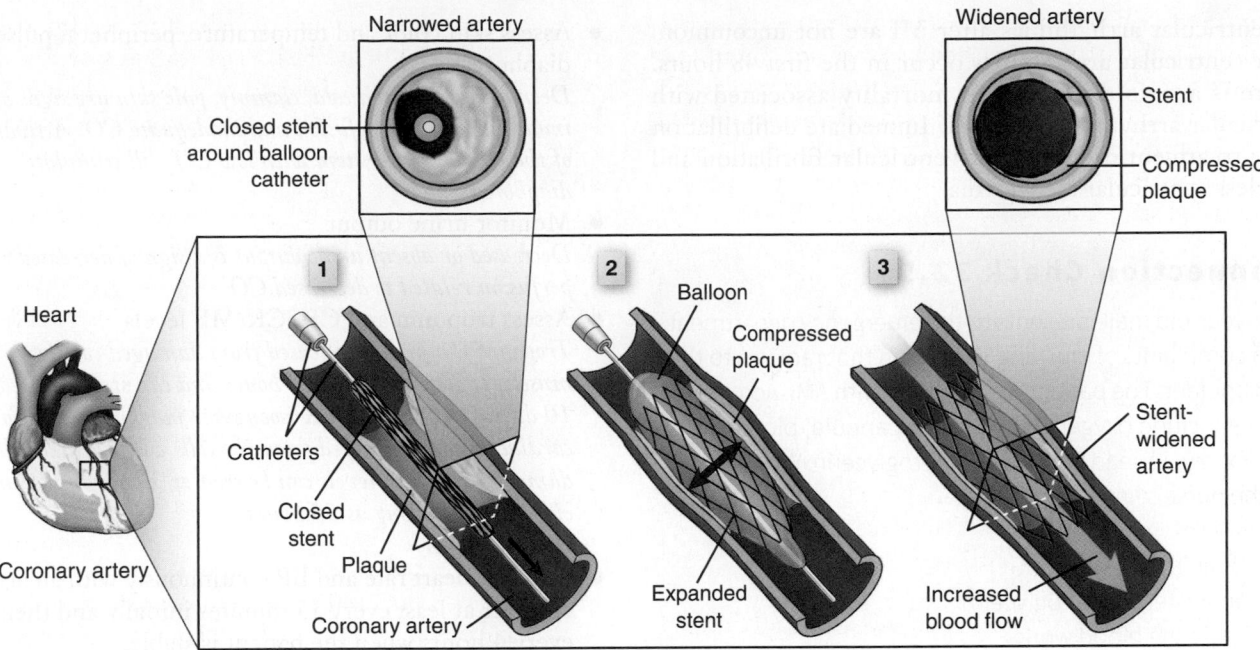

FIGURE 32.10 Stent insertion to open a blocked coronary artery.

is not the first-line intervention after MI because PCI or fibrinolytics are much quicker procedures; they do not involve a long surgical procedure, thus revascularization is accomplished in a timelier fashion. Indications for CABG include unsuccessful PCI or not a candidate for PCI, failure of medical management, or critical left main or three vessel disease.

During CABG, a healthy artery or vein, typically the internal thoracic (mammary) artery or saphenous vein, is grafted to the blocked coronary artery. One end is attached to the aorta, with the other end attached to the blocked coronary distal to the occlusion, thereby bypassing the blocked portion of the artery allowing blood flow to the cardiac tissue (Fig. 32.11). The procedure is most typically done on pump or with cardiopulmonary bypass. Complications associated with CABG include bleeding, dysrhythmias,

MI, stroke, nonunion of the sternum, sternal infection, renal failure because of decreased renal blood flow, or heart failure. Complications of bypass include induction of a systemic inflammatory response resulting in vasodilatory shock, heparin-induced thrombocytopenia, activation of platelets, and the complications associated with cross clamping the aorta during the procedure. An off pump or "beating heart" CABG procedure was developed to avoid the complications related to bypass. This option requires considerable expertise and has not demonstrated consistent improved outcomes.

Secondary Prevention

Cardiac rehabilitation is recommended after an acute cardiovascular event such as MI, percutaneous intervention, or surgical revascularization. It is a supervised exercise program which also provides education regarding diet, weight management, medication purpose and side effects, and psychosocial support. The goals are to improve recovery from the event and improve quality of life. Patients are evaluated by their cardiologist or cardiac surgeon for participation.

Complications

Heart failure is a complication related to MI. When an MI causes a large amount of heart muscle to die, there is decreased left ventricular function. The overall result can be heart failure and is defined as the inability to produce an adequate CO to maintain the body's metabolic demands. Heart failure is discussed in detail in Chapter 30.

Arrhythmias associated with MI include asystole, symptomatic bradycardia, heart block, and ventricular arrhythmias. Asystole, symptomatic bradycardia, and heart block are usually associated with sinoatrial (SA) node dysfunction. This is most common after an inferior wall MI because the right coronary artery supplies the SA node. A temporary pacemaker may be used to prevent asystole.

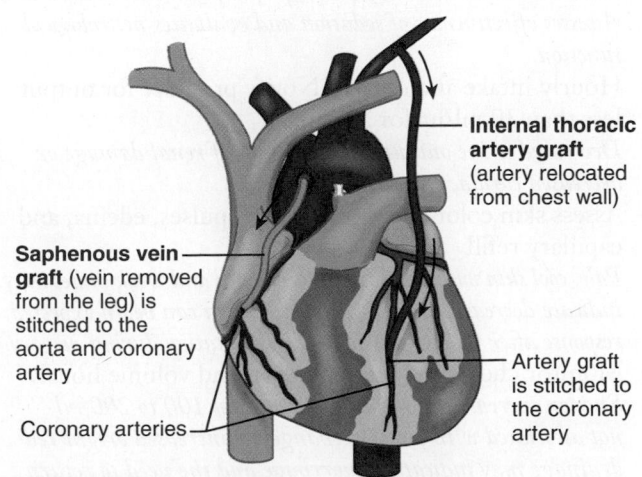

FIGURE 32.11 Coronary artery bypass grafting (CABG).

Ventricular arrhythmias after MI are not uncommon. Most ventricular arrhythmias occur in the first 48 hours. There is a sixfold increase in mortality associated with ventricular arrhythmia after MI. Immediate defibrillation is the treatment of choice for ventricular fibrillation and pulseless ventricular tachycardia.

Connection Check 32.5

A 68-year-old male presents to the emergency department with complaints of crushing chest pain that radiates to the left shoulder. The patient is diagnosed with AMI. Admission orders include oxygen 2 L via nasal cannula, blood work, chest x-ray, 12-lead ECG, and SL nitroglycerin. What should be the nurse's first action?
A. Apply oxygen
B. Obtain the 12-lead ECG
C. Administer the nitroglycerin
D. Obtain the blood work

Nursing Management
Assessment and Analysis
The clinical presentation of MI is related to lack of oxygen delivery to the heart and the resulting decrease in CO. The patient complains of chest pain, shortness of breath, nausea and vomiting, and dizziness. The patient presents with diaphoresis and pallor. Women and older adults may present differently, with women complaining of neck, shoulder blade, and jaw pain as well as abdominal pain. Older adults may present with dyspnea, syncope, weakness, or confusion. Hemodynamics are variable, but typically the patient is tachycardic with a borderline low BP.

Nursing Diagnoses
- **Decreased CO** related to poor cardiac contractility secondary to MI
- **Pain** related to inadequate blood supply by the heart

Nursing Interventions
▪ *Assessments*
- Vital signs and pulse oximetry
  Tachycardia with a borderline low BP and decreased oxygen saturation is a sign of inadequate CO and oxygen delivery.
- Assess characteristics of pain including location, radiation, duration, intensity, precipitating or alleviating factors; use a 1 to 10 pain scale
  Chest pain is an indication of MI. Continued or changing pain characteristics can be indicative of a worsening condition.
- Assess ECG changes
  ST-segment depression is indicative of ischemia. ST-segment elevation is indicative of injury. If present, a Q wave is diagnostic for MI.
- Assess for restlessness
  Restlessness may be found in the early stages, but progression to severe anxiety and sense of doom is a late-stage symptom.

- Assess skin color and temperature, peripheral pulses, diaphoresis
  Decreased pulses and cold, clammy, pale skin are signs of inadequate tissue perfusion and inadequate CO. Activation of the sympathetic system with low CO will stimulate diaphoresis.
- Monitor urine output
  Decreased or absent urine output is a sign of decreased renal perfusion related to decreased CO
- Assess troponin and CK, CK/MB levels
  Troponin is a protein released from damaged cardiac muscle. It elevates within 4 hours and can stay elevated for 10 days. CK/MB, the CK isoenzyme marker specific to cardiac tissue, is released from the cells with cardiac muscle damage. Increased levels can be seen at 3 hours and remain elevated for as long as 36 hours.

Post-CABG
- Monitor heart rate and BP continuously with an arterial catheter at least every 15 minutes initially and then every 4 hours when the patient is stable.
  Tachycardia, bradycardia, hypotension, and hypertension may be signs of decreased cardiac output or compensatory mechanisms.
- Hemodynamic monitoring
  Decreased preload (CVP, PAOP), SvO_2 may indicate a decreased cardiac output leading to poor tissue perfusion
- Continuous cardiac monitoring
  Dysrhythmias are common after CABG.
- Assess heart tones
  Muffled heart tones may indicate tamponade. S3, S4, and crackles may indicate heart failure.
- Monitor breath sounds and continuous oxygen saturation monitoring
  Decreasing saturation may indicate pulmonary complications. Diminished or unilateral absent breath sounds may indicate atelectasis, pleural effusions or pneumothorax.
- Monitor core temperature hourly
  Hypothermia during surgery reduces metabolic rate and risk of organ ischemia. Rewarming may produce hypotension from vasodilation. Core temperatures are most reliable.
- Assess level of consciousness, pupils, and responsiveness
  Assesses effectiveness of sedation and evaluates neurological function.
- Hourly intake and output. Notify provider for output less than 30 ml/hr for 2 hours.
  Decreased urine output may be a sign of renal damage or decreased cardiac output.
- Assess skin color and temperature, pulses, edema, and capillary refill
  Pale, cool skin with delayed capillary refill and weak pulses may indicate decreased cardiac output. Edema can be an expected response after CABG due to fluid resuscitation during surgery.
- Monitor chest tube output, color, and volume hourly
  Sudden increases in output greater than 100 to 200 ml not associated with position changes or increased bright red drainage may indicate hemorrhage and the need to return to the operating room.

- Assess hemoglobin, hematocrit, electrolytes, creatinine and blood urea nitrogen, glucose
  Changes may indicate bleeding, fluid shifts, and renal dysfunction. Tight glucose control is associated with improved outcomes.
- Assess incisions for drainage, warmth, redness, swelling.
  Redness, warmth, swelling, and purulent drainage may indicate infection.

■ Actions

- Administer oxygen
  Oxygen consumption and demand increases; therefore, oxygen supply should be increased.
- Insert two large-bore IVs
  IV access is essential for medication delivery and fluid resuscitation.
- Administer medications as ordered
  Medications are essential to be given in a timely manner:
  - Aspirin and heparin
    Aspirin and heparin are given to prevent new clot formation.
  - Nitroglycerin SL
    Nitroglycerin dilates the coronary arteries, increasing blood flow and decreasing pain.
  - Morphine
    Morphine is a narcotic given for pain relief if nitroglycerin is not effective.
  - Beta blockers
    Beta blockers decrease the sympathetic response to an MI, decreasing cardiac workload and oxygen consumption.
  - Fibrinolytics
    Fibrinolytics work to dissolve clots.
- Continuous ECG monitoring
  Electrocardiogram monitoring is essential to evaluate the evolution of the MI and the effectiveness of treatment and to monitor for dangerous dysrhythmias that can occur.
- Bed rest
  The patient may require bed rest as well as emotional rest to decrease oxygen and cardiac demands.
  Post-CABG
- Maintain tight BP control
  Hypotension may result in graft collapse; hypertension may result in bleeding.
- Administer fluids and medications (vasodilators, vasoconstrictors, inotropes, and diuretics) as ordered
  Maintains hemodynamic stability
- Rewarm patient slowly with warm fluids, blankets, or air flow devices. Prevent shivering.
  Rapid rewarming may cause dysrhythmias and/or hypotension due to vasodilation. Shivering increases oxygen needs.
- Administer pain medication and continuous sedation medications
  Maintains effective sedation and analgesia to decrease anxiety and pain which may potentially increase cardiac workload.
- Pulmonary hygiene while intubated: Reposition frequently, suction as needed. Oral care every 4 hours. Pulmonary hygiene after extubation; Incentive spirometry (IS), cough and deep breathe (C&DB)

every 1 to 2 hours while awake, encourage chest splinting when coughing.
  Helps with weaning toward extubation, oral care helps prevent ventilator associated pneumonia, IS and C&BD reduces risk of hospital acquired pneumonia, improves oxygenation.
- Plan for and initiate early mobility or ambulation
  Reduces complications related to immobility: deep venous thrombosis, pneumonia, constipation, skin breakdown
- Wound care: Initial dressing to be removed or changed by provider, then change daily or as needed.
  Helps prevent wound infection and promotes healing

■ Teaching

- Immediately report signs and symptoms of MI such as chest pain or chest discomfort or increased shortness of breath
  Understanding of the signs and symptoms of MI allows the patient to have earlier intervention, thus decreasing the complications and severity of present or future MIs.
- Purpose, dose, and side effects of medications
  Prescribed medications are to treat the effects of MI and prevent future MIs.
- The American Heart Association "Life's Simple 7":
  1. No smoking of cigarettes or other tobacco products
  2. Maintain a normal body weight
  3. Exercise for at least 150 minutes with moderate-intensity activity, or 75 minutes of vigorous-intensity activity, or a combination of each per week
  4. Eat a healthy diet that follows the current American Heart Association recommendations
  5. Maintain total cholesterol level less than 200 mg/dL
  6. Keep BP less than 120/79 mm Hg
  7. Keep fasting blood glucose less than 100 mg/dL
  Post-CABG
- Signs of infection
  Wound infection requires prompt intervention to promote healing.
- Sternal precautions; do not lift weight over 10 lbs, raise arms overhead, bend at the waist, participate in vigorous activity until cleared by physician
  These activities may interfere with sternal wound healing.
- Participate in cardiac rehabilitation: includes a medical evaluation, exercise training and physical activity counseling, coronary risk factor reduction/secondary prevention, including nutritional counseling and weight management, psychosocial support, and education regarding diet, weight management, purpose of medications, medication side effects, effects on exercise tolerance, and reinforcement for medication adherence.
  Changing modifiable risk factors decreases the patient's risk of repeated MIs.

Evaluating Care Outcomes

A well-managed patient is free from pain and has normal vital signs with an improved SpO$_2$. Signs of decreased perfusion from inadequate CO such as cool extremities, weak pulses, and decreased urine output are resolving. The goals for effective care include resumption of a normal active life free from pain and feelings of anxiety and doom. Myocardial infarction survivors can reduce their risk for repeated MIs through secondary prevention measures such as Life's Simple 7.

CARDIOMYOPATHY

Epidemiology

Cardiomyopathy affects approximately 50,000 people in the United States. Mortality for cardiomyopathy is approximately twice as high in males as in females and nearly twice as high in blacks as in whites. Dilated cardiomyopathy occurs more often in men than women. Hypertrophic cardiomyopathy (HCM) affects women and men evenly. It typically has a familial link. Restrictive cardiomyopathy is the rarest form of cardiomyopathy and affects mostly older adults.

Risk factors for cardiomyopathy are numerous. The major risk factors include diabetes, hypertension, high cholesterol, high-fat diet, obesity, family history of heart disease, sedentary lifestyle, and smoking. Other risk factors include alcohol and cocaine use, chemotherapy medications, end-stage renal failure, genetic/congenital defects, viral infections including HIV, Lyme disease, Chagas disease, nutritional deficiencies such as selenium, thiamine, and calcium, and pregnancy. Cardiomyopathy may not be from one sole cause but may be the result of an accumulation of multiple insults to the heart muscle.

Pathophysiology

Cardiomyopathy is a disorder in which the heart muscle becomes weak. It becomes enlarged, thick, or rigid and may develop structural changes. These changes are associated with inadequate pumping (low CO) and arrhythmias. In rare cases, the muscle tissue in the heart is replaced with scar tissue. These changes result in decreased function of the heart muscle. One measure of function is the *ejection fraction* (*EF*). The EF is the percentage of blood ejected from the ventricle with each contraction. A normal EF is approximately 55% to 65%. Less than 45% usually indicates some disease process weakening the pumping strength of the heart. An EF below 30% represents a severe decrease in cardiac function and represents a patient who is at increased risk for sudden death. There are two major categories of cardiomyopathy, ischemic and nonischemic. Ischemic cardiomyopathy refers to a greatly reduced ejection fraction caused by coronary artery disease such as irreversible loss of myocardium due to MI or possibly reversible contractile ability due to the presence of viable cardiac muscle after MI. The three most common types of nonischemic cardiomyopathy are:

- Dilated cardiomyopathy
- Hypertrophic cardiomyopathy
- Restrictive cardiomyopathy

Dilated cardiomyopathy is the most common type and the third leading cause of heart failure. The disease often starts with the dilation of the muscle in the left ventricle which causes the inside of the chamber to enlarge. The dilated chambers result in poor systolic function impairing contractility, thus decreasing CO. The impaired contractility results in a decreased ejection fraction, typically defined as less than 40%. Eventually, the heart becomes weaker, and heart failure may occur. The problem often spreads to the right ventricle and then to the atria while the disease gets worse. Most often, a specific cause for dilated cardiomyopathy is never identified; however, some factors have been linked with the disease. These include chronic, excessive alcohol consumption, viral infections, or toxins.

Hypertrophic cardiomyopathy (HCM), often referred to as *obstructive hypertrophic cardiomyopathy*, is a condition in which there is excessive myocardial hypertrophy. The heart muscle, typically the left ventricle, thickens, enlarges, and becomes stiff. Contraction is typically not weakened, but filling is impaired creating a diastolic or filling dysfunction. Ejection fraction may be normal. Hypertrophic cardiomyopathy can be the cause of sudden cardiac death (SCD) in young people as a result of life-threatening ventricular dysrhythmias. HCM is considered the most common cause of SCD in young competitive athletes.

Restrictive cardiomyopathy is characterized by stiff ventricular muscle resulting in diastolic dysfunction or impaired filling. Ejection fraction may be normal. In this disease, the normal heart muscle is replaced by fibrosis and scarring. This leads to heart failure and dangerous dysrhythmias. Restrictive cardiomyopathy typically results from another disease such as amyloidosis, sarcoidosis, or hemochromatosis.

Clinical Manifestations

An individual with cardiomyopathy may present with symptoms of angina or heart failure. Angina symptoms include chest pain, dizziness, indigestion, nausea, vomiting, sweating, palpitations, shortness of breath, and unexplained increasing fatigue. Heart failure symptoms include rapid or irregular heart rate, shortness of breath with or without activity, shortness of breath while lying flat, and edema of the legs, feet, and abdomen. Pulmonary congestion is evident due to fluid overload. The patient with fluid overload may present with abnormal heart sounds (gallop or murmur), elevated pressures in the neck (JVD), and an enlarged liver. Other signs of cardiomyopathy include sleeplessness, cough, fatigue, fainting, and loss of appetite.

Connection Check 32.6

The nurse understands which of the following are symptoms of HCM? *(Select all that apply.)*

A. Weakened contraction
B. Poor filling
C. Decreased cardiac output
D. Impaired systolic function
E. Impaired diastolic function

Management

Medical Management

Diagnosis

Diagnostic Testing

Diagnosis of a patient with cardiomyopathy is done through several diagnostic tests. A chest x-ray may show an enlarged heart, as well as the presence of fluid in the lungs. An echocardiogram can estimate the size and motion of the individual chambers of the heart. The heart wall motion may be described as normal, hypokinetic, hyperkinetic, akinetic, or dyskinetic and is graded from mild to severe. An akinetic heart wall has no specific wall movement. A dyskinetic heart wall moves in the opposite direction from where it should be moving. A hypokinetic heart is not moving enough, and a hyperkinetic wall is moving too much. Motion abnormalities help to define the specific cardiomyopathy. Patients with an increased number and severity of impaired wall segments are at increased risk for adverse cardiac events. An echocardiogram can also provide information on ejection fraction.

An ECG is performed to look for electrical disturbances in the heart. The ECG can provide important information about the patient's heart rate and rhythm, as well as problems with conduction of the electrical current from one portion of the heart to another. Cardiomyopathy can lead to dangerous ventricular dysrhythmias.

Right heart catheterization is a procedure in which a catheter is threaded through the chambers of the heart in order to obtain pressure in each individual chamber. These pressures may be used to assess the heart's ability to pump blood through the heart. In addition to pressure readings, a SvO_2 sample and a small biopsy may be obtained.

Cardiac magnetic resonance imaging (MRI) is a technique that uses magnetic and radio waves to create images of the heart. These images may be used in adjunct with the echo to offer a more accurate picture of the size and shape of the heart.

Blood tests may be obtained to evaluate cardiac function. One important blood test is the B-type natriuretic peptide, commonly referred to as the *BNP*. The BNP is a protein released from overstretched ventricular tissue, a common clinical manifestation of cardiomyopathy. A variety of other blood tests are performed to assess end-organ perfusion and specific causes of cardiomyopathy, including chemistry tests to evaluate renal and liver function, thyroid function tests, iron levels, and CBCs to evaluate for anemia.

Treatment

Medications

Medication therapy is an important component in the treatment of a patient with cardiomyopathy. The overall goals for medical treatment are management of the clinical manifestations of heart failure, preventing worsening of the heart function, and reduction of the risks for complications.

Treatment will vary by individual type of cardiomyopathy and may include:

- Angiotensin-converting enzyme (ACE) inhibitors
- Angiotensin-receptor blockers (ARB)
- Beta blockers
- Diuretics

Angiotensin-converting enzyme medications are given to improve the heart's pumping capacity. They reduce afterload or SVR, making it easier for the heart to eject blood. Angiotensin receptor blockers have effects similar to those of ACE inhibitors and are given to those individuals who do not tolerate ACE inhibitors because of its side effects. Beta blockers decrease the sympathetic nervous system response to decreased CO decreasing workload and myocardial oxygen consumption. They have been shown to prevent progression of the disease and improve outcomes. For patients who cannot tolerate an ACE inhibitor and/or ARB, hydralazine and a nitrate may be an alternative. The angiotensin receptor neprilysin inhibitor (ARNI) may be used in place of an ACE inhibitor for patients who do not have improvement in function or who have worsening symptoms. Digoxin, a positive inotrope agent, is not indicated for primary therapy, but may be used to control symptoms such as fatigue, dyspnea, and exercise intolerance. Diuretics reduce fluid accumulation in the lungs that occurs because of the ineffective pumping action of the heart. One diuretic, spironolactone (Aldactone), may help prevent further scarring of heart tissue.

Hypertrophic cardiomyopathy treatment utilizes beta blockers and calcium channel blockers. Some calcium channel blockers improve the filling of the heart by reducing calcium entering the heart during the cardiac cycle, thus decreasing its stiffness. This has the effect of reducing symptoms such as chest pain, breathlessness, and palpitations because CO is improved. Restrictive cardiomyopathy uses a medication regimen aimed at symptom reduction. Diuretics are used in an attempt to control dyspnea and shortness of breath.

Pacemaker Intervention

A biventricular pacemaker can benefit an individual with advanced cardiomyopathy who presents with dyssynchronous ventricular heart function. A pacer wire is placed in both the right and left ventricles in an effort to coordinate the contractions of both ventricles. An implantable cardioverter defibrillator (ICD) is currently recommended for patients with reduced EF (<30%), who are at higher risk for lethal dysrhythmias. This device monitors the heart for lethal ventricular dysrhythmias and delivers a shock if needed. The pacemaker and AICD can be combined into one device, referred to as a *biventricular implantable cardioverter defibrillator*.

For patients with continued symptoms, but who are not candidates for open-heart surgery, septal ablation may be an option. Also called *septal alcohol ablation*, this is a treatment in which a small portion of the thickened heart muscle is destroyed by injecting alcohol through a catheter into the heart muscle. The destroyed muscle is replaced with thin scar tissue, allowing the heart to fill more effectively, thus improving CO.

Surgical Management

Surgical therapies include:

- Septal myectomy
- Surgical ventricular remodeling
- Transmyocardial revascularization (TMR)
- Mechanical circulatory support (MCS) including left ventricular assist device (LVAD)
- Heart transplantation

Septal myectomy is an open-heart surgery in which the surgeon removes part of the thickened, overgrown heart muscle wall (septum) that separates the ventricles. Removing part of this overgrown muscle improves blood flow. Myectomy is used when medications alone do not relieve symptoms. Most people who have undergone a myectomy have no further symptoms.

Surgical ventricular remodeling is an open-heart surgical procedure that reduces the size of the left ventricle to improve the function of the heart. In this procedure, the surgeon either removes a section of the heart muscle or sutures a tuck into the muscle to reduce the overall size of the ventricle. As with the septal myectomy, this procedure reshapes the heart to increase filling capacity and improve heart function.

Despite the increasing success of conventional medical and surgical interventions, many patients with cardiomyopathy have intractable angina that cannot be successfully managed. Transmyocardial revascularization is a surgical procedure that uses CO_2 laser ablation to create transmural channels in the heart muscle to restore myocardial perfusion. The initial premise of this procedure was these channels would offer increased blood supply to the poorly supplied myocardium. This procedure results in a reduction in angina, but research has shown no change in myocardial blood flow. The mechanism of the observed reduction in symptoms is unknown. It has been used as an adjunctive therapy with coronary artery bypass graft to achieve more complete revascularization. Its use, though, is controversial. The DIRECT trial, the only major blinded study of TMR, revealed no benefit of TMR compared with continued medical therapy in patient survival, angina classification, quality of life, duration of exercise, or nuclear imaging.

Placement of an LVAD or heart transplantation may be used for patients with dilated cardiomyopathy. An LVAD is an electrical device that is surgically attached to the patient's ventricle to augment contraction in the weakened heart. Both placement of an LVAD and heart transplantation have an extremely high degree of risk. They are considered only when other medical and surgical means have been exhausted and the patient is at risk for death. These will be discussed in more detail in the cardiogenic shock section.

Complications

Heart failure, the inability of the heart to produce enough cardiac output (CO) to meet the body's metabolic demands, is the main complication of cardiomyopathy. This decrease in CO may be due to problems with filling or contraction. Heart failure is discussed in detail in Chapter 30.

Dysrhythmias are a common complication of cardiomyopathy. Examples include atrial fibrillation and more lethal rhythms such as ventricular tachycardia (V-tach) and ventricular fibrillation (V-fib). Atrial fibrillation decreases CO through loss of the "atrial kick"; the filling force contributed by atrial contraction immediately before ventricular systole to maximize ventricular preload. It also places the patient at risk for stroke because of the formation of clots in the quivering atria. Ventricular tachycardia and V-fib can lead to sudden death. Dysrhythmias are discussed in detail in Chapter 29.

Thrombosis, or clot formation, is a risk due to the sluggish forward flow of blood leading to stasis. Cardiomyopathy patients are at risk for pulmonary embolism (PE), MI, or stroke if clots enter the bloodstream. To reduce the risk of thrombosis, patients are typically prescribed medications such as antiplatelet agents—aspirin or clopidogrel (Plavix)—and anticoagulants such as warfarin (Coumadin) or Factor XA inhibitors such as Rivaroxaban (Xarelto).

Connection Check 32.7

The nurse monitors for which complications in patients with cardiomyopathy? (Select all that apply.)
A. Ventricular dysrhythmias
B. Stroke
C. Pericarditis
D. Pulmonary embolism
E. Pleural effusion

Nursing Management

Assessment and Analysis

Nursing assessment is aimed toward anticipation of heart failure and recognition of the cardiovascular, cerebral, pulmonary, gastrointestinal, and renal effects that may occur as a result. Fatigue, shortness of breath, edema, dizziness, indigestion, palpitations, and loss of appetite are all common presenting symptoms. More dangerous manifestations include ventricular dysrhythmias. While the heart continues to fail to deliver adequate CO, the symptomatology may progress to signs of end-organ damage such as decreases in urine output.

Nursing Diagnosis

- **Decreased CO** related to ineffective cardiac pumping secondary to cardiomyopathy

Nursing Interventions

■ *Assessments*

- Vital signs including oxygen saturation
  Changes in BP and heart rate may indicate worsening disease, decreasing CO or EF. A decreasing oxygen saturation may indicate worsening left heart failure.
- Neurological status
  Increasing fatigue that may progress to lethargy, confusion, and loss of consciousness are signs of decreased CO.
- ECG
  Dysrhythmias may be a sign of decreased CO and are a lethal complication of cardiomyopathy. The ECG can also provide an evaluation of ischemia.
- Lung sounds
  Auscultation of crackles is an indication of the development of pulmonary edema due to left heart failure.
- Chest pain
  Chest pain indicates that the demand for oxygen is higher than the supply, indicating insufficient CO.
- Urine output
  Decreased urine output can be the first sign of decreasing CO because the kidneys receive approximately 25% of the CO.
- Laboratory tests
  - BNP
    An increased BNP is released from overstretched tricular tissue; a sign of heart failure.
  - Renal and liver function tests
    Increased renal and liver function values are a sign of increasingly poor perfusion and inadequate CO.
- Activity tolerance
  Physical activity increases the oxygen demand. Increased fatigue and dyspnea may be signs of worsening heart failure.

■ *Actions*

- Administer medications as ordered:
  - Beta blockers
    Beta blockers decrease the sympathetic nervous system response to decreased CO and decrease the workload of the heart.
  - Diuretics
    Diuretics reduce fluid accumulation in the lungs that occurs because of the ineffective pumping action of the left heart.
  - Antiarrhythmics
    Dysrhythmias are a common complication of cardiomyopathy. Bradyarrhythmias as well as tachyarrhythmias reduce CO and thus decrease tissue perfusion.
  - ACE inhibitors/ARBs
    Angiotensin-converting enzyme inhibitors and ARBs reduce afterload, making it easier for the heart to eject blood.
  - Digoxin
    Digoxin is a positive inotropic agent that can improve the heart muscle contractions, reducing associated heart failure symptoms.
- Provide oxygen
  Increased oxygen supply helps meet the increased oxygen demands.
- Maintain patient positioning as prescribed for particular cardiomyopathy
  Semi- to high-Fowler's position reduces preload and ventricular filling. It also decreases dyspnea. The supine position increases venous return and promotes diuresis.
- Restrict activity and provide a quiet relaxed atmosphere
  A quiet and low-stress environment reduces oxygen and cardiac demands.

■ *Teaching*

- Signs and symptoms of heart failure
  Recognizing symptoms of heart failure can allow the patient to get treatment sooner, possibly preventing hospital admission.
- Medications: purpose, dosages, and potential side effects
  Prescribed medications are to decrease the symptoms associated with cardiomyopathy as well as improve heart function. It is important for the patient to understand the potential side effects to prevent harm.
- Dietary restrictions of fluid and sodium
  Maintaining fluid and sodium restrictions helps decrease volume overload, which helps avoid the development of heart failure.
- Importance of a moderate exercise regimen and understanding the signs of overexertion
  Exercise has been shown to improve symptoms and exercise capacity. Vigorous activity is not recommended with HCM. Patients may be referred to cardiac rehabilitation to exercise in a monitored setting.

Evaluating Care Outcomes

Strict adherence to the medical, dietary, and exercise regimens prescribed may help the cardiomyopathy patient remain free from symptoms of heart failure. Of great importance is the knowledge of when to seek help for worsening symptoms to avoid unnecessary hospitalizations and unwanted complications.

Connection Check 32.8

The nurse questions which order for the patient with cardiomyopathy?
A. ACE inhibitors
B. Beta blockers
C. Diuretics
D. SL nitroglycerin

CARDIOGENIC SHOCK

Cardiogenic shock occurs when the heart muscle is unable to pump adequate CO to meet the body's needs to maintain adequate tissue perfusion. The most common cause of cardiogenic shock is MI, but other causes include decompensation from end-stage congestive heart failure or cardiomyopathy, mechanical complications with acute mitral regurgitation, or rupture of the ventricular wall. It is frequently noted in patients suffering ST-segment elevation MI (5%-10%) and in patients with significant comorbidities. Patients with diabetes are also at increased risk of cardiogenic shock after MI. It is the most common cause of death in patients with MI with a frequency of approximately 7% to 10%.

Pathophysiology

In cardiogenic shock, the heart muscle cannot adequately contract, causing a decrease in cardiac output (CO). The main mechanical defect is a marked reduction in contractility evidenced by a decreased EF at normal systolic pressures. As a result of decreased contractility, left and right ventricular filling pressures are increased, but CO is low. Due to the low cardiac output there is increased oxygen extraction at the tissue level, resulting in a decreased venous oxygen saturation.

Decreased CO leads to the activation of several compensatory mechanisms. These include sympathetic stimulation, which increases the heart rate and cardiac contractility and causes renal fluid retention, augmenting the left ventricular preload. The increased heart rate and contractility increase the myocardial workload and thus the myocardial oxygen demand, worsening myocardial ischemia. Sympathetic stimulation also causes vasoconstriction to maintain systemic BP to increase CO, which also increases SVR. The increased afterload additionally increases cardiac workload. The renin-angiotensin-aldosterone system (RAAS) is also stimulated due to decreased renal perfusion, resulting in vasoconstriction and fluid retention increasing filling pressures. The increased left ventricular volumes combined with poor contractile function contribute to the development of pulmonary edema and hypoxia. This cycle of excessive myocardial oxygen demand combined with inadequate myocardial perfusion worsens myocardial ischemia, ultimately ending in death if the cycle is uninterrupted. Autopsy typically reveals necrosis of more than 40% of the left ventricular cardiac tissue in patients with cardiogenic shock.

Clinical Manifestations

Cardiogenic shock is frequently caused by MI; therefore, the patient may present with clinical symptoms of MI including chest pain, diaphoresis, nausea, and vomiting. These symptoms are the consequence of oxygen-deprived tissue and the compensatory mechanisms that occur as a result of the low CO. Without intervention, clinical symptoms occur including shortness of breath, auscultation of crackles, decreased peripheral pulses, cool pale skin, decreased bowel sounds, decreased urine output, restlessness, and confusion. The initiation of compensatory mechanisms leads to increased heart rate. If a PA line is in place, increased SVR,

increased right and left ventricular end-diastolic volume or pressure, CVP or PAOP respectively, and decreased mixed venous oxygen level are demonstrated. Oxygen deprivation leads to excessive production of lactic acid. Arterial blood gases reveal a metabolic acidosis with an accompanying increase in serum lactate level.

Compensatory mechanisms eventually fail to maintain adequate CO, worsening inadequate organ perfusion. At this time, clinical manifestations include hypotension; tachycardia with weak pulses; tachypnea; cold, cyanotic, and mottled skin; decreased or absent urine output; severely decreased level of consciousness; and severely decreased or absent bowel sounds. Over time, without intervention, multiple organ systems begin to fail. This is evidenced by severe hypotension, bradycardia, hypoxia, liver and pancreas failure leading to hypoglycemia, and hematological changes resulting in emboli, diffuse intravascular clotting (DIC), and severe coagulopathy.

Management

Medical Management

Diagnosis

Laboratory and Diagnostic Testing

Cardiogenic shock is diagnosed after exclusion of other causes of hypotension and shock such as hypovolemia, sepsis, aortic dissection, PE, tension pneumothorax, or cardiac tamponade. Laboratory testing includes cardiac enzymes in conjunction with ECG changes to confirm an AMI. An ABG analysis will assist with the assessment of hypoxia and the presence of metabolic acidosis, which indicates decreased tissue perfusion. Venous oxygen saturation can assist with the evaluation of the adequacy of oxygen supply in relation to tissue oxygen demands. A lactate level may be obtained to assess tissue perfusion. An increased lactate level is an indication of anaerobic metabolism producing increased lactic acid. A metabolic profile including liver function and renal function tests helps assess organ function.

Medications

Treatment priorities include stabilizing oxygenation and initiating medication therapy to increase BP and cardiac output. The focus of medication therapy is to increase BP and CO and decrease cardiac workload. The presence of an arterial line is essential in monitoring the patient's response to medication. A PA catheter can also help to guide management through evaluation of CO, preload, afterload, stroke work indices, and SvO_2. As soon as possible, inotropic medications such as dobutamine hydrochloride (Dobutamine) and epinephrine should be initiated to improve CO. Vasopressor support such as dopamine hydrochloride, norepinephrine (Levophed), or phenylephrine (Neo-Synephrine) should be started to support BP and help maintain an adequate MAP.

Nitroglycerin may be added to decrease preload and afterload. It decreases preload through venous dilation and decreases afterload through arterial dilation. It will also decrease BP, so it should be used with extreme caution. Nitroprusside may also be used with extreme caution to decrease afterload. Diuretics may also be used, again, with caution to decrease filling volumes. Morphine sulfate may also be administered. It may relieve pain due to a myocardial infarction and decrease venous return and preload through its action as a venous dilator.

Treatment

If providing 100% oxygen via a non-rebreather face mask does not adequately improve oxygenation, ventilatory support through endotracheal intubation and mechanical ventilation may be required to decrease the work of breathing and improve oxygenation. Early revascularization through percutaneous coronary intervention has been shown to increase short-term and long-term survival in most patients in cardiogenic shock.

Intra-aortic balloon pump (IABP) therapy may be necessary when the initial medical management does not improve CO enough to maintain adequate tissue perfusion. The primary goal of IABP therapy is to increase myocardial oxygen supply and decrease myocardial oxygen demand. The IABP catheter is inserted into the aorta usually via the femoral artery. Upon placement, the catheter with a balloon at the tip should sit just below the aortic arch, approximately 2 cm from the left SC artery. The IABP moves helium gas in and out of the balloon. It is timed to inflate at the start of diastole and deflate just before systole. As the balloon inflates, it displaces the blood toward the systemic and coronary circulation, which improves coronary and systemic perfusion. While the balloon deflates, it decreases afterload, thus decreasing the workload of the left ventricle (Fig. 32.12). The most common complications from IABP include limb ischemia from clot formation, aortic dissection, bleeding, balloon rupture, infection, thrombocytopenia, and catheter migration.

 Safety Alert **Intra-aortic Balloon Pump**
It is critical to not allow the IABP to remain dormant for longer than a few minutes to reduce risk of clot formation and embolization. The catheter should be monitored regularly for signs of balloon rupture, including brown flecks of blood in the catheter, poor augmentation, or gas leak alarms. Balloon rupture is an emergency and needs immediate intervention. The pump should immediately be placed in standby mode and plans made for immediate removal.

Connection Check 32.9

What action of IABP therapy supports cardiac function?
A. Inflating the balloon during systole, increasing CO
B. Inflating the balloon during diastole, improving coronary circulation
C. Deflating the balloon during diastole, decreasing SVR
D. Deflating the balloon during systole, improving coronary circulation

Surgical Management

The patient in end-stage heart failure or cardiogenic shock who has not improved with inotropic and/or IABP support may be referred for placement of a mechanical circulatory support (MCS) or for heart transplant.

Mechanical Circulatory Support Devices

Mechanical circulatory support devices are mechanical pumps used to assist the ventricles and decrease the workload of the heart. In heart failure or cardiogenic shock, a patient may require an MCS device as a bridge to recovery or to transplantation. Most MCS devices are typically used

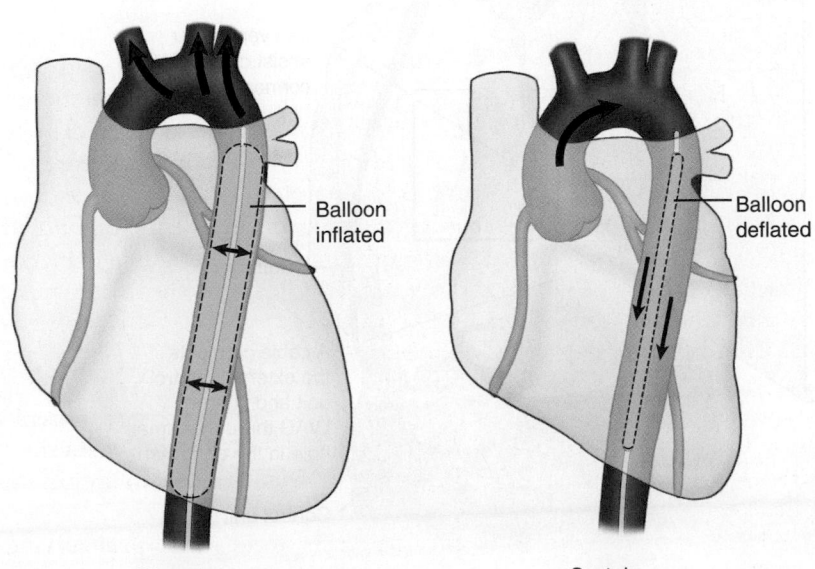

Diastole — Balloon inflated

Systole — Balloon deflated

FIGURE 32.12 Intra-aortic balloon pump; balloon inflated during diastole to push blood into the coronaries, deflated during systole to decrease systemic vascular resistance.

in the left ventricle (LVAD). An LVAD works by pulling blood from the left ventricle into the pump (Fig. 32.13). The pump then ejects the blood into the aorta. A right ventricular assist device (RVAD) works by pulling blood from the right ventricle, then ejecting the blood into the pulmonary artery.

Ventricular assist devices include percutaneous left atrial-to-femoral arterial ventricular assist device (Tandem Heart), a type of ventricular assist device in which a pump returns blood to the femoral artery from the left atrium decreasing the workload of the left ventricle. Another type of ventricular assist device is a percutaneous transvalvular left ventricular assist device (Impella LP 2.5 or Impella CP). This catheter is placed via the femoral artery, retrograde across the aortic valve into the left ventricle to replace the work done by left ventricle. A right ventricular assist device; Impella RP System (Abiomed, United States) provides similar support to patients with refractory right ventricle shock. If the patient is ineligible for a heart transplant, an MCS can be used as long-term or destination therapy.

Extracorporeal membrane oxygenation (ECMO) offers an alternative form of mechanical circulatory support therapy for patients with severe acute respiratory and/or cardiac failure who have a high mortality risk despite optimal conventional treatment. ECMO may be described as a bedside heart-lung intervention. With ECMO, deoxygenated blood is diverted from the vascular system via a central vein and returned to the circulation after being oxygenated outside the body. Indications include respiratory failure and/or cardiogenic shock. Extracorporeal membrane oxygenation is a complex procedure that allows complete support of the patient's respiratory and/or cardiac function at the bedside to allow for recovery and treatment of the underlying process or as a bridge to a more durable device.

Venovenous (VV) ECMO provides respiratory support only. Blood is extracted from cannula placed in the vena cava or right atrium and returned via cannula to the right atrium and provides gas exchange and respiratory support only.

Venoarterial (VA) ECMO provides both respiratory and hemodynamic support. Blood is extracted from a cannula placed in the right atrium and returned via cannula placed in the arterial system, bypassing the heart and lungs.

Total Artificial Hearts

The total artificial heart may be considered a form of heart assist device but is actually a heart replacement device. Many patients in end-stage heart failure have only a few options—immediate heart transplant, two VADs (RVAD and LVAD), or total artificial heart implantation. Criteria for recipients of an artificial heart include end-stage heart failure, life expectancy of less than 30 days, not eligible for a natural heart transplant, and have no other viable treatment options.

Heart Transplantation

Urgent heart transplantation is another option for the patient in cardiogenic shock. This is an option only when all

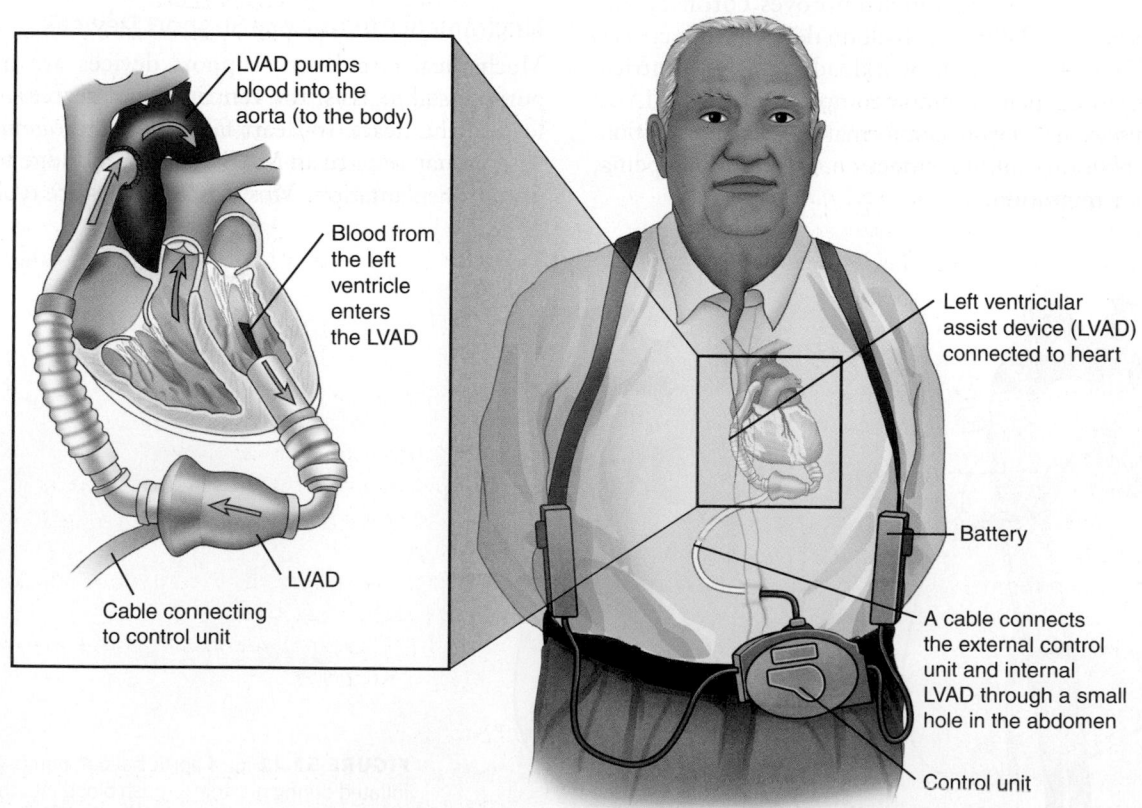

LVAD pumps blood into the aorta (to the body)

Blood from the left ventricle enters the LVAD

LVAD

Cable connecting to control unit

Left ventricular assist device (LVAD) connected to heart

Battery

A cable connects the external control unit and internal LVAD through a small hole in the abdomen

Control unit

FIGURE 32.13 Left ventricular assist device.

other medical and surgical therapies have been exhausted. Unlike an MCS device, a heart transplant replaces the patient's failing heart with a healthy heart received from a donor.

Connection Check 32.10

The nurse understands that a/an _____ is used in the evaluation of cardiogenic shock.
A. PA catheter
B. LVAD
C. RVAD
D. IABP

Nursing Management

Assessment and Analysis

The clinical manifestations in cardiogenic shock are related to the decrease in CO and impaired blood flow to all vital organs: hypotension; tachycardia with weak pulses; tachypnea; cold, cyanotic, and mottled skin; decreased or absent urine output; severely decreased level of consciousness; and severely decreased or absent bowel sounds. Without successful intervention, multiple organ systems begin to fail. Severe hypotension, bradycardia, hypoxia, hypoglycemia, DIC, and severe coagulopathy are possible.

Nursing Diagnosis

- **Altered tissue perfusion** related to inadequate CO

Nursing Interventions

▪ Assessments

- Vital signs and hemodynamic readings
  Hypotension, decreased CO, and increased left ventricular filling volumes are present because of the ineffective contractile ability of the heart. Increased SVR and tachycardia occur as a compensatory mechanism to increase BP and CO. RR is increased to improve oxygenation.
- BP readings in both arms
  BP may have contralateral differences if the patient has the presence of arterial dissection or IABP migration.
- Breath sounds and oxygen saturation
  Decreasing O_2 saturation and/or auscultation of crackles indicate the presence of left heart weakening and pulmonary edema.
- Neurological status
  Decreased level of consciousness occurs as a result of decreased CO.
- Skin color and temperature
  Cold and clammy skin may be a sign of progressing shock.
- Labs to include:
  - ABGs
    Arterial blood gases may reflect a metabolic acidosis due to anaerobic metabolism.
  - Hemoglobin and hematocrit
    Adequate hemoglobin and hematocrit are essential to support oxygenation.

- Metabolic profile
  Metabolic profile data can track organ function through liver function and renal function tests.
- Lactate
  Increasing lactate levels are an indicator of anerobic metabolism.
- SvO_2
  Decreasing SvO_2 indicates increased oxygen utilization at the tissue level due to low CO.

▪ Actions

- Apply 100% non-rebreather oxygen mask
  Maximizing oxygenation is essential
- Anticipate intubation and mechanical ventilation
  Intubation with mechanical ventilation may be required to decrease myocardial workload and improve oxygenation.
- Prepare for invasive hemodynamic monitoring such as arterial, central, and PA catheters
  Invasive monitoring allows more precise evaluation and adjustment of medications.
- Administer inotropic and vasoactive medications as prescribed
  Inotropic medications increase contractility. Vasoactive medications increase BP. Both are done to improve stroke volume and systemic tissue perfusion.
- Administer fluid replacement as prescribed
  Fluid is administered to improve CO and preload only if filling pressures are low.
- Administer diuretics as prescribed
  Diuretics may be administered with caution if left ventricular filling volumes are greatly increased.
- Restrict activity and allow rest periods; treat pain and anxiety
  Restricting activity and decreasing pain and anxiety decrease cardiac workload and oxygen consumption. Morphine for pain also decreases preload with its action as a venous dilator.
- Anticipate the potential placement of an IABP
  IABP helps increase coronary circulation (balloon inflation during diastole) and decrease SVR (balloon deflation during systole)
- If an IABP is in place:
  - Assure the IABP catheter is secured, the head of bed is elevated no more than 30 degrees, and the affected leg is kept straight at all times
    Helps avoid catheter migration
  - Assess catheter tubing for brown flecks or blood
    The presence of brown flecks may indicate balloon rupture.
  - Assess lower-extremity perfusion such as color, temperature, and pulses
    An IABP catheter may cause decreased perfusion to the affected extremity.

▪ Teaching

- Instruct patient on the importance of rest periods
  Increased activity or stress levels cause increased myocardial oxygen consumption and can worsen a shock state.

Box 32.7 *Healthy People 2020*: Cardiovascular Dysfunction and the Goals for 2020

Our nursing care plans and the *Healthy People 2020* goals are intricately linked to promote health and reduce cardiovascular dysfunction. Atherosclerosis is the major cause of the cardiovascular disease discussed in this chapter. The objectives of *Healthy People 2020* put a major focus on decreasing the risk factors for this disease and early identification and treatment of issues. *Healthy People 2020* guidelines also reflect the strong scientific background that supports the benefits associated with eating a healthy diet, maintaining a healthy body weight, smoking cessation, maintaining daily physical activity, and diabetic control. This is essential for myocardial infarction, cardiomyopathy, and ultimately cardiogenic shock.

- Allow family member visitation
  Family visitation can help to decrease a patient's anxiety and stress levels.
- Teach the patient to maintain fluid and sodium restrictions as prescribed
  Maintaining fluid and sodium restrictions decreases the risk of heart failure, which exacerbates the presence of shock.
- Patient will state understanding of symptoms of heart failure to report to his or her provider
  Early treatment of heart failure prevents the progression to shock.

Evaluating Care Outcomes

Quick and effective intervention with inotropic and vasoactive support is essential to return the patient to hemodynamic stability. Careful monitoring of clinical manifestations and hemodynamic status helps evaluate therapeutic interventions. Successful treatment is demonstrated by a satisfactory BP level and cardiac output and adequate tissue perfusion. With strict adherence to dietary and lifestyle changes, the patient may return to activities of daily living, freed from abnormal findings on physical examination, sleeping comfortably, and articulating feelings of control (Box 32.7).

Making Connections

CASE STUDY: WRAP-UP

Post-PCI, an IABP is inserted, and Mr. King is transported to the coronary care unit. A PA catheter and arterial line are placed. The PA line reveals a greatly reduced CO of 2, increased occlusive pressure of 24, increased SVR of 1,800, and decreased SvO_2 of 50%. His

BP remains low at 80/50 mm Hg with a heart rate of 108 bpm. He remains on a norepinephrine and dobutamine drip. He remains intubated and on assist/control on the ventilator with a fraction of inspired oxygen of 60%.

Mr. King requires continuous and extensive monitoring. He remains on the balloon pump and slowly begins to improve. His BP increases to 105/65, and the dose of norepinephrine is decreased. His SVR decreases slightly, and his CO improves to 4. His occlusive pressure decreases to 16 after a 40-mg dose of IV Lasix. After 2 days in the coronary care unit on the balloon pump after PCI, Mr. King begins to turn the corner. His BP is stabilizing, and his CO is within normal limits. His ABGs, pH 7.37, $PaCO_2$ 38, PaO_2 85, and HCO_3^- 24, reveal improved oxygenation and resolution of metabolic acidosis, demonstrating improved systemic blood flow.

Case Study Questions

1. The nurse monitors for which clinical manifestations in the patient diagnosed with MI? *(Select all that apply.)*
   A. Chest pain
   B. Nausea
   C. Diaphoresis
   D. Hypertension
   E. Bounding pulses

2. On arrival to the emergency department, the nurse caring for Mr. King receives several orders from the provider. Which order should the nurse implement first?
   A. Morphine sulfate, 2 mg IV
   B. Nitroglycerin tab SL
   C. Oxygen, 2 L via nasal cannula
   D. Aspirin, 325 mg chewed

3. A treatment goal for Mr. King is to decrease myocardial workload. What order should the nurse anticipate to accomplish this goal?
   A. Norepinephrine IV drip
   B. Dobutamine IV drip
   C. Metoprolol IV push
   D. Aspirin 325 mg PO

4. The nurse caring for the patient with cardiogenic shock incorporates which nursing diagnosis into the plan of care?
   A. Impaired tissue perfusion related to decreased circulating volume secondary to hypovolemia
   B. Impaired tissue perfusion related to decreased circulating volume secondary to peripheral vasodilation
   C. Impaired tissue perfusion related to decreased circulating volume secondary to poor contractile function of myocardial muscle
   D. Impaired tissue perfusion related to decreased circulating volume secondary to interrupted response of the sympathetic nervous system

5. What is the main purpose of the IABP? *(Select all that apply.)*

    A. Deflate during diastole to facilitate myocardial oxygen delivery

    B. Inflate during diastole to facilitate myocardial oxygen delivery

    C. Deflate during systole to decrease SVR

    D. Inflate during systole to increase BP

    E. Deflate during systole to facilitate myocardial oxygen delivery

CHAPTER SUMMARY

Invasive hemodynamic monitoring is important to allow early identification and treatment of the complex medical problems of the critically ill patient. With the use of central venous or PA catheters, the nurse can evaluate the patient's immediate response to treatments including inotropic medications and mechanical support. Invasive monitoring may also be used for transvenous pacemaker insertion, central venous and pulmonary pressure monitoring, volume resuscitation, frequent blood draws, long-term IV antibiotics, medications known to be caustic to peripheral administration, and parenteral nutrition administration. These catheters may also be used when IV therapy is needed, and peripheral veins are not accessible. It is important to remember that IV medications may never be infused through the arterial line for risk of loss of limb.

Pulmonary artery catheters use is decreasing because of questions that have been raised about their precise indications, cost-effectiveness, effect on clinical outcomes, and the extensive training required to accurately interpret the hemodynamic data they provide. The use of a PA catheter needs to be individualized based on patient needs.

Myocardial infarction (MI), cardiomyopathy, and cardiogenic shock are different disease processes that result from destruction of normal heart muscle. Complications arise when the heart is not able to supply enough blood to the other organs of the body. Myocardial infarction refers to the destruction of heart muscle from the lack of oxygenated blood supply. Many patients who develop MI have early warning signs such as fatigue and pain, but these symptoms are frequently ignored or misdiagnosed. Pain is caused by insufficient blood supply to the heart, The gold standard to determine diagnosis of MI is cardiac troponin level elevation. Routine MI admission orders include initial application of oxygen via nasal cannula, blood work, chest x-ray, and 12-lead ECG. Once the diagnosis of MI is made, early patient management involves control of ischemic pain, increasing blood flow to the heart muscle, prevention of clots, decreasing myocardial workload, and maintenance of hemodynamics. Emergency revascularization after MI by angioplasty within 6 hours has been found to have significant survivor benefits. The consequences of MI may include cardiomyopathy and cardiogenic shock.

Cardiomyopathy is a disorder in which the heart muscle becomes weak and may develop structural changes. An individual with cardiomyopathy may present with symptoms of angina or heart failure. Jugular vein distention is a common presenting symptom. Medication therapy is an important component in the treatment and management of a patient with cardiomyopathy. The overall goals for medical therapy are management of symptoms, preventing worsening of heart function, and reduction of risks for complications.

Any disorder that results in the acute deterioration of cardiac function can lead to cardiogenic shock. Cardiogenic shock is a medical emergency; immediate treatment aimed at improving delivery of oxygenated blood, preventing further ischemia, and progression of shock is necessary for any chance of survival.

The most common cause of cardiogenic shock is MI, but other causes include decompensation from end-stage congestive heart failure or cardiomyopathy. Invasive monitoring with arterial and PA catheters can assist in properly managing therapy for the patient in cardiogenic shock. Patient management is a combination of ventilator support and medications. Emergency revascularization helps improve survival. When medical management does not improve cardiac output, adjunct therapy needs to be initiated. Adjunct therapy includes intra-aortic balloon pump or LVAD.

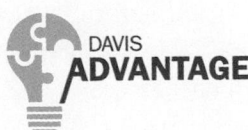

DAVIS ADVANTAGE To explore learning resources for this chapter, go to **Davis Advantage** and find:

– Answers to in-text questions
– Chapter Resources and Activities
– NCLEX®-Style Chapter Review Questions
– Bibliography

Unit VII

Promoting Health in Patients With Hematological Disorders

Chapter 33

Assessment of Hematological Function

Kristy Gorman

Finding Connections

CASE STUDY: EPISODE 1

Follow this patient throughout the chapter.

Marge Starr is a 25-year-old female who presents to the hematology clinic with complaints of generalized fatigue and increased shortness of breath. Ms. Starr is a high school physical education teacher who has noticed that she is having increasing difficulty performing her teaching responsibilities. During the last 2 weeks, she has had to take an afternoon nap after school hours. Ms. Starr schedules an appointment with her nurse practitioner for evaluation of these symptoms…

INTRODUCTION

The hematological system includes the blood, blood cells, lymph, and organs involved with blood formation or blood storage. Blood is a specialized connective tissue that acts as a transport vehicle of materials between the external environment and the body's cells. Blood consists of **plasma** (a clear yellow, protein-rich fluid); solutes (proteins, electrolytes, and organic elements); red blood cells (RBCs), white blood cells (WBCs); and **platelets** (which are fragments of cells). Blood accounts for approximately 7% to 10% of total body weight. The total volume of blood in the average adult is approximately 5 to 6 L, and it circulates throughout the body within the circulatory system.

The hematological system is important in helping the body by circulating oxygen, nutrients, hormones, and metabolic wastes; protecting against invasion of pathogens; maintaining blood coagulation; and regulating fluids, electrolytes, acids, bases, and body temperature. This chapter reviews the physiology of the hematological system and the assessment of hematological status.

OVERVIEW OF ANATOMY AND PHYSIOLOGY

Bone Marrow

Bone marrow is the primary site for blood formation and maturation (**hematopoiesis**). It is involved in the body's immune responses and is one of the largest organs of the body, making up 4% to 5% of total body weight. The bone marrow is a network of flexible connective tissue that produces stem cells (also called pluripotent or *precursor stem cells*). The stem cells are immature, undifferentiated cells that have the ability to become any one of several types of blood cells. Depending on the body's needs, stem cells can begin multilineage differentiation into mature **myeloid** or **lymphoid** stem cells. Lymphoid stem cells produce either T or B **lymphocytes**, which are the main functional cells

of the immune system. Myeloid stem cells differentiate into three cell types: RBCs (**erythrocytes**), WBCs (**leukocytes**), and platelets (**thrombocytes**).

At sites where the bone marrow is hematopoietically active, numerous erythrocytes are produced that make it red, hence the name *red bone marrow*. Red marrow regresses after birth until late adolescence (during active skeletal growth), after which it is located in the lower skull, vertebrae, shoulder and pelvic girdles, ribs, and sternum. Red marrow is gradually replaced by yellow marrow (fat cells) in most of the long bones, including the hands, feet, legs, and arms. Fat occupies approximately 50% of the space of red marrow in the adult. When the demand for red cell replacement increases, as in chronic hemolytic **anemia** (low RBC count), substitution of red marrow for yellow marrow can occur. Self-renewal and differentiation of stem cells are highly regulated processes to ensure homeostasis. Disruption of these processes inevitably leads to abnormal cell growth in the marrow or bone marrow failure.

Connection Check 33.1

The nurse recognizes which statement as correct about blood cell formation?

A. It occurs mostly in the marrow found in flat bones such as the sternum, ribs, and pelvis
B. It occurs mostly in the marrow found in the shaft of long bones
C. It occurs outside the marrow, once it enters the circulatory system
D. It occurs after birth until late adolescence

Blood Cells

Hematopoiesis is defined as the process of formation, development, and differentiation of the formed elements of blood. As previously discussed, all blood cells originate from cells in the bone marrow called pluripotential **stem cells**. Regulatory mechanisms cause stem cells to differentiate into families of parent cells, each of which gives rise to one of the mature, formed elements that are released into the circulation: RBCs (erythrocytes), platelets (thrombocytes), or WBCs (leukocytes) (Fig. 33.1).

The blood cells, or formed elements, are not all true cells because they lack many characteristics and structures of most cells. Platelets, or thrombocytes, are circulating cell fragments that have a cell membrane but no nucleus for cell division. The erythrocyte has no mitochondria available for oxidative metabolism and cellular energy conversion, no ribosomes for regeneration of lost or damaged proteins, and no nucleus to direct cell function and division. Because most blood cells do not divide, they must be constantly renewed by cell division in the bone marrow.

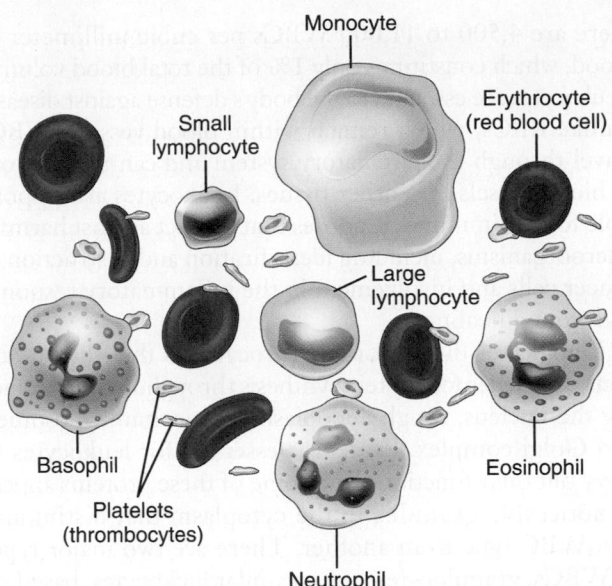

FIGURE 33.1 Formed elements of blood: red blood cells (erythrocytes), platelets (thrombocytes), and white blood cells (leukocytes). Types of white blood cells are lymphocytes, monocytes, neutrophils, eosinophils, and basophils.

Red Blood Cells

Erythrocytes (red blood cells, RBCs) are the most abundant of the formed elements. The erythrocyte is a small, biconcave disk with no nucleus. It has a large surface area and is so flexible that it can move through small capillaries of the circulatory system. The membrane of the red cell is very thin so that oxygen and carbon dioxide gases easily diffuse across. Erythrocytes have two principal functions: (1) to pick up oxygen from the lungs and transport it to systemic tissues and (2) to pick up carbon dioxide from the tissues and deliver it in the lungs. Shifts in the amount, size, shape, or composition of erythrocytes affect their ability to successfully carry out these functions.

The erythrocytes, which are formed in the bone marrow, live approximately 120 days in the circulatory system. The number of RBCs in a human varies with gender, age, and general health, but the normal range is from 3.61 to 5.81 million/mm³ (3.61–5.11 million cells/mm³ in females and 4.21–5.81 million cells/mm3 in males). The number of erythrocytes is controlled through **erythropoiesis** (the selective maturation of stem cells into mature erythrocytes). Differentiation into an erythrocyte begins when the pluripotent stem cell of the marrow becomes an erythrocyte colony-forming unit (ECFU), which has receptors for the hormone erythropoietin (EPO). An ECFU then transforms into an erythroblast when stimulated by EPO. The cell is called a **reticulocyte** when the nucleus shrinks and is discharged from the cell. Reticulocytes (a temporary network composed of ribosome clusters) leave the bone marrow and enter the circulating blood. In approximately 2 days, the last of the ribosome clusters disappear, and the cell is a mature erythrocyte (Fig. 33.2). For normal erythrocyte production, the bone marrow also requires iron, vitamin B_{12}, folic acid,

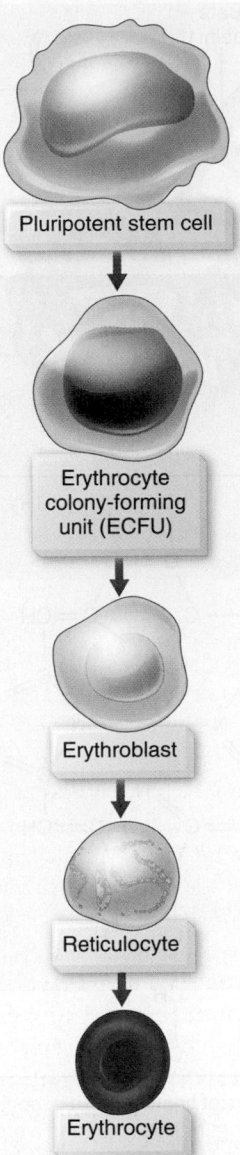

FIGURE 33.2 Erythropoiesis. Steps in the formation of an erythrocyte.

vitamin B_6 (pyridoxine), protein, and other factors. The volume of blood composed of erythrocytes is measured as **haematocrit**, with normal values being 36% to 48% in females and 42% to 52% in males.

The RBCs produce **hemoglobin** (Hgb; the oxygen-carrying component of an RBC), and each normal mature RBC contains thousands of Hgb molecules. Hemoglobin is composed of a pigment (heme) that contains iron (Fe^{2+}) and a protein (globin). The Hgb molecule is made up of four globins with a heme molecule attached to each globin. The heme molecule has iron at its center, which binds with oxygen. This makes Hgb capable of transporting up to four molecules of oxygen; therefore, iron is a significant component of Hgb (Fig. 33.3). Erythrocytes are critical to survival, and a severe deficiency of erythrocytes in the case of major trauma or hemorrhage, can be fatal within a few minutes because of the lack of oxygen.

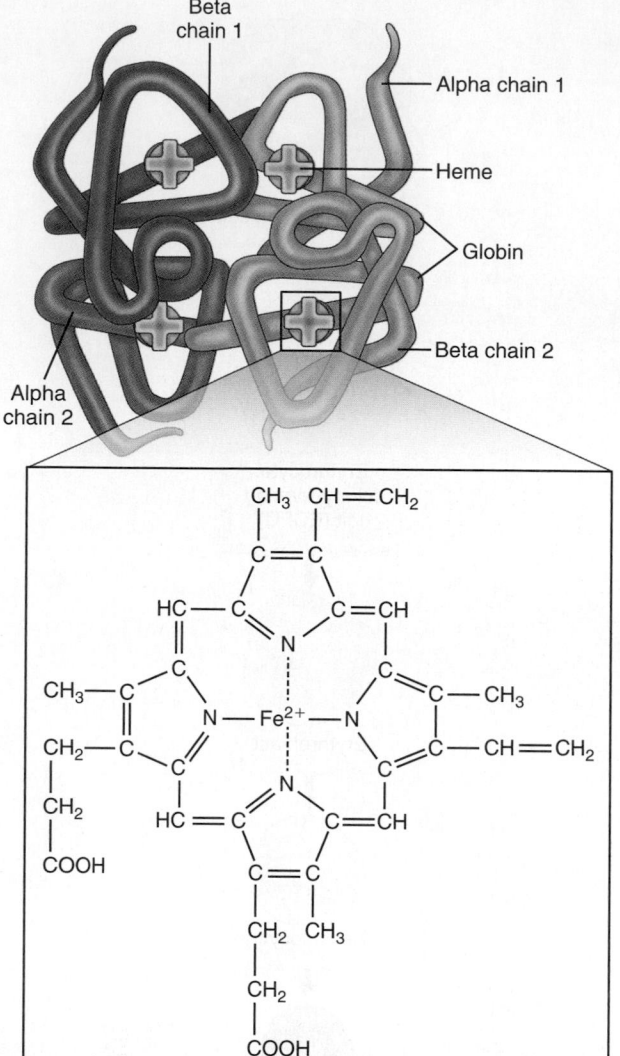

FIGURE 33.3 Structure of hemoglobin. Hemoglobin is composed of a pigment (heme) that contains iron (Fe^{2+}) and a protein (globin). The Hgb molecule is made up of four globins with a heme molecule attached to each globin. The heme molecule has iron at its center, which binds with oxygen.

Connection Check 33.2

What is the role of erythropoietin in the regulation of red blood cells?

A. To make Hgb capable of transporting oxygen
B. To pick up carbon dioxide from the tissues and deliver it to the lungs
C. To decrease RBC production
D. To stimulate RBC production

White Blood Cells

White blood cells, also called *leukocytes*, are components of the body's defense system against infection and disease. Leukocytes are the least abundant formed elements, yet they are required for life to provide protection against infectious microorganisms and other pathogens. On average,

there are 4,500 to 11,000 WBCs per cubic millimeter of blood, which constitutes only 1% of the total blood volume. Leukocytes are essential to the body's defense against disease. Unlike RBCs, which remain within blood vessels, WBCs travel through the circulatory system and can migrate out of blood vessels into other tissues. Leukocytes are responsible for the immune responses that protect against harmful microorganisms, including identification and destruction of cancer cells and involvement in the inflammatory response and wound healing.

Leukocytes differ from erythrocytes in that they retain their organelles for protein synthesis throughout life, including the nucleus, rough endoplasmic reticulum, ribosomes, and Golgi complex. Protein is essential for leukocytes to carry out their functions, and some of these proteins appear as noticeable **granules** in the cytoplasm that distinguish one WBC type from another. There are two major types of WBCs, granulocytes and agranular leukocytes, based on the presence or absence of specific cytoplasmic granules (Fig. 33.4). Those containing specific granules (neutrophils, eosinophils, basophils) are classified as **granulocytes**, and those that lack granules (lymphocytes and monocytes) are classified as **agranulocytes**.

Granulocytes

Granulocytes (neutrophils, eosinophils, and basophils) are spherical and have distinctive multilobar nuclei. They are also distinguished from each other by their relative size and abundance, the size and shape of their nuclei, and the staining properties of their individual granules (Table 33.1). Eosinophils have bright-red granules in their cytoplasm, and basophil granules stain deep blue. Neutrophils have granules that stain a pink to violet hue. Granulocytes play a key role in protecting the body from harmful microorganisms during acute inflammation and infection by means of their individual functions.

Neutrophils

The **neutrophils** comprise 50% to 70% of circulating WBCs. Because they have nuclei that are divided into three to five lobes, they are often called *polymorphonuclear leukocytes* or *PMNs*. Immature (young) neutrophils are called "bands," which have an undivided, horseshoe-shaped nucleus. Mature neutrophils are referred to as "segs" because of their segmented nucleus. An increased need for neutrophils causes an increase in both the segs and the bands. Once the neutrophil matures (segmentation), it is released into the circulation from the marrow to perform its function of **phagocytosis** (engulfing and digesting bacteria). Bands generally account for a small percentage (3%–5%) of circulating granulocytes. An increase in band level is called a **left shift**, which occurs with acute infection, inflammation, or some other significant physical stress (Fig. 33.5). Because they are immature, the bands are not very effective in combating infection.

The neutrophils are primarily responsible for sustaining normal host defenses against invading bacteria and fungi, cell debris, and foreign substances. Neutrophils are phagocytic

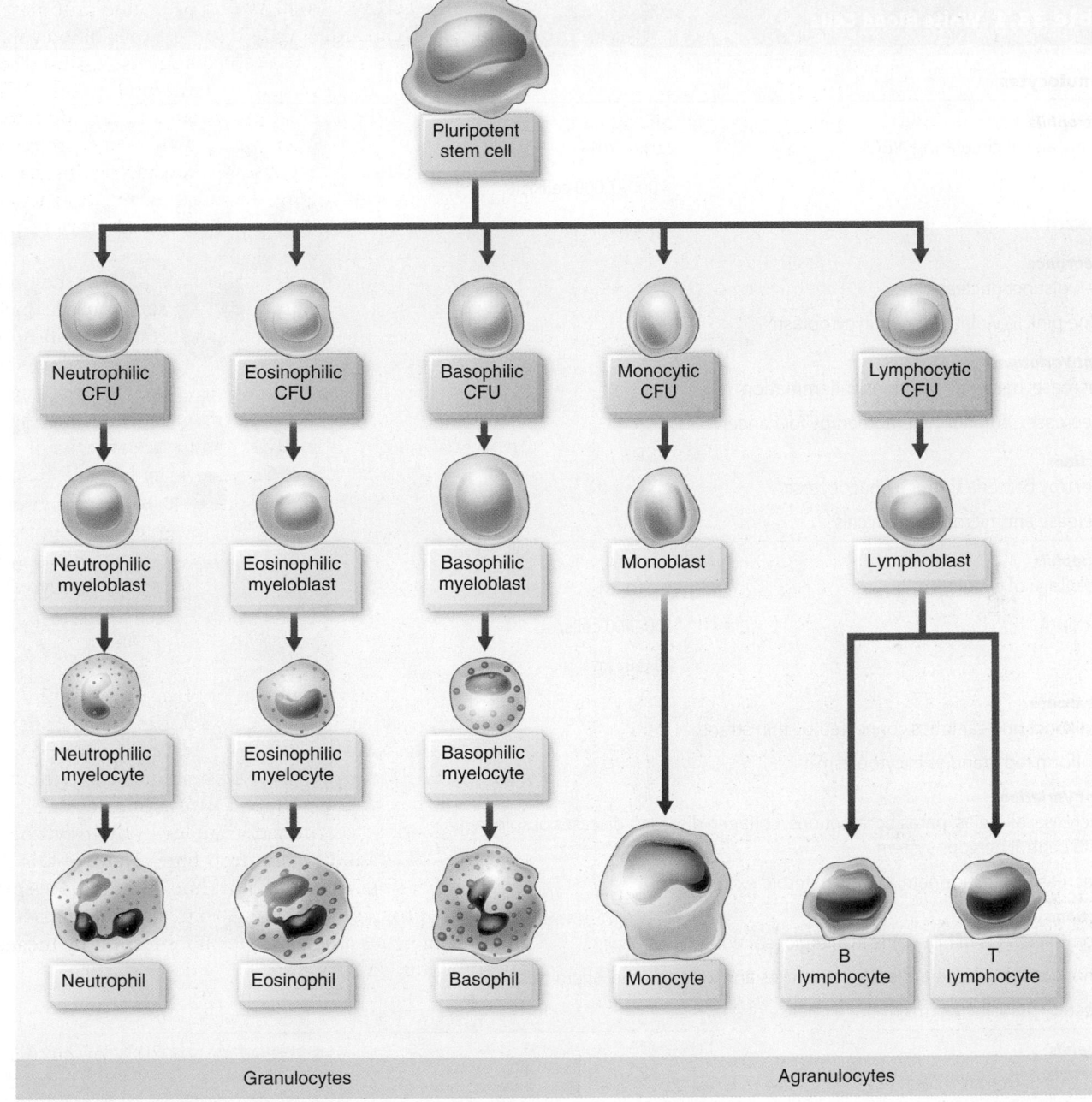

FIGURE 33.4 Leukopoiesis. Stages in the development of white blood cells. The pluripotent stem cell also is the ultimate source of red blood cells and platelet-producing cells (CFU = colony-forming unit).

and are responsible for engulfing and destroying foreign matter and are the first cells to arrive at a site of invasion. Once released from the marrow, neutrophils remain in the circulation for approximately 6 hours before migrating to the invaded tissues.

> **Safety Alert**   Decreased neutrophil counts significantly increase the risk of infection because of a decreased immune response. Protect the patient by using and teaching proper hand hygiene, performing frequent oral care, and limiting visitors.

Eosinophils

Eosinophils constitute 1% to 3% of the total WBCs and have a life span of approximately 3 to 8 hours. Although scarce in the circulating blood, eosinophils are abundant in the mucous membranes of the respiratory, digestive, and urinary systems. The exact functions of eosinophils are unknown, but they do have granules that contain vasoactive amines that may be used to destroy foreign cells invading the body. Eosinophils are involved in hypersensitivity reactions, inactivating some of the inflammatory chemicals released during the inflammatory response. The number of eosinophils increases and migrates to the site of inflammation during allergic reactions, parasitic infections, collagen

Table 33.1 White Blood Cells

Granulocytes

Neutrophils

Percentage of circulating WBCs:	50% – 70%
Cell count:	3,000–7,000 cells/μL
Cell size:	10–16 μm

Appearance
- 3–5 distinct nuclear lobes
- Fine pink to violet granules in cytoplasm

Count Variations
- Increase: bacterial infections, inflammation
- Decrease: radiation, chemotherapy for cancer

Functions
- Destroy bacteria through phagocytosis
- Release antimicrobial chemicals

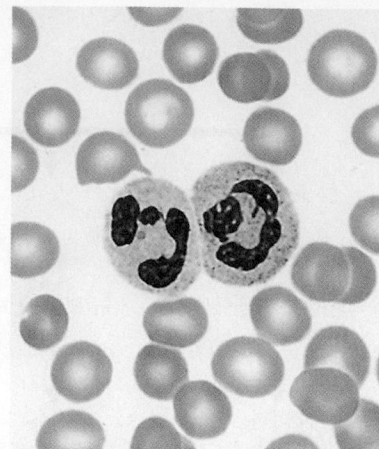

Neutrophils

Eosinophils

Percentage of circulating WBCs:	1% to 3%
Cell count:	100–400 cells/μL
Cell size:	10–16 μm

Appearance
- 2 distinct nuclear lobes connected by thin strand
- Uniform red granules in cytoplasm

Count Variations
- Increase: allergies, parasitic infections, collagen diseases, diseases of spleen and central nervous system
- Decrease: aplastic anemia, corticosteroid excess

Functions
- Combat effects of histamine in allergic reactions
- Phagocytize antigen-antibody complexes and inflammatory chemicals
- Destroy parasitic worms through release of enzymes

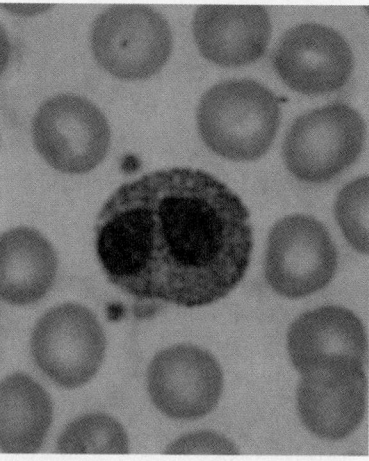

Eosinophil

Basophils

Percentage of circulating WBCs:	0.4% to 1%
Cell count:	20–50 cells/μL
Cell size:	8–10 μm

Appearance
- Two nuclear lobes
- Coarse, abundant blue granules in cytoplasm

Count Variations
- Increase: allergies, inflammatory disorders, infection
- Decrease: alcoholism, anemias, malnutrition, viral infections

Functions
- Release histamine, heparin, and other mediators in inflammation response

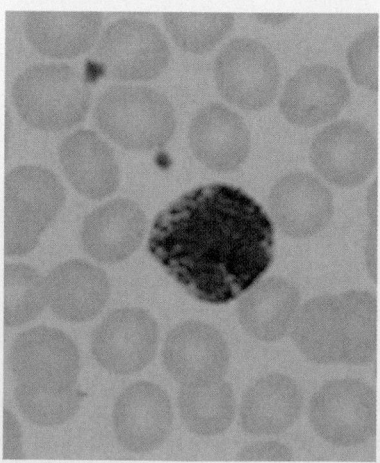

Basophil

Table 33.1 White Blood Cells—cont'd

Agranulocytes

Lymphocytes

Percentage of circulating WBCs: 20% to 35%

Cell count: 1,500–3,000 cells/μL

Cell size: 5–17 μm

Appearance
- Nucleus is round or indented
- Cytoplasm forms sky-blue rim around nucleus

Count Variations
- Increase: diverse infections and immune responses
- Decrease: HIV/AIDS, severe burns, cancer, radiation

Functions
- Mediate immune responses by direct cell attack or through antibodies
- Destroy tumor, virus-infected, and foreign cells
- Reject transplants of foreign tissue

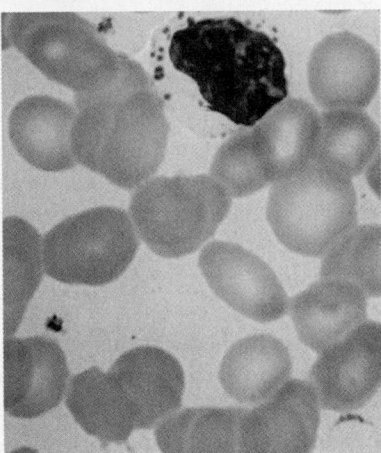
Lymphocyte

Monocytes

Percentage of circulating WBCs: 3% to 8%

Cell count: 100–700 cells/μL

Cell size: 12–18 μm

Appearance
- Kidney or horseshoe-shaped nucleus
- Cytoplasm is abundant and appears blue-gray

Count Variations
- Increase: many viral diseases, chronic inflammation
- Decrease: corticosteroid excess

Functions
- Develop into macrophages in tissues
- Phagocytize bacteria and debris in tissues

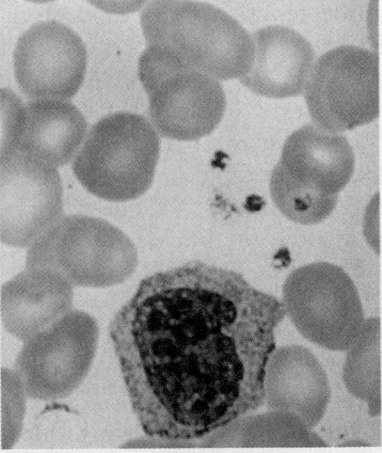
Monocyte

AIDS, Acquired immune deficiency syndrome; *WBCs,* white blood cells.
All blood films with permission from Harmening, D. M. (2009). *Clinical hematology and fundamentals of hemostasis* (5th ed.). Philadelphia, PA: F. A. Davis

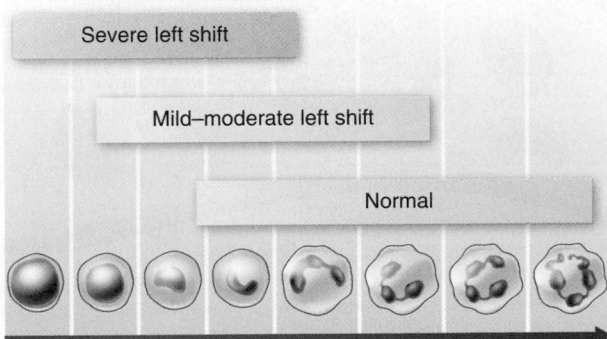
Severe left shift

Mild–moderate left shift

Normal

Increasing neutrophil maturity

FIGURE 33.5 Diagram of left shift. A shift to the left indicates that more immature cells are present in the blood than normal.

diseases, and diseases of the spleen and central nervous system. Containing proteolytic substances that protect the body from parasitic worms in parasitic infections, eosinophils use surface markers to attach themselves to the parasite and then release toxic hydrolytic enzymes that kill the invading organism. Eosinophil counts can increase to more than 30% of baseline in parasitic infections.

Eosinophil counts decrease in conditions such as aplastic anemia (because of bone marrow failure) and infections (because of a significant production of neutrophils). When the body experiences stress, there are changes in adrenal hormones such as cortisol and aldosterone. These increased levels of adrenal steroids suppress the number of eosinophils.

Basophils

Basophils are the least numerous of the WBCs, making up 0.4% to 1% of total WBCs, and have a life span of approximately 7 to 12 hours. Basophils are not phagocytic. Their cytoplasmic granules contain heparin, an anticoagulant; histamine, a vasodilator; and other mediators of inflammation. These chemicals aid in defense mechanisms by making the blood vessels more permeable for neutrophils and clotting proteins to enter the injured site more quickly and efficiently. The basophils are believed to be an integral part of both hypersensitivity and stress responses. Basophils increase in circulation because of pathologic conditions such as inflammatory disorders, all types of infections, and anemias. They also increase as a result of normal physiological and environmental conditions such as exposure to extreme heat or cold, acute stress, and strenuous exercise. Basophils decrease in conditions such as alcoholism, anemias, malnutrition, and viral infections.

Agranulocytes

Lymphocytes

Lymphocytes are essential elements in the immune response and function to produce substances that aid in attacking foreign material. After birth, some lymphocytes are produced in the bone marrow. Differentiation and maturation of lymphocytes occur primarily in the lymph nodes and in the lymphoid tissue of the intestine and spleen after exposure to a specific antigen (see Chapter 18). The ability of lymphocytes to produce antibodies (in the case of B lymphocytes), or cell-surface receptors (in the case of T lymphocytes) that are specific for one of the many millions of foreign entities that may invade the body is essential to acquired immunity. B lymphocytes have the ability to differentiate into **plasma cells**. Plasma cells then produce antibodies, called **immunoglobulins (Igs)** that attack and neutralize antigens produced by bacterial infections. T lymphocytes kill foreign cells directly or release a variety of substances that enhance the activity of phagocytosis by other cells. T lymphocytes are responsible for delayed allergic reactions, rejection of transplants of foreign tissue (e.g., transplanted organs), and destruction of tumor cells.

Monocytes

Monocytes (also called *mononuclear leukocytes*) are leukocytes with a single-lobed nucleus with no granules in the cytoplasm; they are the largest of the leukocytes and account for 3% to 8% of the total leukocytes in the circulating blood. Monocytes enter the blood from the bone marrow and circulate for a short time before they enter the tissues and become tissue **macrophages**. Active in the spleen, liver, peritoneum, and alveoli, macrophages are activated by cytokines released from T lymphocytes and migrate in response to stimuli from bacterial cells. Macrophages remove debris and phagocytize bacteria within the tissues.

Platelets

Thrombocytes, or platelets, are circulating cell fragments of the cytoplasm of large cells in the bone marrow called

megakaryocytes (Fig. 33.6). The production of platelets is a division of hematopoiesis called *thrombopoiesis* (Fig. 33.7). Regulated by the hormone thrombopoietin, some pluripotent stem cells become megakaryoblasts, cells committed to the platelet-producing line. Platelets circulate freely in the blood in an inactive state. After a vascular injury occurs, platelets play an essential part in the control of bleeding. Platelets collect at the damaged site and are activated to begin adhesion and formation of a temporary plug. Their cytoplasmic granules release mediators to activate coagulation factors in the blood plasma and initiate the formation of a stable clot composed of **fibrin** (a fibrous protein).

Platelets have a membrane but no nucleus and cannot replicate. Approximately 25% to 40% of the platelets are stored in the spleen and are released as needed. If not consumed in a clotting reaction, platelets are normally removed by the spleen and live for approximately 7 to 10 days.

Plasma

Blood is made up of plasma (a clear yellow, protein-rich fluid), and the cells and cell fragments suspended in it are RBCs, WBCs, and platelets. Plasma is a complex mixture of water, proteins, nutrients, electrolytes, nitrogenous wastes, hormones, and gases. Plasma is part of the body's extracellular fluid and contains approximately 90% water, 6.5% to 8% proteins, and 2% other small molecular substances. Plasma serves as a transport vehicle for materials carried in the blood (Fig. 33.8).

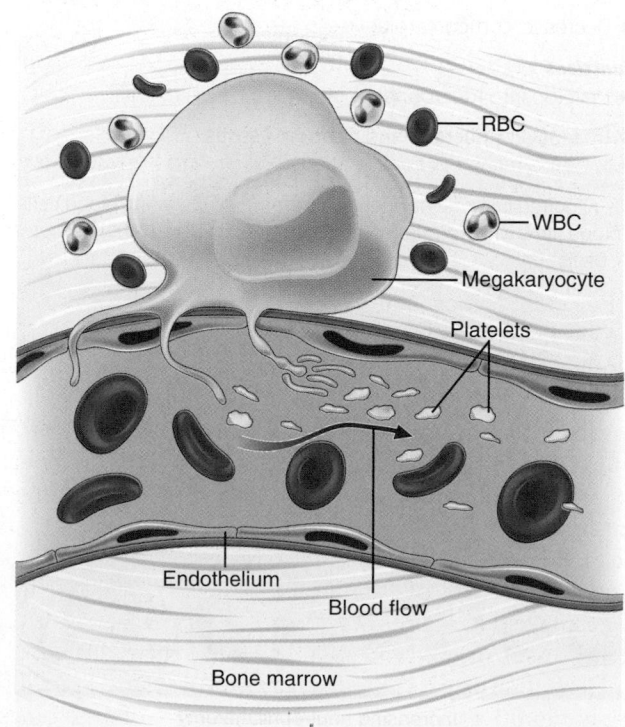

FIGURE 33.6 Platelet production. Thrombocytes, or platelets, are circulating cell fragments of the cytoplasm of large cells in the bone marrow called megakaryocytes.

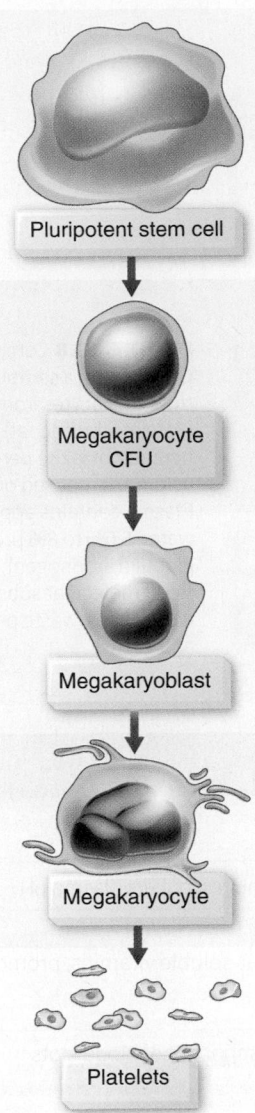

Pluripotent stem cell

Megakaryocyte CFU

Megakaryoblast

Megakaryocyte

Platelets

FIGURE 33.7 Thrombopoiesis. The production of platelets is a division of hematopoiesis called thrombopoiesis and is regulated by the hormone thrombopoietin. Some pluripotent stem cells become megakaryoblasts, cells committed to the platelet-producing line.

Protein, the most abundant plasma solute, plays a variety of roles including clotting, immune defense, and transport of other solutes that contribute to the osmotic regulation of body fluids. There are three major types of proteins in plasma: albumin, globulin, and fibrinogen (Table 33.2). **Albumin**, synthesized in the liver, serves to transport various solutes and buffer the pH of the plasma, and is important in fluid balance by increasing the osmotic pressure of the blood, which prevents the plasma from leaking into the tissues. Low levels of albumin may be the result of inadequate intake (i.e., malnutrition), inadequate production (i.e., liver disease), or excessive loss (i.e., burns, hemorrhage).

Globulins play various roles in solute transport, clotting, and immunity as they are the main proteins of antibodies. There are three main types of globulins, each with different functions: alpha, beta, and gamma. Alpha and beta globulins are made in the liver and are important in transport and

clotting, and gamma globulins are important in immune defense. **Fibrinogen** is an inactive protein that is activated by thrombin (a vitamin K–dependent enzyme) to form fibrin (a sticky protein that forms the framework of a blood clot).

Spleen

The spleen is a coffee bean–shaped, encapsulated organ composed of vascular and lymphoid tissues located in the left upper quadrant of the abdomen (Fig. 33.9). Splenic functions include filtration, host defense, storage, and **cytopoiesis** (formation of cells). The splenic cellular tissue (parenchyma) is composed of two main elements: the red pulp, where filtration occurs, and the white pulp, where immune functions are generated (Fig. 33.10).

The spleen serves as a large filter by removing aged erythrocytes (Fig. 33.11) and plays a part in the removal of abnormal WBCs and platelets. Splenic blood flow is approximately 250 to 300 mL/min. Because the average life span of a normal circulating RBC is 120 days, each red cell averages 1,000 passes through the spleen every day. Normal blood cells pass through the spleen without incident, whereas damaged and aged cells are slowed and trapped. The spleen acts as the major site for clearance from the blood of damaged or aged RBCs, removing approximately 20 mL of senescent (old or dying) RBCs per day. This is facilitated by a group of large phagocytic cells located in the spleen, which ingest and destroy old and defective red cells in a series of enzymatic reactions. The degradation products of RBCs, including iron and amino acids, are recycled.

The spleen also has immunological functions similar to those of other lymphoid organs (e.g., lymph nodes, thymus). Blood passing through the spleen is exposed to all the essential cellular components necessary for both humoral and cellular immune responses. There are follicles within the spleen that aid in antigen production and initiation of T- and B-lymphocyte activities involved in humoral and cellular immune responses. In summary, the spleen filters the blood, produces lymphocytes, and stores blood and platelets.

OVERVIEW OF HEMATOLOGY FUNCTION

Oxygen Delivery

All body tissues rely on oxygen that is transported in the blood to meet metabolic needs. Respiration is a primary function of erythrocytes (RBCs) because they are responsible for producing hemoglobin (Hgb), an oxygen-carrying protein. A Hgb molecule combines loosely with oxygen in the lungs, which allows the transfer of oxygen from Hgb to the tissues (oxygen dissociation). This transfer is important in meeting the body tissues' need for oxygen. The ability of the circulating blood to carry oxygen is dependent on both Hgb levels and the capability of the lungs to oxygenate the Hgb. The number of circulating RBCs is balanced to ensure sufficient RBCs are available for oxygenation. Excessive increases in RBCs raise the blood viscosity, slowing its flow and therefore reducing oxygen transport.

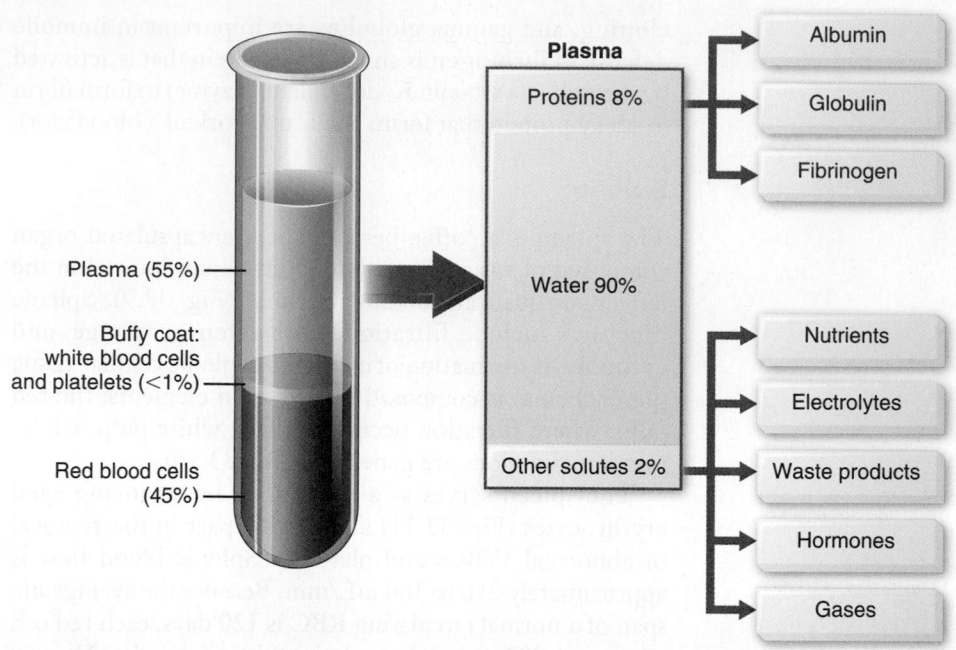

FIGURE 33.8 Components of blood. Centrifuging a sample of blood separates the erythrocytes from the white cells and platelets (buffy coat) and plasma. The hematocrit is the percentage of the volume composed of erythrocytes. Plasma contains approximately 90% water, 6.5% to 8% proteins (albumin, globulin, fibrinogen), and 2% other small molecular substances (nutrients, electrolytes, waste products, hormones and gases).

Table 33.2 Blood Plasma Proteins

Proteins	Functions
*Albumin (60%)**	Maintains osmotic pressure; transports various solutes; buffers plasma pH
*Globulins (36%)** *Alpha (α) globulins, Beta (β) globulins* *Gamma (γ) globulins*	Transport hemoglobin, metal ions, lipids, and fat-soluble vitamins; promote blood clotting Antibodies
*Fibrinogen (4%)**	Activated by thrombin, becomes fibrin; major component of blood clots

*Mean percentage of the total plasma protein by weight

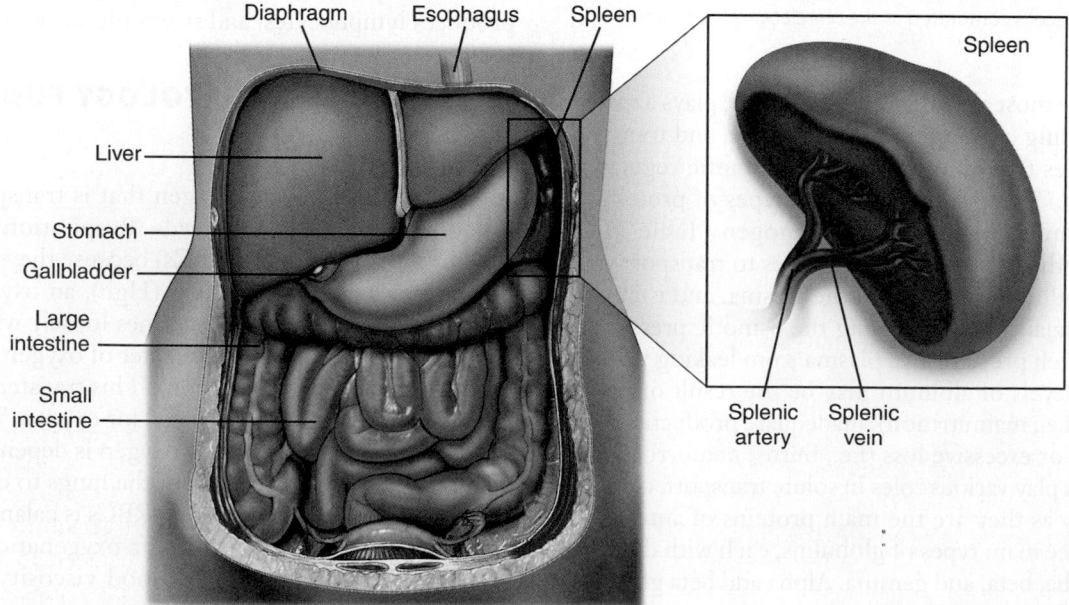

FIGURE 33.9 Spleen location inside the abdomen. The spleen is a coffee bean–shaped, encapsulated organ composed of vascular and lymphoid tissues located in the left upper quadrant of the abdomen.

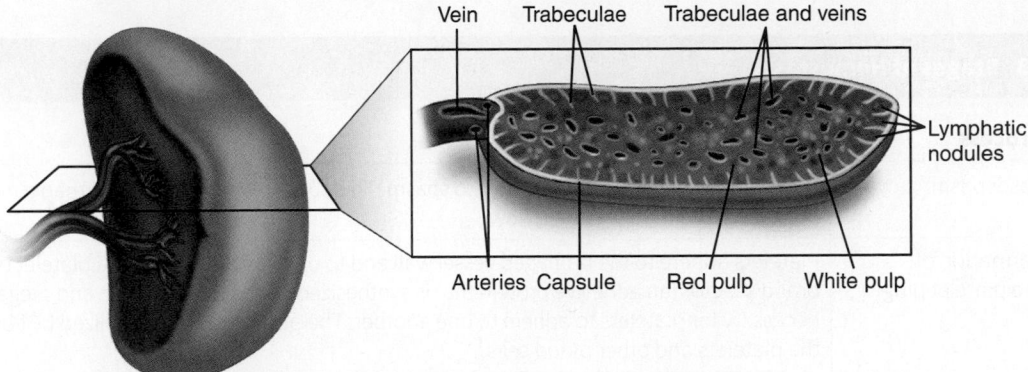

FIGURE 33.10 Splenic architecture. The splenic parenchyma is composed of two main elements: the red pulp, where filtration occurs, and the white pulp, where immune functions are generated.

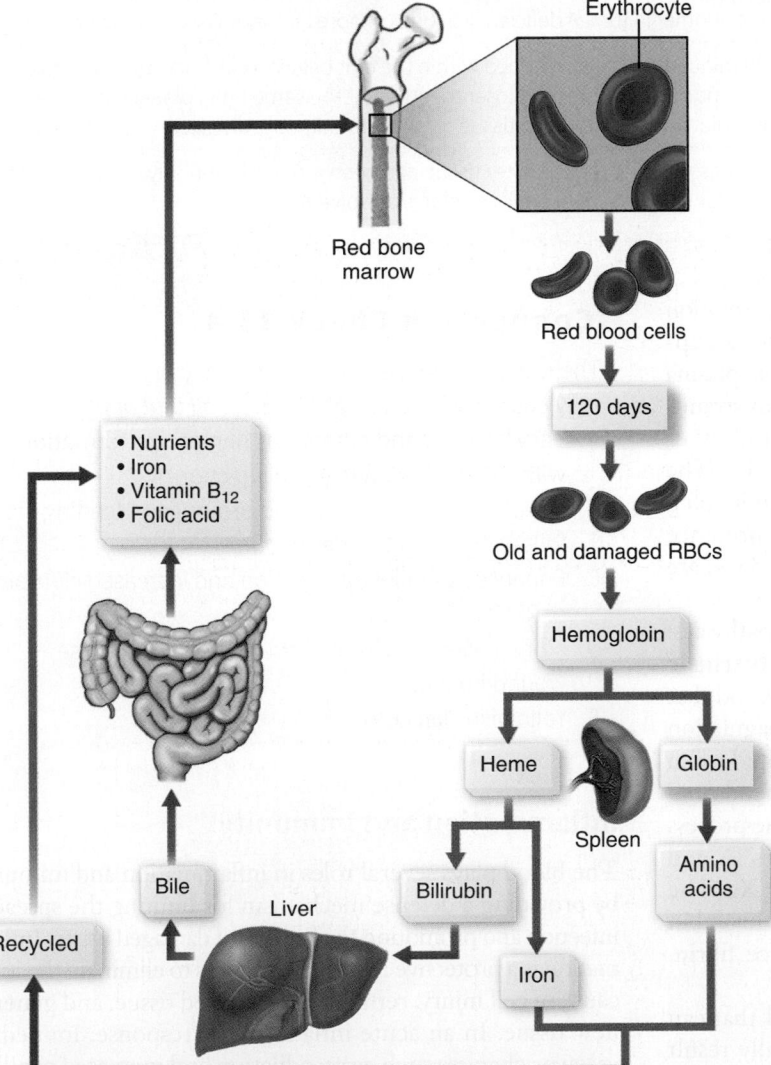

FIGURE 33.11 Life and death of erythrocytes. The average life span of a normal circulating RBC is 120 days. Each red cell averages 1,000 passes through the spleen every day. Normal blood cells pass through the spleen without incident, whereas damaged and aged cells are slowed and entrapped. This is facilitated by a group of large phagocytic cells located in the spleen, which ingest and destroy old and defective red cells in a series of enzymatic reactions. The degradation products of RBCs, such as iron and amino acids, are recycled.

Connection Check 33.3

What is a probable initial assessment finding for a patient with a low hemoglobin count?

A. Increased and bounding peripheral pulses

B. Hypertension

C. Pallor and fatigue

D. Moist mucus membranes

Clotting Cascade

Hemostasis, or blood clotting, is a complex process that stops bleeding. It is also the orderly process (Table 33.3) that balances the production and dissolution of clotting factors and involves (1) vasospasm, (2) formation of a platelet plug, (3) development of a fibrin clot, (4) clot retraction, and (5) fibrinolysis. Hemostasis is normal when it seals a blood vessel to prevent blood loss and hemorrhage.

Table 33.3 **Stages of Hemostasis**

Stage	Process	Description
1	Vasospasm	Damage to a blood vessel causes it to spasm. This spasm, which lasts more than a minute, constricts the vessel and reduces blood flow.
2	Formation of the platelet plug	Platelets adhere to the damaged vessel wall and to one another, forming a platelet plug. Von Willebrand's factor (an adhesive protein that is synthesized by the endothelium and megakaryocytes) is necessary for platelets to adhere to one another. The platelet plug is stabilized by fibrin, which binds the platelets and other blood cells.
3	Clot formation	Coagulation occurs as fibrin forms a meshwork that cements blood components together into an insoluble clot. The process involves two different clotting pathways. The intrinsic pathway is activated by vessel injury; the extrinsic pathway is activated by blood leaking out of the vessel into the tissues. The final outcome is fibrin clot formation. Each clotting factor is activated in sequence; activation of one clotting factor activates another in turn. A deficiency of one or more factors interrupts blood clotting.
4	Clot retraction	After approximately 30 minutes, platelets trapped within the clot begin to contract. This pulls the broken portions of the ruptured blood vessel closer together. At the same time, platelets release growth factors that stimulate cell division and tissue repair in the damaged vessel.
5	Clot dissolution	A process called *fibrinolysis* removes the clot after tissue has been repaired. Fibrinolysis begins within a few days of clot formation and continues until the clot is dissolved.

The blood-clotting cascade is triggered by the formation of a platelet plug, where platelets clump together. It is a stepwise process resulting in the conversion of the soluble plasma protein, fibrinogen, into fibrin. The insoluble fibrin strands create a sticky meshwork that cements platelets and other blood components together to form the temporary clot. The steps of the cascade between the formation of a platelet plug and the formation of a fibrin clot depend on the presence of specific clotting factors. Clotting factors (Table 33.4) are inactive enzymes that become activated in succession.

The coagulation process can be initiated by two pathways: the intrinsic pathway and the extrinsic pathway. **Intrinsic factors** are substances located directly within the blood that first makes platelets clump and then trigger the coagulation cascade (Fig. 33.12). The intrinsic pathway is initiated when the blood is exposed to a stimulus (i.e., damaged subendothelium) and activates factor XII (Hageman factor). The process continues in a chainlike reaction, activating factors IX and XI, in combination with calcium, generating factor Xa. The clotting cascade then continues by converting prothrombin to thrombin, which acts on fibrinogen to produce fibrin, leading to final clot formation.

Extrinsic factors are elements outside the cell that can also stimulate platelet plug formation. They usually result from changes in blood vessels, such as tissue trauma, rather than inside the blood. These changes begin a complex series of chemical reactions that are activated by factor III (tissue thromboplastin) and, in the presence of calcium, are catalysed by factor VII (proconvertin). The binding of calcium causes factor X (thrombokinase) to convert to factor Xa. Just as in the intrinsic pathway, prothrombin is converted to thrombin, then fibrinogen and, ultimately, fibrin. The extrinsic pathway causes clotting to occur more quickly because some of the steps in the intrinsic pathway are bypassed.

Connection Check 33.4

The nurse recognizes that a deficiency in a clotting factor may cause which finding(s)? *(Select all that apply.)*

A. Easy bruising and cutaneous hematoma formation with minor trauma (e.g., an injection)
B. Bleeding from the gums and prolonged bleeding following minor injuries or cuts
C. Enhanced platelet aggregation and increased clumping of RBCs
D. Fibrin molecules form fibrin threads to increase wound healing
E. Yellowish skin color

Inflammation and Immunity

The blood plays several roles in inflammation and immunity by providing a defense mechanism for limiting the spread of infection and promoting the healing of damaged tissue. Inflammation is a protective response that aims to eliminate the initial cause of cell injury, remove the damaged tissue, and generate new tissue. In an acute inflammatory response, immediate vascular changes such as vasodilation and increased capillary permeability occur. This allows the influx of inflammatory cells such as neutrophils and the broad effects of inflammatory mediators (derived from platelets, neutrophils, and macro-phages), which produce fever and other systemic clinical manifestations.

HEMATOLOGICAL ASSESSMENT

Nurses play an important role in identifying hematological disorders. Assessment of this system is generally conducted as part of the general survey of the patient's health or

Table 33.4 Clotting Factors

Factor	Function	Pathway
I. Fibrinogen	Converted to fibrin, clot formation	Common
II. Prothrombin	Converted to thrombin, activates fibrinogen (factor I)	Common
III. Tissue thromboplastin, tissue factor	Activates factor VII	Extrinsic
IV. Calcium ions (Ca⁺⁺)	Intrinsic: Combines with factor IX to activate factor X Extrinsic: Combines with factor III to activate factor VII Common: Combines with factor X to activate prothrombin (factor II)	Intrinsic, extrinsic, and common
V. Proaccelerin, labile factor	Combines with factor X to activate prothrombin (factor II)	Common
VII.* Proconvertin, stable factor	Activates factor X in extrinsic pathway	Extrinsic
VIII. Antihemophilic factor	Activates factor X in intrinsic pathway	Intrinsic
IX. Plasma thromboplastin component, Christmas factor	Activates factor VIII	Intrinsic
X. Stuart-Prower factor	Combines with factor V to activate prothrombin (factor II)	Common
XI. Plasma thromboplastin antecedent	Activates factor IX	Intrinsic
XII. Hageman factor	Activates factor XI	Intrinsic
XIII. Fibrin-stabilizing factor	Cross-links fibrin	Common

*Factor VI designation is no longer used; it was found to be the same substance as activated factor V.

concurrently with focused cardiovascular system assessment. However, unless the nurse specifically focuses on this system, early manifestations of hematological disorders can be missed or attributed to dysfunction of a different body system. Age and gender are important variables when assessing the patient's hematological status because bone marrow and immune activity diminish with age.

History

Nutrition

Dietary pattern can alter cell quality and affect blood clotting. Ask the patient about usual diet, including protein, vitamin, and mineral intake. Diets high in vitamin K, such as raw leafy green vegetables, may increase the rate of blood coagulation. Diets high in fat and carbohydrates and low in protein, iron, and vitamins can decrease the function of all blood cells and potentially lead to different types of anemia (Table 33.5).

Ask about the use of tobacco, alcohol, and other recreational drugs. Chronic alcohol use is associated with nutritional deficiencies and liver impairment, both of which can decrease the ability of the blood to clot. Alcohol (ethyl alcohol, or ethanol) is absorbed readily from the gastrointestinal (GI) tract but cannot be broken down or stored as protein, fat, or carbohydrate. Approximately 90% of the alcohol a person drinks is metabolized by the liver. During metabolism, an excess of an ethanol by product is thought to contribute to the liver damage that

often accompanies increased alcohol consumption. This damage interrupts the synthesis of clotting factors and plasma proteins. A concise patient history can focus on changes related to hematological function, and the nurse should pose the following questions to the patient:

- Have you had any recent changes in energy level?
- Do you have any difficulties maintaining usual daily activities, including recreational activities and sports?
- Have you been experiencing any pain, burning, or tingling sensations? Any changes in skin color or temperature? Any swelling (edema)?
- Have you experienced any bleeding or easy bruising, dizziness, fatigue, or changes in lymph nodes (swelling, pain or tenderness, warmth)?

Past Medical History

Obtain the patient's medical history, being sure to ask about any chronic diseases. Because the liver synthesizes most of the clotting factors, diseases such as hepatitis, cirrhosis, and cancer that alter liver function may result in clotting factor deficiencies. Also, the synthesis of clotting factors II, VII, IX, and X requires vitamin K. The absorption of vitamin K from the diet requires bile, a liver secretion. Cholelithiasis (gallstones) can lead to a clotting deficiency by obstructing the bile duct and, in turn, interfering with bile secretion and vitamin K absorption. Ask about pregnancy because the incidence of gestational thrombocytopenia is observed in 5% to 11% of all pregnancies.

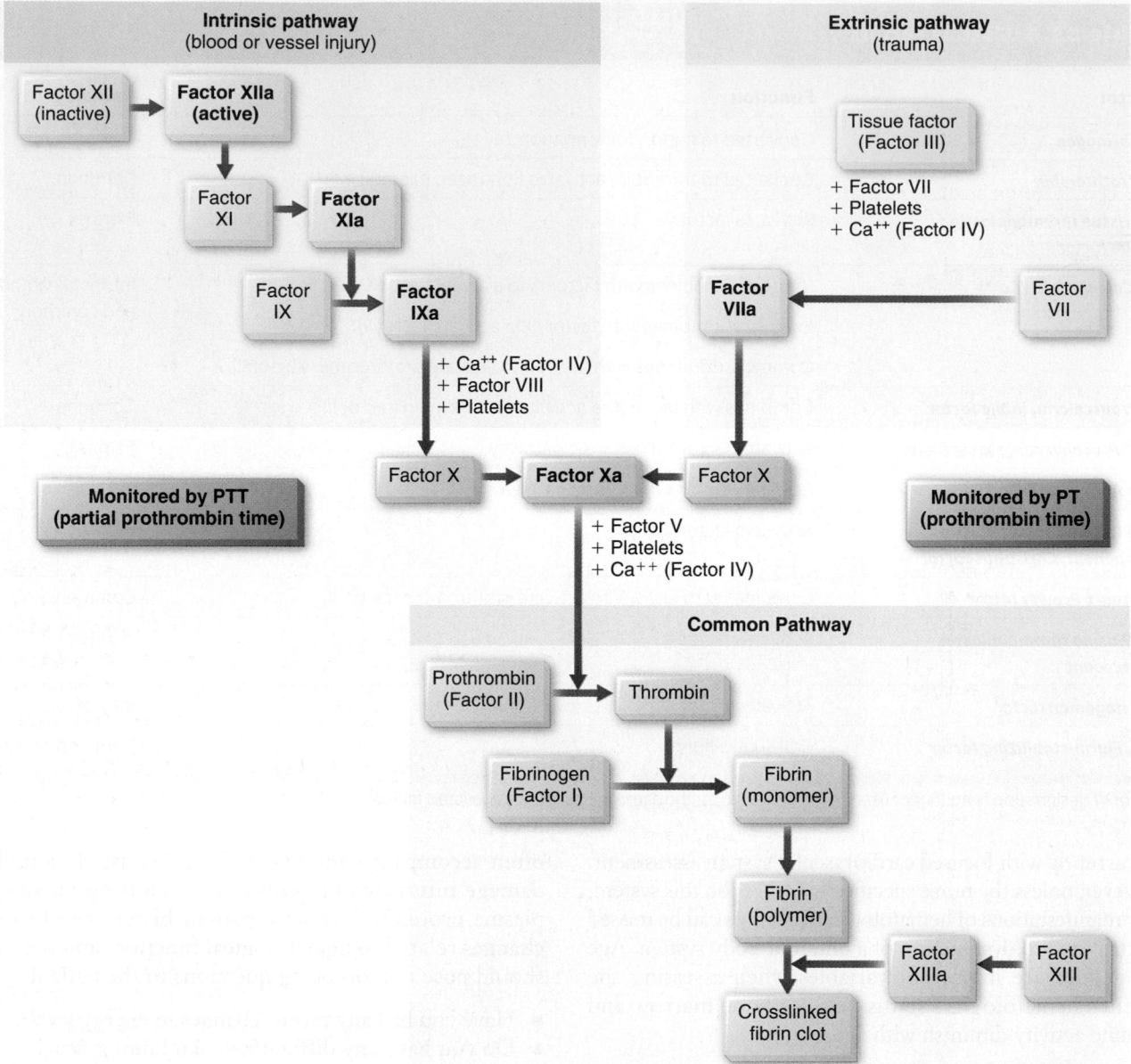

FIGURE 33.12 Clotting pathways. Both the slower intrinsic pathway (on the left) and the more rapid extrinsic pathway (on the right) are necessary to form a stable blood clot. Both pathways come together at factor X activation, which then activates prothrombin (factor II) to thrombin, the final enzyme of the clotting cascade. The intrinsic pathway is measured by PTT (partial thromboplastin time). The extrinsic pathway is measured by PT (prothrombin time).

Medication History

Inquire about current medications, including anticoagulants, aspirin and other salicylates, herbs, nutritional supplements, and nutraceuticals. Some dietary supplements may interact with prescribed medication therapy. For example, goldenseal and green tea may reduce the effect of certain anticoagulants, thus increasing the risk of thromboembolism. Ask about the use of anticoagulants or "blood thinners" such as sodium warfarin (Coumadin), aspirin, or other NSAIDs. If a patient is prescribed any of these medications, there may be a clotting disorder or a health problem that requires further assessment and treatment (Table 33.6). Aspirin can irreversibly inhibit platelet aggregation by inactivation of a crucial cyclooxygenase (COX) enzyme. A 325-mg dose of the medication results in approximately 90% inhibition of COX in circulating platelets. This effect lasts for the life span of platelets (4–7 days). During prolonged aspirin therapy, periodic assessments of Hct, Hgb level, **prothrombin time** (PT), International Normalized Ratio (INR), and renal function are recommended. Also ask the patient about antibiotic use because prolonged antibiotic therapy can lead to coagulopathies, bone marrow depression, or other undesired effects. For example, neutropenia may occur during therapy with penicillins, cephalosporins, or vancomycin. Box 33.1 summarizes selected medications that may predispose the patient to bleeding.

Table 33.5 Sources and Functions of Vitamins and Minerals

Vitamin and Minerals	Food Source	Recommended Dietary Allowance (RDA)	Blood Cell Functions
Vitamins			
Vitamin C (ascorbic acid)	Asparagus, broccoli, sweet and hot peppers, collards, Brussels sprouts, kale, potatoes, spinach, tomatoes, citrus fruits, strawberries	Children: 15 to 75 mg per day depending upon age and gender Adult men aged 19 and older: 90 mg per day Adult women aged 19 and older: 75 mg per day	Facilitates calcium and nonheme (vegetable) iron absorption by increasing the solubility of nonheme iron; synthesizes leukocytes and other immune cell components
Folacin (folic acid)	Liver, legumes, green leafy vegetables	Children: 150 to 300 mcg per day depending upon age Adult men and women: 400 mcg per day	Promotes red cell formation; classified as a hematopoietic vitamin
Vitamin B_6 (pyridoxine)	Meat, poultry, fish, shellfish, green and leafy vegetables, whole-grain products, legumes	Children: 0.5 to 1.0 mg per day depending upon age Adult men aged 14–50: 1.3 mg per day Men over age 50: 1.7 mg per day Adult women aged 14–50: 1.2 to 1.3 mg per day Women older than age 50: 1.5 mg per day	Required for normal development and function of red blood cells; needed for normal synthesis of hemoglobin; classified as a hematopoietic vitamin
Vitamin B_{12} (cobalamin)	Meat, poultry, fish, shellfish, eggs, dairy products	Children: 0.9 to 1.8 mcg per day depending upon age Adult men and women: 2.4 mcg per day	Assists in division and maturity of red blood cells
Vitamin K	Cabbage, cauliflower, cereals, dark green vegetables (broccoli, Brussels sprouts, asparagus), dark leafy vegetables (spinach, kale, collards, turnip greens), fish, liver, beef, eggs	Children: 30 to 75 mcg per day, depending upon age Adult women: 90 mcg per day Adult men: 120 mcg per day	Necessary for formation of prothrombin and other clotting factors in the liver
Minerals			
Calcium	Milk and milk products, fish with bones, greens	1,000 mg before age 50; 1,200 mg after age 50	Bone formation and maintenance; vitamin B absorption; blood clotting
Cobalt	Organ meats, meats	Required in small amounts as a component of vitamin B_{12}	Aids in maturation of red blood cells (as part of B_{12} molecule)
Copper	Cereals, nuts, legumes, liver, shellfish, grapes, meats	Adult men and women: 900 mcg	Catalyst for hemoglobin formation
Iron	Meats, heart, liver, clams, oysters, lima beans, spinach, dates, dried nuts, enriched and whole-grain cereals	Men and postmenopausal women: 8 mg Premenopausal women: 18 mg Pregnant women: 27 mg	Hemoglobin synthesis; cellular energy release (cytochrome pathway); killing bacteria (myeloperoxidase)

Table 33.6 Medications to Treat Clotting Disorders

Medication	Actions
Anticoagulants *Thrombin inhibitors, Vitamin K agonists, indirect factor X inhibitors* • Warfarin sodium (Coumadin) derivatives • Heparin sodium • Trental (pentoxifylline) • Argatroban (Novastan) • Fondaparinux (Arixtra) • Dalteparin (Fragmin) • Enoxaparin (Lovenox) • Dabigatran (Pradaxa)	• Alter the synthesis of blood coagulation factors II (prothrombin), VII (proconvertin), IX (Christmas factor or plasma thromboplastin component), and X (Stuart-Prower factor) in the liver by interfering with the action of vitamin K • Treatment or secondary prevention for deep-vein thrombosis and pulmonary embolism • Prevent new clots from forming; limit or prevent clot extension • Cannot break down existing clot
Fibrinolytics *Thrombolytics – a biosynthetic (recombinant DNA origin) form of the enzyme human tissue-type plasminogen activator (tPA)* • Alteplase • Reteplase • Tenecteplase • Streptokinase	• Break down formed fibrin clots • Give within first 12 hours after onset of ischemic symptoms (e.g., myocardial infarction, thrombotic strokes)
Platelet inhibitors *Platelet glycoprotein (GP IIb/IIIa)-receptor inhibitor* • Clopidogrel bisulfate (Plavix) • Abciximab • Eptifibatide • Tirofiban	• Prevent platelets from becoming active or prevent activated platelets from clumping together • Change platelet membrane, preventing activators from binding to platelet receptor sites • Used for acute ischemic complications of percutaneous coronary intervention, unstable angina, and non–ST-segment elevation myocardial infarction

Physical Assessment

Typically, the physical examination follows a systematic head-to-toe approach. Patient preparation includes clearly explaining the examination as well as proper positioning and draping before and during the examination. During the physical assessment, the nurse is aware and respectful of the patient's feelings (particularly embarrassment and anxiety) as well as providing comfort measures and following appropriate safety precautions. Assess the whole body because blood disorders may cause oxygen delivery to be less than what is needed for normal oxygenation and tissue perfusion in all systems.

Skin, Head, and Neck Assessment

• Inspect the color of the skin and mucous membranes, including observing for pallor or cyanosis or fissures at the corners of the mouth (indicating nutritional deficiencies and/or chronic anemia).
• Palpate for skin temperature, capillary refill, and edema of the extremities.
• Palpate lymph nodes for swelling and tenderness.
• Inspect oral mucous membranes and the skin of the trunk and extremities for erythema, red streaks, petechiae (pinpoint hemorrhagic lesions in the skin), bruising, or purpura (purple rashes caused by blood leaking into the skin).
• A red, swollen, smooth, shiny, and tender tongue (glossitis) may indicate iron deficiency anemia or pernicious anemia.

Respiratory Assessment

• When hematological disorders reduce oxygen delivery, the lungs work harder to increase oxygen delivery.
• Four measures of respiration—rate, rhythm, depth, and sound—reflect the body's metabolic state, diaphragm and chest muscle condition, and airway patency. Knowing a patient's baseline respiratory rate allows detection of changes in the patient's condition.
• Respiratory rates of less than 12 or more than 20 breaths per minute usually are considered abnormal. Report the sudden onset of such rates promptly.
• Many anemias can cause fatigue and shortness of breath at rest or on exertion.

Cardiovascular Assessment

• Obtain the vital signs, including blood pressure (BP), temperature, and apical pulse.

Box 33.1 Medications That May Predispose to Bleeding

Interference With Platelet Production or Function

- Acetazolamide
- Antimetabolite and anticancer medications
- Antibiotics such as penicillin and the cephalosporins
- Aspirin and salicylates
- Carbamazepine
- Clofibrate
- Clopidogrel
- Colchicine
- Dipyridamole
- Thiazide diuretics
- Gold compounds
- Heparin, low molecular weight heparins
- NSAIDs (Acetylsalicylic acid [ASA], ibuprofen, indomethacin, naproxen)
- Quinine derivatives (quinidine and hydroxychloroquine)
- Sulfonamides

Interference With Coagulation Factors

- Amiodarone
- Anabolic steroids
- Warfarin (Coumadin)
- Novel oral anticoagulants such as dabigatran and rivaroxaban
- Heparin, low molecular weight heparins

Decrease in Vitamin K Levels

- Antibiotics
- Clofibrate

- When blood problems reduce oxygen delivery, the heart works harder to facilitate adequate tissue perfusion.
- Use a stethoscope to listen for murmurs, gallops, irregular rhythms, and abnormal BP.
- Systolic BP tends to be lower than normal in patients with anemia.
- Blood pressure may be higher than normal if the patient has too many RBCs.

Renal and Urinary Assessment

- Check the urinary meatus for bleeding or other abnormalities.
- Obtain a clean-catch or catheterized urine specimen for testing as ordered.
- Hematuria is the abnormal presence of gross or microscopic blood in urine. Red blood cells commonly do not appear in the urine without clinical symptoms; however, strenuous exercise can also cause hematuria.

Musculoskeletal Assessment

- Abdominal or bone pain may occur in patients with hyper- or hypoproliferative disorders (i.e., sickle cell anemia, leukemia) or infection.

- Leukemia is a malignant proliferation of white blood cell precursors, or blasts, in bone marrow or lymph tissue, which increases the pressure in the bones.
- Sickle cell anemia causes RBCs to become sickle shaped. The abnormal cells accumulate in capillaries and smaller blood vessels, making the blood more viscous, impairing normal circulation, and causing pain, tissue infarctions, and swelling.
- Assess the range of joint motion and observe for swelling, joint pain, or motion limitation.

Abdominal Assessment

- Advise the patient to empty his or her bladder before the examination to facilitate an abdominal assessment.
- There should be no visible masses. If the abdomen is distended, inquire about changes in bowel patterns and urination.
- Lightly palpate the upper left quadrant of the abdomen for tenderness. The adult spleen is not usually palpable. An enlarged spleen occurs with many hematological problems such as anemia, neutropenia, **thrombocytopenia** (low platelet count), or polycythemia vera (excessive RBC's). Splenomegaly may also occur in conditions such as cirrhosis, hepatitis, mononucleosis, and splenic rupture.
- Palpate gently, as an enlarged spleen may be tender and may rupture easily (Fig. 33.13).

CASE STUDY: EPISODE 2

Ms. Starr's physical examination reveals heart rate 118 beats per minute, BP 90/72 mm Hg, and respiratory rate 26 breaths per minute. Her skin and nailbeds are pale, and her tongue is red and swollen. She is scheduled to have blood samples obtained for complete blood cell count (CBC) with differential. The nurse practitioner also completes a nutritional assessment to determine any possible deficits…

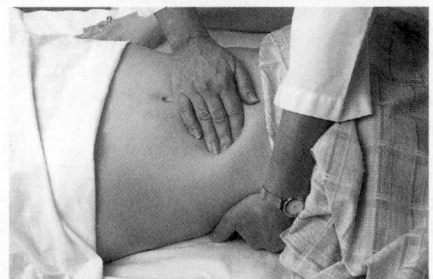

FIGURE 33.13 Palpating for splenomegaly. Palpation of the spleen is best performed with the patient in a supine position with abdomen relaxed. The upper left quadrant is lightly palpated for tenderness. If splenomegaly is noted, palpate gently because the enlarged spleen may rupture with deep palpation.

Connection Check 33.5

When completing a history and physical examination on a patient with a hematological disorder, which action is appropriate?

A. Deeply palpate the spleen to determine the extent of splenomegaly
B. Perform a respiratory assessment after moderate exercise for accurate measurement of depth and rhythm
C. Inspect oral mucous membranes and the tongue for lesions, swelling, and pain
D. Suggest a bone marrow biopsy if the patient reports decreased energy levels

DIAGNOSTIC STUDIES

Laboratory Profile

Table 33.7 presents an overview of the most common diagnostic studies used to assess hematological function.

Complete Blood Count

The most common test used for routine screening of hematological function is the complete blood count (CBC). This diagnostic test provides a highly informative profile of data on multiple blood values, identifying the total number of blood cells (leukocytes, erythrocytes, and platelets) as well as the Hgb, Hct, and RBC indices (mean corpuscular volume [MCV], mean corpuscular hemoglobin [MCH], and mean

Table 33.7 Laboratory Profile

Test	Normal Range for Adults	Significance of Abnormal Findings
Red blood cell (RBC) count	Women: 3.61 – 5.11 million/mm³ Men: 4.21 – 5.81 million/mm³	Increased RBCs (polycythemia or erythrocytosis) can result from: ● High altitude or after increased physical training ● Chronic anoxia ● Polycythemia or erythrocytosis Decreased RBCs can result from: ● Anemia or blood loss ● Abnormal loss of erythrocytes ● Abnormal destruction of erythrocytes ● Lack of needed elements or hormones for erythrocyte production ● Bone marrow suppression
Hematocrit	Women: 36%–48% Men: 42%–52%	Same as for RBC
Hemoglobin	Women: 11.7–15.5 g/dL Men: 14–17.3 g/dL	Same as for RBC
Mean corpuscular volume (MCV)	Women: 78–102 µm³ Men: 78–100 µm³	Increased levels: (*macrocytic*, or larger than normal) pernicious anemia and folic acid deficiencies Decreased levels: (*microcytic*, or smaller than normal) iron-deficiency anemia and lead poisoning
Mean corpuscular hemoglobin (MCH)	25–35 pg/cell	Same as for MCV
Mean corpuscular hemoglobin concentration (MCHC)	31%–37%	Increased levels: (rare) spherocytosis or anemia Decreased levels: iron-deficiency anemia or a hemoglobinopathy
White blood cell (WBC) count	4.50–11.1 10³/mm³	Increased levels: infection, inflammation, autoimmune disorders, and leukemia Decreased levels: prolonged infection or bone marrow depression
Reticulocyte count	0.5%–2.5% of the total RBC count	Increased levels: hemolysis or blood loss; therapeutic response Decreased levels: possible inadequate RBC production (i.e., pernicious anemia) or hypoproliferative bone marrow (hypoplastic anemia)

Table 33.7 Laboratory Profile—cont'd

Test	Normal Range for Adults	Significance of Abnormal Findings
Serum iron (Fe)	30–160 mcg/dL (higher in men)	Increased levels: excess iron; hemochromatosis; liver disorders; megaloblastic anemia
		Decreased levels: iron-deficiency anemia; hemorrhage
Serum ferritin	20–400 ng/mL (lower in premenopausal women)	Same as for iron
Total iron-binding capacity	250–410 mcg/dL	Increased levels: iron-deficiency anemia
		Decreased levels: anemia, hemorrhage, hemolysis; hemochromatosis
Transferrin saturation	20%–50%	Decreased levels: iron-deficiency anemia; hemochromatosis
Platelets	150,000–450,000/µL	Increased levels: thrombocytosis; may indicate polycythemia vera or malignancy; splenectomy (temporary increase)
		Decreased levels: thrombocytopenia; suppressed bone marrow function, autoimmune disease, hypersplenism, or splenomegaly
Hemoglobin electrophoresis	Hgb A: 95%–100% (normal)	Variations indicate hemoglobinopathies
	Hgb A2: 1.5%–3% (normal)	4%–5.8% = beta-thalassemia minor
	Hgb F: Under 1% (normal)	Under 1.5% = Hgb H disease
		2%–5%: beta-thalassemia minor
		10%–90%: beta-thalassemia major
		5%–15%: beta-thalassemia minor
		Homozygous Hgb S:
		70%–98% = sickle cell disease
		Homozygous Hgb C:
		90%–98% = Hgb C disease
		Heterozygous Hgb C: 24%–44% = Hgb C trait
Direct Coombs' and indirect Coombs' test	Negative	Positive findings indicate antibodies to RBCs
Prothrombin time (PT)	10–13 seconds	Prolonged PT may indicate possible deficiencies in clotting factors V and VII; response to oral anticoagulant therapy
		Decreased time may indicate vitamin K excess
Bleeding time	3–8 minutes	Prolonged bleeding time may indicate a platelet function disorder or deficiency of clotting factors
Platelet aggregation	Factor VIII (antihemophilic globulin) 50%–200%	Diminished aggregation may indicate von Willebrand's disease

1 Cubic millimeter (mm³) = 1 microliter (µl).

corpuscular hemoglobin concentration [MCHC]). These laboratory tests, their normal values, and nursing implications are summarized in Table 33.7, as well as other laboratory tests that may be done to evaluate hematological and lymphatic functions.

The RBC count measures circulating RBCs in 1 mm³ of blood and is calculated as the percentage of RBCs in the total blood volume. A low Hct suggests anemia, hemodilution, or massive blood loss. A high Hct indicates polycythemia or hemoconcentration caused by blood loss or dehydration. The Hgb level is the total amount of hemoglobin in the blood, and assessment of Hgb levels measures the severity of anemia or polycythemia and monitors the patient's response to therapy. A low Hgb level may indicate anemia, recent hemorrhage, or fluid retention, causing hemodilution. A high Hgb level suggests hemoconcentration from polycythemia or dehydration.

The CBC can measure other features of the RBCs, including MCV, MCH, and MCHC. Mean corpuscular volume (MCV) expresses the average size of the erythrocytes and indicates whether they are undersized (microcytic), oversized (macrocytic), or normal (normocytic) and is useful in classifying anemias. An elevated MCV indicates the cell is larger than normal (macrocytic) and can be seen in megaloblastic anemias. A decreased MCV indicates the cell is smaller than normal (microcytic) and can be seen in iron-deficiency anemia. Mean corpuscular hemoglobin (MCH), the Hgb-to-RBC count ratio, gives the weight of Hgb in an average RBC. Mean corpuscular hemoglobin concentration (MCHC), the Hgb weight-to-Hct ratio, defines the concentration of Hgb in 100 mL of packed RBCs. It helps to distinguish normally colored (normochromic) RBCs from paler (hypochromic) RBCs.

The platelet count evaluates the function of platelets, or thrombocytes, which promote coagulation and formation of a hemostatic plug in vascular injury. The platelet count also determines the ability of the patient's blood to clot normally. A count lower than 50,000/μL may result in spontaneous bleeding; when the count is lower than 5,000/μL, fatal central nervous system bleeding or massive GI hemorrhage is possible. A decreased count (thrombocytopenia, 80–100/μL) can indicate aplastic or hypoplastic bone marrow, infiltrative bone marrow disease such as leukemia or disseminated infection, or ineffective thrombopoiesis caused by folic acid or vitamin B_{12} deficiency. An increased platelet count (thrombocytosis) can result from hemorrhage, infectious disorders, iron-deficiency anemia, recent surgery, pregnancy, splenectomy, or inflammatory disorders. Whenever the platelet count is abnormal, diagnosis usually requires a CBC, bone marrow biopsy, direct Coombs' test, and serum protein electrophoresis for confirmation.

The WBC count measures all leukocytes present in 1 mm³ of blood, and a WBC count with differential determines the percentages of different types of leukocytes circulating in the blood. The WBC count may increase or decrease significantly in certain diseases but is diagnostically useful when the patient's differential and condition are considered. The purpose of the WBC count is to determine infection or inflammation, to detect and identify various types of leukemia, to determine the need for further tests, such as the WBC differential or bone marrow biopsy, and to monitor responses to antibiotic therapy, chemotherapy, or radiation therapy. An increased WBC count (*leukocytosis*) commonly indicates infection such as an abscess, meningitis, appendicitis, or tonsillitis, or it may result from leukemia and tissue necrosis caused by burns, myocardial infarction, or gangrene. A decreased count (*leukopenia*) signals bone marrow depression that may result from viral infections or from toxic reactions such as those following treatment with antineoplastics (medications that destroy cancer cells), ingestion of mercury

or other heavy metals, or exposure to benzene or arsenicals. It may also indicate influenza, typhoid fever, infectious hepatitis, mononucleosis, measles, or rubella.

Patient Preparation and Nursing Implications

Explain to the patient that the complete blood count (CBC) is used to assess for changes in RBC, WBC, Hct, and Hgb. Inform the patient that there are no dietary restrictions required for the test, and describe that the test requires a blood sample and that slight discomfort may be experienced from the tourniquet and needle puncture. It is important to notify the laboratory and practitioner of medications the patient is taking that may affect test results; it may be necessary to restrict them. Confirm the patient's identity using two patient identifiers according to facility policy. Perform a venipuncture (Box 33.2). A lavender-topped ethylenediaminetetraacetic acid (EDTA) tube is used to collect the blood sample. (Ethylenediaminetetraacetic acid is an anticoagulant that prevents the sample from clotting). The tube is filled and then gently inverted several times to mix the sample and the anticoagulant in the tube. The accuracy of CBC results can be impacted if the specimen collection technique is not correct. For example, the RBC, CBC, Hgb,

Box 33.2 Patient Preparation for Venipuncture

Key Steps

1. Verify the order.
2. Confirm the patient's identity using two patient identifiers according to facility policy.
3. Perform hand hygiene and put on gloves. If the patient has a history of a latex allergy, avoid the use of latex gloves.
4. Explain the procedure to ease anxiety and ensure cooperation.
5. Clean the venipuncture site with an alcohol pad in a back-and-forth motion. Allow the skin to dry before performing venipuncture and then insert the needle into the vein at a 30-degree angle. Continue to fill the required tubes and gently rotate each tube as you remove it to help mix the additive with the sample.
6. Remove the tourniquet as soon as blood flows adequately to prevent stasis and hemolysis, which can impair test results.

Postprocedure Care

1. After gently removing the needle, apply gauze and direct pressure to the venipuncture site until the bleeding stops.
2. Inform the practitioner of abnormal results.

Precautions

1. Handle the sample gently to prevent hemolysis.
2. Send the sample to the laboratory immediately.

Complications

1. May include hematoma at the venipuncture site.
2. Infection may result from poor technique.

and Hct levels may be falsely elevated secondary to venous stasis if the tourniquet is left in place for longer than one minute.

Reticulocyte Count

Reticulocytes are usually larger than mature RBCs because they still contain the network composed of ribosome clusters from the erythroblast precursor cell. Reticulocytes are non-nucleated, immature RBCs that remain in the peripheral blood for 24 to 48 hours while maturing. The reticulocyte count is useful for evaluating anemia, specifically to help distinguish between hypoproliferative and hyperproliferative anemias. The reticulocyte count may also help assess blood loss, evaluate bone marrow response to anemia, and evaluate treatments for anemia. The test involves counting the number of reticulocytes in a whole blood sample, where the value is expressed as a percentage of the total RBC count. A low reticulocyte count indicates hypoproliferative bone marrow (hypoplastic anemia) or ineffective erythropoiesis (pernicious anemia). Pernicious anemia occurs when the body cannot properly absorb vitamin B_{12} from the gastrointestinal tract because vitamin B_{12} is necessary for the proper development of RBCs. To absorb vitamin B_{12}, the body uses a special protein called *intrinsic factor*, which is released by cells in the stomach. When the stomach does not make enough intrinsic factor, the intestine cannot properly absorb vitamin B_{12}; hence, erythropoiesis is disrupted.

An increase in the percentage of reticulocytes indicates that the release of RBCs into the bloodstream is occurring more rapidly than usual. A high reticulocyte count may indicate a bone marrow response to anemia caused by hemolysis or blood loss. The increase in the reticulocyte count is a physiological response to the need for more RBCs.

Patient Preparation and Nursing Implications

Explain to the patient that the reticulocyte count is used to detect anemia or to monitor its treatment. Inform the patient that there are no dietary restrictions required for the test and describe that the test requires a blood sample and that slight discomfort may be experienced from the tourniquet and needle puncture. If the patient is an infant or child, the parents are told that a small amount of blood will be taken from the child's finger or earlobe. It is important to notify the laboratory and practitioner of medications the patient is taking that may affect test results; it may be necessary to restrict them. Confirm the patient's identity using two patient identifiers according to facility policy. Perform a venipuncture. The collection tube is filled completely and then gently inverted several times to mix the sample and the anticoagulant in the tube.

Hemoglobin Electrophoresis

Hemoglobin electrophoresis is the most useful laboratory method for separating and measuring normal and abnormal hemoglobin. The purpose of this test is to help diagnose **thalassemias**, which are a group of inherited autosomal recessive genetic disorders characterized by defective synthesis in one or more of the polypeptide chains needed for Hgb production. They most commonly occur as a result of reduced or absent production of the Hgb alpha or beta chains. This affects Hgb production and impairs RBC synthesis. Hemoglobin electrophoresis may show elevated or normal Hgb A2 levels (beta-thalassemia trait) or elevated Hgb A2 and F levels with reduced or absent Hgb A1 levels (beta-thalassemia major).

Patient Preparation and Nursing Implications

Describe to the patient that hemoglobin electrophoresis evaluates Hgb and explain that no dietary restrictions are required. If the patient is an infant or child, explain to the parents that a small amount of blood will be taken from the child's finger. Confirm the patient's identity using two patient identifiers according to agency policy. Ask whether a blood transfusion has been received within the past 4 months. Perform a venipuncture and collect the sample in a 3- or 4.5-mL EDTA tube (lavender top) that includes an anticoagulant in the tube.

Leukocyte Alkaline Phosphatase

Leukocyte alkaline phosphatase (LAP) is an enzyme produced by normal mature neutrophils. Elevated LAP levels may result from infection, stress, inflammation, pregnancy, steroid use, and leukemia. An elevated neutrophil count without an accompanying elevation in LAP level is associated with chronic myelogenous leukemia. Inform the patient that this test can assist in evaluating for blood disorders. Venipuncture is performed and 1 mL of blood is collected in an EDTA tube.

Coombs Test

A direct Coombs test detects the presence of immunoglobulins (antibodies) on the surface of RBCs that develop through sensitization to antigens (such as Rh factor). This test is performed to diagnose hemolytic disease of the newborn, to investigate hemolytic transfusion reactions, and to aid in the differential diagnosis of hemolytic anemias. Medications such as quinidine, methyldopa, cephalosporins, sulfonamides, hydralazine, levodopa, melphalan, penicillin, rifampin, streptomycin, and isoniazid may cause a false-positive Coombs test result. A positive Coombs test in the neonate indicates that maternal antibodies have crossed the placental barrier and coated the fetal RBCs, causing hemolytic disease of the neonate. In other patients, a positive test result may indicate hemolytic anemia and may help differentiate between autoimmune and secondary hemolytic anemias. A positive test may also indicate sepsis. A weakly positive test may indicate a transfusion reaction in which the patient's antibodies reacted with transfused RBCs that contained the corresponding antigen.

Patient Preparation and Nursing Implications

Describe the purpose of the test and how it is performed. Inform the patient that this test is used in assessing for disorders that break down RBCs. Explain to the patient that no dietary restrictions are needed. Perform the venipuncture and collect the specimen in two 5-mL EDTA tubes.

Iron: Serum Ferritin, Transferrin, Total Iron-Binding Capacity

Serum iron (Fe) levels are measured directly, and blood levels should be drawn in the morning because of a diurnal variation in serum iron, with lower evening values. The patient is instructed to avoid taking any iron supplements for at least 24 hours before the test is performed.

Ferritin is a protein that stores iron in the body. A ferritin level provides information about the body's ability to store iron for later use and is usually performed with iron testing and total iron-binding capacity (TIBC). Low ferritin levels may indicate iron deficiency, chronic GI bleeding, or heavy menstrual bleeding. High levels may indicate alcoholic liver disease, hemochromatosis (excessive iron absorption), hemolytic anemia, Hodgkin's lymphoma, or megaloblastic anemia. Illnesses such as infections, inflammations, and malignant diseases cause increased levels and therefore may make ferritin levels unreliable as an indicator of iron stores.

Transferrin, a plasma protein, transports circulating iron obtained from dietary sources or from the breakdown of RBCs for use in Hgb synthesis or to the liver, spleen, and bone marrow for storage. The purpose of the transferrin level test is to determine the iron-transporting capacity of the blood and evaluate iron metabolism in iron-deficiency anemia. Inadequate transferrin levels may lead to impaired Hgb synthesis and, possibly, anemia. Low serum levels may indicate inadequate transferrin production caused by hepatic damage or excessive protein loss from renal disease. Decreased transferrin levels may also result from acute or chronic infection and cancer. Increased serum transferrin levels may indicate severe iron deficiency.

Total iron-binding capacity measures the amount of iron that appears in plasma if all transferrin is saturated with iron. The TIBC is used with the serum iron to calculate transferrin saturation. As previously discussed, iron is essential to the formation and function of Hgb. In iron deficiency, serum iron levels decrease and TIBC increases, decreasing saturation. In chronic inflammation, serum iron may be low despite adequate body stores, but TIBC may be unchanged or decreased to preserve normal saturation. Iron overload may not alter serum levels until later, but serum iron increases and TIBC remain the same, increasing saturation.

Patient Preparation and Nursing Implications

Blood specimens for serum iron and TIBC are collected in iron-free tubes. Specimens for serum ferritin may be placed in either green- or lavender-top tubes. Check with the laboratory for the total amount needed. Iron must be drawn in the morning, and an overnight fast is recommended. For the transferrin level test, an interfering factor may be hormonal contraceptives and late pregnancy, possibly causing an increase in level.

Clotting Studies: Prothrombin Time, Bleeding Time, International Normalized Ratio, Partial Thromboplastin Time, Platelet Aggregation

Prothrombin Time

Prothrombin time (PT) measures the time required for a fibrin clot to form in a citrated plasma sample after addition of calcium ions and tissue thromboplastin (factor III). The purpose of this test is to evaluate the extrinsic coagulation system (factors V, VII, and X, and prothrombin and fibrinogen) and to monitor response to oral anticoagulant therapy. A prolonged PT may indicate deficiencies in fibrinogen; prothrombin; factors V, VII, or Xl; or vitamin K. It may also result as a therapeutic response from ongoing oral anticoagulant therapy (warfarin, Coumadin; tinzaparin sodium, Innohep). A prolonged PT that exceeds two and one-half times the control value usually indicates abnormal bleeding. More than 1 g per day of salicylates may interfere with the PT value by increasing the value and increasing the risk of bleeding.

Patient Preparation and Nursing Implications

Explain to the patient that the PT test determines whether the blood clots normally. When appropriate, explain that this test monitors the effects of oral anticoagulants; the test will occur daily when therapy begins and will be repeated at longer intervals as the medication results in the desired PT levels. Inform the patient that no dietary restrictions are required. Notify the laboratory and practitioner of medications the patient is taking that may affect test results; they may be restricted. Perform a venipuncture and collect the sample in a 3- or 4.5-mL sodium citrate tube. Gently invert the tube several times to thoroughly mix the sample and the anticoagulant. Remove the needle and apply direct pressure with dry gauze to stop bleeding. Ensure that subdermal bleeding has stopped before removing pressure. If a large hematoma develops at the venipuncture site, monitor pulses distal to the site. Inform the practitioner of abnormal results.

Bleeding Time

The purpose of the bleeding time test is to assess overall hemostatic (clotting) function and to detect platelet function disorders. It is most commonly performed in the patient with a personal or family history of bleeding disorders but is also useful for preoperative screening.

> **⚠ Safety Alert** A bleeding time test is usually not recommended for a patient with a platelet count of less than 75,000 µL because of an increased risk for massive bleeding and ineffective clotting.

Bleeding time measures the duration of bleeding after a measured skin incision. There are three methods of measuring bleeding: template, Ivy, and Duke. The template bleeding time procedure is performed with lancet devices that make two reproducible skin incisions 1-mm deep and several millimeters long. A blood pressure cuff is wrapped around the upper arm and inflated to 40 mm Hg. The drops of blood are blotted with filter paper every 30 seconds until the bleeding stops in both cuts. The average bleeding times of the two cuts is recorded.

Because of these small wounds, the primary hemostatic mechanisms involving platelets and blood vessels can stop the bleeding independently of coagulation reactions. Prolonged bleeding time may indicate disorders associated with thrombocytopenia, such as Hodgkin's disease, acute leukemia, disseminated intravascular coagulation (DIC), hemolytic disease of the newborn, severe hepatic disease (i.e., cirrhosis), or severe deficiency of factors I, II, V, VII, VIII, IX, and XI. Thrombasthenia is a bleeding disorder caused by abnormal platelet function characterized by abnormal clot retraction, prolonged bleeding time, and lack of aggregation of the platelets. Prolonged bleeding time in a patient with a normal platelet count suggests a platelet function disorder (thrombasthenia) and requires additional analysis with clot retraction, prothrombin consumption, and platelet aggregation tests.

> **⚠ Safety Alert** WARNING! If the bleeding does not stop in 15 minutes after the cuts are made, stop the test and maintain a pressure bandage over the incision or puncture sites for 24 to 48 hours to prevent further bleeding. Anticoagulants, NSAIDs, aspirin, and aspirin compounds (prolonged bleeding time) can interfere with this test.

International Normalized Ratio

The **International Normalized Ratio (INR)**, also known as the *INR system*, is performed to measure PT (prothrombin time) and to evaluate the effectiveness of oral anticoagulant therapy (warfarin sodium, Coumadin). Laboratories convert their PT values into an INR, and this test is not used to screen for coagulopathies. For patients receiving warfarin therapy, the therapeutic INR is 2 to 3. For those who are receiving warfarin therapy and have mechanical prosthetic heart valves, the therapeutic INR is 2.5 to 3.5. Increased INR values may be a sign of disseminated intravascular coagulation (DIC), cirrhosis, hepatitis, vitamin K deficiency, salicylate intoxication, uncontrolled oral anticoagulation, or massive blood transfusion. Perform a venipuncture and collect the sample in a 4.5-mL tube with sodium citrate added. Gently invert the tube several times to thoroughly mix the sample and the anticoagulant. Remove the needle and apply direct pressure to the venipuncture site with dry gauze until bleedings stops.

Partial Thromboplastin Time

The purpose of the **partial thromboplastin time (PTT)** or activated partial thromboplastin time (aPTT) is to screen for deficiencies of the clotting factors in the intrinsic pathways and to monitor response to thrombin inhibitor therapy (heparin, argatroban). It is used to evaluate all the clotting factors of the intrinsic pathway (with the exception of platelets) by mixing decalcified plasma (collected in citrate) and a phospholipid substitute (thromboplastin), adding calcium, and determining the time for visible clot formation using an automated system. The reference range of the PTT is 60 to 70 seconds and aPTT is 30 to 40 seconds after adding an activator (that speeds up the clotting time and results in a narrower reference range). For a patient receiving an anticoagulant, the practitioner needs to specify the reference values for the therapy being delivered. A prolonged PTT may indicate an insufficiency of certain clotting factors, the presence of heparin, the presence of fibrin split products, fibrinolysis, or circulating anticoagulants that are antibodies to specific clotting factors.

Inform the patient that this test can assist in evaluating the effectiveness of blood clotting. A venipuncture is performed, and a blood sample is collected in a 7-mL sodium citrate tube. The tube must be filled completely and then inverted several times to mix with contents of the tube. Direct pressure is applied to the venipuncture site until bleeding stops. If a patient is on anticoagulant therapy, additional pressure at the venipuncture site to control bleeding may be needed.

Platelet Aggregation

Platelet aggregation studies are performed in patients who are suspected of having abnormal platelet function, i.e., those who have a prolonged bleeding time and a normal or near-normal platelet count. Platelet aggregation, or the ability of platelets to clump, can be tested by mixing the patient's plasma with a substance called *ristocetin*, and then the degree of aggregation is noted. Aggregation can be impaired with von Willebrand's disease (see Genetic Connections) and with the use of medications such as aspirin, NSAIDs, antineoplastics, and psychotropic agents. Venous blood (4.5 mL) is collected in a sodium citrate tube. The collection tube is completely filled and then gently inverted several times to mix the sample with the sodium citrate. It is important that pressure is applied directly to the venipuncture site until bleeding stops.

Genetic Connections

Von Willebrand's Disease

Von Willebrand's disease (vWD) is a common hereditary platelet disorder caused by a deficiency or dysfunction of von Willebrand factor (vWF). Von Willebrand's disease affects the normal interaction with platelets and impairs primary hemostasis, causing prolonged bleeding (like nosebleeds) and easy bruising. vWD is classified into three major types (types 1, 2, and 3). The disorder is caused by a gene located on chromosome 12 inherited as an autosomal dominant trait (types 1 and 2) or autosomal recessive trait (type 3).

Patients with vWF generally have a normal PT, abnormal platelet function screening test, and prolonged partial thromboplastin time (PTT). A vWF antigen testing helps establish the type of vWD. For most affected patients, vWD is a mild, manageable bleeding disorder in which clinically severe hemorrhage occurs only in the event of trauma or invasive procedures.

The main treatment options for patients with vWD are desmopressin (DDAVP), recombinant vWF, and vWF/factor VIII (vWF/FVIII) concentrates. In addition, antifibrinolytic medications (i.e., aminocaproic acid, tranexamic acid) can be used orally or intravenously to treat mild mucocutaneous bleeding. Patients with possible vWD should be asked about any family or personal history of bleeding problems. Patients should also be asked about the use of medications that might affect coagulation.

Examination of the Bone Marrow

Bone Marrow Aspiration and Biopsy

The purpose of a bone marrow aspiration and biopsy is to diagnose thrombocytopenia, leukemias, granulomas, anemias, and primary and metastatic tumors. This diagnostic study is also performed to determine causes of infection, to help stage diseases such as Hodgkin's disease, to evaluate chemotherapy, and to monitor myelosuppression (Table 33.8).

Table 33.8 Interpretation of Bone Marrow Results

Normal Results	Abnormal Results
• Yellow bone marrow contains fat cells and connective tissue. • Red bone marrow contains hematopoietic cells, fat cells, and connective tissue. • The iron stain, which measures hemosiderin (storage iron), has a +2 level. • Negative Sudan black B stain, which shows granulocytes. • The periodic acid–Schiff (PAS) stain, which detects glycogen reactions, is negative.	• Decreased hemosiderin levels in an iron stain may indicate a true iron deficiency. • A positive iron stain can differentiate acute myelogenous leukemia from acute lymphoblastic leukemia (negative stain). • A positive iron stain may also suggest granulation in myeloblasts. • Increased hemosiderin levels may suggest other types of anemias or blood disorders. • A positive PAS stain may suggest acute or chronic lymphocytic leukemia, amyloidosis, thalassemia, lymphoma, infectious mononucleosis, iron-deficiency anemia, or sideroblastic anemia.

Bone marrow biopsy and aspiration (Fig. 33.14) involve the collection of a soft tissue specimen from the medullary canals of the long bone and interstices of cancellous bone for histological and hematological examination. The procedure is performed by aspiration or needle biopsy under local anesthesia.

- Aspiration biopsy: removal of a fluid specimen from the bone marrow
- Needle biopsy: removal of a core of marrow cells

It is common to perform both methods at the same time to obtain the best possible specimens.

When leukemic cells are identified on bone marrow aspirate smears, special stains are used to explore the interpretation of the abnormal cell population. These stains include the iron stain, which measures hemosiderin (storage iron), the Sudan black B stain, which shows the number of granulocytes, and the periodic acid–Schiff (PAS) stain, which detects glycogen reactions. This microscopic evaluation can be used to distinguish acute myelogenous from acute lymphoblastic leukemias or to subtype myelogenous leukemias.

Patient Preparation and Nursing Implications
Before the Test

- Ensure that the patient has received teaching from the provider performing the procedure, has given informed consent, and that all allergies are documented.

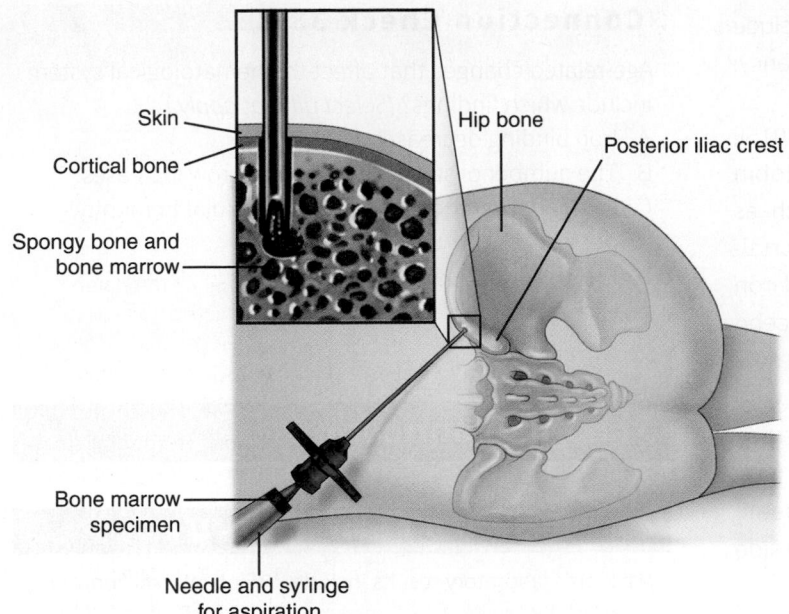

FIGURE 33.14 Bone marrow biopsy and aspiration. The patient is positioned into the prone or lateral decubitus position for biopsy of the posterior iliac crest. The patient may experience feelings of pressure upon insertion of the biopsy needle and a brief, pulling pain will be experienced on removal of the marrow. Some patients can hear a crunching sound or feel a scraping sensation as the needle punctures the bone.

- Assess for bleeding risk, such as medical history, coagulation laboratory results, platelet count, anticoagulant therapy, and other medications or supplements that may interfere with clotting.
- Explain the purpose of the test and the procedure.
- Explain that a blood sample (aspiration) is required before the biopsy for laboratory testing (cells and fluids from marrow).
- Explain which bone site (sternum, anterior or posterior iliac crest, vertebral spinous process, rib, or tibia) will be used. The most common biopsy site is the back of the hip (*posterior superior iliac crest*).
- Explain to the patient that pressure will be felt upon insertion of the biopsy needle and a brief, pulling pain may be experienced on removal of the marrow, caused by the mild suction of the syringe. Some patients can hear a crunching sound or feel a scraping sensation as the needle punctures the bone.
- Tell the patient that the actual test takes only 5 to 10 minutes. If the patient is anxious, use relaxation techniques, or administer a mild sedative, if prescribed, 1 hour before the test.
- Assist the patient to the appropriate position and help maintain a comfortable patient position. If the insertion site is the posterior iliac crest, assist the patient into the prone or lateral decubitus position. If the sample is taken from the sternum or anterior iliac crest, the patient will be supine.
- Encourage deep breaths and relaxation techniques during the procedure.

After the Test

- After aspiration, apply direct pressure over the puncture site according to agency policy for 5 to 10 minutes until bleeding stops. Cover the site with a sterile dressing.

- Instruct the patient to rest for several hours. Report bleeding that completely soaks the dressing or continues for more than 24 hours. Reinforce the dressing, if needed, but do not remove it for at least 24 hours.
- Properly label and promptly transport all specimens to the laboratory.
- Assess for postprocedural pain and provide analgesia as ordered.
- Teach the patient to watch for signs of infection.

AGE-RELATED CHANGES TO THE HEMATOLOGICAL SYSTEM

While the human body ages, the number of cells of the body is gradually reduced. Lean body mass decreases, but fat tissue increases until approximately age 60 years. Bone mass and intracellular fluids also tend to decrease, and normal aging causes a decrease in total body water. With the decrease in total body water, there is less fluid in the bloodstream, so blood volume decreases, with lower levels of plasma proteins. The lower plasma protein level may be related to a low dietary intake of proteins and reduced protein production by the older liver (see Evidence-Based Practice).

Evidence-Based Practice

Older Adults and Anemia

The prevalence of anemia increases with age, with the frequency of anemia doubling in individuals aged 85 years and older compared with individuals aged 65 to 84 years. Additionally, the prevalence of anemia in older people is considerably greater in nursing homes than in other settings. In nursing homes, anemia is present in 48% to 63 % of residents. Various causes that contribute to anemia include iron deficiency, chronic inflammation, renal insufficiency, folate deficiency, and vitamin B$_{12}$ deficiency.

According to a systematic review (Tay & Soiza, 2015), many studies suggest oral iron improves hemoglobin and that this will lead to tangible benefits, such as improved quality of life and lower morbidity and mortality of older adults. The meta-analysis found that oral iron therapy increases hemoglobin levels more than placebo or no treatment. However, intravenous iron may be necessary to treat iron deficiency anemia in patients who have poor iron absorption in the gastrointestinal tract, patients with severe iron deficiency or chronic blood loss, patients who are having treatment with erythropoietin, or patients who cannot tolerate oral iron due to the side effects.

Tay, H. S., & Soiza, R. L. (2015). Systematic review and meta-analysis: what is the evidence for oral iron supplementation in treating anaemia in elderly people? *Drugs & Aging*, 32(2), 149-158. https://doi:10.1007/s40266-015-0241-5

While bone marrow ages, it produces fewer blood cells (Table 33.9). The bone marrow's ability to produce RBCs and WBCs may be decreased. The number of circulating RBCs, along with Hgb and Hct levels, are reduced, and this may contribute to fatigue. Lymphocytes decrease in their number and ability to defend against bacteria, which reduces the ability to fight infection.

Table 33.9 Age-Related Changes in Hematology Results

Test	Age-related Changes
Hematocrit	No normal decline with age
Hemoglobin (Hgb)	No normal decline with age
Reticulocyte count	Slight decrease
Lymphocytes	Both T- and B-cell levels decrease
Albumin	Declines because of a decrease in liver size and enzymes
Serum iron (Fe)	Slight decrease
Iron binding	Decrease
Platelets	No change with age
Sedimentation rate (ESR)	Increase
Vitamin B$_{12}$	Slight decrease

Connection Check 33.8

Age-related changes that affect the hematological system include which findings? *(Select all that apply.)*
A. Iron binding decreases.
B. The number of stem cells in the marrow increases.
C. Lymphocyte function, especially cellular immunity, decreases.
D. Platelet adhesiveness decreases.
E. Hematocrit decreases.

Making Connections

CASE STUDY: WRAP-UP

Ms. Starr's laboratory results include RBC count 3 million/mm^3, Hct 31%, Hgb 9 g/dL, and a decrease in serum ferritin levels. The laboratory results for RBCs, Hct, and Hgb show a decrease in all three values. Combining the laboratory values with vital signs and reported symptoms identifies her disorder. Low Hct and Hgb and low ferritin level combined with her complaints of generalized fatigue and increased shortness of breath and her pale skin and nailbeds, along with red, swollen tongue, suggest iron-deficiency anemia. The decrease in serum ferritin level further supports the differentiation of this anemia. Ms. Starr is prescribed iron supplements and referred to a hematologist for further evaluation.

Case Study Questions

1. The nurse correlates which clinical manifestations with Ms. Starr's diagnosis of iron-deficiency anemia? *(Select all that apply.)*
   A. Decreased temperature
   B. Decreased heart rate
   C. Increased blood pressure
   D. Increased heart rate
   E. Increased respiratory rate

2. Which diagnostic result confirms Ms. Starr's diagnosis of iron-deficiency anemia?
   A. Decreased transferrin saturation
   B. Decreased mean corpuscular volume
   C. Increased total iron-binding capacity
   D. Increased ferritin levels

3. The nurse assesses for which clinical manifestation as a compensatory mechanism for iron-deficiency anemia?
   A. Increased respiratory rate
   B. Increased blood pressure
   C. Decreased temperature
   D. Decreased pulse rate

4. During an assessment of Ms. Starr's mouth, which finding does the nurse correlate with iron-deficiency anemia?

    A. Red, beefy gums

    B. Loss of teeth

    C. Red, swollen, tender tongue

    D. Xerostomia

5. Ms. Starr is scheduled to have a serum iron level in 1 month. The nurse includes which instructions about this test?

    A. "You will need to fast for 12 hours before the test."

    B. "This sample needs to be drawn in the morning."

    C. "Continue to take your iron supplements."

    D. "This test will require three different samples taken at hourly intervals."

nutrients, and other substances in the body. The primary function of RBCs is to transport oxygen to the cells. The primary function of WBCs is to fight infection, destroy foreign matter, and eliminate damaged or abnormal cells in the body. White blood cells are an integral part of the immune system and are necessary for its functioning. Platelets and clotting factors work together in the process of blood clotting and the control of bleeding. The lymphatic system also is involved in the immune response. Blood tests to evaluate the number and types of cells present, their size and shape, and the ability of the blood to clot are the primary diagnostic tests used to evaluate the hematological system. Aspiration of bone marrow may be necessary to provide additional information about blood formation. Nursing care of the patient undergoing diagnostic testing for a possible hematological disorder is both educational, explaining the purpose of the test and any special preparation or expected sensations during the test, and supportive.

CHAPTER SUMMARY

The hematological system is composed of the blood, blood cells, lymph, and organs involved with blood formation or blood storage. Blood is the transport medium for oxygen,

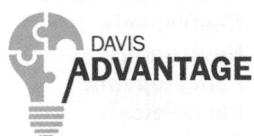

To explore learning resources for this chapter, go to **Davis Advantage** and find:

– Answers to in-text questions

– Chapter Resources and Activities

– NCLEX®-Style Chapter Review Questions

– Bibliography

Chapter 34

Coordinating Care for Patients With Hematological Disorders

Margaret McCormick

LEARNING OUTCOMES

Content in this chapter is designed to assist in:

1. Describing the epidemiology of disorders of the hematological system
2. Correlating clinical manifestations to pathophysiological processes of nonmalignant and malignant hematological disorders:
   a. Iron-deficiency anemia
   b. Vitamin B_{12} and pernicious anemia
   c. Folic acid deficiency anemia
   d. Sickle cell anemia
   e. Aplastic anemia
   f. Glucose-6-phosphate dehydrogenase (G6PD) deficiency
   g. Polycythemia vera
   h. Idiopathic (immune) thrombocytopenia purpura
   i. Leukemia
   j. Malignant lymphoma
   k. Multiple myeloma
3. Describing the diagnostic results used to confirm disorders of the hematological system
4. Discussing the medical management of identified hematological disorders
5. Developing a comprehensive plan of nursing care for patients with nonmalignant and malignant hematological disorders
6. Designing a plan of care that includes pharmacological, dietary, and lifestyle considerations for patients with nonmalignant and malignant hematological disorders
7. Coordinating the interprofessional plan of care for the patient with hematological disorders

ESSENTIAL TERMS

Allogeneic
Anemia
Apoptosis
Autologous
Basophils
Cobalamin
Cryoprecipitate
Eosinophils
Erythrocytes
Erythrocytosis
Erythropoietin
Glossitis
Graft-versus-host disease
Hemarthrosis
Hematology
Hematopoiesis
Hemophilia
Hyperviscosity
Koilonychia
Leukocytes
Leukocytosis

Lhermitte's sign
Lymph
Lymphocytes
Monocytes
Myelodysplasia
Myeloma
Myelosuppression
Neutropenia
Neutrophils
Pancytopenia
Panmyelosis
Pernicious anemia
Phagocytize
Pica
Platelets
Polycythemia
Polycythemia vera
Schilling's test
Thrombocytes
Thrombocytopenia
Thrombocytosis
Thymus

CONCEPTS

- Assessment
- Comfort
- Hematologic Regulation
- Infection
- Medication
- Nutrition
- Oxygenation

Finding Connections

CASE STUDY: EPISODE 1

Follow this patient throughout the chapter.

Mr. William Owens is a 62-year-old male who presents to his healthcare provider with complaints of fatigue, weakness, and shortness of breath on climbing stairs. He also states that he has noticed some bleeding of his gums sometimes when he brushes his teeth but otherwise has been in relatively good health. Mr. Owens has worked in the oil refinery business since he was a teenager. He has a history of smoking one-half to one pack of cigarettes daily for 40+ years, likes to drink beer "with the guys," and has no history of substance use...

INTRODUCTION

Hematology is the study of the blood and the lymphatic system. Blood is composed of plasma (the liquid transporting medium), blood cells, oxygen, nutrients, carbon dioxide, antibodies, and other proteins. **Hematopoiesis** is the production of blood cells in the bone marrow located in flat and irregular bones. The blood cells are red blood cells (RBCs), white blood cells (WBCs), and platelets.

Red blood cells, or **erythrocytes**, are normally round in shape and are without nuclei. The lack of a nucleus makes them malleable and able to squeeze through the small blood capillaries. Red blood cells contain the hemoglobin (Hb) molecule, which bonds with oxygen and becomes oxyhemoglobin in the pulmonary capillaries of the lungs. **Anemia** occurs when there is a reduction in the oxygen-carrying capacity through either fewer RBCs or a reduction in hemoglobin.

There are five different types of WBCs or **leukocytes**: **basophils, eosinophils, neutrophils, monocytes,** and **lymphocytes**. Neutrophils, eosinophils, and basophils are produced in the bone marrow. Neutrophils **phagocytize**, or destroy, pathogens to fight infection, eosinophils respond during an allergic reaction to detoxify the foreign proteins or antibodies, and basophils release histamine in inflammatory reactions. Lymphocytes and monocytes are produced in the lymphatic tissue. Pathogens and dead tissue are phagocytized by monocytes. There are three types of lymphocytes: B cells (produce antibodies to foreign substances), T cells (helper, suppressor, memory, amplifier, delayed hypersensitivity, cytotoxic), and natural killer cells.

The lymphatic system is composed of lymphatic tissue (called *nodes* or *nodules*), lymph (the liquid transporting medium), lymph vessels, the spleen, and the **thymus**. The thymus is a gland located behind the upper sternum that produces T lymphocytes (T cells) and hormones, which mature the immune system. The thymus is larger in infancy and childhood but shrinks with age, and its function is to assist in removing phagocytized pathogens and foreign materials, protect the body from infection, and return fluid to blood vessels to maintain blood pressure. **Lymph** is formed from plasma that is filtered by the blood capillaries and flows through the lymph vessels and lymph nodes. There are three major pairs of lymph nodes: cervical (located in the neck), axillary (located in the underarms), and inguinal (located in the groin). Lymph flows from the left upper quadrant and lower body, through the thoracic duct (in front of the spine), and drains into the left subclavian vein. Lymph from the right upper quadrant enters the right lymphatic duct and drains into the right subclavian vein. The function of the spleen is to produce lymphocytes, monocytes, and certain antibodies. The spleen also phagocytizes old RBCs to form bilirubin.

Platelets or **thrombocytes** are involved with hemostasis, the arresting of the escape of blood from a damaged blood vessel. When a blood vessel is damaged, platelets release serotonin to produce vasoconstriction, becoming sticky and adhering to capillary walls and to one another and forming a platelet plug to stop the initial bleeding. In a series of three stages, platelets release chemicals, or clotting factors, that catalyze the prothrombinase complex to convert prothrombin into thrombin to form a clot. **Thrombocytopenia** is a reduction in the number of platelets, whereas **thrombocytosis** is an increase in platelet production. For normal ranges of blood cells, see Table 34.1.

RED BLOOD CELL DISORDERS

Iron-Deficiency Anemia

Epidemiology

Iron-deficiency anemia (IDA) is considered the most prevalent nutritional deficiency in the world and is highest among non-Caucasian Americans of lower socioeconomic status, especially infants, children, and pregnant women. In the United States, it is highly prevalent among African American and Mexican American women, presumably because of the large numbers of this population with low incomes. It is greater in females than males, especially premenopausal women because of the monthly blood loss with menses. There is an approximate 10% increase of anemia in adults over the age of 65, and this increased incidence of IDA in this population is often a result of the aging process and the increased frequency of chronic diseases. This condition is often referred to as anemia of chronic disease when the specific etiology of the anemia cannot be definitively determined.

Inadequate iron in the diet is often a contributing factor to IDA. Globally, iron intake through food is well below the estimated daily requirement of 8 mg in men aged 19 to 50 years and 18 mg in women, increasing to 22 mg in pregnant females. During periods of blood loss or growth, iron intake may be inadequate to meet the increased demands

Table 34.1 Review of Normal Ranges for Complete Blood Cell Counts (Adult)	
Blood Cell	**Normal Ranges**
Red blood cells (mature, circulating)	Male: 4.21–5.81 million/mm³
	Female: 3.61–5.11 million/mm³
Hemoglobin	Adult (15–64 yr)
	Male 14–17.3 g/dL
	Female 11.7–15.5 g/dL
Hematocrit	42–52% in males
	36–48% in females
Reticulocytes	0.5%–2.5% of total RBC count
White blood cells (total)	4.5–11.1 10³ cells/ mm³
	4,500–11,000 cells/mm³
Neutrophils	59%
	Bands—3%
	Segs—56%
Eosinophils	2.7%
Basophils	0.5%
Lymphocytes	34%
Monocytes	4%
Platelets	150,000–450,000 mm³

One cubic millimeter (mm³) = 1 microliter (µl).

of the body, resulting in a higher incidence of IDA in infants, children, and pregnant women. In lower-socioeconomic areas where lead paint is still present in some buildings, lead poisoning, causing cognitive impairment and developmental abnormalities in children, becomes a concern. Iron-deficiency anemia can result in a condition known as **pica**, causing the iron-depleted individual to ingest nonnutritive substances such as paint, dirt, clay, ice, or laundry starch. Iron replacement resolves this compulsion to eat nonfood items. It is unknown why pica occurs mostly in children and pregnant females.

Iron-deficiency anemia often occurs as a result of hemorrhage and chronic blood loss, for example, heavy menstrual bleeding, certain types of cancer (esophageal, colon, stomach), and ulcerative gastrointestinal problems such as peptic ulcer disease. Poor absorption of iron may be due to celiac disease, Crohn's disease, and the chronic use of medications such as H_2 inhibitors, proton-pump inhibitors, antacids, aspirin, and NSAIDs. Gastrointestinal surgeries such as gastric bypass surgery and partial and total gastrectomy can lead to poor absorption of iron and IDA. In older adults with multiple comorbidities, anemia is frequently a cause for hospitalization and exacerbates many chronic conditions, such as congestive heart failure (CHF) and chronic kidney disease.

Pathophysiology

Every living cell contains iron, and it is essential to the formation of the hemoglobin molecules on RBCs. With an iron deficiency, the body has insufficient hemoglobin to carry adequate oxygen to meet body requirements. Iron also plays a part in adenosine triphosphate production, necessary for glucose metabolism, and DNA synthesis, the basic gene component. The body is able to store iron in the liver as ferritin, and it is transferred to the rest of the body in times of increased demand via the protein transferrin, manufactured in the liver. Simply, IDA occurs when the body has exhausted its iron stores. The sequela of IDA is initiated with the release of cytokines as a response to the acute loss or inflammation that results in a diminished response from the kidneys for production of erythropoietin, increased resistance of the bone marrow to erythropoietin stimulation, and shorter RBC life span.

Greater iron demands occur primarily in periods of growth and development and secondary to pathologic causes. Except in the case of hemorrhage, IDA slowly progresses through several stages from a negative iron balance to iron depletion, deficient erythropoiesis, and finally IDA. Anemia is a late manifestation of iron deficiency.

Clinical Manifestations

As the body's iron stores are depleted, the decreased hemoglobin levels lead to inadequate oxygenation of the body's tissues, or hypoxia. This oxygen deficiency manifests itself as fatigue and pallor, with the onset of tachycardia and tachypnea resulting from the heart and lungs attempting to compensate for the hypoxemia (oxygen deficiency of the blood). As hypoxia increases, the patient may become increasingly short of breath. Iron-deficiency anemia may also affect the rapidly regenerating cells of mucous membranes and the gastrointestinal tract, causing fissures in the corners of the mouth and/or **glossitis**, painful swelling of the tongue, which appears smooth and shiny because of the flattening of the lingual papillae (Fig. 34.1). Spoon-shaped fingernails, or **koilonychias**, are a result of severe, prolonged iron deficiency, which renders the cells of the fingernail soft and malleable. The pressure exerted by ordinary functions such as writing causes the nails to become deformed (Fig. 34.2). Koilonychia is currently an uncommon finding in industrialized countries.

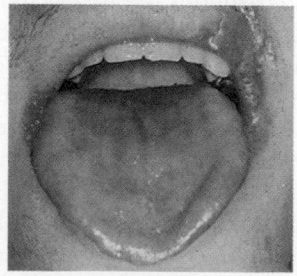

FIGURE 34.1 Glossitis in a patient with iron-deficiency anemia. Note the bright red color, the swelling, and the shiny appearance due to the flattening of the papillae on the tongue.

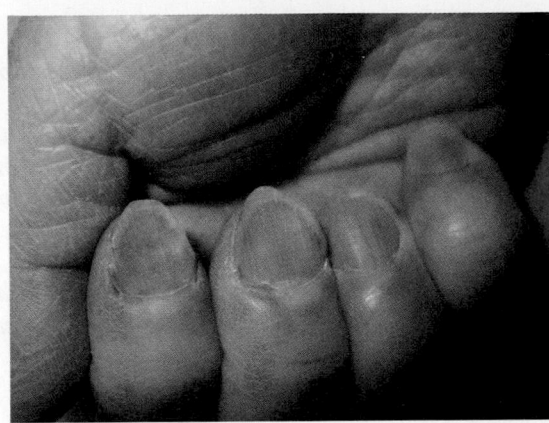

FIGURE 34.2 Koilonychias in a patient with iron-deficiency anemia. Note the spoon shape and thinness of the nail.

Table 34.2 Food Sources of Iron, Vitamin B$_{12}$, and Folic Acid

Foods	Iron	Vitamin B$_{12}$	Folic Acid
Dark green vegetables	X		X
Beets	X		
Dried beans, legumes	X		X
Fortified grains (breads, cereal)	X		X
Meat	X	X	
Seafood		X	
Eggs		X	
Dairy products		X	
Nuts			X
Bran			X
Yeast			X

Management

Diagnosis

The diagnosis of IDA is confirmed by specific blood tests. A complete blood count (CBC) demonstrates decreased hemoglobin and hematocrit levels. Low serum ferritin levels, which reflect the body's iron stores, are a confirmation of IDA. Serum ferritin levels less than or equal to 100 ug/L indicate IDA 100% of the time. Additional diagnostic studies to confirm IDA include serum iron, total iron-binding capacity (TIBC), serum transferrin receptors, and mean corpuscular volume (MCV).

Medical Management

Adjusting the diet to increase iron intake is the easiest and best way to prevent IDA, especially long term. Good dietary sources of iron include meat (especially red meat), dark green leafy vegetables (spinach, broccoli, peas), beets, dried beans, iron-fortified breakfast cereals and breads, and Cream of Wheat (Table 34.2). Ingesting citrus fruits such as oranges or grapefruits increases the vitamin C intake and may improve iron absorption.

If diet alone cannot restore iron levels, then iron supplementation is needed, and this can be done through iron preparations administered orally, intramuscularly, or intravenously. Oral supplementation is the first line of therapy. During iron therapy, patients must be monitored for nausea, abdominal discomfort, constipation, and/or diarrhea. Iron supplementation by parenteral means is indicated only in cases of severe gastrointestinal distress secondary to oral administration, malabsorption disorders, or in acute cases of IDA in which levels need to be increased more rapidly. Parenteral supplementation may be given by intramuscular (IM) or IV routes. In the past, iron dextran was the only IV supplement; however, because it often causes cardiotoxic side effects, and patients need to be closely monitored while infusing, newer formulations of IV iron supplements are now available. These newer solutions do not have major cardiac risks, and although they are much safer to administer to the patient, vital signs still need to be monitored while the iron preparation is being infused.

> **! Safety Alert** Because parenteral iron formulas stain the skin, the Z-track method is used when administering iron intramuscularly. The Z-track prevents leakage of irritating and discoloring medications, such as iron dextran.

Complications

The longer that IDA persists, the greater the clinical manifestations worsen, and this significantly impacts the function and quality of life of the patient. This disorder can adversely affect chronic health conditions such as CHF or chronic renal failure, as well as impair thermoregulation and increase immune dysfunction.

Psychomotor abnormalities and cognitive impairment occur in children with IDA, impairing learning and the ability of the child to function adequately. Iron-deficiency anemia during pregnancy increases the risk for low birth weight, preterm labor, and perinatal and postpartum mortality of the infant and/or mother.

Excessive iron overload may occur in patients but typically is not a result of excessive oral supplement intake. Pica and multiple long-term blood transfusions are usually the causes of iron overload. Clinical manifestations include fatigue, heart palpitations, joint pain, nausea, vomiting, constipation and/or diarrhea, damage to the heart and arteries, and an increased risk of cancer. The health-care provider monitors the folate and TIBC levels when any supplementation is needed.

Nursing Management

Assessment and Analysis

Clinical manifestations of IDA are related to the decreased oxygenation of body tissues. The severity of clinical manifestations is proportional to the severity of iron-store depletion. Clinical manifestations include:

- Decreased hematocrit and hemoglobin levels
- Decreased serum ferritin levels
- Tachypnea
- Shortness of breath
- Tachycardia
- Pallor
- Fatigue
- Blood loss
- Changes in level of consciousness
- Cognitive impairment
- Glossitis
- Physical abnormalities such as spoon-shaped fingernails

Nursing Diagnoses

- **Inadequate tissue perfusion** related to decreased oxygen delivery as a result of decreased iron stores
- **Fatigue** related to inadequate oxygenation to body tissues
- **Activity intolerance** related to impaired oxygen-carrying capacity secondary to IDA

Nursing Interventions

■ Assessments

- Vital signs
  Tachycardia and tachypnea are secondary to the heart and lungs compensating for decreased oxygenation of body tissues caused by decreased iron levels, which leads to decreased hemoglobin levels.
- Serum hemoglobin and ferritin levels
  With an iron deficiency, reflected by low ferritin levels, there is insufficient hemoglobin to deliver oxygen to the body tissues. Decreased hemoglobin and serum ferritin levels indicate IDA.
- Fatigue, pallor, and shortness of breath
  Fatigue, pallor, and shortness of breath worsen with increasingly decreased levels of iron, resulting in inadequate oxygen-carrying capacity.
- Level of consciousness
  Alterations in level of consciousness occur as a result of decreased iron levels that cause decreased oxygenation to the brain. If prolonged IDA is present in a child's developing brain, cognitive impairment could be permanent.
- Blood loss, if present
  The greater the blood loss, the worse the clinical manifestations are as a result of decreasing iron stores and decreased hemoglobin levels leading to inadequate tissue perfusion.

■ Actions

- Increase dietary iron.
  Increasing iron intake through dietary sources increases the body's iron stores and results in increased hemoglobin levels, thus increasing tissue perfusion.

- Increase intake of vitamin C.
  Increasing vitamin C intake may increase iron absorption.
- Administer iron-supplement therapy.
  Iron-supplement therapy is necessary if iron stores need to be increased quickly or if malabsorption disorders are present, which interfere with the body's ability to incorporate iron from dietary sources.
- Minimize blood loss.
  Any obvious hemorrhaging needs to be controlled immediately to minimize blood loss. Excessive bleeding with menstruation may be controlled by various hormonal medications.

■ Teaching

- Dietary sources of iron
  Good dietary sources include meat (especially red), dark green leafy vegetables (spinach, broccoli, peas), beets, dried beans, iron-fortified breakfast cereals and breads, and Cream of Wheat. Many Web sites are available for nutritional information (see Table 34.2).
- Immediately report any signs of bleeding, increasing fatigue, or shortness of breath.
  Most cases of IDA occur over a prolonged period of time. Therefore, clinical manifestations usually present when iron stores have already been significantly decreased.
- Daily iron supplements must be taken as prescribed.
  Iron supplements replace the body's iron stores and increase the production of hemoglobin molecules, leading to improved tissue perfusion. Oral supplements can cause constipation, diarrhea, nausea, or abdominal discomfort. Patients need to be instructed to report these side effects to the healthcare provider. If side effects are too severe, then supplementation via parenteral routes is available.
- Dangers of lead exposure
  In lower-socioeconomic environments, lead paint is still present in many buildings. Exposure to lead can lead to cognitive impairment and developmental abnormalities in children.
- Prenatal teaching about iron intake
  Inadequate iron intake by pregnant women has been linked to lower birth weight, preterm labor, and increased mortality of mother and child.

Evaluating Care Outcomes

Iron-deficiency anemia is a reversible condition that can be managed by increasing dietary iron intake and/or through parenteral supplementation. Elevating iron levels allows the increased production of hemoglobin, which improves the oxygenation of body tissues. As tissue perfusion improves, so do clinical manifestations of fatigue, pallor, and shortness of breath. Heart rate and respiratory rate return to normal as the heart and lungs no longer need to compensate for inadequate tissue perfusion. Normal levels of hemoglobin and serum ferritin confirm the resolution of the anemia. However, children with prolonged IDA may continue to deal with cognitive impairment and developmental abnormalities caused by insufficient oxygenation to the developing brain. These children have special needs that will need to be addressed by other resources.

Connection Check 34.1

Which patient is at greatest risk for developing IDA?

A. A 6-year-old African American boy with no health problems

B. A 15-year-old African American pregnant female

C. A 52-year-old Mexican American female with hypertension

D. A 72-year-old Caucasian male with cardiac disease

Vitamin B₁₂ Anemia

Epidemiology

Vitamin B_{12}, also called **cobalamin**, deficiency occurs either when the body has inadequate sources of vitamin B_{12} or because of malabsorption disorders that make dietary vitamin B_{12} unavailable for body use. Unlike IDA, however, the body does not store vitamin B_{12}, so daily intake is essential. It is estimated that 15% to 25% of older adults have a vitamin B_{12} deficiency that is primarily due to the gradual gastric atrophy and decrease in gastric acid production associated with aging and not necessarily as a result of decreased intake. The slow progression of the anemia and nervous system degeneration in vitamin B_{12} deficiency correlates with a delay in the presentation of clinical manifestations, which may take years to develop.

In addition to older adults, other groups at higher risk for developing a vitamin B_{12} deficiency are individuals with a history of disorders that affect the absorption of vitamin B_{12}. This includes patients with gastrointestinal resections; autoimmune disorders, including AIDS; chronic alcohol use; Crohn's disease; celiac disease; and long-term use of medications that decrease gastric acid secretions, such as proton-pump inhibitors or H_2 blockers. Because vitamin B_{12} is found only in animal proteins, low socioeconomic status and long-term vegetarianism and veganism increase the risk of insufficient vitamin B_{12} intake.

Pathophysiology

Vitamin B_{12} is a coenzyme required for normal function of the central nervous system, formation of red blood cells, and synthesis and regulation of DNA. Cellular metabolism is dependent on vitamin B_{12} because it is essential to the synthesis of fatty acids and energy production. Vitamin B_{12} (also known as *extrinsic factor*) is introduced to the body through dietary sources of animal proteins, including meat, seafood, eggs, and dairy products (see Table 34.2). The parietal cells of the stomach lining secrete a protein-binding substance known as *intrinsic factor* that binds with vitamin B_{12}, leading to absorption in the ileum of the small intestine. **Pernicious anemia** is caused by the lack of intrinsic factor. Although pernicious anemia is often erroneously used as a synonym for vitamin B_{12}–deficiency anemia, in actuality, pernicious anemia is an autoimmune disease that leads to a vitamin B_{12} deficiency because of the inability to absorb vitamin B_{12} without intrinsic factor. Vitamin B_{12} is also

required for the conversion of methylmalonyl coenzyme A, part of the Krebs cycle. It is necessary for the synthesis of certain neurotransmitters and phospholipids needed for normal nervous system function.

Vitamin B_{12} and folate are cofactors essential in DNA synthesis and the methylation cycles of RBCs, part of cellular metabolism. This highly complex process includes converting a folate chain to homocysteine (an amino acid by-product) to methionine, an essential amino acid needed in the methylation cycle. A vitamin B_{12} deficiency traps the folate in the methylation cycle (the methylfolate-trap hypothesis) and leads to increased homocysteine levels that are linked to impaired immune system function, certain cancers (breast, cervical, lung), and a high risk for cardiovascular events such as cerebrovascular accident (CVA) and myocardial infarction (MI). Because of the codependence of vitamin B_{12} and folate on RBC production, it is necessary to determine the specific deficiency that causes the anemia. Supplementation of synthetic folic acid escapes this methylfolate trap, masking the vitamin B_{12} deficiency, and therefore resolves the anemia but has no effect on the neurological symptoms produced by the deficit of vitamin B_{12}. Nitrous oxide administered to a patient with a vitamin B_{12} deficiency interferes with the methylation cycle by destroying methylcobalamin, the form of vitamin B_{12} in human plasma. This leads to impaired RBC production, and a profound postoperative anemia results and can be fatal if the vitamin B_{12} deficiency is not discovered.

Clinical Manifestations

A deficiency of vitamin B_{12} can cause neurological and psychiatric dysfunctions. Demyelination of nerves can lead to spinal cord degeneration, peripheral neuropathy, and altered mental status and is linked to depression. Visual disturbances may occur as a result of nerve atrophy in the eyes. Because of the changes in RBC production related to decreased vitamin B_{12}, the patient may exhibit clinical manifestations observed in other types of anemia, including tachycardia, tachypnea, shortness of breath, dizziness, and fatigue.

With vitamin B_{12} deficiency, the longer the body goes with inadequate levels of vitamin B_{12}, the more severe the neurological deficits become, possibly becoming irreversible. Neurological clinical manifestations include the development of peripheral neuropathy that may progress to spinal cord degeneration. Paresthesias, numbness and tingling in the hands and feet, are usually the first neurological clinical manifestation to occur with vitamin B_{12} deficiency. **Lhermitte's sign** is an electric-shock sensation produced by neck flexion and is rarely observed but may be seen in patients with vitamin B_{12} deficiency. Central nervous system involvement may also lead to confusion, depression, mood swings, impaired taste and/or stinging sensation on the tongue, and impaired sense of balance, particularly in the dark. Dementia resembling Alzheimer's disease can occur in severe cases of vitamin B_{12} deficiency. Visual disturbances may include the inability to distinguish the colors yellow and blue or blindness. Clinical manifestations may also include alternating constipation and diarrhea, anorexia, menstrual irregularities, weight loss, glossitis, low-grade fever, and tinnitus (ringing in the ears). A comparison of clinical manifestations for all RBC disorders is presented in Table 34.3.

Management

Diagnosis

Because of the slow progression of a vitamin B_{12} deficiency and delayed clinical manifestations, the results of a CBC may be the first indication that a problem exists, and further investigation is needed to determine the cause. The diagnosis of vitamin B_{12} deficiency is made based on a history and physical examination and a vitamin B_{12} serum assay blood test. Serum vitamin B_{12} is not low in all individuals with a deficiency because there are inborn errors of vitamin B_{12} metabolism that may cause serum levels to be normal, but low cellular levels may have already resulted in damage. Therefore, the vitamin B_{12} serum assay test has its limitations and has a wide normal range (200 to 1,000 pg/mL). Patients with liver disease, lymphoma, and myeloproliferative disorders may have false-negative results. A more sensitive test for vitamin B_{12} deficiency is to measure the level of methylmalonic acid (MMA), part of the methionine conversion, in the patient's urine or blood. An excess of MMA indicates a lack of vitamin B_{12} in the tissues. Because patients with renal failure, dehydration, or hypovolemia can have falsely elevated serum MMA levels, a urinary MMA test is needed for accurate diagnosis in individuals with these disorders. Other relevant blood tests that may assist in determining vitamin B_{12} deficiency include gastrin levels, intrinsic factor levels, and in rare instances, the **Schilling's test**, a radionuclide 24-hour urine test that indirectly measures intrinsic factor.

Medical Management

Prevention of vitamin B_{12} deficiency is important, and animal proteins provide the only source of vitamin B_{12} in the world. Vitamin B_{12} has not been discovered in any plants. Dietary sources of vitamin B_{12} include meat, seafood, eggs, and dairy products. Long-term vegans/vegetarians or those of low socioeconomic status are at increased risk of deficiency and may need to take a daily supplement of vitamin B_{12}. Oral supplementation of vitamin B_{12} may not be sufficient once the deficiency is profound and the patient has developed clinical manifestations such as fatigue, weakness, and paresthesias. Once severe deficiency is determined, weekly vitamin B_{12} injections are required.

Complications

Vitamin B_{12} deficiency impairs DNA synthesis and the body's ability to produce RBCs. As with any anemic condition, the longer the deficiency lasts, the more pronounced are the clinical manifestations of fatigue, pallor, dizziness, shortness of breath, and impacts on the functional ability of the individual and quality of life. Orthostatic hypotension, especially on standing, may be present.

Table 34.3	Clinical Manifestations of Red Blood Cell Disorders
Red Blood Cell Disorder	**Identifying Clinical Manifestations**
Iron-deficiency anemia	Fatigue
	Pallor
	Tachycardia
	Tachypnea
	Glossitis (smooth, shiny tongue)
	Koilonychia (spoon-shaped nails)
Vitamin B_{12} anemia	Fatigue
	Pallor
	Tachycardia
	Tachypnea
	Shortness of breath
	Dizziness
	Glossitis
	Neurological deficits:
	• Symmetric paresthesia of feet and fingers
	• Lhermitte's sign
	• Confusion
	• Depression
	• Impaired taste
	• Impaired balance
	• Visual disturbances
	• Tinnitus
Folic acid anemia	Fatigue
	Pallor
	Tachycardia
	Tachypnea
	Dizziness
	Mood changes
	Increased bleeding risk
	Neural tube defects in infants born of a woman with folic acid deficiency
Sickle cell anemia	Fatigue
	Pallor
	Tachycardia
	Tachypnea
	Shortness of breath
	Pain in joints, chest, and abdomen
	Fever

Table 34.3 Clinical Manifestations of Red Blood Cell Disorders—cont'd

Red Blood Cell Disorder	Identifying Clinical Manifestations
	Delayed wound healing
	Hand-foot syndrome
	Jaundice
Aplastic anemia	Fatigue
	Pallor
	Tachycardia
	Tachypnea
	Shortness of breath
	Dizziness
	Headache
	Frequent infections
	Bruising
	Nosebleeds
	Gum bleeding
G6PD Deficiency	Fatigue
	Pallor
	Tachycardia
	Tachypnea
	Shortness of breath
	Jaundice
	Dark urine
	Splenomegaly
Polycythemia	Fatigue
	Shortness of breath
	Dizziness
	Headache
	Pruritis
	Facial flushing
	Splenomegaly
	Pruritis
	Vision problems
	Weight loss
	Nosebleeds
	Bleeding gums
	Hypertension
	Thromboembolism

Pregnancy, hyperthyroidism, advanced stages of cancer, and intestinal tapeworms may increase vitamin B_{12} needs despite a normally adequate intake of vitamin B_{12} because of the increased demands of the body as cellular metabolism increases. Supplementation is usually helpful in these cases. Radiation for certain cancers may cause inflammation of the intestines that interferes with vitamin B_{12} absorption.

Nursing Management

Assessment and Analysis

Clinical manifestations of vitamin B_{12} anemia are related to decreased production of RBCs due to impairment of DNA synthesis that leads to overall decreased hemoglobin and hematocrit levels. Patients are assessed for the following clinical presentation:

- Shortness of breath
- Tachypnea
- Tachycardia
- Pallor
- Fatigue
- Dizziness

Neurological clinical manifestations of vitamin B_{12} deficiency are related to the impairment of DNA synthesis necessary for the formation and maintenance of myelin, neurotransmitters, and phospholipids (the principal component of the cell membrane).

- Numbness, tingling, or burning in hands or feet
- Altered mental status (confusion, dementia)
- Depression
- Mood swings
- Coordination and balance
- Impaired taste, stinging sensation on the tongue (can cause glossitis)
- Visual disturbances

Nursing Diagnoses

- **Inadequate tissue perfusion** related to decreased oxygenation as a result of decreased hemoglobin and hematocrit
- **Activity intolerance** related to impaired oxygen-carrying capacity secondary to vitamin B_{12} deficiency
- **Chronic pain** related to inadequate vitamin B_{12} levels as evidenced by peripheral neuropathy

Nursing Interventions

Assessments

- Vital signs
  Vitamin B_{12} deficiency impairs RBC production, with a resulting decrease in tissue perfusion. Tachycardia and tachypnea occur as the heart attempts to compensate for the decrease in tissue perfusion.
- Fatigue, pallor, and shortness of breath
  Fatigue, pallor, and shortness of breath worsen with increasingly decreased levels of RBCs, causing inadequate tissue perfusion.

- Numbness, tingling, or burning of the hands or feet; confusion; mood swings
  Neurological clinical manifestations occur because of the impairment of DNA synthesis of myelin sheath and neurotransmitters.
- Decreased hemoglobin/hematocrit levels, decreased vitamin B_{12} levels, elevated serum and urine MMA levels
  A CBC shows decreased hemoglobin and hematocrit levels. The serum vitamin B_{12} assay is decreased due to the lack of vitamin B_{12} needed for synthesis.
- Fall risk (safety)
  Confusion, dementia, coordination and balance impairment, and visual disturbances make these patients at risk for falls. Paresthesia and tingling (peripheral neuropathy) can affect ambulation, gait, and stability. Severe neuropathy may take time to recover.
- Intake and output
  Constipation, diarrhea, and/or anorexia affect the absorption of vitamin B_{12} and may worsen the problem.

■ Actions

- Ensure adequate vitamin B_{12} intake.
  Ensuring that the patient has an adequate intake of vitamin B_{12} prevents clinical manifestations of anemia and degenerative neurological changes (see Table 34.3).
- Administer vitamin B_{12} therapy.
  Oral supplementation in mild cases of vitamin B_{12} deficiency may be helpful. In more severe cases, supplementation with parenteral therapy is required. Parenteral supplementation may be necessary for patients who lack intrinsic factor and cannot absorb oral supplementation. Vegetarians can prevent or treat this deficiency with oral supplements, vitamins, or fortified soy milk. When the deficiency is due to pernicious anemia or the absence of intrinsic factor, the replacement of vitamin B_{12} involves 1-mg IM injections of cyanocobalamin vitamin B_{12}.
- Monitor use of folic acid.
  Before starting a patient on folic acid, confirm that the patient does not have a vitamin B_{12} deficiency. Folic acid resolves the anemia by escaping the methylfolate trap, but neurological degeneration due to vitamin B_{12} deficiency continues.
- Monitor use of nitrous oxide.
  Nitrous oxide inactivates vitamin B_{12} in the body. Prior to using for anesthesia, confirm that the patient is not vitamin B_{12} deficient.
- Assess pain and activity levels due to peripheral neuropathy.
  Peripheral neuropathy may develop because of vitamin B_{12} deficiency. Increasing pain may interfere with functional abilities. Because position sense, coordination, and balance are affected, physical therapy and occupational therapy should be considered along with the use of assistive devices.

■ Teaching

- Dietary sources of vitamin B_{12}
  Dietary sources of vitamin B_{12} include meat, seafood, eggs, and dairy products.
- Need for vitamin B_{12} supplementation
  Because of the lack of vitamin B_{12} in plants, vegans/vegetarians may need daily oral supplementation. Patients may have a sore tongue and need bland, soft food frequently, along with mouth care.
- Immediately report any clinical manifestations of fatigue, shortness of breath, paresthesias, and confusion.
  Clinical manifestations usually present after prolonged vitamin B_{12} deficiency. Resolution of the anemia does not stop neurological degeneration unless the deficiency is resolved.
- Prenatal teaching
  Pregnancy may increase the demand for vitamin B_{12}. Prophylactic oral supplementation is recommended.
- Radiation for advanced cancers
  Radiation therapy may increase the need for vitamin B_{12} supplementation. Patients with anemia do not respond as well to radiotherapy because of impairment of oxygen transport to cancer cells.
- Actions of acid-reducing medications
  Patients using these medications may develop vitamin B_{12} deficiency because of a decrease in the function of the parietal cells of the stomach, which produce intrinsic factor.

Evaluating Care Outcomes

Vitamin B_{12}–deficiency anemia is reversible. Increasing vitamin B_{12} intake through diet and/or parenteral supplementation resolves the deficit and allows the increased production of RBCs and improves oxygenation of the body's tissues. As tissue perfusion improves, clinical manifestations of fatigue, pallor, and shortness of breath decrease. Heart rate and respiratory rate return to normal because the heart and lungs no longer need to compensate for inadequate tissue perfusion. Normal levels of hemoglobin, hematocrit, and serum vitamin B_{12}, as well as decreased MMA levels, confirm the resolution of the anemia. However, if the vitamin B_{12} deficiency becomes severe and is not treated promptly, degenerative neurological changes may be permanent.

Connection Check 34.2

When a patient with vitamin B_{12} deficiency is counseled about diet, what statement by the patient indicates an understanding of the cause of the anemia?

A. "I know I need to eat more fruits and vegetables."
B. "I have cut out all fried foods in my diet."
C. "I have been eating more organic foods."
D. "I have been having beef or fish at least once a day."

Folic Acid Deficiency

Epidemiology

Folic acid is a water-soluble vitamin (B_9). Folate is the form that is naturally found in foods, whereas folic acid is the synthetic supplementation form, and they are frequently used interchangeably. Folic acid, along with vitamin B_{12}, is necessary for a complex pathway that aids in DNA synthesis and the formation of heme, the iron-containing portion of the hemoglobin molecule. Folic acid deficiency is usually a result of inadequate dietary intake and frequently affects older adults, those with chronic illness, individuals who abuse alcohol, and individuals who go on extreme diets lacking folate. Deficits in folic acid also develop secondary to malnutrition, specific malignancies, Crohn's disease, celiac disease, and malabsorption due to gastrointestinal surgeries or medications. Patients with rheumatoid arthritis who are treated with methotrexate may develop folic acid deficiency secondary to the antagonistic effects of this medication to folic acid; this complication may be managed with folic acid supplementation. Dietary sources of folate include green leafy vegetables, bran, yeast, legumes, and nuts (see Table 34.2). Patients on hemodialysis are at higher risk for developing a folic acid deficiency because it increases folate excretion.

Folic acid deficiency during pregnancy is also linked to fetal neural tube defects and some congenital orofacial abnormalities. The precise mechanism is not completely understood; however, current evidence suggests that folic acid supplementation in pregnancy prevents these defects. It is hypothesized that folate deficiency impairs DNA synthesis during the crucial phase of neurological development of closure of neural tubes. It is recommended that pregnant women take folic acid supplementation of at least 400 mcg daily because this has led to decreased incidence and severity of spina bifida, cleft palate and lip, and other neural tube defects.

In the United States, fortification of cereals and certain grains, such as wheat flour, with folic acid has decreased the incidence of true folic acid deficiency (see Table 34.2). Except in circumstances where there are increased body requirements, such as during pregnancy, in childhood, and in individuals with excessive alcohol use, additional supplementation other than dietary sources is usually not required.

Pathophysiology

Folate, along with vitamin B_{12}, forms a complex pathway that is involved in DNA synthesis and is essential for cell maturation and replication. This is especially important in embryonic neural tube development, in the formation of heme for RBC maturation, and in the synthesis of certain neurotransmitters for brain development and maintenance. Decreases in folate levels delay erythrocyte maturation, thus lowering hemoglobin levels and causing anemia. Folate deficiency is thought to inhibit DNA synthesis to such an extent that during neural tube development, incomplete closure occurs in utero, with resulting congenital anomalies such as spina bifida, anencephaly, and cleft palate and lip. Incomplete synthesis of certain neurotransmitters, particularly in the first few months of life, may cause developmental delays in head growth, spasticity, and speech difficulties and lead to epilepsy. These disorders are a result of decreased transport of folate across the blood–brain barrier.

Folate enters the body through dietary sources or as folic acid supplementation and is absorbed in the jejunum portion of the small intestine. It is not unusual for deficits to occur in the presence of any problem affecting the jejunum, such as in gastric bypass surgery or the Whipple procedure (pancreatic duodenectomy), which is a surgical procedure for specific gastrointestinal cancers. The Whipple procedure involves the removal of the distal segment of the stomach, portions of the duodenum, the head of the pancreas, and the gallbladder and resects the remaining portions, allowing gastric and pancreatic enzymes, as well as bile, to flow into the jejunum for digestion. Specific medications such as oral contraceptives, metformin for type 2 diabetes mellitus, and chemotherapeutic agents (fluorouracil) may interfere with folic acid absorption. Folic acid supplementation may increase the hepatic metabolism of the anticonvulsant phenytoin (Dilantin), which may increase the incidence of seizure activity. It is advisable to correct the folic acid deficiency before initiating the medication because adding the supplement after the patient is on phenytoin may increase the likelihood of seizures.

Chronic alcohol use contributes to folic acid deficiency secondary to malnutrition that is frequently present in these patients. Alcohol also interferes with the absorption of folate. The RBCs in a patient with a history of alcohol abuse demonstrate an abnormal morphology and half the normal life span of 120 days. Alcohol can also damage or kill bone marrow and progenitor (stem) cells, which may lead to **pancytopenia**, an overall decreased proliferation of RBCs, WBCs, and platelets.

Clinical Manifestations

Because of the effects on RBC development, patients with folic acid deficiency present with clinical manifestations consistent with other types of anemia, including pallor, tachycardia, tachypnea, dizziness, and fatigue. Additionally, because of the pancytopenia associated with folic acid deficiency, there are decreased numbers of platelets, increasing the risk of bleeding. It is essential to differentiate between a folate deficiency and a vitamin B_{12} deficiency. The clinical manifestations of folic acid and vitamin B_{12} deficiency are similar because they often coexist. The neurological manifestations of vitamin B_{12} deficiency do not occur with folic acid deficiency but will persist if vitamin B_{12} is not replaced. The neurological symptoms in severe vitamin B_{12} deficiency involving pernicious anemia include psychiatric symptoms and peripheral neuropathy. If sensation is altered, it can affect gait and stability. Patients should avoid excessive heat or cold. Patients with vitamin B_{12} and/or folic acid deficiencies may have fatigue, mood changes, memory difficulties, and weakness. Vitiligo, premature graying of the hair, and glossitis are often seen in patients who have pernicious anemia. Because the folate/vitamin B_{12} codependency affects RBC maturation, folic acid replacement may reverse the anemia, but the neurological degeneration that occurs in vitamin B_{12} deficiencies continues and may become irreversible.

Management

Diagnosis

A CBC confirms the diagnosis of anemia with decreased hemoglobin levels; however, the specific etiology of the anemia must be identified. Serum folate levels may or may not be decreased. Because folate is absorbed in the proximal segment of the small intestine and is quickly available for cell metabolism, serum folate levels should be a fasting blood test; otherwise, the level may be falsely elevated. A more reliable indicator is the RBC folate level. Folate that enters the RBC remains there for the life span of that cell. Thus, an RBC folate level reflects the serum folate level over the past 3 months. However, because 50% of patients with a vitamin B_{12} deficiency also have low RBC folate levels, this is not a definitive test.

Serum MMA and homocysteine levels are the best laboratory tests used to differentiate between anemia caused by a folic acid deficiency and those secondary to a vitamin B_{12} deficiency. Vitamin B_{12} and folate are cofactors in the methylation cycle converting methylmalonyl coenzyme A to homocysteine to methionine as part of the Krebs cycle. In a vitamin B_{12} deficiency, the serum MMA level is more sensitive and is elevated, whereas the homocysteine level remains normal. A folic acid deficiency causes the reverse: The homocysteine level is elevated, whereas serum MMA levels remain normal. Some conditions, such as renal insufficiency, may affect these results, so it is always important to consider the complete clinical presentation and not rely on one test to make a differential diagnosis.

Medical Management

Fortification of cereals and grains with folic acid helps to reduce the incidence of this specific deficiency. In certain patient populations, however, oral supplementation is recommended. Folic acid supplementation is recommended in pregnant women, children in the first year of life, patients with a history of gastrointestinal resections, and individuals with a history of chronic alcohol use. It is recommended that pregnant women consume at least 400 mcg (normal recommendation for adult women) of folic acid daily in order to reduce the occurrence and severity of neural tube defects and some orofacial abnormalities in infants. For patients on certain medications that can interfere with folate absorption, such as oral contraceptives, metformin, and certain chemotherapeutic agents, oral or parental supplementation may be recommended. Short- or long-term supplementation depends on the length of treatment with the medication.

Complications

Folic acid deficiencies interfere with the formation of heme, the oxygen-carrying portion of the hemoglobin molecule. Anemia left unresolved ultimately affects individual function. Folic acid deficiency may also cause neurological clinical manifestations such as confusion or disorientation. However, unlike a vitamin B_{12} deficiency, these clinical manifestations are reversible and resolve with the resolution of the deficiency.

Nursing Management

Assessment and Analysis

Clinical manifestations of anemia are related to incomplete DNA synthesis that affects the formation of heme and the maturation of the RBC, which causes a decreased hemoglobin level.

- Shortness of breath
- Tachypnea
- Tachycardia
- Fatigue
- Pallor
- Dizziness
- Confusion, disorientation
- Decreased hemoglobin
- Elevated homocysteine level with normal serum MMA levels

Nursing Diagnoses

- **Inadequate tissue perfusion** related to decreased oxygenation as a result of decreased hemoglobin and hematocrit
- **Activity intolerance** related to impaired oxygen-carrying capacity secondary to folate deficiency
- **Risk for delayed development** related to incomplete neural tube closure secondary to folate deficiency

Nursing Interventions

■ Assessments

- Vital signs
  Tachycardia and tachypnea are secondary to the heart and lungs compensating for decreased oxygenation of body tissues caused by the reduced production of heme and RBC maturation demonstrated by decreased hemoglobin levels.
- Fatigue, pallor, and shortness of breath
  Fatigue, pallor, and shortness of breath worsen with increasingly decreased levels of hemoglobin causing inadequate tissue perfusion.
- Confusion, disorientation
  Neurological clinical manifestations are caused by decreased oxygenation to the central nervous system.
- Hemoglobin levels, serum folate levels, RBC folate levels, and increased serum homocysteine levels
  Folic acid deficiency causes incomplete DNA synthesis that is necessary for the formation of heme, RBC maturation, and folate levels in the serum and RBCs and influences the metabolic pathway, which results in increased homocysteine levels.

■ Actions

- Ensure adequate folate/folic acid intake.
  Ensuring adequate intake of dietary sources of folate and folic acid through food fortification prevents anemia and neural tube defects (see Table 34.2).
- Administer folic acid supplements.
  Folic acid is the synthetic form for supplementation. Supplementation is needed when the body has increased folate demands, such as in pregnancy, early childhood, or alcoholism.

It is also needed when malabsorption of folate occurs because of disorders such as Crohn's disease, gastrointestinal resections, and the use of medications that interfere with folate absorption.

- Differentiate anemia caused by folic acid deficiency versus vitamin B$_{12}$ deficiency.
  Supplementation of folic acid may reverse the anemia caused by vitamin B$_{12}$ but will not stop the neurological degenerations that occur with vitamin B$_{12}$ deficits. These neurological changes may become irreversible if misdiagnosed.

■ Teaching

- Dietary sources of folate/folic acid
  Good sources include fortified cereals and grains, legumes, green leafy vegetables, bran, yeast extracts, and nuts (see Table 34.2).
- Immediately report any clinical manifestations of fatigue, shortness of breath, dizziness, and confusion.
  Resolution of the anemia through supplementation or blood transfusions is needed to increase tissue perfusion.
- Prenatal teaching
  Because of the strong link between folic acid deficiency and the occurrence of neural tube defects and orofacial abnormalities during embryonic development, it is essential to teach all women of childbearing years the importance of obtaining at least 400 mcg of folic acid daily during the preconception stage and during pregnancy.
- Need for supplementation
  Individuals who have had gastrointestinal resections, such as gastric bypass surgery or a Whipple procedure, need education regarding folic acid supplementation. Individuals on certain anticonvulsants (e.g., phenytoin), oral contraceptives, metformin, and chemotherapeutic agents (fluorouracil, methotrexate) need to be educated about the importance of folic acid supplementation because ordered medications may interfere with the absorption of folate.

Evaluating Care Outcomes

Resolution of the anemia is the most obvious clinical manifestation that the folic acid deficiency has resolved because the DNA synthesis pathway now has sufficient folate to complete the process. The hemoglobin level and serum folate level increase, and clinical manifestations such as fatigue or shortness of breath resolve. If neurological clinical manifestations continue after the hemoglobin returns to normal, assessment for possible vitamin B$_{12}$ deficiency is indicated. Folic acid supplementation during pregnancy usually results in an infant born without neural tube defects or orofacial abnormalities.

Connection Check 34.3

The nurse understands that it is essential for the patient to have which blood test before initiating folic acid supplementation?

A. Vitamin B$_{12}$ level
B. Pregnancy test
C. CBC
D. Liver enzymes

Sickle Cell Anemia

Epidemiology

Sickle cell anemia is the most severe form of the inherited blood disorder sickle cell disease (SCD). The sickle cell trait (SCT) is a genetic mutation that must be present in both parents in order for this form of the disease to manifest in offspring. Parents who carry this gene have a one in four chance of producing a child with sickle cell anemia. Individuals who inherit the SCT from one parent and a normal copy of the gene from the other parent are sickle cell carriers and are said to have only SCT (Fig. 34.3).

Sickle cell disease affects millions of people throughout the world, predominantly descendants from tropical Africa. The rate of inheriting this genetic disorder may be as low as 20% in this population and as high as 40% in some areas. To a lesser extent, this disease affects many descendants of the Middle East and Mediterranean areas (Saudi Arabia, Turkey, Greece, and Italy), certain tribes of India, and Spanish-speaking regions of the Western Hemisphere (South and Central America, Cuba). Caucasians occasionally

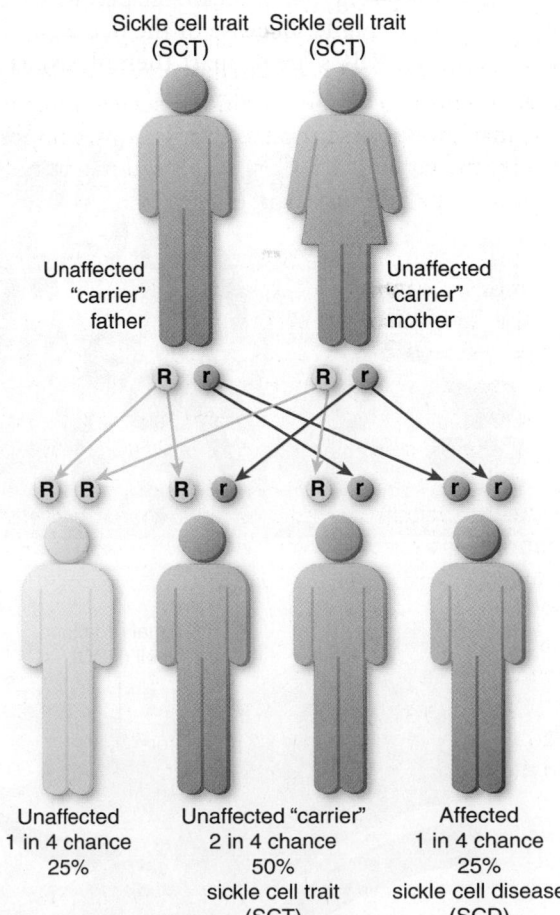

FIGURE 34.3 Diagram of how sickle cell disease is passed from parent to child.
R, dominant gene; *r*, recessive gene.
Blue, not a carrier; *purple*, carrier, but unaffected; *red*, affected.
Note that there is a 25% chance that one of their children will have sickle cell disease.

develop SCD when ancestry may have African descendants. It is estimated that as many as 2 million people in the United States are carriers of the SCT, whereas approximately 72,000 actually have SCD. Statistics show that 50% of children with SCD live to adulthood. Death prior to the age of 20 is usually the result of a sudden, severe crisis rather than the long-term deterioration caused by multiple episodes of thrombosis and infarction causing organ damage. In regions of the world where malaria is endemic, individuals with SCD seem to have some innate protection against this disease. When diagnosed in people with SCD, malaria appears to have a shorter course and be less intense than in those without SCD.

Pathophysiology

Sickle cell disease is a genetic disorder of hemoglobin. A normal RBC is extremely malleable in order to be able to squeeze through minute capillaries to deliver oxygen. In SCD, the RBC goes through a morphological change when it is exposed to decreased oxygen tension. These RBCs become elongated and stiff and lose flexibility. On microscopic examination, these cells are sickle-shaped, thus the name of the disease (Fig. 34.4). Sickle-shaped RBCs carry less oxygen and are fragile. Because of the decreased flexibility and fragility, RBCs break apart (hemolysis) as they pass through the capillary beds. The result is congestion and clumping in the capillary beds and the formation of thrombi (Fig. 34.5). Although the normal life span of an RBC is 120 days, in an individual with SCD, the normal life span is 15 to 20 days.

The hemolysis of the RBCs causes a decrease in the hemoglobin level and thus anemia. Destruction of RBCs also releases bilirubin, causing a rise in the serum bilirubin level. Additionally, possible congestion in the spleen due to the increased RBC fragments that must be phagocytized leads to an enlarged spleen and possible pain.

When the sickling process is rapid and severe, the patient has a sickle cell crisis. There are four types of crises: (1) vaso-occlusive, or painful, crisis (most common type) caused by the obstruction of vessels by hemolyzed cells, leading to tissue hypoxia and pain; (2) aplastic crisis in which the bone marrow ceases to produce RBCs, with a subsequent decrease in the blood reticulocyte count; (3) sequestration crisis caused by a sudden, massive pooling of RBCs in the spleen, with resulting hypovolemic shock and cardiovascular failure; and (4) hemolytic crisis, which results from an increased rate of RBC hemolysis with resultant decreased hemoglobin levels and increased jaundice.

Sickle cell crises are most often precipitated by anything that causes hypoxemia, increasing vasoconstriction and

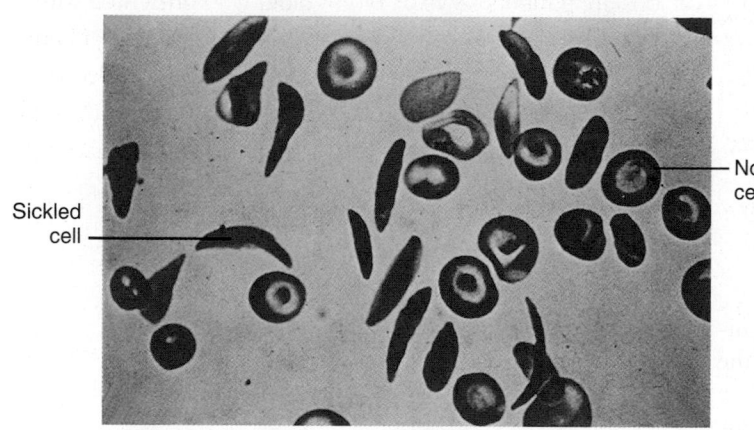

FIGURE 34.4 Peripheral blood smear showing sickled red blood cells. Note the difference between the sickled cells and the normal red blood cells.

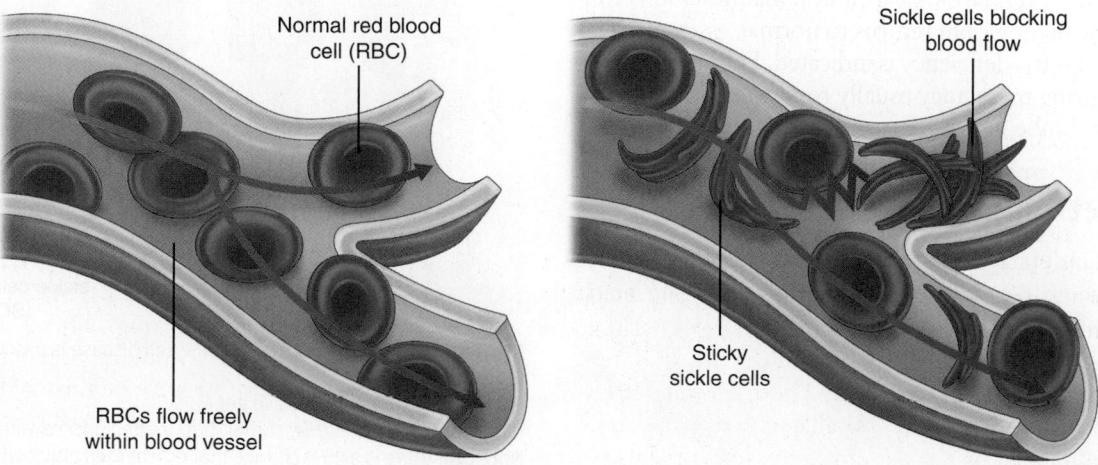

FIGURE 34.5 Sickled cells moving through a capillary and forming a thrombus.

sickling of the RBCs. Precipitating factors include dehydration, cold temperatures, infection, and environments with low oxygen tension, such as depressurized airplane cabins and high mountains. Crises may appear without any apparent reason and usually last several days to a week. They may occur frequently for a period of time and then be dormant.

Clinical Manifestations

The presentation of sickle cell crises is most frequently associated with clinical manifestations related to the anemia, such as fatigue, pallor, and shortness of breath, and the vaso-occlusion of blood vessels resulting in pain and swelling. Any tissue may experience vaso-occlusion and tissue ischemia; however, pain usually occurs in the joints, bones, chest, and abdomen. Ischemic organ damage secondary to the vaso-occlusion causes cerebrovascular, pulmonary, and splenic infarctions; priapism in males (prolonged, painful erection); and kidney and liver damage. Fever may be present even in the absence of infection. Wound healing, especially in the extremities, is often delayed because of impaired circulation and venous stasis. Patients with SCD have an increased risk of developing infections, particularly respiratory infections caused by pneumococcus, pertussis, and *Haemophilus influenzae*.

Clinical manifestations usually do not present until after 6 months of age because the infant is protected by an increased level of fetal hemoglobin in the first few months of life. Long-term organ ischemia can lead to growth and developmental delays. The child with SCD may be smaller than peers. Puberty, with its secondary sexual characteristics, may be delayed, including late menstruation in females. Repeated episodes of crises and infarctions of the bones can lead to uneven development of the fingers and toes, known as hand-foot syndrome, which is characterized as swelling of the dorsal surfaces of the hands and feet, causing pain. Pregnancy, with its increased demand on the body, can be a cause for the exacerbation of SCD. Death is usually the result of CVA, infection, or long-term organ system damage.

Management
Medical Management

There is no cure for SCD, and treatment is aimed at the prevention of crises and symptom management when crises occur. Long-term management is aimed at minimizing complications and organ dysfunction. Providing education to the patient and family is imperative, as is the need for an effective family support system.

During a crisis, oxygen therapy is implemented to reverse the hypoxia caused by decreased hemoglobin and vaso-occlusion of vessels. Aggressive hydration with oral and parenteral fluids increases blood volume and reduces renal vaso-occlusion caused by increased hemolysis of RBCs. Analgesia, usually from opiates, is administered for severe pain (see Evidence-Based Practice). Alternative and complementary treatments for pain management can also be taught and employed by the patient to minimize the use of strong analgesics. Antibiotics for infection are also initiated.

Several promising new treatments for SCD include the use of hydroxyurea, complete blood transfusions, and peripheral stem cell transplantation. Hydroxyurea, a chemotherapeutic agent, increases fetal hemoglobin production and is being used selectively. Hydroxyurea results in fewer episodes of crises and a reduction in acute chest syndrome in patients with frequent and severe sickle cell crises; however, it causes **myelosuppression** (the decreased ability of the bone marrow to produce any type of blood cell) and severe toxic effects. It is also potentially teratogenic (altering fetal development), so patients on hydroxyurea need extensive contraceptive counseling.

Evidence-Based Practice

Acute Pain Management in Adults With Sickle Cell Disease

Sickle cell crises involve vaso-occlusive episodes (VOEs) that cause acute pain in patients with this disorder. Because pain management is such a priority in this situation, this quality improvement study was designed to try to determine why these patients often did not receive rapid pain management. Using a prospective pre-/post-evaluation design, patients 18 years old or older who presented with VOEs in an urgent care center after implementation of an evidence-based standard of care (EBPSC) were involved in this study. The results demonstrated a decrease in the mean time for administration of the first pain medication, as well as significantly increased satisfaction. The findings of this study demonstrate the importance of using an evidence-based approach to creating a positive patient experience.

Kim, S., Brathwaite, R. & Ook, K. (2017). Evidence-based practice standard care for acute paFNn management in adults with sickle cell disease in an urgent care center. *Quality Management in Health Care, 26*(2), 108–115.

An exchange blood transfusion, in which the entire blood volume is exchanged, is also a treatment performed on many patients with SCD. The goal of this treatment is maintaining the sickled hemoglobin to no more than 50% of the total hemoglobin in order to prevent or delay thrombotic episodes, including CVA. Although replacing sickled, diseased cells with healthy ones can prevent clinical manifestations for a short period of time, the patient's bone marrow will continue to produce RBCs that sickle when deoxygenated. Therefore, exchange blood transfusions are not a singular treatment. Patients receiving repeated exchange transfusions have an increased risk of blood transfusion reactions and iron overload. Iron is stored in the liver, and the majority of iron received from a blood transfusion goes into storage. High levels of iron in the liver result in fibrosis and cirrhosis, leading to hepatomegaly and, ultimately, liver failure. Iron-chelating agents such as desferrioxamine may need to be simultaneously administered parenterally with transfusions to bind to the iron and decrease the morbidity of iron overload.

Peripheral stem cell transplantation is being attempted with a human leukocyte antigen (HLA)-matched sibling (one without the sickle cell trait) as the preferred donor, otherwise the best-matched donor available. Transplantation, which at this time provides the only chance of a cure, continues to have a high mortality rate, and the incidence of graft-versus-host disease (GVHD) increases morbidity. **Graft-versus-host disease** occurs when donor bone marrow or stem cells attack the recipient's tissues and occurs if the T cells in the graft (e.g., bone marrow or blood) are mature and can destroy the tissues in the graft recipient. If the recipient's immune system is normal, the grafted T cells are controlled, and no tissue destruction occurs. However, if the immune system is deficient, the grafted T cells remain unchecked and can attack the recipient's tissues, leading to death in some cases. Complications vary in severity but may be severe enough to eventually cause multisystem organ dysfunction and death. Although these treatments have been beneficial in many instances, long-term data are not available on efficacy. Currently, preventive measures such as prophylactic use of penicillin to prevent pneumococcal infection, vaccinations, and maintaining adequate hydration are first-line measures to decrease the incidence of crises.

Emotional support for the patient and his or her family is essential in order for the patient to be able to cope with SCD. Education for the entire family is needed, and genetic testing and counseling may be necessary. Healthcare personnel must be able to recognize if the patient, parents, and/or any other family members need any therapeutic counseling. Patients and family members need to be completely aware of the risk factors that may lead to a sickle cell crisis so that they can try to minimize these risks as much as possible. During a crisis, the patient needs support to decrease the anxiety brought on by the pain and shortness of breath. Patients with sickle cell disease are living longer today, and those who do usually have the strongest support systems.

Complications

Complications of SCD are related to the intermittent episodes of hypoxemia, thrombus formation, and tissue hypoxia resulting in infarction and necrosis. These include acute chest syndrome, CVAs, infection, developmental delays and disabilities, and complications in pregnancy.

Pulmonary infarctions, or acute chest syndrome, are experienced by patients with SCD, and multiple episodes are common because of the recurrent nature of thrombosis and infarction experienced. Clinical manifestations include fever, chest pain, tachycardia, tachypnea, hypoxia, sputum production, increased WBCs, and a pulmonary infiltrate on x-ray that indicates an atypical pneumonia. These infection-related clinical manifestations make acute chest syndrome

different from patients who experience pulmonary infarction due to coronary artery disease. In adults, chest pain may be from infection, pulmonary infarction, or pulmonary fat embolism and has a higher mortality rate. Early diagnosis, rapid assessment, and intervention are related to improved morbidity and mortality.

Cerebrovascular accidents are one of the most serious complications of SCD and historically were thought to be secondary to the vaso-occlusion of small cerebral vessels with resulting tissue ischemia and necrosis. More recent studies indicate that CVAs may also be due to lesions on major blood vessels, particularly the internal carotids and anterior and middle cerebral arteries. Cerebrovascular infarctions are more common in children and older adults, whereas hemorrhagic CVAs occur more frequently in adults in their 20s. The reason for this difference in the type of CVA is still unknown, and patients who have had one CVA are at a higher risk for having subsequent CVAs. Neurological complications, such as cranial nerve palsies, seizures, and extremity paresthesias, may be observed in patients after a CVA.

Infection is the leading cause of hospitalization in patients with SCD; they are prone to infections because of the impaired function of the spleen and phagocytic action. Because pneumonia is common, often caused by the pneumococcus bacterium and *H. influenzae*, annual pneumococcal and flu vaccines are recommended for individuals with SCD. All recommended vaccinations against measles, mumps, and pertussis should be current as well as immunization against hepatitis B. Tuberculin skin testing should be performed every 2 to 3 years but annually in regions where the tuberculosis rate is higher. Osteomyelitis caused by *Salmonella* or *Staphylococcus* is not uncommon. Cuts, sores, and insect bites should be observed carefully because they are potential sources of infection.

Pregnancy can exacerbate SCD because the oxygenation demands of the body are increased. Anemia may also worsen, with subsequently more frequent sickling and crises. Infections, particularly pulmonary, are more common. Obstetrical complications include gestational hypertension, preterm labor, and smaller birth weights. Spontaneous abortions and stillbirths are common. Maternal and neonatal mortality are higher than in the general population. Pregnancy causes a greater need for iron and folic acid, and supplementation is particularly important so that multiple causes of anemia do not occur.

Nursing Management
Assessment and Analysis

Clinical manifestations of sickle cell anemia are related to the sickling RBC leading to decreased oxygen-carrying capacity of hemoglobin, as well as complications of vaso-occlusion. Patients typically present with many of the following clinical manifestations:

- Tachypnea
- Shortness of breath

- Tachycardia
- Fatigue
- Pallor
- Jaundice

The complaint of pain during a crisis is the result of vaso-occlusion of blood vessels and the resulting tissue ischemia and hypoxia. It can also be caused by the clumping of cellular debris from the hemolysis of RBCs, particularly in joints, bones, the chest, and the abdomen. Chest pain, however, can also be caused by pulmonary infiltrates (pneumonia) or pulmonary infarction (emboli in the lung) causing tissue ischemia and also preventing adequate oxygen exchange.

Multiple episodes of crises and infarctions over a period of several years can result in the developmental problems seen in individuals with SCD:

- Hand-foot syndrome
- Delayed puberty with developmental delay of secondary sexual characteristics
- Cognitive impairment, ranging from learning disabilities to mental retardation
- Psychosocial issues

Nursing Diagnoses
- **Impaired tissue perfusion** related to sickling of RBCs with resulting decreased oxygen-carrying capacity and tissue hypoxia
- **Activity intolerance** related to hypoxemia resulting from the sickling RBCs
- **Acute pain** related to clumping of sickled RBCs in the capillary beds, resulting in tissue ischemia
- **Risk for powerlessness** related to frequent sickle cell crises, often for no apparent reason

Nursing Interventions
Assessments
- Vital signs
  Tachycardia and tachypnea are a result of the sickling of RBCs that causes a decreased oxygen-carrying capacity of the hemoglobin molecules. It is also as a result of the decreased life span and increased destruction of RBCs.
- Fatigue, pallor, and shortness of breath
  Fatigue, pallor, and shortness of breath worsen with increasingly decreased levels of hemoglobin and RBCs causing inadequate tissue perfusion and hypoxia.
- Pain, swelling in joints and extremities
  Pain is caused by tissue hypoxia and clumping of cellular debris, particularly in the joints, bones, chest, and abdomen, leading to vaso-occlusion.
- Jaundice
  The decreased life span of RBCs in people with SCD and the increased destruction of those RBCs may cause an increase in serum bilirubin, leading to jaundice.
- Hand-foot syndrome
  Multiple episodes of crises and bone infarctions may lead to uneven growth of the fingers and toes.

- Clinical manifestations of infection
  Fever may be present without infection. However, infection must be ruled out. X-rays to eliminate pneumonia or osteomyelitis may be necessary. Any skin lesions must be assessed for infection. Dental hygiene should not be overlooked as a source of infection.
- Hemoglobin and serum bilirubin levels
  The sickled RBCs have decreased hemoglobin levels, and increased hemolysis of RBCs elevates serum bilirubin.
- Serum iron, vitamin B_{12}, and folate levels
  Because of the lower-socioeconomic status of a large percentage of African descendants globally, malnutrition is a concern. Frequently, patients with SCD also have decreased levels of iron, vitamin B_{12}, and folic acid. These deficiencies complicate the anemia and need to be corrected.
- Psychosocial issues
  Patients with SCD may have anger and/or depression in response to chronic disease. Frequent absences from work may interfere with employment, leading to feelings of guilt or anger.

Actions
- Administer oxygen.
  Oxygen assists in decreasing hypoxia and minimizing the severity of the crisis.
- Provide aggressive hydration.
  Aggressive hydration increases blood volume (easing clumping of debris in capillaries) and flushes the kidneys, minimizing the risk for renal failure.
- Administer pain medication.
  Administering analgesia, usually opiates, helps manage the pain caused by vaso-occlusion.
- Administer blood transfusions.
  Blood transfusions may be needed in cases where the anemia is profound to improve oxygen delivery to the tissues.
- Administer antipyretics.
  Antipyretics help reduce fever if present and decrease the fluid loss associated with temperature elevation and increased metabolic rate.
- Provide supportive measures.
  A sickle cell crisis can be frightening to all involved, the individual with SCD as well as the family. The nurse needs to provide emotional support and be cognizant of the possible need for counseling. Contact additional resources if needed.

Teaching
- Pathophysiology of disease
  Parents need to understand the disease and its unpredictable course. The need for medical intervention early in a crisis can make the difference between a crisis lasting several hours or several days. Timely medical intervention can also minimize potential complications.
- Infection prevention measures
  Because patients with SCD are prone to infection as a result of impaired function of the spleen, the need for updated immunizations and annual flu and pneumococcal vaccines is essential. Good dental hygiene and frequent dental check-ups

and careful monitoring of any cuts, sores, and insect bites are also key to minimizing infections.

- Avoid cold temperatures and wearing tight, restrictive clothing.
  Taking measures that may prevent vasoconstriction may help prevent sickle cell crises.
- Avoid high altitudes and depressurized airplanes.
  Avoiding environments with low oxygen tension may minimize sickling of RBCs and prevent a sickle cell crisis.
- Avoid dehydration.
  Being adequately hydrated helps blood move freely through capillary beds.
- Avoid overexertion.
  It is important for the patient with SCD to take rest periods to avoid undue stress on the cardiovascular system.
- Maintain activities of daily life within prescribed limitations.
  Although care and special considerations need to be taken into consideration, it is still important for the person living with SCD to live as normal a life as possible. Therapy and counseling should be recommended if the patient needs assistance in coping with this chronic disease.
- Risk of more frequent sickle cell crises during pregnancy
  Because of the body's increased demands during pregnancy, exacerbation of the SCD may occur. Pregnant individuals with SCD need to be monitored closely because they have a higher risk of maternal and infant mortality.
- Fetal complications
  Low birth weight, gestational hypertension, preterm labor, spontaneous abortions, and stillbirths are also higher in this population because of increased oxygen demands during pregnancy.
- Genetic counseling
  Because SCD is an inherited disease, genetic counseling is recommended for all individuals with SCD or the SCT.

Evaluating Care Outcomes

Sickle cell disease, a heredity disorder, has no cure. The goals are minimizing episodes of sickle cell crisis, symptom management during times of crisis, and minimization of complications. Providing prompt and appropriate care during a crisis, patient and family education regarding the disease and the importance of prophylactic care, and psychological and genetic counseling when necessary helps the individual with SCD improve quality of life as much as possible. Successful outcomes for a patient with SCD include the ability to live a relatively normal life and minimize sickle cell crises.

Connection Check 34.4

Which activity should be avoided in a patient with sickle cell anemia?

A. Driving to the beach 3 hours away
B. Going to a concert
C. Running in a 5-k race
D. Carpentry work

Aplastic Anemia

Epidemiology

Aplastic anemia, also called hypoplastic anemia, is a rare disease process that develops due to bone marrow depression or damage and is often acquired secondary to infections, including hepatitis and human immunodeficiency virus. It is also associated with treatments using high-dose radiation or chemotherapy for cancer, exposure to toxic chemicals, administration of specific medications (chloramphenicol and gold compounds), and autoimmune disorders. The incidence of aplastic anemia in the United States is estimated to be approximately two to four cases per million people. Although this disease occurs in all age groups, there is a small peak in childhood, usually secondary to inherited marrow dysfunction; a second peak in people between the ages of 20 and 25; and an increased incidence in people older than 60 years of age. The male-to-female ratio is 1:1 in the United States. Although there is an increased incidence in males in Asia, there is no corresponding increased incidence of Asian Americans, suggesting that environmental factors in Asia, rather than heredity or gender, have a role in this increase.

Pathophysiology

The damage to the bone marrow, whether secondary to chemicals or medications or an autoimmune response, results in decreased production of red blood cells, white blood cells, and platelets. In cases where bone marrow damage leads to decreased erythrocytes, granulocytes, and platelets, the condition is known as pancytopenia. Although the exact mechanisms leading to aplastic anemia are not clearly understood, the exposure to infectious agents, chemicals, and other insults to bone marrow leads to a cellular immune response. The result of this response is the production of cytokines that suppress both stem cell growth and development.

Clinical Manifestations

The clinical presentation of aplastic anemia may be insidious or chronic. However, in cases secondary to some type of myelotoxin (poison that directly damages bone marrow), the presentation may be sudden and severe. Similar to other anemias, clinical manifestations of aplastic anemia are typically associated with decreased RBCs and include fatigue, shortness of breath, tachycardia, pallor, dizziness, and headache. Clinical manifestations related to decreased WBCs include increased susceptibility to infections, as well as frequent and prolonged infections. Because aplastic anemia may also lead to thrombocytopenia, the patient may also present with unexplained and increased incidence of bruising, nosebleeds, gum bleeding, and prolonged bleeding from cuts and other injuries.

Management

Medical Management

Diagnosis

Diagnostic testing for aplastic anemia includes a CBC, coagulation tests, iron levels, hemoglobin electrophoresis, and a bone marrow biopsy. The CBC results reveal pancytopenia, including decreased reticulocyte, WBC, and platelet counts.

Due to the potential for thrombocytopenia, coagulation testing is important to evaluate the risk for bleeding. Patients with aplastic anemia are typically treated with blood transfusions, and repeated transfusions may lead to increased iron levels. Hemoglobin electrophoresis is often used in the evaluation of anemias because it is used to identify different forms of hemoglobin (Hgb). In aplastic anemia, there may be an increase in Hgb F, which is normally found in small amounts in adults. Bone marrow results typically demonstrate a lack of hematopoietic cells with a predominance of fat cells.

Treatment

During the diagnostic evaluation phase of aplastic anemia, blood transfusions are a primary treatment. However, the goal of treatment is to minimize transfusions to decrease the sensitization that ultimately increases the risk for bone marrow transplantation rejection. The preferred treatment for aplastic anemia is bone marrow transplantation from an HLA-matched sibling donor. Other treatments focus on stimulating bone marrow with medications such as filgrastim (Neupogen®) and epoetin-alfa (Epogen®), which stimulate the bone marrow production of cells and relieve symptoms. In patients over the age of 60, immunosuppressive therapy is preferred. This therapy is also used in patients with no HLA-matched sibling donor. In patients who develop aplastic anemia secondary to chemotherapy or radiation treatments, Epogen or Neupogen may be used to stimulate bone marrow activity; however, the bone marrow usually recovers once these treatments are completed.

Complications

Aplastic anemia has a high mortality rate of greater than 70%, and these patients are at increased risk of complications associated with pancytopenia. Low RBCs decrease the oxygen-carrying capacity and may result in decreased cellular and tissue perfusion. The patient is at increased risk of hemorrhage and severe infection secondary to decreased platelets and WBCs, respectively. In patients who undergo bone marrow transplantation, there is an increased risk of GVHD.

Nursing Management

Assessment and Analysis

Because aplastic anemia potentially decreases RBCs, WBCs, and platelets, patients are at risk for decreased oxygen-carrying capacity, infection, and bleeding, respectively, the nurse needs to monitor for the following clinical manifestations:

- Shortness of breath
- Tachycardia
- Elevated temperature
- Bruising
- Bleeding gums
- Nosebleeds
- Fatigue
- Pallor
- Dizziness
- Headache

Nursing Diagnoses

- **Activity intolerance** related to decreased oxygen carrying capacity secondary to decreased RBCs
- **Risk for injury** related to decreased platelets secondary to bone marrow suppression
- **Risk for infection** related to decreased WBCs secondary to bone marrow suppression

Nursing Interventions

▪ Assessments

- Vital signs
  Tachycardia and tachypnea are secondary to heart and lung compensation for the decreased oxygen-carrying capacity of RBCs. Temperature may be elevated due to inflammatory or infectious processes.
- CBC results
  Bone marrow suppression caused by aplastic anemia results in pancytopenia, leading to decreased RBCs, WBCs, and platelets
- Bone marrow results
  Aplastic anemia leads to a lack of hematopoietic cells, with a predominance of fat cells.
- Oxygen saturation
  Severe anemia leads to insufficient hemoglobin to carry oxygen; oxygen saturation levels may decrease.
- Signs of bleeding
  Due to decreased platelets, the patient is susceptible to bleeding gums, nosebleeds, and increased time to stop bleeding from trauma, venipuncture, injections, and other causes.
- Fatigue and pallor
  Decreased oxygen to tissues secondary to decreased RBCs leads to fatigue, particularly on exertion, and pallor due to decreased perfusion.
- Dizziness and headache
  Decreased oxygen may lead to dizziness and headache.

▪ Actions

- Provide supplemental oxygen.
  Supplemental oxygen is needed to treat decreased oxygenation and perfusion secondary to decreased Hgb.
- Administer blood products.
  Blood components, including packed red blood cells and platelets, may be required for the treatment of symptomatic pancytopenia.
- Implement bleeding precautions.
  Decreased platelets increase the risk of bleeding, and bleeding precautions include the use of soft toothbrushes and direct pressure to venipuncture and injection sites until bleeding stops, among others.
- Protect from injury.
  Due to pancytopenia, the patient is at risk for decreased tissue perfusion that can result in dizziness and falls. The patient is also at risk for bleeding and infections.

▪ Teaching

- Avoid exposure to potential infection (individuals with acute infection, crowded places, etc.).
  Due to decreased WBCs, the patient is at increased risk of infection, and crowded places may increase the chances of exposure to people with infectious diseases.

- Report all temperature elevations.
  Patients with aplastic anemia may present with a low-grade temperature with an infection due to bone marrow depression that impacts WBC production and maturation.
- Avoid activities with the potential for trauma or injury.
  Potential trauma and injury increase the risk of bleeding due to thrombocytopenia.
- Clinical manifestations of anemia
  Because aplastic anemia is a medical emergency, the patient and family need to be instructed to contact the healthcare provider at the first signs of anemia, infection, and bleeding.
- Nutritional intake
  Adequate nutritional intake enhances immune function and resistance to infection.

Evaluating Care Outcomes

Patients living with aplastic anemia must be constantly vigilant for potential exacerbations. In chronic cases, positive outcomes include stable CBC and platelet counts, with the absence of infection and bleeding. As tissue perfusion is improved, clinical manifestations of tachycardia, shortness of breath, fatigue, and pallor resolve. Healthcare providers managing patients with this disorder need to be attentive to potential complications associated with the administration of specific medications.

Glucose-6-Phosphate Dehydrogenase Deficiency

Epidemiology

Glucose-6-phosphate dehydrogenase (G6PD) is a metabolic enzyme that is important to RBC metabolism because it protects the RBCs from oxidative stresses that can lead to cellular destruction. It is a hereditary disorder that leads to hemolysis when the patient is exposed to specific foods (e.g., fava beans), medications (antimalarial medicines, high doses of aspirin, NSAIDs, and sulfa medications), infection, or stress. In the United States, the incidence of G6PD deficiency is greater in blacks and men. It is estimated that 10% to 14% of African American males in the United States have the gene for this disorder. Similar to patients diagnosed with sickle cell anemia, patients with G6PD have protection against malaria.

Genetic Connections

G6PD Deficiency

Glucose-6-phosphate dehydrogenase (G6PD) deficiency, the most common enzyme disorder in humans, is an inherited recessive X-linked disorder. The mutation is found on the gene locus Xq28, a genetic marker located on the X chromosome.

Pathophysiology

Due to the lack of G6PD, RBCs break down prematurely, resulting in hemolysis. During an acute episode of hemolysis in patients with this disorder, the body continues to produce new RBCs. This deficiency is often the cause of mild to severe jaundice in newborns.

Clinical Manifestations

Patients diagnosed with G6PD deficiency may present with pallor, jaundice, dark urine, fatigue, shortness of breath, tachycardia, and an enlarged spleen. The pallor results secondary to decreased RBCs, and the jaundice and dark urine develop secondary to bilirubin buildup from the hemolysis. The fatigue, shortness of breath, and tachycardia result from the decreased oxygen-carrying capacity of the damaged RBCs. Splenomegaly develops secondary to the elevated numbers of lysed RBCs circulating through the spleen.

Management

Medical Management

Diagnosis

Diagnostic testing for G6PD deficiency includes CBC, reticulocyte count, and blood smear analysis for Heinz bodies (accumulation of degraded Hbg in RBCs). The CBC in patients with this disorder reveals a mild to severe anemia. In patients with G6PD deficiency, the increased reticulocyte count reflects the production of new red blood cells secondary to hemolysis. The blood smear analysis may reveal RBC abnormalities, including the presence of Heinz bodies. Liver enzymes may be elevated in G6PD deficiency due to RBC destruction. Direct DNA testing and sequencing of the G6PD gene are also important to the diagnosis of this disorder.

Treatment

Once definitively diagnosed, prevention is the key to the management and treatment of G6PD deficiency. Avoiding foods and medications that cause hemolysis is indicated. In the case of severe hemolysis, blood transfusions may be necessary because these transfused RBCs are not G6PD deficient and have a normal life span. Folic acid may also be prescribed to support RBC synthesis. Splenectomy may be indicated in patients with an enlarged spleen due to frequent episodes of hemolysis.

Complications

Although rare, adult patients with G6PD deficiency are at risk for severe anemia. There is also a risk of kidney damage secondary to increased circulating lysed RBCs through the renal tubules. In newborns, this deficiency is implicated in prolonged neonatal jaundice and kernicterus, a bilirubin-induced brain disorder.

Nursing Management

Assessment and Analysis

The clinical manifestations of G6PD deficiency are directly related to the RBC lysis that results secondary to the lack of this important enzyme. The nurse monitors for the following in these patients:

- Shortness of breath
- Tachycardia
- Pallor
- Decreased RBCs and Hgb
- Elevated reticulocyte count
- Heinz bodies on the blood smear
- Elevated liver enzymes
- Jaundice
- Dark urine
- Enlarged spleen

With severe anemia, the patient needs to be monitored for cardiovascular deterioration, including a decreased level of consciousness and hypotension.

Nursing Diagnoses

- **Inadequate tissue perfusion** related to decreased circulating RBCs secondary to hemolysis
- **Activity intolerance** related to decreased oxygen-carrying capacity of lysed RBCs

Nursing Interventions
▪ Assessments

- Vital signs
  The G6PD enzyme is required for RBC development, and in its absence, anemia may develop. With the decreased oxygen-carrying capacity of the Hgb, tachycardia and tachypnea may develop as a compensatory mechanism.
- Shortness of breath, pallor, and fatigue
  These clinical manifestations are exacerbated by the decreased oxygen-carrying capacity of the lysed RBCs.
- CBC and reticulocyte count
  Decreased RBCs, hematocrit, and hemoglobin result due to hemolysis. The reticulocyte count may be increased in an attempt to replace the lysed cells.
- Oxygenation saturation
  With severe anemia leading to insufficient hemoglobin to carry oxygen, oxygen saturation levels may decrease.
- Blood smear analysis
  The G6PD deficiency results in RBC abnormalities and the accumulation of degraded Hgb (Heinz bodies). When a Heinz body is identified by macrophages in the spleen, the macrophage engulfs the Heinz body and a small piece of the RBC membrane, resulting in misshapen RBCs, called bite cells, in the RBC analysis.
- Liver enzymes and bilirubin levels
  The excessive amounts of heme released from RBC destruction are catabolized to bilirubin concentrations that exceed the liver's ability to conjugate. This also results in the accumulation of indirect bilirubin.
- Skin color and urine color
  The bilirubin accumulation in the circulation leads to jaundice and dark urine color.

▪ Actions

- Provide supplemental oxygen.
  Supplemental oxygen is needed to treat decreased oxygenation and perfusion secondary to decreased Hgb.
- Implement bleeding precautions.
  Decreased platelets increase the risk of bleeding, and bleeding precautions include the use of soft toothbrushes and direct pressure to venipuncture and injection sites until bleeding stops, among others.
- Administer folic acid.
  Folic acid facilitates RBC production; G6PD places the patient in a state of high RBC synthesis.

▪ Teaching

- Avoid fava beans.
  Because the lack of G6PD leads to hemolysis in response to the ingestion of fava beans, the patient and family need to understand the importance of avoiding this food.
- Avoid medications that increase the risk of crises (aspirin, NSAIDs, etc.).
  Because these medications increase the risk of bleeding, the patient and family are taught to avoid these medications.
- Clinical manifestations of anemia
  Because prevention is so critical to G6PD deficiency management, the patient and family need to understand the importance of immediately reporting signs of anemia.

Evaluating Care Outcomes

In adults with diagnosed G6PD deficiency, preventive measures and knowledge of the disease process are key to the management of this disorder. Avoiding foods and medications that exacerbate this disorder and recognizing the relationship between stress and G6PD deficiency will result in decreased episodes. In stable patients, clinical manifestations of decreased tissue perfusion (tachycardia, shortness of breath, fatigue, and pallor) decrease. Healthcare providers managing patients with this disorder need to be attentive to the potential complications associated with the administration of specific medications.

Polycythemia Vera

Epidemiology

Polycythemia, or **erythrocytosis**, is an increase in the production of RBCs and can be a primary or secondary disorder. Primary polycythemia, or **polycythemia vera** (PV), is a disorder of the bone marrow in which there is an increased production of RBCs that may be accompanied by an increased production of WBCs and platelets. Polycythemia vera has been found to be caused by a mutation in a gene known as the Janus kinase 2, or *JAK2*, gene in 90% of cases. The *JAK2* gene is associated with signal transduction to hematopoietic cells. The reason for this genetic mutation is unknown, and it occurs after birth. According to the National Heart, Lung, and Blood Institute, PV is extremely rare, and only 5 out of 1 million people are diagnosed with this disorder annually. The disorder is found in men more often than women, and most adults are older than 60 years of age at the time of diagnosis. It is exceedingly rare in those younger than 20. Although PV is not hereditary, in some cases there is a familial tendency, indicating that other genetic factors may also be involved. Exposure to radiation has also been associated with an increased incidence of this disorder. In PV, most patients not only exhibit an increase in RBC counts but also an increase in the number of WBCs and platelets.

Secondary polycythemia occurs in response to the body's hypoxic state and may be considered appropriate or inappropriate. Appropriate secondary polycythemia occurs in situations caused by exposure to environments that have low oxygen tension, such as occurs with high altitudes and heavy smoke. The body compensates by producing more RBCs, thus increasing the oxygen-carrying capacity of the blood. This is a temporary response until the body becomes more acclimated to that environment. Inappropriate secondary polycythemia occurs when the body responds to a stimulus in an inappropriate way by secreting additional erythropoietin, which results in increased RBC production. This inappropriate erythrocytosis may occur in kidney disease and certain tumors. In secondary polycythemia, the WBC and platelet counts remain normal in the presence of the increased RBC production compared with PV, in which the number of all blood cells is elevated.

Genetic Connections

Polycythemia

Although most cases of polycythemia are acquired during a person's life, some cases appear to be inherited. Mutations in the *JAK2* and *TET2* genes appear to have a role in the development of this order.

Pathophysiology

In normal hematopoiesis (formation of blood cells), the body's response to a state of hypoxia is to increase RBC production, known as erythrocytosis or polycythemia. This erythrocytosis increases the oxygen-carrying capacity of the blood, and increased production of RBCs thickens the blood, making it more viscous. This **hyperviscosity**, or thickened blood, slows down the circulation of the blood. In a state of polycythemia, the hematocrit is greater than 48% in women and greater than 52% in men. Hemoglobin levels are greater than 16.5 g/dL and 18.5 g/dL in women and men, respectively, and the total RBC count is greater than 6 million/mm^3. Resolution of the hypoxia reverses this process, and normal levels are once again achieved.

In PV, a gene mutation, the *JAK2* gene, stimulates the overproduction of not only RBCs but also WBCs and platelets. Because RBCs have a much larger mass than WBCs or platelets, the increase in RBCs makes the blood

more viscous. As the hyperviscosity increases, circulation slows as the heart labors to pump the thickened blood. Even though there is an increase in the volume of RBCs, the body becomes hypoxic as the hyperviscosity slows oxygen exchange to the tissues.

The erythrocytosis that occurs in appropriate secondary polycythemia is in response to a hypoxic state caused by a low-oxygen-tension environment. **Erythropoietin** is released from the kidneys, which stimulates RBC production in order to resolve the body's perceived oxygen deprivation. At higher altitudes or in mountainous regions, atmospheric pressure is lower than that at sea level. This lower pressure decreases the rate of oxygen exchange because of the difference between atmospheric and alveolar pressures. People exposed to higher altitudes develop appropriate secondary polycythemia to compensate for the lower pressure. This natural erythrocytosis is why many athletes train at higher altitudes—the body's elevated RBC count may give the athlete an "edge" over competitors when competing at lower altitudes due to increased oxygen-carrying capacity. Appropriate secondary polycythemia can also be seen in patients with chronic obstructive pulmonary disease (COPD), patients with heart failure, and patients with a history of heavy cigarette smoking because the body attempts to compensate for the impaired tissue perfusion caused by decreased alveolar function. Certain tumors, such as pheochromocytomas (hypersecreting tumors of the adrenal medulla) and cerebellar hemangiomas, may excrete an erythropoietin-stimulating substance that causes an inappropriate secondary polycythemia.

Clinical Manifestations

Polycythemia vera is a slowly progressive disease and may take years to produce clinical manifestations, which are related to the blood's hyperviscosity, the hypoxic state, and the congestion of organs by the blood cells. The clinical presentation includes shortness of breath, difficulty breathing when lying flat, headache, dizziness, weakness, splenomegaly, and blurred vision. Pruritus (itchiness), especially after a warm bath, and flushing of the face most likely occur as a result of vascular dilation and engorgement of the capillaries from the increased RBCs. The hyperviscosity of the blood and the slowing of blood flow also increase the risk for clot formation. Patients with PV may present with nosebleeds and bleeding gums because the hyperviscosity leads to thrombosis, and fewer circulating platelets are present to form clots in response to injury. Without treatment, patients with PV are at increased risk of death secondary to CVAs, MI, pulmonary embolus, or hemorrhage.

Management

Diagnosis

Because the onset of PV is insidious, the disorder is often discovered during routine blood tests. Complete blood count results include an increased RBC count of greater than 6 million/mm^3, and the hematocrit can exceed 60%. Because splenomegaly is often seen in about 75% of patients, the bone marrow becomes fibrotic and is unable to produce sufficient cells. To make the diagnosis, the World Health Organization (WHO) recommends hemoglobin levels of greater than 16.5g/dL in men and greater than 16.0g/dL in women. In PV, elevated WBC and platelet counts may also be present as a result of the gene mutation's effect on the bone marrow production of blood cells. In secondary polycythemia, the WBCs and platelets remain in the normal range. Other laboratory tests that may aid in diagnosis are an erythropoietin level, blood smear, bone marrow biopsy, and genetic testing. A complete history and physical examination are often keys to diagnosing the cause of the polycythemia.

Medical Management

Treatment of PV is aimed at reducing the hyperviscosity and preventing hemorrhage. Therapeutic phlebotomy involves removing blood to decrease blood volume and viscosity. A unit of blood (350 to 500 mL) is removed weekly until the hematocrit is less than 45%, then only as needed. The patient usually feels more comfortable immediately because this reduces congestion of organs such as the spleen and liver. Repeated phlebotomies may cause iron-deficiency anemia, so serum ferritin levels are monitored as well as CBCs. Phlebotomy, however, does not decrease WBC or platelet levels if elevated in PV, and chemotherapeutic agents such as hydroxyurea or interferon may be given to suppress bone marrow production. Radiation may also be employed to suppress the bone marrow. These treatments may have the undesirable side effect of causing leukemia. Antiplatelet medications, such as anagrelide or low-dose aspirin, may be prescribed to reduce the risk of thrombosis.

When secondary polycythemia is appropriate, treatment of the underlying condition usually resolves the polycythemia. Prevention of secondary polycythemia includes the cessation of activities such as smoking or mountain climbing, which deprive the body of oxygen. Maintaining a healthy lifestyle contributes to preventing conditions that cause polycythemia.

Symptom management in patients with PV is important to maintain quality of life. Regular moderate exercise to improve circulation and decrease thrombosis is emphasized. Medications to minimize itching may be prescribed, as well as interventions focused on avoiding extreme temperatures, taking extra care of the hands and feet, guarding against injury, drinking at least 3 L of fluid daily, avoiding tight clothing, elevating the feet while at rest, and reporting any chest pain or dyspnea.

Complications

The main complications of PV are thrombosis and hemorrhage. As the blood becomes hyperviscous, there is a slowing of blood flow and increased risk of thrombosis. As multiple thromboses occur, injury may result in hemorrhage as the number of circulating platelets available to respond to the injury is decreased. Most deaths in patients with PV are secondary to MI or cerebrovascular attack, followed by other thromboembolic events such as pulmonary infarction. Gastrointestinal hemorrhage occurs because of abnormally formed platelets and a decrease in circulating platelets. Reductions in blood viscosity and volume help to prevent these complications. Abnormal bone marrow scarring may occur from the overproduction of cells, leading to myelofibrosis, which ultimately results in lower-than-normal blood counts of all cells. If the bone marrow begins to grow uncontrollably, acute myelogenous leukemia (AML) occurs. Heart failure is a result of the constant strain on the heart of pumping the hyperviscous blood.

Nursing Management

Assessment and Analysis

Clinical manifestations of polycythemia are related to hyperviscosity, hypervolemia, and engorgement of the capillaries. It is important that the nurse observe for the following in patients with this disorder:

- Shortness of breath, especially when supine
- Fatigue
- Dizziness
- Headache
- Generalized pruritus, especially after a warm bath
- Flushing of the face
- Feeling of fullness in the left upper abdomen (engorged spleen and/or liver)
- Vision problems
- Weight loss

Sudden chest pain, headache, or shortness of breath may be the result of a thromboembolic event, and immediate medical attention is needed.

Nursing Diagnoses

- **Ineffective tissue perfusion** related to hyperviscosity and poor oxygen exchange
- **Activity intolerance** related to impaired tissue perfusion secondary to hyperviscosity and poor oxygen exchange
- **Risk for ineffective coping** related to clinical manifestations of shortness of breath, fatigue, itching, and anorexia

Nursing Interventions

Assessments

- Shortness of breath/dyspnea, especially when supine
  Because of decreased oxygen delivery to the tissues, respiratory effort increases in an attempt to improve oxygen delivery.
- Headache
  Headache is a result of the increased blood volume and hyperviscosity in PV. A sudden, severe headache may be a clinical manifestation of a CVA as the result of clot formation.
- Dizziness
  Dizziness in PV occurs because of impaired tissue perfusion as the blood flow slows secondary to blood hyperviscosity.
- Generalized pruritus, especially after a warm bath
  The itchiness in PV is most likely due to the vascular dilation and capillary engorgement as a result of the increased blood

cell production with resulting increased blood volume. This can be painful due to swelling from the histamine release and increased number of basophils and may be triggered by the exposure to water (aquagenic pruritus).

- Flushing of the face
  Flushing in PV occurs secondary to capillary engorgement caused by the increased blood volume. This plethora causes a ruddy complexion.

- Feeling of fullness in the left upper abdomen
  The abdominal fullness (which may become painful) is due to the organ congestion secondary to the hyperviscosity and increased blood volume.

- Fatigue
  Fatigue occurs because of the increased workload of the heart and poor tissue perfusion secondary to the hyperviscosity. Angina and intermittent claudication can occur.

- Vision problems
  Blurred vision or blind spots occur from poor tissue perfusion or vascular damage to small vessels in the eye secondary to hyperviscosity.

- Weight loss
  The feeling of fullness in the abdomen in the left upper quadrant is caused by organ congestion that leads to abdominal pain, early satiety, and/or anorexia. Patients with elevated hemoglobin and hematocrit should be checked for an enlarged spleen on physical exam by the healthcare provider.

- RBCs, hemoglobin, and hematocrit
  Overproduction of RBCs is a result of stimulation of the bone marrow secondary to either a gene mutation or the body's hypoxic state. This may lead to angina, hypertension, and thrombophlebitis, especially if the patient has cardiac disease.

- Bone marrow biopsy results
  *Examination of the bone marrow shows the **panmyelosis** (overproduction of RBCs, WBCs, and platelets) in PV.*

- Erythropoietin level
  In secondary polycythemia, the hypoxic state stimulates the release of erythropoietin by the kidneys.

- Vital signs during therapeutic phlebotomy
  If blood loss is not too fast, the patient may develop signs of hypovolemia, including hypotension and tachycardia.

- Uric acid level
  The rapid turnover of red blood cells associated with PV may result in an elevated uric acid level. This increase in uric acid can cause gout and kidney stone formation.

Actions

- Obtain routine CBCs.
  If the patient is undergoing therapeutic phlebotomy, blood count checks are done to maintain a hematocrit below 45% in men and below 42% in women. If the patient is on chemotherapeutic agents, CBCs are indicated to monitor the degree of myelosuppression.

- Increase fluid intake.
  Increased fluid intake may reduce the hyperviscosity of the blood.

- Ensure adequate rest.
  Frequent rest periods may be needed to help the patient deal with the increased workload on the heart due to the hyperviscosity and the patient's subsequent shortness of breath.

- Elevate lower extremities when sitting.
  Elevation of the lower extremities aids the circulation in returning to the heart and minimizes the risk of thrombus formation secondary to venous stasis.

- Modify cardiovascular risk factors.
  Obesity, hypertension, diabetes, and smoking can increase the risk of thrombosis, CVA, MI, or deep vein thrombosis (DVT). Avoid restrictive clothing and crossing legs. Encourage smoking cessation. Implement DVT prophylaxis.

Teaching

- Clinical manifestations of severe thromboembolic events
  Patients need to understand the clinical manifestations of MI, CVA, and pulmonary infarction in order to seek immediate medical attention.

- Rationale for aggressive hydration
  Aggressive hydration daily is necessary to minimize hyperviscosity.

- Eat small, frequent meals.
  Small, frequent meals are usually better tolerated because of the abdominal fullness caused by the hyperviscosity and resulting organ congestion.

- Avoid tight, restrictive clothing.
  Tight clothing impairs circulation.

- Avoidance of extreme temperatures of heat and cold
  Itching is worsened by warm baths as a result of capillary engorgement. Cold temperatures cause vasoconstriction. Limit bathing to 30 minutes, and baths should use tepid water. Hot water can also exacerbate symptoms. Avoid vigorous drying off. Use mild soap and apply lotion after bathing. Colloidal oatmeal treatment may be added to bath water to decrease itching.

- Observe bleeding precautions.
  Patients need to observe bleeding precautions because of the risk of hemorrhage from impaired platelet function.

- Routine moderate exercise
  Regular exercise improves circulation and decreases the risk of thrombosis formation.

- Regular laboratory tests
  The CBC must be monitored for sudden changes, which may indicate a status change in the disorder of PV.

- Genetic testing
  Genetic testing may show abnormalities, such as mutations in the JAK2- STAT pathway, that stimulate abnormal cell growth. A positive JAK2 genetic mutation can result in increased cellular bone marrow and a low serum erythropoietin level, which may be hereditary in PV.

Evaluating Care Outcomes

Polycythemia vera is a slowly progressive disorder characterized by elevated RBCs. With proper treatment, complications may be prevented or delayed. Patients need lifelong healthcare attention and need to understand how to deal with the clinical manifestations associated with this disorder. Being able to improve quality of life and prevent major thromboembolic events and hemorrhage is the goal. Resolution of the hypoxic state is the goal in secondary polycythemia.

Connection Check 34.5

Which factor places the patient at a higher risk for developing secondary polycythemia?
A. Type 2 diabetes mellitus
B. History of alcohol abuse
C. Smoking
D. Hypertension

CASE STUDY: EPISODE 2

A physical examination of Mr. Owens shows a well-developed male. His vital signs are as follows: temperature (T) 98.6°F (37.0°C), pulse (P) 102 bpm, respirations (R) 18, blood pressure (BP) 150/92 mm Hg, O_2 saturation 93% on room air. Lungs are clear bilaterally. Heart rate is regular. Bowel sounds are present. The provider orders a chest x-ray, CBC, comprehensive chemistry panel, serum ferritin level, vitamin B_{12} assay, serum folate level, and urinary MMA. The chest x-ray shows some signs of COPD but no infiltrates. The CBC results are as follows: RBC 3.2 million cells/mm³, Hbg 9.4 g/dL, Hct 28.1%, WBC 6.2 × 10³/mm³, platelets 97,000/mm³. Chemistry panel results are within normal range, as are the different serum levels and urinary MMA. The provider subsequently refers Mr. Owens to an oncologist, who orders a bone marrow biopsy, positron emission tomography (PET) scan, and genetic testing…

BLEEDING DISORDERS

Thrombocytopenia

Thrombocytopenia is defined as a reduced number of platelets below the average range of 150,000 to 450,000/mm³. It is not a disease but rather a complication of other disorders or a syndrome as a result of other events occurring in the body. Thrombocytopenia occurs as a result of a decreased production of platelets by the bone marrow or increased platelet destruction. Antibodies that increase platelet destruction may be genetic, acquired, or medication induced. Antiplatelet antibodies bind to the plasma membrane of platelets, causing platelet sequestration and destruction by the mononuclear phagocytes in the spleen and other lymph tissue at a rate that exceeds the abilities of the bone marrow

to produce platelets. In approximately 70% of the cases of idiopathic thrombocytopenic purpura (ITP), there is an antecedent viral disease that precedes the eruption of petechiae or purpura by 1 to 3 weeks. High levels of IgG are found bound to platelets and may represent immune complexes on the platelet surface. Hemorrhagic conditions such as ITP, hemophilia, and disseminated intravascular coagulation (DIC) present with thrombocytopenia and heparin-induced thrombocytopenia (HIT). With all of these disorders, the main complication is the risk for hemorrhage. These hemorrhagic conditions are discussed in this section because of the relationship to platelets and the bleeding potential represented. The risk of developing thrombocytopenia varies throughout the life span of the individual.

Epidemiology

There are numerous causes for thrombocytopenia, including malignancy, infection, certain medications (e.g., sulfa medications), autoimmune conditions (e.g., lupus), and DIC. It is now called immune thrombocytopenia purpura and is the most common autoimmune platelet consumption disorder, and it can be acute or chronic. It may follow a viral infection in children, and pregnancy can induce thrombocytopenia. Approximately 6% to 15% of pregnant women may develop a low platelet count in the final trimester of pregnancy, referred to as gestational thrombocytopenia, that is usually mild and resolves spontaneously during the postpartum phase. Because a low platelet count during pregnancy may be indicative of other diseases, such as ITP, if the patient had thrombocytopenia prior to pregnancy, develops it during the first or second trimester, or presents with a platelet count of less than 75,000 in the third trimester, further evaluation is indicated to rule out ITP.

Acute ITP may occur between the ages of 2 and 6, whereas chronic ITP occurs most often in women between the ages of 15 and 40. Childhood ITP usually presents rapidly and resolves spontaneously within a few weeks to 6 months, whereas chronic adult ITP usually has a more insidious onset and rarely results in remission. The incidence of ITP is estimated at 3.8 million patients in the United States. Risk factors include being of African descent and obese. The female-to-male ratio is approximately 2:1, with the incidence peaking between the ages of 20 to 30 years; however, this ratio becomes about equal after the age of 60 years.

Hemophilia is a group of bleeding disorders in which, although thrombocytopenia may be present, clotting factors VIII (hemophilia A) and IX (hemophilia B or Christmas disease) are inadequate. Hemophilia is a hereditary disorder carried by females on the X chromosome. The manifestation of hemophilia only presents clinically in males, approximately 1 in 5,000 to 7,000. Hemophilia occurs in all ethnic groups. A female carrier of the hemophilia gene has a 50% chance of passing this disorder to any male offspring (Fig. 34.6).

Disseminated intravascular coagulation occurs secondary to severe trauma to the body. Because DIC is not a disease but a result of trauma or severe tissue injury, incidence rates

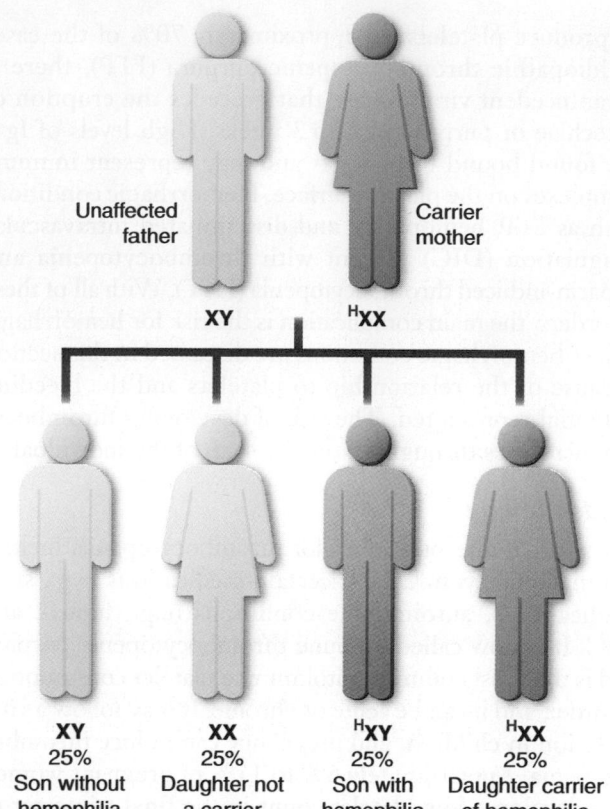

FIGURE 34.6 Hemophilia inheritance pattern. This disorder is inherited from the female but present in the male.

are not measured. Severe trauma may include crush injuries, burns, sepsis, and shock. Obstetrical complications such as abruptio placentae or retained products of conception (placenta or fetal tissue) also cause DIC. Tissue necrosis following extensive abdominal surgery with leakage of intestinal contents may also lead to DIC. Rarely, snakebite, heatstroke, or fat embolism from long-bone fractures lead to DIC. Certain cancers such as leukemia or widespread metastasis may also result in DIC, and there is a high mortality rate with DIC because of multisystem organ dysfunction and hemorrhage.

Heparin-induced thrombocytopenia (HIT) may occur in patients receiving heparin for an existing thrombus or clot. While thrombocytopenia occurs, patients typically do not have bleeding episodes, and additional thrombi occur or the existing thrombus enlarges. There are concerns that the use of heparin to maintain the patency of central lines predisposes patients to the development of HIT.

Pathophysiology

Idiopathic thrombocytopenia purpura usually follows a viral infection or immunization in children. In adults, ITP may be medication induced or secondary to an autoimmune disorder. In all cases, it appears to be an immune system dysfunction in which antiplatelet antibodies are formed, which increases platelet destruction. Rather than the 7- to 10-day life span, the platelets may be destroyed in a matter of hours.

The clotting factors that are lacking in hemophilia interfere with the normal clotting mechanism of the body. The two most common forms are hemophilia A (factor VIII deficiency) and hemophilia B (factor IX deficiency). Minor injuries can result in significant blood loss, and in cases of severe hemophilia, spontaneous bleeding may occur. **Hemarthrosis**, bleeding in the muscles and joints, can be common and eventually disabling as joint deformities occur from repeated bleeding episodes. Severe trauma in a patient may result in the development of DIC. In a complex sequence initiated by the injury, all platelets and clotting factors form multiple thrombi throughout the body secondary to alteration of the body's normal anticoagulant mechanisms. When all the body stores of platelets and clotting factors are exhausted, spontaneous bleeding occurs from nearly every orifice because there are insufficient circulating platelets and clotting factors to stop the bleeding. The multiple emboli cause tissue necrosis, leading to multisystem organ dysfunction.

Heparin-induced thrombocytopenia appears to be the result of an immune response by the body. Although heparin is a natural substance in the body, the administration of exogenous heparin in some patients leads to the body producing antibodies against the "foreign" heparin. It typically occurs 5 to 14 days after the first administration of heparin. In a complex sequela, these antibodies initiate a response that culminates in the formation of new blood clots and a resulting fall in the platelet count as they are consumed (used) to form these thrombi.

Clinical Manifestations

With a reduced number of platelets, easy bruising and petechiae are usually the first clinical manifestations with all forms of thrombocytopenia. Bleeding may occur from the nose, around the gums, or from the gastrointestinal tract. In severe cases, bleeding in vital organs such as the brain may prove fatal.

Management

Diagnosis

The treatment of ITP depends on the level of thrombocytopenia present. If platelet counts remain above 100,000/mm³, an observational strategy is usually employed through routine CBC analyses. A CBC with a manual differential can confirm the diagnosis of thrombocytopenia, which is defined as platelets less than 150,000/mm³. In addition to the CBC, a bone marrow biopsy confirms the diagnosis of ITP. Prolonged prothrombin time, partial prothrombin time, and thrombin time are helpful in diagnosing DIC, as well as a reduced fibrinogen level, elevated fibrin split products, and elevated dimers (cross-linked fibrin fragments). Clotting factors (e.g., factors VIII, IX) may aid in the diagnosis of both hemophilia and DIC. A blood smear is helpful in determining the morphology of the platelets. An additional test, in addition to a CBC to diagnose HIT, is the enzyme-linked immunosorbent assay (ELISA), which is an immunoassay test to determine the presence of the antibodies.

Medical Management

If the thrombocytopenia becomes more profound, treatment with glucocorticoids has proven to be beneficial. Glucocorticoids increase platelet counts by decreasing the antiplatelet antibody production, improving production of platelets by the bone marrow, and decreasing the phagocytosis that is consuming the platelets. In extreme cases, performing a splenectomy has improved platelet counts because the spleen is the primary site of platelet destruction.

In hemophilia cases, depending on the type of hemophilia, replacement of the missing clotting factors is indicated. Replacement of factor VIII resolves bleeding in hemophilia A, whereas factor IX is used in hemophilia B. These clotting factors are delivered intravenously from recombinant DNA products, which do not contain human blood components. For minor injuries, treatment should be obtained as soon as possible with as many as three treatments (one treatment daily). Major traumas need replacement of clotting factors for 7 to 10 days or until healing is assured. Prophylactic treatment with clotting factors may be indicated for some surgeries with factor replacement for up to 7 to 10 days postoperatively. Prompt treatment with clotting factors minimizes complications caused by bleeding, such as joint deformities, which were prevalent prior to factor replacement.

Resolution of the underlying condition that initiates the clotting cascade is imperative in treating DIC, for example, immediate antibiotic therapy to treat the sepsis. Providing supportive care in the form of administering blood, platelets, fresh frozen plasma, and **cryoprecipitate** (plasma product rich in factor VIII) may be employed to maintain hemostasis. These patients are managed in an intensive care setting where they can be closely observed with hemodynamic monitoring equipment. Mortality rates are high in patients who develop DIC, although exact numbers are not known because the cause of death is usually attributed to the underlying disorder.

Stopping the heparin administration is the first step in treating HIT. However, because the formation of additional thrombi occurs frequently in these patients, an anticoagulant is required to prevent further thrombus formation and the production of the antibodies, allowing the platelet count to recover. Warfarin should not be used because it can cause skin gangrene in this population. Three anticoagulants have been approved for use in patients diagnosed with HIT: danaparoid (not available in the United States), lepirudin, and argatroban. Platelet transfusions are discouraged because they may increase thrombus formation.

Complications

Risk of hemorrhage is the major complication of any condition that results in thrombocytopenia, and the severity of the thrombocytopenia determines whether there is a risk of spontaneous bleeding. Although the initial clinical manifestations of thrombocytopenia are ecchymosis and petechiae, as the platelet count decreases, normal activities such as tooth brushing or sneezing may produce spontaneous bleeding. Patients are instructed about bleeding precautions (Box 34.1) when the

---

Box 34.1 Bleeding Precautions for the Patient With Thrombocytopenia/ Bleeding Disorders

1. Use a soft-bristle toothbrush or gauze to clean the teeth. No flossing.
2. Use an electric razor for shaving.
3. Encourage the use of shoes or slippers when out of bed.
4. Maintain a clutter-free environment to minimize bruising.
5. Use a stool softener daily to decrease constipation and straining during bowel movements.
6. Avoid rectal thermometers, suppositories, enemas, and vaginal douches.
7. Avoid sexual intercourse when the platelet count is extremely low.
8. Do not blow nose.
9. When using a knife is necessary, make sure the blade is sharp. More force is required for dull knives.
10. If a laceration occurs, apply direct pressure and/or ice for no less than 5 minutes until bleeding stops.
11. Procedures such as intramuscular injections, arterial sticks, and peripheral blood draws should be kept to a minimum.

---

platelet count drops below 100,000/mm³ and especially when it is below 50,000/mm³. Spontaneous bleeding becomes a real concern when the platelets are less than 20,000/mm³. Transfusions of platelets are usually not given until the platelets are less than 20,000/mm³ because of the risks involved with blood product transfusions; however, if an invasive procedure is being considered, transfusions may be given prophylactically to minimize the risk of bleeding. Close monitoring is indicated in patients with any type of severe trauma in order to detect early manifestations of DIC because early recognition of thrombocytopenia may be key in determining a patient's prognosis.

Nursing Management

Assessment and Analysis

Clinical manifestations of thrombocytopenia are a result of the decreased number of platelets, and the nurse correlates the following findings to this disorder:

- Ecchymosis
- Petechiae
- Nosebleeds
- Bleeding gums
- Black, tarry stools
- Hematuria

Nursing Diagnoses

- **Risk of injury: bleeding** related to decreased number of platelets
- **Risk for effective therapeutic regimen management** related to possible frequent administration of platelets and/or clotting factors
- **Fear** related to hemorrhaging from low platelet count

Nursing Interventions

■ Assessments

- Platelet count
  A decreased platelet count is seen on the CBC. Further testing indicates whether it is due to increased platelet destruction or decreased platelet production. In pregnant patients, monitor liver function tests and platelet count during the pregnancy. Monitor for easy bruising, and report any clinical manifestations of bleeding to the healthcare provider. Watch for excessive postpartum hemorrhage or clots. Place patient on bleeding precautions if the platelet count is below normal, hematocrit is low, or liver function tests are elevated.

- Ecchymosis
  Ease of bruising increases as the number of platelets decreases and tissue injury increases with contact.

- Petechiae/purpura
  Intradermal bleeding occurs as a result of platelet reduction.

- Frank bleeding (nosebleeds; bleeding gums; black, tarry stools; or hematuria)
  Parts of the body where mucous membranes are thin or cells rapidly divide are more prone to bleeding when platelet counts are decreased.

■ Actions

- Implement bleeding precautions (see Box 34.1).
  Due to decreased platelet count, the patient is at increased risk of bleeding from minor injuries, venepuncture, and so forth.

- Minimize blood loss from lacerations or venipuncture.
  If bleeding occurs, apply direct pressure and/or application of ice to cause vasoconstriction to stop bleeding. This includes direct pressure on sites after blood draws and venipuncture.

- Avoid intramuscular injections.
  Intramuscular injections can cause bleeding into the muscle, and the bleeding can be difficult to manage.

- Avoid rectal temperatures, enemas, suppositories, and douches.
  These procedures can tear the thin mucosa of the rectum, anus, and vagina, leading to bleeding.

- Provide a safe environment.
  Keep the patient's room clutter-free to minimize patient injury that leads to bruising.

- Use minimal inflation when assessing blood pressure.
  Overinflation of the blood pressure cuff can cause bruising. Inflate the cuff only until the pulse is obliterated. Avoid automatic blood pressure cuffs.

- Minimize blood draws.
  Blood draws should be kept to a minimum. The use of venous access devices should be considered if frequent blood draws are necessary to prevent the need for multiple venipuncture. Report low platelet counts to the healthcare provider.

■ Teaching

- Instruct patient/family on bleeding precautions (see Box 34.1).
  Teaching patients how to minimize bleeding helps them function with thrombocytopenia or bleeding disorders and to minimize the risk of hemorrhage.

- Instruct the patient to avoid sexual intercourse when the platelet count is less than 50,000/mm³.
  Sexual intercourse during periods of extreme thrombocytopenia can tear the mucous membranes of the vagina or rectum, causing hemorrhage.

- Necessity of frequent CBCs, laboratory tests
  Patients need to understand the importance of frequent CBCs to monitor the thrombocytopenia.

Evaluating Care Outcomes

The goal of patient care is to prevent hemorrhage. The key to managing the thrombocytopenia in ITP, hemophilia, DIC, and HIT is to provide supportive care and treat the underlying condition. Close surveillance is required, along with administration of specific medications or blood products to minimize the risk of bleeding. Patients must demonstrate an understanding of the nature of the condition and the importance of performing interventions to minimize bleeding episodes.

Connection Check 34.6

Which nursing action is indicated for the patient with thrombocytopenia?
A. Avoid intramuscular injections.
B. Encourage the patient to drink plenty of fluids.
C. Place the patient on isolation precautions.
D. Encourage frequent rest periods.

WHITE BLOOD CELL DISORDERS

Leukemia

Epidemiology

Leukemia, a malignant disease or "blood cancer," is a disorder of the bone marrow in which WBCs begin multiplying uncontrollably. There are several types of leukemia, each named for the type of progenitor, or stem, cell from which it evolves. Leukemia is classified as acute or chronic, originating from a lymphoid stem cell (lymphocytes) or myeloid stem cell (granulocytes or neutrophils, erythrocytes, monocytes, and platelets). The four major leukemias are acute myelogenous leukemia (AML), chronic myelogenous leukemia (CML), acute lymphoblastic leukemia (ALL), and chronic lymphocytic leukemia (CLL). Acute myelogenous leukemia and ALL have acute, sudden onsets. Although CML and CLL may be present for years, they eventually degenerate into an acute phase and progress to death if untreated.

Genetic anomalies may be present in some cases, such as CML, also known as chronic myeloid leukemia, in which the presence of the Philadelphia chromosome (abnormal chromosome 22) has been confirmed in more than 90% of patients. Patients with Down's syndrome have also been shown to be at higher risk for developing leukemia because of the association between Down's syndrome and the

Philadelphia chromosome. Down's syndrome is associated with ALL. The Philadelphia chromosome, which is a balanced mutation of chromosome 9 and 22 resulting in the production of bcr/abl kinase proteins, is responsible for the aberrant cell growth seen in CML. However, the Philadelphia chromosome is rarely positive in children with Down's syndrome. Exposure to radiation or benzene has been linked to the development of AML or ALL; there was a high incidence of these acute leukemias following the Hiroshima and Nagasaki bombings in World War II. Patients who have been treated with chemotherapeutic agents and/or radiation therapy are at risk for developing leukemia several years after treatment as a result of possible alterations in bone marrow function. Smoking is also linked to leukemia. In general, leukemia is more prevalent in white males over the age of 60, but its incidence is not limited to age, sex, or race. Acute lymphoblastic leukemia is the most prevalent form of leukemia to occur in childhood.

Pathophysiology

In leukemia, an unknown stimulus mutates either a myeloid or lymphoid stem cell. This single cell clones itself, producing an immature WBC known as a leukemic cell, or blast, which never matures as a result of the mutation. This cloning process becomes uncontrollable, filling the bone marrow with these leukemic cells, which subsequently get pushed into the circulation. This uncontrollable production of WBCs is called **leukocytosis** (Fig. 34.7). Because of the mutation, these WBCs never mature and do not respond to the normal signal that leads to programmed cell death, or **apoptosis**. The bone marrow, spleen, and lymph tissue become congested with the blasts, leading to lymphadenopathies, splenomegaly, and infiltration of the body's mucous membranes and lungs.

Clinical Manifestations

Secondary to the blast congestion, lymph glands in the neck, axillae, or groin and the left upper abdominal quadrant may become swollen and painful. The risk of infection is increased because these leukemic WBCs do not mature; therefore, the number of mature infection-fighting cells, or neutrophils, decreases. This is a condition known as **neutropenia**. Low-grade fevers are commonly observed upon diagnosis in response to minor infections. Major infections such as pneumonia usually do not occur until after chemotherapy initiation, which can cause profound neutropenia where the absolute neutrophil count (ANC) is less than 1,000 mm³.

As leukemia progresses, the bone marrow, which is congested with leukemic cells, is not able to adequately produce RBCs and platelets. Patients often present with clinical manifestations of anemia, including fatigue, pallor, weakness, and shortness of breath, as well as bruising, petechiae,

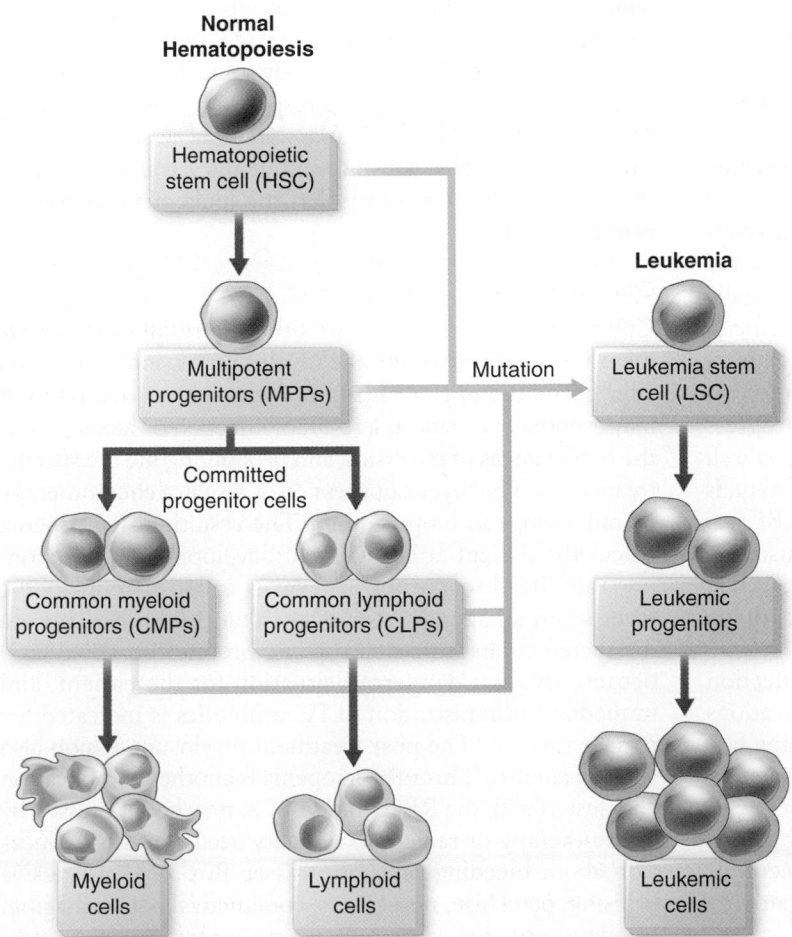

FIGURE 34.7 Normal hematopoiesis compared with the development of leukemic cells.

nosebleeds, and bleeding gums from the decreased number of platelets. Patients often present with low-grade fever in response to exposure to organisms that the immune system can usually handle. Leukemia left untreated is fatal, with infection being the primary cause of death.

Management

Diagnosis

Often a patient presents to the healthcare provider with complaints of flu-like symptoms such as fatigue, low-grade fever, and pallor, although many times a patient is asymptomatic, and a routine CBC reveals the leukemia. A CBC not only reveals the leukocytosis, or increased WBC count, but also demonstrates anemia and thrombocytopenia that occurs as a result of the congested bone marrow. A history and physical examination are performed. Confirmation of the diagnosis of leukemia usually follows a bone marrow biopsy that shows the type of leukemia and extent of the malignancy. Genetic testing can be performed on these cells to determine any chromosomal abnormalities.

Medical Management

Systemic chemotherapy is initiated to destroy the leukemic cells and induce a remission that indicates that the bone marrow is free of leukemic cells and is able to produce healthy blood cells. Remission does not indicate a cure. Radiation therapy is sometimes used as part of this treatment. There are many different chemotherapeutic agents employed today in the treatment of leukemia, and they may be administered solely or in combination regimens. Numerous clinical trials are ongoing, all with the goal of inducing remission.

Treatment strategies consist of two main phases: remission induction and post-remission maintenance. Remission induction includes the initial administration of chemotherapeutic agents. High doses of chemotherapy are given and may be accompanied by radiation therapy. This usually causes the patient to become acutely ill. This is very difficult on the patient, especially if asymptomatic at the time of diagnosis, because the patient may feel the treatment is worse than the disease. Education regarding the progression of the disease and the need for chemotherapy, as well as helping the patient to establish a good support system, is crucial in the early stages of treatment. Routine CBCs to monitor the progression of myelosuppression caused by chemotherapy is indicated to prevent complications. Transfusions of RBCs and/or platelets are usually an aspect of the supportive care for these patients.

In the past, chemotherapy almost always led to infection as a result of the neutropenic state that these medications produce. The advent of granulocyte colony-stimulating factors (GCSFs) has changed this because they are frequently given post-chemotherapy to stimulate the bone marrow to produce neutrophils. Filgrastim (short-acting) and pegfilgrastim (long-acting) are given as subcutaneous injections. In many cases, these medications prevent some patients from developing post-chemotherapeutic infections.

After the induction phase, which may lead to a state of remission or partial remission, the patient usually enters a post-remission maintenance phase of care. Chemotherapy may continue at lower doses and/or less frequently in order to suppress the formation of leukemic cells. This may continue for months or years.

Transplantation is currently the only possibility for a cure from leukemia. Previously, bone marrow transplantation (BMT) was the only type of transplantation, but peripheral stem cell transplantation (PSCT) or hematopoietic stem cell transplantation (HSCT) are now more often used. With both procedures, donor cells are needed to transplant into the bloodstream of the patient, either the patient's own (**autologous**) or from a donor (**allogeneic**). The advantage of PSCT over BMT is primarily one of comfort for the donor. In a BMT, bone marrow is harvested via a large needle inserted into the iliac bone. (The bone marrow biopsy procedure is described in Chapter 33). The stem cells in a PSCT are gathered in a manner similar to donating blood from a peripheral vein. The stem cells are then separated in an apheresis machine (a machine that separates the stem cells from the rest of the blood components), and the blood is returned to the donor minus the stem cells. The success rate of transplantation is approximately the same for both procedures.

A transplantation is not without its potential complications in the form of graft-versus-host disease (GVHD) when donor bone marrow or stem cells attack the recipient. Managing GVHD is complicated and requires maintaining a balance between allowing the body some degree of immune response and suppressing this response to the extent that it can be fatal if the body's immune system successfully destroys the new stem cells. Despite enduring a transplantation, there is also the possibility that the leukemia can return, causing a relapse.

Complications

Complications of leukemia are usually a result of the treatment for the disorder and the myelosuppression that occurs after chemotherapy or radiation. Although the disease itself may eventually be fatal as a result of infection or hemorrhage, the best chances of remission and prolonging life are specific treatments. The myelosuppression, a result of chemotherapy or radiation, can be profound. The resulting neutropenia places the patient at high risk of developing an infection, possibly life threatening. A fever is called a neutropenic fever when a patient's ANC is less than 1,000. Patients are instructed to institute neutropenic precautions (Box 34.2) because this is a dangerous situation for the patient, and immediate administration of IV antibiotics is indicated for patient survival. The post-treatment myelosuppression also leads to anemia. Thrombocytopenia is another complication and, just as with the RBCs and WBCs, may be suppressed by chemotherapy or radiation. Patients need continual education about bleeding precautions (see Box 34.1). Excessive bruising, petechiae, nosebleeds, conjunctival hemorrhaging, bleeding gums, hemoptysis, hematuria, or any gastrointestinal

Box 34.2 Neutropenic Precautions

1. Frequent hand washing or the use of alcohol-based hand sanitizer by the patient and others coming into contact with the patient.
2. Avoid crowds. If the neutropenic patient must go out, a mask is indicated.
3. Avoid obviously sick people, small children, and pets while the neutrophil count is low.
4. Wash all raw fruits and vegetables well before eating. It is best to avoid fruits such as raspberries and blackberries that have little bumps and ridges and cannot be washed well.
5. Monitor temperature daily, and contact the healthcare provider if the temperature is greater than 100.4°F (38°C).
6. For fevers, rigors (shaking chills), and obvious clinical manifestations of illness, seek immediate medical attention. Rapid treatment with IV antibiotics is crucial to prevent sepsis and death.
7. There should not be any live plants or cut flowers in the home environment because they breed bacteria and mold. This also includes while the patient is in the hospital.
8. Avoid standing water in appliances such as humidifiers because this also breeds mold and bacteria.
9. If patients are started on prophylactic antibiotic, antiviral, and antifungal therapies, stress the importance of taking prescribed medications daily and completing the entire course of antibiotics.
10. A patient with neutropenia requires a private room if hospitalized.
11. Avoid rectal temperatures, suppositories, and enemas because of the normal bacteria in the rectum that could enter the bloodstream if there is rectal trauma associated with these interventions.

bleeding needs to be immediately reported to healthcare personnel.

Nursing Management

Assessment and Analysis

Leukemia is usually discovered in a routine CBC because the patient is often asymptomatic. Clinical manifestations that may cause a patient to seek medical attention are a result of the anemia and thrombocytopenia that occur as a result of the bone marrow being clogged with WBCs.

- Leukocytosis
- Neutropenia
- Anemia
- Thrombocytopenia
- Shortness of breath, especially on exertion or lying flat
- Excessive bruising
- Petechiae
- Fatigue
- Pallor
- Dizziness
- Fatigue
- Low-grade fevers in response to minor infections

Nursing Diagnoses

- **Risk for infection** related to immature leukemic cells' inability to fight infection or neutropenia
- **Risk for impaired tissue perfusion** related to the bone marrow's decreased ability to produce adequate RBCs because of the congestion caused by the increased number of leukemic WBCs
- **Risk for bleeding** related to the bone marrow's decreased ability to produce adequate platelets because of the congestion caused by the increased number of leukemic WBCs
- **Risk for compromised family coping** related to the diagnosis of leukemia and lifestyle changes to accommodate treatment

Nursing Interventions

Assessments

- Vital signs
  Low-grade fevers in response to minor infections by cuts, abrasions, sores, and so forth occur because of the decrease in mature neutrophils needed to produce a more pronounced temperature elevation.
- Fatigue, pallor, dizziness, shortness of breath
  These clinical manifestations of anemia occur as a result of decreased erythrocytosis because the bone marrow is congested with WBCs.
- Excessive bruising, petechiae (different from a rash—when you push, petechiae do not blanch)
  These clinical manifestations of thrombocytopenia occur as a result of decreased production of platelets because the bone marrow is congested with WBCs, and there may be spontaneous bleeding into the subcutaneous tissues.
- CBC values
  Leukocytosis of leukemic WBCs occurs from a single mutation. The excessive WBCs clog the bone marrow, resulting in decreased production of RBCs and platelets.

Actions

- Administer chemotherapy as prescribed.
  The patient is started on chemotherapy to destroy the leukemic cells.
- Institute neutropenic precautions.
  The patient needs to take extra precautions to prevent infection due to low neutrophil counts.
- Prophylactic use of antibiotics, antivirals, and antifungals as ordered
  A prophylactic regimen of antibiotics, antivirals, and antifungals is often initiated to provide added protection against infection when the neutrophil count is low.
- Administer IV antibiotics.
  When the ANC is less than 1,000, it is imperative to start IV antibiotics immediately in order to prevent sepsis and possible death.
- Symptom management (nausea/vomiting/diarrhea, ulcerations of the mouth)
  Post-chemotherapy/post-radiation symptom management is continuously assessed to maintain the patient's quality of life.

Antiemetics or antidiarrheal medication are indicated to minimize discomfort as well as to decrease fluid loss.

- Administer ordered blood products.
  The patient may require blood products as cell counts (RBCs and platelets) drop because of the myelosuppression caused by chemotherapy.

■ Teaching

- Neutropenic precautions (see Box 34.2)
  It is essential that the patient/family is instructed in order to prevent a major infection or to initiate treatment immediately upon exhibiting the clinical manifestations of an infection.
- Clinical manifestations of anemia
  In order to minimize the anemia and its complications, education is essential for prompt administration of growth factor or transfusions.
- Manifestations of thrombocytopenia
  It is essential that the patient/family seek medical attention if the patient has any early signs of bleeding.
- Bleeding precautions (see Box 34.1)
  The patient needs to have practical knowledge about how to prevent bleeding when the platelet count is low.
- Diagnosis of leukemia
  The patient/family needs to understand the course that the leukemia takes and why it is important to follow treatment plans as recommended.
- Adverse reactions of chemotherapy or radiation
  The patient/family needs to know what side effects may occur as a result of the treatment regimen in order to notify healthcare personnel of any problems that need to be addressed.
- Possibility of sterility
  Chemotherapy or radiation can render the patient sterile. The patient needs to be educated on alternative methods of family planning, including sperm or egg donation.

Evaluating Care Outcomes

Untreated leukemia is a fatal disorder. The goals of treatment are to induce a remission for the patient and to minimize or prevent complications. Treatments are considered effective when the patient has decreased clinical manifestations of anemia, infection, and bleeding. Prolonging life and improving the quality of life are important considerations in treating patients with leukemia. Symptom management of the chemotherapy and radiation therapy aids in improving the quality of life. At present, a BMT or PSCT is the only chance of achieving a cure for leukemia.

Connection Check 34.7

The nurse correlates which diagnostic result as increasing the risk for infection in the patient with leukemia?

A. WBC 11³/mm³
B. ANC 500 mm³
C. Hbg 8.6 g/dL
D. Platelets 112,000 mm³

LYMPH DISORDERS

Malignant Lymphomas

Malignant lymphomas are divided into two main classifications: Hodgkin's lymphoma, or Hodgkin's disease, and non-Hodgkin's lymphoma (NHL). Hodgkin's lymphoma is characterized by the presence of Reed–Sternberg (RS-H) cells, which are specific giant lymphocytes associated with this disorder. The category of NHL includes all other types of lymphoma, most of which evolve from B- and T-lymphocyte cells. Natural killer cells infrequently develop into lymphomas. The causes of all lymphomas are unknown.

Epidemiology

Hodgkin's lymphoma accounts for approximately 14% of all lymphomas and has a higher survival rate than non-Hodgkin's lymphoma. The incidence of all lymphomas occurs more in men than in women. There is an increased risk in childhood through early adulthood; then the incidence declines until after the age of 55, when it again increases. In the United States, Hodgkin's lymphoma occurs more in those of Caucasian descent, followed by those of African and then Asian descent. There is a higher incidence of Hodgkin's lymphoma in those of higher socioeconomic status, but the reason is unknown. Other risk factors for Hodgkin's lymphoma include infection with the Epstein–Barr virus and being a first-degree relative (parent or sibling) of someone with Hodgkin's disease, both of which suggest possible infectious or familial causes of Hodgkin's disease.

Non-Hodgkin's lymphomas (NHLs) represent approximately 4% of total cancer incidence and account for 4% of cancer-related deaths. An individual has approximately a 1 in 50 chance of developing NHL. The incidence in men is greater than in women, and in the United States, it occurs more in those of Caucasian as compared with African descent. The documented incidence of NHL is higher in industrialized countries than in developing countries. Variations of NHL have different incidences in various geographical areas, and the incidence peaks in preadolescence, then generally occurs again in late adulthood. Causes of NHL are linked to exposure to certain pesticides; therefore, there are higher rates of lymphomas in individuals associated with farming and gardening. Individuals with autoimmune disorders and a history of organ transplantation also have higher rates of NHL. Being infected with HIV/AIDS, the Epstein–Barr virus, human herpesvirus 8, and *Chlamydia* and *Helicobacter pylori* bacteria also increases the risk of developing NHL. Additionally, prior treatment for Hodgkin's lymphoma or with radiation increases the risk of NHL.

Pathophysiology

Malignant lymphomas evolve from a single progenitor, or stem, cell in a lymph node that develops into a solid tumor or mass. As the cancer cells multiply and divide, they spread from the involved lymph node through the lymph system and can eventually affect other lymphoid tissue, including the spleen. When the cancer is left untreated, the involvement of major organs can occur as a result of metastasis or pressure from the mass. The differentiating characteristic of Hodgkin's disease and NHL is the presence or absence of the RS-H cell, a multi-nucleoli cell. The RS-H cell is present in Hodgkin's disease and absent in NHL. The presence of metastasis beyond the lymph node is termed *extranodal lymphoma* and helps determine the treatment and prognosis.

Clinical Manifestations

The clinical manifestations of Hodgkin's disease (HD) and NHL are similar, and patients usually do not seek medical attention until the disease has progressed to the point where systemic involvement has occurred. Clinical manifestations include painless swelling of the lymph nodes in the neck, underarm, and groin; low-grade fevers for no apparent reason; drenching night sweats; unexplained weight loss of more than 10% in less than 6 months; and fatigue. These are known as the "B symptoms" because of the systemic action of the B lymphocytes. Generalized pruritus, or itching, with pronounced excoriation from scratching is present in a large percentage of patients presenting with HD, although the origin is unknown. Another unique feature of HD, which has no known etiology, is alcohol-induced pain at the site of the involved lymph node after a few sips of any alcoholic beverage.

Staging of lymphomas is generally characterized by the classification system established by the World Health Organization (Table 34.4). Staging also is further differentiated between "E" for extranodal and "S" for the involvement of the spleen. Depending on the type of lymphoma, these tumors are usually also classified as indolent (slowly progressive), aggressive, or highly aggressive.

The involvement of major organ groups may also cause further clinical manifestations that cause individuals to seek medical attention. Clinical manifestations of shortness of breath and a feeling of fullness may occur as the enlarging lymph nodes spread to the spleen or liver or compress the vena cava or spine.

Management

Diagnosis

A detailed history and physical examination are the first steps to diagnosing a malignant lymphoma, usually followed by radiological testing that may include a routine chest x-ray, computed tomography (CT) scan, positron emission tomography (PET) scan, or magnetic resonance imaging (MRI). A lymph node biopsy usually provides a definitive diagnosis. Examination of the tissue and determining the presence of the RS-H cells determine whether the patient has HD or NHL. A CBC may show evidence of bone marrow involvement with possible anemia and abnormal WBC count. If bone marrow involvement is suspected, a bone marrow biopsy may be indicated. A lumbar puncture is performed if central nervous system involvement is suspected.

Medical Management

Treatment of malignant lymphomas usually involves the use of chemotherapeutic agents and/or radiation therapy to destroy the tumor cells. Surgical intervention to remove the tumor may also be indicated. If the individual has been diagnosed with an indolent NHL, a wait-and-see approach may be used initially because of the slow growth of the tumor. Stem cell transplantation may be indicated in some patients, but this depends on the type and stage of the disease. The rationale for transplantation is to destroy the mutant lymphoid stem cells with chemotherapy/radiation and then replace them with healthy donor cells. The success of stem cell transplantation in the lymphoma population varies and may depend on the aggressiveness of the underlying disease.

Surgical Management

If a splenectomy is required to treat lymphomas, respiratory problems may occur because of the spleen's proximity to the diaphragm and the need for a high abdominal incision. Pneumonia and atelectasis are possible complications due to postoperative pain and the patient's reluctance to cough and deep breathe. Development of pancreatitis may occur because the tail of the pancreas is near the spleen and may be damaged during surgery. Because of the spleen's role in the immune system, infection is a serious postoperative complication. Overwhelming post-splenectomy infection is a serious complication that has a high mortality rate because sepsis can quickly occur and is usually a result of streptococci, *Neisseria* spp., or influenza. Patients should maintain lifetime vaccinations against these organisms if a splenectomy is performed.

Complications

As the cancer progresses, complications involving major organs and structures can occur, including superior vena cava (SVC) syndrome, spinal cord compression, hypercalcemia, **myelodysplasia** (abnormal blood cell production), severe hepatic or renal dysfunction, hyperviscosity of blood, or venous thrombotic events. Superior vena cava syndrome, spinal cord compression, and hypercalcemia are considered oncological emergencies, and individuals who develop these conditions need immediate medical attention. A splenectomy may be necessary in some patients because of splenic involvement, either as the primary site (tumor in the spleen) or from metastasis of the cancer.

Table 34.4 World Health Organization Staging of Lymphoma

Stage	Description
Stage I	Cancer is limited to a single node.
Stage II	Cancer is found in two or more lymph nodes on the same side of the diaphragm.
Stage III	Cancer is found in lymph groups on both sides of the diaphragm.
Stage IV	Cancer is found in one or more organs in addition to lymph nodes.

In SVC syndrome, the enlarging lymph node compresses the flexible superior vena cava. Edema of the face and one or both arms, shortness of breath, chest pain, or dysphagia develops because there is engorgement in the upper torso and impaired venous return. Compression of the inferior vena cava may occur, but the clinical manifestation of fullness in the abdomen is not as dramatic or life threatening. Thrombosis may occur as venous flow is impeded by the expanding lymph node, slowing blood flow and increasing stasis.

Compression of the spinal cord may result in neurological deficits and paralysis because the expanding tumor may apply pressure on the spinal cord or nerve roots. Neurological deficits and paralysis depend on the location of the spinal cord or nerve root compression. In many cases, immediate radiation or chemotherapy is initiated to reduce the tumor, which decreases the pressure on the spinal cord.

Hypercalcemia is a result of metastasis to the bones that causes bone breakdown (resorption by osteoclasts), and calcium is released into the bloodstream. Hypercalcemia occurs as the serum calcium level exceeds 11 mg/dL, and clinical manifestations range from dehydration and polyuria to decreased neuromuscular activity, confusion, stupor, heart block, and death.

As the bone marrow becomes involved, myelodysplasia (impaired production of RBCs, WBCs, and platelets) occurs. The patient may exhibit clinical manifestations of anemia. White blood cells may be abnormally high or low. In either case, the number of neutrophils is low, and the patient is at risk for infection. Inadequate platelet production places the patient at risk for bleeding. Hyperviscosity can occur as a result of the myelodysplasia or impaired hepatic or renal function and places the patient at a higher risk of developing thrombotic events.

Nursing Management

Assessment and Analysis

Clinical manifestations of malignant lymphomas are a result of the enlarging lymph node(s) and systemic involvement of the B lymphocytes. The nurse monitors for the following clinical manifestations in patients with lymphomas:

- Painless swelling of the cervical, axillary, and inguinal nodes
- Low-grade fevers of unknown origin
- Drenching night sweats
- Unexplained weight loss of greater than 10% in less than 6 months
- Fatigue
- Anemia
- Neutropenia
- Thrombocytopenia

The cause of the generalized pruritus and the alcohol-induced pain in HL is still unexplained.

Nursing Diagnoses

- **Risk for infection** related to bone marrow involvement and adverse effects of treatment

- **Activity intolerance** related to anemia caused by bone marrow involvement
- **Risk for ineffective coping** related to the diagnosis and lifestyle changes to accommodate treatment

Nursing Interventions

▪ Assessments

- Vital signs
  Low-grade fever, drenching night sweats, weight loss, and fatigue are a result of B-cell involvement, which causes systemic clinical manifestations.
- Pain, breathing pattern, face/neck
  Shortness of breath, chest pain, dysphagia, and edema of the face and/or arms may indicate SVC syndrome with resulting venous congestion.
- Neurological status
  The expanding lymphoma may cause spinal cord or nerve root compression.
- Cervical, axillary, and inguinal lymph nodes
  Enlarged lymph nodes are a result of the expanded lymphoma, and the swelling may be painless.
- Skin
  Generalized pruritus/itching can increase the risk of bleeding.
- CBC results
  A CBC may show bone marrow involvement with impaired blood cell production, resulting in decreased RBCs, WBCs, and platelets.
- Lower extremities
  Pain or swelling may occur secondary to thrombus formation if lymphoma compresses veins, slowing blood flow and increasing venous stasis.
- Serum calcium levels
  If metastasis of the lymphoma involves the bones, the resulting bone breakdown releases calcium, causing hypercalcemia.
- Activity tolerance
  Fatigue may develop as a result of the anemia caused by myelosuppression.

▪ Actions

- Administer blood products as ordered.
  Transfusions may be required as blood counts drop because of the myelosuppression that occurs as a result of the treatment regimens.
- Administer chemotherapeutic agents.
  Patients will be started on chemotherapy as a primary treatment of lymphoma.
- Administer IV fluids as prescribed.
  Increased insensitive fluid loss may develop secondary to fevers and drenching sweats. Additionally, in patients with hypercalcemia secondary to bone breakdown, increased fluids decrease the calcium concentration in the kidneys and decrease the risk of calcium-containing renal calculi.
- Symptom management
  Symptom management of the disorder itself, as well as symptoms that may occur as a result of the chemotherapy and radiation, is the focus of nursing care. Easing the discomfort

of itching and the drenching night sweats is important to the comfort of the patient with Hodgkin's disease, as is managing any clinical manifestations of therapy such as nausea and vomiting.

- Obtain routine CBCs.
  Myelosuppression may be a result of chemotherapy or radiation therapy. Hemoglobin and WBC counts need to be monitored closely, as does the platelet count.
- Provide emotional support.
  Emotional support is essential to patients with a cancer diagnosis. Helping them to deal with fears of death and dying and referring them to needed resources are essential to helping them manage the course of the disease.

Teaching

- Disease process
  Knowledge of the disease and its course and treatment helps patients better manage the condition and may improve compliance with ordered interventions.
- Risk of infection
  Patients and family need to understand the importance of good hand hygiene to minimize infection and require instruction to stay away from crowds and obviously sick people when neutrophil counts are low.
- Maintaining treatment schedules
  Chemotherapy and radiation therapy schedules are determined from the results of clinical trials to provide the best chance of remission and/or cure. Patients need to understand the importance of keeping scheduled treatment appointments.
- Encourage frequent rest periods.
  Fatigue may be a result of the anemia caused by bone marrow involvement and/or compounded by the myelosuppression as a result of treatment.
- Dietary intake
  Instruction may be necessary for maintaining adequate nutrition.
- Clinical manifestations of potential complications
  Patients need to understand the importance of seeking immediate medical attention for clinical manifestations, such as shortness of breath, edema of the face and/or arms, chest pain, fevers when neutropenic, or any neurological deficits, that may indicate complications.
- Possibility of sterility
  Chemotherapy or radiation therapy may cause sterility. Those in childbearing years need to be educated about alternative ways of conceiving, including sperm and egg banking.

Evaluating Care Outcomes

Improving the quality of life of patients with malignant lymphomas is the goal of nursing care. Medical and nursing interventions are based on providing patient comfort from the clinical manifestations as well as managing the adverse reactions caused by treating the lymphoma with chemotherapy, radiation, and/or PSCT. The effectiveness of treatments is correlated with normal blood cell counts, sufficient energy to participate in normal activities of daily living, no bleeding, and the absence of infections. Patients and families require education about the various options for managing these clinical manifestations as well as the possible complications of both the disorders and the treatments. When untreated, malignant lymphomas are fatal.

Connection Check 34.8

A patient with lymphoma is beginning the induction chemotherapy regimen. Which information is most essential for the nurse to include in the treatment plan?

A. Advance directives
B. Bleeding precautions
C. Importance of frequent rest periods
D. Neutropenic precautions

Multiple Myeloma

Multiple **myeloma** is a hematologic malignancy involving cells of the immune system that produce antibodies. It is thought that this cancer is caused by an overgrowth of a single clone of stimulated immunoglobulin secreting "B" lymphocytes or plasma cells. The excess antibodies produced by these malignant plasma cells accumulate as extra immunoglobulin or gamma globulin; therefore, multiple myeloma is often referred to as a monoclonal gammopathy.

Epidemiology

Multiple myeloma, an incurable B-cell malignancy, is responsible for approximately 13% of all hematologic cancers, and the incidence is about 5 to 7 cases per 100,000 per year. According to the American Cancer Society, this plasma cell malignancy occurs twice as often in African Americans than Caucasian Americans. Men have a slightly higher risk of developing this type of cancer than women. The average age for developing multiple myeloma is 62 years old, and the risk of developing this type of cancer goes up as people age. Less than 1% of the cases of multiple myeloma are diagnosed in individuals who are younger than 35 years old. In 2018, the American Cancer Society estimated that about 16,400 men and 14,370 women were diagnosed that year. The lifetime risk for an individual living in the United States is about 0.8%. The reported risk factors for developing multiple myeloma include exposure to herbicides, insecticides, petroleum, heavy metals, plastics, and radiation. Individuals with other plasma cell diseases, such as monoclonal gammopathy of undetermined significance (MGUS) or solitary plasmacytoma, are at higher risk of developing multiple myeloma later in life. The survival for this type of malignancy ranges from 1 year to 10 years, with a mean survival of 3 years. The 5-year survival rate, according to the American Cancer Society, is 46.6%.

Pathophysiology

Multiple myeloma arises from an asymptomatic premalignant proliferation of monoclonal plasma cells. The malignant cells of multiple myeloma, plasma cells and plasmacytoid lymphocytes, are the most mature cells of the B lymphocytes. B-cell maturation is associated with a programmed rearrangement of DNA sequences in the process of encoding the structure of mature immunoglobulins. In this disease, there is an overproduction of monoclonal immunoglobulin G (IgG) and immunoglobulin A (IgA) as well as the light chains that are found in the serum or urine using electrophoresis. Interleukin 6 (IL-6), tumor necrosis factor, and interleukin 1b are currently being studied to determine if these cytokines play a role in the growth of myeloma cells and the pathogenesis of multiple myeloma. This neoplastic proliferation of plasma cells involves more than 10% of the bone marrow, and these bone lesions are caused by an imbalance in the function of osteoblast and osteoclasts.

Genetic Connections

Multiple Myeloma

Genomic instability with translocations of the immunoglobulin heavy-chain locus chromosome 14q32 accounts for 50% of the cases. Secondary late-onset translocations and gene mutations are implicated in disease progression. Genetic abnormalities alter the expression of the adhesion molecules on the myeloma cells, resulting in the "up-regulation" of cell-cycle regulatory proteins and anti-apoptotic proteins. Researchers are now examining the microenvironment of tumor cells to determine whether or not they play a role in the development of myelomas. The prognosis for these patients depends on the tumor burden and the proliferation rate of the malignant cells.

Clinical Manifestations

The patient with multiple myeloma often presents to the healthcare provider with a history of fatigue, weakness, bone pain, recurrent infections, weight loss, and paresthesia. Bone pain, particularly back pain, is a common presenting complaint and is secondary to lytic destruction. The weakness, pallor, and fatigue are related to the anemia associated with this disease process. This malignancy is characterized by six cardinal features: lytic bone disease, the presence of a monoclonal antibody protein referred to as the "M" protein, anemia, renal insufficiency, hypercalcemia, and an infectious diathesis or tendency/predisposition to infection.

Management

Diagnosis

The differential diagnosis of multiple myeloma is made when there is a monoclonal plasma cell count greater than or equal to 10%, presence of serum or urine monoclonal proteins, and myeloma-related organ dysfunction. The CRAB criterion is useful when formulating a diagnosis of multiple myeloma and includes *hyperCalcemia* (serum calcium greater than 11.5 mg/dL, *Renal insufficiency* (serum creatinine greater than 2 mg/dL), *Anemia* (hemoglobin less than 10 g/dL or greater than 2 g/dL below the lower limit of normal range), and *Bone disease* (lytic lesions, severe osteopenia, or pathological fractures).

Diagnostic studies include a CBC; electrolytes, including serum calcium; uric acid and creatinine levels; serum and urine protein electrophoresis with immunofixation (detection and typing of monoclonal antibodies or immunoglobulins in serum or urine); quantification of serum and urine monoclonal proteins; and measurement of free light chains. C-reactive protein and beta-2 microglobulin (expression of tumor burden) are also assessed. There is a positive presence of Bence Jones protein due to the excretion of light chains of immunoglobulins in the urine. The excess of light chains is directly toxic to renal structures and is an important aspect of the complications found in multiple myeloma. The diagnostic evaluation may also include bone marrow aspiration, skeletal survey, and bone-density measurements. An MRI may be performed to rule out spinal cord compression if the patient complains of back pain. Multiple myeloma is also suspected if there is a high ratio of total protein to albumin or if the patient presents with spinal cord compression.

Medical Management

First-line therapy includes the use of bisphosphonates, radiation therapy, DVT prophylaxis, dexamethasone, autologous stem cell transplantation, and high-dose chemotherapy (thalidomide, lenalidomide, bortezomib). Thalidomide and lenalidomide were originally used for the treatment of pregnancy-associated morning sickness but were withdrawn from the market due to teratogenicity (damage to the unborn fetus). However, both thalidomide and lenalidomide possess potent activity and are approved for the treatment of patients with newly diagnosed multiple myeloma or heavily pretreated relapsed or refractory multiple myeloma.

Complications

As the disease progresses, complications develop secondary to the underlying pathophysiology as well as to some of the treatment approaches, such as side effects of chemotherapy. Hematologic complications include anemia, bone marrow failure, and bleeding disorders. There is also increased susceptibility to infections, and bone complications include pathologic fractures, spinal cord compression, and hypercalcemia secondary to bone breakdown. Neurological complications may develop, such as spinal cord and nerve root compression and intracranial plasmacytomas (tumor consisting of abnormal plasma cells in the bony skeleton). Renal failure may develop secondary to renal stones and demineralization of bone or the toxic effects of Bence Jones protein on the renal epithelial cells.

Nursing Management

Assessment and Analysis

The clinical presentation of multiple myeloma is related to the multisystem effects of this disease process and often includes the following:

- Bone pain, particularly in the back
- Numbness and tingling associated with neuropathies
- Anemia (normocytic, normochromic)
- Weakness, pallor, and fatigue
- Increased susceptibility to infection
- Hypercalcemia
- Hypercalciuria
- Renal stones

Nursing Diagnoses

- **Acute/chronic** pain related to decreased integrity/destruction of bone
- **Impaired physical mobility** related to pain and possible fracture
- **Risk for infection** related to chemotherapy-related immunosuppression and plasma cell malignancy
- **Risk for injury** related to pathological fractures/decreased integrity of bone
- **Impaired urinary output** related to renal damage
- Fear related to cancer diagnosis

Nursing Interventions
▪ Assessments

- Vital signs
  Tachycardia and tachypnea are secondary to the heart and lungs compensating for decreased oxygenation of body tissues secondary to anemia. Elevated temperature may indicate an infectious process.
- Fatigue, pallor, and shortness of breath
  Fatigue, pallor, and shortness of breath worsen with increasingly decreased levels of hemoglobin causing inadequate tissue perfusion.
- Pain
  Pain, particularly back pain, develops secondary to bone destruction/breakdown.
- Paresthesias
  Nerve root compression may develop secondary to vertebral collapse secondary to bone breakdown.
- Intake and output
  Renal damage may occur secondary to myeloma cast neuropathy or calcium precipitation that results from the bone breakdown.

- Serum and urine calcium
  Bone breakdown may lead to hypercalcemia and hypercalciuria that can result in calcium precipitation in the kidney tubules.
- Serum blood urea nitrogen (BUN) and creatinine
  Damage to the distal and collecting tubules of the kidney may lead to renal insufficiency that elevates both serum and creatinine levels.

▪ Actions

- Administer chemotherapy.
  Destroys the abnormal cells
- Administer bisphosphonate therapy as ordered.
  Bisphosphate therapy reduces bone disease, fractures, and skeletal complications.
- Administer pain medications as ordered.
  Pain may develop related to bone destruction, nerve compression, or renal stones.
- Encourage fluid intake as tolerated.
  Increasing fluid intake can facilitate diluting the elevated serum and urine calcium levels.
- Position patient to facilitate comfort.
  Nerve root and spinal compression may be relieved by positioning that minimizes the compression.
- Encourage ambulation as tolerated.
  Ambulation supports bone activity (buildup) and minimizes the complications of immobility, such as DVT and muscle wasting.

▪ Teaching

- Immediately report any clinical manifestations of fatigue, shortness of breath, dizziness, or confusion.
  Resolution of the anemia through supplementation or blood transfusions is needed to increase tissue perfusion.
- Report any sudden onset of severe pain or new location, especially of back pain, which could indicate a pathological fracture.
  Vertebral collapse or a pathological fracture may present with sudden, severe pain due to damage to nerves and surrounding tissues.
- Report changes in sensation, increased numbness and tingling, or changes in motor function.
  Nerve root compression or spinal cord compression, associated with damage to bone, presents with these clinical manifestations.
- Instruct in the use of nonpharmacological pain management methods, such as music, relaxation, deep breathing, imagery, distraction, and progressive muscle relaxation.
  These nonpharmacologic methods or complementary health approaches may support management, with or without concomitant pain medication administration.

Evaluating Care Outcomes

Symptom management and preventing complications are priorities in evaluating care outcomes for patients with multiple myeloma. Pain that is controlled and the absence of infection are the goals of treatment, as well as facilitating optimal renal function. Patients with multiple myeloma require consistent healthcare follow-up, as well as psychosocial support due to the lack of a cure for this disease. Patients must demonstrate an understanding of the nature of the condition and the importance of performing interventions to minimize complications.

Making Connections

CASE STUDY: WRAP-UP

Mr. Owens has a bone marrow biopsy, which confirms the diagnosis of acute myelogenous leukemia (AML). A repeated CBC with a differential shows Hbg 9.1 g/dL, Hct 27.9%, WBC 9.8×10^3/mm³, and platelets 72,000/mm³, and the ANC is 3.1/mm³. Mr. Owens's oncologist recommends that he immediately start chemotherapy treatment with a regimen of daunorubicin and Ara-C. This regimen is repeated through several cycles, or courses, of chemotherapy. Two weeks after induction of chemotherapy, Mr. Owens's CBC results are Hbg 7.9 g/dL, Hct 23.8%, WBC 5.5×10^3/mm³, ANC 0.6/mm³, and platelets 19,000/mm³. He is given transfusions of packed RBCs, platelets, and an injection of filgrastim (Neupogen), a granulocyte colony-stimulating factor (GCSF), and is started prophylactically on moxifloxacin, acyclovir, and Diflucan. Supportive care with transfusions and growth factors is repeated as indicated by routine CBCs. Six months after chemotherapy induction, Mr. Owens achieves a remission, confirmed by a bone marrow biopsy.

Case Study Questions

1. When a history of Mr. Owens is completed, which factor does the nurse determine is the highest risk for leukemia?
   A. Age
   B. Gender
   C. Worked in an oil refinery
   D. Smoker

2. Which CBC result correlates with a diagnosis of leukemia for Mr. Owens?
   A. RBC 3.2 million cells/mm³
   B. WBC 6.2×10^3/mm³
   C. Hct 28.1%
   D. Platelets 97,000/mm³

3. After Mr. Owens starts chemotherapy treatment, his laboratory results are Hbg 7.9 g/dL, Hct 23.8%, WBC 5.5×10^3/mm³, ANC 0.6/mm³, and platelets 19,000/mm³. Which potential complication is the nurse's first priority?
   A. Anemia
   B. Leukocytosis
   C. Thrombocytopenia
   D. Infection

4. Which statement by Mr. Owens informs the nurse that he needs more education about bleeding precautions regarding his thrombocytopenia?
   A. "I need to buy an electric razor to use for shaving."
   B. "I have an appointment with the dentist to get my teeth cleaned."
   C. "I guess I have to stop walking around barefoot."
   D. "My wife has been after me to clean up my clutter in the family room. I guess I better do that."

5. Mr. Owens should notify medical personnel and/or go to the emergency department immediately if he experiences any of the following symptoms: *(Select all that apply.)*
   A. T 102°F (38.9°C)
   B. Chills
   C. Nosebleed that lasts more than 10 minutes
   D. Diarrhea, three episodes within a 24-hour period
   E. Facial flushing

CHAPTER SUMMARY

Nonmalignant hematological disorders include nonproliferative or decreased production of red blood cells (RBCs), increased destruction of RBCs, or severe blood loss. Anemia indicates hematological dysfunction that requires a determination of etiology and severity, and the cause of the anemia is important and can indicate the type of treatment that is indicated. Nutritional deficiencies leading to a decreased production or life span of the RBCs are evident in iron, vitamin B_{12}, or folic acid deficiency. Destruction of RBCs can be caused by artificial heart valves or genetic mutations. A decreased life span and hemolysis of the RBCs occur in sickle cell disease. Sickle cell disease can result in vasoocclusive crises during hypoxic situations. Blood loss can result from trauma, injury, peptic ulcer disease, polyps, colon cancer, or genetic abnormalities such as hemophilia. Iron-deficiency anemias are often caused by inadequate dietary iron intake of meat, dark green leafy vegetables, dried beans, beets, and iron-fortified breads and cereals. Other causes include hemorrhage (including heavy menstrual bleeding), ulcerative gastrointestinal problems, poor iron absorption, and some gastrointestinal surgeries. Iron is essential to the formation of hemoglobin, and deficiency causes symptoms of anemia. Treatment includes an iron-rich diet or oral supplementation. In cases of poor absorption or gastrointestinal surgeries, supplementation can be delivered in an intramuscular (IM) or IV formulation.

Vitamin B_{12} deficiency occurs because of inadequate dietary intake of meat, seafood, eggs, and dairy products or malabsorption disorders including gastrointestinal resections, autoimmune diseases, alcoholism, Crohn's disease, and long-term use of medications such as proton-pump inhibitors or H_2 blockers. In addition to symptoms of anemia, unresolved vitamin B_{12} deficiency leads to neurological clinical manifestations such as peripheral neuropathy, confusion, depression, impaired taste, impaired equilibrium, and visual disturbances. Treatment includes adequate dietary intake of vitamin B_{12} or supplementation (oral or parenteral) in cases of malabsorption.

Folic acid is provided in the diet from fortified cereals and grains, legumes, green leafy vegetables, bran, yeast, and nuts. Clinical manifestations of folic acid deficiency include symptoms of anemia as well as neural tube and orofacial abnormalities in infants. Short- or long-term supplementation of folic acid depends on the causative factors.

Sickle cell disease is an inherited disorder passed down from parents who each carry the sickle cell gene. Individuals with sickle cell disease often present with sickle cell crises that are precipitated by anything that causes hypoxemia or increases vasoconstriction, leading to the sickling of the RBCs. Clinical manifestations of a sickle cell crisis include fatigue, pallor, and shortness of breath, as well as pain in the joints, bones, chest, and abdomen as the RBCs sickle, causing decreased oxygen-carrying capacity and increased hemolysis of RBCs. Treatment is aimed at the prevention of crises and symptom management, and long-term management is aimed at minimizing complications and organ dysfunction.

Aplastic anemia is a rare disease due to bone marrow suppression that results in pancytopenia. A medical emergency, the mortality rate is greater than 70%. Clinical manifestations develop secondary to decreased production of RBCs, including tachycardia, shortness of breath, fatigue, and pallor. The decreases in WBCs puts the patient at higher risk for infection, and the decreased platelets increase the patient's risk of bleeding. Diagnosed via complete blood count (CBC), reticulocyte count, hemoglobin electrophoresis, and bone marrow biopsy, management of this disease is aimed at replacing blood components, stimulating bone marrow function, and bone marrow transplantation (if there is an available HLA-matched sibling donor). Nursing management focuses on managing tissue perfusion, preventing infection, and monitoring the risk for bleeding.

A lack of glucose-6-phosphate dehydrogenase, a metabolic enzyme that protects RBCs from oxidative stresses that can lead to cellular destruction, results in G6PD deficiency. An inherited recessive X-linked disorder, the diagnosis is made through DNA testing, as well as evaluation of the CBC, reticulocyte count, and blood smear analysis. Clinical manifestations develop secondary to hemolysis that results from the G6PD deficiency and include shortness of breath, tachycardia, pallor, elevated liver enzymes, jaundice, and splenomegaly. Prevention is the key to the management of this disease and focuses on medications and the avoidance of certain foods (fava beans). Nursing management focuses on minimizing the complications associated with decreased tissue perfusion and maximizing oxygenation.

Polycythemia is an increase in the production of RBCs. Clinical manifestations include headache, dizziness, shortness of breath, generalized pruritus, flushing of the face, fatigue, vision problems, and a feeling of fullness in the left upper abdomen. Treatment ranges from doing nothing, when the patient is at higher altitudes, to performing therapeutic phlebotomies to reduce blood volume in order to ease symptoms.

Thrombocytopenia is the decreased production of platelets resulting in clinical manifestations of excessive bruising, petechiae, epistaxis, bleeding gums, black and tarry stool, and/or hematuria. Treatment aims at preventing or minimizing blood loss from hemorrhage. Hemophilia is a hemorrhagic genetic disorder resulting from decreased clotting factors VIII or IX and may include thrombocytopenia. Treatment is aimed at replacement of the missing clotting factor in order to minimize blood loss. Disseminated intravascular coagulation occurs secondary to severe trauma and leads to abnormal thrombosis formation and breakdown, consuming clotting factors and placing the patient at risk of bleeding. Treatment is aimed at providing supportive care and resolution of the underlying condition. Heparin-induced thrombocytopenia (HIT) appears to be an immune response of the body to the administration of heparin occurring 5 to 14 days after introduction, causing the formation of multiple thrombi and spontaneous bleeding. Cessation of heparin administration is the initial step in correcting HIT.

Malignant hematological disorders include two types of white blood cell (WBC) malignancies: lymphoid and myeloid. This can be further divided into the two large groups of leukemia and lymphoma based on the clinical and pathologic presentation. Leukemia is a type of "blood cancer" resulting from an uncontrollable production of WBCs. This extreme leukocytosis results in extremely high WBC counts and decreased RBC and platelet counts due to the congested bone marrow. Clinical manifestations include signs of anemia (fatigue, pallor, shortness of breath, weakness), bruising, petechiae, nosebleeds, bleeding gums, and low-grade temperatures. Leukemia may be classified as acute or chronic, always becoming fatal if left untreated. Treatment includes symptom management and chemotherapy to attempt remission. Transplantation of peripheral blood stem cells or bone marrow is the only chance of a cure at this time.

Malignant lymphomas are a result of the proliferation of lymphocytes, which eventually spread from the originating lymph node to other areas of the lymph system, ultimately metastasizing to non-lymphoid tissue and resulting in death. Lymphomas are classified as either Hodgkin's lymphoma or non-Hodgkin's lymphoma. Clinical manifestations include painless swelling of cervical, axillary, or inguinal nodes; low-grade fever; night sweat; fatigue; unexplained weight loss; and generalized pruritus. Treatment focuses on symptom management and aims at remission induction through chemotherapy/radiation administration. Currently, peripheral blood stem cell or bone marrow transplantation provides the only chances for a cure.

Multiple myeloma is a cancer of the bone marrow in which abnormal plasma cells proliferate. Because plasma cells or mature B lymphocytes normally produce antibodies that are used to fight infection, these abnormal plasma cells reduce the ability of the body's immune system to work properly. When the malignant plasma cells expand, they crowd out the other normal cells usually produced in the bone marrow. This causes infiltrations, destruction of bone, and can metastasize to other organs and lymph nodes. Treatment focuses on the use of chemotherapeutic agents, radiation, or stem cell transplantation to reduce tumor burden, modify bone-related pain, and prevent skeletal-related events such as pathological fractures and spinal cord compression. Renal function is monitored carefully to address fluid and electrolyte balance and prevent damage related to protein and toxins accumulated in the kidneys.

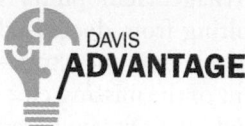

DAVIS ADVANTAGE To explore learning resources for this chapter, go to **Davis Advantage** and find:
– Answers to in-text questions
– Chapter Resources and Activities
– NCLEX®-Style Chapter Review Questions
– Bibliography

Unit VIII

Promoting Health in Patients With Neurological Disorders

Chapter 35

Assessment of Neurological Function

Mallory Trosper

LEARNING OUTCOMES

Content in this chapter is designed to assist in:

1. Identifying key anatomical components of the neurological system
2. Discussing the function of the neurological system
3. Describing the procedure for completing a history and physical assessment of neurological function
4. Correlating relevant diagnostic examinations to neurological function
5. Explaining nursing considerations for diagnostic studies relevant to neurological function
6. Discussing changes in neurological function associated with aging

CONCEPTS

- Assessment
- Cognition
- Medication
- Neurologic Regulation
- Safety
- Sensory Perception

ESSENTIAL TERMS

Adrenergic receptors
Afferent neurons
Alpha receptors
Aqueduct of Sylvius
Arachnoid membrane
Autonomic nervous system (ANS)
Axon
Babinski sign
Basal ganglia
Beta receptors
Blood–brain barrier (BBB)
Brainstem
Cell body
Central nervous system (CNS)
Cerebellum
Cerebrospinal fluid (CSF)
Cerebrum
Cholinergic fibers
Circle of Willis
Corpus callosum
Decussation
Dendrites
Dermatome
Dura mater
Efferent neurons
Enteric system
Falx cerebri
Foramen magnum
Frontal lobe

Glasgow Coma Scale (GCS)
Gray matter
Hydrocephalus
Hypothalamus
Interneurons
Limbic system
Lower motor neurons
Medulla oblongata
Meninges
Midbrain
Mini-Mental Status Examination (MMSE)
Muscarinic receptors
Myelin sheath
Neuroglial cells
Neurons
Neurotransmitters
Nicotinic receptors
Occipital lobe
Parietal lobe
Peripheral nervous system (PNS)
Phrenic nerve
Pia mater
Pons
Reticular formation
Subarachnoid space
Synaptic knob
Temporal lobe
Thalamus
Upper motor neurons
White matter

Finding Connections

CASE STUDY: EPISODE 1

Follow this patient throughout the chapter.

Anthony Smith, a 57-year-old businessman, has been complaining of severe headaches for several weeks. He does not have a history of headaches in the past and is concerned. The headaches do not seem to be correlated with his eating or drinking habits or related to stress, as he has been on vacation for the past week and a half. He made an appointment with his healthcare provider, who recommended he follow up with a neurologist. He has an appointment next week…

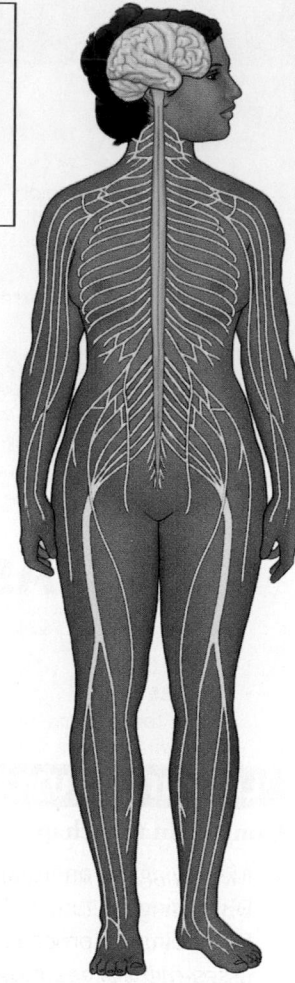

Central nervous system (CNS)
• Brain
• Spinal cord

Peripheral nervous system (PNS)
• Cranial nerves
• Spinal nerves

INTRODUCTION

The nervous and endocrine systems of the body maintain homeostasis and coordination of the body's functions. The focus of this chapter is the neurological system and how it maintains homeostasis and coordination of neurological function. The endocrine system is discussed in Chapter 40. The neurological system works through electrical and chemical messages transmitted from sensory organs to the brain and spinal cord and reciprocating messages transmitted back to target organs and cells. It is divided into two parts (Fig. 35.1):

- The **central nervous system (CNS)**, which consists of the brain and spinal cord
- The **peripheral nervous system (PNS)**, which includes 12 pairs of cranial nerves that originate in the brain, 31 pairs of spinal nerves that originate in the spinal cord, and the **autonomic nervous system (ANS**; Fig. 35.2). The ANS is further divided into the sympathetic and parasympathetic systems. Another segment of the ANS, the **enteric system**, is the "nervous system" of the gastrointestinal (GI) tract. Sometimes referred to as the "second brain," it has autonomous control of the process of digestion. The sympathetic and parasympathetic branches of the ANS are discussed in this chapter.

OVERVIEW OF ANATOMY AND PHYSIOLOGY

Nerve Cell Types and Functions

The nervous system consists of two types of specialized cells, neurons and neuroglia. **Neurons** are impulse-conducting cells that facilitate communication within the nervous system. **Neuroglial cells** are specialized cells that support and protect the neurons.

FIGURE 35.1 The nervous system. The nervous system consists of the central nervous system (brain and spinal cord) and the peripheral nervous system (cranial nerves, spinal nerves, and autonomic nervous system).

Neuroglial Cells

Neuroglial cells are up to 10 times more common than neurons. *Glial* (Greek origin) means "glue," and these neuroglial cells hold the neurons together and provide support, nutrition, and protection. These cells have the ability to multiply, making them a common source for tumor growth in the brain and spinal cord. Neuroglial cells include:

- *Astrocytes*, meaning "stars," provide structure and support. These cells attach to blood vessels, neurons, and the **pia mater**, the innermost layer of the **meninges**, which are the fibrous membrane layers that protect the brain and spinal cord. Astrocytes restrict substances from entering the neurons (the blood–brain barrier [BBB], discussed in detail later in the chapter). Astrocytes also assist in the conduction of impulses and are known to clear cellular debris.
- *Ependymal cells* line the ventricles of the brain and central canal of the spinal cord. They assist in the production of **cerebrospinal fluid (CSF)** and protect the brain from foreign materials that might enter through the bloodstream.

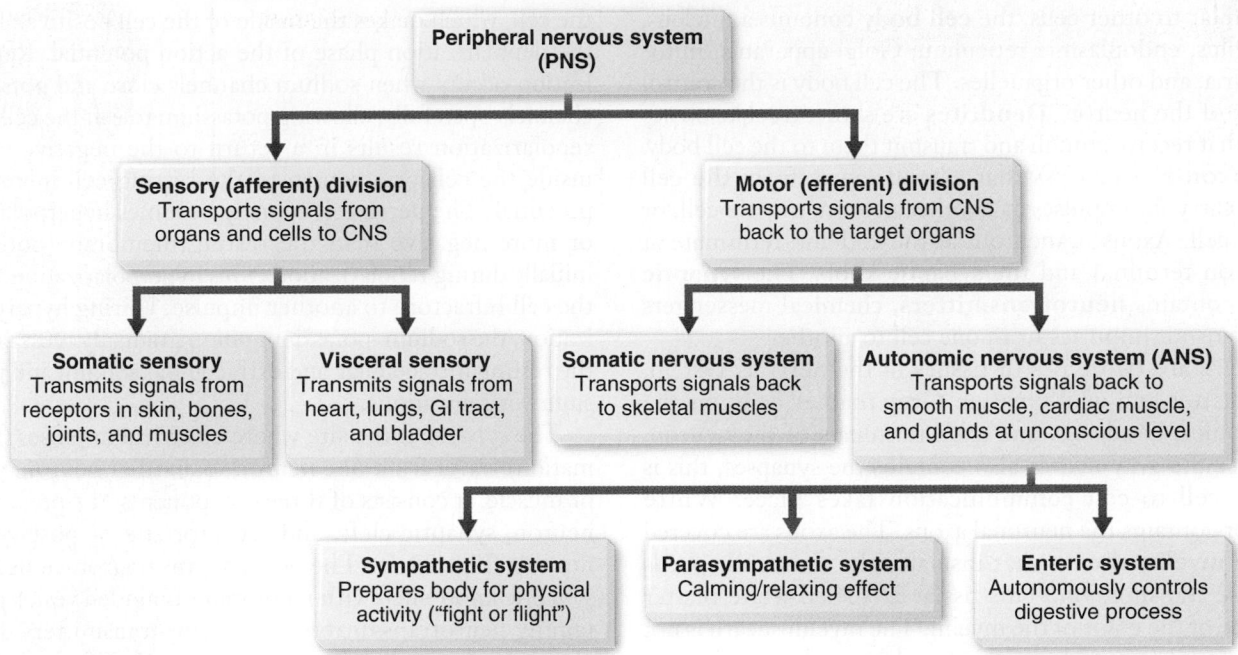

FIGURE 35.2 Functional organization of the peripheral nervous system. The peripheral nervous system includes 12 pairs of cranial nerves that originate in the brain, 31 pairs of spinal nerves that originate in the spinal cord, and the autonomic nervous system that is divided into the sympathetic and parasympathetic systems. The enteric system is the nervous system of the gastrointestinal tract.

- *Microglial cells* are small cells that become phagocytic when they encounter inflammation or debris. They are a means of defense.
- *Oligodendrocytes* are small cells that form myelin sheaths. These sheaths cover the axons of the neurons in the CNS and aid in conduction of impulses.
- *Schwann cells* form myelin sheaths that cover axons in the PNS.

Neurons

Neurons are the specialized communication cells of the brain and spinal cord. They receive stimuli and transmit or conduct information in response to the stimuli. There are three types of neurons: afferent (sensory), efferent (motor), and interneurons. The **afferent neurons** detect sensory stimuli from receptors, such as sensory nerve endings, and transmit them to the CNS. **Efferent neurons** transmit messages from the brain back to the muscles or glands that respond and are considered motor nerves. **Interneurons**, located entirely in the CNS, integrate incoming and outgoing messages, process and store information, and "make decisions" about the body's response to the stimuli. They account for approximately 90% of the body's neurons. Major components of neurons (Fig. 35.3) are:

- The cell body (soma)
- The dendrites
- The axons
- Myelin sheath
- Axon terminal
- Synaptic knob

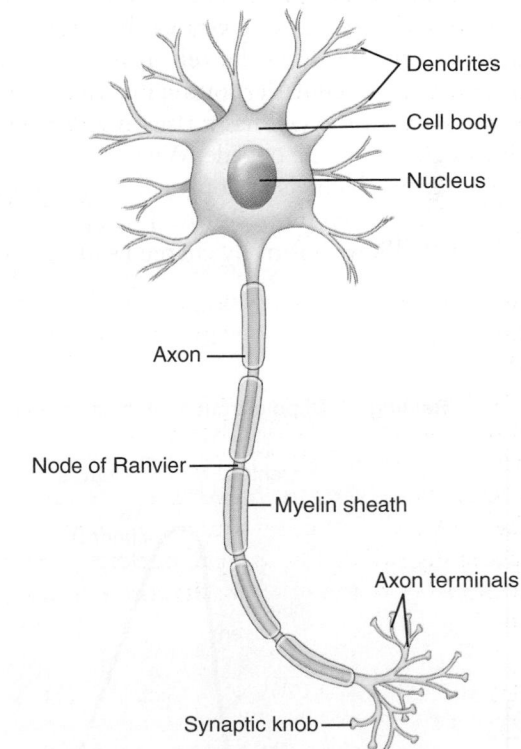

FIGURE 35.3 Structure of the neuron. The cell body is the control center of the neuron and includes a nucleus. Dendrites are short, treelike structures that receive stimuli and transmit them to the cell body. The axon is a process that extends away from the cell body, carrying impulses to another neuron, muscle cell, or organ cell. Axons branch out at the end and terminate at the axon terminal and the synaptic knob. The synaptic knob contains neurotransmitters that transmit impulses from one cell to another.

Similar to other cells, the **cell body** contains a nucleus, nucleolus, endoplasmic reticulum, Golgi apparatus, mitochondria, and other organelles. The cell body is the control center of the neuron. **Dendrites** are short, treelike structures that receive stimuli and transmit them to the cell body. The **axon** is a process that extends away from the cell body, carrying impulses to another neuron, muscle cell, or organ cell. Axons branch out at the end and terminate at the axon terminal and the synaptic knob. The **synaptic knob** contains **neurotransmitters**, chemical messengers that transmit impulses from one cell to another.

There are two types of tissues in the nervous system, gray matter and white matter. **Gray matter** contains the cell bodies, dendrites, and axon terminals of the neuron. Because the gray matter also contains the synapses, this is where cell-to-cell communication takes place. **White matter** contains the neuronal axons. The axons are covered with a **myelin sheath** that insulates the axon and speeds impulse transmission. This tissue is labeled white matter because of the color of the myelin. The myelin sheath is not continuous but is segmented in evenly spaced intervals, with the spaces between the segments called the *nodes of Ranvier*.

Conduction of Nerve Impulses

The action potential of a nerve cell facilitates the transmission of information from a presynaptic neuron to a receptor, which occurs when the action of the sodium–potassium pump creates changes in the electrical balance between the outside and the inside of the cell (Fig. 35.4). Sodium primarily resides extracellularly; potassium is predominantly intracellular. At rest, the cell has a negative charge inside and a positive charge on the outside. When the cell receives a stimulus, sodium channels are opened. Potassium channels also open but much more slowly. The opening of the sodium channels allows positively charged sodium to enter

the cell, which makes the inside of the cell positive. This is the depolarization phase of the action potential. Repolarization occurs when sodium channels close and potassium channels open fully, allowing potassium to exit the cell. This repolarization results in a return to the negative charge inside the cell or a return to the resting cell membrane potential. The nerve cell actually becomes hyperpolarized, or more negative than the resting membrane potential, initially during repolarization. This hyperpolarization makes the cell refractory to another impulse. During hyperpolarization, the sodium–potassium pump gradually reestablishes the resting intracellular and extracellular sodium and potassium concentrations.

The synapse is the site where electrical impulses (information) travel from one neuron to another neuron, gland, or muscle. It consists of three components: the presynaptic neuron, synaptic cleft, and receptor site or postsynaptic neuron (Fig. 35.5). The presynaptic neuron houses the synaptic knob filled with membrane-bounded vesicles containing neurotransmitters. The neurotransmitters diffuse across the synaptic cleft to the receptor site of the receiving neuron, gland, or muscle. The release of neurotransmitters results in the transmission of the electrical impulse and allows cells to communicate with each other.

Neurotransmitters can be excitatory or inhibitory (Table 35.1). Excitatory neurotransmitters open sodium channels, causing depolarization in the postsynaptic membrane, initiating an action potential. Inhibitory neurotransmitters open chloride channels, allowing negatively charged chloride ions into the cell. This causes the postsynaptic membrane to become hyperpolarized, thus refractory to impulses and less excitable. Examples of excitatory neurotransmitters are acetylcholine and norepinephrine. Inhibitory neurotransmitters include gamma-aminobutyric acid (GABA) and dopamine.

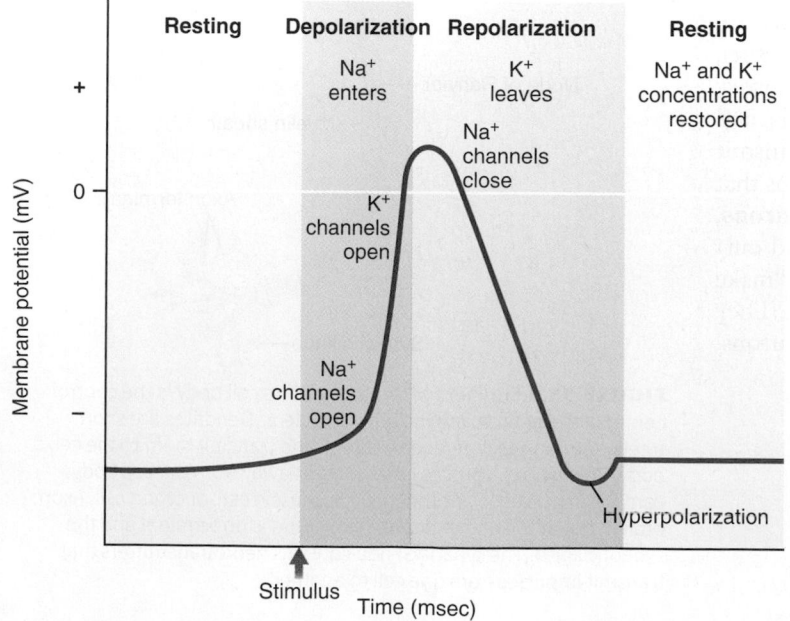

FIGURE 35.4 Action potential. The action potential of a nerve cell facilitates the transmission of information from a presynaptic neuron to a receptor through the action of the sodium–potassium pump. At rest, the cell has a negative charge inside and a positive charge on the outside. When the cell receives a stimulus, sodium channels are opened, allowing positively charged sodium to enter the cell, which makes the inside of the cell positive. This is the depolarization phase of the action potential. Repolarization occurs when sodium channels close and potassium channels open fully, allowing potassium to exit the cell. This repolarization results in a return to the negative charge inside the cell or a return to the resting cell membrane potential.

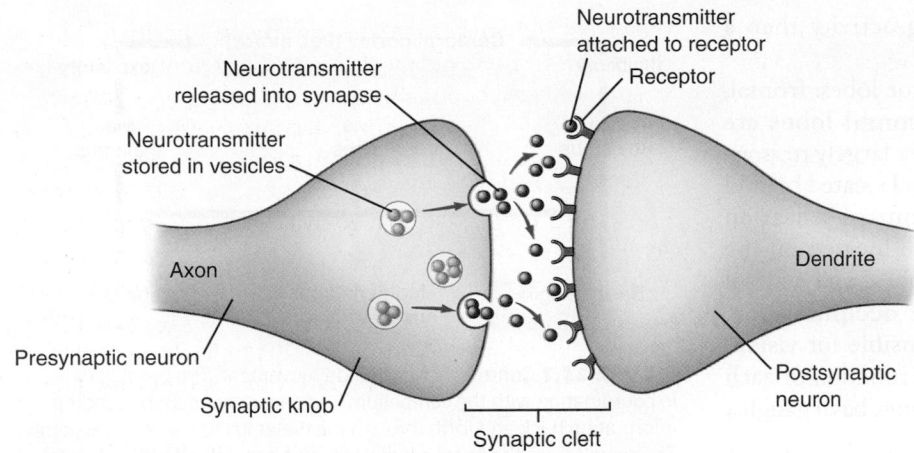

FIGURE 35.5 Structure of a synapse. The synapse is the site where electrical impulses travel from one neuron to another neuron, gland, or muscle, and consists of three components: the presynaptic neuron, synaptic cleft, and receptor site or postsynaptic neuron. The neurotransmitters diffuse across the synaptic cleft to the receptor site of the receiving neuron, resulting in the transmission of the electrical impulse.

Table 35.1 Chart of Neurotransmitters

Neurotransmitter	Class
Acetylcholine	Excitatory
Glutamate	Excitatory
Norepinephrine	Primarily excitatory
Serotonin	Inhibitory
Gamma-aminobutyric acid (GABA)	Inhibitory
Dopamine	Inhibitory

The Central Nervous System

The CNS consists of the brain and spinal cord. The brain is enclosed and protected by the skull; the spinal cord is enclosed and protected by the vertebral column.

Brain

The brain is divided into three parts (Fig. 35.6):

- The cerebrum
- The cerebellum
- The brainstem

Cerebrum

The **cerebrum**, the largest portion of the brain, is covered by a thin layer of gray matter, the cerebral cortex. The majority of the cerebrum is white matter containing myelinated nerve fibers or tracks that carry information or impulses to other areas of the cerebrum and other areas of the brain or spinal column. The longitudinal fissure divides the cerebrum into the right and left hemispheres, which are connected by the **corpus callosum**, a band of thick fibers that facilitates communication between the hemispheres. The surface of the cerebrum has folds (gyri) separated by grooves (sulci). The deeper sulci are called *fissures*. The folds of the cerebrum create a greater surface area that

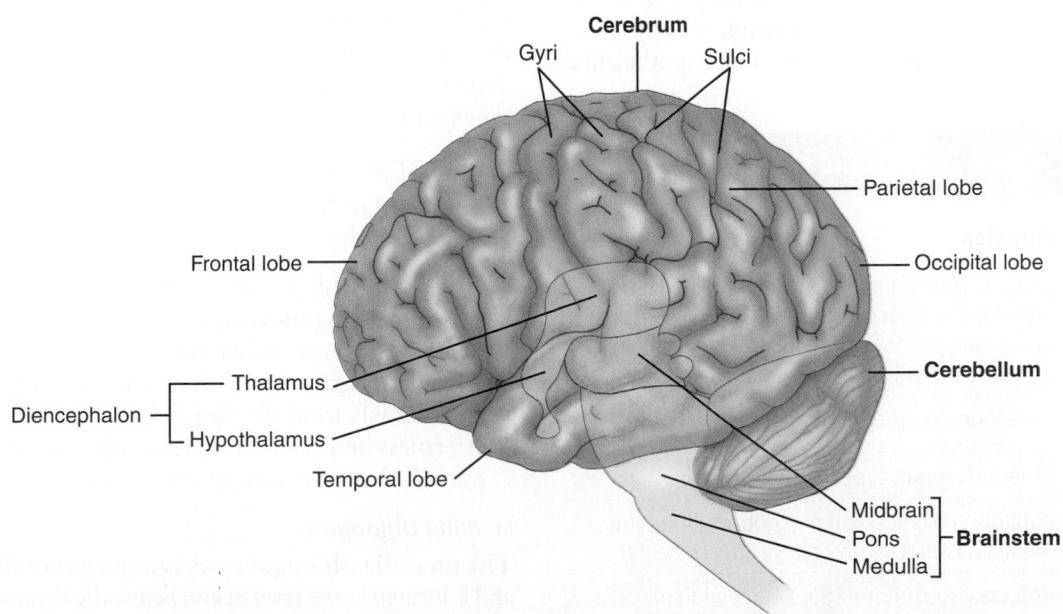

FIGURE 35.6 Structures of the brain. The brain is divided into the cerebrum, the cerebellum, and the brainstem. The cerebrum includes the frontal, parietal, temporal, and occipital lobes. The brainstem includes the midbrain, pons, and medulla.

allows for more information-processing activity than a smooth surface.

The cerebrum is divided into four major lobes: frontal, parietal, temporal, and occipital. The **frontal lobes** are located in the front area of the brain and are largely responsible for motor movement and personality. Located behind the frontal lobes, the **parietal lobes** control sensation and perception. The **temporal lobes** are located on the sides of the brain, beneath the parietal lobes, and control sound recognition and language, and the **occipital lobe**, located at the back of the brain, is responsible for vision. See Table 35.2 for more details about the function of each lobe. The cerebrum also contains the thalamus, basal ganglia, hypothalamus, and limbic system.

Thalamus

The **thalamus** is the relay center for sensory impulses to the cerebral cortex. All information traveling to the cerebral cortex is filtered through the thalamic nuclei. This includes information for pain, temperature, taste, smell, hearing, equilibrium, vision, and touch. The thalamus also relays information from the cerebellum and basal ganglia to the cerebral cortex, and in this way, it helps regulate motor control.

Basal Ganglia

The **basal ganglia**, in coordination with the cerebellum, regulate movement by sending information back and forth through the thalamus to the cerebral cortex (Fig. 35.7). The signals from the basal ganglia are inhibitory, whereas the signals from the cerebellum are excitatory. Coordinated movement is achieved through the balance of both systems operating properly, whereas problems in the basal ganglia result in movement disorders (e.g., Parkinson's disease).

Hypothalamus

The **hypothalamus** is the main regulator for the ANS and sends signals to the brainstem, regulating, among other things, the heart rate and blood pressure. The hypothalamus

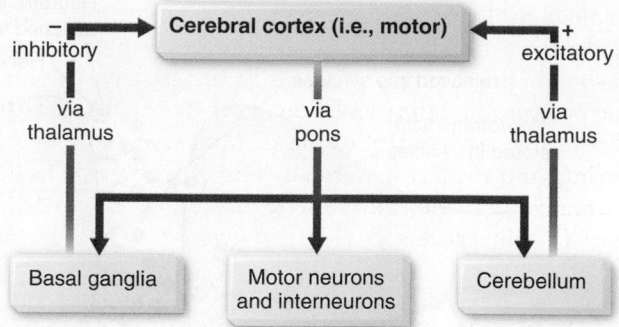

FIGURE 35.7 Control of coordinated movement. The basal ganglia, in coordination with the cerebellum, regulate movement by sending information back and forth through the thalamus to the cerebral cortex. The signals from the basal ganglia are inhibitory, and the signals from the cerebellum are excitatory.

regulates metabolism, reproduction, growth, and stress responses by secreting hormones that control the anterior pituitary gland (discussed in detail in Chapter 40). Additional functions are thermoregulation and the regulation of food and water intake, sleep, memory, and emotional behavior.

Limbic System

The **limbic system** consists of the cingulate gyrus, the hippocampus, and the amygdala. It has a primary role in memory and emotions and also has a center for gratification and aversion. When stimulated, the gratification center produces sensations of pleasure or reward, whereas the stimulation of the aversion center produces objectionable feelings of grief or dread.

Brainstem

The **brainstem** consists of three areas: the medulla, pons, and midbrain. The reticular formation or reticular activating system runs through all levels of the brainstem. All conduction of the motor and sensory tracts is relayed through the brainstem to the cerebellum and cerebrum. Ten of the 12 cranial nerves originate in the brainstem. Any injury or trauma to this area can be life threatening.

Reticular Formation

The **reticular formation** consists of networks of neural cells and has the following functions:

- Motor control, coordination, maintaining balance and posture during movement
- Respiratory and cardiac control
- Pain modulation by providing a route of passage for pain signals from the periphery
- Alertness and sleep by controlling some of the sensory stimuli that reach the cerebral cortex

Medulla Oblongata

The **medulla oblongata** is continuous with the spinal cord and is located at the level of and below the **foramen magnum**, the opening in the skull that allows the spinal cord to connect with the brainstem. All impulses from the brain to

Table 35.2 Cerebral Lobes and Functions	
Lobe	**Function**
Frontal	Motor cortex, voluntary movement; Broca's expressive speech center—dominant hemisphere; personality; behaviors: social, sexual, judgment, and problem solving
Parietal	Sensation interpretation and perception; spatial relationships such as body position; integration of sensory input, especially visual input
Temporal	Auditory sensation and perception; long-term memory; Wernicke's receptive speech center
Occipital	Process visual information; perception of color and shapes

the spinal cord pass through the medulla oblongata. The reticular formation networks located in the medulla oblongata contain the respiratory and cardiac centers. Heart rate, blood pressure, and the regulation of the rhythm and depth of breathing are controlled here. Vomiting, coughing, sneezing, and swallowing are all controlled here as well. Four cranial nerves originate here: glossopharyngeal (IX), vagus (X), spinal accessory (XI), and hypoglossal (XII).

Pons

The **pons** rests above the medulla oblongata below and anterior to the midbrain and relays all impulses between the brain and the spinal cord. Four cranial nerves originate in the pons: trigeminal (V), abducens (VI), facial (VII), and acoustic (VIII).

Midbrain

The **midbrain** contains the nerve pathways between the cerebrum and the medulla oblongata. It also includes the **aqueduct of Sylvius** of the ventricular system, which connects the third and fourth ventricles (discussed in more detail in the following discussion). Cranial nerves III and IV, which control eye movement (oculomotor and trochlear, respectively), originate here.

Cerebellum

The **cerebellum** is located in the base of the brain or posterior fossa, behind the medulla oblongata and pons. Attached to the brainstem by nerve fibers known as peduncles that carry signals to and from the cerebellum, the cerebellum is divided into left and right lobes that are connected by

a narrow structure called the *vermis*. The cerebellum is primarily responsible for coordination of muscle activities, fine motor movement, balance, and equilibrium. Patients with disturbances in the cerebellum usually present with gait and balance issues. The cerebellum also has a role in nonmotor functions such as speech, sensing, and emotion.

Blood Flow in the Brain

Arterial Circulation of the Brain

The arterial circulation of the brain is supplied by the right and left internal carotid arteries and the right and left vertebral arteries. The internal carotid arteries (ICA) are the primary supply of blood to the cerebrum. They divide into the anterior cerebral artery (ACA) and middle cerebral artery (MCA) and are connected to each other by a small anterior communicating artery (ACOM). Ninety percent of all strokes involve the MCA of the brain. The vertebral arteries join to form the basilar artery, which then divides into the posterior cerebral arteries. These supply blood to the occipital lobe, the cerebellum, and the brainstem. Table 35.3 displays which arteries supply circulation to specific areas of the brain and the disorders that result from poor or blocked circulation.

Circle of Willis. The internal carotid arteries and the vertebrobasilar arteries join together via the posterior communicating artery at the base of the brain to form the **circle of Willis** (Fig. 35.8), which is a critical collection of vessels. The ACA, MCA, and posterior cerebral artery all arise from this circle, providing blood flow throughout the brain. If

Table 35.3 Arterial Circulation of the Brain (Circle of Willis)

Name of Artery	Blood Flow to:	Dysfunction With Poor Blood Supply
Middle cerebral artery	Provides blood flow to the lateral aspect of the frontal, temporal, and parietal lobes	Contralateral motor and sensory deficits, speech and language deficits (aphasia)
Internal carotid arteries	Provide blood flow to the anterior portion of the brain	Same as middle cerebral artery (MCA)
Anterior cerebral artery	Provides blood flow to the medial aspect of the frontal and parietal lobes	Contralateral motor and sensory dysfunction
Vertebral artery	Forms three branches: posterior spinal artery provides flow to posterior one-third of dorsolateral spinal cord; anterior spinal artery provides flow to two-thirds of anterior aspect of spinal cord; posterior inferior cerebellar artery (PICA) provides flow to posterior cerebellum	Dizziness, poor balance, ataxia, sensory, coordination deficits, and dysphagia
Basilar artery	Forms two branches: anterior inferior cerebellar artery (AICA) provides flow to the anterior cerebellum; superior cerebellar artery provides flow to superior surface of the cerebellum and portions of the midbrain and pons	Vertigo, diplopia, headache, impaired vision, coma
Posterior cerebral artery	Provides flow to the medial and inferior surfaces of the occipital and temporal lobes	Visual changes

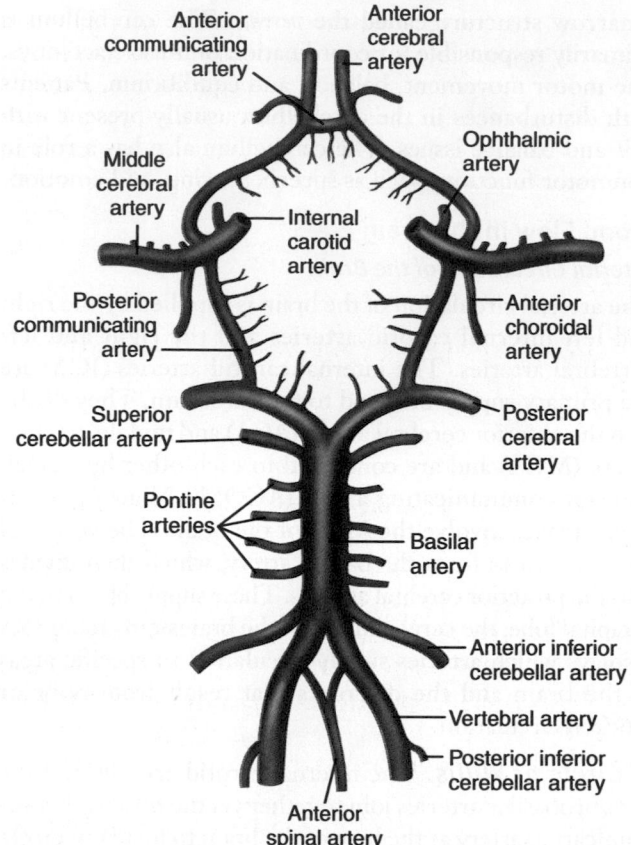

FIGURE 35.8 Cerebral blood supply and the circle of Willis. The anterior cerebral artery, middle cerebral artery, and posterior cerebral artery all arise from the circle of Willis to provide blood flow throughout the brain.

the arteries in the circle of Willis are blocked or ruptured, inhibiting or decreasing blood flow, arterial circulation throughout the brain may be impacted, leading to damage secondary to hypoperfusion and ischemia.

Venous Blood Flow

Venous blood flow or drainage occurs through the dural sinuses, which are venous channels found between the dura mater and the brain. Blood from the deep internal and external veins, as well as CSF from the subarachnoid space, empties into these channels to be transported back to the heart via the internal jugular vein. Unlike other veins in the body, these veins do not have valves.

> **⚠ Safety Alert** The internal jugular vein travels through the neck. For patients with increased intracranial pressure (ICP) due to bleeding or edema, it is imperative to keep the head in proper alignment to allow venous flow or drainage of blood from the brain back to the heart. For sedated patients or those with a decreased level of consciousness (LOC), the nurse may need to provide support to the head to maintain proper alignment that facilitates venous outflow. Increased ICP is discussed in detail in Chapter 39.

The Spinal Cord

The spinal cord is the pathway that carries information to and from the brain and the rest of the body through the spinal nerves of the peripheral nervous system (PNS). Located within and protected by the vertebral column, a series of stacked bony structures, the spinal cord begins at the brainstem and extends to the level of lumbar vertebrae 1 and 2 in adults. It is made up of both gray matter and white matter. The gray matter of the cord containing non-myelinated tissue is responsible for the synaptic transmission of information from cell to cell. In cross section, the gray matter appears as an H within the white matter (Fig. 35.9). The H-shaped area is divided into the posterior, or dorsal, horn and the ventral, or anterior, horn. Nerve fibers that carry impulses into the spinal cord are contained within the dorsal nerve root that enters the cord through the dorsal horn. Nerve fibers that carry impulses out of the spinal cord are contained in the ventral nerve root and exit the cord through the ventral horn. A spinal nerve is a combination of fibers from both the dorsal and ventral nerve roots. Spinal nerves are discussed in detail later in the chapter.

The white matter (myelinated tissue) contains the ascending and descending tracts, which transmit information to and from the brain and target organs or cells. Ascending

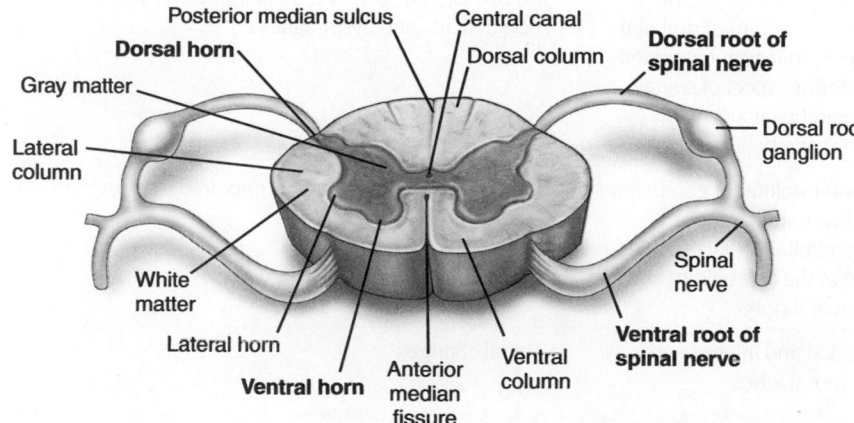

FIGURE 35.9 Structure of the spinal cord. The H-shaped area is divided into the dorsal (posterior) horn and the ventral (anterior) horn. Nerve fibers that carry impulses into the spinal cord are contained within the dorsal nerve root that enters the cord through the dorsal horn. Nerve fibers that carry impulses out of the spinal cord are contained in the ventral nerve root and exit the cord through the ventral horn.

pathways contain sensory neurons and carry impulses up the spinal column to the brain. Descending pathways contain motor neurons and carry impulses down the spinal column to target muscles. Some pathways, during ascent or descent, undergo **decussation** or "crossover" in the spinal column, which results in the right side of the brain controlling the left side of the body, and vice versa. If crossover occurs—if the origin and destination of the track are on opposite sides of the body—they are said to be *contralateral*. If the origin and destination of the track are on the same side of the body, they are said to be *ipsilateral*.

Spinal tracts are named based on the site of origin and termination. The first part indicates the origin, and the second part indicates the termination site. The major ascending tracts are spinothalamic (starts in the spine and ends in the thalamus), spinoreticular, fasciculus gracilis, fasciculus cuneatus, anterior spinocerebellar, and posterior spinocerebellar. Together, they are responsible for pain sensation, temperature, pressure, proprioception, fine touch, and vibration.

The major descending tracts are anterior corticospinal, lateral corticospinal, tectospinal, lateral and medial reticulospinal, and lateral and medial vestibulospinal. Together, they control the conscious movement of the skeletal muscles and subconscious movement and control of balance, muscle tone, and reflexes. They also control head turning in response to auditory or visual cues.

The motor neurons that carry impulses from the brain to the target muscles are divided into upper and lower motor neurons. **Upper motor neurons** originate in the motor area of the cerebral cortex or brainstem and carry motor information down a common pathway and terminate on a lower motor neuron in the spinal cord. The **lower motor neurons** carry the motor information directly to the muscle. Table 35.4 details the major ascending and descending tracts.

Protective Mechanisms

The skull or cranium, vertebrae, meninges, CSF, and blood–brain barrier are protective structures for the brain and spinal cord.

Skull

The skull encases and protects the brain from injury. It is made up of eight cranial bones—two parietal, one occipital, two temporal, one sphenoid, one ethmoid, and one frontal—joined by fibrous joints or suture lines (Fig. 35.10). During infancy, fontanelles or "soft spots" exist to allow for brain growth during early infancy and provide flexibility during delivery for passage through the birth canal. These spaces are covered by a fibrous membrane. The bones gradually grow together, closing the fontanelles at approximately age 2. As discussed earlier, the foramen magnum, an opening in the occipital bone in the base of the brain, is located where the medulla

Table 35.4 Ascending and Descending Tracts

Tract	Function	Decussation
Ascending		
Spinothalamic	Temperature, light pain, pressure, or touch	Yes
Spinoreticular	Pain from injury	Yes
Fasciculus gracilis	Limited trunk position and motion, deep pain, vibration, or touch, level T6 and down	Yes
Fasciculus cuneatus	Limb and trunk position and motion, deep pain, vibration, or touch, level T6 and above	Yes
Anterior spinocerebellar	Proprioception (sensory information regarding position and movement)	Yes
Posterior spinocerebellar	Proprioception (sensory information regarding position and movement)	No
Descending		
Anterior corticospinal	Fine motor control of movement	No
Lateral corticospinal	Fine motor control of movement	Yes
Tectospinal	Reflexive head turning in response to stimuli	Yes
Lateral reticulospinal	Posture and balance, regulation of sensation of pain	No
Medial reticulospinal	Posture and balance, regulation of sensation of pain	No
Lateral vestibulospinal	Posture and balance	No
Medial vestibulospinal	Motor control of head position	Yes

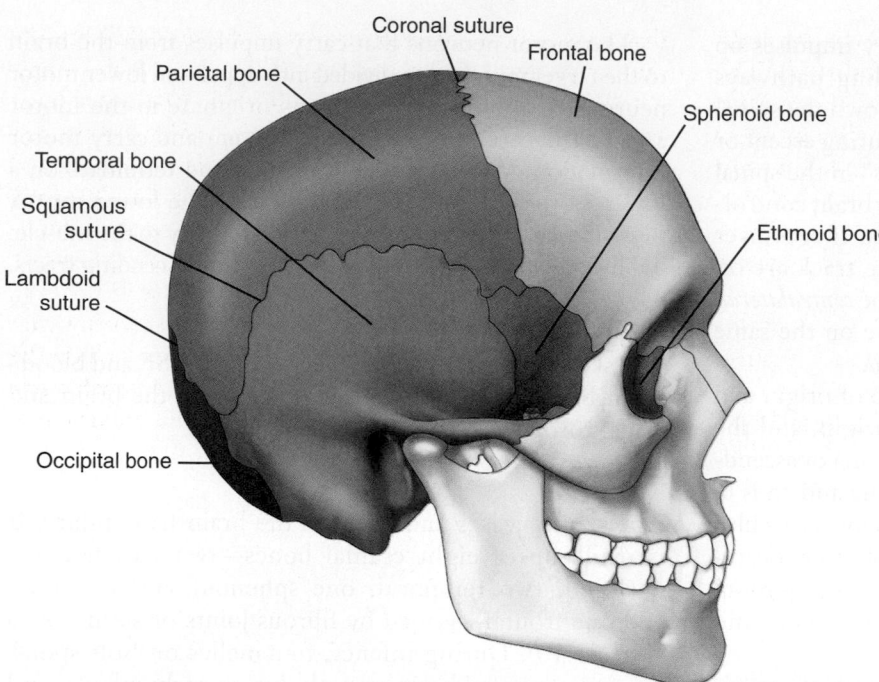

FIGURE 35.10 Cranium. The cranium consists of two parietal, one occipital, two temporal, one sphenoid, one ethmoid, and one frontal bone, joined by suture lines.

oblongata, the lower portion of the brainstem, joins with the spinal cord.

Vertebrae

The vertebrae are the skeletal structures that cover and protect the spinal cord. The vertebrae form a column that provides the head with support, allows flexibility and movement, and maintains the body in an upright position (Fig. 35.11). There are 33 vertebrae: 7 cervical, 12 thoracic,

5 lumbar, 5 sacral (fused), and 4 coccygeal (fused). The vertebrae consist of a body and a vertebral arch composed of a pedicle and a lamina (Fig. 35.12). Extending posteriorly from the vertebral arch are spinous processes. Extending laterally are the transverse processes. These are the points of attachment for ligaments and spinal muscles. The vertebrae are connected by facet joints that allow movement of the vertebral column. Ligaments provide stabilization. Each vertebra has a central canal, the vertebral foramen,

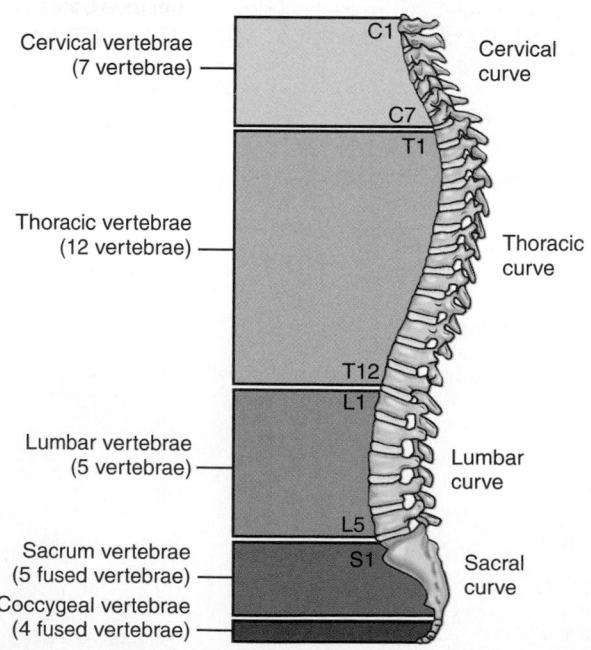

FIGURE 35.11 The vertebral column. The vertebral column is the skeletal structure that covers and protects the spinal cord. There are 33 vertebrae. There are four curves of the vertebral column, the cervical and lumbar concave posteriorly, and the thoracic and sacral concave anteriorly.

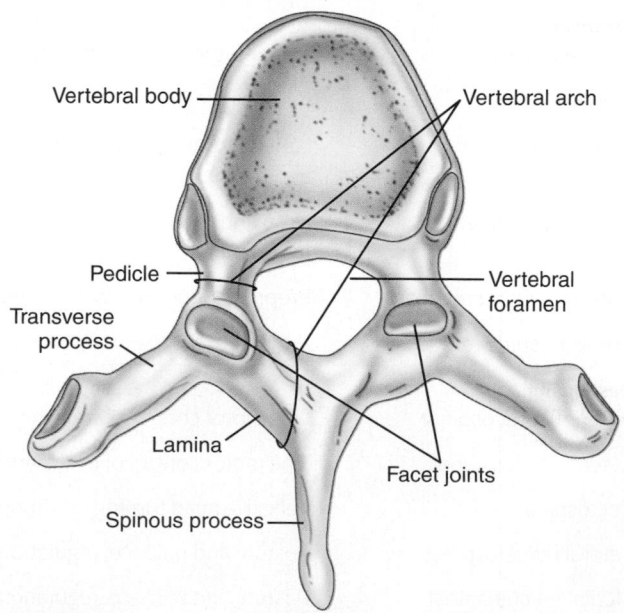

FIGURE 35.12 Vertebral body and curvatures. The vertebrae consist of a body and a vertebral arch composed of a pedicle and a lamina. Vertebrae are connected by facet joints that allow movement of the vertebral column. Each vertebra has a central canal, the vertebral foramen, through which the spinal cord passes.

through which the spinal cord passes. In between the individual vertebrae are discs that act as shock absorbers. The discs are composed of a firm spongy material, the nucleus pulposus, surrounded by fibrous cartilage, the annulus fibrosis. The spinal column is able to support the weight of the body because it has a unique anatomical shape. There are four curves: the cervical and lumbar concave posteriorly, and the thoracic and sacral concave anteriorly.

Meninges

The meninges are fibrous membrane layers that protect the brain and spinal cord (Fig. 35.13). The outermost layer is called the **dura mater** and is a tough, fibrous membrane

that rests against the interior part of the skull. Within the skull, the dura mater consists of two layers: the outer periosteal layer and the meningeal layer. The outer layer stops at the base of the skull. The meningeal layer continues and covers the spinal cord. The meningeal layer folds inward in certain areas to separate portions of the brain. One fold, the **falx cerebri**, separates the right and left cerebral hemispheres (Fig. 35.14). Another fold, the tentorium cerebelli, separates the cerebellum from the cerebrum (see Fig. 35.14). This is sometimes used to define the location of certain structures within the brain. *Supratentorial* structures include the cerebrum and diencephalon (thalamus and hypothalamus). *Infratentorial* structures are the cerebellum and brainstem.

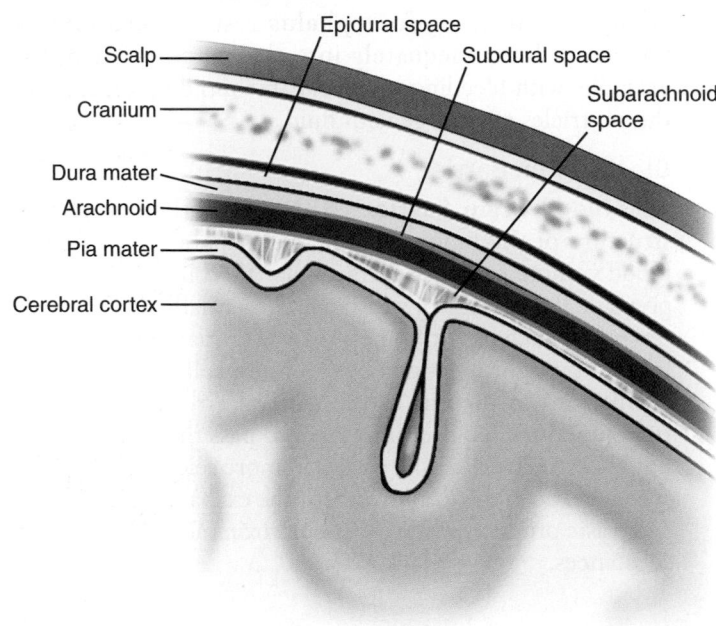

FIGURE 35.13 Meningeal layers and spaces. The meninges protect the brain and spinal cord. The outermost layer is called the dura mater, which is a tough, fibrous membrane that rests against the interior part of the skull. The second layer of the meninges is the arachnoid, which is a very thin layer with a spider-web appearance. The inner membrane is the pia mater, which is a highly vascular membrane that lies in direct contact with the brain. The epidural space is a potential space that exists between the skull and the dura mater. The subdural space sits between the inner dura mater layer and the arachnoid layer. The third space is the subarachnoid space. This is between the arachnoid membrane and the pia mater.

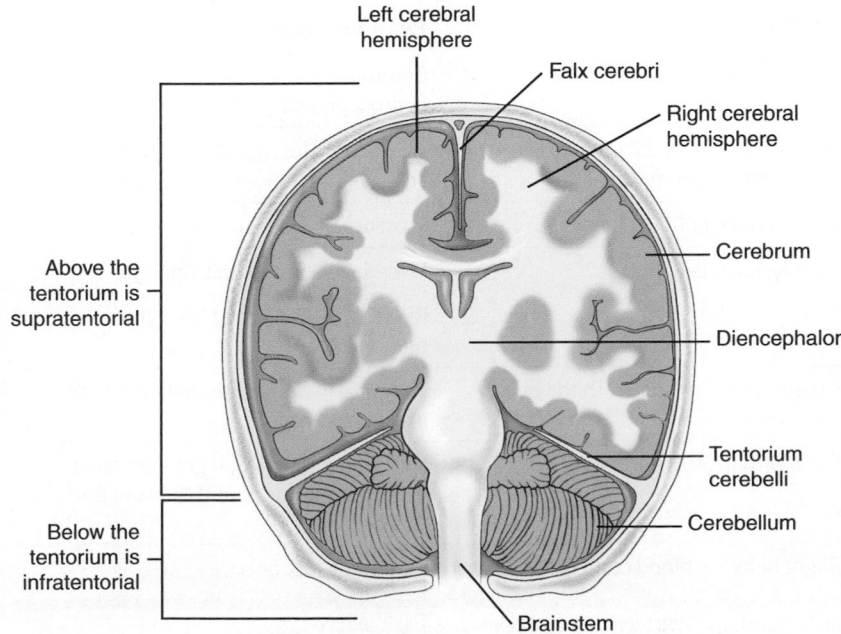

FIGURE 35.14 Falx cerebri and tentorium cerebelli. The falx cerebri separates the right and left cerebral hemispheres. The tentorium cerebelli separates the cerebellum from the cerebrum. Supratentorial structures include the cerebrum and diencephalon (thalamus and hypothalamus). Infratentorial structures include the cerebellum and brainstem.

The second layer of the meninges is the arachnoid. This is a very thin layer with a spider-web appearance. Within this layer are the arachnoid villi, small extensions that protrude through the meningeal layer of the dura mater that facilitate CSF reabsorption (discussed later in the chapter). The inner membrane is the pia mater, which is a highly vascular membrane that lies in direct contact with the brain.

Meningeal Spaces

The meningeal spaces are real or potential spaces between the membrane layers. The epidural space is a potential space that exists between the skull and the dura mater. The middle meningeal artery is located here, and if this artery is torn or damaged by trauma, a hemorrhage can occur. This is called an epidural bleed or hematoma, which is recognized by its rapid accumulation and the onset of neurological symptoms. The subdural space lays between the inner dura mater layer and the arachnoid membrane. If a bleed occurs here, it is more commonly a venous type of hemorrhage. Because of the venous origin, blood accumulates slowly, and clinical manifestations may also develop more slowly. The third space is the **subarachnoid space**. This is between the arachnoid membrane and the pia mater, and much of the CSF flows through this space around the brain and spinal cord. Aneurysmal ruptures often cause bleeding into this space.

Cerebrospinal Fluid

Cerebrospinal fluid is a colorless and odorless fluid that circulates through the ventricles in the brain and into the subarachnoid space. (See Table 35.5 for the characteristics of CSF.) The brain contains four ventricles or chambers: two lateral ventricles, the third ventricle, and the fourth ventricle.

Within each ventricle is a collection of capillaries, the *choroid plexus*. Cerebrospinal fluid is produced in the choroid plexus of the ventricles. Starting in the lateral ventricles, the choroid plexus produces CSF (Fig. 35.15). From there, it flows into the third ventricle, where the choroid plexus adds more fluid. It then flows into the fourth ventricle, with the choroid plexus again adding more fluid. From there, it flows into the central canal that houses the spinal cord or into the subarachnoid space to circulate around the brain, brainstem, and spinal cord, providing cushioning, protection, and nutrition. Approximately 500 mL of CSF is produced daily. CSF is constantly reabsorbed via the arachnoid villi, avenues allowing movement of CSF from the subarachnoid space into the venous system, resulting in only approximately 125 to 150 mL of circulating CSF volume present at any one time. **Hydrocephalus** results when CSF is unable to drain adequately into the venous system, for example, with bleeding in the subarachnoid space, causing the ventricles to enlarge with fluid.

Blood–Brain Barrier

The **blood–brain barrier (BBB)** is another protective structure of the brain. This barrier separates circulating blood volume from the extracellular fluid in the brain and prevents the passage of substances potentially damaging to the brain, such as antibodies, toxins, or macrophages. It is formed by tight junctions between the cells that form the capillaries not present in the general circulation. These tight junctions require substances to pass through the cell, not in between cells. The cells are "more selective" than the spaces between them, allowing for the exchange of nutrients and waste products while excluding toxins and other foreign substances.

Table 35.5 Characteristics of Cerebrospinal Fluid (CSF)

Characteristic	Normal Value	Abnormal Value	Possible Cause
Volume	125–150 mL	Increased with hydrocephalus	Communicating or obstructive hydrocephalus
Pressure	0–15 mm Hg	Increased intracranial pressure (ICP) greater than 20 mm Hg	Hydrocephalus, infection, cyst, cerebral edema
Specific gravity	1.007	Greater than 1.007	Presence of infection, RBCs due to a bleed
Color	Clear	Cloudy, turbulent	Presence of infection with increase in WBCs
		Bloody	RBCs or breakdown of RBCs from hemorrhage
Glucose	Two-thirds of serum value	Greater or less than two-thirds of serum value	Decrease in meningitis, SAH; increase in severe infection
Protein	15–50 mg/dL	Greater than 50 mg/dL	Mild: meningitis, MS; high: tuberculosis meningitis, tumors, and Guillain–Barré syndrome
Blood	None	Slight or heavy blood content	Traumatic tap; SAH

MS, Multiple sclerosis; *RBC,* red blood cell; *SAH,* subarachnoid hemorrhage; *WBC,* white blood cell

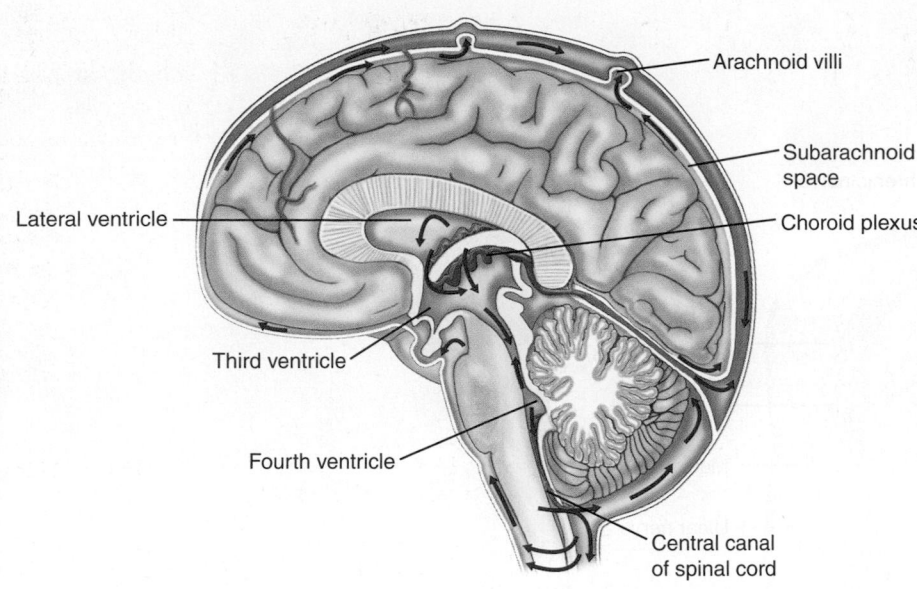

Arachnoid villi

Subarachnoid space

Choroid plexus

Lateral ventricle

Third ventricle

Fourth ventricle

Central canal of spinal cord

FIGURE 35.15 Flow of cerebrospinal fluid. Starting in the lateral ventricles, the choroid plexus secretes CSF. From there, CSF flows into the third ventricle, then into the fourth ventricle. CSF then flows into the central canal that houses the spinal cord or into the subarachnoid space to circulate around the brain, brainstem, and spinal cord, providing cushioning, protection, and nutrition.

Connection Check 35.1

The nurse recognizes that patients with major changes in personality most likely have damage in which lobe of the brain?
A. Frontal
B. Occipital
C. Parietal
D. Temporal

The Peripheral Nervous System

The peripheral nervous system (PNS) is composed of the spinal nerves, the cranial nerves, and the autonomic nervous system (ANS). It consists of sensory nerves that transport signals from organs and cells in the body to the CNS and motor nerves that transport signals back to the target organs. Both are divided into somatic and visceral divisions. The *somatic sensory division* transmits signals from receptors in muscles, bones, joints, and skin. The *somatic motor division* transports signals back to the skeletal muscles to produce a contraction. The visceral sensory division transmits signals from the heart, lungs, GI tract, and bladder. The visceral motor division transports signals back to smooth muscle, cardiac muscle, and glands at an unconscious level. This visceral motor division is also known as the autonomic nervous system (ANS) and is subdivided into the sympathetic and parasympathetic nervous systems.

Spinal Nerves

Spinal nerves transmit information to and from the spinal cord and receptors throughout the body. Because they transmit signals in both directions, they are referred to as *mixed nerves*. There are 31 pairs of spinal nerves: 8 cervical, 12 thoracic, 5 lumbar, 5 sacral, and 1 coccygeal (Fig. 35.16). As discussed earlier, proximal or close to the spinal cord,

each spinal nerve has two points of connection to the cord, the anterior, or ventral, root and the posterior, or dorsal, root. The ventral root transmits motor impulses to the muscle (efferent pathway). The dorsal root carries sensory information to the spinal cord (afferent pathway). Distal to the cord, the spinal nerves divide and form several large branches, which then subdivide further to form *nerve plexuses*—the cervical, brachial, lumbar, and sacral plexuses. The cervical plexus gives rise to nerves that innervate the head and shoulders and, most essential, the **phrenic nerve** that innervates the diaphragm to stimulate respiration. The brachial plexus gives rise to nerves that innervate the neck, shoulder, and arm. The lumbar plexus gives rise to nerves that innervate the thigh and leg. The sacral plexus gives rise to nerves that innervate the posterior thigh, lower leg, and foot. The largest nerve in the body, the sciatic nerve, arises from this plexus and travels down the posterior thigh.

A **dermatome** is an area on the skin that is supplied by a specific spinal nerve (Fig. 35.17) and maps where the nerve fiber provides sensation or feeling. It can be used to determine whether a sensory nerve root is damaged or injured. Dermatomes can be used for nursing assessment following spinal surgery or injury to detect changes in sensation.

Cranial Nerves

The cranial nerves (CN) originate in the brain, except for the olfactory and optic nerves, and transmit signals to receptors in the body. They are identified by Roman numerals and are named in order according to where they arise in the brain, beginning with the anterior or rostral segments, the cerebrum, and working down the brainstem (Fig. 35.18). There are three sensory, five motor, and four mixed (both sensory and motor functions) nerves. Table 35.6 details the cranial nerves and functions. Evaluation of the cranial

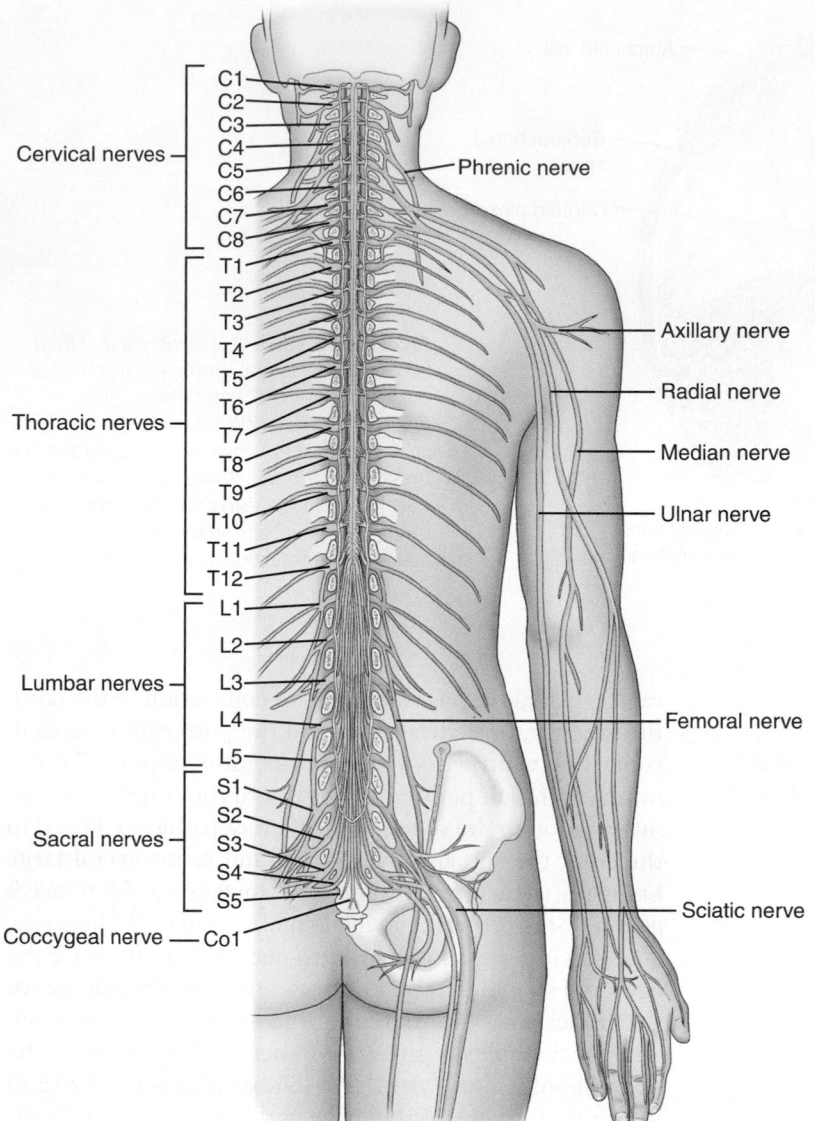

FIGURE 35.16 Spinal nerves. Spinal nerves transmit information to and from the spinal cord and receptors throughout the body. There are 31 pairs of spinal nerves: 8 cervical, 12 thoracic, 5 lumbar, 5 sacral, and 1 coccygeal. The phrenic nerve innervates the diaphragm.

nerves is a critical component of nursing assessment in the patient with disease, injury, trauma, or hemorrhage in the brain.

Autonomic Nervous System

The ANS consists of the sympathetic and the parasympathetic nervous systems. Working in opposition and at an unconscious and involuntary level, the sympathetic and parasympathetic nervous systems regulate the activity of cardiac muscle, smooth muscle, and glands. The effect of each system is regulated by the type of neurotransmitter released at the synapse site and the type of receptor on the target cell.

Sympathetic Nervous System

The sympathetic nervous system is known as the thoracolumbar system because it receives information from the thoracic and lumbar areas in the spinal cord. This system prepares the body for stress or physical activity and is known as

eliciting the "fight-or-flight" response. The neurotransmitter released at the synapse site is typically norepinephrine, and the fibers that secrete norepinephrine are adrenergic fibers. The receptors on the target cells are called *adrenergic receptors*. There are two types of **adrenergic receptors**: alpha and beta. **Alpha receptors** typically have an excitatory effect, producing vasoconstriction that increases blood pressure. **Beta receptors** are usually inhibitory and dilate the bronchioles, which enhances airflow. Beta receptors can also have excitatory effects on cardiac muscle, producing a stronger cardiac contraction and increased heart rate. Both the excitatory effects of increasing heart rate and blood pressure and the inhibitory effect facilitating airflow are necessary for "fight or flight."

Parasympathetic Nervous System

The parasympathetic nervous system is known as the craniosacral system because it receives information from the brainstem and sacral region of the spinal cord. The

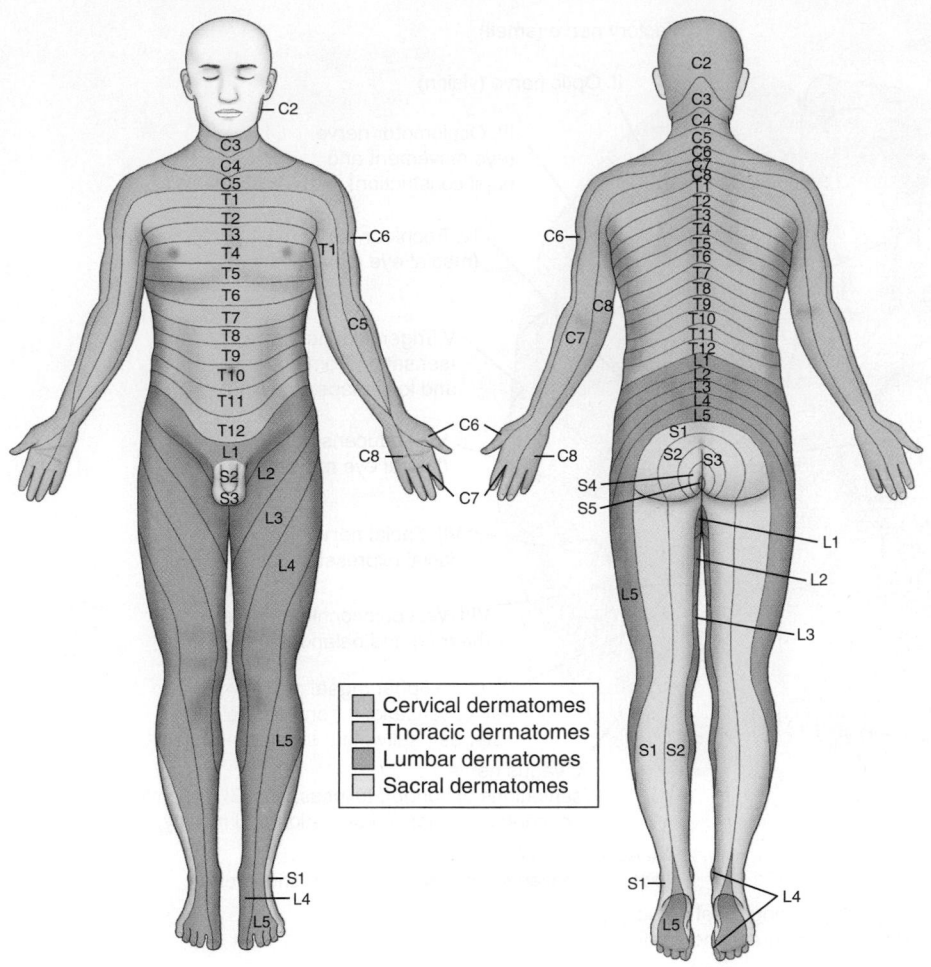

FIGURE 35.17 Dermatome chart. Dermatomes correlate to an area on the skin that is supplied by a specific spinal nerve and maps where the nerve fiber provides sensation or feeling.

Legend in figure:
- Cervical dermatomes
- Thoracic dermatomes
- Lumbar dermatomes
- Sacral dermatomes

neurotransmitter released at the synapse is acetylcholine. The nerve fibers that secrete acetylcholine are called **cholinergic fibers**. There are two types of cholinergic receptors: muscarinic and nicotinic. **Muscarinic receptors**, located on cardiac muscle, smooth muscle, and gland cells, can have excitatory or inhibitory responses depending on the target organ systems. Acetylcholine has an excitatory effect on intestinal smooth muscle but has an inhibitory effect on cardiac muscle. **Nicotinic receptors**, located on skeletal muscle and cells of the adrenal medulla, always have an excitatory effect. See Table 35.7 and Figure 35.19 for the contrasting actions of the sympathetic and parasympathetic nervous systems.

Connection Check 35.2

The nurse correlates which responses as associated with the sympathetic nervous system? *(Select all that apply.)*

A. Increased heart rate
B. Decreased respiratory rate
C. Increase in peristalsis
D. Dilated bronchioles
E. Decreased heart rate

CASE STUDY: EPISODE 2

Mr. Smith continues to have headaches that are not relieved by over-the-counter (OTC) medications. His headaches are intermittent but daily. He has no other symptoms but is experiencing GI upset that he thinks is most likely due to anxiety. He is worried about the headaches and is anxious to have his appointment with the neurologist...

ASSESSMENT

The nurse's ability to perform an accurate neurological assessment requires knowledge of the anatomy and physiology of the nervous system. Neurological changes can happen rapidly and subtly. Early observation, detection, and reporting of changes in the patient's condition are critical in creating positive outcomes for patients. Early detection can promote prompt medical intervention. Due to growing concerns about the potential neurological damage associated with sports injuries, greater attention is being paid to

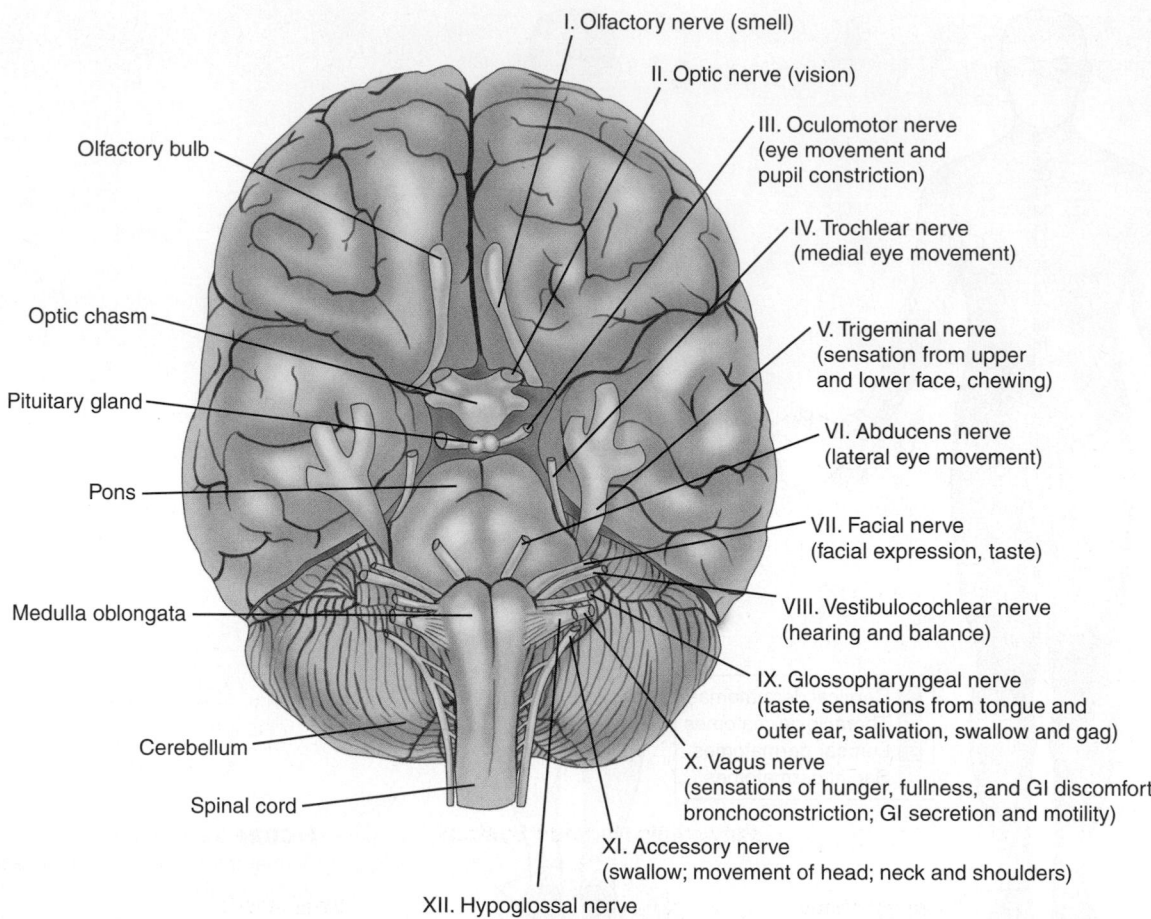

I. Olfactory nerve (smell)

II. Optic nerve (vision)

III. Oculomotor nerve (eye movement and pupil constriction)

IV. Trochlear nerve (medial eye movement)

V. Trigeminal nerve (sensation from upper and lower face, chewing)

VI. Abducens nerve (lateral eye movement)

VII. Facial nerve (facial expression, taste)

VIII. Vestibulocochlear nerve (hearing and balance)

IX. Glossopharyngeal nerve (taste, sensations from tongue and outer ear, salivation, swallow and gag)

X. Vagus nerve (sensations of hunger, fullness, and GI discomfort; bronchoconstriction; GI secretion and motility)

XI. Accessory nerve (swallow; movement of head; neck and shoulders)

XII. Hypoglossal nerve (tongue movement and swallowing)

Olfactory bulb

Optic chasm

Pituitary gland

Pons

Medulla oblongata

Cerebellum

Spinal cord

FIGURE 35.18 The cranial nerves. Cranial nerves are identified by Roman numerals and are named in order according to where they arise in the brain, beginning with the anterior segments, the cerebrum, and working down the brainstem.

Table 35.6 Cranial Nerves and Functions

Number	Name	Composition	Function
I	Olfactory	Sensory	Smell
II	Optic	Sensory	Vision
III	Oculomotor	Motor	Eye movement up, down, lateral, opening of eyelid, pupil constriction
IV	Trochlear	Motor	Medial and downward medial eye movement
V	Trigeminal	Mixed	Touch, temperature, and pain sensations from upper and lower face, chewing
VI	Abducens	Motor	Lateral eye movements
VII	Facial	Mixed	Taste, facial expressions
VIII	Vestibulocochlear (acoustic)	Sensory	Hearing and balance
IX	Glossopharyngeal	Mixed	Taste, touch, pressure, pain, and temperature; sensations from tongue and outer ear; regulation of blood pressure and respiration; salivation, swallow, and gag
X	Vagus	Mixed	Taste; sensations of hunger, fullness, and gastrointestinal discomfort; bronchoconstriction; gastrointestinal secretion, and motility
XI	Accessory	Motor	Swallow; head, neck, and shoulder movements
XII	Hypoglossal	Motor	Tongue movement with speech; food manipulation and swallowing

Table 35.7 **Sympathetic and Parasympathetic Nervous Systems**

	Sympathetic Nervous System	Parasympathetic Nervous System
Primary effect	*Preparation for physical activity—"fight or flight"*	*Calming/relaxing effect*
Neurotransmitter	Norepinephrine	Acetylcholine
Receptor	Adrenergic: ● Alpha-adrenergic ● Beta-adrenergic	Cholinergic: ● Muscarinic (excitatory or inhibitory effect) ● Nicotinic (always excitatory effect)
Actions Eye	Pupillary dilation (α)	Pupillary constriction
Heart	Increased heart rate (β)	Decreased heart rate
Blood vessels	Increased cardiac contractility (β) Vasoconstriction (α) Vasodilation of coronary arteries (β)	Decreased cardiac contractility Vasodilation
Respiratory system	Bronchodilation (β)	Bronchoconstriction
Gastrointestinal system	Decreased gastrointestinal motility (α, β)	Increased gastrointestinal motility
Urinary system	Urinary sphincter contraction	Urinary sphincter relaxation

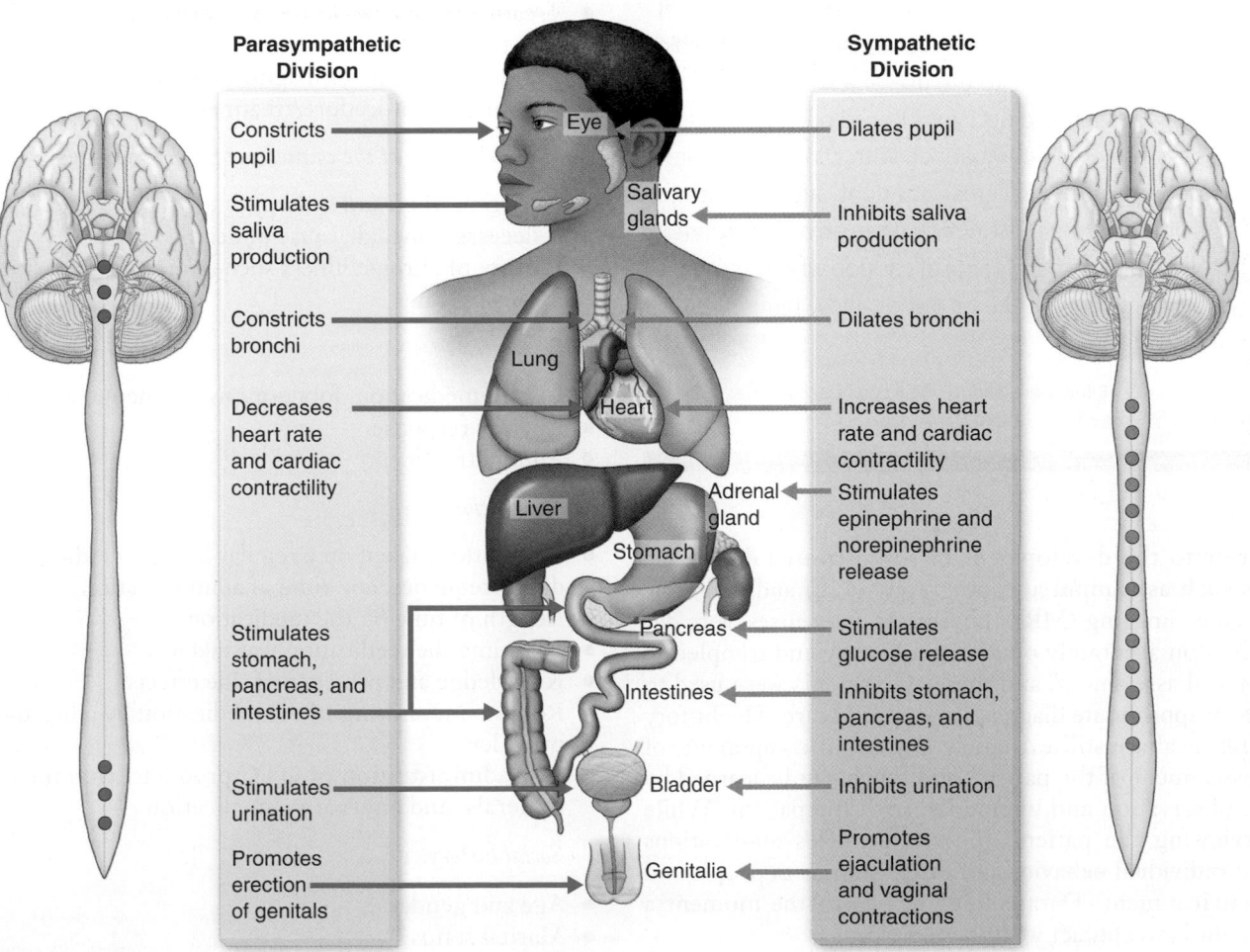

Autonomic Nervous System

FIGURE 35.19 Function of the sympathetic and parasympathetic divisions of the autonomic nervous system (ANS).

potential injuries that involve contact sports like football (see Evidence-Based Practice).

Evidence-Based Practice

Clinical Evaluation of Concussion in Athletes

Due to the incidence of concussive injuries associated with sports injuries, particularly in high school and college male athletes playing football, sideline assessments are often indicated when a player is potentially injured. This literature review included articles identified through searches using PubMed and MEDLINE and initially identified 1,492 articles published between 1965 and 2019 that were further refined to yield a total of 96 papers that included systematic reviews, consensus guidelines, and position statements. Findings revealed some of the complexities related to sideline assessments, particularly in relation to the time-pressured environment that requires rapid evaluation and decision making about the degree of injury and whether the student athlete should be removed from the game. Recommendations focus on the importance of symptom assessment, with priority given to potential cervical spine injury, intracranial bleeding, or other injuries that can present with clinical manifestations associated with a concussive injury. Specific recommendations relate to the use of a standardized assessment approach and decisions based on knowledge of the student athlete in comparison with clinical presentation. When the student seems "not right" after a possible concussive injury, the practitioner, often an athlete trainer, is encouraged to err on the side of caution when determining whether to remove the player or allow him or her to remain in the game.

Putukian, M. (2017). Clinical evaluation of the concussed athlete: A view from the sideline. *Journal of Athletic Training,* 52(3), 236–244.

Prior to the development of sophisticated diagnostic tools such as computed tomography (CT) and magnetic resonance imaging (MRI), physicians and nurses were dependent on accurately obtaining a history and completing a physical assessment, and these assessments were used to make an appropriate diagnosis and plan of care. The history and physical are still extremely important components of the assessment of the patient, and much can be learned by close observation and interaction with the patient. While interviewing the patient, the nurse makes observations about individual behavior and the responses to people and the environment. Data collection begins the moment a nurse initiates contact with the patient.

History and Physical

History

The history is best provided by the patient, but if the patient is unable to provide information, friends or family may be needed. When interviewing, the nurse treats the patient with respect and dignity by conducting the interview process in a nonjudgmental and caring manner, which facilitates establishing a trusting relationship between the nurse and the patient. It is important to be attentive to any subtle cues the patients may provide. The history includes information on regular healthcare, the medical history of the patient and family, chief complaint, allergies, medications, and social history.

Regular healthcare includes:

- Name of the primary healthcare provider
- History of routine health screenings, such as lipid screen, colonoscopy, and mammography
- Status of vaccines, such as tetanus, hepatitis, influenza, and pneumonia
- Alternative healthcare, such as acupuncture and herbal medicines

Medical history includes:

- Chronic illnesses such as diabetes, hypertension, or renal disease
- Treatment for chronic diseases or current problem
- Past trauma/injury
- Recent treatments or diagnostic studies
- Past surgical procedure/treatments

Medical history of the immediate family includes:

- Father, mother, and siblings
- If deceased, include cause of death.
- History of chronic illness such as diabetes, obesity, or hypertension

Allergies:

- List all medication, food, or environmental allergies.
- Allergic response
- Allergy treatment

Medications:

- Medications taken on a regular basis, including name, dose, frequency, and time of administration
- Length of time on the medication
- Last time the medication was taken
- Knowledge and presence of side effects
- Routine monitoring of the medication by a healthcare provider
- Self-administration of OTC products, vitamins, minerals, and alternative medications

Social history:

- Age and gender
- Marital status

- Religion
- Social support networks
- Work history and any environmental risk factors or exposures
- Smoking, alcohol use/abuse, or drug (legal and illegal) abuse

Current history of chief complaint:

- Description of current symptoms that brought the patient to the hospital/clinic, including:
  - Review of time of onset and presentation of symptoms
  - Current treatment of symptoms

Connection Check 35.3

A nurse is performing the initial interview of a patient presenting to the clinic because of neurological complaints. Which actions by the nurse are appropriate? *(Select all that apply.)*

A. Assessment of physical appearance
B. Comprehensive medication list review
C. Reassurance that all will be okay
D. Review of alcohol and drug use
E. Review of risks

Physical

A physical assessment of the neurological system includes establishing the level of consciousness (LOC); determining cognitive function; evaluating mental status; and assessing cranial nerve, motor, cerebellar function, and reflex activity.

Level of Consciousness

The best indicator of neurological deterioration is a change in LOC. Assessing LOC involves identifying patient responsiveness and orientation to person, place, and time. There are different categories that describe LOC: conscious, confused, lethargic, stuporous, obtunded, or comatose (Table 35.8).

Level of consciousness can be assessed using the **Glasgow Coma Scale (GCS)**. The GCS assigns a score for eye-opening, best motor response, and verbal response. The highest possible score is 15, with a score of 8 or less indicating severe neurological issues. When attempting to elicit a response, always begin with the least noxious stimulation, working from central to peripheral. First, call the patient by name. If there is no response, raise the voice to a higher level. If there is still no response, gently shake the patient. If there is no response, a sternal rub can be applied. If there is no response, apply a painful stimulus such as a pinch to the inner arm or nailbed pressure. Be cautious if the patient has other conditions that might make these techniques inappropriate. Table 35.9 details the components of the GCS.

> **! Safety Alert** In order to get an accurate assessment of the patient's response to a stimulus, the command needs to be clear and definitive, such as:
> - Hold up two fingers on your left hand.
> - Wiggle the toes on your right foot.
>
> Avoid commands such as "squeeze my fingers." Hand grasps may be reflexive and may not represent a true response.

Cognitive Function

The **Mini-Mental Status Examination (MMSE)** is a tool that can be used to assess cognitive function. It is a tool that assesses the patient's orientation, attention, calculation, memory, and language abilities. Patients are asked to answer questions, and a correct answer scores 1 point, with a total of 30 points available. A score below 20 is an indication of cognitive impairment (Table 35.10).

Table 35.8 Levels of Consciousness

Level of Consciousness	Definition
Conscious	Awake with appropriate speech and behavior
Confusion	Disorientation, bewilderment, difficulty following commands
Lethargic	Sleepiness; slow and delayed response to stimulus
Obtundation	Somnolence with drowsiness between sleep states, lessened interest in environment, slowed responses to stimulation
Stupor	Minimal movement without stimulus; requires strong vigorous stimulus and then drifts back to unresponsiveness
Coma	Not arousable and unresponsive

Table 35.9 Glasgow Coma Scale (GCS)

Best Eye Opening

Spontaneous	4	Spontaneous, not necessarily to command
To speech	3	Opens eyes only to verbal stimuli
To pain	2	Opens eyes only to painful stimuli
None	1	Does not open eyes

Best Motor Response

Obeys commands	6	Obeys commands
Localizes	5	Purposeful movement to pain
Withdraws (flexion)	4	Withdraws from painful stimuli
Abnormal flexion	3	Flexion in response to pain
Abnormal extension	2	Extension in response to pain
Flaccid	1	No response to pain

Best Verbal Response

Oriented	5	Oriented to person, place, and time
Confused	4	Confused conversation
Inappropriate words	3	Disorganized or random speech
Incomprehensible sounds	2	Moans, mumbles
None	1	No speech

*A patient may be oriented, but if unable to speak because of an artificial airway, T is assigned to the score. For example, a patient who opens eyes spontaneously and obeys commands scores 11 T.

Table 35.10 Mini-Mental Status Examination (MMSE)

Parameter	Questions/Tasks
Orientation	Who are you?
	What is today?
	Where are you?
Attention and calculation ability	Count backward by seven. If this is too difficult, spell a word backward.
Memory ● Immediate ● Recent ● Remote	● Repeat these three words … ● What did you have for breakfast? ● Where did you attend high school?
Language Assess the patient's ability to comprehend and use language	What is this object in my hand?
	Repeat this phrase: "No ifs, ands, or buts."
	Perform this three-stage command: "Take this paper in your right hand, fold it in half, and place it on the floor."
	Follow this written command: Write "close eyes" on a paper; the patient should close his or her eyes.
	Ask the patient to write a sentence. It should contain a noun and verb.
	Ask the patient to copy a design.

These are sample questions. Actual questions will vary from test to test and per facility/agency.

Cranial Nerve Assessment

Cranial nerve assessment is a critical component of the nursing assessment of the patient. It can identify neurological impairment due to disease or trauma to the brain. Table 35.11 details the components of the cranial nerve assessment.

Motor Assessment

A motor assessment is performed to inspect and assess muscle mass and tone as well as strength and equality between the left and right and to note any abnormalities (Box 35.1). The muscle strength of both the upper and lower extremities is assessed. The patient is asked to grasp the hands and squeeze bilaterally. The biceps and triceps are tested by the practitioner grasping the wrists and asking the patient to "pull me toward you" and "push me away." The quadriceps are tested by asking the patient to lift the legs against gravity and then resistance. Plantar flexion is tested by grasping the foot and asking the patient to "step on the gas," and dorsiflexion is tested by asking the patient to pull the "toes to the nose." The practitioner uses the 0-to-5 scale to document the assessment findings. Table 35.12 illustrates scoring of motor strength. Another motor parameter that is assessed is *pronator drift*. This is done by asking the patient to extend both arms out in front of the body, turn the palms upward, and close the eyes. If one arm is weak, the patient's hand pronates and begins to drift downward. This is a positive pronator drift and is a sign of subtle motor weakness.

Sensory System

The sensory system is assessed to determine if the patient can feel or identify specific sensations such as temperature, vibration, superficial or deep pain, proprioception or position sense, and cortical sensory interpretation. This is particularly important when performing a spinal cord assessment. Using the dermatome chart can help determine the area of injury or damage if sensory function has been altered. The patient is instructed to close the eyes while these tests are completed. The practitioner compares findings right to left and proximal to distal.

Table 35.11 Cranial Nerve Assessment

Number and Name	Testing
I Olfactory	Smell aromatic items such as coffee, oranges, vanilla, chocolate
II Optic	Visual acuity—use a Snellen's chart, or ask the patient to read from a book or a newspaper. Assess for peripheral vision (visual fields): The examiner stands 2 feet from the patient. Have the patient cover one eye. With the examiner holding both arms up, the examiner wiggles fingers and moves in from the side, up, down, and toward the patient's nose. The patient states when he or she can see the fingers. Both patient and examiner should see the fingers at the same time.
III Oculomotor	Darken the room. Check pupils by using a flashlight. Ask the patient to look at a stationary object. Bring the light in from the lateral position and shine it directly into the eye (direct reaction). Normal response is constriction. The response should be rapid and the pupils equal in size, shape, and symmetry. After checking both pupils, shine the light into one and look at the opposite eye; that eye should also constrict (consensual reaction). Observe for ptosis (eyelid drooping). Extraocular movements (EOMs) are checked by having the patient follow the examiner's finger while drawing an "H" in the air. The patient should look up, down, laterally, and diagonally.
IV Trochlear	Part of EOM examination: The examiner asks the patient to follow the examiner's finger as it is moved toward the patient's nose (patient appears cross-eyed).
V Trigeminal	Assesses facial sensation for light touch, sharpness, and dullness. The examiner should use fingertips or soft cotton to determine facial feeling, moving to different areas of the face, including the forehead, cheeks, and jawline. Assess motor function by having the patient clench the teeth and then attempt to move the mouth side to side. Ask the patient to open the mouth while the examiner tries to close it.
VI Abducens	Part of the EOM examination: The examination involves asking the patient to follow the examiner's finger by moving the eyes laterally.
VII Facial	Ask the patient to smile, frown, puff cheeks, raise eyebrows, and close eyes tightly and not let the examiner open them.
VIII Vestibulocochlear (acoustic)	Check for hearing by rubbing fingers close to the ear or by whispering. Check balance and ability to walk straight. Check for nystagmus (involuntary and rapid eye movement, generally side to side), usually detected during EOM examination.
IX Glossopharyngeal	Check gag reflex by applying a tongue depressor to the back of the throat. Ask the patient to swallow.
X Vagus	Assess gag and ability to swallow. Check voice for weakness and quality; ask the patient to say "Ah."
XI Accessory	Ask the patient to shrug the shoulder against resistance. Ask the patient to turn the head side to side with resistance. Patient will push while examiner applies pressure.
XII Hypoglossal	Ask the patient to stick out the tongue and move it side to side.

Box 35.1 Abnormalities of the Motor System

- Atrophy: decrease in muscle mass
- Paresis: slight or incomplete paralysis
- Plegia: complete loss of muscle function
- Contraction: shortening or tightening of the muscles
- Involuntary movements: uncontrolled movements
- Spasm: involuntary muscle contraction
- Spasticity: increased muscle tone that creates stiff movement

Light touch and superficial pain are assessed by starting at the feet and working upward. Using a cotton swab snapped in two (the broken tip is used to assess sharp sensation, the soft end to assess dull), the practitioner lightly touches the patient and then asks the patient to state when

Table 35.12 Motor Strength

Score	Description
5	Strong, full ROM against gravity and full resistance
4	Slight weakness, full ROM against gravity and moderate resistance
3	Moderate weakness, full ROM against gravity but not resistance
2	Severe weakness, full ROM but without gravity or resistance
1	Very severe weakness, muscle contraction only
0	No movement

ROM, Range of motion.

he or she feels the stimulus and where he or she feels it. The patient should be able to distinguish between dull and sharp. An open safety pin can be used to assess sharp sensation, but caution must be used to not break the skin. Deep pain is tested only when the patient does not respond to the superficial pain stimulus. Temperature is tested only if peripheral pain is not detected because the same sensory pathways carry pain and temperature. Test tubes filled with hot and cold water or the cool tuning fork can be used to assess this function. The patient's skin is lightly touched while being asked what is being felt.

Vibration is tested by using a tuning fork. Using a 128-Hz tuning fork, the practitioner strikes the forked ends against the heel of the hand, holds the stem, and applies it to the distal extremities such as the toes or feet. Both sides are always compared. The patient is asked to tell the practitioner if the vibrations are felt and when the vibration stops. The tuning fork can also be used to test hearing (acoustic nerve, CN VIII). One technique to assess hearing with a tuning fork involves applying the stem of the vibrating tuning fork to a spot on the mastoid process (prominence of the temporal bone behind the ear) equidistant from both ears. The bones of the skull transmit the impulse to CN VIII, which then transmits the signal to the brain. The sound should be heard in both ears at the same time.

Proprioception is the patient's ability to recognize position with the eyes closed. The examiner holds a digit, toe, or finger on the lateral aspect and then gently moves the digit upward or downward. With eyes closed, the patient should be able to identify whether the position is up or down.

Cortical sensory interpretation is a function of the parietal lobe and involves several tests (Table 35.13). Abnormalities in the sensory system are noted in Table 35.14. Abnormalities in the sensation of pain are noted in Table 35.15.

Cerebellar Assessment

Cerebellar assessment involves evaluating the patient's balance, coordination, gait, and posture. The *Romberg* test is performed to assess balance and involves asking the patient to stand with the feet together, arms at the sides, with the eyes open. The examiner then checks that the patient can do this without swaying. The patient is then asked to close the eyes. If the patient is unable to maintain balance, this is a positive Romberg test and may indicate vestibular or proprioceptive problems. A patient with cerebellar damage may not be able to balance with the eyes open or closed.

Testing for coordination is completed in a variety of ways. A general assessment is done by observing basic activities such as walking, getting up or down from a chair, or reaching for objects. A specific test involves asking patients to move a finger from the nose to the practitioner's finger while the practitioner quickly moves his or her finger to different locations far enough away but close enough so that it can be reached by the patient. Another test of cerebellar coordination involves asking the patient to run the heel of one foot down the shin of the other leg. Assessing gait and posture is another important component of cerebellar testing, and the patient should be able to stand and walk erect, with a steady gait. The practitioner also assesses for length of stride, arm movement, base of gait (how far apart feet are placed), and the ability to turn steadily.

Reflexes

Reflexes are involuntary and automatic responses to stimuli that provide the body with protection and help to adjust to an ever-changing and sometimes dangerous environment. The reflex arc occurs when sensory (afferent) neurons carry a stimulus to the motor neurons in the spinal cord. Motor (efferent) neurons carry the stimulus from the spinal cord to the muscle (a response). A complete neurological

Table 35.13 Cortical Sensory Interpretation		
Name	**Definition**	**Testing**
Stereognosis	The ability to identify an object by its shape by simply holding the object	Place a common object (key or coin) in the patient's hand and ask him or her to identify it.
Two-point discrimination	The ability to distinguish two points separately	Test by using an opened paper clip to provide two points. The points should be about 2 cm apart. The patient should be able to distinguish the two points separately. Use the palms, lips, forearms, shins, soles, and top of the foot. If the patient is unable to distinguish two points, move the paper clip farther apart. Continue to test until the patient states that two points can be felt. The distance is measured. Charts are available that explain acceptable distances for each body part.
Graphesthesia	The ability to identify letters or numbers when drawn on the skin	Ask the patient to close eyes while the examiner draws a letter or number in the patient's palm. The patient should be able to identify it. Neglect of or failure to recognize one side of the body may be noted with patients with issues in cortical sensory function.

Table 35.14 Abnormalities of the Sensory System

Abnormality	Definition
Anesthesia	Absence of sensation; sensations are blocked
Hypoesthesia	Decreased sense of touch or sensation; numbness
Hyperesthesia	Increased sensitivity to touch
Paresthesia	Abnormal feeling of pins and needles; itching, numbness, and tingling

Table 35.15 Abnormalities of the Sensation of Pain

Abnormality	Definition
Analgesia	Complete lack of pain sensation
Hypalgesia or Hypoalgesia	Decreased ability to feel the pain sensation
Hyperalgesia	Hypersensitivity to a painful stimulus

assessment includes evaluating the major deep tendon reflexes. Two major deep tendon reflexes are the biceps and triceps reflexes (Fig. 35.20). The major deep tendon reflexes to be checked are listed in Table 35.16, and the association of reflexes with a cranial nerve assessment is shown in Table 35.17.

Another important reflex to assess is plantar reflex, or the **Babinski sign**. This reflex is noted to have either upward-moving, downward-moving, or mute toes. To test this reflex, the practitioner takes the heel of the reflex hammer, or a sharp object, and stimulates the outside of the sole of the foot (Fig. 35.21), moving inward over the anterior aspect. If the patient's toes flare upward, this is a *positive Babinski*. A negative response is when the toes curl downward.

A positive Babinski is an indication of an upper motor neuron lesion, which indicates damage to the corticospinal tract of the spinal cord. This abnormal reflex finding can occur in patients with multiple sclerosis and traumatic brain injury. Alcohol can cause neuropathy that may elicit mute toes. A negative response is normal in an adult. In an infant, a positive response is elicited and is considered a normal finding because it is a primitive reflex in infants that disappears with the maturation of the CNS.

> **Safety Alert** When caring for hospitalized patients who have neurological deficits, it is important to compare assessments between oncoming and off-going nurses through bedside rounds or reports to establish a baseline. If a change is noted later in the shift, the nurse can be confident of the timing of the change and report it accurately.

Vital Signs and Increased Intracranial Pressure

The heart rate, blood pressure, and respirations are regulated in the brain and brainstem. Changes in vital signs may develop as a result of alterations in cerebral perfusion, disease, trauma or swelling. These vital sign changes are usually late signs of increased intracranial pressure (ICP) or neurological deterioration.

The skull is a hard, bony structure with no ability to expand. Increased ICP occurs when there is a disturbance in the balance of volumes within the brain: brain tissue, CSF, and blood. This can occur because of a mass or lesion, increased blood volume due to a hemorrhagic event, or an increase in CSF due to a blockage or buildup within the CSF drainage system. The Monro–Kellie hypothesis states that the sum of the volumes of the brain—brain tissue, CSF, and intracranial blood—is constant. A change or increase in one should cause a compensatory decrease in one or both of the other two. If the increase in the volume of one of the

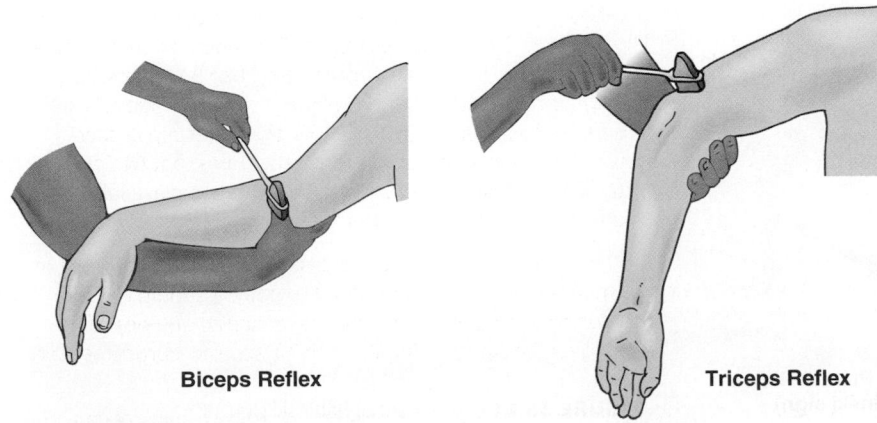

Biceps Reflex **Triceps Reflex** **FIGURE 35.20** Technique for assessment of biceps and triceps reflexes.

Table 35.16 Reflexes

Reflex	Dermatome	Testing
Biceps	C5–C6	Arm flexed, palm down
		Nurse puts finger on tendon and taps finger with hammer
		Normal: elbow flexion
Triceps	C7	Arm flexed, palm toward body
		Tap tendon above elbow
		Normal: elbow extension
Brachioradialis	C5–C7	Arm at rest on thigh
		Tap tendon on forearm between wrist and elbow
		Normal: forearm flexion
Patellar	L3–L4	Flex leg at knee
		Tap tendon below patella
		Normal: knee extension
Achilles	S1–S2	Flex leg at knee
		Tap tendon above heel
		Normal: plantar flexion

Table 35.17 Reflexes Associated With Cranial Nerve Assessment

Reflex	Sensory	Motor	Response
Corneal	V	VII	Blink
Gag	IX	X	Gag
Cough	X	X	Cough
Pupillary	II	III	Pupil constriction

components exceeds the brain's compensatory ability, the ICP increases. This is a medical emergency and requires immediate intervention.

Normal ICP is 0 to 15 mm Hg; measurements greater than 20 mm Hg indicate increased ICP and often require intervention. Patients with increased ICP may demonstrate symptoms of changes in LOC, vomiting, headaches, and seizures. Changes in vital signs are usually late signs of increased ICP. The classic signs of increased ICP are known as Cushing's triad, which is characterized by an elevated blood pressure with a widening pulse pressure, bradycardia, and irregular respirations. In addition to increased ICP, abnormal respiratory patterns can be caused by other brain abnormalities or metabolic disturbances and are described in Table 35.18. Increased ICP is discussed in detail in Chapter 39.

> **⚠ Safety Alert** Changes in the neurological assessment can be very subtle. The patient must be monitored closely for any changes in LOC in an attempt to recognize and intervene appropriately before changes in vital signs occur. Vital sign changes related to increased ICP are late signs of neurological deterioration and may be irreversible.

DIAGNOSTIC STUDIES

Radiographic Procedures

X-ray studies or routine radiographical procedures are non-invasive studies done to assess the skull and spinal column for fractures, compression, stenosis, and malformation and can identify areas of injury or trauma. Patient preparation includes explaining the rationale and expected results of the procedure. The nurse assists the patient with appropriate safe positioning. Close monitoring of the patient who has a suspected cervical–spinal cord injury is essential because of the potential of devastating injury and paralysis if damage to the spinal cord occurs. The patient should be immobilized with a hard collar until a spinal cord injury is ruled out.

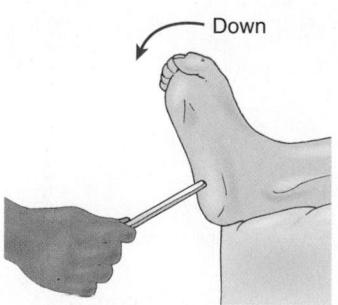

Normal Plantar Reflex

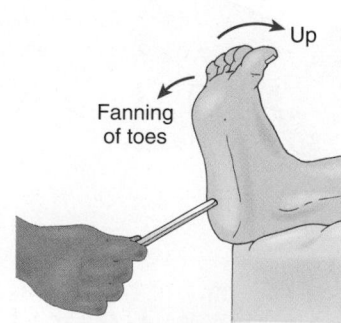

Extensor Plantar Reflex (Babinski sign)

FIGURE 35.21 Assessment of Babinski sign.

Table 35.18 Abnormal Respiratory Patterns

Pattern	Description	Location of Lesion/Injury
Cheyne–Stokes respiration	An increase in rate followed by short periods of apnea	Metabolic disorder; bilateral cerebral or cerebellar lesions
Central neurogenic hyperventilation	Deep, rapid breathing; increase in rate and depth; greater than 25 per minute (can be 40–70 per minute)	Midbrain and upper pons disorder
Apneustic breathing	Slow, deep breathing, then a pause; breath held and released	Disorder of midbrain to lower pons
Cluster breathing; Biot's	Irregular breathing with periods of apnea	Lower pons or upper medulla disorder
Ataxic respiration	Irregular rate and depth with irregular periods of apnea	Upper medulla disorder
Kussmaul's breathing	Rapid and shallow, then deep and labored	Severe metabolic acidosis; diabetic ketoacidosis; renal failure

Computed Tomography

Computed tomography takes cross-sectional images that are viewed as cuts or slices that allow the provider to view the brain, spine, and orbits in a quick, noninvasive manner. A CT scan is used to assess for bleeding, edema, or masses. It is a required screening test for a patient with a suspected ischemic stroke to rule out hemorrhagic stroke prior to receiving thrombolytic (clot-buster) therapy; the presence of a bleed is a contraindication for the administration of thrombolytics. A CT scan is also used to evaluate treatment and monitor for the resolution of injuries. Typically done as a first-step screening procedure prior to MRI or if MRI is contraindicated, the CT scan can be performed with or without contrast. If contrast is necessary, it is given intravenously to help with visualization.

Nursing implications for a CT scan include:

- Providing preprocedure care, including:
  - Explaining the procedure
  - Assessing the potential need to medicate the patient for anxiety (During the examination, the patient is required to lie still on a hard table with the head secured, which may cause feelings of claustrophobia.)
  - Ensuring a patent IV line is in place
  - Checking for allergies to iodine, such as shellfish or dyes, because contrast contains iodine
  - Monitoring blood urea nitrogen (BUN) and creatinine to assess kidney function prior to receiving contrast because it is toxic to the kidney and can impair renal function
  - Assessing for diabetes mellitus and the use of the medication metformin in the management of type 2 diabetes (see Safety Alert)
- Providing postprocedure care, including:
  - Administering IV fluids or increasing the intake of oral fluids to clear contrast medium from the system

- Monitoring for allergic reactions if contrast is administered

> ⚠️ **Safety Alert** Contrast dye is nephrotoxic and can impair renal function. Metformin is cleared primarily through the kidneys, and if it is administered prior to the examination and the administration of contrast, this medication may result in renal impairment. Additionally, metformin levels will remain elevated, potentially resulting in lactic acidosis. Because of this rare and potentially dangerous consequence, metformin must be held 48 hours prior to and after the CT scan or until renal function is determined to be normal via normal BUN and creatinine levels.

Positron Emission Tomography

Positron emission tomography (PET), involves the administration of the radioactive glucose tracer fluorodeoxyglucose (FDG), which detects areas of increased metabolic activity in the body. A PET scan is a very sensitive test for detecting cancer because rapidly dividing cancer cells absorb the tracer (FDG), making them detectable with this imaging. Acute infection can also be identified with the PET scan. Immediately prior to the test, an IV line is inserted, and the tracer is administered.

Nursing implications include:

- Providing preprocedure education, including:
  - No food or drink by mouth is allowed for at least 6 to 12 hours prior to the test to limit metabolic activity related to digestion.
  - No caffeine, alcohol, or tobacco for 24 hours prior to the test because they can interfere with the scan results.

- The patient is instructed to lie very still during the examination to minimize metabolic activity.
- After the tracer has been administered, the patient is instructed to remain quiet in a dark room to allow the tracer to be distributed throughout the body while minimizing metabolic activity.
- Providing postprocedure education, including:
  - Encouraging adequate fluid intake to clear the tracer from the circulation

Magnetic Resonance Imaging

Magnetic resonance imaging (MRI) is a noninvasive and painless imaging study that uses magnetic fields to obtain images. The MRI scan provides three-dimensional images and offers clear visualization and detail of small structures. Images can be obtained with or without contrast, but if used, the contrast is noniodine based, thus limiting issues with allergies and nephrotoxicity. An MRI can be used to assess injuries of the brain and spinal column, as well as to diagnose tumors, infections, and bleeding. It is very useful in the diagnosis of a cerebrovascular accident (CVA), more commonly referred to as stroke.

Nursing implications include:

- Providing preprocedure care, including:
  - Providing patient education about the procedure
  - Screening the patient for the presence of any metal objects, such as keys, watches, credit cards, or phones, prior to the examination. Metal may interfere with the magnetic field and may also be a safety hazard. An implanted device that contains metal, such as a pacemaker, may make the MRI contraindicated because the magnetic field may disable the device.
  - Assessing the potential need to medicate the patient for anxiety. The test requires that the patient lie quietly in a tunnel-like chamber for up to 50 minutes. Velcro straps may be used to hold the patient in position, and the patient may hear loud pounding or pulsating noises because of the operation of the scanner. Patients who are claustrophobic may require sedation. Headsets are typically supplied to provide distracting music.
- Providing postprocedure care, including:
  - Encouraging adequate hydration after the test if contrast is used to facilitate clearance through the kidneys

Magnetic Resonance Angiography

Magnetic resonance angiography (MRA) is a type of MRI that uses the radio-wave signal characteristics of flowing blood to get images of the body's blood vessels. Used to determine the presence of aneurysms, clots, dissections, or vessel stenosis, the MRA is performed in the same fashion as an MRI with the same patient preparation and nursing implications. Contrast may be used in some circumstances. Pre- and postprocedure care is similar to that for the patient undergoing MRI.

Cerebral Angiography

Cerebral angiography is an invasive, intra-arterial, radiological procedure that involves the administration of radiopaque dye through a catheter inserted in an artery, typically the femoral artery. Continuous imaging (fluoroscopy) is done to visualize the cerebral circulation because angiography is an excellent diagnostic test to evaluate cerebral and ocular vessel occlusion, carotid disease, aneurysms, arteriovenous malformations, and other vascular disorders.

Nursing implications include:

- Providing preprocedure education, including:
  - Instructing the patient not take anything by mouth after midnight before the procedure
  - Explaining that the procedure takes approximately 60 to 120 minutes
  - Describing that an IV catheter will be inserted prior to the procedure to provide hydration during and after the procedure to help clear the contrast
  - Teaching that the administration of IV contrast may cause a warm, flushed feeling
- Providing preprocedure care, including:
  - Ensuring informed consent has been obtained
  - Completing a neurological, peripheral pulse, and vital signs assessment before the procedure to establish a baseline from which to evaluate any changes. Ensuring that the patient and family understand that there are risk factors, including the risk for stroke due to the potential for thrombus dislodgement and the risk for impaired peripheral circulation distal to the arterial catheter placement.
  - Assessing for allergies to contrast dye, iodine, and seafood because contrast dye contains iodine. Seafood typically contains iodine.
  - Evaluating renal function parameters (BUN and creatinine) prior to IV contrast administration because contrast is nephrotoxic
  - Assessing for the use of anticoagulants because they place the patient at risk for bleeding during and after the angiogram
  - Administering IV sedation as ordered
- Providing postprocedure care, including:
  - Monitoring vital signs, monitoring neurological status, and assessing puncture site and pulses distal to the catheter insertion site every 15 minutes for the first hour, then every hour as ordered. (It is important to follow agency-specific postprocedure policies.)
  - Maintaining pressure on arterial puncture site for 15 to 20 minutes after removal to avoid bleeding or hematoma formation at the site. Closure devices are now available that eliminate the need for manual pressure to be applied; however, they may not be appropriate for every patient.
  - Ensuring that the patient keeps the leg straight and maintains bedrest for 3 to 12 hours as ordered postprocedure and after catheter removal to avoid bleeding or hematoma formation at the catheter

insertion site. Bedrest time will be dependent on the ability to utilize a closure device versus manual pressure. (It is important to follow agency-specific postprocedure policies.)

- Maintaining IV fluid hydration postprocedure to help clear contrast dye from the circulation
- Monitoring for bleeding, hematoma formation, or infection at catheter-insertion site
- Monitoring renal function (BUN and creatinine levels) postprocedure

Computed Tomography Angiography

Computed tomography angiography is a diagnostic test that combines the technology of a CT scan (cross-sectional images of the brain) and traditional cerebral angiography (enhanced visualization of cerebral vasculature through the IV injection of contrast dye). It is a tool to evaluate cerebral vasculature. Computed tomography angiography is considered less invasive because the contrast is injected into a vein rather than an artery. It is sometimes used if an MRA is contraindicated. The patient preparation and nursing implications are the same as for a CT scan.

Connection Check 35.4

A patient is scheduled for an emergency CT scan because of clinical manifestations of a CVA/stroke. The nurse recognizes which statement as true about the findings of the CT scan?

A. Thrombolytics are contraindicated if the scan identifies a bleed.

B. Thrombolytics are indicated if the scan is positive for a bleed.

C. Thrombolytics are contraindicated if the scan identifies an occlusion.

D. Thrombolytics are indicated if the scan identifies an occlusion.

Electroencephalography

Electroencephalography is an inexpensive, noninvasive procedure that uses 8 to 24 scalp electrodes to trace the spontaneous electrical activity of the brain. It is a diagnostic test for seizure activity and other abnormalities in electrical activity. It can also be used as a part of sleep studies, to evaluate the unconscious patient, or to determine brain death.

Nursing implications include:

- Providing preprocedure education, including:
  - No caffeine consumption for 8 to 12 hours prior to the test; caffeine may alter the results.
  - Wash hair the night before and morning of the test, and avoid the use of hair products prior to the test, to aid in scalp electrode attachment.
- Providing patient support as necessary during the test

Evoked Potentials

An evoked potential is a painless, noninvasive test that measures the speed and size of nerve conduction generated by the nervous system in response to stimuli. Electrodes are attached to the scalp and to different areas of the body depending on the type of test being conducted. The stimulus also varies depending on the test. Visual evoked potentials use visual test patterns as stimuli and are indicated for optic neuritis, masses, or tumors. Auditory brainstem evoked responses are stimulated by sounds and are used to test for CN VIII (acoustic nerve) damage. A somatosensory evoked potential focuses on nerve conduction in the arms and legs and is done with mild electrical stimulation. Somatosensory evoked potential electrodes are typically placed on the wrist (medial nerve) or knee (perineal nerve) and are used for disorders such as multiple sclerosis. Sedation is often required for somatosensory evoked potentials because the electrical stimulus may be painful and to ensure a reliable result.

Nursing implications include:

- Providing preprocedure patient education, including:
  - Wash hair the night before and the morning of the test, and avoid hair products prior to the test, to aid in scalp electrode attachment.
- Offering patient support as necessary during the test

Lumbar Puncture

A lumbar puncture is the most common procedure done to obtain a sample of cerebrospinal fluid (CSF) for analysis and to measure intracranial pressure. Increased pressure may indicate CSF obstruction or overproduction. The presence of abnormalities in glucose or protein as well as a cloudy color may represent infection. The presence of breakdown products of red blood cells, termed xanthochromia, or frank blood may indicate subarachnoid hemorrhage or a traumatic tap, respectively. A lumbar puncture can also be used for the administration of spinal anesthesia and intrathecal medications or to remove CSF to reduce pressure. An invasive procedure, a lumbar puncture requires the insertion of a spinal needle into the L3 to L4 space of the spinal column below the level of the spinal cord. The patient is typically positioned laterally (on the side) in bed, drawing the knees up toward the chest (Fig. 35.22A). This procedure can also be done with the patient leaning across a bedside table with the back arched (Fig. 35.22B).

Nursing implications include:

- Providing preprocedure education explaining the lumbar puncture
- Providing preprocedure care, including:
  - Ensuring that antiplatelet or anticoagulation medications are held prior to the test to reduce the risk of bleeding
  - Checking coagulation studies prior to the test
  - Ensuring that informed consent is obtained
- Providing supportive care as necessary during the test

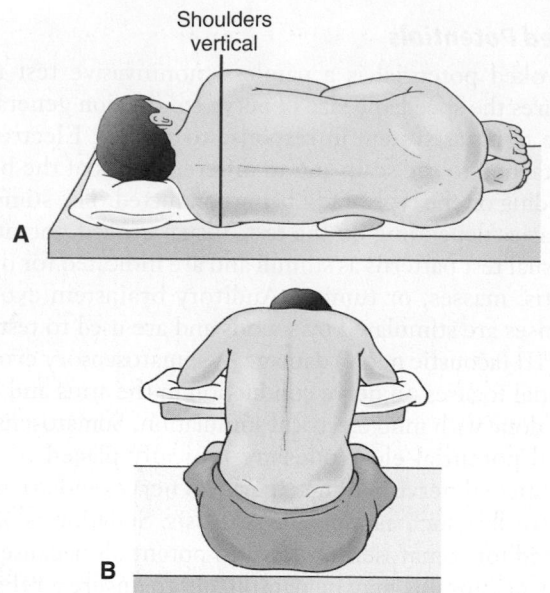

FIGURE 35.22 Positioning for lumbar puncture. A, Patient positioned on side. B, Patient leaning across bedside table.

- Providing postprocedure care, including:
  - Ensuring flat bedrest for 4 to 6 hours after the test to help prevent CSF leakage, which can cause severe headache (see Safety Alert)
  - Encouraging fluids postprocedure to decrease headache intensity if present

> ⓘ **Safety Alert** To avoid post–lumbar puncture headaches, the patient is instructed to lie flat for 4 to 6 hours and stay hydrated. If a headache is severe and prolonged, a "blood patch" can be performed to help seal a CSF leak if present. In this procedure, a small amount of the patient's blood is injected into the site of the puncture, and the resultant clot seals the leak.

Myelography

Myelography/myelogram is an invasive radiographic procedure that involves a lumbar puncture and injection of contrast medium into the subarachnoid space around the spinal cord. X-rays are taken that enable visualization of the entire spinal column to evaluate for lesions, cysts, injury, herniated discs, and masses/tumors. This test is not as commonly performed with the advent of MRI because the MRI can provide similar data.

Nursing implications are similar to those for the lumbar puncture, with the addition of:

- Checking for allergies to contrast dyes, iodine, or seafood because of the administration of contrast during the test
- Ensuring that informed consent has been obtained

- Educating the patient to take nothing by mouth for 4 hours prior to the test
- Ensuring hydration after the test to promote the excretion of contrast dye

Biopsy

Brain biopsies are invasive procedures done to obtain tissue samples for examination and are indicated to rule out or identify infections or abscesses or to identify tumor tissue. Types of biopsies include needle, stereotactic, and open. A needle biopsy involves drilling a small hole into the skull, inserting a needle, and withdrawing a tissue sample. A stereotactic procedure involves the use of specialized computer imaging that utilizes a three-dimensional coordinate system to pinpoint the area to be biopsied. The needle is inserted at the precise location identified through the imaging, and tissue is withdrawn. An open biopsy involves removing bone from the skull in an operative procedure, exposing the tumor or tissue to be biopsied. These procedures are performed in the operating room under sedation or anesthesia. Nursing implications for operating room procedures are discussed in detail in Chapters 15, 16, and 17.

Connection Check 35.5

Which question by the patient having cerebral angiography indicates that teaching has been effective?

A. "This is a fairly simple x-ray test, right?"

B. "Is it unusual if I get hot and flushed when you inject the dye?"

C. "My kidneys have to be in good shape to get this dye, right?"

D. "Is this test to see if an infection is causing my problem?"

PSYCHOSOCIAL CONSIDERATIONS

Neurological events can happen to patients suddenly and without warning, and these occurrences can be devastating to both patients and families. Disease, metabolic disorders, injury/trauma, tumor, hemorrhage, infection, and congenital disorders are all examples of potentially life-altering conditions that affect the neurological system. Deficits can be related to motor, sensation, cognition, and/or speech. Effects can be permanent or temporary, and deficits can be slight or extreme. Aggressive and prolonged rehabilitation may be necessary, and outcomes cannot always be predicted during the early course. Patients and families at first are stunned and confused, and because outcomes are not always predictable, anxiety may develop that can ultimately lead to depression.

Many factors influence how patients and families respond to an event. Age, general health, social status, history of chronic illness, previous life experience, job, and home responsibilities can all affect how a person responds. The event may interfere with life goals (e.g., college, a planned move), future plans, employment and employment opportunities, finances, and social and sexual interactions. Patients may experience altered social roles and body image issues. The nurse must approach the patients and families with a calm and realistic demeanor and may serve as the advocate for the patient and family as they work through the many challenges of the event.

AGE-RELATED CHANGES

Specific age-related changes in the nervous system include motor and sensory changes and alteration of thermoregulation (see Geriatric/Gerontological Considerations). These changes can be subtle and occur over time. Changes in the CNS occur as the brain weight and mass decline with a loss of neurons.

Geriatric/Gerontological Considerations

Neurological Changes

1. Slowed body movements
2. Decreased reaction time
3. Decreased muscle strength and flexibility
4. Decreased sense of touch, smell, temperature, and pain sensations
5. Possible cognitive impairment, such as confusion and/or memory loss—care must be taken to carefully evaluate for other causes of cognitive issues, such as infection.

With aging, there is a natural decline in the availability of neurotransmitters and postsynaptic receptors, which causes a slowing of signal transmission. Voluntary motor movements have decreased functioning. Vascular changes, such as loss of elasticity and stenosis, alter the delivery of oxygen to the brain. The older patient may have compromised thermoregulation because of changes in the ANS, skin, and vasculature. The body temperature may be lower than normal, and therefore a febrile response to infection may not occur.

These changes impact older adults in many different ways. Body movements are slowed, and there is a decreased reaction time to environmental changes. Balance and coordination are impaired and can lead to an increase in falls. There is a decrease in muscle strength, flexibility, and joint function, which may also increase the risk of falls. Polypharmacy, orthostatic hypotension, osteoporosis, and arthritis further complicate the issue. Older adults may need assistive devices to help with safety, and canes and walkers may be used to help stabilize the gait.

Age-related changes also occur in the sensory system, resulting in a decreased awareness of the sense of touch, smell, temperature, and pain sensations. These changes make the older adult more vulnerable to injury. Hearing and eyesight may be impaired, and the loss of smell can lead to a decreased appetite.

Cognitive impairment can occur as a result of the aging process, disease, medications, poor nutrition, and changes in the nervous system. Clinical manifestations range from confusion to disorientation, impulsive behavior, and poor judgment. Memory can also be affected. Caution should be taken in assuming the changes are a "normal" part of aging because these changes can also occur as a result of disease, such as Alzheimer's, uncontrolled diabetes, or even infection. A urinary tract infection left untreated can cause subtle changes in mental status in older patients. A clear diagnosis needs to be made to ensure the best outcome for the patient. Rapid or sudden changes in mental status or cognition should always be evaluated by a provider.

It is critical for the older adult to maintain a healthy lifestyle. Treatment and control of chronic illness, staying active, and participating in new and challenging activities can help maintain a healthy state during the older years. Smoking cessation, healthy eating habits, and exercise can also help. Prevention is the real key for health in this patient population.

Connection Check 35.6

The nurse correlates which clinical manifestations with age-related changes of the nervous system? *(Select all that apply.)*

A. Decreased visual acuity
B. Increased pain sensation
C. Balance problems
D. Dementia
E. Decreased pain sensation

Making Connections

CASE STUDY: WRAP-UP

Mr. Smith keeps his appointment with his neurologist. Upon his arrival, the first part of the assessment process is to complete a comprehensive history and physical examination. Mr. Smith has no significant health history. He exercises regularly, has a healthy diet, and drinks alcohol in moderation. The neurologist next obtains a thorough history of Mr. Smith's chief complaint of headaches, which have been frequent and severe for several weeks and unrelieved with aspirin or Tylenol. There does not seem to be a precipitating event such as diet or exercise, but after close questioning, it seems eating certain foods may be connected. The neurologist continues with the neurological assessment.

Case Study Questions

1. The nurse recognizes which parameter as an important component of the neurological examination for Mr. Smith?

   A. Cranial nerve assessment

   B. Glasgow Coma Scale assessment

   C. Assessing the Babinski sign

   D. Assessing cerebral perfusion pressure

2. The nurse anticipates which as the next step in the assessment process after the neurological examination?

   A. MRI

   B. Evoked potentials

   C. Lumbar puncture

   D. CT scan

3. What information from Mr. Smith's history may make him ineligible for magnetic resonance imaging (MRI)?

   A. History of cerebrovascular accident with residual hemiplegia

   B. History of cardiac dysrhythmias requiring pacemaker

   C. History of seizure disorders controlled by antiepileptic medications

   D. History of deep vein thrombosis requiring anticoagulant therapy

4. Due to Mr. Smith's complaints of persistent headaches, the nurse assesses for other signs of increased intracranial pressure. Which finding may also be associated with increased intracranial pressure?

   A. Change in level of consciousness

   B. Tachycardia

   C. Diaphoresis

   D. Hypotension

5. The nurse's role in the overall patient assessment process includes which of the following actions? (Select all that apply.)

   A. Patient education about the process

   B. Assessing for allergies to seafood

   C. Explaining CT scan test results

   D. Providing reassurance that all will be okay

   E. Checking renal function laboratory values

CHAPTER SUMMARY

The nervous system consists of specialized cells for communication, neurons, and specialized cells for support, neuroglial cells. Transmission of information takes place at the synapse through the action of neurotransmitters. The central nervous system consists of the brain and spinal cord. The brain is divided into three parts: the cerebrum, the cerebellum, and the brainstem. The cerebrum is divided into four major lobes: frontal, parietal, temporal, and occipital, each having a separate and unique function. The cerebellum coordinates muscle activities, controls fine motor movement, and is responsible for balance and equilibrium. The brainstem consists of three areas, medulla oblongata, pons, and midbrain, which are responsible for basic functions such as heart rate and respiration. The spinal cord begins at the brainstem and extends to the level of L1 to L2 in adults. Information is transmitted through ascending and descending tracts to and from the brain to target organs or cells.

The peripheral nervous system (PNS) includes cranial nerves originating in the brain and spinal nerves originating in the spinal cord. The PNS includes the autonomic nervous system that is divided into the sympathetic and parasympathetic systems. The sympathetic nervous system prepares the body for physical activity and is known as eliciting the "fight-or-flight" response. The parasympathetic nervous system prepares the body for rest.

Evaluation of neurological function starts with a complete history and physical examination that is followed by a full neurological head-to-toe assessment, including level of consciousness, mental status, cranial nerves, motor and sensory function, coordination, and reflex activity. Diagnostic studies include computed tomography (CT), CT angiography, positron emission tomography, magnetic resonance imaging, magnetic resonance angiography, cerebral angiography, electroencephalography, evoked potentials, myelography/myelogram, lumbar puncture, and biopsies as indicated.

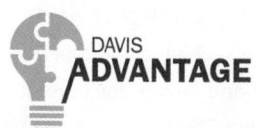

DAVIS **ADVANTAGE** | To explore learning resources for this chapter, go to **Davis Advantage** and find:
– Answers to in-text questions
– Chapter Resources and Activities
– NCLEX®-Style Chapter Review Questions
– Bibliography

Chapter 36

Coordinating Care for Patients With Brain Disorders

Elizabeth Zink

Finding Connections

CASE STUDY: EPISODE 1

Follow this patient throughout the chapter.

James Johnson is a 52-year-old male with a history of hypertension (HTN), type 2 diabetes mellitus (DM), and obesity who has a smoking history of one pack per day for 25 years. Mr. Johnson comes to his provider with a complaint of intermittent headaches that occur in general first thing in the morning. Mr. Johnson tells the provider that his job is very stressful. He says that he generally takes his medication for DM, including metformin (Glucophage) 750 mg, every day regularly but only takes his amlodipine (Norvasc), 10 mg every day, when he can afford the medication. He does not take his furosemide (Lasix), 20 mg every day, because it makes him use the bathroom too often.

Mr. Johnson's blood pressure is 188/92 mm Hg with a heart rate of 95 bpm. He is counseled on the need to take his BP medication, given guidelines for diet and exercise, and prescribed medication to assist with smoking cessation. Mr. Johnson is also given a return appointment in 1 month...

INTRODUCTION

Disorders of the brain impact patients in a variety of ways, and a diagnosis is often frightening depending on how the disorder affects cognition, personality, mobility, and activities of daily living. Many of these disorders are chronic in nature, including primary headaches, seizure disorders, Parkinson's disease, and Alzheimer's disease, requiring lifelong management and coping with exacerbations. Others are more emergent, including primary or metastatic brain tumors, meningitis, and encephalitis, and may be life-threatening emergencies. These patients may present in the emergency department with new onset of complaints or in general medical-surgical settings, outpatient settings, or neuroscience units. This chapter addresses the management of these disorders, with a focus on correlating the pathophysiology of the disorders to the clinical presentations, as well as the rationales for medical and nursing management.

HEADACHE

Headache, also referred to as **cephalalgia**, is the most common manifestation of pain, accounting for more missed days of work and school, and more visits to healthcare providers. Headache also has vast implications in the performance of activities of daily living (ADLs). Headache is classified into two categories: primary and secondary. Primary headaches are not associated with other underlying causes, and the major types of primary headache are tension type, migraine, and cluster headaches. Secondary headaches are caused by an underlying pathology such as infection, neoplasms (tumors), vascular (blood vessel) abnormalities, medication-induced disorders, or idiopathic causes, and typically present with a sudden onset of severe pain.

Epidemiology

Studies indicate that at least 4% of the general population experience chronic daily headaches. One-year prevalence data suggest that 46% to 64% of the population report some type of headache during a lifetime. In the United States, 20% to 40% of the population, 5% to 9% of males, and 12% to 25% of females experience migraine headaches. Ranking of disabilities by the World Health Organization (WHO) places headaches in the top ten ranking for disabling conditions, ranking headaches in the top five for women. The prevalence of tension headaches is in excess of 42%, whereas migraine headaches have been reported in 11% of the population. Cluster headaches, found predominantly in males, with an onset of 30 to 50 years, show an overall prevalence of 0.4% of the population. Of all cluster headaches, 80% are reported as episodic, whereas 20% are classified as chronic.

Pathophysiology

Headaches are the result of the reaction of **nociceptors** (pain-sensitive nerve endings) to triggers, sending messages to the thalamus via the trigeminal nerve (CN V). Headaches (Fig. 36.1) are classified into one of two categories. Primary headaches are those not associated with other underlying disease or organic causes, and secondary headaches are caused by an underlying structural problem such as stroke, tumor, meningitis, or encephalitis (Table 36.1). The **trigeminocervical** complex is a network of neurons relaying pain signals (messages) from the cervical spinal and from the meninges through the trigeminal nerve. This complex has been identified as a potential target for pain-modifying therapies, particularly for migraine headaches.

Clinical Manifestations

Tension headaches may be episodic or chronic in nature. Episodic tension headaches typically occur 10 to 15 days per month, lasting 30 minutes to several days. Chronic tension headaches occur more than 15 days per month during a 3-month period and are generally more severe than episodic headaches. Clinical manifestations include mild to moderate pain that is typically bilateral in the occipital area. Patients often describe the pain as constant pressure to the face, head, and neck, often with sensitivity to light.

Cluster headaches are considered neurovascular headaches. The clinical presentation typically includes severe, unrelenting, unilateral pain in and around the eye. Peak pain is usually within 5 to 10 minutes after onset, continuing in intensity for 1 to 3 hours. They generally occur around the same time for several weeks, more often at night, and reoccur

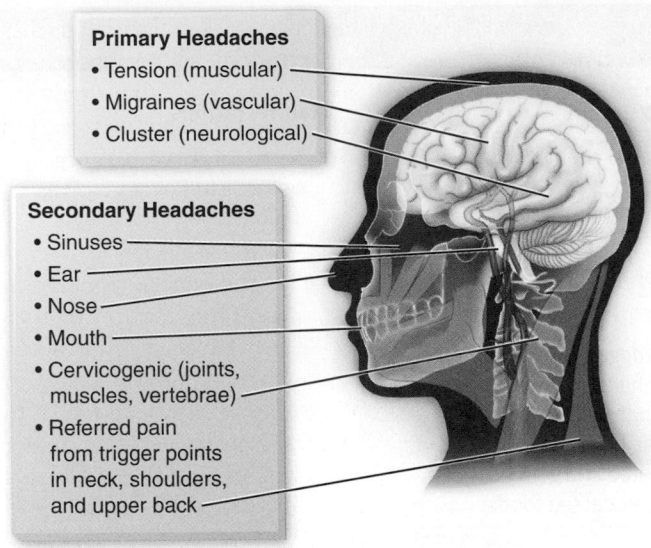

Primary Headaches
- Tension (muscular)
- Migraines (vascular)
- Cluster (neurological)

Secondary Headaches
- Sinuses
- Ear
- Nose
- Mouth
- Cervicogenic (joints, muscles, vertebrae)
- Referred pain from trigger points in neck, shoulders, and upper back

FIGURE 36.1 Classifications and causes of headache.

daily to near daily for weeks to months followed by periods of remission.

Migraine headaches are isolated into four phases. The premonitory phase can occur 24 hours before the headache develops. Clinical manifestations include mood changes, fluid retention, increased urine output, excessive and uncontrolled yawning, and food cravings. Just prior to the migraine, many patients perceive particular sensations referred to as **auras**. Symptoms of auras include but are not limited to flashing lights and muscle weakness. Followed by the headache phase, the pain starts gradually, building in intensity. For some, there is a migraine without the headache pain. Following the headache is the postdromal phase, and during this time, many patients experience confusion and exhaustion. This final period can last for as long as 24 hours before patients feel that they are back to their baseline health. Many of the medications used for the treatment of migraines target specific phases of the migraine headache.

Table 36.1 Pathophysiology of Headaches

	Pathophysiology	Etiology	Manifestations
Tension Headaches Episodic: - 10–15 days per month - Last from 30 minutes to several days	Common anatomical and physiological mechanism: Pain messages are transmitted from the meninges of the brain to the cortex through a mechanism called the trigeminocervical complex	- Jaw clenching - TMJ (temporomandibular joint dysfunction) - Degenerative arthritis of the neck - Forceful/intense	- Most common location is frontal and temporal (sides of head) - Generally bilateral - Occipital (posterior base of head), either one or both sides
Chronic: - Occurring more than 15 days per month over a 3-month period - Generally more severe than episodic headaches	Contractions of the muscles in the neck, face, scalp, and jaw are manifestations of this headache type	- Work or exercise - Poor posture - Lack of sleep - Sleep apnea - Missed meals - Depression - Anxiety	- Pain is mild to moderate - Generally described as a constant pressure to face, head, and/or neck - Often with sensitivity to light - Scalp soreness - Morning headaches when lack of sleep and/or sleep apnea involved - Forceful/intense
Migraine Headaches - Occur most frequently in the morning (especially upon awakening) - Predictable times (menstruation)	The precise pathophysiology is unknown; however, there is an integrated theory involving the hyperexcitation of neurons (cortical spreading depression),	Many triggers: - Changes in weather - Changes in environment - Strong odors, fumes - Tobacco - Motion sickness	- Described as pulsating/throbbing - May be associated with neurological signs such as motor weakness, language disturbances, and pupillary changes

Continued

Table 36.1 Pathophysiology of Headaches—cont'd

	Pathophysiology	Etiology	Manifestations
	the vasodilation of blood vessels leading to the activation of pain receptors, and activation of inflammation in the brain	• Hormonal changes • Hypoglycemia • Flashing lights • Lack of sleep • Stress • Food triggers: aspartame, wine, aged cheeses, monosodium glutamate (MSG), caffeine, caffeine withdrawal, fruits, nuts, fermented and pickled foods, yeast, processed foods	• Some patients experience visual disturbances, such as double vision (diplopia) or seeing spots (floaters)
Cluster Headaches • Most severe form of primary headache • Generally occur around the same time for several (4–8) weeks, more often at night • Occur daily to near daily for weeks to months with long periods of remission • Generally peak 5–10 minutes after onset, continuing in intensity for 1–3 hours • More common in smokers	Trigeminal autonomic (involuntary) cephalalgia	• Cause is unclear • Although also called *histamine headaches*, use of antihistamines to terminate the headaches is unsuccessful • Vascular dilation, extracranial blood flow involving hyperthermia, and increased temporal artery blood flow as proposed mechanisms • Circadian rhythms involving the hypothalamus also speculated as a possible mechanism	• Sudden, extreme pain • One side of the head, behind or around one eye • Agitation and restlessness • Sensitivity to light and sound • Alterations in heart rate and blood pressure • Lacrimation • Stuffy, reddened nose • Ptosis

Connection Check 36.1

The nurse correlates which clinical manifestation to a secondary headache?

A. Sudden severe onset
B. Tense neck muscles
C. Nausea
D. Tingling scalp sensation

Management

Medical Management

Diagnosis

Diagnosis of the specific type or etiology underlying a headache complaint consists of excluding potential causes and depends on the time course of headache occurrence. For example, patients presenting with sudden onset of headache are evaluated for clinical manifestations of meningitis, cerebrospinal fluid (CSF) leak (particularly in patients with a recent history of lumbar puncture or epidural

catheter removal), cerebral aneurysm, cerebral aneurysm rupture, or brain tumor, among other causes. When the time course of headache occurrence is prolonged, the following causes may be considered: sinusitis, opiate dependence and withdrawal, caffeine withdrawal, or over-the-counter medication overuse. One method of tracking and characterizing headache symptoms over a period of time is the use of a headache diary. Patients are instructed to record the time and date of headache occurrence as well as activities, foods, and medications taken in close proximity to the headache, to determine possible triggers and to examine patterns. An example of a diary for headaches is presented in Fig. 36.2.

Review of the headache diary is part of the detailed medical history obtained from the patient, followed by a complete neurological assessment (see Chapter 35 for a description of neurological assessment). In situations in which headaches are atypical, sudden and severe at the onset, or accompanied by neurological deficits, unusual precipitating factors, pain in the neck or jaw upon examination, and in patients older than 50 years of age on presentation, other diagnostic testing is often pursued to assess for a secondary etiology for the headache. Diagnostic tests such as blood

Content/Data:	Examples:
The time the headache started:	
The time the headache ended:	
Were there any auras prior to the start of the headache?	Spots in front of the eyes, odors, ringing in the ears
The location of the headache:	Behind the eyes, back of the neck, temporal
Description of the pain:	• Throbbing • Pressure • Piercing • Stabbing
Intensity of the pain:	Score of 1–10:
Other symptoms:	
Medication taken:	
Other interventions:	• Ice pack • Bedrest • Dark room • Relaxation techniques
Effects of treatment:	
Hours of sleep the previous night:	
Foods eaten before the headache started:	• Caffeine • Diet soda • Artificial sweeteners • Alcohol • Aged cheese • Foods with preservatives: • Sweeteners – Bacon, hot dogs • Chocolate – Chinese food (MSG), cured meats • Ice cream – Processed foods • Salty foods – Citrus fruits • Nuts
Skipped meals:	
Activities before the headache began:	• Exercise • Strenuous activities • Naps
Stressful events:	
Weather changes:	
Menstruation/birth control pills:	

FIGURE 36.2 Headache diary.

tests to assess for infection (e.g., complete blood cell count, blood cultures) and inflammation (C-reactive protein, erythrocyte sedimentation rate), CSF testing, and imaging studies (e.g., computed tomography [CT], magnetic resonance imaging [MRI]) assist in ruling out potential causes of headaches. Cerebrospinal fluid may be obtained via a lumbar puncture to measure pressure (high or low CSF pressures can cause headaches), signs of infection, and inflammation. A CT and/or MRI detects masses, cysts, and irregularities in the vessels or bones of the head. An electroencephalogram

(EEG) measures the electrical activity of the brain and can also assist in the diagnosis of seizures, tumors, inflammation, and brain injury, all of which can lead to headaches. Sleep studies might also be performed to diagnose sleep apnea if a history of obesity, snoring, or fatigue is present.

Treatment

Treatment of tension headaches involves treating any underlying disorders or diseases. Depression and anxiety can cause tension headaches. Counseling and antianxiety and antidepressant medications can aid in the relief of tension headaches. Causes of headaches related to poor posture can be relieved with physical therapy, those related to arthritis can be aided with the use of anti-inflammatory medications, and corrective devices can help alleviate tension headaches caused by temporomandibular joint dysfunction.

Medications

NSAIDs, analgesics, muscle relaxants, and sedatives as well as antidepressants may also assist in alleviating pain for those who suffer from both tension and migraine headaches. Treatment for migraine headaches includes medications used to relieve the clinical manifestations of the migraine (abortive therapy) and those designed to prevent the migraine headache. The use of anti-inflammatory medications can reduce inflammation and ease the pain of migraines. Combination medications, such as those blending acetaminophen with caffeine, can also assist in alleviating symptoms of migraines.

Serotonin, a neurotransmitter, causes vasoconstriction and lowers the pain threshold. Triptan medications such as sumatriptan (Imitrex) increase the levels of serotonin and appear most beneficial during moderate to severe migraine pain. Ergot alkaloid medications such as dihydroergotamine (Migranal) bind to the serotonin receptors on the nerve endings, decreasing transmission of pain messages along the nerve fibers. These medications appear to be most effective during the early phases of migraine headaches.

Many of the medications used in preventive therapy for migraine headaches were initially used for several other conditions. Anticonvulsant medications used to treat seizure disorders, such as lamotrigine (Lamictal) and gabapentin (Neurontin), increase the levels of many neurotransmitters and diminish pain impulses. Antihypertensive medications such as beta blockers (e.g., propranolol [Inderal]) and calcium channel blockers (e.g., amlodipine [Norvasc]) are used for the prevention of migraines. These medications are thought to prevent vasoconstriction or vasodilation in the cerebral blood vessels. Antidepressants are used to treat migraine headaches by increasing serotonin and other chemicals in the brain, such as dopamine and norepinephrine. These medications include selective serotonin reuptake inhibitors such as citalopram (Celexa), paroxetine (Paxil), escitalopram (Lexapro), and fluoxetine (Prozac), as well as serotonin and norepinephrine reuptake inhibitors such as duloxetine (Cymbalta), venlafaxine (Effexor), and Tramadol (Ultram). Tricyclic antidepressants such as amitriptyline (Elavil) and imipramine (Tofranil) are also used in the treatment of migraine headaches.

Lifestyle Modifications and Complementary and Alternative Medicine Therapies

Lifestyle modifications can reduce or prevent headaches. Identifying food triggers and eliminating them from the diet can reduce and prevent migraine headaches. Ensuring steady, regular meals as well as adequate fluid intake and establishing consistent sleep habits can also assist in the relief and prevention of headaches. Riboflavin (vitamin B_2), magnesium, and coenzyme Q10 are also used in the relief and reduction of headaches.

Alternative therapies for the treatment of headaches include biofeedback, massage and gentle exercise of the neck, cognitive behavioral therapy (stress-reduction techniques), meditation, relaxation training, and yoga. Acupuncture and acupressure have also been used in the treatment and prevention of headaches.

Age-Related Considerations

Headaches in children appear to be of shorter duration and are more commonly bilateral in nature. Gastrointestinal disturbances are more prevalent in children with headaches. Dental care and treatment of dental caries, as well as ill-fitting dentures, can be a source of headache. Patients presenting with headaches after age 50 years should be carefully assessed for a vascular cause of headaches such as cerebral blood vessel abnormality (e.g., aneurysm) and stroke.

Complications

Medication Overuse Headaches

Some patients develop chronic daily headaches as a result of excessive use of over-the-counter medications such as acetaminophen and ibuprofen. Daily or near daily use of over-the-counter medications begins a cycle resulting in frequent headaches that cannot be broken unless these medications are stopped. Treatment paradigms may include a sudden withdrawal of these medications while the provider places the patient on medication to prevent headaches or a more gradual withdrawal of the over-the-counter medication.

Status Migrainosus and Hemicrania Continua

Continuous headache syndromes such as status migrainosus and hemicrania continua are debilitating disorders in which patients are unable to experience headache relief and may need to be treated on an inpatient basis. Treatment for these continuous headaches may include IV hydration and pharmacological treatment with dihydroergotamine and antiemetics.

Nursing Management

Assessment and Analysis

The clinical presentation of headache is largely dependent on the etiology and pattern of the clinical manifestations. Patients presenting frequently complain of acute head pain, **photophobia** (sensitivity to light), nausea, vertigo, and aura. A thorough patient history is essential in determining a patient's headache type, the potential causes, and an appropriate treatment plan.

Nursing Diagnoses

- **Acute pain** related to neurovascular dysfunction (vasodilation of cerebral vessels)
- **Knowledge deficit** related to concealment of triggers initiating migraine headache

- **Self-care deficit** related to inability to manage the headaches

Nursing Interventions

Assessments

- Vital signs
  Pain stimulates the autonomic nervous system, resulting in increases in heart rate, blood pressure, and respiratory rate.
- Pain
  Detailed pain assessment may assist in differentiating the type of headache as well as providing important data related to relief measures and pain medication.
- Triggers
  Identifying and managing triggers to headaches is important in decreasing the frequency and severity of headaches.
- Abortive and preventive measures
  Patient identification and management of symptoms at onset may help alleviate the severity of the headache as well as abort the headache.
- Auras
  In patients who experience an aura in advance of the headache, abortive interventions may be implemented earlier to decrease the severity of the headache.

Actions

- Administer prescribed medications
  NSAIDs are prescribed for their anti-inflammatory properties. Caffeine derivatives may be prescribed for patients because they block adenosine and lead to vasoconstriction of blood vessels. Antiemetics may be indicated when headache is complicated by nausea and vomiting.
- Maintain calm, dark, quiet environment
  Excessive noise and lights may trigger and exacerbate pain symptoms by stimulating the sympathetic nervous system.

Teaching

- Importance of adequate sleep
  Sleep and rest are associated with a decrease in headaches associated with stress.
- Take pain medications as prescribed
  Severity of headaches may be better controlled with a timely and appropriate medication regimen.
- Food triggers
  Identifying food triggers and eliminating them from the diet can reduce and prevent migraine headaches.

Evaluating Care Outcomes

Headaches can become a chronic debilitating disorder, and management of headaches requires proper diagnosis and management. Once the patient is familiar with the personal headache history, headache triggers, and best approaches to pain control, episodes of headache are better managed. Lifestyle changes may be required for the best control of headaches in some patients.

Connection Check 36.2

When educating a patient with migraine headaches, the nurse includes which interventions? *(Select all that apply.)*

A. Practice a healthy lifestyle (cease smoking, alcohol in moderation, exercise)
B. Avoid triggers
C. Use techniques such as relaxation and stress reduction
D. Stop taking medications if symptoms subside to decrease tolerance
E. Eliminate all salt and caffeine from the diet

BRAIN TUMORS

Primary Brain Tumors

Primary brain tumors are tumors that originate in the brain and range from slow-growing, benign tumors to highly malignant, aggressive tumors. Primary brain tumors originate from brain cells, brain **meninges** (membranes covering the brain), nerves, and glands (Fig. 36.3). Because of the diversity of these tumors, classification is difficult and is generally based on the type of brain cells involved and the location where the cancer evolves. Tumors are also classified on the basis of the WHO Classification System. They are classified from least aggressive (grade I) to most aggressive (grade IV) depending on the rate of growth and behavior of the cells.

Epidemiology

According to the American Brain Tumor Association, in 2017 approximately 80,000 men, women, and children were diagnosed with a primary brain tumor. This number includes both benign and malignant brain tumors. The American Cancer Society predicted that about 23,880 people (13,270 males and 10,160 females) were diagnosed with a malignant brain or spinal cord tumor in 2018, and approximately 70% of those with a malignant tumor will not survive as a result of their diagnosis. The risk of developing a brain tumor is very low, with the lifetime risk of 1% or less.

Males have a higher incidence, with poorer responses to therapy in comparison with women. The median age at diagnosis for brain tumors is 60 years.

Pathophysiology

Gliomas generally originate in the cerebrum. Glial cells provide the physical structure of the brain and supports the endothelial cells of the blood–brain barrier. Glial cells also provide nutrients and ionic balance and are involved in the repair and scarring processes. Gliomas are inclined to develop along the curved areas of the brain, making the frontal lobes more susceptible. Most commonly found in patients between the ages of 20 and 50 years, gliomas are grade I and II and are slow-growing tumors. Anaplastic gliomas (grade III) are tumor cells out of control, lacking differentiation and/or orientation to one another and to

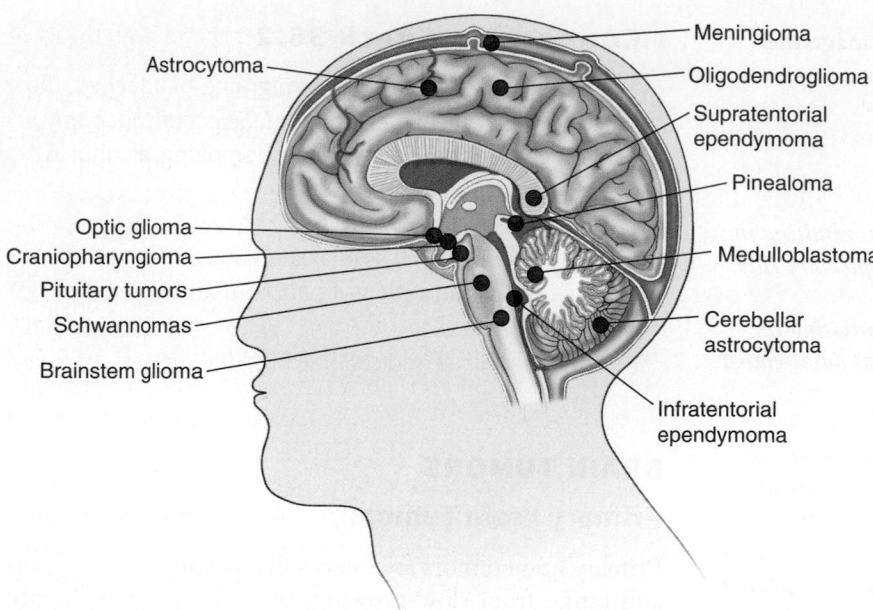

FIGURE 36.3 Location of brain tumors.

surrounding vessels. Glioblastoma multiforme is a grade IV astrocytoma and is the most aggressive and lethal type of tumor, especially when located in or near the brainstem.

Meningiomas are the most common form of brain cancer arising in patients between the ages of 40 and 70 years, affecting females in larger numbers than males. Meningiomas arise from the meninges (layers of the brain). Although 90% of meningiomas are benign, they can still cause devastating damage because they are space-occupying lesions that can increase intracranial pressure (ICP). Additionally, damage may occur based on tumor size or location.

Oligodendrogliomas arise from oligodendrocytes, or oligodendroglia, and their main functions are to provide support and insulation to axons in the central nervous system (CNS), equivalent to the function performed by Schwann cells in the peripheral nervous system. These are slow-growing tumors that generally do not spread to surrounding tissue. Arising from the fatty covering that protects nerves, they generally occur in the cerebrum. Oligodendrogliomas are generally found in middle-aged patients.

Acoustic neuromas (CN VIII) are slow-growing benign tumors that generally do not invade other tissue; however, compression on other cranial verves, (CN V, CN VII, CN IX, and CN X) and tissue (cerebellum and brainstem) can manifest in severe complications. Acoustic neuromas, also known as schwannomas, originate from the protective covering around nerve fibers (CN VIII) at the anatomical location of the cerebellopontine angle. Acoustic neuromas are generally found in adults age 40 to 60 years.

Pituitary tumors are generally found in the anterior lobe of the pituitary, the most common of which is the adenoma, typically a benign tumor. Clinical manifestations of pituitary adenomas are related to hypersecretion of hormones by the pituitary gland, including acromegaly from hypersecretion of growth hormone, amenorrhea-galactorrhea from prolactin

hypersecretion, changes in urine output secondary to changes in antidiuretic hormone secretion, and disorders of the adrenal cortex from hypersecretion of adrenocorticotropic hormone. Pituitary tumors can be found within all age groups. (Management of pituitary tumors is presented in more detail in Chapter 41.)

Metastatic Central Nervous System Disease

Epidemiology

Metastatic tumors are the most common type of brain tumor and metastatic disease in the central nervous system (CNS) occurs in approximately 30% of patients with primary cancers outside of the brain. Primary cancers can spread to the CNS in three common locations, the brain tissue (parenchyma), the spinal cord and the cerebral spinal fluid (leptomeninges) and is then called a metastasis. Metastatic disease in the CNS is most commonly caused by the following primary cancer types: lung, melanoma, renal, breast and colorectal cancer, although other types of cancer may also produce metastases to the CNS.

Pathophysiology

The precise mechanism for cancer cells of a different primary cancer to invade the CNS is not known. Some patients present with metastases to the CNS at the same time that a primary cancer is diagnosed, while other patients present with CNS metastases later in the course of their disease. Primary cancers such as lung cancer are typically a rapidly progressive type of cancer, and therefore it is common to diagnose metastases during the initial presentation.

Clinical Manifestations

Clinical manifestations of brain tumors are dependent on their location in the brain. For example, a meningioma may be attached to the inside of the dura layer of the meninges and may protrude several millimeters into the brain tissue in the frontal lobe, producing no clinical manifestations. A larger meningioma in the same area can cause changes in level of consciousness and cognition secondary to pressure on the frontal lobe. The same type of tumor can also be located in the posterior region of the brain between the cerebellum and pons placing pressure on CN VIII, causing decreased hearing on one side. Brain tumors are often referred to as space-occupying lesions that may cause increased ICP depending on the rate of tumor growth and location (Table 36.2). Malignant brain tumors in particular are associated with swelling as the rapid growth damages brain tissue. Clinical manifestations of increased ICP include **papilledema** (swelling of the optic disk), headache, nausea, and vomiting, decreased alertness, cognitive impairment, personality changes, ataxia, hemiparesis, abnormal reflexes, and cranial nerve palsies. Brain tumors may also be diagnosed during the diagnostic evaluation of patients presenting with new onset of seizure activity.

Management
Medical Management

Chemotherapy and radiation are used in place of or in conjunction with surgery, depending on the type and location of the tumor. The chemotherapeutic agents used to treat brain tumors must have the ability to cross the blood–brain barrier. Some of the chemotherapeutic agents used include carmustine, lomustine, thiotepa, and high doses of methotrexate. Side effects of chemotherapy include fatigue, diarrhea, weight loss, nausea, vomiting (or both), mucositis, hair loss, and sterility. Chemotherapeutic agents also cause neutropenia (decreased white blood cell count), requiring special precautions aimed at increasing vigilance to prevent secondary infections that may be life threatening in the immune-compromised patient. Radiation therapy destroys both tumor and normal cells by damaging cellular DNA. A class of chemotherapeutic agents called *radiosensitizers* are administered to patients in combination with radiotherapy in order to create an environment where cancer cells are more susceptible to radiation. A common medication in this class is temozolomide (Temodar).

Radiation treatment is provided in divided doses, maximizing the recovery of normal cells. Radiation is delivered in a focused manner, concentrating on the affected area. Other technologies such as the CyberKnife are used to direct radiation to the tumor, avoiding healthy brain tissue. Side effects of radiation treatment include fatigue, reddening of the skin (sunburn appearance), headache, swelling, visual changes, neurological disturbances, hearing loss, and facial numbness (Table 36.3). See Chapter 13 for more detailed coverage about the management of patients with cancer. Treatment of brain tumors depends on the cell type of tumor as well as specific genetic characteristics. The

Table 36.2 Presenting Clinical Manifestations of a Brain Mass

Presenting Symptomology	Location of Tumor
Motor weakness	Frontal motor cortex
Sensory loss	Parietal sensory cortex
Speech	Left inferior frontal lobe (Broca's area)
	Left temporal lobe (Wernicke's area)
Loss of vision in one eye	Optic nerve
Bitemporal field cuts	Optic chiasm
Loss of visual field on the same side in both eyes	Optic tract
	Occipital lobe
Loss of upward gaze	Pineal gland
Loss of light reflex	Pineal gland
Bitemporal field cuts with abnormal endocrine function	Suprasellar
Loss of cranial nerves on one side with loss of motor or sensory on contralateral side	Brainstem

Table 36.3 Nursing Interventions for Complications of Radiation Therapy

Intervention	Rationale
Fatigue nutritional supplements (i.e., Boost, Ensure)	Fatigue following radiation therapy is common. Those patients experiencing weight loss are more susceptible; therefore, maintaining weight is important.
Skin utilization of sunscreens, sun-protective covering, skin emollients	Reddened, dry areas of the skin and hair loss are sometimes complications of radiation therapy. Ensuring proper sun protection and relief from dry, itching skin is essential.
Headache/Nausea and vomiting dexamethasone (Decadron), ondansetron (Zofran), dronabinol (Marinol)	Radiation therapy of the brain can cause swelling around the area of the tumor, thereby increasing intracranial pressure, causing headache, nausea, and vomiting. Medications such as dexamethasone (Decadron) are used to reduce swelling. Medications to reduce effects such as nausea and vomiting are important because they can cause dehydration and weight loss and negatively impact quality of life.

World Health Organization (WHO) changed the brain tumor classification system to include both cell type and genetic features.

Surgical Management

Patients undergo biopsies of brain masses to sample the tissue within the mass so that the cells can be examined and a specific diagnosis can be made. Biopsies of brain tissue are performed using advanced radiological techniques that allow the neurosurgeon to map the location of the mass in multiple dimensions. Radiographic images are obtained using CT and MRI scans and are transferred to a computer system that integrates each image into a precise, well-defined coordinate of the area to be biopsied to define an exact location and path for retrieval of brain tissue. This procedure allows for the retrieval of specimens for identification and assists in the determination of an appropriate treatment regimen while minimizing the risk of injury to blood vessels and surrounding healthy brain tissue. The sample of tissue is then examined by a pathologist and a pathological or histological (cellular) diagnosis is made that guides further therapy and treatment planning.

The most common surgical procedure for all types of brain tumors is the craniotomy. During this procedure, a section of the skull is removed (known as a bone flap) to provide access to the brain. In some instances, this can be done to biopsy brain tissue or to excise (remove) a tumor. If the entire tumor cannot be removed, the tumor is debulked, removing as much of the tumor as possible. Following the procedure, the bone flap is then replaced with the use of small plates and screws. Should the bone flap not be returned, the procedure is called a *craniectomy*. When changes in neurological assessment are noted postoperatively and reported to the healthcare provider, they localize the findings to their reference areas in the brain and may order CT imaging to determine whether a structural change has occurred to produce the new findings. A patient's neurological assessment is performed in a serial manner so that the nurse is continually comparing the current assessment with the last one and with the most current baseline.

Complications

Increased Intracranial Pressure

Increased ICP can severely hamper cerebral blood flow, causing decreases in cerebral perfusion pressure (CPP) and leading to secondary injury of the brain via cytotoxic and anoxic injury and herniation of the brain. See Chapter 39 for full coverage of increased ICP.

Bleeding

The risk of intracranial bleeding postoperatively is highly variable and dependent on features of the tumor, location in the brain, proximity of the tumor to blood vessels, and the surgical approach. Patients are typically cared for in high-acuity areas such as an intensive care unit or postanesthesia care unit to facilitate frequent neurological assessments, which are necessary to detect early signs of bleeding that can cause increased ICP. When changes in the neurological assessment are detected, the healthcare team is alerted for further assessment and often radiographical assessment by CT scan is ordered to determine whether there has been a structural change such as bleeding. Bleeding can occur into the area where the tumor was resected, or it can occur above or below the dural covering while blood vessels are manipulated during the surgical approach, which can become disrupted or injured. If postoperative intracranial bleeding is identified, the surgical team determines whether an additional surgical procedure is required or whether medical management can be pursued. The neurological assessment is used to determine how a patient is responding to increased ICP.

Cerebral Edema

The most common type of cerebral edema occurring with neurosurgical procedures and brain tumors is called **vasogenic edema**, in which the blood–brain barrier becomes increasingly permeable. This type of edema is most common after brain tumor resection and is secondary to changes to the usually tightly controlled blood–brain barrier that becomes inflamed and more permeable in the area of the tumor and surgical resection. The time course for cerebral edema after brain tumor resection is variable and is associated with the type of tumor. Serial neurological assessments are used to monitor a patient's response to the surgical procedure, and deterioration of that assessment can be caused by cerebral edema. The edema can be located in and around the area where the tumor was resected or can be located along the path taken by the surgeons to expose and resect the tumor. Emergent treatment for cerebral edema includes osmotic diuretics, hyperventilation, and head positioning (head of bed elevated greater than 30 degrees) (see Chapter 39 for a description of treatment for increased ICP). Management of cerebral edema regarding brain tumors often includes increasing the dose of glucocorticoids as these medications decrease the inflammatory process associated with damage in and around the tumor.

Seizures

Seizures may occur as a presenting sign of a brain tumor and episodically thereafter, or they may occur postoperatively. Locations closer to the upper regions of the brain (**supratentorial,** or above the tentorium) are at greater risk for seizure activity when an abnormality such as a tumor occurs or when tissues are disrupted during a surgical procedure. Immediate treatment of seizures includes administration of benzodiazepines to stop the seizure and antiepileptic medications to prevent recurrence of the seizure (see the subsequent section on seizures for additional information).

Venous Thromboembolism

The occurrence of a malignancy (some brain tumors are malignant), surgical procedure, and immobility place patients with brain tumors at a higher risk of venous thromboembolism (VTE). The nurse ensures that preventive measures such as mechanical VTE prevention devices (e.g., sequential compression devices) and pharmacological prevention (e.g., heparin administered subcutaneously) are applied and administered as ordered.

Nursing Management

Assessment and Analysis

Many of the clinical manifestations observed in the patient with a brain tumor are directly related to the location of the tumor, pressure on adjacent structures, and increased ICP. The clinical presentation often includes:

- Change in level of consciousness
- Headache
- Pupillary changes secondary to compression of CN III
- Vision changes
- Seizure activity
- Elevated blood pressure with widening pulse pressure
- Decreased heart rate
- Nausea and vomiting
- Numbness and tingling

Nursing Diagnoses

- **Impaired tissue perfusion (cerebral)** associated with decreased cerebral circulation secondary to increased ICP
- **Self-care deficit** associated with decreased level of consciousness and neuromuscular dysfunction
- **Fear** associated with the surgical procedure (craniotomy) to remove the brain tumor
- **Risk for infection** associated with the surgical procedure and immunosuppression secondary to chemotherapeutic agents
- **Altered body image** secondary to potential hair loss secondary to chemotherapy, the surgical procedure, and radiation markings

Nursing Interventions

▪ Assessments

- Neurological assessment including level of consciousness, orientation, motor strength, and sensation. Cranial nerve assessment may also be helpful in monitoring a patient's response to a craniotomy (see Chapter 35 for complete neurological assessment, including cranial nerve assessment).
  Vigilant monitoring of the neurological assessment, observing for changes from the patient's preoperative and postoperative baseline, is essential for early identification of potentially life-threatening neurological deterioration. Changes in level of consciousness are the most sensitive indicator of increased ICP and can signal complications of brain tumor resection and craniotomy, such as intracranial bleeding and cerebral edema (swelling). Subtle changes in motor strength on one side of the body when compared with the other are significant when they occur during the recovery period after a craniotomy. The baseline neurological assessment after a surgical procedure should be determined and

agreed upon by the nurse and providers or nurse practitioners caring for the patient to facilitate future comparisons and interpretation. Pupil reaction to light is part of the assessment and changes in reaction are indicative to damage/compression to CN III (oculomotor nerve).

- Vital signs including temperature, blood pressure, heart rate, respiratory rate, and pulse oximetry
  *Changes in vital sign measurements can signal pain (tachycardia), and **Cushing's triad** (decreased heart rate, increased systolic blood pressure, and irregular respiratory rate) occurs late in increased ICP signaling herniation syndrome, a medical emergency.*
- Estimated blood loss
  Estimated blood loss is typically not large in a craniotomy; however, in particular situations, blood loss can be greater than expected, and this should be taken into account during a handoff from the operating room or recovery room.
- Monitor serum electrolytes, particularly serum sodium and glucose
  Serum sodium should be maintained within normal values, and possibly on the high end of normal to prevent fluid moving into cells or interstitium potentially raising ICP. Glucose needs to be monitored because dexamethasone may lead to elevated serum glucose levels.
- Intake and urinary output
  Strict intake and output measurements are necessary in patients who have undergone a craniotomy in which the pituitary gland has been manipulated. These patients are at risk for diabetes insipidus, in which the nurse observes a large urinary output per hour that can rapidly result in an intravascular volume deficit.
- Urine specific gravity and osmolality; serum sodium and osmolality
  In patients who have undergone pituitary surgery, diabetes insipidus can be diagnosed using a combination of conditions including increased urinary output, decreased urine specific gravity (<1.005), an increased serum sodium concentration (>145 mEq/L), and an increase in serum (>280 mOsm/kg) and urine osmolality (<200 mOsm/kg). Increased urine output may decrease blood pressure further, compromising CPP.
- Pain
  Patients may experience postoperative pain associated with the incision and positioning of the head and neck during surgery. Judicious use of opioid medications may be used to treat postoperative pain, balancing the importance of maintaining an adequate neurological assessment. NSAIDs are not preferred for pain control in the postoperative period because of concern for an increase in bleeding risk.

▪ Actions

- Administer glucocorticoids as ordered, dexamethasone (Decadron)
  Postoperatively, patients are given glucocorticoids such as dexamethasone to treat and prevent further local cerebral edema. Dexamethasone has been shown to stabilize cell membranes to prevent the occurrence of cerebral edema.

- Replace urine loss and electrolytes as ordered
  Dehydration can lead to hemodynamic instability (hypotension, tachycardia, dysrhythmias) and decreased cerebral perfusion.
- Elevate head of bed 30 to 45 degrees and maintain head in good alignment
  Promotes venous outflow of blood from the head through the jugular veins in the event of increased ICP
- Administer stool softeners
  Decrease Valsalva and straining, which can increase ICP.
- Administer antiepileptic medications as ordered
  Patients may be administered antiepileptic medications based on tumor location and a history or risk of seizure activity. Some healthcare providers choose to administer antiepileptic medications for a period of time postoperatively with the goal of preventing seizures, which can occur as a result of tissue disruption during the surgical procedure.
- Apply mechanical devices and administer pharmacological prophylaxis of venous thromboembolism as ordered
  The presence of cancer as well as tissue injury during surgery increase a patient's risk of VTE. Pharmacological prophylaxis may not be administered immediately after surgery because of a concern for bleeding risk; however, medication may be initiated further into the patient's hospital course.

■ Teaching

- Tapering of steroids
  It is important to provide clear direction to the patient and family regarding the tapering of the steroid dose during the prescribed number of days. Rapid withdrawal of glucocorticoids can cause an adrenal crisis.
- Monitoring of glucose
  Some patients become hyperglycemic as a result of steroid administration and require home testing of glucose levels while they are receiving glucocorticoids. Typically, this monitoring is temporary until the medication is tapered off.
- Importance of continuing antiepileptic medications and obtaining prescribed blood levels
  Some antiepileptic medications may require serum medication levels to ensure that they are maintained at therapeutic levels.
- Prevention of falls in the hospital and at home
  Because of previous or new motor weakness or visual deficits, patients may have an increased risk of experiencing a fall either in the hospital or at home. Discussions and planning with the patient regarding potential fall or tripping hazards in the hospital and at home are necessary.
- Wear hat or head covering as needed
  Parts of the head may be shaved for the surgical procedure, and with administration of chemotherapy the patient is also at risk for alopecia. Wearing head coverings can decrease heat loss from the head.
- Mouth care secondary to effects of chemotherapy and/or radiation therapy for brain tumor
  Chemotherapeutic agents affect cells that divide quickly, which makes the patient at risk for sores in the mouth. Using a soft toothbrush and non–alcohol-containing mouthwash decreases mouth discomfort.

Evaluating Care Outcomes

The diagnosis of a brain tumor is very stressful to patients and families. Definitive management of brain tumors is based on the location and type of tumor. Vigilant serial monitoring of the neurological assessment compared with the patient's baseline is essential for these patients. Identifying signs of neurological deterioration early is necessary to prompt medical or surgical intervention and to preserve neurological function. Complications such as VTE, seizures, falls, infection, and aspiration should be considered and incorporated into the patient's plan of care and customized to the patient's particular brain tumor type, location, and functional status.

CASE STUDY: EPISODE 2

Mr. Johnson is transported to the emergency department by ambulance. According to his wife, he had a headache the night before, took two aspirin, and went to bed. He awoke during the night and went to the bathroom. She heard a noise and checked on him and found him on the floor, mumbling incoherently and unable to move his left side.

A head CT is done and a CT of his neck to rule out a traumatic injury because of the fall in his bathroom. A right frontotemporal mass is found. Mr. Johnson is admitted to the neurosurgical care unit. The CT identifies a brain tumor, and he is scheduled for a craniotomy. The mass is removed and sent to pathology for identification. He is extubated without difficulty in the operating room following the procedure and admitted to the neurosurgical intensive care unit. Although his speech is slightly slowed, he is able to move his right upper extremity with +5 strength, and his right lower extremity is +4 strength. He is prescribed dexamethasone (Decadron), 4 mg IV or PO every 6 hours for 48 hours...

Connection Check 36.3

Which assessment data does the nurse recognize as the most sensitive indicator of increased ICP?
A. Pupillary
B. Respiratory
C. Level of consciousness
D. Cranial nerves

SEIZURES

Epidemiology

A seizure is an uncontrolled, sudden, excessive discharge of electrical activity resulting in a range of manifestations from changes in behavior to loss of consciousness. Cryptogenic seizures are those of unknown etiology with no association with previous insults to the CNS that are known to increase the risk of seizure activity. **Epilepsy**, a chronic disorder, is characterized by two seizures unprovoked by any immediately identifiable cause occurring more than 24 hours apart.

The type of seizure is determined by the originating source (whether it is partial/focal to a specific location) or if the seizure is generalized (encompassing both sides of the brain) and by loss of consciousness. The International League Against Epilepsy (ILAE) distinguishes three major categories for seizure type based on the presenting feature of the seizure (Fig. 36.4). This new categorization was published by the ILAE in 2017 and seeks to simplify description and categorization of seizures for clinicians and the lay public. A companion glossary of terms in Table 36.4 provides additional detail and description to explain the new classifications.

Pathophysiology

Although no conclusive pathophysiological explanation of cryptogenic seizures has been identified, there are several hypotheses under investigation. It is speculated that the cause of unprovoked seizures involves the genetic or developmental mutation of synapses and of genes coding for sodium channel proteins, causing sodium channels in the brain to remain partly ajar or improperly closed and thereby increasing neuronal hyperexcitability of glutamate. Another possibility involves mutations causing ineffective activity of gamma-aminobutyric acid (GABA), the most common neurotransmitter.

Nonepileptic seizures (Table 36.5) are those provoked by other disorders and conditions and are sometimes described as secondary seizures. Lesions to the brain caused by trauma, surgery, tumors, and strokes can culminate in a seizure disorder. Metabolic syndromes, as well as manifestations of other disease processes, can also cause seizures. Approximately 20% of patients under investigation for epilepsy are in fact diagnosed with psychogenic nonepileptic seizure disorder. While to all appearances the patient appears to be having an epileptic seizure, there are, in fact, no abnormal electrical discharges. Psychogenic nonepileptic seizure disorder is classified as a conversion disorder by the American Psychiatric Association. Young children and babies may experience one seizure during a febrile illness without identification of cause for the seizure or repeated seizure activity.

Clinical Manifestations

The clinical presentation of seizure activity is related to the classification (see Fig. 36.4) and can range from rhythmic jerking of all extremities and loss of consciousness as observed in generalized tonic-clonic seizures to episodes of apparent daydreaming and no loss of consciousness as observed in absence seizures. Partial seizures are typically more localized and may have a loss of consciousness, but this does not occur in all partial seizures. Other clinical manifestations include unilateral, rhythmic muscle movements, **automatisms** (repetitive unconscious movements such as lip smacking, chewing, or swallowing), sudden loss of motor tone, and incontinence.

Seizures can be preceded by a **preictal phase** (just before the initiation of the seizure). During this phase, approximately

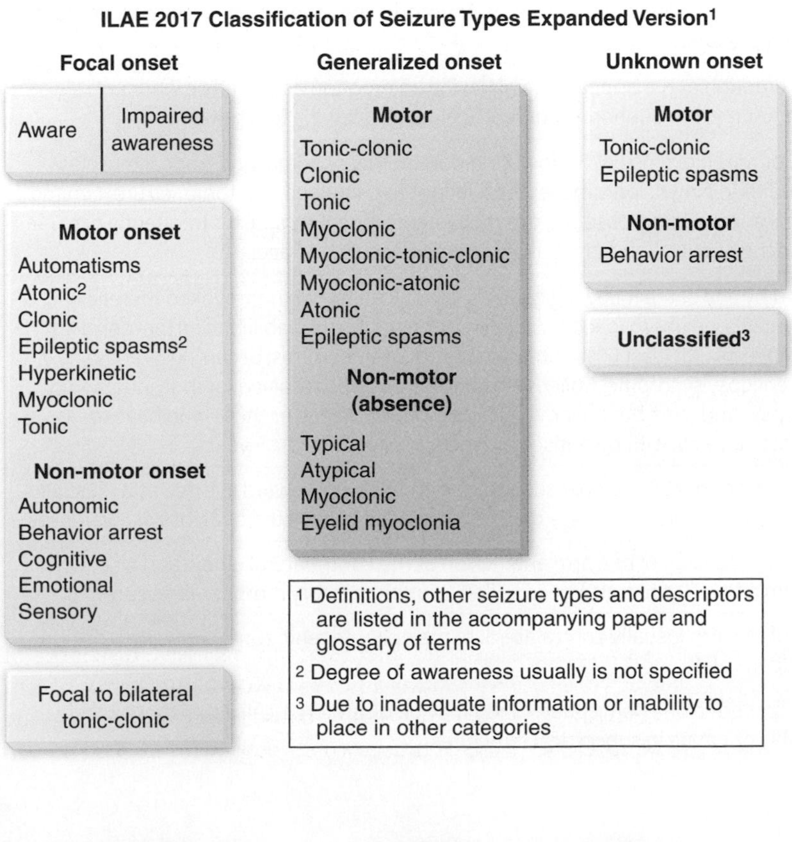

ILAE 2017 Classification of Seizure Types Expanded Version[1]

Focal onset

| Aware | Impaired awareness |

Motor onset
Automatisms
Atonic[2]
Clonic
Epileptic spasms[2]
Hyperkinetic
Myoclonic
Tonic

Non-motor onset
Autonomic
Behavior arrest
Cognitive
Emotional
Sensory

Focal to bilateral tonic-clonic

Generalized onset

Motor
Tonic-clonic
Clonic
Tonic
Myoclonic
Myoclonic-tonic-clonic
Myoclonic-atonic
Atonic
Epileptic spasms

Non-motor (absence)
Typical
Atypical
Myoclonic
Eyelid myoclonia

Unknown onset

Motor
Tonic-clonic
Epileptic spasms

Non-motor
Behavior arrest

Unclassified[3]

[1] Definitions, other seizure types and descriptors are listed in the accompanying paper and glossary of terms
[2] Degree of awareness usually is not specified
[3] Due to inadequate information or inability to place in other categories

FIGURE 36.4 Expanded ILAE 2017 seizure type classification.

Table 36.4 International League Against Epilepsy (ILAE) 2017 Operational Classification of Seizure Types Glossary of Terms

Word	Definition
Absence, typical	A sudden onset, interruption of ongoing activities, a blank stare, possibly a brief upward deviation of the eyes. Usually the patient will be unresponsive when spoken to. Duration is a few seconds to half a minute with very rapid recovery. Although not always available, an EEG would show generalized epileptiform discharges during the event. An absence seizure is by definition a seizure of generalized onset. The word is not synonymous with a blank stare, which also can be encountered with focal onset seizures
Absence, atypical	An absence seizure with changes in tone that are more pronounced than in typical absence or the onset and/or cessation is not abrupt, often associated with slow, irregular, generalized spike-wave activity
Arrest	See behavior arrest
Atonic	Sudden loss or diminution of muscle tone without apparent preceding myoclonic or tonic event lasting ~1–2 s, involving head, trunk, jaw, or limb musculature
Automatism	A more or less coordinated motor activity usually occurring when cognition is impaired and for which the subject is usually (but not always) amnesic afterward. This often resembles a voluntary movement and may consist of an inappropriate continuation of preictal motor activity
Autonomic seizure	A distinct alteration of autonomic nervous system function involving cardiovascular, pupillary, gastrointestinal, sudomotor, vasomotor, and thermoregulatory functions
Aura	A subjective ictal phenomenon that, in a given patient, may precede an observable seizure (popular usage)
Awareness	Knowledge of self or environment
Bilateral	Both left and right sides, although manifestations of bilateral seizures may be symmetric or asymmetric
Clonic	Jerking, either symmetric or asymmetric, that is regularly repetitive and involves the same muscle groups
Cognitive	Pertaining to thinking and higher cortical functions, such as language, spatial perception, memory, and praxis. The previous term for similar usage as a seizure type was psychic
Consciousness	A state of mind with both subjective and objective aspects, comprising a sense of self as a unique entity, awareness, responsiveness, and memory
Dacrystic	Bursts of crying, which may or may not be associated with sadness
Dystonic	Sustained contractions of both agonist and antagonist muscles producing athetoid or twisting movements, which may produce abnormal postures
Emotional seizures	Seizures presenting with an emotion or the appearance of having an emotion as an early prominent feature, such as fear, spontaneous joy or euphoria, laughing (gelastic), or crying (dacrystic)
Epileptic spasms	A sudden flexion, extension, or mixed extension–flexion of predominantly proximal and truncal muscles that is usually more sustained than a myoclonic movement but not as sustained as a tonic seizure. Limited forms may occur: Grimacing, head nodding, or subtle eye movements. Epileptic spasms frequently occur in clusters. Infantile spasms are the best-known form, but spasms can occur at all ages
Epilepsy	A disease of the brain defined by any of the following conditions: (1) At least two unprovoked (or reflex) seizures occurring >24 h apart; (2) one unprovoked (or reflex) seizure and a probability of further seizures similar to the general recurrence risk (at least 60%) after two unprovoked seizures, occurring over the next 10 years; (3) diagnosis of an epilepsy syndrome. Epilepsy is considered to be resolved for individuals who had an age-dependent epilepsy syndrome but are now past the applicable age or those who have remained seizure free for the last 10 years, with no antiseizure medicines for the last 5 years
Eyelid myoclonia	Jerking of the eyelids at frequencies of at least 3 per second, commonly with upward eye deviation, usually lasting <10 s, often precipitated by eye closure. There may or may not be associated brief loss of awareness
Fencer's posture seizure	A focal motor seizure type with extension of one arm and flexion at the contralateral elbow and wrist, giving an imitation of swordplay with a foil. This has also been called a supplementary motor area seizure
Figure-of-4 seizure	Upper limbs with extension of the arm (usually contralateral to the epileptogenic zone) with elbow flexion of the other arm, forming a figure-of-4
Focal	Originating within networks limited to one hemisphere. They may be discretely localized or more widely distributed. Focal seizures may originate in subcortical structures

Table 36.4 International League Against Epilepsy (ILAE) 2017 Operational Classification of Seizure Types Glossary of Terms—cont'd

Word	Definition
Focal onset bilateral tonic–clonic seizure	A seizure type with focal onset, with awareness or impaired awareness, either motor or non-motor, progressing to bilateral tonic–clonic activity. The prior term was seizure with partial onset with secondary generalization
Gelastic	Bursts of laughter or giggling, usually without an appropriate affective tone
Generalized	Originating at some point within, and rapidly engaging, bilaterally distributed networks
Generalized tonic–clonic	Bilateral symmetric or sometimes asymmetric tonic contraction and then bilateral clonic contraction of somatic muscles, usually associated with autonomic phenomena and loss of awareness. These seizures engage networks in both hemispheres at the start of the seizure
Hallucination	A creation of composite perceptions without corresponding external stimuli involving visual, auditory, somatosensory, olfactory, and/or gustatory phenomena. Example: "Hearing" and "seeing" people talking
Behavior arrest	Arrest (pause) of activities, freezing, immobilization, as in behavior arrest seizure
Immobility	See activity arrest
Impaired awareness	See awareness. Impaired or lost awareness is a feature of focal impaired awareness seizures, previously called complex partial seizures
Impairment of consciousness	See impaired awareness
Jacksonian seizure	Traditional term indicating spread of clonic movements through contiguous body parts unilaterally
Motor	Involves musculature in any form. The motor event could consist of an increase (positive) or decrease (negative) in muscle contraction to produce a movement
Myoclonic	Sudden, brief (more than 100 msec) involuntary single or multiple contraction(s) of muscles(s) or muscle groups of variable topography (axial, proximal limb, distal). Myoclonus is less regularly repetitive and less sustained than is clonus
Myoclonic-atonic	A generalized seizure type with a myoclonic jerk leading to an atonic motor component. This type was previously called myoclonic–astatic
Myoclonic-tonic-clonic	One or a few jerks of limbs bilaterally, followed by a tonic–clonic seizure. The initial jerks can be considered to be either a brief period of clonus or myoclonus. Seizures with this characteristic are common in juvenile myoclonic epilepsy
Nonmotor	Focal or generalized seizure types in which motor activity is not prominent
Propagation	Spread of seizure activity from one place in the brain to another, or engaging of additional brain networks
Responsiveness	Ability to appropriately react by movement or speech when presented with a stimulus
Seizure	A transient occurrence of signs and/or symptoms due to abnormal excessive or synchronous neuronal activity in the brain
Sensory seizure	A perceptual experience not caused by appropriate stimuli in the external world
Spasm	See epileptic spasm
Tonic	A sustained increase in muscle contraction lasting a few seconds to minutes
Tonic–clonic	A sequence consisting of a tonic followed by a clonic phase
Unaware	The term unaware can be used as shorthand for impaired awareness
Unclassified	Referring to a seizure type that cannot be described by the ILAE 2017 classification either because of inadequate information or unusual clinical features. If the seizure is unclassified because the type of onset is unknown, a limited classification may still derive from observed features
Unresponsive	Not able to react appropriately by movement or speech when presented with stimulation
Versive	A sustained, forced conjugate ocular, cephalic, and/or truncal rotation or lateral deviation from the midline

From Fisher, R., Cross, J. H., French, J. A., Higurashi, N., Hirsch, E., Jansen, F. E... Lagae, L. (2017). Operational classification of seizure types by the International League Against Epilepsy: Position Paper of the ILAE Commission for Classification and Terminology. *Epilepsia, 58*(4), 522-530.

Table 36.5 Causes of Provoked, Nonepileptic Seizures

Structural (lesions to the brain)	Traumatic injury
	Stroke
	Infarct
Vascular	TIA
Infection	Migraine headache
	Sleep disorders
	Vasculitis
	Hydrocephalus
	Increased intracranial pressure
	HTN encephalopathy
	Eclampsia
	Fever
	Encephalitis/Meningitis
	Renal failure
	Lupus
	Malaria
Inadequate oxygen to the brain (decreased cerebral perfusion, decreased cardiac output)	Arrhythmias
	Carbon monoxide poisoning
	Near drowning
Metabolic	Hypernatremia/Hyponatremia
	Hyperglycemia/Hypoglycemia
	Hypocalcemia
	Hypomagnesemia
	Underactive parathyroid
Substance abuse	ETOH
	ETOH withdrawal
	Cocaine
	Amphetamines
Prescription medications	Antibiotics: ciprofloxacin (Cipro), ceftazidime (Fortaz), cyclosporines (Gengraf)
	Buspirone (Buspar)
	Chlorpromazine (Thorazine)
	Meperidine (Demerol)
	Phenytoin (Dilantin)
	Theophylline (Theo-Dur)
	Overdose of tricyclic antidepressants (amitriptyline)
Toxins	Lead
	Strychnine

ETOH = Ethyl alcohol; *HTN* = hypertension; *TIA* = transient ischemic attack.

20% of those with a seizure disorder may experience what is called an aura. Auras include pleasant or unpleasant odors, visualizations/hallucinations, the sense of "butterflies" in the stomach, a sense of déjà vu, or the intense feeling that a seizure is about to happen.

Following the seizure, there is the **postictal phase**. This is a period after the seizure that lasts 5 to 30 minutes and is an altered state of consciousness. During this phase, the patient can experience drowsiness, confusion, disorientation,

nausea, hypoxia, headache, and migraine. This is the recovery phase of the seizure. Several theories exist to explain this phenomenon including increased ICP secondary to mild **hydrocephalus** (excessive accumulation of CSF in the brain), changes in cerebral blood flow, depletion of neurotransmitters, and alterations in receptor concentrations. Many patients experience exhaustion and depression following the seizure, taking 1 to 2 days for full recovery. During this phase, there may also be diminished short-term memory and poor attention span.

Connection Check 36.4

A patient with a history of seizures experiences lip smacking and daydreams during a seizure with no loss of consciousness. The nurse recognizes these clinical manifestations as associated with which type of seizure?

A. Absence seizure
B. Complex partial seizure
C. Atonic seizure
D. Myoclonic seizure

Management

Medical Management

Diagnosis

Diagnosis of seizures is made via imaging (CT, MRI) and laboratory work-up to rule out causes (lesions, tumors, metabolic and other disorders) and through diagnostics via EEG monitoring for abnormal electrical activity. In some instances, a sleep-deprived EEG may be performed. Stress, such as that found when the individual is deprived of sleep, causes an increase in cortical activity and is a key trigger for seizures. Interviews with the patient also establish any commonalities of the activity (auras, postictal symptoms).

Connection Check 36.5

What is used to diagnose a seizure disorder? (*Select all that apply.*)

A. Electroencephalogram
B. Lumbar puncture
C. Metabolic panel
D. Coagulation studies
E. Electromyogram

Age-Related Considerations

Seizures can be difficult to diagnose in older adults because of their resemblance to other conditions of advanced age such as dementia and Alzheimer's disease. New onset of seizures can generally be attributed to other disorders of cardiovascular and metabolic dysfunction. Because many anticonvulsant medications are cleared by the liver and liver function can decline with age, dosage adjustments must be considered in terms of half-life and toxicity.

Medications

Pharmacological therapy is the major approach to the medical management of seizure disorders (Table 36.6). Antiepileptic drugs (AEDs) or anticonvulsants almost always provide complete control of the seizures. Generally, one medication is prescribed to achieve optimal control. Combinations of medications may be required and are introduced one at a time, with the patient observed for breakthrough seizure activity until the new medication has time to reach therapeutic effectiveness.

In some individuals, maintenance of a state of ketosis can metabolically improve seizure control. The ketogenic diet, high in fat (80%–90%) and low in carbohydrates

and protein, can be calculated with daily monitoring and formulation of meal planning.

Complications

Status Epilepticus

A seizure lasting longer than 5 minutes is a medical emergency, and seizures lasting longer than 30 minutes can cause respiratory failure, brain damage, and death. **Status epilepticus**, seizure activity lasting longer than 5 minutes or two or more seizures without full recovery of consciousness can be caused by head trauma, hydrocephalus, acute drug or alcohol withdrawal, metabolic disturbances, or abrupt withdrawal of anticonvulsive medications. Airway, breathing, circulation (ABC) interventions must be initiated immediately. Patients are intubated, and arterial blood gases are monitored. Peripheral IV access must also be established. Medications such as lorazepam (Ativan) or midazolam

Table 36.6 Medications in the Treatment of Seizures

Medication	Seizure Type	Side Effects	Nursing Intervention
Carbamazepine (Tegretol)	• Secondary tonic-clonic • Complex partial • Simple partial	• Allergy • Dizziness • Ataxia • Blurred/Double vision • Nausea • Behavioral changes • Hepatitis • Aplastic anemia	• Monitor for visual changes • Monitor liver function • Monitor CBC • Do not crush or chew sustained-release capsules
Clonazepam (Klonopin)	• Absence • Myoclonic • Tonic-clonic	• Sedation • Hyperactivity • Aggression • Slurred speech • Increased salivation • Impaired liver function	• Monitor liver function
Gabapentin (Neurontin)	• Partial seizures in those greater than 12 years old	• Somnolence • Fatigue • Dizziness • Ataxia • Weight gain	• Monitor for increased appetite and weight gain • Monitor for dizziness, ataxia
Lamotrigine (Lamictal)	• Partial • Absence • Tonic-clonic • Atonic • Myoclonic	• Somnolence • Dizziness • Nausea • Rash	• Monitor for dizziness • Nausea/Vomiting • Rash can be life threatening when given with valproic acid (Depakote)

Continued

Table 36.6 Medications in the Treatment of Seizures—cont'd

Medication	Seizure Type	Side Effects	Nursing Intervention
Levetiracetam (Keppra)	• Partial • Tonic-clonic	• Fatigue • Ataxia • Loss of appetite • Cough/Runny nose	• Monitor for ataxia • Monitor for loss of appetite
Phenobarbital (Luminal)	• Tonic-clonic activity • Febrile • Partial	• Sedation • Changes in sleep patterns • Inattention • Cognitive impairment	• Monitor for depression, irritability, drowsiness, and cognitive impairment • Utilized less because of high level of sedation
Phenytoin (Dilantin)	• Tonic-clonic activity • Complex partial • Simple partial	• Gingival hyperplasia • Nystagmus • Hirsutism • Ataxia • Folate deficiency • Drug-induced lupus • Rash • Myelosuppression	• Serum levels monitored • Total serum levels: 10–20 mcg/mL • Dilantin (free) levels: 90% bound to protein, which is biologically active at therapeutic range of 1–2 mcg/mL • At high doses can develop nystagmus • Increases levels and prolongs the half-life of Coumadin • Monitor CBC • Monitor for gingival hyperplasia (care with teeth brushing)
Pregabalin (Lyrica)	• Partial	• Dizziness • Blurred vision • Drowsiness • Weight gain	• Monitor for dizziness and drowsiness • Monitor for weight gain
Topiramate (Topamax)	• Partial • Tonic-clonic • Atonic • Myoclonic • Absence	• Somnolence • Fatigue • Anorexia • Difficulty concentrating • Nervousness	• Monitor for ataxia, fatigue, anxiety • Increased risk for renal calculi • Monitor for weight loss
Valproate *Valproic Acid (Depakote)*	• Myoclonic • Absence • Tonic-clonic	• Tremors • Hair loss • Elevated liver enzymes • Liver failure • Pancreatitis • Amenorrhea • Thrombocytopenia	• Monitor for tremor • Monitor for hair loss • Monitor liver function • Monitor complete blood cell count • Monitor coagulation

(Versed), both benzodiazepines, are generally first line in the immediate treatment of seizures, including status epilepticus. To stabilize the patient, a loading dose of phenytoin (Dilantin) or levetiracetam (Keppra) (anticonvulsants) is generally administered along with around-the-clock dosing. When the seizure is refractory to all interventions, patients are placed on high doses of propofol (Diprivan) or placed in a pentobarbital coma. Not only is close monitoring of cardiovascular status required, but continuous EEG monitoring for burst suppression is also initiated.

Surgical Management

Several procedures have been used to treat seizure disorders not managed effectively with pharmacological therapy. Similar to a cardiac pacemaker, the vagal nerve stimulator (VNS) can provide relief for those suffering from refractory simple or complex seizures. It is proposed that stimulation of the vagus nerve (CN X) can effectively control seizure activity via alterations in the release of norepinephrine, increasing the levels of GABA (inhibitory neurotransmitter) and/or by the inhibition of aberrant cortical activity in the reticular activating system.

Implantation of the VNS is generally performed on an outpatient basis. The generator is implanted into a small "pouch" in the left chest below the clavicle. Access to the vagal nerve is then established via an incision in the neck. Either postoperatively or within a 2-week period, the generator is activated and programmed specifically to the patient. The generator is either continuously stimulating the vagus nerve, or the patient carries a small handheld magnet with which he can activate the program with the presence of an aura; thus a seizure can be minimized and extinguished.

Deep brain stimulation is used to treat uncontrolled seizure activity. Electrodes are placed in deep brain structures, including the thalamus, hippocampus, and internal capsule, and are programmed to activate when the seizure activity is sensed. Deep brain stimulation involves implanting electrodes into the brain that release electrical impulses. The therapeutic effect is the reduction of the frequency of seizure activity.

Other surgical approaches to the control of epilepsy in patients unresponsive to medication therapy include **partial corpus callosotomy** (pediatrics), removal of brain tissue that has been identified as containing a seizure focus through surgical excision or laser ablation. These procedures are used for patients with intractable seizures that have been localized to a specific area of the brain. During the partial corpus callosotomy a craniotomy is performed and the connection between the right and left hemispheres of the brain is either disrupted partially or totally severed. This procedure reduces the frequency and severity of the seizures because electrical activity can no longer spread from one hemisphere to the other. Postoperative management is similar to that of the patient undergoing craniotomy for a brain tumor.

Before these surgical procedures, patients are typically evaluated in a dedicated epilepsy monitoring unit, often with surgically placed EEG electrodes on the surface of the brain to specifically identify areas of brain tissue involved in seizure activity. These electrodes are placed during a craniotomy in which the surface of the brain is accessed after a section of the skull is removed, and the electrodes are placed on the surface of the brain. The skull section is replaced similarly to other types of craniotomies, with the connecting wires exposed outside of the surgical wound. The EEG electrodes are connected to an EEG machine for extended monitoring with the goal of identifying a definitive focus of the seizure activity that can be removed. An interprofessional team consisting of neurologists, neurosurgeons, specially trained nurses and EEG technicians care for patients in the epilepsy monitoring unit (EMU).

Nursing Management

Assessment and Analysis

The clinical manifestations of seizure vary widely depending on the etiology of the disorder and the area of the brain involved. Management of seizure activity requires careful observation. Clinical manifestations include:

- Tonic movements
- Clonic movement
- Loss of consciousness
- Aura
- Automatisms
- Loss of motor tone

Nursing Diagnoses

- **Risk for ineffective breathing pattern** related to decreased level of consciousness secondary to the postictal state
- **Risk for injury** related to tonic-clonic motor activity
- **Ineffective coping** related to uncertainty and inability to control the seizures

Nursing Interventions

▦ *Assessments*

- Airway
  During the seizure and postictal state, the patient may have a compromised airway secondary to decreased level of consciousness.
- Vital signs
  Blood pressure, heart rate, and oxygen saturation should be carefully monitored during and after the seizure. Elevations in heart rate and blood pressure may develop during the seizure, and respiratory changes, including airway compromise, may develop after the seizure.
- Seizure activity
  Accurate diagnosis and treatment of seizure activity are facilitated by a detailed description of patient observations immediately before, during, and after the seizure.
- Presence of an aura
  Some patients may experience an aura in advance of a seizure, allowing the patient to assume a safe position.

▦ *Actions*

- Set up suction equipment at the patient's bedside
  The patient may be unable to protect the airway after the seizure activity and may require suctioning of the oral airway.
- Have oxygen available at the patient's bedside
  During the postictal phase, the patient may require supplemental oxygenation to maintain the oxygenation saturation within normal limits for the patient.
- Safety measures (bed in lowest position, suction at the bedside, oral airway at the bedside)
  For the patient experiencing a witnessed seizure, protection includes not forcing any object into the mouth (for fear of biting

tongue, breaking teeth, causing injury, etc.), loosening of restrictive clothing, and turning the patient to the side (preferably to the left side to reduce the risk of aspiration). No attempt should be made to restrain the patient's movement; however, guiding the movement may be necessary to prevent injury.

- Place an IV catheter per orders
  In the event of seizure activity, IV access may be needed to administer medications to stop the seizure activity.
- Document specifics of seizure, observed seizure activity
  Following the seizure, documentation should provide the date, time, and duration of the seizure; a clear description of the seizure; the sequence of the seizure progression; and preictal and postictal observations.

▣ *Teaching*

- Medication regimen
  Control of seizure activity is largely determined by therapeutic levels of prescribed antiseizure medications.
- Medic Alert bracelet
  It is important for patients with seizures to wear a Medic Alert bracelet in the event of seizure activity. This facilitates prompt interventions in the event of a seizure.
- Driving restrictions
  It is important for the patient to research driving restrictions in the state of residence/licensed to drive, as some states restrict driving in patients with seizure disorders. People with a newly diagnosed seizure disorder are required to notify their department of motor vehicles/driving administration.

Evaluating Care Outcomes

Quality of life is closely related to effective control of seizure activity. Compliance with medication, dietary, and activity prescriptions are important to facilitate seizure control. People diagnosed with seizure disorders may also benefit from support and social support to prevent stress and for coping issues related to diagnosis of seizures. Most adult patients diagnosed with seizure disorders are required to take anticonvulsant medications for life.

CASE STUDY: EPISODE 3

Mr. Johnson is postoperative day 2 following his surgery for a right frontotemporal mass. He is alert and oriented, his speech is markedly improved, and his spirits are good. He is seen by speech therapy and passes a swallowing evaluation for a regular diet. Physical therapy is working with him daily. While visiting her husband, Mrs. Johnson begins to scream for help. The nurse finds Mr. Johnson in bed, gurgling, with tonic-clonic movements, and he does not respond to her. He is placed on his left side and given 2 mg of lorazepam intravenously. After 3 minutes, the seizure subsides. The provider comes to the bedside quickly. The nurse tells the provider the details prior to the event, how long it lasted, what the patient was doing during the event, and what was given to control it.

Mr. Johnson is ordered a 1-g bolus of levetiracetam IV and 500 mg IV every 12 hours. An EEG is ordered. The nurse explains to both Mr. and Mrs. Johnson that the potential for seizures postoperatively is high, and the bed should remain in the lowest position with the side rails up...

Connection Check 36.6

A patient with a history of complex partial seizures has a phenytoin (Dilantin) level (free) of 3.1 mcg/mL. The nurse calls the patient and instructs the patient to take which action?

A. Stop the medication and make an appointment for the following week with the provider.

B. Continue the medication and make an appointment right away with the healthcare provider.

C. Take an extra dose now and continue with the current regimen.

D. Skip the next dose and make an appointment right away with the healthcare provider.

MENINGITIS

Meningitis is an inflammation of the **meninges**, the thin covering around the brain and spinal cord. Causes of meningitis include bacterial infection, viral infection, fungal infection, and what is called *aseptic meningitis*. Aseptic causes of meningitis include the use of antibiotics, nonsteroidal anti-inflammatory medications, and **carcinomatosis** (widespread dissemination of cancer throughout the body). Viral meningitis is also considered aseptic meningitis.

Epidemiology

The incidence of meningitis is increased in settings where people live in close proximity, including college dormitories, military barracks, and prisons. In the United States, rates of bacterial meningitis have markedly declined, to a current rate of 0.6 to 4 cases per 100,000 yearly because of the institution of vaccines such as Hib (*Haemophilus influenzae* type b) and conjugate vaccines for *Streptococcus pneumoniae*. The prevalence of meningitis is 10-fold in developing countries. In populations not immunized against mumps, the prevalence of meningitis is 10.9 cases per 100,000, with 30% of those who contract mumps culminating in meningitis. The very young (infants) and those older than 60 years are more predisposed to contracting meningitis.

Pathophysiology

Meningitis is classified as acute or chronic. Acute meningitis indicates a bacterial cause, with the presence of clinical manifestations occurring in hours to days and CSF **pleocytosis** (markedly increased white blood cells). The inflammatory process within the meninges leads to increased turbidity of CSF, leading to sluggish flow of CSF. Acute bacterial meningitis is a medical emergency. Chronic meningitis has an onset of symptoms during weeks to months, with duration of symptoms longer than 4 weeks.

Several routes of entry are responsible for the development of meningitis. Direct inoculation of the organisms responsible for meningitis occurs secondary to traumatic injury and transmission during surgery, procedures such as lumbar punctures, and with monitoring devices such as intraventricular catheters. Transmission also occurs following the colonization or localized infections of bacteria, viruses, fungi, and parasites. This occurs via the skin, the nasopharynx, the respiratory tract (most common), the gastrointestinal and the genitourinary tracts. The organism invades the submucosa, gaining access to the bloodstream and CNS, where the organism begins to seed the CNS. Another means by which transmission occurs is via retrograde neuronal pathways (olfactory and peripheral nerves).

Viral meningitis, an aseptic form of meningitis, is most commonly caused by enterovirus, herpes simplex virus (HSV), herpes zoster, mumps, and measles. A self-limiting form, viral meningitis causes cell necrosis or results in enzymatic or neurotransmitter alterations, depending on the pathogen and cells involved.

Meningitis is a medical emergency because the increased turbidity and sluggish flow of CSF can lead to an increased ICP. While the ICP increases, herniation of the brain can occur because of displacement of brain tissue, CSF, and compression of blood vessels, culminating in severe brain damage, coma, and death. Increased ICP can also be caused by interstitial edema via obstruction of CSF flow and hydrocephalus, cytotoxic edema caused by bacterial release of cytotoxins and neutrophils, which cause cellular swelling, and via vasogenic edema and the increased permeability of the blood–brain barrier.

Clinical Manifestations

The characteristic presentation of meningitis in the adult includes fever, headache, and divergent degrees of altered mental status. The patient may also report **photophobia** (sensitivity to light), chills, nausea, and vomiting. The clinical presentation of meningeal irritation includes nuchal rigidity (neck stiffness) and **opisthotonos** (severe hyperextension of the head with arching of the back). In cases of meningococcal meningitis, a faint petechial rash can develop, which can develop into disseminated intravascular coagulation (DIC).

Connection Check 36.7

Before the start of the semester, what type of meningitis can college-aged students be vaccinated against?
A. Bacterial meningitis
B. Viral meningitis
C. Aseptic meningitis
D. Fungal meningitis

Management

Medical Management

Diagnosis

Examination of CSF via lumbar puncture is the hallmark for the diagnosis of meningitis. Patients with suspicion for space-occupying lesions and new-onset seizures and those with a moderate to severe altered level of consciousness require a CT of the head before the procedure because they are at higher risk for herniation. The opening pressure at the time of the lumbar puncture is recorded, and specimens are tested for glucose, protein, white blood cell count, Gram stain, and culture. Patients with diabetes mellitus may have a higher than normal serum glucose. Therefore, serum glucose is drawn during the time of the lumbar puncture. The rule of thumb is that the CSF glucose level is two-thirds that of the serum glucose (Table 36.7).

Meningitis is also caused by other factors such as pericarditis and myocarditis; therefore, assessment of additional data such as heart murmurs and results of an echocardiogram are analyzed to rule out these causes. Other causes of meningitis include infection from a cochlear implant, conjunctivitis, and exposure to animals and animal bites, requiring investigation.

Table 36.7 Cerebrospinal Fluid Examination in Meningitis

	Glucose	Protein	White Blood Cell Count	Microbiology
Normal values	50–75 mg/dL	14–40 mg/dL	0–5; Lymphocytes	Negative
Aseptic	Normal	Normal to slight ↑	10–30; Lymphocytes	Negative
Bacterial	Less than 40 mg/dL	Higher than 100 mg/dL	100–500 With more than 80% polymorphonuclear (PMN) lymphocytes	Gram stain and culture + for specific pathogens
Viral	Normal	Normal to slight ↑	10–300	Viral isolation, polymerase chain reaction (PCR)

Medications

On the basis of the initial assessment and presumptive diagnosis and before confirmation from microbiological data, broad-spectrum antibiotics are initiated. Treatment for meningitis is dependent on the penetration of the blood–brain barrier by the chosen antibiotic as well as by the type of pathogen itself. Treatment for meningitis generally requires 14 to 21 days of antibiotic treatment. Long-term IV access such as a peripherally inserted central line or other central venous access is typically initiated because of the need for long-term antibiotic therapy.

Complications

Increased ICP is a life-threatening complication of meningitis, and identification and treatment of increased ICP are vital. Early signs of increased ICP are identified during the neurological examination, requiring frequent assessment. The use of dexamethasone to reduce inflammation in the treatment of meningitis remains controversial (see Evidence-Based Practice). Several studies have shown a reduction in hearing loss in those patients with meningitis caused by *H. influenzae.* Irritation of the cerebral cortex can cause seizure activity in the patient with meningitis. Patients with meningitis are also at risk for syndrome of inappropriate antidiuretic hormone (SIADH) and diabetes insipidus (DI).

Evidence-Based Practice

Corticosteroids in the Treatment of Bacterial Meningitis

A Cochrane Review was conducted to examine the outcomes of the use of corticosteroids in the treatment of the inflammatory response in meningitis. The search included studies between 1996 and 2015, and selection criteria included randomized controlled studies (RCTs) of corticosteroids for acute bacterial meningitis. The RCTs were scored for methodological quality, and outcome data were collected, including adverse effects. Separate analyses were completed regarding causative organisms, differences between high-income and low-income countries, and time of steroid administration. Twenty-five studies were located that included 4,121 participants, with 2,511 children, 1,517 adults, and 93 with mixed populations. Findings demonstrated a non-significant reduction in mortality in adults receiving corticosteroids. Analyses of causative organisms demonstrated that corticosteroids reduced mortality in patients with *Streptococcus pneumoniae* meningitis but not in *Haemophilus influenzae.* Corticosteroids were associated with lower rates of significant hearing loss in high-income countries but not in low-income countries. Because corticosteroids significantly reduced hearing loss and neurological sequelae, recommendations from this review support the use of corticosteroids

in patients with bacterial meningitis in high-income countries but not in low-income countries. The use of corticosteroids was not found to reduce overall mortality in the treatment of patients with meningitis.

Brouwer, M. C., McIntyre, P., Prasad, K., & van de Beek, D. (2015). Corticosteroids for acute bacterial meningitis. *Cochrane Database of Systematic Reviews, 6* CD004405. doi: 10.1002/14651858.CD004405.pub4.

Nursing Management

Assessment and Analysis

Many of the clinical manifestations observed in the patient with meningitis are directly related to irritation and inflammation of the meninges that surround the brain and spinal cord. Common clinical findings include:

- Change in level of consciousness
- Headache
- Fever
- Photophobia
- Nausea and vomiting
- Rhinorrhea
- Nuchal rigidity
- **Brudzinski's sign** (involuntary flexion of the hips in response to passive flexion of the neck with the patient in a supine position) (Fig. 36.5)
- **Kernig's sign** (pain in the back of the leg [hamstring] and resistance to movement when the leg is flexed at the hip and then straightened at the knee) (Fig. 36.6)

The neurological examination is the most significant nursing intervention in the care of the patient with meningitis.

Nursing Diagnoses

- **Disturbed sensory perception** related to meningeal irritation
- **Activity intolerance** related to pain and fatigue
- **Ineffective coping** related to the complexity of the treatment regimen to manage meningitis

Nursing Interventions

▪ *Assessments*

- Neurological status
  Because of the risk of increased ICP secondary to increased turbidity of CSF, frequent neurological assessments are essential to recognize subtle signs. Changes in level of consciousness are the earliest sign of increased ICP and should be reported immediately to the healthcare provider.
- Sign of meningeal irritation (nuchal rigidity, Brudzinski's sign, Kernig's sign)
  The inflammatory process in the meninges causes pain upon movement of the neck, and the patient guards the neck. In the patient with a positive Brudzinski's sign, there is involuntary flexion of the hips in response to passive flexion of the neck with the patient in a supine position (ensure no cervical spine injury prior to attempting). To assess the Kernig's sign,

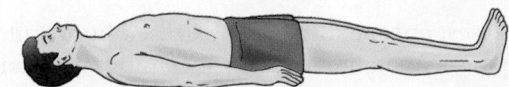

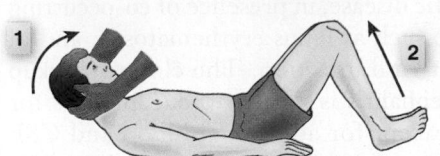

As the neck is flexed, there is stretch on the inflamed meninges, and the knees flex involuntarily to decrease the pain caused by the stretching of the meninges

FIGURE 36.5 Brudzinski's sign.

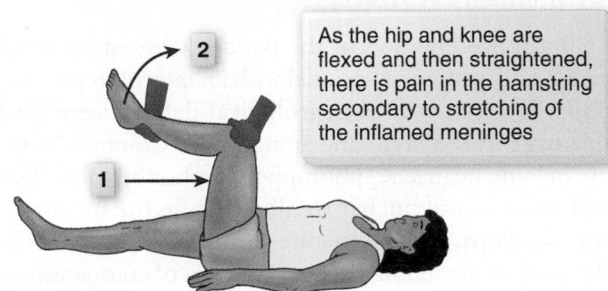

As the hip and knee are flexed and then straightened, there is pain in the hamstring secondary to stretching of the inflamed meninges

FIGURE 36.6 Kernig's sign.

the nurse starts with the patient's hip and knee flexed at a 90-degree angle and then slowly extends (do not force) the knee. Pain behind the knee and repeated pain bilaterally are indicative of a positive sign.

- Vital signs
  Elevated temperature develops secondary to the infectious process. If increased ICP develops, the blood pressure increases with widening pulse pressure and decrease in heart rate.
- Fluid balance
  Monitor blood pressure for signs of hypo/hypertension and heart rate. If the patient develops SIADH, fluid is retained and there may be an increase in blood pressure. With DI the patient has an increased output of dilute urine and is at risk for hypovolemia, hypotension, and tachycardia.
- Headache
  The inflammation of the meninges may lead to headache.
- Cranial nerve assessment: with particular attention to CNs III, IV, and VI
  The eye on the affected side can deviate down and out because of a dilated, light-fixed pupil.
- CSF results
  Treatment of meningitis, particularly bacterial infections, is directed to the specific organism that is isolated in the CSF sample.
- Daily weight
  Changes in fluid volume status correspond to changes in body weight.
- Renal function
  Many antibiotics are cleared by the kidneys, so increases in blood urea nitrogen and creatinine may demonstrate damage to the renal system.
- Vascular assessments
  In the patient who develops DIC, there may be increased bleeding as well as decreased peripheral perfusion.

Actions

- Administer IV fluids
  The patient may have changes in fluid volume status related to increased fluid loss with elevated temperature or development of diabetes insipidus.
- Administer antibiotics as ordered
  Antibiotics should be initiated without delay, and antibiotics that require therapeutic dosing should be monitored judiciously to facilitate their therapeutic goals.
- Decrease environmental stimuli
  Dim the lights, exposure to bright lights from windows (patients may be photo sensitive); and provide quiet environment as these may exacerbate associated with meningitis.
- Maintain head of bed elevated to 30 degrees
  This position increases venous outflow and may decrease intracranial pressure that may be elevated due to turbidity of the CSF.
- Pain management
  Because of associated headache, it is important to implement pharmacological and nonpharmacological interventions to promote patient comfort.
- Implement transmission precautions
  Standard precautions are maintained for all patients. Include droplet precautions (bacterial meningitis per hospital policy).
- Maintain normothermia via antipyretic, cooling baths, and cooling blankets
  Decreases metabolic activity and decreases CNS oxygen demand

Teaching

- Importance of follow-up appointments
  Recovery from meningitis may take weeks to months and requires frequent assessment and evaluation by the healthcare provider.
- Importance of taking full course of antibiotics
  Extended antibiotic therapy may be indicated to lessen the chances of reoccurrence of the infectious process.

Evaluating Care Outcomes

Management of meningitis requires eradication of the infectious organism. During the acute phase, the patient's chief complaints are pain, neck stiffness, and photophobia. Definitive interventions focus on antibiotic therapies and comfort measures. Antipyretics may be indicated with fever. Monitoring for increased ICP is a priority during the acute phase of meningitis. Upon discharge, the patient will be neurologically and hemodynamically stable, and the patient also needs to be knowledgeable of signs of recurrent infection and increased ICP to seek emergent treatment. Compliance with antibiotic therapy after discharge is also a priority because the patient may be discharged while still receiving antibiotic therapy.

ENCEPHALITIS

Epidemiology

Several thousand cases of encephalitis are reported yearly and are primarily caused by enteroviruses such as herpes simplex I and II and arboviruses (transmitted via anthropoid vectors) such as rabies, Lyme disease, and West Nile virus. Herpes simplex virus I causes approximately 10% or 2 million cases in the United States in those from age 20 to 40 years. Herpes simplex virus is the single most rapidly progressing form in the United States. Herpes simplex virus I is contracted via bodily fluids such as oral and nasal secretions, whereas HSV II is sexually transmitted. Primary encephalitis can be sporadic or epidemic. Sporadic forms of encephalitis include HSV, whereas arboviruses such as West Nile virus, St. Louis virus, La Crosse virus, and rabies can be sporadic or epidemic. Encephalitis can also be a complication of an initial virus or reactivation of latent viruses as a result of a compromised immune system, such as varicella-zoster (chickenpox), rubeola (measles), mumps, and rubella (German measles). Most often caused by viral infections, encephalitis can also be caused by bacteria, fungi, and parasitic inoculation. Eastern equine virus is transmitted via horses, humans, and birds and is found primarily in the Eastern United States and Gulf Coast. Western equine virus, predominately found in the Central Plains, involves farming communities. St. Louis virus is seen throughout most temperate regions and throughout the country. West Nile virus, first diagnosed in 1991, is transmitted via the bites of mosquitoes through the bites of infected animals, and Lyme disease is transmitted through the bite of infected ticks.

Pathophysiology

Encephalitis is an acute inflammation of the brain, including the cerebrum, brainstem, and cerebellum, whereas meningitis involves the layers (meninges) covering the brain and spinal cord (myelitis). While the pathogen travels to the CNS, it invades the brain tissues and reproduces, leading to inflammation of the cerebral cortex and white matter. When the inflammation involves both the brain and spinal cord, it is called **encephalomyelitis**.

Acute viral encephalitis can be a life-threatening emergency, quickly leading to increased ICP, coma, and death. Although encephalitis is dangerous in all age groups, those who are very young (infants and children), older adults, and the immunocompromised are most at risk. All forms of encephalitis can take weeks to months to resolve and can leave the patient with debilitating neurological injury and deficits.

In some cases, encephalitis can be caused by an autoimmune response. An immune response causing encephalitis has been known to occur in the presence of cancer, termed paraneoplastic disease, in presence of co-occurring autoimmune disease such as lupus erythematosus, and in response to a recent viral infection. The clinical workup for this type of encephalitis is similar to encephalitis for infectious disease except for additional blood and CSF biomarkers of cancer and specific autoimmune disorders.

Clinical Manifestations

The clinical presentation of the patient with encephalitis includes manifestations associated with an infectious process, including fever, as well as neurological deficits associated with damage to the brain and spinal cord. Common complaints include headache, photophobia, phonophobia (fear of loud noises), and nuchal rigidity. While the infectious process develops, clinical manifestation of increased ICP may be present, including a change in level of consciousness (lethargy, disorientation), as well as focal signs, including muscle spasms and parasthesias.

Management

Medical Management
Diagnosis

Diagnosis of encephalitis follows the procedures and protocol of meningitis, involving examination of the blood and CSF as well as the EEG, CT, and MRI scans. Antivirals are used to treat encephalitis. Acyclovir is used to treat most forms of encephalitis and is considered a prodrug because of its initial administration in a less active form, then metabolized into a more active species after administration. Bioavailability of this medication is low; it also has low solubility in water and is therefore best administered in IV form when high concentrations are required. Ganciclovir (Cytovene) is used in the treatment of encephalitis caused by organisms such as cytomegalovirus (CMV).

 Safety Alert Considered a potential carcinogen, teratogen, and mutagen, ganciclovir, used in the treatment of encephalitis caused by CMV, requires judicious handling.

Connection Check 36.8

The nurse monitors which diagnostic results in the patient with bacterial encephalitis? *(Select all that apply.)*

A. Isolation of CSF via polymerase chain reaction
B. Gram stain and culture of CSF
C. CT
D. MRI
E. EMG

Nursing Management
Assessment and Analysis

The clinical presentation and management of encephalitis is similar to that of meningitis. Typical clinical manifestations include:

- Changes in level of consciousness
- Fever
- Headache
- Photophobia
- Weakness
- Nuchal rigidity

Nursing Diagnoses

- **Ineffective cerebral tissue perfusion** related to hydrocephalus
- **Self-care deficit** related to decreased level of consciousness and weakness
- **Risk for injury** related to decreased level of consciousness

Nursing Interventions
Assessments

- Neurological function
  The infectious process in the CNS may act as a space-occupying lesion and increase ICP, leading to changes in the level of consciousness.
- Vital signs
  Because this is an infectious process, the patient may have an elevated temperature and tachycardia. If ICP is elevated, an increase in blood pressure and widening of pulse pressure may develop.
- Nuchal rigidity, Brudzinski's and Kernig's signs
  Signs of meningeal irritation and involvement of the brain itself can lead to extension into the meningeal layers.
- Cranial nerve assessment with particular attention to CNS III, IV, and VI
  The eye on the affected side can deviate down and out, with a dilated, light-fixed pupil.
- Intake and output
  Fever may increase insensible water loss and some of the antibiotics, and antiviral medications may cause nausea, vomiting, and diarrhea.
- Complete blood counts
  Antiviral medications may cause hematological dyscrasias: granulocytopenia, neutropenia, anemia, and thrombocytopenia.
- Monitor liver function tests (LFTs)
  Antivirals and antibiotics may lead to elevation of liver enzymes due to potential hepatotoxicity.

Actions

- Position patient with head of bed elevated to 30 to 45 degrees with head in good alignment
  This position facilitates venous drainage and minimizes the risk of increased ICP.

- Implement seizure precautions
  Because of the potential for increased ICP as well as the presence of an infectious process in the CNS, the patient's seizure threshold is decreased.
- Encourage oral intake as tolerated
  Because of nausea and vomiting that may occur as side effects of medications, it is important to optimize dietary intake.
- Dim lights and maintain a quiet environment
  These interventions decrease environmental stimuli. Bright lights and loud noises may exacerbate headache. Patients may have photophobia and phonophobia.
- Turn and reposition the patient at least every 2 hours
  Because of limited activity, the patient is at risk of complications of immobility, in particular, skin breakdown.
- Administer stool softeners as needed to prevent constipation
  Limited activity, potential nausea and vomiting, and decreased oral intake increase the chances of constipation; need to minimize Valsalva because of potential to increase ICP

Teaching

- Complications of immobility
  Because the course of encephalitis may lead to an extended hospitalization and bedrest, the patient is at risk for skin breakdown, deep vein thromboembolism, and deconditioning. The recovery process may be extended, and the patient's compliance with interventions to recondition are imperative.
- Importance of follow-up appointments
  Recovery from encephalitis may take weeks to months and requires frequent assessment and evaluation by the healthcare provider.
- Importance of taking full course of antibiotics
  Extended antibiotic therapy may be indicated to lessen the chances of reoccurrence of the infectious process.

Evaluating Care Outcomes

Management of encephalitis requires eradication of the infectious organism. Patients with encephalitis are often critically ill, requiring admission to an intensive care setting. Because of complications associated with increased ICP, the patient's recovery is dependent on secondary injury associated with compression of vital structures. The nurse works with the patient and family to ensure compliance with all prescribed interventions and, before discharge, ensures that they are knowledgeable of reasons to seek medical attention.

PARKINSON'S DISEASE

Epidemiology

Parkinson's disease (PD) is a progressive, neurodegenerative disease of the CNS manifesting primarily in motor dysfunction. Primarily of idiopathic origin, environmental toxins (pesticides and herbicides), brain injury, brain tumors, the use of antipsychotic medication, and a genetic component have all been implicated as possible causes of PD.

Parkinson's disease is found 1.5 to 2 times more often in males than in females and generally begins between the ages of 40 and 70 years. Progression of the disease is escalated in those who are diagnosed at later stages in life. In the United States, the highest prevalence of PD is found within Amish communities. With annual reports of 50,000 new cases per year, it is estimated that more than 500,000 people are afflicted with PD in the United States alone.

Pathophysiology

A motor system disorder, Parkinson's involves the loss of dopamine-producing brain cells in the substantia nigra of the basal ganglia, culminating in a decreased amount of dopamine in the brain. The basal ganglia of the brain consist of several brain structures or collections of neurons (Fig. 36.7): the striatum (caudate, putamen, and globus pallidus), the substantia nigra, and the subthalamic nucleus, all innervated by the dopaminergic system. Motor activity is the result of the release of dopamine and acetylcholine (ACh) and the integration of the basal ganglia, the cerebral cortex, and the cerebellum. With stimulation of the basal ganglia, muscle tone is inhibited and voluntary movement is coordinated and smoothly executed. The coordination of the excitatory messages from the production of ACh in the basal ganglia and the inhibitory messages from dopamine via transport from the substantia nigra to the basal ganglia allow for the control of steady, well-coordinated, fine movement. Deterioration of the substantia nigra decreases the amount of dopamine in the brain. The excitatory ACh neurons continue to proliferate, remaining active while there is a continued loss of dopamine and its inhibitory mechanisms, culminating in the loss of initiation and control of voluntary movement.

Clinical Manifestations

Four discernible symptoms of PD are resting tremors, muscle rigidity, slowness of movement (**bradykinesia**) or loss of movement (akinesia), and postural instability (impaired balance and frequent falls). Other clinical manifestations include mood, cognitive, and behavioral alterations.

Parkinson's disease is characterized by five progressive stages. In the first initial stage, the patient usually presents with unexplained unilateral weakness and upper-extremity tremors. While the patient progresses into later stages, more-pronounced physical disabilities are noted, including a slow, shuffling gait, widening on gait, and postural instability. In the final stages, movements become much slower and rigidity is more pronounced (Fig. 36.8).

Connection Check 36.9

The nurse recognizes that the patient with Parkinson's disease is at risk for which complication?
A. Excessive dry mouth due to autonomic dysfunction
B. Facial twitching secondary to seizure activity
C. Orthostatic hypotension due to involvement of the sympathetic nervous system
D. Flaccid extremities related to the increased levels of dopamine

Management

Medical Management

Diagnosis

Diagnosis of PD is made when two or more cardinal symptoms with asymmetrical presentation, bradykinesia (slow movement), resting tremor, rigidity, and postural instability, are observed in the absence of other causes. There are no specific diagnostic studies to confirm PD, so the presence of progressive decline in motor function accompanied by the tremors and rigidity is typically how the diagnosis is made.

Medications

Pharmacological therapy is initiated when symptoms become difficult or disabling for the patient. Anticholinergics, which can reduce tremors and drooling, may be used in younger patients and include trihexyphenidyl (Artane) and

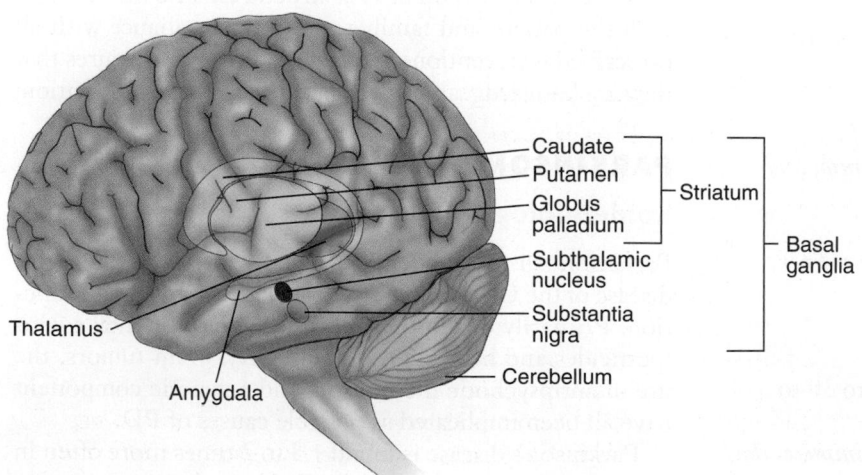

FIGURE 36.7 Sites of damage in Parkinson's disease.

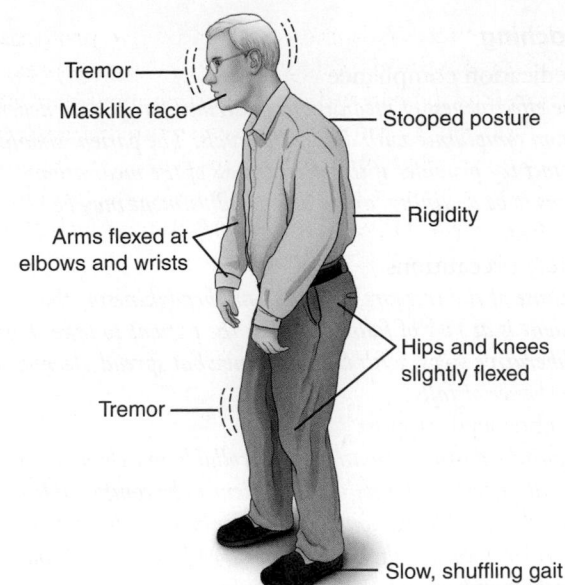

FIGURE 36.8 Clinical presentation of Parkinson's disease.

- Tremor
- Masklike face
- Arms flexed at elbows and wrists
- Tremor
- Stooped posture
- Rigidity
- Hips and knees slightly flexed
- Slow, shuffling gait

burr hole is performed for access and a cylindrical rod or electrode is implanted, allowing the targeted area to receive mild electrical stimulation to reduce tremors and the rigidity associated with PD. Once the probe is confirmed to be in the proper location, a permanent lesion is established in order to destroy the tissue and reduce the tremors and rigidity.

Connection Check 36.10

Which clinical manifestations are included in a diagnosis of Parkinson's disease? *(Select all that apply.)*
A. Flaccidity
B. Total resistance to movement
C. Bradykinesia
D. Tremors
E. Photophobia

---

benztropine (Cogentin). These medications are generally not used in older adults because of side effects including confusion, memory impairment, blurred vision, dry mouth, constipation, and urinary retention.

Dopamine-receptor agonists such as pramipexole (Mirapex) and ropinirole (Requip) are often first-line treatments. Side effects of these medications include nausea and vomiting, urinary frequency, drowsiness, orthostatic hypotension, lower-extremity edema, sleep attacks, and disorders of impulse control (gambling and hypersexuality).

With the progression of PD, levodopa seems to become less effective in the elimination of related motor symptoms. Eventually, the "on" state diminishes, and the "wearing off" state occurs earlier. In this "off" state, the patient with PD becomes stiff and slow and may be unable to move for several minutes. For some, this "on-off" phenomenon is predictable, and it is believed that these fluctuations respond to controlled-release forms of levodopa. For this reason, dopamine precursors such as carbidopa/levodopa (Sinemet) are later used and are most effective in the treatment of bradykinesia, tremors, and rigidity. Recently, an intestinal gel containing levodopa/carbidopa has been introduced as an option for the treatment of motor fluctuations in advanced Parkinson's disease when oral medication is no longer effective. This intestinal gel is administered by an external pump through a percutaneous endoscopic gastric-jejunal tube. These medications can cause side effects consisting of nausea and vomiting, orthostatic hypotension, constipation, arrhythmias, dyskinesias, and dry mouth.

Surgical Management

Stereotactic pallidotomy for control of the clinical manifestations associated with PD involves the opening of the pallidum within the corpus striatum. Locating the specific site is performed via the use of multiple CTs of the head and the stereotactic head ring. Once the location is identified, a

Nursing Management
Assessment and Analysis

The clinical presentation of PD is important to the accurate diagnosis of this neurological disorder. The four cardinal signs include bradykinesia, tremor, rigidity, and postural stability. Other clinical manifestations seen in this disorder include:

- Weakness
- Fatigue
- Masklike face
- Shuffling gait
- Uncoordinated movements
- Widening gait

Nursing Diagnoses

- **Risk for falls** related to ataxia, muscular rigidity, and orthostatic hypotension
- **Risk for constipation** related to decreased mobility and side effects of medications used to treat PD
- **Powerlessness** related to diagnosis of a chronic, progressive disorder

Nursing Interventions
Assessments

- Tremors, rigidity, and bradykinesia
  The coordination of the excitatory messages from the production of ACh in the basal ganglia and the inhibitory messages from dopamine via transport from the substantia nigra to the basal ganglia allow for the control of steady, well-coordinated, fine movement. The lack of balance between ACh and dopamine leads to tremors, rigidity, and bradykinesia.
- Gag and swallow
  Patients with PD may experience difficulty swallowing, manifested by excessive drooling that places the patient at risk of aspiration because of ineffective swallowing.

- Mobility
  Ataxia, bradykinesia, and postural instability are prime symptoms of PD and decrease the patient's physical mobility and ability to complete activities of daily living (ADLs).
- Bowel and bladder function
  Parkinson's disease may impact bowel and bladder functions, making the patient at risk for incontinence and constipation.

▪ Actions

- Administer PD medications as prescribed
  Treatment of PD is primarily aimed at treating the clinical manifestations, so it is important to administer as prescribed to maximize therapeutic effectiveness.
- Implement safety precautions
  Tremors, rigidity, and orthostatic hypotension place PD patients at great risk for falls. The etiology of the disease process and side effects of medications can also cause sleep deprivation. High-risk tasks such as driving can become impaired, requiring ongoing discussion, evaluation, and consensus regarding abilities.
- Facilitate nutritional intake
  Muscles of the face become more involved while PD progresses; the patient may have difficulties with eating, swallowing, and talking. The swallowing difficulties place the patient at risk for aspiration and decreased oral intake.
- Elevate head of bed when eating and drinking
  Impaired swallowing associated with PD increases the risk of aspiration. Elevating the head facilitates the swallow reflex.
- Suction equipment at the bedside
  Because of increased drooling and impaired swallowing, the patient is at risk of aspiration.
- Administer stool softeners and increase fluid intake
  Because of impaired mobility associated with PD, the patient is at risk of constipation and these interventions are aimed to maintain normal bowel function.
- Encourage the patient to participate in self-care activities
  Patients are encouraged to participate in all areas of self-care to their best ability to maintain independence and safety.
- Facilitate interprofessional collaboration with physical therapy, occupational therapy, and speech therapy
  Physical therapists provide exercises and activities that maximize strength, flexibility, and movement. The occupational therapist provides strategies to promote independence and offers accommodations that may need to be made in the home to promote safety and maximize independence in ADLs. The speech therapist completes a swallowing evaluation and makes suggestions to promote safe oral intake. He or she may also have strategies to promote verbal communication.
- Communication
  Difficulties with speech are common in late stages of PD. Continued monitoring and interventions by speech therapy include exercises to improve breathing, swallowing, and speech and identification of assistive devices to assist in communication.
- Consult with social worker
  The social worker can provide information regarding support groups, advocacy groups, and agencies and information about palliative care/hospice care consultation.

▪ Teaching

- Medication compliance
  The effectiveness of medications prescribed for PD are dependent on compliance with dosing intervals. The patient should contact the provider if the effectiveness of the medications seems to be declining, and a dosage adjustment may be required.
- Safety precautions
  Because of the tremors, rigidity, and bradykinesia, the patient is at risk of falls. Teaching the patient to take short, deliberative steps, with the feet somewhat spread, decreases the chance of falls.
- Psychosocial support
  Cognitive dysfunction and uncontrollable muscle movement can all affect the ability of the patient to be comfortable and independent. Depression is not uncommon in this population. Increased responsibilities placed on significant others and family members can be overwhelming.

Connection Check 36.11

What interprofessional team members are involved in the management of the patient with Parkinson's disease? *(Select all that apply.)*

A. Oncologist
B. Speech therapist
C. Occupational therapist
D. Interventional radiologist
E. Physical therapist

Evaluating Care Outcomes

Care coordination and quality of life are important determinants in the evaluation of care for the patient living with PD. Because PD is a progressive, neuromuscular disorder that often ultimately results in loss of motor control and dependence upon others for ADLs, patient and family involvement in decision making about the priorities of care is essential. Patient safety is also a priority; falls are more likely because of postural instability and weakness, and while muscles of the face become more involved, the patient may also have difficulties with eating, swallowing, and talking. Modifications to the living environment are required to ensure patient safety and to maximize independence for as long as possible.

ALZHEIMER'S DISEASE

Epidemiology

A form of dementia involving the gradual progression of the loss of brain function, Alzheimer's disease affects memory, thinking, and behavior. Gradually, there is increasing cognitive decline, leading to severe deterioration. Life expectancy is 2 to 20 years, resulting in death secondary to causes manifested by immobility and organ failure, not from the disease itself. It is estimated that 5.7 million Americans have Alzheimer's disease, 5.5 million older than 65, and approximately 200,000 younger than 65. It is also estimated that 500,000 Americans younger than 65 have some form of dementia, 40% of them with Alzheimer's. Approximately two-thirds of Americans with Alzheimer's disease are women, and there is an increased incidence in older African American adults. Older African-Americans are approximately twice as likely to have Alzheimer's or other dementias in comparison with older whites. Hispanics are approximately one and one-half times as likely to have Alzheimer's or other dementias as older whites. Although Alzheimer's is considered a disease of aging, many older adults do not exhibit clinical manifestations of dementia other than forgetfulness. Early-onset dementia can occur before the age of 65 and progresses rapidly. Those with blood relatives (parents, siblings) who have been diagnosed with dementia appear to be at greater risk. Although discussed as possible risk factors for the development of dementia, neither long-standing hypertension (HTN) or injury to the brain have been proven to cause Alzheimer's disease.

Pathophysiology

Conclusive evidence as to the causes of Alzheimer's does not yet exist. The actual diagnosis of Alzheimer's is made only at autopsy, although several criteria have been formulated for presumptive identification. It is theorized that fragments of protein within nerve cells develop into neurofibrillary tangles obstructing cells, as well as the formation of beta-amyloid neuritic plaques (dying and dead nerve cells), which accumulate within the brain. This results in a decrease in the neurotransmitters that provide the connections between nerve cells within the brain, blocking communication. Mechanisms that elicit the development of these tangles and plaques are unknown; however, several theories have undergone investigation. Restriction of blood flow, destruction of cells by free radicals, and apoptosis (genetically programmed cell death)-inducing factor are several of the theories related to Alzheimer's disease.

Clinical Manifestations

Although many people may develop periods of forgetfulness, there is initially little to no decline in the ability to care for themselves. Forgetfulness is the first symptom of Alzheimer's, which slowly progresses to difficulty with language (vocabulary and fluency), problems with short-term memory such as recent events and conversations, **agnosia** (inability to process sensory information), emotional lability, personality changes, and loss of cognitive skills (abstract thinking, judgment, and calculations). While the disease progresses, there is a loss in ability to perform multiple or complex tasks and difficulty with problem solving. In later stages, the disease progresses to word-finding difficulty and naming of familiar objects, items are misplaced, and the person is easily lost. The person's affect can become flat, with a loss in social skills and changes in personality, and can lead to aggressive, uncontrollable acting out and behavior. The ability to care for oneself can be so limited that the person is bedridden. Death can ensue as a result of infection, pneumonia, falls, malnutrition and dehydration, and multisystem organ failure.

Connection Check 36.12

The nurse recognizes which as the probable cause of Alzheimer's disease?
A. Exposure to environmental toxins
B. CNS trauma
C. Unknown
D. Chronic hypertension

Management

Medical Management

Diagnosis

A confirmed diagnosis of Alzheimer's can be made only on examination of the brain following death. Neurofibrillary tangles and beta-amyloid plaques can be observed microscopically. Presumptive diagnosis is made on the basis of a thorough history and physical examination that includes careful recording of clinical manifestations as well as monitoring the onset, progression, and duration.

Although cognitive impairment can be identified, the cause of the impairment requires careful investigation, especially in older adults, where many other processes can be the cause. Neurological disorders can cause a variety of changes in cognitive ability and include trauma, tumors, stroke, normal-pressure hydrocephalus, vascular abnormalities, and infection. Myocardial infarction, congestive heart failure, arrhythmias, and anemia can also cause cognitive dysfunction in older adults. Metabolic and endocrine disorders such as hyper/hypoglycemia, thyroid dysfunction, renal insufficiency and failure, and hepatic failure, as well as nutritional imbalance, infection, sensory deprivation, and depression can also impinge on cognitive functioning in this population. Additionally, medications and the multiplicity of medications taken as one ages can also affect cognitive function. Utmost care must be taken to diagnose and rule out all possible causes before the speculation of a diagnosis of Alzheimer's disease.

Following the detailed medical history, laboratory data are explored and diagnostic imaging is performed to rule out other causes. Written and oral testing for cognitive function includes mental status, language ability, functional ability, memory, and concentration. Patients also undergo a series of neuropsychiatric testing to rule out depression and delirium.

Medications

Presently, there is no cure for Alzheimer's disease. Although there are several medications approved for Alzheimer's, the foundation of management is physical and emotional support of the patient with Alzheimer's disease and their caregivers. Medications used in the treatment of Alzheimer's disease (Table 36.8) are those that increase the levels of ACh (a neurotransmitter) in the brain by the inhibition of the enzymes acetylcholinesterase and butyrylcholinesterase, which normally break down ACh and butylcholine respectively. This increases communication between remaining neurons. It is also believed that vitamin E, an antioxidant, helps by decreasing the damage caused by free radicals and is often used in combination with other medications.

Nursing Management

Assessment and Analysis

As described earlier, the definitive diagnosis of Alzheimer's disease is made only through autopsy. However, the clinical presentation and deterioration in the patient's cognitive and physical function are routinely used to make an assumption that Alzheimer's disease is present. Clinical manifestations that are associated with this disorder include:

- Forgetfulness that progresses with time
- Short-term memory decline
- Cognitive impairment
- Inability to handle personal finances
- Inability to self-manage medications
- Motor and verbal skill decline

Nursing Diagnoses

- **Acute confusion** related to manifestations of Alzheimer's disease
- **Caregiver role strain** related to the care of the patient with Alzheimer's disease
- **Ineffective coping** related to the diagnosis of Alzheimer's disease

Nursing Interventions

▪ Assessments

- Weight and intake and output
  Patients with Alzheimer's disease may forget to eat and drink while the disease progresses secondary to cognitive decline.
- Bowel and bladder function
  As with other ADLs, as cognition declines the patient may experience incontinence.
- Skin
  Due to cognitive decline and associated decreased mobility, along with incontinence, the patient is at risk for skin breakdown or pressure

Table 36.8 Medications Used to Treat Alzheimer's Disease

Medication	Function	Side Effects
Donepezil (Aricept)	• Inhibits acetylcholinesterase, improving acetylcholinergic function • Treatment of mild-moderate AD • Modest increase in attention, concentration, and mental acuity • Does not slow progression of disease	• May cause bradycardia; monitor HR before administering • Can cause diarrhea, nausea and vomiting, and anorexia; monitor for weight loss and dehydration • Dosing is titrated over several weeks
Rivastigmine (Exelon)	• Inhibits both acetylcholinesterase and butyrylcholinesterase • Treatment of mild-moderate AD • Modest increase in attention, concentration, and mental acuity • Does not slow progression of disease	• May cause bradycardia; monitor HR before administering • Can cause diarrhea, nausea and vomiting, and anorexia; monitor for weight loss and dehydration • Can be administered orally or via transdermal patch
Galantamine (Razadyne)	• Inhibits acetylcholinesterase, improving acetylcholinergic function • Treatment of mild to moderate AD • Modest increase in attention, concentration, and mental acuity • Does not slow progression of disease	• May cause bradycardia; monitor HR before administering • Can cause diarrhea, nausea and vomiting, and anorexia; monitor for weight loss and dehydration • Dosing is titrated over several weeks
Memantine (Namenda)	• Blocks NMDA glutamate receptors, reducing neuronal excitotoxicity • Noncompetitive antagonist of serotonin (5-HT) receptors • Antagonist of different acetylcholine receptors	• Generally well tolerated • Rare instances can cause dizziness, confusion, headache, insomnia, and agitation

AD = Alzheimer's Disease; *HR* = heart rate; *NMDA* = N-methyl-D-aspartate.

- Activities of daily living
  Patients with Alzheimer's disease can gradually lose the ability to feed, bathe, dress, and/or use the toilet themselves.
- Environment and safety
  With cognitive decline, patients may wander and are unable to assess the safety of their surroundings. Additionally, as memory declines, they may forget to take medications as prescribed.
- Coping
  The ability to cope with stress may decline, and the patient may exhibit changes in affect and mood.

▪ Actions

- Encourage/assist with feeding; provide finger foods
  The patient may forget to eat without reminders and assistance secondary to cognitive changes. Finger foods may be easier for the patient to manage and may increase caloric intake.
- Implement safety measures (including maintaining the bed in lowest position, grab bars in the bathroom, clutter-free environment, and eliminating throw rugs)
  Because of the patient's decreased awareness of the surroundings and decreased decision making, the environment must be safe to prevent falls.
- Implement routine toileting practices
  Because of cognitive decline, the patient is at increased risk of incontinence. Establishing a regular schedule of toileting decreases complications associated with incontinence.
- Place a clock and calendar in the patient's room
  Provide orientation to time and date for the patient as cognition declines.
- Provide a routine including walks and other activities
  May require reminders to perform normal ADLs secondary to cognitive decline; maximizes physical mobility and minimizes complications associated with decreased mobility.
- Speak calmly using positive statements and reassurance when the patient is agitated
  The patient may require frequent reminders. A calm approach and tone decrease escalation of the patient's agitation.
- Provide diversionary activities for the Alzheimer's disease patient
  These activities provide stimulation for the patient and facilitate engagement with others.
- Provide the caregiver/family with emotional support
  The cognitive decline of the patient is often difficult for the family to understand, especially if the patient has few other physical clinical manifestations.
- Facilitate activities during the day (no napping) to assist with sleep during the night
  Sleep disturbances may develop in the patient with Alzheimer's disease. Minimizing napping during the day promotes better sleep at night.

▪ Teaching

- Teach families how to care for the patient with Alzheimer's disease
  While the patient's dependence on others increases, the family must be capable of managing the patient's medication, treatments, ADLs, etc.

- Teach family to label all dangerous substances and items and to secure them carefully
  With deterioration in cognitive function, the patient may no longer be capable of recognizing unsafe environmental issues. The patient may not recognize dangerous items.
- Educate family on the potential for monitoring systems that will alert family members should the patient attempt to leave the home
  Provides support to the family if the patient has a tendency to wander; also promotes patient safety
- Provide referral assistance for support groups and for alternative care settings should the need arise
  Depression is common, and assistance and medication might be required.
- Provide location and contact information for support groups, the patient's provider, pharmacist, and social services
  Costs of caring for the AD patient can be very expensive. Social Security and Medicare/Medicaid assistance might be helpful to alleviate the financial stress related to the care of the patient with Alzheimer's disease.

Evaluating Care Outcomes

The diagnosis of Alzheimer's disease is frightening and stressful to both the patient and family. Patient safety and quality of life, as with other progressive neurological disorders, are priorities in the coordination and management of these patients. In addition to physical issues, there are many legal issues related to the care of these patients while their cognitive function declines. Family involvement is essential, particularly in making end-of-life decisions that are consistent with the patient's wishes.

Connection Check 36.13

The nurse recognizes that supplementation with which vitamin has been found to help with symptoms of Alzheimer's disease?

A. Vitamin A
B. Vitamin C
C. Vitamin D
D. Vitamin E

Making Connections

CASE STUDY: WRAP-UP

Postoperative day 7, Mr. Johnson is ready for discharge to acute rehabilitation. The nurse reviews all medications prescribed for Mr. Johnson with him and his wife. These medications include levetiracetam 500 mg bid, amlodipine 10 mg daily, metformin 750 mg daily, glyburide 5 mg daily, and furosemide 20 mg daily. The nurse reiterates the necessity for taking his medication as prescribed. The nurse also introduces Mrs. Johnson to the social worker, and a support group is identified to assist her in caring for herself and her husband once he returns home.

Case Study Questions

1. On Mr. Johnson's initial presentation to the clinic for headache, the nurse assesses him for which clinical manifestations of increased ICP? *(Select all that apply.)*

    A. Confusion

    B. Tachycardia

    C. Clonus

    D. Elevated blood pressure

    E. Incontinence

2. The nurse collaborates with which healthcare team member to arrange for Mr. Johnson to have a swallowing evaluation?

    A. Dental hygienist

    B. Physical therapist

    C. Occupational therapist

    D. Speech therapist

3. What is the rationale for the administration of the dexamethasone (Decadron) to Mr. Johnson postoperatively?

    A. Decreases cerebral edema

    B. Decreases blood pressure

    C. Suppresses seizure activity

    D. Suppresses neuromuscular conduction

4. On the basis of Mr. Johnson's seizure activity, the nurse implements seizure precautions. What equipment does the nurse ask the nursing assistant to place in the room?

    A. EEG machine

    B. Suction equipment

    C. Restraints

    D. Padded tongue blade

5. Which statement by Mr. Johnson indicates the need for further teaching about the levetiracetam?

    A. "I will not drink any alcoholic beverages."

    B. "I will wear a medical alert bracelet."

    C. "I will let my doctor know about all of my prescriptions."

    D. "I can skip a couple of pills if I have a stomach flu."

CHAPTER SUMMARY

Disorders of the brain are characterized by a myriad of clinical presentations that affect a person's physical and cognitive functions. Many of the disorders are chronic and degenerative with no known cure, and care coordination, quality of life, and safety are priorities of care.

Headaches are a common complaint and may represent a specific pathology secondary to different types of headache (migraine, tension, cluster, etc.), or they may be the sign of a more dangerous pathology related to increased intracranial pressure (ICP). Management of pain is largely dependent upon the etiology and a definitive diagnosis. Pain management is a priority, as well as managing triggers or exacerbating factors for headaches.

Primary brain tumors are those tumors that originate in the brain. These tumors range from slow-growing, benign tumors to highly malignant, aggressive tumors. Primary brain tumors originate from brain cells, brain meninges, nerves, and glands. Because of the diversity of these tumors, classification is difficult and is generally based on the type of brain cells involved and the location in which the cancer evolves. Initial management of brain tumors is often focused on the control of ICP and preventing secondary injury due to compression of vital structures in the brain. Metastasis of cancer from various locations in the body to the central nervous system (brain, spinal cord and CSF) is not an uncommon complication of several types of cancer and is the most common type of brain tumor. Brain tumors may be treated surgically or with chemotherapeutic agents and radiation therapy.

Seizures are uncontrolled, sudden, excessive discharge of electrical activity resulting in a range of manifestations from changes in behavior to loss of consciousness. As with headaches, seizure activity may be the primary disorder or may be secondary to changes in the brain caused by brain tumors, trauma, and infectious processes. Control of seizures requires definitive diagnosis of type of seizure and management with appropriate anticonvulsant medications or surgical intervention.

Meningitis is an inflammation of the meninges caused by bacterial infection, viral infection, or fungal infection. There is also an aseptic meningitis secondary to the use of antibiotics and nonsteroidal anti-inflammatory medications and carcinomatosis. Management of meningitis requires eradication of the infectious organism. Compliance with antibiotic therapy after discharge is a high priority.

Encephalitis is an acute inflammation of the brain, including the cerebrum, brainstem, and cerebellum. Although encephalitis is dangerous in all age groups, those who are very young (infants and children), older adults, and the immunocompromised are most at risk. All forms of encephalitis can take weeks to months to resolve and can leave the patient with debilitating neurological injury and deficits. Management of encephalitis focuses on eradication of the infectious agent or the removal of sources of antibodies causing an autoimmune encephalitis, and preventing secondary injury related to potential increased ICP.

Parkinson's disease is a progressive, neurodegenerative disease of the central nervous system manifesting primarily in motor dysfunction. It is a motor system disorder that results secondary to the loss of dopamine-producing brain cells in the substantia nigra of the basal ganglia. Because it is a progressive neuromuscular disorder that often ultimately results in loss of motor control and dependence upon others for activities of daily living, patient and family involvement in decision making about the priorities of care is essential.

Alzheimer's disease is a form of dementia involving the gradual loss of brain function, affecting memory, thinking, and behavior. It is characterized by increasing cognitive decline, leading to severe deterioration. Although conclusive evidence as to the cause of Alzheimer's does not yet exist and the definitive diagnosis of Alzheimer's is made only at autopsy, there are criteria used to establish a presumptive diagnosis. Management of this disorder is focused on slowing the progression of the disorder (if possible), along with a focus on patient safety and quality of life.

The nurse plays an essential role in the management of the patient with a disorder of the brain. Assessment and analysis of subtle changes in the patient's clinical presentation are paramount in preventing secondary and possibly irreversible damage secondary to increased ICP. Because many disorders of the brain are chronic, progressive, and debilitating, working with the family to support the patient is an important nursing role.

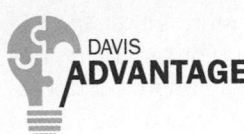

To explore learning resources for this chapter, go to **Davis Advantage** and find:
- Answers to in-text questions
- Chapter Resources and Activities
- NCLEX®-Style Chapter Review Questions
- Bibliography

Chapter 37

Coordinating Care for Patients With Spinal Cord Disorders

Lourdes Carhuapoma

LEARNING OUTCOMES

Content in this chapter is designed to assist in:

1. Describing the epidemiology of spinal cord disorders
2. Correlating clinical manifestations to the pathophysiological processes of:
   a. Low-back pain
   b. Herniated nucleus pulposus
   c. Multiple sclerosis
   d. Amyotrophic lateral sclerosis
   e. Spinal cord injury
   f. Spinal cord tumors
3. Describing the diagnostic results used to confirm spinal cord disorders
4. Discussing the management of:
   a. Low-back pain
   b. Herniated nucleus pulposus
   c. Multiple sclerosis
   d. Amyotrophic lateral sclerosis
   e. Spinal cord injury
   f. Spinal cord tumors
5. Developing a comprehensive plan of nursing care for patients with disorders of the spinal cord
6. Designing a plan of care that includes pharmacological, dietary, and lifestyle considerations for patients with disorders of the spine
7. Explaining the clinical presentation and management of complications associated with disorders of the spinal cord

ESSENTIAL TERMS

Analeptics
Anhidrosis
Annulus fibrosus
Apoptosis
Autonomic dysreflexia
Axial loading
Contralateral
Demyelination
Electromyography (EMG)
Excitotoxicity
Facet joints
Flare
Free radicals
Gardner-Wells tongs
Halo traction device
Herniation
Ipsilateral
Myelin
Neurogenic shock
Nucleus pulposus
Phrenic nerve
Radiculopathy
Sclerosis
Spinal degeneration
Spinal shock
Spinal stenosis

CONCEPTS

- Assessment
- Comfort
- Medication
- Mobility
- Neurologic Regulation
- Nursing Roles
- Oxygenation
- Perioperative
- Safety

Finding Connections

CASE STUDY: EPISODE 1

Follow this patient throughout the chapter.

Cynthia Reynolds is a 38-year-old female who presents to her primary healthcare provider with complaints of intermittent numbness in her left lower extremity and gait imbalance. She is obese with a history of poorly controlled type 1 diabetes mellitus. She is otherwise in good health and has annual check-ups with her healthcare provider. Cynthia reports that she has been trying to get into "better shape" and that she began a home exercise program approximately 3 months ago. She states that she continues to smoke but has "cut down to one-half pack a day"…

INTRODUCTION

The spinal column is the main support for the spinal cord and the nerve pathways that carry information between the brain and the rest of the body. Composed of 33 bony vertebrae, 31 pairs of spinal nerves, 40 muscles, and multiple connecting ligaments and tendons, the spinal cord runs from the base of the skull to the coccyx. The vertebral column is divided into five sections: the cervical spine, thoracic spine, lumbar spine, sacral spine, and coccyx. Between the vertebrae are intervertebral disks that are elastic, fibrous cartilage that keep the spine flexible and protect the vertebrae from injury. The intervertebral disks are the largest avascular structures in the body. The outer layer contains concentric rings of tough fibrous tissue called the **annulus fibrosus**. The central, or inner, portion consists of softer, spongier material and is called the **nucleus pulposus** (Fig. 37.1).

The spinal cord has multiple functions, including somatic (voluntary) and autonomic (involuntary) reflexes, motor control centers, and sensory and motor modulation. The spinal cord is protected by the vertebral column, the spinal meninges, and cerebrospinal fluid (CSF). The spinal meninges are composed of three membranous layers of connective tissue (Fig. 37.2). The outermost layer is the dura mater, the arachnoid is the middle layer, and the innermost layer is the pia mater. The dura mater forms a loose, protective, and nonelastic membrane. The arachnoid is composed of collagen and elastic fibers that form a weblike filmy covering of the spinal cord. The innermost layer, the pia mater, adheres to the brain and spinal cord, and provides support for blood vessels that supply nutrients and oxygen to the brain and spinal cord.

The gray matter of the spinal cord is butterfly-shaped and surrounded by white matter. This serves as the processing center by receiving and integrating information. The gray matter also contains motor neurons that control movement. The white matter surrounds the gray matter and contains the conduction tracts for nerve impulses (Fig. 37.3). These tracts of nerve fibers consist of axons. Axons are the long, thin nerve cell extensions that carry impulses away from the cell body. Most axons are covered with an insulating substance called **myelin** that allows signals to flow freely and quickly. The myelin is whitish in appearance, giving the name "white matter" to this outer section of the spinal cord. Axons carry signals in two directions, up toward the brain (ascending pathways) and down from the brain (descending pathways) within the specific nerve tracts.

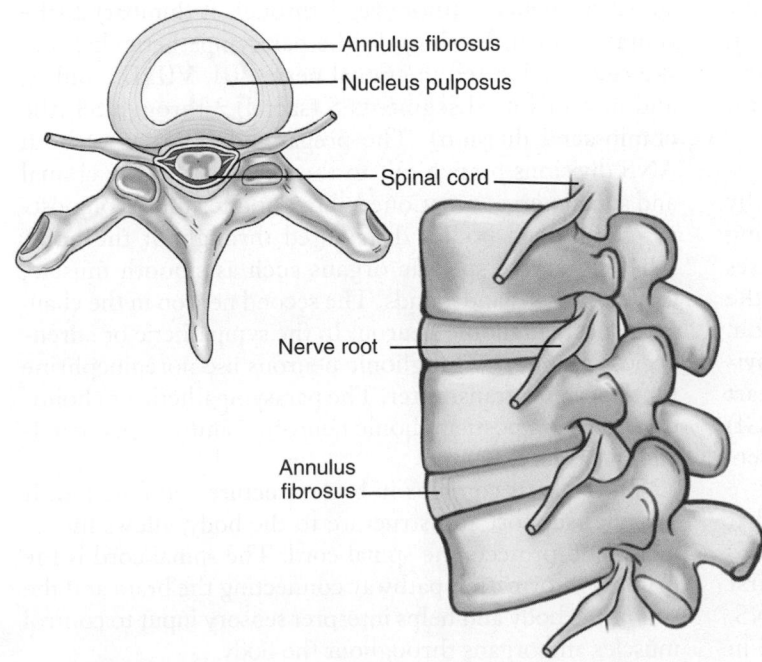

FIGURE 37.1 *A.* Intervertebral disk. *B.* Section of spinal column.

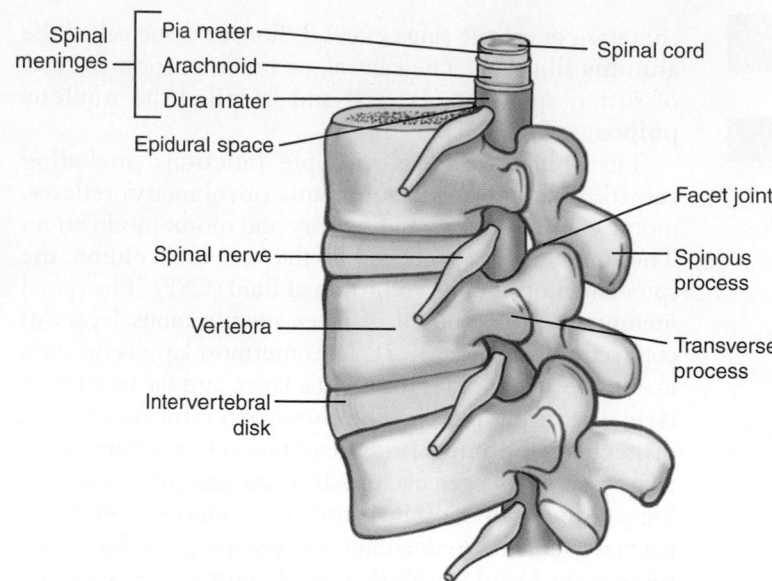

FIGURE 37.2 Spinal cord anatomy.

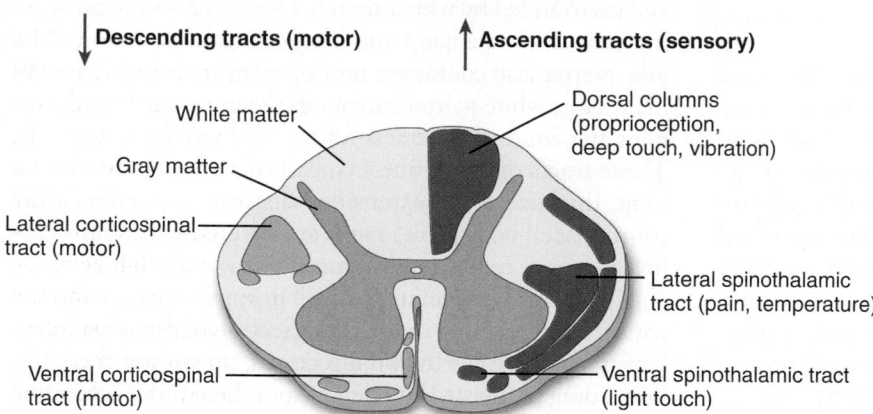

FIGURE 37.3 Spinal cord nerve tracts.

The motor nervous system is divided into the somatic and autonomic nervous systems. The somatic, or voluntary, nervous system controls skeletal muscle and external sensory organs (e.g., skin). It is called *voluntary* because most of the responses can be consciously controlled.

The autonomic nervous system (ANS) has two subdivisions. First, the *sympathetic nervous system* physiologically prepares the body to meet a crisis situation by mobilizing energy stores. The sympathetic nervous system increases the heart rate and blood pressure, dilates the pupil of the eye, shunts blood to muscles, and decreases food digestion. Second, the *parasympathetic nervous system* promotes activities to rebuild the body's energy stores. It slows the heart rate, lowers blood pressure, increases gastrointestinal (GI) tract activity, and shunts blood from the periphery to internal organs.

Both divisions of the ANS have a two-neuron chain that carries information from the central nervous system (CNS) to the periphery. The preganglionic neuron is the first neuron in the chain and has cell bodies located in the CNS. In the sympathetic division, the cell bodies are located in

spinal segments T (thoracic) 1 through L (lumbar) 2 (the thoracolumbar division). In the parasympathetic division, the cells are located in cranial nerves III, VII, IX, and X, and in spinal cord segments S (sacral) 2 through S4 (the craniosacral division). The preganglionic axons of both ANS divisions branch out to the periphery in the cranial and spinal nerves mentioned above and terminate on postganglionic cell bodies distributed throughout the body. They innervate specific organs such as smooth muscle, cardiac muscle, and glands. The second neuron in the chain is the postganglionic neuron. In the sympathetic or adrenergic division, postganglionic neurons use norepinephrine for their neurotransmitter. The parasympathetic or cholinergic division postganglionic neurotransmitter uses acetylcholine as its receptor.

The spine is complex in both structure and function. It provides support and structure to the body, allows movement, and protects the spinal cord. The spinal cord is the primary information pathway connecting the brain and the rest of the body and helps interpret sensory input to control muscles and organs throughout the body.

LOW-BACK PAIN

Epidemiology

According to the National Institute of Neurological Disorders and Stroke, back pain is the second-most common neurological ailment in the United States, equally affecting both men and women. At least 60% to 80% of the population will have an episode at least once in their lifetime. Low-back pain (LBP) often occurs between the ages of 30 and 50, with an annual cost of $50 billion per year spent on treatment alone.

Low-back pain is a common neuromuscular condition, with unpredictable patterns of exacerbation, remission, and recurrence that affect the way the condition is classified, diagnosed, and treated. In 85% of persons with LBP, no cause can be identified, making treatment plans for patients difficult. It may be time limited and harmless, or it can become a chronic condition affecting every aspect of the patient's life. For the majority of persons, LBP does not develop into a chronic, disabling condition; however, approximately 1 in 5 patients report persistent, activity-limiting back pain by 1 year after an acute episode.

Low-back pain often follows injury or trauma but may also be caused by degenerative diseases (Fig. 37.4). These conditions include but are not limited to the following: arthritis, osteoporosis, viral infections, bone diseases, or congenital abnormalities in the spine. Risk factors for LBP include obesity, cigarette smoking, poor posture, stress, poor physical condition, poor sleeping position, and occupations that require heavy lifting. Nicotine in cigarettes is thought to interfere with vital nutrient absorption by the intervertebral disks, leading to disk degeneration.

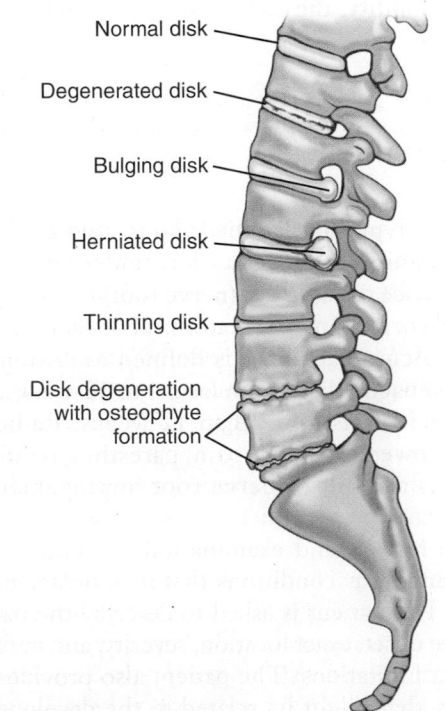

Normal disk

Degenerated disk

Bulging disk

Herniated disk

Thinning disk

Disk degeneration with osteophyte formation

FIGURE 37.4 Types of disk problems.

Connection Check 37.1

The nurse recognizes which factor as placing a patient at the greatest risk for new onset of low-back problems?
A. Sedentary lifestyle
B. Recent long-distance car trip
C. Prolonged standing
D. Cigarette smoking

Pathophysiology

The pathophysiology of LBP remains complex. **Spinal degeneration** (Fig. 37.5) is often associated with aging and involves the loss of normal structure and function of the spine. While water content of the nucleus pulposus decreases, the fibers of the annulus begin to wear out. The body's ability to lubricate facet joints decreases, and they begin to suffer from wear and tear. **Facet joints**, small joints located between and behind each adjacent vertebra, help support and restrict vertebral movement to prevent one vertebra from slipping over the one below. The upper half of the paired facet joints are attached on both sides and on the backside of each vertebra; then they extend downward and project forward or toward the side. The other halves of the joints arise on the vertebra below then project upward, facing backward to engage the downward portion of the upper facet halves. A small capsule surrounds the facet joints, providing a lubricant to the joint, allowing them to slide on each other without a lot of friction. The decrease in the body's ability to lubricate the facet joints results in damage from friction. The decreasing support of facet joints because of weak spinal ligaments also contributes to spinal degeneration. Spinal ligaments are tough bands of fibrous tissue that connect bones and joints. With age, these bands lose strength and elasticity and become more vulnerable to stretching and tearing.

Spinal stenosis refers to constriction of the spinal foramina and canals that can result in pressure on the spinal cord and nerve roots, causing pain. Spinal stenosis often develops as a result of spinal degeneration. While the disks become drier, the bones and ligaments of the spine may grow larger because of arthritis or some other form of chronic inflammation. Other causes of spinal stenosis include a previous herniated disk, spinal cord injury, congenital spinal defect, spinal tumor, or bone disease.

Another factor contributing to LBP is muscle spasm, characterized as the sudden, involuntary contraction of a single muscle or muscle group. Most back muscle spasms are caused by inflammation and soreness because of sudden movement or bending, but they can also result from age-related loss of spinal muscle strength as muscles spasm to protect the worn areas of the spine.

The acute or sudden onset of LBP acts as a warning of ongoing tissue damage. Acute pain is nociceptive and occurs

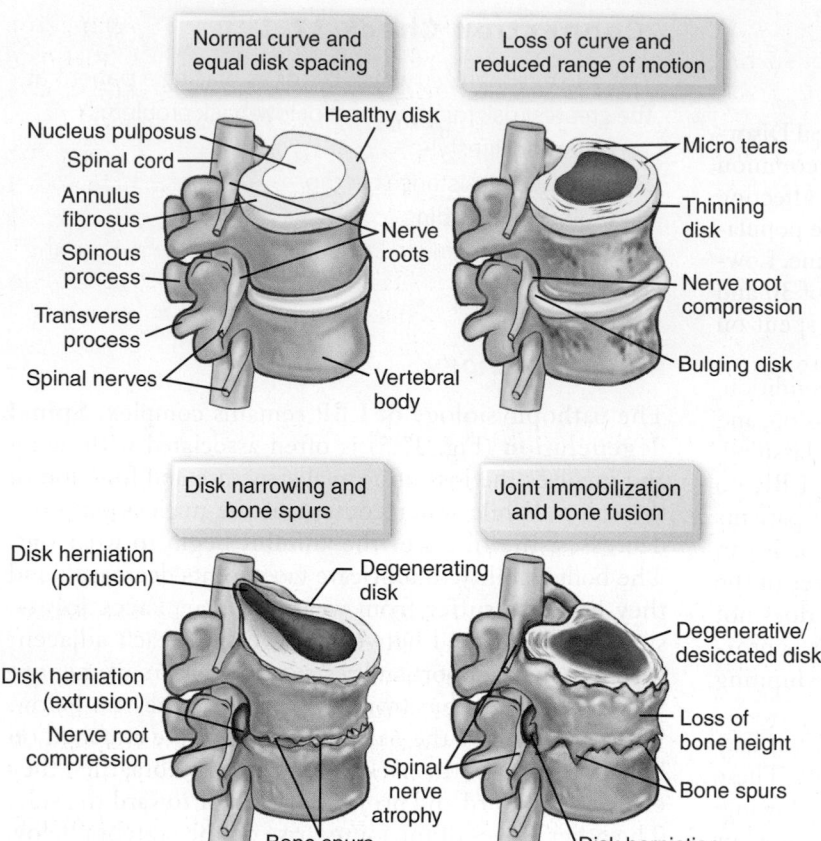

FIGURE 37.5 Spinal degeneration.

secondary to chemical, mechanical, or thermal stimulation of A-delta and C-polymodal pain receptors. Nociceptive pain is the body's normal pain response.

Multiple elements of the lumbar spine are thought to be contributing factors to LBP. Many components of the lumbar spine have sensory innervation that can generate nociceptive signals as responses to tissue-damaging stimuli. Following a nerve injury, sensitization occurs that results in a lowered threshold for activation and an increased response to stimuli. In other words, the nociceptor has an increase in discharge that leads to an increase in pain. Ectopic neuronal pacemakers have been shown to form at various sites along the nerve. They can cause abnormal firing of the nociceptor and result in increased pain. Current theory contends that abnormal or dysfunctional sodium channels are the cause of this ectopic activity. Most chronic LBP cases are thought to involve a combination of nociceptive and neuropathic etiologies. While people age, a decrease is noted in bone strength, in muscle elasticity and tone, and in the disks' ability to cushion the vertebrae.

Clinical Manifestations

The clinical presentation of LBP typically includes dull or acute pain in the lumbar region of the spine that may be exacerbated by movement. Muscle spasms may also be observed and may limit mobility. Decreases in flexibility and

stamina are also possible if pain decreases activity and the patient becomes more sedentary. If there are nerve-related problems, there may also be numbness and tingling or weakness in the leg or foot. As with many spinal disorders that decrease mobility, the patient may also complain of constipation.

Management

Medical Management

Diagnosis

Low-back pain is typically classified and treated according to the clinical manifestations, duration, underlying cause, presence or absence of radicular (nerve root) clinical manifestations, and corresponding anatomical or radiographic abnormalities. Acute back pain is defined as lasting less than 4 weeks, subacute back pain lasts 4 to 12 weeks, and chronic back pain lasts more than 12 weeks. Radicular LBP results in lower-extremity pain, paresthesias, and/or weakness and is a result of nerve root impingement or compression.

A thorough history and examination is completed to identify any dangerous conditions that may be associated with the pain. The patient is asked to describe the pain in detail giving the onset, exact location, severity, and duration with movement limitations. The patient also provides any medical history that might be related to the development of the pain. A physical examination, neurological testing such as **electromyography (EMG)** that measures the electrical impulse within muscle tissue, nerve conduction testing and evoked potentials, and various imaging studies including x-rays, computed tomography (CT), magnetic resonance imaging (MRI), bone scans, or myelograms may be ordered to determine a definitive diagnosis (Table 37.1).

Nonpharmacological and Pharmacological Treatment

Low-back pain treatment options include non-pharmacological and pharmacological interventions. Non-pharmacological treatments include, but are not limited to exercise therapy, superficial heat, acupuncture, massage therapy, meditation/yoga and other complementary and alternative medicine interventions. Pharmacological treatments include acetaminophen, NSAIDS, skeletal muscle relaxants, opioids, systemic corticosteroids, tricyclic antidepressants, and benzodiazepines.

For acute pain or subacute LBP, nonpharmacological treatment options, such as superficial heat and massage therapy, are considered first-line treatment options because acute or subacute LBP is often self-limiting (Box 37.1). For those with acute or subacute LBP unresponsive to nonpharmacological treatment options, nonopioid over-the-counter medications, such as NSAIDs, help reduce swelling and inflammation and may also decrease mild to moderate pain. Nonpharmacological treatment options, such as exercise, interprofessional rehabilitation, acupuncture, or mindfulness-based strategies, are first-line treatment options for patients with chronic LBP pain. In patients with chronic LBP unresponsive to nonpharmacological treatments, NSAIDS are first-line treatment. Muscle relaxants may be prescribed by a healthcare provider to help reduce pain. Medications that block sodium channels may also help reduce pain and include lidocaine, anticonvulsants, and tricyclic antidepressants (Table 37.2). Opioids such as codeine, oxycodone, hydrocodone, and morphine are reserved for the relief of severe pain.

Surgical Management

Other treatments include:

- Interventional therapy – nerve blocks with local anesthetics, steroids, and narcotics injected into affected areas
- Transcutaneous electrical nerve stimulation – mild electrical impulses are sent along nerve fibers to block pain signals to the brain
- Back surgery – if pain is caused by serious spinal pathology related to radicular or spinal cord compression (surgical procedures discussed later in chapter with management of herniated nucleus pulposus.)

Often a combination of medications and adjunctive therapy is used to successfully treat LBP.

Table 37.1 Tests Used to Determine Causes of Spinal Cord Disorders

Test	Definition
Computed tomography (CT scan)	X-rays are passed through the back at different angles, detected by a scanner, and analyzed by a computer. This produces a series of cross-dimensional images that show the shape and size of the spinal canal, its contents, and surrounding structures. This is optimal in visualizing bony structures.
Diskogram	An opaque dye is injected into suspected disks, pictures are taken, and the patient's reaction and image help determine the disk's status.
Magnetic resonance imaging (MRI)	Energy from a powerful magnet produces signals that are detected by a scanner and analyzed by a computer. The resulting cross-sectional images of the spine show the spinal cord, nerve roots, and surrounding spaces. An MRI is optimal in detecting soft tissue damage or disease (e.g., disks between vertebrae or ligaments)
Electromyography	Tests to measure the electrical impulse within muscle tissue. This test indicates if there is old nerve damage that is healing or ongoing nerve injury and findings correlate to the site of damage.
Nerve conduction study	Test to measure the electrical nerve impulse that indicates damage to the nerve. Electrodes are placed on the skin over a nerve that supplies a specific muscle or group. A mild, brief stimulus is delivered through the electrode, and the signal strength and muscle response are measured.
Myelogram	A dye is injected into the spinal column, and an x-ray is taken. This can show pressure on the spinal cord or nerves from herniated disks, tumors, or bone spurs. This procedure requires a lumbar puncture to inject the contrast dye.
X-rays	Radiation beam is passed through the back to produce a two-dimensional picture. X-rays show the structure of the vertebrae and joint outlines.

Box 37.1 Complementary and Alternative Medicine Practices to Treat Low-Back Pain

- Acupuncture – Insertion of small needles or exerting pressure on "energy" points in the body; the patient is supposed to experience a feeling of fullness, numbness, tingling, and warmth.
- Biofeedback – People are trained to control certain bodily processes (heart rate, muscle tension, blood pressure) to improve their health.
- Meditation/Yoga – These can be used as part of a general health regimen, to cope with illness, to improve physiological balance, or to increase relaxation. Techniques include physical postures and breathing techniques, with either a focused attention or an open attitude toward distractions.
- Massage therapy – Consists of alternating levels of concentrated pressure on the areas of spasm; once pressure is applied, it should not vary for 10 to 30 seconds. Massage also leads to increased endorphin levels (chemicals associated with decreased pain and increased euphoria) that are effective in chronic pain management.
- Energy healing therapies – Magnet and light therapy – based on the manipulation of veritable (measurable) energy fields to affect health
- Qi gong – An ancient Chinese discipline involving physical and mental exercises that focus on specific parts of the body
- Whole medical systems that are part of complementary and alternative medicine have evolved over time in different cultures; these include traditional Chinese medicine and Ayurvedic medicine

Nursing Management

Assessment and Analysis

The type, severity, and location of clinical findings associated with LBP are directly related to the underlying cause. This includes pain developing from muscle sprain or strain, nerve root pressure, or arthritis. Clinical findings include:

- Pain in the lower back that may radiate to the extremities
- Numbness and tingling in the extremity (with nerve root injury)
- Muscle spasms
- Decreased mobility/range of motion (ROM)

A thorough evaluation including history and physical examination is completed to identify the cause of LBP.

Nursing Diagnoses

- **Acute pain** related to inflammation, swelling, and strained muscles
- **Impaired mobility** related to pain or discomfort
- **Risk for impaired bowel elimination** related to decreased mobility

Nursing Interventions

Assessments

- Vital signs
  Evaluate for hemodynamic signs of pain including tachycardia, hypertension, and tachypnea.
- Pain
  Pain is secondary to inflammation, swelling, and strained muscles.

Table 37.2 Medications Used to Treat Low-Back Pain

Class of Medication	Examples	Mechanism of Action
Anticonvulsants	Gabapentin (Neurontin), pregabalin (Lyrica), topiramate (Topamax), carbamazepine (Tegretol)	Not proven but are thought to block the sodium channels and decrease formation of ectopic neuronal pacemakers
Tricyclic antidepressants	Amitriptyline (Elavil), nortriptyline (Pamelor), imipramine (Tofranil)	Thought to block the sodium channels and to decrease formation of ectopic neuronal pacemakers
Local anesthetics	Lidocaine	Same as tricyclics
NSAIDs	Aspirin, ibuprofen, ketorolac tromethamine (Toradol), naproxen	Block COX enzymes and prostaglandins throughout the body, thereby decreasing pain and inflammation
Corticosteroids	Prednisone, cortisone, hydrocortisone	They mimic the effects of hormones produced in the adrenal glands; they decrease inflammation by blocking the production of substances that trigger allergic and inflammatory reactions (e.g., prostaglandins)
Opioids	Morphine, codeine, oxycodone	Block the perception of pain by attaching to proteins (opioid receptors) found in the brain, spinal cord and GI tract
Muscle relaxants	Cardisoprodol (Soma), cyclobenzaprine (Flexeril), methocarbamol (Robaxin), metazalone (Skelexin), diazepam (Valium)	Depress the CNS

CNS = Central nervous system; *COX* = cyclooxygenase; *GI* = gastrointestinal.

- Mobility
  Determining how mobility/activities of daily living (ADLs) are affected by pain is important baseline information to follow as different interventions are initiated.
- Numbness and tingling in extremities
  *Low back pain secondary to nerve root compression (**radiculopathy**) causes numbness and tingling in the affected extremities.*
- Bowel function
  Immobility and side effects of some pain medications increase the chance of constipation that can exacerbate pain if the patient strains with defecation.

▩ Actions

- Administer pain medications (see Table 37.2)
  Blocks the perception of pain
- Administer anti-inflammatory medications (see Table 37.2)
  Reduces inflammation and pain to help increase mobility
- ROM
  Increases muscle strength and reduces pain by stretching and strengthening the muscles
- Administer stool softeners as needed
  Decreased mobility, as well as the side effects of some pain medications, increases the risk of constipation. Straining with bowel movements can exacerbate the LBP.
- Increase fluid intake
  Facilitates normal bowel elimination that may be impacted by immobility and side effects of pain medications

▩ Teaching

- Low-back exercises
  Stretching and strengthening muscles facilitates reduction of pain and minimizes future injury. Abdominal strengthening also decreases stress and strain on the low back.
- Take medications as prescribed
  To decrease pain peaks and help promote activity levels
- Nonpharmacological pain relief measures (see Box 37.1)
  To help resume normal functioning without use of medications that can affect thinking and behavior
- Weight control
  Being overweight adds additional stress to back muscles, so being at ideal body weight may decrease pain and complications associated with LBP.

Evaluating Care Outcomes

Patients with LBP can often resume normal functioning with proper treatment, including medications and lifestyle changes such as exercise. Medications are used short term to relieve pain and inflammation, and lifestyle changes are initiated to help decrease the risk of future episodes of LBP. Proper posture, exercise, and use of body mechanics during exercise and work help reduce the patient's risk of re-injury. If the patient experiences clinical manifestations of back pain, these should be reported to the primary care provider.

HERNIATED NUCLEUS PULPOSUS

Epidemiology

While people age, the disks between the vertebrae degenerate and weaken, and the disk becomes more inflexible and more prone to tearing or rupturing with movement. **Herniation**, or leaking out of the interior disk contents into the vertebral areas, is a major cause of severe chronic and recurrent back pain. Ninety percent of herniations occur at the lumbar segments of the spine, especially L4 through L5 and L5 through S1. Herniated disks are most common between age 30 and 45, with males more commonly affected in lumbar disk herniation by a 3:2 ratio. Rarely, a traumatic event such as a fall or a blow to the back can cause a herniated disk. Factors that increase the risk of a herniated disk include age, gender, obesity, smoking, and occupation. Genetics are also suspected of playing a role in disk herniation. Other risk factors include repetitive lifting, pulling, pushing, bending sideways, and twisting. Pain is usually greatest when sitting and decreases when standing.

Pathophysiology

A herniated disk occurs when a weakening of or a tear in the outer fibrous ring (annulus fibrosus) of the intervertebral disk allows the central soft component (nucleus pulposus) to bulge or to be extruded (herniate) outside the disk (Fig. 37.6). Intervertebral disk deterioration occurs over a lifetime as the water-retaining ability of the nucleus pulposus declines. This leads to stiffening of the disk and to the annulus weakening. Herniation of nuclear material into the spinal canal is associated with a significant inflammatory response. Acute nerve root compression, radiculopathy, is responsible for dysfunction, and the type of nerve compressed (motor or sensory) determines the clinical manifestations the patient experiences such as pain, weakness, or numbness.

Clinical Manifestations

Patients with herniated nucleus pulposus typically present with pain caused by the inflammatory process as well as compression to nerve roots. Radiculopathy is nerve root compression and can result in numbness in the affected extremity as well as pain, weakness, and inability to control motor movement in the affected area. The location of the radicular signs can be correlated to the respective dermatome distribution of the spinal nerves.

Connection Check 37.2

In completing the history and physical assessment of a patient with back pain, which finding is most suggestive of a herniated nucleus pulposus?

A. Constipation
B. Numbness in left lower extremity
C. Hyperactive reflexes
D. Hematuria

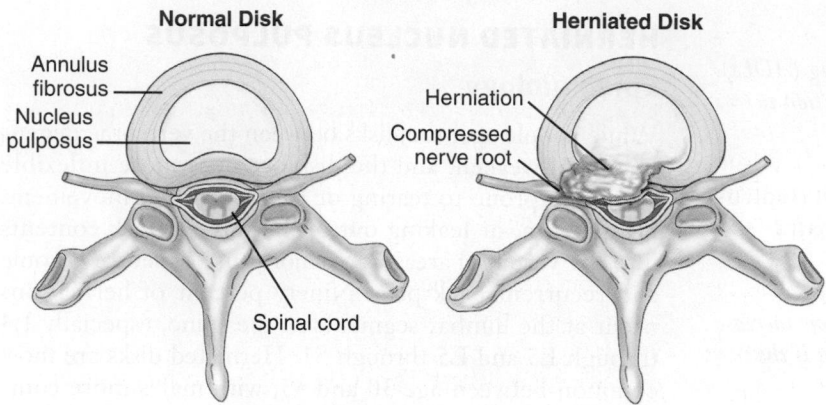

Normal Disk

Annulus fibrosus
Nucleus pulposus

Spinal cord

Herniated Disk

Herniation
Compressed nerve root

FIGURE 37.6 Comparison of normal and herniated disks.

Management

Medical Management

Diagnosis

The healthcare provider performs a complete history and physical, with a focused neurological examination to test reflexes, muscle strength, gait, and the patient's ability to feel touch and vibration. Tests used in diagnosing the herniated disk include imaging studies such as x-rays, CT scans, MRIs, and myelograms. Additional neurological tests used to pinpoint the location of the nerve damage are EMG and nerve conduction studies. See Table 37.1 for full explanations of diagnostic tests.

Treatment

Most patients with a herniated disk show improvement with 1 to 2 months of conservative treatment. This consists of avoiding painful positions and following a regimen of planned exercise and pain medications. Specific exercises include spinal stretching and strengthening, abdominal strengthening, pelvic tilts, and hip stretching. If obesity is a contributing factor, weight loss measures are also indicated.

Medications, including over-the-counter NSAIDs, muscle relaxants, sedatives-tranquilizers, and nerve pain medications such as gabapentin (Neurontin), pregabalin (Lyrica), duloxetine (Cymbalta), and tramadol (Ultram, Ryzolt) and amitriptyline (Elavil) often help relieve pain related to nerve damage. Because of their milder side effects, nerve pain medications are increasingly used as first-line prescription medications for people with herniated disks. Muscle relaxants such as diazepam or cyclobenzaprine also may be prescribed for muscle spasms. Finally, corticosteroids may be given orally or injected directly into the area around the spinal nerves to reduce inflammation and decrease pain.

Physical therapy is used to improve pain and to strengthen muscles. The patient is shown positions and exercises designed to minimize the pain of a herniated disk. While the pain improves, physical therapy advances to a rehabilitation phase of core strength and stability to maximize back health and help protect against future injury. Therapy recommendations include heat or ice, traction, ultrasound, neck or low-back bracing, or electrical stimulation.

Interventions for a herniated disk may be conservative or surgical. Medical management focuses on pain relief, improving function, and preventing future injury. Only approximately 10% of people with herniated disks eventually need surgery to relieve pressure on nerve roots and to stabilize the spine. Surgery is often recommended if the following occurs:

- Conservative treatment fails to improve clinical manifestations.
- Progressive neurological deficits such as weakness develop.
- Problems standing or walking
- Loss of bowel or bladder function

Surgical Management

Several surgical options are used in the treatment of a herniated disk. One procedure is a *laminotomy*, which opens the lamina to decrease pressure on the compressed nerve root or spinal cord. During a *microdiskectomy*, the disk is removed to relieve pressure on the spine or nerve root, and this is often performed as a minimally invasive procedure or in conjunction with a *laminectomy* or partial laminectomy. The partial laminectomy is the surgical removal of part of the lamina and posterior arch of the vertebra. A laminectomy is the surgical removal of the lamina and part of the posterior arch of the vertebra. These procedures are done to remove pressure on the spinal cord or nerve roots and, when done along with the *diskectomy*, to allow the surgeon a better view of the herniated disk. Laminectomies are most commonly used to treat spinal stenosis but can be used to treat other processes such as a herniated disk, traumatic injury, and tumors.

A developing alternative to the diskectomy is artificial disk replacement that involves the surgeon using a manufactured disk to replace a diseased disk. This provides pain relief and restores motion without compromising the spine's anatomical structure.

Spinal fusion is surgery that joins two bones (vertebrae) together. Because fusing permanently joins the two bones together, there is no longer movement between them. Spinal fusion is usually performed along with other surgical procedures such as laminectomy and diskectomy to provide spinal stability. In a spinal fusion, a bone graft (often from the pelvis) or metal hardware is used to join the vertebrae together (Fig. 37.7).

Bone grafts may be obtained from several different places. First, a bone graft from the patient's own body is called an *autograft*. A bone graft may also be obtained from a bone bank. The bone bank is a facility for collecting and storing donated human bone for use in patients requiring a bone *allograft* (bone transplantation between two unrelated people). The third and least common type of graft is the use of a synthetic bone substitute.

Currently, there are several different ways to fuse vertebrae together; bone graft material may be placed over the back part of the spine or placed between the vertebrae, or tiny, hollow metal cages may be placed into the disk space. The cage is filled with the bone graft or a spongelike material that promotes bone growth. Over time, the bone grows through the holes in and around the cage, fusing the vertebrae together. Finally, the vertebrae are often stabilized with instrumentation such as rods, plates, and screws. This decreases movement of the vertebrae and allows the bone grafts to fully heal. Lumbar fusion remains the "gold standard" for treating patients with LBP who have not been helped by conservative measures.

Complications

Because a herniated disk often results in pain or loss of function from mechanical nerve root compression, complications vary depending on the location of the herniated disk. Common complications include:

- Numbness (paresthesias) and weakness
- Loss of bowel and bladder control
- Increased pain - back, arm, leg, neck
- Saddle anesthesia - progressive loss of sensation around areas that would touch a saddle (inner thighs, back of legs, and around the rectum)
- Chronic pain

The development of any of the above complications may require surgical intervention to prevent permanent loss of function.

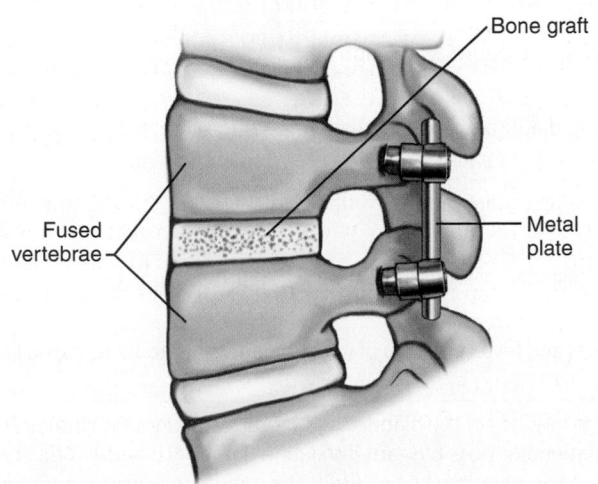

FIGURE 37.7 Lumbar spinal fusion.

Bone graft

Fused vertebrae

Metal plate

Nursing Management

Assessment and Analysis

Clinical manifestations of herniated nucleus pulposus vary depending on the location of the herniated disk. Clinical findings include:

- No symptoms at all
- Arm or leg pain
- Numbness or tingling
- Muscle weakness
- Neck pain
- Extreme constant back pain that shoots down an arm or leg (radicular pain)

Often the pain occurs on one side of the body and may vary widely from a dull ache to a burning or pulsating sensation or a sharp, shooting feeling.

Nursing Diagnoses

- **Pain** related to nerve compression by the protruding disk
- **Impaired physical mobility** related to pain or neuromuscular impairment secondary to the nerve compression and inflammation
- **Self-care deficit** related to pain and physical restrictions secondary to surgical management of herniation of the nucleus pulposus (HNP)
- **Impaired home maintenance** related to pain or physical limitations due to nerve compression, inflammation, or postoperative restrictions

Nursing Interventions

▪ *Assessments*

- Vital signs
  Assess for hemodynamic signs of pain including tachycardia, hypertension, and tachypnea. In patients after back surgery (laminectomy and/or diskectomy), temperature is assessed because elevation may develop related to infection or decreased fluid deficit.
- Pain
  Pain is secondary to compression of the nerve roots by the protruding disk.
- Level of function/mobility
  Baseline of how ADLs/mobility is affected because of pain, or numbness and weakness associated with impaired innervation to muscles
- Muscle tone and strength
  Because of pain, the patient may decrease use of the affected extremity, leading to loss of muscle tone and strength.
- Bowel elimination
  Decreased mobility, as well as side effects of opioid medications, increase the risk of constipation.
- Surgical incision
  The surgical incision needs to be evaluated for approximation, inflammation, and redness that may indicate a postoperative complication
- Urine output
  POUR (postoperative urinary retention) may develop in patients after back surgery due to impaired innervation or

side effects of anesthesia. This complication increases the patient's risk of urinary tract infection and urosepsis.

■ Actions

- Give pain medications as prescribed (see Table 37.2)
  Pain medications are indicated to promote comfort.
- Administer corticosteroids as prescribed
  Corticosteroids decrease the inflammatory process and decrease swelling in the affected area.
- Position of comfort
  Positioning the patient with head of bed elevated 30 – 45 degrees with knees bent helps to decrease strain on back muscles.
- Encourage ROM exercises
  To increase function, prevent contractures, and strengthen core muscle groups
- Increase fluid intake and fiber
  Increasing fluids and high-fiber food decreases the risk of developing constipation.

■ Teaching

- Importance of exercise and mobility
  Core muscle strengthening helps stabilize and support the spine.
- Good posture
  Helps decrease pressure on the spine and disks that will reduce the possibility of reinjury
- Avoid bending at the waist and bend knees with a straight back when lifting

Bending at the waist when lifting can place additional stress on the area of herniation and increase pain. Bending at the knees with the back straight uses the leg muscles to lift and decreases strain on the back muscles.

- Avoid lifting, pulling or pushing objects greater than 5 pounds
  Decreases strain on surgical site and allows bone healing in patients after spinal fusion.
- Review disease process and prognosis
  Helps increase understanding and enhances ability to make informed choices

Table 37.3 provides an overview of postoperative nursing management for patients after laminectomy, diskectomy, or spinal fusion.

Evaluating Care Outcomes

Most patients have improvement with conservative therapy within 2 months. These patients may need to adopt lifestyle changes to prevent re-injury of the spine. The lifestyle changes include a healthy diet, exercise to improve core strength and stability, smoking cessation, and the use of good body mechanics at both work and home. Patients who do require surgical intervention still must make lifestyle changes but must also face the added risks that come from having surgery. Some postsurgical patients may experience a prolonged recovery period before resuming activity levels that were present prior to the herniation and surgery. Most patients recover and go on to lead active lives.

Table 37.3 Nursing Interventions for Surgery for Herniated Nucleus Pulposus

Intervention	Rationales
Assess respiratory status	Changes in respiratory rate and effort may indicate ventilatory impairment.
Monitor vital signs	Hemodynamic signs of pain and hemorrhage include tachycardia, hypotension, tachypnea.
Monitor neurological status	To detect early and subtle changes in motor and sensory examination
Assess pain	Pain occurs secondary to compression of nerve roots and postoperative swelling at site.
Inspect surgical site	To detect signs of infection, hemorrhage, or CSF leak
Maintain the body in good alignment	Promotes stabilization of the surgical site to optimize function
Assist with turning, coughing, and deep breathing	Because of muscle weakness or lack of diaphragmatic innervation, assistance is needed to remove secretions.
Encourage range-of-motion exercises	Increase function, promote strengthening of core muscle groups, and decrease risk of contracture development
Teach importance of following activity level	Dependent on level of injury and stabilization of injured site to prevent further damage
Teach clinical manifestations of infection	Redness, drainage, swelling at the site, and fever are signs of infection and need to be reported to the provider for evaluation and treatment.
Implement bladder and bowel training	Damage to nerves that coordinate the muscles of the bladder and urethra and urination impairs function (urinary retention); assess patient for possible catheterization to empty bladder. Bowel movements may occur on a reflexive basis when the bowel is full. The patient may also experience a permanently relaxed bowel that results in inability to initiate own bowel movement.

CSF = Cerebrospinal fluid.

MULTIPLE SCLEROSIS

Epidemiology

Multiple sclerosis (MS) is a chronic neurological disorder in which the nerves of the CNS (brain and spinal cord) degenerate. The disorder derives its name from the build-up of scar tissue (**sclerosis**) or plaques that form during **demyelination** (destruction of myelin sheath). Multiple sclerosis is classified as an autoimmune disease, in which the immune system mistakenly identifies normal body substances and tissues as foreign and attacks them. Approximately 400,000 people in the United States have MS, with typical onset between 20 and 50 years. It affects more women than men and twice as many Caucasians as any other group. Other risk factors include a positive family history, immunological factors, and certain viral infections. There is a higher prevalence of MS in colder, more northern latitudes.

There are four main types of MS:

1. **Relapsing-remitting:** The most common form of MS, it affects twice as many women as men (typically in their 20s and 30s). Characterized by relapses (exacerbations) during which new clinical manifestations appear and old ones worsen or reappear, these relapses can last days or months. Relapses are followed by periods of remission during which the patient has either a partial or total recovery; this can be slow or almost instantaneous.
2. **Secondary progressive:** The patient who initially had relapsing-remitting develops gradual worsening of the disease. In the early phase, the patient still may experience relapses, but these will progress into a general deterioration. Although some improvement may be seen after a relapse, no real recovery occurs.
3. **Progressive relapsing:** Progressive course with a gradual worsening of clinical manifestations from onset, and the relapses may or may not have recovery.
4. **Primary progressive:** Gradual progression with no remissions; however, there may be temporary plateaus. This form affects men and women equally and typically occurs in the late 30s and early 40s. Initial disease activity is in the spinal cord, not the brain, so these patients are less likely to develop cognitive problems.

Pathophysiology

Myelin is the protective sheath that covers the spinal cord and nerves. It not only protects the nerve, but it also helps the impulses travel along the nerves at a faster rate. These impulses control muscle movements, as well as transmitting sensory data. The CNS contains the blood–brain barrier that separates circulating blood from the brain's extracellular fluid. The barrier is composed of tight junctions between endothelial cells in the CNS vessels that restrict the passage of solutes from the bloodstream. Demyelination is the loss of the myelin sheath (Fig. 37.8). It begins with a breakdown of the blood–brain barrier that allows immune cells (T lymphocytes) to infiltrate and attack the myelin. In MS, the immune system attacks the brain and spinal cord (CNS).

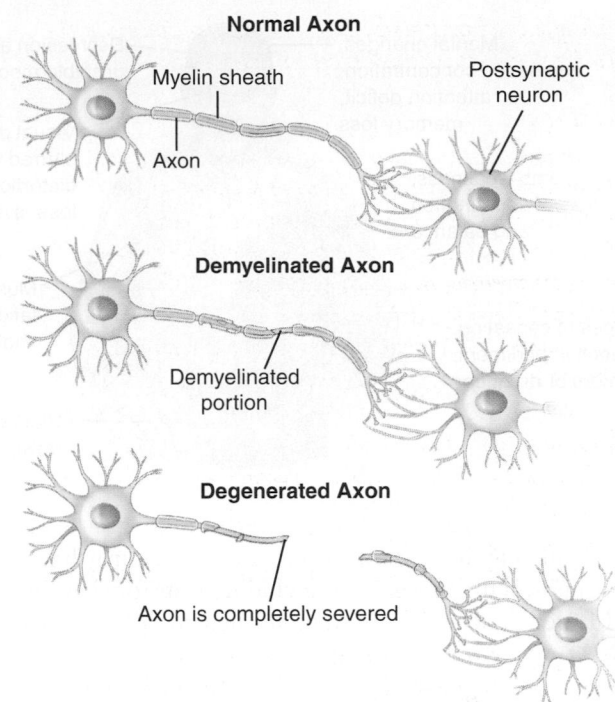

FIGURE 37.8 Comparison of normal and demyelinated axons.

Clinical Manifestations

The resulting inflammation in MS destroys the myelin, resulting in impaired sensation, movement, and thinking. Although nerves can regain myelin, this process occurs more slowly than deterioration in MS. The clinical manifestations and severity are due to the extent of demyelination and the location of scar tissue. Nerve conduction is slowed or irregular due to loss of myelin that facilitates impulse transmission. Depending on the location of the affected nerve fibers, a wide variety of clinical manifestations (Fig. 37.9) may be exhibited, including:

- Numbness or weakness in one or more limbs
- Partial or complete vision loss, often with pain during eye movement (optic neuritis)
- Double or blurred vision
- Tingling or pain
- Electric-shock sensations that occur with head movements
- Tremor, lack of coordination, or unsteady gait
- Fatigue
- Dizziness

Management

Medical Management

Diagnosis

Because clinical manifestations can be intermittent or mimic other diseases and there is no specific test for MS, it can be difficult to diagnose. Therefore, a patient may not be diagnosed for months to years after onset of clinical manifestations. The diagnosis is ultimately made by ruling out conditions with similar clinical presentations. A detailed history, physical, and neurological examination are performed. Blood samples are sent to the laboratory to rule out

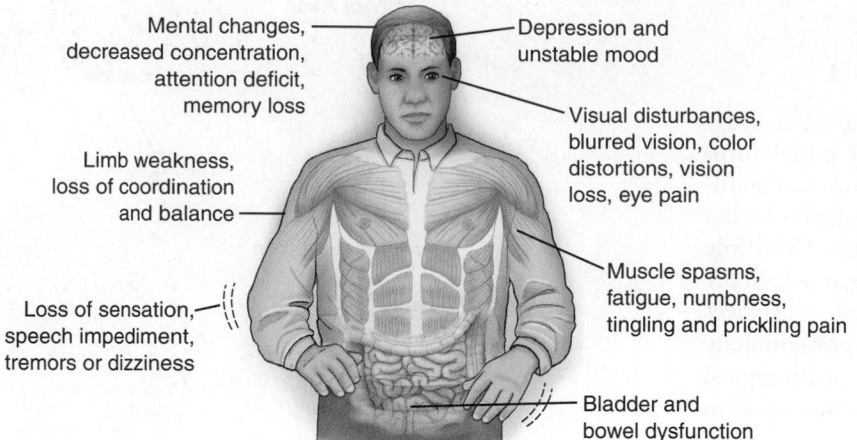

Mental changes, decreased concentration, attention deficit, memory loss

Depression and unstable mood

Visual disturbances, blurred vision, color distortions, vision loss, eye pain

Limb weakness, loss of coordination and balance

Muscle spasms, fatigue, numbness, tingling and prickling pain

Loss of sensation, speech impediment, tremors or dizziness

Bladder and bowel dysfunction

FIGURE 37.9 Clinical manifestations of multiple sclerosis.

other inflammatory or infectious diseases that may have the same clinical manifestations, including tests for vitamin B_{12} and E deficiencies, Lyme titer, antineutrophilic antibodies (ANAs) for autoimmune diseases, angiotensin-converting enzyme for sarcoidosis, HIV/HTLV (human T-lymphotropic virus), erythrocyte sedimentation rate (ESR) for inflammation, rapid plasma reagin (RPR) for neurosyphilis, anticardiolipin antibodies, and lupus anticoagulant for coagulopathy/vascular conditions. A lumbar puncture is often performed to send a CSF sample to be tested for abnormal levels of white blood cells (WBCs) or proteins and to help rule out other causes of these clinical manifestations such as viral infections. Other diagnostic tests include MRI scans to identify brain lesions (plaques), electrophysiological tests, and evoked potentials to examine how quickly impulses are traveling through the nerves. For a definitive diagnosis, the patient must have at least two separate symptomatic events or MRI changes in at least two separate locations.

Treatment

There is no cure for MS. Treatment often focuses on improving the speed of recovery from attacks, reducing the number of attacks, and slowing the progression of the disease. Lifestyle management includes adequate rest, exercise, staying cool, eating a healthy, balanced diet, and relieving stress, because these can all trigger an exacerbation or flare of MS.

Medical management focuses on several areas. First, medications used to modify the disease course include beta interferons (interferon beta-1a [Avonex, Betaseron, and Rebif] and interferon beta-1b [Extavia]), glatiramer (Copaxone), fingolimod (Gilenya), and immunosuppressive agents such as natalizumab (Tysabri) and mitoxantrone (Novantrone). These medications are used to slow the progression of the disease. Second, strategies used to treat attacks include corticosteroids and plasma exchange (plasmapheresis) to decrease the inflammatory and immunologic factors involved in the exacerbation. The final focus is on medications used to treat clinical manifestations. Muscle relaxants such as baclofen (Lioresal and Kemstro) and tizanidine (Zanaflex) decrease spasticity. Physical therapy is used to help strengthen muscles and improve daily function. Medications may also

be prescribed to help reduce fatigue and to treat depression, pain, and bladder or bowel problems. Medications used in the treatment of MS are listed in Table 37.4.

Connection Check 37.3

The nurse correlates which diagnostic result as most conclusive of a diagnosis of MS?
A. MRI changes in at least two separate locations
B. Elevated ESR
C. Elevated WBC
D. Decreased CSF protein levels

CASE STUDY: EPISODE 2

During the assessment, the healthcare provider notes that Cynthia has left lower extremity numbness and previously unnoticed weakness. This is affecting her balance, causing gait ataxia. The healthcare provider also notices increased reflexes in Cynthia's left arm and leg and visual changes in her right eye. An MRI of the brain and spinal cord is ordered to reveal any CNS process that may be present. Because Cynthia has poorly controlled diabetes and because of her upper motor neuron signs (increased reflexes) and leg weakness, the healthcare provider also wants to rule out amyotrophic lateral sclerosis (ALS) as a potential cause of Cynthia's current deficits.

The MRI of the brain and spinal cord reveals lesions or plaques associated with MS. The healthcare provider then orders blood tests and a lumbar puncture to send CSF for testing to rule out other inflammatory or infectious processes. All of these results are normal. Cynthia's CSF results demonstrate increased immunoglobulin G (IgG) synthesis rate and IgG index, which indicate increased rate of IgG production and higher levels when compared to serum levels. These increased IgG levels signify an inflammatory process (MS, infection, cancer, etc.) is occurring within the CNS. Cynthia's

CSF results also show a slight increase in protein and a normal WBC count. The results indicate possible MS.

At her follow-up appointment, the healthcare provider discusses the test results with Cynthia. She is informed that she may have MS, but for a definitive diagnosis, the patient must have at least two separate symptomatic events or MRI changes in at least two separate locations. She has started physical therapy twice a week and reports that her symptoms have improved, and her balance is better. Cynthia has been trying to reduce stress and has continued to lose weight by following a healthy diabetic diet and a supervised exercise program with a trainer at a local gym. She has had several months without any further deficits developing...

Complications

Because MS affects nerves throughout the body, complications can vary. These clinical manifestations may have periods of worsening and have a recovery period with some improvement. Common complications include:

- Muscle stiffness or spasms
- Paralysis, often in the legs
- Problems with bladder, bowel, or sexual function
- Mental status changes – memory loss, problems concentrating
- Depression
- Seizures

Other complications include pressure injuries resulting from immobility, skin breakdown caused by bowel and bladder incontinence, ataxic gait caused by weakness and

Table 37.4 Medications Used to Treat Multiple Sclerosis

Class	Examples	Mechanism of Action
Immunomodulator	Interferon beta-1a (Avonex, Rebif)	Alters the immune response by reducing the body's ability to make antibodies; these antibodies are what attack the myelin; therefore, this slows the attack on myelin and slows disease progression.
Immunomodulator	Interferon beta-1b (Betaseron, Extavia)	See above
Immunomodulator – synthetic protein	Glatiramer (Copaxone), fingolimod (Gilenya)	See above Gilenya is the first oral immunomodulator approved for MS.
Immunosuppressants	Natalizumab (Tysabri), mitoxantrone (Novantrone)	Suppresses body's immune response to prevent leukocytes from attacking each other
Muscle relaxant and antispasmodic	Baclofen (Lioresal, Kemstro), tizanidine (Zanaflex)	Depress CNS to reduce pain and inhibit reflexes at the spinal level to decrease muscle spasm
Corticosteroids	Prednisone, cortisone, hydrocortisone, methylprednisolone sodium succinate (Solu-Medrol)	Mimic the effects of hormones produced in the adrenal glands; decrease inflammation by blocking the production of substances that trigger allergic and inflammatory reactions (e.g., prostaglandins)
Anticholergic; antispasmodics	Oxybutynin chloride (Ditropan)	Inhibits transmission of impulses through parasympathetic nerve fibers
Analeptics	Modafinil (Provigil), Armodafinil (Nuvigil)	Alter neurotransmitters to improve wakefulness
Anticonvulsants	Phenytoin (Dilantin), gabapentin (Neurontin), pregabalin (Lyrica), topiramate (Topamax), carbamazepine (Tegretol)	Not proven but are thought to block the sodium channels and decrease formation of ectopic neuronal pacemakers
Stool softeners	Docusate (Colace)	Absorb water in the large intestine, increasing the bulk of the stool
Antimuscarinics	Tolterodine (Detrol)	Reduces bladder spasms by inhibiting acetylcholine
Laxatives – osmotic	Milk of magnesia, Miralax, lactulose	Pull fluids into the intestine from other tissue and blood vessels; the extra fluid makes the stool softer and easier to pass.
Laxatives – stimulant	Correctol, Dulcolax, Senokot	Irritates the intestinal lining and speeds up how quickly stool moves through the intestines

CNS = Central nervous system; *MS* = multiple sclerosis.

loss of position sense in the legs. Speech defects caused by muscle weakness; mood changes such as depression, euphoria, denial, and forgetfulness may be caused by both medications and the demyelination process.

Nursing Management

Assessment and Analysis

Because MS affects varying nerves throughout the body, the clinical presentation may change with each attack. These clinical manifestations are the direct result of the demyelination process. Often, patients have an "attack" with a partial recovery of the symptoms.

Clinical manifestations include:

- Numbness/weakness
- Complete or partial loss of vision
- Double or blurred vision
- Fatigue
- Dizziness
- Tremor
- Lack of coordination/balance
- Speech problems – especially articulation
- Memory loss

Other clinical manifestations include depression, paranoia, and reduced bowel or bladder control.

Nursing Diagnoses

- **Impaired physical mobility** related to neuromuscular impairment secondary to demyelination
- **Self-care deficit** related to reduced neurotransmission and impaired physical mobility secondary to demyelination
- **Impaired coping, depression** related to the chronic, progressive nature of the disease

Nursing Interventions

▣ *Assessments*

- Neuromuscular function
  Evaluate for changes in clinical presentation or for new symptoms to be addressed as the disease progresses and new areas of demyelination occur.
- Vision/eye movement
  Demyelination of cranial nerves can result in optic neuritis, causing visual changes.
- Skin integrity
  Immobility promotes breakdown as a result of compression of soft tissue between a bony prominence and an external surface. This compromises blood flow and decreases delivery of oxygen and nutrients to cells, resulting in cellular death and injury to the surrounding tissue.
- Ability to perform ADLs
  Evaluate need for assistive devices to decrease the danger of falls.
- Bowel and bladder function
  Impaired innervation to the bladder and bowel may result in incontinence and constipation.

▣ *Actions*

- Encourage ROM exercises
  Increase venous return, prevent stiffness, and maintain muscle strength and endurance.
- Administer interferon beta-1b (Betaseron)
  Interferon beta-1b is used to decrease exacerbations and slow disease progression.
- Administer corticosteroids during exacerbations
  During an exacerbation of MS, typically a result of some type of stress, administration of corticosteroids decreases the inflammatory processes associated with the flare.
- Implement safety measures
  Because of changes in mobility, sensation, and vision, the patient is at increased risk of falls and injury.
- Patch each eye daily as needed in patients with visual deficits and/or diplopia
  Alternating the patching of each eye several times per day improves balance and vision.

▣ *Teaching*

- Take medications as prescribed
  To decrease exacerbations/slow progression; to treat clinical manifestations as needed
- Importance of rest periods and preventing fatigue and overheating
  Fatigue, overexertion, and overheating stimulate MS exacerbations
- Clinical manifestations of MS exacerbation
  To detect early signs of exacerbation to receive early treatment
- Visual scanning
  Because peripheral vision may be decreased in patients with MS, visual environment scanning decreases the risk of injury.
- Check water temperature prior to entering the bathtub or shower
  Decreased sensation secondary to demyelination makes the patient at risk of burn injuries if the water is too hot.
- Maintain ideal body weight
  Impaired immobility may increase weight gain and increased weight is associated with complications with mobility and fatigue in patients with MS.
- Review disease process and prognosis
  To help increase understanding and enhance the patient's ability to make informed choices

Evaluating Care Outcomes

Patients with multiple sclerosis live their lives never knowing when the next exacerbation or attack will occur. Compliance with the medication regimen, specifically Betaseron, helps reduce these exacerbations. Patient and family education are important regarding the medication regimen, the clinical manifestations of exacerbation, and the importance of getting adequate rest and exercise. The goals of care are to keep the patient as active and functional as possible, to provide symptomatic relief, and to provide continued support to the patient and family. Because the problems of

MS are relatively permanent, there is an increased need for personal responsibility and the involvement of supportive family and friends in the patient's care. Most of the patient's time may be spent homebound; therefore, the role in symptom management is central to the most optimal outcomes of needed therapies throughout the course of this illness.

AMYOTROPHIC LATERAL SCLEROSIS

Epidemiology

Amyotrophic lateral sclerosis (ALS), also known as Lou Gehrig's disease, is a rapidly progressing, fatal CNS (brain and spinal cord) disease that affects voluntary muscle control. It is the most common adult-onset motor neuron disease. Amyotrophic lateral sclerosis results in gradual degeneration and death of motor neurons, causing muscle weakness and atrophy, but does not impair the senses or ability to think. Clinical Manifestations usually develop after age 50, and the prevalence of ALS in the United States is 3.9 per 100,000 people. Most people die from respiratory failure within 3 to 5 years of onset of clinical manifestations. Although in most cases the cause is unknown, 10% of cases are caused by a genetic defect (see Genetic Connections).

Genetic Connections

Heritability of Amyotrophic Lateral Sclerosis

On the basis of twin students in Ireland, it is estimated that heritability of amyotrophic lateral sclerosis (ALS) ranges from 61% to 76%. These findings suggest that both genetic and environmental factors have a role in the development of this disease. Findings suggest that genetic variants are important in explaining the role of genetics in ALS. Regional differences noted in this study also suggest that there are both new environmental and genetic risk factors and that larger studies are needed to examine these factors.

Pathophysiology

Motor neurons are located throughout the CNS and serve as controlling and communication links between the nervous system and voluntary muscles. Messages are passed from upper motor neurons (located in the brain) to lower motor neurons (located in the spinal cord) and on to particular muscles. In ALS, both upper and lower neurons degenerate and die. Unable to function, muscles gradually weaken, atrophy, and twitch (**fasciculation**). The progressive degeneration leads to death of the cells, resulting in the brain losing the ability to initiate and

control muscle movement (Fig. 37.10). Eventually, all voluntary muscles are affected, and patients are paralyzed, but sensation is intact. Bulbar ALS, also known as progressive bulbar palsy, is a form of ALS that prominently affects the muscles involved in speech, swallowing, and tongue movements. Amyotrophic lateral sclerosis affects the diaphragm and chest wall, resulting in respiratory failure and the need for placement of an artificial airway (endotracheal tube or tracheostomy) and ventilator support.

Clinical Manifestations

Patient clinical manifestations are often described first as general complaints of muscle cramps or stiffness, muscle weakness on one part of the body first, slurred speech, and difficulty swallowing (dysphagia). The early clinical presentation depends on which part of the body is damaged first. While the disease progresses, the patient experiences weakness and atrophy in other parts of the body. To be diagnosed with ALS, patients must have clinical manifestations of both upper and lower motor neuron damage that cannot be attributed to other causes. Upper motor neuron damage is associated with spasticity, while lower motor neuron damage is characterized by flaccidity.

Connection Check 37.4

The nurse monitors for which complication in the patient with bulbar ALS?
A. Lower back pain
B. Dementia
C. Paresthesias
D. Dysphagia

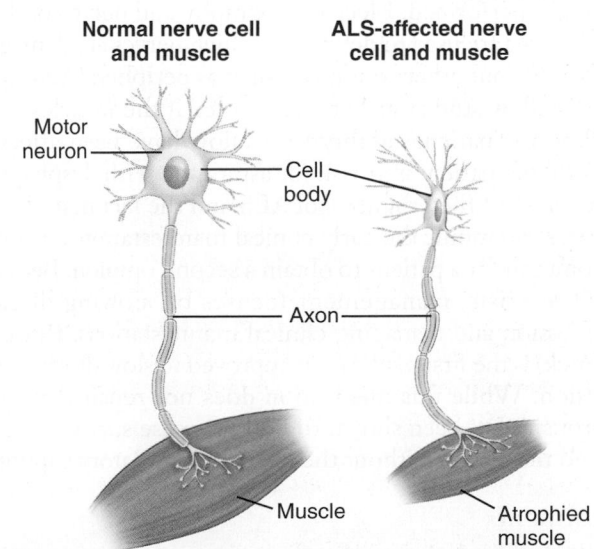

FIGURE 37.10 Comparison of normal and amyotrophic lateral sclerosis (ALS)-affected cell and muscle.

Management

Medical Management

Diagnosis

No single test can be used to diagnose ALS; therefore, a complete history and physical examination must be performed by the healthcare provider. This includes muscle strength and endurance testing to see if weakness, spasticity, atrophy, and hyperreflexia (increased reflexes) are increasing. Other diagnostic tests that may be performed in patients with suspected ALS include:

- B_{12} for deficiency
- RPR for neurosyphilis
- ANAs as a general autoimmune screen
- Thyroid-stimulating hormone for hypothyroidism
- Serum protein electrophoresis/immunofluorescent electrophoresis for protein disorders
- Rheumatoid factor
- ESR as a general inflammatory screen
- Creatine phosphokinase for muscle injury
- Electrolyte panel for imbalances
- Complete blood count and peripheral smear for leukemias/plasma cell dyscrasias
- Anti-MAG and anti-GM1 antibodies for other neuromuscular diseases
- Parathormone for deficiency
- Urinalysis and 24-hour urine for heavy metals
- Serum lead, acid maltase, and hexosaminidase levels for other metabolic-neuromuscular diseases
- Free erythrocyte protoporphyrin for porphyrias

A lumbar puncture is also needed to evaluate CSF protein and cytology.

A CT scan and/or MRI of the neck and head may be performed to rule out other conditions that can mimic ALS (spinal cord tumor, herniated disk, spondylosis, brain tumor, MS, etc.). If there is a known family history of ALS, genetic testing is performed. Electromyography and nerve conduction studies are used to determine which nerves are damaged and to rule out other conditions such as peripheral neuropathy. Swallow studies are ordered to see if the muscles controlling the patient's ability to swallow have been affected because the patient is at risk for aspiration with dysphagia.

Because of the prognosis of ALS and the fact that several diseases can mimic the early clinical manifestations, it is not uncommon for a patient to obtain a second opinion. Because no cure exists, management focuses on slowing disease progression and managing clinical manifestations. Riluzole (Rilutek) is the first medication approved to slow disease progression. While this medication does not repair damaged neurons, it has been shown to both increase survival and to extend the period without the need for ventilatory support.

Treatment

Treatment includes medications for symptomatic relief, such as baclofen for muscle cramps, laxatives and stool softeners for constipation, **analeptics** (CNS stimulants) for fatigue and weakness, and tricyclic depressants for excessive salivation, pain, and depression. See Table 37.5 for examples of medications used to treat ALS.

Often physical, occupational, and speech therapies are used to maximize function. While the disease progresses and muscles weaken, assistive and breathing devices may be used. Nutrition is a very important component of the plan of care. Patients with ALS tend to lose weight, and often a gastric feeding tube must be placed to help meet their nutritional requirements. As the chest and diaphragm muscles weaken, patients need to consider forms of mechanical ventilation requiring a tracheotomy. Patients need to be fully informed about the risks and long-term effects of ventilation.

Complications

Amyotrophic lateral sclerosis is a progressive disease that leads to the inability to move. Complications include aspiration of food or fluid, respiratory failure, pneumonia, pressure injuries, deep vein thrombosis (DVT), pulmonary embolism (PE), constipation, contractures, depression, weight loss, and loss of the ability to care for self. While the patient's physical condition deteriorates, it is important to make decisions about enteral feedings, intubation and mechanical ventilation, as well as end-of-life decisions.

Nursing Management

Assessment and Analysis

The first clinical manifestations of ALS are general complaints because of weakness of the involved muscles. The clinical presentation is directly related to the progressive wasting of the motor neurons and includes:

- Difficulty breathing
- Difficulty swallowing – choking, drooling
- Speech problems – slurring words, slow speech
- Voice changes – hoarseness
- Muscle cramps
- Head drop due to weak neck muscles
- Muscle twitching (fasciculation)
- Increasing muscle weakness – localized to one part of the body then spreads
- Paralysis
- Weight loss
- Tongue atrophy

Although muscle weakness occurs in 60% of patients and is the initial hallmark sign of ALS, clinical manifestations vary with each individual, and can begin in the muscles of the arms, legs, hands, or feet or in the muscles of speech and swallowing. Although everyone with ALS does not experience the same clinical manifestations or progression of the disease, progressive muscle weakness and paralysis are universally experienced.

Nursing Diagnoses

- **Ineffective airway clearance** related to weak cough secondary to motor neuron death and muscle weakness

Table 37.5 Medications Used in the Treatment of Amyotrophic Lateral Sclerosis

Classification	Examples	Mechanism of Action
Benzothiazole	Riluzole (Rilutek)	Decreases glutamate levels, an amino acid that affects the nerves that send messages from the brain to the muscles
Muscle relaxant and antispasmodics	Baclofen (Lioresal, Kemstro), tizanidine (Zanaflex)	Depresses CNS to reduce pain and inhibit reflexes at the spinal level to decrease muscle spasm
Analeptics	Modafinil (Provigil), armodafinil (Nuvigil)	Alter neurotransmitters to improve wakefulness
Antidepressants – tricyclics	Imipramine (Tofranil), amitriptyline (Elavil), nortriptyline (Pamelor)	Contain three fused benzene rings that block the reuptake of norepinephrine and serotonin in the CNS
Laxatives – osmotic	Milk of magnesia, Miralax, lactulose	Pulls fluid into the intestine from other tissue and blood vessels; the extra fluid makes the stool softer and easier to pass.
Laxatives – stimulant	Correctol, Dulcolax, Senokot	Irritates the intestinal lining and speeds up how quickly stool moves through the intestines
Antimuscarinics; anticholinergics	Glycopyrrolate (Robinul)	Inhibits acetylcholine activity on structures innervated by postganglionic cholinergic nerves and on smooth muscles that respond to acetylcholine by blocking cholinergic innervation; results in diminished volume and free acidity of gastric secretions and control of excessive pharyngeal, tracheal, and bronchial secretions

CNS = Central nervous system.

- **Risk for aspiration** related to weakness of muscles of swallowing
- **Ineffective breathing pattern** related to weakness of the respiratory muscles secondary to motor neuron dysfunction
- **Potential for injury** related to impaired physical mobility secondary to motor neuron death and muscle weakness
- **Impaired oral communication** related to dysarthria and tongue atrophy secondary to motor neuron death
- **Ineffective coping** related to the diagnosis of a progressive disease that results in motor paralysis

Nursing Interventions
▪ Assessments
- Airway
  Because motor weakness involves muscles of the face, mouth, and neck, maintaining an intact airway is compromised. Airway compromise is greater as the patient demonstrates weakened cough and impaired swallowing.
- Oxygen saturation
  Motor neuron death and resultant muscle weakness may impair respiratory function and the ability to clear secretions, which leads to decreased oxygenation.
- Motor strength
  While the disease progresses, muscle weakness increases because of neuronal degeneration and cell death.

- Ability to swallow
  Increased risk of aspiration with difficulty swallowing food or fluid because of neuronal degeneration and resultant muscle weakness
- Skin
  Immobility promotes breakdown because of the compression of soft tissue between a bony prominence and an external surface. This compromises blood flow and decreases delivery of oxygen and nutrients to the cells, resulting in cellular death and injury to the surrounding tissue.
- Coping skills
  For current skills that work and to identify support system

▪ Actions
- ROM
  Prevents contracture and strengthens unaffected muscles
- Administer medications to treat clinical manifestations
  To maintain patient's comfort by alleviating muscle cramps, pain, constipation, fatigue, depression, etc.
- Elevate the head of the patient's bed when eating, drinking, or brushing teeth
  Because of impaired swallowing secondary to motor neuron disease, elevating the head of the bed helps prevent aspiration.
- Turn, cough, and deep breathing
  While motor strength declines, the patient needs to be turned and repositioned to promote gas exchange.

- Turn scheduled for every 2 hours
  The patient with ALS is at increased risk for impaired skin integrity because of impaired mobility. The patient can usually let the nurse know when repositioning is needed because of discomfort (as sensation is intact).
- Emotional support
  Because of the progressive nature of the disease, patients require maximum support from staff and family.

■ *Teaching*

- Report increased difficulty swallowing or breathing
  Indicates disease progression as motor neuron death and muscle weakness affect the muscles needed to breathe and swallow
- Disease prognosis and process: need for ventilator
  Discuss so that patient can make informed decisions while still having mild symptoms
- Communication strategies
  To help patient communicate with family and healthcare providers

Evaluating Care Outcomes

Patients with ALS face a difficult future. As a progressive disease, ALS eventually leads to the inability to move and to ventilator dependence. The nurse must help prepare the patient and family for the disabilities that will result from the degeneration, keep the patient comfortable and independent for as long as possible, and help prepare the patient and family for death. The effectiveness of interventions is reflected in the lack of respiratory compromise, stable body weight, and intact skin. The focus of care needs to be supporting the patient and his or her family through this difficult process.

SPINAL CORD INJURY

Epidemiology

Acute spinal cord injury (SCI) is an unexpected catastrophic event that results in the loss of function such as mobility or sensation. Spinal cord trauma may result from either direct injury to the cord or indirectly from damage to surrounding bones, tissues, and blood vessels. The mechanism of this injury may be caused by hyperextension, hyperflexion, rotation and vertical compression (**axial loading**), or penetrating injuries. The incidence of SCI in the United States is approximately 12,000 per year. Currently, approximately 300,000 Americans are living with SCIs, and the cost of care is $4 billion each year.

While spinal cord injuries occur in people of all ages, the majority occur between the ages of 16 and 18, and most commonly affect men. Risk factors include activities such as participating in high-risk physical activities such as speeding and drinking while under the influence of alcohol, substance use, and not using protective gear in sports or recreational activities. In the older population, there is increased risk of spinal cord trauma related to fall-related injuries. Injuries at the C4, C5, C6 and T12 spine levels are most common, with half of the injuries resulting in paraplegia and half in quadriplegia. The leading cause of SCI is automobile accidents (56%), followed by falls (14%), acts of violence/guns (9%), and sports injuries (7%).

Pathophysiology

Spinal cord injury is damage to the spinal cord with resulting functional loss of mobility and/or sensation. Spinal cord injuries result from concussion, contusion, compression, tearing, laceration, transection, or ischemia of the spinal cord. The spinal cord is about 18 inches long, and the nerves within the cord carry messages from the brain to the spinal nerves (*upper motor neurons*) and back. Spinal nerves called *lower motor neurons* branch out from the spinal cord to specific areas of the body. The lower motor neurons have two parts, a sensory portion that carries messages from the body to the brain and a motor portion that carries messages back to the body parts to initiate actions such as muscle movement.

The spinal cord does not have to be severed for loss of functioning to occur. In fact, most injuries leading to spinal column bony fractures result in various types of SCI. Neuron axonal injury occurs as a result of this trauma. The number of axons damaged can vary, allowing some types of injuries to recover and others to result in paralysis. At the moment of injury, affected axons are damaged beyond repair, and the neural cell membranes are ruptured. Blood vessels may sustain trauma resulting in bleeding that, within a short period of time, can spread from the central gray matter to other areas of the spinal cord. Minutes after the initial injury, the spinal cord can swell and fill the entire spinal cavity at the level of injury. This swelling results in anoxia caused by lack of blood flow and oxygen to the spinal cord tissue. While the body loses its ability to self-regulate, blood pressure drops, interfering with the electrical activity of neurons and axons.

The initial trauma of crushing or tearing of axons sets off a biochemical cascade that destroys neurons, demyelinates axons, and triggers an inflammatory response that can result in damage to spinal cord segments above or below the initial injury level. Blood flow changes in and around the injured area of the cord begin to spread, resulting in various movement and sensory changes throughout the body. The reduction in blood flow to the injured cord causes the blood vessels located in the gray matter to leak. Blood flow to the injured area is further reduced while cells lining the still intact blood vessels begin to swell. This combination of decreased blood flow with leaking and swelling vessels prevents the normal delivery of oxygen and nutrients to neurons, resulting in their death.

Additional damage can be caused by overexcitation of the nerve cells with the increased release of neurotransmitters. When spinal cells are injured, neurons flood the injured area with an excitatory transmitter (glutamate) normally used to stimulate activity in neurons. This excessive glutamate results in **excitotoxicity**, a process in which neurons are damaged and destroyed by overstimulation.

Normally, the blood–brain barrier keeps immune system cells from entering the brain or spinal cord. After an SCI, the barrier is broken, and WBCs can invade the surrounding tissue and trigger an inflammatory response characterized by fluid build-up and the arrival of immune cells (neutrophils, T cells, macrophages, and monocytes) to the site. The immune system response may help fight infection and clean up cellular debris, but this may also contribute to the formation of scar tissue within the cord. Another consequence of inflammation is the production of **free radicals**. Free radicals are a by-product of normal cell metabolism and are thought to be involved in degeneration, cancer, and the aging process. In the injured spinal cord, free radicals attack and destroy molecules vital for cell function.

The process of **apoptosis**, or cell death, results in more damage to the spinal cord and further decreases the ability to communicate with the brain. Apoptosis normally helps the body get rid of old, unhealthy cells. The cells shrink and die, and then scavenger cells remove the debris. After an SCI, apoptosis occurs, killing oligodendrocytes (the cells that form myelin) in the damaged area and in adjacent intact areas. The mechanisms of secondary damage (decreased blood flow, inflammation, excitotoxicity, free radical release, and apoptosis) increase the area of spinal cord damage. This increases the resulting deficits the patient experiences as a result of damage to the spinal cord.

Spinal cord injuries are divided into two classifications—complete and incomplete injuries. A complete injury results in a total loss of motor and sensory function below the level of injury. In an incomplete injury, there is incomplete structural damage with some function preserved below the primary injury level. Four types of incomplete injury have been identified (Fig. 37.11):

1. Central cord syndrome
   - Most common
   - Etiology: hyperextension injury with central cord swelling
   - Clinical manifestations: functional motor loss greater in arms than legs, bladder dysfunction, and variable loss of sensation
2. Anterior cord syndrome
   - Etiology: acute anterior compression from bony fragments or acute disk herniation
   - Clinical manifestations: Loss of motor function (paresis or paralysis), pain, temperature, crude touch and pressure below the level of injury; preserved sense of proprioception (position sense), fine touch and pressure, and vibration
3. Posterior cord syndrome
   - Etiology: acute compression
   - Clinical manifestations: loss of proprioception, fine touch and pressure, and vibration; intact pain, temperature, and crude touch and pressure
4. Brown-Séquard syndrome
   - Etiology: hemisection of the spinal cord resulting from penetrating injury (i.e., gunshot or knife injury); may also occur as result of primary ischemia, infection, or hemorrhagic event
   - Clinical manifestations: **ipisilateral** (on the same side as the injury) loss of motor function, proprioception, and vibration; **contralateral** (on the opposite side) loss of pain and temperature

Clinical Manifestations

The level of injury helps predict what parts of the body might be affected. Cervical injuries can result in the inability to breathe (above C4) as the **phrenic nerve** that

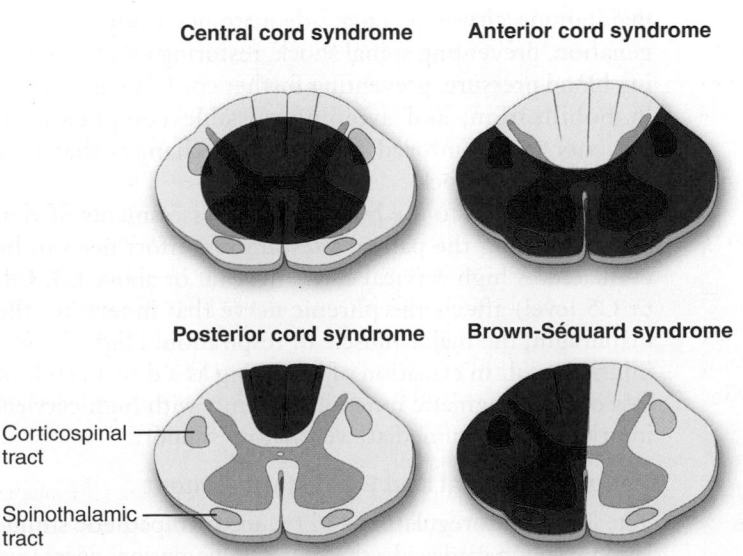

Central cord syndrome **Anterior cord syndrome**

Posterior cord syndrome **Brown-Séquard syndrome**

Corticospinal tract

Spinothalamic tract

FIGURE 37.11 Incomplete spinal cord lesions.

innervates the diaphragm is innervated in this area, and quadriplegia. Thoracic injuries often result in paraplegia and can include poor trunk control. Lumbar and sacral injuries result in decreasing control of legs, bowel and bladder function, and sexual function. See Table 37.6 and Fig. 37.12 for a list of injuries and functional losses. Other effects include chronic pain, low blood pressure, inability to sweat below the level of injury, and decreased temperature control.

Management

Medical Management

Diagnosis

The time between SCI and treatment greatly affects patient outcome. If the patient is admitted with a suspected SCI (associated with trauma to the head or neck), the spine is immobilized (cervical collar, spine backboard) until an examination is performed to identify the level of injury because any significant movement of the spine can result in further damage. A thorough physical and neurological examination, including reflexes, is performed. An x-ray may be performed to look for damage to the vertebrae. If the patient has clinical manifestations of an SCI (inability to move/feel), a CT scan or MRI may be performed to show the location and extent of damage and to reveal problems such as hematomas. The level of injury refers to the vertebra closest to the site of the injury.

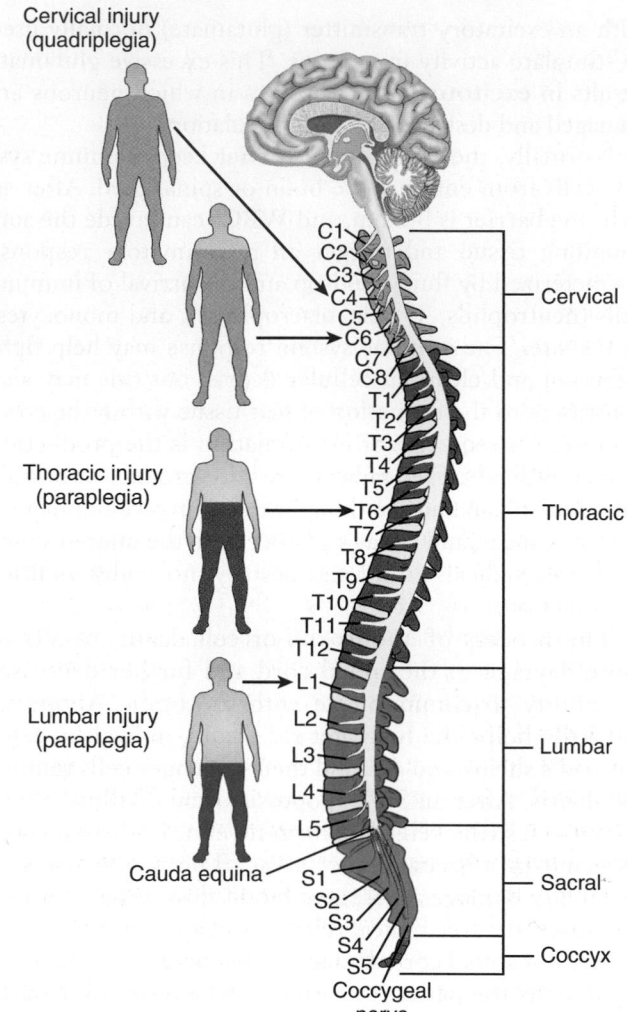

FIGURE 37.12 Spinal cord injury levels.

Table 37.6	Injury Level and Resultant Functional Loss
Injury Level	**Functional Loss**
C1–C4	Quadriplegia with loss of spontaneous respiratory function
C4, C5	Quadriplegia with possible phrenic nerve involvement
C5, C6	Quadriplegia with gross arm movements, phrenic nerve intact
C6, C7	Quadriplegia with biceps intact, diaphragmatic breathing
C7, C8	Quadriplegia with triceps, biceps, and wrist extension intact and some function of intrinsic hand muscles
T1–T5	Paraplegia with trunk and leg involvement, normal arm and hand movement,
T6 – T12	Paraplegia with fair ability to control balance and trunk, little or no voluntary bowel or bladder control
Below L1	Cauda equina injury, variable motor and sensory loss in lower extremities; a reflexive bowel and bladder

Treatment

Currently, there is no way to reverse spinal cord damage. During the acute stage of injury, treatment focuses on maintaining airway patency, adequate breathing and oxygenation, preventing spinal shock, restoring and maintaining blood pressure, preventing further cord damage, spinal immobilization, and avoiding possible complications. Patients are monitored for vital sign changes that may indicate spinal shock.

Before arrival to the hospital, rapid assessments of vital signs including the patient's respiratory effort need to be evaluated. A high cervical cord injury (at or above C3, C4, or C5 level) affects the phrenic nerve that innervates the diaphragm, the major muscle of respiration. High cervical injuries result in cessation of breathing as a direct result of loss of diaphragmatic function. Patients with high cervical injuries require immediate ventilatory support.

Pharmacological and Fluid Management

The loss of autoregulation and reduced sympathetic stimulation result in cardiac dysrhythmias, hypotension, decreased blood vessel tone, and reduced cardiac output. The most profound clinical manifestations are seen in upper thoracic and cervical injuries and in complete SCI. Interruptions to the cardiac accelerator nerves from a cervical SCI can cause the heart to beat dangerously slowly or pound rapidly and irregularly. Medications and even a pacemaker may be required to control the irregular heartbeat.

Loss of vasomotor tone causes blood to pool in vessels and results in low blood pressure. IV fluids, vasopressors, and inotropes are often used to provide adequate fluid resuscitation, increase tone, and increase cardiac output. Several options for volume expansion are commonly used in patients with SCIs. They include crystalloids, colloids, blood products, or a combination of these. Because of fluid shifts after injury, patients with SCIs are at risk for developing pulmonary edema and must be carefully monitored. Vasopressors and inotropes may be indicated in SCIs when the patient remains hypotensive after adequate fluid resuscitation. The vasopressor of choice depends on the patient's hemodynamic profile. Common medications include dopamine hydrochloride (dopamine), norepinephrine bitartrate (Levophed), phenylephrine hydrochloride (Neo-Synephrine), epinephrine, vasopressin (Pitressin), and dobutamine (Table 37.7).

Patients on vasoactive medications must be carefully monitored to prevent complications. High doses of vasopressors and the resultant vasoconstriction can cause decreased perfusion especially in the GI tract, kidneys, and extremities leading to decreased GI motility, impaired renal function, and ineffective peripheral perfusion, respectively.

Current guidelines for the management of acute SCIs no longer recommend the use of corticosteroids for acute SCI. Because there is no strong medical evidence supporting benefits from the administration of corticosteroids, this therapy is avoided because of stronger evidence that the administration of high-dose steroids is associated with harmful side effects, including hyperglycemia and immunosuppression.

Immobilization and Stabilization

After the patient arrives at the hospital, the fracture/dislocation must be reduced early, and spinal immobilization must be obtained to prevent further loss of function, ischemia, pain, and necrosis. Realignment of the spine with traction, a halo device, or surgery is used to achieve optimal function.

A **halo traction** device is used to maintain cervical immobilization for specific types of cervical fractures (Fig. 37.13). The halo traction is made up of a ring around the patient's head attached to a special vest by four rods. Titanium screws are screwed into the skull bone and attached to the halo traction device; weights connect to the halo at the head of the bed over a pulley system. Weights are slowly added, with x-rays taken between each additional weight, until spinal alignment is achieved.

Gardner-Wells tongs are U-shaped tongs used for spinal traction (Fig. 37.14). Pressure-controlled pins are inserted into the skull at opposite ends to permit a longitudinal force to be applied to the axis of the spinal column. The tongs are attached to weights using a pulley system at the head of the bed.

Current management strategies for SCI focus on early surgical intervention if indicated, immobilization, and hemodynamic and respiratory support to prevent secondary injury and optimize recovery.

Connection Check 37.5

Which interventions are indicated to treat the loss of vasomotor tone in the patient with an acute SCI? *(Select all that apply.)*

A. Positive inotropes
B. Corticosteroids
C. Antispasmodics
D. IV fluids
E. Vasopressors

Table 37.7 Summary of Common Vasoactive Medications

Medication	Typical Dose	Receptors	Mechanism of Action
Dopamine	2–10 mcg/kg/min	β_1, β_2, D_1	Vasodilation of renal, mesenteric, and coronary arteries
	5–10 mcg/kg/min	$\alpha_1, \beta_1, \beta_2, D_1$	Increases cardiac contractility, heart rate, and cardiac output; mild vasodilatory effects with preserved dopaminergic activity
	10–20 mcg/kg/min	$\alpha_1, \beta_1, \beta_2, D_1$	Peripheral vasoconstriction; preserved chronotropic and inotropic effects
Epinephrine	2–10 mcg/min	$\alpha_1, \beta_1, \beta_2$	Peripheral vasoconstriction, increased cardiac contractility, smooth muscle relaxation
Norepinephrine	2–30 mcg/min	α_1, β_1	Vasoconstriction and increased cardiac contractility
Phenylephrine	40–200 mcg/min	α_1	Arterial vasoconstriction
Dobutamine	5–15 mcg/kg/min	β_1, Mild β_2	Increased cardiac contractility, mild vasodilation
Vasopressin	0.04 unit/min	V1, V2, V3	Vasoconstriction of vascular smooth muscle

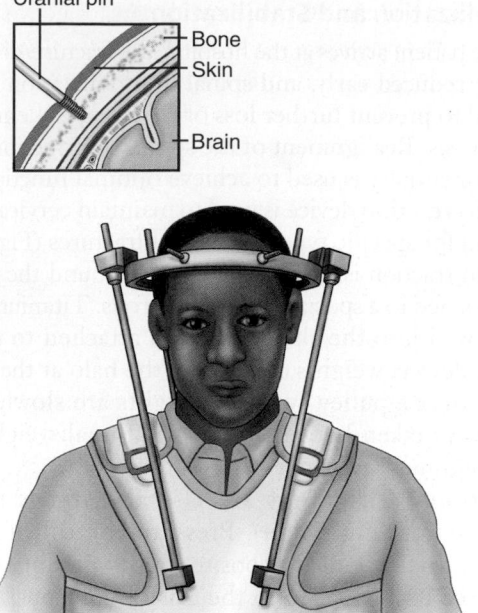

FIGURE 37.13 Halo traction device.

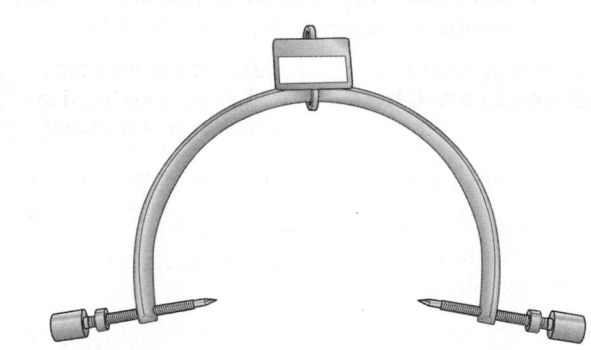

FIGURE 37.14 Gardner-Wells tongs.

Complications

An SCI produces a wide variety of changes in systemic physiology that can lead to a number of complications. These complications are both common and severe and can rival the neurological deficits in their impact on both function and quality of life. Currently, the most common causes of death for patients with SCI are respiratory diseases and cardiovascular events. Depending on the level of injury and the nerves affected, a patient may have multiple potential complications of SCI. The higher the level of injury, the more extensive the disability and the greater the risk of complications.

Spinal Shock

Spinal shock occurs immediately after injury and applies to all phenomena surrounding spinal cord transection. This results in a complete but temporary loss or depression of all or most spinal reflexes as well as sensory, motor, and autonomic activity below the injury level. Depending on the

level of the lesion, hypotension due to sympathetic tone loss is a possible complication. Although the main mechanism of injury that causes spinal shock is usually traumatic in origin and occurs immediately, it can be caused by other mechanisms and progress more slowly. During spinal shock, the brain is unable to transmit signals to muscles and organs, resulting in loss of sensation, movement, and other body functions. Clinical manifestations include flaccid paralysis of all skeletal muscles, absence of deep tendon reflexes, impaired proprioception, decreased visceral and somatic sensations, penile reflex, urinary and fecal retention, **anhidrosis** (absence of sweating), and paralytic ileus. This can last from 24 hours to 1 to 6 weeks, and the return of reflex activity below the level of injury indicates the end of spinal shock.

Neurogenic Shock

Neurogenic shock is a distributive type of shock that occurs in patients with brain, upper thoracic, and cervical injuries and is caused by the sudden loss of the autonomic nervous system signals to the smooth muscle in the vessel walls. This results in loss of vasomotor tone and sympathetic innervation of the heart. The cardiac output decreases because the vessels lose tone, allowing blood to pool in the periphery and blood pressure to fall. In a normal situation, the heart reflexively increases to compensate for the peripheral pooling of blood. In neurogenic shock, the sympathetic pathways to the heart are blocked or damaged, resulting in bradycardia. Clinical manifestations include vasodilation, bradycardia, body temperature instability, and hypotension. Neurogenic shock can be very dangerous and can lead to serious complications such as organ dysfunction and even death if not promptly identified and treated. Treatment often includes fluid, vasopressors, and other medications such as atropine. (See Chapter 14 for a more detailed discussion of neurogenic shock.)

Autonomic Dysreflexia

Autonomic dysreflexia is a syndrome of massive imbalanced reflex sympathetic discharge occurring in 80% of patients with SCI above the T5–T6 level. It most often occurs after the first year of injury but can occur any time after spinal shock subsides. A strong sensory input, such as pain, distended bladder, rapid temperature changes, infection, or a full rectum, is carried into the spinal cord via intact peripheral nerves. This input travels up the spinal cord and evokes a massive sympathetic surge from the intact thoracolumbar sympathetic nerves, resulting in widespread vasoconstriction, causing peripheral arterial hypertension. The brain detects this hypertensive crisis through intact baroreceptors (receptor cells in the bloodstream that relay information about blood pressure to the brain) in the neck and uses two methods to stop its progression. First, the brain attempts to shut down the sympathetic surge by sending descending inhibitory impulses. Unfortunately, these impulses are blocked in the injured spinal cord. Second, the brain attempts to decrease blood pressure by slowing the heart rate via the vagus nerve (parasympathetic). This bradycardia is inadequate, and the hypertension continues. Clinical manifestations include severe headache, hypertension, bradycardia, tachycardia, diaphoresis, and flushing above and pallor below the injury level. Once the inciting stimulus has been removed, reflex hypertension resolves. The most frequent cause of autonomic dysreflexia is a full bladder, and the second most is a full bowel; other causes include tight clothing, GI disturbances, DVT, pressure injury, bladder or kidney infection, temperature extremes, shoes, lying or sitting on a hard object, or a minor injury.

Nursing care of the patient with autonomic dysreflexia includes observing for a rapid rise in blood pressure, often 20 to 40 mm Hg above the patient's baseline: bradycardia; diaphoresis, flushing of the skin above the level of the lesion, chills, and pallor below the lesion level. The patient often reports a severe headache with one or more of the following clinical manifestations: nasal congestion, anxiety, blurred vision, chest pain, or a sense of impending doom. Table 37.8 identifies nursing interventions and their rationale. If the acute episode of autonomic dysreflexia is not identified and treated, the patient may develop seizures, pulmonary edema, myocardial infarction, cerebral hemorrhage, and death.

Halo Brace/Traction Device Complications

Several complications have been identified with the use of halo brace/traction devices to stabilize the head and neck. These include pin infections, skin breakdown, loosening or movement of pins, swallowing problems, and possible dural tears.

Pin site infections occur in approximately 20% of patients with a halo vest. The sites must be frequently assessed for signs of infection and site care provided once a shift and as needed. Pin sites are kept clean using a clean cotton-tipped applicator or gauze soaked with normal saline. A new clean applicator or gauze is used for each pin site. If crusting is noted on assessment, wrap a gauze soaked with normal saline around the pin site for 15 minutes. After removing the gauze, use a clean cotton-tipped applicator to gently remove the crust from the pin site. Ointments and solutions such as hydrogen peroxide should not be used because they can irritate the skin and may cause breakdown at the pin site.

> **⚠ Safety Alert** Pin site loosening is one of the most common complications associated with a halo brace. This can lead to cervical instability and infection. Pin site loosening occurs in as many as 60% of patients with a halo brace. Clinical manifestations that may indicate that the pins are loose include redness, swelling, drainage, site pain, or areas where the skin has pulled away from the site. If no infection is present, the healthcare provider may tighten the pins.
>
> If the pins remain loose, the halo ring may migrate, resulting in a loss of immobilization. The patient often complains of neck pain and that "the vest does not fit correctly/feel the same." Some patients may notice the ability to move their neck. If this occurs, notify the healthcare provider immediately, place the patient in a hard cervical collar (Collar) for spinal immobilization, and prepare for radiological imaging to assess for a change in spinal alignment. The nurse also needs to perform a thorough neurological examination to determine if the patient has worsening or new deficits. The halo will likely be reapplied using new pin sites.

Table 37.8 Nursing Interventions for the Treatment of the Patient With Autonomic Dysreflexia

Intervention	Rationale
Monitor BP closely, at least every 5 minutes	To evaluate treatments and to see if the source of the episode has been found and removed
Administer antihypertensive medications as ordered	To reduce blood pressure if severe or sustained hypertension occurs
HOB at 45 degrees or sit the patient up	Helps reduce blood pressure by allowing blood to pool in lower extremities
Loosen restrictive clothing; remove braces, antiembolism stockings, shoes – look for source of pain from these items	Allows pooling of blood in lower extremities to reduce blood pressure; may be source of episode
Check the bladder; if patient has an indwelling catheter, ensure patency and adequate drainage; if patient does not have an indwelling catheter, perform intermittent catheterization or place indwelling catheter per order; collect sample for UA	This is a possible source of the episode; a urinalysis is sent to assess for a urinary tract or kidney infection.
Check the bowel for impaction	To assess for possible source and remove to terminate episode; a digital rectal examination may be delayed until cardiovascular condition is stabilized because this can exacerbate the hypertension.
Check the patient's body for other sources of noxious stimuli—pressure injuries, wounds, bites, scratches, etc.	To assess for possible source and remove to terminate autonomic dysreflexia episode

BP = Blood pressure; *HOB* = head of bed.

Pressure injuries that develop under the vest portion of the halo brace often result from improper vest size, poor vest application, or insufficient padding. Meticulous skin care and assessment for early signs of skin irritation are key to reducing/preventing breakdown. Other ways to prevent skin breakdown include turning and repositioning every 2 hours and as needed and making sure the vest fits properly and has sufficient padding.

Swallowing difficulties (dysphagia) may occur when the head and neck are placed in an exaggerated extension position. Notify the healthcare provider if the patient complains of swallowing difficulty. The provider may need to adjust the halo to help resolve the problem, or a speech and language pathologist can be consulted to evaluate dysphagia. Other complications are listed by system in Table 37.9.

Surgical Management

Patients with no evidence of external pressure on the spinal cord are transferred to the intensive care unit (ICU) in traction. If there is evidence of spinal cord compression, progressive deficits, compound vertebral fractures, penetrating spinal cord wounds, or bony fragments in the spinal canal, early surgery is performed for decompression and fusion to stabilize the spinal column. Otherwise, patients with neurological evidence of spinal

instability are admitted to the ICU for a comprehensive diagnostic work-up, and neurological monitoring. Surgery, if indicated, is performed depending on the nature of the sustained spinal injury.

Several types of surgery are utilized to stabilize SCIs. Types of surgery include decompression laminectomies, using anterior cervical and thoracic approaches, with fusion in which one or more laminae are removed to allow for cord expansion because of edema. Another approach is the posterior laminectomy and fusion with bone graft to immobilize the neck and prevent further damage to the spinal column, and a posterior approach using either a bone graft or the insertion of rods or other instruments to correct and stabilize the deformities.

Nursing Management

Assessment and Analysis

Spinal cord trauma results in motor and sensory loss below the level of injury. Clinical manifestations vary depending on the location and severity of the cord damage and are caused by loss of innervation at the affected spinal cord level(s).

Cervical cord injuries that occur in the neck result in clinical manifestations that affect the arms, legs, and middle of the body, and include:

- Difficulty breathing
- Loss of bowel and bladder control (see Evidence-Based Practice)
- Numbness
- Weakness or paralysis
- Pain
- Sensory changes
- Spasticity

Thoracic cord injuries occur at chest level, and the following clinical manifestations can occur:

- Loss of normal bowel and bladder control (may include constipation, incontinence, and bladder spasms)
- Numbness
- Sensory changes
- Spasticity (increased muscle tone)
- Pain
- Weakness, paralysis

Lumbar sacral injuries occur at the lower back level; varying degrees of clinical manifestations can occur:

- Loss of normal bowel and bladder control
- Numbness
- Pain
- Sensory changes
- Spasticity (increased muscle tone)
- Weakness and paralysis

Injuries to the cervical or high thoracic spinal cord may also result in blood pressure problems, abnormal sweating, and difficulty maintaining normal body temperature.

Table 37.9 Spinal Cord Injury Complications	
System	**Complications**
Respiratory	Poor cough, atelectasis, pneumonia, ineffective breathing pattern, ARDS
Cardiovascular	Hypotension, bradycardia, decreased cardiac output, venous pooling, impaired tissue perfusion
Neuro/Musculoskeletal	Loss of sensation/function (paralysis), contractures, spasticity, muscle atrophy
Gastrointestinal	Paralytic ileus, septic or necrotic bowel, gastrointestinal bleed, malnourishment, retention, neurogenic bowel, impaction
Genitourinary	Urinary incontinence, urinary tract infection, neurogenic bladder, chronic kidney disease
Skin	Pressure areas leading to skin breakdown and potential pressure injuries

ARDS = Acute respiratory distress syndrome.

Evidence-Based Practice

Catheter-Associated Urinary Tract Infections

Because most patients with spinal cord injuries, multiple sclerosis (MS), and amyotrophic lateral sclerosis (ALS) require either short-term or long-term indwelling urinary catheters, it is important that healthcare staff understand the importance of preventing a catheter-associated urinary tract infection (CAUTI). By knowing and adhering to the CAUTI bundle implemented in their facility, nursing staff members play a pivotal role in decreasing the incidence of CAUTI in their patient population.

Catheter-associated urinary tract infection is the most common type of nosocomial infection, accounting for approximately 40% of all healthcare–associated infections. The current estimated cost of CAUTI can range from $1,200 to more than $2,700 per incident. Research indicates that many CAUTIs are preventable. A multipronged, or bundled, approach to prevent these infections has reduced the risks of CAUTI. Evidence suggests that the following interventions reduce the rate of CAUTI in patients who require short-term indwelling catheterization:

- Using catheters only when medically necessary
- Daily assessments of the need for catheterization and documenting the continued need
- Use reminder systems targeting early removal of catheters
- If appropriate, use external catheters on males
- Consider intermittent catheterization instead of indwelling catheter insertion with the use of a portable ultrasound bladder scanner to check for residual amounts of urine
- Early removal of all unnecessary urinary catheters

Specific nursing interventions that have also been noted to reduce CAUTIs include daily cleaning of the urethral meatus using a perineal cleanser, maintaining a closed urinary drainage system, use of catheter securement devices to prevent movement and urethral traction, maintaining the drainage bag below the level of the bladder, and changing the indwelling catheter only when necessary, not at a routine interval.

John, S., Thomas, M., Cardona, M., Santarina, S. A., Iacono, L., Scanlon, K.,... Rice, K. L. (2015). Staff nurses eliminated catheter-associated urinary tract infections in a neurosurgical intensive care unit. *Journal of Continuing Education in Nursing, 46*(9), 384–386.

Rebmann, T., & Greene, L. (2010). Preventing catheter-associated urinary tract infections: An executive summary of the Association for Professionals in Infection Control and Epidemiology, Inc, elimination guideline. *American Journal of Infection Control, 38*, 644–646.

Nursing Diagnoses

- **Alteration in respiratory function** related to paralyzed muscles, hypoventilation secondary to loss of diaphragm function due to denervation of phrenic nerve
- **Decreased cardiac output** related to loss of vasomotor tone secondary to spinal/neurogenic shock
- **Impaired physical mobility** related to neuromuscular impairment secondary to loss of nerve cells at injured level
- **Fear/anxiety** secondary to loss of motor function and potential for permanent impairment

Nursing Interventions

▣ *Assessments*

- Respiratory function
  Loss of intercostal muscle function results in decreased tidal volume and may lead to hypoventilation; C4 and higher injuries may result in complete loss of diaphragmatic effort.
- Vital signs
  Depending on the level of injury, because of loss of sympathetic input, the patient may experience spinal shock, neurogenic shock, respiratory or cardiac arrest, or autonomic dysreflexia. Patients are unable to regulate temperature, and hypothermia may result because of loss of control of blood vessels.
- Motor function/Sensory level
  Locate specific injury level used to choose and evaluate treatment; used to see if deficits increase or decrease over time
- Pain
  There may be increased pain above the level of injury as a result of damage to the spinal cord or nerve roots.
- Intake and output
  Fluid volume status is important in evaluating the effectiveness of therapies, particularly with spinal shock. Also, with decreased renal perfusion, there is decreased urine output.
- Surgical and/or pin sites
  The sites must be frequently assessed for signs of infection, bleeding, or CSF leak.
- Bowel sounds
  Decreased perfusion to the GI tract can lead to decreased GI motility and paralytic ileus.

▣ *Actions*

- Maintain suction equipment at the patient's bedside
  With decreased cough effectiveness, the patient may require suctioning to clear the airway.
- Facilitate cough effectiveness
  Because of muscle weakness or lack of diaphragmatic innervation, assistance is needed to remove secretions.
- Maintain spinal immobilization and stabilization
  To prevent further injury from an unstable spinal column
- Passive ROM
  Prevents contractures and loss of muscle tone; strengthens unaffected muscles; minimizes risk of developing deep vein thrombosis (DVT)

- Reposition and maintain in good alignment
  Prevents pressure injuries and decreases risk of DVT due to immobility
- Perform routine pin site care
  Pin sites are kept clean using a clean cotton-tipped applicator or gauze soaked with normal saline. A new clean applicator or gauze is used for each pin site. If crusting is noted on assessment, wrap a gauze soaked with normal saline around the pin site for 15 minutes. After removing the gauze, use a clean cotton-tipped applicator to gently remove the crust from the pin site.

▣ Teaching

- Clinical manifestations of respiratory distress
  Because patients with high cervical injuries are at risk of ineffective breathing and cough, they need to recognize these manifestations in order to seek timely treatment
- Clinical manifestations of autonomic dysreflexia
  It is critical that patients and their families understand the clinical manifestations, as well as causes of this potentially life-threatening emergency
- Skin care/management
  To help identify causes of and prevent skin breakdown. In patients who require a wheelchair, they need to be taught to refrain from sitting in one position too long because it can lead to decreased perfusion.

Evaluating Care Outcomes

The primary focus is to get the patient through the acute phase of the spinal cord trauma and to prevent complications. This includes airway management, cardiopulmonary support, maximizing spinal cord perfusion and oxygen delivery, pain relief, and preventing further injury or complications. Nursing management also encompasses pulmonary care (suctioning or assisting with cough), turning to prevent pressure injuries, deep vein thrombus prophylaxis, bowel and bladder training, and management of nutrition, limb edema, and orthostatic hypotension. Once the patient is stable, focus shifts to the rehabilitation phase and the optimal recovery of neurological function. Physical therapy is needed to minimize muscle wasting and to prevent contractures. Spinal cord–injured patients require intense inpatient therapy and are often sent to a facility that specializes in spinal trauma. Throughout the hospitalization, providing emotional support is essential for the patient and family. Assisting with the challenging adjustment to the new onset in alterations of daily living is an important focus for the nursing team in the care of this patient population.

> ⚠ **Safety Alert** Some patients with an established spinal cord lesion depend on manual bowel evacuation (the digital removal of feces) as their routine method of bowel care because they have lost normal bowel function. Manual evacuation is rarely undertaken in the acute setting and may be unfamiliar to nurses. All nursing staff must be aware of the possible risk of autonomic dysreflexia occurring if the patient's bowel becomes distended because of constipation or impaction. Healthcare staff require training in the procedure of manual evacuation to prevent this medical emergency from occurring.

Connection Check 37.6

Which action is the highest priority in the patient who presents with autonomic dysreflexia?
A. Prepare for intubation
B. Initiate vasopressors
C. Remove the stimulus
D. Place a temporary pacemaker

SPINAL CORD TUMORS

Epidemiology

A spinal cord tumor is an abnormal tissue growth (benign or malignant) in or around the spine. Because the spinal column is rigid, any abnormal growth can place pressure on tissues and impair function. Primary spinal tumors originate within the CNS; secondary tumors originate outside the CNS then metastasize or spread to the spine. Approximately 10% to 15% of all primary CNS tumors are found in the spinal cord. The spinal column is the most common site for bone metastases, with a minimum of 30% and as many as 70% of cancer patients having spinal metastasis.

Pathophysiology

The spinal cord consists of nerve bundles that descend from and ascend to the brain carrying electrical impulses that facilitate movement and sensation. A spinal tumor is an abnormal growth of tissue within or surrounding the spine. As this abnormal tissue grows, it causes compression and stretching of the fiber tracts. This results in further neurological deterioration because of the loss of motor and sensory function. Although some spinal tumors can be attributed to exposure to cancer-causing agents, the cause of most tumors remains unknown. This growth can be benign or malignant, primary or secondary.

Spinal tumors are classified in several ways including the area of the spine in which they occur (cervical, thoracic, lumbar), their location in the spine: anterior (front) or posterior (back), and their relationship to the dura (outermost membranous layer surrounding the brain and spinal cord). The types of tumors are based on their relationship to the dura, with extradural located outside the dura, intradural located within the dura, extramedullary located inside the dura but outside the cord, and intramedullary located within the cord. Primary tumors include both malignant and benign tumors (Table 37.10). Secondary spinal tumors

Table 37.10 Table of Primary Central Nervous System Tumors

Type	Origin	Status
Astrocytoma	Cells of tissue that support nerve cells	Most are benign or low-grade malignant tumors.
Ependymoma	Cells lining the center of the spinal cord	Most are benign.
Meningioma	Tissue cells covering the spinal cord (meninges)	Most are benign but can recur and can become malignant based on location and damage to vital structures.
Neurofibroma	Peripheral nerve cells (arise from Schwann cells)	Usually are benign
Sarcoma	Connective tissue cells	Malignant tumors
Schwannoma	Cells that form myelin sheath around peripheral nerve fibers	Benign tumors

are metastases and therefore always malignant. These metastases most often spread from lung, breast, prostate, renal, gland, or thyroid cancer. To prevent permanent spinal cord damage, spinal cord compression must be diagnosed and treated immediately.

Clinical Manifestations

The clinical presentation of a spinal tumor has manifestations similar to low-back pain (LBP) and herniated nucleus pulposus, as well as multiple sclerosis. On the basis of the location of the tumor, the patient may present with back pain that may radiate down the arms or legs. Additional clinical manifestations based on location include numbness and tingling, weakness in the distal extremities, urinary incontinence, and bowel pattern changes. With tumors in the cervical area, the patient may notice loss of manual dexterity and clumsiness.

Management

Diagnosis

To make a correct diagnosis, the healthcare provider completes a through history and physical examination, focusing on back pain and any noted motor or sensory deficits. If the patient has a known primary tumor and develops back pain with deficits such as weakness or tingling, the provider will have a high suspicion of a metastatic process and order radiological testing such as CT or MRI. If the patient does not have a history of tumor, the healthcare provider must rule out other conditions that affect spinal cord function, including bone bruises, muscle spasms, fractured vertebrae, or compression by blood clot, herniated disk, or abscess. Diagnostic students that may be ordered to diagnose a tumor may include a MRI, considered to be the gold standard for examining spinal structures, or myelography with CT if MRI is unavailable. If a primary mass is detected, the patient needs a biopsy to diagnose the type of tumor and a CT of the chest and abdomen (for staging purposes).

Medical and Surgical Management

Although the ideal goal of therapy is to completely remove the tumor, this is complicated by the type and location of the tumor. Removing some tumors may result in permanent nerve damage. Treatment options include:

- Monitoring: often used for small, benign tumors that are not growing or pressing on surrounding tissues; periodic scans are needed to monitor the tumor
- Surgery: usually the first step in treating tumors that can be removed with an acceptable risk of nerve damage; often an option used with benign tumors
- Radiation therapy: used following an operation to eliminate the tumor remnants or to treat inoperable tumors; often first-line therapy for metastatic tumors
- Stereotactic radiosurgery: delivers a high dose of targeted radiation; effective in brain tumors and currently being studied for spinal cord tumors
- Chemotherapy: has not been proven effective for most spinal cord tumors due to issues penetrating the blood brain barrier
- Corticosteroids: to reduce swelling following surgery or during radiation treatments

Complications

Both benign and malignant spinal tumors can compress spinal nerves and cause loss of movement or sensation below the tumor level, spinal instability, changes in bowel and bladder function, and sexual dysfunction. Unless the cause is quickly identified and removed, permanent nerve damage can occur. If the patient requires surgery, other complications include:

- Bleeding or hematoma
- CSF leak
- Meningitis
- Chronic pain
- Injury to CNS tissue
- Spine instability
- Sensory loss

- Sexual dysfunction
- Paralysis
- Infection
- Ventilator dependence
- Wound dehiscence

Nerve damage from spinal cord tumor compression is often permanent, with disabilities continuing after the tumor is removed.

Nursing Management

Assessment and Analysis

Pain in the middle or lower back is the most common symptom of both benign and malignant spinal tumors. Other clinical manifestations are related to the area of the spine involved and may include:

- Back pain radiating to other parts of the body
- Loss of sensation or muscle weakness, often in the legs
- Difficulty walking
- Decreased sensitivity to pain, heat, or cold
- Loss of bladder or bowel function
- Paralysis
- Scoliosis or other spinal deformity

Nursing Diagnoses

- **Impaired physical mobility** related to neuromuscular impairment
- **Acute pain** related to nerve impingement
- **Ineffective coping** related to diagnosis

Nursing Interventions

■ Assessments

- Neurological status
  Locate level of function – sensory and motor to determine necessary interventions as well as to evaluate for signs of deterioration as well as for signs of improvement with treatments.
- Pain
  Patient's pain perception is used to determine an effective pain management plan; may have increased pain above the level of the tumor.
- Bowel or bladder function
  Tumors that compress the spinal cord are associated with dysfunction of bladder and bowel function. The patient may present with incontinence, urinary retention, or constipation.
- Coping skills
  Identify current coping skills that work and the patient's support system.

■ Actions

- Administer medications
  Pain medications to decrease pain, corticosteroid therapy to decrease swelling and inflammation, and medications as ordered for patient comfort
- Increase intake of fluid and fiber in diet
  Fluids and fiber decrease complications associated with bowel constipation that may develop secondary to decreased mobility, pain, and opioid medications.

- ROM exercises
  Prevent contractures and loss of muscle tone; strengthen unaffected muscles
- Reposition every 2 hours and as needed
  To prevent skin impairment and pressure injuries and maintain comfort

Teaching

- Preoperative teaching if scheduled for surgery
  To decrease anxiety level and help promote compliance
- Report clinical manifestations of increased weakness, loss of bowel/bladder function
  May be due to recurrent tumor or spinal cord edema

Evaluating Care Outcomes

The prognosis and outcome depend on the type and location of the tumor and the treatment required. If the tumor is not identified and quickly removed, permanent damage results from the compression on the spinal cord. Risks to the patient can include neurological deficits with clinical manifestations related to the location of the compression site. Some tumors can be safely and completely removed, resulting in full recovery. Often, postoperative radiation therapy follows the removal of tumors. If the tumor is inoperable, radiation therapy is often done as a palliative care measure to control the patient's pain.

Connection Check 37.7

Which intervention is typically the initial treatment of a metastatic spinal cord tumor?
A. Radiation therapy
B. Local chemotherapy into the cord
C. Surgical decompression
D. Corticosteroids

Making Connections

CASE STUDY: WRAP-UP

Six months later, Cynthia again reports left leg numbness and weakness and a new symptom of arm weakness and numbness. A second MRI of the head and spine is completed, revealing new areas of demyelination. Cynthia is formally diagnosed with multiple sclerosis. After a long discussion with her healthcare provider, she agrees to begin Betaseron therapy in hopes of reducing exacerbations and slowing progression of the disease. Cynthia decides to start Avonex intramuscular injections once a week. She is also given a prednisone course to treat her exacerbation, and her clinical manifestations improve within 2 weeks.

Cynthia returns to physical therapy to develop an exercise plan to strengthen her muscles and improve daily function. She may also require medications to treat common complications associated with MS. These include medications to help reduce fatigue, depression, and pain and to help control bowel and bladder problems. Cynthia is given information regarding lifestyle changes to her diet and the importance of continuing her exercises and getting plenty of rest. It is vitally important that she take good care of herself to help try to reduce disease progression and exacerbation. Cynthia is also given the numbers and Web sites of both local and national associations that can provide additional support and information.

Case Study Questions

1. The nurse needs to monitor Cynthia for which complication of MS?
   A. Intolerance to cold
   B. Myopia
   C. Muscle spasms
   D. Tinnitus

2. Which statement by Cynthia indicates that teaching about Avonex has been effective?
   A. "I am so glad I only have to do this once a week."
   B. "I hope that my husband can help since it is three times a week."
   C. "I am glad this medication does not cause the flulike symptoms like Betaseron can."
   D. "There is no increased risk for infections."

3. What exercise modifications need to be included in Cynthia's plan of care?
   A. Increasing weights and repetitions three times a week
   B. Exercising in a warm environment to relax muscles
   C. Low- to moderate-intensity endurance training
   D. High-intensity resistance training

4. The nurse monitors for which clinical manifestations of Cynthia's MS? *(Select all that apply.)*
   A. Blurred vision
   B. Speech problems
   C. Muscle weakness
   D. Bradycardia
   E. Fasciculations

5. Based on her current clinical presentation, the nurse incorporates which problem into Cynthia's plan of care?
   A. Bowel dysfunction
   B. Impaired mobility
   C. Urinary retention
   D. Visual deficit

CHAPTER SUMMARY

At least 60% to 80% of the population will have an episode of low-back pain at least once in their lifetime. Low-back pain often occurs in individuals between 30 and 50 years old with an annual cost of $50 billion per year on treatment alone. Low-back pain/problems often follow injury or trauma. Spinal degeneration is often associated with aging and involves the loss of spinal structure and function. Decreased water content of the disk nucleus results in wear and tear on the annulus and joints. Sudden movement or bending may cause muscle spasm. Patients do not always experience severe back pain with a pulled muscle or bulging disk. A new exercise program with sudden movements could have strained a muscle or caused inflammation in a small area of the spine.

Herniated disks are most common between ages 30 and 45, with males more commonly affected in lumbar disk herniation by a 3:2 ratio. While the disk becomes more inflexible, the possibility of HNP into the spinal canal increases. The resulting nerve compression is responsible for the loss of function, with the type of nerve compressed (motor or sensory) determining the symptom (pain or numbness).

Clinical manifestations of herniated nucleus pulposus vary depending on the location of the herniated disk; often, pain occurs on one side of the body and may vary from a dull ache to sharp, shooting pain. Common clinical findings are no clinical manifestations to, arm or leg pain, numbness or tingling, muscle weakness, and neck or back pain that shoots down one arm or leg. Most patients with a herniated disk have improvement with 1 to 2 months of conservative treatment. This consists of avoiding painful positions and following a regimen of planned exercise and pain medications. Other patients require surgical intervention before they have any improvement of their clinical manifestations, and there are several surgical options used in the treatment of a herniated disk. A laminotomy, surgery in which a large hole is made in the lamina, or a laminectomy, surgical removal of most of the lamina, are often used in conjunction with a diskectomy to remove pressure on the spinal cord or nerve roots. Use of an artificial disk is a developing alternative to the diskectomy. In this new option, the diseased disk is replaced with a manufactured disk; this provides pain relief while allowing the spine's anatomical structure to remain intact.

Currently, the microdiskectomy is the standard procedure used to treat a herniated disk. In this procedure, a small portion of the bone over or the disk material under the nerve root is removed to relieve pressure and to provide room for the nerve to heal. This is done through a small incision, allowing the spinal structure supports to remain intact. Spinal fusion is surgery that joins two bones (vertebrae) together. Because fusing permanently joins the bones together, there is no longer movement between them. Spinal fusion is usually performed along with other procedures such as a laminectomy and diskectomy to provide spinal stability. In a spinal fusion, a bone graft, often from the patient's pelvis, or metal hardware is used to join the vertebrae together.

Multiple sclerosis (MS) is a chronic, degenerative neurological disorder in which the nerves of the central nervous system (CNS) degenerate. There is no cure for MS. Approximately 400,000 people in the United States have MS, with a typical onset between 20 and 50 years of age. Multiple sclerosis is classified as an autoimmune disease. In these diseases, the immune system mistakenly attacks the nerves of the brain and spinal cord, resulting in destruction of the myelin sheath. The myelin sheath covers the spinal cord and nerves, serving as protection and helping relay nerve impulses at a faster rate.

This demyelinating process culminates in impaired movement, sensation, and thinking. Multiple sclerosis is difficult to diagnose because symptoms can be intermittent and can vary depending on the location of the affected nerves. Treatment often focuses on improving the speed of recovery from attacks, reducing the number of attacks, and slowing the progression of the disease. Lifestyle management includes getting plenty of rest and exercise; staying cool; eating a healthy, balanced diet; and relieving stress. Because MS affects varying nerves throughout the body, clinical manifestations change with each attack, and these symptoms are the direct result of the demyelination process. Often, patients have an "attack" with a partial recovery of the clinical manifestations. Common findings include numbness/weakness, complete or partial loss of vision, double or blurred vision, fatigue, dizziness, tremor, lack of coordination/balance, speech problems, and memory loss.

Amyotrophic lateral sclerosis (ALS), also known as Lou Gehrig's disease, is a rapidly progressing, fatal CNS disease that affects voluntary muscle control, and results in gradual degeneration and death of motor neurons. Resulting in muscle weakness and atrophy, ALS does not impair senses or ability to think. In ALS, both upper and lower neurons degenerate and die, leading to gradual muscle weakening, atrophy, and fasciculations. The progressive degeneration leads to death of the cells, destroying the brain's ability to initiate and control muscle movement. Eventually, all voluntary muscles are affected, and patients are paralyzed, resulting in ventilator dependence.

The incidence of spinal cord injury (SCI) in the United States is approximately 12,000 per year, most commonly affecting men aged 16 to 18. Spinal cord trauma may result from either direct injury to the cord or indirectly from damage to surrounding bones, tissues, and blood vessels. Spinal cord trauma is damage to the spinal cord with resulting functional loss such as mobility or feeling. The spinal cord does not have to be severed for loss of function to occur, and in fact, most injuries cause fractures or compressions of the spinal cord that result in damage to the axons. The number of axons damaged can be few to many, allowing some injuries to recover almost completely and others to result in paralysis.

The initial trauma of crushing or tearing of axons sets off a biochemical cascade that kills neurons, demyelinates

axons, and triggers an inflammatory response that can result in damage to segments above or below the initial injury level. Blood flow changes in and around the injured area of the cord begin to spread out and cause problems throughout the body. Spinal cord injuries are divided into two types, complete and incomplete. A complete injury results in a total loss of motor and sensory function below the level of injury. In an incomplete injury, there is incomplete structural damage with some function preserved below the primary injury level. Four types of incomplete injury have been identified: central cord syndrome, anterior cord syndrome, posterior cord syndrome, and Brown-Séquard syndrome. The level of injury helps predict what part of the body might be affected. Cervical injuries can result in inability to breathe and quadriplegia. Thoracic injuries often result in paraplegia and can include poor trunk control. Lumbar and sacral injuries result in decreasing control of legs, bowel and bladder function, and sexual function.

Autonomic dysreflexia, an overactivity of the autonomic nervous system (ANS), occurs in patients after SCI at T5 and above. Autonomic dysreflexia can develop suddenly and, if not promptly treated, can lead to seizures, stroke, and even death. It occurs when an irritating stimulus, e.g., full bladder, is introduced below the level of the SCI. The stimulus sends nerve impulses to the spinal cord, where they travel upward until they are blocked at the level of injury. Because the impulses cannot reach the brain, a reflex is activated that increases sympathetic activity, increasing blood pressure. Nerve receptors in the heart and blood vessels detect the increased blood pressure and send a message to the brain. The brain sends a message to the heart, causing the heartbeat to slow down and the blood vessels above the injury level to dilate. However, the brain cannot send messages below the level of injury and therefore fails to control the blood pressure.

Patients may develop two different shock syndromes after SCI, spinal or neurogenic. Spinal shock occurs immediately after injury and applies to all phenomena surrounding spinal cord transection. This results in a temporary loss or depression of all or most spinal reflex activity below the injury level. Depending on the level of the lesion, hypotension resulting from sympathetic tone loss is a possible complication. Neurogenic shock occurs in patients with upper thoracic and cervical injuries and is caused by the sudden loss of the ANS signals to the smooth muscle in the vessel walls. This results in loss of vasomotor tone and sympathetic innervation of the heart. Clinical manifestations include vasodilation, bradycardia, and hypotension.

A spinal cord tumor is an abnormal tissue growth (benign or malignant) in or around the spine. Because the spinal column is rigid, any abnormal growth can place pressure on tissues and impair function. Approximately 10% to 15% of all primary CNS tumors are found in the spinal cord, and the tumors can be benign or malignant, primary or secondary. Spinal tumors are classified in several ways, including the area of the spine in which they occur (cervical, thoracic, lumbar), their location in the spine: anterior (front) or posterior (back), and their relationship to the dura (outermost layer surrounding the brain and spinal cord).

To prevent damage, spinal cord compression must be diagnosed and treated immediately. A thorough evaluation by the healthcare provider includes a history and physical examination focusing on back pain and any noted deficits. If a patient has a known primary tumor and develops back pain with deficits such as weakness or tingling, the provider should have a high suspicion of a metastatic process. However, if the patient does not have a history of tumor, the healthcare provider must rule out other conditions that affect spinal cord function. The gold standard for examining spinal structures is MRI. Although the ideal goal of therapy is to completely remove the tumor, this is complicated by the type and location of the tumor, because removing some tumors may result in permanent nerve damage.

Because both benign and malignant spinal tumors can compress spinal nerves, and loss of movement or sensation below the tumor level, spinal instability, changes in bowel and bladder function, and sexual dysfunction may result. Unless the cause is quickly identified and removed, permanent nerve damage can occur, and nerve damage from spinal cord tumor compression is often permanent, with disabilities continuing after the tumor has been removed.

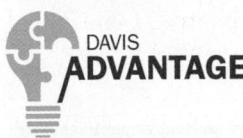

To explore learning resources for this chapter, go to **Davis Advantage** and find:
– Answers to in-text questions
– Chapter Resources and Activities
– NCLEX®-Style Chapter Review Questions
– Bibliography

Chapter 38

Coordinating Care for Patients With Peripheral Nervous System Disorders

Barbara Fitzsimmons

Finding Connections

CASE STUDY: EPISODE 1

Follow this patient throughout the chapter.

Stephanie Jordan is a 45-year-old married female with a 15-year history of myasthenia gravis (MG). She is a math teacher at a private middle school. Over the last week, she developed an upper respiratory infection with a fever of 101.1°F (38.39°C). During this time, she also developed increasing muscular weakness of her legs. Because of her weakness, she has stayed home from work for the past 2 days. This evening during dinner, she experienced marked difficulty with chewing and swallowing. The development of these problems prompted her husband to drive her to the emergency department of the local hospital for an evaluation. Her current medications include pyridostigmine 60 mg every 4 hours while awake, pyridostigmine time-release 180 mg at bedtime, and prednisone 20 mg daily. Following an evaluation in the emergency department, Ms. Jordan is admitted to a neuroscience inpatient unit, where she begins a course of antibiotics for her upper respiratory infection. The provider's plan is also to adjust Ms. Jordan's medications. Her pyridostigmine dose is increased to 90 mg every 4 hours around the clock, and the prednisone is increased to 40 mg daily...

INTRODUCTION

Nurses encounter patients with diseases of the peripheral nervous system (PNS) in a variety of settings. Diseases of the PNS vary in severity from mild to potentially life threatening when patients develop respiratory involvement. These patients may present to the emergency department, general medical-surgical setting, outpatient setting, obstetrics/gynecology department, or neuroscience areas with a new onset of clinical manifestations. Because of the nature of the disorders, nurses need to have an understanding of the pathophysiology of the disorder and treatment so that appropriate care can be planned. Nurses must also be cognizant of the neurological disorder even if the patient is not being admitted for management of the neurological problem because of the potential deterioration of these patients when under stress. This chapter addresses the management of patients with myasthenia gravis (MG), Guillain-Barré syndrome (GBS), and trigeminal neuralgia.

PERIPHERAL NERVOUS SYSTEM

In order to understand the disorders of the PNS, it is important for the nurse to have an understanding of the structures comprising this system. As a review of anatomy, the nervous system is made of two divisions: the central nervous system, or CNS, and the PNS. The CNS includes the brain and spinal cord. In the CNS, oligodendrocytes make the myelin that covers nerve fibers. The PNS is divided into both sensory and motor divisions. The sensory division includes sensory neurons that are responsible for innervating the skin, muscles, joints, and viscera. The motor division includes the motor neurons that control skeletal muscles and the autonomic nervous system (ANS) that innervates smooth and cardiac muscles and glands. The PNS is composed of nerves outside the cranium and vertebral column that include cranial and spinal nerves; **neuromuscular junctions**, which are the synapses between the somatic motor neuron's axon and the muscle; muscles; and the ANS. In the PNS, the **Schwann cells** make the myelin that wraps around the nerves.

Autonomic Nervous System

The ANS is the part of the nervous system that regulates involuntary body functions. The sympathetic division of the ANS is often called the "fight-or-flight system" because it prepares the body to fight or flee from danger. Input is received from the thoracic and lumbar regions of the spinal cord. The sympathetic part of the ANS elevates the heart rate (HR) and blood pressure (BP), increases the respiratory rate (RR), dilates the pupils, shunts blood to the skeletal muscles and skin, and slows digestion. The activity of the sympathetic nervous system mimics the body's response of fleeing a bear in the woods during a walk after a picnic.

Parasympathetic Nervous System

The parasympathetic division is often referred to as the "rest and digest" portion of the nervous system. It is responsible for slowing the HR, lowering the BP, decreasing respirations, shunting blood from the periphery of the body to the internal organs, constricting the pupils, and digesting food. The activity of the parasympathetic nervous system mimics the body's response while resting on the beach on a warm and sunny day after a picnic.

Acetylcholine (ACh) is the neurotransmitter synthesized by parasympathetic neurons. When an action potential is conducted down the axon of the preganglionic autonomic neuron, ACh is the substance released into the synapse between the axon terminal and the membrane of the postganglionic neurons. It crosses the synapse to bind to **nicotinic receptors** (a type of receptor that responds to ACh) of the membrane of the postganglionic neurons, depolarizing that membrane and possibly causing the postganglionic neurons to develop an action potential. An action potential is conducted down the axon of postganglionic parasympathetic neurons as the result of a depolarizing force received from the preganglionic neurons. This causes ACh to be released from the axon terminal into the synapse. Acetylcholine diffuses across the synapse and binds to muscarinic ACh receptors on the parasympathetic end organ. The activity of ACh is terminated by an enzyme called acetylcholinesterase (AChE), the enzyme that breaks down acetylcholine at the neuromuscular junction.

Motor System

The motor division of the PNS involves areas of the brain; descending fiber tracts; and motor neurons involved in producing or altering the movement of skeletal, cardiac, and smooth muscles and in regulating the secretions of various exocrine and certain endocrine glands. On the basis of the motor neurons and effector organs, the motor division can be divided into the somatic and autonomic parts.

The somatic nervous system sends cholinergic motor axons from the spinal cord or brain to the skeletal muscles. Motor fibers from the brain stimulate somatic motor neurons. The axons of these motor neurons travel within the spinal nerves and terminate at the neuromuscular junction. This is the synapse between the somatic motor neuron's axon and the muscle. When a motor neuron depolarizes, ACh is released from axon terminals into the synapse at the neuromuscular junction and binds to nicotinic receptors on skeletal muscles. This causes depolarization, resulting in contraction. Similar to the autonomic fibers described previously, the activity of ACh in the neuromuscular junction is also terminated by the enzyme AChE (Fig. 38.1).

MYASTHENIA GRAVIS

Myasthenia gravis, an acquired **autoimmune** neuromuscular junction disorder that results in the body's immune system attacking healthy cells, is caused by antibodies that are directed toward skeletal muscle nicotinic ACh receptors and muscle-specific kinase (MuSK). The name of the disorder is derived from the Greek term *myasthenia*, referring to muscle weakness, and the Latin term *gravis*, meaning "grave"; hence, MG refers to grave muscle weakness. This chronic neurological disorder is characterized by skeletal muscle weakness that may fluctuate across the day. Patients are typically diagnosed and managed in the outpatient setting. However, periodic inpatient admissions may be required for medication adjustments or when patients experience increased weakness from an infection.

Epidemiology

Myasthenia gravis is a motor disorder characterized by fluctuating, localized skeletal muscle weakness and fatigue. It is an acquired autoimmune disease in which antibodies bind to the ACh receptors on the muscle membrane. It may be made worse by or induced by penicillamine (Cuprimine), used in the treatment of rheumatoid arthritis, but in most cases, MG is idiopathic. The course of the disease may vary from mild, with ocular symptoms of **ptosis** (drooping eyelids) and **diplopia** (double vision), to severe cases with generalized weakness and respiratory involvement.

The prevalence of MG in the United States is 14 to 20 per 100,000 population, for a total of 60,000 cases. Although MG previously was more common in women, it is now more common in men. The average age of onset in women is 20 to 30 years, whereas in men, the onset is 60 to 80 years. For these reasons, it is a disorder affecting younger women and older men. Most patients with MG are over age 50. There are no known risk factors associated with developing the disease.

Pathophysiology

In normal nerve transmission, ACh is produced and secreted in the terminal ends of the motor nerves. Acetylcholine crosses the synaptic clefts and attaches to ACh receptors (AChRs) embedded in the folds of the postsynaptic membrane. This ACh–AChR binding results in depolarization of the end plate. Muscle membrane depolarization quickly occurs, resulting in skeletal muscle contraction.

In MG, circulating anti-AChR antibodies bind with the AChR, resulting in complement-mediated destruction of receptor sites. Postsynaptic membranes lose their folds, and ACh binding is blocked. Sensitivity to normal amounts of ACh is diminished with a reduction of initiating depolarization and therefore muscle contraction. This results in skeletal muscle weakness and fatigability. It is important to realize that in MG, there is an adequate amount of ACh released, but postsynaptic receptor sites are not available.

Myasthenia gravis presents as one of three serotypes: anti-AChR, MuSK, or seronegative MG (SNMG). The

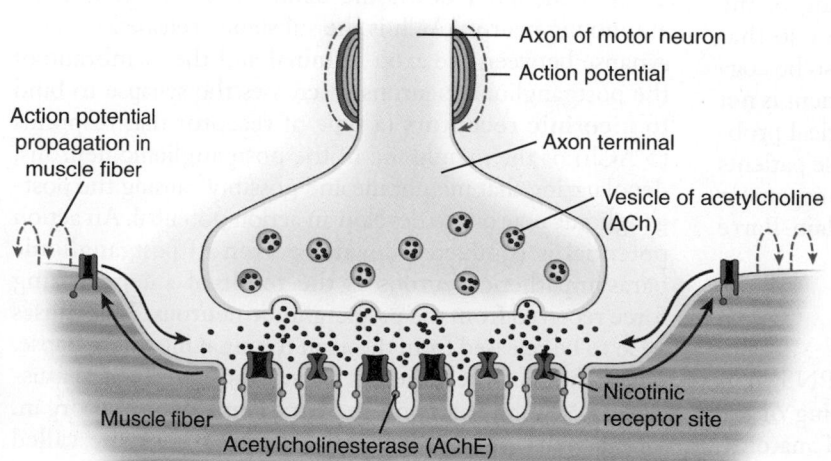

FIGURE 38.1 Action of acetylcholine (ACh) and acetylcholinesterase (AChE) at the neuromuscular junction. When a motor neuron depolarizes, ACh is released from axon terminals into the synapse at the neuromuscular junction and binds to nicotinic receptors on skeletal muscles. This causes depolarization, resulting in contraction. The activity of ACh in the neuromuscular junction is also terminated by the enzyme AChE.

anti-AChR antibody is found in approximately 80% of patients with MG, whereas 10% are MuSK type, and the remaining 10% have no identified circulating antibodies, which is referred to as SNMG.

The thymus gland is an organ of the immune system that produces T cells or T lymphocytes. Seventy percent of patients with MG have thymic hyperplasia (enlarged thymus), whereas 10% have thymoma (tumor of the thymus gland). Although the relationship between MG and thymoma is not clear, it is believed that the thymus gland may give flawed instructions to developing immune cells, eventually resulting in the development of AChR antibodies. This tumor of the thymus gland tends to be benign and enclosed. Patients with thymoma typically have higher levels of antibodies and a more severe disease course. Thymectomy, a surgical procedure for MG patients, is discussed later in this chapter.

Clinical Manifestations

Myasthenia gravis is categorized into ocular, bulbar, or generalized presentations, and patients with MG often seek medical care for muscular weakness and fatigue. Two-thirds of patients with MG present with ocular symptoms, namely, ptosis and diplopia. Many MG patients experience these symptoms within 2 years of disease onset. Ptosis may be unilateral or bilateral. Diplopia is a result of extraocular muscle weakness, and ocular symptoms may worsen with activities that require sustained use of the eye muscles.

Bulbar symptoms are the first to appear in about 16% of MG patients and refer to clinical manifestations involving cranial nerves (CNs; CN IX, CN X, CN XI, and CN XII) that emerge from the medulla of the brainstem (Fig. 38.2 and Table 38.1). The medulla is shaped like a bulb (i.e., tulip bulb), and this is the link to the term *bulbar*. These clinical manifestations include difficulty with phonation, chewing, and swallowing.

Trunk weakness and limb weakness are the initial clinical manifestations in roughly 16% to 20% of MG patients, and typically the patient experiences greater weakness of proximal muscles than distal muscles. Although MG can affect any muscles, the muscles of the neck, deltoids, triceps, wrists, fingers, and ankles are commonly affected. Weakness varies across the day but generally worsens late in the day, and clinical manifestations worsen with sustained muscle use. Patients may complain of difficulty with completing activities of daily living, such as bathing and dressing.

Connection Check 38.1

The nurse recognizes which explanation as the pathophysiological basis for MG?

A. There is an inadequate number of muscarinic receptors.

B. Antibodies to AChRs block neuromuscular junction transmission.

C. Thymomas are present in 80% of patients with MG.

D. There is an abundance of ACh, which binds to viable receptors.

Management

Medical Management

Diagnosis

The diagnosis of MG is based on clinical assessment as well as analysis of diagnostic tests. Serological tests, electromyography, and the edrophonium (Tensilon) test all aid in establishing a diagnosis of MG.

Serological Testing

An assay for AChR antibodies is essential for making a diagnosis of MG. The AChR-binding antibodies are found in roughly 80% of patients with generalized MG but only 55% of patients with ocular MG. The AChR-binding antibody assay is very specific, and positive antibody studies verify MG in the presence of a clinical picture that is consistent with MG. The AChR antibodies compete for the neurotransmitter's ACh binding sites. Additionally, antibodies to

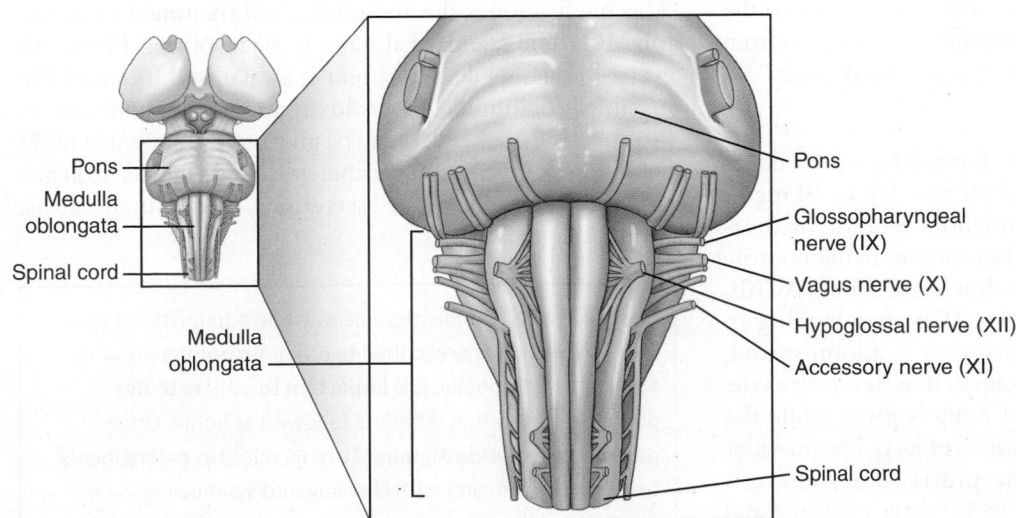

Pons
Medulla oblongata
Spinal cord

Medulla oblongata

Pons

Glossopharyngeal nerve (IX)

Vagus nerve (X)

Hypoglossal nerve (XII)

Accessory nerve (XI)

Spinal cord

FIGURE 38.2 Brainstem with lower cranial nerves (CNs). Cranial nerve IX, CN X, CN XI, and CN XII emerge from the medulla of the brainstem.

Table 38.1 Cranial Nerve Involvement in Myasthenia Gravis

Cranial Nerve	Function
IX (glossopharyngeal)	• Motor fibers control tongue movement, swallowing, and gagging. • Sensory function controls taste, touch, and temperature from the tongue; also has a role in blood pressure control.
X (vagus)	• Innervates organs in the head, neck, and thoracic and abdominal cavities • Key role in function
XI (spinal accessory)	• Controls movement of the head, neck, and shoulders
XII (hypoglossal)	• Controls tongue movement

MuSK are found in about one-third of patients with generalized MG. Patients with MuSK are generally females with prominent bulbar clinical manifestations, shoulder girdle weakness, and respiratory weakness.

Repetitive Nerve Stimulation and Electromyography

Repetitive nerve stimulation is a diagnostic tool used to evaluate neuromuscular transmission and measures muscle action potential after repeated nerve stimulations. With nerve stimulation, immediate stores of ACh at the neuromuscular junction are depleted. This results in a failure to generate an action potential. In MG, there is decreased muscle response with repetitive stimulation.

Single-fiber electromyography is the most sensitive diagnostic tool for detecting an abnormality in neuromuscular transmission. This test requires needles to be placed in the muscle to measure electrical activity. The recording from normal muscles shows two evoked responses from two muscle fibers firing, with minimal fluctuation of the interval between the two. The fluctuation is called "jitter" and is due to the variable time required for neuromuscular transmission from discharge to discharge. In MG, there is increased "jitter."

Tensilon (Edrophonium) Test

Another diagnostic test that is performed by a provider is called the edrophonium or **Tensilon** test. Up to 10 mg of **edrophonium**, a short-acting anticholinesterase medication, is administered via IV push. Edrophonium temporarily improves neuromuscular transmission by inhibiting AChE, which is the enzyme that degrades ACh after binding to the AChR site. Before the medication is administered, the provider focuses on a weak group of muscles, such as the ocular muscles. An initial dose of 2 mg is given while the patient has sustained visual focus on an object. The provider assesses for improvement of the ptosis. If no effect is observed, additional doses of 3 and 5 mg are administered

at 1-minute intervals. Improvement of muscle weakness at 2 to 5 minutes followed by a return to baseline over the next 5 minutes indicates a positive test.

Edrophonium is a rapid-acting AChE inhibitor. This leads to increased levels of ACh at the neuromuscular junction, leading to improved muscle strength in patients with myasthenia. Unfortunately, the activity is not specific to the neuromuscular junction, and ACh accumulates in the parasympathetic ANS as well. This accounts for the majority of the side effects, including bronchospasm, bradycardia, and diarrhea. Increased stimulation of the muscarinic receptors leads to bradycardia in the heart and bronchospasm in the lungs.

Atropine is a muscarinic blocker, and thus the side effects of edrophonium and other AChE inhibitors can be reversed with this medication. Because it works only in the ANS, it will not interfere with the activity at the neuromuscular junction. In short, atropine should be available to reverse any severe bradycardia that may occur during the edrophonium test. This test is best performed in a controlled setting in the hospital, such as an inpatient unit or intensive care unit.

Chest Computed Tomography Scan

A chest computed tomography (CT) scan is routinely performed to evaluate the patient with MG for thymoma. A chest CT scan is more sensitive than plain x-ray films.

Medications

The treatment of MG is individualized to meet the needs of each patient (Table 38.2). The healthcare provider considers the severity of the patient's illness, age, and lifestyle, as well as the financial demands of long-term therapy. Treatments are aimed at (1) symptomatic treatment to increase the availability of ACh, (2) immunosuppression, (3) approaches to alter the immunopathogenic mechanism underlying MG, and (4) immunomodulatory effect with thymectomy.

Pyridostigmine (Mestinon)

Pyridostigmine is a medication that is a reversible inhibitor of AChE. It improves neuromuscular transmission by increasing ACh stimulation of the AChRs that are available. This medication is the accepted initial treatment of choice for MG. The standard dosage is 30 to 60 mg by mouth every 4 hours while the patient is awake, and it is available in tablets or liquid. A pyridostigmine sustained-release formula (180-mg) tablet may be given to the patient at night before sleep. Possible muscarinic side effects include stomach cramps, diarrhea, increased secretions, nausea, bradycardia, and muscle twitches.

> **! Safety Alert**   Pyridostigmine must be administered exactly as prescribed to maintain optimal muscle strength. Additionally, it is important to adhere to the patient's medication schedule followed at home. Often, patients take pyridostigmine 30 to 60 minutes before meals to minimize difficulty with chewing and swallowing.

Table 38.2 Medications Used to Treat Myasthenia Gravis

Medication	Typical Dosage	Nursing Considerations
Pyridostigmine (Mestinon) (anticholinesterase inhibitor) • Oral tablets • Liquid • Sustained release	60-mg tablets every 4 hours while awake 180-mg tablet	Medication should be administered exactly at the prescribed hour; administer 30–60 minutes before meal; monitor for increase in secretions, muscle cramps, and diarrhea.
Prednisone (Deltasone, Prednicot) (corticosteroid)	Low dose: 15–20 mg daily High dose: 60–80 mg daily in controlled setting	Provide education about side effects of steroids: immunosuppression, gastrointestinal bleed, hyperglycemia, weight gain, truncal obesity, and sleep disturbance. Monitor blood glucose levels closely. Patient may require insulin coverage. Confer with provider to provide patient with calcium and vitamin D supplementation to decrease bone loss.

Neostigmine (Prostigmin)

Neostigmine is a shorter-acting AChE inhibitor. This medication is administered intravenously when the patient's oral route is not available because of surgery or other conditions such as Crohn's disease, gastrointestinal bleed, or paralytic ileus. Most acute care facilities have a policy for this medication that limits administration to patients in a monitored setting because of the potential side effects of bradycardia or cardiac dysrhythmias. The IV site needs to be monitored frequently to ensure patency because of the short half-life of neostigmine. Some policies require dual IV access so that a second IV site is available if the first one infiltrates. The provider determines the proper dose conversion to oral pyridostigmine when the patient is ready to resume taking medications orally. The ratio of IV neostigmine is 1 mg equals 60 mg pyridostigmine. The nurse administers the oral pyridostigmine 1 hour before stopping the IV medication. Side effects of this medication are similar to those of pyridostigmine.

Immunotherapy

There are several immunosuppressant medications available to treat MG. These medications are initiated when AChE inhibitors are not adequate in moderately severe MG, and prednisone is the principal medication from this category that is used in MG. The patient may be hospitalized when prednisone is initiated because deterioration may occur in the first few weeks of treatment.

Azathioprine (Imuran) is a steroid-sparing medication that may also be used. It inhibits T-cell and B-cell proliferation through interaction with purine metabolism and nucleic acid synthesis. Another medication that may be used is cyclosporine, which inhibits T helper cell–mediated synthesis of cytokines and other T helper cell–mediated immune reactions. Cyclosporine has been used successfully in patients when steroids and thymectomy have failed. The time to treatment response is approximately 7 months.

Mycophenolate mofetil (CellCept) suppresses both T-cell and B-cell proliferation. This medication is commonly used in the United States. The usual dosage is 1 g twice a day, and adverse effects include diarrhea, anemia, leukopenia, and infections.

Cyclophosphamide (Cytoxan), a chemotherapeutic agent, is also used in the management of MG. At high doses, this medication is used to ablate (destroy) bone marrow and allow the patient's endogenous stem cells to repopulate the immune system with new lymphocytes. This approach allows the patient's immune system to "reboot."

Medications to Be Used With Caution in Myasthenia Gravis

The provider and nurse must be familiar with medications that are contraindicated in MG because some medications have an adverse effect on neuromuscular transmission and may lead to increased weakness. The medications that are contraindicated in MG include some antibiotics, calcium-channel blockers, D-penicillamine, and magnesium. Antibiotics such as streptomycin and polymyxin exhibit a nondepolarizing blocking action on neuromuscular transmission. Calcium-channel blockers and magnesium block calcium, which is necessary for normal neuromuscular transmission.

Aside from IV magnesium sulfate, nurses need to be aware of certain antacids and laxatives that also contain magnesium because they should be avoided in patients with MG. There may be some clinical situations where administration of these medications may be warranted by the patient's clinical condition (i.e., hypomagnesemia). If any of these medications are ordered, the nurse should consult with the provider to determine if increased clinical assessments should be performed (e.g., forced vital capacity).

Patients and families should be educated to inform healthcare providers about these medications when being treated in settings such as the emergency department or surgical setting, where providers may be unfamiliar with MG (Table 38.3).

Additional Therapies

In addition to medication therapies, two additional therapies, IV immunoglobulin (IVIG) and plasmapheresis, are also used in the treatment of MG. These therapies have a quicker onset of action when compared with the immunosuppressant therapies. Their effects are limited to 4 to 6 weeks and are typically used when the patient is hospitalized for exacerbation of MG or prior to surgery. Randomized controlled trials have suggested that IVIG and plasmapheresis are equally effective. The choice of treatment is the provider's decision. Intravenous immunoglobulin is administered by the IV route, whereas plasmapheresis requires the insertion of a dual-lumen catheter.

Intravenous Immunoglobulin

Intravenous immunoglobulin is a concentrated immunoglobulin (Ig) solution primarily composed of IgG that is produced from pooled blood donors. The mode of action is complex, and it inactivates abnormal autoantibodies and suppresses T-cell function. The medication is costly, and a treatment course is approximately $10,000. The total dose administered intravenously over 3 to 5 days is 2 g/kg. This medication is administered slowly, and the rate is carefully titrated. Vital signs are checked frequently, and the patient is monitored for flu-like symptoms (e.g., fever, headache, chills, myalgia). Renal functions, including blood urea nitrogen (BUN) and creatinine, are monitored prior to the initial infusion and then periodically. This medication is carefully administered in patients with diabetes mellitus

or renal insufficiency because renal failure is a potential complication.

For decades, steroids and acetylcholinesterase inhibitors were the mainstay of therapy for patients with MG. In late 2017, a new treatment, eculizumab, was added to the armamentarium of treatments for patients with anti-acetylcholine receptor (AchR) antibody-positive MG. Many of these patients could not tolerate standard treatments. Eculizumab is a monoclonal antibody that is a complement inhibitor. Uncontrolled activation of the complement system plays a major role in the clinical manifestations experienced by patients with MG. Providers must confirm that patients have received a meningococcal vaccine at least 2 weeks before the medication is administered because the risk of meningococcal disease is 1,000-fold to 2,000-fold higher among patients taking this medication. For MG, the medication is administered as an IV infusion of 900 mg/week for the first 4 weeks, 1,200 mg for week 5, and then 1,200 mg every 2 weeks afterward. Adverse effects of the medication include hypertension, nausea, vomiting, diarrhea, and headache. Other medications that inhibit complement are currently under investigation and could potentially change how patients with MG are managed.

CASE STUDY: EPISODE 2

On Ms. Jordan's admission, her examination reveals bilateral ptosis, **dysarthria** (difficulty speaking), and **dysphagia** (difficulty swallowing). Her speech is slurred, and she has difficulty with swallowing secretions. Her vital capacity is 1.3 L. She has diminished strength in all four extremities and requires the assistance of one nurse for ambulation. Her vital signs are as follows: BP 110/70 mm Hg, HR 114 bpm, RR 28, and temperature of 100.3°F (37.9°C). Ms. Jordan requires the insertion of a nasogastric tube for medications, and an infusion of normal saline is initiated for dehydration...

Table 38.3 Medications Known to Exacerbate Myasthenia Gravis

Class of Medications	Names
Antibiotics	Aminoglycosides, ciprofloxacin, clindamycin, telithromycin, ampicillin, erythromycin
Antiarrhythmics	Procainamide, propranolol, timolol, verapamil, quinidine
Neuropsychiatrics	Phenytoin, trimethadione, lithium
Other	Trihexyphenidyl, neuromuscular-blocking agents, magnesium preparations, carbamazepine, oral contraceptives, transdermal nicotine

From Khadilkar, S. V., Yadav, R. S., & Patel, B. A. (2018). Myasthenia gravis. In *Neuromuscular disorders: A comprehensive review with illustrative cases* (pp. 239–260). Singapore: Springer. doi:10.1007/978-981-10-5361-0_22

Plasmapheresis

Plasmapheresis requires the insertion of a large-bore dual-lumen catheter and is usually limited to large medical centers. During plasmapheresis, the patient's blood is removed through the arterial lumen and circulated through the plasmapheresis machine, which removes antibodies that block AChR function. The goal of this treatment is to improve muscle strength. Anticoagulation is required to prevent clotting in the extracorporeal blood during an **apheresis procedure** (a procedure that involves removing whole blood and separating the blood into individual components so that one particular component can be removed). Citrate is the anticoagulant of choice during a plasmapheresis procedure. Citrate is added to the blood when it is outside the body to prevent clotting from occurring. The citrate binds with calcium and effectively blocks the calcium-dependent clotting factor reactions.

The solid blood components, red blood cells, white blood cells, and platelets, are returned through the venous lumen with normal saline and albumin. A total of seven treatments is usually ordered for the patient. Treatments may be done at the bedside, or the patient may be transported to a pheresis center. Because plasmapheresis involves the removal of plasma, medications in the plasma may be removed. Prior to the treatment, the nurse should consult with the provider to determine if any medications should be held. Antihypertensives may increase the chance of hypotension during the treatment, and there is also the potential for plasmapheresis to affect therapeutic levels of medications. Patients are monitored for blood clotting following each session because the procedure can also remove coagulation factors in the blood.

Patients may experience paresthesias from citrate-induced hypocalcemia, and hypotension may occur at the start of the exchange. Patients are asked to report any numbness or tingling, especially around the lips, because these findings are indicative of hypocalcemia. Because the citrate binds with calcium to effectively prevent clotting, the patient has an increased risk of hypocalcemia, and this is the most common side effect of this procedure. The ionized calcium level decreases in the patient as a result of the citrate infusion, the removal of calcium in the patient's wasted plasma, and the calcium-binding properties of albumin. However, these complications may be prevented by adding calcium to the replacement fluid, 5% albumin, or by slowing down the infusion of the citrate during the procedure. If citrate reactions are not treated, they can progress from paresthesias, vibration sensation, nausea/vomiting, and diarrhea to hypotension, chest tightness, tetany, and cardiac arrhythmias.

During plasmapheresis, fluid shifts are caused by removing plasma and replacing the plasma with substitute fluids or 5% albumin, and some patients may experience nausea and vomiting because of these fluid shifts and electrolyte imbalances. The change in intravascular volume and the dilutional effects of the plasma constituent levels may cause hypovolemia. Clinical manifestations of hypovolemia may include dizziness, light-headedness, nausea, diaphoresis, tachycardia, and hypotension. These can be treated by pausing the procedure, placing the patient in a Trendelenburg position if not contraindicated, and administering a saline bolus of fluids. In subsequent procedures, replacement fluids may be adjusted with an increase in colloids and a decrease in crystalloids.

Patients may also experience a vasovagal reaction during or after the plasmapheresis procedure. These patients may experience pallor, sweating, diaphoresis, nausea/vomiting, hypotension, and bradycardia, and the treatment is the same as for hypovolemia. Electrolytes, namely, potassium and calcium, need to be monitored in the patient receiving plasmapheresis.

The pheresis nurse instills heparin in each port of the dual-lumen catheter following the plasmapheresis treatment.

The catheter also needs to be instilled with heparin on nonpheresis days to prevent clotting. The integrity of the line is preserved and clotting prevented by allowing heparin to dwell in the line while it is not in use. Whenever the catheter is accessed, the heparin must first be removed before the line is flushed so that the patient does not receive a bolus of heparin. There is an increased risk of infection and thrombotic complications associated with the plasmapheresis catheter. Of note, this catheter resembles a hemodialysis catheter and should not be confused with a dialysis catheter. A dialysis catheter is a dedicated line specifically used for hemodialysis and is not accessed by nurses outside the dialysis center.

Surgical Management

A surgical approach to the management of MG is thymectomy. Generally, thymectomy is performed within the first 3 years of diagnosis and in individuals less than the age of 65. This surgery is always performed for patients with thymoma. Although there are several approaches to performing this surgery, the standard approach is transsternal extended thymectomy. (These patients require postoperative care similar to that of patients undergoing open-heart surgery). However, transcervical and videoendoscopic procedures, including robotic-assisted surgery, are gaining popularity because of shorter hospital stays and improved cosmetic results. Patients undergoing surgery require IV neostigmine (Prostigmin) because of NPO status and management in an intensive care unit following surgery. Intravenous neostigmine, an IV anticholinesterase medication, is required to maintain muscle strength and respiratory function. Because oral pyridostigmine bromide (Mestinon) is discontinued for surgery, the patient must receive an IV equivalent of the medication.

Complications

It can be extremely difficult to differentiate between worsening of MG and excessive anticholinergic medication in a rapidly deteriorating patient with muscular weakness and potential respiratory failure.

Myasthenic Crisis

Myasthenic crisis is an exacerbation of MG weakness that provokes an acute episode of respiratory failure that is often caused by a respiratory infection from viral or bacterial agents. Weakness may involve the respiratory or bulbar muscles and may affect the patient's ability to protect the airway. Additional features of myasthenic crisis include tachycardia, flaccid muscles, and pale and cool skin. Myasthenic crisis is an emergency that requires prompt recognition and treatment in an intensive care unit for optimal management. The crisis usually lasts for approximately 2 weeks. Intravenous immunoglobulin or plasmapheresis is used to manage the patient throughout the crisis.

Cholinergic Crisis

Another type of crisis that the MG patient may encounter is **cholinergic crisis**. This is due to excessive anticholinesterase medication and is potentially secondary to the patient taking too much of the prescribed MG medication. Features of a cholinergic crisis include muscle bradycardia, **fasciculations** (muscle twitch), sweating, pallor, excessive secretions, and small pupils. It may be difficult to distinguish which crisis, cholinergic or myasthenic, the patient is experiencing because both crises have similar clinical features. The Tensilon (edrophonium) test is useful in distinguishing myasthenic from cholinergic crisis because it has a rapid onset and is short acting. This test may assist the provider in identifying the type of crisis the patient is experiencing and selecting the appropriate treatment course. When Tensilon is administered, if the patient demonstrates muscle strength improvement, it is determined to be a myasthenic crisis. If Tensilon is administered and the patient demonstrates fasciculations and muscle weakness, including the respiratory muscles, it is a cholinergic crisis. Anticholinesterase medications are temporarily discontinued in a cholinergic crisis.

Diet

Patients with MG benefit from the professional evaluation of a speech language pathologist and registered dietitian. Because of the weakness of the oropharyngeal muscles, the patient may have difficulty with chewing and swallowing that increases the risk for aspiration. Modifications are made in the patient's diet so that adequate nutrition is provided and may include thickened liquids or enteral tube feedings.

Connection Check 38.2

During the edrophonium or Tensilon test, a short-acting AChE inhibitor is administered intravenously, and the provider observes the patient for improvement in which function?
A. Level of consciousness
B. Muscle strength
C. Muscle tone
D. Hearing

Nursing Management

Assessment and Analysis

The patient with MG may experience clinical manifestations including respiratory deterioration and muscular weakness. The nurse performs a comprehensive neurological assessment of the patient with MG, including a detailed cranial nerve assessment. The nurse also carefully assesses motor strength to identify muscle weakness. Because of the potential for respiratory weakness, a bedside test known as the *vital capacity* is performed. Vital capacity is defined as the maximum amount of air exhaled following maximal inhalation. A patient has normal respiratory function with a value of 65 mL/kg. When a patient's value falls below 15 mL/kg or generally 1 L, respiratory deterioration may progress

rapidly, and mechanical ventilation will be required. Aside from bedside vital capacity measurements, which the nurse can perform, serial negative inspiratory force and positive expiratory force assessments are performed with the assistance of a respiratory therapist. The patient with MG is assessed for the following clinical manifestations:

- Muscle weakness that increases over the course of the day
- Fatigue
- Ptosis
- Diplopia
- Dysphagia
- Dysarthria

 Safety Alert In patients with MG, it is important to carefully monitor vital capacity measurements. Pulse oximetry is not helpful in determining respiratory deterioration in a patient with MG because the failure is due to weakness of the diaphragm and intercostal muscles. The patient will develop hypoxemia and hypercarbia. Because the patient retains carbon dioxide (CO_2), the provider needs to obtain an arterial blood gas to assess CO_2.

Nursing Diagnoses

- **High risk for ineffective breathing** related to respiratory muscle weakness
- **High risk for aspiration** related to bulbar weakness
- **Fatigue related** to muscular weakness

Nursing Interventions

▪ Assessments

- Assess breath sounds and observe the patient's respiratory effort.
  Obtain vital capacity per provider's order. This is usually obtained immediately prior to a dose of pyridostigmine to obtain a trough value and then 1 hour post-dose to evaluate peak effect.
  If the value is below 1 L, the patient is at risk for respiratory compromise. Notify the provider. Respiratory deterioration may lead to respiratory arrest. Patients often require intubation and mechanical ventilation in an intensive care setting.
- Vital capacity measurement
  Vital capacity is an important respiratory function to monitor. If the value is below 1 L, notify the provider. In MG, the patient develops weakness of the diaphragm and intercostal muscles. Weakness of the respiratory muscles results in diminished forced vital capacity.
- Cranial nerves IX, X, XI, and XII
  Bulbar symptoms are the first to appear in about 16% of MG patients and place the patient at risk for aspiration due to difficulty swallowing.
- Dysphagia
  Weakness of the oropharyngeal muscles places the patient at risk for dysarthria and dysphagia.

- Nutritional intake, intake and output, and daily weight
  Cranial nerve weakness can make it difficult for the patient to chew and swallow. The patient may become fatigued during the meal.
- Dysarthria
  Patients may have a nasal quality to the speech and be at risk for aspiration because of weakness of these muscles. This is related to impairment of CNs V, VII, IX, X, XI, and XII.

■ Actions

- Administer medications at prescribed times and prior to activities requiring swallowing.
  Pyridostigmine must be administered exactly at the prescribed hour to maintain optimal muscle strength. Patients often take pyridostigmine 30 to 60 minutes before meals to minimize difficulty with chewing and swallowing.
- Elevate the head of the patient's bed with eating or drinking.
  Weakness of the oropharyngeal muscles increases the risk of aspiration, and elevating the head of the bed may decrease aspiration.
- Establish effective communication method with the patient.
  Consult with speech language pathology to obtain a picture communication board because verbal communication is impaired by dysarthria.
- Plan meals when medications are at peak levels.
  Timing the meals with peak medication levels decreases the risk of aspiration. Small, frequent meals will help maintain calorie intake. Weight loss may result from poor nutritional intake.
- Offer soft foods and thickened liquids as recommended by the speech language pathologist.
  A temporary feeding tube may be necessary if swallowing is impaired or if the patient deteriorates and requires intubation and mechanical ventilation.
- Plan for rest periods between activities of daily living.
  Use energy conservation techniques, such as sitting while activities of daily living are completed, to minimize fatigue and muscle weakness.

■ Teaching

- Importance of taking medications as prescribed
  It is important to teach the patient to adhere to the medication schedule at home because swallowing may be impaired if eating, drinking, brushing teeth, and other activities are not performed at peak levels of the medications.
- Educate patient to keep medication with him or her at all times. Spare doses should be kept at the place of employment and in the car. When the patient travels, medication should remain with the patient in carry-on luggage.
  The patient should not miss a dose of pyridostigmine bromide because this can lead to muscular weakness.
- Instruct patient to purchase a MedicAlert bracelet and to wear it daily.
  In the event of an emergency, the patient's diagnosis may be rapidly identified by emergency medical service providers.

- Avoid public places such as theaters or concerts in the winter where there are large gatherings of people.
  The patient may be exposed to colds and the flu where there are large gatherings of people, and this increases the risk of exacerbation.
- Obtain vaccines to prevent the flu and pneumonia.
  Vaccines decrease the risk of infection. Respiratory infections may lead to myasthenic crisis that requires hospitalization.
- Prevent fatigue with frequent rest periods. Recognize physical limits, and plan activities during peak energy periods.
  The risk of injury is decreased when activities are scheduled during peak times of medications.
- Do not take any over-the-counter preparations without first checking with the provider.
  Over-the-counter products may have ingredients that are contraindicated in MG.
- Inform the patient and family about resources, such as the Myasthenia Gravis Foundation of America.
  This organization provides detailed education and e-resources for patients and families.

Connection Check 38.3

The nurse assesses for which clinical manifestations in a patient admitted with MG? *(Select all the apply)*.
A. Ptosis
B. Diplopia
C. Hyperventilation
D. Dysphagia
E. Bitemporal headaches

Connection Check 38.4

Which action is critical when administering a pyridostigmine 60-mg tablet to a patient with MG?
A. Administer with milk and crackers to minimize gastrointestinal distress.
B. Administer 2 hours after meals because food slows gastric absorption.
C. Administer 30 to 60 minutes before meals to optimize the strength of the chewing and swallowing muscles.
D. Administer with orange juice because vitamin C facilitates gastric emptying.

Evaluating Care Outcomes

Patients with MG may be successfully managed with cholinesterase inhibitors. The patient and family must be aware of clinical manifestations of crisis and seek medical attention quickly. Patient education plays a crucial role in the successful management of the patient. With adherence to prescribed medications and the treatment plan, patients are able to actively participate in family activities and a career.

It is important for the patient and family to be educated on the disease process and the medications. Not only should the patient be educated about the action of medications required for the management of MG, but the patient should also be knowledgeable about medications to be avoided because they increase weakness. Information about the clinical manifestations of crises are included in a comprehensive teaching plan.

Connection Check 38.5

The patient with MG needs to be educated about medications that should be avoided because they can increase weakness. Which medication should the patient avoid?

A. Acetaminophen
B. Prednisone
C. Azathioprine
D. Maalox

GUILLAIN-BARRÉ SYNDROME

Guillain-Barré syndrome (GBS), another disorder of the PNS, is an acute inflammatory demyelinating **polyneuropathy** (simultaneous neuropathy of peripheral nerves). It often occurs after an infection and leads to a rapidly progressing flaccid paralysis. This syndrome was first identified about a century ago by French neurologists Guillain, Barré, and Strohl. They provided an account of two soldiers who developed acute paralysis with areflexia (absent reflexes) and then recovered spontaneously. It is important that healthcare team members rapidly identify GBS as it presents in the provider's office or emergency department in order to ensure that appropriate treatment is implemented.

Epidemiology

About two-thirds of patients who develop GBS demonstrate clinical manifestations of an infection 3 weeks prior to onset. Respiratory or gastrointestinal infections are the most common sources. *Campylobacter jejuni* is the most frequently identified cause, but cytomegalovirus, Epstein-Barr virus, *Mycoplasma pneumonia*, and *Haemophilus influenzae* are also causes. Guillain-Barré is a syndrome that affects the immune system and attacks the PNS.

Zika is a part of the mosquito-borne group of flaviviruses that are primarily transmitted by mosquitoes. As a virus, Zika had circulated for many decades with no reported epidemics until February 2016 when the World Health Organization declared it a major public health problem. There is recent evidence that supports a link between Zika virus and GBS. Guillain-Barré was the first reported complication of Zika in adults. A recent report suggests that Zika virus should be included in the list of infectious pathogens that can cause GBS. The pathogenesis of Zika virus–associated GBS is unknown. The typical treatment of GBS, which includes plasmapheresis, IVIG, and intensive care can be challenging in remote regions of the world.

The incidence of GBS is about 1 case per 100,000 population, with men and women equally affected. Mortality rates range from 2% to 10% from autonomic dysfunction or complications of immobility and increase with age. Patients are more likely to die if they are over 60 years of age, have a rapidly progressing variant of GBS, develop axonal loss, and require an extended course of mechanical ventilation.

Pathophysiology

Guillain-Barré syndrome is mediated by an immune response with acute lower extremity weakness with areflexia or diminished reflexes developing over several days. An infection usually precedes the development of GBS by about a month. In GBS, the patient's own immune system begins to destroy the myelin that surrounds the peripheral nerves. Destruction occurs between the nodes of Ranvier, which impairs **saltatory (jumping) conduction** and results in the slowing of impulses or a conduction block. There is infiltration of lymphocytes into the peripheral nervous system, which attracts macrophages; the macrophages penetrate the Schwann cell and invade the myelin, resulting in demyelination. Lymphocytes can be seen at points of myelin breakdown on microscopic exam. Axons usually remain intact (Fig. 38.3). In addition to affecting the myelin on cranial and motor nerves, sensory function is often impaired as well.

The patient's immune system produces antibodies in response to a viral or bacterial illness to fight the infection. Antibodies are also produced that attack the myelin of the peripheral nerves. Nerve damage results in numbness and tingling, muscle weakness, paralysis, and potential respiratory compromise.

There are three stages of GBS. The first stage is known as the *acute stage* and starts with the onset of clinical

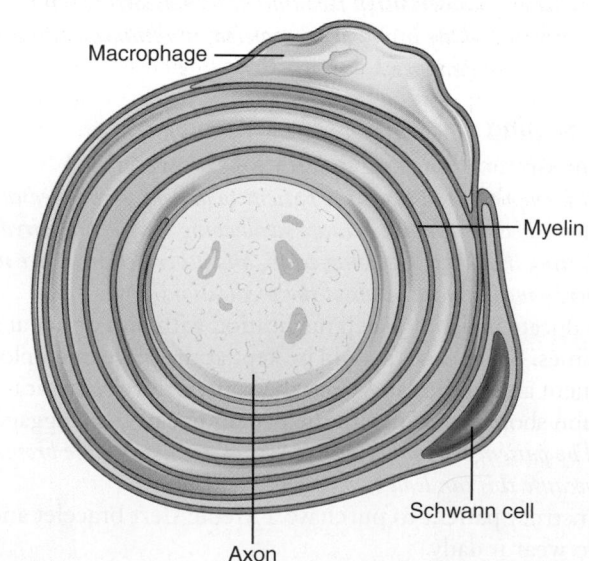

FIGURE 38.3 Guillain-Barré syndrome. Macrophages attach to and destroy myelin, leading to decreased nerve conduction.

manifestations of peripheral nerve **demyelination** (destruction of myelin sheath), edema, and inflammation. This phase lasts approximately 4 weeks. When demyelination ceases, the patient enters the *plateau stage*, which lasts from a few days to weeks. In the *recovery stage*, remyelination and axonal regeneration begin, and there is a gradual improvement in the patient's signs and symptoms.

Clinical Manifestations

Although there are several subtypes of GBS, such as Miller–Fisher syndrome and acute motor axonal neuropathy, the most common form, acute inflammatory demyelinating polyneuropathy, is the focus of this chapter. The patient with GBS develops a symmetrical ascending motor weakness and paralysis that usually starts in the feet and extends to the trunk and arms. (Note: There is an easy way to remember the pattern of weakness in GBS: It starts in the toes, and up it goes.) There may be sensory involvement, and patients may complain of paresthesias and pain that involves the shoulders, back, buttocks, and upper legs. After the first few days of weakness, neurological assessment demonstrates diminished or absent deep tendon reflexes (areflexia). Areflexia is recognized as a key finding in GBS.

Additionally, there may be cranial nerve involvement in 85% of cases of GBS. Cranial nerve VII (facial nerve) is most commonly affected, and the patient may have difficulty with facial expressions such as smiling or frowning. Cranial nerves IX (glossopharyngeal), X (vagus), XI (spinal accessory), and XII (hypoglossal) may also be involved, causing dysphagia. If CN X is affected, the patient may exhibit autonomic dysfunction with possible cardiac dysrhythmias, paroxysmal hypotension, orthostatic hypotension, paralytic ileus, urinary retention, and potential syndrome of inappropriate secretion of antidiuretic hormone (SIADH).

Up to 40% of patients with GBS develop respiratory impairment. Respiratory failure is caused by weakness of the diaphragm and intercostal muscles, and the patient may require intubation and mechanical ventilation to provide respiratory support. The patient's level of consciousness and cognitive function remain intact throughout the course of the illness. The pattern of recovery is the reverse of onset, and the nerves that were affected last are the first to improve.

Connection Check 38.6

What pathophysiological processes occur in the first stage, or the acute phase, of GBS?

A. Peripheral nerve demyelination, edema, and inflammation

B. Depolarization of the spinal nerves

C. Destruction of the myelin-producing oligodendrocytes

D. Regeneration of the myelin sheath

Management

Medical Management

Diagnosis

The patient with GBS is admitted to the inpatient setting for a thorough evaluation. Established diagnostic criteria for GBS include progressive weakness of two or more limbs caused by neuropathy, areflexia, and history of recent viral or bacterial infection. Additionally, a lumbar puncture is performed to obtain cerebrospinal fluid (CSF). Cerebrospinal fluid findings include elevated protein and normal cell count. Electromyography results reveal slowed nerve conduction velocity soon after the patient develops paralysis.

Medications

Management of GBS focuses on supportive care and reducing the severity, potential complications, suffering, and recovery time. Although GBS is an autoimmune disorder, steroids have not been found to help speed recovery. The use of steroids is debatable, and current research is leaning toward patients with GBS *not* receiving corticosteroid therapy.

There are two main approaches used for treatment. These modalities are IVIG and plasmapheresis. Intravenous immunoglobulin therapy can shorten the length of the recovery phase by 50%, and this therapy is recommended for patients who need help to walk within 2 to 4 weeks of clinical presentation of GBS. This treatment may work by several mechanisms, which include blocking of macrophage receptors, the inhibition of antibody production, the inhibition of complement binding, and the neutralization of pathological antibodies. The dosing is 2 g/kg intravenously over 5 days. Typical adverse effects of this medication include flu-like symptoms. Rare adverse reactions are aseptic meningitis and acute renal failure. Fluid overload may occur in patients with heart failure or renal insufficiency.

The American Academy of Neurology recommends plasmapheresis for nonambulatory adult patients with GBS who start treatment within 4 weeks of onset of neuropathic symptoms. Plasmapheresis is also recommended for ambulatory patients who start treatment within 2 weeks of the onset of neuropathic clinical manifestations. This therapy can reduce recovery time, yet requires the insertion of a plasmapheresis catheter, skilled nursing staff, and specialized equipment that may not be available at all healthcare facilities. Plasmapheresis diminishes the length of hospitalization and the need for mechanical ventilation if initiated within the first week of clinical manifestations. There is an increased risk of infection and hemorrhage as a result of the removal of immunoglobulins and clotting factors. Adverse reactions the patient may experience include hypotension, bradycardia, fever, chills, and rash. Additional complications from this treatment include septicemia, pneumonia, cardiac arrhythmias, malaise, bleeding/clotting abnormalities, and hypocalcemia.

Diet

Problems such as immobility, decreased gastric motility, and dysphagia place the patient at risk for inadequate nutrition. A speech language pathologist evaluates the patient for dysphagia and risk of aspiration. During the acute phase of the illness, a dietitian is consulted, and enteral feeding may be initiated to prevent aspiration (see Evidence-Based Practice). Feedings are individualized to meet the patient's caloric needs based on total body weight and laboratory values. Adequate nutrition is key throughout all phases of the illness, especially if the patient is intubated and placed on a mechanical ventilator. Decreased nervous innervation and ventilation support may contribute to muscle atrophy and inhibit the weaning process from the ventilator. Optimal nutrition plays a key role in the patient's recovery and prognosis.

Evidence-Based Practice

Nasogastric Tube Feeding for Patients With Guillain-Barré Syndrome

During the acute phase of Guillain-Barré syndrome (GBS), because of cranial nerve involvement, enteral tube feedings may be ordered to prevent malnutrition and aspiration. The nurse is responsible for insertion of the tube and residual and patency checks for proper positioning. The patient should be evaluated by the dietitian so that feedings meet the caloric and protein needs according to the patient's body weight and laboratory values.

The nurse is responsible for verifying nasogastric tube (NGT) placement after initial insertion, before medication administration, and every 8 hours with continuous enteral feedings. Traditional placement checks are validated by checking a mark at the nose that is placed following NGT insertion, auscultation (insufflation of 30 mL of air), and analysis of gastric contents. The literature supports that insufflation alone is not adequate. Although there are many methods by which tube verification may be accomplished (i.e., pH, enzyme, bilirubin, and carbon dioxide testing), none of these methods allows detection of a tube in the esophagus or gastroesophageal junction. X-ray placement is considered the gold standard. Radiography is the only reliable method to verify the initial placement of blindly inserted small- and large-bore feedings tubes.

Boullata, J. I., Carrera, A. L., Harvey, L., McGinnis, C., Wessel, J. J., Bajpai, S., … Guenter, P. (2017). ASPEN safe practices for enteral nutrition therapy. *Journal of Parenteral and Enteral Nutrition*, 41(1), 15–103.

Complications

In the patient with GBS, respiratory status is monitored in terms of breath sounds and forced vital capacity. Because ventilation is compromised by the loss of motor innervation to the skeletal muscles of respiration, the patient is at risk for respiratory compromise. The airway needs to be maintained, and the patient may require intubation and mechanical ventilation to prevent respiratory arrest.

During the course of GBS, the patient is also at risk for developing complications of immobility. Therefore, subcutaneous heparin may be ordered to prevent venous thromboembolism (VTE). Antiembolism stockings and sequential compression devices also play an important role in VTE prevention. The patient is also at risk for the development of pressure injuries, and a turning schedule should be implemented to prevent skin breakdown. Patients with GBS may perspire because of autonomic manifestations, and the patient's clothing and linens require frequent changes to prevent areas of moisture and to promote skin integrity.

Connection Check 38.7

The nurse correlates respiratory compromise in GBS with which pathophysiological process?
A. Decreased protein in the CSF
B. Progressive limb weakness
C. Diaphragmatic weakness
D. Decreased acetylcholine at the neuromuscular junction

Nursing Management
Assessment and Analysis

It is important for the nurse to perform a thorough baseline assessment of the patient with GBS upon admission so that changes may be noted and the provider alerted. Nursing care is paramount in providing support to the patient during the acute phase of the illness so that complications are averted. Clinical manifestations of the disease include:

- Respiratory muscle weakness
- Skeletal muscle weakness (often ascending)
- Pain
- Autonomic manifestations such as sweating and tachycardia

It is important that complications such as aspiration, VTE, and skin breakdown are avoided so that the patient will be ready to fully participate in rehabilitation. In addition to the physical care the nurse provides, it is important to include the patient in as much decision making as possible. Although weak, the patient remains alert and cognitively intact. Some patients describe the course of their illness as being locked in a body that will not work while being fully aware of their surroundings.

Nursing Diagnoses

- **High risk for ineffective breathing patterns** related to respiratory muscle weakness
- **Pain** related to inflammation early in the acute phase; related to regeneration of sensory nerve fibers later in the course
- **Impaired physical mobility** related to muscle weakness secondary to decreased nerve conduction
- **Anxiety** related to course of illness, immobility, and dependency on others

Nursing Interventions

▪ Assessments

- Perform respiratory assessment with vital capacity measurement.
  Respiratory assessment is a priority because respiratory compromise secondary to weakness of the diaphragm and intercostal muscles may require intubation. Vital capacity measurement is an important function to monitor. The provider should be notified of a value below 1 L. Diaphragmatic weakness results in hypoxemia.
- Cranial nerves VII, IX, X, XI, and XII
  Cranial nerve assessment should be performed to identify deficits. Focus on facial expression, speech, gag, and swallow.
- Motor and sensory assessment
  Motor and sensory impairment may develop related to slowing of impulses or a conduction block secondary to demyelination of peripheral nerves.
- Pain assessment
  Patients often complain of pain. This may be due to sensory nerve fiber involvement.

▪ Actions

- Turn frequently and perform range of motion every shift to maintain joint and muscle integrity.
  Immobility places the patient at risk for contractures, skin breakdown, and VTE.
- Consult with the provider on the need for VTE prevention (subcutaneous heparin, antiembolism hose, sequential compression devices).
  Prolonged immobility leads to venous stasis and the development of VTE.
- Reposition patient frequently.
  Measures are implemented to promote comfort and prevent complications of immobility, including thromboembolism and impaired skin integrity.
- Consult with provider regarding use of analgesics or nonopioids.
  Carbamazepine or gabapentin may be used to relieve neuropathic pain.
- Offer diversions such as music or other relaxation techniques.
  Pain management is addressed with pharmacological as well as nonpharmacological methods.

- Establish a method of communication, and provide a method to call the nurse (e.g., soft call bell).
  Because of limb weakness, the patient may not have the strength to locate and use the call light. A soft squeeze call bell allows the patient to call the nurse with only a gentle squeeze.

▪ Teaching

- Inform the patient and family about the importance of respiratory monitoring in the acute phase.
  Provide encouragement that the disease course lasts several weeks to months and that rehabilitation will assist the patient in returning to premorbid functioning. In addition, it is important to inform the patient and family that recovery from this neurological disorder is possible.
- Educate the patient and family about GBS at each stage of the illness.
  Education allows the patient and family to anticipate that respiratory deterioration may occur. Having this information ahead of time may help to alleviate fear.
- Inform the patient and family about resources, such as the GBS Foundation International (www.gbs-cidp.org).
  Community and other resources provide additional support systems for the patient and family. Respite care may be available through some of these organizations.

Connection Check 38.8

Which nursing intervention is a priority for a patient with cranial nerve impairment from GBS?

A. Perform sensory checks with the neurological examination below the level of the cervical spine.

B. Consult with the provider for initiation of continuous positive airway pressure for breathing.

C. Create a turning schedule with limited time in the side-lying position.

D. Establish effective communication using eye blinks or a communication board.

Evaluating Care Outcomes

The patient with GBS may enter the hospital system through the emergency department and remain in the hospital for several weeks to months. Aside from care in the inpatient setting, the patient may be moved to the intensive care setting for mechanical ventilation. Throughout the course of hospitalization, nursing care focuses on careful monitoring and interventions to avoid complications such as aspiration, skin breakdown, contractures, and VTE that can delay recovery. It is important for the patient to be ready to engage in rehabilitation when stabilized. Family involvement is important to help the patient reintegrate into family activities and work. Some patients recover completely, yet some may have residual numbness and weakness. With proper support and rehabilitation, the patient hopefully returns to baseline functioning within a few months.

TRIGEMINAL NEURALGIA

Patients with trigeminal neuralgia, also referred to as *tic douloureux*, are treated in a variety of healthcare settings ranging from outpatient offices to surgical suites. As a review, the fifth CN is called the *trigeminal nerve*. It emerges from the pons of the brainstem and has three branches, namely, the ophthalmic, maxillary, and mandibular branches. It is a mixed cranial nerve, meaning this nerve has both motor and sensory innervation that is responsible for facial sensation and the strength of the jaw. Trigeminal neuralgia is a pain disorder, and the patient seeks medical attention for relief. It is not unusual for the patient to present to a primary care practitioner with a chief complaint of facial pain (Fig. 38.4).

Epidemiology

There are approximately 15,000 Americans diagnosed with trigeminal neuralgia each year. It is more common in women than in men and rarely affects individuals less than 50 years of age. Risk factors for the development of trigeminal neuralgia are hypertension and multiple sclerosis (MS). In MS, there may be an area of demyelination along the nerve that contributes to the increased incidence. However, for most cases, the cause remains unknown.

Pathophysiology

Trigeminal neuralgia is described by the International Association for the Study of Pain as a sudden, usually unilateral, severe, brief, stabbing, recurrent pain in the distribution of one or more branches of the trigeminal nerve (CN V). In classic trigeminal neuralgia, the etiology is unknown or due to vascular compression. In some cases, it is associated with a tumor, a structural abnormality of the skull base, or MS. The second type of pain is atypical pain, which is a constant burning sensation that covers a more diffuse region of the face.

Clinical Manifestations

Patients with trigeminal neuralgia often report that their pain began spontaneously, whereas others relate that their onset of clinical manifestations followed dental surgery, facial trauma, or a motor vehicle accident. The patient complains of sharp, throbbing, and shock-like pain. Triggers may include touching an area of the skin or an activity such as

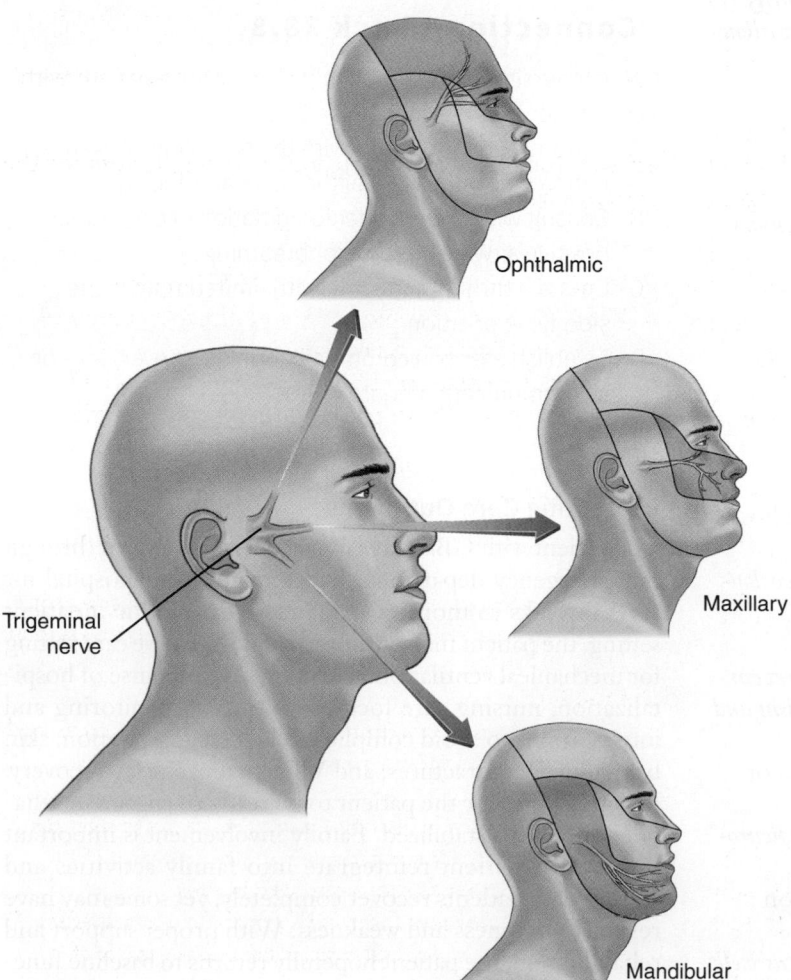

Ophthalmic

Trigeminal nerve

Maxillary

Mandibular

FIGURE 38.4 Branches of the facial nerve (CN V). There are three branches of CN V, and pain manifestations correlate to the sensory distributions of these branches.

brushing the teeth, drinking a beverage, smiling, or talking. Patients may also report that just the breeze from opening the door triggers the pain. Hygiene activities such as brushing the teeth, bathing, and shaving may be neglected because they trigger pain. A patient may have 1 attack per day or as many as 10 to 15 attacks an hour.

Management

Medical Management

Diagnosis

The diagnosis of trigeminal neuralgia is primarily based on the clinical presentation and ruling out other pathophysiological processes, such as direct injury to CN V or tumors. In addition to a comprehensive neurological assessment, including trigeminal reflex testing, a magnetic resonance imaging (MRI) scan of the head is also performed. Blood work may include a sedimentation rate (ESR), antinuclear antibody titer (ANA), or complete blood cell (CBC) count to look for hematological abnormalities.

Treatment

Medications are used in the treatment of trigeminal neuralgia, including the use of antiepileptic drugs (AEDs) such as carbamazepine, oxcarbazepine, or gabapentin. Carbamazepine is the first line of medication therapy used in the treatment of trigeminal neuralgia, and it works by reducing the excitability of neurons by inhibiting neuronal sodium channels. Additionally, baclofen may also be prescribed, particularly in patients with MS, because it works as a muscle relaxant. Although medications can be helpful in abating the pain, some patients do not receive optimal relief and seek surgery. Table 38.4 presents a summary of the surgical approaches for the management of trigeminal neuralgia. Microvascular decompression is the most effective surgical treatment for this disorder; facial pain is usually relieved within 24 to 48 hours, and the patient does not have residual facial numbness.

Connection Check 38.9

The nurse recognizes which class of medications as most effective in the management of trigeminal neuralgia?
A. Anticholinergics
B. Antihistamines
C. Antibiotics
D. Antiepileptics

Nursing Management

Assessment and Analysis

Examination of the cranial nerves identifies the area of the face that is affected. It is important to note the branches of the trigeminal nerve that are affected. Usually the clinical manifestations (e.g., short, stabbing attacks of pain) are unilateral and may correlate to the sensory distribution of a specific CN V branch. The nurse also

Table 38.4 Procedures to Treat Trigeminal Neuralgia

Type of Procedure	Description
Percutaneous rhizotomy	In this procedure, a needle is inserted through the cheek into the foramen ovale. The nerve fibers are damaged or destroyed by radiofrequency, glycerol injection, or balloon compression. Patients will have permanent facial numbness in the region supplied by the branch.
Stereotactic radiosurgery	In this procedure, a single, high-concentrated dose of ionizing radiation is delivered to a precise target at the trigeminal nerve root. This dose of radiation causes a lesion to form, which interrupts pain transmission to the brain.
Microvascular decompression	This is the most invasive procedure. A craniotomy is performed to the suboccipital region. The neurosurgeon performs neurovascular decompression by placing a shredded fluorocarbon resin pad between the vessels and the nerve. The most common vessel to cause compression is the superior cerebellar artery.

assesses for any exacerbating and relieving factors for the patient's pain.

Nursing Diagnoses
- **Pain** related to impairment of CN V function
- **Fear** related to chronic and unpredictable pattern of remissions and attacks of pain
- **Impaired nutrition** related to inability to eat and drink associated with pain of trigeminal neuralgia

Nursing Interventions
Assessments
- Pain, including onset, character, and exacerbating factors
  It is important to identify the pain rating as well as aggravating factors. The pain is believed to be related to irritation of the nerve fibers in CN V.
- Oral intake
  Pain may impair oral intake, so it is important to assess oral intake and fluid-volume status.
- Weight
  If pain significantly interferes with nutritional intake, the patient may have weight loss.
- History of exacerbations and remissions
  Because the time between attacks appears to shorten as the patient ages, it is important to establish any pattern of attacks.

▨ *Actions*

- Administer medications as ordered.
  Medication is taken at prescribed intervals to assist with pain relief. Antiepileptic medications have been found to have an analgesic effect on neuropathic pain.
- Nonpharmacological strategies including meditation, diversional activities, support groups, and acupuncture.
  Suggest meditation or diversional activities.
  Seek a support group so that members may share their experiences.
  Acupuncture has been found to have efficacy similar to that of carbamazepine.
  These interventions are implemented to address pain management through alternative measures. Acupuncture has been found to have efficacy similar to that of carbamazepine in some patients.

▨ *Teaching*

- Identify and avoid exacerbating factors (cold weather, drafts, etc.).
  Because the pain can be severe and interfere with activities of daily living, it is important to minimize factors that cause or exacerbate the pain associated with this disorder.
- The pain from trigeminal neuralgia can affect the patient's quality of life.
  The nurse educates the patient about the medications that are prescribed, including side effects. Although AEDs are used for pain management, the patient should be educated that the indication is neuropathic pain, not epilepsy. The nurse may also suggest alternative methods of hygiene that may not aggravate an attack.

Connection Check 38.10

Which surgical approach is most effective for the patient with trigeminal neuralgia?
A. Stereotactic radiosurgery
B. Cervical decompression
C. Microvascular decompression
D. Percutaneous ablation

Evaluating Care Outcomes

The patient may pursue medical management for trigeminal neuralgia due to the effects of pain on daily activities of daily living and quality of life. If medications do not prove to be effective, the patient may seek surgical evaluation. Proper pain management, either medical or surgical, allows the patient to achieve pain control and have improved quality of life. Inform the patient and family about resources, such as the Facial Pain Association.

Making Connections

CASE STUDY: WRAP-UP

Ms. Jordan demonstrates increasing weakness and requires two nurses to assist her to the bathroom. Her speech remains slurred and is now incomprehensible. The nurse performs a neurological assessment and obtains a forced vital capacity. The vital capacity measurement is 0.8 L. Oxygen saturation is 95% on room air. The provider is notified of the vital capacity, and an arterial blood gas is drawn. The results are pH 7.28, $PaCO_2$ 70 mm Hg, PaO_2 85 mm Hg, HCO_3 25 mEq/L. The patient is moved to an intensive care setting, where she is intubated and placed on a mechanical ventilator. A neostigmine infusion is initiated in order to determine her anticholinesterase requirements during this acute phase of illness. The healthcare provider decides that Ms. Jordan will have five plasmapheresis treatments, and a dual-lumen plasmapheresis catheter is placed. She is scheduled to have her first plasmapheresis treatment performed at her bedside tomorrow.

After three additional plasmapheresis treatments, Ms. Jordan is able to be extubated and returns to the inpatient unit. Her vital capacity at this time is 1.5 L. She completes her final plasmapheresis treatment and is discharged home under the care of her husband. The nurse ensures that Ms. Jordan is knowledgeable of her medications and the importance of taking her medications at the exact time prescribed. Discharge teaching also focuses on clinical manifestations of myasthenic and cholinergic crises.

Case Study Questions

1. Ms. Jordan has been taking prednisone 20 mg daily for management of her MG. What side effects should she be monitored for during her hospitalization? *(Select all that apply.)*
   A. Hyperglycemia
   B. Weight gain
   C. Cardiomegaly
   D. Heart failure
   E. Insomnia

2. The autoimmune dysfunction in MG results from which process?
   A. An overabundance of acetylcholine (ACh)
   B. An inadequate amount of ACh
   C. An inadequate amount of serotonin
   D. Destruction of the postsynaptic membrane

3. While caring for Ms. Jordan, the nurse monitors for which manifestations of a cholinergic crisis? *(Select all that apply.)*
   A. Bradycardia
   B. Angioedema
   C. Diarrhea
   D. Increased heart rate
   E. Decreased saliva

4. During her hospitalization, Ms. Jordan receives plasmapheresis treatments. Following the plasmapheresis treatments, the nurse monitors Ms. Jordan for which complications? *(Select all that apply.)*
    A. Hypotension
    B. Stevens-Johnson syndrome
    C. Galactorrhea
    D. Hypocalcemia
    E. Hypoglycemia

5. After the nurse provides patient education to Ms. Jordan, the patient states that by taking her medications as instructed and planning frequent rest periods in her day, she should expect which outcome?
    A. She will succumb to her disease within 5 years.
    B. Her symptoms will be controlled, and she can consider the disease cured.
    C. She will be able to manage her disease and have quality of life.
    D. She will not develop any respiratory complications.

CHAPTER SUMMARY

The patient with a disorder of the peripheral nervous system (PNS) presents with many challenges and may be encountered in outpatient, inpatient, or intensive care settings. Careful neurological and respiratory assessments allow the nurse to identify deficits in order to prioritize care. It is important that the nurse is able to correlate the pathophysiology of the disorders to the patient's clinical presentation and rationales for treatment modalities.

Myasthenia gravis, an acquired autoimmune neuromuscular junction disorder, is caused by antibodies that are directed toward skeletal muscle nicotinic acetylcholine (ACh) receptors and muscle-specific kinase (MuSK). Patients with MG may be successfully managed with cholinesterase inhibitors. The patient and family must be aware of the clinical manifestations of both myasthenic and cholinergic crises and the importance of seeking medical attention quickly. Patient education plays a crucial role in the successful management of the patient. With adherence to prescribed medications and the treatment plan, patients are able to actively participate in family activities and a career.

Guillain-Barré syndrome (GBS), another disorder of the PNS, is an acute inflammatory demyelinating polyneuropathy. It often occurs after an infection and leads to a rapidly progressing flaccid paralysis due to peripheral nerve demyelination. The management of GBS focuses on supportive care and reducing severity, potential complications, suffering, and recovery time. Although GBS is an autoimmune disorder, steroids have not been found to help speed recovery. The two primary treatment modalities for GBS are intravenous immunoglobulin therapy (IVIG) and plasmapheresis.

Patients with trigeminal neuralgia are treated in a variety of healthcare settings ranging from outpatient offices to surgical suites. This disorder involves the fifth cranial nerve (CN), the trigeminal nerve, which is a mixed CN, meaning this nerve has both motor and sensory innervation that is responsible for facial sensation and the strength of the jaw. Trigeminal neuralgia is a pain disorder, and the patient seeks medical attention for relief. Medications are used in the treatment of trigeminal neuralgia. This includes the use of antiepileptic drugs (AEDs) such as carbamazepine, oxcarbazepine, or gabapentin. Microvascular decompression is the most effective surgical treatment for trigeminal neuralgia, with facial pain typically relieved within 24 to 48 hours, with no residual facial numbness.

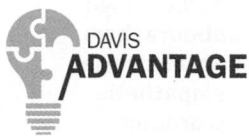 DAVIS ADVANTAGE | To explore learning resources for this chapter, go to **Davis Advantage** and find:
– Answers to in-text questions
– Chapter Resources and Activities
– NCLEX®-Style Chapter Review Questions
– Bibliography

Chapter 39

Coordinating Care for Critically Ill Patients With Neurological Dysfunction

Elizabeth Zink

CONCEPTS

- Assessment
- Cognition
- Medication
- Neurological Regulation
- Oxygenation
- Perioperative

ESSENTIAL TERMS

Agnosia
Aneurysm
Apraxia
Arteriovenous malformation (AVM)
Autoregulation
Basilar skull fractures
Battle's sign
Blood–brain barrier (BBB)
Brain attack
Cerebral autoregulation
Cerebral contusion
Cerebral ischemia
Cerebral perfusion pressure (CPP)
Cerebral vasospasm
Contralateral
Cushing's triad
Cytotoxic edema
Diffuse axonal injury (DAI)
Durotomy
Epidural hematoma
Focal
Hemicraniectomy
Herniation syndromes
Homonymous hemianopia
Horner's sign
Infratentorial
Intracranial compliance
Intracranial pressure (ICP)
Ipsilateral
Ischemic penumbra
Lacunar stroke
Mechanisms of injury
Monro–Kellie doctrine
Subarachnoid hemorrhage
Subdural hematoma
Supratentorial
Sympathetic storming
Transependymal edema
Transtentorial
Triple-H therapy
Uncus
Vasogenic edema

Finding Connections

CASE STUDY: EPISODE 1

Follow this patient throughout the chapter.

   Mr. George Stewart, a 58-year-male, begins slurring his speech, drooling from the left side of his mouth, and leaning to the left side during a meeting at work. His colleagues notify emergency medical services (EMS), and he is transported to the closest hospital. The EMS crew establishes that Mr. Stewart was last witnessed without stroke signs and symptoms at 12:15. He has a history of hypertension, high cholesterol, and smoking. He takes metoprolol (Lopressor or Toprol XL) and simvastatin (Zocor)…

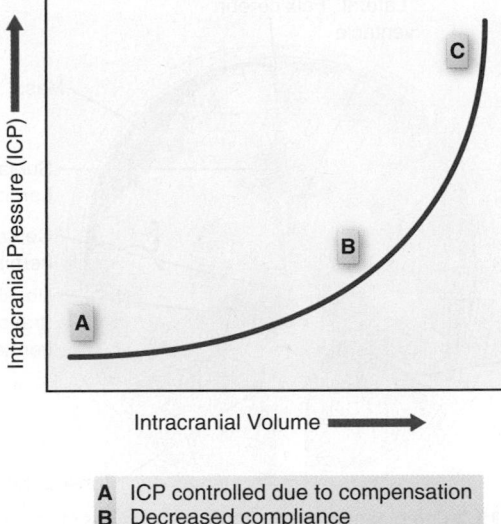

A	ICP controlled due to compensation
B	Decreased compliance
C	Loss of compliance

FIGURE 39.1 Pressure–volume curve. Section A represents an incremental increase in volume where intracranial pressure is maintained and does not increase; this implies that compensation is occurring within the cranial vault to accommodate the increased volume. Section B represents an incremental increase in volume where intracranial pressure begins to rise with the addition of volume, implying a decrease in the ability to compensate for additional volume. Section C represents an incremental increase in volume where intracranial pressure rises disproportionately in response to the continued addition of volume. On this portion of the curve, compliance is extremely limited, and herniation may occur with the continued addition of volume.

INTRODUCTION

The emergent care of patients with injury or disease of the central nervous system requiring intensive care management is a subspecialty of critical care focused on the preservation of neurological function. Patients with disorders of the central nervous system often encounter or present with complications in other body systems; therefore, neuroscience critical care combines interprofessional neurological expertise with general critical care to treat this vulnerable patient population. Acute and critical care nurses working in the neurosciences are experts in performing and trending serial neurological assessments in order to detect neurological deterioration and facilitate rapid medical interventions to prevent further brain injury. Nursing expertise in general critical care and the neurosciences is necessary to optimize patient outcomes.

INCREASED INTRACRANIAL PRESSURE

Pathophysiology and Clinical Manifestations

Increased **intracranial pressure (ICP)** is best illustrated by the **Monro–Kellie doctrine**, which states that three components—brain tissue, blood, and cerebrospinal fluid (CSF)—occupy a rigid box, the skull. When one of these three components increases, the other components must decrease to maintain equilibrium, preventing further injury to the brain through compression of the tissue within the fixed box. The ability of the body to compensate by adjusting the levels of the components is called **intracranial compliance**.

   Brain tissue is composed primarily of water and makes up 80% of the intracranial contents, and blood and CSF each make up 10% of the remaining contents within the cranium. The most common initial method of intracranial compensation involves the displacement of CSF from the cranial vault down through the foramen magnum at the base of the skull and around the spinal cord. The pressure-volume curve (Fig. 39.1) depicts the body's ability to compensate for the addition of one or more of the three intracranial components without a significant increase in ICP until a critical volume is reached (A). At this point, continued accumulation of volume causes a disproportionate increase in ICP referred to as decreased compliance (B). Finally, on the last section of the curve, any addition in volume causes a sustained increase in ICP, which represents a loss of compliance (C). Loss of intracranial compliance leads to cerebral herniation syndrome, in which brain tissue is displaced, and if the displacement is not resolved, the brainstem becomes compressed, eventually causing brain death.

   Cerebral **herniation syndromes** are classified according to the region of tissue that is displaced (Fig. 39.2). The most often recognized signs of cerebral herniation, increased systolic blood pressure (BP) with decreased diastolic BP (widened pulse pressure), bradycardia, and irregular respiratory pattern, actually occur late in the herniation process as the brainstem is compressed and are referred to as "**Cushing's triad.**" Another frequently recognized late sign of increased ICP is a unilateral fixed and dilated pupil. This phenomenon occurs as the bottom portion of the temporal lobe or **uncus** is displaced through the tentorium cerebelli and compresses cranial nerve (CN) III (oculomotor nerve) and is called *uncal* or **transtentorial** (temporal lobes into the tentorium) herniation. Compression of the third cranial nerve produces pupillary dilation on the same side as the cranial nerve compression, or **ipsilateral** to the cranial nerve compression. Motor paresis accompanies pupillary

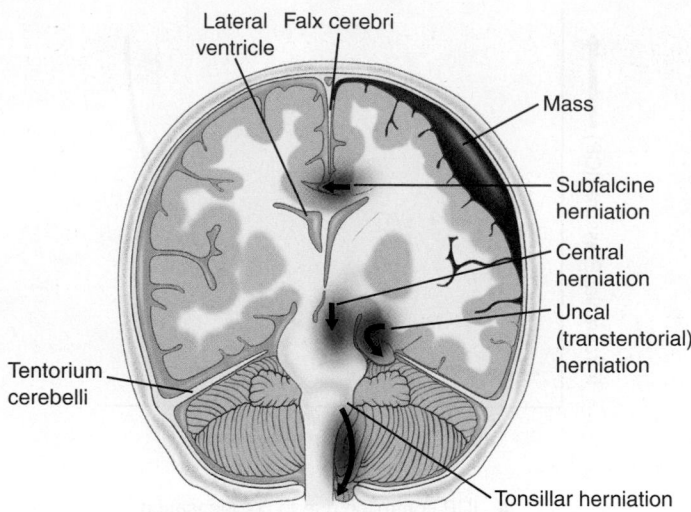

Lateral ventricle
Falx cerebri
Mass
Subfalcine herniation
Central herniation
Uncal (transtentorial) herniation
Tentorium cerebelli
Tonsillar herniation

FIGURE 39.2 Cerebral herniation syndromes: regions of tissue.

dilation on the opposite side, or **contralateral** to the site of herniation. Table 39.1 summarizes the types of cerebral herniation.

There are three types of cerebral edema—vasogenic, cytotoxic, and transependymal—which can impact intracranial pressure (Table 39.2). **Vasogenic edema** occurs when the **blood–brain barrier (BBB)** is disrupted. The BBB is made up of endothelial cells and astrocytes, which form tight junctions around capillaries, reducing the permeability of substances into the brain. Vasogenic edema primarily impacts white matter and is caused by leakage of fluids out of capillaries into the interstitial space. **Cytotoxic edema** does not impact the BBB and primarily involves individual cellular swelling caused by failure of the sodium–potassium pump. **Transependymal edema** is caused by increased pressure in the ventricular system that results in CSF moving into the brain parenchyma.

Table 39.1 Cerebral Herniation Syndromes

	Description	Clinical Manifestations
Subfalcine or cingulate herniation	In this type of herniation, brain tissue is shifted over and underneath the falx cerebri. One of the main concerns in this type of herniation is the risk of compression to the anterior cerebral artery, which could cause a stroke in this region of brain tissue.	Specific clinical manifestations of subfalcine herniation do not exist; however, this type of herniation may be found on a CT scan when evaluating clinical manifestations of increased ICP, such as decreased level of consciousness, unilateral weakness of extremities, or a change in pupillary assessment, and places the patient at risk for further herniation.
Central herniation	Central herniation occurs when the structures of the diencephalon (e.g., thalamus, hypothalamus, pituitary gland) and the tips of both temporal lobes are displaced in a downward direction through the tentorium (portion of the dura that creates a separation between the occipital lobes and the cerebelli), compressing the brainstem.	• Abnormal flexion or extension (posturing) • Bilateral pupillary dilation • Abnormal eye movements such as downward and outward eye movements as cranial nerves controlling eye movements are compressed • Positive Babinski reflex • Coma • Cushing's triad (increased systolic blood pressure, bradycardia, and irregular respiratory pattern)
Uncal herniation	In uncal herniation, an expanding lesion causes the tip of the temporal lobe (uncus) to shift downward and inward toward the midbrain and through the tentorium (portion of the dura that creates a separation between the occipital lobes and the cerebelli), compressing CN III. CN III is innervated by the parasympathetic nervous system, and stimulation of this nerve causes pupillary constriction. Compression of this cranial nerve causes dilation of the pupil and an inability to constrict (fixed and dilated pupil).	• Unilateral dilated pupil • Contralateral motor weakness or flexion/extensor posturing • Positive Babinski reflex • Coma
Tonsillar herniation	Tonsillar herniation occurs, and the bottom portion of the cerebellar hemispheres (tonsils) descends through the foramen magnum, damaging the medulla.	• Abnormal flexion or extension (posturing) • Bilateral pupillary dilation • Positive Babinski reflex • Coma • Cushing's triad (increased systolic blood pressure, bradycardia, and irregular respiratory pattern)

CN, Cranial nerve; *CT,* computed tomography; *ICP,* intracranial pressure.

Table 39.2 Types of Cerebral Edema

	Description	Treatment
Vasogenic edema	Vasogenic edema occurs when the blood–brain barrier (BBB) has been disrupted. The BBB is made up of endothelial cells and astrocytes, which are arranged around capillaries and between the capillary and extracellular fluid. Tight junctions between these cells regulate substances going in and coming out of the brain. For example, bacteria and hydrophilic molecules are not able to pass through the BBB. Active transport mechanisms allow substances such as glucose and some proteins to cross the BBB into the brain. Brain tumors cause disruption of the BBB by production of a substance called *vasogenic endothelial growth factor* (VEGF) that causes separations between the endothelial cells, resulting in increased permeability of the BBB.	Osmotic therapy (mannitol and/or hypertonic saline), hyperventilation, or surgical decompression
Cytotoxic edema	Cytotoxic edema occurs as a result of a decrease in oxygenation where cellular energy reserves are depleted and the sodium–potassium pump fails, causing an influx of sodium and water across the cell membrane. Accumulation of intracellular fluid can cause cell death. In this type of edema, the BBB is intact, and the damage may be reversible if oxygenation is restored.	Same interventions as vasogenic shock
Transependymal edema	This type of cerebral edema is caused by an increase in hydrostatic pressure in the ventricular system associated with hydrocephalus, which results in a leakage of cerebrospinal fluid out of the ventricles and into surrounding brain tissue.	Drainage of cerebrospinal fluid is the primary method of decreasing this type of edema.

Increased ICP is detected by performing serial neurological assessments, including the elements of wakefulness, arousal, cranial nerves, and motor function. The most sensitive indicator of ICP is a decrease in level of consciousness. In order to detect subtle changes in level of consciousness, it is imperative to establish an accurate baseline of functioning from which to judge deterioration. A series of questions that go beyond the basic elements of orientation to person, place, and time help to establish this baseline and include specifics of place or location and specifics about the patient's current state or situation (see Box 39.1 for additional orientation questions).

The clinical presentation of increased ICP may be subtle, particularly in the early stages, and is in sharp contrast to the presentation of cerebral herniation (Table 39.3). The clinical manifestations of increased ICP must be detected early in order to implement treatment and prevent herniation

syndrome. It is important to note that changes in vital signs reflect late changes as herniation occurs.

Intracranial Pressure Monitoring

Intracranial pressure can be monitored using a catheter or sensor placed in one of the lateral ventricles of the brain, in the brain tissue or parenchyma, or in the subarachnoid space (Fig. 39.3). Intracranial pressure monitoring is an additional assessment tool used to trend a patient's response to medical treatments and progression of an intracranial process causing increased ICP (see Table 39.4 for types of ICP-monitoring devices). Recognized guidelines suggest that patients with traumatic brain injury (TBI) and a Glasgow Coma Scale (GCS) score of 8 or less have an ICP monitor placed. Normal ICP is 0 to 15 mm Hg and is typically treated in a stepwise approach when the pressure exceeds 15 mm Hg; however, this threshold is individualized to each patient depending on specific causes of increased ICP. **Cerebral perfusion pressure (CPP)** is a commonly used parameter to indirectly measure cerebral blood flow and is generally maintained above 60 mm Hg. Cerebral perfusion pressure is measured by subtracting ICP from mean arterial pressure (MAP): MAP − ICP = CPP.

There are several different methods of monitoring ICP. The subarachnoid bolt (SAB), one of the oldest methods of ICP monitoring, uses a metal bolt, also referred to as a screw, inserted through a hole drilled in the skull and threaded into place at the inner table of the skull. The dura

Box 39.1 Asking Expanded Orientation Questions

- What state are you in right now?
- What city are you in right now?
- What kind of place are we in right now?
- What floor are we on right now?
- Why are you here today?
- What are your children's/family members' names?

Table 39.3 Increased Intracranial Pressure Versus Cerebral Herniation

	Increased Intracranial Pressure	Cerebral Herniation
Level of consciousness	Progressive confusion and increasing lethargy	Unresponsive
Pupillary assessment	Sluggish reaction and ovoid shape	Unilateral or bilateral pupillary dilation (depending on type of herniation) without reaction
Motor assessment	Focal contralateral motor weakness	Contralateral hemiparesis including flexor or extensor posturing
Vital signs	No change	Cushing's triad (increase in systolic pressure, widening of pulse pressure, bradycardia, and change in respiratory pattern)

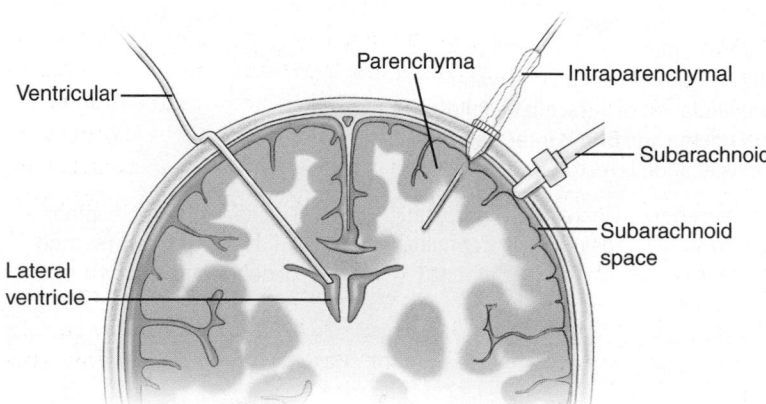

FIGURE 39.3 Intracranial pressure–monitoring devices.

Table 39.4 ICP Monitoring Devices

Monitoring Device	Advantages	Disadvantages
Intraventricular catheter • This device and procedure are also commonly known as a ventriculostomy or external ventricular drain (EVD). • May be connected to a filled transducer system • May have an embedded ICP monitoring sensor/probe	• Ability to monitor pressure and drain CSF • Considered "gold standard" for ICP measurement because of the location of the tip of the catheter in the lateral ventricle • Can be inserted at the bedside or in the operating room (OR)	• Increased risk of infection, particularly when the catheter dwells for greater than 7 days • Measurement drift exists over time when pressure is transduced with a fluid-filled transducer system.
Intraparenchymal sensor/probe • Micro-strain gauge attached to the tip of a small catheter used to measure ICP • Fiberoptic technology used to measure ICP	• Accurate measurement of ICP with less mechanical drift of the measurement over time when compared to devices using a fluid-filled transducer to measure pressure • Can be inserted at the bedside or in the OR	• Inability to drain CSF
Subarachnoid bolt (SAB) • Bolt or screw connected to a fluid-filled transducer system	• Can be inserted at the bedside or in the OR • Lower rate of infection when compared to the IVC because the SAB does not have a fluid reservoir	• Inability to drain CSF • Inaccuracy of measurement due to measurement drift that is inherent with a fluid-filled transducer system

CSF, Cerebrospinal fluid; *ICP,* intracranial pressure.

is incised so that when the bolt is connected to a pressure transducer, pressure is transmitted from the subarachnoid space to the monitor via the transducer. The bolt may be placed in the operating room or at a patient's bedside under sterile conditions. The advantage of this device is that it has a decreased risk of infection when compared to ICP-monitoring systems that also drain fluid. The disadvantages of this device relate to its inability to drain CSF; the system's susceptibility to significant measurement drift (ability to maintain accurate measurements over time); and the risk of the bolt becoming occluded with blood, tissue, or dura. The pressure transducer is typically leveled to the insertion site of the bolt and zero balanced according to specific facility policies. The purpose of leveling the transducer to the insertion site of the SAB is to ensure that pressure is measured near the tip of the device in the brain in order to obtain an accurate reading. The leveling process with the SAB and transducer is similar to the process of leveling a transducer at the phlebostatic axis to measure central venous pressure. Subarachnoid bolt placement is also used in order to introduce probes into the brain parenchyma for monitoring. The bolt in this case provides a secure method for insertion and maintenance of probes that may measure multiple parameters, including ICP, temperature, brain oxygen, cerebral blood flow, and brain metabolism.

Intraparenchymal probes are inserted below the dura into the white matter in one of the frontal lobes of the brain to monitor ICP. The right frontal lobe is often chosen in order to avoid interference with the language center, housed in the left hemisphere for many patients. This type of monitor also may be inserted in the operating room or at a patient's bedside. The technology used in these ICP-monitoring devices is reported to have less measurement drift over time than the SAB, which improves the accuracy of ICP measurement. This type of monitor does not have an external transducer that must be leveled in order to obtain an accurate pressure because the monitor is calibrated prior to insertion. Because of the placement in the brain tissue, CSF drainage is not possible.

The intraventricular catheter (IVC) with external ventricular drain (EVD), or ventriculostomy, is used for monitoring ICP and draining CSF (Fig. 39.4). The tip of the IVC is placed into one of the lateral ventricles in the brain using external landmarks or image guidance in some cases. The catheter is placed under sterile conditions at the bedside or in the operating room and is connected to an external drainage system with a pressure transducer for ICP monitoring. An alternative method of monitoring ICP is to place an intraparenchymal ICP-monitoring probe with the IVC, eliminating the need for attachment of a pressure transducer. The CSF drainage system is leveled to the external auditory meatus of the ear, which approximates the foramen of Monro or the tip of the IVC in the ventricle. Drainage of CSF is controlled by raising or lowering a collection burette above or below this leveling point.

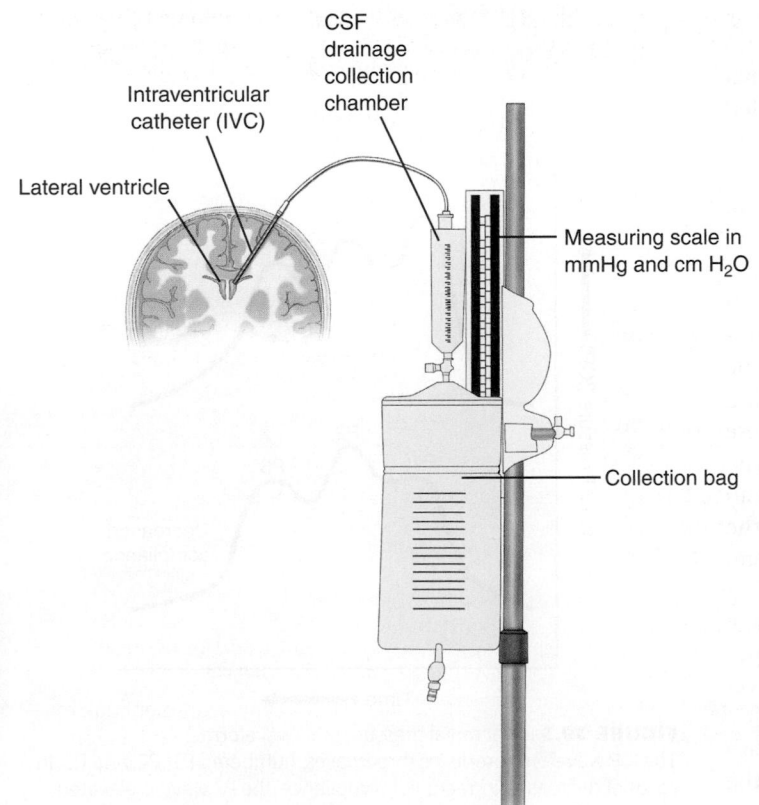

FIGURE 39.4 Cerebrospinal fluid drainage using an external ventricular drainage system (ventriculostomy).

Most external ventricular drains have a measuring scale printed on the device allowing measurements in millimeters of mercury (mm Hg) or centimeters of water (cm H_2O). If the drainage burette is set to 5 mm Hg while leveled at the external auditory meatus, CSF will drain when ICP reaches 5 mm Hg. The CSF can be drained continuously using the method of setting a pressure threshold described previously, or the drain may be closed until ICP reaches a predetermined level, and then the drain is opened to drain at a specific level in relation to the leveling point. When a pressure transducer is attached to the drainage system, a stopcock controls whether CSF is drained or pressure is monitored. An accurate ICP can be monitored only when the drainage system is closed to CSF drainage. The drainage system must be correctly leveled after the head of the bed is repositioned to safely drain CSF. Prior to connection to the patient, the external ventricular drain is flushed with preservative-free normal saline and purged of all air bubbles. Preservative-free saline solution rather than bacteriostatic normal saline is used to flush the system because of a concern for meningeal inflammation, as bacteriostatic saline contains benzyl alcohol. It is important to maintain the system as a closed system to prevent infection.

The drainage system and catheter are generally not changed on a routine basis in order to maintain the sterility of the system. Cerebrospinal fluid cultures may be drawn through a designated port or stopcock located near the insertion point on the head when indicated. The major advantage of the IVC is that it is a monitor and a method of treatment for ICP. The major disadvantages include a higher rate of infection than other methods (approximately 6%) and a risk of bleeding along the catheter tract. A higher incidence of infection in patients with an IVC with external drain may be explained by the connection of the fluid-filled ventricular system to the external environment, which can act as a reservoir for microorganisms.

Complications of CSF drainage include infection, overdrainage of CSF, and introduction of air into the ventricular system if proper leveling is not maintained. If an excessive amount of CSF is drained rapidly through an IVC, a **subdural hematoma** (collection of blood in the subdural space) can result because of contraction of brain tissue that stretches the small bridging blood vessels traversing the space between the dura and brain tissue. When these bridging blood vessels are stretched, tearing can occur, causing a subdural hematoma. Overdrainage of CSF through an IVC may also cause the cerebellar tonsils to "sag" into the foramen magnum, resulting in pressure on the brainstem. Overdrainage of CSF can be prevented by maintaining proper leveling of the drainage system (0 point on drainage system leveled at the external auditory meatus) and proper adjustment of the drainage burette at the ordered level above the external auditory meatus.

It is important to note that ICP values may not always be representative of ICP in all areas or compartments of the brain. For example, most ICP-monitoring devices are placed in the **supratentorial** (above the tentorium cerebelli) space; cerebral edema may cause the **infratentorial** (below the tentorium cerebelli) space to be compartmentalized such that pressures are higher than those measured in the supratentorial space. For this reason, cerebral herniation may occur in the presence of normal ICP.

The ICP waveform produced by all three of the previously described monitoring methods is a pulsatile waveform made up of three waves, numbered P1, P2, and P3 (Fig. 39.5). In cases of decreased intracranial compliance, the P2 wave is elevated above the P1 and P3 waves.

Connection Check 39.1

The nurse is caring for a patient status post-craniotomy for resection of a right frontal tumor. Upon admission, the patient was alert and oriented to person, place, and time and moving all extremities symmetrically, and the cranial nerves were intact. Three hours after admission, the nurse notes that the patient is slower to awaken than during previous assessments, requiring vigorous shaking, and cannot recall location. The patient also exhibits a left pronator drift. What are the nurse's next actions?

A. Notify the patient's provider and prepare the patient for a computed tomography (CT) scan.
B. Record vital signs and prepare to draw blood for serum osmolality.
C. Notify the patient's provider and prepare the patient for a magnetic resonance imaging (MRI) scan.
D. Prepare to hang a fluid bolus and notify the patient's provider.

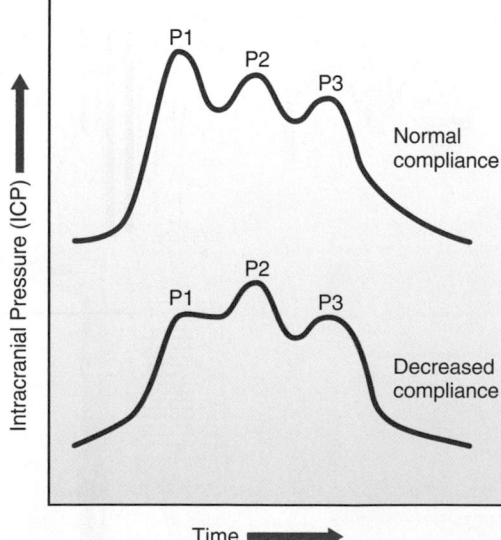

FIGURE 39.5 Intracranial pressure (ICP) waveform. The ICP waveform produces three waves, numbered P1, P2, and P3. In cases of decreased intracranial compliance, the P2 wave is elevated above the P1 and P3 waves.

Management

Medical Management

Treatment of increased ICP is based on decreasing the volume of brain water, blood, or CSF in the intracranial space. The initial approach to the emergency management of increased ICP consists of airway management and therapies to decrease intracranial contents, such as administration of an osmotic diuretic and hyperventilation (see following discussion of specific therapies). Vigilant monitoring of the patient's neurological status is critical during treatment because there may be subtle changes in level of consciousness that may indicate further compromise. Research in the area of additional bedside neuromonitoring technologies, such as brain oxygen probes, digital quantitative pupillary assessment, cerebral blood flow probes, microdialysis probes sampling extracellular fluid metabolites, and cerebral oximetry, is emerging. It is thought that these therapies may complement traditional monitoring methodologies, such as the clinical assessment, ICP, and CPP, and could be helpful in helping the interprofessional team customize therapy to each patient.

Connection Check 39.2

A patient is admitted to the neuroscience intensive care unit (NICU) after a TBI. If the goal of ICP monitor insertion is to measure ICP and drain CSF to control ICP, what device should the nurse anticipate being inserted?

A. Intraparenchymal sensor
B. Epidural sensor
C. Intraventricular catheter
D. Subarachnoid bolt

Diagnosis

Radiographic imaging of the brain, typically a computed tomography (CT) scan, is necessary to determine the cause of increased ICP (e.g., collection of blood, cerebral edema). Laboratory testing such as serum osmolality and arterial blood gas (ABG) testing is necessary to guide medical treatments (Table 39.5).

Table 39.5 Diagnostic Tests Used in the Management of Increased Intracranial Pressure (ICP)

Diagnostic Test	Explanation	Nursing Considerations
Computed tomography* (CT) scan of the head	The CT scan uses x-rays to obtain many cross sections or slices of the head and brain. A computer is used to sequence the delivery and position of x-ray beams and movement of the patient through the machine to allow detailed views of the skull, brain structures and tissue, facial bones, or sinuses depending on the reason for obtaining the CT scan. Reducing the thickness of the cross-sectional images and increasing the number of images enhance the detail of the scan. A disadvantage of the CT scan is the reduced ability to visualize the lower portion of the cerebellum and the brainstem structures (midbrain, pons, and medulla). Magnetic resonance imaging (MRI) is an imaging tool used to visualize these structures (see below for information on MRI). A CT scan is the most common test performed in critically ill patients with a deterioration of neurological status, such as a decrease in level of consciousness, new motor deficit, or new cranial nerve deficit, because the test can be performed quickly. The CT scan is first obtained without the injection of IV contrast material to visualize brain structures and detect bleeding. Images may be obtained after IV contrast is administered if a mass (brain tumor, abscess) is suspected because IV contrast material travels into brain tissue where the blood–brain barrier has been disturbed. A mass is said to "light up" on a	● Transport of a patient with increased ICP is a challenge and must be performed with the right team and the right equipment. Depending on the stability of the patient, providers, nurse practitioners, or respiratory therapists may have to accompany the nurse to ensure continuity of care from the intensive care unit (ICU) to the procedure area. See Evidence-Based Practice Box regarding patient transport for more information on best practice for transporting a critically ill patient. ● If contrast material is expected to be given, risk factors for contrast-induced nephropathy (CIN), such as hypotension, diabetes, and chronic kidney disease, should be assessed and serum creatinine (within 24 hours of test) should be evaluated because contrast can damage the kidney. If a patient is at risk for CIN, strategies to prevent CIN, including prehydration with IV saline, administration of a bicarbonate-based IV solution, or administration of *N*-acetylcysteine (Mucomyst) IV, may be employed. In emergent situations, full assessment of risk factors and prevention strategies may not be undertaken because of the urgency of obtaining needed scans to guide further care. The serum creatinine should be monitored at least once after the contrast administration in the critically ill patient and more often if acute kidney injury is suspected. Typically, an increase in serum

Continued

Table 39.5 **Diagnostic Tests Used in the Management of Increased Intracranial Pressure (ICP)—cont'd**

Diagnostic Test	Explanation	Nursing Considerations
	contrasted CT scan because the blood–brain barrier has been disrupted and contrast material has infiltrated the interstitial space in and around the mass. A noncontrast CT scan must be performed before the administration of contrast if bleeding is suspected because the contrast material and blood appear the same color (white) in the brain tissue, making detection of blood very difficult for a period of time after contrast has been administered.	creatinine of at least 0.5 mg/dL is expected, which will decrease over 24–48 hours. • Because of the exposure to ionizing radiation, a pregnancy test should be performed in women of childbearing age, and the abdomen should be shielded if no alternative to the CT scan exists. • Assess the patient's ability to remain still during the procedure because movement of the head causes decreased clarity (artifact) of the images, which could obscure an abnormality. Patients with increased ICP may be confused, restless, or agitated, requiring sedation or anxiolysis to ensure capture of high-quality images. • Assess the patient's ability to lie flat during the scan. Patients with congestive heart failure or lung disease may not be able to maintain adequate oxygenation while lying flat, as evidenced by decreased oxygen saturation and increases in work of breathing and restlessness. If the patient cannot lie flat for at least 5 minutes, the healthcare team should be made aware to consider another test or a strategy to manage the patient during the test. • Assess allergy to iodine or shellfish because a patient with these allergies may also be allergic to some contrast agents. • Assess the patient's IV access if IV contrast will be administered during the CT; a larger-gauge peripheral IV catheter (typically an 18-gauge) is required for administration of the contrast through a device called *a power injector*. Certain types of central lines called *power injectable lines* may also be able to be utilized for this type of contrast injection.
Computed tomography angiography (CTA)	A CTA scan uses the radiographical technique described above to visualize cerebral arteries, such as the carotid and vertebral arteries, as they enter the skull and join the circle of Willis. The circle of Willis is also visualized. A computer is used to reconstruct the images obtained to create three-dimensional representation of the cerebral vasculature. This type of scan may be obtained if injury to a blood vessel or blockage of the blood vessel is suspected. A CTA scan requires the administration of IV contrast material.	• See above for nursing considerations.
Computed tomography perfusion (CTP) scan	A CTP scan may be used to detect evidence of reduced blood flow (ischemia) to a region of brain tissue supplied by a particular blood vessel; a CTP scan requires the administration of IV contrast material.	• See above for nursing considerations.

Table 39.5 Diagnostic Tests Used in the Management of Increased Intracranial Pressure (ICP)—cont'd

Diagnostic Test	Explanation	Nursing Considerations
Magnetic resonance imaging (MRI)	An MRI scan uses a magnetic field and radiofrequency waves to change the alignment of protons in water molecules, which then release energy (photons) that can be detected by the scanner and sent to a computer for reconstruction of images in different planes and in three dimensions. This type of scan does not utilize ionizing radiation and produces detailed images of soft tissue structures such as the brain, spinal cord, blood vessels, and ligaments. Different protocols containing different scanning modalities can be programmed into the scanner by a technologist to target specific organ systems or disease processes.	• Patients must be screened for metal that may be embedded in and around the eyes (metal workers and welders) or in any other part of the body, including joint implants, cardiac stents, pacemakers, and other implanted devices. If the patient has a history of working with metal, x-rays may be requested by a radiologist to locate or rule out the existence of metal fragments. During MRI, implanted metal can heat up, causing tissue damage. Certain implanted devices, such as a pacemaker or deep brain stimulator (used in patients with movement disorders), may malfunction. Patients may not be able to have MRI because of these factors. An MRI clearance form is often used by MRI technicians to ensure that a patient is safe to be scanned. • Transport of critically ill patients to MRI requires planning because the time to acquire the images is longer than a CT scan, and cardiorespiratory monitoring has to be changed to an MRI-compatible monitoring system. Additionally, IV fluids or other necessary infusions have to be changed to an MRI-compatible infusion pump or lengthened with extension tubing so that the pump does not enter the room. Patients receiving mechanical ventilation must be changed over to an MRI-compatible ventilator. Conventional medical equipment, including cardiac monitors, ventilators, infusion pumps, oxygen tanks, and IV poles, may not enter the MRI scanning room because the strong magnetic field may pull metal equipment into the magnet, which could injure a patient or staff in the room. Many devices do not operate properly in the strong magnetic field. • Assess the patient's ability to remain still during the procedure because movement of the head causes decreased clarity (artifact) of the images, which could obscure an abnormality. Patients with increased ICP may be confused, restless, or agitated, requiring sedation or anxiolysis to ensure capture of high-quality images. Many patients know that they are claustrophobic and require anxiolysis (benzodiazepines are commonly used for this purpose) in order to enter the small scanning tube of the MRI scanner. A pregnancy test should be performed prior to scanning a woman of childbearing age so that appropriate precautions may be applied depending on the stage of pregnancy and in consultation with a radiologist.
Electroencephalogram (EEG)	An EEG records electrical activity in different regions of the cerebral cortex. An EEG is commonly used to detect seizure activity but can also be used to identify areas of abnormal wave patterns indicating brain	• A patient must be completely still for an EEG because any movement, including shivering, is recorded as artifact and obscures the electrical tracing. Some patients may require mild sedation to reduce movement artifact on the

Continued

Table 39.5 **Diagnostic Tests Used in the Management of Increased Intracranial Pressure (ICP)—cont'd**

Diagnostic Test	Explanation	Nursing Considerations
	tissue dysfunction from a variety of causes. Continuous EEG monitoring is frequently used in the ICU to detect seizure activity on an on-going basis and to guide treatment for status epilepticus. An EEG may be used as a test to confirm the cessation of electrical activity in the brain when brain death is suspected. A neurologist with specialized training in the interpretation of EEGs provides an official reading of the EEG tracing.	EEG recording. The EEG technician records the amount of medication given so that the tracing can be interpreted in the context of sedation administration. ● During continuous EEG monitoring, the scalp electrodes are typically placed by an EEG technician, and the patient's head is wrapped in a bandage to keep the electrodes in place. It is important that the nurse inspects the head to ensure that all electrodes are in place so that the EEG recording is continuous.
Serum osmolality	This blood test is used to monitor the diuretic effect of osmotic diuretics such as mannitol (Osmitrol). Osmotic diuretics cause interstitial fluid throughout the body to shift into the vascular space, where it is filtered and eliminated by the kidneys, causing dehydration. This action is necessary to treat edema in the brain; however, severe dehydration, as indicated by a rising serum osmolality, can cause renal failure. Mannitol is typically not given if the serum osmolality reaches 320 mOsm/kg in order to prevent acute kidney injury.	● Ensure that the blood sample for serum osmolality is drawn within 1–2 hours of osmotic diuretic administration.
Serum sodium	Serum sodium is monitored when targeting a specific level of solute concentration (sodium concentration) in the blood with the administration of hypertonic saline solutions. A target above the normal sodium range (135–145 mEq/L) is chosen on the basis of the severity of cerebral edema and the specific disease process. A goal sodium range above 145 mEq/L and typically less than 160 mEq/L is set, and serum sodium is measured every 4–6 hours to ensure that the goal is achieved and not exceeded. Disorders of sodium imbalance occur frequently in the neurosurgical population for reasons that are not clearly understood. Common disorders of sodium imbalance in this population are syndrome of inappropriate antidiuretic hormone (SIADH), diabetes insipidus (DI), and cerebral salt-wasting syndrome (CSW, also called renal salt-wasting syndrome). See Chapter 8 for more information on electrolyte imbalance.	● Serum sodium should not rise by more than 10 mEq/L in 24 hours for patients who have chronic hyponatremia. If sodium levels rise too quickly in a patient with chronic hyponatremia, a disorder called *central pontine myelinolysis* may result. Central pontine myelinolysis causes damage to myelin (the sheath covering neurons to enhance speed of impulse transmission) in the pons, resulting in a decrease in neuronal transmission in the pons. Features of this disorder may include generalized weakness on both sides of the body, quadriplegia in severe cases, lethargy, and paralysis of eye movements. ● In patients with cerebral edema, a decrease in serum sodium may affect the level of consciousness because of an exacerbation of cerebral edema.

Computed tomography (CT) and *computed axial tomography* (CAT scan) refer to the same type of diagnostic examination; *CT scan* is the newer term, and *CAT scan* is the older term. The CT scan is completely known as *computed tomography*, whereas the CAT scan, in full, is *computed axial tomography*. In some references, CAT can also be the acronym for *computerized axial tomography*, but it still refers to the same test.

Medications

The volume of water in brain tissue observed in cerebral edema is reduced by increasing the osmolality of the blood (increasing solute in the blood), thereby changing the osmotic gradient, resulting in diffusion of water from an area of low concentration (brain tissue) to an area of high concentration (the blood). Medications such as mannitol (Osmitrol) and high-concentration sodium chloride solutions (e.g., 3%) are used to increase the osmolality in the blood in order to pull water from the interstitial space of the brain and other tissues into the vascular space. Mannitol pulls water from the interstitial spaces into the vascular space, and then diuresis occurs at the level of the kidney (see Evidence-Based Practice: Mannitol for Treatment of Traumatic Brain Injury). High-concentration sodium chloride solutions pull water from the interstitial spaces into the vascular space without the dramatic fluid shifts caused when osmotic diuretics are utilized. In order to compensate for the systemic dehydration and hypovolemia that occur with the administration of mannitol, IV fluid should be administered to replace losses. It is important to note that there are advantages and disadvantages in using osmotic diuretics and high-concentration sodium solutions; however, studies have not yet demonstrated an advantage of one regimen over the other, which results in differing practices to accomplish the removal of excess fluid volume from brain tissue.

Evidence-Based Practice

Mannitol for Treatment of Traumatic Brain Injury

Mannitol has been used for more than 50 years to manage intracranial pressure (ICP). This study used the Medline, Embase, and PubMed databases to systematically search for randomized controlled studies (RCTs) that focused on the use of mannitol in critical care and perioperative areas. Meta-analyses examined mannitol's effects on ICP, cerebral perfusion pressure (CPP), mean arterial pressure (MAP), brain relaxation, fluid intake, urine output, and serum complications, as well as complications associated with mannitol administration. A total of 55 RCTs were identified, and 7 meta-analyses were conducted. In traumatic brain injury, mannitol was found to cause differences in sodium levels, but it had little impact on MAP when compared with the administration of hypertonic saline. Hypertonic saline was also more effective in leading to satisfactory brain relaxation in patients after craniotomy in comparison to mannitol. Complications associated with mannitol administration included hyponatremia, hyperkalemia, and acute kidney injury. Although the use of mannitol is effective in accomplishing short-term clinical goals, more research is needed, particularly in comparison with hypertonic saline and regarding the long-term outcomes for mannitol.

Zhang, W., Neal, J., Lin, L., Dai, F., Hersey, D. P., McDonagh, D. L., ... Meng, L. (2018). Mannitol in critical care and surgery over 50+ years: A systematic review of randomized controlled trials and complications with meta-analysis. *Journal of Neurosurgical Anesthesiology*. Advance online publication. doi:10.1097/ANA.0000000000000520.

Physical Interventions

Blood volume in the intracranial space may be decreased by raising the head of the bed to greater than 45 degrees to facilitate drainage of venous blood through the jugular venous system. Positioning a patient so that the neck is in a neutral position and hip flexion is minimized also assists in facilitating venous drainage from the head. Further reduction of blood volume in the intracranial space may be accomplished through hyperventilation. Increasing the respiratory rate either through manual ventilation or the use of a resuscitation bag or mechanical ventilator causes an increased clearance of carbon dioxide and constriction of cerebral blood vessels. The consequence of hyperventilation is global cerebral vasoconstriction, which may result in ischemia to uninjured brain tissue. Established guidelines used for the management of patients with severe TBI recommend that arterial carbon dioxide ($PaCO_2$) be maintained in the range of 30 to 35 mm Hg when hyperventilation is employed to decrease ICP. The external drainage of CSF is an effective method for rapidly decreasing increased ICP (see previous discussion). Drainage of CSF may be continuous or intermittent according to the patient's specific needs.

 Safety Alert   Patient Care Activities in Patients With Increased Intracranial Pressure

When caring for a patient with increased ICP, it is important for the nurse to evaluate the patient's response to movements such as turning, side-lying, and lying flat. The optimal position for a patient with increased ICP and *decreased intracranial compliance* (inability to compensate for increase in intracranial contents) is thought to be 45 to 90 degrees with the neck in a neutral position in order to promote drainage of venous blood through jugular veins in the neck. The nurse can evaluate the patient's response by assessing the patient's ICP during a given activity and noting how quickly the ICP value returns to baseline after the activity is completed. Patients may tolerate routine patient care activities such as bathing, turning, and lying flat for diagnostic tests such as x-rays, and other patients may not. In situations where increased ICP does not respond to standard treatments, barbiturates such as pentobarbital can be used to induce a coma, significantly reducing metabolic demands in the brain (Table 39.6). When a barbiturate coma is initiated, other sedatives and analgesic medications are discontinued. Pentobarbital often causes vasodilation of the peripheral blood vessels and myocardial depression, requiring management with vasoactive medication to regulate blood pressure. Advanced hemodynamic monitoring such as a pulmonary artery catheter may also be initiated.

Surgical Management

Refractory increased ICP may also be managed by removing a section of the cranium and dura in order to create space for the swelling brain. This neurosurgical procedure is called a **hemicraniectomy** with a **durotomy** and involves the removal of a section of the skull and opening of the dura. The skull is removed and typically stored in a tissue bank or stored in a tissue pocket within the patient's abdomen. The dura is replaced with a synthetic material that allows for brain tissue expansion and watertight closure of the meningeal layer.

Nursing Management
Assessment and Analysis

Vigilant serial assessments of a patient's neurological status are necessary to identify neurological deterioration that places a patient at risk for increased ICP and cerebral herniation syndrome. Assessments of oxygenation, ventilation, and hemodynamic parameters are necessary to optimize therapy and prevent or mitigate brain injury. Performing a full systems assessment assists the nurse in identifying signs of complications or conditions that may negatively impact the patient with increased ICP, such as respiratory compromise. Assessment of laboratory values such as serum electrolytes and serum osmolality is necessary to detect electrolyte imbalance and dehydration, which can lead to renal insufficiency or failure.

Patients in a barbiturate coma are monitored using ICP monitoring, and in some cases electroencephalogram (EEG) recordings are used to document suppression of electrical activity in the brain. Medication levels may also be monitored, particularly when the dosage is decreased. The ability to elicit a neurological assessment from a patient in a barbiturate coma is limited because of the suppression caused by the medication; therefore, other parameters, such as pupillary size and reaction and corneal reflexes, must be trended. The nurse must ensure that the following safety measures are performed: application of moisture chambers with artificial tears to prevent corneal

Table 39.6 Common Sedatives Used in the Treatment of Increased ICP

Medication	Usual Dosage	Nursing Considerations
Morphine sulfate	Continuous infusion, 2–10 mg/hr and titrated to a pain and sedation scale target	• Patients should have a secure airway (typically an endotracheal tube) in place when any one of these continuous infusions is initiated in order to ensure that retention of carbon dioxide (hypercarbia) does not occur. Hypercarbia causes cerebral blood vessel dilation, resulting in increased cerebral blood volume and increased ICP.
Midazolam (Versed)	Continuous infusion, 2–4 mg/hr and titrated to a sedation scale target	• These infusions should be titrated to the desired effect, either a goal ICP measurement or a specific rating on a validated sedation scale such as the Nursing Instrument for the Communication of Sedation Scale (NICS) or the Richmond Agitation Sedation Scale (RASS).
Fentanyl (Sublimaze)	Continuous infusion, 25–100 mcg/hr and titrated to a sedation scale target	• Propofol infusion syndrome (PrIS) may occur in patients receiving propofol for greater than 48 hours or in patients receiving high doses of propofol (greater than 75 mcg/kg/min). Clinical manifestations of PrIS include acidosis, hyperkalemia, hyperlipidemia, and rhabdomyolysis causing acute kidney injury.
Propofol (Diprivan)	Continuous infusion, 50–200 mcg/kg/min and titrated to a target sedation goal or ICP threshold	• It is important to note that propofol is not an analgesic; therefore, if the patient is suspected to be in pain, it is important to advocate for medication to treat pain in addition to the sedative.
		• These infusions should be titrated to the desired effect, either a goal ICP measurement or a specific rating on a validated sedation scale such as the NICS or RASS.

ICP, Intracranial pressure.
From Brain Trauma Foundation, American Association of Neurological Surgeons, & Congress of Neurological Surgeons. (2017). Guidelines for the management of severe traumatic brain injury, 4th edition. *Journal of Neurosurgery, 80*(1), 6–15.

injury and frequent repositioning to prevent pressure injury.

Continued monitoring of ICP, neurological assessment, and vital signs continues after hemicraniectomy. Nursing and medical management of increased ICP requires the collection and synthesis of many data points in order to adjust and optimize treatment and a positive functional outcome. Clinical manifestations of increased ICP, including subtle changes in level of consciousness, increased blood pressure, decreased pulse rate, widening pulse pressure, changes in respiratory pattern, and pupillary changes, are reported immediately to the healthcare provider in order to ensure prompt intervention to decrease chances of permanent neurological injury.

Nursing Diagnoses

- **Ineffective airway clearance** related to diminished protective reflexes (cough, gag)
- **Ineffective breathing patterns** related to neurological dysfunction (brainstem compression, structural displacement)
- **Ineffective cerebral tissue perfusion** related to cerebral edema, hemorrhage, or hydrocephalus
- **Fluid volume deficit** related to osmotic diuretic administration
- **Ineffective thermoregulation** related to damage to the hypothalamus
- **Interrupted family processes** related to unresponsiveness of the patient; unpredictability of the outcome; prolonged recovery period; and the patient's uncertain residual physical, emotional, and cognitive disabilities

Nursing Interventions

▪ *Assessments*

- Serial neurological assessments every 1 to 2 hours in the critical phase, decreasing in frequency as the risk of cerebral edema and secondary brain injury decreases
  Serial neurological assessments are necessary to trend a patient's response to injury and to detect subtle neurological changes, such as a decrease in level of consciousness or new motor weakness, signaling increased ICP. Changes in level of consciousness are earlier clinical manifestations of increased ICP as compared with changes in vital signs (Cushing's triad) and motor activity. At change of shift, it is important for the oncoming nurse to complete a neurological assessment with the nurse leaving so that subtle patient findings are consistently trended and documented.
- Vital signs and oxygen saturation (SpO$_2$) every 1 to 2 hours
  Trending of vital signs is necessary to detect changes that may signal hemodynamic or neurological instability. In herniation syndrome, the systolic BP rises, and the diastolic remains normal or is lowered, resulting in a widened pulse pressure. The HR is decreased, and the respiratory pattern is irregular. Prompt identification of hypotension and decreased oxygenation (SpO$_2$) is important in preventing further brain injury resulting from decreased perfusion and oxygenation.

- Temperature every 1 to 2 hours
  Temperature elevations may indicate damage to the hypothalamus. Increasing cerebral metabolism may exacerbate existing brain injury by increasing the demand for oxygen and nutrients where there is existing poor blood flow (ischemia).
- Intracranial pressure and CPP every 1 to 2 hours or more frequently if the patient is experiencing an increase in ICP and/or a deterioration of neurological assessment
  Intracranial pressure and CPP are measured frequently in order to trend the values and to rapidly identify trends (increase in ICP and/or decrease in CPP) that require medical interventions in order to prevent herniation syndrome or secondary brain injury due to inadequate cerebral perfusion.
- Cardiac rhythm; serum markers of myocardial injury (creatinine kinase, creatinine kinase specific to cardiac muscle, and troponin)
  Myocardial ischemia, injury, or dysrhythmias may occur as a result of neurological injuries such as TBI or aneurysmal subarachnoid hemorrhage (SAH). The cause of myocardial ischemia is most likely due to a sudden release of catecholamines (epinephrine and norepinephrine) in the body at the time of injury because of activation of the sympathetic nervous system.
- Intake and output every 1 to 2 hours
  Fluid balance may be affected as treatments such as osmotic diuretics are administered. Hypovolemia may result in hypotension that adversely affects cerebral perfusion.
- Serum sodium and/or serum osmolality
  Serum osmolality is monitored after administration of mannitol to quantify the degree of systemic dehydration that has occurred as a result of diuresis. The purpose of monitoring serum sodium is to determine whether a patient is meeting the target to maintain a continuous concentration gradient favoring the pull of water out of the brain tissue. The typical maximum sodium level tolerated is 160 mEq/L.
- Serum electrolytes
  Electrolyte imbalance can occur with osmotic diuresis, and monitoring and replacement of electrolytes are required to prevent complications of electrolyte disturbances such as dysrhythmias and muscle weakness.
- Blood urea nitrogen (BUN) and creatinine
  In patients receiving hypertonic saline, the serum osmolality increases, and the risk of acute renal failure increases as serum osmolality rises above 320 mOsm/kg. Creatinine and BUN are monitored for indications of renal insufficiency.
- Arterial blood gas samples
  Monitoring ABG allows precise measurement of gases dissolved in the plasma and is particularly useful in the patient with increased ICP because it allows evaluation of the PaCO$_2$, which causes vasoconstriction (decreased PaCO$_2$) or vasodilation (increased PaCO$_2$) of cerebral blood vessels. Cerebral vasoconstriction can reduce ICP, and vasodilation of the cerebral blood vessels can increase ICP in brain injury.

- End-tidal carbon dioxide ($EtCO_2$) continuously to guide hyperventilation therapy during treatment of increased ICP

  When hyperventilation therapy is employed, $EtCO_2$ is monitored in order to maintain carbon dioxide in a specified range (30–35 mm Hg). End-tidal carbon dioxide values may be higher or lower than $PaCO_2$; therefore, it is necessary to document the $EtCO_2$ value at the time that a blood sample for an ABG is performed so that a correlation can be made between the $EtCO_2$ and the $PaCO_2$ measured in the arterial blood sample.

◼ Actions

- The head of the bed should be maintained at greater than 30 degrees, with the patient's head in midline. Avoid sharp hip flexion.

  Elevating the head of the bed and ensuring that the head is in midline facilitates drainage of blood from the jugular venous system, decreasing ICP. Avoiding sharp hip flexion ensures that large veins in the abdomen are not compressed, decreasing venous return.

- Avoid placing the patient in a position that allows pressure directly on the operative side after craniectomy.

  Direct pressure on the operative site may lead to injury to brain tissue that is not protected by the bone that has been removed. Additionally, placement on the operative side may increase ICP.

- Perform endotracheal suction only as necessary; pre-oxygenate with 100% oxygen for 1 to 2 minutes prior to suctioning.

  Suctioning a patient with increased ICP can introduce the risk of further elevation of ICP because the act induces coughing, which raises pressure inside the chest and may transiently reduce drainage of blood from veins in the neck, causing a spike in ICP in some patients. Suctioning should be performed when the patient demonstrates mucus in the endotracheal tube or every 4 to 6 hours to maintain patency of the tube. Administering 100% oxygen just prior to suctioning is performed to prevent hypoxia, which can occur during the interruption of mechanical ventilation.

- Administer sedative medications as prescribed.

  Sedation is used in patients with acutely increased ICP to treat pain, anxiety, and restlessness because it decreases ICP when titrated to an appropriate level for a particular patient. When given as a continuous infusion, sedative medications should be interrupted for a time adequate for a patient's neurological assessment to be evaluated. These medications are used judiciously in patients at risk for increased ICP so that subtle changes in the neurological assessment may still be identified.

- Administer osmotic agents (mannitol and hypertonic saline).

  Osmotic diuretics decrease ICP by pulling water from the interstitial spaces into the vascular space, and then diuresis occurs through the distal renal tubules. High-concentration sodium chloride solutions pull water from the interstitial spaces into the vascular space without associated fluid shifts.

- Ensure continuous drainage of CSF through the external ventricular drainage system when applicable.

  Kinks in the ICP monitoring tubing decrease drainage and may result in increased ICP.

- Administer antipyretics and/or implement cooling measures.

  These interventions prevent an increase in cerebral metabolism that accompanies elevated body temperature. Cooling can be achieved using water-cooled blankets or pads, ice packs placed in the axilla and groin, or a centrally placed catheter allowing for cool water to circulate around the catheter (endovascular cooling).

◼ Teaching

- Devices used during the course of treating increased ICP

  Devices such as central lines, ICP-monitoring devices, endotracheal tubes, and gastric tubes may be placed in order to manage patients with increased ICP.

- Medications used to treat increased ICP

  Several medications are used to treat increased ICP, and a patient's routine home medications may be significantly different in the hospital.

- Complications of increased ICP

  Many complications of increased ICP may occur and are closely associated with the primary cause of elevated ICP.

- Rationale for helmet after craniectomy

  As the patient progresses, a helmet is often fitted and placed on the patient's head whenever he or she is out of bed to prevent injury to the unprotected portion of the head.

- Importance of allowing the patient to rest

  Family members need to be instructed on the importance of allowing the patient rest periods because constant stimulation may exacerbate increased ICP.

Evaluating Care Outcomes

The effects of increased ICP on functional outcomes can be diminished with early recognition of deterioration and rapid treatment. Identification and control of the primary problem are also essential. The initial goal in managing increased ICP is to prevent cerebral herniation. The role of the nurse in performing, trending, and communicating neurological assessment findings is critically important to the preservation of neurological function. Positive patient outcomes are related to maximizing neurological function and minimizing the complications associated with increased ICP.

STROKE

Epidemiology

A person experiences a stroke every 40 seconds in the United States, resulting in approximately 6,400,000 Americans living with the effects of a stroke. Each year,

795,000 Americans are diagnosed with a stroke; the majority of these people have a stroke for the first time (610,000), and the remaining 185,000 people have a recurrent stroke. Additionally, 1 in 19 deaths is caused by stroke. The incidence of stroke is greater in men than women until age 55, at which time the incidence of stroke is greater in women than men. Death from stroke is greater in women and African Americans. Particularly concerning is an increase in the incidence of stroke and death rates in minorities aged less than 55 years in the United States. Stroke represents a significant public health threat that must be made a priority by all healthcare providers. Nurses have a unique and important role in their ability to educate patients on stroke risk factors, prevention, and treatment strategies across the continuum of care, from the community to acute care and back into their communities.

The term *stroke* is a general term used to describe a disruption in blood flow to the brain, which can be caused by a blockage of a blood vessel, ischemic stroke, or bleeding into the brain, hemorrhagic stroke. Ischemic strokes comprise 87% of strokes; 10% are caused by intracerebral hemorrhage (ICH), and 3% are caused by aneurysmal SAH (Box 39.2). A significant risk factor for stroke is hypertension, followed by cigarette smoking. Other modifiable risk factors include hypercholesterolemia and illicit drug use (cocaine use is associated with ICH). Major non-modifiable risk factors include age greater than 55, gender, and race. The National Institutes of Health Stroke Scale (NIHSS) may be used to quantify and trend neurological dysfunction in patients presenting with a suspected stroke (Fig. 39.6).

Connection Check 39.3

The nurse recognizes that which patient is at greatest risk for death secondary to stroke?

A. A 36-year-old Caucasian male
B. A 45-year-old Asian male
C. A 56-year-old African American female
D. A 62-year-old Hispanic female

Box 39.2 Types of Stroke

Ischemic Stroke (87%)

Large vessel
Small vessel (lacunar)
Embolic
Cryptogenic

Hemorrhagic Stroke (13%)

Intracerebral hematoma (ICH; 10%)
Subarachnoid hemorrhage (SAH; 3%)

CASE STUDY: EPISODE 3

The EMS crew alerts the hospital during transport about the arrival of a patient with stroke signs and symptoms, and the emergency department (ED) staff notifies the stroke team. Once he arrives in the ED at 12:55, Mr. Stewart is examined, and his stroke signs are quantified using the NIHSS, where he scores 22 points, indicating severe stroke symptoms. Mr. Stewart's time of stroke symptom onset is confirmed to be 12:15. Vital signs are recorded to be BP: 170/90 mm Hg, HR: 80 bpm, rhythm: atrial fibrillation, RR: 14. Two IV catheters are placed, and blood work is drawn to evaluate electrolytes and a complete blood cell (CBC) count. A finger-stick glucose is performed, and the result is 100 mg/dL. An emergent CT scan is arranged, revealing no intracerebral hemorrhage. After discussing the risks and benefits of IV recombinant tissue plasminogen activator (rt-PA) therapy with Mr. Stewart's wife and daughter and evaluating all laboratory work, the stroke team leader orders the following:

- rt-PA 0.9 mg/kg 0.9 mg × 82 kg (weight reported by wife) = 73.8 mg (rounded to nearest whole mg) = 74 mg
- Administer 7.4-mg IV push over 1 minute.
- Administer the remaining 66.6 mg over 1 hour using an infusion pump.

The rt-PA bolus is administered by the nurse at 1:50 p.m., and the continuous infusion is started at 1:52 p.m…

Ischemic Stroke

Pathophysiology and Clinical Manifestations

A sudden blockage of a cerebral blood vessel causes a reduction in the supply of oxygenated blood to the region of the brain fed by the involved artery, resulting in an abrupt onset of clinical manifestations. These clinical manifestations are grouped into stroke syndromes, which can be correlated or localized to a particular cerebral blood vessel (Table 39.7). When blood flow is disrupted, an area of brain tissue suffers irreversible damage, and this is referred to as an infarction (similar to cardiac tissue damage with a myocardial infarction [heart attack]). There is often a zone of tissue surrounding an infarction called the **ischemic penumbra** that contains ischemic tissue that is not irreversibly damaged. The ischemic penumbra is the target of therapies aimed at opening blocked cerebral blood vessels and reestablishing blood flow to ischemic brain tissue, providing the optimal chance for functional recovery. The abrupt nature of stroke symptom onset led to coining of the term "**brain attack**" as a tool to raise the level of urgency surrounding stroke to that of a "heart attack," which has provided a foundation for urging the lay public to seek immediate medical care for myocardial infarction and now stroke symptoms.

Category	Scale Definition		Score
1a. Level of Consciousness (Alert, drowsy, etc.)	0 = Alert 1 = Drowsy 2 = Stuporous 3 = Coma		
1b. LOC Questions (Month, age)	0 = Answers both correctly 1 = Answers one correctly 2 = Incorrect		
1c. LOC Commands (Open/close eyes, make fist/let go)	0 = Obeys both correctly 1 = Obeys one correctly 2 = Incorrect		
2. Best Gaze (Eyes open—patient follows examiner's finger or face)	0 = Normal 1 = Partial gaze palsy 2 = Forced deviation		
3. Visual Fields (Introduce visual stimulus/threat to pt's visual field quadrants)	0 = No visual loss 1 = Partial Hemianopia 2 = Complete Hemianopia 3 = Bilateral Hemianopia (Blind)		
4. Facial Paresis (Show teeth, raise eyebrows and squeeze eyes shut)	0 = Normal 1 = Minor 2 = Partial 3 = Complete		
5a. Motor Arm—Left **5b. Motor Arm—Right** (Elevate arm to 90° if patient is sitting, 45° if supine)	0 = No drift 1 = Drift 2 = Can't resist gravity 3 = No effort against gravity	Left	
	4 = No movement X = Untestable (Joint fusion or limb amp)	Right	
6a. Motor Leg—Left **6b. Motor Leg—Right** (Elevate leg to 30° with patient supine)	0 = No drift 1 = Drift 2 = Can't resist gravity 3 = No effort against gravity	Left	
	4 = No movement X = Untestable (Joint fusion or limb amp)	Right	
7. Limb Ataxia (Finger-nose, heel down shin)	0 = No ataxia 1 = Present in one limb 2 = Present in two limbs		
8. Sensory (Pin prick to face, arm, trunk, and leg—compare side to side)	0 = Normal 1 = Partial loss 2 = Severe loss		
9. Best Language (Name item, describe a picture and read sentences)	0 = No aphasia 1 = Mild to moderate aphasia 2 = Severe aphasia 3 = Mute		
10. Dysarthria (Evaluate speech clarity by patient repeating listed words)	0 = Normal articulation 1 = Mild to moderate slurring of words 2 = Near to unintelligible or worse 3 = Intubated or other physical barrier		
11. Extinction and Inattention (Use information from prior testing to identify neglect or double simultaneous stimuli testing)	0 = No neglect 1 = Partial neglect 2 = Complete neglect		
		Total Score	

FIGURE 39.6 National Institutes of Health Stroke Scale (NIHSS). The NIHSS quantifies and trends neurological dysfunction in patients presenting with a suspected stroke.

Occlusion of large cerebral blood vessels (e.g., carotid arteries, vertebral arteries) by atherosclerotic plaque occurs when the plaque ruptures, causing a blood clot to form and block the vessel (Fig. 39.7), or when atherosclerotic plaque accumulates to a point that it critically narrows and then completely obstructs blood flow. The occlusion of a large cerebral blood vessel can cause ischemia in large areas of brain tissue depending on the location of the occlusion (proximal or distal). These large areas are called *territories*, and the territory name is based on the blood vessel that perfuses that particular area (Fig. 39.8). A territory may contain more than one lobe of the brain.

Table 39.7 Clinical Manifestations of the Most Common Stroke Syndromes

Left Middle Cerebral Artery Syndrome	Right Middle Cerebral Artery Syndrome	Basilar Artery Syndrome
• Weakness of the right face, arm, and leg (arm weakness greater than leg weakness)	• Weakness of the left face, arm, and leg (arm weakness greater than leg weakness)	• Dizziness
• Decrease in sensation on the right side of the body	• Decrease in sensation on the left side of the body	• Ataxia
• Right homonymous hemianopia (loss of vision in the right temporal field of vision and left nasal field of vision, requiring patients to scan an area in order to visualize objects on their right side)	• Left homonymous hemianopia (loss of vision in the left temporal field of vision and right nasal field of vision, requiring patients to scan an area in order to visualize objects on their left side)	• Tinnitus
• Dysphasia—in most patients, the language center of the brain is located in the left hemisphere. Language deficits may involve the motor speech area *(Broca's area)* and cause patients to have difficulty expressing thoughts and to make errors in speech that they are able to detect. Injury or ischemia to the sensory speech area *(Wernicke's area)* results in an inability to process speech input in the brain, causing patients to make errors in speech of which they are unaware.	• Inattention or neglect of the left side	• Nausea and vomiting
		• Weakness on one side of the body that may be ipsilateral to the side of ischemia or injury or contralateral
		• Decrease in sensation on one side of the body that may be ipsilateral to the side of ischemia or injury or contralateral
• Inattention or neglect of the right side		• Difficulty in the articulation of speech
		• Difficulty with swallowing and managing oral secretions

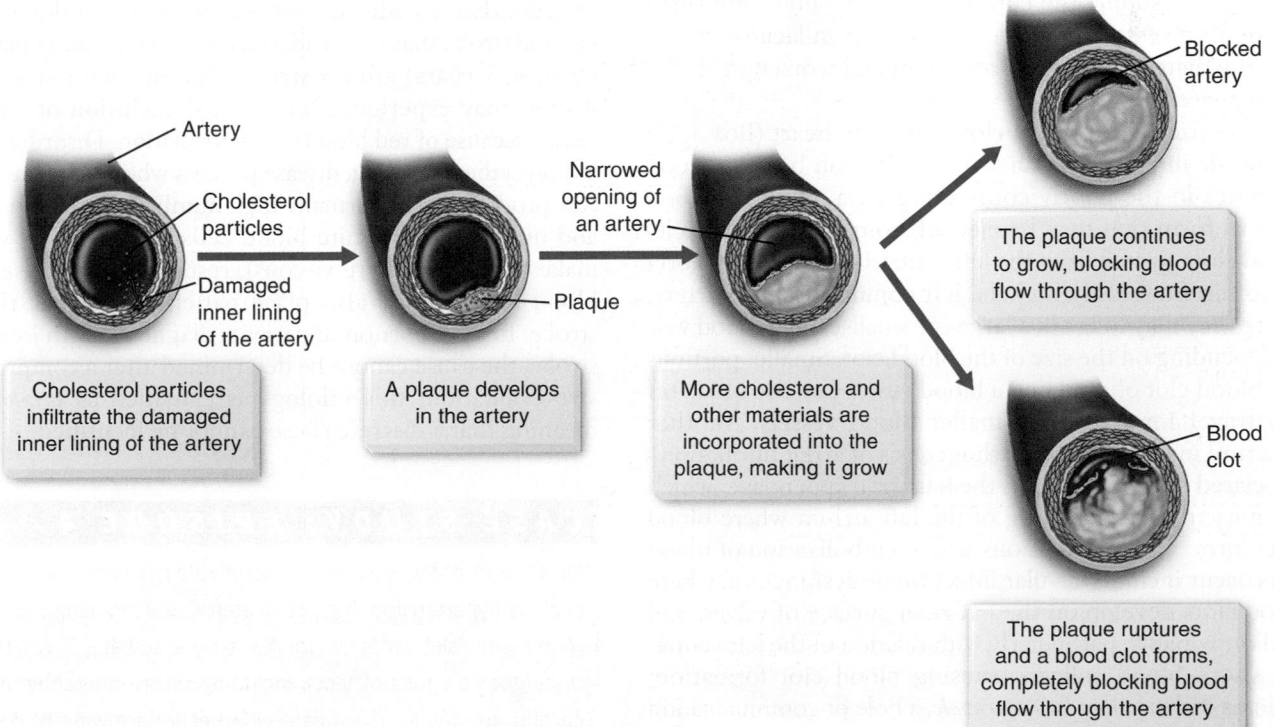

FIGURE 39.7 Development of atherosclerotic plaque that can lead to complete vessel obstruction or rupture.

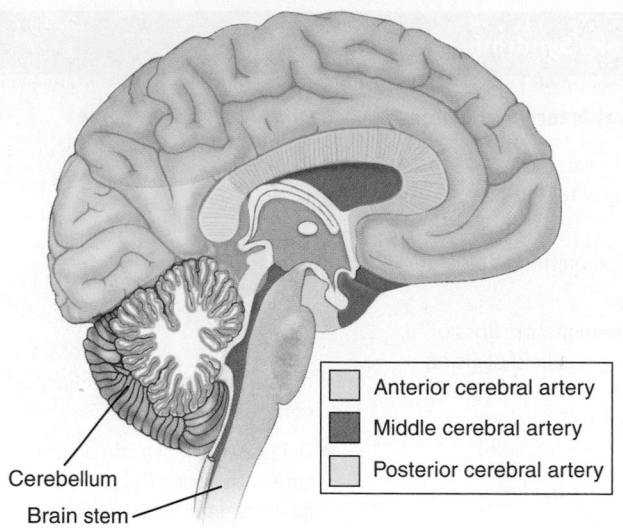

FIGURE 39.8 Territories of the brain. The territory name correlates to the blood vessel that perfuses the specific area.

The occlusion of small intracranial blood vessels supplying the peripheral regions of the brain and deep brain structures cause **lacunar stroke** syndromes, which vary in the severity of functional deficits. A lacunar stroke is a small infarction caused by an obstruction of a small blood vessel or group of small blood vessels. These small blood vessels are also called *perforating blood vessels* because they are the terminal branches of larger arteries. For example, the middle cerebral artery perfuses a large territory of brain tissue in the frontal, temporal, and parietal lobes, spanning the area from the cerebral cortex to the basal ganglia, and the arteries that supply the cortex and basal ganglia are small perforating vessels. Neurological deficits in lacunar stroke may fluctuate between improvement and worsening in the acute phase.

Embolization of blood clots from the heart (Box 39.3) can occur in patients with atrial fibrillation because blood stagnates in the poorly contracting atria, allowing blood clots to form that may be ejected from the left ventricle. Blood clots ejected from the left ventricle travel up the aorta and often flow easily into the left common carotid artery, where they may lodge in a large- or small-caliber blood vessel depending on the size of the blood clot. Smaller portions of a blood clot obstructing a blood vessel can also break off and travel forward into smaller blood vessels. Another structure involved in the pathogenesis of atrial fibrillation–associated cardiac emboli is the left atrial appendage, which is a muscular outpouching of the left atrium where blood clots form. Other conditions where embolization of blood clots occur include valvular infection or dysfunction, where blood clots develop on the irregular surface of valves, and cardiomyopathy, particularly with dilation of the left ventricle where blood collects, causing blood clot formation. Patients with a *patent foramen ovale*, a hole or communication between the right and left atria, are at risk of a clot traveling from the periphery into the heart from the right to the left atrium and then out the left side of the heart through the aorta and ejected toward the brain.

Coagulation disorders causing hypercoagulability represent another significant but less frequent etiology of ischemic stroke that is considered carefully in young patients (aged <55 years) after a stroke. Patients with sickle cell disease may experience mechanical occlusion of a blood vessel because of red blood cell deformation. Disorders such as polycythemia vera (a disease process where the bone marrow produces an abnormally high number of red blood cells and in some cases white blood cells and platelets, which makes the blood more viscous), resulting in increased red blood cell volume, also place patients at higher risk of stroke. In a proportion of patients diagnosed with ischemic stroke, the cause cannot be determined after a comprehensive evaluation; this etiology is classified as *cryptogenic*, meaning that a discrete cause cannot be identified.

CASE STUDY: EPISODE 4

Mr. Stewart possesses several modifiable risk factors for stroke, such as hypertension, high cholesterol, and smoking. His non-modifiable risk factors include his gender and age. This patient undergoes a series of tests, including ultrasonography of the carotid arteries to investigate whether a narrowing of one of the blood vessels leading to the brain may have been the cause of the stroke. Cardioembolic stroke can be attributed to this type of defect. The diagnostic testing regimen after a patient has experienced a stroke is aimed at determining the cause of the stroke, which enables healthcare providers to tailor a secondary prevention program to prevent a recurrence of stroke for a given patient. Education and counseling on smoking cessation are also high priorities for Mr. Stewart...

Management

Medical Management

Diagnosis

Computed tomography (CT) scans and magnetic resonance imaging (MRI) are used, along with the clinical presentation, to guide the diagnostic evaluation of a patient with suspected stroke. Magnetic resonance imaging is more sensitive than CT in patients with strokes that are small or located in the brainstem, and an MRI may be ordered to investigate the caliber and existence of narrowing for the sections of blood vessels within the skull, which cannot be visualized with ultrasound. Carotid duplex scanning is indicated in patients when carotid stenosis or occlusion is the suspected cause of the stroke. Doppler ultrasound allows evaluation of the middle cerebral, intracranial carotid, and vertebrobasilar arteries. An echocardiogram may also be ordered to evaluate current cardiac function and determine whether a cardioembolic source is likely. An injection of agitated saline (agitation causes microbubbles to form) may be used to assist in determining whether the patient has a patent foramen ovale. Laboratory tests include CBC with differential, platelet count, serum electrolytes, BUN, creatinine, and cholesterol level.

Medications

Cerebral blood vessels may be opened or recanalized using IV recombinant tissue plasminogen activator (rt-PA), which allows a blood clot to be dissolved at the site and restores blood flow to ischemic neuronal tissue. Intravenous rt-PA for use in treating patients with acute ischemic stroke is currently the only treatment approved by the U.S. Food and Drug Administration (FDA) for ischemic stroke. In order to receive IV rt-PA, patients must present within 3 hours of stroke symptom onset. In some defined cases, IV rt-PA may be given up to 4.5 hours after stroke symptom onset. See Table 39.8 for inclusion and exclusion criteria used by stroke teams in determining patient eligibility to receive IV rt-PA. In order to mitigate injury to neurons due to ischemia, rt-PA must be given as soon as possible after ischemic stroke but not outside established therapeutic windows. The most significant risk associated with IV rt-PA administration is intracranial bleeding, which occurs in approximately 6.4% of patients receiving IV rt-PA. Administration of IV rt-PA benefits approximately 30% of treated patients, as evidenced by a decrease in or absence of neurological deficits at 90 days after treatment. Adhering strictly to established inclusion and exclusion criteria is associated with a lesser incidence of symptomatic ICH after IV rt-PA.

Another therapy for acute ischemic stroke includes intra-arterial retrieval of the clot or thrombectomy (see Evidence-Based Practice: Treatment of Acute Ischemic Stroke). This intervention involves a cerebral angiogram to locate a vessel occlusion accompanied by the introduction of a stent to ensnare the clot and a suction system to reduce the likelihood of embolization of the clot as it is pulled out of the blood vessel with the stent (also called *endovascular technique*). Performed by an interventional neuroradiologist or other specialist trained in these techniques, this procedure includes the introduction of a catheter into the femoral artery that is then threaded up the aorta and across the aortic arch into the blocked artery (carotid arteries anteriorly and vertebral arteries posteriorly) for direct visualization of the patency or nonpatency of the blood vessel. Dye is injected into the blood vessels through the catheter, and images are obtained in quick succession using x-ray. These procedures require highly specialized teams of physicians and nurses trained in neurointerventional radiology and have the benefit of extending the time window after which a patient is ineligible for a therapy that could recanalize a blood vessel because these procedures may be performed up to 24 hours after the onset of stroke symptoms and identification of the occlusion of a large blood vessel on CT or magnetic resonance angiography. Potential complications of these procedures include damage or rupture of a blood vessel; breakage of the blood clot, which could travel forward and lodge in another blood vessel; and intracerebral hemorrhage. Research has demonstrated a significant recovery benefit when IV r-tPA is administered in combination with endovascular therapy for patients with occlusion of a large-caliber blood vessel (e.g., internal carotid arteries, basilar artery, and middle cerebral arteries). After patients are evaluated for eligibility to receive IV rt-PA and the infusion is initiated, they are then transported for advanced radiographic imaging (either CT angiogram or MR angiogram) to identify a large-vessel occlusion (thrombus). If an occlusion is identified, the patient is transported to the angiography area for thrombectomy while the IV rt-PA continues. Contraindications to these procedures follow the exclusion criteria for IV rt-PA. Traditionally, providers performing these interventions were radiologists with specialized training in cerebrovascular interventions; however, training programs for neurologists and neurosurgeons are emerging, with the intention of increasing patient access to this care, which has historically been available only in large academic medical centers. The Joint Commission, a regulatory body, now accredits primary and comprehensive stroke centers. Primary stroke centers offer access to IV rt-PA, and comprehensive stroke centers offer access to all stroke therapies, including endovascular therapy and neurosurgical services. Research has advanced significantly since 2015, expanding the therapeutic window for treating stroke,

Table 39.8 Inclusion and Exclusion Criteria for the Administration of Tissue Plasminogen Activator (rt-PA)

Inclusion Criteria	Exclusion Criteria 0- to 3-Hour Therapeutic Window	Exclusion Criteria 3- to 4.5-Hour Therapeutic Window

• Measurable neurological deficit using NIHSS
 	
 • No hemorrhage on head CT
 	
 • Time since last time patient was seen to be normal is within 3 or 4.5 hours (if additional exclusions not present) before the IV rt-PA infusion was begun
 	
 • Symptoms present for 30 minutes, not rapidly improving or attributable to another disease (e.g., seizures, migraine)
 	
 • Imaging of head is consistent with an acute ischemic stroke, not hemorrhage or brain tumor
	• Evidence of intracranial hemorrhage on pre-treatment CT scan
	
	 • Minor or rapidly improving clinical manifestations
	
	 • Clinical manifestations of subarachnoid hemorrhage even with normal head CT
	
	 • Active internal bleeding: gastrointestinal or urinary bleeding within last 21 days or known bleeding risk, including but not limited to:
	   • Platelet count less than 100,000/mm³
	   • Heparin during the preceding 48 hours associated with elevated aPTT
	   • Currently taking oral anticoagulants (e.g., warfarin sodium) or recent use with an elevated prothrombin time (PT) greater than 15 seconds or INR greater than 1.7
	
	 • Major surgery or other serious trauma during preceding 14 days
	
	 • Stroke, serious head trauma, or intracranial surgery during preceding 3 months
	
	 • Recent arterial puncture at a noncompressible site
	
	 • Recent lumbar puncture during preceding 7 days
	
	 • Systolic BP greater than 185 mm Hg or diastolic BP greater than 110 mm Hg at the time of administration
	
	 • rt-PA infusion and/or patient requires aggressive treatment to reduce blood pressure to within these limits
	
	 • History of intracranial hemorrhage, neoplasm, arteriovenous malformation, or aneurysm
	
	 • Recent acute myocardial infarction
		• All exclusion criteria for the 0- to 3-hour therapeutic window apply, and additional criteria below are not present
		
		 • Age greater than 80 years
		
		 • Receiving anticoagulants, even if the INR is normal
		
		 • Prior history of stroke and diabetes

aPTT, Activated partial thromboplastin time; *BP,* blood pressure; *CT,* computed tomography; *INR,* international normalized ratio; *IV,* intravenous; *NIHSS,* National Institutes of Health Stroke Scale International; *rt-PA,* recombinant tissue plasminogen activator.

particularly occlusions in large blood vessels such as the internal carotid arteries, the basilar artery, and the middle cerebral arteries. Endovascular therapies are now available to patients who were last known to be well or without symptoms within 24 hours. Intravenous rt-PA can be used concomitantly with endovascular therapy in patients meeting the IV rt-PA therapeutic window (3 hours or 4.5 hours) demonstrating a large-vessel occlusion on radiographic imaging.

Evidence-Based Practice

Treatment of Acute Ischemic Stroke

A systematic literature review and a meta-analysis were conducted to evaluate the treatment effectiveness of endovascular thrombectomy in comparison to best medical care treatment for acute ischemic stroke. Eight studies were identified, representing a total of 2,423 patients, and findings revealed better patient functional outcomes in patients who underwent thrombectomy. Additionally, these patients also demonstrated decreased mortality, with no increased incidence of intracerebral hemorrhage after endovascular thrombectomy.

Balami, J. S., Sutherland, B. A., Edmunds, L. D., Grunwald, I. Q., Newhaus, A. A., Hadley, G., …Buchan, A. M. (2015). A systematic review and meta-analysis of randomized controlled trials of endovascular thrombectomy compared with best medical treatment for acute ischemic stroke. *International Journal of Stroke, 10*(6), 1–11.

The medical management of stroke also includes measures to prevent complications of stroke, including venous thromboembolism (VTE) prophylaxis, management of blood pressure, and control of risk factors for stroke to prevent stroke recurrence. Additionally, a diagnostic work-up aimed at finding the cause for the stroke (Table 39.9) is essential to guide focused treatment. Blood pressure management, particularly in patients who have not received thrombolytic agents, is controversial because of the complex physiology of cerebral blood flow and cerebral autoregulatory dysfunction after stroke. Blood pressure treatment thresholds should be tailored by the provider to a patient's particular stroke type, location, and comorbidities, although blood pressure may be permitted to rise to a systolic goal of 180 to 220 mm Hg in some instances. Hypotension should be avoided in the acute period after stroke. Blood pressure control in acute stroke is based on the concept of **cerebral autoregulation**, which is the protective process by which cerebral blood vessels dilate when systemic blood pressure is reduced and constrict when systemic blood pressure is elevated to maintain

Table 39.9 Diagnostic Testing in Stroke

Diagnostic Test	Rationale
Computed tomography (CT)	• CT scanning is performed in patients with clinical manifestations of stroke in order to determine whether hemorrhage is the cause of symptoms. Radiographical changes associated with ischemic stroke are typically not visualized within the first several hours following a stroke. • A CT scan can be performed with the aid of an IV contrast agent or without (non–contrast-enhanced scan). When initially evaluating a patient with suspected stroke, contrast is not used so that blood can be easily visualized. Intravenous contrast may be helpful in visualizing a mass lesion in the brain (e.g., tumor).
Magnetic resonance imaging (MRI)	• A stroke protocol is performed for patients receiving MRI for suspected stroke, which includes sequences that capture necrotic tissue and areas of the brain that are hypoperfused and directly visualizes the blood vessels to detect blood vessel obstruction or another abnormality such as an aneurysm.
Doppler ultrasound of the carotid arteries	• Doppler ultrasound of the carotid arteries is utilized to detect narrowing of the inner lumen of the carotid vessels by atherosclerotic plaque. Evaluation of the carotid arteries with ultrasound can detect narrowing in the carotid vessels before they enter the skull.
Cerebral angiography	• Four-vessel cerebral angiography is the "gold standard" for visualizing abnormalities such as aneurysms or occlusions in blood vessels as they pass into the skull and brain (intracranial vessels). The right and left carotid and vertebral arteries are entered separately in order to visualize the anterior (carotid arteries) portion of the circle of Willis and the posterior (vertebral arteries) portion of the circle of Willis, including the basilar artery. The femoral artery is typically cannulated for this procedure, although alternative sites such as the brachial artery may be used in specific instances. • Procedures such as angioplasty and stent deployment for narrowed blood-flow–limiting atherosclerotic deposits and coiling of aneurysms are performed using this radiographical modality.
Echocardiography • Transthoracic (TTE)	• Echocardiography is utilized to directly visualize myocardial wall movement and contraction of the chambers of the heart. In stroke, the TTE is utilized to evaluate overall cardiac function as well as the presence of blood clots within the heart that could embolize to the brain. Presence of a patent foramen ovale (PFO) may be revealed on TTE with the assistance of an IV agitated saline injection, where small bubbles may be seen traversing an abnormality in the atrial septum.
• Transesophageal (TEE)	• A TEE may reveal a PFO not found on TTE. A TEE allows better visualization of the left atrial appendage, which may be a source of blood clots, particularly in patients with atrial fibrillation.
Laboratory tests to determine if hypercoagulability is the cause of stroke	• A hypercoagulable state in the blood can cause stroke, particularly in young patients less than 55 years of age. Examples of laboratory tests that may be requested include lupus anticoagulant, anticardiolipin antibodies, protein C activity, protein S activity, and factor V Leiden mutation.

constant blood flow. Cerebral autoregulation is dysfunctional after stroke, making it necessary to implement interventions to protect the brain from abnormally low systemic blood pressure in the absence of this protective mechanism.

Secondary stroke prevention strategies should be individualized for each patient according to specific stroke risk factors. According to stroke center accreditation guidelines, after a stroke, patients should be discharged with antiplatelet therapy, lipid-lowering therapy if indicated, anticoagulation if indicated for atrial fibrillation, and a blood pressure control strategy in patients with hypertension.

Complications

Complications of ischemic stroke can be life threatening in the acute phase and life altering as time progresses. A life-threatening complication of acute ischemic stroke is hemorrhage into the area of infarcted (nonviable or dead) brain tissue, termed *hemorrhagic transformation*, which patients may experience in the absence of thrombolytic therapy or anticoagulation therapy. Hemorrhagic transformation is thought to occur as a result of blood vessel spasm around a blood vessel that has been occluded by a blood clot, which in time resolves, causing the blood clot to break apart and restoring blood flow to surrounding ischemic and infarcted brain tissue. During ischemia, tissues may become friable or fragile, and when normal blood flow or pressure is reestablished, this pressure may cause tissue damage or bleeding.

Cytotoxic edema may occur most often in a stroke occupying a large vascular territory in the brain. Cerebral edema in this situation is caused by the breakdown of intracellular processes due to an inadequate oxygen supply, causing fluid to leak out of cells and into the interstitial space, resulting in edema. As ischemia persists and infarction occurs, cerebral edema may increase, causing increased ICP and placing a patient at risk for cerebral herniation syndrome. Aspiration of food, fluids, or secretions into the lungs is a common complication of stroke because of the decreased level of consciousness, as well as potential impairment of cranial nerves, facial muscles, and function of the palate. Measures to screen for swallowing dysfunction after stroke, early intervention by speech-language pathologists (SLPs), and general aspiration precautions are necessary in preventing this complication.

Chronic complications of stroke may include weakness or paralysis of the extremities and associated risk of muscle contracture. Splinting, passive range of motion, and physical and occupational therapies assist in preserving function and increasing the probability of the return of function to the extremities. Neglect or inattention (also termed **agnosia**) to one side of the body can occur in strokes in the right or left hemisphere; however, this deficit is most characteristic of stroke syndromes in the right hemisphere of the brain. Neglect or inattention of one side of the body occurs on the opposite side of the body from the area of brain injury and causes a patient not to recognize or acknowledge the affected side of the body. Integration of both sides of the body is a major goal in the rehabilitation of patients after stroke. Visual field deficits, such as **homonymous hemianopia** (vision loss on the same side of the visual field in both eyes), commonly occur in stroke and affect an entire side of vision (both nasal and temporal fields; Fig. 39.9).

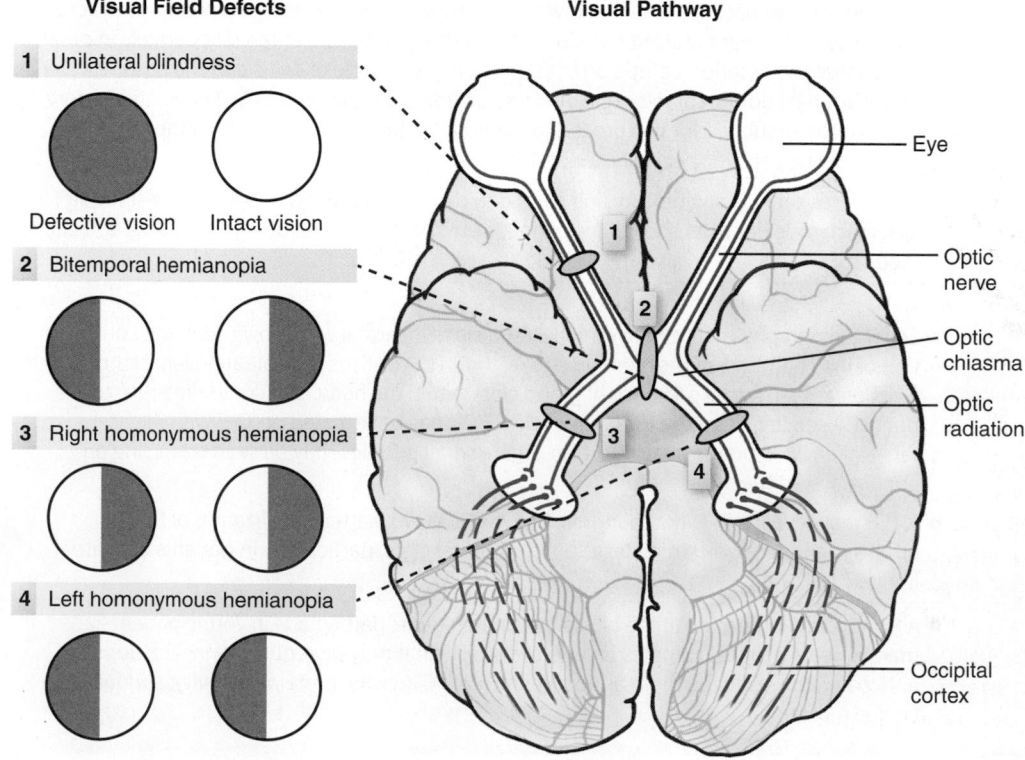

FIGURE 39.9 Visual field defects due to stroke. Visual field deficits, such as homonymous hemianopia, commonly occur in stroke and affect an entire side of vision (both nasal and temporal fields).

Patients with this type of visual field deficit must learn scanning techniques in order to ensure that they are able to visualize an entire visual target. For example, in order to ensure that patients are able to eat their entire meal on a tray or place setting, they must scan the entire space to compensate for the darkened or absent visual fields.

Disorders of speech due to facial muscle or cranial nerve weakness and language are common residual deficits of stroke that often require intensive speech and cognitive therapies. The interprofessional team, including physicians, nurses, and speech therapists, is integral in incorporating strategies into the patient's routine, with the goal of reinforcing learned strategies and adding contextual meaning to the strategies.

Disturbances in the planning of motor activities, or **apraxia**, often occur in strokes that involve the frontal and temporal lobes of the brain. When patients demonstrate a type of apraxia called *ideational apraxia*, they may be able to correctly identify an object such as a comb but proceed to brush their teeth with the comb. Occupational therapists (OTs) work with patients, families, and the healthcare team to develop strategies for recoupling common meanings with objects or activities.

The complication of depression after stroke is important to consider when working with these patients because it can significantly impact recovery and rehabilitation. Depression occurs with an increased incidence in patients with a stroke in the right hemisphere of the brain. Patients should be evaluated at different time points during their recovery phase for depression, which initially could be related to the new situation and residual deficits or body changes that the patient may be experiencing but could potentially become a chronic issue that must be addressed by the interprofessional team.

Hemorrhagic Stroke

Pathophysiology and Clinical Manifestations

Hemorrhagic stroke is separated into three main subtypes: nontraumatic subarachnoid hemorrhage (SAH), intracerebral hemorrhage (ICH), and intraventricular hemorrhage (IVH). **Subarachnoid hemorrhage** is typically caused by a ruptured **aneurysm** (weak, dilated vessel) and less commonly by an **arteriovenous malformation (AVM)**, which is a mass of arteries and veins that is not connected by a capillary network. Cerebral aneurysms occur in 3% to 5% of the general population, and aneurysmal rupture with subsequent SAH makes up approximately 5% of all strokes. Approximately 10% to 15% of patients with aneurysmal SAH die prior to reaching medical care, and mortality for patients treated in the hospital is approximately 50%. Despite intensive treatment, an estimated 50% of SAH survivors have significant, permanent neurological deficits. Risk factors for SAH include hypertension, smoking, heavy alcohol use, use of sympathetic nervous system stimulants such as cocaine, female gender, history of cerebrovascular disease, and postmenopausal state.

A cerebral aneurysm is thought to occur as a result of an inherent weakness or gradually acquired weakness of the medial layer in a segment of a blood vessel. The medial layer in a blood vessel is the muscular layer that adds shape and tone to the vessel; a weakness in a segment of this layer causes an outpouching of the blood vessel through the outermost adventitial layer. Cerebral aneurysms are most often located at bifurcations of blood vessels, and 85% are located in the anterior portion of the circle of Willis (i.e., internal carotid artery, middle cerebral artery, anterior cerebral artery, and anterior communicating artery). The remaining 15% of aneurysms occur in the posterior portion of the circle of Willis (e.g., posterior communicating arteries, posterior cerebral arteries, vertebrobasilar system). Some patients have multiple aneurysms, sometimes making it difficult to discern the source of the rupture. An aneurysm typically ruptures in the thinnest-walled portion of the aneurysm, also called the *dome*. The degree of neurological impairment at onset is quantified using the Hunt and Hess or World Federation of Neurological Surgeons scoring system (Box 39.4). Patients may or may not lose consciousness at the time of aneurysm rupture, which may be related to the size, location, and magnitude of the rupture in the aneurysm. Subarachnoid hemorrhage is characterized by a sudden severe headache, often termed a "thunderclap" headache because of the intensity of the pain experienced at the onset. Subsequent neck stiffness and pain ensue because of the irritation of the meninges, particularly at the base of the skull, where pooling of blood occurs. Photosensitivity may also be associated with meningeal irritation or inflammation.

Nontraumatic intracranial hemorrhage has several causes, the most common of which is hypertension, typically occurring in the deep structures of the brain such as the basal

---

Box 39.4 Grading Scales for Subarachnoid Hemorrhage

Hunt and Hess Grading Scale

Grade I: Asymptomatic or slight headache and neck stiffness

Grade II: Headache and neck stiffness, cranial nerve deficit

Grade III: Headache, neck stiffness, focal motor deficit, lethargy

Grade IV: Stuporous, dense hemiparesis or posturing

Grade V: Comatose, posturing, moribund

Fisher Grading Scale, Determined by Amount of Blood Visualized on Computed Tomography (CT) Scan

Grade 1: No blood on CT scan

Grade 2: Blood layering less than 1-mm thickness

Grade 3: Blood layering greater than 1-mm thickness

Grade 4: Intraparenchymal or intraventricular blood

ganglia and thalamus. Another common cause of intracerebral hemorrhage is oral anticoagulation use (e.g., warfarin [Coumadin] and dabigatran [Pradaxa], apixaban [Eliquis], rivaroxaban [Xarelto]). Intracerebral hemorrhage can also be caused by tumors and AVMs, as well as other disease processes such as Moyamoya disease and amyloid angiopathy (Table 39.10). Intracerebral hemorrhage may be accompanied by extension of the hemorrhage into the ventricular system, leading to IVH. Intraventricular hemorrhage may also occur as a primary site of hemorrhage. Intracerebral hemorrhage is typically managed using medical therapies to manage blood pressure and prevent expansion of the hematoma as well as therapies to reverse coagulopathy and treat increased intracranial pressure (e.g., osmotic therapy, hyperventilation, drainage of CSF).

Medical and Surgical Management

Medical and surgical management of subarachnoid hemorrhage (SAH) aims to prevent and mitigate complications such as aneurysm rebleeding and cerebral vasospasm. **Cerebral vasospasm** occurs in approximately 30% of patients with SAH and causes narrowing of blood vessel segments (refer to the Complications section for a more detailed discussion). Aneurysms are secured either by applying a titanium clip to the neck of the aneurysm during surgery using a microscope or by deploying platinum coils into the aneurysm during angiography, both with the goal of reducing blood flow into the aneurysm (Fig. 39.10). In cases where neither clipping nor coiling the aneurysm is feasible, reinforcement of the aneurysmal wall by wrapping the outside of the aneurysm with synthetic material or muscle during the surgery may be accomplished. Wrapping of cerebral aneurysms is not considered a definitive treatment of the aneurysm because it remains at risk for rupture because blood continues to flow through the weakened aneurysmal vessel wall. The decision to secure an aneurysm by microsurgical technique using clips or by endovascular technique using coils is determined collaboratively by neurosurgeons and neurointerventional radiologists. Factors considered in determining the best treatment for an aneurysm include a patient's overall medical condition and hemodynamic stability and the cerebrovascular anatomy surrounding the aneurysm, such as whether the opening or neck of the aneurysm is wide or narrow or the degree of tortuosity of feeding vessels. Patients with high-grade Hunt and Hess scores (grade 4 or 5), as well as patients with multiple comorbid conditions and with hemodynamic instability at baseline, may be better candidates for aneurysm coiling. Aneurysms with a wide neck and tortuous vascular anatomy may be better candidates for aneurysm clipping. Treatment of other early complications, such as hydrocephalus occurring as blood occludes arachnoid villi, can be accomplished through external ventricular drainage. Management of blood pressure is important in the early period after subarachnoid hemorrhage in order to prevent rebleeding of an aneurysm. Evidence for a precise blood pressure range does not yet exist. The guidelines for the management of SAH recommend management of blood pressure while considering the risk of either hypoperfusion or rebleeding in the period prior to securing the aneurysm.

Surgical management of intracranial hemorrhage above the tentorium cerebelli (supratentorial) has not been shown to improve outcomes unless a hematoma is superficial in location. Surgical evacuation of a hematoma below the tentorium, infratentorial, is generally recommended and supported by recent guidelines because of the risk of brainstem compression and irreversible brain injury. Intraventricular hemorrhage is typically managed with cerebrospinal drainage. Research focusing on the application of thrombolytic therapy

Table 39.10 Causes of Intracerebral Hemorrhage	
Brain tumor	Brain tumors may involve blood vessels and may have a hemorrhagic component. It is often difficult to determine if a mass is underlying an intracranial hemorrhage; therefore, follow-up imaging (e.g., CT, MRI, or angiography) in 1 to several weeks after hemorrhage may be necessary.
Arteriovenous malformation (AVM)	An AVM is a mass of arteries and veins that is not connected by a capillary network. One of the roles of a capillary network is to provide a transition between high- and low-pressure systems. In an AVM, a high-pressure system is connected directly to a low-pressure system, which predisposes the malformation to bleeding. An AVM may not be apparent on initial imaging in the setting of ICH, so follow-up imaging and angiography are required to rule out AVM as a cause for ICH.
Moyamoya disease	Moyamoya disease involves constriction or narrowing of the end of the internal carotid arteries and narrowing of the smaller branches of the arteries in the anterior circulation (e.g., middle cerebral artery, anterior cerebral artery). An arterial network (collateral circulation) develops in response to the narrowing of arteries over time in order to augment blood supply to the affected areas of the brain.
Cerebral amyloid angiopathy	Cerebral amyloid angiopathy (CAA) involves the deposition of beta-amyloid into the walls of blood vessels, rendering them fragile and at risk for damage, resulting in intracerebral hemorrhage. Beta-amyloid is one of the substances thought to play a role in Alzheimer's disease, and in this case, the substance is deposited into blood vessels. Cerebral amyloid angiopathy occurs mainly in older adults.

CT, Computed tomography; *ICH,* intracranial hemorrhage; *MRI,* magnetic resonance imaging.

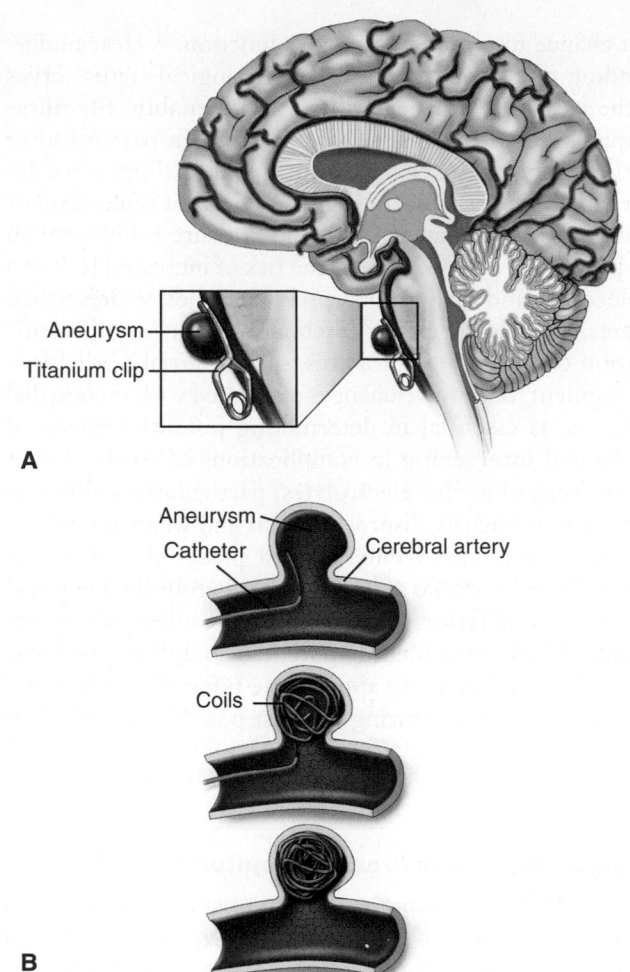

Aneurysm
Titanium clip

A

Aneurysm
Catheter — Cerebral artery

Coils

B

FIGURE 39.10 Methods of securing cerebral aneurysms. *A,* Aneurysm clipping. *B,* Aneurysm coiling. *A,* Aneurysms may be secured by applying a titanium clip to the neck of the aneurysm during surgery using a microscope to reduce blood flow into the aneurysm. *B,* Aneurysms may be secured by deploying platinum coils into the aneurysm during angiography to reduce blood flow into the aneurysm.

to maintain ventricular catheter patency and achieve earlier dissolution of an intraventricular blood clot to improve functional outcome is ongoing.

Complications

Subarachnoid hemorrhage causes neurological and systemic complications such as ischemic stroke, cerebral edema, pulmonary edema, and myocardial ischemia. The morbidity and mortality of patients with SAH are influenced by the management of systemic medical complications, which can cause or exacerbate brain injury. For example, myocardial injury can cause left ventricular failure, resulting in pulmonary edema and hypoxemia that may exacerbate **cerebral ischemia** (insufficient blood flow to the brain to meet metabolic demand).

Cerebral vasospasm causing delayed ischemic neurological deficit is a major complication of SAH, affecting 30% of patients and occurring between days 4 and 14 after the SAH. The peak risk period for cerebral vasospasm occurs from days 5 to 9 after the SAH and is a narrowing of a

segment of a cerebral artery that leads to local cerebral ischemia. Although the precise etiology of cerebral vasospasm is unknown, several postulated causes include an influx of calcium into damaged cells of local tissue and the involved blood vessel, potentially causing local spasm; release and activation of inflammatory mediators in response to endothelial damage, causing vasoconstriction; and adhesion and infiltration of white blood cells across the arterial wall, amplifying the inflammatory response that produces vasospasm.

The clinical manifestations of vasospasm can include confusion, changes in level of consciousness, or new **focal** (localized area) motor weakness, often in a waxing and waning pattern. A new focal motor weakness should be evaluated and treated urgently in a similar manner to an acute ischemic stroke because vasospasm can lead to cerebral infarction. Treatment of vasospasm has historically been centered on hypertension, hypervolemia, and hemodilution, widely known as **triple-H therapy**, with the goal of maintaining arterial patency and preventing cerebral infarction. Hypertension may be accomplished by withholding antihypertensive medications in patients with a history of hypertension or elevating the blood pressure with vasoactive medications. Hypervolemia may be achieved by administering crystalloid or colloidal solutions such as albumin, targeting a hemodynamic parameter that measures or approximates intravascular volume (e.g., central venous pressure, pulmonary artery occlusion pressure [PAOP], global end-diastolic volume). Cardiac output may also be chosen as an endpoint for therapy. The intent of hemodilution is to decrease the viscosity of the blood in order to facilitate flow through often narrowed arteries. Hemodilution may be achieved as hypervolemia is employed, although minimum thresholds for hemoglobin are typically maintained at approximately 30 g/dL with the intent of ensuring adequate oxygen delivery to the brain tissue.

Administration of nimodipine, a calcium-channel blocker, improves outcomes in patients experiencing vasospasm; however, this medication is associated with hypotension, which may necessitate alteration in dosing by increasing the frequency of dosing and decreasing the dose or discontinuing the therapy in some instances. Hypotension in the setting of vasospasm may worsen ischemia caused by the narrowing of the blood vessel. Cerebral angioplasty may be indicated to reestablish blood flow through narrowed arteries in patients who develop focal neurological deficits despite medical therapies to maintain blood flow. In some cases, arterial vasodilators are utilized during cerebral angiography in an attempt to dilate a focal arterial narrowing.

Hyponatremia is a common complication in patients with SAH, which may be caused by syndrome of inappropriate antidiuretic hormone (SIADH) or by cerebral salt-wasting syndrome, also known as renal salt-wasting syndrome. The etiology of sodium and water imbalance in these patients is often difficult to determine because large amounts of fluid, and in some cases large amounts of sodium, are administered, interfering with the results of the serum and urine assays traditionally used in evaluating sodium and water imbalances. Furthermore, SIADH has many potential causes, including medications and mechanical ventilation. The usual treatment of SIADH, focused on fluid restriction, may be problematic in patients with SAH undergoing treatment for cerebral vasospasm with hypervolemic therapy because of the need to maintain adequate blood pressure and intravascular volume. Cerebral salt-wasting syndrome is thought to be a common etiology of hyponatremia in patients with SAH and is characterized by a decrease in sodium accompanied by increased urinary output. The precise physiological mechanism for cerebral salt-wasting syndrome is unknown; however, a postulated mechanism involves the release of atrial natriuretic peptide (ANP) from myocardial cells in response to increased stretch of the myocardium, which occurs with fluid shifts. Treatment of cerebral salt-wasting syndrome includes replacement of fluid losses, sodium replenishment, and administration of fludrocortisone (a synthetic glucocorticoid) to regulate sodium and water reabsorption at the level of the kidney.

Other systemic complications such as myocardial ischemia and infarction, acute left ventricular failure, and acute respiratory distress syndrome (ARDS) may occur secondary to subarachnoid hemorrhage. Patients with SAH require intensive interprofessional, neurological, and general intensive care monitoring in order to optimize functional outcomes.

Connection Check 39.4

A patient is admitted to a unit with a diagnosis of left middle cerebral artery acute ischemic stroke and is not eligible for thrombolytic therapy. The nurse recognizes that this patient is at high risk for which complication?
A. Delirium
B. Aspiration
C. Bronchospasm
D. Palpitations

Connection Check 39.5

The nurse receives a report on a patient in the ICU with an SAH and clarifies that the date of the patient's initial bleed was 4 days before. The nurse needs this information to gauge the patient's risk of which complication of SAH?
A. Hydrocephalus
B. Aspiration
C. Vasospasm
D. Myocardial ischemia

Nursing Management
Assessment and Analysis

Neurological assessment of patients with acute ischemic or hemorrhagic stroke is integral in detecting potentially treatable neurological deterioration rapidly, which allows for the best chance to preserve or restore function. A clear understanding of a patient's baseline neurological status serves as the basis for future assessments and enables the nurse to quickly identify and analyze changes. In patients after hemorrhagic stroke, close monitoring of vital signs, particularly blood pressure, is necessary to prevent rebleeding or expansion of a hematoma. If blood pressure is higher than the prescribed targets, there is the risk of increased ICP and rebleeding, and if the blood pressure is below prescribed targets, there is the risk of cerebral hypoperfusion. Identification of rhythm disturbances, such as atrial fibrillation, ST segment, or T-wave changes associated with myocardial ischemia, is essential in determining potential causes of stroke and intervening in complications of stroke. Close monitoring of serum electrolytes, particularly sodium, is necessary to identify disorders of salt and water imbalance resulting in hyponatremia, which places patients who have suffered a stroke at high risk for cerebral edema and neurological deterioration. Regular assessment of systems enables the nurse to identify potential complications early, track progress, and make appropriate referrals to the interprofessional team, ensuring the best possible outcome for the patient.

> **! Safety Alert** **Blood Pressure Monitoring**
> It is important for the nurse caring for a patient with ischemic or hemorrhagic stroke to closely monitor the patient's blood pressure and ensure that it remains within prescribed limits. When the blood pressure falls below prescribed levels, a reduction in cerebral blood flow may occur, exacerbating ischemia and resulting in a worsening of stroke symptoms. The injured brain is not able to effectively regulate blood flow independently of systemic blood pressure (this usual protective mechanism is called **autoregulation**); therefore, it is important for the nurse to monitor for changes in blood pressure that may require further medical management. Blood pressure values that exceed ordered limits may result in hemorrhage into a region of ischemic or infarcted tissue or place a patient at risk for increased ICP because of an inability of the brain to automatically constrict blood vessels, reducing intracranial blood volume.

Nursing Diagnoses
- **Impaired swallowing** related to lower cranial nerve dysfunction or decreased level of consciousness
- **High risk for impaired gas exchange** related to aspiration
- **Sensory perceptual alterations** related to damage to sensory input areas in the brain and/or integration of sensory inputs
- **Impaired physical mobility** related to hemiparesis

- **Impaired verbal communication** related to decreased perfusion to the speech centers in the brain (Broca's [motor speech] and Wernicke's [sensory speech])
- **Impaired family coping** related to catastrophic illness and uncertain outcome

Nursing Interventions
Assessments

- Serial neurological assessments every 1 to 2 hours
  Changes in level of consciousness are early indicators of increased ICP. Neurological deterioration must be identified quickly in order to mitigate further brain injury. Neurological deterioration during or after IV rt-PA can signal intracranial hemorrhage. When IV rt-PA is administered, neurological assessments, including level of consciousness, motor strength, and pupillary reflexes, are performed every 15 minutes × 6 hours, every 30 minutes × 2 hours, and every 1 hour × 16 hours.
- Vital signs every 1 to 2 hours or more often when administering medications that alter BP. When IV rt-PA is given, the frequency of vital signs is as follows: BP, HR, and RR every 15 minutes × 6 hours, every 30 minutes × 2 hours, and every 1 hour × 16 hours.
  A protective mechanism of the brain, cerebral autoregulation, is dysfunctional after stroke, rendering the brain vulnerable to hypotension because the cerebral blood vessels are not able to automatically dilate, ensuring adequate oxygen delivery to brain tissue. Conversely, high BP can also have negative effects, such as increasing blood volume in the head, resulting in increased ICP. Uncontrolled hypertension after IV rt-PA infusion places a patient at a higher risk for intracranial hemorrhage because of the decrease in fibrinogen caused by rt-PA.
- Neurovascular assessment of the extremity (pulse checks of the dorsalis pedis or posterior tibial artery) used during endovascular therapy must be performed frequently during the first 4 hours after of the procedure.
  Implemented in order to detect arterial clotting due to accessing the artery during the arteriogram
- Puncture site used during the arteriogram is also monitored frequently during the first 4 hours after arterial sheath removal to detect signs of bleeding from the accessed blood vessel.
  The site is assessed for oozing of blood from the puncture site and the presence of a hematoma when palpating the site.
- Electrocardiogram (ECG) and cardiac enzymes
  A possible etiology of ischemic stroke is atrial fibrillation, and continuous electrocardiogram (ECG) monitoring assists in identifying cardiac dysrhythmias. Patients with hemorrhagic stroke, particularly after SAH, may experience myocardial stunning or injury. Trending of 12-lead ECGs and cardiac enzymes allows identification of potential myocardial infarction and/or reversible myocardial stunning.
- Serum electrolytes, particularly sodium
  Hyponatremia is a common complication of ICH, due potentially to SIADH and cerebral salt-wasting syndrome,

which increases the risk for cerebral edema and neurological deterioration.
- Intake and output, cumulative fluid balance
  Accurate accounting of fluid balance is important in evaluating potential sodium and water imbalances as well as approximating volume status, especially in patients with SAH receiving triple-H therapy.

Actions

- Administer rt-PA as ordered.
  Recombinant tissue plasminogen activator (rt-PA) allows a blood clot to be dissolved at the site and restores blood flow to ischemic neuronal tissue. It is administered intravenously for treating acute ischemic stroke and is currently the only treatment approved by the FDA for ischemic stroke. In order to receive IV rt-PA, patients must present within 3 hours of stroke symptom onset. In some defined cases, IV rt-PA may be given up to 4.5 hours after stroke symptom onset.
- Perform bedside swallow screening.
  After a stroke, many patients experience swallowing dysfunction, which places them at risk for aspiration and subsequent pneumonia. The process of swallowing is complex and involves structures in the brainstem, thalamus, and cerebral cortex as well as tongue and facial movements, many of which can be compromised after stroke. Cranial nerves IX, X, XI, and XII, which exit from the medulla in the brainstem, contribute to swallowing and innervate the palate and pharynx, assisting in airway protection. When these cranial nerves have been damaged, aspiration of food or fluid into the lungs can occur.
- Elevate the head of the bed greater than or equal to 30 degrees.
  If a patient is at risk for or is exhibiting clinical manifestations of increased ICP, the head of the bed is elevated to an angle greater than or equal to 30 degrees, and efforts are made to keep the patient's neck in a midline position in order to ensure unobstructed drainage of venous blood from the head, which may decrease ICP.
- Position the head of the bed for patients who have undergone endovascular therapy beginning at 0 to 15 degrees, depending on provider order, and incrementally progressing to 90 degrees before the patient is able to stand.
  Positioning of the head of the bed is important to reduce the incidence of bleeding at the arteriogram access site. The patient is also instructed not to move the affected extremity, typically the leg, for the first 4 to 6 hours after the procedure.
- Place a nasogastric or postpyloric feeding tube for nutrition and medication administration.
  A nasogastric tube or postpyloric feeding tube may be placed to facilitate enteral feeding to allow time for swallowing function to improve or for more formal swallowing evaluation to be completed. A videographical swallowing assessment performed by an SLP is common and enables the practitioner to visualize all phases of the swallowing process to determine the type and extent of swallowing dysfunction that is present. If swallowing dysfunction is thought to be a long-term problem or permanent, a percutaneous endoscopically

placed gastrostomy tube may be placed by a surgeon or gastroenterologist.

- Implement aspiration precautions.
  Specific methods used to prevent aspiration include providing supervision of the patient while eating to observe for clinical manifestations of aspiration or choking, maintaining the head of the bed at least 45 degrees or greater while eating or drinking, reducing distractions to assist a patient in concentrating on eating and drinking, and advocating for evaluation of the patient by an SLP. Some patients require additional measures to prevent aspiration, which are often recommended by an SLP and include tucking the chin when swallowing and thickening liquids with fiber additives. Ensure that patients receive the prescribed therapeutic food preparation, such as a soft or pureed diet. Other members of the healthcare team may be involved in the feeding of patients; therefore, it is critical for the nurse to communicate the appropriate precautions and diet to these team members in order to ensure safety around meals. Patients with dysphagia are typically evaluated by an SLP and may be able to take food and fluid by mouth with a customized plan to prevent aspiration of liquids or solids into the lungs.

- Bleeding precautions are necessary for patients who have received thrombolytics or anticoagulants. Specific precautions include utilizing an electric razor instead of a razor blade for shaving, utilizing a soft toothbrush for oral hygiene, alternating a BP cuff from the left to the right arm to prevent bruising during serial BP measurement, avoiding rectal temperature measurement, and observing strict fall precautions because these patients are at a greater risk for injury related to a fall.
  Patients who have received thrombolytics for acute stroke typically are considered to be at risk for bleeding up to 24 hours after thrombolytic administration because of the inhibition of normal clotting mechanisms (decrease in fibrinogen) caused by rt-PA. Patients receiving anticoagulants are at risk for minor and major bleeding events throughout their course of treatment.

- Provide frequent repositioning, elevate paralyzed or weak limbs to minimize dependent edema, and advocate for evaluation of the patient by OTs and physical therapists (PTs) early.
  Patients with hemiparesis or hemiplegia are at greater risk for the development of pressure injuries because of decreased mobility. Frequent repositioning allows off-loading of pressure from bony prominences (e.g., ankles, heels, ischium, and occiput). Occupational therapists and PTs recommend passive or active range-of-motion regimens and functional splinting, which prevent musculoskeletal and functional complications that can hinder a patient's rehabilitation.

Teaching

- Stroke diagnosis
  Patients and their families should receive information regarding the specific type of stroke and usual course to enable them to become involved in their own care or the care

of their family member. Having specific knowledge of the type of stroke (e.g., hemorrhagic, ischemic) and the causes allows the patient or family to make informed decisions about care and affords them the opportunity to ask further questions.

- Activation of EMS
  Patients and their families should receive information regarding the specific type of stroke and usual course to enable them to become involved in their own care or the care of their family member. Knowledge imparted to patients and families is used as an intervention to increase autonomy and decrease anxiety and stress to the extent that this is possible in this acute circumstance.

- Warning signs and symptoms of stroke
  Knowing the signs and symptoms of stroke may assist a patient or family member in recognizing stroke in his or her own family or in other settings, which improves public health and safety.

- Patient-specific and family risk factors for stroke
  Patients and their families should be aware of the specific risk factors they possess that place them at risk for stroke recurrence. Reviewing family risk factors with other members of the patient's family may help to prevent a first stroke in others. Many risk factors for stroke may be controlled, such as smoking, hypertension, and hypercholesterolemia. Knowledge of the role that these factors play in recurrent stroke may be empowering to patients who must be encouraged to take control of their health in order to prevent recurrent stroke or other conditions such as heart disease.

- Smoking cessation
  Exposure to nicotine due to cigarette smoking causes a decrease in oxygen levels in the blood, which may contribute to blood clot formation and vasoconstriction with each inhalation of smoke. Additionally, nicotine may cause more rapid deposition and accumulation of atherosclerotic plaque. Patients may be more willing to consider smoking cessation after an illness such as stroke.

- Medications for secondary prevention of stroke
  Adherence to medication regimens to reduce BP and hypercholesterolemia and prevent blood clotting is important in instructing patients about their care (Box 39.5). In order to increase adherence to medication regimens, factors such as medication cost and financial resources as well as side-effect profiles should be considered.

Evaluating Care Outcomes

Patients with ischemic and hemorrhagic stroke are highly vulnerable to complications of the disease process, which can be prevented or mitigated by aggressive specialty care targeting the preservation of neurological function. Functional outcomes may not be able to be ascertained in the acute care setting, and preparation of patients for rehabilitation or continued care is necessary to optimize conditions for recovery of function (motor, sensory, and cognitive functions). Implementation, teaching, and reinforcement of secondary stroke prevention measures such as taking

Box 39.5 Medications Prescribed for Secondary Stroke Prevention

Antihypertensives

Used to reduce blood pressure to prevent long-term damage from excessive shear stress and reduce the chance for complications of hypertension, such as intracerebral hemorrhage

- *Beta blockers*
  Metoprolol (Lopressor), labetalol (Trandate)
- *Calcium-channel blockers*
  Diltiazem (Cardizem)
  Amlodipine (Norvasc)
  Verapamil (Calan)
- *Diuretics*
  Hydrochlorothiazide (HCTZ or Aquazide-H)

Lipid-Lowering Medications

Used to reduce the production of cholesterol or the reabsorption of cholesterol, which leads to deposition in blood vessels and eventual blood vessel occlusion

- *Statins*
  Simvastatin (Zocor)
  Pravastatin (Pravachol)
  Atorvastatin (Lipitor)
  Rosuvastatin (Crestor)
- *Niacin*
- *Bile acid sequestrants*
  Ezetimibe (Zetia)

Platelet Inhibitors

Used to prevent platelet aggregation, reducing the risk of blood clot formation, which could cause cerebral blood vessel occlusion

- *Cyclooxygenase inhibitors*
  Acetylsalicylic acid (aspirin)
- *Adenosine diphosphate (ADP) receptor inhibitors*
  Clopidogrel (Plavix)
  Prasugrel (Effient)
- *Combination medications*
  Dipyridamole (Persantine) and aspirin combined into one pill (Aggrenox)

Anticoagulants

Used to prevent clotting in patients with disorders such as atrial fibrillation

- Unfractionated heparin (used as an infusion in the hospitalized patient for short-term anticoagulation)
- Warfarin (Coumadin)
- Dabigatran (Pradaxa)
- Apixaban (Eliquis)
- Rivaroxaban (Xarelto)

antiplatelet therapy and lipid-lowering and antihypertensive medications and follow-up cerebrovascular care after discharge are critical to promoting wellness and preventing stroke recurrence. In addition to rehabilitation services, it is important to consider the psychosocial aspects of the illness affecting patients' position in the family (e.g., main wage earner), their employment, and their need for caregiver support. Evaluation and resources provided by a social worker and case manager are helpful to patients and their families as they transition out of the acute care setting. Nurses caring for patients play a central role in patient outcome along the continuum of stroke care from initial presentation through rehabilitation and discharge to the community.

TRAUMATIC BRAIN INJURY

Epidemiology

Approximately 1.7 million people per year sustain a traumatic brain injury (TBI), with about 52,000 dying from their injury. The human and financial costs of TBI are immense. Many who sustain even a mild head injury suffer long-term effects, such as memory loss and personality changes, that compromise their quality of life. Costs related to TBI are financial and human; many patients are unable to return to previous roles within the family and in their personal and professional lives. The care of a patient with TBI occurs best in environments where seamless continuity and progression of care can occur, from EMS to the ED to the operating room, the critical care unit, acute care unit, rehabilitation unit or facility, and outpatient services. TBI often occurs in conjunction with other systemic injuries that require coordinated, expert management in order to optimize patient outcome. Nurses in acute care, emergency departments, and critical care units play an integral role in anticipatory monitoring of patients and coordinating care for patients with TBI and their families.

Pathophysiology

Types of Head Injury

Traumatic brain injury is classified by the Glasgow Coma Scale (GCS) score into three different categories: mild (GCS 13–15), moderate (GCS 9–12), and severe (≤GCS 8). This disease process is marked by heterogeneity in that there are several possible **mechanisms of injury** (Fig. 39.11), which can cause different injury patterns and damage in the same patient. Concurrent systemic injuries inherent in traumatic events complicate and may exacerbate brain injury. Types of TBI may involve the scalp, skull, meningeal layers, cerebral blood vessels, brain tissue, and neurons (Table 39.11). Often, more than one cranial or cerebral structure is involved in a traumatic injury; for example, a patient may have sustained a frontal contusion as well as a temporal **epidural hematoma**. Traumatic brain injury is further classified into two phases: primary and secondary brain injury. Primary injury occurs with the initial mechanical insult, and secondary injury encompasses all processes that occur subsequent to the initial injury. The role of healthcare providers, from initial encounters with EMS personnel to the ED and critical care units, is to prevent or attenuate the effects of secondary brain injury.

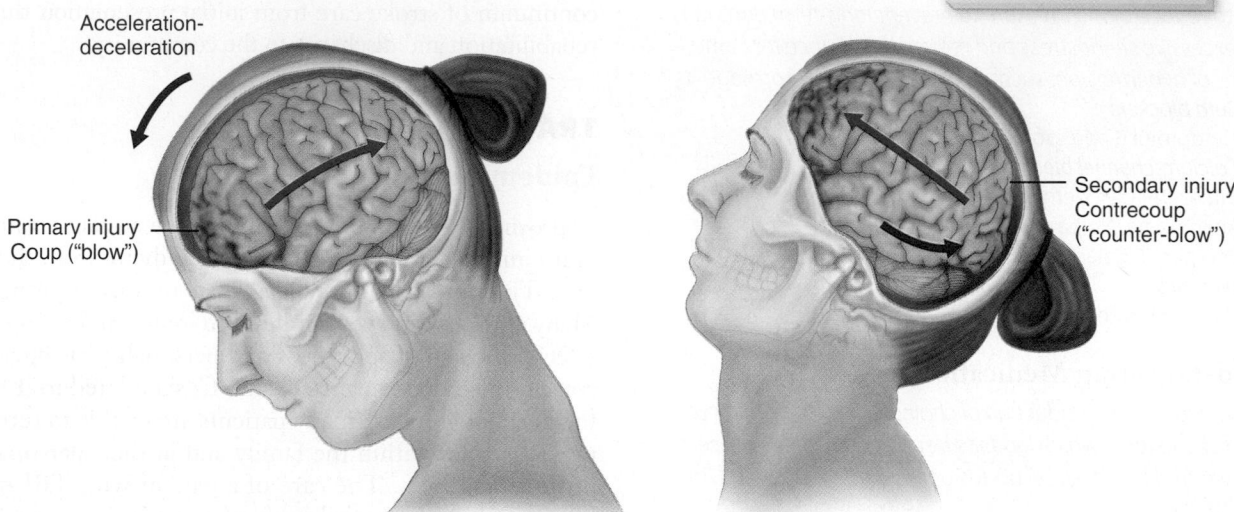

Rotational Forces
- Shearing
- Twisting
- Diffuse axonal injury
- Blood vessel dissection

Contrecoup ("counter-blow")
- Contusion
- Swelling
- Blood clots
- Epidural and subdural hematomas

Acceleration-deceleration

Primary injury Coup ("blow")

Secondary injury Contrecoup ("counter-blow")

FIGURE 39.11 Mechanisms of injury in head trauma. Primary injury occurs with the initial mechanical insult, and secondary injury encompasses all processes that occur subsequent to the initial injury.

Table 39.11 Types of Head Injury

Type of Head Injury	Explanation
Skull fracture	A skull fracture can be linear or displaced. The skull fragments in a displaced fracture can remain in the same plane or can become depressed into the dura or brain tissue. In certain circumstances, these fractures require a surgical procedure to elevate and stabilize the bone (titanium plates and screws may be used). Direct visualization of the dura and underlying structures (e.g., arteries, dural sinuses, brain tissue) is possible in the operating room and is important in identifying additional injury. Fractures occurring at the base of the skull may involve a breach of the dura and subsequent cerebrospinal leak and can damage or impinge cranial nerves and blood vessels that traverse the foramina in the skull base. For example, it is important to evaluate extraocular movements because cranial nerves IV and VI could be damaged if a fracture occurs near the foramen through which they travel.
Penetrating injury	Penetrating injuries occur often as a result of a projectile such as a bullet and can also be caused by a knife or other projectile such as a bomb fragment. Penetrating injuries can cause catastrophic brain injury depending on the location of the injury. In addition to direct tissue damage caused by a bullet or bomb fragment, percussion injury (shock-wave–type force) also causes shearing and stretching injury to neurons, resulting in neuronal injury and death.
Concussion	A concussion is caused by blunt force to the head causing the brain to strike the inside of the skull. Although structural injury does not appear on conventional imaging such as a CT scan, damage has occurred at the cellular level causing an increase in cellular metabolism, resulting in an imbalance between supply of oxygen and glucose and demand because of a decrease in cerebral blood flow. Concussion was once thought to be a relatively benign disorder but has gained recent attention, particularly in athletics, related to the fact that multiple concussions can result in permanent brain injury.
Contusion	A contusion is superficial bleeding that occurs on the surface of the brain (cortex), often at the point of initial impact or "coup" location. Contusions may expand into hematomas and are often associated with cerebral edema. Patients with contusions are often monitored in a setting where they can receive frequent neuro assessments to capture a neurological decline from development of cerebral edema or an expanding hematoma.

Table 39.11 Types of Head Injury—cont'd

Type of Head Injury	Explanation
Epidural hematoma	An epidural hematoma is often caused by damage to an artery traveling in grooves on the inside of the skull when the skull is impacted or fractured. This blood collects in the space between the inside of the skull and the dura, pushing the dura farther away from the skull. Because the dura is tethered to the inside of the skull at the suture lines, the collection of blood is confined in width and expands inward toward the brain, displacing structures laterally and having a convex appearance. When an epidural hematoma is caused by an artery, the speed and force of the blood collection has a rapid effect on ICP and can cause neurological deterioration and coma very quickly. This type of injury typically requires emergency neurosurgery to evacuate the hematoma and decompress the brain structures displaced by the epidural hematoma.
Subdural hematoma	A subdural hematoma is typically caused by damage to a vein or network of veins called *bridging veins*. When the brain moves within the dural covering, small bridging veins that span the inside of the dura to the surface of the brain can be stretched or disrupted, causing bleeding. Blood collects between the inside of the dura and the cortex of the brain and is not confined, so the blood is able to collect in a larger space around the brain. The speed with which the blood collects and the amount are related to the vascular structure that was injured. For example, if a small area of bridging veins is disrupted, blood will begin to collect around the brain but may take some time to cause neurological clinical manifestations. If a larger area of bridging veins or a large venous sinus or an artery is damaged, blood may accumulate more quickly and may cause signs of increased ICP more quickly. There are three types of subdural hematomas: acute subdural hematoma where symptoms occur within minutes to 24 hours after injury; subacute subdural hematoma where symptoms occur within 2 weeks of injury, and chronic subdural where symptoms occur from 2 weeks to months or years after injury. Subacute subdural hematomas are more common in older adults and in patients with a history of alcohol abuse because of cerebral atrophy placing gradual stretch forces on the bridging veins coupled with a high risk of falling. Surgical intervention for subdural hematomas is primarily dependent on the patient's initial neurological status. If neurological status is poor (severe focal neurological deficits or coma), surgery may be performed emergently; however, patients with a mild neurological deficit or absence of neurological deficits may be monitored for neurological worsening and undergo surgery later if necessary.
Intraparenchymal hematoma *Subarachnoid hemorrhage*	An intraparenchymal hematoma is a focal area of bleeding in the brain tissue usually below the cortex. Surgical intervention is typically not performed for this injury because the procedure could cause additional injury, and the blood typically breaks down and is reabsorbed over time. These hematomas are associated with cerebral edema.
Diffuse axonal injury	Diffuse axonal injury (DAI) is caused by rotational and acceleration-deceleration forces and results in direct injury to the axon. Swelling and microscopic hemorrhages can occur. Often, this type of injury occurs deep within the white matter in the area of the reticular activating system, which controls wakefulness. In severe DAI, where many neurons have been injured, patients may not regain consciousness. Treatment for this type of injury does not currently exist. A DAI caused by neuronal injury can be visualized on MRI but may not be visible before 24 hours after injury.

CT, Computed tomography; *ICP,* intracranial pressure; *MRI,* magnetic resonance imaging.

Treatment paradigms, algorithms, and protocols are aimed at preventing or aggressively managing hypotension and hypoxemia in the immediate period after injury because these factors are implicated in increased mortality of patients with severe TBI. The global reduction in cerebral blood flow in the immediate period after TBI associated with cerebral autoregulatory dysfunction places the injured brain at great risk for ischemic injury, as well as injury from biochemical processes accelerated by inflammation.

Injuries to the scalp are of varying severity involving one or more layers of skin and, in some cases, underlying blood vessels. The scalp is a vascular structure, and injuries are typically associated with significant bleeding. Injuries to the scalp warrant careful inspection and palpation for irregularities signifying skull fractures and consideration of concomitant brain injury.

Skull Fractures

The natural function of the skull is to absorb and disperse blunt forces. Skull fractures are separated into two categories, open and closed. An open skull fracture is associated with a disruption of the scalp such that the skull is exposed to the atmosphere. A closed skull fracture may be palpated through the scalp or visualized on x-ray or other radiographical imaging. Skull fractures are further classified as nondisplaced, displaced, or comminuted. Nondisplaced skull fractures must be visualized using radiographical imaging and rarely involve disruption of the meninges because the edges of the fracture are approximated and have not moved from their original position. If a skull fracture is displaced, the edges of the fractured bone are no longer approximated and can be displaced or depressed downward toward the brain; fragments from a comminuted fracture may also be present. The edges of fractured bone or individual bone fragments are often sharp and irregular and can tear the dura mater covering the brain, underlying blood vessels, and venous sinuses, and in some circumstances, these sharp edges can violate the meninges, directly injuring brain tissue. If the dura is damaged, CSF begins to leak, placing a patient at risk for infection and herniation syndrome as intracranial contents shift with the loss of CSF. If a CSF leak is persistent, a catheter may be inserted into the lumbar spine similar to the lumbar puncture procedure; however, the catheter is introduced through the dura and left in place to drain CSF. This catheter is attached to an external CSF drain and is referred to as a lumbar drain. If vascular structures, such as jugular veins and carotid arteries, which traverse the base of the skull through openings called *foramina* and occupy bony ridges on the inside of the skull (middle meningeal artery), are damaged, life-threatening hemorrhage can result (see the following text for descriptions of hematomas).

Fractures of the base of the skull are called **basilar skull fractures** and involve the bony structures at the level of the midface. The major bones in this area are the sphenoid bone, sella turcica (protects the pituitary gland), and inferior portions of the frontal and temporal bones. The hallmark sign of a basilar skull fracture (Fig. 39.12), when the dura has been breached, is the visualization of fluid from the ear (fracture in the middle fossa) or nose (fracture in the anterior fossa). A late sign of a basilar fracture is bruising around the eyes (raccoon's eyes) or the ears (**Battle's sign**; Fig. 39.13). Many blood vessels and cranial nerves traverse the bony structures of the skull base and are vulnerable to injury depending on the location and size of a basilar skull fracture. For instance, the carotid arteries travel through foramina in the sphenoid bone and may be injured, causing clinical manifestations of stroke if a fracture has occurred in that area of the skull base and the carotid artery has been disrupted. Cranial nerves that control the movement of the eyes may also become entrapped or damaged.

Hematomas

An **epidural hematoma** occurs when blood collects in the potential space between the skull and the dura mater (Fig. 39.14). The dura is the tough covering of the brain that covers the brain and spinal cord and is connected to the inside surface of the skull in the suture lines, forming potential compartments or spaces. Potential spaces are collapsed until filled with matter (i.e., fluid or air). When an epidural hematoma occurs, blood fills a particular epidural space or compartment and begins to compress or displace brain tissue inward, causing a concave appearance on radiographical imaging. One of the more common etiologies of an epidural hematoma is an arterial bleed caused by a temporal bone fracture, resulting in disruption of the middle meningeal artery. An epidural hemorrhage is most often caused by an arterial bleed but may also be caused by a venous injury. When an artery is damaged, the flow of blood is very rapid and is under pressure; therefore, the speed with which blood collects and the potential amount can cause a rapid increase in ICP and herniation of brain tissue laterally and then downward if this bleeding is not stopped. An epidural hematoma is a neurosurgical emergency requiring prompt evacuation of the blood clot and repair to the damaged blood vessels. The clinical presentation of an epidural hematoma varies from a comatose state on initial presentation to a lucid (aware of surroundings) state, depending on the size and location of the hematoma as well as the rate and volume of blood collection in the epidural space. Patients with epidural hematomas may initially lose consciousness, regain consciousness and appear lucid, and then very rapidly deteriorate to unresponsiveness with signs of cerebral herniation syndrome. This phased

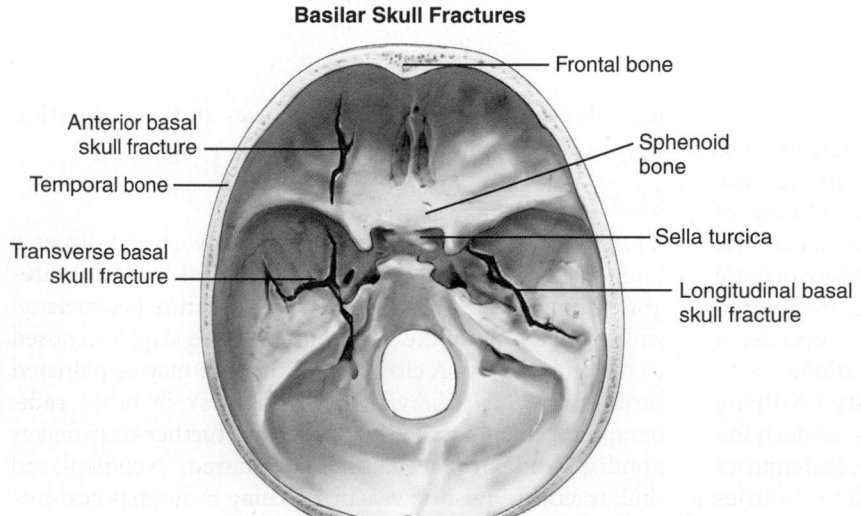

Basilar Skull Fractures

Frontal bone

Anterior basal skull fracture

Temporal bone

Transverse basal skull fracture

Sphenoid bone

Sella turcica

Longitudinal basal skull fracture

FIGURE 39.12 Basilar skull fractures.

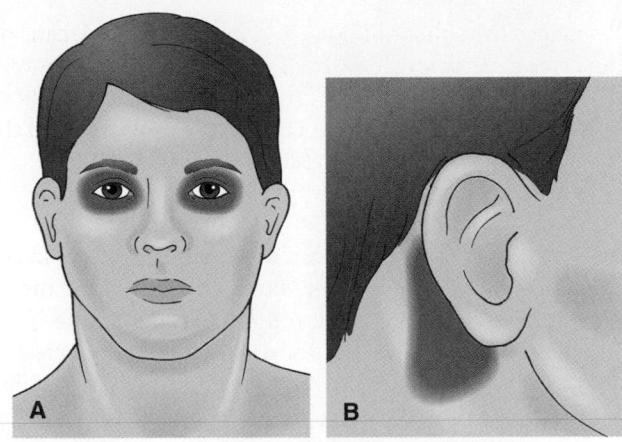

FIGURE 39.13 Late signs of a basilar fracture. *A*, Raccoon's eyes. *B*, Battle's sign.

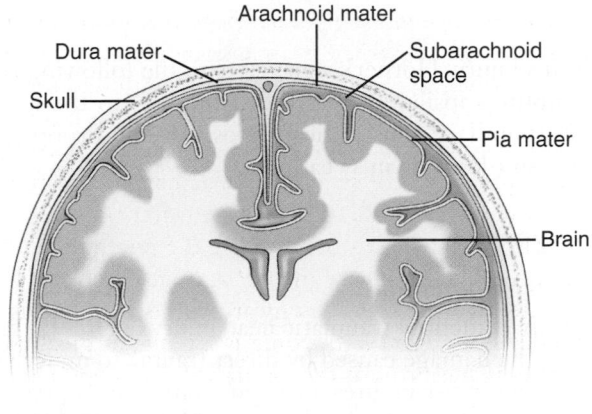

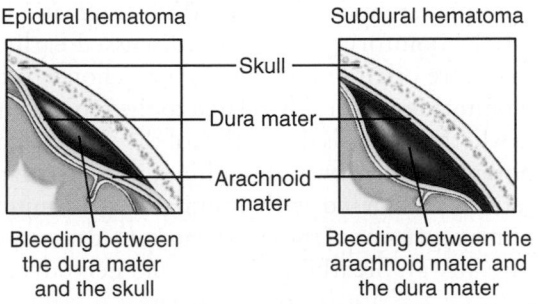

FIGURE 39.14 Hematomas. In an epidural hematoma, blood collects between the skull and dura mater. In a subdural hematoma, blood collects between the arachnoid mater and dura mater.

presentation occurring in a proportion of patients with an epidural hematoma is referred to as the "talk and die phenomenon." Because of the typically rapid accumulation of blood in the epidural space and the tendency for the fluid collection to expand inwardly, compressing brain tissue, this injury is a neurological emergency for which immediate surgical evacuation of the hematoma is the only option.

A **subdural hematoma** refers to a collection of blood beneath the dura and above the arachnoid layer, which is most often caused by venous bleeding but can involve arterial disruption (see Fig. 39.14). The brain is connected to the inner surface of the dura by a network of veins called *bridging veins*. When the head is impacted by a blunt force,

the brain moves within the skull and dural covering. When the brain moves within the dural covering, tension is placed on the bridging veins, causing stretching and tearing and releasing a steady flow of blood around the brain in the subdural space, increasing ICP. Neurosurgical intervention for a subdural hematoma often depends on the clinical stability of the patient and the state of the neurological examination. For instance, if the patient is easily arousable, alert and oriented, and without focal motor deficits, surgical intervention may be deferred while the patient's neurological status is closely monitored.

Contusion

A **cerebral contusion** is a bruise on the surface of the brain that has the potential to transform into a hematoma and is associated with the development of significant cerebral edema. Patients with a cerebral contusion require serial neurological assessments with a high degree of suspicion for neurological deterioration. Neurological assessment is the best means by which to identify increased ICP due to bleeding of the hematoma or cerebral edema and facilitates rapid evaluation and medical intervention, which may be lifesaving.

Neuronal Injury

An increasing body of knowledge exists surrounding neuronal injury during head trauma, which is not easily visualized with the usual radiographical tests such as CT or MRI because the problem is at the cellular level and involves a hypermetabolic state where energy is rapidly consumed and an energy crisis is created, causing cellular injury and death. Magnetic resonance imaging spectroscopy and positron emission tomography (PET) are helping researchers characterize the neuronal responses to head injury across the spectrum of severity from mild to severe. During acceleration, deceleration, or rotational forces, the brain moves within the skull and meninges. **Diffuse axonal injury (DAI)** describes direct injury to neurons due to shearing and rotational forces (Fig. 39.15). The severity of the DAI depends on the location and extent of neuronal injury. For example, if networks of neurons in the area of the reticular activating system are injured, a patient may not have the ability to awaken. Diffuse axonal injury may also be associated with sympathetic dysregulation, also termed **sympathetic storming**, which presents with episodic tachycardia, tachypnea, and hyperthermia and may be accompanied by spontaneous motor posturing (flexor or extensor).

Vascular Injury

Traumatic subarachnoid hemorrhage (SAH) is the most common cause of SAH and is associated with a poor prognosis in patients with TBI. Traumatic SAH is typically focal in location as opposed to aneurysmal SAH, which is more often characterized by diffuse layering of blood in the arachnoid layer (Fig. 39.16). This type of injury occurs as a result of disruption to veins and arteries traversing the arachnoid layer. Local vasospasm may occur as a result of this type of injury, although the local nature of the bleeding

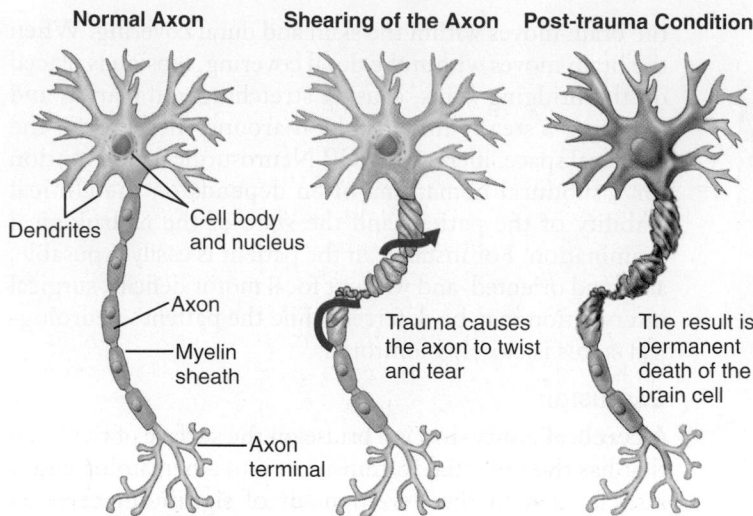

Normal Axon   **Shearing of the Axon**   **Post-trauma Condition**

Dendrites

Cell body
and nucleus

Axon

Myelin
sheath

Axon
terminal

Trauma causes
the axon to twist
and tear

The result is
permanent
death of the
brain cell

FIGURE 39.15 Diffuse axonal injury. Diffuse axonal injury (DAI) is direct injury to neurons due to shearing and rotational forces.

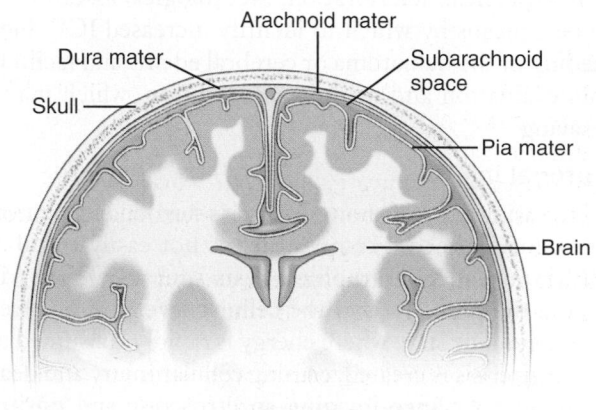

Arachnoid mater

Dura mater

Subarachnoid
space

Skull

Pia mater

Brain

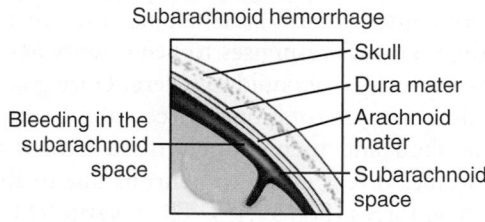

Subarachnoid hemorrhage

Bleeding in the
subarachnoid
space

Skull

Dura mater

Arachnoid
mater

Subarachnoid
space

FIGURE 39.16 Traumatic subarachnoid hemorrhage (SAH). Traumatic SAH is typically focal in location and occurs as a result of disruption to veins and arteries traversing the arachnoid layer.

separates it from the typical course experienced by patients with aneurysmal SAH.

Arterial dissection may occur during head or neck trauma. The extracranial portions of the carotid and vertebral arteries located in the neck are vulnerable to mechanical injury. Arterial dissection is characterized by a disruption or tear to one or more of the blood vessel layers. Disruption of the intima, the innermost layer, can result in clot formation that can occlude the inner lumen of the blood vessel. An intimal tear can also produce a flap of tissue that can occlude an artery, causing an ischemic stroke. Arterial dissection may present with sudden focal neurological changes corresponding to the vascular territory of the involved vessel. Neck pain and the presence of **Horner's sign** are also associated

with this injury. Horner's sign refers to the following triad of symptoms ipsilateral (on the same side) to the injury: miosis (pupillary constriction), ptosis (eyelid droop), and anhidrosis (decrease in sweating).

Management

Medical Management

The management of traumatic head injury focuses on minimizing the damage caused by direct trauma to underlying brain tissue and structures, managing intracranial pressure, and promoting cerebral perfusion. With traumatic head injuries, ICP-monitoring measures (discussed earlier in this chapter) are often implemented. The choice of type of ICP monitoring is typically related to the type of injury as well as whether there is disruption of the skull. Because of the potential for airway, breathing, and circulatory complications associated with traumatic head injuries, emergent management of these patients includes ensuring an effective airway, breathing pattern, and hemodynamic stability.

Diagnosis

Computed tomography of the head is an initial diagnostic test performed in patients with traumatic head injury. Transcranial Doppler studies may also be used to indirectly measure cerebral blood flow and are often used to determine cerebral blood cessation in severe head injuries. Laboratory analysis includes baseline serum electrolytes, complete blood cell count, and coagulation studies. The serum sodium and osmolality are particularly important in the event that hyperosmolar agents are used to decrease ICP.

Treatment

Specific interventions to manage increased ICP include proper positioning as well as the administration of hyperosmolar agents to decrease fluid in the brain (see Increased ICP section earlier in this chapter). Uncontrolled increased ICP ultimately leads to herniation syndrome (see Table 39.1).

Treatment of herniation syndrome is often referred to as a "brain code" due to the rapid nature of resuscitation and the resources required for resuscitation that mirror those of cardiac arrest. Herniation syndrome is treated with the same interventions as increased ICP acutely to decrease ICP and relieve the pressure causing displacement of brain tissue within the skull or through the foramen magnum at the bottom of the cranium.

Surgical Management

Depending on the type of traumatic head injury, various surgical procedures are indicated. With skull fractures, there is a need to debride and clean the wound area as well as to remove any bone fragments that may be at the area of impact. Patients with skull fractures are at risk for infections of the central nervous system, including meningitis and encephalitis (discussed in Chapter 36).

A craniotomy may be indicated in patients with hemorrhagic injuries and typically involves opening of the skull and removal of blood accumulations. Both epidural and subdural hematomas are surgically evacuated to decrease ICP. Surgery is not indicated in patients with diffuse axonal injuries because there is no specific area of blood removal. After surgery, the patients are managed in the ICU, with management of ICP as the priority.

Complications

Patients with TBI may develop complications such as increased ICP, herniation syndromes (discussed earlier in this chapter), meningitis (discussed in Chapter 36) especially with open fractures and dural tears, seizure activity, diabetes insipidus, and syndrome of inappropriate antidiuretic hormone (SIADH). When swelling in the brain places pressure directly on the posterior portion of the pituitary gland or on blood vessels supplying this area, disorders of sodium and water balance can occur. Antidiuretic hormone (ADH) is secreted from the posterior portion of the pituitary gland. Diabetes insipidus occurs in the absence of ADH where urinary output increases rapidly, causing a loss of free water and severe dehydration manifesting as hypernatremia and low urine specific gravity (<1.005). Diabetes insipidus is treated by replacing fluid losses and ADH with an exogenous form, either intravenously, subcutaneously, or intranasally.

SIADH occurs when an excessive amount of ADH is secreted from the posterior pituitary. Traumatic brain injury is associated with disruption of the hypothalamic–pituitary axis, and one possible consequence of this disruption can be SIADH. In contrast to DI, SIADH results in the retention of free water, causing hyponatremia (dilutional) and a normal to low urinary output. The mainstay of treatment for SIADH is restricting the intake of free water; typical restrictions are 1,000 to 2,000 mL per day. Reducing the intake of free water allows urinary output to exceed the amount of free water retained, and serum sodium returns to the normal range. (Both DI and SIADH are discussed in more detail in Chapter 41.)

Nursing Management

Assessment and Analysis

Monitoring for clinical manifestations of increased ICP as well as ensuring effective cerebral perfusion are the priority assessments in the patient after traumatic head injury. It is imperative that the nurse be vigilant to subtle changes in level of consciousness, which may be complicated with the use of medications to induce a barbiturate coma to decrease cerebral metabolism. Vital sign assessments are also important because an effective blood pressure is necessary to facilitate cerebral perfusion in the patient with increased ICP. Serial neurological examinations, including the Glasgow Coma Scale, are aspects of these patients' plans of care. When repeated neurological assessments are performed, a neurological change, such as a change in level of consciousness, subtle motor weakness, or cranial nerve deficit, may be identified early enough to intervene, preventing further damage to the brain.

Nursing Diagnoses

- **Ineffective airway clearance** related to decreased level of consciousness and inability to protect the airway
- **Ineffective cerebral tissue perfusion** related to increased ICP, cerebral edema, hemorrhage, impaired autoregulation, and hyperventilation
- **Risk for impaired thermoregulation** related to damaged temperature-regulating mechanisms in the brain
- **Risk for impaired skin integrity** related to bedrest, hemiparesis, hemiplegia, immobility, decreased level of consciousness, or restlessness
- **Impaired family coping** related to sudden life-threatening illness and uncertain outcome

Nursing Interventions

Assessments

- Serial neurological assessments every 1 to 2 hours in the acute phase of injury
  It is necessary to continually assess the patient with a TBI against an established baseline for signs of increased ICP as well as to monitor for cerebral edema, expansion of a hematoma, or conversion of a contusion to a hematoma.
- ECG and cardiac biomarkers
  Patients with severe TBI may demonstrate ECG findings suspicious for myocardial ischemia and injury due to an initial surge of catecholamines during the sympathetic nervous system response upon initial injury. The release of catecholamines during the initial injury usually results in reversible injury to the myocardium, also referred to as myocardial stunning.
- Vital signs
  Although changes in vital signs are a late sign of increased ICP, it is necessary to trend BP, HR, RR, and temperature as additional pieces of data in analyzing a patient's overall condition. An effective BP is particularly important with increased ICP in order to maintain a therapeutic CPP.

A temperature elevation may be seen with infection (meningitis) or secondary to the area of the brain that controls thermoregulation.

- Seizure activity

  Patients with TBI above the tentorium (supratentorial) and closer to the cerebral cortex are at risk for seizure activity because cellular dysfunction and tissue injury from ischemia may cause a disruption in electrical impulse conduction in the brain, causing disorganized electrical activity, which is a seizure. (Care of patients with seizures is discussed in Chapter 36.)

Actions

- Positioning head of bed greater than 30 degrees with the patient's head in midline, and avoiding sharp hip flexion

  Patients are positioned in the midline with the head of the bed elevated to facilitate drainage of venous blood from the head, decreasing ICP.

- Management of CSF leak: If clear fluid is draining from the ear or nose, it should not be stopped; it should be collected using loosely applied gauze.

  It is important to identify a leakage of CSF because this indicates a breach in the dura and places patients at risk for infection (meningitis or encephalitis). A lumbar drain is placed when a CSF leak is persistent in order to facilitate healing of the dural tear because it reduces pressure on the injured tissue. Drainage may also be tested for glucose in some instances.

- Avoid nasogastric tube placement in patients with a known basilar skull fracture or in patients where the base of the skull has not been visualized on radiographical injury.

  In patients with a basilar skull fracture, placement of a nasogastric tube may cause further disruption of a fracture and places the patient at risk for the tube to invade the cranium. Orogastric tube placement is an alternative.

- Initiate enteral nutrition.

  Current guidelines suggest starting enteral nutrition within the first 72 hours of injury in order to reach an adequate goal rate by 7 days. Patients with severe TBI demonstrate a hypercatabolic state where the body utilizes substrates at a rapid pace, causing utilization and depletion of fat and protein stores. Bedside indirect calorimetry may be helpful in establishing a patient's resting metabolic rate and true caloric needs to optimize his or her nutritional regimen. Indirect calorimetry is performed at the bedside by a respiratory therapist or other credentialed clinician.

- Maintain normothermic temperature (antipyretics and cooling devices as ordered).

  Normal temperature should be achieved and maintained in order to prevent an increase in cerebral oxygen and energy demands, which can worsen metabolic dysfunction in neurons.

- Implement seizure precautions.

  Precautions for seizure activity, particularly generalized tonic-clonic seizure activity, include having suction readily available to clear the airway after a seizure. Common medications to be given during a seizure are benzodiazepines (lorazepam [Ativan]) to stop the seizure activity; antiepileptic medications such as fosphenytoin (Cerebyx), levetiracetam (Keppra), or phenytoin (Dilantin) are administered to prevent further seizures.

- Ensure venous thromboembolism (VTE) prophylaxis with sequential compression devices, graduated compression stockings, and subcutaneous injections of an anticoagulant as prescribed.

  Patients with severe TBI are at an increased risk for VTE and subsequent pulmonary embolus because of tissue or endothelial damage occurring with the traumatic event, immobility, and hypercoagulability caused by the systemic inflammatory response that is activated after a traumatic event (these three factors are known as Virchow's triad).

Teaching

- Specific teaching regarding the patient's injury, coma, and increased ICP

  Families of patients with severe TBI benefit from succinct information regarding the patient's specific type of brain injury and anticipated course. Specific information about a patient's specific type of head injury may empower patients or family members to ask further questions or to take a greater part in their own or their family member's healthcare.

- Orientation to the patient's ICU room and monitoring equipment

  Families should be aware of the purpose of different pieces of monitoring equipment, such as ICP monitors, cardiac monitors, and the ventilator, in order to decrease anxiety and attempt to make them comfortable in the room so that they can accomplish their caregiving role for the patient to the greatest extent possible.

Connection Check 39.6

The family of a patient who sustained a left temporoparietal subdural hematoma and bilateral frontal contusions is visiting the patient for the first time and is asking repeatedly when the patient will awaken. What is the best method for the nurse to use for beginning education with this family?

A. Providing a detailed diagram of the brain and pointing out the functions of each lobe in order to create a foundation from which the family can understand the patient's injury

B. Providing a handout printed from the Internet on severe TBI

C. Assessing the family's level of knowledge and information about the patient's brain injury and providing general information regarding the uncertainty of the outcome in the first several days after TBI

D. Deferring any sharing of information until a formal family conference is held with the medical care team

Evaluating Care Outcomes

Patients with severe TBI have varied responses to brain injury, and treatment depends on the location and severity of the brain injury, comorbid factors, and preexisting health status, as well as the onset of complications. In order to mitigate secondary brain injury and preserve neurological function, the nurse provides anticipatory monitoring of the neurological status and vigilant assessment for potential complications. Educating, supporting, and linking the patient's family with available resources is an essential role of the nurse in promoting family coping.

NEUROGENIC SHOCK

Pathophysiology and Clinical Manifestations

Neurogenic shock, a type of distributive shock causing vasodilation and relative hypovolemia, threatens underlying acute conditions due to hypoperfusion if it is not recognized and treated rapidly. A disruption in sympathetic nervous system stimulation causes an inability of vascular smooth muscle to constrict, resulting in decreased blood return to the heart and decreased cardiac output. Sympathetic nervous system interruption, with unopposed parasympathetic nervous system action, may result in transient, profound bradycardia in some patients. Neurogenic shock occurs as a result of conditions such as spinal cord injury (above the T6 level), stroke in the brainstem, high doses of barbiturates, and anesthesia techniques, both general and regional. In spinal cord injury, neurogenic shock is caused by a disruption of cardiac sympathetic fibers (vasomotor fibers) that exit the spinal cord at the T1 to T6 levels. Disruption of these fibers causes hypotension, bradycardia, and peripheral vasodilation below the level of injury. Additionally, these vasomotor fibers typically oppose the parasympathetic nervous system, preventing sustained bradycardia; however, in this case, the parasympathetic nervous system is unopposed, producing profound bradycardia. When neurogenic shock is caused by general anesthesia or stroke in the brainstem, symptoms of neurogenic shock (hypotension, bradycardia, and peripheral vasodilation) arise from the vasomotor center in the brainstem.

In the absence of pathology causing dysfunction in the sympathetic nervous system, vascular smooth muscle is able to readily constrict, altering the caliber of systemic blood vessels in response to position or systemic volume changes. Vascular tone in neurogenic shock is significantly decreased without the ability to constrict, rendering a patient vulnerable to systemic hypoperfusion. Patients with neurogenic shock typically have warm and dry skin due to systemic vasodilation. Hypovolemia in neurogenic shock is characterized as relative because of the fact that the size of the systemic vasculature has rapidly expanded without a concurrent increase in volume to fill that expanded space. The effects of hypoperfusion in distributive shock are anaerobic metabolism and resultant lactate accumulation, resulting in acidosis, myocardial ischemia, and cerebral hypoperfusion. The clinical presentation includes profound bradycardia, hypotension, changes in level of consciousness, and metabolic acidosis.

Management

Medical Management

The management of neurogenic shock is focused on correcting the primary etiology when possible and treating cardiovascular effects such as hypotension and bradycardia. Intensive cardiovascular support, including fluid resuscitation (boluses of crystalloid to increase stretch of the myocardial fibers in the atria, resulting in an increase in the strength of ventricular contraction and increased cardiac output), vasoactive infusions (e.g., norepinephrine [Levophed], epinephrine [adrenaline], phenylephrine [Neo-Synephrine]), atropine to block vagal (parasympathetic) stimulation, and transcutaneous or transvenous pacing capabilities to treat sustained symptomatic bradycardia, is necessary to prevent systemic complications of shock. If the primary condition cannot be improved, continued cardiovascular support is necessary to maintain adequate systemic perfusion.

Loss of vascular tone is treated with vasoactive agents that have an effect on alpha receptors, such as phenylephrine, norepinephrine, epinephrine, and dopamine (at doses >10 mcg/kg/min). Concurrent fluid resuscitation is undertaken to restore vascular volume and improve systemic perfusion. Episodic bradycardia is treated with parasympatholytic medications such as atropine. Transcutaneous and then transvenous pacing may be utilized to treat repeated episodes of profound bradycardia. Serum lactate levels and arterial blood gases may be utilized to monitor acidosis and judge the effectiveness of resuscitation strategies.

Ongoing treatment of decreased vascular tone may include oral sympathomimetics such as midodrine (Amatine, ProAmatine), which affects the alpha-1 receptors (alpha-1 receptors control vasoconstriction of vascular smooth muscle), causing constriction of the peripheral vasculature. After administration of midodrine, the nurse should see a rise in blood pressure because this medication affects only alpha-1 receptors, and effects on heart rate should not be seen. Vigilant nursing monitoring and care coupled with medical interventions are necessary to prevent multisystem organ failure in neurogenic shock.

Complications

The complication of neurogenic shock is continued systemic hypoperfusion leading to multisystem organ failure. Hypoperfusion in patients with neurogenic shock occurs as a result of massive systemic vasodilation causing a reduction in cardiac output and blood pressure. Bradycardia may also occur, further compromising blood flow to vital tissues and organs because of the disruption of sympathetic outflow, which also contributes to decreased cardiac output and blood pressure.

Nursing Management
Assessment and Analysis

Patients with neurogenic shock require intensive cardiovascular monitoring in order to detect bradycardia, dysrhythmias, and hypotension that result from a disruption in sympathetic innervations. Rapid medical interventions, including administration of atropine, transcutaneous or transvenous pacing, fluid resuscitation, and administration of vasoactive medications, may be employed in the care of a patient with neurogenic shock. Ongoing assessments for patients in neurogenic shock may include monitoring cardiac output, intravascular volume, and other hemodynamic parameters. Mechanical ventilation may also be required in patients with neurogenic shock depending on the underlying cause. Management of common complications such as deep venous thrombosis, pulmonary embolus, and skin breakdown is essential in optimizing outcomes in this patient population.

Nursing Diagnoses

- **Impaired tissue perfusion** related to hypotension, bradycardia, and peripheral vasodilation
- **Risk for fluid volume deficit** due to relative hypovolemia that occurs with loss of vasomotor tone and maldistribution of volume in the vascular space
- **Anticipatory grieving** related to sudden loss of function and accompanying critical illness

Nursing Interventions
■ Assessments

- Vital signs every 1 to 2 hours or more frequently if vasoactive infusions (e.g., norepinephrine [Levophed], phenylephrine [Neo-Synephrine]) are being administered
  Frequent monitoring of vital signs allows for rapid identification of cardiovascular deterioration, such as hypotension or an episode of bradycardia, that may require further intervention, such as titration of vasoactive medications, use of a pacemaker, or administration of atropine (to increase HR).
- Hemodynamic parameters such as central venous pressure (CVP), pulmonary artery occlusion pressure (PAOP), cardiac output/cardiac index (CO/CI), stroke volume (SV), and systemic vascular resistance (SVR) may be measured every 2 to 4 hours or after treatments such as a bolus of IV fluid to evaluate patient response.
  Hemodynamic parameters are measured in order to evaluate a patient's response to medical therapies. For example, the CVP or PAOP is evaluated in order to determine whether an adequate vascular volume or preload has been reestablished. The cardiac output (CO) or cardiac index (CI), which is cardiac output divided by body surface area, is evaluated to determine the overall condition of the vascular system, and systemic vascular resistance is used to quantify the degree of vasoconstriction or vasodilation in the vascular system (see Chapter 32 for further discussion of hemodynamic monitoring).

- Intake and output every 1 to 2 hours.
  Accurate measurement of input and output plays a role in determining whether fluid balance is in excess or if a patient requires additional fluid.
- Physical assessment at least every 4 hours
  Comprehensive physical assessment is integral in detecting multisystem complications that may arise in patients with neurogenic shock, such as ARDS, pneumonia, paralytic ileus, and skin breakdown.

■ Actions

- Raise the head of bed slowly (10–15 degrees per hour) in a systematic manner.
  Because of loss of systemic vasomotor tone, raising the head of the patient's bed may cause orthostatic hypotension because of an inability of the peripheral blood vessels to constrict upon position change. Orthostatic hypotension in this circumstance may cause hemodynamic instability (e.g., lowered BP and cardiac output).
- Assist with the insertion of an arterial line for continuous BP monitoring.
  An arterial line enables continuous monitoring of BP and the ability to set alarm parameters so that hypotension is identified immediately. Frequent blood sampling for ABGs and other laboratory tests is facilitated by the presence of an arterial line.
- Assist with the insertion of a pulmonary artery catheter in situations where cardiovascular dysfunction is severe.
  A pulmonary artery catheter allows for frequent monitoring of preload (measured as CVP and PAOP), afterload (measured as SVR), and contractility (to some extent with cardiac output and stroke volume and right and left stroke work indices) in order to optimize medical therapies on the basis of patient response.
- Administer IV fluids and IV sympathomimetic agents (e.g., phenylephrine [Neo-Synephrine], norepinephrine [Levophed]).
  Fluid resuscitation is undertaken in order to increase vascular volume, which is inadequate compared to the increase in the size of the vascular space due to vasodilation. Administration of sympathomimetics aids in increasing vasomotor tone, which is reflected as an increase in systemic vascular resistance. These strategies used in combination ideally raise cardiac output and restore adequate tissue perfusion.
- Administer atropine.
  Medications such as atropine inhibit the action of the vagal nerve, causing the HR to increase, and treat symptomatic bradycardia.
- Prepare for transcutaneous pacing if a patient does not have transvenous pacing wires in place.
  A temporary pacemaker may be required to manage bradycardia in patients with neurogenic shock because of sympathetic nervous system dysfunction. In some cases where dysfunction of the sympathetic nervous system is irreversible, a permanent pacemaker may be required.
- Implement VTE prophylaxis.
  Patients in neurogenic shock are at high risk for VTE, particularly in cases where the etiology of neurogenic shock

is spinal cord injury. *Pharmacological methods or mechanical devices (e.g., sequential compression devices, pneumatic foot pumps) may be used alone or in combination depending on patient-specific factors.*

■ Teaching

- Explain the specific cause of neurogenic shock and anticipated impact on the patient's immediate and future hospital course.
  There are several causes of neurogenic shock with specific associated implications and factors that impact a patient's overall condition. For instance, in spinal cord injury, neurogenic shock may last for weeks to months or longer, requiring long-term medication management and, in some cases, an implanted pacemaker, whereas a patient in neurogenic shock due to general anesthesia has resolution of clinical manifestations when anesthetics are metabolized.

- Explain the reason for medication therapy.
  Explaining therapeutic measures such as medications that are administered may provide a patient and his or her family a greater sense of control over a traumatic circumstance, where most control is perceived to be exercised by the healthcare team.

- Explain supportive therapies.
  Understanding the rationale behind other supportive therapies may give patients and their families needed information to make necessary decisions regarding care as well as a sense of control in decision making.

Evaluating Care Outcomes

Intensive monitoring of a patient's response to interventions is necessary to establish and maintain adequate tissue perfusion, initially compromised because of systemic hypoperfusion in neurogenic shock. Continuous evaluation of BP, HR, RR, and hemodynamic parameters measuring preload, such as CVP and PAOP, provides valuable information on the effectiveness of interventions. In addition to these physiological parameters, evaluation of mentation can be a sensitive indicator of the adequacy of resuscitation. In patients with a spinal cord injury, an often-irreversible cause of neurogenic shock, decreased vascular tone may be managed with a long-term regimen of oral sympathomimetics and vigilant surveillance of hemodynamic response to different activities, such as transitioning from a lying to a sitting position and transferring from bed to wheelchair. Symptomatic bradycardia may be managed with an implanted pacemaker. See Chapter 37 for a full discussion of spinal cord injury.

Making Connections

CASE STUDY: WRAP-UP

Mr. Stewart is diagnosed with a right middle cerebral artery stroke and carotid stenosis of the right carotid artery (approximately 85% occluded) due to atherosclerosis. Mr. Stewart makes steady progress after evaluations by physical and occupational therapies as well as speech-language pathology. As a strategy to prevent him from experiencing another stroke, he is scheduled for a carotid endarterectomy, a surgical procedure that removes atherosclerotic plaque that has caused extreme narrowing of a blood vessel and stroke. After the carotid endarterectomy, Mr. Stewart is discharged to an acute inpatient rehabilitation facility, where he makes steady progress in regaining the use of his left leg and continues to progress in regaining some function of his left arm.

Case Study Questions

1. The nurse recognizes which findings in Mr. Stewart as modifiable risk factors for stroke? *(Select all that apply.)*
   A. 58 years old
   B. History of hypertension
   C. History of high cholesterol
   D. Male
   E. Tobacco use

2. Which diagnostic study is indicated in Mr. Stewart to evaluate cardiac function and assess for a cardioembolic source of his stroke?
   A. CT scan
   B. ECG
   C. MRI
   D. Ultrasound

3. What is a contraindication to the administration of rt-PA in a patient with suspected ischemic stroke?
   A. Patient who awakens from 6 hours of sleep with symptoms of stroke
   B. Neurological impairment based on the NIHSS
   C. Platelet count of 200,000 mm³
   D. Onset of symptoms 2½ hours before presenting to ED

4. The nurse is monitoring Mr. Stewart after he receives rt-PA. Which clinical manifestation indicates an adverse effect of rt-PA?
   A. Decreasing level of consciousness
   B. Hyperglycemia
   C. Gastroparesis
   D. Productive cough

5. The nurse includes which information in the teaching plan for Mr. Stewart and his family about the management of acute ischemic stroke? *(Select all that apply.)*
   A. Stroke risk factors
   B. Need for annual CT scan
   C. Prevention of aspiration
   D. Prevention of deep vein thrombosis
   E. Importance of BP control

CHAPTER SUMMARY

Care of the critically ill patient with neurological illness focuses on preventing deterioration and, in cases where it cannot be prevented, mitigating the effects of neurological deterioration through rapid identification of complications and aggressive medical interventions. Increased ICP is a common complication of neurological illness such as ischemic and hemorrhagic stroke, central nervous system infection, brain tumors, and intracranial surgery. Decreased level of consciousness is the most sensitive and early indicator of increased intracranial pressure (ICP). When a patient is monitored for increased ICP, the reason for a change in the patient's neurological assessment may not be obvious, but initial treatment and evaluation strategies for increased ICP are the same regardless of the cause. Initial measures such as ensuring a patent airway with adequate oxygenation and ventilation, elevating the head of the bed, administration of osmotic diuretics (if indicated), and preparing the patient for radiographical imaging should be accomplished in rapid sequence.

Patients with ischemic and hemorrhagic stroke require close surveillance of vital signs, particularly BP, to prevent worsening of ischemia or further bleeding depending on the patient's specific stroke diagnosis. Patients who experience a stroke are vulnerable to complications such as aspiration because their ability to swallow after any type of stroke is often impaired. Systematic screening for swallowing dysfunction, appropriate referral to a speech-language pathologist, and implementation of a patient-specific plan for avoiding aspiration help to decrease this morbidity in patients after a stroke. A major complication of subarachnoid hemorrhage is cerebral vasospasm, which occurs most often between days 4 and 14 after the initial hemorrhage, with the peak risk period at 5 to 9 days after initial bleeding. Anticipatory monitoring for clinical manifestations of vasospasm enables timely implementation of a plan of care aimed at preventing cerebral infarction.

Developing and implementing a teaching plan specific to a patient's type of stroke, cerebrovascular risk factors, medications, access to emergency care, and need for continued follow-up care is essential in caring for this population of patients. It is important to take into consideration the patient's or family's learning needs and reported preferences for this important teaching. When teaching specific psychomotor skills for self-administration of medication or other treatments, it is important to include demonstration and return-demonstration activities so that the nurse can be sure that a patient or family member is able to translate verbal or written information into performance of the required activity. During initial encounters with patients and family members, it is important to consider their apparent emotional state as well as their need for information about the event or condition. Assessing the level of knowledge about the situation serves as a foundation to choose specific topics and methods for providing information and education to patients and families.

Traumatic brain injury (TBI) is classified by the Glasgow Coma Scale (GCS) as mild (GCS 13–15), moderate (GCS 9–12), or severe (≤GCS 8). Traumatic injuries to the brain include skull fractures, epidural hematomas, subdural hematomas, contusions, traumatic subarachnoid hemorrhage, and diffuse axonal injuries. Management of these injuries focuses on the management of increased intracranial pressure, maintaining optimal hemodynamic status through the administration of IV fluids and vasoactive medications, and minimizing complications. Recovery from TBI is often a long process, requiring close surveillance of patients and support and teaching for both the patient and families.

Neurogenic shock is caused by several different etiologies, the most well-known of which is spinal cord injury, and is caused when sympathetic innervation is disrupted, resulting in loss of vasomotor tone and possibly bradycardia. Nursing care of the patient with neurogenic shock involves monitoring of the patient's responses to therapies and anticipation of complications that require further intervention to restore hemodynamic stability and maintain patient safety. The nurse should be able to anticipate general medical interventions that may be ordered in the case of deterioration, such as fluid therapy, medications (atropine for bradycardia and vasoactive medications for decreased BP or cardiac output), and cardiac pacing.

Vigilant, skilled, anticipatory monitoring by the nurse caring for critically ill patients with a neurological injury makes a significant impact in preventing complications and restoring or preserving neurological function. These patients allow the nurse to utilize a broad range of nursing skills, such as assessment, teaching, interpersonal, psychomotor, and emergency skills.

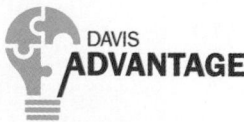

DAVIS
ADVANTAGE
To explore learning resources for this chapter, go to **Davis Advantage** and find:
- Answers to in-text questions
- Chapter Resources and Activities
- NCLEX®-Style Chapter Review Questions
- Bibliography

Unit IX

Promoting Health in Patients With Endocrine Disorders

Chapter 40

Assessment of Endocrine Function

Janice Hoffman

Finding Connections

CASE STUDY: EPISODE 1

Follow this patient throughout the chapter.

Greta Johnson is a 27-year-old female who has been experiencing insomnia, restlessness, and irritability the past several months. Because these symptoms are interfering with her ability to complete her work as a graduate research assistant at a local community college, she presents today to her nurse practitioner for a complete physical. During the initial interview, Greta describes that sometimes she feels as if her "heart is racing" and has noticed palpitations. She has also noted an 8-pound weight loss over the last month despite an increased appetite and food intake ...

INTRODUCTION

The endocrine system includes glands found in various locations in the body and works in conjunction with the nervous system in coordinating many life-sustaining functions associated with metabolism, growth and development, blood glucose control, and sexual functioning.

Endocrine glands include the hypothalamus, pituitary gland, adrenal glands, thyroid glands, parathyroid glands, gonads, and select cells of the pancreas (islet cells) (Fig. 40.1). These glands secrete **hormones** that are chemical messengers that act on specific **target tissues**, resulting in physiological functions. Underproduction and overproduction of selected hormones are the leading causes of endocrine dysfunction. Table 40.1 lists the major endocrine glands and their associated hormones.

Hormones from the endocrine glands are secreted directly into the blood system, compared with hormones secreted from **exocrine** glands that are released through ducts. Exocrine glands include lacrimal, salivary, and sweat glands and the part of the pancreas that secretes pancreatic juices that are released in the small intestine. The function of the endocrine system is directly associated with secretion and levels of circulating hormones, and disorders are classified as primary, secondary, tertiary, and quaternary. Primary disorders involve actual dysfunction of the endocrine gland, secondary disorders refer to dysfunction of the anterior pituitary gland, tertiary disorders refer to dysfunction of the hypothalamus, and quaternary disorders refer to the inability of the target tissue to respond to the hormone.

OVERVIEW OF ANATOMY AND PHYSIOLOGY

The function of the endocrine system is closely linked to the nervous system and is commonly referred to as

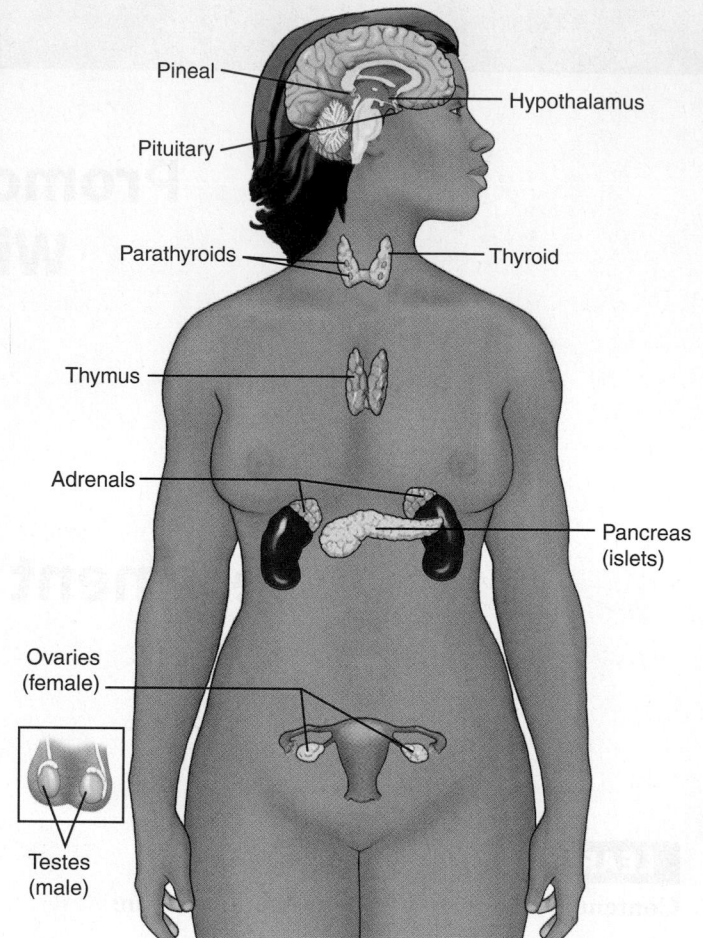

FIGURE 40.1 Major glands of the endocrine system.

neuroendocrine regulation. Both the hypothalamus and pituitary gland play an active role in endocrine function. The secretion of hormones is regulated via signals from the nervous system, levels of hormones in the blood, and other chemical changes in the blood such as glucose, sodium, and potassium levels. Hormonal release is controlled by a **negative feedback system** that increases hormone secretion when circulating levels are decreased. For example, the hypothalamus releases thyrotropin-releasing hormone (TRH) when there are decreased levels of the thyroid hormones; **triiodothyronine** (T3) and **thyroxine** (T4)—circulating in the bloodstream. In turn, the TRH acts on its target gland, the anterior pituitary gland, and thyroid-stimulating hormone (TSH) is released. The target gland for TSH is the thyroid gland, which releases the T3 and T4. While levels of circulating T3 and T4 increase, the feedback to the hypothalamus is to decrease secretion of TRH. Most disorders of the endocrine glands develop secondary to changes in hormone secretion associated with primary disorders (changes in an endocrine gland), secondary disorders (changes in the anterior pituitary gland), or tertiary disorders (changes in the hypothalamus). For example, patients who develop pituitary tumors or sustain injury

Table 40.1 Glands of the Endocrine System

Gland	Hormone	Target	Action
Hypothalamus	Corticotropin-releasing hormone	Anterior pituitary gland	Increases release of adrenocorticotropic hormone
	Gonadotropin-releasing hormone (GnRH)	Anterior pituitary gland	Increases release of follicle-stimulating hormone (FSH) and luteinizing hormone (LH)
	Growth hormone-releasing hormone (GHRH)	Anterior pituitary gland	Stimulates release of growth hormone (GH)
	Growth hormone-inhibiting hormone (somatostatin; GHIH)	Anterior pituitary gland	Inhibits release of GH
	Thyrotropin-releasing hormone (TRH)	Anterior pituitary gland	Stimulates release of thyroid-stimulating hormone (TSH)
	Prolactin-inhibiting hormone	Anterior pituitary gland	Inhibits release of prolactin
Anterior pituitary	Adrenocorticotropic hormone (ACTH)	Adrenal glands	Increases secretion of glucocorticoids and mineralocorticoids
	Follicle-stimulating hormone (FSH)	Ovaries in females	Stimulates maturation of ovarian follicles, ovulation, and estrogen secretion
		Testes in males	Stimulates sperm production
	LH	Ovaries in females	Stimulates secretion of estrogen and progesterone and ovulation
		Testes in males	Stimulates testosterone production
	GH	Tissues and bones	Facilitates growth of bones and tissues through protein synthesis, fat metabolism, and insulin antagonism
	TSH	Thyroid glands	Increases secretion of thyroid hormones (triiodothyronine [T3] and thyroxine [T4])
	Prolactin	Mammary glands	Stimulates production of breast milk
	Melanocyte-stimulating hormone	Melanocytes (melanin-producing cells in the skin and hair)	Increases pigmentation (skin and hair color)
Posterior pituitary	Vasopressin (antidiuretic hormone; ADH)	Distal tubules and collecting ducts in the kidney	Increases water reabsorption
	Oxytocin	Uterus and mammary glands	Stimulates uterine contractions in labor and milk ejection
Adrenal cortex	Glucocorticoids (cortisol)	Liver	Promotes gluconeogenesis (increasing blood glucose)
		Cells of the body	Decreases glucose use
			Promotes protein catabolism
			Promotes fat synthesis
		Bone marrow	Suppresses inflammatory processes
	Mineralocorticoids (aldosterone)	Distal tubules and collecting ducts in the kidney	Promotes sodium reabsorption and potassium excretion by the kidney
Adrenal medulla	Catecholamines (epinephrine and norepinephrine)	Cells of the body	Mimics actions of the sympathetic system

Continued

Table 40.1   Glands of the Endocrine System—cont'd

Gland	Hormone	Target	Action
Thyroid gland	Triiodothyronine (T3)	Cells of the body	Increases metabolic rate
	Thyroxine (T4)		Increases response to catecholamines
	Thyrocalcitonin (calcitonin)	Bones	Decreases osteoclastic (breakdown of bone) activity
		Kidneys	Decreases reabsorption of calcium in the renal tubules
		Intestines	Decreases reabsorption of calcium in the intestines
Parathyroid gland	Parathyroid hormone (PTH)	Bones	Increases osteoclastic (bone breakdown) activity
		Kidney	Increases renal tubule reabsorption of calcium
		Intestines	Increases gastrointestinal reabsorption of calcium (vitamin D required)
Ovaries	Estrogen	Female reproductive organs (primarily controlled by FSH)	Stimulates development of female sex organs and secondary sex characteristics (pubic hair, axillary hair, etc.). In pregnancy, it enhances enlargement of uterus and breasts.
	Progesterone	Female reproductive organs (primarily controlled by LH)	Promotes growth of uterine wall, maintains pregnancy with fertilization, and influences menstruation with no fertilization.
			Stimulates growth of mammary glands.
Testes	Testosterone	Male reproductive organs	Promotes maturation of male sex organs, sperm production, and development of secondary sex characteristics (beard growth, deep voice)
Pancreas	Insulin	Cells of the body	Lowers blood glucose levels by moving glucose into cells
	Glucagon	Liver	Promotes glycogenolysis (increased blood glucose levels by conversion of glycogen to glucose)
		Muscles	Promotes gluconeogenesis (increased blood glucose levels by conversion of amino acids to glucose)

to the pituitary gland secondary to trauma may develop alterations in endocrine function.

Connection Check 40.1

The nurse correlates an increase in the secretion of which hormone with the release of thyrotropin-releasing hormone?
A. Triiodothyronine (T3)
B. Thyroxine
C. Thyroid stimulating hormone (TSH)
D. Thyrocalcitonin

In addition to levels of circulating hormones, the release of hormones is also influenced by intrinsic factors. For example, as part of the stress response, **cortisol** secretion is increased to assist the body in dealing with stresses such as trauma, infection, and disease. Additionally, when patients are prescribed certain medications, such as **corticosteroids** for inflammation, these exogenous agents impact the function of the negative feedback system. Because there are increased circulating levels of corticosteroid, the hypothalamus decreases secretion of corticotropin-releasing hormone. This in turn leads to decreased secretion of adrenocorticotropic hormone

(ACTH) from the anterior pituitary gland, which results in decreased secretion of cortisol from the adrenal cortex. These coordinated activities between the nervous system and endocrine glands assist in maintaining homeostasis.

> **⚠ Safety Alert** Patients who are prescribed cortico-steroids for more than 10 to 14 days require "tapering" of the medication. Because of the effects of the exogenous corticosteroid on the hypothalamus, anterior pituitary, and adrenal cortex, the normal hormonal feedback system is interrupted. Abrupt withdrawal of the exogenous drug may lead to adrenal insufficiency (presented in Chapter 42), which is a medical emergency characterized by decreased blood pressure and hypoglycemia.

Hypothalamus and Pituitary Gland

The hypothalamus and pituitary gland play key roles in the feedback system that regulates homeostasis, and this regulation is commonly referred to as the *hypothalamic-pituitary system* or *complex*. The hypothalamus is a small structure located beneath the thalamus (Fig. 40.2). It is shaped like a flattened funnel and forms the walls and floor of the third ventricle. Hormones produced and secreted by the hypothalamus act directly on other endocrine glands (including the pituitary gland) and are described in Table 40.1. The hypothalamus is connected to the pituitary gland by the **infundibulum**.

Connection Check 40.2

Which hormones are released from the posterior pituitary gland? *(Select all that apply)*.

A. Aldosterone
B. Antidiuretic hormone
C. Follicle-stimulating hormone
D. Luteinizing hormone
E. Oxytocin

The pituitary gland is located at the base of the brain in the sella turcica, which is a depression of the sphenoid bone. Approximately the size of a lima bean, the pituitary gland is approximately 1-3 cm wide and communicates directly with the hypothalamus. The pituitary gland is composed of two lobes, the anterior lobe (adenohypophysis) and the posterior lobe (neurohypophysis), which have distinct functions (Fig. 40.3). The hypothalamus regulates anterior pituitary gland function through the secretion of hormones whose target tissue is the anterior pituitary gland (see Table 40.1).

The anterior pituitary gland secretes two gonadotropins (hormones that stimulate the gonads), follicle-stimulating hormone (FSH) and luteinizing hormone (LH) that have major roles in female and male reproductive functions. Thyroid-stimulating hormone works directly on the thyroid glands located in the anterior neck and is also released from the anterior pituitary gland and stimulates release of thyroid hormones. Adrenal cortical function is also regulated by the release of adrenocorticotropic hormone (ACTH) that stimulates release of **glucocorticoids** and

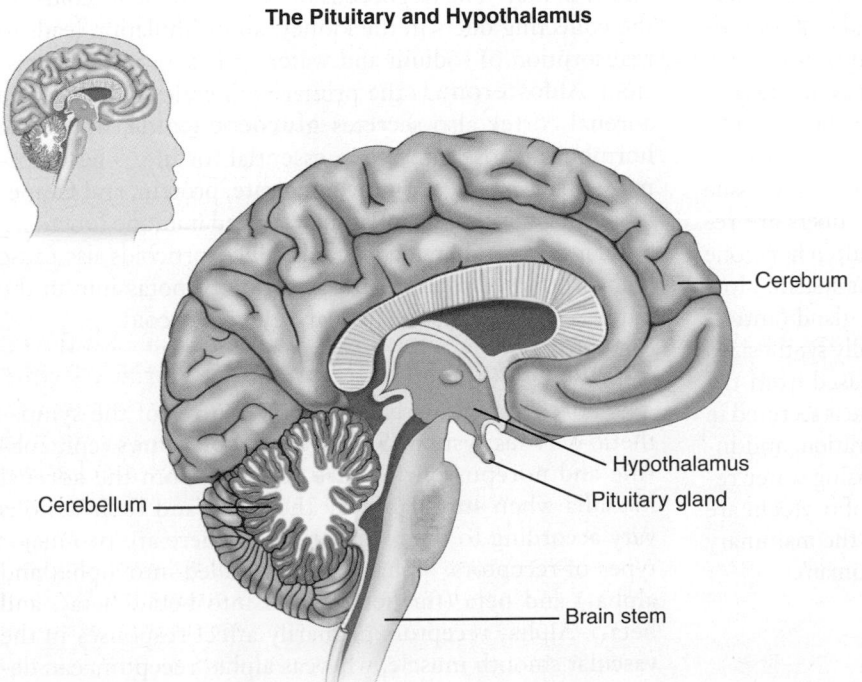

The Pituitary and Hypothalamus

- Cerebrum
- Hypothalamus
- Pituitary gland
- Cerebellum
- Brain stem

FIGURE 40.2 Location of the pituitary gland and hypothalamus.

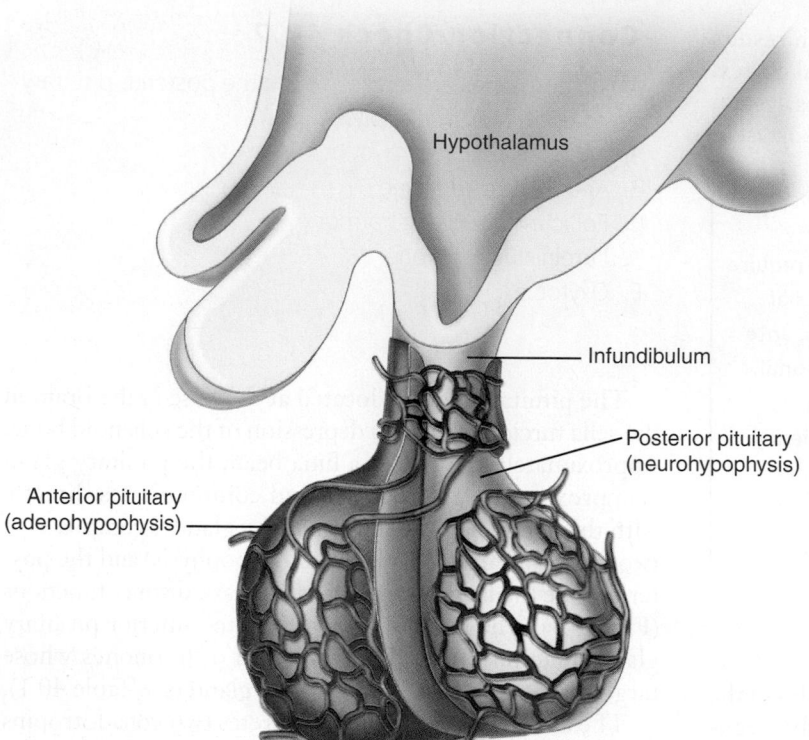

FIGURE 40.3 Anterior and posterior lobes of the pituitary gland.

mineralocorticoids from the adrenal cortex. Prolactin, growth hormone (GH), and **melanocyte-stimulating hormone** are also secreted from the anterior pituitary gland. Prolactin is responsible for milk formation. Growth hormone, also called **somatotropin**, is necessary for maintaining bone density and cartilage growth as well as facilitating protein synthesis. It also increases the use of fatty acids and affects blood glucose levels by decreasing the use of glucose for energy. Growth hormone has an insulin-resistance effect in the peripheral tissue that inhibits the uptake of glucose by muscle and adipose tissue. Melanocyte-stimulating hormone affects skin and hair color. **Melanocytes** are cells of the epidermis that give color to skin through the synthesis of melanin (pigment granules that influence skin color).

The posterior pituitary gland is composed of nerve tissue that arises in the hypothalamus. These nerve fibers are responsible for neuroendocrine reflexes that result in hormone secretion in response to signals from the nervous system. Hormones secreted from the posterior pituitary gland (antidiuretic hormone [ADH] and oxytocin) are actually synthesized in the hypothalamus but are stored and released from the posterior pituitary gland. Antidiuretic hormone is secreted in response to decreased blood pressure, dehydration, and increased serum osmolality and works by increasing water reabsorption in the kidneys. The target tissues of oxytocin are the uterus (causing contractions in labor) and the mammary glands (causing milk release in the lactating woman).

Adrenal Glands

The adrenal glands are located on top of each kidney, and each measures approximately 5-cm long, 1-cm thick, and 3-cm wide (Fig. 40.4). Each adrenal gland has an inner core, the medulla, and a thick outer covering, the cortex, both with distinct endocrine functions (Fig. 40.5).

Adrenal Cortex

The adrenal cortex comprises approximately 90% of the adrenal gland and secretes three types of hormones. The **mineralocorticoids** control fluid balance through their effects on the kidney. The target cells of the mineralocorticoids are the collecting ducts in the kidney, and stimulation leads to reabsorption of sodium and water and excretion of potassium. **Aldosterone** is the primary mineralocorticoid. The adrenal cortex also secretes **glucocorticoids**, which are hormones whose effects are essential for life. These hormones have an effect on carbohydrate, protein, and fat metabolism and suppress inflammatory and immune functions. Similar to the mineralocorticoids, glucocorticoids also cause reabsorption of sodium and excretion of potassium in the kidneys. **Cortisol** is the primary glucocorticoid.

Adrenal Medulla

The adrenal medulla is under the control of the sympathetic nervous system (SNS). **Catecholamines** (epinephrine and norepinephrine) are secreted from the adrenal medulla when stimulated by the SNS, and their actions vary according to the receptor sites. There are two major types of receptors, alpha (further divided into alpha$_1$ and alpha$_2$) and beta (further divided into beta$_1$, beta$_2$, and beta$_3$). Alpha$_1$ receptors primarily affect responses in the vascular smooth muscle, whereas alpha$_2$ receptors can decrease release of norepinephrine and influence blood pressure. Beta$_1$ receptors are located primarily in the heart, and

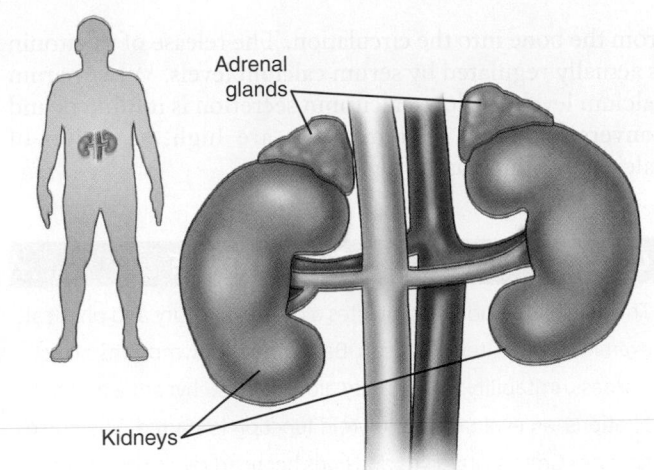

FIGURE 40.4 Location of the adrenal glands.

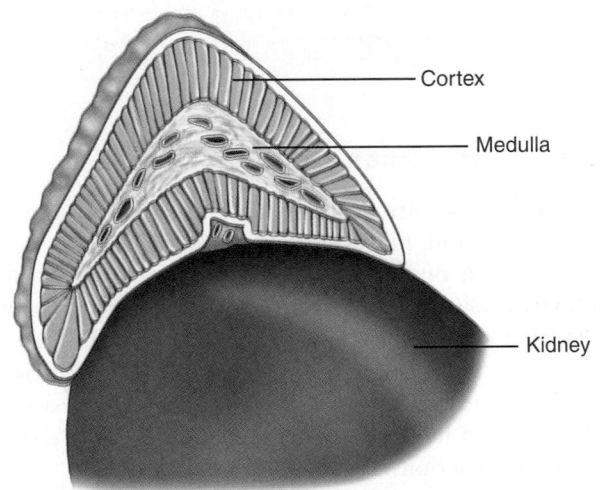

FIGURE 40.5 Adrenal medulla and cortex.

Table 40.2 Catecholamine Effects on Target Tissues

Target Tissue	Receptor	Effects
Lungs	Beta₂	Dilates bronchioles
Heart	Beta₁	Affects chronotropic (rate) activity
		Affects inotropic (contractility) activity
Blood vessels	Alpha	Promotes vasoconstriction
	Beta₂	Promotes vasodilation
Kidneys	Beta₂	Increases renin release
Gastrointestinal (GI) tract	Alpha	Increases sphincter tone
	Beta	Decreases GI motility
Bladder	Alpha	Promotes sphincter contraction
	Beta₂	Relaxes detrusor muscles
Skin	Alpha	Increases sweating
Liver	Alpha	Increases gluconeogenesis and glycogenolysis
Pancreas	Alpha	Decreases release of glucagon and insulin
		Increases release of glucagon and insulin
Eyes	Alpha	Promotes pupil dilation

beta₂ receptors are located in the bronchioles and other sites such as the kidneys. Beta₃ receptors are found primarily in adipose tissue and, when stimulated, enhance **thermogenesis** (heat production). Target tissues for the catecholamines include various types of cells and specific organs of the body; the effects of these hormones are described in Table 40.2. Because epinephrine and norepinephrine are also produced by the SNS, the adrenal medulla and its secretion of these hormones are not essential to life. However, hypersecreting tumors of the adrenal medulla (**pheochromocytomas**), are life threatening and are discussed further in Chapter 42.

Connection Check 40.3

Increased secretion of ADH results in which action?

A. Decreased urine output
B. Increased urine output
C. Decreased serum potassium
D. Increased serum potassium

Thyroid Gland

Located in the anterior neck, the thyroid gland lies directly below the cricoid cartilage (Fig. 40.6). Composed of two lobes, it is connected by a strip of tissue called the *isthmus*. The thyroid gland produces three thyroid hormones, triiodothyronine (T3), thyroxine (T4), and **thyrocalcitonin (calcitonin)**. Production of these hormones requires adequate dietary intake of protein and iodine. Release of T3 and T4 is controlled by the hypothalamic-pituitary system and is based on the circulating levels of these thyroid hormones. When T3 and T4 levels are low, the hypothalamus secretes TRH that stimulates the release of TSH from the anterior pituitary gland. In turn, TSH acts on the thyroid gland, leading to secretion of T3 and T4. While the circulating levels of T3 and T4 increase, the feedback system causes the hypothalamus to decrease release of TRH. Other conditions that increase secretion of TRH, independent of circulating T3 and T4, are cold and stress. The end result is an increase in metabolic activity with both conditions.

Although both T3 and T4 share the same functions, they differ in structure and potency. Most of the circulating T3 and T4 is plasma protein bound. However, it is the free unbound thyroid hormone that is active. For this reason, it is important to assess plasma protein levels (albumin) when assessing

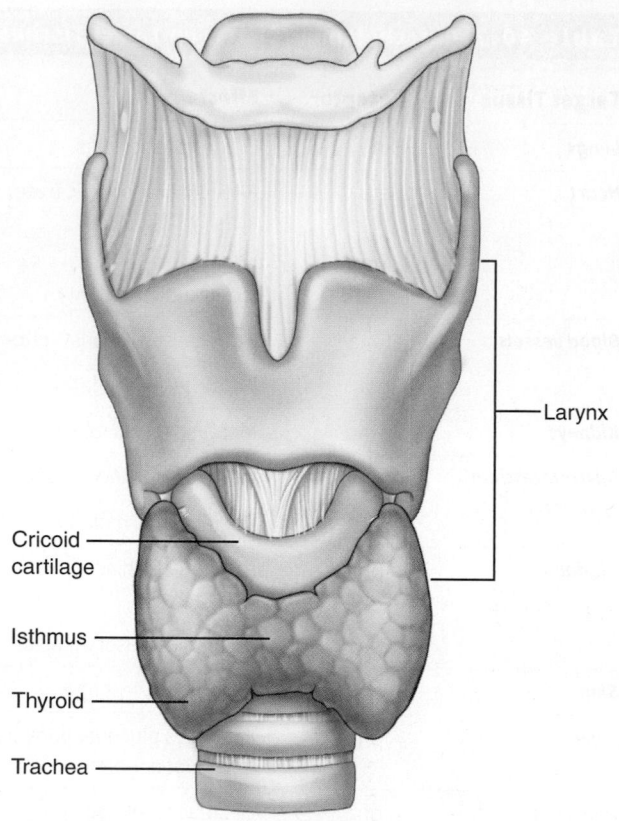

Larynx

Cricoid cartilage

Isthmus

Thyroid

Trachea

Anterior view

FIGURE 40.6 Location of the thyroid gland.

thyroid function, because an increase in free thyroid hormone may occur in the patient with hypoalbuminemia.

Regulation of metabolic activity is controlled by T3 and T4, and secretion of both hormones increases metabolism. Specific actions of T3 and T4 include:

- Increased rate and contractility of the heart
- Increased rate and depth of respirations
- Increased oxygen use
- Increased glucose intake by cells
- Increased glycolysis and enhanced gluconeogenesis
- Increased protein synthesis and catabolism
- Increased mobilization of fatty acids
- Increased oxidation of free fatty acids
- Decreased cholesterol and phospholipids

This overall increase in metabolic activity results in increased heat production in all tissues. The clinical manifestations of thyroid disorder are directly associated with these physiological changes.

Thyrocalcitonin (calcitonin) has a role in the regulation of calcium, along with parathyroid hormone (PTH; **parathormone**) secreted from the PTH glands. Serum calcium and phosphorus levels are lowered by the actions of calcitonin on the bones. Bone **resorption** is a process involving breakdown of bone through **osteoclastic** activity that involves secretion of enzymes and acid that dissolve microscopic bits of bone matrix. Because osteoclastic activity is decreased by calcitonin, there is less calcium released

from the bone into the circulation. The release of calcitonin is actually regulated by serum calcium levels. When serum calcium levels are low, calcitonin secretion is inhibited; and conversely, when calcium levels are high, secretion of calcitonin is increased (Fig. 40.7).

Parathyroid Glands

The PTH glands are usually found partially embedded in the thyroid gland; however, they may also be found above the hyoid bone or near the aortic arch (Fig. 40.8). Measuring approximately 3 to 8 mm in length and 2 to 5 mm in width, they secrete parathyroid hormone (PTH). Secreted in response to low serum calcium levels, the target tissues of PTH include the bones, kidneys, and small intestine.

Parathyroid hormone increases serum calcium through the following actions:

- Increases bone resorption through osteoclastic activity
- Stimulates renal reabsorption of calcium
- Stimulates activation of vitamin D, which increases intestinal reabsorption of calcium.

The action of PTH is opposite to that of calcitonin, secreted by the thyroid gland, because calcitonin decreases serum calcium levels.

Parathyroid hormone also affects phosphorus levels through the following actions:

- Reduces the reabsorption of phosphate from the proximal tubes in the kidneys, leading to a decrease in serum phosphorus levels
- Increases bone resorption, leading to an increase in phosphorus release from the bone
- Increases small intestine absorption of phosphate

The net result of these actions is to lower serum phosphate levels, particularly due to phosphorus loss through the kidneys.

Gonads

Sexual development and function are controlled by hormones secreted from the ovaries and testes. Both the ovaries

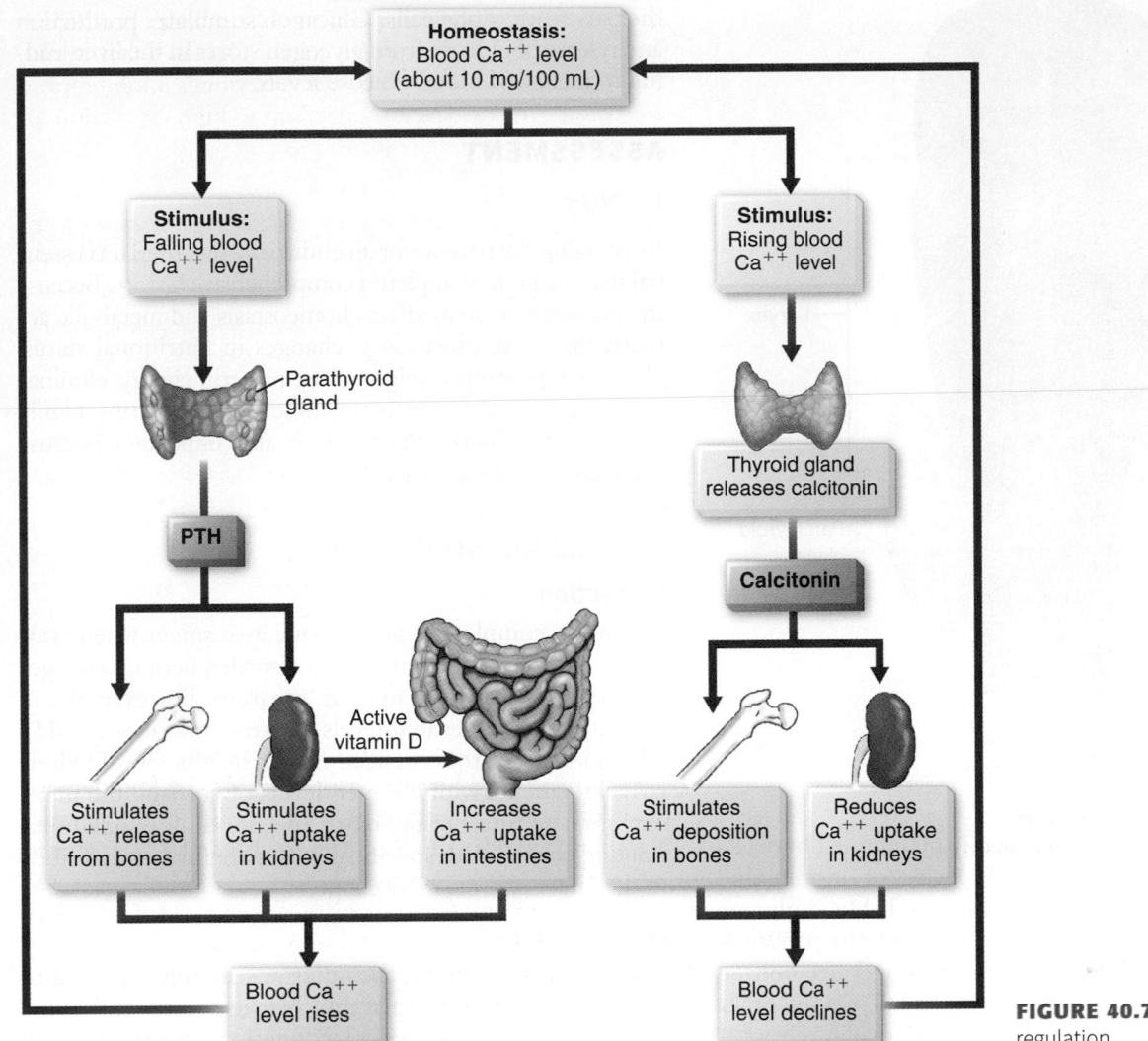

FIGURE 40.7 Overview of calcium regulation.

and testes are controlled by **tropic hormones** released from the anterior pituitary gland based upon secretion of gonadotropin releasing hormone from the hypothalamus. Follicle-stimulating hormone (FSH) and luteinizing hormone (LH) both stimulate maturation of male and female reproductive organs. In the male, FSH and LH stimulate production of **testosterone**, and in the female, these same hormones stimulate production of **estrogen** and **progesterone** that influence development of secondary sexual characteristics, ovarian maturation, and ovulation. These hormones are also required for maintaining normal pregnancy through effects on the cervix, uterine, and breasts. Testosterone in the male is responsible for male sexual characteristics, as well as the production of sperm (see Table 40.1) (these hormones are described in more detail in Unit XV).

Pancreas

The pancreas, located in the upper left quadrant of the abdominal cavity, has both exocrine and endocrine functions (Fig. 40.9). The exocrine function of the pancreas involves the secretion of pancreatic juices into the small intestine

that aid in digestion. Blood glucose control by the islet cells of the pancreas is the endocrine function. Two hormones released by the pancreas play a central role: **insulin**, released from the beta cells of the pancreas, and **glucagon**, released from the alpha cells of the pancreas. To understand diabetes, it is important to understand how blood glucose levels are normally controlled in a healthy person. Glucose arrives in the bloodstream from one of three sources:

- Carbohydrates converted to glucose via digestion, and absorbed through the gastrointestinal tract
- Glucose released from stored **glycogen** in muscles and liver cells
- Glucose newly created (**gluconeogenesis**) in the liver

Once in the bloodstream, the glucose is transported to the target cells. There, insulin facilitates transport of glucose across the cell membrane to the cell's interior. Inside the cell, glucose is metabolized as fuel, releasing energy necessary for normal cellular functioning. Without the effective action of insulin, very little glucose would be able to reach the inside of the cell. Instead, glucose would remain in the bloodstream, and blood glucose levels would rise.

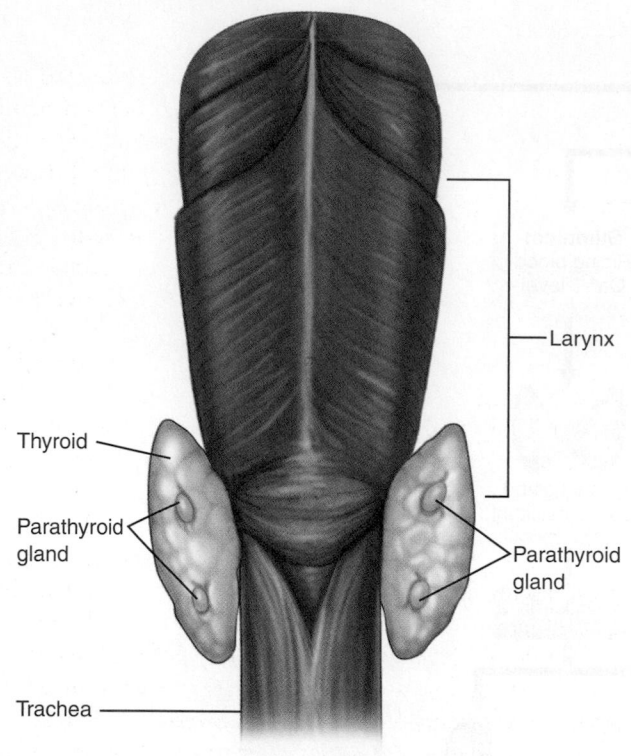

FIGURE 40.8 Location of the parathyroid glands.

A continuous, dynamic balance is maintained between the glucose level in the blood, levels of insulin and glucagon, and cellular uptake of glucose. If blood glucose levels are high, more insulin is secreted by the pancreas. Blood glucose is then driven into the cells and metabolized and as a result glucose levels in the blood fall. On the other hand, if blood glucose levels fall too low, insulin release is suppressed; glucose remains in the bloodstream instead of being driven into the cells. In addition, in response to low blood glucose levels, the hormone glucagon is released from the pancreatic alpha cells. Glucagon stimulates production and release of glucose from glycogen stores in the liver leading to increased blood glucose levels.

ASSESSMENT

History

In assessing the patient for an endocrine disorder, it is essential that the nurse complete a comprehensive history. Because the endocrine system affects homeostasis and metabolic activity, the nurse must assess changes in nutritional status, physical appearance, weight, sleep pattern, energy, elimination pattern, and reproductive function. Evaluating family history for endocrine disorders is also important because some diseases are genetic.

Physical Assessment

Inspection

The nurse completes a head-to-toe assessment when evaluating a patient for an endocrine disorder, because changes in physical appearance may be apparent. For example, in the patient with elevated levels of growth hormone (GH), a broadening of the forehead or jaw may be noted. Similarly, in patients with elevated levels of cortisol, the nurse may note puffiness of the face. (Specific clinical manifestations associated with specific diseases are further described in the endocrine disorder chapters.)

Auscultation

During the assessment, the nurse auscultates the chest to assess cardiac rate and rhythm because some endocrine disorders affect cardiovascular function. In patients with hyperthyroidism, tachydysrhythmias may occur and may be auscultated. Additionally, because of the increased vascularity associated with hyperthyroidism, the nurse also

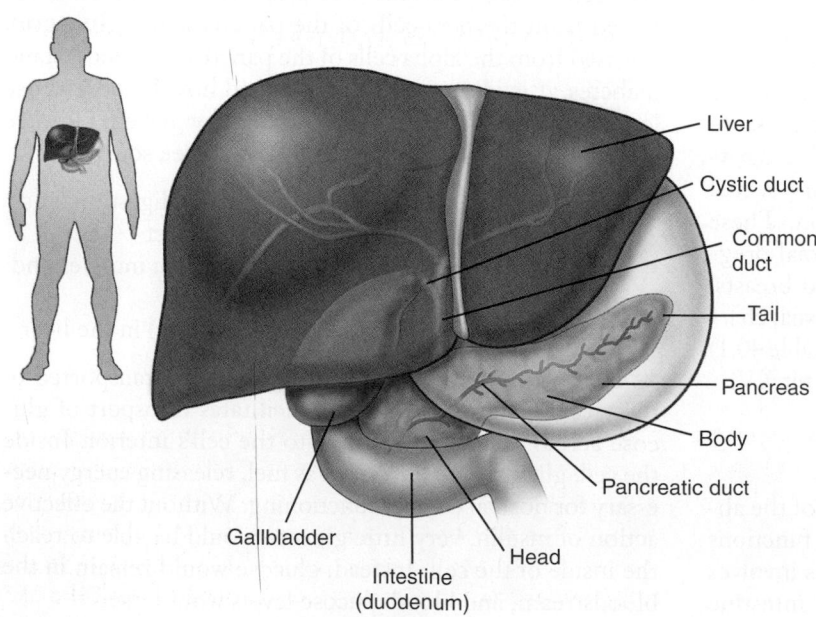

FIGURE 40.9 Location of the pancreas.

listens over the carotid arteries for carotid bruits. Direct auscultation over the thyroid gland may also reveal a thyroid bruit in the patient with hyperthyroidism because of the increased thyroid vascularity associated with this disorder.

Palpation

The nurse uses palpation to assess the testes and the thyroid glands; both are evaluated for size, symmetry, shape, and any nodules or changes in texture. The thyroid gland may be best palpated by standing behind the patient (Fig. 40.10A). The thumbs of both hands are placed on the back of the neck, and the fingers are curved to the front of the neck on either side of the trachea. The patient is asked to swallow, and the nurse locates the isthmus by feeling it rise when the patient swallows. The nurse assesses both the right and left lobes of the thyroid gland. The right lobe is palpated while the patient's head is turned to the right, and the nurse assesses for any irregularities or nodules. The left lobe is similarly evaluated by having the patient turn the head to the left. The thyroid gland may also be assessed from the front. With this approach, the nurse faces the patient and uses the thumbs or fingers to palpate each lobe of the thyroid gland (Figure 40.10B).

Connection Check 40.4

To better locate the isthmus of the thyroid gland in preparation for palpation, the nurse asks the patient to perform which action?

A. "Say 'ah.'"
B. "Touch your chin to your chest."
C. "Look at the ceiling."
D. "Swallow a sip of water."

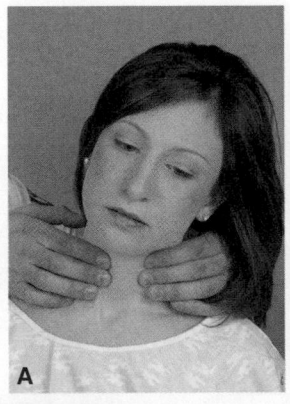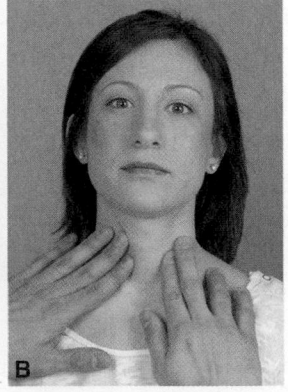

FIGURE 40.10 Palpation of the thyroid gland. A, Posterior approach. The thyroid gland may be best palpated by standing behind the patient. The thumbs of both hands are placed on the back of the neck, and the fingers are curved to the front of the neck on either side of the trachea. The patient is asked to swallow, and the nurse locates the isthmus by feeling it rise when the patient swallows. B, Anterior approach. The thyroid gland may also be assessed from the front. With this approach, the nurse faces the patient and uses the thumbs or fingers to palpate each lobe of the thyroid gland.

DIAGNOSTIC STUDIES

Diagnostic evaluation of the patient with a suspected endocrine disorder includes laboratory assessment of urine and blood samples as well as imaging studies. The specific laboratory tests conducted are associated with the disorder under investigation (Table 40.3). For example, in the patient with suspected diabetes mellitus, blood and urine levels of glucose are measured. In the patient with suspected dysfunction of the adrenal cortex, serum potassium levels are evaluated.

Measurements of circulating hormone levels are also evaluated. In patients with suspected thyroid disease, T3, T4, and TSH levels are assessed (laboratory assessments for specific disorders are presented in Chapters 41 through 44.)

Stimulation and suppression tests are also ordered for patients with suspected endocrine disease. With stimulation testing, a selected hormone is administered to stimulate the target tissue to produce its hormone. Failure of the target to secrete sufficient hormone indicates hypofunction of that gland. Conversely, suppression tests are indicated when there are excess levels of circulating hormone. When levels of circulating hormone do not decrease with suppression testing, hyperfunction of the gland is confirmed.

Imaging Studies

Diagnostic imaging studies are indicated to assess for changes in the size or presence of tumor formation in the glands of the endocrine system. Disorders of the posterior pituitary gland may occur as a result of a pituitary tumor. A pheochromocytoma, a tumor of the adrenal medulla, may be confirmed with imaging studies of the retroperitoneal area. Computed tomography (CT) and magnetic resonance imaging, as well as x-rays are used to confirm abnormalities of the endocrine glands.

Connection Check 40.5

A patient is undergoing a stimulation test to assess adrenal function. After the administration of cortisol, which laboratory result indicates normal function?

A. Decreased blood glucose
B. Decreased serum sodium
C. Decreased serum potassium
D. Decreased serum calcium

AGE-RELATED CHANGES

Changes in endocrine function are associated with aging, and early detection and treatment can minimize long-term consequences. Menopause is an age-related change, but it is also a "normal state" of ovarian hormone deficiency that affects all women as they age. Physiological changes caused by menopause are usually diminished with the use

Table 40.3 Laboratory Tests for Endocrine Disorders

Test	Normal Range for Adults	Significance
Calcium	8.2–10.2 mg/dL	Decreased in hypoparathyroidism
		Increased in hyperparathyroidism
		Decreased by thyrocalcitonin from thyroid gland
Ionized calcium	4.6–5.3 mg/dL	Decreased in hypoparathyroidism
		Increased in hyperparathyroidism
Cortisol	5–25 mcg/dL (morning)	Decreased in hypocortisolism (Addison's)
	3–16 mcg/dL (afternoon)	Elevated in hypercortisolism (Cushing's)
Glucose	65–99 mg/dL	Increased in diabetes mellitus
		Increased in hypercortisolism
Magnesium	1.6–2.6 mg/dL	Decreased in hypoparathyroidism
Phosphorus	2.5–4.5 mg/dL	Increased in hypoparathyroidism
		Decreased in hyperparathyroidism
Potassium	3.5–5.0 mEq/L	Increased in hypocortisolism (Addison's)
		Decreased in hypercortisolism (Cushing's)
Sodium	135–145 mEq/L	Increased in diabetes insipidus (DI)
	(Actual sodium levels may be normal as fluid is retained or lost as the sodium is retained or excreted, respectively.)	Decreased in syndrome of inappropriate antidiuretic hormone (SIADH)
		Decreased in hypocortisolism
		Increased in hypercortisolism
		Decreased in hypoaldosteronism
		Increased in hyperaldosteronism
Free T3 (triiodothyronine)	2.6–4.8 pg/mL	Decreased in hypothyroidism
		Increased in hyperthyroidism
Total T3 (triiodothyronine)	70–204 ng/dL	Decreased in hypothyroidism
		Increased in hyperthyroidism
Free T4 (thyroxine)	0.8–1.5 ng/dL	Decreased in hypothyroidism
		Increased in hyperthyroidism
Total T4 (thyroxine)	4.6–12 mcg/dL	Decreased in hypothyroidism
		Increased in hyperthyroidism
Thyroid-stimulating hormone (TSH)	0.5–8.9 microinternational units (mIU)/mL	Increased in primary hypothyroidism
		Decreased in secondary or tertiary hypothyroidism
		Decreased in primary hyperthyroidism
		Increased in secondary and tertiary hyperthyroidism
Urine specific gravity	1.005–1.030	Decreased with DI
		Increased in SIADH
Vitamin D	20–100 ng/dL	Decreased in hypoparathyroidism
		Variable in hyperparathyroidism

of hormone replacement therapy; however, there are growing concerns associated with these exogenous hormone replacements.

Some of the endocrine changes associated with age are secondary to hypoactive function of endocrine glands secondary to **downregulation** (decreased number of receptors on the surface of the target tissue). Other age-related changes may be associated with an increased incidence of chronic disease. Hormone production, secretion rates, and tissue responsiveness may all decrease with age. Changes may also be associated with compensatory responses to changes in hormone levels; for instance, glucose levels rise with age-related insulin resistance.

Decreased metabolism is associated with decreased appetite, susceptibility to cold intolerance, changes in the quality of sleep, and decreased resting pulse rate and blood pressure. Changes in release of reproductive hormones may lead to problems with sexual functioning, including erectile dysfunction and decreased libido. Patients with decreased glucose tolerance may present with elevated blood glucose levels and weight gain. Decreased synthesis of ADH in the older adult is associated with increased urine frequency and dilute urine, leading to an increased risk of dehydration. Bone density decreases, thinning and drying of the skin, and perineal and vaginal dryness are all associated with advancing age. Although many of these are often associated with aging, it is imperative that a comprehensive evaluation is completed to rule out other causes with these physiological changes.

Connection Check 40.6

The nurse correlates which findings with age-related changes of the endocrine system in a 55-year-old female? *(Select all that apply.)*
A. Breast enlargement
B. Decreased libido
C. Increased sweating
D. Vaginal dryness
E. Insomnia

Making Connections

CASE STUDY: WRAP-UP

The nurse practitioner begins a work-up for thyroid dysfunction for Greta Johnson. On the basis of her clinical presentation, hyperthyroidism is suspected. The laboratory results reveal increased levels of T3 and T4 with decreased levels of TSH. A tentative diagnosis of primary hyperthyroidism is made, and Greta is referred for further evaluation and treatment.

Case Study Questions

1. In assessing a patient with an alteration in thyroid function, the nurse must understand that TRH release is from which structure?
   A. Hypothalamus
   B. Anterior pituitary gland
   C. Posterior pituitary gland
   D. Thyroid gland
2. Which clinical manifestation observed in Ms. Johnson does the nurse correlate with elevated levels of thyroid hormone?
   A. Lethargy
   B. Insomnia
   C. Dry skin
   D. Constipation
3. Which thyroid hormone value does the nurse correlate with primary hyperthyroidism?
   A. Elevated TRH
   B. Elevated TSH
   C. Elevated T3
   D. Elevated thyrocalcitonin
4. The nurse recognizes that the negative feedback system causes which change secondary to increased T3 and T4?
   A. Increased TRH
   B. Decreased TSH
   C. Increased parathormone
   D. Decreased thyrocalcitonin
5. In a patient with a secondary disorder of the thyroid gland, the nurse assesses for changes in function in which structure?
   A. Thyroid gland
   B. Hypothalamus
   C. Posterior pituitary gland
   D. Anterior pituitary gland

CHAPTER SUMMARY

The endocrine system consists of glands located throughout the body that are essential to many vital functions. The hypothalamus plays a major role in endocrine function because of its control of the anterior and pituitary glands. Hormones from the anterior pituitary gland control the function of the adrenal glands, thyroid glands, and reproductive organs. Additionally, GH is controlled by the anterior pituitary gland. The posterior pituitary secretes antidiuretic hormone (ADH) that maintains fluid volume balance by promoting water reabsorption in the kidneys, and sexual hormones.

The adrenal glands are composed of the cortex and medulla, which have independent functions. The adrenal cortex, under the control of hormones from the anterior pituitary gland (ACTH), secretes mineralocorticoids and glucocorticoids. Aldosterone, the primary mineralocorticoid, promotes sodium reabsorption in the kidneys as well as the excretion of potassium. Cortisol, the primary glucocorticoid, has many functions including promoting gluconeogenesis and glycogenolysis that lead to an increase in blood glucose levels. Glucocorticoids have a major role in growth and development as well as anti-inflammatory actions. The adrenal medulla releases catecholamines (epinephrine and norepinephrine) that influence the functions of most body systems.

The thyroid gland secretes hormones that greatly influence metabolic activity (triiodothyronine and thyroxine) and thyrocalcitonin that lowers serum calcium levels. Parathyroid hormone (PTH), secreted by the parathyroid glands, plays a major role in calcium regulation. An increase in PTH increases serum calcium levels, whereas a decrease in PTH lowers serum calcium levels.

Reproductive function is also controlled by the endocrine system. Maturation of both female and male reproductive organs is facilitated by hormones produced from the anterior pituitary glands (follicle-stimulating hormone and luteinizing hormone). Estrogen and progesterone are key to normal female functioning, including controlling the menstrual cycle, facilitating and maintaining pregnancy, and development of secondary sexual characteristics. Testosterone is required for sperm production and development of secondary male sexual characteristics.

The pancreas controls regulation of blood glucose levels and carbohydrate, fat, and protein metabolism through the release of insulin and glucagon. Glucagon increases blood glucose levels through gluconeogenesis and glycogenolysis. Insulin lowers blood glucose levels by facilitating the movement of glucose into cells.

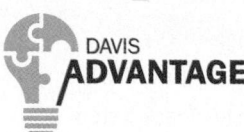

To explore learning resources for this chapter, go to **Davis Advantage** and find:
- Answers to in-text questions
- Chapter Resources and Activities
- NCLEX®-Style Chapter Review Questions
- Bibliography

Chapter 41

Coordinating Care for Patients With Pituitary Disorders

Janice Hoffman

Finding Connections

Carol Andrews makes an appointment with her primary healthcare provider because of a persistent headache, changes in vision, and occasional episodes of nausea. She also complains of enlargement of her hands and feet, requiring her to remove her rings and purchase larger shoes. Her primary healthcare provider orders a series of laboratory studies including serum chemistries and hematology studies. Magnetic resonance imaging (MRI) of the head is also ordered…

INTRODUCTION

The hypothalamus and pituitary glands, described as the hypothalamus-pituitary complex, work together to control many endocrine functions. The pituitary gland, located in the **sella turcica** (a depression of the sphenoid bone), controls many body functions including growth, fluid balance, metabolism, sexual development, and pigmentation. The pituitary gland is composed of two lobes, the anterior lobe (**adenohypophysis**) and the posterior lobe (**neurohypophysis**) that have distinct functions. Hormones secreted by the anterior pituitary gland are controlled by hormones secreted by the hypothalamus (Table 41.1). The hormones released from the posterior pituitary are synthesized in the hypothalamus but stored and released from the posterior pituitary gland.

The anterior lobe of the pituitary gland secretes several major hormones related to metabolic functioning:

- *Adrenocorticotropic hormone* (ACTH) is involved in the synthesis of corticosteroids.
- *Growth hormone* (GH), also known as **somatotropin**, stimulates growth through carbohydrate, protein and fat metabolism.
- *Follicle-stimulating hormone* (FSH) assists in the maturation of the ovaries in females and in spermatogenesis in males.
- *Luteinizing hormone* (LH) is involved in ovulation in females and the production of testosterone in males.

Table 41.1 Hypothalamus and Pituitary Hormones and Actions

Hypothalamus	Anterior Pituitary Gland	Target	Effects
Corticotropin-releasing hormone (CRH) Stimulates release of ACTH	Adrenocorticotropic hormone (ACTH)	Adrenal cortex	Increases secretion of glucocorticoids and mineralocorticoids
Gonadotropin-releasing hormone Stimulates release of FSH and LH	Follicle-stimulating hormone (FSH) Luteinizing hormone (LH)	Ovaries in females Testes in males	Stimulates maturation of ovarian follicles, ovulation, and estrogen secretion Stimulates sperm production
Growth hormone–releasing hormone (GHRH) Stimulates release of GH	Growth hormone (GH)	Tissues and bones	Facilitates growth of bones and tissues through protein synthesis, fat metabolism, and insulin antagonism
Growth hormone inhibiting hormone (GHIH) Inhibits release of GH	Growth hormone (GH)	Tissues and bones	Opposes the effects of GHRH thus decreasing the metabolic effects of growth hormone
Thyrotropin-releasing hormone (TRH) Stimulates release of TSH	Thyroid-stimulating hormone (TSH)	Thyroid gland	Increases secretion of thyroid hormones (triiodothyronine and thyroxine), increasing metabolism
	Posterior Pituitary		
	Vasopressin (antidiuretic hormone; ADH)	Distal tubules and collecting ducts in the kidney	Increases water reabsorption
	Oxytocin	Uterus and mammary glands	Stimulates uterine contractions in labor and milk ejection

- *Prolactin* stimulates the mammary glands for milk production.
- *Thyroid-stimulating hormone* (TSH) controls the secretion of thyroxine (T4) and triiodothyronine (T3) thyroid hormones.

The posterior lobe of the pituitary gland secretes hormones responsible for the following actions:

- **Antidiuretic hormone (ADH)** controls water retention by the kidneys and moderates vasoconstriction and the release of ACTH in the anterior lobe of the pituitary.
- **Oxytocin** plays a major role in circadian homeostasis, the release of breast milk, and cervical changes and uterine contractions during labor and delivery.

Because of the essential role of these hormones, patients with pituitary adenomas are usually followed and treated by a healthcare provider who specializes in managing patients with endocrine disorders both preoperatively and postoperatively.

DISORDERS OF THE ANTERIOR PITUITARY GLAND

Disorders related to the function of the anterior pituitary gland may be caused by an increase or decrease in the secretion of hormones from the hypothalamus or the anterior pituitary gland itself. Primary disorders are related to alterations in function of endocrine glands (for example, the adrenal cortex or thyroid glands), secondary disorders are related to alterations in hormone secretion from the anterior pituitary gland, and tertiary disorders are related to alterations in hormone secretion from the hypothalamus. Patients may present with disorders related to one specific hormone, or in very rare cases, they may present with **panhypopituitarism**. This disorder involves hyposecretion of all hormones from the hypothalamus and has dramatic effects on normal function.

Hypopituitarism

Hypopituitarism is hyposecretion of hormones from the anterior pituitary gland. Because hormones released from the anterior pituitary gland regulate hormone release from the adrenal cortex, thyroid gland, and gonads, alterations in hormonal release affect many body functions. The hyposecretion of growth hormone is also seen with hypopituitarism.

Epidemiology

Hypopituitarism is a rare disorder according to the National Institutes of Health (NIH), affecting fewer than 200,000 individuals in the United States. The etiology of anterior pituitary dysfunction is often secondary to a pituitary tumor or damage to the hypothalamus. Increased intracranial pressure secondary to head trauma, central nervous system (CNS) infections such as meningitis, or brain tumors may also affect perfusion of the hypothalamus and result in damage. Postpartum hemorrhage, resulting in large blood loss and corresponding hypotension, may lead to severe hypoperfusion and infarction of the anterior pituitary. The onset of clinical manifestations of hypopituitarism is gradual and occurs after a majority (70%–90%) of the anterior pituitary is nonfunctional or destroyed.

Pathophysiology

A deficiency of one of the anterior pituitary hormones results in changes in metabolic or sexual function, dependent on which hormone level is decreased. The effects of a decrease in one or more of the anterior pituitary hormones determine the pathophysiology of hypopituitarism. A decrease in adrenocorticotropic hormone (ACTH) leads to a decrease in release of the mineralocorticoids (aldosterone) and glucocorticoids (cortisol) from the adrenal cortex. Likewise, there is a decrease in thyroid hormones secondary to the decreased secretion of thyroid-stimulating hormone (TSH) from the anterior pituitary gland. Alterations in sexual and reproductive functioning are caused by decreased secretion of the gonadotropins, luteinizing hormone (LH) and follicle-stimulating hormone (FSH). There is also a decrease in growth hormone that presents differently according to the age of the patient. In children before the closure of the epiphyses, **dwarfism** (small stature) develops. A lack of growth hormone in adults does not affect bone length but does affect bone density, and osteoporosis (reduction in bone density) may develop.

Clinical Manifestations

The clinical presentation of hypopituitarism is directly related to the hormone involved. Table 41.2 provides an overview of the clinical manifestations.

Connection Check 41.1

The nurse correlates which clinical manifestation to the pathophysiology of decreased ACTH production from the anterior pituitary gland?

A. Hypotension
B. Polyuria
C. Diarrhea
D. Pruritus

Management
Medical Management
Diagnosis

Diagnostic evaluation of hypopituitarism focuses on the particular hormone and target cells/glands affected by the lack of tropic hormone. Hormonal studies conducted to assess for hypopituitarism include the ACTH (Cortrosyn) stimulation test and measurements of TSH, FSH, LH, prolactin, and growth hormone provocative tests. If a tumor of the brain or pituitary is suspected, a head computed tomography (CT) or MRI may be completed. A battery of serum

Table 41.2 Clinical Manifestations Associated With Hypopituitarism

Hormone	Clinical Manifestations
Adrenocorticotropic hormone (ACTH)	Decreased glucocorticoids • Hypoglycemia • Decreased cortisol levels • Decreased ability to handle stress Decreased mineralocorticoids • Hyponatremia • Hypotension • Hyperkalemia
Growth hormone	Decreased bone density Decreased muscle strength Increased risk of bone fractures
Luteinizing hormone	Females • Irregular menses or amenorrhea • Decreased ovulation Males • Decreased testosterone
Follicle-stimulating hormone	Females • Decreased estrogen production • Decreased ovulation Males • Decreased sperm production
Thyroid-stimulating hormone (TSH)	Decreased levels of T3 and T4 • Decreased metabolic rate • Weight gain • Thinning of hair • Decreased libido

studies related to effects on target glands or cells is also performed to assist in a definitive diagnosis based on physical presentation. With suspected abnormalities in growth hormone, manifested by complaints of weakness or pathologic bone fractures, diagnostic evaluation often focuses on "ruling-out" other causes. Direct measurement of growth hormone is difficult because the levels change throughout the course of a day.

Medications

The goals of medical management of hypopituitarism are aimed at restoring target hormone levels to normal levels. Hormone replacement is guided by the specific hormone deficiency. In addition to hormone replacement, supportive therapies such as fluid and electrolyte replacement are the key to managing the patient with hypopituitarism. Hormone replacement may include cortisol, thyroid hormone, testosterone, or estrogen. Management of a decrease in growth hormone is usually focused on the pathophysiological processes associated with decreased bone density and osteoporosis and includes ensuring adequate intake or supplementation with vitamin D and calcium.

Complications

Patients with hypopituitarism may develop life-threatening emergencies, particularly with panhypopituitarism. Lack of ACTH with a resultant decrease in glucocorticoids and mineralocorticoids is a life-threatening emergency because the patient is unable to maintain adequate fluid volume status, which may lead to circulatory collapse (discussed in more detail in Chapter 42). Additionally, a lack of TSH, leading to a decrease in thyroid hormone secretion, may result in a severe decrease in metabolism that affects all body functions and is particularly dangerous in relation to metabolism of medications.

Nursing Management
Assessment and Analysis

Clinical manifestations observed in the patient with hypopituitarism are directly related to the specific hormone deficiency. Common findings may include:

- Hypoglycemia related to decreased secretion of ACTH, resulting in decreased secretion of cortisol
- Decreased ability to cope with stress secondary to decreased secretion of cortisol
- Hyponatremia and hypotension secondary to decreased aldosterone secretion
- Hyperkalemia secondary to decreased aldosterone secretion
- Decreased bone density secondary to decreased growth hormone secretion

Nursing Diagnoses

- **Fluid volume deficit** related to decreased glucocorticoid and mineralocorticoid secondary to decreased secretion of ACTH from the anterior pituitary gland
- **Risk for injury: Falls** related to osteoporosis and weakened bone density associated with decreased growth hormone
- **Impaired mobility** related to increased risk of pathological fractures secondary to decreased bone density

Nursing Interventions
■ Assessments

- Vital signs
  Hypotension and tachycardia develop secondary to decreased secretion of ACTH, leading to decreased secretion of glucocorticoid and mineralocorticoid, resulting in sodium and water loss.
- Changes in fertility
  Decreased testosterone may lead to sterility in males. Decreased LH or FSH may lead to amenorrhea and infertility in females.

- Signs of decreased bone density
  A lack of growth hormone in adults affects bone density, and the patient is at risk for osteoporosis.

■ Actions

- Implement safety measures
  Risk of injury related to falls and pathologic fractures increases secondary to decreased secretion of growth hormone.
- Increase vitamin D and calcium intake
  Treats osteoporosis secondary to decreased growth hormone, vitamin D promotes absorption of calcium in the gastrointestinal tract.
- Hormone replacement
  Supplementation of sex hormones may be administered to treat hypofunction of the gonads.
- Collaborate with physical therapy to maximize mobility
  Osteoporosis increases the risk for falls, and the physical therapist can provide input into safe transfers from bed to chair and measures to decrease the incidence of falls.

■ Teaching

- Signs and symptoms of acute adrenal insufficiency
  Infection, injury, and stress lead to an increased need for ACTH. Because of underlying hypopituitarism, the patient may require exogenous glucocorticoids in the event of stress (physiological or psychological).
- Importance of taking hormone supplements in the morning
  Taking hormone supplements in the morning mimics the normal release of these hormones.

Evaluating Care Outcomes

Patients with hypopituitarism can achieve relatively normal function by complying with prescribed therapy. Replacement hormone therapy based on the specific hormone is combined with supportive treatment to address end gland/target cell effects. Vital signs within normal limits, improved mobility, stable weight, and normal fluid volume status are indicative of stable anterior pituitary function. With appropriate hormone replacement, fertility and conception may be achieved. During periods of stress, such as invasive procedures, the patient needs to be aware of the signs of adrenal insufficiency and the clinical manifestations they should report to their healthcare provider.

Hyperpituitarism

Hyperpituitarism is a disorder related to hypersecretion of hormones from the anterior pituitary gland. As with hypopituitarism, the pathophysiology and clinical presentation are directly related to which hormone levels are elevated secondary to hypersecretion. Hypersecreting tumors of the anterior pituitary gland are often the etiology of hyperpituitarism.

Epidemiology

Hyperpituitarism is usually related to a hypersecreting tumor. The incidence of these types of tumors is higher in females, but there are no differences based on race or ethnicity. These types of tumors may present in children or adults, and there is a genetic association with the tumor development. The patient presentation is consistent with clinical manifestations associated with the oversecreted hormone, and the tumor itself may lead to headaches or visual changes secondary to compression of the optic nerve (CN II) and other structures in the central nervous system.

Pathophysiology

Hyperpituitarism secondary to hypersecretion of hormones leads to specific dysfunction related to the hormone involved. An excess of one of the anterior pituitary hormones results in changes in metabolic or sexual function that are dependent on which hormone level is elevated. The effects of an increase in one or more of the anterior pituitary hormones determine the pathophysiology of hyperpituitarism. An increase in ACTH leads to an increase in release of the mineralocorticoids and glucocorticoids from the adrenal cortex. Likewise, there is an increase in thyroid hormone released secondary to the increased secretion of TSH from the anterior pituitary gland. Alterations in sexual and reproductive functioning are caused by increased secretion of the gonadotropins (LH and FSH). There is also an increase in growth hormone that presents differently according to the age of the patient. In children before the closure of the epiphyses, **gigantism** (large stature) develops. An excess of growth hormone in adults does not affect bone length because of closure of the epiphyses but does affect bone density, and **acromegaly** (thickening of bones, particularly of the hands, feet, and facial bones) may develop (Fig. 41.1).

Clinical Manifestations

The clinical presentation of hyperpituitarism is directly related to the excessive secretion of ACTH, growth hormone, and TSH. Table 41.3 provides an overview of the clinical manifestations. Excessive secretions of LH and FSH are not associated with physiological changes.

Management

Medical Management

Diagnosis

Diagnostic evaluation of hyperpituitarism focuses on the particular hormone and target cells/glands affected by the excess of tropic hormone. Hormonal studies conducted to assess for hyperpituitarism include the ACTH (Cortrosyn) stimulation test and measurements of TSH, FSH, LH, prolactin, and growth hormone provocative tests. If a hypersecreting tumor of the brain or pituitary is suspected, a head CT or MRI may be completed. A battery of serum studies associated with effects on target glands or cells is also performed to assist in a definitive diagnosis based on physical presentation. With suspected increases in growth hormone, the patient presents with increases in the size of the hands and feet and broadening of the facial bones.

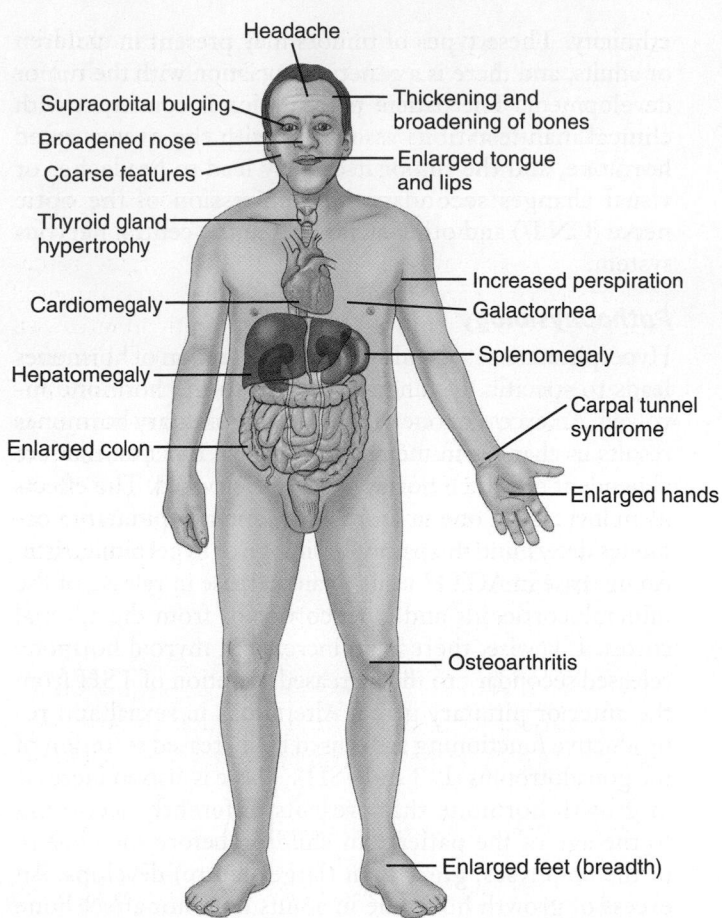

Headache

Supraorbital bulging

Broadened nose

Coarse features

Thyroid gland
hypertrophy

Cardiomegaly

Hepatomegaly

Enlarged colon

Thickening and
broadening of bones

Enlarged tongue
and lips

Increased perspiration

Galactorrhea

Splenomegaly

Carpal tunnel
syndrome

Enlarged hands

Osteoarthritis

Enlarged feet (breadth)

FIGURE 41.1 Characteristics of acromegaly.

Table 41.3 Clinical Manifestations Associated With Hyperpituitarism

Hormone	Clinical Manifestations
Adrenocorticotropic hormone (ACTH)	Increased glucocorticoids
	● Hyperglycemia
	● Increased cortisol levels
	Increased mineralocorticoids
	● Hypernatremia
	● Hypertension
	● Hypokalemia
Growth hormone	Increased bone density
	Coarse facial features
	Menstrual irregularities
Thyroid-stimulating hormone (TSH)	Increased levels of T3 and T4
	● Increased metabolic rate
	● Weight loss
	● Exophthalmos

Medications

The goals of medical management of hyperpituitarism are aimed at decreasing secretion of the involved hormones and treating clinical manifestations secondary to target gland or cell hyperfunction (hyperglycemia, hypertension, etc.). Dopamine agonists (bromocriptine mesylate [Parlodel]) inhibit the release of anterior pituitary hormones. Medications that inhibit release of growth hormone include somatostatin analogs and growth hormone receptor blockers. In some cases, these medications are used to decrease the size of the tumor in advance of surgical removal.

Surgical Management

Hypersecreting tumors of the pituitary gland are surgically removed by a transsphenoidal **hypophysectomy**. The sublabial transseptal approach to a pituitary tumor involves an incision made under the top lip, with entry to the nasal cavity made through the floor of the nose. The nasal septum is moved to the side, and the sphenoid sinus is opened to access the sella turcica and the pituitary gland (Fig. 41.2). A muscle graft is placed after removal of the tumor, and often comes from the patient's thigh. The graft aids in healing and prevents cerebrospinal fluid (CSF) **rhinorrhea** (CSF draining from the nose). Nasal packing is placed after

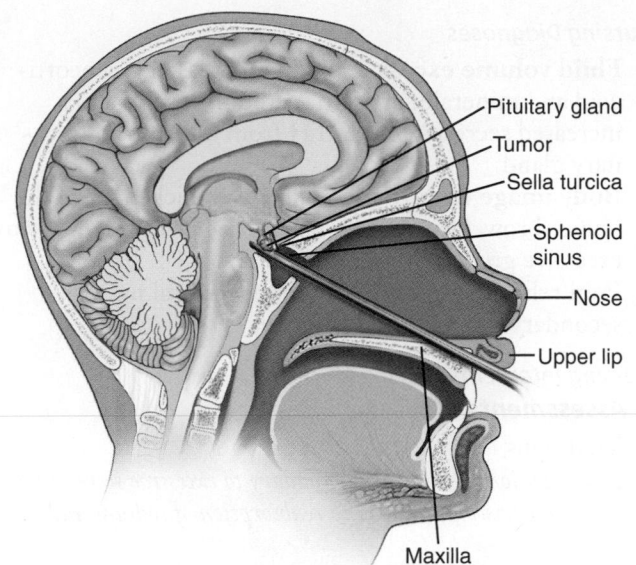

FIGURE 41.2 Sublabial transseptal approach to surgical removal of pituitary tumor. The sublabial transseptal approach to a pituitary tumor involves an incision made under the top lip, with entry to the nasal cavity made through the floor of the nose. The nasal septum is moved to the side, and the sphenoid sinus is opened to access the sella turcica and the pituitary gland.

the incision is closed and a loose dressing is placed below the nares (moustache dressing). Postoperative management of the patient is similar to that for patients undergoing intracranial surgery for other types of brain tumor (discussed in Chapter 36). Postoperatively, these patients must be monitored for increased intracranial pressure, development of diabetes insipidus (presented later in this chapter), meningitis, and cerebrospinal leakage. The patient is instructed to avoid activities that could increase pressure at the incision site, for example coughing, sneezing, and bending over. Smaller pituitary tumors may also be removed via

an endoscopic approach, which poses fewer postoperative complications than the sublabial transseptal approach. This surgical procedure gains access to the pituitary tumor through a fiberoptic device inserted through an incision in the lining of the nose (Fig. 41.3).

Stereotactic radiosurgery, a minimally invasive procedure, is another surgical approach that may be indicated for residual or recurrent pituitary tumors after surgical resection. Delivering high-dose radiation to a precisely targeted area of the brain, the goal is eradication of the tumor with minimal effects to adjacent normal brain tissue. The procedure involves the placement of a stereotactic headframe to allow localization of the target area and immobilization during the procedure. There are minimal complications to this procedure and the patient is typically discharged on the same day, with instruction to monitor pin sites (from the headframe) for bleeding or drainage, and to take acetaminophen for headache.

Connection Check 41.2

The nurse questions which order in the patient who has undergone transsphenoidal hypophysectomy for a pituitary tumor?
A. Offer clear fluids once alert and awake
B. Oxygen 2 L via nasal cannula
C. Maintain head of rhe bed at a 45- to 60-degree angle
D. Apply lip balm prn

Complications
Patients with hyperpituitarism may develop complications related to excess hormone secretion. Excess ACTH with a resultant increase in glucocorticoids and mineralocorticoids leads to hyperglycemia, hypertension, and acromegaly.

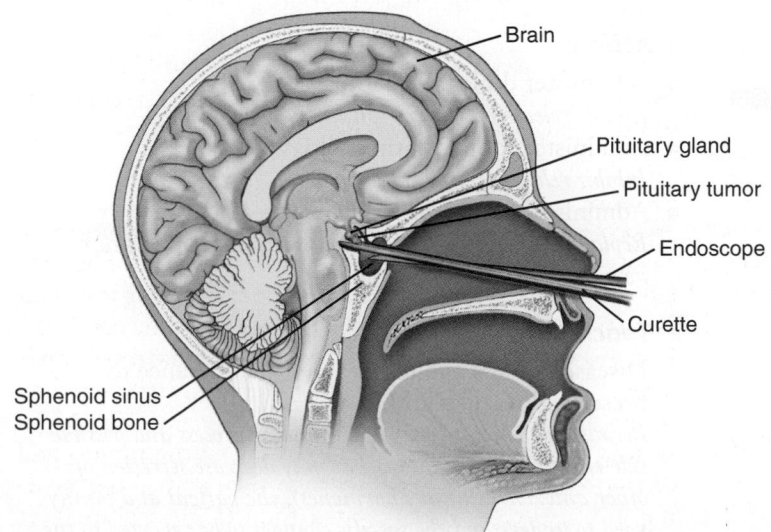

FIGURE 41.3 Endoscopic approach to surgical removal of pituitary tumor. The endoscopic approach gains access to the pituitary tumor through a fiberoptic device inserted into the nostril and then the sella turcica is entered for tumor removal.

Additionally, an excess of TSH leading to an increase in thyroid hormone secretion may result in severe hyperthyroidism and may deteriorate to thyroid storm (discussed in Chapter 43). After transsphenoidal hypophysectomy, the patient is at risk for CSF rhinorrhea that increase the risk of meningitis (see Evidence-Based Practice). Damage to the posterior pituitary gland may lead to disorders of antidiuretic hormone secretion (discussed in the next section of this chapter).

Evidence-Based Practice

Postoperative Cerebrospinal Fluid Leak in Patients With Lower Airway Disease

Cerebrospinal fluid (CSF) rhinorrhea is a potential postoperative complication in patients after transsphenoidal hypophysectomy. This study examined the relationship between postoperative CSF rhinorrhea and lower airway disease (including chronic obstructive pulmonary disease and asthma) in patients after transsphenoidal hypophysectomy. This retrospective review of Healthcare Care and Utilization Project's 2013 National Inpatient Sample compared hospital stays and surgical outcomes in patients with lower airway disease with a disease-free population. Of the patients with lower airway disease in this study, 92% had asthma and had a greater risk for postoperative CSF leak and for the development of diabetes insipidus. Patients with CSF leak had longer hospital stays. Findings from this study recommend perioperative lower airway assessment for patients scheduled for transsphenoidal hypophysectomy to potentially decrease postoperative complications.

Hanba, C., Svider, P.F., Jacob, J.T., Guthikonda, M., Liu, J.K., Eloy, J.A., & Folbe, J.A. (2017). Lower airway disease and pituitary surgery: Is there an association with postoperative cerebrospinal leak? *Laryngoscope,* *127*(7), 1543–1550.

Nursing Management

Assessment and Analysis

Clinical manifestations observed in the patient with hyperpituitarism are directly related to specific hormone excesses. Common findings may include:

- Hyperglycemia related to increased secretion of ACTH, resulting in increased secretion of cortisol
- Hypernatremia and hypertension secondary to increased secretion of aldosterone
- Hypokalemia secondary to increased secretion of aldosterone
- Increased bone density secondary to increased secretion of growth hormone

Nursing Diagnoses

- **Fluid volume excess** related to increased glucocorticoid and mineralocorticoid secretion secondary to increased secretion of ACTH from the anterior pituitary gland
- **Body image disturbance** related to thickening of the bones (brow, facial bones, hands, and feet) secondary to excessive growth hormone secretion
- **Pain** related to compression of peripheral nerves secondary to thickening of bones

Nursing Interventions

▪ Assessments

- Vital signs
  Hypertension may develop secondary to excessive secretion of mineralocorticoid, leading to reabsorption of sodium and water.
- Neurological assessment, including vision
  Pituitary tumors may cause an increase in intracranial pressure. As tumors enlarge and extend beyond the sella turcica, they may compress CN II and CN III.
- Intake and output
  Urinary output may decrease secondary to increased reabsorption of sodium and water. Excessive output of dilate urine may occur if the patient develops diabetes insipidus.
- Daily weight
  Reabsorption of sodium and water secondary to increased mineralocorticoid may lead to increases in weight.
- Serum electrolytes
  Increased secretion of ACTH leads to increased cortisol and aldosterone, leading to sodium retention and potassium loss.
- Changes in size of hands, feet, and bone structure
  Increased secretion of growth hormone leads to thickening of the bones.
- Neurovascular status
  In patients with acromegaly, bone growth may compress peripheral nerves causing numbness, tingling, or pain in the hands and feet

▪ Actions

- Administer dopamine agonists
  Inhibit release of anterior pituitary hormones
- Administer somatostatin analogs
  Inhibit release of growth hormone
- Administer hormone supplements
  Replacement of sexual hormones is required to facilitate normal function and conception.

▪ Teaching

- Disease process and importance of adherence to prescribed medications
  Because of the complexity of the disease process and possible side effects of medications (that may decrease secretion of other anterior pituitary hormones), the patient and family need to understand the specific changes to be reported to the healthcare provider. Collaborate with the pharmacist for medication teaching.

Nursing Interventions for a Patient After Transsphenoidal Hypophysectomy

■ **Assessments**

● Vital signs
Hypotension and tachycardia are seen if the patient develops postoperative DI. Temperature elevation may occur if there is postoperative infection from the surgical incision or secondary to a CSF leak.

● Neurological status
An increase in intracranial pressure secondary to the surgical procedure may lead to changes in the level of consciousness and papillary changes. Visual field changes may develop secondary to postoperative cerebral edema.

● Intake and output
Lack of ADH leads to an increase in excretion of large amounts of dilute urine.

● Mucus membranes and mouth
Because of nasal packing after transsphenoidal hypophysectomy, the patient breathes primarily through the mouth, leading to increased dryness.

● Urine-specific gravity
Urine-specific gravity decreases, usually less than 1.005 secondary to lack of ADH and subsequent excretion of dilute urine.

● Serum sodium and osmolality
Serum sodium and osmolality increase because of increased excretion of water secondary to lack of ADH.

■ **Actions**

● Administer humidified oxygen as ordered
The surgical approach (via the sphenoid) does not allow the patient to breathe through the mouth. The patient is an obligate mouth breather, and humidification facilitates maintaining moist mucous membranes.

● Maintain IV access and administer ordered IV solutions
In patients with a decrease in level of consciousness, IV fluids are usually indicated. The solution ordered is based on the serum sodium level

● Administer desmopressin or vasopressin as ordered
Synthetic ADH is administered to cause water reabsorption in the kidneys.

● Maintain head of the bed at 45 to 60 degrees
Facilitates ease of breathing by dropping diaphragm, and promotes outflow via jugular veins to minimize changes in intracranial pressure

● Provide adequate oral fluids
If the patient is alert and awake, the patient is allowed to drink fluids.

● Provide mouth care
The patient is at risk for fluid volume deficit related to lack of ADH and requires mouth care to minimize complications of dry mucous membranes.

■ **Teaching**

● Signs of meningitis
The surgical approach increases the risk of meningitis, and the nurse needs to monitor for elevated temperature, nuchal rigidity (stiff neck), and photophobia.

● Signs and symptoms of DI: Instruct patient to notify his or her healthcare provider for increased urine output and excessive thirst. Signs and symptoms of fluid overload: Instruct patient to notify his or her healthcare provider for weight gain.
The patient must understand the pathophysiology of this disorder and the importance of fluid volume balance. Overcorrection of DI with DDAVP or Pitressin may lead to fluid overload.

● Use a soft toothbrush after transsphenoidal hypophysectomy
Decreases potential to damage incision line after transsphenoidal activity

● Avoid activities (coughing, sneezing, bending at the waist) after transsphenoidal hypophysectomy
These activities can put strain on the surgical site.

● Report any increase in drainage of clear fluid from the nose after transsphenoidal hypophysectomy
Clear drainage from the nose may indicate a CSF leak that increases risk of meningitis.

Evaluating Care Outcomes

The patient with hyperpituitarism may achieve normal function through the administration of medications that suppress excess hormone secretion, particularly growth hormone. Removal of a hypersecreting tumor of the anterior pituitary with no associated injury to the gland usually results in normal function. Changes in bone structure will not return to normal, but there is no further growth in bone secondary to excessive growth hormone in the adult. After transsphenoidal hypophysectomy, the patient should be neurologically intact with normal fluid and electrolyte balance.

CASE STUDY: EPISODE 2

The result of Carol Andrews' MRI is positive for a pituitary adenoma, and she is scheduled for a transsphenoidal hypophysectomy for removal of the tumor. The operative procedure is uneventful, and she is admitted to the neurosurgical intensive care unit. Postoperative orders include vital signs with neurological assessments every hour, hourly intake and output measurements, head of bed at 45 degrees, oxygen at 35% with humidification via a face tent, a nasal drainage pad to be maintained under the nose and monitored for drainage, and an IV of lactated Ringer's (LR) solution at 80 mL per hour. She has an indwelling urinary catheter and is placed on continuous electrocardiogram monitoring. Laboratory orders include hourly measurements of urine-specific gravity and serum and urine electrolytes every 6 hours…

DISORDERS OF THE POSTERIOR PITUITARY GLAND

Diabetes Insipidus

Epidemiology

Diabetes insipidus (DI) is classified as either central or nephrogenic. Central DI is caused by a decreased secretion of antidiuretic hormone (ADH) from the posterior pituitary gland. Nephrogenic DI occurs when the kidneys are resistant to ADH and are unable to concentrate urine, and this type of DI is observed in patients with chronic renal insufficiency, hypercalcemia, hypokalemia, and interstitial disease of the renal tubules. This chapter focuses on central DI.

Approximately 30% of cases of DI are idiopathic, whereas 25% are secondary to brain tumors, 20% develop after intracranial surgery, and 16% occur after head trauma. Idiopathic DI develops secondary to destruction of the cells of the hypothalamus that produce ADH and is often an autoimmune process. Primary brain tumors leading to DI include craniopharyngiomas (arising near the pituitary gland) and pineal tumors. Postneurosurgical DI varies by type of surgical procedure. In patients undergoing traditional craniotomy, DI is reported in 60% to 80% of the patients, whereas with the transsphenoidal approach (see Fig. 41.1), only approximately 10% to 20% of the patients develop postoperative DI. In some of these cases, particularly in postoperative DI, the disorder is transient.

Pathophysiology

The decrease or absence of ADH in the patient with DI results from lack of production in the hypothalamus. Antidiuretic hormone, stored and released from the posterior pituitary gland, works on the receptor cells in the collecting ducts of the kidney, leading to water reabsorption back into the circulation. With a lack of ADH, the collecting ducts are less permeable to water, and it is excreted as urine. In patients with DI, the lack of ADH leads to excretion of large volumes of very dilute urine.

Clinical Manifestations

The clinical presentation of the patient with DI is dependent on the significance of water loss. Polyuria, polydipsia, and nocturia are the primary clinical manifestations seen in patients with DI. The excessive loss of water leads to hemoconcentration that is observed with elevations in serum sodium and hematocrit. The patient may present with hypotension and tachycardia secondary to hypovolemia. Other signs of fluid volume deficit including thirst, skin tenting, and fatigue may also be observed.

Management

Medical Management

Diagnosis

Diagnostic evaluation of DI includes serum and urine electrolytes, serum and urine osmolality, urine-specific gravity, and CT or MRI of the head (Table 41.4). Urine-specific gravity of less than 1.005 and urine osmolality less than 200 mOsm/kg are key indicators of DI. While the patient loses free water, increases in serum sodium, serum osmolality, and hematocrit develop secondary to hemoconcentration. The water deprivation test is also used in the diagnosis of DI. In this test, all water is withheld, and urine osmolality and body weight are measured hourly. During the test, the patient's weight and urine osmolality are evaluated because normally the withholding of water leads to a urine osmolality 2 to 4 times greater than the serum osmolality. The diagnosis of DI is made when serum osmolality continues to increase and there is no resultant increase in urine osmolality.

Fluid Management and Medications

Management of DI is focused on maintaining adequate fluid volume status. Most patients who are awake and alert are able to replace water loss by drinking fluids. In an emergency or in the unconscious patient, IV fluid administration is indicated. Water losses are replaced with a hypotonic fluid (in relation to the patient's serum osmolality) such as dextrose in water. During IV administration, the patient is monitored for hyperglycemia, volume overload, and correction of hypernatremia. Decreasing the serum sodium by 0.5 mmol/L every hour minimizes the chances of overly rapid correction of hypernatremia.

Desmopressin (DDAVP), a synthetic analog of ADH, is the drug of choice in patients with DI and is available in subcutaneous, intranasal, and oral preparations. There is also a synthetic vasopressin (Pitressin) used to treat DI that is less expensive than desmopressin. Patients receiving either of these medications require frequent monitoring of fluid status, serum electrolytes, and urine output.

Table 41.4 Laboratory Tests For Posterior Pituitary Disorders		
Test	**Normal Range for Adults**	**Significance**
Hematocrit	Male: 43%–49%	Increased in diabetes insipidus (DI)
	Female: 38%–44%	Decreased in syndrome of inappropriate antidiuretic hormone (SIADH)
Serum sodium	135–145 mEq/L	Increased in DI
		Decreased in SIADH
Urine-specific gravity	1.005–1.030	Decreased with DI
		Increased in SIADH

Connection Check 41.3

The nurse correlates which laboratory value as an indication that desmopressin is effective in the treatment of diabetes insipidus (DI)?

A. Serum sodium of 140 mEq/L
B. Serum osmolality of 305 mOsm/kg
C. Urine-specific gravity of 1.004
D. Serum hematocrit of 48%

Complications

The patient with DI may develop dehydration and hypovolemia, progressing to circulatory collapse without adequate fluid administration. Patients with permanent DI who require daily administration of hormone replacement are particularly at risk for hypovolemia. Hemoconcentration secondary to DI also increases the risk for hypernatremia. The clinical presentation of hypernatremia is related to central nervous system dysfunction secondary to shrinkage of brain cells and results in confusion, neuromuscular excitability, seizures, or coma.

Nursing Management

Assessment and Analysis

Because DI is directly related to the lack of ADH, there is loss of free water. Assessment findings include polyuria, urine-specific gravity less than 1.005, and low urine osmolality (especially in relation to serum osmolality). Secondary to hemoconcentration, laboratory analyses reveal an increase in serum sodium, osmolality, and hematocrit. Changes in blood pressure and heart rate are related to the volume of fluid loss. Patients who are awake and alert with an intake thirst mechanism are usually able to maintain fluid volume by drinking adequate fluids.

Nursing Diagnoses

- **Fluid volume deficit** related to loss of free water secondary to lack of ADH
- **Risk for ineffective therapeutic regimen management** related to required administration of desmopressin (DDAVP)
- **Sensory perceptual alteration (vision)** related to compression of CN II and III secondary to pituitary tumor

Nursing Interventions
Assessments

- Vital signs
  Lack of ADH leads to excessive water loss with resulting decrease in blood pressure and increase in heart rate as a compensatory mechanism.
- Intake and output
  Fluid replacement is largely dependent on the volume of urine output secondary to lack of ADH.
- Daily weight
  Increased output of dilute urine, secondary to lack of ADH, leads to decrease in weight.
- Visual acuity
  Growth of the pituitary tumor may compress CN II or CN III.

- Serum sodium and osmolality
  Lack of ADH causes an increase in water excretion leading to the concentration of serum sodium (hypernatremia) and an increase in serum osmolality.
- Urine-specific gravity
  Lack of ADH results in the excretion of large volumes of dilute urine; specific gravity is usually less than 1.005.

■ Actions

- Maintain IV access and administer ordered IV solutions
  In patients with a decrease in level of consciousness, IV fluids are usually indicated. The solution ordered is based on serum sodium level. It is important to maintain vascular access because placement of an IV catheter in a profoundly hypotensive patient is difficult.
- Administer desmopressin or vasopressin as ordered
  Synthetic ADH is administered to cause water reabsorption in the kidney.
- Provide adequate oral fluids
  If the patient is alert and awake and has an intact gag reflex, the patient is allowed to drink fluids.
- Provide mouth care
  The patient is at risk for fluid volume deficient related to lack of ADH and requires mouth care to minimize complications of dry mucous membranes.

■ Teaching

- Importance of taking medications (ADH replacement) as ordered
  Taking the medications (Vasopressin/Pitressin) at the same time daily mimics normal release and supports water reabsorption in the kidneys
- Weigh daily at same time and on same scale
  Weight is directly associated with water loss or gain, and changes of more than 2 lb per day should be reported to the healthcare provider.
- Clinical manifestations of DI
  The patient must understand the pathophysiology of this disorder and the importance of fluid volume balance.
- Clinical manifestations of fluid overload
  Overcorrection of DI with DDAVP or Pitressin may lead to fluid overload.

Connection Check 41.4

The patient experiencing diabetes insipidus (DI) is ordered to receive DDAVP. The nurse monitors for which therapeutic effect of these medications?

A. Increased urine output
B. Increased urine-specific gravity
C. Increased serum sodium
D. Increased serum potassium

Evaluating Care Outcomes

Diabetes insipidus may be transient after head injury or craniotomy, or it may be a permanent disorder. Definitive treatment with synthetic ADH replacement results in water reabsorption and normalization of urine output, urine-specific gravity, and serum electrolytes. Vital signs are normal, output is proportional to intake, and body weight is stable in patients with well controlled DI.

CASE STUDY: EPISODE 3

Approximately 8 hours after Ms. Andrews arrives in the neurosurgical intensive care unit after undergoing transsphenoidal hypophysectomy, the nurse notes that the patient has had 200 to 300 mL/hr urine output for the last 3 hours. Urine-specific gravity is 1.002, and serum electrolyte results include a sodium level of 148 mEq/L and an osmolality of 292 mOsm/kg. The patient's blood pressure is 92/56 mm Hg with a heart rate of 110 bpm. The neurosurgeon is notified, and the patient is started on a Pitressin (vasopressin) IV infusion…

> **⚠ Safety Alert** Fluid administration must be closely monitored in the patient after transsphenoidal hypophysectomy. The administration of hypotonic solutions in the postoperative patient with a normal serum sodium level after transsphenoidal hypophysectomy increases the risk of fluid shifts and can lead to cerebral edema and an increase in intracranial pressure.

Syndrome of Inappropriate Antidiuretic Hormone

Epidemiology

The **syndrome of inappropriate antidiuretic hormone (SIADH)** is a disorder related to an increase in ADH. Because the action of ADH is to reabsorb water in the kidneys, SIADH is characterized by water overload and resultant hyponatremia caused by hemodilution. Causes of SIADH vary and include CNS disorders such as tumors in the brain or neck, side effects of medications such as NSAIDs, psychotropic medications, and bronchogenic carcinoma. There are no specific relationships between the developments of SIADH and race, ethnicity, sex, or age.

Pathophysiology

The excess secretion of ADH in the patient with SIADH leads to reabsorption of water in the kidneys. Hyponatremia develops that is secondary to hemodilution; there is no decrease in total body sodium. The excess ADH results in decreased urine output with an increase in the concentration (increased specific gravity) and osmolality of the urine.

Clinical Manifestations

The clinical presentation of the patient with SIADH is primarily associated with the resultant hyponatremia. Earlier findings include anorexia, nausea, and malaise followed by headache, irritability, confusion, and weakness. While serum sodium levels continue to decrease, the patient may have seizures or become comatose, particularly when serum sodium levels fall below 120 mEq/L. The neurological signs associated with the hyponatremia are related to osmotic fluid shifts in the brain that lead to cerebral edema and increased intracranial pressure.

Management

Medical Management

Diagnosis

Diagnostic evaluation of SIADH includes monitoring and trending urine-specific gravity and serum and urine osmolality and electrolytes (see Table 41.4). Hyponatremia (serum sodium level less than 135 mEq/L) develops, along with a decrease in serum osmolality (<275 mOsm/kg). Urine output decreases, and there are increases in both urine-specific gravity (>1.030) and urine osmolality. This results in a clinical presentation that is unusual. Typically, patients presenting with scant, concentrated urine would have signs indicative of dehydration, including elevated serum sodium, serum osmolality, and urine-specific gravity. However, in patients with SIADH caused by excessive ADH secretion, they present with scant urine output and elevated urine-specific gravity but a decrease in serum sodium and osmolality. This inconsistent clinical presentation is often a key in recognizing the patient with SIADH.

Fluid Management and Medications

Medical management is primarily focused on treating the hyponatremia. The patient is placed on fluid restriction, usually less than 1,000 mL/day. With severe hyponatremia, IV administration of 3% saline may be administered, but this requires very close monitoring because of the hyperosmolarity of this solution and it is typically infused via a central venous access device. Diuretics may be administered to increase urine output. Demeclocycline (Declomycin), a tetracycline derivative, may also be used because it increases water excretion by the kidneys.

Connection Check 41.5

The nurse correlates which finding to a diagnosis of SIADH?
A. Polyuria
B. Polyphagia
C. Decreased urine output
D. Glucosuria

Complications

The primary complications seen in patients with SIADH are related to decreasing serum sodium levels. While the sodium concentration drops below 120 mEq/L, life-threatening complications are likely to occur, including seizures and coma. Because of fluid shifts in the cerebral cortex, cerebral edema and increased intracranial pressure may develop, further exacerbating neurological complications.

Nursing Management

Assessment and Analysis

In the patient with SIADH, the increased reabsorption of water is directly a result of excessive secretion of ADH. Assessment findings include oliguria, increased specific gravity, and increased urine osmolality. The resulting hemodilution secondary to water retention leads to a decrease in serum sodium and osmolality. While water retention increases, the patient may complain of anorexia and nausea, weakness, and headache. While serum sodium levels continue to decrease, the nurse monitors for confusion and irritability. If the serum sodium level drops below 120 mEq/L, the patient is at risk of seizures.

Nursing Diagnoses

- **Fluid volume excess** related to increased water reabsorption secondary to increased ADH secretion
- **High risk for injury** related to cerebral edema and CNS dysfunction
- **Knowledge deficit** related to required fluid restriction

Nursing Interventions

▪ Assessments

- Neurological status
  Fluid overload with resulting hyponatremia may lead to confusion, headache, and changes in level of consciousness.
- Intake and output
  Excess secretion of ADH leads to reabsorption of water in the renal tubules.
- Serum sodium and osmolality
  Serum sodium and osmolality levels decrease secondary to dilution.
- Urine-specific gravity and urine osmolality
  With reabsorption of water in the kidneys, the urine is concentrated, resulting in increased specific gravity and urine osmolality.
- Skin integrity
  Fluid reabsorption may result in skin tautness.

▪ Actions

- Restrict fluids
  Fluids are restricted to concentrate serum sodium. The nurse needs to plan how the fluid will be distributed over the day.
- Administer demeclocycline (Declomycin)
  Demeclocycline increases excretion of water from the kidneys.

- Administer 3% saline as ordered via central IV line
  Hypertonic saline solution to increase serum sodium levels
- Implement seizure precautions
  Risk of seizures increases with hyponatremia, particularly when serum sodium levels fall below 120 mEq/L.

▪ Teaching

- Disease process and management
  Because of complications associated with hyponatremia, it is important for the patient and family to understand the pathophysiology and treatment of SIADH.
- Follow fluid restriction
  It is important that the patient follow restrictions to decrease exacerbating fluid overload.
- Signs of fluid overload
  Signs of fluid overload may be associated with falling serum levels that increase the risk of seizures and other neurological changes.

Evaluating Care Outcomes

Syndrome of inappropriate antidiuretic hormone (SIADH) is managed with the combination of fluid restriction and specific medications that increase serum sodium levels. Stable body weight and relatively equal intake and output are indicative of effective management of SIADH in this patient population. Serum sodium, serum osmolality, urine-specific gravity, and urine osmolality return to normal with effective treatment. The patient and family should be knowledgeable of the signs of water overload and the clinical manifestations they should report to their healthcare provider. Table 41.5 provides a comparison of the clinical manifestations of DI and SIADH.

Table 41.5 Comparison of Diabetes Insipidus and Syndrome of Inappropriate Antidiuretic Hormone

Clinical Manifestations	DI	SIADH
Urine output	Increased	Decreased
Urine-specific gravity	Decreased	Increased
Serum sodium (Na)	Increased	Decreased
Serum osmolality	Increased	Decreased
Hematocrit	Increased	Decreased
Blood pressure	Decreased	May be slightly increased
Heart rate	Increased	No specific change in rate
Pulse	Weak, accelerated	Full, bounding
Thirst	Increased	No specific change

DI, Diabetes insipidus; *SIADH*, syndrome of inappropriate antidiuretic hormone.

Making Connections

CASE STUDY: WRAP-UP

Ms. Andrews responds favorably to the IV Pitressin, and after 24 hours she is started on DDAVP intranasally. Her blood pressure is 110/68 mm Hg with a heart rate of 88 bpm. Urine output has decreased to an average of 50 mL/hr, and IV fluids are discontinued because she is taking oral fluids. Discharge planning is initiated, and she is scheduled to be discharged on the fourth postoperative day. She is discharged on DDAVP. The nurse incorporates teaching about activity restrictions related to transsphenoidal hypophysectomy.

Case Study Questions

1. On review of Ms. Andrews' admission clinical presentation, which clinical manifestations are most related to excessive growth hormone?
    A. Headache
    B. Enlarged hands
    C. Visual changes
    D. Nausea
2. Ms. Andrews is ordered to receive bromocriptine mesylate (Parlodel) for the treatment of her tumor. The nurse correlates which rationale for this medication?
    A. Decreases serum glucose levels
    B. Decreases water reabsorption in the kidneys
    C. Decreases secretion of growth hormone
    D. Decreases secretion of ADH
3. Which laboratory result does the nurse correlate with a diagnosis of diabetes insipidus (DI)?
    A. Serum osmolality, 285 mOsm/kg
    B. Serum sodium, 132 mEq/L
    C. Hematocrit, 32%
    D. Urine-specific gravity, 1.001
4. In providing care to Ms. Andrews after she undergoes a transsphenoidal hypophysectomy, the nurse prioritizes which intervention?
    A. Maintaining the patient in a flat, supine position
    B. Instructing the patient to cough and deep breathe
    C. Monitoring for clear fluid drainage from the nose
    D. Limiting exposure to bright lights

5. The nurse monitors for which therapeutic effect as a result of the administration of Pitressin?
    A. Decreased urine output
    B. Decreased blood pressure
    C. Decreased serum glucose
    D. Decreased thirst

CHAPTER SUMMARY

Disorders of the hypothalamus and pituitary gland adversely affect many normal body functions. Anterior pituitary disorders are classified as hypofunction and hyperfunction, and the clinical presentations of each disorder are directly related to the involved hormones and their target glands or tissues. Hormones secreted from the anterior lobe of the pituitary include adrenocorticotropic hormone (ACTH), follicle-stimulating hormone (FSH), luteinizing hormone (LH), growth hormone (GH), prolactin, and thyroid-stimulating hormone (TSH). The posterior lobe of the pituitary gland stores and secretes antidiuretic hormone (ADH) and oxytocin.

Deficiencies of one of the anterior pituitary hormones results in changes in metabolic or sexual function dependent on which hormone level is decreased. The effects of a decrease in one or more of the anterior pituitary hormones determine the pathophysiology of hypopituitarism. A decrease in ACTH leads to a decrease in release of the mineralocorticoids and glucocorticoids from the adrenal cortex. A decrease in secretion of TSH leads to a decrease in thyroid gland hormone secretion. Alterations in sexual and reproductive functioning are caused by decreased secretion of the gonadotropins (LH and FSH), and decreases in growth hormone affect the strength and integrity of bones and other tissues.

Hyperpituitarism is characterized by excess secretion of one or more of the anterior pituitary hormones. As with hypopituitarism, the pathophysiology and clinical presentation depend on which anterior pituitary hormone secretion is elevated. Treatment of these disorders is guided by the hormones involved. Hypersecretion of growth hormone is characterized by increases in bone density and changes in appearance and size of face, hands, and feet.

Diabetes insipidus develops secondary to a lack of ADH, which results in decreased water reabsorption in the kidney and increased output of large amounts of dilute urine. The urine-specific gravity falls below 1.005, and the patient develops hypernatremia secondary to water loss. Treatment focuses on preventing dehydration and replacing deficient ADH. Daily doses of DDAVP are usually used to treat DI.

Syndrome of inappropriate antidiuretic hormone (SIADH) is a disorder that develops secondary to CNS disorders, most often a tumor, from specific lung cancers, or as a side effect of certain medications. Oversecretion of SIADH leads to increased water reabsorption in the kidneys, resulting in a decrease in urine output, drop in serum sodium level less than 135 mEq/L, and decreased serum osmolality. Treatment focuses on reestablishing normal serum levels because the patient is at risk of seizures, water intoxication, and other neurological complications secondary to hyponatremia. Transsphenoidal hypophysectomy is a surgical approach used to remove pituitary tumors.

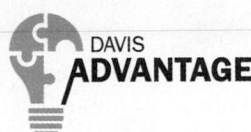

DAVIS
ADVANTAGE

To explore learning resources for this chapter, go to **Davis Advantage** and find:
– Answers to in-text questions
– Chapter Resources and Activities
– NCLEX®-Style Chapter Review Questions
– Bibliography

Chapter 42

Coordinating Care for Patients With Adrenal Disorders

Janice Hoffman

LEARNING OUTCOMES

Content in this chapter is designed to assist in:

1. Describing the epidemiology of adrenal disorders
2. Correlating clinical manifestations to pathophysiological processes of:
   a. Adrenal cortex insufficiency
   b. Adrenal cortex hyperfunction
   c. Pheochromocytoma
3. Describing the diagnostic results used to confirm the diagnoses of adrenal disorders
4. Discussing the medical management of:
   a. Adrenal cortex insufficiency
   b. Adrenal cortex hyperfunction
   c. Pheochromocytoma
5. Explaining the presentation and management of adrenal crisis
6. Developing a comprehensive plan of nursing care for patients with adrenal disorders
7. Designing a plan of care that includes pharmacological, dietary, and lifestyle considerations for patients with adrenal disorders

ESSENTIAL TERMS

Acute adrenal crisis
Adrenal insufficiency
Adrenalectomy
Addison's disease
Aldosterone
Catecholamine
Conn's syndrome
Cortisol
Cushing's disease
Cushing's syndrome
Glucocorticoids
Hyperaldosteronism
Hypercortisolism
Mineralocorticoids
Pheochromocytoma
Virilization

CONCEPTS

- Assessment
- Fluid and Electrolyte Balance
- Medication
- Metabolism

Finding Connections

CASE STUDY: EPISODE 1

Follow this patient throughout the chapter.

Melinda Davis, a 32-year-old female, makes an appointment with her adult nurse practitioner because of changes in her menstrual cycle and concerns about difficulty getting pregnant. Ms. Davis is employed in a day-care center, and she and her spouse have been trying to conceive for approximately 10 months...

INTRODUCTION

One adrenal gland is located on top of each kidney, and each measures approximately 5-cm long, 1-cm thick, and 3-cm wide. Each adrenal gland has an inner core, the medulla, and a thick outer covering, the cortex, both with distinct endocrine functions.

Under the control of the anterior pituitary gland, the adrenal cortex secretes **glucocorticoids** (cortisol), **mineralocorticoids** (aldosterone), and sex hormones (androgens and estrogens). (See Chapters 64–67 for details about the sex hormones.) **Cortisol** is the primary glucocorticoid, and its actions include carbohydrate, fat, and protein metabolism; suppression of the immune response; and control of the body's stress response. **Aldosterone** is the primary mineralocorticoid, and its primary actions are to promote sodium and water reabsorption and potassium excretion in the kidneys. Table 42.1 presents an overview of adrenal gland hormones and their actions.

ADRENAL CORTICAL INSUFFICIENCY

Epidemiology

Adrenal insufficiency may result from destruction of the adrenal glands (primary insufficiency or **Addison's disease**), decreased secretion of adrenocorticotropic hormone (ACTH) from the anterior pituitary gland (secondary insufficiency), or dysfunction of the hypothalamus (tertiary insufficiency). Nonspecific autoimmune destruction of the adrenal gland is the most common cause of primary adrenal insufficiency. Other causes of primary adrenal insufficiency include infectious, cancerous, and traumatic processes that lead to direct insults to the adrenal cortex. Secondary and tertiary adrenal insufficiencies are related to disorders of the anterior pituitary gland and hypothalamus, respectively. Despite the etiology, the clinical presentations of adrenal insufficiency are similar. Females are most often affected by adrenal insufficiency, and it has a peaked incidence in people 30 to 50 years of age.

Connection Check 42.1

The nurse recognizes which patient is at greatest risk for adrenal insufficiency?
A. A 19-year-old male
B. A 35-year-old female
C. A 45-year-old male
D. An 80-year-old female

Pathophysiology

The pathophysiology of adrenal insufficiency may be associated with decreased secretion of corticotropin-releasing hormone (CRH) from the hypothalamus, decreased secretion of ACTH from the anterior pituitary gland, or decreased

Table 42.1 Overview of Adrenal Gland Hormones

Gland	Hormone	Target	Action
Adrenal cortex	Glucocorticoids (cortisol)	Liver	Promotes gluconeogenesis (increasing blood glucose)
		Cells of the body	Decreases glucose use
			Promotes protein catabolism
			Promotes fat synthesis
		Bone marrow	Suppresses inflammatory processes
	Mineralocorticoids (aldosterone)	Distal tubules and collecting ducts in the kidney	Promotes sodium reabsorption and potassium excretion by the kidney
Adrenal medulla	Catecholamines (epinephrine and norepinephrine)	Cells of the body	Mimics actions of the sympathetic nervous system

secretion of glucocorticoids and mineralocorticoids from the adrenal cortex. Patients who are prescribed exogenous corticosteroids for longer than 2 weeks are at risk for acute adrenal insufficiency (**acute adrenal crisis**) if the medications are abruptly discontinued.

Clinical Manifestations

Clinical manifestations of adrenal insufficiency usually present after 90% of the adrenal cortex is destroyed or nonfunctional. While the circulating levels of cortisol and aldosterone fall, the hypothalamus and anterior pituitary gland increase secretion of CRH and ACTH, respectively. Because melanocyte-stimulating hormone (MSH) and ACTH share a progenitor (ancestor) hormone, there is an associated increase in secretion of MSH, leading to a darkened, bronzed hyperpigmentation that accompanies the increased secretion of ACTH (Fig. 42.1).

Secondary to the decreased secretion of cortisol and aldosterone, the patient presents with weakness, weight loss, fatigue, nausea, abdominal pain, gastroenteritis, and emotional lability. Changes in mood include irritability, depression, and inability to concentrate. Hyperpigmentation of the skin and mucous membranes and decreased pubic and axillary hair (secondary to decreased secretion of sex hormones) are also observed. As the loss of sodium and water continues, the patient may develop dehydration and hypotension.

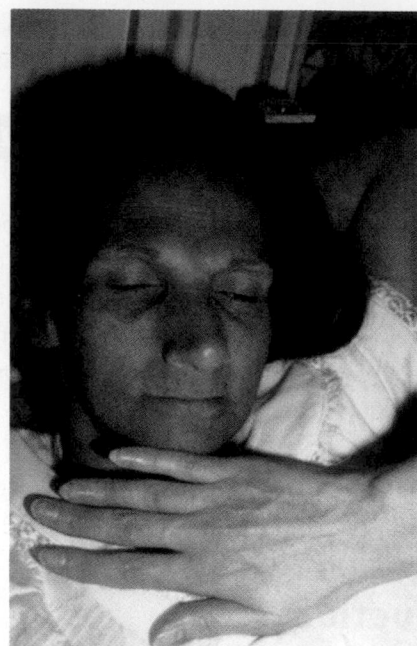

FIGURE 42.1 Darkened, bronzed hyperpigmentation that accompanies the increased secretion of adrenocorticotropic hormone (ACTH) is observed in adrenal insufficiency.

Connection Check 42.2

The nurse correlates which clinical manifestation with the pathophysiology of adrenal insufficiency?
A. Heat intolerance
B. Weight gain
C. Peripheral edema
D. Hypoglycemia

Management

Medical Management

Diagnosis

Diagnostic evaluation of adrenal insufficiency includes tests of the hypothalamic-pituitary axis and adrenal cortex, as well as serum electrolytes (Table 42.2). Hyponatremia and hyperkalemia develop secondary to decreased aldosterone secretion. Direct measurement of serum cortisol levels is performed in the morning because of changes in levels associated with daily activities. Cortisol levels are highest in the morning (between 6 a.m. and 8 a.m.), and levels up to 25 mcg/dL are considered normal. Levels less than 3 mcg/dL are diagnostic for adrenal insufficiency. Serum corticotropin (ACTH) levels may also be obtained, and levels greater than 100 mg/mL are diagnostic of primary adrenal insufficiency. Diagnostic evaluations of the hypothalamic-pituitary axis

Table 42.2 Laboratory Tests for Adrenal Disorders

Test	Normal Range for Adults	Significance
Cortisol	5–25 mcg/dL (morning)	Decreased in hypocortisolism (Addison's)
	3–16 mcg/dL (afternoon)	Elevated in hypercortisolism (Cushing's)
Glucose	65–99 mg/dL	Decreased in hypocortisolism (Addison's)
		Increased in hypercortisolism (Cushing's)
Potassium	3.5–5.0 mEq/L	Increased in hypofunction of the adrenal cortex
		Decreased in hyperfunction of the adrenal cortex
Sodium	135–145 mEq/L	Decreased in hypocortisolism
		Increased in hypercortisolism
		Decreased in hypoaldosteronism
		Increased in hyperaldosteronism

to evaluate secondary and tertiary adrenal insufficiency are presented in Table 42.3.

Imaging studies are also used in the evaluation of adrenal insufficiency. Both computed tomography (CT) and magnetic resonance imaging (MRI) may be used to assess for changes in the size and morphology of the adrenal gland. Shrinking of the adrenal gland is associated with autoimmune destruction, whereas adrenal gland enlargement is often observed with infectious processes.

Medications and Fluid Management

Replacement of cortisol is the definitive treatment for adrenal insufficiency. Patients presenting with acute adrenal insufficiency require emergency stabilization with IV fluids and glucose, along with IV administration of glucocorticoids (cortisol) such as 50 to 100 mg of hydrocortisone sodium succinate (Solu-Cortef) or 4 to 12 mg of dexamethasone (Decadron). One of the advantages of hydrocortisone is that it has both glucocorticoid and mineralocorticoid actions. The patient requires close monitoring, including frequent assessments of vital signs, level of consciousness, and serum sodium, glucose, and potassium levels to ensure an adequate dosage of cortisol. In patients presenting with hyperkalemia, treatment with potassium binding or excreting agents (Kayexalate) are indicated.

Complications

Acute adrenal insufficiency, or adrenal crisis, is a life-threatening emergency that leads to severe hypovolemia and hypotension. Risk factors for adrenal crisis are seen in patients who have underlying adrenal hypofunction and who undergo stressful events such as trauma, surgery, and infections. Because of the decrease in aldosterone and cortisol, the patient loses sodium accompanied by fluid loss.

The patient is also at risk for hyperkalemia and hypoglycemia associated with lack of both mineralocorticoids and glucocorticoids. Patients with primary adrenal insufficiency require additional doses of glucocorticoid during periods of stress such as surgery, trauma, or infection.

Nursing Management
Assessment and Analysis

The clinical manifestations of adrenal insufficiency, whether acute or chronic, are directly related to the actions of the adrenal cortex hormones. The nurse correlates adrenal insufficiency with the following clinical manifestations:

- Hypotension associated with loss of sodium (hyponatremia) and water
- Hypoglycemia associated with decreased cortisol
- Hyperkalemia associated with decreased aldosterone
- Muscular weakness associated with decreased glucocorticoid and hyperkalemia
- Abdominal pain, nausea, weight loss
- Emotional lability

Nursing Diagnoses

- **Fluid volume deficit** associated with sodium and water losses secondary to lack of aldosterone and cortisol
- **Risk for unstable blood glucose level** associated with decreased cortisol secretion from the adrenal cortex
- **Risk for decreased cardiac output** associated with acute adrenal crisis (loss of sodium and water)
- **Body image disturbance** associated with hyperpigmentation secondary to increased secretion of MSH from the anterior pituitary gland

---

Table 42.3 Evaluation of the Hypothalamic-Pituitary Axis in Adrenal Insufficiency

Hypothalamic-Pituitary Axis

Test	Procedure	Results
Corticotropic (Cortrosyn) stimulation test	Cortrosyn, a synthetic corticotropin (form of adrenocorticotropic hormone), 350 mg, is administered intravenously followed by measurement of serum cortisol levels 30 and 60 minutes later.	Cortisol levels of 13–17 mcg/dL are indeterminate. Cortisol levels of less than 13 mcg/dL suggest adrenal insufficiency because Cortrosyn should lead to an increase in cortisol levels. Peak serum cortisol levels greater than 18 mcg/dL exclude the diagnosis of adrenal insufficiency.
Insulin tolerance test	The insulin tolerance test uses hypoglycemic stress to induce cortisol production. The peak serum cortisol response is measured after an insulin challenge of 0.1–0.15 units/kg. The test requires close monitoring of the patient and is contraindicated in patients with a history of seizures or cardiovascular disease.	A cortisol level of less than 18 mcg/dL and a serum glucose level of less than 40 mg/dL suggest adrenal insufficiency.

Nursing Interventions

▪ Assessments

- Vital signs
  Decreased blood pressure occurs secondary to lack of aldosterone, leading to loss of sodium and water. While blood pressure decreases, there is a compensatory increase in pulse rate. Irregular heart rate may also be associated with hyperkalemia.
- Monitor intake and output
  Fluid loss occurs secondary to lack of mineralocorticoid and glucocorticoid, leading to loss of sodium followed by loss of water through the kidneys.
- Serum sodium, glucose, and potassium
  Decreased gluconeogenesis occurs because of lack of glucocorticoid. Lack of glucocorticoid and mineralocorticoid leads to loss of sodium and water and retention of potassium.
- Hematocrit and blood urea nitrogen (BUN)
  Fluid losses lead to hemoconcentration that may increase hematocrit and serum BUN levels.
- Serum cortisol levels
  Random serum cortisol levels of less than 3 mcg/dL or levels of less than 13 mcg/dL with a corticotropic stimulation test suggest adrenal insufficiency.

▪ Actions

- Ensure vascular access for administration of IV fluids containing sodium and glucose
  Loss of water occurs secondary to increased excretion of sodium (direct action of aldosterone). Initiating IV access is complicated with hypovolemia.
- Administer corticosteroid
  Definitive treatment of acute adrenal insufficiency (adrenal crisis) is administration of IV cortisone.
- Maintain safety precautions such as placing the patient's bed in the lowest position and always providing assistance when the patient is getting out of bed
  Postural hypotension may develop secondary to fluid losses, placing the patient at greater risk of falls.

▪ Teaching

- Take oral hormone replacement daily
  Adrenal cortex replacement is required to maintain fluid balance and normal glucose levels.
- Wear medical alert bracelet at all times
  Wearing the medical alert bracelet reduces time to definitive treatment in an emergency situation.
- Clinical manifestations of adrenal insufficiency
  It is important that the patient (and family) is able to detect early signs of adrenal insufficiency because it can deteriorate to adrenal crisis, which is a life-threatening emergency.
- Signs of corticosteroid excess
  Over-replacement of glucocorticoids results in adverse effects including weight gain and osteoporosis.

Evaluating Care Outcomes

Patients with adrenal insufficiency can achieve normal adrenal cortex function with treatment with exogenous corticosteroids. Positive outcomes include vital signs within normal limits, increased energy, stable weight, and emotional stability. During periods of stress, such as invasive procedures, an increase in exogenous corticosteroids is often necessary. It is important for all healthcare providers to be aware of adrenal insufficiency, particularly when prescribing medications such as sedatives, narcotics, or anesthetic agents. The patient and family should be knowledgeable about the clinical manifestations of adrenal insufficiency and what changes require immediate reporting to the healthcare provider.

Connection Check 42.3

A patient has been receiving doses of prednisone for treatment of rheumatoid arthritis for the past 3 months. If this medication is suddenly discontinued, for which complication is the patient at risk?

A. Hypovolemia
B. Hypernatremia
C. Hypothermia
D. Hyperglycemia

ADRENAL CORTEX HYPERFUNCTION

Epidemiology

Adrenal cortex hyperfunction may be secondary to excessive secretion of glucocorticoids (**hypercortisolism**) or excessive secretion of aldosterone (**hyperaldosteronism**). Hypercortisolism is categorized as primary (adrenal cortex disorder), secondary (anterior pituitary gland disorder), or tertiary (hypothalamic etiology). The term *Cushing's* is often used to describe hyperfunction of the adrenal cortex. **Cushing's disease** describes a condition caused by excessive hormone production from an anterior pituitary tumor (70%) producing excessive ACTH or excess hormone secretion from a primary tumor of the adrenal cortex (15%). Approximately 15% of cases of hyperfunction are related to ectopic tumors, usually in the lung, that secrete ACTH. **Cushing's syndrome** is a more broad term and may be used to describe an excess of hormone production (CRH, ACTH, glucocorticoids) or administration of exogenous corticosteroid medications. Despite the etiology, the clinical presentations of hypercortisolism are similar. Females are five times more likely to develop this disorder, and the peak incidence of hypersecreting tumors of the adrenal and pituitary glands is in the 25- to 40-year age range.

Patients may also present with hyperaldosteronism (**Conn's syndrome**). Because the primary actions of aldosterone are sodium and water reabsorption and potassium excretion, hypertension and hypokalemia develop. The incidence of hyperaldosteronism is significantly greater in African Americans than in Caucasians. There is an autosomal dominant pattern of inheritance for primary hyperaldosteronism, with females more at risk than males.

Pathophysiology

Excessive circulating glucocorticoid (cortisol) is the pathophysiological process associated with primary hypercortisolism. Excessive secretion of ACTH from the anterior pituitary gland leads to hypercortisolism through its effects on the adrenal cortex.

Clinical Manifestations

The clinical manifestations of adrenal cortex hyperfunction (Fig. 42.2) are directly related to hypersecretion of these hormones and include hyperglycemia, fluid retention, hypokalemia, abnormal fat distribution, and decreased muscle mass. The maldistribution of fats and changes in muscle are related to the effects that glucocorticoids have on fat and protein metabolism. In female patients, clinical manifestations include **virilization** (male sexual characteristics developing in females), breast atrophy, vocal changes (deepening), and amenorrhea. Overproduction of cortisol also affects the immune system by decreasing inflammatory and immune responses. Lymphocytes are also destroyed

secondary to high levels of circulating cortisol, further placing the patient at risk for infection.

Hyperaldosteronism, usually secondary to a hypersecreting tumor of the adrenal cortex, or hyperplasia, results in increased aldosterone production. Secondary to the action of this hormone, sodium and water reabsorption and potassium excretion are increased. Elevated blood pressure is associated with the sodium and water retention, and cardiac irregularities (atrial or ventricular tachyarrhythmias or appearance of U waves) are secondary to hypokalemia.

Management

Diagnosis of Hypercortisolism

Diagnostic evaluation of hypercortisolism includes assessment of cortisol levels, results of suppression tests, and serum electrolytes (see Table 42.2). Because aldosterone secretion results in both sodium and water reabsorption, there may not be an increase in serum sodium (secondary to water reabsorption); however, the patient does present with hyperglycemia (secondary to glucocorticoid activity) and hypokalemia. Measurement of urinary free cortisol is used as an initial screening tool because it measures urine cortisol during a 24-hour period. The overnight dexamethasone suppression test is another tool to evaluate hypercortisolism, specifically whether the administration of exogenous glucocorticoid (dexamethasone) inhibits the secretion of ACTH that, in turn, decreases stimulation of cortisol release. In this diagnostic study, dexamethasone, 1 mg, is administered at 11 p.m. followed by the collection of a serum cortisol level at 8 a.m. the next morning. The results are based on whether suppression of cortisol secretion occurs secondary to the administration of exogenous glucocorticoid. If the morning level is less than 2 to 3 mg/dL, normal functioning of the hypothalamic-pituitary-adrenal axis is determined. The ACTH level can also be measured, and changes may be secondary to changes in the secretion of CRH from the hypothalamus.

Medical Management of Hypercortisolism

Medical management of hypercortisolism focuses on preventing complications associated with fluid overload, changes in immune status, changes in skin integrity, and changes in body structure. Medications that interfere with ACTH and glucocorticoid production are used in the treatment of hypercortisolism. Aminoglutethimide is an example of a medication that interferes with cortisol production in the adrenal cortex, and cyproheptadine impacts ACTH production. With both types of medications, the nurse must monitor for signs of adrenal suppression including hypoglycemia and hyponatremia. Pasireotide (Signifor), a subcutaneous somatostatin analog, is a medication used to inhibit release of corticotropin in patients with Cushing's disease secondary to a pituitary adenoma.

Surgical Management of Hypercortisolism

Surgical management of hypercortisolism is based on the etiology of the disorder. If the etiology is a pituitary tumor, a transsphenoidal hypophysectomy (discussed in Chapter 41)

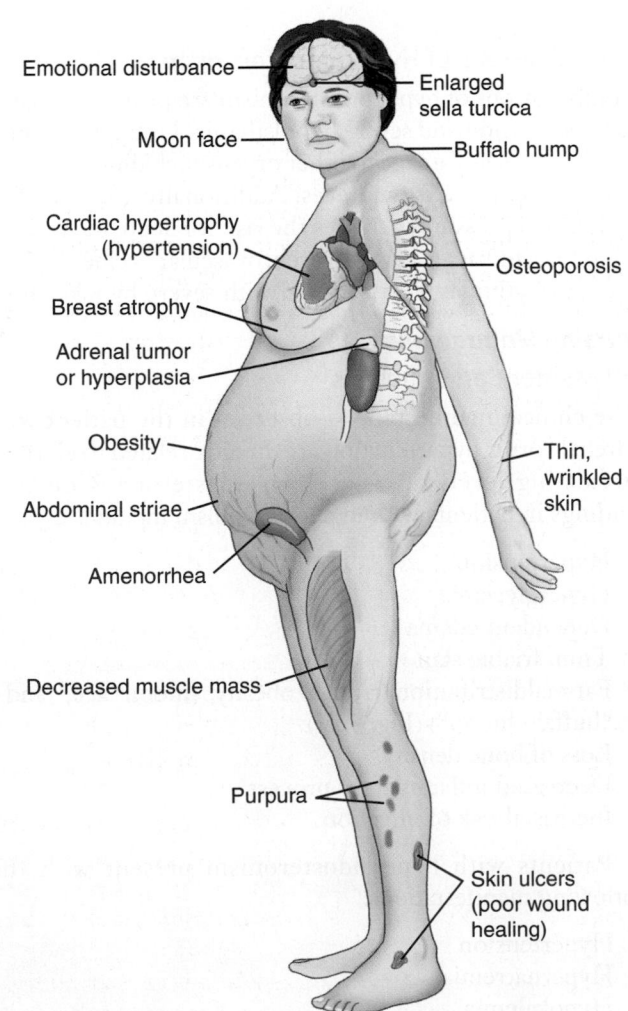

Emotional disturbance
Enlarged sella turcica
Moon face
Buffalo hump
Cardiac hypertrophy (hypertension)
Osteoporosis
Breast atrophy
Adrenal tumor or hyperplasia
Obesity
Thin, wrinkled skin
Abdominal striae
Amenorrhea
Decreased muscle mass
Purpura
Skin ulcers (poor wound healing)

FIGURE 42.2 Clinical manifestations of hypercortisolism.

is performed. With hypersecreting tumors of the adrenal cortex, an **adrenalectomy** (removal of the adrenal gland) may be indicated (presented later in this chapter). Radiation therapy, including stereotactic radiosurgery of the pituitary gland, may also be used in the management of tumors of the pituitary gland (see Evidence-Based Practice).

Evidence-Based Practice

Stereotactic Radiosurgery for Cushing's Disease

Cushing's disease (CD) caused by adrenocorticotropic hormone-secreting pituitary tumors may be treated with stereotactic radiosurgery (SRS). This international, multi-center study examined the control of hypercortisolism (defined as normalization of free urinary cortisol). The cumulative initial control of hypercortisolism was 80% at 10 years, with a 14.5 month mean time to cortisol normalization. The overall rate of hypercortisolism control was 64% in 10 years. The findings of this study support SRS for CD because it frequently controls hypercortisolism but recommend long-term endocrine follow-up after SRS because recurrences can occur.

Mehta, G.U., Ding, D., Patibandia, M.R., Kano, H., Sisterson, N., Su, Y.H., ... Liscak, R. (2017). Stereotactic radiosurgery for Cushing disease: results of an international, multicenter study. *Journal of Clinical Endocrinology & Metabolism, 102*(11), 4284–4291.

Diagnosis of Hyperaldosteronism

Hyperaldosteronism is diagnosed through evaluation of serum electrolytes as well as imaging studies. Elevated serum aldosterone levels as well as hypokalemia and hypernatremia are observed. Because hyperaldosteronism is usually secondary to hypersecreting tumors or hyperplasia, CT, or MRI may demonstrate enlargement or changes of the adrenal cortex.

Medical Management of Hyperaldosteronism

Management aims focus on controlling hypertension, managing hypokalemia, and determining the etiology of hyperaldosteronism. Hypertension is treated with spironolactone (Aldactone), a potassium-sparing diuretic. The patient's potassium and sodium levels are measured closely while on this medication. Potassium supplementation may also be required in treating hyperaldosteronism because loss of potassium is caused by elevated aldosterone.

Surgical Management of Hyperaldosteronism

Surgical management includes an adrenalectomy to remove hypersecreting tumors of the adrenal cortex.

Complications
Complications of Hypercortisolism

Patients with hypercortisolism are at risk for complications associated with excessive cortisol levels. Osteoporosis may develop relative to the effects of cortisol on bone density and can increase the risk of pathological fractures. In patients with hypercortisolism secondary to exogenous corticosteroid therapy, acute adrenal crisis may result with the abrupt withdrawal of this medication. Elevated serum glucose may complicate the management of diabetes mellitus in patients with this disorder. Gastrointestinal bleeding may develop as a result of decreased mucus production in the gastrointestinal tract, decreased blood flow, and release of hydrochloric acid secondary to the effects of cortisol.

> **⚠ Safety Alert** Patients receiving exogenous cortico-steroids (for their inflammatory actions) are often prescribed medications that serve as gastrointestinal prophylaxis. Because of the effects of corticosteroids on the gastrointestinal tract, the patient must be assessed for complaints of gastrointestinal distress and gastrointestinal bleeding.

Complications of Hyperaldosteronism

Complications of hyperaldosteronism are primarily related to hypertension and severe hypokalemia. Untreated hypertension leads to damage to other organs including the heart, vasculature, kidneys, and eyes. Additionally, uncontrolled high blood pressure increases the risk for acute myocardial infarction and acute stroke (cerebrovascular accident). Cardiac dysrhythmias are associated with severe hypokalemia.

Nursing Management
Assessment and Analysis

The clinical manifestations observed in the patient with adrenal cortex hyperfunction are directly related to elevated circulating levels of cortisol or aldosterone. Common findings in patients with hypercortisolism include:

- Hypertension
- Hyperglycemia
- Dependent edema
- Thin, friable skin
- Fat maldistribution (truncal obesity, "moon face," and "buffalo hump") (Fig. 42.2)
- Loss of bone density
- Decreased inflammatory process
- Increased risk of infection

Patients with hyperaldosteronism present with the following manifestations:

- Hypertension
- Hypernatremia
- Hypokalemia
- Headache

Nursing Diagnoses

Hypercortisolism:

- **Fluid volume excess** associated with increased sodium and water reabsorption secondary to excess glucocorticoid secretion
- **Body image disturbance** associated with development of truncal obesity and fat deposition secondary to excess glucocorticoid secretion
- **Risk for infection** associated with immunosuppression
- **Deficient knowledge** associated with diagnosis of hypercortisolism

Hyperaldosteronism:

- **Fluid volume excess** associated with increased sodium and water reabsorption secondary to excess aldosterone secretion
- **Risk for decreased cardiac output** associated with cardiac dysrhythmias secondary to hypokalemia
- **Deficient knowledge** associated with management of hyperaldosteronism

Nursing Interventions

■ Assessments

- Vital signs
  Suppressed immune function secondary to hypercortisolism increases the risk of infection. Small increases in body temperature may be significant, and signs of infection may be masked because of immune suppression. Blood pressure and heart rate may increase secondary to fluid retention.
- Intake and output
  Monitoring is important to evaluate trends once treatment has been started. Urine output should increase and signs of fluid overload should decrease if treatment is effective.
- Serum glucose, potassium
  Glucose levels rise secondary to increased secretion of glucocorticoid. Potassium levels also fall secondary to increased excretion via the kidneys secondary to glucocorticoid and mineralocorticoid activity.
- Daily weight
  Weight gain occurs secondary to fluid retention secondary to sodium and water reabsorption. Peripheral edema may develop.
- Skin
  Thinning skin and increased friability develop secondary to excess cortisol.
- Fat distribution
  Actions of glucocorticoid affect fat metabolism, leading to maldistribution of fat including truncal obesity, moon face, and buffalo hump.
- Muscle mass
  Muscle atrophy develops secondary to altered protein metabolism.
- Wound healing
  Delayed wound healing occurs associated with the suppressed inflammatory response.

■ Actions

- Administer medications that interfere with production/secretion of cortisol
  Decreases secretion of cortisol
- Head of bed elevated 45 degrees
  Decreases work of breathing that may develop secondary to fluid retention
- Turn patient frequently and protect skin from injury
  Thinning of skin along with increased friability of skin accompanied by fluid retention increase the chances of skin injury caused by pressure or friction.

■ Teaching

- Overview of disease process
  It is important that the patient (and family) is able to detect early signs of both hypercortisolism and adrenal insufficiency.
- Importance of taking prescribed medications
  Medications that interfere with cortisol production are key to disease management.
- Modify salt in diet as directed by provider
  Excessive salt intake may further exacerbate fluid retention.

Connection Check 42.4

The nurse monitors for which effects of daily cortisol therapy on a patient's circulating levels of adrenocorticotropic hormone (ACTH) and aldosterone?

A. Decreased ACTH, decreased aldosterone
B. Decreased ACTH, increased aldosterone
C. Increased ACTH, decreased aldosterone
D. Increased ACTH, increased aldosterone

Evaluating Care Outcomes

Patients with hypercortisolism are usually best managed once the etiology of the disorder is determined. If the etiology is a hypersecreting tumor of the pituitary gland or adrenal cortex, surgical intervention (transsphenoidal hypophysectomy, adrenalectomy, or stereotactic radiosurgery) is indicated. The patient should be closely monitored postoperatively and may require lifelong corticosteroid replacement on the basis of the surgical outcome. Stable vital signs and fluid volume status, serum electrolytes within normal limits, and intact skin are expected outcomes with treatment of hyperfunction of the adrenal cortex.

CASE STUDY: EPISODE 2

Ms. Davis is seen by her nurse practitioner about her complaints of inability to conceive and changes in menstrual cycles. During the history, she reports increased swelling of her hands and feet and is unable to wear her wedding ring. Additionally, she has gained approximately 8 pounds in the last month. She complains of increasing fatigue and has noticed that she seems to bruise "just by bumping into things." Her blood pressure is higher than previous measurements. On the basis of these findings, the nurse practitioner orders a complete metabolic panel, abdominal x-rays, cortisol levels, and a dexamethasone suppression test…

PHEOCHROMOCYTOMA

Epidemiology

Pheochromocytomas are rare catecholamine-secreting tumors of the adrenal medulla and, in 50% of cases, are diagnosed only on autopsy. Because of excessive **catecholamine** (epinephrine and norepinephrine) secretion, pheochromocytomas may precipitate life-threatening hypertension or cardiac arrhythmias, leading to sudden death. Occurring in all races, the incidence is higher in Caucasians. In relation to age, the peak incidence is in people 30 to 50 years of age. It is estimated that 25% of pheochromocytomas are familial and specific gene mutations. There are approximately 1,000 cases of pheochromocytoma diagnosed in the United States annually.

Pathophysiology

Pheochromocytomas are catecholamine-secreting tumors of the adrenal medulla and are usually unilateral (Fig. 42.3). The release of the epinephrine and norepinephrine is typically paradoxical, rather than continuous, and leads to vasoconstriction, increased heart rate, increased stroke volume leading to a rise in systolic blood pressure and a widening of pulse pressure. Catecholamine release also stimulates gluconeogenesis, resulting in hyperglycemia.

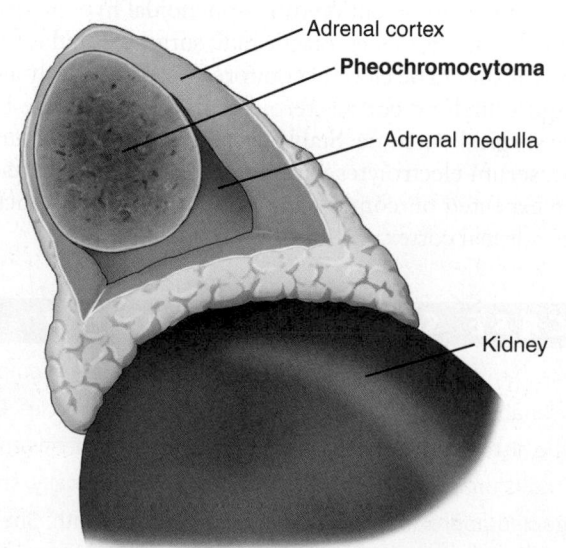

Adrenal cortex

Pheochromocytoma

Adrenal medulla

Kidney

FIGURE 42.3 Pheochromocytoma.

Clinical Manifestations

Clinical manifestations of this disorder are associated with the systematic actions of epinephrine and norepinephrine and include tachycardia, hypertension, severe headaches, palpitations, hyperhidrosis (excessive sweating), hypermetabolism, and hyperglycemia. The severity of attacks correlates to the amount of catecholamine release. Paroxysmal (sudden-onset) hypertension is seen in some patients, with blood pressure elevations in excess of 250/140 mm Hg, posing a life-threatening emergency.

Management

Medical Management

Diagnosis

The classic presentation of pheochromocytoma is marked by a sudden elevation of blood pressure accompanied by other clinical manifestations of catecholamine excess. This clinical presentation, along with specific diagnostic studies, assists in making a definitive diagnosis. Diagnostic assessments for this disorder include measurements of urine and plasma levels of **catecholamines** and catecholamine metabolites as well as imaging studies.

Direct measurements of plasma catecholamines require specific patient preparation to prevent elevations of circulating catecholamines. The patient is placed supine and rests for 30 minutes prior to the test. Additionally, small IV catheters are placed approximately 30 minutes prior to the actual collection of the blood samples. Catecholamine metabolites such as metanephrine and vanillylmandelic acid (VMA) and free catecholamines are also measured in urine. These tests require 24-hour urine collections. Preparation for these tests requires the patient to avoid specific foods, **beverages,** and medications prior to and during the urine collection. The patient is instructed to avoid bananas, chocolate, vanilla, and tea or coffee (including decaffeinated varieties) because these are high in amines and can lead to a false elevation of VMA.

Imaging studies, including CT or MRI scans, are also indicated in the diagnostic work-up for pheochromocytomas. Data from these studies determine whether tumors are unilateral or bilateral. Additionally, imaging data are very important in guiding the surgeon performing the adrenalectomy.

Medications and Monitoring

Patients presenting with signs of hypertension, tachycardia, and other clinical manifestations of pheochromocytoma require bedrest with the head of the bed elevated, usually in a critical care setting. The patient is placed on a cardiac monitor to assess for cardiac dysrhythmias. Pharmacological management focuses on quickly lowering the blood pressure and includes alpha-adrenergic blocking agents or smooth muscle relaxants. Other medications that may be administered include beta-adrenergic blocking agents and calcium channel blockers to decrease blood pressure and heart rate.

Surgical Management

Adrenalectomy is the definitive treatment for pheochromocytoma, and the goals include complete tumor resection, minimal tumor manipulation, and adequate exposure of the adrenal gland to avoid injury to other organs. There are several approaches for adrenalectomy, including open anterior transabdominal, open thoracoabdominal, open posterior or lateral retroperitoneal, lateral transabdominal laparoscopic, and posterior retroperitoneal laparoscopic approaches.

Traditionally, the standard approach in patients with pheochromocytoma was an open transabdominal anterior approach through a bilateral subcostal incision as it provides complete exposure of the abdominal cavity. However, in more recent studies, the laparoscopic approach has demonstrated good outcomes, particularly in medical centers with surgeons and operative teams with significant experience in this approach.

Patient preparation focuses on control of blood pressure and heart rate. Treatment with alpha-adrenergic blockers is started 7 to 10 days prior to the scheduled operative procedure with a goal blood pressure of 120/80 mm Hg or lower in a seated position. A beta blocker may be used to control heart rate but only after blood pressure is lowered. Fluid management is also important during the preoperative phase because of vasodilation secondary to the alpha-adrenergic blockers. During the surgical procedure, the patient is at risk of hypertensive crisis because the vascular pheochromocytoma is manipulated and removed. In the event of an intraoperative hypertensive episode, sodium nitroprusside (Nipride) or alpha-adrenergic blockers are cautiously administered.

Postoperative management of adrenalectomy focuses on monitoring blood pressure, heart rate, and blood glucose levels. Because of the sudden decrease in circulating catecholamines as a result of tumor removal, the patient may develop hypotension or hypoglycemia postoperatively. The patient is also monitored for blood loss due to the vascular nature of the adrenal gland. Several days postoperatively, plasma and urine samples are collected for measurement of catecholamine levels and catecholamine metabolites.

Patients with bilateral pheochromocytomas require bilateral adrenalectomy, and this necessitates lifelong adrenal cortex hormone replacements. These patients are required to take cortisol daily and may require additional doses during episodes of physiological or emotional stress. Patients who undergo bilateral adrenalectomy are at risk for adrenal insufficiency for the remainder of their lives. (Catecholamines from the adrenal medulla do not require replacement because they are also produced in the sympathetic nervous system).

Nursing Management

Assessment and Analysis

The clinical presentation of pheochromocytoma is directly related to the effects of increased levels of circulating epinephrine and norepinephrine:

- Hypertension (often paroxysmal attacks)
- Tachycardia
- Hyperglycemia
- Pounding headaches

Nursing Diagnoses

- **Risk for injury:** Cerebrovascular hemorrhage related to severe hypertension
- **Acute pain:** Headache related to increased levels of circulating catecholamines secondary to the hypersecreting tumor (pheochromocytoma)
- **Risk for injury:** Postoperative hemorrhage related to adrenalectomy

Nursing Interventions

■ Assessments

- Vital signs
  Hypertension and tachycardia develop secondary to excessive circulating catecholamines from pheochromocytoma. In the patient who undergoes adrenalectomy, the patient may develop signs of hypovolemia and shock secondary to hemorrhage.
- Cardiac monitoring
  The patient is at risk of tachydysrhythmias secondary to elevated catecholamines.
- Headache
  Pounding headaches develop secondary to hypertension.
- Plasma catecholamine levels
  Increased secretion of catecholamines from the tumor leads to elevated free plasma levels.
- Plasma and catecholamine metabolite measurements (VMA)
  Elevated levels of catecholamines result in increased levels of catecholamine metabolites.

■ Actions

- Administer sodium nitroprusside (Nipride)
  Quickly decreases blood pressure through direct action on blood vessels, leading to peripheral vasodilation
- Administer alpha-adrenergic blocking agents
  This decreases blood pressure by blocking the alpha-adrenergic effects on blood vessels that lead to vasoconstriction. The blocking action results in vasodilation.
- Administer beta-adrenergic blocking agents
  Beta-adrenergic agents lead to increased chronotropic (rate) and inotropic (force) effects on the heart. Beta-adrenergic blocking agents decrease the heart rate and force of contraction.
- Bed rest with head of bed elevated
  Bed rest decreases secretion of catecholamines and elevating the head of the bed facilitates orthostatic hypotension.
- Maintain calm, quiet environment
  Because of increased circulating levels of catecholamines, it is important to minimize stimuli that could potentially cause stress and additional catecholamine secretion.
- Administer glucocorticoid the morning of surgery for adrenalectomy
  Minimizes the risk of adrenal insufficiency postoperatively caused by the surgical manipulation of the adrenal glands, particularly in the patient undergoing bilateral adrenalectomy.

Teaching

- Clinical manifestations of adrenal insufficiency
  In patients with bilateral adrenalectomy, lifelong cortisol replacement is required. The patient is at risk of adrenal insufficiency, especially during times of physiological or emotional stress.
- Postoperative teaching related to adrenalectomy
  The patient should monitor body temperature as well as surgical site for signs of infection.

Evaluating Care Outcomes

Definitive treatment of pheochromocytoma with adrenalectomy results in complete resolution of this disease process. Because there is the possibility of incomplete resection of the pheochromocytoma or recurrence in patients with a family history of this disorder, patients need to have periodic checks of their blood pressure. Only patients with bilateral tumors requiring bilateral adrenalectomy require lifelong cortisol replacement.

Connection Check 42.5

Which assessment maneuver is contraindicated in the patient suspected of having a pheochromocytoma?
A. Having the patient attempt to touch the chin to the chest
B. Inflating the blood pressure cuff above 200 mm Hg
C. Attempting to dorsiflex the feet
D. Palpating the abdomen

Making Connections

CASE STUDY: WRAP-UP

Ms. Davis returns to the nurse practitioner the following week to review the results of her diagnostic evaluation. Her serum glucose level is 154 mg/dL, and her potassium level is 3.0 mEq/L. Her blood pressure remains elevated, and she has gained another pound in the last week. The abdominal x-rays are suggestive of a mass on the right adrenal gland, and a follow-up CT scan of the abdomen demonstrates a mass on the right adrenal gland. On the basis of this finding and the abnormal results of the dexamethasone suppression test, Ms. Davis is diagnosed with primary hypercortisolism secondary to a hypersecreting tumor and undergoes a right adrenalectomy.

Case Study Questions

1. The nurse correlates primary hypercortisolism to dysfunction of which gland?
   A. Hypothalamus
   B. Anterior pituitary gland
   C. Adrenal cortex
   D. Adrenal medulla

2. The nurse assesses for which clinical manifestations in the patient admitted with primary hypercortisolism? *(Select all that apply.)*
   A. Elevated serum glucose
   B. Elevated serum potassium
   C. Elevated urine-specific gravity
   D. Elevated blood pressure
   E. Elevated temperature

3. Which of the following patients is at greatest risk for primary hypercortisolism?
   A. A 65-year-old male
   B. A 56-year-old female
   C. A 44-year-old male
   D. A 28-year-old female

4. The nurse questions which intervention in the patient diagnosed with hypercortisolism?
   A. Limit salt intake
   B. Limit foods containing potassium
   C. Increase weight-bearing exercises
   D. Avoid use of skin tape

5. The nurse monitors for which complication in Ms. Davis secondary to her hypercortisolism?
   A. Osteoporosis
   B. Hypoglycemia
   C. Muscle loss
   D. Hyperkalemia

CHAPTER SUMMARY

The adrenal glands are composed of a cortex and a medulla that secrete hormones with distinct functions. Disorders of the adrenal cortex may be primary (adrenal cortex), secondary (anterior pituitary gland), or tertiary (hypothalamus) as well as related to hyposecretion or hypersecretion. Adrenal insufficiency is a life-threatening disorder associated with decreased secretion of glucocorticoids and mineralocorticoids, resulting in sodium and water loss, potassium retention, hypoglycemia, muscle loss, weakness, and weight loss. Acute adrenal crisis is a life-threatening disorder that requires emergent hormone (glucocorticoid) replacement.

Hyperfunction of the adrenal cortex may present as excess glucocorticoid secretion (hypercortisolism) or excess mineralocorticoid secretion (hyperaldosteronism). Patients with hypercortisolism present with hyperglycemia, hypokalemia, fluid retention, thinning of the skin, fat maldistribution, increased protein metabolism, and suppressed inflammatory and immune responses. Hyperaldosteronism is characterized by increased sodium and water retention, leading to elevated blood pressure and heart rate as well as hypokalemia.

Pheochromocytomas are catecholamine-secreting tumors of the adrenal medulla leading to profound hypertension, hyperglycemia, and other signs of excess catecholamines.

Blood pressure management is essential to prevent damage to the heart, brain, kidneys, and eyes. Treatment usually involves unilateral adrenalectomy. Postoperatively, the patient must be monitored closely for hemorrhage and hypovolemic shock.

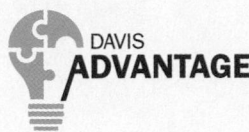

To explore learning resources for this chapter, go to **Davis Advantage** and find:
- Answers to in-text questions
- Chapter Resources and Activities
- NCLEX®-Style Chapter Review Questions
- Bibliography

Chapter 43

Coordinating Care for Patients With Thyroid and Parathyroid Disorders

Janice Hoffman

Finding Connections

Follow this patient throughout the chapter.

Patricia Matthews is a 28-year-old administrative assistant who presents to her family nurse practitioner (FNP) with complaints of weight loss despite "eating all the time," restlessness, insomnia, and changes in her menstrual cycle. On the basis of these findings, the FNP orders diagnostic evaluation of thyroid function and female reproductive hormones…

INTRODUCTION

The thyroid and parathyroid glands are integral to normal body functions. Metabolic activity and rate are primarily under the control of two hormones released from the thyroid glands, **triiodothyronine (T3)** and **thyroxine (T4)**. The release of thyroid hormone is under the control of the anterior pituitary gland (secretion of thyroid-stimulating hormone [TSH]) and the hypothalamus (thyroid-releasing hormone or thyrotropin-releasing hormone [TRH]). Disorders affecting either of these structures can result in hypothyroidism or hyperthyroidism. Serum calcium levels are controlled through the release of **thyrocalcitonin** from the thyroid glands and parathyroid hormone (parathormone [PTH]) from the parathyroid glands (Table 43.1). See Chapter 40 for an overview of the structure, function, and analyses of thyroid and parathyroid glands and hormones. Table 43.2 provides an overview of laboratory tests used to diagnose thyroid disorders.

HYPOTHYROIDISM

Epidemiology

The release of thyroid hormone is under the control of the anterior pituitary gland (secretion of TSH) and the hypothalamus (TRH). Disorders affecting either of these structures can result in hypothyroidism. In the United States, hypothyroidism is largely associated with autoimmune disease, thyroid surgery, or radioactive iodine therapy used in the treatment of hyperthyroidism. **Hashimoto's thyroiditis** is the most common type of hypothyroidism and is caused by an autoimmune response that leads to destruction of the thyroid gland by immunological processes. Hypothyroidism can also be associated with iodine and tyrosine deficiencies because they are needed for the synthesis of thyroid hormone, but they are rarely observed in the United States because of the use of iodized salt. Other causes of primary hypothyroidism include congenital thyroid disorders, autoimmune thyroid destruction, and thyroid cancer. Hypothyroidism is a major cause of **goiter** (enlargement of the thyroid gland; Fig. 43.1) and develops secondary to thyroid gland hypertrophy in an attempt to produce normal amounts of T3 and T4. Women are affected 7 to 10 times more often than men. Hypothyroidism occurs most often in women between the ages of 30 and 60, and the incidence increases with age.

Table 43.1 Overview of Thyroid and Parathyroid Hormones

Gland	Hormone Secreted	Target	Action
Hypothalamus	Thyrotropin-releasing hormone (TRH)	Anterior pituitary gland	Stimulates release of thyroid-stimulating hormone (TSH)
Anterior pituitary	TSH	Thyroid glands	Increases secretion of thyroid hormones (triiodothyronine [T3] and thyroxine [T4])
Thyroid gland	T3	Cells of the body	Increases metabolic rate
	T4		Increases response to catecholamines
	Thyrocalcitonin (calcitonin)	Bones	Decreases osteoclastic (breakdown of bone)
		Kidneys	Decreases reabsorption of calcium in renal tubules
		Intestines	Decreases reabsorption of calcium in the intestines
Parathyroid gland	Parathyroid hormone (PTH)	Bones	Increases osteoclastic (bone breakdown) activity
		Kidney	Increases renal tubule reabsorption of calcium
		Intestines	Increases gastrointestinal reabsorption of calcium (vitamin D required)

Table 43.2 Laboratory Tests for Thyroid Disorders

Test	Normal Range for Adults	Significance
Free T3 (triiodothyronine)	2.6 – 4.8 pg/mL	Decreased in hypothyroidism
		Increased in hyperthyroidism
Total T3 (triiodothyronine)	70–204 ng/dL	Decreased in hypothyroidism
		Increased in hyperthyroidism
Free T4 (thyroxine)	0.8–1.5 ng/dL	Decreased in hypothyroidism
		Increased in hyperthyroidism
Total T4 (thyroxine)	4.6–12 mcg/dL	Decreased in hypothyroidism
		Increased in hyperthyroidism
TSH (thyroid-stimulating hormone)	0.4–4.2 microinternational units/mL	Increased in primary hypothyroidism
		Decreased in secondary or tertiary hypothyroidism
		Decreased in primary hyperthyroidism
		Increased in secondary and tertiary hyperthyroidism

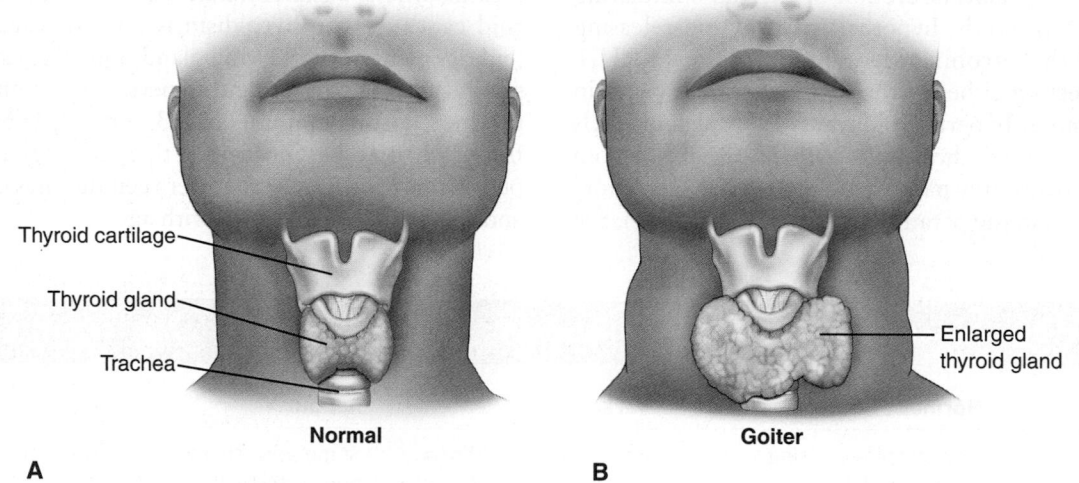

FIGURE 43.1 A. Normal thyroid gland B. Goiter (hyperplasia of the thyroid gland)

Connection Check 43.1

The nurse recognizes that which patient is at greatest risk for hypothyroidism?
A. A 19-year-old male
B. A 35-year-old female
C. A 45-year-old male
D. An 80-year-old female

Pathophysiology

Decreased metabolism is the hallmark of hypothyroidism and affects most body systems. Primary hypothyroidism develops as a result of a disorder of the thyroid gland itself, whereas secondary hypothyroidism is caused by a disorder of the anterior pituitary gland (Fig. 43.2). Tertiary hypothyroidism is associated with a lack of TRH from the hypothalamus.

Clinical Manifestations

The hypometabolic state is characterized by decreased energy, increased sleep, fatigue, weight gain, decreased appetite, and susceptibility to cold temperatures. Patients with hypothyroidism may develop **myxedema**, a condition resulting from an increased deposition of **glycosaminogly-cans** (a type of polysaccharide) in cells and tissues (Fig. 43.3). The increased deposition of glycosaminoglycans causes an osmotic edema and a fluid collection that is associated with

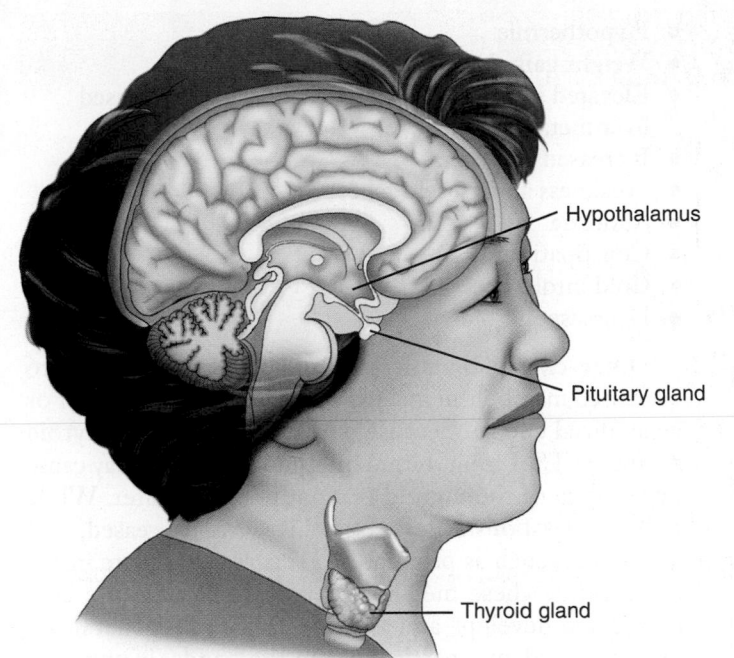

Hypothalamus

Pituitary gland

Thyroid gland

Tertiary:
due to a disorder of
the hypothalamus

Secondary:
due to a disorder of the
anterior pituitary gland

Primary:
due to a disorder of the
thyroid gland itself

FIGURE 43.2 Primary, secondary, and tertiary hypothyroidism.

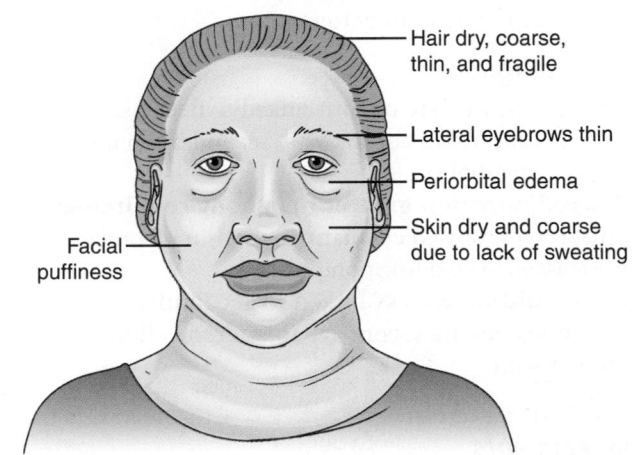

Hair dry, coarse, thin, and fragile

Lateral eyebrows thin

Periorbital edema

Skin dry and coarse due to lack of sweating

Facial puffiness

FIGURE 43.3 Myxedema, related to hypothyroidism.

a generalized nonpitting edema. Cardiac alterations secondary to myxedematous changes include decreased contractility, cardiac enlargement, pericardial effusion, decreased pulse, and decreased cardiac output. Decreased gastrointestinal activity results in constipation and abdominal distention. Skin changes may result over time secondary to cold intolerance, and a lack of sweating may leave the skin dry and coarse. Hair becomes thin and fragile, and hair loss occurs.

Management

Medical Management

Diagnosis

The diagnosis of hypothyroidism is confirmed through analysis of laboratory data, including T3, T4, and TSH. If the etiology is primary hypothyroidism, the TSH level is elevated as a result of the feedback system to the hypothalamus and anterior pituitary gland caused by low circulating levels of thyroid hormones (T3 and T4). In secondary or tertiary hypothyroidism, the TSH may be high or near normal because the disorder is a result of pathophysiology in the anterior pituitary gland or hypothalamus, respectively. When Hashimoto's thyroiditis is suspected, an evaluation of antithyroid antibodies should be performed.

Medications

Replacement of thyroid hormone is the primary treatment for hypothyroidism. The most commonly prescribed medication is levothyroxine (Synthroid). The medication is started at a low dose and increased as needed to treat symptoms of hypothyroidism. Because thyroid hormone affects metabolism, the medication is to be taken in the morning. This replacement therapy is a lifelong regimen, and it is important for the patient to take the medication at the same time every day. Additionally, it is important for the patient to inform all healthcare providers of his or her history of hypothyroidism and the dosage of hormone replacement (see Evidence-Based Practice).

Evidence-Based Practice

Levothyroxine as Primary Treatment for Hypothyroidism

A Medline search was conducted related to the historical evolution and use of levothyroxine as the treatment for hypothyroidism. Although this medication has been used for the treatment of hypothyroidism for over 130 years, this literature confirmed the documented effectiveness and safety of the medication. The studies described refinements in hormone preparation, pharmaceutical production, and regulation of this medication that have contributed to its continued use. According to this study, levothyroxine monotherapy is described in recent guidelines of all major endocrine societies as the first line of treatment for hypothyroidism.

Hennessey, J.V. (2017). The emergence of levothyroxine as a treatment for hypothyroidism. *Endocrine, 55*(1), 6–18.

> **(!) Safety Alert** In patients with a history of cardiovascular disease, the increases in dosage of levothyroxine are made cautiously because sudden increases in cardiac rate and contractility secondary to the medication may lead to angina or congestive heart failure.

Complications

The most severe type of hypothyroidism is termed **myxedema coma** and is characterized by hypoxia and carbon dioxide retention (secondary to hypoventilation), fluid and electrolyte imbalances, and hypothermia. Because of significant decreases in cardiac function, the patient is bradycardic and hypotensive. Additionally, hypoglycemia and hyponatremia develop. Along with significant hypothermia during times of myxedema crises, these patients are particularly sensitive to sedatives, analgesics, and anesthetic agents because metabolism of these medications is significantly slowed, leading to accumulation in the body. Definitive treatment is aimed at replacing thyroid hormone and supportive measures.

> **(!) Safety Alert** Patients with hypothyroidism who are receiving sedatives, hyponotics, or narcotics require close observation because the metabolism of the medication is slower, and respiratory compromise may occur with normal dosages. The dose, as well as the interval between doses, may need to be adjusted in the patient with severe hypothyroidism.

Nursing Management

Assessment and Analysis

Many of the clinical manifestations observed in the patient with hypothyroidism are directly related to the decreased metabolic rate of most body tissues. Common findings include:

- Bradycardia
- Decreased respiratory rate
- Hypothermia
- Weight gain despite decreased caloric intake
- Elevated serum cholesterol secondary to decreased liver metabolism
- Increased sleeping
- Weakness and muscle aches
- Anorexia
- Constipation
- Cold intolerance
- Decrease in libido

Other clinical manifestations not directly linked to decreased metabolism include the development of goiter or generalized edema. Because of decreased levels of thyroid hormone, TSH from the anterior pituitary gland may cause hyperplasia of the thyroid gland leading to goiter. While cellular metabolism decreases, energy is decreased, and metabolites such as proteins and sugars accumulate inside cells. While these metabolites build up inside the cell, myxedema develops and is characterized by generalized nonpitting edema, particularly in the hands, in the feet, between the shoulder blades, and around the eyes. Edema of the tongue and around the larynx results in changes in speech resulting in a husky tone.

Nursing Diagnoses

- **Decreased cardiac output** linked to decreased heart rate and decreased contractility secondary to impaired cardiac metabolism
- **Altered nutrition greater than body requirements** linked to decreased cellular metabolism secondary to decreased thyroid hormone activity
- **Fluid volume excess** linked to accumulation of mucinous edema secondary to altered cellular metabolism

Nursing Interventions

■ *Assessments*

- Oxygen saturation
  Severe hypothyroidism may impair respiratory function, leading to decreased ventilation, which results in lower oxygen saturation.
- Vital signs
  Decreased body temperature, heart rate, respiratory rate, and blood pressure are secondary to the hypometabolic state caused by thyroid hormone deficit.
- Serum calcium levels
  In patients with hypothyroidism secondary to surgical resection/removal of the thyroid gland, damage or removal of parathyroid tissue may lead to decreased serum calcium levels.
- Daily weight
  Decreased cellular metabolism may result in weight gain.
- Skin texture, color, and turgor
  Skin changes are associated with decreased sweating and oil production and are secondary to a hypometabolic state. With severe hypothyroidism, myxedema may develop linked to deposition of metabolites under the skin.

- Bowel elimination
  Patient is at increased risk of constipation secondary to decreased gastrointestinal motility.

■ Actions

- Administer thyroid replacement therapy at the same time every day
  Lifelong thyroid hormone replacement is required in patients with hypothyroidism to increase metabolic activities of most body systems. To mimic the normal circadian rhythm, Synthroid is administered in the morning.
- Administer narcotics and sedatives with caution
  Because of decreased metabolism on medication, secondary to hypothyroidism, the patient must be monitored closely for signs of overmedication such as decreased respiratory rate or difficulty arousing the patient after medication administration.
- Provide warming blankets as needed
  Decreased metabolism results in decreased energy production and cold intolerance. Patients should avoid warming too quickly because it can result in vasodilation and hypotension.
- Turn patient and reposition to promote skin integrity
  Because of myxedema, the skin integrity is altered requiring special actions to prevent pressure.

■ Teaching

- Immediately report chest pain or chest discomfort
  Cardiovascular disease may develop in patients with hypothyroidism. Because of the decreased metabolism of cholesterol, patients with hypothyroidism are at greater risk of elevated cholesterol levels.
- Take thyroid replacement hormones as prescribed; must be taken daily
  Thyroid hormone replacement is required for metabolic activities. Increasing the dose of medication without prescriber input may lead to accelerated cardiovascular function that the heart is unprepared to tolerate because of the long-term effects of hypothyroidism.
- Signs of hypothyroidism and hyperthyroidism
  It is important that the patient (and family) are able to detect early signs of both hypothyroidism (the underlying disorder that could progress to myxedema) and hyperthyroidism (secondary to thyroid hormone supplementation).

Evaluating Care Outcomes

Patients with hypothyroidism can achieve normal thyroid function by complying with the prescribed therapy. Vital signs within normal limits, increased energy, stable weight, and normal skin turgor and texture are indicative of thyroid health in this patient population. During periods of stress, such as invasive procedures, an adjustment in thyroid medications may be indicated. It is important for all healthcare providers to be aware of the hypothyroidism, particularly when prescribing medications such as sedatives, narcotics, or anesthetic agents. The patient and family should be knowledgeable about the signs of hypothyroidism and hyperthyroidism and which clinical manifestations they should report to the healthcare provider.

Connection Check 43.2

The nurse correlates which clinical manifestation to the pathophysiology of hypothyroidism?
A. Cold intolerance
B. Weight loss
C. Insomnia
D. Diarrhea

HYPERTHYROIDISM

Epidemiology

Hyperthyroidism can be present at any age but is most commonly diagnosed in women between the ages of 20 and 40 years; it is also 10 times more prevalent in women. **Graves' disease** is the most common cause of hyperthyroidism and is an autoimmune disorder involving antibodies (thyroid-stimulating immunoglobulins) that bind to the thyroid gland, resulting in the enlargement of the thyroid gland and subsequent hypersecretion of thyroid hormone.

Pathophysiology

Accelerated metabolism is characteristic of hyperthyroidism and affects most body systems. Primary hyperthyroidism is secondary to excess triiodothyronine (T3) or thyroxine (T4) from the thyroid gland. With increased secretion of thyroid-stimulating hormone (TSH) from the anterior posterior gland, secondary hyperthyroidism develops. Tertiary hyperthyroidism occurs as a result of excessive secretion of thyroid-releasing hormone or thyrotropin-releasing hormone (TRH) from the hypothalamus.

Clinical Manifestations

The increase in metabolic rate results in the following clinical manifestations:

- Elevated heart rate, cardiac dysrhythmias, and increased heart sounds
- Thyroid bruit linked to increased blood flow
- Heat intolerance
- Increased gastric activity resulting in increased bowel movements
- Increased appetite
- Weight loss
- Fatigue
- Nervousness
- Insomnia
- Light to absent menses
- Hair loss

Other clinical manifestations include **exophthalmos** (protrusion of the eyeball) and goiter (Fig. 43.4). Exophthalmos is characteristic of hyperthyroidism and results in visual changes. Goiter is also associated with hyperthyroidism and is often the result of hyperplasia of the gland in response to the action of TSH on thyroid tissue.

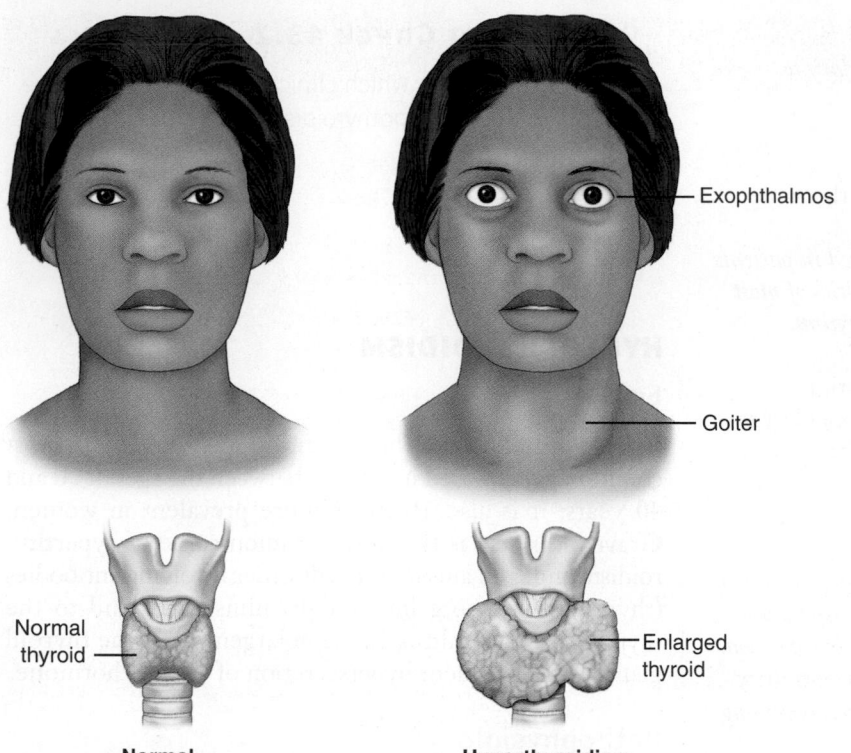

Normal **Hyperthyroidism**

FIGURE 43.4 Exophthalmos and goiter are characteristic of hyperthyroidism.

Management

Medical Management

Diagnosis

Laboratory findings in patients with hyperthyroidism include elevated serum T3, elevated serum T4, and decreased TSH in primary disorders. Table 43.2 provides an overview of diagnostic studies for patients with suspected thyroid disorders. Antibodies to TSH are also evaluated, and high titers are correlated with Graves' disease. In patients with goiter, thyroid scans may be performed to assess the size, position, and function of the gland. The uptake of radioactive iodine (RAIU) is measured after oral administration, and normal uptake varies according to the time of measurement (see Table 43.2). Elevations in RAIU are consistent with a diagnosis of hyperthyroidism.

Treatment

Control of the hypermetabolic state associated with hyperthyroidism is the priority in its management. Although there are specific pharmacological agents used in the treatment of hyperthyroidism, the management of clinical manifestations, particularly in relation to cardiac function and body temperature, is a priority. Nonsurgical treatment focuses on ensuring adequate fluid intake because insensible losses are greater secondary to the hypermetabolic state, monitoring for cardiovascular complications, and promoting a quiet, nonstressful environment. Pharmacological agents that may be used for symptom management include beta-adrenergic blocking agents because these agents slow heart rate and decrease palpitations.

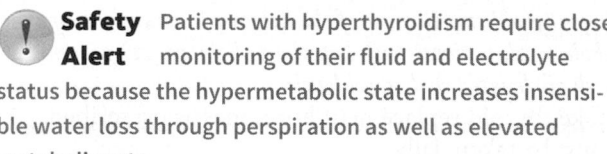

Safety Alert Patients with hyperthyroidism require close monitoring of their fluid and electrolyte status because the hypermetabolic state increases insensible water loss through perspiration as well as elevated metabolic rate.

Medications

For long-term management of hyperthyroidism, antithyroid medications are used, including propylthiouracil (PTU), methimazole (Tapazole), and lithium carbonate (Lithonate). These medications reduce clinical manifestations of hyperthyroidism by interfering either with the formation or release of thyroid hormone. For short-term management, iodine preparations may be administered, particularly to patients before thyroidectomy, to decrease blood flow through the thyroid gland in order to decrease thyroid hormone release. Table 43.3 provides an overview of medications used in treating hyperthyroidism.

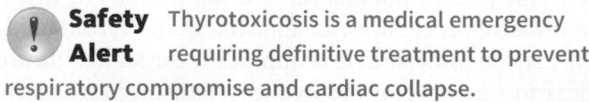

Safety Alert Thyrotoxicosis is a medical emergency requiring definitive treatment to prevent respiratory compromise and cardiac collapse.

Surgical Management

Although most cases of hyperthyroidism are treated successfully with antithyroid medications, surgical management

Table 43.3 Pharmacological Management of Hyperthyroidism

Medication	Actions	Nursing Implications
Propylthiouracil (PTU)	Inhibits the synthesis of thyroid hormone by diverting iodine pathways Interferes with conversion of thyroxine (T4) to triiodothyronine (T3)	• Take the medication at the same time daily, usually in the morning • Monitor weight 2–3 times per week • Teach patient signs of hypothyroidism • Monitor white blood cell count because agranulocytosis may occur
Methimazole (Tapazole)	Inhibits the synthesis of thyroid hormone by blocking the combination of iodine with a protein called thyroglobulin Methimazole also interferes with the conversion of T4 to T3.	• Take the medication at the same time daily, usually in the morning • Monitor weight 2–3 times per week • Teach patient signs of hypothyroidism • Monitor white blood cell count as agranulocytosis may occur
Lithium carbonate (Lithonate)	Lithium is concentrated in the thyroid gland and interferes with thyroid hormone synthesis and can cause formation of thyroid antibodies.	• Monitor for signs of toxicity including vomiting, diarrhea, drowsiness, and lack of coordination • Drink at least 2–3 L of fluids when initially starting the medication • Assess for changes in signs of thyroid dysfunction
Iodine (SSKI - saturated solutions of potassium iodide)	Inhibits the release of thyroid hormone by decreasing vascularity of the thyroid gland	• Assess for signs of iodism including metallic taste, stomatitis, skin lesion, cold symptoms, and severe gastrointestinal distress • Mix solutions in full glass of fruit juice or water • Administer after food to decrease gastrointestinal distress

may be indicated for patients with hypersecreting tumors that are unresponsive to the medications or in patients experiencing tracheal compression due to goiter. Because most patients demonstrate clinical manifestations of hyperthyroidism while being prepared for surgery, it is a priority to establish "normal," or **euthyroid**, function before surgery. This is most often accomplished with iodine preparations to decrease vascularity of the thyroid gland in addition to other

prescribed antithyroid medications, and medications to decrease blood pressure and heart rate, as needed.

For patients with hyperthyroidism, total or subtotal thyroidectomy procedures are performed (Fig. 43.5). With total thyroidectomy, the patient needs to take thyroid replacement hormone for the remainder of his or her life. Potential complications during thyroidectomy include the removal of all parathyroid tissue, resulting in hypoparathyroidism

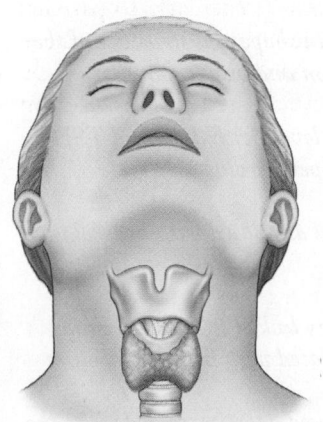

Normal

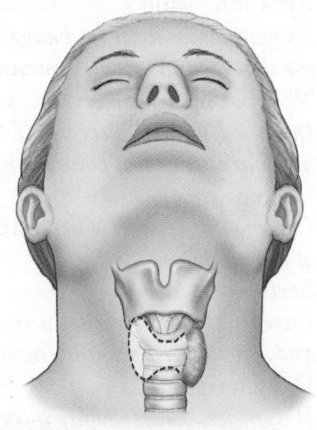

Subtotal Thyroidectomy

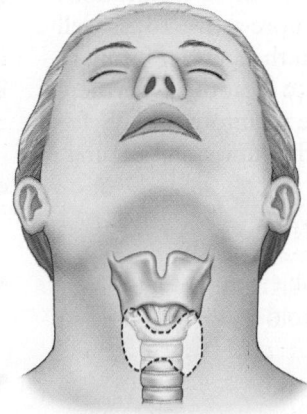

Total Thyroidectomy

FIGURE 43.5 Subtotal and total thyroidectomy.

or damage to the laryngeal nerve that affects swallowing and voice.

Postoperative priorities after thyroidectomy include monitoring for airway compromise, hemorrhage, hypocalcemia secondary to removal of all parathyroid gland tissue, and damage to the laryngeal nerve. Because hemorrhage is most likely in the first 24 hours, it is important to observe for bleeding around the dressing as well as down the back of the neck. Sandbags may be used to help keep the head in proper alignment, and care is used when repositioning the patient to prevent tension on the suture line.

Postoperatively, the patient is positioned in a semi-Fowler's position to ease the work of breathing and to decrease the risk of aspiration of oral secretions associated with lying flat on the back. Humidified air is administered to help decrease the viscosity of secretions, and oral suctioning equipment is maintained at the bedside. A tracheostomy tray is maintained at the bedside because of the risk of respiratory compromise secondary to postoperative swelling, **tetany** (intermittent muscle spasms), and laryngeal damage. Tetany develops secondary to hypocalcemia as a result of damage or removal of parathyroid glands during surgery and results in laryngospasm, making oral intubation difficult or impossible. Suctioning equipment and supplemental oxygen, in addition to the tracheostomy tray, are maintained at the patient's bedside for at least the first 48 hours after surgery.

Assessing for damage to the laryngeal nerve is also a priority in the postoperative period following thyroidectomy. Changes in voice quality, particularly hoarseness or a husky tone, may be indicative of laryngeal nerve damage. Voice assessments are conducted every 1 to 2 hours in the immediate postoperative period to monitor for changes.

Complications

Thyroid storm or **thyrotoxicosis** may develop with poorly managed hyperthyroidism. Clinical manifestations include tachycardia, fever, systolic hypertension, abdominal pain, tremors, and changes in level of consciousness. Airway management and fluid resuscitation are priorities. Antithyroid medications may be administered along with iodine preparations. For management of tachycardia, beta-adrenergic blockers may be administered. Glucocorticoids may also be administered because in high doses these medications decrease the conversion of T4 to the more active T3, as well as decreasing the release of TSH from the anterior pituitary gland. Cooling blankets may be used to treat the hyperthermia. During crisis, the patient must be monitored closely for respiratory complications, cardiac dysrhythmias, and seizures.

Connection Check 43.3

The nurse correlates an increase in which laboratory value to the diagnosis of primary hyperthyroidism?

A. Thyroxine (T4)
B. Thyroid-stimulating hormone (TSH)
C. Serum calcium
D. Serum iodine

Nursing Management

Assessment and Analysis

Because hyperthyroidism accelerates the metabolic rate of almost all cells, the clinical presentation of the patient includes changes in many body systems. The clinical manifestations of hyperthyroidism are directly linked to actions of the excessive thyroid hormones and the associated increase in basal metabolic rate that may increase by 60% to 100%. Clinical presentation includes:

- Weight loss because basal metabolic rate can increase by 60% to 100% in the patient with hyperthyroidism, leading to accelerated use of glucose, fats, and proteins
- Increased gastric motility
- Increased appetite
- Hypoglycemia
- Increased systolic blood pressure; tachycardia that may exacerbate to cardiac dysrhythmias
- Visual changes
- Corneal abrasions (secondary to exophthalmos)

Nursing Diagnoses

- **High risk for decreased cardiac output** linked to tachycardia and dysrhythmias
- **Altered nutrition less than body requirements** linked to increased metabolic rate secondary to elevated thyroid hormone levels
- **Hyperthermia** linked to accelerated metabolic rate secondary to increased circulating thyroid hormones

Nursing Interventions

Assessments

- Vital signs
  Hypermetabolism results in acceleration of the respiratory and cardiovascular systems, leading to elevated heart rate and increased respiratory rate. An elevation in temperature is associated with the hypermetabolic state.
- Intake and output
  Increases in insensible fluid loss develop secondary to the hypermetabolic state, leading to increased respiratory rate, increased diaphoresis, and diarrhea.
- Eyes and vision
  Exophthalmos leads to changes in shape and structure of the eye that lead to eyeball protrusion and visual changes.
- Thyroid hormone levels
  Increased T3 and increased T4 levels with decreased TSH are characteristic of primary hyperthyroidism.
- Goiter
  Common in Graves' disease and associated with hyperplasia of thyroid tissue
- Seizures
  Increased risk for seizure activity linked to hyponatremia and elevated temperature associated with hypermetabolism
- Daily weight
  Weight loss occurs despite increased appetite, secondary to the hypermetabolic state. Use of protein stores leads to loss of muscle mass that contributes to weight loss.

■ Actions

- Administer antithyroid medications as ordered
  Decreases thyroid hormone levels by preventing synthesis of hormone in the thyroid gland or by preventing the conversion of T4 to T3
- Administer iodine preparations
  Decreases vascularity of thyroid tissue resulting in decreased thyroid hormone synthesis and release
- Administer beta-adrenergic blocking agents as ordered
  Used as supportive therapy to treat the associated clinical manifestations of hypermetabolism, including tachycardia, palpitations, and diaphoresis
- Implement cooling measures with elevated temperature
  Temperature elevation and increased insensible fluid loss result secondary to accelerated metabolic rate. Instituting cooling measures decreases risks associated with hyperthermia.
- Administer eye lubricant
  To decrease possible eye dryness and potential for corneal irritation secondary to incomplete eyelid closure with exophthalmos

■ Teaching

- Overview of disease process
  It is important that the patient (and family) are able to detect early signs of both hyperthyroidism (the underlying disorder that could progress to thyroid storm) and hypothyroidism (secondary to thyroid hormone–blocking agents).
- Take the antithyroid medication at the same time every day
  Compliance with antithyroid medications is essential for minimizing complications associated with thyrotoxicosis.
- Consume adequate calories to minimize weight loss
  Weight gain or maintenance of current weight indicates the therapeutic effects of antithyroid medications.

Connection Check 43.4

The patient experiencing thyroid storm is ordered to receive beta-adrenergic agents. The nurse monitors for which therapeutic effect of these medications?

A. Increased respiratory rate
B. Increased appetite
C. Decreased heart rate
D. Decreased bowel sounds

Evaluating Care Outcomes

Patients with hyperthyroidism are usually managed with antithyroid medications. Vital signs within normal limits and stable weight indicate stabilizing thyroid function. The patient and family must be knowledgeable of signs of both hypothyroidism and hyperthyroidism in order to know when to seek healthcare advice. Patients with hyperthyroidism should have an evaluation of thyroid function before undergoing surgical or invasive procedures. Adjustments in antithyroid medications may also be indicated during times

of stress, which can further accelerate the metabolic rate. With proper attention to the treatment plan, patients with hyperthyroidism should be able to maintain a healthy, active lifestyle.

CASE STUDY: EPISODE 2

Ms. Matthews' thyroid hormones (T3 and T4) are elevated, and her TSH is decreased. On the basis of these findings, she is diagnosed with primary hyperthyroidism. The nurse practitioner prescribes the patient to start propylthiouracil (PTU). Ms. Mathews is instructed to ensure that she consumes adequate fluids and monitors her weight weekly. She is scheduled to return to the clinic in 4 weeks...

THYROID CANCER

Patients with thyroid cancer usually present with a nodule on the thyroid gland (Fig. 43.6). According to the American Cancer Society, approximately 53,900 new cases of thyroid cancer were diagnosed in 2018 (40,900 in women and 13,090 in men), and there were approximately 2,060 deaths. The death rate from thyroid cancer has been fairly steady for years and remains very low compared with most other cancers. There are four types of thyroid cancer: papillary, follicular, medullary, and anaplastic. In all types of thyroid cancer other than anaplastic, thyroidectomy is the treatment of choice in the absence of distant metastasis. Following surgery, patients require close monitoring for clinical manifestations of both hypothyroidism and hypoparathyroidism, and their care is similar to that of the patient undergoing thyroidectomy secondary to hyperthyroidism. In patients with anaplastic carcinoma, because of the aggressive nature of this fast-growing tumor, radiation therapy is the treatment of choice. Chemotherapy may be used in patients who are not responsive to radiation therapy. Depending on the diagnosis and treatment of thyroid cancer, coordination between the endocrinologist, surgeon, oncologist, dietitian, social worker, and nurse is essential in promoting health. Often, the overall coordination of this interprofessional care is managed by a registered nurse case manager or care coordinator.

HYPOPARATHYROIDISM

Epidemiology

Hypoparathyroidism is classified as idiopathic (unknown etiology), acquired, or reversible. The most common cause of acquired hypoparathyroidism is secondary to removal of the parathyroid glands during total thyroidectomy or bilateral resection for cancer of the head and neck. Reversible hypoparathyroidism may develop secondary to iodine therapy for hyperthyroidism and with metastasis of malignant tumors. Autoimmune disease is suspected in patients with

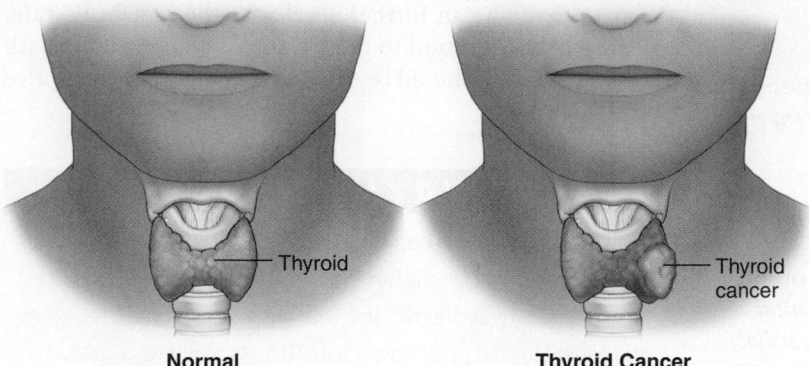

Normal   **Thyroid Cancer**

FIGURE 43.6 Thyroid cancer.

spontaneous presentation of hypoparathyroidism with no identifiable cause. In these cases, antiparathyroid antibodies have been detected in patients with other autoimmune disorders such as diabetes mellitus or adrenal insufficiency. There is also a congenital absence of parathyroid glands known as DiGeorge syndrome; considered an autoimmune disorder, it is usually reversible in children.

Pathophysiology

Hypocalcemia is the primary disorder associated with hypoparathyroidism (Fig. 43.7). Because of a lack of parathyroid hormone (PTH), calcium is not mobilized from the bones, conserved in the kidneys, or absorbed in the small intestines. Vitamin D enters the body in an inactive form through dietary intake or ultraviolet rays and is activated

in the kidneys based on actions of PTH. It is this activated vitamin D that leads to calcium absorption in the intestines. Calcium plays a major role in membrane potential and neuronal excitability and is needed for cardiac, skeletal, and smooth muscle contraction. Table 43.4 provides an overview of diagnostic results seen in parathyroid dysfunction.

Clinical Manifestations

In addition to decreased serum calcium levels, the clinical manifestations of hypoparathyroidism include numbness and tingling around the mouth or in the hands and feet, severe muscle cramps, spasms of the hands and feet, and tetany. Two specific assessments observed in hypocalcemia are Chvostek sign (Fig. 43.8A) and Trousseau sign (Fig. 43.8B) and are associated with an increased risk of tetany that can result in

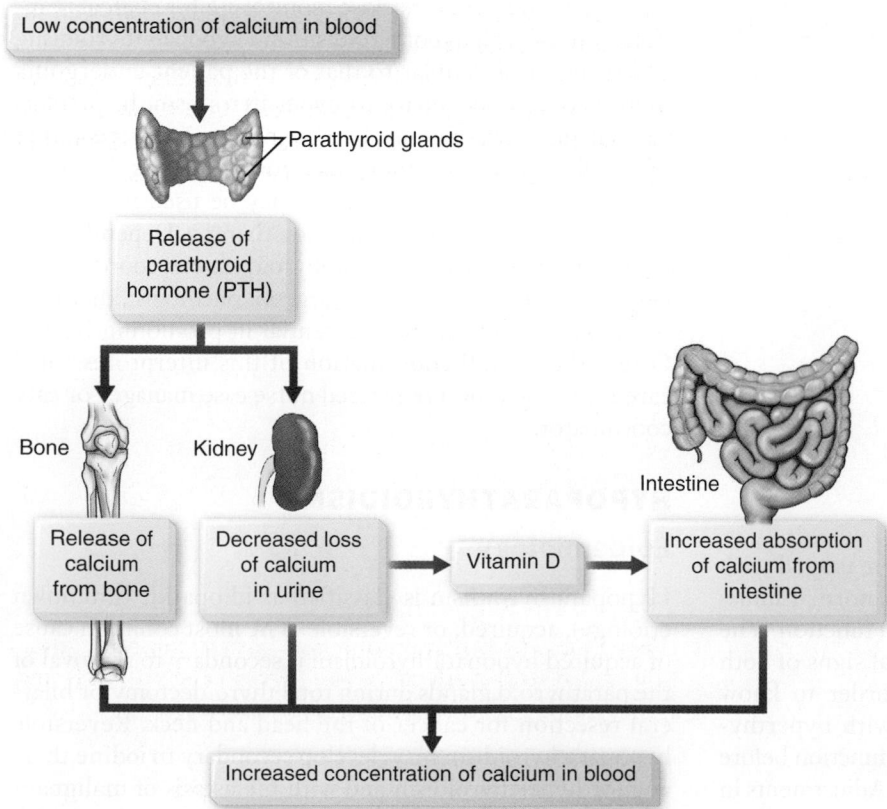

FIGURE 43.7 Actions of parathyroid hormone (PTH). In response to low circulating serum calcium levels, PTH is released from the parathyroid glands and acts on the bones, kidneys, and intestines to increase serum calcium levels. Note that vitamin D is activated in the kidneys and leads to increased calcium absorption in the intestine.

Table 43.4 **Laboratory Tests for Parathyroid Disorders**		
Test	**Normal Range for Adults**	**Significance**
Calcium	8.2–10.2 mg/dL	Decreased in hypoparathyroidism
		Increased in hyperparathyroidism
Ionized Calcium	4.6–5.3 mg/dL	Decreased in hypoparathyroidism
		Increased in hyperparathyroidism
Magnesium	1.6–2.2 mg/dL	Decreased in hypoparathyroidism
Phosphorus	2.5–4.5 mg/dL	Increased in hypoparathyroidism
		Decreased in hyperparathyroidism
Vitamin D		
Vit D 25-hydroxy	30–100 ng/mL	Decreased in hypoparathyroidism
Vit D 1, 25-dihydroxy	18–72 pg/dL	Variable in hyperparathyroidism

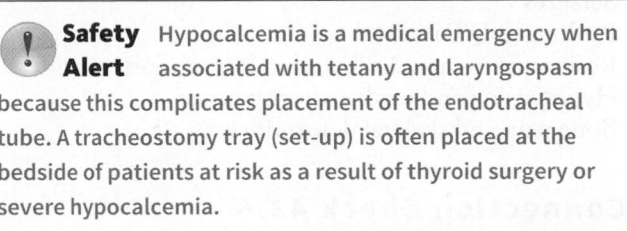

FIGURE 43.8 Assessments for hypocalcemia. A, Chvostek sign; B, Trousseau sign.

laryngospasm and airway compromise (see management of tetany above).

> **⊘ Safety Alert** Hypocalcemia is a medical emergency when associated with tetany and laryngospasm because this complicates placement of the endotracheal tube. A tracheostomy tray (set-up) is often placed at the bedside of patients at risk as a result of thyroid surgery or severe hypocalcemia.

Management

Medical Management

Diagnosis

Diagnostic results consistent with hypoparathyroidism include low serum calcium levels, high serum phosphate levels, and low serum PTH levels. Serum magnesium levels are often evaluated to rule out hypomagnesemia as the cause of hypoparathyroidism, as low serum magnesium levels inhibit synthesis of PTH. Additionally, serum albumin levels are monitored because the majority of serum calcium is plasma protein bound. In the patient with both low serum calcium and albumin, an ionized (free) calcium evaluation is required to determine the extent of the hypocalcemia.

Treatment

Hypoparathyroidism treatment is based on whether the presentation is acute or insidious and focuses primarily on raising serum calcium levels. Intravenous calcium (usually calcium gluconate or calcium chloride) is administered to the patient presenting with acute hypocalcemia and then followed up with oral calcium and vitamin D supplementation. In patients with a history of cardiac disease, IV administration should be slow to minimize hypotension and bradycardia. Chronic hypoparathyroidism is treated with oral calcium and vitamin D based on close monitoring of serum calcium levels.

Connection Check 43.5

The nurse correlates a positive Chvostek sign to hyposecretion of which hormone?
A. Thyroxin (T4)
B. Thyrocalcitonin
C. Parathyroid hormone (PTH)
D. Triiodothyronine (T3)

Nursing Management

Assessment and Analysis

The clinical presentation of hypoparathyroidism is primarily linked to the effects of low serum calcium levels and includes the following findings:

- Decreased serum calcium levels
- Tetany, muscle cramps, carpopedal spasm

- Positive Chvostek and Trousseau signs
- Paresthesias of the hands and feet
- Tingling of circumoral areas
- Seizures
- Prolonged QT interval
- Resistance to digitalis linked to loss of inotropic effect
- Hypotension and cardiac dysrhythmias
- Bone pain and skeletal deformities

Connection Check 43.6

The nurse monitors the calcium levels closely in the patient taking digoxin (Lanoxin) because hypocalcemia may lead to which complication?

A. Elevated heart rate
B. Dysrhythmias
C. Increased cardiac contractility
D. Hypertension

Nursing Diagnoses

- **High risk for ineffective airway clearance** linked to laryngospasm secondary to hypocalcemia
- **Decreased cardiac output** linked to suppressed myocardial contractility secondary to hypocalcemia

Nursing Interventions

■ *Assessments*

- Vital signs
  Hypotension may occur secondary to decreased myocardial contractility and cardiac dysrhythmias.
- Cardiac monitoring
  Hypocalcemia may cause cardiac dysrhythmias secondary to effects on cardiac automaticity.
- Ionized calcium levels
  Ionized calcium is the free and active form of calcium.
- Serum magnesium levels
  Hypomagnesemia interferes with PTH synthesis and contributes to hypocalcemia.
- Acid-base status
  An alkaline pH increases binding of calcium to protein and results in decreased ionized calcium.
- Neuromuscular activity
  Insufficient free, ionized calcium at the neuromuscular junction results in excessive neuronal firing.

■ *Actions*

- Administer calcium replacements
  Raise serum calcium levels. IV calcium is usually administered over 10 to 15 minutes.
- Administer vitamin D
  Vitamin D is needed for calcium absorption from the bowel.

■ *Teaching*

- Medication regimen
  Lifelong supplementation with calcium is necessary secondary to decreased synthesis or secretion of PTH.

- Eat foods high in calcium but low in phosphorus
  Foods high in calcium assist in raising serum calcium levels (Box 43.1). Foods high in phosphorus are to be avoided because phosphorus can bind with calcium in the serum, further decreasing calcium levels.
- Signs of hypocalcemia and hypercalcemia
  This information is needed to prevent complications associated with extremes of either calcium abnormality.

Evaluating Care Outcomes

Compliance with the medication regimen, particularly daily calcium supplements, usually results in stable serum calcium levels. Because of intake of calcium supplements, it is important to ensure that the patient maintains adequate hydration. Equipped with an understanding of the clinical manifestations of both elevated and low calcium levels, the patient and family are knowledgeable about changes that require notification of the healthcare provider.

HYPERPARATHYROIDISM

Epidemiology

Parathyroid adenomas account for 85% of the cases of primary hyperparathyroidism, whereas 15% of cases are secondary disorders associated with hyperplasia of the parathyroid glands. Secondary disorders are most often observed in patients with chronic renal failure or chronic malabsorption of calcium. The incidence of hyperparathyroidism is greatest in people older than 50 years of age and occurs in women more often than men.

Pathophysiology

Hyperparathyroidism causes hypercalcemia secondary to its actions on bone, kidneys, and the bowel. The action of PTH on bone leads to **osteoclastic** (breakdown of bone) activity and bone demineralization, which causes pathological fractures and bone lesions. Osteoclasts are large cells that secrete enzymes and acids to dissolve microscopic bits of bone, and then the minerals and amino acids are reabsorbed

Box 43.1 High Calcium Foods Used in the Treatment of Hypoparathyroidism

Fruits and Fruit Juices
- Calcium and vitamin D–fortified orange juice
- Rhubarb
- Stewed figs

Dark Green, Leafy Vegetables
- Collard greens
- Kale
- Mustard spinach

Soy Products

(resorption). Osteoclastic activity increases release of calcium from the bone and leads to loss of bone density. Increased renal reabsorption of calcium leads to elevated serum calcium levels. Increased calcium levels in the urine filtrate cause hypercalciuria that increases the potential for calcium-containing renal stones. Reabsorption of calcium in the bowel is also increased in patients with hyperparathyroidism.

Patients with chronic renal failure may develop secondary hyperparathyroidism. Decreased serum calcium and inactivated vitamin D develop in early renal failure, and PTH secretion increases in response to the hypocalcemia. Over time, parathyroid gland hyperplasia develops because of low calcium levels. Hyperparathyroidism can be differentiated from other causes of hypercalcemia, such as elevated calcium secondary to malignancy, through intact PTH assays. In hyperparathyroidism, intact PTH levels are intact in 75% to 90% of patients, whereas they are normal in patients with hypercalcemia secondary to malignancy.

Clinical Manifestations

Although some patients with hyperparathyroidism may be asymptomatic, others present with polyuria, anorexia, and constipation associated with elevated serum calcium levels that impact the kidneys and gastrointestinal tract. Cardiac changes associated with elevated calcium levels include a prolonged PR interval and a shortened QT interval due to the shortening of the ST segment. The patient may also develop abdominal pain because hypercalcemia leads to increased secretion of gastrin in the stomach and associated peptic ulcer disease. Other clinical manifestations include lethargy, confusion, muscle weakness, fatigue, and generalized bone pain (secondary to bone demineralization caused by osteoclastic activity).

Management

Medical Management

Diagnosis

Direct measurement of intact PTH is diagnostically definitive for hyperparathyroidism. Diagnostic evaluation of patients with suspected hyperparathyroidism also includes measurements of serum calcium, albumin, phosphorus, and ionized calcium levels. Because serum calcium levels are measurements of serum protein–bound calcium, an evaluation of serum albumin is needed; a low serum calcium level may be associated with a low serum albumin. Measurements of ionized calcium are more accurate because they reflect the active form of calcium. The finding of elevations in both intact PTH and ionized calcium is diagnostic for primary hyperparathyroidism.

Treatment

The treatment of hyperparathyroidism focuses primarily on lowering serum levels. Increased fluid intake is indicated to minimize potential renal injury secondary to elevated serum calcium, and in patients with mild disease, increased oral fluid intake may treat the disorder. More severe cases

of hypercalcemia require IV infusions of normal saline to protect against renal calculi. Patients with hyperparathyroidism are also taught to decrease consumption of calcium-containing antacids and vitamin D. Thiazide diuretics are also to be avoided in patients with hyperparathyroidism because these medications increase reabsorption of calcium in the kidney.

Connection Check 43.7

The nurse prioritizes which nursing diagnosis in the patient after partial parathyroidectomy?

A. High risk for ineffective airway clearance linked to hypocalcemia

B. High risk for ineffective breathing pattern linked to hypercalcemia

C. High risk for hyperventilation linked to hypersecretion of triiodothyronine

D. High risk for airway compromise linked to insufficient iodine stores

---

Nursing Management

Assessment and Analysis

Clinical manifestations of hyperparathyroidism are largely related to elevated serum calcium and include:

- Elevated ionized and serum calcium levels
- Decreased serum phosphorus levels
- Muscle weakness and atrophy
- Low back pain
- Increased incidence of pathological fractures
- Prolonged PR interval
- Shortened QT interval
- Constipation, anorexia, and nausea and vomiting
- Renal stones

Nursing Diagnoses

- **Acute pain** related to pressure in renal tubules secondary to development of calcium-based renal calculi
- **High risk for injury: falls** related to bone demineralization and calcium resorption

Nursing Interventions

■ *Assessments*

- Serum calcium levels
  Excessive PTH leads to release of calcium from the bone, increased renal reabsorption, and increased intestinal absorption, all leading to hypercalcemia.
- Serum phosphorus levels
  Parathyroid hormone increases renal excretion of phosphorus.
- Cardiac monitoring
  Elevated serum calcium may lead to shortening of the QT interval related to decreased depolarization and repolarization of the ventricles.
- Acid-base status
  An acid pH decreases binding of calcium to protein and results in elevated ionized calcium.

■ Actions

- Increase fluid intake to 3,000 mL/day
  Increase fluid administration to decrease incidence of renal calculi. Normal saline is the fluid choice for IV administration.
- Administer furosemide (Lasix) as ordered
  This diuretic medication increases renal excretion of calcium.
- Administer oral phosphates as ordered
  Oral phosphates inhibit calcium loss from the bone and interfere with calcium absorption in the kidneys and bowel.
- Administer calcium chelators
  Binding of calcium decreases the free, activated calcium and lowers serum levels.
- Use a lift sheet in patients with chronic hyperparathyroidism to prevent bone injury
  Sustained hyperparathyroidism results in loss of calcium from the bone and increases the chances of bone trauma and pathological fractures.
- Strain urine with suspected renal calculi
  Confirmation of renal calculi composition is needed to implement corrective therapy.

■ Teaching

- Signs of hypocalcemia and hypercalcemia
  This information is needed to prevent complications associated with the extremes of either calcium abnormality.
- Low-calcium diet
  Decreased consumption of calcium may lead to lower serum calcium levels.
- Increase fluids and fiber to decrease complications of constipation
  Delayed gastric motility secondary to effects of calcium on smooth muscle leads to constipation.

Evaluating Care Outcomes

Hyperparathyroidism is a manageable disease process if patients are compliant with prescribed interventions. Prevention of complications secondary to sustained hypercalcemia is paramount for a healthy lifestyle. In patients who are not responsive to medical management of hyperparathyroidism, a subtotal parathyroidectomy may be performed. Postoperative care for these patients is similar to that for the patient undergoing thyroidectomy.

Connection Check 43.8

The nursing diagnosis "Acute pain related to ureteral pressure and obstruction secondary to calcium-containing renal stones" is most appropriate for the patient with which endocrine disorder?

A. Hypothyroidism
B. Hypoparathyroidism
C. Hyperthyroidism
D. Hyperparathyroidism

Making Connections

CASE STUDY: WRAP-UP

Ms. Matthews returns to the clinic 2 weeks after starting the PTU because she continues to have the same complaints of restlessness and insomnia and has lost another 6 pounds since her last appointment. The nurse practitioner discusses the option of radioactive iodine therapy, but Ms. Matthews refuses because she would like to get pregnant once her hyperthyroidism is controlled. Radioactive iodine therapy is contraindicated in pregnancy because of potential adverse effects to the developing fetus unless the potential benefits of the intervention outweigh the risks to the fetus and mother. She is referred for a surgical consult, and the decision is made for her to undergo a partial thyroidectomy to remove the hypersecreting thyroid tissue.

Case Study Questions

1. Which of Ms. Matthews' demographic variables are consistent with a diagnosis of hyperthyroidism? *(Select all that apply.)*
   A. Age
   B. Socioeconomic status
   C. Occupation
   D. Race
   E. Gender

2. The nurse recognizes that the rationale for the administration of propylthiouracil (PTU) is based on which action of this medication?
   A. Decreases thyroid hormone release from the anterior pituitary gland
   B. Blocks conversion of T4 to T3
   C. Increases TRH release from the hypothalamus
   D. Augments iodine absorption by the thyroid gland

3. The nurse recognizes which rationale for the instructions to Ms. Matthews to increase her intake of fluids secondary to her hyperthyroidism?
   A. There is an increased water loss because of the hypermetabolic state.
   B. There is increased blood flow through the renal system.
   C. There is a decreased availability of TSH.
   D. There is increased water reabsorption in the gastrointestinal tract.

4. What is a nursing priority for Ms. Matthews in preparation for the thyroid surgery?
   A. Maintain weight loss at less than 2 pounds per week
   B. Increase intake of green leafy vegetables
   C. Heart rate within normal parameters
   D. Decrease intake of calcium

5. The nurse recognizes which action of radioiodine therapy that impacts women during their childbearing years?

    A. It interferes with production of estrogen.

    B. It decreases blood flow to the placenta during pregnancy.

    C. It interferes with normal menstrual cycles.

    D. It may adversely impact fetal development.

CHAPTER SUMMARY

Metabolic function is largely under the control of the thyroid glands. The parathyroid glands play a key role in the regulation of calcium and phosphorus levels. Diseases of both of these endocrine glands may manifest as disorders secondary to hypofunction or hyperfunction. Thyroid disorders are classified according to the origin of the hormonal changes: a primary disorder is secondary to changes in the release of the hormones triiodothyronine (T3) and thyroxine (T4) from the thyroid glands, secondary disorders are related to secretion changes of TSH from the anterior pituitary gland, and tertiary processes occur because of changes in secretion of TRH from the hypothalamus. Management of these disorders focus on raising hormone levels or affecting the actions and functions of target tissues.

Hypothyroidism is caused by a decrease in T3 and T4. The clinical presentation of this disorder is characterized by decreased metabolic activity in all cells of the body. Patients with hypothyroidism may exhibit cold intolerance because of decreased metabolic activity. Other clinical manifestations include fatigue, weight gain, bradycardia, dry coarse skin, and sensitivity to narcotics and barbiturates. Severe hypothyroidism, myxedema coma, is associated with significant changes in cardiac function that may result in decreased cardiac contractility and cardiac output.

Hyperthyroidism develops secondary to elevated levels of circulating thyroid (T3 and T4) hormones. Patients with this disorder present with clinical manifestations associated with hypermetabolic activity including tachycardia, restlessness, fatigue, weight loss, and diarrhea secondary to increased gastric emptying. Management of hyperthyroidism focuses on decreasing thyroid hormone levels through medications that decrease synthesis and secretion or surgical procedures that remove the hypersecreting tissue or tumor.

Disorders of the parathyroid glands relate to changes in secretion of parathormone (PTH) and directly affect serum calcium levels. In parathyroid disease, there is a direct relationship between levels of PTH and serum calcium levels; increased PTH leads to increased serum calcium levels, and decreased PTH results in decreased serum calcium levels. Clinical manifestations of hypoparathyroidism include increased neuromuscular transmission, tetany, muscle cramps, and paresthesias of the hands and feet. Management of hypoparathyroidism is focused on increasing serum calcium levels with calcium and vitamin D supplementation. Hyperparathyroidism with resulting hypercalcemia leads to muscle weakness, atrophy, low back pain, and increased incidence of pathological fractures secondary to loss of calcium from bones and an increased incidence of calcium-containing renal stones. Management of hyperparathyroidism is focused on decreasing serum calcium levels through hydration and decreasing intake of calcium.

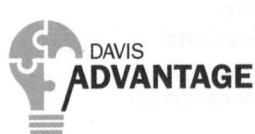

To explore learning resources for this chapter, go to **Davis Advantage** and find:

– Answers to in-text questions

– Chapter Resources and Activities

– NCLEX®-Style Chapter Review Questions

– Bibliography

Chapter 44

Coordinating Care for Patients With Diabetes Mellitus

Susan Renda

LEARNING OUTCOMES

Content in this chapter is designed to assist in:

1. Discussing the epidemiology of diabetes mellitus
2. Describing the pathophysiology of type 1 and type 2 diabetes mellitus
3. Correlating clinical manifestations of type 1 and type 2 diabetes mellitus with the pathophysiology of each disorder
4. Describing the diagnostic studies used to diagnose and monitor diabetes mellitus
5. Comparing indications, administration, actions, and nursing considerations for insulin and oral hypoglycemic agents
6. Explaining complications associated with type 1 and type 2 diabetes mellitus
7. Designing a plan of care that includes pharmacological, dietary, and lifestyle considerations based on the disease process
8. Correlating rationales for nursing interventions with the underlying pathophysiological processes
9. Teaching self-care strategies to patients in relation to the management of diabetes mellitus and pharmacological management

CONCEPTS

- Assessment
- Fluid and Electrolyte Balance
- Medication
- Metabolism
- Nutrition
- pH Regulation

ESSENTIAL TERMS

Basal insulin
Continuous glucose monitoring
Dawn phenomenon
Diabetes mellitus (DM)
Diabetic ketoacidosis (DKA)
Fasting blood glucose
Gestational diabetes
Glucosuria
Glycemic control
Hemoglobin A1c
Hyperglycemia
Hyperosmolar hyperglycemic state (HHS)
Insulin deficiency
Insulin pumps
Insulin resistance
Kussmaul respirations
Metabolic syndrome
Oral glucose tolerance test
Polydipsia
Polyphagia
Polyuria
Prediabetes
Prolonged hyperglycemia
Self-monitoring of blood glucose
Somogyi effect
Type 1 diabetes
Type 2 diabetes

Finding Connections

CASE STUDY: EPISODE 1

Follow this patient throughout the chapter.

Mrs. Edith Simpson is a 63-year-old African American female admitted for unstable angina. She is now 4 days postoperative following a triple cardiac bypass. She has a 15-year history of type 2 diabetes and is managed at home on metformin (Glucophage) and glyburide (Glynase). Her past medical history (PMH) also includes hypertension, hyperlipidemia, and a past surgical history of cholecystectomy. She works as an administrative assistant for the city government. She is married with four grown children. She smoked 1 ppd × 25 years but quit 2 years ago. Her labs indicate an elevated creatinine of 2.2 mg/dL, glomerular filtration rate (GFR) of 27 mL/min/1.73 m^2, white blood cell (WBC) count elevated at 12.5 10^3/mm^3, and a blood glucose of 220 mg/dL…

INTRODUCTION

There are continuous, dynamic, and intricate balancing mechanisms that support the control of circulating fasting blood glucose levels within a tight range of 65 to 99 mg/dL. This level of control occurs despite differences in ages, weight, intake of food, and activity levels. The two hormones primarily responsible for this homeostasis are released by the pancreas: insulin, released from the beta cells of the pancreas, and glucagon, released from the alpha cells of the pancreas.

The normal process of blood glucose level control is as follows (Fig. 44.1):

1. Glucose arrives in the bloodstream from one of three sources:
   - Carbohydrates eaten by mouth, converted to glucose via digestion, and absorbed through the gastrointestinal tract;
   - Glucose released from stored glycogen in muscles and liver cells; or
   - Glucose newly created (gluconeogenesis) in the liver or kidney cells.
2. Once in the bloodstream, the glucose is transported to the target cells.
3. In response to increased blood glucose levels, insulin is released from the pancreatic beta cells.
4. At the target cells, insulin facilitates the transport of glucose across the cell membrane to the cell's interior. Insulin is the key to the cell, allowing glucose to cross the cell membrane to be metabolized (Fig. 44.2).
5. Inside the cell, glucose is metabolized as fuel, releasing the energy necessary for normal cellular functioning.
6. If blood glucose levels are high, more insulin is secreted by the pancreas.
7. When blood glucose is driven into the cells and metabolized, glucose levels in the blood fall as a result.
8. If blood glucose levels fall too low, insulin release is suppressed, and glucose remains in the bloodstream instead of being driven into the cells.
9. In addition, in response to falling blood glucose levels, the hormone glucagon is released from the pancreatic alpha cells. Glucagon stimulates the production and release of glucose from glycogen stores in the liver so that blood glucose levels rise to normal.

When there is a disruption in the production of insulin (**insulin deficiency**) or when there are defects in the effective action of insulin at the cell membrane (**insulin resistance**), glucose cannot effectively cross cell membranes to enter the cell. Instead, glucose remains in the bloodstream, and blood glucose levels rise above normal. The resulting **hyperglycemia** is the hallmark of **diabetes mellitus (DM)**.

Diabetes mellitus is a group of disorders characterized by elevated blood glucose levels and results from defects in insulin production, insulin action, or both. According to estimates from the Centers for Disease Control and Prevention (CDC), over 30 million people in the United States, representing 9.4% of the population, have diabetes. Additionally, 84.1 million adults 18 years or older have prediabetes, which represents approximately 33.9% of the U.S. adult population. In the older adult population, 23.1 million people aged 65 years or older have prediabetes. There are numerous etiologies for these defects, but two types of diabetes, **type 1 diabetes** and **type 2 diabetes**, make up more than 90% of cases.

Another form of diabetes is **gestational diabetes**. It is defined as any degree of glucose intolerance with onset during pregnancy. If the mother's blood glucose is elevated above recommended targets, there is a risk of adverse outcomes to the mother, fetus, and infant. It complicates approximately 7% of all pregnancies, resulting in more than 200,000 cases annually. Women with a history of gestational diabetes have a greatly increased risk of developing type 2 diabetes within 15 years of the birth.

There are other, less common types of diabetes that are due to specific causes. These include:

- Diseases of the exocrine pancreas (such as cystic fibrosis or chronic pancreatitis)
- Surgical removal or resection of the pancreas
- Medication- or chemical-induced elevations in blood glucose levels, such as those that develop secondary to the use of corticosteroids
- Genetic defects in cell function
- Genetic defects in insulin action

The focus of this chapter is type 1 and type 2 DM.

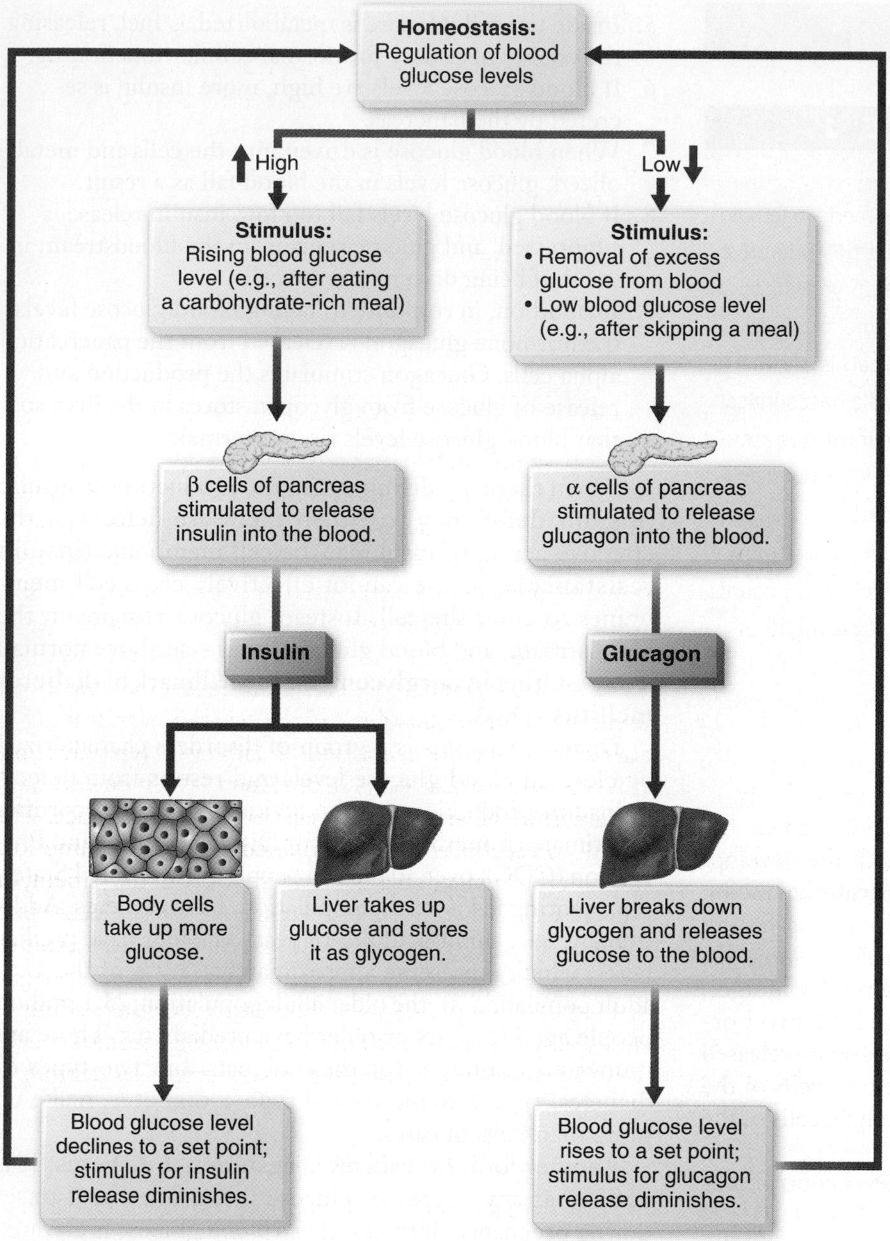

Homeostasis:
Regulation of blood
glucose levels

↑ High   Low ↓

Stimulus:
Rising blood glucose
level (e.g., after eating
a carbohydrate-rich meal)

Stimulus:
• Removal of excess
  glucose from blood
• Low blood glucose level
  (e.g., after skipping a meal)

β cells of pancreas
stimulated to release
insulin into the blood.

α cells of pancreas
stimulated to release
glucagon into the blood.

Insulin

Glucagon

Body cells
take up more
glucose.

Liver takes up
glucose and stores
it as glycogen.

Liver breaks down
glycogen and releases
glucose to the blood.

Blood glucose level
declines to a set point;
stimulus for insulin
release diminishes.

Blood glucose level
rises to a set point;
stimulus for glucagon
release diminishes.

FIGURE 44.1 Glucose homeostasis. Changes
in blood glucose levels are regulated by insulin
and glucagon release from the pancreas. With
increased blood glucose, insulin is released. As
blood glucose levels fall, glucagon is released
to increase blood glucose.

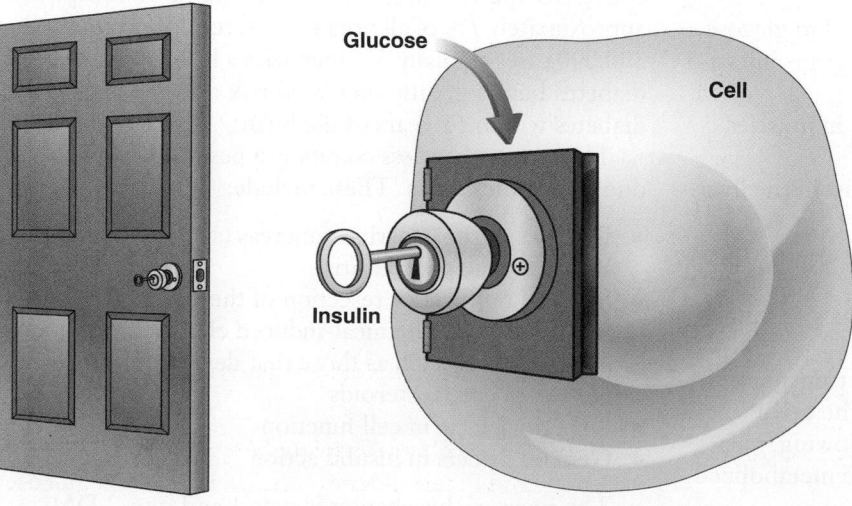

Glucose

Cell

Insulin

FIGURE 44.2 Insulin as the key to the cell. Insulin
facilitates transport of glucose across the cell
membrane to the cell's interior to be metabolized.

TYPE 1 DIABETES MELLITUS

Epidemiology

Although most commonly diagnosed before age 30, type 1 diabetes can occur at any stage of life, even into the eighth and ninth decades. Previously referred to as *juvenile-onset diabetes* because of the typical age of onset, it now affects more than 400,000 children under 14 years of age, with a total of 1.25 million people with type 1 diabetes in the United States. It is the primary cause of diabetes in children under 10 years of age. The prevalence of type 1 diabetes varies by ethnic background, with people of European ancestry having the highest incidence. In adults, type 1 diabetes accounts for 5% to 10% of all diagnosed cases, or 11 to 22 million cases worldwide. The overall incidence of type 1 diabetes is increasing by 2% to 3% each year.

There are both genetic and environmental factors involved in the development of type 1 diabetes. The risk of developing type 1 diabetes increases if family members have type 1 diabetes or other associated autoimmune disorders, such as autoimmune thyroid disease, celiac disease, or Addison's disease. Environmental triggers also play a part in genetically sensitive individuals. Although the specific triggers are not yet fully understood, they are thought to include viruses such as mumps, rubella, and Coxsackie B4; toxic chemicals; exposure to cow's milk with the development of bovine antibodies; and cytotoxins (substances that are toxic to and kill living cells).

Pathophysiology

Type 1 diabetes is typically triggered by an autoimmune process in which the insulin-producing beta cells of the pancreas are destroyed, resulting in an absolute lack of insulin. In children and young adults, this process is usually rapid, with total insulin deficiency occurring within 1 year, after which lifelong insulin therapy is required. If the disease begins in adulthood, the autoimmune destruction of beta cells has a more variable but generally slower time frame. Adult patients with new autoimmune type 1 diabetes, often referred to as late autoimmune diabetes of adulthood (LADA), may retain some insulin-secreting ability for years. Eventually, however, they develop total insulin deficiency. Once beta-cell destruction has progressed to the point of total insulin deficiency, patients with type 1 diabetes require externally delivered insulin (provided via a pump or injection) for the remainder of their lives.

Patients undergoing pancreatic resection as a result of cancer or other diseases of the pancreas may also present with surgically induced diabetes appearing as type 1 diabetes because of a lack of insulin after the surgical procedure. Like patients diagnosed with type 1 diabetes caused by the autoimmune process, these patients will also require lifelong insulin therapy.

Connection Check 44.1

The nurse understands that type 1 DM is caused by which of the following conditions? *(Select all that apply.)*

A. Gestational diabetes
B. A history of mumps or rubella
C. Family history of autoimmune disorders
D. Autoimmune destruction of the beta cells of the pancreas
E. Obesity

Clinical Manifestations

Clinical manifestations caused by the hyperglycemia of type 1 diabetes are evident in many body systems. Predominant features include **polyuria**, **polydipsia**, **polyphagia**, fatigue, and weight loss. Polyuria, increased volumes of urine, is due to an increased concentration of glucose in the urine, or **glucosuria**. Glucose is typically totally reabsorbed in the renal tubules. Hyperglycemia results in glucose excretion in the urine, which creates an osmotic effect that effectively reduces water reabsorption into the renal tubules, leading to excessive volume loss through the kidneys. Hyperglycemia also causes hyperosmolality in the blood, which causes a shift of fluid from the intracellular space to the vascular space. The loss of intracellular water combined with the volume loss through the kidneys creates excessive thirst in the patient, or polydipsia. The lack of insulin necessary to move glucose into the cells leads to the breakdown of proteins and fat as a source of energy. This starvation of the cells leads to polyphagia, increased appetite. Despite an increased appetite leading to consumption of large amounts of food, the continual breakdown of fats and proteins leads to weight loss and fatigue.

Connection Check 44.2

The nurse monitors for which clinical manifestations in the patient newly diagnosed with type 1 DM? *(Select all that apply.)*

A. Polyuria
B. Fatigue
C. Weight loss
D. Polyphagia
E. Decreased appetite

Management

Medical Management

Diagnosis

Type 1 DM in the nonpregnant adult is diagnosed by various methods:

- *Hemoglobin A1c (glycosylated hemoglobin) value.* The HgbA1c test measures the average blood glucose concentration over time by measuring the amount of glucose that binds to red blood cells (RBCs). Reflecting the average life span of an RBC, the test gives an accurate indication of long-term, time-averaged glucose levels over the 6 to 12 weeks prior to the HgbA1c blood draw. When blood glucose concentrations are high, more hemoglobin is affected. On the day the HgbA1c sample is collected, eating, physical activity, or acute stresses do not affect the result, and the test can be done at any time of day and does not require fasting. Because of these characteristics, it is a good tool to monitor the effectiveness of insulin therapy as well as the patient's adherence to the diabetes management plan.

The HgbA1c levels do not show fluctuations, and swings between hypoglycemia and hyperglycemia can be masked in the "average" blood glucose levels. Measurement depends on the RBC survival and the composition of RBC hemoglobin, so HgbA1c results are inaccurate in several clinical situations, such as recent blood loss or transfusions. In addition, it is not accurate in the setting of anemia and treatment with erythropoietin, both of which are common in patients with diabetic renal disease.

- *Fasting blood glucose.* Fasting is defined as no caloric intake for at least 8 hours. Without adequate oral intake, glucagon is released from the pancreas, facilitating the release of glycogen stores from the liver and increasing circulating blood glucose levels. Normally, insulin is released, moving that glucose into the cells, preventing hyperglycemia. Without adequate insulin, hyperglycemia results.
- *Two-hour postprandial (after meals) or the oral glucose tolerance test (OGTT).* This test is performed by asking the patient to consume a beverage containing a glucose load, the equivalent of 75 g of carbohydrate, after fasting for 8 to 12 hours. Blood samples are taken prior to consuming the drink to get a fasting level, then again at 1 hour and 2 hours after consumption. The diagnostic value is based on the blood glucose level 2 hours after consumption.
- *Random blood glucose.* A random blood glucose level of greater than or equal to 200 mg/dL in a patient with classic symptoms of hyperglycemia or hyperglycemic crisis may be indicative of diabetes mellitus.

See Table 44.1 for a summary of the diagnostic laboratory values for diabetes.

Connection Check 44.3

The nurse correlates which laboratory value with the diagnosis of DM?

A. Fasting blood glucose greater than 140 mg/dL
B. Hemoglobin A1c, 5.8%
C. Random blood glucose, 150 mg/dL
D. OGTT, 155 mg/dL

Table 44.1 Laboratory Values Diagnostic for Diabetes Mellitus

Laboratory Test	Value*	Interpretation
Fasting blood glucose OR	Greater than or equal to 126 mg/dL	DM
	100–125 mg/dL	Prediabetes
2-hr postprandial OR	Greater than or equal to 200 mg/dL	DM
	140–199 mg/dL	Prediabetes
Hemoglobin A1c OR	Greater than or equal to 6.5%	DM
	5.7%–6.4%	Prediabetes
Random blood glucose level	Greater than or equal to 200 mg/dL	DM if accompanied by classic signs/symptoms of hyperglycemia

*In the absence of unequivocal signs of hyperglycemia, criteria 1 to 3 should be confirmed by repeated testing on a different day.
DM, Diabetes mellitus.

Treatment

Successful treatment of type 1 DM involves several different strategies, including pharmacological interventions, nutrition management, patient education and self-management, and detection and prevention of complications. Nutrition, patient education and self-management, and detection and prevention of complications are similar for both type 1 and type 2 DM and are discussed under the management of type 2 DM section later in this chapter. The focus here is on the pharmacological interventions for type 1 DM.

Pharmacological Interventions

The primary pharmacological intervention used in the treatment of type 1 DM is insulin administered subcutaneously. Another insulin option is a newer inhaled version of short-acting insulin that may be used in combination with subcutaneous long-acting or intermediate-acting insulin as basal. Oral administration of insulin is not effective because it is broken down and rendered ineffective during the digestive process. The goal of treatment is to maximize **glycemic control**, the maintenance of blood glucose levels within normal ranges, in an effort to prevent the complications of hyperglycemia. In setting glycemic goals, it is important to consider that the closer the goals are to normal ranges, the lesser the risk of complications from diabetes. This has been demonstrated in several large, randomized controlled trials, including the Diabetes Control and Complications Trial/Epidemiology of Diabetes Interventions and Complications (DCCT/EDIC) study and the United Kingdom Prospective Diabetes Study (UKPDS). The recommended guidelines for setting individualized targets focus on weighing the potential risks of hypoglycemia with the benefits of tight glycemic control. Treatment goals should be determined and reassessed periodically on the basis of patient-specific factors such as health status, adverse medication reactions, adherence to treatment, ability to recognize low blood glucose, and patient preferences. If glycemic goals are not met, the patient should be assessed for knowledge; performance skills; and psychosocial, personal, or financial barriers. See Table 44.2 for definitions of glycemic control.

> **⚠ Safety Alert** Insulin is a high-risk medication with a narrow therapeutic margin. Tight glycemic control increases the risk of hypoglycemia in patients who rely on insulin and oral agents that stimulate the release of insulin to manage their diabetes. The benefits of tighter glucose control may not outweigh the risks for some patients. This includes patients with a limited life expectancy, those with comorbidities where a hypoglycemic event will have more serious consequences, or those unwilling or unable to do the monitoring necessary to prevent hypoglycemia. This risk is especially pronounced in patients with a tendency toward hypoglycemia, such as older adults, the malnourished, or those with renal or liver disease.

Blood Glucose Management Plans

Treatment plans that mimic the response of the healthy pancreas to blood glucose levels during the course of a day (Fig. 44.3) are the most effective at maintaining tight glucose control.

The insulin level is never zero because the healthy pancreas always maintains a basal (minimal) level of insulin throughout the day. At mealtimes, there is a sharp increase in insulin secretion in response to the increase in blood glucose levels. The availability of more modern insulin analogs and insulin pumps makes it possible to more closely mimic the actions of a healthy pancreas, creating a physiological approach to diabetes management. An approach using a combination of long-acting or intermediate-acting insulin once or twice a day to provide **basal insulin** is most effective in maintaining tight glycemic control. These approaches include rapid-acting and short-acting insulin taken at mealtimes to cover the incoming carbohydrates, *prandial insulin* or *nutritional insulin*, and a "sliding scale" of additional supplemental or *correctional insulin* to compensate for blood glucose elevations. The need for correctional insulin is determined by a random blood glucose level done via finger stick immediately prior to eating. The prandial and correctional insulins are then administered at the same time prior to eating. In hospitalized patients with questionable or minimal oral intake, prandial and correctional insulins can be given immediately after the meal to confirm adequate carbohydrate intake. This approach best mimics the way the healthy pancreas releases insulin, but it does require

Table 44.2 Glycemic Goals

	American Diabetes Association (ADA)	American Association of Clinical Endocrinologists (AACE)
		All Patients With Diabetes Mellitus: Encourage patients to achieve glycemic levels as near normal as possible without inducing clinically significant hypoglycemia.
Fasting	Target fasting or preprandial blood glucose values to a goal of 70–130 mg/dL for an HgbA1c goal of less than 7%. Target blood glucose readings can be higher or lower depending on individualized HgbA1c goal.	Fasting blood glucose concentration less than 110 mg/dL
2-hour postprandial	Average 2-hour postprandial (after eating) blood glucose value less than 180 mg/dL The 2-hour postprandial blood glucose can be helpful for adjusting mealtime medications.	2-hour postprandial glucose concentration less than 140 mg/dL
HgbA1c	Lowering HgbA1c to below or around 7% has been shown to reduce the microvascular and neurological complications of type 1 and type 2 diabetes. Therefore, for microvascular disease prevention, the HgbA1c goal for nonpregnant adults in general is less than 7%.	A1c less than or equal to 6.5%

HgbA1c, Glycosylated hemoglobin.

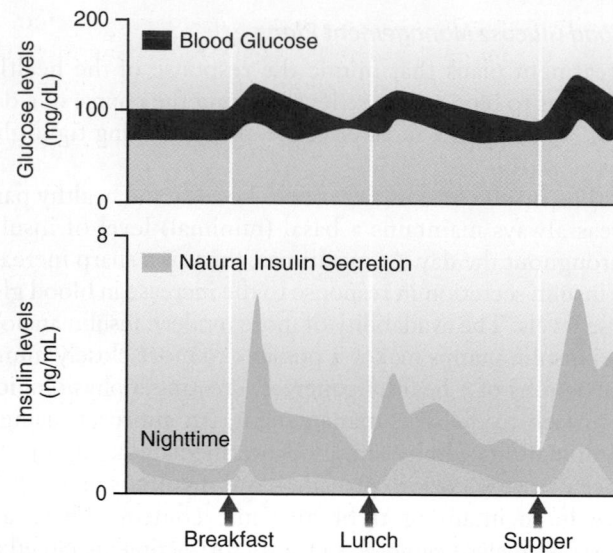

FIGURE 44.3 Normal pancreatic response to glucose levels during the day. Insulin is released as blood glucose levels rise after meals.

multiple blood glucose evaluations (finger sticks) and injections daily. See Table 44.3 for the various types of insulin and Figure 44.4 for the use of long-acting and rapid-acting insulin to mimic normal pancreatic functioning.

Subcutaneous insulin can be drawn up from a vial and administered via needle and insulin syringe, or it can be administered through an insulin pen (Fig. 44.5) or via an insulin pump. If insulin syringes are used, it is important to match the syringe size to the insulin concentration. The most typical insulin concentration is U-100, which means 100 units of insulin per milliliter. U-100 insulin syringes come in several sizes: 1 mL that holds 100 units, 0.5 mL that holds 50 units, and 0.3 that holds 30 units. The patient should choose the insulin syringe size according to his or her insulin dosage. For example, using the small 0.3-mL syringe allows patients who are prescribed very small doses to more accurately draw up their insulin. If insulin requirements are massive because of extreme insulin resistance, a U-500 (500 units per milliliter) insulin

Table 44.3 Types of Insulin

Brand Name	Onset	Peak	Duration	Purpose
RAPID-ACTING*				Prandial insulin used within 0–15 minutes prior to eating or used as correction insulin for blood glucose elevations; used in combination with long-acting insulin
Humalog/Lispro	15–30 min	30–90 min	3–5 hr	Also available in U-200 concentrated form for people requiring larger dosages
NovoLog/Aspart	10–20 min	40–50 min	3–5 hr	
Apidra/Glulisine	20–30 min	30–60 min	1–2.5 hr	
SHORT-ACTING				Prandial insulin used for meals eaten within 30 to 60 min after administration; used in combination with long-acting insulin
Regular Humulin/ Novolin	30–60 min	2–5 hr	5–8 hr	
INTERMEDIATE-ACTING				Covers insulin needs for approximately half the day or overnight; used in combination with rapid-acting or short-acting insulin
NPH	1–2 hr	4–12 hr	18–24 hr	
LONG-ACTING				Basal insulin; used in combination with rapid-acting or short-acting insulin
Lantus, Toujeo, and Basaglar/glargine	1–1.5 hr	No peaks or valleys	20–24 hr	Glargine as Toujeo is U-300, three times the concentration for patients on large dosages.
Levemir/Detemir	1–2 hr	No peaks or valleys	24 hr	
Degludec/Tresiba	1 hr	Steady state achieved at 8 days	24-42 hr	The very long half-life helps maintain glycemic control if dosage is late. Also available in U-200 for people who require large dosages.

*Prandial insulin of choice for both multiple injections and the insulin pump.

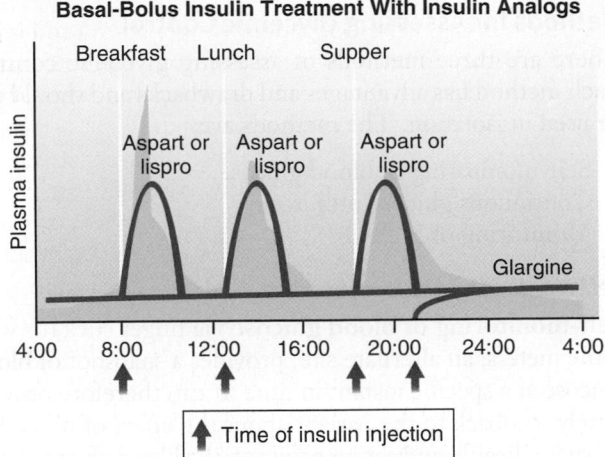

Basal-Bolus Insulin Treatment With Insulin Analogs

FIGURE 44.4 Basal and bolus insulin therapy. Exogenous insulin is administered to coincide with blood glucose spikes after meals.

insulin pump to form a partial closed-loop system in which the pump automatically makes adjustments to the basal rate based on data from the CGM. The patient still counts carbohydrates, checks the glucose level pre-meal, and makes the insulin decision for the meal amount to be delivered.

Evidence-Based Practice

Psychosocial Factors of Insulin Pump Therapy

Insulin pumps are increasingly being used by patients with type 1 diabetes to manage their disease. This systematic review examined psychosocial facilitators and challenges of insulin pump therapy in patients with type 1 diabetes. An integrative literature review was conducted to evaluate the evidence regarding the psychosocial impact of insulin pumps and included literature from January 2005 to February 2017. The systematic search included the CINAHL, Cochrane, Medline, PsycINFO, and Scopus databases. The psychosocial facilitators identified included flexibility and freedom in daily activities and enhanced social situations. Challenges included the demands of the pump therapy, self-consciousness in wearing the pump, fear of pump failure, and hypoglycemia. The findings of this study can be used by healthcare professionals in teaching and preparing individuals for insulin pump therapy.

Payk, M., Robinson, T., Davis, D., & Atchan, M. (2018). An integrative review of the psychosocial facilitators and challenges of continuous subcutaneous insulin infusion therapy in type 1 diabetes. *Journal of Advanced Nursing, 74*(3), 528–538.

concentration is available by special order. In contrast to the insulin syringe and needle, the insulin pen allows the patient to dial in the exact dosage, avoiding the potential errors inherent in measuring and drawing up insulin in the traditional way.

An alternative approach to the administration of insulin is the use of continuous subcutaneous **insulin pumps**. Insulin pumps provide the same delivery of basal and bolus insulin as the multiple-injection technique, but it is provided by a computer-driven device that delivers insulin according to instructions programmed by the patient (Fig. 44.6). The use of the subcutaneous insulin pump has been found to provide better glycemic control, especially in patients with higher hemoglobin A1c levels indicating poor glycemic control with traditional methods. Advantages of the pump include convenience and the ability to deliver more precise dosages. Patients state that it allows a better quality of life and more freedom from the strict restrictions inherent in the traditional insulin administration methods. The disadvantages of insulin pumps are the expense, the need for active participation and learning by the patient in response to glucose levels, the need to "wear" the pump continuously, skin issues around the needle insertion site, and potential complications if the pump malfunctions (see Evidence-Based Practice). A newer form of insulin pump combines continuous glucose monitoring (CGM) with the

Some patients are unable or unwilling to manage the multiple daily blood glucose evaluations and injections or the insulin pump. An alternative treatment plan is twice-daily finger sticks with twice-daily insulin injections. This does not offer the same possibility of tight glycemic control as the other methods, but it is less complicated and easier to manage. The insulin used is typically a mixture

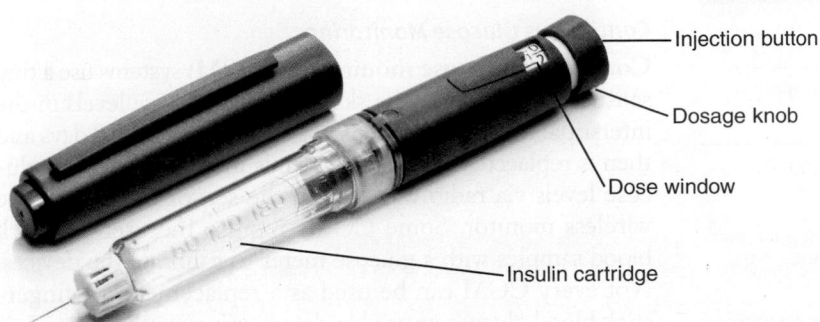

Injection button

Dosage knob

Dose window

Insulin cartridge

FIGURE 44.5 Insulin pen.

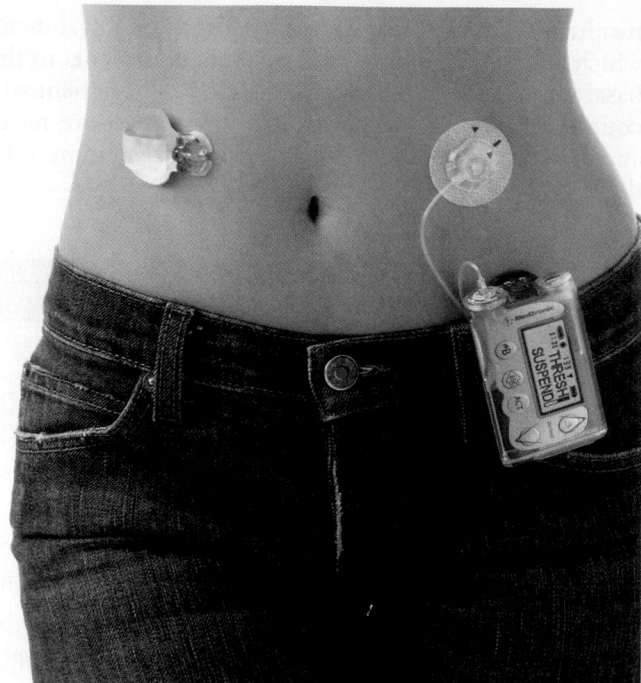

FIGURE 44.6 Insulin pump.

of rapid-acting and long-acting insulin. This insulin can be administered via needle and syringe, or it is also available in an insulin pen. See Table 44.4 for a listing of insulin mixtures.

Connection Check 44.4

The charge nurse is reviewing orders for a newly admitted patient with type 1 DM. It is a priority for the charge nurse to follow up with the provider about which order?

A. NovoLog insulin subcutaneous at bedtime
B. NovoLog insulin subcutaneous 15 minutes prior to meals
C. Basal insulin subcutaneous at bedtime
D. Correctional and nutritional insulin administered immediately after the meal

---

Table 44.4 Premixed Insulin

Brand Name	Composition
Humalog 75/25	75% intermediate-acting insulin and 25% rapid-acting (lispro)
Humulin 70/30 *Novolin 70/30*	70% intermediate-acting insulin and 30% regular insulin
NovoLog 70/30	70% intermediate-acting insulin and 30% rapid-acting (aspart) insulin

Methods for Assessing Glycemic Control

There are three methods of assessing glycemic control. Each method has advantages and drawbacks and should not be used in isolation. The methods are:

- Self-monitoring of blood glucose
- Continuous glucose monitoring
- Monitoring of HgbA1c

Self-Monitoring of Blood Glucose

Self-monitoring of blood glucose via finger stick (or with some meters, an alternate site) provides a snapshot of blood glucose at a specific instant in time. It can therefore provide timely feedback to the patient about the effect of his or her behavior, health, and eating habits on the blood glucose level. In order for this method to be effective, patients must receive instructions on the accurate testing procedure. The most common patient-related error is an inadequate blood sample size. The patient's technique should be observed by a trained observer on the initiation of the plan of care and also should be reviewed annually or as indicated. Patients should be taught the importance of documenting results. With a record of blood glucose levels, food intake, and medication dosage, a diabetes educator can assist the patient in recognizing and interpreting blood glucose patterns. With this information, the patient can learn to adjust insulin dosing, food intake, or exercise and maximize glycemic control. As patients discover what works and what doesn't, they can gain an important sense of control over their blood glucose levels.

The frequency of self-monitoring of blood glucose in patients using insulin should be individualized on the basis of the frequency of insulin injections, hypoglycemic reactions, level of glycemic control, and patient/provider use of the data to adjust therapy. Generally, patients with type 1 DM are advised to check their blood glucose at a minimum of before meals and at bedtime. Patients on insulin pumps often check more frequently, especially during periods of medication adjustment.

Increased frequency of self-monitoring of blood glucose levels is recommended when:

- Therapy is being initiated or actively adjusted
- There is acute or ongoing illness
- There is hypoglycemia unawareness or an increase in hypoglycemic events
- Fasting and/or postprandial blood glucose levels are not consistent with HgbA1c

Continuous Glucose Monitoring

Continuous glucose monitoring (CGM) systems use a tiny sensor inserted under the skin to check glucose levels in the interstitial fluid. The sensor stays in place for 7 to 10 days and then is replaced. A transmitter sends information about glucose levels via radio waves from the sensor to a pager-like wireless monitor. Some CGMs require the user to check blood samples with a glucose meter to calibrate the devices. Not every CGM can be used as a replacement for finger-stick blood glucose or used in determining insulin doses. It is essential that the patient receives education about how to calibrate the device if it is needed and how to interpret the results.

Continuous glucose monitoring devices provide real-time measurements of glucose levels, with levels displayed in 1 to 5 minutes. Users can set alarms to alert them when glucose levels are too low or too high. One form of continuous monitoring is done "on demand" by waving the receiver over the sensor/transmitter and does not have alarms. It is mainly meant to reduce the need for blood glucose sticks. Special software is available to download data from the devices to a computer for tracking and analysis of patterns and trends, and the systems can display trend graphs on the monitor screen. This can provide important information about patterns and trends so that patients can make sense of what is affecting their blood glucose levels. A CGM with alarm functions provides a particular benefit for patients who experience erratic and unpredictable blood glucose drops; the alarm can alert them to take action before the blood glucose drops to dangerous levels.

Hemoglobin A1c Monitoring

Hemoglobin A1c results should be obtained at least twice a year for patients with diabetes and every 3 months if glycemic targets have not been met or if there are treatment changes.

Complications

There are many complications related to both type 1 and type 2 DM. The various complications of long-term hyperglycemia are discussed later in the chapter. The focus here is on acute complications, including diabetic ketoacidosis (DKA), hypoglycemia, the dawn phenomenon, and the Somogyi effect.

Diabetic Ketoacidosis

In **diabetic ketoacidosis (DKA)**, there is inadequate insulin for cells to obtain adequate glucose for normal metabolism. The body attempts to obtain energy by the rapid breakdown of fat stores, releasing fatty acids from adipose tissues. The liver converts the fatty acids into ketone bodies, which can serve as an energy source in the absence of glucose. The ketone bodies, however, have a low pH, resulting in metabolic acidosis. The absence of insulin also results in an increased release of hormones, such as glucagon and cortisol, in response to inadequate glucose transport into the cells. This leads to gluconeogenesis and glycogenolysis, resulting in severe hyperglycemia leading to hyperosmolality and osmotic diuresis, as discussed previously.

The causes of DKA include:

- Intentional or unintentional missed or reduced doses of insulin
- Inadequate insulin due to increased insulin needs secondary to stress or infection
- New onset of type 1 diabetes

Clinical Manifestations. Similar to the initial presentation of DM, the initial patient presentation of DKA is one of polyuria, polydipsia, and polyphagia. The patient becomes dehydrated, and an electrolyte imbalance such as hyperkalemia or hypokalemia may result (see Safety Alert). The increased serum osmolality also results in a shift of fluid from the intracellular to the extracellular space, causing dilutional hyponatremia. The patient is also at risk for hypovolemia secondary to the osmotic diuresis.

Without treatment, the patient abruptly becomes hypotensive and tachycardic because of the volume loss. The patient also develops **Kussmaul respirations**, which are rapid, deep respirations that occur as a compensatory mechanism for the acidosis. There is a fruity, acetone smell to the breath because of the ketone bodies. The patient may complain of nausea and vomiting. Lethargy and coma may ensue without prompt treatment. Figure 44.7 shows the common presenting clinical manifestations of DKA.

Diagnosis. Diagnosis of DKA is based on several factors:

- Blood glucose level greater than 250 mg/dL
- Ketonuria (ketones in the urine)
- Arterial pH of less than or equal to 7.3
- Serum bicarbonate level of less than or equal to 18 mEq/L
- Positive anion gap (Box 44.1)

Treatment. Treatment priorities include:
- Fluid replacement with isotonic normal saline
- Correction of electrolyte imbalances, focusing on monitoring and correction of decreased potassium level if necessary, prior to insulin administration
- Insulin administration, usually by intravenous delivery

Fluid replacement with isotonic normal saline is essential to reverse the dehydration that has resulted from the osmotic

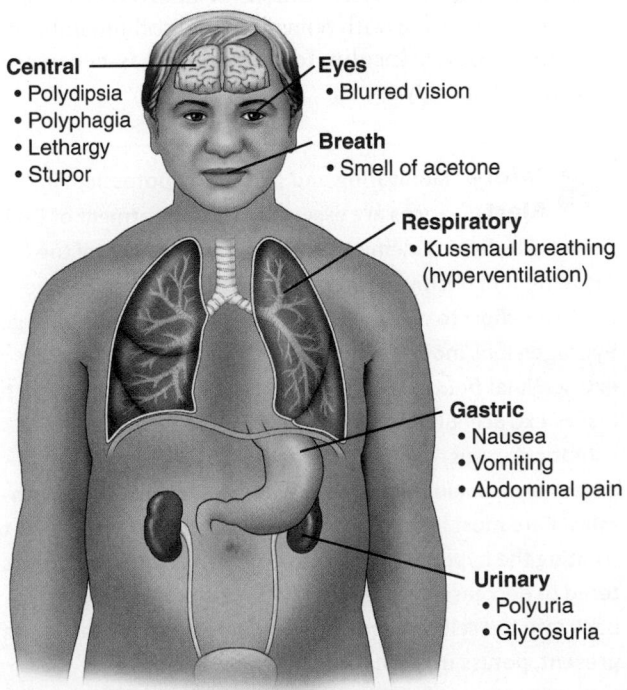

Central
- Polydipsia
- Polyphagia
- Lethargy
- Stupor

Eyes
- Blurred vision

Breath
- Smell of acetone

Respiratory
- Kussmaul breathing (hyperventilation)

Gastric
- Nausea
- Vomiting
- Abdominal pain

Urinary
- Polyuria
- Glycosuria

FIGURE 44.7 Clinical manifestations of diabetic ketoacidosis (DKA).

Box 44.1 Anion Gap

Cations are positively charged ions. The major cations are sodium, potassium, calcium, and magnesium. Anions are negatively charged ions: bicarbonate, chloride, phosphate, and albumin. The anion gap provides an estimation of unmeasured anions in the blood. It is useful in determining the cause of metabolic acidosis. It can also be used as a way of monitoring the response to therapy. The premise of this laboratory analysis is based on the need for electroneutrality in the body; the net positive charge must equal the net negative charge.

The anion gap is calculated using three laboratory values: positively charged sodium, negatively charged chloride, and negatively charged HCO_3. Positively charged potassium is sometimes added to the calculation, but typically the formula is as follows:

$$Anion\ gap = Na^+ - (Cl^- + HCO_3^-)$$

Serum sodium represents approximately 90% of the extracellular cations. Chloride and HCO_3 represent approximately 85% of the extracellular anions. Because of this, the normal anion gap—the normal amount of unmeasured anions—is positive because the sum of the measured serum anions is smaller than the sum of the measured serum cations or sodium in the formula. The normal value of the anion gap is 12 +/– 4.

If there is an addition of a positively charged acid, the anion gap will be altered. Diabetic ketoacidosis results in an elevated anion gap as a result of the accumulation of acids in the serum. The response to treatment can be monitored through evaluation of the anion gap. As the patient improves, the gap should return to normal.

---

diuresis. Monitoring and correcting electrolyte imbalances is essential to avoid the dysrhythmias or neurological complications that can occur with potassium and sodium imbalances (see Safety Alert). Insulin administration is necessary to correct the hyperglycemia.

Safety Alert   Monitoring and correcting potassium imbalances are essential in the treatment of DKA. Initially, hyperkalemia may be present because of the movement of positively charged potassium ions out of the cell in an effort to maintain homeostasis as positively charged hydrogen ions move into the cell as they accumulate in the extracellular fluid. Hypokalemia then ensues as a result of the loss of extracellular potassium in the urine because of the osmotic diuresis. This results in a severe total body loss of potassium, making the patient susceptible to lethal arrhythmias. Care must be taken to monitor potassium levels prior to treating the hyperglycemia with insulin. As insulin is administered to decrease hyperglycemia, potassium will also move back into the cell, worsening hypokalemia. If hypokalemia is present, potassium replacement is a priority.

Connection Check 44.5

The nurse correlates which laboratory values with being diagnostic for DKA? *(Select all that apply.)*
A. Serum bicarbonate of 18 mEq/L
B. Negative anion gap
C. Serum glucose of 350 mg/dL
D. Positive anion gap
E. Arterial pH of 7.36

Hypoglycemia

Hypoglycemia is an important and dangerous complication of the treatment of diabetes. It can present as an acute or even life-threatening emergency due to the potentially devastating effects on the central nervous system. Unlike other tissues of the body that can utilize fatty acids for energy needs, the central nervous system relies solely on glucose for its energy needs. It needs a constant supply to maintain metabolic functioning and avoid cell death.

Hypoglycemia, defined as a blood glucose level of less than 65 mg/dL, results when there is more circulating insulin than is needed to handle the amount of circulating glucose. Surplus insulin can be the result of an overly high dose of insulin administered, overly high dose of the oral agents that stimulate insulin release, or reduced clearance of insulin from the body because of renal insufficiency. Patients are at risk for hypoglycemia when they have a decreased nutritional intake or increased metabolism of glucose through increased exercise. Alcohol can also reduce blood glucose levels by blunting the release of glucose from the liver. Hypoglycemia is more severe when the early signs of low blood glucose are blunted, as in older adults or those who have a change in mental status.

Clinical Manifestations. When blood glucose levels drop below normal levels, the body attempts to raise glucose through the stimulation of the sympathetic nervous system and the release of hormones such as epinephrine, norepinephrine, and glucagon. Symptoms include:

- Anxiety
- Hunger
- Palpitations
- Circumoral paresthesia (numbness around lips)
- Sweating
- Shakiness
- Irritability

If blood glucose levels continue to drop, reaching levels where the central nervous system is inadequately supplied with glucose, symptoms include:

- Difficulty thinking
- Dizziness
- Fatigue
- Sleepiness
- Slurred speech
- Weakness/lack of coordination

If untreated and hypoglycemia progresses further, these symptoms can progress to:

- Seizures
- Coma

If hypoglycemia occurs frequently, the body can lose the early warning signals of sympathetic nervous symptoms. If patients have the accompanying "hypoglycemia unawareness," they will not experience symptoms of low blood glucose until their blood glucose levels fall to the point where the patients are at risk of neurological symptoms. They are then at risk of severe effects such as confusion or loss of consciousness. Individuals with hypoglycemia unawareness should be advised to raise their glycemic targets to strictly avoid further hypoglycemia for at least several weeks to partially reverse hypoglycemia unawareness and reduce the risk of further episodes.

Management of Hypoglycemia. The primary management technique consists of the administration of glucose to raise serum glucose levels. Oral glucose (15–20 g) administration is the preferred treatment for the conscious individual with hypoglycemia, although any form of rapidly absorbed carbohydrate may be used. Juice, soda, honey, jelly, bread, or crackers work well. Carbohydrates that contain fat, such as ice cream or chocolate, are not recommended. Pure glucose is the preferred treatment because fat may retard glucose absorption, prolonging the acute hypoglycemic event. After ingestion of carbohydrate, blood glucose levels should be measured within 15 minutes. If blood glucose levels continue to reflect hypoglycemia after treatment, the treatment should be repeated. Once glucose levels return to normal, the individual should consume a meal or snack to prevent the recurrence of hypoglycemia.

In the hospital setting, if a patient is unable to swallow or absorb oral carbohydrates but has IV access, IV dextrose, 25 to 50 mL of 50% dextrose solution (D50), should be administered. If there is no IV access and the patient is unable to swallow or absorb oral carbohydrates, 1 mg of intramuscular glucagon injection should be administered. Glucagon mobilizes glucose release from stores in the liver.

Glucagon administration is not limited to healthcare professionals. Severe hypoglycemia, where the individual requires assistance from another person and cannot be treated with oral carbohydrates because of confusion combined with the inability to swallow or unconsciousness, should be treated with glucagon. It should be prescribed for all individuals at risk of severe hypoglycemia, and caregivers or family members should be instructed in its administration. Instructions should include calling for emergency help if the glucagon injection is administered and turning the patient on his or her side to avoid aspiration because a side effect of glucagon is nausea and vomiting.

Connection Check 44.6

The nurse should intervene immediately if a patient has which blood glucose level?
A. 200 mg/dL
B. 150 mg/dL
C. 80 mg/dL
D. 40 mg/dL

Dawn Phenomenon and Somogyi Effect

The **dawn phenomenon** and **Somogyi effect** are two other complications of DM that result in increased blood glucose levels in the early morning. They occur more commonly in the patient with type 1 diabetes but are also known to occur in patients with type 2 diabetes. The increased blood glucose levels of the dawn phenomenon result from the naturally occurring release of hormones, such as glucagon, cortisol, and growth hormone, in the early morning. Because the body does not have sufficient insulin to control this glucose surge, blood glucose levels rise. This is most likely reflected in higher fasting blood glucose levels in the morning.

The Somogyi effect is much less common than the dawn phenomenon and results in increased blood glucose levels due to an excessive insulin dosage at night. This can occur in a patient who experiences unrecognized low glucose during the night while sleeping. In that circumstance, blood glucose levels drop, and the body responds in the same way as in the dawn phenomenon, releasing growth hormone, cortisol, and catecholamines in an effort to increase blood glucose by releasing glucose stores from the liver. As stated, both complications result in higher-than-normal blood glucose levels in the morning.

In order to determine what is causing the increased blood glucose levels in the morning, the patient needs to check blood glucose levels in the early morning hours, 2 or 3 a.m., for several nights. If the blood glucose level is low at that early morning time, the high glucose levels later in the morning are most likely due to the Somogyi effect. If the blood glucose level is high or normal at that early morning hour, the increased levels later in the morning are most likely due to the dawn phenomenon.

Nursing Management of Type 1 DM
Assessment and Analysis

The clinical manifestations of type 1 DM are due to the hyperglycemia that results from a lack of insulin secreted by the pancreas. Patients present with polyuria and polydipsia, as well as hemoconcentration in the blood secondary to the increased glucose in the urine, or glucosuria. Both situations create osmotic shifts in fluid, either from the intracellular space to the vascular space or from the renal tubules into the urine. The resultant volume loss triggers the thirst center in the brain, creating polydipsia. Excessive hunger (polyphagia) and fatigue are due to the inability to utilize glucose for cellular metabolism, resulting in the breakdown of fats and proteins.

Nursing Diagnoses

- **Impaired tissue perfusion** related to decreased cardiac output secondary to osmotic diuresis
- **Risk for neurological impairment** related to hypoglycemia

Nursing Interventions

■ *Assessments*

- Vital signs
  Decreased blood pressure and increased heart rate are secondary to the fluid volume deficit created by the osmotic diuresis related to hyperglycemia. Increased respiratory rate, Kussmaul breathing, or hyperventilation with fruity breath odor may be evident in DKA in an effort to compensate for the metabolic acidosis.
- Serum glucose
  Increased glucose levels are due to the lack of secretion of insulin from the pancreas. In a patient already diagnosed with and being treated for type 1 diabetes, increased glucose levels indicate:
  - Inadequate or lack of insulin administration
  - Increased insulin requirements due to stress, such as infection, causing the adrenal release of catecholamines, increasing the hepatic production of glucose
  Decreased glucose levels caused by inappropriate insulin administration, such as too much insulin or insulin given while the patient has inadequate PO intake, can lead to lethargy and coma or death. The brain uses only glucose for cellular metabolism, so it is severely affected by decreased glucose levels.
- Potassium levels
  Potassium levels may be decreased because of the increased volume loss through the kidneys or increased because of the shift of the positively charged potassium out of the cell in an effort to maintain homeostasis when positively charged hydrogen ions move into the cell in the face of acidosis.
- Intake and output
  Increased urine output may be present because of osmotic diuresis secondary to hyperglycemia.
- Carbohydrate intake at meals
  Adequate carbohydrate intake at meals is essential to avoid hypoglycemia related to insulin administration.

■ *Actions*

- Bedside glucose monitoring (finger sticks) done before meals and at bedtime
  Regular finger sticks are done to measure the adequacy of glucose control.
- Administer insulin as ordered.
  - Basal
  - Preprandial
  - Correctional
  Administering rapid-acting insulin before meals, preparing for ingestion of carbohydrates, and correcting for random high glucose levels as determined by self-monitoring

of blood glucose prior to the meal, in combination with longer-acting insulin once a day, will mimic the action of a healthy pancreas, helping to maintain tight glycemic control. In patients with questionable or minimal oral intake, prandial and correctional insulins may be administered together after meals after adequate carbohydrate intake has been confirmed.

- Administration of isotonic IV fluids as ordered
  Intravenous fluids may be necessary to replace the volume lost as a result of osmotic diuresis.

■ *Teaching*

- Signs of hypoglycemia and hyperglycemia
  It is important that the patient (and family) is able to detect early signs of both hypoglycemia (the underlying disorder that can progress to coma or death) and hyperglycemia secondary to inadequate insulin administration.
- Subcutaneous insulin administration:
  - Common sites that provide good absorption (starting with the area of best absorption) include the abdomen, upper arm, thigh, and buttocks.
  - Subcutaneous injection technique
    To ensure injection into the subcutaneous tissue, pinch the skin at the injection site and insert the needle straight in at a 90-degree angle. If the patient is very thin with very small amounts of subcutaneous tissue, the needle should be inserted at a 45-degree angle (Fig. 44.8).
  - Syringe size
    Choose the syringe size (1 mL, 0.5 mL, 0.3 mL) that best matches your insulin dose. The smaller syringes allow for more accurate measurement of smaller insulin dosages. If available, an insulin pen can be used and instructions given to the patient on accurate use and storage.
  - Rotating sites
    Insulin is administered subcutaneously. It is a protein substance. If taken orally, it is broken down in the

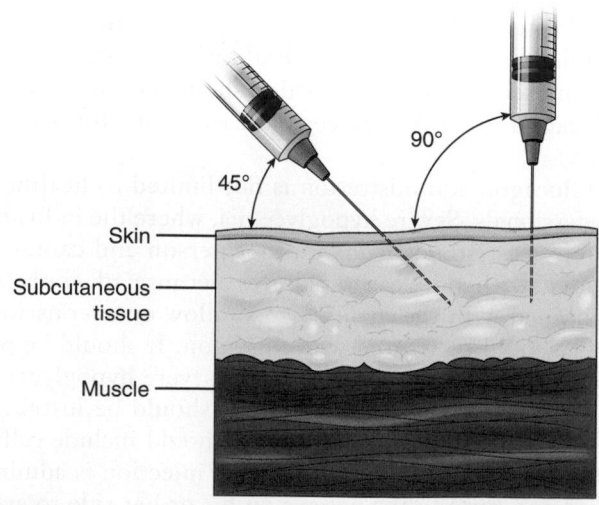

FIGURE 44.8 Subcutaneous injection angles. Subcutaneous injections are usually inserted at a 90-degree angle. In very thin patients with small amounts of subcutaneous tissue, the needle is inserted at a 45-degree angle.

Connection Check 44.9

The nurse recognizes which of the following statements as correct in relation to the pathophysiology of type 2 DM? *(Select all that apply.)*

A. It is due to a relative lack of insulin.
B. It is due to insulin resistance.
C. It is due to an absolute lack of insulin.
D. It remains stable over time.
E. It is due to an autoimmune process that destroys the beta cells of the pancreas.

Clinical Manifestations

Type 2 diabetes mellitus typically has a slower onset than type 1 diabetes. In addition to the three "Ps" of type 1 diabetes—polyuria, polydipsia, and polyphagia—other common clinical manifestations include the following:

- Fatigue
- Poor wound healing
- Cardiovascular disease
- Visual disturbances
- Renal insufficiency
- Recurring infection

For example, recurring yeast infections in women with diabetes may indicate poorly controlled blood glucose levels. Yeast cells are normally occurring flora in the vagina. They are kept in check by the acidic environment present in the vagina. In diabetes, vaginal secretions have more glucose, which produces a nourishing environment for yeast, allowing them to grow and multiply, causing an infection.

Many of these manifestations are due to the microvascular and macrovascular complications of long-term hyperglycemia that are discussed later in the chapter under complications.

Management

Medical Management

Diagnosis

The diagnosis of type 2 DM is done through evaluation of the same laboratory analyses as type 1 DM: HgbA1c levels, fasting blood glucose levels, 2-hr postprandial blood levels, and random blood glucose levels (see Table 44.1). The differentiation between type 1 and type 2 is based more on the situation present at the time of diagnosis rather than on the specific laboratory values. For example, hyperglycemia noted in a physically inactive, overweight adult (BMI >30 kg/m^2) whose blood glucose is initially controlled with oral medications is diagnosed as type 2 diabetes even if insulin is eventually required. This is in contrast to the hyperglycemia noted in a physically active child requiring insulin injections at onset to maintain glycemic control (type 1 diabetes) or the

mother diagnosed with gestational diabetes during pregnancy whose blood glucose levels remain high post-delivery and who is diagnosed with type 2 diabetes. If insulin antibodies were checked, a person with type 2 would be negative, but someone with type 1 diabetes has a strong likelihood of being positive.

Treatment

The treatment of type 2 DM involves a combination of pharmacological interventions and self-management that includes:

- Education
- Monitoring glycemic control
- Nutrition
- Exercise
- Monitoring for complications

Pharmacological Interventions

Pharmacological interventions for type 2 DM include oral medications that increase the production of insulin, lower insulin resistance, slow the absorption of carbohydrates, or help lower blood glucose (Table 44.5). These medications are typically used in combination because of their different mechanisms of action. The combination used depends on the patient's response, with the goal of achieving and maintaining glycemic targets. Intervention at the time of diagnosis with metformin (Glucophage), in combination with lifestyle changes such as diet and exercise, is common. Continuing, timely augmentation of therapy with additional agents, including early initiation of insulin therapy, as a means of achieving and maintaining levels of glycemic control (i.e., HgbA1c <7% for most patients) is recommended.

Another potential medication combination is the use of an oral medication in conjunction with a glucagon-like peptide-1 (GLP-1) receptor agonist. Glucagon-like peptide-1 agonists are incretin mimetics that are injected subcutaneously either once a week or daily depending on the formulation. They lower glucose levels by slowing glucose absorption from the intestine, increasing insulin secretion when blood glucose levels are high and lowering the high glucagon levels sometimes found in people with diabetes after meals. Another side benefit of GLP-1 agonists is the action of decreasing appetite by attaching to an appetite receptor on the hypothalamus, ultimately helping with weight loss.

Many patients with type 2 DM will eventually require insulin therapy because of the typical progressive loss of beta-cell function with the progression of the disease. Initiation of insulin at the time of diagnosis is recommended for individuals presenting with weight loss or other severe hyperglycemic clinical manifestations. Initiation of insulin is also recommended for any patient with an HgbA1c greater than 10%. Patients with type 2 DM can utilize insulin alone or in combination with noninsulin agents. They may be able to maintain glycemic control with one injection a day of basal insulin in combination with an oral agent(s).

Table 44.5　Oral Glucose Control Agents

Medication Class	Mechanism of Action	Dosing	Precautions
Biguanides (metformin)	Decrease glucose production in the liver; increase insulin sensitivity in skeletal muscle	Taken two times a day	Caution in patients with renal impairment; may cause diarrhea
Sulfonylureas	Stimulate the beta cells to produce more insulin	Typically taken once or twice a day	Risk of hypoglycemia
Meglitinides	Stimulate the beta cells to produce more insulin	Taken three times a day before meals	Risk of hypoglycemia
Thiazolidinediones	Decrease glucose production in the liver; increase insulin sensitivity in skeletal muscle	Taken once daily	May increase risk of heart failure; monitor for liver toxicity.
Alpha-glucosidase inhibitors	Slow the breakdown and absorption of sugars and starches	Taken with the first bite of each meal	May cause diarrhea and flatulence. If the patient experiences hypoglycemia, must correct with dextrose or glucose due to slowed absorption of carbohydrates.
DPP-4 inhibitors	Prevent the breakdown of naturally occurring GLP-1, a compound that stimulates insulin release from the pancreas	Taken once daily	May cause nasopharyngitis
SGLT-2 inhibitors	Lower the renal threshold for glucose excretion with blood glucose lowering and weight loss.	Taken once daily	Indicated for people with type 2 diabetes Increase risk of urinary tract and genital infections Reported cases of DKA and acute kidney injury

DPP-4, Dipeptidyl peptidase-4 (DPP-4) inhibitors; *GLP-1,* glucagon-like peptide-1.

However, if the hyperglycemia persists or if the pattern of hyperglycemia shows that they have consistent significant hyperglycemia following meals but not overnight, they may require the addition of prandial insulin as well or adjustment of the other diabetes medications. Increasing numbers of patients with type 2 DM who use prandial and basal insulin are beginning to utilize insulin pumps.

Connection Check 44.10

A nurse is reviewing orders for patients newly diagnosed with type 2 DM. What initial medication orders should be anticipated?

A. Metformin PO twice a day
B. Nutritional insulin subcutaneously prior to meals
C. Basal insulin subcutaneously before bed
D. Correctional insulin subcutaneously after meals

Self-Management

Management of both type 1 and type 2 DM cannot be successful without the individual patient's commitment to behaviors and lifestyle choices on an ongoing basis. Patient behavior strongly impacts hyperglycemia, with education and self-management being critical to successful outcomes. This involves more than adherence to potentially complicated pharmaceutical regimens. It also involves education, meal planning, exercise, self-monitoring of blood glucose, and adherence to a screening program for complications. The information that follows on monitoring glycemic control, education, nutrition, and exercise applies to type 1 and type 2 DM, as well as the management of diabetes in general.

Diabetes Self-Management Education. The goal of diabetes self-management education (DSME) is to empower the person with DM to take responsibility for day-to-day management. It provides the patient with strategies to establish and maintain a healthy lifestyle. According to national standards, all people with diabetes should receive DSME when their diabetes is diagnosed. Education should be individualized and tailored to the patient's needs. Once he or she has completed the initial education, behavioral goals should be set and a follow-up visit schedule planned by the healthcare team and patient. Continuing education may be necessary depending on the patient's needs. Medicare, medical assistance, and most private insurance reimburse for DSME if it takes place in a program that has been accredited by the American Diabetes Association (ADA) or American Association of Diabetes Educators and is implemented by an interprofessional team. To be accredited, the program must cover:

- Describing the diabetes disease process and treatment options
- Incorporating nutritional management into the lifestyle
- Incorporating physical activity into the lifestyle
- Using medication(s) safely and for maximum therapeutic effectiveness
- Monitoring blood glucose and other parameters and interpreting and using the results for self-management decision making
- Preventing, detecting, and treating acute complications
- Preventing, detecting, and treating chronic complications
- Developing personal strategies to address psychosocial issues and concerns
- Developing personal strategies to promote health and behavior changes

A related objective from *Healthy People 2020* is as follows:

- Increasing the proportion of persons with diagnosed diabetes who receive formal diabetes education

Monitoring Glycemic Control

As in type 1 diabetes, assessment of glycemic control is important for several reasons. It allows the provider to determine the effectiveness of treatment and to plan adjustments to medication and follow-up. For the diabetes educator, assessment of glycemic control highlights problem areas in patient self-management so that exploration of patient understanding and appropriate education can occur. Perhaps most importantly, if used in the context of appropriate education and follow-up, it provides feedback to the patient about what is and is not working in the overall treatment plan. As noted earlier in the discussion of type 1 diabetes, glycemic control is assessed through:

- Self-monitoring of blood glucose
- Continuous glucose monitoring
- Monitoring of HbgA1c

See Table 44.2 for glycemic control targets.

Medical Nutrition Therapy

The major goal of medical nutritional therapy is to improve metabolic outcomes by modifying nutrient intake. For patients with diabetes mellitus, approaching normal ranges for blood glucose, blood pressure, and lipids slows the development of each of the chronic complications of diabetes. Meal composition affects glycemic control and cardiovascular risk, so assisting the patient in understanding food choices is an essential piece of diabetes self-management. In addition, deciding what to eat is one of the most common questions asked by patients with diabetes and causes anxiety

and misunderstanding in many situations. Working with a professional to understand and feel comfortable with food choices contributes to improving compliance with an overall diabetes care plan. Individual nutritional guidelines are based on a patient assessment that includes food intake, focusing on carbohydrates; medications; metabolic control (glycemia, lipids, and blood pressure); measurements of height, weight, and body composition; and physical activity.

Carbohydrate Guidelines. Monitoring carbohydrate intake through carbohydrate counting (Box 44.3), exchanges, or experience-based estimation is a key strategy in achieving glycemic control. In insulin-deficient patients, insulin doses should be adjusted to match carbohydrate intake, the insulin-to-carbohydrate ratio. Basal-bolus insulin therapy in conjunction with carbohydrate counting is the most physiological treatment and provides the greatest flexibility in terms of food choices and timing of meals. Patients on insulin who are unwilling or unable to count carbohydrates should use a consistent carbohydrate meal plan.

Box 44.3 Carbohydrate Counting

Carbohydrate counting is a technique useful for managing blood glucose levels. Understanding what foods contain carbohydrate, which raises the blood glucose level, and tracking carbohydrate intake help maintain glycemic targets. Carbohydrate intake recommendations are individualized on the basis of patient size, activity, and medication use. The successful use of this technique requires an understanding of what foods contain carbohydrates and how many carbohydrates they contain.

Foods that contain carbohydrates are:

- Starchy foods and vegetables such as bread, cereal, rice, crackers, potatoes, pasta, dried beans, and corn
- Fruit and juice
- Milk and yogurt
- Sweets and sodas, juice drinks, cakes, cookies, candy, and potato chips
- Nonstarchy vegetables such as greens, carrots, green beans, cucumbers, peppers, broccoli, cabbage, asparagus, mushrooms, onions, and eggplant contain carbohydrates but in much smaller quantities than starchy foods. These are great foods for increasing the quantity in a meal without impacting the glucose as much.

The amount of carbohydrate in food can sometimes be determined by reading labels. If estimating, the following are some examples of foods that contain approximately 15 g of carbohydrate:

- 1 small piece of fresh fruit (4 oz)
- 1 slice of bread (1 oz)
- 1/2 cup of oatmeal
- 1/3 cup of pasta or rice
- 4 to 6 crackers
- 1/2 English muffin or hamburger bun
- 1½ cups of green beans

Carbohydrates should be distributed throughout the day in small meals and snacks. If persons with diabetes choose to consume products containing nonnutritive sweeteners, they should be consumed at levels that do not exceed the acceptable daily intakes. Some of these products contain energy and carbohydrates from other sources that need to be accounted for in the total daily carbohydrate intake. For patients managing their diabetes through diet alone or taking glucose-lowering medications or fixed insulin doses, meal and snack carbohydrate intake should be kept consistent on a day-to-day basis. See Table 44.6 for specific dietary guidelines.

Weight Control

Many individuals with DM are overweight and have insulin resistance. Nutrition therapy often begins with strategies that reduce food intake and increase energy expenditure through physical activity. For patients who are overweight or obese, moderate weight loss (5%–10% of body weight) is associated with significant improvement in insulin resistance, as reflected in metabolic parameters such as blood glucose, blood pressure, and lipid levels. Weight control and diet are essential components of DM management to lower glucose levels and to reduce the risk for cardiovascular disease. Cardiovascular risk is lowest when the BMI is less than 25 kg/m^2. For weight control, patients must balance lower fat and calorie consumption with regular physical activity of 30 minutes on most days.

Physical Activity Recommendations

Both aerobic training and resistance training improve glycemic control. Physical activity also improves insulin sensitivity, blood pressure, and the lipid profile and decreases risks for cardiovascular disease and all-cause mortality. It also helps in the management of depressive symptoms and improves sleep quality. People with diabetes should be advised to perform at least 150 minutes per week of moderate-intensity activity (50%–70% of maximum heart rate) and strength training three times per week, unless contraindicated. Before beginning a program of physical activity more vigorous than brisk walking, people with diabetes should be assessed by a healthcare provider for conditions that might be associated with an increased risk of cardiovascular disease. Of concern are uncontrolled hypertension, severe autonomic or peripheral neuropathy, and preproliferative or proliferative retinopathy or macular edema. In previously sedentary patients whose 10-year risk of a coronary event is likely to be greater than or equal to 10%, a graded exercise test with electrocardiogram monitoring is recommended. In individuals taking insulin or insulin secretagogues (medications that facilitate the release of insulin), physical activity can cause hypoglycemia if the medication dose or carbohydrate intake is not adjusted. Carbohydrate should be ingested if pre-exercise blood glucose levels are less than 100 mg/dL.

Table 44.6 Dietary Guidelines

Food	Guidelines
Carbohydrates	Individualized from a starting point of approximately 45–60 g per meal. Snacks should be <20 g.
Sucrose (table sugar)	If persons with diabetes choose to eat foods containing sucrose, the sucrose-containing foods should be substituted for other carbohydrate foods. Sucrose-containing foods should be eaten in the context of a healthy diet, without excess calorie intake. Labels should be read for "total carbohydrate" content and not just for "sugar" or "sucrose."
Protein	In persons with diabetes and normal renal function, the recommendation for a usual protein intake of 15%–20% of daily food intake does not need to be changed.
	In persons with diabetic nephropathy, referral should be made to dietitians for individualized meal planning.
Fiber	A wide variety of fiber-containing foods, such as legumes, fiber-rich cereals, fruits, vegetables, and whole-grain products, is encouraged. Aim for fiber amounts of 25–50 g per day.
Dietary fat	Total dietary fat should generally comprise less than 30% of daily food intake.
	Dietary saturated fat should be limited to less than 7% of daily food intake. Substitution of monosaturated fats for saturated is encouraged.
	Trans fats (trans fatty acids) should be eliminated.
Alcohol	If adults with diabetes choose to use alcohol, daily intake should be limited to a moderate amount (one drink per day or less for adult women and two drinks per day or less for adult men). A drink is defined as 12 oz of beer, 5 oz of wine, or 1.5 oz of 80-proof distilled spirits.
	Alcohol depresses the release of carbohydrate from the liver and can lower blood glucose. To reduce the risk of hypoglycemia, alcohol is best consumed with food. Check glucose to determine impact of alcohol on blood glucose levels.

Psychosocial Assessment and Care

People with diabetes have a depression rate that is more than twice the rate of people without diabetes. Depression has been identified as one of the most common factors involved in nonadherence to a diabetes treatment plan. The psychosocial assessment should be included as an ongoing part of medical management. Consider a referral to a behavioral specialist if psychosocial issues are a concern.

Monitoring for and Managing Complications

Because the underlying pathophysiology of hyperglycemia involves damage to blood vessels, vascular health and protection are key to avoiding devastating end-organ damage by diabetes. The lifestyle cornerstones of maintaining a healthy weight, healthy eating, and regular exercise improve all diabetes outcomes. In addition to reaching glycemic goals, essential components of vascular health in diabetes include the management of hypertension, hyperlipidemia, and hypercoagulability (antiplatelet treatment) and smoking cessation. In addition to monitoring glycemic control, routine monitoring should also include regular laboratory analysis of coagulation profiles, lipid profiles, renal studies, and dilated eye examinations. Routine monitoring of the skin and feet is essential to avoid wounds and infection, which can potentially lead to amputation.

Connection Check 44.11

The nurse is providing care for a patient newly diagnosed with type 1 diabetes. Which lifestyle modifications need to be included in the plan of care?

A. Limiting exercise, carbohydrate counting, self-monitoring of blood glucose
B. Distributing carbohydrate intake throughout the day, controlling weight, limiting alcohol
C. Carbohydrate counting, self-monitoring of blood glucose, healthcare provider visits as needed
D. Limiting protein intake, distributing carbohydrate intake throughout the day, regular healthcare provider visits

Complications

Hyperosmolar Hyperglycemic State

Hyperosmolar hyperglycemic state (HHS) is a serious metabolic derangement that occurs in patients with DM. The condition is characterized by hyperglycemia, hyperosmolality, and dehydration without significant ketoacidosis. It occurs when there is sufficient insulin to prevent rapid fat breakdown and ketone release. However, there is not enough insulin to prevent severe hyperglycemia. Blood glucose levels can rise to extremes above 600 mg/dL. The resulting extreme hyperosmolality leads to osmotic diuresis. Dehydration can be profound and electrolyte

imbalances severe. Along with dehydration, most patients present with global neurological defects.

It is less common than the other acute complication of DM, diabetic ketoacidosis (DKA), and differs in the magnitude of dehydration, ketosis, and acidosis. Hyperosmolar hyperglycemic state usually presents in older patients with type 2 DM and carries a higher mortality rate than DKA, estimated at approximately 10% to 20%. Hyperosmolar hyperglycemic state most commonly occurs in patients who have some concomitant illness that leads to reduced fluid intake. Infection is the most common preceding illness. Once HHS has developed, it may be difficult to differentiate it from the preceding illness. The diagnosis of HHS is based on the following:

- Blood glucose level of 600 mg/dL or greater
- Serum osmolality of 320 mOsm/kg or greater
- Profound dehydration
- Serum pH greater than 7.4
- Bicarbonate concentration greater than 15 mEq/L
- Low ketonuria and absent to low ketonemia
- Alteration in level of consciousness

Treatment priorities include standard care for dehydration with IV fluid and treatment for altered mental status, including airway management as appropriate. Patients may respond to fluids alone, but IV insulin may be necessary to correct hyperglycemia. See Table 44.7 for the differences between DKA and HHS.

Acute and Long-Term Complications of Hyperglycemia in Both Type 1 and Type 2 DM

Depressed Immune Response. A depressed immune response can lead to infection and poor wound healing, and both are considered acute complications of hyperglycemia. Neutrophil and macrophage phagocytosis of bacteria is impaired, prolonging the inflammatory phase. The proliferative phase is also prolonged as RBCs become less pliable and less able to deliver oxygen to the wound for tissue metabolism and collagen synthesis. Interference with normal wound healing can be particularly important in the surgical, home-health, and long-term care settings. Effects include prolonged hospitalization, increased risk for sepsis, and increased morbidity from the extension of tissue damage. Hyperglycemia is associated with increased rates of:

- Skin and soft tissue infection
- Pneumonia
- Influenza
- Bacteremia/sepsis
- Tuberculosis

Prolonged Hyperglycemia. **Prolonged hyperglycemia** adversely affects blood vessels and nerves. Because the entire body relies on these networks, the long-term effects are extremely widespread.

Vascular Effects. Diabetes can be primarily thought of as a vascular disease, in that the damage done to the lining of blood vessels accounts for much of the damage throughout

Table 44.7 DKA Versus HHS

	DKA	HHS
Occurrence	Most often seen in type 1 DM but can also occur in type 2, especially with severe stress such as infection	Occurs more commonly in older adults in response to stress or infection
Onset	Rapid	Gradual
Laboratory work		
● Blood glucose levels	Greater than 250 mg/dL	Greater than 600 mg/dL
● Arterial pH levels	Less than or equal to 7.3	Greater than 7.4
● Serum bicarbonate levels	Less than 18 mEq/L	Greater than 15 mEq/L
● Urine or serum ketones	+	–
● Effective serum osmolality	Greater than 300 mOsm/kg	Greater than 320 mOsm/kg
● Anion gap	+	–

DKA, Diabetic ketoacidosis; *DM*, diabetes mellitus; *HHS*, hyperosmolar hyperglycemic state.

the body. Complications from diabetes are classified as macrovascular and microvascular. *Macrovascular* complications involve damage to the large arteries that supply the heart and brain. The leading cause of diabetes-related death is cardiovascular disease, with four of five people with diabetes dying from cardiovascular disease. Adults with diabetes die from myocardial infarction about two to four times more often than adults without diabetes. The risk for stroke is two to four times higher among people with diabetes.

Microvascular complications involve damage done to the small blood vessels and result in damage as follows:

- Eyes: The delicate blood vessels that supply the retina are susceptible to damage from prolonged hyperglycemia, resulting in retinal hypoxia. Diabetes is the leading cause of new cases of blindness among adults aged 20 to 74 years. Diabetic retinopathy causes 12,000 to 24,000 new cases of blindness each year.
- Gums: Periodontal disease is more common with diabetes because of the decreased circulation to the gums and increased susceptibility to periodontal bacteria and dental caries. Early tooth loss is a common outcome.
- Kidneys: The vasculature to the kidneys is affected by hyperglycemia. Diabetes is the single leading cause of renal failure requiring dialysis in the United States.
- Peripheral vascular disease (PVD): As many as 36% of patients with diabetes have lower extremity peripheral artery disease based on lower extremity blood pressure readings. In combination with peripheral neuropathy, PVD increases the risk of nontraumatic amputations of the lower extremities. Diabetes is the leading cause of nontraumatic amputation in the United States, with the risk of amputation being

between 15 and 40 times higher for people with diabetes than without.

Neurological Effects. Through mechanisms that currently are incompletely understood, prolonged hyperglycemia damages nerve cells. The results can affect several areas of the body. Typical problems include:

- Diabetic peripheral neuropathy
- Autonomic neuropathy

Diabetic Peripheral Neuropathy. Diabetic peripheral neuropathy results when the nerves to the feet and hands are damaged, but it can also impact other peripheral nerves in the body. Clinical manifestations include numbness, tingling, or pain. Approximately one-third of people with diabetes over the age of 40 have some impaired sensation to their feet. Loss of protective sensation can lead to injury that may not be felt. Infection and amputation are more likely in this setting. The greatest risk is from improperly fitting shoes.

Autonomic Neuropathy. Autonomic neuropathy results when there is damage to the nerves of the autonomic nervous system. Common manifestations are:

- *Diabetic gastroparesis,* which results when the nerves that innervate the stomach are damaged, leading to delayed or erratic emptying of stomach contents into the intestine. Clinical manifestations include symptoms such as bloating, early satiety, nausea, and vomiting. Blood glucose can drop or spike unpredictably if the food reaches the intestine at an unexpected rate.
- Erectile dysfunction
- Orthostatic hypertension
- Urinary problems, such as difficulty starting urination and inability to completely empty the bladder, can result in urinary tract infections.

Nursing Management

Assessment and Analysis

The clinical manifestations of type 2 DM are related to acute changes secondary to hyperglycemia, such as dehydration and electrolyte imbalance. Other manifestations are due to the more long-term effects of hyperglycemia resulting in vessel damage and organ hypoxia, such as fatigue, poor wound healing, recurring infection, cardiovascular disease, visual disturbances, and renal insufficiency.

Nursing Diagnoses

- **Risk for ineffective tissue perfusion** related to macrovascular vessel changes secondary to hyperglycemia
- **Risk for ineffective renal perfusion** related to microvascular changes secondary to hyperglycemia
- **Risk for infection** related to decreased perfusion and sensation in distal extremities

Nursing Interventions

◼ Assessments

- Vital signs
  Decreased blood pressure and increased heart rate are secondary to the fluid volume deficit created by osmotic diuresis related to hyperglycemia. Temperature may be elevated if infection is present.
- Serum glucose
  Increased glucose levels are due to insulin resistance or relative lack of insulin related to body size. In a patient already diagnosed with and being treated for type 2 DM, increased glucose levels indicate:
  - Inadequate self-management, such as poor diet, weight gain, and limited exercise
  - Increased insulin or oral glucose control medication requirements due to stresses, such as infection, causing adrenal release of catecholamines, increasing the hepatic production of glucose
    Decreased glucose levels can be caused by inappropriate administration of insulin or medications that stimulate the release of insulin from the pancreas while the patient has inadequate oral intake or increased activity requiring more circulating glucose.
- Capillary refill in lower extremities
  Decreased perfusion secondary to microvascular changes may manifest as delayed capillary refill.
- Skin assessment, especially lower extremities and feet, looking for breaks in the skin, erythema, trauma, pallor on elevation, dependent rubor, changes in foot size/shape, nail deformities, and extensive callus
  Skin breakdown or wounds may occur unnoticed by the patient because of peripheral neuropathy. Resulting wounds are slow to heal as a result of impaired inflammatory response and tissue hypoxia secondary to vessel damage that occurs secondary to hyperglycemia.
- Intake and output
  Increased urine output may be present because of osmotic diuresis secondary to hyperglycemia.

- WBC count
  An increased WBC count may indicate the presence of infection.
- Serum blood urea nitrogen (BUN) and creatinine levels
  Elevations in serum BUN and creatinine levels are indicative of decreased renal function associated with the microvascular changes that develop in the kidneys secondary to sustained hyperglycemia.
- Spot urine for microalbuminuria
  Elevations of microalbumin are an early indication of microvascular damage to the kidneys from hyperglycemia and/or hypertension.
- Carbohydrate intake at meals
  Adequate carbohydrate intake at meals is essential to avoid hypoglycemia related to insulin administration.

◼ Actions

- Blood glucose monitoring (finger sticks) completed before meals and at bedtime
  Regular finger sticks are done to measure the adequacy of glucose control.
- Administer oral diabetes medications as ordered.
  Oral diabetes medications are administered to increase the production of insulin, lower insulin resistance, or slow the absorption of carbohydrates or in order to lower blood glucose levels.
- Administer insulin as ordered.
  - Basal
  - Preprandial
  - Correctional
    Administering rapid-acting insulin before meals, preparing for ingestion of carbohydrates, and correcting for random high glucose levels as determined by self-monitoring of blood glucose levels prior to the meal, in combination with longer-acting insulin once a day, will mimic the action of a healthy pancreas, helping to maintain tight glycemic control. In patients with questionable or minimal oral intake, prandial and correctional insulins may be administered together after meals after adequate carbohydrate intake has been confirmed.
- Administer isotonic IV fluids as ordered.
  Intravenous fluids may be necessary to replace volume lost due to diuresis.
- Administer antibiotics as ordered.
  Antibiotics may be indicated if infection is present.

◼ Teaching

- Medication education
  Lifelong medication administration is required for cellular metabolism. Increased stress, infection, activity level, increased ingestion of carbohydrates, and decreased PO intake all alter medication requirements. Over time, insulin administration may become necessary.
  Regular blood glucose checks help determine the adequacy of the medication regimen and maintain glycemic targets.
- Regular blood glucose checks via finger sticks, alternate site testing, and CGM
  Regular checks help determine the adequacy of the medication regimen and maintain glycemic targets.

- Healthy lifestyle that includes meal planning and exercise
  Healthy lifestyle choices are essential components in the management of diabetes to help avoid or prolong the development of complications associated with uncontrolled and/or sustained hyperglycemia. Lowering BMI and weight may delay the onset and severity of the long-term complications of DM.
- Signs of hypoglycemia and hyperglycemia
  It is important that the patient and family are able to detect early signs of both hypoglycemia (the underlying disorder that could progress to coma or death) and hyperglycemia secondary to inadequate medication administration.
- Foot care (Box 44.4)
  Meticulous foot care is essential to avoid wounds and infections that could result in amputation due to poor wound healing related to hyperglycemia. The use of therapeutic shoes and evaluation by podiatry can minimize risks.
- Monitoring for complications
  Regular healthcare provider visits are essential to monitor for cardiovascular, renal, visual, and skin complications related to hyperglycemia. Regular healthcare provider visits with routine blood work to monitor cardiovascular and renal functioning, along with annual dilated eye examinations and inspection of the feet and lower extremities, are essential to avoid the complications of long-term hyperglycemia.

Connection Check 44.12

The nurse prioritizes which nursing diagnosis in the plan of care for the patient with type 2 DM?
A. Risk for infection
B. Risk for falls
C. Risk for impaired gas exchange
D. Risk for injury: hyperkalemia

Box 44.4 Foot Care

Foot care education should cover the following:
- Wash feet daily and dry thoroughly, including between the toes.
- Do not soak feet unless specified by a healthcare provider; soaking can unduly break down the skin and make it prone to damage.
- Be careful of hot water.
- Use creams, lotions, or moisturizer but not between the toes to avoid a fungal infection from too much moisture.
- To avoid injury, do not walk barefoot.
- Use caution in cutting nails. Ingrown toenails or other nail problems may require podiatry consultation.

Properly fitting footwear is essential. Check shoes each day for objects that may have fallen inside, excessive wetness, or areas that may cause irritation.

Evaluating Care Outcomes

The patient with type 2 DM can lead a long and healthy life with strict adherence to the treatment regimen. The tight glycemic control necessary to avoid the complications associated with DM is best achieved through active monitoring of blood glucose levels and treatment with glucose control medications and insulin as indicated. Nutrition, patient education, self-management, and detection and prevention of complications are essential components of the successful daily management of diabetes.

Making Connections

CASE STUDY: WRAP-UP

Mrs. Simpson is now 6 days postoperative following her triple cardiac bypass. Her cultures reveal a urinary tract infection, and she is started on Bactrim. Her vital signs are stable, her temperature is within normal limits, and her WBC count is back to normal. During her hospital stay, her diabetes is being treated with subcutaneous insulin. She is given nutritional, correctional as necessary, and basal insulins. Her blood glucose is back within tight glycemic control after an initial increase with the infection. Her urine output is stable, and renal function tests appear to be normal. The plan is to discharge her to home tomorrow.

Case Study Questions

1. The nurse includes which information in the teaching plan for Mrs. Simpson?
   A. Daily insulin administration
   B. Once-a-day blood glucose monitoring
   C. Eliminating fat in her diet
   D. Monitoring for infection
2. Which statement by Mrs. Simpson about her home medication regimen indicates the need for further teaching?
   A. "My kidney problem will not affect my metformin prescription."
   B. "I may need to change from my metformin/glyburide medication therapy because of the problem with my kidneys."
   C. "I will need to be especially careful about low blood glucose."
   D. "I need to be diligent with my self–blood glucose monitoring."
3. Which statement by Mrs. Simpson indicates that teaching has been effective?
   A. "I don't have to worry about my blood pressure now that I've had heart surgery."
   B. "My diabetes is separate from my heart problems."
   C. "My blood glucose may go up if I get another infection."
   D. "I can take two of my glucose pills to make up for a missed dose as long as I check my blood glucose."

4. The nurse recognizes that the management of diabetes is most successful with which action?

    A. A priority focus on medications

    B. A focus on regular healthcare provider follow-up

    C. Patient commitment to self-management

    D. A priority focus on appropriate diet

5. The nurse understands that HHS differs from DKA in which of the following ways? *(Select all that apply.)*

    A. Hyperosmolar hyperglycemic state (HHS) has a more gradual onset.

    B. Diabetic ketoacidosis (DKA) presents with higher serum glucose.

    C. Potassium depletion is a potential complication with HHS.

    D. A positive anion gap is not diagnostic for HHS.

    E. Ketosis is typically not present in HHS.

CHAPTER SUMMARY

Type 1 DM is typically triggered by an autoimmune process in which the insulin-producing beta cells of the pancreas are destroyed, resulting in an absolute lack of insulin. Predominate features include polyuria, polydipsia, polyphagia, fatigue, and weight loss. Diagnosis of type 1 DM is done by one of three methods: fasting blood glucose levels greater than or equal to 100 mg/dL, 2-hr postprandial greater than or equal to 200 mg/dL, and random blood glucose levels greater than or equal to 200 mg/dL in a patient with classic symptoms of hyperglycemia or hyperglycemic crisis.

The primary pharmacological intervention used in the treatment of type 1 DM is insulin administered subcutaneously. An approach using a combination of long-acting or intermediate-acting insulin to provide "basal" insulin; rapid-acting or short-acting insulin subcutaneous or inhaled short-acting taken at mealtimes to cover the incoming carbohydrates, "prandial" insulin; and "correctional" insulin to compensate for blood glucose elevations is most effective in maintaining tight glycemic control. Three methods of assessing glycemic control are:

- Self–monitoring of blood glucose
- Continuous glucose monitoring
- Monitoring of HgbA1c

Complications of type 1 DM include diabetic ketoacidosis (DKA), hypoglycemia, the dawn phenomenon, and the Somogyi effect.

In adults, type 2 DM accounts for about 90% to 95% of all diagnosed cases; thus, it is far more common than type 1 DM. It is caused by defects at the cell membrane that prevent the normal action of insulin, or insulin resistance. Type 2 DM typically has a slower onset than type 1 DM. In addition to the three "Ps" of type 1 DM—polyuria, polydipsia, and polyphagia—other common clinical manifestations include fatigue, poor wound healing, recurring infection, cardiovascular disease, visual disturbances, and renal insufficiency. Diagnosis of type 2 DM is as in type 1 diabetes. Type 1 DM diagnosis may also include a test for insulin antibodies and c-peptide to determine insulin production.

Pharmacological interventions for type 2 DM include oral and injectable medications that increase the production of insulin, lower insulin resistance, or slow the absorption of carbohydrates or medications that help lower blood glucose. These medications are typically used in combination because of their different mechanisms of action.

Management of both type 1 and type 2 DM cannot be successful without the individual patient's commitment to healthy behaviors and lifestyle choices. Education and self-management are critical to successful outcomes. This involves more than adherence to potentially complicated pharmacological regimens. It also involves education, nutrition, exercise, self-monitoring of blood glucose levels, and adherence to a screening program for complications.

Acute complications include hyperosmolar hyperglycemic state (HHS), hypoglycemia in response to medication, and depressed immune response leading to infection and poor wound healing. Prolonged hyperglycemia adversely affects blood vessels and nerves, which can result in the long-term complications of autonomic neuropathy, diabetic peripheral neuropathy, renal failure, blindness, myocardial infarction, or stroke.

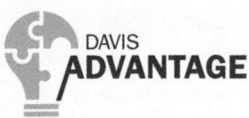

DAVIS **ADVANTAGE** | To explore learning resources for this chapter, go to **Davis Advantage** and find:
- Answers to in-text questions
- Chapter Resources and Activities
- NCLEX®-Style Chapter Review Questions
- Bibliography

Promoting Health in Patients With Sensory System Disorders

Chapter 45

Assessment of Visual Function

Kelley Miller Wilson

LEARNING OUTCOMES

Content in this chapter is designed to assist in:

1. Identifying key anatomical components of the visual system
2. Discussing the function of the visual system
3. Describing the procedure for completing a history and physical assessment of visual function
4. Correlating relevant diagnostic examinations with visual function
5. Explaining nursing considerations for diagnostic studies relevant to the visual system
6. Describing methods to prevent eye trauma and pathology
7. Discussing changes in visual function associated with aging

CONCEPTS

- Assessment
- Inflammation
- Perioperative
- Promoting Health
- Safety
- Sensory Perception

ESSENTIAL TERMS

Accommodation
Amblyopia
Anisocoria
Astigmatism
Convergence
Emmetropia
Enophthalmos
Exophthalmos
Fundus
Hyperopia
Intraocular pressure
Keratomalacia
Miosis
Mydriasis
Myopia
Nystagmus
Orbit
Presbyopia
Ptosis
Pupillary constriction
Red reflex
Refraction
Retina
Sclera
Strabismus
Uvea
Visual acuity

Finding Connections

Melanie McCormick, who is 48 years old, is seeing her nurse practitioner for a routine checkup. Melanie believes she is in excellent health, with "no known chronic diseases." She works full-time as a middle school English teacher, takes no medications, is careful to eat at least four servings of fruits/vegetables daily, and has no significant family history of medical problems. Melanie has been noticing some changes with her vision over the past 5 years that she plans to discuss with her practitioner. Her most common complaints are dry eyes, difficulty reading unless objects are held at arm's length, and "spots" that move in and out of her visual fields on occasion. Melanie contacts her primary healthcare provider for an appointment to have her vision evaluated...

INTRODUCTION

Vision is an important sense, and ensuring eye health is critical to visual acuity. Perhaps one of the most sophisticated systems in the human body, the eye is responsible for taking light, converting it into electrical signals, and then sending it to the brain for processing. One of the five major senses in the body, vision allows awareness and assessment of surroundings, awareness of potential danger, and an appreciation for beauty as well as the ability to work, play, and interact with others.

OVERVIEW OF ANATOMY AND PHYSIOLOGY

Often considered the "window to the brain," the eye is a fascinating structure that encompasses both internal and external frameworks. The adult eyeball is often compared to a Ping-Pong ball in size and shape; it sits in a hollow area of the facial skull called the **orbit** and consists of three layers. The external layer is known as the **sclera**, providing the tough protective outer coating; the middle layer is called the **uvea**, containing such structures as the choroid, the ciliary body, and the iris. The innermost layer is known as the **retina**, which converts light waves into nerve impulses resulting in visual reception. Within the eyeball itself, **intraocular pressure** is needed to keep the eyeball inflated. The following discussion illustrates how the fluid-like substances present in the aqueous and vitreous humors maintain this pressure. The major structures of the eye are diagrammed in Figures 45.1 and 45.2 and consist of internal and external structures.

Internal Structures

Aqueous humor is the clear fluid, similar to water, found in the anterior chamber of the eye. Helping to maintain pressure and nourishing the cornea and lens with oxygen and nutrients, this fluid drains back into the circulation through the canals of Schlemm.

The *canals of Schlemm* are located around the perimeter of the iris, and they allow aqueous fluid to drain back into the bloodstream. The meshwork located along the canals of Schlemm regulates the eye's internal pressure, and blockage of these canals is seen with the eye disease known as glaucoma, which causes an increase in intraocular pressure. This increase in intraocular pressure slowly destroys the

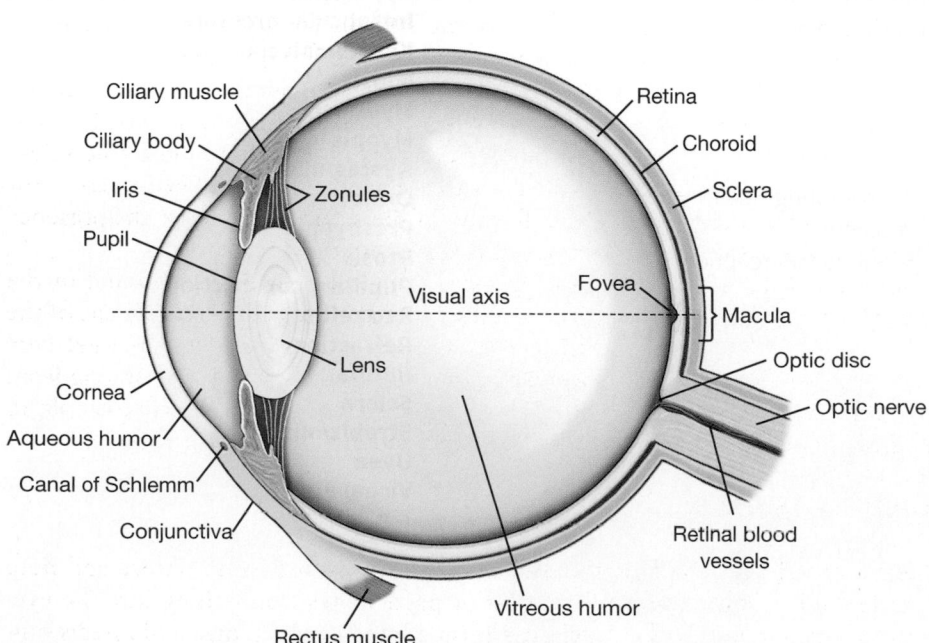

FIGURE 45.1 Internal structures of the eye.

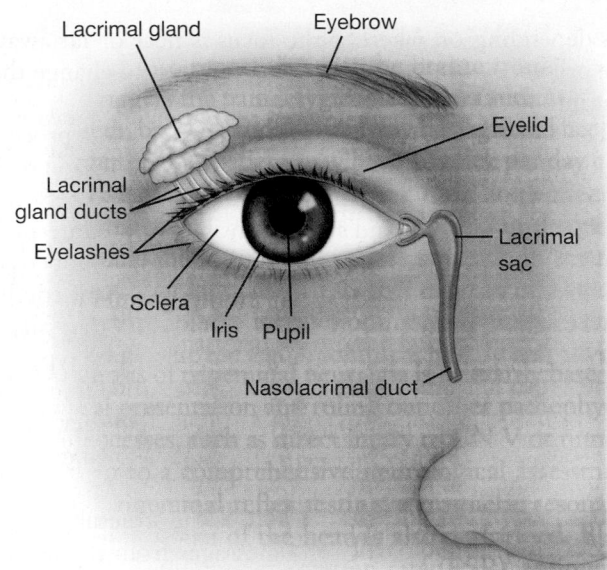

FIGURE 45.2 External structures of the eye.

optic nerve, thus severely restricting or destroying vision. This disorder is discussed in more detail in Chapter 46.

Choroid describes the layer of blood vessels located between the retina and sclera that supplies blood to the retina. The growth of abnormal blood vessels between the retina and the choroid can damage the macula, causing macular degeneration and yielding profound vision loss.

The *ciliary body* is the structure located just behind the iris. It has three main functions, including **pupillary constriction** (allowing change of the lens for eye focus), aqueous humor production (clear fluid that fills the front of the eye), and maintenance of the *lens zonules* (fibers that suspend the lens in place).

Ciliary muscles are the involuntary muscles that change the lens shape to allow the eye to focus on images at different distances. The ciliary muscles change the shape of the lens; they relax and flatten the lens for distance vision. Everyone eventually develops an eye condition called **presbyopia**. With age, this condition involves the ciliary muscles and lens losing their elasticity, causing people over the age of 40 to need "reading glasses" at some point in time.

Conjunctivae function to lubricate the front portion of the eye as well as the eyelids. This clear, thin membrane is the first line of protection for the eye against infection. Inflammation of this layer manifests itself as conjunctivitis, often called "pinkeye."

The *cornea* is the transparent dome that sits on top of the colored portion of the eye that is known as the *iris*. This structure contains no blood vessels and is the first and most powerful lens in the optical system of the eye.

The *fovea* is the central part of the macula that provides the sharpest vision.

The *iris*, or the colored portion of the eye, is actually a ring of muscle fibers located behind the cornea and in front of the lens. The iris contracts and expands, opening and closing the pupil in response to the amount of light present, thus helping to protect the sensitive retina.

Lenses are circular and convex and are located behind the cornea. The lens is responsible for keeping images in focus on the retina. This structure bulges for focus on near objects and flattens for far objects.

The *macula* is the spot seen on an ophthalmic examination and is the most sensitive part of the retina. Located in the central portion of the retina, the macula provides vision for fine work and reading. Degeneration of the macula causes vast decreases in eyesight, often in the 20/200 to 20/800 range.

The *optic disk* is the spot on the retina where the optic nerve leaves the eye; lack of sensory cells here creates a blind spot. Working together, the two eyes cover the blind spot for each other, and the brain is able to fill in the missing information.

The *optic nerve*, cranial nerve II, is often described as the cable connecting the eye to the brain. This substantial nerve carries visual signals from the eye to the brain.

The *orbital muscles* include the six muscles that control eye movements. Four muscles control the movement of the eye when the head is twisted. Weakness or dysfunction of these muscles can lead to conditions such as **nystagmus** (abnormal twitching of the eyes) and **amblyopia** (lazy eye).

The *pupil* is the hole in the center of the iris that allows light to pass. Muscles in the iris control the size of the pupil.

The *retina* is the portion of the eye that converts light rays into electrical signals and then sends them to the brain via the optic nerve. The sides of the retina are responsible for peripheral vision, and the center area of the retina is called the macula.

Retinal blood vessels are visible with an ophthalmoscope upon eye examination and are in the choroid, just beneath the retina. They function to provide nourishment and oxygen to the eye. Abnormalities in these vessels can lead to vision loss in conditions such as diabetic neuropathy and macular degeneration.

The *sclera* is the tough white covering that functions as the outer layer of the eyeball. The sclera is also covered by a clear mucous membrane consisting of cells and an underlying basement membrane of conjunctival tissue. Tiny red lines (blood vessels) are often visible; these blood vessels transport blood to the sclera. Discoloration of the sclera can provide clues to the patient's current health status. For example, yellowing of the sclera can indicate the presence of pathology of the liver or biliary system.

Vitreous humor is the clear, jellylike fluid found in the back portion of the eye that helps maintain the shape of the eye. With age, the vitreous humor changes from a gel-type substance to a liquid and gradually shrinks, separating from the retina. This normal sign of aging can cause people to start seeing "floaters" and dark spots in their vision.

External Structures

Eyelashes and *eyebrows* are protective in nature and help to prevent dust or particulates from falling into the eye. The eyelashes form a screen to keep dust and insects out.

Specialized hairs protect the eyes from foreign particles that could cause injury. Touching the eyelashes triggers the eyelids to blink.

Eyelids function to protect and lubricate the eyes. Oil-producing glands line the inner edge of the eyelid; these oils mix with tears upon blinking, keeping the eyes moist and clean.

Lacrimal glands function to lubricate and prevent dehydration of the cornea. This gland continuously releases tears and other protective enzymes onto the surface of the eye.

Lacrimal sacs are the channels that drain tears and other debris from the eye. The fluid flows down the nasolacrimal duct into the nose, where it functions to help keep the nasal linings moist.

Cranial Nerves

There are four cranial nerves (Table 45.1) that are involved with vision and eye function. These cranial nerves provide the framework for accurate vision to take place. The nerves and their function are listed in the following section.

Connection Check 45.1

In assessing a patient's vision, the nurse recognizes which structures as key to the visual system?
A. Uvea, lacrimal gland, macula
B. Eyeball, cochlea, retina
C. Fovea, retina, macula
D. Rods, ciliary body, aqueous humor

OVERVIEW OF VISUAL FUNCTION

Vision is controlled by the interaction of light and nerve impulses transmitted to the nervous system. As light enters the pupil, it hits the lens. The lens then focuses light rays on the back of the eyeball that is known as the retina. The ciliary muscles attached to the lens change the shape of the lens depending on whether the focus is near or far away. The presence of light on the retina causes it to change the light into nerve signals for the brain to interpret.

The retina uses special cells called *rods* and *cones* to process the light. Each eye contains approximately 120 million rods and 6 to 7 million cones. Rods allow differentiation between black, white, and gray and are responsible for the interpretation of the form or shape of an object. They are not color sensitive, but they do allow for vision in very dark conditions. Cones require more light than rods, and they allow the processing of objects in color. There are three types of cones in the retina. Each cone group is sensitive to one of three different colors—red, green, or blue. Together, these cones can sense combinations of light waves, allowing vision of the millions of colors of the spectrum.

The optic nerve (cranial nerve II) is the structure in the back of the eye that carries the messages from the eye to the brain. The optic nerve serves as the "high-speed Internet" line connecting the eye to the brain that makes the vision process possible.

The four functions of the eye that allow for clear images of objects no matter what the distance are **refraction**, pupillary constriction, **accommodation**, and **convergence**. Refraction refers to the bending of light and is critical to image formation. Refraction errors occur when the bending of light rays by the cornea and lens does not focus the image correctly onto the retina. Whereas **emmetropia** is considered perfect refraction, an eyeball that is too long or too short for the optics of the lens and cornea causes refractive errors (Fig. 45.3).

An irregularly shaped cornea can also have the same effect. Errors in refraction include **myopia** (nearsightedness), **hyperopia** (farsightedness), and **astigmatism**. Myopia results from an eyeball that is too long or when the cornea has too much curve present, thus causing the focused image to fall in front of the retina. Patients with myopic vision have blurred vision of distant objects and therefore have difficulty seeing faraway objects. Hyperopia is the opposite, causing the image to fall behind the retina. These patients have trouble seeing near objects. Astigmatism results from a misshaped cornea. Patients with astigmatism have difficulty seeing fine details either close-up or from a distance. Refractive errors are usually easily corrected with corrective lenses.

The amount of light that is allowed to enter the eye is controlled by pupillary constriction and dilation. The amount of light present and the ability of the retina to adapt to the change affect the degree of dilation. Constriction of the pupil is termed **miosis**, and dilation of the pupil is known as **mydriasis**. In addition to changes in light, medications and eye drops can also alter pupillary dilation and constriction.

Accommodation is the eye's ability to maintain clear vision of an image when an object shifts from distant to near. The changing of the curve of the lens allows this transition to take place. Convergence is the simultaneous inward movement of both eyes toward the center (usually focused

Cranial Nerve	Function
II: Optic	Transports visual information from the retina to the brain and is therefore responsible for vision
III: Oculomotor	Controls pupil constriction as well as eyelid and eyeball movement
IV: Trochlear	Innervates the superior oblique muscles and allows eye movement in a downward and lateral motion
VI: Abducens	Controls lateral movement of the eye

Table 45.1 Cranial Nerves That Control Eye Function

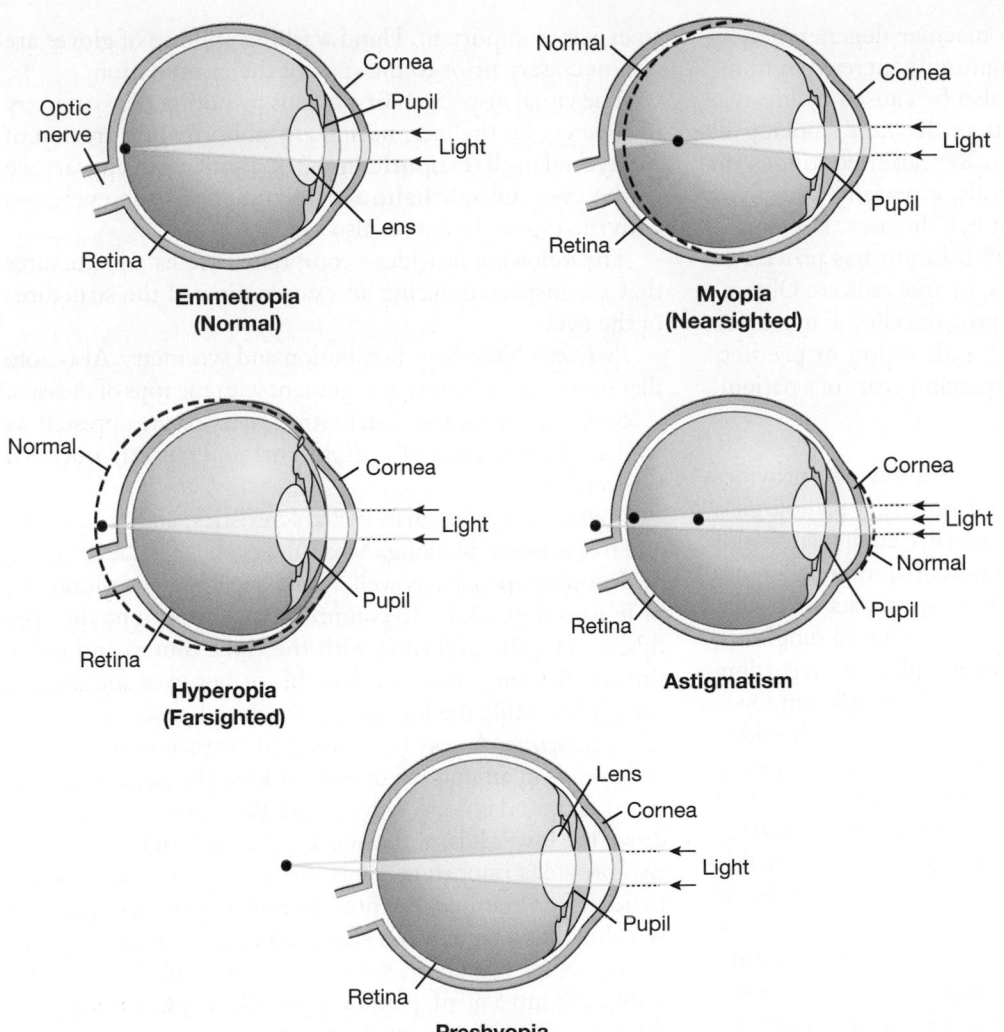

FIGURE 45.3 Refraction and visual disorders.

on the nose) in an effort to ensure the visibility of a single object at close range.

ASSESSMENT

History

Personal History

Obtaining a comprehensive history of the patient's health is essential prior to examination of the eye. Historical information to be gathered includes the patient's living conditions and level of independence; type of occupation; current medications, both prescription and over the counter; allergies to foods and environmental factors; known injury or trauma to the eye; present illnesses; and any past surgical procedures.

Family History

Assessment of the eye also includes questioning the patient about the personal and family history of eye problems. Careful history-taking helps to determine the immediate presence of illness as well as the identification of potential risks for genetic-related illnesses of the eye. Questions such as "Does anyone in your family have vision problems?" and "Does anyone have night blindness, color blindness, or glaucoma?" are important inquiries to make.

Nutritional History

Nutrition plays a role in healthy eyes because vitamins and nutrients impact certain eye conditions. Nutrients such as lutein and beta-carotene are reported to help maintain retinal function. Deficiencies in vitamin A are noted to cause dry eyes, **keratomalacia** (drying of the cornea, which can progress to clouding of the structure), and even blindness. Vitamin C and vitamin E are also known as strong antioxidants that protect the eye against free-radical damage. Free radicals are unbalanced cells in the body that are known to be destructive and are linked to macular degeneration as well as cataract formation; they naturally increase in numbers with advanced age but can also be caused by lifestyle choices. Excessive sun exposure, poor diet, and smoking all increase free-radical production. Research continues on the effects of vitamins and minerals, especially as to their potential use in treating different eye diseases. Replenishment of antioxidants fortified with lutein has proven to decrease the cell destruction caused by free radicals. Obtaining a dietary history from a patient provides clues as to current health issues being encountered with vision or predicts possible difficulties later in the advancing years of a patient.

History of Eye Trauma

Obtaining a complete history of eye trauma also provides clues to the presence of actual and potential pathologies. Assessing the patient's use of protective eye equipment is also important in helping to prevent a potential injury. The use of protective goggles at home and for sports/activities that may cause injury to the eye itself and the use of sunglasses are assessed. Included in the history are questions regarding possible occupational hazards. For example, people employed in steel mills or factories where metals are being shredded are at risk for having tiny, sometimes microscopic pieces of metal embedded in their eyes, particularly if protective goggles are not consistently worn. This leads to the formation of a "rust ring" because the surface of the eyeball is wet, and impaled metallic foreign bodies can quickly begin to rust. Left embedded in the cornea, these metal fragments may result in recurrent corneal erosion. This condition causes substantial pain for patients and occurs as the cornea becomes scratched at random times as the rust penetrates and moves through the cells on the top portion of the cornea.

to expect is important. Hand washing and use of gloves are also necessary prior to the start of the examination.

The visual inspection first begins by noting the symmetry of the eyes on the face, noting any abnormal protrusion of the eyeball itself (**exophthalmos**) or a sunken-in appearance of the eyes (**enophthalmos**). Alignment of the eyebrows with the top of the ears is also assessed.

The following provides a comprehensive list of structures that are inspected during an examination of the structures of the eyes:

Eyebrows: Note hair distribution and symmetry. Also note that the eyebrow is even in alignment with the tops of the ears.

Eyelashes: Note the distribution of eyelashes present as well as the presence of a slight curl and slightly outward projection.

Eyelids: Note the surface characteristics, ability to blink, and frequency of blinking. Assess the eyelids for the presence of drooping (**ptosis**) as well as any swelling, discoloration, or lesions (Fig. 45.4). To comprehensively examine the eyelids, elevate the eyebrows with the right thumb and index fingers. Ask the patient to close his or her eyes and inspect the eyelids while the lids are in this closed position.

Conjunctiva: Assess the color and texture by retracting the eyelids in an upward motion, asking the patient to look up, down, and side to side. Evert the upper eyelids, pull down the lower lids, and inspect. The color of the conjunctiva provides important clues regarding the health of the patient. For example, the presence of very pale conjunctiva is a clue that a patient has a low red blood cell count.

Iris: Note the color, symmetry, size, and shape of the pupil. About 5% of people normally have a noticeable difference in the size of their pupils, which is known as **anisocoria**. The normal pupil size is between 3 and 5 mm.

 Safety **Eye Protection Alert**

- Protective eye equipment, including goggles and prescription protective glasses, should be used for selected contact sports and occupations.
- Ultraviolet protective eyewear should be worn with outdoor sun exposure and with occupations that occur in the outdoors.
- A face shield should be used to protect eyes and face as needed; it should also be used with safety goggles.
- Eye goggles should be worn for grass cutting/trimming/weed whacking as well as chopping wood and using caustic substances that could potentially splash.

Inspection

Prior to any assessment, adequate explanation to the patient regarding the examination that is about to be performed is essential. Instruction on the type of examination and what

---

Connection Check 45.3

What assessment data are most important in completing a history and physical examination of the eye?

A. Family history, current state of health
B. Record of daily food intake, obtaining an accurate weight of the patient
C. Medications taken daily and occupation
D. Use of sun protective glasses on a daily basis and immunization history

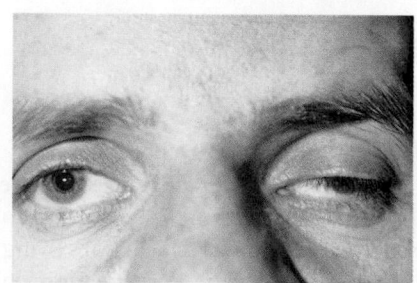

FIGURE 45.4 Ptosis.

Vision Testing

Several relatively simple tests are administered to evaluate the functioning of the eye. Patients who normally wear corrective lenses are tested both with and without their lenses in place.

The Snellen chart (Fig. 45.5), commonly known as the "eye chart," is used to evaluate distance vision. This test is easily completed in a provider's office, clinic, school, or other facility. To complete this test, the chart is usually mounted on a wall or other object 20 feet away from where the patient is standing. There are many variations of this chart, but in general, it includes 11 rows of capital letters. The top row consists of one letter (usually an "E"). The subsequent rows contain letters that get progressively smaller in size. With the patient standing 20 feet from the chart and covering one eye, the provider assists by pointing to the letters. When the last possible letter is completely read, the patient then covers the other eye and is asked to read the chart with the uncovered eye. The patient is asked to continue reading the chart until unable to determine the letter in the row to which the provider is pointing. The provider is then able to determine the patient's "visual acuity" by noting the number assignments in the margin of the chart. A common definition of **visual acuity** is the sharpness or clearness of images perceived; "20/20" vision is considered "normal" vision, meaning the patient at 20 feet reads a letter that most people are expected to be able to read at 20 feet. As an example, a person with 20/40 vision standing 20 feet from a vision chart sees what a normal person sees standing 40 feet from the chart. A person is considered legally blind if the best corrected visual acuity, meaning the best distance vision with eyeglasses or contacts in place, is 20/200 or worse. The Snellen chart vision examination is usually done first with corrective lenses in place and then without corrective lenses being used. Charts are adapted with pictures and other lettering options for pediatric patients and patients unable to read the English language.

Another routine assessment of vision is the Rosenbaum Pocket Vision Screener or Jaeger card. This test assesses for "near" vision and is used with patients who are unable to read without magnification. The card is pocket-size and held 14 inches away from the eyes. The eyes should be tested separately and then together. The value of the lowest line on which the patient can identify at least half of the letters/characters is recorded; "14/14" is considered a normal result, meaning the patient can read at 14 inches what a normal person is expected to be able to read at 14 inches.

An Ishihara chart (Fig. 45.6) is used to assess color vision. People who are color-blind are not able to distinguish red from green or blue from yellow. This chart shows a number figure composed of dots of a single color encircled in a group of dots of a different color. The eyes are tested separately for this test. Failure to determine the number figure present in the inner circle of the chart represents the need for further testing for possible color blindness. The

E	1	20/200
F P	2	20/100
T O Z	3	20/70
L P E D	4	20/50
P E C F D	5	20/40
E D F C Z P	6	20/30
F E L O P Z D	7	20/25
D E F P O T E C	8	20/20
L E F O D P C T	9	
F D P L T C E O	10	
P E Z O L C F T D	11	

FIGURE 45.5 Snellen chart.

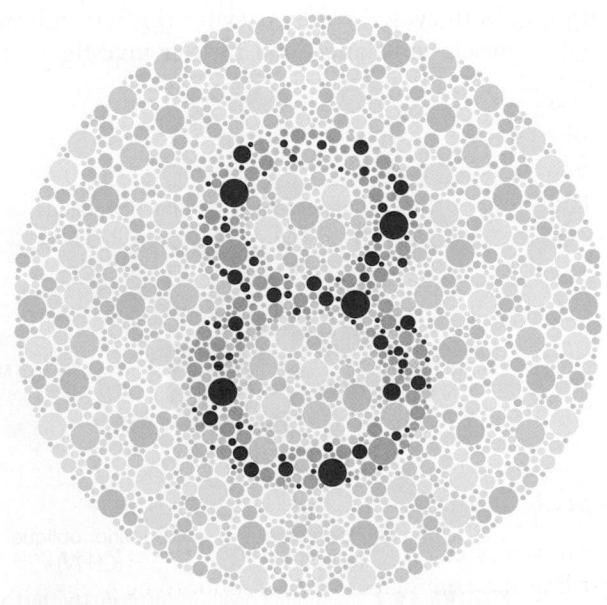

FIGURE 45.6 Ishihara chart.

majority of color blindness occurs in males. Females are carriers of the gene but are not normally affected. Approximately 8% of males and 1% of females are afflicted with this disorder.

The confrontation test is another commonly performed assessment of the eye and is a test of the visual fields that determines the degree of peripheral vision. This test is completed manually or with a computerized machine, similar to what is often seen in departments of motor vehicles when people are briefly eye-tested prior to being issued a driver's license. To complete this test manually, the provider sits facing the patient and asks the patient to look directly into the provider's eyes. The provider covers his or her right eye while asking the patient to cover his or her left. With an extended arm, the provider moves a finger from a nonvisible area to the patient's line of vision. The patient with normal peripheral vision should be able to notice the finger at about the same time the provider does. Repeat this same process having the provider cover the left eye and the patient cover his or her right eye.

The corneal light reflex and the six cardinal positions of gaze (Fig. 45.7) tests are used to assess extraocular muscle function. Cranial nerves III, IV, and VI are also assessed when completing these tests.

The corneal light reflex provides information about the alignment of the eyes. When there are no alignment problems with the eyes, the light reflex is in approximately the same position in both pupils. If, for example, the patient has an irregularity such as **strabismus** (a disorder where the eyes appear to be looking in different directions), the light will appear off-center in the crossed eye. To complete this test, the provider asks the patient to stare straight ahead, often directing the patient to stare at the nose of the provider. As the patient stares at the light object, the provider shines a penlight from a distance of 12 to 15 inches on both corneas. The light should reflect on the shiny surface of the cornea in a symmetric position in both eyes. Asymmetry with this test indicates probable muscle imbalance, and further investigation is warranted.

Assessment of the six ocular movements is done to check eye alignment and coordination. The test is performed on patients older than 6 years of age. To complete this test, the patient is instructed to stand directly in front of the provider with the head held in a fixed position. With a penlight held approximately 12 inches (30 cm) in front of the patient's eyes, the patient is asked to follow the movement of the penlight with his or her eyes only. The penlight should be moved slowly and in an orderly fashion both laterally and medially as is described in Figure 45.7. The penlight movement should be stopped periodically to detect nystagmus.

Pupillary light reflex is the normal, expected constriction of the pupil observed when exposed to bright light. This response is considered a "subcortical reflex arc," meaning the patient has no conscious control over it. Cranial nerve II, the optic nerve, is responsible for the part of the pupillary reflex that senses the incoming light. Cranial nerve III, the oculomotor nerve, is responsible for the pupillary reflex by constriction of the pupil. A direct light reflex (pupillary constriction) occurs when the eye is exposed to bright light. Normally, a consensual light reflex is also seen, meaning there is a simultaneous constriction of the other pupil. To test this reflex, the room should be darkened, and the patient should be instructed to stare straight ahead. The provider then advances the light slowly from the side. The normal response will elicit a constriction of the same-side pupil (ipsilateral; direct light reflex) as well as a simultaneous constriction of the opposite pupil (contralateral; a consensual light reflex).

Connection Check 45.4

The nurse prepares the patient for which common diagnostic evaluations during a visit to an eye care provider?

A. Pupillary light test, ultrasound of the eye
B. Test of peripheral vision, otoscope examination
C. Test for presence of bacteria in the conjunctiva, pupillary light test
D. Snellen eye chart examination, peripheral vision check

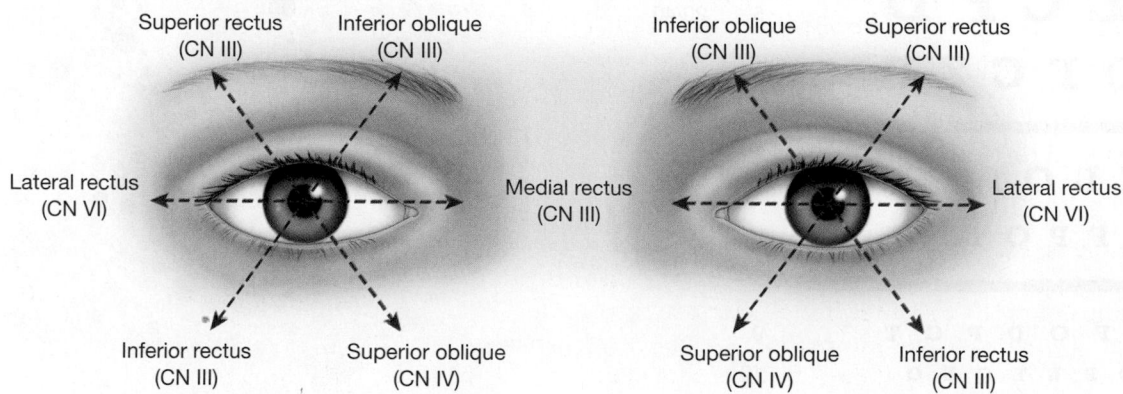

FIGURE 45.7 Six cardinal positions of gaze. This test assesses extraocular muscle function and cranial nerves III, IV, and VI.

DIAGNOSTIC STUDIES

An ophthalmic examination is most commonly completed in the provider's office or clinic setting by a medical doctor (MD) or APRN. Providers who specialize in the evaluation of the eye are ophthalmologists or optometrists. The ophthalmologist is a medical doctor and is trained in all aspects of medical and surgical diagnosis as well as the treatment of eye disorders. An optometrist is a doctor of optometry, allowing for examination and treatment of certain types of visual and eye disorders. Ophthalmic examinations provide very important information about the health of the patient's eyes and also about general health status. Examination of the eye using the ophthalmoscope allows the provider to view the retina as well as other vessels and structures of the eye. The examination usually takes place in a darkened room to allow for pupil dilation, which assists in the examination of the **fundus** (the internal surface of the retina). The patient is asked to stare straight ahead and fix eyes on an object behind the provider. The provider usually places a hand on the shoulder or eyebrow of the patient to assist in determining the distance from the ophthalmoscope. With the ophthalmoscope pressed firmly against the provider's face and starting from 12 to 15 inches away, the provider looks through the hole and moves slowly and steadily toward the patient while slowly advancing the dial on the lens selector dial of the ophthalmoscope to increase the acuity of the visual examination. The provider uses the same eye as the patient is having examined (i.e., the provider places the ophthalmoscope on the right eye and examines the patient's right eye). As the ophthalmoscope is directed inward toward the pupil, a red glow known as the **red reflex** should be visible. The red reflex

is a reflection of light on the retina. The absence of the red reflex could indicate opacity of the lens or cloudiness of the vitreous humor. Cloudiness of the vitreous humor may be the result of the presence of inflammatory cells, cellular debris, and/or blood. Once the retina is visible, the optic disk, optic vessels, fovea centralis, and macula should be visible (Fig. 45.8).

Prior to beginning the ophthalmic examination, the provider explains to the patient the reason for the examination and what to expect. If the patient is in a combative state or unwilling to complete the examination, it is suspended and completed at another time to decrease the potential for injury to the patient and the provider. The nurse is available for questions or postprocedural teaching depending on the results.

Computed Tomography

Computed tomography (CT) scans may be ordered to help diagnose diseases of the eye in the following areas: blood vessels, eye muscles, optic nerve, the presence of an abscess in or around the eye, fractures of the eye socket, and presence of a foreign body in the eye or the eye socket. These scans may be ordered with or without contrast.

Magnetic Resonance Imaging

Magnetic resonance imagining (MRI) gives the provider an image that provides detailed views of the soft tissue with no bone or air contrast. An MRI scan is used most frequently to discover tumors, infection, chronic disease, fractures, changes in the optic nerve, and enlarged eye muscles.

Ultrasonography

Ultrasonography of the eye is done by projecting high-frequency sound waves to produce an image of soft tissue when conditions make it difficult for the provider to see in the eye. (Cataracts and retinal detachment are common conditions that warrant an ultrasound examination by the provider.) This test is often able to be completed in the provider's office. Vitreous hemorrhage and tumors are often discovered using this test.

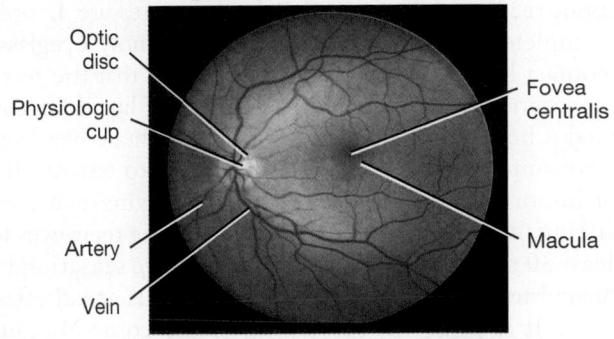

FIGURE 45.8 View of the retina through an ophthalmoscope.

Radioisotope Scanning

Radioisotope scanning is a scan that involves a small amount of various radioactive substances injected into the body with different uptakes to differentiate between normal and malignant tissues. This test is often done to identify tumors and ocular melanomas that are difficult to visualize with some of the less-invasive testing modalities.

Slit-Lamp Testing

Examination of the patient using a slit lamp is often included in a routine ophthalmic examination. This comprehensive test may be conducted to view structures in the posterior portion of the eye as well as for viewing structures such as the optic nerve and retina. Other uses of the slit lamp include diagnosis of cataracts, conjunctivitis, glaucoma, and macular degeneration or to verify the presence of a foreign body. This examination uses an instrument that provides a high-intensity light magnification, making three-dimensional (3D) imaging possible. Eye drops may be used to temporarily anesthetize the eye for this examination, and the patient is required to remove eyeglasses or contact lenses prior to the start of the examination.

Intraocular Pressure Testing

The tonometer is used to measure the pressure inside the eyeball itself. This pressure is known as the intraocular pressure, and the normal range is 10 to 21 mm Hg. Elevation of intraocular pressure decreases the blood flow to the eye structure and can result in catastrophic visual effects. The accumulating pressure within the eye can be caused by an overproduction of aqueous humor or, most commonly, inadequate drainage of the canals of Schlemm in the eye. Often a tonometer is also mounted on the slit lamp so that exact intraocular pressures may be obtained. In order to complete this test, most providers use anesthetizing drops and a yellow-orange dye solution called *fluorescein* (described in the following section) to stain the eye and allow for greater visualization of abnormalities. The test is completed as the patient rests the chin on a support bar and stares straight into an instrument (slit lamp, tonometer, etc.). The provider sits in front of the patient, shines a bright light into the patient's eye, and gently touches the probe to the eye. The tension dial on the instrument thus provides the provider with an accurate reading of the patient's intraocular pressure. In order to complete this test, the patient must remove eyeglasses or contact lenses. The patient is instructed that the test is most accurate when no more than 2 cups of liquid are consumed 4 hours before the test and no alcoholic beverages are consumed for at least 12 hours prior to testing. It is also important to instruct patients receiving eye anesthetizing medication to refrain from rubbing their eyes for at least 30 minutes after the test or until eye sensation has returned to normal. Rubbing an eye that is anesthetized can result in injury or scratching of the cornea because the patient is unable to feel objects that would normally cause pain.

Corneal Staining Test

The corneal staining test is an assessment that uses a yellow-orange dye (fluorescein) placed directly into the eye in the form of a drop or instilled by a piece of blotting paper with dye impregnated on it. After the dye has been inserted into the eye, the patient is asked to blink to help distribute the dye evenly throughout the eye cavity. With the room lights off, a blue light is then held over the open stained eye to detect foreign bodies or scratches that might be present on the cornea. Oftentimes, an anesthetizing medication is also placed in the eye to assist with patient comfort and allow for a more comprehensive examination. Prior to this examination, it is important to instruct the patient on the type of examination being performed, as well as the fact that some of the fluorescein eye stain will remain in the eye and cause a temporary discoloration. If anesthetizing drops are used, instructions to the patient to refrain from rubbing the eye for at least 30 minutes are important to prevent possible eye injury. Table 45.2 outlines important patient teaching related to post–eye examination care. Contact lenses should not be reinserted into the eye until feeling has returned to the eye and the yellow-orange eye color has dissipated, usually 2 to 4 hours after the examination.

Fluorescein Angiography

Performed by a provider or an advanced practice registered nurse, this diagnostic procedure provides detailed images about the internal eye circulation. An IV dye (usually 5 mL of a 10% fluorescein solution) is injected, and photographs are taken in rapid sequence. This test is useful in determining retinal circulation because it identifies problems such as diabetic retinopathy, retinal hemorrhage, macular degeneration, and tumors.

Preparation of a patient for this examination includes patient teaching, safety considerations, placement of a peripheral IV catheter, and administration of eye drops. Patient teaching includes an explanation of the procedure, assessment of any patient allergies, and information that the patient may have slightly yellow skin for a couple hours after the procedure, as well as a green color to his or her urine as the dye is excreted from the body. Instructions to increase the intake of water are also paramount in helping to flush the infused dye out of the body. Ensuring that the patient has a family member or friend to assist with vision needs and transportation home are safety concerns.

Connection Check 45.5

The nurse must consider all of these assessments prior to preparing a patient for diagnostic studies of the eye. Which intervention can be delegated to the technician on the team?

A. Assessing the patient's past medical history
B. Administering preprocedure medications
C. Obtaining an accurate height and weight of the patient
D. Reviewing current medications the patient is taking daily

Table 45.2 Patient Education Related to Eye Examination

Instruction	Rationale
Use eye protection (such as eyeglasses or sunglasses) after the examination is complete.	The anesthetic property of the eye drops blocks the ability to feel foreign objects (which would normally cause pain) entering or touching the eye. (Dust and wind-blown articles are common threats.)
Do not rub the eyes.	The anesthetic property of the eye drops prevents the ability to feel if a foreign substance is present and is being rubbed in the eye. It also makes it difficult for the patient to realize the amount of pressure being exerted with rubbing action, and damage to the eye can result.
Contact lenses should not be reinserted until all feeling has returned to the eye, usually 2 to 4 hours.	Insertion of contact lenses when the eye is anesthetized can result in scratches or damage to the eye because there is no feeling to guide the patient.
No swimming or showering until feeling has returned to the eye, usually 2 to 4 hours	The inability to feel any pain in the eye can result in injury from foreign substances potentially present in swimming pools as well as water forcefully hitting an open eye. The reflex to close the eye to the offending agent is not present.

EYE PROTECTION

The numerous sensitive internal and external structures within the eye itself make eye protection critical for preventing injury or loss of vision. The use of protective goggles at work and at home with high-risk activities is vital. People are often unaware of injuries that can be sustained with everyday activities such as cutting grass, playing sports, unintentional exposure to caustic or corrosive substances, and other everyday at-risk activities. Sunglasses are an important piece of equipment and are often overlooked. Exposure to ultraviolet-B (UV-B) light over time can have damaging effects on the eye. It is now known that there is an association between excessive exposure to UV-B light and the early formation of cataracts. Hand washing is another simple way to prevent injury to the eye by preventing the transfer of toxic or injurious substances directly to the eye. Eye examinations are an important protective measure and are recommended at different intervals depending on the patient's age and health status. In general, it is recommended that patients aged 20 to 39 have a comprehensive eye examination every 3 to 5 years, patients aged 40 to 64 every 2 to 4 years, and patients 65 or older every 1 to 2 years. Prompt treatment for eye concerns should always be acted on to decrease the possibility of permanent damage to these sensitive structures. Patients with chronic diseases such as hypertension and diabetes are also encouraged to keep their diseases well controlled to minimize the possibility of complications.

> **⚠ Safety Alert   Eye Symptoms Needing Further Assessment**
>
> - Sudden loss of vision in any part of the visual field
> - Sudden onset of pain in the eye
> - Flashing lights present
> - Physical trauma/injury to the eye
> - Constant tearing of the eye with or without photophobia

> **Connection Check 45.6**
>
> The nurse recognizes which action as most important to preventing eye trauma?
> A. Wearing protective goggles at home or work as indicated
> B. Keeping hands clean
> C. Refraining from looking directly into light sources
> D. Eating a well-balanced diet

AGE-RELATED CHANGES

Anatomical changes to the eye occur as a natural process as people age. Not all decreases in visual ability are of pathological origin. The most significant age-related changes occur in the lens and the pupil and account for the majority of the visual limitations experienced with advancing age.

As a person advances in age, the pupil becomes smaller and less responsive to light. It is common for people to need more time adjusting from changes in light levels as they age. Loss of lens elasticity is another expected change in the eye that occurs around the age of 45. The loss of elasticity of the lens makes it harder for the lens to bend in order to focus on closely held objects. This loss of lens accommodation is known as presbyopia and makes "reading glasses" necessary for people in this age group and older. Another common expected change that occurs in the eye with aging is the gradual yellowing of the lens. This yellowing tends to absorb and scatter blue light, making it difficult to see differences in shades of blue, green, and violet. Dullness in color perception may become evident. This change in vision may also make it more difficult to navigate where an object ends and the background begins.

Deposits in the vitreous humor, often referred to as "floaters," may become evident in advancing years. These spots may occur as the vitreous humor develops opacities that become visual to the patient as "floaters" and bounce in the visual field. Shrinkage of the vitreous humor may also cause the same clinical manifestations; shrinking is also attributed to advancing age and is considered a normal, expected process.

Some of the other expected changes that occur in the eyes are found in the conjunctiva, the retina, and the eyelids. The conjunctiva becomes more susceptible to chronic inflammation secondary to an increase in eye dryness. The increased dryness can be secondary to hormonal decreases within the body with advancing age in adulthood. The tear glands and conjunctiva may lose the ability to efficiently lubricate the eye and therefore produce "dry eye." The arteries and veins of the retina become narrower with age, thus reducing blood flow and yielding a less responsive light reflex. The eyelids lose elasticity and tone, causing ptosis (drooping), thereby decreasing visual fields.

Connection Check 45.7

The nurse recognizes which findings as expected changes in visual function associated with aging?
A. Presbyopia, decrease in general color perception
B. More narrowed field of vision, otosclerosis
C. Decrease in general color perception, increased tear production
D. Pupillary miosis, presbyopia

Making Connections

CASE STUDY: WRAP-UP

The APRN refers Melanie to an optometrist for further evaluation for glasses or contacts. Melanie will also need to use moisturizing eye drops to ensure that her eyes stay lubricated, obtain and use reading glasses for near vision, and schedule yearly eye examinations to ensure optimal eye health. She is also provided with instructions on vitamins to support eye health.

Case Study Questions

1. Which changes in Melanie's vision are expected age-related clinical manifestations?
   A. Frequent tearing and "spots" in her vision fields
   B. Difficulty reading objects when held at arm's length
   C. Dry eyes and difficulty reading unless objects are held at arm's length
   D. Itching of both eyes and blurry vision

2. Which tests will Melanie's provider order based on her presenting clinical manifestations and history?
   A. Visual acuity test with ophthalmic examination
   B. A CT scan to rule out the presence of tumors or other pathology
   C. Ophthalmic examination using fluorescein to check for foreign bodies
   D. Ophthalmic ultrasound to rule out the presence of cataracts

3. In addition to focused examinations of the eyes, what other data should Melanie's provider assess?
   A. Immunization history
   B. Dietary history
   C. Travel history
   D. Obstetrical history

4. Based on her clinical presentation, Melanie's provider is most likely to offer which suggestion?
   A. Increase the intake of carrots in her diet to help stimulate her visual acuity.
   B. Use lubricating eye drops for 2 weeks, and then return for a follow-up examination.
   C. Get at least 8 hours of sleep at night.
   D. Schedule a follow-up examination with an eye care specialist.

5. What is the rationale for Melanie's provider to perform the Rosenbaum test?
   A. Assesses Melanie's near vision
   B. Assesses Melanie's far vision
   C. Assesses Melanie's peripheral vision
   D. Assesses Melanie's CN IV function

CHAPTER SUMMARY

The visual function of the human body is a spectacular system that contains countless different components. Disruption of any of these key components can result in a loss or interruption of vision. Completing an accurate and comprehensive medical history and eye examination of the patient's visual system, including family history details, is essential for the maintenance of a healthy visual system. Diagnostic testing of the visual system also determines the current level of visual function and provides important baseline information for the future. Predictable changes occur within the eye throughout the life span; these changes are readily visible during physical examination and during certain diagnostic tests related to the eye. The nurse must be keenly aware of the expected changes so that proper patient teaching and instruction can take place. Injury prevention education is another teaching area in which it is essential for the nurse to take an active role with patients, even during routine physical examinations. Providing patients with yearly eye examinations, comprehensive and accurate education, and instruction for injury prevention all help to provide for a lifetime of good vision.

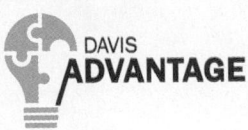

To explore learning resources for this chapter, go to **Davis Advantage** and find:
- Answers to in-text questions
- Chapter Resources and Activities
- NCLEX®-Style Chapter Review Questions
- Bibliography

Chapter 46

Coordinating Care for Patients With Visual Disorders

Kelley Miller Wilson

Finding Connections

CASE STUDY: EPISODE 1

Follow this patient throughout the chapter.

Mike Peterson is a 64-year-old African American architect working in a busy urban architectural firm. Mike has always enjoyed excellent visual acuity, which has been vital to his career reviewing intricate architectural drawings on a daily basis. Lately, Mike has noticed his peripheral vision is decreasing; he is "missing" objects on the left side of his visual field. He plans to visit his provider this week for a physical examination and to discuss this new change in his vision…

INTRODUCTION

The eyes are complex organs that work in conjunction with the brain to provide vision. There are many disorders of the eyes that impact vision, from visual disturbances that are treated with corrective lenses to degenerative disorders that potentially lead to total blindness. Understanding the pathophysiological changes associated with the various disorders provides the basis for the rationales for medical and nursing interventions.

VISUAL ACUITY DISORDERS

Refraction is one of the four functions of the eye that controls clarity of vision no matter what the distance, and there are four refractive errors that occur when the bending of light rays by the cornea and lens does not focus the image correctly on the retina. **Myopia**, nearsightedness, results from an eyeball that is too long or when the cornea has too much curve present, thus allowing the focused image to fall in front of the retina. **Hyperopia**, farsightedness, is the opposite issue, causing the image to fall behind the retina. **Astigmatism** results from a misshaped cornea. Another abnormality known as **presbyopia** occurs almost exclusively with aging and results from the loss of lens elasticity and occurs around age 45. The diagnosis of a visual acuity disorder may be made in a general provider's office or clinic by using a Snellen chart as a general guide. Abnormalities in a visual acuity examination are referred to an eye care professional (ophthalmologist or optometrist) for further assessment and exact diagnosis. The provider also discusses the most appropriate care options available to the patient. All four of these disorders may be successfully treated with prescriptive lenses (eyeglasses or contact lenses).

Epidemiology

Refraction errors affect approximately one-third of persons 40 years or older in the United States. The risk factors and prevalence for each specific refraction error are listed in Table 46.1.

Pathophysiology

The shape of the eye and the role of the cornea provide most of the ability of the eye to focus clearly on objects near and far. The primary disorders of visual acuity are myopia, hyperopia, astigmatism, and presbyopia.

Myopia is a common condition caused by a larger-than-normal eyeball that causes light rays from distant objects to focus before they reach the retina. It may be inherited and is often detected in schoolchildren during routine vision examinations completed at school. Hyperopia commonly occurs when the eyeball is smaller than normal. This size

Table 46.1 Specific Refraction Disorders		
Refraction Error	**Risk Factors**	**Prevalence**
Myopia	Heredity; environmental factors such as reading in dim light and doing excessive amounts of close work may also contribute	Approximately 25% of the U.S. population is known to have myopia, affecting men and women equally.
Hyperopia	Heredity and increased age	Approximately 25% of the U.S. population is hyperopic, with men and women affected equally.
Presbyopia	A normal part of aging	Almost all people experience some degree of presbyopia when they reach their mid-40s.
Astigmatism	Heredity; injury that causes the lens or cornea to become distorted (including trauma, scarring, and surgical procedures involving the structures); persons with keratoconus (a condition where the cornea becomes thin and cone shaped; may be inherited or result from chronic eye rubbing); diabetes	Occurs often with myopia and hyperopia; it is believed that most people have some degree of astigmatism.

distortion causes light rays from near objects to focus improperly on the retina in the back of the eye. Often, babies and young children are slightly hyperopic, a condition that tends to improve as the eye grows.

Astigmatism is a condition that occurs when the lens or cornea (or both) is curved more steeply in an oval instead of a round shape. This distortion often occurs in combination with myopia or hyperopia. The uneven curvature prevents light rays entering the eye from focusing to a single point on the retina.

Presbyopia results from a loss of lens elasticity that occurs in almost all adults around the age of 45. The loss of elasticity of the lens makes it more difficult for the lens to bend in order to focus on closely held objects. "Reading glasses" or handheld magnification is required to visualize properly. Figure 46.1 provides a visual representation of these disorders.

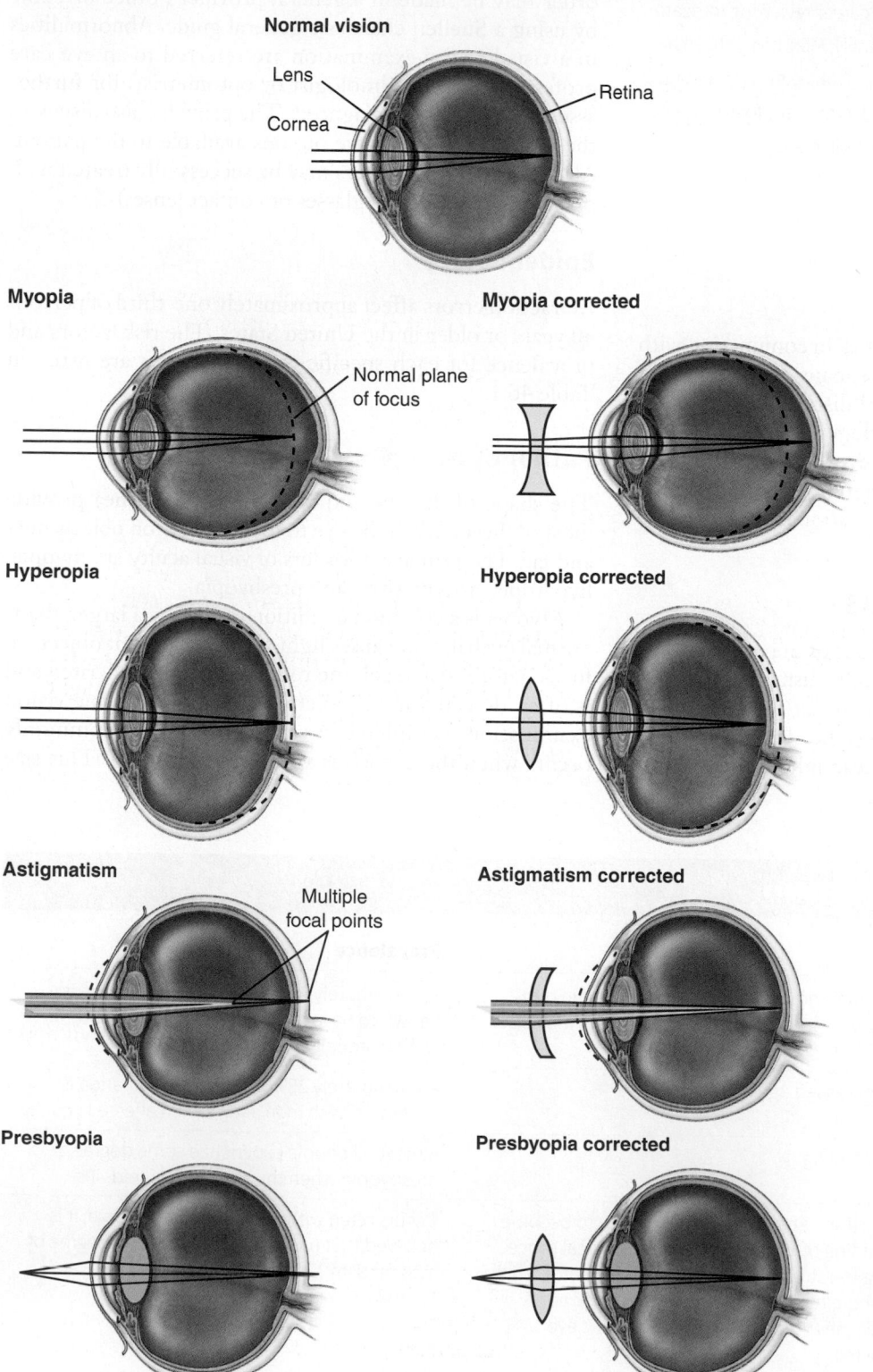

FIGURE 46.1 Refraction and correction of visual disorders.

Clinical Manifestations

The clinical presentations of disorders of visual acuity are directly related to the underlying pathophysiology.

- Myopia causes a person to see near objects more clearly than objects at a distance. The result of this distortion is blurred vision for distant objects.
- Hyperopia occurs when a person can see distant objects more clearly than near objects. Blurred vision of near objects is the symptom associated with this disorder.
- Astigmatism results in visual changes where objects that are near and distant are blurry. Other clinical manifestations include squinting, headaches, and blurry vision.
- Presbyopia, an expected change in vision around midlife, results in the inability to focus on objects held close to the face.

Management

Medical Management

The goals of medical management of disorders of visual acuity focus on maximizing sight through interventions such as corrective lenses. Table 46.2 provides the specific types of correction associated with each disorder. **Orthokeratology** is a nonsurgical option to reshape the cornea that requires the patient to wear a special contact lens that slowly reshapes the cornea and corrects the myopia over time.

Surgical Management

Common surgical treatments for visual acuity disorders include the following (Table 46.3), including different approaches to **keratotomy** (surgical approach involving cutting into the cornea), **keratectomy** (surgical removal of a section or layer of the cornea), and **keratoplasty** (surgical procedure replacement of damaged/diseased corneal tissue with healthy tissue from a donor):

- *Radial keratotomy* is a surgical procedure in which tiny incisions are made in the cornea that cause it to flatten and reduce the refraction disorder (Fig. 46.2A).
- *Photorefractive keratectomy (PRK)* involves removing a portion of the cornea with a laser to change its shape and therefore modify the refractive error (Fig. 46.2B).

Table 46.2 Treatments for Visual Disorders

Condition	Medical Treatment Available
Myopia	Corrective lenses such as glasses or contact lenses
Hyperopia	Convex corrective lenses in eyeglasses or contact lenses
Presbyopia	"Reading glasses" or magnification
Astigmatism	Eyeglasses, contact lenses, or orthokeratology

Table 46.3 Surgical Treatments for Visual Disorders

Condition	Most Commonly Used Surgical Treatment Available
Myopia	Radical keratotomy, photorefractive keratotomy, and LASIK
	Implantable lens known as Phakic Intraocular Lens is another form of treatment to correct myopia.
	This treatment is usually reserved for patients who are unsuitable for LASIK or other vision corrective surgeries.
Hyperopia	Refractive surgery such as LASIK, photorefractive keratectomy, thermal keratoplasty, conductive keratoplasty, and intraocular implants
Presbyopia	Refractive surgery and implanted intraocular lenses (several other therapies are also currently under investigation)
Astigmatism	Refractive surgery, LASIK, photorefractive keratectomy

LASIK, Laser-assisted in-situ keratomileusis.

- *Laser-assisted in situ keratomileusis (LASIK)* involves the use of a laser or a special instrument called a *microkeratome* to create a thin circular flap in the cornea (Fig. 46.2C). The flap is then folded back out of the way, and the surgeon uses the laser to remove some of the corneal tissue. The laser is directed and then uses a cool ultraviolet (UV) light beam to precisely ablate (remove) very tiny bits of tissue from the cornea to reshape it.
- *Laser thermal keratoplasty (LTK)* uses a Holmium laser to reshape the cornea (Fig. 46.2D). The Holmium laser is an infrared or thermal laser that uses heat to shrink the corneal tissue.
- *Conductive keratoplasty* uses radiofrequency energy and does not remove any corneal tissue (Fig. 46.2E). An instrument with a tiny probe on the end is placed at specific points around the peripheral portion of the cornea. These points then emit energy that causes collagen to contract, shrinking the circumference of the cornea and changing the shape of the curve.

Nursing Management

Assessment and Analysis

Treatment of visual acuity disorders varies greatly depending on the diagnosis (Table 46.4). All four visual acuity disorders may be treated medically with corrective eyeglasses or contact lenses. Surgical options are also available for each disorder. Depending on expected results, patient age, and personal circumstances, treatment plans are individualized for the patient.

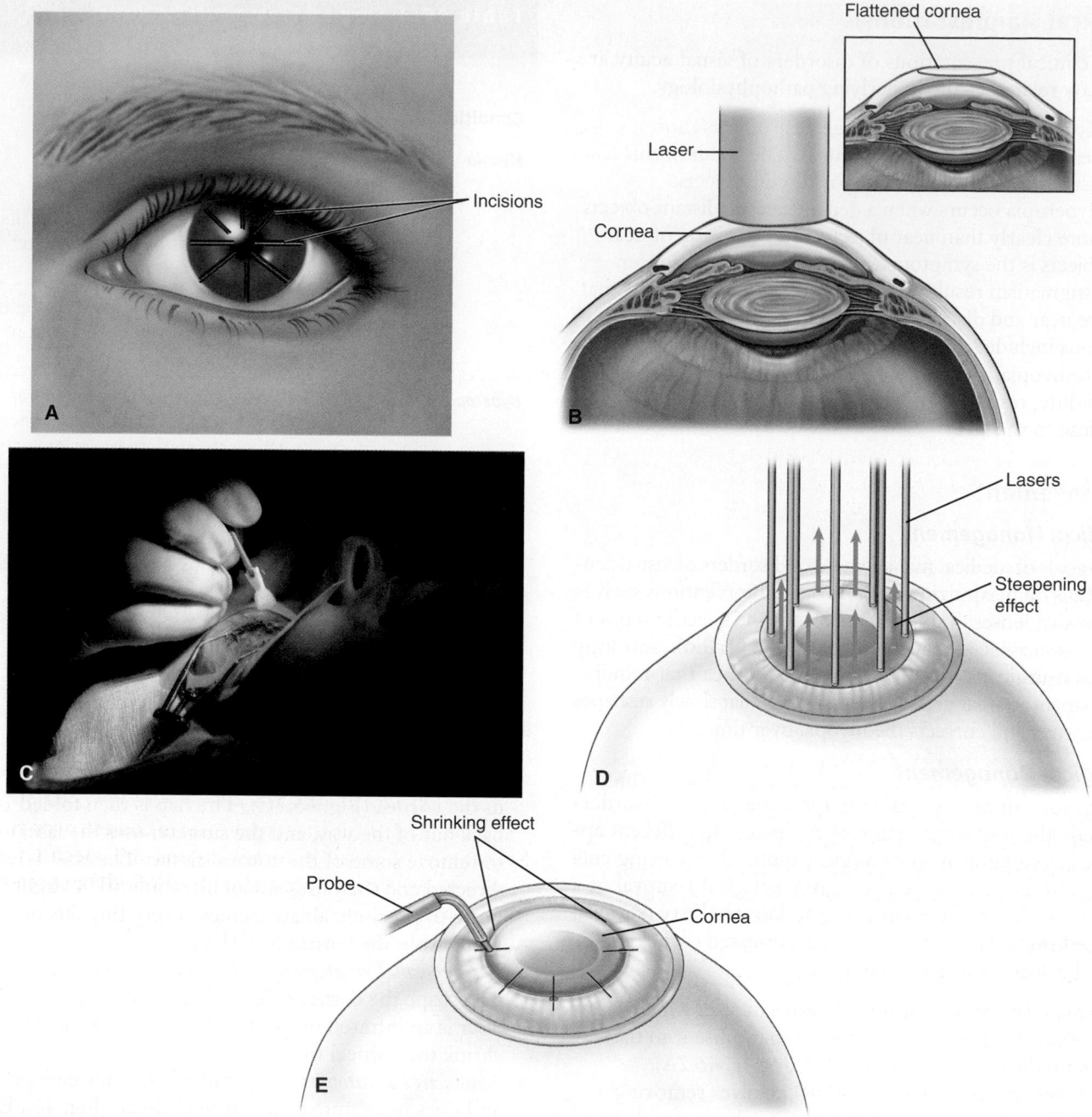

FIGURE 46.2 Common surgical treatments for visual acuity disorders. A, Radial keratotomy is a surgical procedure in which tiny incisions are made in the cornea that cause it to flatten and reduce the refraction disorder. B, Photorefractive keratectomy involves the removal of a portion of the cornea with a laser to change its shape and therefore modify the refractive error. C, Laser in situ keratomileusis (LASIK) uses a laser to create a thin circular flap in the cornea. D, Laser thermal keratoplasty uses a laser to reshape the cornea. E, Conductive keratoplasty uses an instrument with a tiny probe on the end that is placed at specific points around the peripheral portion of the cornea. These points then emit radiofrequency energy that causes collagen to contract, shrinking the circumference of the cornea and changing the shape of the curve.

Nursing Diagnoses

- **Disturbed visual sensory perception** related to refractive disorders of the eye
- **Risk for injury** related to inability to correctly focus
- **Anxiety** related to visual impairment and inability to correctly focus on objects

Nursing Interventions

■ *Assessments*

- Vital signs
  Vital sign changes or fluctuations are not usually directly related to visual acuity disorders. Elevations in pulse and blood pressure are mostly related to pain or anxiety.

Table 46.4 Assessment and Analysis of Visual Disorders

Assessment Data	Analysis/Explanation
Myopia (nearsightedness)	Blurred vision when looking at distant objects, headaches, feeling of eye strain, squinting when looking at objects more than a few feet away
Hyperopia (farsightedness)	Blurred vision when looking at close-up objects, aching eyes or feeling of eye strain, headache during reading
Presbyopia	Holding reading material far away so that letters are clear, blurred vision at normal reading distance, feeling of eye strain or headaches after reading or doing close work (may also occur with myopia and hyperopia)
Astigmatism	Headache, blurred vision at all distances, feeling of fatigue or eye strain

- Eye changes associated with visual acuity changes
  Physical assessment changes center around changes in the corneal shape in myopia, hyperopia, and astigmatism. Presbyopia yields changes in lens elasticity and therefore produces a more elongated lens instead of the expected round shape.
- Diagnostic results
  Diagnostic results for visual acuity disorders center on eye examination and visual acuity changes that are noted on Snellen vision charts or more comprehensive examinations completed by eye care professionals in their office.
- Age-related considerations
  Advanced age increases the risk for all four visual acuity disturbances because the eye begins to undergo predictable changes. Presbyopia, yielding a loss in lens elasticity specifically, is considered a normal process of aging and occurs in midlife around age 45. Routine eye examinations after age 45 are recommended to monitor for any eye changes.

Actions

- Ensure the patient correctly wears corrective lenses (eyeglasses and contact lenses).
  Corrective lenses, both eyeglasses and contact lenses, provide necessary treatment to correct refraction errors.
- Provide adequate lighting to maximize visual acuity.
  Insufficient lighting may place additional strain on the eyes and adversely impact visual acuity.

Teaching

- Importance of wearing corrective lenses, including eyeglasses and contact lenses
  Review with the patient proper care for eyeglasses and proper disinfection, insertion, and storage of contact lenses. Patients wearing contact lenses also need to be instructed to remove lenses at night to prevent eye damage (an exception is contact lenses approved for long-term use).
- Report visual changes or chronic headaches to healthcare provider.
  Patients need to be instructed to notify a healthcare provider for visual disturbances or continued headaches indicating that lens correction may not be sufficient. Yearly follow-up with a provider is recommended for all patients with corrective lenses.

- Postoperative considerations
  Patients should be instructed to notify providers of increased pain, temperature, or other unusual feelings because these could indicate a structural complication or an infection. Follow-up appointments are also very important to ensure that proper healing is taking place. Restrictions on lifting, bending, and Valsalva maneuvers are important instructions for some surgeries to prevent increased intraocular pressure (IOP) from occurring.

Evaluating Care Outcomes

Patients with visual acuity disorders can lead a productive, normal life. The patient requires continued follow-up and monitoring by a healthcare provider to ensure optimal vision as magnification requirements change over time. Knowledge of possible complications and specific postoperative instructions must also be followed for successful treatment.

Connection Check 46.1

The clinic nurse is preparing to check a patient's vision. The nurse knows that nearsightedness or myopia causes light rays

A. from distant objects to focus before they reach the retina.
B. to focus improperly on the retina in the front of the eye.
C. to diverge to focus on the retina.
D. to reflect off the macula.

VISION LOSS RELATED TO OPIOID USE

Epidemiology and Pathophysiology

Opioid use and deaths associated with opioid abuse in the United States have dramatically increased since 2000. An unexpected and devastating result related to IV opioid drug use is endogenous endophthalmitis, an infection transmitted via the bloodstream that multiplies in the choroid, leading to infiltration of the retina and spreading to the vitreous humor. Drug use via injection with non-sterile equipment can result in microbial bloodstream infections that can seed ocular infection, and these infections may be bacterial, fungal, or viral in nature. Despite treatment, nearly 50% of those affected will have no light perception, and the condition can lead to partial or complete blindness.

Clinical Manifestations

Patients with suspected endogenous endophthalmitis present with minimal clinical manifestations, including a red and painful eye, photophobia, floaters, and reduced vision. Most often, patients present with unilateral clinical manifestations, although up to one-third of cases have bilateral involvement. Upon examination, symptomatic patients may have reduced visual acuity, conjunctival injection, corneal edema, and inflammation of the iris and vitreous parts of the eye.

Management

Medical and Surgical Management

A key diagnostic finding associated with endogenous endophthalmitis is the presence of a white infiltrate originating in the choroid and sometimes erupting into the vitreous cavity. Specialized equipment and providers with specialization in eye diseases examine the patient more extensively to make this diagnosis.

Treatment should be initiated as soon as endophthalmitis is suspected and is often started even before a definitive diagnosis is made. Most commonly, treatment begins with prompt intravitreal antibiotic administration, combined with hospitalization, infectious disease consultation, and IV antibiotics.

In determining the best therapeutic approach, the causative organism and the extent of ocular involvement should direct the aggressiveness of therapy. If the ocular lesion is confined to the choroid, systemic therapy with antibiotics or antifungals and close observation may be suitable; if the infection has spread beyond the choroid into the vitreous, then more aggressive intravitreal antibiotic therapy should be considered.

Nursing Management
Assessment and Analysis

Patients often present with local clinical manifestations of an eye infectious process associated with IV opioid use. Treatment plans are individualized for the patient based on the circumstances related to the infectious process.

Clinical manifestations of this disorder include:

- Red, painful eyes
- Photophobia
- Floaters

- Decreased visual acuity
- Corneal edema

Nursing Diagnoses
- **Disturbed visual sensory perception** related to infectious process in the eye secondary to IV opioid use
- **Risk for injury** related to decrease in visual acuity
- **Pain** related to inflammation and infection

Nursing Interventions
■ Assessments
- Vital signs
  Slight elevation in body temperature may be noted with endogenous endophthalmitis secondary to the presence of infection/inflammation. Elevations in heart rate and blood pressure may be associated with anxiety or recent IV drug use.
- Visual changes reported by the patient
  Active infectious processes may cause visual changes. The presence of floaters may also impair visual acuity.
- Eye appearance: Eye assessment changes noted on physical exam
  Redness, tearing, and swelling are objective assessments caused by the infectious process in the eye.
- Diagnostic results for visual acuity changes
  The presence of a white infiltrate originating in the choroid and sometimes erupting into the vitreous cavity

■ Actions
- Administer antibiotics, antifungals, and/or antivirals as prescribed.
  Intravitreal and IV medications treat the infectious process.
- Provide comfort care.
  Cool compresses applied to the affected eye help decrease inflammation of the eye. Sunglasses may offer comfort in bright light conditions.
- Assist with healthcare provider examination by providing adequate lighting and equipment.
  A definitive diagnosis and identification of bacteria or fungus are key to effective treatment.
- Safety considerations if vision is impaired
  Decreased visual acuity increases the risk of falls and other injuries.

■ Teaching
- Activity level
  Instruct patient about any required changes in activity levels based on the provider's instructions and diagnostic findings.
- Hand hygiene
  Clean hands are essential to prevent the transmission of conditions from one eye to another.
- Medication therapy
  It is important that the patient and family understand the importance of taking medications as prescribed and completing all medications to prevent reoccurrence or incomplete treatment. Incomplete treatment can lead to even more serious or complicated infections.

- Relationship between IV opioid use and development of endogenous endophthalmitis
  Drug use via injection with nonsterile equipment can result in microbial bloodstream infections that can seed ocular infection.
- Follow-up treatment
  It is essential that patients follow up with providers with scheduled appointments in order to closely monitor the healing process and any further changes in visual acuity.

Evaluating Care Outcomes

The outcomes of endogenous endophthalmitis are variable and are generally dictated by the aggressiveness of the causative organism. In general, yeasts are associated with the best visual outcomes, bacteria with moderate outcomes, and molds with the worst. Patient compliance with prescribed treatments, especially antibiotic, antifungal, or antiviral therapies, is key to the treatment of this disorder. It is also important that the patient and family understand the connection between IV drug use (opioids) and the development of endogenous endophthalmitis.

CONJUNCTIVITIS

Epidemiology

Conjunctivitis is a nonspecific term used to describe an inflammation of the conjunctivae of the eye. Most commonly known as pinkeye, this condition is usually caused by a wide range of conditions and is present throughout the world. It affects all ages, races, genders, and socioeconomic status groups.

Risk factors for this condition are sporadic or related to epidemic outbreaks. According to a National Health Survey, the prevalence of conjunctivitis in the United States in patients aged 1 to 74 is approximately 13 in 1,000. This study also noted that there are no reliable figures documenting the incidence of conjunctivitis, although it is estimated to be one of the common disorders of the eye. It is estimated that 3% of all emergency department visits are related to eye disorders, and approximately 30% of these are conjunctivitis. In primary care clinics, 2% of visits are related to ocular complaints, with 54% being related to conjunctivitis or corneal abrasions. Following diligent and frequent hygiene practices decreases the chances of transmission of conjunctivitis.

Pathophysiology

The condition termed *conjunctivitis* is described as an inflammation of the conjunctivae of the eye. Although viral conjunctivitis is more common than bacterial, *Streptococcus*, *Staphylococcus*, and *Haemophilus aegyptius are the most common bacterial causes of conjunctivitis*. There are different types of conjunctivitis, and most people in their lifetime will have the unpleasant experience of at least one of them. Diagnosis of conjunctivitis is made based on history, clinical presentation, and physical findings.

Clinical Manifestations

The most common forms of conjunctivitis include the following clinical presentations:

- *Allergic conjunctivitis* is a condition involving inflammation of the conjunctivae secondary to an allergy-causing substance such as pollen or dander. The patient has clinical manifestations including red/pink sclera, intense itching, burning, tearing, and puffy eyelids.
- *Bacterial conjunctivitis* is an infection of the conjunctivae caused by a microbe or bacteria. The microbe often causes a gritty sensation in the eye; patients often describe it as feeling like sand is in the eye. There is also often a purulent eye discharge and matting of the eyelashes upon awakening in the morning.
- *Viral conjunctivitis* is a common condition involving inflammation of the conjunctivae secondary to the presence of a virus. Often seen with common colds, a virus affecting the upper respiratory tract, and sore throats, the eye usually exhibits a watery discharge, and the condition easily spreads from one eye to another.
- *Chlamydial conjunctivitis* is a sexually transmitted infection that is most commonly transmitted through the hand-to-eye spread of infected genital secretions. Chlamydial conjunctivitis may be transmitted during birth from an infected mother to the newborn. The organism causing the infection is *Chlamydia trachomatis*, and the patient usually has clinical manifestations for weeks or months. This specific type of conjunctivitis is known worldwide and in the past was considered to be a leading cause of blindness.
- *Contact lens–related conjunctivitis* is caused by hypersensitivity to one or more of the chemicals used to make the contact lens itself. Contact lens soaking solutions can also cause a hypersensitive reaction, thus yielding conjunctivitis. In addition, this condition is also caused by dirty lenses or debris under the lens in the eye.
- *Mechanical conjunctivitis* involves an irritation of the conjunctival surface caused by mechanical means such as an eyelash, foreign body, or other object of irritation.
- *Traumatic conjunctivitis* results from a direct injury such as a laceration, abrasion, or chemical injury (it is considered a secondary response).
- *Toxic conjunctivitis* typically develops following administration of a medication or direct contact with a corrosive or noxious chemical.

Management

Medical Management

The treatment of conjunctivitis depends on the causative agent. Comprehensive history-taking is essential for determining the type and guides effective patient treatment. The provider may use a slit lamp or other instrument to verify that there is no foreign body present in the eye. In conditions such as chlamydia or other suspected infection, the provider may also take a culture of the conjunctivae for microscopic examination. Visual acuity checks are always performed before treatment and after treatment in the patient with conjunctivitis. Table 46.5 lists the most common treatments for specific types of conjunctivitis.

Nursing Management

Assessment and Analysis

Many clinical manifestations of conjunctivitis (Table 46.6) are similar, and comprehensive history-taking is essential to making the correct diagnosis (Table 46.7). Tearing, itching, and inflammation of the conjunctiva are commonly observed. Incorrect diagnosis can lead to improper treatment.

Nursing Diagnoses

- **Risk for infectious transmission** related to inflammation/infection of the conjunctivae
- **Pain** related to inflammation of the conjunctivae

Nursing Interventions

Assessments

- Vital signs
  A slight elevation in body temperature may be noted with some conjunctival infections of the eye secondary to the presence of infection/inflammation. No other changes in vital signs are expected.
- Appearance of eye
  The sclera is expected to be pink/red/inflamed-looking secondary to the presence of infection/virus or allergen.

Tearing is present secondary to inflammation; purulent discharge may or may not be present depending on whether a bacterial infection is present.

- Diagnostic results
  Diagnosis is based primarily on the physical examination and history. Suspicious bacterial infections may also suggest that the provider swab the eye with a culture swab and send it to the laboratory for microscopic evaluation and incubation.
- Age-related considerations
  This condition affects all age groups, making no one group more at risk than another.

Actions

- Pharmacological therapy
  Specific medications are prescribed on the basis of the etiology and clinical manifestations (see Table 46.5).
- Provide comfort care.
  Cool compresses applied to the affected eye help decrease inflammation of the eye. Sunglasses may offer comfort in bright light conditions. Administration of antihistamine eye drops as prescribed offers some relief from itching of the eye.
- Collaborative care
  Referral to an eye care specialist for visual disturbances or difficult-to-treat clinical manifestations

Teaching

- Hand hygiene
  Clean hands are essential to preventing the transmission of conditions from one eye to another or from one person

Table 46.5 Treatment of Conjunctivitis

Etiology	Treatment
Allergic conjunctivitis	Most common are topical steroid and mast cell stabilizing drops instilled directly into the eye to decrease inflammation and block the release of histamine; topically instilled vasoconstrictor/antihistamine drops to the eye to decrease itching; removal of the allergen if known or if possible; good hand-washing practices
Bacterial conjunctivitis	Administration of antibiotic ointment or drops directly into the eye (rare cases may require systemic antibiotics); good hand-washing practices
Viral conjunctivitis	Cold compresses to the eye for pain relief and decrease in swelling/irritation; eye lubricants and ocular decongestants to help reduce swelling and inflammation; good hand-washing practices
Chlamydial conjunctivitis	Systemic antibiotics in most cases for up to 1 month; good hand-washing practices; medical treatment of the infected partner
Contact lens conjunctivitis	Discontinue wearing of lenses and determine underlying causes (solution allergies, age of lenses, bacterial contamination, trauma); good hand-washing practices
Mechanical conjunctivitis	Removal of trauma-inducing agent; may need antibiotic ointment or drops if significant epithelial disruption is present; good hand-washing practices
Traumatic conjunctivitis	Depends on the cause; usually need corneal staining to determine extent of trauma; may require antibiotic drops/ointment and pressure patch
Chemical-induced conjunctivitis	May require continuous irrigation with normal saline solution; corneal staining examination and antibiotic therapy depending on condition

Table 46.6 Clinical Manifestations of Conjunctivitis

Etiology	Condition	Clinical Manifestations
Bacterial	Acute/chronic bacterial	Tearing, lid crusting, feeling that something gritty is in the eye, purulent discharge, sclera pink/inflamed, eyes may be itchy
Viral	Adenovirus	Tearing, lid crusting, pink and inflamed sclera and conjunctiva, puffy eyelids, itchy
Allergic	Seasonal/dander	Itching, tearing, pink or red inflamed sclera/conjunctiva
Chlamydial	*Chlamydia trachomatis*	Tearing, red/pink conjunctiva and sclera, sticky eye mucous discharge, tearing, photophobia, foreign-body sensation

Table 46.7 Assessment and Analysis of Conjunctivitis

Assessment Data	Analysis/Explanation
Tearing	Initial response that occurs when a foreign substance is present in the eye
Red/Pink sclera	Change in scleral color is secondary to inflammation present on the sclera (mucosal) covering of the eye. This inflammatory process may be caused by bacterial or viral organisms.
Inflamed conjunctivae	Inflammation of the conjunctivae occurs, causing redness or swelling of the conjunctivae secondary to the presence of bacteria or viral organisms in the eye.
Itchy eye	Irritation of the sclera and mucosal linings of the eyelids produces an immune reaction that causes an itching sensation.
Purulent discharge from the eye	Presence of bacteria and the immune system response cause the formation of a purulent drainage to be present in the eye.

to another; conjunctivitis is considered extremely contagious.

- Hygiene at home
  Towels and pillowcases should be changed frequently and isolated from other family members to prevent possible transmission to another person.
- Completion of all prescribed medications
  Completion of all prescribed medication as ordered to prevent reoccurrence or incomplete healing. Incomplete treatments can lead to an even deeper infection in the eye.
- Follow-up care
  It is essential that patients keep follow-up appointments with their provider to verify the healing process and to monitor for any possible visual loss.

Evaluating Care Outcomes

Conjunctivitis is a nuisance for most patients who suffer from this condition. Early diagnosis and definitive treatment offer relief and prevent possible transfer of infection from one eye to another or one person to another. Clinical manifestations of the condition are directly related to the type of conjunctivitis. Most treatments are very effective, and the condition is easily resolved in 10 to 14 days.

Connection Check 46.2

The nurse correlates which clinical manifestations with a diagnosis of viral conjunctivitis? *(Select all that apply.)*

A. Pink or red sclera
B. Presence of upper respiratory symptoms or sore throat
C. Sensation of a foreign body in the eye
D. Watery discharge from the eye
E. Loss of peripheral vision

CORNEAL ABRASION

Epidemiology

One of the most common ophthalmological conditions leading to visits to emergency departments is **corneal abrasion**, and it is estimated to account for more than 10% of eye-related visits to healthcare providers. Contact lens wearers present with this condition more frequently than those who do not wear contact lenses. Two types of abrasions can occur; these are known as superficial and deep. A superficial corneal abrasion is a painful scratch or scrape to the cornea of the eye in which epithelial cells are removed.

Deep corneal abrasions penetrate the Bowman's membrane (the smooth layer of the eye located just under the epithelium) and usually take longer to heal (Fig. 46.3).

The most common risk factors associated with corneal abrasion include:

1. Contact lens wearers
2. Participation in contact sports
3. Presence outdoors in windy conditions without protective eyewear
4. Any abrasive eye injury
5. Dry eye syndrome
6. Abuse of topical eye anesthetics and steroids
7. Autoimmune disorders
8. Recent eye surgeries

There are four common causes of corneal abrasions: trauma, foreign bodies, contact lenses, and spontaneous defect.

Traumatic Corneal Abrasion

A traumatic corneal abrasion is caused by mechanical trauma to the eye resulting in disruption of the epithelial surface. Common causes of this type of abrasion are fingernail scrapes/pokes; animal paws inadvertently hitting the eye surface; pieces of paper or cardboard coming in contact with the eye surface; and makeup applicators (a mascara wand is a common source), hand tools, and branches and leaves coming in contact with the eye surface. Traumatic abrasions are also commonly caused by a foreign body, such as a piece of dust, eyelash, or other small particulate that lodges under the lid, resulting in a scratch to the eye surface.

Foreign Bodies

These disruptions in the corneal epithelium are caused by the removal or spontaneous dislodgment of a foreign substance/object. Common foreign-body abrasions are caused by pieces of rust, wood, glass, plastic, and fiberglass.

Contact Lenses

Removal/insertion of contact lenses and overworn or improperly fitting lenses can cause an abrasion to occur. Improperly cleaned/disinfected lenses can also be the culprit in some corneal abrasions because the dirt/bacteria present can cause an abrasion to develop.

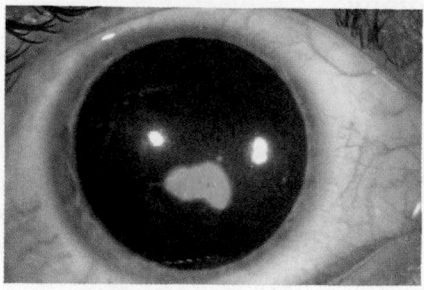

FIGURE 46.3 Corneal abrasion.

Spontaneous Defects

Previous eye abrasions, trauma, or underlying defects make a person more prone to spontaneous abrasions. Dry eyes and underlying chronic illness (e.g., diabetes and autoimmune illness) can make the epithelial cells more prone to a scratch. Persons who have had previous eye trauma, including tears, can develop a spontaneous injury.

Pathophysiology

Corneal abrasions are defined as a disruption of the cornea resulting from physical or chemical trauma. The abrasion is a disruption in the integrity of the cornea that is limited to only the epithelial layers. These abrasions can be very small or very large in size and usually heal within 24 to 48 hours of injury.

Clinical Manifestations

The most common clinical manifestations of corneal abrasions include eye pain (sometimes severe), photophobia (inability to be in the presence of bright light), spasm causing squinting, tearing, blurred vision, and the sensation of a foreign body in the eye.

Management

Medical Management

The medical management of a corneal abrasion includes a comprehensive examination by a healthcare provider. This examination includes a visual acuity test, anesthetizing the eye with an anesthetic agent (commonly tetracaine 1%), corneal staining with fluorescein stain, and visualization under a Wood lamp to confirm the diagnosis of the abrasion. Upon confirmation of the diagnosis, antibiotic eye drops and eye drops to help decrease muscle spasms of the eye may be prescribed. Eye patching is considered controversial and may or may not be used. Tetanus vaccination should be verified and administered if the patient is not considered up to date because any open surface of the body can provide a port of entry for *Clostridium tetani*. Discharge instructions include wearing sunglasses for pain relief and following up with an eye care professional within 24 to 48 hours.

Surgical Management

Most corneal abrasions are treated medically, and unless the patient received an extensive corneal abrasion, treatment is as outlined previously. Extreme corneal abrasions are often diagnosed as deep corneal lacerations and may require surgical exploration and suture placement for repair.

Nursing Management

Assessment and Analysis

The removal of epithelium from the covering of the eye in most cases is extremely painful. The corneal area of the eye has an abundance of nerve cells present that make it almost immediately obvious that an injury has occurred (Table 46.8).

Table 46.8 Assessment and Analysis of Corneal Abrasions

Assessment Data	Analysis/Explanation
Eye pain (can be severe)	Disruption of the epithelial surface of the cornea also disrupts the numerous sensory nerves, resulting in pain.
Tearing	Initial response to eye injury or foreign substance being present in the eye.
Photophobia	This is present because too much light is able to enter the eye with the disruption of the corneal cells.
Redness of the sclera	New blood vessels form, and those present enlarge, to increase blood flow to the eye so that healing can occur.

Most corneal abrasions will heal within 24 to 48 hours after injury and without complication. Clinical manifestations include pain, redness, tearing, the sensation of something in the eye, squinting, and photophobia.

Nursing Diagnoses

- **Pain** related to disruption of epithelial cells on the cornea
- **Disturbed visual sensory perception** related to corneal disruption
- **Risk for infection** related to a tear in epithelial cells of the cornea

Nursing Interventions

Assessments

- Vital signs
  There is no disturbance in vital signs from this injury, although elevations may be noted in heart rate and blood pressure if pain is present.
- Preparation for examination/physical assessment changes
  Prepare the patient for an eye examination. Visual acuity is assessed to verify initial acuity; worsening of these numbers on follow-up examination could indicate the severity of injury. Instillation of tetracaine 1% provides instant pain relief in most instances; instillation of fluorescein eye stain helps to highlight the presence of injury when a UV light (Wood lamp) is shone over the injured eye. This helps the provider verify the presence and extent of injury.
- Diagnostic results
  Diagnostic results are as noted previously and guide treatment.
- Age-related considerations
  This condition affects all ages, and there are no special considerations for age; treatment modalities are considered the same.

Actions

- Pharmacological therapy
  Patients identified as having a corneal abrasion are prescribed medications on the basis of the severity of the abrasion and the amount of pain the patient is experiencing. Pain medication may be over-the-counter preparations, such as acetaminophen, or a stronger prescription-strength medication may be selected by the provider. Antibiotic eye drops are selected according to the degree of abrasion present and the amount of contamination present in the injury. Cycloplegic eye drops such as atropine are sometimes prescribed. These drops dilate the pupil and help decrease the amount of painful muscle spasms in the ciliary body of the eye that can develop after such an injury. Antibiotics are indicated with corneal abrasions that are infected.
- Comfort measures
  Comfort measures are provided to assist the patient in recovery from this injury. Medications taken as prescribed help promote healing and decrease pain from exposed nerve cells and painful muscle spasms of the eye. An eye patch is sometimes recommended and often provides some relief because light is no longer able to reach the eye. Sunglasses are suggested for patients in the presence of bright light to help reduce the photophobic effect of the injury.
- Collaborative care
  Referral to an eye care specialist for severe or difficult-to-heal injuries

Teaching

- Discharge instructions for care at home
  The patient is instructed to follow all discharge instructions provided by the provider, including antibiotic eye-drop instillation to heal/prevent infection, pain medication as ordered to prevent severe pain and to provide comfort, and an eye patch (if ordered) to remain in place with specific time parameters. Eye patches can provide comfort and, in some cases, can add a compression effect to prevent possible bleeding. (Eye-patch placement is controversial, and some providers believe that eye patches can delay healing and therefore do not prescribe patches.) Additionally, the patient is to practice good hand hygiene and keep hands away from the eye to lessen the chance of infection or the possibility of a tear or injury secondary to rubbing the eye. The nurse emphasizes the importance of follow-up appointments so that the chance for permanent injury, including loss of vision, is lessened.

Evaluating Care Outcomes

Patients who suffer a corneal abrasion usually notice significant relief of symptoms within 24 to 48 hours of injury depending on the severity of the abrasion. Medical evaluation, treatment with antibiotic eye drops, pain medication (if indicated), an eye patch (if prescribed by the provider), and verification of tetanus vaccination are all key factors in treating corneal abrasions. Follow-up care appointments with providers are also vital so that assessment of progress and verification of visual acuity may be obtained. Collaborative care with specific eye care professionals is essential for large or complicated abrasions.

Connection Check 46.3

The nurse is developing a teaching plan for the patient with a corneal abrasion and includes which information? *(Select all that apply.)*

A. Hand-washing techniques
B. Steroid eye drops
C. Antibiotic eye drops
D. Comfort measures
E. Anesthetic eye drops

CATARACTS

Cataracts are a common phenomenon that can occur at any time in a person's life but are most commonly seen with advanced age. A cataract is clouding of the eye's crystalline lens. The lens works to focus light onto the retina at the back of the eye, allowing for clear vision both up close and far away. The clouding of this structure decreases vision and leaves patients at risk for injury (Fig. 46.4).

Epidemiology

Cataracts affect nearly 22 million Americans aged 40 and older. By age 80, more than half of all Americans have cataracts, and they are slightly more likely to affect women than men.

Risk factors for cataracts include:

- *Exposure to UV light:* Risk may be higher for those who have had significant sun exposure at a young age. People working in outdoor capacities where sunlight exposure is frequent and intense for long periods of time, such as lifeguards, landscape workers, and sports players, are commonly seen to be at increased risk.
- *Advanced age:* Cataracts are most common after age 60 but can occur at any time.

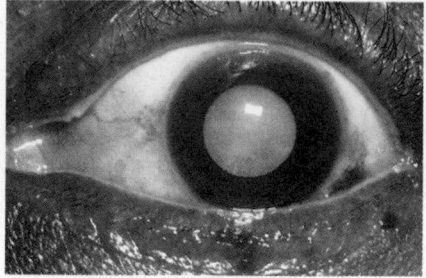

FIGURE 46.4 Cataract.

- *Family history:* Tends to follow family genetic history; those with family members who had cataracts are therefore more likely to develop them at some point in their life.
- *Race and ethnicity:* African Americans have twice the risk of Caucasians. Hispanic Americans are also noted to have a higher risk than Caucasians.
- *Diabetes mellitus and other chronic medical conditions:* Patients with diabetes, both type 1 and type 2, are at a higher risk for developing cataracts and are more likely to develop them at a younger age. It is thought that these cataracts are due to elevated blood glucose levels. Patients with autoimmune diseases are also thought to have a higher risk of developing cataracts because of their chronic steroid use. Patients with certain eye conditions, such as myopia, or patients with previous eye injuries or surgeries are also considered to be at higher risk for cataract development.
- *Obesity:* Being obese may predispose an individual to the development of cataracts.
- *Elevated blood pressure:* High blood pressure may also increase a patient's risk for developing a cataract.
- *Smoking and alcohol use:* Smoking a pack of cigarettes a day may double the risk of developing cataracts.
- *Environmental factors:* Long-term lead exposure is known to cause an increased risk for cataract development similar to an increased exposure to sunlight.

Pathophysiology

The lens is the clear part of the eye that focuses light on the retina for precise, accurate vision. In the normal eye, the light passes through the crystal-clear lens to the retina. The clarity of the lens is necessary for the retina to receive a sharp image. The lens is composed of mostly water and proteins. The specific proteins within the lens produce a chemical reaction to maintain the clarity of the lens. Alteration in the lens proteins occurs over the years as a person ages, yielding a gradual clouding of the lens secondary to the chemical change. Other factors resulting in cataract formation include direct blunt trauma to the eye and glaucoma from diabetes mellitus.

Clinical Manifestations

Clinical manifestations of cataracts include clouded, blurred, or dim vision; increasing night vision difficulty; sensitivity to light and glare; halo vision around light sources; fading or yellowing of colors; and double vision in a single eye. The manifestations change and become more dramatic as the cataract grows larger and distorts more of the patient's vision.

Management

Medical Management

The diagnosis of cataracts is generally completed on physical examination of the patient and includes a visual acuity test and direct ophthalmoscope examination with a slit lamp to observe the eye closely. Opaqueness is often readily seen by the provider during an examination. The most effective treatment of cataracts is surgical removal of the opaque lens. If surgery is not an option for the patient, regular follow-up with the provider is recommended so that progression of the condition may be followed and changes to eyeglass/contact lens prescription may be made as needed to maximize visual acuity.

Surgical Management

One of the most common types of eye surgeries performed in the United States for people over age 65 is for cataract removal. This surgery involves the removal of the clouded lens and its replacement with a plastic lens implant. If a patient is unable to have a replacement lens implanted, then once the cataract is removed, vision correction is achieved with corrective eyeglasses or contact lenses. Surgery is usually done on one eye and scheduled for the other eye, if needed, several weeks later. The procedure is usually done under a local anesthetic in an outpatient setting. Cataract removal also increases the risk of **retinal detachment** (separation of the retina from underlying layer of blood vessels that provide oxygen and nutrition to the eye). Cataract surgery improves vision in up to 95% of patients and prevents blindness.

Surgical Procedures

The two most common surgeries for cataract removal are **phacoemulsification** and extracapsular or intracapsular cataract extraction. The most common procedure in the United States is phacoemulsification (Fig. 46.5).

The procedure is as follows:

1. A local anesthetic is introduced directly into the eye.
2. An incision is then made directly into the eye near the lens by the surgeon.
3. A thin probe is inserted directly into the eye that transmits ultrasound to break up the clouded lens into small fragments.
4. Debris from the procedure is then aspirated out with a suction device.
5. The replacement lens is inserted where the natural lens previously resided.

6. Most incisions are small and seal simultaneously postoperatively and do not require sutures.

The second most common surgical repair for cataracts is the extracapsular or intracapsular procedure (Fig. 46.6). This procedure is generally used in patients with an extremely hard lens and involves:

1. The surgeon makes a small incision under microscopic visualization directly into the eye.
2. The surgeon extracts the clouded lens through the incision.
3. The capsule is left in place to add strength to the structure of the eye and to enhance the healing process.
4. The surgeon then adds a replacement lens, and the incision is sutured closed.

Nursing Management
Assessment and Analysis

Because cataracts affect vision, the clinical presentation of the patient includes specific alterations in the ability to see (Table 46.9). A comprehensive assessment is important to follow the progress of interventions.

Nursing Diagnoses
- **Disturbed visual sensory perception** secondary to opacity of the eye lens
- **Risk for injury** due to clouding of visual fields
- **Anxiety** related to inability to clearly see objects in visual fields

Nursing Interventions
Assessments
- Visual acuity
  Visual acuity test and slit-lamp evaluation are the most common assessments used to diagnose cataracts.
- Diagnostic results
  Visual acuity abnormalities are noted to be present because of increased opacity of the lens. Slit-lamp evaluation provides the provider with direct visualization of the lens and more specific detail about the extent of the opacity present.

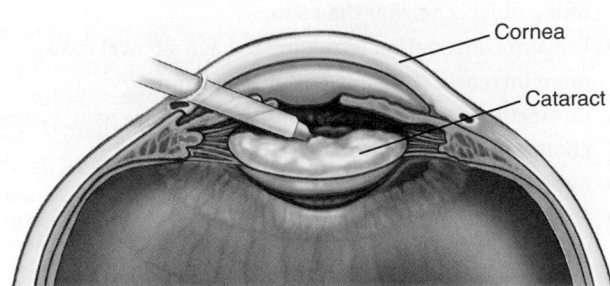

FIGURE 46.5 Phacoemulsification procedure. An incision is made near the lens, and a thin probe is placed that uses ultrasound to break up clouded fragments, which are aspirated out. A replacement lens is then placed.

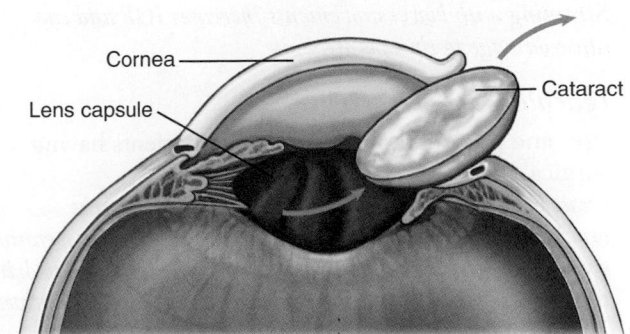

FIGURE 46.6 Extracapsular cataract extraction. A small incision is made, the clouded lens is removed, a replacement lens is placed, and the incision is sutured.

Table 46.9 Assessment and Analysis of Cataracts

Assessment Data	Analysis/Explanation
Visual acuity	Decrease in visual acuity is noted when performing this test secondary to the clouding of the lens distorting the amount of light being able to enter the eye and therefore not allowing an accurate image to form on the retina.
Blurred vision	Clouding of the lens distorts the amount of light that is able to be projected on the retina and causes visual blurring.
Increased difficulty with night vision	Night vision is especially affected because a decreased amount of light is already a factor at night, and with increased clouding of the lens, light entering the eye is further decreased.
Double vision in a single eye	Clouding of the lens may also cause visual distortions to appear, yielding double vision in some cases.

- Age-related considerations
  Yearly eye examinations for patients over age 45 to moni-tor/treat any abnormalities discovered. Changes in the eye lens occur with advancing age, which increases the risk of opacity or cataract formation.

■ **Actions**

- Implement safety measures
  Awareness of loss of vision so that proper safety measures can be implemented. Driving and other activities that require keen eyesight need to be evaluated to prevent possible risk to patient safety.
- Administer eye drops.
  Mydriatic (dilating) and cycloplegic (paralyze ciliary muscles to keep the eye dilated) eye drops are often prescribed in preparation for surgery.
- Elevate the head of the bed 30 to 45 degrees postoperatively.
  Promotes drainage and prevents any increase in IOP
- Position patient on back or nonoperative side.
  Promotes drainage and decreases IOP
- Maintain eye patch as prescribed by the provider.
  The eye patch offers protection, minimizes eye movement, and decreases discomfort.
- Administer stool softeners, as prescribed; increase fiber and fluid intake.
  Straining with bowel movements increases IOP and can cause damage to the operative site.

■ **Teaching**

- Pre- and postoperative teaching for patients having surgical intervention
  Exact preoperative instructions to be obtained from the provider, including NPO status, administration of preoperative eye drops, arrangements for a friend or family member to drive the patient home postprocedure, position changes postoperatively
- Decrease risk factors.
  Protective eyeglasses worn in the presence of sunlight decrease UV ray damage, a known factor in promoting cataract formation.

- Safety concerns
  Talk with the patient and family members regarding current visual impairment and ability to drive. Cataracts decrease visual acuity, creating a safety risk. Discuss safety around the home on stairs and when using kitchen equip-ment and other objects that could cause injury with impaired vision.
- Follow-up appointments
  Discussion with patient regarding importance of follow-up appointments with provider so that condition may be closely monitored for changes
- Accessibility to community agencies
  Referral to local community agencies that can help patients with rides, information, and other services when visual impairment is present (i.e., Prevent Blindness America, EyeCare America)

 Safety Alert **Postoperative (24–48 Hours) Teaching for Patients Having Cataract Surgery**

During the first 24 to 48 hours following cataract surgery, patients should take the following precautions:

- Do not rub or apply pressure to eye.
- Avoid sneezing, coughing, bending over, vomiting, or lifting objects heavier than 5 lb.
- Prevent constipation (straining to have a bowel move-ment increases IOP and can cause bleeding).
- Contact the physician immediately for severe pain, visual change, or increase in eye discharge.
- Avoid eye straining.
- Follow provider's instructions for eye dressing and use of eye shield at bedtime.
- Wipe excess tearing from inner to outer canthus with a clean soft tissue.
- Glasses must be worn if lens implant not inserted by the surgeon.

Evaluating Care Outcomes

Patients with cataracts can lead a normal life. Surgical removal of the cloudy lens in conjunction with prescription eyeglasses can vastly improve preoperative vision. Cloudy vision and inability to see objects clearly pose a great safety risk to patients who are often advanced in age. Detailed postoperative instructions are essential for optimal recovery from this surgery. Continued follow-up with eye care professionals is paramount for any patient suffering from this condition regardless if surgery is performed.

Connection Check 46.4

The nurse suspects a cataract in a 68-year-old Caucasian male patient with lupus based on which information?
A. The patient's history of angina and gender
B. The patient's use of high-dose steroids to treat the lupus
C. The patient's race status and history of high blood pressure
D. The patient's history of long-term exposure to zinc and obesity

GLAUCOMA

Glaucoma is not just a single eye disease but a group of eye conditions that present with increased IOP and result in damage to the optic nerve, leading to loss of vision. High IOP, greater than 21 mm Hg, is most often the culprit. Increased IOP can be the result of inadequate draining of aqueous humor from the canal of Schlemm, or it can be caused by an overproduction of aqueous humor. Early diagnosis is a key factor in minimizing or preventing visual loss.

Epidemiology

Anyone can develop glaucoma, and according to the World Health Organization, it is noted as a leading cause of blindness in the world. According to the National Eye Institute (NEI) at the National Institutes of Health (NIH), it is estimated that as many as 2.2 million Americans have been diagnosed with glaucoma, and approximately another 2 million people have the disease without knowing it.

There are many risk factors known to place patients at increased risk for glaucoma, and it is important to identify those with the highest chance for developing this disease.

Risk factors that increase the chance of developing glaucoma include:

- African American individuals over age 40
- People with a family history of glaucoma
- Everyone over age 60, especially Mexican Americans
- Medical conditions such as diabetes and hypothyroidism
- Patients with myopia
- Prolonged corticosteroid use

Risk factors specific to normal-tension glaucoma include:

- People with family history of this type of glaucoma
- Persons of Japanese ancestry
- Persons with heart disease such as irregular heart rhythm
- More common in women than men

Pathophysiology

Glaucoma causes damage to the optic nerve, resulting in loss of vision and blindness in severe cases. There are five major types of glaucoma: primary open-angle glaucoma, angle-closure glaucoma, normal-tension glaucoma, secondary glaucoma, and pediatric glaucoma.

Primary open-angle glaucoma is the most common form of the disease, affecting approximately 3 million Americans. Most patients have no symptoms or early warning signs. Angle-closure glaucoma is also known as acute glaucoma or narrow-angle glaucoma. In this relatively rare form of glaucoma, the eye pressure rises very quickly.

The clinical manifestations of angle-closure glaucoma include headaches, eye pain, nausea, rainbows around lights at night, and very blurred vision. This form of glaucoma is a medical emergency and requires prompt medical intervention. Eye drops are usually instilled immediately to try to reduce the rising IOP.

Normal-tension glaucoma is also known as low-tension glaucoma or normal-pressure glaucoma. Patients with this type of glaucoma have damage to the optic nerve even though the IOP is not very high. It is not understood why some patients suffer optic nerve damage with IOPs in the "normal" range of 12 to 22 mm Hg, but it is believed to occur either because of a fragile optic nerve (a condition that might be inherited) or a decrease in blood flow to the optic nerve itself (vascular disease including vasospasm and ischemia).

Secondary glaucoma usually results from an eye injury, inflammation, tumor or advanced cases of cataracts, or diabetes. Medications such as steroids, when used chronically, are also noted to cause this type of glaucoma.

Pediatric glaucoma consists of congenital glaucoma (diagnosed during the first year of life), infantile glaucoma (occurring in the first 3 years of life), and juvenile glaucoma (occurring at age 3 through the young adult years). Left untreated, glaucoma continues to progress in a predictable manner. Initially, blind spots occur in the patient's peripheral vision, leading to tunnel vision that may deteriorate to total blindness.

Connection Check 46.5

A 76-year-old patient was recently diagnosed with primary open-angle glaucoma. What part of the past medical history places the patient at risk for developing glaucoma?
A. History of a recent facial trauma
B. Prolonged antibiotic therapy
C. Prolonged corticosteroid usage
D. History of angina

Clinical Manifestations

Clinical manifestations vary by type of glaucoma. In primary open-angle glaucoma, clinical manifestations include gradual loss of peripheral vision, usually in both eyes, and tunnel vision in advanced stages. Acute-angle glaucoma is characterized by severe eye pain, nausea and vomiting, sudden onset of visual disturbance (often in low light), blurred vision, halo vision, and reddening of the eye. Normal-tension glaucoma (also referred to as low-tension glaucoma) is a condition where optic nerve damage and vision loss occur despite having a normal IOP between 12 and 22 mm Hg.

Management

Medical Management

The best prevention for glaucoma is regularly scheduled eye examinations by a qualified provider. (Frequency depends on age, state of health, and presence of known eye pathology.) Medical treatments for glaucoma include medications (early stages) that cause the eye to make less aqueous humor, as well as medications to help drain fluid in the eye, thereby decreasing the pressure in the eye. Commonly used eye-drop medications are included in Table 46.10.

Oral medications may also be prescribed, such as a carbonic anhydrase inhibitor, to help further reduce IOP. These medications work by reducing the production of aqueous humor, leading to a decrease in IOP.

Surgical Management

Surgery is used to treat glaucoma if medications are not effective in treating the disease. The surgeries most commonly used to treat glaucoma include laser trabeculoplasty, filtering surgery, or placements of drainage implants.

Laser trabeculoplasty is used in treating open-angle glaucoma. The patient is given an anesthetic eye drop, and a high-energy laser beam is used to open clogged drainage canals, thereby allowing the aqueous humor to drain more easily from the eye. This procedure is usually performed in the provider's office or eye clinic, and only one eye is treated at a time if both eyes are involved (Fig. 46.7).

Filtering surgery or trabeculectomy is usually done in a hospital or outpatient surgery center under local sedation. The surgeon uses specialized instruments and places an opening in the sclera of the patient, removing a small piece of the trabecular meshwork. This opening allows for the aqueous humor to freely exit the eye and lowers the IOP (Fig. 46.8).

Drainage implants, used most commonly with secondary glaucoma or pediatric glaucoma, commonly take place in a hospital or outpatient clinic. The surgeon inserts a small silicone tube in the eye to help drain the aqueous humor (Fig. 46.9).

Connection Check 46.6

The medical management of glaucoma includes which interventions? *(Select all that apply.)*

A. Beta-blocker eye drops
B. Steroid eye drops
C. Strict bedrest
D. Routine appointments with healthcare provider
E. Antibiotic eye drops

Genetic Connections

Glaucoma

Heredity plays a key role in the development of glaucoma, and genetic factors are believed to account for between 13% and 25% of cases of primary open-angle glaucoma in adults. There are both autosomal-dominant and recessive patterns noted.

Table 46.10 Medications Used in the Treatment of Glaucoma

Type of Compound	Common Medication Names	Desired Effect
Prostaglandin-type medications	Latanoprost (Xalatan), bimatoprost (Lumigan)	Increases the outflow of aqueous humor and thus decreases volume, therefore decreasing intraocular pressures
Beta-blocker medications	Timolol (Betimol, Timoptic), betaxolol (Betoptic), and metipranolol (OptiPranolol)	Reduces the production of aqueous humor, therefore decreasing intraocular pressure
Alpha antagonists	Apraclonidine (Iopidine) and brimonidine (Alphagan)	Reduces the production of aqueous humor and increases drainage
Carbonic anhydrase inhibitors	Dorzolamide (Trusopt) and brinzolamide (Azopt)	Decreases the production of aqueous humor
Miotic or cholinergic agents	Pilocarpine (Isopto Carpine) and carbachol (Isopto Carbachol)	Increases the outflow of aqueous humor
Epinephrine compounds	Dipivefrin (Propine)	Increases the outflow of aqueous humor

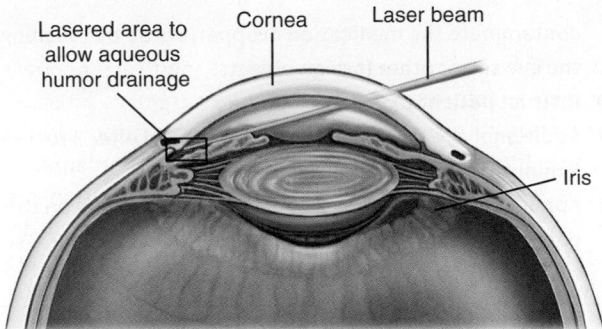

FIGURE 46.7 Laser trabeculoplasty. A high-energy laser beam is used to open clogged drainage canals, allowing the aqueous humor to drain more easily from the eye.

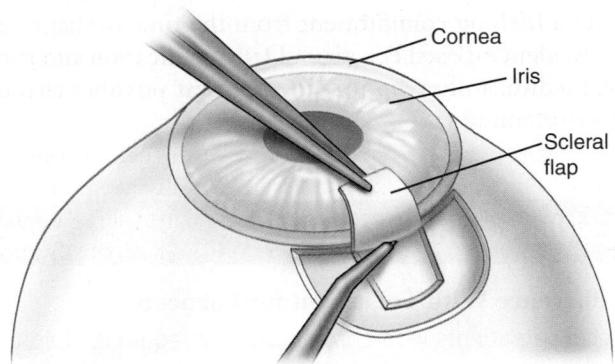

FIGURE 46.8 Filtering surgery or trabeculectomy. The surgeon uses specialized instruments and places an opening in the sclera of the patient, removing a small piece of the trabecular meshwork to allow for the aqueous humor to freely exit the eye.

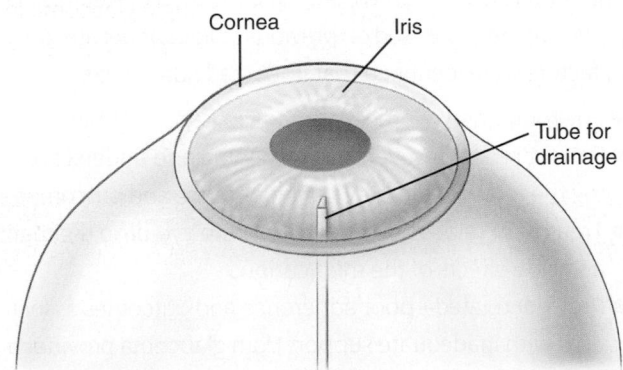

FIGURE 46.9 Drainage implants. The surgeon inserts a small silicone tube in the eye to help drain the aqueous humor.

Nursing Management

Assessment and Analysis

Clinical manifestations of glaucoma are closely related to the damage and complications associated with increased IOP (Table 46.11). Common complaints include decreased visual acuity, nausea and vomiting, and headache. Other clinical manifestations include eye pain and multicolored halos around lights.

Table 46.11 Assessment and Analysis of Glaucoma

Assessment Data	Analysis/Explanation
Vision loss	Can be sudden or gradual and may not be noted until vision loss is more pronounced. Vision loss is associated with pressure on the optic nerve caused by increased IOP, thereby preventing transfer of nerve signals to the brain.
Nausea/vomiting	Increased pressure building in the eye often causes nausea/vomiting in patients.
Headache	Abrupt increase in IOP often causes eye pain, which can be severe.

IOP, Intraocular pressure.

Nursing Diagnoses

- **Disturbed visual sensory perception** related to disturbance in optic nerve function secondary to increased intraocular pressure
- **Anxiety** related to decreasing visual field presence
- **Knowledge deficit** regarding the progressive nature of glaucoma
- **Impaired home maintenance** related to activity restrictions and impaired vision

Nursing Interventions

Assessments

- Physical assessment via ophthalmoscope and use of a tonometer
  Physical examination of patients with glaucoma demonstrates increased ocular pressures in most patients that are verified with a tonometer. Bulging vessels in the internal eye can also be seen on examination with an ophthalmoscope.
- Diagnostic results
  Intraocular pressures registering above the expected 10 to 22 mm Hg are a common finding. Visual acuity tests yield decreases in visual acuity.
- Visual acuity
  Visual acuity tests yield decreases in visual acuity. The patient may describe fogginess of vision.
- Age-related considerations
  Proper screening and routine visual examinations of patients of advanced age can help in the early detection of glaucoma before significant damage is done.

Actions

- Administer medications to decrease IOP.
  Medications are ordered to decrease the production of or increase the outflow of aqueous humor. Table 46.10 describes the actions of and rationales for medications used in the treatment of glaucoma.
- Follow proper procedure for the instillation of eye drops.
  Maintaining aseptic technique is important to proper eye-drop instillation. (The Safety Alert provides a guide for eye-drop instillation.)

- Elevate the head of the bed 35 to 40 degrees.
  Promotes intraocular (aqueous humor) drainage and decreases IOP
- Avoid bending at the waist for the first 48 hours postoperatively.
  Bending at waist may increase IOP.
- Administer stool softeners, and include fluid and fiber intake.
  Constipation or straining to have a bowel movement can increase intraocular pressure.

■ *Teaching*

- Progressive nature of disease process
  Education of patients and family members/significant others regarding the disease process is essential. Education regarding signs/symptoms or when to notify the provider and the importance of follow-up care on a routine basis is essential.
- Medication instructions
  Instructions on the name and type of eye drops are essential for successful treatment and compliance. Provide simple, understandable explanations to prevent the patient from feeling overwhelmed. Instruct the patient not to take any over-the-counter or prescription medications without contacting the eye care provider first (i.e., anticholinergic medications can cause worsening of glaucoma by constricting the drainage of aqueous humor). Due to the frequency of eye-drop administration, a chart of times, eye, and number of drops/dose may be helpful to the patient and family.
- Specific postoperative instructions
  Specific instructions from the patient's eye care provider must be followed precisely. Common instructions that are given include restrictions on strenuous activities, bending at the waist, and lifting of heavy objects (greater than 25 lb) and avoiding constipation for at least the first 2 weeks postoperatively. Lifting heavy objects, bending at the waist, and strenuous activities can increase IOP and cause damage to the newly repaired eye. Constipation or straining to have a bowel movement can increase the chance of postoperative bleeding within the eye. Reporting increased pain or drainage is also an important instruction for postoperative patients.

⚠ Safety Alert Eye-Drop Instillation

When instilling eye drops, the following precautions should be taken:

- Wash hands thoroughly and don nonsterile gloves.
- Verify correct medication/time and number of drops.
- Instruct patient to tilt head back with eyes open and looking upward.
- Retract lower lid downward.
- Invert the medication bottle and gently rest wrist on patient's cheek.
- Gently squeeze bottle and instill prescribed number of eye drops into conjunctival sac, taking care not to contaminate the medication dropper/bottle by touching the eye sac or other foreign objects.
- Instruct patient to gently close eyes.
- Additional eye drops may be administered after 3 to 5 minutes to allow for absorption.
- Application of gentle pressure with a clean tissue on the patient's nasolacrimal duct for 30 to 60 seconds decreases systemic absorption.

Evaluating Care Outcomes

Given the sometimes-insidious disease process of glaucoma, routine examinations and careful, comprehensive patient education are essential to minimize eye damage and promote eye health. The treatment of glaucoma requires a lifelong commitment from the time of diagnosis (see Evidence-Based Practice). Daily medication and routine medical follow-up provide the best possible chance for maintaining vision.

Evidence-Based Practice

Adherence With Treatment for Glaucoma

Because patients with chronic disease requiring lifelong treatment, like glaucoma, may have issues with adherence, this study focused on an evidence-based approach to addressing patient adherence to treatment for glaucoma. The three specific aims included evaluation of risk factors for poor adherence, assessment of whether improved adherence impacted outcomes, and identification of steps to improve adherence. Based on previous studies, four categories of factors were identified that impacted adherence:

- Environmental related—primarily cost of treatments
- Patient related—severity of glaucoma and understanding the relationship between adherence and outcomes
- Treatment related—complexity of the eye-drop regimen and side effects of the medications
- Provider related—poor adherence and outcomes associated with inadequate support from glaucoma provider

The Cochrane review completed included 16 trials that evaluated interventions with adherence. The primary outcome in the review was adherence with prescribed medical management, and secondary outcomes included intraocular pressure (IOP) reduction related to treatment, visual field loss, and quality of life.

The findings of the review revealed that no specific strategy or intervention led to increased compliance. Further studies are needed to evaluate approaches to facilitate better adherence with prescribed medical treatments.

There is also a growing body of research related to other strategies for managing glaucoma, including smartphone technology, minimally invasive surgical interventions (whose outcomes could be compared with more traditional medical management), and different approaches to intraocular medication delivery.

Joseph, A., & Pasquale, L. R. (2017). Attributes associated with adherence to glaucoma medical therapy and its effects on glaucoma outcomes: An evidence-based review and potential strategies to improve adherence. *Seminars in Ophthalmology, 32*(1), 86–90.

CASE STUDY: EPISODE 2

At the appointment with the advanced practice registered nurse, Mike discusses his history, which includes being diagnosed with type 1 diabetes mellitus at age 16. He has no other known chronic illnesses, and his blood glucose is considered in "good control." Mike is diligent about checking his blood glucose before all meals and before bedtime. He does not take any medication on a daily basis other than his insulin injections. Mike does not wear corrective eye lenses except when he is reading. Mike's father died at age 52 of heart failure and complications from diabetes. His mother is 86 years old and without any significant past medical history…

MACULAR DEGENERATION

Macular degeneration is most commonly age related and is a disease that gradually destroys sharp, central vision. Affecting the **macula** (the part of the eye that is responsible for central vision and allows for vision in fine detail), it causes no pain. Macular degeneration is slow to develop in some patients, often causing the patient to be unaware of any changes in vision. In others, it develops at a much faster pace. Patients who have advanced macular degeneration in one eye are at high risk for developing the same condition in the other eye.

Epidemiology

The greatest risk factor for macular degeneration is related to advancing age. According to the study by the NEI at the NIH, middle-aged people have about a 2% risk of developing macular degeneration, but the risk increases to nearly 30% in those patients over age 75. There are also modifiable and nonmodifiable risk factors for this disorder.

Modifiable risk factors include:

- High blood pressure
- High cholesterol
- Obesity
- Smoking
- Decrease in zinc blood levels

Nonmodifiable risk factors include:

- Age (patients over age 60 are at greatest risk)
- Family history of macular degeneration
- Gender (women are more likely than men)
- Race (more common in Caucasians)

Pathophysiology

The macula is a structure in the eye that is located in the center of the retina. The retina converts light and images instantly into electrical impulses and then sends these impulses or nerve signals to the brain via the optic nerve. There are two primary types of macular degeneration: dry macular degeneration and wet macular degeneration (Table 46.12).

Dry Macular Degeneration

Dry macular degeneration, the most common form of macular degeneration, occurs when the light-sensitive cells in the macula slowly start to break down. The dry form of macular degeneration can turn into wet macular degeneration. All people who have wet macular degeneration initially had dry macular degeneration. One of the most common early indications of dry macular degeneration is **drusen bodies**, which are yellow deposits that are located under the retina and are usually found in people over age 60 (Fig. 46.10). Eye examinations that include a comprehensive dilation evaluation usually detect drusen bodies.

There are three phases of dry macular degeneration: early dry macular degeneration, intermediate dry macular degeneration, and advanced dry macular degeneration. In

Table 46.12 Comparison of Wet and Dry Macular Degeneration	
Wet Macular Degeneration	**Dry Macular Degeneration**
• One stage only, which is the most advanced form	• Three stages—early, intermediate, and advanced
• Vision loss in wet macular degeneration	• Vision loss in advanced-stage dry macular degeneration
• All patients with wet macular degeneration had dry macular degeneration first.	• Dry macular degeneration can progress to the wet form even during early-stage dry macular degeneration (no way to tell if or when the dry form of macular degeneration will progress to the wet form of the disease).

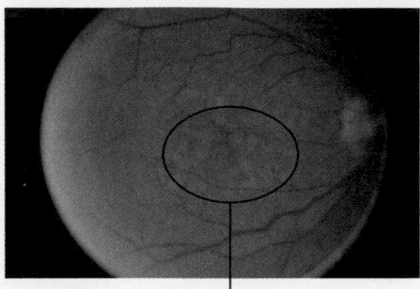

FIGURE 46.10 Dry macular degeneration. One of the most common early indications of dry macular degeneration is drusen bodies, which are yellow deposits that are located under the retina.

early dry macular degeneration, patients present with a few small to medium-sized drusen bodies. There are no other clinical manifestations, and no vision loss occurs. Patients with intermediate dry macular degeneration present with medium-sized drusen bodies, or one or more large drusen bodies are present on examination. Some patients see a blurred spot in the center of their visual field. The patient may require more light for reading and other tasks. Patients with advanced dry macular degeneration have a breakdown of the light-sensitive cells and supporting tissue in the central retinal area. The presence of drusen bodies is also noted on examination. The breakdown can cause a blurred spot in the center of vision that will gradually get bigger and darker, taking up much of the central vision.

Wet Macular Degeneration

Wet macular degeneration occurs when abnormal blood vessels located behind the retina start to grow under the macula (Fig. 46.11). These new networks of blood vessels are known to be very fragile and often leak blood and fluid. The blood and fluid raise the macula from its usual position at the back of the eye, and damage to the macula occurs rapidly.

Clinical Manifestations

Clinical manifestations of macular degeneration include straight lines that appear distorted; absent or distorted central vision; dark, blurry areas or whiteout on center vision;

and diminished or changed color perception. The clinical presentation of macular degeneration is also related to the specific underlying pathophysiology. Dry macular degeneration causes a gradual blurring of the central vision, and the patient may have difficulty recognizing faces. As the condition worsens, a blurred spot may be seen in the center of the visual field; this leads to gradual loss of central vision in the affected eye. Wet macular degeneration usually causes a quick loss of central vision and is also known as advanced macular degeneration. One of the earliest symptoms of this disease is that straight lines begin to appear wavy.

Connection Check 46.7

The nurse recognizes which finding as a complication of macular degeneration?
A. Complete color blindness
B. Disturbance in peripheral vision
C. Blindness
D. Nausea and vomiting

Management

Diagnosis

Changes in central vision (straight-ahead vision), along with advanced age, may raise suspicion with the patient's healthcare provider that the patient has macular degeneration. To assess for possible signs of macular degeneration, the provider completes a comprehensive eye examination, including dilation of the pupils for a better assessment of the back portion of the eye. **Tonometry** examination may also be done to measure the pressure inside the eye. The examination often also includes the use of an **Amsler grid**. This examination is done by asking the patient to look at a grid that resembles a checkerboard (Fig. 46.12). The patient covers one eye and stares at a black dot in the center of the grid. While staring at the dot, patients with macular degeneration may notice that the straight lines appear wavy or

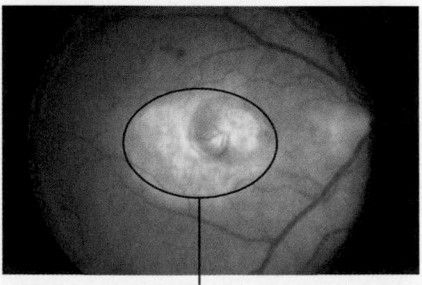

Blood and fluid leakage raises macula

FIGURE 46.11 Wet macular degeneration. Wet macular degeneration occurs when abnormal blood vessels located behind the retina start to grow under the macula and leak blood and fluid that raise the macula from its usual position at the back of the eye.

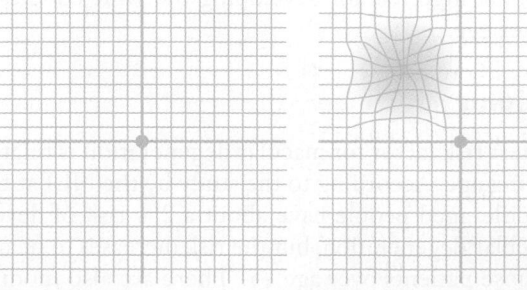

A Normal   **B** Macular degeneration

FIGURE 46.12 Amsler grid. A, Viewed with normal vision. B, Viewed with macular degeneration. The patient covers one eye and stares at a black dot in the center of the grid. While staring at the dot, patients with macular degeneration may notice that the straight lines appear wavy or may interpret that some of the lines are missing.

may interpret that some of the lines are missing. A fluorescein angiogram may also be performed for confirmation of wet macular degeneration. This test requires that a special dye is injected intravenously, and images are taken as the dye passes through the vessels within the retina, identifying leaking blood vessels.

Medical Management

The three most common treatments for macular degeneration are laser surgery, photodynamic therapy, and injections directly into the eye. There is no cure for macular degeneration, and despite treatment, the disease and vision loss may continue to progress.

Dry Macular Degeneration

Once dry macular degeneration reaches the advanced stage, no form of treatment can prevent vision loss. The NEI's Age Related Eye Disease (ARED) study has found that having patients take a specific high-dose formulation of antioxidant and zinc significantly reduces the risk of vision loss. Nutritional recommendations are made when treating a patient with macular degeneration. Recent research provides some foundation that using an ARED formula (vitamin C, vitamin E, beta-carotene, zinc, and copper) can slow the progression of intermediate macular degeneration to the advanced stage. Lutein and zeaxanthin supplements may also produce protective effects.

Wet Macular Degeneration

Two therapies are used for wet macular degeneration.

Photodynamic Therapy

This is a specialized laser treatment for macular degeneration that uses the stimulation/activation of a photosensitive dye by exposure to a light (laser) of a known wavelength that results in the closure of new vessels. The treatment takes about 20 minutes to complete and can be performed in the provider's office. This therapy slows the rate of vision loss, but it does not stop vision loss or restore vision that has already been lost by macular degeneration. The treatment results are often temporary and may require the patient to undergo successive treatments.

Photodynamic therapy uses a medication called verteporfin (Visudyne), a light-activated medication, which is injected directly into the patient's arm. In the presence of oxygen, highly reactive short-lived reactive oxygen radicals are generated. Light activation of this medication results in local damage to the endothelium and therefore results in vessel occlusion. The medication travels through the body and eventually to the blood vessels in the patient's eye and sticks to the surface of new blood vessels. A light is then shined into the patient's eye for about 90 seconds to activate the medication. The activated medication then destroys the new blood vessels, therefore slowing the rate of vision decline. It is important to instruct the patient to avoid exposing skin/eyes to direct sunlight or bright indoor light for 5 days after treatment because the medication is activated by light.

Anti–Vascular Endothelial Growth Factor Therapy

Vascular endothelial growth factor (VEGF) is secreted by oxygen-deprived cells, causing stimulation of the growth of abnormal blood vessels. Anti-VEGF therapy uses injections directly into the eye and is used to treat wet macular degeneration. This medication blocks the effects of the growth factor. The patient will need multiple injections that may be given monthly and that usually involve local anesthesia to the eye. This medication helps slow the progression of vision loss from macular degeneration and in some cases even improves sight.

Surgical Management

Laser surgery uses a light beam to destroy the fragile, leaky blood vessels that are accumulating behind the macula. This high-energy beam of light aimed directly at the new blood vessels destroys them, therefore preventing further loss of vision. Only a small percentage of patients with wet macular degeneration can be treated with this surgery, and there is also concern that laser treatment may destroy healthy tissue as well as impact visual acuity. Surgery is most often performed in the provider's office or eye clinic, and the risk of developing new blood vessels after laser treatment is high. Vision loss may progress despite repeated treatment in some patients.

Nursing Management
Assessment and Analysis

Due to the chances of progressive decrease in visual acuity, assessment for macular degeneration is important. The clinical manifestations of macular degeneration are insidious and result in the loss of sharp, central vision. Table 46.13 describes these changes.

Nursing Diagnoses

- **Disturbed visual sensory perception** related to degeneration of the macula
- **Anxiety** related to loss of vision
- **Risk** for injury related to visual loss

Table 46.13 Assessment and Analysis of Macular Degeneration

Assessment Data	Rationales
Loss of sharp, central vision	Abnormal blood vessels located behind the retina start to grow under the macula. These new networks of blood vessels are usually fragile and often leak blood or fluid, resulting in a loss of sharp, central vision.
Insidious onset	Dry macular degeneration is most common with this onset. Light-sensitive cells slowly begin to break down, causing a gradual blurring; can progress to the more aggressive wet form of macular degeneration.

Nursing Interventions

■ *Assessments*

- Vital signs
  There is no direct effect on vital signs, although a risk factor for the development of macular degeneration is elevated blood pressure.
- Physical assessment/examination
  On physical examination with an ophthalmoscope, yellow spots (drusen bodies) form on the retina. The presence of abnormal vessel leaking is also sometimes seen on ophthalmoscopic examination.
- Visual acuity
  Visual changes develop as abnormal blood vessels located behind the retina start to grow under the macula. These new networks of blood vessels are usually fragile and often leak blood or fluid, resulting in a loss of sharp, central vision. The onset may be insidious.

■ *Actions*

- Safety precautions
  Maintain a safe environment related to increased risk of physical injury secondary to impaired vision
- Provider follow-up
  Routine scheduled follow-up appointments with provider to evaluate for any changes in visual acuity or the presence of other internal changes

■ *Teaching*

- Education regarding diagnosis
  Provide detailed and understandable information regarding patient diagnosis so that patients are able to participate in care and meet expectations for treatment.
- Community resource referrals
  Referral to community services as patient circumstances dictate to help ensure that patient has access to care (i.e., Macular Disease Society, Prevent Blindness America)

Evaluating Care Outcomes

Macular degeneration has no complete cure; the goal of therapy is the preservation of vision. Clinical manifestations of macular degeneration start with a decline in visual acuity along with blurring or distortion of vision. Some of the manifestations may be slow to develop and therefore not initially obvious to the patient. Medical and surgical treatments are available depending on the specific condition.

RETINAL DETACHMENT

Retinal detachment (Fig. 46.13) is a condition that may cause permanent vision loss and is considered a medical emergency, requiring the patient to seek immediate attention by an eye care professional. The retina is a structure within the eye that is light sensitive and sends visual messages to the brain via the optic nerve. Detachment of this structure can happen as it is lifted or pulled from its normal position. Clinical manifestations of retinal detachment experienced by patients may be sudden or gradual. Patients may notice

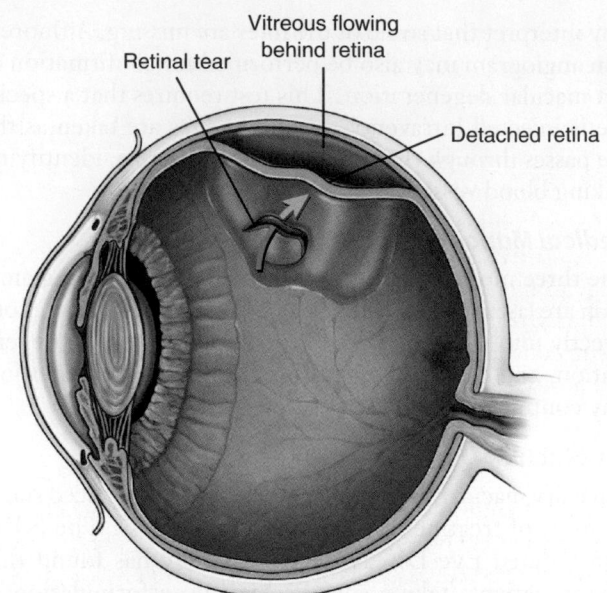

FIGURE 46.13 Retinal detachment. Retinal detachment occurs when there is a separation of the inner layers of the retina from the underlying retinal pigment epithelium.

a sudden or gradual increase in the number of floaters in the visual field, or they may experience light flashes or the appearance of a curtain over the field of vision.

Epidemiology

In the United States, it is estimated that the incidence of retinal detachment is one in 15,000 people. The disease is noted to be more common in patients over age 40 and affects men more often than women and Caucasians more often than African Americans.

Risk factors for retinal detachment include the following:

- Patients who suffer from extreme myopic refraction disturbances
- History of retinal detachment in the other eye
- Family history of retinal detachment
- Patients who have had cataract surgery
- Patients who have suffered eye injuries
- Patients with other eye diseases or disorders
- Presence of systemic diseases such as diabetes mellitus, tumors, sickle cell disease, leukemia, eclampsia, and prematurity

Pathophysiology

Retinal detachment occurs when there is a separation of the inner layers of the retina from the underlying retinal pigment epithelium (choroid). The choroid is known as a vascular membrane containing large branched pigment cells located between the retina and the sclera. Separation of the retina from the retinal pigment epithelium occurs by the following three basic mechanisms:

1. *Rhegmatogenous:* This is the most common form of retinal detachment and occurs when a tear or break in

the retina allows vitreous fluid to move under the retina and separate it from the pigmented cell layer that nourishes the retina.

2. *Tractional:* The least common type of detachment, this condition occurs when scar tissue on the retina's surface contracts and causes the retina to separate from the retinal pigment epithelium.

3. *Exudative:* This form of detachment is usually caused by retinal disease, including inflammatory disorders and injury/trauma to the eye. With this type of detachment, vitreous fluid leaks into the area underneath the retina, but no tears or breaks in the retina are identified.

Clinical Manifestations

Clinical manifestations of retinal detachment experienced by patients may be sudden or gradual. Patients may notice a sudden or gradual increase in the number of floaters in the visual field, or they may experience light flashes or the appearance of a curtain over the field of vision. Patients may describe a painless change in visual acuity or describe their vision as "looking through a veil or cobwebs."

Management

Medical and Surgical Management

Immediate evaluation followed by surgical intervention is noted to be the only effective treatment for retinal detachment. The goal of many treatments is to stop any further progression of vision loss. In most cases, the damage that has already occurred cannot be reversed. The most common and successful treatments are discussed here.

Laser photocoagulation is most often used to repair a retinal tear or hole, and this procedure is usually done as an outpatient and does not require incisions. To perform this procedure, the surgeon directs a laser beam to burn small pinpoint holes on the peripheral retinal surface. The burns create scar tissue that causes the retina to adhere to the underlying tissue (Fig. 46.14).

Panretinal photocoagulation is used for advanced cases of diabetic retinopathy to shrink abnormal new blood vessels that are bleeding into the vitreous. In this procedure, the surgeon places multiple laser burns on the retina, excluding the macula. Two or more sessions are usually required. An advantage of this procedure is that the burns cause new blood vessels to shrink and disappear, thereby preserving central vision. The drawback of this procedure is that it includes some peripheral vision loss.

Cryopexy is an outpatient procedure that is done with local anesthetic and is used to treat tears along the retinal periphery that are difficult to reach with a laser. The surgeon uses intense cold to freeze the area around the tear. The freezing produces inflammation that leads to scarring. The scarring holds the retina in place to the underlying tissue, thereby preventing fluid from passing through the tear.

Pneumatic retinopexy, a treatment for uncomplicated retinal detachment when the tear is located on the upper

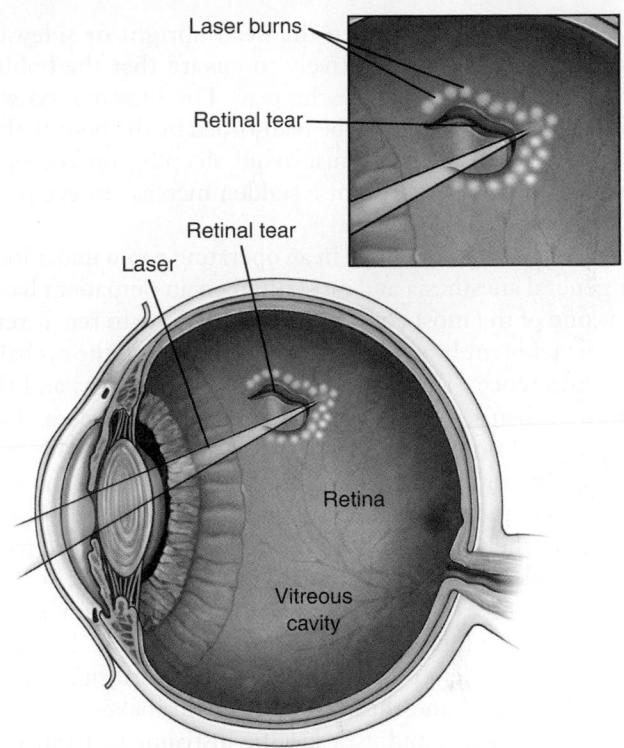

FIGURE 46.14 Laser photocoagulation. A laser beam is used to burn small pinpoint holes on the peripheral retinal surface. The burns create scar tissue that causes the retina to adhere to the underlying tissue.

half of the retina, is an outpatient procedure that is performed under local anesthesia. The surgeon first performs cryopexy around the tear to seal it off. A bubble of gas is then injected into the vitreous cavity; this bubble expands over the next few days, sealing the retinal tear, and evokes a reattachment of the retina to the wall of the eye (Fig. 46.15). Patient positioning is important postop for this procedure.

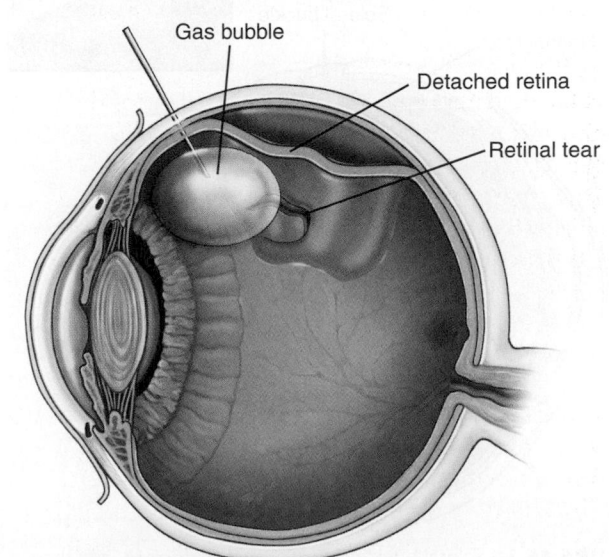

FIGURE 46.15 Pneumatic retinopexy. A cryopexy is performed to seal the tear, and then a bubble of gas is injected into the vitreous cavity. This bubble expands over the next few days, sealing the retinal tear and reattaching the retina to the wall of the eye.

The patient needs to keep the head upright or sideways for a few days postoperatively to ensure that the bubble continues to press against the tear. The injected gas will dissipate from the eye and be reabsorbed by the body within 2 to 8 weeks. Patients must avoid sleeping on the back during this time to prevent a sudden increase in eye pressure or cataract formation.

Scleral buckling is done in an operating room under local or general anesthesia and most often on an outpatient basis. It is one of the most common surgeries done to repair retinal detachment by slightly reducing the size of the eyeball's circumference. The surgery starts with cryopexy, and the surgeon then sews a tiny synthetic band to the sclera. This buckle creation indents the sclera and pushes the wall against the retina. The indentation helps decrease the separation between the retina and underlying layers while also reducing the circumference of the eyeball. Pressure from the "buckle" helps prevent further separation (Fig. 46.16).

Vitrectomy is used to correct retinal detachment as well as to remove a foreign body or repair eye trauma. It is generally an outpatient procedure that may be performed under local or general anesthesia. The surgeon makes tiny incisions in the sclera and uses specific instruments to suction out blood-filled vitreous. A saltwater solution is injected into the eye to help maintain its shape (Fig. 46.17). This surgery is selected for cases where bleeding or inflammation clouds the vitreous and obstructs the surgeon's view of the retina. This procedure is often done in conjunction with

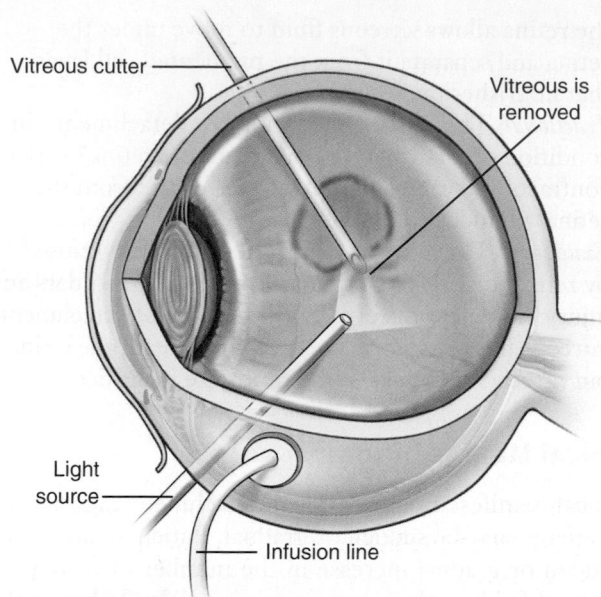

FIGURE 46.17 Vitrectomy. A tiny incision is made in the sclera, and a specific instrument is used to suction out blood-filled vitreous. A saltwater solution is injected into the eye to help maintain the shape of the eye.

other procedures, such as laser photocoagulation, scleral buckle placement, or gas injection.

Nursing Management

Assessment and Analysis

Patients presenting with retinal detachment typically complain of "floaters" in the eye, accompanied by flashing lights. Table 46.14 presents an explanation of these clinical manifestations.

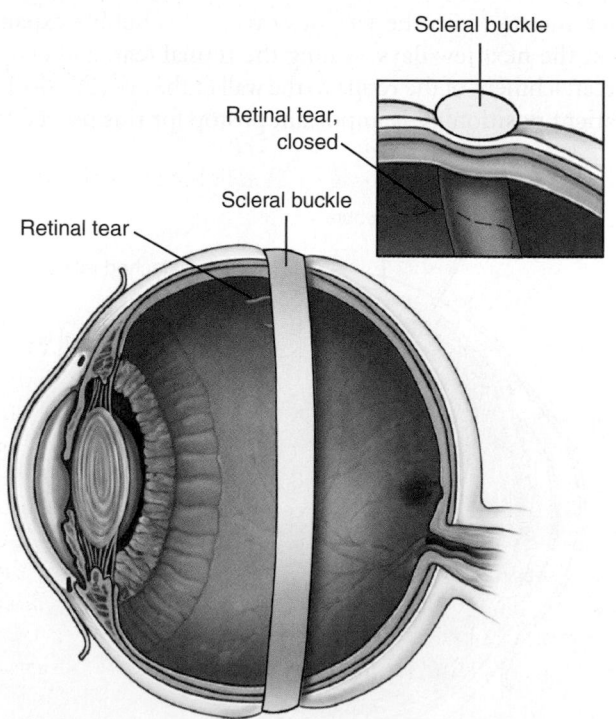

FIGURE 46.16 Scleral buckling. Cryopexy is performed, and then the surgeon sews a tiny synthetic band to the sclera. This buckle creation indents the sclera and pushes the wall against the retina. The indentation helps decrease the separation between the retina and underlying layers while also reducing the circumference of the eyeball.

Table 46.14 Assessment and Analysis of Retinal Detachment

Assessment Data	Analysis/Explanation
"Floaters" present in the visual field (as noted by patient verbal report)	Naturally occurring with advancing age as little bits of debris or tiny specks of tissue appear in visual fields. With retinal detachment, large floaters appear that cause an obstruction of vision.
Light flashes reported by patients	Flashing lights represent the release of an electrical signal from the nerve tissue to the retina, where there is a pulling on the retina from the vitreous gel that separates it from the retina.
Curtain covering visual field as described by the patient	As detachment progresses, visual loss increases to represent what looks like a curtain covering the visual field.

Nursing Diagnoses
- **Disturbed visual sensory perception** secondary to retinal detachment
- **Risk for injury** related to decrease in visual acuity

Nursing Interventions
Assessments
- Visual changes

  Patients may notice a sudden or gradual increase in the number of floaters in the visual field, or they may experience light flashes or the appearance of a curtain over the field of vision.
- Eye assessment changes

  An eye examination is completed by a provider with the use of an ophthalmoscope to view the internal retina of the eye. Abnormal results require further evaluation by an eye care professional who specializes in the treatment of retinal dysfunction.
- Diagnostic results

  The ophthalmoscope examination shows detachment; a dye test also shows the exact locations of the detachment.

Actions
- Assist with healthcare provider examination.

  A complete eye assessment is required to prevent further damage related to potential increased IOP.
- Encourage rest and calm environment.

  The patient should remain in a resting state until a medical evaluation is done to prevent further damage to the eye.
- Loosely cover both eyes.

  Movement of either eye can exacerbate internal eye injury. Because the eyes move together, both eyes must be covered to minimize injury.
- Postoperative positioning

  The patient needs to assume the position ordered by the physician. For example, after pneumatic retinopexy, the patient needs to keep the head upright or sideways for a few days postoperatively to ensure that the bubble of gas, injected into the vitreous cavity during the procedure, continues to press against the tear. The injected gas will dissipate from the eye and be reabsorbed by the body within 2 to 8 weeks. Patients must avoid sleeping on the back during this time to prevent a sudden increase in eye pressure or cataract formation.
- Administer stool softeners and increase intake of fluid and fiber.

  An increase in IOP may develop secondary to straining with bowel movements that can exacerbate the retinal detachment or interfere with reattachment.

Teaching
- Preoperative instructions

  After evaluation, the patient should be given detailed instructions on the type of intervention that is to be done. Patient preoperative teaching is important for patient safety as well as the first step to understanding postoperative instructions. Instructions are usually also given to a family member or friend to decrease the chance of misunderstanding.
- Postoperative instructions

  Postoperative instructions may differ slightly for each provider, but most include eye-patch care (when to leave on/off; how to change); instillation of eye-drop medications (including type of medication, schedule, and how to instill); monitoring for hemorrhage; notifying provider immediately for increased pain or drainage from the eye; prevention of vomiting, sneezing, sudden movement, lifting, or constipation because these may increase IOP and cause detachment to worsen; and no bending over at the waist to prevent an increase in IOP. Most providers also suggest dark glasses (sunglasses) in the presence of bright light to prevent further retinal damage.

Evaluating Care Outcomes

Retinal detachment is a known phenomenon that occurs more readily in females over age 40. Clinical manifestations are gradual or spontaneous and require immediate evaluation by an eye care specialist to minimize permanent visual loss. Treatment often includes surgical intervention directed at preventing further damage to the retina. Strict postoperative instructions provided by the provider must be followed for the best results.

Connection Check 46.8

In providing education about retinal detachment to a newly diagnosed patient, what is the most important information for the nurse to give the patient?

A. This condition is a separation of the retina from the epithelium.

B. Partial detachment does not progress to complete detachment.

C. Retinal detachments are easily treated.

D. Complete detachment yields peripheral visual loss.

EYE TRAUMA

Significant causes of visual loss are related to blunt and penetrating trauma (Table 46.15). Blunt trauma, the more common of the two, occurs when the eye is struck with a finger, fist, racket, tennis ball, or other solid object. These injuries produce damage to the internal eye secondary to the sudden compression and/or indentation of the globe on impact. Penetrating trauma refers to injuries in which the eye is pierced by a sharp object such as a knife or a high-velocity missile such as a piece of metal or a BB pellet. Clinical manifestations of eye trauma are readily visible most of the time but may not be immediately observable on occasion.

Epidemiology

Eye trauma affects people of all ages and races. It is estimated that annually, 2.4 million individuals in the United States experience an eye injury requiring treatment in an emergency

Table 46.15 Common Causes of Trauma to the Eye	
Blunt Trauma to the Eye	**Penetrating Trauma to the Eye**
• Motor vehicle accidents • Assault • Assault with a weapon • Falls	• Assault where there is penetration of the eye with a sharp object • Industrial accidents causing impalement by an object • Any activity or sport where an object can penetrate the eye

department, inpatient/outpatient facility, or healthcare provider's office. Persons under the age of 17 account for nearly 35% of these injuries, with the home being the most common setting.

The most common risk factors for eye trauma include:

• Male gender
• Participation in sports
• Occupation (agricultural, construction, and manufacturing)
• Age group 18 to 45
• Consumption of alcohol

Although this is not a comprehensive list of risk factors, it does address the five most common threats in relation to eye trauma.

Pathophysiology

Blunt trauma may yield an injury where bleeding occurs in the front of the eye between the clear cornea and colored iris. This condition is referred to as a **hyphema** (Fig. 46.18) and can vary in size from microscopic to the total involvement of the eye. Trauma of this nature can also cause damage to the lens, yielding cloudiness or displacement of the lens within the eye. Damage to the retina, causing detachments or tears, is also common with this type of injury.

The most common causes of **blunt eye trauma** include motor vehicle accidents, assaults with weapons, and falls. Periorbital contusion (commonly known as a *black eye*) is the most common injury; although such contusions are

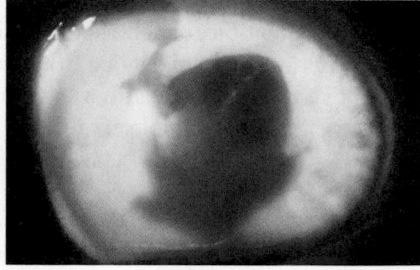

FIGURE 46.18 Hyphema. Bleeding occurs in the front of the eye between the clear cornea and colored iris.

usually benign, a full evaluation should be completed to rule out more serious injury.

Penetrating eye trauma, usually associated with a lack of protective eyewear, can occur at any time. Surface injuries involving the cornea or damage to the eye globe may occur. Corneal damage includes abrasions and lacerations as well as foreign bodies. Globe rupture is an ocular emergency that occurs from either blunt or penetrating trauma. Penetrating injuries to the globe are often caused by penetration with sharp objects.

Clinical Manifestations

The clinical presentation of eye trauma varies widely depending on the type of trauma and the extent of the injury (Table 46.16). Common manifestations of eye trauma include eye pain; edema around the eye; scleral discoloration (redness); changes in vision, including blurred, double, and loss of vision; and excessive tearing.

Management

Medical Management

Diagnosis and Treatment

Medical management of blunt trauma to the eye is possible with some injuries. Rest, eye patching, and special eye drops may be prescribed. Antibiotic eye drops are prescribed to treat or prevent infection, particularly with penetrating eye trauma, and eye drops that dilate may be indicated because dilation can force the inflamed iris to move and keep it from sticking to the underlying lens. Additionally, constriction of the pupil may help to decrease intraocular pressure. Follow-up with an eye care specialist is usually on a frequent basis because close observation of the injury is essential to monitor for proper healing. To prevent further damage, including hemorrhage, patients who present to the provider with a penetrating object in the eye should never have the object removed by anyone other than the eye care professional. Removal of objects without professional guidance can eliminate pressure to the wound and increase bleeding or promote an extrusion of eyeball contents. Computed tomography (CT) scans or x-rays are often done first to observe the extent of the impalement. Verification of tetanus immunization is also part of the medical management.

Surgical Management

Surgical management for eye trauma is dependent on the type of injury that has occurred. Evaluation of the patient by an eye care professional, CT scans, and x-rays to confirm or rule out injury are completed prior to any surgical procedure.

Nursing Management

Assessment and Analysis

The clinical manifestations observed in the patient with eye trauma are directly related to the type and extent of the injury. Table 46.17 includes common findings observed in patients with eye trauma.

Table 46.16 Types of Eye Trauma

Eye Trauma	Treatments
Orbital fracture	Surgical repair usually occurs about 7 days after injury to allow swelling to decrease (exception would be if vision is impaired; may need surgical intervention sooner). Surgical repair involves debridement of the wound and surgically repairing displaced bones, sometimes using mesh or implants to rebuild the orbital area.
Hyphema (blood in the anterior chamber of the eye occurring when blood vessels in the iris rupture and bleed into the clear aqueous fluid of the anterior chamber)	Strict bedrest, head of bed elevated 30–45 degrees, beta-blocker eye drops to control IOP, and mydriatic eye drops to increase patient comfort
Subconjunctival hemorrhage (caused usually by minor trauma, even something as trivial as sneezing or coughing really hard; evaluation by provider to rule out other diagnosis is necessary)	No treatment is needed for this condition; it usually resolves within 2–3 weeks.
Periorbital wounds	Close assessment of these wounds is necessary because it may provide a clue as to other injuries present; elevation of the head and ice/cold packs help decrease swelling.
Globe rupture (results from blunt or penetrating eye injury and results in damage to the sclera of the eye; pain is usually severe, and nausea may be present)	A computed tomography scan is usually done to verify extent/type of injury present; pain medication and antiemetic medications are administered. Prepare for surgery, including making patient NPO. Eye drops should never be administered with a ruptured globe.

IOP, Intraocular pressure; *NPO,* nothing by mouth.

Table 46.17 Assessment and Analysis of Eye Trauma

Assessment Data	Analysis/Explanation
Visual loss	Presence of visual loss occurs in traumatic cases of globe rupture because of a disturbance or loss of vision as the optic nerve is no longer able to receive and transport nerve signals.
Pain	The presence of pain following a traumatic episode indicates an injury to the eye is present. The degree of pain and location of pain depend on the pathology present.
Nausea/Vomiting	Cases involving increased IOP may yield nausea and vomiting in patients secondary to the rise in pressure.

IOP, Intraocular pressure.

Nursing Diagnoses

- **Disturbed visual sensory perception** related to injury to eye structures secondary to trauma
- **Pain** related to traumatic injury to the eye
- **Risk for infection** related to eye injury

Nursing Interventions

Assessments

- Vital signs
  Intraocular pressure may be elevated with certain injuries; pain may cause some elevations in blood pressure, pulse, and respiration.
- Physical changes
  Specific physical changes are seen depending on the injury present and may include bleeding, tearing, swelling, and pain.

- Diagnostic results
  X-ray, CT scan, and magnetic resonance imaging (MRI) scans may be ordered for specific patients to clarify the extent of the injury.
- Age-related considerations include all ages.
  No specific age is immune from eye injury, although it is known to be somewhat more prevalent in the age group of 18 to 25.

Actions

- Cover eyes/stabilize penetrating object.
  Preventing excessive movement of the eye, particularly with an embedded object in the eye, is important to prevent additional injury. Loosely covering both eyes decreases eye movement. Objects penetrating the eye should only be removed by an eye care professional.

- Comfort measures
  Patient may require pain medication to help alleviate the intense pain that is often present in eye trauma patients.
- Positioning
  Specific positioning depends on the type of injury but often requires an elevation of the head of the bed to 30 to 45 degrees to decrease the patient's IOP.
- Maintain a calm, quiet environment.
  Minimizing environmental stimuli promotes rests and minimizes eye movements that can exacerbate the injury and/or increase pain.
- Collaborative care
  Referral to an eye care specialist should be made for any traumatic injury to the eye. The eye care professional may need to perform surgery immediately or follow up with the patient with regular examinations.

▪ Teaching

- Eye care follow-up
  Patient should be instructed on compliance with all follow-up eye examinations. Regular follow-up examinations provide the patient with the best chance for retaining sight.
- Specific instructions
  Patients should understand all postprocedure/postoperative/postmedical treatment for an eye injury. Patient positioning, eye-patch care, medications, and activity restrictions are all paramount in the recovery from eye injuries (all injuries have specific instructions based on the pathology present).

Evaluating Care Outcomes

Traumatic eye injuries vary greatly in their type and degree of injury. Clinical manifestations commonly seen with eye trauma include eye pain, visual disturbances, and visible injury present on presentation. Prompt medical diagnosis with an eye care professional is the key to maintaining visual acuity. Eye injuries take many shapes and forms, and therefore, so do the instructions for care. It is essential that patients receive detailed, easy-to-understand instructions for follow-up in order to have a chance of maintaining vision.

Connection Check 46.9

A patient arrives in the emergency department with a metal object protruding from the eye. What is the priority action for this patient?

A. Remove the metal object right away to prevent any further damage.

B. Apply a tight eye patch to prevent hemorrhage.

C. Assess visual acuity.

D. Instill 1% tetracaine eye drops for pain relief.

Making Connections

CASE STUDY: WRAP-UP

During the appointment, Mike discusses his visual concerns of "missing" objects in his peripheral vision. Immediately, the provider has concerns about a possible eye disease. Mike's age, race, diabetes mellitus (for 50 years), and symptoms make the provider consider glaucoma. Upon ophthalmic examination, the provider is able to identify several bulging blood vessels in the posterior portion of Mike's eye that are concerning. The general provider does not have a tonometer, so intraocular pressure (IOP) may not be evaluated at this time. As one final test, the provider completes a confrontation test with Mike and notes that Mike has several deficiencies in his peripheral field of vision. Mike is then referred to an eye care specialist for further evaluation and diagnosis.

Case Study Questions

1. The nurse correlates which assessment with the presence of bulging blood vessels within the posterior portion of the eye?
   A. Expected changes associated with advancing age
   B. Requires monitoring every 3 to 5 years by the provider
   C. Requires immediate surgical intervention
   D. Can indicate increased IOP

2. The nurse recognizes which patients as at greatest risk for glaucoma?
   A. Patients of Asian descent
   B. Patients with chronic neuromuscular diseases
   C. Patients with diabetes
   D. Patients who have recently undergone cardiac surgery

3. In providing discharge instructions to Mike, what is the rationale for follow-up with an eye care specialist?
   A. Measuring intraocular pressure
   B. Performing a pupillary assessment
   C. Obtaining a complete and accurate visual acuity
   D. Completing testing with an Amsler grid

4. The provider prescribes reading glasses for Mike to treat which disorder?
   A. Glaucoma
   B. Peripheral vision loss
   C. Presbyopia
   D. Increased IOP

5. The nurse expects the provider to prescribe which of the following to treat glaucoma?
   A. Strict bedrest
   B. Low-fat, low-sodium diet
   C. A tight patch to the affected eye
   D. Mydriatic eye drops

CHAPTER SUMMARY

The visual system in the human body is complex and tied to many intricate networks within the eye itself, as well as pathways leading to and within the brain. Changes in visual ability may be gradual or acute but should always involve assessment and evaluation by a healthcare provider. Risk factors and advancing age all play a role in visual dysfunction. Comprehensive knowledge of eye function and disease pathophysiology helps to plan for appropriate treatment and continued care. Thorough, understandable teaching practices by nurses and eye care providers can provide the critical link between visual acuity and visual disruption.

Visual acuity disorders are related to refraction errors and include myopia or nearsightedness, hyperopia or farsightedness, and astigmatism that results from a misshaped cornea. Another abnormality, presbyopia, occurs almost exclusively with aging and results from the loss of lens elasticity; it occurs around age 45. All of these disorders are typically treated with corrective lenses (glasses or contact lenses) or surgical procedures, including radial keratotomy, photorefractive keratectomy, laser-assisted in situ keratomileusis (LASIK), or laser thermal keratoplasty.

Conjunctivitis involves an inflammation of the conjunctivae of the eye and can be secondary to allergies, bacteria, viruses, chlamydia, contact-lens use, mechanical means, or trauma. Clinical manifestations typically include eye irritation, tearing, and discomfort. Treatment is directed to the cause (e.g., antibiotics for infectious conjunctivitis), comfort measures, and protection of vision.

One of the most common eye disorders is corneal abrasions, which are a leading cause of visits to healthcare providers. These abrasions involve a loss of integrity of the cornea, and the patient usually complains of eye pain, photophobia, tearing, spasm, and blurred vision. Management focuses on the administration of antibiotic eye drops and other eye medications to decrease muscle spasms of the eye. Pain and photophobia can be minimized by wearing dark sunglasses.

Cataracts involve a clouding of the eye's lens that decreases vision due to interference with light reaching the retina secondary to the cloudiness. Management focuses on improving vision and is best accomplished by surgical procedures, including phacoemulsification and extracapsular or intracapsular cataract extraction. Lenses that help to maintain the structure of the eye are implanted during the procedure.

Glaucoma is an eye disease that develops secondary to increases in intraocular pressure that results in damage to the optic nerve, leading to loss of vision. Because of either overproduction or inadequate drainage of aqueous humor, intraocular pressure (IOP) increases. Medical management of glaucoma focuses on medications that inhibit aqueous humor production or facilitate drainage through the canal of Schlemm. Surgical procedures to treat glaucoma focus on increasing drainage of aqueous humor, including laser trabeculoplasty, trabeculectomy, and drainage implants. Because of the risk of increased IOP, it is important to teach patients to avoid activities that can potentially increase IOP, including straining with bowel movements and bending at the waist.

Macular degeneration is commonly age related and gradually destroys sharp, central vision due to damage to the macula. Because the degeneration is painless, the onset and progression may be insidious and the diagnosis delayed. Clinical manifestations of macular degeneration include straight lines that appear distorted; absent or distorted central vision; dark, blurry areas or whiteout on center vision; and diminished or changed color perception. Treatment includes laser surgery, photodynamic therapy, and injections directly into the eye. There is no cure for macular degeneration, and despite treatment, the disease and vision loss may continue to progress.

Considered a medical emergency that may cause permanent vision loss, retinal detachment requires immediate attention by an eye care professional. Clinical manifestations may be sudden or gradual and typically include floaters in the visual field as well as light flashes or the appearance of a curtain over the field of vision. Surgical interventions are the only effective treatment, with the goal of stopping further progression of vision loss. Procedures include laser photocoagulation, panretinal photocoagulation, cryopexy, pneumatic retinopexy, scleral buckling, and vitrectomy.

Eye trauma is typically classified as blunt or penetrating injury, and clinical manifestations are associated with the type and severity of the injury. Blunt trauma is often related to motor vehicle accidents, assaults with weapons, or falls, whereas penetrating injuries are often associated with a lack of protective eyewear and sharp objects penetrating the eye. Management is focused on the prevention of further injury, particularly interventions to decrease intraocular pressure and infection.

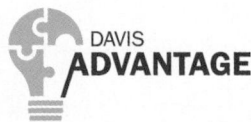

DAVIS ADVANTAGE

To explore learning resources for this chapter, go to **Davis Advantage** and find:
- Answers to in-text questions
- Chapter Resources and Activities
- NCLEX®-Style Chapter Review Questions
- Bibliography

Chapter 47

Assessment of Auditory Function

Kelley Miller Wilson

ESSENTIAL TERMS

Apocrine glands	Ossicles
Audiometry	Otoscope
Cerumen	Ototoxic
Conductive hearing loss	Presbycusis
Decibels	Pure tone audiometry
Electronystagmography	Sensorineural hearing loss
Frequency	Speech audiometry
Hertz	Tinnitus
Hyperacusis	Tympanometry
Mixed conductive-sensorineural hearing loss	Vertigo
Nystagmus	Vestibulocochlear nerve

CONCEPTS

- Assessment
- Comfort
- Medication
- Nursing Roles
- Promoting Health
- Safety
- Sensory Perception

Finding Connections

CASE STUDY: EPISODE 1

Follow this patient throughout the chapter.

Erin Hodge is a 22-year-old waitress who plans to see her provider this week for a physical examination. Erin has always enjoyed excellent health, though she did experience numerous ear infections as a child requiring surgical insertion of pressure-equalizing tubes (tiny tubes surgically inserted in the tympanic membrane to equalize pressure and prevent infectious buildup). Currently, Erin has no known chronic diseases and takes no medication on a daily basis. She has been noticing waxy buildup in her ear canal lately, which she has treated herself using a cotton swab to remove the wax. Erin has not noticed any hearing changes and plans to discuss the recent waxy buildup in her ears with her provider…

INTRODUCTION

The ear is an extraordinary sensory organ that works in conjunction with the brain to interpret sounds. These sounds allow assessment of surroundings, warning of potential dangers, interactions with other people, and appreciation of sounds such as music, work, and play. Many aspects of daily life are affected by the ability to hear. Assessment of the anatomy and physiology of the ear provides essential data about hearing and balance. The interpretation of screening assessments and diagnostic results is also pertinent to providing comprehensive care to patients with hearing disorders.

OVERVIEW OF ANATOMY AND PHYSIOLOGY

Anatomy

There are three parts of the ear that work together to allow hearing and processing of sound. Cranial nerve VIII (the **vestibulocochlear nerve** or acoustic nerve) is responsible for transmitting sound and equilibrium information from the inner ear to the brain. These parts are referred to as the external (outer) ear, the middle ear, and the inner ear (Fig. 47.1).

The external ear consists of the pinna, mastoid process, and external auditory canal, and the major function of this portion of the ear is to funnel sound waves. The middle ear includes the tympanic membrane (eardrum), the malleus, the incus, the stapes, and the eustachian tube. The middle ear has three functions that include conducting sound waves from the outer ear to the inner ear, protecting the inner ear from loud sounds, and equalizing pressure in the middle ear. The inner ear consists of the bony labyrinth, which holds the vestibule and semicircular canal. The cochlea is also housed here and contains the main hearing apparatus. Cranial nerve VIII contains the sensory cells (hair cells) of the inner ear and consists of the cochlear nerve, which carries information about hearing, and the vestibular nerve, which carries information about balance directly to the brain.

The following is a list of structures within the ear and a brief description of their main functions.

- *Pinnae* (also referred to as the *auricles*) are the most visible part of the ear, and their primary function is to collect sounds. Composed of cartilage covered by skin, the pinnae are present on both sides of the face and are embedded in the temporal bone bilaterally at the level of the eye.

- *External auditory canals* are structures 2.5 to 3.0 cm long in the adult that terminate at the eardrum. The canals are lined with glands that secrete **cerumen** (a yellow waxy material). The cerumen lubricates and protects the ear by forming a sticky barrier that helps prevent foreign bodies from reaching the tympanic membrane.

- *Mastoid processes* are parts of the skull that contain spongy bone located just behind the ear. The middle ear and the cochlea portion of the inner ear are embedded in the mastoid bone.

- *Tympanic membranes* (eardrums) are structures that separate the external ear from the middle ear. They are translucent membranes with a pearly gray color and are oval in shape.

- *Eustachian tubes* connect the middle ear with the nasopharynx, allowing for passage of air. These tubes are usually in a closed position but open with swallowing or yawning. Their function is to stabilize the air pressure between the external atmosphere and the middle ear. In children, this tube is flatter in appearance and gradually evolves in the adult to have a more slanted appearance, thereby making drainage more efficient and lessening the chance of infection.

- *Malleus* is the part of the middle ear that is in the shape of a hammer. The function of this structure is to transmit sound vibrations from the eardrum to the incus.

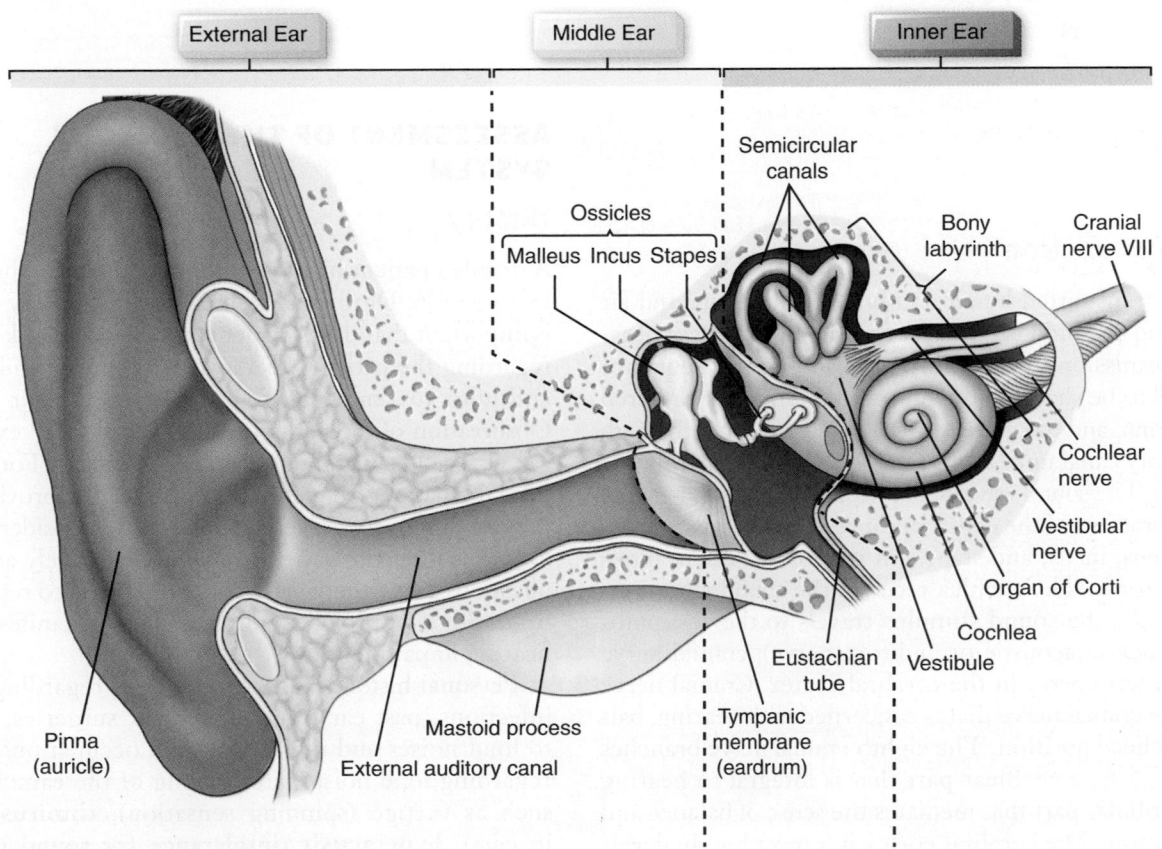

FIGURE 47.1 Anatomy of the ear.

- *Incudes* are the tiny bones that pass vibrations from the hammer to the cochlea.
- *Stapes* are the smallest bones in the human body; they are stirrup shaped and located in the middle ear and are important for transmission of sound to the inner ear.
- *Semicircular canals* are tubes composed of cartilage that contain both fluid and hair cells. The sense of equilibrium is maintained here.
- *Vestibules* are the small, oval-shaped bony chambers located between the semicircular canals and the cochlea. This area contains structures that are important for the sense of balance.
- *Cochlea* are the spiral-shaped, curled tubes located in the inner ear. While sound enters the cochlea, vibrations cause movement of the hairs within the structure, creating nerve signals from cranial nerve VIII that the brain then interprets as sound.
- *Organs of Corti* are located in the cochlea and are the receptors and organs of hearing. They contain hair cells, and while the hairs bend, they change vibrations into electrical impulses that are then carried by cranial nerve VIII to the brain.
- *Bony labyrinth* is the structure that holds the sensory organs for equilibrium and hearing.

Connection Check 47.1

The nurse correlates which anatomical structure as the location of the sensory organs for hearing and equilibrium?
A. Eustachian tube
B. Ossicles
C. Bony labyrinth
D. Tympanic membrane

Auditory Function

Sound is transmitted by air and bone conduction, and air conduction of sound is the most common pathway of hearing. Transmission by air follows the subsequent sequence for sound to be successfully interpreted. Sound is gathered by the pinna, and the waves enter the ear traveling through the auditory canal until they reach the tympanic membrane (eardrum). The sound waves set up vibrations in the eardrum. These vibrations of the eardrum cause the auditory **ossicles** (the malleus, incus, and stapes) in the middle ear to move back and forth. The cochlea receives the sound vibrations next. Finally, the sound stimulus travels to the vestibulo-cochlear nerve (acoustic or auditory nerve), cranial nerve VIII, and terminates in the cerebral cortex. Cranial nerve VIII is the cranial nerve that is concerned with hearing, balance, and head position. The eighth cranial nerve branches into two parts, a cochlear part that is integral to hearing and a vestibular part that mediates the sense of balance and head position. The cerebral cortex is a most highly developed part of the brain that is divided into right and left hemispheres. The temporal lobe of the cerebral cortex is involved with hearing and language.

Bone conduction transmission of sound occurs when the skull bones (commonly tested using the mastoid bone located behind the ear) transport vibrations directly to the inner ear and then to the auditory nerve. The skull transmits high frequencies with less intensity than air, and that is why a person's voice sounds different to them when recorded and played back.

The inner ear, with innervation from cranial nerve VIII, also controls equilibrium and balance. The labyrinth in this portion of the ear constantly provides information to the cerebral cortex of the brain about the body's position in space. It works like an imaginary line to determine verticality or depth. The ears register the angle of the head in relation to gravity. Inflammation of the labyrinth causes the wrong information to be sent to the brain, thus resulting in a staggering gait and a spinning, whirling sensation known as **vertigo**.

Connection Check 47.2

The nurse recognizes which actions as essential functions of the auditory system? *(Select all that apply.)*
A. Transfer of sound waves through the auditory canal
B. Vibration of the eardrum
C. Warming air while it enters the outer ear
D. Balance
E. Secretion of cerumen

ASSESSMENT OF THE AUDITORY SYSTEM

History

A detailed patient history is completed before the physical examination. During assessment of the auditory system, it is important that the provider carefully listen, ask questions regarding the patient's medical history and family history, and note any current medications the patient is taking. Observation of the patient's posture and facial expressions can also yield clues about hearing difficulties. For example, does the patient frequently lean toward the provider when questions are being asked? Other careful considerations include whether the patient is able to accurately answer the questions and if there are frequent requests to repeat questions. Box 47.1 provides common clinical manifestations of hearing impairment.

Personal history includes questions regarding past ear infections, past ear trauma, past ear surgeries, exposure to loud noises and music, possible occupational hazards regarding loud noises, and itching of the ears. Problems such as vertigo (spinning sensation), **tinnitus** (ringing in ears), **hyperacusis** (intolerance for sound levels not normally experienced by others), and difficulty hearing or

Box 47.1 Signs of Hearing Loss

- Frequently asking for instructions to be repeated
- Turning the head or leaning forward to gain clarity on the question being asked
- Loud conversation initiated by the patient
- Failing to respond when spoken to (especially when not looking in the direction of the sound)
- Answering questions incorrectly on a consistent basis
- Raising the volume of the television/radio on a consistent basis
- Avoiding large groups
- Withdrawing from social functions or interactions
- Clinical manifestations of depression

Box 47.2 Assessment of Hearing Function

1. Does anyone in your family have hearing problems? If so, at what age did the hearing difficulties start? Did it affect both ears?
2. Do you notice that it seems that people seem to mumble or speak in a softer voice more than previously?
3. Do you frequently need to ask people to repeat themselves during conversations?
4. Do you have difficulty understanding conversations in a crowded room?
5. Do you often need to increase the volume on electronic items such as televisions or radios?
6. Do you have difficulty hearing conversations on the telephone?
7. Do you sometimes miss the telephone ringing or doorbell ringing?
8. Do family/friends complain about your hearing?

understanding words are also addressed. In addition, history of current health, past illnesses (especially those requiring treatment with known **ototoxic** (causing damage to the ear or hearing) medications, smoking history (nicotine may cause damage to the sensory cells), allergies, and family history provide important information about the auditory system (see Genetic Connections). Questions to accurately and easily assess family history are included in Box 47.2.

Genetic Connections

Hearing Loss

Genetics may have a significant effect on hearing. More than 400 syndromes are linked to hearing loss, and often these disorders are diagnosed in childhood, although some genetic problems lead to progressive hearing loss in the adult years. Common examples of these disorders include the development of hearing loss in adulthood in patients with Down's syndrome. People with the genetic disorder osteogenesis imperfecta have bilateral and progressive hearing loss by their 30s. Other genetic hearing loss–associated syndromes are included in Table 47.1.

Personal Hygiene

The physical examination is an ideal time to assess how the patient cares for and cleans the ears. This is also an opportunity for the nurse to instruct the patient regarding the dangers of using cotton swabs or other foreign objects in the ear canal because inserting foreign objects can cause tissue injury to the sides of the canal, as well as causing cerumen to be moved. Movement of the cerumen by a foreign object places the patient at risk for cerumen impaction, causing changes in hearing, as well as rupture of the eardrum.

Patients who wear a hearing aid require additional assessment. Hearing aids function as an accessory to make sounds more audible; they do not correct hearing loss. The device is designed to amplify and modulate sound for the

Table 47.1 Genetic Causes of Hearing Dysfunction

Syndrome	Characteristics of Hearing Loss
Waardenburg syndrome	Unilateral or bilateral; sensorineural
Branchio-oto-renal (BOR) syndrome	Conductive, sensorineural, or mixed
Neurofibromatosis type 2	Progressive sensorineural loss leading to deafness in many cases
Stickler syndrome	Progressive hearing loss; most usually conductive, though it can be mixed sensorineural
Usher syndrome	Three types: Type I—Profound sensorineural hearing loss with vestibular dysfunction Type II—Progressive sensorineural loss Type III—Progressive sensorineural loss and variable vestibular dysfunction

patient and is specifically designed on the basis of the provider's interpretation of the patient's hearing evaluation/testing. Many different hearing aids are available, and some are designed to be placed in the ear canal itself and others are designed to be placed behind the ear. Wireless technology also has an impact on hearing and advancing hearing aid capability. It is important that the provider continue to assess whether the use of the hearing aid is actually improving the patient's hearing and note when the patient last had a hearing evaluation. Future follow-up plans at predicted intervals should also be discussed with the patient before leaving the provider's office.

Connection Check 47.3

When the nurse assesses a patient regarding the auditory system, which is the most important question to ask?

A. "Do you have any chronic illnesses that require you to take daily medication?"

B. "Have you ever been told that you are tone deaf?"

C. "Did you ever have a foreign body in your ear?"

D. "Do you notice that you have wax in your ears?"

Physical Inspection of the Ear

Before completing the physical examination of the ear, it is important to have the patient sit up straight with the head at the eye level of the provider. Full explanation of how the provider will assess the ear is given to the patient before beginning the examination. Assessment of the ear includes inspection, otoscopic examination, and evaluation of the vestibulocochlear nerve (cranial nerve VIII).

Inspection begins with palpation of the external ear. The provider notes the size and shape of the ears because they should be equal in size bilaterally without swelling or thickening. The color of the ears should be consistent with the facial skin tone of the patient. Inspection for lumps or lesions is also performed. The pinna should feel firm and should be freely moveable without causing any discomfort. Palpation of the mastoid process is also completed at this time, and there should be no swelling or complaint of pain present during the examination.

Examination With an Otoscope

The **otoscope** is used to examine the internal structures of the ear and consists of a light, handle, magnifying lens, and pneumatic bulb (often used with children) to test the movement of the tympanic membrane (Fig. 47.2). To complete the examination, the provider tilts the patient's head away from the examiner. The pinna is pulled up and back in the adult and older child, and the pinna is pulled down on an infant or child younger than 3 years. This important action helps straighten the ear canal and affords better visualization due to the flat anatomical position of the infant's eustachian tube. The pinna is held lightly but firmly, maintaining a steady grip until the examination is complete and the otoscope is removed from the ear canal. The provider holds the otoscope in an "upside-down" position and steadily places the speculum of the otoscope into the ear canal using the hand along the patient's cheek to steady the otoscope. The provider takes care to watch the insertion to ensure safe and easy introduction. On occasion, the provider is unable to see any structures, and a reattempt is made to reposition the otoscope. (If cerumen is present and creating an obstruction, it will need to be removed before a visual examination can be performed.) Once the otoscope is in place, the provider rotates it slowly to visualize the eardrum. The otoscopic examination is usually completed before any hearing tests are conducted.

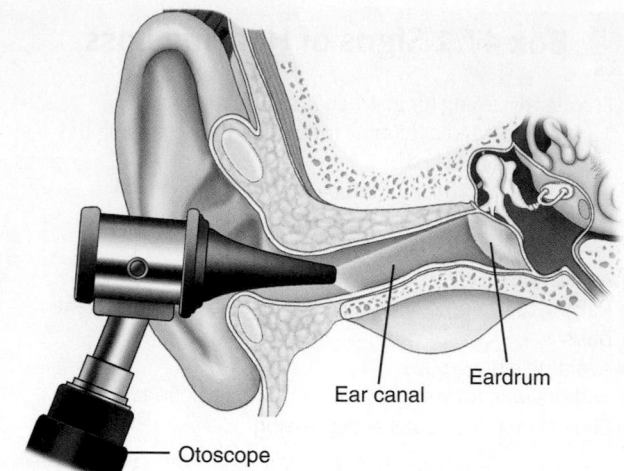

FIGURE 47.2 Otoscopic examination. The otoscope is used to examine the internal structures of the ear.

The otoscopic examination provides a wealth of information about the current status of the ear. Visualization of the external canal is completed while the otoscope is placed in the canal and advanced. Evaluation of the tympanic membrane includes noting the color (red, white, yellow, or gray), translucency (translucent or opaque), and position (retracted, neutral, or bulging) of the drum. Air inflation with a pneumatic otoscope is important to evaluate the mobility of the tympanic membrane. Mobility is assessed by applying positive and negative pressures with a rubber squeeze ball. Any redness, swelling, lesions, or discharge is also documented at the time of examination.

The visual examination of the tympanic membrane is then completed. This is done in a systematic manner. The normal eardrum is shiny, translucent, and pearl gray in color (Fig. 47.3). The cone-shaped light reflex that is elicited is prominent in the anteroinferior quadrant (5:00 in the right eardrum and 7:00 in the left eardrum). This light is the reflection of the otoscope light. The eardrum is flat, slightly pulled in the center, and flutters when the patient swallows or holds the nose. The eardrum is inspected around its entire circumference to ensure that the tympanic membrane is intact (Fig. 47.4). White dense patches may be present on the drum and indicate scarring from repeated ear infections or past ruptures.

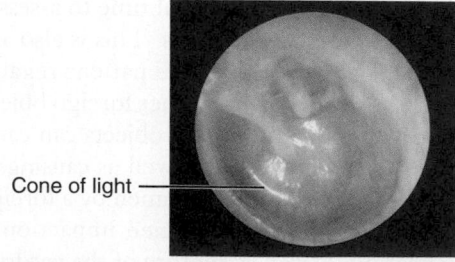

FIGURE 47.3 Normal eardrum on otoscopic examination (left ear). The normal eardrum is shiny, translucent, and pearl gray in color. The cone-shaped light reflex, which is the reflection of the otoscope light that is elicited is noted in the anteroinferior quadrant (7:00 in the left eardrum).

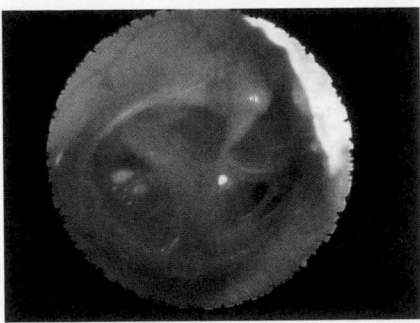

FIGURE 47.4 Perforated eardrum.

CASE STUDY: EPISODE 2

Erin Hodge provides a detailed health, family, and medication history to the nurse provider. Erin's physical examination and simple hearing assessments are all noted as "normal" by the advanced practice nurse and yield no concerns. To complete the examination, the nurse practitioner removes the earwax to increase visualization. Erin notices an immediate improvement in her hearing ability after the wax is removed…

AUDITORY ASSESSMENT

Auditory, or hearing, assessment is completed after the external and otoscopic examination of both ears has been completed. These simple but meaningful tests help identify deficiencies present; however, they cannot determine the extent of the deficiency. Hearing loss is categorized in three ways:

- **Conductive hearing loss** describes a physical obstruction of sound wave transmission.
- **Sensorineural hearing loss** describes a deficit present in the cochlea, cranial nerve VIII, or the brain.

- **Mixed conductive-sensorineural hearing loss** describes profound hearing loss that encompasses both conductive and sensorineural injuries.

Tests used to assess hearing function are detailed in Tables 47.2 and 47.3. Before any testing of a patient's auditory function, a detailed explanation and instructions are given by the provider. Instructions need to be specific to the type of test being conducted.

Diagnostic Studies

In addition to the detailed history and physical examination needed for a thorough evaluation of auditory function, there are also diagnostic studies used to assess hearing and determine underlying pathology.

Audiometry

Hearing acuity is measured through **audiometry**, and this test is most often performed by skilled technicians and nurses with specialized training. This test measures **frequency** (the highness or lowness of tones expressed in hertz; **hertz** is the international unit of frequency defined as the number of cycles per second of a sound). Low pitch is determined by fewer vibrations, and high pitch is determined by a greater number of vibrations. Sound intensity is noted in **decibels** (dB), and threshold is noted as the lowest level of intensity at which pure tones and speech are heard by a patient approximately 50% of the time. Normal conversation is heard at approximately 60 dB; whispers are 20 dB; and very loud, dangerous sounds are considered to be at approximately 110 dB. Documented injury can occur from sounds louder than 85 dB. Audiometric evaluations are often done in special facilities with sound laboratories to ensure that outside distracting noises do not interfere with the testing.

There are two types of audiometry: pure tone and speech. **Pure tone audiometry** generates tones with an audiometer that are presented to the patient at frequencies for hearing speech, music, and other common sounds. The

Table 47.2 **Hearing Tests**	
Test	**Procedure**
Voice test	Simple hearing acuity test performed on both ears at the same time. To perform, the provider stands 1–2 feet away from the patient and asks the patient to cover one ear. The provider whispers a short statement of four words or fewer into the patient's uncovered ear and asks the patient to repeat the words. If the patient is unable to respond or responds incorrectly, repeat the statement choosing new words and in a slightly louder whisper.
Watch test	This simple test is performed to assess high-frequency sounds and is performed with a ticking watch. The watch is held about 5 inches from each ear, and the provider verifies whether a patient is able to hear the ticking. The patient with normal high-frequency hearing is able to hear the watch tones.
Audioscopy	This procedure evaluates hearing ability with a handheld device to assess general tones. The test measures at 40-dB intensity and at frequencies of 500; 1,000; 2,000; and 4,000 cycles per second, or hertz. This test is done in a quiet setting with headphones in place and is most often seen as a screening device in schools or clinics.

Name of Test	How to Perform Test
Weber test	This test is used to distinguish between conductive (bone conduction) and sensorineural (air conductive) hearing loss. To perform this test, activate the tuning fork by holding the stem and striking the two tines with the back of the hand. Place the vibrating tuning fork in the midline of the patient's skull and ask whether the tone sounds the same in both ears or better in one.
Rinne test	This test compares air conduction and bone conduction. The tuning fork is activated as described above. When activated, place the stem of the vibrating tuning fork on the patient's mastoid process, and the patient is asked to indicate when the sound goes away. The tuning fork is then quickly inverted, with the tines located approximately 2 inches from the patient's ear; the patient should still be able to hear the vibrating sound if hearing is normal.

Table 47.3 Hearing Assessment

testing is done by air conduction and bone conduction and determines whether hearing loss is present and, if loss is noted to be present, whether the loss is conductive, sensorineural, or mixed. An increase in air conduction threshold with a normal bone conduction threshold indicates a conductive hearing loss. An elevated threshold for both air and bone conduction thresholds indicates a sensorineural hearing loss, and an increase of air conduction that is greater than an increase in the elevated threshold of bone indicates a mixed hearing loss. In **speech audiometry**, the patient's ability to hear spoken words is measured through a microphone connected to an audiometer. The two components of speech audiometry are the speech reception threshold and speech discrimination. The speech reception threshold determines the softest level at which the patient begins to recognize speech. Speech discrimination determines how well speech is heard and understood when the volume is set at the patient's most comfortable level of hearing.

Connection Check 47.4

Which is the most common examination used to assess a patient's auditory function?
A. Examination using the tuning fork
B. Assessment of all the cranial nerves
C. Examination using the otoscope
D. Evaluation of a written questionnaire

Tympanometry

Tympanometry is completed in healthcare providers' offices and clinics and is performed by technicians, nurses, or other specially trained personnel. Patient preparation centers on educating the patient as to how and why the test will be completed. The equipment used is sensitive and requires delicate handling and usually has single-use earpieces that require disposal and replacement. Tympanometry is performed to assess the mobility of the eardrum and structures of the middle ear because these changes are consistent with presence of fluid in the middle ear. Changes in air pressure are systematically introduced into the external auditory canal at a predictable rate. This test is helpful in distinguishing middle ear pathologic conditions such as otosclerosis, ossicular disarticulation, otitis media, and perforation of the eardrum. Earpieces are placed in the patient's ear before the start of the test, and the machine is able to determine the degree of progression or resolution of serous otitis media.

Electronystagmography

The **electronystagmography** (ENG) test is done to detect both central and peripheral diseases of the vestibular system (the system in the inner ear that is responsible for maintaining balance and orientation in space) in the ear. The ENG detects and records **nystagmus** (involuntary eye movements), because the eyes and ears depend on each other for balance. To perform this test, electrodes are taped to the skin near the eyes, and one or more of the following procedures is completed to stimulate nystagmus. These procedures include caloric testing, changing gaze position, or changing head position. Changing gaze/position is an oculomotor (cranial nerve III) evaluation. This stimulus is initially accomplished with manually controlled objects such as dots placed on walls or ceilings at specific places. Changing head position is a test that is conducted with a rotating drum with stripes and color contrasts as well as a swinging pendulum or metronome. Caloric testing is performed by taking warm or cooler than body temperature water and instilling it directly into the ear. The expected response in a normal patient when any of these procedures are performed is onset of vertigo and nystagmus within 20 to 30 seconds. Movement of the eye is also noted; the eye shows movement toward the water if the water is warm and away from the water if it is cold in caloric testing.

Preparation for this test includes a detailed explanation of the purpose and procedure to the patient. The following teaching points are provided to the patient before the test is performed:

• The patient is to refrain from ingestion of caffeine for at least 24 hours before the test. Caffeine causes stimulation of the central nervous system that can possibly influence testing results.

- The patient is to be NPO for at least 3 hours before the test. Patients may experience nausea and vomiting with this test, and NPO status may help to decrease this sensation.
- Patients with pacemakers should not have this test because pacemaker signals interfere with the sensitivity of this test.
- Patients who normally wear eyeglasses are instructed to bring them to the test. Eyeglasses assist the patient in vision during the testing.
- Patients are informed that reintroduction of fluids after this test is to be gradual to prevent the occurrence of nausea and vomiting.
- Patients might want to consider having a family member drive them home from the test because sometimes nausea, vomiting, or vertigo can continue after testing.

Computed Tomography and Magnetic Resonance Imaging

Detailed visualization of the internal structures of the ear is achieved by either computed tomography (CT) or with magnetic resonance imagining (MRI). A CT scan is noninvasive and completed with or without contrast. Contrast may be ordered because it can improve visibility of internal structures, especially those that may be difficult to see. This test is extremely helpful in diagnosing acoustic tumors, often known as acoustic neuromas.

The MRI is also used for its superior contrast resolution, allowing for very detailed imaging. Patient explanation and teaching by the nurse or the provider are important before this test. Many institutions and healthcare providers also require that a consent be signed by the patient before these tests are completed.

Patient Teaching Before Computed Tomography Scan

1. Explain to the patient about being placed on a table and systematically moved through a shallow tunnel. An IV may be started if the patient is going to receive contrast.
2. Verify that the patient does not have allergies to iodine or other IV dyes.
3. IV contrast, if used, may cause a very warm sensation to the body, which is temporary and disappears shortly after injection.
4. Drink plenty of fluids after the CT scan if IV dye is used to assist in helping the body excrete the IV dye. Instruct the patient that increased urination is to be expected secondary to an increase in fluid volume and the dye's diuretic effect on the kidneys.
5. Certain medications such as metformin (lowers blood glucose) may need to be "held" before and after the CT scan to prevent an increased serum level of the medication and, therefore, a decrease in blood glucose.

Patient Teaching Before the Magnetic Resonance Imaging Scan

1. Instruct the patient on the type of machine being used (MRI machines can be "open" or "closed." Sedation is often needed by patients undergoing "closed" MRIs because many patients become claustrophobic when placed in the MRI machine.)
2. Patients with vascular surgical metal clips are not candidates for MRI because of the presence of the large magnet of this machine. Newer surgical clips that are made from titanium are acceptable for this test.
3. Patients with pacemakers or implantable defibrillators should check with their provider before having any MRI procedure.

Connection Check 47.5

The nurse implements which actions before the patient undergoes diagnostic studies of the ear?
A. Verify the patient's understanding of the scheduled test
B. Request that the nurse technician obtain consent for the test
C. Reassure the patient that the ordered test should be completed
D. Inform the patient that teaching for this procedure is the provider's responsibility

OTOTOXIC MEDICATIONS

The ear is a sensitive organ with many fragile parts. Several categories of medications can prove dangerous to the proper functioning of the ear (ototoxic), and often patients are not aware of this side and adverse effects. The most common categories of medications that pose ototoxic risks are in the following categories (see Chapter 48 for a partial list of specific medications):

- Antibiotics
- Diuretics
- NSAIDs
- Chemotherapeutic agents
- Miscellaneous

This is only a guideline and not all medications in each category pose this risk; medications should be assessed on an individual basis.

Connection Check 47.6

The nurse recognizes which medication as ototoxic?
A. Nonsalicylate pain medications
B. Calcium channel blockers
C. Antibiotics such as gentamicin
D. Beta blockers

HEARING PROTECTION

Protecting the numerous sensory organs of the ear is imperative for the long-lasting health and function of the ear. Evaluation of hearing function is an essential part of the patient's yearly examination. This examination includes the basic screening tools discussed previously as well as more in-depth testing based on the presence of any ear abnormalities. Protection of the ears from excessive noise is facilitated by using earplugs, earmuffs, or other protective equipment. Figure 47.5 provides a graphic representation of decibels ranging from 0 (hearing threshold) to 160 (decibels created by a 12-gauge shotgun). The frequent use of "earbuds" for listening to music and other sounds can pose a serious risk to the ear structures if used well beyond recommended volume levels because damage may be done to sensitive hair cells or other structures within the ear.

Patient education regarding the relationship between volume levels and hearing loss is essential to facilitate awareness of the hazards. Patients with certain pathology and postoperative conditions also need to consider the use of specialized waterproof earplugs for use around and in water conditions. (Most ear-protective equipment is readily available at pharmacies and is often available from employers that have employees who are in the presence of loud noises on a routine basis). The use of cotton swabs or other foreign objects to "clean" out the ear canal is a risky practice because rupture to the eardrum and impaction of wax creating pressure buildup are results that can occur using these objects. Assessing potential needs for protective equipment is an important aspect of the hearing examination, because patient education can prevent possible hearing loss. Box 47.3 provides an overview of risk factors associated with hearing loss.

> **⚠ Safety Alert** Certain measures should be taken to prevent hearing loss. These include yearly hearing evaluation with an annual physical examination; use of earplugs, earmuffs, or other protective equipment in the presence of loud or excessive noise to protect sensitive structures of the ear; limiting use of earbuds for listening to music at levels well beyond recommended sound levels; and use of waterproof earplugs for patients with recurrent ear infections or those with specific pathology requiring earplugs around water conditions. Additionally, cotton swabs should not be used to "clean out" ear canals because of the risk of eardrum rupture or impaction of cerumen.

Connection Check 47.7

The nurse should instruct the patient to perform which action to prevent possible ear trauma?

A. Whisper when possible to prevent ear strain
B. Select earbuds for electronic devices over external earphones
C. Be cautious when taking oral medications
D. Never use a cotton swab or other similar instrument in an attempt to remove wax

AGE-RELATED CHANGES

As with most structures of the body, the ear also undergoes changes while a person ages, including the following changes.

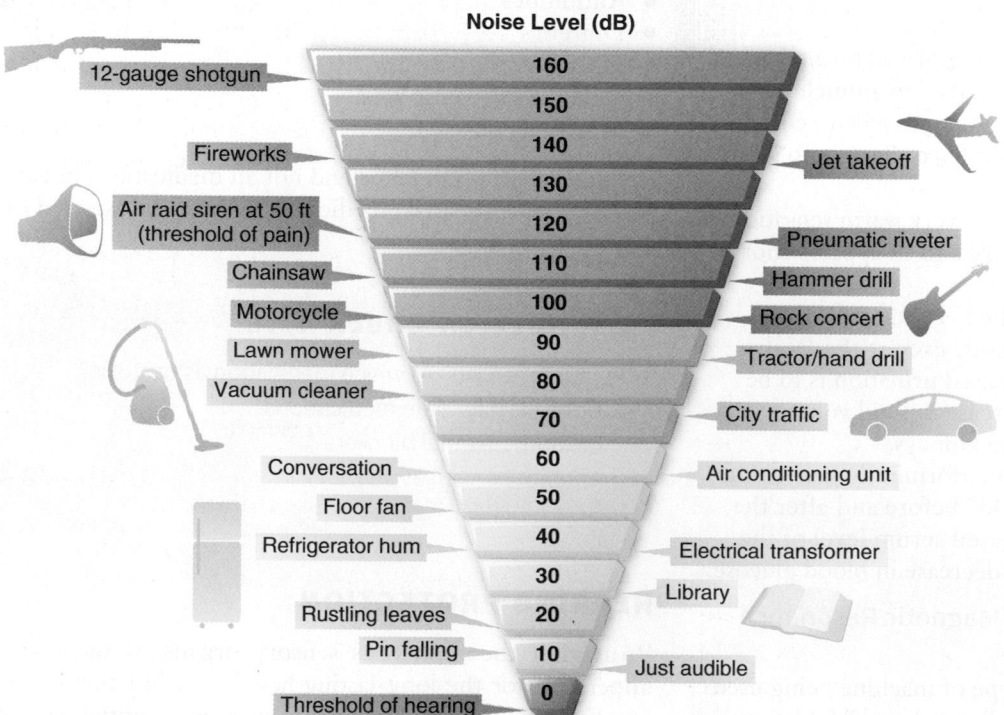

Noise Level (dB)

Left side	dB	Right side
12-gauge shotgun	160	
	150	
Fireworks	140	Jet takeoff
	130	
Air raid siren at 50 ft (threshold of pain)	120	
	110	Pneumatic riveter
Chainsaw		Hammer drill
Motorcycle	100	Rock concert
Lawn mower	90	Tractor/hand drill
Vacuum cleaner	80	
	70	City traffic
Conversation	60	Air conditioning unit
Floor fan	50	
Refrigerator hum	40	Electrical transformer
	30	Library
Rustling leaves	20	
Pin falling	10	Just audible
Threshold of hearing	0	

FIGURE 47.5 Noise levels of common sounds. Volume levels ranging from 0 to 160 dB.

Box 47.3 Risk Factors for Hearing Loss

- Advanced aging
- Repeated infections of the ear
- Medications with ototoxic side effects
- Ear trauma
- Occupations that place the patient in the presence of loud noises
- Tumors of the ear
- Continuous exposure to loud noises

Outer Ear

Cilia lining the ear canal become coarse and stiff, which may decrease hearing because it impedes sound waves from traveling toward the middle ear. Cerumen can also accumulate and oxidize secondary to the coarse, stiff cilia. Atrophy of the **apocrine glands** (glands that produce cerumen) causes the cerumen to become drier. Oxidation causing dryness of the cerumen is a common but reversible cause of hearing loss in older adults. Persons living near busy highways, airports, or other noise-polluted areas also have a greater risk of hearing loss.

Middle Ear

Membrane changes that include stiffening of the tympanic membrane and stiffness or calcification of the ossicles occur with advancing age.

Inner Ear

Presbycusis is a type of hearing loss that occurs with older adults. This loss is gradual and sensorineural (perceptive) in nature and is caused by nerve degeneration in the inner ear or auditory nerve. The onset for this type of hearing loss usually begins at approximately age 50 and then slowly progresses. While this occurs, the patient first notices high-frequency tone loss; it is harder to hear consonants (which are considered high-pitched components of speech). Words may start sounding garbled. Localization of sound, especially in the presence of background noises, is also impaired. Patients aged 70 years or older may also have an increased auditory reaction time, that results in it taking longer for older adults to process and respond to sensory input.

 Safety Alert There are several common age-related changes to be aware of, including atrophy of the apocrine glands that produce cerumen. This can cause dryness of the cerumen, therefore increasing risk of impaction. People between the ages of 50 and 70 years old commonly notice difficulty with hearing, both with frequencies and localized sounds. Constant exposure to loud noises in the home or at work can also increase risk for hearing loss.

Connection Check 47.8

Which findings are expected age-related changes in the auditory system? *(Select all that apply.)*
A. Increase in frequency of ear infections
B. Hearing acuity may decrease.
C. The ability to hear high frequencies is lost first.
D. The tympanic membrane loses elasticity.
E. Increased flexibility of the stapes

Patients with hearing loss may be sensitive to their condition. Because it is important to facilitate effective communication, there are specific strategies that can be implemented with patients with hearing impairment (Table 47.4). Additionally, it should be noted that when patients do not feel well or have decreased energy states, they may not hear as well. It takes energy, concentration, and motivation for patients with hearing impairments to function optimally.

Table 47.4 Effective Communication With Hearing-Impaired Patients

Intervention	Rationale
Face the patient directly when speaking to him or her	Direct visualization of the person talking helps the patient to interpret conversation better by being able to "lip-read" and assess nonverbal communication.
Speak slowly and be attentive to enunciation	Speaking slowly and enunciating all parts of words provides the best chance for hearing-impaired persons to be able to understand spoken communication.
Lower the pitch of voice	Because higher-frequency hearing tones are usually the first tones that are lost, speaking in a lower tone of voice may also help the patient to understand verbal communication.
Take care not to shout	Shouting increases the voice pitch, making it more difficult to understand spoken words; it can also be embarrassing to the patient.

Making Connections

CASE STUDY: WRAP-UP

The provider notes the opportunity for teaching regarding Erin's use of cotton swabs to clean the earwax from her ears. Concern is raised regarding the possibility of inducing trauma to the eardrum or other internal ear structures by use of this foreign object. Erin states that this is the way "everyone" in her family cleans his or her ears, and so she has performed this action for as long as she can recall. The provider concludes Erin's examination with teaching of ear hygiene without the use of introducing objects into the ear canal, thereby possibly preventing trauma or hearing loss to her.

Case Study Questions

1. The nurse recognizes that ear infections are more common in children for which reason?
   A. The immaturity of the hair cells within the ear canal
   B. The increase in wax production in children younger than 5 years
   C. The flat position of the eustachian tube
   D. The immaturity of the immune system

2. What teaching is most important for the provider to provide to Erin during this visit?
   A. Not using cotton swabs or other similar instruments in the ear canal
   B. Ways to remove the waxy buildup from the ear canal
   C. What to do if the patient starts to notice hearing loss
   D. Use of earbuds for listening to music

3. The healthcare provider instructs the patient on which ear protective measures? *(Select all that apply.)*
   A. Earbuds to reduce noise in areas with high-decibel noise levels
   B. Earbuds to help prevent water from entering the ear canal
   C. Headphones to listen to music at medium to high decibelranges
   D. Earplugs to help decrease water from entering the canal while swimming
   E. Wearing earmuffs in the winter

4. Erin does not notice any hearing changes; the provider verifies Erin's ability to hear by using which test?
   A. An MRI for the most definitive testing
   B. Audioscopy
   C. A CT scan of the head
   D. Electronystagmography (ENG)

5. Erin's ability to hear better after her physical examination is directly related to which action?
   A. The removal of the embedded wax from the ear canal
   B. The examination with an otoscope
   C. It is not clear why Erin is hearing more clearly.
   D. The stretching of the ear canal while an otoscopic examination is completed

CHAPTER SUMMARY

The ear and its many structures provide the sounds of life. Without the proper functioning of each of the structures within the ear, hearing is compromised. The auditory system includes the outer ear, middle ear, and inner air. Sound is transmitted by air and bone conduction, and transmission by air is part of the sequence required for successful sound interpretation. Evaluation of auditory system function includes a detailed history, physical examination, hearing ability, bone conduction, as well as CT and MRI scans.

Preventive care is essential when occupational hazards and everyday noise levels pose a risk to well-being. Seeking care from a qualified healthcare provider for routine examinations is also crucial, as well as when unexpected events arise that threaten hearing health. Age-related changes to hearing develop secondary to stiffening of the cilia and tympanic membrane, and dryness of cerumen. Presbycusis may also develop and is associated with a type of hearing loss that is caused by nerve degeneration in the inner ear or auditory nerve.

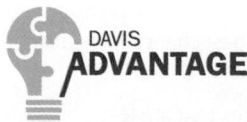
DAVIS ADVANTAGE

To explore learning resources for this chapter, go to **Davis Advantage** and find:
- Answers to in-text questions
- Chapter Resources and Activities
- NCLEX®-Style Chapter Review Questions
- Bibliography

Chapter 48

Coordinating Care for Patients With Hearing Disorders

Kelley Miller Wilson

LEARNING OUTCOMES

Content in this chapter is designed to assist in:

1. Describing the epidemiology of hearing disorders
2. Explaining the pathophysiological process of hearing disorders
3. Correlating clinical manifestations to pathophysiological processes of
   a. Hearing loss
   b. External otitis
   c. Otitis media
   d. Tinnitus
   e. Vertigo
   f. Ménière's disease
4. Describing the diagnostic results used to confirm the diagnoses of selected disorders of the ear
5. Discussing the medical management of selected disorders of the ear
6. Describing complications associated with selected disorders of the ear
7. Developing a comprehensive plan of nursing care for patients with ear disorders
8. Developing a teaching plan for a patient with an ear disorder

ESSENTIAL TERMS

Audiogram
Cholesteatoma
Cochlear implant
Endolymphatic fluid
External otitis
Labyrinthitis
Mastoiditis
Ménière's disease
Myringotomy
Otitis media
Otosclerosis
Ototoxic
Petrositis
Presbycusis
Tinnitus
Tympanometry
Tympanoplasty
Vertigo

CONCEPTS

- Assessment
- Comfort
- Infection
- Medication
- Perioperative
- Promoting Health
- Sensory Perception

Finding Connections

CASE STUDY: EPISODE 1

Follow this patient throughout the chapter.

Margie Newsome, 56 years old, has been experiencing dizziness, nausea, and right-sided hearing loss intermittently for several hours every 2 to 3 days for the past month. Margie takes no medications on a routine basis and has no significant past medical or surgical history, although she does suffer from severe seasonal allergies in the spring. Margie's mother has a past medical history of Ménière's disease, and she wonders if there could be a connection with her symptoms. She plans to see her provider later this week to discuss her symptoms because these occurrences are becoming more frequent...

INTRODUCTION

Nurses in many different settings manage patients and families with alterations in the auditory system, and because this may impact communication, it is important to understand the function of this important sense. Disturbances in the auditory system also impact balance and equilibrium. Loss of hearing and balance poses safety risks and socialization problems and understanding causes and treatments of these disorders allows the nurse to provide patient-centered care.

HEARING LOSS

Many aspects of daily life are affected by the ability to hear, and hearing loss affects not only health but also the overall quality of life. Gradual hearing loss that occurs with advancing age is known as **presbycusis**, a condition that often develops while individuals age. Hearing loss is not expected in younger patients and is an indication of pathology.

Epidemiology

Hearing disorders, although more common with advancing age (usually older than age 60 years), can occur at any time. Several factors are associated with placing a person at higher risk for developing hearing loss:

- Aging (risk increases while age increases)
- Heredity (see Genetic Connections)
- Occupational noises (exposure to loud noises on a regular basis for occupational reasons)
- Recreational noises (exposure to loud noises on a regular basis such as loud music and fireworks)
- Exposure to certain medications
- Illnesses including autoimmune disorders
- Congenital abnormalities

According to the National Institutes of Health, it is estimated that one-third of Americans between the ages of 65 and 75 years have some degree of hearing loss. Hearing loss is noted to be more common in men than in women and is noted to affect nearly half of adults older than 75 years. Box 48.1 summarizes findings from the National Health and Nutrition Examination Survey (NHANES) regarding the prevalence of hearing loss in the United States. Although hearing loss is clearly associated with age and a major health concern in older adults, a decline in hearing loss in adults 20 to 69 years of age was noted in a 2016 NHANES report.

Genetic Connections

Congenital Hearing Loss

Genetic factors are the etiology for more than half of all cases of congenital hearing loss, and most often are either autosomal recessive (both parents carry the recessive gene) or autosomal dominant (one parent has the abnormal gene for hearing loss).

Pathophysiology

In a normally functioning ear, three parts of the ear work in harmony to allow hearing and processing of sound. Sound is gathered by the pinna, and the waves of sound enter the ear by traveling through the auditory canal until they reach the tympanic membrane. The sound waves set up vibrations in the eardrum, thereby causing the middle ear structures to move back and forth. The cochlea then receives the sound vibrations and, finally, the sound stimulus travels to the auditory nerve and the cerebral cortex.

Hearing loss is categorized as conductive, sensorineural, or both, which is termed a *mixed loss*. Conductive loss is most commonly caused by a lesion in one of the main structures (the tympanic membrane, ossicles, inner ear) of the ear. A lesion present in one of these structures prevents

---

Box 48.1 Prevalence of Hearing Loss in the United States

- Eighteen percent of U.S. adults were noted to have speech-frequency hearing loss.
- Men were noted to be at 5.5% higher risk for developing hearing loss than women.
- African Americans were 70% less likely than white subjects to develop hearing loss.
- Increased prevalence was noted among those with smoke exposure or noise exposure, and those with cardiovascular risks.

Data from Centers for Disease Control and Prevention and National Center for Health Statistics. National Health and Nutrition Examination Survey. Hyattsville, MD: U.S. Department of Health and Human Services, Centers for Disease Control and Prevention.

sound from being conducted to the inner ear. Sensorineural hearing loss is the result of a lesion present in either the inner ear (sensory) or the eighth cranial nerve (CN VIII; neural). Sensory hearing loss is sometimes reversible, whereas a neural hearing loss is permanent, and determining the etiology of hearing loss is essential in guiding proper treatment. Neural losses can be life threatening because they often are related to a brain tumor. Mixed loss is a combination of conductive and sensorineural loss involving both the middle and inner ear. This type of hearing loss may be caused by severe head trauma, chronic infection, or a genetic disorder. Table 48.1 describes the common pathologies, manifestations, and types of hearing loss.

Certain medications are known to have the potential to cause damage to some of the sensitive structures of the ear and are said to be **ototoxic**. Common medications with known ototoxic properties include but are not limited to:

- Vancomycin (Vancocin)
- Aminoglycosides (such as gentamicin [Garamycin] and tobramycin [Tobrex])
- Cis-platinum (Cisplatin)
- Acetylsalicylic acid (aspirin)—most common with chronic use or overuse
- Furosemide (Lasix)
- Quinine (Qualaquin)

Clinical Manifestations

Patients with hearing loss begin to exhibit clinical manifestations that provide clues to family, friends, and coworkers that hearing loss is becoming more pronounced. Some of these manifestations of increasing difficulty in hearing include:

1. Turning up the volume on electronics such as televisions and radios
2. Frequently asking others to repeat conversations
3. Withdrawal from conversations
4. Avoiding social situations in which the patient was once an active participant
5. Disturbance in the patient's own quality of speech
6. Intermittently fighting with spouse or family members over hearing-related issues

Management

Medical Management

Diagnosis

Medical management of hearing loss centers on history taking, otoscopic evaluation, and diagnostic testing to determine an accurate diagnosis.

History taking includes assessing onset (gradual or sudden) and duration of clinical manifestations, bilateral versus unilateral loss, history of recent trauma, history of recent infections, and medication history and exploring all past medical/surgical histories. The history needs to focus on any issues in childhood such as delays in talking or difficulty with academics at school because these are associated with hearing loss.

Otoscopic examinations are used to verify the presence and patency of the structures of the external ear as well as portions of the middle ear. The examination includes

Table 48.1 Types of Hearing Loss

Pathology	Clinical Manifestations	Type of Hearing Loss
Obstruction (foreign body, cerumen, external otitis)	Pain, feeling as if ear is "plugged" or has something in it	Conductive
Otitis media	Fluctuating hearing loss, pain, pressure feeling in ear, fever	Conductive
Ear trauma	Pain, bloody drainage, visible blood on otoscopic examination	Conductive
Tumors	Unilateral hearing loss, visible lesion on examination and/or scan	Conductive
Genetic disorders	Positive family history, other genetic abnormalities often present, inability to hear normal sounds	Sensory
Noise exposure	Inability to hear	Sensory
Presbycusis	Progressive hearing loss bilaterally in the presence of a normal neurological examination	Sensory
Tumor of the cerebellopontine angle (acoustic neuromas, meningiomas)	Unilateral hearing loss, tinnitus, facial or trigeminal nerve deficits on occasion with examination	Neural loss
Demyelinating disease (such as multiple sclerosis)	Unilateral loss with clinical manifestations that occur intermittently	Neural loss

assessment for cerumen (wax) impaction; foreign body presence; and acute/chronic infection as well as structural abnormalities.

Pure-tone threshold is an audiological test conducted with air and bone conduction assessment to quantify hearing loss. To complete this test, the patient wears headphones and multiple different frequencies are delivered. An audiometer is used to deliver specific frequencies known as pure sounds at different intensities. Test results are plotted on graphs called **audiograms**.

Speech reception threshold is used to measure the intensity at which speech is recognized by a patient. This test is used to determine the softest level at which the patient is able to recognize speech. Speech discrimination helps to determine the patient's type of hearing loss (conductive, sensorineural, or mixed). This test is done to determine how well the patient hears and understands speech when the volume is set at the patient's most comfortable level of hearing.

A variety of diagnostic tests are used to determine the etiology and type of hearing loss. **Tympanometry** is a test that measures the impedance of the middle ear to the acoustic energy. Commonly used to screen children for the presence of middle ear fluid, this test does not rely on active patient participation. The *acoustic reflex* is a test that notes the response of the stapedius muscle to the presence of loud sound. Computed tomography (CT) scan or magnetic resonance imaging (MRI) scans may also be considered in conjunction with standard hearing testing if bony tumors or bony erosion are suspected. Magnetic resonance imaging angiography is usually conducted if vascular abnormalities are suspected. Standard MRI with gadolinium enhancement is usually performed with patients who present with an abnormal neurological examination and/or when a cerebellopontine-angle lesion is suspected.

Treatment

Treatment of hearing loss is largely dependent on the cause. Infections require antibiotic therapy, and chronic infection may require fluid drainage from the middle ear by **myringotomy** (surgical incision into the eardrum, usually to relieve pressure or drain fluid) and placement of tympanostomy tubes (Fig. 48.1) to ensure continued drainage. Lesions and growths (tumors) may also need to be removed. Autoimmune

disorders are usually treated with corticosteroids to improve hearing function. Patients taking known ototoxic medications are most often advised to discontinue if a less toxic substitute is available.

Hearing aids (Fig. 48.2) may be prescribed to amplify the sound to help patients improve their hearing and facilitate communication capacity. Different types of hearing aids are available to help magnify the sound and require specific fine-tuning with a licensed audiologist or ear care specialist.

Based on the etiology of the hearing loss, surgical procedures may be performed. If hearing loss is secondary to damage to the middle ear, then **tympanoplasty** (surgical reconstruction of the eardrum) may be indicated. There are two types of tympanoplasty, including reconstruction of the eardrum (myringoplasty) and replacement of the ossicles (ossiculoplasty). Before either procedure, the patient must be free of ear infection.

Cochlear implants (Fig. 48.3) are considered for severely hearing impaired or profoundly deaf patients. This treatment involves implanting a small electronic device that is used to provide a sense of sound. The implant includes an external portion that sits behind the ear and an additional portion that is surgically placed under the skin. The implant has several different very sensitive parts that include:

- Microphone: retrieves the sound from the environment
- Speech processor: selects and arranges sounds retrieved from the microphone
- Transmitter and receiver stimulator: receive signals from the speech processor and convert them into electrical impulses
- Electrode array: group of electrodes that collects the impulses from the stimulator and sends them to different regions of the auditory nerve

The cochlear implant does not restore normal hearing but does give profoundly hearing-impaired patients representation of sounds in the environments so that they may understand speech.

Nursing Management
Assessment and Analysis

The clinical presentation of the patient with hearing loss may be insidious in onset, and family or friends may be responsible for the patient seeking out an evaluation of his or her hearing. Clinical manifestations typically observed include:

- Inability to hear at normal tones
- Speaking in a louder tone than others
- Decreased social interactions

See Table 48.2 for an analysis of the clinical manifestations of hearing loss. Because of the increased incidence of hearing loss associated with aging, in providing care to older adults in an acute care setting, there are physical functioning and safety considerations (see Evidence-Based Practice).

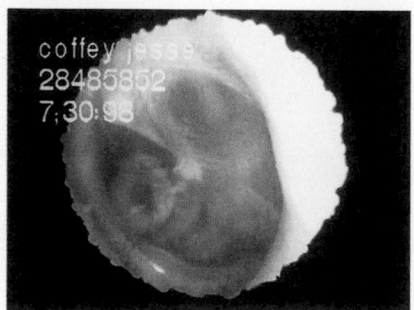

FIGURE 48.1 Tympanostomy tube. Tympanostomy tubes allow continuous drainage from the middle ear in patients with chronic ear infections.

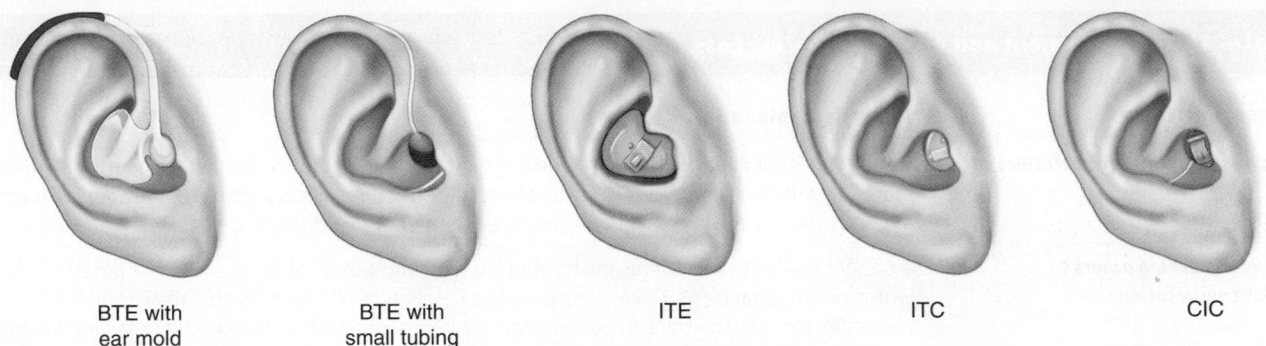

BTE with
ear mold

BTE with
small tubing

ITE

ITC

CIC

FIGURE 48.2 Types of hearing aids. Hearing aids may be in the ear, in the canal, or behind the ear, with or without tubing. BTE–Behind the ear with ear mold; BTE–Behind the ear with small tubing; ITE–In the ear; ITC–In the canal; CIC–Completely in the canal

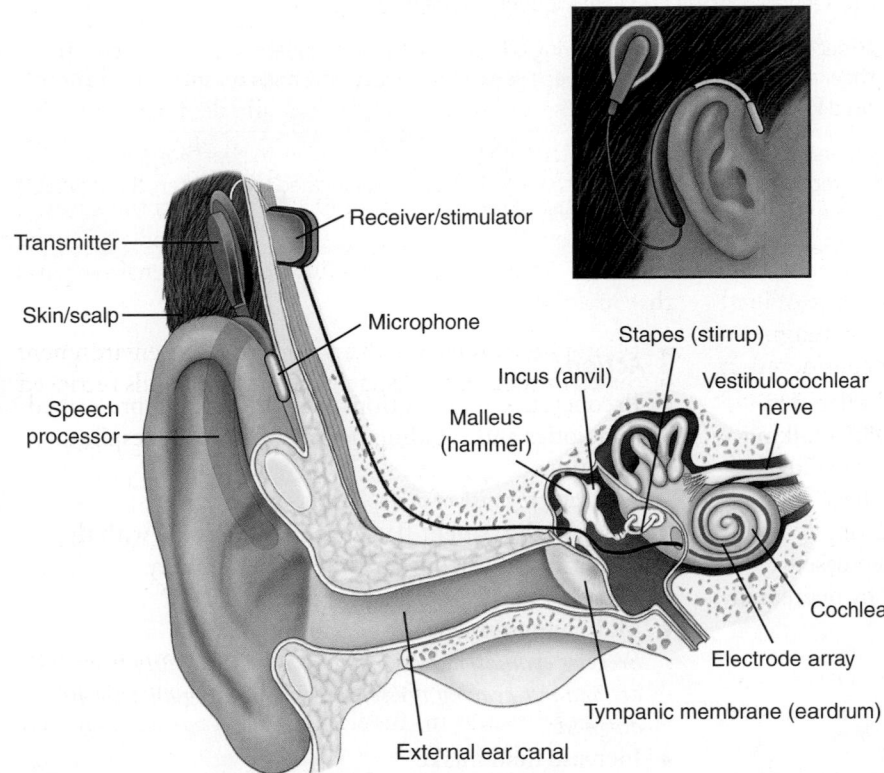

Transmitter

Receiver/stimulator

Skin/scalp

Microphone

Speech
processor

Malleus
(hammer)

Incus (anvil)

Stapes (stirrup)

Vestibulocochlear
nerve

Cochlea

Electrode array

Tympanic membrane (eardrum)

External ear canal

FIGURE 48.3 Cochlear implant. The cochlear implant does not restore normal hearing but does give profoundly hearing-impaired patients representation of sounds to facilitate their understanding of speech.

Evidence-Based Practice

Hearing Impairment and Mobility in Hospitalized Older Adults

Hearing loss is known to increase with advancing age. In older adults admitted to hospitals, this decreased sensory function impacts physical functioning. This study focused on factors from the International Classification of Functioning, Disability, and Health that impact mobility in hospitalized older adults. Based on a secondary analysis of 959 adults age 65 and older admitted to a hospital, findings revealed that hearing impairment, along with other factors including longer lengths of hospital stay and younger age, were associated with mobility decline. Based on the findings of this study the authors recommend development of evidence-based risk determination tools for hospitalized older adults, as well as development of environmental and policy-based interventions to promote physical activity in the hospital.

Chase, J.A., Lozano, A., Hanlon, A. & Bowles, K.H. (2018). Identifying factors associated with mobility decline among hospitalized older adults. *Clinical Nursing Research*, 27(1), 81–104.

Table 48.2 Assessment and Analysis: Hearing Loss

Assessment Data	Analysis/Explanation
Turning up volume on electronics	Commonly seen in patients who are having difficulty with hearing; often one of the first signs that family members notice. While function of hearing structures decreases, compensation of external stimulus takes place in the form of volume adjustments to electronic items.
Frequently asking others to repeat conversation	A patient unable to hear or having trouble interpreting sounds often needs to ask others to repeat words on a regular basis. Decreasing or failing function of structures within the ear makes it necessary for conversations to be repeated. (This can be combined with failing eyesight in older adults that does not allow them to easily read lips.)
Withdrawal from conversation	Patients unable to hear may resort to withdrawing from conversations because they may find their inability to hear both frustrating and embarrassing.
Avoiding social situations	Patients may choose to withdraw from social situations because it is embarrassing and/or too much work to keep asking others to speak louder or repeat conversations.
Disturbance in patient's own quality of speech may become apparent	Speech may become altered because hearing is necessary to make speech sounds correctly. The inability to hear correct sounds makes speech generation inaccurate; patients are unable to hear their own word formations.
Arguing with family members over hearing-related issues	Family members may also become frustrated with the patient's inability to hear "normal" tones as they tire of repeating conversations or hearing electronics at elevated levels. Often, this is what finally drives the patient to seek medical evaluation.

Nursing Diagnoses

- **Disturbed sensory perception**: auditory related to hearing loss as evidenced by head tilting when talking to others, frequently asking others to repeat spoken messages, and verbal report of inability to hear
- **Knowledge deficit** related to cause of hearing loss
- **Impaired social interaction** related to decreased ability to hear conversations as evidenced by decreased participation in social activities

Nursing Interventions

Assessments

- Vital signs
  No expected permanent changes in vital signs occur with hearing loss, although there might be a temporary increase in blood pressure and/or pulse when patients experience periods of frustration associated with decreased hearing ability.
- Changes within the ear structures
  Changes within the ear canal itself may reveal increased drying or drying of the cerumen. The hardened cerumen visible on examination may become impacted and cause some decrease in hearing.
- Diagnostic testing results
  Audiological testing such as assessing pure-tone thresholds, speech discrimination, tympanometry, and acoustic reflex are evaluated with unexplained hearing loss so that proper diagnosis is made.
- Age-related considerations
  Decrease in hearing ability is known to occur in patients approximately age 60 years; presbycusis is a decrease in the ability to hear that is associated with advancing age.

Actions

- Preoperative interventions including taking prescribed antibiotics and avoiding people with upper respiratory infections
  Decreases the risk of postoperative ear injection
- Position the patient flat, turned on the side with the operative side facing up after tympanoplasty
  Decreases the chance of packing being displaced
- Make appointment for hearing evaluation
  Seeking evaluation by a provider with the ability to evaluate and test hearing is essential in providing an accurate diagnosis.
- Increase fluid intake
  In patients with dried cerumen impacting hearing, the increase in fluid intake may decrease the thickening of the ear wax.

Teaching

- Pre-/post-test instructions
  Lack of compliance with pre-/post-testing instructions is often linked to inadequate teaching/instruction from the provider. Comprehensive instructions should be provided to the patient and family members before and after testing.
- Preoperative teaching
  There may be transient hearing loss immediately after surgery because of packing placed into the ear. Avoid forceful coughing because this places increased pressure on the middle ear.
- Postoperative teaching
  Keep the ear and dressing dry to decrease the risk of injection. All dressing changes are performed using sterile technique.

- Use of technology
  Instructions to patients and family members for use of new technology items (hearing aids or other hearing devices) are essential to ensure daily use of items as well as the patient being able to receive maximum benefit from the item(s).
- Noise protection
  Instructions for use of devices to help protect the ears from further injury are essential. Earplugs (or similar noise-blocking devices) are suggested to reduce the presence of loud noises. Use of earbuds or earphones for listening to music is discouraged because of loud sounds directly entering the ear canal in a concentrated form and having a direct effect on the sensitive structures of the inner ear; further hearing loss could then result.
- Avoid using cotton swabs or other devises to remove ear wax
  Damage to tympanic membrane or pushing the ear wax deeper into the ear may be the results of attempts to manually remove cerumen with cotton swab or other sharp devices.
- Follow-up care
  Instructions should be provided on expected follow-up care with the provider to ensure that routine evaluations by providers are completed, thereby lessening the possibility of continued undetected decline in hearing.

Evaluating Care Outcomes

The diagnosis of hearing loss is the first step in obtaining proper treatment. Patients with hearing loss should be fully evaluated by a provider with expertise in speech/hearing disorders to help determine the etiology of their hearing loss. Treatment is therefore based on examination and diagnostic testing results. In many cases, interventions implemented in the home and support offered from technology can help make the patient's hearing dramatically improve.

EXTERNAL OTITIS

External otitis (Fig. 48.4) is a condition commonly referred to as "swimmer's ear" because it is most often related to infectious organisms that are contracted through swimming.

This condition is hallmarked by an inflammation of the outer ear with extension into the ear canal. Inflammation of the skin of the ear canal is caused by either bacterial or fungal agents. External otitis can be acute or chronic, with acute more commonly being bacterial in origin and chronic more often being fungal.

Epidemiology

External otitis has several known factors that have been identified as high risk for developing this uncomfortable condition. The most common risk factors include:

- Recent history of trauma to the painful ear
- Warm temperature climates (water sports season is usually longer, increasing frequency)
- High-humidity climates
- Recent history of swimming
- Hearing aid use

Common in all parts of the world, external otitis occurs annually in four of every 1,000 persons. There is a marked increase in cases of external otitis noted in the summer months, with peaks noted in persons aged 7 to 12 years because this age group is most active with warm weather water sports. Ninety percent of cases are bacterial in nature, and 10% are noted to be resulting from fungal infections.

Pathophysiology

The adult external auditory canal is approximately 2.5 cm in length and is lined with squamous epithelium. This canal functions to transmit sound to the middle ear as well as serving to protect the more proximal structures from foreign bodies. The canal is divided into three sections; the outer third of the canal is primarily cartilage and contains cerumen-producing apocrine glands. The inner two-thirds of the canal is bony in nature and covered with thin skin that is tightly adhered. This inner portion contains no

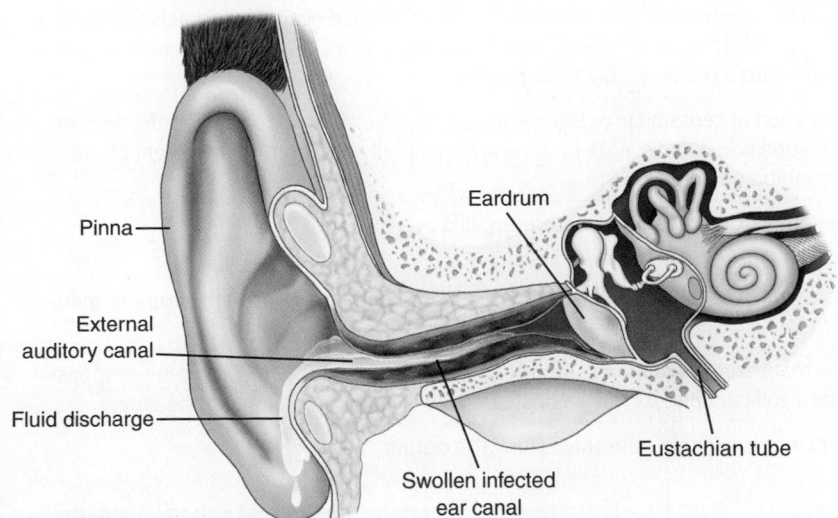

Pinna

External auditory canal

Fluid discharge

Eardrum

Swollen infected ear canal

Eustachian tube

FIGURE 48.4 External otitis ("swimmer's ear"). External otitis is characterized by an inflammation of the outer ear with extension into the ear canal.

apocrine (wax-producing) glands or hair follicles. External otitis develops in swimmers as a result of excessive water exposure yielding a decrease in cerumen. The decrease in cerumen can lead to drying of the external auditory canal resulting in potential skin breakdown, providing an excellent entry port for bacterial or fungal infections. The most common offending bacteria include *Pseudomonas aeruginosa* (50%) and *Staphylococcus aureus* (23%). The most common source of fungal infections is *Aspergillus*, which accounts for 80% to 90% of fungal infections.

Clinical Manifestations

Common clinical manifestations of external otitis include:

- Swelling visualized in and around the external ear
- External ear that is tender to touch
- Pain on movement or pressure to the outer auricle of the ear
- Visualized erythema and/or edema in the ear canal
- Scant clear drainage from the ear canal

Management

Medical Management

Diagnosis

History of presenting clinical presentation, recent activities, or recent trauma to the affected ear are important assessments for the provider to complete. Direct visualization of the external ear structures and otoscopic examination of the internal structures are important and usually help to confirm a diagnosis of external otitis. Table 48.3 identifies the most commonly prescribed topical treatments for patients with this diagnosis.

Treatment

The management of external otitis involves cleaning the ear canal, treating inflammation and infection, and managing pain. Typically managed by topical medications, rather than oral antibiotics, external otitis involves the skin of the ear canal. Fever and pain may be treated with acetaminophen or ibuprofen.

Nursing Management

Assessment and Analysis

Assessment of the external ear provides the first clues as to the type of pathology present as well as the degree of infection involved. The assessment data in Table 48.4 provide a guide for evaluation. Clinical manifestations of otitis media include ear pain that may be exacerbated by movement of the outer ear, edema around the external ear, erythema in the ear canal, elevated temperature, and clear drainage from the ear.

Nursing Diagnoses

- **Pain** related to the infectious process of the external ear as evidenced by verbal report of pain on touch to the external ear, redness/swelling visualized in the external and internal ear canal, and scant amount of drainage exiting from the ear canal

Table 48.3 Treatments for External Otitis

Common Topical Agents	Rationales
2.0% Acetic acid (Vosol) may be ordered with or without steroids	Effective for mild acute external otitis of bacterial or fungal nature. Apply every 4–6 hours; inexpensive and can sting or locally irritate tissues. This agent acidifies, making bacterial growth more difficult, and causes drying of moisture to further inhibit bacterial growth.
2.75% Boric acid or 90% to 95% isopropyl alcohol	Effective for mild acute external otitis of bacterial or fungal origin. Often used as a prophylaxis after swimming because alcohol commonly mixed with 50/50 2% acetic acid evaporates quickly, causing a drying effect in the ear canal. These solutions cause increased drying (evaporation) of moisture, and the acidity component helps to decrease bacterial growth.
Aminoglycosides (such as tobramycin and gentamicin)	Usually an otic preparation of gentamicin or tobramycin; is effective for acute bacterial infections of external otitis. Preparation is instilled every 6 hours and is minimally irritating. These potent broad-spectrum antibiotics inhibit bacterial growth.
Neomycin, polymyxin B, hydrocortisone	Effective for acute external otitis of bacterial nature; applied every 6 hours
Fluoroquinolone with or without steroid	Effective for acute external otitis; applied twice daily; only medication approved with tympanic membrane rupture
Corticosteroids (such as prednisone)	Treats underlying dermatitis/inflammation if present from bacterial invasion. Inflammatory response from bacteria may be significant and requires a decrease in inflammation to enhance healing.
Tolnaftate (Tinactin) or clotrimazole (Lotrimin)	Effective for acute or chronic external otitis that is fungal in nature

Table 48.4 Assessment and Analysis: External Otitis

Assessment Data	Analysis/Explanation
Swelling visualized in and around the external ear	Swelling that is present in the external ear and is visualized is secondary to the inflammation caused by the presence of a bacterial or fungal infection.
External ear that is tender to touch	Inflammatory response created by bacteria or a fungus causes swelling and therefore increased pain on movement of the affected area.
Pain on movement or pressure to the outer auricle of the ear	This pain is secondary to the inflammatory response that is occurring, resulting in swelling and therefore pain on pressure to or movement of the affected area.
Visualization of erythema and edema in the ear canal	The inflammatory response set in motion secondary to the presence of bacteria or fungus causes the erythema/edematous reaction to occur.
Scant drainage from the ear canal	This drainage is secondary to the extra fluid present in the tissues secondary to the inflammation process.

- **Knowledge deficit** related to cause and treatment of external otitis
- **Risk for infection** related to the inflammatory process created by the presence of bacteria/fungi

Nursing Interventions

Assessments

- Vital signs
  Elevations in temperature are sometimes seen in the presence of an ear infection. There may also be an increase in blood pressure and pulse with increased pain.
- Edematous external ear
  The outer ear (auricle) area can be erythemic and swollen; the appearance of the inner canal is often erythemic and edematous with clear drainage sometimes present.
- Pain
  The patient exhibits pain on movement of any part of the external ear or palpation of the ear canal secondary to bacterial or fungal organisms and the inflammatory response.
- Culture and sensitivity of ear drainage
  Culture and sensitivity by swab may be collected to identify the causative organism. Identification of the organism then allows the provider to select the best course of medical treatment.
- Age
  Adults and children are both affected by external otitis. Children may have a slightly higher incidence because they tend to be more active in water-related activities than adults.

Actions

- Pain relief measures
  Pain relief is usually accomplished by over-the-counter (OTC) medications (such as acetaminophen or ibuprofen preparations).
- Comfort measures
  Dry warm heat may provide some comfort when applied to the ear directly.

- Positioning
  Having the patient in a sitting or semi-sitting position with the affected ear on a soft object such as a pillow may provide additional comfort.

Teaching

- Medications
  Instructions for patients and families regarding antibiotic/antifungal eardrops are essential to proper healing. Table 48.5 provides additional instruction on eardrop instillation. Instructions regarding the completion of the entire medication course are imperative so that a reinfection does not occur. Over-the-counter pain medications also require information so that they are administered properly and the patient receives the most comfort.
- Follow-up care
  Instructions to patients or families regarding the necessary follow-up are necessary to ensure that complete and proper healing has taken place.

Evaluating Care Outcomes

Patients generally have a very favorable response to the topical eardrops prescribed and the suggested OTC pain relief medications for the management of external otitis. Summer months yield an increase in cases of external otitis secondary to the increase in water sport activities. On occasion, a patient will present with a very difficult-to-treat infection that requires cultures and additional antibiotic or antifungal treatment.

OTITIS MEDIA

Otitis media (Fig. 48.5) is a common disease process that causes an inflammation of the middle ear canal, most commonly by a bacterial source. This inflammation often leads to a buildup of fluid behind the eardrum, thus leading to bacterial growth and then infection. Otitis media affects adults but is most commonly seen in children because of the smaller and more flattened nature of the eustachian tube.

Table 48.5 Eardrop Administration

Procedure	Rationale
Wash hands and verify the medication ordered *(Donning gloves after washing hands is preferred for the person instilling medication if they are available.)*	Washing hands prevents the accidental introduction of foreign substances into the ear canal. Verifying the medication name/dose/route and time ensures that proper medication and dosing are taking place.
Place bottle of eardrops in warm bowl of water for 3–5 minutes	Placing the eardrop medication bottle in warm water warms the medication to approximate body temperature. Warm eardrop preparations provide more comfort for the patient and prevent the possibility of the patient becoming nauseated.
Tilt the patient's head in the opposite direction of the ear that drops are to be instilled in	Instructing the patient to turn his or her head in the opposite direction ensures that drops are instilled into the canal and they do not just remain on the surface of the outer ear.
Pull the pinna up and back	Pulling the pinna up and back in adults straightens the ear canal and allows the medication to reach all aspects of it.
Instill the correct number of ordered drops of medication down the side of the ear canal	Instilling the medication down the side of the ear canal provides the most comfort for the patient.
Gently move head back and forth two or three times	This repetitive motion ensures that drops are well incorporated into the ear.
Insert a cotton ball into the ear canal	Insertion of a cotton ball into the ear canal serves as a barrier to prevent drops from leaving the canal.
Wash hands and put away supplies	Washing hands after installation of eardrops helps to remove any foreign substances that may have inadvertently gotten on hands (medication or infectious drainage).

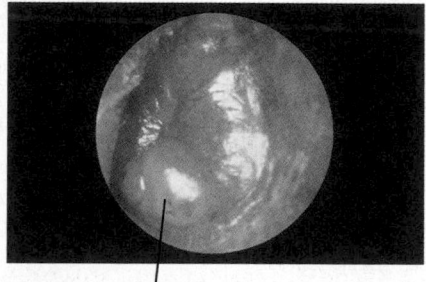

Fluid and inflammation

FIGURE 48.5 Otitis media. Otitis media is characterized by an inflammation of the middle ear, which often leads to a buildup of fluid behind the eardrum.

Epidemiology

Although otitis media can affect anyone, the most commonly identified risk factors for developing the condition are:

- *Anatomical features:* The eustachian tube is flatter in children and other congenital features that can accentuate infection. This flattening of the eustachian tube prevents drainage and makes fluid in the ear more likely to become stagnate or to accumulate.
- *Presence of an upper respiratory infection:* Inflammation from this common illness can cause narrowing of passages in the ear, thereby predisposing the patient to fluid accumulation and infection.

- *History of seasonal allergies:* Inflammation that causes narrowing of passages in the ear tubes, increasing the chance of fluid accumulation and infection
- *Craniofacial abnormalities:* The presence of abnormal bone formations can cause narrowing or obstructions, thereby increasing the risk of infections.
- *Genetic predisposition:* Patients with family members with an identified genetic predisposition for otitis media are at greater risk for this disorder.
- *Smoking in the household:* Smoking can cause chronic inflammation to the airways, thereby increasing a person's risk for otitis media.

Adult-onset otitis media is often secondary to sinusitis, allergies, and being in the presence of cigarette smoke. Exact statistics for the prevalence of these infections are therefore difficult to obtain. An increase in the occurrence of otitis media is found in Native Americans, particularly those of Navajo and Eskimo descent. It is thought that this increase may be caused by an anatomical difference in the ear structure, most notably the eustachian tube, in these races.

Pathophysiology

Acute otitis media is often seen secondary to a viral upper respiratory infection. Under normal circumstances, the middle-ear mucosa absorbs air in the middle ear. In otitis media, the inflammation and secretions can cause an obstruction of the eustachian tube. If air is unable to infiltrate the eustachian tube because of an obstruction, a negative pressure is created that then pulls interstitial fluid into the eustachian tube, creating a serous effusion. The serous effusion provides the perfect medium for microbial growth in the middle ear. Rapid growth of the bacteria becomes overwhelming and yields a middle ear infection otherwise known as otitis media.

Clinical Manifestations

The clinical manifestations of otitis media can be sudden or they may evolve over a couple of days. Some of the most common clinical manifestations are:

- Ear pain
- Tugging or pulling at ears (children)
- Trouble sleeping or lying flat
- Fever (can be quite pronounced in children)
- Fluid or blood draining from the ears (especially with tympanic membrane rupture)
- Hearing loss
- Infants/children often refuse to feed (sucking causes increased ear pain)

Management

Medical Management

Diagnosis

Comprehensive history taking and otoscopic evaluation are essential in determining the origin of clinical manifestations seen in the patient presentation. A comprehensive history includes past medical/surgical history as well as recent history, including exposures to respiratory illnesses. Assessing the patient's home/work environment may also yield clues as to the patient's current state of health. Tympanometry may also be completed by the provider to evaluate for the presence of fluid in the middle ear.

Treatment

On diagnosis of otitis media, oral antimicrobial therapy is the most effective treatment, particularly when effusions are present. The most commonly prescribed medications are noted in Table 48.6. Antimicrobial ear drops are also prescribed with tympanic rupture. Other therapies that are suggested include medications such as analgesics and antipyretics to help with pain and fevers. Decongestants and antihistamines may relieve some of the nasal manifestations of upper respiratory infections; their value in treating otitis media is unclear.

Table 48.6 Antibiotics Used With Otitis Media

Oral Antibiotic Prescribed	Commonly Prescribed Adult Dosage
Amoxicillin trihydrate (Amoxil)	250–500 mg every 8 hours
Amoxicillin and clavulanate potassium (Augmentin)	250–500 mg amoxicillin with 62.5–125 mg clavulanate every 8 hours
Trimethoprim (TMP)/ sulfamethoxazole (SMZ) (Bactrim, Bactrim DS, Septra, Septra DS)	160 mg TMP with 800 mg SMZ twice daily
Cefixime (Suprax)	400 mg daily or in divided doses twice daily
Cefuroxime axetil (Ceftin)	250–500 mg every 12 hours
Cefprozil (Cefzil)	250–500 mg every 12 hours
Azithromycin (Zithromax)	500 mg day 1; then 250 mg on days 2–5

Surgical Management

Surgical treatment for otitis media is usually considered for patients with chronic otitis or frequent reinfections. Tympanocentesis and myringotomy are the surgical interventions most often performed. Tympanocentesis is a diagnostic procedure that provides access for the provider to the middle-ear effusions for culture and evaluation. Myringotomy is a surgical intervention in which a tiny slit is created in the eardrum to relieve pressure caused by fluid accumulation. In many cases, a small plastic tube called a *tympanostomy tube* is inserted into the slit in the eardrum, where it remains for a period of time. Eventually in most cases, the tubes are discarded by the ear and exit the ear through the ear canal. Loss of the ear tubes before the evolution of anatomical changes (in children, the change in position of the eustachian tube) may require an additional surgery to replace the expelled tube.

Complications

The most common complications seen with otitis media include:

- *Chronic suppurative otitis media* occurs when fluid/ pressure builds up and a perforated tympanic membrane occurs with persistent drainage from the middle ear.
- *Facial nerve (CN VII) paralysis* reflects the spread of infection beyond the pneumatized (air-filled) area of the temporal bone and associated mucosa and thereby results in paralysis of this nerve.
- **Labyrinthitis** is an inflammatory disorder of the inner ear labyrinth that occurs as a complication of otitis media, which results in a disturbance in balance and hearing. This complication may be unilateral or bilateral.

Connection Check 48.1

The nurse correlates which complication with a diagnosis of otitis media?
A. Labyrinthitis
B. Mastoiditis
C. Tinnitus
D. Bilateral hearing loss with inability to hear high-pitch tones

Labyrinthitis often results from a benign overgrowth of squamous cell epithelium called a **cholesteatoma** from the middle ear directly into the semicircular canal.

- *Labyrinthine fistula* occurs when an abnormal communication develops between the inner ear and the middle ear or mastoid.
- **Mastoiditis** is the spread of infection to the mastoid bone that causes an inflammation of the mastoid air cells of the temporal bone.
- **Petrositis** develops when there is inflammation of the temporal bone that penetrates deep into the ear.
- *Meningitis* is an inflammation of the meninges which is the outer covering of the brain. Bacteria entering the meninges via the nasopharynx or respiratory tract leads to this potentially life-threatening complication.

Connection Check 48.2

The nurse recognizes which diagnostic test as the best method to confirm the presence of fluid in the ear that increases the patient's risk for developing otitis media?

A. Pure tone audiometry
B. Speech audiometry
C. Tympanometry
D. Acoustic reflex

Nursing Management

Assessment and Analysis

Otitis media presents with many common clinical manifestations that are directly related to pathophysiological changes in the ear. The provider may then use additional assessments to confirm otitis media (Table 48.7).

Nursing Diagnoses

- **Pain** related to inflammation and pressure on the tympanic membrane of the ear as evidenced by verbal reports of pain and nonverbal cues such as guarding or grimacing
- **Knowledge deficit** related to causes and management of otitis media
- **Disturbed sensory perception: auditory** related to scarring and damage secondary to recurrent infections

Nursing Interventions

■ *Assessments*

- Vital signs
  Fever is often present with otitis media secondary to the presence of bacteria and the increase in the body's metabolism (immune system function) in an attempt to overcome the invasion. Pulse and respiratory rate may also be elevated secondary to the body's rise in temperature, as well in response to pain.
- Internal ear
  On otoscopic examination of the ear, fluid may be detected, and the normally pearly grey internal ear is now erythemic and/or edematous. (Examination may be completed with the pneumatic tube placed on the otoscope to assess for movement of the tympanic membrane.)
- Tympanometry results
  This test is often used by the provider to assess for the presence of fluid in the middle ear. The machine notes pressure changes within the ear and documents them on a graph for the provider to evaluate.
- Age-related considerations
  Otitis media can occur at any age but is known to be more prevalent in children secondary to the position of the eustachian tube being more flat. Children and adults with structural deformities of the ear may also be at increased risk.

Table 48.7 Assessment and Analysis: Otitis Media

Assessment Data	Analysis/Explanation
Ear pain	Pain is often one of the first clinical manifestations and is due to the presence of fluid behind the tympanic membrane (causing pressure buildup) and the presence of bacteria, which is creating an inflammatory response.
Difficulty sleeping or lying flat	Lying in a flat position causes an increase in pressure on the tympanic membrane (in cases where fluid is present), and this increased pressure causes an increase in pain.
Fever	The increase in the inflammatory response and the body's own immune response cause an increase in body temperature.
Fluid or blood draining from the ear canal	This is a common clinical manifestation observed when the tympanic membrane has ruptured; infectious fluid and blood are seen exiting through the ear canal.
Hearing loss	Hearing loss can occur with repeated insults to the ear or with a very severe infection that has damaged one of the major structures of the middle ear.

Actions

- Administer prescribed medications
  Commonly prescribed medications are listed in Table 48.7. Medication therapy focuses on management of infection, pain, and pressure.
- Position of comfort
  Assisting the patient to a sitting or semisitting position helps to keep increased pressure off the tympanic membrane and results in a decrease in pain for the patient.
- Pain/fever
  Over-the-counter pain medications are often advised to help increase patient comfort from pain or fever. Common OTC medications for pain/fever include acetaminophen (Tylenol) and ibuprofen (Motrin).

Teaching

- Antibiotic therapy
  It is essential that patients understand to complete all prescribed oral medication as ordered and not to stop when "feeling better." Incomplete courses of medication put patients at risk for a reinfection or a resistant infection called a "super infection."
- Medication instructions
  Patients are to be given instructions about OTC medications for pain and discomfort to ensure proper dosage and time intervals
- Avoid getting water into the ear
  Getting water into the ear can exacerbate the risk of infection and increase pressure and pain
- Follow-up care
  Patients need to be given specific instructions regarding follow-up care with the provider. Follow-up is key to determining the resolution of the infection and to assess for any possible complications from the infectious process.

Safety Alert The reoccurrence of otitis media is increased if the patient does not complete the full course of antibiotic therapy. After the antibiotics are completed, follow up with the healthcare provider is important to verify absence of infection. Pain and pressure are exacerbated with the patient in a flat position; elevating the head of bed facilitates drainage and decreases pain.

Evaluating Care Outcomes

Otitis media can be very painful for patients, but use of antibiotics, pain medication, positioning, and provider follow-up usually provide curative results within a relatively short period of time. Patients' and family members' ability to follow instructions for treatment provide the best results in the quickest amount of time. Additionally, teaching to minimize risk factors of reoccurrence of otitis media facilitates positive patient outcomes.

Connection Check 48.3

The medical management of the patient with otitis media includes which priority interventions?

A. Administration of oral antibiotics
B. Administration of steroids
C. Use of anesthetizing eardrops such as tetracaine
D. Administration of decongestants to prevent eardrum rupture

---

Connection Check 48.4

The nurse recognizes that which priority assessments are included in the evaluation of a patient with a hearing disorder? *(Select all that apply.)*

A. CN III assessment
B. CN VII assessment
C. Complete and comprehensive history
D. Otoscopic examination
E. Diagnostic audiogram

TINNITUS

Tinnitus (Fig. 48.6) is most commonly described as a noise or ringing in the ears and is a relatively common affliction that is often a manifestation of an underlying disorder. Common causes include age-related hearing loss, ear injury, or circulatory system disorders. The clinical manifestations are often annoying and make it difficult to cope with the recurrent ringing or noise in the ears.

There are two types of tinnitus: subjective and objective. Subjective tinnitus is defined as sounds that are heard only by the patient and is the most common form. The cause is thought to be secondary dysfunction of the middle or inner ear or a dysfunction of the vestibulocochlear nerve (CN VIII). Objective tinnitus is defined as sounds that the provider may actually hear on examination of the patient. The cause is usually secondary to muscle contractions, blood vessel bruit, or inner-ear bone conduction disturbance.

Epidemiology

Certain known risk factors have been identified as associated with the development of tinnitus and include:

- *Advanced age:* Hearing loss that occurs at approximately age 60 years can cause tinnitus.
- *Exposure to loud noises:* Common loud noises that can affect a patient's hearing include construction equipment, portable music devices with earbuds, and firearms. Short-term exposure to loud sounds, such as attending a loud music concert with resulting tinnitus, usually resolves in a matter of hours. Long-term exposure tends to cause permanent tinnitus.

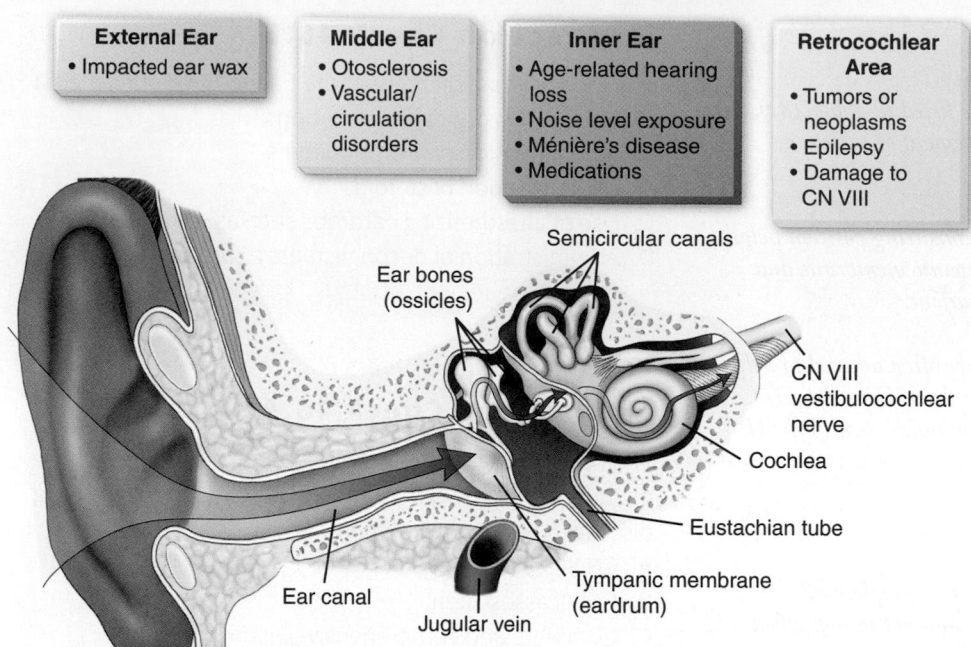

FIGURE 48.6 Causes associated with tinnitus. The pathophysiology of tinnitus can be associated with structural changes in the auditory system

- *Earwax blockage:* Obstruction of the eardrum can induce pressure and hearing loss with development of tinnitus.
- *Genetics:* **Otosclerosis**, or stiffening of the middle ear bones, can cause tinnitus, and this etiology is often seen within families.
- *Medications:* Many prescription and OTC medications increase the risk of tinnitus, including salicylates, NSAIDs, and selected antihypertensive, antidepressant, and chemotherapeutic ears. The relationship between these medications and the development of tinnitus is thought to be cochlear changes.

> ⚠️ **Safety Alert** Tinnitus is associated with salicylate toxicity which is the reason patients are instructed to follow dosing directions with these medications. Even with normal doses of these medications, tinnitus has been reported in some patients.

Connection Check 48.5

The nurse recognizes which risk factors for the development of tinnitus?
A. Overuse of medications containing salicylate
B. Family history of chronic respiratory infections
C. Involvement in water sports activities
D. History of migraine headaches

A marked increase of tinnitus is observed in both sexes at approximately the age of 40 years and peaks again between the ages of 65 and 79 years. A decline in clinical manifestations usually begins around age 80 years. Overall, males have a slightly higher incidence than females, but it is thought this might be secondary to occupational noises that are present in predominantly male-oriented occupations. Nearly 36 million Americans have constant tinnitus, and nearly half of the normal population has suffered from intermittent tinnitus.

Pathophysiology

Because tinnitus is a clinical manifestation and not a disease process, its pathophysiology may be secondary to many different disorders. Tinnitus can be caused by disorders of the outer, middle, or inner ear. Frequently, tinnitus occurs because there is a disruption of the background noise that is always present, making the body more aware of the sounds present within the ear itself that are part of normal body function. Table 48.8 describes some of the common pathologic causes associated with tinnitus.

Clinical Manifestations

The most common bothersome sensations of sound described by patients, when no sound is actually present, include ringing, buzzing, roaring, clicking, whistling, and hissing sounds in the ear. These sounds may be present consistently or intermittently.

Management

Medical Management

Diagnosis

Because tinnitus is defined as a clinical manifestation and not a disease, it is imperative that the healthcare provider try to discover the underlying cause of the clinical presentation. Determining the underlying cause leads to the most effective treatment for the patient. Obtaining a comprehensive

Table 48.8 Etiology of Tinnitus

Etiology	Explanation
Ménière's disease	Abnormal (usually increased) inner ear fluid, pressure, or composition can result in tinnitus.
Stress and depression	Tinnitus often worsens with increased states of stress or depression, which is thought to be secondary to vasoconstriction and increased adrenaline secondary to stress.
Temporomandibular joint (TMJ) dysfunction	TMJ is considered a somatic tinnitus and is thought to be caused by the sensory input from the jaw that interacts with the hearing pathways.
Head/Neck injuries	Neurological damage from head/neck injuries can affect the inner ear or cranial nerves, thus yielding tinnitus.
Acoustic neuroma	Benign tumor that develops on cranial nerve VIII, usually unilaterally, that can result in tinnitus
Head/Neck tumors	Tumor pressing on vessels in the head and neck that can cause a tinnitus sensation
Atherosclerosis	Buildup of cholesterol deposits may cause vessels close to the middle ear to lose some elasticity making flow more turbulent, therefore creating tinnitus.
Elevated blood pressure	Elevated blood pressure and factors contributing to elevated blood pressure, such as stress, alcohol consumption, and caffeine, make tinnitus more noticeable.
Medications	Certain antibiotics, cancer chemotherapies, diuretics, quinine, and salicylates are all well-known medications that can cause tinnitus to occur.
Vitamin B$_{12}$ deficiencies	A deficiency in this vitamin is known to cause the clinical manifestations of tinnitus as well; it is thought to be secondary to microvascular compression.

medical and surgical history is an important starting point and includes assessment for the following findings:

- Impacted earwax
- Otosclerosis
- Vascular problems such as circulation disorders
- Ménière's disease
- Medication list from patient
- Noise level exposures
- Damage to CN VIII from trauma or previous surgical procedure
- Presence of tumors
- Epilepsy or history of seizure disorders

Treatment

The healthcare provider often prescribes medications aimed at reducing the clinical manifestation and not as a curative treatment. The medications most frequently prescribed for tinnitus include:

- Alprazolam (Niravam, Xanax)
- Anticonvulsant medications (phenytoin, carbamazepine)
- Antihistamines (diphenhydramine)
- Acamprosate (Campral)
- Niacin (vitamin B complex)
- Gabapentin (Neurontin)
- Tricyclic antidepressants (nortriptyline; usually reserved for the more severe cases)

Treatment also includes identifying potential triggers for tinnitus in order to minimize or avoid exposure. New research points to possible sound therapy with or without counselling as possible treatments for tinnitus.

Nursing Management
Assessment and Analysis

Nursing management of tinnitus focuses on the careful ability of the provider to assess the clinical manifestations, as well as the present and past medical/surgical history. Additionally, correlating the assessment data with the underlying pathophysiologic changes facilitates a more comprehensive approach to the management of tinnitus (Table 48.9).

Nursing Diagnoses

- **Disturbed sensory perception: auditory** related to dysfunction of the ear or neurological system as evidenced by ringing, buzzing, or other abnormal sound sensations in the ear
- **Anxiety** related to abnormal sounds present in the ears

Nursing Interventions
■ *Assessments*

- Vital signs
  There is no significant effect of tinnitus on vital signs other than increased anxiety from the clinical manifestations, which may cause an increase in blood pressure, pulse, or respirations.
- Physical assessment
  Changes in physical condition are dependent on whether there is an identifiable cause of the tinnitus. The presence of brain tumors may yield very noticeable neurological assessment changes, whereas medication-induced tinnitus yields no detectable changes at all in assessment.
- Character of tinnitus sounds
  Based on the etiology, the sounds associated with tinnitus are different. For example, with atherosclerosis, the buildup of

Table 48.9 Assessment and Analysis: Tinnitus

Assessment Data	Analysis/Explanation
Impacted earwax	Earwax that is impacted in the ear canal can cause a disturbance in air conduction and pressure within the ear and therefore cause tinnitus to occur.
Otosclerosis	This condition, which relates to abnormal bone growth in the middle ear, can create conduction disturbances that lead to tinnitus.
Vascular/circulation disorders	Abnormal or disturbances in circulation flow can create sound similar to a bruit, resulting in a tinnitus sound.
Ménière's disease	Disturbance in the canals located within the inner ear can create these abnormal tinnitus sounds.
Medications (such as salicylates or those containing salicylates)	Medications can cause tinnitus sounds to occur; some occur with prescribed usage, and some occur with overuse.
Noise levels	High noise levels can cause short-term tinnitus to occur (such as after a loud concert), or it can be long term with repetitive daily exposure to loud noise (such as construction equipment or fireworks). Tiny hairs lining the ear canal are often damaged from these loud noises and cause the tinnitus sounds to occur.
Cranial nerve VIII damage	Damage to the vestibulocochlear nerve from trauma, tumor, illness, or a previous surgical procedure can cause the ringing or buzzing sounds of tinnitus to occur.
Presence of tumors or neoplasms	Any abnormal growth can create an obstruction (large or small) and generate abnormal sounds to occur in the ear, thus yielding tinnitus.

cholesterol deposits may cause vessels close to the middle ear to lose some elasticity making flow more turbulent and creating tinnitus, while with CN VIII tumors, the pressure on the nerve causes the abnormal sounds.

- Diagnostic results
  An MRI/CT scan may be ordered in an attempt to locate a cause for the clinical manifestations of tinnitus. Careful history taking is one of the most important clues in diagnosing tinnitus.
- Age-related considerations
  Tinnitus clinical manifestations tend to occur with advancing age; 40 years is when clinical manifestations often begin to occur; peaking at ages 65 to 79.

■ Actions

- Administer medications as prescribed
  Medications have specific rationales and indications in the treatment of tinnitus. Most are used to decrease the problem as opposed to curing it.
- Discontinuation of possible tinnitus-causing medications
  Discontinue medications that have tinnitus as a possible side effect if another suitable substitute is available. This may require consultation with the healthcare provider.
- Discontinuation of portable music devices that require the use of earbuds or earphones
  Earbuds/earphones are known to aggravate patients who have tinnitus; discontinuing the use of these items may cause some improvement in tinnitus clinical manifestations

■ Teaching

- Diary of clinical manifestations
  Instructing patients to keep a diary of clinical manifestations may help to identify a causative agent. This diary should

include date/time/symptoms experienced to see if an identifiable trend is present.
- Medication instructions
  Instructions should be given regarding any new medications being prescribed and about any well-known medications that can aggravate tinnitus (such as medications containing salicylates).

Evaluating Care Outcomes

Success of treatment of tinnitus usually depends on the ability to discover the definitive cause of the clinical manifestations. Abolishment of clinical manifestations is then geared toward treating the pathology itself. In many cases, treatment of the underlying pathology results in reduction or remission of the clinical manifestations of tinnitus.

VERTIGO

Vertigo is a clinical manifestation that evokes a feeling of illusory movement and like tinnitus, is not a specific disorder. Transient feelings of spinning and dizziness are experienced by nearly everyone at one time or another; however, patients with a documented diagnosis of vertigo exhibit these feelings on a regular basis. Senses of swaying or tilting are also common.

Epidemiology

Several risk factors are associated with an increasing possibility of developing vertigo:

- Medications (including salicylates, anticonvulsants, antihypertensive medications, and tranquillizers)

- Head injury
- Upper respiratory tract viral infection
- Cerebral vascular disease
- Advanced age; older than age 60 years
- Family history of vertigo
- Presence of another disease such as Ménière's disease, labyrinthitis
- Presence of tumor
- Migraine headaches

According to the National Institutes of Health statistics, approximately 40% of people in the United States experience feeling dizzy at least once during their lifetime. Prevalence is also noted to be slightly higher in women and increases with age.

Pathophysiology

Abnormalities in the semicircular canals (canals within the ear that contain fluid that allow a person to know the position in space) or the central nervous system (CNS) structures that process signals from the semicircular canals are thought to be responsible for the spinning sensation experienced by patients with vertigo. Disorders of the inner ear and CN VIII are termed *peripheral disorders*, whereas disorders of the vestibular nuclei and their pathways to the brain are considered *central disorders*. The visual, vestibular, and proprioceptive systems provide input to the CNS about problems with balance. Disturbances in any of these body systems can result in vertigo and are often related to specific pathologic conditions.

Connection Check 48.6

The nurse correlates the pathology of hearing disorders with which change in function?
A. An abnormality in the auricle
B. Disturbances in the semicircular canals
C. Disturbances in CN IX
D. Disturbances in CN VIII

Clinical Manifestations

Clinical manifestations of vertigo include a spinning sensation at rest or with minimal movement, imbalance, light-headedness, nausea and vomiting, and hearing loss.

Management

Medical Management

Diagnosis

Because vertigo is typically an episodic disorder, not a specific disorder, a comprehensive history is the primary approach to diagnosis. Due to vertigo being a clinical manifestation observed in disease processes such as CN VIII tumors, head injury, and Ménière's disease, other diagnostic studies, including CT, MRI, and hearing tests may also be completed as part of the evaluation.

Treatment

Treatment goals for vertigo focus on treating the cause of the vertigo. If a vestibular disorder has been identified, the most effective vestibular nerve suppressants include the following medications:

- *Diazepam (Valium)*, 2 to 5 mg orally every 6 to 8 hours; this medication depresses all levels of the CNS and is most effective for acute episodes.
- *Meclizine (Antivert)*, 25 to 50 mg orally three times daily; this medication decreases excitability of the inner ear labyrinth and blocks conduction of inner ear vestibular-cerebellar pathways.
- *Prochlorperazine (Compro)*, 10 mg intramuscularly (IM) four times daily or 25 mg rectally; this medication, usually used to treat nausea, blocks postsynaptic mesolimbic dopaminergic receptors in the brain and decreases stimuli to the brainstem reticular system.
- *Scopolamine (Buscopan)*, 0.6 mg orally every 4 to 6 hours or by patch as ordered by the provider; this medication blocks the action of acetylcholine at parasympathetic sites in smooth muscle, secretary glands, and the CNS.
- *Glycopyrrolate (Robinul)*, 1 to 2 mg orally two to three times daily; this medication blocks the action of acetylcholine at the parasympathetic sites.
- Vertigo secondary to Ménière's disease may also include dietary modifications that lower sodium in the diet and the addition of a potassium-sparing diuretic.

In addition to pharmacological management, slowly changing body position may greatly decrease clinical manifestations of vertigo.

Complications

Vertigo can have a profound effect on activities of daily living in patients, including the ability to operate an automobile independently, maintain employment outside the home, and many simple daily activities. Injuries from falls are not uncommon and may be of particular concern to older adults, who can suffer catastrophic effects from a fall. Depression and anxiety are other common complications that arise while patients often begin to feel desperate and at times helpless.

Nursing Management

Assessment and Analysis

Nursing management of patients with vertigo involves comprehensive assessment in an attempt to identify possible causes (Table 48.10). The clinical presentation includes complaints of sensations of spinning, that may be accompanied by dizziness and nausea.

Nursing Diagnoses

- **Disturbed sensory perception** associated with disturbance in the body's equilibrium system as evidenced by verbal report of dizziness, sensations of spinning, history of falls or accidents, and clumsy behavior
- **Anxiety** associated with changes in sensations of homeostasis

Table 48.10 Assessment and Analysis: Vertigo

Assessment	Analysis/Explanation
Spinning sensation at rest or with minimal movement	The spinning sensation, even at rest, is caused by an abnormality of the semicircular canals within the inner ear; usually related to tiny debris being present in the inner ear that interferes with balance or equilibrium
Imbalance	The imbalance sensation that occurs when there is a suspected disturbance with the vestibular system; often with tiny debris being present for unknown reasons
Light-headedness	Light-headedness is associated with the vestibular system.
Nausea/Vomiting	Feelings of nausea and vomiting are a direct result of the imbalance or spinning sensation that occurs in the body.
Hearing loss	The occurrence of hearing loss with vertigo is usually a clinical manifestation of another pathology being present such as a tumor or damage from a traumatic event.

- **Risk for injury** associated with imbalance and disturbances of equilibrium

Nursing Interventions

Assessments

- Vital signs
  There is no specific disturbance in vital signs noted with vertigo other than possible increases in blood pressure, pulse, or respiratory rate secondary to anxiety.
- Balance
  Physical assessment usually reveals difficulties with patients maintaining balance or the sense of proprioception caused by changes in the inner ear or CNS.
- Diagnostic results
  CT or MRI scans as well as other diagnostic tests are often ordered to determine pathophysiology and to evaluate nerve conduction.
- Age-related considerations
  Increase in age has been noted with vertigo, but it can happen at any age and is dependent on pathology.

Actions

- Administer prescribed medications
  Rationales and indications are specific to each agent and are aimed at decreasing dizziness and other clinical manifestations
- Minimize frequency and speed of position changes
  Patients with vertigo can benefit from limiting position changes to decrease feelings of dizziness.
- Decrease intake of salt, nicotine, alcohol, and aspartame in the diet
  Omissions from the diet are thought to be helpful, though the exact rationales are not well understood. Decreasing salt intake probably decreases vertigo based on its impact on fluid retention and blood pressure. Limiting salt intake is particularly important in the patient with hypertension who experiences vertigo. Avoiding caffeine is most likely associated with the stimulant effects of caffeine. Aspartame may have a toxic effect on the inner ear and brain.

- Reduce stress
  Decrease in stress is also thought to decrease CNS excitability and therefore decrease clinical manifestations of vertigo.
- Complementary and alternative therapies
  Ginkgo biloba and ginger are also cited as possible remedies in treating clinical manifestations of vertigo, although no real explanation has been given as to how these substances work to decrease vertigo.

Teaching

- Change positions slowly
  Instructions to plan slow, methodical position changes help to decrease vertigo in patients. Decreasing the clinical manifestations of vertigo with changing position may also decrease the patient's risk of falling.
- Safety
  Instructions to patient and family members regarding potential falls are important. Clutter-free environments and use of assistive devices (such as a cane or walker) to steady patients when walking also are advisable in an attempt to prevent falls.
- Medication/dietary
  Compliance with dietary modifications and medications is increased if the patient understands the indications and rationales.

Connection Check 48.7

The nurse includes which information in the teaching plan for a patient suffering from vertigo?

A. Addressing safety issues

B. Administering antipyretics as ordered

C. Taking a hot shower when clinical manifestations are severe

D. Maintaining strict bed rest for 24 to 48 hours after clinical manifestations appear

Safety Alert **Safety Considerations for Patients With Vertigo**

Patients with vertigo are at risk for falling and should take safety precautions including changing positions slowly, maintaining a clutter-free environment, and limiting intake of medications and other substances such as nicotine and alcohol that can exacerbate the vertigo.

Evaluating Care Outcomes

Vertigo is a very challenging clinical problem that has many possible etiologies. Finding the cause of the vertigo is often key to management and providing effective treatment. Medications may help lessen the effects of vertigo but may have undesirable side effects. Safety is a key concern because falls are noted to happen because of the disturbance in sense of balance. With proper treatment and management, patients with vertigo should be able to lead healthy, active lives.

MÉNIÈRE'S DISEASE

Ménière's disease is a disorder of the inner ear that affects the patient's balance and hearing. First described by French physician Prosper Ménière in 1861, this well-known disease is most noted for three clinical manifestations: unilateral sensorineural hearing loss, tinnitus, and vertigo. The patient usually describes these symptoms occurring as an "attack" that can last for several hours to several days.

Epidemiology

Patients typically seek healthcare when the clinical manifestations of tinnitus, vertigo, and hearing loss continue with no specific cause. The risk factors associated with this disorder include the following:

- Head injury
- Middle ear infection
- Syphilis
- Allergies
- Alcohol abuse
- Fatigue
- Respiratory infection
- History of recent viral illness
- Smoking
- Certain medications

Ménière's disease is a disorder known to affect 615,000 people in the United States, with more than 45,000 new cases diagnosed each year. Studies indicate that whites and those of European descent are affected most often, females more often than males, and the peak age range is between the ages of 40 and 60 years.

Pathophysiology

Although the exact cause of Ménière's disease is unknown, several correlations have been made about the disease. It is known to occur most often with infections, during periods of high stress, after traumatic injury, and with allergens. The clinical presentation of Ménière's disease is characterized by a clinical triad of vertigo, tinnitus, and hearing loss. These patients also exhibit an excess of **endolymphatic fluid** (lymph fluid within the ear) in the inner canals of the ear, which causes an obstruction of the inner canal system, and may lead to distention of this portion of the inner ear. This disruption leads to vertigo because of damage to the vestibular system. Decreased hearing from dilation of the cochlear duct that stimulates development of tinnitus is also observed in patients with Ménière's disease (Fig. 48.7).

Clinical Manifestations

The clinical presentation of Ménière's disease varies from daily to rare clinical manifestations and may have an onset with or without warning. Severity of episodes also varies

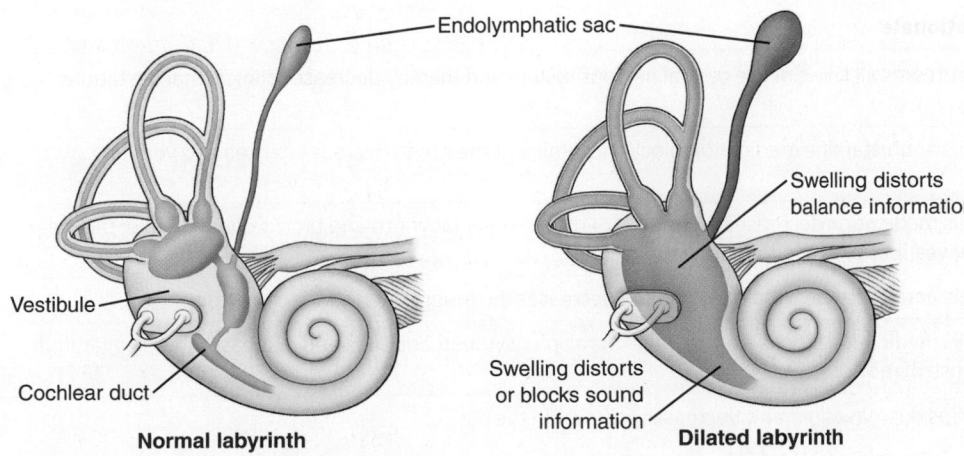

Endolymphatic sac

Swelling distorts balance information

Vestibule

Cochlear duct

Swelling distorts or blocks sound information

Normal labyrinth

A Normal inner ear

Dilated labyrinth

B Inner ear with Ménière's disease

FIGURE 48.7 Ménière's disease. A, Normal inner ear; B, Inner ear with Ménière's disease. An excess of endolymphatic fluid in the inner canals of the ear (B) causes an obstruction of the inner canal system in Ménière's disease.

and is usually unilateral. Clinical manifestations of Ménière's disease include the following:

- Vertigo
- Nausea and vomiting
- Sweating
- Increase in clinical manifestations with sudden movements
- Unilateral and sometimes bilateral hearing loss
- Tinnitus
- Diarrhea
- Headaches
- Abdominal pain
- Uncontrollable eye movements

Management

Medical Management

Although there is no known cure for Ménière's disease, diagnosis is based on clinical presentation and ruling out other disorders, and treatment is aimed at providing symptomatic relief. Clinical manifestations may be relieved with medications and dietary changes including low-sodium diets in an attempt to decrease the amount of total body fluid. It is thought that this decrease in fluid also decreases the fluid present in the semicircular canals of the ear and therefore relieves pressure in the inner ear. Balance testing (Romberg's test) can also provide useful information. Medications used in the management of Ménière's disease are listed in Table 48.11.

Other supportive measures that can help alleviate clinical manifestations in patients with Ménière's disease include:

- Low-sodium diet
- Avoiding sudden movements
- Avoiding bright lights

- Ensuring at least 8 hours of sleep per night
- Acupuncture
- Regular daily exercise
- Limit caffeine and alcoholic beverage intake

Some of these measures are effective because they also decrease fluid in the body. They also work by decreasing the CNS stimulation, leading to a decrease in the likelihood of developing clinical manifestations of Ménière's disease.

Surgical Management

Surgical intervention may also be considered for those with severe (unrelenting) Ménière's disease. Vestibular nerve transection helps control vertigo without damaging hearing. Surgically instilling gentamicin directly into the middle ear can also help decrease vertigo symptoms in some patients. A more radical surgery reserved for very severe cases includes removal of part of the inner ear called a *labyrinthectomy*. Although this surgery also improves the clinical manifestations of vertigo, complete hearing loss in the ear on the affected side is a result of the procedure.

CASE STUDY: EPISODE 2

Margie's provider performs comprehensive current and past medical histories, as well as a complete physical examination. Although nothing is apparent on physical examination, the provider is surprised to learn that Margie has been suffering from severe seasonal allergies and that she has a parent who suffers from Ménière's disease. The provider refers Margie to an otolaryngologist for further evaluation…

Table 48.11 Medications for Treatment of Ménière's Disease

Medication	Rationale
Diazepam (Valium) or other benzodiazepines	Depresses all levels of the central nervous system and thereby decreases clinical manifestations.
Promethazine (Phenergan) or other antiemetic medication	This antihistamine medication blocks histamine at the site to decrease nausea and vomiting.
Meclizine (Antivert) or other antihistamine	This medication decreases excitability of the inner ear labyrinth and blocks conduction of the inner ear vestibular cerebellar pathways.
Dimenhydrinate (Dramamine)	This antihistamine affects the ear and decreases the exaggerated sense of motion.
Scopolamine (Isopto)	This medication blocks acetylcholine at the parasympathetic sites and decreases the exaggerated sense of motion.
Diuretics such as furosemide (Lasix)	Helps decrease fluid and decreases pressure in the ear

Nursing Management

Assessment and Analysis

The clinical presentation of Ménière's disease presents a challenging examination for the provider. Focused assessments are performed to identify possible clues to the disease (Table 48.12).

Nursing Diagnoses

- **Disturbed sensory perception** related to Ménière's disease as evidenced by dizziness, balance or gait disturbance, nausea/vomiting, and tinnitus
- **Risk for injury** related to equilibrium/balance disturbances
- **Ineffective coping** related to vertigo and impaired hearing

Nursing Interventions

■ Assessments

- Vital signs
  Specific vital sign changes are not noticed until there are secondary changes due to other processes such as anxiety or infection that may lead to increases in temperature, blood pressure, pulse, and respiratory rate.
- Positive Romberg's test
  Patients may exhibit a positive Romberg's test on examination (meaning they have a disturbance in balance) and may also have nystagmus. Sensations of dizziness and strange sounds may be experienced by the patient.

- Caloric test
  The caloric test evaluates the patient for the presence of nystagmus, which is often present in Ménière's disease.
- MRI/CT scans
  Magnetic resonance imaging/CT scans are often performed for patients presenting with balance/vertigo/tinnitus issues to rule out the presence of tumors or other structural abnormalities.

■ Actions

- Medications
  Rationales and indications are specific to each agent and are aimed at decreasing the clinical manifestations. Specific medications and rationales are presented in Table 48.12.
- Limit sodium intake
  Decreasing sodium intake minimizes fluid retention and can minimize the excess endolymphatic fluid associated with Ménière's disease
- Positioning of patient
  Positioning the patient in a way that minimizes frequent or vigorous head turns is helpful in decreasing vertigo by decreasing fluid movement within the vestibular system of the inner ear.
- Safety measures
  Take care to prevent falls, including decreasing clutter present in rooms. Use of a cane or walker may also help provide stability with ambulation.

Table 48.12 Assessment and Analysis: Ménière's Disease

Assessment Data	Analysis/Evaluation
Vertigo	Membranous portion of the labyrinth is encased by bone necessary for hearing and balance; it is filled with fluid called *endolymph*, and a disturbance in the volume of fluid may be responsible for the clinical manifestations of vertigo.
Nausea/Vomiting	The disturbance in balance that occurs with the endolymph can cause feelings of nausea and vomiting.
Sweating	Overstimulation of cranial nerve VIII is thought to be the cause of sweating.
Increase in clinical manifestations with sudden movement	Sudden movements can increase clinical manifestations because of the movement of the endolymph.
Unilateral or bilateral hearing loss	Hair cell death in the inner ear has been reported with Ménière's disease and provides a possible reason for the hearing loss.
Tinnitus	Extra or unusual sounds may be heard because of the increase in endolymph within the labyrinth.
Diarrhea	Overstimulation of the sympathetic nervous system may cause diarrhea.
Headache	Overstimulation of the sympathetic nervous system is thought to be a possible cause of headache in Ménière's disease.
Abdominal pain	Overstimulation of the sympathetic nervous system resulting in increased secretion of gastric acid is thought to be a causative agent.
Uncontrollable eye movement	This uncontrollable movement, known as nystagmus, is a clinical manifestation that occurs as the eyes are controlled by input from the labyrinth of the ear; the disturbance in the labyrinth system that occurs with Ménière's disease can cause nystagmus to occur.

- Collaboration with neurology or otolaryngology providers
  Collaboration with other specialty providers can help to ensure that patient-centered, comprehensive care is provided.
- Acupuncture
  Although this is a nontraditional method of treating disease in the Western world, positive effects on balance and nausea symptoms have been demonstrated with this alternative therapy.

■ Teaching

- Disease process
  Teaching patients and family members about the disease itself helps to decrease anxiety and increase compliance with the medical regimen.
- Testing (pre- and post-testing)
  Instructions for pre- and post-testing are necessary for patients and family members so that compliance may be achieved and anxiety decreased.
- Medications
  Information regarding specific new medications should be provided to the patient and family members to increase compliance.
- Safety
  Information regarding the use of assistive devices (canes /walkers) should be provided so that patients may decrease the risk of falling.
- Follow-up care
  Instructions to the patient and family regarding all necessary follow-up care because frequent regular evaluations provide the best possible control of clinical manifestation in patients with Ménière's disease

Evaluating Care Outcomes

Ménière's disease is a disorder characterized by varied clinical manifestations that range in severity and also in time frame of attacks. A definitive diagnosis is the key to addressing the clinical manifestations and effectively managing this disease process. Treatments depend on the severity of the illness as well as the frequency of attacks. Because there is no known cure for this disease, the goal in most cases is to control the clinical manifestations. Medications, patient teaching, and follow-up care help the patient achieve the best possible outcomes.

Connection Check 48.8

The nurse correlates which clinical manifestations in the patient with Ménière's disease being received from the emergency department?

A. Fever greater than 101°F (38.3°C)
B. Seizures with nystagmus
C. Bloody drainage from the ear canal
D. Vertigo and tinnitus

Making Connections

CASE STUDY: WRAP-UP

At Margie's initial appointment with the otolaryngologist, the provider is concerned about her symptoms of nausea, dizziness, and right-sided hearing loss that have been occurring on such a regular basis. On the basis of the clinical manifestations and physical examination, including the Romberg's test, a tentative diagnosis is made of Ménière's disease and Margie is started on a low-sodium, caffeine-restricted diet and Antivert and Phenergan. An MRI of the head is also ordered to evaluate for a tumor on CN VIII.

Case Study Questions

1. The provider is most concerned with which clinical manifestations that could represent early presentation of Ménière's disease?
   A. Seasonal allergies and right-sided hearing loss
   B. Her age and episodic nausea
   C. Her dizziness and right-sided hearing loss
   D. Seasonal allergies and nausea

2. The provider is concerned about what other aspect of Margie's history?
   A. Her mother's past medical history of Ménière's disease
   B. Her severe seasonal allergies
   C. Her hearing loss on one side only
   D. Her age

3. What is the priority nursing consideration for Margie?
   A. Making sure that her allergies do not progress to asthma
   B. Implementing safety measures
   C. Providing medication to help suppress nausea
   D. Reassuring her that symptoms will be relieved after allergy season

4. Assuming that Margie is diagnosed with Ménière's disease, what is the next step in her care?
   A. Referral to an ear, nose, and throat specialist
   B. A STAT CT scan to definitively diagnose Margie
   C. Administration of medications to stimulate the CNS
   D. Antibiotic therapy to determine if the symptoms are infection related

5. What does the nurse teach Margie about surgical intervention for patients with Ménière's disease?
   A. It is a well-known cure
   B. It may be considered for those with severe, unrelenting disease.
   C. There is no surgical intervention for this disease.
   D. It is only about 25% effective

CHAPTER SUMMARY

Hearing disorders are not only associated with the ability to hear sounds but also with the body's sense of equilibrium. Hearing loss is categorized as conductive, sensorineural, or mixed. Presbycusis is a term referring to hearing loss that occurs with advancing age. Although the clinical presentations of the different disorders are similar, the underlying pathophysiology of these disorders varies. Hearing loss may have specific etiologies associated with structural changes in the ear and may be enhanced by hearing aids or other technologies such as cochlear implants. Health screening and noise prevention measures are also important interventions associated with maintaining auditory system function.

Inflammatory conditions such as external otitis and otitis media are typically associated with pain and discomfort in the affected ear. Usually short term and self-limiting, these disorders are successfully treated with appropriate antibiotics. Permanent changes in hearing are not common with these disorders unless the inflammation or infection becomes recurrent and results in damage to the ear structures.

Tinnitus and vertigo are disorders with multiple etiologies and are often the clinical manifestations associated with tumors on or around CN VIII, or disorders such as Ménière's disease. Expert evaluation should be initiated without delay in instances in which patients' hearing, balance, and equilibrium are affected. Based on the specific diagnosis, there are common treatment modalities including decreasing sodium and caffeine in the diet.

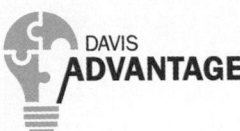
DAVIS
ADVANTAGE

To explore learning resources for this chapter, go to **Davis Advantage** and find:
- Answers to in-text questions
- Chapter Resources and Activities
- NCLEX®-Style Chapter Review Questions
- Bibliography

Unit XI

Promoting Health in Patients With Integumentary Disorders

Chapter 49

Assessment of Integumentary Function

Mary Donnelly

LEARNING OUTCOMES

Content in this chapter is designed to assist in:

1. Identifying key anatomical components of the integumentary system
2. Discussing the function of the integumentary system
3. Describing the procedure for completing a history and physical assessment of integumentary function
4. Discussing changes in integumentary appearance and function associated with aging
5. Correlating relevant diagnostic examinations to integumentary function
6. Explaining nursing considerations for diagnostic studies relevant to integumentary function

CONCEPTS

- Assessment
- Infection
- Medication
- Nursing Roles
- Promoting Health
- Skin Integrity

ESSENTIAL TERMS

Albinism
Alopecia
Apocrine sweat glands
Braden scale
Cryosurgery
Dermis
Ecchymosis
Eccrine sweat glands
Epidermis
Erythema
Hirsutism
Keratin
Keratinocytes
Langerhans cells
Merkel cells
Melanocytes
Onycholysis
Petechiae
Primary lesions
Pruritus
Sebaceous glands
Secondary lesions
Subcutaneous tissue
Vitiligo

Finding Connections

INTRODUCTION

The integumentary system, including the skin, hair, and nails, comprises the protective coating that guards the body from injury. Because the skin is the largest and most visible organ, alterations in integumentary appearance and function may signal underlying pathologies of other body systems. Careful assessment and interpretation of skin, hair, and nail abnormalities as well as expedient implementation of nursing interventions sustain the body's protective shield.

OVERVIEW OF ANATOMY, PHYSIOLOGY, AND FUNCTION

The skin layers include the **epidermis** and **dermis** (Fig. 49.1). The five major functions of the skin are protection, temperature regulation, vitamin D metabolism, sensation, and excretion. Providing protection from the external environment, as well as to underlying structures and organs, the skin is essential to homeostasis. Supporting temperature regulation, the skin also plays a role through facilitating heat loss or heat conservation through the skin. Vitamin D metabolism is another major function of the skin, because the epidermis is the major source of vitamin D for the body. Activated in the epidermis by ultraviolet (UV) light, vitamin D enters the circulation and works in the gastrointestinal system to facilitate calcium absorption. Sensation is controlled in the dermis, the location of many nerve receptors that communicate with the central nervous system. The

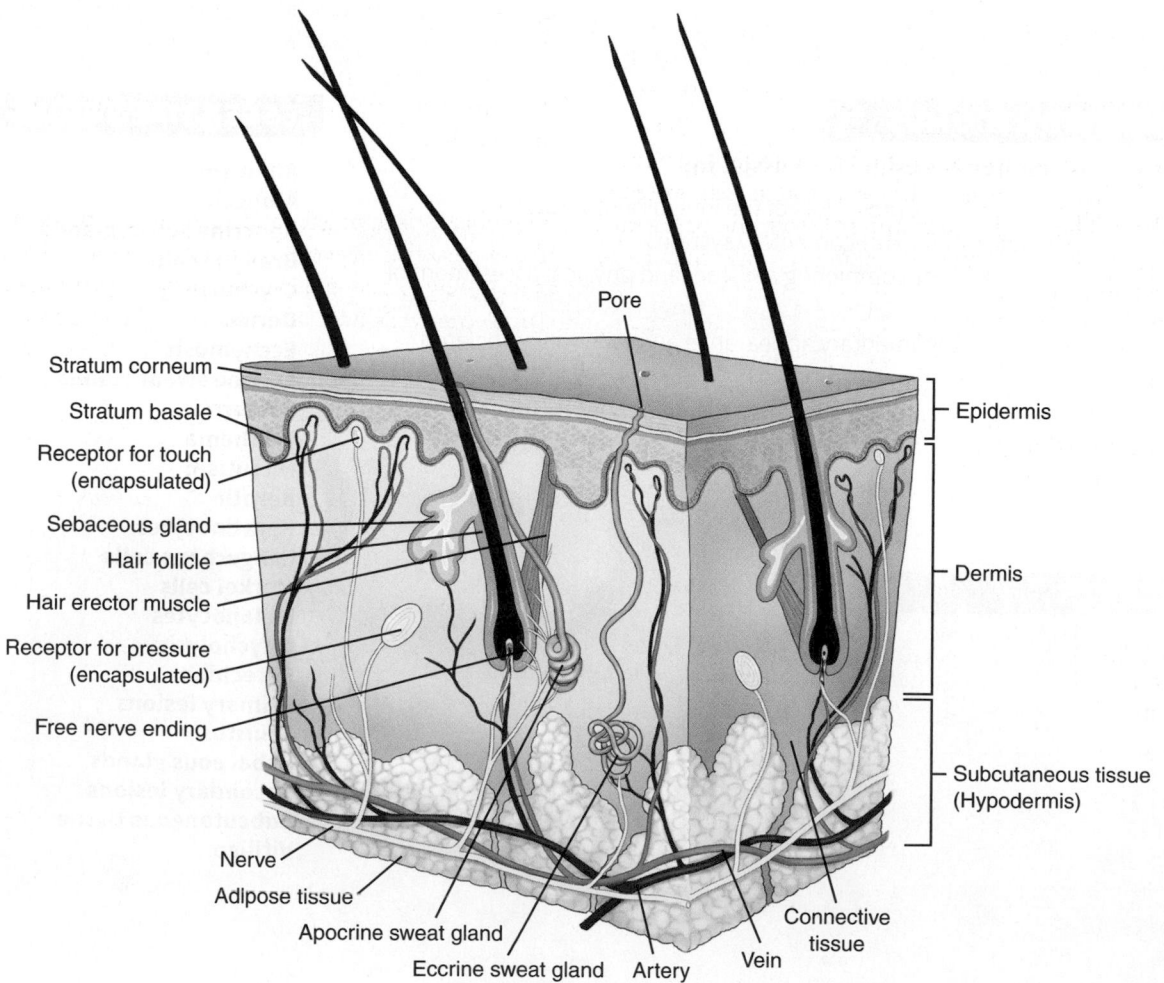

FIGURE 49.1 Anatomy of the skin.

role of the skin in excretion is linked to losses of fluid through the sweat glands; the evaporation of water through the skin also aids in cooling the body. **Eccrine sweat glands** cover most of the body's surface and **apocrine sweat glands** are present in hair follicles of the armpits and genitalia.

Skin

The integumentary system comprises approximately 15% of the body's total weight and requires 33% of the body's blood volume for optimal function. During times of decreased cardiac output, highly acute illness, and long-term chronic illness, the skin is highly susceptible to damage. Several factors place the skin at increased risk for damage, including reduced mobility, decreased perfusion and oxygenation, increased skin moisture and temperature, friction and shear, decreased sensory perception, hemodynamic instability, vasoactive medications, intensive care unit length of stay, surgery, and overall health status. Pressure from medical devices, such as urinary catheters, intravenous lines, endotracheal and nasogastric tubes can cause pressure injuries. Therefore, careful skin assessment and evidence-based interventions to promote adequate skin tissue perfusion represent essential nursing responsibilities.

Epidermis

The outermost skin layer is called the *epidermis* (Fig. 49.2) and protects the body by forming a barrier that resists pathogen invasion. Five compact sections of **keratinocytes** at various stages of maturation compose the epidermis. Keratinocytes are stratified epithelial cells that produce **keratin**, which is a waterproof fibrous protein that protects skin and hair. These cells push upward from the basement membrane to the skin surface during a cycle that lasts approximately 1 month.

The innermost layer, referred to as the *stratum basale*, is composed of newly formed, actively replicating basale keratinocytes, whereas the outermost level, the *stratum corneum*, contains approximately 25 layers of flattened, dead keratinocytes that slowly slough away. In addition to protective keratinocytes, the epidermis houses dendritic structures

called **Langerhans cells, melanocytes,** and Merkel cells. Langerhans cells migrate to the epidermis from the bone marrow, making them the outermost cells of the immune system. Langerhans cells ingest foreign substances that enter the body through the skin, then present the antigen to the immune system's T cells. The T cells then orchestrate the inflammatory response to destroy the pathogen if required. The epidermis is anchored to the dermis by rete ridges that point downward into the dermis (Fig. 49.3). This structural feature creates a more secure bond between the two skin layers.

The epidermal layer also contains melanocytes and Merkel cells. **Melanocytes** produce melanin, which is the pigment that prescribes skin color and protects underlying skin structures from UV damage. Under normal circumstances, melanocytes are present in a 1:36 ratio with basale keratinocytes. Each melanocyte has a dendritic structure that allows melanin to be transported through and released into the group of 36 keratinocyte cells. Differences in the appearance of skin color result from variations in melanocyte activity rather than the number of melanocyte cells present. Darker skin tones reflect increased melanin production from that individual's melanocytes. **Merkel cells** are mechanosensitive cells that are innervated by slowly adapting type 1 (SA1) afferent neurons that detect light touch stimuli. Merkel cells are touch-sensitive cells that transduce mechanical stimuli through cation channels. The sense of touch assists in gathering information about the external environment and in accomplishing skilled movements.

Dermis

The dermis is approximately 2 to 4 mm thick and encases blood vessels, nerves, immune system cells including macrophages and mast cells, dermal proteins including collagen and elastin, hair follicles, and sweat and **sebaceous glands** (glands that secrete sebum, which lubricates the hair follicles to the skin and hair). Each of these structures supports the five functions of the skin. Table 49.1 provides an explanation of how each structure correlates to specific functions.

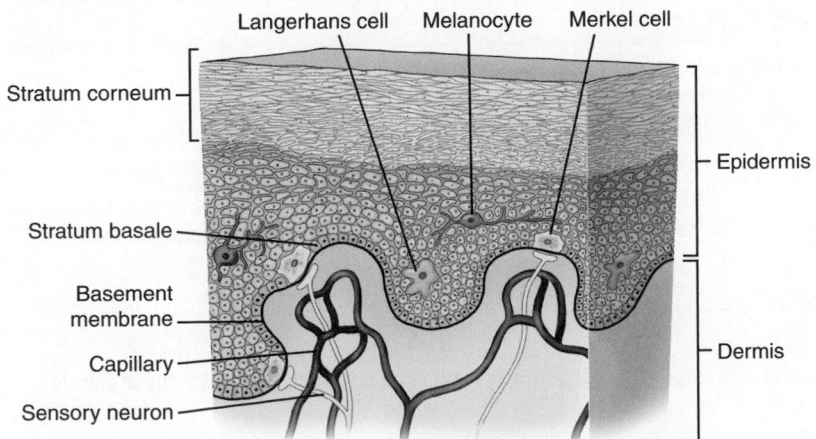

FIGURE 49.2 Epidermis.

Langerhans cell Melanocyte Merkel cell

Stratum corneum

Stratum basale

Basement membrane

Capillary

Sensory neuron

Epidermis

Dermis

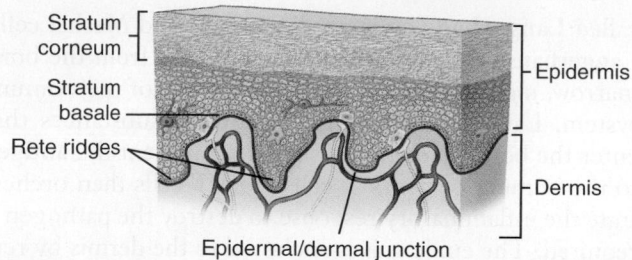

FIGURE 49.3 Rete ridges. The epidermis is anchored to the dermis by rete ridges that point downward into the dermis that creates a secure bond between the two skin layers.

Subcutaneous Tissue

Below the two skin layers lies the **subcutaneous tissue** or hypodermis, which contains adipose tissue, connective tissue, nerves, and blood supply. The adipose tissue located in this layer surrounds and insulates the deeper structures including organs, muscle, and bone. Distribution of adipose tissue varies depending on gender, genetic predisposition, and lifestyle habits.

Hair

In addition to having significant cosmetic importance, hair reduces heat loss and shields the skin from sun exposure. Although distribution varies, hair is present on most of the body. Both hair and hair follicles are composed of keratinocytes. Hair follicles are anchored in the dermis and then protrude into the epidermis. The hair itself is referred to as a *root* when contained within the follicle, and the portion that emerges from the follicle is referred to as the *shaft* (Fig. 49.4).

Extension of the hair shaft cycles between growth and rest. During the hair growth cycle, dead keratinocytes are tightly packed together within the follicle to be pushed toward the skin surface. This process results in lengthening of the hair shaft. During the resting cycle, active accumulation of keratinocytes is absent. However, the hair follicle holds onto the hair shaft, which minimizes hair loss during the resting cycle. Usually, the growth phase follows a resting phase, and the time frame varies depending on the hair's location. Complete death of a hair follicle results in baldness or **alopecia**, and causes include heredity, stress, and illness.

Nails

Nails protect the tips of the fingers and toes. They are composed of a hard keratin and have a slow but continuous growth process. Beneath the skin, the nail matrix houses constantly dividing basale keratinocytes that form the nail root (Fig. 49.5). The nail body refers to the visible portion that adheres to the nail bed. The condition of the nails reflects general health, state of nutrition, occupation, and habits of self-care. Coloration of the nail bed provides

Table 49.1 Structure and Function of the Dermis	
Structure	**Function**
Blood vessels	Supply nutrients, white blood cells, and oxygen for skin maintenance and healing and remove waste products
	Support temperature regulation via dilation and constriction
Nerves	Allow for recognition of pain, pressure, temperature, and touch
Skin immune system: Langerhans cells (epidermis), macrophages and mast cells (dermis)	Recognizes and reacts to invading pathogens using the inflammatory response
	Langerhans cells are located in the epidermis. They are the outermost immune system cells and detect initial pathogen invasion.
	Macrophages and mast cells are located in the dermis. Macrophages destroy bacteria while mast cells mediate the inflammatory response using histamine.
Dermal proteins: Collagen and elastin	Sustain resiliency; collagen creates tensile strength, and elastin provides elastic recoil
Hair follicles	Enclose the hair shaft
	In the presence of epidermal skin damage, cells within the hair follicle replicate to heal the injury.
Glands: Sebaceous and sweat	Sebaceous glands produce sebum, which exits from the hair follicle. Sebum is a lipid-rich substance that moisturizes hair and skin.
	Eccrine sweat glands cover most of the body's surface. They produce a water and salt mixture that evaporates to cool the body.
	Apocrine sweat glands are present in hair follicles of the armpits and genitalia. Secretions from these glands contribute to body odor.

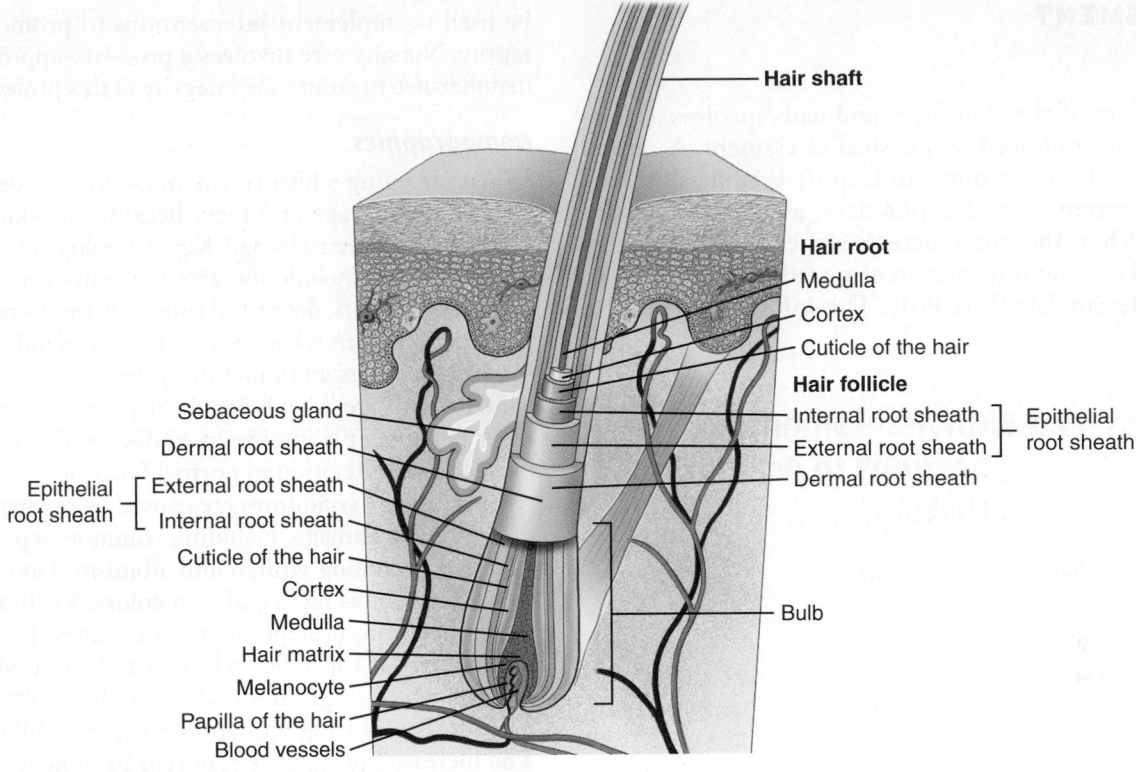

FIGURE 49.4 Structure of the hair follicle.

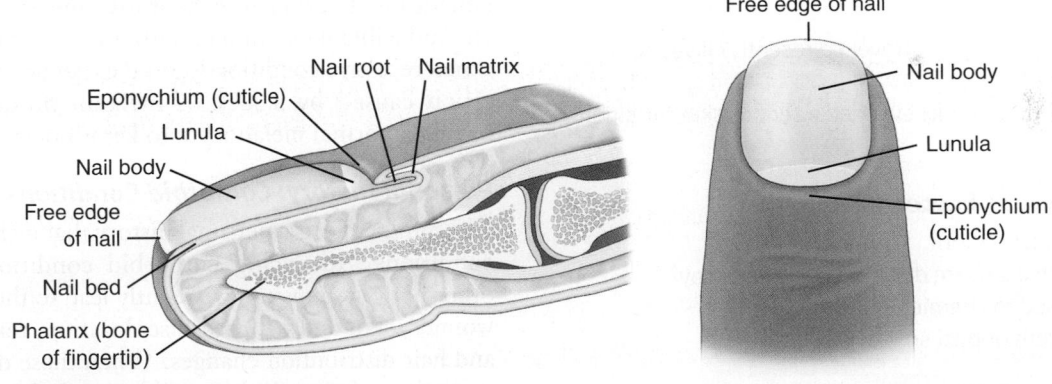

FIGURE 49.5 Structure of the nail.

information about the perfusion status of the body's most distal locations.

Connection Check 49.1

Which properties of the epidermal and dermal layers contribute to wound healing? *(Select all that apply.)*

A. The 30-day maturation time of epidermal keratinocytes
B. Eccrine gland sweat production
C. Melanocytes in a 1:36 ratio with keratinocytes
D. Presence of Langerhans cells, macrophages, and mast cells
E. Blood vessels in the dermis and subcutaneous tissue

Connection Check 49.2

Which statement accurately describes the skin's protective capabilities?

A. The epidermis can resist damage when exposed to continuous moisture.
B. Melanocytes always provide adequate protection to underlying structures from UV exposure.
C. Langerhans cells, located in the epidermis, often provide the initial signal to the immune system that pathogen invasion has occurred.
D. Temperature is regulated by blood vessels and sweat glands.

ASSESSMENT

History

Examination of the skin, hair, and nails involves a thorough history followed by physical assessment. A careful evaluation allows the nurse to identify existing skin conditions, current skin care practices, and individual risk factors. When the nurse detects a specific alteration in normal skin function, pertinent questions are posed to collect relevant data (Box 49.1). This information can also be used to implement interventions to promote skin integrity. Nursing care involves a proactive approach to skin maintenance to ensure the integrity of this protective organ.

Demographics

When obtaining a history, the nurse gathers demographic data, including age and race, because the skin's primary functions are affected by age. Key physiological skin changes in older adults include increased fragility caused by thinning of skin layers, decreased subcutaneous tissue, decrease in excretion from sebaceous and sweat glands, and fewer sensory receptors and immune system cells. These factors contribute to aged skin being more prone to damage. With older patients, it is important to discuss skin changes that present as an alteration in normal function.

Specific skin conditions are caused by pigmentation disorders or sun damage, including common depigmentation disorders including vitiligo and albinism that affects individuals of various races and skin colors. **Vitiligo** describes a confined type of depigmentation caused by the loss of melanocytes at a specific body area and affects all races and has a genetic background with more than 30% of affected individuals reporting vitiligo in a parent, sibling or child. The increased prevalence reported in some countries and among darker skinned persons results from a dramatic contrast between vitiligo macules and dark skin. The skin phototype (SPT) is determined by the combination of genetically determined constitutive melanin pigmentation and inducible melanin pigmentation. **Albinism** is an autosomal recessive condition leading to generalized depigmentation caused by a lack of melanin production despite having a normal melanocyte to keratinocyte ratio.

Personal History: Comorbid Conditions

The nurse collects a personal history that includes comorbid conditions. Advancing comorbid conditions that affect other body systems can frequently lead to the emergence of wounds, skin and nail bed discoloration, textural changes, and hair distribution changes. When these deviations from normal are detected, the common underlying pathology is inadequate oxygen and nutrient delivery to the integumentary system. However, common conditions including diabetes mellitus, cardiovascular disease, respiratory disease, liver and kidney disease, and obesity each have a specific pathophysiology that results in an alteration in skin tissue perfusion. A patient with one or more of these complicated illnesses frequently experiences a disruption in skin integrity. Refer to Table 49.2 to explore how common comorbidities affect integumentary appearance.

According to *Healthy People 2020*, diabetes mellitus, cardiovascular disease, and cancer are widespread disease processes that impact many Americans. Each of these conditions has a unique pathophysiology that impacts overall body function. Because the skin is the body's most visible organ, evidence of damage caused by these diseases may be observed during assessment of the integumentary system.

> ## Box 49.1 Skin Assessment: Questions to Ask During a History
>
> ### Health History/Medications
>
> Tell me about your disease history.
> Tell me about your allergies.
> When was the last time you had a health examination?
> What medications do you take (including herbal remedies)?
> Have you had any recent changes to your medication regimen?
>
> ### Family History
>
> Has anyone in your family or household experienced recent skin changes?
> Has anyone in your family travelled recently? If yes, to where?
> Has anyone in your family ever had a serious skin condition or skin reaction?
>
> ### Environmental Factors
>
> What is your occupation?
> How much sun exposure do you receive each day?
> Are you exposed to chemicals at work?
> Are you a current or past smoker?
>
> ### Social History
>
> What is your normal bathing routine?
> What skin care products do you use?
> Do you have someone at home who regularly looks at your skin?
>
> ### Focused Skin Assessment Questions
>
> Tell me about the skin changes that you have noticed.
> When did you notice the area, at what location, and how has it changed?
> Describe how the affected area feels (examples include itching, burning, pain, tingling, numbness).
> How has the discomfort changed since it first began?
> How have you treated the area, and what has been effective?

Adapted from Ball, J. W., Dains, J. E., Flynn, J. A., Solomon, B. S., & Stewart, R. W. (2018). Skin, hair, and nails. In *Seidel's guide to physical examination* (pp. 114–165). St. Louis, MO: Elsevier.

Table 49.2 **Prevalent Diseases and Associated Skin Complications**

Disease Process	Associated Skin Complications	Relationships Between Disease Process and Skin Complications
Type 2 diabetes mellitus (DM)	Pain Numbness of extremities Increased risks for wounds Diabetic foot ulcers (DFUs) Increased incidence of bacterial and fungal skin infections	Type 2 DM is a complex disease that alters the function of many body systems. Nerves do not require insulin for glucose transport and are particularly vulnerable to the pathologic effects of chronic hyperglycemia. Advanced glycation end products contribute to demyelination, nerve degeneration, and delayed conduction. Peripheral neuropathy affects as many as 50% of individuals with diabetes. Decreased blood supply results from vascular changes and autonomic dysfunction, which decreases the supply of white blood cells to open wounds. Chronic hyperglycemia impairs both the innate and adaptive immune responses. DFUs are caused by trauma to the site. Neuropathy makes it difficult for people to recognize that a wound is present. Failure to identify the presence of wounds or skin abnormalities because of neuropathy in combination with high levels of glucose in the bloodstream makes patients with type 2 DM prone to infection.
Heart disease: Coronary artery disease (CAD)	Hypoperfusion to integumentary system Acute: Pale pink, blue, or purple discoloration of nail beds, fingers, toes, feet, and mucous membranes Chronic: Finger clubbing Complications of immobility	The ability of the heart to function as an adequate pump to supply organs and tissues with adequate blood volumes becomes suboptimal when CAD damages the heart muscle. For patients who require invasive therapies such as mechanical ventilation, intra-aortic balloon pumps, extracorporeal membrane oxygenation, or other types of invasive monitoring after a major myocardial infarction are at risk for pressure injury as a result of immobility. Activity intolerance for patients with advanced congestive heart failure may lead to pressure injury.
Peripheral vascular disease affects lower extremities	Arterial insufficiency: Pain, pale to blue discoloration, dry skin, shiny skin, alopecia, dry wounds near toe tips that are very difficult to heal unless blood flow is restored Venous insufficiency: Edema, dermatitis, itching, hemosiderin staining, wet wounds from ankle to mid-calf	Atherosclerosis in systemic blood vessels leads to inadequate blood flow to lower extremities. Symptoms are related to the lack of oxygen to the tissues. Most often, dysfunction of venous valves in the lower extremities is the underlying problem in venous insufficiency. Blood pools in the legs because the valves are not able to close properly to prevent backflow.
Cancer	Wounds with excessive pain, odor, drainage, bleeding, and itching Skin inflammation caused by radiation (radiation dermatitis) Incontinence-associated dermatitis Complications of immobility	Tumors from internal structures may become visible outside the body. One example is a fungating breast tumor. These tumors often have complicated symptoms that require interprofessional management. Skin damage from radiation therapy occurs because radiation is very harmful to all rapidly reproducing cells including those in the skin layers. The extent of damage ranges from an erythematous rash to full-thickness wounds. Chemotherapy agents, nutritional deficiencies, and a high-acuity illness may lead to incontinence of urine and/or stool. Generalized weakness caused by therapies and end-of-life situations may lead to the formation of skin problems caused by immobility, such as pressure injury.

Personal History: Medications

Commonly used medications frequently have side effects that affect skin appearance and function. For example, corticosteroid therapy leads to thin, fragile skin that tears easily because the medication interferes with the formation of the epidermis and collagen production. The Safety Alert below lists commonly used medications that have the potential to cause mild skin irritation to full-thickness necrosis. Collecting a complete medication history assists with identifying whether a specific medication or a combination of medications has contributed to the skin abnormality.

 Safety Alert **Medications That May Disrupt Skin Integrity**

Antibiotics: Ampicillin, amoxicillin, penicillin, polymyxin B, sulfonamides, tetracyclines

Anticoagulants: heparin, warfarin, enoxaparin, rivaroxaban, apixaban

Cardiac medications: angiotensin-converting enzyme inhibitors, amiodarone, beta blockers, calcium-channel blockers, hydralazine, lipid-lowering agents

Chemotherapy: Doxorubicin, rituximab, infliximab, vinca alkaloids

Other: allopurinol, anticonvulsants, antiepileptic, antimalarials, glucocorticoids, NSAIDs, opiates, oral contraceptives, radiocontrast media, steroids

---

Family History

After discussing the patient's current skin conditions and personal history, the nurse inquires about family history. It is important to collect data about skin, hair, and nail conditions affecting family members because many conditions are genetically linked. Also, skin, hair, and nail conditions can be caused by infective organisms transmitted among people living within close quarters, such as bacterial, viral, or fungal infections, scabies, or lice.

Diet

Consumption of adequate amounts of protein, carbohydrates, fats, vitamins, and minerals is required to maintain a healthy integumentary system. If a patient lacks sufficient intake of nutrients, it is often visible in the appearance of the skin, hair, and nails. When wounds exist, whether surgical or caused by another etiology, the need for protein, B vitamins, vitamins A and C, fats, carbohydrates, iron, and zinc increases during the healing process. Therefore, diet is a key component to address when developing a plan for patients who have developed or are at risk for developing skin disorders. The nurse evaluates the adequacy of nutrition through reviewing results of plasma protein levels (Table 49.3) and body mass index (BMI) (Table 49.4).

Table 49.3 Plasma Protein Guidelines

Protein Type	Normal	Malnutrition
Serum albumin	3.4–5.1 g/dL	Less than 3.5 g/dL
Serum prealbumin	19.5–35.8 mg/dL	Less than 19.5 mg/dL
Transferrin	230–390 mg/dL	Less than 100 mg/dL

Table 49.4 Defining Body Mass Index

Body Mass Index (BMI)	Weight Classification
Less than 18.5 kg/m²	Underweight
18.5–24.9 kg/m²	Normal weight
25–29.9 kg/m²	Overweight
Greater than or equal to 30 kg/m²	Obese

Environmental Factors

Occupational exposures, lifestyle habits, and sun exposure impact skin integrity. Chemical exposures in the workplace or at home can lead to skin inflammation or chemical burns. Allergic contact dermatitis is a T cell–mediated hypersensitivity reaction to a substance after repeated exposures. Depending on the strength of the allergen, a skin reaction may take days to years to emerge. Common substances that cause allergic contact dermatitis include latex, topical ointments, plant products, chemicals, dyes, cleaning agents, metals, personal care products, and fragrances.

Lifestyle habits such as tobacco use and travel may impact skin integrity. Smoking leads to vasoconstriction of blood vessels. Chronic vasoconstriction can be very damaging to vasculature and surrounding skin layers, causing dryness, cracking, and increased risk for wound development and even tissue necrosis. Travel to areas of the world without access to preventive healthcare may lead to exposure to unusual infectious skin disorders.

The sun's ultraviolet rays (UVRs) expose the skin and its structures to radiation that quickens the skin's aging process. In addition, excessive exposure to the radiation from UVRs can disrupt the normal function of the DNA of various skin cells. For example, sun-damaged skin has 50% fewer Langerhans cells, which impacts the immune system's ability to identify pathogen invasion in the epidermis. Ultimately, the risk for developing skin cancers, including melanoma, is much higher for patients who have experienced frequent sunburns. Because environmental factors are frequently modifiable, educating the patient or caretaker regarding preventive measures may minimize the risk for injury.

Because of Ms. Bloom's advanced age, her skin is at increased risk for dryness caused by the physiological changes associated with aging. The patient reports a latex allergy that causes redness but denies any serious skin reactions in the past. She has struggled with being overweight since her late-30s, and her current BMI is 28 kg/m². Ms. Bloom denies any recent dietary changes or any travel outside the country. She lives with her husband, and they are retired. Ms. Bloom reports spending a lot of time working outdoors in her garden, and she regularly wears sunscreen. Her daily skin care regimen includes bathing and moisturizing her skin once a day, and she reports using a new fragrance spray for approximately 2 weeks…

Physical Assessment

After conducting a thorough history, the nurse performs a comprehensive, head-to-toe inspection of the integumentary system. The assessment is conducted in a well-lit area while the patient is minimally clothed. Visual inspection and manual palpation are used to detect abnormalities. The nurse observes for visual inconsistencies in the color, moisture, and presence of lesions and palpates the tissue to identify atypical findings in relation to temperature and texture.

When abnormalities are detected, the nurse considers the cause of the condition. Etiologies may stem from endogenous sources such as comorbid or hereditary conditions or exogenous sources including pressure or incontinence. By first determining the cause, the nurse is able to individualize problem-specific solutions to prevent further skin deterioration.

For patients who are acutely or chronically ill, all skin surfaces are inspected because deviations from the normal color and texture of the skin, as well as the development of lesions or wounds, may be correlated to the onset of new complications of the illness. The nurse pays particular attention to changes in the color, temperature, and texture of pressure points including the occiput, scapula, sacrum, ischium, ankles, and heels. The risk for pressure injury development escalates when these patient populations develop decreased sensory perception, increased moisture on the skin, decreased level of activity, decreased mobility or ability to reposition the body, inadequate nutritional intake, and increased friction and shear.

After inspection and palpation, the nurse documents observations regarding the following characteristics:

- Color and temperature
- Moisture
- Integrity
- Cleanliness
- Tissue changes
- Vascular markings
- Lesions

The nurse uses the findings of an in-depth skin assessment to formulate a plan of care to promote skin integrity. Also, the patient or caregiver is educated about ways to improve the daily skin care regimen. Ultimately, these initiatives promote comfort as well as amplify the skin's ability to resist deterioration.

Color

Under normal circumstances, skin color is determined by circulatory status and genetic predisposition. When evaluating skin color, the nurse collects information regarding recent or gradual changes in skin tone. Frequently, variations in skin color may correlate with changes in blood flow or the presence of inflammation. Refer to Table 49.5 for common skin color variations, including the cause and significance. The nurse also palpates for a change in skin temperature when color change is present. A cooler temperature of the affected tissue can indicate decreased perfusion, whereas warmer temperatures may reveal increased circulation or inflammation.

When changes in color, temperature, or both are noted, further assessment is needed to identify the cause. For patients with decreased mobility or highly acute conditions, the nurse regularly inspects pressure points for redness and texture change. These patients are at higher risk for pressure-related skin damage, which often begins with red discoloration. Blanchable **erythema** (redness of the skin) describes reddened skin discoloration over a bony prominence that turns white when the site is palpated. This characteristic indicates that blood vessels at the site have dilated to reperfuse tissues that received inadequate blood flow while the site was exposed to excessive pressure. However, if the erythematous area does not blanch when pressure is applied, deep tissue damage is probable. Blanching occurs when normal red tones of the light-skinned patient are absent. When assessing for pressure injuries in dark-skinned individuals, dark skin may not show the blanch response. Instead, after applying light pressure, an area darker than the surrounding skin or one that is taut, shiny, or indurated is noted. Check for localized changes in temperature and texture of the skin, and request the patient to report any change in sensation.

Moisture

The level of moisture present in the skin assists the nurse in predicting whether a patient is at risk for skin breakdown. Excessively dry skin lacks adequate lubrication, which increases the potential for fissures and cuts. In addition, dry skin is less pliable, thus increasing the risk for damage caused by shearing and friction. Conversely, moist skinfolds create an optimal environment for yeast and bacterial invasion. Moisture caused by incontinence, gastric drainage, or other caustic substances can lead to skin irritation that may result in wound development. For both excessively dry and moist

Table 49.5 Skin Color Abnormalities

Color	Cause	Location	Significance
Pallor: Acute	Decreased blood flow Low hemoglobin levels	May be generalized or isolated to specific body regions	May indicate: Anemia, restricted blood flow (arterial insufficiency), shock
Pallor: Nonacute	Genetic predisposition	Generalized	Albinism
Erythema (red)	Increased blood flow	May be generalized or isolated to specific body regions	May indicate: Fever, inflammation, infection, pressure-related injury
Cyanosis (blue)	Poor perfusion Deoxygenated hemoglobin	Often localized to finger and toe tips, lips, mucous membranes	May indicate: Exposure to cold temperatures, heart failure (acute or severe chronic)
Yellow	Liver disease – Jaundice (icterus)	Generalized or isolated to sclera	May indicate: Increased bilirubin levels, increased hemolysis of red blood cells, increased carotene consumption
	High levels of carotene	Palms, soles, and face	
Yellow: Nonacute	Genetic predisposition	Generalized	Varies on the basis of ethnicity
Brown	Hemosiderin from RBCs becomes trapped in dermal layers	Ankle-to-calf region	Indicates chronic venous insufficiency
	Increased melanin production	Hormones cause darkening of the nipples, areola, genitalia, and face	Occurs during pregnancy
Brown: Nonacute	Genetic predisposition	Generalized	Varies on the basis of ethnicity

skin, gentle cleansing techniques using products that contain skin protectants are used to minimize friction and protect the epidermis.

Increased moisture and humidity on the skin disrupt the stratum corneum's ability to function as a water-resistant layer. Incontinence of urine, stool, or both may lead to incontinence-associated dermatitis (IAD), which is an inflammation of the skin caused by exposure to urine and/or stool. The condition leads to erythema, swelling, and skin breakdown that may be mild to severe. Table 49.6

Table 49.6 Strategies to Promote Moisture Balance of the Skin

Problem	Intervention	Rationale
Excessive dryness	Hydrate with emollients to soften skin	Soft, supple skin resists damage inflicted by pressure, shear, and friction.
Excessive moisture	Apply a moisture barrier	Barrier products offer a protective layer that shields the epidermis from damage caused by moisture.
	Avoid diaper use	Diapers trap moisture and humidity against the skin, thus increasing the potential for development of skin lesions.
	In chronic or severe cases of incontinence, consider containment measures	In severe cases, removing the presence of urine and stool using the least-invasive method should be considered to minimize skin damage.

provides effective moisture management strategies that can prevent serious and painful skin complications.

Integrity

Skin integrity refers to the degree of intactness of the skin. Commonly, hospitalized persons face problems such as excessive moisture or dryness, **pruritus** (itching), skin tears, puncture sites, abrasions, edema, blistering, and immobility, and all of these conditions threaten skin integrity. The nurse examines the overall condition of the patient to implement etiology-based management strategies to minimize further skin deterioration.

Many factors can disrupt skin integrity (Table 49.7). When a skin condition is detected, the nurse documents the location, size, color, lesion characteristics, distribution, moisture and drainage, clinical manifestations of infection, and subjective findings. Subjective symptoms such as pruritus and burning may have many underlying causes, but early management helps minimize further skin deterioration. Once this information has been collected, members of the interprofessional team, which may include the primary healthcare provider; specialized physician teams such as dermatology, infectious disease, gastroenterology, and rheumatology; the wound ostomy continence nurse; and the primary nurse, can identify the underlying cause and develop a strategy to promote healing.

Cleanliness

Poor self-care and hygiene habits such as the inability to clean the skin regularly because of functional, psychological, or economic causes can lead to a variety of problems that range from mild discomfort to full-thickness skin breakdown. These patients are at risk for localized and systemic infection as well as discomfort. Observation of self-care by the nurse provides the opportunity to evaluate the patient's functional status and helps identify areas for health-related education.

Tissue Changes

Many classifications for wound descriptions exist depending on the underlying wound etiology. When wounds emerge, they have the potential to penetrate through skin layers, subcutaneous tissue, and muscle into the bone. When describing skin damage in general, the terms "partial thickness" and "full thickness" may be used. In a partial-thickness wound, skin breakdown is limited to the epidermis and superficial dermis. These tissues are capable of healing by regeneration, whereas a full-thickness wound pervades through the dermal layers into subcutaneous tissue and muscle and may even expose bone. These wounds heal by scar formation, which has only 80% of the strength of normal skin. Refer to Chapter 50 for details about wound classifications.

Vascular Markings

Vascular markings arise from malformations in a blood vessel that are visible on the skin. Spider angiomas (Fig. 49.6) and cherry angiomas (Fig. 49.7) are benign findings, whereas a port-wine stain (Fig. 49.8) is present at birth and may lead to dermal deformity with increased age. If an individual develops low platelet counts (thrombocytopenia) or severe systemic infection, microvascular dysfunction can lead to hemorrhage beneath the skin that has a red to purple discoloration. **Petechiae** are pinpoint-sized, nonblanching, red to purple flat lesions (Fig. 49.9). **Ecchymosis** refers to bruising that results from larger areas of hemorrhage under the skin.

Lesions

In order to describe skin conditions using a uniform approach, the nurse uses a classification system. When

Table 49.7 Factors That Disrupt Skin Integrity	
Factors	**Causes**
Skin infections	Fungal, bacterial, and viral pathogens
Mechanical	Friction, shear, immobility, adhesives, abrasion injuries
Chemical	Urine, stool, gastric fluids, caustic chemicals, soaps with high pH
Inflammatory conditions	Lupus, Crohn's disease, allergen exposure

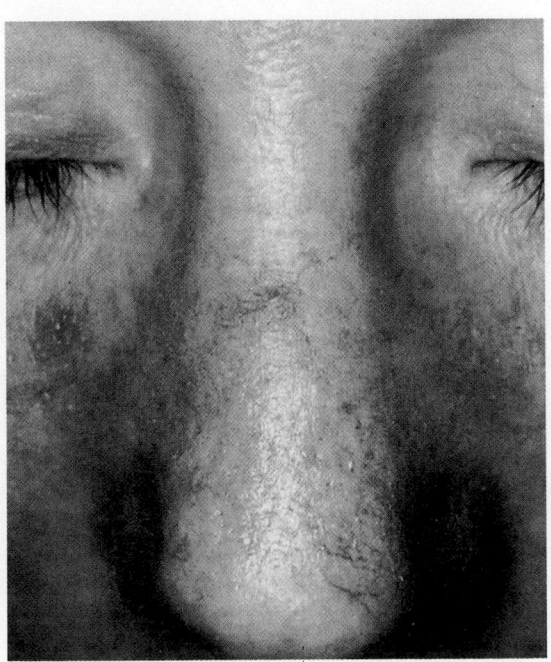

FIGURE 49.6 Spider angioma.

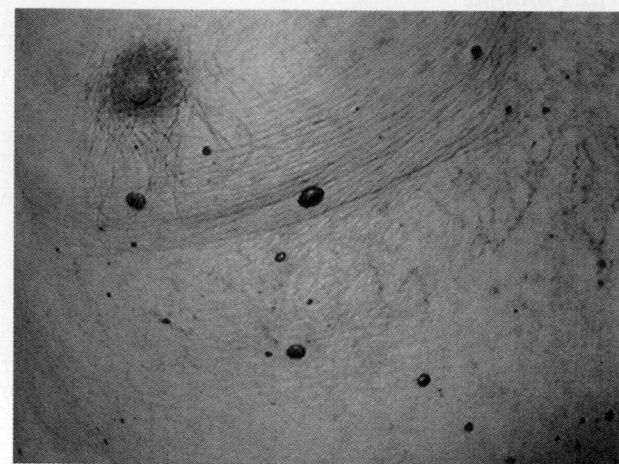

FIGURE 49.7 Cherry angioma.

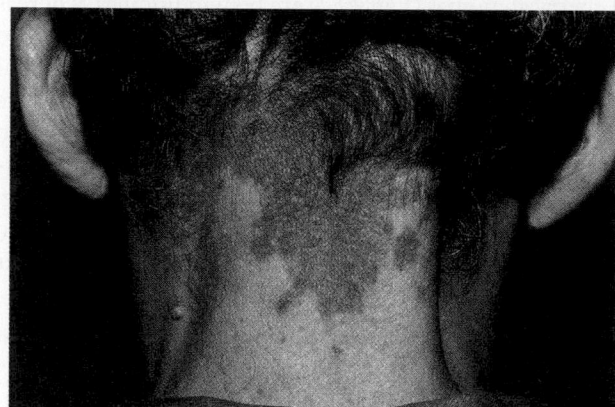

FIGURE 49.8 Port-wine stain.

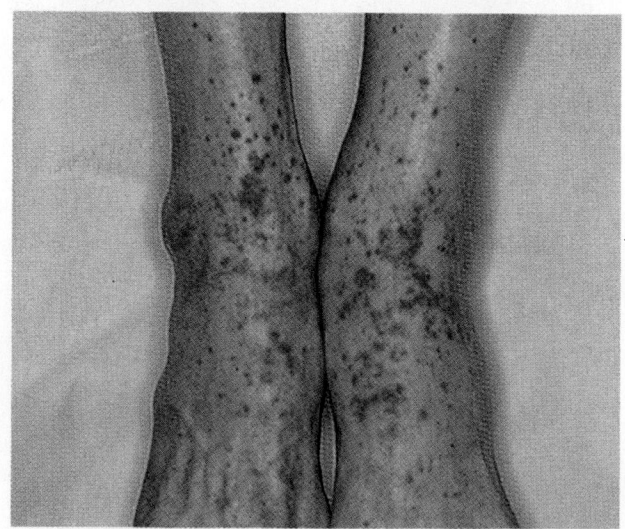

FIGURE 49.9 Petechial rash.

characteristics of lesions are documented, the anatomical location, type of lesion, color, distribution, and arrangement are identified. **Primary lesions** may emerge as a direct result of an infectious disease process, an allergic reaction, or an environmental cause. In addition, birthmarks are considered to be primary lesions and most often present as macules or patches. Primary lesions are described in Table 49.8. **Secondary lesions** describe a transformation of the primary lesion that may be caused by manual disturbance of the site that may develop secondary to itching or picking at the lesion, the treatment method implemented, or advancement of the underlying disease. Terms such as *clustered and coalesced* may be used to describe lesions that are grouped together or merge together. Secondary lesions are described in Table 49.9. Distribution refers to the extent and pattern of the lesions, and Table 49.10 provides an overview for commonly used terminology. The nurse describes in detail the arrangement of lesions when there are multiple affected areas.

Screening for Malignancies of the Skin

Nevi, or moles, are circumferential, benign epidermal or dermal growths that are less than 1 cm in size and more common in patients with lighter skin tones. During skin assessment, the nurse evaluates these sites for cancerous cell changes. Guidelines from Table 49.11 offer an efficient way to identify when moles require evaluation from a skin care expert.

Assessment of Dark Skin

Genetic predisposition and the level of activity of the melanocytes determine skin color, and when these factors produce darker skin tones, the assessment of erythema, cyanosis, and pallor becomes very difficult to visually detect. Specifically, erythema often appears as a deeper shade of the patient's natural skin color, and cyanosis and pallor may be noticeable only when assessing mucosal membranes or capillary refill. Therefore, the nurse uses information gathered from the patient's history and physical inspection and palpation to make an accurate assessment.

The nurse first questions the patient about normal skin appearance to better identify skin variations that may require further investigation. Visual inspection assists in identifying skin areas with an appearance that is inconsistent with the patient's natural skin tone. The nurse uses touch to detect temperature variations and the presence of edema, induration, or pain. If areas of suspected injury are noted, an interprofessional treatment approach is implemented.

For patients in acute and long-term care settings, research supports using a proven risk assessment tool such as the Braden scale to predict risk for subtle skin changes caused

Table 49.8 Primary Skin Lesions

Lesion	Characteristics and Size	Examples	
Macule 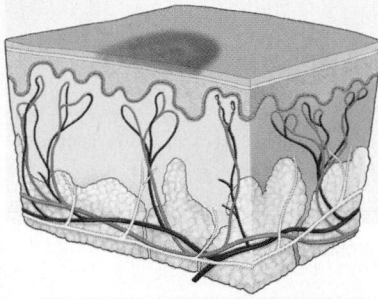	• Circumscribed • Flat • Nonpalpable • Shade other than skin color • Less than 1 cm in diameter	• Freckles • Flat moles • Petechiae	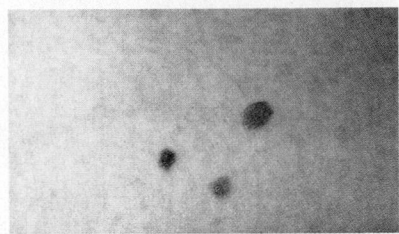 Flat moles
Patch 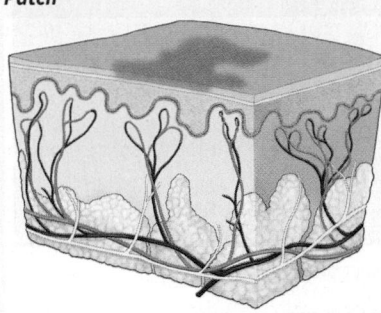	• Irregularly shaped macule • Greater than 1 cm in diameter	• Port-wine stain • Mongolian spots • Vitiligo	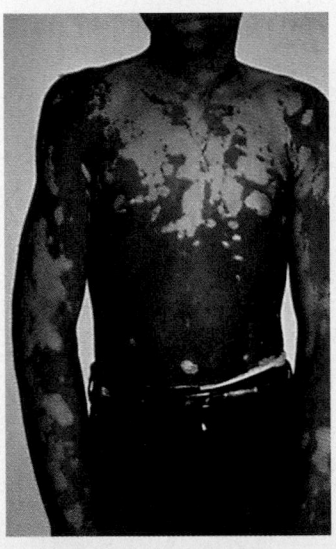 Vitiligo
Papule 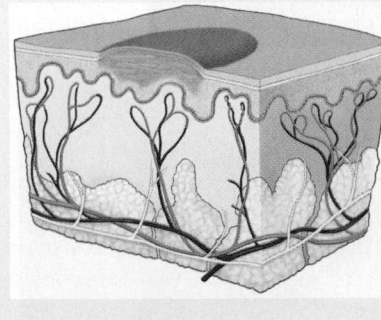	• Circumscribed • Elevated • Palpable • Firm • Located in epidermis or dermis • Less than 1 cm in diameter	• Elevated moles • Lichen planus • Warts	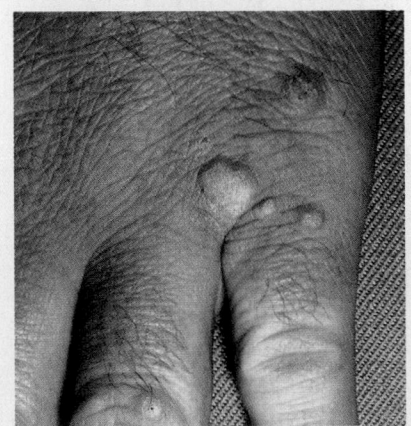 Warts

Continued

Table 49.8 Primary Skin Lesions—cont'd

Lesion	Characteristics and Size	Examples	
Plaque 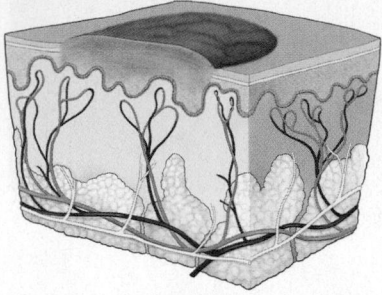	• Flat • Elevated • Firm • Rough • Greater than 1 cm in diameter	• Atopic dermatitis • Psoriasis • Mycosis fungoides • Eczema	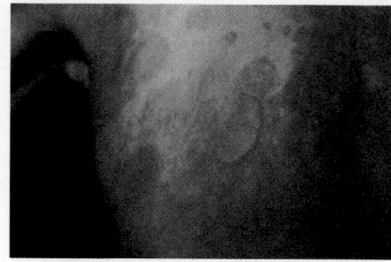 Mycosis fungoides
Wheal 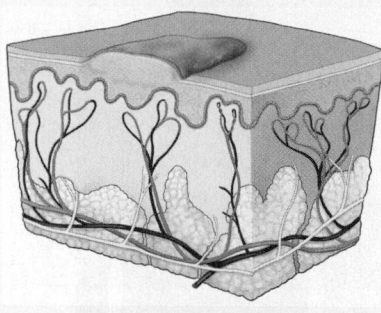	• Irregularly shaped • Elevated • Solid • Frequently pale red in color • Caused by edema • Size varies	• Insect bites • Allergic reaction	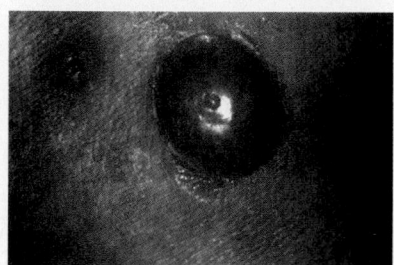 Insect bites
Nodule 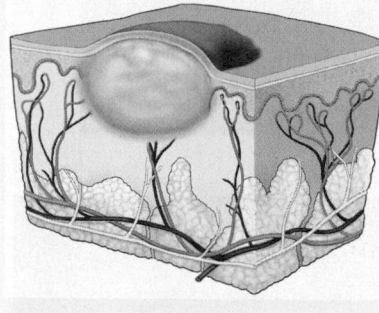	• Circumscribed • Elevated • Palpable • Firm or soft • Located in the dermis or hypodermis • 1–2 cm in diameter	• Lipoma	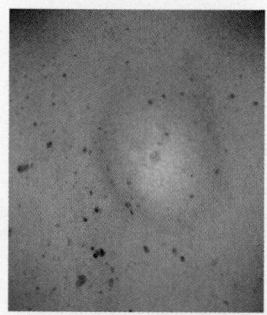 Lipoma
Tumor 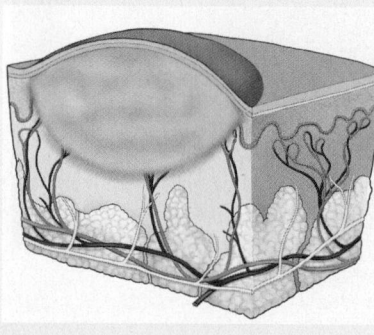	• Variable in shape • Elevated • Solid • Located in the dermis • Greater than 2 cm in diameter	• Lipoma • Cancer • Benign growth	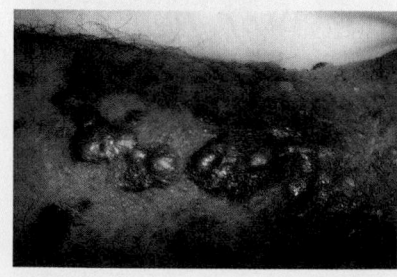 Lymphoma

Table 49.8 Primary Skin Lesions—cont'd

Lesion	Characteristics and Size	Examples	
Cyst 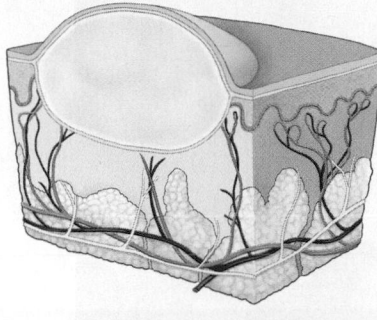	• Circumscribed • Elevated • Filled with liquid or solid substance • Located in dermis or hypodermis • Size varies	• Epidermoid cyst • Sebaceous cyst	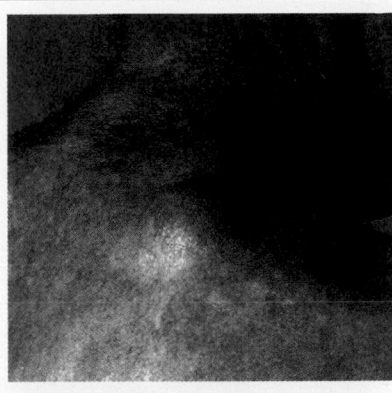 Epidermoid cyst
Vesicle 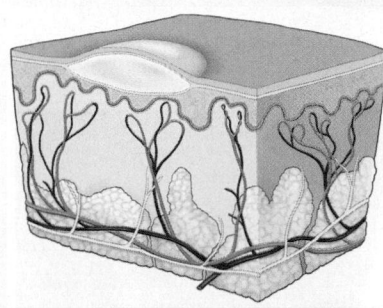	• Circumscribed • Elevated • Filled with serous fluid • Located in epidermis • Less than 1 cm in diameter	• Small blister • Varicella • Herpes zoster • Herpes simplex	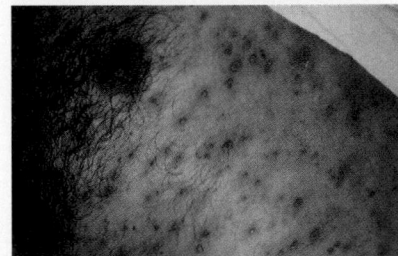 Varicella (Chickenpox)
Bulla 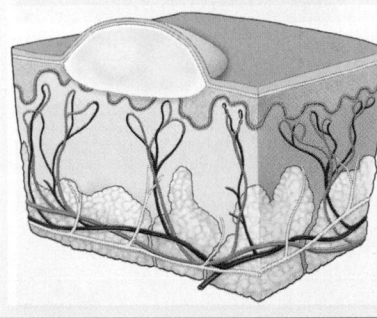	• Same characteristics as vesicle • Greater than 1 cm in diameter	• Large blister • Partial-thickness burns • Pemphigus	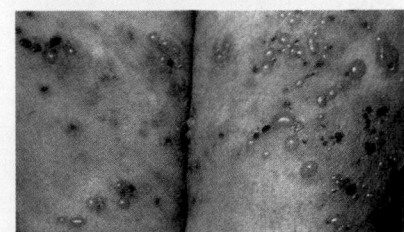 Pemphigus vulgaris
Pustule 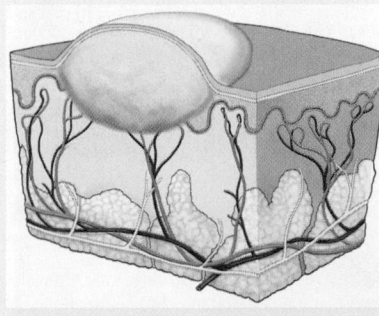	• Same characteristics as vesicle • Filled with purulent fluid • Size varies	• Acne • Folliculitis	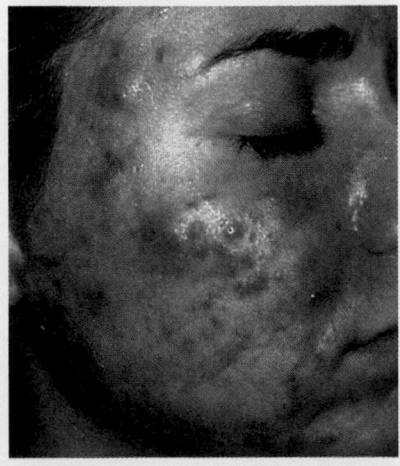 Acne

Table 49.9 Secondary Skin Lesions

Lesion	Characteristics and Size	Examples	
Scale 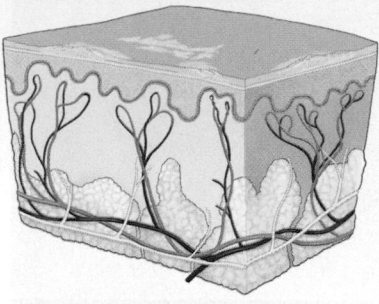	• Irregular shape • Flakes of stratum corneum • May be dry or oily • Size varies	• Skin flaking after a medication rash	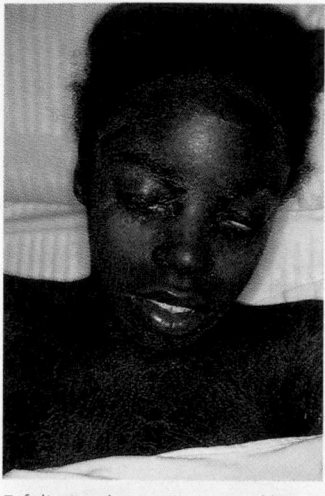 Exfoliative dermatitis caused by medication reaction
Lichenification 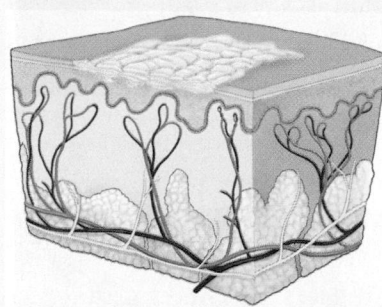	• Irregular shape • Excessive manipulation (i.e., scratching) causes epidermis to become rough and thick • Size varies	• Chronic dermatitis	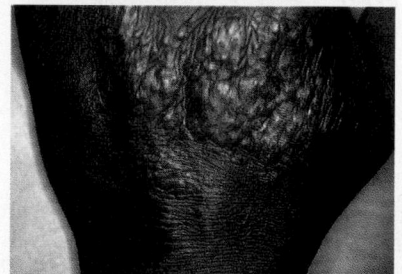 Lichen simplex chronicus
Excoriation 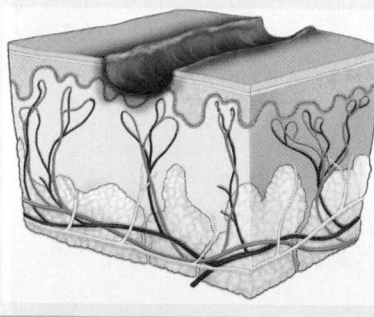	• Linear • Hollowed-out appearance • Wound bed is dry • Size varies	• Abrasions from scratching	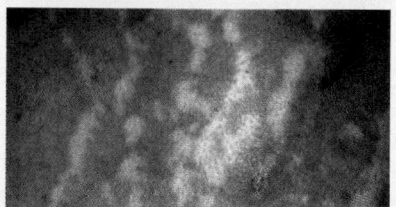 Linear excoriation from uremic pruritus
Fissure 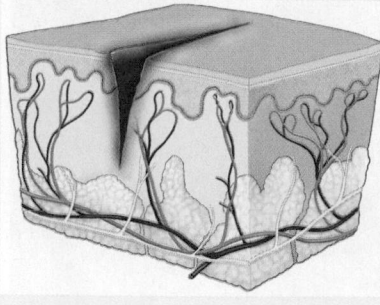	• Linear • Cracked tissue that may extend into dermis • Wound bed may be moist or dry • Size varies	• Athlete's foot	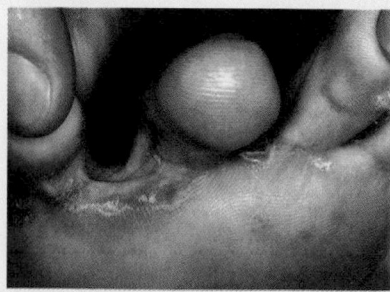 Athlete's foot

Table 49.9 Secondary Skin Lesions—cont'd

Lesion	Characteristics and Size	Examples	
Erosion 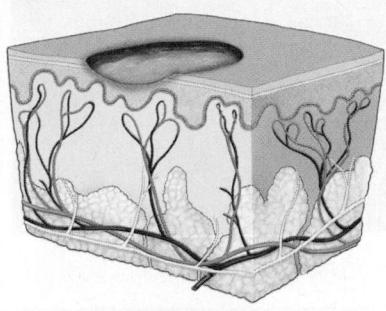	• Circumscribed • Limited to epidermis • Red, moist, and concave wound bed • Heals without scar formation • Size varies	• Open vesicles or bullae	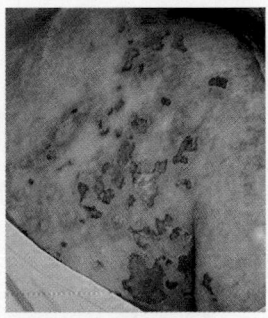 Pemphigus vulgaris open bullae
Ulcer 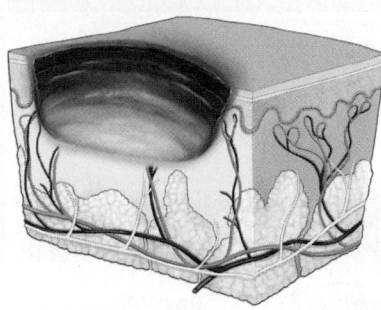	• Shape varies • Depth varies – may extend into fascia or down to tendon or bone • Cause varies – frequently associated with immobility, excessive moisture, highly acute illness that minimizes perfusion to skin • Heals by scar formation • Size varies	• Pressure injury	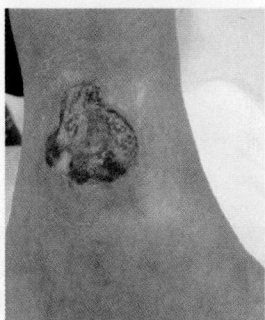 Leg ulcer
Crust 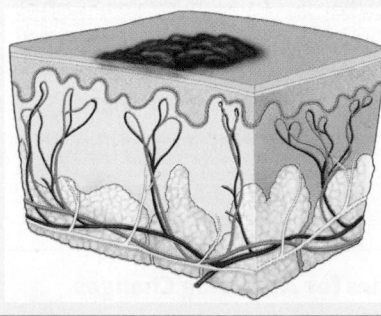	• Shape varies • Dried exudate from a wound bed (serum, blood, or pus) • Color varies depending on source of exudate • Size varies	• Scab • Eczema • Impetigo	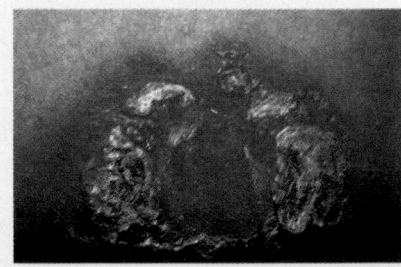 Impetigo
Atrophy 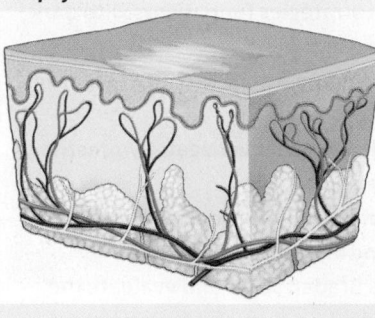	• May be localized or generalized • Describes thinning epidermis, dermis, or both • Skin appears thin and tears easily • Size varies	• Skin in older adults • Striae	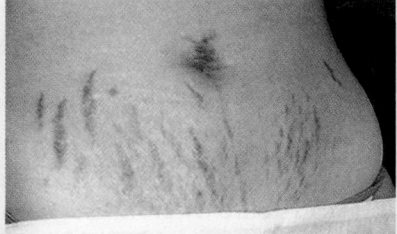 Stretch marks

Continued

Table 49.9 Secondary Skin Lesions—cont'd

Lesion	Characteristics and Size	Examples	
Scar	• Shape varies • Fibrous connective tissue that fills into wound bed that extends into the dermis and below • Scar tissue has 80% of the tensile strength of normal skin tissue, so the site is at increased risk for future damage • Size varies	• Healed wounds • Surgical sites	 Surgical site

Table 49.10 Terms to Describe Distribution and Arrangement of Skin Lesions

Distribution	
Localized	Limited to a small area
Regional	Distributed across a specific body part
Generalized	Distributed across numerous body parts
Arrangement	
Annular	Ring-shaped
Iris/Target lesions	Concentric rings
Linear	In a line
Polymorphous	Presenting in several different shapes
Zosteriform	Follows a dermatome
Satellite	Outlying lesion near a larger area of lesions

Table 49.11 Guidelines for Abnormal Skin Growths

Characteristic	Normal Finding	Possible Malignancy
Shape	Symmetrical	Asymmetrical
Border	Regular	Irregular or blurring edges
Color	No color variation	Mixture of shades or colors
Diameter	Less than 6 mm	Greater than 6 mm and evolving or expanding

by immobility, moisture, and inadequate nutrition. The National Pressure Ulcer Advisory Panel has stated that nursing home residents with darkly pigmented skin have increased incidence of pressure injury in comparison to Caucasian residents. Difficulty with identifying the initial color change associated with tissue damage in darker skin leads to a delay in pressure injury identification and initiation of treatment.

> **Safety Alert** **Guidelines for Assessing Changes in Dark Skin**
>
> The following assessment strategies for patients with dark pigmented skin should be used:
> 1. Gather subjective information from the patient regarding normal skin appearance.
> 2. Use inspection and palpation to investigate symmetrical differences in skin tone and texture.
> 3. Use touch to detect increased heat, edema, bogginess (excessive softness), and induration.
> 4. Complete the patient's Braden score and evaluate the level of mobility to guide the selection of preventive measures.

5. Pay particular attention to skin covering pressure points and areas where the patient reports increased pain or discomfort.
6. Document findings upon completion of the skin assessment and closely monitor for any change in the patient's normal skin appearance.

Braden Scale

In all healthcare settings, nurses must be knowledgeable about the risk of pressure injury as well as prevention strategies. The **Braden scale** is a commonly used tool that assists the nurse with identifying patients who are at risk for pressure-related skin damage. This tool requires the nurse to evaluate specific parameters for each patient: sensory perception, moisture, activity, mobility, nutrition, friction, and shear. Scores can range from 6 to 23, with a score of 1 or 2 in the mobility category as the most sensitive indicator for risk of pressure injury. Lower total scores indicate higher overall risk for developing alterations in skin integrity. Refer to Chapter 50 for further details about Braden scoring.

When a patient has a Braden score of 18 or lower, the nurse uses clinical decision-making skills to implement prevention strategies that address specific patient needs. Prevention measures are nurse-centered interventions that aim to redistribute pressure and include manual turning and repositioning for patients with decreased mobility, chair seat cushions that redistribute pressure, keeping the head of the bed lower than 30 degrees when patients are not at risk for aspiration, and heel protection. Certified wound ostomy continence nurses (CWOCNs) specialize in evaluating risk, recommending prevention and treatment strategies, and teaching patients, families, and staff about pressure injuries in many healthcare settings. See Box 49.2 for the CWOCN's job description.

Hair Assessment

Color, cleanliness, quantity, thickness, texture, and distribution and lubrication of the patient's hair are evaluated during the skin assessment. Before physical assessment and palpation, the nurse questions the patient about recent or gradual changes in the texture or pattern of hair on all body surfaces. Underlying illness, nutritional deficits, medications, stress, and unhealthy dieting may cause hair loss or textural changes.

Regular and thorough hair hygiene helps to minimize discomfort and skin irritation. If a patient complains of discomfort, the nurse evaluates the area for abnormalities such as lesions, erythema, dandruff, and the presence of lice infestation. When the scalp is assessed, it is important to inspect for irregularly shaped moles or skin growths because patients are not able to independently visualize this body surface.

Box 49.2 Role of the Certified Wound Ostomy Continence Nurse

Wound Ostomy Continence Nurses Function in the Following Ways:

- Provide consultation that reflects best practices for managing patients with wounds of various etiologies, urostomies, colostomies, ileostomies, fistulas, and continence problems
- Suggest specialized devices for pressure redistribution to help prevent formation of or minimize deterioration of wounds affected by pressure
- Participate in educating staff, patients, and families about wound, skin care, and ostomy management strategies
- Conduct research to further the body of knowledge related to wound, ostomy, and continence issues

Adapted from Wound Ostomy and Continence Nursing Society. http://www.wocn.org/

The quantity, quality, and distribution of hair have a wide range of normal variations, and the nurse focuses on gathering information about any deviations from the individual's usual hair characteristics. For example, decreased amounts of hair and increased dryness of skin on the lower extremities indicate ischemic skin changes usually associated with arterial disease. Although gradual hair loss can be part of the normal aging cycle, many etiologies and medications can contribute to hair loss. Alopecia is the general term used to describe hair loss (Fig. 49.10), and the degree and pattern of loss varies on the basis of etiology (Table 49.12). **Hirsutism** describes excessive male-pattern hair growth in women (Fig. 49.11). An example is a female with male hair patterns on the face, chest, areolae, lower back, linea alba, and buttocks. Causes include ovarian disorders such as polycystic ovary syndrome, adrenal gland disorders, and long-term glucocorticoid therapy that leads to Cushing's syndrome. Because hair is often viewed as a cosmetic feature, the nurse focuses on changes in the pattern and texture of the hair that may be a sensitive subject for the patient.

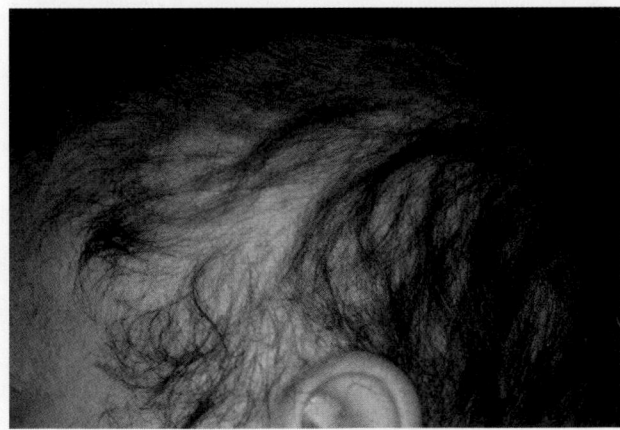

FIGURE 49.10 Alopecia secondary to chemotherapy.

Table 49.12 Causes of Alopecia

Focal (Localized) Hair Loss	Etiologies
	• Genetic predisposition
	• Scarring
	• Postmenopausal state
	• Inflammatory disorders
	• Localized radiation therapy
	• Androgen medications including anabolic steroids, tamoxifen, nortestosterone contraceptive pills

Global (Diffuse) Hair Loss	Etiologies
	• Postpartum state
	• Surgery
	• High fever
	• Nutrient deficiency and unhealthy diets
	• High-acuity illness
	• Emotional stress
	• Radiation therapy to the head
	• Heavy metal poisoning
	• Medications including angiotensin-converting enzyme inhibitors, anticoagulants, antiparkinsonian and antiseizure agents, beta blockers, birth control pills, histamine blockers
	• Chemotherapy including alkylating agents
	• Chronic disease states including renal or liver failure, thyroid disease, autoimmune disease (i.e., lupus, inflammatory bowel disease)

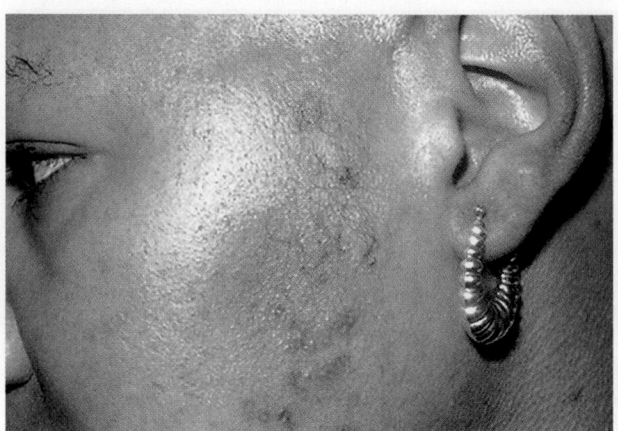

FIGURE 49.11 Hirsutism of face.

Nail Assessment

Systemic illness, local infection, or occupational exposures contribute to variations in nail color, shape, consistency, and lesion formation. Because there are many causes for nail abnormalities, the key nursing intervention is to collect a thorough history about the disorder, ascertain whether changes are acute or chronic, and document findings. An interprofessional approach is frequently used to determine the etiology and manage treatment for nail disorders. The color, shape, and consistency of nails, along with the presence and characteristics of lesions, provide important information about the nails and overall health status.

Color

The color of the nail beds provides information about perfusion status as well as chronic illness. Normal capillary refill time (CRT) is less than 2 seconds. Common variations in nail bed coloration and their causes are listed in Table 49.13.

Shape

A normal nail adheres to the nail bed, is surrounded on three sides by the nail folds, and is slightly convex in shape. Alterations in nail shape often indicate chronic disease states.

Consistency

The consistency of the nail should be firm, and the underlying nail bed color should be visible. Overly thick nails are often a result of advanced age, infection, or heredity as well as **onycholysis**, which refers to the nail plate detaching from the nail bed. Additional variations in nail consistency are described in Table 49.13.

Lesions

Nail bed and nail fold lesions may be associated with a wide variety of skin conditions (Table 49.14). When nail conditions are present, bacterial or fungal pathogens may exacerbate the condition. Skin cancers such as squamous cell carcinoma and melanoma may become visible under the nail bed or on folds surrounding the nail.

CASE STUDY: EPISODE 3

Overall, Ms. Bloom's skin has a healthy appearance. All of her nail beds are pale pink and display CRT of less than 2 seconds. She appears to have adequate moisture balance as evidenced by the absence of cracks, excessive dryness, or scabs. Skin, hair, and nails are clean and well-groomed. Hair distribution is appropriate on the basis of age and gender. The rash is located below the neck on her anterior chest wall and measures 6 cm × 8 cm × 0 cm, which correlates to the length times width times depth. The site has erythema with a well-defined border and increased warmth in comparison with surrounding skin. Within the 6 cm × 8 cm × 0 cm erythematous area, there are scattered, serous-filled, intact vesicles that are localized to the chest. The affected area appears to have increased moisture, but there are no localized signs of infection. Ms. Bloom reports a low-grade fever, pruritus, and burning. The provider orders the collection of a sterile swab culture of a vesicle base to rule out an infectious source…

Connection Check 49.3

Which clinical finding requires additional investigation by the nurse?
A. CRT less than 2 seconds
B. New-onset petechial rash
C. A macule with symmetrical shape, regular border, and uniform color
D. Pale or cyanotic nail bed after exposure to cold temperatures

---

Table 49.13 Variations in Nail Color, Shape, and Consistency

VARIATIONS IN NAIL COLOR

Color	Significance	
Yellow	Yellow nail syndrome is associated with lymphedema and chronic respiratory diseases	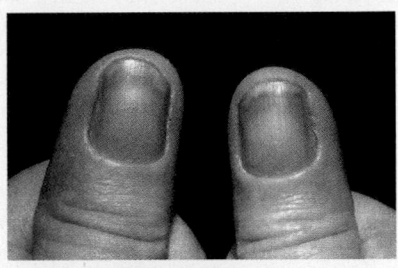 Yellow nail syndrome
White (opaque)	Abnormal keratinization of nail matrix that may be caused by cirrhosis, inflammatory bowel disease, or heredity	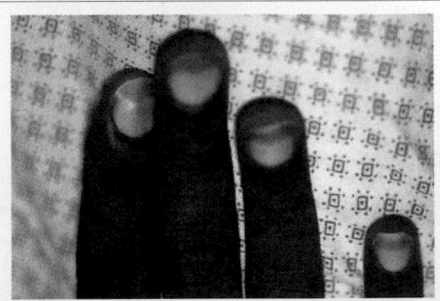 Half-and-half nails of chronic renal disease
Partially opaque nails	Terry's nails, white, ground glass appearance, may be associated with chronic diseases including congestive heart failure, end-stage renal disease, liver disorders, and diabetes mellitus	
Cyanotic	Decreased perfusion, respiratory failure, or cold temperatures	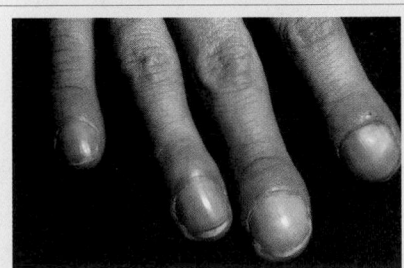 Blue (cyanotic) nails with clubbing

Continued

Table 49.13 Variations in Nail Color, Shape, and Consistency—cont'd

Color	Significance	
Longitudinal red to brown lines	Splinter hemorrhages that may indicate bacterial endocarditis or nail trauma	Splinter hemorrhages caused by bacterial endocarditis

VARIATIONS IN NAIL SHAPE

Shape	Significance	
Spoon shape (Koilonychia)	Nails become concave in shape, which may indicate iron-deficiency anemia, sulfur protein deficiency, hyperthyroidism, idiopathic or hereditary cause	Koilonychia
Nail clubbing	Enlarged fingertip caused by the expansion of the soft tissues surrounding the nail, which may be associated with long-standing cardiopulmonary conditions, liver disease, gastrointestinal tract diseases	Late clubbing

VARIATIONS IN NAIL CONSISTENCY

Consistency	Significance	
Brittle nails	Nails are very dry and crack easily; common conditions include diabetes mellitus, hypothyroidism, malnutrition, and gout	Brittle nails
Pitting	Multiple small depressions are present in the nail bed; commonly associated with psoriasis, lichen planus, rheumatoid arthritis, and eczema	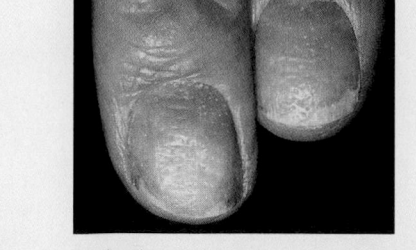 Pitting in psoriasis

Table 49.13 Variations in Nail Color, Shape, and Consistency—cont'd

Consistency	Significance	
Transverse or Beau's lines	Horizontal grooves in the nail plate that may indicate severe illness, malnutrition, high fever, or chemotherapy treatment	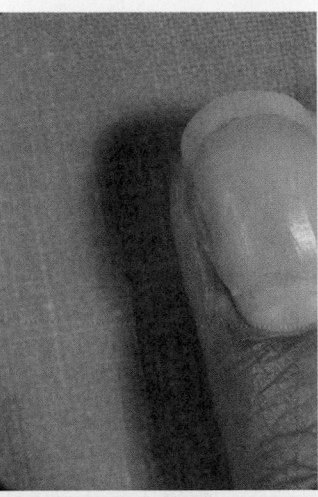 Beau's Lines

Table 49.14 Nail Lesions

NAIL LESIONS ASSOCIATED WITH SKIN ABNORMALITIES

Skin Disease	Appearance	
Psoriasis	Nails become thin and rough with dry, flaky lesions present on nail folds	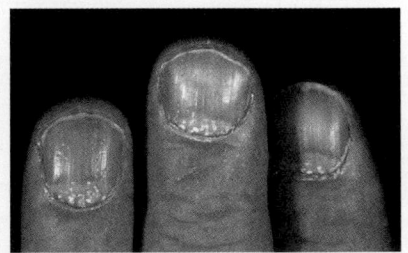 Psoriasis
Chemical or allergic dermatitis	Damaged nail plate with surrounding skin inflammation associated with an exogenous agent	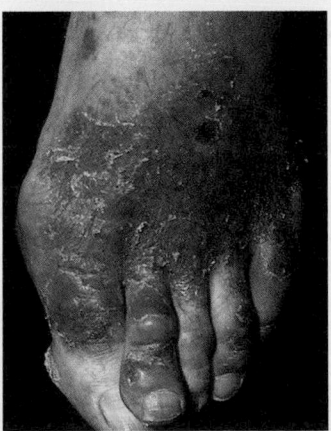 Allergic dermatitis

Continued

Table 49.14 Nail Lesions—cont'd

COMMON INFECTIONS THAT CAUSE NAIL LESIONS

Infective Agent	Presentation
Paronychia (bacterial)	Skin infection of the nail fold
Onychomycosis (fungal)	Nails appear yellowed, thick, and inflamed and grow in an unusual shape

Bacterial paronychia

Onychomycosis in a patient with diabetes

AGE-RELATED SKIN CHANGES

The performance of the five basic functions of the skin (protection, temperature regulation, vitamin D metabolism, sensation, and excretion) becomes less efficient as the body ages. In older adults, the skin becomes increasingly fragile, takes longer to heal, and is more prone to age-related skin conditions (Table 49.15).

Structurally, the vascularity of the dermis decreases, which leads to slower healing rates and a thinner dermis. In addition, the cycle of maturation of the epidermis begins to slow by approximately 50%, and this delay interrupts wound contraction. Flattening of the rete ridges weakens the strength of the epidermal-dermal junction, thus increasing the risk for skin tearing even with minor trauma. Collagen and elastin begin to steadily break down, which weakens the tensile strength of the skin. These structural changes cause the skin to function less effectively as a barrier and increases the risk for damage.

In addition to structural changes that affect the skin's protective ability, there are changes that occur in the immune system cells found in the skin. With age, the quantity of Langerhans and mast cells decreases, and this negatively impacts the body's ability to recognize and mobilize an immediate inflammatory response to pathogen invasion. Additionally, fewer active melanocytes increase the risk for sun-related skin damage.

Temperature regulation and excretion become less efficient because of decreased subcutaneous tissue, fewer sweat glands, and reduced vascularity. These changes increase the risk for exposure-related injury such as heat stroke and hypothermia. Older individuals also develop a decreased perception of injury because fewer sensory receptors are present in the skin layers. Hair and nail growth rates decrease as well. See Geriatric/Gerontological Considerations for an overview of specialized skin care for older patients because of their increased susceptibility to complications from alterations in skin integrity.

Table 49.15 Common Age-Related Skin Conditions

Condition	Appearance	Description	Medical Management
Xerosis	Skin appears rough and scaly; it may be erythematous and cracked Frequently located on extremities (Fig. 49.12)	Dry skin that is very uncomfortable. Patients often describe pruritus or burning.	Mild, pH-balanced soaps are used for bathing. Limit bathing time to 10 minutes and use warm water. Twice daily use of moisturizers is encouraged.
Eczema	Erythema, weeping, crusting, scales, and severe pruritus (Fig. 49.13)	Skin inflammation (or dermatitis) that may become chronic with scratching and rubbing	Topical steroids
Psoriasis	Thick, flaky, silvery skin covering circumferential red patches; skin, hair, and nails may be affected (Fig. 49.14)	These lesions emerge from overproduction of epidermal cells. These sites may not be pruritic.	Topical steroids
Herpes zoster (shingles)	Blistering and erythema along a dermatome (Fig. 49.15)	Results from resurgence of varicella virus. Subjective symptoms include burning and pain.	Lidocaine patch to affected area Antiviral medications

Geriatric/Gerontological Considerations

Skin Care Considerations for Older Adults

- Identify risk factors for impaired skin integrity as a result of immobility, chronological age, malnutrition, incontinence, compromised profusion, immunocompromised status, chronic medical conditions such as diabetes mellitus, spinal cord injury, or renal failure.
- Use mild, pH-balanced soaps for cleansing.
- Limit number of complete baths to two to three per week and alternate them with partial baths. Excessive bathing depletes aging skin of moisture and increases dryness.
- Bathe with warm water (between 90° F [32.2°C] and 105° F [40.8°C]), and limit bathing time to approximately 10 minutes.
- Apply moisturizers twice a day to prevent skin from drying out.
- Avoid skin care products that contain allergens such as lanolin, latex, and dyes.
- When incontinence is present, clean skin immediately after incontinence episode. Use skin barrier creams to shield skin from frequent exposure to moisture.
- During hospitalization, implement skin preservation measures including daily skin moisturizing, assist with frequent repositioning, and consider pressure redistribution devices for older adults with decreased mobility.
- Ensure fluid intake within cardiac and renal limits to a minimum of 1,500 mL per day.

Connection Check 49.4

The nurse is teaching skin care guidelines to the caretaker of a 79-year-old incontinent female who has a total Braden score of 14 with a score of 2 in the mobility category. What are appropriate educational priorities? *(Select all that apply.)*

A. Gently cleanse and dry the skin immediately after an incontinence episode
B. Use a toileting schedule to minimize episodes of incontinence
C. Aggressively clean the patient's skin after an incontinence episode
D. Assist the patient with repositioning at least every 2 hours
E. Use diapers for stool and urine containment

DIAGNOSTIC STUDIES AND NURSING CONSIDERATIONS

Laboratory Studies

Tissue Culturing

When a skin infection is suspected, microscopic examination of the tissue allows for identification of the pathogen. Methods of tissue collection vary depending on the lesion's characteristics but include the swab culture, needle aspiration culture, and biopsy. The method for collection varies depending on the appearance and extent of the affected area. Once the infective organism has been identified, the

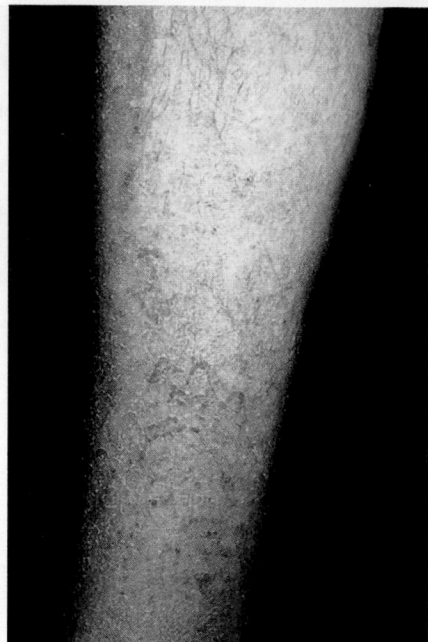

FIGURE 49.12 Xerosis (dermatitis).

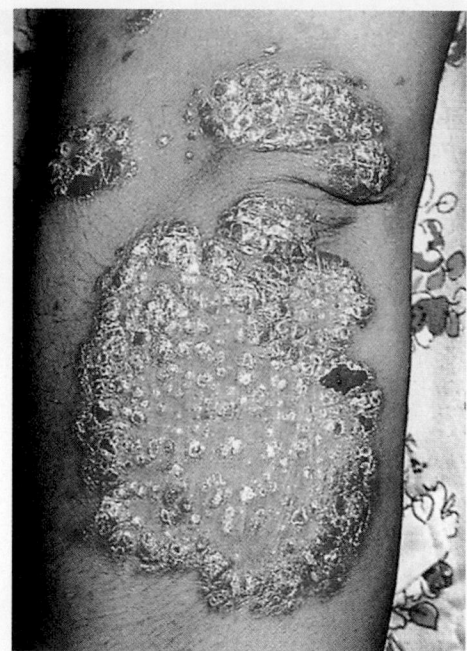

FIGURE 49.14 Psoriasis vulgaris: elbow.

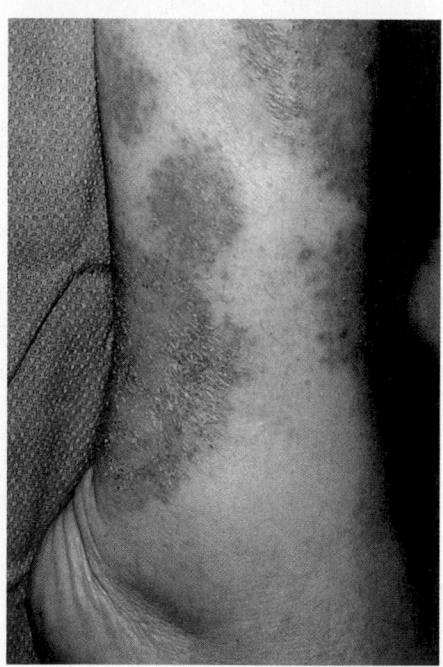

FIGURE 49.13 Eczema.

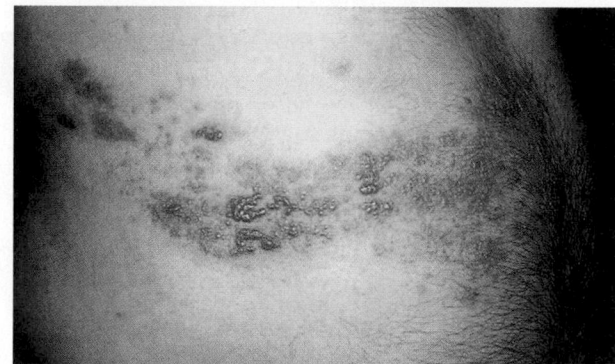

FIGURE 49.15 Varicella-zoster virus infection.

culture also determines the appropriate medication for treatment.

- Swab cultures collect fluid from the most superficial tissue layers. Although this process has minimal risk factors for bleeding or additional infection, it represents the least accurate type of culture. Swab cultures identify the correct infecting organism approximately 60% of the time.
- Needle aspiration cultures pinpoint the types of infective organisms that have invaded tissues surrounding the wound bed. This process involves inserting a needle into the periwound to aspirate fluid from surrounding tissues.

- Biopsy examines deeper layers of the skin for infecting organisms and represents the gold standard for wound culture. Types of tissue biopsy are discussed later in the chapter.

Nurses are responsible for obtaining a swab culture specimen (Box 49.3). Needle aspiration cultures and biopsies require advanced practice skills because of the use of sharp instruments to remove tissue, and these specimens are collected only by an advanced practice registered nurse or healthcare provider.

Diagnostic Studies

In addition to tissue surveillance by way of culturing, additional laboratory and diagnostic evaluations may be ordered to ensure appropriate treatment for patients who are suspected of having a more serious skin infection. These include:

1. Complete blood count (CBC) to evaluate for infection. This test can also help reveal if the infection is an acute occurrence.

Box 49.3 How to Obtain a Swab Culture (Levine Technique)

1. Evaluate the wound bed to locate a 1-cm² area of clean, viable wound tissue.
2. Prepare to use sterile technique and a sterile collection tube to obtain a specimen.
3. Clean the entire wound bed using a nonantiseptic solution such as normal saline to remove surface residue.
4. Moisten the sterile swab with normal saline.
5. Rotate swab with gentle pressure within a 1- to 2-cm² area of clean wound tissue for 5 seconds. The goal is to express fluid from the deeper layers of the wound into the entire swab.
6. Place the swab into the sterile container without touching other surfaces on the skin or the tube to reduce the risk of contamination.
7. Label the specimen with patient identifiers, wound site, and time collected.
8. Send the specimen to the laboratory without delay to reduce risk for contamination.

Adapted from Bryant, R. A., & Nix, D. P. (2012). *Acute & chronic wounds: Current management concepts* (4th ed.). St. Louis, MO: Mosby Elsevier.

2. Chemistry screening to evaluate protein status (albumin) as well as the accumulation of waste products in the blood (lactate, blood urea nitrogen, creatinine)
3. Blood cultures to identify whether the organism has entered the circulatory system.
4. Doppler ultrasound to evaluate blood flow through vessels. Skin infections may cause severe soft tissue swelling that occludes blood flow or contributes to clot development.

Significance of Abnormal Values

An abnormal value indicates that a skin infection is present, and Table 49.16 provides an overview of common skin infections. Treatment often involves topical and systemic medications; however, surgical tissue debridement may be indicated for severe, rapidly spreading conditions.

Fungal Infection

Fungal skin lesions often manifest as erythematous coloration, well-defined edges, scaling, pustules, papules, plaquelike distribution, and satellite lesions (Fig. 49.16). These rashlike lesions may emerge on any moist skin surface, and patients frequently report itching and burning from the affected area.

If pustules are present, an intact pustule should be removed and placed in a sterile container for analysis. The roof of the lesion is inspected for fungal characteristics. Skin scraping may be used in the absence of pustules; however, the test results may not be as accurate. During diagnostic evaluation of a fungal specimen, a potassium hydroxide (KOH) preparation is most frequently used because it partially dissolves the keratin protein so that the fungal cells become perceptible in the specimen.

Table 49.16 Categories of Skin Infections

Categories	Etiologies
Fungal infections	Candidiasis
	Dermatophytoses (tinea)
Bacterial infections	Folliculitis
	Intertrigo (inflammation on skin surfaces that rub together)
	Abscess
	Cellulitis
	Necrotizing fasciitis
Viral infections	Varicella
	Herpes simplex virus
	Herpes zoster
	Rubella
	Measles
	Human papillomavirus

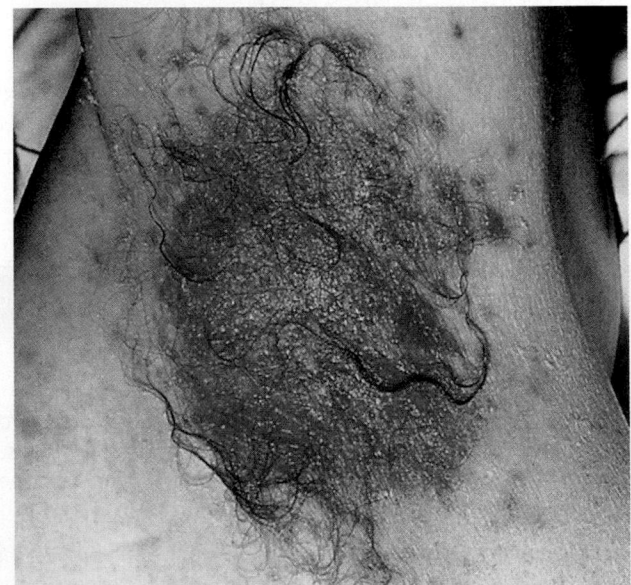

FIGURE 49.16 Cutaneous candidiasis.

Bacterial Infection

Bacterial skin conditions may range from a mildly uncomfortable pustule on a hair follicle to insidious infections that destroy the skin and fascia of an entire extremity. Because there are many types of bacterial skin infections with a variety of clinical presentations, culture or biopsy is very effective in the identification of the causative organisms. When intact fluid-filled lesions are present, the swabbing technique may be used to absorb aspirate from the wound base of vesicles, pustules, or bullae that may be cultured.

Viral Infection

Viral skin lesions often have a vesicular appearance and may be highly contagious. The primary method for culturing is gentle scraping of the vesicle base using a scalpel. When the affected area is on a mucous membrane, the site may be swabbed and sent for culture. If viral skin infections are severe, additional diagnostic testing may be indicated.

Patient Preparation

In preparation for a swab specimen or removal of a blister or pustule, the provider reinforces that the purpose of specimen collection is to assess for tissue infection. Obtaining consent and discussing possible complications are the responsibilities of the healthcare provider. Before the culture is completed, it is essential that the nurse ensures that the patient understands what to expect from the procedure.

Ideally, the specimen is collected before any antiseptic cleansers, topical or systemic antifungal, antibiotic, or antiviral medications are used for treatment. This helps ensure a representative specimen and ultimately helps identify the most effective pharmaceutical treatment. This guideline may not be realistic if the patient is severely ill, and in these cases, the safety of the patient takes precedence over tissue sample collection. Initially, the nurse ensures that the patient is stable before proceeding to specimen collection. A pain management plan must be in place and discussed with the patient before starting the procedure.

Nursing Implications

Nurses are frequently responsible for educating the patient about the skin condition and cause, treatment, and prevention. Also, nursing staff may be required to collect cultures using the swabbing technique described in Box 49.3.

Skin Biopsy

Skin biopsy is a key diagnostic tool that allows for microscopic examination of skin conditions or infections. Shave, punch, and excisional biopsies are commonly used techniques, and these techniques differ in the amount and depth of tissue removal. Biopsy is indicated for ulcers and nodules ensuring that all skin layers are scrutinized. When skin biopsy is completed in a timely fashion, it assists with diagnosis as well as identification of an appropriate treatment.

- Shave biopsy is used to collect superficial tissue samples of the epidermis and dermis. A sterile blade is used to remove a small piece of skin tissue, and healing occurs through tissue regeneration.
- A punch biopsy, which is the most frequently used technique, removes a circular, continuous section that contains epidermis, dermis, and upper layers of subcutaneous tissue. The sample is approximately 3 to 4 mm wide, and local analgesia is administered. Closure of the site may require minimal suturing.
- An excisional biopsy removes a relatively large, deep section of tissue. This technique may be used to remove an entire lesion, so sutures, a graft, or even a flap may be required to close the area.

Significance of Abnormal Values

After a skin biopsy, the specimen is analyzed. Common abnormal diagnoses include skin cancer, benign growths, bacterial or fungal infection, or inflammatory lesions. Table 49.17 provides information about common treatment plans. Removal procedures include excision, freezing with

Table 49.17 Treatment for Abnormal Biopsy Results

Laboratory Result	Treatment
Malignant growth: 　**Melanoma** 　**Basal cell carcinoma** 　**Squamous cell carcinoma**	Treatment involves surgical removal of the lesion as well as removal of 5–6 mm of healthy tissue surrounding the lesion to ensure safe margins. Depending on the size and extent of the affected area, surgical removal may be done at one time or over multiple visits.
Benign growth	Lesion may be removed on the basis of patient preference. If the lesion has the potential to become cancerous, the site is excised.
Bacterial infection	Completing a Gram stain of the biopsy helps to determine whether the infective agent is gram-positive or gram-negative. On the basis of this information, broad-spectrum antibiotics are started. When the organism has been isolated, the antibiotic choice may be re-evaluated. Also, a complete blood count, ultrasound, and/or blood cultures may be appropriate to evaluate the systemic response to infection.
Fungal infection	Potassium hydroxide preparation is used to reveal the fungal infection. Depending on the extent of the affected area, systemic antifungal medications may be added to a topical antifungal treatment.
Inflammatory lesions	There are many causes for inflammatory lesions that range from internal sources such as lupus or inflammatory bowel disease to external sources that trigger a contact dermatitis. Treatment must be guided by the underlying etiology. This requires blood work and additional diagnostic testing.

Sources: DiGiulio, M., Jackson, D., & Keough, J. (2013). *Medical-surgical nursing demystified: A self-teaching guide.* New York, NY: McGraw Hill; American Academy of Dermatology guidelines. (2015). Biopsy and pathology. Retrieved from https://www.aad.org/education/clinical-guidelines

liquid nitrogen (**cryosurgery**), a type of surgery that involves the use of extreme cold to destroy abnormal tissues, laser removal, and topical creams.

Patient Preparation

When preparing a patient for skin biopsy, the provider ensures that the patient understands what to expect during the procedure. Before the procedure, patients are questioned about recently ingested medications and bleeding abnormalities so that patients with increased risk for bleeding are managed safely. The pain management plan that is appropriate for the type of biopsy being completed is explained, as well as the most common risks associated with this procedure, including infection and scarring.

Before skin layers are removed via biopsy in the severely acute, immunocompromised, and chronically ill patient populations, the individual patient risk factors and goals for care are considered and discussed with the interprofessional team. Ultimately, these surveillance techniques can increase the patient's risk for infection because the process creates a wound bed and provides an entry site for additional pathogens.

Nursing Implications

Removal of the skin tissue sample is performed by a specially prepared healthcare provider. Nursing responsibilities focus on monitoring and supporting the patient's response to the procedure. After the procedure, the nurse ensures that the patient understands the general biopsy site care instructions (Box 49.4). Depending on the extent and depth of the tissue removed, site care instructions may require individualization.

The comprehensive assessment of the integumentary system provides an overview of the overall health status, as well as specific data related to the status of the skin, nails, and hair. Table 49.18 provides guidelines related to providing care to patients with impaired skin integrity.

Connection Check 49.5

A patient presents with a new-onset, erythematous rash that contains intact pustules. Subjective symptoms include itching and burning. Which diagnostic evaluation is most helpful in determining the underlying etiology?

A. Excisional biopsy
B. Skin scraping
C. Sterile collection of pustule roof
D. Cryosurgery

Connection Check 49.6

The nurse questions which intervention in the stable patient with the nursing diagnosis "Impaired skin integrity related to draining skin lesions on right lower extremity"?

A. Place patient on isolation precautions
B. Obtain a swab specimen from wound bed after cleansing with a non-antiseptic solution
C. Educate patient about wound and skin treatment regimen
D. Administer broad-spectrum antibiotic before obtaining a culture

Box 49.4 Biopsy Site Care Instructions

1. Leave the initial dressing in place for the rest of the day. A small amount of pink or red drainage is normal.
2. Change the dressing daily until the site has healed (usually 1–2 weeks). Healing is defined as the absence of open wounds.
3. When performing site care, wash and dry your hands. Wash the site with soap and water, then dry thoroughly. Cover with a Band-Aid or dressing and change it daily.
4. If erythema, edema, increased pain, or drainage develops, clean the site with hydrogen peroxide and cover it with the dressing. Contact the provider who collected the biopsy for further instructions.
5. Showering is permitted the day after the biopsy. While the site is healing, avoid activities that require full immersion in water such as swimming or soaking in a bath.

Adapted from Johns Hopkins Medicine, Patient Instructions for Biopsy Site Care; www.hopkinsmedicine.org.

Table 49.18 Evidence-Based Practice Guidelines for Impaired Skin Integrity Interventions

Intervention	Rationale
• Identify patients at risk for impaired skin integrity due to immobility, age, malnutrition, incontinence, compromised perfusion, immunocompromised status, chronic medical condition, such as diabetes mellitus, spinal cord injury, or renal failure.	Targeting risk variables can focus assessment on particular risk factors to guide prevention and interventions
• Assess site of skin impairment and determine cause of wound, lesion, pressure injury, or skin tear	The cause of the wound must be determined before appropriate interventions can be implemented

Continued

Table 49.18 Evidence-Based Practice Guidelines for Impaired Skin Integrity Interventions—cont'd

Intervention	Rationale
• Use a validated risk assessment tool such as the Braden scale to identify individuals at risk for skin breakdown due to pressure	Targeting variables can focus assessment on particular risk factors and guide prevention and care
• Inspect and monitor skin and high-risk areas such as bony prominences at least once a day for color changes, erythema, swelling, warmth, pain or other sign of infection, or changes in sensation	Systematic inspection can identify impending problems early
• Monitor the patient's skin care practices, type of cleansing agent, temperature of water, and frequency of skin cleaning. Cleanse the skin gently with pH-balanced cleansers.	Cleansing should not compromise the skin
• Individualize skin care plan according to the patient's skin condition and needs and preferences	Avoid harsh cleansing agents, hot water, extreme friction or force, or cleansing too frequently
• Monitor the patient's incontinence status and minimize exposure to moisture from perspiration or wound drainage.	Moisture may contribute to pressure injuries development by macerating the skin
• Evaluate for use of support surfaces (specialty mattresses, beds, chair cushion, or other devices	Pressure reducing devices limit risk of skin breakdown due to decreased tissue perfusion
• Assess nutritional status	Optimizing nutritional intake, including calories, fatty acids, protein, vitamins is needed to promote wound healing
• Interprofessional collaboration should be used for assessment and management	Collaboration promotes consistency, decreases costs, and reduces errors. The added expertise from all team members benefits not only the patient but the caregivers. Healthcare professionals involved in the care of patients must be willing and able to work together toward positive patient outcomes

Making Connections

CASE STUDY: WRAP-UP

On the basis of information gathered in the history and physical assessment, this rash is characteristic of an allergic contact dermatitis brought on by the recent change in the patient's fragrance. The nurse teaches Ms. Bloom to discontinue the new fragrance and explains how the rash may progress. Explaining that the contact with the new spray led to an acute allergic contact dermatitis, the nurse describes that the rash will most likely develop into vesicles opening into erosions that will then crust and eventually flake off.

Case Study Questions

1. Which skin layers have been affected by Ms. Bloom's allergic contact dermatitis?
   A. Dermis only
   B. Epidermis only
   C. Both epidermis and dermis
   D. Subcutaneous tissue

2. When a sterile swab specimen is collected, which statement best describes the correct technique?
   A. Rotate swab with gentle pressure within a 1- to 2-cm^2 area of nonviable wound tissue
   B. Saturate swab with drainage found in the base of the wound
   C. Rotate swab with gentle pressure within a 1- to 2-cm^2 area of clean wound tissue
   D. Clean the wound with an antiseptic solution before obtaining the specimen

3. What information is important to include regarding site care instructions for the healing rash?
   A. Clean skin with an abrasive surface to remove dried substances
   B. Moisturize the drying rash with emollients to soften and gently remove crusts
   C. Manually drain the vesicles
   D. Avoid showering while rash persists

4. The nurse recognizes which description as indicative of a vesicle?
   A. Less than 1 cm in diameter, circumscribed, elevated, serous-filled
   B. Size varies, circumscribed, elevated, pus-filled
   C. Less than 1 cm in diameter, circumscribed, elevated, palpable, firm
   D. Greater than 1 cm in diameter, flat, elevated, firm, rough

5. The nurse correlates which surveillance cell, present in the epidermal layers, as introducing the allergen to the T cells?
   A. Macrophage
   B. Merkel cells
   C. Mast cells
   D. Langerhans cells

CHAPTER SUMMARY

Water-resistant keratinocytes form the epidermis, hair, and nails, whereas the dermis contains blood vessels, nerves, immune system cells, dermal proteins, hair follicles, and sweat and sebaceous glands. All of these structures contribute to the integumentary functions of protection, temperature regulation, vitamin D metabolism, sensation, and excretion.

Comprehensive assessment of integumentary function requires collection of the patient's history followed by inspection and palpation. Integumentary assessment varies depending on the patient's presenting complaint. For example, in an ambulatory practice, the assessment may be focused on a new-onset skin condition that is confined to a specific body area, whereas in the inpatient setting with the complications of acute or chronic illness and immobility, the skin assessment should be conducted on all body surfaces at regular intervals in addition to the Braden scale to predict risk for pressure injury.

Depending on the setting and the extent of the skin condition, the history may include demographic data, comorbidities and medication history, family history, diet, and environmental factors such as occupational and sun exposure. The assessment of the skin, hair, and nails often occurs because of a change or deterioration in appearance or function; therefore, gathering the patient's subjective report represents a key assessment component. Important physical assessment guidelines for the skin include color, temperature, moisture, overall integrity, cleanliness, tissue loss, vascular markings, and lesions. For hair, it is important to observe for cleanliness, quantity, quality, and distribution. In the presence of nail abnormalities, the nurse evaluates for variations in color, shape, consistency, and lesion formation.

Skin changes that occur normally with aging lead to a slow deterioration in overall structure and function of the integumentary system. Specifically, aged skin has decreased vascularity, tensile strength, and immune cell surveillance; slower healing rates; and less-efficient temperature regulation and excretion mechanisms. When these natural skin changes are combined with excessive exposure to chemicals or sun, comorbidities that affect perfusion to skin layers, and medications that have skin-related side effects, serious complications may develop. Potential problems include pain-producing lesions, excessive hair growth or loss, wounds with delayed healing, alterations in the patient's body image, and infection.

Infectious sources may be fungal, bacterial, or viral in origin. Laboratory studies, which may include culture, site biopsy, CBC, chemistry screening, blood cultures, and ultrasound, may be used to identify the pathogen. Treatment varies depending on the extent and severity of the infection or other abnormality such as cancer. Nurses are responsible for collecting swab specimens, managing pain, monitoring the patient during specimen collection, and teaching the patient and family about expectations during the procedure and postprocedure site care. Any technique that requires a sharp instrument to remove the specimen should be completed only by an advanced practice nurse or provider.

Although the body maintains a healthy state, the skin, hair, and nails protect internal structures and support homeostasis. Conversely, during times of prolonged acute and chronic illness, these protective tissues may succumb to skin failure. The white paper published by the National Pressure Ulcer Advisory Panel recognizes that not all pressure injuries are preventable, especially in those at the end of life who are frail. If a terminal pressure injury develops and the healing process cannot be re-established in someone with a terminal illness, at the end of life, or in the critically ill person, then the primary goal should no longer be wound closure. Palliative wound care as a concept is still developing, and it is not restricted to hospice care; nor does it imply that curative treatments should not be implemented and cannot be effective. Instead, the primary goals should shift to symptom management.

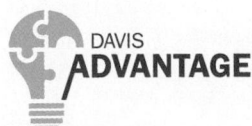

DAVIS ADVANTAGE | To explore learning resources for this chapter, go to **Davis Advantage** and find:
- Answers to in-text questions
- Chapter Resources and Activities
- NCLEX®-Style Chapter Review Questions
- Bibliography

Chapter 50

Coordinating Care for Patients With Skin Disorders

Catherine Ratliff

LEARNING OUTCOMES

Content in this chapter is designed to assist in:

1. Discussing the epidemiology of disorders of the skin
2. Correlating clinical manifestations to pathophysiological processes of:
   a. Bacterial skin infections
   b. Herpes simplex
   c. Fungal infections
   d. Psoriasis
   e. Skin trauma
   f. Pressure injuries
   g. Skin cancer
   h. Reconstructive surgery
3. Describing the diagnostic results used to confirm the diagnoses of skin disorders
4. Discussing the medical management of:
   a. Bacterial skin infections
   b. Herpes simplex
   c. Fungal infections
   d. Psoriasis
   e. Skin trauma
   f. Pressure injuries
   g. Skin cancer
   h. Reconstructive surgery
5. Describing complications associated with skin disorders
6. Developing a comprehensive plan of nursing care for patients with skin disorders
7. Designing a plan of care that includes pharmacological, dietary, and lifestyle considerations for patients with skin disorders
8. Describing the process and stages of wound healing

CONCEPTS

- Assessment
- Cellular Regulation
- Infection
- Medication
- Perfusion
- Promoting Health
- Skin Integrity

ESSENTIAL TERMS

Abrasion
Actinic keratosis
Angiogenesis
Basal cell carcinoma
Braden scale
Cellulitis
Debridement
Dermatophyte
Eschar
Excoriation
Exudate
Folliculitis
Fournier's gangrene
Full thickness
Furuncle
Granulation tissue
Herpes simplex virus (HSV)
Herpetic whitlow
Laceration
Maceration
Melanoma
Methicillin-resistant *Staphylococcus aureus* (MRSA)
Methicillin-sensitive *Staphylococcus aureus* (MSSA)
Mucocutaneous
Necrotizing fasciitis
Neoangiogenesis
Onycholysis
Onychomycosis
Partial thickness
Phases of wound healing
Pressure injury
Primary intention
Psoriasis
Quantitative tissue biopsy
Secondary intention
Shearing forces
Skin tear
Slough
Squamous cell carcinoma
Telangiectasias
Tertiary intention
Tinea
Tunneling
Undermining

Finding Connections

CASE STUDY: EPISODE 1

Follow this patient throughout the chapter.

Martin Parker is a 42-year-old man with a 20-year history of T-10 paraplegia from a skiing accident who presents with a left ischial pressure injury measuring 2 cm (L) × 3 cm (W) × 10 cm (D). His wound started about 5 years ago after a furuncle (boil) was opened and drained. He had debridement surgery in the past but was disappointed when this created a larger wound that still has not healed. He has never been told that he has osteomyelitis (bone infection) before. He is currently packing gauze in his wound and changing the dressing one or two times daily. There is undermining of 2 cm from 6 o'clock to 10 o'clock around the wound edge. Wound edges are rolling inward (epibole). The base of the wound is not visible. When probing the wound, the nurse feels exposed, rough bone. Exudate is thick, yellow, and malodorous. The packing in the wound is saturated, as is the secondary dressing over the top of the wound. The periwound skin is intact, and erythema extends greater than 5 cm from the wound's edge. No induration or hardness is palpated along the periwound skin. He has had night sweats over the past three nights but has not taken his temperature.

Mr. Parker has no comorbidities. He is on a strict bowel regimen where he uses an enema every other day to be continent of bowel movements. He catheterizes himself several times a day. He is an accountant and spends much of his time in his wheelchair. He has a pressure-reducing cushion on his wheelchair but does not do his "push-ups" as often as he should. He does not have a specialty mattress at home. Mr. Parker has a very supportive wife...

INTRODUCTION

The skin is the largest organ of the body and consists of two main layers: the epidermis (outer layer) and the dermis (inner layer). The primary function of an intact epidermis is protection, whereas the main function of the dermis is to provide strength, support, blood, and nutrients to the epidermis. Lastly, the subcutaneous tissue, which is composed of adipose tissue (fat), connective tissue, blood vessels, lymphatic vessels, and nerves, lies beneath the dermis. This layer helps to anchor the dermis to the underlying structures, provides insulation for temperature regulation, and provides cushion-like protection or padding for the skin and underlying structures.

The natural flora on the surface of the skin helps protect against harmful microorganisms. However, penetration of the skin from repeated exposure to environmental hazards, trauma, or chronic disease weakens the skin's protective function, increases the likelihood of skin breakdown, and places the patient at risk for infection. This chapter focuses on skin infections, selected skin disorders, skin trauma, and skin cancers. Additionally, reconstructive surgery for patients with a history of skin disorders is presented.

BACTERIAL SKIN INFECTIONS

Skin and soft tissue infections are categorized according to the depth of infection, tissues involved, and interventions necessary to resolve the infection (Box 50.1). The U.S. Food and Drug Administration classifies skin and soft tissue infections as uncomplicated or complicated. Uncomplicated skin and soft tissue infections include superficial **cellulitis** (a diffuse spreading infection of the dermis and subcutaneous tissues; Fig. 50.1), **folliculitis** (inflammation of the hair follicles; Fig. 50.2), impetigo (Fig. 50.3), **furuncles** (boils), simple abscesses, and minor wound infections. These infections usually respond to antibiotic therapy alone or surgical drainage with or without antibiotic therapy. Alternatively, complicated skin and soft tissue infections involve the invasion of deeper tissues by microorganisms, which usually requires considerable surgical **debridement** (removal of dead or infected skin to facilitate healing), as well as infections that occur in the presence of a systemic disease process that may affect the patient's response to therapy. As with most complicated skin and soft tissue infections, necrotizing soft tissue infections are wounds that contain dead, or necrotic, tissue that provides an optimum medium for bacterial growth and require surgical intervention. These infections can involve the dermis and subcutaneous tissues (necrotizing cellulitis), the fascia (**necrotizing fasciitis**), and the muscle. However, it is often difficult to determine the depth and severity of the infection at presentation. Thus, identifying tissue involvement, classifying the infection, and directing treatment can be challenging.

Table 50.1 lists commonly occurring uncomplicated skin and soft tissue infections, the causative organisms, a description of the infection, the presenting clinical manifestations, and the usual treatment. It is important to understand that treatment modalities can change significantly depending on the age of the patient and the strain of bacteria. Additionally, treatment varies for immunocompromised patients or those with other comorbidities.

Epidemiology

Uncomplicated skin and soft tissue infections occur in many settings, involve different bacteria, and are usually mild to moderate in severity. Most skin and soft tissue infections are caused by gram-positive bacteria such as *Staphylococcus aureus* and *Streptococcus pyogenes*.

Methicillin-resistant *Staphylococcus aureus* (MRSA) infections are categorized as either community acquired (CA-MRSA) or healthcare acquired (HA-MRSA), with

Box 50.1 Superficial Surgical Site Infections

The CDC defines a superficial surgical site infection as meeting the following criteria: infection occurring within 30 days after the operative procedure, involving only skin and subcutaneous tissue of the incision, and the patient has at least one of the following:

- Purulent drainage from the superficial incision
- Organisms isolated from an aseptically obtained culture from the superficial incision or subcutaneous tissue
- Superficial incision that is deliberately opened by a healthcare provider and is culture-positive or is not cultured and the patient has at least one of the following clinical manifestations: pain or tenderness, localized swelling, erythema, or heat (A culture-negative finding does not meet this criterion.)
- Diagnosis of a superficial incisional surgical site infection by the healthcare provider

The CDC defines a deep incisional surgical site infection as meeting the following criteria:

- Infection occurs within 30 or 90 days after the operative procedure, involves deep soft tissues of the incision (e.g., fascial and muscle layers), and the patient has at least one of the following clinical manifestations:
  - Purulent drainage from the deep incision
  - A deep incision that spontaneously dehisces (opens or separates) or is deliberately opened or aspirated by a healthcare provider and is culture-positive or is not cultured and the patient has at least one of the following clinical manifestations: fever (greater than 100.4°F [38°C]) or localized pain or tenderness (A culture-negative finding does not meet this criterion.)
  - An abscess or other evidence of infection involving the deep incision that is detected on anatomical or histopathological examination or imaging study

Organ/space surgical site infections must meet the following criteria:

- Infection occurs within 30 or 90 days after the procedure and involves any part of the body deeper than the fascial/muscle layers that is opened or manipulated during the operative procedure, and the patient has at least one of the following clinical manifestations:
- Purulent drainage from a drain that is placed into the organ/space (e.g., closed suction drainage system, open drain, T-tube drain, CT-guided drainage)
- Organisms isolated from an aseptically obtained culture of fluid or tissue in the organ/space
- An abscess or other evidence of infection involving the organ/space that is detected on gross anatomical or histopathological examination or imaging study

CDC, Centers for Disease Control and Prevention; *CT,* computed tomography.

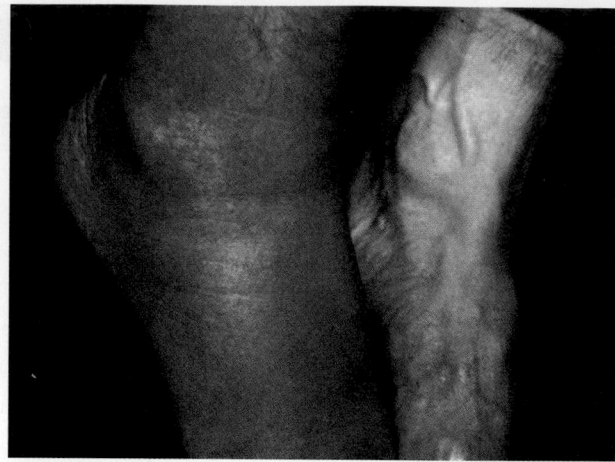

FIGURE 50.1 Cellulitis.

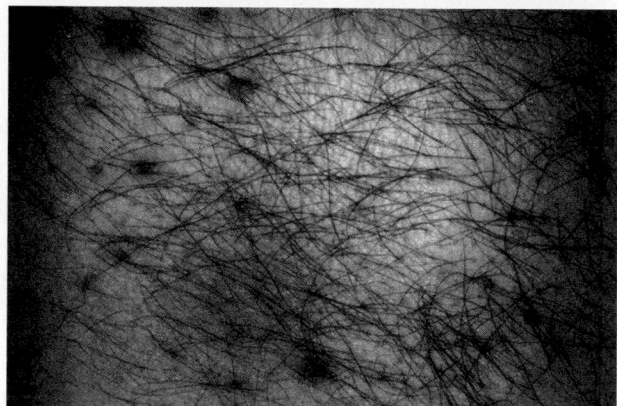

FIGURE 50.2 Folliculitis.

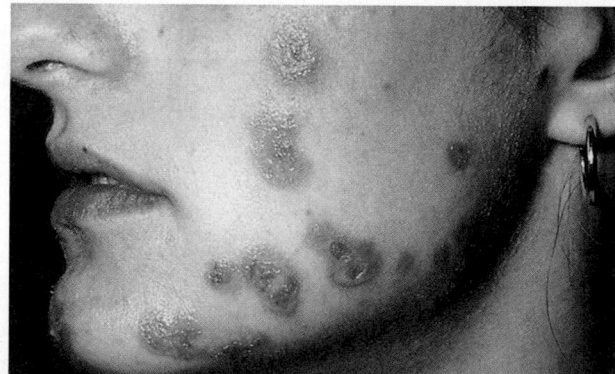

FIGURE 50.3 Impetigo.

Approximately 80% of CA-MRSA cases are uncomplicated skin and soft tissue infections in the form of cellulitis, folliculitis, impetigo, or an abscess.

The risk of MRSA infection after surgery is generally low but affects up to 33% of patients after certain types of surgery. Postoperative MRSA infections can occur as surgical site infections, chest infections, or bloodstream infections (BSIs; bacteremia). The incidence of MRSA surgical site infections varies from 1% to 33% depending on the type of surgery performed and the carrier status of the

CA-MRSA being more common. Community-acquired MRSA begins as a localized skin infection from a break in the skin among healthy individuals who have not been hospitalized. Community-acquired MRSA and HA-MRSA are transmitted through direct contact with colonized skin or the surface of a shared item where MRSA is present.

Table 50.1 Uncomplicated Skin and Soft Tissue Infections

Infection	Causative Organism(s)	Description	Clinical Manifestations	Treatment
Impetigo	MSSA Group A strep	Contagious, localized, inflammatory skin infection	Vesicles, pustules, honey crusted sores on face or extremities without systemic symptoms	Topical mupirocin (Bactroban) ointment For those with limited lesions
Folliculitis	MSSA CA-MRSA *Staphylococcus aureus*	Superficial inflammation and infection of hair follicles	Multiple or single pustules with hair follicle in center on any skin bearing hair	Moist heat; topical mupirocin (Bactroban) ointment Clindamycin 1% lotion or gel; alternatively, benzoyl peroxide 5% wash may be used when showering for 5 to 7 days. Treatment for MRSA usually requires two oral antibiotics.
Furuncle ("boil")	MSSA CA-MRSA	Infection of hair follicle that extends through dermis into subcutaneous tissue and forms a small abscess	Inflammatory nodule with overlying pustule with hair follicle in the center; outbreaks can occur in families or settings with close personal contact (sports); chronic furunculosis with nasal colonization of MRSA	Small: moist heat Large: incision and drainage and systemic antibiotics Furunculosis: mupirocin (Bactroban) ointment intranasally
Carbuncle	MSSA	A furuncle that extends into adjacent follicles	Coalescent inflammatory lesion; pus drains from multiple follicles; typically on back and neck	Incision and drainage; systemic antibiotics
Cellulitis	Most commonly: Group A strep CA-MRSA MSSA	Diffuse infection of the dermis and subcutaneous tissue; usually occurs through breaks in the skin	Painful, edematous, warmth with poorly demarcated borders of erythema on any part of the body; usually unilateral; lymphadenitis; lymphangitis; fever may be present	Systemic antibiotics
Cutaneous abscess	Polymicrobial	Collections of pus within the dermis and subcutaneous tissues	Painful, fluctuant red nodules surrounded by a ring of erythema	Incision and drainage Systemic antibiotics

CA-MRSA, Community-acquired methicillin-resistant *Staphylococcus aureus*; *MRSA*, methicillin-resistant *S. aureus*; *MSSA*, methicillin-sensitive *S. aureus*.

individuals concerned. The optimal prophylactic antibiotic regimen for the prevention of MRSA after surgery is not known. There is currently no evidence to suggest that using a combination of multiple prophylactic antibiotics or administering prophylactic antibiotics for an increased duration is beneficial to people undergoing surgery in terms of reducing MRSA infections. Treatment of MRSA infections includes antibiotics that are known not to have resistance against MRSA bacteria. Prevention strategies that have been reported to decrease the rate of surgical site infection include decolonization of *S. aureus* carriers with either

mupirocin ointment alone or in combination with chlorhexidine gluconate baths.

Complicated skin and tissue infections and necrotizing soft tissue infections are usually polymicrobial. In complicated (non-necrotizing) skin and soft tissue infections, gram-positive bacteria such as **methicillin-sensitive Staphylococcus aureus** (MSSA) and *S. pyogenes* are isolated about 50% of the time. However, anaerobes and gram-negative bacteria such as *Pseudomonas*, Enterobacteriaceae, and clostridial species can also be cultured. Similarly, aerobic bacteria such as streptococci, enterococci, staphylococci, and anaerobic bacteria such as *Bacteroides* and *Peptostreptococci* have been cultured out of necrotizing soft tissue infections. The published mortality rate of necrotizing soft tissue infections ranges from 25% to 70%.

Factors influencing the patient's susceptibility to infection include acute or chronic skin ulcerations, fungal infections, venous stasis disease and alterations in venous drainage, obesity, arterial compromise to the skin, lymph node resection, and immunocompromised state. Additional factors that put individuals at risk for necrotizing soft tissue infection, such as necrotizing fasciitis, include diabetes mellitus, trauma, alcohol or injection drug use, and the use of nonsteroidal anti-inflammatory medications because of their immunosuppressant effect.

Methicillin-resistant *S. aureus* infections are frequently associated with poor hygiene, overcrowded living conditions, skin-to-skin contact, sharing of contaminated objects, previous infection with MRSA, and trauma. It is important to understand, however, that CA-MRSA can cause infection in otherwise young and healthy individuals. Inanimate objects are common reservoirs for CA-MRSA. Overcrowded conditions and person-to-person contact potentiate its transmission. Therefore, demographic groups at higher risk of MRSA infections include children, young adults, minorities, low-socioeconomic groups, homosexual men, athletes, prisoners, day-care workers, and tattoo recipients. Methicillin-resistant *S. aureus* typically colonizes in the anterior nares of the patient and can cause recurrent infections in the patient and exposure of others to the bacteria. The prevalence of nasal MRSA colonization in the general population of the United States is 20% to 40%. Up to 80% to 90% of patients with MRSA bacteremia and surgical site infections have nasal colonization of the bacteria.

Pathophysiology and Clinical Manifestations

Non-necrotizing cellulitis occurs when microorganisms, especially streptococcal and staphylococcal species, find a portal of entry through breaches in skin integrity. Initial presentation of bacterial skin infections can include erythema, warmth, edema, and localized pain. Cellulitis is identified by rapidly spreading erythema, warmth, localized pain, and edema with possible inflammation of regional lymph nodes.

Necrotizing soft tissue infections are very serious, potentially life-threatening infections that spread rapidly and destroy a significant amount of tissue. They can penetrate and spread throughout the dermis, subcutaneous tissues, fascia, and muscle. Necrotizing infections involving the fascia are more common because of the fascia's poor blood supply and limited immune function, which allow pathogens to spread rapidly along the fascial plane. Initially, systemic manifestations of necrotizing soft tissue infections may be mild. However, if they are left untreated, more severe manifestations such as fever, tachycardia, pain that

is disproportionate to physical findings, disorientation, lethargy, and hypotension may signal a worsening, systemic infection. In necrotizing fasciitis, palpation of the erythematous skin can yield firmness to the underlying tissues. Furthermore, necrotizing infections eventually lead to edema and vascular occlusion that causes ischemia, tissue necrosis with resulting loss of feeling to the involved area, and sepsis. The most common sites of necrotizing infections are the abdomen, lower extremities, and perineum. **Fournier's gangrene** is the descriptive name given for necrotizing fasciitis of the genital or perineal area. Table 50.2 describes the clinical manifestations of uncomplicated and complicated skin and soft tissue infections.

Management

Medical Management

There are no guideline indications for the duration of skin and soft tissue infection therapy. In general, short-course therapy for uncomplicated skin and soft tissue infection is the standard of care. The treatment duration for complicated skin and soft tissue infection is variable and depends on the patient (influenced by immunological status, comorbidities, age, etc.), the severity of the infection, and the causative agent.

Table 50.2 Clinical Manifestations of Bacterial Skin Infections

Uncomplicated SSTIs	Complicated SSTIs
Usually no systemic symptoms	Systemic symptoms: fever (or hypothermia), hypotension, tachycardia, confusion/disorientation, sepsis
Localized signs: erythema/cellulitis, furuncles, pustules, folliculitis, cutaneous abscess, purulent drainage if open wound	Spreading area of cellulitis with swelling of regional lymph nodes
Localized increased warmth to surrounding tissues	Edema, ischemia, tissue necrosis with resulting anesthesia to the involved area
Mild to moderate pain	Moderate pain to pain that is disproportionate with clinical manifestations
No changes in blood work	Blood work: elevated white blood cell count, elevated C-reactive protein
	Later stages: bullae, skin ecchymosis; CT scan shows gas in subcutaneous tissues

CT, Computed tomography; *SSTI,* skin and soft tissue infections.

Diagnosis

Patients who present with systemic clinical manifestations of infection require an aggressive approach to management. The initial diagnostic evaluation includes blood culture and sensitivity, complete blood count with differential, serum electrolytes, and C-reactive protein to monitor inflammation and the effects of treatment. Marked abnormalities in these results accompanied by hypotension require immediate hospitalization for fluid resuscitation, surgical evaluation, and the initiation of broad-spectrum systemic antibiotics. Some infectious organisms can produce gas in the subcutaneous tissues. If this is suspected, identification of the gas by computed tomography (CT) scan and immediate surgical exploration and debridement are performed.

Blood cultures, needle biopsies, and punch biopsies are usually not necessary for localized skin and soft tissue infections such as cellulitis. With an infection such as cellulitis, antibiotic therapy directed against staphylococci and streptococci is usually effective. Table 50.1 further summarizes the medical treatment of uncomplicated skin and soft tissue infections.

Nasal colonization of MRSA has been associated with recurrent MRSA skin and soft tissue infections, and there is a high correlation between nasal swab cultures positive for MRSA and wound infections resulting from MRSA. Most systemic antibiotics do not reach adequate concentrations to treat intranasal MRSA. Therefore, patients with MRSA-positive nasal cultures and new or recurrent skin and soft tissue infections resulting from MRSA may be treated empirically with 2% mupirocin (Bactroban) topical ointment to each naris twice daily for 5 days. Some acute care institutions also include bathing patients with a chemical antiseptic.

For hospitalized patients with complicated skin and soft tissue infections (defined as patients with deeper soft tissue infections, surgical/traumatic wound infections, major abscesses, cellulitis, and infected ulcers and burns), in addition to surgical debridement and broad-spectrum antibiotics, empirical therapy for MRSA should be considered pending culture data. For patients with recurrent skin and soft tissue infections, decolonization strategies should be offered in conjunction with ongoing reinforcement of hygiene measures. These strategies may include nasal decolonization with mupirocin twice daily for 5 to 10 days and topical body decolonization regimens with a skin antiseptic solution (e.g., chlorhexidine) for 5 to 14 days or dilute bleach baths.

Patients with open wounds present a slightly different dilemma about whether or not to culture the wound. There is no need to culture a wound in the absence of clinical manifestations of infection, as there can be a plethora of organisms on the surface of chronic wounds. There is a high suspicion for infection if there is necrotic tissue or a foreign body present, the wound is large and deep and has been open for a long time, or the wound is frequently contaminated with stool or urine. In the absence of clinical manifestation of infection, the quantity of organisms is believed to be the best indicator of infection. Wound tissue is the best specimen for quantitative tissue cultures because it reflects the number of bacterial organisms within the tissue and not on the surface of the wound. A **quantitative tissue biopsy**, an invasive test in which a piece of tissue below the surface of the wound is obtained and sent for quantitative Gram stain and culture, is considered the gold standard in identifying wound pathogens. Infection is present if the quantitative culture is greater than or equal to 10^5 colony-forming units per gram of tissue and/or beta-hemolytic streptococci are present. Many practitioners revert to the surface swab culture because it is quick, noninvasive, cost-effective, and less painful to the patient (Box 50.2). Many times, a quantitative swab culture is adequate for the identification and treatment of wound infection, and some investigators report a correlation of findings with tissue biopsy. Wounds that include necrosis or **eschar** (brown or black, thick, leathery, devitalized tissue) require debridement of this tissue to reveal viable tissue for culturing.

Complications

A major complication of skin and soft tissue infections is the overuse and misuse of systemic antibiotics. Treating infections without guidance from cultures not only puts the patient at risk for side effects from the medications but can also exacerbate the problem of antibiotic resistance. Some providers resort to using antibiotics when some uncomplicated skin and soft tissue infections can be treated simply with warm compresses or incision and drainage without follow-up antibiotics. However, incorrect wound-culturing techniques can lead to further complications, such as misidentification of the virulent bacteria, worsening infection, and bacteremia (bacteria in the bloodstream). It is important that practitioners learn the appropriate technique in performing swab cultures so that patients are not exposed to the wrong antibiotic or put at increased risk of pain and infection with an unnecessary, invasive biopsy.

Complicated soft tissue infections, such as necrotizing soft tissue infection, present another set of complications because it is often not possible to diagnose these infections on initial presentation. An experienced practitioner must use clinical judgment to aggressively guide treatment. Immediate surgical debridement of infected tissue is paramount to the patient's prognosis. Delay in treatment can lead to a significant amount of tissue loss, a multitude of future surgeries, and/or death. Of course, with any invasive procedure, the patient is put at even greater risk of infection with surgical debridement.

Nursing Management
Assessment and Analysis

The clinical manifestations observed in patients with bacterial skin infections are related to the bacteria involved, the depth and composition of tissues involved, the temporal association

Box 50.2 Swab Culture Technique for Wound Cultures

General Guidelines

1. Debride the wound to access viable tissue if necrosis or eschar is present. Do not culture purulent material, necrotic debris or tissue, drainage, or hard eschar.
2. Thoroughly clean the wound prior to culturing by wiping or irrigating the wound with sterile water or saline to remove surface debris or exudate.
3. Follow standard precautions for infection control according to facility policies for hand hygiene and use of gloves, gowns, masks, eye protection, or face shields depending on any anticipated exposure.

Prepare Equipment and Supplies

1. Obtain appropriate culture supplies; swab collection and transport systems from the laboratory: two-swab system for aerobes and Gram stains and one-swab system for anaerobes.
2. Gather supplies to clean/prepare the wound, collect the culture, and redress the wound: drape to set up the field, hand sanitizer, gloves, sterile saline (without preservatives), sterile 4 × 4 gauze, and wound dressing.

Clean and Prepare the Wound

1. Wash hands and apply clean gloves.
2. Remove the soiled wound dressing and discard in an approved receptacle.
3. Remove gloves and wash or clean hands with hand sanitizer.
4. Apply clean gloves.
5. Thoroughly irrigate the wound with sterile normal saline (preservative-free).
6. Wipe the surface of the wound vigorously with sterile 4 × 4 gauze moistened with sterile saline (preservative-free) to remove surface contaminants.
7. Gently blot excess saline from the wound bed with dry, sterile gauze.
8. Assess and measure the wound.
9. Remove gloves and wash hands.

Obtain Swab Culture

1. Wash or clean hands with hand sanitizer.
2. Apply gloves.
3. Select culture swab for anaerobic specimen. If the wound bed is dry, moisten the swab with the culture medium or sterile saline (preservative-free).
4. Rotate the swab tip over a 1 cm × 1 cm area of viable tissue at or near the center of the wound for 5 seconds, applying sufficient pressure to cause tissue fluid to be expressed from the wound bed.
   - Immediately insert the culture swab into the transport tube or container.
   - Use caution to avoid contaminating the swab or the outside of the transport tube or container.
5. Repeat step 4 to obtain a second specimen for aerobic/Gram stain from the same clean tissue site using the second swab system.
6. Redress the wound.
7. Discard the used supplies in approved receptacles.
8. Remove gloves and wash hands.
9. Label the culture specimen with complete information: date, time, location of wound, site/source of the specimen, reason for the culture, relevant symptoms, antibiotic use, and history of MRSA. Request quantitative processing of the sample.
10. Place the culture in a laboratory biohazard transport bag (or per hospital or facility procedure) and immediately send the specimen to the laboratory (within 2 hours).
11. Document the procedure.

MRSA, Methicillin-resistant *Staphylococcus aureus*.

of clinical manifestation onset and presentation to the health-care provider, existing comorbidities of the patient, and the age of the patient.

Open wounds are always considered contaminated. Microorganisms are present in the contaminated wound, but the body's immune system is able to keep the number of microorganisms at a minimum. A wound infection is a contaminated wound in which the body's immune system cannot contain the microorganisms, so they continue to multiply. **Exudate** (wound drainage) that contains pus, odor, erythema, inflammation, and increased pain occurs in response to an infection. The characteristics of wound exudate (Table 50.3) denote infection with specific bacteria.

Table 50.3 Wound Exudate

Exudate and Characteristics	Significance
Serosanguinous	
• Appears blood-tinged, straw to amber colored, reflecting presence of serum and red blood cells	• Normal during first 48 hours after injury
Purulent	
• Creamy yellow pus	• Colonization with *Staphylococcus*
• Greenish-blue with a fruity odor	• Colonization with *Pseudomonas*
• Beige pus with fishy odor	• Colonization with *Proteus*

Source: Spear, M. (2012). Wound exudate: The good, the bad, and the ugly. *Plastic Surgical Nursing, 32*(2), 77–79.

Connection Check 50.1

The nurse in the emergency department is triaging patients. Which patient requires immediate attention?

A. A 16-year-old with a laceration that was sutured closed 3 days ago and now has erythema extending 2 cm beyond the suture line

B. A 30-year-old patient with an open sacral pressure injury with exposed bone with purulent exudate

C. A 48-year-old patient with an indurated, erythematous area on his thigh who is complaining of 10/10 pain and has had a fever for 24 hours

D. A 60-year-old patient with diabetes mellitus who has a nail embedded in his foot because he could not feel it in his shoe

Nursing Diagnoses

- **Acute or chronic pain** related to pressure and edema secondary to the wound infection
- **Impaired tissue integrity** related to the open wound
- **Risk for imbalanced fluid volume** related to fluid loss secondary to the open wound and potential surgical debridement.
- **Risk for infection** related to insufficient knowledge of modes of transmission

Nursing Interventions

Assessments

- Vital signs
  Hypotension, tachycardia, hyperthermia or hypothermia, disorientation, lethargy, and disproportionate pain can indicate worsening infection or sepsis. Decreased intravascular volume leads to hypotension and tachycardia.

- Wound and skin
  It is important to establish a baseline of the appearance of the wound or skin to help guide treatment.
- Pain
  Pain disproportionate to the appearance of the wound may indicate underlying infection or tissue damage.
- Complete blood count (CBC) results
  An elevated white blood cell count is indicative of an infectious process.
- Culture results (wound, nares, blood)
  An appropriately performed swab culture of the wound helps guide antibiotic treatment. There is a high correlation of MRSA colonization of the anterior nares and recurrent MRSA infections. Blood cultures are warranted with systemic clinical manifestations to guide treatment.
- Nutritional status
  Adequate nutrition status facilitates wound healing, particularly protein and fluid intake.

Actions

- Administer antibiotics based on culture results.
  Appropriately treat infections using results from the culture and sensitivity to eliminate infection and decrease the risk of antibiotic resistance.
- Wound care as prescribed
  Providing care, including cleansing the wound, dressing changes, and minimizing irritation and pressure, is important to wound healing.
- Surgical evaluation
  Surgical evaluation is necessary for complicated skin and soft tissue infections and if a necrotizing infection is suspected to determine the specific treatment required.

Teaching

- Hand washing
  Hand hygiene greatly reduces the levels of bacteria present on the skin and is the most important factor in preventing the transmission of infection.
- Wound care
  Educating caregivers and patients about clinical manifestations of infection and appropriate application and removal of dressings improves clinical management and outcome.
- Clinical manifestations of infection
  Early recognition of the clinical manifestations of infection may facilitate earlier treatment, prevent complications, and decrease morbidity.

Evaluating Care Outcomes

With the correct antibiotics verified by wound cultures, patients with bacterial skin infections can usually be successfully treated with antibiotics and wound care as needed in the outpatient setting. Care of the patient and family includes teaching about wound care, clinical manifestations of infection, and infection transmission. A rapid and thorough evaluation is essential to a positive prognosis with necrotizing soft tissue infections. Upon initial presentation and follow-up, a wound or cellulitic area that is causing pain out of proportion to the injury should be immediately referred for a surgical evaluation. With aggressive therapy including surgical debridement and specialized wound care, patients with necrotizing soft tissue infections can recover.

HERPES SIMPLEX VIRUS

The Greeks first discovered **herpes simplex virus (HSV)** more than 2,000 years ago and used the term *herpes* to describe something "creepy or crawly." Today, HSV is the most common viral infection diagnosed in developed countries and has become a public health concern. Herpes simplex virus infections exist as two types: type 1 (HSV-1) and type 2 (HSV-2). An HSV-1 infection causes a recurring oral mucosal lesion or "cold sore," and HSV-2 is the cause of genital herpes (GH). Recently, however, researchers have found an increasing incidence of GH attributed to HSV-1.

Epidemiology

Both HSV-1 and HSV-2 are common, lifelong viral infections usually acquired and transmitted asymptomatically through body fluids or skin-to-skin, skin-to-mucosa, or mucosa-to-mucosa contact. Herpes simplex virus-1 can be transmitted without sexual contact, and orolabial lesions typically occur at a young age most likely because of the sharing of utensils or cups during childhood. Herpes simplex virus-1 infections are usually found on the face, oral cavity, lips, and skin. Herpes simplex virus-2 can cause painful anogenital lesions and is one of the most prevalent sexually transmitted infections (STIs). However, most people infected with HSV-2 do not know that they have it and can shed the virus intermittently within the genital tract. Therefore, most GH infections are transmitted by someone who is asymptomatic or unaware of the presence of the infection. Traditionally, HSV-2 was considered the sole cause of GH; however, recent studies show an increased prevalence of GH attributed to HSV-1, likely because of orogenital sexual contact.

Additionally, HSV-1 and HSV-2 can cause a **herpetic whitlow** (painful lesion on the fingers), which occurs when the herpes virus is introduced through breaks in the skin, commonly on the fingers of healthcare workers. Those with active herpetic lesions on the body are also at high risk. Although both viruses can cause a herpetic whitlow, approximately 60% are thought to be caused by HSV-1.

Between 60% and 95% of all adults are believed to be infected with the HSV-1, and it has been identified as the cause of GH in 71.2% of all subjects. In young adults 18 to 24 years old, HSV-1 was found to be the cause of GH in 79.6% of the cases compared to 31.8% of adults aged 25 years and older. Conversely, HSV-2 was found to be the cause of GH in 66.7% of the cases, compared to 20.6% of adults aged 18 to 24.

The Centers for Disease Control and Prevention reported that 16.2% of people in the United States between the ages of 14 and 49 are infected with GH. In general, women are twice as likely as men to be infected, and blacks are three times more likely than whites. The prevalence of HSV-2 among African Americans is 41.8%, and more specifically, there is a prevalence of 48% among African American women. These statistics are based on the number of people who tested positive for HSV-2 antibodies, which are present only if the person is infected with the virus. Although not everyone infected with the HSV-2 virus becomes symptomatic, the virus can still be transmitted to others.

Genital herpes infections caused by HSV-1 show slightly different statistics. Positive predictors for genital HSV-1 infections include being white and having receptive oral and anal sex. Herpes simplex virus-1 is more frequently the cause of GH in women, those under 25, and homosexual men. Most likely, this is related to increased orogenital contact. Those in a monogamous relationship for at least 2 months and who participated in orogenital sex were more likely to have HSV-1 as the cause of GH. Conversely, those with multiple partners over 6 months had a greater likelihood of having HSV-2 infections.

Pathophysiology and Clinical Manifestations

Herpes simplex viral infections can occur on the skin, mucous membranes, central nervous system, and genital tract. There are two phases of reactivity of the herpes virus, primary and secondary infections. A primary HSV infection describes the first time an individual is infected with the herpes virus. Primary infection can occur through direct contact with an individual with HSV who is asymptomatic; is in a prodromal (early) stage of the disease; or has active oral or genital infections, secretions, or lesions. Clinical manifestations of primary infection occur within 2 weeks of viral transmission and can include fever; malaise; myalgias; anorexia; irritability; cervical or inguinal lymphadenopathy; and lesions that can involve the lip, face, mucous membranes of the mouth, pharynx, or genitals. Many times, the primary infection is asymptomatic and can be transmitted unknowingly. Once HSV penetrates the skin or mucous membrane, the virus travels down the peripheral sensory neurons to the ganglia, where it remains dormant until a trigger incites an active lesion.

Secondary (or recurrent) HSV infections occur following an exogenous or endogenous trigger that reactivates the dormant virus. Triggers are individually specific but commonly occur in response to ultraviolet (UV) light exposure, febrile illnesses, and stress, for example. The virus is then transferred from the ganglia back to the initial site of inoculation via the peripheral nerve. Typically, the secondary infection is milder than the primary infection and is usually preceded by a prodrome of a burning, itching, or tingling sensation where the lesion eventually occurs. An area of redness first appears on the lips or genitals followed in about 2 days with the appearance of multiple fluid-filled vesicles. The pain usually subsides once the vesicles rupture. The number of lesions and the nature of the outbreak depend on the individual's immune status at the time, and in general, genital recurrences occur more frequently than oral recurrences. Recurrences of GH caused by HSV-1 occur less frequently than those caused by HSV-2.

Management

Medical Management

Diagnosis

Because many primary HSV infections are asymptomatic and lack the classic, painful vesicular lesions, a diagnosis based on clinical presentation alone is nonsensitive and nonspecific. The prognosis and type of clinical counseling a patient needs are dependent on accurate identification of the type of GH infection confirmed by laboratory analyses (HSV-1 or HSV-2). Virological and type-specific serological testing are also available.

Virological testing is appropriate for a patient seeking medical attention because of the presence of **mucocutaneous** (a region of the body where mucosa transitions to skin) lesions or ulcers. Viral culture and polymerase chain reaction (PCR) testing are preferred for the individual with active lesions; however, their sensitivity decreases as the lesions start to heal. Polymerase chain reaction testing is preferred for detecting HSV in spinal fluid. A negative viral culture or PCR test does not negate infection because viral shedding can be intermittent. The cytological Tzanck's smear (examines skin scrapings smeared onto a slide) and cervical Pap smear (examines cervical scrapings smeared onto a slide) are both nonspecific methods of diagnosis, and their results are not reliable.

Serological type-specific glycoprotein G–based assays obtained from capillary or serum blood samples accurately distinguish HSV-1 from HSV-2. These tests are ordered by providers for those patients who have recurrent genital symptoms with negative HSV cultures, a clinical diagnosis of GH without laboratory confirmation, a partner with GH, a person presenting for STI testing with a history of multiple sex partners, persons with HIV, or homosexual men. False-negatives can occur during the early stage of infections because the sensitivities for the HSV-2 antibody can vary and seroconversion can take up to 12 weeks. Although the specificity of the type-specific test is greater than 96%, false positives still occur. Therefore, repeated, confirmatory testing is helpful, especially if GH acquisition is suspected of being recent (within 12 weeks of exposure). Screening for HSV in the general population is not warranted.

The presence of type-specific HSV-2 antibodies implies that the individual acquired GH through anogenital sexual contact, and it is necessary to provide the appropriate education and counseling for individuals who are seropositive for HSV-2. It is more difficult to interpret the serological presence of HSV-1 antibodies because most people who are seropositive for HSV-1 contracted it during childhood and may be asymptomatic. The presence of HSV-1 antibodies does not distinguish the anogenital form of HSV-1 from the orolabial infection. It is important to understand that individuals with HSV-1 antibodies remain at risk of acquiring HSV-2 and should be offered the same education and counseling to include the natural history of GH, sexual and perinatal transmission, and methods to reduce transmission. Moreover, the sex partners of patients with GH benefit from education and counseling as well.

Treatment

The basis of medical treatment of GH is systemic antiviral chemotherapy. Treatment can be directed at first or recurrent episodes as well as daily suppressive therapy, and options need to be discussed with the patient. In counseling patients, it is important to stress that the medications do not eradicate the latent virus. Also, decreased frequency and severity of recurrences are based on continued use of suppressive therapy. Additionally, suppressive therapy has shown to decrease the risk of transmitting HSV-2 to sexual partners. Three antiviral medications, acyclovir, valacyclovir, and famciclovir, tested in randomized trials, have shown clinical benefit in the treatment of GH. Because the bioavailability of IV acyclovir is greater than the oral route, IV acyclovir is utilized for patients with severe disease or those who encounter complications of HSV, such as disseminated infection, pneumonitis, encephalitis, or hepatitis.

Complications

One of the most significant complications of HSV infections is its effect on quality of life due to the psychosocial stress of a diagnosis of GH. Patients report feeling isolated, devastated, and embarrassed because of this diagnosis and fear transmitting the virus to others. Infection with HSV-2 is a major risk factor for the acquisition and transmission of HIV as well. Also, because of a loss of skin integrity, open epithelial lesions carry the risk of secondary bacterial infections.

The most devastating time to acquire GH is during pregnancy because the complication of disseminated neonatal herpes carries a mortality rate of up to 30%. Because the viral load is much greater during a primary HSV infection, the greatest risk of maternal transmission occurs among women who acquire a primary infection in the third trimester of pregnancy as opposed to those with recurrent disease. It takes approximately 12 weeks for the neonate to passively acquire maternal antibodies, and when the mother is infected in the final trimester of pregnancy, immunity may not be developed in time to protect the neonate during delivery. Antiviral medications have been shown to be safe for use during pregnancy and should be prescribed for women who contract GH in the first or second trimesters. Cesarean sections are generally recommended for women presenting with primary GH lesions at delivery and in the last 6 weeks of pregnancy because of high viral shedding that can affect the neonate.

Nursing Management
Assessment and Analysis

Clinical manifestations of symptomatic primary HSV infections can include fever; malaise; myalgias; anorexia; irritability; cervical or inguinal lymphadenopathy; and painful lesions that can involve the lip, face, mucous membranes of the mouth, pharynx, or genitals. As previously discussed, however, HSV infections can also be asymptomatic.

Connection Check 50.2

Which statement made by a patient who is currently asymptomatic with an HSV-2 infection indicates the need for more education about the disease?

A. "It's okay to have intercourse with my partner as long as we use a barrier method of protection and I take my antiviral medications."

B. "It's more likely that I could spread the HSV-2 infection if I have sexual relations when I have open ulcers and pain."

C. "When I get pregnant, I will be certain to tell my gynecologist about my HSV-2 infection."

D. "I understand that I could still transmit the virus if I don't have symptoms."

Nursing Diagnoses

- **Acute pain** related to primary or secondary HSV infections
- **Risk for infection** related to open HSV lesions
- **Deficient knowledge** related to unfamiliarity with safe sex practices and characteristics of HSV transmission
- **Risk for social isolation** related to new diagnosis of HSV genital infection

Nursing Interventions
■ Assessments

- Pain and fever
  The prodromal period may include fever, malaise, and headache, and the patient's understanding of prodromal symptoms may help the patient recognize the onset of an outbreak.
- Oral cavity lesions (questions about sore throat, dysphagia, anorexia, mouth pain)
  Oral lesions cause outbreaks that range from painful to severe and even life-threatening to infants, children, and adolescents.
- Genital lesions
  The appearance of lesions may provide additional information about the stage of the disease process.
- Sexual history
  Understanding the number of partners, use of barrier protection, participation in oral or anal intercourse, dysuria, dyspareunia (painful intercourse), and history of other STIs helps to guide treatment and counseling.

- Skin and mucous membranes for presence and appearance of lesions
  Secondary bacterial skin infections can occur with open HSV lesions.
- Knowledge of HSV and transmission of the virus
  Patients must understand that HSV-1 can cause genital lesions through orogenital contact and that an individual with genital HSV-1 can still contract HSV-2. Knowledge about transmission increases the likelihood of safe sex practices and may decrease anxiety related to the new diagnosis.
- Assess serum human chorionic gonadotropin (hCG) levels.
  To assess for pregnancy
- Ability to cope with diagnosis of HSV
  Counseling is warranted because of the psychosocial stress of a new diagnosis of GH.

■ Actions

- Perform viral cultures and/or serological testing.
  Viral cultures can be performed on open lesions; serological testing is necessary to differentiate HSV-1 and HSV-2 infections.
- Administer antiviral medications as indicated.
  Antiviral medications can decrease the frequency and severity of outbreaks.
- Administer analgesic medications as indicated and warm sitz baths for comfort.
  Over-the-counter analgesics and warm water soaks can provide symptomatic relief of pain from open lesions.
- Collaborate with interprofessional team for psychological support.
  Counseling is warranted because of the psychosocial stress of a new diagnosis of GH.

■ Teaching

- Actions of antiviral medications
  Taking the antiviral medications does not cure HSV and does not reduce the risk of transmitting the virus but may decrease the frequency and severity of outbreaks.
- Safe sex practices
  There is a decreased incidence of HSV-2 infections with those who use condoms. Patients should be educated not to have sexual intercourse during an outbreak even with condom use because of the high incidence of transmitting the virus during that time.
- Considerations related to HSV infection during pregnancy
  Pregnant women must be educated about the risks of acquiring HSV during pregnancy. Genital herpes acquired during pregnancy includes the complication of disseminated neonatal herpes that carries a mortality rate of up to 30%. Because the viral load is much greater during a primary HSV infection, the greatest risk of maternal transmission occurs among women who acquire a primary infection in the third trimester of pregnancy as opposed to those with recurrent disease. It takes approximately 12 weeks for the neonate to passively acquire maternal antibodies.

Evaluating Care Outcomes

To prevent transmission of the virus, it is paramount to teach safe sex practices to individuals with or without an HSV infection, including the use of a condom as well as not engaging in sexual contact during an outbreak. Teenagers and young adults must be made aware of the risk of contracting HSV-1 through orogenital sex. Referring an individual for counseling with a new diagnosis of HSV may be essential in helping him or her cope with feelings of isolation, depression, and anger and can help him or her develop and maintain social and intimate relationships.

FUNGAL INFECTIONS

Fungal infections in humans are quite common and are caused by two different types of fungi: **dermatophytes** (aerobic fungi) and yeasts. Clinically, the impact of fungal infections ranges from mild to fatal, and the clinical manifestations vary by infection site and depend on the patient's immune response.

Epidemiology

Fungal infections can spread directly from person to person, through animal contact, or indirectly through contact with inanimate objects that hold skin scales from infected hosts. Dermatophytes are aerobic fungi that infect the stratum corneum (the top, dead layer of the skin) and survive on keratin and therefore cannot survive on mucosal surfaces. Typically, a fungal infection with dermatophytes presents asymmetrically on the patient, affecting one foot or one hand. Because fungal infections proliferate in warm, moist environments, the groin, feet, axillae, and skinfolds are primary places for infection. The Latin word **tinea**, meaning worm, is used to describe fungal infections caused by dermatophytes and precedes the anatomical location of the infection. For example, tinea pedis describes a fungal infection of the foot, or athlete's foot, and tinea capitis involves the head. Synonyms used to describe dermatophyte infections include *dermatophytosis*, *tinea*, and *ringworm*. Table 50.4 describes the diagnosis and treatment of some common fungal skin infections. In the community setting, yeast, or *candidiasis*, most commonly causes oral or vaginal thrush. However, nosocomial invasive fungal or *Candida* infections affecting the critically ill and immunocompromised patients can have devastating consequences.

The incidence and prevalence of fungal infections vary among populations and environmental exposure. Greater than 4 million healthcare visits per year are related to superficial fungal infections, and the most common types are tinea pedis and **onychomycosis** (fungal infection of the nails). The majority of healthcare visits per year are for onychomycosis (23.2%), followed by fungal infections of the skin (20.4%) and, lastly, the feet (18.8%). Generally, risk factors for dermatophytosis include the presence of fungal infections in the family, male gender, farmers and manual laborers, and the use of immunosuppressive medications.

Prevalence rates of tinea pedis range from 25% to 70% over the lifespan, making it the most commonly occurring dermatophyte infection, especially among athletes. Onychomycosis has been shown to be more prevalent with advancing age, likely because of decreased vascular flow, difficulty in grooming nails and maintaining foot hygiene, frequent nail injuries, and diabetes. Approximately 72% of those older than 45 are affected, and it is more frequently found among men, likely because of men's greater participation in manual labor and sports, which require tight-fitting shoes. Fungal scalp infections are found more frequently among those of lower socioeconomic status.

Candida, or yeast, causes a broad range of infections that range from those easy to treat in an outpatient setting to significant and fatal infections that occur among the acutely sick and critically ill populations. Three out of four women will experience a vulvovaginal yeast infection, and half of all women will have more than one in a lifetime. Risk factors include tight-fitting or synthetic-fiber clothing, douching too frequently, and contamination with bacteria from the rectum because yeast thrives in warm, moist environments on the skin and mucous membranes of the gastrointestinal tract and vagina. These infections are usually treated with an over-the-counter antifungal medication (such as Monistat) for 1 to 7 days.

The more significant *Candida* infections that occur among hospitalized patients may be related to the medical treatment of other diseases or infections. In the United States, 12% of all hospital-acquired bloodstream infections (BSIs) are caused by *Candida*. This may be due to several factors, including increased empirical use of antimicrobials; a large population of immunocompromised patients due to cancer, organ transplants, and chemotherapy; an increase in survival of the sickest patients; and invasive procedures. Additional risk factors include *Candida* colonization, renal failure, severity of illness, and the need for total parenteral nutrition. Among intensive care unit (ICU) patients, mortality rates of *Candida* BSIs range from 38% to 75%. The increasing incidence of hospitalizations involving candidemia has led to longer lengths of hospital stay and additional costs.

Pathophysiology and Clinical Manifestations

Dermatophytes, which reproduce by the formation of spores, cause superficial cutaneous fungal infections and do not spread beyond the epidermis. Found living in soil, on animals, and on humans, dermatophytes are aerobic fungi that feed on the dead keratin of the skin, hair, and nails. Areas that are occluded, such as the toe spaces, are most at risk of infection, and an identifiable characteristic of dermatophyte infections is an active, raised border. Yeasts, on the other hand, multiply by budding and thrive in warm, moist environments on the skin and mucous membranes of the gastrointestinal tract and vagina. Fungal infections may present as scaling rashes, plaques, vesicles, or pustules. Table 50.4 reviews common fungal infections and their clinical manifestations.

(Text continued on page 1111)

Table 50.4 Common Fungal Infections

Name	Site	Clinical Manifestations	Diagnosis	Medical Management
Tinea capitis	Scalp	• Scaling of scalp, alopecia, broken hair at scalp line	• Physical findings: scaling, adenopathy, alopecia, pruritus • KOH microscopy	• Oral antifungals to penetrate hair shafts Example: terbinafine (Lamisil) • Topical antifungal medications, such as itraconazole, terbinafine, and fluconazole
Tinea corporis	Body	• Annular patches or plaques with advancing, raised border and central clearing	• Clinical appearance • KOH microscopy A fungal culture, used as an adjunct to KOH for diagnosis, is more specific than KOH for detecting a dermatophyte infection. If clinical suspicion is high, yet the KOH result is negative, a fungal culture should be obtained.	• Topical antifungals for infections • Topical azoles (i.e., ketoconazole, clotrimazole, miconazole, and allylamines) (i.e., terbinafine) • Topical therapy should be applied to the lesion and at least 2 cm beyond this area once or twice a day for at least 2 weeks.

Continued

Tinea cruris (jock itch)

Groin

- Sharply delineated, symmetrical red to reddish-brown plaques with central clearing; border with pustules or vesicles; pruritic; scrotum spared

- Evaluate feet because the same dermatophyte causes tinea pedis.
- Differentiate from *Candida* intertrigo, which does not have central clearing.

- Topical antifungal (terbinafine [Lamisil], butenafine [Lotrimin])
- Topical antifungal agents of the imidazole or allylamine family

Tinea faciei

Face

- Annular rash with raised margins
- Pruritus

- Clinical appearance Tinea faciei is the most frequently misdiagnosed entity among cutaneous fungal infections. The atypical clinical features support the separation of this disease from tinea corporis.
- KOH microscopy The surface scrapings are obtained from the border of the lesions where the more severe inflammatory reaction occurs and where more fungal elements are present.

- Topical antifungals (butenafine [Lotrimin], clotrimazole [Mycelex])
- Topical antifungal agents (i.e., ciclopirox and terbinafine)

Table 50.4 Common Fungal Infections—cont'd

Name	Site	Clinical Manifestations	Diagnosis	Medical Management
Tinea pedis	Feet	• Maceration of interdigital skin of feet • Diffuse dry scaling of soles of feet	• Clinical appearance • KOH microscopy if needed	• Keep feet dry and ventilated. • Topical antifungal (terbinafine [Lamisil]) • Severe: oral antifungal
Tinea versicolor (pityriasis versicolor)	Upper chest, back, upper arms	• Scaly patches of different colors (erythematous, hypo- or hyperpigmented)	• Wood's lamp • KOH microscopy	• Topical antifungals (terbinafine [Lamisil] or ketoconazole [Nizoral]) • Selenium sulfide shampoo (Selsun Blue) • Oral "azole" antifungals for resistant or recurrent infections • Over-the-counter (OTC) remedies include clotrimazole (Lotrimin, Mycelex) and miconazole (Lotrimin). Another OTC option is selenium sulfide shampoo 1% (Selsun Blue) or 1% ketoconazole shampoo (Nizoral).
Onychomycosis (tinea unguium)	Nails	• Yellow, brittle, thick nails with subungual hyperkeratosis	• Clinical appearance • KOH microscopy	• Topical antifungals effective with debridement • Oral antifungals (terbinafine [Lamisil], itraconazole [Sporanox], fluconazole [Diflucan] Topical therapy: • Ciclopirox olamine 8% nail lacquer solution

- Efinaconazole 10% topical solution (the first FDA-approved topical triazole for toenail onychomycosis)
- Tavaborole 0.5% topical solution, an oxaborole solution (boron-containing compound)
- Topical treatments may be useful to prevent recurrence in patients cured with systemic agents.

Oral therapy:

- Terbinafine
- Itraconazole

Nonpharmacological approaches include the following:

- Laser treatment
- Photodynamic therapy
- Mechanical, chemical, or surgical nail avulsion
- Chemical removal with a 40%–50% urea compound used with very thick nails
- Removal of the nail plate as an adjunct to oral therapy

Oral thrush (oropharyngeal candidiasis) 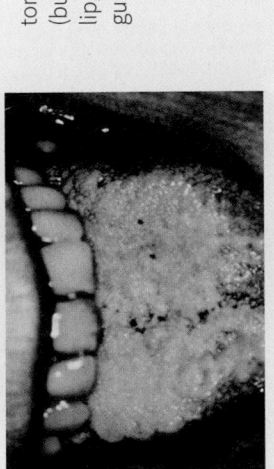	Mouth: tongue, inner cheek (buccal mucosa), inner lip, and occasionally gums (gingiva)	• Creamy white plaques on erythematous mucous membranes • Thick white coating of tongue, inner cheeks, inner lips, or gums	• Clinical signs and symptoms • Visual inspection of the area	• Oral antifungal liquids (swish and swallow) or lozenge such as Nystatin • May be either treated topically (i.e., nystatin) or ingested in liquid form (i.e., fluconazole)

Continued

Table 50.4 Common Fungal Infections—cont'd

Name	Site	Clinical Manifestations	Diagnosis	Medical Management
Vulvovaginal candidiasis	Vagina and vulva	• Thick, cottage cheese–like vaginal discharge • Pruritus	• Clinical signs and symptoms Take a sample of the vaginal secretions and look at the sample under a microscope to see if an abnormal number of *Candida* organisms are present.	• Topical and intravaginal antifungals
Intertrigo	Skinfolds: worsened by heat, moisture, lack of air Common inflammatory condition affecting areas of skin that are in contact with each other (intertriginous zones, i.e., groin, armpits, under breasts) Caused by combination of frictional rubbing, increased temperature, and moisture	Maceration from moisture; erosions from skin surfaces rubbing together; erythema; itching and burning; satellite lesions	• Clinical signs and symptoms	• Eliminate causative factors when possible: separate skinfolds; keep skin dry. • Topical antifungal powder (nystatin)

FDA, U.S. Food and Drug Administration; *KOH*, potassium hydroxide.

Management

Medical Management

Diagnosis

The diagnosis of tinea infections is usually made with a focused history, physical examination, and potassium hydroxide (KOH) microscopy, but sometimes Wood's lamp examination, fungal culture, or histological tissue evaluation is necessary to confirm the diagnosis. Potassium hydroxide microscopy, which has a 76.5% sensitivity and an 81.6% negative predictive value, makes it more sensitive than a fungal culture. To perform KOH microscopy, the scraping of skin from the affected area is placed on a slide and viewed through a microscope after adding a drop of 10% to 20% KOH solution. The presence of hyphae confirms the diagnosis. A Wood's lamp examination that uses a UV light held close to the skin in a darkened room is helpful in diagnosing tinea versicolor. This fungus fluoresces a pale yellow to white. Otherwise, a Wood's lamp usually is not helpful in diagnosing fungal infections because there is a declining number of infections that still fluoresce under UV light. Table 50.4 provides additional detail regarding diagnoses of fungal infections.

Treatment

Antifungal agents are the primary agents used to treat fungal infections, and Table 50.4 provides an overview regarding the medical management of common fungal infections. Healthcare providers often prescribe ineffective antifungal therapies because of a lack of knowledge of the medications and incorrect diagnoses. Not every antifungal medication is the same, and what is an appropriate treatment for one infection may not be for another. Therefore, research recommends better healthcare provider education concerning the diagnosis, management, and prevention of fungal skin infections.

Prevention

Generally, the prevention of fungal skin infections requires avoidance of the causative factors, which include wearing tight shoes for prolonged periods, moisture and perspiration, contact of surfaces with bare skin, and sharing of contaminated personal items. Meticulous hand washing and eliminating the sharing of personal items are the primary methods of preventing infection transmission. For hospitalized patients, prevention of superficial fungal infections can be achieved by keeping skinfolds dry and clean, frequent turning of bed-bound patients to enhance airflow, and timely cleansing and drying of incontinence and wound exudates.

Complications

Complications of fungal infections occur when they are not treated promptly and are allowed to proliferate, especially in the critically ill and immunocompromised patient. Prompt diagnosis of *Candida* infections in an ICU is difficult because of the time needed for finalization, thus delaying treatment and increasing the risk of mortality. Because of the high mortality rate of an invasive *Candida* infection, many prediction tools have emerged. For example, the *Candida* colonization index requires the acquisition of surveillance cultures from multiple patient body sites a few times per week up to daily while the patient is in the ICU. The *Candida* colonization index is the ratio of the number of body sites that grow the same species of *Candida* divided by the number of body sites tested. A *Candida* colonization index of 0.5 identifies patients who are colonized and are at great risk of developing invasive candidiasis. This guides clinicians to promptly treat patients at greatest risk with antifungal medications and reduce morbidity from candidemia. Other risk identification scales consider admitting diagnoses, use of corticosteroids or other immunosuppressive medications, antibiotic use, parenteral nutrition, and the presence of an invasive central venous catheter.

Connection Check 50.3

A mother brings in her 8-year-old child because of a new rash of annular patches, raised borders, and central clearing. What should be done first?

A. Obtain a scraping of the rash for KOH microscopy.

B. Explain to the mother that this is probably tinea corporis and an antifungal ointment will successfully treat it.

C. Obtain a focused history to include medications, activities in which the patient partakes, and any history of skin disorders or fungal rashes.

D. Explain to the mother that the rash will subside on its own.

Nursing Management

Assessment and Analysis

Nursing assessment and care of the skin are crucial in the diagnosis and treatment of fungal skin infections. Clinical manifestations include rashes, plaque formation, pustules, and vesicles. Patients at increased risk require enhanced surveillance because of immunocompromise, alterations in skin integrity, and obesity (particularly with moist skinfolds), which increase the risk of fungal infections.

Nursing Diagnoses

- **Impaired comfort** related to fungal skin infections as evidenced by pruritus
- **Risk for infection transmission** related to colonization of fungus as diagnosed by rash, KOH microscopy, and/or cultures
- **Risk for impaired skin integrity** related to moisture on skin secondary to incontinence and diaphoresis

Nursing Interventions

Assessments

- Assess skin, paying close attention to creases and moist environments and noting any treated or untreated fungal infections.

  Particular attention needs to be given to creases and moist environments. Macerated skin from moisture and a dark environment support successful penetration and proliferation of fungi. A patient with tinea pedis many times will have tinea cruris because of contamination when putting on clothing. The development of skin and eye lesions is sometimes the only clue to finding that the cause of sepsis is a Candida *infection.*

- Pruritus

  Pruritus is a side effect of some fungal infections and can exacerbate skin breakdown.

- Current and recent medications

  Antibiotic use increases the risk of fungal infections.

- Liver function

  Oral antifungal agents can cause liver damage, requiring the assessment of liver function results.

- Health history

  Assessment of the history of fungal infections may help identify colonization; certain populations are more susceptible to fungal infections (see Epidemiology section).

Actions

- Meticulous hand washing before and after patient contact

  Hand washing is the most important way to decrease the transmission of fungi.

- Perform cultures as needed.

  Surveillance cultures in an ICU can identify the risk of Candida *bloodstream infections and decrease morbidity and mortality.*

- Administer antifungal medications as prescribed.

  Prompt treatment with the correct antifungal medications can decrease morbidity and mortality. Applying antifungal medications appropriately treats the infection and alleviates symptoms such as pruritus.

- Cleanse incontinent episodes as soon as they occur and keep the perineum as dry as possible; change moist bed linens and gowns.

  Fungal infections thrive in dark, moist environments.

- Separate skinfolds with gauze or other dressings and keep dry to decrease the risk of intertrigo.

  Intertrigo is caused by skinfolds rubbing together and **maceration** *(soft, white skin secondary to constant exposure to moisture) of moist tissue, allowing invasion of fungi.*

- Meticulous cleanliness and application of antifungal medications

  In the presence of infection, cleanliness decreases the proliferation of infection and increases healing.

Teaching

- Avoid tight-fitting clothes, shoes, and communal washing (wear shower shoes).

  Women with tight-fitting clothes are more susceptible to vulvovaginal Candida *infections. Tight-fitting shoes hold*

the web spaces between toes closed, increasing temperature and moisture. The transmission of fungi can occur from inanimate objects.

- Clinical manifestations of fungal infections

  Understanding the clinical manifestations will allow for prompt treatment.

- Complete antifungal infection medications as prescribed.

  The complete eradication of the fungal infection requires the patient to complete the entire course of antifungal medications. Stopping the medications once clinical manifestations are gone may lead to recurrent infection.

Evaluating Care Outcomes

Treating fungal infections in the community has a high success rate as long as the correct antifungal medication is prescribed. Educating the patient about clinical manifestations and causes of fungal infections can decrease occurrences and the severity of the infection. For the hospitalized patient, keeping the skin and skinfolds dry and cleaning incontinence episodes as soon as they occur is an appropriate goal to decrease the incidence of fungal infections. The healthcare provider must keep in mind that critically ill and immunocompromised patients with a fungal infection of the skin are at high risk of developing a bloodstream infection that could prove to be fatal. Therefore, close monitoring of the patient's status, including vital signs and blood work, is essential in his or her care.

PSORIASIS

Psoriasis is a lifelong inflammatory disorder characterized by exacerbations and remissions of raised, scaling, erythematous plaques usually seen on the extensor surfaces of the body. Although there is no cure for psoriasis, there is a variety of treatments available that can control symptoms.

Epidemiology

Psoriasis is an immune disorder that causes chronic inflammation of the skin characterized by thick, raised red patches covered with silvery, flaking scales. Essentially, the etiology of psoriasis is unknown. Infections, medications, stress, trauma, and hormonal changes are some of the things that can aggravate the disease. Patients with psoriasis fare better in warmer climates with sun exposure because UV radiation kills rapidly proliferating skin cells.

It is difficult to establish the true incidence and prevalence of psoriasis because not everyone seeks medical help for the disease. In previous studies, psoriasis was found to affect as many as 7.5 million people, or about 2% of the population. Its prevalence varies with ethnicity, and it is less common in people of Asian or African descent. Seventy-five percent of patients in some studies reported a moderate to severe form of the disease with plaques affecting 3% or more of the total body surface area. Men and women are equally likely to develop psoriasis, and the mean age of onset is 28, with a range of 15 to 35 years. Onset of psoriasis before age 30 is linked with more severe cutaneous manifestations, serious psychosocial impact, and a family history of the disease. Up to 30% of those with psoriasis develop psoriatic arthritis, a complication that causes inflammation, pain, and stiffness of the joints.

Pathophysiology and Clinical Manifestations

Although the cause of psoriasis remains unknown, current research suggests that it results from an interaction of multiple genes, the immune system, and environmental influences (see Genetic Connections: Psoriasis). Epidermal thickness with increased vascularity and increased inflammation are the main pathological aspects of psoriasis. New epithelial cells are continually made in the basal layer of the epidermis, and it takes approximately 28 days for these new cells to reach the surface of the skin and shed. In psoriasis, this process is accelerated for unknown reasons, and more skin cells are made than are actually shed, and these cells form the scaly plaques on the surface of the skin. Also, the dermal capillaries become tortuous and dilated (Fig. 50.4), causing the red appearance of the skin under the scaly plaques, and these abnormal capillaries are the last aspect of psoriasis to resolve after treatment. Although psoriasis can occur anywhere on the body, psoriatic plaques are most often seen on the elbows, knees, legs, palms, soles of the feet, scalp, trunk, and face. There are several forms of psoriasis including plaque, guttate, and erythrodermic.

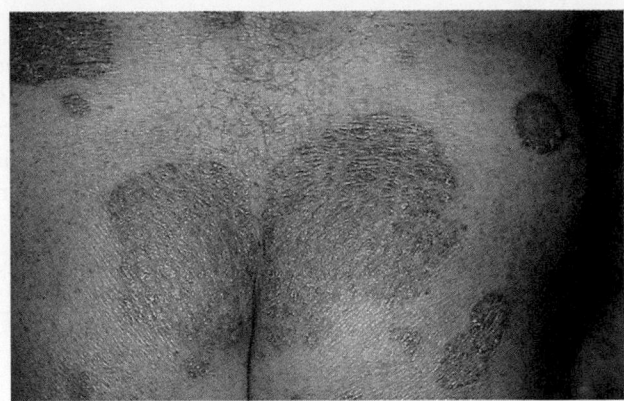

FIGURE 50.4 Psoriasis.

Genetic Connections

Psoriasis

The occurrence of psoriasis is multifactorial. Genetic, age, behavioral, and environmental factors are associated with the development of the disease. In at least 30% of cases, a genetic predisposition is recognized. Research demonstrates that monozygotic (identical) twins have a higher concordance rate for psoriasis (70%) as opposed to dizygotic (fraternal) twins (20%). Seventy-one percent of children with psoriasis have a positive family history of the disease, and in families where both parents have the disease, psoriasis is found among half of the siblings. Therefore, it is important to ask about family history of a patient who presents with clinical manifestations of psoriasis.

The most common type of psoriasis is plaque psoriasis, affecting approximately 80% to 90% of those with the disease. Patients with this type of psoriasis present with well-circumscribed, thick, reddened papules or plaques, often covered with silvery scaling flakes. In guttate psoriasis, small plaques 2 to 10 mm in diameter appear in a centripetal distribution (starting from the face and extremities and moving toward the trunk). Many times, this is the initial presentation of psoriasis in children. Up to 33% of patients with guttate psoriasis eventually develop chronic plaque psoriasis. *Erythroderma*, another form of psoriasis, can involve most or all of the skin. Erythroderma can occur when psoriatic plaques become confluent and extensive or may be an indication of unstable psoriasis exacerbated by infection, medications, or corticosteroid withdrawal. This may lead to the skin's inability to thermoregulate, causing hypothermia and heart failure.

Psoriasis is not always limited to the skin. Psoriatic arthritis (PsA) is a common manifestation of psoriasis, and there is evidence to suggest that there is a genetic component to PsA. It is believed that the genetic susceptibilities of the host interact with environmental and other random factors to precipitate the disease. Psoriatic arthritis usually involves the joints of the hands and spine. Additionally, nail involvement is common and presents as pitting, **onycholysis** (lifting of the nail away from the nail bed), and splinter hemorrhages under the nail.

Management

Medical Management
Diagnosis

There are no laboratory tests specific for psoriasis. Plaque psoriasis is usually diagnosed on the basis of a patient's clinical manifestations. However, some forms of psoriasis mimic other skin disorders, such as bacterial and fungal infections, making it sometimes necessary for a dermatologist to perform a skin biopsy for a definitive diagnosis. If PsA is suspected, serum inflammatory markers such as C-reactive protein and an erythrocyte sedimentation rate (ESR) usually are elevated. Rheumatoid factor usually is not found in PsA, and this can help differentiate PsA from rheumatoid arthritis.

Treatment

Because there is no cure for psoriasis, the goal in treating this disorder is to reduce the clinical manifestations, control the disease, and improve quality of life. Therefore, it is important to complete a thorough skin assessment to note the location and extent of the lesions, as well as to ascertain what the patient's goals of treatment are. There are several therapies available, including topical creams and ointments and UV light therapy, as well as systemic medications (Table 50.5).

> ⚠️ **Safety Alert** Phototherapy for psoriasis requires exposure to UVA (long wave ultraviolet A) or UVB (short wave ultraviolet B) light rays and needs to be performed in a controlled environment under the clinical expertise of a dermatology provider. Medications such as antibiotics and over-the-counter supplements can sensitize the patient to phototherapy, causing burning of the skin and increasing the patient's risk of skin cancer.

Complications

In addition to the side effects of medications, patients with psoriasis are at high risk of developing other diseases (i.e., cancer, cardiovascular disease, Crohn's disease, diabetes, metabolic syndrome, uveitis, and liver disease). It is important to understand the patient's risk of developing these comorbidities when counseling patients and considering therapies to manage the disease. As previously mentioned, PsA occurs in approximately 30% of those individuals diagnosed with psoriasis. Those with PsA experience pain, soft tissue swelling, and limitations in movement for 6 weeks or longer, and this can be a debilitating consequence of psoriasis.

Research demonstrates an increased risk of malignancy among patients with psoriasis. Non-melanoma skin cancer; lymphoma; and cancer of the lung, larynx, pharynx, liver, pancreas, female breast, penis, vulva, bladder, and kidney are among the most common malignancies found to develop. **Basal cell carcinoma** (abnormal, uncontrolled cancer cells in the skin's basal cells) and **squamous cell carcinoma**

Table 50.5 Treatments for Psoriasis

Treatment	Rationale
Topicals	
• Moisturizing ointments, gels, creams	• For mild to moderate psoriasis: moisturizing plaques minimize scaling, decrease itching, keep the skin hydrated
• Coal tar: creams and shampoos	• Suppresses cell division and decreases inflammation; applied twice daily
• Corticosteroids	• Fast acting; decrease inflammation and itching; vasoconstrictive to decrease redness; prevent formation of new lesions
• Vitamin D analogues (calcipotriene, calcitriol)	• Inhibit proliferation of keratinocytes to decrease plaque formation; added benefits if used with topical corticosteroids
• Retinoids (vitamin A)	• Diminish proliferation of keratinocytes and decrease inflammation
• Salicylic acid (in combination with other topical therapies)	• Decreases scaling and softens plaques
Phototherapy	
• Narrow-band ultraviolet therapy (NB-UVB) phototherapy	• Inhibits cellular turnover and downregulates local immune system function; treatments measured in seconds of exposure; has synergistic effect when used with methotrexate
• PUVA photochemotherapy: uses oral psoralens to sensitize cells to ultraviolet A (UVA) radiation; can be combined with other therapies	• Same effects as NB-UVB but also penetrates dermis to decrease inflammation
Biologics	
• Immunomodulatory medications (e.g., Humira, Enbrel, Remicade)	• Inhibit the effects of immune system components; for moderate to severe psoriasis in individuals who have not responded to other therapies; require careful monitoring for serious side effects
Traditional systemic medications	
• Methotrexate, cyclosporine, acitretin	• Inhibits the enzyme involved in rapid cell growth; requires careful monitoring

(cancer cells that arise from the flat squamous cells that make up the epidermis) seem to be related to the treatment exposures during phototherapy. In addition to therapy-related malignancies, patients with psoriasis who choose to smoke or consume large quantities of alcohol have a greater risk of developing cancers of the oral cavity, esophagus, liver, pancreas, lung, kidney, and breast.

Research also suggests that patients with psoriasis may be at greater risk of developing cardiovascular disease. This may be related to the chronic inflammation of psoriasis that results in high levels of circulating oxidants, which stimulate the formation of atherosclerotic lesions in blood vessel walls. Therefore, prudent monitoring of cardiovascular risk factors such as obesity, increased cholesterol and triglycerides, and hypertension should occur in patients with psoriasis.

Some forms of psoriasis are associated with recent streptococcal infections among patients who complained of sore throat symptoms 1 to 2 weeks prior to the psoriatic eruption. Additionally, patients with psoriasis are at increased risk of systemic infections, mainly related to the immuno-suppressant therapies used to treat the disease. Therefore, immunizations against influenza and pneumonia are highly recommended.

Lastly, psoriasis can have a significant impact on an individual's quality of life. Depression leading to suicidal ideation occurs in more than 5% of those with psoriasis. Studies confirm that worry and anxiety occur in more than 30% of patients with psoriasis, and interpersonal difficulties affect every aspect of relationships. Persistent stress occurs when patients practice avoidance behavior because they believe they are being judged on the basis of physical appearance due to this skin disorder. Not only does this stress and worry have a negative impact on the success of treatment, but it can further exacerbate the disease. Therefore, it is essential to consider not only the physical but also the psychosocial implications of psoriasis when caring for these patients.

Connection Check 50.4

An 18-year-old with psoriatic plaques on the elbows, knees, and legs has been successfully treated with a combination of therapies including phototherapy. Because the patient is an avid soccer player and expects to receive a college scholarship next year, which information is the most important aspect to teach at this time?

A. The importance of knowing the clinical manifestations of PsA (soft tissue swelling, limitations of movement) because as many as 30% of those who have psoriasis develop PsA

B. The importance of adhering to the medication regimen

C. The importance of finding a support group to help cope with stress and anxiety that can develop as a response to treatment and can exacerbate the disease

D. The importance of using sunscreen while outside

Nursing Management
Assessment and Analysis

Psoriasis significantly affects the quality of life of the individual patient and the family. The effects of the disease are not necessarily proportionate with the extent of the disease on the individual. Psoriasis can lead to psychosocial stress, poor self-esteem, financial worries, increased pain and discomfort, and infection. A baseline skin assessment is necessary to identify the location, quality, and amount of plaques and areas of infection and to evaluate the effectiveness of treatment. Clinical manifestations of psoriasis include thickening of the epidermis related to silver-white scales over red, circumscribed, thickened plaques. Patients with psoriasis are at higher risk of developing non-melanoma skin cancer and PsA that can lead to impaired mobility and restrict activities of daily living. More than 50% of patients diagnosed with psoriasis complain of physical pain as well as physical irritation and itching.

Because there is a high rate of psoriasis within families, it is important to obtain a detailed family history from those patients presenting with clinical manifestations of psoriasis. Assessment also focuses on conditions that increase the risk of psoriasis, including immunocompromise or immunosuppression and impaired skin integrity. Because of the skin changes associated with psoriasis, patients often manifest issues around personal appearance, leading to an increased risk of depression, anxiety, obsessive behavior, and difficulty expressing emotions such as anger. Depression and low self-esteem are associated with psoriasis and can be so debilitating that patients contemplate suicide. Pathological anxiety and worry occur because of the effects of avoidance behavior. Stress and anxiety have deleterious effects on the response to treatment and can exacerbate the disease.

Nursing Diagnoses

- **Impaired skin integrity** related to chronic skin inflammation and pruritus
- **Chronic pain** related to chronic skin inflammation, psoriatic plaques, and arthritis
- **Disturbed body image** related to altered appearance secondary to thick, scaling plaques on the skin

Nursing Interventions
Assessments

- Vital signs
  Vital signs can be affected by infection (increased temperature, increased heart rate, decreased blood pressure with sepsis).
- Pain
  Patients with psoriasis have increased levels of discomfort, pain, and itching associated with inflammation of the skin.
- Skin
  Baseline and ongoing skin assessments help guide and evaluate the effectiveness of treatment; skin infections are noted with erythema, increased warmth, and purulent drainage.
- Mood, affect
  Mood and affect are a reflection of emotional well-being.

■ *Actions*

- Administer ordered medications.
  The specific actions of medications, although they do not cure psoriasis, minimize symptoms and may minimize exacerbations.
- Monitor for side effects of treatments.
- Topical preparations
  Staining of skin, hair, nails, and clothes can occur with topical treatments.
  Skin atrophy can occur with prolonged use of topical corticosteroids.
  Disease can worsen after discontinuing strong topical corticosteroids.
  Increased serum calcium levels and photosensitivity may occur with vitamin D analogues.
  Skin irritation may occur with retinoids.
  Systemic toxicity may occur if used in conjunction with oral salicylates.
- Phototherapy
  Itching, burning, erythema, stinging, increased risk of skin cancer, abdominal fullness, flulike symptoms, nasal congestion
- Biologics (immunomodulatory medications such as Humira, Enbrel, and Remicade)
  Infections, injection site reactions, rash, tuberculosis, cancers of the bladder or skin, neurological reactions, hypertension, malignancies, fever, chills
- Traditional systemics (methotrexate, cyclosporine, acitretin)
  Infection, fever, chills, nausea, infertility, photosensitivity, severe allergic reactions, difficulty breathing, liver or kidney damage, hypertension, hair loss
- Provide emotional support
  Low self-esteem may occur on the basis of patients' sense of altered body image because of plaques.
- Referral to counseling for psychosocial dysfunction
  Psoriasis can have a negative impact on quality of life, leading to high levels of anxiety, depression, anger, and possibly suicidal thoughts.
- Administer analgesics as ordered for control of pain.
  Some patients require analgesic medication for the pain caused by psoriasis.
- Encourage patient and family to join a psoriasis support group.
  Local support group information and many online resources are found on the National Psoriasis Foundation Web site (www.psoriasis.org). Support groups can help patients cope with the disease.

■ *Teaching*

- Proper hand washing before and after application of topical medications
  To avoid staining and unnecessary absorption of medications as well as diminish the transmission of bacteria
- Clinical manifestations of adverse reactions to specific therapies
  Explanations of adverse reactions helps the patient understand the treatments.

- Signs of skin infection (purulent drainage, erythema, increased warmth)
  Understanding the clinical manifestations allows for more timely treatment.
- To limit the amount of sunlight exposure while taking systemic therapies
  Photosensitivity can occur in response to systemic therapy.
- For phototherapy: daily examination of skin to look for signs of overexposure (erythema, tenderness on palpation, blisters)
  Phototherapy should be held and reevaluated because of the increased risk of skin cancer, pain, and infection if patients experience signs of overexposure.

Evaluating Care Outcomes

Address emotional and psychological stress because physical clinical manifestations have proven to be crucial in the management of psoriasis. Providing emotional support, allowing the patient to verbalize concerns, and referral to the appropriate providers and support groups can improve overall quality of life. Educating the patient and family about medication side effects, including frequent skin assessment during phototherapy, is essential for the patient's health and safety.

Connection Check 50.5

The nurse correlates the use of KOH testing with the definitive diagnosis of which skin disorder?
A. Bacterial infections
B. Herpes simplex
C. Fungal infections
D. Psoriasis

SKIN TRAUMA

Traumatic injuries to the skin are the result of external sources and are classified as acute wounds. There are many types of traumatic skin injuries, including lacerations, abrasions, excoriations, friction blisters, skin tears, pressure injuries, and burns. Pressure injuries are discussed in more detail later in this chapter, and burns are discussed in Chapter 51.

Epidemiology

Laceration

A **laceration** is a break in the skin caused by penetration of a sharp object or high **shearing forces** that exert a diagonal force on the skin, causing damage. The wound edges of abrasions may be smooth or jagged. Lacerations are superficial (near the skin surface) or extend into the deeper tissues such as the nerves, muscle, bone, or tendon. Lacerations that are superficial and do not involve the underlying tissues are usually treated in the primary healthcare provider's office.

Abrasion

Abrasions, occurring as a result of friction and shear from external forces, are usually minor injuries involving only the epidermis. Some abrasions involve part or all of the dermis. An example of an abrasion is a grazing or scraping injury to the skin of the knee of a patient who fell on concrete. Minor abrasions do not usually require treatment by healthcare personnel, leading to difficulty in determining incidence and prevalence rates because these injuries are not consistently reported.

Excoriation

An **excoriation** is a superficial abrasion. It can be self-induced through repetitive scratching and is usually linear in appearance. Excoriations are commonly seen in disorders of the skin that cause pruritus (itching), such as insect bites, scabies, dermatitis (inflammation of the skin from an allergic reaction), and chicken pox (varicella-zoster virus). The term *excoriation* is also used to describe the loss of epithelium in response to prolonged exposure to urine and feces in an individual who is incontinent. Urine and feces alter the pH of the skin, causing it to become more alkaline, which supports bacterial proliferation, leading to skin breakdown in the perineal area, also known as incontinence-associated dermatitis (IAD). More than 200 million people worldwide are affected by urinary incontinence. Approximately 35% of the older adults in acute care facilities and 41% of those in long-term care facilities experience IAD.

Friction Blisters

Friction blisters commonly occur on the feet of long-distance runners or on individuals with poor-fitting shoes, as well as on the palms of athletes who play racquet sports. Friction is a force that is applied parallel to a surface, resulting in a rubbing motion. This causes the cells of the epidermis to separate, and increased hydrostatic pressure causes plasma-like fluid to accumulate between the cells. Moisture on the surface increases the risk of blistering. Most commonly, blisters occur on the feet and palms where the skin is thick; however, blisters can occur on other parts of the body because of the external forces of friction and shear. Up to 39% of marathon runners experience friction blisters on the feet.

Skin Tears

Skin tears are traumatic wounds usually caused by minor trauma that primarily affect older adults. Minor trauma in this population includes injuries involving wheelchairs (25%), bumping into objects (25%), transfers (18%), falls (12.4%), and tape removal. In the United States, more than 1.5 million skin tears occur among institutionalized older adults. Approximately 80% of these skin tears occur on the upper extremities, whereas other common areas include the lower extremities, back, and buttocks. In addition, premature infants who have immature skin, as well as individuals who are critically ill, are also at risk of developing skin tears. Payne and Martin developed a skin tear classification scale that assists in the diagnosis and treatment of skin tears (Table 50.6). The Skin Tear Audit Research (STAR) Classification System, which was developed in Australia, is another skin tear classification system that includes three categories and two subcategories of skin tears.

Pathophysiology and Clinical Manifestations

The explanation of the pathophysiology of skin trauma and the acute wound must include a discussion of the structure and function of the skin, a definition of wound tissues, wound healing, and the influence of age. There are many functions of the skin, including protection from bacterial invasion and external elements; perception of the environment through

Table 50.6 Payne-Martin Skin Tear Classification

Category	Description
Category I	Skin tear without tissue loss: The epidermal flap either completely covers the dermis or covers the dermis to within 1 mm of the wound margin.
	Ia: Linear type
	Ib: Flap type
Category II	Skin tears with partial tissue loss
	IIa: Scant tissue loss: Partial-thickness wound in which less than or equal to 25% of the epidermis flap is lost and greater than or equal to 75% of the dermis is covered by the flap.
	IIb: Moderate to large tissue loss: Partial-thickness wound in which greater than or equal to 25% of the epidermal flap is lost and greater than or equal to 25% of the dermis is exposed.
Category III	Skin tears with complete tissue loss: Epidermal flap is absent.

Adapted from Payne, R., & Martin, M. (1993). Defining and classifying skin tears: Need for a common language. *Ostomy Wound Management, 39*(5), 16–26.

the senses of touch, pain, temperature, and pressure; retention of water; absorption; thermoregulation; immune surveillance; and metabolism of vitamin D. However, once the surface of the skin is breached, homeostasis is disturbed, and skin functions become less effective. Aging can impact wound healing because of structural changes of the skin (see Geriatric/Gerontological Considerations).

Geriatric/Gerontological Considerations

Wound Healing

The functions of the skin and its ability to heal are significantly affected by the aging process. Epidermal thinning occurs with aging and makes the skin more susceptible to external mechanical forces such as friction, shear, trauma, and moisture. The rete ridges are epidermal finger-like projections that reach and "lock" into the dermal layer. With aging, the rete ridges flatten between the dermal-epidermal junction, making it more susceptible to tearing injury from external shearing forces. Additionally, aging skin is a less effective barrier against water loss and infection because the dermis thins by about 20% and causes a decrease in the number of dermal cells, blood vessels, nerves, and collagen. Older adults are also subject to loss of subcutaneous tissue, which results in loss of the insulating properties and mechanical protection of the skin. This leads to alterations in sensation, thermoregulation, and moisture retention in the skin of older adults, making them more susceptible to traumatic injuries such as skin tears, excoriations, and pressure injuries.

A cascade of healing is set into motion in response to traumatic injury of the skin. **Partial-thickness** skin loss describes a wound where damage extends through the epidermis and into the dermis but not through the dermis. This can be a shallow laceration, abrasion, or excoriation. Because the hair follicles originate in the dermis, not all of them are destroyed in a partial-thickness wound. Each hair follicle is surrounded by epidermal cells that proliferate and migrate along the wound bed within the first 24 hours of injury. Repair of the dermis takes longer because **neoangiogenesis** (growth of new blood vessels) must occur while collagen fibers build to help contraction of the wound and full re-epithelialization.

Full-thickness skin trauma involves the epidermis, dermis, subcutaneous tissues, and possibly muscles, tendons, or bones and can occur as a result of a deep laceration or ulcer. The four **phases of wound healing** are initiated when a full-thickness injury occurs. The four phases of wound healing are hemostasis, inflammatory, proliferative, and maturation (Table 50.7; Fig. 50.5). After the immediate injury, platelets and other clotting factors are activated and aggregate to form a clot, stopping hemorrhage at the site

Table 50.7 Four Phases of Wound Healing

Phase	Actions
Hemostasis (immediate)	Activation of platelets and clotting factors
	Fibrin deposition
	Platelet release of cytokines
	Fibroblasts activate production of collagen
Inflammatory (from 24 hours to 2 weeks)	Surrounding vasculature begins to "leak" in response to mast cells.
	Neutrophils phagocytize bacteria and remove foreign material.
	Fluid escapes into the wound and causes edema.
	Macrophages remove additional bacteria, residual foreign bodies, and necrotic tissue.
	Macrophages secrete growth factors and cytokines that activate the synthesis of collagen and lay down extracellular matrix.
Proliferative	Angiogenesis
	Epithelialization
	Fibroplasia with formation of granulation tissue
	Collagen deposition
	Wound contraction
Maturation (up to 2 years)	Decreased fluid within wound
	Decreased metabolic rate
	Reorganization of collagen fibers
	Continued collagen synthesis and degradation

of blood vessel damage as part of the hemostasis phase. Fibrin is deposited in the wound and functions as a provisional matrix to stabilize the wound site. Then, platelets release cytokines, which initiate the wound-healing process and play a key role in the progression of the wound-healing cycle. The cytokines recruit additional cells such as fibroblasts that activate the production of collagen, which is essential in repairing the extracellular matrix.

The main function of the inflammatory phase of wound healing is to remove debris within the wound. This phase begins within the first 24 hours after injury and can last up to 2 weeks for an acute wound. In response to mast cells, the surrounding vasculature begins to leak neutrophils (white blood cells) into the area of injury to phagocytize bacteria and remove foreign materials. Along with the neutrophils, fluid also escapes into this area and causes swelling. Additionally, monocytes attracted to the wound site become macrophages and are stimulated to remove any additional bacteria, residual

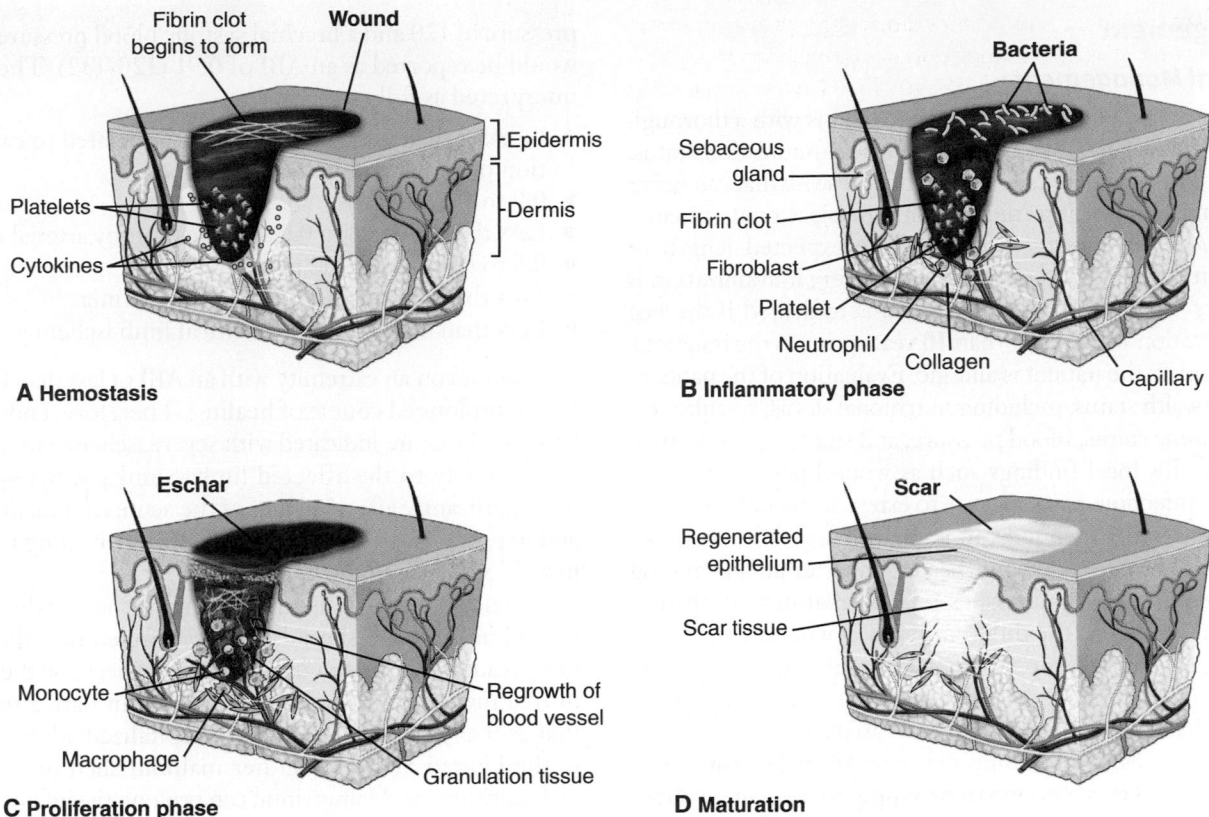

FIGURE 50.5 Four phases of wound healing. A, Hemostasis. B, Inflammatory. C, Proliferative. D, Maturation.

foreign bodies, and necrotic tissue. Lastly, macrophages secrete growth factors and cytokines that activate fibroblasts, which synthesize collagen and lay down the extracellular matrix. The clinical characteristics of the inflammatory phase include edema, erythema, heat, and pain. The wound bed during this phase may have visible necrotic (dead) tissue.

The third phase of the wound-healing cycle is the proliferative phase. The four major steps of this phase are **angiogenesis** (growth of new blood vessels from previously existing ones), epithelialization, granulation (growth of new tissue), and collagen deposition with tissue formation. During the proliferative phase, the number of macrophages decreases and fibroblasts proliferate, secreting collagen to replace the provisional fibrin matrix and provide a strong extracellular matrix. While the macrophages are synthesizing collagen, keratinocytes emerge to help with re-epithelialization. Endothelial cells are activated to initiate angiogenesis, which increases blood supply to the new tissue. As the capillary bed is laid down, the wound fills with **granulation tissue** and appears beefy red, shiny, and granular. During this time, the metabolic rate of the tissue is higher and requires adequate nutrition and oxygenation to properly heal the wound.

In the maturation or remodeling phase, which is the final phase of wound healing, granulation tissue matures into a scar. There is decreased fluid within the wound, decreased metabolic rate and cell densities, and an increase and reorganization of collagen fibers, resulting in increased tensile strength of the wound. Collagen synthesis and degradation continue during this phase for up to 2 years. Still, the tensile strength of the scar tissue becomes only 80% of that of normal tissue, making it more susceptible to tissue breakdown and trauma.

Connection Check 50.6

The nurse is admitting a patient to the unit who is a paraplegic and has a history of healed sacral pressure injuries, verified by the large scars on the sacrum. What action should the nurse take first?

A. Apply a moisturizing lotion to the sacrum.

B. Place a dressing such as a silicone foam dressing over the scars.

C. Place the patient in a sitting position to keep pressure off the sacrum.

D. Help the patient choose the most nutritious foods on the menu.

Connection Check 50.7

In completing a skin assessment, the nurse correlates erythema, redness, and warmth with which phase of wound healing?

A. Hemostasis

B. Inflammatory

C. Proliferative

D. Maturation

Management

Medical Management

Medical management of skin trauma begins with a thorough wound and medical history, including immunization status. Tetanus is a potentially life-threatening disease that can occur following penetrating injury with an object contaminated with *Clostridium tetani* bacteria. The expected length of immunity to the *C. tetani* bacteria following immunization is 10 years. Therefore, tetanus toxoid is indicated if the last immunization was greater than 10 years prior to the traumatic injury, unless the patient is allergic. Evaluation of the patient's overall health status, including nutritional status, vascular status, immune status, blood pressure, and smoking, is essential. Additionally, local findings such as wound perfusion, tissue viability, infection, and exposure to external mechanical forces are considered. A wound can contain many different types of tissues over the course of healing, and an understanding of the types of wound tissues guides treatment decisions. Table 50.8 explains the different types of wound tissue.

Adequate blood supply to an extremity and ultimately to the wound is needed for healing to occur. Disease states such as diabetes mellitus, peripheral vascular disease, anemia, arteriosclerosis, and cardiopulmonary disorders can affect the blood, oxygen, and nutrient supply to an acute wound. The ankle-brachial index (ABI) is the ratio of the systolic blood pressures obtained at the ankle and in the arm and is a sensitive, noninvasive indicator of arterial perfusion to the lower extremities. For example, an ankle systolic blood pressure of 120 and a brachial systolic blood pressure of 132 would be reported as an ABI of 0.91 (120/132). The ABI is interpreted as follows:

- Greater than 1.3: abnormal, usually related to calcification of vessel wall
- 0.9 to 1.3: normal
- Less than or equal to 0.9: lower extremity arterial disease
- 0.6 to 0.8: borderline perfusion
- Less than or equal to 0.5: severe ischemia
- Less than or equal to 0.4: critical limb ischemia

A wound on an extremity with an ABI of less than 0.8 may have a prolonged course of healing. Therefore, endovascular procedures are indicated with severe ischemia to improve blood supply to the affected limb. Similarly, hypotension can significantly affect healing of the acute wound. Smoking and hypothermia should be avoided while healing to maximize blood flow to the wound.

Nutritional status is another important indicator of wound healing and should be incorporated into the treatment plan to promote wound healing and decrease the length of treatment. The Nutrition Screening Initiative reported that as many as 40% to 60% of hospitalized adult patients in the United States are either malnourished or at risk of malnourishment. Malnutrition can prolong the inflammatory phase of wound healing by decreasing fibroblast proliferation, collagen formation, and angiogenesis. Unfortunately, the biochemical data on which many clinicians still rely, such as serum albumin and prealbumin levels, can be significantly

Table 50.8	Definition of Tissue Types
Tissue Type	**Definition**
Granulation tissue 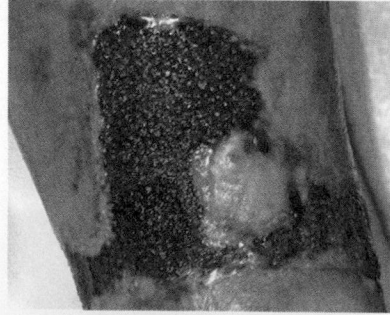	Red/pink moist granular tissue composed of new blood vessels Healthy, healing tissue
Hypergranulation tissue 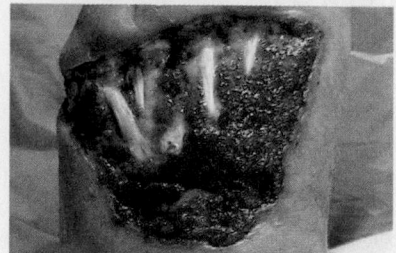	Hyperplasia of granulation tissue recognized by its friable red appearance usually in response to a prolonged inflammatory phase

Table 50.8 Definition of Tissue Types—cont'd

Tissue Type	Definition
Necrotic tissue 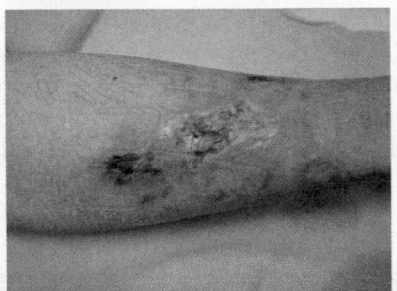	Dead or avascular or devitalized tissue
Eschar 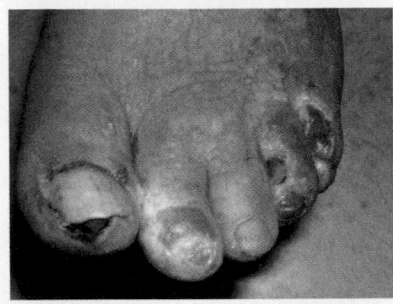	Thick, leathery, devitalized tissue; black or brown; hard, soft, or boggy Loose or firmly attached to wound bed
Slough 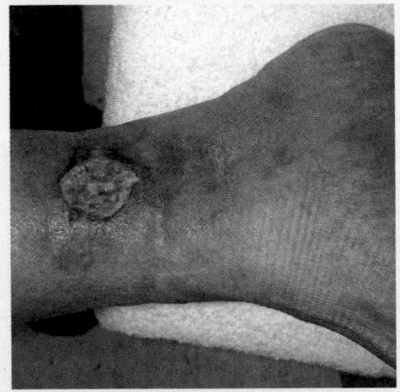	Soft, moist devitalized tissue that may be white, yellow, tan, green May be loose, stringy
Macerated tissue 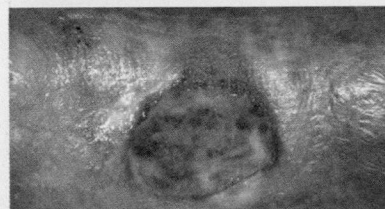	Softened tissue in response to prolonged exposure to moisture

affected by numerous confounding factors, including hydration status, medications, alterations in metabolism, and inflammation, making them an unreliable reflection of nutritional status.

Nutrition screening uses valid and reliable tools to quickly ascertain an individual's risk of malnutrition, and the anthropometric measurements of weight, height, and body mass index (BMI) are utilized as part of these tools. Additionally, significant unwanted weight loss and any significant recent illnesses are also indicators utilized in some nutrition screening tools (see Chapter 55 for the Malnutrition Universal Screening Tool [MUST] from the British

Association of Parenteral and Enteral Nutrition; referral to a nutritionist for a complete nutritional assessment is initiated when an individual scores 2 or higher on the MUST).

The immune status of a patient plays an important role in the ability to heal. For patients with immune deficiencies such as AIDS, treatment with prophylactic antibiotics is considered. If possible, immunosuppressant medications, such as steroids, should be weaned to the lowest possible dose. When it is not possible to wean patients from steroids, providers use high doses of vitamin A to counteract the steroids' detrimental effects. Vitamin A works by boosting the immune response and enhancing the early inflammatory phase of wound healing.

Identifying infection is another important part of wound management, and culturing a wound by surface swab or punch biopsy assists with antibiotic selection and guides treatment. The surgical management of a traumatic wound involves debridement (removal) of necrotic (dead) tissue to decrease the bioburden (bacteria living on the wound surface) of the wound, thereby decreasing the risk of infection. Table 50.9 provides an overview of the different methods of debridement.

Table 50.9 Overview of Debridement Methods

Method	Considerations	Contraindications
Surgical/sharp Necrotic tissue is removed using a scalpel, scissors, forceps, or curette.	Urgent need for debridement	Malignant wounds
	Highly selective	Patients with clotting/bleeding abnormalities
	Rapid results	Ischemic tissue
	Pain unless the patient has neuropathy; analgesia often needed	Unstable patient status
	Risk of hemorrhage/complications	Underlying dialysis fistula, prosthesis, or arterial bypass graft
	Cost; use of special equipment	Caution with wounds involving hands and face
	Requires patient consent	Caution with immunocompromised patients
	Requires special training and expert comfort level (including anatomical knowledge)	
	Must distinguish between necrotic and healthy tissues	
	Can be done bedside	
	May require the need for operating room and systemic anesthetics for extensive procedures	
	Anticoagulant therapy	
Autolytic Endogenous enzymes present in wound fluid interact with moist dressing to soften and remove necrotic tissue.	Need for minor or moderate debridement	Some dressings cannot be used with infected wounds
	Patient has a decreased or minimal risk of wound infection	Exposed tendon/bone
	Performed in any setting	Friable skin
	Can be used with other methods	Deep, extensive wounds
	Selective	Severe neutropenia
	Safe, easy to use	Immunocompromised patients
	Painless and soothing when dressing in place	
	Slow	
	Risk of maceration to surrounding skin	
	Removal of some dressings may be painful	
	Odor	

Table 50.9 Overview of Debridement Methods—cont'd

Method	Considerations	Contraindications
	Secondary dressing is needed for some types of primary dressings	
	Absorptive dressings can dehydrate the wound bed	
Mechanical Wet-to-dry: Moist dressing is applied to wound, allowed to dry, and removed with force.	Larger wounds	Clean wounds
	Nonsurgical candidates	
	Nonselective	
	Painful	
	Frequent dressing changes required, can be done up to three times a day; non–cost-effective	
	May macerate surrounding skin	
	Bleeding	
	Dressing fibers stick to wound bed and can cause a foreign body reaction	
	May dispense bacteria when removed	
	Traditional more than a modern accepted practice	
	Increases circulation to wound bed	
Hydrotherapy: Moving water dislodges loose debris.	May macerate periwound skin	Clean wounds
	Time-consuming	Presence of diabetic neuropathy
	May cause trauma to wound bed and lead to bacterial contamination of wound and environment	
	Labor-intensive	
	Theoretical risk of fluid embolism or promotion of infection with irrigation	
	Healthcare professional needs personal protective equipment because of aerosolization	
	Can impede venous blood flow in legs	
	Bed-bound patients	
Pulsed lavage: Irrigation combined with suction		Clean wounds
Maggot larvae (*Lucilia sericata*, green bottle fly) Consume necrotic tissue and bacteria	Psychological distress	Allergies to adhesives, fly larvae, eggs, soybeans
	Allergic reaction	Patients with bleeding abnormalities
	Potential for increased pain in ischemic wounds	Deep, tunneled wounds
	Time-consuming	
	Selective	
	Rapid	
	Costly	

Continued

Table 50.9 Overview of Debridement Methods—cont'd

Method	Considerations	Contraindications
	May be painless	
	Decrease bacterial load	
	Bedside use	
	Can be used for various wound types, including infected wounds	
Enzymatic Enzymes degrade and remove necrotic tissue.	Patient on anticoagulants	Clean wound
	Can be used on infected wounds	Allergy to component of the enzyme preparation
	Cost-effective	
	Bedside use	
	Can be selective	
	Decreased wound trauma	
	Cost varies	
	Daily or twice-a-day application depending on type of enzyme	
	Sting/inflammation around wound with some enzymes	
	Not used with heavy metal salts (silver and mercury)	
	May need cross-hatching of eschar	
	Clinicians need to document in patient's medication record because enzymes are prescribed medications.	
	Match type of enzyme used to type of nonviable tissue in the wound.	

Source: Kirshen, C., Woo, K., Ayello, E., & Sibbald, R. (2006). Debridement: A vital component of wound bed preparation. *Advances in Skin and Wound Care, 19*(9), 511–512.

Controlling or eliminating external factors, such as exposure to urine and feces, and decreasing the mechanical forces of friction and shear are necessary in the healing and prevention of traumatic skin injury. Cleansing incontinent episodes as soon as possible and using moisture barrier creams such as zinc pastes can reduce the exposure of the perineal skin to the detrimental effects of urine and feces. Shearing exerts a diagonal force on the skin, causing an opposing motion of the internal tissue layers against bone, leading to damage to deeper structures such as blood vessels, muscle, and subcutaneous fat. Friction, on the other hand, inflicts a parallel force on the skin, damages the superficial layers, and occurs when one surface slides across another. Keeping the head of the bed at less than 30 degrees minimizes the forces of friction and shear by limiting the ability of the body to "slide down" the surface of the bed. Friction also plays a role in the development of traumatic foot blisters, which can be minimized with properly fitting shoes, appropriate socks, and utilization of gel soles in the shoes.

Surgical Management

Surgical approaches to the management of traumatic skin injuries vary depending on the nature of the wound itself. There are three different surgical closure approaches: primary intention, secondary intention, and tertiary intention (Table 50.10; Fig. 50.6). Prior to wound closure, necrotic tissue must be removed because it provides a medium on which bacteria can multiply, leading to infection. **Primary intention** is the approach used with typical surgical incisions with well-approximated edges that are closed with sutures or staples. With **secondary intention**, the wound is left open and allowed to fill in with granulation tissue. Often, these wounds are packed with gauze and changed daily. The healing process with secondary intention can be slow, and scar tissue is more pronounced. **Tertiary intention** often

Table 50.10 Types of Wound Closure

Intention (Closure)	Unique Characteristics	Key Points
Primary	Clean, minimally contaminated 6–8 hours old	May close with tape, staples, sutures, glue
Secondary	Animal bites Abscess cavities, ulcers	No sutures Delayed skin coverage, grafts
Tertiary	Too contaminated to close	Must clean, debride, and observe 4–6 days before suturing

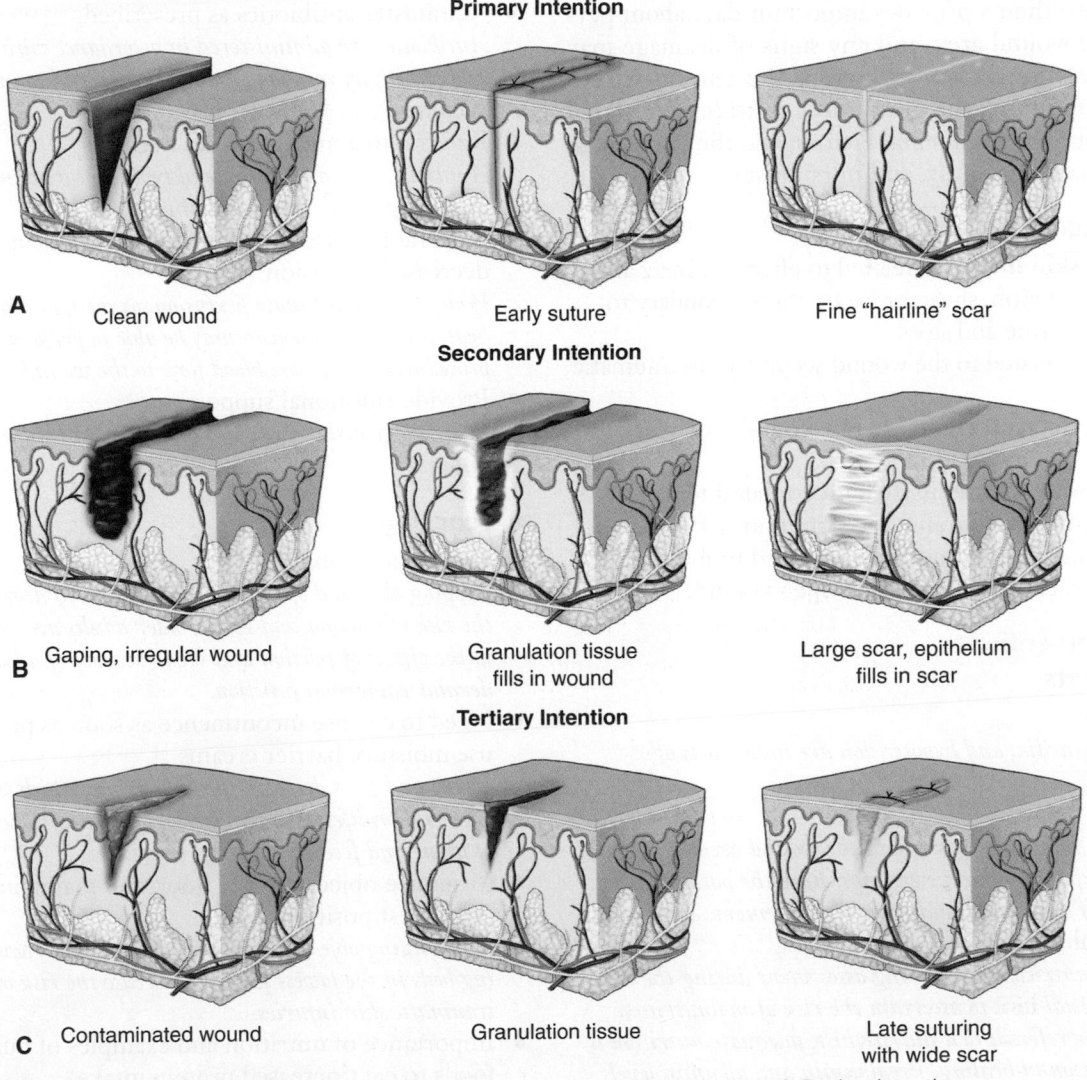

FIGURE 50.6 Types of wound closure. A, Primary intention. B, Secondary intention. C, Tertiary intention.

uses skin grafts for wound closure, after a period of observation following initial surgical debridement.

Complications

As with any breach in the integrity of the skin, patients with traumatic skin injuries are at high risk for infection. Clinical manifestations of infection include increasing erythema, increased temperature of surrounding tissues, odor, purulent drainage, increased swelling, increased pain, and fever. Depending on the depth of the injury, an individual can be at further risk of damage to underlying structures of muscle, tendon, bone, and nerve, requiring deep lacerations to be explored down to the wound bed to determine the involvement of these structures. Additionally, pain from a traumatic skin injury can range from mild to severe and must be treated accordingly. Lastly, scarring from skin injuries that are on the face or other apparent surfaces can be psychologically traumatic and can affect self-image and interpersonal relationships.

Nursing Management

Assessment and Analysis

Specific assessments include the overall health and nutritional status, skin integrity, mobility, and hydration status of the patient. In addition to a comprehensive physical assessment, the nurse examines and documents the characteristics of the actual area of skin trauma, as well as the surrounding tissue. Assessment of color, temperature, edema, and erythema provides important data about perfusion to the wound area, and any signs of drainage may indicate infection. When managing the patient with a traumatic skin injury, the nurse must consider associated patient factors; environmental factors; and the knowledge base of the patient, family, and nursing staff.

Nursing Diagnoses

- **Impaired skin integrity** related to effects of mechanical irritants of friction, shear, or excoriation secondary to exposure to urine and stool
- **Acute pain** related to the wound secondary to traumatic skin injury
- **Risk for infection** related to the wound secondary to traumatic skin injury
- **Risk for body image disturbance** related to the wound secondary to traumatic skin injury
- **Risk for imbalanced nutrition** related to increased metabolic rate secondary to the open wound

Nursing Interventions

■ Assessments

- Vital signs
  Fever, tachycardia, and hypotension are indications of infection.
- Pain
  Pain occurs related to pressure in the wound area, as well as potential exposure of nerve endings. Rate the patient's pain on a scale of 0 to 10 to guide pain management.
- Nutritional status
  Perform a nutritional screening assessment during the patient's initial visit to ascertain the risk of malnutrition and need for referral to a nutritionist; adequate nutrition is needed for wound healing. Prealbumin and albumin levels may provide data about the overall nutrition status. The MUST score is effective in guiding nutritional assessment and management.
- Skin
  Conduct a baseline skin assessment, including measurement of wounds, to guide treatment and evaluation of interventions; observe for clinical manifestations of infection (increased erythema, temperature, swelling, increased pain, odor, purulent drainage).

- Peripheral vascular status
  Wounds need adequate perfusion to heal, and cool, pale skin is indicative of decreased perfusion.
- Fluid volume status
  Adequate perfusion is dependent on ideal fluid volume status. Dehydration can exacerbate alterations in skin integrity.

■ Actions

- Perform wound care as prescribed (including cleansing and using appropriate dressings).
  Cleansing decreases the bacterial burden, and moist wound-healing products support adequate healing.
- Administer pain medications as prescribed.
  Nerve endings can be exposed in open wounds, causing pain.
- Administer antibiotics as prescribed.
  Antibiotics are administered in accordance with the culture and sensitivity results to lower the bacterial count and support healing.
- Referral to a nutritionist as needed
  A nutritionist can recommend types and amounts of foods that can promote wound healing.
- Referral for vascular evaluation with documented decreased perfusion
  Wounds need adequate perfusion, oxygen, and nutrients to heal; a vascular surgeon may be able to perform reperfusion procedures to increase blood flow to the wound.
- Provide emotional support.
  Body image disturbance can occur with a traumatic skin injury.

■ Teaching

- Proper positioning
  Keeping the head of the bed at less than 30 degrees decreases the risk of friction and shear; older adults are more prone to the effects of friction and shear because of a flattened dermal-epidermal junction.
- Need to cleanse incontinence as soon as possible and use moisture barrier creams
  Urine and feces decrease the pH of skin, which supports bacterial proliferation; barrier creams minimize the effects of urine and feces on perineal tissue.
- Minimize objects on the floor, and maintain the bed in the lowest position.
  Minimizing objects on the floor in patients' rooms and keeping beds in the lowest position decrease the risk of falling and traumatic skin injuries.
- Importance of nutrition and examples of nutritious foods to eat (increased protein intake)
  Wounds require adequate nutrition to heal.
- Utilize mobility aids as prescribed, and ask for assistance.
  Minimizing falls reduces the risk of traumatic skin injuries.

Evaluating Care Outcomes

Acute traumatic wounds usually heal without consequence. Educating the patient and family about the clinical manifestations of infection is important in managing wounds. Additionally, because aging skin is at even greater risk of trauma, awareness of potential environmental hazards can minimize traumatic injuries. Ensuring that wheelchairs are in good repair, floors are clear from clutter, beds are kept in their lowest position, and patients are positioned with the head of the bed at less than 30 degrees when possible are ways to minimize environmental risks. Lastly, evaluating and maximizing nutrition for a patient with an open wound supports wound healing.

Connection Check 50.8

Which position is best to reduce the risk of skin tears in an immobile, older adult patient?

A. In a side-lying position
B. Foot of the bed elevated to no greater than 15 degrees
C. In a chair with feet on the floor
D. Head of the bed elevated no greater than 30 degrees

PRESSURE INJURIES

Pressure injuries are a common health problem among individuals who are physically limited or bedridden. A pressure injury is localized damage to the skin and underlying soft tissue, usually over a bony prominence or related to a medical or other device. The injury can present as intact skin or an open ulcer and may be painful. The injury occurs as a result of intense and/or prolonged pressure or pressure in combination with shear. The tolerance of soft tissue for pressure and shear may also be affected by microclimate, nutrition, perfusion, comorbidities, and the condition of the soft tissue.

Ultimately, the nurse's goal is to limit pressure and shearing to prevent pressure injury development. However, for the patient with an existing pressure injury, the goals are wound management and the prevention of further tissue breakdown and infection.

Epidemiology

Pressure injuries are a significant clinical issue that spans across all ages and all healthcare settings. In the United States, the 2.5 million people treated annually for pressure injuries in acute care facilities are three times more likely to be transferred to a long-term care facility. Of those people treated annually, as many as 60,000 may die from complications. Most pressure injuries occur in individuals over age 65. However, people of all ages are susceptible to pressure injuries depending on comorbid conditions such as diabetes, dementia, malnutrition, and immobility.

The prevalence of pressure injuries in the United States is estimated to be 10% to 18% in acute care facilities, 2.3% to 28% in long-term care, and up to 29% in home care. The incidence of pressure injuries is estimated to be 0.4% to 38% in acute care, 2.3% to 23.9% in long-term care, 0% to 17% in home care, and 0% to 6% in rehabilitative care. The Agency for Healthcare Research and Quality (AHRQ)

continuously monitors and studies the incidence, significance, complications, and costs associated with the management of patients with pressure injuries, and the National Pressure Ulcer Advisory Panel (NPUAP) serves as the source for public policy, education, and research to support improved patient outcomes.

Not only is the cost of treating pressure injuries exorbitant, but they also significantly affect the patient's quality of life. Estimates indicate that the annual cost of treating pressure injuries in the United States runs between $9.2 billion and $15.6 billion. This includes increases in length of stay and treatment regimens related to infection, pain, support surfaces, and decreased functional ability. Pressure injuries increase the risk of mortality in the older adult population and those in ICUs by 25% to 33%. In patients admitted to the hospital with pressure injuries as the primary admission diagnosis, the mortality rate is 1 in 25 patients, whereas admissions with pressure injuries as a secondary diagnosis has a death rate of 1 in 8 patients.

Factors that increase a patient's susceptibility to the development of pressure injuries are multifactorial and include the following:

- Impaired or decreased mobility and decreased functional status with exposure to increased forces of pressure and shear
- Increased age
- Comorbid conditions such as end-stage renal disease, anemia, or diabetes mellitus
- Use of steroids
- Impaired blood flow as in atherosclerosis or lower extremity peripheral arterial disease
- Cognitive impairment
- Urinary or fecal incontinence
- Undernutrition, malnutrition, and deficits in hydration
- History of previous pressure injuries because the tensile strength of scars over healed pressure injuries is diminished and prone to repeated breakdown
- Terminal illness

Pressure injuries are an added burden to caregivers and are viewed by laypeople as preventable. Although pressure injuries are not always the result of improper care or poor-quality care, their development not only casts a negative reflection on the institution in which the patient stays but is also viewed as clinical negligence that may lead to litigation. Pressure injuries are a major litigation issue across healthcare settings, and judgments as high as $312 million for a single case have been awarded.

Pathophysiology and Clinical Manifestations

The discussion of the pathophysiology of pressure injuries must include an explanation of the extrinsic factors of pressure and shear that lead to development. Pressure is exerted when tissue is compressed between the surface on which the patient lies and the bony prominences of the body. This causes a decrease in capillary blood flow, leading to decreased perfusion of a localized area of the body, potentiating tissue ischemia and death. On average, intracapillary pressure is estimated at 32 mm Hg, whereas pressure exerted on a localized area of the body from a hard surface can reach up to 300 to 500 mm Hg depending on weight and surface area exposed. Lying flat in bed causes pressures of 50 to 94 mm Hg to be exerted on the heels, sacrum, and scapulae. This level of pressure exceeds the pressure necessary to keep the capillaries open (32 mm Hg), causing ischemia of the tissues. The intensity of the pressure and the duration of time that the skin is exposed to that pressure inversely correlate to pressure injury. In other words, a pressure injury can develop in less time with a higher intensity of pressure or in a longer period of time with a lesser degree of pressure. Therefore, the use of pressure-redistribution surfaces and frequent repositioning of the patient are equally important. Pressure-related tissue damage is not only associated with the surface involved but also the type of tissue involved. The epidermis and the dermis can withstand a lengthier exposure to ischemia without incurring irreversible damage. Therefore, tissue injuries related to pressure may be first manifested in the muscle and subcutaneous fat and characterized by a change in the color, temperature, or consistency of intact skin.

Most pressure injuries occur over bony prominences; however, they can occur on any body surface or related to a medical or other device. Commonly, the occiput (back of the head), ears, scapulae, sacrum and coccyx, ischium and buttocks, greater trochanters of the hips, and the heels of the feet are affected. An individual who sits for prolonged periods of time is exposed to higher pressures in the coccyx and ischial areas (and possibly the heels or even the lateral surfaces of the feet if a wheelchair is not adjusted to the patient's body). In the lying positions, the scapulae, sacrum, greater trochanters, heels, occiput, and ears are typically affected. Kyphosis of the spine can also lead to increased pressure and tissue breakdown on the back. Wrinkles in bedsheets or pads beneath the patient can increase pressure and potentiate the development of a pressure injury. Medical device–related pressure injuries result from the use of devices designed and applied for diagnostic or therapeutic purposes. The resultant pressure injury generally conforms to the pattern or shape of the device. The injury should be staged using the staging system. For example, a pressure injury can occur on the external nares related to the presence of a nasogastric tube or on the glans of the penis due to pressure exerted from an indwelling urinary catheter. Mucosal membrane pressure injury is found on mucous membranes with a history of a medical device in use at the location of the injury. Due to the anatomy of the tissue, these ulcers cannot be staged.

Further complications of pressure include reperfusion injury, impaired lymphatic function, and mechanical deformation of cells. With ischemia, affected tissues reduce their metabolic needs to reduce further damage caused from hypoxia. During reperfusion of this ischemic area, the oxygenated blood carrying white blood cells to the area releases inflammatory factors in response to the injury. These inflammatory factors include free radicals, which lead to further cell damage. Lymphatic function is impaired during ischemia, which leads to an accumulation of metabolic waste products, further potentiating tissue death. Lastly, alterations of tissues and cells related to pressure cause cellular membranes to rupture, leading to irreversible tissue damage.

In addition to pressure, the extrinsic forces of shear also play a role in the development of pressure injuries. Shearing forces exert a diagonal impact, and the damage occurs internally in response to the opposing motions of bone and subcutaneous tissues (Fig. 50.7). Shear and pressure usually occur together, causing significant damage first to muscle and subcutaneous tissues and later to skin. The collagen and elastic fibers of the skin increase tensile strength and make it less susceptible to shearing forces. Shear occurs when an older adult, for example, slides down in bed or while sitting up in a chair. When this occurs, blood vessels in the dermis become contorted, diminishing blood flow and perfusion, leading to ischemic damage to the tissues. Keeping the head of the bed at less than 30 degrees and minimizing the amount of time the patient is kept in a chair can diminish the effects of shear. Additionally, increased moisture from incontinence and perspiration causes maceration and inflammation, increasing the risk of skin breakdown. Utilizing draw sheets; cleaning incontinence episodes as soon as they happen; utilizing barrier ointments on the perineal skin; and maintaining dry, clean sheets or surfaces can diminish the damaging effects of moisture.

Connection Check 50.9

The nurse recognizes that pressure injury is most probable in which areas in the patient positioned in a supine position? *(Select all that apply.)*

A. Occiput

B. Nares

C. Behind the knees

D. Sacrum

E. Heels

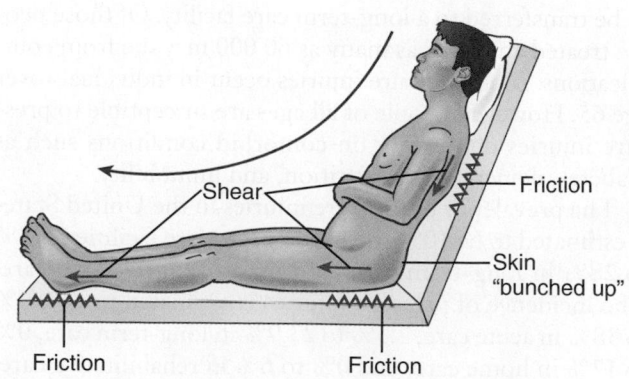

FIGURE 50.7 Shearing forces and friction that can damage skin.

Historically, there are four stages of pressure injuries. However, in 2007, the NPUAP revised its classification to include two additional categories: unstageable injuries and deep tissue injury. The NPUAP redefined the definition of pressure injuries during the NPUAP 2016 Staging Consensus Conference. Table 50.11 presents the pressure injury staging system.

Management

Medical Management

Admission to any care setting requires a thorough head-to-toe physical examination, including meticulous evaluation of the patient's skin as well as a wound history. Skin and risk assessments are conducted upon admission and at regular

---

Table 50.11 Pressure Injury Classification

Stage/Category	Description	
Stage 1 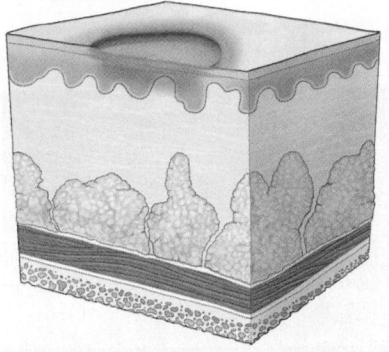	**Non-blanchable erythema of intact skin** Intact skin with a localized area of non-blanchable erythema, which may appear differently in darkly pigmented skin. Presence of blanchable erythema or changes in sensation, temperature, or firmness may precede visual changes. Color changes do not include purple or maroon discoloration; these may indicate deep tissue pressure injury.	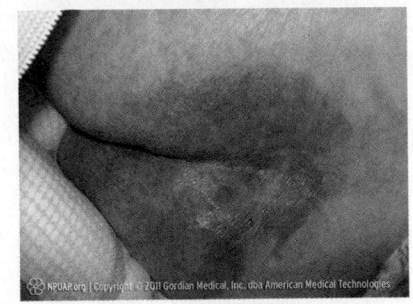
Stage 2 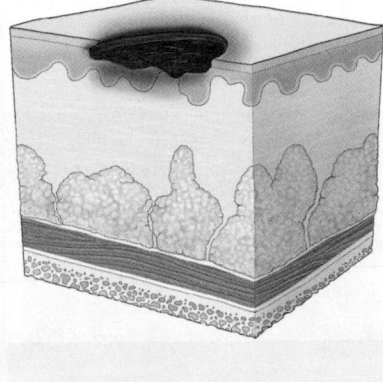	**Partial-thickness skin loss with exposed dermis** Partial-thickness loss of skin with exposed dermis. The wound bed is viable, pink or red, and moist and may also present as an intact or ruptured serum-filled blister. Adipose (fat) and deeper tissues are not visible. Granulation tissue, slough, and eschar are not present. These injuries commonly result from adverse microclimate and shear in the skin over the pelvis and shear in the heel. This stage should not be used to describe moisture-associated skin damage (MASD), including incontinence-associated dermatitis (IAD), intertriginous dermatitis (ITD), medical adhesive–related skin injury (MARSI), or traumatic wounds (skin tears, burns, abrasions).	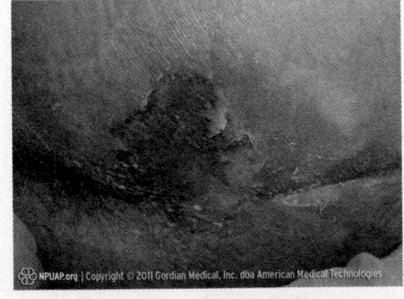
Stage 3 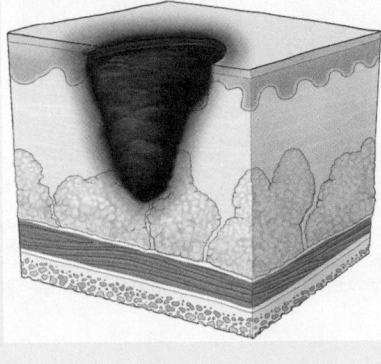	**Full-thickness skin loss** Full-thickness loss of skin, in which adipose (fat) is visible in the ulcer and granulation tissue and epibole (rolled wound edges) are often present. Slough and/or eschar may be visible. The depth of tissue damage varies by anatomical location; areas of significant adiposity can develop deep wounds. Undermining and tunneling may occur. Fascia, muscle, tendon, ligament, cartilage, and/or bone are not exposed. If slough or eschar obscures the extent of tissue loss, this is an unstageable pressure injury.	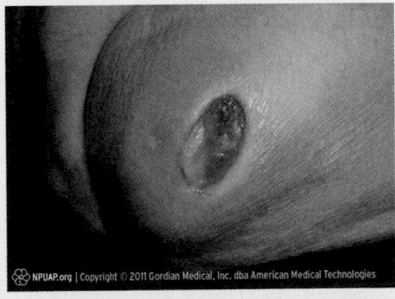

Continued

Table 50.11 Pressure Injury Classification—cont'd

Stage/Category	Description	
Stage 4 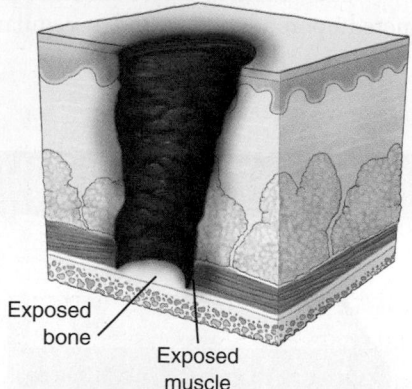 Exposed bone / Exposed muscle	**Full-thickness skin and tissue loss** Full-thickness skin and tissue loss with exposed or directly palpable fascia, muscle, tendon, ligament, cartilage, or bone in the ulcer. Slough and/or eschar may be visible. Epibole (rolled edges), undermining, and/or tunneling often occur. Depth varies by anatomical location. If slough or eschar obscures the extent of tissue loss, this is an unstageable pressure injury.	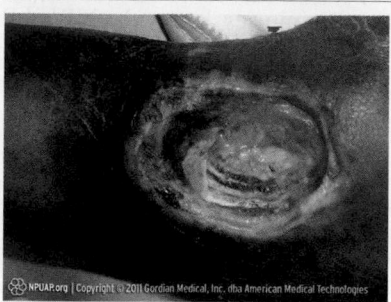
Unstageable 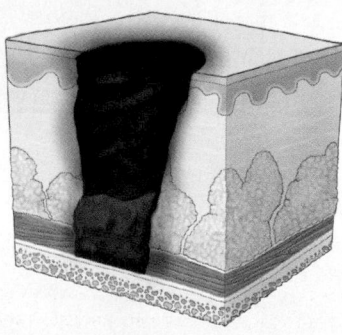	**Obscured full-thickness skin and tissue loss** Full-thickness skin and tissue loss in which the extent of tissue damage within the ulcer cannot be confirmed because it is obscured by slough or eschar. If slough or eschar is removed, a Stage 3 or Stage 4 pressure injury will be revealed. Stable eschar (i.e., dry, adherent, intact without erythema or fluctuance) on the heel or ischemic limb should not be softened or removed.	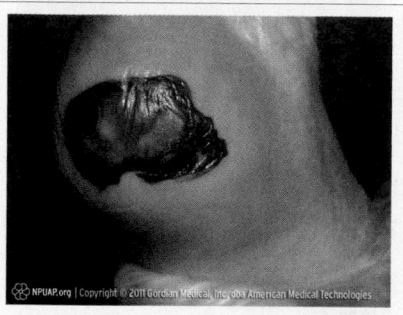
Deep tissue pressure injury (DTPI) 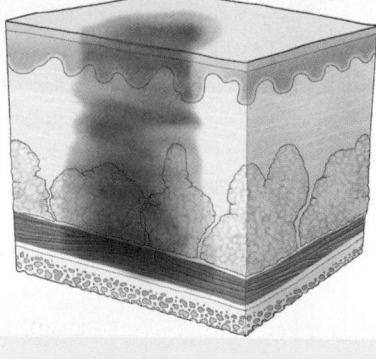	**Persistent non-blanchable deep-red, maroon, or purple discoloration** Intact or non-intact skin with localized area of persistent non-blanchable deep-red, maroon, purple discoloration or epidermal separation revealing a dark wound bed or blood-filled blister. Pain and temperature change often precede skin color changes. Discoloration may appear differently in darkly pigmented skin. This injury results from intense and/or prolonged pressure and shear forces at the bone–muscle interface. The wound may evolve rapidly to reveal the actual extent of tissue injury or may resolve without tissue loss. If necrotic tissue, subcutaneous tissue, granulation tissue, fascia, muscle, or other underlying structures are visible, this indicates a full-thickness pressure injury (unstageable, Stage 3 or Stage 4). Do not use DTPI to describe vascular, traumatic, neuropathic, or dermatological conditions.	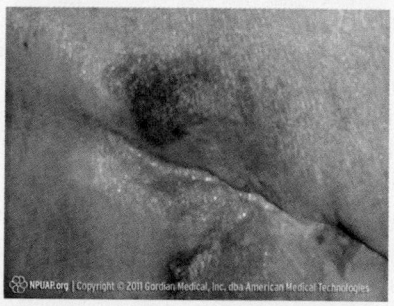

From National Pressure Ulcer Advisory Panel. (2016). *NPUAP pressure injury stages.* Retrieved from http://www.npuap.org/resources/educational-and-clinical-resources/npuap-pressure-injury-stages/

intervals according to the institution's policies, with documentation placed in the patient's chart. Although there are no specific regulations mandating a minimum standard for skin assessments, the Centers for Medicare and Medicaid Services recommended five key parameters to be addressed: temperature, moisture-balance status, color, turgor, and integrity. Any evidence of pressure on the body of the patient admitted to a healthcare facility must be documented as part of the admission skin assessment, or the institution can be held legally responsible for its development and may not receive reimbursement for its treatment. When skin integrity is compromised on admission, a licensed provider must document its etiology and description in the patient's record.

Pressure injury risk assessments are important in identifying patients at greatest risk of pressure injury development. The **Braden scale**, the most widely utilized pressure injury risk assessment tool, guides clinicians in medical management decisions to modify treatment parameters and reduce a patient's pressure injury risk. A score of 15 to 18 = mild risk, 13 to 14 = moderate risk, 10 to 12 = high risk, and 9 or below = very high risk. Decisions regarding support surfaces, nutrition, and the need for physical and occupational therapy, for example, are protocols that can be initiated on the basis of the Braden scale (Fig. 50.8; Box 50.3) score (dependent on institution policy).

Support Surfaces

To diminish the effects of pressure, attention to the surface on which the patient lies and/or sits is essential to pressure injury treatment. Various redistributing surfaces are used in pressure injury prevention and treatment, including overlays, mattresses, integrated bed systems, and chair cushions. The goal of these support surfaces is to redistribute pressure, reduce shear, and control heat and humidity (microclimate). Because of a lack of consistent recommendations about support surfaces for the prevention and management of pressure injury, in 2015 the Wound, Ostomy and Continence Nurses Society developed an algorithm for support-surface selection to assist clinicians in selecting support surfaces. This is thought to be the first evidence-based algorithm that provides clinical guidelines for support-surface selection based on individual patient needs (see Evidence-Based Practice).

> **⚠ Safety Alert** It is important to maintain regular turning schedules, proper positioning, and the use of lift sheets for reduction of friction and shear for patients at risk for pressure-related injury, even if they are on a redistributing support surface. Additionally, nurses must be educated about the specifications of each surface. For example, placing too many linens on surfaces that provide pressure redistribution through inflation and deflation of the mattress may obstruct airflow and reduce the efficacy of the support surface.

Evidence-Based Practice

Selecting Support Surface for Pressure Injuries

The use of support surfaces is an effective intervention for the prevention and treatment of pressure injuries. Because of a paucity of evidence to guide healthcare professionals in the selection of support surfaces, the Wound, Ostomy and Continence Nurses Society (WOCN) led the development of an evidence-based and consensus-based algorithm. A task force of clinical experts was assembled to review the literature around the use of support surfaces to manage pressure injuries, to develop specific recommendations for the algorithm, to draft the algorithm, and to establish the face validity of the tool. Based on the work of the task force, 20 "key opinion leaders" reviewed the draft algorithm, reached consensus on the supporting evidence, and revised the draft and evaluated its content validity. The results demonstrated a strong content validity index (CVI) for the algorithm, which is thought to be the first evidence-based algorithm to guide clinical decisions about the implementation of support surfaces in the management of pressure injuries. It is the hope of the WOCN that this algorithm is used in facilities across the United States to provide additional data about the effectiveness of this tool.

McNichol, L., Watts, C., Mackey, D., Beitz, J., & Gray, M. (2015). Identifying the right surface for the right patient at the right time: Generation and content validation for the algorithm for support surface selection. *Journal of Wound, Ostomy and Continence Nursing, 42*(1), 19–37.

Pressure-redistributing support surfaces are a type of durable medical equipment used for patients with pressure injuries. A major distinction between support surfaces is that some are powered and others are nonpowered. They are categorized into the following three groups, and insurance coverage is based on the specific type of surface prescribed:

- *Group 1 support surfaces* are generally designed to either replace a standard hospital or home mattress or as an overlay placed on top of a standard hospital or home mattress. These are static surfaces that do not require electricity. Products in this category include mattresses, pressure pads, and mattress overlays (foam, air, water, or gel) and are meant to disperse pressure over a larger area. These are appropriate for patients at risk of developing a pressure injury or those with a stage 1 or 2 pressure injury. For Medicare reimbursement of Group Support 1 surfaces, the following criteria must be met:
  - The patient is completely immobile or has limited mobility (i.e., cannot independently make changes in body position significant enough to alleviate pressure).

Braden Scale for Predicting Pressure Sore Risk

Patient's name_____ Evaluator's name _____ Date of Assessment_____

Sensory Perception Ability to respond meaningfully to pressure-related discomfort	**1. Completely Limited** Unresponsive (does not moan, flinch, or grasp) to painful stimuli, due to diminished level of consciousness or sedation OR limited ability to feel pain over most of body.	**2. Very Limited** Responds only to painful stimuli. Cannot communicate discomfort except by moaning or restlessness OR has a sensory impairment which limits the ability to feel pain or discomfort over $1/2$ of body.	**3. Slightly Limited** Responds to verbal commands, but cannot always communicate discomfort or the need to be turned OR has some sensory impairment which limits ability to feel pain or discomfort in 1 or 2 extremities.	**4. No Impairment** Responds to verbal commands. Has no sensory deficit which would limit ability to feel or voice pain or discomfort.	
Moisture Degree to which skin is exposed to moisture	**1. Constantly Moist** Skin is kept moist almost constantly by perspiration, urine, etc. Dampness is detected every time patient is moved or turned.	**2. Very Moist** Skin is often, but not always moist. Linen must be changed at least once a shift.	**3. Occasionally Moist** Skin is occasionally moist, requiring an extra linen change approximately once a day.	**4. Rarely Moist** Skin is usually dry, linen only requires changing at routine intervals.	
Activity Degree of physical activity	**1. Bedfast** Confined to bed.	**2. Chairfast** Ability to walk severely limited or non-existent. Cannot bear own weight and/or must be assisted into chair or wheelchair.	**3. Walks Occasionally** Walks occasionally during day, but for very short distances, with or without assistance. Spends majority of each shift in bed or chair.	**4. Walks Frequently** Walks outside room at least twice a day and inside room at least once every two hours during waking hours.	
Mobility Ability to change and control body position	**1. Completely Immobile** Does not make even slight changes in body or extremity position without assistance.	**2. Very Limited** Makes occasional slight changes in body or extremity position but unable to make frequent or significant changes independently.	**3. Slightly Limited** Makes frequent though slight changes in body or extremity position independently.	**4. No Limitation** Makes major and frequent changes in position without assistance.	
Nutrition <u>Usual</u> food intake pattern	**1. Very Poor** Never eats a complete meal. Rarely eats more than $1/3$ of any food offered. Eats 2 servings or less of protein (meat or dairy products) per day. Takes fluids poorly. Does not take a liquid dietary supplement OR is NPO and/or maintained on clear liquids or IV's for more than 5 days.	**2. Probably Inadequate** Rarely eats a complete meal and generally eats only about $1/2$ of any food offered. Protein intake includes only 3 servings of meat or dairy products per day. Occasionally will take a dietary supplement OR receives less than optimum amount of liquid diet or tube feeding.	**3. Adequate** Eats over half of most meals. Eats a total of 4 servings of protein (meat, dairy products) per day. Occasionally will refuse a meal, but will usually take a supplement when offered OR is on a tube feeding or TPN regimen which probably meets most of nutritional needs.	**4. Excellent** Eats most of every meal. Never refuses a meal. Usually eats a total of 4 or more servings of meat and dairy products. Occasionally eats between meals. Does not require supplementation.	
Friction and Shear	**1. Problem** Requires moderate to maximum assistance in moving. Complete lifting without sliding against sheets is impossible. Frequently slides down in bed or chair, requiring frequent repositioning with maximum assistance. Spasticity, contractures or agitation leads to almost constant friction.	**2. Potential Problem** Moves feebly or requires minimum assistance. During a move, skin probably slides to some extent against sheets, chair, restraints or other devices. Maintains relatively good position in chair or bed most of the time but occasionally slides down.	**3. No Apparent Problem** Moves in bed and in chair independently and has sufficient muscle strength to lift up completely during move. Maintains good position in bed or chair.		

Total Score [ ]

FIGURE 50.8 The Braden scale.

Box 50.3 Braden Scale Scoring

Mild risk:	15 to 18
Moderate risk:	13 to 14
High risk:	10 to 12
Very high risk:	9 or below

- The patient has a pressure injury of any stage on the trunk or pelvis.
- The patient has at least one of the following conditions:
  1. Impaired nutritional status
  2. Fecal or urinary incontinence
  3. Altered sensory perception
  4. Compromised circulatory status
- *Group 2 support surfaces* are generally designed to either replace a standard hospital or home mattress or as an overlay placed on top of a standard hospital or home mattress but are powered surfaces (require electricity or battery). Products in this category include the active support surface, integrated bed system, nonpowered, overlay, powered, reactive support, and replacement mattress. Most of these products allow the nurse to adjust the air mattress supportive pressure by alternating the inflation and deflation of air cells, which is recommended for patients with stage 3 and 4 pressure injuries. Additionally, low-air-loss mattresses are similar to air-permeable pillows that remain inflated and have a drying effect on tissues. The use of these mattresses is recommended for patients with stage 1 or 2 injuries who are not improving on static surfaces and for patients with stage 3 and 4 pressure injuries. For Medicare reimbursement of group support 2 surfaces, the following criteria must be met:
- The patient has multiple stage 2 pressure injuries located on the trunk or pelvis that have failed to improve over the last month, and the patient has been on a comprehensive injury treatment program for at least the past month (minimum of 30 days) that included each of the following:
  1. Use of an appropriate group 1 support surface
  2. Regular assessment by a nurse, physician, or licensed healthcare practitioner
  3. Appropriate turning and positioning
  4. Appropriate wound care
  5. Appropriate management of moisture/incontinence
  6. Nutritional assessment and intervention consistent with the overall plan of care
- The patient has large or multiple stage 3 or 4 pressure injuries on the trunk or pelvis.
- The patient had a recent myocutaneous flap or skin graft for a pressure injury on the trunk or pelvis (surgery within the past 60 days), and the

patient has been on a group 2 or 3 support surface immediately prior to a recent discharge from a hospital or nursing facility (discharge within the past 30 days).
- *Group 3 support surfaces* are complete bed systems, known as air-fluidized beds, which use the circulation of filtered air through silicone beads. These systems are considered dynamic surfaces and require electricity. Air-fluidized (or high-air-loss) mattresses contain silicone-coated beads that liquefy with the infusion of air into the bed, which reduces moisture and has a cooling effect. These support surfaces are indicated for stage 3 and 4 pressure injuries or for patients with multiple pressure injuries. Group 3 support surfaces are covered only if the patient is bedridden or chair-bound with stage 3 or stage 4 pressure injuries that would require institutionalization without the use of an air-fluidized bed. Additionally, the patient must have been treated conservatively for at least a month without progression of wound healing that included repositioning to relieve pressure over bony prominences (usually every two hours) and the use of a group 2 support surface.

Connection Check 50.10

A 78-year-old patient fractured a hip 1 week ago and is now being admitted to a rehabilitation facility for physical therapy because of difficulty ambulating. During the admission skin assessment, the nurse notes an area of nonblanchable erythema on the sacrum. What is the nursing priority at this time?

A. Order a redistributing mattress for the patient's bed.

B. Consult the nutritionist for a complete nutritional assessment.

C. Perform and document the admission skin and risk assessments.

D. Apply a hydrocolloid dressing over the area to protect it from further trauma.

Nutrition

Adequate nutrition plays a significant role in healing pressure injuries, and patients require supplementary nutritional support (Table 50.12). Appropriate amounts of calories, protein, fluids, vitamins, and minerals are necessary for tissue repair and the prevention of pressure injuries. Evaluating a patient's nutritional status with the use of a nutrition screening tool is done on the patient's first visit to any healthcare setting, and a referral to a nutritionist is generated for those deemed to be at risk. Decreased collagen formation and fibroblast proliferation are effects of undernutrition and protein-energy malnutrition that prolong the inflammatory phase of wound healing. Undernutrition, a deficiency in energy and protein, can be reversed solely with the administration of nutrients and significantly impacts the body's

Table 50.12 Nutritional Assessment Relevant to Pressure Injuries

Nutritional States	Definition and Characteristics
Undernutrition	Protein and energy deficiency
	Consequences can be reversed completely with the administration of nutrients.
	Contributing conditions include increased dependence on others for eating, decreased oral intake of food and fluids, unintentional weight loss, and aging.
Protein-energy malnutrition (PEM)	Wasting with excessive loss of lean muscle mass
	Results from untreated undernutrition and can be reversed with administration of nutrients
	Increased morbidity and mortality
Cachexia	Loss of muscle and weight loss with or without loss of fat mass
	Is a metabolic syndrome associated with underlying illnesses
Hypermetabolism	Increased metabolic rate causing an increased need for calories in response to trauma, severe illness, infection, or pressure injuries, for example
	Energy pulled from glycogen stores first, then visceral protein stores
	Results in anorexia, muscle wasting, decreased nitrogen retention, impaired albumin synthesis

Data from Posthauer, M. E., Banks, M., Dorner, B., & Schols, J. M. G. A. (2015). The role of nutrition for pressure ulcer management: National Pressure Ulcer Advisory Panel, European Pressure Ulcer Advisory Panel, and Pan Pacific Pressure Injury Alliance white paper. *Advances in Skin & Wound Care, 28*(4), 175–188.

ability to heal and fight infections. Hypermetabolism, which occurs as a result of trauma, severe illness, or infection, utilizes calories rapidly. The body compensates for insufficient energy during a hypermetabolic state by stealing energy from visceral protein stores to maintain organ functioning. As a result, anorexia, muscle wasting, decreased nitrogen retention, and impaired albumin synthesis occur.

Box 50.4 includes recommendations from the NPUAP's white paper on the role of nutrition in pressure injury management.

Wound Care

Pressure injury wound assessment includes staging the injury; evaluating wound tissues, the topography of the wound, and wound exudate; and measuring wound dimensions. Wound measurements are performed on admission and at intervals according to institutional policies. Measurements must include length (head to toe), width (widest perpendicular to the length), and depth (measured at 90 degrees to the wound surface). A circumferential assessment for **undermining** (tissue destruction or pressure injury extending under the wound edges, making the injury larger at its base than at the skin surface) and inspection and measurements of **tunneling** (a passageway under the skin surface that is also known as a sinus tract that results in dead space that can increase the risk for abscess formation) are included in each wound assessment.

The selection of wound-care products is based on the characteristics of the wound (wound type, tissue type, exudate characteristics, location, and bacterial profile) as well as patient-related factors (activity level, compliance, caregiver, and level of consciousness). Primary wound dressings are applied directly to the wound bed, and their removal should not be traumatic in order to avoid damage to new granulation tissue. Secondary dressings are applied over the top of primary dressings and serve to protect the wound and to secure the primary dressing. Table 50.13 presents the different types of wound dressings available. (Refer to Table 50.8 for the definitions of different tissues found in wounds and Table 50.9 for debridement methods.)

Debridement

Wound debridement removes necrotic tissue, reducing the risk of infection and facilitating healing. There are many different types of wound debridement, including surgical, autolytic, mechanical, maggot, and enzymatic (see Table 50.9). Necrotic tissue within the wound bed impairs granulation tissue development and keeps the wound in the inflammatory phase of wound healing. If conservative measures such as local wound care, including conservative debridement methods (autolytic, mechanical, maggot, and enzymatic), are not successful in removing the necrotic tissue, surgical/sharp wound debridement may be warranted. Surgical/sharp debridement can occur in an inpatient setting, outpatient setting, or operating room, depending on the extent and goals of debridement, and requires anesthetic medications (local or general). Healing by secondary intention or reconstructive flap surgery may be required following surgical debridement of pressure injuries.

A comprehensive wound assessment and physical examination are necessary to evaluate for any potential contraindications to surgical/sharp debridement. Because wound healing requires adequate oxygenation, wounds with poor

Box 50.4 National Pressure Ulcer Advisory Panel Advisory Panel White Paper Recommendations

Macronutrient Requirements:

- Energy: Energy (kilocalories) is provided by the macronutrients of carbohydrates, fats, and protein. Increased energy is needed to overcome the effects of a hypermetabolic state that is created by pressure injuries. Carbohydrates are the main source of fuel for collagen synthesis. Thirty to 35 kilocalories per gram of body weight per day is recommended for patients with pressure injuries.
- Protein: All phases of wound healing require adequate amounts of protein for collagen synthesis, fibroblast production, and cell multiplication. The recommended daily allowance (RDA) of protein for healing wounds is 1.2 to 1.5 g per kilogram of body weight. Higher levels of protein in older adults can potentiate renal disease and cause dehydration.
- Amino acids: Amino acids are the precursors to protein. The amino acids of arginine and glutamine are essential during periods of stress such as pressure injury healing.
- Fluids: Vitamins, minerals, glucose, and other minerals rely on fluids for bodily dispersion. Fluid needs are individualized according to health status and healing needs. Therefore, the nutritionist evaluates and calculates each patient's needs. It is important to monitor fluid status by observing mucous membranes, skin turgor, weight, urine output, and serum sodium. Also, fluid need calculations must include the loss of fluids with heavily exuding wounds.

Micronutrient Requirements:

The need for micronutrients increases with pressure injuries.

- Ascorbic acid (vitamin C): Ascorbic acid is essential in collagen formation, capillary strength, immune function, and tissue repair and regeneration. If the patient is unable to consume the RDA of vitamin C by ingesting fruits and vegetables, vitamin supplementation is initiated.
- Zinc: Zinc is needed for collagen formation and protein synthesis. A patient with prolonged poor dietary intake and highly exuding pressure injuries is at risk for zinc deficiency. Zinc supplementation should not exceed 40 mg per day and should only be given to those who show signs of zinc deficiency, including loss of appetite, abnormal taste, impaired immune function, and impaired wound healing. Too much zinc can impair healing and inhibit the effects of copper, possibly causing anemia.
- Copper: Copper is essential for collagen cross-linking and red blood cell formation. If the diet does not contain adequate foods rich in copper (nuts, seafood, whole grains, legumes), providing a multivitamin with 100% of the RDA of copper is sufficient.

Adapted from Posthauer, M. E., Banks, M., Dorner, B., & Schols, J. M. G. A. (2015). The role of nutrition for pressure ulcer management: National Pressure Ulcer Advisory Panel, European Pressure Ulcer Advisory Panel, and Pan Pacific Pressure Injury Alliance white paper. *Advances in Skin & Wound Care, 28*(4), 175–188.

perfusion due to peripheral vascular disease should not be debrided unless surgical revascularization occurs first. Additionally, patient-centered concerns, such as pain and postdebridement expectations, must be addressed and consent given prior to any invasive procedure.

Comorbidities

The Braden scale addresses the extrinsic factors of pressure, friction, and shear, as well as mental status, mobility, nutrition, and incontinence, all of which contribute significantly to the development of pressure injuries. However, the medical management of comorbid diseases such as peripheral vascular disease, diabetes, congestive heart failure, incontinence, and end-stage renal disease must be optimized for successful wound healing to take place.

Complications

As with any open wound, infection is the main complication. Assessing for local clinical manifestations of wound infections (erythema, increased warmth, swelling, increase in injury size or depth, increased pain, purulent exudate, and odor) should occur on a regular basis. Swab cultures can be helpful, but punch biopsies with culture can help identify bacteria in deeper tissues such as muscle and bone (osteomyelitis). If osteomyelitis is suspected, evaluation with x-ray, computed tomography (CT) scan, or magnetic resonance imaging (MRI) is recommended. If the bone is exposed, the patient is diagnosed clinically with osteomyelitis, making further scanning unnecessary at that point to confirm infection. Imaging may be necessary to observe the structural integrity of a joint. C-reactive protein levels and ESRs are elevated with infection and inflammation. As infection and inflammation are treated, these values decrease, making them important indexes to assess the effectiveness of treatment. Patients who are immunocompromised and/or have extensive wounds are at greater risk of infection. Therefore, vigilant monitoring for systemic clinical manifestations of infection (fever, increased white blood cell count) helps to identify bacteremia (bacteria in the blood) or sepsis (systemic infection).

Pressure injuries on the sacrum, coccyx, ischium, and trochanters are at risk of fecal and urine contamination in a patient who is incontinent. Depending on the severity of the injury and potential surgical interventions, a temporary diverting colostomy may be recommended to avoid contamination of the site with feces and/or urine until the injury or surgical site is completely healed. Once healing is complete, the temporary colostomy can be re-anastomosed at the patient's request.

In addition to the obvious physical manifestations of pressure injuries, a patient may also experience body image disturbances related to a chronically open wound. Lifestyle changes related to the pressure injury, such as changes in employment status, can put a financial strain on the family and interpersonal relationships. Caregivers can feel overwhelmed because of the physical and psychosocial needs of the patient with a pressure injury. Lastly, the chronic pain of an open wound can lead to feelings of hopelessness and fear.

Table 50.13 Types of Wound Dressings

Product Category	Description	Function	Appropriate Use	Advantages	Disadvantages
Alginate	Composed of calcium alginate (seaweed component)	Forms a gel-like substance when coming into contact with exudate; provides hemostasis	Moderate to heavy exudate	Painless removal; exudate management; moldable to wound surface; maintains moist environment	Most wound dressings are expensive, but topical dressing selection is based on wound characteristics and dressing functions; wound must be moist for gelling to occur and for avoidance of traumatic removal. Require secondary dressing
Collagens	Pads, gels, or particles of collagen; usually derived from bovine or porcine sources; usually contain cellulose or alginate for absorption	Promote deposition of collagen; stimulate granulation tissue	As primary dressing in minimal to heavily exuding wounds; can pack into tunnels	Absorbent, nonadherent; usually dissolve in wound bed; moldable	Require secondary dressing
Nonadherent contact layers	Thin, nonadherent sheets placed in wound bed	Protection of wound bed; covering of topical ointments when applied to wound bed	Primary dressing for protection of wound bed and to keep topical ointments in contact with wound bed (and not absorbed by outer dressing)	Are porous and allow exudate to pass through for absorption on other dressings; protect new granulation tissue; can be applied over topical ointments	Not recommended for dehydrated wounds or viscous exudate; require secondary dressing
Foams	Semipermeable, nonadherent, absorptive dressing made of open-cell, medical-grade expanded polymer	Absorption; maintain moist environment; insulate wound	Moderate to heavy exudate. Absorption of minimal to heavy exudate, nonadherent	Nonadherent; waterproof outer layer; provide bacterial barrier; good for hypergranulation	Will dry out wounds without enough exudate; not for autolytic debridement
Hydrocolloids	Composed of carboxymethylcellulose, gelatin, pectin, elastomers, and adhesives that are hydrophilic and turn into a gel when exudate is absorbed	Debridement, absorption, protection; occlusive wafer-type dressing; can be adhesive or nonadhesive	To protect intact or newly healed skin from further exposure to friction and shear; scant to minimal exudate; to assist in debridement of necrotic tissue	Provide autolysis with necrotic wounds; are moldable; extended wear times; good bacterial barrier	Can dislodge with friction and shear or with heavy exudate; not for use on infected wounds

Hydrogels	Contain mostly water in a polymer gel base; come in gel or sheet form	Autolytic debridement of necrotic tissue/eschar; Stage 3 or 4 pressure injuries	Cooling and soothing to patient; provide hydration to promote autolytic debridement	Not for heavily exuding wounds; will dehydrate if not covered (consider using a contact layer between hydrogel and secondary dressing); can cause maceration
Hydrofibers	Consist of highly absorptive, soft, woven fiber layers (made from sodium carboxymethylcellulose)	To absorb moderate to heavy exudate; partial to full thickness; can use in infected, necrotic, or granulating wounds	Nonadherent; highly absorptive; easy application and removal; good for packing deep wounds	May require a secondary dressing
Semipermeable films	Thin sheets of polyurethane with an adhesive	Shallow wounds with minimal to no exudate; can be placed over bony prominences for protection from mechanical trauma	Transparent nature allows wound/skin inspections; can be used as a secondary dressing; bacterial barrier Act as a semiocclusive; also allows the exchange of gases, vapors; *not for infected wounds*	Nonabsorptive; adhesive can damage healthy skin
Gauze	Usually a cotton or synthetic mesh of fibers Also antimicrobial gauze sponges and dressing rolls	Used for packing deep wounds, mechanical debridement, primary or secondary dressings; delivery of topical agents	Absorption; mechanical debridement	Can cause mechanical trauma to granulation tissue upon removal; painful removal; decreases temperature of wound; frequent dressing changes
Hydrofera Blue	Bacteriostatic dressing (made of Hydrofera polyvinyl alcohol sponge, methylene blue, gentian violet)	Used with diabetic ulcers, postsurgical incision sites, large abrasions, burns, and trauma wounds Protects against infection by inhibiting the growth or reproduction of bacteria Protects wounds from harmful microorganisms	Highly absorptive dressing that absorbs bacteria-laden exudates away from the wound bed and physically binds endotoxins to the dressing	Does not inhibit the activity of enzymatic debriders Absorption capacity superior to many silver-impregnated dressings and equal to that of high-absorbency foams

All of these dressings are expensive except for gauze. This is not an all-inclusive list; there are many other products.

Nursing Management

Assessment and Analysis

The treatment of pressure injuries is multifactorial and requires an interprofessional approach to patient care that includes nursing, medicine, nutrition, social work, physical and occupational therapies, and pain services. The nurse's role is critical in the treatment and prevention of pressure injuries. It is essential to assess and accurately document the findings of the skin, wound, and risk assessments in the patient care record. In addition to following wound-care protocols of the institution, the nurse must also recognize the clinical manifestations of local and systemic infections.

The assessment of the patient with pressure injuries requires the nurse to complete a thorough skin assessment, along with an evaluation of nutritional status, fluid volume status, and activity and mobility. In the patient presenting with an existing pressure injury, detailed and consistent documentation of the wound appearance is required to monitor for signs of healing or deterioration.

Nursing Diagnoses

- **Impaired skin integrity** related to trauma secondary to exposure to pressure, friction, and shear
- **Acute and/or chronic pain** related to skin trauma, wound infection, and/or wound treatment
- **Imbalanced nutrition, less than body requirements**, related to hypermetabolic state secondary to the open wound
- **Depression** related to sense of loss as evidenced by forced lifestyle changes (loss of job, strained relationships) secondary to non-healing pressure injury
- **Risk for infection** related to the open wound

Nursing Interventions

■ Assessments

- Vital signs
  Vital signs reflect systemic status related to infection and hydration status. An elevated temperature may be indicative of infection. With sepsis, tachycardia and hypotension may also develop.
- Pain
  Pressure injuries may cause pain because of edema and pressure in the area, as well as the exposure of nerve endings with large wounds.
- Functional assessment
  A functional assessment provides data on the patient's mobility status, how many hours/day the patient sits or lies down, and typical activities of daily living (including type of work). It is also important to ask what kind of bed and/or wheelchair surface the patient uses.
- Skin
  Admission skin and risk assessments identify patients at risk of developing pressure injuries and those who already have existing signs of pressure.

- Pressure-prone areas
  Depending on positioning, different areas are at increased risk for pressure and decreased perfusion. Patients who are supine are at increased risk of pressure to the occiput, scapulae, sacrum, ischium, and heels.
- Risk assessments (Braden scale)
  Admission assessments identify which patients are refusing treatment and provide the basis of their refusal, help define initial care approaches, and provide documentation, which must occur every 48 hours in acute care, weekly in long-term care, and on every home-care visit.
- Wounds
  Wound assessments should include location, injury stage, wound measurements (length, width, depth), tissue type, the presence of infection, exudate, and a description of periwound skin.
- Nutritional status
  The AHRQ recommends nutrition screening upon patient admission with referral to a nutritionist if found to be at risk of malnutrition. Wound healing requires increased protein, nutrients, and hydration.
- Past medical history
  History of previous pressure injuries increases the risk of new injury, as well as potentially resulting in delayed wound healing.
- Serum albumin and prealbumin
  Nutritional status is important to skin integrity and wound healing. Decreased serum albumin and prealbumin may indicate nutritional deficits.
- Blood values of C-reactive proteins and ESRs
  These values are elevated in infection and inflammation and are good indexes to monitor resolution.

■ Actions

- Positioning to decrease pressure on bony prominences
  Skin breakdown starts to occur within 2 to 6 hours of the onset of pressure. Repositioning is essential for the immobile patient to reduce pressure over bony prominences and pressure injury risk. Reassessment of pressure-prone areas during repositioning helps to guide repositioning treatment plans.
- Keep the head of the bed at 30 degrees or less.
  Keeping the head of the bed at 30 degrees or less decreases the effects of shearing forces by minimizing the patient sliding down in the bed.
- Utilize draw sheets to reposition the patient.
  Draw sheets decrease the effects of friction by not allowing the patient's skin to be dragged along the surface of the bed.
- Control moisture, and cleanse the patient immediately after incontinence.
  Urine and feces irritate the epidermis, increasing susceptibility to skin breakdown.
- Apply moisture barrier ointment to skin subject to incontinence.
  Increased moisture on the skin causes maceration, increasing susceptibility to skin breakdown.
- Obtain appropriate bed surfaces.
  Bed surfaces should be selected according to the patient's clinical presentation and to redistribute pressure.

- Wound care: cleansing, dressings
  Wound care should be done according to wound-dressing recommendations and clinical evaluation; wound dressings should be chosen according to the needs of the wound.
- Documentation of wound progression with each dressing change or at least weekly
  Wound documentation provides the status of the effectiveness of therapies and can guide further treatment decisions.
- Nutritionist referral
  Nutritionists develop a diet plan specific to meet the needs of the patient with open pressure injuries.
- Administer antibiotics as prescribed for infections.
  Infection inhibits wound healing.
- Physical therapy/occupational therapy referrals
  Rehabilitation therapies maximize a patient's functional status to allow the patient to be an active participant in his or her care.
- Provide emotional support to the patient, and refer to social work if needed.
  Patients with a chronic wound can experience a decreased quality of life as a result of depression.
- Provide emotional support to caregivers, and refer to social work if needed.
  Caregivers can experience role strain when caring for a person with a chronic illness.

Teaching

- Importance of turning and repositioning
  Patient and family compliance increase with teaching about the relationship between the lack of movement and pressure injury development.
- Nutritional requirements
  Adequate wound healing requires adequate nutrition. The patient needs to consume an adequate intake of proteins and carbohydrates.
- Importance of adequate fluid intake
  Fluid status is associated with normal skin turgor, and dry, scaly skin increases the risk for loss of skin integrity.
- Clinical manifestation of infection
  Early recognition of infection is important to minimize the risk of systematic involvement.

Evaluating Care Outcomes

Prevention of pressure injuries is an important nursing intervention, and surveillance and assessment of risk factors contribute to decreasing the incidence. Pressure injury diagnosis, management, treatment, and prevention require an interprofessional approach to care. Initial and consistent ongoing skin assessment is crucial to the management of pressure injuries. It is essential to include the patient, family, and caregivers in the treatment plan. Careful assessment of risk factors, skin, wound, and nutrition guide the clinical decision-making process. Uncomplicated wound healing and prevention of further tissue damage are the ultimate goals in treating pressure injuries.

CASE STUDY: EPISODE 2

Mr. Parker undergoes extensive wound debridement to remove necrotic tissue and bone. Initially, he does not want to undergo reconstructive surgery for fear of a larger wound that will not heal. Advanced wound-care products applied by highly specialized nurses are used to attempt wound closure by secondary intention.

After 1 year without wound closure, Mr. Parker and his wife decide that he will undergo debridement and myocutaneous flap reconstructive surgery for his ischial pressure injury. He does well perioperatively and is transferred to a rehabilitation hospital, where a low-air-loss mattress is used along with complete avoidance of lying or sitting on the surgical site for 4 weeks. A small area of the incision dehisces. However, with local wound care and continued off-loading of the site over the next 2 weeks, the area heals…

SKIN CANCER

The most common form of cancer in the United States is skin cancer. The most common types of skin cancers are categorized into two groups, **melanoma** and non-melanoma.

Epidemiology

Non-melanoma skin cancers include basal cell and squamous cell carcinomas. **Actinic keratoses** are atypical keratinocytes found in the epidermis and represent the most common form of precancerous lesions. Approximately 2.2 million people are diagnosed each year with a form of non-melanoma skin cancer in the United States. Furthermore, basal cell carcinomas are the most common form of cancer occurring in human beings, accounting for approximately 75% of all diagnosed skin cancers. In contrast, melanoma skin cancers account for less than 2% of all diagnosed cancers in the United States each year but account for the vast majority of skin cancer deaths. Both basal cell and squamous cell carcinomas have a higher incidence among the solid organ transplant population, most likely because of immunosuppression therapy. In the United States, men are diagnosed with melanomas of the skin at a higher rate. The overall lifetime risk for being diagnosed with melanoma is about 2.4% (or 1 in 40) for whites, 0.1% (or 1 in 1,000) for blacks, and 0.5% (1 in 200) for Hispanics.

Ultraviolet damage to the DNA of keratinocytes increases with extended time in the sun and is a major contributing factor to the development of skin cancers. Therefore, there is an increased risk of developing melanoma with advancing age because of prolonged sun exposure over time. Melanoma is currently the most common cancer affecting women aged 25 to 29 and the second most common cancer diagnosed in women aged 30 to 34. Use of tanning salons is a causative theory of the development of this cancer among these age groups. Survival rates associated with melanoma skin cancer are dependent on the staging of the cancer, which reflects tumor depth, early recognition, and treatment directly related to prognosis. Actinic keratosis is diagnosed in more than 10 million people per year worldwide and represents the most common skin condition treated by dermatologists. The cumulative effect of sun exposure correlates with an increased incidence of actinic keratosis. Therefore, the incidence of actinic keratosis increases after age 40. About a quarter of these lesions regress spontaneously, but 0.1% to 10% develop into squamous cell carcinomas. Individuals with less melanin (e.g., those with fair skin; blond or red hair; and blue, green, or gray eyes) are more prone to developing actinic keratosis. Additionally, the chances of having this type of cancer are greater with increased proximity to the equator.

The main modifiable risk factor associated with skin cancers and premalignant lesions is exposure to UV radiation (Box 50.5), with those who spend much time in the sun (either for work or for pleasure) at greatest risk. Although people with fair skin are at greatest risk, darker-skinned populations still carry a risk of developing skin cancers (see Genetic Connections: Skin Cancer). Additionally, occupational exposure to some carcinogens can increase the risk.

Genetic Connections

Skin Cancer

The genetic risks for the development of melanoma of the skin include skin type, number of nevi and having atypical nevi, and having a family history of skin cancer.

Pathophysiology and Clinical Manifestations

Ultraviolet radiation from sunlight is composed of UVA and UVB rays. Ultraviolet radiation is the main cause of all types of skin cancers. Ultraviolet B rays do not penetrate deep into the skin and are responsible for sunburns that occur from prolonged periods in the sun. Ultraviolet B rays cause direct damage to DNA within the skin cells, whereas UVA rays penetrate deeper into the skin and are responsible for indirect damage that disrupts the cellular membranes. Researchers hypothesize that UV radiation energy is absorbed by the DNA of the epidermal cells and mediates immune suppression, leading to the development of cancerous cells.

Box 50.5 Patient Education for Skin Cancer Prevention

The American Cancer Society recommends the phrase "slip, slop, slap … and wrap" to remember ways to reduce the risks of getting skin cancer (slip on a shirt, slop on sunscreen, slap on a hat, and wrap on sunglasses to protect the eyes and skin around the eyes).

- Limit time spent in the sun between the hours of 10 a.m. and 4 p.m. when UV rays are strongest.
- Wear clothing to protect as much of the skin as possible. If light can be seen through the clothing, then UV rays can still get through. Some companies are now making lightweight fabrics that provide UV ray protection.
- Use sunscreen with an SPF of at least 30, applied thickly. Sunscreens do not provide total protection.
  - An SPF of 30 means that you are exposed to 1 minute of UV radiation for every 30 minutes spent in the sun.
  - Reapply often for best protection (at least every 2 hours and more frequently with swimming).
- Wear a hat with at least a 2- to 3-in. brim to protect the eyes, ears, forehead, nose, and scalp.
- Wear sunglasses that block UVA and UVB radiation to decrease your chances of eye disease.
- Avoid tanning beds.
- Be especially diligent in using these guidelines in protecting children.
- Examine your body (front and back) monthly, and keep a map of your current skin spots; seek medical advice if any lesion has the following characteristics (ABCDE):
  - A: Asymmetry
  - B: Border irregularity
  - C: Color variation (areas of brown, tan, black, blue, red, white, or any combination)
  - D: Diameter is greater than 6 mm
  - E: Elevation or enlargement of the lesion

SPF, Sun protection factor; *UVA,* ultraviolet A; *UVB,* ultraviolet B.

Actinic Keratosis

Actinic keratoses are considered precancerous lesions. Formed by atypical keratinocytes (epidermal squamous cells), they proliferate in the epidermis. Without treatment, they evolve into squamous cell carcinoma.

- **Clinical features:** Skin-colored to reddish-brown macules, papules, or plaques; range from a few millimeters up to 2 cm; usually occur as multiple lesions
- **Body distribution:** Sun-exposed areas (particularly cheeks, temples, forehead, anterior and posterior neck, ears, backs of hands, and forearms)
- **Clinical course:** May begin as erythematous, scaly plaques that exfoliate with toweling off or the rubbing of clothes during the day; induration at the base, cutaneous horn, ulceration, or pain may indicate transformation to squamous cell carcinoma.

Squamous Cell Carcinoma

Squamous cell carcinoma (Fig. 50.9) is mostly attributed to cumulative exposure to UVB rays over an extended period of time and is a cancer that arises from epidermal squamous cells (keratinocytes). These atypical squamous cells intermix with the normal squamous cells and can invade the underlying dermis (Fig. 50.10). Squamous cell carcinomas can cause significant damage to adjacent tissue and can metastasize within a few months. Many times, actinic keratoses are within or adjacent to the squamous cell carcinomas.

- **Clinical features:** Crusted papules and plaques that can become indurated and ulcerated. Larger lesions can become painful and bleed. Also, squamous cell carcinomas can arise from chronically open wounds, burn scars, or leg ulcers because of chronic inflammation.
- **Body distribution:** Sun-exposed skin, especially the top of the head, neck, and lips
- **Clinical course:** Can invade fatty tissue beneath the dermis and spread via the lymph nodes to other parts of the body (although this is not that common); recurrence rate within 3 years is 18%.

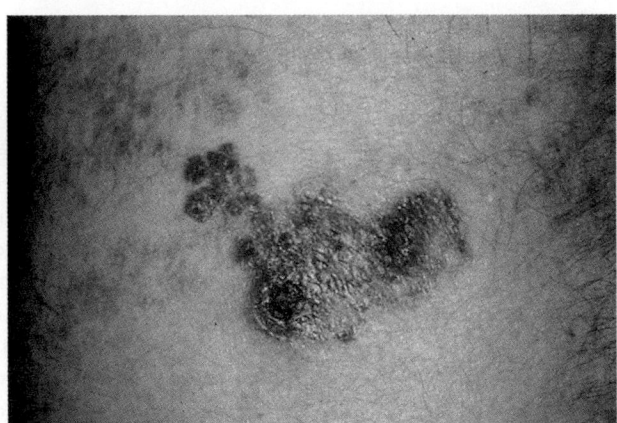

FIGURE 50.9 Squamous cell carcinoma.

Basal Cell Carcinoma

Basal cell carcinomas (Fig. 50.11) arise from the basement membrane of the epidermis. Although these are rarely metastatic, they can significantly damage adjacent tissue secondary to large excisions and damage vital structures.

- **Clinical features:** Pearly, translucent, flesh-colored papules; superficial **telangiectasias** (broken blood vessels) are usually visible; may have rolled edges or ulcerations
- **Body distribution:** Sun-exposed areas, especially head, neck, and trunk
- **Clinical course:** Usually not metastatic but can become locally invasive; recurrence rate after excision is 44% in 3 years.

Malignant Melanoma

The most serious of all skin cancers are malignant melanomas (Fig. 50.12) that originate from melanocytes found in the basement membrane of the epidermis. There are several different stages of malignant melanomas, depending on the thickness and depth of the tissue.

- **Clinical features:** Appearance can follow the ABCDE rule (see Box 50.5):
  - A: Asymmetric appearance
  - B: Irregular borders
  - C: Variation of color (brown, black, tan, blue, red, white, or any combination)
  - D: Diameter greater than 6 mm
  - E: Elevation or an evolving, enlarging, and changing existing lesion
- **Body distribution:** Anywhere on the body, especially where there are existing moles; upper back, lower legs, soles of feet, and palms of hands in dark-skinned individuals
- **Clinical course:** Favorable outcome if diagnosed and treated early; rapid metastasis can occur; 5-year survival rate of 91% and 10-year survival rate of 89%

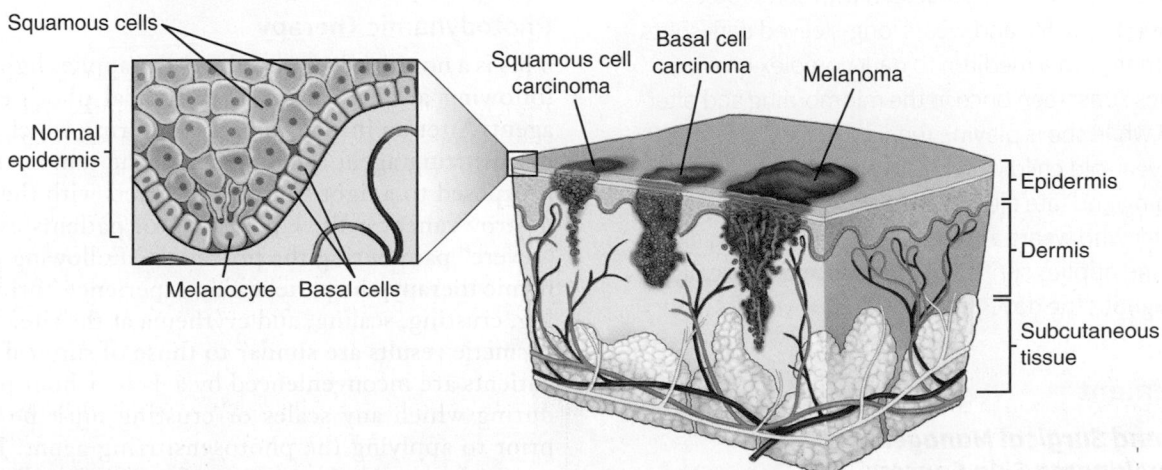

FIGURE 50.10 Atypical squamous cells intermix with the normal squamous cells and can invade the underlying dermis, causing squamous cell carcinomas, basal cell carcinomas, and melanomas.

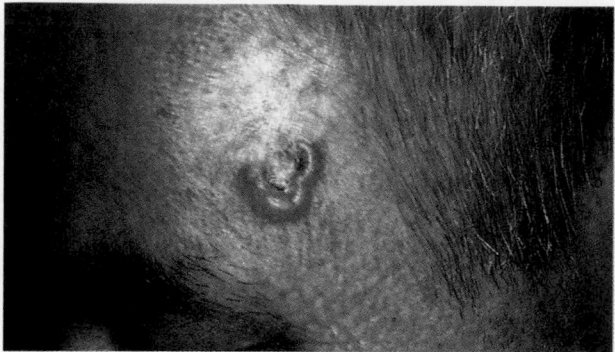

FIGURE 50.11 Basal cell carcinoma.

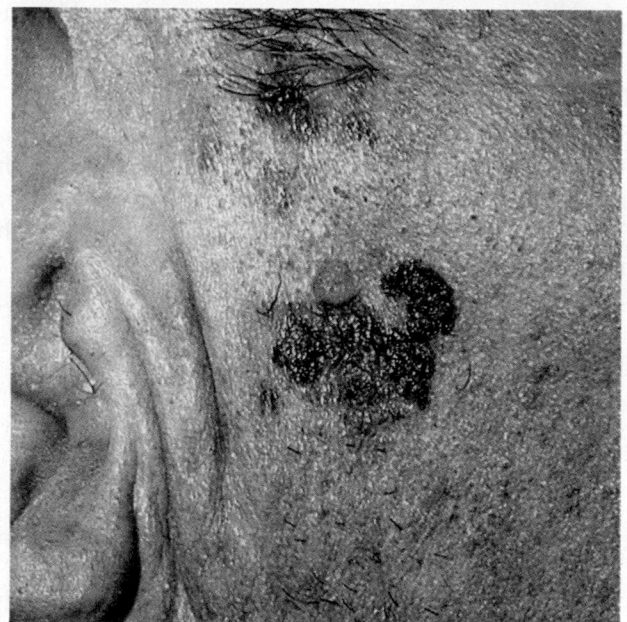

FIGURE 50.12 Malignant melanoma.

Connection Check 50.11

Which individual is at greatest risk for developing skin cancer?

A. A fair-skinned, blue-eyed teenager who works outside in the summers, uses sunscreen with sun protection factor (SPF) of 50, and wears long-sleeved dark shirts

B. A woman with a medium to dark complexion who applies sunscreen once in the midmorning and afternoon while she is playing tennis

C. A 10-year-old child who plays outside in the early morning and late afternoons and uses SPF 30

D. A surfer who wears a wet suit with long sleeves and legs and applies sunscreen to his face periodically throughout the day

Management

Medical and Surgical Management of Non-melanoma Skin Cancers

Management of non-melanoma skin cancers is dependent on size, location, recurrence risk factors, age, and the patient's current state of health.

Surgical Excision

Skin cancers with well-defined margins (surrounding structures are not involved) can be treated with surgical excision. In 95% of the cases of low-risk tumors, excision of the tumor with a 4-mm (millimeter) margin is successful. Not only does surgical excision provide a high cure rate, but also the cosmetic results of surgical excision are preferred over radiotherapy. Excised tissue is sent for biopsy.

Curettage and Electrodesiccation

The curettage and electrodesiccation treatment method is appropriate for low-risk, smaller lesions. After the patient receives a local anesthetic, a sharp curette (or scoop) is used to scrape away friable tumor tissue until the firm base of the tumor is felt by the surgeon. Electrodesiccation denatures the proteins in the dermis and destroys the tumor's base. This method can minimize damage to surrounding tissues, and three treatment sessions are usually needed for complete removal. Successful outcomes are operator dependent. Healing is by secondary intention, cosmetic results are good, and the method is cost-effective.

Mohs' Micrographic Surgery

Considered the "gold standard" for the treatment of non-melanoma skin cancers, Mohs' micrographic surgery is a highly specialized surgical approach completed only by surgeons specifically trained in this procedure. The surgeon excises horizontal sections of the tumor, leaving a minimal margin of normal tissue. Each layer of tissue is histologically examined by frozen section and microscopically analyzed during surgery. Excision continues until all residual tumor is removed. This allows the surgeon to explore all of the margins to reduce the risk of incomplete excision or removal of too much tissue, possibly causing unfavorable cosmetic outcomes.

Photodynamic Therapy

This is a noninvasive procedure that applies light therapy following an application of a topical photosensitizing agent. After an incubation period during which the photosensitizing agent accumulates in the tumor, the tumor is exposed to a light source that reacts with the agent to destroy cancer cells. Up to 20% of patients experience "severe" pain during the procedure. Following photodynamic therapy, the patient may experience burning, itching, crusting, scaling, and erythema at the site. Although cosmetic results are similar to those of surgical excision, patients are inconvenienced by a 4- to 5-hour procedure during which any scales or crusting must be removed prior to applying the photosensitizing agent. Photodynamic therapy is advantageous for patients who are poor surgical candidates because of other comorbidities or for those who have large or multiple lesions that can be treated at one time.

Cryotherapy

Liquid nitrogen is used for cryotherapy. It creates temperatures between −50°F (−45.6°C) and −60°F (−51.1°C), which freeze the vasculature, leading to cell death and tissue destruction. The freezing of the tissues is nonselective, and the microcirculation becomes impaired, causing pain that usually requires local anesthesia. As the tissues thaw, patients experience increased tenderness. In the days following the procedure, the patient may experience blistering and sloughing at the site, requiring local wound care. **Slough** is soft, moist devitalized tissue that may be white, yellow, tan, or green. Healing occurs with minimal scarring.

Radiotherapy

Radiotherapy is appropriate for use in patients who are poor surgical candidates because of their health or the site and extent of the tumor. In cases of aggressive squamous cell carcinoma, radiotherapy is an additional treatment following surgical excision. Radiotherapy is external-beam radiation delivered in fractionated doses from an x-ray machine. It is contraindicated for previously irradiated areas and some non-melanoma skin cancers. Because of side effects, such as alopecia, skin atrophy, and the development of telangiectasias, it is recommended that this therapy not be used on patients under 50 years of age.

Topical Chemotherapy

Topical chemotherapy with 5-fluorouracil is used in the treatment of multiple actinic keratoses or for superficial widespread basal cell carcinoma that would take multiple surgical procedures for complete removal. This therapy occurs over several weeks, and the lesions become inflamed, begin to crust, drain, and eventually erode away. Patients are educated about the appearance of the lesions during therapy and that post-therapy cosmetic results are usually effective.

Medical and Surgical Management of Malignant Melanoma

Treatment of malignant melanomas consists of excision with a 5-mm margin of unaffected tissue and biopsy, including a sentinel lymph node (the first lymph node to which cancer is likely to spread) biopsy. The outcome of treatment depends on the staging of the tumor and lymph node involvement. Tumors confined to the epidermis have a better prognosis postoperatively. With positive lymph nodes, a complete lymphadenectomy is indicated.

Metastatic melanoma is incurable, having a median survival of 7.5 months following initial diagnosis. Immunotherapy with interferon alpha and interleukin-2 provides a treatment option, although with only modest benefits. The desired effect of immunotherapy is to stimulate the antitumor response of the immune system and inhibit tumor growth and metastases. Further research is under way to develop more effective therapies for the treatment of metastatic melanoma.

Connection Check 50.12

What should the nurse teach the patient to expect during and following cryosurgery for the removal of a basal cell carcinoma?

A. "You may experience some discomfort during and immediately after the procedure. Local wound care may be required because of minor skin sloughing in the next few days."

B. "You will not have any pain with this procedure and need to see your provider only if complications develop."

C. "You may experience some discomfort during the procedure, but there is no follow-up care required."

D. "You will receive a local anesthetic just prior to the procedure. In the next few days, you may experience burning and itching at the site."

Complications

In addition to the physical complications of the treatments, the psychosocial aspects of skin cancers can have far-reaching effects on both the patient and family. The impact of the diagnosis of melanoma does not necessarily correlate with the stage and severity of the prognosis. Many times, patients are angry with themselves for not finding the cancerous lesion earlier or for not changing their lifestyle to reduce the risk of melanoma. Also, there may be financial concerns for the families during treatment. Patients with melanoma respond well to a straightforward approach of honesty and clarity in diagnosis and prognosis discussions and prefer to be involved in the decision making and treatment plans. Anxieties about treatment progress and risk of recurrence are diminished with regular follow-up and education. Research demonstrates that patients with melanoma may benefit from the support of a psychological healthcare professional.

Nursing Management

Assessment and Analysis

Thorough assessment and history-taking skills are essential in identifying risks for skin cancers. Physical changes in the appearance of skin, as well as a review of risk factors and exposures, are important to an accurate diagnosis and treatment plan. Clinical manifestations are associated with the type of cancerous lesion. Care for the patient following medical or surgical interventions includes psychosocial support and an understanding of community resources.

Nursing Diagnoses

- **Alterations in body image** related to altered pigmentation, scarring, and surgical excisions secondary to skin cancer
- **Acute pain** related to treatments for skin cancer
- **Risk for infection** related to treatments for skin cancer

- **Fear** related to the threat to well-being secondary to diagnosis of skin cancer

Nursing Interventions

▪ *Assessments*

- Skin

  Recent changes in size, color, or sensation in moles, birthmarks, or scars are significant signs potentially related to skin cancer. Significant sunburns with blistering are risk factors for skin cancer. Spending prolonged periods of time in the sun during peak sun intensity increases the risk of skin cancer. Regular use of sunscreen is important to assess. Skin that has sustained significant injury in the past is more prone to skin cancer development.

- Work history

  Work environments that require outdoor work increase exposure to the effects of UV radiation.

- Family and personal history

  A risk factor of skin cancer includes a positive family history.

- Psychosocial history

  Skin cancers can provoke fear related to the diagnosis and prognosis.

▪ *Actions*

- Provide pain medication as prescribed for postprocedural pain.

  Some treatments of skin cancer involve surgical excision or topical therapies that can disrupt the skin, causing pain.

- Provide emotional support.

  A diagnosis of skin cancer can evoke fear and concern over alterations in body image, prognosis, and finances.

- Refer to social work or psychologist

  Skin cancers can provoke fear related to the diagnosis and prognosis, and referral for counseling is indicated.

▪ *Teaching*

- Limit sun exposure.

  Exposure to the sun is directly related to the development of skin cancer. There are specific actions that can minimize exposure, including the application of sunscreen and wearing hats and long sleeves, as well as limiting exposure during the times when the sun is brightest.

- Sunscreen use

  The SPF of sunscreen should be at least 30 (with an explanation that SPF 30 means the patient is fully exposed to harmful UV rays for 1 minute of every 30 minutes in the sun). Sunscreen should be applied thickly and reapplied at least every 2 hours or more frequently if swimming or exercising.

- Skin self-examinations

  Skin self-examinations should be performed monthly, looking at both anterior and posterior surfaces as well as the top of the head, soles of the feet, and palms of the hands.

- Wound care for postoperative incisions or effects of other skin cancer treatment

  Education about proper wound care decreases the risks of infection and promotes healing.

- Information about different types of skin cancer

  Because not all skin cancers have the same prognosis, education about the specific types of skin cancer may alleviate concerns.

- Providing patients and families with contact information for local chapters of the American Cancer Society

  Support groups can help patients cope with a new diagnosis of skin cancer.

Evaluating Care Outcomes

Treatment for skin cancers begins with teaching about risks and ways to prevent the development of skin cancers. Certainly, the prognoses of actinic keratosis, basal cell carcinomas, and most squamous cell carcinomas are much better than those for patients with malignant melanoma. Education for patients treated for actinic keratosis and basal carcinomas includes an explanation of prognosis as well as ways to decrease risk factors. Emotional support and connecting the patient and his or her family with appropriate community resources significantly helps the patient with a new diagnosis of melanoma.

RECONSTRUCTIVE SURGERY

Reconstructive surgery is performed by a plastic/reconstructive surgeon following trauma, surgical debridement of a wound, excision of cancerous lesions, or repair of congenital defects (such as a cleft lip or palate) to repair or improve functional deficits.

Epidemiology

More than 5 million reconstructive surgeries are performed each year in the United States. There are two distinct groups of patients who require reconstructive surgery: those who need surgery because of congenital defects or disfiguring birthmarks and those who need surgery because of trauma, excisions of tumors, infections, or chronic wounds.

The most common reconstructive surgeries performed by plastic surgeons were for cancer reconstruction and wound repair and closure. Tumor removal and repair accounted for approximately 90% of these reconstructive procedures. Additional reconstructive surgeries include scar revision, laceration repair, dog bite repair, hand surgery, burn care, breast reconstruction, and microsurgery.

Pathophysiology

The plastic surgeon performs primary closure of the wound with minimal scarring if the edges of the wound are fairly straight. For wider wounds, surgical debridement and healing by secondary or tertiary intention may be required. Healing by tertiary intention includes the use of skin grafts, myocutaneous (skin, subcutaneous tissues, and muscle), fasciocutaneous (skin, subcutaneous tissues, and fascia), and free muscle flaps.

Management

Medical Management and Complications

Medical management of the postoperative reconstructive surgical wound involves diligent assessment skills. As with any surgery, reconstructive surgery runs a high risk of infection. A close assessment of the surgical site and donor sites of skin grafts and free tissue transfers for erythema, increased warmth, purulent drainage, approximation of the incision line, swelling, increased pain, and local lymphadenopathy is essential. For flaps and free tissue transfer, hematoma formation, induration, and signs of decreased vascularity are indications that may require further surgical interventions. Additionally, attention to frequent laboratory values such as CBC values and serum electrolyte panels is essential in monitoring for hemorrhage, fluid and electrolyte imbalances, and infections. Antibiotics may be ordered prophylactically for initial treatment; however, culture and sensitivity information must be evaluated and antibiotic therapy targeted to treat any identified pathogens. Lastly, nutrition must be optimized for healing to occur.

Nursing Management

Assessment and Analysis

Nursing care of the patient undergoing reconstructive surgery extends from the preoperative to the postoperative periods. The nurse focuses on diligent assessment of the wound as well as any graft sites and is attentive to signs of infection, decreased perfusion, and delayed wound healing. Additionally, elevations in white blood cell count must be reported to the provider. Fluid and electrolyte status, as well as nutritional intake, are also important parameters to follow in the patient after reconstructive surgery. Wound care, psychosocial needs, pain management, and astute assessment skills are critical in managing the reconstructive surgical patient.

Nursing Diagnoses

- **Acute pain** related to injury/inflammation at surgical and donor sites
- **Risk for infection** related to the surgical incision or open wound
- **Risk for ineffective peripheral tissue perfusion** related to failure of microvascular anastomoses of the flap
- **Risk for imbalanced nutrition (less than body requirements)** related to hypermetabolic state of wound healing
- **Risk for deficient fluid volume** related to hypermetabolic state of wound healing, fluid loss during surgery

Nursing Interventions

▪ Assessments

- Vital signs
  Elevated temperature and heart rate may be indicative of infection.
- Pain
  Postoperative pain is likely after reconstructive surgery because of the debridement, surgical exploration, and reanastomosis.

Uncontrollable pain may indicate complications, including inflammation, infection, dehiscence, and rejection.
- Baseline and ongoing wound/surgical incision assessments
  Assessment of the wound/surgical incision is necessary for evaluation of infection, perfusion, bleeding, and potential graft rejection.
- Intake and output
  The surgical patient is at risk for fluid volume deficit related to blood loss and increased metabolic demands that increase insensible fluid loss.
- CBC
  Because the postoperative patient is at risk for hemorrhage, the patient is assessed for decreases in hematocrit and hemoglobin, and elevated white blood cell counts are indicative of infection.
- Serum electrolytes
  The postoperative patient is at risk for dehydration that can lead to elevated serum sodium levels and third spacing that requires monitoring of albumin levels.
- Medication history
  Anticoagulants and antiplatelet medications must be stopped several days before surgery to avoid excessive bleeding.

▪ Actions

- Administer pain medications according to prescriptions.
  Pharmacological pain interventions are essential for the management of moderate to severe pain.
- Assist patient in identifying alternative methods of pain control to supplement medications: distraction, imagery, relaxation, application of heat and cold.
  Alternative methods of pain control can give the patient a sense of self-control and active participation in his or her care.
- Obtain nutrition referral for nutrition assessment.
  The hypermetabolic state of wound healing requires supplementation of protein, energy, carbohydrates, fluid, and vitamins and minerals.
- Obtain a specialty bed if reconstruction was for a pressure injury.
  Specialty beds can reduce the effects of pressure on the new flap. Pressure can compromise blood flow to the flap and cause more tissue destruction.
- Position patient so that he or she is not lying on the newly reconstructed surgical area.
  Positioning the patient appropriately can reduce or eliminate pressure on the surgical area.
- Provide emotional support to the family/caregivers.
  Caregivers can experience anxiety and apprehension about their abilities to provide care to the patient.

▪ Teaching

- Importance of following prescribed diet
  The hypermetabolic state of wound healing requires supplementation of protein, energy, carbohydrates, fluid, and vitamins and minerals.

- Clinical manifestations of infection and decreased tissue perfusion to patient and family
  Rapid and early assessment for infection or decreased tissue perfusion of the flap is essential to prevent further injury, including graft failure.
- Expected progression of healing
  Anxiety can be diminished if the patient and family/caregivers understand what to expect.
- Wound care
  Patients with wounds healing by secondary intention require wound care throughout the wound-healing process.
- Appropriate methods of off-loading, such as push-ups while sitting in the wheelchair and repositioning while lying down
  Wheelchair push-ups (patient lifting body weight up off of wheelchair surface) every 15 minutes and repositioning while lying down every 2 hours diminish the effects of pressure.

Evaluating Care Outcomes

The patient undergoing reconstructive surgery has many needs during the perioperative period. Success rates of skin grafts, muscle flaps, and free tissue transfer flaps can be tenuous and vary by the location of the flap, health status of the patient, presence of preoperative infections such as osteomyelitis, and postoperative care. Patients undergoing debridement with closure by secondary intention need dressing changes throughout the healing phase and will likely go home with an open wound. The patient and family/caregivers require support to help them meet the physical and psychosocial demands of wound healing and the prescribed course of treatment. The goal of treatment is a well-healed wound and improved functional status of the patient.

Making Connections

CASE STUDY: WRAP-UP

Mr. Parker's wife has been his advocate and support throughout his hospitalization and treatment. She diligently makes certain all of the necessary therapies are in place and that he is adhering to orders. Mr. Parker receives nutrition counseling and physical and occupational therapies while in the rehabilitative hospital, helping him to maintain his upper-body strength, which is needed for transfers in and out of bed and his wheelchair. Also, he adheres to the recommendation of doing "push-ups" (paraplegic patients in wheelchairs should lift their bodies off the surface of the wheelchair cushion every 15 minutes). He has a pressure-redistributing cushion on his wheelchair and a specialty mattress in his home. He is able to return to work and lives a full life without an open wound, something he has not done for more than 6 years.

Case Study Questions

1. The nurse is preparing to admit Mr. Parker to the rehabilitation unit following his hospital stay for his myocutaneous flap surgery. Which action should be the priority in preparing for his arrival?
   A. Having his favorite food available to help him maintain a healthy nutritional status
   B. Having a bed available for his wife to spend the night
   C. Having the appropriate mattress on his bed to redistribute pressure
   D. Having advanced wound dressings for highly exuding wounds available

2. Which priority should be implemented early in the treatment plan for Mr. Parker?
   A. Maintaining upper-body strength
   B. Performing full passive range-of-motion exercises to his lower extremities three times daily
   C. Maintaining his contact with work e-mail to facilitate his eventual return to work
   D. Getting out of bed to his wheelchair and going outside

3. In what position is Mr. Parker at least risk of increasing pressure to the ischial muscle flap?
   A. Lying on his left side
   B. Lying on his right side
   C. Sitting up in bed at a 60-degree angle
   D. Sitting up in bed at a 45-degree angle

4. The nurse is teaching Mr. Parker about wound healing. Which statement by him indicates that the teaching was effective?
   A. "I will deeply massage my muscle flap daily to increase circulation and speed healing."
   B. "I will make sure I get a mattress overlay at home so that I don't need to worry about changing positions during the night."
   C. "I will be sure to increase my intake of lean meats and proteins."
   D. "I will go on a diet when I'm discharged because I've gained so much weight over the past few years."

5. Which activity could compromise the healing of Mr. Parker's new flap? *(Select all that apply.)*
   A. Smoking
   B. Wheelchair "push-ups"
   C. Incontinence
   D. Participating in physical therapy
   E. Increased fluid intake

CHAPTER SUMMARY

The skin is the largest organ of the body and serves important functions in relation to protection, sensation, and temperature regulation. Specific functions include protection from bacterial invasion and external elements; sensation of the environment through the senses of touch, pain, temperature, and pressure; retention of water; absorption; thermoregulation; immune surveillance; and metabolism of vitamin D. Disorders of the skin may be related to local damage or trauma or indicative of systemic disease.

Skin infections may be bacterial, viral (herpes simplex), or fungal in origin, and each has characteristic clinical manifestations. Treatment is based on identifying the specific pathogen and administration of targeted antibiotics and other therapies. Patients with skin infections may also manifest issues related to stigma and body image disturbance because of the skin infections, requiring sensitivity by the healthcare team.

Similar to patients with skin infections, patients with psoriasis may also have concerns related to body image because of the chronic nature of this disorder. Psoriasis is a lifelong inflammatory disorder that is characterized by exacerbations and remissions of raised, scaling, erythematous plaques usually seen on the extensor surfaces of the body. Although there is no cure for psoriasis, there are various treatments available that can control clinical manifestations.

Traumatic injuries to the skin are the result of external sources and are classified as an acute wound. There are many types of traumatic skin injuries, including lacerations, abrasions, excoriations, friction blisters, skin tears, pressure injuries, and burns. Clinical manifestations vary depending on the size and depth of the trauma as well as injury to underlying structures, including blood vessels, muscles, and bones. Wound healing is important in reestablishing skin integrity and has four phases—hemostasis, inflammatory, proliferative, and maturation—and each phase has specific clinical manifestations that reflect whether the healing is proceeding normally.

Patients in many healthcare settings are at risk for damage to the skin related to pressure, and because of the complexity and cost in the treatment of complicated pressure injuries, surveillance and prevention are primary nursing considerations. Pressure injuries are a common health problem among individuals who are physically limited or bedridden and include localized injury to the skin and/or underlying tissue, usually over a bony prominence, as a result of pressure or pressure in combination with shear. Complications of pressure injuries include infection, both local and systemic. The nurse's goal is to limit pressure and shearing to prevent pressure injury development. Treatment includes different approaches, including support surfaces to decrease or alleviate pressure, ointments, dressings, and surgical debridement.

Skin cancer is the most prevalent type of cancer, and exposure to the sun is one of the primary risk factors. Ultraviolet damage to the DNA of keratinocytes increases with extended time in the sun and is a major contributing factor to the development of skin cancers. Non-melanoma skin cancers include basal cell and squamous cell carcinomas. The most serious of all skin cancers is malignant melanoma that originates from melanocytes found in the basement membrane of the epidermis. Treatment for skin cancers may be complex, including surgical excision, cryotherapy, radiotherapy, topical chemotherapy, and photodynamic therapy. As with other skin disorders, patients with skin cancer may have to deal with body image disturbances.

Reconstructive surgery is performed by a plastic/ reconstructive surgeon following trauma, surgical debridement of a wound, excision of cancerous lesions, or repair of congenital defects (such as a cleft lip or palate) to repair or improve functional deficits. There are two distinct groups of patients who require reconstructive surgery: those who need surgery because of congenital defects or disfiguring birthmarks and those who need surgery because of trauma, excisions of tumors, infections, or chronic wounds.

The skin and its structures serve as a protective barrier against microbial invasion and environmental exposures, and skin disorders cause a compromise in the skin's integrity, thereby facilitating the risk of infection and injury to the patient. Nursing interventions can provide fortification of the mechanical barrier of the skin through education, support, and proactive recommendations. Once skin breakdown occurs, however, nurses must be able to assess, implement, and evaluate the patient before, during, and after treatment. This requires knowledge of skin infections, wound healing, and therapies used in treating patients with skin and soft tissue disorders.

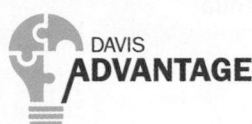

DAVIS ADVANTAGE | To explore learning resources for this chapter, go to **Davis Advantage** and find:
- Answers to in-text questions
- Chapter Resources and Activities
- NCLEX®-Style Chapter Review Questions
- Bibliography

Chapter 51

Coordinating Care for Patients With Burns

Kelly Krout and Carrie Cox

LEARNING OUTCOMES

Content in this chapter is designed to assist in:

1. Discussing the epidemiology of burn injuries
2. Explaining the pathophysiological processes associated with burn injuries
3. Describing classifications of burn injuries
4. Correlating the pathophysiological changes with clinical manifestations seen in patients with superficial, partial-thickness, and full-thickness burns
5. Discussing the appropriate diagnostic examinations for patients with burn injuries
6. Explaining the medical and surgical management of patients with burn injuries
7. Developing comprehensive plans of care for patients with burn injuries
8. Designing a plan of care that includes pharmacological, dietary, and lifestyle-based considerations for patients with burn injuries

CONCEPTS

- Assessment
- Comfort
- Fluid and Electrolyte Balance
- Infection
- Medication
- Nutrition
- Oxygenation
- Perfusion
- Promoting Health
- Skin Integrity

ESSENTIAL TERMS

Allograft
Autograft
Burn excision
Burn shock
Compartment syndrome
Contracture
Cultured epithelial autograft (CEA)
Debridement
Deep partial-thickness burn
Donor site
Eschar
Escharotomy
Fasciotomy
Full-thickness burn
Hydrotherapy
Lund and Browder
Meshed graft
Myoglobinuria
Rule of nines
Sheet graft
Split-thickness skin graft
Superficial burn
Superficial partial-thickness burn
Systemic inflammatory response syndrome (SIRS)
Total body surface area (TBSA)
Xenograft
Zone of coagulation
Zone of hyperemia
Zone of stasis

Finding Connections

CASE STUDY: EPISODE 1

Follow this patient throughout the chapter.

Joe Smith is a 40-year-old male weighing approximately 220 lb (100 kg) who presents to the hospital's emergency department with burns to his face, anterior trunk, and bilateral upper extremities. He has singed nasal hairs and carbonaceous sputum but is reporting no difficulty swallowing or breathing. He sustained the burn while throwing gasoline on a brush fire. He has no past medical history and is currently taking no medications. The patient has been placed on 100% oxygen and has two large-bore peripheral IV catheters. The burns are pale and dry, and the patient is not complaining of any pain except around the edges of the wounds...

INTRODUCTION

Patients with burns are optimally managed at a burn center, where they have the advantage of an interprofessional team of healthcare providers skilled in the specialized treatment of burn injuries. Currently in the United States, there are only 68 burn centers verified by the American Burn Association. Burn center referral criteria established by the American Burn Association are listed in Box 51.1. Because of the limited number of burn centers, the majority of patients receive their initial care at local hospitals prior to transfer to a specialized burn center. For this reason, it is essential for healthcare providers with no specialized education in burn care to have a basic understanding regarding the stabilization and initial management of this patient population.

INCIDENCE AND EPIDEMIOLOGY

According to the latest data released in October 2018 by the National Fire Protection Agency (NFPA), 1,319,500 fires were reported in the United States in 2017, which resulted in 3,400 civilian deaths and 14,670 civilian injuries. (These statistics are updated annually and are available at www.nfpa.org/News-and-Research.) As a result of these fires, property damage was estimated at $23 billion, which is a large increase from previous years and attributed to the wildfires in northern California. The United States has the tenth-highest fire death rate of the 25 industrialized nations. Notably, the southern United States has the highest fire incident rate per thousand people (4.6) and the highest civilian death rate per million population (12.7). The Midwest has the highest civilian injury rate per million population (49.1), whereas the western United States has the highest property loss per capita rate ($46.9).

Box 51.1 American Burn Association's Burn Center Referral Criteria

A burn center may treat adults, children, or both.

- Partial-thickness burns equal to or greater than 10% of the total body surface area
- Burns that involve the face, hands, feet, genitalia, perineum, or major joints
- Full-thickness burns in any age group
- Electrical injury, including lightning injury
- Chemical injury
- Inhalation injury
- Burn injury in patients with pre-existing medical conditions that may complicate management, prolong recovery, or affect mortality
- Any patients with burns and concomitant trauma (e.g., fractures) in which the burn injury poses the greatest risk of morbidity or mortality. In such cases, if the trauma poses the greater immediate risk, the patient's condition may be stabilized initially in a trauma center before transfer to a burn center. Provider judgment will be necessary in such situations and should be in concert with the regional medical control plan and triage protocols.
- Burned children in hospitals without qualified personnel or equipment for the care of children
- Burn injury in patients who require special social, emotional, or rehabilitative intervention

Questions concerning specific patients can be resolved by consultation with the burn center provider.

Outdoor fires (e.g., fields, vacant lots, trash, wildfires) account for approximately 47% of all property fires. Residential and non-residential structure fires combined account for another 38% of fires. However, residential (one- and two-family homes, including manufactured homes, apartments or other multi-family housing) structure fires account for 76% of all structure fires. Finally, vehicle fires account for 15% of the total number of fires. The largest percentage (78%) of deaths occurs on residential properties, with the majority of these being in one- and two-family homes (67%). Vehicles account for the second-largest percentage of fire deaths at 13%.

The two most commonly reported etiologies for burn injury are fire/flame and scald injuries. Admissions to burn centers show admission cause as 43% fire/flame, 34% scald, 9% contact, 4% electrical, 3% chemical, and 7% other. Scald injuries are most prevalent in children under the age of 5, whereas fire/flame dominates all other age groups. The leading cause of both residential and non-residential structure fires is cooking (80.2%), with fires caused by heating being the second-leading cause (9.6%). The two leading causes that result in fatalities and/or injuries for residential fires are cooking- and smoking-related incidents. Some examples include grease burns, scald injuries, flame burns, and falling asleep while smoking.

The majority of fire-related fatalities and injuries occur in people between the ages of 20 to 69 years. This age group accounts for more than half of the fire injuries reported in the United States. According to data collected by the NFPA, men are 1.6 times more likely to die in fires than females, and data collected by the American Burn Association demonstrate that men account for nearly 68% of all patients admitted to burn centers. Although the exact reasons for this are unknown, possibilities include the greater likelihood of men participating in risk-taking behavior and the more high-risk occupations of men. Men also suffer more injuries trying to extinguish fires and rescuing people. Approximately 30% of all fire deaths in females occurs in women 70 years old and older, and this may be due to the fact that women have a longer life expectancy than men and are often performing the majority of the cooking. By contrast, male fire deaths are higher in the age range of 40 to 59. Notably, older adult females have twice the number of fire injuries when compared with older males.

People with limited physical and mental abilities, especially older adults, are at a much higher risk of fire death. Older adults (ages 65 and over) have a risk of dying in a fire that is 2.5 times higher than that of the population as a whole. This risk increases to 3.4 times for those ages 85 and over. As the baby boomers enter retirement age, a corresponding increase in fire deaths and injuries among older adults is likely. In the past, children under the age of 5 were also considered to be at high risk of death due to fire. However, for children ages 4 or younger, the risk of fire death was 30% less than that of the general population. The risk of death for this age group was greater than for older children because as children mature and their cognitive and social abilities develop, the risk of fire death drops sharply. For children ages 5 to 9, the fire death risk was 60% less than that of the general population. For those aged 10 to 14, the risk of fire death was 70% less, dropping even further to 80% less for 15- to 19-year-olds.

Other factors that influence the risk of fire death or injury are related to socioeconomics. The lower-socioeconomic population groups have the highest risk of fire injury or death, whereas the wealthiest have the lowest. Closely tied to income is education level, with those living below the poverty line for extended periods of time experiencing higher fire death rates. African Americans and American Indians/Alaska Natives also have higher fire death rates per capita than the national average, with African Americans accounting for 20% of the total fire deaths while only making up 13% of the U.S. population.

To reduce the incidence of burn injuries, many burn centers are involved in community prevention activities. These activities focus on the higher-risk population groups, including children and older adults. See Box 51.2 for burn injury prevention strategies. In addition, *Healthy People 2020* calls for a reduction in the incidence of residential fire deaths (Box 51.3).

PATHOPHYSIOLOGY

Classifications

Burns are generally classified in terms of etiology, depth of tissue damage, **total body surface area (TBSA)** involved, and severity.

Burn Etiology

A burn injury results when the tissues of the body are damaged by a heat source. The heat source may be thermal, electrical, chemical, or the result of radiation.

Thermal

Thermal burns can be the result of a flash, scald, or contact with hot objects or flames, and common causes include house fires, car fires, cooking accidents, or injuries as a result of careless smoking. Associated accelerant use (e.g., gasoline, kerosene, or propane) may increase the severity of the burn and associated inhalation injury because this adds a chemical insult in addition to the thermal injury. Contact burns are also thermal in nature and are often associated with cooking or heating incidents. Scald injuries are most prevalent among the young and may be associated with accidents or even abuse. The two factors that determine the depth of a thermal injury are the temperature to which the skin is heated and the duration of contact with the heat.

Electrical

Electricity has many devastating effects on the body and may result in a wide spectrum of injuries, ranging from mild to lethal. Electrical injuries account for approximately 4% to 5% of admissions to burn centers in developed countries and up to 27% of admissions to burn centers in developing countries. Of these, 61% are a result of work-related accidents such as gas and electric workers injured while working on breaker boxes or overhead power lines. These burns related to work on power lines are the fourth-leading cause of traumatic work-related deaths. Electrical injuries are associated with an overall increase in the length of hospital stay, morbidities, and number of required surgeries. This is due to the fact that electrical injuries often are linked to other types of ensuing trauma due to subsequent falls and the potential cardiac injury. In addition, as electricity passes through the body, it has the potential to cause damage to multiple organs, which then must also be addressed and treated in conjunction with any burns that have occurred. Electrical burn injuries can be associated with extensive burns that may even require amputation. Patients may present with cardiac and/or neurological problems as well as associated trauma and/or flame burns.

Electrical injury may occur by direct contact with the source, by an arc between two objects, or as a result of a flame injury caused by ignition of the surroundings. The effects of electricity on the body depend on certain factors, including the type and strength of the current, the duration of contact, the pathway of flow through the body, and local

Box 51.2 Burn Prevention Strategies

Burn Prevention Inside the Home

- Install and maintain working smoke alarms on each level of the home and inside each sleeping area. Each month, check that they are working, and change the batteries every 6 months unless the alarm is hardwired into the home or has a 10-year lithium battery.
- Install and maintain working carbon monoxide detectors on each level of your home.
- Develop and practice a home fire escape plan. Make sure everyone in the home knows the meeting place and knows never to return into a burning home for any reason.
- Keep all windows and doorways free of clutter in case of the need to escape quickly.
- Keep a flashlight and telephone near the bedside.
- Keep a working fire extinguisher on each level of the home and know how to use it properly.
- Never set the water heater above 120°F (48.9°C).
- Teach children how to stop, drop, and roll.
- Keep matches and lighters out of the reach of children.
- Never leave a child unattended in a bathtub or near a fire/fireplace.
- Never smoke in bed or while drowsy.
- Never smoke while receiving oxygen therapy.
- Never leave burning candles unattended, and try not to burn candles on low surfaces for risk of being knocked or bumped.
- Always exercise caution while cooking, and do not leave anything unattended on the stove.
- Avoid wearing long sleeves or flowing clothing while cooking.
- Never let a child play near the stove/oven while cooking. Always turn pot handles inward and use the rear burners when possible.
- Never use the kitchen oven as a means to heat the home.
- Avoid running electrical cords under carpets.
- Avoid using space heaters in the bedroom or while asleep.
- While a space heater is in use, there should be a minimum of 3 feet of clearance around the heater in all directions.
- Avoid falling asleep while using a heating pad.
- Be sure to use proper protection and ventilation while working with chemicals in the home, including cleaning products. Read all product labels carefully before use.
- Never store flammable liquids inside the home or near a source of heat.

Burn Prevention Outside the Home

- Always store flammable liquids outside the home in clearly labeled, airtight containers in well-ventilated areas (such as a garage or shed).
- Never refill a hot engine (i.e., lawnmower or weed whacker). Wait until thoroughly cooled before refilling with gasoline.
- Never use flammable liquids to start a campfire or grill.
- Never throw flammable liquids onto an already burning fire.
- Use caution with campfires, and do not leave children unattended around the fire.
- Fireworks should be used only by adults and with extreme caution.
- Be careful of overhead and underground electrical wires while working outside.
- If downed electrical wires are found, do not touch! Call the local electric company to report immediately.
- Caution children never to play near or on electrical boxes or climb trees with electrical wires passing through the branches.
- Always use sunscreen with an SPF of at least 30 when outdoors, and be sure to reapply often. Consider a wide-brimmed hat and sunglasses.

SPF, Sun protection factor.

Box 51.3 *Healthy People 2020*

As of 2007, the incidence of residential fire deaths was down to 0.95 deaths per 100,000. The *Healthy People 2020* goal set by the surgeon general focuses on a 10% improvement in incidence for 2020.

- Goal (IVP-28): Reduce the incidence of residential fire deaths to 0.86 death per 100,000 people.

tissue resistance. The epidermis is the body's best insulation, but once breached, the body acts as a volume conductor. Bone is more resistant to the flow of electricity, and the electricity tends to flow along the top of the bone, often damaging the overlying muscles, nerves, and vessels. Consequently, deep muscle injury may be present even when skin and superficial muscle may appear uninjured.

When a person comes into contact with alternating current, the body often becomes part of the circuit. In alternating current, the movement of an electric charge sporadically changes direction, creating a tetany effect, or involuntary state of muscle contraction that interferes with the person's ability to easily break free from the source. This muscle contraction enables the electric current to flow continuously back and forth between the person and the source, which may either throw the person or draw the person into continual contact with the source. As a result, the current may pass through the body for a greater period of time, exacerbating the severity of the associated injury. Direct current is a one-directional, constant flow of electricity. In the United States, direct current injuries occur from lightning strikes, contact with car or boat batteries, and contact with railway train lines. Electrical current also disrupts the electrical activity of the body and may result in immediate cardiac and/or pulmonary arrest on scene.

The common household electric circuit carries a charge of 120 volts. High-voltage injuries occur when a person comes into contact with 1,000 volts or greater. These types of injuries are often work related and are more common in men. Patients who sustain high-voltage injuries often present with very deep burns and sequela from associated trauma. Flash injuries and/or flame burns may also occur as a result of possible ignition of clothing. The hands and mouth are the most frequently injured sites for low-voltage electrical injuries in children as they may have oral contact with electrical cords or sockets. Surgical management and extensive rehabilitation may be required for the best functional outcomes.

Chemical

Chemical burns account for approximately 3% of all burn center admissions and occur in both the industrial and household settings. The three subclasses of chemical burns include acids, alkalines, and organic compounds. Some examples of chemical burns include those caused by cement, gasoline, lime, hydrofluoric acid, and bleach. The extent of a chemical injury is dependent on many factors, including the agent, the mechanism of action, the concentration and volume of the agent, and the duration of contact with the agent.

Radiation

Radiation burns are the least common type of burn injury, and the severity of complications is dependent on the type, dose, and length of exposure. These injuries are often associated with the industrial use of ionizing radiation, nuclear accidents, and therapeutic radiation treatment. Sunburn is also considered a radiation burn because it is caused by ultraviolet radiation and is the most common type of radiation burn seen in healthcare settings. Localized radiation injuries often appear similar in nature to thermal burns because they are characterized by erythema, edema, blisters, and pain. Prolonged full-body exposure to ionizing radiation often causes nausea, vomiting, diarrhea, fatigue, headache, and fever.

Connection Check 51.1

The nurse recognizes which etiology as consistent with a thermal burn?
A. Direct current
B. Scalding
C. Exposure to organic compounds
D. Ionizing radiation

Burn Depth

Burns are classified according to the depth of tissue damage: superficial, partial-thickness, or full-thickness injuries. Figure 51.1 presents an overview of burn depth in relation

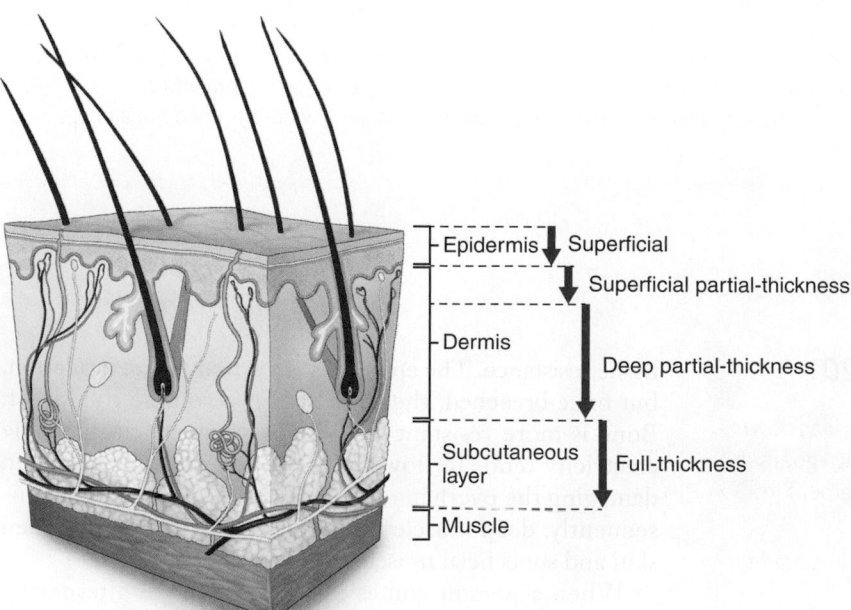

FIGURE 51.1 Burn depth in relation to skin anatomy.

to skin anatomy. Determination of the exact depth of the burn is often impossible on initial inspection, even for the most experienced burn-care provider. This is because burn wounds frequently evolve or "declare themselves" within the first 24 to 72 hours, and it is essential to frequently reassess the burn injury to ensure appropriate resuscitation and treatment. The traditional classification terms of first-, second-, and third-degree are not used in the burn community because they do not give an accurate or descriptive representation as to the true extent of injury. These terms are replaced with the burn-depth classification system, including superficial, superficial partial thickness, deep partial thickness, and full thickness. See Table 51.1 for a summary of burn-depth classifications.

Superficial

Superficial burns affect only the epidermal layer of the skin and are characterized by mild erythema and hypersensitivity, which typically resolve in 24 to 72 hours. Sunburn is the most common type of superficial burn injury (Fig. 51.2). These types of burns heal quickly, typically do not require medical intervention or admission to a burn center, and do not usually result in scarring.

Superficial Partial Thickness

A **superficial partial-thickness burn** involves the epidermis and the superficial or minimal layers of the dermis (Fig. 51.3). Because of the exposed nerve endings located within the dermal layer of the skin, these burns are often very painful. The patient is extremely sensitive to touch and even to air currents when the wound dressing is removed and the burn is exposed. Superficial partial-thickness burns often have wet, weeping blisters and are pink in color. The capillary refill time on areas of open blisters remains normal. Despite the destruction of the entire epidermis, superficial partial-thickness burns usually heal in 1 to 2 weeks with minimal to no scarring. Depending on the location and extent of the superficial partial-thickness burn, medical management and admission to a burn center may be warranted for wound care and pain management. Treatment of superficial and minor partial-thickness burns is highlighted in Box 51.4.

Deep Partial Thickness

A **deep partial-thickness burn** involves the epidermis and extends into the deeper portions or bottom layers of the dermis (Fig. 51.4). The patient often reports varying areas of pain and decreased sensation. Deep partial-thickness burns appear waxy and do not have the characteristic weeping blisters that are seen in superficial partial-thickness injuries. This is due to the fact that the entire epidermis and the majority of the dermis have been damaged. The burn may appear light pink or cherry red in color, and capillary refill is decreased or absent. The challenge with a deep partial-thickness burn is determining the true extent of the injury and whether it will heal without requiring surgical intervention. It is essential to engage in close observation of the burn wound to monitor for potential progression from a deep partial-thickness to a full-thickness burn injury. The majority of these types of burns take more than 2 weeks to heal, during which time the risk of infection is paramount because patients with burn injuries are immune-compromised

Table 51.1 Burn-Depth Assessment

Burn Depth	Tissue Involvement	Wound Characteristics	Pain Assessment	Healing
Superficial	Minimal damage to the epidermis	Dry, no blisters; pink or red; blanches easily	Hypersensitive	3–7 days with no scarring
Superficial partial thickness	Entire epidermis and minimal damage to the dermis	Blisters that may be closed or open and weeping; pink or red; mild edema; blanches easily	Hypersensitive	7–14 days with no scarring
Deep partial thickness	Entire epidermis and deeper layers of the dermis	Blisters that may be closed or open; waxy appearance; cherry red, mottled, or pale in the center; edema; sluggish or no blanching	Hypersensitive around the wound edges but may be sensitive to pressure only in the center	Healing may take 3–6 weeks and may leave some scarring, or the wound may have to be surgically excised and grafted.
Full thickness	Destruction of entire epidermis and dermis have; may involve subcutaneous fat, muscle, and/or bone	Dry, leathery; pale, white, brown, tan, black, charred; no blanching; may be contracted if muscle involvement	No pain in the center of the wound but may be sensitive to pressure	Will not heal without surgical excision and grafting

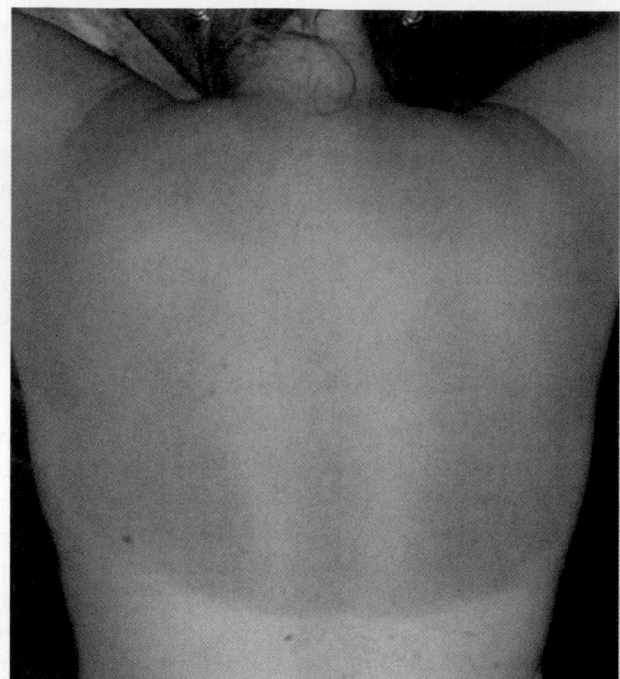

FIGURE 51.2 Superficial burn.

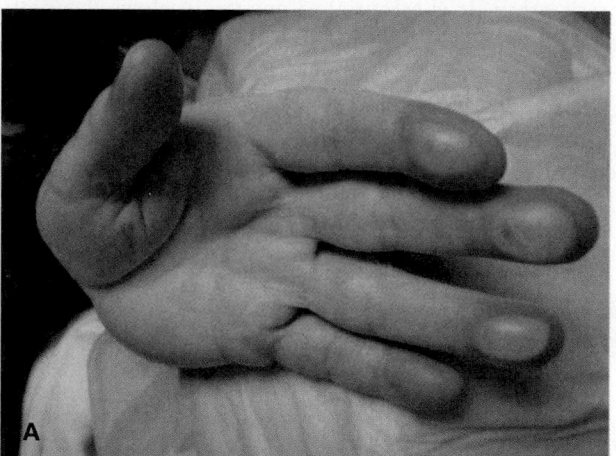

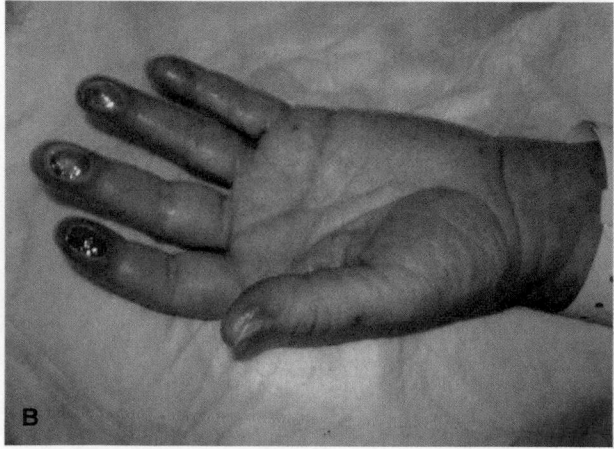

FIGURE 51.3 Superficial partial-thickness burn. A, Pre-debridement of blisters. B, Post-debridement of blisters.

Box 51.4 Care of the Superficial and Minor Partial-Thickness Burn

Although other mechanisms may cause a superficial burn injury, it is quite common to see this type of burn from the sun. In a true superficial burn, no blisters are noted. If blisters appear, the burn is then considered partial thickness. Minor partial-thickness injuries are commonly seen from scalding liquids. Care of the superficial and minor partial-thickness burn wound is outlined here.

Superficial

- Do *not* apply ice or submerge in ice water.
- May apply a cool compress or run under cool water.
- A dressing should not be required because there are no open blisters.
- Lotion should be applied liberally once or twice per day.
- Choose lotion that is aloe based and/or fragrance-free.
- Ibuprofen, acetaminophen, or aspirin may be taken as necessary for pain and discomfort.
- Drink plenty of fluids to rehydrate.
- Rest.

Partial Thickness

- If one to three quarter-sized or smaller blisters appear, try not to open (pop) the blisters. This allows for a moist healing environment, decreased risk of infection, and less discomfort for the patient.
- If the blister or blisters are broken, wash the area with a mild antiseptic soap and warm water.
- Apply a thin layer of bacitracin ointment and cover with a nonadherent bandage.
- The wound should be thoroughly cleansed and the dressing changed at least once per day.
- The patient may continue with his or her usual activities of daily living; however, dependent extremities should be elevated to prevent edema and encourage venous return.
- The patient should be aware of any clinical manifestations of infection, such as fever, increased pain, redness or swelling, purulent drainage, or red streaks radiating from the wound. If noted, the patient should see his or her primary care provider right away.
- It is encouraged that the patient follow up with his or her primary care provider.

without the skin as a barrier to infection. Unfortunately, burns are not an exact science, and the burn surgeon decides whether to operate or to try to let the burn heal on its own.

Full Thickness

A **full-thickness burn** involves destruction of the epidermis, the dermis, and portions of the subcutaneous tissue (Fig. 51.5). All epidermal and dermal structures are destroyed, including hair follicles, sweat glands, and nerve endings. Full-thickness burns do not heal spontaneously. As a result

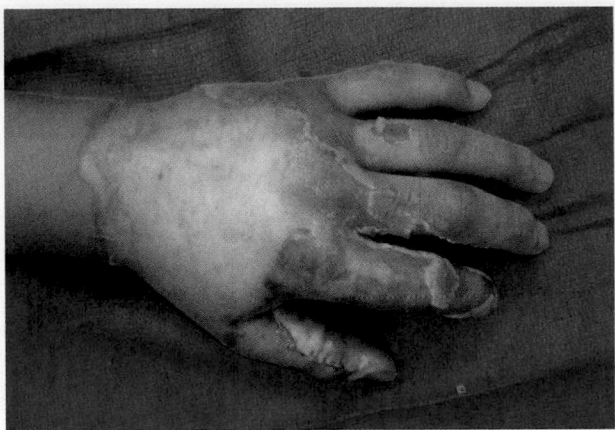

FIGURE 51.4 Deep partial-thickness burn (blisters debrided).

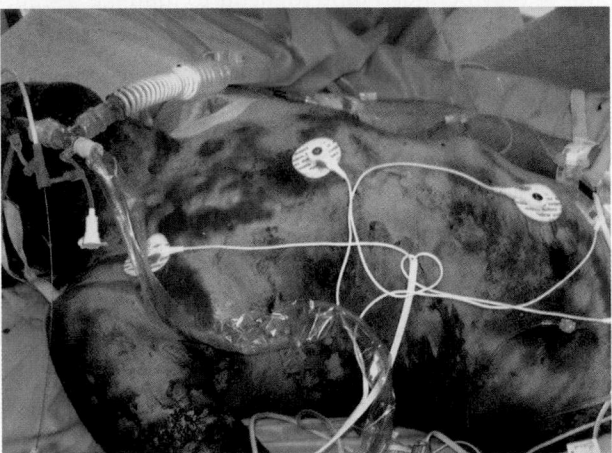

FIGURE 51.5 Full-thickness burn.

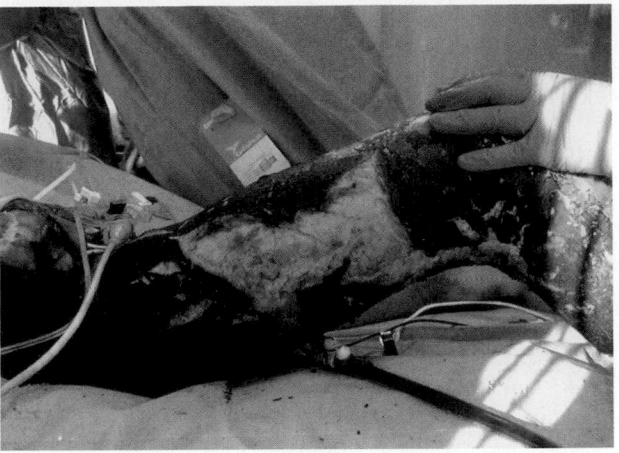

FIGURE 51.6 Full-thickness burn with muscle and bone involvement.

of the extensive damage to the nerve endings, full-thickness burns are often insensate. This absence of pain is often misleading for patients, and many do not comprehend the severity of their injury. Full-thickness burns generally have no blister formation. Although full-thickness burns may take on a variety of colors, they are always very dry and feel like leather to the touch. This full-thickness burn tissue is often referred to as **eschar**. The charred appearance associated with full-thickness injuries is not common. Because all epithelial elements and structures are destroyed, full-thickness burns do not heal spontaneously and require skin grafting. Burns that extend beyond the subcutaneous layer into muscle and/or bone are also considered full thickness, as shown in Figure 51.6.

Connection Check 51.2

The nurse correlates which clinical manifestation with superficial partial-thickness burns?

A. Eschar
B. Dry, leathery appearance
C. Blisters
D. Waxy appearance

Total Body Surface Area Percentage

Expressed as a percentage, total body surface area (TBSA) determination is essential to guiding adequate fluid resuscitation and treatment. Both over- and underestimation of the size of the burn can have significant effects on outcome. Underestimation can result in inadequate resuscitation, which may cause shock and organ failure. Overestimation can put the patient at risk for complications such as pulmonary edema due to the excess fluid given during resuscitation. Adult Patients are resuscitated at injuries of 20% or greater TBSA. The three most common methods for determining TBSA are the rule of palm, the **rule of nines**, and the **Lund and Browder** classification.

Rule of Palm

The size of the patient's hand, including the fingers, accounts for approximately 1% TBSA. This quick method of determining burn size is particularly useful in pre-hospital settings for very small and/or very large burns, scattered burns, and in mass-casualty situations where time is of the essence.

Rule of Nines

The "rule of nines" is the most commonly used method in pre-hospital settings for making a determination of the percentage of TBSA burned. With this method, the adult body surface areas are broken down into 9% or multiples thereof. This division is modified in infants and children because of the large surface area of the child's head and the smaller surface area of the lower extremities. One concern with the rule of nines is that it assumes all physically mature persons, regardless of weight and body shape, have the same distribution of body surface area percentages. The rule of nines diagram is displayed in Figure 51.7.

Lund and Browder Classification

In the hospital setting and in the majority of burn centers, the most widely accepted and accurate method of determining the percentage of TBSA burned is the Lund and

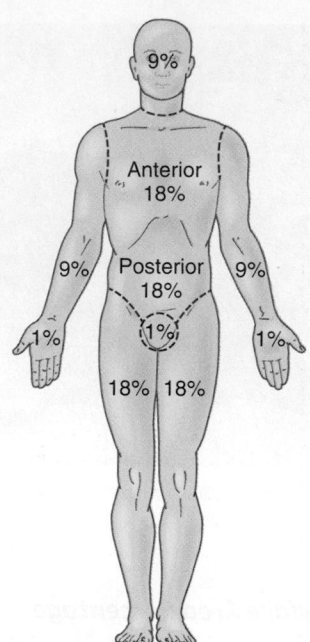

FIGURE 51.7 Rule of nines for determination of total body surface area (TBSA) burn size. This is expressed as a percentage.

Browder classification. Measurements, which take into account surface area related to age, are assigned to each body part. The Lund and Browder classification chart has come into question because it does not account for the altered body mass distribution in obese patients, and future revisions are currently being considered by burn experts. Only partial- and full-thickness burns are recorded on the Lund and Browder chart because superficial burns are not taken into account during resuscitation. The Lund and Browder chart is not completed until a full and thorough **debridement** (removal of damaged tissue) of the burn wound has been completed because this TBSA percentage provides the basis for determining the amount of fluid resuscitation. A visual representation of the Lund and Browder diagram is displayed in Figure 51.8.

Severity

There are several other factors that play an important role in determining the severity of a burn and directly impact overall patient outcome. These factors include the presence of an inhalation injury, patient age, past medical history, and presence of concomitant injury, as well as the anatomical location of the burn injury. Of these factors, the two that are of greatest significance in the determination of survival and that warrant further discussion include age and past medical history. Even very small burns can prove fatal to older adults because of the inability to tolerate the aggressive fluid resuscitation and surgical management required. As the baby boomer generation enters into retirement, patient age and past medical history will continue to play a key role in patient decisions and outcomes (see Geriatric/Gerontological Considerations).

Geriatric/Gerontological Considerations

Burn Care in Older Adults

Managing the care of older adults with burn injuries can present many challenges for the burn team. Common age-related changes in this population put them at a much higher risk of burn injury. These changes include reduced mobility, decreased vision, decreased sense of smell, reduced coordination and strength, and decreased sensation. These normal changes can place older adults at a much higher risk of a severe burn injury because they may have difficulty escaping the fire or removing the source of heat.

Once a burn injury has been sustained, the older adult patient may be much more difficult to manage because of pre-existing medical conditions, decreased immune function, poor nutritional status, decreased pulmonary and/or cardiac function, and poor social support. The skin of the older adult patient is also much thinner and less elastic, which can affect the depth of the injury and the ability of the burn wound to heal. In fact, eschar separation in a full-thickness burn wound is normally delayed in the older adult patient, and many patients are simply not candidates for the operating room because of pre-existing medical conditions. For this reason, older adult patients often have prolonged and complicated hospitalizations and recoveries. Early wound excision and grafting are recommended if they can be tolerated by the patient. The goal is prompt closure of wounds and prevention of infection by decreasing the hospital stay as much as possible.

Anatomical Changes

The functional outcome of the patient is directly related to the depth of the burn injury, with full-thickness burns resulting in the most significant anatomical skin changes. Skin that has been grafted after a full-thickness burn injury can become severely scarred, and normal movement and appearance are usually significantly impaired. The localized tissue response to the burn can be illustrated by the concentric zones of burn injury, as displayed in Figure 51.9, with each zone representing the localized tissue response. The **zone of coagulation** is the area that had the most contact with the heat source and is the location of the most severe damage. The tissue undergoes protein coagulation, eschar is often present, and the patient often reports no pain within this area because all nerve cells are destroyed. The **zone of stasis** immediately surrounds the zone of coagulation and is characterized by damaged cells and impaired circulation. It is this area of the burn that is most at risk for conversion if the patient does not receive adequate resuscitation. Improper resuscitation or under-resuscitation may

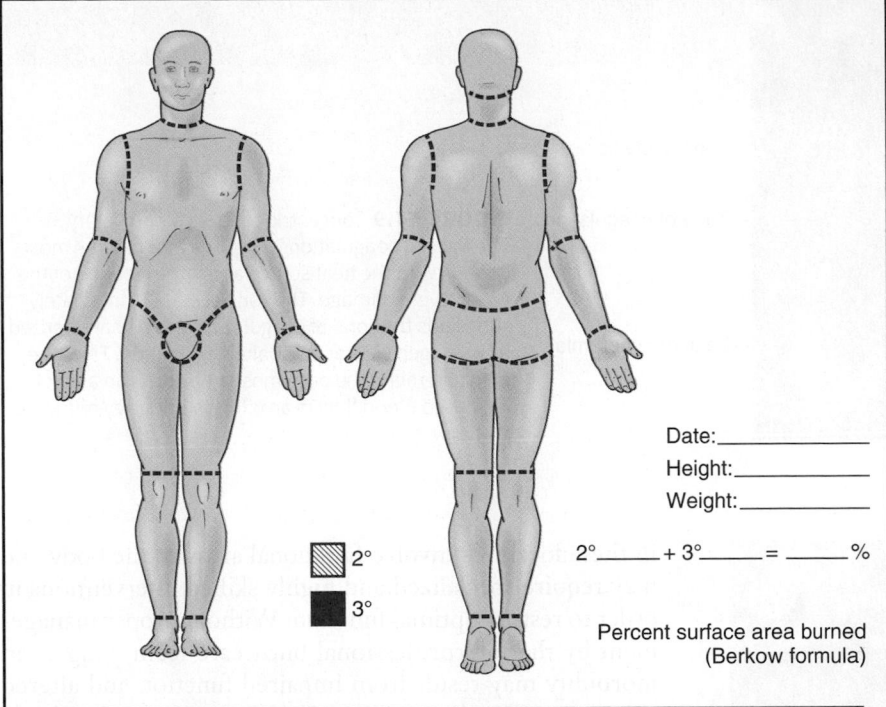

Date:_____

Height:_____

Weight:_____

☒ 2°

■ 3°

2°_____ + 3°_____ = _____%

Percent surface area burned
(Berkow formula)

Area	0–1 Year	1–4 Years	5–9 Years	10–14 Years	15 Years	Adult	2°	3°
Head	19	17	13	11	9	7		
Neck	2	2	2	2	2	2		
Ant. Trunk	13	13	13	13	13	13		
Post. Trunk	13	13	13	13	13	13		
R. Buttock	2.5	2.5	2.5	2.5	2.5	2.5		
L. Buttock	2.5	2.5	2.5	2.5	2.5	2.5		
Genitalia	1	1	1	1	1	1		
R.U. Arm	4	4	4	4	4	4		
L.U. Arm	4	4	4	4	4	4		
R.L. Arm	3	3	3	3	3	3		
L.L. Arm	3	3	3	3	3	3		
R. Hand	2.5	2.5	2.5	2.5	2.5	2.5		
L. Hand	2.5	2.5	2.5	2.5	2.5	2.5		
R. Thigh	5.5	6.5	8	8.5	9	9.5		
L. Thigh	5.5	6.5	8	8.5	9	9.5		
R. Leg	5	5	5.5	6	6.5	7		
L. Leg	5	5	5.5	6	6.5	7		
R. Foot	3.5	3.5	3.5	3.5	3.5	3.5		
L. Foot	3.5	3.5	3.5	3.5	3.5	3.5		
Total								

FIGURE 51.8 Lund and Browder classification.

cause the burn to become deeper because of limited blood flow, causing the zone of stasis to convert into the zone of coagulation, as shown in Figure 51.10. The outermost area is termed the **zone of hyperemia** and is generally an area of increased blood flow in an effort to bring key nutrients for tissue recovery. This area usually sustains minimal injury and recovers spontaneously within 1 to 2 weeks. The full extent of damage may not be evident for 24 to 72 hours post-injury because it may take that long for burns to reveal the true depth of injury.

Connection Check 51.3

The nurse correlates which zone of burn injury as the most susceptible to sustained injury because of insufficient fluid resuscitation?

A. Zone of stasis

B. Zone of conversion

C. Zone of hyperemia

D. Zone of coagulation

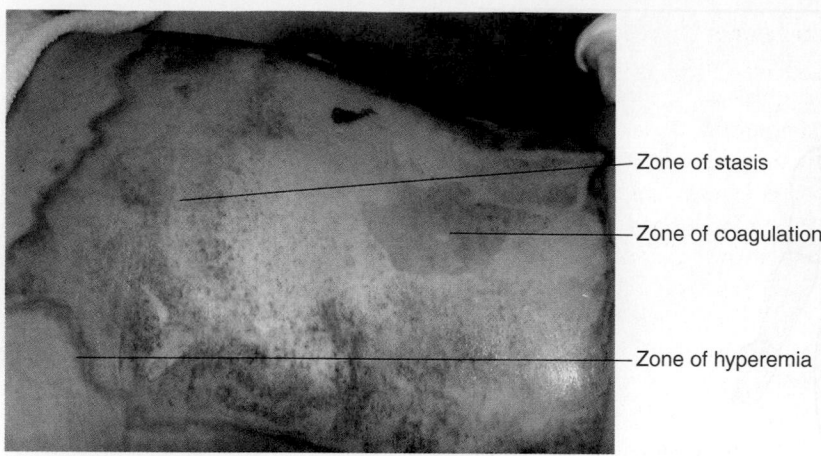

—Zone of stasis

—Zone of coagulation

—Zone of hyperemia

FIGURE 51.9 Concentric zones of a burn injury. The zone of coagulation is the area that had the most contact with the heat source and is the location of the most severe damage. The zone of stasis immediately surrounds the zone of coagulation and is characterized by damaged cells and impaired circulation. The zone of hyperemia is the outermost area and is an area of increased blood flow in an effort to bring key nutrients for tissue recovery.

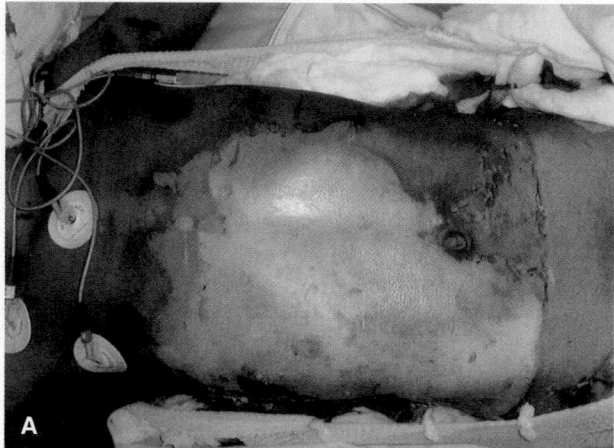

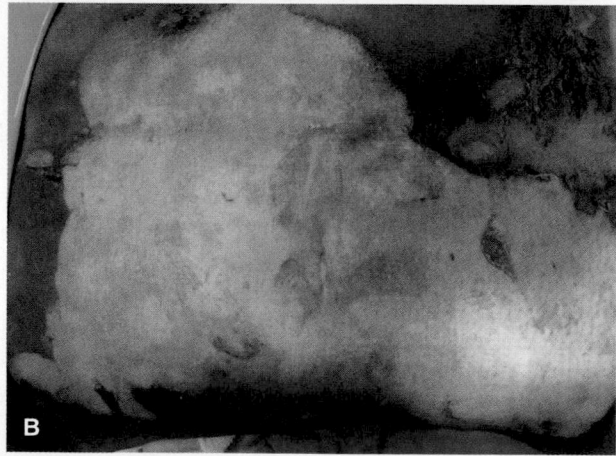

FIGURE 51.10 Burn wound conversion. A, Chest and abdomen post-burn day 1. B, Chest and abdomen post-burn day 2.

Functional Changes

The location of a burn injury plays an important part in determining the level of care required and in the functional changes that may result. According to the American Burn Association, referral criteria to a burn center involve injuries to specific areas of the body, including the face, hands, feet, genitalia, and perineum and burns over major joints. Burns

in these locations involve functional areas of the body and may require specialized and highly skilled interventions in order to restore optimal function. Without proper management by the interprofessional burn-care team, long-term morbidity may result from impaired function and altered appearance. Survivors of large burns often require multiple and sometimes lifelong plastic and reconstructive surgical procedures in order to maintain proper function and range of motion.

Connection Check 51.4

The nurse recognizes that burns to which body areas meet the criteria for referral to a burn center because of the increased risk of functional changes? *(Select all that apply.)*
A. Chest
B. Perineum
C. Elbows
D. Face
E. Hands

SYSTEMIC EFFECTS OF MAJOR BURN INJURIES

Burns that are less than 20% TBSA produce a localized tissue response. Burns that are greater than 20% TBSA are considered major burn injuries and produce both localized and systemic responses. All body systems are affected by the release of cytokines and other mediators into the systemic circulation.

Respiratory

Inhalation injuries, defined as the toxic effects of heat and the chemical products of combustion on the lungs and in the airways, are present in 10% to 20% of patients admitted to burn centers and significantly increase morbidity and mortality. In order to minimize complications and decrease the overall mortality rate, rapid diagnosis and management of inhalation injuries are critical (Box 51.5). Recognizing an inhalation injury is particularly important because it has been recognized as the third most important factor, after extent/depth of burn and patient age, in determining mortality. Inhalation injuries should always be considered when the patient was injured or trapped within an enclosed space, such as in a house or car, or there are burn injuries of the face, neck, or chest.

There are three main types of airway inhalation injuries: inhalation injury above the glottis, inhalation injury below the glottis, and carbon monoxide poisoning. Inhalation burns are most commonly limited to the upper airway above the glottis (nasopharynx, oropharynx, and larynx) and are usually thermal or chemical in nature. Because of the protective response of the respiratory tract, the majority of heat absorption and tissue damage occurs above the glottis and vocal cords. These above-the-glottis burns are associated with injury to the nose, throat, and mouth, and because swelling can occur within minutes to hours of injury, emergent intubation may be required to maintain the airway. Inhalation injury below the glottis is almost always chemical in nature and is rarely caused by heated air alone. This type of severe inhalation injury is most common in patients with prolonged exposure to smoke, such as those rendered unconscious by fire. Wheezing and tracheobronchitis may be seen in the first minutes to several hours post-injury.

Most fatalities that occur at the scene of a fire are due to carbon monoxide poisoning. Because carbon monoxide binds to the hemoglobin molecule with an affinity 200 times greater than that of oxygen, tissue hypoxia results when carbon monoxide levels are above normal. In cases of suspected carbon monoxide poisoning, oxygen measurement by pulse oximeter is useless because the determination between the oxygen and carbon monoxide molecules saturating the hemoglobin is not possible. Normal carboxyhemoglobin levels are less than 2% but may be as high as 5% to 10% in heavy smokers. Although carbon monoxide may cause a cherry red discoloration of the skin in patients with carbon monoxide levels at 40% or higher, this manifestation is seen only in approximately 50% of cases. More common clinical manifestations observed in patients with carbon monoxide poisoning include headache, confusion, nausea, dizziness, vomiting, and dyspnea. These clinical manifestations are usually seen when carbon monoxide levels reach approximately 30%. Table 51.2 provides a listing of clinical manifestations in relation to the percentage of carbon monoxide levels.

Patients with an inhalation injury may present with facial burns, singed nasal and facial hairs, carbon in their sputum, redness of the oral pharynx, inability to swallow, and tachypnea. The respiratory epithelium may be damaged as a result of inhaled gases and particulate matter. Mucus production and impaired ciliary function may result, which ultimately may lead to cell death and sloughing of the respiratory tract. Anxiety and agitation may ensue if the patient begins to experience respiratory distress. Clinical manifestations of respiratory distress may include stridor, progressive hoarseness, rales, rhonchi, and/or retractions of the lower rib cage. Endotracheal intubation should be considered if the patient presents with any of these clinical manifestations.

Cardiovascular

Initially, the greatest threat to a patient with a major burn injury is **burn shock**, which is a combination of distributive and hypovolemic shock. This type of shock results secondary to a massive fluid shift. Electrolytes, water, plasma, and proteins leak out of the intravascular space and into the interstitial space because of the increase in capillary permeability, which results from the body's initial inflammatory protective mechanism. The large fluid loss within the intravascular space increases the viscosity of the blood, which results in sluggish blood flow, decreased oxygen delivery, and overall decreased cardiac output. Because of the increased viscosity of the blood, the patient initially presents with an elevated hematocrit.

Generally, fluid leakage occurs during the first 8 to 36 hours after the injury, with maximum shifting peaking at approximately 24 hours post-burn. If fluid resuscitation

---

Box 51.5 Physical and Clinical Manifestations of an Inhalation Injury

- Facial burns
- Singed nasal and facial hairs
- Carbonaceous sputum (soot), hypersecretion
- Naso- or oropharynx erythema
- Excessive agitation/anxiety (hypoxia)
- Tachypnea, intercostal retractions, flaring nostrils
- Inability to swallow
- Hoarseness, grunting, brassy voice
- Rales, rhonchi, diminished breath sounds

Table 51.2 Clinical Manifestations of Carbon Monoxide Poisoning

Carbon Monoxide (%)	Clinical Manifestations
5–10	Mild headache and confusion
11–20	Severe headache, flushing, vision changes
21–30	Disorientation, nausea
31–40	Irritability, dizziness, vomiting
41–50	Tachypnea, tachycardia
Greater than 50	Coma, seizures, death

is not adequate, the burn patient begins to demonstrate clinical manifestations of shock, including hypotension, tachycardia, reduced urinary output, and altered mental status. Figure 51.11 provides an overview of the pathophysiological changes occurring during burn shock. If the state of shock continues to progress without proper fluid resuscitation and management, the patient will begin to decompensate, resulting in multisystem organ failure and potentially death.

In the post–burn shock phase, which begins approximately 24 to 48 hours after injury, the capillaries begin to regain integrity. Burn shock slowly begins to resolve, and the fluid gradually returns to the intravascular space. Urinary output continues to increase secondary to patient diuresis, and blood pressure and cardiac output begin to normalize.

Fluid and Electrolytes

The two electrolytes of most concern during the burn shock phase are potassium and sodium. Initially, hyperkalemia may result because of the release of potassium from damaged cells into the vascular space. As fluid shifts continue, potassium and sodium begin to leak out of the intravascular spaces, and hypokalemia and hyponatremia may result.

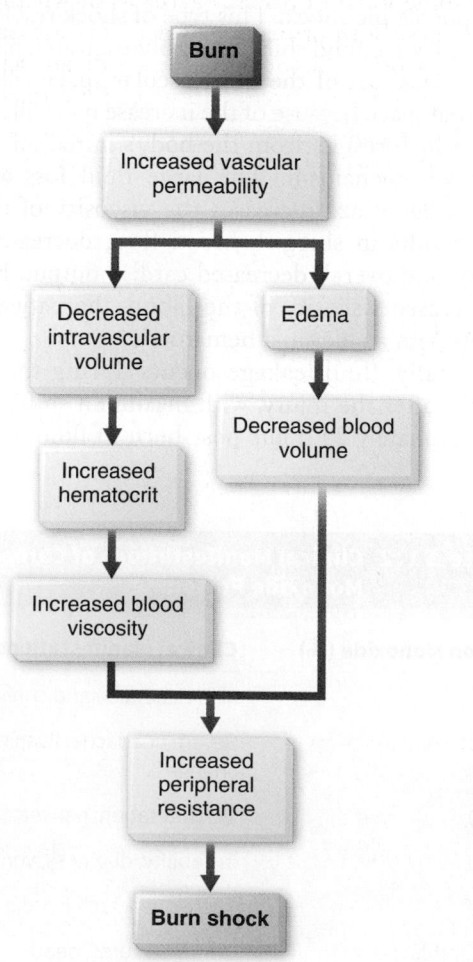

FIGURE 51.11 Pathophysiology of burn shock.

Although potassium and sodium are of utmost importance, all electrolytes are closely monitored, and replacement therapy is initiated as warranted. It is extremely important to account for evaporative fluid loss that may occur through the burn wound, as this amount may be as great as 5 L per day and continues until all wounds are closed.

Renal

Because of the initial decrease in circulating blood volume, renal function may also be impaired secondary to decreased renal perfusion. Destruction of red blood cells results in free hemoglobin being released into the body following a major burn injury. If the patient has sustained muscle damage as a result of the burn injury, myoglobin may also be present in the bloodstream. When fluid resuscitation and resulting blood flow are inadequate, myoglobin and hemoglobin have the potential to occlude renal tubules, causing acute tubular necrosis. This is most commonly seen with electrical injuries.

Gastrointestinal

The patient with a burn injury often has complications of the gastrointestinal system secondary to a decrease in both nutrient absorption and gastrointestinal motility. Paralytic ileus is not seen as frequently in the burn population because of the increased use of prokinetic agents and early initiation of enteral nutritional support. A nasogastric tube is placed in patients with large burns for both long-term feeding access and to relieve initial gastric distention, nausea, and vomiting. Patients with burns who have suffered a significant injury and require massive fluid resuscitation are at risk for developing abdominal compartment syndrome secondary to massive resuscitation volumes.

Metabolic

A burn injury causes an array of physiological alterations within the body, placing the patient in a constant hypermetabolic state for up to 1 to 3 years post-injury. Burn injuries often double the normal resting energy expenditure and greatly increase the patient's caloric needs. Because the nutritional needs are constantly fluctuating for the patient with burn injuries, determining caloric needs is a dynamic and ongoing process. Factors affecting the metabolic rate in patients with burns include age, gender, infection, concomitant trauma, pain, surgery, sleep, and ambient temperature. Without additional nutritional support in patients with large burn injuries, particularly those with a burn greater than 20% TBSA, wound healing is impaired. Even patients who can feed themselves often require supplementary caloric support and/or enteral feeding because of their hypermetabolic state. Nutrition is so important that many burn centers continue to enterally feed patients up to and throughout their entire operative procedures (see Evidence-Based Practice: Impact of Enteral Feeding in Morbidity and Outcomes in Patients With Burns).

Evidence-Based Practice

Impact of Enteral Feeding in Morbidity and Outcomes in Patients With Burns

Due to the hypermetabolic state that develops in patients with severe burn injuries, there is increased focus on meeting the nutritional needs in this patient population. This study examined current evidence regarding whether early enteral nutrition impacts patient outcomes in patients with major burn injuries. Data sources included Medline, Embase, and the China National Knowledge Infrastructure throughout May 2018 and only included randomized controlled trials that reported patient outcomes. In total, 958 articles were reviewed, with seven randomized controlled trials enrolling 527 participating included in the final analysis. For purposes of this study, enteral nutrition was described as a standard formula starting within 24 hours of the burn injury or admission to the intensive care unit. The findings of the study supported previously reported improvements in clinical outcomes in those patients who received early enteral nutrition. Specific findings included preservation of gut integrity, fewer gastrointestinal hemorrhages, less infectious complications, and reductions in both organ failures and sepsis. Reduced lengths of hospital stays were also associated with early enteral nutrition in this patient population.

Pu, H., Doig, G. S., Heighes, P. T., & Allington, M. J. (2018). Early enteral nutrition reduces mortality and improves other key outcome in patients with major burn injury: A meta-analysis of randomized controlled studies. *Critical Care Medicine, 46*(12), 2036–2042.

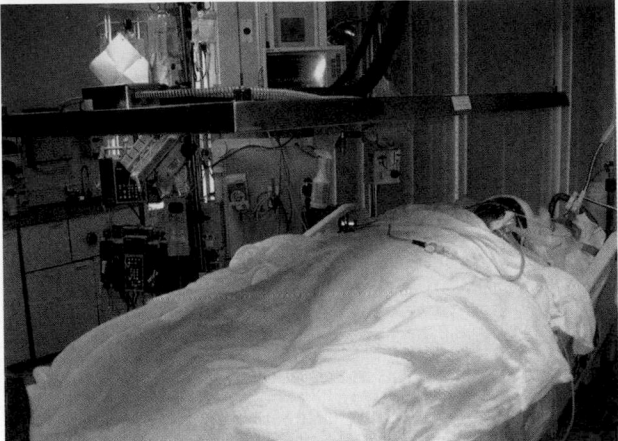

FIGURE 51.12 Specialized heating equipment in the burn intensive care unit.

burn wounds. The loss of skin integrity is compounded by the release of abnormal inflammatory factors, which alter the patient's underlying metabolic profile. As a result of these alterations, patients with extensive burns develop **systemic inflammatory response syndrome (SIRS)**. The term *SIRS* relates to the exaggerated inflammatory response that occurs in the body after injury and may precede the development of sepsis. All patients with extensive burns exhibit some form of SIRS regardless of whether or not sepsis ensues. Burn professionals demonstrate expertise in recognizing other factors that may indicate sepsis, such as a change in mental status, increased fluid requirements, decreased urine output, and a decline in respiratory function. (See Chapter 14 for more discussion of shock and sepsis.)

Sepsis

The skin is the body's largest protection barrier, and once it is breached, the patient is continuously at risk for infection. If the patient survives the first 24 hours after the initial burn injury, sepsis is usually the leading cause of death (see Evidence-Based Practice: Infection and Sepsis in Patients With Burns). Current medical definitions regarding sepsis are not applicable in the burn population because many patients with burns may demonstrate all of the criteria of sepsis without actually having an infection and/or being septic.

Massive amounts of body heat may be lost through open wounds as a result of impaired thermoregulatory function. Once the patient loses skin, it is impossible for the body to successfully regulate temperature. Because of this, it is essential to maintain a high ambient temperature within the patient's room and within the operating room. This is particularly essential when the wounds are exposed. Many burn centers have specialized heating equipment to assist in patient warming (Fig. 51.12). This equipment may include heat shields located in the ceiling above the patient's bed that may be lowered, as well as additional space heaters that are often placed in the room. Many of the newer or newly remodeled burn centers now have radiant heat under the flooring and behind the walls in each patient room.

Immunological

Patients with burn injuries are at high risk for infection and sepsis because of loss of the protective function of the skin, altered immunological defenses, and the presence of open

Evidence-Based Practice

Infection and Sepsis in Patients With Burns

A panel of experts in burn care came together in 2007 to develop a consensus for definitions concerning infection and sepsis among burn patients. This definition is still relevant today. The panel defined sepsis in patients with burns as "a change in the burn patient that triggers the concern for infection."

The triggers include at least three of the following clinical manifestations:

A. Temperature greater than 102.2°F (39°C)
B. Progressive tachycardia and tachypnea
C. Thrombocytopenia, low platelet count (does not apply until 3 days after resuscitation)
D. Hyperglycemia
E. Insulin resistance
F. Enteral tube feed intolerance characterized by large amounts of residual tube feeding

In addition to these indicators, documented incidence of an infection or clinical response to antimicrobials is also required to make a definitive diagnosis of sepsis in the patient with burns.

Pu, H., Doig, G. S., Heighes, P. T., & Allington, M. J. (2018). Early enteral nutrition reduces mortality and improves other key outcomes in patients with major burn injury: A meta-analysis of randomized controlled studies. *Critical Care Medicine, 46*(12), 2036–2042.
Greenhalgh, D., Saffle, J., Holmes, J., Gamelli, R., Palmieri, T., Horton, J., … Latenser, B. (2007). American Burn Association consensus conference to define sepsis and infection in burns. *Journal of Burn Care and Research, 28*(6), 776–790.

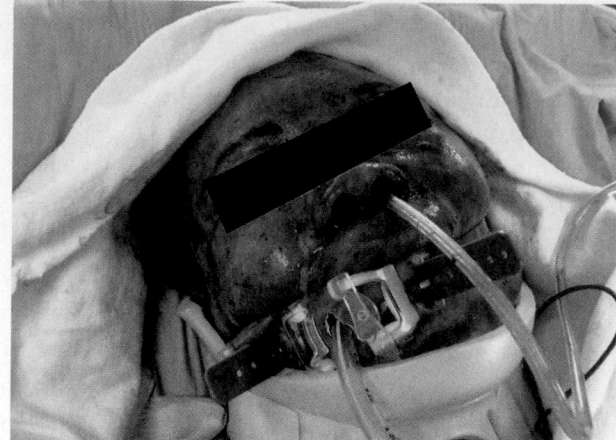

FIGURE 51.13 Inhalation injury characterized by edema around the nose and mouth with soot present in the nares. Endotracheal and nasogastric tubes in place.

Infection control is a high priority when dealing with the patient who has suffered a burn injury. Approximately 28% to 65% of these patients die as a result of sepsis. The majority of burn centers employ multiple infection control strategies and techniques, including contact precautions for all patient interactions; disposable equipment, including blood pressure cuffs, stethoscopes, electrocardiogram (ECG) leads; and antibiotic-coated urinary and central line catheters. Although the prevention of infection in the patient with burns may be impossible, every method should be employed to reduce the overall risk.

SPECIAL CONSIDERATIONS IN THE PATIENT WITH BURNS

Inhalation Injuries

An inhalation injury can exist in the presence or absence of a cutaneous burn (Fig. 51.13). Regardless of the TBSA percentage burned, an inhalation injury increases the overall mortality rate because the patient often develops pneumonia or hypoxemia and requires lengthy ventilatory support. Although inhalation injuries can significantly increase morbidity and mortality, there are few standards for diagnosis, treatment, and the measurement of outcomes. Chest x-rays performed on admission are often normal in patients with an inhalation injury, and as a result, a fiberoptic bronchoscopy examination is recommended for definite diagnosis because this study can reveal damage to the respiratory tract and lungs that is not evident on chest x-ray. It is

important that patients are observed closely for approximately 24 hours post–burn injury because of the insidious onset of inhalation injuries.

Patients with burns rarely exhibit immediate signs of respiratory distress; therefore, it is essential to monitor for less obvious indicators of an inhalation injury, including a change in voice (such as hoarseness), anxiety, and/or confusion. It is also important to note whether the burn injury occurred outside or inside because confinement in a burning environment increases the risk of sustaining an inhalation injury. At any time that airway patency is questionable, early intubation is recommended. Delay may result in severe airway obstruction, at which time intubation may become extremely challenging and may require an emergent tracheostomy. As a result of upper airway edema, an endotracheal tube that becomes dislodged may be almost impossible to replace. It is essential to secure the patient's endotracheal tube with umbilical twill or commercially prepared endotracheal tube holders and not adhesive tape because tape does not stick to the burned face and does not allow for swelling. An emergency tracheostomy tray is maintained at these patients' bedsides in the event of unplanned extubation.

Connection Check 51.5

The nurse correlates which clinical manifestations with the possibility of an inhalation injury? *(Select all that apply.)*
A. Facial burns
B. Singed nasal hairs
C. Soot in the sputum
D. Hoarseness
E. Eschar

Because of the risk of carbon monoxide poisoning associated with inhalation injuries, treatment requires immediate application of 100% oxygen by mask, which is maintained until carboxyhemoglobin levels are below 10%. The half-life of carbon monoxide in the blood is approximately 30 minutes to 1 hour on 100% oxygen as opposed to 4 hours on room air. Because the majority of patients with burns are placed on 100% oxygen at the scene, it is important to note that measurement of carbon monoxide levels may be a poor indicator of injury because the majority of the carbon monoxide may have been dissipated by the time the patient arrives at the hospital.

Electrical Injuries

The American Burn Association describes electrical injuries as "the grand masquerader" because the extent of tissue damage is not always apparent on the surface of the skin. Burn healthcare professionals are making efforts to move away from the terms *entrance* and *exit points* because the two may be difficult to distinguish. Instead, the term *contact points* is used when describing electrical injuries (Fig. 51.14). The patient's entire body is assessed for contact points, with close attention paid to the scalp because contact points may be hidden by the hair.

In addition to burn wound management, there are additional priorities to consider when caring for patients with electrical injuries. In 15% of patients experiencing electrical injuries, there is also associated physical trauma secondary to the patient falling or being thrown. Patients with electrical burns should be placed in a cervical collar until cervical spine films are cleared for possible injury. Other priorities when managing patients with electrical injuries include cardiac monitoring, fluid resuscitation, neurological assessment, renal management, and maintenance of peripheral circulation.

Continuous cardiac monitoring is recommended for at least 24 to 48 hours for patients presenting with a documented cardiac arrest or dysrhythmia and/or extremes in burn size and age. It is important to obtain a baseline ECG to track any cardiac abnormalities that may arise. Neurological assessments are completed on a regular basis to monitor for any changes in level of consciousness. Fluid

resuscitation is calculated based on the TBSA of the burns. However, it is important to remember that this calculation is just a starting point for fluid resuscitation because there may be extensive damage to internal structures underneath the skin's surface that are not obvious with external assessment. Urine output is closely monitored for signs of **myoglobinuria**, which indicates muscle damage and manifests as red or tea-colored urine. If myoglobin is suspected, a urinalysis is performed. Myoglobin can occlude renal tubules and cause acute tubular necrosis; thus, it is important to maintain a urine output of 1 mL/kg/hr for patients with electrical injuries.

Chemical Injuries

Early recognition and immediate initiation of continuous irrigation to the affected area is crucial when dealing with chemical burns (Fig. 51.15). The three most common classes of chemicals that cause burn injuries are acids, alkalis, and organic compounds. It is important to note that alkali burns tend to penetrate deeper, causing liquefaction necrosis of the underlying tissue requiring a lengthy irrigation period. Organic compounds, such as gasoline, are also of importance because of their ability to systemically absorb into the body, causing renal and hepatic damage. Tar and asphalt burns are also common injuries but are thermal and not chemical in nature and require immediate cooling rather than removal. Refer to Table 51.3 for additional information on each chemical classification.

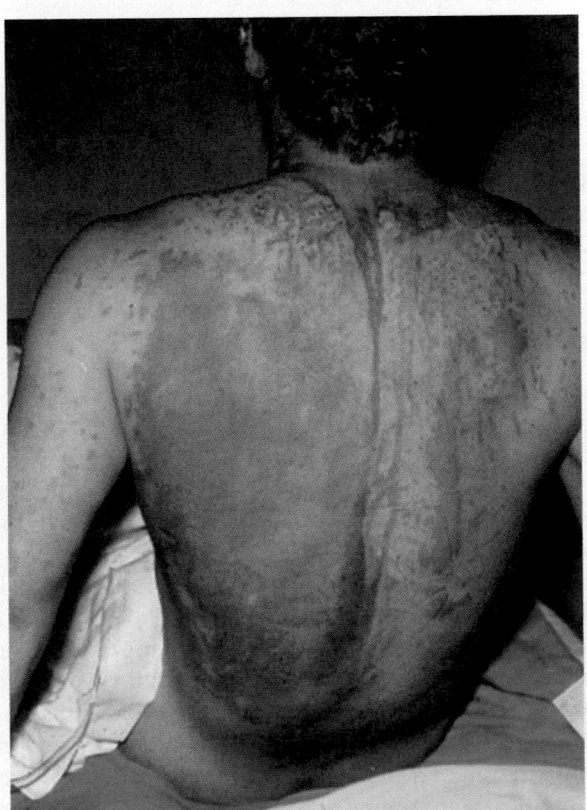

FIGURE 51.15 Chemical injury to the back.

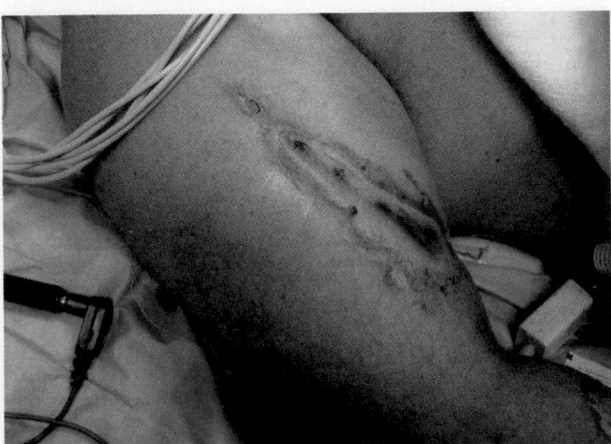

FIGURE 51.14 Contact point associated with electrical injury.

Table 51.3 Mechanisms of Action of Chemical Burn Injuries

Acids	Alkalis	Organic Compounds
Protein donor that releases hydrogen ions and can reduce pH to values as low as 0; results in coagulation of proteins and possible full-thickness injury	Protein acceptor that strips hydrogen ions from protonated amine and carboxylic groups. This increases pH values above neutrality and may cause liquefaction necrosis. This allows for deeper tissue penetration and often results in full-thickness injury.	Act by dissolving the lipid membrane of cells and disrupting the protein structure of the cell, which may result in full-thickness injury. This also allows for systemic absorption, which may lead to hepatic and renal damage.
Examples: bathroom cleaners, drain cleaners, rust removers, glass etching, home swimming pools	Examples: oven cleaners, drain cleaners, wet cement, fertilizers, heavy industrial cleaners	Examples: phenols, creosote, and petroleum products (gasoline)

The use of personal protective equipment by all healthcare team members is crucial when managing suspected chemical injuries to ensure that no one else is injured or affected by the chemical. Initial treatment of chemical burns involves the removal of saturated clothing, brushing off the skin if the agent is in powder form, and continuous irrigation with copious amounts of water. The use of a neutralizing agent is usually not recommended because of the exothermic (heat-producing) reaction that occurs. Irrigation continues until the patient reports a decrease in pain, the patient's temperature can no longer tolerate further irrigation, or the patient is transferred to a burn center. Chemical injuries to the eyes are flushed continuously until an ophthalmologist can complete a full examination.

> **⚠ Safety Alert** Protect yourself! It is imperative that healthcare workers ensure that the scene is safe and protect themselves using the appropriate personal protective equipment when a chemical injury is suspected.

Escharotomies and Fasciotomies

Any circumferential burn to an extremity is at risk for developing **compartment syndrome**. As fluid seeps from the intravascular spaces into the interstitium, pressure within the tissues continues to rise and confines swelling inside muscle compartments, resulting in compartment syndrome. Involved extremities are elevated, and pulses in both burned and unburned extremities are assessed and compared on an hourly basis. Clinical manifestations of compartment syndrome include progressive diminishing of the pulse, numbness, tingling, and complaint of pain with flexion and/or extension. This pain is often not proportional to the extent of the injury and is unrelenting despite appropriate administration of pain medication. Compartment syndrome is a medical emergency and requires immediate surgical intervention in order to salvage the limb.

In full-thickness burns, eschar acts as a tourniquet, and as fluid resuscitation continues, vascular compromise may result. Pulses are monitored on an hourly basis in all affected extremities. In some patients, if it is difficult to palpate pulses, a Doppler may be required to assess peripheral circulation. Other assessments include skin color, temperature, sensation, and capillary refill. It is imperative that the nurse monitor for progressive diminution of pulses and report these data to the healthcare provider rather than waiting until pulses are completely absent. An **escharotomy** (surgical incision through eschar) is performed to relieve the pressure (Fig. 51.16) and should extend only through the eschar and into the immediate subcutaneous fat. This procedure may be performed at the bedside using a scalpel or an electrocautery device. In circumferential burns to the chest, pulmonary function may be restricted because of the inability of the chest wall to expand with ventilation. The chest wall escharotomy (Fig. 51.17) is considered a medical emergency and in rare instances may be performed by scene first responders after consultation with a burn center. See Figure 51.18 for common escharotomy sites.

A **fasciotomy** is performed when the burn extends into the muscle and is more commonly seen in patients who have sustained an electrical injury and have developed

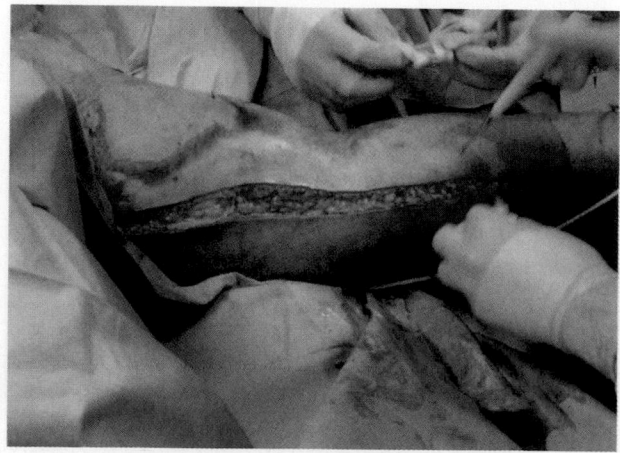

FIGURE 51.16 Upper extremity escharotomy.

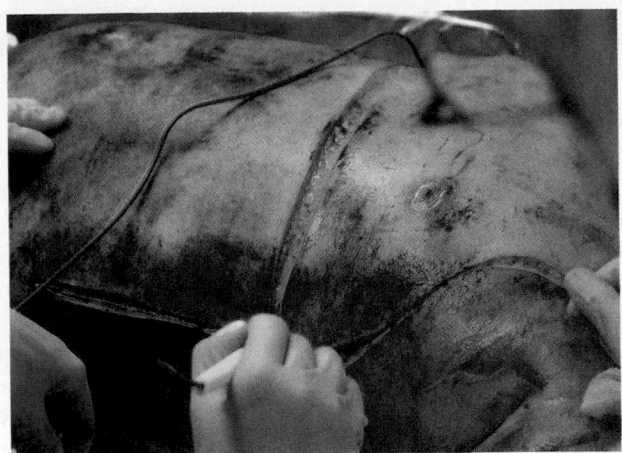

FIGURE 51.17 Chest wall escharotomy.

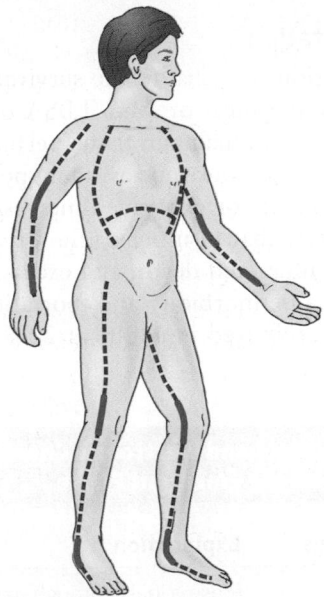

FIGURE 51.18 Preferred escharotomy sites. Patient should be placed in anatomical position (palmar surface up), and mid-medial and mid-lateral incisions are made for each extremity, extending the length and depth of the eschar only. The chest wall should have an H-type pattern, with all efforts to avoid the axilla because it contains many lymph nodes, vessels, and nerves. The connecting horizontal line should be placed roughly at the patient's diaphragm.

compartment syndrome. A fasciotomy is an incision that extends through the subcutaneous fat and muscle fascia, allowing for expansion of the muscle compartment. Fasciotomies are done by the provider under sterile conditions in the operating room.

MANAGEMENT OF BURN INJURIES

Although other areas of medicine are traditionally delineated into separate medical and nursing tasks and priorities, burn care is an exception. Burn treatment is based on an interprofessional team approach including physicians, registered nurses, advanced practice registered nurses, physician assistants, wound-care technicians, intensivists, clergy, environmental services, physical therapists, occupational therapists, clinical nutritionists, social workers, case management, psychologists, psychiatrists, respiratory therapists, research coordinators, community outreach educators, child life specialists, and outpatient management services. The primary goal of this extensive team is to return the whole patient to his or her highest level of function, including the physical, psychological, social, and vocational aspects of his or her life. Members of the interprofessional burn team work closely together to ensure an optimal outcome during the emergent phase by focusing on the following priorities. Burn management has traditionally been organized into three phases: the emergent (resuscitative) phase, the intermediate phase, and the rehabilitative phase. Care among the phases is not static, and the nursing and medical priorities in each phase may overlap. Although the rehabilitative phase is listed last, planning for rehabilitation and functional outcome starts immediately upon admission.

Emergent Phase

Medical Management

Although the emergent phase does not officially begin until the patient reaches the hospital, it is vital that basic burn care be initiated at the scene. The initial priorities for emergency personnel on scene include stopping the burn process, airway management, fluid resuscitation, and prevention of hypothermia. Although the receiving registered nurse is given a comprehensive patient report, it is essential that two key pieces of information are provided in the handoff: the circumstances surrounding the injury and the total amount of fluid the patient received during transport. Primary and secondary survey recommendations in the emergent phase are outlined in Box 51.6.

During the emergent phase, the primary goal is to resolve immediate life-threatening issues resulting from the burn injury. These priorities include baseline diagnostic evaluation, airway management, fluid resuscitation, pain management, prevention of hypothermia, and initiation of wound care.

Diagnostic Studies

To determine the patient's baseline condition and identify pre-existing illnesses, basic laboratory studies and radiographical examinations are necessary for all patients with burn injuries. Specific diagnostic studies include complete blood count (CBC), serum glucose, creatinine, blood urea nitrogen (BUN), prothrombin time/activated partial thromboplastin time (PT/aPTT), international normalized ratio (INR), complete metabolic panel (CMP), arterial blood gases (ABGs), ECG, chest x-ray, and a toxicology screen. A serum carboxyhemoglobin level is obtained on all patients with suspected inhalation injuries, and bronchoscopy is indicated for a definitive diagnosis. For electrical injuries, it is important to obtain a baseline ECG and troponin and creatine kinase-MB (CK-MB) levels. Patients with concomitant trauma require additional diagnostic and

Box 51.6 Primary and Secondary Survey of the Burn Patient in the Emergent Phase

Primary Survey Assessment Includes:

Airway and C-spine stabilization
- Maintain a patent airway (may require intubation).
- Consider cervical spine immobilization if warranted.

Breathing
- Provide high-flow 100% oxygen by mask.

Circulation
- Elevate extremities (*no* pillow under head).
- Remove tight jewelry or clothing.
- Neurovascular checks with circumferential burns and electrical burns to extremities

Disability
- Neurological examination

Expose and examine
- Extent and depth of burn wounds and possible associated trauma

Fluid resuscitation
- Insert a minimum of two large-bore peripheral IV lines and start Lactated Ringer's.

Secondary Survey Assessment Includes:

- Circumstances of the injury
  - Cause of burn injury?
  - Exact time of burn injury?
  - Enclosed space?
  - Associated trauma (electrical)?
  - Length of time before rescue?
  - Chemicals involved?
  - Use of accelerant?
- Medical history, current medications, allergies, and vaccinations
- Last food and fluid intake documentation
- Complete "head-to-toe" physical examination
- Determine the extent and depth of burn injury (calculate TBSA percentage)
- Cover the wounds with a clean, dry sheet
- Maintain core body temperature
- Pain medication, IV narcotics preferred
- Tetanus status (considered current if received within the previous 5 years)
- Initial laboratory values/tests: CBC, CMP, PT/aPTT, urinalysis, surveillance cultures
  - ABG and carboxyhemoglobin level for suspected inhalation injury
  - 12-Lead ECG and CK-MB/troponin for electrical injury
- Fluid resuscitation calculation and IV fluid rate adjustment

It is important to note that burn wound care does not begin until the patient is stabilized. The immediate concern is for airway, breathing, and circulation, followed by fluid resuscitation and prevention of hypothermia.

ABG, arterial blood gas; *CBC,* complete blood count; *CMP,* complete metabolic panel; *CK-MB,* creatine kinase-MB; *ECG,* electrocardiogram; *PT/aPTT,* prothrombin time/activated partial thromboplastin time; *TBSA,* total body surface area.

radiographical examinations. Common laboratory findings and electrolyte changes are displayed in Table 51.4.

Airway Maintenance

The assessment of the patient's airway takes top priority. A nonrebreather mask is placed on all patients with burn injuries, and 100% oxygen is administered. Patients at risk for intubation include those with facial burns, changes in voice (such as hoarseness), carbon noted in the sputum, and with injury associated with a fire in an enclosed space. If intubation is warranted, the most experienced person performs the procedure, and special care is taken to secure the endotracheal tube, especially if facial burns are present. It is essential to secure the patient's endotracheal tube with umbilical twill or commercially prepared endotracheal tube holders and not adhesive tape because tape does not stick to the burned face and does not allow for swelling.

Fluid Resuscitation

Fluid resuscitation is crucial to the survival of the patient who has suffered a burn of 20% TBSA or greater. The overall objective is to maintain tissue perfusion and organ function while at the same time avoiding potential complications of inadequate or excessive fluid resuscitation. It is important to note that insufficient fluid resuscitation can lead to organ failure and death, and excessive amounts of fluid can also cause morbidity and mortality. Intravenous resuscitation is initiated in adults at 20% TBSA, and if

Table 51.4 Fluid and Electrolyte Changes in the Emergent Phase

Clinical Findings	Explanation
Generalized dehydration	Plasma leaks through damaged capillaries (third spacing) and into interstitial spaces.
Reduction in blood volume	Secondary to third spacing, blood pressure falls, and cardiac output is diminished.
Decreased urinary output	Secondary to fluid loss and decreased renal blood flow
Hyperkalemia	Massive cellular trauma causes the release of potassium into extracellular fluid.
Hyponatremia	Large amounts of sodium are lost to third spacing, wound drainage, and shifting into cells as potassium is released.
Metabolic acidosis	Loss of bicarbonate ions accompanies the loss of sodium.
Elevated hematocrit	Plasma is lost to extravascular spaces, leaving the remaining blood very viscous.

possible, it is recommended to consult with a burn center prior to the initiation of resuscitation. The fluid of choice for resuscitation is lactated Ringer's. Intravenous access is essential and should be obtained as soon as possible. Ideally, two large-bore, preferably No. 20 gauge or larger, peripheral IV catheters are placed through unburned skin. However, if no such areas exist, the IV lines can be inserted through burned tissue but must be well secured. If obtaining a peripheral IV catheter is extremely difficult, an intraosseous line is also acceptable. Major burn injuries often require the placement of a central venous catheter because of the large volumes of fluid that need to be administered during the emergent phase.

There are numerous resuscitation calculations and/or formulas available for burn resuscitation; however, most burn centers throughout the United States follow Advanced Burn Life Support (ABLS) guidelines. These guidelines are based on the patient's age, weight in kilograms (kg), %TBSA burned, and whether electrical injury was involved. the guidelines require 2 to 4 mL of lactated Ringer's per kilogram of body weight multiplied by %TBSA burned. Half of the total volume is given in the first 8 hours postburn, and the remaining half is given over the next 16 hours. It is important to note that the resuscitation begins from the time the burn injury occurred. For example, if emergency services personnel (EMS) were unable to obtain an IV line on the scene and the patient arrives at the emergency department 2 hours post-injury, fluid volume should be adjusted, and the initial 8-hour volume now must be infused over 6 hours. For adults and children age 15 or greater, fluid resuscitation should be initiated at 2 mL per kilogram; for children age 14 or younger, including infants, resuscitation should be initiated at 3 mL per kilogram; and for electrical injuries in *all* ages, resuscitation should be initiated at 4 mL per kilogram. An example calculation of the fluid-resuscitation formula is provided in Box 51.7. Some providers choose to introduce the use of colloids prior to the 24-hour

resuscitation mark or after the 24-hour mark. This decision is often based on patient response to resuscitation and laboratory values. Examples of colloids given include albumin or plasma.

During fluid resuscitation, an indwelling urinary drainage catheter is placed in the bladder to closely monitor urine output because this is the most reliable indicator of adequate fluid resuscitation. Urine output should be maintained at 0.5 mL/kg/hr. If myoglobin is present in the urine, output should be maintained at 1 mL/kg/hr until clearing of the urine occurs to prevent the development of acute renal failure. Diuretics are not indicated during the emergent phase, and if urine output drops, the rate of fluid administration is increased. Other parameters that are monitored (as listed in Table 51.5) during fluid resuscitation include heart rate, blood pressure, central venous pressure, serum chemistries, hemoglobin, and hematocrit.

The calculated fluid volume is the starting point in the fluctuating fluid-resuscitation process. Patients with inhalation injuries, electrical injuries, associated trauma, and/or alcohol and drug dependencies may require higher volumes of fluids related to pre-existing medical conditions or poor health. If there is a delay in starting fluid resuscitation, patients usually require higher volumes of fluid. It is also important to note that some patient populations, such as older adults, children, and those with pre-existing cardiac disease, may be very sensitive to fluid and should be closely monitored for signs of fluid volume overload. Inadequate fluid resuscitation, which results in inadequate blood flow, may also result in conversion of the burn wound within the first 24 to 72 hours, as shown in Figure 51.10.

Box 51.7 Fluid-Resuscitation Example

Patient weight: 70 kg
TBSA burned: 50% flame burn

The patient is a young healthy adult with no pertinent past medical history.

Resuscitation Calculation:

2 mL × 70 × 50 = 7,000 mL of lactated Ringer's in the first 24 hours

First 8 hours: 3,500 mL, rate = 438 mL/hr

Calculate from time of injury.

Next 16 hours: 3,500 mL, rate = 218 mL/hr

TBSA, Total body surface area.

Table 51.5 Indications of Adequate Fluid Resuscitation

Urine output	0.5 mL/kg/hr
	1 mL/kg/hr if myoglobin present
Systolic blood pressure	Greater than 100 mm Hg
Heart rate	Less than 120 bpm
Central venous pressure (CVP)	5–10 mm Hg
Pulmonary	Lungs sound clear, blood pH within normal range (7.35–7.45)
Gastrointestinal	Abdomen soft, non-tender; no nausea, vomiting, or ileus; bladder pressure less than 10 mm Hg
Level of consciousness	Clear; alert; and oriented to person, place, and time (keep in mind any narcotics that may have been administered for pain)

Connection Check 51.6

Using the resuscitation guidelines, the nurse determines that a patient requires a total of 12 L of fluid in the first 24 hours post-injury. How much of the total volume needs to be given within the first 8 hours?
A. 4,000 mL lactated Ringer's
B. 6,000 mL lactated Ringer's
C. 8,000 mL lactated Ringer's
D. 10,000 mL lactated Ringer's

Connection Check 51.7

When hemodynamic status is monitored in a patient with a burn injury, what amount of urine output indicates adequate fluid resuscitation?
A. 0.5 mL/kg/hr
B. 1 mL/kg/hr
C. 2 mL/kg/hr
D. 3 mL/kg/hr

Prevention of Hypothermia

Hypothermia is commonly seen in patients with burns because the skin, their primary insulation, is no longer intact. It is imperative to keep the patient covered at all times and to closely monitor his or her temperature, especially in the emergency department, where patients are typically exposed for assessments. The ambient room temperature is usually increased to decrease heat loss in patients with significant burn injuries.

Wound Care

Typically, the burn wound is not the first priority during the emergent resuscitative phase because more life-threatening issues often take precedence. Although the burn wound is covered with clean, dry blankets to prevent hypothermia, the initiation of wound care may be delayed for several hours until the patient is stabilized because there are more life-threatening concerns for the patient at this point.

Pain Management

A burn is one of the most painful injuries an individual can sustain. Intravenous narcotics, such as morphine sulfate (morphine), are used for the initial management of pain. The intramuscular route of administration is avoided because there may be impaired medication absorption due to an edema formation and decreased peripheral perfusion. Pain medication is administered intravenously in doses no larger than those needed to manage pain. The nurse monitors closely for signs of respiratory depression when giving large doses of pain medication. Although morphine sulfate (morphine) is commonly used, other types of narcotics may also be used, including fentanyl (Sublimaze) and hydromorphone (Dilaudid).

Connection Check 51.8

The nurse recognizes which diagnostic test as most sensitive in a patient with a suspected electrical burn injury?
A. Arterial blood gas
B. CK-MB levels
C. Echocardiogram
D. Serum carboxyhemoglobin

Connection Check 51.9

Which intervention is the priority for the patient during the emergent phase of burn management?
A. Application of silver sulfadiazine cream
B. Use of clean, dry sheets and warm blankets
C. Initiation of wet normal saline dressings
D. Maintaining the injured area open to air

Medications

In addition to pain management, patients with burn injuries are given a variety of other pharmacological therapies. Medications are given to treat common concerns or potential complications facing the burn patient, including anticoagulation therapy, nutritional support, gastrointestinal motility, anxiety, and depression. See Table 51.6 for a listing of medications commonly used in patients with burn injuries.

Nursing Management
Assessment and Analysis

During the emergent phase, the priority assessments focus on immediate life-threatening injuries, including airway management, particularly with suspected inhalation injury; fluid volume status; temperature control; and pain management. Clinical manifestations during this phase may include:

- Facial burns
- Naso- or oropharynx erythema
- Hoarseness, grunting
- Carbonaceous (soot) sputum
- Dyspnea
- Wheezing
- Tachypnea
- Intercoastal retractions and flaring nostrils
- Elevated carboxyhemoglobin levels
- Tachycardia
- Hypotension
- Confusion, agitation, changes in level of consciousness
- Decreased urine output
- Hypothermia
- Headache
- Complaints of pain

Nursing Diagnoses

- **Ineffective airway clearance** related to airway edema secondary to injury from heat and/or chemicals

Table 51.6 Medications in Burn Care

Medication Type and Name	Medication Purpose
Analgesia	Pain management
Morphine sulfate (morphine)	
Hydromorphone (Dilaudid)	
Fentanyl (Sublimaze)	
Ketamine (Ketalar)	
Oxycodone (OxyContin, Tylox)	
Methadone (Dolophine)	
Nonsteroidal anti-inflammatory medications (ibuprofen or naproxen sodium)	
Sedation	Induce sedation and decrease anxiety
Haloperidol (Haldol)	Antipsychotic and sedative effects
Lorazepam (Ativan)	Helps reduce anxiety
Diazepam (Valium)	Helps reduce anxiety and treat alcohol withdrawal
Midazolam (Versed)	Short-acting amnesic effects
Propofol (Diprivan)	Short-acting hypnotic agent
Dexmedetomidine hydrochloride (Precedex)	Initial sedation in mechanically ventilated patients
Anticoagulation Therapy	Both promote venous return and decrease risk for thromboembolism
Enoxaparin (Lovenox)	
Heparin	
Nutritional Support	Provide essential nutrients
Multivitamins	Promote wound healing
Zinc sulfate (zinc) and ferrous sulfate (iron)	Promote hemoglobin formation and cell integrity
Oxandrolone (Oxandrin)	Preservation of lean body mass and promotion of weight gain
Gastrointestinal Support	Promote gastrointestinal function
Ranitidine (Zantac)	Decreases stomach acid and risk of ulceration
Esomeprazole (Nexium)	Decreases stomach acid and risk of ulceration
Pantoprazole (Protonix)	Decreases stomach acid and risk of ulceration
Aluminum/Magnesium antacid (Mylanta, Maalox)	Neutralizes stomach acid
Nystatin (Mycostatin)	Prevents overgrowth of yeast in oral mucosa
Metoclopramide (Reglan)	Promotes stomach emptying and decreases nausea
Polyethylene glycol 3350 (MiraLAX) Docusate sodium (Senokot)	Laxative agents for use in constipation

- **Impaired gas exchange** related to carbon monoxide poisoning, smoke inhalation, and upper or lower airway obstruction
- **Risk for fluid volume deficit** related to hypovolemia due to third spacing of fluids and inadequate fluid resuscitation

- **Altered tissue perfusion** related to decreased cardiac output
- **Risk for hypothermia** due to altered skin integrity
- **Risk for infection** due to loss of skin's protection and the burn injury

- **Acute pain** secondary to the burn injury
- **Anxiety** related to fear surrounding the burn injury

Nursing Interventions

■ *Assessments*

- Breath sounds, respiratory rate, and indicators of inhalation injury
  Edema and irritation of the airway may develop secondary to damage caused by heat and chemical irritants as evidenced by hypoxemia, rhonchi, stridor, change in voice (hoarseness), and/or dyspnea. Inhalation injuries may impair respiratory function, leading to decreased ventilation and changes in rate and effort, resulting in lower oxygenation.
- Oxygen saturation, ABGs, and carboxyhemoglobin levels
  The oxygen molecules may be saturated by carbon monoxide instead of oxygen, which is evident only through measurement of carboxyhemoglobin levels. Carbon monoxide binds to the hemoglobin molecule with an affinity 200 times greater than that of oxygen; tissue hypoxia results when carbon monoxide levels are above normal. Results of ABGs also provide information related to the acid-base status of the patient.
- Face and neck for burns, singed nasal and/or facial hair, and singed eyebrows/eyelashes
  Edema and irritation of the airway may develop secondary to damage caused by heat and chemical irritants as evidenced by hypoxemia, rhonchi, stridor, change in voice (hoarseness), and/or dyspnea.
- Upper airway
  Damage and irritation caused by the heat and chemical irritants in smoke may cause the airway to appear red and edematous. The mouth and/or airway may also appear black because of soot.
- Changes in voice, hoarseness, and swallowing difficulty
  Damage for the heat and chemical irritants in smoke may cause edema and irritation, resulting in changes in the voice, hoarseness, and/or difficulty swallowing.
- Vital signs
  Blood pressure may be low and pulse elevated secondary to potential hypovolemia due to significant fluid losses and shifts. The pulse may also be elevated secondary to increased work of breathing with inhalation injuries, pain, and fear/anxiety. Because of impaired skin integrity, temperature may be decreased. Patient shivering further accelerates the patient's metabolic rate and may exacerbate tachycardia.
- Urine output
  Indicators of inadequate resuscitation and development of hypovolemia may be evidenced by urine output less than 0.5 mL/kg/hr.
- Pain
  Pain will be noted in areas of partial-thickness burns because nerve endings are exposed.
- Anxiety
  Patient anxiety levels may be high because of the appearance of the burn wound and exposure to trauma.

- Burn wound size and depth
  Although wound treatment is not a priority in this phase, estimations of %TBSA burned and wound depth are required to determine fluid resuscitation.

■ *Actions*

- Place patient on 100% humidified oxygen or assist with intubation if necessary.
  Immediate intervention is necessary for respiratory distress and to provide humidified oxygen and assist in the clearing of carbon monoxide. The half-life of carbon monoxide while on 100% oxygen is 30 minutes to 1 hour compared with 4 hours breathing room air.
- Trend ABG values and carboxyhemoglobin levels.
  Increasing $PaCO_2$ and decreasing PaO_2 and oxygen saturation may indicate the need for intubation. As carboxyhemoglobin levels lower, weaning of oxygen support (FiO_2) to a minimal level to sustain oxygenation is indicated.
- Elevate the head of the bed to allow for better oxygenation.
  Raising the head of the bed decreases the work of breathing by lowering the diaphragm.
- Maintain emergency airway (intubation and tracheostomy) trays at the bedside.
  Inflammation and edema secondary to airway injury may make endotracheal intubation difficult or impossible. In patients with an endotracheal tube in place, a tracheostomy tray should be maintained at the bedside in the event of an unplanned extubation.
- Assist with intubation as necessary.
  Delaying intubation may result in edema and possible airway obstruction.
- Ensure securement of the endotracheal tube if the patient is intubated.
  If the tube is dislodged, it may be impossible to reinsert due to the edema. In addition, the securement device will require adjustment (e.g., twill) as the edema continues to worsen/decrease.
- Monitor mechanically ventilated patients closely for signs of respiratory compromise.
  Close monitoring of mechanically ventilated patients allows for early detection of respiratory distress.
- Place two large-bore IV catheters and begin fluid resuscitation with lactated Ringer's.
  Adequate fluids are necessary to prevent hypovolemic shock from developing as a result of massive fluid loss and fluid shifts. Lactated Ringer's is an isotonic fluid that supports intravascular volume.
- Roughly estimate the %TBSA burned and patient weight in kilograms.
  A quick estimation of the %TBSA burned and patient weight guides the determination of fluid to be administered in the first 24 hours on the basis of the resuscitation formula.
- Cover wounds with a clean, dry sheet.
  Minimizes evaporative heat loss and decreases the risk of hypothermia

- Institute warming measures in the form of blankets or other external heat sources.
  Minimizes evaporative heat loss and prevents the development of hypothermia

■ *Teaching*

- Immediately report difficulty breathing and/or swallowing.
  Respiratory distress may develop quickly or may be delayed in patients with an inhalation injury.
- Instruct patient to cough and deep breathe every hour.
  Assists in clearing airway and mobilizing secretions
- Signs of inhalation injury
  Because the signs of inhalation injury may be insidious, it is important that the patient and family be able to recognize early signs of compromised airway and breathing difficulties.
- Explain all procedures to the patient and family in clear and simple terms.
  Understanding helps alleviate fear and anxiety in the patient, which may result in tachycardia and hypertension.
- Importance of maintaining a warm environment
  Decreases risk of heat loss and development of hypothermia
- Risk factors that increase chances of infection
  Because of loss of skin integrity, the patient is at increased risk of infection, so family members must follow instructions regarding gloves, gowns, and hand washing.

Evaluating Care Outcomes

At the end of the emergent phase, the anticipated outcomes include the absence of respiratory distress, appropriate fluid resuscitation manifested by stable vital signs and adequate urine output, temperature regulation, and effective pain management. In the event of inhalation injuries, stabilization of the airway and sufficient oxygenation are positive outcomes during this emergent phase. The nurse anticipates adequate urine output with an expected outcome of 0.5 mL/kg/hr, with the recognition that any decrease in urine output below the recommended level must be immediately reported to the provider. Because patients with burns lose the ability to effectively manage their temperature, the nurse anticipates normothermia with appropriate interventions. Adequate pain management and lessened anxiety are also expected outcomes of management during the emergent phase.

Intermediate Phase

Medical Management

The burn patient enters into the intermediate phase after resuscitation and stabilization have been achieved. This phase usually begins 48 to 72 hours after the initial burn injury. Within the intermediate phase, the management priorities shift to wound healing and closure, pain management, ensuring optimal nutrition, and continued prevention of infection. Although the focus moves away from the life-threatening priorities of the emergent phase, continued assessment and management of respiratory and circulatory status are essential during the intermediate phase.

Wound Care

Hydrotherapy

Wound-healing practices vary greatly among facilities and burn centers. **Hydrotherapy** is the favored cleansing method within most burn centers because it allows for thorough wound cleansing and uses water during dressing changes to assist in the removal of residual topical agents and necrotic tissue. In the past, hydrotherapy involved total immersion into a tank or tub of water. More recently, burn centers have begun using portable shower trolleys covered with disposable plastic liners to help prevent the spread of infection and cross-contamination. For patients who cannot tolerate extensive hydrotherapy, burn wound care may be done at the bedside.

Clean Technique and Infection Control

It is important to note that burn wound care is a clean, not a sterile, procedure. Sterile technique involves employing techniques to reduce exposure to microorganisms, such as using a sterile field and sterile instruments and gloves. Clean technique involves using techniques to reduce the overall number of microorganisms, such as preparing a clean field and using clean gloves and instruments. Burn wound care is extensive, physically exhausting, and time-consuming, with some dressing changes lasting up to 2 to 4 hours. Often, these dressing changes occur in patient rooms where the temperature is usually set as high as 90°F (32.2°C) to prevent the risk of hypothermia.

During every dressing change, it is essential that both the nurse and physician assess the burn wound for progression of healing and evidence of infection. The dressing change is also the ideal time for the physical and occupational therapists to assess the wound, as well as to observe the patient's function and range of motion.

Topical Medicines and Wound Dressings

There are numerous variations of topical medications and wound dressings that are used on burn wounds. The choice of the agent and dressing depends on wound depth, location of the injury, presence of infection, and provider preference. The most commonly used topical medications and dressings for wound management are outlined in Table 51.7, and a common application is displayed in Figure 51.19. Special care is taken when wrapping fingers and toes because they must be dressed individually to prevent *webbing* (the growing together of the skin between the fingers and toes) and maintain full range of motion (Fig. 51.20).

Mechanical and Enzymatic Debridement

The preferred method of wound cleansing involves the use of a mild soap or chlorhexidine and water along with gentle debridement of the burn wound (Fig. 51.21). The three kinds of debridement are mechanical, enzymatic, and surgical. While cleansing, removal of the loose tissue is important to allow for proper visualization of the burn wound and is

Table 51.7 Topical Medications and Wound Dressings

Antimicrobial Agent	Effective Against	Wound Indication	Application	Benefits	Disadvantages	Nursing Considerations
Silver sulfadiazine (Silvadene)	Broad-spectrum and *Candida* coverage	Partial- and full-thickness burn wounds	1/4-in.-thick application with roll gauze to cover; dressing changes every 12 hours	Cooling effect when applied; easy, painless application	May cause transient leukopenia; may also cause a wound film on partial-thickness burns, making it hard to assess healing	Avoid in patients with a documented sulfa allergy. Avoid application to face.
Bacitracin	No gram-negative or fungal coverage	Partial-thickness burn wounds and grafts	Thin layer applied with a nonadherent gauze and an outer roll gauze; dressing changes every 24 hours	Easy, painless application; only once-per-day dressing change	Not as effective on full-thickness burn wounds because of minimal penetration of eschar	Best choice for use on a face, but left open to air. Use bacitracin ophthalmic ointment near and around eyes.
Mafenide acetate 10% cream or 5% solution (Sulfamylon Cream or Slurry)	Broad-spectrum, effective against *Pseudomonas* but has little anti-fungal coverage	Cream used on full-thickness burns to ears only; solution used on partial-thickness burn wounds and grafts	Cream is applied 1/16 in. thick and left open to air. Solution is applied to nonadherent gauze and roll gauze. Cream is changed every 12 hours; solution dressings are changed every 24 hours and may be wet down at 12 hours.	Cream penetrates eschar. Solution is only a once-per-day dressing change.	Solution is a wet-type dressing and may not be used on initial large burn wounds because it may cause hypothermia.	Some patients may complain of stinging upon application to partial-thickness burn wounds. Frequent sensitivities noted.
Silver sheeting products (Acticoat, Silverlon, Mepilex)	Broad-spectrum, effective against MRSA and fungus	Partial-thickness burn wounds, Stevens–Johnson syndrome (SJS), and patients with toxic	Some products are a wet application with sterile water and roll gauze. Dressing changes every	Dressing needs to be changed only every 4–7 days.	Expensive. Burn wounds often need to be observed daily. Solution is a wet-type dressing and may not be used on initial large burn	This is best used in the patient with SJS/TEN as the dressing change process is extremely painful and wounds do not need to be

Table 51.7 Topical Medications and Wound Dressings—cont'd

Antimicrobial Agent	Effective Against	Wound Indication	Application	Benefits	Disadvantages	Nursing Considerations
		epidermal necrolysis (TEN), donor sites	3–7 days; wet down with sterile water every 12 hours. Some products are applied dry and not wet down.		wounds because it may cause hypothermia.	observed daily. May also be of good use in the outpatient setting. Some patients may complain of stinging upon application. Do not use with normal saline because it will deactivate silver.
Enzymatic cream (collagenase)	No antimicrobial effects and thus is often mixed with other ointments and/or creams	Full-thickness burn wounds (specifically digests collagen in necrotic tissue without harming intact tissue)	Thin layer applied with a nonadherent gauze and an outer roll gauze; dressing changes every 24 hours	Easy, painless application; only once-per-day dressing change; may help penetrate and soften eschar for debridement		Considered for use in patients with full-thickness burn wounds who are not candidates for the operating room because of age or medical condition; also considered for use in very small areas of full-thickness burns in an attempt to heal without surgery.

MRSA, Methicillin-resistant *Staphylococcus aureus*.

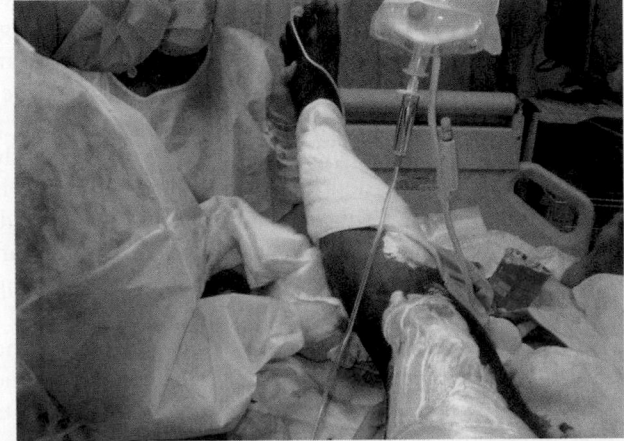

FIGURE 51.19 Silver sulfadiazine and roll gauze.

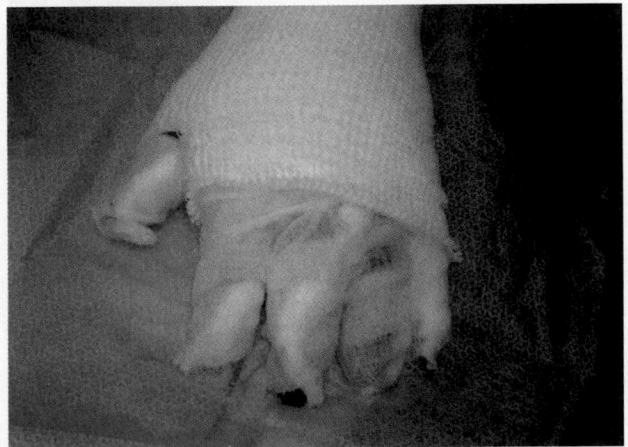

FIGURE 51.20 Dressing applied to hand. Note that each finger is wrapped loosely and individually.

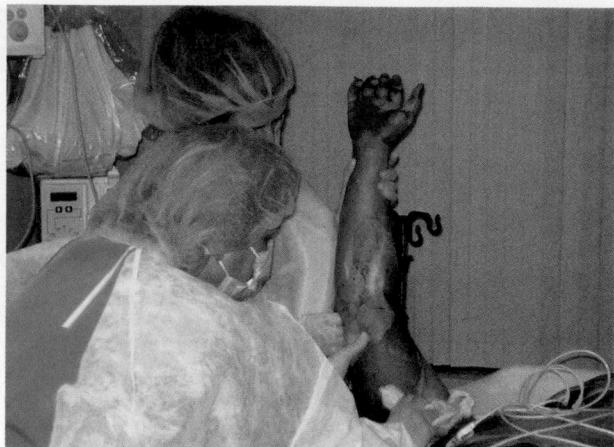

FIGURE 51.21 Wound cleansing with normal saline and chlorohexidine solution and roll gauze.

accomplished through the use of tweezers and scissors and is often aided by the removal of gauze dressings and hydrotherapy. An example of a partial-thickness wound pre- and post-debridement is shown in Figure 51.22. Enzymatic debridement involves the application of a proteolytic ointment that hastens eschar separation and wound healing. Enzymatic debridement is often reserved for patients with

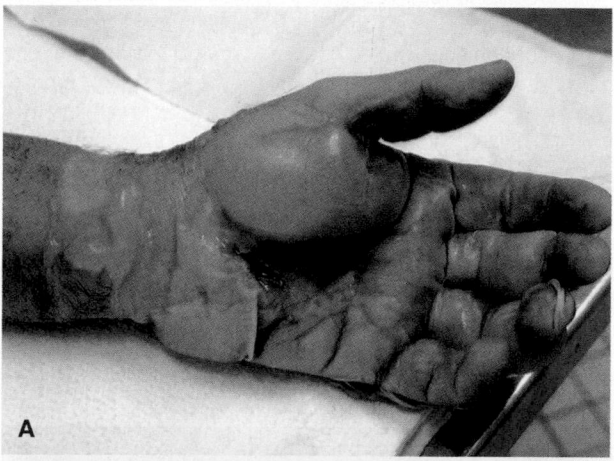

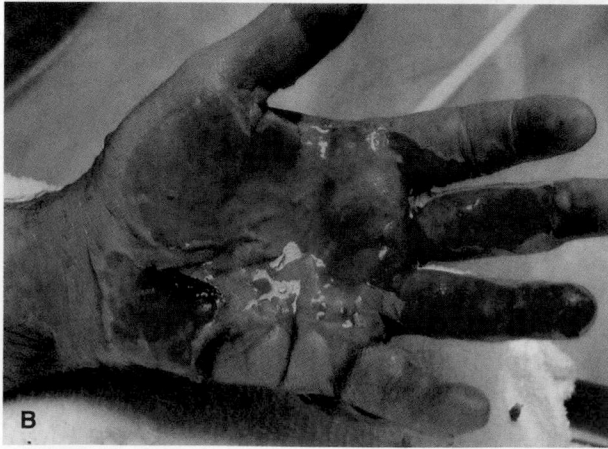

FIGURE 51.22 Wound debridement of a partial-thickness burn. A, Pre-debridement. B, Post-debridement.

deep partial-thickness wounds where signs of healing are evident. This type of debridement is also considered in patients with full-thickness burns who may not be candidates for surgery. If mechanical and enzymatic debridement are not effective, surgical debridement is necessary.

Surgical Debridement and Wound Closure

Early excision and grafting of burns decrease the length of hospital stay and greatly increases the survival rates of these patients. **Burn excision** is considered as soon as the patient is hemodynamically stable and able to tolerate the procedure. It is not uncommon for the patient with a large full-thickness burn to be taken to the operating room for excision and grafting within 24 to 48 hours of admission. Types of skin substitutes and grafts are described in Table 51.8.

The ideal replacement for lost skin is **autograft** because it is the patient's own skin and will not be rejected by the body. The epidermis and a partial layer of the dermis (**split-thickness skin grafts**) are harvested from an unburned area, known as the **donor site**. The most common donor site is the thigh because of the ability to obtain a continuous donor sheet of skin. However, in patients with large burns, any site on the body may be utilized, including the scalp and scrotum if necessary. Once healed, donor sites may be re-harvested numerous times. These split-thickness skin grafts are then applied to the excised wound in the form of a sheet or **meshed graft**. **Sheet grafts** are often utilized on exposed areas of the body, such as the face and hands, because they give a more seamless and cosmetic appearance due to the fact that the grafts are not meshed. Skin grafts are meshed (have holes placed in them that allow for expansion) when unburned skin is in short supply in order to provide maximal wound coverage and closure. A mesh expansion ratio of 1:2 upward to 1:4 is commonly utilized. Examples of meshed and sheet autografts are presented in Figure 51.23. In some instances, the burn surgeon may choose to apply a small full-thickness skin graft to allow for the best function in certain anatomical areas, such as the eyelids.

In extensive burns where there is not enough unburned tissue to harvest, **allograft** (cadaver skin) is often utilized. With the placement of allograft as a temporary covering, there is decreased evaporative loss of heat and better pain control for the patient, and it provides a barrier against bacterial growth. Allograft, as seen in Figure 51.24, is only a temporary covering and is eventually rejected by the body and is replaced by the patient's own skin. When allograft is not available, **xenograft** (pig skin) may also be considered. In some developing countries where allograft and xenograft are not readily available, things such as fish skin are being sterilized and used for temporary burn wound coverage.

Another alternative to consider with massive burns is the use of **cultured epithelial autograft (CEA)**. This technique is considered only in the most severely burned patients where there is no other alternative because the patient remains very vulnerable to infection, and the CEA skin is extremely fragile. Cultured epithelial autograft involves a biopsy taken from an area of unburned skin and then sent

Table 51.8 Types of Skin Substitutes and Grafts

Graft	Source	Coverage	Benefits	Drawbacks
Autograft	Patient's own unburned skin May be meshed to cover larger areas or placed as a sheet on faces and hands for a smoother, more cosmetic appearance	Permanent	This is the ideal coverage for all patients' burns and has the highest chance of wound closure.	May be delicate if meshed widely before application. Staple removal may be tedious.
Cultured epithelial autograft (CEA)	Patient's own skin sample is sent to a laboratory, where the epidermis is grown in larger patches.	Permanent	Is a good choice in patients with large burns of 70% or more TBSA burn who do not have enough unburned skin to use as donor for autografting	Is extremely expensive, very fragile, and susceptible to infection once applied. Dermal layer will never regenerate.
Integra (artificial skin)	Two-layer man-made silicone membrane used to replace dermis and is covered with autograft	Permanent	May provide a functional dermis and better chance of wound closure	High risk for infection of the Integra and subsequent graft loss
Allograft	Cadaver skin	Temporary	Used as a temporary covering once eschar is removed to help close and protect wound	Will eventually reject and have to be replaced by permanent grafting
Xenograft	Pig (most common) or bovine (cow) skin	Temporary	Used as a temporary covering once eschar is removed to help close and protect wound	Will eventually reject and have to be replaced by permanent grafting

TBSA, Total body surface area.

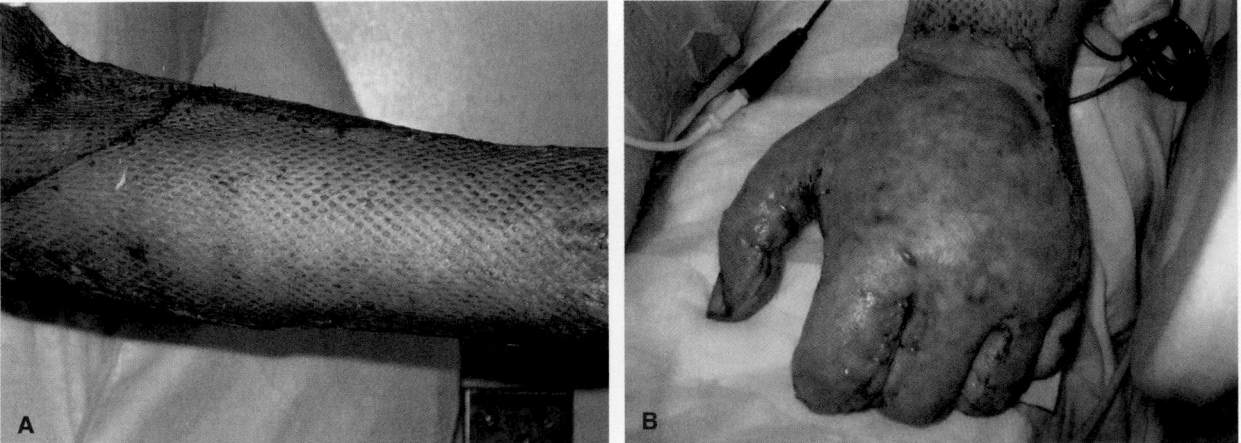

FIGURE 51.23 Autograft. A, Meshed autograft to the forearm. B, Sheet autograft to the hand/fingers.

to a laboratory where, over a 2-week period, epithelial cells are grown in the laboratory and attached to petroleum-impregnated gauze. Excision of the burn wound is not delayed while waiting for the CEA, and ideally, the wound is excised, and an allograft is placed as a temporary covering. Cultured epithelial autograft is extremely delicate because it involves the growth of only the epidermal layer. After the placement of the CEA, the patient is often placed in traction, which allows elevation of extremities and pressure relief. These patients then require extensive one-on-one nursing care that focuses on time-consuming wound healing and infection control. It is for this reason that CEA is utilized only in burn centers. Examples of CEA are shown in Figure 51.25.

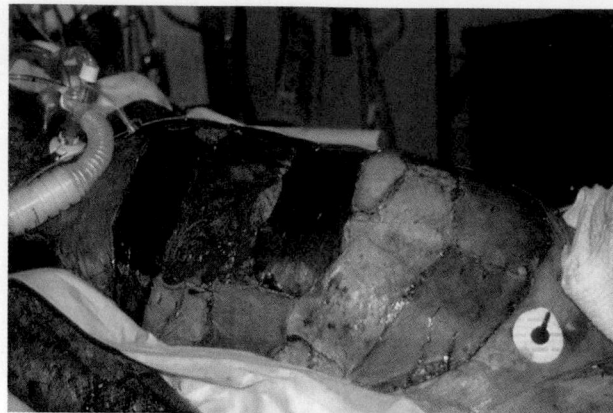

FIGURE 51.24 Allograft.

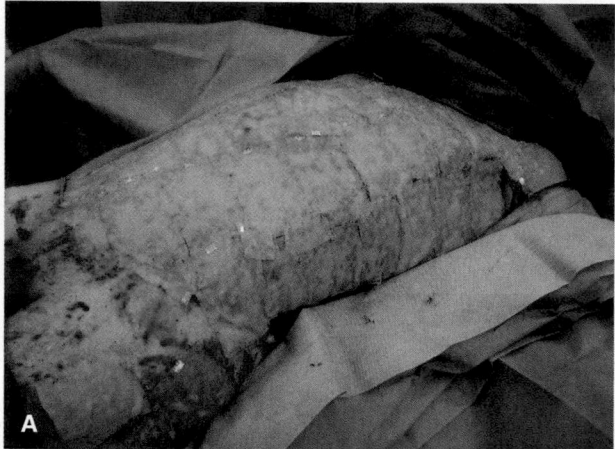

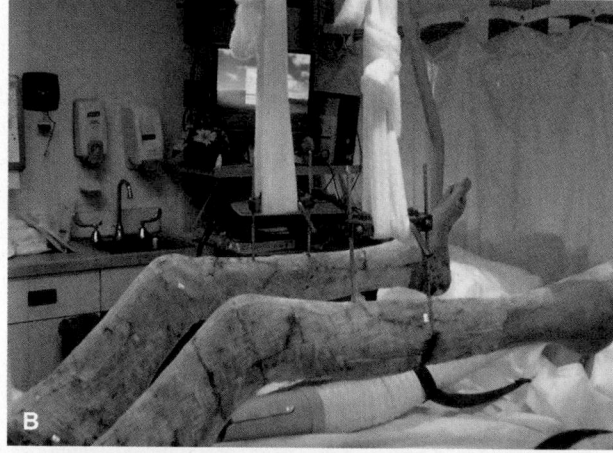

FIGURE 51.25 Cultured epithelial autograft (CEA). A, CEA to abdomen. B, CEA to lower extremities that are placed in traction.

CASE STUDY: EPISODE 2

It has been determined that Joe Smith's wounds are full thickness. Current wound management includes silver sulfadiazine cream twice a day. The surgeon has determined that the patient requires surgery. Medical and nursing priorities continue to focus on pain management and infection prevention...

Pain Management

Burn pain continues to be managed aggressively throughout the emergent phase and well into the intermediate and even rehabilitative phases. The multifaceted pain experienced by the burn patient includes background, procedural, and breakthrough pain. *Background pain* is the underlying pain from the primary injury that is continuous and ongoing. *Breakthrough pain* is pain related to specific episodes associated with activities of daily living (ADLs), such as walking. *Procedural pain* is associated with therapeutic activities such as wound care and physical therapy. Inadequate and inconsistent management of pain is well documented in the burn literature, and pain is whatever the burn patient says it is. Although the pain is aggressively managed and patient comfort is a priority, the patient needs to actively participate in the plan of care and particularly in the rehabilitation process. Because of the large doses of pain medication that are administered, the patient is optimally treated at a burn center, where his or her pain can be effectively managed by the interprofessional team.

The pain management plan of care is individualized and includes both pharmacological and nonpharmacological methods of pain management. Recommended IV narcotics, usually used during dressing changes, include morphine sulfate (morphine), fentanyl (Sublimaze), ketamine, and/or hydromorphone (Dilaudid). Intravenous narcotics are continued while the pain is severe and unrelenting; however, all efforts are made to transition to oral pain medications as soon as tolerated. It is important to differentiate between pain and anxiety because they are treated differently. In addition to pain management, patients are often given anxiolytics for anxiety related to wound-care procedures, appearance changes, and fear. However, these medications are indicated only once the pain is under control. In addition, pain medication is given on a scheduled basis instead of on an as-needed (prn) basis because this helps to better manage the pain over time and hopefully prevents it from becoming intolerable.

> **!** **Safety Alert** When giving large doses of IV pain medication, especially during dressing changes, ensure that proper ventilatory support and emergency equipment are immediately available.

Nutritional Support

Nutrition plays a significant role in the outcomes of the patient with major burn injuries. Large burn injuries place the patient in a prolonged hypermetabolic and catabolic state, resulting in an increased caloric need to assist in wound healing. Early enteral nutrition is associated with a reduction in ileus and stress ulcers because it reduces the inflammatory mediators released by the body. Once a person has sustained a burn of approximately 20% or greater, it is difficult to consume the amount of calories and protein needed for wound healing, and nutritional supplementation is often required because of the fact that his or her metabolic rate is greatly increased as a result of the burn injury. Nutritional supplementation is most often achieved through the placement of a nasogastric tube, where feedings can be given continuously or intermittently in the form of a bolus. In large burn injuries, longer nutritional support is required, and the placement of a duodenal feeding tube is often recommended to help prevent aspiration and allow for feeding up to and during procedures. Supplemental vitamins and minerals are also often administered to promote wound healing. Total parenteral nutrition is not often utilized among patients with burns because of its complication rates, including an increased risk for infection and hyperglycemia.

Prevention of Infection

Prevention of infection after burn injury is challenging. The most common cause of death after the emergent phase is infection resulting in sepsis and multisystem organ failure because these patients have lost the largest protective barrier, the skin. Infection control practices vary widely among burn units, and prevention and outbreak control represent major challenges. Prophylactic antibiotics are not recommended because of the potential of breeding antibiotic-resistant pathogens, and instead, treatment is based on positive culture results. Cross-contamination among patients with burn injuries is common, and as a result, isolation guidelines are widespread practices among burn centers. Proper hand-washing technique continues to be one of the most effective methods of preventing the spread of infection. Some burn centers require the use of contact precautions when entering all patient rooms. Regardless of the type of infection control method employed, it is essential that all members of the healthcare team, as well as family and visitors, are knowledgeable about and adhere to all standards.

Connection Check 51.10

The nurse anticipates supplementary feeding via a nasogastric tube in a patient for which reasons? *(Select all that apply.)*

A. Hypermetabolic state.
B. Multiple open wounds.
C. Increased heat loss.
D. Increased caloric needs.
E. Burn greater than 20% TBSA.

Nursing Management
Assessment and Analysis

As the patient progresses into the intermediate phase after successful resuscitation, the priorities expand to wound management and infection control. The patient continues to require close observation of respiratory status and hemodynamic stability. The nurse monitors for the following

additional clinical manifestations during the intermediate phase:

- Wound color and consistency
- Wound drainage
- Eschar
- Responses to therapeutic interventions
- Graft sites
- Pain
- Weight
- Serum total protein and albumin
- Infection

Nursing Diagnoses

- **Risk for infection** related to impaired immune response and loss of skin integrity
- **Altered nutrition less than body requirements** related to hypermetabolism and burn injury
- **Acute pain** related to exposure of nerve endings in wound bed and wound-care procedures
- **Anxiety** related to painful wound-care procedures
- **Self-care deficit** related to impaired mobility due to the burn injury
- **Powerlessness** related to hospitalization and inability to care for self

Nursing Interventions
■ *Assessments*

- Vital signs
  An elevated heart rate may be secondary to sustained hypovolemia, as well as pain and anxiety. Respiratory rate and blood pressure may also be elevated secondary to pain and anxiety. Temperature may be elevated with an infection. The patient also needs to be assessed for hypothermia, particularly with large burns that can lead to increased loss of heat through the open wounds.
- Daily weight
  Increased metabolic rate may result in weight loss.
- Daily caloric intake
  Increased metabolic rate results in an increased caloric need to assist in wound healing.
- Total protein and albumin levels
  Assessment of nutritional status includes monitoring total protein and albumin levels. Normal serum total protein is 6 to 8 g/dL, and serum albumin is 3.4 to 5.1 g/dL. Adequate albumin also supports oncotic pressure that promotes fluid remaining in the intravascular space.
- White blood cell counts
  Loss of the protective mechanisms due to burn injuries increases the risk of infection, and an elevated white blood count may indicate a wound infection.
- Wounds for signs of healing and clinical manifestations of infection
  If the burn wound is not showing any evidence of healing, surgery may be indicated, or a change in the wound-care regimen may be warranted. With the loss of the skin as a protective barrier, the patient remains at constant risk for infection resulting from the invasion of microorganisms.

- Pain and anxiety
  Pain associated with daily dressing changes places the patient at risk for tachycardia and hypertension.
- Participation in plan of care and ADLs
  It is important for the patient to be actively involved in the plan of care and to understand the rationales for all interventions.

■ Actions

- Time medication administration so that the patient receives the full benefit during wound-care procedures.
  Procedural pain is often the most intense pain associated with a burn injury, and medication must be timed to allow for maximum absorption, as well as to time the most painful procedures during the peak effectiveness times of medications.
- Give pain medication on a scheduled basis instead of on an as-needed (prn) basis.
  Assists in effectively managing pain and allows a steady state to develop within the body; also ideally provides the patient with more consistent pain relief
- Explore the effectiveness of nonpharmacological pain relief techniques, such as music therapy and guided imagery.
  Nonpharmacological techniques have been shown to assist in the reduction of procedural burn pain and anxiety.
- Calorie counts and encouragement of oral intake
  Maintenance of caloric needs is essential in determining whether adequate nutrition is provided for wound healing.
- Wound care
  Daily wound care and assessment are essential for wound healing and the prevention of infection.
- Assist with ADLs and compliance with rehabilitation exercises.
  Even though the patient's injury location may present a challenge, encouragement of self-performance of ADLs and rehabilitation exercises is essential for rehabilitation therapy.

■ Teaching

- Instruct patient to request additional pain medication when needed and not to delay until the pain is intense.
  If pain becomes intolerable, it can be difficult to assist the patient in achieving a tolerable pain level.
- Provide information to patient and family about the natural progression of burn wounds, grafts, and/or donor sites.
  Providing information can help to reduce misconceptions and anxiety related to surgery and recovery.
- Provision of a rehabilitation plan and discussion of the importance of doing ADLs and rehabilitation therapy
  Providing a rehabilitation plan and encouragement of self-performance of ADLs helps prevent complications associated with decreased mobility and provides a sense of self-control.
- Education on the importance of nutrition and provision of a diet plan
  Maintenance of caloric needs is essential for wound healing, performance of daily activities, and the rehabilitation regimen.

Evaluating Care Outcomes

During the intermediate phase, there are several additional priorities for the nurse to focus on, including outcomes related to adequate nutrition, pain management, wound healing, and infection control. Stable body weight and normal albumin and total protein levels are indicative of improving nutritional status. Effective pain management is supported by stable vital signs, as well as the patient reporting adequate comfort. Additionally, the patient is comfortable enough to participate in ADLs and understands the importance of asking for pain medications prior to pain becoming intolerable. The effectiveness of wound management is determined by evidence of the healing of burn injuries as well as no signs of infection. Stable vital signs, including normal heart rate and blood pressure, are consistent with adequate fluid volume status and pain management. Normal temperature and normal white blood cell counts support a lack of infection.

Rehabilitative Phase

Medical Management

The last phase in the burn process is the rehabilitation phase. This stage begins from the time the patient is admitted to the burn center and may last for several years, even extending well beyond discharge. All members of the interprofessional team are essential during this phase; however, rehabilitative and psychological support are of primary importance.

Not only is a burn injury physically painful, but dealing with the long-term emotional consequences is also often difficult. The patient with a burn injury may endure many psychological and emotional challenges throughout his or her lengthy course of treatment and recovery. The patient may experience posttraumatic stress disorder (PTSD), body image disorder, anxiety, and/or depression. To ensure that these issues are effectively managed, the interprofessional team at a burn center must include mental health professionals. Psychologists, psychiatrists, and advanced practice mental health nurse practitioners and clinical specialists are often involved, and many patients may require both emotional and pharmacological interventions for mental health issues. Although the patient may suffer emotional consequences as a result of the burn injury, the family members and loved ones are also often affected by this traumatic experience. Psychological and emotional support and/or counseling are geared toward the patient as well as the family. Nurses often have the most contact with the patient and his or her family and play a key role in the provision of support. Many burn centers have specialty support groups for survivors of burn injuries and their families.

Although survival rates for patients with major burn injuries are increasing, it is essential to return the patient to his or her highest level of function and mobility. Physical and occupational therapists are important members of the interprofessional team and begin working with the burn patient immediately upon admission. Modalities including range of motion, positioning, splinting, ambulation, and

ADLs are implemented as soon as the patient is physiologically stable. Once the patient is discharged, physical and occupational services continue in the home, at a rehabilitation facility, or in an outpatient setting. In some cases, these patients require rehabilitation therapy for several hours a day up to 5 days a week for many months after their injury.

Complications

One of the most devastating sequelae associated with burn injuries is the development of **contractures**. There are several contributing factors to the development of contractures, including the extent, depth, and location of the burn. Contractures are characterized as permanent tightening of the skin that may involve underlying muscles and tendons and result in limited mobility. The patient's personal motivation and compliance with therapy regimens play important roles in the development of contractures. Contractures are especially devastating in the pediatric population because burned or grafted skin is unable to expand as the child grows. Splinting is the most common method used to help prevent the formation of contractures (Fig. 51.26). Splints are placed by rehabilitation therapists to maintain range of motion and function of the involved joints. It is especially important to employ the use of splints when a burn injury crosses over a major joint, such as the elbow or knee.

Scarring is another major concern when dealing with a burn injury. Any area that has been grafted will have some element and degree of scarring. As burn wounds mature over the course of months to years, hypertrophic scarring can result. Burns to the face and hands that have caused scarring are particularly traumatic to the patient and may result in appearance changes and disfigurement. As patients progress to discharge, they are measured and fitted for specialty pressure garments (Fig. 51.27). The purpose of these garments is to apply continuous and uniform pressure over the area of burn to prevent hypertrophic scarring. These garments are to be worn 23 hours a day for up to a year or more after injury in some patients. Specialty face masks may also be utilized to help prevent scarring.

Nursing Management

Assessment and Analysis

The rehabilitative phase is the longest and may last several years depending on the TBSA affected, the severity of the burns, and the complexity of the treatments. Just as in the two previous phases, the patient must be monitored for infection, nutritional status, and pain during this phase. Additionally, the priorities expand to promoting greater mobility, flexibility, comfort, and psychosocial health. During this phase, the nurse observes for the following clinical manifestations:

- Pain/discomfort
- Contractures
- Scarring
- Disfigurement

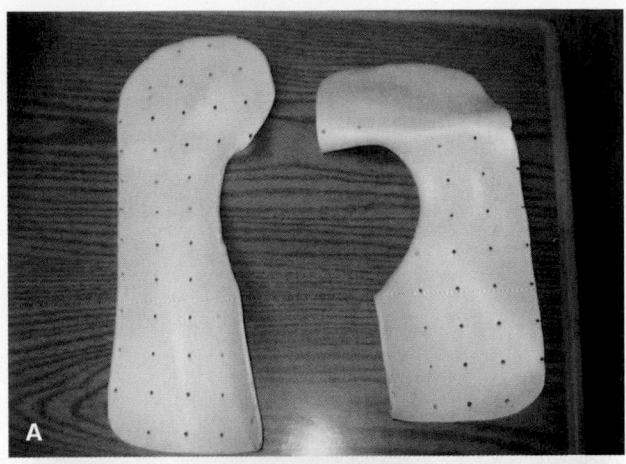
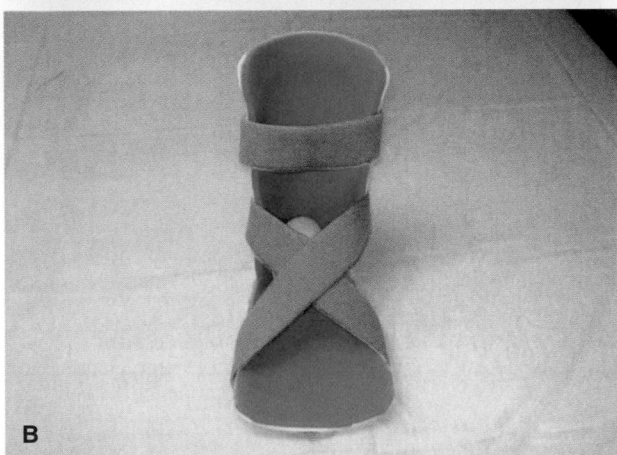
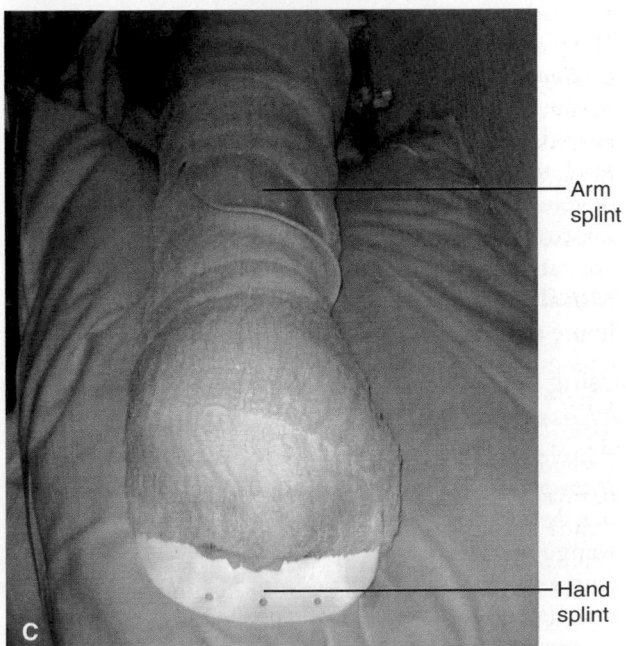

FIGURE 51.26 Splints. A, Hand splints. B, Foot splint. C, Hand and arm splints with burn dressings.

- Limited mobility
- Altered/depressed mood
- Flat affect
- Fear
- Anxiety

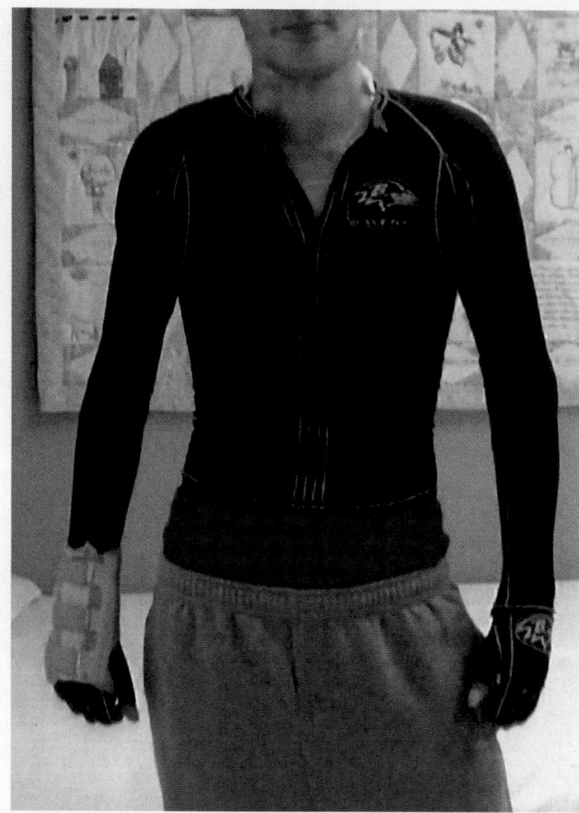

FIGURE 51.27 Full-body pressure garment.

Nursing Diagnoses

- **Activity intolerance** related to pain when exercising because of the burn injury
- **Impaired physical mobility** related to pain on movement and potential scar and contracture development
- **Disturbed body image** related to altered physical appearance
- **Moral distress** related to anticipation of discharge to home and/or a rehabilitation center

Nursing Interventions

▣ Assessments

- Pain level
  If the patient is in pain, participation in physical activities may be impaired, further complicating recovery.
- Range of motion
  In the patient with extensive scarring and/or contracture development, the mobility of joints may be limited, requiring specific strengthening and flexibility exercises.
- Compliance with treatment and the rehabilitation regimen
  Helps to prevent tightening of the skin and the development of contractures and scarring
- Assess readiness for integration into society.
  Many patients have anxiety about pending discharge and perceive difficulties with returning to society.

▣ Actions

- Splinting and encouragement of rehabilitation exercises and ADLs
  Essential to help prevent development of contractures and maintain joint function
- Include psychology in patient treatment decisions.
  Burn patients may deal with multiple associated sequelae, including PTSD, nightmares, and body image disorder.
- Provide community resources for support upon discharge, including psychological support.
  Community resources for burn survivors may be difficult to find but can provide essential social and psychological support.

▣ Teaching

- Teach patient and family the importance of and how to apply pressure garments and/or face masks.
  Prevent hypertrophic scarring
- Teach patient and family about burn prevention, sun protection, and prevention of hyperthermia.
  Patients with burns may be lacking sweat glands, and new skin and/or grafted skin is sensitive to sunlight.

Evaluating Care Outcomes

The focus during the rehabilitative phase is to return the patient to the highest functioning level, and expected outcomes include pain management, prevention of complications, improvements in mood, and increasing independence with activities of daily living. The nurse plays an integral role in assisting and encouraging the patient during physical and occupational therapy treatment regimens. It is important for the patient and family to verbalize and demonstrate an understanding of therapy routines because noncompliance can quickly lead to contractures and loss of function. The nurse also works closely with the patient and the psychologist to effectively manage and deal with the possible psychological sequelae, which may include body image disorder, nightmares, and PTSD.

OTHER CONDITIONS TREATED IN A BURN CENTER

Burn center referrals are not always limited to treating typical burn injuries, and patients with various disease processes that involve the integumentary system, underlying soft tissue, and/or muscle are treated and managed at burn centers. Some of the conditions and disease processes treated at burn centers include Stevens–Johnson syndrome (SJS), toxic epidermal necrolysis (TEN), erythema multiforme, purpura fulminans, staphylococcal scalded skin syndrome, bullous pemphigoid, necrotizing fasciitis, calciphylaxis, scleroderma, and frostbite.

Stevens–Johnson Syndrome and Toxic Epidermal Necrolysis

Although both Stevens–Johnson syndrome and toxic epidermal necrolysis (TEN) have been related to multiple etiologies, the most common causes are an adverse medication reaction, viral infection, or reaction to the staphylococcal toxin. In both disorders, the epidermis separates from the dermal layer and sloughs. Stevens–Johnson syndrome (SJS) may involve less than 30% TBSA, whereas TEN may involve greater than 30% TBSA. In both conditions, slough to the oral mucosa, conjunctiva, vaginal canal, gastrointestinal tract, and urethral lining may also occur. The mortality rate associated with TEN ranges from 25% to 80% and is usually due to septicemia, which leads to multiple organ failure. The lesions associated with SJS and TEN are extremely painful and hypersensitive. Immediate concerns focus on protection of the airway because of the oral lesions and inability to control oral sloughing and bleeding. Endotracheal intubation may be required. A definitive diagnosis is confirmed through biopsy. Because of the complexity of this type of condition, in which treatment often includes electrolyte replacement, nutritional support, expert wound care, strong infection control practices, and extensive rehabilitation, these patients are often best managed at a burn center.

4. The nurse anticipates that the donor site(s) for Mr. Smith will be from which area?
   A. Upper extremities
   B. Thigh
   C. Scalp
   D. Chest

5. What are nursing priorities for Mr. Smith during the rehabilitative phase? *(Select all that apply.)*
   A. Prevention of contractures
   B. Sustaining oxygenation
   C. Compliance with physical and occupation therapy regimens
   D. Psychological readiness for integration into society
   E. Fluid resuscitation

Making Connections

CASE STUDY: WRAP-UP

Joe's surgery is successful, and he is prepared for discharge to home. During discharge teaching, the nurses discuss the importance of proper nutrition to promote wound healing, as well as monitoring for signs of infection. The nurse ensures that Joe has appropriate referrals for psychological and rehabilitative therapy.

Case Study Questions

1. On the basis of the initial burn wound description, what depth of injury has this patient sustained?
   A. Superficial
   B. Superficial partial thickness
   C. Deep partial thickness
   D. Full thickness

2. Using the rule of nines, what is the approximate size of Mr. Smith's burn injury?
   A. 80% TBSA
   B. 65% TBSA
   C. 40% TBSA
   D. 24% TBSA

3. On further assessment, Mr. Smith's estimated TBSA is determined to be 45%, and his weight is 220 lb. Using the resuscitation formula, the nurse calculates what volume to be administered during the first 24 hours?
   A. 9,000 mL lactated Ringer's
   B. 14,000 mL lactated Ringer's
   C. 18,000 mL lactated Ringer's
   D. 21,000 mL lactated Ringer's

CHAPTER SUMMARY

Because of the limited number of burn centers within the United States, it is essential that all healthcare providers possess the basic burn-care knowledge required in the initial management of patients with burns. As a result of the resource-intensive nature of caring for patients with burns, they are best managed in burn centers, where they can be cared for by an interprofessional specialty team of providers. It is important that healthcare providers are familiar with American Burn Association transfer criteria.

Burns are generally classified in terms of etiology, depth of tissue damage, total body surface area (TBSA) involved, and severity. Special considerations must be given to patients who sustain inhalation, electrical, and/or chemical injuries because specialized treatment may be warranted. Burn injuries may be superficial, partial thickness, or full thickness in depth. The TBSA of the burn can be determined using various methods, including the rule of palm and the rule of nines. Burns that are 20% TBSA or greater are considered major burn injuries and produce both localized and systemic responses within the body. All body systems are affected by a major burn injury. Rapid and adequate fluid resuscitation is essential to prevent the development of hypovolemic shock.

The management of a burn injury can be broken down into three phases: the emergent, intermediate, and rehabilitative phases. In the emergent phase, the focus is on airway management, fluid resuscitation, and prevention of hypothermia. The intermediate phase focuses on wound healing, pain management, ensuring optimal nutrition, and continued prevention of infection. The rehabilitative phase begins the day the patient is admitted to the burn center and often lasts for many years, even extending well beyond discharge.

Burn injuries can be physically and emotionally devastating for both the patient and the family. Caring for this unique population of patients even presents physical and emotional challenges to members of the burn healthcare team. Many recent studies are investigating the effects of burnout and emotional exhaustion among healthcare providers, especially those working with the burn population. Special emphasis also needs to be placed on education regarding the location of community resources to assist patients in both the prevention and management of burn injuries.

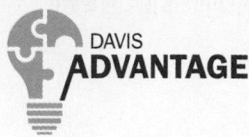

DAVIS ADVANTAGE | To explore learning resources for this chapter, go to **Davis Advantage** and find:
- Answers to in-text questions
- Chapter Resources and Activities
- NCLEX®-Style Chapter Review Questions
- Bibliography

Unit XII

Promoting Health in Patients With Musculoskeletal Disorders

Chapter 52

Assessment of Musculoskeletal Function

Kelley Miller Wilson

Finding Connections

CASE STUDY: EPISODE 1

Follow this patient throughout the chapter.

Twenty-four-year-old Abby Ridgeway recently graduated from a prestigious Midwestern college where she was a 4-year scholar athlete on the school's championship women's soccer team. Since graduation, Abby has been playing on a weekly intermural coeducational soccer team with a talented and competitive group of young adults. Last Tuesday evening during one of the games, Abby, in uncontested pursuit of the ball, extended her left leg to keep the ball in play. Almost as soon as she extended her leg, she felt a "pop" followed by instant unyielding pain, the kind that every soccer player dreads. After being assisted to a standing position, Abby was unable to bear any weight on the injured left leg. Assisted by teammates, Abby was taken to the closest emergency department (ED) for medical evaluation…

OVERVIEW OF ANATOMY AND PHYSIOLOGY

Bones

The musculoskeletal system, the second largest system of the body, is an amazing group of structures performing in perfect precision, allowing for movement, protection of vital organs, production of blood cells in the marrow, support for standing erect, and finally, a reservoir for essential minerals in the bones. The skeleton forms the framework of the human body and consists of 206 bones. These bones support the integumentary system of the body and allow for upright posture and weight bearing. Even though bones are made up of minerals, resulting in a hard structure, they contain both living and nonliving tissues. The portion of the bone that contains living tissue includes the blood vessels, nerves, **collagen** (predominant protein in the connective tissue),and living cells. The living cells contain **osteoblasts** (cells that help form bone) and **osteoclasts** (cells that help demineralize and destroy old bone).

Bones are generally classified in two ways, by structure (composition) or by shape. Classification by bone shape includes long bones, short bones, flat bones, irregular bones, and sesamoid bones. Long bones (Fig. 52.1), often weight-bearing bones, are cylindrical in shape with rounded ends. Examples of long bones found in the human body include the femur located in the upper leg, the tibia and fibula located in the lower leg, the humerus located in the upper arm, and the radius and ulna located in the lower portion of the arm. Long bones also serve as levers for muscles. Short bones found in the body are defined as being as wide as they are long (Fig. 52.2). The primary function of short bones is to provide stability with little movement. Examples of these bones are the carpals and tarsals located in the wrist and foot. Flat bones are another type of bone found abundantly in the human body (Fig. 52.3). Flat bones are strong flat plates of bone with the purpose of protecting vital organs. Examples of flat bones include the sternum (breast bone), the cranium (skull), and the ribs. In adults, the highest numbers of red blood cells are formed in these flat bones. The irregular bones (Fig. 52.4) are bones that do not fall into any specific category because of their nonuniform shape. Examples

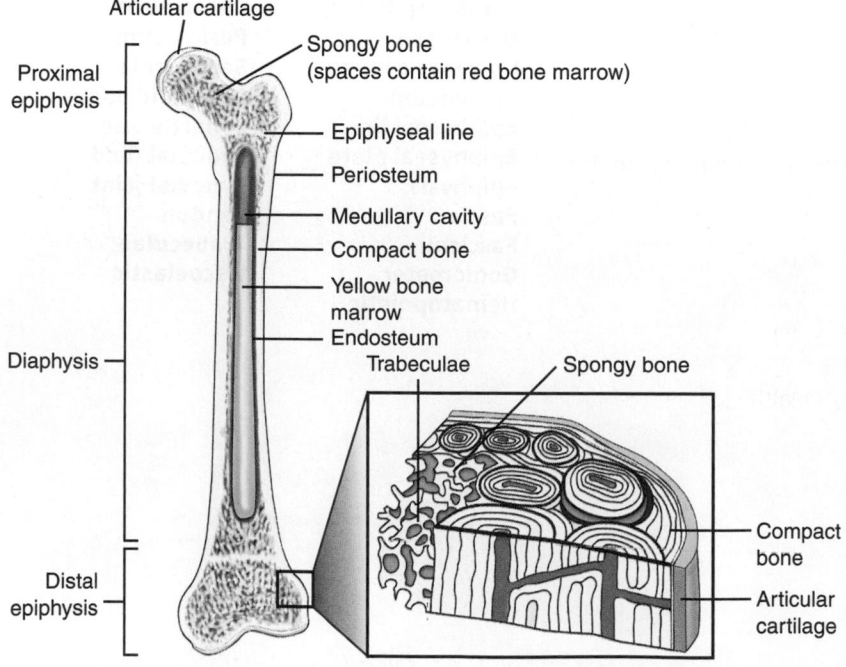

FIGURE 52.1 Long bone.

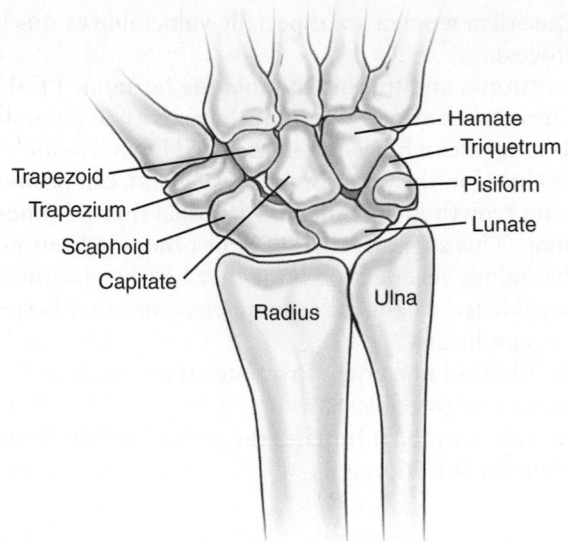

FIGURE 52.2 Short bones. Examples are carpal bones in the wrist.

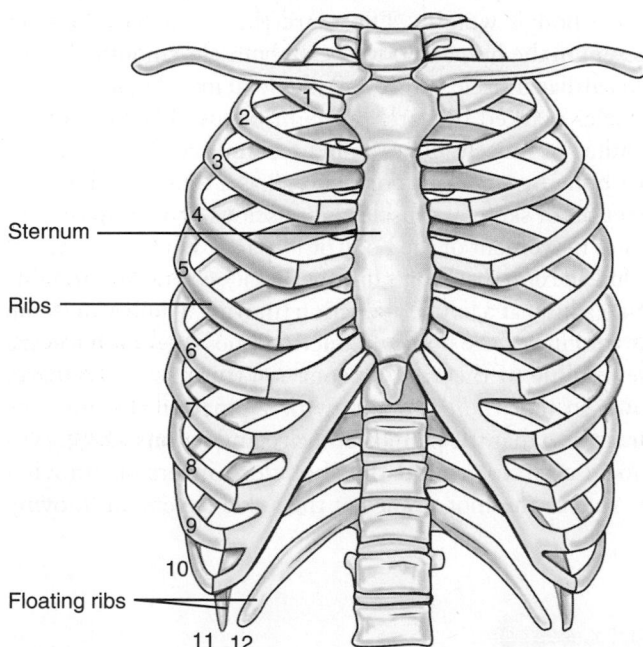

FIGURE 52.3 Flat bones. Examples are the protective bones of the chest and sternum.

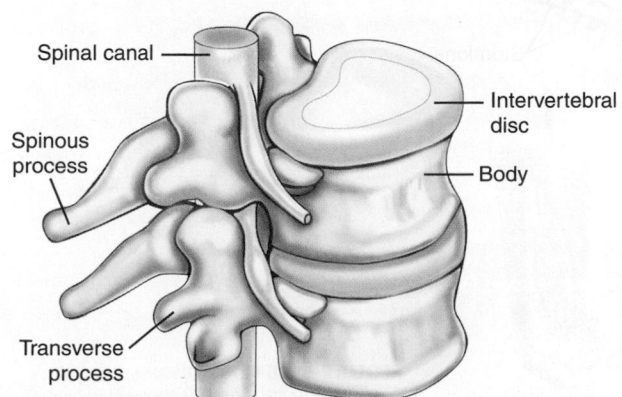

FIGURE 52.4 Irregular bones. Example is the vertebral body.

of irregular bones are the vertebrae and the mandible (lower jaw). Finally, **sesamoid bones** are short and irregular bones embedded in a tendon. The most commonly cited example of a sesamoid bone is the patella (kneecap), which sits within the patellar or quadriceps tendon (Fig. 52.5).

Bones of different shapes contain different portions of osseous tissue known as *compact* and *spongy* bone. Compact bone is dense and looks smooth. Microscopically, compact bone contains the canals and passageways that serve as conduits for nerves, blood vessels, and lymphatic vessels. Spongy bone, on the other hand, is composed of small latticelike pieces and therefore has more open space. The lattice pieces, called **trabeculae**, form an open network that is filled with bone marrow, which functions to produce essential blood cells of the body. Two types of marrow are present in the bones of healthy individuals, red and yellow marrow. Red marrow consists mainly of **hematopoietic** tissue, whereas yellow marrow is made up mainly of fat cells. Hematopoietic tissue contains specialized cells that give rise to the formation of blood cells. Red blood cells, platelets, and white blood cells are all produced in the red marrow. Yellow marrow stores fat that the body may use in cases of extreme starvation. Yellow marrow also may transform into red marrow in cases of severe blood loss or anemia.

Long bones, which are similar in structure to many of the bones in the human body, typically have the following structures (see Fig. 52.1):

- **Diaphysis:** This is the shaft, which is made up of the long portion of the bone. It is constructed of a thick compact bone that surrounds the medullary cavity in adults. The medullary cavity contains fat known as the yellow marrow.
- **Epiphysis:** This is known as the end portion of the bone. A thin layer of compact bone forms the exterior portion of the bone, and the interior of this portion of the bone contains spongy bone.

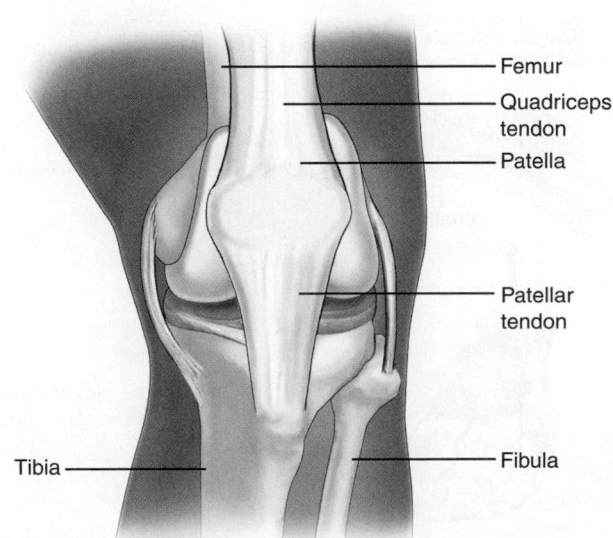

FIGURE 52.5 Sesamoid bone. Example is the patella or "knee cap."

- **Epiphyseal plate:** In the bones of younger patients, **cartilage** is present at the junction of the diaphysis and the epiphysis, which allows growth to occur and the bones to lengthen.
- **Epiphyseal line:** This is a remnant of the epiphyseal plate; the cartilage that is present is converted to bone after puberty so that no further bone growth is possible.
- **Periosteum:** This is the tough outer surface of the bone (diaphysis). It consists of connective tissue, primarily of bone-forming cells known as osteoblasts. This portion of the bone also provides an insertion or anchoring point for tendons and ligaments.
- **Endosteum:** This is the internal bone surface that is covered with a delicate connective tissue membrane.
- **Articular cartilage:** This is where the long bones articulate at the epiphyseal surfaces. The bony surfaces are covered with a specialized cartilage called **hyaline cartilage,** which cushions the bones' ends and absorbs stress during joint movement.

Bones consist of both inorganic and organic substances. The organic components consist of cells and the bone matrix. The inorganic substances consist of mineral salts, most notably calcium phosphate. Calcium salts are present in the form of very tiny crystals, which help to create the hard quality of the bone.

Hormonal Influences

Several hormones have been identified as factors that influence bone growth and loss. The specific hormones and their roles in creating this influence include:

- Estrogen: Induces a chemical in osteoclasts that causes them to self-destruct and slow the rate of bone destruction. Menopause with the associated loss of estrogen makes women more prone to bone loss. Asian and Caucasian women are especially vulnerable to this process.
- Calcitonin and thyroid-stimulating hormone (TSH): These two hormones inhibit the activity of osteoclasts. Recent research has found that TSH, a hormone produced in the anterior pituitary gland, can promote bone growth independent of its usual thyroid functions. This suggests that TSH or other medications that mimic its effect on bone may be a key factor for possible treatments of **osteoporosis** or other bone loss conditions.
- Parathyroid hormone: Promotes the activity and number of osteoblasts
- Growth hormone: Initiates the growth of bone until adult size is achieved

Muscles

Muscles are structures that contract and help produce movement. Muscles account for approximately 40% to 50% of the body's weight. There are three types of muscles present in the human body: skeletal muscle, smooth muscle, and cardiac muscle (Fig. 52.6). Skeletal muscles are striated muscles marked by dark and light bands. They consist of bundles of muscle fibers called **fasciculi** and are attached to a bone by a fibrous cord known as a tendon. The main function of skeletal muscles is conscious or voluntary control of movement of the body or its parts. These movements include flexion (bending a limb at a joint), extension (straightening a limb at a joint), abduction (moving a limb away from the midline of the body), adduction (moving a limb toward the midline of the body), pronation (turning the forearm down so that the palm is down), supination (turning the forearm so that the palm is up), circumduction (moving the arm in a circle around the shoulder), inversion (moving the sole of the foot inward at the ankle), eversion (moving

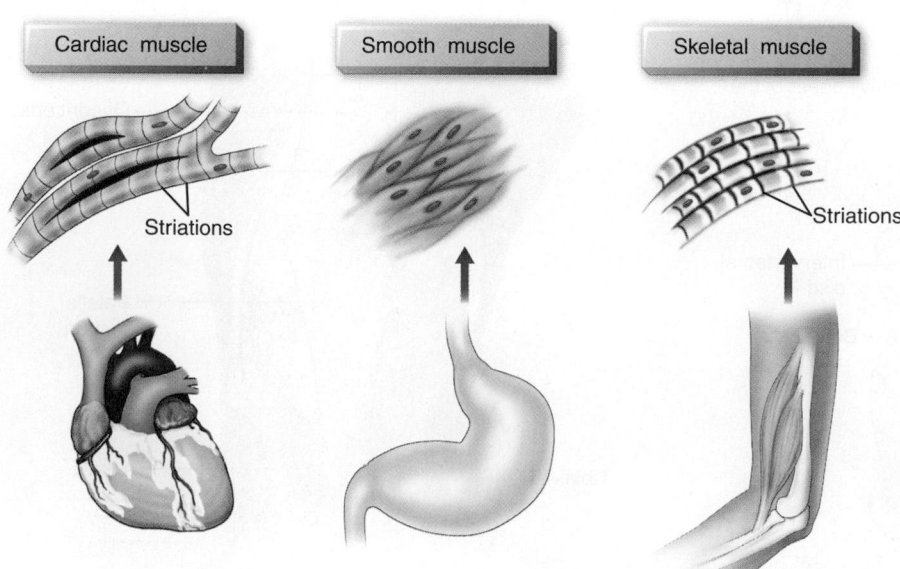

FIGURE 52.6 Muscle tissues; cardiac striated muscle, striated skeletal muscle, and smooth muscle.

the sole of the foot outward at the ankle), rotation (moving the head around a central axis), protraction (moving a body part forward and parallel), retraction (moving a body part backward and parallel to the ground), elevation (raising a body part), and depression (lowering a body part) (Fig. 52.7).

Smooth muscle, or nonstriated muscle, is involuntary. Smooth muscles are under control of the autonomic nervous system, which controls contractions of organs and blood vessels automatically. This specific muscle tissue is found in the walls of hollow organs such as the stomach, esophagus, blood vessels, and bronchi. Stimulation is by involuntary neurogenic impulses. Examples of this action include moving food along the esophagus or constricting/dilating blood vessels.

Cardiac muscle is a highly specialized striated muscle that can contract without neural stimulation because of

the property of **automaticity**. Automaticity allows cardiac tissue to set a contraction rhythm through the presence of pacemaker cells. Cardiac muscle can also be stimulated to increase or decrease the contraction rate through input from the autonomic nervous system. Cardiac muscle tissue is highly resistant to fatigue, allowing it to beat continuously throughout a lifetime because of the presence of a large number of mitochondria, myoglobin (oxygen-carrying protein found within the muscle), and an excellent blood supply. These properties allow for continuous aerobic metabolism. The properties of cardiac muscle cells are discussed in detail in Chapter 28.

Joints

Joints are defined as a place of union between two or more bones. They permit mobility, provide mechanical support, and are an essential part of the musculoskeletal system. Joints are often referred to as either nonsynovial (Fig. 52.8) or synovial (Fig. 52.9). **Nonsynovial joints** are joined by fibrous tissue or cartilage and are immovable. **Synovial joints** are freely moveable because of the lubricating liquid called **synovial fluid** that fills the joint space. Synovial joints are enclosed in a joint cavity where the two bones meet. It is the presence of synovial fluid that prevents friction and allows for freedom of movement. The synovial joints are also covered with a layer of cartilage that lines the entire inner surface of the joint space. **Cartilage** is an avascular structure that receives its necessary nutrients from the synovial fluid while it is circulated during joint movement. The cartilage also provides additional cushion to the joint to allow for unencumbered and comfortable movement. Another structure that helps reduce friction with movement is a **bursa**. Not a part of synovial joints but frequently found close to them, a bursa is a fluid-filled sac lined with synovial tissue. It acts as a cushion between tendons, skin, or ligaments

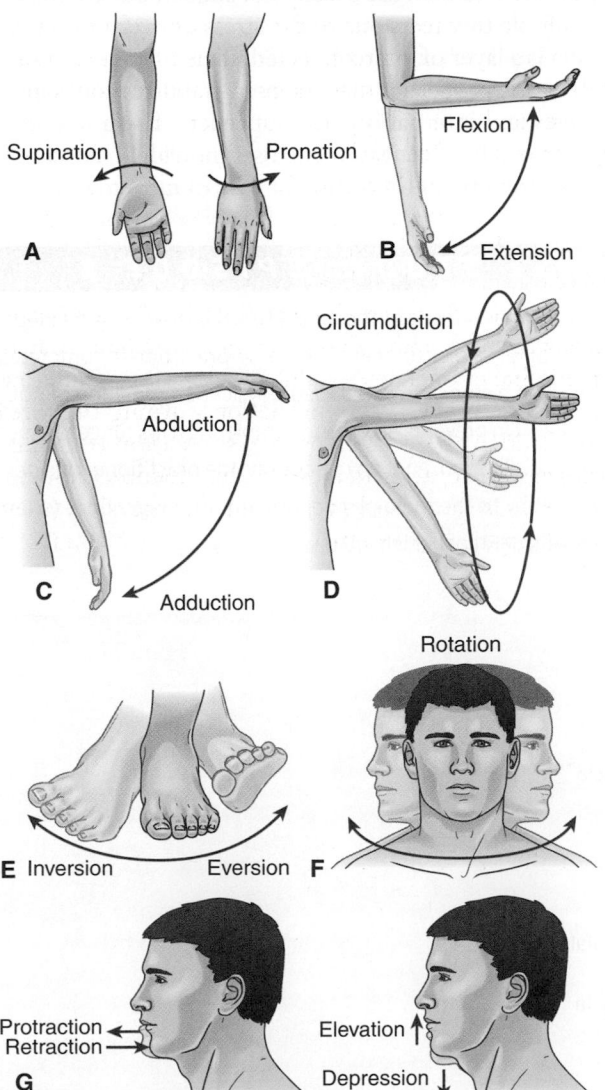

FIGURE 52.7 Skeletal muscle movements. A, Supination and pronation; B, Flexion and extension; C, Abduction and adduction; D, Circumduction; E, Inversion and eversion; F, Head rotation; G, Protraction, retraction, elevation, and depression.

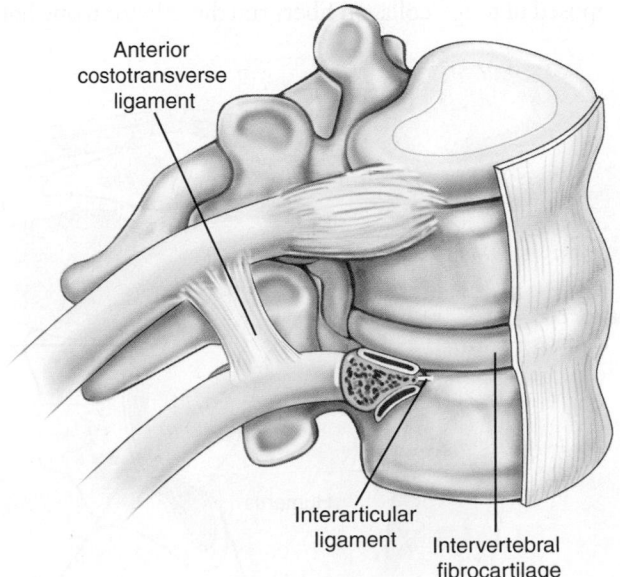

FIGURE 52.8 Nonsynovial joint. Example is vertebral body.

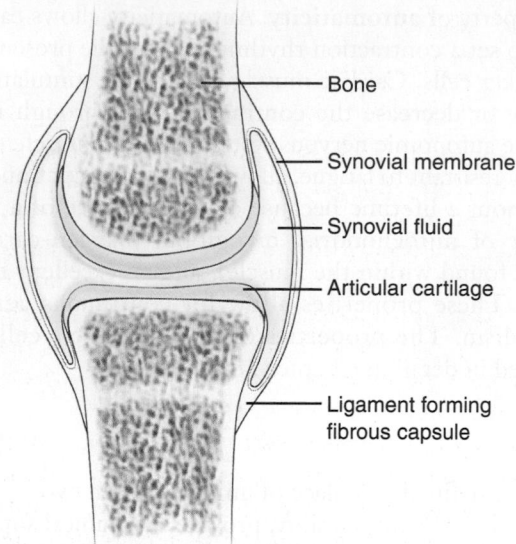

FIGURE 52.9 Synovial joint. Examples include elbow, wrist, and knee.

and bones to facilitate the friction-free movement between soft and hard (bone) structures (Fig. 52.10).

Joints may also be classified functionally. There are three specific classifications to consider when referring to skeletal joints. These functional descriptions include:

- **Synarthrosis:** These joints permit little or no mobility (e.g., skull sutures).
- **Amphiarthrosis:** These joints permit slight mobility (e.g., vertebrae).
- **Diarthrosis:** These joints permit a variety of movements (e.g., the shoulder).

Ligaments, Tendons, and Fascia

Ligaments are fibrous connective tissues present at joints to help provide stability to the joint. These fibrous bands composed of tough collagen fibers run directly from one bone to another to reinforce the joint and help prevent undesired directional movements (Fig. 52.11). To prevent joints from becoming too loose or unstable, ligaments are arranged in crossing patterns. Ligaments are also **viscoelastic**, which means they gradually lengthen when under tension and return to their original shape when the tension is removed. However, ligaments do not generally retain their original shape when stretched past a certain point for a prolonged period of time. This has strong implications for dislocated joints. The longer a bone remains outside a socket, as happens with a dislocation, the greater the potential for permanent damage from this overstretching of the ligaments, which can increase the risk of more frequent dislocations. Broken or torn ligaments result in joint instability; surgical intervention may be necessary to return the joint to proper functioning.

Tendons are fibrous connective tissues that connect muscle to bone or structures such as the eye. Where ligaments provide stability, tendons facilitate movement (Fig. 52.12). Injuries to a tendon are usually not sudden but are the result of multiple tiny tears due to the stress of overuse over time. **Fascia** is a layer of interconnected fibers of connective tissue with elastic properties that encloses, stabilizes, and separates muscles and internal organs. Superficial fascia lies directly under the skin. Deep fascia encloses individual muscles, providing strength and allowing for ease of movement.

CASE STUDY: EPISODE 2

Shortly after arriving at the local ED, Abby is seen by the department's nurse practitioner. The nurse practitioner completes a thorough history and a modified physical examination of Abby's left leg. Pain prevents Abby from completing a full range of motion (ROM) evaluation. After an initial x-ray, the practitioner decides to send Abby to the radiology department for magnetic resonance imaging (MRI) of her left knee...

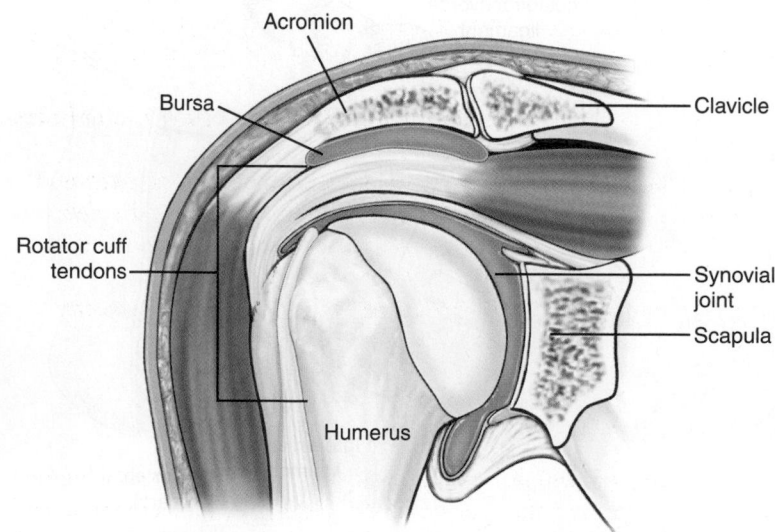

FIGURE 52.10 Bursa provides a cushion between tendons, skin, or ligaments and bones.

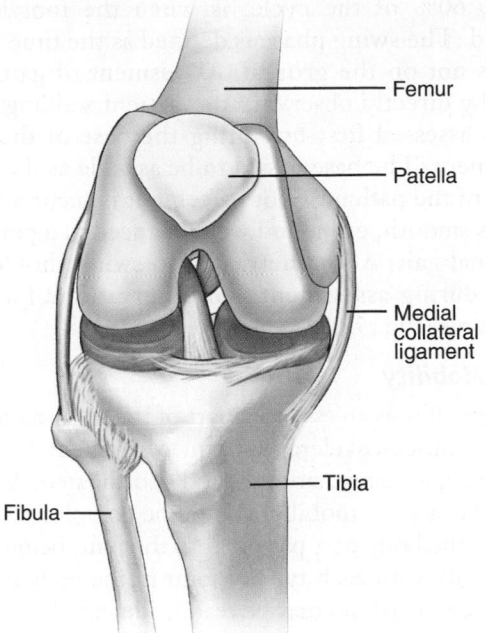

FIGURE 52.11 Medial collateral ligament of the knee provides joint stability and protection against undesired directional movement.

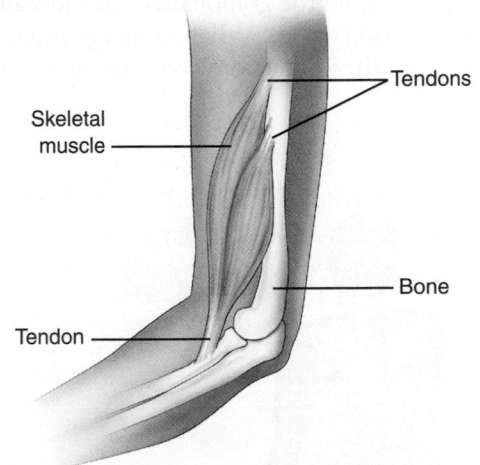

FIGURE 52.12 Tendons connect muscle to bone and facilitate movement.

Connection Check 52.1

The nurse understands which of the following are considered the key components of the musculoskeletal system?

A. Bones, ligaments, smooth muscle, and joints
B. Bones, tendons, ligaments, and cardiac muscle
C. Bones, muscle, joints, and ligaments
D. Bones, skeletal muscle, tendons, and ligaments

ASSESSMENT

Past Medical History and History of Present Illness

As with any thorough assessment of a system of the human body, one of the first parts of the examination process is always obtaining the patient's history. Past medical history may have implications for current injury or disease. For example, a shoulder dislocation in the past may predispose a person for future dislocations. Hormonal disturbances may have implications with calcium balance. Also, patients with Down's syndrome are known to experience accelerated aging, which has musculoskeletal implications.

The aim of gathering the history of the present illness or chief complaint is to gain a clear description of the current problem so that proper treatment may be initiated. Some conditions of the musculoskeletal system may be managed by a primary care practitioner, whereas others require the expertise of a specialist and interprofessional team. The interview of patients presenting with musculoskeletal difficulties includes asking the patients to recite:

- Location of pain including quality of pain (sharp, stabbing, dull, throbbing, continuous); time frame associated with pain (when did the pain start); factors that make the pain better/worse
- Presence of swelling? Note time swelling was first noticed and any increase/decrease of swelling.
- Stiffness? Note location, duration, and degree of stiffness present.
- Deformity? Note any change from the uninjured state of the affected area.
- Weakness? Note the presence of weakness and measure the degree of weakness present. Has the weakness increased or resolved since the injury?
- Instability of the affected area? Is there instability present? If so, note the degree of instability present by recording the specific current level of functioning of the injured area.
- Loss of function? Is there an inability of the affected area to function in a manner that it previously did?
- Are there color or temperature changes present with the affected area?
- Is there any altered sensation present such as numbness or tingling?
- Are there any other associated symptoms or past medical history that could impact the injury? Is there any significant family past medical history related to this type of injury?
- How have the symptoms responded (if at all) to any treatment that has been administered?

Physical Assessment

After a complete and thorough interview has been obtained from the patient or designee of the patient, a complete and thorough focused physical assessment must take place. A physical examination begins with a general inspection of the posture, gait, joint mobility, and skin. It involves looking for symmetry of movement, involuntary movements, deformity, swelling/edema, discoloration, and hypertrophy/atrophy. Palpation is also an important part of the physical examination to assess muscle tone and strength, range of motion, sensation, skin temperature, and quality of pulses. The examination is usually completed in a sequential order and notes any pain or discomfort present without stimulus and/or evoked during the process.

Posture

Posture is the position in which minimum stress is placed on each joint in the body. In 1949, the American Academy of Orthopaedic Surgeons defined good posture as a state of muscular and skeletal balance that protects the supporting structures of the body against injury or progressive deformity. Good posture maintains the body's alignment in sitting, standing, and prone and supine positions; poor posture causes compensation on other bones, joints, and muscles, which can result in damage to a structure. To assess the posture of a patient, the patient should stand comfortably erect as appropriate for age. A plumb line (imaginary or actual) should be drawn through the anterior ear, shoulder, hip, patella, and ankle. Curvature of the spine as well as the length, symmetry, and movement of the extremities should be noted (Fig. 52.13).

Gait

Gait is described as the patient's ability to demonstrate an erect stance and swing phase with walking. The stance phase, 60% of the cycle, is when the foot is on the ground. The swing phase is defined as the time when the foot is not on the ground. Assessment of gait must be done by directly observing the patient walking. Normal gait is assessed first by noting the base of the walking movement. The base is said to be as wide as the shoulder width of the patient. Foot placement is accurate, and the walk is smooth, even, and well balanced in a patient with a normal gait. A symmetrical arm swing should also be noted during assessment and observation of a patient's gait status (Fig. 52.14).

Joint Mobility

Joint mobility is an essential part of the assessment process for the musculoskeletal system. Movement for joints is deliberate, accurate, smooth, and coordinated. Assessment of ROM or joint mobility should be completed while stabilizing the body part proximal to the joint being assessed. Familiarity with each type of joint in the body is essential so that abnormalities may be readily identified. Joint motion is not expected to cause pain or discomfort upon movement. A **goniometer** is an instrument that is used to measure the angles that a patient is able to achieve with the movement of each specific joint (Fig. 52.15). To use the goniometer, the provider extends the joint being assessed to a neutral or zero-degree position. The zero-degree point of the goniometer is centered on the joint. With the limb kept at a zero-degree line on the goniometer, the moveable arm is used as a measuring device. When using the goniometer for assessment, flex the joint and measure the angle of greatest flexion.

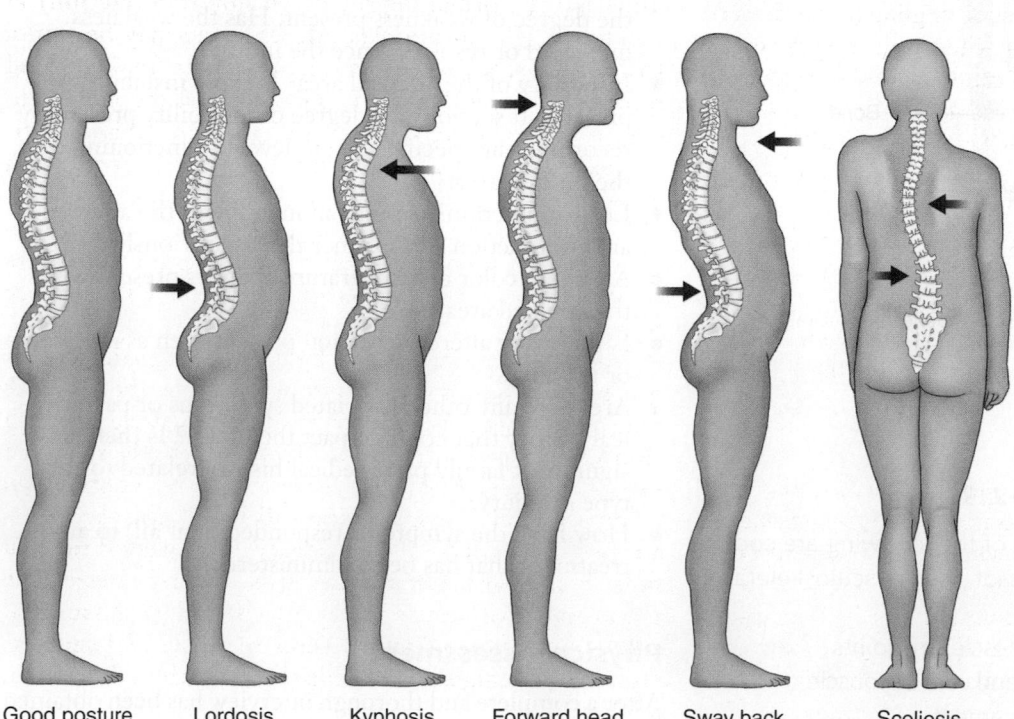

Good posture   Lordosis   Kyphosis   Forward head   Sway back   Scoliosis

FIGURE 52.13 Assessing postures.

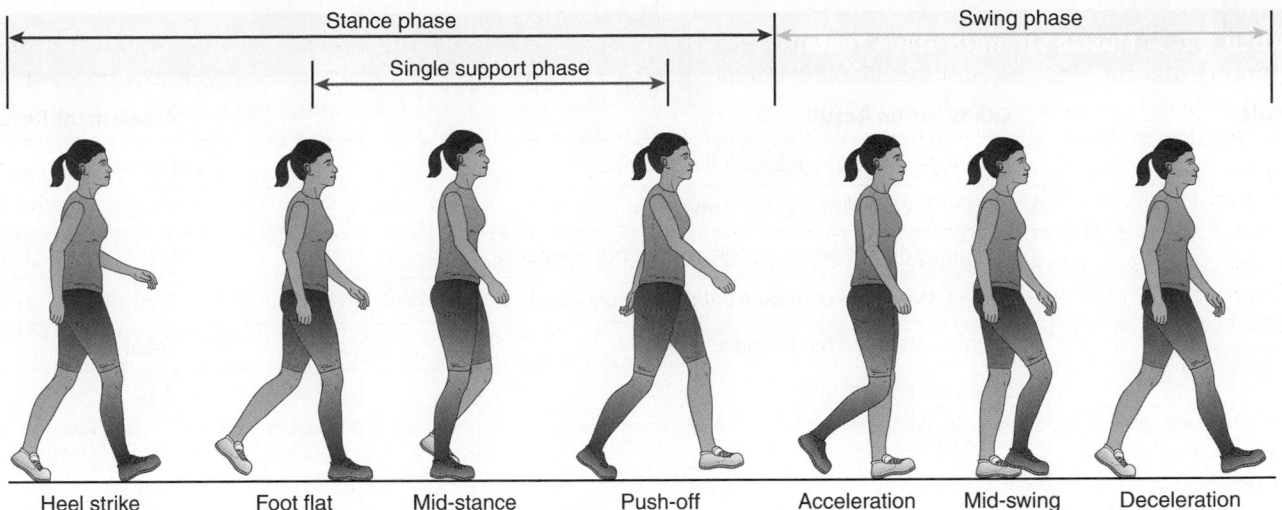

FIGURE 52.14 Assessing for normal walking gait.

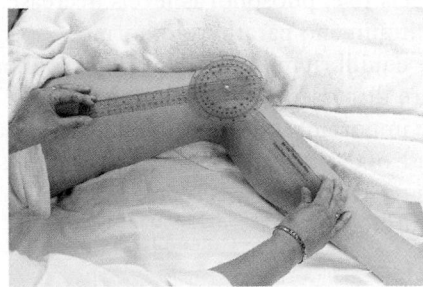

FIGURE 52.15 Goniometer to assess joint mobility.

Sensation

Evaluation of sensation is another key indicator regarding skeletal bone function. Numbness or tingling (**paresthesia**) is an abnormal assessment finding when evaluating the musculoskeletal system. Paresthesia often indicates damage to a sensory nerve by pressure or fracture and often resolves after treatment of the injury has been initiated. Assessing the patient's ability to determine the presence of a stimulus is also important. The pinprick test may be used. With the use of a paper clip or other specific instrument designed specifically for this purpose, a stimulus is applied to assess whether the patient is able to feel the stimulus equally and symmetrically near the suspected area of injury. The inability to feel sensation is an indicator that sensory nerve damage may be present.

Pulse Assessment

An assessment of pulses in the patient's extremities is a standard part of the physical examination. It is particularly important to assess the pulses when injury or suspected injury is present. Pulses indicate whether blood flow is adequate to an extremity. Pulse assessment is done using two fingers and avoiding the use of the thumb because it has its own pulse, which may be misleading. It is important to assess the pulse rate, rhythm, depth, and symmetry.

Muscle Tone and Strength

Tone is the normal degree of tension (contraction) in voluntary relaxed muscles. Muscle tone may be found to be increased or decreased. Assessing for increased tone is usually a bit easier to detect. Ask the patient to completely relax all muscles, or "go limp." The practitioner then takes the extremity and moves it through a full ROM. It is expected in a normal examination that the practitioner will note a mild, even resistance to movement. Notations should be made for any extra or involuntary movements of the muscles if they are present.

Muscle strength is tested by having the patient resist force as the practitioner attempts to move the patient's body part against the direction of pull. Muscle strength should be equal bilaterally. Muscle strength is graded on a 0 to 5 scale, with 0 representing no contraction of muscle and 5 representing full ROM against resistance. A grade of "5" is considered to represent normal muscle strength. Oftentimes, it is easier to determine the presence of muscle weakness when there is a normal side present from which to compare. Table 52.1 summarizes the grading scale for muscle strength evaluation in adults.

Table 52.1 Muscle Strength Grade Table

Grade	Examination Result	Assessment Result
5	Full range of motion against full resistance	Normal
54	Full range of motion against some resistance	Good
53	Full range of motion against gravity but not resistance	Fair
52	Full passive range of motion but not against gravity or resistance	Poor
51	Slight contraction but no movement	Trace
50	No visible contraction	Zero

Connection Check 52.3

The assessment of the musculoskeletal system begins with which of the following?
A. Comprehensive assessment of medical history
B. Comprehensive assessment of pain
C. Comprehensive assessment of movement
D. Comprehensive assessment of bone integrity

Connection Check 52.4

Comprehensive assessment of ROM by the practitioner provides what information?
A. Detailed information regarding tendon function
B. Information regarding muscle strength and tone
C. Information regarding the health of the joint space
D. Information regarding the condition of the ligaments

 Safety Alert If you suspect an acute bone injury:
- Immobilize the extremity
- Control bleeding if present
- Elevate above the level of the heart, if possible
- Apply ice/cold packs to extremity with cloth covering tissue to prevent possible frozen tissue injury
- Refer for emergency medical evaluation

DIAGNOSTIC STUDIES

Laboratory Studies

Bones are the major source of calcium in the body. Adequate calcium levels are essential for bone health. Assessing calcium levels through blood tests is an important indicator of bone integrity or density. Low calcium levels are an indicator of increased fracture risk. In addition to calcium, phosphorus and vitamin D levels are all common laboratory values used to assess bone health. Vitamin D works in the body to promote the gastrointestinal absorption of calcium and phosphorus. In a healthy individual, calcium and phosphorus have an inverse relationship, meaning that while calcium levels rise, phosphorus levels decrease. The hormones calcitonin and parathyroid hormone work together to keep the equilibrium of calcium and phosphorus. These concepts are discussed in detail in Chapter 40. Estrogens also play an important role in stimulating osteoblast activity. The decrease of estrogens with menopause increases fracture risk. Assessing estrogen levels is primarily done through an analysis of urine.

Imaging Studies

X-Ray

Obtaining images of a part of the musculoskeletal system is often needed to find a specific injury or confirm the presence of an abnormality. These images assist the practitioner in assessing the full extent of the injury/abnormality that is present so that effective treatment may be initiated.

Preparation of Patient/Nursing Implications

- Removal of clothing or jewelry from the site to be x-rayed because they can potentially obscure the image.
- Proper shielding of the patient is required to limit the degree of radiation exposure. Lead aprons are applied to cover the ovaries or testes. Thyroid glands are also covered in an attempt to prevent potential damage to these sensitive structures.

Computed Tomography

A computed tomography (CT) scan combines a series of x-ray views from different angles to produce cross sectional images of bones and soft tissues within the body. The addition of contrast material can be used to identify blockages or other blood vessel abnormalities. Computed tomography scans are done to diagnose muscle and bone disorders including tumors and fractures. Computed tomography–guided biopsy may also be completed for selected patients with known tumors. Abnormal values are defined as any fracture, break in bone surface, or presence of other structure that is not expected to be there, for example, neoplasms.

Preparation of Patient/ Nursing Implications

- Patient education regarding test to be performed
- If contrast is to be used, see Safety Alert

 Safety Alert There are several nursing implications important to be aware of for any imaging study:

- Assess pregnancy status. Fetuses are susceptible to injury from x-rays or imaging studies.
- Assess for allergies
- Assure consent has been signed if required for procedure
- Many imaging studies require the administration of IV contrast to improve visualization of structures. Contrast dye is nephrotoxic and can also have a negative impact if administered to a patient receiving metformin. If contrast dye is to be used, the nurse should:
  - Ensure insertion of IV if IV contrast is to be administered
  - Assess for allergies to contrast dye
  - Assess patient's renal status
  - Verify whether the patient is taking metformin. Contrast medium can greatly increase the level of metformin in the blood. In addition to the potential of hypoglycemia, increased levels can also increase the patient's chances of developing lactic acidosis. Metformin should be stopped before the procedure and held for 48 hours after the procedure.
- Encourage fluids after the examination if contrast dye is used

---

Magnetic Resonance Imaging

Magnetic resonance imaging is a radiological imaging test that uses a magnetic field and radio wave energy to create pictures of internal structures of the body. The pictures from an MRI often provide more detail than those from other imaging methods. It is used to diagnose disk disease, tumors, osteomyelitis, and ligamentous tears. The scanner is typically a long tube-like structure. Many patients have difficulty with the claustrophobic feeling they experience from being in a closed spaced. These patients may require sedation to complete the MRI. Open MRI machines are available in some areas and allow the patient to complete the examination in the open, thereby limiting feelings of claustrophobia.

Preparation of Patient

- Patient education regarding the loud banging sounds that will be heard during the examination
- No food or drink for 8 hours before the test for patients having an MRI of the abdomen or pelvis
- Ensure that there is a family member or friend to drive the patient home after the test if sedation is administered

Nursing Implications

- Assessment of the potential for claustrophobia
- Assess the patient for any metal objects such as hairpins, earrings, pacemaker, metal clips (surgically implanted), metal heart replacement valves, and intrauterine device. External metal objects need to be removed because they might interfere with the magnetic imaging. The decision to do the test with internal metal in place is made on an individual basis, but MRI may de-program pacemakers.
- Assess for the presence of any medication patches. A burn at the site may occur if the patch is left in place.

Arthrogram

An arthrogram is a series of images taken of a joint after contrast medium has been injected. After administration of local anesthetic, a radiologist or orthopedic provider uses fluoroscopy or ultrasound to accurately inject the appropriate quantity of contrast into the joint. This procedure allows for visualization of soft tissue structures of a joint: the tendons, ligaments, muscles, cartilage, and joint capsule. An abnormal result can reveal degenerative changes in the cartilage, a partial or complete tear, an enlarged or ruptured joint capsule, or a joint cyst. Pieces of bone, cartilage, tumor, or tissue may also be seen in the joint space with this examination.

Preparation of Patient

- Education regarding the procedure
- Remove objects or clothing from the joint area

Nursing Implications

- Verify whether the patient is taking any anticoagulants including aspirin
- Ensure "time-out" taken by staff before the start of the procedure to confirm the right patient, right procedure, and right anatomical location
- Provide post procedure instructions and information regarding joint pain for 1 to 2 days after the procedure

Bone Mineral Density Studies

Radiological examinations using CT scans, dual-energy x-ray absorptiometry (DEXA) scans, and ultrasound can assess bone density or the amount of calcium and other minerals in the bone. The most common test is the DEXA scan. Low bone density is an indicator of the presence of osteoporosis and increased fracture risk. The bones most often used for this test are located in the spine, the hip, the hand, the foot, and the forearm. The test is painless for the patient and takes less than 30 minutes in most cases. This test is done to both identify patients with osteoporosis and to monitor treatment progress.

Results for bone scans are reported in T scores and Z scores. A T score is a determination of bone density compared with what is expected in a healthy young (approximately 30-year-old) adult of the same sex. A Z score is a comparison of what is expected for a patient of the same age, sex, weight, and racial origin. Because a low bone mineral density is more common in older adults, the Z score can be misleading when diagnosing osteoporosis. A low Z score, –2 or lower, may suggest that something other than aging is causing abnormal bone loss and requires close examination by the practitioner. The determination of osteoporosis is typically done through the T score. Table 52.2 illustrates the interpretation of T score results for osteoporosis.

Preparation of Patient/Nursing Implications
- Patient education regarding test and potential results
- Notify the practitioner of any recent examination completed that required contrast because contrast material can sometimes interfere with accurate test results

Bone Scan

A bone scan is a diagnostic scan to find damage to bones, disease (such as cancer), infection, or trauma. A radioactive material, a tracer, is injected IV. The tracer travels through the body and after approximately 3 hours is absorbed into the bones. The bone images are then completed. Areas that show little or no amount of tracer appear as dark or "cold" spots. These areas of "cold" spots define areas with a lack of blood supply to the bone and may indicate the presence of cancer. "Hot spots" are areas where the tracer accumulates in the bone. These spots are often attributed to fractures that are healing, bone infection, or diseases of bone metabolism. Hot spots, as cold spots, may also indicate bone cancer and need further evaluation.

Preparation of Patient
- Patient education regarding the test. If the patient is breastfeeding, the nurse needs to instruct the patient to use formula and discard the breast milk for the next 48 hours until radioactive tracers are removed from the body.
- Ensure insertion of IV
- Verify that the consent for the test has been signed

Nursing Implications
- Verify that the patient has not had a procedure or taken a medication with bismuth in the last 72 hours because this can interfere with the test
- Increase fluids post-test to help excrete the radioactive tracer from the body

Table 52.2 Interpretation of Bone Density Study Results

T Score	Interpretation
–1 and greater	Bone density within normal limits
–1 to –2.5	Indicates a sign of osteopenia, a condition that may lead to osteoporosis
–2.5 and below	Indicates presence of osteoporosis

Electromyography

Electromyography (EMG) is a diagnostic test that assesses the health of motor neurons and muscle. Motor neurons transmit electrical signals to the muscles that make them contract. Using tiny needle electrodes that are strategically placed on the muscles, the EMG machine translates these signals into graphs or numbers that the practitioner interprets. This test takes approximately 30 to 60 minutes and is done to distinguish nerve dysfunction, muscle dysfunction, or problems with nerve-to-muscle signal transmission. It is expected that an EMG recording will show no electrical activity when a muscle is at rest. Abnormal electrical activity seen in muscles at rest may indicate a problem with the nerve supply to the muscle. Abnormal wave lines with muscle contractions may indicate a muscle or nerve problem such as amyotrophic lateral sclerosis, inflammation, or other muscle problems.

Preparation of Patient
- Education regarding the test:
  - There is a possibility of slight pain on needle insertion.
  - Slight bruising at the site where the electrodes were placed may occur.
  - Shower before the test and do not apply any lotions to allow for better electrode contact.
  - Do not eat or drink foods or fluids that contain caffeine 2 to 3 hours before the test.

Nursing Implications
- Verify that the patient does not have a pacemaker or bleeding disorder
- Verify medications patient is taking because some may interfere with muscle contraction
- Assess for pain during and after testing

Arthroscopic Examination

Arthroscopy is a surgical procedure that allows a practitioner to view the inside of a joint through an instrument called an arthroscope (Fig. 52.16). This procedure is used to diagnose, repair, and remove loose or foreign materials in the joint. It may also be used to monitor the progress of a previously diagnosed disease. Abnormal findings during an arthroscopic examination include abnormal color/shape of the ligaments and cartilage, the presence of growths or cysts, evidence of joint dysfunction such as arthritis, and the presence of infection.

Preparation of Patient
- Education regarding the procedure
- Standard preoperative protocols according to the institution
- Ensure consent has been signed

Nursing Implications
- Assess patient medications; special concern with anticoagulants and aspirin because these increase the risk of postoperative bleeding
- Assess pregnancy status

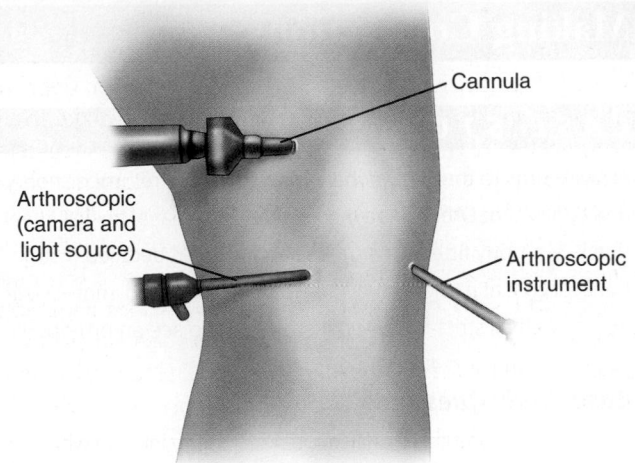

FIGURE 52.16 Arthroscopic surgery allows visualization inside of the joint to diagnose, repair, and/or remove loose or foreign materials.

- Verify last time the patient had food or drink. Patients can be at risk for aspiration if food/drink is ingested less than 12 hours before surgery.
- Ensure that "time-out" is taken by staff before the start of the procedure to confirm the right patient, right procedure, and right anatomical location
- Verify that the patient has not had a test such as an arthrogram in the previous 10 days on the affected joint. Contrast may cause inflammation and cause difficulty with visualization of the joint.
- Discharge instructions to include:
  - Apply ice to site for the first 1 or 2 days; do not apply ice directly to the skin—use a towel between the skin and ice
  - Elevate leg
  - Follow provider advice regarding weight bearing
- Ensure that there is a family member or friend to drive the patient home after discharge

Arthrocentesis

Arthrocentesis is a clinical procedure where fluid is aspirated from a joint (Fig. 52.17). This procedure is done for diagnostic reasons as well as for pain relief. The most common reason for an arthrocentesis is to diagnose gout, arthritis, and synovial infections. This test may be done under guided fluoroscopy or with no imaging guidance at all. Abnormal results for this test include greater than expected amounts of fluid present, abnormal color of joint fluid (i.e., red or cloudy), or purulent fluid.

Preparation of Patient
- Education regarding the procedure
- Positioning of the patient to assure best access to joint to be examined

Nursing Implications
- Assess whether patient is taking any medications, especially anticoagulants or aspirin

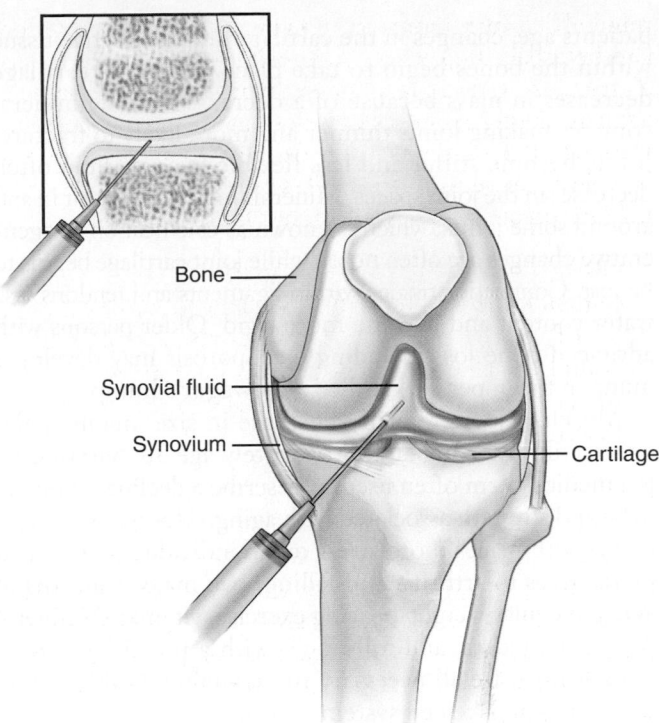

FIGURE 52.17 Arthrocentesis; a procedure to aspirate fluid from a joint for diagnostic reasons as well as for pain relief.

- Ensure "time-out" before the start of the procedure to verify right patient, right procedure, and right anatomical location
- Postprocedure instructions from the practitioner to include the application of ice to the wound for the first 24 hours postprocedure; do not apply ice directly to the skin—use a towel between the skin and ice

Connection Check 52.5

The nurse anticipates which follow-up test after a postmenopausal woman presents with a tibial fracture confirmed by x-ray?

A. Bone scan
B. Arthrogram
C. EMG
D. DEXA scan

AGE-RELATED CHANGES OF THE MUSCULOSKELETAL SYSTEM

Obvious changes with the musculoskeletal system while people age include changes in bone density, posture, and gait. From age 30, bone density begins to diminish. The loss of bone density accelerates in women after menopause because of loss of estrogen. These are not always obvious bone changes that occur in mass or density. Also, while patients age, changes in the cartilage and connective tissue within the bones begin to take place. The joint cartilage decreases in mass because of a decrease in bone mineral content, making joints thinner and more likely to fracture. Joints become stiffer and less flexible because fluid often decreases in the joint spaces. Minerals may also deposit in and around some joints, which is known as calcification. Degenerative changes are often noted while joint cartilage begins to be lost. Connective tissues within ligaments and tendons lose water content and become more rigid. Older persons with advanced bone loss including osteoporosis may develop a hump in the upper back, called a **Dowager's hump**.

Muscle fibers gradually decrease in size, number, and contractility starting at approximately age 30. **Sarcopenia** is a medical term often used to describe a decline in muscle mass and strength associated with aging. This identified loss of strength places more stress on an individual's joints and predisposes to arthritis and falling, two major concerns of aging. Regular weight-bearing exercise, vitamin D/mineral supplementation, and follow-up with a practitioner on a regular basis are all necessary to maintain a healthy, functional musculoskeletal system.

 Safety Alert The following things can be done to help prevent falls in older adults:

1) <u>Exercise regularly:</u> Regular exercise increases joint flexibility, muscle strength, and balance.

2) <u>Review medications:</u> Identification of over-the-counter and prescription medications that may increase dizziness or drowsiness, which predisposes patients to a fall, is essential for safety.

3) <u>Yearly eye examinations:</u> Yearly eye examinations maximize vision and decrease the possibility of falls due to visual impairment.

4) <u>Home safety review:</u> Review the home environment to assess for tripping hazards from rugs and furniture; placement of grab bars in bathrooms around toilets, baths, or showers; and the presence of railings and adequate lighting. Attention to these items can decrease the risk of a fall in the home.

Connection Check 52.6

What are the most important supplements for bone health for patients of advancing age?

A. Calcium and vitamin D
B. Omega-3 fish oil and vitamin D supplements
C. Phosphorus and calcium
D. Phosphorus and omega-3 fish oil supplements

Making Connections

CASE STUDY: WRAP-UP

Abby returns to the ED after her MRI. Results are returned shortly and confirm that Abby has a medial meniscus tear of her left knee. She is promptly fitted for crutches and is given detailed instructions for care at home that include ice, elevation, and immobilization as well as strict follow-up instructions to see an orthopedic surgeon in the next 48 hours.

Case Study Questions

1. Signs and symptoms of an acute knee injury include which of the following?
   A. Pain that is transient
   B. Inability to bear weight
   C. Loss of popliteal pulse
   D. An unsteady gait

2. The ED nurse anticipates the orthopedic surgeon will perform which diagnostic procedure for further analysis of Abby's injury?
   A. Bone scan
   B. X-ray
   C. Arthroscopy
   D. Arthrocentesis

3. Abby's nurse in the ED provides discharge instructions that include which of the following?
   A. Exercise the joint as tolerated
   B. Follow-up with her primary care doctor after swelling has decreased
   C. Ice, elevation, and follow-up with an orthopedic surgeon within 48 hours
   D. Application of warm packs and keeping the leg in a dependent position as often as possible

4. The nurse should intervene if she notices that Abby has which of the following?
   A. Increased pain after immobilization and ice application
   B. Worry about her soccer career
   C. Her leg elevated above the level of her heart
   D. Developed some nausea

5. Which statement by Abby indicates that the discharge teaching has been ineffective?
   A. "Elevation and application of ice to the knee will help decrease swelling."
   B. "Crutches are optional and should be used only if needed."
   C. "Follow-up with an orthopedic surgeon within 48 hours is essential."
   D. "Take pain medication and immobilize the leg."

CHAPTER SUMMARY

The musculoskeletal system, the second largest system of the body, is a group of structures performing in perfect precision allowing for movement, protection of vital organs, production of blood cells in the marrow, support for standing erect, and finally, a reservoir of storage for essential minerals in the bones. The skeleton forms the framework of the human body and consists of 206 bones. These bones support the integumentary system of the body and allow for upright posture and weight bearing.

Muscles are structures that contract and help produce movement. There are three types of muscles present in the human body: skeletal muscle, smooth muscle, and cardiac muscle. The main function of skeletal muscle is movement of the body or its parts under conscious or voluntary control. Smooth muscle is involuntary muscle under the control of the autonomic nervous system which controls contractions of organs and blood vessels automatically. Cardiac muscle is specialized striated muscle that can contract without neural stimulation because of the property of automaticity. Automaticity allows cardiac tissue to set a contraction rhythm through the presence of pacemaker cells.

Joints are defined as a place of union between two or more bones. They permit mobility and provide mechanical support. Ligaments are present at joints to help provide stability to the joint. These fibrous bands composed of tough collagen fibers run directly from one bone to another to reinforce the joint and help prevent undesired directional movements. Tendons are fibrous connective tissues that connect muscle to bone or structures such as the eye.

As with any thorough assessment of a system of the human body, the first step is obtaining the patient's history. After a complete and thorough interview has been obtained from the patient or designee of the patient, a complete and thorough focused physical assessment must take place. A physical examination includes a general inspection of posture, gait, symmetry, joint mobility, bone assessment, and sensation. Inspection includes noting the presence of symmetry, involuntary movements, deformity, swelling/edema, discoloration, hypertrophy/atrophy, and posture/alignment. Palpation is also an important part of the physical examination to assess muscle tone and strength as well as presence of bone integrity. A final part of the physical assessment is radiographical diagnostic studies such as x-rays, CT scans, or MRI. Specialized musculoskeletal studies include arthroscopic examination, electromyography, bone scan, and bone mineral density studies.

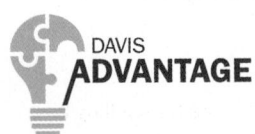

To explore learning resources for this chapter, go to **Davis Advantage** and find:
- Answers to in-text questions
- Chapter Resources and Activities
- NCLEX®-Style Chapter Review Questions
- Bibliography

Chapter 53

Coordinating Care for Patients With Musculoskeletal Disorders

Regina Twigg

LEARNING OUTCOMES

Content in this chapter is designed to assist in:

1. Describing the epidemiology of musculoskeletal disorders
2. Correlating clinical manifestations to pathophysiological processes of:
   a. Muscular dystrophies
   b. Osteoporosis
   c. Paget's disease
   d. Osteomyelitis
   e. Scoliosis
   f. Total joint replacement
   g. Bone cancer
3. Describing the diagnostic results used to confirm the diagnoses for musculoskeletal disorders
4. Discussing the medical management of:
   a. Muscular dystrophies
   b. Osteoporosis
   c. Paget's disease
   d. Osteomyelitis
   e. Scoliosis
   f. Total joint replacement
   g. Bone cancer
5. Developing a comprehensive plan of nursing care for patients with musculoskeletal disorders
6. Designing a plan of care for patients with musculoskeletal disorders that includes pharmacological, dietary, and lifestyle considerations
7. Coordinating the interprofessional plan of care for the patient undergoing joint replacement surgery

ESSENTIAL TERMS

Arthroplasty
Bone mineral density (BMD)
Bone remodeling
Cobb's angle
Dual-energy x-ray absorptiometry (DEXA) scan
Dystrophin
Muscular dystrophy (MD)
Osteoblastic
Osteoblasts
Osteoclastic
Osteoclasts
Osteomyelitis
Osteopenia
Osteoporosis
Osteosarcoma
Osteotomy
Paget's disease of the bone (PDB)
Scoliosis
Spinal instrumentation
Spinal stabilization
Thoracic-lumbar spinal orthotic (TLSO)
Total joint replacement (TJR)

CONCEPTS

- Assessment
- Cellular Regulation
- Infection
- Medication
- Mobility
- Nutrition
- Perioperative
- Promoting Health

Finding Connections

CASE STUDY: EPISODE 1

Follow this patient throughout the chapter.

Eileen Doherty is a 55-year-old female patient who presents to her healthcare provider with complaints of increasing difficulty in walking and increasing pain in her lower back. She shows early signs of kyphosis in her posture. She is currently on no medications and states she takes a multivitamin and calcium "when she remembers them." Eileen has annual checkups with her healthcare provider, and despite her relatively good health, she is concerned about the recent pain and resulting limitations on her activity level...

INTRODUCTION

Musculoskeletal disorders are important to discuss because they impact our ability to move and thus affect our ability to perform activities of daily living. Weakness, pain, or infection affects our movement and/or bone strength, at times limiting our ability to walk. Although not life threatening, foot problems (Table 53.1) or foot pain is a common complaint with many causes. As with other musculoskeletal disorders, however, they can negatively impact our ability to move freely.

This chapter discusses disorders resulting in muscle weakness, weakened bone, disorders that are the result of infection, and musculoskeletal problems that result in pain.

MUSCULAR DYSTROPHIES

Epidemiology

Muscular dystrophy (MD) is a disease with many different subtypes that affect certain muscle groups, are age specific in relation to presenting symptomatology, have variations in severity, and are caused by a defect in different genes. They are classified as an inherited group of progressive myopathic (muscle) disorders that are caused by imperfections in normal muscle function. The primary symptoms are progressive muscle weakening and wasting of skeletal or voluntary muscle groups. Muscular dystrophy can appear at any age from infancy until middle age and beyond. The type of MD and its severity are partially determined by age at onset. Some people with MD have rapidly progressive muscle weakness and wasting and die young, in their 20s. Others experience mild, slowly progressing symptoms and have a normal life span.

Overall, the different types of MD affect more than 50,000 Americans. The most severe forms of MD are Duchenne and Becker. Duchenne muscular dystrophy (DMD) is the most well-known form and is the most common in children. It occurs in one of every 7,250 males between the ages of five and 24. The prevalence for females

Table 53.1 Foot Disorders

Disorder	Description	Symptoms	Management
Hallux valgus (Bunion)	A deformity or lateral deviation in the first metatarsophalangeal joint	Pain at the affected joint	Conservative treatment includes wearing footwear that provides adequate space, foot padding, splinting, foot exercises, and nonsteroidal anti-inflammatories. Surgery is an option if pain or functional disability progress.
Plantar fasciitis	Inflammation of the plantar fascia, the thick band of tissue that connects your heel to your toes	Stabbing heel pain that is typically worse with the first steps in the morning, decreasing in severity while the foot loosens up	Conservative therapies include physical therapy, night splints that stretch the calf and arch of the foot, orthotics, and nonsteroidal anti-inflammatories
Morton's neuroma	A neuroma or thickening of nerve tissue that occurs between the third and fourth toes	Pain, tingling, burning, or numbness, and/or a feeling that something is inside the ball of the foot or something is bunched up in the shoe under the ball of the foot	Conservative treatment includes padding to support the metatarsal arch, icing the affected area, orthotics, nonsteroidal anti-inflammatories, or injections of cortisone or local anesthetics into the affected area
Flatfoot (pes planus)	Loss of metatarsal arch	Pain in the foot primarily in the heel or arch	Treatment includes orthotics to provide arch support, stretching exercises, and a structurally supportive shoe

is three per 100,000. Approximately two-thirds of all cases have a genetic component, and the remaining one-third of the reported cases are found to be caused by new genetic mutations. Becker MD is also primarily prevalent in males and typically occurs in childhood. Myotonic dystrophy is the most common form of MD found in adults. The inherited X chromosome link is the only known associated risk factor (see Genetic Connections: Muscular Dystrophy).

Genetic Connections

Muscular Dystrophy

The Duchenne and Becker muscular dystrophies (MDs) are caused by a mutation to the dystrophin gene. Dystrophin is a protein responsible for muscle repair. Persons affected by MD are lacking the dystrophin gene, thereby resulting in the inability to repair muscle. Both Duchenne and Becker MDs are inherited X-linked recessive traits; the gene responsible for these conditions is located on one of the two sex chromosomes, the X chromosome. Because males have only one X chromosome, one altered gene can cause the disorder. Females have two X chromosomes. The gene mutation has to be present on both to cause the disorder. Because of this, MDs are far more common in boys. Females can be carriers but are not typically affected by the disease. The diagnosis of MD usually includes genetic testing. Genetic counseling is recommended for those with a family history of MD.

Connection Check 53.1

The nurse recognizes which patient is at greatest risk for development of DMD?
A. Female at birth
B. Male at birth
C. Female at adolescence
D. Male at adolescence

Pathophysiology

The Duchenne and Becker muscular dystrophies (MDs) are caused by a mutation to the dystrophin gene. **Dystrophin,** a protein responsible for muscle repair, is located on the plasma membrane of muscle fibers and provides reinforcement and stabilization of the glycoprotein complex (a molecule that contains carbohydrate and protein). In the absence or reduction of dystrophin, the glycoprotein complex is digested by proteases, which causes degeneration of the muscle fibers resulting in muscle weakness. The primary commonalities among all the MD disorders are progressive

muscle weakness, muscle wasting, and increased muscle enzyme serum levels. With the wasting and breakdown of muscles, serum enzymes such as creatine kinase (CK), lactate dehydrogenase (LD), alanine aminotransferase (ALT), aspartate aminotransferase (AST), and aldolase are elevated and are used in clinical practice to measure the extent of damage and/or deterioration.

Clinical Manifestations

There are nine subgroups of the MDs. Each has a distinct clinical presentation; however, all present with progressive muscle weakness and all typically present with chronic pain, most notably in the lower back and legs. See Figure 53.1 for areas of muscle weakness associated with each subgroup of MD.

The nine subgroups of MD are as follows:

- Duchenne
- Becker
- Myotonic
- Facioscapulohumeral
- Limb-girdle
- Oculopharyngeal
- Congenital
- Distal
- Emery-Dreifuss

With progressive deterioration and weakness to the facial, limb, respiratory, and cardiac muscles, the ultimate result is muscular damage. This is caused primarily by the lack of the key protein (dystrophin) to maintain the integrity of the muscle fibers as well as the ability to repair muscle tissue while it breaks down and/or deteriorates. Muscle bulk is reduced, resulting in fat and excessive scar tissue. Because of progressive muscle wasting and weakness, falls are often associated with MD, which puts patients at risk for fractures. Progressive deterioration of facial muscles is associated with problems with dental hygiene, speech clarity, and articulation. As a result of immobility, gastrointestinal (GI) dysfunction is often associated with MD. The most life-threatening result of this progressive deterioration is the cardiopulmonary compromise that occurs as a result of the development of cardiomyopathy. Cardiomyopathy, a form of heart disease that presents with weakened heart muscle and decreased pumping ability, results in arrhythmias, shortness of breath, and extreme fatigue. Refer to Table 53.2 for a summary of the subtypes of MD.

Connection Check 53.2

The nurse recognizes that which of the following pathophysiological manifestations are associated with MD? *(Select all that apply.)*
A. Decreased tissue oxygenation
B. Decreased blood flow to muscles
C. Degeneration of muscle fibers
D. Decrease in enzyme activity
E. Increased muscle bulk

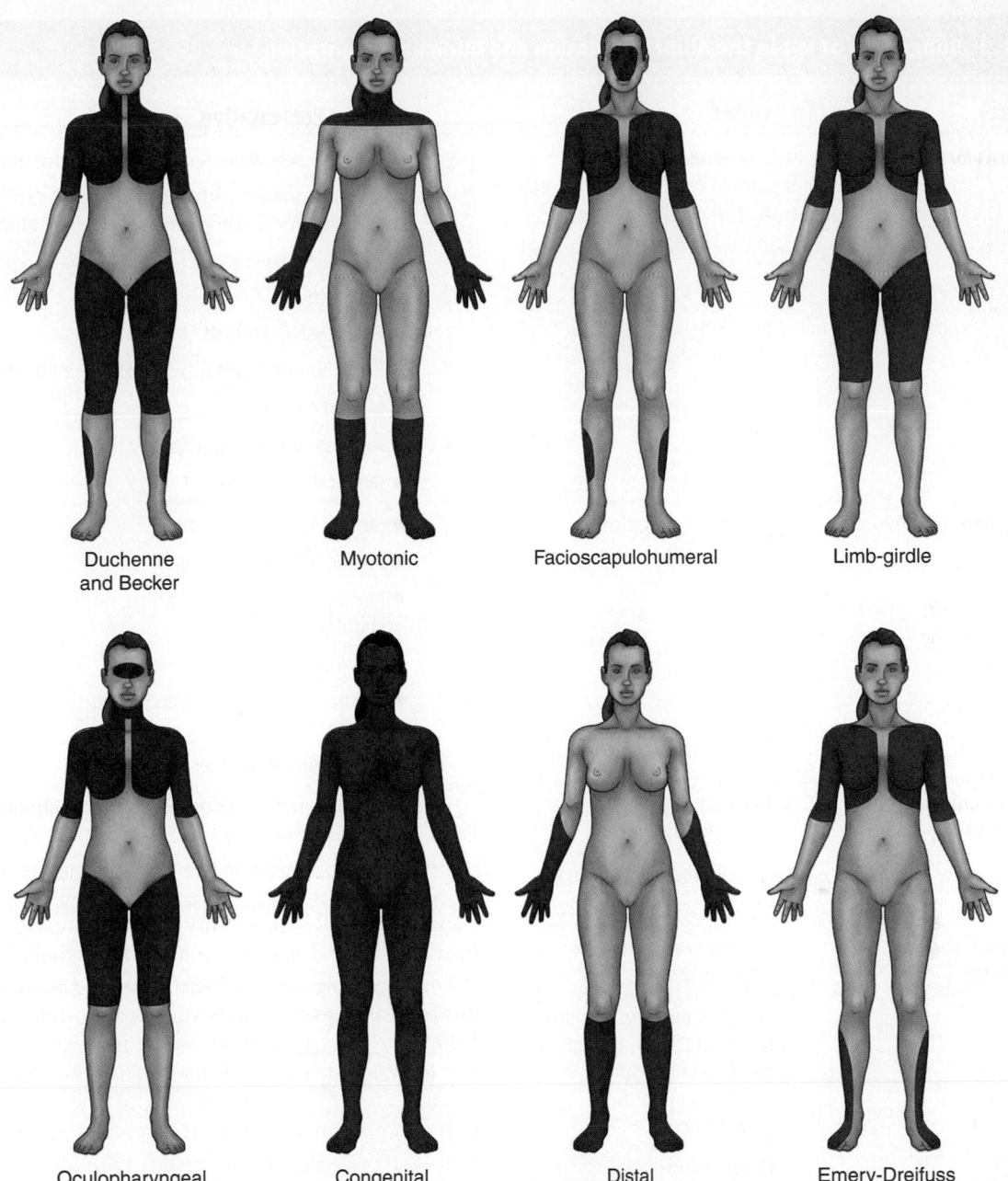

FIGURE 53.1 Main areas of muscle weakness in different subtypes of muscular dystrophy.

Management

Medical Management

Diagnosis

Diagnosis of MD usually begins with a preliminary review of serum muscle enzymes such as CK, which is usually an early sign of the disease and requires frequent and close monitoring. Other serum enzymes such as LD, ALT, AST, and aldolase are elevated and are frequently evaluated in clinical practice to monitor for muscle wasting and/or deterioration. Recent literature supports monitoring serum creatinine levels as a differential diagnosis between Duchenne and Becker MD, as well as a prognostic indicator of severity of disease progression. Other diagnostic studies such as chest x-ray, electrocardiogram, computed tomography (CT), and electromyography are frequently warranted to determine the extent of muscle wasting or the presence of cardiopulmonary compromise associated with the disease.

The Muscular Dystrophy Association and Center for Disease Control and prevention suggest early screening, diagnosis, and intervention. A definitive diagnosis for MD is often difficult secondary to the fact that the clinical presentations for all MDs are similar in nature. Among the medical community, the gold standard is the muscle biopsy in which a small piece of muscle tissue is extracted and examined for changes in the structure of the muscle cells. If MD is present, changes are visible, and the biopsy can begin to detect the form of MD present in the tissue sample. The diagnostic criteria for nearly all MDs now incorporate genetic testing (see Genetic Connections: Muscular Dystrophy).

Table 53.2 Subgroups of MD in the Adult Population and Clinical Presentation

Type	Onset	Clinical Presentation
Duchenne muscular dystrophy (DMD)	2–4 years of age	<ul><li>Limb muscle weakness (proximal more than distal)</li><li>Positive Gowers' sign (muscle weakness of the proximal muscles, more commonly seen in lower limbs)</li><li>Calf enlargement</li><li>Leg pain</li><li>Progressive scoliosis</li><li>Equinovarus (clubfoot) deformities of the feet</li><li>Mental retardation</li><li>Progressive cardiomyopathy</li><li>Respiratory failure</li></ul>
Becker muscular dystrophy (BMD)	Delayed onset, slower progression 5–25 years of age	<ul><li>Similar symptoms as DMD</li><li>Milder, slower progression</li><li>Muscle wasting affecting hips, pelvic area, thighs, and shoulders</li><li>Calves enlarged</li><li>Cardiac involvement less common, but if present more severe</li><li>Mental retardation less common</li></ul>
Emery-Dreifuss muscular dystrophy (EDMD)	Delayed onset, slower progression Usually seen by 10 years of age	<ul><li>Wasting and weakness of muscles in shoulders, upper arms, and calf</li><li>Contractures in neck, elbows, and heels early in disease</li><li>Cardiac involvement that leads to need for pacemaker</li></ul>
Oculopharyngeal muscular dystrophy (OPMD)	Usually seen mid-40s to 50 years of age French-Canadian families or family of French-Canadian descent and Hispanic residents of northern New Mexico Progression is slow	<ul><li>Ptosis</li><li>Weakness of the facial muscles and pharyngeal muscles</li><li>Dysphagia</li></ul>
Limb-girdle muscular dystrophy (LGMD)	Progression variable Severe disability 10 years postdiagnosis Usually seen in mid-20s to 30s	<ul><li>Upper extremity and neck weakness</li><li>Lower extremity and hip muscle weakness</li></ul>
Facioscapulohumeral muscular dystrophy (FSH or FSHD) *Also known as Landouzy-Dejerine*	Manifestations usually appear in adolescence, but onset and severity are widely variable	<ul><li>Weakness and deterioration around eyes, mouth, and upper shoulders</li><li>Lower extremity weakness with later signs of weakness to abdominal and occasionally hip muscles</li></ul>
Myotonic	Most common form in adults	<ul><li>Prolonged spasm or stiffening of muscles after use</li></ul>
Congenital	Present at birth Progress slowly	<ul><li>Severe contractures</li></ul>
Distal	Rare Progresses slowly Affects fewer muscles	<ul><li>Muscle weakness and wasting in the distal extremities</li></ul>

Treatment

The medical management of MD focuses on the prevention of progressive deterioration of the disease, supportive measures to assist maximization of functional capacity, and pain management. There is no specific cure or pharmacological intervention. Glucocorticoid therapy is frequently the medication of choice in conjunction with supportive and collaborative care; however, practitioners need to be cognizant of the correlation of high dose steroid usage and increased propensity to obesity. Glucocorticoids such as prednisone have been shown to decrease the rate of muscle deterioration and increase restorative functional abilities. The pharmacodynamic principle of this therapy focuses on reduction of inflammation and regulation of metabolic pathways of proteins, carbohydrates, and fats, which thereby results in a decrease of enzyme activity and reduced muscle destruction. Many patients and healthcare providers support an integrative therapy regimen that includes the use of supplements such as coenzyme Q10, carnitine, amino acids (glutamine, arginine), anti-inflammatory medications, and antioxidants (fish oil, vitamin E, green tea extract) in addition to corticosteroid therapy. In addition to steroid therapy, pain management is primarily done with medications such as Tylenol, aspirin, or ibuprofen.

The psychosocial management of MD is even more complicated and intensive. Often, the stress associated with psychosocial management of MD exceeds that of the physical aspects of the disease. Supportive care is necessary on multilevel and multisystem perspectives. The focus is adapting to the deterioration of physical capacities and overall changes in roles and functional abilities. A referral to the Muscular Dystrophy Association (MDA) for supportive services and genetic counseling information is medically recommended.

Complications

Spinal deformity and neuromuscular deterioration causing weakness of the trunk and lower extremities are severe complications of MD. With the development of **scoliosis** (curvature of the spine) and overall thoracic-lumbar changes, respiratory and cardiac compromise can develop. Total contact orthotic devices that support the trunk assist with minimization of spinal deformity and support cardiovascular function to prevent cardiac compromise that can occur with progressive MD. Ineffective cardiovascular and pulmonary functions are additional life-threatening complications that result with progressive MD.

Nursing Management

Assessment and Analysis

Many of the clinical manifestations observed in patients with MD are directly linked to the progressive muscle weakness and wasting that occur at a neuromuscular level. Common findings include:

- Weakness that affects the proximal before the distal limb muscles
- Difficulty with running, jumping, and walking up stairs
- Lumbar lordosis (excessive inward curvature of the lumbar spine)
- Calf enlargement
- Cardiomyopathy, especially involving the atrioventricular (AV) node
- Later cardiovascular disease associated with cardiomyopathy, such as heart failure (left ventricular)
- Respiratory compromise
- Falls leading to fractures
- Depression

Nursing Diagnoses

- **Impaired physical mobility** associated with decreased muscle tone in the lower extremities as evidenced by the inability to walk independently
- **Risk for dysphagia** associated with decreased facial movement and/or cranial nerve VII dysfunction
- **Risk for falls** associated with decreased muscle tone in the lower extremities
- **Risk for decreased cardiac output** associated with AV node dysfunction
- **Risk for ineffective breathing patterns** associated with lumbar posture deformity

Nursing Interventions

■ *Assessments*

- Vital signs—heart rate, blood pressure, and pulse oximetry (SpO_2)
  Increased heart rate, decreased blood pressure, and decreased SpO_2 may indicate deterioration of cardiovascular and respiratory status.
- Forced vital capacity
  The amount of air exhaled during a forced exhalation, FVC, has a predictive value in assessing pulmonary function.
- Chest x-ray
  Changing chest x-ray indicates potential for respiratory compromises due to changes in skeletal structure.
- Laboratory enzymes
  Increased CK, LD, ALT, AST, and aldolase lactic levels indicate muscle deterioration and break down.
  Increased serum and 24-hour urine creatinine clearance levels indicate differential diagnosis and severity of muscle deterioration and disease progression.
- Electrocardiogram
  Atrioventricular node disturbances indicate changes in cardiac electrical activity and can be indicative of cardiac compromise.
- Functional level
  Decreases in functionality may indicate worsening progression of the disease, requiring more orthopedic and/or cardiovascular support.
- Pain
  Pain that is in control helps keep the patient active, which maximizes function and decreases immobility, which can lead to potential contractures or deformities

in the muscles that result from shortening of muscle tissue.

Actions

- Administer corticosteroid therapy as ordered
  Shown to decrease the rate of muscle deterioration and increase restorative functional abilities. The pharmacodynamic principles of this therapy focus on decreasing inflammation and regulating the metabolic pathways of proteins, carbohydrates, and fats, which thereby decreases enzyme activity and reduces muscle destruction.
- Pain management—administer aspirin, ibuprofen, Tylenol as ordered for pain control
  Managing pain is essential to maintaining mobility as much as possible.
- Range-of-motion exercises
  Maximize function and decrease potential contractures
- Put patient on fall precautions
  Because of increasing weakness, the patient is at increased risk for falls and fractures.
- Collaborative care with occupational therapy, physical therapy, and rehabilitative medicine team
  Coordinated care with an interprofessional team helps maximize comfort, mobility, and function.

Teaching

- Reinforce exercises and physical and occupational therapy regimens
  Assist with comfort and mobility and delay further deterioration and contractures
- With family members, recognize signs of caregiver burden
  Most patients with MD are cared for at home even as they progress to a very dependent ventilator dependent state as a result of cardiopulmonary compromise. Increasing dependency on family members can cause caregiver strain and burden. Family members should be taught to recognize these symptoms and recognize the need to contact supportive services such as the MDA to provide respite care when needed.
- Genetic counseling (see Genetic Connections: Muscular Dystrophy)
  Highly recommended by the MDA

Evaluating Care Outcomes

The ultimate outcome for the patient with MD is to promote and maintain optimal levels of function and comfort and a prescribed quality of life within the limitations of the disease (see Evidence-Based Practice). Supportive and collaborative care for both the patient and the family is an essential component of nursing care for the MD population, promoting maximal wellness in the patient and controlling caregiver burden. Disability is the greatest fear; thus, supportive and psychiatric care are essential to the holistic nursing approach for this patient population.

Evidence-Based Practice

Muscular Dystrophy Surveillance, Tracking, and Research Network

The Center for Disease Control and Prevention (CDC) supports the Muscular Dystrophy Surveillance, Tracking, and Research Network (MD STARnet) with the provision of funding in an effort to collect data about persons affected by MD. This surveillance and monitoring program is aimed at improving the quality of life and care for those living with the disease. Most programs collect information on persons with MD who are treated in hospitals, clinics or via medical specialists. MD STARnet is the only research-based program that monitors and gathers information from all persons affected with MD who live in the United States. This large-scale research program can provide more data and healthcare information based on the enormity of numbers which can help move the research for MD forward in the future.

Centers for Disease Control and Prevention, National Center for Health Statistics. (2018). MD StarNET Data and Statistics. Retrieved from www.cdc.gov/ncbddd/musculardystrophy/data.html

CASE STUDY: EPISODE 2

Eileen Doherty has returned to her healthcare provider with complaints of increasing pain in her lower back and the "feeling like I could fall" while walking. Her kyphotic posture appears to be worsening, and when her height is measured, it is noted that she has a decrease from 5 ft 3 in. to 5 ft 2.5 in. over the course of the year. She remains on her medication regimen of multivitamins and calcium and states she has begun to take Aleve (naproxen) for pain. She is very concerned about her fear of falling, increasing level of pain, and decreasing level of function…

OSTEOPOROSIS

Epidemiology

Osteoporosis is a chronic condition that results in deterioration of bone tissue and density, increasing a patient's risk for fractures. It is the most common bone disease in humans and creates a major public health concern for the future. The International Osteoporosis Foundation (IOF) estimates that osteoporosis effects 75 million people in Europe, United States and Japan. The National Osteoporosis Foundation (NOF) estimates that 9.9 million Americans have osteoporosis and approximately 43.1 million have a low bone density. One in two women and one in five men older than 50 years of age will sustain an osteoporotic fracture and 50% of all postmenopausal women will sustain an osteoporotic fracture. Of these women, 25% will exhibit clinical signs of vertebral deformity and 15% will develop a hip fracture in their lifetime. Approximately one-third of men who experience a hip fracture as a result of osteoporosis will die within 1 year after sustaining the fracture. The NOF states that all ethnic backgrounds are affected by osteoporosis; however, 20% of non-Hispanic, Caucasian, and Asian women aged 50 years and older are estimated to have osteoporosis. Of these women, 52% have a low bone density score. The statistics for men are 7% of non-Hispanic, Caucasian, and Asian men aged 50 years and older are estimated to have osteoporosis, and 35% of these are estimated have a low bone density. Additionally, 33.6 million Americans have low bone density of the hip, which increases the risk for osteoporosis. Caucasian small-framed women with a lower body weight have the highest risk factor for the development of osteoporosis.

The annual cost for osteoporotic fractures in the United States is $19 billion, and in 2025 that cost is estimated to rise to $25.3 billion. Those who sustain an osteoporotic hip fracture have an estimated mortality in excess of a 10% to 20% death rate within a year. Osteoporosis-related fractures are associated with a heavy economic burden, with more than 432,000 hospital admissions, 2.5 million medical office visits, and more than 180,000 admissions to long-term care facilities. These statistics and financial costs are estimated to continue to grow while the population continues to age.

The risk factors for osteoporosis are defined as primary and secondary. Primary risk factors are those that are non-modifiable, such as age or race, and lifestyle choices such as sedentary lifestyle, not enough calcium intake, or smoking. Secondary risk factors include other disease states that are associated with an increased risk such as Cushing's disease or medication use such as steroids (Table 53.3). Although not totally understood, Down's syndrome is also associated with an increased risk of osteoporosis, potentially associated with the accelerated aging associated with that syndrome.

Table 53.3 Primary and Secondary Risk Factors for Osteoporosis

Primary Risk Factors	Secondary Risk Factors
Genetics	*Medications*
● Age (older than 50 and postmenopausal)	● Corticosteroid therapy for more than 3 months
● Gender (females greater than males)	● Anticonvulsants
● Race (Caucasian or Asian)	● Heparin therapy
● Family history	● Thyroid hormones
● Smaller body frame (< 58 kg)	
Nutrition	*Disease pathology*
● Low calcium intake	● Cushing's disease
● Low vitamin D intake	● Hypogonadism or premature menopause
● High potassium intake	● Malabsorptive issues (Crohn's, celiac disease, gastric surgery, etc.)
● Inadequate calories	
Lifestyle	
● Sedentary lifestyle	● Chronic liver disease
● Cigarette smoking	● Inflammatory bowel disease
● Excessive alcohol consumption (more than three glasses per day)	● Rheumatoid arthritis
	● Hyperthyroidism
	● Hyperparathyroidism
	● Previous fracture
	Other
	● Parental history of hip fracture
	● Recurrent falls
	● Prolonged immobilization

Connection Check 53.3

Which of the following is a risk factor associated with osteoporosis?
A. African American
B. Weight greater than 58 kg
C. Hispanic
D. Weight less than 58 kg

Pathophysiology

Bone is a living, growing tissue that constantly forms new bone while replacing older bone through a process called **bone remodeling**. It is maintained by two types of bone cells, osteoclasts, and osteoblasts. **Osteoclasts** break down bone by adhering to the surface of the bone and secreting acids and enzymes directly into the bone cavity; **osteoblasts** rebuild the bone by synthesis and mineralization of the new bony matrix within the bone cavity. It is thought to be a preventive measure by removing older bone and replacing with newer bone. Bone loss (**osteopenia**) occurs when bone resorption or **osteoclastic** activity is greater than bone rebuilding or **osteoblastic** activity, which ultimately results in a decreased bone mineral density (BMD). The resulting bone loss causes changes in the skeletal structure and results in an increased risk for fractures.

Bone mineral density (BMD) peaks between 25 and 30 years of age; then, as a result of aging and other associated risk factors, bone remodeling is altered. Some important factors to note that occur with aging are 1) a decrease in calcitonin levels, a hormone that decreases osteoclastic activity; 2) a decrease in estrogen levels, which results in the inhibition of bone formation; and 3) an increase in the parathyroid hormone, which increases osteoclastic activity and bone turnover. All of these changes produce a decrease in the BMD; hence, the bones become more porous, brittle, and fragile, thereby increasing the risk for fractures (Fig. 53.2). Trabecular, or cancellous (spongy), bone loss is thought to occur first, which is then followed by loss of the compact (cortical) bone. Most frequently noted areas of bone loss are associated with vertebral changes of the lumbar spine and hip fractures, and Colles' fracture of the wrist.

Clinical Manifestations

Osteoporosis is also frequently referred to as the "silent disease" secondary to the fact that patients are not diagnosed until a fracture occurs after an unremarkable fall or strain. Fragility fractures most often occur in the spine, hip, and distal radius. Because of this, it is important to understand the risk factors of this disease. Prevention is the key modifying factor to incorporate into the medical care for patients at risk for osteoporosis.

Management

Medical Management

Diagnosis

Universal recommendations call for annual height measurements with a preferred wall-mounted stadiometer. The gold standard assessment for osteoporosis is BMD measurements for women over the age of 65 or men over 70 and for

postmenopausal women and men 50 to 69 with a high risk-factor profile. They are obtained through a **dual-energy x-ray absorptiometry (DEXA) scan**. A DEXA scan gives precise measurements at clinically relevant skeletal points within the body, which highlight areas for future fracture risks. The DEXA scan reports T scores of the standard deviation above or below the mean for healthy young individuals. A low BMD, one that is 2.5 standard deviations or more below the mean for a young adult person, is highly correlated with an increased risk for fractures. A BMD that is low but not at the level of osteoporosis is indicative of **osteopenia**, a precursor to osteoporosis (Table 53.4).

Another assessment tool, quantitative computed tomography (QCT) measures volumetric bone density of the spine and hip and can identify cortical and trabecular bones distinctly. This tool is not recommended for screening but for research and diagnostic management. The literature also supports the use of ultrasonography as a good predictor for fractures and osteoporosis risk for both men and women. The major limitation with this diagnostic tool is associated with limited precision.

Although there is no definitive laboratory test to confirm osteoporosis, biochemical markers are helpful in providing insightful information associated with the status of bone remodeling. Biochemical markers of bone remodeling reflect the overall rate of bone resorption and formation. Some of the biochemical markers that are used to monitor effectiveness of treatment are bone-specific alkaline phosphatase, osteocalcin, N-telopeptide (NTX), and C-telopeptide. Numerous other laboratory studies (serum and/or urine calcium, vitamin D, phosphorous, serum alkaline phosphatase, hematocrit, erythrocyte sedimentation rate (ESR), and urine hydroxyproline excretion) can be used to rule out secondary osteoporosis and/or other metabolic bone disorders such as Paget's disease or osteomalacia. Additionally, tests such as protein measurements can be done to rule out hyperthyroidism.

Another important step in assessing osteoporosis is fracture risk assessment screening. The most widely used tool is the Fracture Risk Assessment Tool, or FRAX, which was

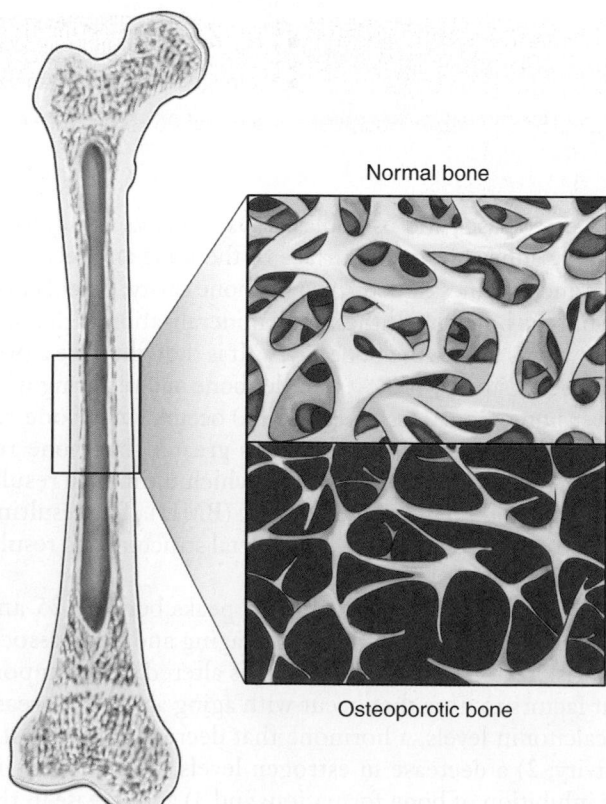

Normal bone

Osteoporotic bone

FIGURE 53.2 Bony changes indicative of osteoporosis.

Table 53.4 WHO Criteria for Diagnosis of Osteoporosis

Classification	Score
Normal	BMD within 1 SD of young normal adult, T-score –1.0 or higher
Low bone mass, or osteopenia	BMD between 1 and 2.5 SDs lower than that of a young normal adult, T-score between –1.0 and –2.5
Osteoporosis	BMD more than 2.5 SDs lower than that of a young normal adult, T-score –2.5 or lower

WHO, World Health Organization; *BMD*, bone mineral density; *SD*, standard deviation.

developed by the World Health Organization's Collaborating Centre for Metabolic Bone Disease. The FRAX uses clinical risk factors with or without BMD to assess a person's 10-year risk for the development of fractures. This tool collects information on numerous key issues and associated clinical risk factors and then calculates a 10-year probability for hip and any one of four major osteoporotic fractures. The medical convenience of the FRAX tool is the ability to link directly to the National Osteoporosis Guideline Group algorithms and guidelines for clinical management. The FRAX tool is not used for patients under the age of 40 and over the age of 90 years.

Because of the silent nature of the disease, x-rays are not commonly used for osteoporosis screening and assessment. It is estimated that a change of greater than 25% to 40% in demineralization of the bone would need to be evident to be detected via x-ray.

Treatment

Prevention and early screening are the treatment focus for osteoporosis. The NOF advocates for a comprehensive approach to the management of osteoporosis. Weight loss and muscle-strengthening exercises to reduce the incidence of falls and fractures are highly recommended. Additionally, a healthy lifestyle that includes weight bearing exercise that helps build and maintain strong bones, and avoidance of smoking and excessive alcohol intake (more than three drinks per day) are endorsed by the surgeon general as a means for prevention of osteoporosis.

Medications

Pharmacological intervention is focused on preventing and slowing the progression of bone loss. The first line of prevention is safe and inexpensive with the use of calcium and vitamin D. The recommended dose of calcium either via dietary consumption or via supplements varies by age; however, 1,200 mg/day is the recommended daily intake for adults 51 years of age or older. The average person ingests between 600 and 700 mg per day; therefore, supplementation is necessary to maintain serum calcium levels required to support and maintain skeletal function. Higher doses of calcium (1,200 to 1,500 mg per day) have been shown to have limited benefit and are correlated with a higher incidence of the development of kidney stones and cardiovascular disease. Vitamin D helps with calcium absorption within the intestines and assists with the maintenance of adequate serum calcium levels that are imperative for bone health, muscle performance, and decreased risk for falling. The recommended intake for vitamin D is 800 to 1,000 international units (IU), which can be ingested from dietary sources such as vitamin D–fortified milk, cereals, egg yolks, saltwater fish, and liver. Sunlight for 15 minutes per day also helps with vitamin D and calcium absorption. Other pharmacological options for prevention and/or treatment of osteoporosis are listed in Table 53.5. The NOF endorses the Food and Drug Administration (FDA)–approved medications for the prevention of osteoporosis and decreased fracture risks; however, the organization does encourage practitioners to assess the potential

Table 53.5 Pharmacological Interventions for Treatment of Osteoporosis

Class and Mechanism of Action	Generic/Trade Name	Method of Administration	Special Considerations
Bisphosphonate Impedes bone resorption by inhibiting osteoclastic activity, thereby absorbing calcium phosphate in bone	Alendronate (Fosamax or Fosamax Plus D)	Daily or weekly tablet (must be taken on empty stomach)	All bisphosphonates can cause GI disturbance, dysphagia, and inflammation of esophagus
	Ibandronate (Boniva)	Monthly tablet (on an empty stomach) or IV infusion every 3 months	
	Risedronate (Actonel or Actonel with Calcium)	Daily or weekly tablet (must be taken on empty stomach)	
	Zoledronate (Reclast, zoledronic acid)	Annual IV infusion	Zoledronate has been shown to have higher risk for development of atrial fibrillation
Calcitonin Decreases osteoclastic activity in bone, decreases mineral release and collagen breakdown in bone, and assists with renal excretion of calcium	Miacalcin or Fortical	Intranasal spray daily; subcutaneous injection available	Can cause rhinitis and rarely epistaxis

Continued

Table 53.5 Pharmacological Interventions for Treatment of Osteoporosis—cont'd

Class and Mechanism of Action	Generic/Trade Name	Method of Administration	Special Considerations
Estrogen/Hormone therapy Estrogen assists with bone remodeling and osteoclastic activity	Estrace, Estraderm, Premarin	Varied methods of administration	Risk for MI, stroke, breast cancer, PE, and DVT
Estrogen agonist/antagonist (formally known as selective estrogen receptor modulators, or SERMs) Assists with bone remodeling and osteoclastic activity	Raloxifene	Daily tablet	DVT
Parathyroid hormone Parathyroid hormone is thought to protect against gonadotropin-releasing hormone agonist-related bone loss	PTH (1-34), Forteo	Subcutaneous injection daily	Leg cramps, dizziness
Parathyroid hormone analog Increases bone density and strength	Abaloparatide (Tymlos)	Periumbical subcutaneous injection daily	Dizziness or tachycardia
Dual-acting bone agent Decreases osteoclastic activity and increases osteoblastic activity, thereby balancing bone turnover, increasing bone formation/remodeling	Strontium ranelate	Daily soluble sachet	Non-FDA approved
Monoclonal activity Inhibits osteoclastic function, formation, and survival, thereby reducing osteoclastic bone resorption	Denosumab	Subcutaneous injection every 6 months	Non-FDA approved Can be used with patients that cannot take bisphosphonates or patient with reduced renal function Causes infections

DVT, Deep vein thrombosis; *FDA,* Food and Drug Administration; *GI,* gastrointestinal; *IV,* intravenous; *MI,* myocardial infarction; *PE,* pulmonary embolism.

benefits versus risk with each individual patient. The NOF recognizes but does not endorse those non-FD-approved medications for the treatment and prevention of osteoporosis.

Complications

The complications of osteoporosis surround the skeletal changes that occur as a result of bone loss and lack of bone remodeling. Patients with osteoporosis are more at risk for falls, which incurs a greater risk for fractures, specifically vertebral compression fractures and hip fractures. All fractures in older adults can result in a higher incidence of prolonged hospitalization and ultimately death.

Nursing Management

Assessment and Analysis

Many of the clinical manifestations observed in the patient with osteoporosis are directly associated with a decrease in

bone resorption and bone building, which lead to osteopenia (bone loss) and osteoporosis. Common findings include:

- "Dowager's hump" (kyphosis of the dorsal spine)
- Loss of height (loss as great as 2 to 3 in. [5–7.5 cm])
- Back pain (sharp or acute)
- Pain increased with activity and relieved with rest
- Restriction of movement, especially in the thoracic and lumbar regions
- Fear of falling (known as "fallophobia") and/or history of previous falls
- Previous fractures

Other clinical manifestations such as constipation, abdominal distention, and reflux esophagitis are associated with the decrease in movement and spinal deformity. Potential respiratory complications are due to curvature of the spinal column and decreased chest excursion.

Nursing Diagnoses

- **Risk for trauma** associated with bone loss and the potential for falls and/or fractures
- **Impaired physical mobility** associated with pain and musculoskeletal changes

Nursing Interventions

▣ *Assessments*

- Fall risk
  Age and change in skeletal structure (bone loss and decrease in BMD) can result in deformity and disability, which are correlated with the potential for falls and resulting fractures
- Pain
  The presence of pain decreases mobility and optimal functioning.
- Nutritional status
  Adequate ingestion of protein, magnesium, vitamin K, calcium, vitamin D, and trace elements is essential for bone formation and remodeling.
- Assess level of activity and exercise
  Exercise is an integral part of prevention and management for osteoporosis and pain control. Strive for an active lifestyle.
- Body image disturbance
  Skeletal changes can cause issues associated with posture (kyphosis), decrease in limb length (specifically lower extremities), and difficulty with clothing fitting appropriately. Physical appearance can change and cause issues associated with self-esteem.

▣ *Actions*

- Administer one of the following medications as ordered
  - Bisphosphonates
    Impedes bone resorption by inhibiting osteoclastic activity, thereby absorbing calcium phosphate in bone
  - Calcitonin
    Decreases osteoclastic activity in bone, decreases mineral release and collagen breakdown in bone, and assists with renal excretion of calcium
  - Estrogen/Hormone therapy
    Estrogen assists with bone remodeling and osteoclastic activity
  - Estrogen agonist/antagonist
    Assists with bone remodeling and osteoclastic activity
  - Parathyroid hormone
    Parathyroid hormone is thought to protect against gonadotropin-releasing hormone agonist-related bone loss
  - Parathyroid hormone analogs
    Parathyroid hormone analog is thought to increase bone density and strength; thereby reducing fracture risk.
  - Dual-acting bone agent
    Decreases osteoclastic activity and increases osteoblastic activity, thereby balancing bone turnover, increasing bone formation/remodeling
  - Monoclonal activity
    Inhibits osteoclastic function, formation, and survival, thereby reducing osteoclastic bone resorption

- Support exercise program/Implement steps to correct or supplement underlying physical and functional deficits
  Exercises for strengthening abdominal and back muscles are essential to the promotion of function and safety. Low intensity weight bearing exercise such as walking is effective. Improved posture, balance, and strengthened muscle tone will enable the patient to move safely, promote functional capability, and decrease risk for falls.
- Provide training for safe movement with activities of daily living
  This patient population is at great risk for falls with transfers and lifting. Use assistive devices when appropriate.
- Contact home health agency for a home environmental safety evaluation
  High risk for falls and fractures, so home environment needs to be evaluated for environmental and safety hazards

▣ *Teaching*

- Take medication as prescribed
  Many of the bisphosphonates need to be ingested first thing in the morning on an empty stomach. They can cause GI disturbances, esophagitis, and visual disturbances. These side effects need to be reported to provider as soon as possible.
- Instruct patient in weight reduction if necessary
  Weight loss has been shown to decrease stress on the skeletal structure.
- Instruct patient to incorporate adequate ingestion of vitamin D and calcium
  Medications may cause a decrease in calcium levels. Calcium helps with collagen synthesis and bone formation, thereby assisting with maintaining bone health. Vitamin D facilitates calcium absorption in the GI system.

Evaluating Care Outcomes

Patients with osteoporosis can live a functional and safe lifestyle if best practice standards are followed and maintained. The evaluative outcomes focus on early identification of the risk for fracture and/or osteoporosis. Education and support for patients with dietary and lifestyle issues, as well as education and discussion surrounding bone-sparing medications such as bisphosphonates are essential. Persistence with a healthy lifestyle and monitoring of the treatment regimen have been shown to be highly effective.

PAGET'S DISEASE

Epidemiology

Paget's disease is the second-most common bone disease with approximately 1% to 2% of the white adult male population older than 50 years of age being affected. Results obtained via autopsy approximate 3% to 3.7% of the patients older than 40 years of age were affected. Prevalence increases with age, with approximately 8% of the male gender and 5% of the female gender affected in their eighth decade of life. It is most commonly associated with men of

Caucasian, European, Dutch, and/or British descent. For reasons not completely understood, the disease is most common in the United Kingdom, specifically Lancashire towns.

Genetics have been linked to 15% to 40% of the known cases of Paget's disease. It is most commonly associated with an autosomal dominant trait that is more pronounced in the fifth to sixth decade of life. Also, research from the University of Pittsburgh School of Medicine has linked a gene from the measles virus with Paget's disease. It is thought that having measles during childhood is an environmental trigger for the disease.

Pathophysiology

Paget's disease of the bone (PDB), also referred to as *osteitis deformans,* is a bone metabolism disorder associated with accelerated bone remodeling, resulting in bone that is structurally abnormal. The skeletal areas most commonly affected are the skull, femur, tibia, pelvic bones, and vertebral column. Because of the insidious nature of the disease, a confirmed diagnosis is not known until a fracture develops or occurs.

As discussed in osteoporosis, bone is constantly renewed through the process of remodeling maintained by two types of bone cells, osteoclasts and osteoblasts. Osteoclasts break down bone by adhering to the surface of the bone and secreting acids and enzymes directly into the bone cavity; osteoblasts rebuild the bone by synthesis and mineralization of the new bony matrix within the bone cavity. With PDB, the osteoclasts increase in size and number, escalating resorption of bone. Consequently, osteoblasts add to new bone at an increased rate, which leads to enlarged bony structures that are disorganized in structure and reduced in mechanical strength, leading to patients at risk for the development of deformities and fractures. There are three characteristic phases of pagetic bone: initial (incipient-active), mixed, and inactive. In the initial phase, there is a hyperactive bone resorptive process in place that leads to architecturally disorganized bones and deformities. The mixed phase is classified with the coexistence of bone osteolysis (increased vasculature to bone) and sclerosis in which osteoblastic cells are more proliferative, resulting in lamellar (remodeled) bone that is functionally disorganized. Last is the inactive phase, which results in a disorganized bony structure that displays an increased fibrous connective tissue with increased blood vessels. This leads to a hypervascular state and ultimately osteosclerotic bone; bone that is disorganized and brittle.

Clinical Manifestations

Paget's disease is initially asymptomatic. As it progresses, clinical manifestations of PDB vary according to the severity, extent, and site of bony involvement. The two main clinical characteristics of PDB are pain and deformity in the affected bony site. Additionally, fractures, bone tumors, neurological

disease, and cardiac disease, from related dysfunction with calcium and phosphate imbalance can also occur. Atypical clinical manifestations of PDB are an increase in pain with weight-bearing and an increase in nocturnal pain.

Management

Diagnosis

Diagnosis of PDB is difficult secondary to the asymptomatic nature of the disease. It is estimated that 80% of all PDB patients are asymptomatic. The diagnosis is made incidentally via radiographical examination or via routine laboratory chemistry screening that reveals an increase in serum alkaline phosphatase. Specific clinical indicators for the medical team to focus on are previous fractures, deformities, pain, and familial history of PDB. The pain may arise directly at the pagetic lesion but more commonly from the complications of the bone deformities, causing nerve impingement and/or degenerative issues associated with the disorganized bony structure.

The first step in clinical diagnosis of PDB is a comprehensive history and physical examination with measurements of serum concentrations of alkaline phosphatase, calcium, and urine hydroxyproline excretion. Diagnosis is highly speculative with an elevated serum alkaline phosphatase, normal serum calcium, and no evidence of hepatobiliary disease. Biochemical assay of bone turnover is important for both diagnostic and treatment purposes. Radiographical and nuclear examinations are performed and reveal changes within the bony structure and deformities. Thermography, a noninvasive and painless imaging technique that uses an infrared camera to detect increased temperature variations on the body's surface, can be used to reveal increased blood flow, thus increased temperature in the affected bony area. A bone scan is the most sensitive test for pagetic bone, revealing focal areas of increased activity ("hot spots") that are highly suspect of PDB. Computed tomography is most helpful in a differential diagnosis, especially when associated with **osteosarcoma** (primary bone tumor). A bone biopsy may be ordered in the event that osteosarcoma is suspected in a pagetic bone; however, it is not reliable for the diagnosis of PDB.

Medical Management

Medical management of PDB is dependent on the following factors: presence or absence of symptoms of active disease, distribution of the pagetic bone, metabolic activity of a pagetic lesion, and potential consequences of bony overgrowth at the site of diagnosis. On the basis of these findings, management is either surgical or nonsurgical. The goal of treatment is focused on reduction of pain and increased functional mobility with a decreased risk for fractures.

Medications

There is no effective treatment of Paget's disease. Medication therapy is focused on pain management and functional outcomes. Analgesic therapy is needed for pain control and can span from mild to moderate with the use of aspirin-based products to nonsteroidal analgesics such as ibuprofen. Opioid analgesia is used with severe pain.

Calcitonin was the first therapeutic treatment used for PDB. Calcitonin decreases osteoclastic activity in bone, decreases mineral release and collagen breakdown in bone, and assists with renal excretion of calcium. Unfortunately, long-term management of Paget's disease is difficult with this medication alone. Problems include medication side effects (nausea, flushing, and rash) and the need for regular subcutaneous injections. Patients also may develop resistance to this medication.

The development of oral and IV bisphosphonates has improved the medical outcome for patients with Paget's disease. Treatment with bisphosphonates is recommended for patients with bone pain or other symptomatic active bone disease such as PDB. Bisphosphonates decrease osteoclastic activity, thereby suppressing bone resorption. The bisphosphonates have been shown to suppress bone resorption within days to weeks as evidenced by a decrease in urine hydroxyproline, as well as a decrease in serum alkaline phosphatase, which reveals a suppression of bone formation. Oral etidronate (Didronel) was the first bisphosphonate used with a 50% reduction in disease activity noted. Presently, it is used less, secondary to the fact that the therapeutic doses required for effective management have been linked to side effects such as bone demineralization. The six newer nitrogen-containing bisphosphonates (zoledronic acid, pamidronate, risedronate, alendronate, ibandronate, and neridronate) are the primary agents used for the initial treatment of PDB. These medications suppress bone remodeling without causing demineralization of the bone (see Table 53.5). Zoledronic acid is the preferred medication of choice and is administered via an intravenous infusion over 15 to 20 minutes in a secluded line not to be mixed with other medications. The rationale for this choice is due to the medication tolerance and a documented prolonged remission of Paget's disease. Zoledronic acid is not recommended by the United States FDA for patients who have a creatinine clearance less than 30 to 35 mL/min. Major issues with the oral bisphosphonates, risedronate (Actonel) and alendronate (Fosamax), medications also used in the treatment of osteoporosis, are the poor absorptive issues and mild (GI) issues with oral ingestion. Patients must be instructed to take these medications on an empty stomach and monitor for symptoms such as diarrhea, nausea, and dyspepsia. Additionally, because of the renal toxicity of these medications, any patients with renal dysfunction are not eligible candidates for this therapeutic intervention. IV therapy such as with pamidronate (Aredia) and zoledronic acid (Reclast) has been shown to be highly effective; however, serum calcium, phosphorus, and 25-hydroxyvitamin D (calcidiol) should be monitored during treatment. To reduce the risk for hypocalcemia, it is recommended enhanced supplementation with calcium and vitamin D be given 8 weeks before initiating this therapy in patients whose 25-hydroxyvitamin D level is 20 ng/mL (50 nmol/L)

or less. Supplementation of calcium and vitamin D is warranted post treatment on the basis of serum laboratory results. Pamidronate is well tolerated and easy to administer in a hospital and/or outpatient setting; however, recent studies have shown that some patients develop a resistance to the medication, resulting in treatment inefficacy.

Surgical Management

Surgical management of PDB is focused on the secondary degenerative changes of the bony structure such as in the case of osteoarthritis (OA). Surgical intervention can span from joint replacement to spinal decompression and stabilization. Another option is **osteotomy**. Osteotomy is a surgical removal of damaged or deformed bone. This procedure can be corrective for skeletal deformities such as bowleg knee (varus) or knock-knee (valgus) (Fig. 53.3) that occur naturally or as a result of PDB. Surgical spinal decompression, removal of bony substances that are causing nerve impingement, and **spinal stabilization** (surgically inserted rods, pins, and pedicle screws that maintain spinal column structure) can be used with the ultimate goal of maintaining skeletal structure and function and preventing vertebral column pain and/or possible paralysis and/or paresthesias. The primary goal for surgical intervention is reduction of pain and maximizing functional outcome. Nonsurgical management is recommended before surgical intervention.

Complications

In patients with advanced PDB, deformities and pain occur. Frequently, there are skeletal changes such as bowing of long bones (especially in the tibia, "saber tibia") and enlargement of the skull, which can cause impingement on the auditory nerve resulting in deafness, enlargement of the mandible leading to a protrusion of the chin (prognathism), and enlargement of the maxilla and cheekbones causing dental problems. The ultimate effect of PDB is to structurally weaken bones, which puts the patient at an increased risk for fractures. These fractures are most commonly seen in the tibia and femur as small stress fractures. Secondary degenerative changes are associated with PDB.

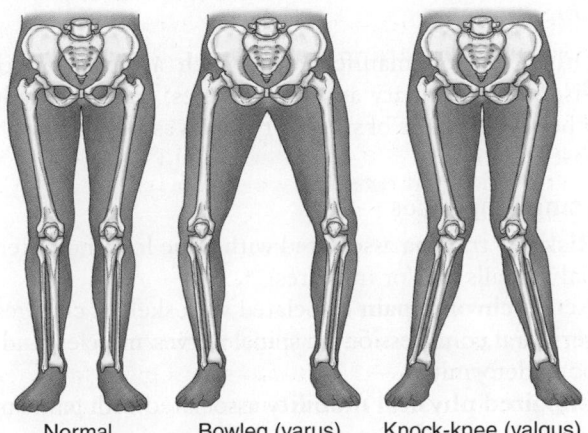

Normal   Bowleg (varus)   Knock-knee (valgus)

FIGURE 53.3 Bow-leg and knock-knee.

The most serious complication of PDB is the development of primary bone tumors, such as the rare but serious osteosarcoma. The prevalence of osteosarcoma in PDB is estimated to be less than 1%; however, it can be found in those patients aged 70 years or greater. The nature of the correlation between the two diseases is unknown but is thought to be linked to aggressive osteoblastic activity that is found most commonly in those patients affected by Paget's disease.

Connection Check 53.4

Medical management for Paget's disease is based on which of the following characteristics? (Select all that apply.)

A. Presence of symptoms of active disease
B. Distribution of the pagetic bone
C. Metabolic activity of a pagetic lesion
D. Absence of symptoms of active disease
E. Decreased calcium and phosphorous levels

Nursing Management

Assessment and Analysis

Many of the clinical manifestations observed in the patient with Paget's disease are directly associated with an increase in bone loss affected by excessive or overactive osteoclasts, which leads to disorganized skeletal structure. Common findings include:

- Generalized pain, especially in the lower back, and bone pain
- Inclination or deformity of long bones and cranial bones
- Spinal curvature
- Spinal cord compression and neurological impairment
- Fissures of the cortex
- Complete or incomplete fractures
- Deafness and/or paralysis of other cranial nerves
- Increased heat in the skin overlying the affected bone
- Osteosarcoma

Other clinical manifestations such as hyperparathyroidism, gout, urinary and renal stones, and heart failure may be seen because of secondary issues associated with the disease pathology.

Nursing Diagnoses

- **Risk for trauma** associated with bone loss and potential for falls and/or fractures
- **Acute/chronic pain** associated with skeletal changes, vertebral compression on spinal nerves/muscles, and bone deformity
- **Impaired physical mobility** associated with pain and musculoskeletal changes

Nursing Interventions

■ *Assessments*

- Pain
  Pain control helps keep the patient comfortable and promotes optimal levels of functioning and mobility.
- Weight
  Weight reduction helps with reduction of stress on bones that might be weakened or misaligned.
- Serum calcium levels
  Serum calcium levels may be lowered due to the treatment with some bisphosphonates.
- Fall risk and gait disturbances
  Assess for varus (bowlegged) knees and valgus (knock-knee) knees, which put patients at greater risk for gait disturbances and falls.
- Body image disturbance
  Skeletal changes can cause issues associated with hearing and eating as well as bowing of the tibia, which result in difficulty with activities of daily living. Physical appearance can change and cause issues associated with self-esteem.

■ *Actions*

- Administer bisphosphonates as ordered
  Bisphosphonates disable osteoclasts, thereby slowing bone resorption and increasing bone-building activity.
- Administer supplemental calcium and vitamin D as ordered
  Calcium levels may be lowered with treatment with bisphosphonates. Supplemental calcium is suggested as well as vitamin D to facilitate GI absorption of calcium.
- Administer analgesic therapy as prescribed
  Controlling pain within tolerable levels assists with maximal level of function.
- Apply thermal therapy as ordered from rehabilitative services
  Thermal therapy (hot and/or cold) has been shown to reduce pain and increase functionality.
- Support exercise program/Implement steps to correct or supplement underlying physical and functional deficits
  Exercises for strengthening abdominal and back muscles are essential to the promotion of function and safety. Improved posture, balance, and strengthened muscle tone will enable the patient to move safely, promote functional capability, and decrease risk for falls.
- Provide training, orthotic shoes, braces, and other supportive measures including a physical therapy consult for safe movement with activities of daily living
  Patient population is at great risk for falls with transfers and lifting; use assistive devices when appropriate.
- Contact home health agency for a home environmental safety evaluation
  High risk for falls and fractures, so home environment needs to be evaluated for environmental and safety hazards

■ *Teaching*

- Take pain analgesic medication as prescribed
  Adequate pain control facilitates active participation in daily activities. Caution: Opioids are highly addictive and can cause constipation, drowsiness, and respiratory depression. Patients should not drink alcohol or operate heavy machinery (car) while taking opioids.
- Take bisphosphonate medication as prescribed
  Many of the bisphosphonates need to be ingested first thing in the morning on an empty stomach. They can cause GI disturbances, esophagitis, and visual disturbances. These side effects should be reported to provider as soon as possible.
- Instruct patient to incorporate adequate ingestion of vitamin D and calcium
  Medications may cause a decrease in calcium levels. Calcium helps with collagen synthesis and bone formation, thereby assisting with maintaining bone health. Vitamin D facilitates calcium absorption in the GI system.

Evaluating Care Outcomes

Typically Paget's disease is found in the gerontological patient population; however, an accurate, inclusive family and personal history, in combination with a comprehensive history and physical examination, is the first line of assessment for this metabolic bone disease. Careful management of pain and discomfort is essential to a well-managed plan of care. Additionally, overall fracture reduction is maintained with careful screening by both physical and occupational therapies. This screening is essential for identification of gait disturbances, assessment of fall risk, and completion of a home safety assessment.

OSTEOMYELITIS

Epidemiology

The incidence and prevalence for osteomyelitis are directly linked to the mechanism of infection; hematogenous or nonhematogenous. Hematogenous, or endogenous, **osteomyelitis** is a result of infectious spread from another area of the body via the bloodstream. Nonhematogenous, or exogenous, osteomyelitis is a result of an open fracture and/or trauma to the bone. Acute hematogenous osteomyelitis is more commonly seen in children and those less than 1 year of age, accounting for approximately 85% of all documented cases. Nonhematogenous osteomyelitis is more commonly associated with adults and open surgical fractures or trauma. Open fracture or trauma is reported to have between a 2% and 16% incidence of osteomyelitis. It is most common with metaphysis of long bones, such as within the femur, tibia (19%–26%), or humerus, with the lower more commonly affected. Trauma is the leading causative factor, which tends to affect males between the ages of 18 to 30 years; however, osteomyelitis can be linked to other causative factors such as implanted surgical devices and puncture wounds.

Osteomyelitis is classified into one of three categories: 1) acute infection, which is less than 2 weeks; 2) subacute infection, which is from 2 weeks to 3 months; or 3) a chronic infection, which lasts longer than 3 months. The prevalence of chronic osteomyelitis averages 5% to 25% for patients undergoing treatment for an acute osteomyelitic infection. Diabetes and foot puncture prevalence statistics for chronic osteomyelitis can range as high as 30% to 40%. The overall incidence of osteomyelitis is approximately 2%.

Pathophysiology

The pathophysiology for acute and/or chronic osteomyelitis is complex and not clearly understood; however, the principles of virulence of a bacterium, patient immune status, underlying patient pathology and type, and location and vascularity of the bone are highly correlated. In both acute and chronic osteomyelitis, the process begins with an invasion of the bone and surrounding tissue by one or multiple bacterial pathogens. This leads to inflammation and an increase in the vascularity to the region that ultimately results in edema. Within days to weeks, a thrombus occurs in the vessel, which leads to ischemia and slow necrosis of the affected area and bone. Once necrotic bone is present, the healing is delayed, and a superimposed infection or abscess is highly probable. This results in a cycle of more inflammation and infection. The ultimate clinical hallmark is bone necrosis and the development of sinus tracts between the bone and skin (Fig. 53.4).

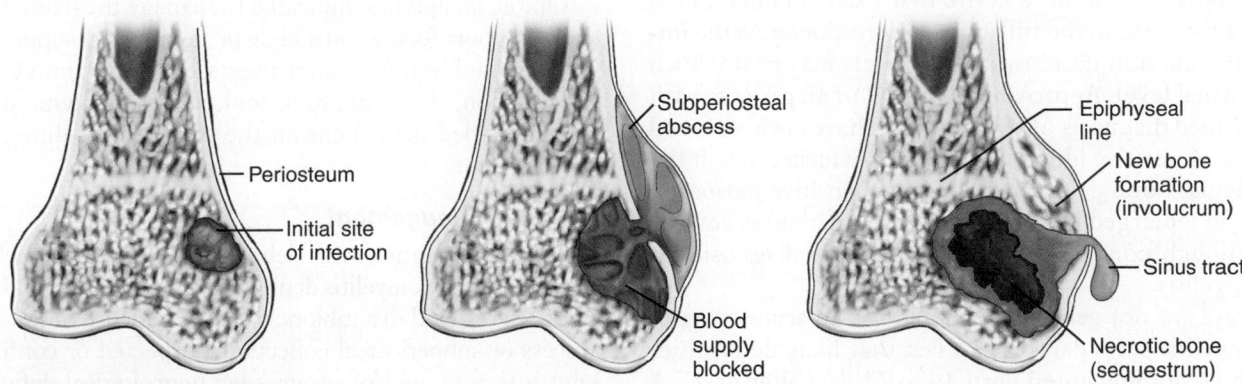

FIGURE 53.4 Abscess and sinus tract formation in osteomyelitis.

Exogenous osteomyelitis can be from trauma and/or surgery in which the spread is via direct inoculation from a fracture or open wound or contagious spread from a contiguous wound. Endogenous is caused by the spread of an infection from one area of the body to another because of infections in adjacent soft tissue and joints or indirect inoculation. Older adults are affected by contiguous osteomyelitis in which skin infections spread to bone. This can be polymicrobial or monomicrobial and is seen in such cases of decubitus ulcer, affected total joint arthroplasties, and other vascular insufficiencies. They account for approximately 34% of the documented cases. *Staphylococcus aureus*, coagulase-negative staphylococci, and aerobic gram-negative bacilli are the most common pathogens found in contiguous osteomyelitis.

Clinical Manifestations

Clinical manifestations of acute osteomyelitis include pain not relieved by rest, swelling, tenderness and warmth at the site, fever, nausea, chills, and a general feeling of being unwell or malaise. Manifestations of chronic osteomyelitis include constant bone pain, edema, tenderness, erythema, and warmth at the site. Occasionally, especially in children, there is an absence of the classic osteomyelitis manifestation of fever, pain and increased inflammatory markers. The absence of these symptoms does not rule out osteomyelitis, which warrants a more aggressive diagnostic evaluation.

Management

Medical Management

Diagnosis

Diagnosis of osteomyelitis can be difficult secondary to the fact that many serum laboratory tests are nonspecific. Also, radiographical studies often show normal function rather than pathology. A white blood cell (WBC) count, ESR, blood cultures, and C-reactive protein (CRP) levels are the initial steps for diagnosis of osteomyelitis. White blood cells are elevated in infection. The ESR and CRP level are indicators of inflammation. The WBC count and ESR are commonly elevated in osteomyelitis. The CRP level is normally elevated in the first 7 days of infection as a direct response to the inflammatory response. As the initial inflammation decreases, CRP levels may trend down to a normal level. Approximately 50% of all patients with a confirmed diagnosis of osteomyelitis have positive blood cultures. A positive blood culture with evidence of soft tissue edema, bone degeneration, and a positive periosteal elevation (enlarged bone due to pus formation) is considered enough conclusive data to confirm a diagnosis for osteomyelitis.

X-rays are not generally ordered for an acute onset of osteomyelitis secondary to the fact that bony deformities are not commonly noted until 14 to 21 days after onset. A bone scan is the test of choice for acute osteomyelitis when the x-ray is negative for definitive changes. An increased uptake of a radioisotope to the infected bone can detect an infection within 2 to 3 days of onset. A bone scan can result in a false-positive result of osteomyelitis due to many confounding variables (increase or decrease in bone metabolism, bone injury, decreased blood flow, septic arthritis, cancer). Therefore, multiple tests are performed for a definitive diagnosis. Computed tomography scans and magnetic resonance imaging (MRI) are useful tools to evaluate the diagnosis, but bone biopsy is the gold standard for conclusive diagnosis for osteomyelitis. An open (preferred) approach or needle aspirate can be used for this procedure. A positive biopsy (infectious bone) is conclusive for both acute and chronic osteomyelitis.

Medications

Due to the complex nature of osteomyelitis, a collaborative medical management team is highly recommended. The medical management of osteomyelitis requires clinically appropriate antibiotic therapy and surgical debridement and incision of the infected and/or necrotic tissue and bone. The antibiotic regime is based on culture and sensitivity results. Age, renal function and health status are important criteria in the antibiotic selection. In the event that laboratory and diagnostic data is not available, a broad spectrum antibiotic should be initiated. The initial line of treatment is antibiotic IV infusions over a course of 4 to 6 weeks from the time of the final surgical debridement or surgical cleaning of the wound. Betalactam antibiotics, such as penicillin and cephalosporin, are the first-line options unless Methicillin-resistant staphylococcus aureus (MRSA) is suspected. In the event that MRSA is present, or an allergy to penicillin is present, intravenous vancomycin is the medication of choice. Fluoroquinolones are an alternative choice for staphylococcus infections and have been shown to be highly successful because of their high bone-penetrating ability. The IV infusion is typically started in the hospital and is often managed in the home post initial treatment. Dependent on laboratory results, some patients can move from IV infusions to oral antibiotic therapy, but IV infusion is strongly supported. Additional intraoperative antibiotic bead placement with severe and/or chronic osteomyelitis has been shown to be therapeutic and effective.

Opioid analgesia is indicated to manage the pain. Nutritional support focuses on a high-protein diet to support and aid in wound healing. Supplements such as vitamin C, zinc sulfate, iron, thiamine, folic acid, and a multivitamin are recommended dependent on the patient's baseline nutritional status.

Surgical Management

Surgical intervention with debridement is required when a patient with osteomyelitis demonstrates one of the following: failure to respond to antibiotic therapy, evidence of soft tissue abscess or subperiosteal collection, suspected or confirmed joint infection, and/or progressive neurological deficits or spinal instability in the case of vertebral osteomyelitis. In the event that a patient has known or suspected infected orthopedic hardware, surgical removal is often warranted. In the most extreme cases, a surgical amputation is performed to promote healing and vascular supply to healthy tissue and bone proximal to the infection.

Complications

In the absence of appropriate therapy and medical management, osteomyelitis is associated with disabling and life-threatening complications such as sepsis, potentially resulting in amputation. Squamous cell carcinoma has been reported with chronic osteomyelitis, along with other tumors such as fibrosarcoma, myeloma, lymphoma, plasmacytoma, angiosarcoma, and rhabdomyosarcoma. Prompt diagnosis and early treatment with antimicrobial therapy are essential.

Nursing Management
Assessment and Analysis

Many of the clinical manifestations observed in the patient with osteomyelitis are directly associated with the pain and the extent of the infection within the bone and the surrounding tissue. Common findings include:

- Fever (> 101°F [38.3°C]), especially when a bloodstream-borne infection is present
- Pain, defined as constant, localized, and pulsating tenderness, swelling, erythema, and warmth at the affected area
- Irritability, general malaise, lethargy
- Difficulty moving joints near the affected area
- Difficulty bearing weight on the affected area
- Poor perfusion to the area as demonstrated by venous stasis ulcers
- Stiff back (vertebral involvement)

Nursing Diagnoses

- **Acute/chronic pain** associated with inflammation
- **Impaired physical mobility** associated with pain and inflammation
- **Peripheral neurovascular dysfunction** associated with impaired perfusion to affected extremity
- **Risk for disturbance to body image** associated with skeletal changes and bone deformities.

Connection Check 53.5

John, a 28-year-old man, has been recently diagnosed with osteomyelitis following an open reduction internal fixation to his tibia fracture. What is the most appropriate nursing diagnosis for John?

A. Hypotension associated with tibia fracture
B. Infection associated with tibia fracture
C. Fear associated with tibia fracture
D. Pain associated with tibia fracture

Nursing Interventions
Assessments

- Temperature, pulse, and blood pressure
  Elevated heart rate, decreased blood pressure, and febrile (fever) state may indicate an infection.
- Pain
  Increased pain may indicate activation of the inflammatory process. Pain unusual to the illness can be indicative of infection. Additionally, difficulty moving joints, stiffness, and overall pain near the affected joint area are signs of infection.
- Wound assessment
  Redness, heat, purulent drainage, pain, and edema are all signs of wound infection.
- Neurovascular assessment
  Weak pulses, pallor, pain, paresthesia, and/or paralysis indicate impaired circulation, which requires prompt intervention to avoid disabling complications due to decreased blood flow to the affected area.
- Laboratory tests—WBC, ESR, CRP
  Increased WBC, ESR, and CRP are indications of infection and inflammation.
- Blood cultures, wound cultures
  Positive blood cultures and/or wound cultures definitively diagnose infection and determine the appropriate antibiotic coverage.

Actions

- Administer IV antibiotics as ordered
  Because of the severity of the infection and the potentially disabling complications, IV antibiotics are indicated and continued for 4 to 6 weeks.
- Administer analgesic therapy as prescribed
  Pain that is controlled within a tolerable level helps the patient achieve a maximal level of function.
- Apply thermal therapy as ordered
  Thermal therapy (hot and/or cold) has been shown to reduce pain and increase functionality.
- Apply gentle range-of-motion exercises to the joints above and below the affected site
  Exercises for strengthening and flexibility help promote function and prevent contractures
- Provide training for safe movement with activities of daily living
  Patient population is at great risk for falls with transfers and lifting; use assistive devices when appropriate.
- Provide nutritional support
  Adequate ingestion of vitamin C, zinc, iron, thiamine, folic acid, and protein can help with wound healing and eliminating infection.
- Contact home health agency for home infusion antibiotic therapy
  Long-term antibiotic infusion therapy can safely be managed in the home with the assistance of a home infusion nurse.

▪ *Teaching*

- Take pain analgesic medication as prescribed
  Pain control is essential to encourage mobilization. Caution: Opioids are very addicting and can cause constipation, drowsiness, and respiratory depression. Patients should not drink alcohol or operate heavy machinery (car) while taking opioids.
- Take prescribed antibiotics
  Complete a full prescription to avoid a rebound or resistant infection.
- Instruct patient on nutritional therapy to incorporate high-protein diet
  A high-protein diet helps with tissue and wound healing.

Evaluating Care Outcomes

Overall evaluation of care outcomes for osteomyelitis is focused on control of pain, resolution of infection, and limb preservation. Adherence to the IV antibiotic regimen is essential to avoid complications such as bone abscess, fracture, bacteremia, delayed bone healing, gangrene, and ultimately amputation. Early recognition and prompt treatment are essential for effective clinical management and reduction of potential complications. A well-managed patient has pain and infection under control and retained limb functionality.

SCOLIOSIS

Epidemiology

Scoliosis is not a diagnosis but rather a description of the structural alteration that is noted by a curvature of the spine greater than a 10° curvature that is normally associated with rotation and compression; identified through the measurement of Cobb's angle (described below). While the median age of the population rises, so does the incidence of lumbar scoliosis in those 40 years of age and older. Caucasians have a higher incidence (11.1%) than African American (3.14%), and gender does not seem to be a factor, with males equal to females. The prevalence of adolescent idiopathic scoliosis, which is defined as greater than a 10° Cobb's angle, is 2% to 3%. Risk factors associated with scoliosis are smoking; obesity; older age; occupations that require heavy physical work; sedentary lifestyle; psychologically strenuous work; and persons who have a lower educational level.

Pathophysiology

There are three main categories of scoliosis: neuromuscular, congenital, and idiopathic. Neuromuscular scoliosis occurs in patients with neurological musculoskeletal problems such as cerebral palsy, myelomeningocele, muscular dystrophy, or leg discrepancy. Congenital scoliosis is asymmetry in the vertebral column secondary to a congenital anomaly. Idiopathic scoliosis has no distinct etiology and is defined by exclusion and age of presentation. The actual cause is unknown; however, the pathophysiological process is rather clear in its presentation. As the degree of curvature in the vertebral column increases, damage to the vertebral bodies occurs. A curvature of greater than a 50° Cobb's angle causes instability within the spinal column. Greater than a 60° angle causes significant compromise to the thoracic region, resulting in cardiopulmonary compromise.

Clinical Manifestations

In scoliosis, there is a sideways curvature of the spine greater than 10%. Pain may be present, but other causes of pain should be ruled out before being attributed to scoliosis. Clinical manifestations of scoliosis include:

- Sideways curve in the spine
- Uneven shoulders
- One shoulder blade that appears more prominent than the other
- Uneven waist
- One hip higher than the other
- Signs of cardiopulmonary compromise with severe scoliosis such as tachypnea, tachycardia, shortness of breath, and decreased oxygen saturation

Management

Medical Management

Diagnosis

Clinical diagnosis of scoliosis is done with visible inspection, radiographical imaging, and quantifying the curvature. **Cobb's angle** is the measurement used to evaluate the amount of curvature in the spine. This is done by identifying the upper and lower vertebra most affected by the curve, drawing perpendicular lines from each, and measuring their angle of intersection (Fig. 53.5).

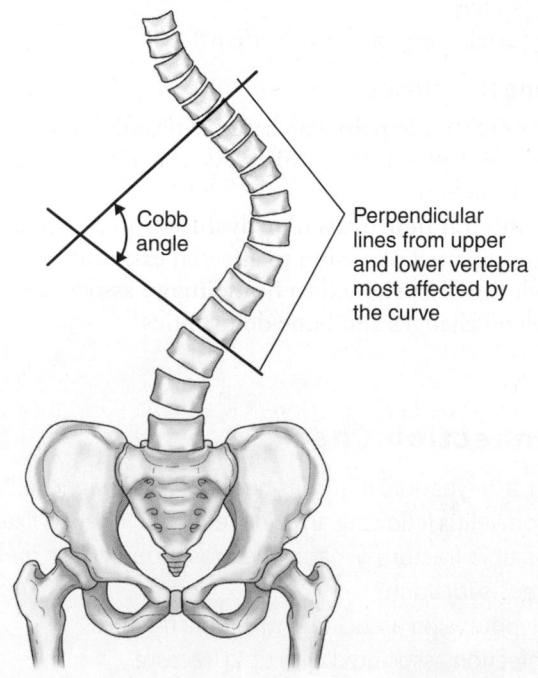

Cobb angle

Perpendicular lines from upper and lower vertebra most affected by the curve

FIGURE 53.5 Cobb's angle; diagnostic for scoliosis. The intersection of perpendicular lines drawn from the upper and lower vertebrae most affected by the curve.

The first step in diagnosis is the identification of the underlying etiology and assessment of the severity of the curvature and the risk for progression. A comprehensive history and physical examination include when the deformity was first noted, rate of progression, pain, associated symptoms, and cardiopulmonary dysfunction. For the adolescent and adult populations, assessment of asymmetry of the iliac crest and posterior inferior iliac spines is palpated bilaterally. This is done with the patient in the standing position with hips and knees fully extended. Leg discrepancy is noted on palpation and many times on visual inspection. Simple inspection while standing behind the patient may reveal subtle differences such as discrepancy in shoulder height or scapulae, waistline asymmetry, and a difference in arm length. The patient's head may not appear aligned over the sacrum while leaning to one side or another. The Adams forward bend test (observe the patient from the back as he or she bends forward until the spine is parallel to the horizontal plane) reveals a thoracic or lumbar prominence on one side. Kyphosis, spinal curvature making the patient seem hunched over, may be visible when standing to the side of the patient. A scoliometer is used to determine the quantification of trunk rotation. Lastly, radiographical studies are required to confirm the diagnosis, type, and severity of scoliosis; Cobb's angle, and to evaluate skeletal maturity.

Treatment

Medical treatment for scoliosis in the adult population with a curvature of less than a 50° Cobb's angle is treated conservatively with thermal therapy, physical and occupational therapies, a progressive exercise regimen, and pain management. Pharmacological intervention is focused on comfort and pain relief. Pain management ranges from mild (aspirin) to moderate (nonsteroidal analgesia) to severe (opioid analgesia). Thermal therapy is used to reduce pain, promote comfort, and assist with spinal flexibility. A growing body of research has shown that exercise can reverse the signs and symptoms of spinal deformity and prevent further progression within adolescents and adults.

Surgical Management

Surgical intervention may be required with a Cobb's angle greater than 50°. It is considered only after conservative treatment has been shown to be unsuccessful. Surgery is done via **spinal instrumentation** and/or spinal fusion. Spinal instrumentation involves placing steel rods on either side of the spine. They are attached to the spine with hooks or pedicle screws in an effort to straighten the curve both side to side and front to back, decrease pain, and promote skeletal flexibility. The latest evidence supports the insertion of pedicle screws based on the primary advantages of improved coronal correction: correction of the sideways curve, decreased rates of pseudarthrosis, lower failure rate for surgical implants, and the overall ability to correct the curvature of the spine in three planes.

Postoperatively, a total contact orthotic (TCO) device, a **thoracic-lumbar spinal orthotic (TLSO)**, is worn by the patient for stabilization purposes. The TLSO brace is a custom-fitted orthotic device that stabilizes the spine to prevent instability and flexion or rotation that could subsequently injure the thoracic-lumbar column.

Nursing Management

Assessment and Analysis

Many of the clinical manifestations observed in the patient with scoliosis are linked to the curvature of the vertebral column. Common findings include:

- Pain from degenerative changes within the vertebral column (usually thoracic and/or lumbar region)
- Kyphosis
- Asymmetry of hip and shoulder height
- Prominence located on the thoracic rib or scapula region on one side
- Asymmetry in leg length
- Cardiopulmonary compromise with a severe Cobb's angle

Nursing Diagnoses

- **Acute/chronic pain** associated with curvature of the thoracic and/or lumbar column
- **Impaired physical mobility** associated with lumbar pain
- **Risk for impaired cardiopulmonary dysfunction** associated with compromise to the thoracic cavity
- **Risk for falls** associated with impairment of the vertebral column
- **Risk for pathologic fractures** associated with destruction of the bony matrix
- **Body image disturbance** associated with change to posture

Nursing Interventions

▪ *Assessments*

- Vital signs
  Tachypnea, tachycardia, shortness of breath, and decreased oxygen saturation may indicate cardiopulmonary compromise with severe scoliosis.
- Pain
  Pain frequently accompanies scoliosis. Increased pain indicates inadequate pain interventions or further progression of the disorder.
- Assess safety hazard during ambulation and transfers
  Increased curvature of the vertebral column can cause balance and gait disturbances.

▪ *Actions*

- Administer pain medication as ordered
  Adequate pain management helps the patient achieve maximal functional mobility.
- Maintain orthotic device
  Orthotic devices such as a TCO/TLSO may be used with/without spinal instrumentation to help with posture and pain relief.

- Apply thermal therapy as ordered
  Thermal therapy (hot and/or cold) has been shown to reduce pain and increase functionality.

■ *Teaching*

- Information on analgesic medication
  Pain control is essential to encourage mobilization. Caution: Opioids are addicting and can cause constipation, drowsiness, and respiratory depression. Patients should not drink alcohol or operate heavy machinery (car) while on opioids.
- Teach patient and family how to care for TCO/TLSO brace
  The patient must wear the brace at all times, unless prescribed differently by the practitioner. The patient generally needs help with washing and changing clothes because of brace limitations.
- In the event of a fall, report to provider immediately
  For the patient postspinal instrumentation, subluxation or misalignment can occur with falls.
- Maintain level of activity and exercise as prescribed by provider and physical therapy
  Exercise is an integral part of the prevention and management of scoliosis and pain control. Strive for an active lifestyle.

Evaluating Care Outcomes

Overall evaluation of care outcomes for scoliosis is focused on pain control and reduction in curvature and rotation of the spinal column. A well-managed patient has pain under control and has functional mobility. This patient wears a TLSO brace as prescribed, and exercises and pursues weight reduction to decrease disease progression.

Connection Check 53.6

What is considered a nursing priority for a patient with scoliosis?
A. Maintain bedrest
B. Encourage exercise
C. Restrict fluids
D. Restrict pain medication

JOINT REPLACEMENT

Epidemiology

Total joint replacement (TJR), also referred to as **arthroplasty**, is most commonly associated with the joints of the hip and the knee but may also include any and all joints within the body. Other common areas are the shoulder, elbow, ankle, and wrist. This is a surgical procedure designed to repair articulating surfaces with a synovial joint. A new smooth surface is restored. The life span for the replacement is typically 10 to 15 years.

According to the Centers for Disease Control and Prevention (CDC), due to the aging population and the increased incidence of overweight Americans (one-third of all Americans), the need for joint replacement surgery is expected to grow exponentially. The CDC revealed that from 2000 to 2010 the number of joint replacements increased from 138,700 to 310,800 in the 45 and older population with approximately 310,800 total hip replacements. Additionally, the incremental increase was seen in younger age groups and a decrease was evident in the older population. The largest age group was that of the 55 to 64 years of age, with an increase of triple over this period of time. Financially, the average length of stay in the hospital for joint replacement surgery decreased from 5 days to 4 days from 2000 to 2010, which equates to a financial cost saving. From a gender perspective, approximately 18.1% of men and 20.1% of women have joint replacement surgery. *Healthy People 2020* focuses on prevention of disorders that increase the need for joint replacement by stressing weight reduction and smoking cessation.

Pathophysiology and Clinical Manifestations

Osteoarthritis (OA) is the leading clinical indication for TJR (Fig. 53.6). Joint cartilage consists of a matrix of proteoglycans and collagen. In OA, there is a decrease in the proteoglycans, which are responsible for the management of the fluid within the joints. The result is a loss of cartilage strength and functionality. Normal cartilage is bluish-white in color. With OA, there is a slow change to translucent color to opaque to yellow-brown in appearance. The result of these changes is the erosion of cartilage and bone with a reduction and narrowing of the joint space and a production of bone spurs (osteophytes). With progression of the disease, fissures, pitting, and ulcerations develop, and there is an increase in the thinning of the cartilage. The inflammatory response produces cytokines (enzymes) such as interleukin-1, which enhance the deterioration. The normal body compensatory mechanisms cannot overcome the rapid degeneration. The result is joint destruction, dysfunction, and deformity, which leads to immobility, pain, muscle spasm, and localized inflammation. Joint replacement involves the removal of the damaged area of the bones with replacement prosthesis. The replacement joint may be a partial or complete prosthesis.

Management

Medical Management
Diagnosis

Diagnosing or determining the need for TJR is based on deformity, tissue destruction, and loss of function of a specific joint. Joint changes, stiffness, pain that limits normal activities, and associated muscle atrophy are common indicators to be evaluated. The need for joint replacement is confirmed through radiographical studies such as an x-ray (Fig. 53.7) and MRI that reveal structure and joint pathology associated with the clinical indices for a joint replacement.

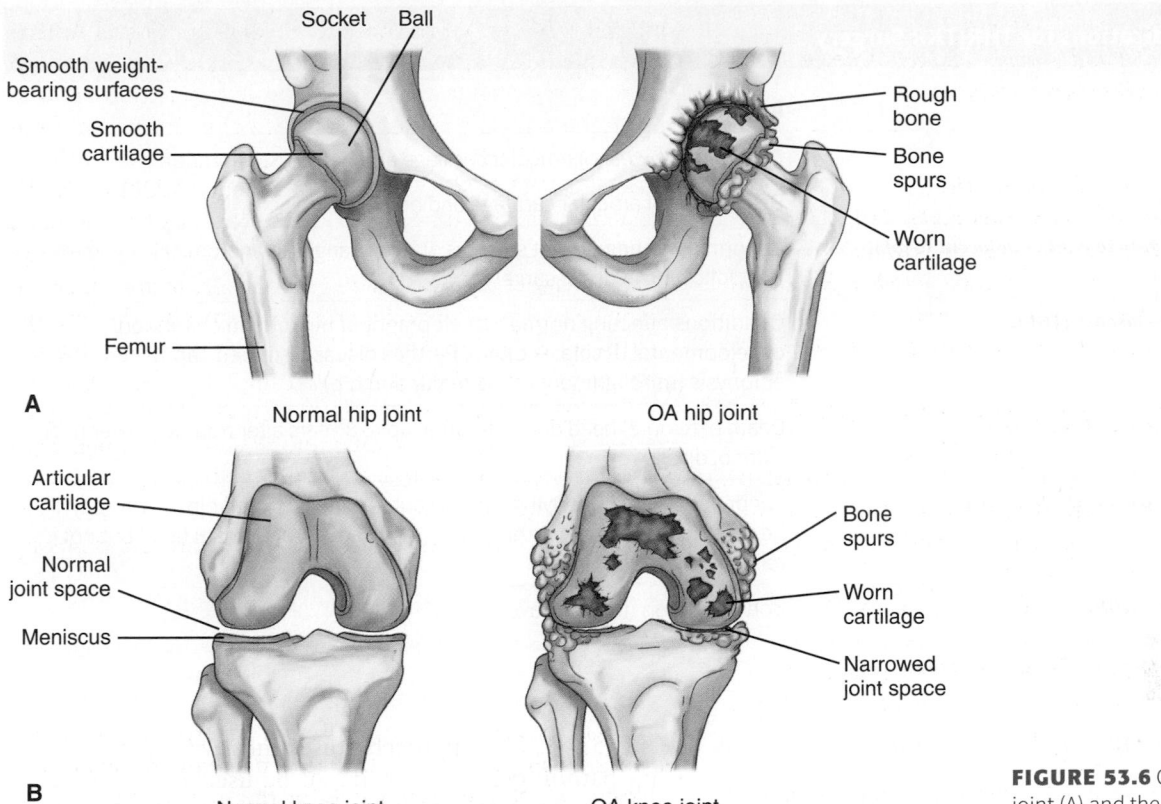

FIGURE 53.6 Osteoarthritis of the hip joint (A) and the knee joint (B).

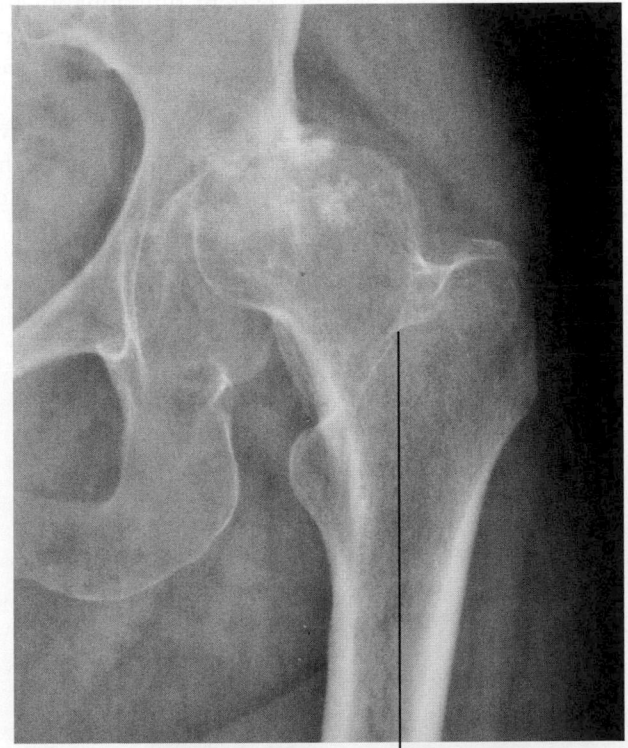

Narrowed joint space due to loss of cartilage

FIGURE 53.7 X-ray of severe osteoarthritis of the hip.

Treatment

The initial medical management before joint replacement is focused on weight management, activity modification, nonsteroidal therapy, and the use of joint supplements such as glucosamine and chondroitin. When the conservative approach is unsuccessful, joint replacement is frequently recommended. The National Institute for Health and Care Excellence states that a total hip replacement (THR) or a total knee replacement (TKR) can be considered once self-management, exercise, and analgesia are no longer effective in relieving pain during activities of daily living. Other clinical indicators for THR and TKR surgeries are described in Table 53.6.

Surgical Management

Surgical management of joint replacement includes resurfacing of the joint and/or a complete or partial replacement of the joint. Today, most prostheses are made of a cobalt-chrome polished ball with a polyethylene cup or socket on the corresponding surface area (ball and socket). For both THR and TKR, the procedure can be done utilizing an uncemented or a cemented approach with the use of polymethylmethacrylate cement. The cemented approach uses glue or cement to attach the prosthesis to the bone and is usually used for older patients with a life expectancy of 20 years and who are unlikely to require revision surgery.

Table 53.6 Indications for THR/TKR Surgery

Clinical Condition	Indication
Osteoarthritis	Degenerative wear of articular cartilage and bony cyst formation
Rheumatoid arthritis	Destruction of articular cartilage and bony erosions
Previous injury or surgery to joint or adjacent to joint	Abnormal wearing of joint surfaces due to changes in anatomical alignment of joint following injury or surgery
Previous childhood hip disease (THR)	Conditions affecting normal development of hip joint in childhood: developmental dysplasia of hip; Perthes disease, slipped capital femoral epiphysis (misalignment of the femur and hip)
Avascular necrosis of femoral head (THR)	Death of femoral head due to trauma (up to 8 years after traumatic event), or alcohol disease
Intracapsular fractured neck of femur (THR)	For patients with underlying osteoarthritis in the fractured hip, a THR may be used instead of hemiarthroplasty (replacement of femoral head but not relining of acetabulum)
Ankylosing spondylitis (THR)	Bony ankylosis (loss of movement) of hip joint

THR, Total hip replacement; *TKR,* Total knee replacement.

The cement acts as a filler in between bone and prosthesis providing a stable fixation.

Uncemented prosthetics are secured by placing a hole in the bone(s) that is anatomically correct to hold the device in place. The prosthetic joint is coated with hydroxyapatite, which allows for bone ingrowth into the surface of the prosthesis creating a stable bond. This type of surgical approach is used for the younger, more active patient population, allowing for an increase in joint movement and subsequent ease of removal in the event that a revision is required at a later date.

A newer alternative approach for the younger, more active patient population is referred to as *joint resurfacing*

(Fig. 53.8). This approach is used mostly for patients with hip pathology; however, it can be used for other joints such as a knee and shoulder. For patients with hip pathology, the surgical approach involves shaving the femoral head with preservation of the femoral neck and the insertion of a metal cup and metal socket. Surgical and recovery times are greatly reduced, and patient functionality and outcomes are optimized. This approach can also be done with the knee with a unicondylar or partial knee replacement (Fig. 53.9).

Joint replacement has a traditional or minimally invasive surgical approach. The approach varies according to the surgeon. The traditional surgical approach is an incision of

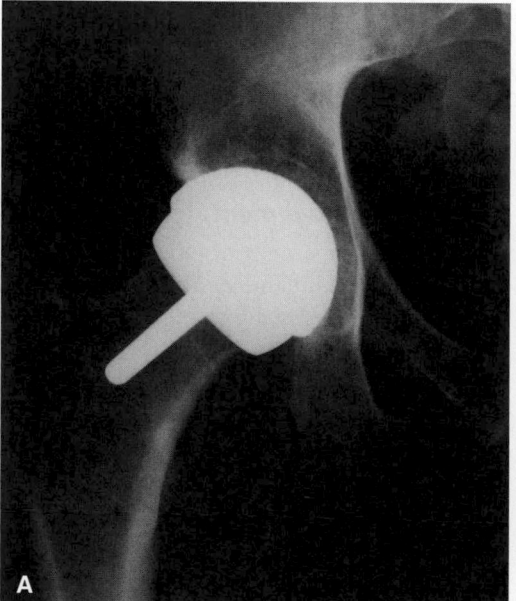
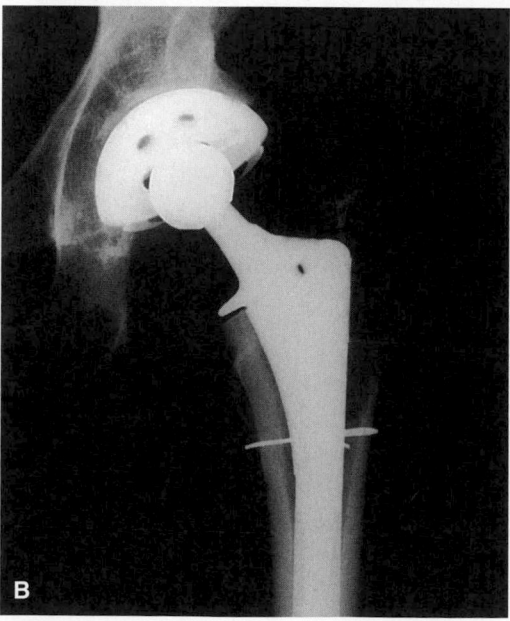

FIGURE 53.8 Hip replacement. A, Hip resurfacing; preserving the femoral bone; B, Total hip replacement.

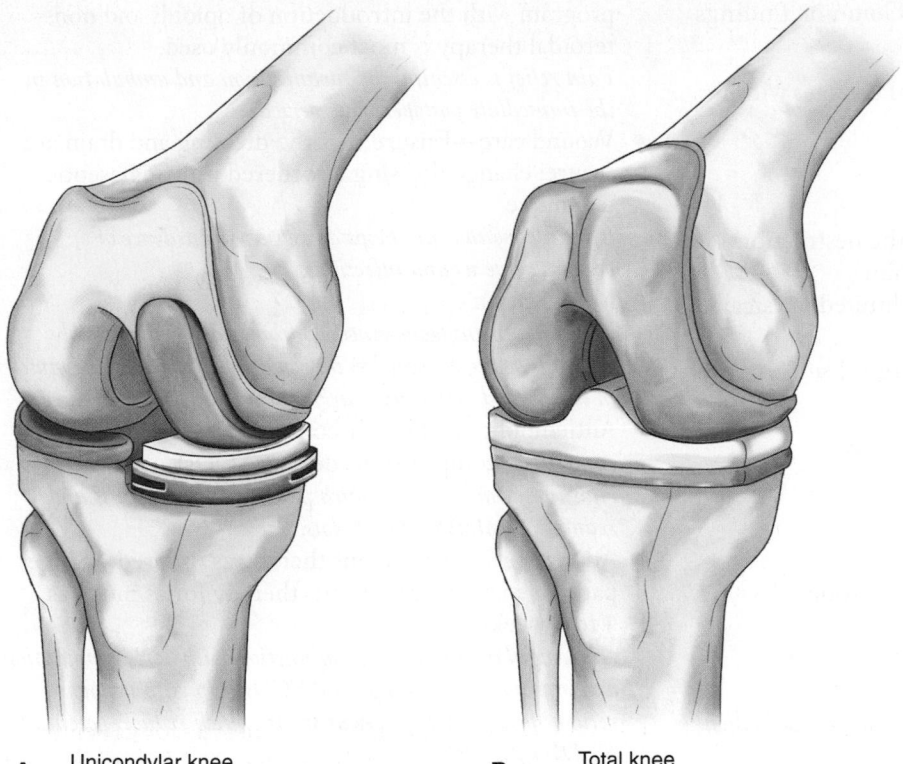

A Unicondylar knee replacement

B Total knee replacement

FIGURE 53.9 Knee replacement. A, Unicondylar or partial knee replacement; B, Total knee replacement.

approximately 20 to 30 cm in length with staples and/or sutures postoperatively. A longitudinal versus lateral approach causes less damage to the muscle and a shorter incision. Staples are more frequently used for hip surgery because of faster rates of closure and improved wound healing time. The use of a semipermeable dressing rather than tape has been shown to decrease the incidence of skin blistering, promoting optimal conditions for healing and reduction in surgical site infections. A drain is placed during surgery to prevent hematoma formation and allow for autologous blood donation within the first 6 hours of surgery. Because of the potential of a large amount of blood loss during TJR surgery, the addition of this autologous transfusion device has been of great clinical benefit.

A minimally invasive surgical approach is an incision of approximately 10 cm or less. The major advantage of this surgery is reduction in complications such as tissue trauma, which promotes faster healing and quicker recovery. Recent studies have shown an increase in patient satisfaction with this approach; however, the visualization of the joint is limited from a surgical perspective. Because of the relative newness of this surgical approach, outcome statistics are limited. Independent of the surgical technique used, the overall goal for joint replacement remains to allow the patient's bone to grow into the joint and keep the prosthesis securely in place.

Complications

The most immediate postoperative complications are hypotension, bleeding, and hypovolemia due to excessive blood loss during surgery. Wound site infection is another potential complication. Intraoperative and postoperative adherence to asepsis with washing hands, proper emptying and cleaning of the drain, and monitoring of temperature and WBC count are simple measures to help prevent wound site infection. Additionally, prophylactic antibiotic therapy is considered protocol until the drain has been removed. The critical complication that is of concern in TJR is dislocation and/or subluxation or partial dislocation. This is where the prosthesis has become loose and is no longer in alignment within the joint. This condition is immediately recognizable because of asynchrony in leg length or abnormal rotation of the hip. This causes severe pain and the inability to bear weight on the affected joint and/or extremity. The most lethal complication is that of a deep vein thrombosis (DVT) and potential pulmonary embolism (PE).

Connection Check 53.7

Which symptom is an appropriate indication for TJR?
A. An inability to perform activities of daily living without pain
B. A desire to participate in contact sports without pain
C. A knee injury that may restrict aggressive skiing
D. A hip injury that restricts a prior running routine

Nursing Management

Assessment and Analysis

Many of the clinical manifestations observed in the patient requiring a joint replacement are associated with the degenerative changes within the joint. Common findings include:

- Pain from deterioration and structural changes within the affected joint and extremity
- Loss of mobility and joint function

Nursing Diagnoses

- **Acute/chronic pain** associated with the destruction and/or deterioration of the affected joint
- **Activity intolerance** associated with limited physical mobility and progressive pain
- **Risk for infection** associated with surgical site complication

Nursing Interventions: Preoperative and Postoperative Nursing Management

■ *Assessments*

Preoperative Assessments

- Presurgical screening; ECG, metabolic profile, coagulation studies, complete blood count
  Ensuring that patients have been adequately screened for anaesthesia risk correlates with a decreased level of cardiopulmonary compromise and improved pain satisfaction postoperatively.
- Pain management
  Assessment of pain tolerance and acceptable level of pain is crucial to early mobilization and ambulation in the early postoperative period.

Postoperative Assessments

- Vital sign assessment
  Hypertension, tachycardia, and tachypnea postoperatively may indicate problems with perfusion and oxygenation. Hypotension and tachycardia may signal hypovolemia and blood loss.
- Temperature
  Increased temperature may indicate a postoperative infection, which may compromise the new prosthetic joint.
- Pain level
  Assessment and management of pain is crucial to early mobilization and ambulation in the early postoperative period.
- Laboratory assessment
  A decrease in hemoglobin and hematocrit postoperatively due to blood loss hinders oxygen-carrying ability. The patient may require a blood transfusion.
- Neurovascular assessment
  Weak pulses, pallor, paresthesia, paralysis, pulselessness, and pain indicate neurovascular dysfunction compromising the new joint.
- Monitor wound drainage
  Excessive bloody drainage may indicate a "bleeder" that needs to be evaluated. Thick, purulent drainage may indicate infection.

■ *Actions*

Postoperative Actions

- Administer pain medication as ordered—Patient-controlled analgesia with a 24- to 48-hour weaning

program with the introduction of opioids and nonsteroidal therapy is most commonly used.
Pain relief is essential for mobilization and ambulation in the immediate postoperative period.
- Wound care—Ensure that the dressing and drain are secure; change dressing as ordered utilizing aseptic technique
  Effective wound care helps decrease the incidence of postoperative wound infections.
- Mobilization
  Early movement postoperatively from bed to chair, possibly within 6 hours, is needed to improve and strengthen the muscles in the affected extremity. Early movement facilitates recovery.
- Antiembolic stocking or compression stocking with sequential compressions device (SCDs)
  Aids in venous return, which prevents venous stasis and reduces potential for blood clots.
- Administer anticoagulant therapy as ordered—Some patients may remain on this therapy for as much as 4 to 6 weeks.
  Anticoagulant therapy in conjunction with early ambulation and antiembolic stockings and SCDs help with venous return, prevention of venous stasis, which reduces potential for DVT and PE.
- Continuous passive motion (CPM) machine with TKR
  Some physiotherapists use a CPM machine, which gently flexes and extends the knee (TKR) continuously. The CPM is thought to slowly help increase range of motion, but the evidence does not support its routine use.
- Maintain proper positioning and turning schedule
  Abduction pillows prevent dislocation and internal rotation of the affected extremity with a THR. A turning schedule prevents pressure on heels and other bony prominences, which reduces the risk for decubitus ulcers for any type of joint replacement surgery.

■ *Teaching*

- Preoperative education about the procedure
  Research has shown that those patients who have a greater understanding of the procedure and the level of importance report a higher level of outcome and lower level of pain postoperatively.
- Postoperative education
  - Take pain analgesic medication as prescribed
    Pain control is essential to encourage mobilization. Caution: Opioids can cause constipation, drowsiness, and respiratory depression. Patients should not drink alcohol or operate heavy machinery (car) while on opioids.
  - Anticoagulation teaching
    - Administration of anticoagulant therapy and signs and symptoms of DVT
      Low molecular weight heparin subcutaneous injections are most commonly used in the home setting. Patient and family teaching should focus on the need to continue the prescribed medication until further notice to prevent DVT. Signs and symptoms of DVT such as pain, warmth, and tenderness at the

site of the clot should be reported to the provider immediately.

- Bleeding precautions while on anticoagulation
  Avoid use of electric razors, use soft toothbrushes, no flossing, and avoid high risk for injury activities such as football.
- Diet
  If on warfarin for anticoagulation limit or maintain consistent intake of foods high in vitamin K such as green vegetables; these foods interfere with the efficacy of warfarin
- Home management
  Need to reinforce teaching for hip flexion less than 90 degrees for approximately 2 to 3 months. Encourage usage of a raised toilet seat and pull bar in the bathroom (toilet and shower) to prevent flexion of 90 degrees and to prevent falls. Remove scatter rugs around the house and encourage use of slip socks or shoes at all times to prevent patient falls. Avoid crossing the leg over midline to prevent hip abduction and venous stasis as DVT prophylaxis. Use assistive walking devices such as a walker or crutches if recommended by physical therapy.

Evaluating Care Outcomes

Total joint replacement therapy and outcomes are focused on reduction in pain and restoration of functional outcomes. With adequate assessment, wound care, positioning, and careful movement, the immediate postoperative goals of prevention of hypovolemia, surgical site infection, and dislocation of the prosthesis can be achieved. A return to independent activity without limitation in movement and functionality is possible by strictly following activity restrictions, then exercising as directed by the provider and physical therapist. Weight loss and a healthy diet are also necessary for a good result.

BONE CANCER

Bone cancer is subdivided into two classifications: benign bone cancers, which are noncancerous and often asymptomatic, and malignant, which are cancerous in nature and originate either from a primary or secondary source. Primary bone tumors are more prevalent between the ages of 10 and 30 years and are generally seen only in a small percentage of the population. Secondary or metastatic lesions are more often diagnosed in the older patient population.

Osteochondroma, a benign bone tumor, is the most common form of bone cancer and is seen at the end of a long bone, such as the knee or shoulder. Ewing's sarcoma, a primary bone cancer, is most common in children and is the most malignant and deadly of all the bone cancers. Other bone tumors associated with the adult population are chondrosarcoma, fibrosarcoma, and rhabdomyosarcoma. Chondrosarcomas, tumors of the hyaline cartilage, affect the pelvis and proximal femur area. These neoplasms are generally characterized by dull pain and swelling of the lower extremity. Chondrosarcomas generally have a better prognosis then osteosarcomas and are found predominantly

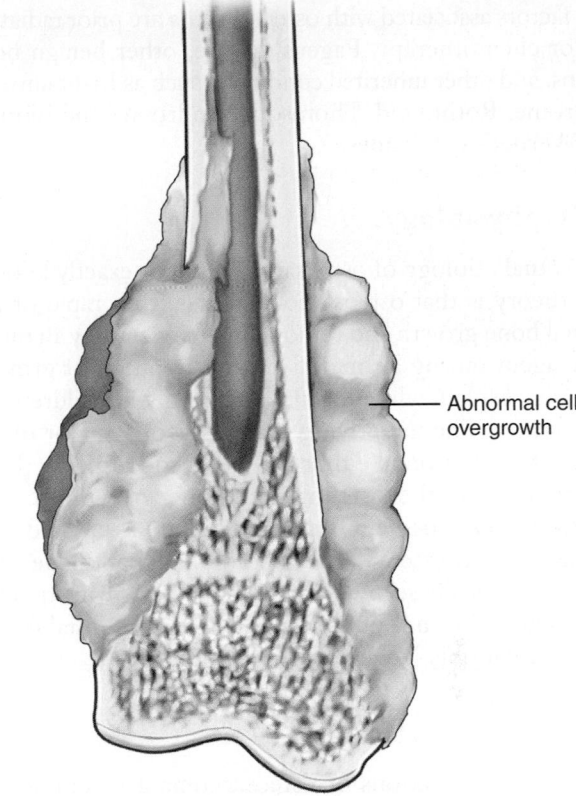

Abnormal cell overgrowth

FIGURE 53.10 Osteosarcoma; abnormal and undifferentiated cell growth around the bone.

in people of middle to older years of age. Fibrosarcoma, a tumor of the fibrous connective tissue, is a rare primary malignancy in which there is abnormal fibroblast cell division, which leads to lack of cellular control and subsequent invasion of local tissue and migration to other sites in the form of metastasis. Rhabdomyosarcoma is a malignant tumor that originates from normal skeletal muscle cells. The cause is unknown. It is very rare in adults, and only 350 to 400 cases are diagnosed each year in children under the age of 21. This section on bone cancer will predominantly focus on osteosarcoma, which is the most prevalent primary malignant tumor in the adult population.

Epidemiology

Osteosarcoma is rare, accounting for only 1% of all cancers diagnosed annually in the United States; however, it is the fifth most common malignancy among adolescents and young adults. Approximately 750 to 900 new cases of osteosarcoma (Fig. 53.10) are diagnosed yearly in the United States. Of these statistics, 400 cases arise in children and young adults less than 20 years of age. Osteosarcoma is found twice as often in males than in females between the ages of 10 and 30 years. Peaks for osteosarcoma are also seen in the older population because of a link between osteosarcoma and Paget's disease. The overall prognosis for that group is very poor. Metastasis of osteosarcoma is typically to the lungs and, if it occurs, can be seen within 2 years from the time of diagnosis and ultimately results in death.

Risk factors associated with osteosarcoma are prior radiation and/or chemotherapy, Paget's disease, other benign bone lesions, and other inherited conditions such as Li-Fraumeni's syndrome, Rothmund-Thomson's syndrome, and Bloom's and Werner's syndromes.

Pathophysiology

The actual etiology of osteosarcoma is not exactly known. One theory is that osteosarcoma arises from rapid or abnormal bone growth and remodeling triggered by an oncogenic agent during a time of cell proliferation or growth. This may explain why it occurs commonly in children and adolescents. The underlying pathology of a tumor of the bone is a disruption in either the osteolytic response (bone destruction) or the osteoblastic (bone growth) activity within the bone tissue. Osteosarcomas are associated with a production of osteoid or immature malignant bone cells. They are typically seen where the bone is growing quickly, such as near the ends of the long bones in the distal femur, the proximal tibia, or the proximal humerus.

Clinical Manifestations

Clinical manifestations of osteosarcoma are common to those of other musculoskeletal health problems, sometimes delaying diagnosis. The following manifestations may be present primarily at the tumor site:

- Pain worse with motion and unrelieved by rest
- Pain may result in a limp
- Swelling
- Redness
- Decreased range of motion
- Fracture

Management

Medical Management

Diagnosis

The primary evaluative tool is a comprehensive history and physical examination focusing on the musculoskeletal system. The past medical history focuses on exposure to previous radiation and/or chemotherapy. Following the history and physical, diagnostic studies including CT, bone scans, myelography, arteriography, MRI, bone biopsy, and biochemical analyses of the blood and urine are recommended. Serum alkaline phosphatase, LD, and ESR levels are frequently elevated with osteosarcomas due to the increased enzyme activity at the level of the muscle, the deterioration of bone, and the inflammatory response. With metastasis from the breast, kidney, or lung to the bone, elevated calcium levels are frequently noted. Computed tomography is not definitive in diagnosis but is helpful with assessing for metastasis. Magnetic resonance imaging is superior to CT due to the ability to define the extent of soft tissue involvement, neurovascular compromise, joint and marrow involvement, and the presence of metastasis. The definitive diagnostic study is a bone biopsy done to determine cell histology and cancer stage and confirm the diagnosis.

Treatment

The primary objective of medical management is to destroy or remove the tumor. The ultimate goal for treatment is limb salvation, survival, and maintenance of quality of life. Treatments can range from radiation therapy (if radiosensitive) to chemotherapy to surgical incision. Radiation therapy, such as brachytherapy (internal radiation) or external radiation treatment, is used if the tumor is radiosensitive. In the case of primary bone tumors, radiotherapy is used to destroy or to reduce the size of the tumor so that chemotherapy and/or surgical excision can be used for treatment. Radiation therapy can be scheduled for one session or for multiple sessions depending on the radioactive treatment response and the tumor's cellular structure.

Chemotherapy is another treatment alternative. Again, the goal is to reduce and/or destroy the bony tumor to prevent metastasis. Essential to the successful eradication of bone tumors via chemotherapy is early identification and treatment. Treatment must be initiated when the disease burden is low. Most osteosarcoma tumors, as well as other bone tumors, use a multimodality treatment approach: multiple chemotherapeutic agents and/or a combination of radiation and surgical intervention.

Pain control is another significant goal of treatment. Treatment includes nonsteroidal anti-inflammatories, such as acetaminophen, but commonly narcotics are necessary to manage pain.

Surgical Management

Surgical management of bone cancers is focused on resection of the cancerous mass and limb salvation. For most bone cancers, radical resection, removal of the mass, the entire muscle, bone, and other surrounding tissues that have direct involvement with the lesion, is performed. The focus of this surgical approach is limb salvation and prevention of metastasis. In the event of large bone resection, TJRs with prosthetic implants as well as other surgical procedures (allograft, vascular grafting) may be required.

Complications

In the absence of appropriate therapy and medical management, neoplasms of the bone are associated with disabling and life-threatening complications such as amputation and death. In the event that destruction of the tumor is not evident and tumor growth and spread are probable, resection of the entire bone is deemed medically appropriate. Other complications after surgery include delayed wound healing, osteomyelitis and wound infections, and hypercalcemia.

Nursing Management

Assessment and Analysis

Many of the clinical manifestations observed in the patient with bone cancer are directly associated with the pain and the extent of the cancer to the bone and surrounding tissues and organs. Most common sites of involvement are the distal femur, proximal tibia, proximal humerus, and middle and proximal femur (occasionally the jaw with Paget's disease). Common findings include:

- Localized pain, typically over several months' duration
- Pain frequently noted with incurrence of injury (may come and go over time)
- Soft tissue mass that is large and tender on palpation

Other clinical manifestations such as fever, malaise, and weight loss are associated with metastasis and are not normally seen with primary bone cancer diagnosis.

Nursing Diagnoses

- **Acute/chronic pain** associated with the destruction of bone
- **Impaired physical mobility** associated with pain and inflammation
- **Peripheral neurovascular dysfunction** associated with impaired perfusion
- **Ineffective tissue perfusion** associated with inflammation
- **Grieving** associated with impaired body image (possible loss of limb)
- **Risk for pathologic fractures** associated with destruction of the bony matrix

Nursing Interventions

■ *Assessments*

- Respiratory rate/level of consciousness
  Bone cancer requires aggressive pain management; a decrease in respiratory rate or level of consciousness may indicate overmedication.
- Pain assessment
  Regular pain assessment provides a baseline and is an indicator of effective/ineffective pain management.
- Neurovascular assessment
  Weak pulses, pallor, pain, paresthesia, paresis, and/or paralysis indicates a compromise in neurovascular status that may be caused by compartment compromise (increased pressure in the tissues surrounding the mass) resulting in loss of muscle, tissue, nerves, and bone.
- Palpation of mass
  A palpable mass with swelling, pain, and tenderness may indicate a progression of tumor growth and metastasis.
- Assess level of activity, exercise, and independent function
  Independence versus dependence is a potential problem for patients with bone cancer. Pain and the disability caused by osteosarcoma may limit the ability to perform activities of daily living independently.

■ *Actions*

- Administration of pain medication as ordered
  Pain is extensive and requires aggressive pharmacological intervention. Monitor vital signs of patient for opioid-induced respiratory depression.

- Work with healthcare team to support long-term pain relief, pharmacological and nonpharmacological
  The most effective pain management approach helps the patient maintain a functional status as well as provides a plan for procedures that may be necessary to manage increasing pain.
- Prepare and support the patient for radiation treatment if warranted; be sure patient is free from moisture, deodorant, or creams
  Moisture, deodorant, or creams may cause radiation skin irritations and burns.
- Administer chemotherapeutic therapy as ordered
  The goal of chemotherapy is to reduce or destroy tumor cells.
- Support and position the affected extremities with gentle range of motion and exercises to the joints above and below the affected site
  Bone tumors weaken the bone, causing extreme pain on movement. Exercises for pain relief and external supports are used for additional support, comfort and safety.
- Apply thermal therapy as ordered from rehabilitative services
  Thermal therapy (hot and/or cold) has been shown to reduce pain and increase functionality.

■ *Teaching*

- Take pain analgesic medication as prescribed
  Adequate pain management is essential to promote maximal independent functioning. Caution: Opioids are addictive and can cause constipation, drowsiness, and respiratory depression. Patients should not drink alcohol or operate heavy machinery (car).
- Teach patient about radiation therapy
  Radiation therapy can cause localized skin irritation, blisters, and burns. No creams, talcum powder, or emulsion agents should be used before radiation treatment. Also, general malaise can be seen with some radiation treatments.
- Teach patient to eat a diet rich in protein
  A high-protein diet helps with tissue and wound healing.
- Provide training for safe movement with activities of daily living
  The patient population is at great risk for pathologic fractures causing falls. Use assistive devices when appropriate.
- Patient understanding of disease process and symptom management, onset and course of injury and illness
  Patient understanding of the disease process, course of illness, and symptom management is essential for early diagnosis and treatment of the disease.

Evaluating Care Outcomes

Limb salvation and prevention of metastasis are the essential components of a well-managed patient with osteosarcoma. Effective pain management facilitating an optimal level of independence are paramount for patient comfort. Early recognition of symptoms is of key importance because it allows early initiation of treatment with radiation, chemotherapy, and/or surgical excision.

Connection Check 53.8

A patient is postoperative day 1 following a surgical procedure after a recent diagnosis of osteosarcoma to his tibia. The nurse recognizes the patient has good understanding of his diagnosis by which statement?

A. "The doctors opened my bone to take a biopsy for the diagnosis."

B. "The doctors opened my bone to take the tumor out and all the tissue around it."

C. "The doctors opened my bone to remove dead bone."

D. "The doctors opened my bone to clean out the infected area."

Making Connections

CASE STUDY: WRAP-UP

Ms. Eileen Doherty demonstrates classic signs of osteoporosis (vertebral changes noted as kyphosis, or "dowager's hump"). She states she has noticed that her pants seem longer. She complains of back pain and increased difficulty with simple activities of daily living such as short walks. Initial diagnostic results for Ms. Doherty reveal an elevated ESR, decreased serum calcium level, and a –2.5 T score for BMD study. These results are consistent with primary osteoporosis. The healthcare provider orders Ms. Doherty to begin bisphosphonate therapy with ibandronate (Boniva) by mouth.

Case Study Questions

1. Ms. Doherty demonstrates the need for more teaching by which of the following statements?
   A. "I don't need to take calcium or vitamin D anymore."
   B. "I know I need to develop an exercise plan."
   C. "I may need to remove a lot of the small throw rugs around the house."
   D. "I know I will need to follow up on a regular basis."

2. The nurse understands which screening tool will help evaluate home safety?
   A. FRAX
   B. Medication
   C. Dietary
   D. Activity

3. Ms. Doherty's greatest risk factor for the development of osteoporosis is which of the following?
   A. A low BMD
   B. A high BMD
   C. A low FRAX
   D. A high QCT

4. The nurse understands which of the following is an important teaching point for Ms. Doherty?
   A. Boniva must be taken on an empty stomach.
   B. Boniva is taken once a week.
   C. Boniva may cause joint pain.
   D. Boniva is taken instead of calcium.

5. The nurse understands which of the following is implicated in the development of osteoporosis?
   A. An increase in calcitonin level
   B. A decrease in estrogen level
   C. A decrease in the parathyroid hormone
   D. A decrease in phosphorus level

CHAPTER SUMMARY

Muscular dystrophies (MDs) are classified as an inherited group of progressive myopathic (muscle) disorders that are caused by defects in normal muscle function. The Duchenne and Becker muscular dystrophies (MDs) are caused by a mutation to the dystrophin gene; a gene responsible for muscle repair. In the absence or reduction of dystrophin, there is degeneration of the muscle fibers resulting in muscle weakness. The primary commonalities among all the MD disorders are progressive muscle weakness, muscle wasting, and increased muscle enzyme serum levels.

Osteoporosis is a chronic condition that results in deterioration of bone tissue and density, which results in an increased risk for fractures. The most widely used fracture risk assessment tool is the FRAX (Fracture Risk Assessment Tool). Assessment is primarily done through BMD measurements obtained through a dual-energy x-ray absorptiometry (DEXA) scan. Intervention is focused on preventing and slowing the progression of bone loss with the use of calcium and vitamin D. Although other medications are available, the primary treatment is the administration of bisphosphonates.

Paget's disease of the bone (PDB), also referred to as *osteitis deformans*, is a bone metabolism disorder that is associated with accelerated bone remodeling. Osteoclasts increase in size and number, escalating resorption of bone. Consequently, osteoblasts add to new bone at an increased rate, which leads to enlarged bony structures that are disorganized in structure and reduced in mechanical strength, leading to patients at risk for the development of deformities and fractures. The skeletal areas most commonly affected are the skull, femur, tibia, pelvic bones, and vertebral column. There is no effective treatment of Paget's disease. Medication therapy is focused on pain management and functional outcomes. Bisphosphonates are used to help manage the bone remodeling.

Osteomyelitis is defined as a localized infection of the bone. Hematogenous, or endogenous, osteomyelitis is a result of infectious spread from another area of the body via the bloodstream. Nonhematogenous, or exogenous, osteomyelitis is a result of an open fracture and/or trauma to the bone. Clinical manifestations include pain not relieved by rest, swelling, tenderness, erythema and warmth at the site, fever, nausea, chills, and malaise. Chronic osteomyelitis results in constant bone pain and swelling, tenderness, and warmth at the site. The initial line of treatment is antibiotics. Opioid analgesia is indicated to manage the pain. The priority nursing diagnosis is infection.

Scoliosis is not a diagnosis but rather a description of the structural alteration that is noted by a curvature of the spine greater than a 10° curvature (Cobb's angle) that is normally associated with rotation and compression. Conservative treatment includes thermal therapy, physical and occupational therapies, a progressive exercise regimen, and pain management. Pharmacological intervention is focused on comfort and pain relief. A Cobb's angle greater than 50° may be managed surgically via spinal instrumentation and/or spinal fusion. A nursing priority with scoliosis is to provide pain relief to enable the patient to maintain adequate exercise levels.

Total joint replacement (TJR) is most commonly associated with the joints of the hip and the knee. Our aging population and the increased incidence of overweight Americans (one-third of all Americans), is expected to exponentially increase the need for joint replacement surgery. Osteoarthritis is the leading clinical indication for TJR. A total hip replacement (THR) or a total knee replacement (TKR) can be considered once self-management, exercise, and analgesics are no longer effective in relieving pain during activities of daily living.

Bone cancer is subdivided into two classifications: benign bone cancers, which are noncancerous and often asymptomatic, and malignant, which are cancerous in nature and can originate from either a primary or secondary source. The cause of primary bone cancer, osteosarcoma, is not exactly known. One theory is that osteosarcoma arises from rapid or abnormal bone growth and remodeling triggered by an oncogenic agent during a time of cell proliferation or growth. Clinical manifestations include pain, redness, warmth, and deformity around the tumor site. The primary objective of medical management is to destroy or remove the tumor. Surgical management of bone cancers is focused on resection of the cancerous mass and limb salvation. Treatments can range from radiation therapy to chemotherapy to surgical incision.

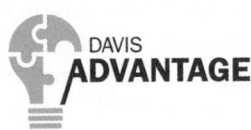

To explore learning resources for this chapter, go to **Davis Advantage** and find:
– Answers to in-text questions
– Chapter Resources and Activities
– NCLEX®-Style Chapter Review Questions
– Bibliography

Chapter 54

Coordinating Care for Patients With Musculoskeletal Trauma

Susan Kulik

LEARNING OUTCOMES

Content in this chapter is designed to support the learner in:

1. Describing the epidemiology of various types of musculoskeletal trauma
2. Identifying the clinical manifestations in the pathophysiological processes of:
   a. Strains and sprains
   b. Fractures
   c. Amputations
   d. Meniscus injuries
   e. Carpal tunnel syndrome
3. Describing the diagnostic results used to confirm the specific type of musculoskeletal trauma
4. Explaining the effective medical management of:
   a. Sprains and strains
   b. Fractures
   c. Amputations
   d. Meniscus injuries
   e. Carpal tunnel syndrome
5. Developing a comprehensive plan of nursing care for patients with musculoskeletal trauma
6. Designing a plan of care that includes pharmacological, dietary, and lifestyle considerations based on patients with musculoskeletal trauma
7. Explaining the clinical presentation and management of complications associated with musculoskeletal trauma

ESSENTIAL TERMS

Amputation
Carpal tunnel syndrome (CTS)
Closed reduction
Compartment syndrome
Dislocation
External fixation
Fat emboli
Fracture
Hypovolemia
Internal fixation
Malunion
Neuromas
Neurovascular compromise
Nonunion
Open reduction
Phantom limb pain
Rhabdomyolysis
Sprain
Strain
Traction
Traumatic amputation
Venous thromboemboli (VTE)

CONCEPTS

- Assessment
- Comfort
- Inflammation
- Medication
- Mobility
- Perfusion
- Perioperative
- Promoting Health

Finding Connections

Follow this patient throughout the chapter.

Zachary White is a 29-year-old male driver involved in a head-on motor vehicle collision. He was ejected from his vehicle, and his right leg was trapped under the vehicle until the medics arrived on scene. He is awake, alert, and yelling because of the severe pain in his right leg. On closer inspection, he has an open right femur fracture that is bleeding profusely and is missing a chunk of muscle. The EMS placed Zachary's right leg in a Hare traction splint, start two large-bore IV lines, and transported him to the emergency department.

Zachary's breath smells of alcohol, and his family member states that he was at a college party. He has no medical history and is not allergic to any medications…

INTRODUCTION

Musculoskeletal conditions and injuries are not just conditions of older age; they are relevant across the life span. Between 60% and 77% of unintentional injuries reported in the United States are due to musculoskeletal trauma. Approximately 20 to 27 million musculoskeletal injuries occur annually in the United States, with **strains** and **sprains** the most prevalent, followed by **fractures**. These injuries often yield negative effects on patients' mobility and sensation and subsequently impair their performance of activities of daily living (ADLs). Nurses must be knowledgeable and prepared to provide appropriate care for patients with musculoskeletal injuries.

STRAINS AND SPRAINS

Epidemiology

Strains and sprains consistently occur from sporting injuries in athletes of all ages, but they are also caused by accidents at home, at work, and during recreation. Ankle sprains are the most frequently occurring orthopedic injury and are responsible for 40% of all athletic injuries, totaling five million annually. The frequency of ankle sprains can be ranked highest among the sports of basketball, ice-skating, and soccer. Another common injury, an anterior cruciate ligament (ACL) tear, a severe strain, occurs mostly from noncontact injuries from sports that involve twisting and jumping. Basketball, football, soccer, and gymnastics generate the highest number of ACL tears. Women are nine times more likely than men to sustain an ACL tear because of several biomechanical and neuromuscular factors. Women have a greater degree of valgus knee torques (knock-knee),

have less muscular strength, and have more knee laxity (flexibility), which puts them at higher risk of ACL injury. There are an estimated 80,000 to 100,000 ACL repair surgeries annually in the United States.

Pathophysiology and Clinical Manifestations

A strain is an injury to muscle or tendon tissue. Tendons connect muscles to bones. A strain is the tearing or stretching of a muscle or tendon, often resulting from overextension, overexertion, or overstretching. Strains can be categorized according to their severity:

- First-degree/mild strains demonstrate minimal inflammation and pain. Symptoms can last for several days, but range of motion (ROM) remains unaffected.
- Second-degree/moderate strains result from actual tearing of the muscle and tendon fibers. This injury is often painful, with severe muscle spasms, extensive inflammation, and ecchymosis that appear several hours or days after the initial injury. Symptoms can last for several weeks.
- Third-degree/severe strains include the rupture of the muscle or tendon, causing considerable internal bleeding, pain, inflammation, and ecchymosis. Surgical repair may be needed if there is extensive tearing in the muscle or tendon.

A sprain is an injury to ligaments. Ligaments are segments of connective tissue that secure bones to bones and bones to cartilage. As in tendons, a sprain is defined as the stretching or tearing of a ligament resulting from overextension, overexertion, or overstretching (Fig. 54.1). Sprains are also classified similar to strains on the basis of severity:

- First-degree/mild sprains demonstrate stretching and/or minimal tearing of ligament fibers. Edema and pain may be evident, but joint function remains intact, and patients are able to ambulate with slight discomfort.
- Second-degree/moderate sprains result from a moderate amount of tearing in the ligament fibers. The joint remains intact, and the ligament is not completely torn. Increased swelling, ecchymosis, pain, and altered weight-bearing mobility are evident in these patients.
- Third-degree/severe sprains include the complete tearing of a ligament, which renders the patient unable to ambulate because of joint instability. Symptoms include severe pain, ecchymosis, and edema.

Connection Check 54.1

The nurse recognizes that the stretching or tearing of a muscle or tendon occurs in which condition?

A. Strains
B. Dislocations
C. Fractures
D. Sprains

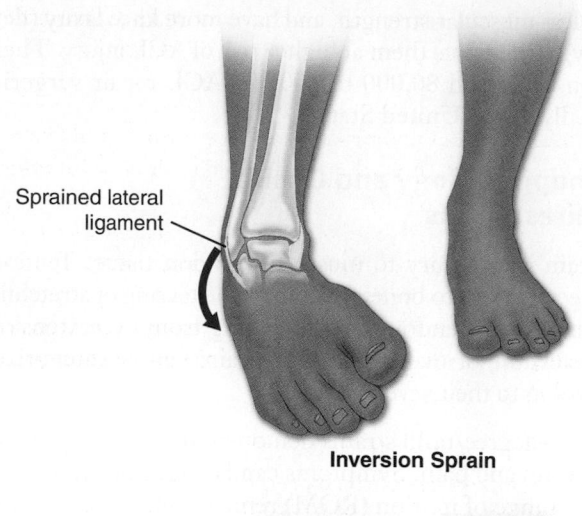

Inversion Sprain

Sprained lateral ligament

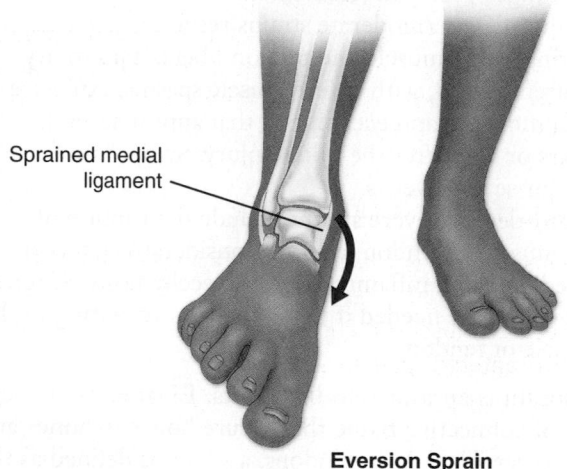

Eversion Sprain

Sprained medial ligament

FIGURE 54.1 Inversion and eversion sprains caused by ankle rotation.

Management

Medical Management

Diagnosis

The diagnosis of sprains and strains is based on a thorough history and physical examination of the affected area and is often confirmed by radiography, ultrasound, or magnetic resonance imaging (MRI). Ultrasounds are low cost and highly effective in identifying strains and sprains, but an MRI may be more definitive in the final diagnosis.

Treatment

Treatment of first- and second-degree strains and sprains involves **RICE**, a common acronym referring to the treatment plan for strains and sprains:

- **R**est the injured extremity for as long as 72 hours to allow the ligaments or tendon time to heal.
- **I**ce applied for no longer than 30 minutes three to five times per day for 24 to 72 hours after injury. This promotes vasoconstriction and decreases bleeding and fluid collection in the injured area.
- **C**ompression by means of an Ace wrap or similar compression dressing to minimize further swelling,

which can delay healing. The dressing should be wrapped tightly but not enough to alter neurovascular function. Ensure that circulation, movement, and sensation remain intact.

- **E**levate the affected area to minimize dependent swelling.

Functional supports in the form of braces may be used for 4 to 6 weeks and are preferred versus immobilization. Exercise therapy programs may be prescribed and consist of neuromuscular and proprioceptive exercises. In addition to the therapies mentioned previously, NSAIDs are usually prescribed to minimize pain and inflammation.

Third-degree strains may require surgical repair of the torn tendon or muscle. Surgical repair typically involves an open incision and the use of thick suture material to reattach the torn muscle and tendons. Occasionally, either a graft from the patient's healthy tendon or a donor graft can also be used for surgical repair. Third-degree sprains may necessitate the need for arthroscopic surgical repair. Arthroscopic surgery uses small scopes to visualize and repair the injured area. Musculoskeletal allografts are gaining popularity for ligamentous reconstruction by orthopaedic surgeons while their safety and efficacy continue to improve. Postoperative treatment for strains and sprains involves immobilization of the affected extremity for 4 to 6 weeks and physical therapy.

Complications

There can be numerous complications from strains and sprains, such as chronically unstable joints, bursitis, tendinitis (Box 54.1), and frequent reoccurrence. Strains and sprains

---

Box 54.1 Bursitis and Tendinitis

Definitions

Bursitis is an inflammation of the bursa, a sac located between bone or muscle or tendon that contains lubricating fluid to decrease friction with movement. Tendinitis is an inflammation of the tendon. Both are more common in people older than 40 because age makes tendons less elastic and more prone to tearing.

Causes

Both conditions are typically caused by overuse, repetitive minor impact, or a sudden, more significant impact to the affected area. Areas typically affected include the elbow, hip, shoulder, or knee.

Symptoms

Pain in the affected area occurs in both conditions.

Treatment

Avoidance of activities that aggravate the irritation, rest for the affected area, and anti-inflammatory medications are methods of treatment for both conditions.

can cause significant alterations in patient mobility, limiting function and the ability to perform self-care. Additionally, patient noncompliance with therapeutic treatment regimens can cause future disability, increased risk for repeated injuries, and the need for surgical intervention. Although extremely rare, **compartment syndrome**, excessive pressure in a compartment of the body due to bleeding or edema which impedes blood flow resulting in severe tissue damage in the affected area, can develop in patients with sprains and strains.

Nursing Management
Assessment and Analysis

Close examination of the affected extremity typically reveals swelling, ecchymosis, and deformity due to strain, tearing, or rupture of the ligaments, tendons, or muscles. Patients may also exhibit intolerance to palpation and be unable to bear weight on the injured side.

Nursing Diagnoses
- **Acute pain** associated with the physical injury
- **Altered peripheral tissue perfusion** associated with edema and vessel damage
- **Impaired physical mobility** associated with the injury

Nursing Interventions
■ Assessments
- Physical assessment of injured extremity via inspection and palpation: palpate the injured extremity noting the six Ps to include **p**ain, **p**ressure, **p**aralysis, **p**allor, **p**aresthesia, and **p**ulselessness. Complete the neurovascular assessment by checking movement and sensation.
  Inspection and palpation are done to assess circulation, movement, and sensation in the injured area. The presence of the six Ps may indicate neurovascular compromise of the injured area and may necessitate immediate medical intervention to prevent permanent damage. Extreme pain may indicate the presence of a fracture.
- Patient history of injury
  Appropriate medical management is dependent on an accurate patient history to include determination of a chronic versus acute injury.

■ Actions
- **R**est the injured extremity
  Minimizing activity promotes healing.
- **I**ce applied to the injury
  Cryotherapy causes vasoconstriction, which decreases further bleeding and inflammation.
- **C**ompression via ace wrap
  Compression reduces the inflammation that causes pain and delays healing.
- **E**levation
  Elevation decreases edema, which eases pain and promotes mobility of the injured area.
- Administer anti-inflammatory and analgesia medications as ordered

Inhibit prostaglandin (mediators of pain and inflammation) formation, which can reduce pain and inflammation

■ Teaching
- Immediately report any worsening symptoms in the injured area, to include continued pain, loss of function, loss of mobility, or loss of sensation
  Alterations in circulation, movement, and sensation can signal the need for further medical intervention.
- RICE therapy
  Compliance with the prescribed treatment regimen ensures appropriate healing and the return of the injured limb to normal function.

Evaluating Care Outcomes

Severe strains and sprains may require surgical intervention and lengthy postoperative treatment regimens that include physical therapy. Optimal recovery is possible with compliance with physical therapy–suggested exercises. A well-managed patient should return to normal function with compliance with the treatment protocol.

Connection Check 54.2

The nurse identifies which pathophysiological finding in a third-degree sprain?
A. Stretched muscle or tendon fibers
B. Torn/ruptured ligaments
C. Torn/ruptured muscle or tendon fibers
D. Stretched ligaments

CASE STUDY: EPISODE 2

Zachary demonstrates classic symptoms of an open, displaced femur fracture. The emergency department provider immediately consults with the orthopedic surgeon, and 45 minutes later, Zachary is taken to the operating room. After significant irrigation of the open right femur fracture, the surgeon conducts an open reduction with placement of an external fixator...

FRACTURES
Epidemiology

The incidence of fractures in the United States is on the rise, with an estimated six million fractures occurring annually. Fractures most often occur in the young and in the older population because both groups have bone that is porous and contains areas of weakness. Fragility fractures in older adults are a result of progressive decrease in bone density and bone strength. They also frequently suffer from chronic bone disorders that increase the risk of pathologic fractures. These chronic bone disorders are Cushing's syndrome, osteoporosis, osteogenesis imperfecta, neoplasms, anorexia, and Paget's disease. These diseases significantly weaken bones, decrease load-carrying capacity and tolerance to force, increase the patient's susceptibility to fractures, and further prolong the healing process. Fractures in young people between the ages of 12 and 21 are typically the result of high-energy trauma. Examples of high-energy trauma include motor vehicle collisions, contact sports, and bicycle accidents. Fractures in people 65 years or older are usually caused by low-energy trauma, for example, fractures from falling.

Pathophysiology and Clinical Manifestations

Bone is classified as dense, irregular connective tissue made up of osteoblasts and osteocytes. Bones provide support and structure, assist the body in movement, and protect vital organs. When excessive force is placed on bones, they fracture. A **fracture** is defined as a disruption, or break, in the continuity of a bone. There are numerous classifications of fractures that can occur throughout the body (Fig. 54.2).

Types of Fractures

- *Complete.* The disruption spans across the width of the bone, causing bone fragments.
- *Incomplete.* The disruption occurs through part of the bone cortex; however, there is no displacement of bone fragments.
- *Closed (simple).* Fracture that is contained within the skin
- *Open (compound).* Disruption in which pieces of bone protrude through the skin, creating an external wound that exposes the fracture site. Open fractures are graded on the basis of their severity.
  - Grade I. Presence of a puncture wound, minimal injury to the soft tissues, and vasculature remains intact
  - Grade II. Puncture wound, fragments of broken bone, moderate skin and muscle contusions, and significant wound contamination
  - Grade III. Severe damage to soft tissues, nerves, muscles, and blood vessels. The open fracture site is considered extremely contaminated and contains numerous comminuted fractures.

Fracture Patterns

- *Avulsion.* Caused by the overstretching and tearing of a tendon or ligament, separating a small segment of bone at the insertion site
- *Comminuted.* Fracture that has several disruptions producing shattered bone fragments within the fracture site
- *Compression.* Fracture caused by excessive force along the axis of cancellous (spongy internal layer of bone) bone, leading to the bone collapsing on itself; representative in vertebral compression fractures from falls of significant heights
- *Depressed.* Disruptions in which fragments of bone are forced inward; frequently seen in facial and skull fractures involving blunt trauma
- *Displaced.* Malalignment of bone fragments at the fracture site

- *Greenstick.* An incomplete disruption in which one side of the bone is bent and the other is fractured; generally seen in children because of the flexibility of their bones
- *Nondisplaced.* Bone fragments are well approximated within the site of disruption.
- *Oblique.* The fracture line occurs usually at a 45-degree angle across the cortex of the bone.
- *Spiral.* The fracture wraps around the shaft of the bone.
- *Impacted.* Segments of bone are wedged into each other at the fracture line.

Management

Diagnosis

The diagnosis of fractures is based on a thorough history of how the injury occurred, a physical assessment, and is confirmed by radiography or computed tomography (CT). When the patient's history is obtained, it is important to note the specific mechanism of force that caused the injury. Other imperative information includes the patient's medical history and any chronic illnesses, medications, and potential substance abuse. Medications and substance abuse can impair mental judgment and function and contribute to motor vehicle accidents and falls, thus producing bone fractures and other traumatic injuries. If a chronic illness is suspected as having a major role in the injury, a bone scan and MRI may be needed to confirm the diagnosis.

Treatment

Definitive treatment of fractures is highly dependent on their type and location and may require either surgical or nonsurgical intervention. Table 54.1 describes various fractures and their treatment. In the case of open fractures with contaminated wounds, antibiotics are implemented to prevent osteomyelitis and other wound infections. Effective pain management is an important aspect in treating fractures. Narcotics and anti-inflammatory medications are effective in controlling pain and inflammation. These medications allow the patient to gradually regain movement and function of the injured area. After definitive treatment, movement and function are key in preventing muscle atrophy and contractures.

Nonsurgical Management

Nonsurgical treatment of a fracture, or a **closed reduction**, is the most frequent type of nonsurgical fracture treatment in which the fractured bone segments are manually manipulated and realigned while the patient is under general anesthesia. General anesthesia is needed to ensure complete muscle relaxation for proper bone realignment. After closed reduction, the realigned bone is typically placed in a cast or a splint. Splints are a form of nonrigid immobilization to maintain alignment of bone fragments. Casts are rigid immobilization devices constructed of fiberglass or plaster for use on weight-bearing extremities. Adjunctive therapies include ultrasound and electromagnetic stimulation. Percutaneous autologous bone marrow grafting has been used

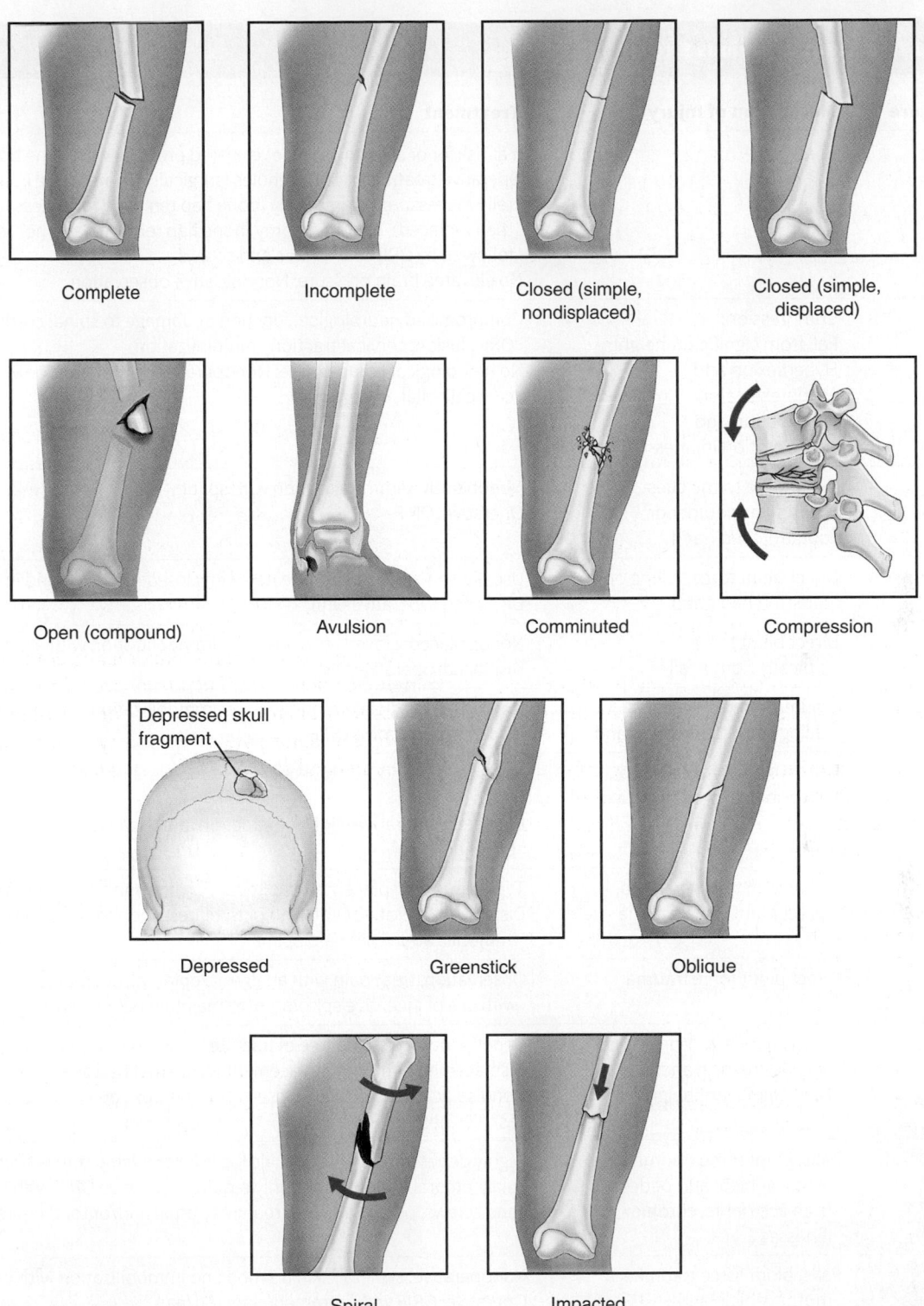

FIGURE 54.2 Types of fractures.

with nonunions, and treatment has demonstrated increased healing rates.

Surgical Management

Surgical repair of fractures includes an **open reduction** with **internal fixation** or **external fixation**. Open reduction requires a surgical incision that enables the surgeon to accurately visualize the wound and ensure proper realignment. Internal fixation requires the use of plates, screws, rods, and other hardware to realign the fractured bone segments. Irrigation and debridement might be needed for open fractures that are contaminated with dirt and foreign matter. External fixation is the application of a series of rods and pins to the area surrounding the fracture,

Table 54.1 Fractures of Various Sites

Type of Fracture	Mechanism of Injury	Treatment
Skull	Blunt force	If at risk for or showing signs of elevated pressure within the brain: Operative treatment via Burr holes (surgically created hole in the skull to relieve pressure), craniotomy (bone flap removed for access to brain tissue then replaced), or craniectomy (bone flap removed and not replaced) followed by ORIF with plates and screws No elevated brain pressure: Nonoperative observation
Spinal	Compression: Fall from significant heights Hyperflexion and hyperextension: Acceleration and deceleration injuries	Compromised neurological function or damage to spinal cord: Operative ORIF, fusion, cervical traction, immobilization No neurological compromise: Nonoperative immobilization with a stiff cervical collar, observation
Clavicle	Blunt force to the chest, falling on shoulder or outstretched hand	Nonoperative: immobilization with splint Operative: ORIF
Humerus	Direct blunt force, falling on outstretched hand	Usually nondisplaced and treated with closed reduction and immobilization Displaced: Operative ORIF
Elbow	Direct blunt force typically from a fall	Nondisplaced: closed reduction and immobilization with a cast Displaced: operative ORIF
Forearm (radius and ulna)	Trauma, direct force, and falling on outstretched hand	Nondisplaced: closed reduction and immobilization with a cast/splint Displaced: operative ORIF
Wrist	Fall on outstretched hand, direct blunt force trauma	Nondisplaced: closed reduction and immobilization with splint/cast, pressure dressing Displaced: operative ORIF with traction, pins/screws, or application on an external fixator
Metacarpal/ Phalanges	Fall on outstretched hand, direct blunt force trauma	Typically nondisplaced: closed reduction, immobilization with splint/cast Displaced: operative ORIF with pins, plates, and screws followed by immobilization with cast/splint
Rib	Direct blunt force trauma	Observation, treat pain with analgesia/epidural, deep breathing exercises with use of incentive spirometry to maintain pulmonary hygiene
Pelvic	Crush injuries, motor vehicle crashes, and falls from significant heights	Dependent on type/degree of fracture Displacement: emergent placement of external fixator and/or ORIF Nondisplaced/Less severe: Observation, bedrest, analgesia, and ambulation as tolerated
Hip	Falls, blunt force trauma, motor vehicle and pedestrian accidents, chronic illnesses	Highly dependent on the specific location of the fracture within the acetabular/femoral region; commonly requires operative ORIF with nails, plates, and screws; potentially also requires partial and/or total hip replacement
Femur	Falls, blunt force trauma, motor vehicle and pedestrian accidents	Nonoperative: skeletal/skin traction and immobilization with cast/brace Operative: ORIF with intramedullary rod/nail
Tibia/Fibula	Direct blunt force trauma, stepping torsion/rotation of leg and ankle	Nondisplaced: Closed reduction and immobilization with cast/splint Displaced/open: application of external fixation and/or ORIF with plates and screws followed by immobilization with cast/splint
Metatarsal/ Phalanges	Crush injuries and blunt force trauma	Typically nondisplaced: closed reduction, immobilization with splint/cast Displaced: operative ORIF with pins, plates, and screws followed by immobilization with cast/splint

ORIF = Open reduction and internal fixation.

creating an external frame to stabilize and align the displaced fragments. External fixators are frequently used when there is significant soft-tissue damage at the fracture site (Fig. 54.3).

Traction

Traction can be used in conjunction with any of the other previously mentioned forms of fracture treatment. Traction involves the use of weights and force to reduce the fracture and relieve muscle spasms.

- *Skeletal traction.* Pins, tongs, screws, and wires are surgically secured to the bone, and weight is then applied to provide realignment (Fig. 54.4A). Cervical traction is an example of skeletal traction in which a halo device, or Crutchfield tongs, is applied to stabilize the cervical fracture.
- *Skin traction* uses a flexible harness, boot, or belt to secure the extremity while 5 to 10 lb of weight is applied to relieve muscle spasms and maintain the length of the bone (Fig. 54.4B). Buck's traction is a form of skin traction commonly used for femur and hip fractures.

Connection Check 54.3

The nurse correlates which diagnostic result for an older adult with a suspected pathologic fracture?

A. Decreased bone density
B. Increased osteocytes
C. Hypertension
D. Coagulopathy

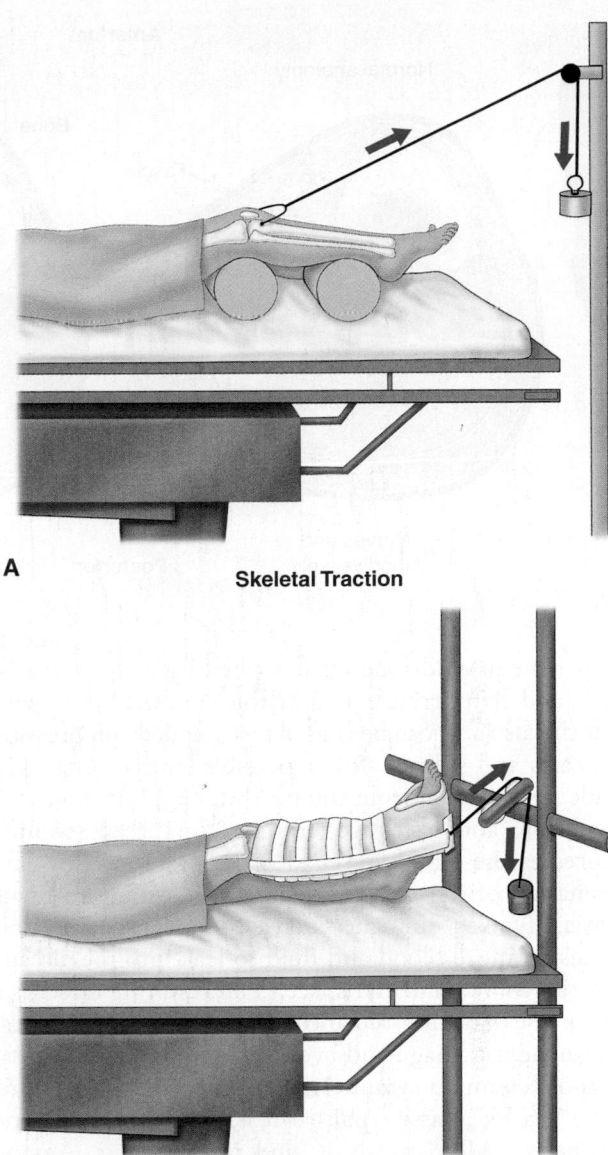

A   Skeletal Traction

B   Skin Traction

FIGURE 54.4 Types of traction. A, Skeletal traction; B, Skin traction.

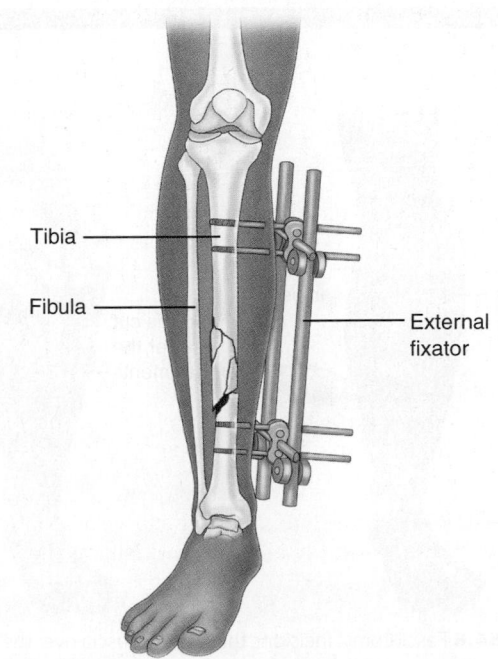

Tibia
Fibula
External fixator

FIGURE 54.3 External fixation for an open tibial fracture.

Complications

Neurovascular compromise is a complication due to any source of decreased blood flow and oxygenation to the tissues. One cause is the severing of blood vessels and nerves surrounding the bone by sharp bone fragments created by a fracture. The use of traction and immediate fracture reduction is vital in preventing further damage to the neurovasculature. Joint **dislocation** in which the displaced bones compress the nerves and vessels is another cause of neurovascular compromise, and the joint should be realigned as soon as possible. Compartment syndrome is a rare but serious complication which, when undetected, can cause permanent loss of the affected limb due to neurovascular compromise caused by increased pressure in the extremity (Fig. 54.5). Compartments are composed of muscles, nerves, and blood vessels. These compartments are surrounded by tough connective tissue linings called *fascia*.

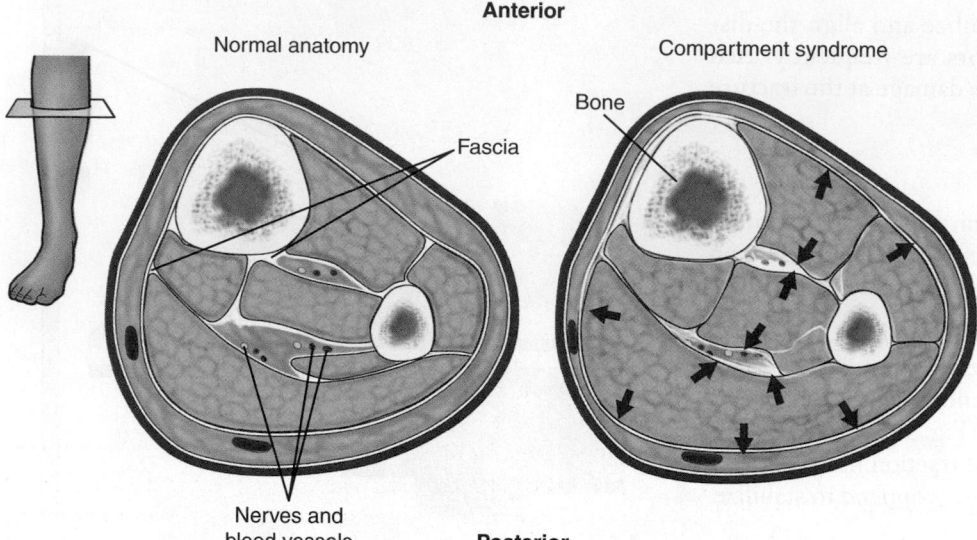

FIGURE 54.5 Compartment syndrome: increased pressure in the compartment causing compression of nerves and blood vessels.

Compartment syndrome occurs when there is increased edema and hemorrhage within the compartment space under the fascia. It can be caused by extended compression from casts and splints. Other possible sources of edema include hemorrhage from the initial injury, burns, venous thrombosis, and excessive exercise. Increased swelling compresses the blood vessels, restricting blood flow and oxygenation of the muscles and nerves, leading to tissue hypoxia. Hypoxia stimulates increased capillary permeability, causing more blood and fluid to leak into the already restricted compartmental space. The resulting effect is a vicious cycle of neurovascular compression that can progress to permanent damage and eventual loss of the extremity. The most common symptoms of compartment syndrome are the "six Ps"; passive **p**ain at rest, along with **p**ressure, **p**aresthesia, **p**allor, **p**aralysis, and **p**ulselessness. Among the six Ps of compartment syndrome, pallor, paralysis, and pulselessness are considered to be late findings. Once compartment syndrome is suspected, the nurse should immediately notify the provider to relieve the pressure on the extremity (see Evidence-Based Practice). If caused by pressure from a cast, the provider will remove the cast immediately. An immediate fasciotomy is indicated in the case of internal pressure from edema. A fasciotomy is a procedure in which the surgeon makes incisions on both the medial and lateral aspects of the extremity down through the fascia, relieving the compartment pressure (Fig. 54.6).

bleeding disorders, and bone fractures. The nurse must perform frequent neurovascular examinations that include the assessment of both the affected and unaffected limbs. Key findings indicative of compartment syndrome include pain out of proportion to the injury and pain with passive movement in the affected limb. Direct compartment pressure can be measured with a Stryker device. A pressure within 30 mm Hg of the diastolic pressure or an absolute pressure greater than 30 mm Hg is diagnostic for compartment syndrome. An immediate fasciotomy is indicated to preserve extremity function.

Kistler, J. M., Ilyas, A. M., & Thoder, J. J. (2018). Forearm compartment syndrome: evaluation and management. *Hand Clinics, 34(1)*, 53-60.

Evidence-Based Practice

Compartment Syndrome

Compartment syndrome is a serious condition that, if untreated, can lead to the loss of the affected limb. Causes of compartment syndrome include burns, vascular injuries, penetrating trauma, insect bites, IV infiltration, animal bites,

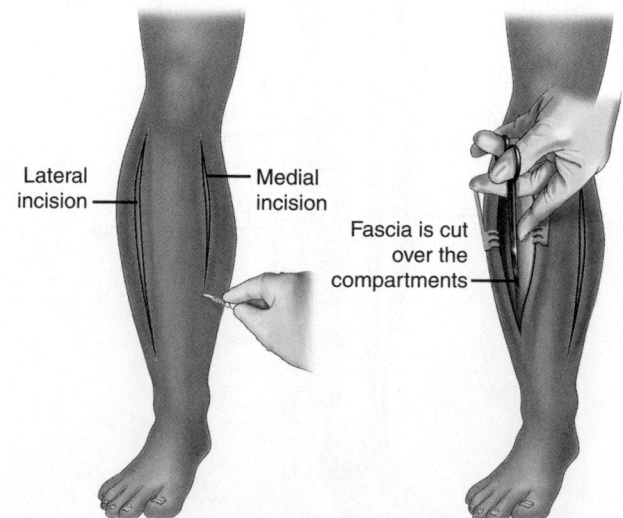

FIGURE 54.6 Fasciotomy: incisions through the fascia over the affected compartment to relieve pressure.

Venous thromboemboli (VTE) is another possible complication. VTE develop in the large vessels of the extremities because of extended periods of immobility, traumatic injuries, cardiac disease, long surgeries, obesity, smoking, and use of oral contraceptives. Venous thromboemboli can be perpetuated by musculoskeletal trauma, specifically fractures involving the upper and lower extremities. Clots can develop in large vessels and hinder circulation or can break apart and travel to the pulmonary arteries and become *pulmonary emboli* (Fig. 54.7). Pulmonary emboli clog the pulmonary vasculature hindering gas exchange, impairing oxygenation, and potentially leading to respiratory failure and patient death. Patients experiencing a pulmonary embolism exhibit dyspnea, tachycardia, abnormal breath sounds, pleuritic chest pain, cyanosis, anxiety, and altered mentation. Chapter 27 discusses pulmonary emboli in detail.

Fat embolism syndrome is a rare complication after orthopedic injury and surgery. **Fat emboli** frequently manifest in long bone fractures where particles of the exposed fatty bone marrow have migrated into the systemic circulation. The particles then mobilize throughout the body and clog smaller blood vessels, producing generalized petechiae: small or pinpoint round spots that appear red or purple on the skin. Much like VTE, fat emboli can travel to and lodge in the pulmonary artery and become pulmonary emboli. As a result, patients experience symptoms of respiratory distress, acute confusion, and restlessness potentially leading to respiratory failure and patient death.

> **Safety Alert** It is imperative that the nurse immediately identify patients with long bone fractures and recognize that they are highly susceptible to developing life-threatening fat emboli. The nurse should conduct frequent assessments of the patient's respiratory status and report any abnormal findings immediately.

Traumatic rhabdomyolysis is a potential complication from injuries that result in compression and tissue ischemia, such as crush injuries. Crush injuries produce continued compression of muscle tissue that restricts blood flow and precipitates tissue ischemia. Tissue ischemia catalyzes a vicious cycle of further inflammation, increased capillary permeability, and the release of more fluid and intracellular contents into the compartment and circulatory system. Myoglobin is an intracellular oxygen-binding protein found in skeletal muscle. It is one of the many intracellular components that spill out of dead muscle cells. Once in the circulatory system, myoglobin travels to the kidneys and is lodged in the nephrons. As a result, the kidneys are unable to effectively filter the proteins and fall victim to acute tubular necrosis and renal failure. Symptoms of rhabdomyolysis include severe flank plan and dark tea-colored urine. Patients who have experienced crush injuries must have regular monitoring of their serum myoglobin and renal function levels. If rhabdomyolysis is present, fluid resuscitation is indicated to help "flush" the myoglobin through the kidney. Rhabdomyolysis is frequently complicated by multiple electrolyte disorders including hyperkalemia, hypophosphatemia, and hypo/hypercalcemia.

Hypovolemia is a potential complication due to the loss of blood that may occur with the fracture. Fractures produce sharp shards of bone that can sever adjacent blood vessels, causing severe exsanguination. Open fractures can generate significant amounts of blood loss that must be controlled as early as possible. Although not immediately visible, internal hemorrhaging from closed fractures must also be rapidly assessed and treated. The presence of large hematomas at the site of injury can signify internal bleeding. Close monitoring of vital signs is essential. The pelvis is highly vascular and a potential fracture site where patients can quickly hemorrhage and decompensate into hypovolemic shock (Fig. 54.8). Table 54.2 notes various fracture sites and their potential blood loss.

Infection is a common complication associated with fractures. All open fractures are deemed contaminated and can cause a bone infection called *osteomyelitis*. If undetected, bacterial infections can develop into gas gangrene and tetanus. Other potential sources of infection are external fixators, internal hardware from surgical repair, and hospital-acquired nosocomial infections. Patients with a wound/bone infection can exhibit delayed wound healing, purulent drainage, erythema, fever, and elevated white blood cell counts. Infection can be prevented through strict aseptic wound care and frequent assessments.

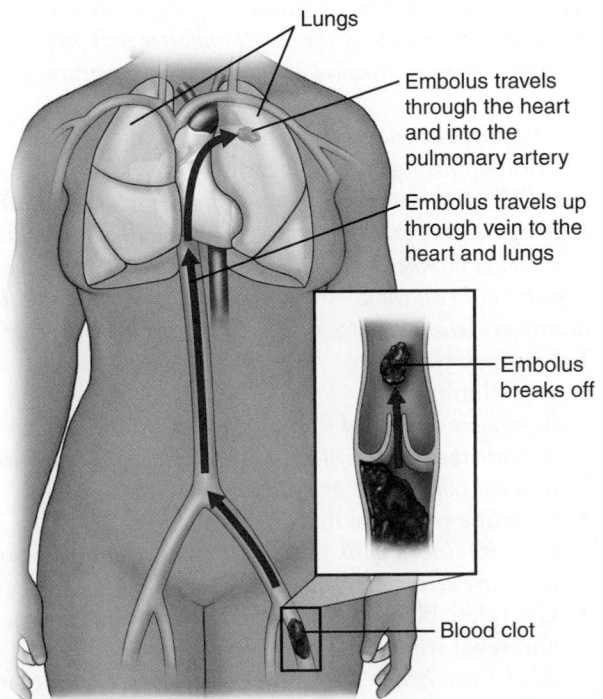

Lungs

Embolus travels through the heart and into the pulmonary artery

Embolus travels up through vein to the heart and lungs

Embolus breaks off

Blood clot

FIGURE 54.7 Pulmonary emboli.

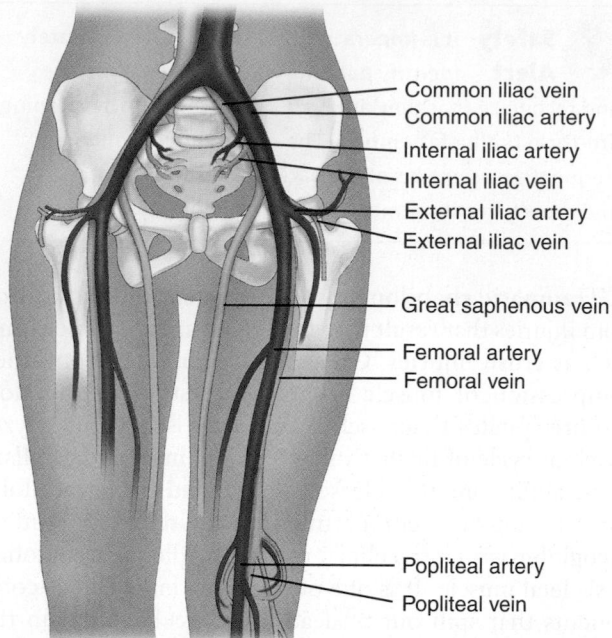

Common iliac vein
Common iliac artery
Internal iliac artery
Internal iliac vein
External iliac artery
External iliac vein

Great saphenous vein

Femoral artery
Femoral vein

Popliteal artery
Popliteal vein

FIGURE 54.8 Blood supply in the pelvis. The pelvis is highly vascular causing it to be a fracture site where there can be extensive blood loss.

Table 54.2 Potential Blood Loss per Fracture Site

Fracture Site	Potential Blood Loss (mL)
Humerus	500–1,500
Elbow, radius, ulna	250–750
Pelvis	750–6,000
Femur	500–3,000
Tibia, fibula	250–1,000

Malunion and **nonunion** are also possible complications of fractures. Both can cause significant impairment to mobility. Malunion occurs when fractures fail to heal in the correct anatomical alignment. It can be the result of inadequate fracture reduction and immobilization, misalignment during fracture reduction, or the premature removal of splints and casts. Severe traumatic fractures that are comminuted with many bone fragments are at high risk for malunion.

Nonunion refers to a fracture that has failed to heal. Nonunion is further categorized into septic nonunion and aseptic nonunion. Septic nonunion is precipitated by infection, whereas aseptic nonunion can be due to older age, anemia, use of tobacco and nicotine, diabetes, and medications that suppress healing such as NSAIDs, steroids, and aspirin. Surgical treatment of malunion and nonunion typically includes bone grafting, either from the patient or by using cadaver and donor bone, and/or the application of bone growth stimulators.

Nursing Management
Assessment and Analysis

Close examination of the affected extremity typically reveals swelling, ecchymosis, and deformity due to bone misalignment and the resultant bleeding and inflammatory process. Hemorrhage may be evident with an open fracture in which the bone fragments have severed the blood vessels. Pain may or may not be present at the fracture site, but patients frequently exhibit pain when the affected site is manipulated on examination.

Nursing Diagnoses

- **Acute pain** associated with muscle spasms and trauma
- **Activity intolerance** associated with immobility
- **Impaired mobility** associated with limb immobilization
- **Impaired skin integrity** associated with the presence of a cast, splints, and traction

Nursing Interventions
Assessments

- Vital signs
  Excessive bleeding leads to symptoms of hemorrhagic shock: low blood pressure, tachycardia, and tachypnea. Tachycardia, tachypnea, and decreased pulse oximetry with chest pain may indicate pulmonary embolus. An elevated temperature may indicate infection.

- Physical assessment of the site of injury via inspection and palpation. Palpate the injured extremity noting the six Ps: **p**ain, **p**ressure, **p**aralysis, **p**allor, **p**aresthesia, and **p**ulselessness. Complete the neurovascular assessment by checking movement and sensation.
  The presence of one or several of the six Ps may indicate neurovascular compromise that can lead to hemorrhage, compartment syndrome, infection, or permanent loss of function. The absence of the six Ps indicates that proper treatment is being provided and that there is no neurovascular compromise.

- Verify proper positioning, application, and stability of traction/splinting/immobilization devices
  Immobilization, traction, casts, and splints secure the fractured bone segments to promote healing. Occasionally, immobilization devices become loose, compromise circulation, or move out of position. Frequent assessment is needed to ensure that the devices are secure and are not hindering the healing process.

- Laboratory tests
  - Myoglobin
    Myoglobin is released from damaged muscle and may indicate the presence of rhabdomyolysis, which may lead to renal compromise or failure.
  - Creatine phosphokinase (CPK)
    CPK is released with any muscle breakdown, increased levels are seen with rhabdomyolysis
  - Complete blood count (CBC), metabolic profile, and renal studies
    Rhabdomyolysis is frequently complicated by multiple electrolyte disorders including hyperkalemia, hypophosphatemia, and hypo/hypercalcemia as well as renal

failure. Blood loss and infection are potential complications of fractures. A complete blood count (CBC), metabolic profile, and renal studies are used to detect signs of infection (increased white blood cell count), blood loss (decreased hemoglobin and hematocrit), electrolyte disturbances (metabolic profile) and indications of renal failure (increased blood urea nitrogen [BUN] and creatinine).

- Urine appearance
  Urine may be tea colored in rhabdomyolysis because of ruptured blood cells that clog the nephrons. Acute kidney injury is the most serious and even life-threatening complication of rhabdomyolysis.
- Intake and output
  All fractures result in blood loss. Adequate volume replacement is necessary to prevent hypovolemic shock. Blood loss from drains, incisions, and wounds should be monitored closely. Also, hypovolemia and rhabdomyolysis may result in decreased urine output.

▪ Actions

- Maintain pulmonary hygiene
  Incentive spirometry exercises and coughing and deep breathing expands alveoli, helping maintain adequate alveolar gas exchange
- Administer analgesia as ordered
  Administration of scheduled narcotic and anti-inflammatory medications inhibits prostaglandin formation, thus reducing pain and allowing the patient to reestablish function and mobility.
- Administer antibiotics as ordered
  Reduce the risk of infection, especially in patients with open fractures
- Administer anticoagulants as ordered
  Patients with fractures are highly susceptible to VTE and pulmonary emboli.
  Anticoagulants help prevent blood clots and emboli.
- Wound/Pin care
  Providing daily pin site and wound care using strict aseptic technique reduces the risk of infection and promotes healing.
- Elevation
  Elevating the affected extremity above the level of the heart minimizes pain and edema.
  *If a crushing injury is suspected, do not elevate the limb because elevation reduces arterial pressure.
- Apply ice
  Promotes therapeutic vasoconstriction and decreases edema and pain
- Range-of-motion exercises and ambulation using available assistive devices
  Ambulation and movement as soon as ordered prevent muscle atrophy and contractures, promote function and mobility, and promote healing and strength. Early ambulation as possible helps prevent VTE through the action of muscle contraction, which discourages blood from pooling. Assistive devices are very helpful in allowing the patient to perform self-care. (Box 54.2)

Box 54.2 Assistive Devices

Assistive devices facilitate the patients' performance of activities of daily living, promote patient independence, prevent complications associated with immobility, and enhance the patient's feelings of self-esteem and self-worth. Some of the commonly used assistive devices related to mobility and ambulation include canes, walkers, wheelchairs, crutches, over-bed trapeze devices, and prosthetic limbs.

- Repositioning
  Patients in traction, casts, and other immobilization devices have an increased risk of skin breakdown and decubitus ulcers. Provide the patient with a trapeze that is set up to encourage mobility while in bed.
- Provide hydration and nutrition
  Metabolic demands increase during bone and wound healing. Extra protein, calcium, and vitamins A/D/C are needed for adequate bone repair. Adequate fluid intake is essential to ensure adequate "flushing" of the kidneys to prevent the complications of rhabdomyolysis. Iron supplements may be required for the treatment of anemia after surgery.
- Positive feedback and encouragement
  Empower the patient to continue with treatment/rehabilitation and boost self-confidence

▪ Teaching

- Treatment process
  Providing a clear explanation of all available treatment options enables the patient to make knowledgeable healthcare decisions and take an active role in their care.
- Overview of healing process
  Patient and supportive family members need to understand the healing process in order to be compliant with the treatment protocol. Healing may take months or years to complete (Box 54.3).
- Consume adequate calories and vitamins to promote healing
  Metabolic demands increase during bone and wound healing. Extra protein, carbohydrates, calcium, and vitamins A/D/C are needed for adequate bone repair. Vitamin D supplementation promotes bone healing. Extra fiber and fluids are needed to avoid constipation caused by narcotic analgesics.
- Appropriate use of analgesia
  Effective pain control enables the patient to perform self-care, ambulate, and reestablish independence.
- Wound care via aseptic technique
  Prevents infection, promotes skin integrity, and expedites healing
- Exercise and ambulation using assistive devices
  Exercise and ambulation allows for the earliest return to normal activities and discourages muscular atrophy, contractures, and loss of function. Mobility may be dependent on the

Box 54.3 Healing of Fractures

Fractured bones undergo a healing process that can extend from 6 months to a year. Healing is a five-stage process that begins within 24 hours of the initial injury.

- Stage 1: A hematoma forms around the fracture site within 24 to 72 hours of the initial injury.
- Stage 2: The hematoma undergoes a transformation to granulation tissue, which provides the basis for bone healing. This stage occurs 72 hours to 14 days after the initial injury.
- Stage 3: Granulation tissue develops into a callus (fibrocartilaginous tissue bridging the gap of the fracture) at 2 to 6 weeks. During this stage, the callus initiates the fusion of the bone segments.
- Stage 4: The callus is reabsorbed and converted into bone tissue 3 weeks to 6 months from the initial injury.
- Stage 5: Final stage of bone repair for mechanical function; this typically happens at 4 to 6 weeks and can last as long as a year.

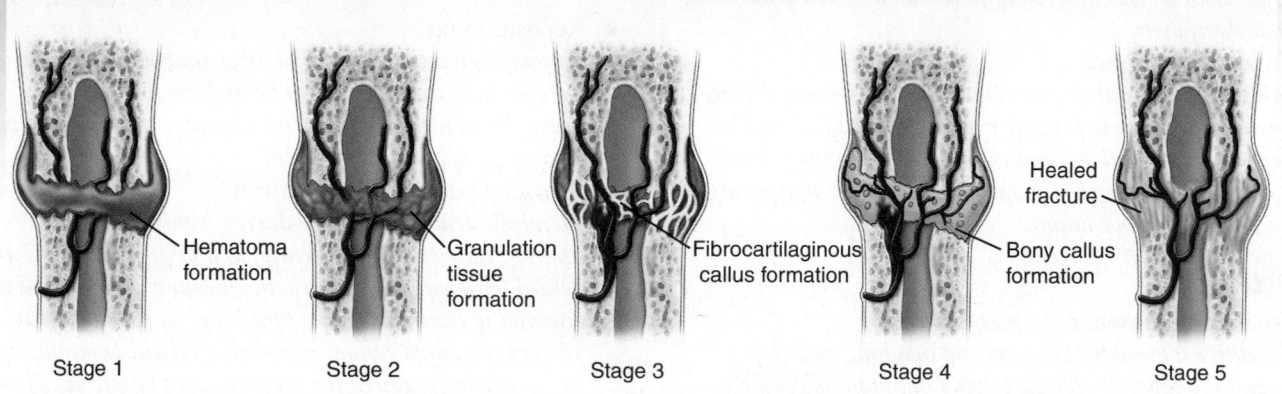

| Stage 1 | Stage 2 | Stage 3 | Stage 4 | Stage 5 |

Hematoma formation — Granulation tissue formation — Fibrocartilaginous callus formation — Bony callus formation — Healed fracture

---

proper use of assistive devices such as canes, walkers, and wheelchairs.
- Proper use of slings, splints, casts, and traction devices
  Fosters bone healing, minimizes complications that can cause malunion or non-union
  (see Box 54.4)
- Self-care activities
  Patient, family, and support members need to collaborate to allow patient to perform self-care with the least assistance needed.

Connection Check 54.4

A patient has returned from the postanesthesia care unit after having surgery to have an external fixator placed for an open tibia fracture with extensive soft tissue damage. What should the nurse do immediately?

A. Conduct a neurovascular assessment
B. Elevate the extremity
C. Perform pin site care
D. Remove the dressing and assess the wound

Evaluating Care Outcomes

The ultimate goal for the patient with a bone fracture is to return to normal activity and function as soon as possible. Most patients are able to return to their preinjury status and regain normal function within 6 to 12 months of the initial injury. This may be dependent on the severity of the fracture and need for surgery, presence of fracture-related

complications, and compliance with the treatment regimen. A well-managed patient:

- Is free from infection
- Uses analgesic intervention as prescribed
- Does not exhibit any neurovascular compromise such as compartment syndrome or VTE
- Complies with and actively participates in nutrition, activity, and exercise protocols
- Maintains stable vital signs, intake and output, and perfusion

AMPUTATIONS

Epidemiology

Amputations occur for various reasons in people of all ages. They can be traumatic or elective in nature. Risk factors for **traumatic amputations** include blunt force trauma obtained in motor vehicle crashes, motorcycle crashes, accidents where the patient is caught between two objects, and pedestrian versus vehicle injuries. This accounts for 1% of all trauma patients. Risk factors also include engaging in risk-taking behaviors, gunshot wounds, industrial jobs requiring the use of power tools, and the use of lawn mowers and snow blowers. The conflicts in Iraq and Afghanistan precipitated thousands of traumatic amputations among military professionals because of improvised explosive devices. Amputations of the upper extremities are more frequently seen in motor vehicle crashes, whereas lower extremity amputations generally occur because of motorcycle crashes and pedestrian injuries.

Box 54.4 Cast Care

Cast Care Dos and Do Nots

DO	DO NOT
Do keep the cast clean and dry at all times.	Do not pull out any padding from under the cast.
Do cover the cast with a plastic bag or cast cover for bathing or showering.	Do not get the cast wet. For casts that were applied using water resistant cast padding, you may shower or swim in a pool only, but must dry the lining of the cast after you finish with a cool air hair dryer to prevent skin breakdown.
Do use a hair dryer on cool air setting to dry the cast if it gets wet by blowing air under the cast.	Do not allow the patient to place any objects inside the cast.
Do contact the provider if there is any red skin irritation, blisters or sores around the edges of the cast or inside the cast.	Do not apply powder or deodorant to itching areas. Notify the provider if there is persistent itching.
Do cover rough edges of the cast with tape to prevent skin irritation.	Do not trim or break off any rough edges around the cast.
Do elevate the cast above the heart if increased swelling, pain, numbness, tingling or change in color or circulation are noted. If this does not relieve the symptoms, notify the provider.	Do not rest the heel of the leg cast on a pillow or bed. Keep the heel floating off the surface by elevating the leg with a pillow or blanket roll under the calf to prevent sores.
Do contact the provider if the cast is damaged, cracked, or extremely wet. The cast will need to be changed.	

Elective amputations are typically due to vascular compromise secondary to chronic illnesses such as peripheral vascular disease, diabetes, neoplasms, and infections. Risk factors for elective amputations include noncompliance with the diabetic treatment regimen, smoking, and venous stasis ulcers.

Pathophysiology and Clinical Manifestations

Amputation is the severing, or removal, of part of the body, generally involving the extremities. In traumatic amputations, high-energy trauma mutilates and destroys soft tissues, blood vessels, nerves, and bones of the extremities. The amputation can occur at the time of injury or is necessary immediately after injury to preserve life. Elective amputations are caused by disorders that lead to ischemia and eventual cell death. This lack of tissue perfusion prevents distribution of oxygen throughout the affected extremity. Cell death occurs from lack of oxygenation; necrotic tissue begins to form and creates an open wound. The open wound acts as a portal of entry for bacteria that thrive in low-oxygen environments, such as *Clostridium perfringens*. While the bacteria spread and migrate through the body, they secrete toxins that stimulate a systemic response leading to gangrene (an anaerobic infection caused by *C. perfringens)* and sepsis. Without immediate amputation, tissue ischemia migrates proximally through the limb and ultimately leads to overwhelming sepsis and multiple organ dysfunction.

Management

Medical Management

Traumatic Amputations

Due to the life-threatening nature of traumatic amputations, it is imperative to immediately control the bleeding and replace the blood lost from the injury. A tourniquet should be applied to the remaining portion of the limb to stop both arterial and venous bleeding. The tourniquet can remain in place for as long as 6 hours before the tissue becomes necrotic. Typically, patients with traumatic amputations also demonstrate polytrauma based on the same mechanism of injury. As a result, a rapid but thorough injury assessment should be conducted on the patient's arrival to the hospital. A coagulation panel and CBC can establish the need for immediate blood transfusion. A serum lactate level, an indicator of anaerobic metabolism, helps determine the level of hypoxemia and gauge the success of resuscitative efforts. To preserve life and maintain limb function in traumatic amputations, salvage surgery may be required to control hemorrhage, reattach limbs (Box 54.5), or remove/reconstruct the damaged tissue.

Elective Amputations

All possible medical interventions to reestablish perfusion are used before performing elective amputations. Radiography is used to determine the extent of bone damage or infection, whereas venograms and arteriograms are done to assess the level of peripheral circulation. Cultures and sensitivities isolate infective organisms in the wound and allow for accurate implementation of antibiotics. Medical interventions include hyperbaric therapy (100% oxygen administered under pressure in a hyperbaric chamber), percutaneous transluminal angioplasty (insertion of a balloon-tipped catheter into the affected artery that can be expanded to open the artery and restore blood flow), and anticoagulant therapy. In the case of neoplasms of the bone, resection of the tumor and bone grafting can often eliminate the need for surgical amputation. Once all other efforts have been exhausted, elective amputations are performed to salvage the remaining function of viable tissue.

Box 54.5 Care for Limb Reattachment

Recent advances in microsurgery have improved patient outcomes in the reattachment of severed extremities. Successful reattachment is highly dependent on the proper care of the amputated body part. Warm ischemia time, the time the severed extremity remains at body temperature after the loss of blood supply, should be limited. The limb should be cleansed with isotonic fluids (normal saline or lactated Ringer's solution), wrapped in a clean towel, and placed in a container then placed on ice. It is important to not place the extremity directly in ice. For a major traumatic amputation, replantation is not recommended if warm ischemia time is more than six to eight hours. For a digit, more than 10-12 hours is generally considered to be too long, but successful digit transplantation has been seen after a delay of 94 hours.

Prosthetic devices now allow amputee patients to resume near-normal function. Current prosthetic technology and design use state-of-the-art muscle and nerve sensors that allow the patient to perform both fine and gross motor movements. Patients are often fitted and sized for a prosthesis before their elective amputation surgery.

 Safety Alert Traumatic amputations cause serious disruptions in muscle, bone, and blood vessels. As a result, these patients have a significant risk of succumbing to hemorrhagic shock. The nurse should:
- Immediately assess the wound for active hemorrhaging
- Place a pressure bandage or tourniquet and monitor for effectiveness
- Obtain a CBC and type and crossmatch for immediate blood transfusion according to the provider's orders
- Prepare the patient for surgery to repair the severed extremity

Connection Check 54.5

The nurse correlates which of the following critically low laboratory results with a traumatic amputation?
A. Hemoglobin (Hgb): 7.0 g/dL
B. Glucose: 60 mg/dL
C. BUN: 10 mg/dL
D. WBC: 4,000 10³/mm³

Complications

Hemorrhage in traumatic amputations is caused by the destruction of large blood vessels within the extremity, leading to severe bleeding and consequent hypoperfusion. If the bleeding is not immediately controlled with a pressure dressing or tourniquet, the patient further decompensates into hypovolemic shock and death.

Infection in older patients with peripheral vascular disease who are undergoing elective amputations is a potential complication. These patients are at an increased risk for developing infections of the tissue and bone. Osteomyelitis is an infection of the bone that can quickly progress to sepsis in geriatric patients. Infection is also a problem in traumatic amputations because large open wounds are often contaminated with dirt and debris.

Contractures may occur in the residual limb because of the loss of bone, nerves, and muscle. Contractures are most often seen in patients with lower-extremity amputations and are manifested by lack of movement and exercise in the residual limb. These can be avoided by encouraging the patient to perform active ROM exercises and participate in physical therapy.

Phantom limb pain is a common complication of amputations which produces numbness, tingling, and a sharp burning pain perceived as manifesting in the removed limb or in the distal aspect of the remaining limb. The pain typically weakens over time but can be exacerbated by touching the residual limb. Weather changes, stress, nervousness, exhaustion, and further sickness can also exacerbate the pain. Different theories exist on the exact mechanism behind phantom limb pain. A frequently cited theory is that inflamed nerve fibers in the stump of the amputated extremity still send pain signals to the brain. The most prevalent theory presently is that when the nerves are severed during the amputation process, sensory function of the lost limb relocates to the spinal cord and brain cortex, causing the continued sensation of pain from the amputated extremity. The administration of antidepressant and anticonvulsant medications such as gabapentin has demonstrated effectiveness in treating phantom limb pain. Mirror therapy has also been successful in treating phantom limb pain by reversing the relocation of sensory nerve function through visual feedback.

Neuromas are clumps of nerve axons in the distal end of the residual limb that have regenerated after surgical amputation. Neuromas mostly occur in upper-extremity amputations but can develop in any residual limb. The development of neuromas is often inevitable and interferes with the proper fit and use of prosthetic devices, frequently requiring additional surgery for removal.

Nursing Management

Assessment and Analysis

In traumatic amputation, close examination of the affected extremity typically reveals extensive damage to blood vessels, bone, nerves, muscles, and other soft tissue due to high-energy blunt force trauma. Massive blood loss before hospital arrival leads to signs of shock such as tachycardia and hypotension. Patients with traumatic amputations also experience polytrauma, which can cause life-threatening issues with the airway and breathing. Because of the severity of the injury, patients often experience significant pain.

Preoperatively, elective amputations often exhibit signs of infection, absent circulation, severe pain, and lack of movement because of necrotic muscle and tissue.

Nursing Diagnoses

- **Acute pain** associated with surgery and phantom limb pain
- **Chronic pain** associated with surgery and phantom limb pain
- **Ineffective tissue perfusion** associated with edema and impaired arterial circulation
- **Impaired skin integrity** associated with delayed healing and prosthesis rubbing
- **Ineffective coping** associated with change in body image
- **Impaired physical mobility** associated with amputation, weakness, and musculoskeletal impairment
- **Grieving** associated with loss of the body part and future lifestyle changes
- **Self-care deficit** associated with deficient knowledge of stump care and rehabilitation
- **Risk for**:
  - **Infection** associated with invasive surgery
  - **Fluid volume deficit** associated with surgical disruption of hemostasis
  - **Bleeding** associated with the vulnerable surgical site

Nursing Interventions

■ Assessments

- Vital signs
  Hypotension and tachycardia may occur secondary to hemorrhage and sepsis. Increased temperature is an indication of infection. Decreased SpO_2 indicates problems with oxygenation.
- CBC
  Hemorrhage in traumatic amputation causes loss of red blood cells (RBCs), and low hemoglobin and hematocrit.
- Pulses, temperature, color, movement, and sensation of affected extremity
  Weak pulses, pale color, a cool temperature, and limited movement or sensation indicate inadequate blood flow and tissue perfusion in the affected limb that may indicate the potential need for elective amputation.
- Pain
  Phantom limb pain is a common side effect due to remapping of impulses from the amputated extremity to the spinal cord, causing continued pain sensations.
- Wound/incision site
  Warm, red tissue with purulent drainage is a sign of wound infection.

■ Actions

- Insert large bore IV
  The massive blood loss associated with traumatic amputation necessitates IV blood and fluid resuscitation.
- Transfusion of IV fluids and blood products as ordered
  Replace fluid and blood lost in traumatic amputation

- Administer analgesia as ordered
  Improved pain control promotes movement, function, increasing the ability to participate in rehabilitation.
- Alternative pain management techniques
  Alternative pain management modalities such as TENS unit or CAM therapies are synergistic in conjunction with analgesic medications.
- Refrain from using a pillow under the remaining portion of the lower extremity
  Prevents the development of flexion contractures that can occur if a pillow is left under the extremity
- Application of ice for no longer than 15 to 20 minutes
  Promotes vasoconstriction and decreases painful edema
- Nutrition: maintain adequate intake and output
  The increased metabolic demands of healing require additional protein and carbohydrates.
- Range of motion
  Strengthens muscles and prevents contractures in the residual limb fostering improved self-care
- Application of rigid splint
  Minimizes edema by compressing residual limb for a better fit into the prosthesis

■ Teaching

- Medication regimen
  Adequate pain control allows the patient to ambulate and perform self-care. Taking antibiotics as prescribed promotes wound healing and decreases the risk of superinfection and the development of antibiotic-resistant organisms.
- Nutrition and hydration
  Sufficient dietary intake of proteins and carbohydrates allows for adequate healing of bone, muscle, and skin. Increasing dietary fiber and maintaining hydration prevents narcotic-associated constipation.
- Wrap limb with compression dressing (Fig. 54.9)
  - Figure-eight technique
  - Start 1 to 3 days postoperatively
  - Wrap from distal to proximal position
  - Start with minimal tension, then increase gradually
  - Rewrap two to three times per day
  - Keep wrapped unless bathing
  - If pain occurs, the wrapping is probably too tight
    Limb wrapping decreases edema and aids in the correct fitting of the prosthesis on the residual limb.
- Wound care
  Wound care often continues after discharge from the hospital. Using the aseptic technique minimizes the risk of infection.
- Signs and symptoms of infection
  Patients need to know and identify early signs of infection: increased or purulent drainage, redness, warmth, or increased temperature, and seek medical attention as necessary.
- ROM exercises
  Prevent contractures and strengthen muscles for movement and function
- Community support resources
  A case manager or social worker can coordinate resources to allow the patient to resume rehabilitation and self-care

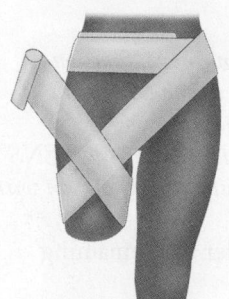 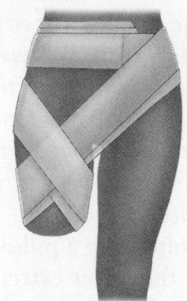 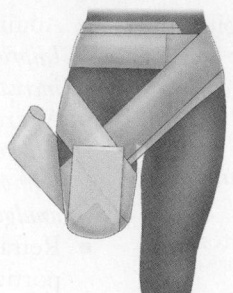 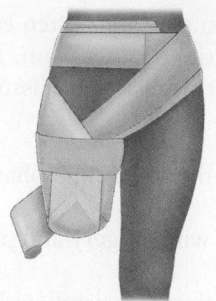 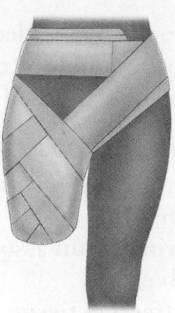

FIGURE 54.9 Procedure for wrapping the residual limb to prevent edema and provide compression.

1. Hold the bandage roll at your waist with one hand. Use the other hand to roll the bandage all the way around your waist.
2. Turn the bandage so that it goes down toward the floor. Roll it diagonally down your thigh, and continue to the back of your limb. Stretch the bandage slightly while you wrap your limb.
3. Roll the bandage around to the front of your limb. Roll it diagonally up your thigh, to your waist. Roll it all the way around your waist again, in the same direction as the first time.
4. Repeat these steps until the bandage covers the top of your thigh to the end of your limb. Overlap the bandage as you wrap so you cover new skin each time. If you need to use more than one bandage, secure each bandage with a clip or tape before you apply another one.
5. When you are finished, secure the last bandage. Try to end the bandage in a place that is not in a skin fold or at your hip.

activities at home with the use of various assistive devices. Organizations composed of other amputee patients can offer additional encouragement and emotional support.

- Collaborate with the physical therapist and prosthetist-orthotist
  These professionals can promote adaptation to new lifestyle and help ensure prosthesis fit. They can also serve as a resource for any prosthesis-related issues.

Connection Check 54.6

A patient with diabetes who had an elective below-the-knee amputation returns to the unit for IV antibiotic care on postoperative day 3. On closer examination, the nurse notices the patient has a pillow under the residual limb. What should the nurse do in this situation?

A. Leave the pillow in place to prevent dependent edema
B. Remove the pillow to prevent contractures
C. Remove the pillow to prevent VTE
D. Leave the pillow to promote circulation

Evaluating Care Outcomes

Patients with amputations who are compliant and actively participate in home care and rehabilitation can expect to lead productive lives once discharged from the hospital. Adjusting to a traumatic amputation is more difficult than adjusting to a planned one. The nurse can help to provide anticipatory counseling to help prepare for an emotional reaction. The presence of strong family and support systems is instrumental in helping the patient make a smooth transition home from the hospital. A well-managed patient is free from evidence of infection, has acceptance of body image and limits of physical mobility, and is knowledgeable in the use of prosthetic devices to ambulate and function as independently as possible.

MENISCUS INJURIES

Epidemiology

Meniscus injuries occur in patients of all ages and genders. Acute meniscus injuries occur on average in 61 out of 100,000 people. Men are more than twice as likely as women to sustain a meniscus injury of the knees. Risk factors for meniscus injuries include congenital abnormalities, chronic joint diseases such as rheumatoid arthritis and osteoarthritis, ligament deficiencies, and insufficient quadriceps muscle control. Athletes participating in football, soccer, skiing, basketball, and baseball have an increased risk of developing meniscal injuries. Contributing factors of meniscal tears include overuse of the joint, failure to stretch and warm up, poor quadriceps muscle development, and abnormal alignment of the knee joint.

Pathophysiology

The menisci are semilunar-shaped wedges of cartilage positioned between the tibia and femur of both knee joints (Fig. 54.10A). They serve to cushion, protect, and stabilize the knee joint from shock during flexion and movement. There is a lateral and a medial portion of each meniscus. Medial menisci are "C" shaped and positioned on the medial aspect of the knee. They are torn when excessive twisting, or rotational, force is applied to a knee that is bent. The medial aspect is larger in size and more apt to tear than the lateral meniscus. The lateral meniscus is more "U" shaped and is located on the lateral aspect of the knee joint. Lateral menisci tear when the lateral compartment of the knee slides or subluxates forward, which impinges the meniscus between the tibia and femur. Meniscus tears (Fig. 54.10B) frequently accompany more severe knee injuries such as ACL tears.

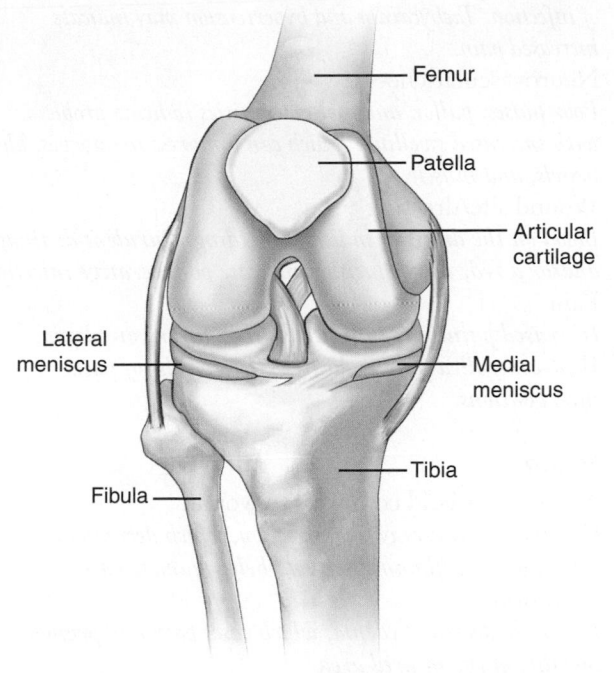

A

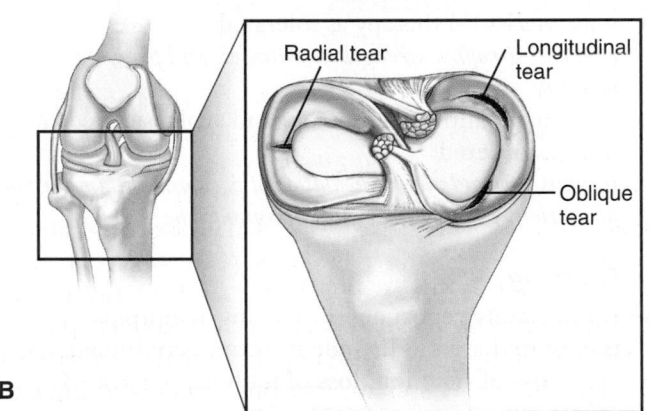

B

FIGURE 54.10 Menisci. A, Normal menisci; B, Radial, longitudinal, and oblique meniscal tears.

Clinical Manifestations

Pain experienced at the time of menisci injury is variable and is typically followed by an insidious onset of effusion, increased fluid in the joint, during the next day. Patients may experience mechanical symptoms, such as catching, locking, clicking, or instability, and usually report medial or lateral pain. An effusion combined with joint line tenderness is one of the most sensitive and reliable signs of meniscal tear.

Management

Medical Management

Diagnosis

The diagnosis of meniscus injuries is based on physical examination using either the McMurray's test, in which the knee is supported and flexed while the lower leg is rotated internally and externally (Fig. 54.11), or Steinman's test, in which the knee is flexed and extended. A positive result is indicated when either test reveals an audible/palpable

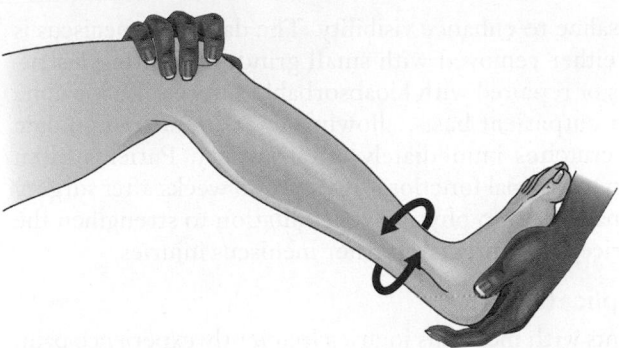

FIGURE 54.11 McMurray's test. With the knee supported and flexed, the lower leg is rotated internally and externally. An audible/palpable "click," an inability to extend the knee, or the presence of pain is a positive test.

"click," an inability to extend the knee, or the presence of pain. Radiography may be needed to rule out degenerative joint diseases. An MRI can further help isolate and characterize the extent of the tear.

Treatment

Treatment of meniscus tears is dependent on the size and severity of the tear. Smaller tears often heal within a few months and are treated with limited rest, ice, and administration of NSAIDs. Total immobility and resting of the affected joint is not recommended because it may cause muscle atrophy, stiffness, and further movement problems. Patients are encouraged to continue daily activities as tolerated.

Surgical Management

Surgery in the form of an arthroscopic surgical repair of meniscus tears, or meniscectomy, may be indicated for small tears that have not healed with conventional treatment or for large unstable tears. Arthroscopic surgery involves the insertion of small fiber-optic scopes through small incisions in the knee (Fig. 54.12). The joint is insufflated or irrigated

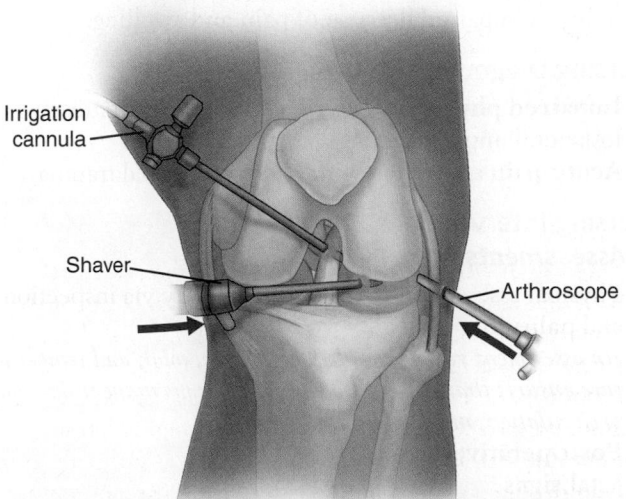

Arthroscopic instruments are inserted through small incisions in the knee; the knee is infused with saline and the damaged tissue is removed with small grinding or shaving instruments.

FIGURE 54.12 Arthroscopic surgical repair.

with saline to enhance visibility. The damaged meniscus is then either removed with small grinding/rotating instruments or repaired with bioabsorbable sutures. This is done on an outpatient basis, allowing the patient to ambulate with crutches immediately after surgery. Patients often return to normal function within 6 to 8 weeks after surgery and may undergo physical rehabilitation to strengthen the quadriceps and prevent further meniscus injuries.

Complications

Patients with meniscus injuries frequently experience pain, immobility, and the inability to carry out everyday activities. If left untreated, meniscus tears can lead to permanent joint damage and immobility.

Connection Check 54.7

The nurse prioritizes which nursing diagnosis in the patient immediately after arthroscopic surgical repair of the medial meniscus injury?

A. High risk for ineffective airway clearance associated with general anesthesia

B. High risk for ineffective breathing associated with intubation

C. Self-care deficit associated with pain, edema, and immobility

D. Pain associated with inflammation

Nursing Management

Assessment and Analysis

Patients often present complaining of "popping" or "clicking" when they bend their knee. They may also describe pain to the anterior or posterior aspect of the knee joint. Close examination of the affected knee may reveal swelling, warmth, and an accumulation of fluid within the joint. Mobility is impaired because of pain and swelling.

Nursing Diagnoses

- **Impaired physical mobility** associated with musculoskeletal impairment
- **Acute pain** associated with musculoskeletal trauma

Nursing Interventions

▪ *Assessments*

- Physical assessment of injured extremity via inspection and palpation
  An assessment revealing adequate pulses, color, and temperature ensures that there is no emergent or permanent damage to circulation, movement, and sensation.
  Postoperative
- Vital signs
  Tachycardia and hypotension may result because of hypovolemia due to hemorrhage. Increased temperature is an indicator

of infection. Tachycardia and hypertension may indicate increased pain.

- Neurovascular check
  Poor pulses, pallor, and cool extremities indicate problems with increased swelling, which can compress the nerves, blood vessels, and muscle.
- Wound site/dressing
  Blood on the dressing indicates bleeding. Purulent drainage and/or a red, warm incision indicate postoperative infection.
- Pain
  Increased pain may indicate further injury or edema. Well-controlled pain indicates effectiveness of pain interventions.

▪ *Actions*

- Apply ice or cold compress to wound
  Cryotherapy causes vasoconstriction, which decreases further bleeding and inflammation and helps manage pain.
- Elevation
  Elevation decreases edema, which eases pain and promotes mobility of the injured area.
- Exercise/ROM therapy as tolerated
  Prevents atrophy, strengthens muscles, and promotes mobility
- Administer anti-inflammatory and analgesia medications as ordered
  Inhibits prostaglandin (mediators of pain and inflammation) formation reducing pain and inflammation

▪ *Teaching*

- Immediately report any worsening symptoms to the injured area to include infection, continued pain, loss of function, loss of mobility, or loss of sensation
  Alterations in circulation, movement, and sensation can signal the need for further medical intervention.
- Pain management
  Compliance with the prescribed treatment/medication regimen supports the ability to participate in activities of daily living (ADLs) and rehabilitation facilitating the return of the injured limb to normal function.
- Wound care
  Wound care often continues after discharge from the hospital. Using aseptic technique minimizes the risk of infection.
- Exercise/Physical therapy/Rehabilitation therapy
  Promotes ambulation, muscle strength, and return to pre-injury functioning

Evaluating Care Outcomes

A well-managed patient has pain under control and actively participates in the prescribed rehabilitation plan, promoting a return to preinjury functioning. Patients may occasionally exhibit some long-term stiffness or soreness dependent on weather and activity.

Connection Check 54.8

The nursing diagnosis "ineffective peripheral tissue perfusion associated with deficient knowledge of aggravating factors" applies to which fracture patient with the highest risk of developing VTE?

A. A 30-year-old female on oral contraceptives who smokes one pack of cigarettes per day

B. A 40-year-old male who ambulates four times a day with a walker

C. A 70-year-old diabetic female who attends rehabilitation once a day

D. A 20-year-old male who smokes 10 cigarettes per day and ambulates with crutches

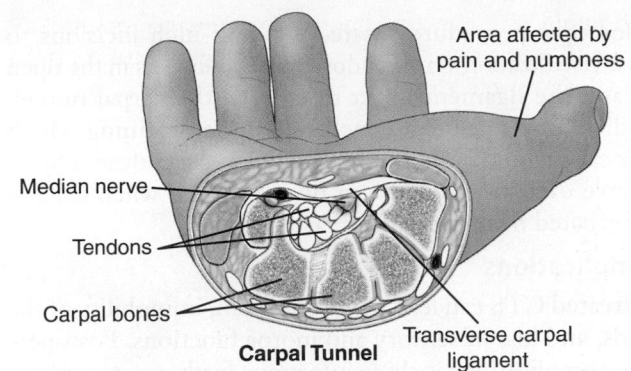

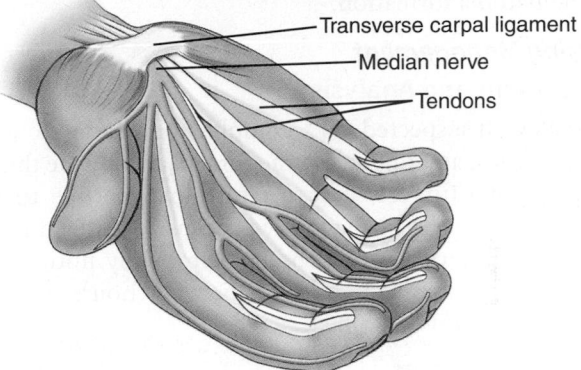

FIGURE 54.13 Carpal tunnel syndrome: inflammation in the carpal tunnel produces pressure on the median nerve causing pain, numbness, and tingling.

CARPAL TUNNEL SYNDROME

Epidemiology

Carpal tunnel syndrome (CTS) is the most frequent compression neuropathy of the hands. Risk factors for CTS include age, type of employment, and gender. Higher occurrences are noted in patients who have jobs requiring repetitive motions of the hands and wrists such as computer operators, musicians, construction workers, and factory workers. Women are four to five times more likely to get CTS than their male counterparts, partially because of the smaller size of the carpal tunnel in women. Factors that precipitate CTS include pregnancy, congenital malformations, hormone therapy, trauma to the hand or wrist, and other idiopathic causes. This syndrome usually occurs in adults.

Pathophysiology and Clinical Manifestations

The carpal tunnel is an area located between the carpal bones of the wrist. The tunnel contains the median nerve, tendons, and ligaments. Repetitive motions of the wrist elicit inflammation of the tendons and ligaments (Fig. 54.13). Inflammation compresses the median nerve causing sharp pain, numbness, and tingling of the hand. Grip strength may be decreased, and over time there is atrophy of the muscles. Symptoms initially occur intermittently at night, then progress if not treated.

Management

Medical Management

Diagnosis

Diagnosis starts with a detailed patient history. The history includes the patient's occupation, factors responsible for generating the wrist pain, and medical history. The Phalen's test aids in diagnosis of CTS and is performed by having the patient relax his or her hand in the flexed position for

60 seconds or by placing the back of the hands together while flexing both wrists. This compresses the median nerve. Patients with CTS experience numbness and tingling during the Phalen's test. Tinel's sign, tapping the median nerve over the carpal tunnel at the wrist, will also elicit paresthesia over the median nerve region of the wrist. Nerve conduction studies and electromyographies are frequently ordered to determine the severity of CTS and rule out any potential spinal cord lesions or tumors. Cervical spine radiography eliminates any possible cervical disorders that could cause radiating pain in the hands. Occasionally, MRI and ultrasound may be used to isolate the cause of CTS.

Treatment

Treatment of CTS can be done with conventional nonoperative measures such as modifying the work environment to eliminate repetitive motion and promote ergonomics. Ultrasound therapy, NSAIDs, steroid injections, night splinting, and acetaminophen are other treatment options.

Surgical Management

Surgical intervention called *carpal tunnel release surgery* is often performed as an outpatient procedure to decrease pressure on the median nerve. There are two types of surgical decompression of the median nerve: open release and endoscopic. Open release is a procedure that creates a 2-inch incision in the wrist, allowing visualization. The transverse carpal ligament is then cut to enlarge the carpal tunnel. The endoscopic procedure creates two half-inch incisions to allow visualization via an endoscopic camera. As in the open release, the ligament is cut to enlarge the carpal tunnel. Studies have not been conclusive in determining which surgical method is the most beneficial. A synovectomy to remove excess synovium can be performed when CTS is exacerbated from rheumatoid arthritis.

Complications

Untreated CTS can lead to chronic pain, immobility of the hands, and loss of sensory and motor functions. Postoperative complications include infection, further nerve injury, and hematoma formation.

Nursing Management

Assessment and Analysis

Patients with suspected CTS complain of pain in the wrist and numbness and tingling in the fingers; mostly the thumb and first two fingers. These symptoms are due to the compression of the median nerve because of inflammation caused by repetitive motions. Patients may notice that the symptoms diminish, or weaken, a few hours after the repetitive motion is stopped.

Nursing Diagnoses

- **Alteration in rest: sleep pattern disturbance** associated with pain
- **Acute/chronic pain** associated with inflammation and pressure on the median nerve
- **Impaired physical mobility** associated with neuromuscular impairment

Nursing Interventions

▪ Assessments

- Patient work or activity history
  A work or activity history of repetitive movements such as computer or assembly-line work puts patients at risk for CTS.
- Physical assessment of injured extremity via inspection and palpation
  Numbness and tingling during the Phalen's test or paresthesias with a Tinel's test may indicate CTS caused by compression of the median nerve.
- Pain, paresthesia
  Pain is caused by inflammation and edema, resulting in compression of the median nerve.

▪ Actions

- Splinting at night or with symptoms
  Immobilizes the joint, decreasing irritation and inflammation on the median nerve
- Exercise/ROM therapy as tolerated
  Prevents atrophy, strengthens muscles, and promotes mobility
- Administer anti-inflammatory medications as ordered
  Inhibits prostaglandin (mediators of pain and inflammation) formation reducing pain and inflammation
- Collaborate with occupational therapist
  An occupational therapist can evaluate the work area and make recommendations for modifications to eliminate causative factors.

▪ Teaching

- Immediately report any worsening symptoms to the injured area to include infection, continued pain, loss of function, loss of mobility, or loss of sensation
  Alterations in circulation, movement, and sensation can signal the need for further medical intervention.
- Exercise/physical therapy
  Promotes movement, muscle strength, and return to preinjury functioning
- Pain management
  Compliance with the prescribed treatment/medication regimen supports the ability to participate in activities of daily living (ADLs) and rehabilitation facilitating the return of the injured limb to normal function.
- Work/activity modifications; stop the activity responsible for CTS or modify how activity is performed
  Eliminates the cause of CTS, prevents further recurrences

Evaluating Care Outcomes

A well-managed patient is compliant in their treatment protocol, which includes their medication regimen, use of splints, workplace modification, and undergoing surgical intervention if necessary. This patient is often successful in obtaining symptomatic relief of CTS and is able to return to normal preinjury functioning.

Making Connections

CASE STUDY: WRAP-UP

Zachary is admitted to the ward from the operating room at 0600 in the morning. Frequent nursing assessments noting the six Ps are performed to assess neurovascular function. Laboratory testing to include serum myoglobin and CPK are ordered. His urine remains clear yellow, ruling out the presence of rhabdomyolysis. His pain is controlled with PO oxycodone. His provider's orders include the provision of adequate hydration and nutrition and an order for physical therapy to evaluate his readiness for exercise and ambulation using assistive devices. If he continues to improve, he will be discharged to home soon.

Case Study Questions

1. Zachary has undergone placement of an external fixator for an open displaced femur fracture. Immediately following surgery, he begins to exhibit dyspnea, pleuritic chest pain, anxiety, and tachycardia. The nurse suspects which complication?

   A. Pneumothorax

   B. Deep vein thrombosis

   C. Fat embolism

   D. Myocardial infarction

2. Following the surgical procedure for an open displaced femur fracture, what action does the nurse frequently perform?

    A. ROM exercises

    B. Neurovascular assessments

    C. Dressing changes

    D. Pain assessments

3. The nurse monitors for which common symptom of compartment syndrome?

    A. Passive pain at rest

    B. Pain with movement

    C. Pallor

    D. Paresthesia

4. Because Zachary has lost a significant amount of blood, what complication should the nurse monitor for?

    A. Bradycardia

    B. Hypotension

    C. Metabolic alkalosis

    D. Hyperkalemia

5. The nurse monitors Zachary for which signs of rhabdomyolysis?

    A. Bloody urine and abdominal pain

    B. Anuria, nausea, and severe flank pain

    C. Low serum myoglobin, fever, and severe headaches

    D. Elevated serum myoglobin, tea-colored urine, and severe flank pain

CHAPTER SUMMARY

A strain is the tearing or stretching of a muscle or tendon. A sprain is defined as the stretching or tearing of a ligament. Strains and strains are categorized according to their severity. Treatment of first- and second-degree strains and sprains involves RICE: rest, ice, compression, and elevate. NSAIDs are usually prescribed to minimize pain and inflammation. Third-degree injuries may require surgical repair.

A fracture is defined as a disruption, or break, in the continuity of a bone. There are numerous classifications of fractures that can occur throughout the body. Types of fractures include complete, incomplete, closed (simple), or open (compound). Effective pain management and definitive surgical or nonsurgical treatment is indicated depending on the type and location of the fracture. Venous thromboemboli, fat emboli, neurovascular compromise, and compartment syndrome are complications of fractures. Neurovascular assessments should be completed frequently on these patients.

Amputation is the severing, or removal, of part of the body, generally involving the extremities. There are two types of amputations, traumatic and elective. In traumatic amputations, high-energy trauma mutilates and destroys soft tissues, blood vessels, nerves, and bones of the extremities. Traumatic amputations involve massive hemorrhage due to the high-energy destruction of blood vessels. Elective amputations are due to disease, diabetes, peripheral vascular disease, and neoplasms that hinder tissue perfusion and lead to ischemia and eventual cell death. Hemorrhage and infection are complications to be monitored for in these patients.

Medial menisci are torn when excessive twisting, or rotational, force is applied to a knee that is bent. Lateral menisci tear when the lateral compartment of the knee slides or subluxates forward, which impinges the meniscus between the tibia and femur. Contributing factors of meniscal tears include overuse of the joint, failure to stretch and warm up, poor quadriceps muscle development, abnormal alignment of the knee joint, and congenital abnormalities. Small tears can be treated with limited rest, ice, and administration of NSAIDs. Small tears that have not healed with conventional treatment or large unstable tears require arthroscopic surgical repair.

The carpal tunnel is an area located between the carpal bones of the wrist. The tunnel contains the median nerve, tendons, and ligaments. Repetitive motions of the wrist elicit inflammation of the tendons and ligaments. Inflammation compresses the median nerve causing sharp pain, numbness, and tingling of the hand. Treatment of CTS can be done nonoperatively with measures such as modifying the work environment to eliminate repetitive motion and promote ergonomics. Surgical intervention, carpal tunnel release surgery, is performed to decrease pressure on the median nerve.

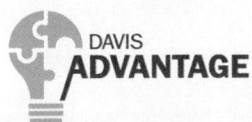

DAVIS ADVANTAGE | To explore learning resources for this chapter, go to **Davis Advantage** and find:
– Answers to in-text questions
– Chapter Resources and Activities
– NCLEX®-Style Chapter Review Questions
– Bibliography

Unit XIII

Promoting Health in Patients With Gastrointestinal Disorders

Chapter 55

Assessment of Gastrointestinal Function

Jana Goodwin

Finding Connections

CASE STUDY: EPISODE 1

Follow this patient throughout the chapter.

Martin Jhanes is a 70-year-old male patient who presents to his healthcare provider complaining of worsening heartburn that has persisted over the last 3 months. He also reports nausea, decreased appetite, abdominal bloating, frequent belching, and gas. He states that there is "burning pain" in his stomach until he eats. Symptoms persist despite dietary changes and treatment with over-the-counter antacids and H_2 antagonists, which have worked in the past. He reveals that his last bowel movement was several days ago. He reports having difficulty with bowel movements since he retired last year. He noticed that his stool was darker than usual but thought it was from the Pepto-Bismol that he had taken. He denies laxative use or abuse. Mr. Jhanes also reports feeling tired and complains of light-headedness when moving from a sitting to a standing position. The patient has a past medical history significant for hypertension, myocardial infarction, and hypercholesterolemia. He reports drinking a glass of wine with dinner every night and being a former smoker. Mr. Jhanes states that he smoked about one pack of cigarettes per day for 20 years. He currently takes lisinopril (Zestril) 20 mg PO daily, clopidogrel (Plavix) 75 mg PO daily, and atorvastatin (Lipitor) 10 mg PO daily. He has not taken any medication in 2 days...

INTRODUCTION

The gastrointestinal system is responsible for intake, digestion, and elimination of food and fluids, and proper functioning is key to adequate nutrition. Consisting of two divisions, it is divided into the alimentary tract and accessory organs. Normal intake is through the mouth; however, in patients with disorders that affect the ability to eat or swallow, nutrition may be delivered directly to the stomach or small intestine. Digestion begins in the mouth and continues in the stomach and small intestine. The large intestine is primarily responsible for reabsorption of fluids and electrolytes and elimination of waste products. Equally important to the normal function of the gastrointestinal system is the role of the accessory organs that include the teeth, tongue, salivary glands, liver, gallbladder, and pancreas. Normal functioning of the gastrointestinal system also includes actions of the nervous and endocrine systems.

OVERVIEW OF ANATOMY AND PHYSIOLOGY

The gastrointestinal tract, also known as the alimentary tract, begins with the esophagus and ends with the anus

(Fig. 55.1). Responsible for the digestion and absorption of nutrients and expelling of metabolic wastes, the tract consists of the mouth, pharynx, esophagus, stomach, small intestine, and large intestine. Additionally, the teeth, tongue, salivary glands, liver, gallbladder, and pancreas are involved in the digestive process.

The Mouth

The process of digestion begins in the mouth, where the mechanical and chemical breakdown of food occurs. The mechanical breakdown of ingested food occurs through the process of **mastication** (chewing). Saliva, which contains amylase, lipase, and lysozyme, is excreted from a group of glands: parotid, sublingual, and submandibular glands (Fig. 55.2). Amylase is responsible for the chemical breakdown of carbohydrates, whereas lipase chemically digests fat. Digestion of protein actually occurs in the stomach. Lysozyme has antimicrobial properties that destroy the cell wall of bacteria in the mouth. **Deglutition**, or swallowing, consists of two phases and involves the pharynx, esophageal muscles, and the following cranial nerves (CNs), CN V (trigeminal), CN VII (facial), CN IX (glossopharyngeal), and CN XII (hypoglossal). The **buccal** (mouth) phase involves the tongue and the pharyngeal muscles, and the esophageal phase involves the palate and esophageal muscles. Peristaltic movement of the esophagus moves the bolus of food into the stomach.

The Esophagus

The esophagus (Fig. 55.3) is a hollow muscular tube that extends from approximately the vertebral levels of C6 to T7. It is positioned inferior to the pharynx and posterior to the trachea and passes through the diaphragm via a space known as the esophageal hiatus and then connects to the stomach. The external musculature of the esophagus is skeletal muscle in the upper one-third, skeletal/smooth mix in the middle third, and smooth muscle in the lower third. The mucosa of the esophagus consists of nonkeratinized stratified squamous epithelium. The peristaltic movements push the food bolus downward as the esophagus constricts above the bolus and dilates below the bolus.

The Stomach

The esophagus extends through the diaphragm and connects to the stomach. In normal digestion, the lower esophageal sphincter protects the esophageal mucosa from the regurgitation of partially digested food and the acid produced in stomach. Specialized cells secrete chemicals essential to the digestive functions of the stomach:

- *Mucous cells:* Secrete mucus that protects the stomach lining
- *Parietal cells:* Secrete hydrochloric acid that aids in the conversion of food to **chyme** (partly digested semiliquid food), as well as convert gastric lipase and pepsinogen

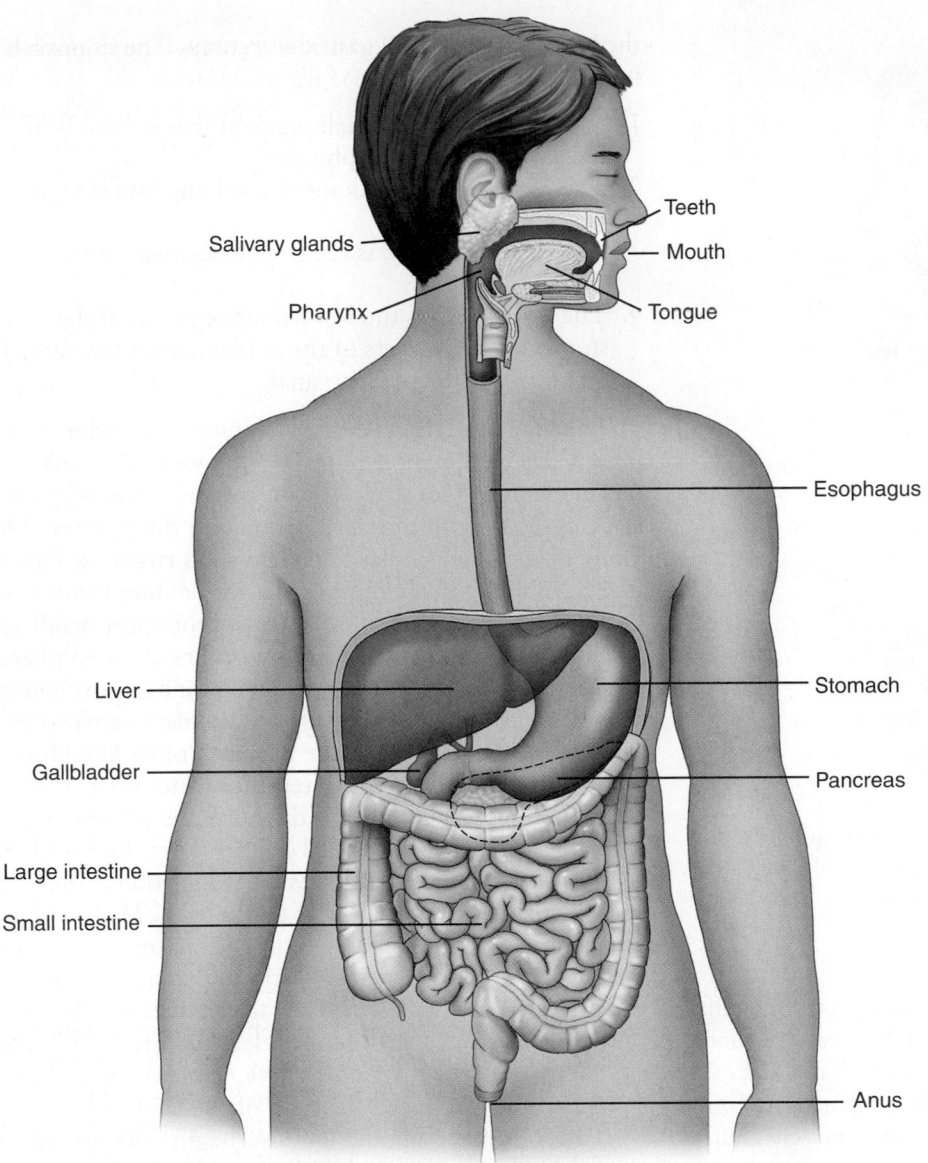

FIGURE 55.1 Gastrointestinal system.

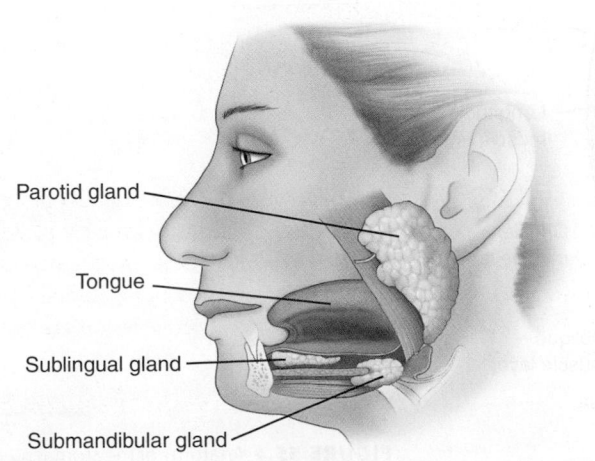

FIGURE 55.2 The mouth and salivary glands. The parotid, sublingual, and submandibular glands, located in the mouth, produce saliva and begin digestion in the mouth.

to active forms. The parietal cells also secrete **intrinsic factor**, a chemical needed for the absorption of vitamin B_{12}, an important component of hemoglobin synthesis.

- *Chief cells:* Secrete the enzymes gastric lipase, which digests approximately 15% of dietary fat, and pepsinogen, which is responsible for protein digestion
- *Enteroendocrine cells:* Secrete hormones needed for digestion:
  - *Gastrin:* Stimulates secretion of hydrochloric acid and enzymes, and intestinal motility
  - *Serotonin:* Stimulates gastric motility
  - *Histamine:* Stimulates secretion of hydrochloric acid
  - **Somatostatin**: Inhibitory hormone that delays emptying of the stomach, reduces absorption in the small intestine, and inhibits secretions from the gallbladder and pancreas

Gastric motility is influenced by smooth muscle regulated by the sympathetic and parasympathetic nervous systems.

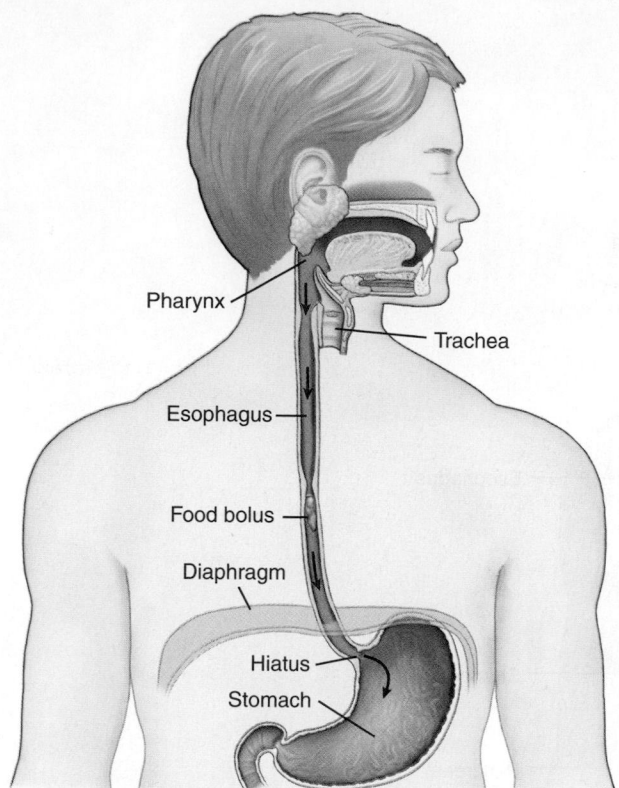

Pharynx

Trachea

Esophagus

Food bolus

Diaphragm

Hiatus

Stomach

FIGURE 55.3 Esophagus. The esophagus extends through the diaphragm and connects to the stomach. In normal digestion, the lower esophageal sphincter protects the esophageal mucosa from the regurgitation of partially digested food and the acid produced in the stomach.

Swallowing stimulates the swallowing center in the medulla oblongata to signal the stomach to stretch to receive food. Before meals, the stomach has a volume of 50 mL but can hold up to 4 L at its fullest. Peristaltic contractions controlled by the pacemaker cells of the smooth muscle churn

the food and mix it with gastric secretions. The stomach has four landmark areas (Fig. 55.4):

1. The *cardiac area* is a small segment that is 3 cm below the gastroesophageal sphincter.
2. The *fundic area* is the dome-shaped uppermost segment of the stomach.
3. The *corpus*, or body, is the largest segment of the stomach.
4. The *pyloric area* is the lowermost segment of the stomach that consists of the antrum, a narrow funnel that leads to the pyloric canal.

The small area right beyond the canal is the pylorus, and it connects to the duodenum. The passage of chyme into the duodenum is controlled by the pyloric sphincter, which is a ring of smooth muscle surrounding the pylorus. The lining of the stomach has folds known as **rugae** that allow for stretching of the lining in order to facilitate absorption.

Through the hormonal and neurological feedback systems, gastric secretion activity occurs in three phases (Fig. 55.5). In the cephalic phase, mental and sensory stimuli activate the vagus nerve (CN X) to stimulate gastric secretion. In the gastric phase, the presence of carbohydrates, fat, and partially digested protein stimulates the release of acetylcholine, histamine, and the hormone gastrin. These chemicals stimulate the parietal cells to secrete hydrochloric acid and intrinsic factor, whereas the stimulation of the chief cells results in the secretion of pepsinogen. Hydrochloric acid converts pepsinogen to pepsin, the enzyme responsible for the digestion of proteins. Lastly, in the intestinal phase, the presence of chyme stretches the duodenum. Initially, the duodenal stretch leads to the release of intestinal gastrin and stimulation of the vagus nerve, which stimulates the stomach. However, the presence of the acid and semidigested food in the duodenum also begins the inhibitory

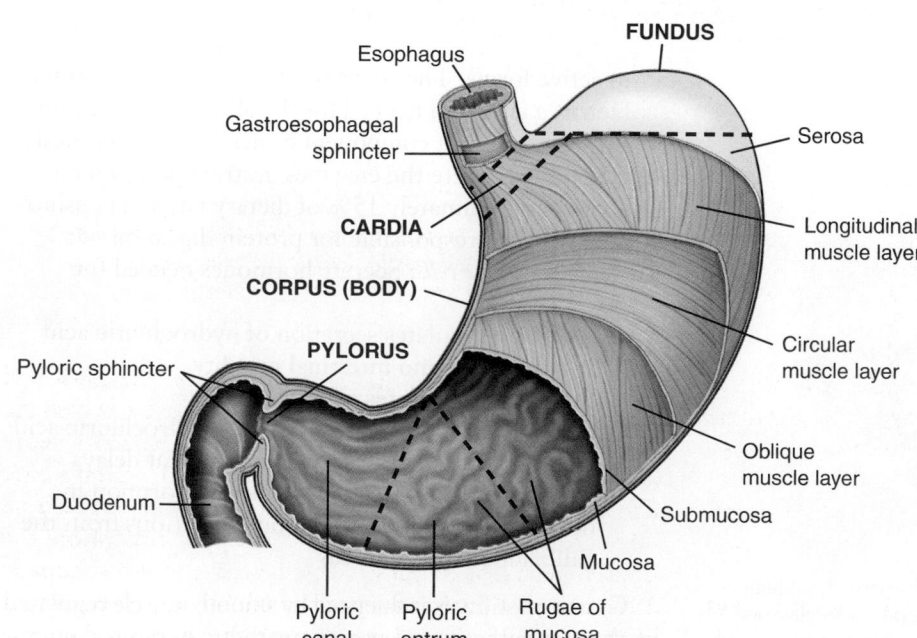

Esophagus

FUNDUS

Gastroesophageal sphincter

Serosa

CARDIA

Longitudinal muscle layer

CORPUS (BODY)

Circular muscle layer

PYLORUS

Pyloric sphincter

Oblique muscle layer

Duodenum

Submucosa

Mucosa

Pyloric canal

Pyloric antrum

Rugae of mucosa

FIGURE 55.4 Anatomy of the stomach. Note the four major landmarks of the stomach: the cardia, fundus, corpus (body), and pylorus.

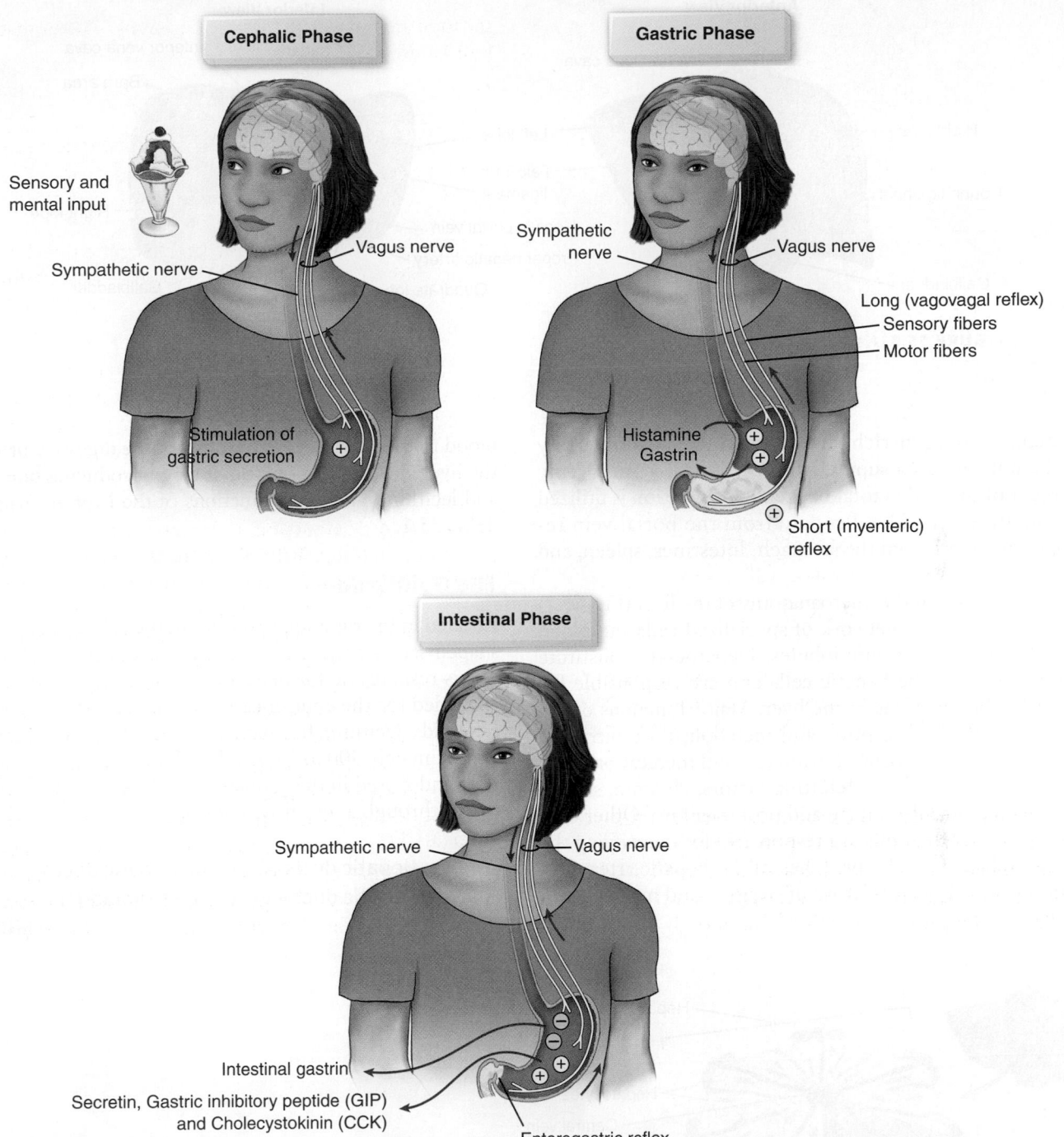

FIGURE 55.5 Phases of gastric secretion. In the cephalic phase, mental and sensory stimuli activate the vagus nerve (CN X) to stimulate gastric secretion. In the gastric phase, the presence of carbohydrates, fat, and partially digested protein stimulates the release of acetylcholine, histamine, and the hormone gastrin. In the intestinal phase, the presence of chyme stretches the duodenum.

phase. Signals from the medulla stimulate the sympathetic and parasympathetic nervous systems, which inhibit gastric activity. The secretion of secretin and cholecystokinin also inhibits gastric motility and enzyme secretion.

The Liver

After the skin (integumentary system), the liver is the second largest organ of the body and typically weighs 1 to 1.5 kg.

Attached beneath the diaphragm, the liver is positioned largely across the right upper quadrant and extends into the left upper quadrant. It is segmented into four lobes separated by ligaments that suspend the liver under the rib cage and diaphragm in the abdominal cavity (Fig. 55.6). The inferior view of the liver has two grooved areas where the inferior vena cava, hepatic vein and artery, common hepatic duct, and gallbladder are positioned. Twenty-five percent of the cardiac output flows through the dual blood supply

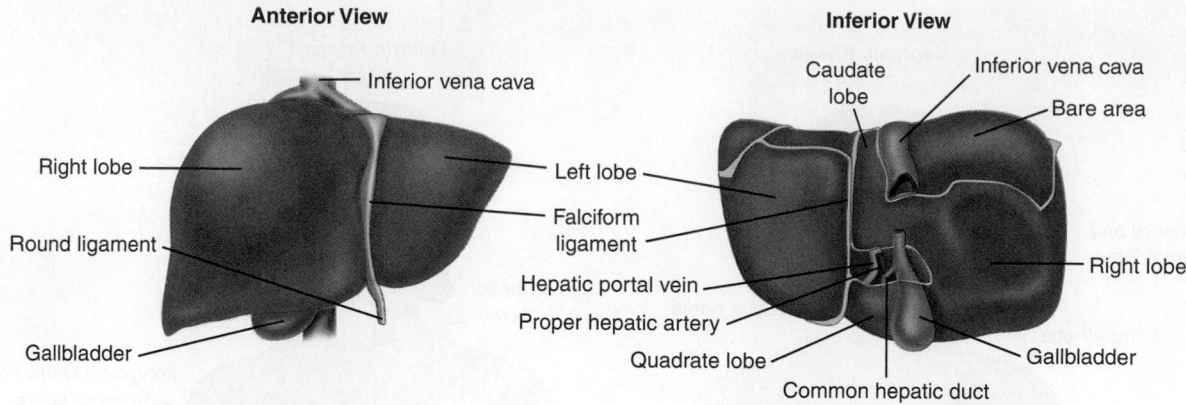

FIGURE 55.6 Liver. Anatomical features of the liver.

system, an oxygen-rich supply from the hepatic artery and a nutrient-rich supply from the portal vein. Twenty percent of the body's total oxygen consumption is utilized by the liver. The blood supply from the portal vein receives nutrients from the stomach, intestines, spleen, and pancreas.

A closer look at the microanatomy of the liver (Fig. 55.7) reveals an intricate network of specialized cells and blood vessels known as hepatic lobules. Hepatocytes constitute the majority of the hepatic cells and are responsible for many of the functions of the liver. Major functions of the liver include (1) absorption and metabolism of nutrients; (2) degradation of toxins, hormones, and medications; and (3) synthesis of proteins (clotting factors, albumin, several clotting factors, fibrinogen, and prothrombin). Other cells known as **Kupffer cells** are responsible for detoxifying the blood of bacteria. The branches of the hepatic artery and portal veins supply a mixture of oxygen- and nutrient-rich blood to the hepatocytes. In terms of the digestive process, the liver aids in the digestion of fat by producing bile acids and lecithin. The other functions of the liver are listed in Table 55.1.

The Gallbladder

Located in the right upper quadrant, the gallbladder, a pear-shaped sac, is attached to the inferior portion of the liver and is responsible for bile storage and concentration. Bile is needed for the emulsification of fat. Bile contains phospholipids (lecithin), bile pigments (bilirubin), and bile salts; approximately 500 to 1,000 mL of bile is excreted from the liver and stored in the gallbladder. Bile leaves the liver and passes through a ductal system (Fig. 55.8):

Hepatic ducts→Common hepatic duct→
Cystic duct and into the gallbladder

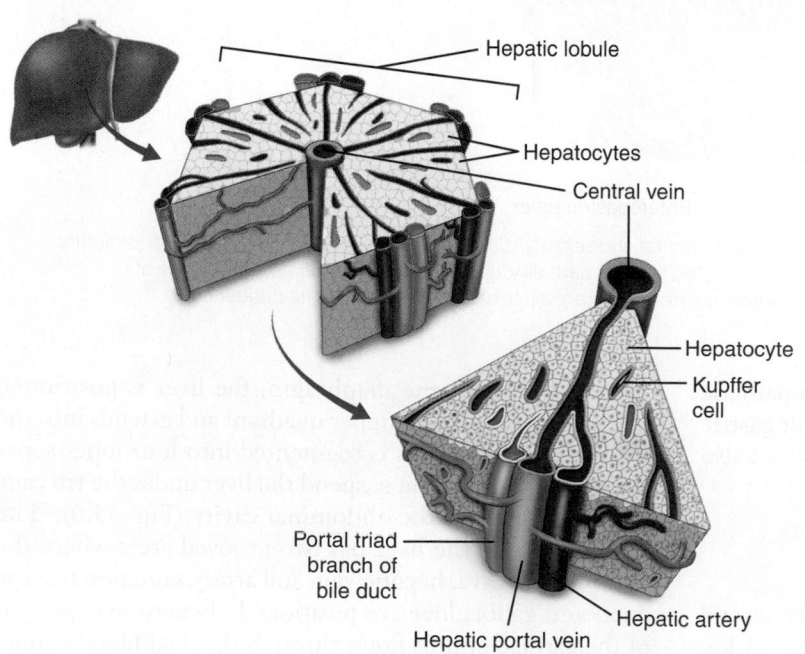

FIGURE 55.7 Liver microanatomy includes an intricate network of specialized cells and blood vessels known as hepatic lobules.

Table 55.1 Functions of the Liver

Gastrointestinal Process	Liver Function
Digestion	Emulsification of fat
	Absorption of dietary fat
Vitamin and mineral metabolism	Storage of vitamins A, B_{12}, D, ferritin
	Excretes excess calcium
Protein metabolism	Deamination and transamination of amino acids
	Converts ammonia to urea
Carbohydrate metabolism	Conversion of dietary fructose and galactose to glucose
	Conversion of lactic acid to pyruvic acid or glucose-6-phosphate
	Storage and release of glycogen
	Synthesizes glucose from fat and amino acids when glycogen stores are low
Lipid metabolism	Synthesis of fat, cholesterol, and phospholipids
	Produces ketone bodies, VLDL, and HDL
Plasma protein synthesis	Synthesizes blood plasma proteins: albumin, fibrinogen, prothrombin
Detoxification	Detoxifies alcohol and medications that are metabolized in the liver; deactivates thyroxine and metabolizes bilirubin and excretes it as bile pigment
Phagocytosis	Aids in the elimination of bacteria in the blood

HDL, High-density lipoprotein; *VLDL,* very low-density lipoprotein.

After the ingestion of a meal, bile exits the gallbladder via the cystic duct that communicates with the bile duct. The terminal end of the bile duct connects with the terminal end of the pancreatic duct to form the hepatopancreatic ampulla in the pancreas. This ampulla connects with the duodenal papilla, which contains the hepatopancreatic sphincter (sphincter of Oddi) that opens during digestion and releases bile to the small intestine to emulsify the dietary fat.

The Pancreas

The pancreas is a gland that is 12 to 15 cm in length and is positioned inferior to the stomach in the right upper quadrant (see Fig. 55.8). It has three landmark areas: the head, which is surrounded by the duodenum; the body; and the tail. The pancreatic duct is in the middle of the pancreas and extends from the tail to the head, where it joins the bile

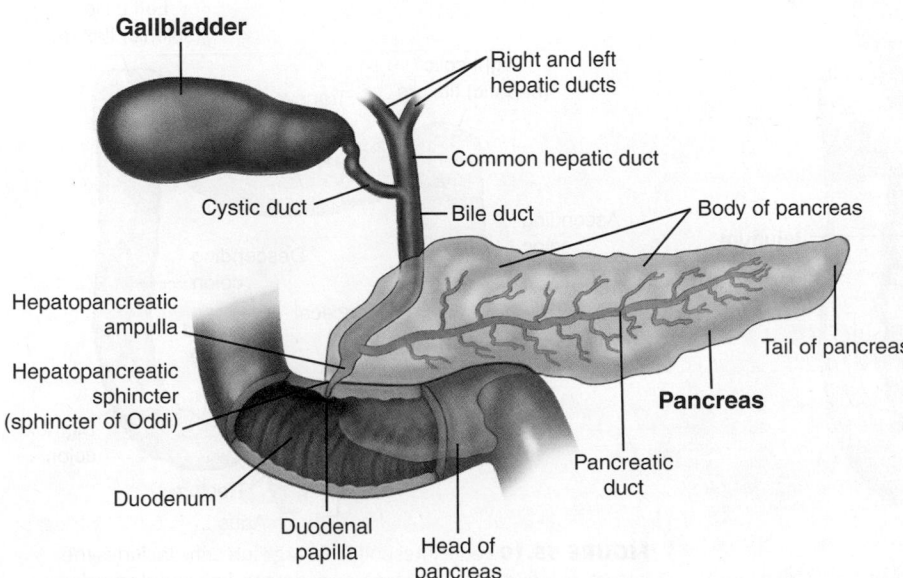

FIGURE 55.8 The gallbladder and pancreas. The gallbladder is a pear-shaped organ located in the right upper quadrant. The pancreas is a gland that is positioned inferior to the stomach in the right upper quadrant. The terminal end of the bile duct connects with the terminal end of the pancreatic duct to form the hepatopancreatic ampulla in the pancreas.

duct. The pancreas has both endocrine and exocrine functions. As an endocrine gland, it produces insulin and glucagon. As an exocrine gland, the pancreas secretes 1,200 to 1,500 mL daily of a liquid known as pancreatic juice that contains water; sodium bicarbonate; proenzymes needed for protein digestion; and the pancreatic enzymes needed for carbohydrate (amylase), fat (lipase, phospholipase A, and cholesterol esterase), and DNA and RNA (deoxyribonucleases, ribonucleases) digestion. The digestion of these nutrients is essential to cellular metabolism. The release of these enzymes is secreted through the acinar cells of the pancreas and is regulated by neural and hormonal feedback systems. Acetylcholine stimulates the release of pancreatic enzymes during the cephalic phase. These pancreatic enzymes are stored in the duodenum and released as the chyme arrives. **Cholecystokinin** is released from the jejunum and duodenum when gastric acid, long fatty chains, and certain amino acids are present. The release of cholecystokinin stimulates the release of pancreatic enzymes that contract the gallbladder and relax the hepatopancreatic sphincter for the release of bile into the duodenum. Lastly, **secretin** is released from the small intestine in response to the presence of the acidic chyme in the small intestine. The release of secretin stimulates the liver and pancreas to release sodium bicarbonate, which neutralizes the acidic chyme and protects the intestinal lining.

The Small Intestine

Protein, carbohydrate, and fat digestion and absorption occur in the small intestine (Fig. 55.9). The small intestine has a diameter measuring 2.5 cm, beginning at the end of the pyloric sphincter and ending at the ileocecal junction and filling most of the abdominal cavity. The small intestine is divided into three components: the duodenum, jejunum, and ileum. Chyme leaves the stomach via the pyloric canal and connects with the duodenum, the first and shortest (10 in.) segment of the small intestine. Measuring 8 ft in length, the rich blood supply and muscular intestinal wall of the jejunum make it the thickest portion of the small intestine, where digestion and absorption occur. As the longest portion of the small intestine, the 12-ft ileum occupies the lower portion of the abdominal cavity and connects to the large intestine at the ileocecal valve. Pancreatic enzymes and bile pass through the bile duct and the pancreatic accessory duct and are released into the duodenum. Pancreatic amylase and intestinal enzymes break down carbohydrates into monosaccharides. The lining of the small intestine has **villi**, fingerlike projections that increase the absorption of nutrients. Each villus has **goblet cells** that secrete mucus and enterocytes, which aid in absorption. This process results in only indigestible fibers entering the large intestine.

The Large Intestine

Semiliquid chyme leaves the small intestine through the ileocecal valve and enters the last segment of the digestive tract, the large intestine (Fig. 55.10). Because most nutrients are absorbed in the small intestine, the function of the large intestine is fluid and electrolyte reabsorption and elimination. Measuring 6 ft in length, the large intestine includes the cecum, colon, and anal canal. The cecum is pouchlike and receives the semiliquid chyme from the small intestine. Here, vitamins A, D, E, and K; sodium; and water are reabsorbed, creating semiformed stool. The appendix, a 2- to 7-cm narrow-ended tube, is attached to the end of the cecum. The exact role of the appendix is unknown, but the tube is filled with lymphocytes.

The transformation of waste from a semiliquid state to formed stool occurs in the colon. The colon is divided

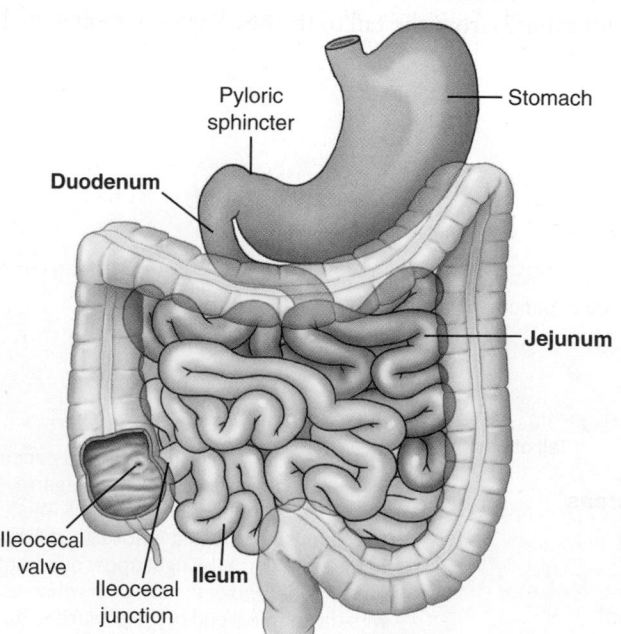

FIGURE 55.9 The small intestine. The small intestine is divided into three components: the duodenum, jejunum, and ileum.

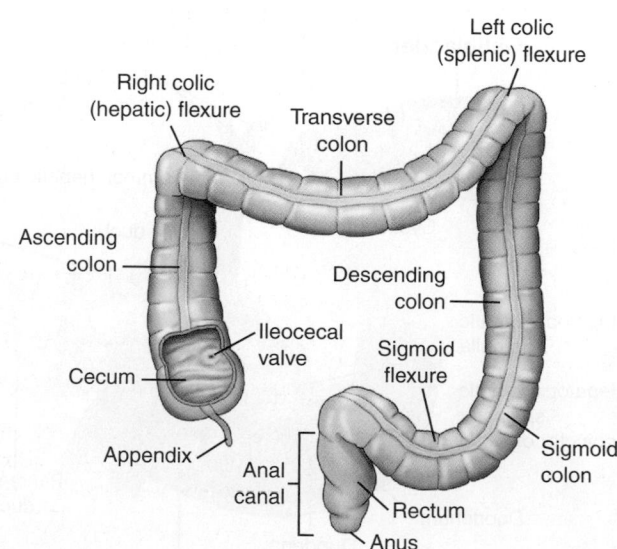

FIGURE 55.10 Large intestine. The large intestine includes the cecum, colon (ascending, transverse, descending and sigmoid sections), and the anal canal terminating in the anus.

into four sections: ascending, transverse, descending, and sigmoid. The ascending colon begins in the right lower quadrant at the ileocecal valve and extends to the hepatic flexure in the right upper quadrant. Here, the stool is in a semiliquid state. Following the ascending colon is the transverse colon, which extends from the right hepatic flexure in the right upper quadrant to the left splenic flexure in the left upper quadrant. The descending colon then extends from the left splenic flexure in the left upper quadrant to the sigmoid colon in the left lower quadrant. The last portion of the colon, the sigmoid, connects the descending colon and rectum. The rectum is 15 cm long and sits in the pelvic cavity. Finally, the anal canal is the last 3 cm of the digestive tract. It includes internal and external anal sphincters to regulate the passage of stool, which consists of bacteria, bilirubin, and indigestible fiber. The presence of bacteria is the cause for flatus and represents 30% of fecal content.

Connection Check 55.1

The nurse recognizes that an impairment of which CN makes a patient at risk for aspiration due to ineffective swallowing?

A. Trochlear
B. Trigeminal
C. Vagus
D. Accessory

Connection Check 55.2

Patients experiencing diarrhea are at risk for which alteration in absorption?

A. Decreased chyme absorption
B. Increased chyme absorption
C. Decreased potassium absorption
D. Increased potassium absorption

ASSESSMENT

History

The gastrointestinal assessment is included in either the routine physical or a problem-focused examination. The comprehensive assessment of any patient begins with a thorough history. It is important for the nurse to assess the patient's level of understanding and ability to communicate to ensure a reliable health history account. Additionally, the nurse must conduct a culturally sensitive and relevant interview while avoiding stereotyping. Asking questions about cultural practices may provide insight into eating habits as well as general healthcare practices (Table 55.2).

In the routine assessment, patients are initially asked broad, general questions regarding their health history and practices followed by specific questions in response to the patient's response. However, in problem-focused examinations, a history of the present illness is developed by initially asking patients very specific questions based on

---

Table 55.2 Health History of the Gastrointestinal System

Data	Questions
Dietary practices	Who prepares the food in your home? Do you fast for cultural or religious reasons? Do you have any dietary restrictions due to religious or cultural practices? How often do you eat? What do you consider to be healthy or unhealthy foods? Do you use food to treat illnesses? Any food intolerances? Any food allergies?
Nutrition	Do you take vitamins? Any history of vitamin deficiencies? Completion of a food frequency questionnaire. Completion of nutritional screening tool. (MUST, Figure 55-11)
Oral health	Do you see a dentist? How often per year? Do you have a history of dental caries or cavities? Do you wear dentures? Do you have gum disease? Have you been treated for oral candidiasis or oral cancer? Do you have difficulty swallowing or suffer with chronic hoarseness?
Preventive health	What are your exercise habits? Have you had Hepatitis vaccines? Have you had a colonoscopy or sigmoidoscopy? What were the results?
Weight changes	Have you had any unexplained weight loss or weight gain? Do you diet frequently? Any binging or purging? Do you ever make yourself vomit?
	Any **hematemesis** (blood in emesis)/**hemoptysis** (blood in sputum)? Calculate body mass index (BMI)?
Appetite changes	Have you had increased hunger or thirst? Any early feeling of fullness?
Stool changes	How often do you have a bowel movement? When was your last bowel movement? Have you noticed any changes in color, consistency, or odor? Have you noticed any bright red blood? Have you noticed undigested food? Any laxative use? Frequent flatus?
Pain	Where is the pain? How often do you have pain? When do you have pain? What have you done to relieve the pain? What are the characteristics of your pain? Do you experience pain before or after eating meals? Do you experience pain with defecation?

their reported symptoms and then moving to broader general questions about health. It is also essential to collect a thorough medical, surgical, family, and social history. This information can aid in determining the overall gastrointestinal health of the patient (Table 55.3). For example, cardiac, psychiatric, neurological, and endocrine disorders can impact the function of the gastrointestinal system. Further, it is important to obtain a thorough family history to assess genetic risk factors for cancer screening. Lastly, determining the patient's medication regimen is necessary to ascertain the effects, as well as side effects, of medications on the gastrointestinal system.

A nutritional assessment aids in understanding the patient's behaviors and practices specific to food intake and impact on the gastrointestinal system and includes a thorough nutritional history, physical assessment, and serum studies. Questions focus on weight or appetite changes, loss of appetite (**anorexia**), or binging or purging practices. Ascertaining perceptions on what is considered healthy eating and a healthy weight provides information on assessing risk factors for malnutrition. The Malnutrition Universal Screening Tool (MUST), from the British Association of Parenteral and Enteral Nutrition, may be used for a complete nutritional assessment (Fig. 55.11). A referral to a nutritionist for a complete nutritional assessment is indicated for a MUST score of two or higher. Other key questions focus on amounts and types of foods eaten, accessibility to healthy foods, known nutritional deficiencies, and changes in bowel patterns. The patient is also asked about the characteristics of stool: color, frequency, consistency. Presence of blood in the stool can be described as bright blood in the stool (**hematochezia**) or black, tarry stool (**melena**).

The physical assessment includes both a head-to-toe assessment and anthropometric measurements, including height, weight, body mass index (BMI), waist circumference, body composition, skinfold measurements, and circumference measurements. If possible, it is recommended that actual height and weight measurements be taken, as opposed to using stated values by the patient, because the calculation of BMI is based on height and weight measurements. Waist circumference is an important nutritional measurement because excess adipose fat along the waist increases the risk for type 2 diabetes mellitus, elevated blood lipids, hypertension, and cardiovascular disease. Body composition measurements, completed through a variety of techniques with varying reliability, provide data about fat mass, muscle mass, and body fat percentage. Skin calipers, biometrical impedance, and dual-energy x-ray absorptiometry (DEXA) scans are examples of techniques to measure body composition, and due to the variability in measurements, body composition is usually trended over time. Skinfold measurements are used to estimate subcutaneous body fat, and circumference measurements of the calf and midarm may be used as another approach to body composition analysis. Based on the patient's current health status, all of these anthropometric measurements may not be available. In these situations, it is important to collect as much data as possible and use the findings, in conjunction with the nutritional assessment and laboratory findings, to determine the patient's nutritional assessment.

Specific diagnostic studies that are helpful in determining nutritional status include serum albumin, prealbumin, and transferrin. Normal serum albumin is 3.4 to 5.1 g/dL, and levels less than 3.5 g/dL are indicative of altered nutritional status and are associated with increased morbidity and mortality in older adults. Prealbumin (normal range 12–42 mg/dL) is considered a more accurate indicator of plasma proteins when compared with albumin, and decreased levels are also associated with increased morbidity and mortality in older adults. Due to transferrin's role in iron binding and transport, transferrin levels are also important to nutritional assessment, and levels range from 215 to 365 mg/dL in males to 250 to 350 mg/dL in females.

Table 55.3 Questions to Assess the Gastrointestinal System

Pertinent History	Questions
Social history	Do you smoke? Do you use street drugs?
	Do you use prescription or over-the-counter (OTC) medications? Do you use herbals? Do you drink alcohol? Recent antibiotic use?
	Any recent international travel?
Medical history	Do you have a history of previous heart attacks, chest pain? Parkinson's disease, sickle cell disease? Sjögren's syndrome?
	Do you have a history of diabetes, multiple sclerosis? Crohn's disease? Irritable bowel disorder? Gastroesophageal reflux disease (GERD)?
	Do you have a history of anorexia nervosa? Bulimia? Depression? Familial adenomatous polyposis? Celiac disease?
Surgical history	Any history of previous abdominal surgeries?

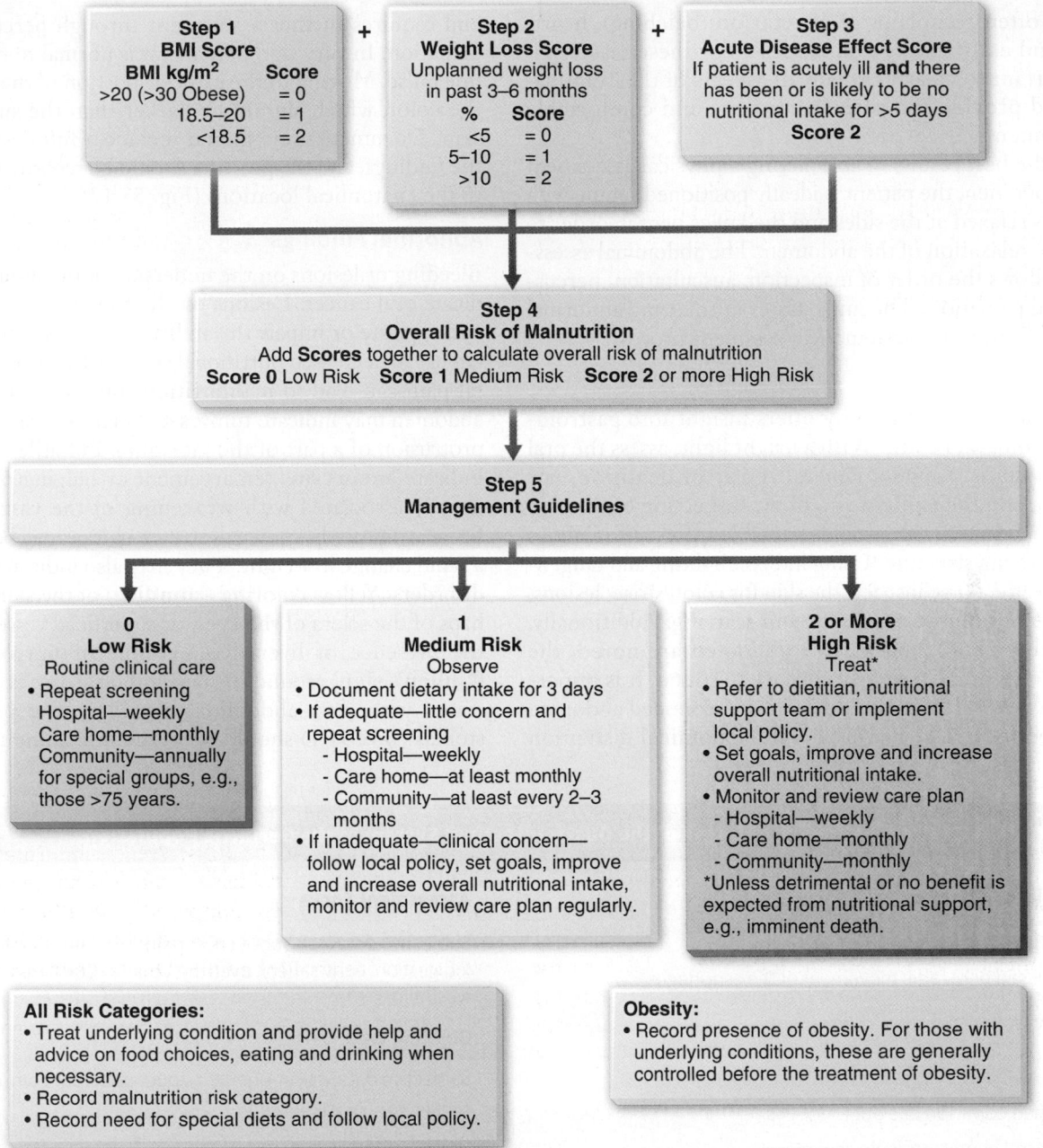

Step 1
BMI Score

BMI kg/m²	Score
>20 (>30 Obese)	= 0
18.5–20	= 1
<18.5	= 2

+

Step 2
Weight Loss Score
Unplanned weight loss
in past 3–6 months

%	Score
<5	= 0
5–10	= 1
>10	= 2

+

Step 3
Acute Disease Effect Score
If patient is acutely ill **and** there
has been or is likely to be no
nutritional intake for >5 days
Score 2

Step 4
Overall Risk of Malnutrition
Add **Scores** together to calculate overall risk of malnutrition
Score 0 Low Risk   **Score 1** Medium Risk   **Score 2** or more High Risk

Step 5
Management Guidelines

0
Low Risk
Routine clinical care
• Repeat screening
Hospital—weekly
Care home—monthly
Community—annually
for special groups, e.g.,
those >75 years.

1
Medium Risk
Observe
• Document dietary intake for 3 days
• If adequate—little concern and
repeat screening
  - Hospital—weekly
  - Care home—at least monthly
  - Community—at least every 2–3
    months
• If inadequate—clinical concern—
follow local policy, set goals, improve
and increase overall nutritional intake,
monitor and review care plan regularly.

2 or More
High Risk
Treat*
• Refer to dietitian, nutritional
support team or implement
local policy.
• Set goals, improve and increase
overall nutritional intake.
• Monitor and review care plan
  - Hospital—weekly
  - Care home—monthly
  - Community—monthly
*Unless detrimental or no benefit is
expected from nutritional support,
e.g., imminent death.

All Risk Categories:
• Treat underlying condition and provide help and
advice on food choices, eating and drinking when
necessary.
• Record malnutrition risk category.
• Record need for special diets and follow local policy.

Obesity:
• Record presence of obesity. For those with
underlying conditions, these are generally
controlled before the treatment of obesity.

FIGURE 55.11 Malnutrition Universal Screening Tool (MUST).

Decreased levels of transferrin are associated with infection, kidney disease, and hepatic damage, as well as indicative of insufficient protein in the diet in patients with malnourishment.

Physical Examination

Focused on the collection of objective data, the physical examination includes a direct assessment of the oral cavity; direct assessment of the skin; and an indirect assessment of the underlying structures: the intestinal tract, liver, kidney, spleen, and abdominal arteries. A review of diagnostic testing findings may provide additional information about physical assessment findings. For example, in the patient with **hepatomegaly** (enlarged liver), the laboratory results may reveal elevated liver function tests (LFTs). Before proceeding with the actual examination, it is important to consider information collected during the health history. Individual preferences, along with religious, cultural, or geriatric considerations, may require the nurse to alter the approach to the examination. Some people, based on cultural or religious reasons, are uncomfortable with exposing the abdominal area or are sensitive to touch, which can lead to contraction of the underlying musculature in the abdomen, giving the false appearance of abdominal rigidity. Additionally, in assessing the older adult, it is important that the nurse recognize age-related changes to the gastrointestinal system. For example, with changes in the esophagus, the patient often complains of **eructation** (belching), heartburn, and early satiety (Table 55.4). For these reasons, it is important to clearly explain all aspects of the examination and provide the patient a private and comfortable environment.

For the best results in completing a physical assessment of the abdomen, the patient is ideally positioned supine with the arms relaxed at the sides and the knees bent in order to promote relaxation of the abdomen. The abdominal assessment follows the order of inspection, auscultation, percussion, and palpation. The nurse notes normal and abnormal findings during this systematic assessment process.

Inspection

Inspection of the oral cavity offers insight into gastrointestinal and oral health. With a bright light, assess the oral mucosa, gums, tongue, general repair of dentition, jaw strength, and the ability to swallow. Inspection of the skin over the abdomen can provide valuable information about the underlying structure. Using indirect lighting and tangential views, the nurse inspects the skin for color, striae, lesions, presence of superficial vessels, and scarring. Additionally, the contour and shape of the abdomen are noted; the abdomen should be slightly concave to round. It is important to assess for fullness at the sides. A rounded abdomen from obesity can be confused with abdominal distention

and requires further assessment through percussion and palpation. In very thin patients, it is normal to note a midline pulse. Moving to the exterior portion of the anus, note the color, which should be darker than the surrounding skin. Documentation should include a full description of the findings, and the position should be recorded according to the anatomical locations (Fig. 55.12).

Abnormal Findings

Bleeding or lesions on the underside of the mouth may indicate oral cancer. Lesions on the tongue can impair taste and appetite or impair the ability to swallow and may contribute to decreased nutritional status. Missing teeth or dental pain can lead to malnutrition. Bulging masses on the abdomen may indicate tumors or **hernias** (displacement or protrusion of a part of the intestine). Pulsatile masses may indicate **aneurysms** (enlargement or bulging of an artery usually associated with weakening of the vascular wall). Striae, commonly known as stretch marks, may be seen with a rapid change in weight. They may also indicate endocrine disorders. Yellow coloring (**jaundice**) of the skin, and perhaps of the sclera of the eyes, or superficial vessels indicate the presence of liver disease. Blue or purple coloring (**Cullen's sign**) around the periumbilical area is often associated with intra-abdominal bleeding. The presence of stomas (Box 55.1) should be noted, including their color

---

Table 55.4 Normal Biological Changes of the Gastrointestinal System in the Geriatric Population

Age-Related Changes	Assessment Focus
• Esophageal stiffening • Decreased peristaltic movement of the esophagus • Decreased gastric emptying	**Subjective data:** Ask about chest pain, eructation, heartburn, indigestion, early satiety, over-the-counter GERD treatment, weight loss **Objective data:** Weight
• Decreased bile synthesis • Widened common bile duct • Increased cholecystokinin secretion	**Subjective data:** Ask about right upper quadrant pain, early satiety, decreased appetite **Objective data:** Inspection of the skin. Palpation of the abdomen
• Distention and dilation of pancreatic ducts • Decreased weight of the pancreas • Decreased sensitivity of pancreatic B cells to glucose • Decreased lipase production	**Subjective data:** Ask about diabetes symptoms: Thirst? Frequent urination? Increased appetite? Right upper quadrant or right shoulder pain. Color and consistency of stool. **Objective data:** Weight (loss); serum blood glucose levels
• Decrease in number and size of hepatic cells • Decrease in liver enzyme activity and cholesterol synthesis	**Subjective data:** Ask about medications (prescribed, OTC, and herbals), alcohol intake **Objective data:** Percuss and palpate abdomen
• Decreased peristalsis • Decreased mucus secretion in the large intestine • Decreased elasticity of the rectal wall • Decreased sensation of rectal wall distention • Decreased percentage of water weight	**Subjective data:** Ask about frequency of bowel movements. Bloating? Urgency or straining? Incontinence? Laxative use? Medication use? Dietary practices? **Objective data:** Auscultate bowel sounds, percuss and palpate abdomen, assess rectal area for hemorrhoids

GERD, Gastroesophageal reflux disease; *OTC,* over the counter.

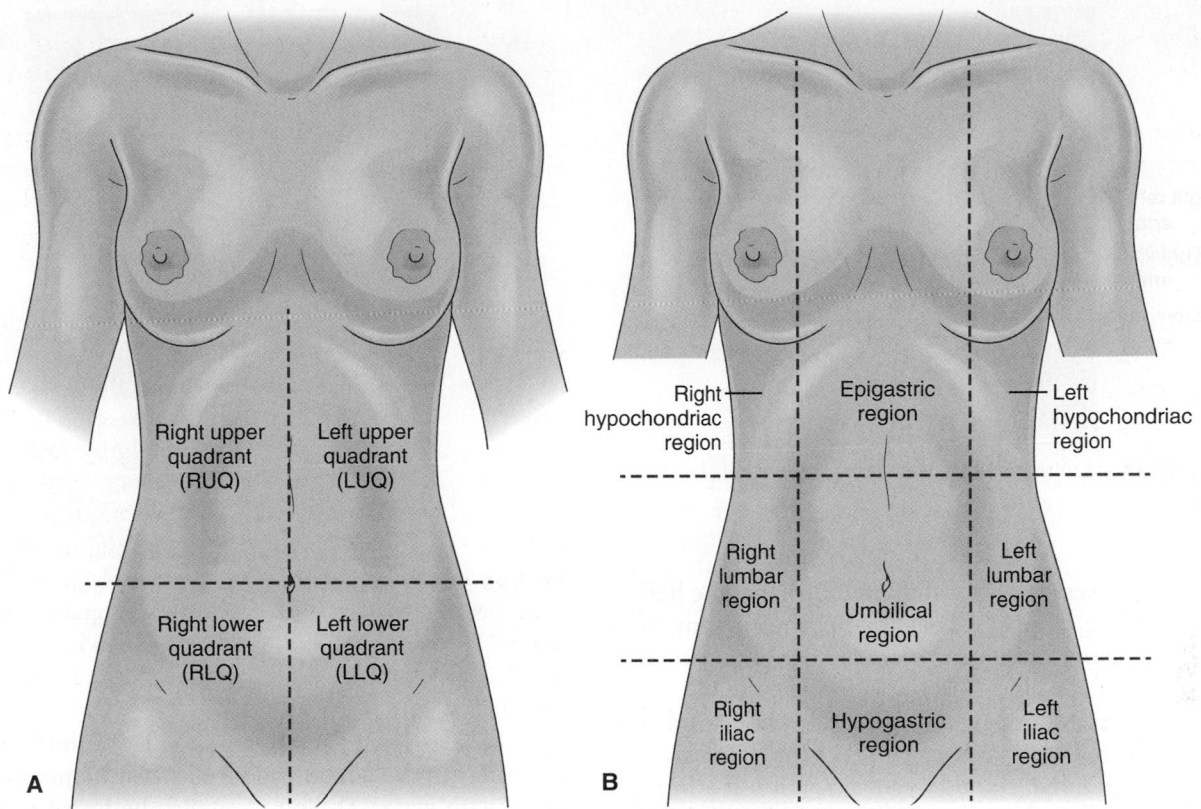

FIGURE 55.12 Abdominal assessment according to anatomical locations. A, The four quadrants of the abdomen. B, The nine regions of the abdomen.

Box 55.1 Assessment of a Stoma

Inspection of an Ostomy: The Three "Ss"

In a patient with an ostomy, several key areas should be assessed and documented:

Skin: The surrounding skin color of the stoma should be consistent with the rest of the abdomen. Any lesions or excoriations should be described and documented.

Stoma: Assess the stoma for color and consistency. The stoma should be pink and moist.

Stool: Consistency of stool is dependent on the location of the stoma. For instance, an ostomy located in the ileum will pass semiliquid stool, whereas the stool from the sigmoid colostomy will be formed.

and size. Visible swollen, protruding veins underlying the skin of the anus are indicative of **hemorrhoids**.

Auscultation

The purpose of auscultation is to indirectly assess bowel sounds and the vascular integrity of the arteries. Typically in the assessment process, percussion and palpation occur prior to auscultation. However, manipulation of the abdomen can result in an inaccurate interpretation of bowel sounds as being hyperactive, so auscultation is completed after inspection. The diaphragm of the stethoscope is considered best for high-pitched sounds such as bowel sounds. The stethoscope should be placed lightly on the abdomen. Bowel sounds are normally present in the right lower quadrant at the ileocecal valve and are the starting point for auscultation. Moving in a counterclockwise position, the nurse listens in each quadrant, paying close attention to the quality of pitch and sound made by the intestines. Normal bowels sounds can range from low- to high-pitched gurgling, and the frequency of bowel sounds occurs at a rate of 5 to 30 times per minute. A commonly held practice in determining the absence of bowel sounds is to auscultate each quadrant for a minimum of 5 minutes. More recent studies suggest that this practice yields low specificity and sensitivity in determining the absence of bowel sounds. It is important to take into consideration all the assessment findings before determining absence. The frequency of intestinal movement and quality of sound can be influenced by several factors, including the timing of food intake, mobility, medications, neurological disorders, and electrolyte imbalance. Hypoactive bowel sounds can be caused by anesthetics, opioids, and anticholinergic medications, as well as conditions such as **constipation** or **ileus** (absence of normal gastrointestinal motility). Conversely, hyperactive bowel sounds can be secondary to the actions of cholinergic medications or infectious and inflammatory bowel disorders.

The abdominal arteries, including the abdominal aorta, renal, iliac, and femoral arteries (Fig. 55.13), can

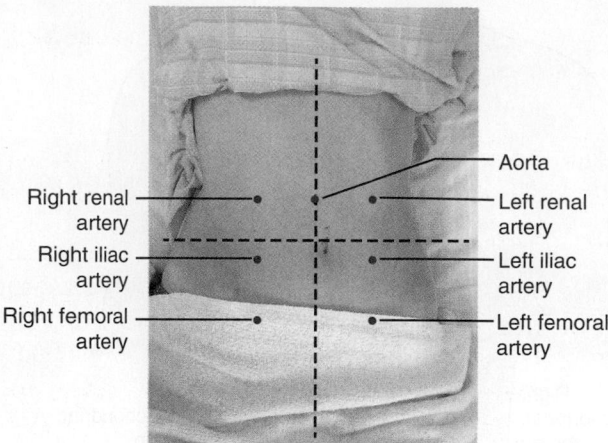

FIGURE 55.13 Auscultation sites for assessing abdominal vascular sounds.

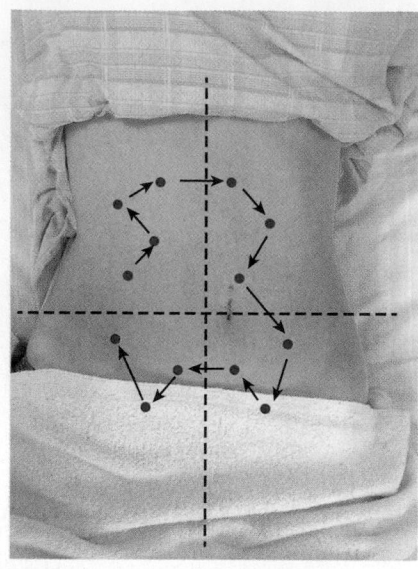

FIGURE 55.14 Percussion sites. Percussion of the abdomen is performed by moving in a clockwise fashion starting in the right upper quadrant.

be indirectly assessed in the abdomen by using the bell of the stethoscope, which is best for hearing low-pitched sounds like **bruits** (abnormal sounds heard upon auscultation of blood vessels). The whooshing sound of a bruit may indicate partial obstruction of the vessel, and it is never considered a normal variant to hear a bruit in the abdomen. The nurse should avoid palpation if a bruit is auscultated and report the finding to the healthcare provider.

Abnormal Findings

Hypoactive bowel sounds can be a later indicator of obstruction, whereas hyperactive bowel sounds can be an early indication of obstruction, diarrhea, or inflammatory bowel disorders. Absent bowel sounds may indicate paralytic ileus caused by mechanical or neurological dysfunction. Bruits can indicate an arterial obstruction.

Percussion

The size of the organs is ascertained through percussion and palpation. Accurate percussion and interpretation require a quiet environment and a skilled practitioner. Nursing students and novice registered nurses often find this skill difficult because of the inability to distinguish between tympany and dullness and the need for proper placement of the fingers on the abdomen. Fingernail length should be short to avoid pinching or scratching the patient. The patient should be supine with the legs partially bent, allowing for the abdominal muscles to be in a relaxed position. To perform this assessment, the nurse places the nondominant hand parallel to the abdomen and firmly places an outstretched finger on the abdomen. Striking the outstretched finger with a finger from the dominant hand, the nurse continues this motion, moving in a clockwise fashion (Fig. 55.14). Percussion over the intestinal area should elicit a drumlike sound known as **tympany**. This sound is similar to the sound heard when percussing a balloon filled with air and should be the predominant sound of the abdomen because air rises in the intestines when patients are in a supine position. Percussion over the liver

or stomach should elicit dullness, a flat sound. This sound is similar to the sound produced when tapping a balloon filled with water. Dullness can also be heard in an obese abdomen, over the intestinal tract when filled with fecal matter, over a full bladder, or in the presence of fluid accumulation in the abdomen, or **ascites** (Fig. 55.15).

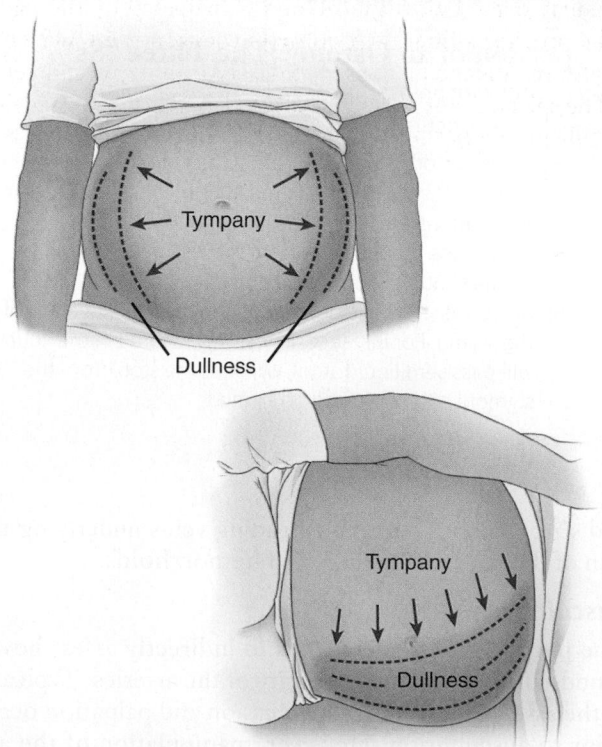

FIGURE 55.15 Abdominal distention from ascites. Percussion over the intestinal area should result in a sound known as tympany. Dullness can be heard in the presence of ascites.

Abnormal Findings

Tympany can be the predominant sound when abdominal gas is present. The presence of fluid can displace air, and dullness can be the dominant sound. This can also indicate constipation.

Palpation

As stated previously, the purpose of palpation is to evaluate the underlying structures (Fig. 55.16) as well as to assess for abdominal tenderness and abdominal tone. The starting point for palpation is away from any areas of discomfort stated by the patient. *Light palpation* (Fig. 55.17) begins by slightly pressing the pads of the fingers into the abdomen and gliding them over the abdomen in small, incremental, circular movements clockwise around the abdomen. During palpation, it is important to note the abdominal tone and any areas of tenderness. Palpating large abdomens in obese patients can be difficult because of the increased pressure met against the palpating hand. Using the bimanual technique can improve the assessment. Again, it is important to note that pulsating masses should never be palpated.

Deep palpation (Fig. 55.18) is a technique that allows the practitioner to assess the size and consistency of the liver, kidney, and spleen. However, it is a skill typically performed by advanced practice nurses or providers.

The *hooking technique* (Fig. 55.19) is also an advanced practice skill used to assess the edge of the liver. Standing to the left of the patient and placing the fingers under the 12th rib as shown in the figure, when the patient inhales, the liver's edge may come below the rib and be palpated by the pads of the provider's fingers. A normal liver span is 6 to 12 cm. *Hepatomegaly* is the term used to describe an enlarged liver.

The spleen is not normally palpated, but in splenomegaly, the spleen moves beneath the costal margin and is felt on palpation (Fig. 55.20). **Organomegaly** is the term used to describe generalized enlargement of organs.

Abnormal Findings

A rigid abdomen can indicate pain, guarding, or **peritonitis**, which is inflammation of the peritoneal cavity. A mass may indicate a tumor, aneurysm, or hernia.

CASE STUDY: EPISODE 2

The physical examination reveals the following: vital signs: T 97.8°F (36.5°C), pulse 115 bpm, respirations 18, supine BP 130/80 mm Hg, standing 100/60 mm Hg. Abdomen soft, round, slightly distended, and tender. Hypoactive bowel sounds present in all four quadrants. No superficial vessels or lesions present. Generalized tympany with dullness noted in left lower quadrant on percussion. Skin warm, dry, flaky, and intact. No palpable masses present. Fecal occult blood testing results are pending...

Connection Check 55.3

The nurse places the patient in which position for a gastrointestinal assessment to promote relaxation of the abdominal muscles?

A. Sitting upright with arms relaxed in the lap and feet on the floor
B. Semirecumbent with knees extended and arms at the sides
C. Side lying with arms above the head and knees flexed
D. Supine with arms at the side and knees flexed

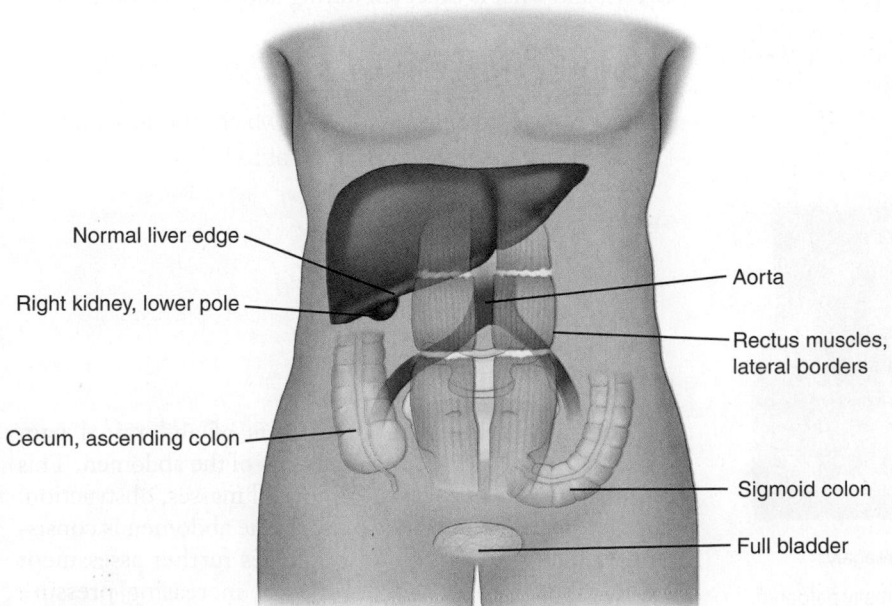

Normal liver edge
Right kidney, lower pole
Cecum, ascending colon

Aorta
Rectus muscles, lateral borders
Sigmoid colon
Full bladder

FIGURE 55.16 Normal palpable structures. The purpose of palpation is to evaluate the underlying structures of the abdominal cavity.

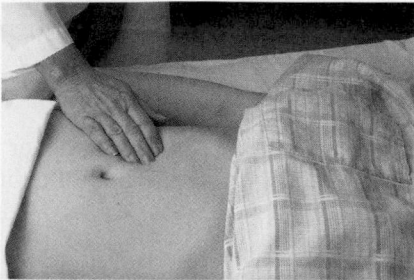

FIGURE 55.17 Light palpation. Light palpation begins by slightly pressing the pads of the fingers into the abdomen and gliding them in small, incremental, circular movements clockwise around the abdomen.

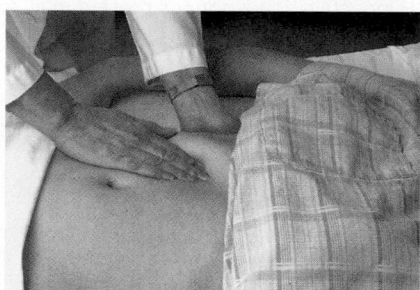

FIGURE 55.18 Deep palpation. This is a technique that allows the assessment of the size and consistency of the liver, kidney, and spleen.

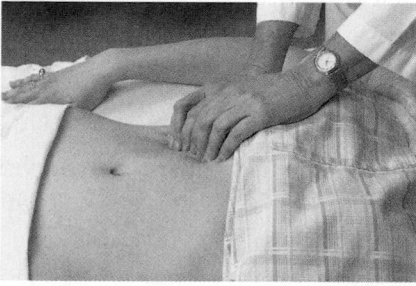

FIGURE 55.19 Hooking technique. This technique is used to assess the edge of the liver. The practitioner stands to the left of the patient and places the fingers under the 12th rib, as shown in the figure. When the patient inhales, the liver's edge may come below the rib and be palpated by the pads of the fingers.

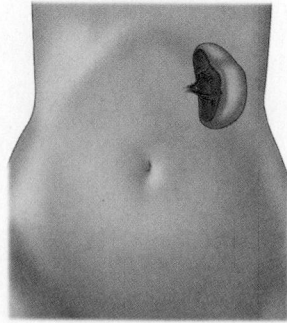

Normal spleen   Splenomegaly

FIGURE 55.20 Splenomegaly. The spleen is not normally palpated, but in splenomegaly, the spleen is felt on palpation.

DIAGNOSTIC STUDIES

Diagnostic testing is essential to the comprehensive assessment of gastrointestinal function. The results of diagnostic tests are correlated with the patient's clinical presentation and the healthcare practitioner's physical assessment findings to develop an accurate diagnosis. Laboratory results are also vital in establishing a baseline, as well as in determining the patient's response to treatment.

Laboratory Studies

Assessment of gastrointestinal function includes various types of serum, urine, and stool analyses (Table 55.5). A complete blood count (CBC) provides important information about potential blood loss through assessment of the red blood cell count, hemoglobin, and hematocrit, and the white blood cell count is indicated for evaluation of inflammatory or infectious processes. A serum chemistry panel is obtained to assess for electrolyte imbalances associated with impaired absorption or excretion. As described previously, serum albumin, prealbumin, and transferrin levels provide data regarding nutritional status. With suspected liver disease, a prothrombin time is important to assess clotting because this test measures the time required for prothrombin to be converted to thrombin and may be prolonged because of impaired synthesis of clotting factors in the liver. Additionally, liver function tests (LFTs) are evaluated with suspected hepatic dysfunction. Urine analysis is indicated in patients with suspected pancreatitis because urine amylase is elevated in this disorder. In patients with complaints of changes in bowel pattern, stool samples are collected for occult blood.

Patients may be apprehensive while awaiting test results. To avoid delays in treatment or inaccurate results, nurses must be knowledgeable and aware of all aspects of the diagnostic study, including patient education and preparation. Patients should understand the purpose of the test, possible side effects, and what is expected during and after the procedure.

Connection Check 55.4

The nurse correlates an increase in which laboratory value with the diagnosis of acute pancreatitis?
A. Serum sodium
B. Serum amylase
C. Serum potassium
D. Serum creatinine

Imaging Studies

Patients presenting with complaints of abdominal pain typically undergo a routine plain x-ray of the abdomen. This diagnostic study may reveal abnormal masses, obstruction, or strictures. The presence of air in the abdomen is consistent with an obstruction and requires further assessment because perforation can occur with increasing pressure behind the obstruction. Routine plain x-rays require no

Table 55.5 Diagnostic Testing for Gastrointestinal Function

Gastric Analysis	Teaching	Pre-/Intra-/Posttest	Results
After a period of fasting, gastric fluid is obtained through a nasogastric tube or during endoscopic procedure. The fluid is used to: • Measure gastric acidity • Assess for presence of: • Blood • Bacteria • Medications	Patients must be NPO from 8–12 hours Patients should refrain from caffeine and alcohol intake at 24 hours prior to test.	**Pretest** Patient education Remove loose dentures before test Assess patient medication intake **Intratest** Monitor for patient distress during nasogastric insertion **Posttest** Monitor vital signs after procedure Patient education on reporting symptoms associated with post-procedural complications, further treatment, or lifestyle modification options	Gastrin levels Increased levels can occur with duodenal ulcers, Zollinger–Ellison syndrome (ZES), hypersecretion of antral gastric cells, resection of small intestines Decreased levels can occur with adrenal insufficiency, rheumatoid arthritis, thyroid toxicosis, pernicious anemia, chronic renal failure, and atrophic gastritis Cultures should be negative for *Mycobacterium*
Stool analysis			
Stool is collected to assess for presence of: • Blood (gross and occult) • Fecal leukocytes • Bacteria (*Clostridium difficile*) • Mucus • Parasites • Fat	Patient education on rationale for test and specimen collection methods	**Pretest** Analysis and studies should be done prior to the administration of antibiotics, antidiarrheal medications, laxatives. Stool specimen should not be collected from the toilet. Patient education on specimen collection. **Posttest** Patient education on contact isolation if *C. difficile* cultures are positive.	Presence of blood may indicate gastrointestinal cancer, inflammatory disorders, or hemorrhoids. Presence of *C. difficile* is an indication of pseudomembranous colitis. Presence of mucus Bloody (colon cancer and inflammatory disorders) Clear (spastic constipation) Increased fat (steatorrhea) may indicate malabsorption or pancreatic disorders.
Liver function tests			
Alanine aminotransferase (ALT) Normal value: Male: 13–40 units/L Female: 24–36 units/L	Patient education on rationale for test and specimen collection methods	Collected in red-top tube Previous intramuscular injections may cause ↑ levels	↑ levels Hepatitis Cirrhosis Obstructive jaundice Pancreatitis Cholestasis Severe burns

Continued

Table 55.5 Diagnostic Testing for Gastrointestinal Function—cont'd

Gastric Analysis	Teaching	Pre-/Intra-/Posttest	Results
Albumin Normal: 3.4–5.1 g/dL	Patient education on rationale for test and specimen collection methods	Collected in gold-, gray-, or red-top tube	↑ levels Dehydration ↓ levels Malnutrition Thyroid disorders Liver disorders Hypervolemia Genetic hypoalbuminemia
Aspartate aminotransferase (AST) Normal value: Male: 20–40 units/L Female: 15–35 units/L	Patient education on rationale for test and specimen collection methods		↑ levels Hepatitis Cirrhosis Liver cancer Skeletal muscle trauma/diseases Severe burns Acute pancreatitis Acute hemolytic anemia ↓ levels Acute renal disease Beriberi Chronic renal dialysis Diabetic ketoacidosis
Bilirubin Normal: Total bilirubin: 0.3–1 mg/dL Indirect bilirubin: 0.2–0.8 mg/dL Direct bilirubin: 0.1–0.3 mg/dL	Patient education on rationale for test and specimen collection methods		↑ levels (conjugated) Gallstones Extrahepatic duct obstruction Dubin–Johnson syndrome ↑ levels (unconjugated) Hemolytic jaundice Large-volume blood transfusion Sepsis Hemolytic anemia Pernicious anemia Sickle cell anemia Transfusion reaction

preparation except an explanation. In the patient with severe, acute abdominal pain, positioning may be difficult because the patient may experience increased pain secondary to peritoneal irritation when placed in a supine position.

Ultrasonography

Using a Doppler, sound waves are transmitted to a particular organ. The sound waves are converted to an electronic image to provide a real-time depiction of the soft tissue structure. As a diagnostic procedure, ultrasonography can detect any size and structural abnormalities of the underlying abdominal cavity organs and vessels. The abdominal cavity is also evaluated for the presence of ascites. The liver and pancreas can be visualized to detect cysts, tumors, or masses. The gallbladder and kidneys can be further visualized for stones. As a therapeutic intervention, ultrasonography can be utilized to place stents in obstructed areas. Ultrasonography is the preferred method of visualization of abdominal structures in patients who cannot tolerate contrast dye (Table 55.6).

Barium Studies

Barium studies consist of a series of x-rays and are ordered to examine the integrity and patency of the gastrointestinal tract; these studies can be diagnostic or therapeutic. Preparation for barium studies typically requires the patient to follow a special diet the day before the test (clear liquids) and then nothing by mouth after midnight. A laxative or enema may also be prescribed for the night before the study. Patients are typically given barium, a radiographic opaque liquid, to drink. However, if there is a concern about possible perforations anywhere along the gastrointestinal tract, a water-soluble liquid, gastrografin, is administered. With the use of fluoroscopy, patients are then taken through a series of time-sensitive x-rays. There are several studies that can be performed: an upper gastrointestinal series,

which visualizes the esophagus, stomach, and duodenum; a small bowel series, which visualizes the small intestine; and lastly, the barium enema, which visualizes the colon. Regardless of the type of barium study performed, the nursing interventions are similar (Table 55.7).

Table 55.6 Abdominal Ultrasonography

Types of Ultrasonography	Abnormal Findings
Gallbladder	Polyps
	Tumor
	Gallstones
Liver	Tumor
	Abscess
	Intrahepatic dilated bile ducts
Pancreas	Tumor
	Cysts
	Pseudocysts
	Abscess
	Inflammation
Bile ducts	Gallstone
	Dilation
	Stricture
	Tumor
Abdominal aorta	Aneurysm
Abdominal cavity	Ascites
	Abscess

Table 55.7 Types of Barium Studies

Barium Study	Description	Rationale	Special Considerations	NPO	Significance of Findings
Swallow	More thorough view of the esophagus	Dysphagia	Barium related Fecal impaction Administer ↑ fluid intake Laxative	8–12 hours prior to study	Strictures Stenosis Varices Muscular weakness Tumors
Upper GI	Visual of lower esophagus, stomach, duodenum	Dyspepsia Dysphagia Epigastric pain	Barium related Fecal impaction Administer ↑ fluid intake Laxative	8–12 hours prior to study	Ulcers Gastric Duodenal Cancers/tumors Esophageal

Continued

Table 55.7   Types of Barium Studies—cont'd

Barium Study	Description	Rationale	Special Considerations	NPO	Significance of Findings
					Gastric
					Duodenal
					Diverticulum
					Duodenal
					Esophageal
					Hiatal hernia
Small bowel follow-through (SBFT)	Visual of small intestine Patient drinks barium	Nausea, vomiting	Barium related Fecal impaction Administer ↑ fluid intake Laxative	8–12 hours prior to study	Small bowel obstruction, malabsorption disorders
Small bowel enema (SBE)	Visual of small intestine Patient given an enema	Provides better visualization than SBFT	Barium related Fecal impaction Administer ↑ fluid intake Laxative	8–12 hours prior to study	Small bowel obstruction, malabsorption disorders
Barium enema	Visual of colon	Persistent diarrhea Bloody stools Fistulas	Barium related Fecal impaction Administer ↑ fluid intake Laxative	8–12 hours prior to study	Polyps Tumors Inflammatory bowel diseases Intussusception

Safety Alert   Postprocedural Care

Increased fluid intake and/or enemas are necessary to prevent constipation and impaction in patients who undergo barium studies.

Connection Check 55.5

The nurse monitors for which complication in the patient who has undergone a barium enema?

A. Fluid overload
B. Dehydration
C. Diarrhea
D. Constipation

Endoscopy

Endoscopy is the general term used to describe the procedure in which a fiberoptic scope is used to visualize the gastrointestinal tract. Endoscopic studies can serve three purposes: diagnostic, curative, or palliative. Patients are sedated with a narcotic and a sedative. The pre- and postprocedural nursing interventions are similar and are outlined in Table 55.8.

Safety Alert   Endoscopy Procedural Care

After an upper endoscopy, the nurse monitors for the return of swallow before providing oral intake to decrease the risk of aspiration. After a lower endoscopy, anticoagulants and aspirin (acetylsalicylic acid, or ASA) are usually held temporarily due to the risk of bleeding.

Evidence-Based Practice

Preferred Colorectal Cancer Screening Recommendations

Patient Population	Test
Male or female age 50 at average risk	Colonoscopy every 10 yrs. Fecal immunoassay test (FIT) annually **OR** Alternative colorectal cancer screening: • Flexible sigmoidoscopy every 5 to 10 years • Computed tomography (CT) colonography every 5 years • FIT-fecal DNA every 3 years
African Americans beginning at age 45	Colonoscopy every 10 years or FIT annually **OR** Alternative colorectal cancer screening: • Flexible sigmoidoscopy every 5 to 10 years • CT colonography every 5 years • FIT-fecal DNA every 3 years
Persons who have had consistent screening and remain negative can consider stopping screening at age 75 or life expectancy of less than 10 years.	Colonoscopy every 10 years or FIT annually **OR** Alternative colorectal cancer screening: • Flexible sigmoidoscopy every 5 to 10 years • CT colonography every 5 years • FIT-fecal DNA every 3 years
Persons who have not had a colonoscopy may consider screening up to age 85. Consider comorbidities.	Colonoscopy every 10 years **OR** Alternative colorectal cancer screening: • Flexible sigmoidoscopy every 5 to 10 years • CT colonography every 5 years • FIT-Fecal DNA every 3 years

Family History of Colorectal Cancer (CRC) or Advanced Adenomas

Patient or family history of CRC or advanced adenoma in first-degree relative < age 60 or 2 first-degree relatives	Colonoscopy every 5 years beginning at age 40 years **OR** 10 years younger than age at diagnosis of youngest affected relative
Patients with adenomas without known history of hereditary nonpolyposis colorectal cancer (HPNCC)	• Advise genetic testing or counseling for patients with more than 100 adenomas • Annual flexible sigmoidoscopy or colonoscopy until colectomy is deemed best treatment • Patients with retained rectum after subtotal colectomy • Flexible sigmoidoscopy every 6 to 12 months

Continued

Evidence-Based Practice—cont'd

Those affected or a known first-degree relative with HNPCC	Colonoscopy every 1–2 years beginning at age 20–25 years until age 40 years, then consider annually 2–5 years before the youngest age of diagnosis of CRC in the family if diagnosed before age 25 years. • Women should consider screening for endometrial cancer beginning at age 30–35. • Consider screening for gastric cancer beginning at age 30–35. • Consider screening for urinary cancer beginning at age 30–35.

U.S. Preventive Services Task Force, Bibbins-Domingo, K., Grossman, D. C., Curry, S. J., Davidson, K. W., Epling, J. W., … Siu, A. L. (2016). Screening for colorectal cancer: US Preventive Services Task Force recommendation statement. *JAMA, 315*(23), 2564–2575.
United States Preventive Services Task Force. (2016). *Final recommendation statement colorectal cancer screening*. Retrieved from https://www.uspreventiveservicestaskforce.org/Page/Document/RecommendationStatementFinal/colorectal-cancer-screening2#consider; Rex, D. K., Boland, C. R., Dominitz, J. A., Giardiello, F. M., Johnson, D. A., Kaltenbach, T., … Robertson, D. J. (2017). Colorectal cancer screening: recommendations for physicians and patients from the U.S. Multi-Society Task Force on colorectal cancer. *Gastroenterology, 153,* 307–323.

Table 55.8 Types of Endoscopic Studies

Study	Description	Rationale	Special Considerations	NPO Status	Significance of Findings
Small bowel endoscopy	Visualization of the jejunum and ileum	Gastrointestinal bleeding Abdominal pain		12 hours	Upper gastrointestinal bleeding
Esophagogastro-duodenoscopy	Visualization of the esophagus, stomach, and duodenum	Suspected upper gastrointestinal bleeding, dysphagia Epigastric pain	Monitor return of gag reflex Vital signs	8–10 hours prior to study	Peptic ulcers *Helicobacter pylori* infection Gastritis Hiatal hernia Esophageal • Varices • Strictures • Tumors
Endoscopic retrograde cholangiopan-creatography	Visualization of pancreatic and biliary ducts	Jaundice Right upper quadrant pain Elevated • Amylase • Lipase • Serum alkaline phosphatase	Should not be performed during acute illness phase of pancreatitis	8–12 hours prior to study	**Common bile duct** • Gallstones • Tumor • Strictures • Cysts **Pancreatic duct** • Chronic pancreatitis • Pseudocysts
Colonoscopy (see Evidence-Based Practice)	Visualization of colon from anus to cecum	Colon cancer screening +Fecal occult blood testing Abnormal sigmoidoscopy	Bowel prep 24 hours prior to colonoscopy	6–8 hours prior to study	Colon cancer Benign polyps Crohn's disease Diverticular disease arteriovenous malformations

Table 55.8 Types of Endoscopic Studies—cont'd

Study	Description	Rationale	Special Considerations	NPO Status	Significance of Findings
		Lower gastrointestinal bleeding Family history of familial nucleus polyposis			
Sigmoidoscopy	Visualization of the sigmoid colon, rectum, and anus	Lower gastrointestinal bleeding Colon cancer Tumors Screening family history of polyps Abdominal pain Persistent or chronic intermittent diarrhea Constipation	The following medications may need to be stopped temporarily ● Aspirin ● Clopidogrel ● Warfarin	Clear liquid meal	Colitis ● Ulcerative ● Pseudomembranous Crohn's Polyps Intestinal ischemia

AGE-RELATED CHANGES

The gastrointestinal system has a large functional reserve capacity, and aging generally has minimal effects on gastrointestinal function (see Table 55.4). Digestion and absorption of nutrients are usually normal in older adults, and changes in function are primarily secondary to changes associated with the rate of new cell growth, as in other body systems. As smooth muscle tone decreases in the gastrointestinal system, contractions responsible for propelling food along weaken, and the movement of food through the digestive system is slower. This usually presents as constipation and may be accompanied by hemorrhoids if the constipation is chronic and requires straining when having bowel movements. If there is weakening of the cardiac sphincter related to aging, esophageal reflux may develop, and the patient may present with "heartburn." Cancer rates, particularly stomach and colon, increase with age. Loss of bone mass and changes in calcium regulation may also be associated with tooth loss in older adults that impacts nutritional intake and digestion.

Connection Check 55.6

The nurse recognizes which clinical manifestation as a normal age-related variant in an older adult?

A. Diarrhea
B. Melena
C. Constipation
D. Anorexia

Making Connections

CASE STUDY: WRAP-UP

The healthcare provider orders the following diagnostic tests for Mr. Jhanes:

• CBC with differential
• Electrolyte panel
• Fecal occult blood test
• Abdominal flat x-ray
• Esophagogastroduodenoscopy (EGD)

The results of Mr. Jhanes's diagnostic tests are as follows:

Hgb 7 g/dL

HCT 21%

BUN 30 mg/dL

Creatinine 2.0 mg/dL

The EGD reveals a gastric ulcer, and a biopsy is sent to the laboratory for *Helicobacter pylori*.

On the basis of these results, Mr. Jhanes is referred back to his primary healthcare provider for treatment of the gastric ulcer.

Case Study Questions

1. On the basis of the assessment findings of the case study, which requires immediate follow-up by the registered nurse?

   A. Reported bowel movement several days ago

   B. Missed dose of lisinopril

   C. Hypoactive bowel sounds present in all quadrants

   D. BP 130/80 mm Hg, standing 100/60 mm Hg

2. Which subjective and objective data support the order for fecal occult blood testing? *(Select all that apply.)*

   A. Reports of stool darker than usual

   B. Reports of feeling tired and complaints of light-headedness when moving from a sitting to a standing position

   C. Clopidogrel (Plavix) 75 mg PO daily

   D. Skin warm, dry, flaky, and intact

   E. Heart rate 115 bpm, respirations (R) 18, supine BP 130/80 mm Hg, standing 100/60 mm Hg

3. Which statement by Mr. Jhanes regarding the endoscopic procedure indicates that further teaching is required?

   A. "I can eat solid foods 3 hours prior to the procedure."

   B. "I can eat solid foods 12 hours prior to the procedure."

   C. "I cannot eat or drink 1 hour prior to the procedure."

   D. "I can return to my normal diet after the procedure."

4. Mr. Jhanes returns to the unit after an endoscopic gastro-duodenoscopic procedure. The nurse will prioritize the interventions in which order?

   A. Vital signs, focused physical assessment, start diet, and discontinue IV fluids

   B. Focused physical assessment, vital signs, discontinue IV fluids, and start diet

   C. Discontinue IV fluids, vital signs, focused physical assessment, and start diet

   D. Start diet, discontinue IV fluids, focused physical assessment, and vital signs

5. The biopsy results are positive for *H. pylori*. Which statement by the patient indicates understanding of these results?

   A. "There is no cure for this disease, and I will have it for the rest of my life."

   B. "I hope that I don't pass this on to my wife."

   C. "I think I contracted this infection from eating shellfish."

   D. "I will need to take antibiotics to get rid of the infection."

CHAPTER SUMMARY

The gastrointestinal system includes the mouth, pharynx, esophagus, stomach, and small and large intestines, as well as the salivary glands, liver, gallbladder, and pancreas. Primary functions of the gastrointestinal system include the intake, digestion, metabolism, and elimination of food and fluid. Additionally, certain hormonal homeostatic actions are dependent on the normal function of the gastrointestinal system.

The process of digestion begins in the mouth, where the mechanical and chemical breakdown of food occurs. Deglutition involves the pharynx, esophageal muscles, and cranial nerves (CNs) V, VII, IX, and XII. This is a two-phase process: the buccal phase involves the tongue, and the pharyngeal-esophageal phase involves the palate and esophageal muscles. Peristaltic movement of the esophagus moves the bolus of food into the stomach.

The esophagus is a hollow muscular tube that extends from approximately the vertebral levels of C6 to T7. The peristaltic movements push the food bolus downward as the esophagus constricts above the bolus and dilates below the bolus. The esophagus extends through the diaphragm and connects to the stomach. In normal digestion, the lower esophageal sphincter protects the esophageal mucosa from the regurgitation of partially digested food and the acid produced in the stomach. Specialized cells in the stomach secrete hydrochloric acid, enzymes, and hormones. Gastric motility is controlled by smooth muscle, pacemaker cells, and the autonomic nervous system.

Protein, carbohydrate, and fat digestion and absorption occur in the small intestine. Bile and pancreatic enzymes are released into the duodenum to break down the chyme for digestion. The thickest part of the intestine, the jejunum, digests and absorbs the nutrients. The small intestine is lined with villi, which aid in the absorption of the nutrients.

Indigestible fiber in the form of semiliquid chyme passes through the ileocecal valve into the large intestine, where fluid and electrolyte reabsorption and elimination occur. Entering into the cecum, vitamins (A, D, E, and K), sodium, and water are absorbed, and the stool becomes semiformed. As the stool passes through the colon, it becomes formed and passes through the rectum to the anal canal.

The liver, gallbladder, and pancreas are considered accessory organs of the gastrointestinal tract. Attached beneath the diaphragm, the liver is positioned largely across the right upper quadrant and extends into the left upper quadrant. The liver is responsible for detoxification of blood; metabolism of medications, as well as carbohydrate, protein, and fat; vitamin storage; production of bile acids and lecithin; and synthesis of fibrinogen and prothrombin.

The gallbladder is attached to the inferior portion of the liver and is responsible for bile storage and concentration. Lecithin, bilirubin, and bile salts are excreted from the liver through a ductal system and stored in the gallbladder. The terminal ends of the bile and pancreatic ducts form the hepatopancreatic ampulla in the pancreas. The pancreas is inferior to the stomach in the right upper quadrant. As an endocrine gland, the pancreas produces insulin and glucagon, and as an exocrine gland, it secretes sodium bicarbonate; proenzymes; and pancreatic enzymes needed for carbohydrate, fat, and DNA and RNA digestion.

Diagnostic tests are essential to a comprehensive gastrointestinal assessment. Diagnostic studies relevant to the gastrointestinal system include serum studies, radiographical examinations, and endoscopic evaluations. Because nurses are often directly involved in the pre- and postprocedure care of these patients, knowledge of the anticipated complications and providing support to patients while awaiting results are important.

Assessment of oral health, nutritional status, and gastrointestinal function is important because there are structural and functional problems that can impair nutrition, digestion, and elimination and lead to systemic dysfunction. A comprehensive history, physical examination, and review of diagnostic study results provide essential data for the diagnosis, treatment, and management of gastrointestinal disorders. Additionally, age-related changes should be taken into consideration during the history and physical. In order to obtain an accurate assessment, it is important to remember the order in which an abdominal assessment is conducted: inspection, auscultation, percussion, and palpation.

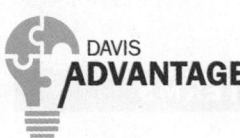

To explore learning resources for this chapter, go to **Davis Advantage** and find:
- Answers to in-text questions
- Chapter Resources and Activities
- NCLEX®-Style Chapter Review Questions
- Bibliography

Chapter 56

Coordinating Care for Patients With Oral and Esophageal Disorders

Cindy Fox

Finding Connections

Follow this patient throughout the chapter.

Juan Rodriguez is a 50-year-old man presenting to his healthcare provider for a clinic appointment. Mr. Rodriguez has what appears to be a small ulcer on the side of his tongue. It has been there for 2 weeks, and it is painful and not healing. Mr. Rodriguez has been smoking two packs of cigarettes per day since he was 20 years old, and he admits to drinking bourbon before he goes to bed at night. Mr. Rodriguez has not been to a dentist for 5 years, and he has a notable oral fetor (foul breath). His medical history includes hypertension, gastroesophageal reflux disease (GERD), and depression. Medications prescribed to him include nortriptyline, triamterene, and omeprazole (Prilosec). Mr. Rodriguez has been divorced for the last 15 years and lives with his girlfriend. Mr. Rodriguez works as a mechanic and supplements his income by working temporary jobs when he can find work…

INTRODUCTION

The oral cavity (mouth) and the esophagus are part of the upper gastrointestinal (GI) tract. The oral cavity extends from the lips to the anterior tonsils and is responsible for mastication, chewing, taste, breathing, and articulation of speech. The esophagus is a muscular hollow canal 25 cm long and 2 cm in diameter extending from the pharynx to the stomach, and it transports food from the pharynx to the stomach.

The structures of the oral cavity and the esophagus are vulnerable to injury, infection, trauma, and cancer. According to *Healthy People 2030*, many cancers are preventable by eliminating risk factors such as tobacco products, physical inactivity, obesity, and exposure to ultraviolet light. Diseases of the oral cavity and esophagus are particularly vulnerable to lifestyle choices. Screening and prevention are key elements in the elimination of diseases of the oral cavity. Unfortunately, screening for disorders of the esophagus in most cases occurs after clinical manifestations occur and the disease has progressed.

Health disparities contribute to the risk of developing cancer. The most prevalent factor influencing inequity in healthcare is socioeconomic status (SES). Because SES is primarily based on income, education level, occupation, social status within the community, and place of residence, it has a greater influence than race or ethnicity on an individual acquiring education, health insurance, and a safe/healthy work environment. Based on *Healthy People 2020*, socioeconomic status also influences behavioral risk factors such as smoking, level of physical activity, obesity, and the likelihood of participating in cancer screenings.

ORAL AND ESOPHAGEAL DISEASES

Stomatitis

Epidemiology

Oral **stomatitis** is an inflammatory condition affecting the oral mucosa, dentition, and periosteum. Known risk factors for stomatitis are:

- Viral infections
- Bacterial infections
- Fungal (*Candida albicans*) infections
- Irritants (alcohol, tobacco, mouthwash)
- Radiation therapy (7–14 days after starting treatment)
- Chemotherapy (peaks 6–12 days after last dose)
- Allergic (metal, medications, dental material, cosmetics, gum, foods)
- Vitamin deficiency (vitamin B complex, folate, zinc, iron)
- Systemic disease (chronic kidney disease, inflammatory bowel disease)

Stomatitis occurs in about 40% of patients receiving chemotherapy. The rate and severity of occurrence are higher in females than in males. When chemotherapy and radiation therapy are given in combination (chemoradiation), the risk of developing stomatitis is compounded, and up to 90% of these patients develop stomatitis. Measures to decrease the severity of stomatitis and to promote healing include frequent mouth care, hydration, using artificial saliva, and avoiding food that is very hot or that has rough edges. Factors that affect the rate and severity of stomatitis include:

- Age
- Nutrition
- Type of cancer
- Chemoradiation
- Oral hygiene

Connection Check 56.1

The nurse recognizes which risk factors for the development of stomatitis? *(Select all that apply.)*

A. High-fiber diet
B. Radiation therapy
C. Past history of skin cancer
D. Poor dental hygiene
E. Smoking

Pathophysiology and Clinical Manifestations

Stomatitis (also known as oral mucositis) presents as a painful inflammation and ulceration of the lining of the mouth that may also include the lips, pharynx, tongue, gingiva, esophagus, roof and floor of the mouth, buccal mucosa, and other mucous membranes anywhere along the GI tract. The most commonly affected locations are the tongue and buccal area (Fig. 56.1).

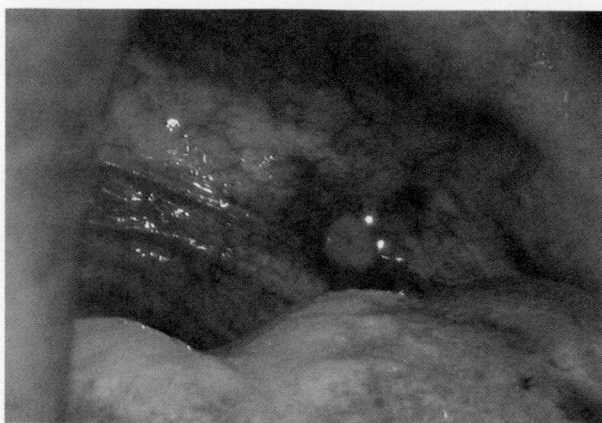

FIGURE 56.1 Oral mucositis. Stomatitis presents as a painful inflammation and ulceration in the mouth.

These sores are painful and increase the risk of bleeding, as well as local and systemic infections. Stomatitis is classified as primary or secondary and is determined by the cause of the inflammation. For the purposes of this chapter, the information presented is limited to stomatitis occurring in the oral cavity.

- Primary stomatitis occurs most often, and the most common types are aphthous stomatitis or canker sores that present as painful, small oral ulcers, herpes simplex stomatitis, and traumatic ulcers.
- Secondary stomatitis usually occurs as the result of viral, bacterial, or fungal infections in patients with suppressed immune systems, often secondary to radiotherapy and/or chemotherapy.

Depending on the severity, stomatitis can alter the quality of life. Swallowing and speaking can become painful, and tissue damage resulting from stomatitis can lead to local or systemic infections.

Recurrent aphthous ulcers (RAUs) are the most common lesion affecting the oral cavity, with up to 66% of the population affected. These lesions occur as single or multiple rounded, flat, painful ulcers and are usually white or yellow and surrounded by inflamed tissue. Eating, drinking, and oral hygiene may be interrupted. Recurrent aphthous ulcers are classified as minor, major, or herpetiform. Minor RAUs occur in 70% to 85% of the cases, are less than 1 cm, occur as one to five ulcers at a time, and last up to 14 days. Major RAUs represent 10% of all cases and are the most severe of the cases. Major RAUs are over 1 cm; are found on the lips, tongue, soft palate, and pharynx; can last about 6 weeks; and may produce scarring. The herpetiform type accounts for up to 10% of the cases and presents as recurrent outbreaks of small, deep, painful ulcers. Several ulcers can appear simultaneously, measuring 2 to 3 cm, and can merge together to form larger ulcerations.

The etiology of RAUs is not known, but a number of factors are known to predispose an individual to this disease. These factors include genetic factors; streptococcal infections; decreased immunity; stress; trauma; food allergies;

endocrine imbalances; and deficiencies of iron, vitamin B_{12}, and folic acid.

Another common cause of stomatitis is related to an oral fungal infection known as **candidiasis**, moniliasis, thrush, or yeast infection (Fig. 56.2). *Candida albicans* is normally present in the mouth. Infrequently, oral candidiasis is caused by *Candida glabrata* or *Candida tropicalis* yeasts, which are also present in the oral cavity. Common factors contributing to candidiasis include:

- Radiation therapy
- Chemotherapy
- Long-term use of antibiotics
- Steroids
- Certain antidepressant medications
- Diabetes
- Malnutrition
- Dementia
- Denture colonization
- Poor oral hygiene
- Dry mouth
- Decreased immune function
- Anxiety and stress

Oral candidiasis often presents with redness and cracking at the corners of the mouth, or there may be a red, smooth area near the middle of the tongue. A white coating of the tongue is usually called thrush and is also secondary to oral candidiasis (see Fig. 56.2).

Older adults in long-term care and residential facilities with self-care and cognitive deficits often have poor oral hygiene, contributing to an increased risk for oral infections. In addition, older adults are more prone to developing candidiasis because of their decreased immune function and other risk changes related to the aging process. Early identification and assessment of patients at risk for stomatitis facilitate appropriate treatment and prevention of complications.

Patients undergoing chemotherapy and radiation therapy are at risk for developing stomatitis. In severe cases, patients who are receiving chemotherapy may need to have a dose reduction or a delay in treatment if clinical manifestations of stomatitis become severe. Normally, the cells that line the GI tract undergo rapid division, and old cells undergo rapid replacement by new cells. Chemotherapy destroys mucous membrane cells faster than new ones can develop. The result is the formation of painful sores in the

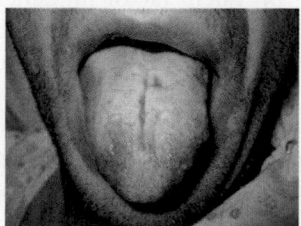

FIGURE 56.2 Oral candidiasis. The white coating of the tongue is called thrush and is secondary to oral candidiasis.

mouth. When chemotherapy and radiation therapy are given in combination (chemoradiation), stomatitis is more severe. A number of scales used to rate stomatitis exist. These scales are used to grade symptoms in order to manage patient care and can also be used to quantify data for research. An example of an oral stomatitis grading scale is listed in Table 56.1.

Xerostomia (dry mouth) can increase the risk of contracting candidiasis and developing stomatitis, and it is a clinical manifestation of several diseases, as well as a side effect of many different medications. Patients receiving radiation to the oral cavity are prone to develop oral complications. Xerostomia is also a side effect of radiotherapy, occurring up to 78% of the time in patients receiving significant radiation exposure to the salivary glands. Patients with xerostomia have decreased, thickened, or no saliva, causing them to experience difficulty with eating, swallowing, talking, and tasting. Xerostomia can be temporary or permanent, and up to 57% of patients remain symptomatic 1 year or more after completing radiotherapy.

Saliva keeps the oral cavity moist, and it helps with taste, swallowing, and speech. Saliva also helps prevent dental caries (tooth decay) by washing away bacteria, plaque, and food debris, and it also decreases the acidity in the oral cavity that can lead to the erosion of enamel on the surface of the teeth. Patients with xerostomia are at risk for developing dental caries and require a thorough dental prophylaxis at least twice per year.

Other causes of xerostomia include removal of the salivary glands, dehydration, diabetes, Sjögren's syndrome (autoimmune disorder affecting the salivary and lacrimal glands), cystic fibrosis, HIV, and rheumatoid arthritis. Common types of medications that can cause xerostomia include cold and allergy medications, psychiatric medications, and pain relievers. Interventions to relieve the effects of xerostomia include frequent mouth care, use of medications to promote saliva production (pilocarpine), lubricants, moistening agents, and sipping water throughout the day. Patients with xerostomia should avoid foods with excessive amounts of sugar, alcohol, tobacco, and caffeine to prevent further irritation or dryness of the oral cavity. Prevention,

patient education, and early treatment are important in order to decrease the risk of complications in these patients.

Management
Medical Management
Management of stomatitis includes prompt diagnosis through frequent assessment of the oral cavity before, during, and after chemotherapy and radiation therapy. Preventive measures include oral mouth rinses every 4 hours or more frequently and at bedtime using a solution of 1 teaspoon of salt or sodium bicarbonate (baking soda) per pint of water, or a saline and sodium bicarbonate mixture. Benefits of oral rinses include removal of loose particles and hydration of oral tissue. In particular, sodium bicarbonate thins oral mucus and decreases acidity and yeast growth. Topical analgesics and anesthetics may be prescribed to relieve lip or mouth pain, and moisturizers should be applied to the lips and oral membranes as needed to prevent dryness and cracking. Patients are encouraged to see the dentist for a thorough oral cleaning and examination at least 1 month prior to chemotherapy or radiotherapy in order to prevent oral cavity complications.

Complications
Patients with stomatitis are at an increased risk for pain because of inflammation and ulcerations of the oral mucosa. Due to the painful ulcerations in the mouth, they may demonstrate **dysphagia** (difficult swallowing) or **odynophagia** (painful swallowing). Patients who are unable to eat require parenteral or enteral feedings to maintain nutritional requirements. In severe cases of stomatitis, open lesions and edema may result in airway obstruction as well as oral and systemic infections with the spread of bacteria, viruses, and other infectious agents.

Stomatitis interrupts the function and the integrity of the oral cavity, which affects quality of life. Patients may experience interruptions in treatments and dose adjustments related to the mucotoxic side effects of the therapies, thus affecting therapeutic outcomes in patients receiving radiation and chemotherapy.

Table 56.1 Oral Stomatitis Grading Scale

	Grade 1	Grade 2	Grade 3	Grade 4	Grade 5
Functional/ symptomatic	Able to eat a normal diet with minimal symptoms	Symptomatic but can eat a modified diet	Symptomatic and unable to eat or drink by mouth	Symptoms are life threatening	Death
Clinical examination	Redness of mucosa	Patchy oral ulcerations	Confluent oral ulcerations that bleed with minor trauma	Tissue necrosis with significant bleeding; life-threatening consequences	Death

Source: Perry, M. C., Doll, D. C., & Freter, C. E. (2012). *The chemotherapy source book* (5th ed., p. 204). Philadelphia, PA: Lippincott Williams and Wilkins.

Nursing Management

Assessment and Analysis

Diagnosis of stomatitis is based on physical examination, patient history, and clinical presentation. Chemotherapeutic agents, radiotherapy, steroids, and decreased immune function are associated with this disorder. Patients with stomatitis have a higher risk of contracting opportunistic infections from viruses, bacteria, and other organisms because of impaired immune function and inadequate nutrition. Determination of the offending irritant is important so that it can be avoided in the future and treatment plans are not interrupted. Common assessment findings include:

- Dry, red, swollen, and cracked oral mucosa
- Mouth ulcers
- Recurrent aphthous ulcers (canker sores)
- Open, bleeding mouth sores
- Pain
- Presence in inflammation or irritations in other mucosal areas (vagina, rectum, esophagus)

Nursing Diagnoses

- **Acute pain** related to swollen, cracked, ulcerated oral mucosa
- **Risk for infection** related to impaired nutritional status and impaired integrity of oral mucosa
- **Imbalanced nutrition, less than body requirements** secondary to decreased oral intake related to dysphagia or odynophagia
- **Impaired oral mucous membranes** related to effects of chemotherapy/radiation therapy or deficiencies in providing routine oral care
- **Knowledge deficit** related to postprocedural understanding or inability to follow treatment plan
- **Impaired swallowing** related to abscess/infection and immunosuppressive therapies

Nursing Interventions

▪ Assessments

- Vital signs
  Temperature may be elevated if there is infection associated with the stomatitis. Fluid volume deficit may lead to increased pulse rate and decreased blood pressure.
- Oral mucosa
  Bleeding or ulcerated oral mucosa occurs from a number of causes, including nutritional deficiencies, exposure to radiation, chemotherapy, irritants, allergic responses, and pathogenic organisms. Assessing the cause and the severity of the oral mucosa impairment determines the treatment plan.
- Nutritional intake
  Patients with painful oral lesions avoid eating and drinking and experience dysphagia and weight loss.
- Weight
  Due to pain in the mouth and difficulty swallowing, the patient may have insufficient caloric intake to maintain an ideal weight.

- Intake and Output
  Fluid intake may be compromised due to oral ulcerations as well as difficulty swallowing.

▪ Actions

- Implement aspiration precautions.
  Viscous lidocaine can decrease the gag reflex for a short period of time. Suction equipment should be in place, and the head of the bed (HOB) should be elevated at least 45 degrees.
- Administer prescribed medications.
  Antimicrobials (antibiotics, antifungals, topical and immune modulators) are used to treat stomatitis-related infections.
  - Antimicrobials: tetracycline syrup and minocycline swish and swallow
    Topical and oral antimicrobial medications provide systemic and topical therapy for relief of infection-related symptoms.
  - Antiviral medications: acyclovir (Zovirax) IV and acyclovir PO/topical
    For herpes simplex stomatitis, IV acyclovir (Zovirax) is given to patients who have impaired immune function. Patients with intact immune function may receive acyclovir in topical or oral form.
  - Antifungal medications: nystatin ice pop or troche (lozenge)
    Nystatin (Mycostatin) swish-and-swallow suspension provides both local and topical applications.
  - Viscous lidocaine, Campho-Phenique mouthwash, triamcinolone in benzocaine (Kenalog in Orabase) topically, and with dexamethasone elixir: swish and expectorate.
    For relief of local discomfort, viscous lidocaine, topical triamcinolone in benzocaine (Kenalog in Orabase), and dexamethasone elixir are used to swish and expectorate and are often used for RAUs. Other medications used for the treatment of RAUs include antibiotics, multivitamins, low-level laser therapy (LLLT), and a variety of combined therapies.
- Administer water-soluble lubricants for the lips and mouth.
  Lanolin-based creams and ointments are most effective for moisturizing and softening dry, chapped lips.

▪ Teaching

- Mouth care after each meal and as needed, using a soft-bristled toothbrush
  Frequent gentle mouth care cleanses the mouth of pathogens and prevents further infection. Frequent mouth rinsing with warm saline or sodium bicarbonate (baking soda) solution promotes comfort and gentle cleansing and rinses pathogens from the oral cavity.
- Discourage the use of alcohol-containing mouthwash and lemon-glycerin swabs.
  Mouthwashes containing alcohol can further dry and irritate the oral mucosa, and lemon-glycerin swabs can irritate sore, inflamed oral tissue.

- Dentures and other oral appliances should be removed if patient experiences severe stomatitis or oral pain. *Dental appliances can cause irritation and ulcerations of oral tissues and increase the risk of infection. Dentures should not be worn if oral injury exists. Daily cleaning with a commercial denture cleaner, brushing, and rinsing after each meal to prevent colonization of pathogenic organisms and infection.*
- Encourage regular dental checkups *Dental examinations provide thorough cleaning and expert assessment of the oral cavity to screen for complications and pathology.*
- Encourage saline mouth rinses every 4 hours and as needed. *A dry mouth puts patients at risk for oral complications.*
- Dietary choices influence pain and healing. *Foods and fluids that are high in protein or vitamin C promote healing. Foods that cause irritation are those that are spicy, salty, hot, hard, and acidic and have sharp edges.*

Evaluating Care Outcomes

Stomatitis is a preventable disease process except when related to radiation and chemotherapy. In the latter instance, symptoms may be unavoidable but lessened with prompt recognition of clinical manifestations and early therapeutic interventions. Oral hygiene, including cleaning of dental appliances and feeding utensils, and the maintenance of an adequate nutritional status are paramount in the prevention or management of stomatitis. With appropriate treatment, the patient should have stable vital signs, fluid volume status, and weight.

Hiatal Hernia

The esophagus carries food from the oropharynx to the stomach, and its function is essential in maintaining adequate nutrition and nourishment to the body. The esophagus is a hollow muscular tube that carries food from the oral cavity to the stomach. The esophagus has three types of layers, the mucosa, the submucosa, and the muscularis propria, each with different functions and tissue types. The esophageal mucosa has an inner and an outer layer. The outer layer is the epithelial layer, and it is made of squamous cells. The inner layer, the lamina propria, is the mucosal layer under the epithelium, and it is made of connective tissue. The next layer is called the *submucosa*, and it is found in some parts of the esophagus. The submucosa contains glands that secrete mucus. The innermost layer, located under the submucosa, is a thick muscular band called the *muscularis propria*. This muscular layer rhythmically contracts as it pushes food through the esophagus to the stomach.

The upper esophageal sphincter is located at the upper portion of the esophagus. This muscle relaxes to allow food and fluids to pass into the esophagus. The lower portion of the esophagus that connects to the stomach is called the **gastroesophageal junction (GEJ)**. Below the GEJ is a muscular area called the **lower esophageal sphincter (LES)**. The purpose of this sphincter is to allow food from the esophagus to enter the stomach and to prevent contents from the stomach from entering the esophagus.

The diaphragm normally has an opening (esophageal hiatus) that allows the distal end of the lower esophagus to pass through it. The thoracic cavity is above the diaphragm, and the abdominal cavity is below the diaphragm. The lower esophageal sphincter (LES) is located at the gastroesophageal junction (GEJ) near the lower end of the esophagus. The pressure in the LES is considerably higher than the pressure in the thoracic cavity. The ability of the LES to maintain higher pressures is due in part to its anatomical placement in the abdomen and the acute angle formed as the esophagus enters the stomach (angle of His).

Epidemiology

The incidence of hiatal hernia increases with age as supportive structures weaken over time. Approximately 60% of those affected are 50 or older, and of those affected, 9% are symptomatic. There are two main types of hiatal hernia; 95% are the "sliding" type, and 5% are the "rolling" type. Ninety-six percent of patients who have Barrett's esophagitis (complication of GERD) have a hiatal hernia that is 2 cm or more in size.

The prevalence of hiatal hernia is more common in Western countries as opposed to rural African countries because of the lack of dietary fiber and the "unnatural" sitting position (causes straining) used for defecation. These factors can cause increased intra-abdominal pressures that push the stomach through the esophageal hiatus. Other risk factors include obesity, pregnancy, and smoking.

Pathophysiology and Clinical Manifestations

A hiatal hernia occurs when a portion of the stomach protrudes upward through the esophageal hiatus (opening in the diaphragm that the esophagus passes through) and into the thoracic cavity. The two major types are type 1 and type 2 hernias (Fig. 56.3). A type 1 hiatal hernia (sliding type) is usually acquired through an ongoing process of disruption to the GEJ. The consequences of years of wear and tear typically occur after age 50 from the repetitive stresses of deep inspiration, Valsalva maneuvers, positional changes, acid reflux, and vomiting compounded by pregnancy and obesity, eventually compromising the integrity of the hiatus. As the competence of the GEJ becomes impaired, reflux occurs, and the ability of the esophagus to clear the acid becomes compromised. **Strictures** (esophageal narrowing) and lower esophageal mucosal rings (Schatzki's rings) may develop secondary to this esophageal mucosal damage from GERD and lead to dysphagia. Another manifestation of a type 1 hiatal hernia is the development of Cameron lesions. These lesions are described as single or multiple gastric erosions and/or ulcerations typically visualized at the level of the diaphragmatic hiatus on upper endoscopic examination.

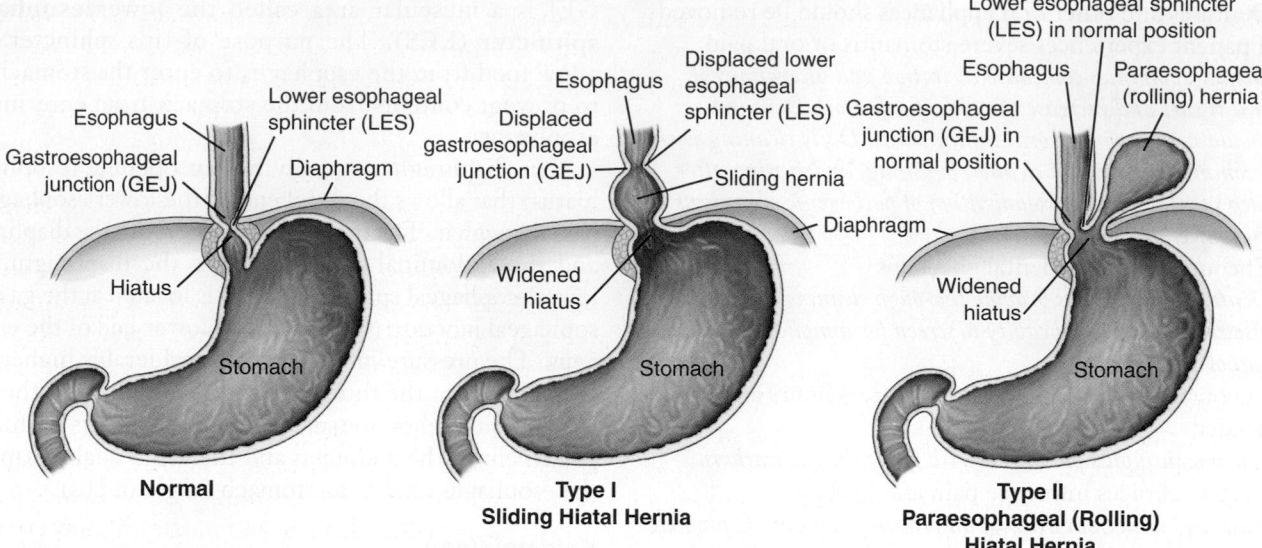

FIGURE 56.3 Type 1 and type 2 hiatal hernias. Type 1 (sliding) hernias involve a widening of the hiatal tunnel that allows part of the cardiac portion of the stomach to herniate upward, which allows stomach acids and enzymes to come into contact with esophageal tissue. Type II (rolling) hernias involve the fundus and sometimes part of the greater curvature of the stomach rolling through the esophageal hiatus.

Cameron lesions are usually found incidentally and represent a source of obscure gastrointestinal bleeding in patients with type 1 hiatal hernias. Mechanical trauma at the level of the diaphragmatic hiatus in combination with mucosal injury from gastric acid and/or NSAID use may cause Cameron lesions. With type 1 hernias, there is a widening of the hiatal tunnel that allows part of the cardiac portion of the stomach to herniate upward, which allows stomach acids and enzymes to come into contact with esophageal tissue, putting the patient at risk for the development of a premalignant condition known as **Barrett's esophagus**. The hernia slides in and out through the esophageal hiatus into the chest as a result of a weakened diaphragm. Most of these hernias are asymptomatic, and the size of the hernia influences the likelihood of developing reflux disease. A type 1 hiatal hernia is mainly an acquired condition and can be caused by trauma, hereditary weakness in the surrounding muscles, or a congenitally large hiatus. Clinical manifestations typically include:

- Heartburn
- Regurgitation
- Chest pain
- Dysphagia
- Belching

Type 2 (rolling type), or paraesophageal, hernias are thought to occur because of an anatomical defect that causes improper anchoring of the stomach below the diaphragm. The GEJ remains in its normal anatomical position, but the fundus and sometimes part of the greater curvature of the stomach roll through the esophageal hiatus. Variable degrees of herniation can occur, with some type 2 hernias being quite small. In rare cases, the whole stomach can herniate above the diaphragm and into the chest. Reflux is not usually present because the LES remains secured below the diaphragm. Clinical manifestations of type 2 hernias usually include:

- Feeling full after eating
- Feeling breathless after eating
- Feeling of suffocation
- Chest pain that feels like angina
- Increased symptoms when lying flat

Connection Check 56.2

The nurse correlates which clinical manifestation with a type 1 hiatal hernia?

A. Heartburn
B. Hematemesis
C. Feeling of suffocation
D. Anorexia

Management

Medical Management

The following commonly performed tests are used to determine the cause of upper abdominal pain and to diagnose hiatal hernia:

- Upper abdominal x-ray
- Endoscopy
- Barium swallow with fluoroscopy (most specific diagnostic test)
- Esophagogastroduodenoscopy, or EGD (views the esophagus and stomach lining)

Medications are used for the symptoms of heartburn and acid reflux. Most people who have a hiatal hernia do not experience these symptoms, but if they do, they may require medication management or surgery.

- Antacids are used to neutralize stomach acid and are usually obtained over the counter. Common antacids are Mylanta, Maalox, Gelusil, Rolaids, and Tums. Common side effects include diarrhea and constipation.
- Proton pump inhibitors and H_2-receptor antagonists are prescribed to treat GERD (Table 56.2).

Some complementary medicine practitioners report that a hiatal hernia can be reduced or corrected by using massage to push the stomach back into its normal position below the diaphragm. Currently, there is no evidence or clinical trials to prove the efficacy of these claims, and further research is needed to investigate the efficacy of this practice.

Surgical Management

Surgery for hiatal hernia is the treatment of choice when the benefits outweigh the risks for the patient. Hiatal hernias tend to progressively become larger over time. Usually, asymptomatic type 1 hiatal hernias are treated medically, but larger symptomatic type 1 hernias may be treated surgically. If left untreated, type 2 hernias have the potential to enlarge to the stage of becoming a giant intrathoracic stomach, in which at least one-third of the stomach is herniated into the chest cavity. At this stage, clinical manifestations of substernal pain, pressure, and gastric ulcers may develop as a result of displacement of the stomach into the thoracic cavity. Patients may present acutely with strangulation of the stomach from acute gastric volvulus. Gastric volvulus is a surgical emergency. The pathology of gastric volvulus is demonstrated as an abnormal rotation of all or part of the stomach around one of its axes. The most common cause of gastric volvulus is paraesophageal hiatal hernia. Clinical manifestations may include abdominal or chest pain, early satiety, dysphagia, GI bleed, gastric outlet obstruction, and retching without vomiting. It may be difficult or impossible to place a nasogastric tube. The significance of this pathologic change is that hemorrhage, ischemia, necrosis, and perforation may occur. Prompt surgical intervention is necessary to prevent irreversible damage and mortality. Surgery is the treatment of choice for type 2 (paraesophageal) hernias even in the absence of symptoms because of the potential risk of incarceration and strangulation if left untreated. There is a higher recurrence rate for type 2 hernias than for type 1 hernias because the tissues of the hiatus encounter more impairment with type 2 hernias.

Nissen fundoplication and laparoscopic antireflux surgeries are frequently used to treat type 2 hernias. The open Nissen fundoplication is a surgical procedure whereby the surgeon wraps part of the stomach around the distal esophagus to stabilize it and to reinforce the LES (Fig. 56.4).

Table 56.2 Comparison of H₂-Receptor Antigen Antagonists and Proton Pump Inhibitors

H₂-Receptor Antigen Antagonists (H₂RAs)	Proton Pump Inhibitors (PPIs)
H₂-receptor blockers reduce acid production longer than antacids but are slower to take effect.	PPIs block production of acid and allow the esophagus to heal.
H₂RAs decrease acid production of parietal cells in the stomach lining by blocking histamine-2 at one of the first steps of acid production.	PPIs block the last step in gastric acid secretion and stop the acid pumps in the stomach. PPIs are more effective in suppressing gastric acid secretion than H₂RAs.
Used to treat *Helicobacter pylori* in combination with antibiotic therapy; also used to treat gastroesophageal reflux symptoms	Used to treat gastroesophageal reflux symptoms
Common H₂-blockers include cimetidine (Tagamet HB), famotidine (Pepcid AC), nizatidine (Axid AR), or ranitidine (Zantac 75). Stronger prescription-strength H₂-blockers are available.	Over-the-counter (OTC) PPIs include lansoprazole (Prevacid 24HR) and omeprazole (Prilosec OTC). Prescription-strength PPIs are available.
Patients may develop a tolerance.	Tolerance is unlikely.
Cimetidine can interact with warfarin, phenytoin, and theophylline with long-term use.	PPIs can interfere with the absorption of ketoconazole, ampicillin, iron, and digoxin.
H₂RAs have an onset of action of 1 hour and a duration of about 12 hours.	PPIs have a delayed onset of action and a duration of action lasting up to 24 hours.
H₂RAs are frequently used as a step-down treatment for patients with uncomplicated GERD symptoms after PPI-induced symptom relief. H₂RAs have few side effects and are well tolerated.	Long term use is linked to a reduction of micronutrient absorption, gastrointestinal and pulmonary infections, osteoporosis and bone fractures, heart and kidney disease, and dementia.

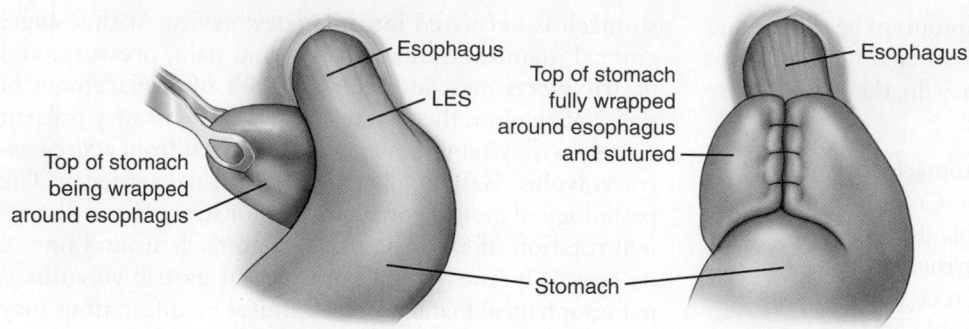

FIGURE 56.4 Nissen fundoplication. Laparoscopic Nissen fundoplication is the gold standard for the treatment of a hiatal hernia and is performed through several small incisions in the abdomen.

Gastropexy (attachment of the stomach below the diaphragm to prevent reherniation) is used after reduction if the stomach is unusually movable after reduction is performed. Other surgical procedures for type 2 hernias include:

- **Herniotomy** (surgical removal of the herniated sac)
- **Herniorrhaphy** (repair of the hiatal defect)
- Antireflux procedure
- Reduction (attachment of the stomach below the diaphragm to prevent reherniation)

Laparoscopic Nissen fundoplication (LNF) is the gold standard and is performed most often for hiatal hernia repair. The surgeon performs the surgery through several small incisions in the abdomen. Advantages vary with these types of surgeries. Patients with advancing age and significant comorbidities are often better candidates for the minimally invasive laparoscopic surgery rather than open surgery. There are fewer complications and shorter hospital stays with minimally invasive laparoscopic surgery. The disadvantage of laparoscopic repair is that the recurrence rates are higher than with open surgical procedures. Postoperative complications include infection, bleeding, atelectasis, pneumonia, obstructed nasogastric tube, gas bloat syndrome, and temporary dysphagia.

Complications

The most common complication of type 1 (sliding) hernias is gastroesophageal reflux, or GERD. Reflux occurs when there is chronic exposure of the LES to the low pressure of the thorax. Reflux symptoms increase with coughing, obesity, ascites, and positional changes such as bending and lying supine.

Supradiaphragmatic volvulus (abnormal 180-degree twisting of the stomach above the diaphragm) and obstruction are rare complications of a type 2 (rolling) hiatal hernia. Iron-deficiency anemia is a later symptom seen in some adults with type 2 hernias that present as slow bleeding from gastric mucosal folds caused by gastric ulcers and erosions.

Nursing Management

Assessment and Analysis

A hiatal hernia is often asymptomatic and is usually found incidentally when a patient is being evaluated for another problem. Large hiatal hernias can cause gastroesophageal reflux with clinical manifestations of heartburn and noncardiac chest pain. Typically, the clinical manifestations of hiatal hernia are worse after meals because of the displacement of stomach contents into the thoracic cavity. Lifestyle changes such as weight reduction, sleeping with the HOB elevated, avoiding the use of tobacco or alcohol, and stress control can help reduce clinical manifestations. Medications are prescribed to relieve GERD symptoms, but surgical intervention may be necessary. Clinical manifestations of hiatal hernia include:

- Heartburn
- Regurgitation
- Dysphagia
- Eructation (belching)
- Breathlessness
- Feeling of suffocation
- Chest pain
- GERD
- Iron-deficiency anemia (related to volvulus)

> **! Safety Alert** Gastrointestinal and cardiac symptoms are similar, and it is important to assess the patient, notify the healthcare provider, and perform an electrocardiogram if the patient complains of chest pain or shortness of breath.

Nursing Diagnoses

- **Impaired swallowing** related to esophageal narrowing
- **Anxiety** related to impaired breathing
- **Pain** related to damage secondary to exposure of esophageal tissue to gastric acid
- **Knowledge deficit** related to the therapeutic regimen

Nursing Interventions

■ **Assessments**

- Breathlessness, feelings of suffocation, chest pain, palpitations
  Respiratory symptoms and asthma-like symptoms are a result of aspirating stomach contents and occur mostly while sleeping. After eating a large meal, patients may experience a feeling of breathlessness or chest pain if the hernia interferes

with lung expansion. Palpitations develop secondary to irritation of the vagal nerve.

- Dysphagia

  Strictures and lower esophageal mucosal rings are common causes of dysphagia, related to esophageal mucosal damage from GERD. Schatzki's rings are narrow areas, less than 1.3 cm, and can also occur congenitally. These rings are located at or near the GEJ where normal mucosal epithelium transitions from columnar cells to squamous cells. Incarcerated or strangulated paraesophageal or mixed paraesophageal hernias are causes of dysphagia.

- Clinical manifestations of GERD, heartburn

  A hiatal hernia can cause the LES to weaken. This causes reflux of gastric contents into the esophagus, resulting in irritation, inflammation, and pain.

- Nausea and vomiting

  Persistent nausea and vomiting in patients with a hiatal hernia who are unresponsive to antiemetic medications may indicate gastric volvulus. This strangulation can lead to GI tract or esophageal obstruction.

- Eructation

  Air escapes from the stomach and into the esophagus, and occasionally, reflux material is brought up into the mouth.

- Iron-deficiency anemia

  Herniated gastric pouches and folds from paraesophageal hernias (with erosions and ulcerations) are a cause of chronic blood loss that may lead to anemia.

▪ Actions

- Medication management:
  - Antacids

    Neutralize or buffer stomach acid
  - Histamine receptor agonists

    Acid production is decreased (see Table 56.2).
  - Proton pump inhibitors

    Acid production is blocked (see Table 56.2).
  - Prokinetic medications

    Gastric emptying is increased with prokinetic medications such as Reglan. Long-term use is not recommended because of the possibility of psychotropic or neurological side effects such as tardive dyskinesia.

- Position the patient supine on the right side, and elevate the HOB at least 30 degrees after meals.

  Lying on the right side promotes gastric emptying, and the elevated HOB position promotes peristalsis and uses gravity to return gastric refluxate from the esophagus to the stomach.

▪ Teaching

- Educate the patient to limit the following foods and substances: spicy/fatty foods, caffeine, chocolate, carbonated beverages, acidic foods, peppermint, alcohol, caffeinated beverages, and certain medications (if possible), such as calcium channel blockers, anticholinergic medications, and smooth muscle relaxers.

  These foods, substances, and medications are associated with decreasing LES pressure, which allows gastric reflux from the stomach into the esophagus.

- Encourage the patient to eat meals 2 hours before lying supine.

  Eating large meals causes delayed gastric emptying and leads to gastric reflux.

- Educate the patient to wear nonrestrictive clothing.

  Tight clothing causes an increase in intra-abdominal pressure, which weakens the LES and contributes to GERD.

- Educate the patient and family about maintaining a normal weight.

  Obesity increases intra-abdominal pressure, increasing the hiatal hernia and GERD.

- Educate the patient on proper positioning after eating.

  Compliance increases with sound understanding of instructions as well as the rationale.

- Conduct postoperative education for patients after laparoscopic Nissen fundoplication (LNF) (see Box 56.1).

  Large paraesophageal hernias are surgically repaired to prevent obstruction or strangulation. Postoperative care after LNF begins preoperatively. Complications are less frequent with LNF procedures than with an open surgical approach.

Evaluating Care Outcomes

Lifestyle changes and medication management often effectively relieve the clinical manifestations of hiatal hernia. Surgical intervention is recommended for large or symptomatic hernias. Patients need to receive education aimed at reinforcing dietary and lifestyle choices and reduction of risk factors that exacerbate the symptoms of hiatal hernia. Nursing education postoperatively focuses on pain management, airway management, respiratory management, and nutritional support.

Gastroesophageal Reflux Disease

Gastroesophageal reflux disease (GERD) is a chronic disorder that describes a variety of clinical manifestations, with or without tissue damage, caused by acid reflux from the stomach (or duodenum) into the esophagus. Reflux occurs when the LES is weak or relaxes inappropriately, causing the pressure gradient between the LES and the stomach to be lost. Gastroesophageal reflux disease usually occurs in association with hiatal hernia, but herniation of the gastric mucosa does not occur with GERD. Gastroesophageal reflux disease can be caused by a temporary or sustained decrease in LES competence. Certain foods and substances can also affect LES tone. Gastroesophageal reflux disease is one of the most common diseases of Western civilization, with many factors contributing to the development of GERD. Lifestyle choices are the primary determinants related to acquiring GERD, and a variety of treatments and surgeries are available for the management of GERD.

All people at some point will experience "physiological" gastroesophageal reflux. Esophageal motility and gravity facilitate esophageal clearance, and adequate emptying of gastric contents acts as a physiological means to prevent gastroesophageal reflux. Saliva is rich in bicarbonate, and it

Box 56.1 Postoperative Patient Education After Laparoscopic Nissen Fundoplication

- Follow a soft diet for about 1 week until swallowing improves. Avoid foods that are not easy to swallow. Take small bites and eat slowly.
- Avoid activities that cause air to be swallowed. Examples are drinking carbonated beverages, lemonade, and punch; sucking on sweets; chewing gum; and using a straw.
- Notify the healthcare provider for chest pain or difficulty breathing that gets worse with time.
- Continue antireflux medication regimen unless notified otherwise by a healthcare provider.
- Driving is allowed after 1 week and after narcotic pain medications have been discontinued.
- Walking is encouraged.
- No heavy lifting.
- After surgery, the doctor usually changes the original surgical dressing after 2 days. Steri-Strips are left intact and usually fall off in about 10 days. Keep them clean and dry and do not peel them off.
- Wash incisions with soap and water and pat them dry with a clean towel.
- Observe incisions for redness or drainage, and report any of these symptoms to the healthcare provider.
- Notify the healthcare provider for a fever greater than 101°F, or 38.3°C. Patients older than 65 years: report temperature above 100°F, or 37°C. Report nausea, vomiting, and severe bloating or unusual pain.
- Bring a list of questions to the first postoperative appointment, usually within 4 weeks after surgery.

Seek medical care emergently for:

- Feeling very full, with inability to vomit or burp
- Thick drainage that has a foul odor coming from incisions
- Difficulty swallowing
- Abdomen that feels hard and painful
- Gauze that becomes soaked with blood
- Stools that are black, bloody, or tarry
- Vomiting up blood or "coffee grounds" emesis
- Difficulty breathing and feeling light-headed
- Coughing up blood, new chest pain when breathing in
- An arm or leg that is painful, swollen, warm, and red

coats the esophageal epithelium. Production of mucus, prostaglandins, and epithelial growth factors helps to protect the esophageal mucosa. Anatomically, the structures that form the high-pressure zone at the lower esophagus include the intra-abdominal esophagus, the phrenoesophageal ligaments, the gastric mucosal "rosette," and the esophageal hiatus. This high-pressure zone forms a physiological sphincter called the LES. Pressures are higher at the gastroesophageal junction (GEJ), and gastric luminal pressures are lower. This prevents the reflux of gastric contents from the stomach. The angle of His (cardioesophageal junction)

and physiological factors work together to control the amount and frequency of gastric reflux into the esophagus.

Epidemiology

Gastroesophageal reflux disease results from the backward flow of gastroduodenal contents (refluxate) into the esophagus and/or adjacent organs, producing a variety of clinical manifestations that may or may not cause tissue damage. Chronic in nature, GERD is a highly prevalent disorder in Western countries, with about 10% to 20% affected, whereas the prevalence in Asian countries is 5%. Sanitation practices and chlorination of the water supply have influenced the low prevalence of *Helicobacter pylori* (HP) in Western countries. The lower prevalence of GERD in undeveloped countries is thought to be related to lifestyle, dietary habits, and the presence of HP, a gram-negative bacterium commonly associated with gastric ulcers and stomach cancer. *Helicobacter pylori* has been found to decrease gastric acid secretion, but because it is a class 1 carcinogen, steps have been taken to eradicate this organism.

There are many factors that are associated with a decrease in LES pressures that influence transient or chronic gastroesophageal reflux; common examples include:

- Hiatal hernia
- LES hypotension
- Loss of esophageal motility
- Increased compliance of the hiatal canal
- Increased states of gastric secretion
- Eating large meals
- Delayed emptying of gastric contents
- Obesity
- Pregnancy
- Ascites
- Tight belts or girdles
- Presence of a nasogastric tube

Pathophysiology and Clinical Manifestations

Gastroesophageal reflux disease results when there is a retrograde flow of GI contents into the esophagus, resulting in inflammation. Gastroesophageal reflux disease is the result of many different factors; some of these factors are the result of esophageal motility dysfunction, anatomical or diaphragmatic defects, or increased intra-abdominal pressure. The most common cause of GERD is from the relaxation of the LES, allowing gastric reflux into the esophagus.

Refluxed material in the esophagus normally returns to the stomach with the help of gravity, peristalsis, and saliva. When the esophagus is inflamed or injured, the ability of the esophagus to clear refluxed material becomes slower, resulting in an extended period of exposure of the esophagus to refluxed material from the stomach. Each episode of acid reflux results in hyperemia (increased blood flow), erosion (ulceration), and possible minor bleeding to the esophagus. During reflux, other gastric substances such as pepsin and bile may be present. These substances, like acid, are caustic to the esophageal epithelium.

Management

Medical Management

Diagnostic Tests

Twenty-four-hour ambulatory esophageal pH monitoring involves continuous measurement of gastric pH by monitoring and recording the pH of the stomach through a catheter that is placed in the nose and terminates at the distal esophagus. The patient keeps a diary of symptoms and activities. pH monitoring is a useful diagnostic tool used in patients with atypical symptoms.

The esophagogastroduodenoscopy (EGD) test evaluates esophagitis and monitors Barrett's esophagitis. During this test, biopsy samples can be taken and strictures can be dilated. Strictures occur as a result of fibrosis and scarring related to injury from acid exposure. Over time, strictures can lead to dysphagia.

Esophageal manometry or motility testing is the gold standard for the assessment and measurement of esophageal motor activity. During this test, catheters filled with water are inserted into the nose or mouth and withdrawn slowly while readings of LES pressure and peristalsis are taken. Esophageal manometry is used infrequently to diagnose GERD, and when used for this purpose, it is inconclusive except when used in conjunction with patient history, barium radiology, or endoscopy.

Connection Check 56.3

In preparing a patient for esophageal manometry, which content does the nurse include in preprocedure teaching?

A. This test measures the acid content in your stomach.
B. This test measures the pressure and action of the esophagus.
C. This test allows a sample of the esophagus to be obtained.
D. This test is used only in patients with diagnosed hiatal hernia.

Medications

Medication management for the treatment of GERD focuses on any or all of the following:

- Inhibiting gastric acid secretion
- Increasing gastric emptying
- Protecting the lining of the stomach

Because gastroesophageal reflux disease is a chronic disease, it requires long-term management and maintenance in most cases. About 80% of patients who discontinue treatment relapse within 1 year. Side effects of some of these medications require additional attention. For example, the long-term use of protein pump inhibitors (PPIs) is associated with hip fractures, and metoclopramide (Reglan) is associated

with tardive dyskinesia. The categories of medications used to treat GERD include:

- Antacids (increase gastric pH)
- Histamine receptor antagonists (decrease gastric acid production; short acting)
- Prokinetic medications (increase gastric emptying)
- Proton pump inhibitors (decrease gastric acid production; long acting)

Endoscopic Treatments

The Stretta procedure involves the use of radiofrequency energy through an endoscope by using needles positioned near the GEJ. This procedure reduces pain by decreasing vagus nerve activity. The endoluminal gastroplication is an endoscopic procedure whereby the LES is tightened with sutures.

Surgical Management

A small number of patients with GERD will require surgery. Patients who have not responded favorably to medical treatment or who have developed complications are surgical candidates. When indicated, the gold standard for surgery is laparoscopic Nissen fundoplication.

Complications

When damaged esophageal tissue heals, the body sometimes substitutes columnar epithelium (Barrett's epithelium) for the normal squamous cell epithelium of the lower esophagus. Barrett's epithelium is more resistant to acid than squamous cell epithelium, but it has a high propensity for malignancy. After exposure to gastric acid, fibrosis and scarring may occur in response to the healing process. Strictures may develop and lead to progressive dysphagia.

Nursing Management

Assessment and Analysis

The clinical presentation of GERD is related to the effect of gastric reflux material on the esophagus. The effects of GERD range from mild irritation to cancer-causing cellular changes. Common clinical manifestations of GERD include:

- Heartburn (dyspepsia)
- Severe atypical chest pain
- Odynophagia (painful swallowing)
- Hemorrhage
- Dental caries
- Aspiration pneumonia
- Chronic cough
- Morning hoarseness
- Adult-onset asthma
- Laryngitis
- Pharyngitis
- Bronchitis
- Regurgitation

Nursing Diagnoses

- **Acute/chronic pain** related to physical injury as evidenced by esophageal irritation

- **Risk for aspiration** related to inadequate LES function
- **Impaired swallowing** related to stricture or inflammation
- **Imbalanced nutrition, less than body requirements** related to decreased intake secondary to dysphagia and pain

Nursing Interventions

▪ **Assessments**

- Respiratory symptoms: aspiration pneumonia, chronic cough, morning hoarseness, night-time wheezing, adult-onset asthma, laryngitis, pharyngitis, bronchitis with long-term regurgitation

  Respiratory symptoms occur with aspiration of acid reflux into the tracheobronchial tree, larynx, pharynx, nose, and mouth (especially when supine). Gastroesophageal reflux disease is a causative factor in the development of adult-onset asthma.

- Regurgitation

  Occurs when acid reflux reaches the level of the pharynx, leaving a sour taste in the mouth. If the patient is supine, regurgitation can lead to aspiration.

- Severe atypical chest pain

  Caused by esophageal spasms or stimulation of esophageal pain receptors. Pain may be so severe that it lasts for 2 hours, and it can radiate to the neck. Pain increases when supine, bending, or performing a Valsalva. The etiology of chest pain needs to be determined to rule out cardiac causes.

- Hemorrhage

  Associated with erosion and necrosis of the esophagus from chronic acid reflux

- CBC

  Chronic erosion of the esophageal tissue may lead to bleeding that results in decreased hematocrit and hemoglobin.

- Dyspepsia

  Reflux of gastric contents into the esophagus occurs most often as a result of excessive relaxation of the LES, leading to inflammation and ulceration of the esophagus. Minor bleeding from capillaries may occur with erosion.

- Dysphagia and odynophagia

  The damage from the refluxate causes inflammation and ulcerations in the esophagus. When healing occurs, scarring occurs with the development of strictures or rings, causing esophageal stenosis and difficulty swallowing.

- Signs of Barrett's esophagus

  Metaplasia of columnar epithelium from squamous cells in the lower third of the esophagus results from chronic acid reflux into the esophagus. Columnar cells, like the cells found in the stomach, are resistant to the damaging effects of stomach acid; however, these cells, not normally seen in the esophagus, have a propensity for dysplasia, thus becoming adenocarcinomas.

- Dental caries

  Eructation of acid reflux into the oral cavity leads to the destruction of tooth enamel and decay.

- Water brash

  A production of excessive saliva in response to reflux, leading to the sense of fluid in the throat, is termed water brash.

There is no sour taste, and acid is not present. Patients who exhibit water brash may or may not have esophageal injury.

- Eructation, flatulence, or bloating

  Occurs when eating a large meal and with abdominal distention, causing increased intra-abdominal pressure. The LES pressure decreases and allows gastric refluxate to enter the esophagus.

- Nausea

  Nausea occurs as a result of stomach acid and bile that reflux into the esophagus from the stomach, usually after eating.

- Globus (sensation that there is a lump in the throat)

  Gastric refluxate into the larynx and pharynx resulting from GERD

- pH of gastric aspirate

  Acid refluxate from the stomach has a pH of 1.5 to 2.0, whereas the normal pH of the esophagus is 6.0 to 7.0.

▪ **Actions**

- Medication management:
  - Antacids

    Neutralize or buffer stomach acid
  - Histamine receptor agonists

    Acid production is decreased (see Table 56.2).
  - Proton pump inhibitors

    Acid production is blocked (see Table 56.2).
  - Prokinetic medications

    Gastric emptying is increased with prokinetic medications such as Reglan. Long-term use is not recommended because of the possibility of psychotropic or neurological side effects such as tardive dyskinesia.

- Position the patient on the right side with the HOB elevated 6 to 12 inches.

  Lying on the right side promotes gastric emptying, and elevating the HOB promotes peristalsis and uses gravity to return gastric refluxate from the esophagus to the stomach. Sleeping in this position also decreases reflux at night.

- Provide 4–6 meals per day.

  Eating three larger meals per day increases pressure in the stomach and delays gastric emptying. Eating four to six smaller meals decreases pressure.

▪ **Teaching**

- Educate the patient to limit the following foods and substances: spicy/fatty foods, caffeine, chocolate, carbonated beverages, acidic foods, peppermint, alcohol, and certain medications (if possible), such as calcium channel blockers, anticholinergic medications, and smooth muscle relaxers.

  These foods, substances, and medications are associated with decreasing LES pressure, which allows gastric reflux from the stomach into the esophagus.

- Avoid smoking and alcohol.

  Both smoking and alcohol may lead to a decrease in LES pressure, increasing the risk of reflux.

- Avoid NSAIDs and aspirin.

  Both NSAIDs and aspirin can irritate the lining of the esophagus.

- Encourage the patient to eat meals 2 hours before lying supine.
  Eating large meals causes delayed gastric emptying and leads to gastric reflux.
- Educate the patient to wear nonrestrictive clothing
  Tight clothing causes an increase in intra-abdominal pressure, which weakens the LES and contributes to GERD.
- Educate the patient and family about maintaining ideal body weight.
  Obesity increases intra-abdominal pressure, increasing the hiatal hernia and GERD.

Evaluating Care Outcomes

Positive healthcare outcomes in patients with GERD are primarily a result of lifestyle choices. Individuals with GERD are frequently asymptomatic, and the disease remains undetected. Many patients ignore minor symptoms and choose to self-medicate, seeking medical attention when symptoms become advanced. It is essential that patients seek medical attention if they develop clinical manifestations of GERD in order to obtain relief and to prevent complications. Patients with GERD require education about lifestyle changes involving diet modification and adherence to medication regimens in order to maintain an optimal quality of life and to avoid complications. Surgical candidates today usually undergo minimally invasive laparoscopic surgery or endoscopic procedures in order to treat GERD.

ORAL CANCER

Epidemiology

In the United States, 3% of all new cancers are oral cancers. In 2018, the estimated number of new cases in the United States was 51,540, and the estimated number of deaths was 10,030 (see Evidence-Based Practice: Rising Incidence of Oropharyngeal Cancer). Men are affected two to four times more than women are, and the risk of developing oral cancer increases with age. The average age of diagnosis is 62. African American and Caucasian individuals are about equally affected. Oral cancer accounts for 25% of all head and neck cancers. Patients who survive 5 to 10 years have a 20-times higher risk of developing a second cancer.

Evidence-Based Practice

Rising Incidence of Oropharyngeal Cancer

- The incidence of oral cancer, including cancers of the tonsils and base of the tongue, continue to increase in North America and Western Europe, with up to 70% of new cases being related to HPV.
- The suspected cause of the rising incidence of oropharyngeal cancer is related to increasing numbers of sexual partners and oral sexual practices with exposure to human papillomavirus (HPV).

- Human papillomavirus 16 accounts for most of the oropharyngeal squamous cell carcinomas (OSCCs) in the United States and Europe.
- By the year 2020, it is expected that the incidence of HPV-related OSCC will surpass the incidence of HPV-related cervical cancer.
- Patients with HPV-positive oropharyngeal cancer are not necessarily heavy cigarette smokers and alcohol users.
- Patients who have OSCC and who are HPV positive have an overall survival rate of 95%, whereas an HPV-negative patient can expect a 62% survival rate at 2 years.
- Preliminary evidence shows that the HPV vaccine is effective in preventing cervical HPV infections, but data showing effectiveness in preventing oral HPV infections are lacking.

Gooi, Z., Chan, J. Y., & Fakhry, C. (2016). The epidemiology of the human papillomavirus related to oropharyngeal head and neck cancer. *The Laryngoscope, 126*(4), 894–900.

Malignancies of the lip are most commonly seen because of intense exposure to the sun, excessive alcohol consumption, and pipe or cigarette smoking (Fig. 56.5). Of the lip carcinomas, about 95% are **squamous cell carcinomas (SCCAs)**. Of these, 85% occur on the lower lip, 5% occur on the upper lip, and 5% affect both lips. Basal cell carcinomas occur most often on the lower lip and are usually slow growing initially, with metastasis occurring in later stages. Outcomes regarding carcinoma of the upper lip are less favorable because 95% of these tumors are squamous cell carcinomas that tend to grow rapidly and metastasize. Basal cell carcinomas tend to grow slowly and become invasive over time. These lesions usually appear as ulcerations or lesions on the outer border of the lip. The average age for carcinoma of the lip is 60 to 65, the male–female ratio is 30:1, and Caucasians are more commonly affected than African Americans.

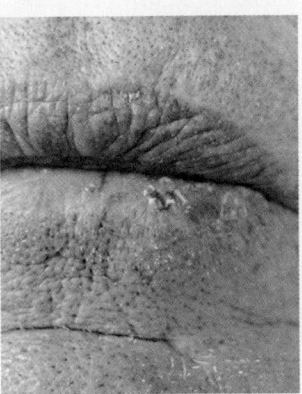

FIGURE 56.5 Squamous cell cancer of the lip. Ninety-five percent of lesions on the lip are squamous cell carcinomas.

Cancer of the oral cavity is primarily SCCA and is staged in relation to the following locations of the mouth:

- Lip
- Anterior two-thirds of the tongue
- Buccal mucosa
- Floor of the mouth
- Hard palate
- Upper and lower gingiva

Risk factors for oral cancer include:

- Habitual tobacco use
- Habitual alcohol use
- Poor oral hygiene
- Mechanical irritation from dental appliances
- Use of mouthwash with high alcohol content
- Chewing betel nut
- Herpes simplex virus (HSV-1)
- Human papillomavirus (HPV-2, 11, and 16)
- Mutations (related to the *p53* gene, *EGFR* gene, or TGF-alpha)
- Abnormalities such as nonhealing ulcers, **leukoplakia** (white patches), or **erythroplakia** (red patches)

The majority of malignant tumors of the oral cavity are SCCAs because the oral cavity is lined with squamous epithelium. About 90% of SCCAs are related to nicotine and alcohol abuse, and almost 75% of these malignant tumors develop between the base of the ridge that forms the borders of the lower jaws containing the sockets of the teeth (alveolar ridge) and the border of the tongue (Fig. 56.6). This location is the drainage area of the oral cavity. The significance of this location, also known as the "gutter area" of the mouth, is that the oral mucosa in this area is more likely to come into contact with carcinogenic and irritating substances, and tumors in this area have a propensity for metastasis.

Basal cell carcinoma is the second-most-frequent oral cancer but is considerably less common than SCCA. It primarily occurs on the lips. Initially, basal cell cancer causes very few clinical manifestations, and it appears as a raised scab that later looks like an ulcer with a raised, pearly border. Basal cell carcinomas do not metastasize but can aggressively invade the skin of the face. The Oral Cancer Foundation presents information about oral cancer, including video and audio clips and a pictorial gallery, as well as links that provide current information about oral cancer.

Pathophysiology

Most malignancies of the oral cavity are SCCAs (Fig. 56.7) arising from squamous epithelium lining the oral cavity. Other types of oral cancers include verrucous carcinoma (Fig. 56.8), which is a low-grade SCCA that rarely metastasizes. Minor salivary glands are potential sites of adenocarcinoma, adenoid cystic carcinoma, mucoepidermoid carcinoma, and polymorphous low-grade carcinoma.

Premalignant Lesions

Leukoplakia

Leukoplakia is the most prevalent premalignant lesion occurring on the lips and in the oral cavity, often found incidentally. These lesions occur from long-term irritation to oral mucous membranes, causing a thickening of the keratin layer of the dermis (Fig. 56.9).

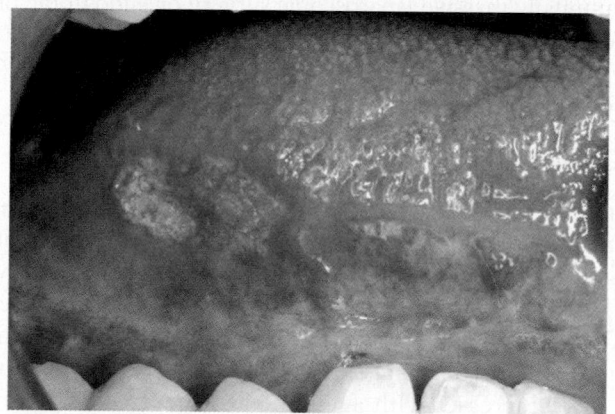

FIGURE 56.7 Squamous cell carcinoma of the tongue. Malignancies of the oral cavity are squamous cell cancers arising from squamous epithelium lining the oral cavity.

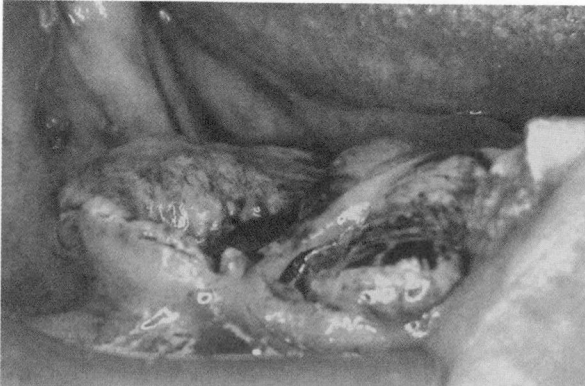

FIGURE 56.6 Cancer of the floor of the mouth. Malignant tumors develop between the base of the ridge that forms the borders of the lower jaws containing the sockets of the teeth and the border of the tongue.

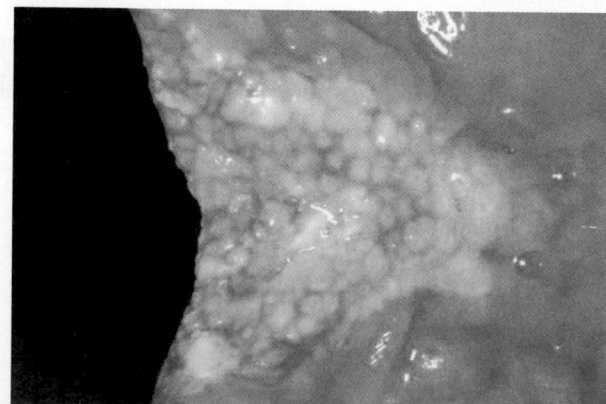

FIGURE 56.8 Verrucous carcinoma. Verrucous carcinoma is a low-grade squamous cell cancer that rarely metastasizes.

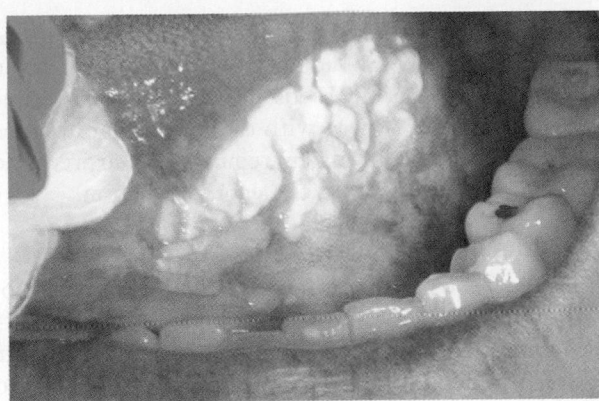

FIGURE 56.9 Leukoplakia. Leukoplakia manifests as slightly raised, sharply rounded white plaques.

Leukoplakia presents as nonremovable (by rubbing), slightly raised, sharply rounded white plaques. Irritants such as pressure from dental prostheses, cheek chewing, and tobacco and alcohol abuse are risk factors for the development of leukoplakia. These irritants also increase the risk for development of cancerous changes to existing plaques. Other abnormalities include infection of these plaques and development of cancerous changes. Leukoplakia can be present anywhere on the oral mucosa and occurs most often in adults over 40. Men are two times more likely than women to develop leukoplakia, primarily because of smoking. Upon visual examination, it is not possible to determine if these lesions are carcinoma in situ or invasive carcinoma because of similar morphological appearances. Owing to the potential for malignant degeneration, leukoplakia lesions require examination through biopsy and surgical removal. Leukoplakia lesions of the tongue or lips are most likely to develop into cancer and should always be examined and biopsied. Leukoplakia has the potential of malignant degeneration and the morphological likeness to carcinoma in situ and invasive carcinoma.

Erythroplakia

Erythroplakia is less common than leukoplakia, and it can occur in combination with leukoplakia. Located on the mucosal surface of the floor of the mouth, tongue, palate, or mandibular mucosa, these macular lesions are red because of increased vascularity and are velvety in appearance. Erythroplakia is often asymptomatic but may cause complaints of a sore, burning sensation. Erythroplakia lesions are highly suspicious for malignancy and require biopsy. Disruption from the basement membrane to the surface of the epithelium occurs, with mild to moderate dysplasia resulting from the erythroplakia. Dysplasia that fills the entire epithelium is termed carcinoma in situ. Further dysplasia to the basement membrane becomes invasive carcinoma.

Clinical Manifestations

The clinical presentation of cancer of the oral cavity usually affects the floor of the mouth or the tongue. Patients are often asymptomatic in the early stages, but later clinical manifestations of oral cancer include:

- Oral bleeding
- Raised area on the lip or in the mouth
- Oral ulcer with poorly defined margins, mucosal lesion, or nodule
- White and/or red patches in the oral cavity
- Increasing pain that radiates to the ear and neck
- **Dysarthria** (difficulty speaking)
- Dysphagia
- Difficulty chewing
- Oral fetor (odor)
- Regional lymph node involvement
- Weight loss
- Poor-fitting dentures

Management

The management of oral cancer depends on the size, location, and stage of the cancer and the patient's current and potential level of function related to the side effects of treatment. After an interprofessional work-up, patients review their treatment options and make decisions on the basis of individualized counseling and informed consent.

The prognosis among oral carcinomas is variable. Factors influencing the prognosis and treatment options include tumor site, extent of involvement, and histological differentiation of the lesions. In order to determine prognosis and an appropriate treatment regimen, the tumor, nodes, metastasis (TNM) classification is a tool used for consistent documentation purposes. HPV-positive patients have a much better prognosis than HPV-negative patients even when classified with stage 4 head and neck cancer. Even patients with multiple positive lymph nodes who are HPV positive have a favorable prognosis for cure. The *Cancer Staging Manual* (8th ed.) of the American Joint Committee on Cancer (AJCC) gives a more accurate prediction of survival for patients newly diagnosed with head and neck cancer using separate scales for patients based on HPV status.

Diagnostic Tests

Laboratory tests include:

- Complete blood count (to monitor for anemia, infection and bleeding risk)
- Chemistry profile (to monitor fluid, electrolytes, renal and nutritional status)
- Liver function tests (to rule out metastasis to the liver)

Imaging studies include:

- Computed tomography (CT) scan to evaluate bone involvement
- Magnetic resonance imaging (MRI) to evaluate soft tissue involvement
- Chest x-ray to rule out metastasis

Rationale for Tests

In order to determine correct diagnosis and staging, special tests and examinations are performed. These tests include:

- Examination of the oral cavity and oropharynx under anesthesia
- Direct laryngoscopy
- Tumor mapping
- Positron emission tomography (PET) to check for metastasis
- Panorex films (an x-ray that provides a full view of the upper and lower jaws, teeth, temporomandibular joints) of the mandible to rule out invasion of the mandible

Medical Management

Oral cavity tumors and the treatment modalities for these tumors can potentially affect the integrity of the oral mucosa and the patient's ability to eat, speak, and breathe. Medical management includes:

- Airway management
- Removal of the source of irritation
- Radiotherapy
- Chemotherapy
- Chemoradiation
- Surgical removal (treatment of choice) using scalpel, laser, or cryoprobe
- Retinoids (vitamin A derivative)
- Beta-carotene (antioxidant that converts to vitamin A)

Radiation Therapy

Radiation therapy (radiotherapy) can be the primary treatment for oral cancer or can be used after surgery to destroy areas of cancer that were not possible to remove surgically. Radiotherapy delivery is by external beam radiation or interstitial implantation (brachytherapy). *External beam radiation* reaches the tumor site by passing through the mucous membrane outside of the tumor. The regimen for radiotherapy is usually 5 days per week for 6 to 9 weeks. Monitoring of radiation doses allows for careful dose monitoring in order to limit the amount of radiation to the brain and spinal cord. *Interstitial implantation* (used for small non-infiltrating lesions) involves the placement of radioactive seeds close to the tumor bed. These seeds emit low levels of radiation and are permanently implanted. In early-stage lesions involving the floor of the mouth or anterior tongue, implanted radiation seeds can be curative. Interstitial implantation increases the dosage of radiation because of its close proximity to the tumor; in addition, after external beam radiation, interstitial implantation further boosts the radiation dose with less exposure of radiation to surrounding structures. Methods of radiation delivery include seeds, needles or wires, and radiation catheters or through a mold of radioactive material placed over a lesion for a prescribed amount of time. Patients receiving interstitial radiation, with the exception of seeds, require hospitalization during treatment with radiation precautions in place. The reason that patients receiving radioactive seeds do not require hospitalization is that the seeds emit low levels of radiation and pose no risk to others, with the exception of pregnant women and small children who require specific precautions and are more sensitive to the effects of radiation.

Medications

Oral cancer is treated with medications alone or in combination with surgery or radiotherapy. The benefit of medications alone or as an adjunct to surgery or radiation continues to be under investigation. Types of medications include chemotherapeutic agents and agents that target and block growth factors (GFs). Epidermal growth factor (EGF) is one of the GFs associated with oral cancers. Growth factors are hormone-like substances normally found in the cells of the human body. Oral cancer cells grow more quickly because they have more GF receptors than normal, healthy tissue. More than a dozen medications recently received U.S. Food and Drug Administration (FDA) approval, including cetuximab (Erbitux) and erlotinib (Tarceva); these medications target and block EGF receptors.

Intensity-modulated radiation therapy (IMRT) is a three-dimensional conformal radiotherapy that involves a highly precise type of external beam radiation therapy that uses software/hardware to deliver radiation to a specific location while sparing surrounding structures unaffected by the cancer. The use of IMRT results in improved quality of life as seen by decreased rates of xerostomia (dry mouth).

Chemotherapy may be given prior to or in combination with radiation therapy. Deep, infiltrating lesions of the anterior tongue may be treated with surgery, radiotherapy, and chemotherapy or a combination of therapies (concomitant therapy). Surgery, radiation, and chemotherapy are standard treatments for infiltrating lesions of the upper gingiva and hard palate. Other types of oral cancers require radiation and/or surgical interventions.

Patients undergoing radiation therapy may experience the following side effects:

- Skin irritation to the treated area
- Fatigue
- Nausea
- Weight loss
- Stomatitis (mucositis)
- Xerostomia from damage to the salivary glands
- Loss of taste
- Erythema and moist desquamation of the skin
- Laryngeal edema
- Bone pain

With the use of IMRT, a type of external radiation therapy that delivers radiation doses more effectively and with less damage to healthy cells than external beam radiation, fewer side effects occur (see Evidence-Based Practice: Proton Therapy).

Evidence-Based Practice

Proton Therapy

Proton therapy is a newer form of external beam radiation that is specifically shaped to the dimensions of the tumor site. Proton therapy uses a precise beam of radiation to kill cancer cells. The beam is aimed at various levels, and it is specifically shaped to the dimensions of the tumor. The procedure is painless, is noninvasive, and produces very little side effects.

Frank, S. J., Blanchard, P., Lee, J. J., Sturgis, E. M., Kies, M. S., Machtay, M., … Fuller, C. D. (2018, April). Comparing intensity-modulated proton therapy with intensity-modulated photon therapy for oropharyngeal cancer: The journey from clinical trial concept to activation. *Seminars in Radiation Oncology, 28*(2), 108–113.

Chemotherapy for oral cancer may be given as a neoadjuvant therapy (the first treatment before surgery and/or radiation therapy) or as an adjuvant therapy (the first treatment after surgery and/or radiation therapy). Chemoradiation treatments may be given during clinical trials for oral cancer. Common side effects of chemotherapy include:

- Xerostomia
- Taste disturbance
- Anorexia
- Nausea and vomiting
- Stomatitis
- Fatigue
- Hair loss
- Hearing loss
- Diarrhea and/or constipation
- Low red and white cell counts

Connection Check 56.4

Which statement by the patient undergoing external beam radiation indicates the need for further teaching?

A. "My grandchildren will not be able to visit because I will be radioactive."

B. "This therapy will hopefully decrease the size of the tumor."

C. "I will have daily radiation treatments for several weeks."

D. "At least this procedure is not painful."

Surgical Management

Surgical management of small, noninvasive lesions requires treatment under local or general anesthesia in an ambulatory clinic setting. Other options for the management of smaller lesions include carbon dioxide laser, cryotherapy (extreme application of cold), and photodynamic therapy. Factors that influence surgical intervention of oral cancers include tumor size, location, invasion into bone, and lymph node metastasis. Large tumors require external surgical removal, and the most advanced tumors may require composite resections. Extensive oral surgeries include single or combinations of glossectomy (partial or total), partial mandibulectomy, or neck dissection (removal of lymph nodes in the neck and possible removal of muscle, veins, and nerves).

Complications

Complications of oral cancer include infiltration to muscles and underlying tissue, resulting in difficulty eating or talking. Lymphatic spread varies with tumor site. Common sites for metastasis are the lungs, liver, and bone. Surgery and radiation therapy are the primary treatment modalities for oral cancer. After surgery for oral cancer, the following complications may occur:

- Infection
- Facial edema
- Weight loss
- Difficulty/inability talking
- Dysphagia

Rare but severe complications of radiotherapy include:

- Hearing loss
- Osteoradionecrosis (bone death from radiation)
- **Trismus** (difficulty opening the mouth)
- Carotid artery rupture

Nursing Management
Assessment and Analysis

Oral cancer has an effect on many daily functions, including swallowing, chewing, and talking. Tumors may become invasive, rapidly growing into underlying muscles and interfering with the ability to speak, eat, and talk. The goals of pain management are to optimize quality of life and to increase the ability to perform the activities of daily living. Treatments for oral cancer, such as surgery and medication management, chemotherapy, and radiotherapy, also can have debilitating and sometimes disfiguring side effects as well. Common manifestations related to the presentation and management of oral cancer include:

- Dysphagia
- Oral bleeding
- Impaired nutritional status
- Weight loss
- Anorexia
- Dysarthria
- Oral or lip lesions that do not heal in 2 weeks
- Leukoplakia
- Oral fetor
- Poor-fitting dentures
- Xerostomia

Nursing Diagnoses

- **Risk for ineffective airway clearance** related to ineffective cough and swallow secondary to postoperative edema

- **Imbalanced nutrition, less than body requirements**, related to difficult or painful swallowing or inability to swallow
- **Impaired verbal communication** related to surgeries affecting quality of speech
- **Acute or chronic pain** related to surgery, malignancy, or treatment
- **Anxiety** related to impaired breathing, cancer diagnosis, or treatment course

Nursing Interventions

■ *Assessments*

- Ability to swallow
  Impaired swallowing due to pain or edema interferes with adequate oral fluid and nutritional intake. This provides important data needed to determine the best diet according to the patient's ability to chew and swallow.
- Fluid intake
  Fluid intake is also compromised based on mouth pain and dysphagia.
- Nutritional intake
  Data collection related to overall caloric intake, as well as intake of carbohydrates, proteins, and fats, enables the nurse to make appropriate nutritional recommendations in collaboration with the nutritionist.
- Weight
  Weight loss trends are an indicator of metastasis. Other causes of weight loss are related to edema from oral lesions causing difficulty swallowing and chewing.
- Albumin and total protein levels
  Decreased nutritional status is indicated with decreased serum levels of albumin and total protein.
- Clinical manifestations of oral mucosal irritation or infection, irritation from dental appliances, oral lesions, bleeding, difficulty swallowing or chewing, lesions, and nodules
  The purpose of an oral cavity assessment is to inspect the condition of the oral mucosa and identify the presence of infection, the level of hygiene practices, and the presence of lesions and to determine the potential for or presence of malignant processes.
- Lymph nodes
  Enlarged cervical lymph nodes indicate metastasis.
- Psychosocial adjustment
  Adjustments to the disease process, treatments, and side effects may require consultation with the palliative care team, social worker, or chaplain.

■ *Actions*

- Airway management
  Airway management promotes adequate air exchange by removing secretions either by encouraging coughing and deep breathing or by suctioning. Ineffective airway clearance may result in some patients with an enlarged tumor or who have undergone surgical procedures to the oral cavity. Other associated oral cavity findings include edema, inflammation, and thick and tenacious secretions.

- Aspiration precautions
  Aspiration precautions help identify those patients who are at risk and to identify specific preventive measures to prevent aspiration. Specific actions taken to prevent aspiration include assessment of the patient's ability to swallow; providing thickened liquids; performing respiratory assessment; pulmonary toilet; elevating the patient's HOB as high as possible, at least 30 degrees; and providing elixir forms of medications when possible.
- Maintain emergency bedside equipment at all times.
  Maintain suction setup, oxygen setup, pulse oximetry (nearby), and an oral airway at the HOB for ineffective airway clearance.
- Provide oral care.
  Due to xerostomia, as well as soreness of the mouth, frequent oral care is needed to decrease chances of further irritation from food particles and to provide comfort.
- Administer steroids as prescribed.
  Decrease oral edema and improve airway and breathing.
- Provide cool mist via oxygen test as needed.
  Cool mist provides humidification and lessens the complications of xerostomia.
- Nutritional consult
  All patients with oral cancer should have a nutritional consult upon admission in order to ensure optimal caloric intake and to identify disease-specific nutritional risks and individual dietary preferences.

■ *Teaching*

- Aspiration Precautions
  Encouraging the patient to eat small amounts of food and not to talk while eating decreases the risk of aspiration.
- Avoid tobacco products and alcohol intake.
  Use of tobacco products and excessive alcohol intake increase the risk of oral cancer.
- Provide nutritional education to the patient.
  As a result of chemotherapy, changes in taste may occur, such as a metallic taste, and aversions to certain foods may occur, especially meats. Encourage high-protein foods and the use of gravies, sauces, herbs, and seasonings to make foods more palatable.
  Collaborate with the nutritionist to teach patients and families about patients' nutritional needs and how to assess whether patients are getting adequate nutrition. Liquid nutritional supplements are ordered for nutritionally depleted patients.
- Oral hygiene and assessment education
  The patient/family needs to inspect the oral cavity daily to identify any redness, irritation, or signs of infection. Additionally, frequent mouth rinsing, particularly after eating, can ease discomfort and decrease food retained in the oral cavity.
- Management of xerostomia
  Patients receiving chemoradiation are at increased risk for oral complications such as stomatitis, oral infections, and xerostomia. These patients must be diligent in performing their regimen of oral hygiene, including frequent mouth rinses to rinse away oral pathogens and to maintain adequate

hydration. Radiation to the oral cavity affects the production of saliva from the salivary glands, as seen by a decrease in or absence of the secretion of saliva.

- Frequent sips of water or saliva substitutes
  These help to decrease the symptoms of xerostomia. Salivary dysfunction is temporary or permanent as a result of radiotherapy and permanent if the salivary glands are surgically removed.

Evaluating Care Outcomes

Prevention is the key to reducing the number of patients diagnosed with oral cancer, and it is achieved through decreasing risk factors. The screening provided through regularly scheduled dental examinations provides a mechanism for prevention and early recognition of oral cancer and premalignant lesions so that patients can expect more favorable outcomes related to quality of life and prognosis. Most often, an oral cancer diagnosis occurs when the disease is at an advanced stage. This delayed diagnosis results in patient and family education focusing on treatment modalities such as surgery, radiation, and/or chemotherapy and the side effects or changes that occur as a result of these treatments.

CASE STUDY: EPISODE 2

Mr. Rodriguez has received his biopsy results. He has squamous cell carcinoma on the right side of his tongue. The PET scan results are negative for distant metastasis, and Mr. Rodriguez is scheduled to go to the dentist for a full mouth extraction due to severe gingivitis and tooth decay. He will have a right hemiglossectomy with a right modified radical neck dissection soon after his tooth extraction, and he will receive IMRT about 4 weeks later…

ORAL TRAUMA

Epidemiology

Oral trauma includes injury to specific bones of the face, including nasal, mandibular, and maxillary fractures, as well as soft tissue injuries in and around the mouth. The severity of injuries ranges from minor soft tissue injuries to complicated fractures and is usually the result of blunt or penetrating injuries. The causes of oral trauma include automobile accidents, athletic activities (boxing, basketball, baseball, etc.), and physical altercations. As the population ages, there is an increased incidence of facial trauma in older adults (over 60 years of age), most often secondary to falls.

Pathophysiology

The pathophysiology of oral trauma is directly related to the location and severity of the injury. Of primary concern is potential direct damage to the oral cavity that can lead to

partial or complete airway occlusion. Because of the rich blood supply to the face, the patient is at risk of significant blood loss, and with oral hemorrhage, this can further compromise the airway. Because of normal flora in the mouth, infection may develop after traumatic injuries to the oral cavity. Injuries to the maxilla may occur and are classified as Le Fort I (horizontal maxillary fracture of the alveolar process with the teeth contained with the detached fragment, passing through the alveolar ridge, lateral nose, and inferior wall of maxillary sinuses), Le Fort II (pyramidal fracture that passes through the posterior alveolar ridge, lateral wall of the maxillary sinuses, inferior orbit rim, and nasal bones), and Le Fort III (fracture that passes through the nasofrontal suture, maxilla-frontal suture, orbital wall, and zygomatic arch; Fig. 56.10).

Clinical Manifestations

Clinical manifestations of oral trauma include:

- Increased respiratory rate
- Stridor (noisy breathing)
- Shortness of breath
- Decreased oxygen saturation
- Hypercarbia (elevated carbon dioxide levels)
- Elevated heart rate
- Changes in level of consciousness
- Oral bleeding
- Swelling and edema
- Loss of teeth
- Pain

Management

Medical Management

Initial emergency management is directed at establishing and maintaining the airway and controlling bleeding. The patient may require an emergent tracheostomy on the basis

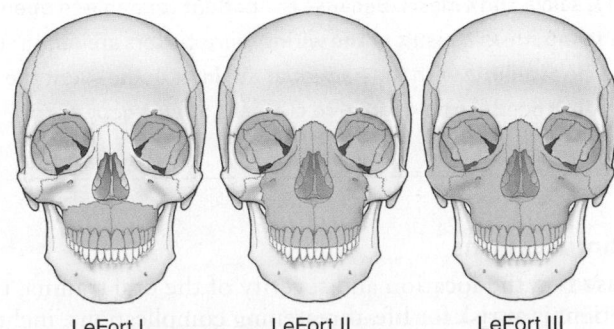

FIGURE 56.10 Types of Le Fort fractures. Le Fort I fractures are horizontal maxillary fractures of the alveolar process with the teeth contained with the detached fragment, passing through the alveolar ridge, lateral nose, and inferior wall of maxillary sinuses. Le Fort II fractures are pyramidal fractures that pass through the posterior alveolar ridge, lateral wall of the maxillary sinuses, inferior orbit rim, and nasal bones. Le Fort III fractures pass through the nasofrontal suture, maxilla-frontal suture, orbital wall, and zygomatic arch.

of a clinical presentation that reveals that the patient cannot maintain an effective airway. Because most facial injuries are related to some type of trauma, the patient is typically evaluated in an emergency department, where IV access is established. Diagnostic studies include:

- Complete blood cell count
- Serum chemistry analysis
- Arterial blood gas analysis
- Facial x-rays
- Facial CT or MRI

Because of the increased risk for infection, broad-spectrum antibiotics are ordered. Consultations with neurosurgeons, oral surgeons, and dentists are often initiated to determine specific interventions.

Surgical Management

Surgical stabilization of the facial fracture is typically indicated, and one of the following procedures may be performed:

- Open reduction internal fixation is indicated with extensive facial fractures and includes the placement of plates and screws that provide jaw stability.
- Fixed occlusion of the fracture involves the use of wires to immobilize the jaw in a fixed, mouth-closed position. This procedure is indicated when there is a need to replace and realign damaged teeth. The wires are usually maintained in place for 6 to 12 weeks to allow adequate healing of the bones (see Safety Alert).
- Microplating surgical procedures may be performed that use bone substitutes to foster repair of the facial fractures.
- Inner maxillary fixation is used to stabilize mandibular fractures. This procedure aligns the bites and also uses wires to keep the mouth closed for healing.

> **⊘ Safety Alert** Patients with wired jaws are at risk for airway compromise, particularly with managing saliva and emesis. Because the patient is unable to open the mouth as a result of the wiring, wire cutters are required to be available with the patient at all times in the event the mouth needs to be opened to clear the airway or perform other lifesaving maneuvers.

Complications

Based on the location and severity of the oral trauma, the patient is at risk for life-threatening complications, including airway compromise, aspiration of teeth, infection, and the inability to consume adequate nutrition. Even with successful surgical restoration, the patient may continue to have issues with pain, temporomandibular joint (TMJ) function, and disfigurement. With extensive facial trauma, the patient may develop a cerebrospinal leak, with an increased risk of meningitis.

Connection Check 56.5

In caring for a patient who sustained a Le Fort fracture, the nurse monitors for which complications? *(Select all that apply.)*
A. TMJ pain
B. Esophageal strictures
C. Airway obstruction
D. Infection
E. Dyspepsia

Nursing Management
Assessment and Analysis

Facial trauma is a medical emergency that requires prompt assessment and definitive treatment. The priority assessments focus on ensuring an intact airway and effective breathing pattern. Clinical manifestations of oral trauma include alterations in respiratory rate and rhythm, bleeding and swelling in and around the mouth, difficulty managing oral secretions (potentially related to impaired swallowing), disfigurement, changes in level of consciousness, and visual disturbances.

Nursing Diagnoses

- **Risk for ineffective airway clearance** related to bleeding and swelling in and around the mouth
- **Risk for bleeding** related to increased vascularity of the face and mouth
- **Risk for infection** related to normal flora in the mouth, as well as risk of wound contamination with a facial fracture
- **Imbalanced nutrition**, less than body requirements, related to impaired ability to eat/drink secondary to facial trauma

Nursing Interventions
▪ *Assessments*

- Oral airway
  Because of the increased risk of soft tissue edema and bleeding, the patient remains at risk for airway compromise, including after surgical interventions. Increased swelling can lead to partial or complete airway obstruction.
- Respiratory rate and quality
  The patient may hypoventilate because of airway compromise, and this increases the risk of hypercapnia. Respiratory stridor is indicative of airway obstruction.
- Oxygen saturation
  Because of trauma in and around the mouth, as well as possible breathing impairment, the patient is at risk of decreased oxygenation.
- Arterial blood gas values
  The patient is at risk for hypoxemia and hypercarbia secondary to hypoventilation associated with facial trauma and edema
- Temperature
  Because of flora in the mouth and nose along with possible bone disruption, the patient is at increased risk of infection that is manifested by an increase in temperature.

- Serial complete blood count (CBC)
  Because of the increased vascularity of the face, the patient may have significant blood loss. Serial assessments of CBC may allow earlier confirmation of hemorrhage. The white blood cell count needs to be monitored due to risk of infection.
- Serial serum electrolytes
  Due to decreased nutritional and fluid intake, the patient is at risk for electrolyte disturbances.
- Daily weights
  Oral intake may be limited or totally prohibited during the emergent phase, leading to decreased nutritional intake.

Actions

- Maintain wire cutters with the patient at all times if jaw is wired.
  Wire cutters are required in the event the patient experiences respiratory compromise, requiring the mouth to be opened.
- Provide oral humidification.
  The patient is at risk for dry mouth and thickened secretions because of the decrease in normal humidification and the filtering actions of the nose and mouth. Even if the patient does not require supplementation oxygen, supplemental humidification may be required.
- Elevate the head of the bed 30 to 45 degrees.
  This position decreases the risk of aspiration, facilitates breathing, and promotes gas exchange.
- Administer antibiotics as ordered.
  The patient has an increased risk of infection because of oral trauma.
- Provide diet as ordered.
  The patient may be on tube feedings or soft oral diet. Even with jaw wiring, patients may be able to have oral intake via a syringe or straw. Adequate nutrition is essential to wound healing.
- Provide frequent mouth care.
  Rinsing the mouth after meals is important to decrease the risk of injection and promote wound healing.

Teaching

- Have wire cutters with patient at all times.
  The patient or a family member must be able to cut the wires in the event the patient experiences respiratory distress. If the wires have to be cut, the patient is also instructed to immediately notify the healthcare provider because the wires may need to be replaced.
- Mouth care after each meal
  To decrease risks of inflammation and infection
- Signs and symptoms of infection
  Because of the increased risk of infection related to oral trauma, it is important that the patient report a temperature elevation, increased oral swelling, pain, or a change in oral secretions.

Evaluating Care Outcomes

Patients experiencing oral or facial trauma require emergent stabilization and treatment, usually followed by weeks or months of follow-up care and monitoring. Once the oral trauma has stabilized, the patient requires close surveillance for infection, impaired wound healing, decreased nutritional intake with associated weight loss, and issues related to change in appearance. Stable weight, lack of infection, and wound healing are indicative of successful outcomes.

ESOPHAGEAL CANCER

Esophageal cancer develops in the mucosal layer of the esophagus and grows outward into the submucosal and muscular layers, and it occurs in any part of the esophagus. The types of cells that normally line the esophagus are squamous cells. There are two main types of esophageal cancers, SCCAs and adenocarcinomas. Less than 1% of esophageal cancers include small-cell neuroendocrine cancers, lymphomas, and sarcomas. Recent trends in North America and Western Europe show the incidence of esophageal adenocarcinoma taking the lead over SCCAs. This trend lends itself to the prevalence of GERD in developed countries. Patients are usually asymptomatic until the tumor has occluded 50% of the esophageal lumen and metastasis has occurred to the lung, liver, bone, stomach, cervical lymph nodes, or other sites. Overall 5-year survival rates range from 5% to 30%. Palliative care treatment options exist for patients diagnosed in the later stages of the disease.

Epidemiology

Esophageal cancer accounts for 1% of all new cancer cases in the United States, and the estimated number of new cases in 2018 was 17,290, with 13,480 being males and 3,810 being females. Of these cases, the estimated number of deaths for 2018 was 15,850, with 850 being males and 3,000 being females. The incidence of esophageal cancer in adults is greatest between the ages of 45 and 70. The rate of incidence of esophagus adenocarcinoma (EA) is higher in Caucasians than in Asians and African Americans, whereas the incidence of esophageal squamous cell carcinoma (ESCC) is highest in Asians. The rates are very high in parts of China, Iran, and Southern Africa, suggesting an association between either genetics or environment.

Nonmodifiable risk factors of esophageal cancer include age, sex, and race, whereas modifiable risk factors include the use of alcohol and tobacco. The risk of developing esophageal cancer increases 18 times for those who drink more than 13 oz of alcohol per day, and the amount of alcohol consumed on a consistent basis has a direct effect on the cancer risk. Cigarette smokers are two to six times more likely to develop esophageal cancer than nonsmokers, and the combination of smoking and heavy alcohol use increases the risk for esophageal cancer 44 times. The following factors also influence the risk of developing esophageal cancer:

- Nutritional deficiency (molybdenum, zinc, and vitamin A)
- Barrett's esophagus (columnar cells in the lower esophagus)

- GERD (long term, untreated)
- Obesity
- Lye strictures (esophageal narrowing caused by lye ingestion)
- Esophageal diverticula
- Achalasia (decreased esophageal smooth muscle relaxation)
- Tylosis (esophageal callus formation)
- Obesity (associated with hiatal hernia and GERD)

Pathophysiology

The majority of tumors occurring in the upper two-thirds of the esophagus are usually SCCAs. The use of alcohol and tobacco products increases the risk of squamous cell esophageal cancer more so than adenocarcinoma, with more than half of the cases of squamous cell esophageal cancer associated with smoking. Esophageal adenocarcinoma is mostly found in the lower one-third of the esophagus, mainly at the GEJ and cardiac (first part of the stomach) portion of the stomach. When reflux of gastric acid occurs over a long period of time, the squamous cells lining the lower one-third of the esophagus are replaced with columnar cells (gland cells that normally line the stomach and small intestine). This metaplastic transformation is known as Barrett's esophagus and is a known cause of esophageal adenocarcinoma. Esophageal cancer grows rapidly, spreading to nearby lymph nodes and into the esophageal lumen, causing thickening and invasion of neighboring tissue. More than 50% of esophageal cancers metastasize, with the most common sites being the liver, lung, bone, and stomach. Patients are usually asymptomatic until the tumor is large and well advanced. By the time patients seek medical attention, these fast-growing tumors have progressed to later stages. Another factor contributing to late diagnosis is that there is no preventive screening for esophageal cancer.

Heavy alcohol consumption and tobacco use are primary risk factors linked to SCCA of the esophagus, especially when used together. The compounds found in tobacco smoke may be responsible for genetic mutations commonly found in esophageal tumors. A mutation of the *Tp53* gene is usually present in patients with advanced adenocarcinoma. Long-standing alcohol and tobacco use increase the ability of these substances to damage suppressor genes and overexpress the oncogenes that cause esophageal disease (see Evidence-Based Practice: Gene Mutation and Carcinogenesis).

Evidence-Based Practice

Gene Mutation and Familial Clustering
- Mutations of three genes have been associated with the development of esophageal disease.
- Mutations of the *MSR1, ASCC1,* and *CTHRC1* genes have been associated with Barrett's esophagus (BE) and

adenocarcinoma and accounted for 11% of cases in the study population.
- In the past 40 years, there has been a six-fold increase in esophageal cancer in Western countries.
- Individuals having no siblings with BE or esophageal adenocarcinoma (EA) have a 3.2% baseline risk of developing BE or associated cancers.
- The risk of developing BE or EA increases with the number of siblings who are affected:
  With one sibling affected, the risk goes up to 9.1%.
  With two siblings affected, the risk goes up to 26.6%.

Contino, G., Vaughan, T. L., Whiteman, D., & Fitzgerald, R. C. (2017). The evolving genomic, landscape of Barrett's esophagus and esophageal adenocarcinoma. *Gastroenterology, 153*(3), 657–673.

There is a strong causal relationship with GERD and adenocarcinoma. Patients with adenocarcinoma are seven times more likely to have GERD symptoms than patients who do not have adenocarcinoma. Patients with chronic, severe GERD are at least 43 times more likely to develop esophageal adenocarcinoma. There is no relationship between GERD and SCCA.

Clinical Manifestations

Progressive dysphagia is the most common symptom of esophageal cancer, indicating a large late-stage cancer in most cases. When patients experience difficulty swallowing, the tumor has narrowed the lumen of the esophagus to about half its diameter. Other clinical manifestations include hemoptysis (coughing up blood), pain or a burning sensation in the middle of the chest, painful swallowing as food or fluids reach the tumor, vomiting, weight loss, anorexia, hoarseness, and melena. Hypercalcemia may develop related to metastasis of the esophageal tumor to the bones, production of hypercalcemic substances by the tumor tissue, or release of a parathyroid hormone–related protein (PTHrP). Esophageal cancers do not usually produce clinical manifestations until the disease has advanced and recovery is unlikely.

Management

Medical Management

Screening

Currently, screening for esophageal cancer in the general population is nonexistent. Careful screening and follow-up for high-risk patients, such as those with Barrett's esophagus, are monitored closely for malignancy with scheduled endoscopies. These patients are treated medically or surgically according to the degree of esophageal dysplasia.

Diagnostic Tests

- A *barium swallow* identifies irregularities in the surface of the wall of the esophagus and is one of the first tests done to diagnose esophageal cancer. A barium swallow can also diagnose a tracheoesophageal fistula. These fistulas occur when a tumor invades the tissue between the esophagus and the trachea, creating a hole connecting them, increasing the patient's risk of food or fluid traveling from the esophagus to the trachea.
- *Computed tomography scans* are used to determine how far the cancer has spread in the esophagus and to assess for spread to the lymph nodes and nearby organs. Patients may receive oral or IV contrasts before a CT scan to visualize various structures and to identify tumors. Decisions to perform surgical interventions are determined according to CT scan results. When performing a CT-guided needle biopsy, a radiologist guides a biopsy needle toward a mass to obtain a tissue sample for evaluation.
- *Positron emission tomography* scans detect areas of metastasis and can even detect small collections of cancer cells that are not detectable with other diagnostic studies. Radioactive glucose is administered intravenously and then concentrates in cancers. A scanner is used to detect the radioactive deposits.
- *Endoscopic ultrasonography* is performed by placing a small ultrasound probe in the esophagus. The probe produces sound waves that penetrate into normal tissue and abnormal tissue. These sound waves are converted into a picture that shows how much the tissue and nearby lymph nodes are affected by the cancer.
- *Endoscopy* is used to diagnose esophageal cancer, and there are two different approaches. An *upper endoscopy* is performed by inserting an endoscope through the patient's mouth, the esophagus, and to the stomach. The esophageal wall is observed, and a biopsy can be performed on tissue that appears abnormal. A *bronchoscopy* is performed using an endoscope to view the trachea and the bronchi in order to detect abnormal tissue in these areas. Therapeutic procedures and collection of tissue specimens can be obtained.
- *Thoracoscopy and laparoscopy* are performed by a healthcare provider who passes a scope and instruments through a tube and into the chest or the abdomen of the patient. Lymph nodes and other organs located near the esophagus are viewed, and tissue samples for biopsy are taken to determine potential areas of metastasis. *Biopsies* may be performed with several of these diagnostic tests and involve removing tissue samples that appear to be cancerous or abnormal. These tissue samples are observed under a microscope, and if cancer cells are present, the grade and the type are determined.

Complementary and Alternative Medicine

Complementary and alternative therapies can promote relaxation and relieve muscle tension that contributes to the sensation of pain. Yoga, meditation, spirituality, and religion are used to relieve pain in some individuals with esophageal cancer. Massage and vibration are used for muscular relaxation, which decreases the perception of pain by decreasing pain signal transmission. Other complementary and alternative therapies used for chronic pain include imagery, aromatherapy, music, and humor. These therapies have been used as adjuncts or in place of medical or surgical interventions (see Chapter 12).

Surgical Management

In rare cases, esophageal cancer is discovered when it is localized to the esophagus, and surgery can be curative. Esophageal tumors, lymph nodes, and surrounding tissue are surgically removed depending on the stage of the cancer. Most often, palliative surgical interventions are done to restore patients' ability to swallow and to maintain optimal nutrition.

An open esophagectomy is a surgical procedure that involves the removal of all or part of the esophagus and the neighboring lymph nodes (Fig. 56.11). When a portion of the upper or middle esophagus is removed, most of the esophagus is removed, and the stomach is pulled up and connected to the esophagus in the neck area. If the stomach cannot be used to replace the esophagus in the neck, then a piece of intestine

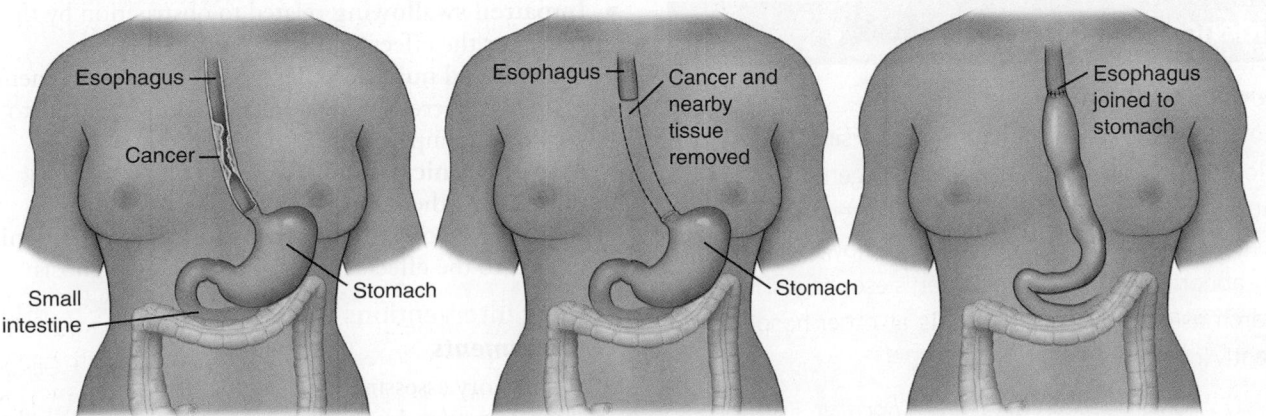

FIGURE 56.11 Esophagectomy. A part of the esophagus with the cancer is removed, and then the stomach is connected to the remaining esophagus in the upper chest or the neck.

is used to form a new esophagus. When the cancer is in the distal esophagus or the gastroesophageal juncture, parts of the stomach and esophagus are removed, and the stomach is connected to the remaining esophagus in the upper chest or the neck. Treatment regimens include surgery combined with chemotherapy and/or radiation therapy. In some cases, a minimally invasive esophagectomy is performed laparoscopically for small cancers through several small incisions.

Endoscopic Treatments

Several endoscopic interventions are also indicated in the management of esophageal cancer. *Endoscopic mucosal resection (EMR)* involves the removal of the esophageal lining with instruments attached to an endoscope. Endoscopic mucosal resection is used to remove precancerous (dysplastic) lesions and small, singular esophageal cancers. Proton pump inhibitors are used after EMR to prevent recurrence. *Photodynamic therapy* is used to treat dysplasia, early esophageal cancer, and recurrence of esophageal cancer. This therapy uses light to activate a chemical that can kill cancer cells. *Laser ablation* is performed using a laser through an endoscope to destroy cancer cells. It is also used to relieve esophageal obstruction and improve swallowing. Liquid nitrogen therapy (cryotherapy ablation) has also been used to destroy abnormal cells with Barrett's esophagus (see Evidence-Based Practice: Cryotherapy Ablation). *Radiofrequency ablation* is used to treat dysplasia in areas of Barrett's esophagus. A balloon is passed into the area of Barrett's esophagus and inflated until the balloon comes in contact with the inner lining of the esophagus. High-powered energy is applied to destroy the cells in the inner lining. Normal cells should replace the Barrett's cells, and afterward, the patient remains on acid-blocking medications. Follow-up with periodic endoscopy and biopsies is done to monitor for further changes to the esophageal lining. *Argon plasma* coagulation is used to clear the esophagus when the patient is having difficulty swallowing, and it is similar to laser ablation. *Electrocoagulation* is used to remove the tumor with electrical current and occasionally is used to clear the esophageal blockage.

Evidence-Based Practice

Cryotherapy Ablation

A pilot study was conducted at the University of Maryland Medical Center (UMMC) using liquid nitrogen (cryotherapy ablation) to remove the abnormal cells seen in Barrett's esophagus. This endoscopic procedure showed regression of the abnormal cells found in Barrett's esophagus. Further research using larger clinical trials at other hospitals is currently in progress.

University of Maryland Medical Center. (2015). *Cryotherapy*. Retrieved from http://www.umm.edu/gi/cryotherapy.htm

Complications

Complications of esophageal cancer include risks related to treatment for the disease in addition to risks associated with advanced disease. Complications associated with surgical interventions include dysphagia caused by strictures at the surgical site of anastomosis, heartburn related to disturbance or loss of the LES pressure allowing reflux of acid and bile into the esophagus, and frequent nausea and vomiting due to decreased stomach emptying from nerve involvement related to the surgical procedure. The patient may also develop *dumping syndrome* due to partially digested food entering the small intestine too quickly and causing distention and diarrhea. Radiation therapy also has the potential for complications, including blistering and ulceration of the skin and fatigue. Gastrointestinal complications include stomatitis, nausea and vomiting, and diarrhea. In addition to complications associated with chemotherapy discussed in the oral cancer section, specific side effects associated with the chemotherapeutic medications commonly given for esophageal cancer include diarrhea associated with the administration of 5-FU, nerve and renal impairment associated with cisplatin administration, and cardiac toxicities seen with the administration of doxorubicin and epirubicin.

Nursing Management

Assessment and Analysis

Many of the clinical manifestations observed in the patient with esophageal cancer are related to cellular changes that lead to obstruction of the esophageal lumen. Common findings include:

- Dysphagia (with or without hiccups)
- Pain (throat, back, or chest)
- Hoarseness
- Chronic cough
- Weight loss
- Hypercalcemia
- Gastrointestinal bleeding
- Anemia
- Coughing up blood

Nursing Diagnoses

- **Impaired swallowing** related to obstruction by the tumor or the effects of radiotherapy
- **Imbalanced nutrition**: Less than body requirements related to decreased nutritional intake secondary to swallowing impairment
- **Acute/chronic pain** related to the physical injury (pressure of the tumor mass in the esophagus)
- **Ineffective coping and compromised family coping** related to the effects of the disease and prognosis

Nursing Interventions

▪ *Assessments*

- Respiratory assessment
  Aspiration related to dysphagia can cause adventitious breath sounds and decreased oxygenation. As the cancer progresses, infiltration of the tracheobronchial tree or development of a

tracheoesophageal fistula may occur, with eventual lung metastasis. Other respiratory symptoms may be due to aspiration and regurgitation of undigested food particles.

- Nausea and vomiting
  Nausea and vomiting occur from the interruption of normal peristalsis by the tumor. Patients with dysphagia who experience vomiting are at risk for aspiration. Postoperative nausea and vomiting can occur because of decreased gastric emptying and vagal nerve involvement.

- Hoarseness or cough
  A hoarse cough is related to tumor involvement with the larynx or recurrent laryngeal nerve, aspiration pneumonia, or a tracheoesophageal fistula.

- Painful swallowing (odynophagia)
  Dull, substernal pain that may radiate occurs when esophageal cancer is so large that food is blocked from passing into the stomach. Pain occurs a few seconds after swallowing as food reaches the area of blockage where the tumor is located.

- Dysphagia and hiccups together
  Difficulty swallowing progressively increases over a few months. Patients will usually eat softer foods as the dysphagia starts; they may avoid meat, bread, and raw vegetables because these foods get stuck in the throat more easily. Eventually, liquids can become difficult to swallow.

- Weight loss
  Patients are at risk for nutritional deficiency when food becomes stuck in the esophagus because of the increasing size of the tumor. Dysphasia is a late symptom that indicates a large esophageal cancer. Weight loss occurs because of problems with swallowing and the associated pain. Additionally, the increase in metabolism from the cancer adds to the weight loss.

- Hematocrit and hemoglobin
  There is an increased risk of bleeding as tumors invade the esophageal tissues. Bleeding from the tumor can appear in stool or emesis, causing anemia. Stools may appear black (melena).

- Serum calcium levels
  Elevated calcium levels are seen in patients with advanced squamous cell esophageal carcinoma. Potential causes of the increased calcium levels are bone metastasis, production of hypercalcemic substances by the tumor tissue, or release of PTHrP.

- Liver enzymes and jaundice
  Elevated liver enzymes and jaundice are indicators of liver metastasis or alcohol-related liver disease.

- Psychosocial adjustment
  Adjustments to the disease process, treatments, and side effects may require consultation with the palliative care team, social worker, or chaplain.

▪ Actions

- Maintain the HOB greater than 30 degrees, and provide suction and oxygen equipment.
  Esophageal obstruction from tumor growth increases the risk of aspiration. Measures to prevent aspiration help to prevent respiratory complications.

- Collaborate with the nutritionist.
  The patient may require calorie counts, soft diet/thickened liquids, nutritional supplements. Food and fluids prevent

weight loss and promote healing. Collaboration with a nutritionist ensures an individualized diet plan to maintain optimal nutrition. Thickened or soft foods are easier to swallow, and nutritional supplements between meals increase caloric intake. Following esophagogastrostomy, provide six small meals low in complex sugars and high in protein and fat to prevent dumping syndrome (diarrhea after eating).

- Provide six small meals per day, low in complex sugars and high in protein and fat, for patients after esophagogastrostomy.
  Smaller meals along with a decrease in complex sugars and foods high in protein and fat delay gastric emptying and prevent dumping syndrome (diarrhea after eating).

- Collaborate with speech and language pathologist.
  Speech and language pathologists treat problems with swallowing and can teach the patient and family strategies to increase the effectiveness of swallowing and decrease aspiration.

▪ Teaching

- Lines, tubes, and incisions
  Patients will receive information about their surgery preoperatively to psychologically prepare for what they will experience postoperatively. Patients undergoing esophageal surgery can expect to see chest incisions, drains, a jejunostomy tube (for enteral tube feeding), a nasogastric tube for decompression of the stomach, an IV line, and possibly a chest tube.

- Preoperative care for esophageal surgery; smoking cessation 2 to 4 weeks before surgery
  Smoking cessation improves respiratory outcomes postoperatively.

- Coughing, deep breathing, incentive spirometry, turning every 2 hours, and early ambulation
  This is the highest postoperative priority in patients who have undergone esophagectomy to promote prevention of respiratory complications.

- Pain management: monitoring duration, quality, and intensity
  Teach the patient and family the use of alternative pain techniques and to request pain medication when anticipating painful events. Nonpharmacological measures enhance the patient's perception of pain control. Pain management teams use specific patient reports to adjust pain regimens.

- Enteral or parenteral nutrition support may be necessary up to 3 weeks after surgery.
  Patients need to remain NPO to prevent postoperative complications and to allow surgical incisions time to heal.

- Dental screening
  Preoperative dental examinations and oral care four times per day will help prevent postoperative infection.

- Postoperative nutritional education: The patient is instructed to sit upright and eat six to eight small meals per day with fluids in between meals.
  The size of the stomach is considerably smaller. Diarrhea resulting from interruption of vagal nerve fibers can occur 20 minutes to 2 hours after eating. Imodium can be given before meals to manage diarrhea.

Evaluating Care Outcomes

Esophageal cancer is usually diagnosed in later stages because symptoms occur when the tumor has invaded deep into the layers of the esophagus and distant metastasis has occurred, thus decreasing survival. Currently, the only screening method used is endoscopy, but this is used when patients have suspicious symptoms or precancerous conditions such as Barrett's esophagus. The most important outcome for patients who have esophageal cancer is that the patient maintains a stable weight and receives adequate nutrition. Treatment goals aim to slow the progression of the disease, and overall, there is about a 20% chance of 5-year survival. Surgery, radiation therapy, and chemotherapy are used to treat esophageal cancer. Patient education that focuses on avoiding lifestyle choices such as alcohol and tobacco use and maintaining a healthy weight is important in order to inform patients of how these behaviors impact the disease process. Often, newly diagnosed patients enter into palliative care regimens, with the possibility of a cure being unlikely.

ESOPHAGEAL TRAUMA

Because of its anatomical position in the thoracic cavity and its close proximity to the oropharynx, the esophagus is the most common site for GI trauma. Direct effects of esophageal trauma may cause impairment of swallowing and nutrition, and indirect trauma may occur to the lungs or the mediastinum. Excessive force applied to the esophageal mucosa may cause it to rupture or perforate. Perforation can cause respiratory impairment, shock, or sepsis (most likely related to GI contents spilling into the thoracic cavity) and gastric acid entering the mediastinal cavity. High mortality rates are associated with esophageal perforation.

Epidemiology

The most common causes of esophageal trauma are from diagnostic and therapeutic interventions (iatrogenic) performed while passing endoscopic instruments through the esophagus. Diagnostic endoscopy carries a complication rate of 0.1%, and therapeutic endoscopic procedures have a complication rate of 10% to 15%. Other epidemiological facts about esophageal trauma include the importance of early treatment and determining the etiology, severity, and location of the trauma. Factors that contribute to morbidity and mortality secondary to esophageal trauma are related to the amount of time from diagnosis to intervention. Mortality doubles 24 hours after the injury. Esophageal perforations have a 12% to 36% survival rate if diagnosed and surgically treated within 24 hours, and after 24 hours, the mortality rate increases to 30% to 50%. The location of the injury is also important because the mortality varies by site; cervical injury mortality is 6%, thoracic mortality is 27%, and abdominal mortality is 21%. Spontaneous perforation of the esophagus has a 30% to 40% mortality, iatrogenic injuries have a 15% to 20% mortality, and direct trauma has a 5% to 10% mortality.

There are various and multicausal factors related to esophageal trauma that include:

- Blunt injuries
- Ingestion of caustic agents
- Endoscopic procedures
- Chronic vomiting
- Straining
- Seizures
- Foreign objects
- Instruments/tubes
- Ulcers
- Complications of esophageal surgery
- Open penetrating wounds

There are approximately 25,000 chemicals today known to cause chemical burns when ingested. These substances are classified by how they damage protein. See Table 56.3 for examples.

Pathophysiology and Clinical Manifestations

The pathophysiology of esophageal trauma is related to the cause of the trauma, and there are many factors that cause esophageal trauma. Common causes of esophageal trauma include ingestion of caustic substances, blunt injuries, open penetrating wounds, foreign-body ingestion, instrumentation

Table 56.3 Caustic Substances That Cause Chemical Burns When Ingested

Category of Caustic Agent	Examples of Common Caustic Substances
Oxidizing agents	Bleach, peroxide, etc.
Corrosives	Sulfuric acid, hydrochloric acid, etc.
Reducing agents	Ferrous ion, sulfite compounds, etc.
Desiccants	Calcium sulfate, silica gel, etc.
Vesicants	Sulfur, mustard, nitrogen mustard, etc.
Protoplasmic poisons	Hydrozoa acid, etc.

and tube placement, and spontaneous esophageal rupture and Mallory–Weiss syndrome.

Ingested caustic substances cause severe pain to the mouth, pharynx, and chest (behind the sternum and the epigastric area), and corrosive white crusts or chemical burns form in the mouth. Other clinical manifestations include gagging, excessive salivation (sialorrhea), glottic edema, dyspnea, aspiration pneumonia, hemorrhage, mediastinitis, peritonitis, and tracheoesophageal fistula. Long-term effects include wasting, long esophageal strictures, and progressive dysphagia. Progressive clinical manifestations occurring after 24 to 48 hours include damage to the kidney, liver, and possibly the central nervous system (CNS) secondary to toxic effects of the ingested substance; shock; and circulatory collapse.

Sulfuric acid is in many drain-cleaning products, and in adults, the most common cause of sulfuric acid ingestion is suicidal intentions. Strong acids have a pH of less than 2. The pH of an acid is less than 7 and greater than 0 on a 0-to-14 scale, with 7 being neutral, and the closer to 0, the stronger the acid. Many factors influence the degree of injury from caustic ingestion, but the major determinant is the amount of time that the chemical is in contact with the tissue. Ingestion of acids causes severe coughing and gagging, allowing the acid to make contact with the glottis and airway structures. Severe chemical epiglottitis and airway compromise can occur. Aspiration pneumonia is an unlikely side effect in conscious patients, but when it does occur, it increases the risk of death.

Alkalis tend to cause more harm to the esophagus and cause less injury to the stomach. Conversely, because of the resistant nature of squamous cell epithelium to acid, these acids cause more harm to the stomach and less to the esophagus. The esophagus is more sensitive to alkali substances. Alkalis with a pH greater than 11.5 tend to penetrate deeply into esophageal tissue and cause adjacent tissue damage. These burns tend to occur in areas of anatomical narrowing.

Treatment for ingestion of caustic agents includes analgesics, hydration, management of shock, nutritional support, tracheostomy, and high-dose steroids. Regularly scheduled endoscopy studies provide information to regulate steroid therapy and to develop a treatment plan. Dilation of esophageal strictures may be performed after 2 weeks.

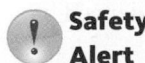 **Safety Alert** The following procedures are contraindicated in patients who have ingested a caustic substance:

- *Emetic administration* can reintroduce the caustic substance to esophageal tissue.
- *Neutralizing agents* are not useful because the damage already occurred upon exposure to the caustic substance.
- *Nasogastric tube insertion* via blind placement can lead to esophageal perforation or induce vomiting and cause reexposure to the caustic substance.
- *Activated charcoal* is not beneficial and can interfere with endoscopy testing.

Blunt injuries most often result from motor vehicle accidents. Esophageal tears can result from the impact of the driver's chest forcefully making contact with the steering wheel. Over time, localized necrosis to the esophageal wall occurs, and fistulas can develop. Clinical manifestations of esophageal trauma from blunt injuries include coughing upon swallowing. Esophageal rupture to the lower one-third of the esophagus is usually from blunt trauma. Surgical intervention is required to repair tears, fistulas, and esophageal ruptures. Open penetrating wounds occur most often in the cervical region of the spine, resulting from sharp objects that penetrate the neck or the upper chest. Common clinical manifestations include food or saliva coming from the wound. Minor wounds are treated by placing a feeding tube for 4 to 6 days in order to control mucosal damage and promote healing. Surgical management is used to treat large, open, penetrating wounds.

Foreign-body ingestion in adults usually occurs unintentionally. Some commonly ingested objects include fish or chicken bones, glass shards, parts of false teeth, nails, needles, and large fruit stones. Prisoners have been known to swallow cutlery. Foreign bodies typically lodge in the upper esophageal sphincter. Clinical manifestations associated with foreign-body ingestion include marked dysphagia, odynophagia, swelling of the neck, severe coughing, and neck stiffness. Pain is localized to the neck and retrosternal area. Severe pain in the back and behind the sternum indicates possible mediastinitis. Impacted foreign objects can cause necrosis to the wall of the esophagus, mediastinitis, pleuritis, peritonitis with abscess formation, and possible surgical emphysema. About 95% of small foreign bodies pass through the digestive tract and leave the body later in the stool. The patient's feces should be checked for up to a week or more to assess for the passage of the foreign body.

Instrumentation and tube placement are common causes of iatrogenic esophageal perforation. Instrumentation using esophagoscopy, especially during stricture dilation, can cause perforation. Placement of nasogastric and endotracheal tubes can also cause perforation. The most common sites of iatrogenic perforation are at the three sphincters, areas of esophageal stenosis, and the pyriform sinus.

Spontaneous esophageal rupture (Boerhaave's syndrome) occurs with sudden increased intraesophageal pressure related to vomiting or stenosis. This disorder is common in patients with alcohol abuse or chronic vomiting. The clinical presentation of Boerhaave's syndrome includes hematemesis, severe pain behind the sternum or between the shoulder blades, left upper quadrant pain, hypotension, pallor, dyspnea, and circulatory collapse. Treatment for Boerhaave's syndrome requires open surgical intervention with thoracotomy and antibiotic therapy.

Mallory–Weiss syndrome occurs from severe vomiting that infrequently causes a fatal hemorrhage in the esophagus or the GEJ. This disorder is often associated with chronic alcohol abuse, but other causes can be malignant tumors and hyperemesis gravidarum developing during pregnancy. Clinical manifestations include pallor, tachycardia, and possible shock. Bleeding usually resolves in 24 to 48 hours. Endoscopic or surgical intervention is necessary if bleeding does not resolve. This condition is rarely fatal.

Management

Medical Management

Therapeutic interventions for the treatment of esophageal trauma focus on control of any bleeding, wound management and drainage, prevention of infection, and providing nutrition. Interventions vary in relation to the cause, location, size, and degree of injury; contamination; duration of time from the injury; and the presence of other associated injuries. The clinical manifestations of esophageal trauma are often vague in relation to the amount of trauma and the potential for complications. Common clinical manifestations of esophageal trauma include pain, fever, dyspnea, and crepitus. Diagnostic tests include:

- Chest x-ray
- Chest CT
- Contrast esophagography

Medications used to treat esophageal injuries include broad-spectrum antibiotics, high-dose corticosteroids, opioid or nonopioid analgesics, and topical analgesics.

Surgical Management

The purpose of surgical management is to control bleeding, remove damaged tissue, repair wounds, resect part of the esophagus with gastric pull-through, or replace the esophagus with a bowel segment.

Complications

Complications of esophageal trauma include risks related to surgical or endoscopic procedures, straining, and injury. Esophageal rupture is a serious complication that is caused by external trauma or instrumentation of the esophagus, increased pressure within the esophagus from vomiting or retching, diseases of the esophagus, and corrosive esophagitis. Other complications related to esophageal trauma include:

- Infection
- Abscesses
- Subcutaneous emphysema in the neck
- Pneumothorax
- Shock
- Sepsis
- Respiratory impairment
- Esophageal mucosal burns
- Esophageal strictures
- Aspiration pneumonia
- Hemorrhage

Nursing Management

Assessment and Analysis

Management of the patient with esophageal trauma centers around the type of injury and the assessment of clinical manifestations related to the injury so that complications can be reduced or eliminated. Addressing any threat of cardiopulmonary complications is the top priority, followed by prevention of other complications, such as hemorrhage and infection, and maintaining nutritional support. Patients receive nothing by mouth (NPO) while diagnostic tests are performed to confirm the extent of the injury. Common manifestations related to the management of the patient with esophageal trauma are presented according to the type of injury.

Exposure of caustic substances in the oral cavity causes local epithelial trauma that can cause corrosive crusts or chemical burns in the mouth. Gagging, sialorrhea, glottis edema, dyspnea, hemorrhage, mediastinitis, peritonitis, tracheoesophageal fistula, perforation, kidney and liver damage, CNS damage, shock, circulatory collapse, and death are all possible consequences. Without prompt intervention, these clinical manifestations can occur as a result of accidental or intentional ingestion of a caustic substance.

Food and saliva present in a mediastinal wound can require placement of a feeding tube or surgical intervention. Patients remain NPO to allow the esophagus to heal. Irritation, mucosal ulceration, bleeding, obstruction, perforation, and death are all possible. Clinical manifestations of foreign-body ingestion include impaction of food or an object in the esophagus, usually bone fragments or meat in the esophagus. Esophageal impaction is a serious condition, and it can progressively lead to death.

Symptoms of Boerhaave's syndrome include spontaneous esophageal rupture, usually from vomiting. It can occur with a sudden increase in intraesophageal pressure and is often associated with alcohol abuse or chronic vomiting. Signs include hematemesis, pain behind the sternum and between the shoulder blades, left upper quadrant pain, hypotension, pallor, dyspnea, and circulatory collapse.

Symptoms of Mallory–Weiss syndrome occur from a tear in the esophageal mucosa or in the GEJ, usually brought on by excessive alcohol ingestion. Often, clinical manifestations resolve without treatment within 10 days. Signs include hematemesis, bloody stools, pallor, tachycardia, possible shock, and rarely death.

Nursing Diagnoses

- **Impaired swallowing** related to esophageal trauma as evidenced by coughing, gagging, or vomiting
- **Imbalanced nutrition**: Less than body requirements related to the inability to ingest food as evidenced by inadequate caloric intake
- **Acute pain** related to esophageal trauma as evidenced by unacceptable pain score or autonomic responses (changes in respirations, heart rate, and blood pressure, and diaphoresis)
- **Impaired oral mucous membranes** related to caustic ingestion as evidenced by chemical burns or ulcerations

Nursing Interventions

■ Assessments

- Airway, breath sounds, and oxygenation
  Dependent on the location of the esophageal trauma, the airway can be compromised by esophageal rupture with gastric contents and acid spilling as well as esophageal tissue edema.

- Vital signs

  Pulse rate, respiration, and blood pressure may be elevated with pain. With hemorrhage, sepsis, or shock, there may be a decrease in blood pressure with a compensatory increase in heart rate. Leakage from anastomosis sites of postoperative patients may produce clinical manifestations of early shock that include fever, tachycardia, and tachypnea.

- Chest pain

  Chest pain may be caused by esophageal trauma or damage by gastric secretions or ingestion of caustic agents.

- Level of consciousness

  Changes in level of consciousness are associated with septic or shock states.

- Serum electrolytes
  - Serum albumin

    Albumin levels below 2.5 g/dL indicate severe protein depletion.

  - Transferrin

    Transferrin is needed for iron transfer, and it usually decreases with albumin.

  - Serum potassium levels

    Serum potassium is lost in gastric secretions, particularly if the patient requires nasogastric suctioning.

- Complete blood count

  The red blood cell count may decrease secondary to blood loss or with malnutrition. The white blood cell count increases with the inflammation and infection associated with esophageal trauma.

- Daily weights

  Weight loss may occur related to decreased intake secondary to esophageal trauma.

■ Actions

- Low intermittent esophageal and gastric suction

  Gastric and esophageal suctioning allow the esophageal mucosa to rest and heal. Low, intermittent suction provides less trauma to the mucosa than constant suction.

- Keep patient NPO.

  Esophageal rest for more than a week allows time for the injury to heal.

- Provide nutrition.

  Total parenteral nutrition (TPN) provides calories and protein while the patient is NPO to promote healing nutrients.

- Administer antibiotics.

  Due to potential contamination by food or bacteria, broad-spectrum antibiotics are indicated to prevent or treat infection.

- Administer high-dose corticosteroids

  Suppresses inflammation and help prevent esophageal strictures

- Pain management

  Opioid and nonnarcotic analgesics are prescribed for pain. Topical analgesics and anti-inflammatory agents are used to treat burns to the oral mucosa.

■ Teaching

- Explain procedures, tests, medications, and discharge instructions.

  Compliance is greater when the patient understands all teaching as well as the rationale for ordered interventions.

- Signs of infection

  Because of esophageal trauma and risk of leakage, the patient should be taught to monitor temperature and site (as applicable) for signs of redness, tenderness, or drainage.

- Monitor weight.

  Due to the potential for impaired nutrition, it is important that the patient closely monitors for weight loss.

Evaluating Care Outcomes

Esophageal trauma has many causes and can lead to significant changes in nutritional intake. The management of esophageal trauma can be a serious and often fatal medical emergency that may require surgical intervention. Measures taken to control bleeding, infection, and airway management are necessary to prevent progressive complications. Prompt recognition and prevention of potential complications are of vital importance in obtaining favorable outcomes.

Connection Check 56.7

The nurse includes which information in the discharge teaching plan for the patient who sustained esophageal trauma?

A. Take ordered antibiotics until your temperature is normal.

B. Limit pain medications to times of severe pain.

C. Check your temperature every other day.

D. Notify your provider if increased drainage from the injured area is noted.

Making Connections

CASE STUDY: WRAP-UP

Mr. Rodriguez's 2-year survival rate is 95% because he is HPV positive. If he were HPV negative, his 2-year survival rate would have been 65%. He has just reached his second year with an uneventful recovery from surgery and radiation therapy. He is eating, drinking, and talking well. His weight is proportionate to his height. He stopped smoking 2 years ago using Chantix. He stopped drinking bourbon but says that he drinks a six-pack of beer each week with his friends. He continues to have a supportive relationship with his girlfriend, and they are planning to get married. Mr. Rodriguez has not had a raise in salary for 2 years, and he does not always have enough money to buy his medications. He ran out of Prilosec, and he says that is why his heartburn (he has GERD) is worse; he tries to stay away from spicy foods and fatty foods, but he drinks five cups of coffee each day. He sleeps with his head elevated at least 30 degrees, and he says this helps decrease his heartburn at night.

Case Study Questions

1. What type of collaborative care referral is of highest priority for Mr. Rodriguez before starting radiation therapy?

   A. Substance abuse consult

   B. Dental consult

   C. Nutrition consult

   D. Homehealth care referral

2. The nurse is screening Mr. Rodriguez for his risk of developing secondary stomatitis. What information in his history indicates the highest risk for developing secondary stomatitis?

   A. He is on amitriptyline, and he rinses his mouth after each meal with antiseptic mouthwash.

   B. He is on omeprazole (Prilosec), and he recently adopted a cat.

   C. He started radiation therapy 10 days ago, and he is on a methylprednisolone dose pack for poison ivy.

   D. He is on triamterene, and his roommate recently moved out.

3. Mr. Rodriguez reflects back on what may have contributed to the development of his tongue cancer. What risk factors did Mr. Rodriguez have? *(Select all that apply.)*

   A. He drank bourbon every day.

   B. He smoked cigarettes.

   C. He had poor oral hygiene.

   D. He consumed a high-fat diet.

   E. He had a sedentary lifestyle

4. Which statement made by Mr. Rodriguez indicates a need for interprofessional consultation to address his risk of Barrett's esophagus?

   A. "I have cut back to drinking a six-pack of beer each week."

   B. "I cannot afford to take Prilosec for my GERD."

   C. "I could not afford to take my antibiotic when they told me I had *H. pylori*."

   D. "My girlfriend tells me that I have bad breath."

5. What statement by Mr. Rodriguez indicates the need for additional teaching about the prescribed Prilosec (Omeprazole)?

   A. "I should take this medication when I eat spicy food."

   B. "I need to take this medication everyday to be effective."

   C. "This medicine works by decreasing the acid in my stomach."

   D. "This medication helps heal inflammation in my esophagus."

CHAPTER SUMMARY

The oral cavity is the entry point of the digestive system, and it houses the structures for breathing, chewing, tasting, and articulation. Impairment of the oral mucosa interrupts vital functions as well as sensory and social functions that allow individuals to interact and enjoy a satisfying quality of life. The cells of the mouth are especially vulnerable to injury and infection.

Stomatitis is a painful disorder that causes inflammation and ulceration of the lining of the mouth, making the delicate tissue of the oral mucosa susceptible to local and systemic infections. The causes of stomatitis are variable, ranging from infectious agents to medications, cancer treatments, irritants, vitamin deficiencies, diseases, and allergic causes. Good oral hygiene and optimal nutrition are essential in limiting the severity and complications related to stomatitis.

Hiatal hernia results from a weakened gastroesophageal junction (GEJ). Sliding hernias are often small and cause few or no symptoms. Larger sliding hernias cause symptoms related to gastroesophageal reflux disease (GERD). Chronic inflammation caused by GERD puts the patient at risk for development of Barrett's esophagus and adenocarcinoma. Type 2 paraesophageal hernias, or rolling hernias, occur when structural abnormalities allow part of the stomach to roll through the esophageal hiatus, forming a pouch of stomach above the diaphragm and next to the esophagus that can be small or large. Paraesophageal hernias left untreated can become larger over time, and the following complications can include the development of a giant intrathoracic stomach, volvulus, incarceration, and strangulation. Surgical candidates include patients with sliding hernias who are not responding to medical treatment and patients with large paraesophageal hernias.

Medication management for both hiatal hernia with reflux and GERD consists of antacids, histamine-2-receptor agonists, proton pump inhibitors, and prokinetic medications. Patients with sliding hernias usually have symptoms of GERD. Lifestyle changes such as weight control and avoiding foods and substances that decrease lower esophageal pressure can decrease the development of GERD and Barrett's esophagus.

The majority of oral cancers are squamous cell carcinomas (SCCAs). Lifestyle choices related to alcohol use, tobacco, and poor oral hygiene are well-known causes. Oral cancer does not usually present with clinical manifestations until it has progressed to later stages. The treatments for oral cancer have functional and quality-of-life implications. The prognosis of oral cancer is determined by location, size of the tumor, and metastasis using the TNM clinical classification.

Oral trauma may be a life-threatening emergency because of the risk of airway compromise secondary to soft tissue edema and bleeding in the mouth. Once the airway and bleeding are controlled, these types of injuries require surgical stabilization followed by comprehensive follow-up care. The patient must be monitored for airway stability, nutritional intake, and potential risk for infection.

Esophageal cancer, like oral cancer, is usually asymptomatic until later stages, with a poor outcome for recovery. The esophagus is lined with squamous cells. Cancers of the esophagus typically are either SCCA or adenocarcinoma. Squamous cell carcinoma usually affects the upper two-thirds of the esophagus, whereas adenocarcinoma affects the lower one-third of the esophagus, usually at the GEJ. The development of adenocarcinoma is related to GERD. Disruption of esophageal function affects the ability of the patient to acquire adequate nutrition and maintain a healthy weight.

Surgery, radiation therapy and chemotherapy, and endoscopic and minimally invasive procedures are used to manage esophageal cancer.

Esophageal trauma interferes with the patient's ability to swallow and to obtain nourishment. Most of these injuries occur accidentally, but some are self-inflicted. Outcomes of esophageal trauma are related to early treatment, the etiology of the trauma, and the severity and location of the trauma. Esophageal rupture or perforation can lead to circulatory collapse, shock, hemorrhage, and death. Surgical and endoscopic procedures are used to treat esophageal trauma.

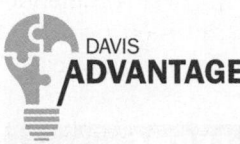

To explore learning resources for this chapter, go to **Davis Advantage** and find:
- Answers to in-text questions
- Chapter Resources and Activities
- NCLEX®-Style Chapter Review Questions
- Bibliography

Chapter 57

Coordinating Care for Patients With Stomach Disorders

Kristy Gorman

Finding Connections

CASE STUDY: EPISODE 1

Follow this patient throughout the chapter.

Mrs. Sharon Taylor is a 37-year-old graphic designer. Over the last several months, she has had increased episodes of a burning sensation near the midline in the epigastrium and back. Her pain has been alleviated after eating. Mrs. Taylor has had recent episodes of pain waking her up a few nights a week. Mrs. Taylor schedules a visit to her advanced practice registered nurse (APRN). While she describes the pain pattern to her provider, the provider gathers additional information. On the basis of her history, the provider refers Mrs. Taylor to an internist who orders an endoscopy. The provider explains that the endoscopy allows visualization of the esophageal, gastric, and duodenal mucosal linings, as well as allowing tissue samples to be obtained for biopsy during the procedure…

INTRODUCTION

The stomach is part of the upper gastrointestinal (GI) system that is responsible for much of the digestive process. The stomach receives food from the esophagus and acts as a reservoir that permits eating large amounts of food at intervals of several hours. Food contained in the stomach is mixed, churned, and transported into the duodenum. The first stages of protein and carbohydrate digestion occur in the stomach. Very few substances are absorbed across the gastric mucosa (stomach lining), but water and alcohol are absorbed.

A person's nutritional status depends not only on the type and amount of intake but also on proper gastric functioning. Although only a few diseases affect the stomach, they can be very serious and in some cases life threatening. The most common disorders include **gastritis** (inflammation of the gastric lining), gastroenteritis, peptic ulcer disease (PUD), and gastric cancer, and each of these disorders can affect digestion and nutrition.

The gastric mucosa in the stomach wall contains many deep glands (Fig. 57.1), and these glands contain parietal (oxyntic) cells, which secrete hydrochloric acid and intrinsic factor, and chief (zymogen, peptic) cells, which secrete pepsinogens (Fig. 57.2). These secretions aid in the digestion and absorption of nutrients. Several of the glands open on a common chamber called the *gastric pit* at the surface of the mucosa. Mucus is secreted along with bicarbonate by mucous cells on the surface of the epithelium, creating a viscoelastic and highly alkaline gel to lubricate and protect the GI tract wall. Important mediators of these protective mechanisms include nitric oxide, intrinsic nerves, peptides, and prostaglandins. Prostaglandins exert their effect through improved mucosal blood flow, decreased hydrochloric acid

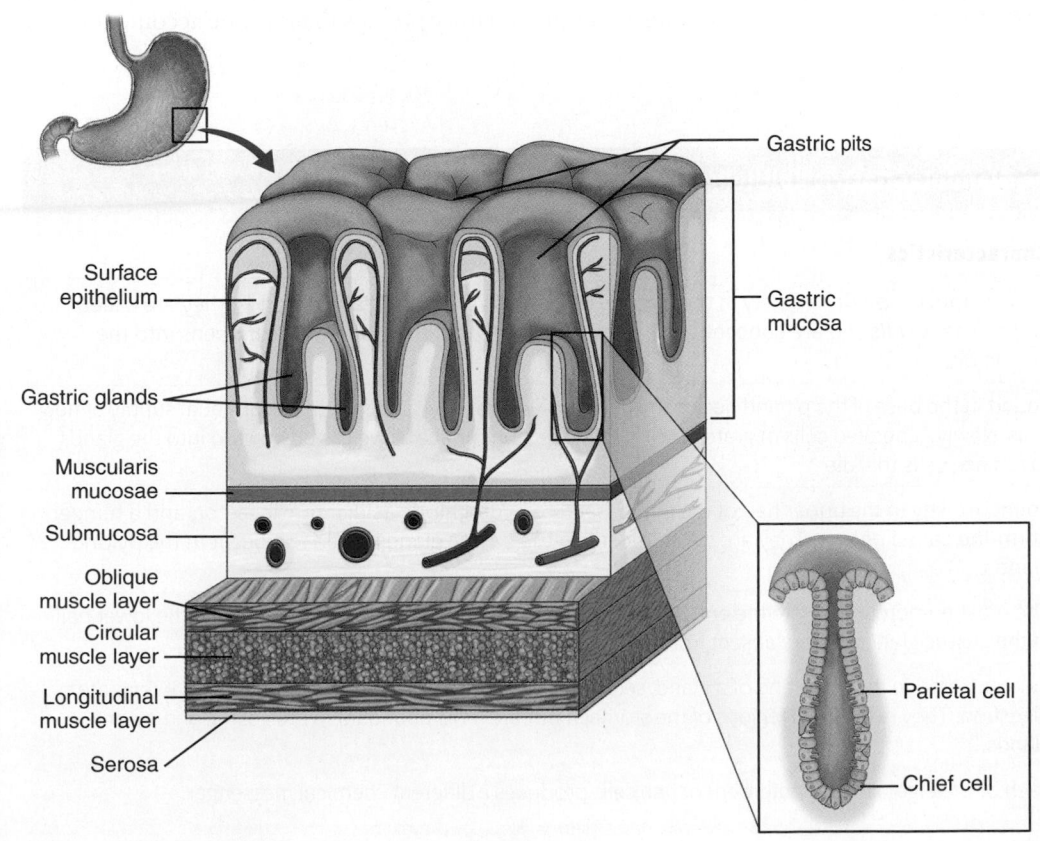

Gastric pits

Surface epithelium

Gastric mucosa

Gastric glands

Muscularis mucosae

Submucosa

Oblique muscle layer

Circular muscle layer

Longitudinal muscle layer

Serosa

Parietal cell

Chief cell

FIGURE 57.1 Microscopic anatomy of the stomach wall.

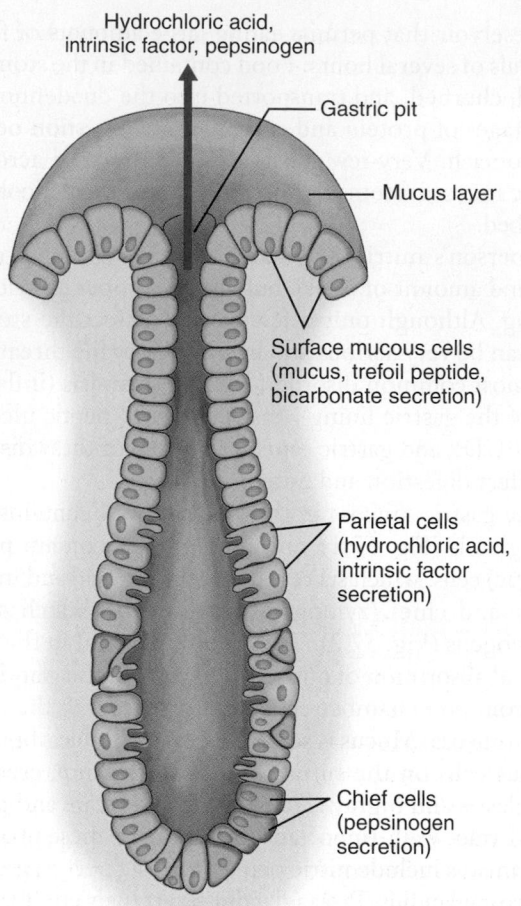

Hydrochloric acid, intrinsic factor, pepsinogen

Gastric pit

Mucus layer

Surface mucous cells (mucus, trefoil peptide, bicarbonate secretion)

Parietal cells (hydrochloric acid, intrinsic factor secretion)

Chief cells (pepsinogen secretion)

FIGURE 57.2 Structure of a gastric gland from the fundus and body of the stomach. These acid- and pepsinogen-producing glands are referred to as "oxyntic" glands in some sources.

secretion, increased bicarbonate secretion, and enhanced mucus production. The epithelial cells in the mucosal layer of the stomach have a high turnover rate and are replaced every 4 to 5 days. Because of the regenerative abilities of the mucosal layer, injury to this layer heals rapidly without leaving scar tissue (Table 57.1).

GASTRITIS

Gastritis is a localized or patchy inflammation of the gastric mucosa and may be acute (lasting several hours to a few days) or chronic, resulting from repeated exposures to irritating agents or recurring episodes of acute gastritis. When the gastric mucosa is damaged by agents such as aspirin, nonsteroidal anti-inflammatory drugs (NSAIDs), ethyl alcohol, or bile salts, this barrier is disrupted, and hydrogen ions move into the tissue. While the hydrogen ions build up in the mucosal cells, intracellular pH (acidity) decreases, enzymatic reactions deteriorate, and cellular structures are disrupted. Aspirin and NSAIDs inhibit prostaglandin synthesis, which also disrupts the integrity of the mucosal surface. Hydrochloric acid can then diffuse back into the mucosa and injure small vessels. This causes edema, hemorrhage, and ulceration of the stomach's lining.

Types of Gastritis

As described earlier, gastritis may be acute, lasting several hours to a few days, or chronic, resulting from repeated exposures to irritating agents or recurring episodes of acute gastritis. **Acute gastritis** is characterized by an acute mucosal inflammatory process that may be accompanied by

---

Table 57.1	Cell Types in the Glandular Gastric Epithelium

Types of Cells	Characteristics
Mucous cells	Secrete mucus, predominately in the cardiac and pyloric glands. In gastric glands, they are called *mucous neck cells* and are concentrated in the narrow neck of the gland where it opens into the gastric pit.
Regenerative (stem) cells	Found in the base of the pit and neck of the gland, divide rapidly, and produce a continual supply of new cells. Newly generated cells migrate upward to the gastric surface as well as downward into the glands to replace cells that die.
Parietal cells	Found mostly in the upper half of the gland; secrete hydrochloric acid, intrinsic factor, and a hunger hormone called *ghrelin*. They are found mostly in the gastric glands, but a few occur in the pyloric glands.
Chief cells	The most numerous. Secrete the enzymes gastric lipase and pepsinogen. They dominate the lower half of the gastric glands but are absent from cardiac and pyloric glands.
Enteroendocrine cells	Concentrated in the lower end of a gland; secrete hormones and paracrine messengers that regulate digestion. They occur in all regions of the stomach but are most abundant in the gastric and pyloric glands.
	Each of the eight kinds of enteroendocrine cells produces a different chemical messenger.

hemorrhage into the mucosa. Early clinical manifestations may include a thickened, reddened mucous membrane with extrusive rugae, or longitudinal folds. Various degrees of mucosal necrosis and inflammatory reaction occur in acute gastritis, and in severe cases, sloughing of the surface mucosa may lead to acute GI bleeding.

Chronic gastritis is prolonged, persistent, or intermittent inflammation of the gastric mucosa and is characterized by patchy, diffuse inflammation of the mucosal lining of the stomach. The presence of chronic inflammatory changes eventually leads to atrophy of the glandular epithelium of the stomach. The major types of chronic gastritis include *Helicobacter pylori* gastritis (the most common), autoimmune gastritis, and **atrophic gastritis** which is a type of chronic gastritis that is seen most often in older adults. *H pylori* infection, which is prevalent in approximately half of the world's population, is known to be a key cause of chronic gastric inflammation that progresses to atrophy, characterized by total loss of fundal glands, minimal inflammation, thinning of the gastric mucosa leading to atrophy, and abnormal cellular changes. These alterations can lead to peptic ulcers and gastric cancer. The combination of bacterial factors, environmental insults, and the host immune response that drives the initiation and progression of mucosal atrophy, metaplasia, and dysplasia, leads toward gastric cancer.

Epidemiology

Acute gastritis may be caused by chronic ingestion of irritating foods and alcohol or a complication of acute illnesses including traumatic injuries, such as burns, severe infection, hepatic, renal, or respiratory failure, or major surgery. Endotoxins released from infecting bacteria such as staphylococci, *Escherichia coli*, and *Salmonella* can lead to gastritis by immune cell infiltration and cytokine production. Bacterial and viral infections are often considered food poisoning because contaminated food is the usual route of entry.

Overuse of aspirin and other NSAIDs is a high risk factor for acute gastritis, with risk factors including alcohol, cytotoxic agents, caffeine, corticosteroids, and antimetabolites. Acute gastritis is also caused by local irritation from radiation therapy and ingestion of poisons (e.g., dichlorodiphenyltrichloroethane [DDT], ammonia, mercury, and carbon tetrachloride).

Erosive or stress-induced gastritis (a severe form of acute gastritis) is a complication of conditions such as shock, severe trauma, or major surgery and is most likely due to inadequate gastric mucosal blood flow during periods of intense physiological stress. Adequate mucosal blood flow is important to maintain the mucosal barrier and to buffer any back-diffused hydrogen ions. When blood flow is inadequate, these processes fail, and mucosal breakdown occurs.

Pathophysiology

The most common cause of gastritis is *H pylori*. Other causes of gastritis include alcohol, NSAIDs, Crohn's disease, tuberculosis, and bile reflux. These agents cause injury by different mechanisms. In general, the infectious and inflammatory causes result in immune cell infiltration and cytokine production, which damage mucosal cells. Irritating agents such as alcohol, aspirin, and bile generally work to disrupt the mucosal barrier, causing mucosal damage by back diffusion of hydrogen ions. This process allows gastric juices to come into contact with the gastric tissue, producing mucosal reddening, edema, and superficial surface erosion. Ulceration may occur and can lead to hemorrhage.

Connection Check 57.1

The nurse is screening patients for their risk of developing acute gastritis. The nurse should consider which patient at greatest risk?

A. A 25-year-old woman who has a vegan diet
B. A 32-year-old man who takes ibuprofen daily
C. A 77-year-old man who smokes
D. An 80-year-old woman who takes low-dose aspirin daily for atrial fibrillation

Chronic gastritis and prolonged inflammation of the stomach may be caused either by chronic local irritation or by the bacterium *H pylori*. Chronic gastritis has also been associated with the presence of antibodies to parietal cells and intrinsic factor. The intrinsic factor is critical for absorption of vitamin B_{12}. When body stores of vitamin B_{12} are depleted, hemoglobin cannot be synthesized and **pernicious anemia** results.

The most common form of chronic gastritis is caused by *H pylori* infection. *Helicobacter pylori* has an estimated rate of infection of over half of the world's population and could reach up to 70% in developing countries and up to 20% to 30% in industrialized countries. The incidence of *H pylori* increases in people older than 60, and transmission is likely person-to-person by vomitus, saliva, feces, or inadequately treated drinking water. *Helicobacter pylori* may also come from contaminated food that has not been washed well or cooked properly.

It is not known for certain how *H pylori* spreads, so prevention is difficult. Vaccines are under development to prevent or even cure *H pylori* infection. To help prevent infection, it is advised that people wash their hands with soap and water after using the bathroom and before eating, eat food that has been washed well and cooked properly, and drink water from a clean, safe source.

Helicobacter pylori is a spiral-shaped, gram-negative microorganism that can colonize the highly acidic human stomach. *H pylori* has multiple flagella, which assist in migrating deep within the gastric and duodenal mucosa. The bacteria have the ability to sense pH and produce large amounts of urease, which buffers the acidity of the environment. Urease catalyzes the hydrolysis of urea to create ammonia and ammonium ions, resulting in the pH elevation of the environment. By creating a neutral environment, *H pylori* reduces the viscoelasticity of the mucus, in turn permitting it to swim freely to penetrate the mucous layer and attach to epithelial cells beneath, where it can cause inflammation over the course of lifelong infection. The reduction in the viscoelasticity impacts the integrity of the mucous layer, compromising its function as a protective barrier against acid. The persistent inflammation extends deep into the mucosa, causing destruction of the gastric glands, metaplasia (cellular changes), and atrophy (cell loss). The mechanism of atrophy has been shown to be directly related to effects of bacterial toxins and the cytokine environment within the gastric mucosa. More virulent bacterial strains and a permissive host immune response are strongly associated with atrophy and progression to severe disease.

Clinical Manifestations

The clinical presentation of gastritis is associated with the damage to the gastric mucosa and typically includes epigastric pain, nausea and vomiting, weight loss, decreased appetite, and changes in color of the stool. Pain may be exacerbated with the ingestion of spicy foods. With atrophic gastritis, there may be no symptoms. In patients with acute gastritis or exacerbations of chronic gastritis, there may be evidence of dehydration or upper GI bleeding. With significant fluid or blood loss, the patient may develop signs of hypovolemic shock including pallor, tachycardia, and hypotension.

Management

Medical Management

Diagnosis

The diagnosis of gastritis cannot be based exclusively on clinical manifestations. The gross endoscopic diagnosis of gastritis correlates poorly with histological findings and is somewhat useless as a diagnosis without confirmatory biopsy. Additionally, there is poor correlation between clinical presentation and histological gastritis.

An upper GI x-ray series or endoscopy and histological examination of a tissue specimen obtained by biopsy may be useful for ruling out disorders that can suggest gastritis, such as gastric polyps and gastric neoplasms. If hemorrhage is suspected, stools may be tested until they are negative for **occult** (hidden) blood. Fecal occult blood can be detected by simple tests (e.g., guaiac, Hematest, Hemoccult) that cause color changes in samples of feces in the presence of blood.

Urea breath testing can be used to detect active infection with *H pylori*. A baseline breath test is first obtained. The patient then drinks a urea solution that contains a special carbon atom. *Helicobacter pylori* secretes an enzyme, urease, which breaks down the urea, releasing the carbon. Blood carries the carbon dioxide (CO_2) to the lungs, and it is expelled in the breath. The amount of CO_2 is compared to the baseline sample. A positive urea breath test reveals low levels of exhaled carbon-13. Other tests for *H pylori* infection include serological testing and fecal antigen testing.

Treatment

Collaborative care for the patient with acute gastritis is directed toward supportive care for relieving the clinical manifestations and removing or reducing the cause of discomfort. Healing is spontaneous and may occur within a few days. Gastrointestinal rest should be provided by 6 to 12 hours of NPO status, then slow reintroduction of clear liquids (broth, tea, gelatin, carbonated beverages), followed by ingestion of heavier liquids (cream soups, puddings, milk), and finally a gradual reintroduction of solid food. It is also important to eliminate irritating foods such as caffeine and spicy foods. If nausea and vomiting threaten fluid and electrolyte balance, IV fluids and electrolytes are ordered.

Medications are used to relieve pain and discomfort. Medications that block and buffer gastric acid secretions for pain relief are usually prescribed, including proton pump inhibitors (PPIs) and H_2-receptor antagonists. Proton pump inhibitors act by inhibiting H^+/K^+-ATPase enzyme in the gastric parietal cells. It is this enzyme that is responsible for the production of hydrochloric acid in the stomach. Esomeprazole, lansoprazole, or pantoprazole 30 to 60 mg intravenously twice daily may be given initially, increased as necessary to maintain intragastric pH greater than 4.

Antacids are generally aluminum- or magnesium-containing compounds that decrease gastric acidity by neutralizing the acid (Maalox, Mylanta). They also have been shown to heal ulcers successfully by binding bile acids, inhibiting pepsin, promoting growth of new blood vessels in injured mucosa, increasing local prostaglandin synthesis, and binding growth factors, which increases their concentration at areas of mucosal injury. Sucralfate (Carafate) may also be prescribed. Sucralfate has no effect on gastric pH but provides a physical barrier to prevent mucosal damage by gastric acid. It does this by binding to the granulation tissue in exposed ulcer beds. The combination of antacids and sucralfate should be avoided because of the potential formation of a solid mass. Patients with chronic gastritis may require long-term parenteral or oral vitamin B_{12} supplementation for the prevention or treatment of pernicious anemia.

Although they are not routinely recommended unless a life-threatening consequence ensues, there are a wide variety of treatment regimens available for eradicating infections in individuals with clinical manifestations of disease attributable to *H pylori*. The success of *H pylori* cure depends on the type and duration of therapy, patient compliance, and factors such as antibiotic resistance. There are various treatment regimens for *H pylori* eradication, and most include the combination of a PPI with two antibiotics for 7 to 14 days. Using combinations of antimicrobial agents reduces the risk of antibiotic-resistant *H pylori* strains. Triple therapies are recommended as first-line treatments. Quadruple therapy is recommended as second-line treatment when triple therapies fail (Table 57.2).

Table 57.2   Common Treatment Regimens for *Helicobacter pylori*

Treatment Regimen	Eradication Rates (%)	Comments
Triple Therapy Proton pump inhibitor (PPI) *plus* Clarithromycin 500 mg twice daily or metronidazole 500 mg twice daily *plus* Amoxicillin 1 g twice daily for 7–14 days	73–86	Often used as first-line therapy; in the United States, recommendation is to treat for at least 10 days
OR		
PPI *plus* Clarithromycin 500 mg twice daily *plus* Metronidazole 500 mg twice daily for 7–14 days	70–85	May be used as first-line therapy in penicillin-allergic patients
Quadruple Therapy Bismuth subsalicylate 525 mg four times daily *plus* Metronidazole 250 mg orally four times daily *plus* Tetracycline 500 mg orally four times daily *plus* PPI twice daily (or ranitidine 150 mg orally twice daily) for 10–14 days	75–90	Usually used as second-line therapy in patients who fail to respond to triple therapy
Levofloxacin-Based Triple Therapy PPI twice daily *plus* Levofloxacin 250–500 mg twice daily *plus* Amoxicillin 1 g twice daily for 10 days	60–80	Often recommended for second-line or rescue therapy
Sequential Therapy PPI twice daily *plus* Amoxicillin 1 g twice daily for the first 5 days followed by PPI twice daily *plus* Clarithromycin 500 mg twice daily and tinidazole 500 mg twice daily for the next 5 days	83–98	Overall eradication rate greater than 90%; recommended for second-line or rescue therapy but may also be considered for initial therapy

From Greenberger, N., Blumberg, R., & Burakoff, R. (2016). *Current diagnosis & treatment gastroenterology, hepatology, & endoscopy* (3rd ed.). New York, NY: McGraw-Hill; Crowe, S. (2014, June). Treatment regimens for *Helicobacter pylori*. Retrieved from www.UpToDate.com

Diet

The patient's daily caloric needs, food preferences, and eating pattern must be taken into consideration. The patient is instructed to avoid spicy foods and other foods noted to exacerbate symptoms. Bland, nonspicy diets and smaller frequent meals have been known to minimize gastric distress. The patient is also warned to avoid aspirin. If clinical manifestations persist, the patient may take antacids. The patient is also advised to be sure that foods and water are safe, to protect themselves against exposure to toxic substances (e.g., lead and nickel), and to quit smoking.

Connection Check 57.2

The nurse recognizes that the treatment of *H pylori* includes which medications? *(Select all that apply)*.

A. PPIs
B. Antiemetics
C. Antibiotics
D. NSAIDs
E. Antacids

Surgical Management

In the rare patient requiring surgical intervention for severe hemorrhagic gastritis, the options include vagotomy (surgery to sever the vagus nerve to reduce secretion of acid within the stomach), partial or total **gastrectomy** (removal of the stomach), or **pyloroplasty** (enlarging the pylorus opening). Such surgery is necessary only if more conservative measures have failed to control the bleeding. Surgical interventions are discussed in further detail in the Peptic Ulcer Disease section.

Nursing Management

Assessment and Analysis

Gastritis is a condition in which the stomach lining is inflamed and refers specifically to abnormal inflammation in the stomach lining. Many people with gastritis have no symptoms. Those who are symptomatic may experience dyspepsia—upper abdominal discomfort or pain, nausea, or vomiting. Clinical manifestations include:

- Epigastric pain
- Nausea and vomiting
- Decreased appetite
- Weight loss
- Changes in color of the stool

Nursing Diagnoses

- **Acute pain** related to irritated stomach mucosa
- **Anxiety** related to treatment
- **Deficient knowledge** about dietary management and the disease process
- **Risk for deficient fluid volume** related to insufficient fluid intake and excessive fluid loss subsequent to vomiting

Nursing Interventions

▪ Assessments

- Vital signs
  Increased heart rate and decreased blood pressure are caused by fluid volume deficit from vomiting or blood loss.
- History of presenting signs and symptoms
  Heartburn, indigestion, and nausea and/or vomiting are clinical manifestations of gastritis. Dyspepsia (heartburn) may occur after ingestion of certain medications (aspirin/ NSAIDs) or alcohol. Gastritis caused by endotoxins (food poisoning) has an abrupt onset.
- Laboratory assessment for *H pylori*
  Breath and stool analyses are non-invasive ways to test for H pylori. Carbon-13 urea breath test determines the presence of bacteria. Enzyme-linked immunosorbent assay (ELISA) stool testing can detect the H pylori antigen in a fresh stool specimen.
- Serum electrolytes
  In the patient with vomiting, the serum potassium may be low due to loss in the vomitus. With fluid deficit, the serum sodium may be elevated.
- Intake and output
  Pain and decreased appetite may limit the patient's intake of food and fluid, and fluid loss may lead to dizziness, tachycardia, and hypotension.

▪ Actions

- Administer IV fluids as prescribed
  Fluid replacement is prescribed in patients with severe fluid loss. If nausea and vomiting threaten fluid and electrolyte balance, IV fluids and electrolytes are ordered.
- Administer H_2-receptor antagonists as prescribed
  H_2-receptor antagonists block gastric secretions.
- Administer antacids as prescribed
  Antacids are used as buffering agents to correct the pH balance of the acidic gastric environment.
- Administer PPIs as prescribed
  Antisecretory agents (PPIs) can be used to suppress gastric acid secretion.

▪ Teaching

- Immediately report **hematemesis** (vomiting of blood)
  Hemorrhagic gastritis may lead to vomiting of blood. The vomited blood can be bright red or can have a dark "coffee grounds" appearance. Immediate correction of blood loss may be required to prevent hemorrhagic shock and is dependent on the amount of blood loss and the rate of bleeding.
- Take medications as prescribed
  It is important to take medications as prescribed, even if the symptoms are relieved, until discontinued by the prescriber. Teach patients not to take other over-the-counter medications if they are taking related prescribed medications, and it is best to review these medications with their healthcare provider.
- Avoid medications and other irritants that are associated with gastric episodes
  Read all over-the-counter drug labels that may contain NSAIDs or aspirin. Limit intake of food and spices that

cause gastric episodes, such as caffeine, citrus juices, or hot spices. A bland, nonspicy diet combined with smaller, more frequent meals may prevent distress.

- Follow prescribed dietary teaching regarding types of foods and how to introduce back into the diet. *Gastrointestinal rest should be provided by 6 to 12 hours of NPO status, then slow reintroduction of clear liquids, followed by ingestion of heavier liquids, and finally a gradual reintroduction of solid food. It is also important to eliminate irritating foods such as caffeine and spicy foods.*

Evaluating Care Outcomes

The patient can recover in approximately 1 day because of the ability of gastric mucosa to repair itself. The patient's appetite may be diminished for approximately 2 to 3 days. Patients with gastritis can achieve full recovery by complying with the prescribed therapy and avoiding irritating substances such as caffeine, alcohol, and NSAIDs. Expected outcomes include vital signs within normal limits, decreased pain, report of less anxiety, and compliance with the therapeutic regimen. The patient and family should be knowledgeable of the signs of gastritis and what clinical manifestations should reported to their healthcare provider.

Connection Check 57.3

The nurse recognizes which gastric disorder as a complication of inadequate mucosal perfusion secondary to intense physiological stress?
A. Erosive gastritis
B. Chronic gastritis
C. Duodenal ulcers
D. Esophageal reflux

GASTROENTERITIS

Gastroenteritis is a self-limiting illness of the digestive system in which inflammation of the lining of the stomach and small intestines produces watery diarrhea, abdominal pain or cramping, nausea or vomiting, and sometimes fever. Most cases are infectious, although gastroenteritis may occur after ingestion of medications and chemical toxins (e.g., metals, plant substances). Gastroenteritis may also be called the "stomach flu", traveler's diarrhea, or food poisoning.

Epidemiology

Infectious gastroenteritis may be caused by ingestion of a virus, bacteria, or parasite. Viruses are the leading cause of acute gastroenteritis in the United States. Viral spread may be transmitted from person to person by fecal-oral route of contaminated food and water, or by airborne transmission, as in norovirus. The viruses most commonly implicated are Norovirus and Rotavirus. Other viruses that may cause gastroenteritis include adenoviruses, echoviruses, and coxsackieviruses. Many types of bacteria cause foodborne illnesses, and the most generally implicated are *Staphylococcus aureus*, *Salmonella*, *Shigella*, *Clostridium botulinum*, *Clostridium perfringens*, *Campylobacter* and *Escherichia coli*. Bacteria may cause gastroenteritis by several mechanisms:

- *Salmonella* and *Campylobacter* – ingesting raw or undercooked poultry, seafood, unpasteurized milk
- *Campylobacter* - ingesting raw or undercooked chicken and unpasteurized milk; also may be transmitted by dogs or cats with diarrhea
- *Salmonella* - ingesting undercooked eggs and by contact with reptiles, birds, or amphibians.
- *Shigella* - transmitted person to person by fecal-oral route or foodborne

Organisms such as *E coli* and *Clostridium* species are normal enteric flora found in the large intestine. Pathogenic strains can cause gastroenteritis, and *E Coli* O157:H7 is the strain that causes the most severe illness. Parasites such as *Ascaris*, *Enterobius*, and *Trichinella spiralis*; *Giardia* and *Cryptosporidium* may cause gastroenteritis. It is typically acquired via person-to-person transmission (often in day care centers) or from ingesting contaminated water.

Other causes of gastroenteritis may include adverse effects from antibiotics, enzyme deficiencies, food allergens and ingestion of toxins, such as poisonous plants or metals. Studies suggest that the use of acid-suppressing medications such as proton pump inhibitors (PPIs) may increase the risk of developing gastroenteritis by reducing the acidic environment that provides an initial defense against gastrointestinal infections. Proton pump inhibitor therapy is also suggested to be a risk factor for the development and recurrence of *C difficile* colitis as well as increasing the risk of *Campylobacter* gastroenteritis.

Pathophysiology

The bowel reacts to the various causes of gastroenteritis with increased luminal fluid that cannot be absorbed. This causes abdominal pain, vomiting, severe diarrhea, followed by the depletion of intracellular fluid resulting in dehydration and electrolyte loss. Studies of rotaviruses found the virus attaches and enters mature enterocytes at the tips of small intestinal villi, causing structural changes to the small bowel mucosa. Consequently, maldigestion of carbohydrates occurs causing an accumulation in the intestinal lumen. This leads to malabsorption of nutrients and a concomitant inhibition of water reabsorption.

Bacterial gastroenteritis is less common than viral, but also results in diarrhea from various causes. Certain bacteria produce enterotoxins, exotoxins, or spread by mucosal invasion.

- Enterotoxins (produced by *E coli* and *C difficile*) adhere to the intestinal mucosa but do not invade. These toxins stimulate adenylate cyclase, which produces hypersecretion of fluid and electrolytes, resulting in watery diarrhea.

- Exotoxins are produced by bacteria such as *Staphylococcus aureus*, *C perfringens*, and *Bacillus cereus*. These toxins generally cause nausea, vomiting, and diarrhea within 12 hours of ingestion of contaminated food. Symptoms usually resolve within 36 hours.
- Mucosal invasion occurs with bacteria such as *Shigella*, *Salmonella*, *Campylobacter*, *Clostridium difficile*, some *E coli* subtypes that invade the mucosa of the small bowel or colon and cause small ulcerations, bleeding, protein-rich fluid excess, and secretion of electrolytes and water. The resulting diarrhea contains WBCs and RBCs and sometimes gross blood.

The *Giardia intestinalis* parasites adhere to or invade the intestinal mucosa, causing nausea, vomiting, diarrhea, and general malaise. The infection can become chronic and cause a malabsorption syndrome.

Clinical Manifestations

The clinical presentation of gastroenteritis includes diarrhea, nausea, vomiting, anorexia, abdominal distention and discomfort, poor skin turgor, dehydration, hyperactive bowel sounds, decreased blood pressure and dry mucus membranes. *Clostridium botulinum* and some chemicals affect the nervous system, causing clinical manifestations such as headache, tingling or numbness of the skin, blurred vision, weakness, dizziness, and paralysis.

Management

Medical Management

Diagnosis

Diagnosis is made by clinical evaluation or by stool culture, although PCR (assays used to screen for specific organisms), and immunoassays are increasingly used. Stool testing is guided by assessment findings and the organisms that are suspected based on patient history and epidemiologic factors (e.g., immunosuppression, exposure to a known outbreak, recent travel, recent antibiotic use). Cases are typically stratified into

- Acute watery diarrhea (most likely viral)
- Subacute or chronic watery diarrhea (may be parasitic)
- Acute inflammatory diarrhea without blood and presence of WBCs (may indicate bacterial)
- Acute inflammatory diarrhea with blood (test for *E coli* and *C difficile*)
- Diarrhea with gross blood (test for amebic dysentery, shigellosis, and *E. coli* O157:H7 infection; rule out ulcerative colitis via sigmoidoscopy)

A gram stain of a stool culture (by direct rectal swab), or blood culture may be performed to show the causative bacteria. The stool is checked for ova and parasites. Performing a rapid antigen testing of stool identifies rotavirus infection.

Treatment

Supportive treatment, including oral or IV rehydration is all that is needed for most patients. Antidiarrheal agents such as Loperamide hydrochloride (Imodium) may be used if fever is absent and stools are free of blood and *C difficile* or *E coli* O157:H7 infection is not suspected. Oral bismuth subsalicylate may be given for relief of abdominal cramping. Antibiotics are prescribed only in select cases and should not be given until stool culture results are known. An antiemetic may be beneficial if the patient is vomiting.

Diet

Initially, clear liquids are prescribed as tolerated. Oral glucose-electrolyte solutions, broth, or bouillon may prevent dehydration or treat mild dehydration. Even if vomiting, encourage the patient to take frequent small sips of such fluids; vomiting may subside with volume replacement. Gradually reintroduce foods starting with bland and easy-to-digest foods. Caffeine and milk products should be avoided.

Nursing Management

Assessment and Analysis

Patient history focuses on severity of diarrhea and dehydration. The onset, frequency, quantity, and duration of diarrhea and vomiting are key factors in assessing patient status. Data regarding oral intake, urine output, and weight loss is collected and the patient is asked about recent travel history (including cruise ships), eating history, and day care history. Ruling out other diagnoses is important. Mucus or gross blood in the stool almost always indicates bacterial or parasitic infection.

Nursing Diagnoses

- **Acute Pain** related to inflammation
- **Diarrhea** related to GI dysfunction, infection, and toxins
- **Dysfunctional Gastrointestinal Motility** related to diet, food intolerance, nutritional status, toxins or ingested contaminated material, and treatment regimen

Nursing Interventions
▪ *Assessments*

- Vital signs, including orthostatic measurements
  Decreased intravascular fluid volume due to loss of body fluid causes a drop in blood pressure and elevated heart rate. Orthostatic vital signs are performed to assess for fluid volume deficit. Tachycardia with hypotension occurs with hypovolemia.
- Abdomen for distention
  Distention occurs when increased fluid and gas can't pass freely through the GI tract.
- Bowel sounds and bowel elimination pattern
  Hyperactive bowel sounds can be characterized as loud, gurgling, splashing, or rushing; they're higher pitched and occur more frequently than normal bowel sounds. Hyperactive bowel sounds follow sudden nausea and vomiting.

- Serum electrolytes, BUN, and creatinine
  Evaluates hydration and acid-base status in patients who appear seriously ill. Potassium and other electrolytes may be lost with severe diarrhea. Severe dehydration and acidosis are life-threatening.
- Intake and output
  The patient is at risk of fluid loss due to vomiting and diarrhea associated with the gastroenteritis. Tracking intake (including oral fluids, IV fluids and flushes, IV medications, tube feedings and flushes, and liquid medications, as well as fluid output, including urine, liquid stool, vomitus, blood, and drainage from tubes), provides important data regarding fluid status.
- Perineal skin status
  Skin breakdown and infection may result from diarrhea.
- Skin and mucous membranes for signs of dehydration
  Decreased skin turgor occurs with moderate to severe dehydration. Other findings include dry oral mucosa, dry and furrowed tongue, and increased thirst.
- Pain level and effectiveness of interventions
  It is important to recognize the characteristics (type, severity, onset, etc) and duration of the pain to guide ongoing assessment and determine the possible causes.

▪ Actions

- Perform hand hygiene
  Meticulous hand hygiene is practiced to prevent spread of the contagion. Use alcohol-based hand rub (ABHR) on hands before and after direct patient contact, before donning and after removing gloves, after contact with body fluids, mucous membranes, nonintact skin, or wound dressings if hands aren't visibly soiled. Wash hands with soap and water when hands are visibly soiled with blood or another body fluid or after potential exposure to C difficile, Bacillus anthracis, or Norovirus.
- Administer IV fluids if the patient is unable to tolerate clear liquids; if IV fluids are needed, ensure patent IV access.
  The patient is at risk of fluid and electrolyte imbalance due to vomiting and diarrhea. Vomiting may subside with volume replacement.
- Administer prescribed medications, such as antidiarrheals
  Antidiarrheals, such as loperamide, decrease peristalsis and decreases the number of bowel movements.
- Give clear liquids or oral rehydration solutions
  Replaces lost fluids and electrolytes.
- Allow uninterrupted rest periods.
  Provide bed rest with convenient access to a toilet or bedpan.
- Apply venous thromboembolism (VTE) prophylaxis
  Decreased intravascular volume, along with decreased mobility, increase the risk for thromboembolism
- Provide meticulous perineal care, including sitz baths if indicated
  Performing warm sitz baths three times per day will relieve anal irritation
- Provide frequent oral care, including lip emollients
  Fluid deficit increases the risk of dry oral mucous membranes and cracked lips.

▪ Teaching

- Include the patient's family or caregiver in teaching
  Compliance with teaching often increases when patient and family are both included in the teaching
- Dietary modifications
  Clear liquids initially and then progressing the diet as the nausea, vomiting, and diarrhea subside.
- Preventive measures, especially when traveling
  Explain that traveler's diarrhea is caused by inadequate sanitation and occurs after bacteria-contaminated food or water is ingested.
- Proper food preparation
  Bacteria can contaminate food at any time during growth, harvesting or slaughter, processing, storage, and shipping. Foods may also be contaminated with bacteria during food preparation in a restaurant or home kitchen. Bacteria multiply quickly when the temperature of food is between 40 and 140 degrees. Thoroughly cooking food kills bacteria.
- Preventive measures
  Rotavirus immunization is part of the recommended infant vaccination schedule. To prevent recreational waterborne infections, people should not swim if they have diarrhea. Infants and toddlers should have frequent diaper checks and should be changed in a bathroom and not near the water. Swimmers should avoid swallowing water when they swim.

Evaluating Care Outcomes

Effective outcomes are demonstrated when the patient consumes the prescribed diet without diarrhea, nausea or vomiting. The patient exhibits balanced intake and output and demonstrates no further signs of fluid volume loss. The patient identifies pain intensity on a pain scale and rates the pain consistently. The patient has normal laboratory values and stable vital signs. Preventive measures include the patient identifying causative factors of gastroenteritis and demonstrating prevention behaviors.

PEPTIC ULCER DISEASE

An **ulcer** in the GI tract may be defined as a break in the lining of the mucosa, with considerable depth and involvement of the submucosa. **Erosions** are breaks in the surface epithelium that do not have measurable depth. The term **peptic ulcer disease (PUD)** is used broadly to include ulcerations and erosions in the stomach and duodenum from a variety of causes. This is because pepsin, which is proteolytic in acidic solution, plays a major role in causing the mucosal breaks regardless of the cause of the provoking agent (e.g., *H pylori*, aspirin, or an NSAID).

Types of Peptic Ulcers

There are two major forms of peptic ulcers: **duodenal ulcers** and **gastric ulcers**, both of which are chronic. Duodenal ulcers make up approximately 80% of peptic ulcers, affect the proximal part of the small intestine following a chronic course, and are characterized by remissions and exacerbations (with complications that necessitate surgery in approximately 5% to 10% of patients). Chronic gastric ulcers tend to occur in the lesser curvature of the stomach, near the pylorus.

Epidemiology

Peptic ulcer disease is very common in the United States, with approximately 4.5 million individuals (new cases and recurrences) affected per year. The majority of peptic ulcers occur in people between 25 and 64 years of age, and the lifetime prevalence of PUD in the United States is equal among men and women. An estimated 15,000 deaths per year occur as a consequence of complicated PUD (e.g., GI hemorrhage, abdominal or intestinal infarction, perforation, and penetration).

In the past, stress and anxiety were thought to be causes of PUD, but research has shown that the principal risk factors of PUD are *H pylori* infection and NSAID use. Infection with the gram-negative bacterium *H pylori* may be acquired though ingestion of contaminated food and water. Familial tendency (such as type O blood) has been reported as a predisposing factor but now is thought to stem mainly from intrafamilial infection with *H pylori*. There is also a connection between peptic ulcers and certain medical conditions such as chronic obstructive lung disease and chronic renal failure, but the cause is unclear. Other causes include exposure to irritants, trauma, psychogenic factors, and normal aging. Alcoholic beverages stimulate gastric acid production, and high concentrations of alcohol to the gastric mucosa cause mucosal injury. Cigarette smoking may predispose people to PUD and may interact with *H pylori* and NSAIDs to increase mucosal injury. Smoking also impairs ulcer healing and increases ulcer recurrence. Studies demonstrate that cigarette smoke and the active ingredients in cigarettes are associated with death of mucosal cells, inhibition of cell renewal, decreased GI mucosa blood flow, interference with the mucosal immune system, and promotion of tumor growth. In rare cases, peptic ulcers are found in patients with a gastrin-secreting tumor causing profound acid secretion as part of Zollinger-Ellison syndrome (Box 57.1).

Pathophysiology

Peptic ulcers occur mainly in the gastroduodenal mucosa because this tissue cannot withstand the digestive action of gastric acid (hydrochloric acid) and pepsin. Erosions result from the corrosive action of acid gastric juice on a vulnerable epithelium caused by an imbalance between mucosal defenses and acid/peptic injury. A damaged mucosa cannot secrete enough mucus to act as a barrier against gastric acid. Depending on the circumstances, the ulcer may penetrate only the mucosal surface, or it may extend into the smooth muscle layers. Healing of the smooth muscle layers involves replacement with scar tissue. The mucosal layers that cover the scarred muscle layer have the ability to regenerate; however, the regeneration is often imperfect, which contributes

Box 57.1 Risk Factors for Peptic Ulcers

- *Helicobacter pylori* infection
- NSAID and aspirin use
- Excessive smoking and alcohol ingestion
- Other medications (e.g., potassium chloride, concomitant use of steroids with NSAIDs, bisphosphonates, sirolimus, mycophenolate mofetil, fluorouracil)
- Neoplasia
- Acid hypersecretory disorders (e.g., Zollinger-Ellison syndrome)
- Hyperparathyroidism
- Crohn's disease
- Sarcoidosis
- Myeloproliferative disorder
- Systemic mastocytosis
- Other rare infections (e.g., cytomegalovirus, herpes simplex, tuberculosis)
- Critically ill patients with severe burns, head injury, physical trauma, or multiple organ failure

Source: Greenberger, N., Blumberg, R., & Burakoff, R. (2016). *Current diagnosis & treatment gastroenterology, hepatology, & endoscopy* (3rd ed.). New York, NY: McGraw-Hill.

to repeated episodes of ulceration. An ulcer may penetrate the outer wall of the stomach or duodenum, but this is rare (Fig. 57.3).

In a peptic ulcer resulting from *H pylori*, acid is not the dominant cause of bacterial infection but contributes to the consequences. *Helicobacter pylori* releases a toxin that promotes mucosal inflammation and ulceration, stimulating the release of cytokines and other mediators of inflammation that contribute to mucosal damage. Damage to gastroduodenal mucosa allows for decreased resistance to bacteria, and thus infection from *H pylori* bacteria may occur.

Peptic ulcer disease resulting from NSAIDs has both topical and systemic origins. Damage to the cells may occur when NSAIDs diffuse across the mucosal layer and into epithelial cells because they also inhibit the production of prostaglandins that protect epithelial cells in the GI tract from acid-related damage. Inhibition of prostaglandin synthesis increases gastric acid and pepsin secretion, decreases bicarbonate, reduces gastric mucosal blood flow, and decreases mucus production. This disrupts the integrity of the mucosal surface, allowing gastric acid to diffuse back into the mucosa and injure small vessels, leading to edema, hemorrhage, and ulceration of the stomach's lining.

Clinical Manifestations

The clinical presentation of PUD depends on ulcer location and patient age. Many patients (particularly older adults) have few or no clinical manifestations. Pain is the most common symptom. Burning epigastric pain aggravated by fasting and improved with food or antacids (which neutralize the acid) is a symptom complex associated with a *duodenal ulcer*. Pain may also awaken the patient from sleep because of nocturnal gastric acid secretion.

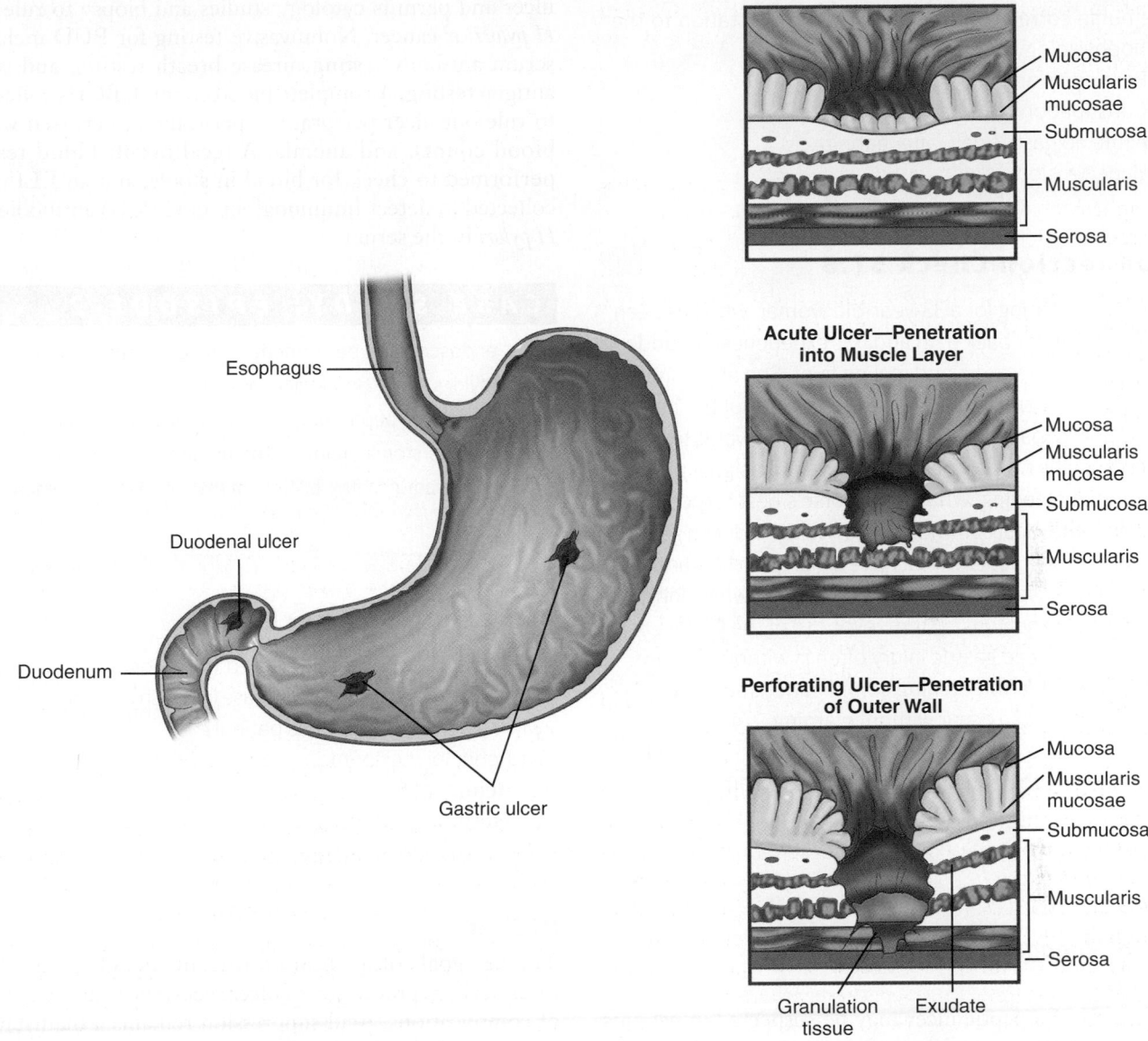

Erosion—Penetration of Only the Mucosal Surface
- Mucosa
- Muscularis mucosae
- Submucosa
- Muscularis
- Serosa

Acute Ulcer—Penetration into Muscle Layer
- Mucosa
- Muscularis mucosae
- Submucosa
- Muscularis
- Serosa

Perforating Ulcer—Penetration of Outer Wall
- Mucosa
- Muscularis mucosae
- Submucosa
- Muscularis
- Serosa
- Granulation tissue
- Exudate

- Esophagus
- Duodenal ulcer
- Duodenum
- Gastric ulcer

FIGURE 57.3 Peptic ulcers. Erosions result from the corrosive action of acid gastric juice on a vulnerable epithelium caused by an imbalance between mucosal defenses and acid/peptic injury. A damaged mucosa cannot secrete enough mucus to act as a barrier against gastric acid. Depending on the circumstances, the ulcer may penetrate only the mucosal surface, or it may extend into the smooth muscle layers as an acute ulceration. The ulcer may also penetrate the outer wall of the stomach or duodenum and perforate the outer wall.

With a *gastric ulcer*, pain is triggered or worsened by eating, usually occurring shortly after meals with little or no relief from antacids. It is believed that the pain occurs when the increased acid content of the stomach and duodenum erodes the lesion and stimulates the exposed nerve endings. Contact of the lesion with acid stimulates a local reflex mechanism that also initiates contraction of the adjacent smooth muscle.

The pain is usually located over a small area near the midline in the epigastrium near the xiphoid and may radiate below the costal margins into the back or, rarely, to the right shoulder. Superficial and deep epigastric tenderness and voluntary muscle guarding may occur with more extensive lesions. An additional characteristic of ulcer pain is periodicity,

as the pain tends to recur at intervals of weeks or months. During an exacerbation, it occurs daily for a period of several weeks and then remits until the next recurrence.

> **Safety Alert** Do not make assumptions about pain. Acute pain may be indicative of a complication, such as perforation (sudden, intense epigastric pain and rigid abdominal muscles), or it may be totally unrelated to peptic ulcer disease (e.g., pancreatitis, coronary heart disease, or gallbladder disease). The nurse needs to ensure a comprehensive evaluation of the pain, particularly with an acute onset.

Connection Check 57.4

The nurse correlates which clinical manifestation to the pathophysiology of a gastric ulcer?
A. Pernicious anemia
B. Constipation
C. Acute epigastric pain after eating
D. Hypertension

Connection Check 57.5

The nurse is caring for a 33-year-old woman who has been taking aspirin for back pain and has experienced a sudden episode of tachycardia and feeling faint. She also vomited coffee-ground emesis and passed a tarry stool but has no complaints of pain or heartburn. The patient wants to know why there was no sign of pain as a warning signal prior to the sudden bleeding. What is the nurse's best response?
A. Pain is the most common sign of NSAID-induced gastric injury, so the patient must have a high pain tolerance.
B. NSAIDs cause damage to epithelial cells, which inhibit the enteric nervous system response of the GI tract.
C. NSAID-induced gastric injury often is without symptoms, and life-threatening complications such as GI bleeding can occur without warning.
D. NSAIDs have anti-inflammatory and analgesic effects, preventing the patient from feeling any pain as a warning sign.

Management

Medical Management

Diagnosis

A diagnosis of a peptic ulcer may be suspected in patients presenting with epigastric pain but needs to be differentiated from other conditions with similar clinical manifestations, such as gastroesophageal reflux disease, biliary tract disease, hepatitis, pancreatitis, abdominal aortic aneurysm, gastroparesis, functional dyspepsia, neoplasia, mesenteric ischemia, and myocardial ischemic pain. Although peptic ulcers can be diagnosed during upper endoscopy, laboratory and radiological tests may help narrow the diagnosis. Some patients with peptic ulcers are anemic because of acute bleeding or chronic blood loss. Liver function tests and levels of amylase and lipase are evaluated for hepatitis and pancreatitis. An abdominal ultrasound may reveal gallstone disease or an abdominal aortic aneurysm. An electrocardiogram and measurement of cardiac enzymes may be used to evaluate myocardial causes of pain. Lastly, an upper GI and small bowel x-ray series with upright and lateral decubitus views showing free air indicates perforation.

Because of its increased sensitivity and specificity, upper GI endoscopy is the preferred procedure for evaluation of PUD, as compared with barium upper GI x-rays.

Endoscopy or esophagogastroduodenoscopy confirms the ulcer and permits cytology studies and biopsy to rule out *H pylori* or cancer. Noninvasive testing for PUD includes serum antibody testing, urease breath testing, and stool antigen testing. A complete blood count (CBC) is collected to rule out ulcer perforation, peritonitis (increased white blood count), and anemia. A fecal occult blood test is performed to check for blood in stools, and an ELISA is collected to detect Immunoglobulin G (IgG) antibodies to *H pylori* in the serum.

CASE STUDY: EPISODE 2

The endoscopy is performed at an outpatient clinic near Mrs. Taylor's home 2 weeks after visiting her APRN. The endoscopy reveals several peptic ulcers. A tissue sample is taken from Mrs. Taylor's stomach lining. The tissue sample is positive for *H pylori*, a gram-negative bacterium that infects the stomach…

Connection Check 57.6

A 67-year-old male is suspected of having a peptic ulcer. The nurse monitors for a decrease in which diagnostic value with GI hemorrhage in this patient?
A. Reticulocyte count
B. Hematocrit
C. Prothrombin time
D. IgG antibodies to *H pylori*

Medications

The key goals of medication therapy include pain relief, ulcer healing, prevention of ulcer recurrence, and reduction of complications. Acid suppression remains a mainstay in healing both duodenal and gastric ulcers and in preventing recurrence. Therapy in patients who are *H pylori*–positive with active or previously documented ulcers is focused on eradicating *H pylori* infection and healing the ulcer. The objective of therapy in patients with NSAID-induced PUD is to heal the ulcer and remove the offending agent.

Antacids neutralize gastric acid, whereas the use of H_2-receptor antagonists decreases acid production. H_2-antagonists such as ranitidine, nizatidine, cimetidine, or famotidine block gastric acid secretion stimulated by histamine, gastrin, and acetylcholine. Patients with peptic ulcers or those who must continue NSAID therapy for some other disorder should be treated with PPIs such as omeprazole, lansoprazole, or pantoprazole for as long as the NSAID is used. Proton pump inhibitors block the final stage of hydrogen ion secretion by blocking the action of the gastric parietal cell proton pump. Other agents can be used to enhance mucosal defenses. Misoprostol, a prostaglandin E analog, has been shown to prevent gastric mucosal damage in chronic users of NSAIDs. Sucralfate

(Carafate) is more commonly used because it acts locally to enhance mucosal defenses. Sucralfate selectively binds to necrotic ulcer tissue and serves as a barrier to acid, pepsin, and bile and can directly absorb bile salts.

Diet

The patient with PUD should avoid dietary irritants such as spices, alcohol, and caffeine. Consuming six small meals or small hourly meals is encouraged, along with intake of adequate fluids. If GI bleeding is evident, the patient should have nothing by mouth. Discourage smoking because it slows the rate of healing and increases the frequency of relapses.

Surgical Management

With the increased effectiveness of medications to treat PUD, surgical treatment is usually only required with nonhealing and bleeding ulcers. Minimally invasive procedures involving endoscopic approaches allow ulcers to be removed or bleeding controlled. More conventional surgical interventions are indicated for perforation, lack of response to conservative treatment, suspected cancer, or other complications. Gastric cancer must always be considered in patients with a gastric ulcer or gastric outlet obstruction. Surgery for PUD is dependent on type, location, and extent of the ulcer. Today, most patients having a procedure for PUD undergo oversewing of a bleeding ulcer, or patch of a perforated ulcer, or distal gastrectomy. Major operations include bilateral vagotomy, pyloroplasty, and gastrectomy (Fig. 57.4). The parietal cell vagotomy is safe (mortality risk less than 0.5%) and causes minimal side effects. The vagotomy severs the vagal nerve supply to the proximal two-thirds of the stomach, where the majority of the parietal cells are located, and preserves the vagal innervation to the antrum and pylorus and the remaining abdominal viscera. The parietal cell vagotomy decreases total gastric acid secretion by approximately 75%, and GI side effects are rare. Considerations for PUD surgery should include whether *H pylori* infection is present, the need for NSAID therapy, previous treatment, and the

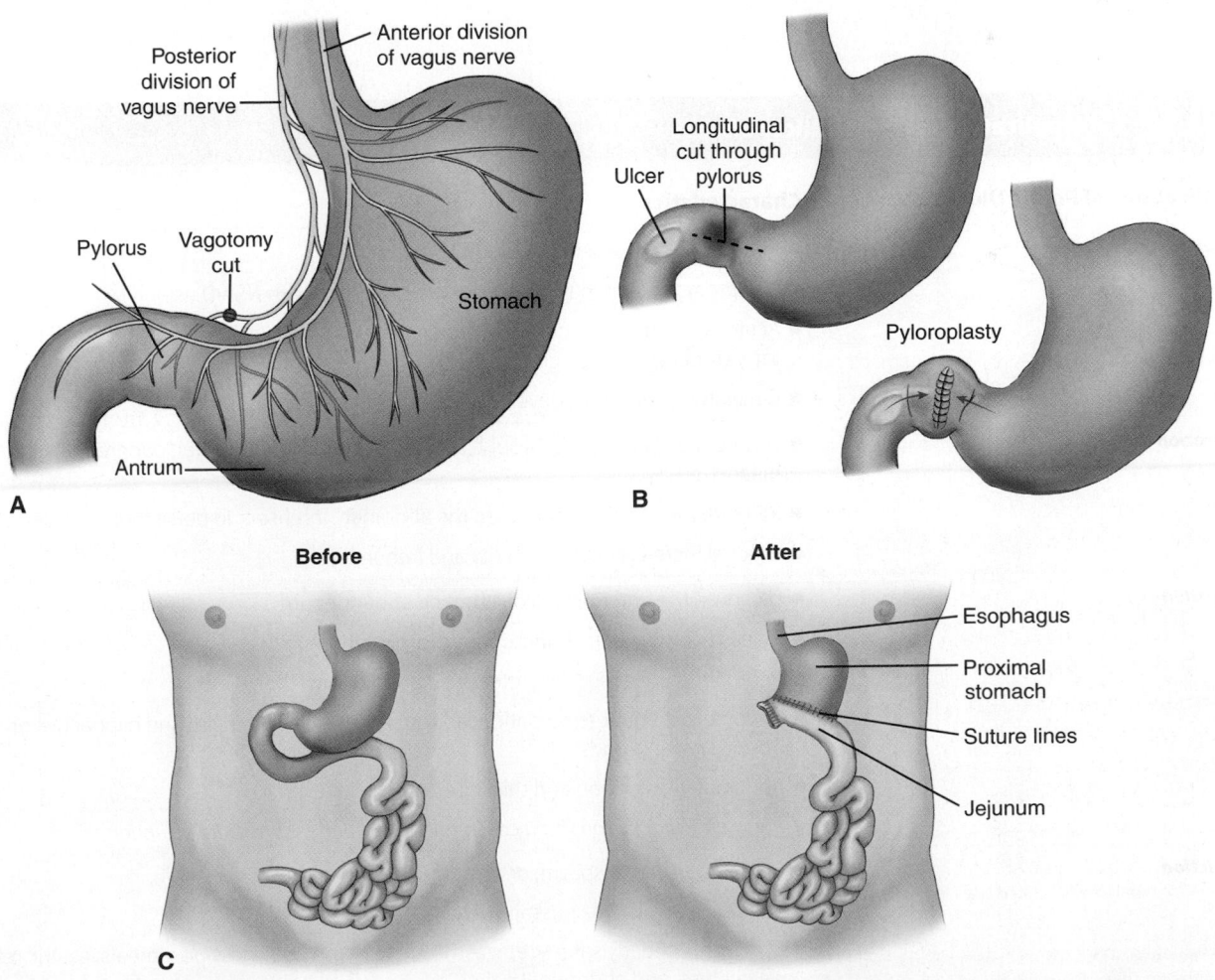

FIGURE 57.4 Various types of operations currently popular for treating duodenal ulcer disease. A, Bilateral vagotomy; The vagotomy severs the vagal nerve supply to the proximal two-thirds of the stomach, where the majority of the parietal cells are located, and preserves the vagal innervation to the antrum and pylorus and the remaining abdominal viscera. B, Pyloroplasty; Enlarging the pylorus opening to allow stomach contents to empty more easily. C, Distal gastrectomy. Involves removing a section of the stomach with reattachment to the jejunum.

likelihood of future compliance with treatment. Pyloroplasty involves enlarging the pyloric opening allowing the stomach to empty more easily and is usually only performed after conservative medical treatments have failed. The distal gastrectomy involves removing the section of the stomach that is developing ulcers and attaching it to the jejunum.

Connection Check 57.7

The nurse monitors for which clinical manifestations in the patient diagnosed with a duodenal ulcer? *(Select all that apply.)*

A. Intermittent abdominal pain, which is relieved after eating and taking antacids but becomes worse at night
B. Nausea and vomiting
C. Right upper quadrant tenderness and is positive for occult blood in stool
D. Complaints of heartburn or regurgitation and vomiting
E. Bloating and flatulence

Complications

The most common complications of PUD are GI hemorrhage, abdominal or intestinal infarction, perforation and penetration into attached structures, obstruction, and peritonitis. There is also an increased risk of gastric **adenocarcinoma**, a malignant tumor arising from glandular tissue, in patients with *H pylori*. Hemorrhage is caused by bleeding from granulation tissue or erosion of an ulcer into an artery or vein. A tear in the mucosa at the gastroesophageal junction (Mallory-Weiss syndrome) can occur as a result of severe vomiting, trauma, or seizures (Table 57.3; Box 57.2).

Peritonitis is defined as inflammation and infection of the serosal membrane that lines the abdominal cavity and contained organs. Bacteria invade the peritoneum after inflammation and perforation of the GI tract. Protein-filled fluid and electrolytes accumulate in the peritoneal cavity causing the peritoneum to become inflamed and edematous. The inflammation may be localized as an abscess, or diffuse extending throughout the peritoneum.

Table 57.3 Complications of Peptic Ulcer Disease

Complications of Peptic Ulcer Disease	Characteristics
Gastrointestinal bleed	• May be sudden, severe, and without warning • Symptoms of pain may not be present (common with NSAID use) • Acute hemorrhage: sudden weakness; dizziness; cold, moist skin; passage of loose, tarry stools and coffee-ground emesis • Circulatory shock may develop depending on amount of blood loss
Penetration	• Ulcer crater penetrates through adjacent organs: small bowel, pancreas, liver, or biliary tree • Referred pain to sites other than the abdomen, intense and persistent • Gradual increase in pain severity and frequency
Perforation	• Ulcers on the anterior wall of stomach or duodenum • Release of gastrointestinal contents into peritoneum • Peritonitis causes sudden, intense epigastric pain • Abdomen is tender to palpation, abdominal muscles are rigid, and hypoactive or absent bowel sounds • Abdominal distention and third spacing • *Perforation is a serious medical condition requiring immediate attention*
Obstruction	• Caused by edema, spasm, or contraction of scar tissue • Interference with free passage of gastric contents • Symptoms of early satiety, epigastric fullness and heaviness post meals, gastric reflux, weight loss, and abdominal pain • Severe obstruction: vomiting of undigested food

Box 57.2 Gastrointestinal Bleeding

Hematemesis, the vomiting of blood, is the hallmark of upper gastrointestinal bleeding. Bright red blood in the emesis is indicative of active bleeding. Coffee-ground emesis indicates older blood that has had time to be reduced by acid in the stomach. Melena is black, tarry stools with a foul odor due to the degradation of blood in the small intestine and colon.

Nursing Management

Assessment and Analysis

Collection of patient history includes causes and risk factors for gastritis and PUD, with careful attention to aspirin and NSAID use. The physical examination includes:

- General appearance and height and weight relationship
- Abdominal examination including shape and contour
- Bowel sounds and tenderness to palpation
- Presence of obvious or occult blood in vomitus and stool

The patient with PUD may be asymptomatic or may experience periods of exacerbation and remission of clinical manifestations, with remissions lasting longer than exacerbations. Clinical manifestations may include:

- Left epigastric pain described as heartburn or indigestion accompanied by feeling of fullness or distention
- The pain usually is rhythmic and frequently occurs when the stomach is empty—between meals and at 1 or 2 o'clock in the morning.
- Increasingly severe and constant localized abdominal pain that increases with movement and respirations may indicate progressing peritonitis.
- Possible referral of pain to the shoulder or thoracic area
- Anorexia, nausea, and vomiting
- Inability to pass stools and flatus
- Hiccups

Because epigastric pain can also signal myocardial infarction, a 12-lead electrocardiogram is performed, and the patient is placed on telemetry to monitor for any dysrhythmias. Nursing care priorities include reducing discomfort, maintaining nutritional status, and preventing or rapidly identifying and intervening for potential complications. In a patient admitted with an acute bleed related to PUD, the immediate priorities of care are restoring blood volume and cardiac output.

Nursing Diagnoses

- **Acute pain or chronic pain** related to physical (gastric and/or duodenal mucosal) injury
- **Deficient knowledge** about prevention of symptoms and management of PUD

- **Disturbed sleep pattern** related to discomfort
- **Risk for deficient fluid volume** related to loss of blood

Nursing Interventions

■ Assessments

- Vital signs
  Vital signs including orthostatic measurements; increased heart rate and decreased blood pressure are caused by fluid volume deficit from vomiting. Orthostatic vital signs are performed to assess for fluid volume deficit. Loss of blood volume may cause orthostatic hypotension with syncope or dizziness upon standing. Orthostatic changes are present if there is a decrease of more than 20 mm Hg in systolic blood pressure, a decrease of 10 mm Hg in diastolic blood pressure when going from a supine to an upright position.
- Gastric pH as ordered, check emesis, and feces for occult blood
  The gastric Ph provides data regarding the acidity of gastric secretions. Monitoring for occult blood helps identify slow bleeding or recurrent hemorrhage.
- Use of alcohol or other medications, including aspirin and other NSAIDs
  NSAIDs break down the gastric mucosal barrier and result in local gastric mucosal injury. Alcohol is irritating to the gastric mucosal. Cigarette smoking is associated with death of mucosal cells, inhibition of cell renewal, and decreased GI mucosa blood flow.
- Serum electrolytes and blood urea nitrogen (BUN)
  Electrolytes are lost through vomiting, gastric drainage, and diarrhea. Careful monitoring is essential to identify possible shock and to intervene at an early stage. Serum potassium levels may be decreased with vomiting. Digestion and absorption of blood in the GI tract may cause elevated BUN levels.
- Pain, including exacerbating and relieving factors.
  Food can act as an antacid by neutralizing gastric acid for approximately 30 to 60 minutes. Afterward, gastric acid secretion may increase. Foods that increase pain should be avoided.
- Diet, including pattern of food intake, eating schedule, and foods associated with pain
  This helps increase patient awareness and identifies whether nutrient intake is adequate.
- CBC
  If the patient is experiencing GI bleeding, hemoglobin and hematocrit values may be low. The WBC count may be elevated with inflammation or infection.
- Blood culture and/or peritoneal fluid culture
  A positive culture for the offending organism will guide the choice of antibiotic or antifungal therapy.
- Weight
  In the patient with increased pain or early satiety, intake of nutrients may be decreased, and the patient may exhibit weight loss.

- Clinical manifestations of abscess formation, including persistent abdominal tenderness and fever.
  An abscess may lead to fistula formation, septicemia, respiratory compromise, bowel obstruction, shock, and/or liver failure.

■ Actions

- Maintain IV infusions and administer blood products as prescribed
  IV fluids and blood products are given to restore blood volume and oxygen-carrying capacity.
- Administer prescribed medication therapy
  Pain relief can be achieved by giving prescribed medications such as PPIs before breakfast and antacids 1 to 3 hours after meals. Interventions for PUD related to H pylori are aimed at reducing pain related to the infection and promoting healing of the gastric mucosa.
- Administer medications to reduce gastric acidity as ordered
  Reducing the acidity of gastric secretions reduces the risk of bleeding.
- Assist with gastric lavage, as indicated for GI bleeding; irrigate the nasogastric tube with room temperature saline as ordered
  Irrigation helps remove irritating blood from the gut and may slow bleeding.
- Prepare the patient and his family for upper endoscopy or surgery as planned
  Endoscopy or emergency surgery may be performed to repair the bleeding site or sclerose bleeding vessels.
- Limit food intake after the evening meal; eliminate bedtime snacks
  Eating before bed can stimulate gastric acid and pepsin production, increasing the chance of night-time pain.
- Document and report complaints of anorexia, fullness, nausea, vomiting, or symptoms of dumping syndrome
  Problems with gastric emptying may be associated with PUD or surgery to treat PUD. It is important to monitor and report symptoms because a change in therapy or food intake may be necessary. Dumping syndrome develops secondary to concentrated, partially digested food entering the small bowel rapidly, causing abdominal distention.
- Pain documentation to include location, character, timing and relationship to meals, and measures that relieve or aggravate the pain;
  Monitoring for changes in pain is important in evaluating outcomes of therapies and to inform preventive measures.

■ Teaching

- Take medications as prescribed
  H_2-receptor antagonists block gastric secretions. Antacids are used as buffering agents to correct the pH balance of the acidic gastric environment. Antisecretory agents (PPIs) can be used to suppress gastric acid secretion. Teach patients not to take other over-the-counter medications if they are taking related prescribed medications.
- Avoid eating within two hours of bedtime.
  Eating late increases the production of gastric acid that may irritate gastric lining
- Advise patients to avoid risk factors such as overuse of aspirin and NSAIDs, spicy foods, and beverages that contain caffeine
  Such foods and fluids have stimulatory effects on gastric acid secretion.

Evaluating Care Outcomes

Indicators that the patient with PUD has decreased pain include expressed feelings of increased comfort and pain control. The patient reports pain at a level of three or lower on a 0 to 10 scale. The patient consumes the prescribed diet without nausea or vomiting. The patient demonstrates no further signs of fluid volume loss.

> ### Connection Check 57.8
> The nurse incorporates which information into the teaching plan for a patient diagnosed with a duodenal ulcer?
> A. "You will probably have increased pain after eating."
> B. "Smoking cigarettes can make the PUD worse."
> C. "Antacids are not usually effective for the pain."
> D. "Eating bland foods will aid in healing."

GASTRIC CANCER

Gastric cancer is cancer of the GI tract classified according to gross appearance (polypoid, ulcerating, ulcerating and infiltrating, or diffuse; Fig. 57.5) and is one of the most common forms of cancer worldwide. The prognosis is dependent on the stage of the disease at the time of diagnosis, and the 5-year survival rate is approximately 23%.

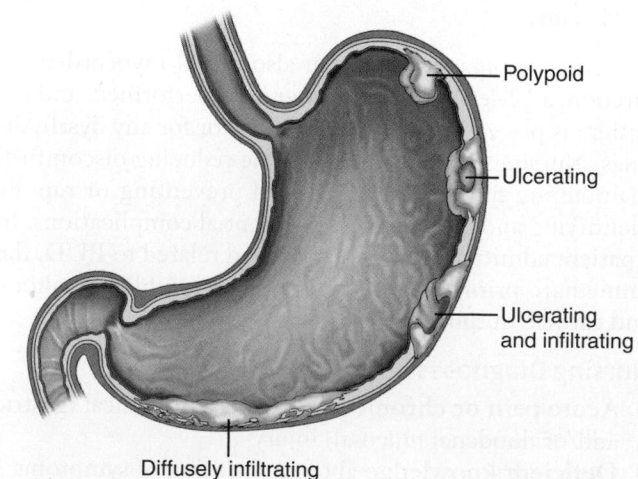

FIGURE 57.5 Gross appearance of gastric cancer. Gastric cancer is classified according to gross appearance noted as polypoid, ulcerating, ulcerating and infiltrating, or diffusely infiltrative.

Epidemiology

The incidence of gastric cancer varies widely, being highest in Hispanics, African Americans, and Asian Americans. It is more common in lower socioeconomic groups and affects males two times more often than females. Gastric cancer represented the leading cause of cancer-related mortality in the United States until the 1930s, and it was the leading cause of cancer-related deaths worldwide until the late 1980s, when lung malignancies peaked in occurrence. Although the overall incidence of stomach cancer in the United States has declined in the past 75 years, it is the second leading cause of cancer mortality worldwide.

Causes of gastric carcinomas are unknown. Diet appears to be a significant factor, with a diet rich in foods with additives such as smoked foods, pickled vegetables, and salted fish and meat increasing the risk of gastric cancer. Dietary nitrates are also proposed as a possible cause of gastric cancer. Gastric bacteria, more common in the **achlorhydric** (low hydrochloric acid) stomach of patients with atrophic gastritis, convert nitrate into nitrite, a proven carcinogen. The reduced consumption of nitrate-rich preserved foods has been suggested as a cause of the dramatic decrease in gastric cancer seen in North America and Western Europe.

The risk of gastric cancer is greater in patients with low gastric acidity (**achlorhydria**), such as those with severe atrophic gastritis associated with intestinal metaplasia and pernicious anemia. Chronic atrophic gastritis is by far the most common precursor for gastric cancer, and the prevalence of atrophic gastritis is higher in older age groups but can occur in people younger than 40 years of age.

Other related factors include chronic inflammation of the stomach, high alcohol consumption, smoking, family history, and *H pylori* infection. Patients with *H pylori*–associated ulcers have a three- to six-fold increased risk of gastric malignancy later in life. Because *H pylori* infection has been shown to cause gastric cancer, its elimination forms the cornerstone of eradication of gastric cancer. Many patients with *H pylori* infections have already developed atrophic gastritis, which is the precursor disorder to gastric cancer (see Evidence-Based Practice).

Evidence-Based Practice

Gastric Cancer and *Helicobacter pylori*

Helicobacter pylori is associated as a risk factor for development of gastric cancer. In an effort to more clearly explain the relationships between *H pylori* and gastric cancer, a prospective, double-blind, placebo-controlled, randomized trial was conducted on 470 patients who had undergone endoscopic resection of early gastric cancer or high-grade adenoma. The patients were randomized into two groups; one receiving *H pylori* eradication therapy with antibiotics, and the other receiving a placebo. The two

outcomes measured were metachronous gastric cancer detected on endoscopy one year after treatment, and improvement in glandular atrophy in a 3-year follow up examination. Findings demonstrated that patients with early gastric cancer in the treatment group had lower rates of cancer as well as improvement in the grade of gastric atrophy.

Choi, I.J., Kook, M.C., Kim, Y.I, Cho, S.J., Lee, J.Y., Kim, C.G., Park, B. & Nam, B. (2018). *Helicobacter pylori* therapy for the prevention of metachronous gastric cancer. *The New England Journal of Medicine*, 378(12), 1085–1095.

Pathophysiology

A gastric adenocarcinoma is a malignant epithelial tumor that infiltrates the mucus-producing cells of the stomach and is most frequently found in the distal portion (pylorus and antrum). Gastric carcinogenesis is a multifactorial and multistep process, starting from chronic gastritis and progressing over many years to atrophy, intestinal metaplasia, dysplasia, and eventually adenocarcinoma. The risk of developing gastric cancer correlates best with the severity and extent of atrophic gastritis and gastric atrophy. Inadequate acid secretion in patients with atrophic gastritis creates an alkaline environment that allows bacteria (e.g., *H pylori*) to multiply and act on nitrates in food. Nitrates interact with amino acids in the stomach to form carcinogenic nitrosamines. The nitrosamines are converted to nitrites, which are a major risk factor for gastric cancer.

Approximately 95% of gastric cancers are adenocarcinomas, commonly classified as an *intestinal type* and a *diffuse type*. The intestinal type is associated with chronic atrophic gastritis, severe intestinal metaplasia and dysplasia, and tends to be less aggressive than the diffuse type. The diffuse type is associated with an invasive growth pattern in dispersed clusters of uniform-sized malignant cells that infiltrate the submucosa, causing thickening of the stomach wall (arising beneath normal-appearing epithelium). Metastases occur early because of the rich blood and lymphatic supplies to the stomach.

Clinical Manifestations

Unfortunately, stomach cancers often are asymptomatic until late in their course, and the disease is often quite advanced, and metastases are usually present at the time of diagnosis. Clinical manifestations, when they do occur, are essentially nonspecific and include indigestion, anorexia, weight loss, vague epigastric pain, vomiting, and an abdominal mass. The patient may experience ulcer-like pain unrelieved by antacids, typically occurring after meals. Because these symptoms are vague, patients and healthcare providers tend to dismiss symptoms or treat the patient for acid disease, which makes early detection difficult. While the disease progresses, the patient may be anorexic and cachectic at the time of diagnosis. An abdominal mass may be palpable, and erosion of the gastric tumor into a large perigastric vessel may cause life-threatening hemorrhage. Massive hematemesis or **melena**, black tarry stools with a foul odor due to the degradation of blood in the small intestine and colon, are uncommon, but secondary anemia may occur after occult blood loss.

Management

Medical Management

Diagnosis

Diagnosis of gastric cancer is accomplished by a variety of techniques including barium x-ray studies, endoscopic studies with biopsy, and cytological studies of gastric secretions. Barium x-rays of the GI tract with fluoroscopy show changes that suggest gastric cancer, including a tumor or filling defect in the outline of the stomach, loss of flexibility, and atypical gastric mucosa with or without ulceration. A chest x-ray may reveal metastasis.

Esophagogastroduodenoscopy is the visual examination of the lining of the esophagus, stomach, and upper duodenum using a flexible fiber-optic endoscope. This procedure identifies the cancer and helps rule out other diffuse gastric mucosal abnormalities by allowing direct visualization. Biopsy of visible gastric mucosal lesions can be obtained to determine the presence of cancer cells. Computed tomography (CT) and endoscopic ultrasonography may be used to determine the spread of a diagnosed stomach cancer. This allows evaluation of the depth of the tumor and presence of lymph node involvement for staging of the cancer.

Laboratory studies such as CBC may reveal anemia, evidenced by low hematocrit and hemoglobin values. Patients may have macrocytic or microcytic anemia associated with decreased iron or vitamin B_{12} absorption. Liver function study results (e.g., bilirubin and alkaline phosphatase) may be elevated with metastatic spread of the cancer to the liver. Carcinoembryonic antigen radioimmunoassay may be elevated. A stool guaiac may test positive.

Medications

There are no specific medications for gastric cancer. Radiation and chemotherapy have not shown to be useful as primary treatment methods in stomach cancer because the disease is often widely spread to other abdominal organs upon diagnosis, and they are typically used for palliative purposes or to control metastatic spread of the disease. Antiemetics such as ondansetron, dronabinol, or metoclopramide are common regimens for nausea and vomiting control secondary to side effects of the therapy. Opioid analgesics are used for pain management, and vitamin supplementation is given for deficiencies.

 Safety Alert Nausea and feelings of early satiety are common side effects of chemotherapy, which may impair nutrient consumption, indicating a need to institute enteral or parenteral feedings. Early nutrition screening and assessment can help to identify and minimize nutritional problems. It is important for data to be both subjective and objective when assessing the ability to consume adequate nutrients.

Surgical Management

Gastric dysplasia is the universal precursor to gastric adenocarcinoma. Patients with severe dysplasia should be considered for gastric resection if the abnormality is widespread or multifocal. In patients with early stages of gastric cancer, laparoscopic surgery (minimally invasive surgery) plus adjuvant chemotherapy (anthracycline such as 5-fluorouracil) or radiation may be a curative option. However, long-term survival rates with surgery alone remain suboptimal for all but the earliest gastric cancer.

Complications

Dumping syndrome, also known as rapid gastric emptying, is the most common complication after a partial gastrectomy. Alterations in the gastric anatomy after surgery or interference in its extrinsic innervation following a vagotomy may alter gastric emptying. After pyloric resection or bypass, concentrated **chyme** (partially digested food) may enter the small bowel rapidly, causing abdominal distention, inappropriate gut hormone release, and rapid glucose absorption. Early clinical manifestations (15-30 minutes after a meal) include dizziness, tachycardia, pallor, sweating, diarrhea, and palpitations. Signs of late dumping (1-3 hours after a meal) include symptoms of hypoglycemia such as weakness, sweating, and dizziness. Both can be life-threatening. Dumping syndrome is managed primarily by planning dietary intake to allow smaller boluses of undigested food to enter the intestine. Meals are small and more frequent. Liquids and solids are taken at separate times instead of together to facilitate adequate nutritional intake. Other complications of gastrectomy include wound infections, leaking of anastomotic sites, strictures, and internal bleeding.

Nursing Management

Assessment and Analysis

Patients with early gastric cancer may have no clinical manifestations. However, the main clinical manifestations of early gastric cancer may include:

- Indigestion (heartburn)
- Abdominal pain/discomfort, initially relieved by antacids or nutrition changes
- Feeling of fullness
- Epigastric, back, or retrosternal pain
- Anorexia

While the tumor grows, these signs and symptoms become more severe and do not improve with dietary changes or antacids. Clinical manifestations of advanced gastric cancer include:

- Nausea and vomiting
- Obstructive symptoms
- Iron-deficiency anemia
- Palpable epigastric mass
- Enlarged lymph nodes
- Weakness and fatigue
- Weight loss
- Metastasis

Nursing Diagnoses

- **Pain** related to the tumor mass
- **Anxiety** related to the disease and anticipated treatment
- **Fear** related to well-being or potential death
- **Imbalanced nutrition: less than body requirements** related to early satiety or anorexia leading to decreased intake

Nursing Interventions

■ *Assessments*

- Physical examination, assessing for signs of metastasis
  Carefully assess the patient's abdomen for distention and/or a palpable mass, which may suggest hepatomegaly from metastasis. Percuss to detect ascites. Also palpate the patient's lymph nodes, especially the supraclavicular and axillary nodes. Hard, enlarged lymph nodes result from metastasis. Examine the patient for other assessment findings that depend on the extent of disease and location of metastasis.
- Hematocrit and hemoglobin
  With advanced disease, hematocrit and hemoglobin levels may be decreased because of anemia secondary to hematemesis or melena. Macrocytic or microcytic anemia results from decreased vitamin B$_{12}$ absorption due to lack of intrinsic factor
- Serum electrolytes
  Electrolytes are lost through vomiting, gastric drainage, and diarrhea. Serum potassium levels may be decreased with vomiting. Digestion and absorption of blood in the GI tract may cause elevated BUN levels.
- Bilirubin and alkaline phosphatase
  Abnormal bilirubin and alkaline phosphatase occur with advanced disease and hepatic metastasis.
- A modified oral glucose tolerance test with hematocrit measurement
  Blood glucose levels between 120 and 180 minutes after drinking the solution, an increase in hematocrit of more than 3 percent at 30 minutes, and a rise in pulse rate of more than 10 beats per minute after 30 minutes confirms dumping syndrome.
- Comprehensive pain assessment
  Include location, characteristics, onset/duration, frequency, quality, intensity or severity, and precipitating factors. A pain management plan is developed on the basis of the patient's response to pain.

- Early signs of dumping syndrome
  Symptoms include vertigo, increased heart rate, syncope, sweating, pallor, and palpitations. Early manifestations of dumping syndrome may occur within 30 minutes of eating and are a result of the rapid emptying of contents into the small intestine. Late dumping syndrome occurs 90 minutes to 3 hours after eating and is caused by excessive insulin release. Both can be life threatening. Alterations in the gastric anatomy after surgery or interference in its extrinsic innervation following a vagotomy may alter gastric emptying. After pyloric resection or bypass, concentrated chyme may enter the small bowel rapidly, causing abdominal distention, inappropriate gut hormone release, and rapid glucose absorption.
- Patient's level of anxiety (moderate, severe, or panic) and the reality of the threats represented in the patient's current situation
  The level of anxiety and the reality of the perceived threat influence what type of intervention is appropriate. A patient in panic may need medical intervention, whereas those with moderate or severe anxiety are often managed by counseling and teaching new coping skills.
- Assess the possible need for end-of-life care
  Gastric cancer and its treatment may cause debilitating adverse effects. Hospice programs can help both the patient and family learn symptom management and coping techniques.

■ *Actions*

- Encourage the patient to eat small, frequent portions of nonirritating foods that are high in protein and calories along with dietary supplements
  Meals must be nutritionally adequate to promote healing. Adding vitamins and minerals, calories, or other nutritional components may be needed for the patient who is unable to eat a nutritionally adequate diet. Total parenteral nutrition may be necessary to maintain weight and nutrition and allow the GI tract to heal.
- Encourage the patient and family to verbalize feelings, concerns, and fears related to the diagnosis, prognosis, and treatment
  Because disease is usually advanced at the time of diagnosis, provide grief counseling and refer the patient and family to cancer support groups or hospice services as appropriate.
- Prepare the patient and family physically and emotionally for surgery as indicated
  Surgical resection is the preferred method for treating gastric cancer and may include total gastrectomy and partial gastrectomy. Surgery may be curative or palliative. Palliative resection may improve the quality of life if the patient is suffering from obstruction, hemorrhage, or pain.

■ **Teaching**

- Provide information to both the patient and family or caregiver.
  Review the disorder, diagnostic testing, and treatment, including surgery and combination chemotherapy
- Discuss medications to be included in the chemotherapy plan
  Include drug names, dosages, routes of administration, expected results, and frequency of administration
- Provide information approximately pain and precipitating factors
  The patient will be able to monitor discomfort and when to intervene as appropriate.
- Teach the patient and family about high-calorie, high-protein meals
  Meals must be nutritionally adequate to promote healing.
- Teach the patient and family about nutritional supplements
  Additional vitamins and minerals, calories, dietary fiber, and other supplements may be added to the diet of a patient with inadequate food intake.
- Provide information about the signs of Dumping Syndrome and what can make this more likely to happen
  The patient is more likely to have this problem if they had surgery to take out all or part of the stomach. High sugar foods may cause the stomach to empty too fast. Avoid foods such as sweetened cereals, donuts, cakes, rolls, pastries, candies, cookies, soda, juice, or syrup.
- Teach the patient relaxation techniques and coping strategies
  Relaxation techniques help reduce stress and promote healing. Techniques include deep breathing, guided visualization, and progressive relaxation.

Evaluating Care Outcomes

The major goals for the patient with gastric cancer include absence of infection, stable weight, reduced anxiety, optimal nutrition, relief of pain, and adjustment to the diagnosis. Expected outcomes for the patient include consuming prescribed diet without nausea or vomiting, expressing feelings of decreased anxiety, and verbalizing pain and effectiveness of comfort measures.

Making Connections

CASE STUDY: WRAP-UP

Mrs. Taylor's treatment of the peptic ulcers and infection includes two antibiotics, a PPI, and bismuth salts. She is instructed to take the entire course of her medications and to follow up with the internist in 6 months for a repeated endoscopy. The provider explains that failure to be compliant with the medication regimen may cause antibiotic resistance and persistent infection.

Case Study Questions

1. The nurse is monitoring Mrs. Taylor, who has been diagnosed with a peptic ulcer. Which assessment finding most likely indicates perforation of the ulcer?
   A. Bradycardia
   B. Numbness in the legs
   C. Sudden and severe epigastric pain
   D. Nausea and vomiting

2. Mrs. Taylor is scheduled for a vagotomy and asks the nurse about the purpose of this procedure. Which response by the nurse is most accurate?
   A. Diminishes stress reactions
   B. Heals the gastric mucosa
   C. Reduces the stimulus to acid secretions
   D. Decreases food absorption in the stomach

3. The nurse is monitoring for the early clinical manifestations of dumping syndrome. Which findings are consistent with this complication?
   A. Sweating and pallor
   B. Bradycardia and indigestion
   C. Double vision and chest pain
   D. Abdominal cramping and pain

4. The nurse is reviewing the medication record regarding Mrs. Taylor's PUD. Which medication, if noted on the patient's record, will the nurse question?
   A. Rabeprazole sodium (AcipHex)
   B. Furosemide (Lasix)
   C. Indomethacin (Indocin)
   D. Propranolol hydrochloride (Inderal)

5. The healthcare provider has ordered a blood test for *H pylori*. How does the nurse prepare the patient for this diagnostic test?
   A. Instructing the patient not to consume food or liquids after midnight
   B. Giving an oral suspension of glucose 1 hour before the test
   C. Explaining that a small dose of radioactive isotope will be used
   D. Telling the patient that no special preparation is needed

CHAPTER SUMMARY

Gastritis is an inflammation of the gastric mucosa caused by any of several conditions, including infection (*Helicobacter pylori*), medications (NSAIDs, alcohol), stress, and autoimmune disorders (atrophic gastritis). Many cases are asymptomatic, but dyspepsia and GI bleeding sometimes occur.

Diagnosis is by endoscopy. Treatment is directed at the underlying cause, although it often includes acid suppression and, for *H pylori infection*, antibiotics.

Gastroenteritis is an inflammatory process of the digestive system. Infectious gastroenteritis is typically caused by ingestion of a virus, bacteria, or parasite, with viruses the leading cause of acute gastroenteritis. Clinical manifestations include vomiting and diarrhea that my lead to dehydration and hypovolemia. Definitive treatment is based on identification of the cause of the gastroenteritis. Nursing priorities include monitoring fluid and electrolyte status, administering treatments focused on elimination of the causative agent, as well as treating the diarrhea, and ensuring adequate hydration and nutrition.

Hematemesis is vomiting of red blood and indicates upper GI bleeding. Coffee-ground emesis results from bleeding that has slowed or stopped and indicates older blood that has had time to be reduced by gastric acid in the stomach. Patients with chronic blood loss may present with clinical manifestations of anemia (e.g., weakness, easy fatigability, pallor, chest pain, dizziness). Patients with less significant degrees of bleeding may simply have mild tachycardia (heart rate > 100 bpm). Orthostatic changes in pulse (a change of > 10 bpm) or blood pressure (a drop ≥ 10 mm Hg) often develop after acute loss of greater than or equal to 2 units of blood.

Helicobacter pylori is a common gastric pathogen that causes gastritis, peptic ulcer disease (PUD), and gastric cancer. Infection may be asymptomatic or result in varying degrees of dyspepsia. Diagnosis is by urea breath test and testing stool samples. Treatment is with a proton pump inhibitor plus two antibiotics.

A peptic ulcer is defined as an erosion of the GI mucosa, typically in the stomach (gastric ulcer) or the proximal region of the duodenum (duodenal ulcer), that may penetrate only the mucosal surface, or it may extend into the smooth muscle layers. Virtually all ulcers are caused by *H pylori* infection or NSAID use. Symptoms typically include burning epigastric pain that is often relieved by food. Diagnosis is by endoscopy and testing for *H pylori*. Treatment involves acid suppression, eradication of *H pylori* (if present), and avoidance of NSAIDs.

The etiology of gastric cancer is multifactorial, but *H pylori* plays a significant role. Symptoms include early satiety, obstruction, and bleeding but are likely to occur late in the disease. Diagnosis is by endoscopy, followed by CT and endoscopic ultrasound for staging. Treatment is mainly surgery; chemotherapy may provide a temporary response. Long-term survival is poor except for those with local disease. Gastric cancer is often diagnosed late in the disease because symptoms may be vague or nonexistent. Encourage all patients with complaints of dysphagia, a sensation of gastric fullness, or heartburn to seek medical evaluation.

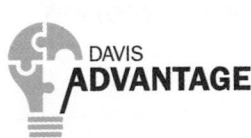

To explore learning resources for this chapter, go to **Davis Advantage** and find:
- Answers to in-text questions
- Chapter Resources and Activities
- NCLEX®-Style Chapter Review Questions
- Bibliography

Chapter 58

Coordinating Care for Patients With Intestinal Disorders

Vickie M. Lester

CONCEPTS

- Assessment
- Bowel Elimination
- Cellular Regulation
- Comfort
- Digestion
- Infection
- Inflammation
- Medication
- Nutrition
- Perfusion
- Safety

ESSENTIAL TERMS

Abdominoperineal resection
Abscess
Anastomosis
Colectomy
Colostomy
Cullen's sign
Diverticulum
Dyspepsia
Ecchymosis
Eructation
Familial adenomatous polyposis (FAP)
Fecalith
Fissure
Fistula
Gluten
Grey Turner's sign
Hemicolectomy
Hereditary nonpolyposis colorectal cancer (HNPCC) or Lynch syndrome
Herniorrhaphy
Ileostomy
Kock (Koch) pouch
McBurney's point
Metastasis
Narcotic bowel syndrome
Ostomy
Proctocolectomy
Rovsing's sign
Stoma
Strictures
Tenesmus
Turner's sign

Finding Connections

CASE STUDY: EPISODE 1

Follow this patient throughout the chapter.

Jack Conner is a 17-year-old male who has been experiencing abdominal pain and has recently noticed blood in his stool. He has been awakening at night frequently to have bowel movements, all grossly bloody and watery. He has only recently let his parents know of these problems, and an appointment is made with his primary healthcare provider. Jack is a high school senior who is involved in theatre and choir activities in school…

INTRODUCTION

The intestinal system is composed of the small and large intestines. The main functions of the intestinal system are digestion, absorption, and elimination of waste products. The small intestine is approximately 20 ft (6 m) in length and extends from the pylorus to the ileocecal valve, which connects the small intestine to the large intestine. The small intestine's primary function is digestion and absorption of nutrients across the intestinal wall into the circulation. Enzymes are secreted throughout the small intestine to aid in the breakdown of food into absorbable nutrients. There are three sections to the small intestine:

- Duodenum—attaches to the pylorus and is approximately 10 in. (25 cm) long
- Jejunum—approximately 8 ft (2.5 m)
- Ileum—approximately 12 ft (3.5 m)

The large intestine is approximately 5 to 6 ft in length (1.5–1.8 m) and extends from the ileocecal valve to the anus. The large intestine's primary function is absorption of water. There is also some absorption of electrolytes, although not to the extent of absorption in the small intestine. Feces is formed in the large intestine where microorganisms break down proteins that were not absorbed in the small intestine. It also serves as a reservoir for feces until defecation. The large intestine is divided into three sections:

- Cecum—approximately 2 to 3 in. (5–8 cm)
- Colon
  - Ascending colon—located on the right side of the abdomen extending upward, bending at the hepatic flexure to become the transverse colon
  - Transverse colon—located horizontally across the abdomen from the hepatic flexure to the splenic flexure, becoming the descending colon
  - Descending colon—lies on the left side of the abdomen from the splenic flexure extending downward to the sigmoid colon

  - Sigmoid colon—the lower "S-shaped" curve extending to the rectum
- Rectum—approximately 7 to 8 in. (17–20 cm) extending to the anus

The vermiform appendix is located behind the cecum and is approximately 3 to 4 in. (8–10 cm) long. It is an accessory organ of the intestinal system but has no known function.

INTESTINAL DISORDERS

Hernias

Epidemiology

A hernia is a protrusion of abdominal contents through an area of weakened muscle in the abdominal cavity and is one of the oldest recorded afflictions of mankind. Hernias can be congenital or acquired and typically occur because of weakened abdominal muscles accompanied by increased abdominal pressure. There are approximately 700,000 inguinal hernia repairs performed in the United States each year with an estimated direct annual cost of $2.5 billion. Inguinal hernias are more common in men, whereas femoral hernias are more common in women. Ventral or incisional hernias develop in previous surgical incision sites usually as a result of infection or the patient had poor wound healing after surgery. Approximately 10% to 15% of patients with abdominal incisions develop a ventral hernia. Indirect inguinal hernias are the most common type and occur only in men. Risk factors for developing a hernia are obesity, smoking, excessive wound tension, malnutrition, pregnancy, and certain medications such as immunosuppressive agents.

Pathophysiology

Although a hernia can occur anywhere in the body, it most frequently occurs in the abdominal cavity, with the intestines protruding through an abnormal opening (Fig. 58.1). If the contents can easily be placed back into the abdominal cavity manually or by lying down, it is known as reducible. If the contents cannot be placed back into the abdominal cavity, it is known as irreducible or incarcerated. In patients with an incarcerated hernia, it can become strangulated, affecting intestinal flow and/or blood supply. If the blood supply is obstructed, it is then known as a strangulated hernia, and the patient may present with symptoms of an intestinal obstruction.

Common causes of hernias may include straining (straining to urinate or have a bowel movement), lifting heavy objects, sudden twists, pulls or muscle strain, weight gain, and chronic cough. Another cause may be a weakened area of abdominal muscle due to a previous abdominal surgery. While people age, muscular tissues become infiltrated and replaced by adipose and connective tissue, which also increases the risk of development of a hernia.

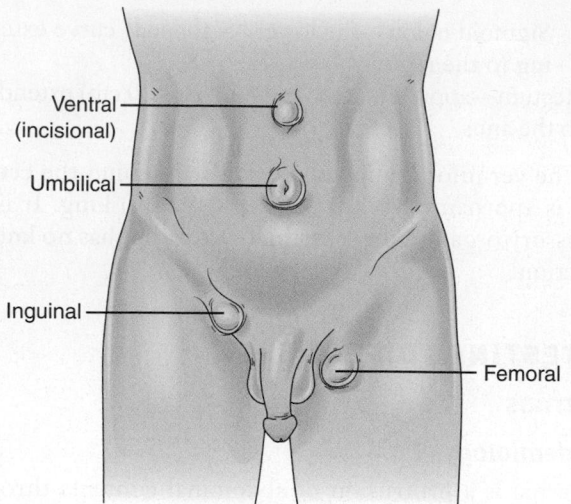

FIGURE 58.1 Types of hernias. Inguinal hernias occur between the abdomen and the thigh and protrude through weakened muscles of the lower abdomen through the inguinal canal. Femoral hernias form due to fat enlargement in the femoral canal causing the pull of contents from the peritoneum into the hernia sac. Femoral hernias typically present below the inguinal ligament. Umbilical hernias are due to increased abdominal pressure and are typically caused by the omentum or peritoneal fat that incarcerates into the hernia. Ventral hernias form from a previous abdominal surgical incision and usually manifest as a bulge along the incision.

Types of Hernias

Inguinal

Approximately 96% of groin hernias are inguinal, and they are more common in males than females. In the groin between the abdomen and the thigh, intra-abdominal fat or part of the small intestine protrudes through weakened muscles of the lower abdomen through the inguinal canal. There are two types of inguinal hernias.

Indirect Inguinal Hernia. Also known as congenital hernias, indirect inguinal hernias develop in the womb. In the male fetus, the spermatic cord and testicles normally descend through the inguinal canal into the scrotum. If the inguinal ring does not close normally after birth, the muscle is weak causing fat or intestine to slide through this weakness. In the female fetus, the female organs or small intestine slides into the groin through the weakened abdominal muscles. Although indirect inguinal hernias are congenital, they may not become obvious until later in life.

Direct Inguinal Hernia. This type of hernia occurs only in males, and it is due to connective tissue degeneration that causes weakened muscles in adulthood. Fat or small intestine slides through the weakened muscle into the groin. The most common symptom of groin hernias is a feeling of heaviness or discomfort that is most noticeable when straining or lifting. The pressure is released when the patient stops straining or lies down. If the patient is experiencing significant pain, incarceration or strangulation should be suspected. Inguinal hernias typically present above the inguinal ligament and extend below it.

Femoral

Approximately 4% of groin hernias are femoral. Femoral hernias are more common in females than males. Fat in the femoral canal enlarges and pulls contents from the peritoneum into the hernia sac. Forty percent of femoral hernias present as an incarcerated or strangulated hernia and must be treated as an emergency. Femoral hernias typically present below the inguinal ligament.

Umbilical

Umbilical hernias occur more frequently in women than men and are due to increased abdominal pressure, usually related to obesity or multiparity (giving birth to more than one child). It is typically the omentum or peritoneal fat that incarcerates (constricts blood flow) into the hernia. Umbilical hernias can also be congenital and appear in infancy. Many congenital umbilical hernias close in the first 12 to 18 months of life, and surgical repair is rarely recommended until a child is approximately 3 years old.

Ventral or Incisional

Ventral hernias form from a previous abdominal surgical incision. They may be due to inadequate healing from an infection, inadequate nutrition, smoking, immunosuppressive medications, connective tissue disorders, or obesity. The highest incidence occurs with midline abdominal wound incisions, with upper abdominal incisions having a higher incidence than lower abdominal incisions. Abdominal wound dehiscence can also lead to a ventral hernia. With ventral hernias, the patient complains of a bulge in the abdominal wall along an old incision site.

Clinical Manifestations

Patients with hernia typically present with a bulge or visible swelling, often associated when coughing or bearing down. Other clinical manifestations include an ache that radiates into the area of the hernia. Strangulation clinical manifestations include abdominal distention, nausea, vomiting, pain, fever, and tachycardia. This is a medical emergency, and the patient must be prepared for surgery immediately to prevent the development of gangrene.

Management

Diagnosis

Hernias are typically diagnosed based on physical examination alone, but if this is not definitive, a herniography (a radiographical examination of a hernia after the introduction of a contrast medium), ultrasound, computed tomography (CT) scan, or magnetic resonance imaging (MRI) can confirm the diagnosis. A CT scan or MRI may be needed to differentiate between inguinal and femoral hernias.

Surgical Management

The most common treatment of hernias is surgery. If the patient is a poor surgical risk, a truss, or binder, may be applied. A truss is a firm pad held in place against the hernia by a belt that reduces the hernia and prevents contents from protruding through the weakened muscle. The truss may be unilateral or bilateral, and the hernia must be reduced prior to the application of the truss. There are also similar products for other types of hernia. The surgical procedure to repair a hernia is called a **herniorrhaphy**. Often the patient may have a synthetic or biological material, called *mesh*, placed to reinforce the area of weakness and prevent recurrence of the hernia. When mesh is used during the surgical repair, the procedure is called a *hernioplasty*. The mesh reinforces the defective area and enhances a lower incidence of recurrence. Herniorrhaphy may be performed through laparoscopic surgery or through an open laparotomy. Surgical repair using laparoscopy generally has a shorter recovery time. Many hernia repairs are now performed on an outpatient basis. If the hernia has strangulated, the surgery is more extensive, and the patient will be hospitalized. A temporary **colostomy**, a surgically created opening on the abdomen in which the large intestine is connected for the elimination of fecal matter, may be required in extensive surgeries.

Postoperative management of the patient undergoing surgery for hernia repair is similar to the care of patients undergoing any other abdominal surgery with the exception of encouraging the patient to cough. Coughing places pressure on the site of repair and increases the incidence of recurrence of the hernia. The patient should be instructed to splint the surgical area when coughing to provide support.

Complications

Complications of hernias include strangulation of the intestine, which impedes intestinal flow and the blood supply to the intestines. This can result in intestinal obstruction and/or necrosis of bowel tissue. A bowel resection may be necessary. Complications related to surgery with general anesthesia to correct hernias include nausea, vomiting, urinary retention, sore throat, and headache. As with any surgery requiring anesthesia, early ambulation and deep breathing prevent complications such as pneumonia and venous thromboembolism (VTE). Recurrence of the hernia can occur, requiring the patient to undergo another surgery for repair. Wound infections can occur, but they are rare unless the patient has undergone an extensive surgery.

> **⚠ Safety Alert** The patient with a strangulated hernia may present with clinical manifestations of an intestinal obstruction. This is an emergency, and the patient must be prepared for immediate surgery to prevent gangrene from developing. Strangulation signs and symptoms include abdominal distention, nausea, vomiting, pain, fever, and tachycardia.

Nursing Management

Assessment and Analysis

The clinical manifestations of hernias are closely related to their location and type of hernia. The clinical presentation of hernia typically includes:

- Bulging or swelling at the site of the hernia
- Ache that radiates in the area of the hernia
- Feelings of fullness or pressure in the area of the hernia

In the case of a strangulated or incarcerated hernia, the patient may present with painful engorgement of the hernia, nausea, vomiting, and abdominal distension.

Nursing Diagnoses

- **Acute pain** related to the surgical incision
- **Knowledge deficit** related to postoperative care and home care

Nursing Interventions

▪ Assessments

- Vital signs
  Increased heart rate and respirations may be indicative of pain and/or bleeding. Elevated temperature may be indicative of infection.
- Pain
  Pain results from the surgical incision and manipulation of abdominal contents during the surgical repair. Adequate pain management allows the patient to resume normal activities sooner.
- Intake and output
  Urinary retention is a complication as a result of the effects of general anesthesia. If the surgery is performed in an outpatient setting, the nurse should have the patient urinate and measure this recording before discharge. If the patient is admitted to the inpatient facility, intake and output should be measured for 24 hours to ensure that the patient is not retaining urine.
- Surgical site
  The surgical site should be well-approximated. Swelling or drainage may be indications of early infection.

▪ Actions

- Deep breathing and early ambulation
  Promote lung expansion and prevent atelectasis and VTE
- Administer pain medications as needed
  Pain medication is essential for the patient to recover to an optimal level and to prevent complications such as atelectasis and VTE. Pain results from the surgical incision and manipulation of abdominal contents during the surgical repair. Adequate pain management allows the patient to resume normal activities sooner.
- Give patient prescription for pain medication prior to discharge
  The patient will require pain medications at home, and this will promote the patient to return to normal activities of daily living.

- Apply ice pack to scrotum and elevate scrotum
  The ice pack and elevation are used to reduce swelling; a scrotal support may also be used to reduce swelling and elevate the scrotum.
- Begin diet with clear liquids, advancing diet as tolerated to patient's preoperative diet
  Nausea and vomiting are common after anesthesia, and the patient should exercise steps to prevent nausea and vomiting.

■ Teaching

- Coughing is discouraged.
  Coughing causes undue pressure on the surgical site and can possibly lead to recurrence of the hernia. If coughing is necessary, the surgical site should be splinted with pillows to prevent pressure on the site.
- Avoid heavy lifting for several weeks
  Heavy lifting can place undue pressure and straining on the surgical site and lead to reoccurrence of the hernia.
- Pain management techniques
  The patient will be discharged with a prescription for pain medication. The nurse should teach the patient about the medication and to avoid driving or operating machinery while taking this medication. If the pain is unrelieved by the medication, this should be reported to the healthcare provider.
- Observe incisions for redness, swelling, heat, and drainage, which indicate infection. The patient should report fevers, chills, and increasing pain to their healthcare provider.
  These are clinical manifestations of infection and should be reported to the healthcare provider as soon as possible.

Evaluating Care Outcomes

Patients recovering from hernia repair surgery return to their previous level of functioning within 6 to 8 weeks after surgery depending on the extent of the surgical repair. The patient who is experiencing surgery for a recurrence of a previous hernia repair may require a longer healing time. Like other postoperative patients, outcomes include stable vital signs, absence of infection, and normal bladder and bowel function. In the event a patient is a poor surgical candidate, outcomes focus on patient comfort and ensuring a clear understanding of the clinical manifestations of strangulation.

Connection Check 58.1

The nurse correlates strangulated hernias with which finding?
A. Impede blood flow of the intestines
B. Result from pressure on an old surgical incision
C. Lead to bouts of diarrhea
D. A hernia in which contents can be placed back into place

Hemorrhoids

Epidemiology

Hemorrhoids are swollen or dilated veins in the anorectal area. Simply, they are varicose veins of the rectum. They may be caused or precipitated by straining during defecation, prolonged constipation, heavy lifting, prolonged standing and sitting, portal hypertension (as in cirrhosis), increased intra-abdominal pressure, pregnancy, obesity, and heart failure. It is a common disorder that affects both men and women but is more frequently reported by women.

Pathophysiology

Hemorrhoids are internal (lying above the dentate line) or external (lying below the dentate line). The anus is approximately 4-cm long, with the dentate line approximately in the center. Internal hemorrhoids cannot be seen on visual inspection (Fig. 58.2). Hemorrhoids can become prolapsed or protrude through the anal canal. A strangulated hemorrhoid is trapped by the anal sphincter, compromising blood flow to the vein in the hemorrhoid. Hemorrhoids may also become thrombosed or clotted.

A standard grading system is used for the grading of internal hemorrhoids according to severity of prolapse and serves as a guide for treatment:

- Grade I: The hemorrhoids do not prolapse.
- Grade II: The hemorrhoids prolapse on defecation but reduce spontaneously.
- Grade III: The hemorrhoids prolapse on defecation and must be reduced manually.
- Grade IV: The hemorrhoids are prolapsed and cannot be reduced manually.

The grading system, however, does not account for other factors such as size, number of hemorrhoids, pain, bleeding, and any other comorbidities the patient may have.

Clinical Manifestations

Approximately 40% of hemorrhoids are asymptomatic. Bleeding is almost always painless and is observed as bleeding during a bowel movement and usually associated with

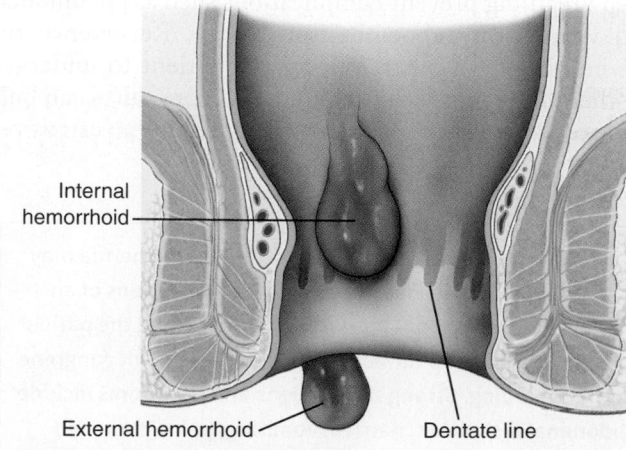

FIGURE 58.2 Hemorrhoids. Hemorrhoids are internal (lying above the dentate line) or external (lying below the dentate line).

internal hemorrhoids. External hemorrhoids are associated with itching, irritation, and pain of the rectal area. Clinical manifestations of hemorrhoids include pain and pruritus in the rectal area. Bleeding may occur and is usually seen on the toilet tissue but may also be streaked in the stool. The hemorrhoid may be prolapsed or protruding from the rectum. Some hemorrhoids may prolapse during defecation and spontaneously return after defecation. Pain symptoms may range from mild to severe.

Management

Medical Management

External hemorrhoids are diagnosed by visual inspection. Internal hemorrhoids are diagnosed by digital examination, anoscopy (procedure involving a small, tubular instrument inserted into the anal canal for inspection), and sigmoidoscopy. Treatment of hemorrhoids is usually conservative and involves relief of symptoms and associated pain. Cold packs and sitz baths (warm water baths covering the hips and buttocks) three or four times a day reduce some swelling and decrease pain. If conservative therapy does not alleviate symptoms within 3 to 5 days, the patient needs to be referred to a primary care provider. The patient is encouraged to consume adequate fluid and fiber intake to decrease constipation associated with hemorrhoids. Stool softeners may also be recommended. Topical nitroglycerin (0.4%) ointment may be used to decrease pain caused by thrombosed hemorrhoids as well as topical nifedipine. There are a number of over-the-counter preparations available in creams and suppositories used to treat hemorrhoids. A variety of combinations of ingredients are available for the treatment of hemorrhoids and are listed in Table 58.1.

Surgical Management

Surgical intervention is seldom required for external hemorrhoids unless the hemorrhoid is thrombosed (internal or external). In this situation, surgical evacuation may be done in the provider's office. Patients seen within 48 to 72 hours after thrombosis occurs may benefit from surgical incision and evacuation.

Patients with grade IV and some with grade III may require definitive treatment with surgery. Surgery is usually done on an outpatient basis. Several surgical techniques are used:

- *Rubber-band ligation*—this is the most widely used technique. The hemorrhoid is identified by using an anoscope. A rubber band is placed around the base of the hemorrhoid, which constricts circulation, causing the hemorrhoid to slough off in 2 to 4 days.
- *Bipolar, infrared, and laser coagulation*—this technique uses bipolar current or infrared or laser light, which causes coagulation and necrosis of the hemorrhoid, leaving fibrosis in the submucosal layer.
- *Sclerotherapy*—involves injecting a sclerosing agent (an agent that causes formation of scar tissue) directly into the hemorrhoid, which causes an inflammatory reaction leading to the vessel drying up and disintegrating.
- *Cryosurgery*—uses liquid nitrogen to freeze the hemorrhoid. This procedure is usually associated with intense pain and is not the first method of choice.
- *Hemorrhoidectomy*—excision of the vein. The area may be left open to heal by secondary intention, or it may be closed with sutures. Closing the area with sutures is less painful for the patient but has a higher risk of infection.

Complications

Complications following surgery for hemorrhoids include infection, pain, urinary retention, fecal impaction, damage to the sphincter, bleeding, and abscess formation, which involves a localized collection of pus. Although infection is rare, it is something the patient needs to be aware of. Fecal impaction occurs as a result of inadequate pain management, with the person being afraid to have a bowel movement, or as a result of opiate usage. The patient will likely have the fecal impaction manually removed under anesthesia. Urinary retention occurs because of rectal spasms and pain.

Nursing Management

Assessment and Analysis

Clinical manifestations of hemorrhoids include rectal pain and itching that may be accompanied by bleeding. The management is based on severity of clinical manifestations, location and response to conservative therapy.

Table 58.1 Medications Used for the Treatment of Hemorrhoids

Ingredient/Classification	Examples of Medications	Action
Local anesthetics	Benzocaine, dibucaine, lidocaine	Provide temporary relief from burning, itching, and pain
Protectants/Emollients	Cocoa butter, lanolin, white petroleum, zinc oxide, mineral oil, cod liver oil, or shark liver oil	Form physical barrier on the skin to prevent irritation of the perianal region
Astringents	Calamine, zinc oxide, witch hazel	Promote skin dryness, which helps relieve itching, irritation, and inflammation
Corticosteroids	Hydrocortisone	Reduce inflammation

Nursing Diagnoses
- **Acute Pain** associated with inflammation in the rectal area
- **Knowledge deficit** associated with the care of hemorrhoids and/or postoperative care
- **Risk for altered bowel elimination: constipation** associated with fear of pain with bowel movements

Nursing Interventions

▪ Assessments
- Vital signs
  A fever may be indicative of an infection and should be reported to the healthcare provider. An increased heart rate and/or respirations may be indicative of pain.
- Visual inspection of rectal area
  The rectal area may appear reddened secondary to itching. Postoperatively, it may appear swollen from manipulation during surgery. There should not be significant drainage or bleeding.
- Frequency and character of bowel movements
  The patient often tries to avoid having a bowel movement due to painful defecation, particularly after surgery because of the increased pain associated with bowel movements. This can lead to constipation and should be avoided because this will further increase pain and perhaps bleeding at the surgical site.
- Bowel habits postoperatively compared with preoperative pattern
  If the patient becomes constipated after surgery, this can lead to increased pain with each subsequent bowel movement.
- Pain
  Pain results secondary to the surgical procedure, and associated inflammation. Adequate pain management allows the patient to resume normal activities sooner.
- Intake and output
  Urinary retention may occur because of rectal spasms and pain.

▪ Actions
- Administer pain medications
  The first bowel movement after surgery may be painful, and the patient needs to take an analgesic prior. Fainting has occurred during bowel movements early after surgery because of the intensity of the pain along with vagal stimulation.
  - Local anesthetics
    Provide temporary relief from burning, itching, and pain
  - Astringents
    Promote skin dryness, which helps relieve itching, irritation, and inflammation
  - Corticosteroids
    Reduce inflammation
  - Protectants/emollients
    Form physical barrier on the skin to prevent irritation of the perianal region
- Provide cold packs and sitz baths
  These interventions are used to reduce swelling and pain

- Administer laxatives
  Bulk laxatives (hydrophilic psyllium) require the use of increased fluids, or they can result in constipation. If the patient has not had a bowel movement within 3 days after surgery, a mild laxative may be ordered.
- Apply local moist heat
  Local moist heat can be used to provide comfort but should be avoided in the immediate postoperative period because of an increased risk of bleeding.

▪ Teaching
- Care of surgical site
  The area should be washed gently and patted dry to keep the surgical area free from contaminants that may cause infection.
- Measures to prevent constipation
  Prevention of constipation is imperative during the postoperative period because the patient may avoid having a bowel movement in fear of increasing pain. Include good sources of fiber; include whole grain and raw vegetables and fruits. Regular bowel habits are important for the patient in the postoperative period for avoiding constipation. Increasing fluids and fiber in their diet helps prevent constipation. Over-the-counter stool softeners such as docusate sodium may also be used. The use of narcotic analgesics may increase the chances of developing constipation.
- Avoid straining to have a bowel movement and avoid sitting for long periods of time
  Straining and sitting for long periods of time can increase inflammation and pain associated with hemorrhoids.
- Avoid stimulant laxatives
  Stimulant laxatives should be avoided because they are irritating and habit-forming.
- Nonpharmacological methods of reducing pain
  Cold packs and sitz baths alleviate some pain associated with hemorrhoids. The use of sitz baths can be used for cleansing as well as having a soothing effect, and they can be used three or four times a day and after bowel movements.
- Contact the healthcare provider if unable to urinate
  Urinary retention may occur because of rectal spasms and pain.

Evaluating Care Outcomes

The patient who has undergone surgery for hemorrhoids usually returns to a normal level of functioning within just a few weeks. Because hemorrhoid surgery is usually performed on an outpatient basis, the patient and family need to demonstrate understanding of what is normal in the recovery process as well as of what is abnormal. The patient should demonstrate adequate pain management to prevent constipation without adding to the chances of constipation with narcotic analgesics. The patient and family acknowledge the importance of contacting the healthcare provider if the patient is not able to urinate after discharge.

Connection Check 58.2

Which interventions are considered conservative treatments for hemorrhoids? *(Select all that apply.)*

A. Hemorrhoid creams and ointments
B. Sitz baths
C. Over-the-counter analgesics
D. Cryosurgery
E. Rubber-band ligation

Irritable Bowel Syndrome

Epidemiology

The exact cause of IBS is unknown. The mucosal lining of the bowel remains essentially unchanged with symptoms. Other names that may be used for IBS include spastic colon, nervous digestion, and spastic colitis, and is characterized by areas of bowel spasm and dilation (Fig. 58.3). It is associated with other conditions such as fibromyalgia, chronic fatigue syndrome, gastroesophageal reflux disease, functional dyspepsia, noncardiac chest pain, depression, anxiety and somatization.

Irritable bowel syndrome (IBS) is a functional disorder of the intestines of unknown etiology with no known cure. It occurs twice as often in women as in men, and often clinical manifestations worsen with a woman's menstrual cycle, suggesting a hormonal component. It is most often diagnosed between the ages of 30 and 50 years, and accounts for approximately 25-50% of all referrals to gastroenterologists. The prevalence of IBS in North America is estimated to be 10% to 15%.

Pathophysiology

Irritable bowel syndrome is a complex and often misunderstood functional disorder characterized by abdominal pain and altered bowel habits for which no other pathophysiological cause can be found. There are four sub-types of IBS:

1. IBS-C (constipation dominant)
2. IBS-D (diarrhea dominant)
3. IBS-M (mixed, or alternating from diarrhea to constipation)
4. IBS unclassified (meets IBS diagnostic criteria but cannot be accurately categorized with the other 3)

Although the exact cause of IBS is unknown, there are many theories regarding the pathophysiology of this disorder, as well as an area of intense research. Possible theories include:

- *Gastrointestinal motility*: Motility abnormalities are noted in some patients with IBS. There have been observations involving increased frequency and irregularity of luminal contractions, prolonged transit time in IBS-C (causing too much water to be absorbed in the small intestine), and increased motor response in IBS-D (causing too little water being absorbed in the small intestine). However, no predominant pattern of motor activity has emerged as a marker for IBS.

- *Visceral hypersensitivity*: Increased sensation and sensitivity to intestinal activity have been noted in patients with IBS. The enteric nervous system extends from the esophagus to the anus and contains as many neurons as the spinal cord. One chemical mediator, 5-hydroxytryptamine (5-HT), or serotonin, may be implicated in IBS. Approximately 95% of serotonin is found in the gastrointestinal tract. Serotonin levels have been found to be increased in patients with IBS. Serotonin is released into the gastrointestinal tract initiating an intestinal reflex. The visceral hypersensitivity also has an exaggerated response to various stimuli in the gastrointestinal system such as balloon-distention studies.

- *Intestinal inflammation*: Increased numbers of lymphocytes have been noted in both the large and small intestines in patients with IBS. Increased numbers of mast cells have also been noted in the terminal ileum, jejunum, and colon of IBS patients. There has been a correlation between abdominal pain and the presence of activated mast cells in proximity to colonic nerves.

- *Postinfectious*: Often the patient with IBS may report previous long-lasting infectious gastroenteritis causing increased intestinal permeability, low-grade inflammation, and increased flatulence due to bacterial fermentation.

- *Bacterial overgrowth*: There have been conflicting reports in the research as to the possibility of small intestinal bacterial overgrowth as being a possibility for IBS and continues to be an area of ongoing research.

- *Food sensitivity*: Certain foods may precipitate abdominal pain in patients with IBS.

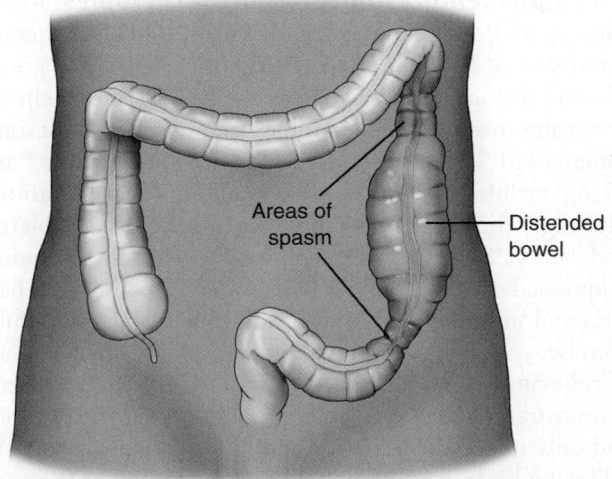

Areas of spasm

Distended bowel

FIGURE 58.3 Irritable bowel syndrome. Irritable bowel syndrome is characterized by areas of bowel spasm and dilation.

- *Carbohydrate malabsorption*: Although still under investigation, fructose, sorbitol, and lactose contribute to gastrointestinal symptoms such as flatus, pain, bloating, belching, and altered bowel habits.
- *Gluten sensitivity*: A few studies have explored the possibility of an overlap between celiac disease and IBS-D. These patients respond to gluten-free diets. Celiac disease should be ruled out, however.
- *Genetics*: A genetic component has been noted for some patients with IBD, although research is ongoing.
- *Psychosocial dysfunction*: Anxiety and depression may play a role in patients with IBS. A history of physical and/or sexual abuse has also been implicated. Stress has been shown to alter gastrointestinal motility in both IBS as well as in patients with normal bowel habits.

Clinical Manifestations

The clinical presentation of IBS includes diarrhea, constipation, flatus, and abdominal pain that may vary based on classification. Patients most often report left lower quadrant pain accompanied by abdominal distension and alternating bouts of diarrhea and constipation. The pain increases after eating and is relieved with bowel movements. Due to the pain and abdominal cramping, the patient may become anorexic with noticeable weight loss.

Management

Treatment for IBS is symptom-based. No one treatment is effective for all patients with IBS, and therefore treatment is highly individualized. A trusting and therapeutic relationship must be established. It is not life threatening, but symptom management may be a lifelong struggle. There are many clinical trials under way, and therefore treatment recommendations are limited. Patients are encouraged to keep a diary of diet, episodes of stress, and triggers associated with the onset of symptoms.

Medical Management

Diagnosis

There are no diagnostic tests that show a definitive diagnosis of IBD. However, a number of tests may be performed to rule out other pathophysiological causes for concern. These tests may include flexible sigmoidoscopy, colonoscopy, CT scan, lactose intolerance tests, stool cultures, and blood tests. After organic causes have been ruled out, the Rome IV or Manning Criteria are used to make the diagnosis of IBS.

The Rome IV Diagnostic Criteria for Functional Gastrointestinal Disorders is one of the most common diagnostic instruments. The patient must have had recurrent abdominal pain or discomfort at least 1 day per week in the last 3 months associated with two or more of the following:

- Improvement with defecation
- Onset associated with a change in frequency of stool
- Onset associated with a change in form (appearance) of stool

The Manning Criteria is another tool used in the diagnosis of IBS. The more clinical manifestations the patient has, the greater likelihood of being diagnosed with IBS.

- Pain relieved with defecation
- More frequent stools at the onset of pain
- Looser stools at the onset of pain
- Visible abdominal distention
- Passage of mucus
- Sensation of incomplete evacuation

Based on clinical presentation and results of these two tools, an individualized management plan is developed.

Treatment

Medications used to treat IBS are listed in Table 58.2. The focus of medical management is on controlling spasm, minimizing diarrhea, releasing neurotransmitters to promote peristalsis, and addressing depression. Cognitive-behavioral therapy, relaxation, stress management, acupuncture, hypnosis, and Chinese herbs have also been noted to be successful in the treatment of IBS. A diet high in fiber may help control symptoms associated with IBS because a bulkier stool reduces tension on the sigmoid colon.

Dietary Modification. The patient with IBS is encouraged to maintain a food diary and note any foods that trigger symptoms. A diet low in fermentable oligo-, di-, and mono-saccharides and polyols (FODMAPs) are noted to improve symptoms for IBS. These short-chained carbohydrates are poorly absorbed and cause some abdominal bloating. Examples of foods that should be avoided include fructose, apples, pears, mangoes, cherries and wheat. Patients eliminate FODMAPs from their diet for 6 to 8 weeks. After resolution of symptoms, they are gradually re-introduced to determine tolerance for specific foods. Patients should also be encouraged to avoid gas-producing foods. Some patients benefit from avoiding lactose, as well. Nonceliac gluten sensitivity (NCGS) has been thought to affect IBS-D patients but the evidence has been inconsistent.

Complementary and Alternative Therapies. Relaxation techniques, acupuncture, hypnosis, and hypnotherapy can decrease IBS symptoms. Probiotics (types of "good" bacteria that are thought to improve health) often help the symptoms in some patients. It has been suggested that some patients with IBS may not have enough "good bacteria," and taking probiotics may help ease clinical manifestations. Although the benefits of probiotics are not completely understood, there have been some general benefits including suppressed growth or epithelial binding by pathogenic bacteria and improved function of intestinal barriers. Regular exercise, yoga, massage, or meditation may be effective ways of relieving stress and anxiety. Some Chinese herbs have demonstrated some relief but should be used with caution and only under the advice of the healthcare provider. The following herbs have demonstrated some relief of IBS:

- Peppermint (*Mentha piperita*) and fennel (*Foeniculum*) are natural antispasmodics and have anti-inflammatory

Table 58.2 Medications Used for Treatment of Irritable Bowel Syndrome

Classification	Medications	Action
Antispasmodic agents	Dicyclomine (Bentyl, Antispas)	Anticholinergic and antimuscarinic components that block acetylcholine, relaxing smooth muscle spasm and GI motility; inhibit gastric secretion
Antidiarrheals	Loperamide (Imodium)	Slow bowel transit, enhance water absorption, and strengthen anal sphincter tone, resulting in fewer stools but does not relieve pain
	Diphenoxylate hydrochloride (Lomotil)	Decreases motility, propulsion, and secretions
Guanylate cyclase agonists	Linaclotide (Linzess) for IBS-C despite treatment with osmotic laxatives	Stimulates intestinal fluid secretion and transit
Serotonergic agents	Tegaserod* (Zelnorm) for IBS-C in female patients	Agonist activity causes release of other neurotransmitters and results in increased peristalsis, increased intestinal secretion, and decreased visceral sensitivity
	Alosetron** (Lotronex) for refractory IBS-D in female patients	Limits gastrocolic reflexes, which can slow transit time and improve muscle tone
Selective type-2 chloride channel (CIC-2) activator	Lubiprostone for IBS-C in women	Increases fluid secretion in the small intestine and is believed to enhance colonic motility by increasing intraluminal volume
Antidepressants		Low doses of antidepressants have been shown to decrease pain
Selective serotonin reuptake inhibitors (SSRIs)	Paroxetine (Paxil); fluoxetine (Prozac); sertraline (Zoloft)	SSRIs inhibit serotonin uptake and may increase pain threshold while decreasing transit time
Tricyclic antidepressants (TCAs)	Amitriptyline (Elavil); imipramine (Tofranil); nortriptyline (Pamelor); desipramine (Norpramin)	TCAs block norepinephrine reuptake and are believed to slow transit time and improve pain tolerance

GI, Gastrointestinal; *IBS,* irritable bowel syndrome; *IBS-C,* irritable bowel syndrome with constipation; *IBS-D,* irritable bowel syndrome with diarrhea.
*Tegaserod was pulled from the market in March 2007 because of increased risk of heart attack and stroke in patients with a previous history of or risk factors for cardiovascular disease. It is currently available only through the FDA's Emergency Investigational New Drug protocol.
**Alosetron was pulled from the market in 2000 after cases of ischemic colitis and severe constipation were reported. It can be prescribed for women with severe IBS-D if the clinician enrolls in a special program and is intended for severe cases of IBS-D who have not responded to other treatments.

properties. They relax smooth muscle in the intestines and help expel gas.

- Herbal teas such as chamomile (*Chamaemelum nobile*) have gentle antispasmodic properties.
- Ginger—helps control nausea and expel gas

> **⚠ Safety Alert** There is a reported increase in the use of herbal remedies in recent years. Medicinal herbs are classified as dietary supplements and are not regulated as medications in the United States. When patients choose to self-administer herbal remedies, teaching must be provided to make them aware that many herbal remedies can interfere with medications they are taking, and the healthcare provider should be consulted. Patients are taught to obtain information related to the herbal

medication of their choice from reputable sources. Some online sources include:

- Natural Medicines Comprehensive Database
- Natural Medicines Research Collaboration
- ConsumerLab
- Medline Plus Drugs and Supplement Directory
- National Institutes of Health National Center for Complementary and Alternative Medicine Herb Fact Sheets
- NIH Office of Dietary Supplements

Complications

Complications associated with IBS often involve psychosocial concerns such as social isolation related to frequent diarrhea. Patients can be referred to support groups to develop strategies to manage changes in physical functioning caused by IBS, such as spasm, constipation and diarrhea. If certain food groups are avoided because of onset of symptoms, patients may not be receiving all the nutrients they need. Clinical manifestations may overlap with other conditions, and it is important that other causes be ruled out before making a diagnosis of IBS. Fluid volume deficit and hypokalemia are also complications when the patient has bouts of frequent diarrhea.

Nursing Management
Assessment and Analysis

Patients can often associate foods that may trigger symptoms and keeping a diary can assist in identifying these trigger foods. Patients often associate a stressful situation with the onset of symptoms, and the diary helps to identify these sources of stress and find better ways of dealing with them. Patients with IBS may also complain of anxiety, sleep disturbances, and difficulty concentrating. A thorough pain assessment is necessary to rule out a pathophysiological cause of pain.

Clinical manifestations for IBS include intermittent abdominal pain and altered bowel habits. The most frequent complaint of abdominal pain is in the left lower quadrant with relief after defecation. Other clinical manifestations may include abdominal distention and bloating, anorexia, excessive flatulence, **dyspepsia** (heartburn), **eructation** (belching), a continual urge to defecate, and a sense of incomplete evacuation. Nausea and increased pain may be associated with meals. For the patient with IBS-D, there may be mucus in the stool but not blood. In the patient with IBS-D, nocturnal diarrhea is uncommon and is usually indicative of an organic disease. The patient usually appears well and does not exhibit significant weight loss.

Nursing Diagnoses

- **Chronic pain** related to spasms and increased motility
- **Ineffective coping** related to the psychosocial effects of IBS
- **Ineffective health maintenance** related to living with a chronic disease

Nursing Interventions
■ Assessments

- Vital signs
  Elevated heart rate and blood pressure may develop secondary to severe pain. Fever may develop secondary to dehydration, inflammation or infection.
- Intake and output
  With frequent bouts of diarrhea, the patient is at increased risk of fluid volume deficit.
- Serum electrolytes
  The patient is at risk of hypokalemia during bouts of diarrhea. Additionally, the serum sodium and blood urea nitrogen may be elevated secondary to dehydration.

- Pain
  The most frequent complaint of abdominal pain is in the left lower quadrant with relief after defecation and is most likely due to the intestinal spasm and dilation.
- Bowel pattern
  Patients with IBS may have constipation, diarrhea, or a combination of both.
- Weight
  The patient is at risk of weight loss, particularly during exacerbations of IBS.
- Psychosocial assessment
  Because onset of symptoms is often associated with stress, a thorough psychosocial assessment can reveal triggers.

■ Actions

- Administer ordered IV solutions
  Based on the degree of fluid volume deficit that results from diarrhea, IV replacement fluids are ordered. A common solution is 0.45NS with potassium supplementation.
- Establish a trusting relationship
  Irritable bowel syndrome is often thought of as a psychological illness rather than a physical illness. A therapeutic, trusting relationship is necessary for the patient to have an open relationship with the caregiver, providing empathy and support.
- Avoid foods that exacerbate clinical manifestations of IBS
  Caffeine and alcohol increase gastrointestinal motility and irritate the gastrointestinal mucosa. Indigestible carbohydrates such as beans produce increased gas, leading to abdominal discomfort.
- Establish a regular bowel routine
  Drinking six to eight glasses of water per day helps to regulate stool frequency. Increase physical activity to promote GI motility.
- Implement complementary and alternative medicines that may relieve symptoms
  Complementary and alternative therapies often help relieve symptoms associated with IBS but should be used only under the advice of the provider.
  - Peppermint (*Mentha piperita*) and fennel (Foeniculum) are natural antispasmodics and have anti-inflammatory properties. They relax smooth muscle in the intestines and help expel gas.
  - Herbal teas such as chamomile (*Chamaemelum nobile*) have gentle antispasmodic properties.
  - Ginger—helps control nausea and expel gas
- Make appropriate referrals to
  - Dietitians
  - Psychological counseling
  - Support groups
    Irritable bowel syndrome is a complex disease of unknown etiology that requires an interprofessional approach including a dietitian, case manager, and psychiatric approaches.

■ Teaching

- Avoid trigger foods that exacerbate clinical manifestations
  Trigger foods that cause the patient to have symptoms are different for every patient. Common foods that seem to

trigger abdominal discomfort include caffeine, alcohol, eggs, wheat products, and beverages containing sorbitol or fructose. Caffeine and alcohol may irritate the gastrointestinal tract. Lactose intolerance is common. These foods may increase gastrointestinal motility, leading to increased abdominal pain and/or diarrhea.

- Keep a diary
  The diary can assist the patient in identifying sources of stress and trigger foods that exacerbate symptoms.
- Consume regular meals and drink 8 to 10 cups of liquid per day
  Regular meals enhance the promotion of regular bowel habits. Adequate fluid intake helps regulate stool consistency and frequency.
- Encourage regular exercise and 7 to 8 hours of sleep each night
  Regular exercise and adequate sleep are important for both regular bowel habits and managing stress and anxiety.
- Smoking cessation techniques
  Smoking has also been associated with IBS, and patients therefore should be taught about the effects of smoking and offered smoking cessation counseling. Nicotine increases gastrointestinal motility, which can lead to increased pain and/or diarrhea.

Evaluating Care Outcomes

Irritable bowel syndrome remains a mysterious and often complex syndrome of unknown etiology, with varying effects on different individuals, making it difficult to manage. Expected outcomes in the management of IBS include stable vital signs and weight, decrease in clinical manifestations, and patient's understanding and adherence to nutritional and activity recommendation to manage this chronic disease. Another desired outcome in the care of the patient with IBS is establishing a trusting relationship because these individuals often feel as if the healthcare provider sees them as having a psychological illness rather than a physical illness.

Connection Check 58.3

The nurse recognizes which findings as diagnostic for IBS?
A. Rome IV and/or Manning Criteria
B. CT scan of the abdomen shows inflammatory process
C. Blood urea nitrogen and creatinine are elevated
D. Patient has abdominal pain and a psychiatric diagnosis

Inflammatory Bowel Disease

Epidemiology

Inflammatory bowel disease (IBD) is an umbrella term for two very similar chronic diseases of the gastrointestinal tract: Crohn's disease and ulcerative colitis. It is estimated that 1.6 million Americans currently suffer from IBD in America. The incidence of IBD is higher in the United States, Canada, the United Kingdom, Sweden, and Norway, with Canada having the highest incidence in the world. The

risk is higher among Ashkenazi Jewish populations of Europe and American Jews of European descent. Diagnosis can occur at any age but is more likely to occur between the ages of 15 and 35. The annual estimated financial burden (direct and indirect costs) of IBD in the United States is $14.6 billion to $31.6 billion. Traditionally, IBD has been considered a predominately Caucasian disease, but the incidence among African Americans is steadily increasing.

Pathophysiology

The exact cause of IBD is unknown, but it has been linked to genetic predisposition, environmental conditions, and defects in immune regulation. This genetic predisposition may manifest as an overactive immune response to bacteria located in the gastrointestinal tract. It may then be triggered by an environmental response such as infection, medication, or smoking. Whereas the immune system usually attacks foreign invaders, in people with IBD, the immune response has an inappropriate response in the intestinal tract causing inflammation. The inflammation affects the ability to absorb nutrients resulting in diarrhea and weight loss in some patients.

There have been some studies to examine dietary influences in the development of IBD. Some trigger foods which may be implicated include hypersensitivity to cow's milk in infancy and refined sugar intake, particularly in Crohn's disease. Dietary fiber has been noted to possibly decrease the risk of Crohn's disease but not ulcerative colitis.

Clinical Manifestations

Inflammatory bowel disease is chronic in nature, and the severity ranges from mild to severe, with periods of remission and exacerbations. Exacerbations often are precipitated by physical or emotional stress. Although there are similarities, there are also many differences between Crohn's disease and ulcerative colitis (Fig. 58.4). Similarities include persistent diarrhea; abdominal pain or cramps; fever; weight

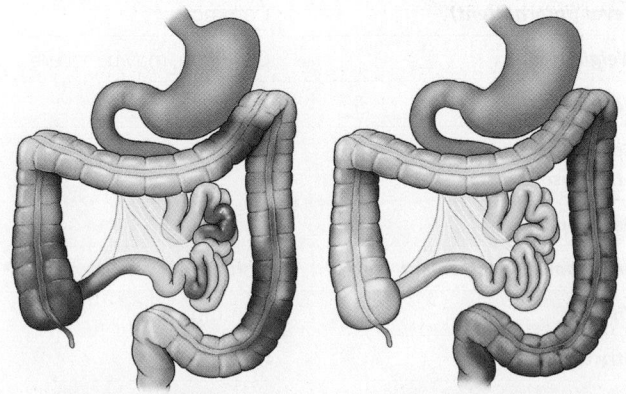

Crohn's Disease   **Ulcerative Colitis**

FIGURE 58.4 Inflammatory bowel disease. Crohn's disease manifests patchy involvement throughout all layers of the bowel. It may skip areas of the bowel and can occur anywhere in the gastrointestinal tract from mouth to anus. Ulcerative colitis begins in the rectum and proceeds in a continuous, diffuse pattern toward the cecum.

loss; fluid imbalances; malnutrition; mouth ulcers; anemia; blood from the rectum; joint, skin, or eye irritations; and delayed growth. Extraintestinal manifestations seen in IBD include uveitis (intraocular inflammatory disorder), sclerosing cholangitis (inflammation of the hepatic ducts), nephrolithiasis (renal stones), cholelithiasis (gallstones), joint disorders, skin disorders, and oral ulcerations. Table 58.3 demonstrates differences between Crohn's disease and ulcerative colitis, with a focus on the anatomical and functional differences. Patients with Crohn's disease are at higher risk for cancer of the small bowel, whereas patients with ulcerative colitis

are at higher risk for colon cancer after having the disease for a long period of time. Although there is no medical cure for either disease, a **colectomy** (removal of the large intestine) cures ulcerative colitis in the gastrointestinal tract. However, having a colectomy does not cure the extraintestinal manifestations associated with ulcerative colitis. Patients with Crohn's disease who undergo surgical resection of diseased sections of the bowel are at increased risk of reoccurrence at the sites of the **anastomoses**, the area where the two sections of the bowel were reattached after removal of diseased bowel.

Table 58.3 Comparison of Crohn's Disease and Ulcerative Colitis

Characteristic	Crohn's Disease	Ulcerative Colitis
Region/Location affected	Terminal ileum (most common), sometimes colon with patchy involvement throughout all layers of the bowel, skip lesions; can occur anywhere in the GI tract from mouth to anus	Colon, rectum; begins in the rectum and proceeds in a continuous, diffuse pattern toward the cecum
Distribution of lesions	Transmural, all layers	Mucosa and submucosa only of the colon
Characteristic stool	Loose, semiformed	Frequent, watery, with blood and mucus
Number of stools per day	5–6 soft, loose, nonbloody	10–20 liquid, bloody
Granuloma	Common	Occasional
Fistula, fissure, abscess	Common	Rare
Stricture, obstruction	Common	Rare
Malabsorption, malnutrition	Yes	Not common or minimal incidence
Etiology	Unknown	Unknown
Peak incidence age	15–35 years	15–25 years and 55–65 years
Complications	Fistulas, nutritional deficiencies	Hemorrhage, nutritional deficiencies
Need for surgery	Frequent	Infrequent; cure with colectomy
Fever (intermittent)	Common	During acute attacks
Weight loss	Common, may be severe	Rare
Tenesmus	Rare	Common
Cobblestone appearance of mucosa	Common	Rare
Pseudopolyps	Rare	Common
Small bowel involvement	Common	Minimal, only backwash into ileum
Fistulas	Common	Rare
Strictures	Common	Occasional
Anal abscess	Common	Rare
Perforation	Common (transmural)	Common (toxic megacolon)
Recurrence after surgery	Common at site of anastomosis	Cure with colectomy

GI, Gastrointestinal.

Patients with IBD usually present to the healthcare provider with abdominal pain, diarrhea, fluid and/or electrolyte imbalances, and weight loss.

CASE STUDY: EPISODE 2

Mr. Conner presents to his primary care provider with complaints of abdominal pain and bloody stools (12–14 stools per day). He describes that he has been having bright red blood in his stools for 6 months with abdominal pain that began shortly thereafter. On examination, abdominal pain is diffuse in location and sharp in character. A stool sample reveals watery consistency with blood streaks and "pus" or "droplets of fat" floating on top of the stool along with spasms of the anal sphincter and persistent desire to empty the bowel. On the basis of his clinical presentation, a colonoscopy is scheduled…

Crohn's Disease

Crohn's disease can affect any portion of the gastrointestinal tract from mouth to anus, although it is more common in the terminal ileum and colon. It is transmural, affecting all layers of the bowel. It is not uniform in appearance and is noted for having skip lesions with normal-appearing bowel between lesions. The lesions cause deep ulcerations between layers of edematous tissue, creating a cobblestone appearance. With each exacerbation, the intestines become more scarred, which then leads to less ability to absorb nutrients. Because Crohn's disease is transmural, it may actually penetrate the bowel wall, leading to complications such as fistulas, abscesses, and peritonitis. **Fistulas** are abnormal tracts between two or more body areas; patients with Crohn's disease may develop anovaginal and rectovaginal fistulas. Strictures and adhesions are also common. Diarrhea is less severe than in ulcerative colitis. Stools are typically soft or semiliquid and do not usually contain blood unless there has been a perforation. Nutritional deficits arise from the inability to absorb nutrients, and electrolyte disturbances are common. Abdominal pain is usually worse in the right lower quadrant.

Ulcerative Colitis

Ulcerative colitis affects the large intestine and involves only the mucosa and submucosa. The disease spreads uniformly beginning at the rectum and spreading upward toward the cecum. The small intestine is rarely involved. Diarrhea is common, often with more than 20 stools per day with losses of several liters of fluid per day. Blood, mucus, and pus are common with ulcerative colitis. Another clinical manifestation includes abdominal pain and tenderness that is worse in the left lower quadrant. Patients may manifest **tenesmus** which involves spasms of the anal sphincter and persistent desire to empty the bowel. Additionally, a lesion called a *crypt abscess* releases secretions that result in purulent discharge from the bowel mucosa.

Abscesses may form in ulcerated areas. Scar tissue is common, interfering with absorption of nutrients. Whereas there is no known cure for Crohn's disease, a total colectomy is a surgical cure for ulcerative colitis.

Indeterminate Colitis

In rare cases, healthcare providers are unable to determine if the patient has ulcerative colitis or Crohn's disease and are therefore given the diagnosis of indeterminate colitis. This resembles ulcerative colitis more than Crohn's disease.

Management

The primary goals of treatment are to rest the bowel and control the inflammation. Other goals are to combat infection, correct malnutrition, alleviate stress, provide symptomatic relief, and improve quality of life. The treatments include medications, surgery, and correction of nutritional deficits and involve many psychosocial needs. Although IBD cannot be cured with medication, there are medications to help control the disease and treat or prevent exacerbations. The medications most often used to treat IBD are listed in Table 58.4.

Diagnosis

Colonoscopy, sigmoidoscopy, and barium enema are commonly used in the diagnosis of both Crohn's disease and ulcerative colitis. The colonoscopy findings may assist in differentiating Crohn's disease and ulcerative colitis. In the patient with Crohn's disease, the colonoscopy detects early mucosal changes including inflammation, stricture, and fistulae. In ulcerative colitis, findings from colonoscopy include swollen, friable bowel mucosa with multiple ulcerations. Barium enema results may provide data regarding the depth of disease involvement. In patients with IBD, additional diagnostic tests include complete blood count, serum electrolytes, serum albumin, and stool samples for pathogens. However, in rare cases the healthcare provider is unable to determine whether the patient has Crohn's disease or ulcerative colitiis (Indeterminate Colitis).

Medical Management

Fluid and electrolyte management is crucial for the patient with ulcerative colitis. When the bowel is inflamed, and the patient is exhibiting severe diarrhea, absorption of fluids and nutrients is compromised. The patient is encouraged to rest frequently to decrease bowel motility.

Medications

The patient with IBD is taught the importance of adhering to prescribed medication management (see Table 58.4). Medications often have unpleasant side effects, which should be reported to the provider prior to discontinuation of use.

Nutrition

Malnutrition is common with IBD and can lead to many other complications such as poor wound healing, decreased muscle mass, and a decreased immune system. Dietary considerations are highly individualized depending on which portion of the bowel is affected. Nutritional abnormalities

Table 58.4 Medications Used to Treat Inflammatory Bowel Disease

Classification	Medications	Action
5-Aminosalicylates	Sulfasalazine (Azulfidine, Azulfidine EN-Tabs), mesalamine (Asacol, Pentasa, Rowasa, Canasa, and Lialda), olsalazine (Dipentum), and balsalazide (Colazal)	Block production of prostaglandins and leukotrienes to decrease inflammation. May be given orally or rectally to reduce inflammation. These medications are contraindicated if patient is allergic to aspirin. Sulfasalazine is contraindicated in patients allergic to sulfa. These medications are effective in both achieving and maintaining remission. They are used primarily to treat ulcerative colitis. They are effective in 2–4 weeks after initiation.
Antimicrobials	Metronidazole (Flagyl, Protostat) and ciprofloxacin	Help control clinical manifestations in Crohn's disease but ineffective in ulcerative colitis. They are also used to treat secondary infections. They reduce small intestinal bacterial overgrowth and reduce flares.
Glucocorticoids	Dexamethasone (prednisone) and budesonide (Entocort)	Decrease inflammation but should be given for short periods of time during exacerbations and tapered appropriately because of long-term side effects. These medications are effective in achieving remission but not maintaining. Steroids must be used with caution because they also impair immune resistance, which then causes a decrease in healing of fistulas and abscesses. Budesonide (Entocort) is a newer nonsystemic steroid that has fewer side effects and is useful in treating exacerbations but not useful during remission.
Biologic therapies	Biologic therapies used include infliximab (Remicade), certolizumab (Cimzia), adalimumab (Humira), and natalizumab (Tysabri)	Alter a person's immune response. They alter an inflammatory protein called tumor necrosis factor (TNF). Although these medications have been traditionally used as second-line agents, some providers are recommending them earlier in treatment. This group of medications has many toxic side effects such as blood dyscrasias, infection, pancreatitis, and digestive intolerance and should be used with caution.
Immunomodulators	Azathioprine (Imuran), mercaptopurine (Purinethol), cyclosporine (Sandimmune, Neoral, and Gengraf), and methotrexate	Modifies the activity of the immune system to decrease inflammation; may be used for long-term therapy
Antidiarrheals	Diphenoxylate hydrochloride and atropine sulfate (Lomotil) and loperamide (Imodium)	Provide symptomatic relief and bowel rest. These medications must be used with caution because they can cause colon dilation.

can be caused by a number of problems including malabsorption, decreased food intake, medications, and/or intestinal losses. The patient may need to be hospitalized for bowel rest and receive total parenteral nutrition (TPN). In Crohn's disease, monthly B_{12} injections may be necessary because of the inability of the ileum to absorb this nutrient. Other nutritional deficits include zinc, potassium, magnesium, and vitamins. Liquid vitamin preparations are usually necessary because tablets or capsules may be excreted intact because of the frequency of diarrhea. Albumin levels are frequently used to determine nutritional status, but other factors may alter albumin levels such as inflammation, infection, or cancer. There is also no gold standard for measuring vitamin and mineral deficiencies. Being aware of the clinical manifestations associated with vitamin deficiencies helps guide treatment. Foods to avoid include milk, gluten, caffeine, cocoa, chocolate, citrus juices, cold or carbonated drinks, nuts, seeds, popcorn, and alcohol.

Complementary and Alternative Medicines

Complementary and alternative medicines (CAMs) are estimated to be used by 30% to 50% of patients with IBD, although patients are often reluctant to mention this to their provider for fear of being judged because some providers may not have adequate knowledge of CAMs. some examples of CAMs being used include marijuana, turmeric and curcumin, fish oil, probiotics, aloe vera, *Androphigus paniculata* (e.g., India echinacea), *Boswellia* (e.g., frankincense), *Tripterygium wilfordii* Hook F (thunder god vine), wheat grass, and wormwood. Research data vary widely, recommendations are inconsistent and these herbs are not regulated by the Food and Drug Administration (FDA).

Other therapies include acupuncture and moxibustion, mind-body therapies, and exercise.

Psychosocial Management

Although there is no evidence to suggest that IBD is a psychosomatic illness, exacerbations may occur during times of emotional or physical stress. Poor quality of life has been implicated in many studies because of the chronic nature of the disease. The inability to control clinical manifestations can disrupt lives because patients fear of being away from home because of the frequency of diarrhea. Eating is frequently associated with the onset of abdominal pain, causing mealtimes to become unpleasant. A thorough assessment of support systems, stress-producing factors, and coping mechanisms is essential. Studies have shown that patients often have maladaptive coping skills that affect peers, family, and others.

When caring for patients with IBD, it is important to consider their stage of growth and development at the time of diagnosis as the average age when diagnosis is made is generally 15 to 35 years of age. Patients with IBD are concerned with how others view them, and this impacts self-esteem. There may be a perceived, or actual, loss of independence, sense of control, privacy, body image, healthy self, peer relationships, self-confidence, productivity, and ways of expressing sexuality, therefore increasing risk of depression. There is also the problem of embarrassment in using public bathrooms and shame with the individuals with ostomies. Depression and anxiety are common in the patient with IBD and should be treated accordingly. Patients often do not discuss these concerns with their healthcare provider, and therefore it often goes untreated. Pharmacological and nonpharmacological treatments may be necessary. Continuous follow-up by the primary care provider is also necessary.

Surgical Management

Surgery for Crohn's disease is reserved for patients for whom medical management has failed and/or who experience complications from the disease. These complications may include strictures, abscesses, intestinal obstruction, perforation, hemorrhage, or cancer. When a diseased portion of the bowel is removed, it frequently recurs in another section of the bowel. Nevertheless, surgery does not cure Crohn's disease.

Patients with ulcerative colitis for whom medical management has failed or who have experienced complications may undergo a colectomy and be cured of the disease but not of the extraintestinal manifestations. Many patients with ulcerative colitis undergo surgery. An example of a patient for whom medical management has failed may include therapy that includes excessive long-term side effects such as high-dose corticosteroids. Having a colectomy for those patients for whom medical management has failed has demonstrated an improved quality of life. The standard procedure for ulcerative colitis is an ileal pouch anal anastomosis (IPAA). The entire colon and rectum are removed, a pouch is created to collect waste, and the patient is able to defecate normally. Patients with ulcerative colitis may undergo a **proctocolectomy** with permanent ileostomy, which includes the removal of the colon and rectum and permanent closure of the anus. The ileostomy is permanent. Another procedure includes the creation of a continent ileostomy (**Kock or Koch pouch**) after proctocolectomy. A portion of the ileum is used to create a reservoir that can be catheterized to remove stool. Pouch failure is more common in patients with indeterminate colitis. Box 58.1 provides an overview of surgical options for patients with ulcerative colitis.

Complications

Patients with inflammatory bowel disease have the potential for many complications in both the gastrointestinal tract and extraintestinal structures. Perineal abscesses and fistulas occur in up to one-third of patients with Crohn's disease, and strictures and fistulas are more common in the patient with Crohn's disease. Extraintestinal complications include joint swelling and pain, ankylosing spondylitis, osteoporosis, kidney stones, eye inflammation, mouth sores, and skin lesions. During inflammation, the patient may experience fever, anorexia, and malaise. Anal **fissures**, tears in the anal wall, or painful ulcers develop secondary to severe bouts of diarrhea. Intestinal obstruction occurs secondary to inflammation and edema. Fibrosis and scarring over time may also cause narrowing of the bowel, leading to an obstruction. Malnutrition frequently develops because of malabsorption of nutrients, severe diarrhea, and anorexia due to the fear that eating may cause an exacerbation of symptoms. In Crohn's disease, the small bowel is affected most often, and malabsorption is more common in this population. Anemia from hemorrhage and malnutrition may lead to patients needing blood transfusions and patients are often prescribed iron supplements to treat anemia.

Surgical complications may include anal canal strictures, pelvic sepsis, pouch failure, fecal incontinence, pouch dysplasia/cancer, sexual dysfunction, and female infertility. Chronic pouchitis is a complication associated with the IPAA procedure in approximately 20% of patients in the first year and 50% after five years. Early clinical trials suggest one probiotic preparation may be effective in the prevention of recurrent pouchitis. This preparation, VSL#3, contains four *Lactobacillus* species, three *Bifidobacterium* species, and one strain of *Streptococcus salivaris* subspecies *thermophilus*.

Fistulas are more common with Crohn's disease. The presence of a fistula can often cause other complications such as sepsis, skin irritations, and malnutrition, dehydration, and fluid and electrolyte imbalances. Fistulas are very difficult to treat, and collaboration with a wound and ostomy nurse is essential. Surgery is often necessary to repair some fistulas. Bowel rest and TPN are frequently used for the treatment of fistulas. Types of fistulas that may occur include:

- Enterocutaneous fistula (between skin and intestine)
- Enteroenteral fistula (between intestine and intestine)
- Enterovesicular fistula (between bowel and bladder)
- Enterovaginal fistula (between bowel and vagina)

Box 58.1 Surgical Options for Ulcerative Colitis

- Proctocolectomy with permanent ileostomy—the colon and rectum are removed, and the anus is closed. The ileostomy is permanent.
- Proctocolectomy with continent ileostomy (Kock pouch)—the colon is removed. The distal portion of the ileum is used to create a pouch, which serves as a reservoir for stool. The patient then must insert a catheter into the pouch several times a day to eliminate the stool.
- Abdominal colectomy with ileoanal anastomosis—the colon is removed, and the ileum is sutured to the anal canal. Leakage of stool is a problem for these patients.
- Colectomy, mucosal proctectomy, and ileal pouch-anal canal anastomosis (IPAA)—performed in a two-step procedure. In the first procedure, the colon and rectal mucosa are removed. An ileoanal reservoir is created by using a portion of the ileum. A temporary ileostomy is created. After the pouch heals (usually in 2–3 months), a second surgery is performed, and the ileostomy is reversed; the pouch serves as a reservoir for stool. The patient then has normal continence of the bowel.

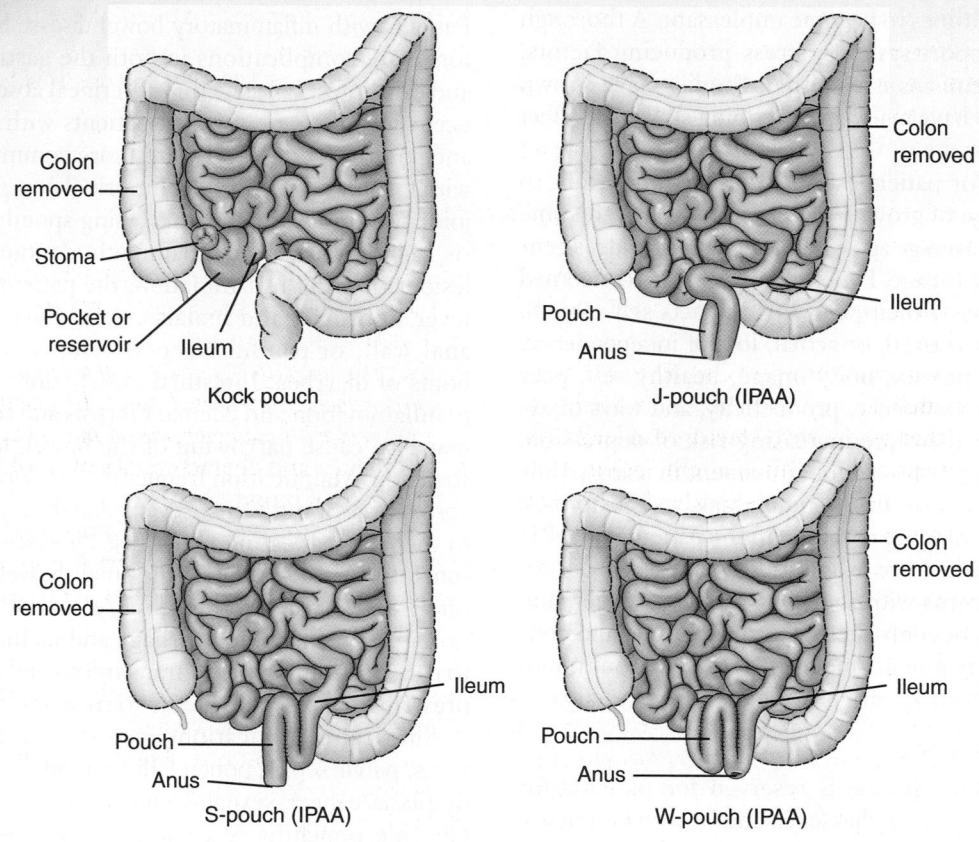

Skin irritation and excoriation often occur because of intestinal secretions being rich in enzymes; protection of the skin is of utmost importance. The skin may come in contact with intestinal secretions through fistulas and **ostomies**, surgical openings in an organ, such as an **ileostomy** (opening in the ileum) and colostomy (opening in the colon). The anus can also become irritated from frequent diarrhea. Toxic megacolon (colonic dilation of greater than 5 cm) occurs more commonly in ulcerative colitis and requires emergency colectomy. It usually occurs during an acute exacerbation. Bacterial overgrowth contributes to toxic megacolon. Perforation of the bowel with possible peritonitis can also occur because of the deep ulcerations in the intestines. **Strictures** or narrowing of the bowel usually occur because of fibrosis and scar tissue and require surgery

to correct. Fluid and electrolyte losses caused by excessive diarrhea can lead to fluid and electrolyte disturbances and must be treated accordingly, with magnesium and potassium being of particular importance.

Short bowel syndrome can occur if more than 100 cm of small bowel is removed because absorption is greatly affected. The jejunum is where most carbohydrate and protein absorption takes place, and the ileum is where absorption of fats, fat-soluble vitamins, and B_{12} takes place. If the jejunum alone is removed, the ileum assumes the function of fat absorption. The removal of the ileum accounts for more complications because it is responsible for the absorption of fats, vitamins, bile salts, and B_{12}. Patients having 50% to 70% of the small intestine removed experience malabsorption but can usually be managed with dietary modification, oral nutrition supplements, and medications. If removal exceeds 75% of the small intestine, the patient requires long-term TPN or intestinal transplantation. Whether or not the colon is left intact also plays a role in the treatment of short bowel syndrome. The colon absorbs water, electrolytes, and fatty acids although in smaller amounts. Short bowel syndrome may leave the patient TPN dependent.

Although much less common, pulmonary complications may occur. Inflammation of the trachea, bronchi and bronchioles may develop before or after bowel resection. IBD-associated serositis (inflammation of serous membrane such as the pleura, pericardium or peritoneum) may occur as pleural effusions or pericarditis. Pulmonary necrobiotic nodules are a rare extra-intestinal manifestation of Crohn's disease. These are lung nodules that can cavitate and are composed of inflammatory cells with necrosis. Pulmonary complications appear to be associated with medications used to treat IBD.

Chronic abdominal pain affects many patients with IBD, many of whom are treated with narcotic pain relief medications. Many of these patients also experience an overlap of IBS-IBD, which has also been associated with the clinical manifestations of chronic abdominal pain. Pain management for the patient with IBD can prove to be a challenge. Narcotics slow intestinal activity and should be used with caution. Stress and other psychosocial factors can lead to an increased pain perception in this patient population. Chronic narcotic use in these patients can lead to narcotic bowel syndrome. Thought to be underdiagnosed, **narcotic bowel syndrome** is characterized as chronic, intermittent, and cramping abdominal pain associated with the effects of the narcotic analgesic wearing off. The patient therefore takes additional narcotics to relieve the pain, and this leads to a vicious cycle of chronic abdominal pain. Narcotic bowel syndrome often goes undiagnosed for long periods of time. It is estimated that about 4% to 6% of people using long-term opioids develops the syndrome. There must be an established trusting relationship between the patient and the healthcare provider because the patient may go elsewhere for treatment seeking more pain medications which may cause the situation to become worse. Treatment involves weaning the patient off all narcotic pain medications. The patient may be placed on long-acting narcotics to assist with treatment of withdrawal. Antidepressant and antianxiety medications may also be used to treat symptoms associated with withdrawal. Nonpharmacological therapies should also be initiated.

Nursing Management

Assessment and Analysis

Assessment of intake and output and daily weights will help determine nutritional status of patients with suspected IBD. Frequent diarrhea leads to extreme losses of fluids and potassium, or hypokalemia. Patients with IBD are often victims of social isolation because of the fear of incontinence in public or having the need to be close to a bathroom at all times. Moreover, patients with IBD often report exacerbations as related to a stressful event. Clinical manifestations include persistent diarrhea, abdominal pain or cramps, fever, weight loss, fluid imbalances, mouth ulcers, anemia, melena, as well as extraintestinal manifestations including uveitis, sclerosing cholangitis, nephrolithiasis, cholelithiasis, joint disorders, and skin disorders.

Nursing Diagnoses

- **Deficient fluid volume** associated with diarrhea
- **Diarrhea** associated with intestinal inflammation and malabsorption of nutrients
- **Imbalanced nutrition**: less than body requirements related to the inability to absorb nutrients secondary to inflammation
- **Ineffective coping** associated with chronic disease

Nursing Interventions

▪ Assessments

- Vital signs
  With significant fluid loss, the patient may develop signs of decreased fluid volume including a low-grade fever, elevated heart rate, and decreased blood pressure.
- Nutritional intake
  Assisting the patient to maintain an intake diary will assist in monitoring nutritional status. Frequent diarrhea is associated with malabsorption of nutrients.
- Frequency and characteristics of stools and note any presence of blood
  Excessive losses result in complications such as fluid and electrolyte imbalances. Blood may be noted in the stool of the patient with ulcerative colitis but is unusual with Crohn's disease.
- Intake and output
  Patients often do not attempt to eat or drink in fear of exacerbating clinical manifestations. Urine output should be monitored for at least 30 mL/hr to provide information regarding renal perfusion.
- Daily weight
  Weight is the best measure for nutritional needs.
- Fluid and electrolyte status
  Patients tend to lose many electrolytes through diarrhea, particularly potassium and magnesium.
- Psychosocial assessment and support systems
  The patient frequently is a victim of social isolation because of fears of incontinence and/or frequent trips to the bathroom.

▪ Actions

- Encourage smaller frequent meals
  Decreases gastric motility
- Encourage the patient to engage in mealtimes with family
  Mealtimes often become unpleasant experiences, and patients often isolate themselves from the rest of the family.
- Encourage periods of rest
  Help decrease gastric motility and conserve energy
- Establish a therapeutic relationship
  Helps develop trust between patient and healthcare provider

- Make appropriate referral to interprofessional team
  Inflammatory bowel disease is a complex disease and requires a team approach including a case manager, dietitian, and any local support groups.
- Pain management
  Positioning and maintaining a quiet environment may promote comfort. Pain medications may be ordered; if administered, monitor for side effects like constipation.
- Provide meticulous skin care
  The patient having frequent diarrhea needs special attention to the rectal area because the feces contain enzymes that may cause excoriation to the skin surrounding the anus.

■ Teaching

- Importance of adequate nutrition
  Malnutrition due to malabsorption is common with the patient with IBD. Adequate nutrition is required for healing and maintaining a stable weight. A daily multivitamin may be prescribed, but vitamins with iron may be controversial due to poor tolerance and may worsen symptoms. Reducing fiber and fat intake during exacerbations, drinking plenty of fluids, and avoiding milk and milk products during exacerbations are also important to the patient's teaching.
- Indications, actions and side effects of prescribed medications, which may vary (see Table 58.4)
  If the patient has a good knowledge of his or her medications, compliance will increase.
- Importance of regular follow-ups and annual colonoscopy
  Regular follow-ups and colonoscopy are necessary because cancer can develop, particularly with ulcerative colitis.

Evaluating Care Outcomes

Inflammatory bowel disease affects individuals in varying degrees, making it difficult to determine exact evaluation criteria for all patients. The patient with IBD should have a good understanding of the importance of maintaining a healthy weight because malnutrition is a common problem. Demonstrating stable vital signs, fluid and electrolyte balance, and stable weight are important outcomes. The patient who has failed medical management may undergo surgery to control clinical manifestations of the disease. Ulcerative colitis is typically more receptive to treatment and can be cured with surgery. Crohn's disease is much more difficult to treat, and patients experience varying levels of success to treatments.

Celiac Disease

Epidemiology

Celiac disease is a genetic autoimmune disorder that damages the small intestine. It is related to eating foods containing gluten found in wheat, barley and rye. Gluten is not only found in foods, such as bread and pasta, but also in some hair and skin care products. It can be very serious, causing long-lasting problems, particularly with malabsorption. Some people may have gluten sensitivity with some of the same clinical manifestations while not having celiac disease, while others may have an allergy to wheat while not having celiac disease. It is important to recognize that if a person cannot have gluten in their diet, it does not necessarily mean they have celiac disease.

Celiac disease is more common in Caucasians, especially in those of European descent, and females. It also has familial tendencies, with heritability estimates ranging from 57% to 87%. It is more common in people with Down syndrome, Turner's syndrome, and Type 1 diabetes. It is estimated that 1 of every 141 people in America are affected, with many undiagnosed.

Pathophysiology

When people with celiac disease eat gluten, they experience an immune reaction that attacks the small intestine causing inflammation and leading to damage to the intestinal villi, lengthening of intestinal cysts, and mucosal lesions. Because the small intestine is where most absorption takes place, these intestinal changes can lead to malabsorption/malnutrition issues. Left untreated, patients can develop other autoimmune disorders such as type 1 diabetes, dermatitis herpetiformis, and autoimmune thyroiditis. There are rare cases of patients who continue to have symptoms and trouble absorbing nutrients even while maintaining a gluten-free diet. These individuals have refractory celiac disease. The intestines are severely damaged, and the patient may need to receive total parenteral nutrition (TPN) to meet their nutritional needs.

Clinical Manifestations

The clinical presentation of celiac disease in adults is related to intestinal mucosal damage that causes diarrhea (often foul smelling, light in color and frothy), steatorrhea, flatulence, weight loss, and other signs of malabsorption. The patient may also present with fatigue and weakness related to malabsorption and malnutrition. In severe cases of celiac disease that is associated with longstanding impaired absorption, severe abdominal pain and increased bleeding tendencies may be observed. Celiac disease is often difficult to diagnose because the clinical manifestations are similar to other diseases such as irritable bowel syndrome (IBS) and lactose intolerance, and the patient must be persistent in getting the correct diagnosis.

Some patients present with atypical symptoms and only minor gastrointestinal complaints. These patients may exhibit symptoms of anemia, dental enamel defects, osteoporosis, arthritis, neurological symptoms, infertility, and increased transaminases. Although they do not exhibit the same gastrointestinal symptoms, they can have severe mucosal damage and a biopsy is necessary. Approximately 20% of patients diagnosed in childhood recover completely with a gluten-free diet and continue to have latent disease into adulthood. They remain asymptomatic and regain normal villous architecture, but still require regular follow-ups.

Peripheral neuropathies have been noted in up to 50% of patients with celiac disease which can be associated with vitamin deficiencies and does not seem to improve with a gluten-free diet.

Management
Medical Management
Diagnosis

Diagnosis of celiac disease is done through blood tests for antibodies against gliadin, genetic tests and biopsy. Gliadin is a water-soluble glycoprotein in the gluten of wheat. Gluten is a group of proteins found in barley, oats, rye and wheat that give flour its stickiness. The most sensitive test for celiac disease is antitissue transglutaminase antibody (anti-tTG), IgA by enzyme-linked immunosorbent assay. A finding of greater than 10 unit/mL is consistent with a diagnosis of celiac disease. Other diagnostic studies, primarily aimed at determining the degree of malabsorption and malnutrition, include CBC, serum electrolytes, coagulation profile, and liver function tests.

Treatment

The only treatment for celiac disease is lifelong adherence to a gluten-free diet. Ingesting even a small amount can trigger intestinal damage. Following the gluten-free diet can still take months to several years to heal the intestine in the adult patient, but approximately 70% of patients see improvement within 2 weeks of being gluten-free. Once the intestines are healed, new villi grow and absorption from food is restored. One of the issues with following a gluten free diet is the presence of gluten in products that are not typically associated with these grains, such as salad dressings, puddings, sausage, and soy sauce.

Because some medications may contain gluten, patients should consult their healthcare provider or pharmacist as to any medications, prescription or over-the-counter, that may contain gluten. They usually contain only minimal amounts and may be taken without causing symptoms. While some skin and hair products may contain gluten, it is important to know that this can transfer from hand-to-mouth unknowingly, making it important to read labels.

Management of celiac disease includes six key elements and can be remembered by using the acronym, CELIAC:

- **C**onsult a dietician
- **E**ducation about the disease
- **L**ifelong adherence to gluten-free diet
- **I**dentify and treat malabsorption and malnutrition
- **A**ccess support groups (like the Celiac Foundation)
- **C**ontinue management through an interdisciplinary team

Patients with latent celiac disease are not advised to be on a gluten-free diet but should be monitored. If clinical manifestations develop, a biopsy is indicated.

Dietary advice for all patients with celiac disease includes:

- No foods containing wheat, rye, or barley in all forms
- Soybean flour, tapioca flour, rice, corn, buckwheat, quinoa, and potatoes are safe
- Distilled alcoholic beverages, vinegars, and wine are safe
- Beer, ales, lagers, and malt vinegars should be avoided
- Oats may be introduced with caution as the research is mixed

After initiation of the gluten-free diet, the patient is monitored at 4 to 6 weeks for a complete blood count (CBC), vitamin B_{12}, iron studies, liver enzymes, and serologic tests: IgA anti tissue transglutaminase (tTG) or IgA (or IgG) deamidated gliadin peptide (DGP). Serum IgG antigliadin and IgA endomysial antibody levels fall when the patient adheres to a strict gluten-free diet.

Complications

Malnutrition and malabsorption are the most common complications of celiac disease because most absorption of nutrients takes place in the small intestine. Complications associated with changes to the intestinal mucosa and the malabsorption include anemia, osteopenia, and osteoporosis.

Nursing Management
Assessment and Analysis

Because of the damage to the intestinal mucosa associated with the immune response to gluten, the patient presents with gastrointestinal complaints. The clinical manifestations are directly related to the intestinal wall changes and include:

- Diarrhea
- Flatulence
- Abdominal bloating (due to distension secondary to fluids and gas)
- Steatorrhea
- Weakness, fatigue
- Weight loss
- Anemia
- Orthostatic hypotension
- Hypocalcemia

Nursing Diagnoses

- **Imbalanced nutrition: less than body requirements** associated with the inability to absorb nutrients
- **Knowledge Deficit** associated with gluten-free diet
- **Risk for dysfunctional gastric motility** associated with inadequate absorption of nutrients

Nursing Interventions
▪ *Assessments*

- Vital signs
  Due to diarrhea, there is an increased fluid loss that may lead to signs of hypovolemia, including decreased blood pressure, orthostatic hypotension, and tachycardia. The temperature may be elevated due to the inflammatory process or fluid volume deficit.
- Serum electrolytes
  There may be increased loss of potassium due to the diarrhea, and decreased absorption of calcium due to intestinal mucosal damage. With hypocalcemia, the patient may demonstrate Chvostek or Trousseau signs.
- CBC
  Anemia may develop secondary to malabsorption of key nutrients, as well as potential intestinal bleeding due to mucosal wall destruction.
- Intake and output
  Diarrhea leads to an increased loss of fluids through the bowels. Urine output may be decreased due to hypovolemia.

- Stool characteristics
Diarrhea develops secondary to damage to the surface of the intestinal wall. The diarrhea may be watery, frothy, light in color, with a foul odor
- DXA (Dual energy x-ray absorptiometry)
The patient is at risk of osteopenia and osteoporosis secondary to malabsorption of calcium
- Current knowledge of the gluten-free diet
Assessment of the patient's current knowledge needs to be established before beginning any teaching. Gluten may be in foods and products that the patient does not associate with this protein found in wheat, rye, and barley.

■ Actions

- Refer patient to a dietician knowledgeable in celiac disease for gluten-free diet teaching
It is always important to involve other members of the healthcare team with more expertise in an area in order to enhance the patient's knowledge
- Refer to support group for celiac disease
Support groups help the patient to learn more about the disease as well as coping strategies used by others
- Develop a trusting relationship
A trusting relationship is necessary in all patient encounters and assists the patient in sharing important information with a non-judgmental approach
- Encourage patients to ask about gluten-free choices when dining out
If gluten-free choices are not on the menu, the patient can help encourage the restaurant to include these choices in the future

■ Teaching

- Use dishwasher for plates, utensils, pans, etc. exposed to gluten
Use of the dishwater eliminates gluten residue that may be on others' plates, utensils, etc.
- Diet adherence to the gluten-free diet
A lifelong commitment to a huge change in their diet can be very difficult for many patients; particularly if they only had mild symptoms
- Read food labels
It is important to know how to read food labels and recognize if gluten is a part of the food choice
- Importance of consistent follow up with primary healthcare provider
Because celiac disease is a chronic condition, the patient needs to be monitored for subtle signs of the disease in order to minimize complications.
- Gluten-free resources (applications include Allergy Eats Mobile, Dine Gluten Free, and Find Me Gluten Free)
Patients who are knowledgeable are more likely to be compliant with dietary restrictions. The applications also allow more flexibility in finding restaurants where gluten options are available.

Evaluating Care Outcomes

After the patient has reportedly been adhering to a gluten-free diet and is without clinical manifestations, it is still important to follow-up as recommended by the provider for serum laboratory tests confirming that the gluten-free diet is alleviating the inflammation associated with the disease. The dietary changes require a lifelong commitment and the success is monitored by serial anti-tTG levels. If the patient is noncompliant and/or the clinical manifestations persist, it is important to continue educating the patient as to the long-term effects of the chronic inflammation in the small intestine as well as the inability to absorb nutrients properly. Patients with well-managed celiac disease demonstrate stable weight, normal bowel movements, and stable electrolytes.

Diverticulitis

Epidemiology

A **diverticulum** is a small, pouchlike protrusion or herniation, most often occurring in the gastrointestinal tract, particularly the colon. It is more common in Western industrialized societies and is more common in older people. It occurs most frequently in the left colon and is thought to be related to the lack of fiber in the diet, obesity, and lack of physical activity (see Evidence-Based Practice: Diverticulitis and Whole Fiber). In Africa and Asia, the incidence is much lower, and it tends to affect the right side of the colon more frequently as well as younger populations. It is also less common in vegetarians. The incidence increases with age, with diverticulitis found in 30% to 50% of adults over the age of 60 and increasing to 65% by age 85. Men are more affected than women in younger patients, whereas females are more affected in older patients. Risk factors for diverticulosis include increasing age, obesity, smoking, low-fiber diet, heredity, and some medications (NSAIDs, acetaminophen, oral corticosteroids, and opiates). There has also been an association between eating red meat and high-fat diets with the risk of diverticular complications.

Evidence-Based Practice

Diverticulitis and Whole Fiber

It has been previously reported that patients with diverticular disease should not consume whole pieces of fiber such as seeds, corn, and nuts, and this continues to be a routine practice in patients with diverticular disease. The rationale was that these undigested fragments can become lodged in the diverticulum and induce an episode of diverticulitis. Pemberton (2018) states that this theory is unproven.

Pemberton, J. H. (2018). Acute colonic diverticulitis: Medical management. Retrieved from https://www.uptodate.com/contents/acute-colonic-diverticulitis-medical-management

Pathophysiology

Diverticulitis is generally extraluminal, occurring on the outside of the colon, and is often referred to as an *outpouching* (Fig. 58.5). Diverticulosis is the presence of diverticula that are noninflamed. Many patients with diverticulosis are asymptomatic and may not even know they have the condition. Diverticulitis is an inflammation and/or infected diverticula. Diverticulitis most often occurs in the colon, most commonly in the sigmoid colon.

When a patient has diverticula, the colon wall thickens and becomes rigid. Without adequate fiber intake, more water is absorbed from the stool. This slows transit time and makes it more difficult for the stool to pass through the colon. This then causes increased intraluminal pressure from constipation and straining, which is thought to lead to the formation of diverticula. Dietary fiber is thought to act by producing a larger, bulkier stool that results in a wider-bore colon, which is less likely to develop diverticula.

Diverticula seem to occur at points of weakness in the intestinal wall. Food can become entrapped in the diverticula, and when it mixes with normal bacterial flora, this leads to decreased blood supply, forming a mass called a **fecalith** or dried, hard, concrete-like stool. The diverticular wall is eroded by increased intraluminal pressure or hard, dried food particles. This process leads to inflammation and/or infection. This inflammation can spread to other areas of the intestine. Diverticulitis most often occurs in the sigmoid colon. Because the sigmoid colon is the segment with the smallest diameter, increased intraluminal pressure may predispose this area to more frequent herniation. Diverticulitis may be acute or chronic. In chronic diverticulitis, the bowel can become scarred, leading to narrowing of the lumen, and the patient may develop an intestinal obstruction. In a small number of patients with diverticulitis, it is difficult to distinguish from carcinoma because both may show focal thickening of the bowel wall, or it may even resemble inflammatory bowel disease (IBD). Diverticulitis may lead to stricture formation that also has the appearance of cancer. Biopsy is required to make the differential diagnosis.

Clinical Manifestations

Patients with diverticulitis complain of abdominal pain over the area that is involved, usually the sigmoid colon. They may experience fever or leukocytosis, and often a palpable mass is felt over the involved area. The patient may complain of increased flatus, anorexia, abdominal bloating/distention, and diarrhea or constipation. Stools may contain mucus and blood. Bleeding occurs because of inflammation near areas of blood vessels and may range from minor to severe. Older adult patients, however, may present afebrile with a normal white blood cell (WBC) count and minimal abdominal tenderness. The first sign that may appear in the older adult patient is a change in mental status. Baseline temperature is often decreased from normal in the older adult. Therefore, one of the most common signs of infection may not be apparent in the older adult, and the patient may present with increased confusion, falling, and anorexia. If perforation has occurred, the patient may present with clinical manifestations of sepsis. If the pain is more generalized over the abdomen, peritonitis may have developed, and if peritonitis has occurred, the patient displays profound guarding with widespread rebound tenderness.

Management

Medical Management

Diagnosis

The most common diagnostic tests are plain flat-plate abdominal x-rays, but the diagnosis is usually confirmed with a CT scan. The CT scan also helps differentiate from other sources of abdominal pain and complicated cases of

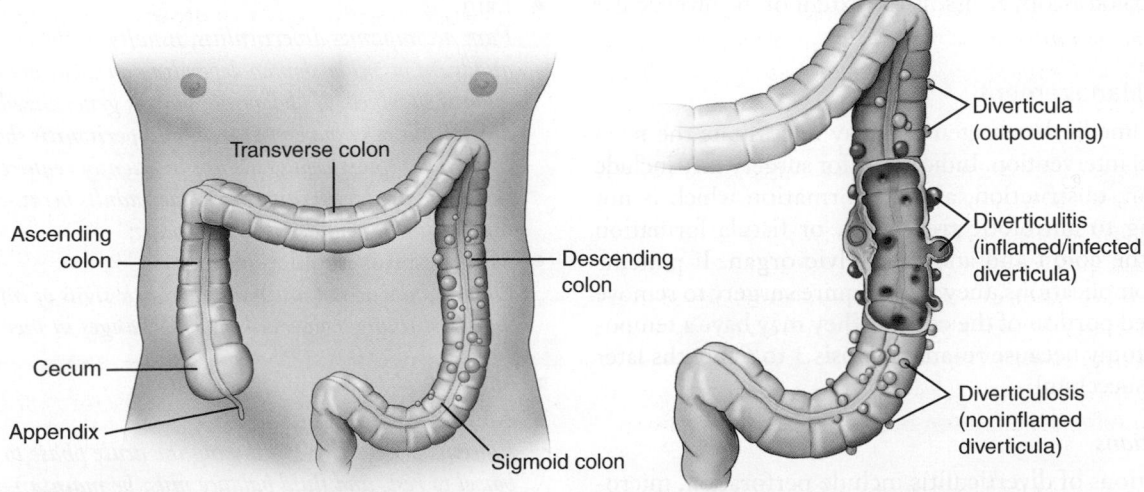

FIGURE 58.5 Diverticulitis. Diverticulitis is generally extraluminal, occurring on the outside of the colon, and is often referred to as an outpouching. Diverticulosis is the presence of diverticula that are noninflamed. Diverticulitis is an inflammation and/or infected diverticula.

diverticulitis. The white blood cells (WBCs) are monitored for elevations initially associated with inflammation and possible infection but should decrease with treatment. The urinalysis may show a few red blood cells (RBCs) if the ureter is near a perforated diverticulum. The patient with suspected diverticulitis should not have a barium enema because of the risk of rupturing the diverticula.

Treatment

Uncomplicated diverticulitis may be treated on an outpatient basis with broad-spectrum antibiotics for 7-10 days but should be reassessed after 2-3 days of therapy. The patient is advised to consume a clear liquid diet until symptoms subside, and then the diet should then be advanced slowly as tolerated. Common antibiotics used to treat diverticulitis include: Ciprofloxacin and metronidazole, trimethoprim-sulfamethoxazole and metronidazole, amoxicillin-clavulanate, Augmentin or Moxifloxacin. The patient should be admitted to the hospital for fever higher than 102.5°F (39°C), microperforation (few air bubbles outside the colon or confined to the pelvis), immunosuppression, significant leukocytosis, severe abdominal pain or diffuse peritonitis, advanced age, significant comorbidities, intolerance of oral intake, noncompliance or failed outpatient treatment. There are no dietary restrictions in acute uncomplicated diverticulitis, although limiting to a clear liquid diet for 2 to 3 days is common, while advancing as tolerated.

If the patient is admitted to the hospital, IV fluids are started, and nothing is given by mouth (NPO) to allow the bowel to rest. The patient may have a nasogastric (NG) tube for bowel decompression and will receive parenteral antibiotics. Laxatives and enemas should be avoided because they increase intestinal motility. Pain medications may be given as needed, and opiates are frequently needed. Inpatients may be discharged as clinical manifestations resolve and should complete a course of 10 to 14 days of antibiotics, and then have a follow up examination. After clinical manifestations completely resolve, the patient is recommended to have a colonoscopy to assess the extent of the diverticular disease.

Surgical Management

Failure of medical management may necessitate the need for surgical intervention. Indications for surgery may include perforation, obstruction, abscess formation which is not responding to antibiotic treatment, or fistula formation between the colon and another pelvic organ. If patients develop complications, they may require surgery to remove the diseased portion of the colon. They may have a temporary colostomy because re-anastomosis 3 to 6 months later is usually successful.

Complications

Complications of diverticulitis include perforation, microperforation, abscess and fistula formation, bowel obstruction, and bleeding. Inflammation can also result in fistulas to other organs.

Nursing Management

Assessment and Analysis

Fever often accompanies diverticulitis, ranging from a low-grade fever to 101°F (38.3°C) due to inflammation. Tachycardia often accompanies increased temperature. Pain accompanies diverticulitis, usually in the left lower quadrant or midabdomen depending on what area of the colon is involved. If abdominal pain is generalized, the diverticula may have ruptured, and peritonitis should be suspected. Altered bowel habits often accompany diverticulitis with constipation, diarrhea, or both. The patient may also complain of increased flatus and anorexia. Stools may contain mucus or blood. An elevated WBC is indicative of infection. However, it is not unusual for the patient with diverticulitis to initially present with a normal WBC.

Nursing Diagnoses

- **Acute pain** related to inflammation and distention of the colon
- **Knowledge deficit** related to the need to consume adequate fiber in the diet

Nursing Interventions

■ Assessments

- Vital signs
  Fever often accompanies diverticulitis, ranging from a low-grade fever to 101°F (38.3°C) because of inflammation. Tachycardia often accompanies increased temperature secondary to an increase in insensible fluid loss due to fever.
- Serum potassium levels
  If the patient has intermittent NG suction, potassium loss increases and requires monitoring and replacement if levels are below 3.5 mEq/L.
- Intake and output
  Fluid volume status may be impacted by NG suction and decreased intake. Important to monitor urine output to determine renal perfusion.
- Pain
  Pain accompanies diverticulitis, usually in the left lower quadrant or midabdomen depending on what area of the colon is involved. If abdominal pain is generalized, the diverticula may have ruptured, and peritonitis should be suspected. Opioid analgesics are frequently required but should be used with caution in older adults because of the mental status changes that may occur.
- Mental status in older adults
  Older adults do not always show classic signs of infection. The first changes observed may be changes in mental status.

■ Actions

- Administer IV fluids
  Patients are often NPO during the acute phase to allow the bowel to rest, and fluid balance must be maintained.
- Administer ordered antibiotics
  Diverticulitis is a localized infection. Antibiotics are administered until pain, inflammation, infection, and fever subside.

- Nasogastric tube to low intermittent suction
  Gastric decompression decreases gastric motility and allows the bowel to rest until inflammation decreases.
- Provide oral care
  Oral cavity may be dry due to insensible fluid loss, as well as increased mouth breathing in the patient with an NG tube. Apply lip balm to dry, cracked lips.

■ Teaching

- Dietary recommendations
  The nurse should teach patients about increasing fiber from raw fruits and vegetables in their diets. Without adequate fiber intake, more water is absorbed from the stool. This slows transit time and makes it more difficult for the stool to pass through the colon. This then causes increased intraluminal pressure from constipation and straining, which is thought to lead to the formation of diverticula. But it is also important to note that patients should not increase their fiber during acute phases, and the diverticulitis should be resolved.
- Avoid straining, bending, and lifting.
  These activities increase intra-abdominal pressure, which can lead to further outpouching of the diverticula.
- Weight reduction
  Obesity has been linked to increased intra-abdominal pressure, which is a risk factor for diverticulitis.
- Complete antibiotic therapy as prescribed
  Adherence to antibiotic therapy is crucial, and the nurse should stress to the patient who is being treated in the outpatient setting about the importance of taking all of the medication as prescribed. Rebound infection can occur when the prescribed dose of antibiotics is not taken.

Connection Check 58.4

A patient is admitted to the hospital for treatment for diverticulitis. The nurse recognizes which interventions appropriate for this patient?

A. High-fiber diet, ambulate frequently, IV fluids, pain medications

B. Antibiotics, IV fluids, NPO, NG tube, pain medications

C. Laxatives, enemas, diet, pain medications

D. Surgery with follow-up physical therapy

Evaluating Care Outcomes

Uncomplicated diverticulitis may be managed on an outpatient basis. Frequently, however, the patient is admitted to the hospital for antibiotic therapy and bowel rest. The patient will be free of abdominal pain and fever prior to discharge from the hospital. Maintaining adequate fiber in the diet may decrease recurrence or the severity of bouts of diverticulitis.

Appendicitis

Epidemiology

Appendicitis is an acute inflammation of the vermiform appendix. Affecting males more than females, appendicitis is a common condition that occurs more frequently in the 10- to 19-year-old age group. When it does occur in older adults, it usually ruptures and is much more serious, and mortality is higher in this age group. There are no particular risk factors or preventive measures.

Pathophysiology

The appendix is a small hollow appendage that extends off the cecum, and although it is made of lymphatic tissue, it has no known function. Appendicitis usually occurs as a result of a fecalith or other foreign body blocking the opening, leading to inflammation and subsequent infection. Other, less common causes may include malignant tumors, twisting and kinking of the appendix, edema of the bowel wall, adhesions, and other infections.

When the opening to the appendix becomes blocked, the mucosa begins to secrete fluid, leading to venous engorgement that increases intraluminal pressure and restricts blood flow. Subsequently, bacterial invasion occurs, and an abscess may develop if this process occurs slowly. Gangrene can occur in as little as 24 to 36 hours and is life threatening. Perforation can occur in as few as 24 hours, but the risk increases after 48 hours and can result in peritonitis, and this, too, is life threatening.

Clinical Manifestations

The patient with appendicitis presents with periumbilical abdominal pain, often with complaints of anorexia, nausea, and vomiting. While the inflammatory process progresses, pain is shifted to the right lower quadrant of the abdomen and becomes more severe and steady in the area of **McBurney's point** (Fig. 58.6). When applying and releasing pressure to this area, if the patient notes increased pain when pressure is released, this is called *rebound tenderness* and is another indication of appendicitis. Another sign of appendicitis is **Rovsing's sign**, which presents when palpation of the left lower quadrant of the abdomen elicits pain in the right lower quadrant. The WBC may have a moderate

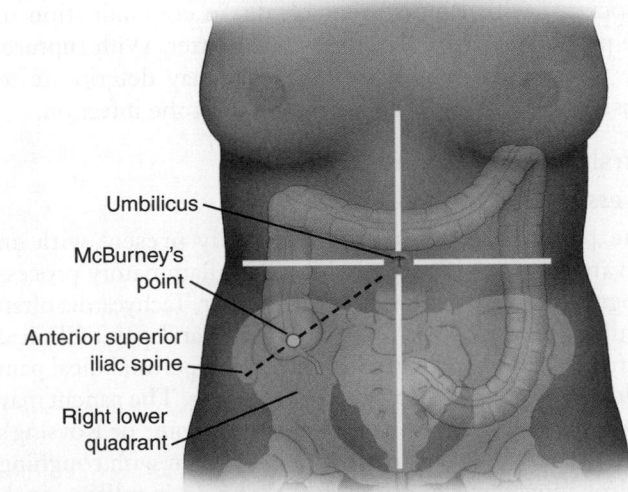

FIGURE 58.6 McBurney's point. Located in right lower quadrant of the abdomen, pain increases at McBurney's point with appendicitis.

Umbilicus

McBurney's point

Anterior superior iliac spine

Right lower quadrant

increase with acute appendicitis (10,000–18,000/mm³), and if the WBC is elevated to greater than 20,000/mm³, a perforated appendix should be suspected. In the event of perforation, the patient may exhibit signs of sepsis, including elevated temperature, tachycardia, and decreased blood pressure.

Management
Diagnosis

Appendicitis is commonly diagnosed based on clinical presentation and specific physical assessment findings. An ultrasound may reveal an enlarged appendix, but a CT scan is the most commonly used diagnostic test. Other diagnostic testing includes CBC and serum electrolytes.

Surgical Management

There is no medical management for acute appendicitis. A surgical consult should be obtained as soon as possible, and the patient needs to be prepared for the operating room for removal of the appendix (appendectomy). Laxatives and enemas should be avoided because they can increase intra-abdominal pressure that may result in perforation of the appendix.

The surgeon may perform the appendectomy with laparoscopy, where several small incisions are made, and the laparoscope is placed. If the appendix is suspected of being ruptured and/or peritonitis is suspected, a laparotomy with a larger abdominal incision is made. If there are no complications after the appendectomy, the patient may be discharged from the postanesthesia care unit (PACU) or the following day. If complications develop after the appendectomy, such as peritonitis or abscesses, the patient is admitted to the hospital to receive parenteral antibiotics for several days depending on the severity of the infectious process.

Complications

The major complications secondary to appendicitis are associated with rupture that results in contamination of the peritoneal cavity with intestinal matter. With rupture, the patient develops peritonitis that may deteriorate to sepsis and requires IV antibiotics to treat the infection.

Nursing Management
Assessment and Analysis

The patient may or may not initially present with an elevated temperature, but while the inflammatory process progresses, the patient will develop a fever. Tachycardia often results because of the fever, fluid loss, and pain. Clinical manifestations may begin with cramping periumbilical pain followed by anorexia, nausea, and vomiting. The patient may exhibit pain in the area of McBurney's point or Rovsing's sign. If the patient expresses increased pain with coughing and/or movement and indicates that pain is relieved with bending the right hip or knees, further assessment for

perforation and peritonitis is required. An abrupt change in the character of the pain and a change in blood pressure and/or pulse may also indicate perforation. The patient with appendicitis will likely have an elevated WBC count and a left shift in the differential (indication of increased number of immature white blood cells associated with inflammation and infection).

Nursing Diagnoses

- **Acute pain** associated with inflammation of the appendix
- **Risk for deficient fluid volume** associated with increased fluid loss (fever and vomiting)
- **Knowledge deficit** associated with preoperative and postoperative care

Nursing Interventions
▪ Assessments

- Vital signs
  A fever may not be present initially but will develop as inflammation increases. Tachycardia may also be present because of the fever.
- Intake and output
  Because of potential vomiting and fever, the patient is at risk for fluid volume deficit. During the surgical procedure, anesthesia depresses the nervous system and the ability to assess the patient's need to urinate. Urinary retention is more common with lower abdominal surgeries because of spasms and/or guarding related to pain. If the patient is being discharged from the PACU, it is imperative that the patient urinate before discharge.
- White blood cell count and differential
  The patient with appendicitis will likely have an elevated WBC count with a left shift in the differential.
- Pain
  The patient with appendicitis experiences pain, particularly in the right lower quadrant. Changes in pain, particularly if abrupt, may indicate perforation.
- Rebound tenderness
  When applying and releasing pressure to McBurney's point, the patient notes increased pain when pressure is released; this is an indication of appendicitis.

▪ Actions

- Make sure the patient is NPO
  Because surgical intervention is the definitive treatment for appendicitis, the patient must have nothing by mouth during the diagnostic work-up in the event the patient must emergently go to the operating room
- Administer prescribed IV fluids
  Because of an increase in fluid loss secondary to vomiting and fever, IV fluids are maintained preoperatively and postoperatively to maintain fluid balance.
- Prepare patient for operating room
  There is no medical treatment for appendicitis. The patient needs to be prepared for the operating room for removal of

the appendix. Ensure that the surgical consent form is signed prior to the patient receiving any sedatives or narcotics.

- Provide comfort measures
  While the patient is prepared for the operating room, ice may be applied to the right lower quadrant to impede blood flow to the area, which slows the inflammatory process. The nurse should never apply heat, however, because this increases blood flow and inflammation to the area and may cause the appendix to rupture. Analgesics may be prescribed preoperatively but are generally with-held until a diagnosis is made to prevent masking of clinical manifestations. Postoperatively, the patient requires opioid analgesics.

- Position patient supine with head of bed elevated 30° to 45° with knees flexed or side-lying with knees flexed.
  This position decreases the strain (pull) on the abdominal muscles and may decrease pain secondary to inflammation in the peritoneal cavity

- Advance diet as tolerated after surgical procedure
  Once bowel sounds have returned, begin diet with clear liquids, advancing as tolerated while assessing for nausea and/or vomiting

▨ Teaching

- Turning, coughing, deep breathing, and incentive spirometer 10 times every hour while awake
  Promotes lung expansion and prevents atelectasis and helps mobilize any secretions to be expectorated

- Early ambulation
  Promotes circulation and prevention of VTE and improves respiratory function

- Take full course of antibiotics despite lack of fever or pain
  The patient may have antibiotics prescribed, particularly if the appendix ruptured prior to surgery. Emphasize the importance of completing all antibiotics, even if having no symptoms.

- Teach wound care if appropriate
  If the appendix ruptured, the incision will be left open by the surgery to heal by secondary intention. Wound care usually involves a moist saline dressing two to three times a day. The patient/family should be taught to change the dressing before discharge. A home health referral should be included in the discharge planning to assist the patient and family at home with the dressing changes and assess for any complications that may arise.

> **⊙ Safety Alert** If the patient is suspected of having appen-dicitis, the nurse should never apply heat because this increases blood flow and inflammation to the area and may cause the appendix to rupture.

Connection Check 58.5

The nurse is caring for a patient in the emergency depart-ment with abdominal pain, fever, nausea, and vomiting. The patient is suspected of having appendicitis. What inter-vention may the provider order to confirm diagnosis?

A. Flat-plate x-ray of the abdomen, chemistry panel

B. CT scan, complete blood count (CBC), abdominal assessment for rebound tenderness

C. Administer a laxative to see if symptoms improve

D. Colonoscopy, esophagogastroduodenoscopy (EGD), and endoscopic retrograde cholangiopancreatogram (ERCP)

Evaluating Care Outcomes

The patient who has had surgery for appendicitis without rupture is usually discharged from the PACU on the first postoperative day. Most patients have an uneventful recov-ery, and can resume normal activities in 2 to 4 weeks. If the appendix has ruptured, the patient is admitted to the hospital and treated with antibiotics and wound care. The family is involved in wound care, and a home health nurse is ordered to monitor progress of healing and assist the family with wound care. Expected outcomes include stable vital signs, CBC within normal limits, and demonstrated understanding of postoperative and discharge teaching.

COLORECTAL CANCER

Epidemiology

Colorectal cancer involves cancer of the rectum and large intestine. It is the third most common form of cancer and second leading cause of death in the United States. In 2018, the American Cancer Society estimated that there would be 97,220 new cases of colon cancer and 43,030 new cases of rectal cancer, with a combined death of 50,630 in the United States. The incidence has steadily decreased in the United States, probably attributable to increased awareness and better screening techniques. Most colorectal cancers are found in the distal portion of the large intestine. The incidence has increased, how-ever, in right-sided colon cancers, primarily in the cecum in the United States and internationally for reasons that are unclear. This could be associated with better screen-ing for left-sided colon cancers and removal of polyps during colonoscopy. Death rates have been decreasing for more than 2 decades, also attributable to better screen-ing methods and removal of polyps during colonoscopy before they can progress into cancer. Colorectal cancer affects men slightly more than women, with African Americans having the highest incidence and mortality with no clear reason. With early detection, it is now one of the most curable of all cancers. The United States has one of the highest survival rates from colorectal cancers.

Risk factors for developing colorectal cancer during one's lifetime include personal or family history of colorectal cancer (first-degree relative), history of adenomatous polyps, inflammatory bowel disease (IBD) for 10 years or more, familial adenomatous polyposis, hereditary non-polyposis colorectal cancer (HNPCC) or Lynch syndrome, physical inactivity, obesity (body mass index $\geq$ 30 kg/m²), high-fat diets and consumption of red meat ($\geq$ seven servings a week) and processed meats, cigarette use, and alcohol intake ($\geq$ four drinks per week). Another factor associated with increased risk is inadequate intake of fruits and vegetables, although it is unclear whether diets high in fiber seem to help. People with type 2 diabetes also have a 30% increased risk for development of colorectal cancer compared with people without diabetes. The risk of developing colorectal cancer increases with age, and the incidence is higher in industrialized countries. Risk factors are just that—risk factors. It does not necessarily mean the disease will develop, and many people with no known risk factors also get the disease. Most colorectal cancers are sporadic rather than familial (see Genetic Connections).

Genetic Connections

Hereditary Aspects of Colorectal Cancer

Heredity accounts for about 5% to 10% of all colorectal cancers. **Familial adenomatous polyposis (FAP)** is an autosomal dominant disorder that accounts for less than 1% of all colorectal cancers. Numerous colonic adenomas appear during childhood. Thousands of adenomas develop by late childhood or early adulthood. If left untreated, nearly 100% of these individuals will develop colon cancer by the age of 40 to 45. Treatment involves a total colectomy, usually in their late teens or early 20s. **Hereditary non-polyposis colorectal cancer (HNPCC)**, or **Lynch's syndrome**, is an autosomal dominant syndrome and accounts for 3% to 5% of all colonic adenocarcinomas. Lynch's syndrome is characterized by early age onset and predominance of right colon tumors. Patients with the gene for Lynch's syndrome are also at risk for developing extracolonic malignancies including carcinoma of the endometrium, ovary, stomach, small bowel, pancreas, upper renal tract, and hepatobiliary tract. They have a lifetime risk of colon cancer of approximately 80% to 100%, usually before age 45. Affected women also have a higher risk of developing endometrial cancer. Once Lynch's syndrome or FAP is diagnosed, genetic testing is performed on all offspring so close surveillance can be implemented with early intervention in order to prevent colorectal cancers from developing.

There have been several studies associated with what are known as protective factors for colorectal cancers. There is some evidence that diets high in fruits and vegetables, regular physical activity, regular use of aspirin or other NSAIDs, and hormone replacement therapy in postmenopausal women may have protective properties for colorectal cancer. Research continues on the effectiveness of the administration of folic acid, vitamin B_6, calcium, magnesium, garlic, fish consumption, and statin medications, but there is no clear evidence to support either at this time.

Pathophysiology

Most colorectal cancers are adenocarcinomas, which are a type of cancer that originates in glandular cells of internal organs. **Metastasis** (spread of the cancer) can occur by direct extension to adjacent organs, through the lymphatic system or the bloodstream. The most common area of metastasis is to the liver, but colorectal cancer can also metastasize to the lungs, brain, bones, and adrenal glands. Seeding may also occur during resection when the cancer calls break off from the tumor into the peritoneal cavity. A surgeon experienced in resection of colon cancer uses special techniques to prevent this from occurring. Box 58.2 illustrates common diagnostic tests for colorectal cancer.

Clinical Manifestations

In the very early stages of colorectal cancer, the symptoms are insidious and may be ignored by the patient until the disease is advanced. Clinical manifestations vary according to where the cancer is located in the intestine. Unexplained weight loss and fatigue may be the first signs for any location of the cancer. Other clinical manifestations may include a change in bowel regularity and/or the appearance of stool, blood in the stool (red or black depending on location), abdominal pain and/or distention, and a sensation of pressure as with incomplete evacuation after a bowel movement, along with clinical manifestations of anemia. The patient's presentation progresses to clinical manifestations of intestinal obstruction as the cancer increases in size. Specific to the area in which the primary tumor is located, clinical manifestations include (Fig. 58.7):

- Ascending colon: vague abdominal pain and/or cramping, change in bowel habits, anemia, and fatigue
- Transverse colon: pain, clinical manifestations of obstruction, change in bowel habits, anemia, and fatigue
- Descending colon: pain, change in bowel habits, bright red blood in stool, and clinical manifestations of intestinal obstruction
- Rectum: blood in stool, change in bowel habits, rectal discomfort, and feeling of incomplete evacuation

Box 58.2 Diagnostic Studies for Colorectal Cancer

- Fecal occult blood test (FOBT) or fecal immunochemical test (FIT) and digital rectal examination (DRE)—stool sample is collected and placed on a special slide and tested for hidden blood. A DRE is performed by the provider.
- Lower GI series—a tube is inserted into the rectum, and the large intestine is filled with barium. The patient is asked to change positions several times in order to evenly distribute the barium. X-ray pictures and/or video are taken. The barium is constipating, so care should be taken to advise the patient to take appropriate measures to prevent constipation.
- Double-contrast barium enema—takes place after the patient has expelled most of the barium from the intestine. The remaining barium clings to the intestinal wall. The intestine is then inflated with air, and additional x-ray images are taken.
- Sigmoidoscopy—a flexible tube with a light and camera at the end is inserted into the rectum and colon up to the transverse colon. The camera transmits images to a computer screen. Biopsies can be taken from the rectum and sigmoid colon for further examination.
- Colonoscopy—a long, flexible tube with a light and camera on the end is inserted into the full length of the colon. The provider has the ability to view the entire colon as well as to remove polyps and take biopsies as deemed necessary. The patient receives sedation for the procedure.
- Virtual colonoscopy—performed in either the computed tomography (CT) scanning department or magnetic resonance imaging (MRI) (most commonly CT scanning). A tube is inserted into the rectum. For CT, carbon dioxide is administered to enlarge the colon for better viewing. For MRI, a contrast medium is given through the rectum to expand the large intestine. Cross-sectional images are produced and processed to create three-dimensional, computer-generated images of the large intestine. Sedation is not required for the procedure.
- Fecal DNA testing—colorectal cancers contain abnormal DNA that is shed in the stool. If this test is positive, it should be followed with a colonoscopy.
- Wireless capsule endoscopy—known as the pill camera, - is a pill approximately the size of a vitamin. The patient swallows the pill with the camera within the pill, and the camera captures video throughout the GI tract. It takes approximately 8 hours to pass through the GI tract while images are recorded on a portable device. The images are transferred from the portable device to a computer. This technique is most useful with cancers of the small bowel that are difficult to detect through traditional endoscopy.

DNA, Deoxyribonucleic acid; *GI,* gastrointestinal.

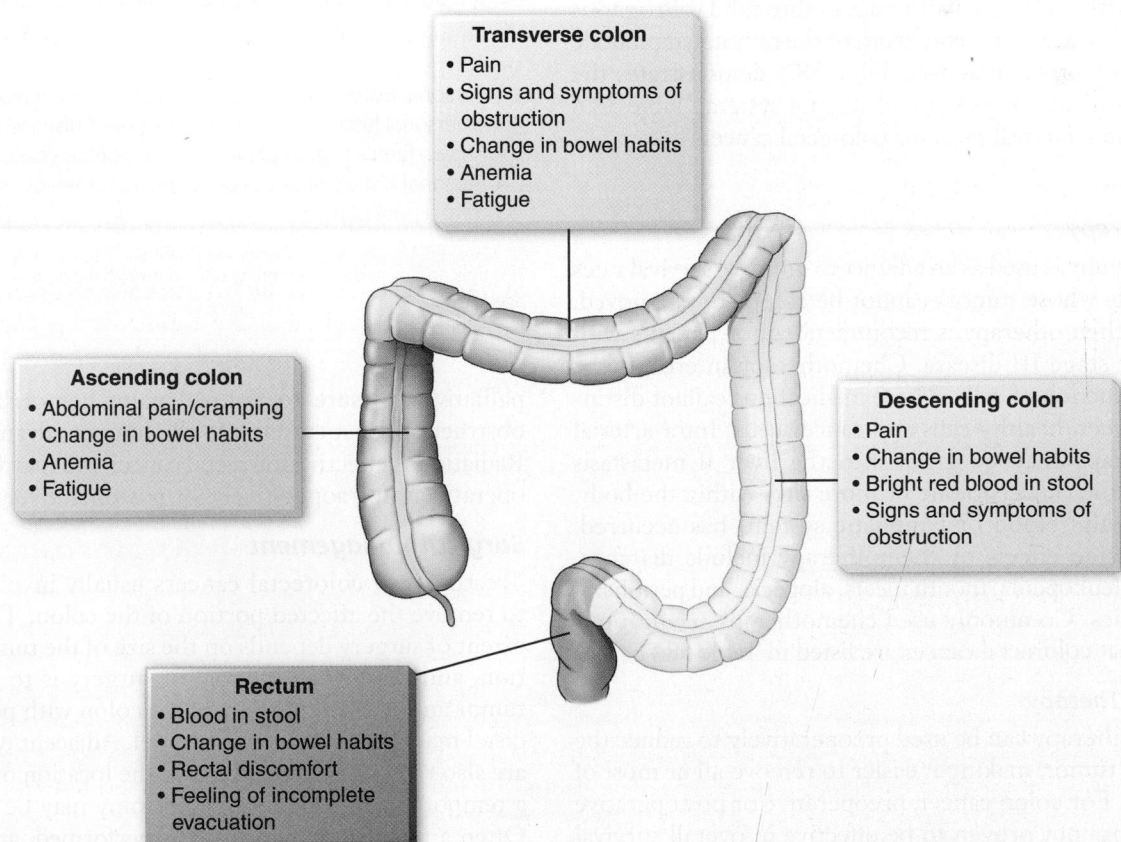

FIGURE 58.7 Colorectal cancer tumor clinical manifestations based on anatomical location of the tumors.

Management

Medical Management

Diagnosis

Colonoscopy is the gold standard for colorectal cancer screening. With the use of colonoscopy, biopsies can be taken, and polyps removed during the procedure. There are studies that demonstrate that colonoscopy is overutilized in some populations and underutilized in others. Individuals have different risk factors for colorectal cancer, and the recommendation for colonoscopy is based on the patient's risk factors, rather than age alone. Colonoscopy is far more expensive than some of the other screening methods as well as more invasive. Recommendations for screening for colorectal cancers are included in Box 58.3. For more specific guidelines related to age, race and other comorbidities, refer to Chapter 55 Evidence-Based Practice: Preferred Colorectal Cancer Screening Recommendations.

Other diagnostic studies that may be evaluated with suspected colorectal cancer include a serum carcinoembryonic antigen (CEA), CBC, CT, MRI, and abdominal x-rays. An elevated CEA indicates overexpression of an oncofetal glycoprotein that is normally expressed by mucosal cells, the CBC results may demonstrate anemia due to blood loss and elevated WBC secondary to inflammation or infection, and CT, MRI, or abdominal x-rays may provide information about abdominal obstruction.

The most common method of staging colorectal cancer is with the TNM (tumor-node-metastasis) classification system, which is further classified into stages I through IV. Prognosis worsens with larger size and depth of the tumor, lymph node involvement, and metastasis. Table 58.5 demonstrates the TNM classification system and staging system. Table 58.6 demonstrates survival rates for colorectal cancer.

Treatment

Chemotherapy

Chemotherapy is used as an adjunct to improve survival rates for patients whose tumors cannot be completely removed. Adjuvant chemotherapy is recommended for patients with stage II or stage III disease. Chemotherapy interrupts the DNA production of cells. These medications cannot distinguish between healthy cells and cancer cells. Intra-arterial chemotherapy may be given into the liver if metastasis (spread of the cancer to one or more sites within the body, usually by the blood or lymphatic system) has occurred. Common side effects of chemotherapy include diarrhea, mucositis, leukopenia, mouth ulcers, alopecia, and peripheral neuropathies. Commonly used chemotherapy medications used to treat colorectal cancer are listed in Table 58.7.

Radiation Therapy

Radiation therapy can be used preoperatively to reduce the size of the tumor, making it easier to remove all or most of the tumor. For colon cancer, preoperative or postoperative radiation has not proven to be effective in overall survival rates, but it can be effective in providing regional or local control of the disease. Radiation can also be used as a

---

Box 58.3 Screening Recommendations for Colorectal Cancers

People With Average Risk

Age 45–75

Stool-based tests (options)
- High-sensitivity fecal occult blood test (FOBT) annually
- Highly sensitive guaiac-based fecal occult blood test (gFOBT) every year
- Multi-targeted stool DNA test (MT-sDNA) every 3 years

Visual (structural) exams of the colon or rectum (options)
- Flexible sigmoidoscopy (FSIG) every 5 years
- Virtual colonoscopy every 5 years
- Colonoscopy every 10 years

Age 76–85

Do not screen routinely* The decision would be made based on patient's overall health and prior screening history

Age older than 85

Do not screen*
People with risk factors such as inflammatory bowel disease, Familial adenomatous polyposis (FAP), and Lynch's syndrome should follow their provider's recommendations.

People at Increased or High Risk

Screening might need to begin before age 45 and be screened more often and/or get specific tests for these individuals

- Strong family history of colorectal cancer or certain types of polyps
- Personal history of colorectal cancer or certain types of polyps
- A personal history of inflammatory bowel disease
- Known family history of hereditary colorectal caner
- Personal history of radiation to the abdomen or pelvic area to treat a prior cancer

*Complications seen with screening often outweigh the benefits for persons aged 76 to 85.

---

palliative measure to control pain, hemorrhage, bowel obstruction, or metastasis to the lung in advanced disease. Radiation is effective for rectal cancer and may be used preoperatively, intraoperatively, or postoperatively.

Surgical Management

Treatment of colorectal cancers usually involves surgery to remove the affected portion of the colon. The type and extent of surgery depends on the size of the tumor, its location, and its stage. The goal of surgery is to remove the tumor and affected portion of the colon with proximal and distal margins of the normal bowel. Adjacent lymph nodes are also removed. Depending on the location of the tumor, a temporary or permanent colostomy may be performed. Often a temporary colostomy is performed, and at a later time after healing has taken place, an **anastomosis** (attachment of one end to the other) is performed to reconnect the

Table 58.5 American Joint Committee on Cancer's Tumor-Node-Metastasis Classification of Colorectal Cancer

T	Primary Tumor
T_x	Primary tumor cannot be evaluated because of incomplete information
T_{is}	Carcinoma in situ; cancer is in the earliest stage and has spread; involves only the mucosa
T_1	Tumor has grown beyond the mucosa into the submucosa
T_2	Tumor has grown through the submucosa into the muscularis propria (outer muscle layer)
T_3	Tumor has grown through the muscularis propria into the outer layers but not into neighboring organs or tissues
T_{4a}	Tumor has spread completely through the serosa (visceral peritoneum), the outermost layer of the intestine
T_{4b}	Tumor has spread completely through the serosa (visceral peritoneum), the outermost layer of the intestine, and into nearby tissues or organs
N	**Lymph Node Involvement**
N_x	Lymph nodes cannot be assessed because of incomplete information
N_0	No lymph node involvement is found
N_{1a}	Cancer is found in one nearby lymph node
N_{1b}	Cancer is found in 2–3 nearby lymph nodes
N_{1c}	Cancer is found in fat near lymph nodes but not in the lymph nodes themselves
N_{2a}	Cancer is found in 4–6 nearby lymph nodes
N_{2b}	Cancer is found in 7 or more nearby lymph nodes
M	**Metastasis**
M_0	No distant metastasis is seen
M_{1a}	Cancer has spread to 1 distant organ or set of distant lymph nodes
M_{1b}	Cancer has spread to more than 1 distant organ or set of lymph nodes, or it is in parts of the abdominal cavity
	Stage Grouping
0	T_{is}, N_0, M_0: The cancer is in its earliest stage; known as carcinoma in situ or intramucosal carcinoma
I	T_{1-2}, N_0, M_0: Cancer has grown into submucosa or muscularis propria, but it has not spread to nearby lymph nodes or distant sites
IIA	T_3, N_0, M_0: The cancer has grown into the outermost layers but has not gone through them and has not spread to lymph nodes or distant sites
IIB	T_{4a}, N_0, M_0: Cancer has grown through the wall of the colon or rectum but has not grown into other tissues or organs; it has not spread to lymph nodes or distant sites
IIC	T_{4b}, N_0, M_0: Cancer has grown through the wall of the colon or rectum and grown to nearby tissues or organs; it has not spread to lymph nodes or distant sites
IIIA	T_{1-2}, N_1, M_0: The cancer has grown through the submucosa and may have grown into the muscularis propria; it has spread to 1–3 nearby lymph nodes or into areas of fat near the lymph nodes; it has not spread to distant sites or T_1, N_{2a}, M_0: The cancer has grown into the submucosa and has spread to 4–6 nearby lymph nodes; it has not spread to distant sites
IIIB	T_{3-4}, N_1, M_0: The cancer has grown into the outermost layers of the colon or rectum or through the visceral peritoneum; it has spread to 1–3 lymph nodes or areas of fat near lymph nodes; it is not in distant organs or T_{2-3}, N_{2a}, M_0: The cancer has grown into the muscularis propria or into the outermost layer of the colon or rectum; it has spread to 4–6 nearby lymph nodes but not to distant sites or T_{1-2}, N_{2b}, M_0: The cancer has grown into the submucosa or into the muscularis propria and spread to 7 or more lymph nodes; it has not spread to distant sites

Continued

Table 58.5   American Joint Committee on Cancer's Tumor-Node-Metastasis Classification of Colorectal Cancer—cont'd

T	Primary Tumor
IIIC	T_{4a}, N_{2a}, M_0: The cancer has grown through the wall of the colon or rectum and has spread to 4–6 nearby lymph nodes but has not spread to distant organs or T_{3-4a}, N_{2b}, M_0: The cancer has grown through the visceral peritoneum and is in 7 or more lymph nodes but has not reached nearby organs or distant sites or T_{4b}, N_{1-2}, M_0: The cancer has reached nearby tissue or organs and at least 1 lymph node or fat near lymph nodes but has not spread to distant sites
IVA	Any T, Any N, M_{1a}: The cancer has spread to 1 distant organ or set of lymph nodes (liver, lung, etc.)
IVB	Any T, Any N, M_{1b}: The cancer has spread to more than 1 distant organ or set of lymph nodes or it has spread to distant parts of the peritoneum

Table 58.6   Colorectal Cancer 5-Year Survival Rates*

Stage	Colon	Rectal
I	74%	74%
IIA	67%	65%
IIB	59%	52%
IIC	37%	32%
IIIA	73%	74%
IIIB	46%	45%
IIIC	28%	33%
IV	6%	6%

*Survival rates were better for some stage III cancers than some stage II cancers, but the reasons are unclear.

Table 58.7   Commonly Used Chemotherapy Medications for Colorectal Cancer

Medication	Action
5-Fluorouracil (5-FU) with leucovorin (LV)	Cell-cycle-specific, interfering with the synthesis of DNA and RNA, causing their death
Capecitabine (Xeloda)	Converted in tissue to 5-FU, which inhibits DNA and RNA synthesis by preventing thymidine production, causing death of rapidly replicating cells
Oxaliplatin (Eloxatin)	A platinum-based antineoplastic agent; binds to DNA and RNA miscoding information and/or inhibiting DNA replication, and cells die
Bevacizumab (Avastin)	An antiangiogenesis medication that reduces blood flow to the tumor cells, depriving them of nutrients needed for replication
Irinotecan (Camptosar)	Inhibits the enzyme topoisomerase I required for DNA replication, causing cell death by damaging DNA produced during the S phase of cell synthesis
Cetuximab (Erbitux)	Cetuximab (Erbitux)—a monoclonal antibody that binds to protein to slow cell growth

colon to the rectum to allow for normal defecation. It may be possible to preserve sphincter function in some rectal cancers. Common surgical procedures are:

- **Colectomy**—excision of part of or all of the colon
- **Hemicolectomy**—excision of half or less of the colon (may be right or left)
- **Abdominoperineal resection**—the affected colon and affected rectum are removed, and the anus is closed. The colon is removed through an abdominal incision, and the rectum is removed through a perineal incision. The ileostomy is permanent.

Complications

Based on the timing of diagnosis, location of the cancer, as well as the treatment, the patient may develop complications related to colorectal surgery. For patients undergoing chemotherapy, complications include fatigue, increased risk of infection, and anemia. Radiation enteritis may develop and lead to diarrhea, blood in the stool, and weight loss. Postoperative complications include blood loss, anastomoses, infection, and incisional dehiscence. Metastasis is also a potential complication for colorectal cancer, particularly when the cancer is more advanced when diagnosed.

Nursing Management
Preoperative Patient

The patient with colorectal cancer undergoes a variety of emotions, and it is important to include family members whenever possible with assessment and teaching. Nursing management includes teaching, preparation for treatments, and emotional support.

Assessment and Analysis

Assess the patient's current knowledge of the disease and treatment. A comprehensive understanding of the location, type, severity, and classification of the cancer is key to providing holistic nursing care. It is also important to correlate the clinical manifestations and diagnostic study results with the definitive diagnosis. The clinical presentation is closely associated with the location of the tumor, and includes unexplained weight loss, fatigue, blood in the stool, and clinical manifestations of anemia. Assess any support systems the patient has because the patient will need this support from family and friends through surgery and afterwards at home.

Nursing Diagnoses

- **Knowledge deficit** related to surgery for colorectal cancer
- **Fear** related to the potential outcome of surgery for colorectal cancer

Nursing Interventions
▨ Assessments

- Vital signs
  Vital signs measure physiological function and provide a baseline for after surgery.
- Serum electrolytes and CBC values
  It is important that the patient's serum electrolytes are within normal limits prior surgery. The CBC provides baseline data about hemoglobin and hematocrit, as well as the WBC that may be elevated due to inflammation or infection
- Current knowledge of disease and pre-/postoperative care
  The nurse should reinforce any teachings given by the surgeon, such as the incision and any drains that may be present after surgery. The knowledge of what to expect postoperatively helps to alleviate concerns and fears associated with the surgery.

▨ Actions

- Bowel prep (if ordered)
  The patient will likely receive a thorough "bowel prep" prior to surgery to minimize bacterial growth and prevent contamination with feces during surgery. The most common method of bowel prep or cleansing is polyethylene glycol solution (e.g., GoLYTELY). An antibiotic may also

be given prior to the incision, also to reduce the risk of infection (see Evidence-Based Practice: Mechanical Bowel Preparation).
- Establish a therapeutic relationship
  A therapeutic relationship enhances the trust of the patient and decreases anxiety and fears.
- Ensure the surgical consent form is signed and witnessed
  This is a legal requirement for all invasive procedures. The consent form must be signed prior to the patient receiving any type of sedative, hypnotic, narcotic, or anesthetic agent

▨ Teaching

- Preoperative teaching related to ostomy care (Box 58.4)
  With adequate preoperative teaching, it is more likely the patient will be compliant with the treatment regimens, and to have less anxiety and fear of what to expect. If the patient has adequate preoperative teaching related to ostomy care, the patient demonstrates better adjustment postoperatively. If the patient is expected to have an ostomy performed during surgery, a preoperative consultation is necessary with the wound ostomy continence nurse (WOCN).
- Pain
  Teach the patient about methods of pain management postoperatively, such as patient-controlled analgesia (PCA), epidural anesthesia with the progression to oral pain medication. Knowledge of how pain will be managed postoperatively decreases anxiety and fears.

Evidence-Based Practice

Mechanical Bowel Preparation

There is growing evidence that bowel surgery can safely be performed without mechanical bowel preparations. Because of the time required, as well as the side effects of bowel preparations, including fluid and electrolyte loss and patient issues with tolerating the ordered medications, there is evidence the bowel can be adequately prepared immediately before the surgical procedure.

Bhat, A. H., Parray, F. Q., Chowdri, N. A., Wani, R. A., Thakur, N., Nazki, S. & Wani, I. (2016) Mechanical bowel preparation versus no preparation in elective colorectal surgery: A prospective randomized study. *International Journal of Surgery Open 2 (2016) 26-30.* http://dx.doi.org/10.1016/j.ijso.2016.02.010
Rollins, K. E., Javanmard-Emamghissi, H. & Lobo, D. N. (2018). Impact of mechanical bowel preparation in elective colorectal surgery: A meta-analysis. *World Journal of Gastroenterology, 24 (4), 519-536.* http://dx. doi.org10.3748/wjg.v24.i4.519

Postoperative Patient

Nursing management of the patient undergoing surgery for colorectal surgery is similar to that for other general abdominal surgeries.

Box 58.4 Ostomy Care

A colostomy is a surgically created opening on the abdomen in which the large intestine is connected for the elimination of fecal matter into an appliance specifically designed for this purpose. If the entire colon is removed, the opening is connected to the ileum of the small intestine and is called an ileostomy. If the patient has an ostomy (colostomy or ileostomy), the color and integrity need to be assessed frequently. The stoma should be reddish pink and moist. There is usually some edema initially, which subsides with time. Common locations of stomas according to ostomy location are demonstrated in Figure 58.8. The appliance is secured in place to minimize skin exposure to the stool. Slight bleeding from the stoma is not initially unusual. If the stoma begins to show signs of ischemia (dark red, purplish, or black color) or unusual bleeding, the provider should be notified immediately. The skin around the ostomy site should be inspected frequently and assessed for leakage. Leakage around the appliance into the surgical incision is a risk for infection. The ostomy will begin to function within 2 to 4 days postoperatively. It is important to note any gas being expelled from the appliance, as well as stool. The appliance needs to be emptied when there is gas or if it is one-third to one-half full of stool to decrease the risk of the appliance detaching from the skin. Stool appearance is initially liquid.

The final consistency of the stool is dependent on the location of the ostomy (Fig. 58.9). The closer the ostomy is to the small intestine, the more liquid the stool. The patient with an ileostomy needs to be monitored more closely for fluid and electrolyte balance depending on the amount of drainage noted. The ostomy is described according to location and can be placed in any section of the colon or at the ileum. Stool consistency is generally described as:

- Ileostomy—liquid to semiliquid
- Ascending colostomy—semiliquid
- Transverse colostomy—semiliquid to semiformed
- Descending colostomy–semiformed
- Sigmoid colostomy—formed

Self-care of the ostomy by the patient is far more successful if initial teaching is implemented before the surgery, if possible. Occasionally, a patient undergoes surgery under emergent conditions, and therefore, preoperative teaching is not possible. If the surgery is planned, the patient should have a consult with the wound ostomy continence nurse (WOCN) prior to surgery, who will discuss fears and concerns associated with having an ostomy. The WOCN provides educational materials that patients can review prior to having surgery and answer any questions. The WOCN marks the abdomen for the best possible placement of the ostomy based on the contour of the abdomen in lying, sitting, and standing positions. The WOCN also assesses the presence of any skin folds, creases, bony prominences, and scars, as this allows for optimal placement and best fitting of an appliance after surgery.

Assessment and Analysis

Vital signs measure physiological functions and should be within the range of preoperative levels. After anesthesia, it is important to note the patient's ability to arouse and orientation to surroundings. Change in level of consciousness is often the first sign of other complications. The patient is better able to participate in activities to prevent postoperative complications if pain is adequately treated. Postoperatively, pain in the surgical area is expected. The bowel sounds will be severely diminished or absent, which is expected postoperatively due to surgical manipulation. The CBC may demonstrate mild anemia, and the WBC is elevated due to inflammation, and is monitored for infection. In the case of an ostomy, assessment of the stoma is important to ensure that there is adequate perfusion to the stoma.

Nursing Diagnoses

- **Acute pain** associated with the surgical incision
- **Potential for infection** associated with interruption of primary defenses (skin) and indwelling tubes and drains
- **Risk for imbalanced fluid volume** associated with the response to abdominal surgery
- **Knowledge deficit** associated with postoperative care
- **Disturbed body image** associated with the ostomy

Nursing Interventions

Assessments

- Vital signs at least every 4 hours
  A mild elevation in temperature may be expected in the first 48 hours because of the inflammatory response to surgery. A marked elevation in the first 48 hours is usually related to atelectasis. After the first 48 hours, the patient should continue to be assessed for infection. Elevations in heart rate and decrease in blood pressure are indicative of decreased fluid volume status.
- Hemoglobin and hematocrit
  Monitor hemoglobin and hematocrit daily while patient is hospitalized because this may indicate bleeding and/or nutritional deficits. It is important to compare preoperative levels to postoperative levels while noting the estimated blood loss in surgery.
- White blood cells
  WBC is monitored every day for the first few days. A mild elevation can be expected in the first 48 hours because of the inflammatory response. Later an elevation may indicate infection or other complication
- Nausea and vomiting
  Anesthesia and manipulation of the bowel decrease peristalsis, and bowel sounds may be absent for 1 to 3 days after surgery. The patient will not have anything to eat or drink after surgery (NPO), with IV fluids and electrolyte replacements given as needed. The patient may have an NG tube for stomach decompression postoperatively, and it must be frequently assessed for patency. The NG tube remains in place until bowel function returns.

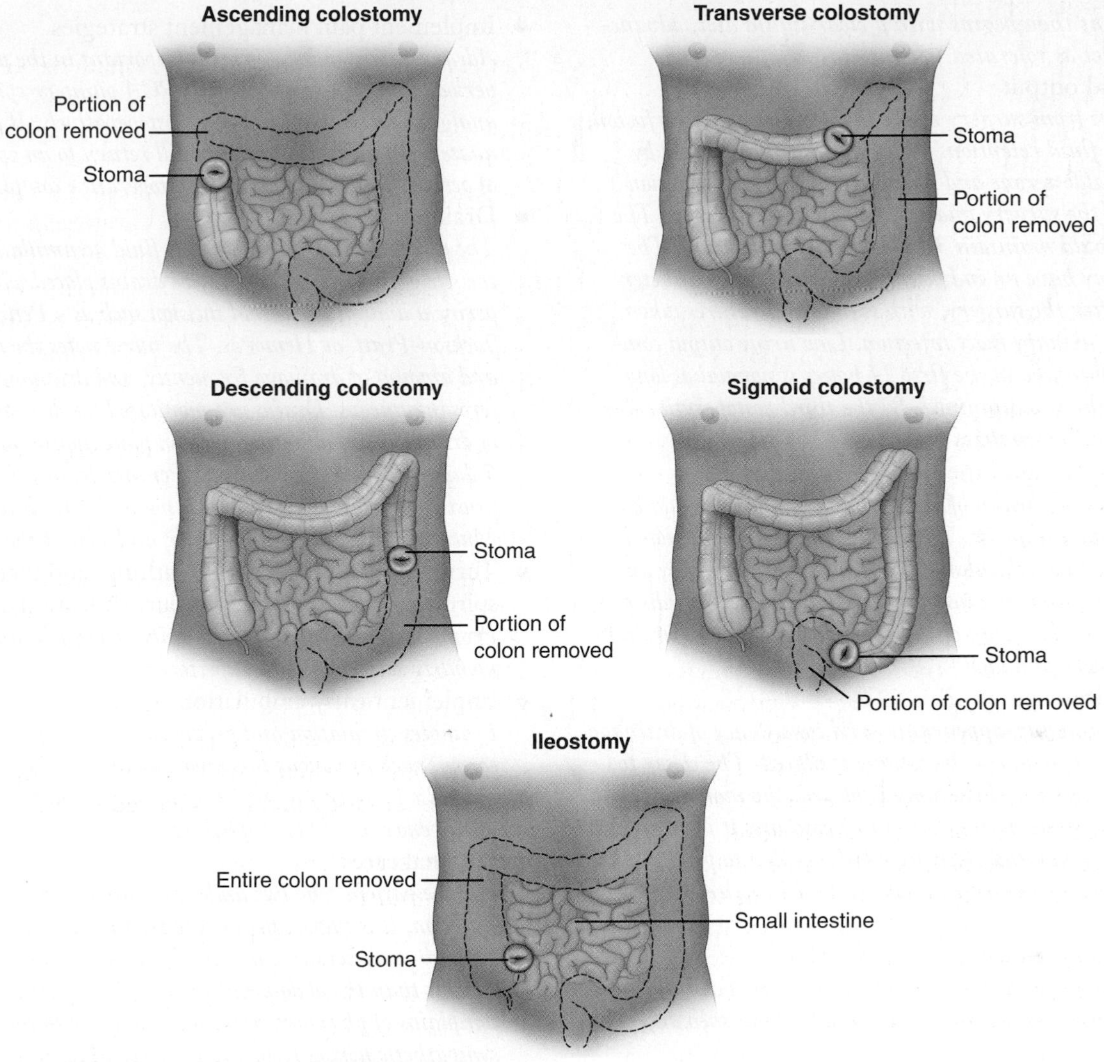

Ascending colostomy

Portion of colon removed

Stoma

Transverse colostomy

Stoma

Portion of colon removed

Descending colostomy

Stoma

Portion of colon removed

Sigmoid colostomy

Stoma

Portion of colon removed

Ileostomy

Entire colon removed

Small intestine

Stoma

FIGURE 58.8 Common locations of stomas.

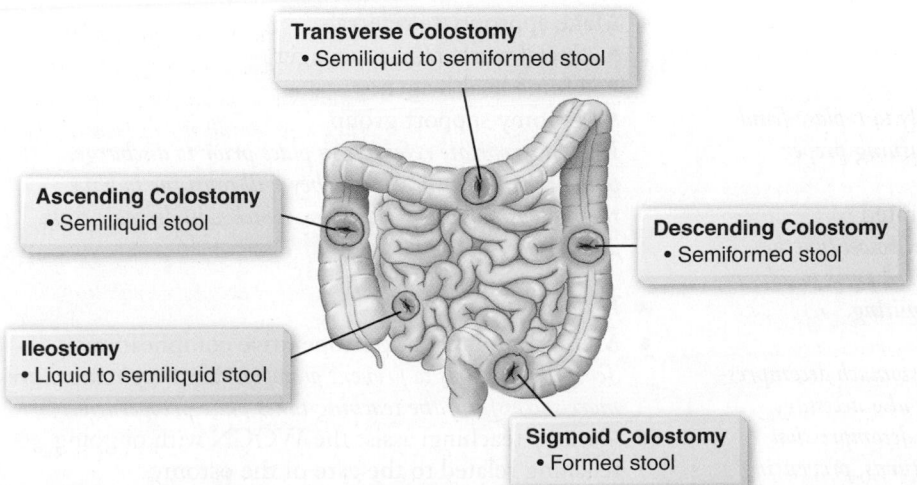

Transverse Colostomy
• Semiliquid to semiformed stool

Ascending Colostomy
• Semiliquid stool

Descending Colostomy
• Semiformed stool

Ileostomy
• Liquid to semiliquid stool

Sigmoid Colostomy
• Formed stool

FIGURE 58.9 Stool consistency based on the location of the ostomy.

The patient then begins with a clear liquid diet, advancing the diet as tolerated.

- Intake and output
Fluid losses from surgery result in decreased renal perfusion, leading to fluid retention. The lower output is caused by increased aldosterone and antidiuretic hormone secretion because of the surgery and associated stress associated. The patient should maintain 30 mL/hr of urine output. The patient may have an indwelling urinary (Foley) catheter in place after the surgery, with standard measures taken to prevent urinary tract infection. Low urine output compared with intake in the first 24 hours is normal as long as 30 mL/hr is maintained. By the third postoperative day, urine output normalizes

- **Stoma** (opening of the ostomy), if applicable
Determines the health of the stoma. The stoma should be reddish pink and moist. There may be some edema noted initially, which will subside in a few days. There may also be slight bleeding or serosanguineous drainage. Any discolorations could be a sign of necrosis and should be reported to the healthcare provider.

- Ostomy drainage
The type, amount, appearance, and consistency of drainage will differ as to where the ostomy is placed. The closer to the small intestine the ostomy is placed, the more liquid the stool. For the patient with an ileostomy, it is important to monitor fluid and electrolyte balance due to potential losses of potassium (see Evidence-Based Practice: Passive Drains).

- Abdominal/perineal dressing/incision
Incisions and dressings should not have excessive drainage noted because this could indicate complications such as bleeding.

- Pain
Adequate pain management is necessary for the patient to return to an optimal level of functioning and to prevent postoperative complications.

Actions

- Administer IV fluids
IV fluids are maintained postoperatively to replace fluid losses in surgery and to assist in maintaining proper fluid balance.

- Maintain NPO/Advance diet as tolerated
Prevention of nausea and vomiting until bowel function returns. Return of bowel sounds is required prior to advancing the diet to minimize nausea and vomiting.

- Nasogastric tube care
The patient may have an NG tube for stomach decompression, and measurement of this output is also necessary. Nasogastric tubes that allow for gastric decompression remain in place until bowel function returns, preventing nausea and vomiting from occurring. It is important to ensure that there is consistent drainage, as lack of output from the drain may indicate an obstruction. Without adequate decompression and drainage, there may be pressure on the surgical site.

- Implement pain management strategies
Adequate pain management is important in the postoperative period. The patient may have a PCA pump or epidural analgesia for the first few days postoperatively. If pain is adequately controlled, the patient will return to an optimal level of activity sooner and prevent postoperative complications.

- Drain management
The placement of drains prevents fluid accumulation near the site of surgery. There may be drains placed within the perineal and/or abdominal incision such as a Penrose drain, Jackson-Pratt, or Hemovac. The nurse notes the appearance and amount of drainage frequently, and drainage is usually serosanguineous. Drains are monitored for decreasing amount of drainage and are usually left in place approximately 3 to 5 days. When the dressing of a Penrose drain is changed, care must be taken to make sure it is not accidentally dislodged. Make a note of the amount, color, and odor of the drainage.

- Turning, coughing, deep breathing, and incentive spirometer 10 times every hour while awake
Promotes lung expansion, prevents atelectasis, and helps mobilize secretions to be expectorated

- Implement early ambulation
Promotes circulation and prevention of postoperative complications such as venous thromboembolism (VTE). The patient may also be receiving anticoagulation therapy with heparin or Lovenox for VTE prophylaxis.

- Perianal care
For the patient who has undergone an abdominoperineal resection, it is important to note that the perineal incision is much more sensitive and a greater source of pain for the patient than the abdominal incision. The patient often complains of phantom rectal sensation due to the fact that sympathetic nerves responsible for rectal control are not severed during surgery. The area should be inspected frequently for drainage and abscess (localized collection of pus) formation. Sitz baths may be ordered for comfort and gentle cleansing of the perineal area.

- Make appropriate referrals
  - Social worker/case manager
  - Home health agency
  - Ostomy support group
With appropriate referrals in place prior to discharge, patients can be assured that they will continue to have their needs met after discharge, which will decrease fears and anxiety.

Teaching

- Methods to prevent postoperative complications
Teaching methods to prevent postoperative complications are more successful if the teaching takes place preoperatively.

- Ostomy teaching: assist the WOCN with ongoing teaching related to the care of the ostomy
If the patient has adequate preoperative teaching related to ostomy care, the patient demonstrates better adjustment postoperatively. If the patient is expected to have an ostomy performed during surgery, a preoperative consultation is necessary with the WOCN.

Evidence-Based Practice

Passive Drains

Surgeons often use a type of drain in the patient near the site of incision to prevent fluid collection, which may cause an infection. Drains may be active or passive. Examples of passive drains include Penrose drains, Foley catheter, Word catheter, and Malecot catheter. They are called *passive* because they rely on gravity to drain. Active drains may be further subdivided into open or closed systems. An example of an open system is a Salem sump, which is connected to suction into a canister at the bedside. The Jackson-Pratt drain is referred to as a closed system and works by negative pressure. A disadvantage of the open system is the potential for bacterial contamination. Most surgeons prefer closed systems with negative pressure, such as the Jackson-Pratt drain.

Numata, M., Godai, T., Shirai, J., Watanabe, K., Ingaki, D., Hasegawa, S., Masuda, M. (2014). A prospective randomized controlled trial of subcutaneous passive drainage for the prevention of superficial surgical site infections in open and laparoscopic colorectal surgery. *International Journal of Colorectal Disease, 29*(3), 353–358.

Evaluating Care Outcomes

There is a direct relationship between outcomes and how well the patient was prepared for the surgery and/or treatment related to colorectal cancer. The outcomes for the patient with colorectal cancer depends on the extent of the disease and treatment regimen. At discharge the patient demonstrates stable vital signs, adequate hematocrit and hemoglobin, no signs of infection, positive bowel sounds, ability to care for surgical incision site and ostomy (as required), and pain management strategies. The patient requires follow-up care for return of normal bowel function, as well as adaption to the diagnosis and treatment.

> **⚠ Safety Alert** If the stoma begins to show signs of ischemia (dark red, purplish, or black color) or unusual bleeding, the provider should be notified immediately. This is a sign that there is little or no blood flow to the stoma.

Connection Check 58.6

The nurse is caring for a patient with colorectal cancer who just had a total colectomy with placement of a permanent ileostomy. Which nursing diagnosis is a priority for the immediate postoperative period?

A. Disturbed body image
B. Acute pain
C. Potential for infection
D. Knowledge deficit

ABDOMINAL TRAUMA

Epidemiology

Abdominal trauma may result from blunt trauma in which there is no penetrating injury or from a penetrating injury caused by a stabbing or a gunshot wound. The most common cause of blunt trauma is motor vehicle crashes, with motor vehicle crashes and pedestrian versus automobile accidents accounting for more than 75% of all cases of blunt abdominal trauma. Any abdominal organ may be injured, but the spleen & liver are the most common organs.

With abdominal stab wounds, the liver is the most often injured organ. Although stab wounds are approximately three times more prevalent than gunshot wounds, morbidity and mortality are less. Abdominal trauma from gunshot wounds is associated with approximately 90% of mortalities from penetrating abdominal injuries.

Pathophysiology

Abdominal trauma may be the result of blunt trauma or penetrating injury between the diaphragm and the pelvis. Blunt trauma may occur as a result of a motor vehicle accident, falls, assaults, or contact sports. Although injury may not be immediately obvious, there may be significant internal organ damage. Blunt trauma involves concussive and compression forces that result in tears and hematomas of solid organs, as well as deceleration forces that can lead to organ rupture secondary to intraluminal pressure changes. Bleeding and organ damage may also develop secondary to stretching and tears along ligaments that support organs secondary to these deceleration injuries.

Penetrating trauma may be caused by gunshot wounds or stabbing wounds. Any organ within the abdominal cavity has the potential for injury as a result of either injury, but the liver is the most commonly injured organ. The foreign object penetrates the abdominal cavity and may result in profuse bleeding that may deteriorate to hemorrhagic shock.

Hypovolemic shock can occur rapidly. Trauma to solid organs, such as the liver and spleen, causes hemorrhage when injured. Hollow organs, such as the stomach, urinary bladder, and intestines, may cause peritonitis when their contents (undigested food, urine, or feces) spill into the abdominal cavity.

Clinical Manifestations

Once the trauma patient's airway, breathing, and circulation have been thoroughly assessed, then the patient needs to be evaluated for signs of hemorrhage, shock, and peritonitis. The clinical manifestations vary widely according to the organ of injury, and assessment includes the presence, location, and quality of any pain experienced by the patient. Often with abdominal trauma, there are obvious injuries, including bruising, penetrating injuries, abrasions, lacerations, discolorations, and asymmetry. **Ecchymosis** (bruising) around the umbilicus (**Cullen's sign**) or the flank areas

(**Turner's sign** or **Grey Turner's sign**) may indicate intra-abdominal and/or retroperitoneal hemorrhage and should be reported to the provider immediately. With the loss of bowel sounds, peritonitis should be suspected. Auscultation of bruits over the abdomen may indicate renal artery, arterial, or aortic damage. Abdominal trauma is often associated with other injuries, such as bone fractures and head injuries.

Management

Medical Management

Diagnosis

Laboratory tests include baseline serum chemistries, CBC, and urinalysis. The hemoglobin and hematocrit may or may not be abnormal initially as fluids are being lost along with the red blood cells. Once fluid resuscitation has begun, a change will then be noted in the hemoglobin and hematocrit if the patient is bleeding internally, as the remaining RBCs will be diluted. Urinalysis is assessed for the presence of blood in the urine. The patient should also be typed and cross matched for the possibility of a blood transfusion. Based on the stability of the patient, x-rays and CT or MRI scans may be completed to fully determine the severity of the trauma. If the patient is able to travel to radiology, a CT scan is performed to identify specific areas of injury. Healthcare providers must be attentive to potential spinal cord injuries when transferring to radiology and patients should be accompanied by a provider familiar with the care of the trauma patient.

Diagnostic peritoneal lavage (DPL) may be used to diagnose intra-abdominal bleeding. The provider inserts a catheter into the abdominal cavity. Fluid is allowed to enter the abdominal cavity and is then allowed to drain. If the fluid that drains out of the abdomen appears bloody, the patient is prepared for emergency surgery. Another diagnostic tool used to evaluate trauma patients is the focused abdominal sonography for trauma (FAST), which can be used to scan the abdomen in 3 to 5 minutes, noting any free fluid in the abdominal cavity. The FAST scan is recommended versus DPL if ultrasound is available.

Treatment

Medical management is totally dependent on the nature of the injury or injuries. Large-bore IV lines are inserted, and fluid resuscitation is initiated for volume expansion. A nasogastric tube may be inserted for gastric decompression. The trauma patient's condition can change rapidly and requires vigilant observation. An indwelling urinary catheter may be inserted to observe for hematuria as well as to closely monitor urinary output in the immediate postoperative period.

Surgical Management

The patient may be transported emergently to the operating room for an exploratory laparotomy to determine and treat the injuries. With bowel perforation or laceration, the injury is surgically explored and repaired, and the patient is started on antibiotics due to increased risk of peritonitis.

Complications

Complications of abdominal trauma are directly related to the injury to internal organs. Hemorrhagic shock may develop, particularly secondary to penetrating trauma. Peritonitis, potentially leading to septic shock, may develop with intestinal damage that allows fecal material to enter the peritoneal cavity. Ischemic bowel and paralytic ileus may also occur secondary to the traumatic event. With significant blood loss, accompanied with sepsis, the patient may develop adult respiratory distress syndrome and disseminated intravascular coagulopathy.

Nursing Management

Nursing care of the abdominal trauma patient is based on protocols from Advanced Trauma Life Support that follows the ABCDE pattern: Airway, Breathing, Circulation, Disability (Neurological status), and Exposure.

Assessment and Analysis

Airway management is the priority to ensure a patent airway, as chest injuries are often associated with abdominal trauma. The abdominal trauma patient's vital signs can change very quickly based on the amount of fluid loss, and the nurse should be trained in emergency management. Clinical manifestations of abdominal trauma are based on type (blunt or penetrating) of trauma, as well as organs and structures involved. Based on the severity of the trauma, clinical presentation of abdominal trauma may include:

- Tachycardia
- Tachypnea
- Pain
- Bruising
- Abrasions
- Lacerations
- Discoloration
- Cullen's sign
- Turner's sign
- Absence of bowel sounds

The patient can deteriorate quickly with large blood and fluid losses, and hypovolemic shock and death can occur rapidly.

Nursing Diagnoses

- **Risk for ineffective airway clearance** associated with trauma
- **Risk for deficient fluid volume** associated with blood loss
- **Acute pain** associated with tissue damage caused by abdominal trauma

Nursing Interventions

■ *Assessments*

- Airway
  It is important to assess airway clearance because the patient may have blood and/or vomitus in the oral cavity.

Establishment of a patent airway is the priority because other injuries are likely with abdominal trauma and require adequate oxygenation and perfusion of vital organs.

- Vital signs including oxygen saturation
Vital signs can change very quickly with abdominal trauma. Respiratory rate and effort may increase with airway obstruction. Heart rate increases and blood pressure decreases with significant blood loss. Pulse may increase with pain.

- Level of consciousness using the Glasgow Coma Scale
Determines patient's level of consciousness because there may be associated head injury with motor vehicle accidents. The level of consciousness may also decrease with profound hypovolemia associated with blunt trauma to the abdominal cavity.

- Clinical manifestations of hypovolemic shock
Hypovolemic shock and death can occur rapidly and are manifested by decreased blood pressure, increased pulse, diminished peripheral pulses, decreased skin temperature, and decreased urinary output.

- CBC and urinalysis
The hemoglobin and hematocrit need to be monitored because values may decrease as fluid resuscitation is started in patients with blood loss. Low values also are indicative of the degree of blood loss from the injury.

- Serum electrolytes
Baseline serum electrolytes are particularly important in patients who may require nasogastric decompression because potassium loss occurs with NG suctioning.

- Urinalysis
Urinalysis is assessed for the presence of blood in the urine.

- Bowel sounds
With damage to the abdominal organs, there may be a decrease or complete absence of bowel sounds.

- Area of injury
Observe for signs of internal bleeding (Cullen's and Turner's signs) with blunt abdominal trauma. Assess for entry and exit wounds with gunshot wounds. Observe area of stabbing, and if the instrument is still in the patient's body, do not remove and allow the physician to manage the weapon.

■ Actions

- Administer supplemental oxygen
With trauma, particularly with the risk of hypovolemia, supplemental oxygen increases oxygen delivery to maximize organ perfusion

- Insert large-bore IV and administer IV fluids
Administration of IV fluids rapidly may prevent the patient from hypovolemic shock.

- Do not remove object protruding from wound
Removing objects may increase the risk of bleeding.

- Control bleeding
Promotes hemodynamic stability

- Administer antibiotics
Prophylactic antibiotics are typically initiated with abdominal trauma secondary to the risk of internal damage that may lead to peritonitis

- Consult with primary provider regarding need for Type and Cross match
With the increased chance of bleeding with abdominal trauma, it is important to have blood ready for transfusion as the patient's condition warrants.

■ Teaching

- Explain to the patient and family all procedures regardless
The patient has many fears and is generally unfamiliar with hospital and trauma protocols. Patient confidence and cooperation is enhanced by understanding of what is happening in the ED, OR, PACU, and inpatient unit.

- Keep family informed about the patient's condition
Families are often subject to being overlooked in the trauma setting and should be kept informed of the patient's condition.

- Nutrition and diet
Based on the type of injury, the patient may require dietary modifications. With significant damage to the gastrointestinal tract, the patient may require long-term total parenteral (TPN) or enteral nutrition.

- Wound care
Based on the extent of the surgical procedure, the patient may have tubes, drains, or an ostomy. Patient teaching encourages independence in postoperative care.

- Clinical manifestations of infection
Due to the increased risk of peritoneal contamination with abdominal trauma, the patient needs to acknowledge the signs and symptoms of infection and to report immediately to their provider.

Evaluating Care Outcomes

The outcome is largely dependent on the nature and extent of the injuries. The priorities are physiological stability as evidenced by stable vital signs, hematocrit and hemoglobin within acceptable parameters, no clinical manifestations of infection, adequate pain management, and stable weight. The patient is independent in care requirements for the postoperative wound, and any associated equipment (for example, ostomy).

> **! Safety Alert** Clinical manifestations of hypovolemic shock are restlessness, anxiety, cool clammy skin, confusion, weakness, pale color, tachypnea, tachycardia, and hypotension. If the patient experiences abdominal trauma and displays these clinical manifestations, the nurse should keep the patient calm and warm, elevate lower extremities (unless contraindicated by other injuries), maintain a patent airway, and maintain IV access.

Connection Check 58.7

A patient has just been brought to the emergency department by emergency medical services after a motor vehicle accident. What is the first thing the nurse should do?

A. Ask the patient if he or she is in pain
B. Mental status examination and vital signs
C. Ask the patient to move all extremities
D. Order laboratory tests

Making Connections

CASE STUDY: WRAP-UP

A colonoscopy shows that Jack has multiple ulcerative lesions in the descending colon. His upper gastrointestinal endoscopy is negative. The wireless capsule endoscopy is negative. His vital signs are: temperature is 100.5°F (38°C); pulse is 133; respiratory rate is 24; blood pressure is 122/75 mm Hg; pain score is 7/10 (0–10 pain scale). His weight is 62 kg (136.4 lb), and his height is 165.5 cm (65.2 in.). His hemoglobin is 7.6 g/dL, and his hematocrit is 21.2 %. Jack's diagnosis is ulcerative colitis.

Jack Conner undergoes surgery for his ulcerative colitis. He had the first of two surgeries: colectomy, mucosal proctectomy, and ileal pouch-anal canal anastomosis. Jack has a temporary ileostomy. He will return to the hospital in 2 to 3 months to have the ileostomy reversed.

Case Study Questions

1. What clinical manifestations does Jack display that are consistent with a diagnosis of ulcerative colitis? *(Select all that apply.)*
   A. Bloody stools
   B. Constipation
   C. Belching
   D. Chest pain
   E. Dysphagia

2. What diagnostic tests does the nurse expect to be ordered for Jack on the basis of these symptoms?
   A. CBC, MRI, electrolytes, stool analysis
   B. CT scan, MRI, chemistry panel, ERCP
   C. Colonoscopy, CBC, wireless capsule endoscopy, upper GI endoscopy
   D. BUN, creatinine, ultrasound, chest x-ray

3. What other priority information may the nurse assess in order to care for Jack?
   A. Psychosocial history, family history, vital signs, previous bowel history
   B. Vaccine history, medication history, heart rate
   C. Orientation status, ability to participate in sports, blood pressure
   D. Cranial nerves, sensation, skin assessment

4. Which information does the nurse include in the teaching to Jack related to his diagnosis of ulcerative colitis?
   A. "Decrease fluid intake to decrease diarrhea."
   B. "Spread out your meals to six times per day."
   C. "Avoid foods high in potassium."
   D. "Increase your intake of simple sugars for energy."

5. On the basis of the above information, what will the nurse consider a priority to notify the provider?
   A. Height and weight
   B. Temperature
   C. Blood pressure
   D. Hemoglobin and hematocrit

CHAPTER SUMMARY

Hernias typically occur because of weakened abdominal muscles accompanied by increased abdominal pressure. Types of hernias include inguinal, femoral, umbilical, and ventral. Inguinal hernias occur most often in males, whereas femoral hernias occur most often in females. Indirect inguinal hernias are the most common and occur only in males. They are commonly repaired with surgery that may include using a mesh material to minimize reoccurrence of the hernia. A hernia is usually self-limiting and surgical repair is an elective procedure unless the hernia becomes strangulated, causing blood supply to be compromised.

Hemorrhoids may be internal or external. If conservative treatment fails, there are several surgical options. Conservative treatments include sitz baths, oral analgesics, and hemorrhoid ointments and creams. Hemorrhoids can become quite painful, requiring analgesic usage, but are usually self-limiting, although surgery may be necessary with perforations or excessive bleeding.

Irritable bowel syndrome (IBS) is a complex illness in which there is no pathologic cause, which is characterized by abdominal pain and changes in bowel habits and characteristics of the stool. There are three types: diarrhea dominant (IBS-D), constipation dominant (IBS-C), and mixed (IBS-M). There are many psychosocial issues surrounding the patient with IBS. Social isolation is a common problem with IBS-D because of the frequency of needing to locate restrooms while in public. Treatments vary according to the severity of the syndrome and the type of syndrome the patient experiences.

Inflammatory bowel disease is a term used for ulcerative colitis and Crohn's disease. Although there are many similarities, there are many differences as well. Surgery for either type depends on the severity of the disease and failure to maintain remission with medication. Surgery for Crohn's disease often causes a flare at the site of anastomosis and is reserved for severe cases in which medical management fails. Surgery for ulcerative colitis can result in cure of the disease itself but does not cure the extraintestinal complications that often coincide with the disease. Inflammatory bowel disease requires an interprofessional team because there are many physical, as well as psychosocial factors impacting the disease. A dietitian should be utilized because he or she can manage the many nutritional deficits resulting from frequent gastrointestinal losses.

Celiac disease is a genetic autoimmune disorder associated with gluten sensitivity. Patients with this disorder typically present with diarrhea, flatulence, abdominal bloating, weakness, fatigue, and weight loss. Treatment is based on lifelong adherence to gluten-free diet, and support groups and networks are available to support the patient and family in this goal.

Diverticulitis is a term used to describe inflammation of diverticula. Diverticula are small pouchlike herniations in the colon. If stool is trapped in the diverticula, inflammation can result. Treatments are based on severity and may include outpatient antibiotics or inpatient care requiring gastric decompression as well as IV antibiotics.

Appendicitis is a common disorder that affects 5% to 12% of the population. It occurs more often in adolescents and young adults, affecting males more than females. The only treatment is surgical removal of the appendix.

Colorectal cancer rates and deaths are decreasing in the United States because of improvements in diagnosis and treatment. Compared with other cancers, colorectal cancers have improved significantly in survival rates as a result of increased public awareness and early interventions. Treatment of colorectal cancer includes surgical procedures, including colectomy and ileostomy, often with chemotherapy and/or radiation therapy.

Abdominal trauma is divided into two groups: blunt trauma (caused by things such as vehicle accidents and sports injuries) and penetrating trauma (caused by things such as gunshot wounds and stabbings). Surgical intervention is typically required for abdominal trauma, and based on the area of injury the patient is at risk for hemorrhage and infection.

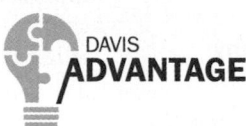

To explore learning resources for this chapter, go to **Davis Advantage** and find:
- Answers to in-text questions
- Chapter Resources and Activities
- NCLEX®-Style Chapter Review Questions
- Bibliography

Chapter 59

Coordinating Care for Patients With Hepatic Disorders

Sandy Swoboda

LEARNING OUTCOMES

Content in this chapter is designed to assist in:

1. Describing the epidemiology of hepatic disorders.
2. Correlating clinical manifestations with pathophysiological processes of:
   a. Hepatitis
   b. Cirrhosis
   c. Liver cancer
   d. Liver trauma
3. Describing the diagnostic results used to confirm the diagnoses of hepatic disorders
4. Discussing the medical management of:
   a. Hepatitis
   b. Cirrhosis
   c. Liver cancer
   d. Liver trauma
5. Developing a comprehensive plan of nursing care for patients with hepatic disorders
6. Designing a plan of care that includes pharmacological, dietary, and lifestyle considerations for patients with hepatic disorders

CONCEPTS

- Assessment
- Clotting
- Fluid and Electrolyte Balance
- Infection
- Inflammation
- Medication

ESSENTIAL TERMS

Alpha-fetoprotein
Ascites
Asterixis
Cholangiography
Cholangitis
Cholestasis
Cirrhosis
Disseminated intravascular coagulation (DIC)
Ecchymosis
Esophageal varices
Epistaxis
Hemochromatosis
Hepatic encephalopathy
Hepatitis
Hepatocytes
Hepatomegaly
Hepatosplenomegaly
Hepatorenal syndrome (HRS)
Icterus
Jaundice
Laënnec's cirrhosis
Petechiae
Portal hypertension
Pruritus
Sclerotherapy
Sengstaken-Blakemore tube
Splenomegaly
Spontaneous bacterial peritonitis (SBP)
Thrombocytopenia
Transjugular intrahepatic portosystemic shunt (TIPS)
Urticaria

Finding Connections

CASE STUDY: EPISODE 1

Follow this patient throughout the chapter.

Harold Green, a 56-year-old unemployed male, presents to the clinic with anorexia, generalized weakness, malaise, and weight loss. He has type 2 diabetes mellitus, treated with metformin XR 1,500 mg once per day. His medical history includes IV drug use, and currently he describes drinking two to three beers per day with his friends while looking for work…

INTRODUCTION

The liver is located under the diaphragm in the right upper quadrant (RUQ) of the abdominal cavity and receives approximately 25% of the cardiac output via the hepatic portal vein and the hepatic artery. The portal vein carries deoxygenated nutrient-rich blood from the small intestines, and the hepatic artery delivers oxygen-rich blood from the general circulation. The liver serves several functions including blood storage, blood filtration, production of bile, synthesis of clotting factors (prothrombin and factors II, VII, IX, and X), removal of clotting factors to prevent clotting, and metabolism of carbohydrates, fats, and protein. The liver also serves to detoxify the blood and is a storage area for vitamins A, D, E, and K and iron. Hepatic dysfunction occurs when the liver is no longer able to perform its usual functions. Several conditions such as **hepatitis** (inflammation of the liver), **cirrhosis** (chronic liver disease characterized by inflammation and irreversible scarring), liver trauma, and liver cancer all impair the ability of the liver to perform its routine functions (Box 59.1).

Box 59.1 Healthy People 2020

Healthy People 2020 initiatives for liver disorders focus on health promotion and prevention, healthy lifestyles, education, and vaccination. Specific goals of *Healthy People 2020* for patients with hepatitis and cirrhosis include interventions to reduce hepatitis A, hepatitis B, and new hepatitis C infections; increased education to the population about hepatitis and knowledge about infection; and efforts to reduce the number of deaths associated with cirrhosis.

Source: U.S. Department of Health and Human Services, http://www. healthypeople.gov

HEPATITIS

Epidemiology

The incidence and prevalence of hepatitis is worldwide, and the risk for developing hepatitis is generally associated with individual behavior and exposure. There are several viruses that cause hepatitis, and transmission is either through fecal-oral contamination or directly through blood and body fluid exposures. Other risk factors for hepatitis include alcohol abuse, exposure to some prescription and over-the-counter (OTC) medications, toxins, or autoimmune diseases (Box 59.2). In autoimmune hepatitis, an immune system response causes inflammation of the liver, which can be classified as type 1 or type 2. Type 1 autoimmune hepatitis occurs most frequently in females during adolescence, and these patients usually have other autoimmune disorders such as type 1 diabetes, Graves' disease (hyperthyroidism), ulcerative colitis, or proliferative glomerulonephritis. Type 2 autoimmune hepatitis is less common and affects girls between the ages of 2 and 14.

Connection Check 59.1

The nurse recognizes which patient is at greatest risk for type 1 autoimmune hepatitis?
A. A 45-year-old postmenopausal female
B. A 30-year-old female with a history of hyperthyroidism
C. A 16-year-old female with type 1 diabetes mellitus
D. A 12-year-old female with autism

Approximately two billion people worldwide have been infected with the hepatitis virus, and almost 350 million people live with a chronic infection. Twenty-five percent of adults with chronic hepatitis will develop cirrhosis or liver cancer because of chronic infection with the virus (cirrhosis is discussed later in the chapter). The introduction of

Box 59.2 Risk Factors for Hepatitis

Medications
- Statins
- Anabolic steroid
- Azathioprine
- Methotrexate
- Isoniazid
- Valproic acid
- Tetracyclines
- Phenytoin
- Acetaminophen

Toxins
- Industrial chemicals
- Carbon tetrachloride
- Phosphorus
- Mushrooms

vaccines for hepatitis A and hepatitis B has greatly decreased the incidence of these types of viral hepatitis.

Pathophysiology

Hepatitis is inflammation of liver cells most commonly caused by a virus that impairs its ability to function normally. This inflammation limits the ability of the liver to detoxify substances, limits the production of proteins and clotting factors, and alters the ability to store vitamins, fats, and sugars. Modes of transmission of viral hepatitis include contact with blood, blood products, semen, saliva, and mucous membranes; direct contact with infected fluids or objects; or through the fecal-oral route with contaminated water or food such as shellfish. Patients with hepatitis may experience a mild or severe illness that can be acute or chronic.

The viruses of hepatitis are classified according to letters ranging from A to G, each of which differs in its incubation period, mode of transmission, and other characteristics. The most common hepatitis viruses are hepatitis A, B, and C. The major viral types of hepatitis and routes of transmission are found in Table 59.1. Diagnosis of type is made by using a specific serological profile.

Clinical Manifestations

Clinical manifestations of hepatitis include abdominal pain, irritability, **pruritus** (itching of the skin), malaise, fever, nausea, vomiting, **jaundice** (yellowish skin color), and laboratory abnormalities such as elevated liver enzymes (aspartate aminotransferase- [AST] and alanine transaminase [ALT]), elevated bilirubin (total and direct), elevated serum ammonia, and decreased albumin. Pruritus is excessive itching on the body, especially in the hands and feet, caused by accumulation of bile salts under the skin that cannot be processed by the liver

Patients can also exhibit jaundice (**icterus**) or yellowing of the skin or sclera (Fig. 59.1). Jaundice occurs secondary to the liver's inability to metabolize and excrete bilirubin (hepatocellular jaundice), resulting in elevated bilirubin levels in plasma. Bilirubin is a by-product of the breakdown of red blood cells that is filtered through the liver and stored with bile. Bile acids normally secreted by the liver make stool its brown color. With an obstruction in the liver, these bile acids are not excreted in the stool, resulting in clay-colored stools. This also leads to increased excretion of conjugated bilirubin in the urine producing a dark amber color. Obstructive jaundice may be caused by scarring, edema, stone formation, and any obstruction that interferes with the normal process of bile flow through the bile ducts.

In general, symptoms of hepatitis can be mild or severe and vary from patient to patient according to the degree of liver involvement. Patients may present with common flulike symptoms.

Fulminant viral hepatitis is a severe, rapidly progressive, life-threatening form of acute liver failure that includes neurological decline (encephalopathy, insomnia, somnolence, and impaired mentation), gastrointestinal (GI) bleeding, coagulation disorders, **thrombocytopenia** (low platelet

Table 59.1 Types of Hepatitis

	Hepatitis A	Hepatitis B	Hepatitis C	Hepatitis D	Hepatitis E	Hepatitis G
Route of transmission	Fecal-oral, contaminated water or food	Percutaneous or mucosal Blood, body fluids, needles or sharp instruments	Percutaneous or mucosal Blood, body fluids, needles or sharp instruments	Percutaneous or mucosal In conjunction with hepatitis B, blood, body fluids, or sharp instruments	Fecal-oral, contaminated water or food	Infected blood or blood products
Source of virus	Feces, contaminated water or food	Blood, body fluids	Blood, body fluids, needles or sharp instruments	Blood, body fluids, needles or sharp instruments	Feces	Infected blood or blood products
Incubation period	15–50 days	45–60 days	2–25 weeks	2–8 weeks	2–8 weeks	Unknown
Acute or chronic	Acute	Chronic	Chronic	Acute	Acute	Acute
Available vaccine	Yes	Yes	No	Prevented with HBV vaccine	No	No
Treatment	Symptomatic	Interferon and antivirals	Interferon and antivirals	Interferon and antivirals	Symptomatic	Symptomatic

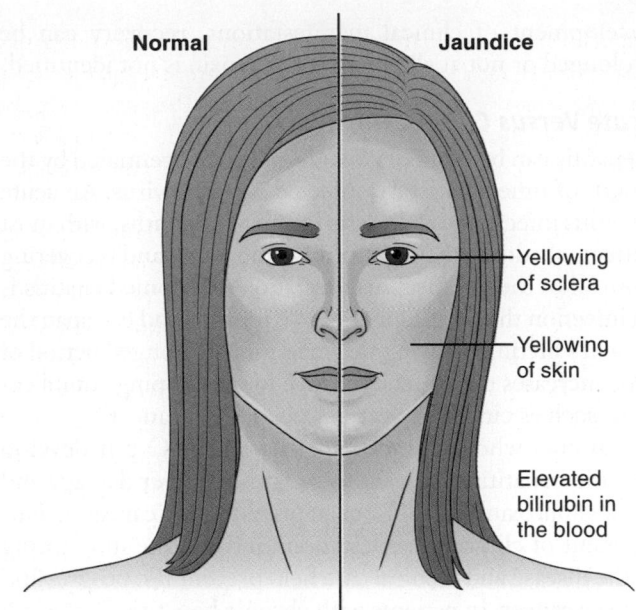

FIGURE 59.1 Jaundice. Patients exhibit jaundice or yellowing of the skin or sclera due to inflammation of the liver. Jaundice is secondary to the liver cells' inability to excrete bilirubin resulting in elevated circulating bilirubin.

Normal / Jaundice
— Yellowing of sclera
— Yellowing of skin
Elevated bilirubin in the blood

count of less than 150,000 mm³), fever, oliguria, edema, and **ascites** (accumulation of fluid in the peritoneal cavity secondary to low serum albumin levels). (Ascites is discussed in more detail in the section on Cirrhosis).

Hepatic encephalopathy presents with impaired mentation, altered levels of consciousness, confusion, somnolence, and insomnia due to the accumulation of toxins in the bloodstream that are normally cleared by a healthy liver. In severe hepatic failure, the liver is unable to metabolize waste secondary to severe inflammation, and because the **hepatocytes** (liver cells) are not functioning properly. Additionally, due to scarring of the liver, blood bypasses the liver and is not detoxified. As a result, waste products accumulate, specifically ammonia, causing changes in mental status. Additional complications of liver failure include the inability of the liver to produce clotting factors, resulting in coagulation disorders and thrombocytopenia.

Types of Hepatitis

Viral Hepatitis

Hepatitis A is the most common type of hepatitis and is primarily spread through the oral route from food, water, or shellfish that has been infected with the virus. It can also be spread through close contact with infected persons such as in households and day care centers, with an increased incidence in the presence of unsanitary conditions. Hepatitis A is an acute infection lasting as long as 8 weeks and has several phases. The first phase can last for about a week and presents with abrupt onset of fever with anorexia, nausea, vomiting, malaise, abdominal pain, myalgia, diarrhea, **urticaria** (pale red, raised bumps on the skin), cough, and

hepatosplenomegaly (enlarged liver [**Hepatomegaly**] and/or spleen [**Splenomegaly**]). Clinical manifestations of later phases include clay-colored stools and a rise in serum bilirubin levels, and jaundice may occur 4 to 30 days after onset of infection. Clinical manifestations in patients with hepatitis A are usually mild, and some patients are completely asymptomatic. The most definitive diagnosis of hepatitis A is through a blood test for the presence of anti-hepatitis A immunoglobulin M (IgM anti-HAV), which can be elevated for as long as 6 months.

Hepatitis B is spread by blood and body fluids or secretions such as semen. The virus can be spread through mucous membranes, contact with infected fluids, during childbirth, or through skin puncture with contaminated needles or other instruments. Patients infected with hepatitis B can have acute or chronic infections and are considered infectious as long as antigens are present in the bloodstream. There is a vaccine for hepatitis B that is required for all healthcare personnel. This vaccine is a multiseries injection given at specified intervals, with several vaccines currently available. Recommendations for intervals for children and adults are available from the CDC (Centers for Disease Control and Prevention), WHO (World Health Organization) and local state and governing bodies. The dose given is dependent on the specific vaccine and age of the individual. In the United States, local laws and requirements vary, however, hepatitis A and B vaccines may be required for entry into day-care, elementary, and middle schools.

Chronic hepatitis B infection is present in more than 350 million people globally and accounts for one-third of the cases of liver cirrhosis and one-half of all cases of hepatocellular carcinoma (HCC). Risk factors for hepatitis B include sexual contact with infected persons, multiple sex partners, male homosexual sex, injection drug use, hemodialysis, blood transfusions, and occupational exposure. Acute hepatitis B occurs after an incubation period of 4 to 10 weeks, and chronic hepatitis B is diagnosed by detectable serum HBV (hepatitis B virus) DNA levels and persistent elevation of ALT and AST levels. High-risk patients with hepatitis B should be screened every 6 to 12 months for HCC. Screening includes an ultrasound and a serum **alpha-fetoprotein** (protein produced by the liver) level as a marker for liver cancer. Because patients with a chronic hepatitis B infection can still spread the virus to others, it is important to educate patients about screening and vaccination of close family members and sexual partners to prevent the spread of infection.

Hepatitis C (previously known as non-A non-B) is spread through blood or body fluids and from mother to child during childbirth. A significant number of cases of hepatitis C occur from sharing of contaminated needles by IV drug users and unintended needlesticks in the healthcare environment. Other risk settings include tattoo and body piercing establishments because of the chance of contact with blood. Infection with hepatitis C can be acute or chronic, and approximately 85% of acute cases develop chronic infection, with cirrhosis developing within 20 to 30 years of diagnosis. Studies examining the spread of hepatitis C and specific genotypes indicate that Baby Boomers, those born in the United States between 1940 and 1965, may also be at increased risk for hepatitis C as a result of medical interventions in which glass and metal syringes were re-used. Medical management of hepatitis C is available with established cure rates, but treatment is costly. There is currently no vaccine for hepatitis, but there is ongoing research. Hepatitis C is the most common indication for liver transplantation.

Evidence-Based Practice

Hepatitis C: Implications to Public Health

Hepatitis C, a global public health issue, is a leading cause of liver cirrhosis and hepatocellular cancer. Several studies on vaccine development, including peptides, recombinant protein, DNA, and viral vectors have been conducted. The search for vaccine for this disease is ongoing.

Ghasemi, F., Rostami, S., & Meshkat, Z. (2015). Progress in the development of vaccines for hepatitis C virus infection. *World Journal of Gastroenterology*, *21(42)*, 11984.

Hepatitis D infection is not common in the United States and occurs only in people who are infected with the hepatitis B virus because it requires the hepatitis B antigen to replicate. It is spread through contact with infectious blood and is most commonly found in patients who are IV drug users, receiving hemodialysis, and have received multiple blood transfusions. There is no vaccine for hepatitis D.

Hepatitis E is caused by the hepatitis E virus that is transmitted via the fecal-oral route primarily through water that is contaminated in areas of poor sanitation. This is rare in the United States, and there is currently no vaccine for hepatitis E. Patients with this type of hepatitis exhibit clinical manifestations similar to those of hepatitis A; the disease has a rapid onset and is self-limited. Almost all patients with hepatitis E develop jaundice.

Hepatitis G was discovered in 1996 and is known to be transmitted by infected blood or blood products, making patients with hemophilia and those who require blood transfusions at greatest risk. Patients who are infected with hepatitis B or C virus can often be infected with hepatitis G. Little is known about the frequency of hepatitis G, and currently there is no vaccine.

Nonviral Forms of Hepatitis

Nonviral forms of hepatitis are caused by ingested, inhaled, or injected toxins or medications. Patients with nonviral forms of hepatitis have clinical presentations similar to those of viral hepatitis such as anorexia, nausea and vomiting, jaundice, and **hepatomegaly** (an enlarged liver). Diagnosis includes a detailed history and physical examination and a history of exposure to potential toxins. If it is determined that the patient has been exposed to a liver toxin and the toxin is removed, recovery can be rapid. However, if there is a prolonged time period between exposure to the toxin and the

development of clinical manifestations, recovery can be prolonged or not at all possible if the toxin is not identified.

Acute Versus Chronic Hepatitis

Hepatitis can be acute or chronic and is differentiated by the length of time a patient is infected with the virus. An acute hepatitis infection usually lasts less than 6 months, with most patients shedding the virus in this time frame and recovering from all of their clinical manifestations. Chronic hepatitis is an infection that lasts longer than 6 months and can span the patient's lifetime. Having the virus for a prolonged period of time increases the patient's chance for developing complications such as cirrhosis, liver failure, or liver cancer.

Patients who contract hepatitis B and C can develop chronic hepatitis that leads to progressive liver damage and causes approximately 80% of all primary liver cancers. Management of clinical manifestations and routine monitoring of the disease and medical care help prevent the progression to liver cancer. In patients with chronic hepatitis C, the risk for liver cancer is decreased for patients on antiviral therapy because this therapy prevents the virus from reproducing, thus slowing the progression of liver damage. The treatment course and antiviral medication choice are based on the age of the patient, severity of illness, adverse reactions, medication tolerance, viral load, ALT level, and the patient's compliance with the medication regimen.

Management

Medical Management

Diagnosis

Laboratory and diagnostic testing include assessments that determine the extent of liver damage and guide diagnosis. Diagnostic test results and a thorough physical examination are important in the determination of the cause of the patient's clinical manifestations. Most of these tests are collected as routine blood samples and require no specific preparation. Table 59.2 provides an overview of some of the most important laboratory tests used to evaluate liver function.

Monitoring AST and ALT levels along with the clinical presentation of the patient provides information about whether these elevations are associated with the liver solely or with another major organ. (Often abnormalities in a liver panel may not be associated specifically with the liver). An AST level that is extremely high (usually 10 times the normal range) indicates acute hepatitis most often caused by a virus but can also be associated with exposure to medications or other hepatotoxins. These levels usually remain elevated for 1 to 2 months but can take as long as 3 to 6 months to return to normal. Liver enzymes are measured serially over time to monitor recovery or worsening of the disease. Ratios of AST to ALT can help determine whether the liver disease is viral in origin or associated with a toxin or alcohol exposure.

Two laboratory values that indicate abnormalities of bile flow are the GGT (gamma glutamyl transferase) and alkaline phosphatase. Specifically, GGT is a protein that

Table 59.2 Diagnostic Testing for Liver Disorders

Test	Normal Results
ALT Alanine transaminase	Males: 13–40 units/L Females: 24–36 units/L
AST Aspartate transaminase	Males: 20–40 units/L Females: 15–35 units/L
Alkaline phosphatase (Total)	Males: 35–142 units/L Females: 25–125 units/L
Alkaline phosphatase (Liver Fraction)	0–93 units/L
GGT Gamma glutamyl transferase	Males: 0–30 units/L Females: 0–24 units/L
LDH Lactate dehydrogenase	90–176 units/L
Bilirubin, total	0.3–1 mg/dL
Bilirubin, indirect	0.2–0.8 mg/dL
Bilirubin, direct	0.1–0.3 mg/dL
Albumin	3.4–5.1 g/dL
Ammonia	15–60 mcg/dL
Coagulation tests • Prothrombin time • Activated partial thromboplastin time (aPTT)	 10–13 seconds 25–35 seconds
Platelets	150,000–450,000 mm³

is found in the liver and bile ducts, and high levels of this enzyme can indicate inflammation, injury, or blockage of the bile ducts, more commonly known as **cholestasis**. Alkaline phosphatase is an enzyme found in the bone, intestines, liver, and bile ducts and when elevated indicates a blockage of bile flow that can be caused by gallstones or scarring in the biliary tree.

Serum albumin measures the amount of protein that is made by the liver. A low serum albumin may be an indicator of liver damage and malnutrition. Bilirubin is a by-product of the breakdown of red blood cells that is filtered through the liver. There are two measurements of bilirubin, direct and indirect. Indirect bilirubin, or unconjugated bilirubin, measures the serum level of bilirubin before it gets to the liver. Once it is in the liver, it is changed (conjugated) to direct bilirubin while it binds to certain sugars. The direct bilirubin is then released into the bile and stored in the gallbladder. When the liver is unable to conjugate the bilirubin because of dysfunction, levels are elevated, and patients develop jaundice.

Lactate dehydrogenase (LDH) is a test for an enzyme that is produced by many organs in the blood as the result of tissue damage. It is not used solely to help determine liver disease but is a test used in conjunction with those listed previously to determine the presence and severity of liver dysfunction.

Medications

Approved therapeutic agents for use in patients with hepatitis include oral antiviral agents for viral suppression. Postexposure prophylaxis for hepatitis A exposure should be considered if the source of exposure was serologically confirmed or the source of exposure had infectious hepatitis A. Use of immune globulin is recommended if exposure to the source of hepatitis A was less than 2 weeks. The hepatitis A vaccine is also recommended.

Pegylated interferon injections also work toward viral suppression. Vaccination for hepatitis B is recommended for all children as well as adults in high-risk categories. Table 59.3 lists these medications with mechanism of action, side effects, and treatment response. Most oral agents used to treat hepatitis B are given daily for as long as 1 year or longer to slow or stop the growth of the virus. Injections of the interferons can be weekly or multiple times a week for 6 to 12 months. Patients undergoing medical treatment are followed serially over time to monitor liver function tests (LFTs) and treatment response.

Table 59.4 provides an overview of vaccines available for hepatitis A and B; there are no vaccines for the other types of hepatitis.

Diet and Activity

Diet recommendations for patients with hepatitis are similar to a healthy diet, low in fat and high in fruits, vegetables, and whole grains. Adequate oral intake is also important to ensure the hydration. Eating a low-fat diet decreases indigestion due to the liver's inability to process bile, which emulsifies dietary fat. If liver tissue is damaged, it is unable to store large amounts of glycogen for energy, and eating small, frequent meals helps the liver restore glycogen reserves. Small, frequent meals also provide nutrition in the anorexic patient with hepatitis who does not feel like eating. Patients should avoid alcohol and any medication that is toxic to the liver such as acetaminophen. Vitamin supplements of A, D, E, and K are also beneficial.

There is no recommended exercise program for patients with hepatitis and no specific exercise is restricted. Activities such as walking and resistance training, as well as low-impact aerobics help maintain strength and minimize fatigue. It is important for patients to maintain a good balance of proper rest and exercise. The patient should alternate periods of rest with low-level exercise, and as fatigue resolves, activity can be increased.

Connection Check 59.2

In reviewing diagnostic results of a patient with suspected hepatitis, the nurse correlates which result as consistent with hepatitis A?

A. Prolonged prothrombin time (PT)

B. Decreased white blood cell count

C. Presence of IgM anti-HAV

D. Detectable serum HBV DNA

Table 59.3 Approved Agents for Use in Patients With Hepatitis

	Approved Agent	Mechanism of Action	Side Effects	Treatment Response
Hepatitis A	None			
Hepatitis B	Oral agents: tenofovir, entecavir, lamivudine, telbivudine. All oral agents are given once a day for 1 year or longer.	Viral suppression and remission	Oral agents: limited side effects	Based on serial monitoring of liver enzymes
	Injections: Interferon-alpha: injection several times a week (6–12 months) Pegylated interferon: weekly injection (6–12 months)	Viral suppression	Injections: flulike symptoms, depression, headaches, fatigue, thyroid problems	
Hepatitis C	Pegylated interferons Ribavirin Combination therapy • peginterferon with ribavirin • interferon with ribavirin Interferon therapy lasts 12–8 months. Ribavirin therapy lasts 48 weeks	Viral suppression	Pegylated interferons: flu-like symptoms, depression, headaches, fatigue, thyroid problems	Serum test for presence of hepatitis C
	Harvoni (sofosbuvir + ledipasvir) is a polymerase inhibitor 8–12 weeks of treatment	Direct acting antiviral	Severe form of anemia Fatigue, headache, nausea, diarrhea, insomnia, weakness	

Table 59.4 Vaccines for Hepatitis

Hepatitis Vaccine	Description
Hepatitis A vaccine	Recommended for healthcare workers, restaurant workers, food handlers, persons traveling to areas with endemic hepatitis A, children and workers in child care, and those with risky behavior such as illegal injected drug users and persons with chronic liver disease. One injection followed by a booster dose 6–12 months later. Vaccine is considered effective for 15–20 years. Protection from the vaccine usually occurs 2–4 weeks after vaccination.
Hepatitis B vaccine	Recommended for everyone including newborns. Vaccine is given as a series of three injections over 6 to 12 months. Vaccine is considered effective for 15 years or longer.

Surgical Management

Liver Transplantation

Hepatitis C–related cirrhosis is the most common reason for liver transplantation. Currently, liver transplantation occurs primarily from a cadaver donor through a procedure known as an *orthotopic liver transplant*. In this procedure, the native diseased liver is removed, and a cadaver donor liver is transplanted in its place. A living donor liver transplant can occur, in which a lobe of the liver, usually the right lobe, is removed from a donor and transplanted to the recipient after the recipient's diseased liver has been removed. Patients undergoing these procedures require intense patient education, support, and long-term medical management.

The major complications after liver transplant are organ rejection and infection. Organ rejection typically presents between days 4 and 10 postoperatively and is characterized by fever, RUQ pain, tachycardia, changes in bile, and jaundice. To reduce the risk of rejection after liver transplantation, the patient is placed on immunosuppression medications such as cyclosporine and tacrolimus. These medications also increase the patient's risk of infection. In the first postoperative year, approximately 80% of patients develop at least one postoperative infection, and these infections are the primary reason for critical illness and death in patients after liver transplantation.

Nursing Management

Assessment and Analysis

Many of the clinical manifestations observed in the patient with hepatitis are directly associated with the inability of the liver to perform its normal functions because of inflammation. Common findings include:

- Elevated temperature associated with inflammation
- Elevated LFTs
- Jaundice
- Fatigue
- Decreased appetite

Nursing Diagnoses

- **Activity intolerance** associated with fatigue, fever, flu-like symptoms
- **Acute pain** associated with edema of liver
- **Altered nutrition (less than body requirements)** associated with decreased liver metabolic function secondary to loss of appetite, nausea, and vomiting
- **Altered thought processes** associated with elevated serum ammonia levels secondary to liver dysfunction
- **Knowledge deficit** associated with the disease process

Nursing Interventions

▪ Assessments

- Vital signs
  Elevation in temperature and pulse associated with infectious process
- Serum liver enzymes
  Elevated levels of liver enzymes indicate that liver injury is present and liver enzymes have entered the bloodstream.
- Serum bilirubin
  Bilirubin is a by-product of red blood cell breakdown, and the liver is responsible for removing bilirubin in the blood. Total bilirubin and direct, or conjugated, bilirubin levels are elevated because of inflammation and obstruction of the liver by hepatitis.
- Color of skin, sclera
  Yellow pigmentation of the eyes and skin occurs because of increased levels of bilirubin in the blood. Deep jaundice may result in a greenish tint to the skin due to by-products of bilirubin conversion.
- Nutritional intake
  Loss of appetite occurs because of abdominal fullness or the lack of desire to eat foods the patient previously enjoyed as a result of indigestion. This occurs frequently with fatty foods and alcohol.
- Daily weight
  Monitors nutritional intake and evaluates weight loss associated with decreased nutritional intake. Anorexia may develop secondary to abdominal distention and obstruction. An increase in body weight may be secondary to ascites.
- Intake and output
  Fluid volume status, either overload or depletion, may occur. Fluid overload is often associated with ascites that develops

secondary to damage to liver by the inflammatory and infectious processes seen with hepatitis.

- Signs of organ rejection in the patient after liver transplantation
  In patients who undergo transplantation for cirrhosis, organ rejection may occur within the first 10 days after the procedure and may include RUQ pain, changes in bile drainage, fever, tachycardia, and jaundice.

▪ Actions

- Administer medications as ordered (see Table 59.3)
  Administer medications as ordered for management of specific hepatitis type if indicated.
- Provide small, frequent meals and supplements (as needed)
  Because of decreased appetite and feelings of fullness, small, frequent meals and nutritional supplements are encouraged to promote adequate nutrition.
- Administer antiemetics
  Antiemetics decrease symptoms of nausea and vomiting associated with the virus, which may occur for a prolonged time. Use caution; some antiemetics (phenothiazines) are metabolized by the liver and should not be used.
- Promote balance between physical activity and rest
  Rest decreases metabolic demands on the liver
- Encourage rest periods between walking and physical activity
  Maintains strength and conditioning

▪ Teaching

- Nutritional teaching
  Importance of balanced nutrition to promote energy and small, frequent meals to increase nutritional intake while minimizing the negative effects of eating. Patients with clinical manifestations of hepatitis such as nausea and vomiting tend to limit food intake. It is important to stress calorie intake and proteins in moderate doses because the liver processes protein; vitamins and minerals with a balanced diet or supplements; limit fat intake because the liver may not be able to make enough bile to process fats. Small, frequent meals are indicated because the liver cannot store glycogen for energy because of inflammation. Hydration is important to manage symptoms including dizziness, fatigue, skin and mucous membrane dryness and side effects of any medications. Alcohol and caffeine should be avoided as they may cause dehydration.
- Good hand hygiene before and after meals and use of the bathroom to decrease transmission from fecal-oral route
  Practice good hand hygiene before and after eating and after using the toilet to decrease transmission from the fecal-oral route
- Avoid behaviors (needle sharing, unprotected sex) that contribute to transmission
  Avoiding behaviors that expose patients to the virus decreases transmission. Mode of transmission of the diagnosed form of hepatitis must be included in the discharge teaching.

- Importance of vaccinations to prevent hepatitis A and hepatitis B

  The hepatitis A vaccine can prevent hepatitis A. It is recommended for healthcare workers, food handlers, child-care workers, and travellers to endemic hepatitis A areas. It is a series of two injections (initial injection and booster 6–12 months later). The vaccine is effective for as long as 20 years. The hepatitis B vaccine can prevent hepatitis B and the serious consequences of HBV infection, including liver cancer and cirrhosis. The hepatitis B vaccine is usually given as a series of several injections. This vaccine series gives long-term protection from HBV infection. It is recommended for everyone.

- Safe public water supply, sewage

  Consider the water source and whether the public water supply is safe from sewage. Infected fecal matter can transmit hepatitis A.

Evaluating Care Outcomes

Hepatitis is a manageable disease process when patients have a clear understanding of the disease and are compliant with interventions and therapies. Expected outcomes include stable vital signs, stable weight, and comprehensive understanding of the risk factors, transmission, and treatment of hepatitis. Additional outcomes include decrease in liver function test values while the infection is resolving. Lifestyle activities that contribute to liver disease should be altered or eliminated to slow the progression of the disease. Knowledge of diet, nutritional intake, activity tolerance, and compliance with medical interventions are necessary. Patients require serial follow-up and monitoring of symptoms and should take a proactive role in their self-care.

CIRRHOSIS

Epidemiology

Cirrhosis, the end result of most chronic liver diseases, accounts for approximately 35,000 deaths annually in the United States and is the ninth leading cause of death. Between 1999 and 2016, annual deaths from cirrhosis increased by 65%, with the largest increases associated with alcoholic cirrhosis among people between the ages of 25 to 34. Most patients with cirrhosis die in their 50s and 60s because the liver has had many years of exposure to viruses, toxins, or medical conditions that have led to cirrhosis. Hepatitis C is the leading cause of chronic hepatitis and cirrhosis, followed by alcoholic liver disease.

Risk factors that predispose a patient to develop cirrhosis include chronic infection with hepatitis A, B, or C, followed by chronic alcoholism, biliary disease, accumulation of fat in the liver, and some autoimmune diseases. Improving health habits and refraining from risky behaviors such as needle sharing and unprotected sex, refraining from consumption of alcohol, and receiving vaccination for hepatitis are steps that can be taken to help prevent cirrhosis.

Cirrhosis of the liver is caused by several different factors including viruses, alcohol, biliary disease, accumulation of fat in the liver cells, genetic and autoimmune diseases, and other causes. The most common causes are chronic infections with hepatitis B and C viruses and alcohol use. Alcohol-induced cirrhosis (also known as **Laënnec's cirrhosis**) is now the second most common form of cirrhosis in the United States and results from chronic alcoholism and malnutrition. In this type of cirrhosis, fibrosis occurs around the central veins and portal areas. Patients may develop vascular or arterial spider angiomas on the abdomen. These numerous small vessels look like spider legs and are common with alcoholic cirrhosis. Some patients develop reddened palms known as *palmar edema* or liver palms.

Another cause of cirrhosis is postnecrotic or micronodular cirrhosis, which involves bands of scar tissue in the liver due to previous acute viral hepatitis or exposure to hepatotoxins. Biliary cirrhosis is defined by scarring of the liver tissue around the bile ducts and lobes of the liver because of chronic biliary obstruction and infection or **cholangitis** (inflammation of the common bile duct). Patients with biliary cirrhosis commonly develop severe itching, or pruritus, because of retention of bile salts. Other causes of cirrhosis include nonalcoholic steatohepatitis (NASH), which is commonly found in obese patients. This is caused by the accumulation of fat in the liver cells, which leads to inflammation of the liver cells and over time results in cirrhosis. Nonalcoholic steatohepatitis can be diagnosed by a liver biopsy.

Genetic causes of cirrhosis include Wilson's disease and **hemochromatosis** (iron overload). In Wilson's disease, there is an abnormality of a protein that causes excessive accumulation of copper in the liver leading to chronic inflammation. Similarly, in patients with hemochromatosis, there is an abnormally high accumulation of iron, which leads to chronic liver inflammation and cirrhosis. Treatment of these patients is aimed at decreasing levels of copper and iron, respectively.

An autoimmune diagnosis of cirrhosis is more common in women, caused by an abnormal immune system that causes progressive inflammation and dysfunction of the liver. Other causes of cirrhosis can be associated with exposure to hepatotoxins, medications, parasites, and cardiac dysfunction. Some patients with severe long-term right-sided heart failure develop what is known as *cardiac cirrhosis*, which causes decreased oxygenation of the liver cells, leading to liver cell death.

Pathophysiology

Cirrhosis of the liver (Fig. 59.2) is a chronic disease that causes cell destruction and fibrosis or scarring of hepatic tissues. Functional liver cells die, and damaged liver cells regenerate into nodules of liver cells that are surrounded by fibrous tissue. The blood supply to this area is abnormal and occurs through a thick capillary network surrounding

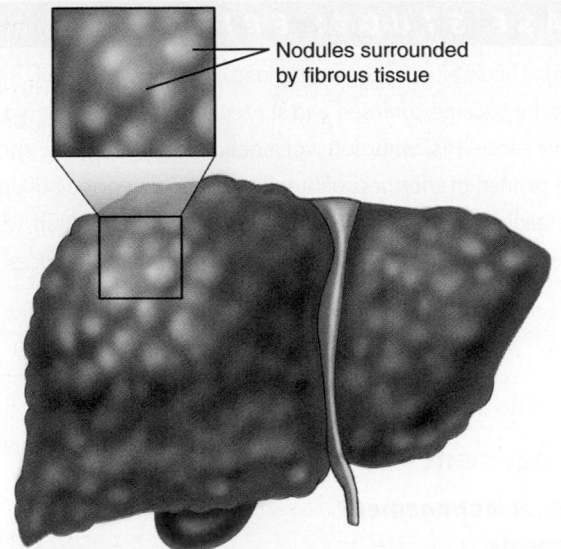

FIGURE 59.2 Cirrhosis. Cirrhosis causes cell destruction and fibrosis or scarring of hepatic tissues. Functional liver cells die, and damaged liver cells regenerate into nodules of liver cells that are surrounded by fibrous tissue.

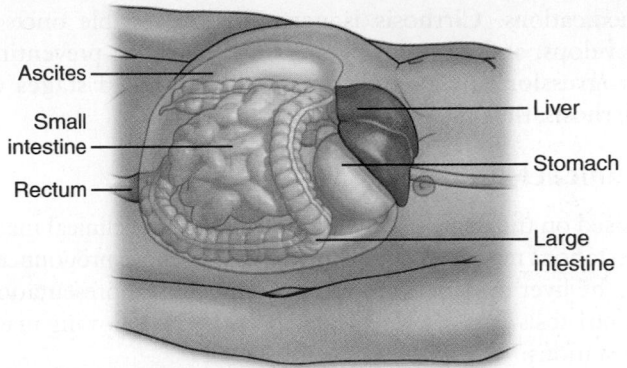

FIGURE 59.3 Ascites. Ascites is the accumulation of protein-rich fluid in the abdominal cavity, and if the accumulation of ascitic fluid is greater than 500 mL, the patient develops an increase in abdominal girth, abdominal pain, and bloating.

these nodules. In a normal healthy liver, approximately 85% of blood flow occurs through the portal vein in contrast to a cirrhotic liver, where blood flow is dependent on the hepatic artery. This irreversible chronic injury to functional liver cells results in liver cell necrosis, altered liver structure and function, and leads to alterations in blood and lymph flow, resulting in hepatic insufficiency and hypertension in the portal vein.

Alteration of blood flow to the liver results in **portal hypertension** (an increase in the pressure in the veins that carry blood through the liver) and shunting of blood around the liver, bypassing the liver cells. While the blood reaches the liver from the stomach, intestines, spleen, and pancreas, it travels through the portal vein branching into the liver. Because these vessels are blocked by the scarring of the liver, blood cannot flow freely and blood backs up, causing an increase in pressure that leads to the enlargement of the veins in the esophagus, skin of the abdomen, and veins in the rectum and anus (hemorrhoids). This shunting of blood around the liver causes increased pressure in the surrounding vessels resulting in **esophageal varices** and gastric varices (abnormally dilated and weak veins), which may result in upper GI bleeding.

Other pathophysiologic changes that develop secondary to altered blood flow include ascites, coagulopathy, and hepatic encephalopathy. Ascites is the accumulation of protein-rich fluid in the abdominal cavity (Fig. 59.3) and is associated with a poor quality of life, increased risk of infection, and a poor long-term outcome. Some patients with ascites develop pleural effusions because of the exchange of fluid across the diaphragm to the pleural space surrounding the lungs. Because the liver synthesizes most of the coagulation cascade factors and fibrinolytic proteins, liver disease impacts the synthesis of clotting factors and coagulation mechanisms, leading to prolonged or excessive bleeding. Patients with

significant liver disease are thrombocytopenic and have a prolonged PT. Some patients may exhibit significant bleeding, leading to **disseminated intravascular coagulation (DIC)**. In DIC, small blood clots form inside blood vessels, which in turn disrupt blood flow to organs and disrupt normal coagulation leading to excessive bleeding from the GI tract, pulmonary system, wounds, and any skin puncture sites such as IV sites.

Hepatic encephalopathy is characterized by numerous disturbances in the central nervous system, including changes in motor function, to changes in levels of consciousness ranging from restlessness and confusion to seizures and coma. Patients with hepatic encephalopathy can be staged (Table 59.5) based on the severity of their clinical presentation. The main cause of hepatic encephalopathy is the accumulation of ammonia and toxins in the blood that are normally detoxified by the liver. These accumulated toxins lead to altered neurological status. Other causes of encephalopathy include dehydration, excessive diuresis, infection, surgery, fever, and exposure to sedatives or antianxiety

Table 59.5 Stages of Hepatic Encephalopathy

Stage	Clinical Manifestations
1	Patients have slurred speech, tremors, lethargy and euphoria, reversal of day and night sleep patterns
	Asterixis, impaired writing, impaired decision making, poor coordination
2	Increased drowsiness, disorientation, inappropriate behavior, mood swings, agitation
	Asterixis, fetor hepaticus (sweet fecal smell of the breath)
3	Severe confusion, difficult to awaken, slurred speech
	Asterixis, increased deep tendon reflexes, rigid extremities
4	Coma, nonresponsive to painful stimulus

medications. Cirrhosis is generally irreversible once it develops, and treatment generally focuses on preventing progression and complications. In advanced stages of cirrhosis, the only option is a liver transplant.

Clinical Manifestations

Based on the degree of liver involvement, the clinical manifestations may vary and get progressively more pronounced as the liver dysfunction worsens. The clinical presentation of cirrhosis (Fig. 59.4) typically includes the following manifestations:

- Shortness of breath
- Jaundice
- Increased abdominal girth
- Abdominal pain and bloating
- Enlarged spleen
- Elevated liver enzymes
- Increased risk of bleeding
- Thrombocytopenia
- Prolonged PT
- Hemorrhoids
- Elevated serum ammonia levels
- Changes in level of consciousness
- Changes in motor function
- Hyponatremia
- **Asterixis** (flapping tremor of the hand when wrist extended)

CASE STUDY: EPISODE 2

Several hours after Mr. Green attended a cookout with family members, he became confused and started saying things that did not make sense. His confusion worsened the following day, and he complained of shortness of breath and had an episode of upper GI bleeding. He was admitted to the hospital for a work-up, which revealed high serum ammonia levels and esophageal varices…

Management

Medical Management

Diagnosis

Laboratory and diagnostic testing includes assessments that determine the extent of liver damage to guide diagnosis (Table 59.6). Diagnostic test results and a comprehensive physical examination are important to determine interventions.

There are several diagnostic studies that are performed to determine the severity of liver failure.

- *Diagnostic ultrasound and computed tomography (CT)* scans are noninvasive tests to determine abnormalities of the liver.

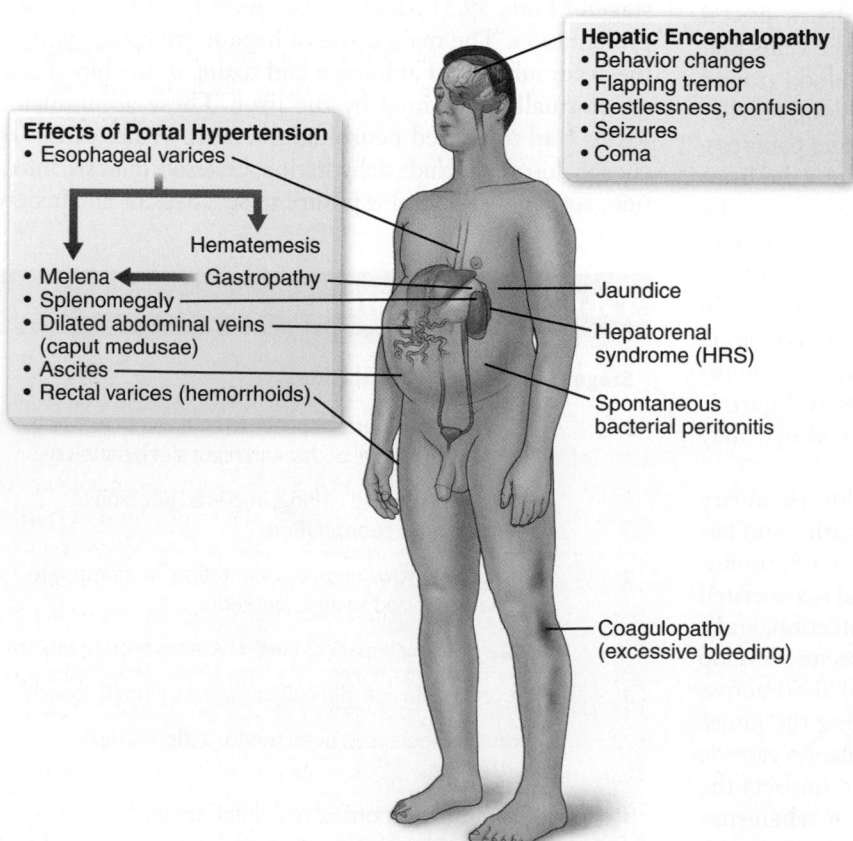

Hepatic Encephalopathy
- Behavior changes
- Flapping tremor
- Restlessness, confusion
- Seizures
- Coma

Effects of Portal Hypertension
- Esophageal varices
  - Hematemesis
- Melena ← Gastropathy
- Splenomegaly
- Dilated abdominal veins (caput medusae)
- Ascites
- Rectal varices (hemorrhoids)

Jaundice

Hepatorenal syndrome (HRS)

Spontaneous bacterial peritonitis

Coagulopathy (excessive bleeding)

FIGURE 59.4 Clinical presentation of cirrhosis.

Table 59.6 Abnormal Laboratory Values With Liver Disease		
Test		**Result**
ALT	Males: 13–40 units/L	Elevated
	Females: 24–36 units/L	
AST	Males: 20–40 units/L	Elevated
	Females: 15–35 units/L	
Alkaline phosphatase (Total)	Males: 35–142 units/L	Elevated
	Females: 25–125 units/L	
Alkaline phosphatase (Liver Fraction)	0–93 units/L	Elevated
Bilirubin, total	0.3–1 mg/dL	Elevated
Bilirubin, direct	0.1–0.3 mg/dL	Elevated
Albumin	3.4–5.1 g/dL	Decreased
Ammonia		Elevated
Coagulation tests		
• Prothrombin time	10–13 seconds	Prolonged
• Activated partial thromboplastin time (aPTT)	25–35 seconds	Prolonged
Platelets	150,000–450,000 mm³⁻	Decreased

ALT, Alanine transaminase; *AST,* aspartate transaminase.

- *Esophagogastroduodenoscopy (EGD)* is a minimally invasive procedure that uses an endoscope to visualize the GI tract from the esophagus to the duodenum to evaluate for esophageal varices or bleeding.
- *Percutaneous transhepatic portal angiography* is used to visualize the portal venous system and liver biopsy. Endoscopic retrograde cholangiopancreatography (ERCP) is a technique that combines endoscopy and fluoroscopy to visualize the biliary system to diagnose and treat causes of obstruction in the biliary tree.
- *Percutaneous transhepatic cholangiography* is a radiological test that uses a contrast medium injected into the bile duct of the liver to visualize the biliary tract and identify obstruction that, if identified, can be treated with the insertion of drains or stents.
- *Liver biopsy* is an invasive procedure done to collect a sample of liver tissue to determine the severity of liver disease (Fig. 59.5). This can be done percutaneously, transvenously, or directly in the operating room

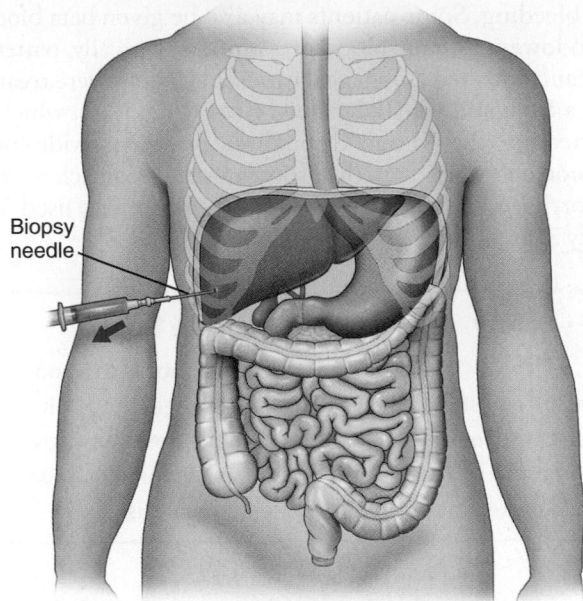

FIGURE 59.5 Liver biopsy. Liver biopsy is an invasive procedure done to collect a sample of liver tissue to determine the severity of liver disease.

through the abdomen. Patients who undergo liver biopsy are usually maintained on bedrest for several hours postprocedure, sometimes with a 5- to 10-lb sandbag over the biopsy site. Careful monitoring is required after the procedure associated with the risk of hypotension and bleeding (see Safety Alert).

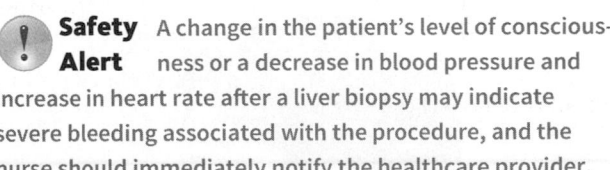

> **Safety Alert** A change in the patient's level of consciousness or a decrease in blood pressure and increase in heart rate after a liver biopsy may indicate severe bleeding associated with the procedure, and the nurse should immediately notify the healthcare provider.

Treatment

Ascites requires restriction of sodium intake to less than 2 g per day and administration of diuretics to increase salt and water excretion. Patients receive a combination of diuretics such as spironolactone and furosemide. In patients with end-stage liver disease, often secondary to cirrhosis, it is necessary to perform routine and frequent paracentesis for ascites that requires removal of several liters of fluid to relieve patient's clinical manifestations of abdominal bloating and pain and shortness of breath. With removal of fluid, the patient may develop hypotension requiring close monitoring

Treatment of portal hypertension involves symptom management and controlling complications of bleeding. Patients may undergo endoscopic procedures such as banding or **sclerotherapy** (a procedure used to shrink veins). Banding involves placing bands around the varices to block the bleeding, and sclerotherapy involves the injection of a solution into the bleeding varices to make them shrink to stop bleeding. Some patients may also be given beta blockers to lower systemic blood pressure. Historically, patients with uncontrolled esophageal variceal bleeding were treated with a **Sengstaken-Blakemore tube** (Fig. 59.6), which is inserted into the GI tract through the nose to provide compression and traction in the esophagus and stomach to stop hemorrhage. This modality of treatment is rarely used (see Safety Alert).

> **⚠ Safety Alert** **Sengstaken-Blakemore Tube**
> A Sengstaken-Blakemore tube is a temporary measure and should not be left in place longer than 24 hours. It can cause mucosal ulcerations, and the tube can migrate up out of the stomach and cause airway obstruction. Scissors should be kept at the bedside for emergency use.

Management of patients with hepatic encephalopathy includes avoiding protein overload, decreasing bacterial production of ammonia, and correcting fluid and electrolyte imbalances. Patients should eat small, frequent meals to prevent protein loading. To reduce the bacterial production of ammonia, patients usually receive neomycin and lactulose. Neomycin is a broad-spectrum antibiotic that destroys bacteria normally present in the GI tract, decreasing protein breakdown and production of ammonia. Lactulose promotes the excretion of ammonia in the stool and can be given

orally or via rectal enemas. These treatments can cause diarrhea and altered fluid and electrolytes; therefore, it is important to monitor fluid volume status and electrolyte values. Patients also receive vitamins A, B complex, C, and K, as well as folic acid to correct abnormalities.

Surgical Management

In some cases of cirrhosis, patients with ascites require surgical intervention that includes the placement of a shunt between the portal venous system and the systemic venous system to reduce portal pressure to reduce fluid accumulation. This type of shunt is known as a **transjugular intrahepatic portosystemic shunt** (TIPS) (Fig. 59.7). Cirrhosis is also an indication for liver transplantation (see Liver Transplantation).

Complications

In addition to complications associated with ascites, portal hypertension, coagulopathies, and hepatic encephalopathy, patients with cirrhosis are also at risk for hyponatremia, hepatorenal syndrome, and spontaneous bacterial peritonitis. The significant changes in liver function secondary to the pathophysiologic changes of cirrhosis often results in liver failure.

Hyponatremia (low serum sodium) is often seen in patients with advanced cirrhosis. This complication is associated with an impairment in the kidneys' ability to excrete free water, resulting in retention of water that is disproportionate to retention of sodium. On review of laboratory results, these

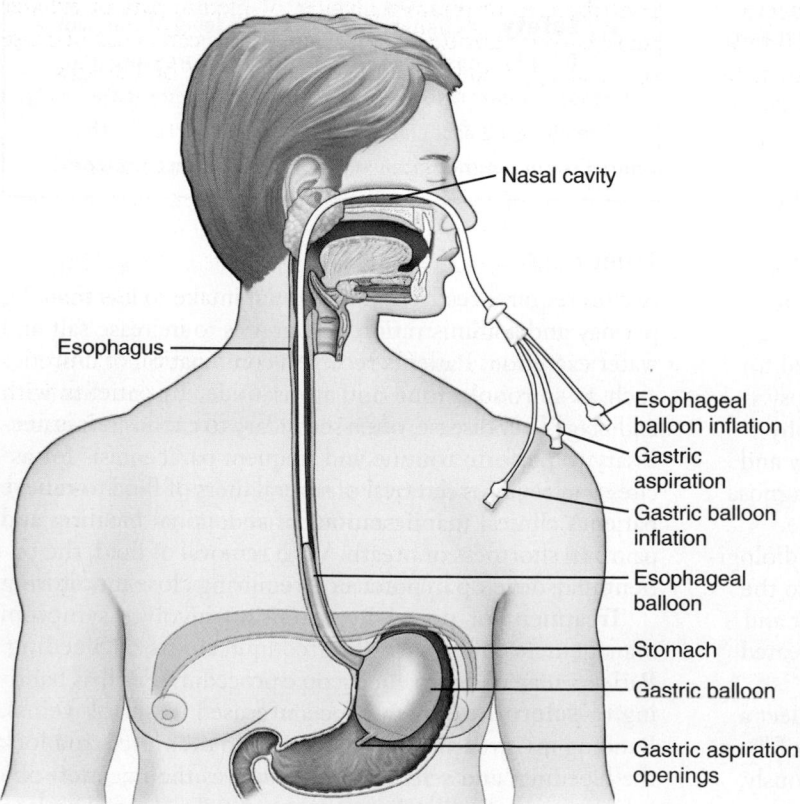

- Nasal cavity
- Esophagus
- Esophageal balloon inflation
- Gastric aspiration
- Gastric balloon inflation
- Esophageal balloon
- Stomach
- Gastric balloon
- Gastric aspiration openings

FIGURE 59.6 Sengstaken-Blakemore tube. A Sengstaken-Blakemore tube is inserted into the gastrointestinal tract through the nose to provide compression and traction in the esophagus and stomach to stop hemorrhage.

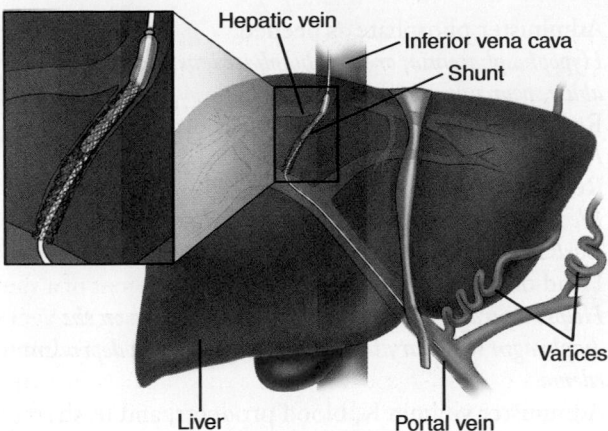

FIGURE 59.7 Transjugular intrahepatic portosystemic shunt (TIPS). The transjugular intrahepatic portosystemic shunt involves the placement of a shunt between the portal venous system and the systemic venous system to reduce ascites accumulation by decreasing portal pressure.

patients demonstrate hyponatremia and decreased serum osmolality.

Some patients with cirrhosis develop **hepatorenal syndrome (HRS)** which is characterized as rapid deterioration of kidney function as a result of altered blood flow to the kidneys. The mortality associated with HRS is high, and the only long-term treatment is liver transplantation. Patients with HRS may have normal urine output or oliguria, and the diagnosis is usually based on abnormal laboratory values such as elevated serum creatinine and blood urea nitrogen (BUN) levels.

Spontaneous bacterial peritonitis (SBP) is the development of peritonitis in the abdomen that can occur in patients with chronic cirrhosis, and clinical manifestations include fever, abdominal pain, encephalopathy, or acute hemodynamic decompensation. Diagnosis of SBP is confirmed with a diagnostic paracentesis (Fig. 59.8) and culture

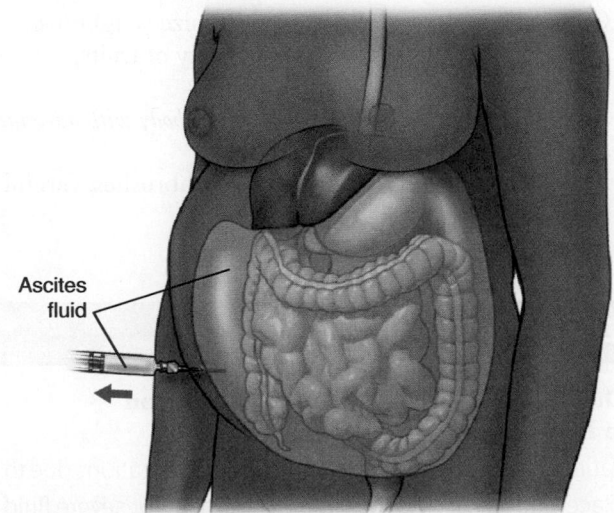

FIGURE 59.8 Paracentesis. Paracentesis is an invasive procedure done to remove fluid from the abdominal cavity to ease patient symptoms, as well as to collect samples for laboratory analysis.

of the ascitic fluid. Patients with SBP usually have cultures positive for *Escherichia coli* (43%), *Streptococcus* species (23%), or *Klebsiella pneumoniae* (11%). Patients are generally treated with a short course of antibiotic therapy; however, some patients are treated for prolonged periods of time prophylactically.

Nursing Management
Assessment and Analysis

Many of the clinical manifestations observed in the patient with cirrhosis are directly associated with the inability of the liver to perform its normal functions. Common findings include:

- Shortness of breath
- Decreased blood pressure
- Petechiae, bruising, and bleeding
- Altered mental status
- Asterixis
- Elevated liver enzymes
- Jaundice
- Dark amber urine
- Increased abdominal girth and bloating
- Decreased serum albumin levels
- Spider angiomas
- Palmar erythema
- Pruritus (secondary to accumulation of bile salts)

Other clinical manifestations associated with cirrhosis include acid-base disorders including respiratory alkalosis and metabolic alkalosis. Elevated serum ammonia levels, hyperventilation, and hypoxemia due to ascites or bacterial infection contribute to respiratory alkalosis while the patient exhales more carbon dioxide. Metabolic alkalosis can occur because of vomiting, fluid loss, diarrhea, and the use of diuretics.

Nursing Diagnoses

- **Fluid volume excess** associated with water and sodium retention secondary to decreased plasma protein (albumin)
- **Fluid volume deficit** associated with third spacing of peritoneal fluid (ascites), coagulation abnormalities, variceal bleed
- **Altered nutrition, less than body requirements**, associated with altered liver metabolism of nutrients, impaired absorption of fat-soluble vitamins, B vitamins, insufficient intake
- **Impaired skin integrity** associated with compromised nutrition, edema, decreased immune status, and accumulation of bile salts
- **Risk for injury: Bleeding** associated with coagulopathy

Nursing Interventions
Assessments

- Respiratory status, shortness of breath
  Adventitious breath sounds, decreased breath sounds, and increased respiration rate may indicate pulmonary fluid overload or inability to lower the diaphragm because of ascites.

- Vital signs
  Blood pressure may be elevated because of fluid volume excess, but blood pressure may be low because of fluid shift out of the vascular space secondary to decreased oncotic pressure due to low serum albumin.
- Peripheral edema secondary to fluid retention (see Evidence-Based Practice: Outpatient Treatment of Fluid Retention in Patients with Cirrhosis)
  Fluid shift into tissues associated with retention of sodium and water, decreased albumin
- Abdominal girth
  Increased girth due to accumulation of fluid (ascites) in the peritoneal cavity secondary to fluid shifts caused by loss of intravascular plasma proteins
- Bleeding gums, **ecchymosis** (bruising), and **epistaxis** (nosebleed), and **petechiae** (small, round spots on the skin as a result of bleeding)
  Complications of decreased clotting factors and vitamin K deficiency
- Skin, sclera, urine, and stool color;
  Signs of jaundice (yellowish skin and sclera) along with dark urine and clay-colored stools are associated with increased bilirubin levels due to the inability of the liver to produce bile or because bile flow is blocked.
- Mental status
  Signs of anxiety, behavioral or personality changes, lethargy, stupor, asterixis indicate hepatic encephalopathy secondary to elevated ammonia levels
- Intake and output
  Fluid status requires vigilant monitoring due to risk of fluid retention secondary to ascites, diarrhea, and potential blood loss.
- Daily weight
  Increased weight indicates fluid retention.
- Acid-base disorders
  Elevated serum ammonia levels, hyperventilation, and hypoxemia contribute to respiratory alkalosis. Metabolic alkalosis can occur because of vomiting and fluid loss, diarrhea, and the use of diuretics.
- Signs of organ rejection
  In patients who undergo transplantation for cirrhosis, organ rejection may occur within the first 10 days after the procedure and may include RUQ pain, changes in bile drainage, fever, tachycardia, and jaundice.

■ Actions

- Administer diuretics
  Diuretics help decrease fluid overload and edema.
- Administer electrolyte replacements such as potassium
  Maintain electrolytes within normal range. Potassium levels may be low associated with vomiting, diarrhea secondary to treatment for elevated ammonia levels, the use of diuretics, or low dietary intake of potassium-rich foods.
- Administer magnesium as needed
  Hypomagnesemia in patients with a history of alcohol abuse is a result of poor nutrition and diarrhea.

- Administer phosphate as needed
  Hypophosphatemia, or low phosphate levels, due to alcohol abuse, poor nutrition, use of diuretics
- Restrict sodium and fluid intake as ordered
  Prevents fluid accumulation and edema
- Restrict protein intake
  Elevated amounts of protein in the diet can raise ammonia levels and lead to hepatic encephalopathy.
- Head of bed elevation and leg elevation
  Helps respiratory status by decreasing pressure on the diaphragm secondary to ascites and minimizes dependent edema
- Administer vitamin K, blood products, and fresh frozen plasma as ordered
  Corrects coagulation disorders secondary to liver's inability to synthesize clotting factors
- Promote rest periods between activities; sit down while bathing, dressing
  Decreases metabolic demand on liver, decreases oxygen demand, and prevents fatigue

■ Teaching

- Overview of disease process and dietary restrictions (protein, sodium, fluid)
  Promotes knowledge of signs and symptoms of disease and promotes understanding of the importance of following dietary guidelines to prevent progression of the disease process
- Lifestyle changes:
  - No alcohol intake
    If alcohol is the cause of cirrhosis, remove alcohol from diet and refer to support groups
  - Educate about medications that are metabolized in the liver such as acetaminophen (Tylenol) and over-the-counter herbs and supplements
    These medications can cause further liver damage.
- Seek routine care for liver disease
  Encourage patient to be proactive in disease process and to monitor laboratory values and progression of disease.
- Consume adequate calories to minimize weight loss, eating a well-balanced diet with plenty of fruits, vegetables, and whole grains
  Helps prevent malnutrition and provides body with adequate energy
- Need for care with hygiene, soft toothbrushes, careful flossing, electric razors
  Minimize risk of bleeding

Evidence-Based Practice

Outpatient Treatment of Fluid Retention in Patients With Cirrhosis

Patients with cirrhosis often require hospitalizations due to exacerbations of fluid retention. Treatment for severe fluid retention in patients with cirrhosis is more cost-effective when performed in an outpatient setting, and it decreases preventable rehospitalizations. This literature review examined outpatient evidence-based interventions used in patients with cirrhosis with fluid retention and included 17 manuscripts (nine randomized controlled trials with a total of 1,694 patients, one meta-analysis that included five randomized controlled trials with 330 patients, and three cohort studies with 86 patients). There were also 2,115 articles from a systematic review and another 110 articles from a literature review. Six primary interventions that can be safely implemented in an outpatient setting were identified and include daily weights, sodium restrictions, diuretics, albumin infusions and paracentesis, placement of transjugular intrahepatic portosystemic shunt (TIPS), and telephone management. Because cirrhosis is a chronic disease, managing exacerbations of fluid retention in an outpatient setting decreases rehospitalizations and is more cost-effective than admission to an acute care facility.

White, A. (2014). Outpatient interventions for hepatology patients with fluid retention: A review and synthesis of the literature. *Gastroenterology Nursing, 37*(3), 236–244.

Evaluating Care Outcomes

Cirrhosis is a manageable disease process when patients have a good understanding of the disease and are compliant with interventions and therapies (see Evidence-Based Practice: Outpatient Treatment of Fluid Retention in Patients With Cirrhosis). Expected outcomes include stable vital signs, stable weight, decreased abdominal girth, and absence of bleeding tendencies. Lifestyle activities that contribute to liver disease need to be altered or eliminated to slow progression of the disease. Knowledge of diet, nutritional intake, activity tolerance, and compliance with medical interventions are necessary. Patients require routine follow-up and monitoring of symptoms and should take a proactive role in their self-care. If the disease progresses to end-stage symptoms and patients require hospitalization at the end of life, education and interventions associated with the need for intensive care unit (ICU) management, potential transplantation, and/or palliative care can be explored.

Connection Check 59.3

Elevated ammonia levels can lead to hepatic encephalopathy. Which provider order best reduces this risk in patients with cirrhosis?

A. Administer furosemide and spironolactone
B. Administer antibiotics
C. Restrict protein intake
D. Restrict caloric intake

Connection Check 59.4

In a patient with cirrhosis, the nursing diagnosis "Risk for injury and bleeding associated with prolonged clotting factors" is most appropriate associated with which disorder?

A. Pruritus
B. Vitamin K deficiency
C. Hyponatremia
D. Ascites

LIVER CANCER

Epidemiology

Worldwide, more than 700,000 people are diagnosed with liver cancer annually. Liver cancer is more common in sub-Saharan African countries and in Southeast Asia. In 2018, in the United States, it was estimated that more than 42,000 men and women will be diagnosed with liver and intrahepatic bile duct cancer, with more than 30,000 deaths. Patients may also develop liver cancer secondary to metastasis from other areas. The incidence of hepatocellular carcinoma (HCC) more than doubled between 1995 and 2015, with the increase among African Americans even higher. The mortality rate also increased to approximately 4.7 per 100,000 between 2010 and 2015.

Pathophysiology

Hepatocellular carcinoma is the most prevalent type of primary liver cancer, accounting for 85% to 90% of cases. Secondary liver cancer most often metastasizes from the colon, with more than half of patients diagnosed with colorectal cancer developing liver cancer. Risk factors for primary liver cancer include diseases that cause long-term inflammation of the liver including chronic infection with hepatitis B or C, or a several-year history of heavy alcohol drinking (defined as more than two alcoholic drinks a day for several years). Because of the inflammation, necrosis, fibrosis, and ongoing liver regeneration associated with chronic disease, cirrhotic changes occur and increase the risk of HCC development. Other risk factors include autoimmune disorders, hemochromatosis, obesity, a history of diabetes, or as a by-product of mold found in certain foods. Hemochromatosis is the excess build-up of iron in the body and can be a genetic disorder or a result of massive transfusions, chronic alcohol use, or hemolytic anemia. Obese patients tend to accumulate fat in the liver, which leads to chronic liver damage, inflammation, and nonalcoholic steatohepatitis (NASH). A by-product of the mold *Aspergillus flavus* found in peanuts, soy, rice, corn, and wheat stored in hot and humid environments can cause genetic mutations in the liver and has been associated with liver cancer in China and Africa. Liver cancer is usually fatal within 6 to 12 months of diagnosis, and for some patients the only cure is a liver transplant.

Clinical Manifestations

Liver cancer is often asymptomatic until the liver becomes enlarged or the patient demonstrates clinical manifestations of liver dysfunction. Because the tumor typically impairs normal functions of the liver, patients exhibit abdominal pain, weight loss, anorexia, weakness, fatigue, jaundice, and ascites. The prognosis for patients with primary liver cancer is poor because patients are usually asymptomatic and are not diagnosed until late in the disease process. If diagnosed early, aggressive surgery can be successful if the tumor is small and slow growing and the liver is otherwise healthy. However, in many patients, liver tumors may be undetected on physical examination because of the location of the liver in the abdomen.

Management

Medical Management

Diagnosis

Routine screening for liver cancer is indicated in high-risk patients, including those with cirrhosis, viral hepatitis, hemochromatosis, alpha-1-antitrypsin deficiency, and a history of chronic alcohol use. Cross-sectional imaging studies every 6 to 12 months are recommended in patients with cirrhosis, along with assessment of alpha-fetoprotein measurements. This aggressive screening has resulted in 30% to 50% increases in diagnosis of HCC as compared with those patients who are not screened. In patients with suspected metastasis to the liver, ultrasound and contrast CT scans of the liver are useful in identifying tumor growth. Full body scans may also be indicated if the site of the original cancer has not been determined. A liver biopsy may also be performed to determine the type and stage of the cancer.

Treatment

Some patients may undergo a combination of chemotherapy and radiation, but radiation alone is ineffective at slowing tumor growth. Selective internal radiation therapy is considered for patients with liver cancer that cannot be treated surgically and includes delivering radiation directly into the liver via a catheter placed in the hepatic artery by an interventional radiologist. Systemic chemotherapy may be used for liver cancer but is generally ineffective. Hepatic arterial infusion allows for a more direct, targeted approach to delivery of chemotherapeutic agents to the liver. This procedure involves placement of a catheter into the hepatic artery by an interventional radiologist. An advantage to this approach is fewer side effects as compared with systemic administration of chemotherapy. Transcatheter arterial chemoembolization is another treatment for liver cancer that involves cannulation by an interventional radiologist of the feeding artery of the tumor. High doses of chemotherapy are administered via the catheter, and then the artery is occluded with gel foam of coils to prevent systemic toxicity. Ablation procedures are also used with liver tumors, including radiofrequency ablation that uses energy waves to heat and kill tumor cells. Liver cancer is also treated with cryotherapy, which uses liquid nitrogen to freeze and kill tumor cells.

Surgical Management

Surgical options for treatment of cancer are dependent on the degree of normal liver function and whether it is a primary or secondary cancer; surgical options for metastatic disease are typically palliative for symptom relief of pain and distention. In patients with small, single liver tumors with normal liver function, a partial hepatectomy may be performed to remove the tumor. Liver transplantation may also be an option in patients with small, single primary liver cancer.

Connection Check 59.5

The nurse assesses for which clinical manifestations in the patient diagnosed with liver cancer? *(Select all that apply.)*

A. Periumbilical pain
B. Anorexia
C. Hemoptysis
D. Fatigue
E. Jaundice

Nursing Management

Assessment and Analysis

The clinical manifestations in patients with liver cancer are directly associated with the degree of liver dysfunction and include:

- Pain in the RUQ with extension to the back or shoulder
- Fluid accumulation in the peritoneal cavity (ascites)
- Anorexia
- Weakness
- Shortness of breath
- Jaundice of skin, sclera
- Elevated serum liver enzymes, bilirubin

Nursing Diagnoses

- **Pain** associated with pressure caused by the presence of the tumor
- **Activity intolerance** associated with fatigue and weakness
- **Risk for ineffective coping** associated with changes in health status and chronic disease

Nursing Interventions

■ *Assessments*

- Shortness of breath
  Fluid accumulation in the peritoneal cavity pushes up on the diaphragm and causes shortness of breath. Patients can experience hypoxia from intrapulmonary arteriovenous shunting and commonly develop pleural effusions.

- Vital signs
Increased respiratory rate and shortness of breath due to increased pressure on the diaphragm; elevated fever usually associated with infection
- Pain
Pain in the upper abdomen on the right side that may extend to the back or shoulder is associated with tumor size and location.
- Abdominal swelling and bloating
Ascites or protein-rich fluid accumulation in the peritoneal cavity occurs because of impaired sodium and water retention due to inflammation of the liver resulting in decreased production of plasma proteins (albumin) and to the presence of the tumor.
- Weakness and feelings of extreme tiredness
Associated with poor nutritional intake secondary to abdominal fullness and lack of appetite
- Weight loss
Decreased appetite causes poor nutritional intake.
- Appetite and feelings of fullness, nausea, and vomiting
Gastrointestinal symptoms can be associated with size of the tumor, accumulation of ascites, and compression on the stomach, leading to feelings of early satiety and decreased appetite
- Skin color and eyes
Jaundice develops, causing yellowish skin and scleral yellowing secondary to elevated bilirubin levels due to tumor obstructing bile ducts.
- Urine color
Increased serum bilirubin levels being filtered by the kidneys leads to dark, amber urine
- Abdominal girth measurements daily
Measure and document abdominal girth daily at the level of the umbilicus (standardized location) to determine fluid accumulation
- Liver enzymes and look for trends in laboratory values
All liver enzymes can be elevated because of abnormal functioning of the liver.

Actions

- Administer pain medications such as NSAIDs, narcotics via oral route, IV, subcutaneous, topical patches, or narcotic-coated lollipops
Provides symptomatic relief. The use of pain therapy is patient specific; some patients respond to nonsteroidal anti-inflammatory medications, whereas others require topical patches. Combinations of therapies may be indicated depending on the severity of the patient's symptoms.
- Nerve blocks
Nerve blocks may be used and are injected locally directly into the nerves of the abdomen to provide relief of pain.
- Administer antibiotics and antipyretics
Antibiotics may be used if the patient has an infection. Antipyretics are used to treat temperature elevations.

- Apply elastic wraps/bandages or support stockings to lower extremities and elevate the legs
These actions help prevent edema and promote venous return. Leg elevation increases venous return and prevents peripheral edema.
- Restrict fluid intake; sodium restriction and protein restriction
Fluid restriction helps prevent edema, sodium restriction prevents accumulation of salts, and sodium retention and protein restriction may prevent symptoms of encephalopathy.

Teaching

- Provide education on the importance of eating and maintaining an exercise regimen.
Proper diet and exercise teaching helps to maintain nutrition and strength and range of motion and conditioning. Importance of limited salt intake is particularly important.
- Provide patient education about procedures, diagnostic tests, interventions, or treatments (see Box 59.3)
Describe different treatment regimens to patients once ordered to help them understand the procedures.
- Teach patient about therapies used to control pain, alleviate symptoms for palliative therapy
Controls and relieves symptoms of pain and discomfort and improves quality of life

Evaluating Care Outcomes

The prognosis for patients with liver cancer depends on the age of the patient, the stage of the cancer, and whether or not it is primary or secondary liver cancer. Once a patient has been diagnosed, the course of treatment is determined for either cure if diagnosed early in the disease or treatment of symptoms. Surgical options may be curative or palliative to control pain due to tumors. Preventing complications of fluid retention and decreased nutritional intake are important care outcomes for these patients and their families.

Evidence-Based Practice

Liver Cancer

Studies of patients taking metformin for diabetes have shown a decreased risk of certain cancers. The impact of these studies has been scrutinized based on treatment duration, and patient factors. However, in 2018, results from a review of a national Veteran Health Administration database found a decreased incidence of liver cancer in patients receiving metformin compared with other solid tumors. Future clinical studies examining the possible protective effects of metformin should be conducted.

Murff, H.J., Roumie, C.L., Greevy, R.A., Hackstadt, A.J., McGowan, L.E.D., Hung, A.M., Grijalva, C.G. & Griffin, M.R. (2018). Metformin use and incidence cancer risk: evidence for a selective protective effect against liver cancer. *Cancer Causes & Control, 29*(8), 823–832.

Box 59.3 Complementary Therapy for Patients With Liver Cancer

Relaxation techniques: Listening to soft music, learning breathing techniques to breathe more slowly, or massage may help patients relax.

Acupuncture or acupressure: Based on traditional Chinese medicine, acupuncture involves the use of fine needles to specific points on the body to aid in healing and decrease pain. Acupressure uses touch pressure in the same manner without the use of needles.

LIVER TRAUMA

Epidemiology

The liver is the most vulnerable organ to trauma in the abdominal cavity because of its size, vascular structure, and location near the ribs. The right lobe of the liver is more susceptible to injury than the left lobe because of the proximity of the ribs. In trauma, injuries to the liver can include lacerations, contusions, hematomas, bile leaks, and bleeding.

In the United States, liver trauma is more common in males and accounts for approximately 15% to 20% of blunt abdominal injuries. The primary causes are associated with motor vehicle accidents or injuries associated with occupation, sports, or fighting. Blunt trauma accounts for approximately 70% of injuries and is usually associated with motor vehicle accidents. The steering column of a car can cause trauma to an entire lobe of the liver, the seat belt can cause liver trauma, and mountain bike accidents can cause severe hematomas. Other blunt injuries can be attributed to crush injuries, blast injuries, and direct-force blunt injury from a blow to the abdomen by a hard object such as a baseball bat. Penetrating injuries such as gunshot wounds, shrapnel, and stab wounds also cause trauma to the liver and are more prevalent in urban areas. Hemorrhage is the most common cause of death in patients with liver trauma.

One caveat about liver trauma is that the patient may have other injuries in addition to a liver injury. These include abdominal and retroperitoneal injuries (60%), thoracic injuries (18%), extremity injuries (12%), and head injuries (10%). Pelvic fractures, long bone fractures, and soft tissue injuries are also common. The mortality rate associated with concomitant injuries of the liver, abdomen, and head is approximately 70%.

Pathophysiology

The outcome of patients with liver injury is dependent on the mechanism of injury, the presentation of the patient on admission to the hospital, the patient's age, the severity of the injury, concomitant injuries, and shock state. Because of the vascularity of the liver, any type of trauma increases the risk of hemorrhage. Additionally, damage to the hepatocytes may lead to signs of liver dysfunction seen with other liver disorders.

Clinical Manifestations

Whether the patient sustains blunt or penetrating liver trauma, significant blood loss may occur, leading to severe hypotension despite fluid resuscitation. Clinical manifestations of shock may develop, including decreased blood pressure, tachycardia, tachypnea, decreased level of consciousness, pallor, and cool skin. Urine output may be decreased, and with associated trauma to the kidney or bladder, there may be frank blood in the urine. Patients may complain of RUQ pain and guarding and rebound tenderness of the abdomen may be observed. While blood and fluid accumulate in the abdominal cavity, there is dullness to percussion accompanied by abdominal distention and peritoneal irritation. Bowel sounds are most likely diminished, and the lack of sounds does not necessarily correlate with hemorrhage. If bowel sounds are heard in the chest cavity, this may indicate a diaphragmatic tear, and special attention is made to breathing patterns.

Management

Diagnosis

Historically, most liver injuries were treated surgically. However, evidence shows that almost 86% of liver injuries have stopped bleeding by the time surgical exploration is performed, and 67% of operations performed for blunt abdominal trauma are nontherapeutic. In general, as part of an abdominal trauma work-up, patients undergo an abdominal CT scan. This diagnostic intervention has reduced the incidence of exploratory surgery. In trauma situations, abdominal, chest, and cervical x-rays are also performed to rule out other injuries. Approximately 80% of adults and 97% of children are treated conservatively by using careful follow-up imaging studies. Other diagnostic tests indicated for patients with liver trauma include a complete blood count (CBC) to monitor for both blood loss and infection, coagulation profile, serum electrolytes, LFTs, and drug and alcohol screens. Because of the risk of hemorrhage, the patient is also typed and crossmatched for blood products.

Medical Management

Patients who present with a potential liver injury require fluid resuscitation, frequent monitoring of vital signs and complete blood count, and blood transfusions depending on the severity of bleeding. Conservative, nonsurgical management includes hemodynamic monitoring for shock, close observation for changes in the abdominal examination, increased pain, serial hemoglobin and hematocrit testing, and CT scans. Patients are initially on bed rest and then have activity restrictions for as long as 6 weeks with no strenuous activity and no contact sports. Liver function tests

(LFTs) are monitored over time and can be elevated initially in response to trauma to the liver.

Surgical Management

Operative management is used to control excessive bleeding or bile leaks. Operative procedures include suturing, cautery, removal of a damaged portion of the liver (hepatic resection) or packing around the liver. If packing is used to control bleeding, the patient may have to return to the operating room several times for packing removal and re-exploration of the wound.

Complications

Immediately after the injury, the risk of hemorrhagic or hypovolemic shock is high. Because patients with liver trauma often have concomitant injuries to the abdomen or other body systems, they are also at risk for other complications including atelectasis, pneumonia, abscess, fistulas, transfusion-related acute lung injury, peritonitis, and sepsis. Because of damage to the liver, the patients often have issues with albumin synthesis, blood coagulation, resistance to infection, and nutritional deficits. In rare cases, liver transplantation is utilized as salvage therapy with massive tissue destruction.

Nursing Management

Assessment and Analysis

Clinical manifestations observed in the patient with liver trauma are associated with the severity of the injury and blood loss. Common findings include:

- Increased respiratory rate
- Tachycardia
- Low blood pressure
- Abdominal pain and guarding due to the injury
- Low hematocrit and hemoglobin
- Tense, firm abdomen due to bleeding into the peritoneal cavity
- Elevated liver enzymes

Early assessment and intervention in patients with abdominal trauma lead to appropriate management and facilitate positive patient outcomes.

Nursing Diagnoses

- **Risk for fluid volume deficit** due to bleeding
- **Ineffective breathing pattern** associated with abdominal pain
- **Risk for infection** associated with products of liver metabolism entering the abdominal cavity leading to peritonitis

Nursing Interventions

▪ Assessments

- Monitor vital signs (VS) and clinical manifestations of shock
  Frequent measurement of VS determines hemodynamic status. Elevated pulse rate and decreased blood pressure may indicate bleeding or shock state because of the highly vascular

nature of the liver. Respirations may be elevated or altered because of pain.

- Abdominal guarding/tenderness and RUQ
  The RUQ is a common site of pain for trauma to the liver; worsening pain may indicate peritonitis. Peritonitis or inflammation can occur from tissue trauma and leakage of bile or blood into the abdominal cavity from trauma.
- Serial hemoglobin or hematocrit (H&H)
  Measures the extent of bleeding and blood loss and determines the need for fluid or blood replacement. Trending changes in H & H may indicate continuing internal hemorrhage
- Serum LFTs
  Alterations in LFTs may indicate the inability of the liver to function normally.
- Nausea and vomiting
  The nausea and vomiting occurs because of inflammation of the peritoneal cavity and may be an early, subtle sign of peritonitis.
- Abdominal girth
  Abdominal enlargement may be due to bleeding in the abdominal cavity.
- Urine output
  Decreased perfusion to the kidneys associated with hypovolemia results in decreased production and is a sign of decreased renal perfusion.

▪ Actions

- Fluid resuscitation as ordered
  Maintains hemodynamic stability and promotes organ perfusion
- Administer blood products as ordered
  Transfusion maintains adequate hemoglobin concentration. In the absence of typed and crossmatched blood, blood type O negative may be administered.
- Administer antibiotics as ordered
  Injuries to the liver may result in infectious processes in the peritoneal cavity (penetrating knife injuries or associated intestinal injury), and antibiotics are used to destroy the organisms.
- Activity restrictions
  Patients should have no strenuous activity for 6 weeks after injury, including no contact sports and no heavy lifting or straining to allow for healing.

▪ Teaching

- Educate patient about diagnostic studies such as CT scan
  Computed tomography scans identify the location of an injury, fluid collections, and bleeding; although CT is the preferred diagnostic test, some institutions may use ultrasound.
- Take prescribed vitamins and iron supplements
  Because the liver is a storage area for vitamins A, D, E, and K and iron, the patient with liver trauma requires supplementation with these vitamins and iron. Additionally, iron is needed for synthesis of hemoglobin.

- Importance of activity restrictions
  Recovery from liver trauma may take 6 to 8 weeks and strenuous activity should be avoided to allow the liver to heal.
- Patient education about abdominal signs and symptoms of increased pain, tenderness
  Some patients with liver trauma may develop future complications such as liver abscesses because of undiagnosed injury or a delay in the healing process.

Evaluating Care Outcomes

Liver trauma is a result of an injury to the liver via either blunt or penetrating trauma. It is important to serially monitor a patient with trauma to the abdomen for liver damage, which may not occur immediately after the traumatic event. Therefore, close abdominal assessments, serial hematocrit and hemoglobin levels, and frequent hemodynamic monitoring are important. The outcome of patients with liver injury is dependent on the mechanism and severity of injury, the presentation of the patient on admission to the hospital, age, and other injuries sustained at the time of the liver injury. Patients can recover well from injury with prompt intervention. It is important to monitor for concomitant complications such as atelectasis, pneumonia, and abscess formation.

Connection Check 59.6

Which statement by a patient diagnosed with liver trauma indicates understanding of the prescribed plan of care?
A. "I will need a liver transplant."
B. "I will need a blood transfusion."
C. "I am at increased risk for infection."
D. "I will never be able to drink alcohol again."

Making Connections

CASE STUDY: WRAP-UP

Mr. Green is admitted to the unit for further follow-up. On physical examination, he is responsive to questions and is oriented to person and time but not place and is mildly confused. His blood pressure is 91/43 mm Hg, and his heart rate is 100 bpm. He complains of slight shortness of breath with a respiratory rate of 24. His oxygen saturation is 94% on 2-L nasal cannula. He is afebrile. His abdomen is very large and distended, and the nurse notes the presence of veins throughout the abdomen. He complains that his clothes are too tight and that it is hard to lie flat on his back; he has to sit in a semi-upright position. His arms and legs are covered with scarring from his former

IV drug use. His pupils are reactive and equal, and his sclera are slightly yellow as is his skin. He states that his urine is very dark.

Diagnostic tests reveal:
- Chest x-ray indicates small bilateral pleural effusions
- Electrocardiogram reveals sinus tachycardia
- LFTs elevated greater than 4 times the normal range (AST = 220 IU/L; ALT = 185 IU/L)
- Bilirubin levels are twice the normal range (total bilirubin = 2.8 mg/dL; direct bilirubin = 1.0 mg/dL)
- Prolonged INR (international normalized ratio)
- Elevated serum ammonia levels
- Low albumin levels 3 g/dL

Mr. Green is diagnosed with liver failure.

Case Study Questions

1. What clinical manifestation does Mr. Green display that is consistent with a diagnosis of liver failure?
   A. Yellow sclera
   B. Arm and leg scars from IV drug abuse
   C. Tachycardia
   D. High blood pressure

2. Which clinical manifestation experienced by Mr. Green will be relieved by paracentesis?
   A. Jaundice
   B. Dyspnea
   C. Diarrhea
   D. Decreased urine output

3. Which order will the nurse anticipate for Mr. Green?
   A. Increase iron intake
   B. Strict bedrest
   C. Placement of an indwelling urinary catheter
   D. Restrict sodium to 2 g per day

4. Which information does the nurse include in teaching Mr. Green about his diagnosis of liver failure?
   A. "Avoid foods high in fat"
   B. "Avoid foods high in protein"
   C. "Need for oxygen when he is discharged"
   D. "Need for antihypertensive medications"

5. Based on Mr. Green's most recent clinical presentation, which finding is the priority that the nurse needs to communicate to the healthcare provider?
   A. Temperature
   B. Worsening mental status
   C. Inability to lie flat
   D. Blood pressure

CHAPTER SUMMARY

The liver serves several functions including blood storage, blood filtration, production of bile, synthesis of clotting factors (prothrombin and factors II, VII, IX, and X), and metabolism of carbohydrates, fat, and protein. The liver also serves to detoxify the blood and is a storage area for vitamins A, D, E, and K and iron. Hepatic dysfunction occurs when the liver is no longer able to perform its usual functions. Several conditions such as hepatitis, cirrhosis, liver trauma, and liver cancer all impair the ability of the liver to perform its routine functions.

Hepatitis is inflammation of liver cells most commonly caused by a virus that limits the ability of the liver to detoxify substances, limits the production of proteins and clotting factors, and alters the ability to store vitamins, fats, and sugars. Modes of transmission of viral hepatitis include contact with blood, blood products, semen, saliva, and mucous membranes; direct contact with infected fluids or objects; or through the fecal-oral route with contaminated water or food.

Patients with hepatitis can have a mild or severe illness, which can be acute or chronic. The viruses of hepatitis are classified according to letters ranging from A to G, each of which differs in its incubation period, mode of transmission, and other characteristics. The most common hepatitis viruses are hepatitis A, B, and C.

Cirrhosis of the liver is a chronic disease that causes cell destruction and fibrosis or scarring of hepatic tissues. Functional liver cells die, and damaged liver cells regenerate into nodules of liver cells, which are surrounded by fibrous tissue. This irreversible chronic injury to functional liver cells results in liver cell necrosis and altered liver structure and function, leading to alterations in blood and lymph flow, resulting in hepatic insufficiency and hypertension in the portal vein. Alteration of blood flow to the liver results in portal hypertension and shunting of blood around the liver that leads to increased pressure in the surrounding vessels and esophageal and gastric varices, which may result in upper GI bleeding. Cirrhosis is generally irreversible, and treatment generally focuses on preventing progression and complications. In advanced stages of cirrhosis, the only option is a liver transplant.

Liver cancer is classified as either primary or secondary. Primary liver cancer (hepatocellular carcinoma) originates from the liver, and secondary liver cancer originates from other areas of the body and metastasizes to the liver. Risk factors for primary liver cancer include diseases that cause long-term inflammation of the liver, including chronic infection with hepatitis B or C or a several-year history of heaving drinking (defined as more than two alcoholic drinks a day for several years). Other risk factors include autoimmune disorders, hemochromatosis, obesity, and a history of diabetes or as a by-product of mold found in certain foods. The prognosis for patients with liver cancer depends on the age of the patient, the stage of the cancer, and whether or not it is primary or secondary liver cancer. Once a patient has been diagnosed, the course of treatment is determined for either cure if diagnosed early in the disease or treatment of the symptoms if more advanced and considered incurable.

Liver trauma is a result of an injury to the liver via either blunt or penetrating trauma. The right lobe of the liver is more susceptible to injury than the left lobe because of its proximity to the ribs. In trauma, injuries to the liver can include lacerations, contusions, hematomas, bile leaks, and bleeding, and it is important to serially monitor a patient with trauma to the abdomen for liver damage, which may not occur immediately after the traumatic event. Close abdominal assessments, serial hemoglobin and hematocrit values, and frequent hemodynamic monitoring are important. Patients can recover well from injury with prompt intervention. It is important to monitor for concomitant complications such as atelectasis, pneumonia, and abscess formation.

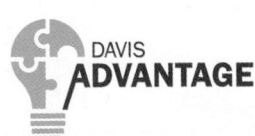

To explore learning resources for this chapter, go to **Davis Advantage** and find:
- Answers to in-text questions
- Chapter Resources and Activities
- NCLEX®-Style Chapter Review Questions
- Bibliography

Chapter 60

Coordinating Care for Patients With Biliary and Pancreatic Disorders

Sandy Swoboda

Content in this chapter is designed to support the learner in:

1. Describing the epidemiology of biliary and pancreatic disorders
2. Correlating clinical manifestations to pathophysiological processes of:
   a. Cholecystitis
   b. Acute pancreatitis
   c. Chronic pancreatitis
   d. Pancreatic cancer
3. Describing the diagnostic results used to confirm the diagnoses of biliary and pancreatic disorders
4. Discussing the medical management of:
   a. Cholecystitis
   b. Acute pancreatitis
   c. Chronic pancreatitis
   d. Pancreatic cancer
5. Developing a comprehensive plan of nursing care for patients with biliary and pancreatic disorders
6. Designing a plan of care that includes pharmacological, dietary, and lifestyle considerations for patients with biliary and pancreatic disorders

CONCEPTS

- Assessment
- Cellular Regulation
- Inflammation
- Medication
- Nutrition
- Safety

ESSENTIAL TERMS

Acalculous
Amylase
Autodigestion
Bile
Biliary
Calculous
Cholangiogram
Cholecystitis
Cholecystokinin
Choledocholithiasis
Cholelithiasis
Common bile duct
Cullen's sign
Endoscopic retrograde cholangiopancreatography (ERCP)
Gallstones
Gastrojejunostomy
Grey Turner's sign
Hepaticojejunostomy
Hepatobiliary iminodiacetic acid (HIDA) scan
Lipase
Lithotripsy
Murphy's sign
Necrosectomy
Pancreaticoduodenectomy
Pancreaticojejunostomy
Pleural effusion
Pseudocyst
Ranson's criteria
Sphincter of Oddi
Sphincterotomy
Steatorrhea
Trypsin
Vagotomy
Whipple procedure

Finding Connections

CASE STUDY: EPISODE 1

Follow this patient throughout the chapter.

Tony Edwards presents to the emergency department with severe, acute epigastric pain and nausea and vomiting. He describes the pain as sudden and radiating to the back. His heart rate is 110 bpm, blood pressure is 108/65 mm Hg, respiratory rate (RR) is 18, and temperature is 100.2°F (37.9°C). His abdomen is tender. Laboratory values include white blood cell count (WBC) $10.7 \times 10^3/mm^3$, blood urea nitrogen (BUN) 23 mg/dL, creatinine (Cr) 1.2 mg/dL, serum lipase level 250 U/L, amylase 3,500 U/L, alanine transaminase (ALT) 190 U/L, aspartate aminotransferase (AST) 150 U/L, total bilirubin 0.4 mg/dL, and albumin 3.3 g/dL. His sclerae are slightly yellow…

INTRODUCTION

The **biliary** system includes the gallbladder and bile ducts. The cystic duct (from the gallbladder) and the hepatic duct (from the liver) join to form the **common bile duct**. The primary purpose of the biliary system is to transport bile from the liver, where it is produced, to the gallbladder, where it is stored, and then to the duodenum, where it aids in the digestion of fats. **Bile** is a digestive enzyme that helps break down fats. Biliary disease occurs when the gallbladder or ducts become inflamed, infected, or cancerous, impairing the ability of the gallbladder to function normally. Several disorders, such as cholecystitis, pancreatitis, and pancreatic cancer, impair routine biliary functions.

CHOLECYSTITIS

Epidemiology

Cholecystitis is the inflammation of the gallbladder caused by an obstruction of bile flow and is classified as either **calculous** cholecystitis (presence of gallstones) or **acalculous** cholecystitis (without stones). **Gallstones** are hard deposits formed from bile contents that often cause obstruction of ducts in and around the gallbladder. Approximately 20 million people in the United States have gallstones, also known as **cholelithiasis**, and more than 500,000 cholecystectomies (removal of the gallbladder) are done annually. The incidence of gallstones and cholecystitis increases with age, and gallstones are more common in women than men and also more common in people of European descent than in people of African American descent. One approach to remembering signs and symptoms associated with gallstones is the five Fs (fair, fat, female, fertile, and over forty years of age). Risk factors for gallstones include obesity or rapid

weight loss, weight-loss surgery, eating large amounts of foods with saturated fats, pregnancy (because of elevated progesterone levels), genetics (members of the Pima and Chippewa tribes may have increased risk), and some medications (estrogen, octreotide, and cholesterol-lowering medications).

Pathophysiology

Gallstones are hard deposits that form in the gallbladder and are generally classified into three categories: cholesterol stones (the most common type), pigmented (formed from excess bilirubin), and mixed stones (combination of both types). Gallstones vary in size and can be very small like a pea or as large as a softball. Patients can have multiple stones or a single stone, and gallstones are most commonly found blocking the cystic duct or the common bile duct (Fig. 60.1). The medical term for gallstones in this location is **choledocholithiasis**.

Acalculous cholecystitis is associated with biliary stasis, where there is a slowing or stopping of the flow of bile either from decreased contractility of the gallbladder or spasms in the **sphincter of Oddi**. Because this sphincter controls the release of digestive enzymes into the duodenum, opening only in response to oral intake, when not working properly, it contributes to biliary stasis. The exact mechanism of acalculous cholecystitis is not well understood. Some believe the presence of endotoxin in sepsis can cause necrosis, hemorrhage, and ischemia to the gallbladder or that it inhibits the release of **cholecystokinin**, a peptide hormone activated when eating that causes the gallbladder to contract and release bile, leading to biliary stasis. Several causes of acalculous cholecystitis are found in Box 60.1.

Patients with noncomplicated cholecystitis related to gallstones recover within 1 to 4 days after onset of clinical manifestations, and the disease has only a 4% mortality rate. However, approximately 25% of patients with cholecystitis develop a complication, some requiring emergent surgery (12% of cases). Complications such as perforation or gangrene can lead to a critical illness and carry a mortality rate of up to 60%, usually due to sepsis.

Clinical Manifestations

The clinical presentation of acute cholecystitis ranges from no physical findings to pain and tenderness in the right upper quadrant (RUQ), sometimes with rebound tenderness or guarding, fever, and tachycardia. The pain associated with cholecystitis is due to the release of cholecystokinin, which causes the gallbladder to contract. Pain can be described as colicky pain, which is intermittent and radiating to the back, and this is related to the movement of the gallstones through the bile ducts as the bile flows. There are several small valves in the ducts, and the colicky pain is due to the movement of stones through these areas. Radiation to the back is related to the innervations of the gallbladder. Forty percent of patients have a palpable fullness in the RUQ, and

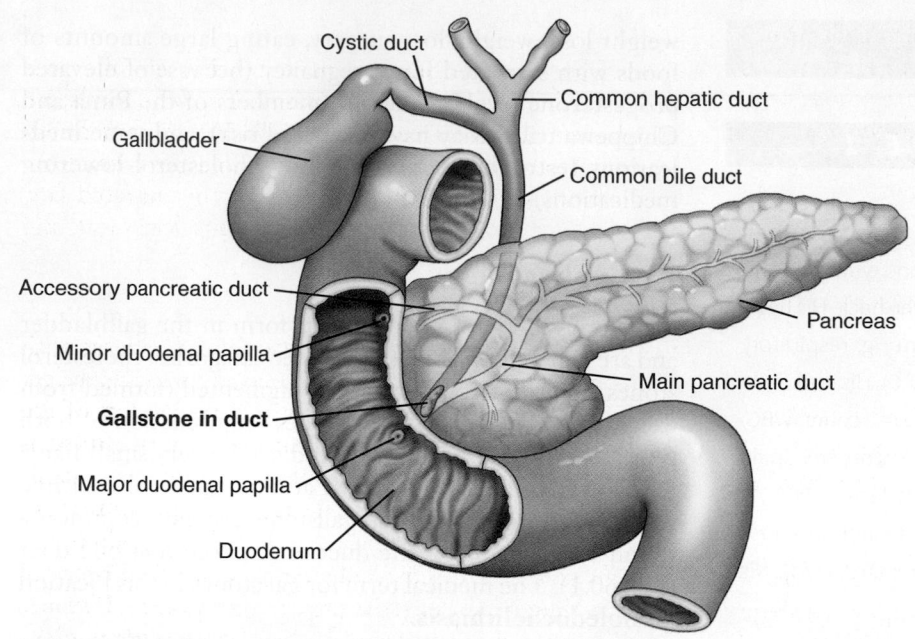

FIGURE 60.1 Gallstone in the common bile duct. Gallstones are most commonly found blocking the cystic duct or the common bile duct.

Box 60.1 Causes of Acalculous Cholecystitis

- Abdominal surgery
- Severe trauma
- Long-term IV nutrition (> 1 month)
- Prolonged fasting
- Sickle cell disease
- Diabetes mellitus
- Endotoxin
- AIDS
- *Salmonella* infection
- Cytomegalovirus

some patients exhibit a positive **Murphy's sign**, which is pain on palpation of the RUQ upon deep inspiration. To test for the presence of a positive Murphy's sign, the examiner's fingers are placed on the RUQ of the abdomen, and then the examiner gently presses down while asking the patient to take a deep breath. The test is positive if the patient has pain upon deep inspiration. Some patients with gallstones may be jaundiced because of the impaired bile flow. Sometimes, cholecystitis is difficult to diagnose because not all patients exhibit specific localized clinical manifestations, and the pain can be general. It is common for older adults and patients with diabetes to present with vague symptoms.

Management

Medical Management

Diagnosis

There are several different tests that are utilized to determine the presence of gallstones. It is also important for the nurse to be aware of patient allergies to iodine or radiopaque substances because these may be used for some of the procedures. This includes monitoring for allergic reaction to any diagnostic agent used. Diagnostic tests include:

- Abdominal x-ray is occasionally used to detect calcified gallstones
- Abdominal ultrasonography is a noninvasive test that is most commonly used to determine the presence of gallstones and acute cholecystitis. A thickened gallbladder is indicative of cholecystitis.
- Computed tomography (CT) visualizes the entire abdomen and can detect the presence of gallstones.
- The **hepatobiliary iminodiacetic acid (HIDA) scan** is a nuclear medicine scan that uses a radioactive tracer to study the production and flow of bile, visualizing the liver, gallbladder, bile ducts, and small intestine.
- **Endoscopic retrograde cholangiopancreatography (ERCP)** allows visualization of the common bile duct where gallstones can be removed. In patients with acalculous cholecystitis who are a high operative risk, a percutaneous drain can be placed. Patients who undergo ERCP should not eat or drink anything the night before the procedure but can take their cardiac and blood pressure medications the morning of the examination with a small amount of water. Patients are sedated for the test and need to have someone drive them home. After the ERCP, the patient goes to the postanesthesia care unit (PACU) to allow time for recovery from the sedation. It is important that the nurse observe the patient after the ERCP for a potential systemic inflammatory response syndrome (SIRS) caused by the manipulation of the bile ducts and potential bacterial translocation.
- Cholecystography is a rarely used diagnostic procedure that is a radiographic test of the gallbladder after the

patient orally takes radiopaque dye, which collects in the gallbladder and is excreted by the liver.

- **Cholangiogram** is commonly used in the operating room to image the biliary tree. A radiopaque dye, usually containing iodine, is injected intravenously, which outlines the bile ducts and gallstones.

Additional diagnostic studies used in the diagnosis of cholecystitis included a complete blood count and liver function tests. Significant findings associated with this diagnosis include:

- Elevated WBC due to inflammation
- Elevated liver enzymes, including AST, ALT, lactate dehydrogenase (LDH), and alkaline phosphatase (ALP), as well as bilirubin because of blockage of bile flow in the bile ducts

Treatment

Historically, extracorporeal shock wave therapy or **lithotripsy** was commonly used to dissolve gallstones. Patients would sit in a tub of water, and high-energy sound shock waves were directed through the water toward the stones to break them up into smaller pieces that would then pass through the bile duct. This treatment modality was used in conjunction with oral agents to help dissolve the gallstones. Lithotripsy is used for the treatment of small gallstones; however, the current preferred method of intervention for gallstones is laparoscopic surgery, which is one of the most common surgeries performed in the United States (see Surgical Management).

Medications

Treatment of a patient with acute cholecystitis includes nothing by mouth (NPO) status, IV hydration, correction of electrolyte and fluid imbalances, pain management, and IV antibiotics as indicated. The use of antibiotics in these patients is typically a short course with broad-spectrum medications. Patients are NPO to prevent the release of cholecystokinin, which is activated when eating and causes the gallbladder to contract and release bile, which leads to pain. Morphine is usually contraindicated for pain management because it can cause the sphincter of Oddi to spasm, which results in pain. Narcotics such as meperidine (Demerol) can be used for severe pain management. Acetaminophen or nonsteroidal medications such as ibuprofen or naproxen can also be used for pain management in patients with less severe pain.

In some cases, oral agents are used to dissolve the gallstones; these natural bile acids are provided to reduce the size and number of gallstones. Effective medications include ursodiol, Actigall, and chenodiol, which work best in small-sized stones that have a high cholesterol content. The drawback to some of these medications is that patients may need to take the medications for up to 2 years, which can be very expensive, and if the patient stops taking them, the stones usually reappear. Because treatment is prolonged, many patients are noncompliant with this therapy.

Diet

Several foods contribute to the formation of gallstones and should be avoided. Fatty foods such as fried foods, ice cream, dairy products, red meats, and heavy alcohol should be restricted because they promote gallstone formation. Patients are advised to choose foods low in saturated fats, including rice, potatoes, pasta, yogurt, fruits, lean meat, and whole grains.

Surgical Management

Several surgical options for the treatment of patients with cholecystitis are available, and the intervention is dependent on the presentation of the patient and the severity of the clinical manifestations. The standard surgical treatment is a laparoscopic cholecystectomy. If the patient has complications such as a perforated gallbladder or peritonitis, an open surgical procedure may be indicated. Open cholecystectomy may also be indicated if the patient has a history of previous abdominal surgeries or is morbidly obese. If stones are present in the common bile duct, surgeons may place a T-tube, or biliary drainage tube, into the common bile duct to monitor bile drainage. This tube exits the patient's abdomen through the skin and is connected to a closed drainage system. This tube may stay in place for up to 2 weeks after surgery. Bile output should not exceed 500 mL in the first 24 hours.

Laparoscopic cholecystectomy uses several small incisions (up to 1/2 in. long) in the abdominal cavity. Carbon dioxide gas is inserted to create space in the abdomen, and the surgical instruments and a laparoscope (a small thin telescope, camera, and surgical equipment) are placed through the incisions to remove the gallbladder. This procedure involves general anesthesia and can be done on an outpatient basis or may require the patient to stay in the hospital overnight.

During the immediate postoperative period, the patient recovers from anesthesia in the postanesthesia care unit (PACU), where the nurse monitors vital signs, pain, neurological status, nausea and vomiting, and the surgical site for distention, bleeding, or bruising. Once the patient is awake and following commands, clear liquids are given slowly in small amounts to prevent nausea and vomiting. After the first 12 hours of liquids and no nausea, vomiting, or abdominal cramping, patients can gradually introduce small amounts of solid foods and maintain a low-fat diet. Discharge instructions include incision care (keep Band-Aid or dressing on for first 24 hours and then remove), recognizing signs and symptoms of infection, signs of jaundice (yellow eyes or skin), pain medication instruction, constipation prevention, activity level (encourage walking and normal activity within a week, such as driving, working, and light lifting of less than 10 pounds), and no driving while taking narcotics. It is important to teach the patient that it is okay to take a shower after the first 48 hours and get the incision a little wet in the shower, but patients should not let the water pressure flow directly on the incision, which can increase chances of infection at the incision site. The patient should not soak in a tub, pool, or hot tub for up to 1 week. Pain after a laparoscopic cholecystectomy can occur at the incisions and sometimes in one or both of the shoulders because of irritation of the diaphragm from the carbon dioxide gas given during the surgery.

Postoperative care of the T-tube requires assessment of the characteristics of the drainage (color, consistency, and amount), routine emptying of the contents of the drainage bag, skin care, and routine flushing with appropriate preservative-free solution as ordered. Patient teaching includes information about care, biliary drainage, clinical manifestations of obstruction, color of urine and stool (if bile is being drained outside of the body), and infection.

Open cholecystectomy is the removal of the gallbladder through an open incision in the abdomen and is performed under general anesthesia. This was the most common means of removal of the gallbladder prior to the development of laparoscopy. This procedure is indicated for patients with previous abdominal surgeries because of scarring and adhesions, morbid obesity, or peritonitis. About 5% of laparoscopic procedures are converted to open procedures if there is an injury to a blood vessel, difficulty removing or visualizing the gallbladder, or other reasons as determined by the surgeon during the procedure.

Postoperative care after open cholecystectomy includes monitoring vital signs, pain, neurological status, and the abdomen for signs and symptoms of distention, bleeding, or bruising. Once the patient is passing flatus, clear liquids are introduced, and the diet is advanced to regular if the patient has no nausea or vomiting. Pain management via patient-controlled analgesia or as needed, pulmonary interventions to encourage lung expansion, coughing and deep breathing to prevent pneumonia and atelectasis, and walking are encouraged. Discharge teaching includes signs and symptoms of infection, prevention of constipation, low-fat diet, and activity levels. If a T-tube is present, routine care and teaching of T-tube management are necessary. The patient is typically in the hospital for several days after open cholecystectomy.

Nursing Management
Assessment and Analysis

The most common symptom of acute cholecystitis is abdominal pain. Pain can be described as colicky pain, which is intermittent and radiating to the back. Physical examination includes RUQ tenderness, fever, and elevated heart rate. Upon physical examination, the patient may have a positive Murphy's sign, and this is elicited during deep palpation of the abdomen. Pain occurs when the inflamed gallbladder touches the peritoneum during deep inspiration. When this test is performed, it is not unusual for patients to quickly hold their breath or stop breathing when they experience the pain from this test. Patients also have elevated liver enzymes, bilirubin, and WBC because of obstruction and inflammation.

Nursing Diagnoses

- **Acute pain** related to obstruction and edema related to gallstones
- **Fluid volume deficit** related to nausea, vomiting, and increased insensible fluid loss
- **Imbalanced nutrition, less than body requirements**, related to nausea and vomiting
- **Knowledge deficient** regarding condition, prognosis, treatment regimen, self-care, and discharge needs

Nursing Interventions

■ Assessments

- Vital signs
  Fever and tachycardia may represent inflammation due to gallstones. Elevated respiratory rate may occur because of anxiety and pain, the rate may be shallow and rapid because of pain, and blood pressure may be low as a result of dehydration/inflammatory response.
- Serum electrolytes
  These measure imbalanced electrolytes due to dehydration from nausea and vomiting and lack of oral intake and include BUN and creatinine (elevated). In the patient with nasogastric tube suctioning, the serum potassium should be monitored closely because this electrolyte is lost with nasogastric suctioning.
- Serum WBC
  Inflammation leads to an elevated WBC count.
- Liver enzymes, bilirubin
  Liver enzymes (AST, ALT, LDH, ALP) and bilirubin are elevated because of blockage of bile flow in the bile ducts.
- Skin turgor
  Decreased skin turgor indicates dehydration.
- Pain (onset, duration, exacerbating and relief factors)
  Pain can be intermittent and colicky. Pain can be severe epigastric and in the RUQ with radiation to the back, mid-shoulder/scapula, or in the chest. The onset is fast, commonly within 1 hour of eating a high-fat meal, and common at night.
- Abdominal assessment: distention, bowel sounds; Murphy's sign
  Palpation may reveal rebound tenderness, muscle guarding, or rigid abdominal muscles due to pain.
- Stool
  Steatorrhea (presence of excess fat in stool or oily stools), *clay-colored stools due to blockage of bile flow*
- Daily weight
  Provides information in regard to fluid gains or losses
- Intake and output
  Provide data about fluid volume status and prevent dehydration
- Nutritional intake
  Determines diet history, fat intake, foods that can contribute to symptoms

■ Actions

- Maintain NPO status.
  NPO status prevents gallbladder contraction that releases bile to break down nutrients; these contractions cause pain because of the inflamed gallbladder.

- Administer ordered antibiotics.
  A short course of antibiotics may be given to reduce inflammation and treat infection.
- Administer ordered bile acid reducers.
  Bile acid reducers help dissolve gallstones.
- Administer analgesics as ordered.
  Analgesics decrease the patient's symptoms of pain. Avoid morphine due to spasm of the sphincter of Oddi.
- Administer antiemetic as ordered.
  Antiemetics decrease symptoms of nausea and vomiting, which may occur for a prolonged time due to abdominal pain and obstruction.
- Promote bedrest in semi-Fowler's position.
  Avoid lying flat because this makes the pain worse, particularly with peritonitis, by stretching the abdominal muscles when supine. Repositioning helps alleviate abdominal pain and pressure.
- Nasogastric tube (NGT) to low suction (intermittent or continuous is ordered based on type of tube)
  An NGT is used to decompress the stomach and remove gastric secretions.

■ *Teaching*

- Postoperative instructions
  Discharge teaching includes signs and symptoms of infection, prevention of constipation, low-fat diet, and activity restrictions (encourage walking and normal activity within a week, such as driving, working, and light lifting of less than 10 pounds), and no driving while taking narcotics.
- T-tube management
  The patient needs to monitor the insertion site for inflammation and drainage. The T-tube bag should be emptied when one-half to two-thirds full to decrease the pull on the insertion site.
- The patient should avoid a diet high in saturated fats.
  Obtaining a diet history can help identify foods that contribute to symptoms. Bile breaks down fats; thus, a diet high in fat requires activation of bile for breakdown and increases pain. Stress small, frequent meals.
- Disease clinical manifestations, progression, diagnostic procedures, and interventions
  Patient education about the disease improves overall management and health. It is important that the patient recognize and report symptoms that may indicate relapse or complications, including pain, chills, fever, jaundice, dark urine, and light (clay-colored) stools.

Evaluating Care Outcomes

Cholecystitis is a manageable disease process. It is important to educate patients about this disease and its clinical manifestations and help them develop a plan for prevention. Timely and accurate diagnosis facilitates definitive treatment that focuses on pain management and medical and/or surgical management. Absence of pain and vital signs and fluid status within normal limits, as well as normalizing liver enzymes and WBC count are all indicators of recovery from this disease process.

Connection Check 60.1

The nurse recognizes which as risk factors for cholecystitis? *(Select all that apply.)*
A. Obesity
B. Male
C. Female
D. African American descent
E. European descent

Connection Check 60.2

The nurse correlates which clinical manifestation with cholecystitis?
A. Retroperitoneal pain
B. Absence of bowel sounds
C. Diarrhea
D. RUQ pain

ACUTE PANCREATITIS

Epidemiology

Pancreatitis is a disease characterized by inflammation of the pancreas and is classified as acute or chronic. In acute pancreatitis, patients usually present with life-threatening conditions that require hospitalization, frequently in the intensive care unit (ICU). Acute pancreatitis is an inflammation of the pancreas that can be mild to severe and affect people of all ages. Patients with a mild case of pancreatitis have no end-organ dysfunction and have a low mortality rate (<1%). Mild pancreatitis is self-limiting, and 85% of patients fully recover. Patients with severe acute pancreatitis may develop SIRS and end-organ dysfunction. Severe acute pancreatitis has a mortality rate of 15% to 30%. More frequent in males than females, acute pancreatitis occurs over all age spans, and the risk of pancreatitis is two to three times higher among African Americans than Caucasians. Chronic pancreatitis is defined as persistent inflammation that causes scarring and damage to the pancreas and surrounding tissue.

The most prevalent causes of acute pancreatitis are gallstones and alcohol. Alcohol consumption accounts for approximately one-third of all cases of pancreatitis and is more commonly found in men because of the increased frequency of heavy alcohol consumption in males. Gallstone pancreatitis is due to the presence of gallstones obstructing the bile duct or located near the area where the bile duct and pancreatic duct empty into the duodenum (Fig. 60.2), both causing alteration in the flow of bile and pancreatic enzymes and leading to inflammation of the pancreas. Gallstone pancreatitis is more common in women than men, and the incidence increases with every decade of life. Cannabis has recently been identified as a possible risk factor due to toxin release in a small number of reports. Other causes of pancreatitis are presented in Box 60.2.

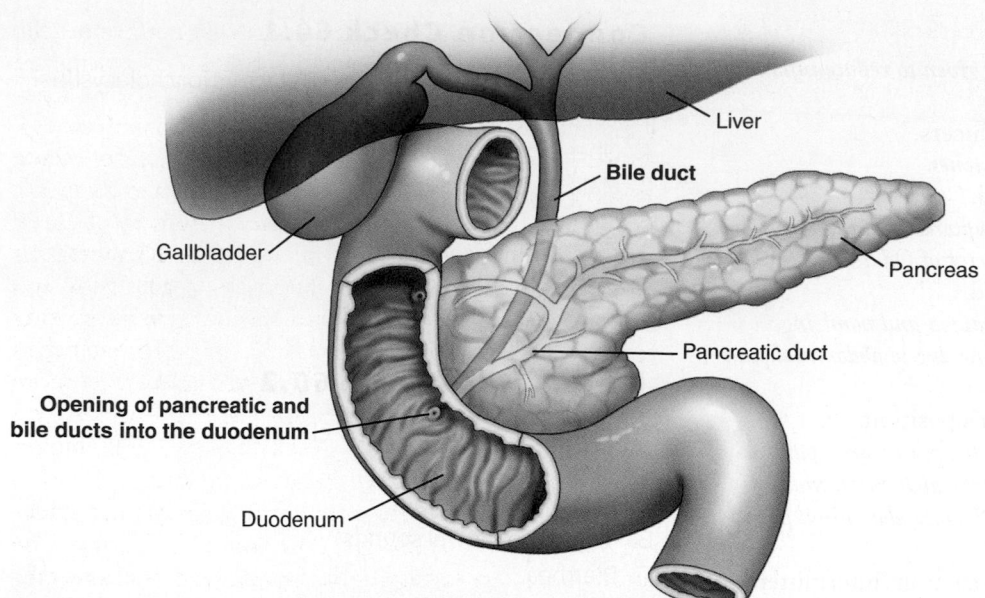

FIGURE 60.2 Diagram of pancreatic and bile duct openings. Gallstones obstruct the bile duct or the area near where the bile duct and pancreatic duct empty into the duodenum. They both cause alteration in the flow of bile and pancreatic enzymes, thus leading to inflammation of the pancreas.

Box 60.2 Causes of Acute Pancreatitis

- Alcohol
- Gallstones
- Trauma
- Medication reactions
- Hypertriglyceridemia
- Hypercalcemia
- Bile duct abnormalities or obstruction (tumor)
- Surgery
- Infectious organisms
- Parasites
- Spider bites
- Scorpion stings
- Idiopathic (unidentified cause)
- Pancreas divisum (congenital anomaly where pancreatic duct is divided into two parts)

Pathophysiology

Acute pancreatitis is the third-leading cause of gastrointestinal (GI) disorders that require hospitalization, and the cost of care in the United States for this disease and its complications is more than $2 billion annually. Acute pancreatitis is a reversible process involving inflammation of the pancreas secondary to the release of pancreatic enzymes that "autodigest" the pancreas, peripancreatic tissues, and adjacent areas. **Autodigestion** occurs when the pancreatic enzymes digest the pancreas and surrounding tissue. Acute pancreatitis may occur as an isolated event, or it may be recurrent. The exact mechanism of the release of the pancreatic enzymes is not well known, and pancreatitis has a variety of causes ranging in severity from mild to severe and life threatening.

Clinical Manifestations

Patients with acute pancreatitis present with sudden onset of epigastric pain that is felt in the upper left quadrant or mid-abdomen and can radiate to the back or shoulder blades. This pain is usually characterized as being deep and very sharp and becomes more intense within minutes of eating foods high in fat content. The pain can be constant and severe and last for several days, and some patients complain of severe pain when lying flat or bending forward. Pain can also be associated with nausea, vomiting, and anorexia. Patients with alcoholic pancreatitis may not have symptoms of pain for several hours or days after binge drinking. The general clinical presentation of patients with pancreatitis includes abdominal fullness from gas or bloating, hiccups, indigestion, fever, tachycardia, and hypotension.

Management

Medical Management

Diagnosis

Physical examination reveals a tender abdomen with localized guarding and rebound tenderness. The presence of **Cullen's sign** (periumbilical bruising) and **Grey Turner's sign** (flank bruising) are infrequent findings and indicate retroperitoneal hemorrhage. Grey Turner's and Cullen's signs usually take 24 to 48 hours to develop and can be a predictor of acute pancreatitis with pancreatic necrosis and retroperitoneal or intra-abdominal bleeding.

Laboratory tests used in the diagnosis of pancreatitis include a metabolic panel, hematology studies, and specific tests of pancreatic enzymes such as serum amylase and serum lipase. **Amylase** is an enzyme that aids in the digestion of carbohydrates, and **lipase** is an enzyme that aids in the digestion of fats. Patients can exhibit elevated BUN, AST, ALT, and WBC (Table 60.1). Elevated BUN indicates

Table 60.1 Common Laboratory Values Associated With Acute Pancreatitis

Serum Laboratory Test	Level	Rationale
Albumin	Decreased	Due to poor nutrition
Amylase	Rapid increase	Pancreatic enzyme
AST	Elevated	Common in bile flow obstruction
ALT	Elevated	Common with gallstone pancreatitis
Calcium	Decreased	Due to fat necrosis, hypoalbuminemia, and malnutrition, all common in alcoholic pancreatitis
Direct bilirubin	Elevated	Mostly seen with biliary obstruction
Lipase	Elevated	Pancreatic enzyme
WBC	Elevated	Due to inflammation

ALT, Alanine transaminase; *AST*, aspartate transaminase; *WBC*, white blood cell count.

impaired kidney function suggestive of hypovolemia or a hypercatabolic state. Monitoring elevations in BUN early in the course of the disease may provide an indicator of mortality from pancreatitis. Elevated AST indicates damage to liver cells, and elevated ALT is indicative of gallstone pancreatitis. Elevated serum lipase is the most specific test for pancreatitis because lipase is produced only by the pancreas. Patients with gallstone pancreatitis may have elevated serum bilirubin, serum amylase, and serum liver enzymes—AST, ALT, ALP, and LDH—related to gallstones obstructing bile flow. Elevated WBC counts are an indicator of inflammation.

Diagnostic imaging tests for pancreatitis include abdominal CT scans, abdominal magnetic resonance imaging (MRI), and abdominal ultrasound. The purpose of these diagnostic tests is to evaluate for the presence of an inflamed pancreas, gallstones, and bile duct obstruction or distention.

Connection Check 60.3

The most specific laboratory result in the patient with acute pancreatitis is an elevation in which laboratory value?

A. Serum bilirubin
B. Serum lipase
C. Serum trypsin
D. Serum lactase

There are several scoring systems to determine the severity of pancreatitis. Four such scoring mechanisms are the Ranson's criteria, the APACHE II score (Acute Physiology and Chronic Health Evaluation), the Balthazar CT severity index, and the Bedside Index Severity of Acute Pancreatitis (BISAP). Most commonly used is the **Ranson's criteria**, which are a means to measure the severity of illness and the likelihood of mortality in patients with pancreatitis (Table 60.2). The patient is evaluated upon admission and then again within the first 48 hours according to the scoring criteria. If at 48 hours the patient has a score of greater than or equal to 3, severe pancreatitis is likely, and with a score less than 3, severe pancreatitis is unlikely. The mortality rate associated with the score is found in Box 60.3. The higher the overall score, the higher the mortality rate.

The APACHE II score is an illness severity score calculated on the basis of the first 24 hours of ICU stay. The score is based on demographic factors (age, immunosuppression, chronic health status) and physiological factors (fever, mean arterial pressure, heart rate, oxygenation status, serum electrolytes [sodium, potassium, creatinine, hematocrit, and WBC count], and Glasgow Coma Scale score).

Computed tomography with contrast is the standard for the diagnosis of pancreatic necrosis or fluid collections around the pancreas and is used for scoring the severity of pancreatitis. The Balthazar index is calculated from the results of a CT scan and ranges from 0 to 10 on a point system given the extent of the inflammation of the pancreas and surrounding pancreatic tissue and the presence of pancreatic necrosis. The grading of the pancreas is given a letter grade of A through E, representing the range from normal pancreas to inflammatory changes to peripancreatic fluid collections. Necrosis of the pancreas is scored based on the percentage of the pancreas with necrosis with an overall higher percentage correlating with a higher severity of illness and poor outcome.

Table 60.2 Ranson's Criteria

At Admission	At 48 Hours
Age greater than 55 years	Hematocrit decrease greater than 10%
WBC greater than 16 10³/mm³	BUN increase greater than 5 mg/dL after fluid resuscitation
LDH greater than 350 IU/L	Calcium less than 8 mg/dL
AST greater than 250 IU/L	PaO₂ less than 60 mm Hg
Glucose greater than 200 mg/dL	Base deficit greater than 4 mg/dL
	Fluid sequestration greater than 6 L

AST, Aspartate transaminase; *BUN*, blood urea nitrogen; *LDH*, lactate dehydrogenase; *WBC*, white blood cell count.

> ### Box 60.3 Mortality Associated With Ranson's Score
>
> - Score 0–2: 2% mortality
> - Score 3–4: 15% mortality
> - Score 5–6: 40% mortality
> - Score 7–8: 100% mortality

The BISAP score is calculated based on several patient factors, including age, mental status, BUN, presence of pleural effusions, and SIRS criteria (points for fever range, respiratory status, WBC). A score of 0 to 2 indicates a mortality rate of less than 2%, and 3 to 5 points is associated with a mortality rate of greater than 15%.

Treatment

Specific interventions for the treatment of acute pancreatitis traditionally include NPO status to prevent the release of pancreatic enzymes responsible for autodigestion of the pancreas; however, evidence of early initiation of enteral feeding helps protect the gastrointestinal mucosal barrier. Patients are given IV hydration and pain medications. IV fluid administration includes several liters of fluid initially followed by a high rate of maintenance fluid at approximately 200 to 300 mL/hr continuously to maintain intravascular volume. Crystalloids, either normal saline or lactated Ringer's, are the most common fluids used, and some evidence suggests that a combination of crystalloids and colloids should be used. If the patient receives several liters of IV fluid, it is imperative to monitor the patient for clinical manifestations of overhydration that can lead to pulmonary edema. If the patient has severe acute pancreatitis with end-organ involvement (heart, lungs, kidneys), the patient needs to be managed in the ICU because of the potential for hypovolemic shock, pulmonary compromise, renal failure, and GI bleeding. Aggressive supportive therapy is crucial to the recovery of these patients because they may require medications to decrease inflammation and surgical procedures to resect areas of necrotic pancreas. In general, IV antibiotics are not given to patients with acute pancreatitis related to fever because the fevers are secondary to inflammation of the pancreas, not infection. If the patient has necrotic pancreatitis, IV antibiotics are indicated (explained later in this chapter). If pancreatitis is caused by gallstones, the patient generally undergoes a cholecystectomy.

The specific cause of pancreatitis (biliary obstruction, alcohol) also determines the medical management. Gallstone-induced pancreatitis leads to the removal of the gallbladder (cholecystectomy) for acute treatment and to prevent recurrence of pancreatitis. Laparoscopic cholecystectomy is performed if the patient is stable and inflammation has resolved. Endoscopic **sphincterotomy** to dislodge gallstones may alternatively be performed. In this procedure, an endoscope is placed into the ducts in the opposite direction of bile flow, and the sphincter or muscles of the bile and pancreatic ducts are cut to remove gallstones or blockages. This is usually done after an ERCP. If pancreatitis is alcohol induced, it is important to monitor and treat the patient for alcohol withdrawal, which includes agitation, hallucinations, tachycardia, fever, diaphoresis, and possible nausea and vomiting. Treatment may include sedation, hydration, and nutrition.

Medications

Medications used in the treatment of acute pancreatitis include opioid analgesics for pain, anticholinergics to decrease secretions, histamine blockers, pancreatic enzymes, and antibiotic therapy. Table 60.3 includes a list of common medications for patients with acute pancreatitis.

Prophylactic antibiotics for acute pancreatitis have been controversial for the last five decades. Several randomized controlled trials and retrospective studies have examined the practice of prophylactic antibiotics. Some studies have suggested that there is a lower incidence of peripancreatic infection with the use of antibiotics; however, the routine use of antibiotics as prophylaxis against infection in severe acute pancreatitis is not recommended. Because the mortality associated with acute pancreatitis is primarily due to infectious complications, the use of antibiotics for this disease has been common, but the evidence does not support routine antibiotic use because no difference in outcome was found between patients treated with antibiotics versus those who received a placebo. If antibiotics are utilized, it is important that the antibiotics chosen penetrate the pancreatic tissue to treat the infection.

Diet

Historically, patients with severe acute pancreatitis were managed with IV fluids and parenteral nutrition, avoiding the use of enteral nutrition in an effort to "rest" the inflamed

Table 60.3 Approved Agents for Acute Pancreatitis

Type of Agent	Rationale
Opioid narcotics: morphine sulfate	Treats pain
Anticholinergic agents	Decreases intestinal motility and decrease pancreatic enzyme release
Spasmolytics	Relaxes smooth muscle and relax sphincter of Oddi
H₂ (Histamine) antagonist or proton pump inhibitor	Decreases gastric acid secretions
Pancreatic enzymes	Aids in digestion of fats and proteins; taken with meals
Antibiotics	Treats acute necrotizing pancreatitis
Octreotide	Decreases secretion of enzymes

pancreas and prevent the release of pancreatic enzymes. New guidelines advocate for the initiation of early enteral feeding; however, the optimal timing and formulations require more study. Patients with mild forms of acute pancreatitis usually begin oral intake within a few days of their first onset of pain and do not require parenteral nutrition (see Evidence-Based Practice: Enteral Nutrition in Acute Pancreatitis).

Evidence-Based Practice

Enteral Nutrition in Acute Pancreatitis

Patients with acute pancreatitis often require supplemental nutrition during the acute phases of this disease. According to a meta-analysis that suggested that enteral nutrition was related to improved outcomes when compared with parenteral nutrition, a Cochrane Database review was conducted to compare different formulations of enteral nutrition, as well as the effectiveness of probiotics in the management of acute pancreatitis. The review yielded 15 trials that represented 1,376 participants. Although there were no conclusive findings related to different formulations of enteral nutrition or the use of probiotics in relation to outcomes, patients with acute pancreatitis who were treated with enteral nutrition as opposed to no nutritional support did demonstrate improved survival. Further studies are needed to examine differences in outcomes of different enteral nutrition formulations and the efficacy of probiotics.

Poropat, G., Giljaca, V., Hauser, G., & Atimac, D. (2015). Enteral nutrition formulations for acute pancreatitis. *Cochrane Database of Systematic Reviews, 3,* CD010605. doi:10.1002/14651858.CD010605.pub2

Complications

Necrotizing pancreatitis occurs in approximately 20% of all patients with acute pancreatitis and is associated with a high rate of complications and a high mortality rate of up to 50%. Necrotic pancreatitis may present 1 or more weeks after the initial onset of acute pancreatitis and is diagnosed by CT scan, which shows the presences of air and gas surrounding the pancreas. Necrotizing pancreatitis is caused by activation of pancreatic enzymes that basically "eat through" the tissue of the pancreas (like acid disintegrates nylon) and enter the peritoneal cavity and surrounding tissue, causing extensive peripancreatic tissue breakdown, inflammation, and hemorrhage from the rupture of surrounding blood vessels. Patients with necrotizing pancreatitis can develop sepsis, shock, and multiple-organ failure.

There are two types of pancreatic necrosis, sterile and infected. Sterile pancreatic necrosis describes areas of necrosis that are free of bacteria, and infected pancreatic necrosis relates to necrosis that is caused by bacteria. The

type of necrosis is determined through a needle biopsy and culture. Patients with necrotizing pancreatitis are treated medically on the basis of clinical presentation. Interventions may include drainage or surgical intervention that involves debridement of the necrotic tissue and infected debris via the step-up approach. If the culture is positive, the patient is treated with antibiotics. Common organisms include *Pseudomonas, Escherichia coli, Klebsiella, Enterococcus, Proteus, Staphylococcus aureus,* and *Candida* species.

Patients with necrotizing pancreatitis usually undergo a surgical procedure that can include pancreatic resection, open abdominal resection with open packing and serial debridements every 2 to 3 days, or **necrosectomy** (resection of necrotic tissue) with lavage or drainage. The currently recommended intervention for this is the step-up approach, which is a minimally invasive approach to the surgical management of this disease that involves percutaneous catheter drainage. This approach eliminates the need for necrosectomy in 35% to 50% of patients when compared with the traditional approach. More recently, an endoscopic step-up approach has been developed and demonstrates promising results (see Evidence-Based Practice: Endoscopic or Surgical Step-Up Approach to Necrotizing Pancreatitis).

Evidence-Based Practice

Endoscopic or Surgical Step-Up Approach to Necrotizing Pancreatitis

The surgical step-up approach to management of necrotizing pancreatitis has replaced open surgery over the last decade. In this multicenter, randomized trial, 418 patients were recruited to participate and were assigned to either the surgical or endoscopic step-up approach. The endoscopic approach involved ultrasound-guided transluminal drainage, followed by necrosectomy, as indicated. Although the endoscopic step-up approach did not demonstrate significant differences in reducing major complications or death, the rate of fistulas and length of hospital stay were lower in the endoscopy group. The findings from this study may result in a shift to the endoscopic approach as the preferred treatment.

Van Brunschot, S., Van Grinsen, J., Van Santvoort, H. C., Bakker, O. J., Besselink, M. G., Boermeester, M. A., ... Fockens, P. (2018). Endoscopic or surgical step-up approach for infected necrotising pancreatitis. *Lancet, 391,* 51–58.

Pancreatic hemorrhage is a rare complication that occurs in 1% to 3% of patients with acute pancreatitis as a result of pancreatic enzymes causing microrupture of the vascular system surrounding the pancreatic bed. Patients experience increased pain, decreased blood pressure, and elevated heart rate. Abdominal examinations may reveal Grey Turner's sign or Cullen's sign. If an active bleed is diagnosed, patients undergo embolization to stop the hemorrhage.

Pancreatic **pseudocysts** are encapsulated areas of fluid that contain pancreatic enzymes and pancreatic tissue. Pseudocysts usually form within 4 to 6 weeks after an episode of acute pancreatitis and can vary in size and number and usually resolve spontaneously over a period of several weeks. Some patients may require percutaneous drainage. If a pseudocyst becomes infected, it is known as a pancreatic abscess, and the patient requires either percutaneous drainage or necrosectomy (excision of necrotic tissue) to drain or debride the infected fluid collection and surrounding tissue. Patients with infected pseudocysts primarily present with chills, fever, nausea, vomiting, and abdominal pain. It is important to carefully monitor for complications such as rupture and impending shock.

The incidence of pleural effusion in patients with acute pancreatitis is about 20%. A **pleural effusion** is the abnormal accumulation of fluid between the layers of the pleura in the lung and can occur in pancreatitis because of impaired capillary permeability or inflammation. Pleural effusions are typically located in the left lung because of the proximity of the pancreas to the left hemidiaphragm but occasionally can be bilateral. Some patients with pleural effusion may complain of shortness of breath, hiccups, or pleuritic chest pain related to the presence of the pleural effusion. The effusions are filled with exudates (high protein and blood) and have high amylase levels (> 30 times normal) if tested.

Nursing Management

Assessment and Analysis

The classic presentation of acute pancreatitis is the sudden onset of acute unbearable abdominal pain. Other common clinical manifestations include:

- Elevated heart rate and respiratory rate, and low blood pressure
- Pain
- Elevated serum lipase, amylase, and glucose values
- Hypocalcemia
- Steatorrhea, clay-colored stools
- Hypovolemia
- Hypoxia
- Pleural effusion
- Clinical manifestations of Adult Respiratory Distress Syndrome (ARDS)
- Multiple organ dysfunction

Abnormal vital signs include tachycardia and hypotension due to intravascular volume depletion. Patients have elevated third-space volume loss due to capillary leak or loss of fluid into the interstitial space and out of the intravascular spaces. This volume loss requires IV fluid resuscitation. If this volume loss is not replenished, patients can develop shock and multiple organ dysfunction. Laboratory analysis shows elevated liver enzymes and bilirubin, along with elevated white blood count. Calcium levels are low because of the accumulation of fatty acids, which chelate calcium salts, causing soapy deposits in the abdomen. Stools are clay colored due to the blockage of bile into the duodenum.

Hypoxia occurs in patients with pancreatitis because of intrapulmonary shunting caused by the collapse of small alveoli in the dependent airways, whereby blood in the pulmonary system is not ventilated, and no gas exchange occurs. It is typical to see a patient with pancreatitis have a room air PaO_2 less than 75 mm Hg (normal PaO_2 is 80–95 mm Hg). Respiratory insufficiency can lead to acute respiratory distress syndrome (ARDS), a complication that leads to a mortality rate of more than 50%. ARDS is an acute lung injury caused by inflammation of the lungs, causing stiffness and the inability to exchange oxygen.

Nursing Diagnoses

- **Acute pain** related to inflammation, edema, and distention of the pancreas and surrounding tissue
- **Ineffective breathing pattern** related to pain, pulmonary infiltrates, pleural effusion, and atelectasis
- **Imbalanced nutrition, less than body requirements**, related to decreased food intake and increased metabolic demands

Nursing Interventions

■ *Assessments*

- Vital signs
  Fever and tachycardia may represent inflammation. An elevated respiratory rate may occur because of anxiety and pain, the rate may be shallow and rapid as a result of pain, and blood pressure may be low because of dehydration and fluid shifts secondary to the inflammatory response.
- Oxygen status
  The patient's PaO_2 may be decreased because of alveoli collapse and pleural effusion.
- Pain location, intensity, duration
  Pain located in the RUQ (head of pancreas) or LUQ (tail of pancreas) is related to autodigestion of the pancreas due to leaking of pancreatic enzymes into tissue surrounding the pancreas, leading to edema, distention of the pancreas, and peritoneal irritation. Localized pain may indicate pseudocyst or abscess formation.
- Abdominal assessment
  Palpation may reveal rebound tenderness, muscle guarding, or rigid abdominal muscles.
- Grey Turner's and/or Cullen's signs
  Grey Turner's sign is bruising noted on the flank due to leaking of exudate stained with blood into the flank area; Cullen's sign is bruising around the umbilicus. Bruising in these areas indicates hemorrhage, severe inflammation, and tissue damage.
- Serum lipase and amylase
  Elevated lipase and amylase are due to inflammation of the pancreas, which interrupts its normal structure and function. Serum lipase levels are a useful diagnostic

biomarker in pancreatitis because levels can remain elevated for up to 2 weeks. Elevated amylase levels that are three times normal are indicative of acute pancreatitis. These levels are elevated within 12 hours of the onset of inflammation, and elevation can last approximately 4 days.

- Serum glucose
  Glucose elevations due to the digestion of the pancreas, which leads to decreased production and availability of insulin
- Serum calcium, Trousseau sign, or Chvostek sign
  - *Hypocalcemia: assess for neuromuscular irritability when calcium levels are low because of the accumulation of fatty acids, which chelate calcium salts, causing soapy deposits in the abdomen.*
  - *Trousseau sign: hand spasms with inflation of the blood pressure cuff 20 mm Hg above the patient's systolic blood pressure (SBP) for 3 to 5 minutes. Under these ischemic conditions, the nerves become irritable, and spasms result.*
  - *Chvostek sign: facial twitching. Tapping the skin over the facial nerve anterior to the external auditory meatus produces Chvostek sign. In a patient with acute hypocalcemia, ipsilateral contraction of the facial muscles occurs.*
- Stool color
  Steatorrhea, clay-colored stools due to obstruction of bile flow
- Nutritional intake
  Patients exhibit loss of appetite because of pain; in alcoholic pancreatitis, patients may be malnourished at baseline.
- Daily weight, monitoring of fluid intake and output
  Daily weights and intake and output monitor fluid volume status and prevent dehydration. Hypovolemia (intravascular) occurs because of third-space losses in the retroperitoneum from autodigestion of the pancreas and capillary leak; these fluid shifts can impact weight, and with significant ascites formation, the weight increases as the fluid retention increases.

■ Actions

- Maintain NPO status.
  Maintaining NPO status decreases the secretion of digestive enzymes and prevents the contraction of the gallbladder and the release of cholecystokinin.
- NGT to low suction, as ordered
  Decompresses stomach, prevents abdominal distention
- Administer ordered medications.
  - Administer analgesics.
    Analgesics decrease the patient's symptoms of pain.
  - Administer antiemetics.
    Antiemetics decrease symptoms of nausea and vomiting, which may occur over a prolonged time.
  - Administer histamine blockers.
    Histamine blockers to decrease acid secretion and inhibit pancreatic enzyme activity

- Administer sedatives and anti-anxiety medications.
  Sedatives and antispasmodics help decrease spasms and subsequent enzyme secretions.
- Promote bedrest in semi-Fowler's position or fetal position.
  Bedrest decreases the stimulation of pancreatic secretions and resulting pain. The semi-Fowler's position relieves abdominal pressure and tension, and the fetal position is generally most comfortable.
- Encourage coughing and deep breathing.
  These help to prevent atelectasis and improve oxygenation. Patients commonly have pleural effusions.

■ Teaching

- Appropriate diet and intake of small, frequent meals and vitamin supplements
  A diet history can help identify foods that can contribute to symptoms. Oral intake should be limited initially to small amounts (fist-sized) and then slowly advanced as the pain subsides. Decreased pain is an indicator of decreased inflammation. Initial foods to eat after an illness with pancreatitis include carbohydrate-containing foods because they stimulate the pancreas less. Avoid fat- and protein-rich foods, which increase pancreatic enzyme stimulation.
- Abstain from alcohol.
  Alcohol consumption accounts for approximately one-third of all cases of pancreatitis.
- Abstain from smoking.
  Smoking is associated with pancreatic cancer and with interfering with the healing needed by the pancreas; smoking can adversely impact the healing process.
- Disease symptoms, progression, diagnostic procedures, and interventions
  Patient education about the disease improves overall management and health and provides details that the patient needs to report to the healthcare provider.

Evaluating Care Outcomes

Acute pancreatitis is a serious, often life-threatening disorder that requires vigilant nursing management. Because of the potential for sepsis and hypovolemia, monitoring of fluid and electrolytes, as well as complete blood count, is a priority for evaluating the effectiveness of the treatment plan. Pain management and nutritional status are also indicators of how the disease process is progressing. Positive outcomes of acute pancreatitis include stable vital signs, stable weight, serum electrolytes within normal limits, decreased pain, and decreases in liver enzymes.

Patients diagnosed with acute pancreatitis may be hospitalized for weeks and require transitional care (home care, skilled nursing facility, etc.) that focuses on reestablishing their weight and muscle mass, as well as understanding the disease process and lifestyle changes that may be required (abstaining from alcohol and smoking, dietary restrictions, etc.).

CASE STUDY: EPISODE 2

Tony Edwards has been in the hospital for 1 day and was transferred to the medical ICU this morning for worsening symptoms. On physical examination, he is restless and slightly combative. His blood pressure is 91/43 mm Hg, and his heart rate is 100 bpm. He is short of breath, with a respiratory rate of 24. His oxygen saturation is 85% on room air. His temperature is 38.5°C (101.3°F). His abdomen is distended, and he has severe pain. He screams that the staff members are trying to kill him by keeping him in the hospital, and all he wants to do is go back to his friend's house and continue to party. He states that he drinks a "ton of beer" whenever he feels like it and occasionally uses marijuana. His arms and legs are covered with tattoos and some scarring from his former IV drug use. His pupils are reactive and equal, and his sclera are slightly yellow, as is his skin. He states that his urine "looks like really dark iced tea." Tony is diagnosed with acute pancreatitis secondary to his alcoholic binge over the weekend…

CHRONIC PANCREATITIS

Epidemiology

The most common cause of chronic pancreatitis is heavy, prolonged alcohol use. Other causes are listed in Box 60.4. Chronic pancreatitis is commonly diagnosed between ages 30 and 40 and is more common in men than women. According to the National Institutes of Health, chronic pancreatitis is the seventh most commonly diagnosed digestive disease in the United States, with an annual cost of more than $3 billion. Alcohol-related pancreatitis is more common in men, whereas gallstones and autoimmune disorders are more common in women. The prevalence of chronic pancreatitis increases with age, with most patients diagnosed at around age 62. African Americans have a two- to three-times-higher risk of chronic pancreatitis when compared with Caucasians. One of the primary differences between acute and chronic pancreatitis is that the chronic form is not reversible, and over time, both the exocrine and endocrine functions of the pancreas are altered.

Pathophysiology

Chronic pancreatitis is inflammation of the pancreas that occurs when digestive enzymes autodigest the pancreas and surrounding tissues for a prolonged period of time. Because of inflammation and scarring, the pancreas is unable to make the digestive enzymes necessary for the digestion of proteins and fats or the hormones necessary to regulate glucose (insulin and glucagon). Fibrosis of the pancreas secondary to the chronic inflammation is associated with chronic pancreatitis and further contributes to the loss of normal pancreatic function.

Box 60.4 Causes of Chronic Pancreatitis

- Heavy alcohol use
- Hereditary disorders of the pancreas
- Cystic fibrosis
- Hypertriglyceridemia
- Hyperlipidemia
- Hypercalcemia

Clinical Manifestations

Patients with chronic pancreatitis have upper abdominal pain, which can spread to the back and feels worse after eating or drinking. Pain is often constant and prevents the patient from normal daily activities and is often described as recurring epigastric and LUQ pain. The pain is exacerbated by alcohol consumption and overeating. Other clinical manifestations include nausea, vomiting, weight loss, diarrhea, pale or clay-colored stools, and steatorrhea or oily stools. Patients may complain of losing weight despite normal eating patterns. Weight loss occurs because the pancreas is no longer secreting pancreatic enzymes to digest food, leading to decreased absorption of nutrients and malnourishment.

Management

Medical Management

Diagnosis

The diagnostic work-up of chronic pancreatitis includes abdominal CT, ultrasound, or ERCP to visualize the pancreas, as well as to verify structural or obstructive changes. Other diagnostic tests include laboratory analysis of amylase and lipase levels, which are usually elevated, as well as elevations of serum alkaline phosphatase and bilirubin that are associated with chronic pancreatitis secondary to obstructive processes. As the disease progresses and impairs endocrine functions of the pancreas, serum glucose levels are monitored because increased levels are associated with chronic pancreatitis due to the lack of insulin.

Treatment

Treatment of patients with chronic pancreatitis includes pain management, IV fluid replacement, electrolyte management, nutritional support, and insulin therapy to treat elevated blood glucose levels. Pancreatic enzyme replacement therapy (PERT) is used to treat the malnutrition and malabsorption associated with chronic pancreatitis and provides amylase, lipase, and protease. In many cases, patients with chronic pancreatitis are cared for in the ICU, and GI prophylaxis with histamine blockers or proton pump inhibitors may be prescribed secondary to increased gastric acid secretion. In patients with significant weight loss secondary to this disorder, total parenteral nutrition may be required.

Heavy tobacco use and alcohol consumption are associated with chronic pancreatitis; therefore, patient education includes modification of these risk factors.

Surgical Management

In some patients, surgical resection may provide symptomatic relief of pain; however, surgical intervention is not always appropriate for patients with chronic pancreatitis, and the risks are high (see Evidence-Based Practice: Comparison of Endoscopy and Surgical Approach in the Treatment of Obstructive Chronic Pancreatitis). Surgical procedures for pain relief include the Puestow procedure, which opens the pancreatic ducts and redirects the flow of pancreatic enzymes into the intestine, or resection of the head of the pancreas. Laparoscopic draining may be indicated in patients with abscesses or pseudocysts. Because of the irreversible nature of chronic pancreatitis, these surgical procedures address issues related to pain, inflammation, and obstruction and are not curative.

Evidence-Based Practice

Comparison of Endoscopy and Surgical Approach in the Treatment of Obstructive Chronic Pancreatitis

Patients with chronic pancreatitis often require treatment for the pain caused by obstructions in the pancreas secondary to structural changes and damage to the pancreas. Both endoscopy and surgical interventions have been used to treat the pain. To assess for differences in treatment modalities, a Cochrane Database review was completed. Three trials were identified, two of which compared endoscopy with surgical intervention and included 111 participants and another trial with 32 participants that compared surgical intervention with conservative therapy. Patients who underwent surgical intervention had better pain relief, improved quality of life, and preservation of exocrine function when compared with endoscopy. Additionally, surgical patients demonstrated better pain relief and pancreatic function when compared with patients receiving conservative therapy. Because of the low numbers of participants, additional trials need to be conducted to further compare surgical interventions with both endoscopy and conservative therapy in patients with painful obstructive chronic pancreatitis.

Ahmed, A. U., Pahlplatz, J. M., Nealon, W. H., van Goor, H., Gooszen, H. G., & Boermeester, M. A. (2015). Endoscopic or surgical intervention for painful obstructive chronic pancreatitis. *Cochrane Database of Systematic Reviews, 3*, CD007884. doi:10.1002/14651858.CD007884.pub3

Nursing Management

Assessment and Analysis

Chronic pancreatitis is characterized by pain and weight loss and is an irreversible disease process. In addition to constant, burning pain that is characterized by exacerbations of intense, unrelenting pain, other clinical manifestations include:

- Anorexia
- Nausea and vomiting
- Constipation
- Flatulence
- Steatorrhea (fatty stools)
- Elevated amylase, lipase, serum bilirubin, and alkaline phosphatase
- Elevated blood glucose levels

Nursing Diagnoses

- **Acute pain** related to inflammation and obstruction of the pancreas
- **Imbalanced nutrition, less than body requirements**, due to malabsorption and altered secretion of pancreatic enzymes
- **Hopelessness** related to the chronic, progressive, irreversible nature of chronic pancreatitis

Nursing Interventions

▪ Assessments

- Vital signs
  Pulse rate, respiratory rate, and blood pressure elevations are associated with episodes of pain exacerbations.
- Serum blood glucose levels
  With decreased insulin production/release with endocrine dysfunction, serum glucose levels are elevated.
- Amylase and lipase levels
  Elevations of these pancreatic enzymes are associated with chronic pancreatitis.
- Serum bilirubin and alkaline phosphatase
  Obstruction of the bile ducts leads to increases of both bilirubin and alkaline phosphatase.
- Weight
  Because of malabsorption secondary to the altered secretion of pancreatic enzymes, the patient with chronic pancreatitis is at risk of weight loss.
- Pain
  Chronic pancreatitis is characterized by persistent, recurring episodes of epigastric and LUQ pain secondary to inflammation and obstruction.
- Abdomen
  Tenderness of the abdomen may be observed. Palpation may reveal a mass in the LUQ that may indicate a pseudocyst or abscess.
- Skin color
  Jaundice may be observed with obstruction of the bile ducts.
- Stool
  Steatorrhea may develop with progressive pancreatic insufficiency, as well as clay-colored stools with bile obstruction.

■ *Actions*

- Administer pancreatic enzymes (PERT).
  These medications contain amylase, lipase, and protease to enhance the absorption of nutrients.
- Provide GI prophylaxis as ordered.
  Histamine blockers or proton pump inhibitors may be prescribed to treat the increased gastric acid secretion associated with chronic pancreatitis.
- Provide rest and a calm environment.
  These interventions decrease strain on the already-diseased pancreas and may decrease the secretion of acids in the stomach, which can exacerbate chronic pancreatitis.
- Implement pain-relief measures.
  Pain may be managed with the administration of opioids initially and then with nonopioids when the pain is less intense.
- Collaborate with a dietitian to ensure adequate nutrition.
  The patient may require increased caloric intake or parenteral nutrition as a result of alterations in absorption. A low-fat diet is often prescribed because of difficulty breaking down fats, resulting in steatorrhea.

■ *Teaching*

- Avoid alcohol.
  Alcohol further exacerbates the dysfunction of the pancreas.
- Do not chew pancreatic enzymes.
  These medications are available as extended-release or enteric-coated formulations, so they need to be swallowed whole to receive a therapeutic dose.
- Limit fat in the diet.
  Malabsorption of fat is associated with chronic pancreatitis, and fat is limited in the diet, particularly in patients with steatorrhea.
- Avoid intake of irritating foods/beverages (coffee, caffeine).
  This may increase gastric distress.
- Referral to support groups such as Alcoholics Anonymous or Al-Anon
  Chronic pancreatitis is a progressive, irreversible disease, and avoiding the use of alcohol minimizes further damage to the pancreas. Additionally, participation in support groups may be therapeutic and may provide suggestions and recommendations for dealing with this chronic disorder.

Evaluating Care Outcomes

Chronic pancreatitis is a progressive, irreversible disease that results in pain, malabsorption, and weight loss. Effectiveness of disease management is related to pain management and minimizing weight loss secondary to the administration of opioid and nonopioid medications. Additionally, a decrease in steatorrhea is associated with the actions of pancreatic enzyme replacement. Patient and family involvement are important in minimizing the exacerbations of chronic pancreatitis by avoiding alcohol intake and seeking out support groups to deal with this incurable disease.

PANCREATIC CANCER

Epidemiology

Pancreatic cancer is the fourth most common cause of cancer-related deaths in the United States. In 2017, the American Cancer Society reported that over 50,000 people were diagnosed with pancreatic cancer. Approximately 23% of patients survive to 1 year after diagnosis, and only 5% survive to 5 years. Almost 80% of patients with cancer of the pancreas have unresectable tumors because the diagnosis occurs late in the disease process.

There is no reliable screening test for the early detection of pancreatic cancer, and clinical manifestations are usually vague and similar to those of other GI disorders. The 5-year survival rate for early surgical resection of a small pancreatic tumor that has no lymph node involvement can reach 40%, but this is uncommon because patients are usually diagnosed late in the disease process due to the vagueness of the clinical presentation. The majority of pancreatic cancers are adenocarcinomas and develop in the exocrine portion of the pancreas. An adenocarcinoma is a malignant tumor that grows on the epithelial cells of an organ. The most common pancreatic cancer is ductal adenocarcinoma (75%–93%), most frequently found in the head of the pancreas. Adenocarcinomas are fast growing and spread to other local organs, primarily the stomach, duodenum, gallbladder, liver, and intestines. Metastasis occurs through the invasion of the lymph and vascular systems and can spread to the lung, peritoneum, and spleen. Other types of pancreatic cancers include those that occur in the endocrine tissues of the pancreas, and these tumors produce hormones and are named according to the hormones they produce, such as insulinoma (insulin-producing tumor) and glucagonoma (glucagon-producing tumor).

The exact cause of pancreatic cancer is not known, but there is a high association with behaviors such as cigarette smoking (smokers are twice as likely as nonsmokers to develop pancreatic cancer); diets high in fat; and consumption of meat, fried foods, refined sugars, and nitrates, all of which are modifiable risk factors. There is also a higher risk of pancreatic cancer in patients with diabetes, chronic pancreatitis, or a family history of pancreatic cancer and people of Ashkenazi Jewish descent. Some evidence suggests that patients with diabetes mellitus that is diagnosed later in life (after age 50) are at increased risk for pancreatic cancer.

The risk for pancreatic cancer increases with age, and it is commonly diagnosed in people over the age of 60 years. People of African American descent are more likely to develop pancreatic cancer than people of European descent, and men are more likely to develop pancreatic cancer than women. Because cigarette smoking doubles the risk of pancreatic cancer and is associated with diagnosis at an early age, it is important to teach the patient to quit smoking because this is one of the leading preventable causes of pancreatic cancer. Some occupational exposure to toxins such as gasoline derivatives and other chemicals may predispose a patient to the risk of pancreatic cancer.

Pathophysiology

Pancreatic tumors may be primary or metastatic, usually originating in the lung, breast, thyroid, kidneys, or skin. Because of the rapid growth of adenocarcinomas in the pancreas, both exocrine and endocrine functions deteriorate as the tumor invades the pancreatic tissue. Pancreatic tumor, because of the proximity of other GI organs, may metastasize to the stomach, duodenum, gallbladder, and intestine. Cancer that invades the tail and body of the pancreas may metastasize to the liver via the splenic vein, and the patient may present with an abdominal mass and hepatomegaly.

Clinical Manifestations

The clinical presentation of the patient is directly related to the degree of pancreatic damage secondary to tumor growth and, as described earlier, may not manifest until significant damage has occurred. Pain, jaundice (associated with obstruction of the bile duct), fatigue, and weight loss are the most frequently observed clinical manifestations. The pain is typically described as dull pain in the epigastric area and back.

Management

Medical Management

Diagnosis

The clinical evaluation of pancreatic cancer includes an ultrasound, CT scan, MRI, and/or an ERCP to determine the presence of a mass. The definitive diagnosis for pancreatic cancer is through histopathology. Tissue samples are collected by a fine-needle biopsy or excisional biopsy through a laparotomy. Patients may also undergo angiography to determine the involvement of vessels surrounding the pancreas. Once diagnosed, the tumor is staged according to the size, extent, lymph node involvement, and metastases, and the course of treatment is determined.

Laboratory Values

There is no single blood test available for the early diagnosis of pancreatic cancer, but several routine laboratory results may be abnormal. Although these tests are not specifically diagnostic for pancreatic cancer, they include elevated amylase, elevated total and direct bilirubin, and elevated liver enzymes. Fecal fat, trypsinogen, **trypsin** (an enzyme that aids in digestion of proteins), and lipase may indicate how the pancreas is functioning and the need for pancreatic enzyme supplementation.

Treatment

Several clinical trials have been performed to test and develop a vaccine that is used to treat patients who have pancreatic cancer, but no vaccine is available to prevent pancreatic cancer. The current evidence for the use of adjuvant therapy recommends combined chemotherapy and radiation. External beam radiation to the tumor and surrounding tissue over a 6-week period concurrent with 5-fluorouracil chemotherapy for up to 4 months help to improve long-term survival.

Surgical Management

The stage of the cancer and the location of the tumor determine whether surgical intervention is an option. Surgical resection is potentially curable; however, only a small percentage of patients qualify for surgical resection because of the latent nature of the clinical presentation. If the cancer has spread to distant lymph nodes or there is metastasis to the liver, the cancer is generally unresectable. Patients may undergo surgery to relieve symptoms (palliative surgery), but excision of the tumor is not possible. A celiac nerve block can be performed to decrease the pain associated with the tumor's compression of the celiac nerves surrounding the aorta. If a patient has a localized tumor, several surgical interventions are possible. If the tumor is located in the head, neck, or uncinate process of the pancreas, the patient can undergo the **Whipple procedure** or **pancreaticoduodenectomy** (Fig. 60.3).

There are several modifications of this procedure, but in general, the head of the pancreas, distal stomach, spleen, gallbladder, common bile duct, portions of the duodenum, proximal jejunum, and lymph nodes are resected. If the tumor is in the body or tail of the pancreas (Fig. 60.4), the patient undergoes a distal pancreatectomy (removal of the tail and part of the body of the pancreas) and splenectomy. A **pancreaticojejunostomy** (anastomosis of the pancreas to the jejunum), **hepaticojejunostomy** (anastomosis of the hepatic duct to the jejunum), or **gastrojejunostomy** (anastomosis of the stomach to the jejunum) may also be done to reconstruct the GI tract. A **vagotomy** (surgical resection of the vagus nerve) is done to decrease acid secretion in the stomach and decrease peptic ulcer formation.

Postoperatively, patients who undergo these procedures should be monitored for exocrine insufficiency (lack of digestive enzymes to properly digest food) and insulin-dependent diabetes mellitus. In addition, patients will have an NGT that is not to be manipulated (see Safety Alert). Pain management via PCA, pulmonary interventions to encourage lung expansion, coughing and deep breathing to prevent pneumonia and atelectasis, and abdominal assessment are all postoperative standards of care.

> ⚠ **Safety Alert** After a Whipple procedure or pancreaticoduodenectomy, NGTs are maintained postoperatively to decompress the stomach, prevent bloating, and remove gastric acid secretions to minimize pressure on the surgical site. These NGTs are placed intraoperatively and are not to be manipulated in any way. A **DO NOT MANIPULATE NGT** sign is placed on the wall above the patient's head. These NGTs are not to be repositioned, irrigated, or checked for placement because these actions can cause a breakdown of the anastomotic site. If a patient removes the NGT, it is not to be replaced by the nursing staff. A member of the surgical team is to be notified.

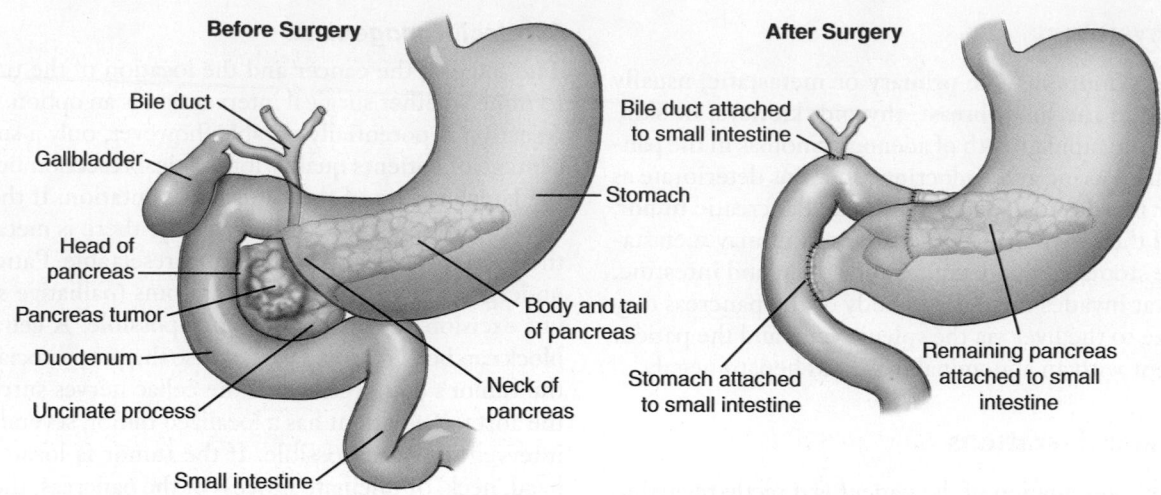

Before Surgery

Bile duct
Gallbladder
Head of pancreas
Pancreas tumor
Duodenum
Uncinate process
Small intestine
Stomach
Body and tail of pancreas
Neck of pancreas

After Surgery

Bile duct attached to small intestine
Stomach
Remaining pancreas attached to small intestine
Stomach attached to small intestine

FIGURE 60.3 Pre– and post–Whipple procedure. In the post–Whipple procedure, note that the head of the pancreas, distal stomach, spleen, gallbladder, common bile duct, portions of the duodenum, proximal jejunum, and lymph nodes have been resected.

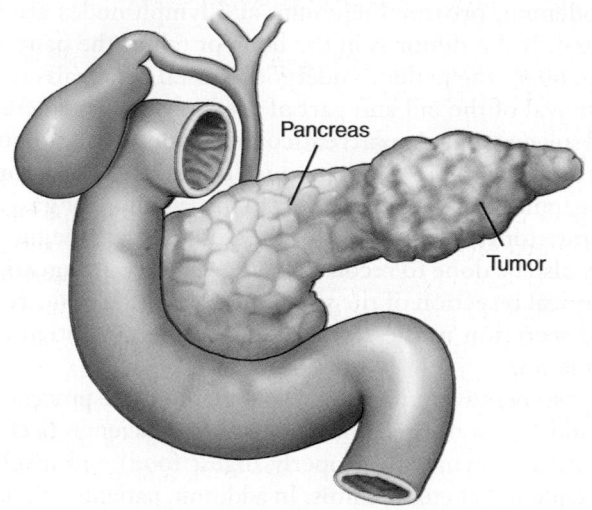

Pancreas
Tumor

FIGURE 60.4 Pancreatic tumor. Pancreatic tumors often develop in the body or tail of the pancreas.

Connection Check 60.4

The nurse receives a patient from the operating room after he undergoes a Whipple procedure. The nurse recognizes that this procedure is indicated for the patient who has which disorder?

A. Acute pancreatitis
B. Peritonitis
C. Cholecystitis
D. Pancreatic cancer

Nursing Management
Assessment and Analysis

Patients with pancreatic cancer present with nonspecific clinical manifestations that can be attributed to a variety of GI disturbances. Pain, jaundice, fatigue, anorexia, and weight loss are primary clinical manifestations, with vague, nonspecific abdominal and epigastric pain common. Pain is described as dull and intermittent that sometimes increases in intensity with eating and movement. Jaundice, which occurs in 80% of patients, develops in a pattern that is first seen in the mucous membranes, then the palms of the hands and eventually becomes generalized. Patients may complain of pale, greasy stools, which is attributed to a tumor that blocks digestive enzyme release. Other clinical manifestations include pruritus starting with the palms of the hands and then generalized and dark-amber urine due to the accumulation of bilirubin.

Nursing Diagnoses

- **Pain: acute or chronic** related to the pressure caused by the pancreatic mass
- **Imbalanced nutrition:** less than body requirements related to malabsorption and anorexia
- **Anxiety** related to the cancer diagnosis

Nursing Interventions
Assessments

- Vital signs
  Tachycardia may be related to fever and pain. Elevated blood pressure may be related to pain and anxiety. Fever may be related to infection due to blocked bile ducts.
- Fluid intake and output
  Daily intake and output monitor fluid volume status and prevent dehydration. With the development of ascites, there may be a fluid shift from the intravascular space.
- Serum glucose
  Elevated because of impaired insulin secretion due to tumor or due to removal of pancreas, which secretes insulin
- Weight
  Weight loss due to anorexia due to presence of tumor and malabsorption

- Muscle mass
  Cachexia (weight loss) secondary to loss of muscle mass is common because of decreased appetite and altered protein metabolism.
- Pain location, intensity, duration
  It is important to note the location, intensity, and duration of pain that is caused by the pancreatic tumor compressing surrounding organs and nerves. Pain may radiate to the back because of the compression of nerves.
- Abdomen
  Distention and enlargement of the abdomen are common in advanced disease because of the presence of ascites.
- Skin color
  Jaundice due to tumor obstruction of bile flow
- Pruritus
  Accumulation of bile salts under the skin causes itching.
- Postoperative assessment
  Postoperatively monitor vital signs, pain, glucose, NGT output, abdominal assessment, and surgical site.

Actions

- Provide intravenous fluids.
  Hypovolemia occurs because of third-space losses in the retroperitoneum from autodigestion of the pancreas and capillary leak.
- Maintain NPO status.
  Maintain NPO status until the return of GI function postoperatively, then slowly introduce a diet with clear liquids, and then advance to a regular diet to decrease strain on the surgical site.
- NGT to low suction
  Decompresses stomach because postoperative abdominal distention and decreased GI tract motility can place strain on the surgical anastomosis
- **NEVER** manipulate NGTs.
  NGTs are placed by the surgeon, and manipulation can increase the risk of anastomotic breakdown.
- Administer insulin.
  Pancreatic cancer affects the ability of the pancreas to produce and secrete insulin, leading to hyperglycemia.
- Encourage coughing and deep breathing and the use of an incentive spirometer or flutter valve every hour while awake.
  Prevents atelectasis, improves oxygenation, prevents postoperative pneumonia
- Administer analgesics and antiemetics as ordered.
  Pain management postoperatively for incisional pain and discomfort; preoperative pain management for pain caused by tumor compression
- Nutritional supplements
  These help to improve calorie input, prevent weight loss, and promote postoperative surgical wound healing. These include high-calorie, high-protein supplements.

Teaching

- Postoperative care: what to expect after surgery, pain management
  Informs the patient and improves compliance with prescribed interventions

- Medication regimens
  It is important for the patient to be knowledgeable of the mechanism of actions as well as the side effects of the ordered mediations. Pain medications may increase the risk of constipation and increase pressure and discomfort in the abdominal cavity.
- Diet and nutrition
  Nutritional supplements are prescribed to increase calorie intake to maintain weight and promote healing after surgery. Megestrol acetate (Megace) may be given as an appetite stimulant.
- Signs and symptoms of hyperglycemia and hypoglycemia
  With compression and damage to the pancreas, the production and secretion of insulin and glucagon may be impaired, leading to hyperglycemia or hypoglycemia.
- Disease symptoms, progression, diagnostic procedures, and interventions
  Patient education about the disease and disease progression improves symptom management and increases compliance with the prescribed interventions.
- Coping skills, palliative care, and support groups (Box 60.5)
  Support groups and networks provide additional information for patient and family.

Evaluating Care Outcomes

The diagnosis of pancreatic cancer generally occurs in a late stage of the disease, and often the patient does not have a prolonged life expectancy. With patients who are surgical candidates, it is imperative they are aware of the postoperative requirements and restrictions. Because a diagnosis of pancreatic cancer carries a devastating prognosis, it is important for the healthcare providers to direct the patient to and encourage the use of support systems and self-help books. Encouraging the patient to be knowledgeable about the disease, treatment, interventions, and restrictions is important.

Box 60.5 Complementary Alternative Medicine for Pancreatic Cancer

No alternative treatments are effective for the treatment of pancreatic cancer. There are alternative therapies a patient might want to consider to help with the management of the signs and symptoms of the disease. These include activities or therapies that help with coping, including exercise, relaxation techniques, art therapy, and meditation. It is important to teach the patient with a terminal illness to develop his or her immediate support system with friends and family members and encourage talking about the diagnosis and relying on surrounding support systems. Support groups may be encouraged, and self-education about the disease and end-of-life care or hospice should be addressed.

Connection Check 60.5

The nurse assesses for which finding in a patient with a positive Cullen's sign?
A. Periumbilical bruising
B. Rebound tenderness
C. RUQ pain with radiation to shoulder
D. Flank bruising

Connection Check 60.6

The nurse should question the administration of which medication in the patient admitted with cholecystitis?
A. Acetaminophen
B. Demerol
C. Ibuprofen
D. Morphine

Making Connections

CASE STUDY: WRAP-UP

Tony's condition continues to worsen. His abdominal pain is excruciating, he is delirious, and he develops hypovolemic shock with a blood pressure of 80/40 mm Hg and heart rate of 125 bpm. Because of the hypovolemic shock, fluid resuscitation is started in an attempt to increase his blood pressure.

Diagnostic tests reveal:
- Chest x-ray indicating left pleural effusions, atelectasis
- Electrocardiogram revealing sinus tachycardia
- Elevated serum lipase and amylase

Tony is intubated and placed on a mechanical ventilator and started on broad-spectrum antibiotics for the treatment of acute pancreatitis and hypovolemic shock. He is closely monitored for necrotizing pancreatitis and sepsis.

Case Study Questions

1. Tony's pain continues to worsen. What is the rationale for the healthcare provider to more likely prescribe meperidine (Demerol) for pain instead of morphine?
   A. Meperidine can be given intravenously or intramuscularly.
   B. Morphine is not absorbed in the pancreas.
   C. Morphine causes spasms in the sphincter of Oddi.
   D. Meperidine is better tolerated in patients with substance abuse.

2. What laboratory finding is the primary diagnostic indicator for pancreatitis?
   A. Elevated blood urea nitrogen (BUN)
   B. Elevated serum lipase
   C. Elevated aspartate aminotransferase (AST)
   D. Elevated lactate dehydrogenase (LDH)

3. In reviewing the prescriptions for Tony's acute pancreatitis, what order would the nurse anticipate?
   A. Maintenance of NPO status
   B. Oral fluid restriction
   C. Low-fat diet
   D. Regular diet

4. During the physical examination of Tony, what clinical manifestation correlates with his diagnosis?
   A. Constipation
   B. Steatorrhea
   C. Clear lung sounds throughout all lung fields
   D. Diarrhea

5. Tony is ready for discharge. What should be included in his discharge teaching about pancreatitis?
   A. Education about alcohol restriction
   B. Education about smoking cessation
   C. Education about a low-carbohydrate diet
   D. Education about vaccines

CHAPTER SUMMARY

Disorders of the gallbladder and pancreas are common and lead to admissions to acute care facilities. Cholecystitis, inflammation of the gallbladder, is most typically caused by obstruction of the bile duct by gallstones. The clinical presentation of cholecystitis includes acute right upper quadrant pain, often accompanied by clay-colored stool and darkened urine secondary to elevated serum bilirubin. Cholecystectomy is often required, as well as diet modifications.

Pancreatitis may be acute or chronic and may lead to serious complications. Acute pancreatitis may result in actual autodigestion of the pancreas and is associated with complications such as necrotizing pancreatitis and sepsis. Patients with acute pancreatitis present with a sudden onset of epigastric pain in the upper left quadrant or mid-abdomen, often accompanied by radiation to the back or shoulder blades. Pain is worsened within minutes of eating foods high in fat content and can be constant and severe and last for several days. Some patients complain of severe pain when lying flat or bending forward. Pain can also be associated with nausea and vomiting and anorexia. Medical management includes bowel rest, fluid administration, and monitoring for complications. Chronic pancreatitis is a progressive, irreversible disease that results in pain, malabsorption, and weight loss. Effectiveness of disease management is related to pain management and minimizing weight loss secondary to the administration of opioid and nonopioid medications. Avoiding alcohol intake and seeking out

support groups to deal with this incurable disease are key aspects of the care of patients with this disorder.

Pancreatic cancer is often considered a terminal disease secondary to late diagnosis. The clinical presentation typically includes nonspecific symptoms such as pain, jaundice, and anorexia. Abdominal and epigastric pain is common, vague, and sometimes nonspecific. Surgical interventions are indicated in the absence of metastatic disease. If there is evidence of metastatic disease, medical management is primarily symptomatic and palliative.

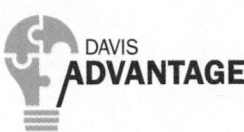

DAVIS
ADVANTAGE

To explore learning resources for this chapter, go to **Davis Advantage** and find:
- Answers to in-text questions
- Chapter Resources and Activities
- NCLEX®-Style Chapter Review Questions
- Bibliography

Unit XIV

Promoting Health in Patients With Renal Disorders

Chapter 61

Assessment of Renal and Urinary Function

Sarah Tarr

LEARNING OUTCOMES

Content in this chapter is designed to assist in:

1. Identifying key anatomical components of the renal and urinary systems
2. Discussing the function of the renal and urinary systems
3. Describing the procedure for completing a history and physical assessment of the renal and urinary systems
4. Correlating relevant diagnostic examinations with renal and urinary system function
5. Explaining nursing considerations for diagnostic studies relevant to renal and urinary system function
6. Discussing changes in renal and urinary system function associated with aging

CONCEPTS

- Assessment
- Fluid and Electrolyte Balance
- Infection
- Medication
- pH Regulation
- Urinary Elimination

ESSENTIAL TERMS

Afferent arterioles
Antidiuretic hormone (ADH)
Anuria
Bladder
Bowman's capsule
Bruit
Collecting tubule
Continence
Creatinine
Distal convoluted tubule (DCT)
Dysuria
Efferent arterioles
Glomerular filtrate
Glomerular filtration rate (GFR)
Glomerulus
Kidney
Loop of Henle
Major calyces
Micturition
Minor calyx
Nephron
Nocturia
Oliguria
Papillae
Polyuria
Proximal convoluted tubule (PCT)
Pyramids
Renal pelvis
Renin
Ureter
Urethra

Finding Connections

Reginald Jones is a 72-year-old African American male patient who presents to his healthcare provider with complaints of recent weight gain, swelling in his hands and feet, voiding only small amounts of urine, and fatigue. His wife accompanies him and reports that he is "just not himself" and "sometimes seems dazed." Mr. Jones has a history of depression and borderline hypertension, which at this time are not being treated with any medications. His last visit to a healthcare provider was more than 2 years ago. Mr. Jones and his wife are concerned about these recent changes and his overall health...

OVERVIEW OF ANATOMY AND PHYSIOLOGY

The renal system is composed of the two kidneys. The urinary system is composed of two ureters, the urinary bladder, and the urethra. The two systems work together to help maintain homeostasis in the human body. For example, urine is formed as blood is filtered through the kidneys. The bladder then provides storage, and the ureters and urethra act as passages for urine to exit the body; thus, the function of excreting wastes from the body is complete.

The kidneys perform the following functions essential to the maintenance of homeostasis in the human body: (1) excretion of wastes, (2) regulation of fluid and electrolyte balance, (3) regulation of acid-base balance, (4) regulation of blood pressure, (5) secretion of erythropoietin for red blood cell (RBC) production, and (6) activation of vitamin D. The urinary system provides for the storage and passage of urine, promoting **continence** and facilitating voiding. This chapter will first examine the anatomy and physiology of the kidneys and then examine the anatomy and physiology of the urinary system structures.

Renal Anatomy

Kidney Gross Anatomy

The **kidneys** are bean-shaped organs located retroperitoneally (behind the abdominal contents), one on each side of the spinal column (Fig. 61.1). The kidneys are held in place by connective tissue known as the renal fascia. The left kidney is typically located slightly higher than the right kidney because of the position of the liver. Each kidney is approximately 4 to 5 in. (10 to 12 cm) long, 2 to 3 in. (5 to 7 cm) wide, and 1 in. (2.5 cm) thick, and each weighs approximately 4 to 6 oz. An adrenal gland, an endocrine organ, sits atop each kidney (see Chapter 40).

Each kidney is surrounded by multiple layers of subcutaneous and connective tissue that provide support and protection. The outermost layer of the kidney is termed the *renal capsule* (Fig. 61.2). This thin, fibrous tissue serves to protect the organ and absorb shock. The capsule covers the distal surface of the kidney and extends to the medial portion of the kidney, termed the *hilum*. The hilum is the indented part of the kidney and is the location at which the renal artery and nerves enter the organ and the renal vein and ureters exit.

The inner tissue of the kidney, the parenchyma, lies beneath the renal capsule and contains the functional layers of the organ. When the parenchyma is viewed as a cross

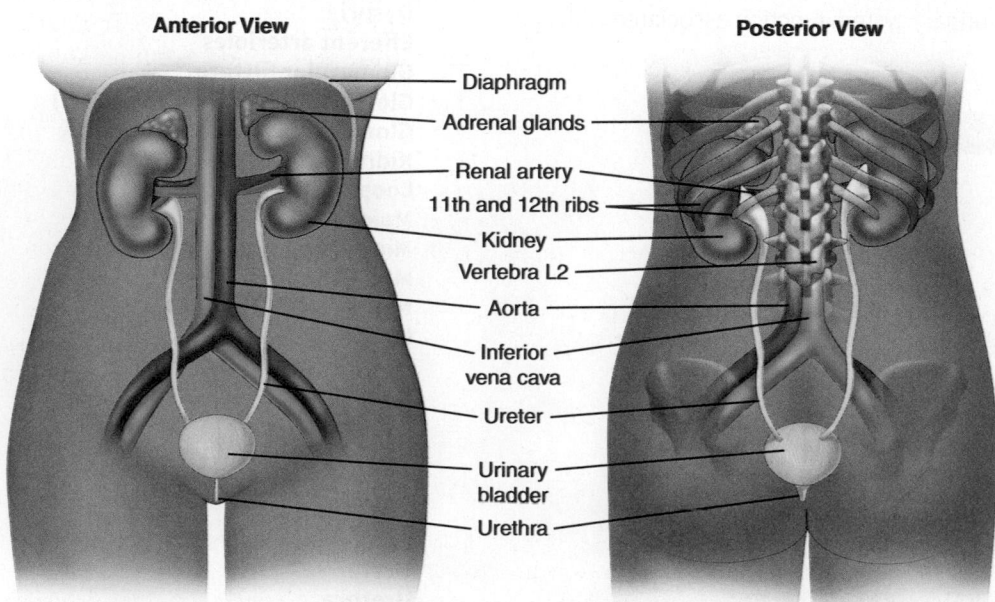

FIGURE 61.1 The renal and urinary systems: anterior and posterior views.

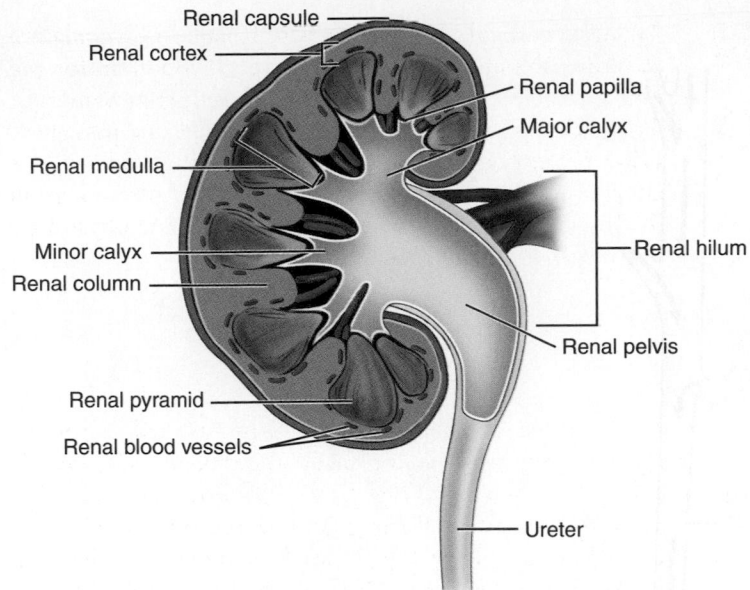

FIGURE 61.2 Gross anatomy of the kidney.

section, the tissue layer lying directly beneath the renal capsule is the cortex. The medulla is the innermost layer of tissue and is composed of multiple **pyramids**. Each kidney contains approximately 12 to 18 pyramids. Each pyramid is separated by tissue known as renal columns.

The narrow tips of the renal pyramids are the **papillae**. The papillae empty urine into the calyces, cuplike collection structures. A small cluster of these structures is known as a **minor calyx**. Minor calyces widen moving toward the hilum and merge to form **major calyces**, which empty into the larger collection sac known as the **renal pelvis**. The renal pelvis can store only a small volume of urine, approximately 3 to 5 mL. The renal pelvis narrows to become the ureters. Urine flows through the gross structures of the kidney via the following route: from the papillae of the pyramids into the minor calyces, the major calyces, the renal pelvis, and the ureters en route to the bladder.

Kidney Microscopic Anatomy

A **nephron** is the functional unit of the kidney. Approximately 800,000 to 1.2 million nephrons are contained within each kidney. It is here that the work of filtering the blood to remove wastes and produce urine occurs. Nearly 80% of nephrons in the kidneys are known as cortical nephrons, meaning they are short in length and are fully contained within the cortex region of the organ. The remaining 20% of nephrons are juxtamedullary nephrons and contain structures that lie deep within the medulla of the kidney.

Each nephron is composed of the following: a **glomerulus**, a **Bowman's capsule**, and a tubular system (Fig. 61.3). A glomerulus is a collection of semipermeable capillaries responsible for filtering blood. The Bowman's capsule is the structure surrounding each glomerulus. The tubular system is composed of the **proximal convoluted tubule (PCT)**, the **loop of Henle**, the **distal convoluted tubules (DCTs)**, and a **collecting tubule**. The PCT emerges from the

Bowman's capsule and winds until straightening into the loop of Henle. The loop of Henle is composed of a descending and an ascending limb, each of which is responsible for reabsorbing different substances in the process of urine formation. The DCT is a continuation of the ascending limb of the loop of Henle that thickens and continues twisting until it widens further into a collecting tubule.

Blood Supply

The kidneys receive 20% to 25% of the total cardiac output, a flow rate of approximately 1,200 mL of blood per minute. The renal artery, a branch of the abdominal aorta, enters each kidney at the hilum and delivers blood to the kidney. As the renal artery enters the kidney, it branches into several segmental arteries, which then branch into interlobar arteries. The interlobar arteries travel through the renal columns between the pyramids, moving outward toward the renal cortex tissue. As the interlobar arteries approach the renal cortex, they divide, forming arcuate arteries and then cortical radiate arteries.

The branches formed off these cortical radiate arteries are the **afferent arterioles**. The afferent arterioles form a collection of capillaries that direct blood flow to the glomeruli of the nephrons, where the process of urine formation begins. Capillaries within the glomeruli then merge into the **efferent arterioles** to transport blood away from the glomeruli and into the peritubular capillaries. This collection of capillaries drains blood into the venous system. The renal vein then carries blood away from the kidneys and drains into the inferior vena cava (see Figs. 61.3 and 61.4).

Renal Physiology

The kidneys perform several functions essential to the maintenance of homeostasis in the human body: (1) urine formation and the excretion of wastes, (2) regulatory functions such

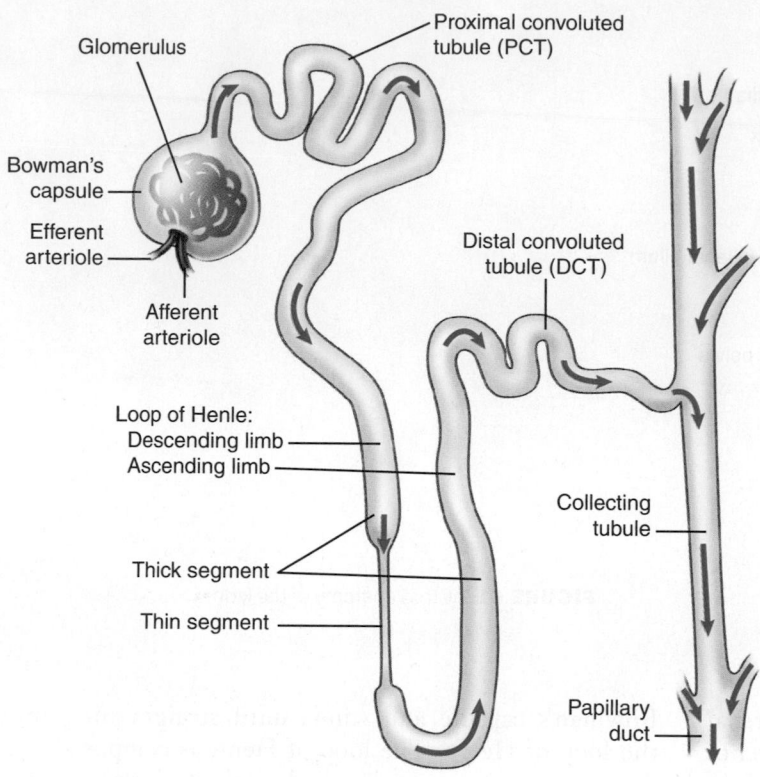

FIGURE 61.3 Anatomy of a nephron.

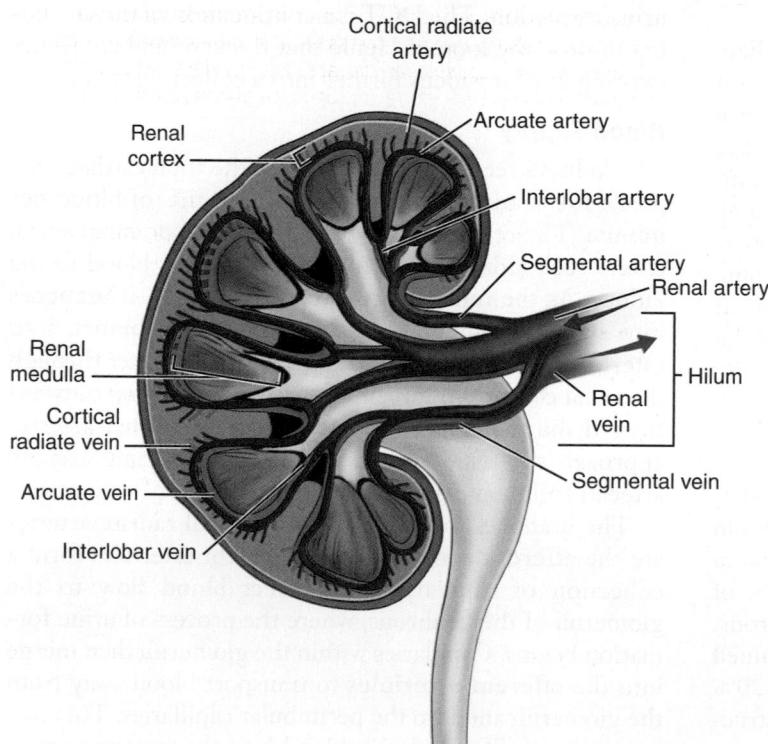

FIGURE 61.4 Renal circulation. The renal artery delivers blood to the kidney. As the renal artery enters the kidney, it branches into segmental arteries, then into interlobar arteries. The interlobar arteries travel through the renal columns between the pyramids, moving outward toward the renal cortex tissue. As the interlobar arteries approach the renal cortex, they divide, forming arcuate arteries and then cortical radiate arteries.

as regulation of fluid and electrolyte balance and acid-base balance, and (3) hormonal functions such as renin production that helps regulate blood pressure, secretion of erythropoietin for RBC production, activation of vitamin D, and the production and release of bradykinin and prostaglandins (PGs).

Urine Formation

Urine is formed through the continuous processes of filtration, reabsorption, secretion, and concentration (Fig. 61.5). Each of these processes is discussed in the following subsections.

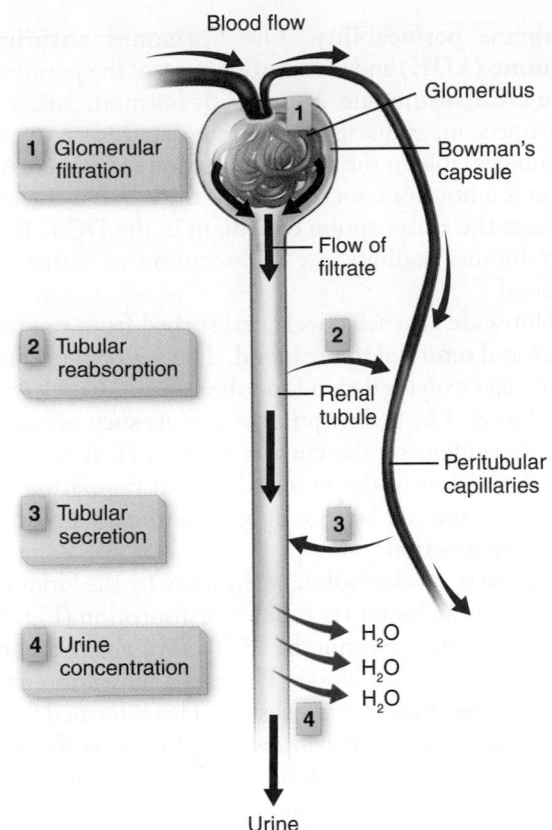

FIGURE 61.5 Steps of urine formation.

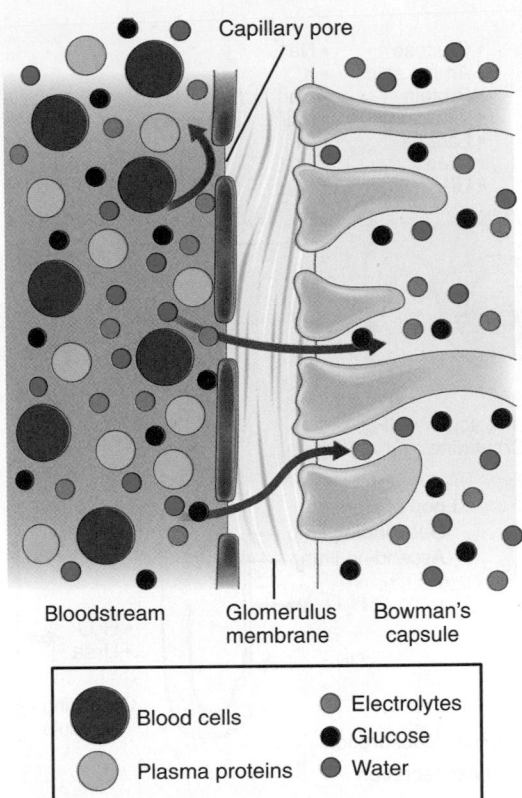

FIGURE 61.6 The glomerular filtration membrane. As blood enters the capillaries of the glomerulus, glomerular filtrate is formed via hydrostatic pressure. It moves across the glomerular membrane and into the Bowman's capsule. The filtrate contains electrolytes, water, and small particles such as urea nitrogen, creatinine, and glucose.

Glomerular Filtration

Glomerular filtration begins as blood is filtered across the semipermeable membrane of the glomerulus (Fig. 61.6). The membrane filters particles primarily by their size. The capillary pores do not normally allow large particles such as plasma proteins and blood cells to pass through the membrane. However, in conditions that increase the capillary membrane permeability (i.e., diabetes mellitus and renal failure), plasma proteins and blood cells may escape through the membrane and into the urine.

When blood enters the capillaries of the glomerulus, **glomerular filtrate** is formed via hydrostatic pressure, which forces electrolytes, water, and small particles such as urea nitrogen, **creatinine**, and glucose from the blood across the glomerular membrane and into the Bowman's capsule. The glomerular filtrate or ultrafiltrate then flows from the Bowman's capsule into the PCT, where it is termed *tubular filtrate*.

The amount of blood filtered by the glomeruli in a set amount of time is the **glomerular filtration rate (GFR)**. The normal GFR is approximately 125 mL/min. This rate of filtration results in an average of 180 L of filtrate per day! Although a large volume of filtrate is produced, the reabsorption that occurs beyond the glomerulus returns much of this volume to the body. In a healthy adult, approximately 1 to 3 L of filtrate is actually excreted as urine each day.

The rate of glomerular filtration is dependent on several factors, including systemic blood pressure, blood flow, and volume. The kidneys have some ability to change the pressure within the glomerular capillaries through the dilation and constriction of the afferent arterioles that direct blood into the glomerulus and the efferent arterioles that guide blood away from the glomerulus. The constriction of the afferent arterioles or dilation of the efferent arterioles results in decreased pressure within the glomerular capillaries and a decreased filtration rate. Dilation of the afferent arterioles or constriction of the efferent arterioles results in the opposite, increased glomerular capillary pressure and an increased filtration rate. This regulatory mechanism enables the kidneys to maintain a constant GFR despite global changes in blood pressure. This is a powerful compensatory mechanism, but it cannot typically compensate for systolic blood pressures below 70 mm Hg. Pressures at or below that level result in a decreased GFR.

Tubular Reabsorption

Tubular reabsorption is the second phase of urine production. It is the movement of water and solutes from the tubular filtrate back into the blood (Fig. 61.7). These processes occur throughout the length of the tubular system and are accomplished through both active and passive transport. Different from glomerular filtration, which occurs nonselectively based on particle size, the kidneys allow for selective reabsorption of certain substances to occur within the tubular

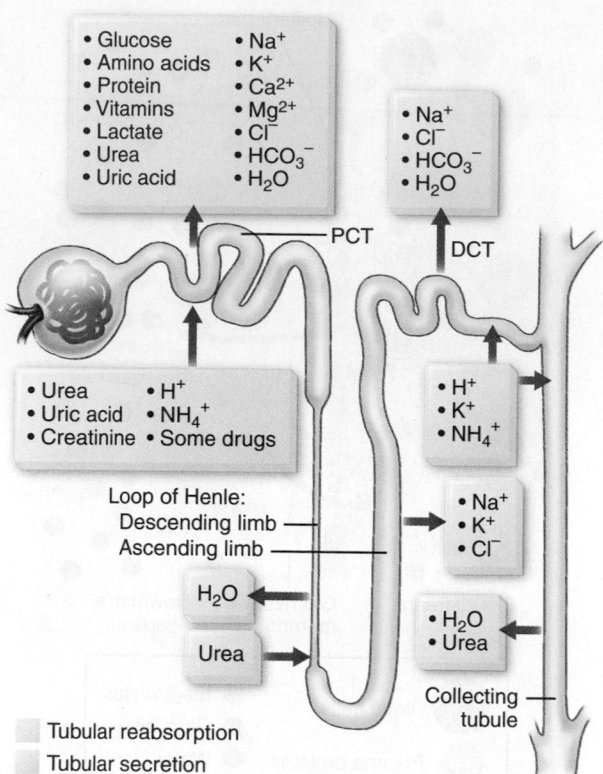

FIGURE 61.7 Tubular reabsorption and tubular secretion of solutes throughout the renal tubule.

membrane permeability. The hormones **antidiuretic hormone (ADH)** and aldosterone control the permeability of the DCT membrane. Antidiuretic hormone, also known as vasopressin, is discussed in great detail later regarding the kidneys' role in the regulation of water balance. Aldosterone is a hormone secreted from the adrenal cortex that increases the reabsorption of sodium in the DCT. Because water follows sodium, the reabsorption of water is also increased.

Solutes are also selectively reabsorbed from the tubular filtrate and returned to the blood. The reabsorption rate of specific electrolytes depends on the level of that electrolyte in the blood. The reabsorption of a solute such as bicarbonate is dependent on the current serum pH. A more thorough discussion of the kidneys' role in regulating water, electrolyte, and pH balance appears in the later section on regulatory function.

Glucose is another solute reabsorbed by the kidneys and returned to the blood via tubular reabsorption (Fig. 61.8). Transport proteins within the PCT move glucose from the filtrate back into the blood. There is a maximum amount of glucose the kidneys can reabsorb. This is termed the *renal threshold* or *transport maximum* for glucose reabsorption. The typical value associated with the renal threshold for glucose is 220 mg/dL, meaning that at blood glucose levels of 220 mg/dL or less, all glucose is bound to the transport proteins and returned and reabsorbed in the blood. At higher levels, the transport proteins become saturated, resulting in the presence of glucose in the filtrate and subsequently in the urine. A patient with uncontrolled or undiagnosed diabetes mellitus will therefore at times test positive for glucose in the urine, termed glycosuria.

system. To avoid dehydration, up to 99% of the glomerular filtrate is reabsorbed and returned to the blood, mainly in the PCT. The PCT is responsible for reabsorbing approximately 65% of the glomerular filtrate. Reabsorption of water can also occur in the DCT depending on the

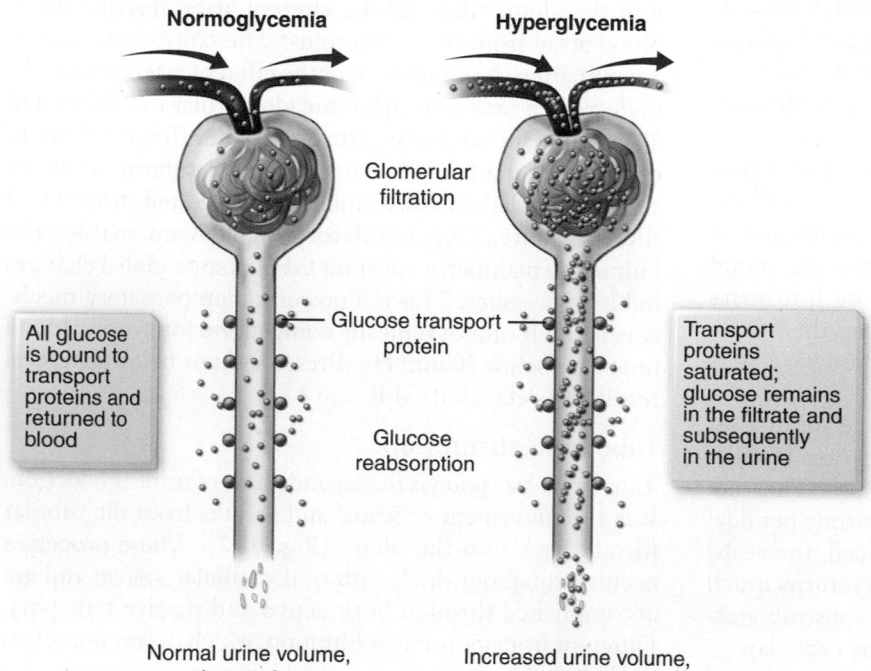

Normal urine volume, glucose-free

Increased urine volume, with glycosuria (glucose in urine)

FIGURE 61.8 Renal threshold for glucose transport. A serum glucose over 220 mg/dL results in incomplete reabsorption and resulting glycosuria.

Tubular Secretion

Tubular secretion is the third phase of urine formation and is the movement of solutes from the blood into the filtrate. Substances move from the capillaries into the renal tubule cells and then into the urine to be excreted from the body. Substances secreted in this fashion include potassium ions (K^+) and hydrogen ions (H^+). Both are secreted back into the filtrate in quantities necessary to maintain stable electrolyte and blood pH levels. This is discussed in more detail later in the chapter and is illustrated in Figure 61.7.

Urine Concentration

Following tubular secretion, the urine must be concentrated prior to its excretion from the body. Without the kidneys' ability to concentrate the urine, the body would quickly experience dehydration due to significantly large volume losses. The loop of Henle plays a significant role in this final step of urine formation. The descending portion of the loop is permeable to water and is responsible for reabsorbing the additional water required to concentrate the urine. The role of the kidneys in maintaining a homeostatic balance of water within the body is discussed further in the next section.

Regulatory Function

Water Balance

Water accounts for approximately 50% to 60% of the body weight of the average adult. Two-thirds of this water is found in the intracellular fluid (ICF), whereas the majority of the remaining water is found outside the cells in the extracellular fluid (ECF). Water found in the ECF is distributed throughout the plasma, lymph, and interstitial fluid (tissue fluid). Small quantities of water (2%) are also found in the cerebrospinal fluid (CSF), the gastrointestinal (GI) tract, the respiratory tract, and the vitreous humor of the eye. The kidneys are the primary organs responsible for maintaining water balance within the body.

For this fluid balance to be maintained, the kidneys must ensure that the volume of water taken into the body is equal to the volume of water lost from the body (Fig. 61.9). Water is taken into the body through consumed liquids and foods. Water is also present in the body as a product of metabolism. Water losses occur through perspiration (water from sweat glands), urination, defecation, cutaneous transpiration (water loss through the epidermis), and exhalation.

Osmolality is a measure of the concentration of solutes, including electrolytes and ions, contained in the blood. Typically, the osmolality of the fluid inside the cells and the fluid outside the cells is nearly equal because water is allowed to pass freely along the cell membrane. When less water is taken into the body, serum osmolality increases because the solutes are more concentrated as a result of the decrease in water content. Likewise, when excess water is taken into the body, serum osmolality decreases because the excess water dilutes the concentration of solutes.

When serum osmolality is altered, several mechanisms are activated to restore homeostasis. The hypothalamus is

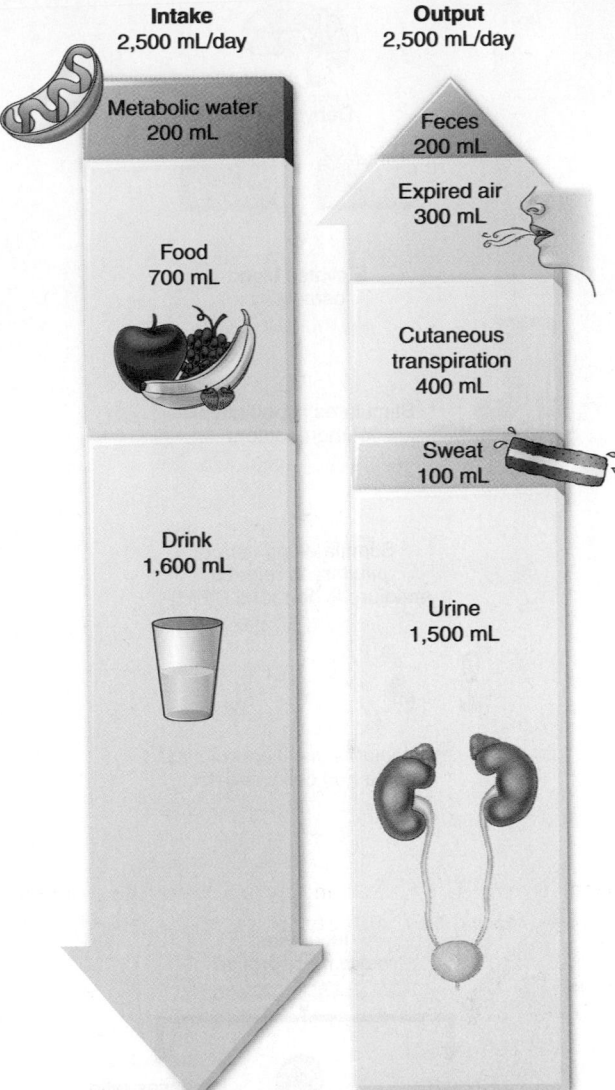

FIGURE 61.9 Normal mechanisms of fluid intake and output.

capable of detecting changes in the osmolality of blood. When serum osmolality increases because of dehydration, the brain is stimulated to produce the sensation of thirst. In addition, increased osmolality triggers the release of ADH from the posterior pituitary gland. Antidiuretic hormone regulates water balance by altering the permeability of the tubular membrane, making it more permeable to water and resulting in the increased absorption of water. These mechanisms, along with the production of more-concentrated urine, result in a decrease in serum osmolality. The action of ADH is illustrated in Figure 61.10.

Conversely, when excess water is taken into the body, osmolality decreases, and the secretion of ADH is suppressed. The kidneys then produce more dilute urine to rid the body of excess water and to restore serum osmolality. These mechanisms of regulating water balance enable the kidneys to control the volume and concentration of urine independently from fluid intake. Therefore, the kidneys are able to prevent dehydration when fluid intake is low and prevent volume overload when fluid intake is excessive. The

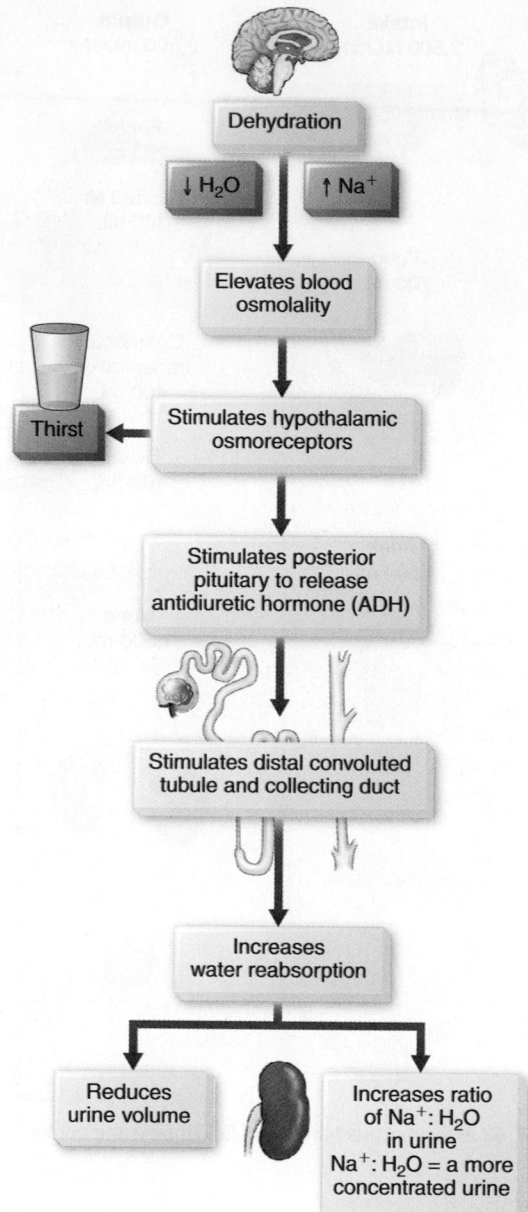

FIGURE 61.10 Action of antidiuretic hormone (ADH).

role of the kidneys in maintaining water balance is invaluable. When the kidneys lose this regulatory capacity, homeostasis is altered, and all body systems are affected. Complete loss of this regulatory function can result in death.

Electrolyte Balance

The kidneys also control the composition of the blood by reabsorbing and secreting electrolytes to maintain levels within normal ranges. The PCT is responsible for reabsorbing up to 80% of the electrolytes contained in the filtrate. Figure 61.7 illustrates the locations throughout the tubule at which various solutes, including electrolytes, are reabsorbed and secreted.

The rate of reabsorption and secretion of each electrolyte is dependent on the concentration of that electrolyte in the serum. To explain, when a higher-than-normal electrolyte

level is detected, the kidneys act by increasing the secretion of this electrolyte. Likewise, when a specific electrolyte level is lower than normal, the kidneys increase the reabsorption of that electrolyte to restore homeostasis.

As an example, the release of the hormone aldosterone from the adrenal cortex is stimulated when serum levels of sodium are decreased (hyponatremia), causing increased reabsorption of sodium (Na^+) in the distal tubule (Fig. 61.11). As a result, sodium is reabsorbed, increasing serum sodium levels. Water is also reabsorbed. Aldosterone is also secreted in instances of elevated potassium (hyperkalemia), resulting in the excretion of K^+. This is one mechanism by which the kidneys exert control of specific electrolyte levels. The rates of reabsorption and secretion of other electrolytes, including

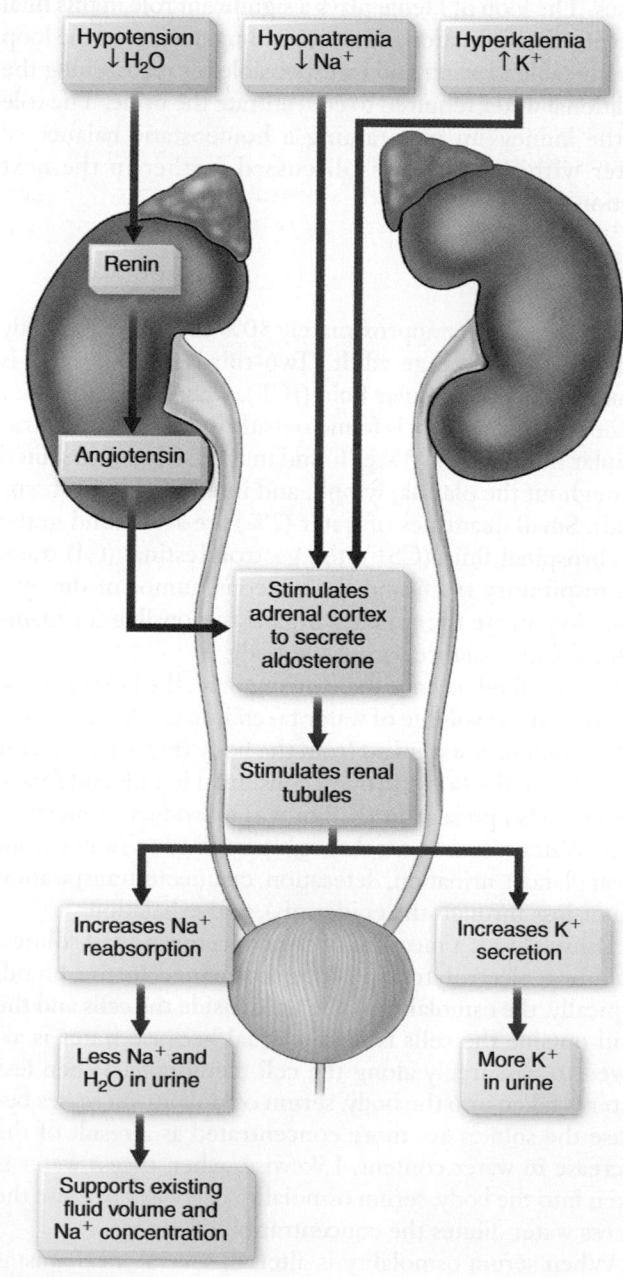

FIGURE 61.11 Action of aldosterone secretion.

calcium and phosphate, are also partially controlled by hormonal action on the kidney. Both calcium and phosphate are reabsorbed mainly in the PCT. Their reabsorption and secretion are regulated by parathyroid hormone and calcitonin. These hormones are discussed in detail in Chapter 40.

Acid-Base Balance

To maintain homeostasis, the pH of the blood must constantly remain between 7.35 and 7.45. A serum pH (H^+ levels) less than 7.35 is termed *acidosis*, and a serum pH greater than 7.45 is termed *alkalosis*. Three bodily mechanisms work to maintain normal serum pH levels: an acid-base buffer system, regulation by the respiratory system, and regulation by the renal system. The role of the kidneys in regulating the acid-base balance is invaluable because cells within the body cannot survive and function properly when pH is not maintained within the normal range.

In instances of acidosis, the kidney tubules excrete H^+ and reabsorb bicarbonate ions (HCO_3^-) to increase serum pH to a normal level. In cases of alkalosis, the kidney tubules reabsorb H^+ and excrete HCO_3^- to decrease pH to a normal level. Although the renal regulation of pH balance is the last mechanism to activate when the serum pH is altered, its response exerts the most control in restoring the pH to a normal level; the kidneys are the only organs with the capability to fully excrete H^+ from the body.

Hormonal Function

In addition to producing urine and regulating water, electrolyte, and acid-base balance, the kidneys are responsible for producing hormones, including renin, erythropoietin, activated vitamin D, bradykinin, and PGs.

Renin

Renin aids in blood pressure regulation within the body. It is produced and released when receptors in the kidneys sense a decrease in blood flow, volume, or pressure. Renin is also released when decreased levels of sodium in the renal blood supply are detected. Upon its release, renin interacts with angiotensinogen released from the liver to produce angiotensin I, which, with the aid of angiotensin-converting enzyme (ACE) secreted from the lungs, results in the formation of angiotensin II (Fig. 61.12). Angiotensin II constricts blood vessels, resulting in increased blood pressure. In addition, angiotensin II stimulates the adrenal glands to release aldosterone. Aldosterone causes increased sodium reabsorption and subsequent water reabsorption in the DCT.

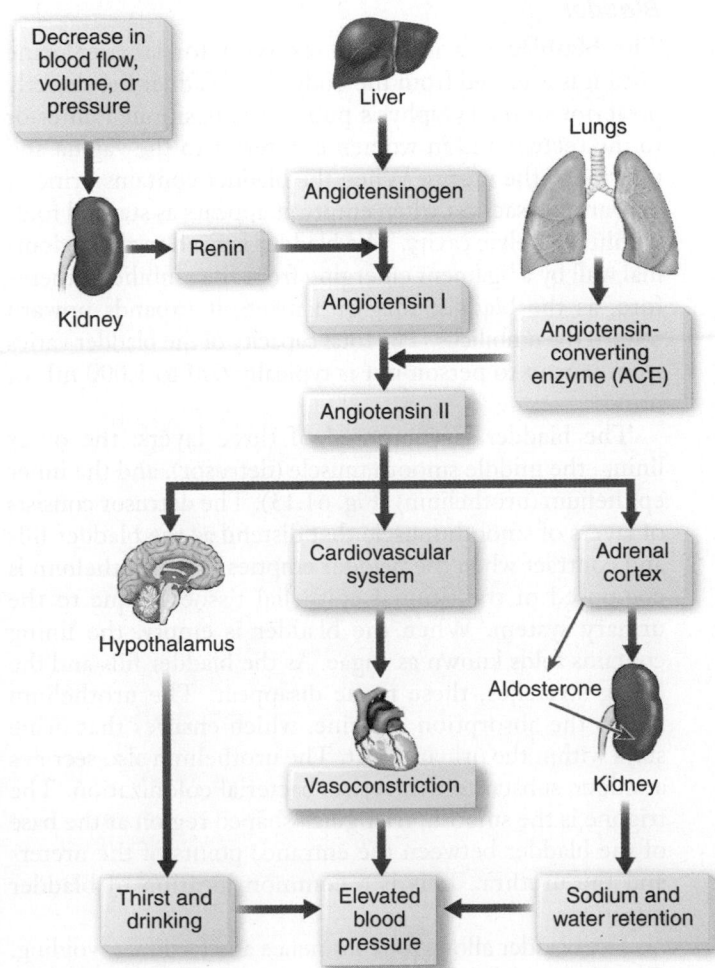

FIGURE 61.12 Renin-angiotensin-aldosterone system (RAAS).

This regulatory mechanism is termed the *renin-angiotensin-aldosterone system*. Angiotensin II also stimulates the hypothalamus to stimulate thirst.

Erythropoietin

Erythropoietin is a hormone produced exclusively by the kidneys in response to decreased renal blood flow and hypoxia. Erythropoietin stimulates the bone marrow to produce RBCs. In cases of renal impairment and failure, erythropoietin is produced in insufficient quantities, and a resulting anemia occurs.

Vitamin D

Although obtained through diet and exposure to ultraviolet radiation, vitamin D must be activated in order to be useful to the body. The steps required for activation begin in the liver, where vitamin D is converted to calcidiol, then continues in the kidneys, where calcidiol is converted to its active form, 1,25-dihydroxycholecalciferol or calcitriol. The activated form of vitamin D is required for calcium to be absorbed in the GI tract. A patient with renal impairment can have deficiencies in activated vitamin D and, as a result, decreased serum calcium levels. Because of the inverse relationship of calcium and phosphate, serum phosphate is typically increased in patients with renal impairment (discussed in detail in Chapter 62).

Prostaglandins

Prostaglandins are hormones produced by various tissues of the body. They typically affect the tissues surrounding their site of production. The kidneys specifically produce prostaglandin E_2 and prostacyclin. These PGs function within the kidneys to trigger vasodilation, resulting in increased blood flow to the kidneys and increased sodium and water excretion. Prostaglandins synthesized in the kidneys may also play a role in lowering systemic blood pressure as a result of decreasing vascular resistance. As the quantity of functional kidney tissue decreases in renal failure, the production of PGs also decreases. The absence of the vasodilating effects of PGs may be a contributing factor to the development of hypertension often associated with renal failure.

Bradykinin

Bradykinin is a hormone released by the kidneys in response to the presence of PGs, ADH, and angiotensin II. It increases the permeability of the capillary membrane to certain solutes and dilates the afferent arteriole to ensure adequate reabsorption of solutes and blood flow to the kidneys.

Connection Check 61.1

The nurse expects to observe which of the following altered laboratory values in a patient diagnosed with renal failure?

A. Decreased calcium

B. Increased calcium

C. Decreased phosphorus

D. Increased hematocrit

Urinary System Structures

Ureters

A **ureter** is a small, hollow, muscular tube through which urine travels from the renal pelvis of the kidney to the bladder. Each ureter is approximately 10 to 12 in. (25.4 to 30.5 cm) long, and one is associated with each kidney. The ureter is composed of three layers: an inner mucous membrane, a middle layer of smooth muscle, and an outer layer of fibrous tissue. The narrowing where each ureter joins the renal pelvis is known as the ureteropelvic junction. Each ureter joins the bladder on its posterior side at the ureterovesical junction. Because these areas represent locations of narrowing in the ureter lumen, they are common sites for the obstruction of urine flow related to urinary stones, or calculi.

Urine moves one way through the ureters and into the bladder as a result of the peristaltic contractions of the smooth muscle fibers of the ureters. These contractions occur as stretch receptors within the renal pelvis detect increased urine volume. Urine is prevented from backflowing into the kidneys when the pressure in the bladder increases (i.e., with coughing or voiding) because the muscles of the bladder and urethra contract to close off the lumen.

Bladder

The **bladder** is a muscular reservoir for storing urine until it is excreted from the body. The bladder lies directly posterior to the symphysis pubis. It is positioned anterior to the rectum and in women is anterior to the vagina and inferior to the uterus. When the bladder contains urine, it appears as a sac; yet when empty, it appears as stacked folds within the pelvic cavity. The bladder is fixed to the abdominal wall by a ligament emerging from the umbilicus; therefore, as the bladder fills with urine, it expands upward toward the umbilicus. The total capacity of the bladder varies from person to person but is typically 600 to 1,000 mL of urine.

The bladder is composed of three layers: the outer lining, the middle smooth muscle (detrusor), and the inner epithelium (urothelium) (Fig. 61.13). The detrusor consists of layers of smooth muscle that distend as the bladder fills and contract when the bladder empties. The urothelium is composed of transitional epithelial tissue unique to the urinary system. When the bladder is empty, the lining contains folds known as rugae. As the bladder fills and the lining stretches, these rugae disappear. The urothelium resists the absorption of urine, which ensures that urine stays within the urinary tract. The urothelium also secretes a unique substance that resists bacterial colonization. The trigone is the smooth, triangular-shaped region at the base of the bladder between the entrance points of the ureters and the urethra. This is a common location of bladder infections.

The bladder allows for continence and facilitates voiding. Continence is the ability to voluntarily control the emptying

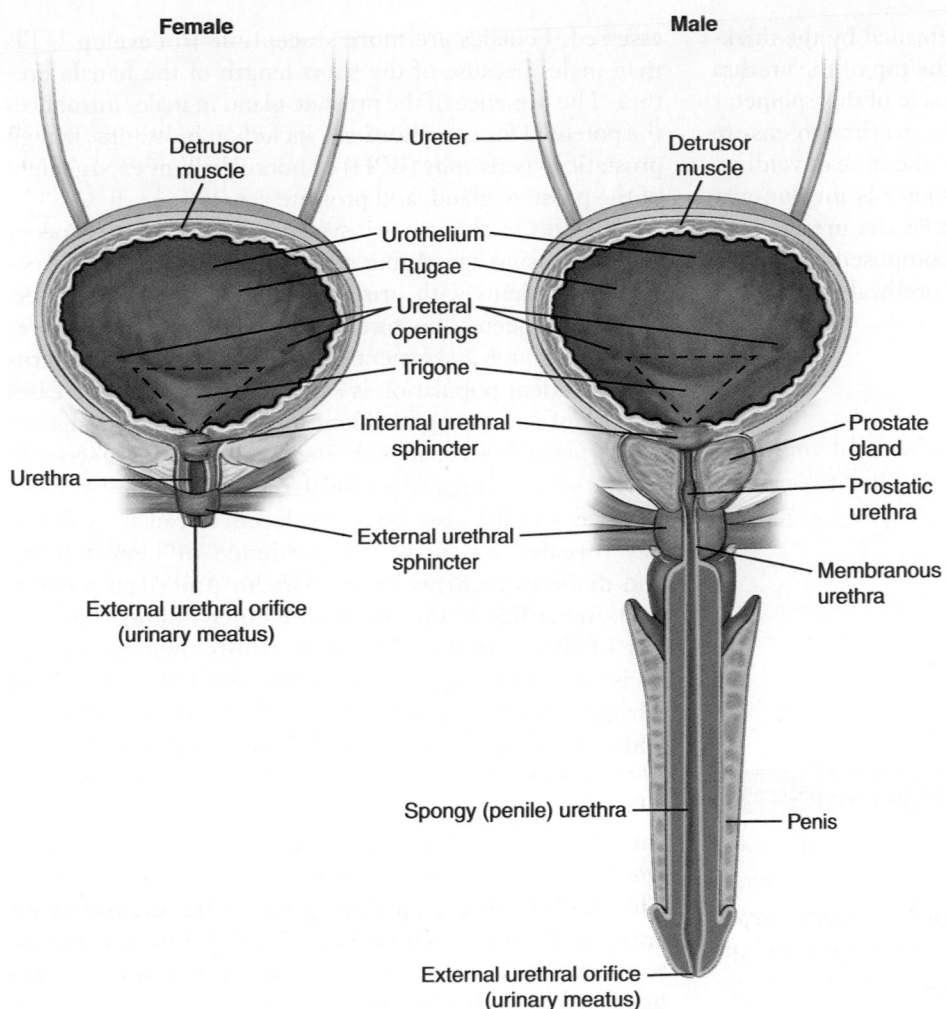

Female

Male

- Detrusor muscle
- Ureter
- Detrusor muscle
- Urothelium
- Rugae
- Ureteral openings
- Trigone
- Internal urethral sphincter
- Prostate gland
- Prostatic urethra
- Urethra
- External urethral sphincter
- Membranous urethra
- External urethral orifice (urinary meatus)
- Spongy (penile) urethra
- Penis
- External urethral orifice (urinary meatus)

FIGURE 61.13 Layers and anatomy of the bladder and urethra.

of the bladder. **Micturition**, voiding, is the act of releasing urine from the body. Micturition is a learned response coordinated by the brain and the spinal nerves that innervate the bladder.

As the bladder fills with urine, stretch receptors in the bladder are stimulated, sending impulses to the sacral spinal cord (S2 to S4) and the brain, triggering the urge to void. If the time to void is suitable, the brain transmits signals to nerves along the thoracolumbar (T11 to L2) and sacral spine to relax the muscles of the bladder neck, sphincter, and pelvic floor. As these muscles relax, the bladder contracts, and urine is released from the body.

If the time to void is not suitable, inhibitor impulses in the brain are stimulated. Signals are transmitted to the thoracolumbar and sacral spinal nerves to contract the muscles of the sphincter and pelvic floor, resisting increasing bladder pressure. The contraction of these muscles temporarily inhibits voiding. Typically, the urge to urinate occurs when the bladder is distended with 200 to 250 mL of urine. The average adult voids five to six times each day.

Medical conditions or trauma involving the brain, spinal cord, or nerves innervating the muscles of the bladder, sphincter, or pelvic floor can affect the normal functioning

of the bladder. This can result in a lack of continence, also called *incontinence*, and/or difficulty voiding. Such conditions include multiple sclerosis, paraplegia, quadriplegia, spina bifida, and diabetes mellitus. Medications affecting nerve pathways can also alter the functioning of the bladder. Classes of medications known to have the potential to affect bladder function include opioid pain medications, some antihypertensives, certain antidepressants, some antiemetics, and antihistamines.

Urethra

The **urethra** is a narrow muscular passage extending from the neck of the bladder to the urinary meatus, the opening at the end of the urethra through which urine exits the body. The length of the urethra varies in males and females. The average length of the male urethra is 8 to 10 in. (20.3 to 25.4 cm) long. The male urethra extends from the bladder neck through the prostate gland and continues for the length of the penis. The average female urethra is only 1 to 2 in. (2.5 to 5.1 cm) long. The short length of the female urethra allows for bacteria to more easily invade the urinary tract, explaining the increased incidence of urinary tract infections (UTIs) in females when compared with males.

The internal urethral sphincter is formed by the thickening of the detrusor muscle around the top of the urethra as it exits the bladder. The smooth muscle of this sphincter contracts, maintaining closure of the urethra to ensure that urine remains in the bladder until the time of voiding. Control of the internal urethral sphincter is involuntary. The external urethral sphincter encircles the urethra as it enters the pelvic floor. Because it is composed of skeletal muscle fibers, control of the external urethral sphincter is voluntary.

Connection Check 61.2

The nurse is caring for an older adult with intermittent urinary incontinence. The nurse recognizes that the incontinence is a result of which structure failing to contract to keep urine in the bladder until micturition?

A. The detrusor muscle
B. The external urethral sphincter
C. The urethra
D. The internal urethral sphincter

CASE STUDY: EPISODE 2

Mr. Jones has presented with complaints of decreased appetite, fatigue, 10-lb weight gain over 2 months, changes in mental status, and urinating "only small amounts of urine." Vital signs reveal that Mr. Jones is hypertensive, and his laboratory values reveal elevated BUN, creatinine, potassium, phosphorus, and decreased calcium. A physical assessment reveals a lethargic gentleman with obvious pallor and peripheral edema in his extremities.

The provider orders a renal ultrasound and a computed tomography (CT) scan to assess for obstructions within the urinary tract. Both the ultrasound and the CT scan are negative for masses or obstructions, leading the provider to diagnose Mr. Jones with renal insufficiency likely related to uncontrolled hypertension…

ASSESSMENT

History Collection

Demographics and Personal Data

Collecting a subjective patient history is a critical component of assessing the functioning of any body system. When the renal and urinary systems are evaluated, essential demographic data to be collected include gender, age, race, socioeconomic status, occupational history, and dietary and personal habits.

Because of the variations in the anatomy of the male and female urinary systems, each gender is predisposed to unique complications that should be considered and assessed. Females are more susceptible to develop UTIs than males because of the short length of the female urethra. The presence of the prostate gland in males introduces the potential for complications, including prostatitis, benign prostatic hypertrophy (BPH) or nonmalignant enlargement of the prostate gland, and prostate cancer.

Changes in the urinary system and its function occur with increasing age. Aging adults are more prone to experience problems with urination, including incontinence, urgency, frequency, nocturia, and urinary retention. Therefore, a thorough assessment of urinary elimination patterns of this patient population is essential. Aging also increases the risk of developing bladder cancer. For a further discussion of age-related changes in the renal and urinary systems, see the section titled "Age-Related Changes."

Race should also be considered because evidence has revealed an increased incidence of hypertension and diabetes mellitus in the African American population. According to the National Kidney Foundation, one out of three African American adults over the age of 65 is affected by hypertension, and more than 3 million African Americans have diabetes. Both hypertension and diabetes are precursors to the development of renal dysfunction.

Socioeconomic status should also be assessed when evaluating renal function. Research has revealed relationships among those with low socioeconomic status, low levels of education, and lack of access to healthcare and the development of chronic conditions that increase the risk of renal complications. Low socioeconomic status has also been linked with a higher incidence of bladder cancer. This may be due in part to the associations of low socioeconomic status with occupational exposure to specific chemicals and to an increased rate of smoking, factors that increase the risk of developing bladder cancer. Occupational history should be assessed because some occupations result in exposure to chemicals known to be damaging to the kidneys. Exposure to chemicals such as aromatic amines and hydrocarbons is known to increase the risk of bladder cancer. Individuals employed as textile workers, hairdressers, painters, and manufacturers of rubber and leather products have a high incidence of bladder cancer.

A thorough review of dietary intake should occur. Consumption of foods high in protein, dairy products, and salt may lead to an increased development of renal calculi. Inadequate fluid intake also increases the risk of developing UTIs, renal calculi, and even renal failure. A dietary review may also reveal changes in appetite and taste sensation that are sometimes present in patients with renal failure.

Smoking history should be assessed because smoking is the primary risk factor for the development of bladder cancer. Smokers have more than a five-fold increase in the risk of developing bladder cancer when compared with nonsmokers. Educating patients regarding the need for smoking cessation and providing them with strategies for cessation are essential responsibilities of the healthcare team, including the nurse.

Personal and Family Health History

Patients should be questioned about their overall health status. Alterations in the functioning of the renal and urinary systems can produce systemic effects. Complaints of fatigue, changes in weight, excessive thirst, and signs of fluid retention are symptoms that warrant further investigation of the functioning of the renal and urinary systems. As mentioned previously, chronic conditions such as diabetes and hypertension can compromise blood flow to and through the kidneys, resulting in renal complications. The patient should be asked about a personal history of such conditions. A personal history of neurological deficits, urological cancers, frequent UTIs, and trauma to the urinary tract should also be assessed. Because conditions such as diabetes and hypertension have a hereditary component, it is vital to assess the family history of the patient for the presence of these conditions. The family history should also be reviewed for the presence of kidney disease, urological failure, and frequent UTIs.

Because the urinary and reproductive systems are closely related, a brief sexual and reproductive history should be collected. Alterations in urinary function do not specifically alter the functioning of the reproductive system but can affect the level of self-confidence required for sexual relationships. The patient with urinary system alterations such as frequency or incontinence may find it difficult to feel pleasure in a sexual relationship because of embarrassment, fear, and lack of self-confidence. Nurses should be prepared to provide education regarding management of the urinary system alteration and to support the patient to pursue the desired sexual relationship.

Medication Use

It is essential to collect a thorough history of a patient's current and past use of over-the-counter (OTC) medications, prescription medications, vitamins, and herbal supplements. Many classes of medications are known to affect the normal functioning of the urinary system. Medications such as diuretics increase the quantity and frequency of urine output. Medications, including some chemotherapeutic agents, phenazopyridine (Pyridium), and nitrofurantoin (Macrodantin), are known to alter the color of urine. Classes of medications used to treat neurological and musculoskeletal disorders can affect the normal functioning of the muscles and nerves controlling bladder contraction and relaxation. This may lead to urinary incontinence, urinary retention, and other difficulties in voiding.

Many classes of medications are also known to be toxic to the kidneys. Such medications are termed *nephrotoxic*. See the Safety Alert for a partial list of substances with nephrotoxic potential. A patient prescribed these medications must be closely monitored for complications related to nephrotoxicity.

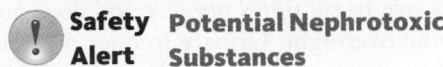

Safety Alert **Potential Nephrotoxic Substances**

Antibiotics
Acyclovir (Zovirax)
Amikacin (Amikin)
Amphotericin B (Amphocin)
Bacitracin (BACiiM)
Cephalosporins
Gentamicin (Garamycin)
Kanamycin (Kantrex)
Neomycin (Neo-Fradin)
Penicillins
Rifampin (Rifadin)
Streptomycin
Sulfonamides
Tetracycline (Vibramycin)
Tobramycin (Tobrex)
Vancomycin (Vancocin)

Analgesics
Cyclooxygenase-2 (COX-2) inhibitors
Nonsteroidal anti-inflammatory drugs (NSAIDs; e.g., aspirin, ibuprofen)
Salicylates

Other Medications
Antiretrovirals
ACE inhibitors
Benzodiazepines
Contrast media
Cyclosporine (Sandimmune)
Diuretics
Lithium (Lithobid)
Methotrexate (Rheumatrex)
Tacrolimus (Prograf)

Substances
Cocaine
Gold
Heroin
Lead
Mercury

Renal and Urinary Assessment

When specifically assessing the renal and urinary systems, question the patient regarding any changes in the appearance (clarity and color) or odor of urine, the pattern of urination, and the ability to voluntarily control voiding. A change in the color of urine may be a result of medications, overhydration, dehydration, or the presence of blood in the urine (hematuria). Urine typically smells slightly of ammonia. Changes in the odor of urine may be caused by medications, hydration status, or the presence of infectious organisms.

A patient's pattern of urination should be thoroughly assessed in regard to frequency, flow, and amount. The average adult voids five to six times per day and does not regularly need to void overnight. Urinary frequency refers to the sensation of needing to void more than normal but voiding only small amounts of urine each time. **Nocturia** describes the increased need to urinate at night. The patient should also be questioned regarding any changes in the flow of urination. **Dysuria**, pain or discomfort with urination, may indicate an obstruction or infection. Difficulty starting the flow of urine despite the sensation to void, termed *hesitancy*, may be indicative of age-related changes in the male prostate gland.

Patients typically do not know the normal quantity of their urine output. However, they can usually convey if there have been increases or decreases in the amount of urine output. Any change in the volume of urine output warrants further investigation. **Anuria** is a total urine output of less than 100 mL in 24 hours. **Oliguria** is a decreased amount of urine output, 100 to 400 mL in 24 hours. **Polyuria**

describes excess quantities of urine output. The significance of these and other urinary system abnormalities is presented in Table 61.1.

The mode by which a patient voids must also be assessed. Most patients void spontaneously; however, some patients may eliminate urine via self-catheterization or indwelling drainage devices as a result of previous alterations in the functioning of the renal and/or urinary system or other body systems. Patients requiring the use of such devices to void are at an increased risk of developing UTIs and should be closely monitored for signs and symptoms of infection.

Patients should also be questioned regarding their ability to voluntarily control voiding. Changes in the ability to voluntarily control micturition can occur with age and during pregnancy, postpartum, and postoperative recovery. A patient may report incontinence, urgency, retention, and/or hesitancy. See Table 61.1 for a description and the clinical significance of such subjective complaints.

Table 61.1 Renal and Urinary System Assessment Abnormalities

Finding	Definition	Clinical Significance of Abnormal Finding
Anuria	Less than 100-mL urine output/24 hr	End-stage renal disease, acute renal failure, urinary tract obstruction
Dysuria	Difficulty or pain with urination	Urinary tract infection, cystitis (bladder infection)
Enuresis	Involuntary urination at night	Lower urinary tract disorder
Frequency	Increase in incidence of voiding, usually urinating only small amounts with each void	Bladder inflammation, excessive fluid intake, urinary retention
Hematuria	Presence of blood in the urine	Cystitis or other inflammation in the urinary tract, calculi, cancers of the urinary tract, renal disease, bleeding disorders, medications such as anticoagulants
Hesitancy	Difficulty starting the flow of urine	Urethral obstruction, enlargement of the prostate gland (benign or malignant)
Incontinence	Inability to voluntarily control micturition	Bladder infections, trauma to the external sphincter, neurogenic bladder, trauma to the nerve innervating the urinary tract structures
Nocturia	Frequent urination at night	Heart failure, renal disease, bladder obstruction, consumption of excessive fluids late at night
Oliguria	Decreased urine output; less than 400-mL urine output/24 hr	Shock, end-stage renal disease, acute kidney injury, severe dehydration, blood transfusion reaction
Polyuria	Increased urine output; greater than 2,000-mL urine output/24 hr	Excessive fluid intake, diabetes insipidus, diabetes mellitus, diuretic medications, diuresis phase of chronic renal failure
Renal colic	Pain radiating to the perineal or groin area	Ureter spasm during passage of calculi, ureter obstruction
Retention	Inability to completely empty the bladder of urine	Normal finding briefly after childbirth, pelvic surgery, and removal of indwelling catheter
		Prolonged/abnormal related to neurogenic bladder, obstruction or stricture of the urethra
Urgency	Sudden onset of the urge to void immediately	Medications, pelvic organ prolapse, cystitis, UTI

UTI, Urinary tract infection.

Physical Examination

Following the collection of subjective data, a physical examination of the patient should occur. In addition to the specific assessment of the renal and urinary systems, physical assessment data of all body systems should also be collected. Vital signs and weight provide valuable baseline information on overall health status. A patient's mental status and level of consciousness should be noted because cognitive changes may reflect renal dysfunction. Auscultation of the lungs is also vital in assessing the body's overall fluid status.

When the renal system is assessed, the location of the kidneys can be estimated using the costovertebral angle (CVA) as a landmark. The CVA is formed by the lower border of the 12th rib and the spine. When assessing the renal and urinary systems, begin with inspection. Auscultation should follow and precedes palpation and percussion because these techniques amplify bowel sounds and diminish abdominal vascular sounds.

Inspection

Because alterations in the renal and urinary systems affect all other body systems, begin with an inspection of the skin, oral mucosa, abdomen, and extremities. Depending on subjective reports by the patient, an inspection of the urethral meatus may also be necessary. When inspecting, assess for the presence of the following abnormal changes:

Skin: poor skin turgor, rough texture, pallor, yellow-gray color, flank bruising
Mouth: ammonia breath odor, stomatitis (inflammation and ulceration of oral mucosa)
Abdomen: uneven contour, unilateral lower abdominal mass, striae (stretch marks)
Extremities: edema
Urethral meatus: bloody or purulent discharge, skin lesions or rashes, obvious tissue trauma

Auscultation

With the patient supine, auscultate over the abdominal aorta and each renal artery with the bell of the stethoscope (Fig. 61.14). When auscultating, listen for a **bruit** (a turbulent or whooshing sound produced by an increase in the volume of blood traveling through a vessel or a decrease in the diameter of a blood vessel). The presence of a bruit indicates altered blood flow to the kidneys and warrants further investigation.

Palpation

With the patient in the supine position, lightly palpate in all four abdominal quadrants. Instruct the patient to report any discomfort or tenderness upon palpation. The bladder is typically not palpable unless distended with urine. If filled with urine, the bladder is sensitive to palpation and feels round and firm.

To palpate the kidneys, position one hand under the patient's flank between the rib cage and the iliac crest (Fig. 61.15). Position the other hand over the abdomen,

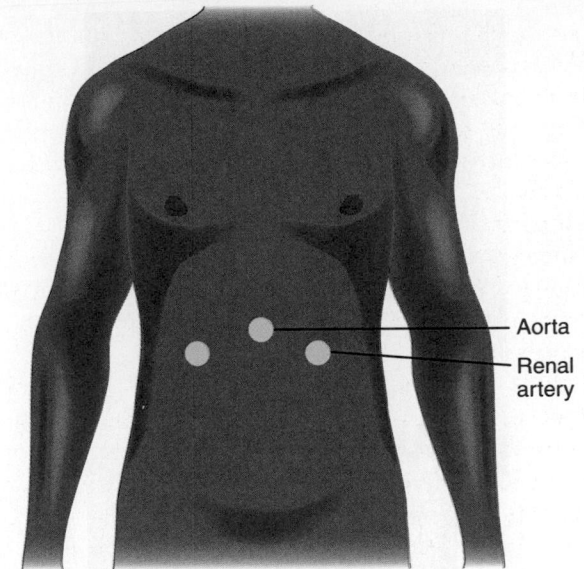

FIGURE 61.14 Auscultation of renal vessels. If a bruit is heard, it may indicate altered blood flow to the kidneys.

Aorta
Renal artery

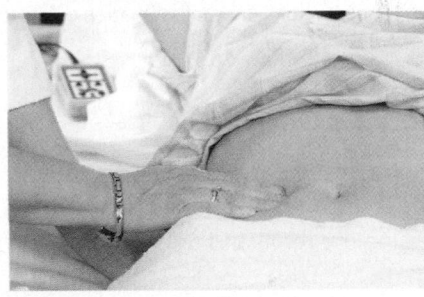

FIGURE 61.15 Palpation of the kidneys; position one hand under the patient's flank between the rib cage and the iliac crest. Position the other hand over the abdomen, just below the rib cage. Ask the patient to take a deep breath, and use your lower hand to raise the flank while the upper hand palpates.

just below the rib cage. Ask the patient to take a deep breath and use the lower hand to raise the flank while the upper hand palpates. The lower pole of the right kidneys is occasionally palpable in some patients. The left kidney is positioned deeper than the right and is typically not palpable.

Percussion

While the patient remains supine, percuss over the symphysis pubis upward toward the umbilicus. Dullness is the sound elicited over a distended bladder. A bladder containing little to no urine produces no sound upon percussion.

Assess for flank tenderness utilizing fist percussion over each kidney at the CVA (Fig. 61.16). Have the patient return to a sitting position and position yourself behind the patient. Place one hand flat over the CVA. Form a fist with the other hand and strike it against the dorsal surface of the flattened hand. This blow to the flank area should not elicit pain or tenderness. If the patient reports pain or tenderness, it is suggestive of kidney inflammation or infection.

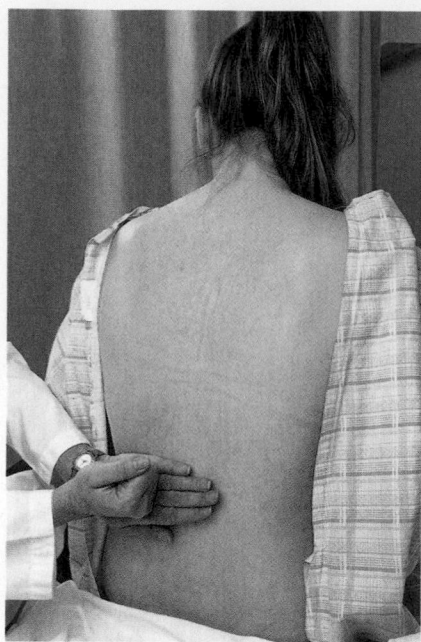

FIGURE 61.16 Percussing for costovertebral angle tenderness. Pain or tenderness is suggestive of kidney inflammation or infection.

Connection Check 61.3

The nurse is assessing a patient for a routine physical examination. Which of the following are *normal* findings when assessing the renal and urinary systems? *(Select all that apply.)*

A. Inability to palpate the kidneys
B. CVA tenderness upon percussion
C. Absence of a renal artery bruit
D. Purulent drainage from the urinary meatus
E. Tympanic sounds over an empty bladder upon percussion

DIAGNOSTIC STUDIES

A variety of diagnostic studies can be utilized to further assess the structure and function of the kidneys and urinary system. Such studies are classified as blood tests, urine tests, and radiographical tests. We present several diagnostic studies of each class throughout the following sections.

Laboratory Studies

Blood Tests

Blood tests are routinely performed to assess kidney function. The most commonly utilized blood tests include serum creatinine, BUN, and BUN/creatinine ratio. Additional values that reflect the functioning of the kidneys include uric acid and bicarbonate. Electrolyte values including sodium, potassium, phosphorus, and calcium are also monitored as a reflection of kidney function.

The patient should be educated regarding the indication for the blood test and should be informed of the results and their significance. There is no specific patient preparation required for these blood tests. Obtaining a sample of blood for the tests involves little risk to the patient. Abnormal results should be closely monitored.

Serum Creatinine

Creatinine is the end product of protein and muscle breakdown in the body. Creatinine is filtered by the kidneys and excreted into the urine. No commonly occurring medical condition other than renal dysfunction causes an increase in the serum creatinine, making it the most reliable indicator of kidney function, specifically reflecting glomerular function.

The normal range for serum creatinine in adults is 0.5 to 1.2 mg/dL. Males typically have slightly higher levels than females because of their larger muscle mass. Muscle mass and the resulting amount of creatinine produced in the body decrease with age; however, creatinine clearance also decreases, resulting in relatively stable creatinine levels in healthy aging adults. A patient with little muscle mass may present with slightly decreased creatinine levels.

An increase in the serum creatinine level does not occur until approximately 50% of the kidneys' function has been lost. Hence, any increase in the serum creatinine indicates impairment in the renal system and warrants immediate investigation and intervention. An increased creatinine level can be attributed to causes such as acute and/or chronic kidney injury or disease, cancer, diabetic nephropathy, shock, congestive heart failure, and consumption of a high-protein diet. A decreased creatinine level can be attributed to the loss of muscle mass or certain medications, including some classes of antibiotics (e.g., aminoglycosides and cephalosporins) and lithium carbonate.

Blood Urea Nitrogen

Urea nitrogen is a by-product of protein metabolism that occurs in the liver. The kidneys are responsible for filtering it from the blood. Serum BUN is a measure of the renal excretion of urea nitrogen.

The normal range for BUN in adults is 8 to 21 mg/dL. Increased BUN can occur not only in cases of renal dysfunction but also with liver disease, dehydration, infection, consumption of a high-protein diet, GI bleeding, steroid use, and trauma. Decreased BUN can be indicative of severe liver damage, malnutrition, consumption of a low-protein diet, or fluid volume excess. An elevated BUN is not diagnostic of renal dysfunction but certainly indicates it as a possibility. The hydration status of the patient should also be considered when interpreting the results of serum BUN. Serum creatinine should also be assessed in a patient with an elevated BUN.

Blood Urea Nitrogen/Creatinine Ratio

A BUN/creatinine ratio can be utilized to assess if the cause of elevated BUN is renal or nonrenal in nature. The normal ratio of BUN to creatinine is in the range of 10:1 to 20:1. In cases of hypovolemia or hypotension, the serum BUN rises more quickly than the serum creatinine level. This results in an increased ratio of BUN to creatinine. Likewise, a decreased ratio can occur in instances of fluid volume excess. When both the BUN and creatinine levels are increased and the ratio remains normal, renal dysfunction is likely.

Uric Acid

Purines are compounds that naturally occur in cells of the body and are also taken into the body in dietary sources (e.g., organ meats, anchovies, sardines, shellfish, asparagus, beans, mushrooms, spinach). Uric acid is formed as a by-product of purine metabolism. Excess uric acid is then excreted into the urine. Uric acid values are dependent upon kidney function, the rate of purine metabolism, and dietary intake of foods containing purines.

Normal uric acid values for adults are in the range of 3.5 to 8 mg/dL. Values greater than 12 mg/dL are critical and warrant immediate intervention. Excess uric acid is termed *hyperuricemia*. It can result in the development of gout—inflammatory arthritis that is caused by uric acid crystals in the joints and in severe cases can cause renal damage. Increased uric acid can occur as a result of renal failure, multiple myeloma, malnutrition, leukemia, lymphoma, metastatic cancers, and alcoholism. Some medications, including acetaminophen (Tylenol), furosemide (Lasix), and aspirin, are also known to cause hyperuricemia when used long term.

Decreased uric acid can occur as a result of burns, pregnancy, folic acid anemia, and Wilson's disease. Medications such as allopurinol (Zyloprim), Rasburicase (Elitek), azathioprine (Imuran), and warfarin (Coumadin) are known to decrease uric acid levels.

Bicarbonate

Bicarbonate values are typically reported as a component of arterial blood gas results. Bicarbonate ions (HCO_3-) are alkaline and serve as buffers in the bloodstream to maintain pH in the normal range of 7.35 to 7.45. The kidneys regulate the concentration of HCO_3- in the blood by altering the rate of excretion and production of the ions on the basis of serum pH. Because the ions are alkaline, an increase in the amount of bicarbonate ions increases the serum pH, resulting in metabolic alkalosis. Likewise, a decrease in the amount of HCO_3- lowers the serum pH, resulting in a state of metabolic acidosis.

The normal range for bicarbonate in adults is 22 to 26 mEq/L. Increases in bicarbonate levels can occur as a result of severe vomiting or gastric suctioning, excess loss of potassium, or excess administration of bicarbonate. A decrease in bicarbonate levels can occur in renal failure as the kidneys lose their ability to produce HCO_3- to buffer the blood. Decreased bicarbonate levels can also occur as a result of diabetic ketoacidosis, severe diarrhea, malnutrition, and burns.

Electrolytes

The serum concentrations of several electrolytes are regulated in part by the kidneys. Therefore, these electrolyte values can be examined as a reflection of the functioning of the kidneys.

Sodium (Na^+) is the primary cation in the ECF. Sodium exhibits water-retaining effects. In adults, the normal range for sodium is 135 to 145 mEq/L. In the late stages of renal failure, a patient's sodium balance can be altered as fluids accumulate in the body because of the kidneys' decreasing ability to filter and excrete properly.

The kidneys are responsible for excreting the majority of the body's K^+ and maintaining it in the narrow range of 3.5 to 5.0 mEq/L. Potassium is typically one of the first electrolyte values to reflect an alteration in kidney function. As kidney function declines, potassium values typically increase above the normal level, termed *hyperkalemia*. Hyperkalemia can lead to cardiac dysrhythmias and therefore requires immediate recognition and intervention.

Phosphorus (PO_4) is the primary anion in the ICF. The significant majority of phosphorus in the body exists as phosphate and is found along with calcium in the bones and teeth. Phosphorus and calcium are inversely related, meaning that as one increases, the other decreases. The normal range for phosphorus in adults is 2.5 to 4.5 mEq/L. Because the kidneys are responsible for excreting phosphorus from the body, as kidney function decreases, the phosphorus levels increase. This is known as hyperphosphatemia.

Calcium is the main mineral in teeth and bones. As noted earlier, in cases of declining kidney function, calcium levels decrease (hypocalcemia) as phosphate levels increase. The normal range for calcium in adults is 8.2 to 10.2 mg/dL. Hypocalcemia also occurs as kidney function declines because the kidneys are unable to produce quantities of vitamin D sufficient for calcium to be absorbed from the GI tract.

Urine Tests

Various urine tests can be utilized to assess the functioning of the renal and urinary systems. The most commonly performed urine tests include bedside urine dipsticks, urinalysis, culture and sensitivity, composite urine collection, creatinine clearance, and urine cytology.

Bedside Urine Dipsticks

Urine can be tested at the bedside to assess the specific gravity; the pH; and the presence of protein, glucose, bilirubin, blood, and ketones. This testing method can provide the healthcare team with current information that may be needed to direct immediate treatment decisions for a patient. Commercially available dipsticks include a color-coded chart corresponding to a grading scale to be used when interpreting results. To yield accurate results, a fresh sample should be used for testing, and the dipsticks should be stored in a dry, sealed container. Follow institution policy and manufacturer guidelines for performing dipstick testing and reporting results.

Urinalysis

A urinalysis provides an overall examination of urine to provide baseline data or to monitor specific characteristics of the urine. The most precise urinalysis results are obtained by collecting urine from the patient's first void of the day.

To obtain accurate urinalysis results, the sample should be sent to the laboratory within 1 hour of collection. If not analyzed within an hour, RBCs hemolyze, bacteria multiply, casts disintegrate, and the pH becomes increasingly alkaline. Although not ideal, if the sample cannot be sent to the laboratory within 1 hour, it should be refrigerated until it can be sent.

Urinalysis results include data on multiple characteristics and components of the urine. These characteristics and components are briefly examined in the following subsections. The normal range of findings and the significance of abnormal findings in adults are outlined in Table 61.2.

Color, Turbidity, and Odor

Some basic information about the urine can be gleaned simply by observing the urine. Urine should appear yellow in color because of the pigment urochrome. The range of the yellow color varies depending on hydration status. Urine should appear clear, without turbidity (cloudiness). Normal urine smells faintly like ammonia but should not smell foul.

Specific Gravity

The specific gravity is a measure of the concentration of solutes contained in the urine. It reflects the ability of the kidneys to concentrate and dilute the urine effectively.

Table 61.2 Normal Urinalysis Results and Significance of Abnormal Findings

Component	Normal Findings for Adults	Clinical Significance of Abnormal Findings
Color	Pale yellow	*Clear or pale* indicates dilute urine related to excess fluid intake. *Dark amber* indicates concentrated urine related to dehydration and presence of bilirubin. *Red/brown* indicates blood, myoglobin, or bilirubin in urine. *Other colors* may occur as a result of foods or medications.
Turbidity	Clear	*Cloudy* indicates the presence of bacteria, pus related to infection, or sediment.
Odor	Faint odor of ammonia	*Foul* indicates the presence of bacteria related to infection, dehydration, or the effects of some foods and medications.
Specific gravity	1.005–1.030	*Increase* indicates diabetes mellitus, dehydration, or fever. *Decrease* indicates renal insufficiency, diabetes insipidus, or diuretic use.
Osmolality	250–900 mOsm/kg (24-hr collection)	*Increase* indicates diabetes mellitus, dehydration, or fever. *Decrease* indicates renal insufficiency, diabetes insipidus, or diuretic use.
pH	4.5–8	*Altered* indicates changes in renal function, infection, or certain medications and can also be related to the freshness of the sample.
Protein	2–8 mg/dL	*Increase* indicates stress, strenuous exercise, fever, septicemia, lead, mercury, or high-protein diet. *Persistently increased* indicates acute or chronic renal disease.
Glucose	Negative	*Presence* indicates undiagnosed or uncontrolled diabetes mellitus or decreased renal threshold for glucose.
Ketones	Negative	*Presence* indicates diabetic ketoacidosis, high-protein diet, or anorexia nervosa.
Bilirubin	Negative	*Presence* indicates hepatic biliary obstruction or liver disease.
Red blood cells (RBCs)	0–4/ (hpf)	*Slight increase* is normal with presence of an indwelling urinary catheter or during menstruation. *Significant increase* indicates bleeding disorders, cystitis, tumor, calculi, or trauma.
White blood cells (WBCs)	0–5/hpf	*Increase* indicates presence of inflammation, urinary infection, or fever.
Casts	Few or none	*Increase* indicates the presence of bacteria, kidney disease, or urinary calculi.
Bacteria	Less than 1,000 colonies/mL	*Increase* indicates possibility of UTI or contamination during sample collection.

hpf, High-powered field; *UTI*, urinary tract infection.

Osmolality

Osmolality provides further information regarding the concentration of solutes in the urine. It is a more precise measure of the kidneys' ability to concentrate and dilute the urine than specific gravity.

pH

The normal range for urine pH is wide and is affected by many factors. A pH value of 7.0 is neutral, so less than 7.0 is acidic, and a pH value greater than 7.0 is alkaline.

Protein

Proteins are not typically contained in the urine because they are large and are not permitted to cross intact glomerular membranes. The presence of protein in the urine is termed *proteinuria*. Transient conditions such as infection and inflammation increase the permeability of the glomerular membrane, allowing some protein molecules to enter the urine. When proteinuria is identified in such cases, subsequent urinalyses should be obtained after resolution of the infection or inflammation to ensure that the urine is then negative for proteins. Proteinuria that persists indicates abnormalities in glomerular filtration and requires further assessment.

Glucose

Glucose does not appear in the urine until the renal threshold has been reached at serum glucose levels of approximately 200 mg/dL. At glucose levels less than 220 mg/dL, the PCT of the nephron can reabsorb glucose, and none is present in the urine.

Ketones

The partial metabolism of fatty acids in the body produces ketones. Normally, there are no ketones contained in the urine. In situations when fat is burned as energy in place of glucose, as in diabetes, ketones are produced and are present in the urine.

Bilirubin

Bilirubin is formed during the breakdown of hemoglobin and is not typically present in the urine. Bilirubin in the urine, bilirubinuria, causes the urine to appear dark amber to brown in color.

Red Blood Cells

Red blood cells are not normally present in the urine and are indicative of bleeding within the renal and/or urinary system. The presence and number of RBCs are assessed using microscopic examination.

White Blood Cells

Small numbers of white blood cells (WBCs) can be present in urine samples because of perineal contamination during voiding. The presence and number of WBCs are assessed using microscopic examination.

Casts

Casts are molds formed around the outside of particles such as RBCs, WCBs, proteins, or bacteria. They are not present in the absence of these particles. Casts are often described by the particle they surround (e.g., RBC cast, WBC cast). Casts are also assessed by microscopic examination.

Bacteria

Urine can easily be contaminated during collection, so the presence of bacteria in a urinalysis does not definitely confirm a UTI. If urinalysis results indicate an increased presence of bacteria, a urine culture should be obtained to confirm the diagnosis and to isolate the infectious organism.

Culture and Sensitivity

Culturing urine is useful to identify the number and type(s) of bacteria present. Sensitivity testing involves combining bacteria isolated in the urine with various classes of antibiotic medications to determine which are most effective at stopping the multiplication of the bacteria. Culture and sensitivity testing provides healthcare professionals with data useful when planning the best course of treatment for UTIs. Careful medication selection is crucial because medication resistance has become an increasing problem in managing UTIs and many other infections.

Urine to be tested for culture and sensitivity should be collected using a clean-catch technique (Box 61.1) and should be placed in a sterile specimen container. This ensures that the bacteria identified are not present because of contamination of the urine sample. It typically takes 48 to 72 hours to isolate any bacteria present. Bacteria commonly

---

Box 61.1 Patient Education: Collecting a Clean-Catch Urine Sample

Clean-catch urine samples are required for urine cultures to ensure that any bacteria found in the urine are not there as a result of contamination. Patients should be instructed to complete the following steps to provide a clean-catch sample:

1. Wash hands.
2. Remove cap from sterile specimen container, ensuring not to touch the inside of the lid or container.
3. <u>Males</u>: Use enclosed towelette(s) to wipe the head of the penis.
   <u>Females</u>: Spread the labia with one hand and use the other hand to wipe from front to back with the enclosed towelette(s).
4. Begin urinating a small amount into the toilet. Without stopping the flow of urine, place the cup into the stream of urine and collect enough urine to fill the cup. Finish urinating into the toilet.
5. Securely attach the cap onto the sterile container, ensuring not to touch the inside of the lid or container.

isolated in culture samples include *Escherichia coli*, enterococci, *Klebsiella*, and streptococci.

Composite Urine Collection

Composite urine collection involves collecting all urine voided for a defined period of time ranging between 2 and 24 hours. Such specimens can be used to measure the quantity of specific components of the urine including electrolytes, minerals, creatinine, protein, and glucose. Collection begins by discarding the first voided urine of the time period. All other urine should be saved, and the sample should be refrigerated or kept on ice for the duration of collection. At the completion of the collection period, the patient is asked to void, and the final urine should be added to the sample. All urine must be saved to ensure the accuracy of the results.

Creatinine Clearance

Creatinine clearance testing of the urine is a type of composite urine collection. This test is a reliable indicator of GFR. Creatinine clearance measures the amount of creatinine excreted from the body during a defined time period. Urine is typically collected for 24 hours, but shorter collection periods may also be ordered. A blood sample testing for creatinine is required and can be obtained at any point during the urine collection period. The urine and blood samples are compared, and the creatinine clearance is calculated using one of several established mathematical formulas. Creatinine clearance is sometimes used to ensure adequate dosing of medications. The normal range for creatinine clearance in adults is 88 to 137 mL/min. Values are generally slightly lower in females than males. Decreased creatinine clearance occurs as a result of renal impairment and as a result of muscle wasting.

Urine Cytology

Urine collected for cytological examination is used to identify any abnormal cells present in the urine. Abnormal cells are often present in the urine with bladder cancer. For this reason, examination of the urine is used as a diagnostic tool and a treatment marker in patients with bladder cancer. A urine sample other than the first void of the day should be collected and sent to the laboratory for microscopic analysis within 1 hour of collection.

Imaging Studies

A variety of radiographical studies are available to examine the renal and urinary systems. Regardless of the study, nursing responsibilities include patient education, patient preparation, and monitoring for complications during and after the study. The patient should be educated on indications for the study, preparation for the study, what to expect during the study, possible complications, and any required follow-up care.

Many radiographical studies require the patient to complete bowel preparation the evening prior to the procedure. This eliminates feces and flatus in the bowel so that the view of the urinary tract is not obstructed by a distended colon. Agents commonly used for bowel preparation include enemas, magnesium citrate, bisacodyl (Dulcolax), and castor oil. Bowel preparation agents such as Fleet enemas and magnesium citrate should be used cautiously in patients with known renal dysfunction. Patients may also be instructed to take in nothing by mouth (NPO status) for an ordered period of time prior to the procedure.

Bedside Sonography

Portable ultrasound scanners provide a noninvasive means of estimating the volume of urine contained in the bladder. This technology can be used to assess for the presence of urine remaining in the bladder after voiding (postvoid residual) or to determine if there is a need for intermittent catheterization in a patient who is not independently voiding. This study can be completed at the bedside independently by the nurse. It requires no preparation of the patient and results in no discomfort or risk to the patient.

Conductive gel is placed over the symphysis pubis, and the probe is positioned above the pubic bone, pointing downward toward the coccyx. Bedside scanners are typically equipped with icons that indicate the accuracy of the probe placement. The scanner displays the estimated volume of urine contained in the bladder. For the most accurate results, the scan should be completed twice, and the results should be averaged. Large volumes of urine in the bladder following voiding or in a patient who is unable to spontaneously void indicate the need for catheterization.

X-ray

An x-ray of the kidneys, ureters, and bladder (KUB) is a simple abdominal x-ray taken with the patient lying in the supine position. It reveals the size and anatomy of the renal and urinary system structures and can also reveal masses, obstructions, and calculi within the kidneys and urinary tract. The test requires no preparation of the patient and results in no discomfort or significant risk to the patient. If possible, x-rays should be avoided during pregnancy.

Intravenous Urography

Intravenous urography is also termed *IV pyelography*. This test requires the administration of radiographical dye (contrast) via an IV line with the patient in the supine position. The contrast is circulated within the venous blood and upon reaching the kidneys is filtered by the glomeruli and is then excreted in the urine. Following the injection of dye, x-rays are performed at specific time intervals. A final x-ray is taken after the patient voids to measure the volume of any residual urine in the bladder. Intravenous urography reveals the size and anatomy of the KUB as well as any tumors, cysts, calculi, and obstructions within the urinary tract.

Nursing Implications
Preprocedure

- Instruct the patient to complete bowel preparation the evening prior to the procedure and to remain NPO for approximately 8 hours prior. Before the procedure, the nurse should confirm that the patient has completed the bowel preparation as ordered and has remained NPO for the prescribed time.

- Instruct the patient that the study lasts approximately 30 to 45 minutes and results in no discomfort. The patient should be told that he or she may feel a brief flushing sensation of the body and a salty taste in the mouth during the injection of the contrast.
- Ensure signed informed consent has been obtained after education regarding the indication and potential risks of the procedure
- Assess the patient's baseline serum creatinine prior to the study because of the nephrotoxic potential of the contrast. Caution should occur when utilizing contrast in patients of increased age and those with known renal dysfunction.
- Question the patient regarding any allergies to the contrast dye to be injected during the procedure. See the Safety Alert for patients receiving IV contrast.

Postprocedure
- Instruct the patient to increase fluid intake following the study to ensure adequate excretion of the contrast.
- Monitor the patient for changes in urine output, irritation at the IV site, and delayed signs of reaction to the contrast (e.g., rash, dyspnea, tachycardia). If there is a concern for changes in renal function related to the contrast, subsequent serum creatinine laboratory tests may be ordered.

> **⚠ Safety Alert** **Nursing considerations for patients receiving IV contrast for radiographical studies:**
>
> - Confirm the presence of signed informed consent.
> - Assess patient for a history of allergies to contrast, iodine, and shellfish.
>   - Patients with a history of these allergies may be premedicated with steroids.
> - Confirm the presence of emergency medications and equipment at the bedside.
> - Review baseline serum creatinine as evidence of renal function.
> - Review patient history for the presence of renal dysfunction.
> - Educate the patient regarding the flushing sensation and salty taste he or she may notice during contrast administration.
> - Ensure the patency of the IV.
> - Assess the patient for signs of a delayed reaction to contrast (e.g., rash, dyspnea, tachycardia)
> - Ensure that the patient increases fluid intake following the study.
> - If warranted, monitor subsequent serum creatinine laboratory values.

Renal Ultrasound

A renal ultrasound can be utilized to identify masses, cysts, and obstructions within the kidneys. Conductive gel is applied to the patient's skin, and an external probe is moved across the abdomen. Ultrasound images are produced as sound waves enter the body and are reflected back. The patient is exposed to no radiation, and the technology is noninvasive, making it a safe procedure with no risk to the patient. Ultrasound can be used to determine kidney size. Kidneys that are smaller than normal may be reflective of chronic kidney disease, and kidneys that are larger than normal may be reflective of a polycystic process or an obstruction. Ultrasound technology can also be used to differentiate between renal cysts and tumors. The patient may be ordered to drink up to 24 oz of fluid 1 hour prior to the study without voiding until completion of the ultrasound. No other preparation of the patient is required. There is no specific monitoring required during or following the study.

Computed Tomography

A CT scan produces three-dimensional images of the renal and urinary system structures as well as the surrounding tissues. Although not commonly a first-line diagnostic test, a CT scan may be used to further examine findings from studies such as x-rays or ultrasounds. Unlike ultrasounds, CT scans are capable of detecting slight variances in densities, providing more specific diagnostic results related to kidney size, tumors or other masses, renal vessels, and obstruction.

Nursing Implications
Preprocedure
- Instruct the patient to remain NPO for several hours prior to the procedure if required by the institution.
- Ensure signed informed consent has been obtained after education regarding the indication and potential risks of the procedure. Patient education includes the requirement to lay completely still while the scanner rotates around the body. If the patient is anxious or unable to follow such instructions, sedation or anxiolytic agents may be required. The scan lasts approximately 10 to 15 minutes.
- Assess allergies and baseline renal function because CT scans can be performed with or without IV contrast. Contrast may be withheld in a patient with known renal dysfunction.

Magnetic Resonance Imaging

Magnetic resonance imaging (MRI) varies from x-rays and CT scans in its use of magnetic forces rather than ionizing radiation to produce images for diagnostic testing. Magnetic resonance imaging is known for its ability to reveal contrasts between soft tissues of the body. For this reason, it is useful in examining the tissue of the kidneys to assess for abnormalities.

Nursing Implications

Preprocedure

- Educate the patient:
  - The procedure is painless but can last for up to 90 minutes.
  - Remove any metal objects, including jewelry, removable metal dental devices, hearing aids, glasses, and body piercings.
  - The machinery used for MRI is a cylinder surrounded by a large magnet. The patient lies on a moveable examination table and is slowly guided through the cylinder.
  - A patient with known claustrophobia or a patient who is unable to lie still for other reasons may require sedation or anxiolytic medications prior to the MRI. Open MRI equipment is available for use in patients who are claustrophobic, obese, or unable to lie still for other reasons.
- Ensure signed informed consent has been obtained after education regarding the indication and potential risks of the procedure.
- Assess for the presence of pacemakers and some other types of implanted medical devices because MRI is contraindicated in patients with these devices present.
- Assess allergies and baseline renal function because MRI is infrequently performed with IV contrast.

Cystography and Urethrography

Diagnostic tests utilizing cystography are termed *cystograms*. For this procedure, contrast dye is injected into the bladder via a urinary catheter or a cystoscope, and a thin, lighted instrument is inserted into the urethra and slowly advanced into the bladder. Cystography can be used to assess the bladder for abnormalities, including calculi and masses. It can also be used to examine the bladder if trauma is suspected. A similar test can be performed to assess for trauma to the urethra and is termed a *urethrogram*. A specific type of this diagnostic test, a voiding cystourethrogram (VCUG) can also be performed to determine if vesicoureteral reflux is present. A VCUG requires the patient to void after the bladder is filled with contrast while x-rays are taken. If reflux is present, urine is backflowing from the bladder into the ureters and/or kidneys, increasing the patient's risk of developing kidney infections.

Nursing Implications

Preprocedure

- Educate the patient regarding the indication and risks of the procedure. The insertion and use of the urinary catheter or cystoscope should be thoroughly explained.
- Ensure that informed consent has been obtained.
- Assess for allergies to contrast, iodine, and shellfish. Because the contrast does not enter the bloodstream, there is no danger of nephrotoxicity.

Postprocedure

- Monitor the patient for signs and symptoms of infection because the instrumentation used increases the risk of infection.
- Educate the patient on signs and symptoms of infection and adequacy of urine output once discharged.

Arteriography

Arteriography, or angiography, involves visualizing the renal vasculature to assess for strictures, bleeding, renovascular hypertension, and other vascular abnormalities. An arteriogram requires placement of a catheter into the femoral artery. The catheter is then advanced to the level of the renal arteries, and IV contrast is injected to highlight any vascular abnormalities.

Nursing Implications

Preprocedure

- Educate the patient regarding the indication of the study and its potential risks; also, educate the patient about the bowel preparation that should occur the evening prior to the angiogram and the need to remain NPO after midnight.
- Ensure that signed informed consent has been obtained.
- Assess for allergies to contrast, iodine, and shellfish. See the related Safety Alert for further nursing considerations related to the use of IV contrast for radiographical studies.

Postprocedure

- Apply manual pressure to the femoral site following removal of the femoral catheter until the bleeding has stopped. A pressure dressing should then be placed over the site, and the nurse should assess the site frequently per institutional policy for bleeding.
- Monitor vital signs frequently.
- Monitor color, temperature, and pulses distal to the femoral site every 30 to 60 minutes to assess for signs of the development of a thrombus or hematoma, which can occlude distal blood flow.
- Instruct the patient to lie with the affected leg straight for the prescribed time, usually 8 to 12 hours.

Renography (Kidney Scan)

A kidney scan is an additional diagnostic test that can be utilized to assess renal blood flow. A radionuclide is injected intravenously and is absorbed by the kidney tissue. An external probe is then placed over the kidney to detect radiation emissions. Images of the kidney are produced by these emissions. The study is useful in determining kidney size, general blood flow through the kidneys, glomerular and tubular filtration, and urinary excretion. Signed informed consent should be obtained following patient education about the indications and risks of the study. A kidney scan requires no specific patient preparation or monitoring during or after the procedure.

Renal Biopsy

A renal biopsy involves removing a tissue sample via a small percutaneous (through the skin and other tissue) site using CT or ultrasound guidance while the patient is sedated and lying in the prone position. Renal biopsies are useful in ruling out malignant processes and diagnosing renal abnormalities that have not been successfully diagnosed with other diagnostic tests.

Nursing Implications

Preprocedure

- Educate the patient regarding the procedure and its associated risks.
- Ensure that a signed informed consent has been obtained.
- Ensure that the patient has been NPO for 4 to 6 hours prior to the procedure and has stopped taking aspirin, warfarin (Coumadin), and other agents that may affect the ability of the blood to clot normally prior to the procedure.
- Send a type and screen and coagulation laboratory values, including a platelet count, prothrombin time, and activated partial thromboplastin time, to the laboratory prior to the study because of the risk of bleeding.
- Obtain baseline vital signs and monitor vital signs frequently during the biopsy.

Postprocedure

- Apply manual pressure to the site until bleeding has stopped. A pressure dressing should then be applied, and the nurse should monitor the site frequently per institutional policy for bleeding.
- Assess hematocrit and hemoglobin levels postprocedure because bleeding can sometimes occur internally with no external indications. Signs of internal bleeding include flank pain, decreased urine output, decreased blood pressure, and other signs of hypovolemia and shock.
- Assure the patient remains on bedrest for up to 24 hours following the renal biopsy.
- Educate the patient regarding the following:
  - Some local discomfort may occur at the site of the biopsy, but pain radiating to the abdomen and flank should be reported.

- Increase fluid intake following the biopsy to prevent clot formation in the urinary tract, which could obstruct the flow of urine.
- The most common complication following a renal biopsy is hematuria. This typically resolves within 48 to 72 hours following the procedure. Inform the patient that within this time period, hematuria is an expected finding, but notify the healthcare provider of hematuria occurring beyond 72 hours after the procedure. The patient should also be told to notify the provider of the presence of clots in the urine or any difficulties with voiding.
- Avoid heavy lifting for 1 week following the procedure.
- Do not resume taking anticoagulant medications until instructed by the healthcare provider.

Cystoscopy

Cystoscopy is a surgical procedure utilized to diagnose and/or treat bladder problems. A cystoscope is a tubular, lighted device that is inserted through the urethra while the patient is sedated and in the lithotomy position. As a diagnostic tool, it can be used to assess for bladder trauma, urethral trauma, or urinary tract obstructions. Cystoscopy can also be used to remove an enlarged prostate gland, bladder tumors, or renal calculi. Cystoscopy can be performed utilizing local or general anesthesia.

Nursing Implications

Preprocedure

- Educate the patient regarding the indication of the study and its potential risks; also, educate the patient about the bowel preparation that should occur the evening prior to the cystoscopy and the need to remain NPO after midnight.
- Ensure that signed informed consent has been obtained.
- Assess baseline vital signs before the administration of anesthesia and at frequent intervals throughout and immediately following the procedure.

Postprocedure

- Assess urine volume to ensure adequate output.
- Educate the patient regarding the following:
  - Expected findings following cystoscopy include urinary frequency and pink-tinged urine. Gross bleeding and/or clots in the urine are not normal and should be reported to the healthcare provider.
  - Mild analgesics and topical measures such as warm, moist heat and sitz baths may be used to manage the discomfort following the procedure.
  - Monitor for signs and symptoms of infection (e.g., fever, chills, dysuria) and report these to the healthcare provider immediately should they occur

Connection Check 61.5

The nurse is caring for a patient receiving IV contrast for a renal CT scan. Nursing responsibilities related to the administration of IV contrast include which of the following? *(Select all that apply.)*

A. To assess for allergies to contrast, iodine, and seafood prior to the study

B. To educate the patient to increase fluid intake following the study

C. To obtain an order for NPO status following the study

D. To ensure that IV contrast is administered only through a central line

E. To assess the patient's baseline creatinine value prior to the study

AGE-RELATED CHANGES

The renal and urinary systems undergo many changes with increasing age. Both systems experience anatomical and physiological changes that are reflected as changes in subjective and objective assessment findings and laboratory results (see Geriatric/Gerontological Considerations). Although baseline renal function may remain stable with age, the kidneys are less tolerant of insult. Therefore, damage to the kidneys caused by disease processes or medications can be much more significant in the geriatric population.

Geriatric/Gerontological Considerations

Renal and Urinary System Age-Related Changes and Assessment Findings

- Kidneys decrease in size → Kidneys less palpable on examination
- Number of nephrons decreases, nephrons lose functioning, glomerular membrane thickens → ↓GFR, ↑BUN and creatinine
- Blood flow to kidneys decreases → ↓GFR, ↑BUN and creatinine
- Changes in loop of Henle → Decreased ability to concentrate urine, decreased effect of ADH and aldosterone, urinary frequency, risk for dehydration
- Loss of muscle tone and elasticity → Risk for urinary incontinence
- Decreased bladder capacity → Urinary frequency, urgency, incontinence
- Enlargement of prostate gland → Urinary hesitancy, frequency, straining, slow urine stream, urinary retention

ADH, Antidiuretic hormone; *BUN,* blood urea nitrogen; *GFR,* glomerular filtration rate.

The kidneys decrease in mass by up to 10% each decade starting at approximately age 50. The number of glomeruli also begins to decline around the age of 50. The decreased number of glomeruli coupled with the thickening of the glomerular membrane results in decreased filtering capacity. It is estimated that by the seventh decade of life, between 30% and 50% of glomeruli have lost their function. This is typically manifested as a decrease in GFR and sometimes an increase in BUN and creatinine levels. By approximately age 65, the GFR of an otherwise healthy adult is 65 mL/min, half of the normal value for GFR. The GFR decreases more rapidly in adults with chronic conditions that affect the kidneys, such as diabetes mellitus and hypertension. The decrease in GFR affects the speed at which the kidneys are able to eliminate medications from the body. Therefore, GFR is an important consideration when planning the dosage and administration schedules of many medications in the geriatric population.

Blood flow to the kidneys also decreases with age. This decrease in blood flow is intensified in the presence of alterations in the vascular system such as atherosclerosis and hypertension, which are often associated with aging. Decreased blood flow to the kidneys also contributes to the decrease in the GFR.

Changes in the functioning of the loop of Henle and the kidney tubules coupled with a decrease in the effectiveness of ADH and aldosterone result in a decreased ability to concentrate the urine. Consequentially, the aging adult produces less-concentrated urine and experiences more frequent urination. These factors explain the common finding of nocturnal polyuria in the geriatric population. The total water content of the body also decreases with age. The decreased effect of ADH and the production of less concentrated urine place the aging adult at an increased risk for dehydration.

The structures of the urinary system also undergo changes related to increasing age. In females, the bladder, vagina, and pelvic floor muscles lose tone and elasticity, which contributes to an increased occurrence of urinary incontinence. This can be further intensified in women who previously lost muscle tone and elasticity during pregnancy and childbirth.

The capacity of the bladder in both sexes decreases with age by up to 50%. This results in the need for more frequent urination and increased occurrence of urinary urgency and, at times, urinary incontinence.

A majority of men experience changes in their urination patterns related to enlargement of the prostate gland. Enlargement of the prostate gland not related to a malignant process such as cancer is termed *benign prostatic hypertrophy* (BPH). Benign prostatic hypertrophy causes the urethra to be compressed and results in urinary hesitancy, frequency, straining to urinate, slow urine stream, and urinary retention (BPH is discussed in Chapter 66).

As a whole, aging adults experience a higher incidence of UTIs. Urinary tract infections are the most common bacterial infection in the geriatric population. In women, the increased incidence can be partially attributed to age-related changes in the pH of vaginal secretions that make the environment more conducive to bacterial growth. In men, alterations in the flow of urine related to BPH can alter the ability of bacteria to be eliminated efficiently from the urinary tract. The increased occurrence of urinary retention in both sexes results in higher-than-normal postvoid residuals, which may also explain the increased incidence of UTIs in the geriatric population.

Connection Check 61.6

The nurse caring for an 86-year-old female patient who presents with nocturnal polyuria incorporates which priority nursing diagnosis into the plan of care?
A. Risk for deficient fluid volume
B. Risk for sleep deprivation
C. Risk for excess fluid volume
D. Risk for urge urinary incontinence

Making Connections

CASE STUDY: WRAP-UP

At the completion of a thorough health history, physical assessment, and collection of laboratory studies, the following pertinent data have been collected:

- 72-year-old African American male
- Decreased appetite, fatigue, 10-lb weight gain over 2 months, changes in mental status, urinates "only small amounts of urine"
- Personal medical history: "borderline hypertension"
- BP 188/92 mm Hg, HR 94 bpm, R 22, T 98.2°F (36.8°C), O_2 saturation 94% on room air
- Follows commands, yet appears lethargic; +2 nonpitting, bilateral pedal edema; pallor with poor skin turgor
- Creatinine: 1.8 mg/dL
- BUN: 40 mg/dL
- BUN/creatinine ratio: 15:1
- Potassium: 5.5 mEq/L
- Phosphorus: 3.9 mEq/L
- Calcium: 8.2 mg/dL

Mr. Jones is admitted to a medical unit for further monitoring and treatment of hypertension and his newly diagnosed renal insufficiency.

Case Study Questions

1. The nurse has received the following provider orders for Mr. Jones, who was recently admitted to the medical unit. Which order should the nurse plan to implement first?
   A. Administer 40 mg furosemide (Lasix) IV daily.
   B. Implement fluid restriction less than 1,500 mL/24 hr.
   C. Monitor urine specific gravity with each void.
   D. Instruct patient to follow a low-sodium diet.

2. The provider orders a basic metabolic panel to be drawn 12 hours after Mr. Jones's admission. When the results are reported, the nurse recognizes that which of the following laboratory values should be reported to the provider most urgently?
   A. Creatinine 1.9 mg/dL
   B. Calcium 8.0 mg/dL
   C. Potassium 5.7 mEq/L
   D. Phosphorus 4.2 mEq/L

3. The nurse caring for Mr. Jones should implement which of the following priority nursing interventions? *(Select all that apply.)*
   A. Strict monitoring of intake and output
   B. Frequent monitoring of vital signs
   C. Administer supplemental oxygen
   D. Safety/fall precautions
   E. Obtain daily weights

4. The nurse caring for Mr. Jones incorporates which of the following priority nursing diagnoses into the plan of care?
   A. Risk for falls
   B. Risk for imbalanced fluid volume
   C. Impaired urinary elimination
   D. Readiness for enhanced knowledge

5. Which statement by Mr. Jones indicates that the discharge teaching by the nurse has been effective?
   A. "I should carefully monitor and record my weight each day."
   B. "If I am feeling well, I do not have to take my blood pressure medications regularly."
   C. "If I have aches and pains, I should take over-the-counter Motrin."
   D. "I should try to increase the amount of potassium I take in by eating at least one banana every day."

CHAPTER SUMMARY

The renal system is composed of two kidneys. The functions of the renal system include removing wastes from the bloodstream, regulating blood pressure and red blood cell production, activating vitamin D, and maintaining the balance of fluids, electrolytes, and acids and bases.

Each kidney contains nearly a million nephrons, which are the functional units of the kidneys. Through the continuous processes of filtration, reabsorption, secretion, and concentration, nephrons move wastes from the blood into the urine while maintaining a careful balance of fluids and electrolytes.

The urinary system is composed of two ureters, the urethra, and the urinary bladder. The function of the urinary system is to store urine and to allow for the excretion of urine from the body. Micturition occurs as a result of the coordination of signals from the brain and spinal nerves that innervate the bladder. Continence is the learned ability to control urination and can be affected by medications, trauma, and comorbid conditions.

Assessment of the renal and urinary systems should include the collection of a subjective health history and an objective physical examination. Data related to gender, age, race, socioeconomic status, occupational history, past medical history, and dietary and personal habits should be obtained from a health history. A physical examination should occur following the sequence of inspection, auscultation, palpation, and percussion.

A variety of laboratory and diagnostic tests can be utilized to evaluate the structure and function of the renal and urinary systems. Serum laboratory values, including creatinine, BUN, and electrolytes, can be obtained to assess the function of the renal system. Urine tests can also be used to evaluate renal function. Radiographical studies, including ultrasounds, x-rays, and computed tomography scans, can be used to evaluate the structure of the kidneys, ureters, bladder, and renal vasculature.

The kidneys and urinary system structures undergo changes with increasing age. The size of the kidneys and the number of nephrons decrease with aging, resulting in slowed kidney function. Females may experience a loss of muscle tone of the urinary system and its supportive structures, causing an increased risk of urinary incontinence. Males may experience enlargement of the prostate gland and associated urinary frequency, hesitancy, and urinary retention. Patients of advanced age are also at an increased risk of experiencing dehydration and developing UTIs.

Nursing roles in caring for clients with potential alterations in the renal and urinary systems include monitoring vital signs and intake and output data, collecting a health history and physical examination, evaluating laboratory results, and monitoring the client during and following radiographical procedures. The nurse also has a responsibility in assisting clients to maintain normal functioning of the renal and urinary systems by teaching healthy dietary and lifestyle habits in addition to the need for preventive healthcare screenings.

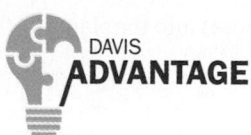

DAVIS **ADVANTAGE** | To explore learning resources for this chapter, go to **Davis Advantage** and find:
- Answers to in-text questions
- Chapter Resources and Activities
- NCLEX®-Style Chapter Review Questions
- Bibliography

Chapter 62

Coordinating Care for Patients With Renal Disorders

Vinciya Pandian

Finding Connections

CASE STUDY: EPISODE 1

Follow this patient throughout the chapter.

Doris Flood is a 35-year-old woman who presents to the clinic with complaints of abdominal and left flank pain. She is currently not on any medications except for a multivitamin daily. Ms. Flood complains of increased frequency of voiding, an urgency to void, and the presence of cloudy urine. She also complains that she has noticed abdominal distention over the last year. Vital signs reveal a temperature of 101°F (38.3°C) (orally) and a blood pressure of 180/100 mm Hg...

INTRODUCTION

The kidneys play a critical role in the overall function of the body. The kidneys remove waste, help maintain fluid and electrolyte balance, and help regulate the acid-base balance of the body. Adequate functioning of the kidneys is essential to an individual's health and well-being. Patients with compromised renal function may present with a variety of clinical manifestations. If the kidneys are not functioning properly and adequate treatment is not implemented promptly, acute illness occurs, and death is inevitable. This chapter discusses specific disorders of the kidneys and renal system.

POLYCYSTIC KIDNEY DISEASE

Epidemiology

Polycystic kidney disease (PKD) is one of the most common genetic disorders in the world, affecting approximately 1 in 600,000 people in the United States and 12.5 million people worldwide. Polycystic kidney disease represents about 10% to 15% of chronic renal disorders. It is a progressive kidney disorder causing excessive growth of fluid-filled cysts in the kidneys, often leading to complications over time. There are two forms of PKD, childhood and adult. Polycystic kidney disease in infancy and childhood is less common. It is caused by an autosomal-recessive disorder, and its course is rapid and progressive, leading to severe lung and liver dysfunction and **end-stage renal disease (ESRD)**, causing death during infancy or childhood. The adult form is autosomal-dominant polycystic kidney disease (ADPKD), which is relatively common. It affects 1 in 540,000 people in the United States and has a 50% chance of genetic inheritance. Autosomal-dominant polycystic kidney disease is a multisystemic disorder characterized by cysts that are not limited to the kidneys but may also be present in the liver, spleen, and pancreas. Adult PKD lies dormant for many years and usually appears between the ages of 30 and 40 years. The prevalence of PKD is the same for men and women and involves both kidneys.

Connection Check 62.1

The nurse recognizes that genetic counseling is appropriate for which patient?
A. A child with frequent urinary tract infections
B. An adult with frequent urinary tract infection
C. An adult with autosomal-dominant polycystic kidney disease
D. An adult with metastatic renal cancer

Pathophysiology

Polycystic kidney disease is a genetic disorder that manifests in the cortex and medulla of both kidneys and appears as large, thin-walled, fluid-filled cysts ranging from millimeters to centimeters in diameter (Fig. 62.1). Cysts develop as a result of a repeated cell-division process within the renal tubule known as a cystogenic process that occurs many times over the life of the patient with PKD. Progressive expansion causes emerging cysts to separate from the parent tubule, leaving an isolated sac. The cysts become large and compress the

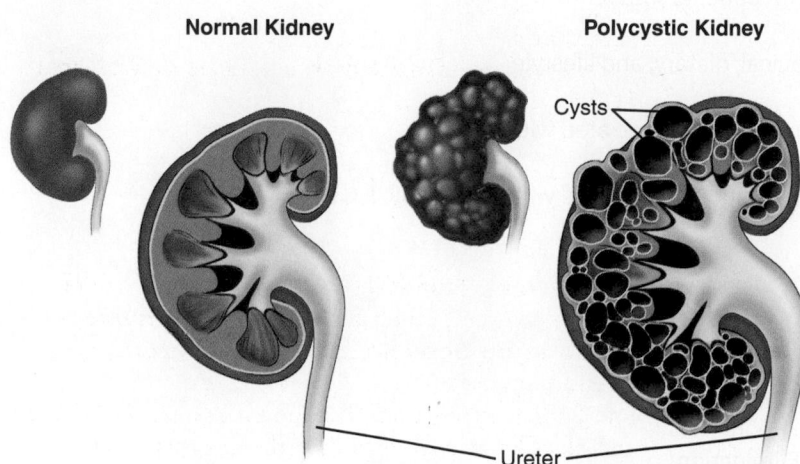

Normal Kidney **Polycystic Kidney**

Cysts

Ureter

FIGURE 62.1 Polycystic kidney disease.

surrounding tissue, destroying the underlying renal tissue. The compression of the underlying tissue reduces the blood flow and subsequent nutrient supply to the renal tissues, which are highly sensitive to reduced blood and nutrients.

Clinical Manifestations

Polycystic kidney disease generally has no clinical manifestations in the early stages. The symptoms become apparent as the cysts enlarge. The first symptom to appear is hypertension as a result of damage to the surrounding renal structures caused by the enlargement of the cysts. Hematuria also occurs because of the rupture of the cysts. The patient may complain of lower back or flank pain, headaches, or pain in the abdominal area. The patient also may initially manifest clinical manifestations of urinary tract infection (UTI), increase in urinary frequency, or urinary calculi (stones) that cause severe pain as a result of obstruction to urinary flow. Physical examination on palpation may reveal bilaterally enlarged kidneys, increased abdominal girth, and costovertebral angle tenderness. The disease progresses to ESRD in about 50% of patients by age 60. The remaining 50% of patients have mild to moderate symptoms and generally die from complications such as infection or impaired renal function.

Management

Medical Management

Diagnosis

The diagnosis of PKD is generally made based on clinical manifestations and patient and family history. Laboratory tests such as urinalysis reveal blood (hematuria) or bacteria in the urine. Definitive diagnosis is determined by abdominal ultrasound, magnetic resonance imaging (MRI), IV pyelogram (IVP), or computed tomography (CT) scan. Diagnostic imaging can reveal other complications related to PKD, such as cysts on the liver and other abdominal organs. A renal ultrasound, a less invasive and less expensive method of diagnosing PKD, can also assist in the visualization of cysts.

Connection Check 62.2

The nurse understands that which diagnostic study is most specific in identifying PKD?
A. Abdominal x-ray
B. Serum creatinine level
C. Urinalysis
D. Computed tomography scan

Treatment

PKD frequently progresses to ESRD because of the renal impairment caused by the cysts. The enlarged cysts obstruct and compress surrounding tissue, causing a reduction in renal circulation. The impairment of renal circulation causes renal failure, resulting in decreased clearance of

wastes and inadequate fluid, electrolyte, and acid-base balance. Patients who progress to severe PKD will require treatment consistent with that of ESRD: **hemodialysis (HD)** or **peritoneal dialysis**.

Other treatment goals for PKD include managing UTIs, pain, and hypertension. Managing UTIs requires regular checkups and immediate treatment as the clinical manifestations of infection become evident. Antibiotics are necessary to control the spread of infection up to the kidney. Pain can be managed with nonnarcotic pain medications such as acetaminophen and opiate narcotic pain medications such as morphine. Severe pain may require nephrectomy as a palliative measure. Hypertension is managed with medications such as angiotensin-converting enzyme (ACE) inhibitors or angiotensin-receptor blockers. Lifestyle changes such as proper diet, exercise, and smoking cessation are also recommended. All treatments described are intended to manage symptoms. **Renal transplant** may be considered as the only curative measure.

Complications

Common complications of PKD include severe hypertension, renal calculi, recurrent UTIs, hematuria, and heart-valve abnormalities. People with PKD are also at high risk for developing life-threatening aneurysms in the aorta or cerebral circulation. Additionally, PKD can lead to the development of cysts in the liver and the gastrointestinal tract. The cysts that form in the liver destroy surrounding tissues and impair the normal functioning of the liver in degrading waste products of digestion. The cysts in the intestines can cause diverticulosis or an outpouching of the intestines. The most common complication of PKD is renal failure and is characterized by the inability of the kidneys to remove waste products and excess fluid from the circulation. Renal failure is discussed in detail later in this chapter.

Nursing Management

Assessment and Analysis

The clinical manifestations observed in patients with PKD typically appear as a result of the enlargement and rupture of the cyst. Typical findings of PKD include:

- Hypertension
- Hematuria
- Pain or heaviness in the back, abdomen, or flank area
- Headaches
- UTI
- Urinary calculi
- Palpable, bilaterally enlarged kidneys

Nursing Diagnoses

- **Excess fluid volume** related to the inability of the kidneys to excrete fluid and excessive fluid intake
- **Risk for infection** related to alteration in urinary elimination pattern
- **Ineffective therapeutic regimen management** related to lack of knowledge regarding the disease process

Nursing Interventions

Assessments

- Vital signs
  Increased temperature may be present because of infection. Hypertension is present because of changes in the renal tissue caused by the cysts. Increased heart rate may be present as a result of infection and pain.
- Oxygenation
  Anemia associated with chronic kidney disease may impair oxygen exchange at the cellular level, which results in lower oxygen saturation.
- Daily weight
  An increase in sodium and water retention may result in weight gain.
- Laboratory values
  - Hemoglobin/hematocrit
    Anemia is associated with chronic renal disease because of the decreased production of erythropoietin, a protein produced in the kidneys necessary for red blood cell (RBC) production.
  - Plasma creatinine level/blood urea nitrogen
    Impairment in renal function may affect the renal clearance of waste products. Evidence of impairment in renal clearance is seen as an elevation in serum creatinine and BUN levels.
  - Plasma sodium level
    Patients with PKD may retain sodium, which causes fluid retention and predisposes the patients to hypertension, fluid overload, and heart failure.
  - Plasma potassium level
    Patients with PKD may have an elevated potassium level as a result of the impaired renal elimination of potassium.
  - Plasma calcium level
    Patients with PKD may have low calcium levels because of renal damage impairing the conversion of vitamin D to its active form, which allows the GI absorption of calcium from the diet.
  - Plasma phosphorus level
    Patients with PKD may have elevated phosphorus levels because of impaired renal clearance of phosphates.
  - Urinalysis/urine cultures
    Patients with PKD are at high risk for UTIs due to the compression of the tissue by the cysts impairing elimination. Careful monitoring of the clinical manifestations of a UTI is necessary to ensure prompt treatment and avoid the ascension of the infection to the renal structures.

Actions

- Diet modification consistent with impaired renal function, specifically low potassium, phosphorus, protein, and sodium
  Diet modification is essential to prevent severe complications from eating foods high in protein, potassium, and phosphorus that the kidneys cannot excrete adequately. Excess sodium intake can cause fluid retention.
- Fluid restriction
  Fluid restriction is important in the care of the patient with PKD and renal failure. Excess fluid intake may

not be excreted, and fluid overload and heart failure may occur.

- Administer antihypertensive agents as ordered.
  Uncontrolled hypertension is a significant complication of PKD because of the damage to the renal tissue by the enlarged cyst that compresses the surrounding tissue, reducing perfusion to the tissues. Complying with prescribed antihypertensive agents is required for patients with PKD to reduce elevated blood pressure, which is a risk factor for heart disease and stroke.
- Administer antibiotics as ordered.
  Prompt administration of antibiotics is essential to control the spread of a UTI up to the renal system.
- Administer pain medication as ordered.
  Pain medications may be necessary to manage the pain associated with PKD.

Teaching

- Immediately report clinical manifestations of infection.
  Patients with PKD are at high risk for UTIs due to the compression of the tissues by the cysts impairing elimination. Prompt attention is necessary to halt the spread of infection to the renal tissue.
- Follow prescribed dietary restrictions.
  Following required prescribed dietary restrictions is required to avoid the serious metabolic complications that are associated with renal failure.
- Follow prescribed antihypertensive therapy.
  Following prescribed medications is essential to avoid uncontrolled high blood pressure that can lead to heart disease or stroke.
- Follow prescribed antibiotics for diagnosed UTIs.
  Following prescribed antibiotics is important in order to prevent the spread of infection to the renal tissue and to prevent antibiotic resistance.

Evaluating Care Outcomes

The goal of treatment for patients with PKD is to prevent complications. Complying with prescribed medications such as antihypertensives to maintain normal blood pressure and the use of antibiotics to treat UTIs is essential to the treatment plan for PKD. Diets restricting sodium, potassium, fluid, and phosphorus are necessary if renal failure is present. Vital signs within reasonable limits and the absence of infection are indicative of maintaining health for patients with PKD.

CASE STUDY: EPISODE 2

Continued evaluation of Ms. Flood reveals an increase in abdominal girth and tenderness in the costovertebral area with palpation. Urinalysis reveals cloudy urine and hematuria. Ms. Flood has the classic signs of PKD as evidenced by left flank pain, increased frequency, urgency, hematuria, and abdominal distention combined with hypertension. The diagnostic test IVP confirms the diagnosis. The healthcare provider implements measures to prevent ESRD…

PYELONEPHRITIS

Epidemiology

Pyelonephritis is one of the most common renal diseases. The incidence is roughly 12 to 13 cases annually per 10,000 population in women and 2 to 3 cases per 10,000 in men. Young women are most often affected, probably reflecting sexual activity in that age group and the associated increased susceptibility to UTIs. Infants and older adults are also at increased risk as a result of anatomical variations and hormonal status.

The major risk factor associated with pyelonephritis is multiple pre-existing UTIs, treated or untreated. These infections may be caused by:

- Vesicoureteral reflux, which is a retrograde flow of urine from the bladder to the ureters
- Obstructions such as benign prostatic hypertrophy (BPH), a stricture, or a urinary stone
- A long-term indwelling urinary catheter
- Pregnancy is implicated in the development of acute pyelonephritis, known as pregnancy-induced acute pyelonephritis, as a result of the physiological changes associated with pregnancy, specifically hormonal changes and anatomical changes that lead to the retention of urine
- Sexual activity in women

Pathophysiology

Pyelonephritis is an inflammation of the renal parenchyma and urinary collecting system. The most common cause is a bacterial infection that occurs as a result of contamination of the urinary meatus with bacteria found in the GI tract that ascend via the ureters to the renal tissue (Fig. 62.2).

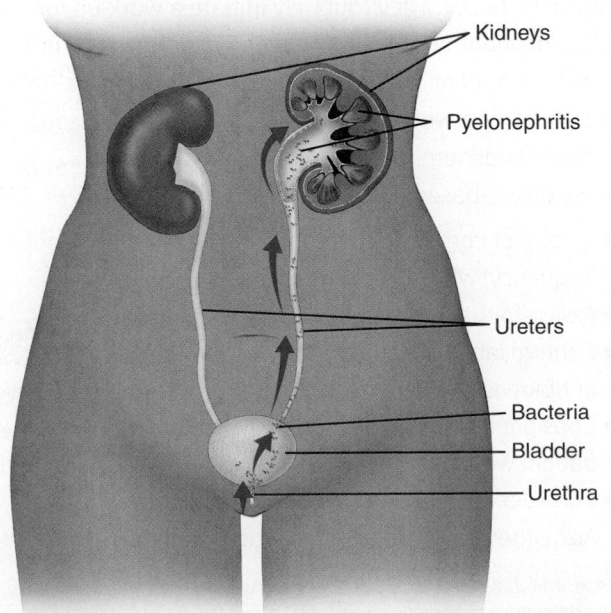

FIGURE 62.2 Pyelonephritis: an infection typically caused by bacteria migrating up the ureter to the kidney.

An inflammatory process occurs as a result of the bacterial invasion of the renal parenchyma. Acute pyelonephritis usually begins in the renal medulla and spreads to the renal cortex. Although many viruses and bacteria can cause pyelonephritis, the bacterium *Escherichia coli* is the most common cause. Other causative agents include fungi, protozoa, and viruses.

Clinical Manifestations

Clinical manifestations include signs of infection, which include fever, chills, nausea, and vomiting. Back or flank pain is also typically present. Costovertebral tenderness and enlarged kidneys are noted by palpation on physical examination. Patients may also present with clinical manifestations of a UTI, such as frequent and painful urination, and hematuria. The presence of fever, acute dysuria, new or worse urinary urgency or incontinence, gross hematuria, and suprapubic or costovertebral pain are more discriminating symptoms among the elderly for diagnosing pyelonephritis.

Connection Check 62.3

The nurse correlates which clinical manifestations with the pathophysiology of acute pyelonephritis? *(Select all that apply.)*
A. Nausea and vomiting
B. Hematuria
C. Flank pain
D. Fever
E. Abdominal pain

Management

Medical Management

Diagnosis

Pyelonephritis may be diagnosed by history and physical examination combined with laboratory results. Laboratory testing includes urinalysis, urine culture, blood cultures, and complete blood count (CBC). Urinalysis can show pyuria, bacteriuria, and hematuria. White blood cell (WBC) casts may be present in the urine, and a complete WBC count shows leukocytosis (increased WBCs) with an increase in immature neutrophils (bands); this is referred to as a "shift to the left." A shift to the left typically indicates acute infection. Once the urinalysis is obtained and shows infection, a urine culture must be conducted to identify the specific pathogen and medication sensitivities. Blood cultures are usually obtained before starting antibiotic therapy. Histological examination of renal tissue, if done, reveals inflammation of the renal cells.

Imaging studies may be necessary in cases that present insidiously, more subtly, or gradually. A CT scan or ultrasound may reveal renal structures that are reduced in size or hydronephrosis, (edema or retained fluid in the kidney) sometimes due to obstruction. Pathology shows loss of functioning nephrons, infiltration of parenchyma with inflammatory cells, and fibrosis.

Treatment

Hospitalization allowing treatment with IV antibiotics is usually appropriate for patients suffering from pyelonephritis, which is especially true for pregnant women because of the concern for premature labor with treatment. Elderly or severely ill patients with comorbid conditions (e.g., diabetes, immunodeficiency, or lung disease) also benefit from hospitalization to manage or prevent potential complications. Outpatient treatment may be acceptable for patients with mild to moderate illness and those who can be stabilized with oral antibiotics and adequate hydration and discharged under close supervision. Patients with frequent infections may be treated prophylactically on low-dose antibiotics. Unfortunately, long-term antibiotic use can lead to antibiotic resistance, which poses a challenge in finding effective treatment over time.

Medications

Medications used in the management of pyelonephritis are typically antibiotics. Management varies depending on the severity of symptoms. The treatment includes outpatient treatment with oral antibiotics or short-stay hospitalization with IV antibiotics with the possible continuation of oral antibiotics upon discharge from the hospital. Broad-spectrum antibiotics combined with an aminoglycoside are typically used. Trimethoprim-sulfamethoxazole (Bactrim) is commonly used because of its effectiveness and low cost in comparison to other antibiotics, but it is contraindicated in patients with a sulfa allergy. Other antibiotics used for pyelonephritis include fluoroquinolones such as ciprofloxacin (Cipro). Caution should be used when antibiotics such as trimethoprim-sulfamethoxazole and the fluoroquinolones are used because these antibiotics are contraindicated in children and child-bearing women as a result of the teratogenic effect on bone growth. Urine culture and sensitivity testing are essential in selecting antibiotics that will eliminate the pathogen and avoid the use of stronger antibiotics that will increase the risk of antibiotic resistance.

Supportive Interventions

In addition to antibiotic therapy, supportive measures may be necessary, such as fluid replacement. Patients are encouraged to drink at least eight glasses of fluid daily. Intravenous fluids may need to be administered during hospitalization if the patient requires fluid replacement to help "flush out" the kidneys and bladder or if the patient is dehydrated as a result of vomiting. Nonsteroidal anti-inflammatory drugs or narcotic analgesics can be administered to reduce pain. Antipyretic medications can be prescribed to help reduce elevated temperatures that may be associated with the infection. Specific urinary analgesics such as phenazopyridine (Pyridium) help to relieve the symptoms associated with ailments of the lower urinary tract. Drinking cranberry

juice was once believed to increase the acidity of urine, creating an environment that is not conducive to pathogen growth. More recent research indicates it may prevent bacteria from sticking to the urinary tract structures. Regular use is associated with less frequent UTIs in some patients, but it is not a cure or prevention for everyone. Intake of large amounts of vitamin C may also inhibit the growth of bacteria by acidifying the urine.

Complications

Recurrent infections or poorly treated pyelonephritis can lead to scarring, **chronic kidney disease (CKD),** or permanent damage. It may also progress to urosepsis. The bacteria can migrate to the bloodstream from the urinary tract, releasing endotoxins that initiate the inflammatory cascade—releasing cytokines and initiating the complement cascade. Widespread inflammation alters metabolism and can cause multisystem organ failure as a result of septic shock. Changes in mental status, fever, tachycardia, tachypnea, hypotension, **oliguria**, and leukopenia are the early signs of urosepsis (see Evidence-Based Practice). Sepsis is discussed in detail in Chapter 14.

Evidence-Based Practice

The Association of Urinary Tract Infections and Neuropsychiatric Disorders, Including Delirium, in the Elderly

Urinary tract infections (UTIs) account for an estimated 25% of infections among the elderly. Delirium is prevalent in up to 30% of the elderly population in the United States. For many years, delirium was perceived as a symptom of UTI in the elderly, causing providers to note UTI as a causative factor. They routinely initiate a work-up for UTI when delirium occurs and frequently find bacteriuria and initiate treatment. One systematic review identified a strong correlation between UTI and neuropsychiatric disorders, including delirium.

Evidence-based nursing recommendations:

- Assess for common symptoms of UTI (dysuria, urgency, frequency) when delirium is present.
- Assess for patient baseline cognitive function.
- Confirm laboratory results before administering antibiotics.
- Consider all plausible etiologies when caring for a patient with delirium.
- Consider the presence of comorbidities (e.g., Alzheimer's dementia, neurological deficit).

Chae, J. H. J., & Miller, B. J. (2015). Beyond urinary tract infections (UTIs) and delirium: a systematic review of UTIs and neuropsychiatric disorders. *Journal of Psychiatric Practice, 21*(6), 402–411.

Surgical Management

Emergency surgery may be indicated for patients who experience fever persisting longer than 48 hours or positive blood culture results. These clinical manifestations may be indicative of an abscess or/and obstructing calculi, requiring surgical intervention. Surgery may also be indicated in cases where a structural anomaly is potentially causing an obstruction that is the cause of the infection.

Nursing Management

Assessment and Analysis

The clinical manifestations observed in patients with pyelonephritis are related to the inflammatory process that occurs because of the infection. Symptoms include low back or flank pain. The patient may complain of bladder spasms and burning during urination. Other urinary symptoms include frequency, urgency, hesitancy, and nocturia. Urine is noted to be hematuric, cloudy, and foul-smelling. Older women may experience nonspecific urinary symptoms such as dysuria or urinary incontinence. In addition to the pain and urinary symptoms, the patient also exhibits the following symptoms:

- Fever
- Chills
- Nausea and vomiting
- Anorexia

Nursing Diagnoses

- **Infection** related to an impaired urinary elimination
- **Ineffective therapeutic regimen management** related to inadequate knowledge of the disorder

Nursing Interventions

■ Assessments

- Assess vital signs.
  Hyperthermia is a response to infection to kill the microorganisms. Poorly treated infection may result in hypotension and tachycardia as a result of the vasodilation that occurs in the inflammatory response.
- Assess pain level.
  Back, flank, or groin pain is a diagnostic indicator of pyelonephritis. Continued pain assessment helps evaluate pain-control efforts.
- Laboratory analysis
  - Assess urinalysis and urine culture
    Urine tests are the primary diagnostic tool for pyelonephritis. The urinalysis would indicate pyuria, bacteriuria, and hematuria. A urine culture will help identify the pathogen.
  - Complete WBC count
    A complete WBC count reveals leukocytosis and immature cells, indicating infection.
  - Blood cultures
    Positive blood cultures indicate septicemia, an infection within the bloodstream.

■ Actions

- Administer prescribed antibiotics as ordered.
  Administering prescribed antibiotics is important in eradicating the pathogen. Following the prescribed antibiotic regimen helps to reduce antibiotic resistance.
- Administer prescribed pain medications.
  Following the prescribed medications helps in providing comfort to the patient.
- Provide adequate hydration, PO or IV as ordered.
  Adequate hydration is important in maintaining good urine flow to avoid urine stasis. Hydration may also be necessary to maintain adequate circulating volume in the face of vasodilation associated with inflammation.

■ Teaching

- Explain the disease condition to the patient and family.
  It is important that the patient and family can detect early signs and symptoms of pyelonephritis in order to obtain treatment in the early stages, avoid the use of more aggressive antibiotic therapy, reduce antibiotic resistance due to lack of knowledge regarding prescribed medication regimen, and prevent further complications such as chronic pyelonephritis.
- Instruct the patient and family on how to avoid UTIs (Box 62.1).
  Instructing the patient and family on avoidance of frequent UTIs helps to prevent complications such as chronic

---

Box 62.1 Teaching Measures to Reduce the Incidence of Urinary Tract Infections

Teaching the patient and family measures to reduce the incidence of urinary tract infections should include:

1. The importance of taking antibiotics as prescribed. Tell the patient and family that symptoms may improve in 1 to 2 days; however, the prescribed antibiotic medication regimen should be completed.
2. Proper hygiene, including instruction on the careful cleansing of the perineal area with soap and water with bathing and after defecating, moving back the folds of the labia, and cleaning the area from front to back with each cleaning, especially after urination
3. The importance of emptying the bladder before and after sexual activity in order to avoid the risk of pathogens entering the urinary tract
4. Urinating regularly throughout the day, suggesting a micturition frequency of every 3 to 4 hours
5. The importance of adequate fluid intake. A full eight glasses of water per day is recommended.
6. Avoiding the use of vaginal douches, harsh soaps, bubble baths, powders, and sprays in the perineal area
7. The signs and symptoms of urinary tract infection, such as frequency, urgency, hesitancy, change in urine color (e.g., cloudy appearance), pain on urination, and fever
8. The use of unsweetened cranberry juice for the prevention of urinary tract infection

pyelonephritis, possible renal failure from frequent infections as a result of scarring and damage of the renal parenchyma, and antibiotic resistance to the repeated use of antibiotics.

- Take prescribed medications as ordered.
  Taking the prescribed medications is important in eradicating the pathogen and preventing antibiotic resistance and providing appropriate pain relief and comfort. Instruct the patient regarding the change in the color of the urine to orange when using phenazopyridine (Pyridium).
- Instruct the patient and family on the importance of rest.
  Rest is important for the restorative process during illness.

Evaluating Care Outcomes

With proper treatment, follow-up care, and prevention, the prognosis for pyelonephritis is good, and complications such as damage to renal structures, scarring, and chronic pyelonephritis can be avoided. A well-managed patient does not experience the symptoms associated with pyelonephritis, such as burning or pain on urination, urinary frequency, hesitancy, urgency, nocturia, and hematuria. Self-care efforts and compliance with treatment are evident from improvements in symptoms and reductions in recurrent infections.

ACUTE GLOMERULONEPHRITIS

Epidemiology

Glomerulonephritis is an inflammation of the **glomeruli** of the kidney. It is the third-leading cause of renal failure in the United States. It is caused by autoimmune disorders, such as Goodpasture's syndrome or lupus, vasculitis (blood vessel inflammation), or an infection such as *Streptococcus*. Glomerulonephritis is typically classified as acute or chronic based on the presentation of symptoms. Acute glomerulonephritis develops acutely, typically as a result of a complication from an infection, and can be found in patients across the life span but is most often seen in children and young adults. Chronic glomerulonephritis can result from some of the same causes as acute or may be genetic. It develops more slowly with fewer symptoms and may result in irreversible damage. It may also result from unresolved acute glomerulonephritis. The prognosis of the disease is based on the causative agent and the extent of damage to the glomeruli and surrounding renal structures and functions. Risk factors associated with glomerulonephritis are infections such as recent strep infections, immune diseases such as lupus, vasculitis, hypertension, and diabetes.

Pathophysiology

Glomerulonephritis is an inflammation of the glomeruli within the Bowman's capsule of the kidney triggered by an immunological mechanism. The glomerulus is a key structure in the nephron consisting of a network of capillaries and is where the first step of filtration and urine formation takes place.

There are two types of antibody-induced immunological conditions affecting the glomerulus in glomerulonephritis.

In type 1, the antibodies produced are specific for antigens within the glomeruli and glomerulus basement membrane (GBM). As a result of that interaction, immunoglobulins and complement are deposited along the basement membrane.

In type 2, the antibodies react to antigens not specific to the glomerulus but still deposit immune complexes along the GBM. Both type 1 and type 2 result in the accumulation of antigens, antibodies, and complement in the glomeruli and GBM, which ultimately results in injury to the glomerular membrane and a decrease in effective filtration through the glomeruli. There is an overall decrease in the **glomerular filtration rate (GFR)** and an increase in permeability to larger-size proteins.

Connection Check 62.4

What is the etiological process in glomerulonephritis?
- A. Tubular necrosis caused by bacteria and antibody reactions
- B. Deposition of immunological complexes and complement along the GBM
- C. Deposition of bacteria and immunological components within the loop of Henle
- D. Destruction of proteolytic enzymes contained in the GBM

Clinical Manifestations

As a result of the increased permeability, protein and blood are seen in the urine as well as WBCs and casts. Patients present edematous, with decreased urine output and hypertension. Renal laboratory tests such as BUN and creatinine are elevated.

Management

Medical Management

Diagnosis

Diagnostics of glomerulonephritis include a complete medical history and physical examination and laboratory tests. A urinalysis may reveal the presence of WBCs, RBCs, proteins, and casts. Other laboratory tests include the CBC and differential, which would demonstrate increased WBCs and serum chemistries indicating increased serum BUN and creatinine levels. Decreased albumin and complement levels would also be present. Decreased complement components indicate an immune-mediated response. The diagnosis of acute post-streptococcal glomerulonephritis is made based on a history of group A beta-hemolytic streptococci infection in the throat or a skin lesion. Erythrocyte casts in the urine also suggest acute post-streptococcal glomerulonephritis.

Treatment

Treatment is based on the cause of the disease and symptom management. It involves medications and supportive care. Medications focus on antibiotic treatment, most specifically penicillin for post-streptococcal glomerulonephritis if the infection is actively present. Diuretics and other antihypertensives may need to be added to treat hypertension. The edema is treated with the restriction of sodium and fluids. If the BUN is elevated, reductions in dietary protein may be necessary to reduce the buildup of metabolic waste. Corticosteroids are not always recommended but may be indicated to modulate the inflammatory response triggered by an immunological mechanism. Plasmapheresis may also be considered to reduce the immune-triggered inflammation. Plasmapheresis is an extracorporeal separation of the blood components to filter out immune complexes created as a part of the immunological response. The filtered plasma is discarded while the red blood cells and a replacement colloid such as donor plasma are returned to the patient. Lastly, rest is the most important means of restoration and symptom relief.

Complications

Ninety-five percent of patients with glomerulonephritis recover if the condition is treated early in the course of the illness, but if untreated or if the patient is unresponsive to treatment, acute or chronic kidney disease may develop. A rapidly progressive form of glomerulonephritis can progress to renal failure within weeks to months.

Nursing Management

Assessment and Analysis

The clinical manifestations of glomerulonephritis are present because of the damage to the GBM. They include:

- Hematuria
- Oliguria
- Periorbital edema
- Peripheral edema of lower extremities
- Generalized body edema
- Ascites
- Abdominal or flank pain
- Hypertension

Nursing Diagnoses

- **Impaired urinary elimination** related to effects of damage to the glomerular membrane
- **Ineffective therapeutic regimen management** related to lack of knowledge regarding the treatment regimen

Nursing Interventions

Assessments

- Vital signs
  Hypertension is a common finding because of fluid retention associated with glomerulonephritis. Hypertension is a risk factor for cardiovascular disease, stroke, and renal failure.
- Daily weights
  Weight gain is associated with sodium and water retention.
- Intake and output
  Measuring intake and output of fluids is essential in assessing the accumulation of fluids. Increases in fluid retention can develop because of the potential sodium retention associated

with renal impairment. Fluid retention is a risk factor for elevated blood pressure and heart failure.

- Measuring abdominal girth or extremity size
  Measuring abdominal girth and extremity size is important in assessing fluid retention. Fluids tend to pool in dependent areas such as the abdomen or extremities.
- Skin condition
  Edema can increase the risk of skin breakdown.
- Monitor dietary intake
  A patient with glomerulonephritis has the potential for malnourishment from the excessive loss of protein in the urine because of the damage of the glomeruli. Excess sodium intake can cause fluid retention, resulting in elevated blood pressure and heart failure. Protein intake may need to be limited if the BUN is elevated and there are no signs of malnutrition.
- Laboratory analysis
  - Renal function tests
    BUN/creatinine should be monitored to track renal function.
  - WBC count
    Elevations in WBC indicate infection.
  - Urinalysis
    Protein and RBCs can be found in the urine because of damage in the GBM.

Actions

- Administer antihypertensives as ordered.
  Diuretics are used to combat sodium and fluid retention. Other antihypertensives such as ACE inhibitors may be prescribed to control blood pressure adequately.
- Administer corticosteroids as ordered.
  Corticosteroid agents may be indicated to modulate the inflammatory response triggered by the immunological mechanism.
- Maintain low- to moderate-protein diet
  Care must be taken to limit protein intake if the BUN is elevated, but a low- to moderate-protein diet may be needed to treat protein loss through the urine.
- Dietary sodium and fluid restriction
  Sodium and fluid restriction is necessary to prevent fluid retention, which can cause elevated blood pressure and heart failure.

Teaching

- Overview of the disease process
  It is important for the patient and family to understand the disease process and the signs and symptoms associated with glomerulonephritis.
- Prescribed medications
  It is essential for the patient and family to understand the medications and their side effects and to report the side effects to the healthcare provider. Medication adherence must be emphasized.
- Dietary restrictions
  It is important for the patient and family to understand the salt and water restrictions and the rationale for the restrictions. The amount of protein intake must be followed

as prescribed in order to obtain the necessary amount in the event of protein loss.

- Avoid infections.
  The patient and family should be instructed on avoiding exposure to infectious diseases, especially if on corticosteroids.

Evaluating Care Outcomes

Evaluating care is based on improvements in kidney function and the symptoms associated with glomerulonephritis. Monitoring serum BUN, creatinine, and electrolytes is important in assessing the condition of the patient. Patient teaching can be evaluated by the patient's verbalization of information regarding the condition. A well-managed patient has a blood pressure within normal limits, no edema, and renal function within normal limits.

RENAL CANCER

Epidemiology

Renal cancer or kidney cancer is one of the most common cancers in the United States. The United States is projected to have about 63,000 new cases of renal cancer per year. Approximately 14,000 people die from renal cancer per year. Renal-cell carcinoma (adenocarcinoma) is the most common type of renal cancer and occurs more often in males 50 to 70 years old than in females. African Americans and American Indians/Alaskan Natives have slightly higher rates of renal cancer for unknown reasons. The use of cigarettes, pipes, and cigars poses a high risk for the development of renal cancer. Chewing tobacco and other forms of smokeless tobacco such as snus or snuff constitute a significant source of cancer-causing nitrosamines that can increase the risk for several types of cancers, including renal cancer. A familial association has been linked to first-degree relatives and the incidence of renal cancer. Other risk factors associated with adenocarcinoma are obesity; hypertension; exposure to certain substances, such as asbestos, some herbicides, cadmium, and gasoline; certain medicines, such as diuretics; and a cystic disease that occurs with ESRD.

Connection Check 62.5

Which of the following risk factors has been associated with renal cancer?
A. Aspirin use
B. Alcohol abuse
C. Use of artificial sweeteners
D. Cigarette smoking

Pathophysiology

Renal cancers are usually found in the cortex or pelvis of the kidney. Malignant tumors in the kidney are more frequent than benign tumors. Kidney tumors compress underlying tissues, reducing circulation to the renal structures and damaging underlying tissues. This compression can lead to compromised renal functioning or renal failure. Thirty percent of malignant tumors have metastasized by the time of diagnosis. Locations of metastasis include the long bones, lungs, and liver. Extension of cancer into the renal vein and vena cava is common.

Clinical Manifestations

Most patients are asymptomatic initially in the course of the disease. The eventual stretching, compressing, and invading of tumors within the renal structures can cause the classic triad, which includes a flank mass, flank pain, and hematuria. Other symptoms include weight loss, fatigue, hypertension, fever that is not related to infection, and anemia. If there is compression of the testicular vein due to the mass, there may be a varicocele, an enlargement of the venous plexus in the scrotum, present.

Connection Check 62.6

The nurse recognizes that which patient has the highest risk of renal cancer?
A. A 76-year-old African American female
B. A 50-year-old Caucasian male
C. A 24-year-old Caucasian male
D. A 50-year-old African American male

Management

Medical Management

Diagnosis

Several studies are needed to diagnose renal cancer. Ultrasound is widely used to differentiate between a solid mass, tumors, and cysts. Other tests for diagnosing renal cancer include angiography, percutaneous needle aspiration, CT scan, and MRI. Radionuclide isotope scanning is used to detect metastasis. Urine cytology testing shows the presence of neoplastic or atypical cells. Renal biopsy is sometimes utilized to look for cancerous tissue cells. Once diagnosed, cancer can be staged to aid in treatment decisions. Robson's system of staging renal carcinoma is one staging system utilized (Fig. 62.3).

Medications

Biological immunotherapy such as cytokines, interleukin-2, or interferon can be used to boost the immune system to aid in the destruction of cancer cells. Some targeted medications can be used to block the growth of cancer cells. These therapies can shrink cancer in a small number of patients. Unfortunately, renal cancer cells are resistant to chemotherapy, and thus chemotherapy is not the standard medical treatment.

Surgical Management

Treatment of renal carcinoma usually involves surgery. The typical treatment for renal cancer is radical nephrectomy for patients with type I and type II staging and particular

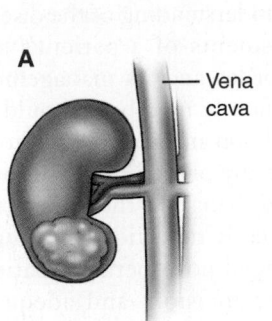
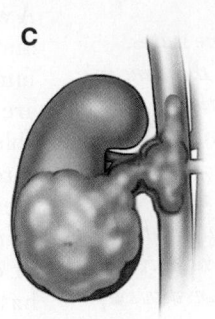
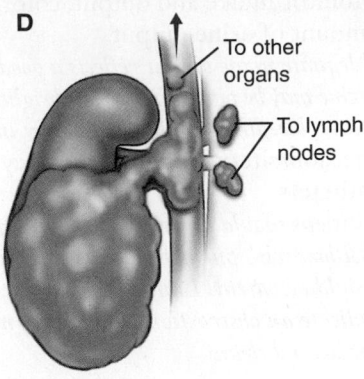

Stage I
Limitation to renal capsule

Stage II
Involving the perirenal fat but confined to the fascia with metastasis to adrenal glands

Stage III
Regional lymph node, renal vein, and vena cava involvement

Stage IV
Involving metastases to other sites in the body

FIGURE 62.3 Robson's system of staging renal carcinoma.

stage III tumors. Radical nephrectomy involves removal of the affected kidney, adrenal gland, and surrounding tissues, such as the fascia, part of the ureter, and the draining lymph nodes. With early detection, renal cancer has shown a 60% to 70% 5-year survival after undergoing radical nephrectomy. If an early or small-stage cancer, partial nephrectomy or nephron-sparing surgery is considered for treatment. In this procedure, the surgeon attempts to remove just the tumor. When metastasis involves the lungs and long bone or the tumor is inoperable, radiation therapy is used as a palliative measure. Metastatic renal cancer has a survival rate of 3% to 10% at 5 years.

Complications

The complications of renal cancer involve the disease process as well as the treatment. By compressing and stretching the tissues, renal cancer causes pain and reduces the circulation needed by the tissues. The renal system is highly sensitive to reductions in circulating oxygenated blood and nutrients. If untreated, the reduced circulation can cause end-stage renal failure. If the tumor is not identified in the early stages and treatment initiated, the overall prognosis of the condition is reduced, and the survival rate is poor.

Nursing Management
Assessment and Analysis

Early symptoms of renal cancer are rare in occurrence. The following symptoms can be seen as a result of the size of the mass and compression of the renal tissues:

- Hematuria
- Flank or abdominal pain
- Palpable mass
- Weight loss
- Fever
- Hypertension
- Anemia
- Fatigue

Nursing Diagnoses

- **Acute pain** related to renal cancer
- **Impaired urinary elimination** related to obstruction of tissues secondary to the tumor
- **Ineffective therapeutic regimen management** related to lack of knowledge regarding the disease process

Nursing Interventions
■ *Assessments*

- Vital signs
  Hypertension may accompany renal cancer. Tachycardia may be an indicator of pain.
- Pain
  Pain is commonly present because of the size of the mass and compression of the underlying tissue. Assessing pain identifies the need for and effectiveness of pain-control measures. Nurses must assess both objective signs of pain, such as a number from 1 to 10, and other nonverbal signs, such as facial grimaces, tense body position, elevated blood pressure, and rapid pulse or respirations.

Preoperative assessment

- Knowledge
  Assess the knowledge of the patient and family regarding the disease condition so that they can make informed decisions regarding care and treatment.
- Full systems assessment
  Documentation of a full nursing assessment and a plan of care is necessary for baseline comparison data for the postoperative phase.

Postoperative assessment

- Vital signs
  Accurate assessment of vital signs is crucial to assess recovery. Hypotension and tachycardia may reflect dehydration after surgery and the need for fluid replacement. Increased temperature may indicate surgical site infection. Decreasing SpO_2 may indicate postoperative atelectasis.

- Monitor intake and output, color, consistency, and amount of urine output.
  Adequate urine output reflects a good fluid volume status. Urine may be pink initially, but bright red blood in the urine indicates bleeding. Cloudy urine may indicate infection.
- Incision/site/wound care/patency of tubes and catheters
  Incisions should be clean, dry, and intact. Red or warm incisions with purulent drainage indicate infection. Drains should be patent. Limited drainage through drains may indicate an obstruction, which may need to be cleared to keep the wound clean.

■ Actions

- Administer medication as ordered.
  Biological immunotherapy such as cytokines, interleukin-2, or interferon can be used to boost the immune system to aid in the destruction of cancer cells.

Postoperative

- Administer pain medication as ordered.
  Adequate pain control is necessary for the healing process, reducing stress, and allowing the patient to move freely, cough, and breathe deeply, lessening respiratory complications.
- Administer IV hydration as ordered/encourage PO hydration as ordered.
  Adequate hydration postoperatively is necessary to maintain circulating volume.
- Encourage respiratory exercises.
  Coughing and deep breathing, the use of incentive spirometry, and position changes and ambulation are necessary to prevent respiratory complications.
- Appropriate care of catheters, stents, nephrostomy tubes, or drains
  Maintain patency of all drainage tubes; label and document for clarity and communication among providers; maintain gravity drainage as appropriate to prevent backflow of drainage, which increases the risk of infection.
- Perform wound care as ordered.
  Change dressing as ordered. Inspection of the site for the presence of redness, swelling, edema, or drainage is important and, if present, indicates infection.

■ Teaching

- Teach the patient and family about the condition and any procedures or diagnostic tests.
  Explain to the patient and family any anticipated tests or procedures; provide instruction regarding the disease process. Providing instructions can help to alleviate stress and improve recovery.
- Teach the patient and family regarding medications.
  Provide information on prescribed medications, including purpose, dose, scheduling, and potential adverse effects, to facilitate compliance with the medication regimen.
- Provide appropriate resources for counseling regarding the disease process, tests and procedures, changes in body image, and financial concerns
  Appropriate resources and counseling help alleviate stress and grief. Grief can affect the outcome of care procedures.

Evaluating Care Outcomes

A well-managed patient has an understanding of the disease and treatment options. Assessments of a patient's and family's knowledge of the disorder and its management are essential. The patient and family members should be able to report changes in the condition and adverse symptoms throughout the illness and after any procedures. Improvements in elimination patterns and changes in the color of the urine should be monitored for early detection of changes or complications. A well-managed postoperative patient has good pain control, a clean incision, and adequate elimination free from blood or signs of infection.

RENAL TRAUMA

Epidemiology

The incidence of **renal trauma** correlates with the number of motor vehicle collisions, violent crimes, and other accidents that involve speed or poor judgment in an action that may result in damage to the kidneys. This includes any falls, automobile accidents, sports activities, gunshot wounds, stabbings, or significant traumatic injuries, especially if they involve the abdomen, flank, or back. Pelvic fractures can cause perforation and tearing of the tissues in the renal system. A sharp blow may cause contusions, tearing, or rupture of the kidney. The kidneys are vulnerable to injury because of the lack of bone to protect the area as compared to other organs such as the heart, which is protected by the rib cage. Most accidents involve males less than 30 years of age and represent blunt-force trauma.

Pathophysiology and Clinical Manifestations

The extent of the injury depends on the mechanism of injury, the force, and the speed of the impact. Injuries to the renal system can range from contusion or hematoma to a shattered kidney. Renal trauma is graded according to the extent of the injury (Table 62.1). Urinary output can be reduced or absent as a result of the trauma depending on the damage to the renal system. Hematuria may be present when trauma occurs in the kidney, bladder, or urethra. The amount of hematuria does not necessarily predict the degree of damage to the renal system from the trauma. If bleeding is extensive, clinical manifestations of shock may be present. The patient may complain of back or flank pain; extensive bruising may be present.

Management

Medical Management

Diagnosis

Diagnosis of the injury to the renal system is determined by imaging studies such as ultrasound, CT scan, IVP, MRI, or renal arteriography. Both kidneys should be assessed and the findings compared. Urine is evaluated for the presence of blood. A CBC and serum chemistry levels are also

Table 62.1 Renal Trauma Grading

Grade	Description
1	Hematuria, contusions, normal imaging studies
2	Nonexpanding hematomas, superficial lacerations
3	Renal lacerations greater than 1 cm in depth not involving the collecting system
4	Renal lacerations or fracture extending into the collecting system
	Injuries of the renal artery or vein—controlled hemorrhage
	Expanding hematomas compressing the kidney
5	Shattered kidney—severe fracture so that kidney is fragmented
	Laceration or thrombus of the renal artery or vein

From the American Association for the Surgery of Trauma (AAST) classification. Retrieved from http://www.aast.org.

obtained to reveal complications of the injury, such as the extent of bleeding or damage to renal function.

Connection Check 62.7

The nurse providing care for the patient post–motor vehicle accident with a suspected injury to the renal system anticipates which of the following orders?
A. Perform an electrocardiogram (ECG).
B. Send a urinalysis to the laboratory.
C. Administer diuretics.
D. Administer antihypertensives.

Treatment

Management is based on the extent of the injury. Treatment focuses on stabilizing the patient and surgically repairing any perforations or lacerations. Initial treatments focus on controlling bleeding, preventing shock, and promoting urinary drainage. These treatments include careful monitoring of vital signs, intake and output, and hematocrit levels to assess bleeding. Pain assessment is important and can indicate such conditions as urethral colic or obstruction. Surgery may be required to control severe bleeding; however, small areas of bleeding may be allowed to heal by rest until the hematuria resolves. If the kidneys are intact, rest and observation may be indicated.

Surgical Management

A small percentage (9%) of injuries require surgical exploration to determine the extent and type of damage. Approximately 11% of these patients require nephrectomy. Nephrectomy is indicated in cases of severe bleeding due to damage of the kidney itself or severe renovascular injury.

Complications

The most significant complication to consider when taking care of the patient with an injury to the renal system is the extent of damage to the function of the kidney. Bleeding is also a major concern when an injury to the renal system occurs. In rare cases, renal shattering can occur, leading to major renal vascular laceration. As a result, the patient experiences significant hemorrhage, which may be life threatening.

Connection Check 62.8

Prior to the patient's CT scan, which information should be obtained from the patient or family member?
A. A family history of CT scans
B. Time of patient's last meal
C. List of patient's allergies
D. Time of last pain medication

Nursing Management

Assessment and Analysis

Clinical manifestations are based on the extent of renal trauma. They include:

- Gross hematuria
- Flank pain
- A palpable flank mass
- Back/flank bruising
- Hypotension and tachycardia with severe blood loss

Nursing Diagnoses

- **Acute pain** related to renal trauma
- **Impaired urinary elimination** related to trauma or blockage of the ureters or urethra

Nursing Interventions

Assessments

- Vital signs
  Changes in vitals can provide valuable information regarding the patient's overall status. Hypotension and tachycardia may indicate blood loss.
- Pain
  Nursing interventions focus on assessing the need for pain control and the effectiveness of pain-relief measures. Increased pain may indicate the severity of the injury.
- Urine output and color
  Oliguria may indicate an obstruction. Hematuria may indicate extensive damage and bleeding.
- Laboratory values
  - Urinalysis
    A urinalysis may reveal microscopic blood that is not immediately apparent.
  - Renal function
    Baseline renal function should be established to determine changes as time progresses.
  - Hemoglobin/Hematocrit
    Decreasing hemoglobin/hematocrit may indicate bleeding.

- Knowledge
  Assess the knowledge of the patient and family regarding the trauma, medication, procedures, or surgery so that they can make informed decisions regarding care and treatment.

■ Actions

- Administer pain medications as necessary.
  Adequate pain control is necessary for the healing process, reducing stress and promoting the patient to move freely, cough, and breathe deeply, lessening respiratory complications.
- Administer fluids as ordered.
  Adequate hydration is necessary to maintain circulating volume, especially if bleeding is present.
- Provide incision care as ordered.
  If surgery has occurred, inspection of the site for the presence of redness, swelling, edema, or drainage is essential to evaluate healing. Complications such as infection or bleeding may be apparent.
- Encourage rest.
  Rest may be the preferred treatment to allow the kidneys to heal if surgery is not indicated.

■ Teaching

- Teach the patient and family about the condition and any procedures or diagnostic tests.
  Explain to the patient and family any anticipated tests or procedures; provide instruction regarding the disease process. Providing instruction can help to alleviate stress and improve the recovery process.
- Teach the patient and family regarding medications.
  Provide information on prescribed medications, including purpose, dose, scheduling, and potential adverse effects.

Evaluating Care Outcomes

Evaluating nursing outcomes is based on monitoring the patient's condition through vital signs and the amount of bleeding. Fluid replacement or blood transfusions may be necessary to maintain homeostasis. A well-managed patient has vital signs within reasonable limits, minimal bleeding, and adequate urinary output and good pain control.

RENAL FAILURE

Renal failure is the partial or complete inability of the kidneys to filter waste products and water from the blood through glomerular and tubular filtration. The function of the kidneys is essential to the entire body. If the kidneys fail to function properly, the remainder of the organ systems will be affected, and multisystem organ failure will occur. **Acute kidney injury (AKI)** is a rapid, acute disease process that, in most cases, is reversible if addressed in a responsive and timely manner. However, if AKI is not addressed immediately, chronic kidney disease (CKD) is inevitable.

Chronic kidney disease usually develops more slowly than AKI and can occur over months to years. The treatment for CKD is long-term dialysis or a renal transplant for survival. Advances in technology, interventions, and medication therapies have improved the life expectancy of individuals with CKD. Careful monitoring of CKD and compliance by the patient with the treatment plan can improve outcomes.

ACUTE KIDNEY INJURY

Epidemiology

Acute kidney injury is a condition characterized by an acute, rapid loss of renal function. Evidence indicates that the incidence of AKI is increasing, particularly among hospitalized patients with acute illness or those undergoing major surgery. Recent data suggest 2,000 to 3,000 cases annually or 200 to 300 cases per million population annually. The increase in incidence might be partially attributable to higher sensitivity in classification. Other causes could be increased incidence of cardiovascular disease and diabetes mellitus and an expanding list of modifiable risk factors, such as sepsis, administration of contrast media, and exposure to nephrotoxins. Also, an aging population increases the incidence of AKI. Older adults are more vulnerable to AKI because of the decline in the number of nephrons with aging.

Pathophysiology

Acute kidney injury is defined as rapid and progressive azotemia, an accumulation of nitrogenous waste products such as urea, nitrogen, and creatinine and progressive increases in potassium. Oliguria may be present and is defined as a reduction of urine output to 400 mL per day. Uremia may be present and is defined as a renal function decline that involves multiple body systems. Fifty percent of AKI cases are nonoliguric. Patients with nonoliguric failure generally recover much more quickly than oliguric patients and have fewer complications. Oliguric patients are at an increased risk for CKD if circulating fluid volume is not returned to normal. The causes of AKI vary, but there are three major categories: prerenal, intrarenal, and postrenal (Fig. 62.4).

Prerenal Causes

Prerenal causes, the most common cause of AKI, are a result of external factors (those that are not related to the anatomical structures of the urinary system) that reduce renal blood flow and lead to decreased glomerular perfusion and filtration. Decreased renal perfusion affects the clearance of waste products, also known as azotemia. Hypovolemia, decreased cardiac output, decreased peripheral vascular resistance, and vascular obstruction can affect circulation. The renal system senses the decrease in perfusion, which stimulates the renin-angiotensin-aldosterone system (RAAS). The RAAS is a compensatory mechanism that conserves sodium and water in order to maintain blood pressure. The result is low urine output with an increase in BUN and creatinine (ratio of > 10:1) and an inability of the kidneys to conserve sodium. If renal perfusion remains compromised and compensatory mechanisms fail, then

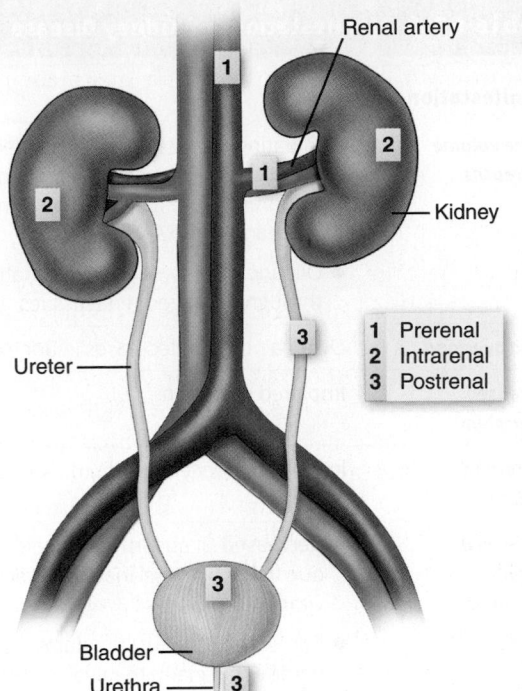

FIGURE 62.4 Causes of acute kidney injury. Prerenal causes include external factors that reduce renal blood flow. Intrarenal causes involve direct damage to the renal system. Postrenal causes involve mechanical obstruction of the lower urinary tract.

intrarenal damage to renal tissue may occur. Prerenal conditions account for 60% to 70% of the conditions leading to intrarenal damage. If assessment and treatment occur quickly, the intrarenal damage is typically resolved once the cause is removed.

Intrarenal Causes

Intrarenal causes of AKI involve direct damage to the renal parenchymal tissues, resulting in impaired nephron functioning. The **nephron** is the functional unit of the kidney, and any direct assault to the nephron significantly compromises the perfusion and filtration of waste products. The damage occurs as a result of prolonged ischemia, exposure to nephrotoxins such as aminoglycoside antibiotics, contrast dye used in imaging studies, hemoglobin released from hemolyzed RBCs, or myoglobin released from necrotic muscle cells. Nephrotoxins cause crystallization or damage to the epithelial cells of the tubules. Hemoglobin and myoglobin block the tubules and cause renal vasoconstriction. Acute glomerulonephritis and acute tubular necrosis (ATN) are also causes of AKI.

Acute tubular necrosis is an intrarenal condition caused by ischemia, nephrotoxins, or pigments and accounts for 90% of all intrarenal cases. The ischemia of the basement membrane and tubular epithelium seen in ATN results in a decreased GFR. Acute tubular necrosis is reversible if it is identified early and appropriate measures are taken. In most cases, nephrotoxic agents such as aminoglycoside antibiotics are the causative factors, and removal of these substances aids in reversing the disease process.

Postrenal Causes

Postrenal causes involve mechanical obstruction of the lower urinary tract (the ureters, bladder, and urethra). As the urine leaves the kidneys, flow is obstructed at some point at the ureters or below, causing reflux into the renal pelvis, impairing kidney function. Postrenal causes include BPH, prostate cancer, calculi, trauma, and tumors. Postrenal causes account for fewer than 5% of all cases, and the potential associated intrarenal damage is typically reversible if the obstruction is removed quickly. If the obstruction is not removed, AKI occurs.

Connection Check 62.9

Which is a prerenal cause of AKI?
A. Acute glomerulonephritis and neoplasms
B. Septic shock and nephrotoxic injury from medications
C. Pyelonephritis and calculi formation
D. Hypovolemia and myocardial infarction

Phases of Acute Kidney Injury

Acute kidney injury may progress through four phases: the initiating, or onset, phase when kidney injury first occurs; the oliguric phase when urine output decreases because of renal tissue damage; the diuretic phase when the healing begins; and the recovery phase when renal function begins to improve.

Initiating Phase

The initiating, or onset, stage is the beginning phase of the insult, continuing until signs and symptoms appear. This phase can last for hours to days. Triggering events typically arise from prerenal conditions that result in an approximate 25% decrease in circulating volume, resulting in an equal decrease in tissue oxygenation. Compensatory mechanisms cause the release of angiotensin II, aldosterone, norepinephrine, and antidiuretic hormone to preserve the blood flow to essential organs. Vasoconstriction occurs along with sodium and water retention. A decrease in urine output accompanied by a high specific gravity of urine and a low urine sodium concentration are observed in the initiating phase. If the prerenal cause is corrected, the condition is reversible.

Oliguric Phase

A clinical manifestation of the oliguric phase is a urine output below 400 mL per day. Oliguria in this phase, in contrast to the oliguria seen in prerenal failure or in the initiating phase before intrarenal damage occurs, is characterized by urine with a fixed specific gravity (between 1.007 and 1.010) and a high sodium concentration (> 40 mEq/L [> 40 mmol/L]). A high sodium concentration with a fixed specific gravity indicates intrarenal damage that does not respond to the compensatory mechanisms of RAAS. Complicating the diagnosis is the fact that 50% of patients may not exhibit oliguria, allowing more damage to occur before disease detection.

Also in this phase, there are increases in BUN/creatinine, electrolyte abnormalities, acidosis, and fluid overload as a result of reduced GFR. This phase may last up to 14 days or longer depending on the initiation of definitive treatment such as dialysis. The longer the oliguric phase lasts, the poorer the prognosis.

Diuretic Phase

This phase occurs when the cause of AKI has been corrected. There is an osmotic diuresis resulting from high urea levels. Urine output can increase from 1 to 3 L to 3 to 5 L a day. The patient may experience severe fluid loss as a result of increased urination, leading to dehydration and causing electrolyte imbalances. This phase can last from 1 to 3 weeks. As this phase ends, acid-base, electrolytes, BUN, and creatinine levels begin to normalize.

Recovery Phase

The recovery phase begins as the kidney begins to return to its regular excretory function. During this stage, the basement membrane is restored, and the GFR increases up to 70% to 80% of normal. Fluid and electrolyte balance normalize. The recovery phase can last from several months to 1 year.

Clinical Manifestations

Clinical manifestations include signs of volume overload due to decreased urine output, such as edema, pulmonary edema and shortness of breath, heart failure and jugular vein distention, hypertension, and dysthymias; chest pain; or pressure. Electrolyte imbalances include increased potassium, phosphorous, BUN/creatinine; decreased calcium, sodium, and pH; and metabolic acidosis (Table 62.2). Patients may suffer from anorexia, nausea, constipation, or diarrhea. Patients may become confused and lethargic, and with severe fluid and electrolyte imbalances, they may suffer seizures or coma.

Connection Check 62.10

When the patient is in the diuretic phase of AKI, the nurse must monitor which serum electrolyte imbalance?
A. Hypokalemia and hyponatremia
B. Hypokalemia and hypernatremia
C. Hyperkalemia and hyponatremia
D. Hyperkalemia and hypernatremia

Management

Medical Management

The goals of managing AKI are to eliminate the cause, prevent complications, and assist the patient in recovery. It is primarily supportive and involves ensuring adequate circulating volume, correcting fluid overload, and correcting biochemical abnormalities. Assessment of adequate hydration is essential for maintaining appropriate intravascular

Table 62.2 Manifestations of Kidney Disease

Manifestation	Cause
Urine volume decreases	• Initiating phase—urine output decreases because of decreases in circulating volume and the resulting compensatory mechanism of RAAS • Oliguric phase—decreased filtration through damaged renal tissues
Fluid overload	Overload due to decreases in urine output
Increased potassium	Impaired excretion
Decreased sodium	Inability to conserve sodium
Decreased calcium/ increased phosphorus	• Decreased GI absorption of calcium due to the kidneys' inability to activate vitamin D • Decreased calcium stimulates the parathyroid gland to release parathyroid hormone, which stimulates the release of calcium and phosphorous from bone. • Decreased phosphorus clearance
Metabolic acidosis	• Decreased acid excretion • Increased loss of bicarbonate • Increased production of nonvolatile acids such as lactic acid or phosphoric acid
Anemia	Impaired erythropoietin production
Increased BUN	Impaired clearance, dehydration, increased protein intake and breakdown
Increased creatinine	Impaired clearance—the best indicator of renal failure

BUN, Blood urea nitrogen; *GI*, gastrointestinal; *RAAS*, renin-angiotensin-aldosterone system.

volume and cardiac output. Assessment includes monitoring of blood pressure, heart rate, urine output, and clinical signs such as the quality of pulses, skin color, temperature, and respiratory status. Fluid intake and output must be carefully and closely monitored and documented.

Medications

Diuretic therapy may be used, including loop diuretics such as furosemide (Lasix) or bumetanide (Bumex), and an osmotic diuretic (mannitol) to treat fluid overload. Nephrotoxic agents such as contrast dyes should be avoided or used with extreme caution. Treatment of hyperkalemia, an essential component of care, is discussed under "Complications."

Nutrition

Nutritional therapy is an important element of supportive care for patients in AKI. The goal of nutrition for patients in AKI is to provide calories to prevent catabolism despite the restrictions required to prevent electrolyte and fluid disorders and azotemia. If the patient does not receive proper nutrition and calories, then catabolism of body protein will occur, which causes urea, phosphate, and potassium levels to increase. Adequate carbohydrate, protein, and fat are necessary components of the diet. Potassium and sodium are strictly regulated. Sodium is restricted to prevent edema, hypertension, and congestive heart failure; potassium is restricted to avoid the cardiac complications of hyperkalemia.

Dialysis

Dialysis may need to be considered in the short term to allow recovery of the renal tissue while preventing possible life-threatening disorders. Indications for dialysis include:

- Severe volume overload resulting in heart failure or severe respiratory distress
- Elevated potassium level with ECG changes
- Severe metabolic acidosis
- Altered mental status
- Pericarditis, pericardial effusion, and cardiac tamponade

Dialysis is discussed in detail later in the chapter.

Complications

Hyperkalemia is a severe complication in AKI because of the risk of life-threatening cardiac arrhythmias (see Safety Alert).

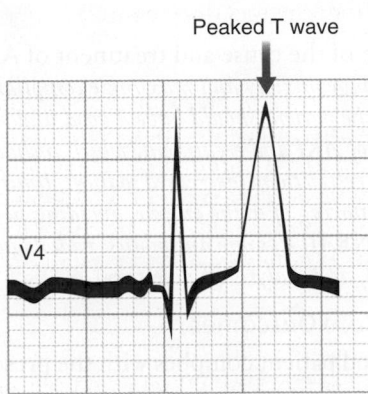

Serum Potassium	ECG Effects
Normal	
>6.0 mEq/L	Peaked T waves
>7.5 mEq/L	Long PR interval, Wide QRS duration, Tall T waves
>9.0 mEq/L	Absent P waves, Sinusoidal wave

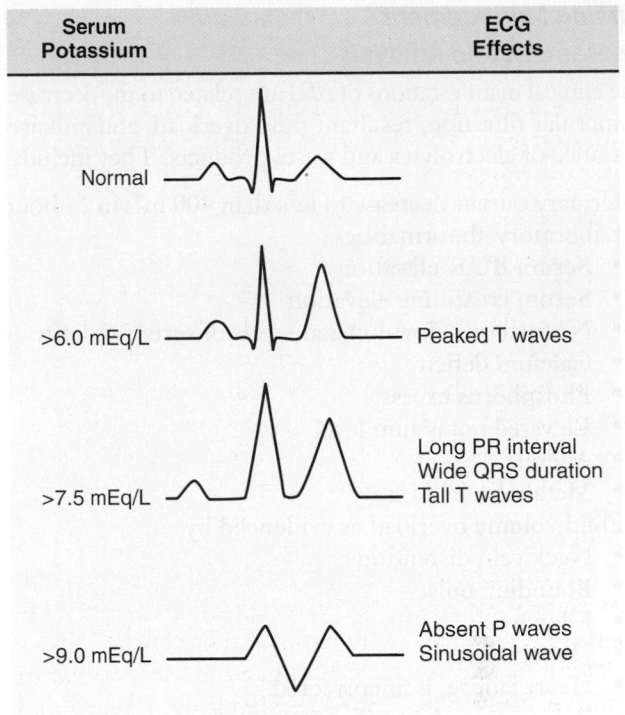

Hyperkalemia is a medical emergency because it can lead to cardiac arrest. The primary goals of medical management include:

- Stabilize the myocardial cell membrane through the administration of IV calcium gluconate or calcium chloride. Calcium chloride is more concentrated than calcium gluconate but can cause severe irritation and pain when given intravenously.
- Enhance cellular uptake of potassium.
  - Administration of IV glucose followed by IV regular insulin. Insulin facilitates the intracellular movement of potassium. *Glucose is given first to avoid the hypoglycemia that could result from IV insulin administration.*
  - Administration of albuterol, a beta agonist, facilitates the intracellular movement of potassium.
  - Administration of bicarbonate stimulates an exchange of hydrogen ions and potassium ions, moving potassium into the cell.
- Enhance total body elimination of potassium.
  - Administration of PO (or per rectum) sodium polystyrene sulfonate (Kayexalate), which binds with potassium and facilitates elimination in the stool. The patient should be monitored for water and sodium retention because of the fluid shifts that result from this treatment. Kayexalate should never be given to a patient with paralytic ileus because the fluid shift creates a risk of necrotic bowel.
  - Administration of IV furosemide (Lasix), a loop diuretic, facilitating the elimination of potassium in the urine.
- Emergent hemodialysis (HD)

 Safety Alert Hyperkalemia

Hyperkalemia decreases the threshold necessary to generate an action potential, which can result in life-threatening dysrhythmias such as ventricular fibrillation, ventricular tachycardia, or asystole. The initial indication of hyperkalemia on ECG is peaked T waves. Worsening hyperkalemia is indicated by a widening of the QRS complex, the loss of the P wave, and finally the presence of the sine wave.

Peaked T wave

V4

Nursing Management
Assessment and Analysis

The clinical manifestations of AKI are related to the decreased glomerular filtration, resultant fluid overload, and impaired clearance of electrolytes and waste products. They include:

- Urinary output decrease to less than 400 mL in 24 hours
- Laboratory abnormalities
  - Serum BUN elevation
  - Serum creatinine elevation
  - Normal or below-normal levels of serum sodium
  - Calcium deficit
  - Phosphorus excess
  - Elevated potassium level
  - Anemia
  - Metabolic acidosis
- Fluid volume overload as evidenced by
  - Neck vein distention
  - Bounding pulse
  - Edema
  - Hypertension
  - Heart failure, if uncorrected
  - Pulmonary edema, if uncorrected
  - Pericardial and pulmonary effusion
- Lethargy
- Stupor

Nursing Diagnoses

- **Excess fluid volume** related to renal failure and fluid retention
- **Fatigue** related to anemia, metabolic acidosis, and uremic toxins
- **Potential complications:** dysrhythmias arising from electrolyte imbalances
- **Potential complications:** metabolic acidosis related to the inability to excrete H^+, impaired HCO_3^- reabsorption, and decreased synthesis of ammonia

Nursing Interventions

■ Assessments

- Vital signs
  Hypotension and tachycardia may be present initially, reflecting a hypovolemic state causing the AKI. Later, hypertension will be present because of fluid overload.
- Urine output
  Urine output is decreased initially because of decreased circulating volume. Later, it will be decreased because of impaired clearance.
- Laboratory values
  - BUN/creatinine
    Increased because of the reduced clearance
  - Potassium
    Increased because of the reduced clearance
  - Sodium
    Decreased because of the kidney's inability to conserve sodium
  - Hemoglobin/hematocrit
    Decreased because of the kidney's decreased production of erythropoietin

- Calcium/phosphorus
  Calcium is decreased because of the kidney's inability to activate vitamin D. Phosphorus is increased because of the release of parathyroid hormone (PTH) in response to low calcium, releasing both calcium and phosphorus from the bone.
- Arterial blood gasses
  Metabolic acidosis due to inadequate clearance of acid, increased loss of bicarbonate, and increased production of nonvolatile acids
- Oxygenation and breath sounds
  Breath sounds may reveal rales due to fluid overload and pulmonary edema decreasing oxygenation and SpO_2.
- Peripheral vascular system
  Signs of fluid overload include edema and jugular vein distention.

■ Actions

- Manage fluid balance.
  Initially, cautious fluid administration may be necessary to ensure adequate circulating volume. Later, fluid restriction may be necessary to ease or prevent complications of fluid overload.
- Administer diuretics as ordered.
  Diuretics are necessary to relieve fluid overload.
- Administer potassium-lowering therapy as necessary.
  Elevated potassium can cause lethal dysrhythmias.
- Positioning, ambulation, cough, and deep-breathing exercises
  Positioning or ambulation as the patient tolerates eases the work of breathing and prevents complications of immobility such as atelectasis and pneumonia.
- Weigh the patient daily.
  Increased weight may reflect fluid overload. Weight is used to make the dialysis plan (discussed under "Dialysis" later in the chapter).
- Skin care
  Edema decreases tissue perfusion and increases the risk of decubitus. Keep the skin clean and dry, and change the patient's position frequently.
- Monitor and document food intake.
  Monitoring food intake provides information regarding nutrition status, which is important for the healing process. Consult with a dietitian to assist the patient and family with food preparation for special diets such as reduced sodium and potassium.

■ Teaching

- Knowledge of the cause and treatment of AKI
  To help manage anxiety and maximize compliance with treatment, the patient should have a good understanding of the cause of AKI and treatment, which includes fluid and dietary restrictions (decreased sodium, limited protein), careful monitoring of urine output, avoiding nephrotoxic substances (NSAIDs, some antibiotics, radiological contrast dye, alcohol), and dialysis (if necessary).

Evaluating Care Outcomes

A well-managed patient complies with the prescribed treatment regimen and returns to normal urine excretion with the elimination of waste products from the circulation through proper glomerular membrane perfusion and filtration. Complications such as heart failure, prolonged hypertension, pulmonary edema, dysrhythmia, or renal failure are avoided. The patient has a complete recovery.

CHRONIC KIDNEY DISEASE

Epidemiology

Chronic kidney disease (CKD) is a worldwide public health problem with a steadily increasing incidence and prevalence. One in seven Americans has CKD. The absolute prevalence of CKD is anticipated to increase by 60% from 484,995 in 2005 to approximately 785,000 by 2020, according to data from the U.S. Renal Data System. The absolute incidence is anticipated to increase by 41% by 2020. Data from 2010 and 2015 reveal an incidence of 120,253 in 2010 and 132,978 in 2015. The prevalence is higher for individuals 60 or older. Rates are higher in African Americans and Native Americans than in Caucasians and are higher in men than in women. The most common causes of CKD are diabetes and hypertension. Other risk factors include hyperlipidemia; smoking; the use of recreational drugs and NSAIDs; obesity; glomerulonephritis; and other disorders such as PKD, lupus, and atherosclerosis.

> **Connection Check 62.11**
>
> The risk factor or factors most often associated with CKD include which of the following? *(Select all that apply.)*
> A. Hypertension
> B. Diabetes mellitus
> C. Malnutrition
> D. Peripheral vascular disease
> E. Smoking

Pathophysiology

Chronic kidney disease is the progressive, irreversible loss of kidney function. It is characterized by slow increases in BUN and creatinine. Different from AKI, it has a longer, more insidious onset and is typically caused by a long-term disease or medical comorbidities such as hypertension, diabetes, lupus, PKD, and pyelonephritis (Table 62.3).

Table 62.3 Acute Kidney Injury Versus Chronic Kidney Disease

	Acute Kidney Injury (AKI)	Chronic Kidney Disease (CKD)
Etiology	Usually caused by an event that leads to kidney injury: • Dehydration • Hypovolemia • Surgery • Infection • Medications • Injury or trauma	Usually caused by a long-term disease that leads to decreased renal function over time: • Uncontrolled diabetes • Uncontrolled hypertension • Malnutrition • Polycystic kidney disease
Clinical features	Rapid onset may be reversible; symptoms may develop at the time of the event that causes the injury: • Electrolyte imbalances • Oliguria • Azotemia • Hypertension • Decreased GFR • Fluid retention	Slow onset, chronic disorder; may be asymptomatic until very little renal function remains: • Anemia • Calcium and vitamin D deficiency • Oliguria • Azotemia • Hypertension • Decreased GFR • Fluid retention • Uremia
Laboratory values	• Sudden increases in BUN and creatinine levels • Increased urine specific gravity • Sudden reduced GFR	• Slow increases in BUN and creatinine • Decreased serum calcium • Decreased hemoglobin and hematocrit • Increased serum phosphate • Increased urine protein

BUN, Blood urea nitrogen; *GFR,* glomerular filtration rate.

It may also be the result of poorly managed AKI. Chronic kidney disease may be asymptomatic until very little renal function remains. Advanced stage kidney disease is referred to as end-stage renal disease (ESRD).

Clinical Manifestations

Chronic kidney disease has a devastating effect on every system in the body (Fig. 62.5). Alterations in sodium and fluid balance result in hypertension, heart failure, and pulmonary edema. Altered potassium excretion can result in lethal arrhythmias. Impaired metabolic waste elimination results in uremia and GI symptoms such as nausea, vomiting, and anorexia and neurological symptoms such as a headache, lethargy, fatigue, confusion, and ultimately, without treatment, seizures and coma. Altered calcium and phosphorus levels result in bone breakdown and osteodystrophies or defective bone development. Decreased acid clearance and bicarbonate production result in metabolic acidosis. Endocrine and reproductive dysfunctions occur, such as infertility, amenorrhea, hyperparathyroidism, and thyroid abnormalities.

Decreased production of erythropoietin results in chronic anemia.

Management

Medical Management
Diagnosis

The diagnosis of CKD is based on consistently elevated serum creatinine levels and decreased creatinine clearance, both of which are impacted by the GFR. Another key indicator is the persistent presence of protein/albumin in the urine. Urinalysis can also detect RBCs, WBCs, protein, casts, and glucose. See Table 62.4 for a listing of laboratory values in CKD. Imaging studies such as renal ultrasound, CT scans, and a renal biopsy can provide additional information on the status of kidney structure and function.

Chronic kidney disease can be staged based on GFR and protein in the urine, with six stages delineated by GFR and three stages delineated by albuminuria or the albumin-to-creatinine ratio (ACR). This staging provides guidance for the detection and management, including risk stratification for complications, of CKD (Table 62.5). For example, a patient with G6 and A3 has a very high risk for all-cause mortality.

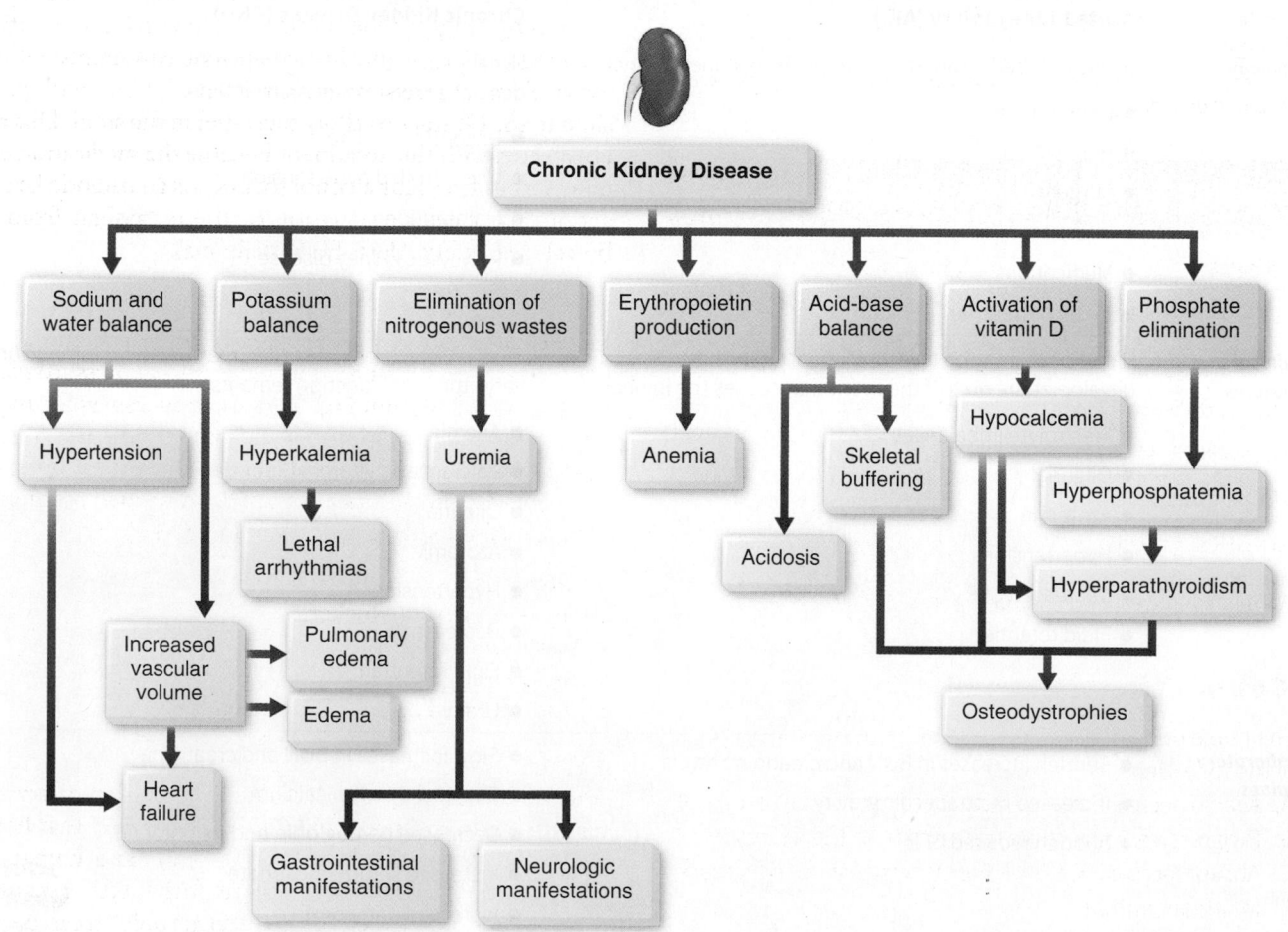

FIGURE 62.5 Clinical manifestations of chronic kidney disease.

Table 62.4 Laboratory Values Related to Renal Failure

Test	Normal Value	Value in Renal Failure
Creatinine	0.5–1.2 mg/dL	Increased
BUN	8–21 mg/dL	Increased
Serum sodium	135–145 mEq/L	Normal or decreased
Serum potassium	3.5–5.0 mEq/L	Increased
Serum phosphate	2.5–4.5 mg/dL	Increased
Serum calcium	8.2–10.2 mg/dL	Decreased
Serum CO_2	23-29 mEq/L	Decreased
Arterial pH	7.35–7.45	Decreased
Hemoglobin	Male 14–17.3 g/dL	Decreased
	Female 11.7–15.5 g/dL	
Hematocrit	Male 42–52%	Decreased
	Female 36–48%	
Urine protein	6–8 g/dL	Increased
Creatinine clearance	88–137 mL/min	Decreased

BUN, Blood urea nitrogen.

Table 62.5 Stages of Chronic Kidney Disease

G Stages	A Stages
G1 = GFR >90 mL/min	A1 = ACR <30 mg/g
G2 = GFR 60–89 mL/min	A2 = ACR 30 to 299 mg/g
G3a = GFR 45–59 mL/min	A3 = ACR >300 mg/g
G3b = GFR 30–44 mL/min	
G4 = GFR 15–29 mL/min	
G5 = GFR <15 mL/min	

ACR, Albumin-to-creatinine ratio; *GFR,* glomerular filtration rate;

Connection Check 62.12

The nurse understands that CKD is characterized by which of the following?

A. A rapid decrease in urine output with a CKD-elevated BUN
B. Progressive, irreversible destruction to the kidneys
C. Abrupt increasing creatinine clearance with a decrease in urinary output
D. Confusion and somnolence leading to coma and death

Treatment

Once the patient has developed CKD, measures to remove the waste products should be immediately implemented. Removal of waste products is managed through renal replacement therapies (RRTs), which are discussed in detail later in the chapter. Secondary but essential goals are to support the remaining function of the kidneys, treat the patient's clinical manifestations, and prevent any complications. Preventive and maintenance therapies focus on managing and controlling hyperkalemia, hypertension, anemia, dyslipidemia, and renal osteodystrophies, which involves managing phosphate levels, hyperparathyroidism, and hypocalcemia. Medication and nutrition management are also key factors.

Hyperkalemia

Elevated potassium levels can be lethal and must be addressed immediately to avoid serious complications. Potassium can be cleared via dialysis or by managing diet—restricting foods high in potassium in the diet—and when acutely elevated, medication therapy may be necessary to reduce the serum potassium level. Acute hyperkalemia may require IV calcium gluconate to stabilize the cardiac membrane. Intravenous glucose and insulin, albuterol, or bicarbonate may be administered to stimulate the movement of potassium into the cell. Intravenous furosemide is administered to improve clearance through the kidneys.

Sodium polystyrene sulfonate (Kayexalate), a cation-exchange resin, is another treatment commonly used to lower elevated serum potassium levels. It binds with potassium in the GI tract to allow excretion in the stool. Diarrhea is expected with this treatment because the medication contains sorbitol, a sugar alcohol that exerts an osmotic laxative action that causes evacuation of the potassium from the bowel (see Safety Alert: Hyperkalemia).

Hypertension

Hypertension must be managed both before and after a diagnosis of renal failure. The target blood pressure should be around 130/80 mm Hg. Treatment measures for hypertension include weight loss for obese patients; lifestyle changes such as exercise, avoidance of alcohol, smoking cessation, and diet modification; and prescribed medication compliance. Medication therapy includes:

- Diuretics
- Beta-adrenergic blockers
- Calcium channel blockers
- ACE inhibitors
- Angiotensin-receptor blocker agents

Anemia

Anemia is caused by the decreased production of erythropoietin by the kidney. Guidelines recommend that hemoglobin levels should be 11 to 12 g/dL and hematocrit should be 33% to 36% for patients with CKD. Because of recombinant DNA technology, erythropoietin can be produced and administered intravenously or subcutaneously.

Improvements in hemoglobin levels can be noted in 2 to 3 weeks, which is reflected in improved cardiac performance and exercise tolerance and an enhanced quality of life. Hypertension can emerge as a complication of erythropoietin because it increases whole-blood viscosity.

Oral iron supplements may be needed if the ferritin concentrations fall below 100 ng/mL. Constipation is a side effect of oral iron supplements, requiring stool softeners. If iron levels are not increased with oral supplements, then parenteral iron injection may be used. Supplemental oral folic acid (1 mg daily) is also given because folic acid is removed with dialysis. Folic acid enhances the formation of RBCs.

Blood transfusions are an option but should be used only if the patient is actively bleeding and is symptomatic with dyspnea, excess fatigue, tachycardia, palpitations, or chest pains. Undesirable effects of transfusions include the suppression of erythropoiesis, which is stimulated in the face of hypoxia, and because each unit of blood contains about 250 mg of iron, there is a possibility of iron overload.

Dyslipidemia

Because of alterations in lipoprotein metabolism in CKD, dyslipidemia is another complication with CKD. Recommendations for patients with CKD include a goal of lowering low-density lipoproteins (LDLs) below 100 mg/dL (2.6 mmol/L) and maintaining a triglyceride level below 200 mg/dL (2.25 mmol/L). Statins are the most effective medications for lowering LDL cholesterol levels. Fibrates (fibric acid derivatives) are the most effective medications for lowering triglyceride levels. They can also increase high-density lipoproteins (HDLs).

Renal Osteodystrophy

Monitoring this condition is done through x-rays, bone scans, bone biopsy, and bone densitometry. Treatment options for osteodystrophies include managing phosphate and calcium levels. Phosphate management includes limiting dietary phosphorus, administering phosphate binders, and controlling hyperparathyroidism. Phosphorus intake is restricted to less than 1,000 mg per day. Phosphate binders are used to bind phosphate in the GI tract, which allows it to be excreted in the stool. Phosphate binders must be administered with each meal to be effective because most phosphorus is absorbed within 1 hour after eating. Constipation is a common complaint with phosphate binders, so stool softeners may need to be added to the medication regimen. Some phosphate binders contain aluminum. Because dementia and bone disease have been associated with excessive aluminum intake, preparations that contain aluminum should be used with extreme caution. Also, magnesium-containing antacids that can be used as phosphate binders should be avoided in CKD because magnesium is solely excreted via the kidneys.

Hyperparathyroidism. Secondary hyperparathyroidism occurs because of the excessive parathyroid stimulus due to decreased calcium levels in CKD. Calcimimetic agents are used to control hyperparathyroidism by increasing the sensitivity of the calcium receptors in the parathyroid glands. As a result, the parathyroid glands detect calcium at lower serum levels and decrease PTH secretion. Parathyroid hormone and alkaline phosphatase levels should be monitored. If the renal osteodystrophy remains after treatments with pharmacological agents, the next option for decreasing the synthesis and secretion of PTH is subtotal parathyroidectomy. In severe cases, a total parathyroidectomy may need to be performed to control the condition.

Hypocalcemia. Hypocalcemia is present in CKD because of the inability of the GI tract to absorb calcium in the absence of activated vitamin D. Management of hypocalcemia includes vitamin D and calcium supplementation. Regular monitoring is essential because hypercalcemia may occur if hyperparathyroidism and the release of calcium from bone are not controlled. Hypercalcemia can cause increased cardiac irritability and mortality in patients with end-stage renal disease. If hypercalcemia exists, substances containing calcium should be avoided.

Managing Medications

Chronic kidney disease can cause delayed and decreased elimination of medications, leading to potentially toxic accumulation of medications in the circulatory system. Medication dosages may need to be adjusted according to the kidney's level of function. Agents that pose concerns regarding toxicity include digitalis preparations, antibiotics, and pain medications. Demerol is an example of a pain medication to be avoided in CKD. Demerol is contraindicated because it is metabolized to normeperidine in the liver, which the kidneys excrete. If serum levels of Demerol become elevated in the CKD patient, seizures can occur. Nonsteroidal anti-inflammatory drugs should also be avoided with CKD patients; NSAIDs block the synthesis of the renal prostaglandins that promote vasodilation, and this can worsen renal hypoperfusion. Acetaminophen can be substituted for NSAIDs in patients with renal failure. If more potent pain medications are required, oxycodone with acetaminophen and morphine sulfate may be considered.

Certain medications, such as aminoglycosides, penicillin, and tetracyclines, can be nephrotoxic, thus requiring adjustments to the frequency or dose for safety. Adjustments are based on trough and peak serum blood levels.

Medication administration times may need to be changed for patients on dialysis. Some water-soluble medications are filtered out in dialysis, resulting in a decreased therapeutic benefit of the medication for the patient. Medications typically prescribed in the morning may need to be given after dialysis. Also, antihypertensives or cardiac medications may need to be given after dialysis to avoid the hypotensive events that may occur because of fluid shifts during dialysis.

Nutrition

A dietician should be consulted for nutritional education and guidance. The recommendations for diet should be individualized to meet the needs of the patient and the degree of renal failure. Dietary proteins are restricted in patients with CKD because urea nitrogen and creatinine are end products of protein metabolism. A diet that is low in protein (0.6–0.8 g/kg of body weight per day) and low in phosphorus and that is supplemented with amino acids can slow the progression of renal failure. Once the patient starts dialysis, an increase in protein intake may be allowed (1.2–1.3 g/kg of ideal body weight [IBW] per day) because protein loss is high in dialysis.

Sufficient calories from carbohydrates and fats are needed to minimize the catabolism of body protein and to maintain body weight. The required intake of carbohydrates and fats should be 30 to 35 kcal/kg of body weight per day. For individuals with malnutrition or inadequate caloric intake, commercially prepared products are available that are high in calories and low in protein, sodium, and potassium. Such preparations include Nepro, Microlipid, Sumacal, Suplena, and Polycose. Amino acid preparations may also be supplemented (Amin-Aid).

Water restrictions are based on urine output and insensible water losses. Insensible losses through sweat and respiration account for about 600 mL of water per day. Adding the previous day's urine output and the insensible water loss together gives the replacement amount for the next day for patients not receiving dialysis. Careful monitoring of all liquid intake is important, including items such as gelatin and ice cream that are liquid at room temperature. The fluid replacement must be distributed throughout the day to lessen the patient's feelings of thirst. Adjustments must be made to fluid intake to maintain weight gains of no more than 1 to 3 kg between dialysis treatments.

Sodium and potassium restrictions are important and depend on the ability of the kidneys to excrete these electrolytes. Sodium may be restricted to between 2 and 4 g depending on the degree of edema and hypertension. Patients and families are instructed to avoid high-sodium foods such as cured meats, pickled foods, canned soups and stews, frankfurters, cold cuts, soy sauce, and salad dressings. Salt substitutes should be avoided because of high potassium chloride content. Dietary restrictions for potassium range between 2 and 4 g (39 mg = 1 mEq). High-potassium foods that should be avoided include oranges, bananas, melons, tomatoes, prunes, raisins, deep green and yellow vegetables, beans, and legumes.

Phosphate should be limited to 1,000 mg per day. Foods that are high in phosphate include dairy products (milk, ice cream, cheese, and yogurt) and some puddings. Most foods that are high in phosphate are also high in calcium, so restricting phosphate also restricts calcium.

Surgical Management

Renal transplantation is a surgical option for a patient in ESRD. Renal transplantation is not considered a cure but is thought to improve the quality of life. The need for dialysis is removed; dietary and fluid restrictions are not eliminated but are reduced. Patients do need to remain compliant with a lifelong treatment plan that involves continued vigilant treatment for comorbidities such as hypertension, diabetes, and heart disease as well as lifelong immunosuppressive therapy.

Recipients who are in good health except for the primary kidney disease and are between the ages of 5 and 50 years have the best outcome and prognosis for transplant. The complications associated with the primary renal disease, such as retinopathy due to uncontrolled hypertension or diabetes, usually improve with the transplantation.

Although the science surrounding renal transplant is rapidly evolving, there are several absolute contraindications. Some of these relate to disease states that may hinder successful transplant over time, such as untreated or metastatic cancer, or refractory coronary artery or heart disease. Other contraindications are psychosocial issues such as persistent drug abuse or severe psychiatric disease that may hinder compliance with the very complicated lifelong treatment regimen.

The transplantation procedure involves placing the donated kidney in the lower abdominal cavity (iliac fossa) of the recipient. The renal artery of the donor kidney is connected to the external iliac or hypogastric artery and the renal vein to the external iliac vein. The ureter is connected to one of the recipient's ureters or directly to the urinary bladder (Fig. 62.6).

There are three types of donors:

- Deceased or cadaveric donors
- Living related donors
- Living unrelated donors

The most common form of donation is cadaveric. Donors are matched to potential recipients via a national registry. Success is tied to close blood and antigen matching. An ideal deceased donor is young, between 10 and 39 years old, with no medical conditions known to affect the kidneys, such as hypertension; had normal kidney function; and had no infectious or malignant conditions that could be transmitted to the recipient through the act of organ donation. Unfortunately, the number of patients in need of a kidney transplant is increasing, so critical review and evaluation of the ideal donor are ongoing. An issue with cadaveric donation is the amount of "cold ischemia time." **Cold ischemia time** is the amount of time the kidney is separated from a blood supply, chilled, and transported for transplantation. Cold ischemia time is sometimes associated with a delay in the function of the transplanted kidney or poor overall transplantation results. Living donors are another option and are considered beneficial for several reasons: living related donors tend to have better compatibility, the surgery for both types of living donor types can be scheduled for a time most beneficial to all, and there is limited "cold ischemia time."

Treatment post-transplantation involves continued management of the existing comorbidities and the suppression of the immune system to minimize the risk of rejection. Rejection is minimized with immunosuppressive medications.

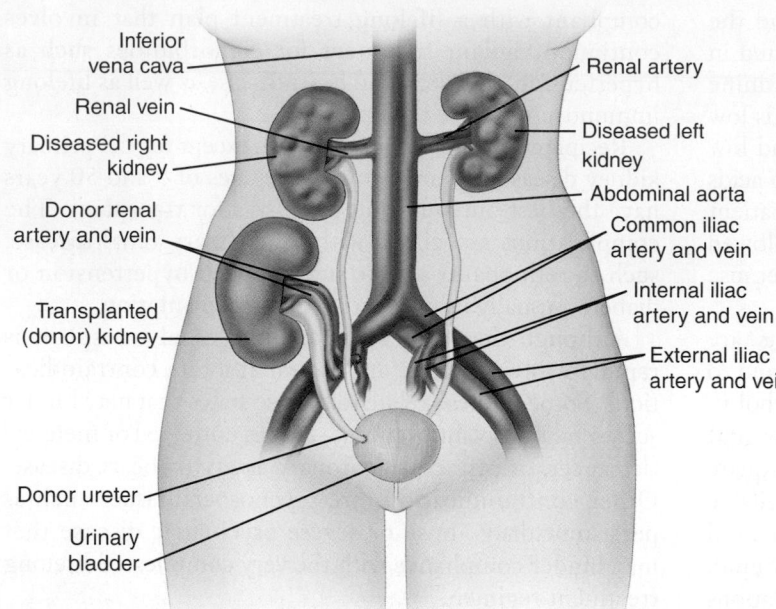

Labels on the figure:
- Inferior vena cava
- Renal vein
- Diseased right kidney
- Donor renal artery and vein
- Transplanted (donor) kidney
- Donor ureter
- Urinary bladder
- Renal artery
- Diseased left kidney
- Abdominal aorta
- Common iliac artery and vein
- Internal iliac artery and vein
- External iliac artery and vein

FIGURE 62.6 Placement of the transplanted kidney. The donated kidney is placed in the lower abdominal cavity. The renal artery of the donor kidney is connected to the external iliac or hypogastric artery and the renal vein to the external iliac vein. The ureter is connected to one of the recipient's ureters or directly to the bladder.

Complications

There is a risk of rejection even if immunosuppressive therapy is used. Hyperacute rejection occurs within minutes to hours after the graft; accelerated rejection occurs within 2 to 4 days. Both conditions result in graft failure and necessitate graft removal. Acute rejection, the most common and treatable form, occurs during the first 3 months after the transplant. The clinical manifestations of acute rejection may include fever, swelling, and tenderness over the graft site; decreased urine output; and a rise in the serum creatinine level. Increased doses of immunosuppressive medications are used to manage episodes of rejection. Chronic rejection is another primary cause of graft loss. The presenting manifestations associated with chronic rejection are progressive azotemia, proteinuria, and hypertension. These are evidence of progressive renal failure.

Other complications associated with renal transplantation include hypertension as a result of rejection, renal artery stenosis, and renal vasoconstriction. Some patients develop glomerular lesions and may have manifestations of nephrosis. Hypertension and altered blood lipids increase the risk of death from myocardial infarction and stroke following transplant.

Long-term immunosuppression is associated with complications such as viral, bacterial, and fungal infections of the blood, lungs and central nervous system (CNS). Tumors may appear with carcinoma in situ of the cervix, lymphomas, and skin cancers. The risk of congenital anomalies is increased in infants whose mothers have undergone immunosuppressive therapy. Corticosteroid use may lead to bone problems, GI disorders such as ulcer formation, and cataract formation.

Nursing Management
Assessment and Analysis

The clinical manifestations reflect the derangements of all body systems seen with CKD. They include hypertension, heart failure, and pulmonary edema because of alterations in sodium and fluid balance. Also present are GI symptoms such as nausea, vomiting, and anorexia and neurological symptoms such as a headache, lethargy, fatigue, and confusion due to impaired metabolic waste elimination. Altered calcium and phosphorus levels result in bone breakdown and osteodystrophies. Endocrine and reproductive dysfunctions occur, such as infertility, amenorrhea, hyperparathyroidism, and thyroid abnormalities. Anemia is a result of the decreased production of erythropoietin.

Nursing Diagnoses

- **Excess fluid volume** related to renal failure and fluid retention
- **Disturbed thought processes** reflecting the effects of uremic toxins on the CNS
- **Fatigue** related to anemia, metabolic acidosis, and uremic toxins
- **Potential complications:** dysrhythmias arising from electrolyte imbalances

Nursing Interventions
■ *Assessments*

- Vital signs/SpO$_2$
  Hypertension may indicate fluid overload due to inadequate water removal.
  Oxygen saturation may be decreased in the presence of fluid overload/pulmonary edema.

- Assess pulmonary, cardiac, and peripheral vascular systems.
  Rales may be present on auscultation because of fluid retention. Peripheral edema and neck vein distention may be present because of fluid retention.
- Monitor laboratory values.
  - Serum potassium
    Hyperkalemia may be present in CKD because of decreased glomerular filtration.
  - Serum sodium
    Serum sodium may be increased or decreased depending on volume status.
  - Serum calcium and serum phosphate
    Calcium levels are decreased due to the loss of vitamin D activation. Phosphate and calcium levels are inversely related. Decreases in calcium levels stimulate the parathyroid gland to release parathyroid hormones, increasing phosphate. Phosphate is also increased due to inadequate clearance in the kidneys.
  - Hemoglobin and hematocrit
    Hemoglobin and hematocrit levels are decreased because of the decreased production of erythropoietin.
  - Arterial pH
    Metabolic acidosis may be present because of decreased hydrogen ion excretion and decreased bicarbonate production.

Post-transplant

- Vital signs/SpO$_2$/temperature/pain
  Hypotension may be present post-transplantation if there is excessive bleeding. Decreased oxygenation may be present if the patient develops atelectasis or pneumonia. Increased temperature may signal an infection. Increased or poorly managed pain may contribute to the patient's inability to do respiratory exercises to prevent pulmonary complications.
- Incision
  Assess for redness, warmth, or drainage that may indicate infection or acute rejection.
- Renal function tests
  Poor renal function may indicate rejection.
- Monitor intake and output.
  Urine output may be increased due to the improved clearance of BUN, which acts as an osmotic diuretic, and because of the IV fluids received in the operating room.

■ Actions

- Maintain cardiac monitor.
  Cardiac monitoring is necessary to assess for ECG changes that might indicate hyperkalemia.
- Weigh the patient at the same time each day in the morning before dialysis; use the same scale and record and maintain the same clothing with weights
  The weight of the patient provides accurate information regarding fluid status. Weight gain/loss guides the dialysis treatment plan; it helps in identifying the amount of fluid to be removed.

- Restrict fluids and sodium.
  Fluid and sodium restrictions are necessary because of the kidney's inability to remove excess fluid, placing the patient at risk of volume overload.
- Administer prescribed medications as directed.
  - Medication used to treat hyperkalemia
    It is essential to maintain potassium within normal ranges to avoid potentially lethal cardiac dysrhythmias.
  - Antihypertensives
    Antihypertensives are necessary to control hypertension.
  - Phosphate binders
    Phosphate binders bind phosphate in the GI system, allowing for excretion in the stool.
  - Calcium supplementation
    Calcium supplementation is used when necessary to maintain normal calcium levels.
  - Calcimimetic agents
    Calcimimetic agents manage secondary hyperparathyroidism by increasing the parathyroid gland's sensitivity to calcium, thus decreasing the release of PTH.
  - Synthetic erythropoietin
    Synthetic erythropoietin replaces reduced erythropoietin levels that occur in CKD, helping maintain adequate hemoglobin and hematocrit levels.
  - Folic acid and ferrous sulfate
    Replacement may be necessary to support RBC production. They are water-soluble vitamins that are lost during dialysis.
  - Stool softeners
    Constipation is a side effect of many of the medications used in CKD, and so stool softeners help treat constipation.
- Skin care
  Edema decreases tissue perfusion and increases the risk of decubitus ulcers.
- Proper positioning
  Maintaining a semi-Fowler's position eases the work of breathing by facilitating the diaphragm to lower on inspiration.
- Renal diet; adequate protein levels
  Adequate caloric intake is necessary to avoid protein breakdown, which worsens the accumulation of nitrogenous wastes.

Post-transplant

- Administer medications as ordered.
  - Immunosuppressive medications
    Immunosuppressive medications help prevent rejection.
  - Pain medication
    Adequate pain control allows the patient to participate in care, perform respiratory exercises, and ambulate as soon as possible to prevent respiratory complications.

■ Teaching

- Do not miss dialysis appointments.
  Missing scheduled dialysis may result in acute and lethal fluid and electrolyte complications, especially hyperkalemia.

- Dietary restrictions
  Adequate protein and limited salt and fluid are necessary to support the caloric needs of the body and reduce the occurrence of volume overload.
- Clinical manifestations of CKD and complications
  The patient must know when to seek help in order to avoid the complications of CKD.
- Avoid nephrotoxic substances such as NSAIDs, contrast media, nephrotoxic antibiotics, and alcohol.
  Avoidance of nephrotoxic substances is essential to avoid the complications of CKD.
- Daily weight
  Weight is an excellent indicator of fluid volume status.

Post-transplant

- Teach the patient and family the importance of taking immunosuppressive agents as prescribed.
  Immunosuppressive medications preserve the life of the transplanted kidney. The medications will be taken for the remainder of the patient's life.
- Teach the patient and family to avoid exposure to potentially infectious environments or persons as much as possible.
  Teach the patient and family the importance of avoiding contact with potentially infectious environments or persons because of the risk of infection due to the lifetime of immuno-suppressive therapy.

Evaluating Care Outcomes

Patients with CKD can be well managed with meticulous care and compliance with the treatment regimen. A well-managed patient maintains a regular dialysis schedule and is compliant with diet and medications, avoiding the complications associated with CKD.

RENAL REPLACEMENT THERAPIES

Renal replacement therapies (RRTs) are artificial processes for removing waste and water from the body when the kidneys are no longer functioning adequately. Renal replacement therapy techniques include intermittent hemodialysis (HD), commonly referred to as hemodialysis; continuous hemofiltration and HD, also referred to as **continuous renal replacement therapies (CRRTs)**; and peritoneal dialysis (PD). Hemodialysis and PD are processes in which blood is separated from a dialysis solution by a semipermeable membrane. Hemodialysis uses an artificial membrane; PD uses the peritoneal membrane. Solutes and water move across the membrane by diffusion (Fig. 62.7), or movement across a concentration gradient, supported by the addition of dialysate to the circuit, and by filtration, which is the movement of water driven by a hydrostatic pressure gradient. Continuous renal replacement therapy is a process where blood flows through a filter, and solute and fluid removal is accomplished via filtration, diffusion, or convection—the movement of solutes through the membrane via the force of fluid or water movement.

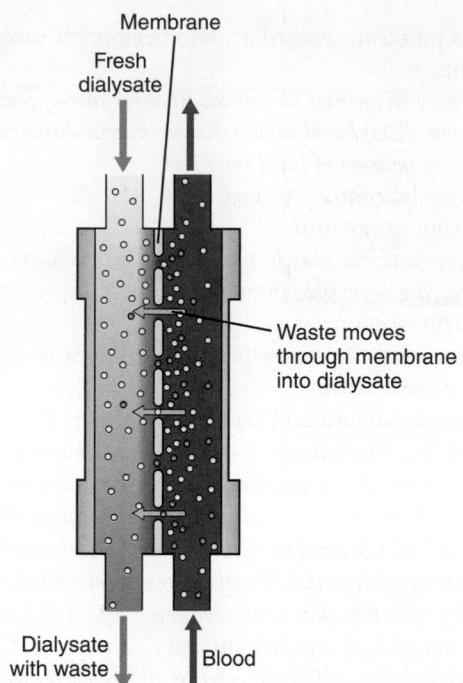

FIGURE 62.7 Solute and water movement across the semipermeable membrane. Solutes and water move across the membrane, driven by diffusion, or movement across a concentration gradient, supported by the addition of dialysate to the circuit, and by filtration, which is the movement of water driven by a hydrostatic pressure gradient.

Dialysis is indicated for AKI or ESRD characterized by the following:

- Presence of severe fluid and electrolyte imbalances
- Elevated serum creatinine
- Elevated serum potassium levels
- Acidosis
- Presence of uremic manifestations
- Patients with GFR less than 10 mL/min

The most common forms of RRT for ESRD are intermittent HD and PD. Hemodialysis can be performed in outpatient centers, inpatient hospital settings, and sometimes in home settings. Peritoneal dialysis is generally performed in the home, but patients often receive PD while hospitalized or as outpatients. The morbidity and mortality of the two types of dialysis are comparable; however, the patient's condition, desire, and ability to manage dialysis at home; work situation; and proximity to a dialysis center may influence a decision to pursue either form. Continuous renal replacement therapies are typically indicated for acutely ill patients; these therapies manage acid-base balance, electrolyte levels, and fluid balance slowly and continuously in a hemodynamically unstable patient.

Hemodialysis

Vascular Access

There are generally three types of vascular access for HD (Fig. 62.8). Intravenous vascular access may be secured using a central venous double-lumen catheter in the subclavian

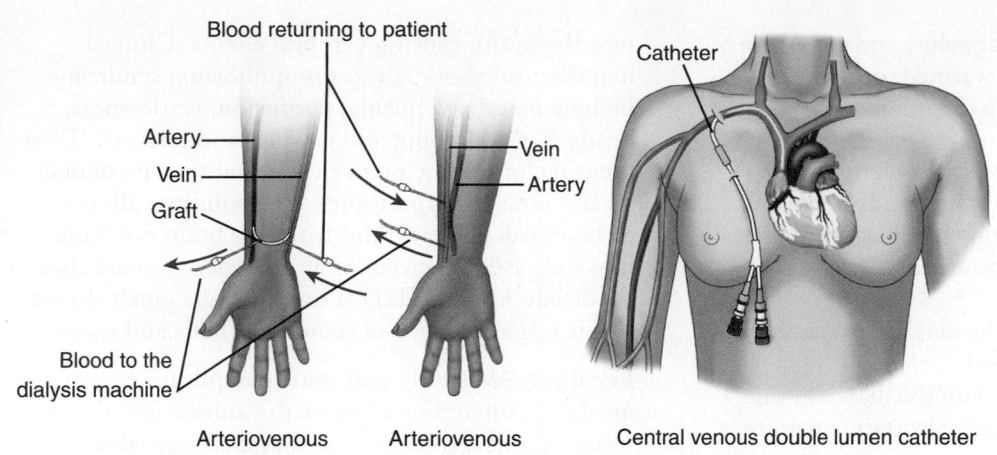

FIGURE 62.8 Options for vascular access for hemodialysis. A central venous double-lumen catheter is typically used for short-term treatment. An AV fistula is a surgical anastomosis of an artery and vein. An AV graft is created by inserting a prosthetic graft between an artery and vein.

or internal jugular vein. This type of access is typically used for the short term, such as treating a patient with AKI with intermittent HD or when waiting to secure long-term access for HD via **arteriovenous (AV) fistula** or **arteriovenous (AV) graft**. An AV fistula is created by surgical anastomosis of an artery and vein, typically the radial artery and cephalic vein, in the nondominant arm. After the procedure, the fistula is allowed to mature to become suitable for dialysis. Maturing the AV fistula occurs when the low-pressure vein becomes accustomed to the higher pressures generated in the artery, which allows adequate blood flow for dialysis. The "matured" fistula appears large—bulging and tortuous under the skin. Maturation can require weeks to months, so advanced planning is needed, or, as noted previously, a central venous catheter may be used in the short term.

An AV graft, another option for dialysis, is created by inserting a prosthetic graft between an artery and vein, typically in the nondominant arm. Arteriovenous graft access can be used more quickly than the fistula but does not last as long and is more prone to infection; thus, it is not the preferred option for access. On assessment, a functional AV fistula or graft has a palpable pulsation, a thrill, and a bruit on auscultation.

Hemodialysis Process

Hemodialysis is a life-sustaining procedure for a patient with AKI or ESRD. Hemodialysis uses the processes of diffusion and filtration to remove waste products, electrolytes, and excess water from the body (Fig. 62.9). Patients generally undergo dialysis three times per week, 3 to 5 hours for each treatment. The exact duration and the number of sessions per week depend on the individual's status—renal function, weight, serum electrolyte, BUN/creatinine levels, and general health of the patient. The process involves several steps:

1. Blood is pumped from the body through the vascular access device to a dialyzer.
2. In the dialyzer, the blood moves past an artificial semi-permeable membrane.

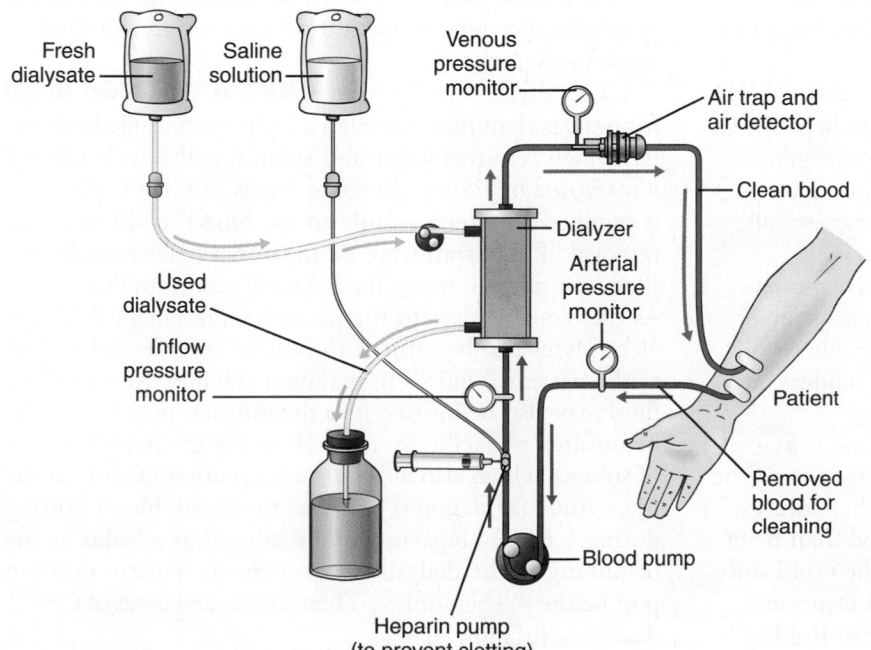

FIGURE 62.9 Hemodialysis. Blood is removed from the body and pumped through a dialyzer. Dialysis fluid is pumped through the dialyzer in the opposite direction of the blood to provide a concentration gradient for the removal of wastes. Blood is then returned to the body.

3. A dialysate solution with similar solute concentration as normal extracellular fluid is warmed to body temperature and pumped along the other side of the membrane.
4. Solute molecule movement across the membrane is determined by a concentration gradient, from an area of higher to lower concentration via diffusion. Waste products such as urea and creatinine diffuse across the membrane into the dialysate.
5. Bicarbonate may be added to the dialysate to make corrections for acidosis if present.
6. Negative pressure is maintained on the dialysate side to allow excess fluid removal via hydrostatic pressure, a process known as filtration.
7. Heparin is added to the circuit to prevent clotting.
8. Saline may be added to help prevent clotting and facilitate flow through the dialyzer.
9. The "cleaned" blood is returned via the vascular access device.

Complications

Systemic complications of HD can occur during or after dialysis and include:

- Hypotension due to the rapid removal of fluid from the vascular compartment or vasodilation. The patient may display light-headedness, nausea, vomiting, seizures, vision changes, and chest pain from cardiac ischemia. The treatment is to decrease the rate of fluid removal and to replace fluid intravenously with normal saline (0.9% saline solution).
- Muscle cramps, headache, nausea, dizziness, and malaise are common during and after dialysis as a result of the rapid removal of electrolytes and water. Treatment includes reducing the filtration rate or infusing a normal saline bolus.
- Bleeding may occur because of the altered platelet function associated with uremia and the use of heparin during the dialysis procedure.
- Systemic infection is a concern. Patients on chronic HD have a higher risk of developing hepatitis B, hepatitis C, cytomegalovirus, and HIV infections than the general population. Multiple blood transfusions, immune system depression, and underlying disease processes all contribute to the risk of infection.
- Dialysis-associated dementia is a progressive, potentially incurable neurological complication associated with long-term dialysis. It is thought to be due to aluminum, which is present in phosphate binders in the dialysate or the PO phosphate binders.
- Dialysis disequilibrium syndrome develops as a result of very rapid changes in the composition of the extracellular fluid. Urea, sodium, and other solutes are removed more rapidly from the blood than from the cerebrospinal fluid and the brain. The rapid shift of fluid and substances can create a high osmotic gradient in the brain, resulting in a shift of fluid into the brain, causing cerebral edema. Clinical manifestations of dialysis disequilibrium syndrome include nausea, vomiting, confusion, restlessness, headaches, twitching and jerking, and seizures. Treatment includes slowing or decreasing the rate of dialysis and infusing hypertonic saline solution, albumin, or mannitol to draw fluid from the brain cell back into the systemic circulation. In order to avoid this syndrome, the first HD is usually done much slower and is less aggressive in removing fluids and solutes.

Localized AV fistula and graft complications can also occur. Infection and clotting or thrombosis are the most common shunt problems. Aneurysms may also occur. *Staphylococcus aureus* septicemia is commonly associated with contamination of the fistula. Infection and thrombosis can lead to systemic manifestations such as septicemia and embolization.

Continuous Renal Replacement Therapy

Continuous renal replacement therapy is indicated for acutely ill patients with AKI or patients with severe fluid overload who are hemodynamically unstable. It is recommended in critically ill patients because it limits the risk of complications associated with the rapid rate of fluid and solute loss, such as the hypotension that complicates intermittent HD. Vascular access for CRRT is accomplished through the double-lumen catheter described for short-term HD or a single-lumen central venous line in combination with an arterial line. In CRRT, fluid and solute removal is slow and continuous and can be adjusted hourly depending on how the patient is tolerating the procedure. The mechanisms used for solute and fluid removal are similar to HD, diffusion via a concentration gradient and filtration via hydrostatic pressure. Continuous renal replacement therapy adds solute removal via convection, which is the movement of solutes through the membrane via the force of fluid or water movement.

Generally, the process for CRRT is as follows: Blood from the patient flows through a highly permeable hemofilter, which removes water and solutes, collectively termed *ultrafiltrate* or *filtrate*. In some forms of CRRT, dialysate is pumped countercurrently to the blood to aid in solute removal. The ultrafiltrate drains into a collection device. Blood continues through the filter and returns to the patient. As the blood returns to the patient, replacement fluid and electrolytes can be infused to replace volume and solutes as the patient requires to maintain stability. Replacement fluid may also be infused into the infusion port before the hemofilter to facilitate convection for greater clearance of solutes, which also aids in the prevention of clots in the filter. Anticoagulation is also used to prevent blood clotting during CRRT. Heparin may be infused as a bolus at the beginning of the dialysis or through the heparin infusion port before the hemofilter. There are several types of CRRT described in Table 62.6.

Table 62.6 Types of Continuous Renal Replacement Therapy (CRRT)

Type of CRRT	Vascular Access	Purpose	Requirements	Limitations
Slow continuous ultrafiltration (SCUF)	Double-lumen central venous catheter (venovenous [VV]) or arterial/ venous access	Slow fluid removal via filtration	Requires a pump to generate pressure to drive blood through the circuit with VV access; does not use dialysate or replacement fluid	Low filtration rates; requires extensive monitoring
Continuous arteriovenous hemofiltration (CAVH)	Arterial and central venous access	Slow fluid and solute removal via convection and filtration	Does not require a pump—difference between mean arterial pressure and venous pressure drives blood through the filter; requires replacement fluids prior to filter; does not use dialysate; may use replacement fluids after the filter to aid in maintaining patient stability	Low solute removal due to lack of diffusion; unreliable blood flow in critically ill, hypotensive patients; increased risk of embolus; requires extensive monitoring
Continuous arteriovenous hemofiltration with dialysis (CAVHD)	Arterial and central venous access	Slow fluid and solute removal via diffusion and filtration	Does not require a pump—difference between mean arterial pressure and venous pressure drives blood through the filter; uses dialysate fluid to increase solute removal; may use replacement fluids after the filter to aid in maintaining patient stability	Unreliable blood flow in critically ill, hypotensive patients; increased risk of embolus; requires extensive monitoring
Continuous venovenous hemofiltration (CVVH) (Fig. 62.10)	Double-lumen central venous catheter	Slow fluid and solute removal via convection and filtration	Requires a pump to generate pressure to drive blood through the circuit; does not use dialysate; requires replacement fluid prior to the filter; may use replacement fluids after the filter to aid in maintaining patient stability	Low solute removal due to lack of diffusion; requires extensive monitoring
Continuous venovenous hemofiltration with dialysis (CVVHD)	Double-lumen central venous catheter	Slow fluid and solute removal via diffusion and filtration	Requires a pump to generate pressure to drive blood through the circuit; uses dialysate fluid to increase solute removal; may use replacement fluids after the filter to aid in maintaining patient stability	Requires extensive monitoring

Peritoneal Dialysis

Peritoneal dialysis is another life-sustaining treatment for a patient with ESRD. It offers increased patient control and flexibility with the option of home treatment. Peritoneal dialysis requires a shorter training period for the patient and can be performed independently by the patient or a family member. Typically, PD involves fewer dietary restrictions and greater mobility for the patient. The clearance of metabolic wastes is slower but more continuous. It avoids rapid fluctuations in extracellular fluid composition and associated symptoms. Peritoneal dialysis is indicated for patients who desire more control, who have vascular access problems, or who respond poorly to HD with hemodynamic

instability. Older patients and ESRD patients with diabetes may be more easily managed with PD.

In PD, the highly vascular membrane of the peritoneal cavity is used as the dialyzing layer (Fig. 62.11). Fluid and solute removal occurs via diffusion and filtration. The PD process consists of fill, dwell, and drain phases. In the fill phase, room-temperature, sterile dialysate is instilled into the peritoneal cavity via a permanent indwelling PD catheter, typically made of silicone rubber tubing. The fluid remains in the abdomen for a predetermined "dwell time." Metabolic waste products and excess electrolytes diffuse into the dialysate while it remains in the abdomen. Water diffusion is controlled using dextrose in the dialysate as an

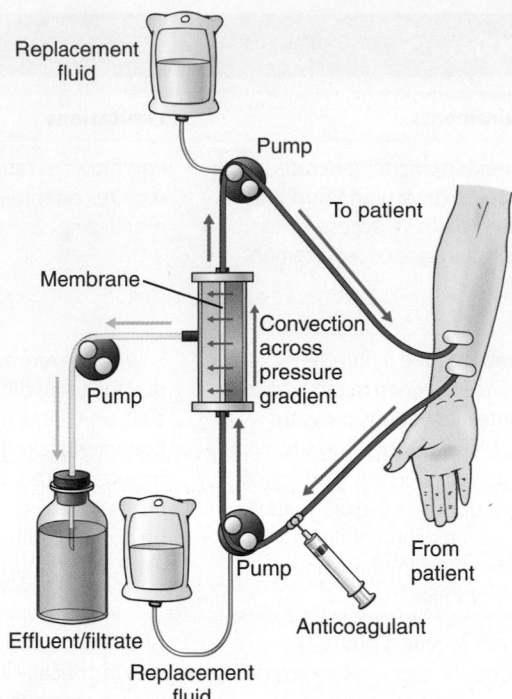

FIGURE 62.10 Continuous venovenous hemofiltration. Blood is pumped from the patient and flows through a highly permeable hemofilter that removes water and solutes. Blood continues through the filter and returns to the patient. As the blood returns to the patient, replacement fluid and electrolytes can be infused to replace volume and solutes as the patient requires to maintain stability.

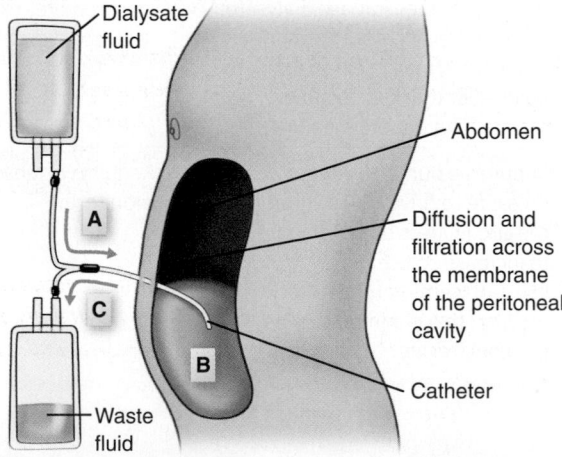

FIGURE 62.11 Peritoneal dialysis (PD). The PD process consists of the (A) fill, (B) dwell, and (C) drain phases.

osmotic agent. Gravity then drains the fluid out of the peritoneal cavity into a sterile bag.

There are several forms of PD: continuous, automated, and intermittent:

Continuous ambulatory peritoneal dialysis (CAPD). With CAPD, dialysate is infused into the abdomen four or five times a day with a dwell time of 4 to 6 hours. Patients may be ambulatory during the dwell time. With CAPD, it is not necessary to wake up and perform dialysis tasks during the night; patients typically sleep with the solution in the abdomen at night. Additionally, CAPD does not require any machines.

Automated peritoneal dialysis. Automated peritoneal dialysis uses a cycler to perform multiple overnight exchanges, specifically programmed to meet individual patient needs. A typical pattern calls for 30-minute cycles, 10 minutes for each phase, for 8 to 10 hours during the night. This method allows the patient to be dialysis-free during the day.

Intermittent peritoneal dialysis. The intermittent regimens typically consist of multiple short dwells utilizing automated technology. Intermittent peritoneal dialysis calls for 30 to 40 exchanges weekly. Typically, the patient has 30- to 60-minute exchanges, allowing approximately 15 minutes of drain time.

Contraindications

Contraindications for PD include:

- History of multiple abdominal surgeries or chronic abdominal conditions such as pancreatitis or diverticulitis
- Recurrent abdominal wall or inguinal hernias
- Obesity with large abdominal wall
- Pre-existing back problems or vertebral disease
- Severe chronic obstructive pulmonary disease

Complications

Peritonitis and Catheter Infection

Peritonitis can result from contamination of the dialysate or tubing or from bacteria in the intestine migrating into the peritoneal cavity. Peritonitis is usually caused by *S. aureus* or *Staphylococcus epidermidis*. The primary clinical manifestation of peritonitis is a cloudy peritoneal effluent with an increased WBC count. Antibiotics can be given orally, intravenously, or intraperitoneally. Repeated infections warrant removal of the PD catheter and a switch to the use of HD. Catheter site infection can also be caused by *S. aureus* or *S. epidermidis* (from skin flora) and is usually treated with antibiotics. Clinical manifestations of infections of the catheter exit site include redness at the site, tenderness, and drainage. If the infection is not treated properly, then subcutaneous tunnel infections usually result in abscess formation and may cause peritonitis, necessitating catheter removal.

Abdominal Pain

Abdominal pain and distention may be caused by intraperitoneal irritation from the low pH of the dialysate solution and generally subside in 1 to 2 weeks. Pain can also result from the tip of the catheter resting against the bladder, bowel, or peritoneum; accidental infusions of air; infusing the dialysate too rapidly; or infusing the dialysate at less than room temperature. Changing the catheter's position and attention to correctly infusing the solution may help solve these problems.

Hyperglycemia and Increased Triglyceride Levels

Glucose in the dialysate can be absorbed into the bloodstream, causing hyperglycemia. Serum triglyceride levels may also increase with PD because continuous absorption of glucose results in increased insulin secretion, which stimulates the hepatic production of triglycerides. Dietary and insulin administration modifications may be necessary.

Outflow Problems

Outflow problems occur because of mechanical interruptions in the flow of the dialysate or ultrafiltration. Interruptions may be caused by kinks in the catheter, an omentum (a fold of peritoneum) compressing the catheter, or migration of the catheter out of the peritoneal cavity. Catheter repositioning or replacement may be required. Constipation or a full colon may also cause these problems, requiring some form of cathartic.

Respiratory Compromise

Atelectasis, pneumonia, and bronchitis may occur from a repeated upward displacement of the diaphragm, resulting in decreased lung expansion. The longer the dwell time, the higher the risk of developing pulmonary complications. Frequent repositioning, deep-breathing exercises, and elevating the head of the bed can help prevent respiratory complications.

Protein Loss

The peritoneal membrane is permeable to plasma proteins, amino acids, and polypeptides, which may result in an excessive protein loss. A positive nitrogen balance can be maintained with adequate protein intake.

Connection Check 62.13

The nurse understands that CRRT is indicated for which of the following patients?

A. A hospitalized but hemodynamically stable patient
B. A hospitalized, hemodynamically unstable patient
C. A hospitalized ESRD patient being discharged home soon
D. A hospitalized ESRD patient who is stable but in an intensive care setting

Nursing Management

Nursing Interventions

■ *Assessments*

- Vital signs
  Blood pressure and heart rate are indicators of fluid volume status that are changing during the dialysis procedure. Hypotension may occur with aggressive fluid removal.
- Oxygenation/respiratory status
  Decreased oxygenation may occur with fluid volume overload, with decreased respiratory effort, or during dwell time in PD. Abnormal findings such as gallops, murmurs, rales, shortness of breath, and tachypnea can indicate fluid volume overload.
- Temperature
  Increased temperature is an indicator of infection. All forms of dialysis increase the risk of infection through the presence of multiple IV lines or a PD catheter.

- Daily weight at the same time every day
  Weight gain or loss is a good indicator of fluid volume status and helps guide dialysis treatment.
- Filtrate appearance
  Pink or bloody filtrate in any form of dialysis indicates bleeding. Cloudy filtrate in PD indicates infection.
- Laboratory values
  - Coagulation studies; hemoglobin/hematocrit
    Bleeding risk is higher with all forms of dialysis because of the need for heparinization.
  - WBC count
    Infection is a risk with all forms of dialysis.
  - Electrolytes and renal studies
    Dialysis produces changes in electrolytes and renal studies, which may require changes in the dialysis procedure or dialysate composition.
- Nutritional intake
  Sodium and water restriction may be necessary to optimize dialysis. Protein intake may need to be increased because of protein loss during dialysis.
- Specific assessments by the type of dialysis
  - HD
    - Frequent assessment of bruit/thrill
      A patent AV fistula or graft has a palpable pulsation, a thrill, and a bruit or whooshing sound on auscultation caused by the flow of blood. A normally functioning graft has a low-pitched bruit. A turbulent bruit is indicative of an increased force, mostly due to stenosis. Absence of thrill or bruit is indicative of a nonfunctional AV fistula or graft.
    - Neurological assessment
      The rapid shift of fluid and substances can create a high osmotic gradient in the brain, resulting in a shift of fluid into the brain causing cerebral edema (dialysis disequilibrium syndrome). Dialysis-related dementia, primarily caused by aluminum in the dialysate or phosphate binders, may occur.
    - Systems assessment post-dialysis
      Muscle cramps, headache, nausea, dizziness, and malaise are common during and after dialysis as a result of the rapid removal of electrolytes and water.
  - CRRT
    - Frequent/hourly vital signs
      Continuous renal replacement therapy is typically performed in critically ill patients who may become unstable during dialysis.
    - Hourly assessment of the volume of filtrate
      Increases of filtrate may require modifications of the procedure to maintain hemodynamic stability. A decrease in filtrate may indicate a clot or obstructed filter, necessitating a change in the CRRT tubing and filter.
  - PD
    - Abdominal girth
      Measure the abdominal girth and record in order to make comparisons for future assessments.
    - Monitor outflow.
      Decreased outflow may indicate a kinked or malpositioned catheter, which may require repositioning of the catheter, turning the patient to the side, or gentle abdominal massage.

Actions

- Perform dialysis as prescribed.
  - HD
    - Specially trained HD staff perform hemodialysis.
      Specialized training is required because of the risk of complications with HD, one being hypotension caused by rapid fluid shifts.
    - Avoid any procedures, blood draws, IV insertion, or blood pressure readings in the arm with the HD access.
      Use of the extremity of the vascular access site for any procedures, blood pressure readings, or venipuncture can increase the risk of thrombus formation and infection.
    - Hold medications that may be dialyzed out or cause complications during the procedure until after the HD session.
      Some antibiotics or anticonvulsants may be lost in dialysis. Water-soluble vitamins are also lost during dialysis. Antihypertensives or vasoactive medications may cause hemodynamic instability during the procedure and should be held as ordered, especially if the patient is known to be hemodynamically unstable during dialysis.
  - CRRT
    - Continuous renal replacement therapy requires intensive nursing support to perform and document hourly functions of fluid maintenance, including replacement and dialysate infusions if utilized; measuring of the filtrate; and monitoring of lines, circuits, and vital signs.
      Fluctuations may require changes in the dialysis protocol, such as decreasing fluid removal, or changes in dialysate or replacement fluid.
  - PD
    - Perform instill, dwell, and drain functions.
      This process allows for the removal of water and solutes.
    - Warm dialysate to body temperature.
      Body-temperature dialysate helps prevent hypothermia and discomfort.

Teaching

- Teaching regarding disease process and dialysis
  Teaching the patient and family regarding the importance of dialysis is essential. Compliance with dialysis, whatever form the patient is receiving, is life sustaining.
- Assistance with social service and counseling services
  Assist the patient and family in accessing social services and counseling. Patients undergoing dialysis of any form require extensive support services to assist with adaptation to their condition. The patient and family may need help coping with the loss of function of the kidney, the change in body image, and the thoughts regarding dependency on the dialysis machine.
- Teach patient and family about troubleshooting for possible problems during PD.
  Teach the patient and family the techniques of instillation, dwelling, and draining, such as warming dialysate; slowing instillation if necessary; increasing the height of bag to foster instillation; checking the tubing for kinks and removing kinks to facilitate instillation and drainage; repositioning the patient for proper instillation, dwelling, and drainage; and checking abdominal dressings for dampness and changing if needed to prevent infection.

Evaluating Care Outcomes

Dialysis does not cure renal failure but is a life-sustaining treatment. Well-managed patients can lead close-to-normal lives—able to work, relax with friends and family, and eat with some limitations—as long as they remain compliant with the prescribed dialysis treatment regimen. Strong emotional support is necessary to adapt to the changes in lifestyle and body image.

Making Connections

CASE STUDY: WRAP-UP

Doris Flood's diagnosis of PKD is confirmed by IVP. Her blood pressure remains elevated at 178/102 mm Hg. Laboratory testing reveals a BUN of 30 mg/dL and creatinine of 2.5 mg/dL, indicating renal impairment is already occurring. Ms. Flood is complaining of abdominal pain and continued urinary frequency and burning during urination. She expresses extreme anxiety over this diagnosis.

Ms. Flood's provider orders antibiotics to treat the UTI. She is started on an ACE inhibitor, captopril, for her hypertension. Ms. Flood and her provider begin discussions on how to treat her renal insufficiency. A social worker is contacted to help her obtain the resources necessary to manage her medical condition adequately. The nurse talks with her about her anxiety and helps her explore options to deal with this new diagnosis.

Case Study Questions

1. The nurse monitors for which clinical manifestation in Ms. Flood, who is newly diagnosed with PKD?
   A. Hypotension related to fluid shifts
   B. Bradycardia related to fluid overload
   C. Hypertension related to decreased renal perfusion
   D. Tachycardia related to fluid loss

2. The nurse includes which information in the teaching plan about the management of PKD?
   A. "Your blood pressure will normalize when we successfully manage your PKD."
   B. "Your UTI will not recur if you finish your antibiotic prescription."
   C. "Staying on your antihypertensive medication is necessary to control your blood pressure."
   D. "This disease is reversible if you closely follow your provider's orders."

3. The nurse providing care for Ms. Flood should include which activity in the plan of care?
   A. Providing cranberry juice at meals to reduce the risk of UTIs
   B. Frequent range-of-motion exercises to reduce stiffness due to inactivity
   C. Encourage fluids to maintain adequate volume and perfusion to the kidneys
   D. Restrict fluids to reduce the risk of fluid overload
4. The nurse caring for Ms. Flood incorporates which priority nursing diagnosis into the plan of care?
   A. Pain related to irritation on urination secondary to UTI
   B. Imbalanced nutrition related to excessive loss of protein in the urine
   C. Decreased cardiac output related to dysrhythmias secondary to electrolyte imbalance
   D. Impaired perfusion related to decreased circulating volume secondary to diuresis
5. Which statement by Ms. Flood indicates that teaching has been effective?
   A. "I'm glad we can control this disease with medications."
   B. "I'm glad we caught this early so I won't need dialysis forever."
   C. "Getting a new kidney will help even if I develop the cysts again."
   D. "I have a choice between hemodialysis and peritoneal dialysis."

CHAPTER SUMMARY

Polycystic kidney disease (PKD) is one of the most common genetic disorders. It appears as large, thin-walled, fluid-filled cysts on the kidneys. The cysts become large and compress the surrounding tissue, destroying the underlying renal tissue. The disease progresses to end-stage renal disease (ESRD) in about 50% of patients by age 60, requiring treatment consistent with ESRD—hemodialysis (HD) or peritoneal dialysis (PD). Other treatment goals for PKD include managing UTIs, pain, and hypertension.

Pyelonephritis is an inflammation of the renal parenchyma and urinary collecting system. Clinical manifestations include signs of infection, such as fever, chills, and nausea/vomiting. Antibiotics are typically used in the management of pyelonephritis.

Glomerulonephritis is an inflammation of the glomeruli of the kidney. There is an overall decrease in the glomerular filtration rate and an increase in permeability to larger-size proteins. Treatment is based on the cause of the disease and symptom management, such as diuretics and other antihypertensives to treat hypertension; edema is treated with sodium and fluid restriction, and inflammation/infection is treated with antibiotics.

Renal or kidney cancer is one of the most common cancers in the United States. Malignant tumors in the kidney are more frequent than benign tumors. Kidney tumors compress the underlying tissues, reducing circulation to the renal structures and damaging underlying tissues. This compression can lead to compromised renal functioning or renal failure. The typical treatment for renal cancer is radical nephrectomy.

The kidneys are vulnerable to injury and renal trauma because of the lack of bony structures to protect the area where they are located compared to other organs such as the heart, which the rib cage protects. The extent of the injury depends on the mechanism, the force, and the speed upon impact. Management is based on the extent of the injury. Treatment focuses on stabilizing the patient and surgically repairing any perforations or lacerations. Surgery may be required to control severe bleeding; however, if the kidneys are intact, rest and observation may be indicated.

Acute kidney injury (AKI) is a condition characterized by an acute, rapid loss of renal function. It is defined as rapid and progressive azotemia, an accumulation of nitrogenous waste products such as urea nitrogen and creatinine, and progressive increases in potassium. Prerenal causes of AKI are external to the genitourinary system that reduce renal blood flow and lead to decreased glomerular perfusion and filtration. Intrarenal causes of AKI involve direct damage to the renal system. Postrenal causes involve mechanical obstruction of the lower urinary tract. The goals of managing AKI are to eliminate the cause and prevent complications. Management is primarily supportive and involves ensuring adequate circulating volume, correcting fluid overload, and correcting biochemical abnormalities. Dialysis may need to be considered in the short term to allow recovery of the renal tissue while preventing possible life-threatening disorders.

Chronic kidney disease (CKD) is the progressive, irreversible loss of kidney function. Different from AKI, it has a longer, more insidious onset and is typically caused by a long-term disease or medical comorbidities. The diagnosis of CKD is consistent with elevated serum creatinine levels, decreased creatinine clearance determinations, and increased protein in the urine. It has profound effects on all body systems. Chronic kidney disease is managed through renal replacement therapies (RRTs) and supportive care to treat the patient's signs and symptoms and prevent any complications. Renal transplantation is a surgical option for a patient with ESRD. Renal transplantation is not considered a cure but is thought to improve the quality of life—the need for dialysis is removed, and dietary and fluid restrictions are not eliminated but are reduced.

Renal replacement therapies are artificial processes for removing waste and water from the body when the kidneys are no longer functioning. Renal replacement therapy techniques include intermittent HD, commonly referred to as hemodialysis; continuous hemofiltration and HD, also referred to as continuous renal replacement therapies (CRRTs); and PD. Intermittent HD uses the processes of diffusion and filtration to remove waste products, electrolytes, and excess water from the body. Continuous renal replacement therapy is indicated for acutely ill patients in AKI or patients with severe fluid overload. It is recommended in critically ill patients because it limits the risk of complications due to the rapid rate of fluid and solute loss, such as the hypotension that complicates intermittent HD. Peritoneal dialysis uses the highly vascular membrane of the peritoneal cavity as the dialyzing layer. Fluid and solute removal occurs via diffusion and filtration. It offers increased patient control and flexibility with the option of home treatment.

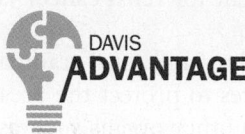

To explore learning resources for this chapter, go to **Davis Advantage** and find:
– Answers to in-text questions
– Chapter Resources and Activities
– NCLEX®-Style Chapter Review Questions
– Bibliography

Chapter 63

Coordinating Care for Patients With Urinary Disorders

Kristen Ann Farling and Joanne Walker

LEARNING OUTCOMES

Content in this chapter is designed to assist in:

1. Describing the epidemiology of urinary disorders
2. Correlating clinical manifestations with pathophysiological processes of:
   a. Urinary tract infections
   b. Urolithiasis
   c. Incontinence
   d. Bladder cancer
3. Describing the diagnostic results used to confirm the diagnosis of urinary disorders
4. Discussing the medical management of:
   a. Urinary tract infections
   b. Urolithiasis
   c. Incontinence
   d. Bladder cancer
5. Developing a comprehensive plan of nursing care for patients with urinary disorders
6. Designing a teaching plan that includes pharmacological, dietary, and lifestyle considerations for patients with urinary disorders

CONCEPTS

- Assessment
- Cellular Regulation
- Comfort
- Fluid and Electrolyte Balance
- Infection
- Medication
- Perioperative
- Safety
- Urinary Elimination

ESSENTIAL TERMS

Adjuvant
Calculus
Clean intermittent catheterization (CIC)
Cystitis
Detrusor muscle
Dysuria
External urethral sphincter
Functional incontinence
Hematogenous
Hematuria
Immunotherapy
Internal urethral sphincter
Micturition
Neoadjuvant
Nephrolithiasis
Overflow incontinence
Pessary
Precision medicine
Pyelonephritis
Reflex incontinence
Stress incontinence
Targeted therapy
Ureterolithiasis
Ureteropelvic
Urge incontinence
Urothelium

Finding Connections

CASE STUDY: EPISODE 1

Follow this patient throughout the chapter.

Heather Tomlinson is a healthy 24-year-old sexually active female who presents with a 3-day history of urinary frequency, dysuria, and urgency. She denies fever, chills, or vomiting but has mild nausea. She is married and the mother of a 1-year-old daughter. Her family history is significant for heart disease and kidney stones. Physical examination reveals a well-nourished female in no distress. Mild suprapubic tenderness is noted but no costovertebral angle tenderness (tenderness on the back in the area over the kidneys). VSs: T 98.9°F (37.2°C), P 75 bpm, R 18, BP 118/78 mm Hg. Urinalysis reveals cloudy yellow urine, urine dip TNTC (too numerous to count) white blood cells, small amount of red blood cells, positive nitrites, and a large number of bacteria. A urine culture is submitted, and results are awaited...

URINARY TRACT INFECTIONS

Epidemiology

Urinary tract infections (UTIs) account for 8 million doctor visits and more than 100,000 hospital admissions each year. The annual cost of treating UTIs is estimated to be $1 billion. Urinary tract infections occur more frequently in females than males. As men age, however, their risk for UTIs increases because of prostatic enlargement. More than 50% of females will have at least one UTI in their lifetime (see Evidence-Based Practice). The most common age groups for UTIs in women are those in the 18-to-30-year range (thought to be due to honeymoon **cystitis** and pregnancy) and older women. Sexual activity, diabetes, poor hygiene, estrogen deficiency, recent catheterizations, and foreign objects such as kidney or bladder stones increase the risk of developing a UTI. Conditions causing incomplete bladder emptying, such as pelvic organ prolapse, also increase the risk for UTI because of retained urine acting as a reservoir for bacteria. If the infection is isolated to the lower urinary tract or bladder, it is referred to as *cystitis*, and if it involves the upper urinary tract or kidneys, it is referred as **pyelonephritis**.

Evidence-Based Practice

Treatment and Prevention of Recurrent Lower Urinary Tract Infections in Women

A rapid review of the literature was conducted to evaluate the science addressing the treatment and prevention of recurrent urinary tract infections (UTIs) in women, defined as more than two UTIs in 6 months or more than three UTIs in 1 year. After evaluation of original research, systematic reviews, meta-analyses, and practice guidelines, an algorithmic approach was developed. The algorithm proposes the use of prophylactic antibiotics after patient assessment for complicating factors and education regarding behavioral changes such as better control of glucose in diabetes, discontinuing the use of cleansers that disrupt normal flora, voiding before and after sexual activity, and avoiding sequential anal and vaginal intercourse.

Smith, A. L., Brown, J., Wyman, J. F., Berry, A., Newman, D. K., & Stapleton, A. E. (2018). Treatment and prevention of recurrent lower urinary tract infections in women: a rapid review with practice recommendations. *The Journal of Urology, 200*(6), 1174-1191.

Connection Check 63.1

The nurse recognizes which patient is at greatest risk for a UTI?

A. A 35-year-old sexually active male
B. A 23-year-old sexually active female
C. A 50-year-old sexually active female
D. An 18-year-old sexually active male

Pathophysiology

A UTI occurs when bacteria enter the sterile bladder, causing inflammation. The most common way for bacteria to gain entrance to the bladder is through the urethra. A **hematogenous**, or blood-borne, infection is less common. Females are at risk for developing a UTI because of their short urethra and its close proximity of the vagina and rectum. This proximity allows vaginal and fecal flora to migrate to the urethra, causing a UTI. Men are less likely to develop a UTI because of their long urethra that deters migration of bacteria to the bladder.

Clinical Manifestations

Clinical manifestations of a UTI include bladder irritability or **dysuria** (painful urination), urinary frequency, urgency, urinating in small volumes, gross **hematuria** or microhematuria, and suprapubic pain. If systemic symptoms such as fever, nausea, vomiting, and flank pain are present, the infection has potentially migrated to the kidney and is classified as pyelonephritis.

Management

Medical Management

Diagnosis

Diagnosis of a UTI is based on clinical manifestations and aided by urinalysis. A urine culture may be done when necessary or in the case of a complicated UTI. A visual inspection of the urine specimen may reveal bloody and/or cloudy urine. Urinalysis demonstrates leukocytes, nitrites, hemoglobin, and bacteria. Leukocytes or white blood cells (WBCs) and red blood cells (RBCs) are present in the urine because of the inflammatory and infectious process associated with an infection. Nitrites are present because some bacteria convert nitrate to nitrite. Urine culture reveals greater than 100,000 bacteria. *Escherichia coli*, *Enterobacter*, *Pseudomonas aeruginosa*, and *Klebsiella pneumoniae* are common offenders. *E coli*, a common intestinal bacterium, is responsible for 80% of all uncomplicated UTIs.

Treatment

Treatment is primarily through medications. First-line treatment is antimicrobial therapy. The choice of antibiotic is dependent on urine culture sensitivities but, typically, an uncomplicated UTI—women who are not pregnant, do not have diabetes and are afebrile—can be treated empirically with a 3-day course of antibiotics. Trimethoprim/sulfamethoxazole (Bactrim DS) and ciprofloxacin (Cipro) are common antibiotics prescribed because of their efficacy in treating urogenital pathogens. A complicated UTI—diabetic, febrile, male gender—is typically treated with 7 to 10 days of antibiotics. In addition to antibiotics, bladder analgesics such as phenazopyridine (Pyridium) can be used to decrease dysuria, frequency, and urgency. Urinalysis and a urine culture can be obtained after completing antibiotics to verify the infection has been treated appropriately.

Complications

Complications of a UTI include drug resistance or pyelonephritis and renal abscess. Drug resistance is possible when the patient does not complete antibiotics as prescribed. This resistance makes it difficult to find an appropriate antibiotic when/if the infection returns. Untreated or incomplete treatment of a UTI potentially allows for bacteria to migrate to the kidneys, causing pyelonephritis or renal abscess.

Surgical Management

Surgical management of a UTI is reserved for patients with known risk factors for infections (bladder or kidney stones) or anatomical defects allowing for incomplete bladder emptying (pelvic organ prolapse in women or an enlarged prostate in men). An example of pelvic organ prolapse is a cystocele, which occurs when the walls between the bladder and vagina are weakened, allowing the bladder to descend into the vagina (Figure 63.1). This change in anatomy prevents the bladder from emptying completely, leading to UTIs. Surgical interventions such as colporrhaphy correct the defect in the vaginal wall, allowing the bladder to empty effectively, thus decreasing the risk of UTIs. Similarly, men with an enlarged prostate can also retain urine and develop UTIs (Figure 63.2). Surgical interventions for this condition, such as a transurethral resection of the prostate, remove excess prostatic tissue, allowing for complete bladder emptying.

Nursing Management

Assessment and Analysis

Most patients' physical examination is benign. When present, clinical manifestations of a UTI are due to the inflammatory process that occurs because of the infection. Assess the patient for the following:

- Fever
- Dysuria
- Urinary frequency
- Urinary urgency
- Gross hematuria
- Cloudy urine
- Malodorous urine

Physical examination findings of suprapubic tenderness, costovertebral tenderness, or fever may indicate pyelonephritis. Assess vital signs for temperature elevation, tachycardia, and low blood pressure, which can be indicative of an infection requiring hospitalization for fluid status monitoring and IV antibiotics.

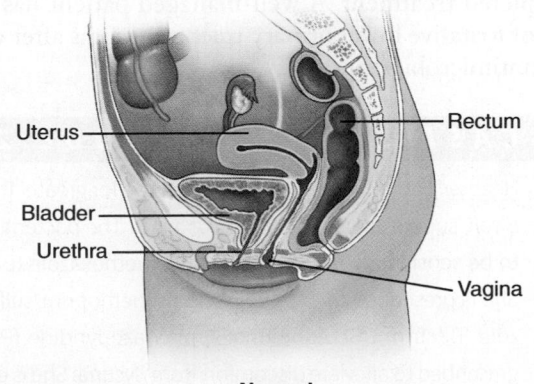
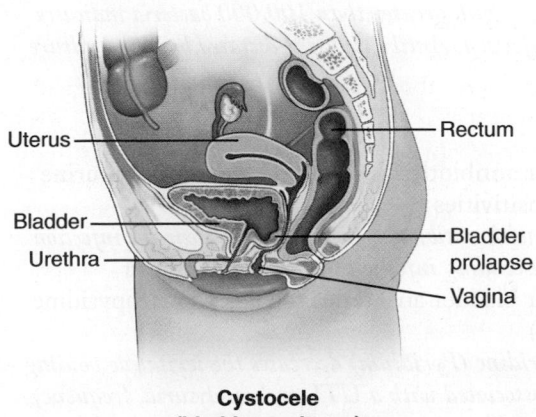

Normal

Cystocele (bladder prolapse)

FIGURE 63.1 Cystocele (bladder prolapse). The walls between the bladder and vagina are weakened, allowing the bladder to descend into the vagina.

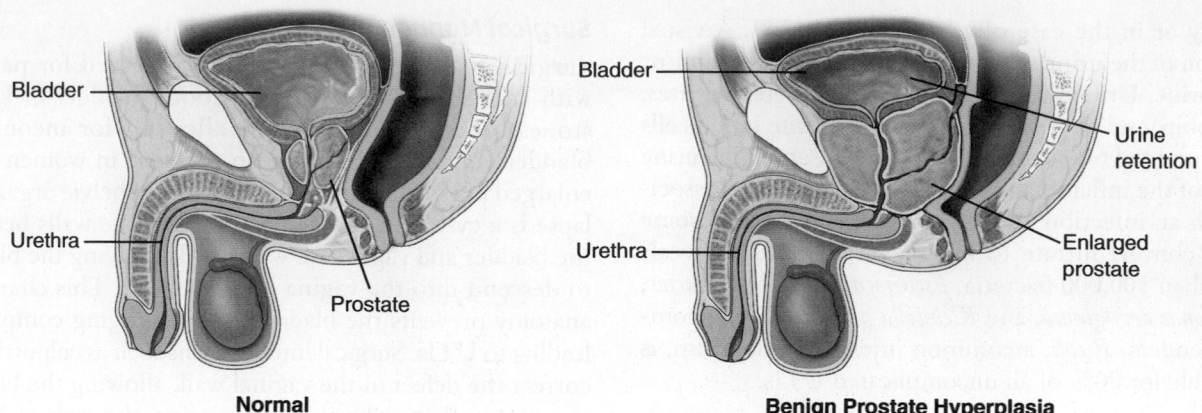

FIGURE 63.2 Benign prostatic hyperplasia (enlarged prostate) can cause urinary retention, which increases the risk for urinary tract infection.

Nursing Diagnoses

- **Altered urinary elimination** associated with irritation of bladder mucosa
- **Knowledge deficit** associated with the infection
- **Acute pain** associated with inflamed bladder mucosa

Nursing Interventions

■ *Assessments*

- Vital signs
  Elevated temperature, elevated heart rate, and decreased blood pressure may indicate upper urinary tract involvement and dehydration or a patient developing a systemic infection.
- Urinary symptoms
  Dysuria, urinary frequency, urgency, and gross hematuria are signs of a possible UTI.
- Abdominal examination
  Suprapubic tenderness can indicate lower tract infection, and costovertebral tenderness can indicate upper tract infection.
- Urinalysis
  The presence of hematuria, leukocytes, nitrates, and cloudy urine indicates infection.
- Urine culture
  Urine culture with greater than 100,000 bacteria indicates an active infection. Antibiotic use is dictated by urine culture sensitivities.

■ *Actions*

- Administer antibiotics as ordered, dependent on urine culture sensitivities
  Treatment with antibiotics, if indicated to clear the infection and avoid ascending infection such as pyelonephritis
- Administer bladder analgesics such as phenazopyridine (Pyridium)
  Phenazopyridine (Pyridium) decreases the irritative voiding symptoms associated with a UTI, such as dysuria, frequency, and urgency. Phenazopyridine (Pyridium) is used only short term (3 days) to avoid masking continued symptoms of a UTI.

■ *Teaching*

- Report elevated temperature, flank pain, nausea, and vomiting
  Fever, flank pain, nausea, and vomiting despite antimicrobial therapy may indicate spread of infection, antibiotic resistance, and the need for either hospitalization or a change in antibiotics.
- Increase fluid intake
  Increase fluids to prevent dehydration and to flush urine of bacteria.
- Signs and symptoms of a UTI
  Early treatment of infection decreases morbidity.
- UTI prevention
  Wipe front to back and urinate before and after intercourse to prevent migration of bacteria to the bladder.
- Medication education
  Complete all antibiotics as prescribed. Untreated or incomplete treatment of a UTI may cause pyelonephritis or renal abscess or drug resistance. Educate patients that phenazopyridine (Pyridium) turns the urine an orange/red color.

Evaluating Care Outcomes

The health of the kidneys is protected by early and completed treatment. A well-managed patient has resolution of irritative lower urinary tract symptoms after completing antimicrobial therapy.

CASE STUDY: EPISODE 2

Heather's urine culture results are positive for greater than 100,000 *E coli*, supporting the diagnosis of a UTI. The bacteria are shown to be sensitive to trimethoprim/sulfamethoxazole (Bactrim DS). She is prescribed a 7-day course of trimethoprim/sulfamethoxazole (Bactrim DS). Additionally, phenazopyridine (Pyridium) is prescribed to alleviate discomfort from dysuria. She is encouraged to increase her water intake…

UROLITHIASIS

Epidemiology

Urolithiasis is calcifications in the urinary system, commonly referred to as *kidney stones*. They can occur in the kidneys, ureter, and bladder, with renal stones being the most prevalent. **Nephrolithiasis** refers to a **calculus** in the kidney; **ureterolithiasis** refers to a calculus in the ureter. Urinary stones affect 12 per 10,000 persons in the United States, occur more frequently in males, and affect Caucasians more than African Americans. Stones appear more frequently in the southeastern United States and summer months, thought to be because of humidity, sweating, and decreased water consumption leading to dehydration. Family history increases one's risk of stones as do dietary habits such as increased sodium intake. Industrialized countries have a higher incidence of stones, thought to be due to high dietary protein intake. A person who develops urinary stones is at an increased risk of developing subsequent stones, with 10% of first-time stone formers developing another stone within 10 years.

Connection Check 63.2

The nurse understands which population is at increased risk for developing urinary stones?
A. Black females living in Florida
B. White males living in Georgia
C. Black males living in New York
D. White females living in Oregon

Pathophysiology

Urinary stones occur when microscopic crystals in the urinary tract aggregate together, causing a stone (calculus) to occur. Just as a small piece of sand can cause a pearl to develop in an oyster, tiny crystals in the urine can accumulate to form a stone. The majority of stones (80%) are calcium, and the remaining 20% are a combination of cystine, uric acid, and xanthine. Dehydration contributes to stone formation by allowing solutes to accumulate in the concentrated urine. Common places for a stone to obstruct include the **ureteropelvic** junction as the urine exits the kidney, the lower third of the ureter as it crosses the iliac vessels, and the ureterovesical junction as the urine flows into the bladder (Fig. 63.3).

Clinical Manifestations

The major clinical manifestation of urinary stones is severe pain when the stone lodges in the ureter, causing distention and obstruction of urine flow. Pain associated with urinary stones is usually colicky, with concomitant nausea and vomiting. The location of the stone influences the location of the pain, with upper ureteral stones causing referred pain to the flank and lower ureteral stones causing lower abdominal, genital pain along with irritative voiding symptoms. Gross hematuria and microhematuria

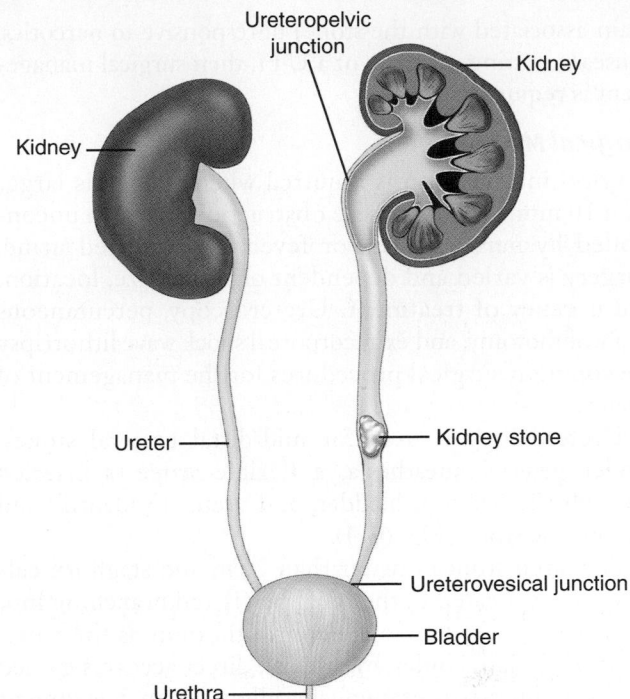

FIGURE 63.3 Kidney stone in the ureter.

can be present with any stone location and occur in 95% of patients.

Management

Medical Management

Diagnosis

The diagnostic modality of choice for urinary stones is a noncontrast, stone survey computed tomography (CT) scan. A CT scan is a quick, noninvasive imaging modality with high sensitivity and specificity. In addition to identifying calculi, CT can assess for obstructive uropathy such as hydronephrosis. Hydronephrosis, or swelling of the kidneys, occurs when urine flow is blocked, allowing urine to accumulate in the kidney. A kidney ureter bladder (KUB) plain film or x-ray is quick and inexpensive but does not detect radiolucent stones such as uric acid stones. Ultrasound is recommended in children and pregnant females because of the lack of radiation exposure.

Treatment

Fifty percent of stones less than 5 mm pass spontaneously. For patients with small, less than 5-mm stones, minimal pain, and no hydronephrosis or infection, the opportunity to pass the stone on their own, a trial of passage, is the first-line treatment. Narcotics and/or nonsteroidal anti-inflammatory medicine along with antiemetics are used during this trial of passage. Alpha-adrenergic blockers such as tamsulosin (Flomax), doxazosin (Cardura), and terazosin (Hytrin) can be used to relax the musculature of the lower ureter and aid in stone passage. If the stone does not pass after 4 to 6 weeks or if the patient develops renal colic (pain associated with the stone) unresponsive to narcotics, nausea/vomiting, or signs of a UTI, then surgical management is required.

Surgical Management

Surgical intervention is required when a stone is larger than 10 mm, causing severe obstruction and pain uncontrolled by narcotics and/or fever with infected urine. Surgery is varied and dependent on stone size, location, and urgency of treatment. Ureteroscopy, percutaneous nephrolithotomy, and extracorporeal shock wave lithotripsy are common surgical procedures for the management of stones.

Ureteroscopy is used for mid/distal ureteral stones. Under general anesthesia, a flexible scope is inserted through the urethra, bladder, and ureter to identify and remove the stone (Fig. 63.4).

For large stones greater than 2 cm and staghorn calculi, stones located in the renal pelvis and branching into the calyces, percutaneous nephrolithotomy is the treatment of choice. Under anesthesia, direct access is gained to the kidney percutaneously, allowing an instrument called a *nephroscope* to identify and remove the offending stone (Fig. 63.5).

Extracorporeal shock-wave lithotripsy (ESWL) can be used for both renal and ureteral stones less than 2 cm. Extracorporeal shock-wave lithotripsy is a noninvasive procedure that utilizes shock waves to break up stones into small pieces, allowing the patient to pass stone fragments. Under conscious sedation and with the assistance of fluoroscopy, the offending stone is identified and fragmented with shock waves. Contraindications to ESWL include pregnant females and patients with uncorrected bleeding disorders (Fig. 63.6).

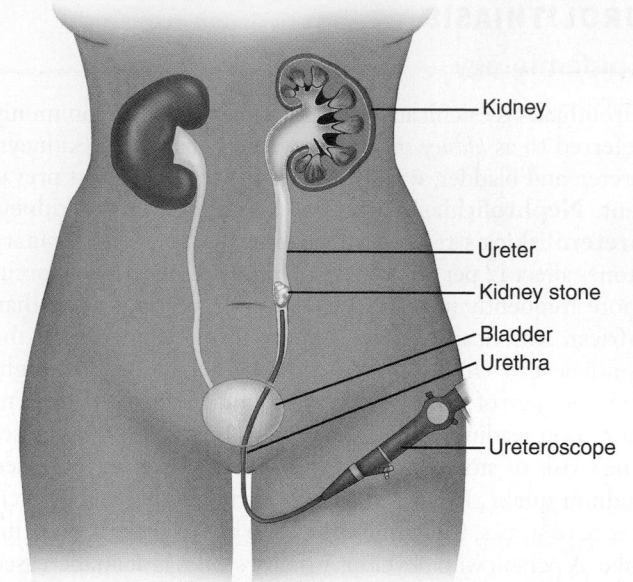

FIGURE 63.4 Ureteroscopy: a flexible scope is inserted through the urethra, bladder, and ureter to identify and remove the stone.

Complications

Untreated stones can lead to pyelonephritis, urosepsis, and irreversible renal damage. A rise in renal function indicators such as blood urea nitrogen and creatinine (BUN/Cr) indicates that aggressive treatment of the kidney stone is required to avoid these complications. A ureteral stent or nephrostomy tube may be necessary to allow drainage of urine from the obstructed kidney. A ureteral stent is a thin, flexible tube inserted into the ureter to facilitate urine drainage from the kidney. A nephrostomy tube is inserted through the skin into the kidney to allow urine drainage.

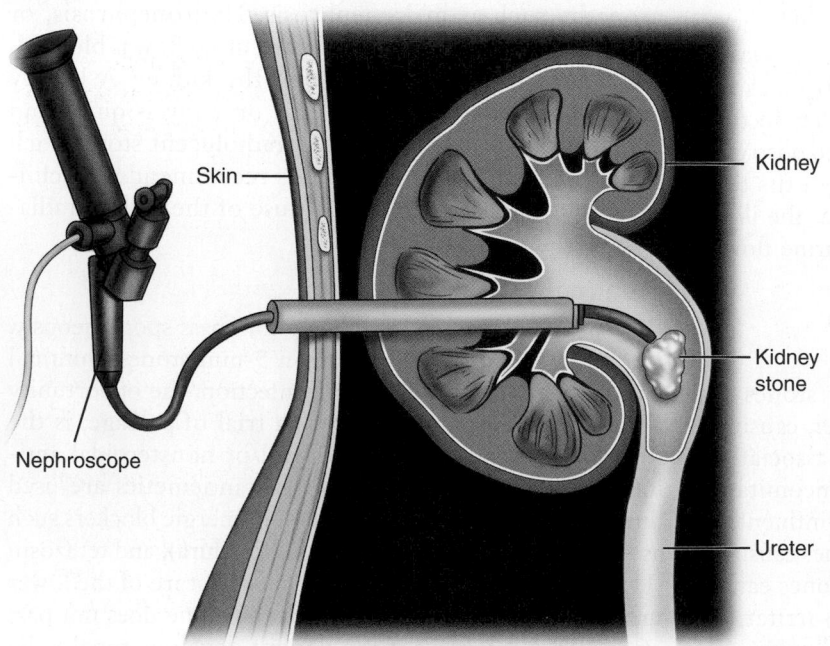

FIGURE 63.5 Percutaneous nephrolithotomy: direct access is obtained to the kidney percutaneously, allowing a nephroscope to identify and remove the offending stone.

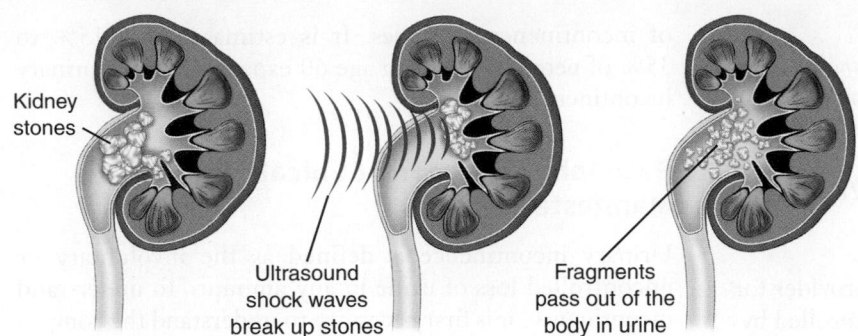

Kidney stones

Ultrasound shock waves break up stones

Fragments pass out of the body in urine

FIGURE 63.6 Extracorporeal shock-wave lithotripsy (ESWL) to crush kidney stones.

> **Safety Alert** If a trial of passage is prescribed, it is imperative that the patient either confirms passage of the stone with actual stone fragments collected while straining urine or that a KUB or CT scan confirms passage of the stone. A retained, asymptomatic ureteral stone can insidiously obstruct the flow of urine, resulting in potential loss of kidney function.

Nursing Management

Assessment and Analysis

The prominent clinical manifestation of urolithiasis is pain. It is due to the stone lodging in the ureter causing inflammation, distention, and blockage of urine flow. Renal colic is the severe, intermittent pain associated with a kidney/ureteral stone. Patients with renal colic have a difficult time finding a comfortable position because of the pain. Patients may be pacing, trying to alleviate the pain. This is in contrast to patients with other types of severe pain who sit or lie as still as possible because movement exacerbates the pain.

Nursing Diagnoses

- **Acute pain** associated with inflammation and obstruction of the kidney
- **Altered elimination** associated with the obstruction
- **Risk for infection** associated with the obstructed stone

Nursing Interventions

■ *Assessments*

- Vital signs
  Increased heart rate and respiratory rate may be due to pain. Elevated temperature and low blood pressure can be caused by dehydration, infection and sepsis, and complications of untreated stones indicating a need for more aggressive therapy.
- Pain or renal colic—severe, intermittent pain associated with a kidney/ureteral stone
  Evaluation of pain helps determine the location of the stone and is necessary to evaluate effectiveness of the therapy. Renal stones cause flank pain and may radiate to the scrotum in men and the vulva in females. Midureteral stones can present with abdominal pain. Lower ureteral stones can present with

lower abdominal pain, referred pain to the genitalia, and irritative voiding symptoms.
- Nausea and vomiting
  Kidney obstruction can cause nausea and vomiting because of severe pain and irritation of the gastric nerve.
- Urine pH
  Acid stones are formed in acid urine.
- Urine culture
  A positive urine culture indicates the need for aggressive management with antibiotics, stone removal, and possible hospitalization.
- Complete blood count and serum chemistries
  Elevated WBC count may indicate antibiotics are required. Monitor BUN/Cr to assess renal function. The BUN may be elevated if dehydrated, and the Cr may be elevated in acute obstruction of the kidney with resulting renal damage.
- Urine output/color
  Minimal urine output should be between 30 and 50 mL/hr. Decreased urine output may indicate dehydration or an obstructed kidney. Gross hematuria may be present and, if present, ranges from iced-tea color to fruit punch. Aggressive stone removal is indicated for thick urine, "ketchup" consistency, or blood clots.

■ *Actions*

- Administer analgesics such as hydromorphone (Dilaudid) or morphine sulfate (morphine) as ordered
  Kidney stones can cause severe pain because of inflammation, irritation, distention, and blocked urine flow.
- Administer antiemetics as ordered
  Kidney stones can cause nausea and vomiting because of gastric nerve irritation.
- Administer alpha blockers as ordered
  Tamsulosin (Flomax), doxazosin (Cardura), or terazosin (Hytrin) helps dilate/relax the lower ureter and allows for ease of stone passage. A common side effect is light-headedness, and patients should be educated to rise slowly from a seated position to avoid orthostatic hypotension.
- Maintain fluid status; encourage PO fluids or administer fluids IV as ordered.
  Hydration to facilitate urine production and flow is paramount in kidney stone management. If the patient is unable to stay hydrated despite antiemetics, hospitalization for IV fluids may be required.

- Strain urine
  Collect stone and send for stone analysis. Stone analysis helps dictate patient education and prevention of future stones.
- Insert Foley catheter if the patient is unable to void
  Urine retained in the kidney or bladder puts the patient at risk for pyelonephritis, urosepsis, and irreversible renal damage.

■ *Teaching*

- Trial of passage patients: Strain urine, call provider for fever, chills, nausea/vomiting, or pain uncontrolled by pain medicine
  - *Straining urine is important to confirm passage of the stone with actual stone fragments.*
  - *The symptoms may indicate obstruction and/or infection and the need for hospitalization.*
- Kidney stone prevention: hydration, low-sodium diet, increase dietary intake of citrate, decrease dietary intake of oxalate
  - *Hydration is paramount in the prevention of kidney stones. Encourage urine output of 2 L a day and monitor urine color. If urine is clear yellow, this shows adequate hydration, and if urine is amber, this indicates the need to increase fluids.*
  - *A low-sodium diet can prevent stones by decreasing the risk of dehydration associated with a high-sodium diet.*
  - *Increase dietary intake of citrate found in lemons and lemonade. Citrate prevents the formation of stones.*
  - *Avoid foods high in oxalate, such as rhubarb, chocolate, tea, coffee, and nuts. These foods can increase the risk of stones.*

Connection Check 63.3

Which statement by the patient indicates teaching about tamsulosin (Flomax) has been effective?
A. "Will this medicine help my nausea?"
B. "So, this medicine will help me pass the stone by relaxing the muscles?"
C. "I need to take this medicine so I don't get an infection."
D. "This medicine is for my pain."

Evaluating Care Outcomes

The avoidance of kidney stone formation is accomplished by adequate hydration, following dietary restrictions, and careful monitoring. If a stone is present, kidney function can be preserved through careful assessment of urine and appropriate management with hydration. A well-managed patient is free from pain, is afebrile, and has adequate amounts of clear yellow urine.

INCONTINENCE

Epidemiology

Urinary incontinence is a growing public health problem that affects approximately 20 million Americans. While the percentage of our aging population increases, the incidence of incontinence increases. It is estimated that 15% to 35% of people older than age 60 experience some urinary incontinence.

Pathophysiology and Clinical Manifestations

Urinary incontinence is defined as the involuntary or uncontrolled loss of urine in any amount. To understand incontinence, it is first necessary to understand the components of the normal **micturition** (urination) cycle. It involves a complex interplay between the sympathetic and parasympathetic nervous systems. The parasympathetic nervous system provides motor stimulation to the bladder and mediates bladder contraction. The sympathetic nerves mediate bladder storage by stimulating contractions in the bladder neck and proximal urethra, blocking urine flow. While the bladder slowly fills with urine from the kidneys via the ureters, the stretching of the **detrusor muscle** (or bladder muscle) slowly increases. Stimulation from the sympathetic nervous system maintains closure of the **internal urethral sphincter** preventing contraction of the detrusor muscle, allowing the bladder to fill. When the detrusor muscle reaches a certain threshold of distention, sensory nerves on the bladder wall are stimulated. This sensation is perceived as fullness, and the signal is transmitted to the spinal cord, to S2–S4, the portion of the spinal cord known as the *sacral micturition center*, by way of the pelvic nerve. The message is also transmitted to the brain via the spinal cord. The brain then sends the message back through the spinal cord via parasympathetic fibers (sympathetic activity is inhibited) to initiate detrusor muscle contraction. At the same time, the internal urethral sphincter relaxes (an involuntary action) to initiate voiding, or emptying, of the bladder. If perceived as an appropriate time to void, the **external urethral sphincter** is voluntarily relaxed, allowing urine to flow into the urethra.

There must be intact neural pathways for normal bladder function. Injuries or lesions at the level of S2 to S4 or below generally result in an areflexic (flaccid) bladder, resulting in retention with overflow. Injuries above this level often result in a hyperreflexic bladder, resulting in uncontrolled spontaneous voiding. Types of incontinence include **stress incontinence**, **urge incontinence**, mixed (combination of stress and urge), **overflow incontinence**, **reflex incontinence** or **functional incontinence**. Types, causes or risk factors, and manifestations are outlined in Table 63.1.

Management

Medical Management

The first step in the management of urinary incontinence is a realization on the part of the patient that incontinence is not a normal part of the aging process and that it is often treatable and always manageable. The nurse plays a key role in the management process throughout, beginning by

Table 63.1 Types of Incontinence

Incontinence Type	Causes/Risk Factors	Manifestations
Stress incontinence	● More common in women ● Childbirth, which causes stretching and relaxing of pelvic floor muscles, ligaments, and urethra ● Postmenopausal women ● Smoking, obesity	● Urine leakage occurs when abdominal pressure increases: laughing, coughing, lifting, exercising
Urge incontinence	● Exposure to bladder irritants such as caffeine, artificial sweeteners, or nicotine	● Strong urge to urinate followed by uncontrolled leakage
Mixed (combination of stress and urge)	● Combination of previous	● Combination of above
Overflow	● Flaccid/enlarged bladder due to obstruction (e.g., enlarged prostate), spinal cord injury, stroke, diabetes, neurological diseases	● Frequent urination
Functional	● Inability to get to the toilet or communicate the need to do so	● Patient is continent but environmental factors lead to loss of urine in inappropriate areas
Reflex	● Disorders that affect the nervous impulse for voiding such as multiple sclerosis, brain tumors, or stroke	● Bladder muscle contracts on its own, urethral sphincters exhibit varying control

encouraging the patient to seek help/evaluation and helping to reduce the self-imposed stigma that many patients feel.

Diagnosis

Diagnosis starts with a thorough history. This history should include questions about medical, urological, voiding, neurological, and reproductive history. The patient should be questioned as to management routines and patterns of incontinence and voiding characteristics. A voiding diary may provide much useful information. A physical should include a thorough neurological assessment and examination of the genitalia.

Laboratory Testing/Imaging Studies

Laboratory testing begins with urine culture and urinalysis, which may rule out infection and/or illness such as uncontrolled diabetes mellitus as factors. Blood tests associated with renal function, such as BUN/Cr, reveal the effects of bladder function on the upper urinary tracts.

Imaging studies may include plain x-rays or films of the kidneys, ureters, and bladder (KUB), IV pyelogram (an x-ray of the renal system with IV contrast solution to facilitate imaging), or a voiding cystourethrogram (VCUG). A VCUG uses contrast dye injected into the bladder to enable visualization of the voiding process. Ultrasound tests provide useful information about the urinary tract without exposing the patient to radiation. Urodynamic studies measure the transport, storage, and elimination functions of the urinary tract. An element of urodynamic testing is uroflowmetry, which tests the urinary flow rate in milliliters per second.

A cystometrogram (CMG) assesses the bladder's filling and storage function. It graphically represents bladder pressure compared with volume while the bladder is filled with liquid. Often, a CMG is coupled with a sphincter electromyogram. Electrical signals from the periurethral muscles are graphically recorded by placing electrode patches on the external area (perineal and perianal). A pressure-flow analysis combines data from the previous tests with measurement of the urine flow pattern.

Treatment

The primary goal of treatment, when possible, is to prevent or stop urinary leakage. If this is not possible, containment with scrupulous skin care and odor control becomes the new objective. Another goal of equal importance is prevention or reduction of damage to the upper tracts or the kidneys, manifested by deteriorating renal function. Management is based on the type of incontinence and is done with medications, nonsurgical measures, or surgical measures if the medications or nonsurgical means have not worked. Medications indicated in the management of incontinence are noted in Table 63.2.

Nonpharmacological and nonsurgical measures include measures to strengthen the pelvic floor such as Kegel exercises. Kegel exercises consist of contracting and relaxing the pubococcygeus muscles that form part of the pelvic floor in an effort to improve muscle tone. Specifically, Kegel exercises are used for strengthening the **external urinary sphincter**, which is under voluntary control. Other nonsurgical means are treatments that alter the angle of the structures that affect bladder and urethral pressure such as a pessary. A **pessary** is a device that fits into the vagina to

Table 63.2 Medications Used to Treat Incontinence

Medication	Purpose
Anticholinergics Oxybutynin (Ditropan); tolterodine (Detrol); darifenacin (Enablex); trospium (Sanctura); salifenacin (Vesicare); and fesoterodine (Toviaz)	Used to calm an overactive bladder. Anticholinergics block nervous stimulation from the parasympathetic nervous system to help relax and control bladder muscle contractions
Topical estrogen	Used in stress incontinence in peri and postmenopausal women to help restore tone in the urethra and vaginal areas
Tricyclic antidepressant Imipramine (Tofranil)	Used to treat mixed-urge and stress incontinence; decreases bladder contractility and has an antispasmodic effect on the bladder
Alpha-adrenergic blockers Tamsulosin (Flomax), alfuzosin (Uroxatral)	Used in issues of urge or overflow in men - useful in enlarged prostate issues. Promote urethral relaxation, relaxes bladder neck and muscle fibers in the prostate
Beta-3 adrenergic agonist Mirabegron (Myrbetrig)	Used to treat frequent and/or urgent uncontrolled urination; relaxes bladder muscles

BPH, Benign prostatic hyperplasia.

support the bladder in an attempt to control incontinence and support bladder emptying (Fig. 63.7). **Clean intermittent catheterization (CIC)** is another technique used to manage incontinence. Clean intermittent catheterization involves the intermittent placement of a catheter through the urethra into the bladder. This is done to completely empty the bladder in an effort to prevent UTIs or kidney damage due to urinary retention. A CIC also helps establish voiding patterns and may eliminate the frequent feelings of needing to void.

Surgical Management

Surgical interventions include procedures that tighten the pelvic floor and provide support to the urethra; a suburethral sling used for stress incontinence, or a procedure to increase bladder capacity; augmentation cystoplasty. There are several types of suburethral slings; a bladder neck or pubo-vaginal sling with support at the bladder neck and proximal urethra and a midurethral sling with support at midurethral level. These slings prevent urethral descent and urine leakage during physical activity or stress when abdominal pressure increases. Severe stress incontinence after prostate cancer treatment in men can be treated with an artificial urinary sphincter. This is a surgically implanted device; a cuff, balloon and pump, which supports the function of the urinary sphincter by restricting flow from the bladder via the saline filled cuff around the urethra. When appropriate to void, the man squeezes the pump located in the scrotum, allowing the saline to flow from the cuff into the balloon, releasing the pressure to allow urination. See Table 63.3 for a listing of interventions based on incontinence type.

Complications

Complications of urinary incontinence include skin changes associated with exposure to a moist environment. Poorly managed incontinence may also lead to renal disease secondary to retention and/or incomplete emptying, which results in backflow of infected urine.

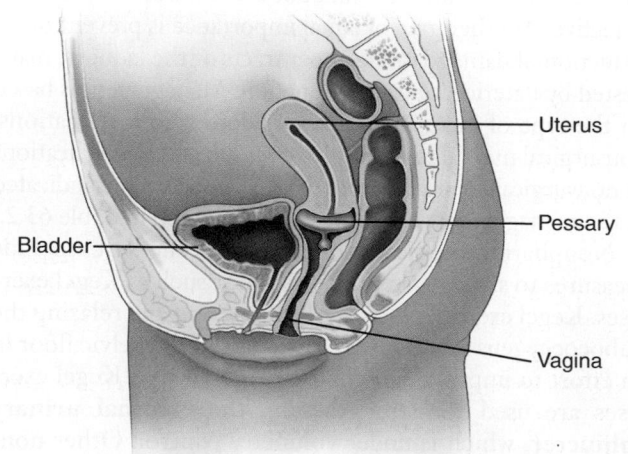

FIGURE 63.7 Pessary: a device that fits into the vagina to support the bladder in an effort to control incontinence.

Connection Check 63.4

The patient with stress incontinence is prescribed Kegel exercises. The nurse tells the patient that Kegel exercises will help:
A. Strengthen the detrusor muscle
B. Strengthen the posterior urethral valves
C. Strengthen the internal sphincter
D. Strengthen the external sphincter

Table 63.3 Interventions Based on Incontinence Type

Type of Incontinence	Nonsurgical Measures	Surgical
Stress	• Pelvic floor exercises, e.g., Kegel • Pessaries	• Suburethral sling • Artificial urinary sphincter • Collagen injection (periurethral) to strengthen the muscles around the urethra
Urge	• Eliminate bladder irritants such as nicotine or coffee • Prompted voiding—voiding at predetermined intervals • Fluid control; adequate intake without large volumes at one time, stop intake 2 hours before sleep • Clean intermittent catheterization (CIC) when antispasmodics are used in doses high enough to paralyze the detrusor muscle • Biofeedback	• Augmentation cystoplasty to increase bladder capacity
Reflex incontinence and dyssynergia (incoordination of the detrusor muscles and the external urethral sphincter)	• CIC • Reflex voiding (for men)—using a condom catheter and a leg bag to collect the urine—allowing the bladder to spasm and empty on its own	• Augmentation cystoplasty
Overflow incontinence (retention)	• CIC • Indwelling catheter • Double voiding—void and then wait 3-5 minutes and void again • Fluid control—adequate intake—spread out during waking hours—stopping 2 hours before bed	• Correction of underlying obstruction
Total or continual incontinence	Containment devices and skin protection, such as diapers and skin barrier ointments	• Correction of structural anomaly • Urinary diversion
Functional	Nursing measures to alleviate functional aspects of leakage, such as timed toileting or mobility devices	• As indicated by concomitant causes of incontinence

Nursing Management

Assessment and Analysis

The clinical manifestations of incontinence vary depending on the causative factors. Some patients have stress incontinence associated with physical activity due to sphincter incompetence. Others have incontinence associated with urinary retention issues secondary to obstructions such as benign prostatic hypertrophy.

Nursing Diagnoses

- **Alteration in urinary elimination** associated with lack of control
- **Knowledge deficit** associated with incontinence skin care and management
- **Alteration in body image perception** associated with incontinence or "wetting" episodes

Nursing Interventions

■ *Assessments*

- Vital signs
  Increased temperature, rapid pulse, and decreased blood pressure may indicate infection with urinary retention as a possible etiological factor
- Assessment of what precipitates urinary incontinence
  Determining the cause, such as stress or urge incontinence, impacts treatment.
- Urinalysis
  White blood cells, nitrates, proteinuria, and hematuria may indicate infection.
- Urine culture
  A urine culture identifying specific bacteria identifies the presence of an infection and dictates antibiotic treatment.

- Voiding diary
  Determining incontinence patterns is essential to outlining management options.

◼ Actions

- Administer medications as ordered on the basis of incontinence assessment results
  - Anticholinergics/Antispasmodics
    Block impulses from the parasympathetic nervous system to relax and control the bladder.
  - Tricyclic antidepressants
    Decreases bladder contractility and has an antispasmodic effect on the bladder
  - Alpha-adrenergic blocking agents
    Promote urethral relaxation; aid in issues of urinary retention
  - Topical estrogen
    Restore tone in urethra and vaginal areas
  - Beta-3 Adrenergic Agonist
    Relaxes bladder muscles

◼ Teaching

- Medications
  Understanding the medications and side effects used in the treatment plan helps ensure compliance.
- Technique for CIC
  Clean intermittent catheterization is a fairly easy but awkward procedure. Adequate teaching with a return demonstration helps ensure effective technique at home.
- Voiding diary
  The voiding diary helps determine the type of incontinence and the effectiveness of therapy.

Evaluating Care Outcomes

The well-managed patient has been assessed for type of incontinence, and appropriate interventions have been implemented. The incontinence has been resolved or managed through containment and skin barrier products, and the patient is able to carry out normal activities of daily living. The patient is clean, odor-free with intact skin, and has a management plan in place that considers mobility, skin integrity, and maintenance of urological health.

BLADDER CANCER

Epidemiology

Bladder cancer is the fourth most common cancer among men and the eighth most common among women. The incidence of bladder cancer has increased by 50% from the mid-1950s to the mid-1990s. According to the American Cancer Society, in 2017 in the United States there were 79,030 new cases of bladder cancer and 16,780 deaths. Smoking is the most important risk factor for bladder cancer in the United States. Other risk factors include aromatic amine exposure from the rubber and chemical industries, polycyclic aromatic hydrocarbon exposure from the coal and aluminum industries, chronic infection

or inflammation from chronic catheter use, or incomplete bladder emptying. In some third-world countries, schistosomiasis, a parasitic infection, is the leading risk factor.

Pathophysiology and Clinical Manifestations

Tumor formation in bladder cancer is attributed to genetic changes in target cells. Target cells are normal cells of the body that have undergone some alteration, synthesize abnormal proteins, and then undergo malignant changes. The process is thought to be caused by the activation of oncogenes (genes that when altered promote the uncontrolled proliferation of cancer cells) that act in one of two ways: by inactivation of tumor suppression genes or by activation of genes that cause cells to grow in a rapid, random manner.

The tumor, nodes, metastasis (TNM) staging system is a widely used system for staging all types of cancer (Fig. 63.8). Bladder cancers are classified as non-muscle invasive cancer (T1), affecting the inner lining of the bladder (**urothelium**), or muscle invasive cancer (T2–T4), which means the cancer has extended through the urothelium and into the detrusor muscle. Painless hematuria is the most common presenting symptom of bladder cancer.

Management

Medical Management

Diagnosis

Early detection and treatment increase survival rates. A thorough history and physical are essential first steps in reaching a diagnosis of bladder cancer. The history should

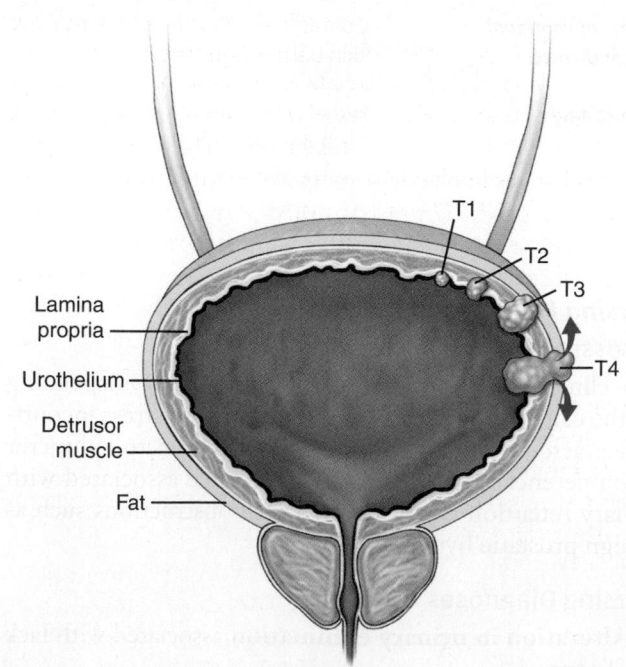

FIGURE 63.8 The stages of bladder cancer. Superficial (T1) cancer affects the urothelium or lining of the bladder. Invasive (T2–T4) is when the cancer has extended through the urothelium and into the detrusor muscle.

include careful questioning associated with risk factors such as smoking and exposure to second-hand smoke. There are a number of tests that are helpful in determining a diagnosis of bladder cancer. Urine cytology is a screening test but has only 40% accuracy. Blood and urine tests may be done to look for tumor markers. Urine cultures are done to rule out infection as a cause of symptoms. Cystoscopy, or examination of the bladder with a scope, is used to make a definitive diagnosis. This is coupled with a biopsy of any lesions that are discovered during the examination. Imaging studies (CT, magnetic resonance imaging, positron emission tomography, ultrasound) may be used to determine whether there is spread of the cancer outside of the bladder.

Treatment

Drug therapy for low-grade bladder cancers consists of topical therapy or installation of solutions into the bladder, intravesical therapy. This can be either intravesical immunotherapy or chemotherapy. Intravesical immunotherapy, such as bacille Calmette-Guérin (BCG), is aimed at "jump-starting" the body's own immune defenses to battle the invasion of cancer. Intravesical chemotherapy instills medications given to kill actively growing cancer cells.

Although topical chemotherapy has long been a mainstay in the treatment of non-invasive bladder cancers, systemic **immunotherapy** is relatively new in the treatment of later-stage bladder cancer. In a healthy individual, "checkpoint" molecules keep the immune system from attacking the body's normal cells. Cancer cells avoid being attacked by the immune system by using these checkpoint molecules. Systemic immunotherapy targets checkpoint molecules. Examples of drugs in this category are atezolizumab (Tecentriq), durvalumab (Imfinzi), avelumab (Bavencio), nivolumab (Opdivo) and pembrolizumab (Keytruda).

New advances in high-grade metastatic bladder cancer management and treatment may be classified under the broad title of **precision medicine**. Diagnostic testing may identify genetic changes in bladder cancer cells and allow more accurate/precise prediction of individual prognosis. Those individuals with cancers that are likely to recur are candidates for **targeted therapy**. Targeted drug therapy is directed at changes in cells that cause them to become cancer: examples include lapatinib (Tykerb) and erlotinib (Tarceva). This therapy may also target blood vessels that carry nutrition to the cancer cells using antiangiogenesis drugs. Examples of these drugs are bevacizumab (Avastin); sorafenib (Nexavar); cabozantinib (Cometriq); and pazopanib (Votrient). Gene therapy is another new treatment using lab-modified viruses that are instilled into the bladder and infect cancer cells.

> ⚠ **Safety Alert** Bacille Calmette-Guérin is a live, weakened bacterium. To ensure that others are not infected by the bacteria, after voiding following treatment, the patient should pour 2 cups of bleach into the toilet and allow it to sit for 20 minutes before flushing.

Surgical Management

The surgical interventions for low-grade bladder cancers consist of excision or removal of the tumor through fulguration or laser ablation. Fulguration destroys the tumor by using high-frequency electrical current, and laser ablation destroys tissue by irradiating it with a laser beam.

Prior to treatment, a biopsy is done to determine the depth of invasion. Intravesical chemotherapy may be given before surgical excision (**neoadjuvant**) or after surgical excision (**adjuvant**). Radiation is indicated postoperatively.

Muscle-invasive bladder cancers require more extensive and life-altering treatments. There are surgical, nonsurgical, and combined approaches. One approach, a "bladder preservation" procedure; excision of the tumor or partial cystectomy (partial bladder removal), may be combined with radiation and/or chemotherapy. Chemotherapy is indicated to downgrade tumors preoperatively or to help eradicate cancer that has spread beyond the bladder either grossly (visible to the eye) or microscopically through the lymphatic system. Radiation is indicated postoperatively in those patients who have solid tumor recurrence after cystectomy.

Another approach for surgical management of invasive bladder cancer, radical cystectomy, combined with neoadjuvant chemotherapy, is considered to be the definitive approach. It offers the best chance of cure or extension of the disease-free state. In male patients, the procedure is called a *radical cystoprostatectomy* and involves removal of the bladder, prostate, seminal vesicles, lower ureters, and in some cases, the urethra. In female patients, the procedure is called a *radical cystectomy* or *anterior exenteration*. Generally, the structures removed are the bladder, uterus, ovaries, fallopian tubes, anterior wall of the vagina, lower ureters, and often the urethra. These procedures also involve pelvic lymph node dissection in both male and female patients. There is controversy as to how extensive this dissection should be, and it varies from a wide, all-encompassing excision to excision of the sentinel lymph node.

This radical surgery requires reconstruction of the urinary tract. This may be accomplished in one of three ways, all of which use segments of the gastrointestinal tract to provide reconstruction for the removed portion of the urinary tract. The ileal conduit uses a short (15-cm) segment of ileum to provide a viaduct for the exit of urine from the body through a stoma on the abdomen. The orthotopic neobladder uses 20 to 30 cm of small intestine to create a bladder that is anatomically in the same position as the native bladder and uses the patient's external sphincter for continence. The third option, a neobladder with catheterizable stoma and an internal pouch to collect urine, requires clean intermittent catheterization (CIC) and is the option most fraught with complications. Table 63.4 outlines options for urinary tract reconstruction.

Table 63.4 Summary of Urinary Tract Reconstruction Options

	Ileal Conduit	Orthotopic Neobladder	Neobladder With Continent Catheterizable Stoma
Advantages	• Simplest "tried and true" procedure • Fewest complications	• No external pouch • Most closely resembles "normal" urination	• No external pouch • Stoma often placed in umbilicus, not visible
Disadvantages	• External pouch, stoma • Adhesives may cause skin irritation • Lifelong equipment (pouches, drainage bag) required	• May require intermittent catheterization • May require physical therapy for sphincter training • May not achieve continence	• Stoma may not be continent • Strictures at skin level may occur • Catheter required to empty the internal pouch at regular intervals
Bowel used	• 10–15 cms of terminal ileum	• 30 cm of ileum	• Ileum and cecum, possibly appendix

Connection Check 63.5

The nurse understands that non-muscle cancers affect only:

A. Muscle and surrounding fat
B. The urothelium, or inner lining of the bladder
C. Structures adjacent to the bladder
D. The lobes of the prostate

Complications

Complications may be associated with the disease process or treatment. Disease process complications include bleeding from friable tumors in the bladder or pain caused by impingement of other organs by the tumor. Treatment-related complications include lasting side effects from chemotherapy, such as peripheral neuropathy, or hemorrhagic cystitis from radiation. Complications from surgery include bowel obstruction, fistula formation, hernia development in the surgical site, and complications/disadvantages specific to the type of reconstruction of the urinary tract (see Table 63.4).

Nursing Management

Assessment and Analysis

The clinical manifestations noted in patients with bladder cancer are typically associated with treatment side effects and the emotional factors associated with the diagnosis. Fatigue and poor nutritional intake may be associated with chemotherapy or antibiotic side effects such as lowered hemoglobin and hematocrit, nausea, and oral thrush. Decreased appetite and a flat affect may be associated with depression secondary to poor prognosis and a change in body image. Painless hematuria, which may be gross or microscopic, is the most common presenting symptom of bladder cancer. The patient may have irritative voiding symptoms (frequency, urgency, nocturia), which may be due to the presence of the tumor in the bladder.

Nursing Diagnoses

- **Knowledge deficit** associated with disease, diagnostics, and management options
- **Alteration in elimination pattern** associated with the effects of treatment on a continuum from irritative symptoms to reconstruction of the urinary tract

Nursing Interventions

■ *Assessments*

- Vital signs
  Increased pulse and decreased blood pressure may indicate blood loss postoperatively. Increased pulse, decreased blood pressure, and increased temperature may indicate infection.
- Urinalysis
  Hematuria may be present in bladder cancer.

■ *Actions*

- Administer medications as ordered:
  - Intravesical immunotherapy
    Immunotherapy is used to aid the body's natural defense against tumor growth.
  - Intravesical chemotherapy
    Chemotherapy is used to destroy the tumor cells.
  - Immunotherapy
    Systemic immunotherapy targets checkpoint molecules to allow for destruction of cancer cells.
  - Targeted therapy
    Targeted drug therapy is directed at changes in cells that cause them to become cancer or target blood vessels that carry nutrition to the cancer cells
- Continuous bladder irrigation (CBI)
  Continuous bladder irrigation may be used after tumor excision or biopsy to clear blood and clots from the bladder and prevent obstruction.
- Accurate intake and output
  Accurate bladder intake and output recording is essential to determine whether clots have cut off the flow of urine. (If CBI is in place, true urine output = total fluid output minus amount of irrigant instilled.)

■ *Teaching*

● Bladder cancer, treatment and outcome
A cancer diagnosis is frightening. Increasing a patient's knowledge helps him or her feel a measure of control and increases compliance.

Evaluating Care Outcomes

The well-managed patient with bladder cancer has an effective pain management plan in place, is disease-free or symptom controlled, and is aware of the treatment course and options. Anxiety is at an acceptable level as self-reported or reported by significant others. There is an awareness of how to access support through peer and professional groups.

Making Connections

CASE STUDY: WRAP-UP

Heather understands the importance of completing her antibiotics as directed to prevent bacterial resistance. She is encouraged to increase her fluid intake to flush her urine and to call her provider for fever or flank pain or if her symptoms do not improve after completing the antibiotics. She is provided with education on how to prevent future UTIs, such as wiping front to back after using the toilet and urinating after sexual intercourse.

Case Study Questions

1. Which statement by Heather regarding new flank pain indicates teaching has been effective?
   A. "I'll call the doctor for pain medicine if the flank pain comes back."
   B. "Does new flank pain mean I might have an infection in my kidneys?"
   C. "New flank pain means the infection has spread to my gallbladder."
   D. "This pain may mean the infection could involve my reproductive system."

2. Which action by Heather indicates the need for further teaching about her prescribed medicines?
   A. Heather calls in a panic because her urine is an orange color.
   B. Heather is scheduling her follow-up appointment even though her dysuria resolved with phenazopyridine (Pyridium).
   C. Heather states her understanding that phenazopyridine (Pyridium) should be taken no more than 3 days.
   D. She reports her symptoms have improved but continues to take her trimethoprim/sulfamethoxazole (Bactrim DS) as prescribed.

3. The nurse recognizes Heather's urinalysis is suspicious for a UTI by the presence of the following: *(Select all that apply.)*
   A. Ketones
   B. White blood cells
   C. Bacteria
   D. Bilirubin
   E. Protein

4. Which statements are true regarding UTIs? *(Select all that apply.)*
   A. Urinary tract infections are more common in women because of the close proximity of the urethra, vagina, and rectum.
   B. Sexual intercourse does not increase the risk for UTIs.
   C. It is more common for males to develop a UTI because of the length of the urethra.
   D. Sexual intercourse increases the risk for a UTI.
   E. Flank pain is a symptom of lower UTIs.

5. The nurse understands which common signs indicate a lower UTI? *(Select all that apply.)*
   A. Fever
   B. Dysuria
   C. Frequency
   D. Hematuria
   E. Nausea

CHAPTER SUMMARY

Urinary tract infections occur more frequently in young women but can affect older men and women as well. Irritative voiding symptoms such as frequency, urgency, dysuria, and suprapubic pain are signs of a UTI, and diagnosis is made on the basis of urinalysis and urine culture results. Treatment of UTIs is based on urine culture sensitivities, and repeated urine cultures should be obtained after completion of antibiotics to verify that the infection has been eradicated.

Approximately 8% of Americans will develop a kidney stone in their lifetime. Kidney stones frequently occur in the southeastern United States, and risk factors for urolithiasis include poor fluid intake, diet high in sodium and protein, and family history. Patients with urolithiasis can develop severe pain, and the size and location of the stone helps dictate treatment options. If the patient has a concurrent UTI, surgical intervention may be required.

Urinary incontinence, defined as the involuntary or uncontrolled loss of urine in any amount, affects as many as 25 million Americans, both men and women. Incontinence is a symptom of other pathology. Careful assessment is necessary to determine the type of incontinence, eliminate the causative factors, and formulate the disease-specific treatment plan. In part because of our aging population (baby boomers), incontinence is one of the fastest-growing public health problems.

Bladder cancer incidence has increased by 50% in the last 40 years. In the United States, cigarette smoking is the most important risk factor, which has implications for public health education by nurses. Treatment for bladder cancers ranges from intravesical instillations of chemotherapeutic agents for superficial and low-grade cancers to bladder removal and urinary tract reconstruction for muscle-invasive or high-grade cancers.

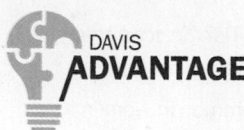

To explore learning resources for this chapter, go to **Davis Advantage** and find:
- Answers to in-text questions
- Chapter Resources and Activities
- NCLEX®-Style Chapter Review Questions
- Bibliography

Promoting Health in Patients With Reproductive Disorders

Chapter 64

Assessment of Reproductive Function

Valerie Bader

LEARNING OUTCOMES

Content in this chapter is designed to assist in:

1. Identifying key anatomical components of the reproductive system
2. Discussing the function of the reproductive system
3. Describing the procedure for completing a history and physical assessment of reproductive function
4. Correlating relevant diagnostic examinations to reproductive function
5. Explaining nursing considerations for diagnostic studies relevant to reproductive function
6. Discussing changes in reproductive function associated with aging

CONCEPTS

- Assessment
- Female Reproduction
- Inflammation
- Male Reproduction
- Pregnancy

ESSENTIAL TERMS

Androgens
Breast
Cervix
Clitoris
Ejaculation
Epididymis
Estrogen
Fallopian tubes
Fertile
Follicle-stimulating hormone (FSH)
Gonad
Gravida (G)
Labia majora
Labia minora
Luteinizing hormone (LH)
Menarche
Menstruation
Mons pubis
Oocyte
Ovaries
Ovulation
Parity
Penis
Perineum
Progesterone
Prostate gland
Scrotum
Seminal vesicles
Sperm
Spermatogenesis
Testes
Testosterone
Uterus
Vagina
Vas deferens
Vulva

Finding Connections

FEMALE REPRODUCTIVE SYSTEM

The main goal of the reproductive system is to ensure species survival through the creation of life. To accomplish reproduction, the female reproductive system manages the following: (1) the secretion of sex hormones; (2) the production of ova (eggs); and (3) maintenance of an environment for fertilization, embryonic and fetal development, and expulsion of the fetus when it has physiologically matured and can survive extrauterine life.

Anatomy of the Female Reproductive System

The anatomy of the female reproductive system includes both external female genitalia and internal reproductive organs. External female genitalia are collectively referred to as the *vulva*, and includes two structures not directly involved in reproduction, the urethral meatus and the perineal body (the central tendon of the perineum that provides support to the pelvic floor). The internal female reproductive organs are directly responsible for reproduction and both produce and respond to female sex hormones.

External Female Genitalia

The external female genitalia or **vulva** consists of the **mons pubis, labia majora, labia minora, clitoris, vestibule,** and the **perineum**: the area between the **vagina** and **anus** (Fig. 64.1). The mons pubis is located anterior to the vaginal opening and is composed of a firm pad of adipose tissue that protects the symphysis pubis during sexual intercourse. After puberty, the mons pubis is covered by coarse hair in the shape of an inverted triangle. The labia majora consist of two folds of dense adipose tissue that extend directly from the mons pubis. The labia majora provide a protective covering for the labia minora. They can vary in size and appearance depending on age and childbearing status. The labia majora are 7 to 8 cm in length, 2 to 3 cm in width, and 1 to 1.5 cm in thickness and are somewhat tapered in the posterior portion.

The labia minora consist of two smaller folds of connective tissue, covered by skin without hair follicles. The skin of the labia minora is rich in sebaceous glands, which lubricate the area, and nerve endings, which make this tissue very sensitive. The labia minora have a pink to reddish color and can vary greatly in appearance depending on age, race, and parity. Anteriorly, the labia minora converge to form the frenulum of the clitoris. Posteriorly, the labia minora meet to form the fourchette, which is a bandlike area of skin that may tear during vaginal childbirth, or trauma. The fourchette is directly anterior to the anus.

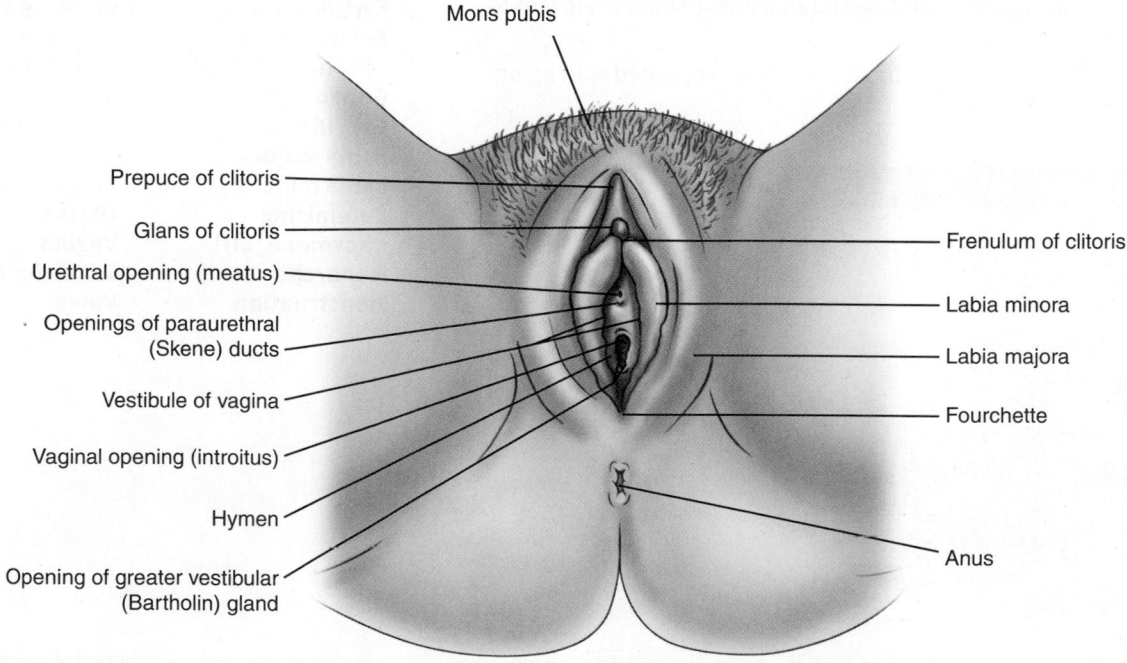

Mons pubis

Prepuce of clitoris

Glans of clitoris

Urethral opening (meatus)

Openings of paraurethral (Skene) ducts

Vestibule of vagina

Vaginal opening (introitus)

Hymen

Opening of greater vestibular (Bartholin) gland

Frenulum of clitoris

Labia minora

Labia majora

Fourchette

Anus

FIGURE 64.1 Female external genitalia.

The clitoris, at the anterior junction of the labia minora, consists of erectile tissue that extends through both sides of the labia minora. Together, the clitoris and labia minora are anatomically homologous structures to the male penis. The clitoris especially is very well innervated, which heightens sensitivity and erotic sensation. The clitoris, like the penis, enlarges with sexual stimulation. The area of skin that surrounds the hood of the clitoris is called the *glans clitoris*. The glans clitoris is the exposed portion of the clitoris. It is located at the anterior junction of the labia minora and together with the labia minora plays a vital role in sexual sensation.

The vaginal vestibule is located medially to the labia minora. It is composed of the external urethral orifice, vaginal introitus, hymen, if present, and Skene's and Bartholin's glands. The majority of the vestibule is occupied by the vaginal orifice called the *introitus*, the opening of the vagina, which may be covered by the hymen. The hymen is a thin membrane that can completely or partially cover the vaginal orifice if present. The vestibular bulbs consist of two elongated masses of erectile tissue on either side of the vaginal orifice. The vestibular bulbs become engorged with blood during sexual arousal, causing narrowing of the vaginal orifice during intercourse. This narrowing applies pressure on the penis during intercourse and thus increases stimulation of the penis. The vestibular bulbs are analogous to the corpus spongiosum of the penis.

The urethral orifice, or meatus, is posterior to the clitoris and anterior to the vaginal opening. This is the site of micturition, or voiding. On either side of the urethral meatus are the Skene's glands, also referred to as the *paraurethral glands*. These glands are mucus-secreting glands embedded in the urethral wall. The Skene's glands are anatomically homologous structures to the male prostate gland. The Bartholin's glands, or greater vestibular glands, are located just inside the vaginal opening. The Bartholin's gland secretes mucus that helps to lubricate the vagina and introitus during intercourse.

Connection Check 64.1

The patient asks the nurse in which part of her vulva do orgasms occur. The nurse understands the principal location of sexual pleasure for women is which of the following?
A. Clitoris
B. Hymen
C. Vagina
D. Introitus

Internal Female Genitalia

The internal female genitalia consist of the vagina, cervix, uterus, fallopian tubes, and ovaries (Fig. 64.2). The **vagina** is a tube that serves as a passageway for menstrual flow, sexual intercourse, and childbirth. The entrance is marked by the introitus and extends to the uterine cervix. The walls of the vagina are approximately 7.5 cm anteriorly and 9 cm posteriorly and are lined with a mucous membrane called the *vaginal mucosa*. Vaginal mucosa is composed of stratified squamous epithelium and has a pink to reddish color with tiny palpable folds called *rugae*. The rugae unfold, and the cells of the vagina enlarge during pregnancy, both of which allow the vagina to expand dramatically during childbirth and accommodate the birth of the fetus. The vagina is directly adjacent to the bladder anteriorly, and the rectum posteriorly. Normal vaginal discharge is composed of mucoid cervical secretions, desquamated vaginal wall epithelium, and normal bacteria.

The uterine **cervix**, located in the deepest part of the vagina, contains a narrow opening into the uterus which is

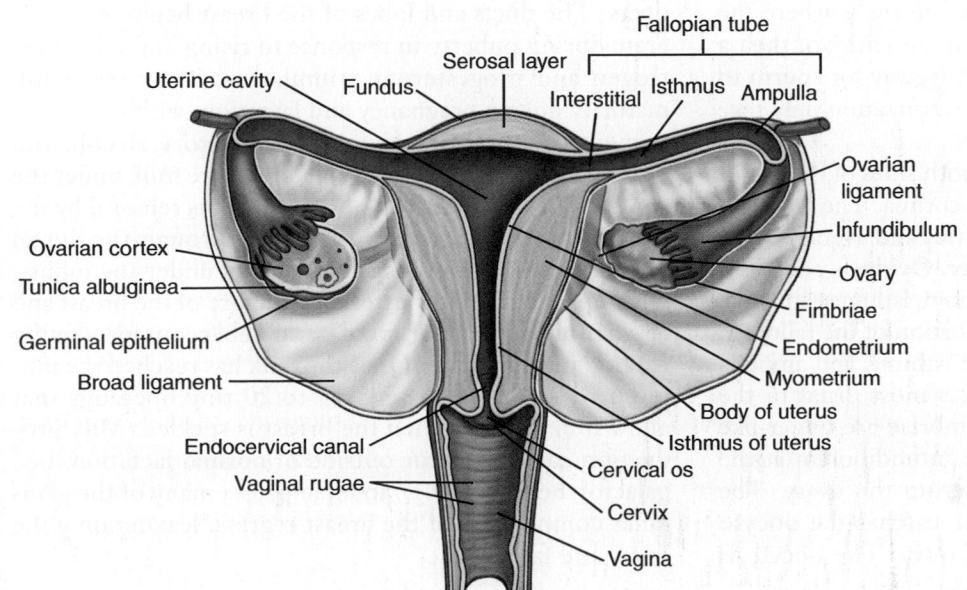

FIGURE 64.2 Internal female reproductive genitalia.

called an *os*. The cervix can be visualized by using both a speculum, which is inserted into the vagina, and a light source. On visual examination, a nulliparous (a woman who has not given birth) woman's cervix appears smooth with a small circular os, whereas the cervical os of a woman who has given birth appears more like a slit. The outer portion of the cervix, which protrudes into the upper vagina, is covered by stratified squamous epithelial tissue. The endocervical canal, to which the os opens, can be 2 to 4 cm in length and is lined with columnar epithelial tissue. The squamocolumnar junction is the area where the columnar epithelium of the endocervical canal, and the squamous epithelium of the external os meet. The cells of the squamocolumnar junction are sampled for the Papanicolaou (Pap) smear, because this area is where cervical cancer occurs.

The **uterus**, also called the *womb*, is shaped like an inverted pear. It is a thick-walled, hollow, muscular organ, located between the bladder and the rectum. The uterus is suspended in the pelvis by a series of ligaments and is usually positioned in an anteverted posture, tilting slightly anteriorly. The uterus is divided into three distinctive areas: the cervix; the lower uterine segment or isthmus; and the upper uterine segment, at the top of which is the dome-shaped fundus. The size of the uterus varies, depending on age and **parity** (viable pregnancies) but is approximately 7.3 cm in length, 4 cm in width, and 3.2 cm in height for nulliparous women. The uterus has several layers: the outermost layer of the uterine wall is called the serosal layer, the middle muscular layer is called the myometrium, and the inner layer that grows and sheds with each menstrual cycle is called the *endometrium*. The term **menstruation** refers to the shedding of the endometrial lining each month while a woman is fertile. The middle layer of the uterus, or myometrium, has muscle fibers arranged in three layers: each layer of cells is aligned at an angle to the other layers. When the uterine muscle contracts, arterioles that are perpendicular to the layers of muscle cells are closed off, and bleeding is controlled. This action prevents continuous haemorrhage during childbirth. The uterus is where the fertilized ovum, or zygote grows into an embryo, then a fetus. The uterus also provides a passageway for **sperm** to travel to the fallopian tubes, where fertilization may take place.

The **fallopian tubes** grow from both sides of the top of the uterus, an area referred to as the cornua. The fallopian tubes, or oviducts, extend to the ovaries and average 10 to 14 cm in length and 1 cm in diameter. Oviducts consist of four anatomical sections: the interstitium, isthmus, ampulla, and infundibulum. The interstitial portion of the fallopian tube is closest to the uterus, and the isthmus and ampulla are midsection. The infundibulum is most distal to the uterus and closest to the ovaries. Fimbriae are finger-like projections extending out from the infundibulum at the very end of the fallopian tube covering the ovary. The fimbriated end of the fallopian tube catches the **oocyte** (immature ovum) released by the ovary. The oocyte is then swept toward the ampulla by the movement of ciliated columnar epithelium cells and muscular tubal contractions. The ampulla is the site of fertilization of the oocyte by the sperm. A pregnancy that implants outside the uterus, in the fallopian tube, causes severe pain and internal haemorrhage.

The **ovaries** are located on either side of the uterus in the upper pelvic cavity in an area called the *ovarian fossa*. They are suspended by the ovarian ligament anteriorly and the broad ligament posteriorly that runs between the pelvic sidewall and the uterus. Ovaries are shaped like a large almond and are grey in color: a normal ovary measures as large as 1.5-cm by 2.5-cm and 4-cm long. The ovaries are the female gonad; ovarian follicles, the site of oocyte or egg development, are located within the ovaries. The ovaries are the site where female sex hormones (**estrogen and progesterone**) are produced. At birth, a woman has over a million oocytes present in each ovary, of which approximately 300 mature and are released during the reproductive years.

Breasts

Breast tissue consists of a series of glands, lobes, ducts, and fibrous and fatty tissue (Fig. 64.3). They are attached to the chest wall by the fascia covering the pectoralis major muscle and serratus anterior muscles. Cooper's ligaments connect the fascia of the two muscles and form support for the breasts that lie between the second and sixth rib and extend from the sternum to the midaxillary line. Fibrous and fatty tissue forms the majority of the breast's volume and provides support for the underlying ducts and lobes. The variations in breast size and shape can be attributed to the amount of dense fibrous and fatty tissue and are greatly affected by pregnancy, lactation, and age.

Each breast contains approximately 15 to 20 lobes of glandular tissue; mammary glands that produce milk after childbirth. Lobes connect to the nipple through extensive ducts. The ducts and lobes of the breast begin to proliferate during puberty in response to rising and falling estrogen and progesterone stimulation. They reach full maturity during pregnancy and lactation, with the development of more extensive lobes, secretory alveoli, and ducts. During lactation, the alveoli secrete milk under the stimulation of prolactin, a hormone that is released by the anterior pituitary gland. Milk flows through the ductal system to the lactiferous sinus directly under the nipple. The nipple is the most external structure of the breast and is surrounded by the areola and sebaceous-producing Montgomery's glands. Once the milk has reached the nipple, it is expelled through 15 to 20 tiny openings that allow milk to flow when the breast is suckled. Milk production can also occur outside of normal lactation, i.e., galactorrhea (Box 64.1). In menopause, many of the glandular components of the breast regress, leaving only the ducts and fatty tissue.

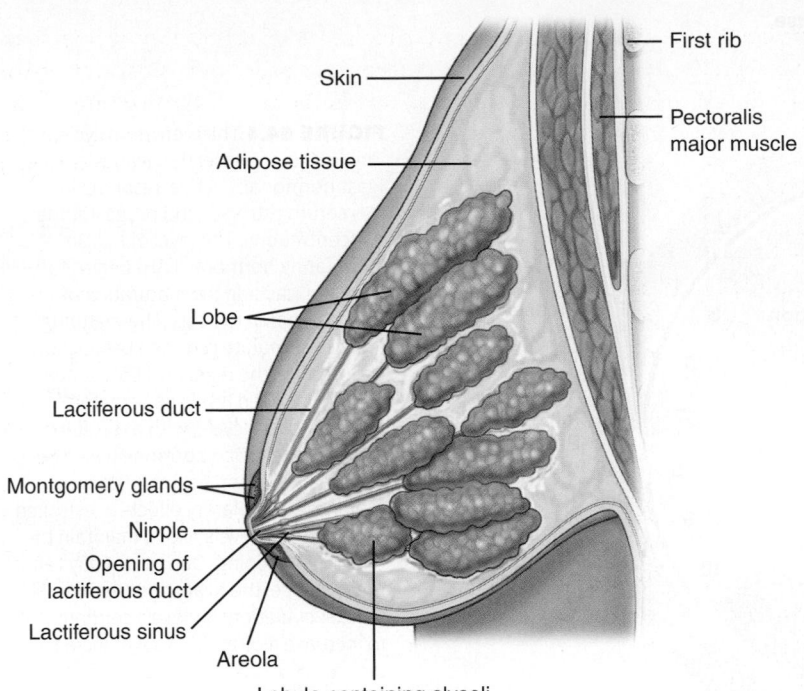

FIGURE 64.3 Breast anatomy.

Physiology of the Female Reproductive System

The Menstrual Cycle

Menarche is characterized by the first episode of menstrual bleeding. The first menses is an indication that the female has reached puberty, which is preceded by increased production of progesterone and estrogen secreted by the ovaries. The age of onset of menses can vary but typically occurs between the ages of 12 and 13. Each month after menarche, **follicle stimulating hormone (FSH)** produced in the pituitary gland stimulates the ovary to develop a mature oocyte, and **luteinizing hormone** stimulates the release of the mature oocyte. If fertilization of the oocyte fails to occur, then the endometrial lining, which had thickened to support a fertilized egg, sheds in a process called *menstruation*. This monthly cycle is controlled by hormonal secretions of FSH and **luteinizing hormone (LH)** from the anterior pituitary and the release of estrogen and progesterone from the ovaries.

The menstrual cycle can be divided into three distinct parts: the follicular or proliferative phase, the secretory or luteal phase, and the menstrual or ischemic phase (Fig. 64.4). The follicular phase is when the ovaries are the least hormonally active, resulting in low serum estrogen and progesterone concentrations. During the follicular phase, the level of FSH begins to increase, causing the maturation of the developing follicles, the site of oocyte development. One of these follicles will eventually become the dominant follicle, which is released during **ovulation**. The maturing follicles stimulate estrogen production, which in turn suppresses the release of FSH. This is an example of the negative feedback system controlled by the hypothalamus (Box 64.2). Follicle-stimulating hormone is required for the initial recruitment and maturation of the dominant follicle, but LH is needed for the completion of follicle maturation and, ultimately, the release of the oocyte, also known as *ovulation*.

Estrogen levels peak on the 12th day of the cycle, resulting in a surge of LH. This is the beginning of the luteal phase. During this time, the endometrial lining begins to thicken under the stimulatory effects of estrogen. Progesterone levels rise to maintain the endometrial lining. As a result of the LH surge, the ovary releases a mature follicle approximately 1 to 2 days after the surge. Once ovulation has occurred, LH levels continue to increase, along with a slight increase in serum FSH concentration. If fertilization does not occur, there are gradual decreases in LH, which lead to decreases in progesterone and estrogen production.

Box 64.1 Galactorrhea

Galactorrhea is the production of milk from the breast that occurs outside of normal lactation. This can be a sign of underlying pathology and should be evaluated. Galactorrhea usually affects women of reproductive age but has also been seen in males and infants. There are several causes, which range from sexual stimulation of the breast, abnormalities in hormonal levels, and pituitary adenoma. Galactorrhea can resolve spontaneously, and in some cases the cause may not be known. The evaluation for galactorrhea usually includes a physical examination, serum hormone testing, and imaging if necessary.

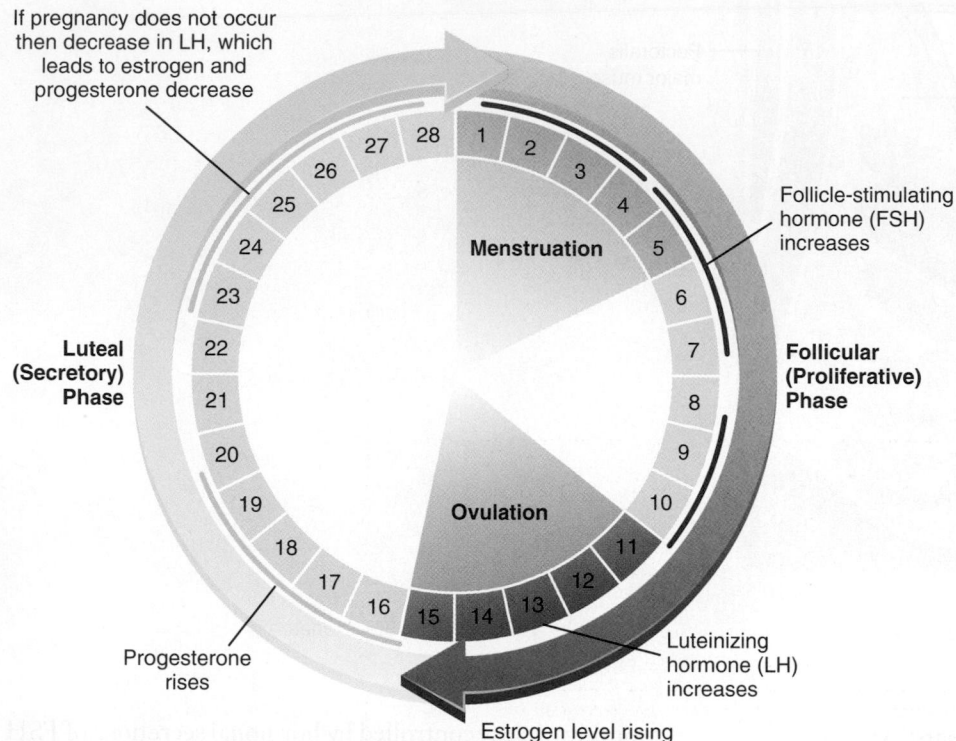

FIGURE 64.4 The menstrual cycle. The follicular phase: the ovaries are the least hormonally active, resulting in low serum estrogen and progesterone concentrations. The level of follicle-stimulating hormone (FSH) begins to increase, causing the maturation of the developing follicles. The maturing follicles stimulate estrogen production, suppressing the release of FSH. Luteal phase: Estrogen levels peak on the 12th day of the cycle, with a resultant surge of luteinizing hormone (LH). The endometrial lining begins to thicken under the stimulatory effects of estrogen. Progesterone levels rise to maintain the endometrial lining. One to two days after the LH surge, the ovary releases a mature follicle: ovulation. LH levels continue to increase along with a slight increase in serum FSH concentration. Ischemic phase: If fertilization does not occur, there are gradual decreases in LH, leading to decreases in progesterone and estrogen production leading to sloughing off of the endometrial lining; menstruation.

Box 64.2 Hypothalamic-Pituitary-Gonadal Regulation of the Menstrual Cycle

Secretions of gonadal hormones are under the direct control of the hypothalamus. The hypothalamus secretes gonadotropin-releasing hormone (GnRH) that stimulates the anterior pituitary gland to secrete follicle-stimulating hormone (FSH) and luteinizing hormone (LH). Increasing levels of GnRH cause increases of FSH, which promotes proliferation and maturation of ovarian follicles. The maturing follicle then begins secreting estrogen. The rising level of estrogen suppresses the release of FSH in a negative feedback loop. At the same time, inhibin, an additional hormone, is also secreted by the maturing follicle. This hormone blocks the secretion of GnRH and FSH. As the cycle progresses, estrogen promotes proliferation or growth of the lining in preparation for implantation.

LH is primarily responsible for the completion of follicle maturation and ultimately ovulation. Once ovulation has occurred, the corpus luteum secretes progesterone that sustains endometria lining and the embryo until the placenta begins to produce progesterone.

Ultimately, the drop in estrogen and progesterone leads to sloughing off of the endometrial lining, known as *menstruation* or the *ischemic phase* (Fig. 64.5).

The average menstrual cycle occurs every 28 days. The onset of menses is considered day one of the menstrual cycle. The normal cycle length varies considerably from female to female but should occur every 21 to 35 days, lasting 2 to 8 days in duration. The average blood loss ranges from 20 to 80 mL. Abnormalities in frequency, volume loss, and duration are discussed in Chapter 65.

Ovulation

Ovarian follicles are the site of oocyte development. The immature oocyte lies within a primordial follicle surrounded by granulosa and theca cells. During follicle development, under the stimulation of estrogen, the granulosa and theca layer nourishes and protects the follicle until it reaches maturity. Ovulation, the release of a mature oocyte from the dominant follicle, occurs as a result of the LH surge. The area on the ovary where the follicle ruptures to release the egg transforms itself. Facilitated by LH, the follicle walls collapse inward, forming the corpus luteum. The fully developed corpus luteum continues to secrete estrogen as well as progesterone, which helps prepare the endometrium for implantation of the pre-embryonic morula (early-stage embryo). Should fertilization occur, the levels of both estrogen and progesterone increase under the direct stimulation of human chorionic gonadotrophic, a glycoprotein hormone secreted from the corpus luteum on the ovary during early pregnancy. The progesterone secreted by the corpus luteum continues to maintain the embryo until the placenta develops and begins to secrete progesterone.

Few primordial follicles reach maturity. The body reabsorbs the follicles that fail to reach maturity in a process called *atresia*. The lifetime allocation of follicles is present in the ovaries prior to birth. During intrauterine development,

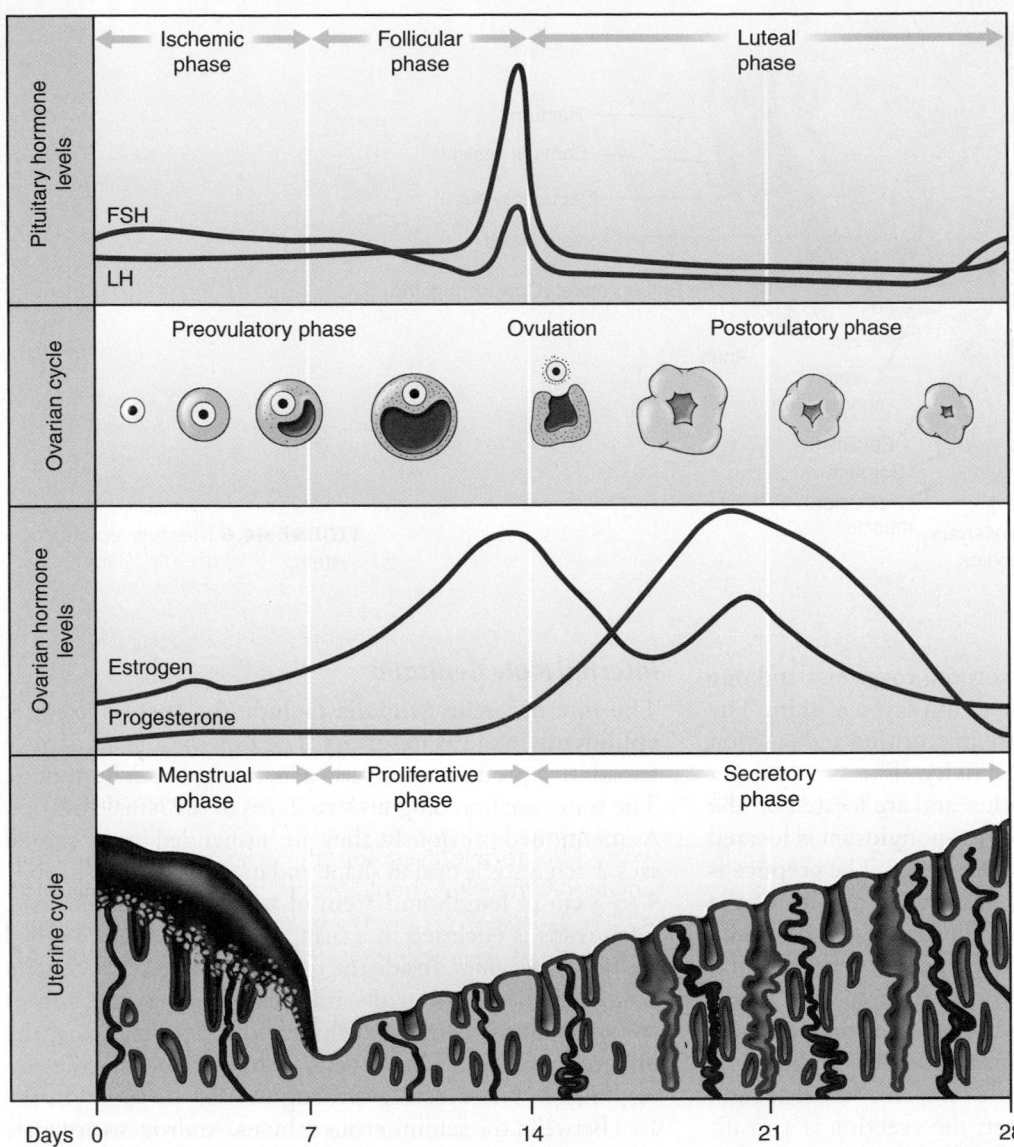

FIGURE 64.5 Hormonal control of the menstrual cycle.

the human ovarian reserve consists of several million follicles at approximately 5 months of gestational age. After birth, there is a decline in the follicular count from 4 million to 2 million. At the onset of menses, it is estimated that only 300,000 to 400,000 follicles remain. During the reproductive years of a normal female, approximately 500 mature follicles are released from the ovaries. Further decline in follicle count occurs as the female ages. When the finite store of ovarian follicles has been depleted, decreasing secretion of estrogen and progesterone causes the commencement of menopause. Menopause is discussed in Chapter 65.

Connection Check 64.2

The nurse understands the luteal phase of the menstrual cycle is accompanied by what hormonal changes?

A. Low levels of estrogen and progesterone
B. Increased levels of progesterone and estrogen
C. Increased levels of estrogen and LH
D. Increased levels of FSH and estrogen

MALE REPRODUCTIVE SYSTEM

The organs of the male reproductive system are specialized for the following functions:

- To produce, maintain, and transport sperm and protective fluid, semen
- To discharge sperm within the female reproductive tract
- To produce and secrete male sex hormones

Anatomy of the Male Reproductive System

The anatomy of the male reproductive systems includes both external and internal male genitalia (Fig. 64.6). They can be further delineated into primary reproductive organs, the testes, and secondary organs, the ducts, glans, and penis. There are also supportive components of the male reproductive system, the **scrotum** and spermatic cords.

External Male Genitalia

External male genitalia include the penis and scrotum. The **penis** (glans penis) is a long cylindrical structure with three

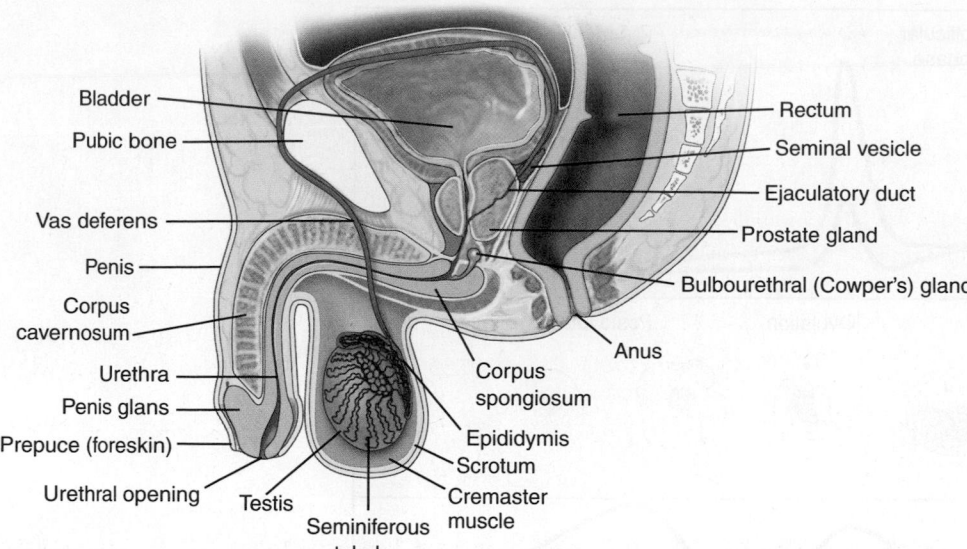

FIGURE 64.6 The male reproductive system.

columns of erectile tissue, two corpora cavernosa and one corpus spongiosum, covered by a thin layer of skin. The primary functions of the penis are micturition and ejection of seminal fluid during sexual activity. The two corpora cavernosa run parallel to each other and are located on the dorsal side of the penis. The corpus spongiosum is located on the ventral side and houses the urethra. The prepuce is an area of loose skin (foreskin) that covers the tip of the glans in the uncircumcised male. The skin can be retracted to reveal a slit-like opening called the *meatus* of the urethra, where both urine and seminal fluid are released. The frenulum is a connective tissue membrane of foreskin extending from the urethra on the ventral side of the penis. It prevents excessive retraction of the foreskin. Sexual arousal causes the penis to become erect; the erection is a result of increased blood flow to the glans from a series of large venous sinuses. During intercourse, semen is forced through the ejaculatory duct in a process called **ejaculation**. Ejaculation occurs during orgasm, which provides a great sense of pleasure.

The **scrotum** is a loose protective pouch suspended between the penis and anus. The scrotum contains two lateral compartments that house the testes. After adolescence, the scrotum is sparsely covered with hair and has a darker pigmentation than the adjacent skin. The function of the scrotum is to protect and support the testes. The scrotal wall has tiny skin folds called rugae; below the rugae is an underlying muscle called the *cremaster muscle*. The cremaster muscle can cause minute fluctuations in the scrotal size. The changes in size allow for regulation of the temperature within a testis. The temperature must be approximately two degrees below body temperature to produce sperm. When the body's temperature is elevated, the muscles relax to lower the scrotum, moving farther from the body. Alternatively, when the body's core temperature is lower, the muscles contract, bringing the scrotum closer to maintain heat and sperm viability.

Internal Male Genitalia

The internal male genitalia include the **testes**, urethra, **epididymis**, and **vas deferens**. The testes are a pair of male gonads that produce sperm and generate male sex hormones. The testes are homologous structures to the female ovaries. As mentioned previously, they are suspended in the scrotal sacs. Each testis is oval in shape and measures approximately 4 to 5 cm in length and 3 cm in width in the adult male. Each testis is enclosed in a firm, fibrous membrane called the *tunica albuginea*. Inside the testes are lobules that contain long, coiled seminiferous tubules, which is the site of **spermatogenesis**; the development of spermatozoa, the mature sperm cell. The Leydig, or interstitial cells that are responsible for secreting **androgens** can be found in the area between the seminiferous tubules. Androgens are male sex hormones, the primary one being **testosterone**. Testosterone is responsible for the development of primary and secondary sex characteristics in males. Testosterone in the embryonic stages causes undifferentiated gonads, ducts, and external genitalia to develop into the testes, scrotum, ducts, glands, and penis. Without the initial presence of testosterone, the genitalia develop in a female form. The testicular arteries (gonadal arteries) branch off the abdominal aorta. They are paired arteries that supply blood to the testes.

Sperm forms in the seminiferous tubules, then moves through a series of ducts—the epididymis, vas deferens, ejaculatory duct, and urethra—that ultimately transport the sperm outside the body. The epididymis is very long, measuring about 20 feet in length. It is a tightly coiled duct lying just outside each testis connecting the efferent ducts to the vas deferens, providing storage and a site of maturation of sperm. Sperm that has matured exits the epididymis through the vas deferens.

The vas deferens is a straight, fibromuscular tube connecting the left and right epididymis with the **seminal vesicles** to form the ejaculatory ducts. During ejaculation, the smooth muscle in the vas deferens wall contracts, propelling sperm forward into the ejaculatory ducts. They pass through the prostate and empty into the urethra.

There are three glands in the male reproductive system: the seminal vesicles, prostate, and bulbourethral or Cowper's glands. Their primary function is to add fluid and provide nutrients to the sperm to increase viability. The seminal vesicles are two saclike glands located on the posterior base of the bladder. They are approximately 5 cm in length. The convoluted structure is attached to the vas deferens near the base of the urinary bladder. They produce a thick alkaline fluid that makes up 65% to 75% of the seminal fluid. This fluid contains proteins, enzymes, fructose, mucus, vitamin C, flavins, phosphorylcholine, and prostaglandins. High fructose concentrations provide nutrient energy for the spermatozoa as they travel through the female reproductive system.

The **prostate gland** is a walnut-sized gland that is located below the bladder surrounding the urethra and ejaculatory ducts. The prostate consists of five lobes enclosed by a fibrous capsule. It stores and secretes a thin, milky, slightly alkaline fluid that promotes sperm motility along with protecting the sperm from acidic fluids, which can be found in both the male urethra and the female vagina.

Bulbourethral, or Cowper's, glands are pea-sized glands posterior to the prostate on either side of the urethra. These glands are responsible for the secretion of a gelatinous seminal fluid called *pre-ejaculate*. This fluid helps to lubricate the urethra for spermatozoa to pass through and also flushes out any residual urine or foreign matter, which decreases sperm viability. The lubrication also aids with penetration during intercourse. The urethra, a tubular structure approximately 8-mm long, connects the bladder and ejaculatory ducts to the outside of the body.

Physiology of the Male Reproductive System

Spermatogenesis

Spermatogenesis is the process of sperm production. Spermatogenesis begins at puberty as a result of stimulation from the anterior pituitary's gonadotropic hormones, LH and FSH. Luteinizing hormone, also called interstitial cell-stimulating hormone (ICSH), is the hormone responsible for the production of testosterone inside the Leydig, or interstitial, cells. Interstitial cell-stimulating hormone works synergistically with FSH to stimulate sperm production.

The testes contain primitive sex cells called *spermatogonia*. The spermatogonia are located in the seminiferous tubules. Inside the walls of the seminiferous tubules are Sertoli's cells ("nurse cells"). These cells form a protective envelope around the immature sperm cell. They are stimulated by FSH and secrete nutrients that aid in the process of meiosis and the development of mature sperm. As nutrients become depleted, the hormone inhibin is secreted from the Sertoli's cells, sending a signal to the anterior pituitary to slow the release of LH. As with female hormonal control, this is a negative feedback loop that helps control the production of sperm (Figure 64.7).

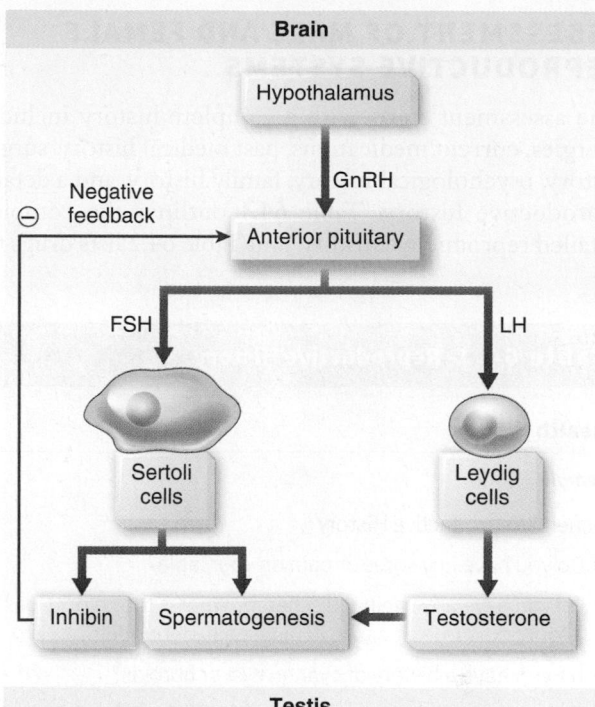

FIGURE 64.7 Hormonal control of spermatogenesis. Luteinizing hormone (LH) facilitates the production of testosterone inside the Leydig cells. Sertoli's cells are stimulated by FSH and secrete nutrients that aid in the process of meiosis and the development of mature sperm. While nutrients become depleted, the hormone inhibin is secreted from the Sertoli's cells, sending a signal to the anterior pituitary to slow the release of LH.

Connection Check 64.3

The negative feedback loop involved in spermatogenesis is facilitated by what hormone?
A. ICSH
B. LH
C. FSH
D. Inhibin hormone

CASE STUDY: EPISODE 2

Cindy's reproductive history reveals she is a G2 P1011. She has not had a period for the last 3 months. In addition to her fatigue, she also complains of cold intolerance and a noticeable increase in weight. She could possibly be pregnant despite her negative home test. Laboratory testing to be done includes serum pregnancy tests along with prolactin, FSH, and LH. A laboratory sample for thyroid-stimulating hormone (TSH) is also sent to evaluate her fatigue, cold intolerance, and recent weight gain which may be signs of hypothyroidism. Speculum and bimanual examinations are done. A Pap smear is obtained along with cultures for gonorrhea and chlamydia. The remainder of her examination is unremarkable...

ASSESSMENT OF MALE AND FEMALE REPRODUCTIVE SYSTEMS

The assessment starts with a complete history including allergies, current medications, past medical history, surgical history, psychological history, family history, and a detailed reproductive history. Table 64.1 outlines the complete, detailed reproductive history, and Table 64.2 lists drugs that can affect reproduction. Transitional Care lists birth control options.

Physical Examination of Female Genitalia

The physical examination of the female genitalia consists of external and internal assessments. External examination of female genitalia includes inspection of the mons pubis,

---

Table 64.1 Reproductive History

Health History

Female

General Reproductive History

- Do you have any sores or pain on your labia?
- Do you have any vaginal discharge? What is the color? Does it have a foul odor? Does it cause itching, pain, or burning?
- Do you have a history of ovarian cyst or fibroids?
- Have you had a Pap smear? If yes, have they all been normal?
- Family history of breast, ovarian, uterine, or cervical cancer

Menstrual History

- When was your last menstrual period (LMP), or are you menopausal?
- Age of first menses (menarche)
- Cycle frequency? (every 21-35 days within normal limits [WNL])
- How many days are your cycles? (2-8 days is WNL)
- How heavy is the flow? (pad/tampon count)
- Do you have premenstrual symptoms?
- Do you have painful periods?
- Do you have bleeding between your periods?

Pregnancy History

- Pregnancy history, including number of pregnancies, number of living children (see Box 64.3)

Sexual History

- Are you sexually active?
- Are you satisfied with your sex life?
- Do you have painful intercourse?
- Do you bleed after intercourse?
- What age did you begin your sexual experiences? Please be specific, oral vs. penetration.
- What is your sexual preference? Male, female, both, or other?
- How many partners have you had in the last 12 months? In the last two months?
- How many partners do you currently have?
- Assess contraceptive use
- Do you have a history of any sexually transmitted infections? HIV, hepatitis B, hepatitis C, herpes, syphilis, gonorrhea, chlamydia, *Trichomonas*, warts?
- Assess strategies to protect from sexually transmitted infections.

Male

General Reproductive History

- Any painful lesions, sores, or discharge from your penis?
- If discharge, what color is it? How long have you had it? Does it have an odor?
- Do you have any problems with your scrotum or testes?
- Have you noticed any lumps, bumps, or swelling of the scrotum?
- Have you ever been told you have a hernia?
- Family history of prostate cancer

Sexual History

- Are you sexually active?
- Are you satisfied with your sex life?
- Do you have painful intercourse?
- What age did you begin your sexual experiences? Please be specific, oral vs. penetration.
- What is your sexual preference? Male, female, both, or other?
- How many lifetime partners have you had?
- How many partners do you currently have?
- Contraceptive use? Do you use condoms?
- Do you have a history of any sexually transmitted infections? HIV, hepatitis B, hepatitis C, herpes, syphilis, gonorrhea, chlamydia, *Trichomonas*, warts?
- Assess strategies to protect from sexually transmitted infections.

Box 64.3 Determining Pregnancy History

Gravida (G) = The total number of pregnancies regardless of duration.
Parity (P) = The numbers of past pregnancies that have gone to viability and have been delivered. Parity can be further delineated by using (TPAL): T = Full Term, P = Preterm, A = Abortions: spontaneous or induced, L = Living Children. An example = A woman who has one child born at 40 weeks and one spontaneous abortion is a G2 P1011.
Descriptive terms include:

- A nulliparous woman (nullip) has not given birth previously; also refers to a woman who has given birth to a baby unable to survive outside the womb
- A primigravida is in her first pregnancy.
- A primiparous woman (primip) has given birth once.
- A multigravida has been pregnant more than once.

labia majora and minora, inguinal area, and perineum. Careful attention is paid to areas of inflammation, lesions, asymmetry, and palpable masses.

A breast examination is also performed. Breast examination is first done with the patient in a seated position. A visual inspection is done to assess the breasts for symmetry; it is common for one breast to be larger on the dominant side. Skin color, texture, vascularity, abnormal skin lesions, and dimpling should all be assessed. The patient is then asked to place her arms at her side, above her head, leaning forward, and finally, placing her hands on her hips. These various maneuvers are used to detect abnormalities that can be a sign of abnormal pathology. Next, attention is focused on the clavicular and axillae areas, which are palpated for

lymph node enlargement. The patient is then asked to lie in the supine position with one arm behind her head. The breast should be palpated with a light, medium, and firm circular motion making sure to palpate all the layers of the breast down to the chest wall. Assess the nipple and areola for masses and discharge. If discharge is observed, document color, consistency, and whether discharge is bilateral or unilateral. Discharge can be a sign of underlying pathology and should be investigated. Use the moment to assess the patient's knowledge of self–breast examination. If the patient is knowledgeable, then reinforce the pertinent normal findings and timing of monthly breast examinations.

Internal examination is done manually (bimanual examination) and with the speculum. The speculum examination is done to visualize the vagina and cervix. The patient is supine, with her legs in the dorsal lithotomy position with her feet comfortably resting in the stirrups. Place a drape across the patient's lower abdomen to provide coverage. The drape should provide coverage but should not obscure the external genitalia. The patient should be informed of the examiner's actions at all times; each step should be announced before it is performed. The patient should also be informed that she may stop or pause the examination at any point.

The speculum should be warmed by lukewarm water or a heating pad and lubricated to provide comfort upon insertion. The labia minora are gently spread apart with the examiner's nondominant hand, and the speculum is inserted below the meatus to avoid stimulation of the urethra. Inform the patient that she may experience a little pressure as the speculum is advanced. Once the speculum is inside, assessment of the vaginal mucosa and vaginal secretions and cervix is completed.

The bimanual examination can provide very valuable information. The examiner places the two lubricated fingers of the dominant hand into the vagina until the cervix is

Table 64.2 Drugs Affecting Reproduction

Women	Men
• Steroids can hamper the pituitary's ability to produce follicle-stimulating hormone and luteinizing hormone.	• Supplemental testosterone and anabolic steroids have a negative effect on sperm production.
• Antihypertensives such as Aldomet may raise prolactin levels, hampering ovulation.	• Alcohol may decrease testosterone production and increase estrogen production.
• Medications targeting the central nervous system, such as antiseizure medications or tranquilizers, may negatively impact prolactin levels and ovulation.	• Tetrahydrocannabinol, the main ingredient in marijuana, decreases sperm production.
• Thyroid medications may interfere with ovulation.	• Long-term opiate use decreases testosterone production, decreasing quantity and quality of sperm.
	• 5-Alpha-reductase inhibitors used to treat prostate enlargement decrease semen and sperm volume.
	• Alpha blockers used to treat prostate enlargement can negatively impact ejaculation.
	• Selective serotonin reuptake inhibitors (SSRIs) have a negative impact on the movement of sperm.

Transitional Care

Birth Control Options

Method	Advantages/Disadvantages
Birth control pills:	
• Combination pills (progestin and estrogen combination)	• Mainstay of birth control pills (99% effective) • Risk of blood clot formation
• Progestin only	• Decreased risk of clot formation • Must be taken at the exact same time every day to be effective • No placebo pills—all pills are active
Vaginal ring (NuvaRing): A flexible plastic ring placed in the vagina that delivers estrogen and progestin; remains in place for 3-4 weeks and then is removed for a week to allow for menstruation	• Do not have to remember to take a pill every day • Risk of blood clot formation
Diaphragm/Cervical cap: Dome-shaped rubber barrier method **used in combination with spermicide;** inserted into the vagina and covers the cervix	• 85% to 95% effective • Eliminates blood clot risk of birth control pills • Inserted prior to sexual activity; must remain in place 6 hours after sex
Intrauterine device (IUD):	
• ParaGard: Surgically implanted device that continuously releases copper that lines the uterus, creating an environment toxic to sperm • Mirena: Surgically implanted device that releases progestin	• 99% effective • Once implanted, may remain in place for approximately 5 years • May cause pain and heavy bleeding for several months after insertion • Risk of serious side effects such as uterine perforation
Patch: Hormone (estrogen)–releasing patch that is placed on an arm, back, or buttocks that remains in place for a week; replaced once a week for 3 weeks then left off 1 week to allow for menstruation	• 99% effective • Delivers 60% more estrogen than birth control pills, resulting in higher blood clot risk especially in women who smoke
Implant (Implanon, Norplant): A small rod (matchstick size) device inserted under the skin of the upper arm that releases progestin	• 99% to 100% effective • Effective as long as 3 years • May cause irregular bleeding
Injectables (Depo-Provera): Intramuscular injection of progestin given every 12 weeks	• 99% effective • Requires an injection every 12 weeks
Condom	• Protects against sexually transmitted infection • 98% effective when used correctly • Oil-based lubricants such as Vaseline may create holes in the condom, eliminating its effectiveness

reached. The other hand is placed on the lower abdomen to aid in palpation during the examination. Uterine size, position, mobility, and tenderness can be assessed with this technique. Careful attention is given to the presence of cervical motion tenderness because this is a sign of pelvic inflammatory disease. Afterward, attention is turned to the assessment of the adnexal area, the fallopian tubes and ovaries. They are assessed for the presence of a mass and tenderness. Normal ovaries are often not palpable.

A rectovaginal examination is not routinely performed. It is used to assess specific areas of concern such as pelvic pain, pelvic masses, and rectal symptoms. Stool guaiac testing, an assessment for bleeding from the gastrointestinal tract, may also be done with this examination. The examination is accomplished by placing one finger in the vagina and the other in the rectum. The examiner must change gloves between the bimanual examination and rectal examination to avoid cross-contamination of the rectum and vagina.

Physical Examination of Male Genitalia

Examination of the male external genitalia includes both inspection and palpation and can be performed with the patient in the lying or standing position. The general consensus is to perform the examination while the patient is standing. The examiner is seated directly in front of the patient. As with the female examination, the male should be given a verbal explanation of all aspects of the examination before it occurs. The male patient is also assured that he may stop or pause the examination at any time. With gloved hands, the examiner assesses the pubic hair, general appearance of the penis, and scrotum. Next, the penis is inspected for lesions, scars, or swelling. The presence or absence of foreskin is assessed. If foreskin is present, it is retracted to assess hygiene and inflammation. The glans is compressed to assess for drainage or discharge, paying careful attention to the color and odor of the discharge. Palpation of the penile shaft for tenderness and masses is done next. Visually inspecting the scrotum is done by lifting each scrotal sac and assessing all aspects of the skin. A visual scanning of the scrotum may reveal large scrotal masses, undescended testes, and the inguinal bulges of a hernia. Masses in the scrotum should be transilluminated in a dark room with a powerful light source. The results of the transillumination examination are quite informative because most benign masses easily allow light to pass through. Palpation of the scrotum and its contents may reveal the presence, size, position, and shape of the testicles. Visually assess the inguinal region for rashes, inflammation, or lesions. Ask the patient to bear down to assess for asymmetry or bulge. The right and left inguinal regions are palpated by using the index finger to check for lymphadenopathy (enlargement of the lymph nodes).

The internal examinations of the prostate and anus are done together. First, a visual inspection of the perineal and anal sphincter is done to assess for lesions, masses, or hemorrhoids. A digital rectal examination is done to assess the size of the prostate. It should be performed on all males older than 50 years and any male complaining of difficulty initiating urination or frequency.

DIAGNOSTIC STUDIES

Diagnostic studies include imaging and surgical procedures to assess the male and female reproductive systems. They include mammography, ultrasound, magnetic resonance imaging (MRI), colposcopy, laparoscopy, hysteroscopy, dilation and curettage, endometrial biopsy, and hysterosalpingography.

Mammography is a screening tool used to detect tumors in the breast less than 5 mm in diameter in asymptomatic women, which may not be palpable on clinical breast examination. The mammography uses x-ray films of the breast taken from various angles to detect abnormalities in breast tissue. Ultrasonography is a noninvasive imaging modality that uses high-frequency sound waves that pass through tissue. It records the pattern of the sound waves as they bounce off the organs. Waves are converted into images that assess structures' size, location, shape, contour, and position. It is usually the first-line testing to assess pelvic abnormality because it is inexpensive and readily available. It is valuable for screening for both men and women.

Magnetic resonance imaging is noninvasive imaging that uses a powerful magnet and radiofrequency to obtain cross-sectional images of body tissue. It is a screening tool used for both men and women. This modality is superior to computed tomography in producing images in any plane. It cannot be used to image bones, bone density, calcification, or calcium stones and therefore is used solely to visualize soft tissue.

Colposcopy is used to evaluate the mucosa of the cervix and/or vagina. It is most often used after there has been an abnormal Pap smear that revealed an underlying lesion or precancerous cells. Colposcopy provides direct visualization and magnification of the mucosal layer of the vagina or cervix with a colposcope, a low-power binocular microscope. During the procedure, a dilute solution of acetic acid is used to remove mucus and to enhance visualization of the columnar epithelium. In addition, Lugol's solution, an iodine-based solution, may be used to assess vaginal and cervical tissues. Normal vaginal tissue has a high glycogen content and stains brown with the application of Lugol's solution. Suspicious or abnormal tissue does not absorb the stain and may appear lighter in color. If abnormal areas are observed, endocervical biopsies are taken from the cervix.

Laparoscopy is an invasive procedure that allows direct visualization of the female anatomy by use of a fiber-optic scope inserted through a small incision on the abdominal wall. The abdomen is distended with CO_2 to increase visualization.

Hysteroscopy is an invasive surgical procedure that allows for direct visualization of the endometrial cavity via fiber-optic scope inserted through the cervix via the vagina. The hysteroscopy can be interventional as well as diagnostic, allowing resection of endometrial polyps and intracavitary fibroids.

Dilation and curettage (D&C) is an invasive surgical procedure that dilates the cervix to allow passage of a curette for endometrial sampling or removal of products of conception.

Endometrial biopsy can be done via D&C or noninvasively in the doctor's office. It provides a sampling of the endometrial lining. It is indicated if there is abnormal uterine bleeding or to assess for infection. Biopsies are also indicated in men to rule out cancers of the reproductive system.

Hysterosalpingography is an x-ray procedure used to assess the uterus and fallopian tubes. A small catheter is placed through the cervix. A contrast solution is then instilled via the catheter after which an x-ray of the pelvis is performed to assess the flow of the contrast through the uterus and fallopian tubes. See Table 64.3 for a description

Table 64.3 Significance, Patient Preparation, and Nursing Implications of Diagnostic Studies of the Reproductive System

Study	Significance of Abnormal Findings	Patient Preparation	Nursing Implications
Mammography	May show areas of concern for breast cancer that may require further imaging and biopsies	Instruct patient to avoid the use of cream, deodorant, and lotions.	Inform the patient that the results may not be available for a few days and that her provider will contact her with the results.
Ultrasound	May show tumors, abscess, thickened endometrial stripes, and congenital anomalies Ultrasound may also be used to assess breast tissue and guide a biopsy if an abnormality is detected on a mammogram. In men, ultrasound can detect tumors or abnormal tissue i.e. – in the scrotum.	A full bladder may be required for this test if assessing the female pelvis. Undress from the waist down. If a transvaginal approach is to be used, explain how the probe will be inserted in the vagina.	Inform the patient that results are usually available within hours of the testing; however, the practitioner will have to review them before a management decision is made.
Magnetic resonance imaging	May show anatomical anomalies, tumors, abscess, inflammation, atrophy, bleeding, or hemorrhage	Explain to the patient that this test requires that the patient lie still while the images are taken. It may also require administration of IV contrast. Remove all jewelry. Assess pregnancy status.	1. Inquire about implanted metal in the body, which may prevent the patient from participating in the study. 2. Assess for claustrophobia; provide supportive care. 3. Confirm allergies before administrating contrast.
Colposcopy	May show precancerous cells, human papillomavirus-related changes of the cervix	Encourage the patient to empty her bladder. Patient should avoid placing anything in the vagina for at least 24 hours before the procedure. If the patient is menstruating, the procedure may need to be rescheduled because heavy bleeding makes visualization of the cervix and vaginal mucosa difficult. Assess pregnancy status prior to the procedure.	1. Informed consent must be signed before the procedure. 2. Confirm patient's allergy; Lugol's solution is contraindicated in patients with an iodine or shellfish allergy. 3. Recognize that the patient may be anxious regarding the procedure and may have additional questions before and after the procedure. 4. Provide adequate pain medication after the procedure. 5. Review postprocedure expectations along with signs and symptoms that require further evaluation.
Laparoscopy	May show possible pathology, ovarian cyst, fibroids, endometriosis, tubal abscess	NPO the night before surgery. Prep the surgical site for the procedure. Confirm right site, right patient, and right procedure. Assess pregnancy status prior to procedure.	1. Ensure patient understands surgical procedure. 2. Informed consent must be signed before the procedure. 3. Ensure patient understands anesthesia and pain control methods. 4. Discharge teaching should include at least 2 days of rest postoperatively. The risk of bloating and abdominal pain should be discussed with the patient as the result of the instillations of CO_2 into the abdomen.

Table 64.3 Significance, Patient Preparation, and Nursing Implications of Diagnostic Studies of the Reproductive System—cont'd

Study	Significance of Abnormal Findings	Patient Preparation	Nursing Implications
Hysteroscopy	Uses direct visualization of the endometrial cavity; allows surgical removal of fibroids and polyps that are in the cavity	NPO the night before surgery. Prep the surgical site for the procedure. Confirm right site, right patient, and right procedure. Assess pregnancy status prior to procedure.	1. Ensure patient understands surgical procedure. 2. Informed consent must be signed before the procedure. 3. Discharge teaching should include at least 2 days of rest postoperatively. 4. Nothing in vagina for 4 weeks after procedure.
Dilation and curettage	Can assess for molar pregnancy (when what should have been fetal tissue becomes an abnormal growth in the uterus), endometrial cancer, and other abnormalities of the endometrial lining	NPO the night before surgery. Prep the surgical site for the procedure. Confirm right site, right patient, and right procedure. Assess pregnancy status prior to procedure.	1. Ensure patient understands surgical procedure. 2. Informed consent must be obtained. 3. Discuss normal postoperative bleeding (pad counts). The patient may experience cramping that should respond to NSAIDs.
Endometrial biopsy	Assess for possible endometrial cancer or endometritis	Assess pregnancy status prior to procedure.	1. Ensure patient understands procedure. 2. Informed consent must be obtained. 3. Explain that some cramping and vaginal bleeding may occur after the procedure; cramping should respond to NSAIDs.
Hysterosalpingogram	May reveal blocked or dilated fallopian tubes or abnormalities in the uterine cavity	Assess pregnancy status prior to the procedure.	1. Ensure patient understands procedure. 2. Assess allergies to iodine and other contrast materials. 3. Informed consent must be obtained. 4. Explain that some cramping and vaginal bleeding may occur after the procedure; cramping should respond to NSAIDs.

NPO, Nothing by mouth.

of the diagnostic studies, abnormal findings, and nursing implications for patient preparation.

Laboratory Testing

Laboratory assessment includes the Pap test (cervical cytology), wet preparations (wet preps), and cervical, vaginal, rectal, and genital cultures. The Pap test is effective in detecting cancerous or precancerous cells in the cervix. The American Congress of Obstetricians and Gynecologists (ACOG) recommends women have cervical cytology done regularly starting at age 21. The Pap test should be done every 3 years between the ages of 21 and 29 provided that all results are within normal limits. Women ages 30 through 65 can be screened every 5 years with Pap and human papillomavirus (HPV) cotesting or a Pap test alone every 3 years. The decision to test for HPV should be made by the patient and her provider. The American Cancer Society recommends discontinuing screening for cervical cancer in low-risk women at age 65. There are certain populations of women who may require earlier or more frequent screening, depending upon risk factors. An example of a high-risk population for cervical cancer is women with HIV. The Office on Women's Health from the U.S. Department of Health and Human Services recommends a Pap test twice annually the first year of diagnosis of HIV and annually thereafter. It is important to note that even if a cervical cancer screening is unwarranted, annual assessment of external and internal genitalia may be performed.

A wet prep refers to a microscopic examination of secretions obtained from the vagina during the speculum examination. The sample is placed on a slide, mixed with saline and covered with a slip, then visualized microscopically to detect common vaginal infections such as *Trichomonas, Candida,* and bacterial vaginosis.

Serum blood tests looking at hormone levels of FSH, LH, total estrogen, progesterone, and testosterone are important to determine normal functioning. Serum testosterone testing is used if there are complaints of decreased libido, erectile dysfunction, or impotence in men. Human chorionic gonadotropin, a hormone produced by the placenta, can be assessed to confirm pregnancy and help quantify gestational age.

Men have been advised to have a prostate-specific antigen (PSA) test done to screen for prostate cancer annually. Prostate cancer is one of the leading causes of mortality for men older than 50. Prostate-specific antigen is a protein produced by the prostate gland and may be considered a tumor marker. Increased levels of PSA have been associated with a 25% to 60% increase in prostate cancer risk. Recently, that recommendation for annual testing has come under review because of questions of accuracy. There have been instances of men with elevated PSA levels who do not have cancer, resulting in unnecessary biopsy and treatment. There are also instances of men who have normal PSA levels who do have prostate cancer, resulting in inadequate treatment. Routine testing should be done after conversations with the provider, taking into account age, patient history, and any other pertinent factors.

AGE-RELATED CHANGES IN THE FEMALE AND MALE

Aging in the female is marked by several external and internal changes. Approximately four years before their last menstrual cycle, women begin to notice more irregularity in their menstrual cycles and decreased bleeding during menses. Some women with uterine fibroids or obesity actually experience increased bleeding. Twelve months after the final menstrual cycle, a woman is considered postmenopause. When a woman enters postmenopause she can no longer achieve a pregnancy. Also, during menopause, estrogen and progesterone decrease significantly, and FSH levels become elevated. The decrease in estrogen leads to the classic symptoms of perimenopause and menopause: hot flashes, bladder symptoms, decreased pelvic support, vaginal atrophy, shrinking of the labia minora and majora, and decreased clitoral size and sensitivity. Subsequently, some women experience an increased incidence of vulvovaginitis (infections of the vulva and vagina), urinary symptoms, dyspareunia (painful intercourse), and decreased libido. Cardiovascular disease risk increases after menopause and is the leading cause of death for women older than 50. This increased risk is associated with the decline in circulating estrogen as well as other risk factors such as hypertension (HTN), obesity, diabetes, and sedentary lifestyle. Bone loss also accelerates after menopause, leading to osteoporosis in some women.

The male reproductive ability remains throughout the lifespan, but normal sexual function requires a biopsychosocial process that relies on multiple factors to function properly. With advancing age, there is an increase in erectile dysfunction,

benign prostatic hyperplasia, prostate cancer, and other chronic illnesses that may cause sexual dysfunction. Additionally, psychosocial illness and its subsequent treatment may also play a role in decreased libido and erectile dysfunction. All complaints of erectile dysfunction and urinary abnormalities should be investigated because they may be a symptom of an underlying disorder or malignancy.

Connection Check 64.4

Assessment of the male and female reproductive systems includes: *(Select all that apply.)*
A. Reproductive history
B. Electrocardiogram
C. Abdominal CT scan
D. Physical examination
E. Laboratory markers such as PSA

Making Connections

CASE STUDY: WRAP-UP

Cindy's serum studies are unremarkable except for a slightly elevated TSH level. Her pregnancy test is negative. She restates her desire to get more information about long-term birth control (see Transitional Care). She is encouraged to follow up with her primary care provider regarding her slightly elevated TSH level because it may indicate hypothyroidism, which would account for her fatigue, cold intolerance, irregular menses, and weight gain. It could also affect her ability to get pregnant should she wish to. Cindy should also take medroxyprogesterone, 10 mg daily for five days to stimulate shedding of the endometrial lining. When the endometrial lining builds up without shedding, a cancer can develop. The menses following the medroxyprogesterone treatment will likely be very heavy, and Cindy should be forewarned about this.

Case Study Questions

1 The nurse includes which information in the teaching plan for Cindy? *(Select all that apply.)*
   A. Follow up with your primary care provider if this fatigue and cold intolerance continues.
   B. The use of condoms as a birth control method
   C. The use of an at-home pregnancy test is a satisfactory way to confirm pregnancy.
   D. Make an appointment with your primary care provider within 2 weeks.
   E. The reason for the medroxyprogesterone treatment and what to expect.

2. Which statement by Cindy indicates teaching has been effective?

   A. "I wish condoms were more effective. I don't like to take pills."

   B. "I'll make an appointment to see my provider soon to follow up on the TSH levels."

   C. "This thyroid problem won't affect me if I want to get pregnant."

   D. "I'm feeling better. I don't need to see my doctor."

3. The nurse includes which of the following in the discussion about birth control?

   A. Progestin-only birth control pills increase the risk for blood clots.

   B. Intrauterine devices protect against sexually transmitted disease.

   C. Condoms are very effective when used correctly.

   D. Hormone releasing patch lowers blood clot risk.

4. Cindy begins to have very heavy bleeding with her periods. She is scheduled for a hysteroscopy for evaluation. Which statement by Cindy indicates teaching has been effective?

   A. "I'll be able to resume normal activities the same day as the test."

   B. "I'll have to abstain from sex for a few days after the test."

   C. "I'm glad I will be able to eat and drink prior to this test."

   D. "This is a test that can be done in the doctor's office."

5. Cindy understands the hysteroscopy is being done to evaluate her for which of the following?

   A. The presence of fibroids

   B. An HPV infection

   C. A molar pregnancy

   D. The presence of an abscess

CHAPTER SUMMARY

The anatomy of the female reproductive system includes both external and internal female genitalia. They can be further delineated into primary reproductive organs (ovaries) and secondary organs (uterus, fallopian tubes, and the breasts). The external female genitalia consist of the mons pubis, labia majora, labia minora, clitoris, vestibule, and perineum. The internal female genitalia consist of the vagina, cervix, uterus, fallopian tubes, and ovaries.

The menstrual cycle can be divided into three distinct parts: the follicular or proliferative phase, the secretory or luteal phase, and lastly the menstrual or ischemic phase. It is regulated by the hypothalamic and pituitary glands and gonadal hormonal secretions of GnRH, FSH, estrogen, and progesterone.

While the female ages, her fertility declines, culminating in menopause, which is the cessation of menstruation. Along with the loss of fertility are several age-related changes that occur to the external and internal female anatomy. These changes can affect a women's sexual health as well as result in alteration of body self-image. The nurse understands that it is important to recognize the various stages and phases of female reproductive health so that she may educate her patient regarding normal anatomy and physiology.

The organs of the male reproductive system are specialized for the following functions: to produce, maintain, and transport sperm and protective fluid, semen; to discharge sperm within the female reproductive tract; and to produce and secrete male sex hormones. The anatomy of the male reproductive systems includes both external and internal male genitalia. They can be further delineated into primary reproductive organs, the testes, and secondary organs, the ducts, glans, and penis. The internal male genitalia include the testes, urethra, epididymis, and vas deferens. External male genitalia include the penis and scrotum.

The assessment of male and female reproductive systems starts with a complete history including allergies, current medications, past medical history, surgical history, psychological history, family history, and a detailed reproductive history. The female physical examination includes an internal speculum and manual examination and breast examination. Examination of the male external genitalia includes both inspection and palpation. The internal examination of the prostate and anus is done to check for prostate enlargement.

Diagnostic studies include imaging and surgical procedures to assess the male and female reproductive systems. They include mammography, ultrasound, MRI, colposcopy, laparoscopy, hysteroscopy, dilation and curettage, and endometrial biopsy. Laboratory assessment includes the Pap smear, wet preparations (wet preps), and cultures. Serum blood tests looking at hormone levels of FSH, LH, total estrogen, progesterone, and testosterone are important to determine normal functioning. Men should have a PSA test done to screen for prostate cancer and testing for testosterone levels.

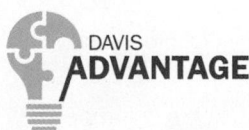

DAVIS ADVANTAGE

To explore learning resources for this chapter, go to **Davis Advantage** and find:
- Answers to in-text questions
- Chapter Resources and Activities
- NCLEX®-Style Chapter Review Questions
- Bibliography

Chapter 65

Coordinating Care for Female Patients With Reproductive and Breast Disorders

Amy S. D. Lee

LEARNING OUTCOMES

Content in this chapter is designed to assist in:

1. Describing the epidemiology of reproductive disorders
2. Correlating clinical manifestations to pathophysiological processes of:
   a. Breast cancer
   b. Dysmenorrhea
   c. Endometriosis
   d. Menopause
   e. Fibroids
   f. Ovarian cancer
   g. Uterine cancer
   h. Cervical cancer
3. Describing the diagnostic results used to confirm the diagnoses of reproductive disorders
4. Discussing the medical management of:
   a. Breast cancer
   b. Dysmenorrhea
   c. Endometriosis
   d. Menopause
   e. Fibroids
   f. Ovarian cancer
   g. Uterine cancer
   h. Cervical cancer
5. Developing a comprehensive plan of nursing care for patients with reproductive disorders
6. Designing a teaching plan that includes pharmacological, dietary, and lifestyle considerations for patients with reproductive disorders

ESSENTIAL TERMS

Aromatase inhibitor
Breast cancer type 1 susceptibility protein (BRCA1)
Breast cancer type 2 susceptibility protein (BRCA2)
Breast conservation therapy
CA 125
Ductal carcinoma in situ (DCIS)
Dysmenorrhea
Dysplasia
Endocrine therapy
Endometriosis
Hormone therapy (HT)
Human papillomavirus (HPV)
Invasive breast cancer
Leiomyoma
Lobular carcinoma in situ (LCIS)
Mastectomy
Menopause
Menorrhagia
Metastasis
Prostaglandins
Sentinel node
Tamoxifen
Vasomotor symptoms

CONCEPTS

- Assessment
- Cellular Regulation
- Comfort
- Female Reproduction
- Medication
- Nutrition

Finding Connections

CASE STUDY: EPISODE 1

Follow this patient throughout the chapter.

Karen Sims is a 43-year-old female patient who presents to her healthcare provider complaining of noticing a "knot" in her right breast recently in the shower. It is not painful and does not seem to change with position or palpation. She had a mammogram at age 40 that was normal, but she has not had one since. She takes combination oral contraceptive pills (OCPs) for birth control and is otherwise in relatively good health. She is clearly worried about the knot in her breast and presents for evaluation…

BREAST CANCER

Epidemiology

Cancer of the breast almost exclusively occurs in women. Breast cancer affects tens of thousands of American women yearly, and although breast cancer survival rates have increased significantly, it remains the second most common cause of cancer-related deaths in women. The single greatest risk factor for breast cancer is a woman's age. While a woman ages, her risk of breast cancer increases. American women aged 80 to 85 are 15 times more likely than women aged 30 to 35 to develop breast cancer. Ethnicity modifies the effect of age, although ethnicity alone does not have consistent risk elevation. African American women younger than 50 have a higher risk of developing breast cancer, whereas those older than 50 have a lower risk than Caucasian women of the same age. Hispanic women in North America have a lower incidence of breast cancer than Caucasian women, whereas Asian women in North America have the same risk as Caucasian women. However, Asian women living in Asian countries have a very low risk of breast cancer. There currently exists no accepted explanation for these differences.

Women with higher numbers of ovulatory cycles in their lifetime also carry a higher risk of breast cancer. Those with early menarche and late menopause have a 30% to 50% increase in breast cancer risk. Lack of pregnancy and live childbirth before the age of 30 nearly doubles the breast cancer risk. Only pregnancies resulting in a live birth lower the breast cancer risk. Seventy percent to 80% of breast cancer simply occurs by chance and cannot be traced to any family member but family history, particularly in first-degree relatives, can be a risk factor for breast cancer. Five percent to 10% of breast cancers are caused by known genetic mutations (see Genetic Connections). Women with a family history not associated with a known genetic mutation have a lifetime risk below 30%. Fifteen percent to 20% of breast cancers are associated with a family history but are likely also a result of environmental factors in the setting of genetic susceptibility. Benign, noncancerous breast disease that is proliferative; those with quickly growing cells such as hyperplasia, have an increased breast cancer risk of as much as 70%. Benign breast disease that is nonproliferative is not associated with any increased risk. Other factors associated with the risk of breast cancer include excessive alcohol use, inactivity, obesity, and the use of hormones.

Genetic Connections

Genetic Testing to Assess Breast Cancer Risk

Genetic testing provides an opportunity for women to learn whether they have a family history of breast cancer caused by an inherited gene mutation. The two gene mutations that have been currently identified are the BReast CAncer gene (BRCA)1 and BRCA2. Genetic carriers of these mutations have a 50% to 85% lifetime risk of breast cancer and a 45% risk of ovarian cancer by age 70. Genetic testing for BRCA1 and BRCA2 can be done with a simple blood test. It has been widely publicized, but this testing is indicated only for certain people at high risk, including women with a:

- History of breast cancer before age 50
- History of triple negative breast cancer (hormone receptor–negative)
- History of ovarian cancer
- Personal or family history of bilateral breast cancer
- Family history of breast cancer diagnosed before age 45
- Family history of ovarian cancer

This test is not indicated in women with a low risk of gene mutation, such as women who are the only person in their family with breast cancer, no family history, or when the breast cancer diagnosed in the family occurred after age 50.

Pathophysiology

Cancer is a condition in which the cells of the body grow and divide abnormally and uncontrollably. The cells can invade nearby tissues and spread to other areas through the bloodstream and lymphatic system. Breast cancer can be divided into a series of categories or stages associated with size, spread to lymph nodes, and distant spread of the breast tumor to other tissues called **metastasis** (Fig. 65.1). The first stage, stage 0, includes the in-situ lesion of **ductal carcinoma in situ (DCIS)**. Ductal lesions occur in and are limited to the lining of the milk ducts. **Lobular carcinoma in situ (LCIS)**, lobular lesions occurring in the lobules where milk is produced, were included in stage 0 in past staging models but are now not considered cancer. Both DCIS and LCIS place the patient at higher risk of developing

invasive breast cancer. Invasive lesions are those that spread to other areas or organ systems (see Evidence-Based Practice).

Evidence-Based Practice

Breast Cancer Staging

In 2018, the American Joint Commission on Cancer (AJCC) updated the breast cancer staging guidelines. Early guidelines included tumor size (T), lymph node involvement (N), and distant spread or metastasis (M); the T, N, M characteristics. The updated guidelines include cancer characteristics such as tumor grading or how much the abnormal cells look like normal cells, hormone receptor (estrogen and progesterone) status, *HER2* status (a gene that can play a role in the development of breast cancer) which looks at the amount of HER2 protein produced by the cancer cells, and a oncotype DX score; a genomic test that analyzes the gene activity that can affect how cancer is likely to develop and respond to treatment. Including these new factors is more complex but more accurately matches treatment. For instance, a tumor with stage 2 characteristics but hormone-positive cancer will have a different plan of treatment than a hormone receptor–negative tumor, thus the stage and treatment may change; downgraded in this example. The following table is not comprehensive but provides examples of staging.

Giuliano, A. E., Edge, S. B., & Hortobagyi, G. N. (2018). Eighth Edition of the AJCC Cancer Staging Manual: Breast Cancer. *Annals of surgical oncology, 25*(7), 1783-1785.

Stage I

Tumor 2 cm or less with no lymph node spread and no distant metastasis.

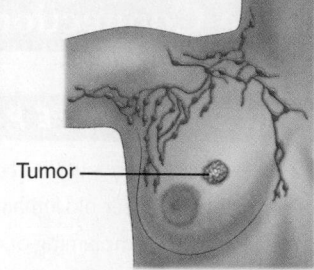

Tumor

Stage II

Tumor may increase in size with possible spread to nearby lymph nodes; no distant metastasis.

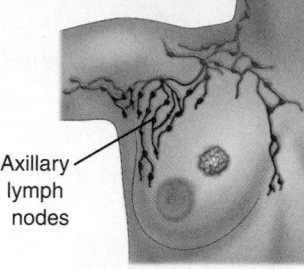

Axillary lymph nodes

Stage III

Tumor may increase in size with possible spread to lymph nodes, chest wall, or skin; no distant metastasis.

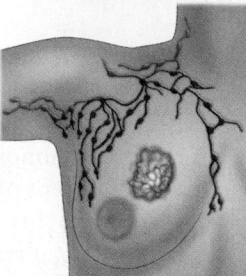

Stage IV

Tumor of any size with direct extension to chest wall or skin and with distant metastasis.

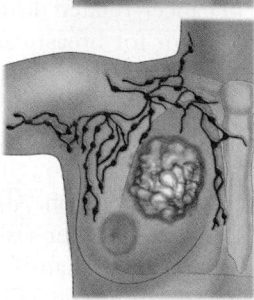

FIGURE 65.1 Four stages of breast cancer.

Evidence-Based Practice

Stage	Description	Lymph node	Metastasis	Hormone status
Stage 0	In situ lesions (DCIS)	No	No	
Stage IA	Tumor up to 2 cm	No	No	
Stage IB	No tumor in breast or tumor less than 2 cm	Yes – less than 2 mm	No	But if hormone receptor–positive staged and treated as IA
Stage IIA	No breast tumor	Yes – greater than 2 mm	No	
	Tumor less than 2 cm	Yes	No	
	Tumor 2-5 cm	No	No	But if HER2 , HR + staged and treated as IB

Evidence-Based Practice—cont'd

Stage	Description	Lymph node	Metastasis	Hormone status
Stage IIB	Tumor 2-5 cm	Yes	No	But if HER2+, HR+ staged and treated as IB
	Tumor greater than 5 cm	No	No	
Stage IIIA	Tumor any size	Yes – 4-8 lymph nodes	No	But if HR+, HER2+ staged and treated as IB
	Tumor >5cm	Yes		
Stage IIIB	Tumor any size and spread to chest wall	Yes – 9 lymph nodes	No	But if HR+, HER2+ staged and treated as IIA
	Inflammatory breast cancer	Yes	No	
Stage IIIC	Tumor any size and spread to chest wall	Yes – 10 or more lymph nodes	No	But if HR+, HER2+ or – staged and treated as IIIA
Stage IV	Tumor of any size	Yes	Yes	

Clinical Manifestations

Clinical manifestations vary depending on the type of breast cancer. Most commonly, the presence of a new mass or lump is noted. Cancerous masses are typically hard, irregular, and painless but may be soft or rounded and tender. There are sometimes changes in the shape of the breast or swelling. There may be skin changes such as peeling, flaking, pitting, dimpling, or redness. There may also be changes in the nipple such as inversion, thickening of the tissue, or drainage.

CASE STUDY: EPISODE 2

Ms. Sims' breast examination reveals a palpable 2-cm mass in the right breast. The mass is not mobile and is nontender. There are no nodes felt in the adnexa or adjacent areas. There is no nipple discharge. The patient is referred for diagnostic mammography and ultrasonography of the palpable mass…

Management

Medical and Surgical Management

Diagnosis

Diagnostic tests for breast cancer include mammography, ultrasonography, magnetic resonance imaging (MRI) and, if necessary, biopsy. Patients may have breast cancer detected as part of routine screening mammography or mammography with MRI (currently recommended screening for high-risk women), or they may present with a specific complaint that leads to the discovery of the tumor through diagnostic imaging. Once mammography detects a suspicious area, ultrasonography may be used to further define the area.

Ultimately, the area will be recommended for biopsy if it is deemed suspicious on imaging. Biopsy results will be definitive for diagnosis. Table 65.1 outlines the different types of biopsy.

If the initial diagnostics indicate the tumor may be invasive, sentinel node biopsy may be indicated. This evaluation may help determine the extent or stage of the breast cancer. The **sentinel node(s)** is the first lymph node to which cancer cells travel if they are to spread. In breast cancer, these nodes are generally found in the axilla but may be more central if the cancer is in the center of the chest. Injecting a radioactive substance or blue dye near the tumor and tracking it to the first node determines the sentinel node(s). Research has demonstrated that if the sentinel lymph node(s) is found to be free of cancer, it may not be necessary to proceed with the removal of further nodes or an axillary lymph node dissection (which generally removes 20–40 nodes). If the sentinel nodes have cancer cells present, a more complete removal of the lymph nodes is necessary for evaluation, and axillary lymph node dissection may be completed.

Once a diagnosis is made, laboratory data that may be obtained include a complete blood count (CBC) with platelets, liver function tests, and a chest x-ray. A baseline bone scan and liver scan may be obtained if the patient is found to have skeletal symptoms or abnormal liver function tests. Computed tomography (CT) of the abdomen and a bone scan may also be performed if the disease is clinically felt to be stage II or higher.

Treatment

Medical and surgical management varies depending on the category or staging of the cancer. Treatment options include surgery, chemotherapy, and radiation. Surgery alternatives are **breast conservation therapy**, also referred to as *lumpectomy*, or total **mastectomy** (Figs. 65.2 and 65.3).

Table 65.1 Types of Breast Biopsy

Biopsy Type	Description
Fine-needle aspiration	If the mass is palpable, the needle is guided to the mass through feel. If the mass is not palpable, the needle is guided to the mass through mammographic imaging, ultrasound, or magnetic resonance imaging (MRI). Once the needle is in the mass, a sample is suctioned out into a syringe. This is repeated several times. Local anesthesia may or may not be used.
Core needle	Similar to fine-needle aspiration except it uses a wider needle with a cutter that removes a larger sample. Local anesthesia may or may not be used.
Vacuum-assisted	Uses mammographic imaging, ultrasound, or MRI to locate the mass. A biopsy probe is introduced through a small skin incision. A vacuum device pulls tissue through the probe, where a rotating cutting device removes the sample and delivers it to a collection area. The probe can be repositioned to sample several areas. Sutures are not required. Done under local anesthesia.
Surgical excision	If the mass is palpable, an incision is made across the breast and the mass is accessed. If the mass is less than 2.5 cm, it is usually removed completely. If the mass is larger, a portion is removed for evaluation. If the mass is not palpable, it is first located through imaging and then "marked" by a hooked wire that is inserted into the mass and left to guide the surgeon to the mass. The surgical excision is the same as for a palpable mass. Sutures are required for closure of the incision. Local or general anesthesia may be used.

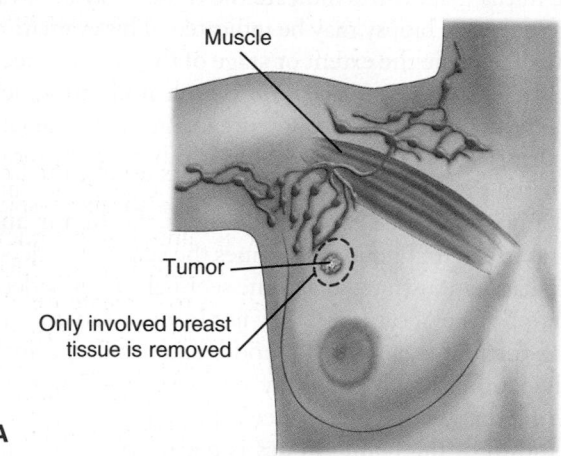

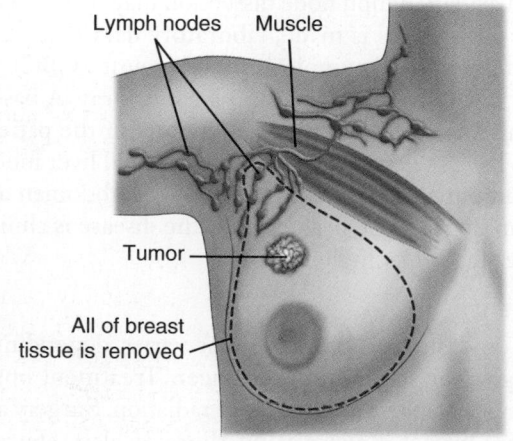

FIGURE 65.2 Breast cancer surgery. A, Breast conservation or lumpectomy. B, Modified radical mastectomy.

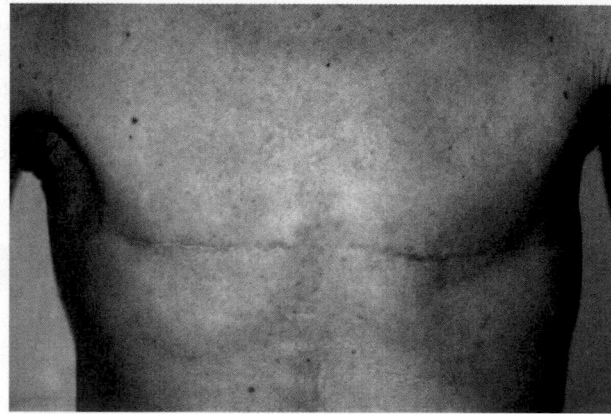

FIGURE 65.3 Chest after mastectomy.

Chemotherapy options include adjuvant chemotherapy, which is administered after surgery to destroy any remaining cancer cells, or neoadjuvant chemotherapy, which is administered prior to the surgical procedure in an attempt to shrink the tumor. Table 65.2 describes treatment options available for breast cancer.

Treatment for In Situ Lesions

Lobular carcinoma in situ (LCIS) is not considered a precursor for invasive breast cancer and therefore has no recommended treatment. Care of the patient with LCIS is directed at risk-reduction strategies because these women are at an increased risk of developing invasive breast cancer. Ductal carcinoma in situ (DCIS) requires surgical treatment. Lesions thought to be large (more than 4 cm) require mastectomy. Even though lymph node dissection or sentinel

Table 65.2 Breast Cancer Treatment Options

Treatment	Description
Breast conservation surgery (lumpectomy)	Removes only the involved breast tissue and a minimal surrounding margin with the best possible cosmetic preservation of the breast. An option in early-stage disease or advanced disease that has been reduced by chemotherapy. Used in conjunction with postoperative radiation and chemotherapy.
Modified radical mastectomy	Removal of the entire breast tissue. An option in early-stage disease or more advanced disease that has been reduced by chemotherapy. Used in conjunction with chemotherapy and may or may not require postoperative radiation.
Axillary lymph node staging	Removal of axillary lymph nodes. Done with invasive breast cancer and some noninvasive. Recent advances allow for removal of only the first lymph node from the tumor (sentinel node). Other nodes are then removed only if the sentinel node is positive.
Chemotherapy	Drugs used to treat cancer. May be used prior to surgery or after.
Radiation therapy	Radiation directed at the tumor and surrounding tissue to treat cancer. Typically done after surgery for lumpectomy or inflammatory breast disease, for recurrence, or for palliation in advanced disease.

node evaluation is not usually indicated in DCIS, patients with large lesions may benefit from nodal assessment because of the risk of invasive disease. Lesions of intermediate size that can be removed with clear margins (no cancer shown in the margin of tissue around the tumor) can be considered for mastectomy or breast conservation therapy. Breast conservation therapy is done in conjunction with radiation therapy. After adequate counseling, the choice of treatment is largely left up to the patient. Patients with very small DCIS lesions may, on an individual basis, be offered excision of the lesion without radiation therapy. Tamoxifen (Nolvadex), antiestrogen therapy, has been shown to reduce the risk of local recurrence in women undergoing breast conservation therapy and therefore may be offered in these patients.

Treatment for Early-Stage Invasive Cancers

Cancers smaller than 1 cm with a clinically negative axilla are preferably treated with surgical excision. Patients with larger tumors that have significant comorbidities or no spread to the axillary nodes may also be referred for surgical excision. Multiple trials have demonstrated that mastectomy and breast conservation therapy are equivalent, and therefore the patient is offered both of these options. If mastectomy is chosen, immediate reconstruction may be considered.

Radiation therapy is recommended for patients undergoing breast conservation therapy. Radiation therapy is also recommended for those choosing mastectomy if four or more lymph nodes are found to be positive. It may also be selectively used in those stage II patients with one to three positive nodes. Patients with tumors at least 1 cm in size or with axillary node involvement are recommended to have cytotoxic (toxic to cells) adjuvant chemotherapy. If patients are found to have cancers that are hormone receptor–positive, **endocrine therapy (aromatase inhibitor** or **tamoxifen)** is also recommended after completion of cytotoxic therapy. Postmenopausal patients with tumors between 1 and 2 cm without nodal involvement may be offered endocrine therapy alone, but all premenopausal patients should be offered chemotherapy.

Treatment for Intermediate-Stage and Advanced-Stage Cancers (Operable)

Preoperative neoadjuvant chemotherapy is usually the first line of treatment for intermediate-stage and advanced-stage operable cancers unless the patient has underlying comorbidities that preclude the use of chemotherapy. After chemotherapy, the tumor is reassessed to evaluate for the potential of breast conservation therapy as a result of tumor response to the chemotherapy. Preoperative chemotherapy has been shown to increase the success rate of breast-conserving surgery. Chemotherapy is recommended after surgical treatment in all patients. This is followed by or done concurrently with radiation therapy. If the tumor is hormone receptor–positive, endocrine therapy is offered for 5 to 10 years. Breast reconstruction may be done in those undergoing mastectomies, but it is often preferable for reconstruction to be delayed until after completion of radiation therapy.

Treatment for Locally Advanced and Inoperable Cancers

Patients with inoperable breast cancers may undergo neoadjuvant chemotherapy as initial treatment. If the tumor responds to chemotherapy and becomes operable, the next step is to undergo modified radical mastectomy. If the cancer responds dramatically, the patient can be offered breast conservation therapy. If the tumor does not respond to initial chemotherapy, the patient may be switched to another chemotherapy regimen before surgery is attempted. All patients should be offered postoperative chemotherapy and radiation to the breast or chest wall. In these cases, immediate breast reconstruction is not encouraged.

Treatment for Local Recurrence and Systemic Metastases

If the recurrence of the tumor is confined to the breast alone, a course of curative therapy is begun. In patients who have undergone initial breast conservation therapy, a complete mastectomy is the next step. If the tumor is not initially operable, chemotherapy may be considered. When the patient has not previously undergone radiation, surgical excision is done followed by chemotherapy and radiation. If the patient has undergone an initial mastectomy, surgical excision can be attempted, although the disease is often too advanced for this option. In this situation, chemotherapy can be initiated followed by surgery once the disease is under control. If this patient has not previously had radiation, then radiation may follow. Patients who have metastases to one or more organ systems have quality and quantity of life as focuses of treatment, as current approaches do not appear to be curative. Therapeutic benefit has to be weighed against toxic effect.

Complications

Treatment does sometimes have complications. Immediate postoperative complications are the same as those for any surgery. Wound infection and dehiscence are of initial concern as well as the usual immobility side effects of surgery such as pulmonary embolism and pneumonia. Once acute surgical recovery has occurred, complications of surgery stem from scarring and lymph node effects. The most common long-term complaints are shoulder immobility, pain, and lymphedema.

Lymphedema occurs because of the removal of the axillary lymph nodes and subsequent scarring, resulting in disruption of lymph drainage from the arm. The result is swelling of the arm. Sentinel lymph node evaluation and minimization of lymph node dissection have led to lowered incidences of lymphedema (Fig. 65.4).

Once chemotherapy has begun, the patient may experience a variety of side effects associated with the cytotoxic drugs. The most common chemotherapy side effects are hair loss, nausea, vomiting, mouth pain, diarrhea or constipation, peripheral neuropathy, rash, and nail changes. Decreased white blood cell count with possible subsequent fever and increased risk for infection is also a complication. Chemotherapy may also result in premature ovarian failure. In a young woman, this has significant implications for future estrogen-related health issues, including bone loss and loss of fertility. There is also a possible long-term risk of myelodysplastic syndrome (dysfunctional blood cells) and acute leukemia for some chemotherapeutic agents.

Finally, radiation therapy has some very predictable side effects. These include some redness with patchy desquamation (shedding of the outer skin layers) of the treated skin. The skin may also itch but usually does not have a "burning" sensation. Breast swelling and discoloration may continue for 6 months after treatment but usually resolves in 12 to

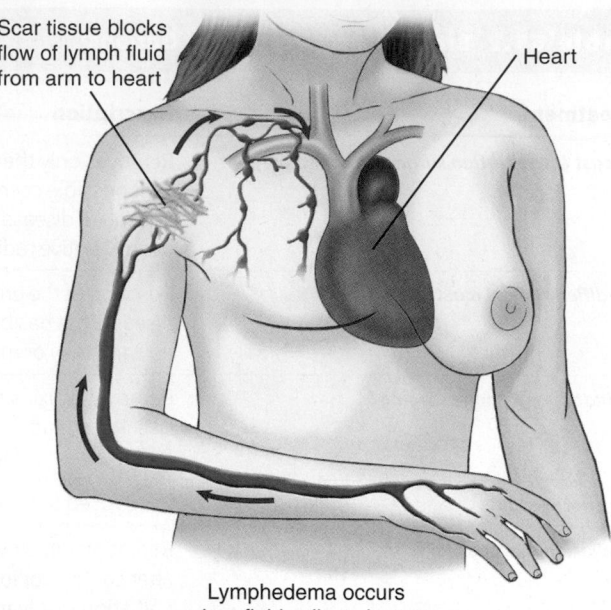

Scar tissue blocks flow of lymph fluid from arm to heart

Heart

Lymphedema occurs when fluid collects in arm

FIGURE 65.4 Lymphedema. Scar tissue can prevent the flow of lymph fluid, resulting in edema in the affected extremity.

18 months. Pneumonitis, a nonproductive cough with a chest x-ray demonstrating an infiltrate in the radiated area, may develop in some patients 6 weeks to 6 months after treatment completion. Evidence also exists to show that significant radiation to the myocardium may lead to latent (15–20 years) cardiac morbidity and mortality. There is an increased risk of other cancers in women treated with radiation for breast cancer. However, the incidence of these malignancies is suggested to be clinically insignificant.

Nursing Management

Assessment and Analysis

Assessment of the breast cancer patient is dependent on the point in time of diagnosis and treatment. Initial clinical manifestations are associated with the presence of a tumor, noting a lump in the breast, or other signs such as skin and nipple changes. Later manifestations are associated with treatment. Due to the killing of all rapidly dividing cells, chemotherapy may result in hair loss, nausea, vomiting, mouth pain, diarrhea or constipation, peripheral neuropathy, rash, and nail changes as well as a decreased white blood cell count. Lymph node removal may result in lymphedema or swelling of the arm on the affected side due to blockages in lymph flow. Radiation causes skin changes such as irritation, redness, itchiness, or burning. Breast swelling may be present as well as nonproductive cough with lung an infiltrate.

Nursing Diagnoses

- **Pain/Discomfort** associated with surgery, scarring, and radiation irritation of the skin
- **Risk for infection** associated with surgical procedure, lowered white blood cell count
- **Nutrition**: altered, less than body requirements associated with nausea/vomiting

- **Body image disturbance** associated with loss of breast, loss of hair

Nursing Interventions

■ *Assessments*

- Vital signs
  Elevated blood pressure and rapid pulse can be a sign of pain or anxiety. Elevated temperature and pulse are also indicative of infection.
- Pain
  Patients should verbalize their pain on a rating scale to help understand their pain level and to ensure adequate treatment.
- Daily weight
  Weights will give an idea of the nutritional status of the patient. Drastic weight loss indicates a nutritional deficit.
- Intake and output
  Intake and output allows evaluation for tolerance of oral liquids and foods and an evaluation of vomiting.
- Wound evaluation
  Good wound evaluation detects the early signs of infection such as redness, warmth, and increased or purulent drainage.
- Skin evaluation
  Inspect any radiated skin for radiation side effects such as irritation, redness, itchiness, or burning.
- Monitor complete blood count (CBC) and metabolic profile
  Due to its cytotoxic effects, chemotherapy may result in decreased white blood cell counts, decreased hemoglobin and hematocrit, and elevations in liver enzymes.
- Assess mood and nonverbal cues
  These patients are at great risk for psychological issues. Patients with depression are often withdrawn or offer other nonverbal cues that indicate pain, depression, and anxiety.

■ *Actions*

- Give chemotherapeutic drugs as ordered
  Chemotherapy is indicated for invasive breast cancer.
- Give pain medications as ordered
  Provides pain relief allowing the patient to more fully participate in activities of daily living
- Give antiemetics as ordered
  Help to relieve nausea and vomiting, promoting adequate nutritional intake
- Have the patient cough and deep breathe postoperatively
  Prevents atelectasis and pneumonia
- Keep the wound clean and dry
  Aids in wound healing and helps prevent infection
- Encourage verbalization
  It is important to actively involve patients in their care. Encouraging verbalization and communication is part of that process.

■ *Teaching*

- Explain the treatment course
  Patients will be less anxious if they are educated about what to expect, and what their planned treatment involves.
- Medications and treatment side effects
  Patients should understand the side effects of radiation and chemotherapy as well as potential treatment options.
- Wound care
  Teach the patient to keep the wound clean and dry. Report any signs of infection or dehiscence immediately.
- Nutritional counseling
  Help patients develop a nutrition plan to maintain adequate weight and hydration.
- Support groups
  Give patients a list of support groups and other resources to help them cope.
- Breast cancer screening with mammography:
  - Women ages 40-44 may begin annual screening
  - Women ages 45-54 should have annual screening
  - Women ages ≥55 can maintain yearly or move to biannual; screening should continue as long as the woman is in good health.
  - Clinical breast examination is not recommended
    The goal of screening is to detect breast cancer early

Evaluating Care Outcomes

With adequate treatment, many women are able to survive breast cancer today. Those with advanced-stage cancer are still able to achieve prolongation of their life while balancing quality of life. The patient undergoing treatment for breast cancer will have immediate needs associated with surgery, chemotherapy, and radiation. The well-managed patient should be able to manage any nausea and vomiting in a way that allows her to maintain adequate nutrition and weight. Her surgical sites should heal without infection. Scarring and lymphedema should be kept to a minimum through appropriate therapy. The psychological support provided throughout treatment helps to manage anxiety and depression.

Connection Check 65.1

Ms. Brown has been diagnosed with LCIS. The nurse will help Ms. Brown schedule which procedure?
A. Chemotherapy
B. Radiation
C. Mammogram
D. Surgery

DYSMENORRHEA

Epidemiology

Dysmenorrhea, or difficult monthly menses, is one of the most common gynecological complaints among younger women. It is the leading cause of school and work absence in young women. The majority of dysmenorrhea is associated with normal menstrual cycles and has no associated pelvic pathology. This is considered primary or functional dysmenorrhea. Dysmenorrhea is less common in the first few years after menarche but becomes more commonplace as regular ovulatory cycles are established. The severity of symptoms tends to be worse in those with early menarche, longer menses, and heavier menses. Cigarette smoking may also increase dysmenorrhea, likely because of nicotine-related vasoconstriction. Only 10% of dysmenorrhea is found to correlate with pelvic pathology such as endometriosis and is considered secondary dysmenorrhea. Endometriosis is discussed later in this chapter.

Pathophysiology

In primary dysmenorrhea, a buildup of fatty acids in the phospholipids of the cell membranes occurs after ovulation. The high level of omega-6 fatty acids in the Western diet contributes to a high level of omega-6 fatty acids in the cell wall phospholipids. Just prior to menses, progesterone levels in the body begin to fall. During this time, the omega-6 fatty acids, especially arachidonic acid, are released, causing the release of **prostaglandins** and leukotrienes in the uterus. Prostaglandins and leukotrienes cause an inflammatory response in the uterus that results in several common complaints.

Clinical Manifestations

Abdominal cramping is the most common symptom of dysmenorrhea. However, women may also complain of other symptoms including headache, nausea, and vomiting. Symptoms are acutely associated with the onset of menses, generally continue for 24 to 48 hours, and occur cyclically.

Management

Medical Management

Medications are the primary means of management for dysmenorrhea. The mainstay of treatment is non-steroidal anti-inflammatories (NSAIDs). NSAIDs result in the reduction of the production of prostaglandins. This causes decreased uterine contractions and therefore fewer symptoms. NSAIDs should be initiated 1 or 2 days prior to the onset of menses and continued until symptoms resolve (usually 1–2 days after menses start). Combined oral contraceptive pills (OCPs) that contain both estrogen and progesterone are also used to treat primary dysmenorrhea. Their action of limiting endometrial growth reduces the amount of endometrium available for prostaglandin and leukotriene production. Also, by prohibiting ovulation, they interfere with ovarian progesterone secretion. There are other pharmacological approaches that are similar to OCPs, but they are administered differently. They include transdermal patches (Ortho Evra patch), vaginal rings (Nuva-Ring), injections (Depo-Provera), and intrauterine (IUD) devices (Mirena). Typically, they are either a combination of both estrogen and progesterone or progesterone alone that inhibit ovulation and/or limit endometrial growth, thus decreasing the symptoms associated with dysmenorrhea.

Some nonpharmacological approaches such as herbal preparations, transcutaneous nerve stimulation (TENS), heat therapy, physical activity, and dietary supplementation with omega-3 fatty acids have been shown to improve the symptoms of primary dysmenorrhea.

Surgical Management

Surgical treatment may be indicated if NSAIDs or other hormonal approaches have not been effective. If after 6 months of medical treatment no relief has been achieved, then laparoscopy is indicated to evaluate for endometriosis. Uterine anomalies should also be considered. If symptoms are suspicious for an anomaly, imaging and surgical management may be indicated.

Nursing Management

Assessment and Analysis

Dysmenorrhea is generally cyclic, timed to the menstrual cycle. The symptoms are associated with prostaglandins and leukotrienes released during menses that cause an inflammatory response in the uterus resulting in abdominal cramping. The symptoms sometimes also include headache, nausea, and vomiting.

Nursing Diagnosis

- **Pain, acute** associated with cyclic dysmenorrhea

Nursing Interventions

■ **Assessments**

- Vital signs
  Pain may result in increased blood pressure and pulse.
- Pain
  The pain of dysmenorrhea may be very mild or can be quite debilitating. Treatment options may change depending upon pain levels.

■ **Actions**

- Provide nonpharmacological interventions: heat, acupuncture, herbal preps, exercise, TENS, omega-3 supplementation as ordered
  These interventions have been shown to result in relief of dysmenorrhea through localized relaxation, release of natural endorphins, increased pelvic blood supply, and production of less potent prostaglandins and leukotrienes.
- Give NSAIDs as ordered
  These medications are the first-line treatment in dysmenorrhea because they inhibit prostaglandin production.
- Administer hormonal methods as ordered
  Drugs such as oral contraceptives and other devices that contain a combination of estrogen and progesterone are effective in the treatment of dysmenorrhea through the limiting of endometrial growth, thereby allowing less production of prostaglandins and leukotrienes.

■ **Teaching**

- Counsel on possible nonpharmacological interventions
  Patients need education on the possible relief demonstrated with these methods.
- Educate on how to take prescribed medications
  NSAIDs and hormonal therapy should be taken as prescribed for best results.
- Maintain a menstrual calendar
  Patients can chart symptoms and medication administration in relation to their menstrual cycles. This can aid in diagnosis, timing of treatment, and effectiveness of medications. Dysmenorrhea is usually cyclic and worse during the first 2 days of the cycle.

Evaluating Care Outcomes

Patients with dysmenorrhea can be managed with NSAIDs, hormonal suppression, or both. A well-managed patient has her pain well controlled with no interference in her everyday activities.

Connection Check 65.2

Ms. Green is a 16-year-old who has missed 2 days of school each month this year because of painful menses. She has seen her healthcare provider for treatment. The school nurse is reinforcing the prescribed treatment of oral contraceptives and NSAIDs. The nurse teaches Ms. Green to do which of the following?

A. Take her OCPs every other day

B. Take the NSAIDs at the onset of symptoms and then as needed

C. Start NSAIDs 2 days prior to menses and continue on schedule until symptoms resolve

D. Stop the oral contraceptives if she has any vaginal bleeding

ENDOMETRIOSIS

Epidemiology

Endometriosis results when uterine endometrial glands exist and grow outside the uterine cavity or endometrium, often resulting in pain. Endometriosis is the most common cause of secondary dysmenorrhea. There is an apparent hereditary link to endometriosis. Patients with a first-degree relative with endometriosis are five- to tenfold more likely to have endometriosis. Monozygotic twins have a 75% concordance rate for endometriosis. Patients with bleeding disorders also demonstrate an increased risk for endometriosis.

Pathophysiology

Endometriosis development depends on abnormal hormonal activity associated with the interaction of the enzyme aromatase, an enzyme involved in the synthesis of estrogen. Endometriosis tissues have an increased amount of aromatase in them that is not found in normal endometrium. The aromatase leads to a rise in the local production of estrogen. The increase in local estrogen results in prostaglandin activity that contributes to even higher aromatase levels and even more estrogen production. Also implicated is a deficiency in 17-B hydroxysteroid dehydrogenase type 2 in the tissue that inhibits the inactivation of estradiol (the most potent estrogen) to estrone (the least potent estrogen), further raising local estrogen levels in the tissues.

In endometriosis, endometrial tissue is found outside the uterus implanted on other body structures. The majority of endometriosis implants are found in the pelvis (Fig. 65.5). The ovaries are the most likely sites for implants. Other sites in the pelvis may include the pelvic peritoneum, the cul-de-sac: a pouch between the rectum and uterus, uterosacral ligaments, pelvic lymph nodes, cervix, uterus, vagina, vulva, colon, and appendix. Less likely but possible sites include the umbilicus, surgical scars, bladder, kidneys, lungs, and extremities. Many theories have been postulated to explain this phenomenon, such as the possibility of retrograde menstruation in which endometrial tissue is shed up into the pelvis out of the fallopian tubes during menstruation. The finding of endometriosis implants in premenarchal girls questions this theory. Other possible theories include deficient cell-mediated immunity leading to impaired removal of endometrial cells from aberrant locations, "multipotential" cells in other areas with the ability to transform into endometrial cells, and the spread of endometrial cells through the blood and lymph systems.

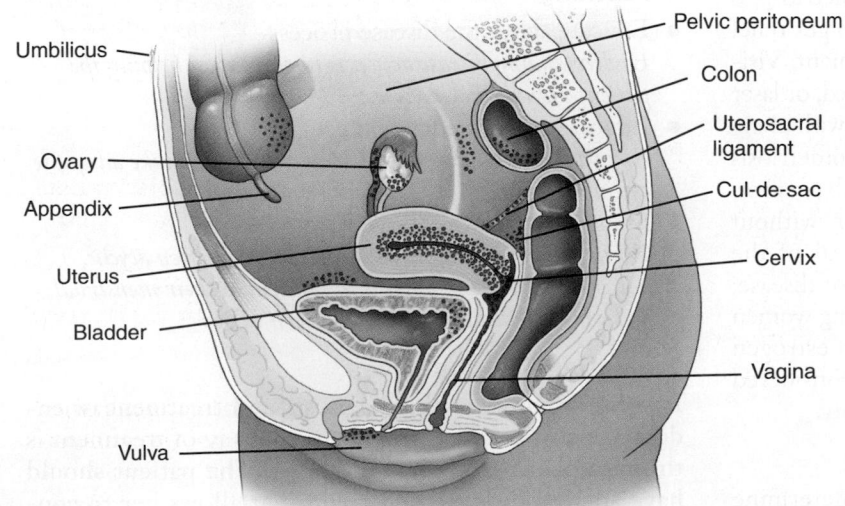

FIGURE 65.5 Common sites of endometriosis implants.

Clinical Manifestations

The overall accumulation of estrogen and prostaglandin in the endometriosis tissues results in inflammation and pain that can be both cyclic and acyclic. Typical symptoms include dysmenorrhea, excessive bleeding during menses, pain during intercourse, and infertility.

Management

Medical Management

Diagnosis

Diagnosis of endometriosis is through laparoscopy with biopsy of suspicious lesions. Oral contraceptives are the first line of treatment of endometriosis. If these fail, other pharmacological approaches should be used. Gonadotropin-releasing hormone (GnRH) agonists result in a systemic hypoestrogenic state that impairs the action of the endometriosis. Another pharmacological option is aromatase inhibitors that block local estrogen biosynthesis that occurs outside of the ovaries. They are generally administered in combination with a progestin, a combination oral contraceptive, or a GnRH analog. Aromatase inhibitors are still under investigation for the treatment of endometriosis and are typically reserved for severe, refractory pain.

> **Safety Alert** All agents that lead to hypoestrogenism (such as GnRH agonists and aromatase inhibitors) can cause bone loss. Any patients receiving these agents should receive hormonal add-back therapy such as norethindrone acetate, the female hormone progestin, and counseled to maintain adequate dietary calcium and vitamin D intake as well as practice appropriate weight-bearing exercise.

Surgical Management

The most common surgical treatment for endometriosis is laparoscopy. Patients are five times more likely to get relief from surgical management than medical management. Visible endometriosis implants can be excised, cauterized, or laser vaporized. It is common after surgery to follow up with pharmacological management to prevent further endometriosis recurrence. In extreme cases, it may be necessary to perform hysterectomy (removal of the uterus) with or without oophorectomy (removal of the ovaries). Removal of the ovaries has been associated with less recurrence of disease, but the risk associated with ovarian removal in young women (younger than age 40) associated with the loss of estrogen must be weighed carefully. This should also be considered very cautiously in young women who desire fertility.

Complications

The location of the endometriosis implant will determine the complications associated with this process. The most common complications are implants in the pelvis that lead to inflammation and scarring resulting in chronic pelvic pain and infertility. In the rare cases in which the implants are located in other areas, the results will be pain, inflammation, and scarring. Another complication, catamenial pneumothorax, is a condition in which endometrial implants on the lungs result in cyclic pneumothorax associated with the menstrual cycles.

Nursing Management

Assessment and Analysis

The symptoms of debilitating chronic pain, excessive bleeding, and infertility are the result of the increased vicious cycle of increased aromatase, increased estrogen, and inflammation.

Nursing Diagnoses

- **Pain, chronic** associated with inflammation and scarring of endometrial implants
- **Risk for infertility** associated with hormone irregularities and tissue scarring

Nursing Interventions

■ **Assessments**

- Vital signs
  Blood pressure and pulse may be elevated in the patient in pain.
- Pain scale rating
  Endometriosis may cause very little pain or may be completely debilitating. It is important to know how much pain the patient is experiencing to evaluate the extent of the disease and efficacy of treatment.

■ **Actions**

- Administer medications as ordered: pain medications, GnRH agonists
  Pain medications may be necessary in the patient with chronic pelvic pain. Gonadotropin-releasing hormone agonists lead to a hypoestrogenic state and decreased symptoms.

■ **Teaching**

- Educate about the disease process
  Understanding disease action is important in helping the patient manage her disease.
- Educate about medication use
  Any patient receiving a GnRH agonist should take adequate calcium and vitamin D for bone protection.
- Maintain a menstrual calendar
  While understanding that endometriosis is often acyclic, patients can chart symptoms in relation to their menstrual cycles to determine whether a pattern exists.

Evaluating Care Outcomes

It is important that the diagnosis and treatment of endometriosis be made early. The mainstay of treatment is through pharmacological methods. The patient should have adequately controlled pain that allows her to continue to function normally in all of her daily activities.

Early intervention will optimally minimize infertility and chronic pelvic pain.

Connection Check 65.3

The nurse is taking care of Ms. Davis, a 19-year-old with significant pelvic pain not associated with her menstrual cycles. After 6 months of oral contraceptive use and NSAIDs, she has had no relief. The nurse understands the next course of treatment indicated includes:

A. Narcotics

B. Laparoscopy

C. Hysterectomy

D. Oophorectomy

MENOPAUSE

Menopause is considered to have occurred after 12 months of no vaginal bleeding, or amenorrhea. All women will eventually go through menopause while they age. The menopausal transition initiates with the irregularity of menses and ends after 12 months of amenorrhea. The time from the beginning of menstrual irregularity until after 12 months of amenorrhea is referred to as *perimenopause*. Once 12 months of amenorrhea has occurred, *postmenopause* is considered to have commenced. Menopause occurs on average at the age of 50 to 51.

Pathophysiology

Menses is dependent on estrogen and progesterone production from the ovaries. Menopause occurs while the ovaries fail and their estrogen production declines. If the ovaries fail to produce estrogen through the process of ovulation, menses slowly become irregular and finally disappear completely while the uterine lining becomes thin and atrophic.

Clinical Manifestations

The most common symptoms of menopause are **vasomotor symptoms** such as hot flashes (Box 65.1). Other potential clinical manifestations or complications include bone loss, osteoporosis, increased fracture risk, central weight gain leading to cardiovascular disease, dyslipidemia, and type 2 diabetes mellitus.

Management

Medical Management
Diagnosis

Diagnosis of menopause is typically based on symptoms as described above and menstrual evaluation. It is important to rule out other etiologies for amenorrhea such as hypothyroidism as it can result in many of the same symptoms as menopause. Other etiologies to consider are pregnancy,

Box 65.1 Common Vasomotor Symptoms of Menopause

- Hot flashes
- Night sweats
- Joint pain
- Vaginal atrophy leading to vaginal dryness and painful intercourse and urinary dysfunction
- Sleep disturbance
- Anxiety
- Moodiness
- Depression
- Cognitive changes

hyperprolactinemia, other thyroid diseases, medication use, hypoglycemia, malignancies, and pheochromocytomas.

Laboratory Tests

Laboratory tests include follicle-stimulating hormone (FSH) levels. In response to ovarian failure, the pituitary increases production of FSH in an attempt to make the ovaries respond and ovulate. Perimenopausal women and postmenopausal women demonstrate varying elevations of FSH. Women in the perimenopause period may have periodic elevations of FSH followed by periods of normal levels. Therefore, measurement of FSH can be misleading and should be evaluated with caution. Pregnancy testing, prolactin levels, a thyroid panel, CBC, and a metabolic panel are other laboratory tests that can assist in ruling out other etiologies of amenorrhea described above.

Medications

Estrogen therapy is the most effective treatment for the symptoms of menopause but should be used with caution because its use is associated with varying increased risk of breast cancer and cardiovascular events. There appears to be an increased risk of breast cancer in women using estrogen and progesterone combined and less in women using estrogen alone. This is thought to be due to an increase in breast density that results in difficulty reading mammograms. This risk increases with prolonged use. Also, women who began estrogen and progesterone use in the first 10 years of menopause showed no significant increase in cardiovascular events, but this was not true for those who started **hormone therapy (HT)** once they were past the first 10 years of menopause.

With an understanding of these risks, recommendations for HT include treating women with significant vasomotor symptoms for the shortest duration required. The lowest possible effective dose should be initiated in recently menopausal women with moderate to severe symptoms who are in good cardiovascular health. Therapy should not generally extend beyond 4 to 5 years. In women with an intact uterus who require the addition of progestin to protect the uterus from hyperplasia (or overgrowth of the tissue that lines the uterus that can lead to cancer) that can occur with the use of estrogen alone, it is best to minimize the dose and duration of that medical therapy. For the minority of women who continue to have severe symptoms, HT may be continued after trials of alternative therapies and a complete risk versus benefit evaluation.

Treatment for genitourinary atrophy includes the use of vaginal estrogen therapy. This can be used with little systemic effect and is the preferred method of treatment. Moderate to severe vaginal symptoms can be treated with local estrogen in the form of vaginal tablets, creams, or rings. Patients with mild atrophy may opt to try vaginal moisturizing agents and lubricants.

If the woman is not able to take estrogen or simply chooses not to, there are several off-label medications and treatments that are used. Selective serotonin reuptake inhibitors (SSRIs), selective norepinephrine reuptake inhibitors (SNRIs), clonidine, and gabapentin have all been shown to be somewhat effective. Selective serotonin reuptake inhibitors should be avoided in women with breast cancer on tamoxifen therapy because they reduce tamoxifen metabolism. Black cohosh is one of the most commonly used herbal treatments, but it has been shown to be ineffective in trials.

Complications

Several overall health concerns result from the hypoestrogenic state of menopause. Bone loss leading to osteoporotic fracture is a direct result of declining systemic estrogen levels. Increased abdominal fat and weight gain associated with menopause may contribute to a higher risk of cardiovascular disease (CVD) due to insulin resistance, hyperlipidemia, and hypertension. Cardiovascular disease is the leading cause of death and disability in women worldwide. This risk increases significantly with age and menopause.

Nursing Management

Assessment and Analysis

Assessment of the menopausal patient focuses on symptomatology due to decreased estrogen levels. The most common symptoms include hot flashes; vaginal atrophy–related symptoms such as vaginal dryness, painful intercourse, and urinary dysfunction; sleep disturbances; mood changes; joint pain; and memory decline.

Nursing Diagnoses

- **Fatigue** associated with sleep disturbances
- **Impaired memory** associated with estrogen loss
- **Sexual dysfunction** associated with vaginal atrophy

Nursing Interventions

▪ *Assessments*

- Vital signs
  Hypertension in the postmenopausal woman is a sign of CVD.
- Menstrual calendar
  Menopause is defined as occurring after 12 months of amenorrhea.

- Weight
  Postmenopausal weight gain may contribute to CVD, insulin resistance, hyperlipidemia, and hypertension.
- Laboratory review
  FSH will be elevated in menopause as the pituitary increases production of FSH to make the ovaries respond and ovulate. Prolactin, thyroid-stimulating hormone, CBC, and chemistry panel are frequently drawn to eliminate other etiologies for patient symptoms.

▪ *Actions*

- Administer estrogen and progesterone as ordered
  Replacement of hormones no longer released because of menopause produces the most effective relief of symptoms.
- Administer other therapies as ordered such as SSRIs, SNRIs, gabapentin, and clonidine if hormonal therapy is contraindicated
  Some nonhormonal medications have been found to be effective in the relief of menopausal symptoms for reasons not completely understood. SSRIs are thought to be effective because they play a role in regulating body temperature.
- Discuss alternative methods of relief
  Cooling therapies may help with hot flashes; naps may assist with sleepless nights, as well as reassurance that symptoms are usually self-limiting.

▪ *Teaching*

- Educate on the pros and cons of HT
  Hormone therapy is controversial and is recommended only for short-term use in symptomatic patients because of increased cancer and CVD risk.
- Teach patients the etiology of symptoms
  Patients may find comfort in knowing the majority of symptoms are short term.
- Educate patients on alternative treatments for vaginal symptoms
  Educate on lubricants or estrogen creams for the vagina to decrease symptom of painful intercourse.
- Educate on the importance of adequate calcium and vitamin D intake as well as regular weight-bearing exercise
  With the loss of estrogen, women are at increased risk for decreased bone density and fracture—calcium, vitamin D, and weight-bearing exercises help maintain bone health.

Evaluating Care Outcomes

A well-managed menopausal patient has symptoms under control through the use of hormonal therapy if indicated or the use of SSRIs, SNRIs, clonidine, or gabapentin. This patient maintains a healthy diet and weight, exercises regularly and takes calcium and vitamin D supplementation. It is important that women begin these healthy behaviors at a young age and continue in menopause to protect their bone and cardiac health.

FIBROIDS

Epidemiology

Fibroids are reported to occur in as many as 70% to 80% of women. They are more prevalent in African American women, occurring in as many as 75% of women of that race. They are more prevalent in white women than in Asians. They are also more common in women who have never been pregnant, those who started menstruating at an early age, and those who were older at the time of their first term pregnancy. Black women who have had children do not appreciate the same risk reduction as white women. Fibroids are more likely in obese women in general but also in nonobese women with polycystic ovarian syndrome. Diabetes mellitus and hypertension have also shown a correlation to a higher incidence of fibroids.

Pathophysiology

Fibroids or uterine **leiomyomas** are the most common solid benign tumors of the female pelvis and are the leading cause of hysterectomy. The tumors originate from the muscular tissue of the uterus, but their etiology is not completely understood. They are defined by their location in the uterus. Submucous fibroids are found inside the uterus and distort the uterine cavity. Intramural fibroids are found within the muscle wall of the uterus but do not distort the cavity or extend to the subserosal surface. Fibroids that extend out of the outer, subserosal surface of the uterus are called *subserosal*. These may extend off the uterus completely in a pedunculated fashion (Fig. 65.6). Fibroids are dependent on the ovarian production of estrogen and progesterone for growth. Therefore, growth will generally occur in the reproductive years with a decline in growth once menopause has been achieved.

Clinical Manifestations

Many fibroids are completely asymptomatic. The most common symptoms are vaginal bleeding and pelvic pressure. Women may experience heavy menses associated with an overall increase in uterine and endometrial size, or they may experience **menorrhagia** (prolonged irregular bleeding) associated with endometrial distortion from submucosal fibroids. This is the most common complaint because

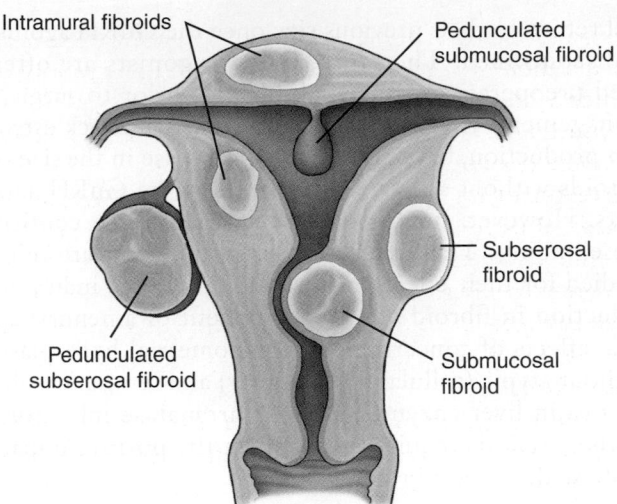

FIGURE 65.6 Fibroids. Submucosal, intramural, subserosal, and pedunculated subserosal that extend off of the uterus.

it often results in significant anemia. Significant pelvic pressure and bulk can result in dyspareunia (painful intercourse), dysuria, and difficult defecation.

Management

Medical Management

Diagnosis

The diagnosis of fibroids is often suspected when a patient presents for menorrhagia or pressure symptoms. Pelvic mass may be felt on pelvic examination, but imaging is key in the diagnosis of fibroids. Transabdominal or transvaginal ultrasound is 90% to 100% sensitive in the detection of fibroids. Color Doppler studies help identify the vascularity of the fibroid.

Magnetic resonance imaging assists in the anatomical delineation, further identifying the site, size, and depth of muscular invasion of the fibroid. Any other reasons for pelvic mass and uterine bleeding should also be thoroughly evaluated to verify the diagnosis.

Treatment

Medical treatment of fibroids is primarily focused on hormone therapy (HT) for reduction of symptoms. Estrogen and progestin combination pills and progestin-only formulations are used for the control of bleeding and dysmenorrhea. Evidence suggests that their relief in fibroid patients tends to be short term. Also, there is some concern that hormonal use could stimulate fibroid growth and should be monitored closely if used. Tranexamic acid is an antifibrinolytic drug that can be taken for five days with the onset of menses to decrease overall blood loss. Gonadotropin-releasing hormone (GnRH) agonists induce a false menopause state that results in size reduction of the fibroids and decreased bleeding. The bone loss and menopausal symptoms associated with this type of drug lead to a suggestion of a limit of 6 months of use. The effect with a GnRH agonist is temporary, and the fibroids will return to their previous size once the GnRH agonist is discontinued. Therefore, GnRH agonists are often used preoperatively to shrink fibroids prior to surgical management. Aromatase inhibitors, which block estrogen production, have also shown a decrease in the size of fibroids without as many side effects as the GnRH agonists. However, further research is needed to confirm these findings. Finally, antiprogesterone agents are being studied for their effect on fibroids. Early data indicate a reduction in fibroid size with a benefit of amenorrhea. Side effects of concern include endometrial hyperplasia without atypia (cellular abnormality) and temporary elevations in liver enzymes. As with aromatase inhibitors, further study is required to confirm the positive impact of these drugs on fibroids.

Surgical Management

Surgical options are the primary tool utilized in the management of fibroids. Hysterectomy, or surgical removal of the uterus, is the most common treatment for fibroids. It is the only definitive treatment that ensures no recurrence and complete resolution. It is permanent and eliminates all future fertility as well. Hysterectomy may be performed via laparotomy, an open abdominal incision; transvaginally (removal of the uterus through the vagina); or laparoscopically, a procedure done through several small incisions that allow introduction of instruments and a camera, with or without robotic assistance. Vaginal and laparoscopic hysterectomies offer lower complications, shorter hospital stays, and quicker recovery.

If fertility is a priority, then myomectomy is an option. Myomectomy is a surgical procedure to remove the visible and accessible fibroids and then repair the uterus to its prefibroid state. Myomectomies are traditionally performed through laparotomy, but in certain patients with trained skilled surgeons, a myomectomy may be able to be performed laparoscopically. As with hysterectomy, laparoscopy generally results in less blood loss, decreased hospital stays, and quicker recovery.

Interventional radiologists may perform a procedure called a *uterine artery embolization* (UAE). In this procedure, the uterine arteries are accessed through the femoral arteries. An embolizing material is introduced into the uterine arteries, which results in devascularization (cutting off the blood supply) and subsequent degeneration of the fibroids (Fig. 65.7). Minor complications include vaginal discharge, fibroid expulsion, and hematoma. When compared with patients undergoing other surgical procedures, UAE patients had shorter hospital stays and a quicker recovery. Concerns do exist over the effect of UAE on premature ovarian failure. Also, there are few data demonstrating the safety of pregnancy after UAE. Therefore, the current recommendation is that women should not become pregnant after undergoing this procedure.

Another approach uses MRI-focused ultrasound therapy to penetrate and destroy the fibroid. Adverse effects include

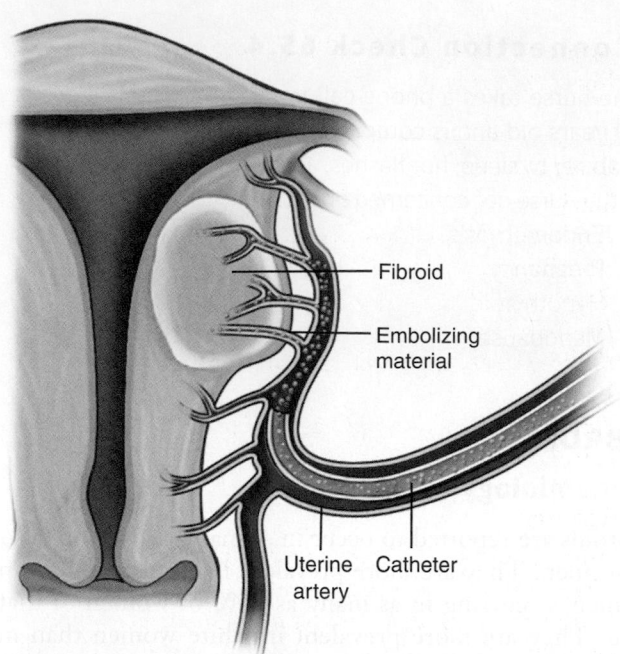

FIGURE 65.7 Uterine artery embolization. Embolizing material is infused into the uterine artery to cut off blood flow to the fibroid.

heavy menstrual bleeding, continued pain, nausea, and leg and buttock pain due to sono effect on the sciatic nerve. The sciatic nerve pain will eventually resolve. The procedure is costly and can treat only one fibroid at a time. Women wishing to conceive in the future are not advised to pursue this approach.

Complications

In rare cases, fibroids may become so large as to cause pathologic compression on adjacent structures such as the ureters, resulting in compromised renal function. Patients may become so anemic that blood transfusion is required. The least common but most concerning issue is distinguishing the fibroid from a leiomyosarcoma, a dangerous malignant tumor that often appears similar to a benign fibroid on examination and imaging. Consideration must be given to this option when evaluating fibroids or uterine tumors.

Nursing Management

Assessment and Analysis

Patients with fibroids present with symptoms such as heavy or prolonged vaginal bleeding due to increased uterine size from the fibroids or bleeding of a submucosal fibroid. They may also have pelvic pressure due to the bulk of the fibroids putting pressure on other organs in the pelvis.

Nursing Diagnoses

- **Risk for activity intolerance** due to anemia, vaginal bleeding, and pelvic pressure
- **Impaired urinary elimination** due to pressure from fibroids
- **Chronic pain** associated with pelvic pressure from fibroids

- **Acute pain** associated with the surgical procedure for fibroid treatment

Nursing Interventions

■ Assessments

- Vital signs
  Hypotension and tachycardia will reflect symptomatic anemia. Pain may cause tachycardia.
- Pain scale
  Pain assessment can help evaluate fibroid development and the adequacy of pain management.
- Pad count
  Evaluating the number of pads used can help to quantify the actual amount of vaginal bleeding.

■ Actions

- Administer blood transfusion as ordered
  The significantly anemic patient may acutely need blood to maintain intravascular volume and oxygen carrying capacity.
- Administer nonsurgical methods of treatment if chosen
  Gonadotropin-releasing hormone agonists induce a false menopause state that results in size reduction of the fibroids and decreased bleeding; estrogen and progesterone therapy are used for the control of bleeding and dysmenorrhea; and aromatase inhibitors block estrogen production, decreasing the size of fibroids.
- Administer medications for pain relief as ordered
  Pain medications may be necessary in the preoperative or postoperative patient. Degenerating fibroids can be quite painful.

■ Teaching

- Treatment options
  The patient should make a well-informed choice about treatment on the basis of her age, health, and fertility desires.

Evaluating Care Outcomes

The well-managed patient should have controlled vaginal bleeding that does not result in anemia or interference with normal activity. This patient understands the risks and benefits of all treatment options and chooses the one that best meets her needs based on age, health, and fertility desires.

Connection Check 65.5

Ms. Harris has large uterine fibroids that are causing her pain and heavy bleeding. The nurse is educating her on her treatment options. Which option is considered the only definitive treatment for fibroids?

A. Uterine artery embolization
B. Hysterectomy
C. Lupron administration
D. Myomectomy

OVARIAN CANCER

Epidemiology

Ovarian cancer is the fifth most common cancer found in women. Approximately 70% to 75% of the cases are not discovered until the late stages (stage III or IV) of the disease. As a result, ovarian cancer causes the most deaths of any gynecological malignancy. If diagnosed in stage I, the 5-year survival rate is more than 73%. However, if diagnosed in stage III or IV, the 5-year survival rate falls to 21% and less than 5%, respectively.

There appears to be a hormonal influence on the development of ovarian cancer. A history of breastfeeding, pregnancy, and oral contraceptive use bestows a protective effect as does the use of progesterone alone as hormone replacement therapy. Conversely, long-term hormone replacement with estrogen only or estrogen/progesterone combination increases the risk of ovarian cancer. Androgens (primarily male hormones such as testosterone) are suspected to have a negative effect on ovarian cancer. This is evidenced by the fact that obesity and polycystic ovarian syndrome, states that have higher circulating androgens, appear to carry a greater risk. Elevated gonadotropin levels (FSH/LH) found in menopause do not appear to cause malignant lesions but may promote the growth of an existing tumor. Other factors that may be implicated but not completely understood are age of first menses, age of menopause, infertility history, and the use of ovarian-stimulating drugs. Other women considered high risk for developing ovarian cancer are those with a family history, those with *BRCA1* or *BRCA2* gene mutations, or those with hereditary nonpolyposis colorectal cancer (HNPCC) syndrome. It is uncommon to find ovarian cancer in a woman younger than 40, but the incidence increases from that point forward. Most cases are diagnosed in women in their 70s.

Pathophysiology

As with breast cancer, ovarian cancer is a condition where the cells of the body grow and divide abnormally and uncontrollably. The cells can invade nearby tissues and spread to other areas through the bloodstream and lymphatic system. Staging of ovarian cancer is established by the International Federation of Gynecology and Obstetrics (FIGO) and is based on operative findings. Table 65.3 outlines staging of ovarian cancer. Fig. 65.8 illustrates ovarian cancer.

Clinical Manifestations

The symptoms experienced prior to diagnosis of ovarian cancer tend to be vague and nonspecific. Symptoms that should cause one to consider ovarian cancer are bloating, pelvic or abdominal pain, early satiety or problems with eating, and urinary urgency or frequency. In later-stage ovarian cancer, ascites or excessive fluid in the abdominal cavity is present. Often patients and providers alike dismiss the

Table 65.3 Federation of Gynecology and Obstetrics Staging of Ovarian Cancer

Stage	Description
Stage I A, B, C	Growth limited to one or both ovaries; staging increases if it extends to a surface tumor and there are malignant cells in ascites or peritoneal washings
Stage II A, B, C	Involves one or both ovaries with extension to the pelvis; staging increases as there is extension to the uterus, fallopian tubes, or to other pelvic tissues and there are malignant cells in ascites or peritoneal washings
Stage III A, B, C	Involves one or both ovaries with peritoneal metastasis limited to or beyond the pelvis and/or positive retroperitoneal or inguinal lymph nodes; staging increases as abnormal cells are noted on the abdominal peritoneal surfaces and there is abdominal metastasis increasing in size
Stage IV	Involves one or both ovaries and has distant metastasis

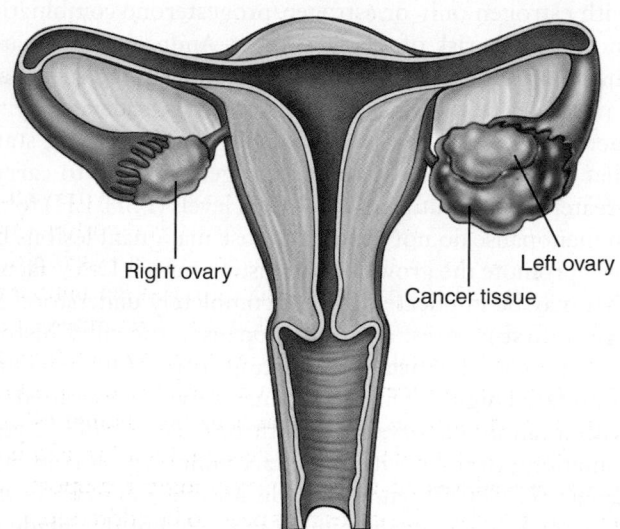

Right ovary Left ovary Cancer tissue

FIGURE 65.8 Ovarian cancer.

symptoms as associated with common nonpathologic etiologies. As a result, most ovarian cancers are diagnosed in the advanced stages. It is important for both patients and healthcare providers to recognize the symptoms of ovarian cancer and be diligent in investigating the etiology.

Management

Medical and Surgical Management

Diagnosis

There are no recommended screening tests for ovarian cancer. If ovarian cancer is suspected, the biochemical marker **CA 125**, a blood test, may be ordered. CA 125 levels will rise in the presence of ovarian cancer, but there is no established expected rise, and many other conditions such as diverticulitis, endometriosis, cirrhosis of the liver, and uterine fibroids may also cause the levels to rise. CA 125 levels are normal in 50% of early ovarian cases as well.

Radiographical tests include pelvic ultrasonography or CT to visualize the ovaries. In women who are at particularly high risk for developing ovarian cancer (BReast CAncer

Gene [BRCA] 1 or BRCA2 positive, family history, or HNPCC syndrome), CA 125 levels and pelvic ultrasounds may be used together for screening. However, this approach is not recommended in the general population because studies have shown that the overall benefit of earlier detection through these methods does not demonstrate a significant overall effect on mortality. It may actually lead to more invasive harm with minimal yield because of aggressive surgical intervention for ultimately benign lesions. Biopsy of an ovarian mass is not generally recommended because of the potential for spread during biopsy. Definitive diagnosis is made through surgical removal of a suspected mass followed by total specimen pathology.

Surgical Treatment

Surgical management of a suspected ovarian carcinoma traditionally consists of surgical staging and debulking of the tumor. The debulking procedure attempts to remove as much of the tumor bulk as possible. In addition to removal of the mass, the staging procedure includes peritoneal washings (saline solution is rinsed into the abdomen and pelvis and then removed and sent for cytology), peritoneal biopsies (removal of samples of the peritoneal enclosure of the abdomen for pathology), omentectomy (removal of samples of the omental tissue surrounding the bowels), and lymphadenectomy (removal of lymph nodes for pathology to determine spread). Most procedures also include removal of the uterus, both ovaries, and fallopian tubes. However, in rare situations in the woman wishing to retain her fertility with very early-stage malignancy, this may be deferred and only the involved ovary is removed.

Medications

Medical management with chemotherapy follows surgical debulking. Standard chemotherapy is typically administered through IV methods, but recent trials have shown intraperitoneal (IP) chemotherapy to be superior to IV administration. However, IP chemotherapy tends to carry a higher toxicity risk. Another more recent medical option is to give chemotherapy prior to surgery. This can complicate diagnosis of histological or cell type of the tumor because chemotherapy tends to alter the composition of the tumor. This is important because histological subtype is an important factor to consider when determining which chemotherapeutic agent is most effective for treatment. For this reason, optimal initial debulking remains the standard of care in the majority of patients.

Nursing Management

Assessment and Analysis

Symptoms of ovarian cancer tend to be vague and nonspecific and are often not reported until the cancer is advanced. Even when reported, they are frequently dismissed as benign in etiology. The common symptoms due to the presence of the tumor are bloating, difficulty eating or early satiety, pelvic or abdominal pain, and urinary frequency or urgency.

Nursing Diagnoses

- **Ineffective coping** associated with the cancer diagnosis
- **Acute pain** associated with surgery
- **Altered nutrition**, less than body requirements secondary to cancer and chemotherapy

Nursing Interventions

Assessments

- Symptom assessment
  Ovarian cancer should be considered when bloating, difficulty eating, abdominal pain, or urinary frequency or urgency is present.
- Vital signs
  Elevated blood pressure and pulse are signs of pain. Elevated temperature can indicate infection.
- Abdominal girth
  A manifestation of later-stage ovarian cancer is ascites.
- Weight
  Weight loss may be associated with nutritional deficits associated with cancer and chemotherapy, whereas weight gain can be an indicator of fluid retention.
- Diagnostic tests; CA 125 levels and imaging
  CA 125 levels may be elevated in ovarian cancer but should be evaluated with other indicators as CA 125 can be elevated in other conditions. Pelvic ultrasound or CT may visualize the tumor.
- Chemotherapy side effects
  The chemotherapy for ovarian cancer treatment is often toxic with many side effects. They include nausea, vomiting, diarrhea, and constipation. Hair loss is common as well as a decrease in white blood and red blood cells. It is important to evaluate for these side effects and treat them as able.
- Psychological evaluation
  Be aware of the potential of anxiety and depression associated with this diagnosis and offer support and counseling as necessary.

Actions

- Give pain medications as ordered
  Pain medications help the patient to maintain comfort and participate in activities of daily living.

- Give chemotherapeutic agents as ordered
  Adjunct therapy to surgery with ovarian cancer
- Give antiemetics as ordered
  Nausea and vomiting are common with chemotherapy. Antiemetics are very important in treatment as they help the patient maintain a nutritional balance.

Teaching

- Educate all women on the symptoms of ovarian cancer
  Symptoms are vague and nonspecific. It is extremely important that women recognize them early and providers investigate them thoroughly.
- Discuss methods to ease chemotherapy side effects
  Patients should use all prescribed methods and any complementary methods to combat the side effects of chemotherapy and ease the treatment of this disease. Poorly controlled side effects may delay or hamper treatment, cause nutritional deficiencies, and put the patient at risk for infection.
- Provide information on support groups or counselors
  This is a difficult disease with a poor prognosis. Patients can find help through support groups and counselors.

Evaluating Care Outcomes

Optimal management includes awareness of even the vaguest symptoms of ovarian cancer and immediately reporting them. It is imperative that women be taught the early symptoms. Once diagnosed, the patient will need support throughout the operative and chemotherapeutic phases of treatment, both physically and mentally. A well-managed patient undergoing chemotherapy is receiving adequate antiemetics to control nausea. Nutritionally, the patient is eating enough calories to maintain adequate weight for healing. Hair loss and body image are addressed through psychological support, and ultimately end-of-life issues may need to be addressed.

Connection Check 65.6

A nurse working in a clinic has received phone calls from several patients. It is a priority for the nurse to suggest immediate follow-up for the female patient complaining of which of the following?

A. Urinary frequency at night
B. Chest discomfort after spicy meals
C. Difficulty eating due to feeling full and bloated
D. Pain with the onset of menses

! Safety Alert   Transgender Males and Gynecologic Care

It is important for transgender males to receive appropriate gynecologic care and recommended preventive screening exams (breast, pap, and pelvic exams). Transgender males continue at risk for gynecologic disorders but often delay seeking this care. Increased sensitivity and knowledge by the medical staff and nurses to the unique needs and concerns of this population can aid in providing these services.

UTERINE CANCER

Epidemiology

Uterine cancer, or endometrial cancer, is the most common gynecological cancer in the United States. There is a 2.6% lifetime risk for women living in developed nations. Uterine cancer primarily occurs in postmenopausal women, with the highest incidence between the ages of 55 and 65. The median age at diagnosis is 61. Most cases are sporadic and multifactorial in nature; 2% to 5% are associated with a hereditary gene alteration called hereditary nonpolyposis colorectal syndrome (HNPCC).

The greatest risk factors for the most common endometrial cancers (type I, endometrioid) are unopposed estrogen exposure and obesity. Unopposed estrogen exposure may be the result of estrogen therapy in the absence of progesterone replacement or therapeutic tamoxifen use. Endogenous sources of elevated estrogen levels that may result in endometrial cancers include obesity, cirrhosis, estrogen-producing tumors, and anovulation. A less common but more aggressive type of uterine malignancy (type II, serous/clear cell) is a malignancy with aging and genetic/molecular changes. Serous carcinomas occur more commonly in African Americans.

Pathophysiology

As with other cancers, uterine cancer is a condition in which the cells of the body grow and divide abnormally and uncontrollably. The cells can invade nearby tissues and spread to other areas through the bloodstream and lymphatic system. Approximately 80% of endometrial carcinomas are endometrioid adenocarcinomas that consist of malignant glandular cells that look very much like the cells of the uterine lining. They are commonly early stage and grade and are associated with estrogen stimulation associated with obesity. Approximately 10% of endometrial carcinomas are serous and clear cell carcinomas. Associated with endometrial atrophy, they tend to be diagnosed in women 5 to 10 years older than those with endometrioid carcinomas. With early diagnosis, endometrioid carcinomas have an 88% overall survival rate. Serous carcinomas and clear cell carcinomas have a much poorer prognosis, with 18% to 27% overall survival rates for serous carcinomas and 42% overall survival rates for clear cell carcinomas. Uterine sarcomas, cancers that arise from muscle and support tissue of the uterus, account for 3% to 5% of all uterine cancers (Fig. 65.9). Metastatic or recurrent uterine cancer of any histology is considered incurable and in the advanced stage has a median survival of approximately 1 year. Table 65.4 outlines FIGO tumor staging for uterine cancer.

Clinical Manifestations

The most common symptom of endometrial cancer is vaginal bleeding. Postmenopausal women with vaginal bleeding and premenopausal women with irregular or heavy bleeding who have risk factors or who have been unresponsive to

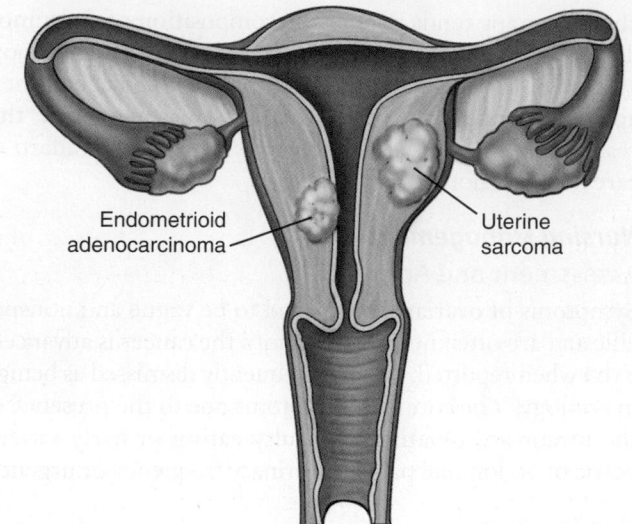

FIGURE 65.9 Uterine cancer.

Table 65.4 Federation of Gynecology and Obstetrics Tumor Staging for Uterine Cancer

Stage	Description
Stage I A, B, C	Endometrial cancer confined to the corpus, the main body of the uterus; staging increases as there is invasion of the myometrium
Stage II A, B, C	Endometrial cancer involves the corpus and the cervix but has not extended outside the uterus; staging increases as there is invasion of the cervical stroma
Stage III A, B, C	Endometrial cancer extends outside the uterus but is confined to the true pelvis; staging increases as there is invasion of the visceral peritoneum, fallopian tubes, vagina and there are metastases to pelvic and/or para-aortic lymph nodes
Stage IV A, B	Endometrial cancer involves the bladder or bowel mucosa or has metastasized to distant sites; staging increases with distant metastases

medical treatment should undergo evaluation for endometrial cancer.

Management

Medical and Surgical Management

Diagnosis

Diagnosis can be done through biopsy, pelvic ultrasound, and in some cases, surgical dilation and curettage (D & C: scraping the lining of the uterus for a tissue sample). Endometrial biopsy is 99% sensitive in detecting high-grade endometrial carcinomas. Pelvic ultrasound also aids in the detection of an abnormally thickened endometrium that may be associated with the development of endometrial cancer. Patients with a negative endometrial biopsy and normal pelvic ultrasound who continue to have abnormal bleeding may be candidates for surgical D&C to ensure adequate uterine sampling.

Treatment

The initial treatment is the surgical removal of the uterus, fallopian tubes, and ovaries. As in ovarian cancer, other procedures include obtaining abdominopelvic washings for cytology (saline solution is rinsed into the abdomen and pelvis and then removed) to check for cancer cells and performing pelvic and aortic lymphadenectomy (removal of lymph nodes for pathology to determine spread). Omentectomy (removal of samples of the omental tissue surrounding the bowels) and peritoneal biopsies may also be performed. The FIGO tumor staging then guides treatment. For example, early stage I disease can be treated with surgery that is often curative, not requiring further treatment.

Adjuvant therapy (additional therapy after surgery) is determined on the basis of staging or risk. Typically, radiation treatment is the choice of therapy. Chemotherapy is the first-line management for those with high risk or higher-stage disease, but response continues to be modest. Despite a good survival rate in early-stage patients, patients with advanced or recurrent endometrial cancer have an overall poor survival rate. Once primary chemotherapy has failed, there is no accepted second-line agent for treatment. Chemotherapy resistance is not uncommon and presents challenging treatment dilemmas. Metastatic and recurrent disease is considered incurable and has poor survival rates of only about 1 year. Optimal sequencing with chemotherapy and radiation continues to be investigated.

Nursing Management

Assessment and Analysis

Identification of the patient at risk is critical in assessment of the patient when evaluating for uterine cancer. Patients with uterine cancers will often present with abnormal vaginal bleeding. The most common age at presentation is between 55 and 65. Once the possibility of uterine cancer is considered, pelvic ultrasound and endometrial biopsy are critical for further assessment.

Nursing Diagnoses

- **Acute pain** associated with the surgical staging procedure
- **Nausea** associated with chemotherapy
- **Ineffective coping** associated with the cancer diagnosis

Nursing Interventions

▪ Assessments

- Vital signs
  Blood pressure and pulse may be elevated in the patient in pain. Temperature elevations are a sign of infection.
- Daily weight
  Weight loss reflects fluid loss and nutritional deficits. Nausea and vomiting from chemotherapy treatment are often implicated in weight loss. Weight gain may be reflective of fluid retention.
- Intake and output
  Intake and output allows for evaluation of the patient's fluid balances as well as nutritional deficits.
- Pain scale
  Pain scales allow patients to identify and adequately treat their pain.
- Abnormal vaginal bleeding
  Abnormal vaginal bleeding is the most common symptom in uterine cancer.
- Patient age
  Most uterine cancers occur between the ages of 55 and 65.

▪ Actions

- Administer pain medications as ordered
  Pain medications are important to relieve the acute pain associated with surgical intervention as well as the chronic pain associated with the disease and its treatment. Adequate pain management allows the patient to participate in activities of daily living.
- Administer chemotherapy as ordered
  Chemotherapy after surgery is often indicated, but a positive response is limited.
- Provide comfort measures for the chemotherapy patient
  The patient undergoing chemotherapy may experience side effects of nausea, vomiting, or stomatitis. Assist these patients with comfort measures including antiemetics, mouth rinses with salt water or mouthwash, and complementary therapies.

▪ Teaching

- Educate about disease prevention
  Obesity and unopposed estrogen are the most common risk factors for uterine cancer. Encourage patients to maintain a healthy weight and exercise regularly. Any patients on estrogen therapy who have an intact uterus should be on replacement progesterone as well. Patients on tamoxifen should be closely monitored for endometrial hyperplasia.
- Discuss chemotherapy comfort measures
  It is important that the patient undergoing chemotherapy also receive medications for nausea. Avoiding hot or spicy food, anti-inflammatories, and mouth wash preparations may help stomatitis. Complementary therapies may also be used to relieve the common side effects of chemotherapy.
- Provide psychological support resources
  Support groups, image centers, and counselors are all important resources to have readily available for the patient undergoing treatment for cancer.

Evaluating Care Outcomes

Nutritional needs are paramount with a patient undergoing treatment for uterine cancer. The well-managed patient is able to maintain adequate weight and nutritional status while optimally achieving most of her normal daily functions. The majority of endometrial cancer is diagnosed in the early stage and frequently is cured with surgery alone. Education regarding the need for routine long-term follow-up is important. Psychological support resources should be available and easily accessed.

Connection Check 65.7

The nurse is most concerned about Ms. James, a 60-year-old female patient, when she calls complaining of which of the following?

A. Vaginal itching
B. A foul vaginal discharge
C. Hot flashes at night
D. Vaginal bleeding

CERVICAL CANCER

Epidemiology

Cervical cancer is the 13th most common cancer in women in the United States. It is in the top 10 cancers among black women, American Indian or Alaska Native, and Hispanic women. The highest incidence is in women 50 to 79 years of age and in Hispanic women. Approximately half of cervical cancer cases are diagnosed in the late stages of the disease. Diagnosis in later stages occurs more frequently in women older than 50, black women, and women who have not had a Pap smear for longer than 5 years.

Cervical cancer rates in the United States and other developed nations have declined significantly since the introduction of the Pap smear in the mid-20th century. The lowest users of Pap smears today are uninsured women, smokers, obese women, women older than the age of 65, Asians or Pacific Islanders, and recent immigrants. A majority of cervical cancer cases worldwide occur in underdeveloped countries. Approximately 85% of cervical cancer deaths occur in these countries.

Nearly 100% of cervical cancer tests are positive for infectious **human papillomavirus (HPV)**. Although women may be infected with HPV and never develop cervical cancer, it is almost always the cause of cervical cancer. Associated risk factors for HPV include early sexual activity, multiple sexual partners, low socioeconomic status, and immunosuppression. Other risk factors that are thought to be possible contributors are herpes simplex virus type 2, smoking, douching, poor nutrition, and oral contraceptive use.

⚠️ **Safety Alert** It is important to counsel patients to avoid the modifiable risk factors for HPV. They include early sexual activity, multiple sexual partners, smoking, douching, and poor nutrition. It is also important to encourage young women to get vaccinated against HPV. The Centers for Disease Control and Prevention (CDC) currently recommends vaccination for children aged 11 or 12. Two HPV vaccines are now available as prevention; however, they are ineffective against an existing virus.

Pathophysiology

Cervical cancer is a slow-developing disease that begins with early cervical **dysplasia**, or abnormal cell maturation (low grade progressing to high grade), that only develops into invasive cancer if left untreated. Early detection of dysplasia allows for removal of the dysplastic cells and prevention of cervical cancer.

Clinical Manifestations

There are no recognizable symptoms of cervical dysplasia. Most dysplasia is not even visible to the eye of the trained provider. Vaginal bleeding is the most common symptom of invasive cervical cancer. Sexually active women may experience postcoital bleeding. In women who are not sexually active, it is not uncommon to be completely asymptomatic until the disease is very advanced.

Management

Medical and Surgical Management

Diagnosis

Almost all cervical cancers are preventable with adequate routine screening. The mainstay of cervical cancer screening is the Pap smear. Human papillomavirus testing is also frequently being used as an adjunct to the Pap smear. Screening guidelines include the following:

- Women should have their first Pap smear at age 21.
- Women between ages 21 and 30 with normal Pap smears should have Pap smears every 3 years. Human papillomavirus (HPV) testing is not indicated as a screening test in women in that age group but should be sent reflexively if atypical cells are detected on the Pap smear of any age group.
- A Pap smear with HPV cotesting is preferable in women between the ages of 30 and 65. If both Pap and HPV tests are negative, cotesting may be repeated every 5 years.
- Those with risk factors such as HIV, immunosuppression, diethylstilbestrol exposure, or a history of dysplasia or cervical cancer may need more frequent Pap smears.
- Women who have had a total hysterectomy for benign cause and with no history of cervical intraepithelial neoplasia (CIN 2; abnormal cells found on the cervix caused by HPV) in the preceding 20 years should not have any further Pap smears.
- Women older than 65 with no history of CIN 2 in the last 20 years and either three consecutive negative Pap smears or two consecutive cotests in the last 10 years with the last one done within 5 years may discontinue Pap smears.

If the Pap smear reveals dysplasia or atypical cells with the presence of HPV, the patient is referred for colposcopy and cervical biopsy. Colposcopy involves swabbing the cervix with an acetic acid solution or a Lugol's solution and then looking at it with a lighted magnifying device that allows for abnormal areas to be easily identified. Once abnormal tissue is identified, a sample or biopsy of the tissue is obtained for pathology (Fig. 65.10). Cervical biopsy is diagnostic for dysplasia or cancer.

Radiological evaluation is an important step prior to treatment. Magnetic resonance imaging is accepted as the best measurement of tumor volume. Positron emission tomography scanning is helpful in identifying distant metastasis. If cervical cancer is diagnosed, FIGO staging is used but can be somewhat difficult because it may understage the patient. Its value is still under investigation, but tumor stage may be a prognostic indicator along with the patient's age, presence of anemia, and any other patient comorbidities.

Surgical Treatment

Surgical management is used in the early stages of cervical cancer. Radical trachelectomy (removal of the uterine cervix only) is performed, particularly in women who desire to retain their fertility. In women without a desire for fertility, a radical hysterectomy with lymph node dissection is frequently performed. Those with recurrent cervical cancer are evaluated closely to determine the extent of the disease. If the cancer is truly confined to the pelvis, exenteration or removal of all pelvic organs can be curative. Patients must be thoroughly counseled about the surgery. The mortality rate is around 5%, and the morbidity rate is close to 70%. The patient is ultimately left with a colostomy and urinary diversion.

Medical Treatment

Medical management in the form of chemoradiation is routine in women with higher-stage disease after radical surgery. In chemoradiation, chemotherapy is administered at the same time as radiation because it is thought that chemotherapy makes the cancer cells more susceptible or sensitive to radiation. Radiation is generally achieved through localized brachytherapy (internal radiation placed directly into or next to the tumor) but may also be done through generalized pelvic radiation. Chemoradiation may also be used in those women with recurrent cervical cancer if they have not received radiation previously. If the patient has previously been radiated, the only choice of treatment is chemotherapy alone. Five-year survival rates depend on the stage at diagnosis. Those with localized disease have a 92% 5-year survival rate compared with 58% for those with regional disease and 17% for those with distant disease.

Nursing Management

Assessment and Analysis

Cervical cancer usually exhibits no symptoms until it is very advanced; thus, assessment of the cervical cancer patient must focus on prevention, early diagnosis, and treatment. The importance of routine screening cannot be overstated.

Nursing Diagnoses

- **Ineffective health maintenance** associated with lack of Pap screening
- **Ineffective coping** associated with the cancer diagnosis
- **Acute pain** associated with the surgical procedure
- **Nausea** associated with chemoradiation administration

Nursing Interventions

Assessments

- Vital signs
  Elevated blood pressure and pulse are symptoms of pain and anxiety.
- Pap smear results
  Pap smear is the screening tool to identify cervical cell change associated with dysplasia and cancer.
- Intake and output
  Patient intake and output can help reveal nutritional deficits or fluid retention.
- Daily weights
  Patient weight is also an indicator of nutritional status and fluid retention. If the patient is suffering nausea and vomiting, weight may be a valuable indicator of nutritional status.
- Pain scale
  Patients may use a pain scale to indicate their subjective level of pain and evaluate treatment.

Actions

- Refer for colposcopy/biopsy
  Abnormal Pap results require further investigation with colposcopy and biopsy.
- Give pain medications as ordered
  Patients with good pain relief will heal better and will be more able to participate in activities of daily living.

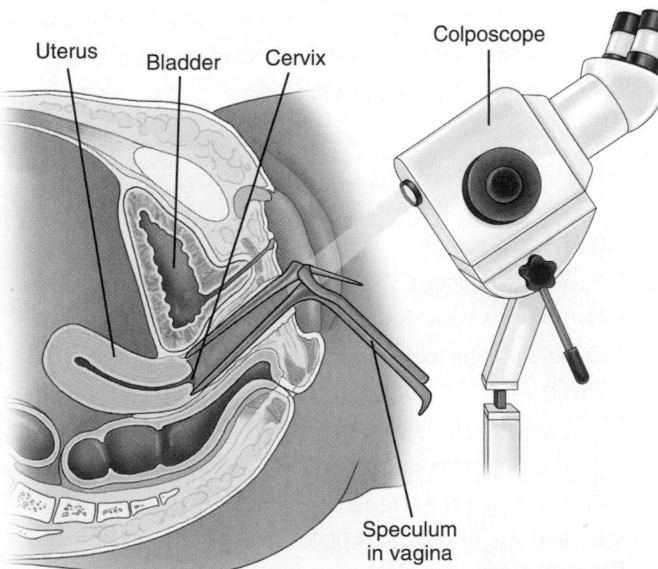

FIGURE 65.10 Colposcopy. The colposcope is inserted through a speculum into the vagina. The cervix is swabbed with an acetic acid solution allowing abnormal tissue to be identified and sampled for biopsy.

- Give antiemetics as ordered
  A common side effect of surgery and chemoradiation is nausea/vomiting.
- Give support/offer resources
  Patients with a cancer diagnosis often have psychological concerns and feel comforted by support. Offer resources for support groups, counselors, or image centers.

■ Teaching

- Educate on the need for routine screening
  Educate all women to seek routine Pap screening and to follow up on any recommended interventions. Cervical cancer can be successfully treated if found early.
- Provide information on support groups
  Patients with a cancer diagnosis often have psychological concerns and may benefit from a support group or counselor.

Evaluating Care Outcomes

With screening and early intervention, cervical cancer is an almost completely preventable disease. Women must be properly educated and provided with the resources to seek screening and treatment. Once cancer is diagnosed, a well-managed patient has her pain under control and her nutritional needs maintained throughout surgery and chemoradiation to facilitate healing. Psychological support is vital for the woman enduring cervical cancer.

Connection Check 65.8

A 25-year-old patient presents to the clinic for her annual gynecological examination. Her last Pap smear was at the age of 21. What should she have today?
A. Breast examination, pelvic examination, and Pap smear
B. Breast examination, pelvic examination, and Pap smear with HPV cotesting
C. Breast examination, pelvic examination, and HPV testing
D. Breast and pelvic examinations only

Making Connections

CASE STUDY: WRAP-UP

Ms. Sims's imaging suggests a lesion suspicious for malignancy. Biopsy of the mass confirms invasive cancer of the right breast. On the basis of imaging, clinical examination, and biopsy, it is felt to be a stage I breast cancer. Ms. Sims is referred to a breast surgeon, radiation oncologist, and medical oncologist for management and treatment.

Ms. Sims consults with her physicians. Because she is stage I, she is offered breast conservation versus mastectomy. After careful consideration, she chooses breast conservation. Because her tumor is more than 2 cm, she requires 3 to 6 months of chemotherapy after surgery. Once chemotherapy is complete, she will undergo radiation therapy as recommended for all breast conservation patients. Stains of her tumor also reveal that her tumor is estrogen positive. She will take tamoxifen (Nolvadex) for 5 years. She will require life-long follow-up with mammograms.

Case Study Questions

1. The nurse at the breast center is educating Ms. Sims on her options. She explains that if she chooses breast conservation therapy, her next step in treatment after surgery will be which of the following?
   A. Chemotherapy followed by radiation
   B. Radiation followed by chemotherapy
   C. Chemotherapy and physical therapy
   D. Follow-up surgery 6 months later

2. The nurse has received a set of orders for Ms. Sims. Which order should the nurse call the provider to verify prior to implementation?
   A. Pain medication
   B. Oral contraceptives
   C. Tamoxifen
   D. Stool softener

3. The nurse taking care of Ms. Sims in the postoperative area should be most concerned about the surgical wound if the assessment includes which of the following?
   A. Bloody drainage saturating the dressing
   B. Serosanguineous drainage on the dressing
   C. Redness under the surgical tape
   D. Tenderness at the incision site

4. The nurse in the postoperative area assesses Ms. Sims for pain. The pain assessment should include which of the following? *(Select all that apply.)*
   A. Pain scale
   B. Heart rate
   C. Extremity pulse check
   D. Blood pressure
   E. Wound drainage

5. Ms. Sims has begun radiation treatments. The nurse in the radiation center monitors Ms. Sims for what important side effect?
   A. Swelling of the affected arm
   B. Opening of the surgical wound
   C. Infection of the surgical site
   D. Redness, itching, and irritation of the radiated skin

CHAPTER SUMMARY

With adequate treatment, many women are able to survive breast cancer today. Those with advanced-stage cancer are still able to achieve prolongation of their life while balancing quality of life. Treatment is generally a combination of surgery, chemotherapy, and radiation. The degree of each is determined by the stage of the cancer.

Dysmenorrhea is the most common gynecological complaint for young women and can greatly interfere with their lives each month. Ninety percent of cases of dysmenorrhea have no associated pelvic abnormalities. The majority of cases will easily respond to treatment with NSAIDs, hormonal suppression, or both. Women may also find relief in nonpharmacological approaches as well. After 6 months of failed treatment for dysmenorrhea, laparoscopy should be performed to evaluate for endometriosis.

Endometriosis occurs when endometrial tissue implants outside the uterus. The ovaries are the most common location for the implants, but they may also be found throughout the pelvis and even outside the pelvis. Biopsy through laparoscopy must be done to confirm a suspected diagnosis. Endometriosis is an estrogen-dependent disorder, and therefore treatment stems on control of estrogen levels in the body. First-line treatment is continuous oral contraceptives followed by medications such as GnRH agonists that decrease circulating estrogen. Surgical treatment first attempts to excise or cauterize the endometriosis but ultimately may result in hysterectomy. In the most extreme cases, hysterectomy must be accompanied by oophorectomy to achieve a beneficial result.

Although the actual average age of menopause is 50 to 51, symptoms may begin much earlier and may persist for several years. In a minority of women, symptoms may persist well into their 70s and may be detrimental to overall quality of life. It is important that patients receive care, education, and treatment to make symptoms manageable and controllable. Although HT is the most effective symptom relief medication, its controversial effect on breast cancer and cardiovascular health has led to recommendations that it be used only short term and only in women who are very symptomatic. Those with only vaginal symptoms may use vaginal estrogen therapy, which has little to no systemic absorption. As women continue to age, the long-term issues of hypoestrogen begin to emerge such as poor bone health.

Patients with asymptomatic fibroids may be monitored and managed expectantly in the low-risk patient. The most common symptoms patients complain of are heavy vaginal bleeding and pelvic pressure. The most common and only definitive treatment to ensure no recurrence is hysterectomy. However, patients who desire to maintain fertility and preserve their uterus may opt for a procedure that just removes the fibroid, myomectomy.

Patients with ovarian cancer are frequently in the advanced stages by the time they are diagnosed. The prognosis is generally poor. Early detection is key in better outcomes for these patients. Unfortunately, no screening test currently exists for the general population. Women must be aware of the vague symptoms of ovarian cancer which include pelvic or abdominal pain, difficulty with urination, and difficulty eating and report them immediately to their provider. Providers must thoroughly investigate these complaints before deciding that they are attributable to other benign causes. If ovarian cancer is suspected and confirmed, the patient will undergo surgery and chemotherapy.

Uterine or endometrial cancers are the most common of all the gynecological cancers. The majority of endometrial cancer is diagnosed in the early stage and frequently is cured with surgery alone. Most patients present with vaginal bleeding that should be evaluated with pelvic ultrasound and endometrial biopsy. Once a diagnosis is made, FIGO recommends surgical removal of the uterus, ovaries, and fallopian tubes in addition to pelvic washings and lymphadenectomy. If the patient has a higher-risk or higher-stage malignancy, she will undergo both chemotherapy and radiation. Higher-risk and higher-stage cancers carry a poorer prognosis, whereas metastatic and recurrent cancers are considered noncurable, with an average of 1-year survival.

Cervical cancer is the 13th most common cancer in women in the United States. There are no recognizable symptoms, but vaginal bleeding is the most common complaint. Almost all cervical cancers are preventable with adequate routine Pap smear and HPV screening and early intervention if diagnosed. Treatment consists of surgical excision and, in advanced stages, chemoradiation.

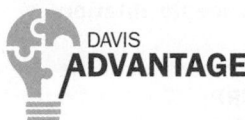

DAVIS
ADVANTAGE

To explore learning resources for this chapter, go to **Davis Advantage** and find:
– Answers to in-text questions
– Chapter Resources and Activities
– NCLEX®-Style Chapter Review Questions
– Bibliography

Chapter 66

Coordinating Care for Male Patients With Reproductive and Breast Disorders

Shari Lynn

Finding Connections

Follow this patient throughout the chapter.

Scott Andrews is a 65-year-old male patient who presents to his healthcare provider with a complaint of difficulty urinating. He complains of pain with urination and occasional blood-tinged urine. He states that he has an increased urgency to urinate and wakes up three to four times during the night to urinate. He also complains of occasional incontinence…

BENIGN PROSTATIC HYPERPLASIA

Epidemiology

Benign prostatic hyperplasia (BPH), an enlarged prostate, is noted in about 50% of men 51 to 60 years of age and 90% of men over the age of 80. It equally affects men of all races. BPH is not a form of cancer. A patient can have BPH and prostate cancer simultaneously or independently of each other.

Pathophysiology

The prostate gland is a normal part of the male anatomy. It is about the size of a walnut and surrounds the urethra. Its primary function is to assist in controlling urine flow. It also mixes sperm with prostatic fluid and seminal fluid to be ejaculated during orgasm. Around the age of 25, the prostate begins to grow. This growth is not completely understood. One theory related to enlargement of the prostate is a change in the balance between estrogen, which is present in small amounts in males, and testosterone. Other theories implicated in the development of BPH include an accumulation of the male hormone dihydrotestosterone (DHT) and a high intake of calories, protein, calcium, and polyunsaturated fats. When this gland does become enlarged, it pinches the urethra, interfering with the flow of urine from the bladder (Fig. 66.1).

Connection Check 66.1

Which of the following is true of BPH?
A. It is a form of metastatic cancer.
B. Benign prostatic hyperplasia is not a form of cancer.
C. Males as young as 25 years old are equally at risk.
D. Benign prostatic hyperplasia is a precursor to testicular cancer.

Clinical Manifestations

The clinical manifestations of BPH are related to **lower urinary tract symptoms (LUTS)**. Those manifestations include difficulty starting the flow of urine even with straining, a weak stream of urine, multiple interruptions during urination, and dribbling once urination is complete. Symptoms related to changes in the bladder include urgency, frequency, the feeling that the bladder has not completely emptied after urination, and frequent awakening at night to urinate. As the bladder becomes more sensitive to the retention of urine, incontinence may result. The patient may experience bed-wetting and the inability to respond quickly enough to the need to urinate. A urethral obstruction or enlarged prostate that is left untreated may result in **bladder outlet obstruction (BOO)**, which includes acute urinary retention (AUR), bladder infection, bladder stones, and increasing pressure in the kidney, possibly resulting in hydronephrosis or postrenal acute kidney (AKI) injury or pyelonephritis (Table 66.1).

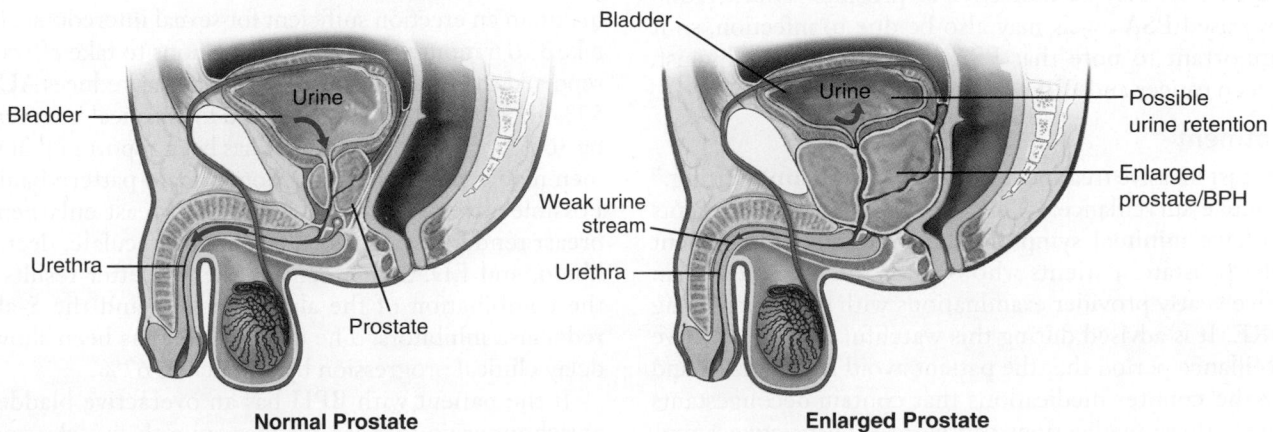

FIGURE 66.1 Normal and enlarged prostate.

Table 66.1 Complications of Benign Prostatic Hyperplasia

Clinical Manifestation/ Complication	Cause
Acute urinary retention	Blockage of urethra by enlarged prostate, obstructing urine flow
Urinary tract infection (UTI)	Secondary to urinary stasis
Bladder stones	Crystallization of mineral deposits in concentrated urine due to obstructed urine flow
Bladder damage	Stretching and weakening of the bladder wall muscles from incomplete emptying, resulting in the bladder no longer contracting properly
Kidney damage	Increased pressure in the kidney secondary to urinary retention and backflow of urine, causing hydronephrosis (swelling of urine-collecting structures in the kidney) and postrenal AKI
	Pyelonephritis–UTI migrating from the bladder to the kidney

AKI, Acute kidney injury.

Management

Medical Management

Diagnosis

Diagnosis is made on the basis of the symptoms. It is confirmed with a **digital rectal examination (DRE)**. The enlarged prostate can be palpated on examination. A urinalysis is done to rule out the presence of an infection causing symptoms. In addition, the **prostate-specific antigen (PSA)** level is checked. This is a protein produced by the prostate gland and may be considered a tumor marker. An elevated PSA may be indicative of prostate cancer. However, raised PSA levels may also be due to infection, so it is important to note that PSA levels do not distinguish between cancer and BPH.

Treatment

The least invasive treatment for BPH is "**watchful waiting**," or "active surveillance." This approach is used in patients who have minimal symptoms and minimal enlargement of the prostate. Patients who opt for this treatment plan receive yearly provider examinations with evaluation using a DRE. It is advised during this watchful waiting or active surveillance period that the patient avoid tranquilizers and over-the-counter medications that contain decongestants because these medications can worsen obstructive symptoms. In addition, patients should avoid excess fluids in the

evening to decrease the chances of **nocturia** (waking up to void).

Connection Check 66.2

The nurse realizes that which clinical manifestation is an expected finding of BPH?
A. Increased urinary output
B. Swelling of the penis and scrotum
C. Frequent nocturia
D. Tea-colored urine

Medications

Pharmacological management may also be a treatment option for BPH. Many types of medications are currently being used to treat BPH. The two major classes of drugs are 5-alpha reductase inhibitors and alpha-adrenergic blockers. It is not possible to predict which medication will work best for any particular patient; however, these medications appear to improve symptoms in 35% to 40% of men taking them. Alpha blockers act on the alpha receptors in the prostate, causing the smooth muscles of the prostate to relax. Relaxation of these muscles decreases the constriction of the urethra. It may take 2 weeks to 4 months to notice symptom improvement. The patient needs to be aware of adverse effects, such as headache, nasal congestion, dizziness, drowsiness, postural hypotension, reflex tachycardia, and retrograde or delayed ejaculation.

The other class of medications is the 5-alpha reductase inhibitors, which act as antiandrogens. Testosterone affects prostate growth and development. 5-Alpha-reductase converts testosterone into DHT. Dihydrotestosterone stimulates the growth factors that encourage prostate hyperplasia while concurrently reducing the rate of cell death in the prostate. This imbalance results in enlargement of the prostate. The 5-alpha-reductase inhibitors prevent testosterone from being converted to DHT, which causes enlarged tissues to shrink, thus reducing obstruction of the urethra. Fortunately, this medication does not affect levels of circulating testosterone, which reduces the chance of **erectile dysfunction (ED)**, the inability to achieve or maintain an erection sufficient for sexual intercourse. It can take 3 to 6 months for these medications to take effect. It is reported that the use of these medications reduces AUR by 57% to 59% and reduces the need for surgical intervention by 36% to 55%. In addition, it has been reported that some men may experience a reduction in male-pattern baldness. Possible adverse effects include rash, breast enlargement, breast tenderness, reduced volume of ejaculate, decreased libido, and ED. Some men experience better results with the combination of the alpha blockers and the 5-alpha-reductase inhibitors. The combination has been shown to delay clinical progression by as much as 67%.

If the patient with BPH has an overactive bladder, an anticholinergic to relax bladder smooth muscle, such as oxybutynin, may be added.

Alternative Therapies

If medication is not an effective treatment and the patient is not a surgical candidate, then obstruction of the urethra secondary to prostate enlargement and incontinence can be managed through intermittent catheterization of the bladder or the use of an indwelling catheter. The indwelling catheter can stay in place and be changed monthly or per protocol.

Other alternative therapies that have been used in treating BPH include saw palmetto (*Serenoa repens*), African plum (*Pygeum africanum*), Cernilton, and South African star grass (*Hypoxis rooperi* and some species of *Pinus* and *Picea*). Saw palmetto is reported to be used by approximately 2 million men in the United States. The long-term effects and safety of this herbal remedy are unclear. Some studies have shown that there were mild to moderate reductions in urinary symptoms. African plum has not been compared to pharmaceutical therapy but has been shown to reduce symptoms of BPH in comparison to placebo. South African star grass has been shown to improve urinary symptoms of BPH due to beta-sitosterols, substances that may bind to the prostate to reduce inflammation. The effectiveness and safety have not been studied over the long term. Cernilton (from ryegrass pollen, *Secale cereale*) has been shown to reduce urological symptoms; however, long-term effects have not been studied.

Surgical Management

Transurethral Resection of the Prostate

If pharmacological treatment is not effective and the patient is a surgical candidate, there are other possible interventions. One of these is a **transurethral resection of the prostate (TURP)** (Fig. 66.2). This has been the most common surgery for BPH for many years and is usually used to treat smaller prostates. In this procedure, a lighted scope known as a resectoscope is passed into the urethra. A small cutting tool is used to remove the entire inner prostate, leaving the outer layer. Symptoms are usually relieved quickly, resulting in a stronger flow of urine. A catheter may remain in place after surgery for 3 to 5 days to drain the bladder. Recovery from the TURP may include a risk of bleeding and infection. The patient is permitted only light activity immediately postoperatively.

Transurethral Incision of the Prostate

Another procedure is the **transurethral incision of the prostate (TUIP or TIP)**. This procedure is used for the patient with a small to moderately enlarged prostate. During the TUIP/TIP, instruments are inserted through the urethra as in the TURP, but the prostate is not removed. The surgeon makes two small incisions into the prostate, which relieves compression of the urethra and opens up the channel. The result is an easier passage of urine.

Open Prostatectomy

For the patient with a very large prostate who is experiencing complications such as bladder stones or bladder damage, the surgeon may perform an open prostatectomy. This procedure is performed approximately 200,000 times a year in the United States. During this procedure, an incision is made in the patient's lower abdomen to access and remove the prostate gland. This procedure carries a higher risk of complications such as incontinence, impotence, and retrograde ejaculation (ejaculation that does not result in semen exiting the body but reverses and deposits it in the bladder).

Laser Surgery

Another option is laser surgery for men with a smaller or moderately large prostate gland. This therapy uses high-energy lasers to annihilate and/or remove overgrown prostate tissue. Several laser procedures include ablation procedures that burn away prostate tissue and enucleation procedures that remove the prostate tissue that is restricting

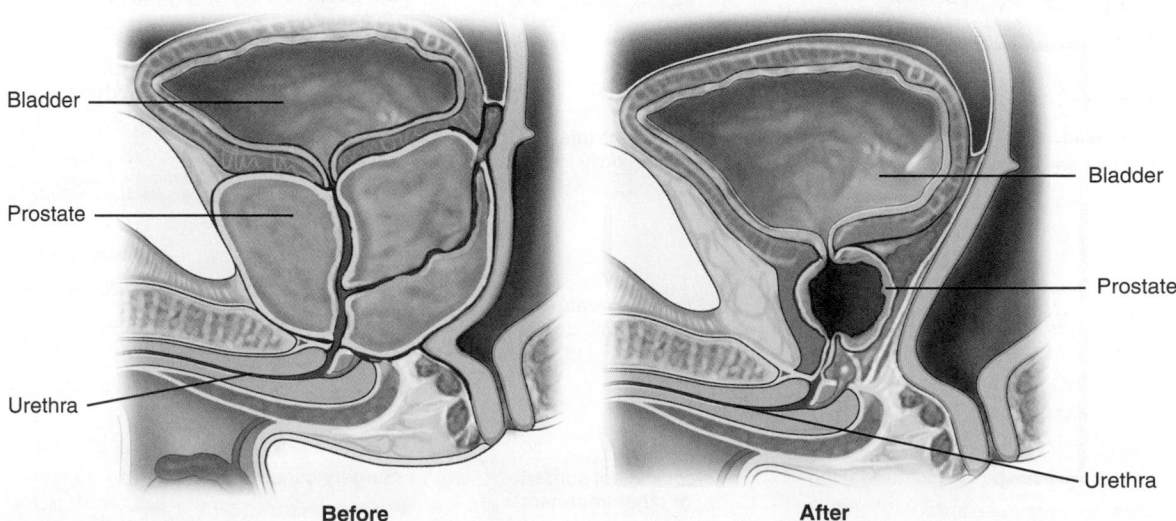

Before **After**

FIGURE 66.2 Changes in the prostate gland after a transurethral resection of the prostate (TURP). The entire inner prostate is removed, leaving just the outer layer, easing the flow of urine.

the flow of urine and prevent tissue regrowth. Laser surgery usually results in immediate symptom relief and has a lower risk of adverse effects than the TURP procedure. This may be used for men who are taking anticoagulants because there is usually less bleeding.

Transurethral Microwave Therapy

A **transurethral microwave therapy (TUMT)** is a minimally invasive procedure in which an electrode is passed through the urethra into the area of the prostate. The electrode produces microwave energy that heats the inner portion of the prostate, destroying the tissue and causing the gland to shrink. Ease of urine flow is restored. Irritating adverse effects may last for weeks so symptom relief may take some time to occur. This procedure is usually reserved for small prostates.

Transurethral Needle Ablation

Transurethral needle ablation (TUNA) is an outpatient procedure. A lighted cystoscope is passed through the urethra allowing visualization to place needles into the prostate. Once the needles are in place, radio waves pass through the needles to heat and destroy the prostate tissue that is constricting the urethra. This procedure results in scarring of the prostate tissue, causing it to shrink and open. Men who receive this procedure may not notice symptom relief immediately. It is a good choice if there is a concern about excess bleeding.

Prostatic Stents

Prostatic stents may also be used. These stents are placed in the urethra to keep it open. Tissue growth on the metallic stent anchors it in place. If a plastic stent is used, it needs to be changed every 4 to 6 weeks. Stents are not usually considered a long-term treatment because of potential adverse effects of pain upon urination and urinary tract infections (UTIs). This is usually only an option for men who cannot take medication and are not surgical candidates.

Water-Induced Thermotherapy and Transurethral Ethanol Ablation

Two of the more recent procedures are water-induced thermotherapy and transurethral ethanol ablation of the prostate. Water-induced thermotherapy is a 45-minute procedure done using topical anesthesia. Hot water is used to cause coagulation necrosis of the prostate tissue that is compressing the urethra. Transurethral ethanol ablation of the prostate involves the injection of ethanol into arterioles and venules. The ethanol creates a necrotic area secondary to thrombotic occlusion. This necrosis stops the hyperplastic overgrowth of prostatic tissue. Additional evaluation is needed for these two procedures. See Figure 66.3 for a flowchart of treatment options.

Nursing Management
Assessment and Analysis

The clinical manifestations of BPH are caused by the obstruction of urine flow due to an enlarged prostate. They include difficulty starting the flow of urine, a weak urine stream, multiple interruptions during urination, and dribbling once urination is complete. Other symptoms include urgency, frequency, the feeling that the bladder has not completely emptied after urination, and nocturia.

Nursing Diagnoses
- **Disturbed sleep pattern** related to nocturia
- **Risk for infection** related to urinary stasis

Nursing Interventions
■ *Assessments*
- Urinary symptoms
  Subjective data from the patient regarding the extent of urinary symptoms assist in diagnosis and aid in determining treatment options. Mild symptoms that do not interfere with

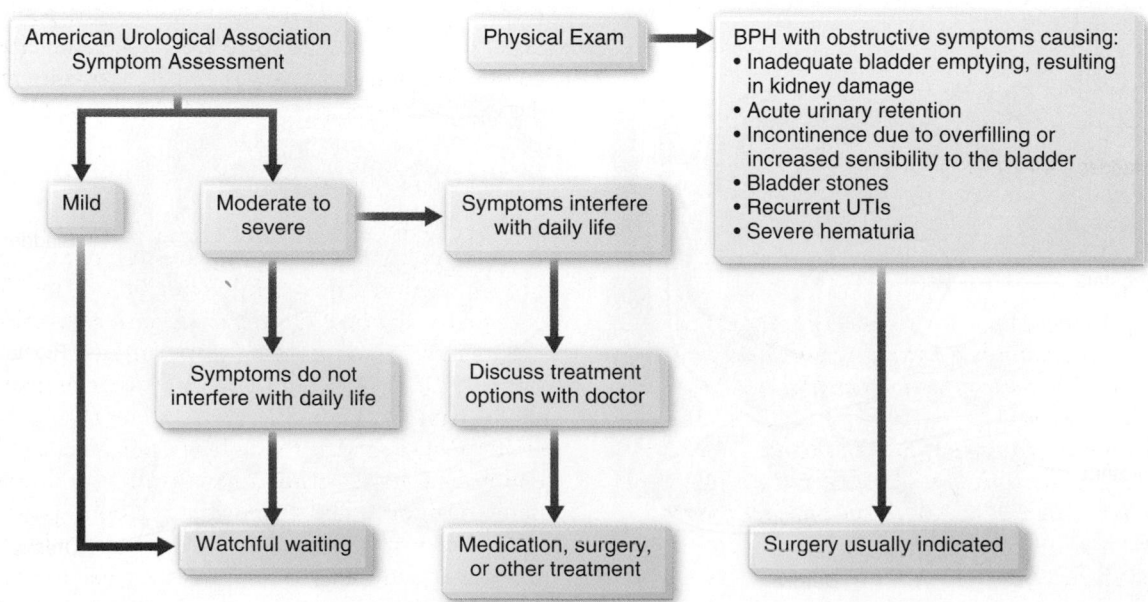

FIGURE 66.3 Treatment options for benign prostatic hyperplasia.

activities of daily living may require only watchful waiting. More severe symptoms that interfere with activities of daily living, such as nocturia and an inability to empty the bladder, may require more aggressive treatment.

- Temperature

  An increase in temperature may indicate a UTI secondary to urinary stasis.

- Focused abdominal examination

  A distended abdomen may signify bladder distention, thus indicating the patient's inability to empty the bladder and risk for a UTI.

- Bladder scan

  Use of a bladder scanner to check postvoid residual (PVR) to determine the ability of the patient to empty his bladder and discovering any urinary stasis that may lead to infection

- Urinalysis

  The results will determine a possible infection from urinary stasis or related LUTS.

Actions

- Catheterization

  To check for PVR and to relieve distended bladder, decreasing the risk of bladder damage

- Administer medication therapy: 5-alpha-reductase inhibitors and/or alpha-adrenergic blockers as ordered.

  5-Alpha-reductase inhibitors limit the production of DHT, a substance that encourages prostate hyperplasia. Alpha-adrenergic blockers relax the smooth muscle of the prostate.

Teaching

- Watchful waiting

  Explanation of the term "watchful waiting," including recognition of worsening symptoms, and when to seek further treatment help alleviate anxiety and ensure that the patient seeks treatment when necessary.

- Decrease liquid intake in the evening.

  Decreased fluid intake in the evening may decrease nocturia.

- Medication therapy education

  Understanding the possible adverse effects of medications and contraindications with other medications and food assists the patient in making choices about what medication therapy is best.

- Follow-up

  Stressing the importance of follow-up with the provider results in better care of the patient as well as more prompt recognition of worsening symptoms and the need for possible further intervention.

- Information regarding surgical options

  Printed information given to the patient allows the patient to make better-informed choices should surgery become a necessity.

- Care of surgical/invasive treatment sites

  Care of any surgical sites using aseptic technique decreases the risk of infection and assists in healing.

Connection Check 66.3

A patient's orders include the placement of a catheter as a temporary treatment of his BPH. The nurse understands that rationales for this intervention is which of the following? *(Select all that apply.)*

A. Exact monitoring of intake and output

B. Retrieving a sterile sample for urinalysis

C. To evaluate PVR volume

D. To facilitate complete emptying of the bladder

E. To avoid unnecessary surgical procedures

Evaluating Care Outcomes

Patients with BPH are usually managed with watchful waiting and medication therapy. A well-managed patient understands the importance of compliance with the medication regimen, limiting fluid intake at night, and following up with the provider if symptoms worsen. This patient has less urinary retention, a strong urine stream, and decreased nocturia. With the proper interventions and education, the patient can live a normal life with BPH.

ERECTILE DYSFUNCTION

Epidemiology

According to the National Institutes of Health, there are an estimated 30,000,000 men in the United States who suffer from chronic erectile dysfunction. The incidence increases with age, affecting 61% of males 40 to 69 years of age and 77% of males over the age of 70. Erectile Dysfunction is projected to affect 32,000,000 males throughout the world by the year 2025. The most common causes of ED include cardiovascular disease, smoking, obesity, stroke, spinal cord injury, diseases of the neurological system, diabetes, liver disease, kidney disease, low levels of testosterone, prostate and/or rectal surgery, Peyronie's disease (curvature of the penis occurring during erection secondary to scar tissue), adverse effects of medication, and psychological issues. Substance abuse disorder is implicated in problems of ED in up to 25% of cases.

Pathophysiology and Clinical Manifestations

Erectile dysfunction is the inability to achieve or maintain an erection sufficient for sexual intercourse. An erection occurs when the penis fills with blood, making it firm enough to penetrate the vagina. A normal erection typically occurs in response to sexual stimulation. There is an inhibition of the sympathetic nervous system and an activation of the parasympathetic nervous systems (PNS). In response to stimulation of the PNS, nitric oxide is released from the endothelial lining in the cavernosum blood vessels in the penis forming cyclic guanosine monophosphate (cGMP). This causes smooth muscle relaxation, allowing the arterial blood to rush into the corpus cavernosum, which compresses venous return, causing the penis to become tumescent or engorged with blood. In the older male, any number of these actions may be compromised due to decreased perfusion of the penis, atherosclerosis of the arteries, decreased endothelial function, decreased production of nitric oxide and decreased androgen production.

Connection Check 66.4

A patient is complaining of an inability to achieve an erection. The nurse realizes this may be related to a personal medical history of which condition?

A. Crohn's disease
B. Hepatitis C
C. Migraines
D. Diabetes

Management

Medical Management

Diagnosis

Diagnosis is made on the basis of patient complaint. A careful assessment may reveal causative factors, such as diabetes, cardiovascular disease, or low levels of testosterone. Erectile dysfunction is managed according to the cause of the problem.

Medications

Medication therapy is one of the first forms of medical management of ED. Medications include **phosphodiesterase type 5 (PDE-5) inhibitors** such as sildenafil (Viagra), vardenafil (Levitra), avanafil (Stendra) and tadalafil (Cialis). The PDE-5s inhibit the breakdown of the cGMP, the substance that causes smooth muscle relaxation, vasodilation, and increased blood flow that leads to an erection. This allows for an erection to develop. These medications do not have an effect on how long the erection lasts or the size of the erection. They do not work in the absence of sexual stimulation. These medications are not recommended in the patient who is taking nitrates for other cardiac issues or alpha blockers for BPH because these medications together can cause sudden hypotension. Some other adverse effects of these medications can include headache, facial flushing, effects in color vision, and nasal congestion. The medication chosen to treat an individual is related to the patient's sexual activity and personal choice. These medications come in pill form and are convenient to use.

Another treatment option is alprostadil pellets, known as **medicated urethral system for erection (MUSE)**. The pellets are placed in the urethra with the use of an applicator. Once the pellet is in place, the patient massages the penis for approximately 10 minutes, allowing the medication to coat the urethra and promote absorption. Alprostadil is a prostaglandin E_1, which causes increased blood flow to the penis through vasodilation. The male is encouraged to urinate before application of the pellet because this improves the action of the medication. Adverse effects include a burning sensation in the urethra and a risk for

hypotension. Effects of this medication on the fetus are not clear, so the patient must be counseled to use a barrier method of contraception so as not to risk pregnancy in his partner.

Another treatment for ED is intracavernosal injection, which requires the male to deliver the medication via injection directly into the corpus cavernosa of the penis. After injection of this medication, the male attains an erection in 5 to 20 minutes, which lasts 30 to 60 minutes. There is the rare chance of priapism, which is an erection lasting more than 3 hours. The challenge with this medication is the ability of the man to self-inject. An adverse effect related specifically to this form of medication is penile scarring from repeated injections. In addition, this medication is contraindicated in men who are taking anticoagulants because of the increased risk of bleeding. Also, because the man has now created an opening in the penis at the injection site, there is an increased risk of contracting a sexually transmitted infection or a bloodborne infection.

Another treatment option is a vacuum device. This option involves a cylinder placed over the penis using subatmospheric pressure to draw the penis into the tube, creating an erection. A constriction band is then put in place to keep the blood in the penis. It should be noted that the temperature of the penis will be cooler. Although some men may find it cumbersome to have to work the device, it does not have the adverse effects of medications.

Surgical Management

If medication therapy or the vacuum device is not successful, there is the option of surgery to place an implant or penile prosthesis. An inflatable tube is placed in the penis with the inflation bulb in the scrotum. The male compresses the bulb to inflate the tube, creating an erection. There is a 90% success rate with the implant.

> **Safety Alert** An erection lasting more than 3 hours, priapism is a rare occurrence with oral medication as well as intracavernosal injection but can occur with any of these treatment options. Priapism is a medical emergency, requiring immediate treatment by a physician or in the emergency department so as not to risk permanent impotence.

Psychosocial Management

In addition to all methods, there is also psychosexual counseling for possible psychogenic issues that may be affecting the ability of the man to achieve an erection. Even if the reason for ED is organic, there is still a psychological aspect. Regardless of the intervention, men may still have anxiety regarding the success of the intervention, anxiety related to performance, and anxiety related to the response of their partners.

Nursing Management

Assessment and Analysis

Erectile dysfunction can present when there is neurological or vascular damage interfering with the coordination of the brain, nervous system, and hormonal activity required to cause the blood vessels in the penis to become engorged, causing an erection and allowing vaginal penetration.

Nursing Diagnoses

- **Ineffective sexual patterns** related to altered body function or structure/surgical procedure
- **Risk for situational low self-esteem**

Nursing Interventions

▣ *Assessments*

- Health history
  Cardiovascular disease, diabetes, low testosterone levels, and trauma are health problems that may lead to ED.
- Emotional state, performance anxiety
  Unstable emotions, embarrassment, or performance anxiety may increase the problem of or be a causative factor of ED.

▣ *Actions*

- Administer medications as ordered—PDE-5 inhibitors.
  The PDE-5s inhibit the breakdown of cGMP, a substance leading to smooth muscle relaxation, vasodilation, and increased blood flow essential for the development of an erection.
- Emotional support
  Creating a nonjudgmental, relaxed atmosphere reduces patient anxiety and creates a relationship of trust.

▣ *Teaching*

- Education regarding contributing factors
  Teaching patients that smoking and obesity can contribute to ED may give the patient an incentive to stop smoking and/or control his diet.
- Medications—PDE-5 inhibitors, alprostadil (pellets)
  Do not take ED medications with nitrates because of the potential for a sudden drop in blood pressure. Recognize the risk of priapism and the need to treat it as a medical emergency to avoid permanent impotence.
- Medications—intracavernosal injections
  Ensure the patient understands the increased risk of infection and priapism.
- Education regarding other options to treat ED
  Patients should make the decision as to what option best meets their needs. They then need careful instruction on the use of a penile pellet implantation, a penile injection, or a vacuum device. This should be done in a compassionate and nonjudgmental way to help overcome fear and possible embarrassment.

Evaluating Care Outcomes

Patients with ED are often embarrassed regarding discussion of the subject. It is important to create an atmosphere that is professional and nonjudgmental, allowing the patient to feel comfortable discussing his concerns. A well-managed patient is educated regarding treatment options and associated contraindications such as the concurrent use of alpha blockers and nitrates due to the dangers of sudden hypotension. Appropriate and educated use of medications or other modalities may allow normal, healthy sexual functioning.

Connection Check 66.5

A patient is experiencing ED. He has a history of angina treated with nitroglycerin when necessary. His understanding of his possible medical treatment is indicated by which statement?

- A. "I guess I'm not bad enough yet to need Viagra."
- B. "I understand Viagra can make my blood pressure higher."
- C. "Can Viagra increase my chest pain?"
- D. "So I guess Viagra is out of the question because it might drop my blood pressure."

PROSTATE CANCER

Epidemiology

Prostate cancer is globally one of the most commonly diagnosed cancers in men. Of males diagnosed with prostate cancer, 81% have localized prostate cancer, with a smaller percentage having regional or metastasized cancer. The 5-year survival rate for men who are diagnosed with local prostate cancer is 100% as opposed to 28.7% for those found to have distant metastatic cancer. African American males have a greater incidence of prostate cancer and have a greater chance of dying from the disease than Caucasian men. The lowest rates are found in American Indian and Alaska Native males. Most males diagnosed with prostate cancer are over 65 years of age; however, there has been an increase in the number of men under the age of 55 years.

Although the absolute cause of prostate cancer is not known, studies have related diagnosis to genetic and environmental factors. Risk factors include family history. Other risk factors are believed to be diets high in red meat and consumption of calcium as well as a high body mass index (BMI). There is evidence to show that a diet that consists of vegetables, vitamin E, lycopene, selenium, and antioxidants may play a protective role against the development of prostate cancer.

Pathophysiology

Prostate cancer is a slow-growing cancer (Fig. 66.4). Tumors that develop in the prostate tend to develop on the periphery of the gland, which does not obstruct the flow of urine; hence, they go unnoticed until there is associated pain. Prostate cancer most commonly can metastasize to the lymph nodes, bone, rectum, and bladder. It may be curable when localized but responds to treatment even when widespread. In cases where the cancer has metastasized to the bone, patients may still experience an extended survival rate.

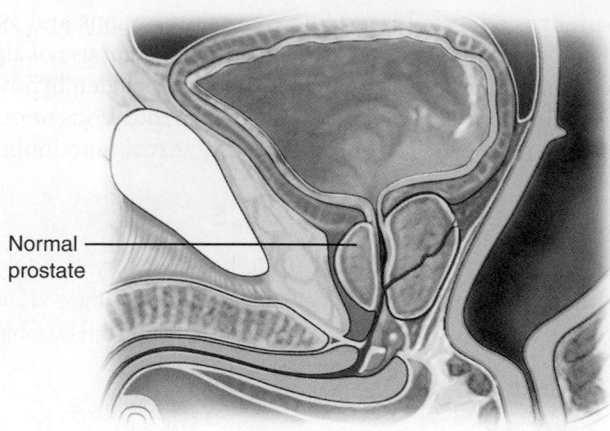 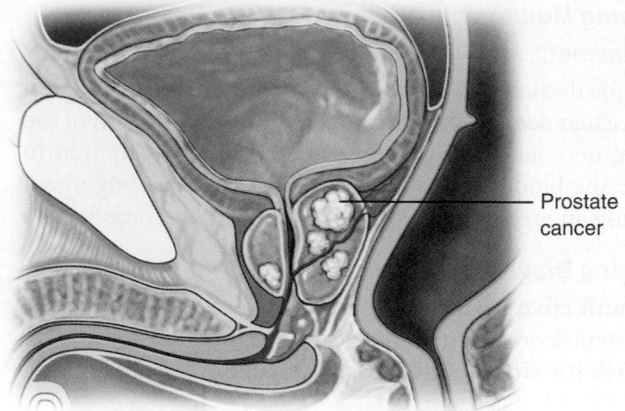

Normal prostate

Prostate cancer

FIGURE 66.4 Appearance of the normal prostate compared with prostate cancer.

Clinical Manifestations

In the early stages, prostate cancer may not cause any signs or symptoms, but as it advances, symptoms may develop. They may vary on the basis of local or invasive disease. Infrequently, symptoms similar to the symptoms of BPH may develop, such as trouble urinating or a weak stream of urine. Table 66.2 lists the clinical manifestations of prostate cancer.

Management

Medical Management

Diagnosis

Diagnosis of prostate cancer is controversial. The American Cancer Society recommends that men have digital rectal examinations (DREs) beginning at the age of 50 on an

Table 66.2 Presenting Symptoms of Localized Prostate Cancer	
Local Disease	**Locally Invasive Disease**
● Asymptomatic	● Hematuria
● Elevated PSA	● Dysuria
● Weak urinary stream	● Perineal and suprapubic pain
● Hesitancy	● Erectile dysfunction
● Sensation of incomplete emptying of the bladder	● Incontinence
● Frequency	● Loin pain or anuria resulting from obstruction of the ureters
● Urgency	● Symptoms of renal failure
● Urge incontinence	● Hemospermia (blood in the semen)
● Urinary tract infection	● Rectal symptoms, including tenesmus (rectal pain or cramping, a sensation of incomplete defecation)

PSA, Prostate-specific antigen.

annual basis. The recommendation changes to age 45 for African American men and/or those with a family history of prostate cancer. Additionally, the prostate-specific antigen (PSA) test has been the gold standard for the detection of early prostate cancer for years. Prostate-specific antigen is a protein produced by the prostate gland and may be considered a tumor marker. Commonly, men were advised to get the PSA test on an annual basis. The critical cutoff point for PSA screening is 4 ng/mL; however, some studies suggest that this is too high. A man with a PSA of 4 to 10 ng/mL has a 20% to 25% chance of being diagnosed with prostate cancer. Men with a reading greater than 10 ng/mL increase their chances to approximately 60%. Levels of PSA are also affected by age. A PSA of 5 ng/mL may be considered a normal reading for a man who is 73 years old; however, a reading of 3.9 ng/mL may indicate a red flag in a man who is 50 years old. Because of these differing predictive values, this practice is now being questioned. Annual testing is resulting in overdiagnosis and overtreatment of prostate cancer as well as underdiagnosis. There have been many instances of men with elevated PSA levels who do not have cancer as well as those with normal readings who do have cancer. Some providers now look at serial PSAs from month to month as opposed to just one reading.

Guidelines for prostate cancer screening have been updated to include "informed decision making" (Box 66.1) before taking a routine screening test. Men who are of average risk for prostate cancer are advised to begin discussing prostate cancer with their healthcare provider by the age of 50 or by the age of 40 to 45 if they are African American or have a family history. For men who decide to go forward with screening, recommendations include a PSA with or without a DRE. A DRE may be suggested if PSA results are borderline. If the PSA is 4.0 ng/mL or greater, this should be followed by further evaluation. A PSA between 2.5 and 4.0 ng/mL should result in an individualized risk assessment, which includes race, family history, results of previous biopsies, and a DRE. For those men who have a PSA less than 2.5 ng/mL, the recommendation is continued testing every other year. Although these guidelines exist, it is important

Box 66.1 Important Discussion Points Regarding the Decision-Making Process of Prostate Screening and Treatment

- There is conflicting evidence that screening may reduce the risk of death.
- PSA and DRE can give a false-positive or a false-negative result.
- If prostate cancer is present, the PSA will detect it earlier than no screening at all.
- Abnormal screening results may result in biopsies, which are painful and can cause complications such as bleeding or infection.
- The treatment of prostate cancer can lead to complications such as erectile dysfunction, incontinence, and bowel problems, to name a few.
- Immediate treatment of prostate cancer is not always necessary.

DRE, Digital rectal examination; *PSA,* prostate-specific antigen

is the tumor, nodes, metastasis (TNM) classification used with other cancers. The score is based on T—the size and location of the tumor, N—spread to lymph nodes, and M—presence of metastasis (Table 66.3; Fig. 66.6).

Connection Check 66.6

A patient does not understand how he can be diagnosed with late-stage prostate cancer because he has never had any difficulty urinating. What is the appropriate answer the nurse may provide?

A. Tumors of the prostate often develop near the edges of the prostate, so they do not interfere with urination.

B. The tumor has already metastasized away from the urethra, so it does not interfere with urination.

C. There is interference with urination only when there is an underlying urethral stricture.

D. Tumors of the prostate do not interfere with urination in the early stages of the disease.

to note that there is no absolute value below which a man can be assured he does not have prostate cancer.

If abnormalities are found on the DRE and PSA, the next step is a prostatic biopsy. This involves taking a small tissue sample via needle from the prostate for analysis. This can be done in a provider's office with local anesthetic. If found to be positive, the tissue is staged using various scoring systems and staging methods. One of the scoring systems is the Gleason scoring system (Fig. 66.5). This system differentiates the diagnosis of prostate cancer into five different grades. In grade 1, the tissue is well differentiated and most likely results in the best prognosis. This patient has the greatest chance of a cure. A grade 5 classification is a poorly differentiated cancer with a poor prognosis. Tissue samples from two different sites are graded separately, and both scores are added together. The highest score possible on the Gleason scale is a 10 if each of the two sites tested is graded as a 5. An alternative scoring system

Treatment

Treatment options for prostate cancer include radiation, cryotherapy, ablative hormone therapy, chemotherapy, and surgery.

Radiation

Radiation may be a nonsurgical option for those patients who would like to avoid surgery. Radiation may also be used after surgery if there is evidence that the cancer has metastasized. The two options for radiation treatment include the use of external-beam radiation that is aimed at the tumor or the surgical implantation of small radioactive pellets into the prostate called brachytherapy. The external-beam radiation involves high-energy radiation that precisely targets the prostate tumor. This can also include the associated lymph nodes. This therapy is time-consuming because treatments are repeated at least five times a week for 8 weeks. External-beam radiation therapy can also be delivered using the CyberKnife technology. CyberKnife is a robotic assisted

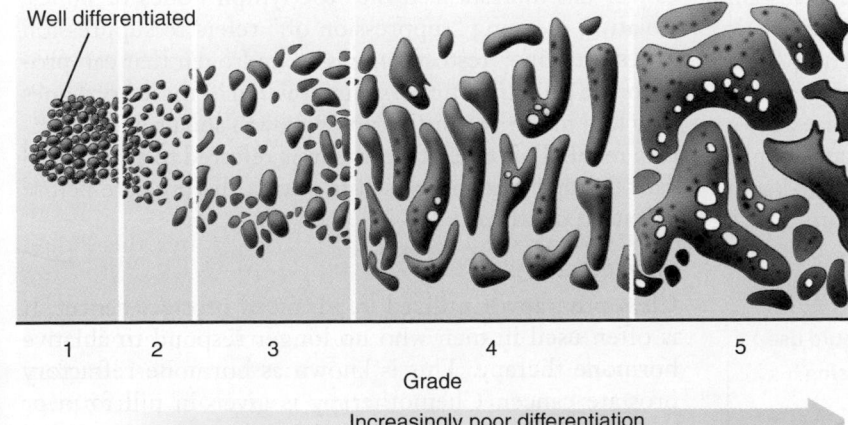

FIGURE 66.5 Cell type appearance and grading with the Gleason scoring system. Scoring ranges from grade 1, where the tissue is well differentiated, to grade 5, reflecting poorly differentiated cancer and a poorer prognosis.

Table 66.3 Stages of Prostate Cancer Using TNM Classification

TNM Classification	Definition
T1	Incidental (impalpable and not detected by ultrasonography)
T2	Locally confined to the prostate
T3	Locally extensive
T4	Fixation onto or invasion of neighboring organs
N0	No regional lymph node metastasis
N1	Metastasis in single regional lymph node less than 2 cm in largest dimension
N2	Metastasis in single regional lymph node greater than 2 cm but less than 5 cm in largest dimension
N3	Metastasis in regional lymph node greater than 5 cm in largest dimension
M0	No distant metastasis
M1	Distant metastasis
M1a	Metastasis in nonregional lymph nodes
M1b	Metastasis in bone
M1c	Metastasis in other sites

TNM, Tumor, nodes, metastasis.

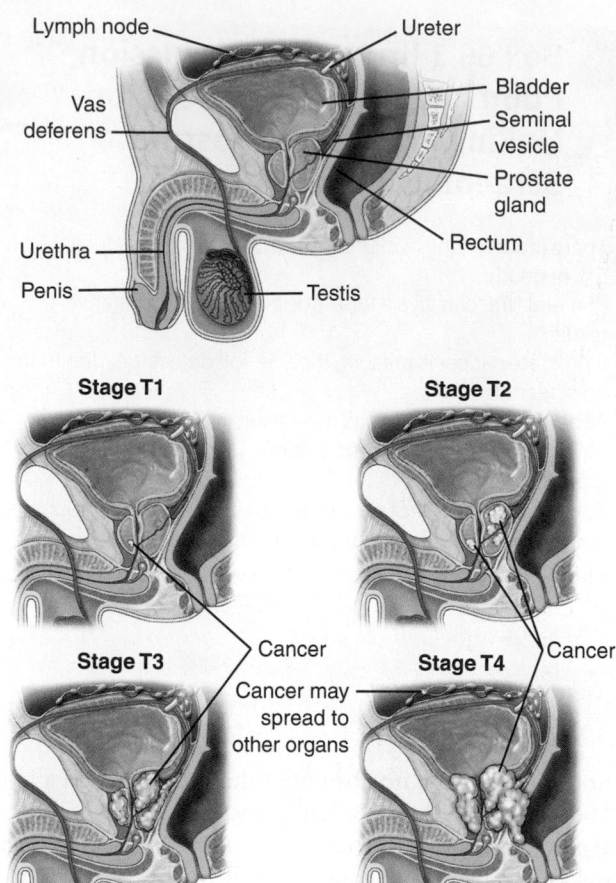

FIGURE 66.6 Tumor, nodes, metastasis (TNM) staging of prostate cancer. T1 = impalpable; T2 = locally confined to the prostate; T3 = locally extensive; T4 = fixation onto or invasion of neighboring organs.

system that allows the delivery of high doses of radiation with precise accuracy. Treatment may be completed with four or five sessions; it is much more efficient when compared with conventional external-beam radiation therapy.

Brachytherapy is a procedure that places radioactive seeds or pellets in the prostate through the perineum. In this way, the therapy can be targeted at a very precise area. The pellets are left in place permanently. They gradually lose reactivity over time. The patient is instructed to abstain from sex for 2 weeks, and at the end of the 2 weeks, he is instructed to wear a condom to protect his partner from radiation exposure. This method is more convenient for the patient because it is often outpatient surgery with a short recovery time. It is used with cancer that has not metastasized outside the prostate. Both external-beam radiation and brachytherapy may result in incontinence and/or impotence.

> **Safety Alert** A man receiving brachytherapy should use a condom during sex to avoid exposing his partner to radiation.

Cryotherapy and Ablative Hormone Therapy

Cryotherapy is another treatment for prostate cancer. Liquid nitrogen is delivered into the prostate through the perineum using metal probes to freeze the prostate. This is an early-stage treatment or is used when other treatments have failed. It is not used often because it has a low success rate; usually needs to be repeated; and may result in impotence, incontinence, and rectal complications.

Ablative hormone therapy is often used in men whose cancer has metastasized into the lymph nodes or bones. Ablative, meaning "suppression of," refers to suppression of testosterone. Testosterone is an androgen that can promote the growth of tumors. Suppression of these hormones may lead to the slowing of tumor growth and provide symptom relief. This type of treatment is referred to as neoadjuvant therapy when it is used to shrink the prostate before radiation treatment.

Chemotherapy

Chemotherapy is utilized in advanced prostate cancer. It is often used in men who no longer respond to ablative hormone therapy. This is known as hormone-refractory prostate cancer. Chemotherapy is given in pill form or intravenously and is given in cycles with a treatment period followed by a rest period. These cycles vary from daily to weekly or every 3 to 4 months.

Surgical Management

Surgical options include the radical prostatectomy. In this procedure, the patient's prostate and seminal vesicles are removed under general anesthesia. If deemed necessary, the surgeon may remove pelvic lymph nodes. There are various surgical techniques for performing the radical prostatectomy. In the open retropubic technique, the surgeon removes the prostate and lymph nodes through a single abdominal incision. A newer method is the laparoscopic technique in which the surgeon removes the prostate and lymph nodes through a few small abdominal incisions. A variation on this is the robot-assisted prostatectomy in which the surgeon directs the laparoscopic procedure from a console. An additional surgical procedure is the perineal approach, in which the incision is made between the scrotum and the anus. The choice of surgical approach is usually the surgeon's preference. Some surgeons feel that the perineal approach causes less pain; however, this technique does not allow access to the lymph nodes that drain the prostate. The radical prostatectomy almost always results in impotence, but a newer procedure, the nerve-sparing prostatectomy, attempts to keep the nerves intact that control erection.

Nursing Management

Assessment and Analysis

The clinical manifestations of prostate cancer are typically not evident until the disease has been present for a long period of time. It is a slow-growing cancer developing on the periphery of the prostate gland, so it does not obstruct the flow of urine, which allows it to go unnoticed until there is associated pain. The pain is due to obstruction of urine flow and bladder distention resulting from compression of the urethra.

Nursing Diagnoses

- **Risk for infection** related to surgical intervention/pharmacological intervention
- **Sexual dysfunction** related to the disease process/surgical intervention

Nursing Interventions

▪ Assessments

- Risk factors
  African American men, men 55 or older, men with a family history of prostate cancer, and men with a diet low in fruits and vegetables are at higher risk for prostate cancer.
- PSA levels
  A PSA level of 4 ng/mL or greater requires further assessment.
- DRE results
  A large, palpable prostate on examination combined with a high PSA level requires further assessment.
- Urinary symptoms
  Obstruction of urine flow, a weak stream, and a distended bladder may indicate an enlarged prostate that requires further assessment—PSA and DRE.

▪ Actions

- Administer medication therapy as ordered:
  - Ablative hormone therapy
    Ablative hormone therapy suppresses androgens, which promote tumor growth, thus slowing tumor growth.
  - Chemotherapy
    Targeted chemotherapy to destroy cancer cells once ablative hormone therapy is no longer effective

Postop surgical care
- Aseptic wound care after prostatectomy
  Reduces risk of infection and promotes healing
- Manage bladder irrigation, if present.
  Bladder irrigation helps remove blood clots to ensure the free flow of urine
- Administer stool softeners.
  To prevent straining during bowel movements

▪ Teaching

- Education regarding disease process
  It is important the patient understands the disease and treatment process to improve compliance and potential positive outcome.
- Brachytherapy
  Keep the patient and significant other safe by explaining the importance of abstention from sex for 2 weeks following the start of treatment and then condom use to protect the patient's partner from radiation.
- Chemotherapy/radiation
  Explain possible adverse effects of chemotherapy/radiation so that the patient may be better prepared as to what to expect.
- Signs of infection
  Teach the patient the signs and symptoms of possible postsurgical infection, such as fever, increasing pain, swelling, bleeding, nausea, vomiting; instruct the patient to contact the healthcare provider or go to the emergency department if symptoms are severe.
- Prevention
  Instruct the patient as to possible causes and preventions of prostate cancer. An increased prostate cancer risk is associated with a high consumption of calcium or the ingestion of greater than seven multivitamins a week. Prostate cancer prevention includes increased consumption of foods with selenium, such as oysters, tuna, whole-wheat bread, or sunflower seeds.

Evaluating Care Outcomes

Prostate cancer responds well to treatment. It may be curable when localized but responds to treatment even when widespread. A well-managed patient demonstrates proactive behaviors such as regular screening, avoiding high consumption of calcium and high-dose multivitamins, and eating foods containing selenium. This patient articulates good understanding of the disease process and treatment options. The best outcomes include good response to treatment with normal sexual functioning, normal urination, and no incontinence.

TESTICULAR CANCER

Epidemiology

The incidence of testicular cancer diagnosis has increased over the last 20 years. This increase involves environmental and genetic factors. A male with a brother who has been diagnosed with testicular cancer is 8 to 10 times more likely to be diagnosed as well. A male whose father was diagnosed with testicular cancer has a four- to six-times-greater chance of being diagnosed. There is also an increased risk in males with Down's syndrome and testicular dysgenesis syndrome. The occurrence of testicular cancer is highest in Caucasian men and lowest among African American men. Cryptorchidism (undescended testicle) is one of the greatest risk factors for testicular cancer. Of men who receive a diagnosis of testicular cancer, the expected cure rate is 95%, and in patients with metastatic cancer, the expected cure rate is 80%.

Pathophysiology

Testicular cancer may be localized or metastasized to other locations. Testicular tumors usually spread through one of three routes. First, they may spread through the testicular wall into the blood supply or tubes that transport sperm, metastasizing into adjacent tissue. The second route is through the lymph nodes to the back of the abdomen. A tumor on the right side tends to spread to the right side of the abdomen. Tumors on the left side tend to spread to the back of the abdomen. Metastasis through the lymph nodes is the most common mode of transportation. The third mode of transportation involves the spread of cancer via the bloodstream to more distant organs, such as the brain, lung, and bone.

There are various types of testicular cancer. The most common types that account for the majority of testicular cancers are seminoma and nonseminoma, such as embryonal carcinoma, teratocarcinoma, and teratoma. Seminoma is a slow-growing cancer usually found in men in their 30s and 40s. Seminomas are usually in the testis but can spread to the lymph nodes. This type of cancer is very sensitive to radiation. A nonseminoma cancer generally occurs in men in their teens to 40s. It tends to grow and spread more quickly. It is not uncommon to have more than one type of testicular cancer in a given testicle (Fig. 66.7).

Clinical Manifestations

Testicular cancer usually presents as a painless mass; however, some patients may complain of pain, swelling, or hardness in the scrotum. The patient may complain of discomfort ranging from acute testicular pain, dull abdominal pain, and dull ache in the scrotum to a heavy or firm feeling in the scrotum. The mass may also present with swelling and redness. Where there is metastasis, the patient may present with gastrointestinal symptoms; pain in the lumbar region of the back; gynecomastia

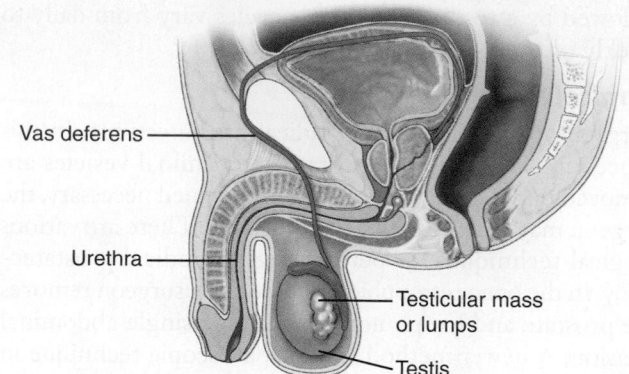

FIGURE 66.7 Mass associated with testicular cancer.

(breast enlargement); and respiratory symptoms including dyspnea, cough, and hemoptysis.

Management

Medical Management

Diagnosis

Diagnosis of testicular cancers is done through a combination of physical assessment, ultrasonography, and laboratory results. Physical assessment reveals a mass and swelling in the testicle or scrotum. There may be patient report of pain. Self-examination may be the first evidence of a lump, which is best done in a warm shower. The use of ultrasound is an important diagnostic tool to identify a mass as testicular cancer as opposed to an infection, collection of fluid, testicular torsion, or hernia. In a small percentage of patients, testicular cancer is not detected as the primary site until patients first present with symptoms such as pain in the abdomen, back, or bones; cough or difficulty breathing; and neck mass and/or swelling of breast tissue. Some testicular cancers produce tumor markers, which are proteins released by the tumors that can be detected by blood tests. Two of these common tumor markers are alpha-fetoprotein and human chorionic gonadotropin. Once the tumors are removed, these tumor marker laboratory values should decrease. If they do not, there may be other tumors present. If testicular cancer is in fact present, the tumor is classified through staging to assess the best treatment options. Staging is based on x-ray, computed tomography (CT) scans, microscopic examination, and on surgical findings. Testicular cancer staging is similar to prostate cancer staging using the TNM system (Table 66.4).

Treatment

Treatment typically depends on the type of tumor. For all types, it starts with the removal of the affected testicle, including the blood supply to that testicle, through an abdominal incision. Surgery for seminomas may be followed by radiation and/or chemotherapy. Nonseminomas that grow more quickly are not responsive to radiation. Treatment for them involves the removal of the affected testicle, including the blood supply, and removal of lymph nodes. Surgery is followed by chemotherapy.

Table 66.4 Staging of Testicular Cancer

Stage	Meaning
T0	No evidence of primary testicular cancer
T1	Tumor confined to the testicle
T2	Tumor invading outside the capsule of the testicle
T3	Tumor invading the tubes that transport sperm
T4	Tumor invading blood vessels that supply the testicles
T4B	Invades the scrotum
N0	No tumor in any lymph nodes
N1	Less than six nodes positive for cancer, no nodes greater than 2 cm
N2	More than six positive nodes, any node greater than 2 cm
N3	Masses, disease, and lymph nodes in the back
N+	Tumor has spread to multiple sites outside the lymph nodes

Nursing Management

Assessment and Analysis

The clinical manifestations of testicular cancer are due to the mass or lump present in the testes. The patient may complain of a heavy or full feeling in the scrotum, a dull ache in the scrotum, or abdominal pain.

Nursing Diagnoses

- **Ineffective health maintenance** related to lack of knowledge regarding self-care secondary to the disease process/surgical intervention
- **Risk for infection** related to surgical intervention/ pharmacological intervention

Nursing Interventions

▨ Assessments

- Physical assessment
  Lumps, swelling, and redness in the scrotum are symptoms of testicular cancer that require further assessment.
- Vital signs/temperature
  Hypotension and tachycardia may reflect volume loss postoperatively. An increased temperature may be a sign of a postoperative infection.

▨ Actions

- Wound care
  Maintaining aseptic technique while cleaning and dressing the surgical wound is essential in preventing infection.
- Administer chemotherapeutic agents as ordered.
  Chemotherapy is indicated to destroy cancer cells in both seminoma and nonseminoma testicular cancer.

▨ Teaching

- Signs of infection
  Teach the patient the signs and symptoms of possible postsurgical infection, such as fever, increasing pain, swelling, bleeding, nausea, and vomiting; instruct the patient to contact a healthcare provider or go to the emergency department if symptoms are severe.
- Chemotherapy
  Educate the patient as to the possible effects of chemotherapy, including the possibility of decreased testosterone production and increased risk of cardiovascular disease, such as angina and myocardial infarction.
- Retroperitoneal lymph node resection
  If retroperitoneal lymph node resection is performed, inform the patient that this procedure may result in nerve damage, affecting ejaculation.
- Sperm storage
  Encourage the patient to bank sperm before treatment should the patient wish to preserve potential fertility.
- Follow-up
  There is an increased risk for recurrence in the patient with testicular cancer, and the patient should be encouraged to see his primary care provider for a minimum of 10 years after treatment because 10 years is the most common time frame for recurrence.

Evaluating Care Outcomes

Testicular cancer has an excellent survival rate. The cure rate when testicular cancer is diagnosed early without metastasis is 90% to 100%, depending on the type of tumor and metastatic state. With adequate education and screening, testicular cancer can be diagnosed early, resulting in a successful treatment plan. Planning ahead and "banking" sperm will allow the possibility of a family in the future.

Connection Check 66.7

A patient is diagnosed with testicular cancer. In educating the patient, the nurse realizes that the best treatment is which of the following?
A. Watching and waiting to see if the cancer metastasizes
B. Chemotherapy and then rechecks every 6 months
C. Concentrated radiation to the testicle and lymph nodes
D. Removal of the affected testicle

MALE BREAST CANCER

Epidemiology

Male breast cancer is a rare disease, 100 times less common than in females. Men have a breast cancer risk of 1/1,000. The American Cancer Society stated there were approximately 2,360 new cases of invasive breast cancer in men diagnosed in 2014. It is also estimated that male breast cancer would cause approximately 430 deaths. Male breast cancer is usually diagnosed later in life, with the mean age of diagnosis in the 60s. The rates of male breast cancer are higher in North America, Europe, and Africa. There is a lower incidence in Asia.

There are many risk factors associated with male breast cancer. These risk factors include advanced age between 60 and 70 and a mutation in the **breast cancer type 2 susceptibility protein (BRCA2)** gene or **breast cancer type 1 susceptibility protein (BRCA1)** gene, with *BRCA2* being the more predominant cause. Other risk factors include a family history of breast cancer, excessive alcohol consumption, testicular disorders such as cryptorchidism or mumps orchitis (inflammation of the testes), working in a hot environment and/or working with gasoline, and previous exposure to radiation. Risk factors also include hormonal imbalance related to obesity, liver disease, Klinefelter's syndrome (a genetic condition resulting from an extra "X" chromosome, resulting in smaller-than-normal testicles and lower production of male sex hormones), and hormonal treatments such as estrogen treatment for prostate cancer or estrogen-related medications used in a sex-change procedure (Box 66.2).

Pathophysiology

Men possess a small amount of breast tissue that cannot produce milk. It is nonfunctioning tissue that is located in the area directly behind the nipple on the chest wall. Breast cancer in men is the uncontrolled growth of abnormal cells of that breast tissue. Because of this small amount of breast tissue, cancer spreads more easily to the nipple, skin, and muscle. Men are typically diagnosed with ductal carcinoma, the most commonly occurring form, which consists of infiltrating ductal carcinoma and ductal carcinoma in situ (DCIS). Other forms include inflammatory breast cancer, or Paget's disease of the nipple. Infiltrating ductal carcinoma occurs when abnormal cells spread beyond the lining of the ducts. **Ductal carcinoma in situ (DCIS)** occurs when abnormal cells are found in the lining of the duct in the breast. Inflammatory breast cancer occurs when cancer cells block lymph vessels in the skin, resulting in a breast that appears warm, swollen, and red. Lastly, **Paget's disease** of the nipple occurs when a tumor grows from ducts beneath the nipple and into the surface of the nipple. Lobular carcinoma, which can occur in women, is rare in men.

Clinical Manifestations

Clinical manifestations of breast cancer in men are similar to those in females, but because of the smaller amount of breast tissue, it is easier to feel a developed mass. Symptoms include a swelling or lump in the breast area, a dimpling of the skin or nipple, erythema, discharge from the nipple, and/or inversion of the nipple. Inflammatory breast cancer results in red, warm, and swollen breast tissue.

Management

Medical and Surgical Management
Diagnosis

A physical examination that includes a clinical breast examination is completed, checking for lumps or unusual appearance or drainage. Ultrasonography and magnetic resonance imaging (MRI) can be used to visualize internal abnormalities. An estrogen and progesterone receptor test determines the amount of estrogen and progesterone receptors that exist in the cancer tissue. The results of this test give information on whether the cancer may respond to hormone therapy. The **human epidermal growth factor receptor 2 (HER2)** test measures the amount of HER2 growth factor that is present in the cancer tissue. This growth hormone signals cell growth. Cancer cells may produce this growth factor in excess, causing excessive growth of cancer cells. The results of this test determine if monoclonal antibody therapy may halt cancer growth. Additional tests, including sentinel lymph node biopsy, chest x-ray, CT scan, bone scan, and positron emission tomography (PET) scan, are used to determine if metastasis to other body parts has occurred. If breast cancer is found to be present, the tumor is classified through staging to assess the best treatment options. Table 66.5 lists tumor staging.

Box 66.2 Nursing Care of Transgender Patients

There are barriers to the ability of transgender patients to receive healthcare. These barriers include feeling uncomfortable disclosing their identity to the healthcare provider; lack of resources and knowledge of providers; lack of financial resources and insurance; physical barriers, including hospital room assignments as they relate to gender; precision in electronic medical documentation; and accurate references in evaluating lab results. It is important for the provider to understand proper vocabulary, such as *transgender, transmale, transfemale, transsexual,* and so forth. Attention to anatomy and physiology is important for proper treatment. Because hormonal therapy is undertaken by a large part of the transgender population, understanding the effects of these hormones on the body and possible interactions with medications prescribed for male reproductive disorders is vital in treating patients. For example, a biological male who is transitioning to a female and receiving estrogen with decreasing levels of testosterone will need to be monitored closely as treatment progresses. Estrogen may cause an increased risk of cardiovascular events, which may also be affected by medications administered for benign prostatic hyperplasia, prostate cancer, and/or testicular cancer. It is equally important to address the psychological needs of transgender patients as they move forward in attaining comprehensive healthcare.

Markwick, L. (2016). Male, female, other: Transgender and the impact in primary care. *Journal for Nurse Practitioners, 12*(5), 330–338.

Table 66.5 Male Breast Cancer Staging

Stage	Definition
Stage 0 (carcinoma in situ)	
• Ductal carcinoma in situ (DCIS)	• Abnormal cells present in lining of breast duct but without metastasis
• Paget's disease of the nipple	• Abnormal cells in nipple only
• Lobular carcinoma in situ (LCIS)	• Abnormal cells in lobules of breast
Stage I	Tumor of less than 2 cm in diameter with no lymph node involvement
Stage II	Tumor of up to 5 cm in diameter with or without lymph node involvement
Stage III	• Tumor of greater than 5 cm in diameter • May involve proximal lymph nodes and lymph nodes above the collarbone
Stage IV	Metastasis to other areas, such as bone, brain, liver, and/or lungs

Treatment

Male breast cancer treatment correlates with the stage of cancer diagnosed. Treatment options include surgery, chemotherapy, hormone therapy, and radiation therapy. Surgical options include a lumpectomy or breast-conserving surgery or mastectomy. Lumpectomy is rarely used in men due to the small amount of tissue that enables easy cancer spread to the nipple, requiring removal of all breast tissue for successful treatment. Surgery usually involves a mastectomy. Depending on the stage of cancer, there are several options for mastectomy. A simple mastectomy involves the removal of the entire breast, including the nipple but not the lymph nodes. A modified radical mastectomy involves the removal of the breast and axillary lymph nodes. With a large, fast-growing, and spreading tumor, a radical mastectomy is indicated. This procedure involves the removal of the breast, axillary lymph nodes, the lining over the chest muscle, and possibly part of the chest muscle.

Chemotherapy can be used prior to or after surgery. Adjuvant chemotherapy (chemotherapy after surgery) is used as insurance against the possible presence of cancer cells not readily seen in an effort to lower the risk of a recurrence. Neoadjuvant chemotherapy is used prior to surgery to shrink the tumor to allow for more complete excision. Hormone therapy is used when the tumor is hormone receptor–positive, meaning the cancer grows in response to the hormone estrogen. Although estrogen is usually thought of as a female hormone, it is also present

at lower levels in men. Antiestrogen medications block estrogen from binding to estrogen receptors on breast cancer cells, slowing their growth. Hormonal therapy is not effective on tumors that are hormone receptor–negative.

Radiation may also be used to kill cancer cells or keep them from growing. Internal radiation or brachytherapy and external radiation are options. External radiation employs the use of an external beam to shrink or kill cancer cells or decrease symptoms. Internal radiation involves implanting radioactive substances concealed in seeds, catheters, wires, and needles directly into or near the cancer. Radiation is largely used when breast-conserving surgery is done, so, as noted previously, it is rarely used in men.

Targeted therapy uses medications or other substances to specifically attack cancer cells without attacking normal cells. An example of this form of treatment is monoclonal antibodies. These antibodies are created from a single type of immune cell. They attach to the substances on cancer cells. By attaching to the cells, antibodies kill cancer cells, stop them from growing, or keep them from spreading. The monoclonal antibodies are delivered through infusion.

Connection Check 66.8

The nurse understands that neoadjuvant chemotherapy is utilized in which of the following ways?
A. After surgery as insurance against reoccurrence of the tumor
B. Prior to surgery to help facilitate complete excision of the tumor
C. Prior to surgery as insurance against recurrence of the tumor
D. After surgery to eliminate any obvious remaining tumor cells

Nursing Management
Assessment and Analysis

The clinical manifestations of breast cancer are due to the mass or lump present in the breast tissue. Symptoms include a swelling or lump in the breast area, a dimpling of the skin or nipple, erythema, discharge from the nipple, and/or inversion of the nipple. Clinical manifestations of inflammatory breast cancer are due to blockage of lymph vessels and include red, warm, and swollen breast tissue.

Nursing Diagnoses
- **Ineffective health maintenance** related to lack of knowledge regarding self-care
- **Risk for infection** related to surgical intervention/pharmacological intervention

Nursing Interventions
Assessments
- Physical assessment

  A lump in the breast, dimpling or discharge from the nipple, nipple inversion, and redness may indicate the presence of a tumor. Red, warm, and swollen breast tissue may indicate inflammatory breast cancer.

Postoperatively

- Vital signs

  An increase in temperature may indicate an infection. A decrease in blood pressure may indicate bleeding or hypovolemia postoperatively.

  An increase in pulse may indicate bleeding, hypovolemia, pain, or anxiety.

- Incision

  Check for bleeding, color, edema, and approximation of the suture line to determine the status of the wound. A clean, well-approximated incision with minimal to no serous sanguineous drainage indicates a healing wound.

- Pain

  Request a pain scale rating to assess the need for pain medication, and determine the efficacy of treatment.

▣ Actions

- Administer medications as ordered.

  Depending on the tumor staging, chemotherapy may be given preoperatively to shrink the tumor to facilitate complete excision, or it may be given postoperatively to kill any possible remaining cancer cells.

- Change dressing.

  Change dressing as ordered by the provider. Observe for redness, bleeding, odor, discharge, swelling, and approximation. Aseptic technique assists in preventing an infection.

- Empty drain at the surgical site.

  Empty the drain; record the color and amount of drainage. Proper documentation allows the surgeon to determine when the drain can be removed.

- Administer pain medication per order.

  Managing pain makes the patient more comfortable and allows better participation in essential postoperative activities, such as coughing and deep breathing and ambulation.

▣ Teaching

- Care of suture site

  Discuss dressing changes and proper cleaning techniques.

- Signs and symptoms of infection

  Discuss signs of infection, such as fever, chills, nausea, vomiting, purulent discharge, or increased redness, so that the patient recognizes when it is necessary to call the provider.

- Breast self-examinations

  Continue or start self–breast examinations to monitor for reoccurrence.

- Follow-up appointment with provider

  Keep appointments with the surgeon to monitor the progress of healing.

- Provide emotional support and resources.

  Creating a nonjudgmental, relaxed atmosphere reduces patient anxiety and creates a relationship of trust and acceptance; give the patient information on resources for support.

Connection Check 66.9

The nurse would question which order in a patient with receptor-negative male breast cancer after radical mastectomy?

A. Administer antiestrogen therapy PO.

B. Empty drain every 4 hours and prn.

D. Administer pain medication every 4 hours prn.

E. Instruct on proper self–breast examination.

Evaluating Care Outcomes

A clean, dry wound without swelling, redness, drainage, or pain and with well-approximated wound edges indicates good surgical site healing. A well-managed patient knows what to expect regarding the care of the surgical site and signs of infection, as well as all resources available to help with emotional coping. The ability to articulate fears and anxieties regarding the cancer and the ability to return to the previous lifestyle and work indicate the beginning of emotional healing.

TESTICULAR TRAUMA

Epidemiology

Testicular trauma is an uncommon event even though the testicles are a vulnerable target. Approximately 85% of testicular trauma is from blunt trauma, whereas penetrating trauma accounts for 15%. Blunt trauma result from sports injuries, a kick to the groin, motor vehicle accidents, or falls and injury resulting from the straddling of an object. Sports injuries are the most common cause of injury. Penetrating trauma may be a result of stab wounds, gunshot wounds, animal bites, self-mutilation, or emasculation. Testicular injuries are more commonly found in males 25 to 40 years old.

Pathophysiology

The testes are the male sex glands located behind the penis in the scrotum. They are essential in the production of sperm and testosterone. The testes are surrounded by connective tissue called the *tunica vaginalis* and are covered by a fibrous capsule called the *tunica albuginea*. When there is testicular rupture, the integrity of the tunica albuginea is altered, resulting in bleeding into the tunica vaginalis, referred to as a *hematocele*. Bleeding into the scrotal wall results in a scrotal hematoma.

Categories of Injury

There are three basic categories related to testicular injury: blunt trauma, penetrating trauma, and degloving trauma. Blunt trauma refers to testes that receive an impact from an object of significant force. This trauma can be from a baseball injury or a kick to the groin. This kind of injury has also been seen in mountain bikers from the force of the bike seat or as a result of motorcycle accidents. Occasionally, blunt trauma results in the dislocation of a testicle. In this case, the testicle has moved to a location other than its normal anatomical position. Dislocation can involve one or both testicles. Penetrating trauma to the testes may be secondary to stabbings or gunshot wounds.

Degloving injuries, also called *avulsion injuries*, occur when the skin of the scrotum is sheared off. This most typically occurs from accidents incurred while operating heavy machinery such as industrial or farming accidents. Degloving trauma is the least likely of the three trauma categories to occur.

Connection Check 66.10

The emergency department nurse receives a report from a field provider regarding a patient being transported to the hospital after a groin injury sustained during a football game. The nurse prepares for which type of trauma?

A. Blunt trauma

B. Degloving trauma

C. Penetrating trauma

D. Retrograde trauma

Management

Medical and Surgical Management

Management starts with a thorough history and physical exam. Essential information includes the mechanism of injury. Scrotal ultrasound is helpful in determining the extent and nature of the injury. Blunt injuries occur most often and can often be treated conservatively if there is no rupture of the tunica albuginea. This treatment includes nonsteroidal anti-inflammatory drugs (NSAIDs), support of the scrotum, ice packs, and bedrest for 24 to 48 hours. If the injury has resulted in epididymitis (inflamed testicle) or a UTI, treatment involves antibiotics. Immediate surgical exploration may be necessary if Doppler studies or ultrasonography suggests internal trauma that may result in atrophy and necrosis. Initial management requires debridement and irrigation. Injury to the epididymis or vas deferens may be repaired using microsurgery. Removal of the testicle, orchiectomy, is rarely necessary unless there is irreparable damage to the testis.

If degloving is involved, the favored method of repair is primary closure using the remaining intact scrotal skin. If there is not sufficient skin for primary closure, the testis may be relocated to another body area, such as the subcutaneous tissue of the thigh, while allowing time for the tissue injury to heal. The temperature of the thigh is approximately 10° lower than the core body temperature, which promotes sperm production while allowing time for the damaged tissue to heal. Scrotal reconstruction can then begin in about 4 to 6 weeks. If neither of these options is possible, the testicles may remain exposed and be treated with daily dressings until enough granulation tissue forms that can be combined with a split-thickness graft for coverage. Successful reimplantation if testicular amputation has occurred is possible using microvascular techniques to restore vascularization if treatment is received within 8 hours of amputation. With any testicular surgery, antibiotics are given preoperatively and postoperatively. The patient may have drains inserted intra-operatively to decompress the surgical site, facilitating drainage, and decreasing swelling and pressure. Bleeding and infection are major risks in this type of injury.

Nursing Management

Assessment and Analysis

The clinical manifestations of testicular trauma are the result of either blunt or penetrating trauma. They are pain, swelling, bleeding, and infection. Degloving injury can result in significant loss of tissue and potential loss of testicular function.

Nursing Diagnoses

- **Risk for infection** related to surgical intervention/ pharmacological intervention
- **Anxiety** related to the threat to biological integrity

Nursing Interventions

■ *Assessments*

- Physical assessment
  Bleeding, swelling, or skin evulsion of the testicles indicate blunt, penetrating, or degloving testicular trauma.
- Pain
  A testicular injury typically results in intense pain. Assessing pain level and duration helps determine the extent of injury and the adequacy of treatment.
- Temperature
  An increased temperature is a sign of infection, which is especially important in penetrating or degloving injury.
- Wound assessment
  Assess for signs of wound infection, such as redness, warmth, or purulent drainage.

■ *Actions*

- Conservative treatment for minor trauma with NSAIDs, scrotal support, ice packs, and bedrest
  Conservative treatment allows time for the swelling to decrease and the tissue to heal.
- Wound care
  Dress wound using aseptic technique to prevent infection.
- Administer antibiotics as ordered.
  Antibiotics may be ordered to prevent or treat infection.
- Monitor drain output.
  Excessive drainage may indicate bleeding, which may require repair. Discolored or malodorous drainage may indicate infection.

- **Compassion and support**
  Offer emotional support to help the patient emotionally deal with this injury.

■ *Teaching*

- **Care related to nonsurgical intervention**
  Teach the patient how to care for scrotal injury by explaining proper dosing of NSAIDs; the use of a scrotal sling or folded towels to elevate the scrotum; the use of ice packs, including the use of a towel between the skin and the ice pack; and the importance of rest to assist in recovery.
- **Postsurgical care**
  Teach the patient how to care for the surgical area, especially keeping it clean and dry to decrease the chance of infection.
- **Drains**
  Teach the patient and/or significant other how to manage the care of drains, should the patient be discharged with drains in place, to encourage independence.
- **Worsening symptoms**
  Teach patient to call the provider when signs and symptoms of a worsening condition occur, such as fever, redness, a heavy feeling in scrotal area, swelling, bleeding, nausea and vomiting, and increasing pain.

Evaluating Care Outcomes

A well-managed patient experiencing testicular trauma has pain under control and understands the necessary treatment to aid in recovery. The patient with minor trauma is resting, using ice and scrotal support to decrease swelling. The patient who required a surgical repair is healing well and free from infection.

Making Connections

CASE STUDY: WRAP-UP

After assessment of his symptoms and education, Scott agrees to a blood draw for PSA levels, a urinalysis, and a DRE. Based on the results of the DRE, a PSA of less than 2 ng/mL, and urinalysis within normal limits, Scott is told the best intervention at this time is "watchful waiting." He is told that if his symptoms worsen, he may be prescribed medication therapy such as 5-alpha-reductase inhibitors or alpha-adrenergic blockers. The nurse provides patient education focusing on watchful waiting and the importance of future provider follow-up.

Case Study Questions

1. Scott's initial complaint is of problems urinating. He is diagnosed with BPH. He understands BPH causes this symptom because the enlarged prostate exhibits which of the following?
   A. Often swells when the patient has a full bladder
   B. Obstruction to the flow of urine
   C. Can easily be injured secondary to blunt trauma
   D. Is sensitive to diets high in potassium

2. Scott has been told by his provider that the best approach for his diagnosis of BPH at this time is "watchful waiting." The nurse explains that watchful waiting is appropriate because of which of the following?
   A. He has minimal symptoms and minimal prostate enlargement.
   B. He is too old to require surgical intervention.
   C. The provider wants to monitor lymph node involvement.
   D. His PSA levels were too high in combination with a negative DRE.

3. The nurse recognizes more teaching is necessary by which of the following statements?
   A. "I guess I need to plan on yearly follow-ups."
   B. "I'll call for an appointment if my symptoms get worse."
   C. "I'm glad I'll be able to take my decongestants for my allergies."
   D. "I'm glad medications are not necessary at this point."

4. If Scott is given a prescription for an alpha blocker such as Flomax, he will be educated as to how this medication works. This education will include which of the following statements?
   A. The medication relaxes the muscles of the prostate, allowing easier urination.
   B. The medication relieves discomfort associated with urination.
   C. The medication lowers PSA levels.
   D. The medication dilates the urethra, allowing easier urination.

5. Scott is told to report any additional pain, fever, nausea, and/or vomiting to his provider for which of the following reasons?
   A. An enlarged prostate can cause a spike in fever.
   B. Nausea and vomiting can be related to dilation of the prostate gland.
   C. The combination of these symptoms with BPH may be a sign of cancer.
   D. Urine stasis from lack of bladder emptying may cause a UTI.

CHAPTER SUMMARY

Benign prostatic hyperplasia (BPH) affects 50% of men age 51 to 60 years of age and 90% of men over the age of 80. Frequent nocturia is a common complaint. Although "watchful waiting" is often the treatment with BPH, if left untreated, the patient may develop urinary retention, a urinary tract infection (UTI), bladder stones, bladder damage, and kidney damage. If severe urinary retention develops, catheterization may be indicated to fully empty the bladder. Patients need to be educated to be able to recognize worsening symptoms to avoid complications.

Erectile dysfunction is the inability to achieve or maintain an erection sufficient for sexual intercourse. Causative factors include diabetes, cardiovascular disease, or low levels of testosterone. There are several treatment options, but the most common is medication therapy in the form of PDE-5 inhibitors. Erectile dysfunction can be treated surgically with a penile implant as well as with other nonsurgical options, such as medications injected into the penis or pellets inserted into the urethra that cause vasodilation that stimulates blood flow.

Prostate cancer is the cause of approximately 9% of cancer-related deaths in the male population. Regular screening should be done for patients at risk for prostate cancer because it is relatively symptomless in the early stages. Tumors develop on the edges of the prostate, so they do not interfere with urine flow initially. Although the prostate-specific antigen (PSA) test has always been the gold standard for the diagnosis of prostate cancer, it is now being questioned because annual testing is resulting in overdiagnosis and overtreatment of prostate cancer as well as underdiagnosis. Some providers now look at serial PSAs from month to month as opposed to just one reading. Patients need to be educated as to what the results of the PSA mean for them in particular according to their age and other risk factors.

The prevalence of testicular cancer is low; the expected cure rate is 95%, and in patients with metastatic cancer, the expected cure rate is 80%. The disease is more prevalent in Caucasian males and less prevalent in African American males. The survival rate after a patient has been treated for testicular cancer is good. Treatment for all types starts with the removal of the affected testicle, including the blood supply to that testicle. Slow-growing testicular cancers are treated with radiation and/or chemotherapy following surgery. Faster-growing tumors do not respond to radiation and so are treated with chemotherapy and the removal of lymph nodes postoperatively.

Male breast cancer is a rare disease affecting less than 1% of the population and is usually diagnosed in men between the ages of 60 and 70. Breast cancer in men is the uncontrolled growth of abnormal cells of the breast tissue. Because there is a small amount of breast tissue in a man, cancer spreads more easily to the nipple, skin, and muscle. It is treated in the same way female breast cancer is treated, using chemotherapy, radiation, and surgery, depending on what stage the breast cancer is when diagnosed.

Testicular trauma, although the testes are seemingly in a vulnerable position, is an uncommon event. The three categories of testicular trauma include blunt trauma (e.g., from a kick to the groin), penetrating trauma (e.g., from a knife wound), and degloving trauma (e.g., from a heavy machinery accident). Degloving trauma is the least common. Most blunt testicular trauma requires treatment with NSAIDs, bedrest, ice, and scrotal support. For the more severe testicular traumas, secondary to penetration or degloving, surgery is required.

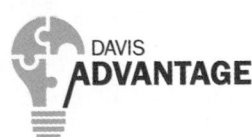
DAVIS
ADVANTAGE | To explore learning resources for this chapter, go to **Davis Advantage** and find:
- Answers to in-text questions
- Chapter Resources and Activities
- NCLEX®-Style Chapter Review Questions
- Bibliography

Chapter 67

Coordinating Care for Patients With Sexually Transmitted Infection

Lynn McDonald

Finding Connections

CASE STUDY: EPISODE 1

Follow this patient throughout the chapter.

Keisha Pritchard is a 24-year-old female who presents to her OB/GYN healthcare provider for her annual checkup. Her medical history consists of sexual activity since 13 with a history of 11 partners, chlamydia (treated at a clinic 1 year ago), smoking (one-half pack a day), and drinking (every weekend while partying). She also states she does not use condoms because she does not like how they feel. She states she knows her current male partner is "clean" because she asked him. She attends school at a local college...

INTRODUCTION

Sexually transmitted infections (STIs), also referred to as sexually transmitted diseases (STDs), are a worldwide epidemic. Sexually transmitted infections are contagious (viral, bacterial, or parasitic) and may cause physical, emotional, and psychological burdens with the capability of causing catastrophic sequelae. They are mainly transmitted from person to person by intimate contact but can be spread congenitally or via bloodborne pathogens. Sexually transmitted infections have also been linked to the acquisition and transmission of HIV. Common STIs, such as the human papillomavirus (HPV), *Chlamydia*, gonorrhea, pelvic inflammatory disease (PID), syphilis, and genital herpes, are discussed in this chapter.

HUMAN PAPILLOMAVIRUS

Epidemiology

Human papillomavirus is a very common STI of the anogenital tract. There are more than 100 known types of HPV, with 40 types linked to the lower genital tract of males and females. Human papillomavirus is well recognized as the precursor to cervical cancer. Additional evidence is being revealed as to its role in the development of cancers of the vulva, vagina, anus, penis, and some head and neck cancers. Infection with HPV, specifically HPV 6 and HPV 11, is also responsible for other diseases, such as juvenile respiratory papillomatosis and genital warts.

Globally, the incidence of HPV in females is highest in sub-Saharan Africa (24%), Latin America and the Caribbean (16%), Eastern Europe (14%), and South East Asia (14%). In the United States, the prevalence of any type of HPV in females is 39%, and 20.4% of females are infected with an **oncogenic** (implicated in the formation and development of cancerous tumors) type of HPV. Human papillomavirus is very common in women under 30, and approximately 75% to 80% of females will acquire HPV by the age of 50.

Human papillomavirus exposure is typically temporary and has little long-term significance. However, exposure to oncogenic HPV increases the risk for cervical cancer for women who are past the age of 30. Worldwide, cervical cancer is the fourth-leading cause of cancer in women and the second-leading cause in women aged 15 to 44 years. Because the prevalence of HPV in cervical cancer overwhelms the incidence in other cancers, this section focuses primarily on females and HPV and how HPV relates to cervical lesions and cancer.

Connection Check 67.1

The nurse recognizes that which virus leads to an increased risk for cervical cancer?

A. Cytomegalovirus
B. Herpes simplex virus
C. Human parvovirus
D. Human papillomavirus

All HPV strains are transmitted by direct skin contact during vaginal, anal, and oral sexual intercourse; therefore, risk factors are related to sexual behavior. They include multiple sexual partners (within the year and lifetime), sexually active unmarried females, and onset of sexual intercourse at an early age. In addition to risk factors, there are several cofactors that aid in the **pathogenesis** (origin and development of disease) and progression of HPV. These are immunosuppressive conditions (e.g., HIV), chronic conditions requiring long-term immunosuppressive therapy (e.g., transplant recipients), oral contraceptives, smoking, and STIs, particularly herpes and chlamydia. These risk factors are associated with an increased risk for cervical cancer; however, not everyone exposed to high-risk HPV will develop cervical cancer.

Pathophysiology

The different types of HPV are grouped into "low-risk," "intermediate-risk," and "high-risk" strains. "Low-risk" strains cause 90% of condyloma acuminata (condylomas), or genital warts. Low-risk strains are not commonly known to lead to cervical cancer. The estimated **incubation period** (exposure to infection time) is 3 weeks to 8 months. Genital warts may appear as soft, fleshy, flat, raised lesions that may resemble cauliflower in appearance and usually occur in clusters. Common sites are the penis, vulva, vagina, perineum, and anal region (Fig. 67.1).

Certain intermediate-risk and high-risk strains have been known to lead to cervical cancer. There are 14 different high-risk strains in total, and all are considered oncogenic. Specifically, the high-risk strains HPV 16 and HPV 18 are linked to 70% of squamous cell carcinomas of the cervix. The majority of patients who have oncogenic HPV usually have **subclinical** disease or are in the early stage of a disease that does not show symptoms.

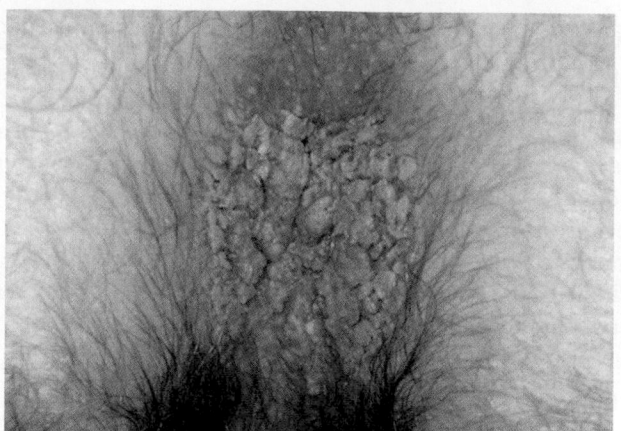

FIGURE 67.1 Condylomata acuminate, or genital warts, in the perianal region; they resemble cauliflower in appearance.

High-risk HPV is a double-stranded deoxyribonucleic acid (DNA) virus that invades the cells through microabrasions of the basal epithelium in the epithelial tissue of the cervix, making the host susceptible to attack. As HPV slowly replicates, it begins to occupy more of the basal membrane. In the beginning stages of infection, low-grade squamous intraepithelial lesion (LSIL), otherwise known as cervical intraepithelial neoplasia I (CIN I), occupies one-third of the epithelium. If the infection persists, it may develop into CIN II (two-thirds of the epithelium) or CIN III (the full thickness of the epithelium). Both CIN II and III can be referred to as *high-grade squamous intraepithelial lesions (HSILs)*. High-grade squamous intraepithelial lesions may take several years to develop (up to 20 years) depending on the host's immunity and ability to fight off infection.

Clinical Manifestations

Typically, HPV infections cause no symptoms, hence the need for adequate screening. Females with nononcogenic HPV may experience symptoms of genital warts. Most patients who have genital warts claim they do not have other associated symptoms, but genital warts can be painful and bothersome. Some patients complain of itching, burning, and tenderness. Genital warts may also cause emotional distress.

Management

Medical Management

Diagnosis

The Papanicolaou (Pap) test remains the most cost-effective tool to screen females for cervical cancer. It is the first-line test to detect an abnormal growth in the cervix or vagina. In this test, cells are scraped from the surface and internal opening of the cervix. The cells are examined under a microscope to view for abnormalities (**cytology**). When used routinely at scheduled intervals, the Pap test has proven to be an effective tool to detect preinvasive cervical cancer.

Human papillomavirus DNA testing, an evaluation of cells scraped from the cervix, is used to detect high-risk oncogenic HPV. It can be used as a reflex check in females who are diagnosed with **atypical** (abnormal) cells on a Pap test. In females over 30 years, HPV testing is recommended as a routine addition to the Pap test as a co-test. Human papillomavirus testing should not be used in lieu of Pap testing. A **colposcopy** is a magnified examination of the cervix, vagina, and vulva. A colposcopy and biopsy may be indicated if the cytological specimen (Pap) is abnormal and if high-risk HPV DNA is detected. Current guidelines (www.acog.org) suggest that cervical cancer screening should begin at 21 years of age because cervical carcinoma is relatively rare under the age of 20 years. Also, females under the age of 21 who are exposed to oncogenic HPV are highly likely to clear the infection.

Medical Management of Nononcogenic HPV

Treatment is not recommended for HPV in the absence of genital warts or lesions. If genital warts are diagnosed, largely by way of visual inspection, treatment is done to remove the warts, but it is not clear if removal clears the HPV infection. Recommended treatments for genital warts include creams (imiquimod ([Aldara] 5% cream), gels (podofilox 0.5% solution or gel), or ointments (sinecatechins 15%) applied directly to the affected area. They work by modifying or enhancing the immune response to the wart or by breaking down the skin on the wart. Another option, cryotherapy, may be a first-line clinician therapy to treat genital warts. Cryotherapy destroys the wart through thermal-induced **cytolysis** (breakdown of cells). Surgical excision is also an option. The warts may be surgically removed at a single visit; however, reoccurrence is possible.

 Safety Alert Special precautions about genital warts and pregnancy:
- The safe administration of the creams, gels, and ointments used to treat warts has not been established in pregnant females and therefore should be avoided.
- If the pelvic outlet is obstructed by genital warts, a cesarean section may be indicated.

Medical Management of Oncogenic HPV

Providers take several factors into consideration in the management of cervical warts and lesions associated with high-risk oncogenic HPV strains: age, size, location and stage of the disease, pregnancy, probability of compliance, cost, skill level, and resource availability. Invasive procedures are one option but may be performed only after the HSIL has been diagnostically proven with colposcopy and biopsy. Once the lesion is confirmed as HSIL, the provider will decide which procedure is most appropriate for the patient. Table 67.1 lists the common procedures to manage HSIL.

Table 67.1 Common Procedures and Definitions for Management of HSIL

Procedure	Definition
Loop electrosurgical excision procedure	This procedure employs a wire loop that transmits a painless current to the affected abnormal cervical tissue.
Ablation	These procedures burn or freeze abnormal cervical tissue. The most common procedures are cryosurgery (freezing) and laser ablation (beam of light used to irradiate abnormal cells).
Excision	This procedure involves the resection of abnormal tissue. The most commonly done procedure with advanced cervical lesions is cold knife conization (CKC). This procedure involves biopsy of the cervix by obtaining a cone-shaped sample; CKC may be done to diagnose cancers of the cervix or uterus or to treat CIN.
Laser conization	This procedure utilizes a beam of light to excise abnormal cervical tissue.

CIN, Cervical intraepithelial neoplasia; *HSIL,* high-grade squamous intraepithelial lesion.

Prophylaxis

Prophylactic HPV management in the form of a vaccine is recommended for females and males. The Advisory Committee on Immunization Practices (ACIP) of the Centers for Disease Control and Prevention (CDC) recommends routine vaccination with the **human papillomavirus 9-valent vaccine** (see Evidence-Based Practice: Human Papillomavirus Vaccination).

Evidence-Based Practice

Human Papillomavirus Vaccination

The Advisory Committee on Immunization Practices (ACIP) recommends vaccination for female and males with the human papillomavirus 9-valent (9vHPV) vaccine to prevent HPV-associated cancers and disorders, such as cervical, vulvar, vaginal, and other HPV-related malignancies; precancerous HPV-related lesions; and genital warts in females and genital warts and penile, anal, and HPV-associated oral pharyngeal cancers in males. Current ACIP guidelines for females and males include a two-dose vaccination between the ages of 9 and 14 and three doses between the ages of 15 and 26. Females can be vaccinated through the age of 26 years, and males can be vaccinated through 21 years. Special populations include children with a history of sexual abuse. This population should begin the vaccination series at 9 years old. Men who have sex with men (MSM) and transgender persons can be vaccinated up through 26 years old. The ACIP also recommends three doses of the vaccine for individuals with immunocompromising conditions such as HIV, B-lymphocyte antibody deficiencies, and

transplantation. The administration of the 9vHPV vaccine has been proven to significantly reduce the risk of cervical cancer in women by 90%.

Bernstein, H. H., Bocchini, J. A., & Committee on Infectious Diseases. (2017). Practical approaches to optimize adolescent immunization. *American Academy of Pediatrics, 139*(3), e20164187. doi:10.1542/peds.2016-4187

Practices.Meites, E., Kempe, A., & Markowitz, L. E. (2016). Use of a 2-dose schedule for human papillomavirus vaccination—Updated recommendations of the Advisory Committee on Immunization Practices. *Morbidity and Mortality Weekly Report, 65*(49), 1405–1408. doi:10.15585/mmwr.mm6549a5

Nursing Management
Assessment and Analysis

Clinical manifestations arc not clearly defined in HPV. Some patients have no symptoms; others complain of burning, itching, or pain associated with genital lesions or warts.

Nursing Diagnosis
- **Ineffective health maintenance** related to deficient knowledge regarding self-care, treatment prevention, and spread of disease

Nursing Interventions
Assessments
- Pain
  May be an indication of a worsening condition or complication
- Presence of genital warts
  Genital warts are a common manifestation of HPV.

Actions
- Administer mild analgesia prn as ordered after treatment to remove or manage HSIL.
  Provides pain relief and comfort

▪ *Teaching*

- Educate the patient on prevention, manifestations, transmission of STIs, reducing the number of partners, and the use of barrier methods.
  Safe sex will help to decrease transmission of HPV to another person and thus the overall prevalence.
- Encourage healthy practices (e.g., healthy diet, limit drinking, no smoking) and routine gynecological and primary care.
  Improve health outcomes and well-being
- Encourage completion of the full series of HPV vaccinations.
  Vaccination will reduce the risk of the acquisition of HPV-related cancers and disease.
- Instruct the patient to report any history of infection to partners.
  The partner may be at risk and/or may need to be treated. Early treatment can reduce complications of infection.
- Instruct the patient on the appropriate application of gels, creams, or ointments as indicated for genital warts.
  Proper application will maximize benefit and minimize adverse effects.
- Call provider if experiencing worsening pain and/or vaginal discharge.
  May be an indication of a worsening condition or complication

Evaluating Care Outcomes

Many females and males are exposed to HPV; however, because of its slow progression and effective treatment modalities, patients do not have to succumb to complications related to that exposure. A well-managed patient receives the appropriate vaccinations, practices safe sex, limits partners, has good health habits (e.g., annual pelvic examinations), and is aware of when to contact the provider.

SYPHILIS

Epidemiology

Syphilis is complex chronic infection that has the ability to acutely or chronically infect every organ of the body in a very subtle manner. It is classified into four stages: primary, secondary, latent (early and late), and tertiary. The tertiary stage is also classified as cardiovascular and gummatous. Neurosyphilis (central nervous system [CNS]) has been classified at times as tertiary but can be present at any stage. The World Health Organization (WHO) estimated that more than 12 million persons are infected with syphilis annually. The CDC reported 88,042 new cases (all stages) and reported 27,814 primary and secondary syphilis cases in the United States in 2016. It is transmitted through genital and oral sexual intercourse and congenitally from mother to fetus. Populations most at risk are persons 25 to 29 years of age and homosexual men. The CDC reported a surge of 17.6% in primary and secondary syphilis and an increase of 27.6% in congenital syphilis. Females are screened routinely during antepartum visits. Similar to those of other STIs, risk factors include unprotected sexual intercourse, multiple sexual partners, men who have sexual intercourse with men (MSM), transgender women, sex workers, incarcerated individuals, and individuals with a history of HIV (see Evidence-Based Practice: The Care of Transgender Men and Women). Infants are at increased risk when they have a mother who has been exposed to syphilis.

Evidence-Based Practice

The Care of Transgender Men and Women

The term *transgender* relates to a person who identifies with a sex that differs from the one assigned at birth. Transgender women (trans-women) identify as women but have male genitalia. Correspondingly, transgender men (trans-men) identify as men but have female genitalia. Gender expression differs from sexual orientation. Trans-male or trans-women may engage in sexual relations with either men, women, or both. Trans-women may not undergo genital affirmation surgery but can engage in oral, vaginal, and anal relations with a functioning penis. Trans-men who have a vagina and cervix will continue to be at risk for bacterial infections, human papillomavirus (HPV), and cervical cancer. Clinicians should assess and screen appropriately for asymptomatic and symptomatic sexually transmitted infections (STIs) and human immunodeficiency virus (HIV)–related risks in relation to the individual's anatomical features and sexual practices.

Luzzati, R., & Maurel, C. (2015). Transgender identity and sexually transmitted diseases including HIV. In C. Trombetta, G. Liguori, & M. Bertolotto (Eds.), *Management of gender dysphoria* (pp. 337–344). Milano, Italy: Springer. 20171217140706435997486
Poteat, T. (2017). *Transgender people and sexually transmitted infections (STIs)*. Retrieved from http://www.transhealth.ucsf.edu 20171214200819560475468
20180108114251177343029

Pathophysiology and Clinical Manifestations

Syphilis is an ulcerative genital disease caused by the anaerobic spirochete *Treponema pallidum*. This bacterium invades the mucous membranes and becomes systemic by entering the blood and lymphatic system. The CNS is invaded early in the disease. The incubation period is 1 week to 3 months. Primary syphilis initially manifests as a chancre. A chancre is a painless, hard lesion that can develop into a painless open lesion, located at the site of exposure. The most common sites are the vulva, vagina, anus, penis, rectum, lips, and oral pharynx (Fig. 67.2).

Chancre lesions will last 3 to 6 weeks with or without treatment. **Lymphadenopathy** (abnormally large lymph nodes, usually a result of a disease) often occurs in combination with the chancre or in secondary syphilis. If the patient

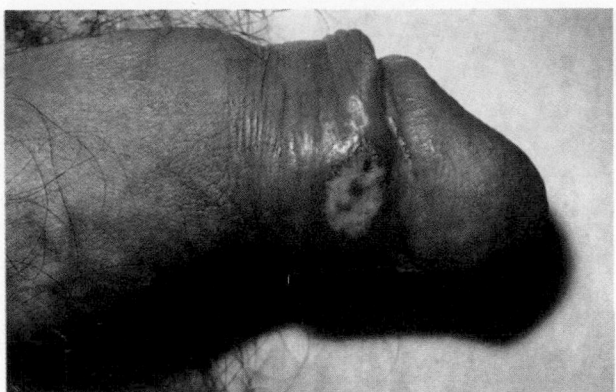

FIGURE 67.2 Primary chancre of syphilis: a large ulceration on the penis.

with primary syphilis does not receive adequate treatment, the infection will travel systematically and progress to secondary syphilis.

Secondary syphilis is marked by a rash and/or mucous membrane lesions. These rashes or lesions may overlap the time period when the chancre is still healing or appear weeks later. A maculopapular rash may develop on the palms, soles, buttocks, and upper thighs (Fig. 67.3). These rashes may appear macular (flat discolored spot), papular (elevated, hard skin that does not contain pus), or pustular (skin that contains pus) or a combination of all. Lesions called *condylomata lata* (warty growths on the skin) may also develop at this time, along with mucous patches in the mouth. These lesions are considered infectious (Fig. 67.4).

Other symptoms may include fever or malaise, alopecia, joint pain, and headaches. The infection may involve the kidney and liver (nephritic syndrome, hepatitis), but this is rare. The primary and secondary periods are the most infectious stages.

Early **latent** (hidden) syphilis develops after the secondary symptoms reduce in intensity, typically 1 year after exposure. The late latent period is considered greater than 1 year after exposure. In the latent period, the risk of sexual transmission is low. Within the late latent period,

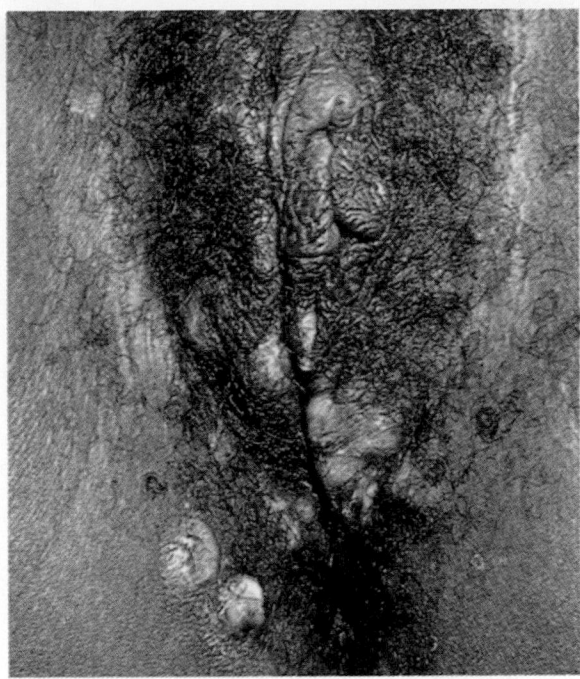

FIGURE 67.4 Secondary syphilis condylomata lata; wart-like growths in the perianal region.

three situations may occur: (1) the patient spontaneously resolves the infection, (2) the patient remains in a latent state, or (3) the patient progresses to late or tertiary syphilis. Late or tertiary syphilis may develop in one-third of patients with syphilis without treatment. There are three types of tertiary syphilis: neurosyphilis, cardiovascular syphilis, and gummatous syphilis (skin and subcutaneous tissues).

Neurosyphilis is an infection in which *T. pallidum* invades the CNS. Neurosyphilis can manifest in four forms: asymptomatic, general paresis, meningovascular, and a syndrome called *tabes dorsalis*. Asymptomatic is the most common form of neurosyphilis. In this form, there are cerebrospinal fluid (CSF) abnormalities without symptoms of nervous system damage. In general paresis neurosyphilis, there is a combination of psychiatric and neurological findings. Patients can present with decreased mental function or mood and personality changes. Meningovascular or syphilitic meningeal infection may result in fibrosis or thickening of cerebral vessels, causing sudden-onset stroke, hemiplegia, or abnormal CSF findings. *Tabes dorsalis*, a late stage of neurosyphilis, involves a slow degeneration of the spinal cord leading to loss of sensation, loss of peripheral reflexes, progressive ataxia, and finally, paralysis.

Cardiovascular syphilis and gummatous syphilis are rare forms of tertiary syphilis. Cardiovascular syphilis damages the aortic musculature. Gummatous syphilis, composed of rubberlike lesions, occurs in the skin, bones, or internal organs. Both are rare because of the widespread use of penicillin but have an increased incidence in patients with HIV. See Table 67.2 for common manifestations of syphilis.

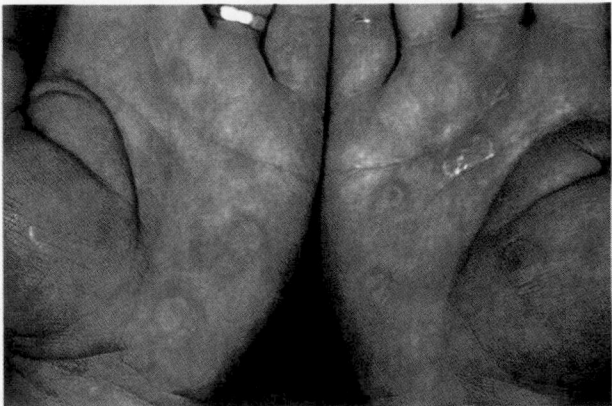

FIGURE 67.3 Maculopapular rash on palms that occurs with secondary syphilis. This rash can appear macular, papular, and/or pustular on the palms, soles, or trunk.

Table 67.2 Common Manifestations of Syphilis

Syphilis Stage	Details
Primary Genital ulcer Chancre: firm, round, and painless	The first symptom occurs on average at 21 days or 10–90 days. The chancre lasts 3 to 6 weeks. Ulcers and chancres appear where syphilis enters the body. Without treatment, the infection progresses to secondary stage.
Secondary Skin rashes: lesions (including palms and soles), macular, papular, pustular Mucous patches: painless, silvery ulcerations of mucous membrane with surrounding erythema Condyloma lata: large, raised, gray or white lesions Generalized lymphadenopathy Fever (low-grade), malaise, anorexia, arthralgias, and myalgias Central nervous system: headache, meningitis, cranial neuropathies Other: Renal: glomerulonephritis, nephritic syndrome Liver: hepatitis Bone and joint: arthritis	A rash can appear when the primary chancre is healing or several weeks after the chancre has healed. Symptoms can go away with or without treatment. However, without treatment, the infection progresses to the latent or possibly tertiary stage.
Latent (hidden) No signs or symptoms	Early latent—infection occurred within the past 12 months. Late latent—infection occurred more than 12 months ago. Detected through serological tests Can continue in this stage for years
Tertiary Cardiovascular: Aortic regurgitation Aortic aneurysm Neurosyphilis: Seizures Hemiparesis or hemiplegia Impaired proprioception and vibratory sensation Visual changes Ataxia Urinary and fecal incontinence Cranial nerve involvement (II–VII) Stroke	This stage is rare. Early neurological manifestations may occur within the first few months or years of infection. Late neurological manifestations may occur 10–30 years after the infection was first acquired. Death can occur due to damage to internal organs.

Table 67.2 Common Manifestations of Syphilis—cont'd

Syphilis Stage	Details
Optic atrophy	
General paresis	
Personality changes	
Hyperactive reflexes	
Decreased memory	
Slurred speech	
Gummata: rubbery nodules or ulcers of pink, fleshy tissue located in the skin, mucous membranes, bones, eyes, respiratory system or gastrointestinal system	
Tabes dorsalis: syphilitic myelopathy causing a loss of coordination of movement	

Management

Medical Management

Diagnosis

The diagnosis of syphilis is confirmed by serological (blood testing) and microscopic testing. The most commonly used serological procedure is done in two stages, the nontreponemal and treponemal-specific tests. Nontreponemal tests look for indirect markers of infection, such as biomarkers released as a result of cellular damage due to the spirochetes of syphilis. Examples include the rapid plasma reagin (RPR) and Venereal Disease Research Laboratory (VDRL) tests. Treponemal tests look for direct markers of infection, such as antibody production. Examples include fluorescent treponemal antibody absorption (FTA-ABS), *T pallidum* particle agglutination assay (TP-PA), and various enzyme immunoassays (EIAs). These nontreponemal and treponemal-specific tests cannot be used individually because they both have limitations that may produce false-positive results.

Darkfield microscopy is a quick traditional method of testing for primary and secondary syphilis. It may not be used as often if serological testing is available. Darkfield microscopy works by "brightening up" an object against a dark background. This form of microscopy can illuminate the slim bacterium *T pallidum* that is not readily visible utilizing other types of stains. In order to obtain a specimen for microscopy, the lesion is cleaned with saline-soaked gauze, and then a slide is pressed firmly on the exudates and viewed. The combination of serological testing and the examination of the CSF obtained through a lumbar puncture is the current method to definitively diagnose neurosyphilis.

Medications

The main medication used for all stages of syphilis is penicillin. Patients who are allergic to penicillin may use other approved medications; however, these alternatives may not be as effective. They include ceftriaxone, tetracycline, and doxycycline. Patients who are allergic may undergo desensitization for treatment with penicillin. Desensitization is a procedure where, under close observation in the hospital, a penicillin dose is slowly administered after the administration of both methylprednisone (anti-inflammatory) and diphenhydramine (antihistamine) to counteract the potential reaction. Pregnant women with a penicillin allergy would go through desensitization because there are no alternatives to penicillin in the treatment of syphilis while pregnant.

Connection Check 67.2

The nurse understands that which of the following are correct about syphilis? *(Select all that apply.)*

A. A chancre is a common symptom in tertiary syphilis.
B. Neurosyphilis invades the CNS and may occur at any stage of syphilis.
C. The most infectious stages of syphilis are the primary and secondary stages.
D. Latent infections are detected primarily by visual inspection.
E. Penicillin G is the preferred treatment for all stages of syphilis.

Nursing Management

Assessment and Analysis

The clinical manifestations of syphilis vary depending on the stage of the disease, as illustrated in Table 67.2. The initial manifestation is a chancre sore. Without treatment, the disease can progress into secondary and tertiary stages. The symptoms worsen as the disease progresses. In the second stage, skin rashes may appear, along with fever and symptoms of malaise. In the tertiary stage, gummatous disease may produce extensive tissue damage and disfigurement. In addition, profound damage to the cardiac system or CNS may result in valvular problems, seizures, issues with mobility, and eventually paralysis.

Nursing Diagnoses

- **Risk for loss of cognitive function** related to infection with syphilis
- **Situational low self-esteem** related to the clinical manifestations of syphilis
- **Impaired mobility** related to spinal cord damage

Nursing Interventions

▣ *Assessments*

- Vital signs, particularly temperature
  Increased temperature is a sign of infection. Monitoring temperature helps to evaluate the course of infection and response to treatment.
- Presence of chancre
  Initial manifestation of primary syphilis
- Skin
  The presence of a diffuse rash or mucous patches is indicative of secondary syphilis.
- Neurological status
  Neurological changes such as mood swings, confusion, seizures, and balance issues are indicative of neurosyphilis.
- Serology tests
  Positive tests are indicative of the presence of syphilis; the response to treatment may be monitored by decreasing markers of infection in the serology tests.

▣ *Actions*

- Administer penicillin as ordered.
  Penicillin is the most effective antibiotic in the treatment of syphilis.

▣ *Teaching*

- Educate the patient on the importance of seeking and maintaining treatment.
  Treatment is essential to avoid progression of the disease to secondary or tertiary stages.
- Educate the patient on prevention, manifestations, transmission of STIs, reducing the number of partners, and barrier methods.
  Safe sex can help decrease the transmission and occurrence of syphilis.
- Instruct the patient to report any history of infection to sexual partners.
  The partner may be at risk and/or may need to be treated. Early treatment can reduce untoward complications of infection.

Evaluating Care Outcomes

Even with the discovery of penicillin, syphilis continues to be a global health concern, particularly with the growing epidemic of HIV/AIDS. Effective treatment for halting progression to the later stages is possible with early diagnosis and management. A well-managed patient is compliant with the treatment plan, practices safe sex, and is aware of when to contact the provider. Similar to other STIs, syphilis screening should be part of routine screening for those at risk because this infection may present asymptomatically.

GENITAL HERPES

Epidemiology

Genital herpes is a common, chronic STI caused by herpes simplex virus 1 (HSV-1) and herpes simplex virus 2 (HSV-2). National estimates reveal that the prevalence of HSV-1 is 47.8% and that of HSV-2 is 11.9% among individuals aged 14 to 49, with a total adolescent and adult population ratio of 1 to 5. The majority of genital herpes is caused by HSV-2. Globally, the prevalence of HSV-2–related genital herpes present in persons aged 15 to 49 is 417 million. Estimates reach over a billion within the same age range when including the cases of genital herpes caused by either HSV-1 or HSV-2.

Risk factors for genital herpes are similar to those for other STIs. They include a history of other STIs, early age of sexual intercourse, MSM practices, multiple partners, low socioeconomic status, and immune-compromised individuals. Herpes simplex virus 2 is more commonly diagnosed in females than males because the female genitalia are more susceptible to skin breaks. Genital herpes is more easily transmitted from males to females than from females to males.

Pathophysiology

Genital herpes is a highly contagious infection caused by HSV. Entry can occur through minute breaks such as a scratch or abrasion through uninfected skin. The herpes simplex virus travels from the site of infection (skin or mucous membrane) via the lymphatic, blood, or ascending nerves to the sacral ganglion cells and remains latent until it becomes reactivated and travels down many different sensory nerve fibers. Herpes antibodies develop after the initial infection.

Generally, genital herpes is transmitted by direct skin-to-skin contact during the **prodromal** stage of infection (onset of the infection). Infection can occur through oral-to-oral, oral-to-genital, genital-to-genital, or anal contact. Transmission can also occur during childbirth when the child is passing through the birth canal. The virus may shed from persons with or without symptoms. The majority of patients are unaware they are infected; therefore, transmission to others may occur unknowingly. Others may not recognize the infection as herpetic and therefore may not take necessary precautions to prevent transmission to others.

Clinical Manifestations

HSV outbreaks occur episodically. Between outbreaks, HSV lies dormant in the sacral area in the CNS. It becomes reactivated as a result of stressors or triggers. Triggers for the onset of these outbreaks can be due to physical factors (e.g., immunosuppression, ultraviolet radiation, fatigue, menses) and psychological factors (emotional and psychological stress). The frequency, severity, and duration of these episodes may vary from patient to patient. Females tend to have more severe symptoms than males. Outbreaks or episodes also tend to decrease over time. The primary or initial outbreak presents as one or several clear vesicles, or blisters, that erupt in the genital area. The vesicle then ruptures and forms a painful ulcer several days later. The ulcer may last up to 2 to 4 weeks if untreated (Fig. 67.5). Table 67.3 displays common symptoms observed in males and females.

Psychosocial Impact of Genital Herpes

Genital herpes is a chronic condition that may affect quality of life. The frequency and severity of the pain can change the general well-being of an individual, especially when clustered with other symptoms. Psychosocially, genital herpes may have implications that can lead to depression, withdrawal from relationships, poor coping skills and self-confidence, shame, guilt, and perceived poor body image. Patients may feel or be stigmatized or stereotyped as one who is promiscuous and/or one who made a poor decision, making them unwilling to disclose the chronic infection to new sexual partners. At the same time, these individuals are concerned they may transmit the infection to others. This can lead to overall detrimental effects on quality of life.

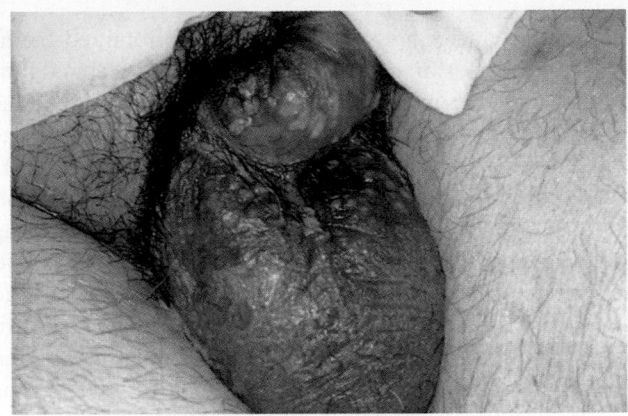

FIGURE 67.5 Genital herpetic ulcers. Clear vesicles, or blisters, in the genital area.

Management

Medical Management

Diagnosis

Diagnosis of HSV infection can begin clinically through visual inspection of the oral, genital, and anal areas. Cell culture and polymerase chain reaction (PCR) testing are the preferred methods for those who seek medical treatment for the HSV ulcers or lesions. In order to obtain a culture from an ulceration, the top layer is removed, and the sample is retrieved from the underside. Fluid from a ruptured vesicle can be collected and sent off in a culture medium. Results are most accurate within 24 to 48 hours from the time the vesicle or ulcer appears. Culture sensitivities are low; therefore, the PCR assay is the more sensitive test to

Table 67.3 Manifestations of Genital Herpes

Common Site for Genital Herpes	Other Symptoms That May Occur With Vesicles	Prodromal Signs
Females: Cervix Vulva/Perineum Legs Buttocks Anus	• Fever • Headache • Dysuria • Myalgias—pain in the muscles • Burning and tingling	• Itching • Burning • Tingling or an abnormal sensation prior to presence of a vesicle or ulcer
Males: Penis Prepuce (penile) (foreskin) Scrotum Anus Buttocks Thighs Inside urethra	• Itching localized to groin area • Swollen lymph nodes in groin area • Flu-like symptoms	• Itching • Burning • Tingling or an abnormal sensation prior to presence of a vesicle or ulcer

detect HSV antibodies. Samples may be obtained from a vesicle or ulcers, skin or mucous membranes, or spinal fluid. Type-specific laboratory confirmation is necessary because the vesicles or ulcers may be missed or may resemble another type of infection. A surface protein, glycoprotein (GgG) is an accurate serology test that elicits type-specific antibody responses; HSV-specific glycoprotein G1 is used to diagnose HSV-1, and HSV-specific glycoprotein G2 is used to diagnose HSV-2. Immunoglobulin M (IgM) testing for HSV-1 or HSV-2 is not useful because it is not type-specific, and its antibodies may be detectable during recurrent genital or oral episodes. Both type-specific virology and type-specific serology testing should be available in the clinical setting for prognostic and counseling implications; however, routine serological testing of asymptomatic individuals is not recommended because it may heighten the risk of false-positive test results.

Medications

Medication therapy consists of antiviral medications to suppress the infection and provide symptom relief. Antiviral medications can also help to decrease the duration and severity of the infection. Currently, there is no cure for genital herpes.

Primary therapy is used to treat all newly diagnosed outbreaks in a patient. Fever, malaise, and a headache may accompany the genital lesion outbreak. Treatment may help to lessen the severity and duration of symptoms. *Episodic therapy* is used to treat symptoms that occur intermittently. Episodic therapy is most effective when treatment begins in the prodromal stage or within the first 24 hours. *Suppressive therapy*, regular daily dosing with an antiviral, is used to reduce the incidence of outbreaks by 70% to 80%. Suppressive therapy may be encouraged for individuals who have six or more outbreaks in a year. Because the incidence of outbreaks tends to lessen with time, the provider should have frequent communication with the patient to determine the continued necessity of suppressive therapy.

Nursing Management

Assessment and Analysis

The clinical manifestations of genital herpes are a result of HSV traveling down sensory pathways typically to the genital area in response to a physiological or psychological trigger or stress. As a result, a vesicle or painful blister appears that may last days to weeks. Prodromal symptoms such as itching or altered sensation may occur prior to the appearance of the blister, indicating the beginning of an outbreak. Along with the physical pain, psychological discomfort or embarrassment may result.

Nursing Diagnoses

- **Ineffective sexual pattern** related to abstinence from sexual activities until acute infection subsides; change in reproductive potential
- **Situational low self-esteem** related to expressions of shame or guilt

Nursing Interventions

■ *Assessments*

- Skin of buttocks and genital area
  The presence of clear vesicles or blisters indicates a herpes outbreak.
- Frequency of outbreaks
  Therapy is dictated by the frequency of outbreaks; six or more outbreaks in a year may indicate a need for suppressive therapy.

■ *Actions*

- Administer antiviral medications as ordered.
  Prompt initiation of medication in the prodromal stage helps decrease the severity and duration of the outbreak.
- Refer patient to support groups for counseling if needed.
  Group support is beneficial to expose the patient to others who have coped with infection and to help the patient validate and share feelings.
  Counseling is beneficial to help attain or nurture a healthy psychosocial makeup.

■ *Teaching*

- Educate the patient on prevention, manifestations, transmission of STIs, reducing the number of partners, and barrier methods.
  Safe sex can help decrease the transmission and occurrence of genital herpes.
- Instruct the patient to report any history of infection to sexual partners.
  The partner may be at risk and/or may need to be treated. It is important that the patient understand that genital herpes transmission is possible even when symptoms are not evident.
- Start treatment as soon as prodromal symptoms occur.
  Prompt treatment may decrease the severity and duration of an outbreak.
- The importance of abstinence during symptomatic episodes
  Abstinence during an acute outbreak can help reduce transmission to sexual partners.
- Educate patient on means to help alleviate symptoms.
  - Warm salt baths prn
    Assist with drying up the lesions and ease physical discomfort due to pain or itching from the vesicles or ulcers
  - Ice to the affected area
    May aid in relieving discomfort
  - Loose-fitting clothing
    Increased airflow may help ease discomfort and promote healing.

Evaluating Care Outcomes

Genital herpes is a non–life-threatening, incurable infection that can have physical and psychological consequences. A well-managed patient understands that effective management requires prompt treatment as soon as prodromal symptoms are evident. This patient understands that normal, healthy sexual relationships are possible with appropriate safe-sex practices, abstinence during acute outbreaks, and proper treatment with antivirals.

Connection Check 67.3

Which statement is correct when providing discharge instructions to a patient with genital herpes?

A. Genital herpes is an infection that is always symptomatic.

B. Genital herpes is a mildly contagious infection.

C. Genital herpes is an infection that can be cured by antivirals.

D. A person can transmit HSV to others without displaying any symptoms.

CHLAMYDIA TRACHOMATIS

Epidemiology

Chlamydia trachomatis (chlamydia) is the most common sexually transmitted bacterial infection. It is a urogenital infection that primarily infects the urethra and cervix. It is transmitted through vaginal, anal, or oral sexual intercourse via bodily secretions. Transmission may occur during childbirth, from mother to child, and may lead to conditions such as conjunctivitis, pharyngitis, and pneumonia. Globally, the WHO reports there are more than 131 million cases annually. Although cases are felt to be underreported, the CDC estimated approximately 1.6 million new cases annually in the United States in 2016. The frequency and morbidity of *Chlamydia* infections are reported to be greater in females. Simultaneous *Chlamydia* infection often occurs with gonorrhea, but the incidence of chlamydia is greater.

Risk factors for *Chlamydia* include age, particularly 25 years or younger; low socioeconomic status; multiple sexual partners; history of STIs; unmarried status; immature cervix; and a diagnosis of mucopurulent inflammation of the cervix. Three groups at high risk are sexually active females under the age of 25, persons over the age of 25 who frequently engage in sexual intercourse with a new partner, and MSM. The CDC recommends that these groups be screened annually.

Pathophysiology and Clinical Manifestations

C trachomatis, the bacteria that causes chlamydia, is an **obligate intracellular bacterium** that cannot grow outside a living cell; it needs the metabolism of the host to reproduce. The incubation period is between 7 and 21 days. Its cellular walls resemble gram-negative bacteria.

Connection Check 67.4

The nurse recognizes that which patient is at the greatest risk for *C trachomatis*?

A. An 18-year-old single female

B. A 45-year-old married female

C. A 60-year-old single female

D. A 30-year-old married male

Most individuals who contract chlamydia have no symptoms; only 5% to 30% of females and 10% of males develop symptoms. Table 67.4 displays the female and male manifestations of chlamydia.

Management

Medical Management

Diagnosis

The diagnosis of chlamydia is made through a swab specimen taken from the vagina, cervix, penis, urethra, rectum, or other involved orifice. It is done utilizing a highly sensitive assay called the *nucleic acid amplification test (NAAT)*. To obtain a urethral specimen from a male, the swab is placed in the urethral meatus about 2 to 3 cm. Samples from females should be taken from the vagina or endocervix. If a urine sample is obtained, the most sensitive sample is obtained during the first void in the morning. Many reports describe the coexistence of *Chlamydia* infection with gonorrhea; therefore, patients should be routinely tested for both infections simultaneously. Individuals diagnosed with chlamydia should be rescreened in 3 months after completion of prescribed therapies because there is a high risk for reinfection.

Medications

Medication therapy consists of doxycycline or azithromycin as first-line treatment of *C trachomatis* for nonpregnant females, males, and HIV-infected individuals. Azithromycin is administered in one dose, in contrast to doxycycline,

Table 67.4 Manifestations of Chlamydia	
Clinical Symptoms in Females	**Clinical Symptoms in Males**
• Dysuria—painful urination	• Dysuria
• Dyspareunia—painful sexual intercourse	• Urethral discharge (clear or cloudy)
• Lower abdominal pain	• Meatitis—inflammation of the urinary meatus
• Abnormal vaginal bleeding (postcoital/after sexual intercourse or intermenstrual/between menses)	• Proctitis or rectal discharge (clear or cloudy)
• Vaginal discharge (clear or cloudy)	
• Cervical abnormalities (friable, tender, inflamed)	
• Proctitis (inflammation of the rectum or anus) or rectal discharge (clear or cloudy)	
Rectal infections may occur in both females and males: discharge, anal itching, soreness, bleeding and painful bowel movements	

which is administered twice daily for 7 days. For this reason, azithromycin is the medication of choice for patients at risk of noncompliance with lengthy medication regimens; however, both medications are equally effective. If doxycycline is chosen, it is important to warn against excessive sun exposure. Erythromycin is an alternative medication used to treat pregnant females.

 Safety Alert   Expedited Partner Therapy

Expedited partner therapy (EPT) is the clinical practice of providing a prescription to the partner of a patient diagnosed with chlamydia or gonorrhea without completing a physical exam on the partner. The purpose of EPT is to prevent reinfection, halt the spread of the disease, and lessen long-term sequelae to the female reproductive system. Quick partner treatment provides another strategy for partner notification. Providers advise their patients to inform their partners to get tested or treated. Expedited partner therapy increases the number of partners treated and decreases the likelihood of reinfection by 29%. Expedited partner therapy is available in most states and many countries throughout the world and shows promise as a public health initiative in decreasing chlamydia and gonococcal infections at a population level.

Centers for Disease Control and Prevention 2017 Expedited Partner TherapyCenters for Disease Control and Prevention. (2017, July 3). *Expedited partner therapy*. Retrieved from https://www.cdc.gov/std/ept/default.htm 201801081142511773430229

Complications

If left untreated in females, the *Chlamydia* infection may travel to the uterus and fallopian tubes and cause a condition called pelvic inflammatory disease (PID). This condition is addressed later in this chapter. In males, if the *Chlamydia* infection spreads, it may travel to the epididymis, causing **epididymitis** (inflammation of the epididymis), a rare condition, or prostate gland infection. Further complications in women include infertility, tubal abscesses, ectopic pregnancy, chronic pelvic pain, and **Fitz–Hugh–Curtis syndrome** (perihepatitis, or inflammation of the peritoneal covering of the liver). Other complications include **Reiter's syndrome**, also known as reactive arthritis. This is a rare autoimmune arthritic condition that causes **urethritis**, or inflammation in the urinary genital tract, and conjunctivitis, an inflammation of the mucous membranes lining the eyes.

Nursing Management
Assessment and Analysis

Both females and males may be asymptomatic for chlamydia; however, dysuria is a symptom that may occur. Females may experience lower abdominal pain and painful intercourse because of inflammation caused by the infection.

Males may present with inflammation and infection of the urinary meatus.

Nursing Diagnosis
- **Risk of infection**: Risk factors: insufficient knowledge to avoid exposure to pathogens; unsafe sex practices

Nursing Interventions
■ *Assessments*
- Monitor vital signs, particularly temperature.
  Increased temperature may signal infection. Monitoring temperature helps to evaluate the course of infection and response to treatment.
- Monitor current signs/symptoms of STI.
  Symptoms, when present, indicate active infection. Monitoring helps in the evaluation of response to treatment.
- Urinary function
  Dysuria in both males and females is a clinical manifestation of chlamydia.
- Pain during intercourse
  Painful intercourse may occur with a Chlamydia *infection.*
- Unusual vaginal bleeding or discharge from urinary meatus
  Bleeding or discharge is a manifestation of a Chlamydia *infection.*

■ *Actions*
- Administer antibiotics as ordered.
  Antibiotics such as azithromycin, doxycycline, and erythromycin are the treatment of choice for chlamydia.

■ *Teaching*
- Educate the patient on prevention, manifestations, transmission of STIs, reducing the number of partners, and barrier methods.
  Safe sex can help decrease the transmission and occurrence of chlamydia.
- Instruct the patient to report any history of infection to sexual partners.
  The partner may be at risk and/or may need to be treated. Early treatment can reduce untoward complications of infection.
- Educate the patient on the importance of taking the entire prescribed therapy.
  The patient may develop resistance to the antibiotic if the entire regimen is not completed.
- Call the provider if experiencing worsening pain and/or vaginal discharge.
  May be an indication of a worsening condition or complication
- Encourage healthy practices (routine gynecological and primary care, healthy diet, no drinking or smoking).
  Improve outcomes and well-being
- Instruct the patient on the importance of getting retested for chlamydia in 3 months.
  Reinfection is common.

Evaluating Care Outcomes

Successful management of the patient with chlamydia requires prompt diagnosis and treatment with appropriate antibiotics. A well-managed patient completes the entire prescribed therapy and understands that safe-sex practices are essential in limiting reoccurrence and transmission to sexual partners.

NEISSERIA GONORRHOEAE

Epidemiology

Neisseria gonorrhoeae (gonorrhea) is the second most common bacterial STI, after chlamydia. Like chlamydia, gonorrhea tends to be underdiagnosed and underreported. Globally, the WHO reports there are more than 78 million cases annually. The CDC reported a total of 468,514 gonorrhea cases in 2016. Although rates have decreased from those reported in the 1990s, the national rate increased to 145.8 cases per 100,000 population in 2016. The CDC reports an increase in incidence with younger persons, with the highest rates in males and females aged 20 to 24. The CDC also reports an increase in incidence in MSM and in populations in endemic areas of the United States where the infection is routinely seen.

Risk factors are similar to those of chlamydia: age, particularly under 25 years old; low socioeconomic status; multiple sexual partners; history of STIs, including PID; and unmarried status. The CDC suggests that high-risk groups be screened annually.

Pathophysiology and Clinical Manifestations

Gonorrhea is transmitted through genital-to-genital, oral-to-genital, and anal-to-genital contact. Perinatal transmission (mother to infant) during delivery may also occur. It is caused by the bacterium *Neisseria gonorrhoeae*, also known as gonococcus, a gram-negative intracellular diplococcus. These gonococci attach to the surface of columnar mucosa epithelial cells. Local invasion occurs and attacks the mucosal surfaces of the genitourinary tract, eyes, throat, and rectum. The gonococci replicate and invade host immune cells, leading to dissemination and systemic infection. The incubation period for females is usually less than 10 days. For males, the incubation period is usually within a 14-day period. Approximately 50% of females and males experience clinical manifestations. See Table 67.5 for the female and male clinical manifestations of gonorrhea.

Management

Medical Management

Diagnosis

The diagnosis of gonorrhea is made through the NAAT assay. It is the most sensitive and specific test to detect gonorrhea in women. The test is costly, but the results are

Table 67.5 Manifestations of Gonorrhea

Clinical Manifestations in Females	Clinical Manifestations in Males
• Vaginal discharge	• Dysuria (which occurs before purulent discharge)
• Intermenstrual bleeding	
• Anorectal discomfort	• Copious purulent urethral discharge (gold standard manifestation for gonococcal urethritis)
• Dysuria	
• Cervicitis—inflammation of the cervix	• Rectal pain, bleeding, or purulent discharge

Rectal infections may occur in both females and males; manifestations include discharge, anal itching, soreness, bleeding, and painful bowel movements.

available rapidly. Samples can be obtained from the vagina, cervix, and urine. All samples from the male or female must be immediately placed into the proper medium and transported promptly to the laboratory. Diagnosis may also be made by culture. The results are extremely sensitive for males and females who are symptomatic but are less sensitive in those who are asymptomatic. In addition to detecting gonococci, the culture test has the added benefit of detecting antibiotic resistance. The culture test is less expensive than the NAAT, with a turnaround time of 48 hours. The collection procedure is similar to that for obtaining chlamydia cells.

Gram staining may be used to test the urethra in males. It is a highly sensitive and specific test and is considered positive if polymorphonuclear leukocytes with intracellular gram-negative diplococci are present (Fig. 67.6); however, stains demonstrate low sensitivity for males who are asymptomatic. Concomitant infection with chlamydia may occur; therefore, testing should be done for both.

Connection Check 67.5

The nurse recognizes that which statements are true of gonorrhea? *(Select all that apply.)*

A. Gonococci are viruses caused by *N gonorrhoeae*.

B. Concomitant infection with chlamydia can occur; therefore, test for both.

C. Gonorrhea remains localized to an expectant mother; therefore, there is a very low risk of vertical transmission to the infant.

D. The NAAT is effective in the detection of genitourinary infection with *N gonorrhoeae*.

E. A hallmark symptom in males with gonorrhea is copious purulent urethral discharge.

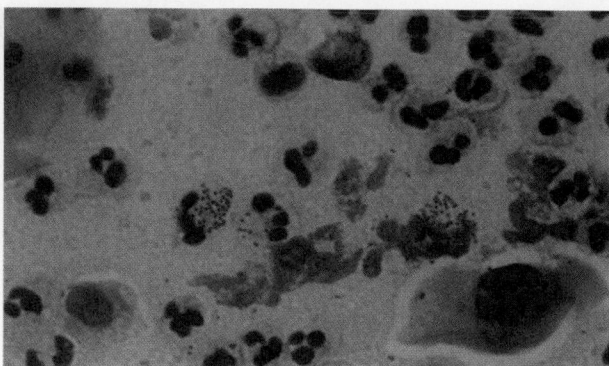

FIGURE 67.6 Gram stain of urethral discharge from a male patient with gonorrhea shows gram-negative intracellular diplococci.

Medications

Quinolone-resistant strains of gonorrhea have been detected worldwide. As a result, a classification of antimicrobial medications called *fluoroquinolones* should not be administered to patients to treat gonorrhea. Instead, the CDC recommends a dual treatment of two medications to treat gonorrhea (see Safety Alert). One is an antimicrobial classification of medications called *cephalosporins*. Ceftriaxone is a *cephalosporin*, administered intramuscularly or intravenously. The second medication is a semisynthetic macrolide antibiotic called azithromycin. Azithromycin is also used to treat several bacterial infections other than STIs. Infectious disease consultation should be considered for those individuals who experience treatment failure due to antibiotic resistance.

⚠ Safety Alert **Antibiotic-Resistant Gonorrhea**

With the global increase in the incidence of gonorrhea has come the rise of antimicrobial-resistant cases. Over the years, certain gonorrhea strains have developed resistance to microbials such as penicillin, tetracycline, and fluoroquinolones. This led to extended-spectrum cephalosporins (cefixime or ceftriaxone) as a treatment option. However, many global countries reported cephalosporin resistance. The macrolide antibiotic azithromycin was administered to patients who could not tolerate cephalosporins. When used alone, some patients developed azithromycin resistance. The CDC identified the dual (two-medication) therapy for treatment (ceftriaxone and azithromycin) for gonorrhea with the aim of delaying the appearance of gonorrhea strains resistant to either medication. The combination of these two medications has been shown to be successful in the treatment of gonorrhea. New medications continue to be studied and evaluated for possible dual-therapy use in the future.

Centers for Disease Control and Prevention. (2015). *Gonococcal Isolate Surveillance Project (GISP)*. Retrieved from https://www.cdc.gov/std/gisp

---

Complications

Complications in females include PID, pelvic abscesses, ectopic pregnancy, infertility, and Fitz–Hugh–Curtis syndrome. In males, epididymitis and, in rare cases, infertility may occur. Disseminated gonococcal infection may lead to systemic complications such as arthritis, tenosynovitis (common), and skin lesions. Rare complications include endocarditis and meningitis.

Nursing Management

Assessment and Analysis

The clinical manifestations of gonorrhea are similar to those of chlamydia. Unusual vaginal bleeding, dysuria, rectal pain, vaginal or urethral drainage in females and dysuria, rectal pain, gonococcal urethritis, and urethral discharge in males are caused by inflammation due to the infectious process.

Nursing Diagnosis

- **Risk of infection**: Risk factors: insufficient knowledge to avoid exposure to pathogens; unsafe sex practices

Nursing Interventions

▪ Assessments

- Monitor vital signs, particularly temperature.
  Increased temperature may signal infection. Monitoring temperature helps to evaluate the course of infection and response to treatment.
- Monitor current signs/symptoms of STI.
  Symptoms indicate active infection. Monitoring helps in the evaluation of the response to treatment.
- Urinary function
  Dysuria in both males and females is a clinical manifestation of gonorrhea.
- Rectal pain
  Rectal pain is a common clinical manifestation of gonorrhea in both males and females.
- Vaginal bleeding or discharge from the urinary meatus
  Bleeding and discharge are manifestations of gonorrhea infections.

▪ Actions

- Administer antibiotics as ordered.
  Antibiotics such as ceftriaxone and azithromycin are the treatment of choice for gonorrhea.

▪ Teaching

- Educate the patient on prevention, manifestations, transmission of STIs, reducing the number of partners, and barrier methods.
  Safe sex can help decrease the transmission and occurrence of gonorrhea.
- Instruct the patient to report any history of infection to sexual partners.
  The partner may be at risk and/or may need to be treated. Early treatment can reduce untoward complications of infection.

- Educate the patient on the importance of taking the entire prescribed therapy.
  The patient may develop resistance to the antibiotic if the entire regimen is not completed.
- Call the provider if experiencing worsening pain and/or vaginal discharge.
  May be an indication of a worsening condition or complication
- Encourage healthy practices (routine gynecological and primary care, healthy diet, no drinking or smoking).
  Improve health outcomes and well-being
- Instruct the patient on the importance of getting retested for gonorrhea in 3 months.
  To check for reinfection

Evaluating Care Outcomes

Gonorrhea is a common bacterial infection, especially in high-risk groups. Many findings report that males and females continue to engage in risky sexual practices and therefore should be tested routinely. Partners of those infected should also be tested and treated accordingly. Successful management of the patient with gonorrhea requires prompt diagnosis and treatment with appropriate antibiotics. A well-managed patient completes the entire prescribed therapy and understands that safe-sex practices are essential in limiting reoccurrence and transmission to sexual partners.

CASE STUDY: EPISODE 2

During her physical examination by her OB/GYN provider, Keisha complains of lower abdominal pain. On examination, the provider notes that Keisha has mucopurulent discharge coming from her cervix, along with uterine tenderness. The provider sends NAAT cervical swabs for gonorrhea and chlamydia and performs a Pap test and a wet prep that immediately show the presence of white blood cells (WBCs). Serology is sent for HIV, syphilis, and hepatitis. As part of his work-up, the provider sends Keisha for a transvaginal ultrasound…

PELVIC INFLAMMATORY DISEASE

Epidemiology

According to the National Health and Nutrition Examination Survey (NHANES), of U.S. women aged 18 to 44, 2.5 million have experienced a diagnosis of PID in their lifetime; however, the accurate number may be higher because of unreported cases. This leads to approximately 60,000 hospitalizations, 106,000 outpatient visits, and frequent emergency visits annually. Overall, the trend in the prevalence of PID has decreased within the United States and other resource-rich countries within the last decade.

The risk factors for PID are similar to those for other STIs and include unprotected sexual intercourse, sexual intercourse at 25 years old or younger, oral contraceptive use, multiple sexual partners, and previous history of PID. Bacterial vaginosis, douching, sexual intercourse during menses, and intrauterine devices may contribute to the onset of PID by causing a disturbance in the cervical barrier that may aid in the movement of bacteria through the pelvic cavity.

Pathophysiology

Pelvic inflammatory disease is an acute infection that originates from the vagina or cervix and ascends to the upper genital tract, infecting the uterus, fallopian tubes, and ovaries. Pelvic inflammatory disease is a polymicrobial infection caused by an STI such as chlamydia or gonorrhea or by other pathogenic microorganisms that comprise the normal vaginal flora (Fig. 67.7; see Evidence-Based Practice: Another Bacterial Infection Associated With PID).

Evidence-Based Practice

Another Bacterial Infection Associated With PID

There is growing evidence that *Mycoplasma genitalium*, a slow-growing sexually transmitted pathogenic bacterium, is associated with pelvic inflammatory disease (PID). This bacterial infection is seen in 0.4% of young adults. In males, *M genitalium* may cause urethritis (inflammation of the urethra) and is linked to nongonococcal urethritis (NGU) and nonchlamydial urethritis. Persistent and recurrent urethritis attaches itself to the epithelial cells. In women, *M genitalium* can be detected in the cervix and/or endometrium of women with PID. This infection in women is typically asymptomatic. *M genitalium* may cause PID and tubal infertility but not as often as chlamydia. There is no current diagnostic test approved by the U.S. Food and Drug Administration (FDA) available in the United States. However, with the advent of the nucleic acid amplification test (NAAT), more studies are being conducted to understand the pathogenicity (cause of disease) of this organism. Treatment is dependent on the symptoms associated with urethritis and cervicitis (inflammation of the cervix) or PID.

Centers for Disease Control and Prevention 2015 Sexually Transmitted Diseases Treatment Guidelines, 2015.Centers for Disease Control and Prevention. (2015). Sexually transmitted diseases treatment guidelines, 2015. *Morbidity and Mortality Weekly Report, 64*(3), 1–140. Retrieved from http://www.cdc.gov 20171217160447762587428

Muonz, J. L., & Goje, O. J. (2016). *Mycoplasma genitalium*: An emerging sexually transmitted infection. *Scientifica, 2016*(7537318), 1–5. doi:10.1155/2016/7537318 2018060914163895 3178763

Sethi, S., Zaman, K., & Jain, N. (2017). *Mycoplasma genitalium* infections: Current treatment options and resistance issues. *Infection and Drug Resistance, 2017*(10), 283–292. doi:10.2147/IDR.S105469

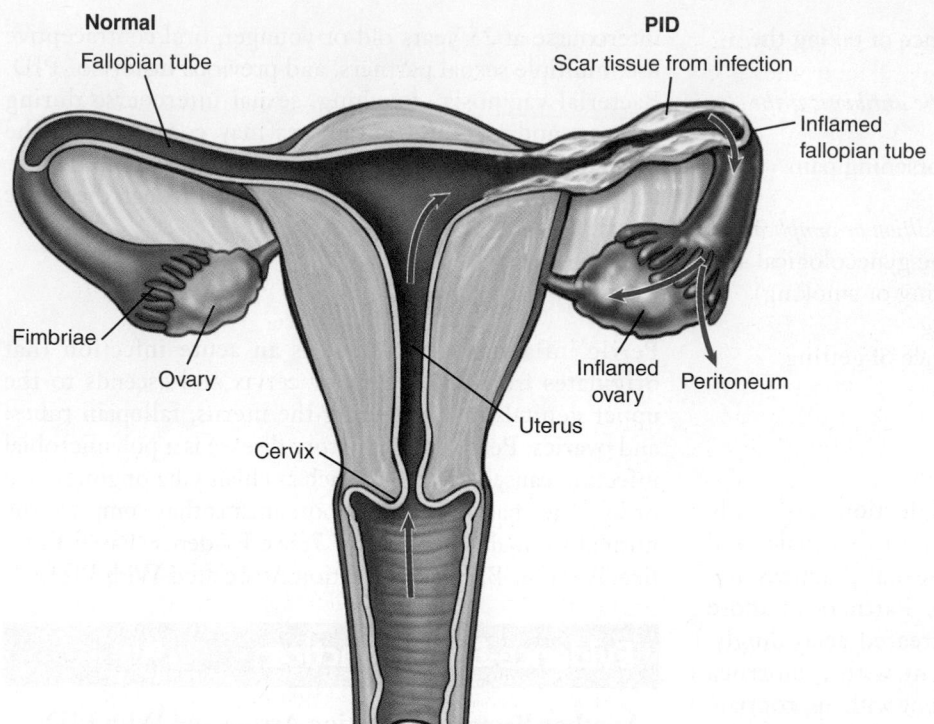

Normal

Fallopian tube

Fimbriae

Ovary

Cervix

Uterus

PID

Scar tissue from infection

Inflamed fallopian tube

Inflamed ovary

Peritoneum

FIGURE 67.7 Normal female anatomy (L) and female anatomy with pelvic inflammatory disease and its sequelae (R).

Clinical Manifestations

Clinical manifestations of PID include:

- Lower abdominal pain
- Uterine tenderness
- Adnexal tenderness, which is pain in the ovaries or fallopian tubes noted during examination
- Cervical motion tenderness

Management

Medical Management

Diagnosis

Pelvic inflammatory disease is a challenge to diagnose due to the variety of symptoms and the subtle or lack of symptoms the patient may experience. Additionally, the clinical manifestations that present with a diagnosis of PID may have other causes, which should be ruled out. Diagnosis is primarily done through clinical observation of the presence of lower abdominal pain in combination with one or all of the clinical manifestations indicative of PID. Additional criteria that can reinforce a diagnosis of PID are the following:

- Oral temperature greater than 101°F (<38.3°C)
- Abnormal cervical or vaginal mucopurulent discharge or cervical friability
- Abundance of WBCs on saline microscopy of vaginal fluid
- Elevated C-reactive protein level
- Elevated erythrocyte sedimentation rate
- Laboratory-confirmed diagnosis of chlamydia or gonorrhea

Radiological imaging such as transvaginal ultrasound and magnetic resonance imaging (MRI) can be used as an aid in diagnosing PID if the clinical determination is uncertain. Other procedures used to diagnose PID are endometrial biopsy and laparoscopy. Doppler studies may be used if a pelvic infection is suspected. Laparoscopy, once viewed as the gold standard for diagnosis, detects limited symptoms of PID, such as **salpingitis** (inflammation of the fallopian tube). This procedure is difficult to justify given the variety of symptoms that can occur with PID in addition to salpingitis. Also, it can be costly and may promote increased procedural risks, such as infection, bleeding, and organ injury.

Treatment

Treatment of PID should be initiated as soon as the diagnosis is strongly suspected. Treatment may be done on an inpatient or outpatient basis. Inpatient hospitalization is considered for the following reasons:

- If the patient does not respond well to or tolerate oral antibiotics
- Pregnancy
- Severe illness
- Differential diagnoses such as tubo-ovarian abscess (TOA) or appendicitis
- Suspected ectopic pregnancy

Hospitalized patients should receive parenteral or IV antibiotic treatment for a minimal of 24 hours and should be changed to oral antibiotics when clinical symptoms improve. Outpatient treatment includes both a single intramuscular dose of ceftriaxone and oral antibiotics such as metronidazole or doxycycline. It is important to educate patients to abstain from alcohol when taking metronidazole because of the potential of serious side effects. Both parenteral and oral regimens have comparable efficacies.

Complications of PID

The complications of PID are chronic pelvic pain, infertility, and ectopic pregnancy. Occasionally, females with PID may be diagnosed with a TOA, an inflammatory mass involving the fallopian tubes, ovaries, and neighboring organs. A ruptured TOA can lead to peritonitis (inflammation of the peritoneum) or sepsis and is considered a surgical emergency. Ultrasound or computed tomography (CT) may be used to diagnose TOA. Patients with TOA should be hospitalized for at least 24 hours for treatment with parenteral antibiotics. After discharge, oral antibiotics are continued.

Connection Check 67.6

The nurse recognizes that which of the following statements are true of PID? *(Select all that apply.)*

A. Pelvic inflammatory disease is an acute infection that routinely descends from the upper genital tract to the cervix or vagina.

B. If the patient is diagnosed with PID and is pregnant, inpatient admission should be considered.

C. Symptoms such as lower abdominal pain and elevated blood pressure are specific criteria for PID.

D. Laparoscopy is the only definitive test to diagnose PID.

E. A tubo-ovarian abscess is a severe complication of PID.

Nursing Management
Assessment and Analysis

The clinical manifestations of PID—lower abdominal pain, uterine and adnexal tenderness, and abnormal purulent vaginal discharge—are due to the inflammation occurring in the upper genital tract. Other manifestations are related to the inflammatory process, such as elevated temperature and increased C-reactive protein and sedimentation rates, both markers of inflammation.

Nursing Diagnoses

- **Acute pain** related to biological injury, inflammation, edema, congestion of the pelvic tissues
- **Anxiety** related to the disease/infectious process

Nursing Interventions
▪ *Assessments*

- Pain
  Lower abdominal pain with uterine or adnexal tenderness may be present because of the upper genital tract inflammation.
- Unusual vaginal bleeding or discharge
  Bleeding or discharge is due to irritation and inflammation in the genital tract.
- Temperature
  A fever may be due to the acute inflammatory process.

- Sexual practices
  Multiple partners and unprotected sex expose the patient to pathogens and thus increase the risk of STIs and PID.
- Birth control
  The presence of intrauterine devices disturbs the cervical barrier and allows for the movement of pathogens into the upper genital tract, as does douching.
- Previous STI or PID
  Repeated STIs or previous PID is a risk factor for PID.

▪ *Actions*

- Administer antibiotics as ordered.
  Prompt antibiotic treatment is necessary to prevent long-term sequelae from PID.

▪ *Teaching*

- Educate the patient on prevention, manifestations, transmission of STIs, reducing the number of partners, and barrier methods.
  Safe sex can help decrease the occurrence of PID.
- Avoid douching, tub baths, tampon use, and sexual intercourse during active infection.
  Avoid activities that may bring bacteria into the upper genital tract.
- Educate the patient on the importance of taking the entire prescribed therapy.
  The patient may develop resistance to the antibiotic if the entire regimen is not completed.
- Call the provider if experiencing worsening pain and/or vaginal discharge.
  May be an indication of a worsening condition or complication

Evaluating Care Outcomes

Safe-sex practices can help decrease the occurrence of STIs and PID. A well-managed patient receives early intervention that includes proper diagnosis, the establishment of an effective antibiotic regimen, and suitable follow-up and maintenance to avoid the potential complications of PID.

 Safety Alert **Adolescents and STIs**

Young people 15 to 24 years old account for nearly half of the 20 million reported STI cases. Vulnerable adolescents engage in risky behavior for affection, social status, and sexual desire. They can be easily influenced by the media and/or peer pressure. Some adolescents possess a false sense of invincibility and denial because they do not see the deleterious and potentially life-long effects resulting from the infections. Engagement in these risky sexual behaviors can lead to unfavorable outcomes. Schools, youth-serving programs, family, the community, and online and mobile technologies should support and promote positive, healthy behavioral changes, preferably before the onset of sexual intercourse. Counselors and health professionals should be readily available to promote healthy communication between adolescents and their parents. Educational content should be all-inclusive and developmentally appropriate to promote abstinence. It should discuss the myths and harmful effects of acquiring an STI, risk factors, and sexual and non-sexual strategies that can limit contraction and transmission.

Making Connections

CASE STUDY: WRAP-UP

On completion of Keisha's physical assessment and radiology test, the provider diagnoses her with PID. She is given an intramuscular shot of ceftriaxone and sent home with a prescription for oral doxycycline and metronidazole to be taken for 14 days. Keisha's nurse educates her about the medications and provides information on steps to make positive lifestyle changes related to drinking, smoking, and unhealthy sexual practices. Keisha is asked to return within 3 days to check the status of symptoms and to obtain the results of her test.

Keisha returns in 3 days as requested. She states that she is feeling much better, which is confirmed by a clinical examination by her provider. All results are negative except for chlamydia. Keisha is informed that the chlamydia can be treated with doxycycline, so no additional antibiotics are necessary. Keisha is very interested in making some lifestyle changes because the diagnosis of PID has really scared her. The nurse provides Keisha with community resources, the number to the local health department, and informative Web sites to assist her in making these modifications for better health. She is asked to return in 3 months to be retested for at-risk STIs.

Case Study Questions

1. Keisha is diagnosed with chlamydia during her recent examination. The nurse is aware that this infection can transcend the upper genital tract and lead to which clinical manifestations if untreated?
   A. Leg/calf tenderness, adnexal tenderness, pelvic tenderness
   B. Heavy menses, abdominal pain, fatigue
   C. Elevated C-reactive protein, positive rapid plasma reagin (RPR), elevated erythrocyte sedimentation rate (ESR)
   D. Uterine tenderness, abdominal pain, cervical motion tenderness

2. Keisha is diagnosed with PID. If left untreated, what complication is she at risk for developing?
   A. Uterine prolapse
   B. Polycystic ovary syndrome
   C. Infertility
   D. Endometriosis

3. Keisha is prescribed metronidazole (Flagyl) as part of the medications she needs to take after discharge. When addressing this medication, what should the nurse explain?
   A. "This medication should be taken only on an empty stomach."
   B. "This medication should be refrigerated."
   C. "When you take this medication, alcohol should be avoided."
   D. "When you start feeling better, this medication can be discontinued."

4. The nurse provides recommendations for which healthy lifestyle changes for Keisha? *(Select all that apply.)*
   A. Avoid sexual intercourse while under the influence of drugs or alcohol.
   B. Limit the number of sexual partners.
   C. Utilize condoms if engaging in sexual activity.
   D. Seek out reputable Web sites to become properly informed about STIs.
   E. Abstain from sexual intercourse.

5. Which statements by Keisha indicate that teaching has been effective? *(Select all that apply.)*
   A. "I know I should eat well and limit sexual activity for a while."
   B. "I can expect my symptoms to improve within 3 days."
   C. "There is no point in telling my boyfriend; I can't give him PID!"
   D. "I should call my provider if I experience a fever, increased abdominal pain, vaginal discharge, or nausea and vomiting."
   E. "Because I was prescribed doxycycline, I know I should avoid prolonged exposure to sunlight."

CHAPTER SUMMARY

Human papillomavirus (HPV) is a very common sexually transmitted infection (STI) of the anogenital tract. Risk factors are related to sexual behavior, including early onset of sexual activity, multiple partners, and unprotected sex. Females with nononcogenic HPV may experience symptoms of genital warts. Oncogenic HPV is the precursor to cervical cancer. The Papanicolaou (Pap) test is the most used tool to screen females for cervical cancer. Human papillomavirus DNA testing, an evaluation of cells scraped from the cervix, is used to detect high-risk oncogenic HPV and is routinely ordered in women 30 years and older.

Syphilis is classified into four stages: primary, secondary, latent (early and late), and tertiary. Syphilis is most infectious during the primary and secondary phases. Latent phases are not contagious, but if not treated, severe complications can occur. The tertiary stage is a rare complication of syphilis developing 10 to 30 years after the initial infection. This stage may affect a multitude of organs, causing tissue damage and disfigurement, cardiovascular damage, and central nervous system (CNS) changes. However, neurosyphilis can occur at any stage. The risk factors are similar to those of other STIs and include early onset of sexual activity, multiple partners, and unprotected sex. The therapy for all stages of syphilis is penicillin.

Genital herpes is a common, chronic, and at-present, incurable STI caused by herpes simplex virus 1 (HSV-1) and herpes simplex virus 2 (HSV-2). The risk factors for genital herpes are similar to those of other STIs. The clinical manifestations include an outbreak of clear vesicles or blisters in the genital area that rupture and form a painful ulcer several days later. Medication therapy consists of antiviral medications used to suppress the infection and provide symptom relief.

Chlamydia trachomatis (chlamydia) is the most common sexually transmitted bacterial infection. The majority of individuals who contract chlamydia do not have symptoms.

The complications include infertility, tubal abscesses, ectopic pregnancy, chronic pelvic pain, and Fitz–Hugh–Curtis syndrome (perihepatitis, or inflammation of the peritoneal covering of the liver). Medication therapy consists of doxycycline or azithromycin as first-line treatment.

Neisseria gonorrhoeae (gonorrhea) is the second most common bacterial STI, after to chlamydia. They commonly occur together. The clinical manifestations include vaginal discharge, intermenstrual bleeding, anorectal discomfort, dysuria, and cervicitis—inflammation of the cervix. Medication therapy consists of a combination of ceftriaxone (injection) and azithromycin (orally).

Pelvic inflammatory disease (PID) is an acute infection that originates from the vagina or cervix and ascends to the upper genital tract—the uterus, fallopian tubes, and ovaries. The risk factors for PID are similar to those of other STIs. The clinical manifestations of PID include lower abdominal pain, uterine tenderness, and adnexal tenderness. The treatment of PID is IV or oral antibiotics, which should be initiated as soon as the diagnosis is strongly suspected. The complications of PID are chronic pelvic pain, infertility, and ectopic pregnancy.

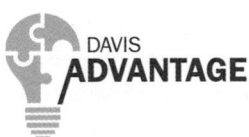

DAVIS
ADVANTAGE | To explore learning resources for this chapter, go to **Davis Advantage** and find:
- Answers to in-text questions
- Chapter Resources and Activities
- NCLEX®-Style Chapter Review Questions
- Bibliography

Unit XVI

Promoting Health in Special Populations

Chapter **68**

Managing Care for the Adult Patient With Obesity

Alice Moore

LEARNING OUTCOMES

Content in this chapter is designed to assist in:

1. Describing the epidemiology of obesity.
2. Describing the pathophysiology of obesity
3. Correlating clinical manifestations to pathophysiological processes of obesity
4. Describing the diagnostic results used to confirm the diagnosis of obesity
5. Discussing the medical management of obesity
6. Describing complications associated with morbid obesity
7. Developing a comprehensive plan of nursing care for patients with obesity
8. Developing a teaching plan for a patient with obesity

ESSENTIAL TERMS

Anastomosis
Anorexigenic
Bariatrics
Basal metabolic rate
Body mass index (BMI)
Dumping syndrome
Energy expenditure
Leptin
Obesogenic
Satiety

CONCEPTS

- Assessment
- Medication
- Metabolism
- Nutrition
- Perioperative

Finding Connections

CASE STUDY: EPISODE 1

Follow this patient throughout the chapter.

Lauren Wiley is a 34-year-old who was diagnosed with obesity 15 years ago. She has tried various dietary and exercise programs along with pharmaceutical options. Lauren describes that her weight is interfering with her ability to walk and participate in social activities with her family. She is currently 5 ft 6 in. tall and weighs 256 lb. She presents to her primary care provider to discuss a referral to a bariatric surgeon for weight loss…

CLASSIFICATIONS OF BODY WEIGHT

The degree to which a person has excess adipose tissue is classified in terms of being overweight and obese. **Body mass index (BMI)** is routinely used to classify body weight and correlates with total body adiposity. Body mass index is calculated by weight in kilograms divided by height in meters squared.

$$BMI\ (kg/m^2) = \frac{Weight\ (kilograms)}{Height\ (meters)^2}$$

Table 68.1 lists body weight classifications based on the National Institutes of Health (NIH) criteria.

In addition to BMI, waist circumference and overall health risks are important in the management of patients who are overweight or obese. Increased waist circumference correlates with abdominal adiposity. Subcutaneous and intra-abdominal adiposity significantly increases morbidity. In adults with a BMI of 25 to 34.9 kg/m², a waist circumference of greater than 102 cm (40 in.) in men and greater than 88 cm (35 in.) in women denotes an increased relative risk of obesity-related risk factors. The presence

Table 68.1 Classification of Body Weight

NIH Classification	BMI (kg/m²)
Underweight	Less than 18.5
Normal weight	18.5–24.9
Overweight	25.0–29.9
Obesity (class 1)	30.0–34.9
Obesity (class 2)	35.0–39.9
Extreme obesity (class 3)	Greater than 40.0

BMI, Body mass index; *NIH,* National Institutes of Health.

of obesity-related diseases, obesity-associated conditions, cardiovascular risks, and other risks increases the need for weight reduction in patients who are overweight and obese. Due to this growing prevalence of obesity, **bariatrics**, the medical specialty that focuses on the causes, prevention, and treatment of obesity, has expanded over the last decade.

Connection Check 68.1

Using the NIH classification for BMI, the nurse identifies the patient with a BMI of 32 kg/m² as which category?
A. Overweight
B. Class 1 obesity
C. Class 2 obesity
D. Extreme obesity

EPIDEMIOLOGY

Prevalence

Obesity has reached epidemic levels in the United States. According to the Center for Disease Control and Prevention, in 2017, the obesity prevalence rates in all states revealed that more than 20% of adults are obese. States ranged from 20% or less of the state population in Colorado and Hawaii to 35% or more in seven other states (Alabama, Arkansas, Iowa, Louisiana, Mississippi, Oklahoma, and West Virginia). In 2015–2016, 39.8% of adult Americans, approximately 93.3 million people, were considered obese; this is an increase from the 2011–2013 percentage of 34.9%. It is estimated that in 2013, of those persons categorized as obese, 41%, or 33.7 million people, were categorized as class 2 obesity or higher. On the basis of current trends, it is projected that 42% of all American adults will be obese by 2030.

Effects of Long-Term Obesity

Obesity increases mortality and significantly increases morbidity. Obesity and obesity-associated conditions significantly increase hospital length of stay and overall healthcare costs. Medicare and Medicaid finance 42% of the total medical costs attributed to obesity. In 2013, Medicaid paid nearly 11%, or $8 billion, of the cost to treat conditions associated with severe obesity and predicted an increase of $941 in annual per-capita medical expenditures for moderately obese adults and an increase of $1,980 for severe obesity. Annual hospital costs are $160 million higher in patients who are obese and undergo the most common nonbariatric surgical procedures compared with their normal-weight counterparts.

Impact on Mortality

Obesity causes a marked decrease in life expectancy, and the all-cause mortality (death from any cause) risk increases in patients with a BMI of greater than 30 kg/m². In the United States, the all-cause mortality rate is 20% higher in adults with obesity compared to adults with normal weight. The effect of a high BMI on mortality also increases with age. Class 2 and class 3 obesity in adults aged 45 to 64 is associated with premature death of at least 7 years from all-cause mortality and 10 years from cardiovascular disease–specific mortality.

Impact on Morbidity

Obesity is linked to numerous chronic health conditions, and there is a strong association between obesity and its major comorbidities. Type 2 diabetes mellitus (DM) is the most prevalent, with the overlap between type 2 DM and obesity being about 50%. Heart disease is the second most prevalent and is associated with metabolic syndrome, which is defined as central obesity, high serum triglyceride levels, lower serum high-density lipoprotein, elevated total cholesterol levels, hypertension, and elevated fasting blood glucose. These top two are followed by other comorbidities such as airway obstruction, chronic kidney disease, nonalcoholic fatty liver disease, infertility issues, gastroesophageal reflux disease (GERD), cancer, increased medication prescription for pain relief, and psychiatric disorders.

Obesity also increases the risk of stroke and obstructive sleep apnea. Gastrointestinal conditions such as GERD, cholelithiasis, and nonalcoholic fatty liver disease are increased in patients with obesity. Osteoarthritis is increased in non–weight-bearing and weight-bearing joints, suggesting that the disease of obesity itself rather than solely mechanical trauma causes the increase in osteoarthritis. Increased BMI is associated with a decreased glomerular filtration rate with progression to chronic kidney disease. Obesity increases the risk of cancer and also increases the likelihood of dying from cancer. Reproductive abnormalities are also seen. Obesity is associated with a decrease in psychosocial aspects of health, such as well-being and quality of life, and is related to an increase in social stigmatization and discrimination. Having a diagnosis of more than one comorbidity is highly associated with obesity and an increasing BMI category.

PATHOPHYSIOLOGY

The regulation of body weight is a complex interplay between appetite and **energy expenditure**. The hypothalamus is signaled by hormones, metabolites, and neural pathways to regulate appetite. Figure 68.1 displays the complex mechanisms that contribute to appetite. The majority of energy expenditure is in the form of basal metabolism, or the amount of energy required to maintain vital organ function, also referred to as the **basal metabolic rate**. **Leptin**, a hormone produced by fat cells, plays a major role in body weight. Two major roles of this hormone are communicating **satiety** (the feeling of being satisfied with the amount of food eaten) to the hypothalamus and regulating energy expenditure or balance. In addition, energy expenditure comes from an increase in physical activity or exercise and the metabolic requirements of metabolizing and storing food, along with thermogenesis, which varies according to chronic caloric intake levels. Weight gain occurs when the intake of caloric nutrients exceeds energy expenditure.

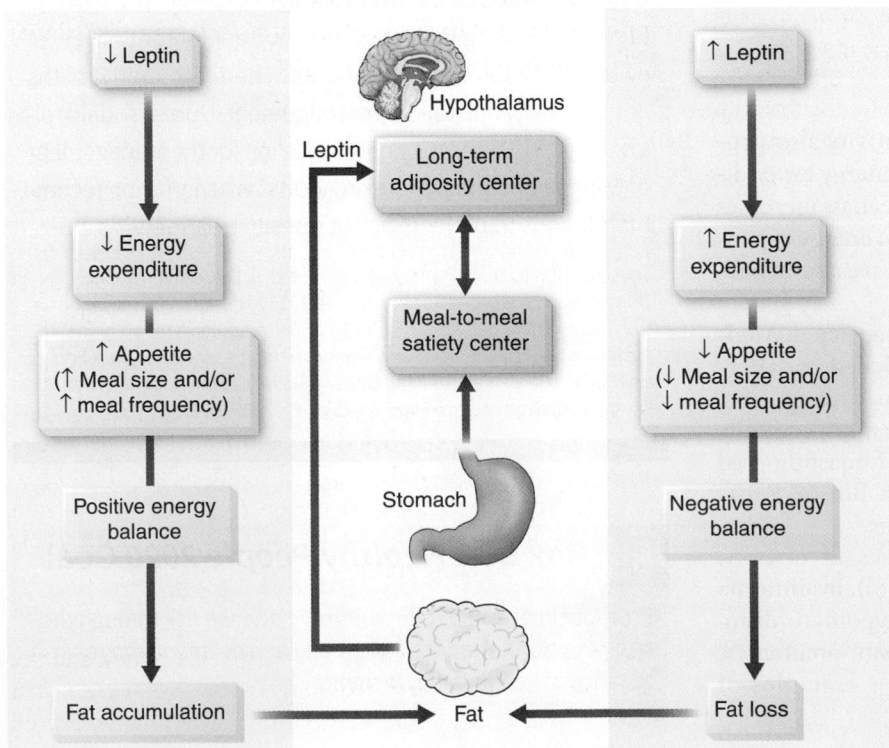

FIGURE 68.1 The complex mechanisms that contribute to appetite. The regulation of body weight is a complex interplay between appetite and energy expenditure. The hypothalamus is signaled by hormones, metabolites, and neural pathways to regulate appetite. Leptin communicates satiety to the hypothalamus and regulates energy expenditure or balance. The majority of energy expenditure is in the form of basal metabolism. Energy expenditures also come from an increase in physical activity or exercise and the metabolic requirements of metabolizing and storing food, along with thermogenesis. Weight gain occurs when the intake of caloric nutrients exceeds energy expenditure.

Obesity is a complex disease in which genetic, environmental, biochemical, and behavioral factors intertwine, and most patients with obesity have more than one factor contributing to their disease. Genetic factors are well documented and contribute to more than 50% of variations in BMI. People with relatives who are obese are more likely to develop obesity. Identical twins, regardless of whether they are raised together or apart, are likely to have similar BMIs. Specific genetic mutations have been found and have led to an increased understanding of obesity. Most of the genetic defects identified affect appetite, such as leptin and melanocortin-4 receptor mutations. Genetic polymorphisms have been linked to obesity in several populations. The discovery of these mutations has led to increased understanding of the powerful biological nature of appetite and has resulted in obesity being seen as a medical condition as opposed to a moral failing.

Environmental factors have a significant role in obesity. **Obesogenic** environments, those that cause obesity, coupled with genetic factors likely account for the majority of the increase in obesity. Increased availability and access to high-calorie, high-fat foods have led to increases in caloric consumption. Other environmental factors, such as automation, have led to a decrease in energy expenditure because the availability and preparation of food require much less activity.

Connection Check 68.2

In correlating contributing factors with the pathophysiology of obesity, which factor is considered environmental?
A. Increased appetite
B. Automation
C. Growth hormone deficiency
D. Obese family members

Behavioral factors such as physical inactivity also promote obesity. In addition to an increase in energy expenditure from physical activity, increased muscle mass increases the basal metabolic rate and helps to increase energy expenditure. Binge eating and compulsive eating are also behavioral factors that promote obesity.

Biochemical alterations can be genetic or acquired. Medication therapy is one cause of acquired biochemical alteration. Many medications are obesogenic and increase appetite. The precise actions of these medications are not specifically understood, although these medications are frequently used to treat conditions in patients with obesity. Box 68.1 lists commonly prescribed obesogenic medications.

There are also many secondary causes of obesity. Cushing's disease (hypersecretion of cortisol), insulinoma (insulin-secreting tumor of the pancreas), hypothyroidism, polycystic ovarian syndrome, hypogonadism, pregnancy, and growth hormone deficiency are a few examples of secondary disorders.

Box 68.1 Obesogenic Medications

- Hypoglycemic agents
- Antihypertensive medications
- Hormones
- Antihistamines
- Anticonvulsants
- Antipsychotics
- Antidepressants

Connection Check 68.3

The nurse correlates which clinical manifestations with the pathophysiology of obesity? *(Select all that apply.)*
A. Increased waist circumference
B. Increased basal metabolic rate
C. Binge eating
D. Joint pain
E. Yellowish skin

MANAGEMENT

Medical Management

Clinical practice guidelines on the identification, evaluation, and treatment of adults who are overweight or obese direct the management of obesity (Box 68.2; see Evidence-Based Practice: Clinical Practice Guidelines for Obesity Treatment).

Evidence-Based Practice

Clinical Practice Guidelines for Obesity Treatment

Clinical practice guidelines are important for the delivery of evidence-based care to patients. There are many myths about obesity and obesity management. Nurses should follow the "2013 AHA/ACC/TOS Guideline for the Management of Overweight and Obesity in Adults" when making recommendations to patients about obesity treatment.

Jensen, M. D., Ryan, D. H., Apovian, C. M., Ard, J. D., Comuzzie, A. G., Donato, K. A.,. . .Obesity Society. (2014). 2013 AHA/ACC/TOS guideline for the management of overweight and obesity in adults: A report of the American College of Cardiology/American Heart Association Task Force on Practice Guidelines and The Obesity Society. *JAMA: Journal of the American College of Cardiology, 63*(25 pt. B), 2985–3023.

Box 68.2 *Healthy People 2020* Goal

Promote health and reduce chronic disease risk through the consumption of healthful diets and achievement and maintenance of healthy body weights.

Laboratory Testing

Laboratory testing in obesity is aimed at the identification of secondary causes and comorbid risk factors, and specific tests are selected on the basis of the results of the history and physical examination. Because of the prevalence of concomitant disease, laboratory testing may include screening for diabetes mellitus, dyslipidemia, thyroid dysfunction, and fatty liver disease. Initial laboratory tests include fasting blood glucose or hemoglobin A1C, liver function tests, fasting lipoprotein panel, and thyroid-stimulating hormone (TSH). Elevations in TSH may point to primary hypothyroidism, whereas decreased TSH and decreased triiodothyronine and thyroxine may indicate secondary hypothyroidism. In patients with physical characteristics of Cushing's disease, 24-hour urine collection for urinary free cortisol excretion should be performed to assess for excessive cortisol secretion leading to weight gain.

Diagnostic Testing

Diagnostic testing is seldom indicated to diagnose or treat obesity, and a thorough history and physical examination usually determine whether further diagnostic testing is necessary. Diagnostic tests are used to evaluate for comorbidities of obesity. An overnight sleep study is used to test for sleep apnea. A right upper quadrant ultrasound tests for fatty liver disease. Transvaginal ultrasonography is used to evaluate for ovarian cysts. An electrocardiogram (ECG) or echocardiogram may be used for patients with obesity who have a high risk of cardiovascular disease.

Accurate ECG lead placement is important in all patients, but particular attention is needed in performing a 12-lead ECG in patients with obesity. Patient size can obscure landmarks and result in improper lead placement. Electrocardiogram abnormalities, such as T-wave abnormalities, left axis deviation and low QRS voltage, can be seen in obesity in the absence of clinical symptoms.

It is important to note the impact of obesity on radiological testing. Computed tomography (CT), magnetic resonance imaging (MRI), fluoroscopy, and plain radiograph tables all have weight limits, typically 350 to 450 lb. A 2008 survey found that one-quarter of all U.S. emergency departments were unable to obtain CT imaging for patients greater than 350 lb, and two-thirds were not able to obtain MRI studies. More than 90% of emergency departments were unable to perform CT or MRI studies on patients greater than 450 lb. In addition, excess abdominal adiposity obscures organs and traditional landmarks, making the diagnosis of many conditions more difficult. Because of attenuation through excess adipose tissue in ultrasound, plain radiographs, and nuclear medicine, CT is the preferred imaging modality for patients with obesity. The utility of ultrasonography in the morbidly obese is severely limited.

Treatment

Weight-Loss Therapy

All adults with a BMI greater than or equal to 30 kg/m^2 should be assisted with developing weight-related goals and treatment. Those with a BMI greater than or equal to 25 kg/m^2 or with a high-risk waist circumference and greater than or equal to two other risk factors should also begin weight-loss therapy.

Diet Therapy

Diet modification, increased physical activity, and behavior therapy are the mainstays of all weight-loss regimens. Diet therapy is developed and individualized between the healthcare provider and the patient. A calorie reduction of 500 to 1,000 calories daily (kcal/day) results in a 1- to 2-lb (2.2- to 4.4-kg) weight loss weekly if the patient is currently maintaining a stable weight. Very low–calorie diets, those less than 800 kcal/day, are used only in limited circumstances and only under the supervision of a healthcare practitioner in a medical setting where frequent monitoring can be accomplished because of the potential risk for complications.

Physical Activity

Physical activity is important for all adults. Long-term goals of 30 minutes of moderate-intensity exercise on most, if not all, days of the week are recommended. Increased physical activity in patients with obesity can increase daily energy expenditure and increase the basal metabolic rate by increasing lean body mass.

Behavioral Therapy

Behavioral therapy combined with diet and physical activity is recommended. Self-monitoring via food logs, stimulus control, social support, and cognitive restructuring is encouraged. Patients with obesity can find Internet, as well as face-to-face, weight-loss programs that offer behavioral therapy. A psychological evaluation may be considered if there is a suspected eating disorder.

Medications

Pharmacotherapy should be considered in patients with a BMI greater than or equal to 30 kg/m^2 or with a BMI greater than or equal to 27 kg/m^2 with one or more obesity-associated comorbidities whose weight-loss attempts have been unsuccessful in the past. It should be employed only in the presence of diet, exercise, and behavioral therapy and requires close observations by a healthcare provider. The potential risks of medication treatment should be weighed against the benefits, and a thorough health examination should take place prior to starting any pharmacotherapy.

The majority of weight loss occurs within the first 6 months of starting a medication. Several medications currently available for the long-term treatment of obesity include orlistat; lorcaserin; phentermine-topiramate extended release; bupropion-naltrexone extended-release tablet; and liraglutide, a daily injectable.

Orlistat (Xenical, Alli) inhibits pancreatic lipase, thereby reducing dietary fat absorption. The prescription brand of orlistat (Xenical) is supplied in a 120-mg capsule and should be taken three times per day with any meal that contains fat. The over-the-counter version of orlistat (Alli) is supplied in a 60-mg capsule. Orlistat causes a modest increase in weight loss of 5 to 7 pounds over a year period. Persons who take the medication may also report the lowering of blood pressure and are less likely to develop type 2 diabetes. Common side effects of the medication include significant gastrointestinal symptoms, including increased flatus, loose and oily stools, abdominal cramping, and nausea. Rare cases of liver injury, a serious side effect, have been reported, and symptoms include dark urine, itching, light-colored stools, loss of appetite, or jaundice. Because of the mechanism of action, it may also decrease the absorption of fat-soluble vitamins (A, D, E, and K) and beta-carotene. Patients are instructed to take a multivitamin 2 hours before or after taking orlistat. It is contraindicated in patients with cholelithiasis, hepatic disease, pancreatic disease, or malabsorption syndrome.

Lorcaserin (Belviq) affects chemicals in the brain that help to regulate appetite and increase the feeling of fullness after eating so that less food is eaten. Lorcaserin is taken twice daily, and the expected weight loss is 3% to 5% of an individual's weight. Common side effects include headache, dizziness, nausea, fatigue, constipation, and dry mouth. Lorcaserin is contraindicated in patients with severe depression and cardiac or valvular disease.

Phentermine/topiramate-extended release (Qsymia) is a combination medication. Phentermine is approved by the U.S. Food and Drug Administration (FDA) to suppress appetite for up to 12 weeks. Topiramate is approved for the treatment of seizures and migraines, and weight loss was observed to be a side effect associated with decreased appetite and enhanced satiety. Phentermine/topiramate is taken once daily and produces the most weight loss, as much as 9% of initial weight. To minimize side effects, the combination of phentermine/topiramate contains lower dosages of each medication than if used alone. Common side effects include altered taste, numbness, tingling, insomnia, dizziness, and anxiety. Because phentermine/topiramate may cause birth defects, females must use a reliable form of birth control and receive pregnancy tests on a monthly basis during treatment.

Bupropion-naltrexone (Contrave) is a combination medication typically used as a second option in the treatment of obesity. It was approved by the FDA in September 2014 as an adjunct to diet and exercise in patients with a BMI of greater than 30 kg or greater than 27 kg in the presence of at least one weight-related comorbidity. The initial dose is one tablet daily for 1 week, which is then increased to two tablets twice daily by week 4. It is approved for up to 12 weeks and results in the loss of approximately 5% to 6% of body weight. Common side effects are headache, insomnia, vomiting, dizziness, and dry mouth. It can raise blood pressure, and cardiovascular effects have not been yet established. It contains bupropion, an antidepressant, and the FDA recommends counseling in patients aged 18 to 24 for risks of suicidal ideations.

Liraglutide (Saxenda) is the only FDA-approved injectable medication for weight loss. It is an adjunct to a reduced-calorie diet and increased physical activity for chronic weight management in adults with a BMI of greater than 30 kg or greater than 27 kg with at least one weight-related comorbid condition. Dosing is done through daily injection, with the initial dosing titrated up by weekly increments to the target dose of 3 mg to reduce the gastrointestinal (GI) side effects of nausea and vomiting. The mechanism of action is via slowing gastric emptying. It is contraindicated in patients with medullary thyroid cancer (MTC). Common side effects of liraglutide include headache, nausea, diarrhea, and an increase in the resting heart rate.

Phendimetrazine (Bontril PDM), diethylpropion (Tenuate), benzphetamine (Regimex), and phentermine (Adipex-P, Lomaira) are available for short-term treatment of up to 12 weeks for obesity. They decrease appetite, also known as an **anorexigenic** effect. They may also increase satiety, and through these mechanisms, patients may experience weight loss. Because of their sympathomimetic effects, these medications should be used with caution in patients with hypertension and are contraindicated in patients with cardiovascular disease, hyperthyroidism, arrhythmias, agitation, insomnia, or glaucoma. Common side effects include insomnia, headache, dry mouth, and irritability. Because of the chronic nature of obesity, these medications are not strongly supported by treatment guidelines. Patients often develop tolerance within several weeks.

Safety Alert Patients with cardiovascular or heart valve disease should be monitored closely for adverse effects if prescribed lorcaserin or phentermine/topiramate for weight loss. Phendimetrazine, diethylpropion, benzphetamine, and phentermine are contraindicated in patients with cardiovascular disease because of their sympathomimetic effects.

Connection Check 68.5

In administering orlistat to a patient for weight loss, the nurse recognizes which as the mechanism of action of this medication?

A. Reducing fat absorption
B. Suppressing appetite
C. Increasing satiety
D. Accelerating metabolic rate

Surgical Management

Bariatric Surgery

Diet, physical activity, behavioral therapy, and pharmacotherapy are ineffective in many patients with obesity. Bariatric surgery, a procedure intended to lead to weight loss, is an option for patients who have a BMI greater than or equal to 40 kg/m². Patients with a BMI of 35 to 39.9 kg/m² with comorbidities or a significant reduction in quality of life should also be considered for surgery (see Evidence-Based Practice: Bariatric Surgery). In 2011, a total of 340,768 bariatric surgeries were performed worldwide. The American Society of Metabolic and Bariatric Surgery estimated that the number of surgeries in the United States grew from 158,000 in 2001 to 228,000 in 2017, with approximately 59.39% of these procedures being sleeve gastrectomy (Box 68.3).

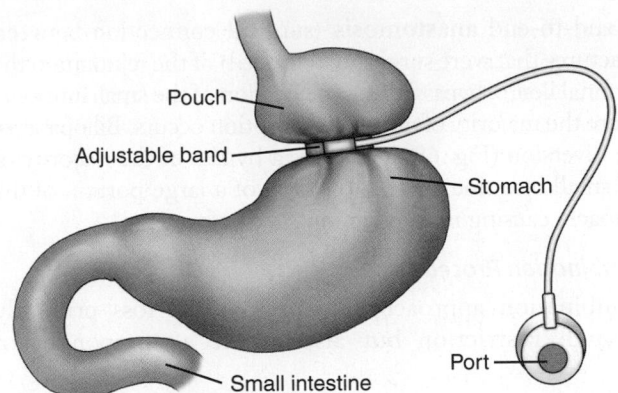

FIGURE 68.2 Adjustable gastric banding (AGB). Laparoscopic AGB involves placement of a silicone band around the fundus of the stomach, causing a restriction in the amount of food intake.

Evidence-Based Practice

Bariatric Surgery

The Cochrane Collaboration performed a systematic review of 22 bariatric surgery studies in 2014. The review indicated that bariatric surgery results in greater weight loss than conventional treatment and that body mass index (BMI) was on average 6 kg/m² lower 2 years after surgery. In addition, patients had improvements in quality of life and management of diabetes mellitus.

Colquitt, J. L., Pickett, K., Loveman, E., & Frampton, G. K. (2014). Surgery for weight loss in adults. *Cochrane Database of Systematic Reviews, 8.* doi:10.1002/14651858.CD003641.pub4

Types

Bariatric surgical procedures include restrictive, malabsorptive, and combination techniques. Most procedures are performed openly or laparoscopically, dependent on the surgeon's expertise and the patient's history of abdominal surgery, degree of obesity, and other medical conditions. More than 90% of the procedures are performed laparoscopically.

Restrictive Procedures

Restrictive procedures cause weight loss by reducing gastric capacity and include adjustable gastric banding (AGB), sleeve gastrectomy, and gastric plication. Laparoscopic AGB (Fig. 68.2) involves the placement of a silicone band

around the fundus of the stomach, causing a restriction in the amount of food intake. The band can be adjusted by a healthcare provider to decrease or increase the amount of restriction by injecting saline through a subcutaneous port in the abdominal wall. During a sleeve gastrectomy, most of the greater curvature of the stomach is removed, creating a smaller, sleeve-like tube. The remaining stomach is approximately 25% of its original capacity. Gastric plication, a new procedure, is still considered investigational. This procedure involves infolding of the greater curvature of the stomach to create gastric restriction.

Malabsorptive Procedures

Although malabsorptive procedures are no longer commonly performed and account for only 2% of the surgeries performed worldwide, there are many patients who had these procedures in the past and require regular follow-up care. These procedures induce weight loss through decreased nutrient absorption; jejunoileal bypass and biliopancreatic diversion are examples of these procedures. Jejunoileal bypass (Fig. 68.3) is

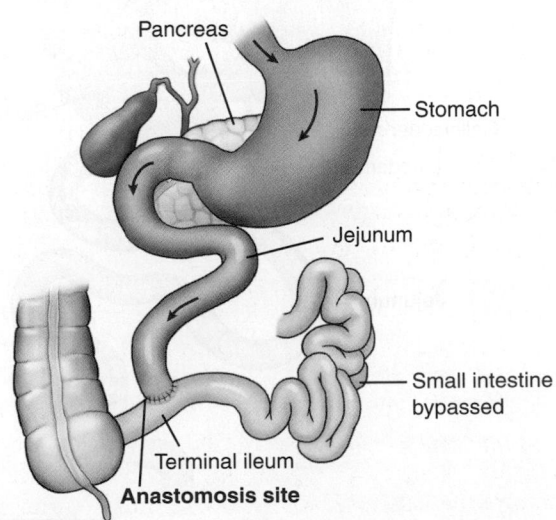

FIGURE 68.3 Jejunoileal bypass procedure (JIB). A jejunoileal bypass is an end-to-end anastomosis of the jejunum to the terminal ileum, bypassing a large portion of the small intestine, causing malabsorption.

Box 68.3 Health Disparities

Obesity is more prevalent among middle-aged, rural, economically and educationally disadvantaged, and racial/ethnic minority populations, yet these patients are unlikely to have bariatric surgery.

an end-to-end **anastomosis** (surgical connection between structures that were surgically removed) of the jejunum to the terminal ileum, bypassing a large portion of the small intestine, where the majority of nutrient absorption occurs. Biliopancreatic diversion (Fig. 68.4) involves a bypass of the majority of the small intestine and the removal of a large portion of the stomach, causing malabsorption.

Combination Procedures

Combination approaches induce weight loss primarily through restriction but also create a component of malabsorption. The Roux-en-Y gastric bypass (RYGB; Fig. 68.5) is a combination procedure that involves the creation of a restrictive 30-mL gastric pouch and bypass of a portion of the small intestine, causing mild malabsorption. The Roux-en-Y gastric bypass is the most commonly performed (46.6%) bariatric surgery worldwide.

Complications

Recent data show that the 90-day mortality rate after bariatric surgery is 0.11%, and the 30-day mortality rate is 0.09%. Several other studies have shown a mortality rate consistently under 1%. With the improvement in surgical techniques, mortality rates have steadily declined and are significantly less than those for other commonly performed surgical procedures.

As with all surgeries, there are complications, and they vary depending on the type of surgery. Overall, short-term life-threatening complications of bariatric surgery include pulmonary embolism, infection, and anastomosis leak. Long-term complications and side effects include band slippage, obstruction, hernia, esophageal erosion, ulcers, acid reflux, vitamin deficiency, osteoporosis, anemia, and **dumping syndrome**. Dumping syndrome is the result of stomach contents being rapidly "dumped" into the small intestine and occurs because of this rapid delivery of large amounts of osmotically active solids and liquids into the duodenum. The following clinical manifestations are often observed with this syndrome:

- Nausea
- Vomiting
- Abdominal pain, cramps

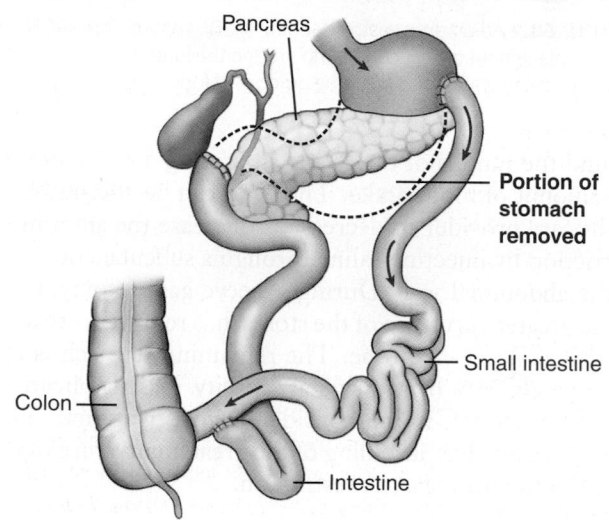

FIGURE 68.4 Biliopancreatic diversion (BPD). Biliopancreatic diversion involves a bypass of the majority of the small intestine and removal of a large portion of the stomach, causing malabsorption.

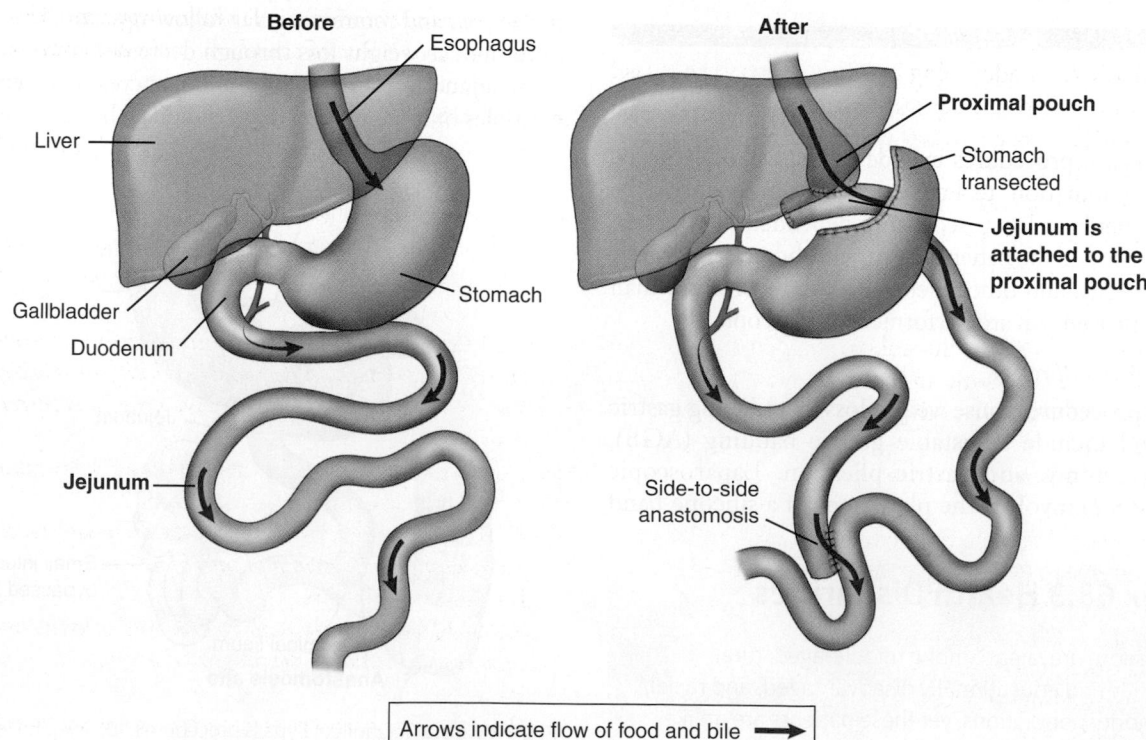

Arrows indicate flow of food and bile ➞

FIGURE 68.5 Roux-en-Y gastric bypass (RYGB). Roux-en-Y gastric bypass is a combination procedure that involves the creation of a restrictive 30-mL gastric pouch and bypass of a portion of the small intestine, causing mild malabsorption.

- Diarrhea
- Dizziness, light-headedness
- Bloating, belching
- Fatigue
- Heart palpitations, rapid heart rate

> ⚠ **Safety Alert** Tachycardia, fever, hypotension, and abdominal pain should be reported immediately because they may be signs of anastomosis leak, a life-threatening complication associated with infection and sepsis.

CASE STUDY: EPISODE 2

Ms. Wiley is referred to a bariatric surgeon by her primary care provider. Other than her obesity, Ms. Wiley also has mild hypertension and chronic joint pain. She is referred to an information session on bariatric surgery, and after this session, she decides to have laparoscopic RYGB surgery. The surgery is planned for the following week…

Connection Check 68.6

The nurse assesses for which clinical manifestations of dumping syndrome in the patient after bariatric surgery? *(Select all that apply.)*

A. Nausea
B. Increased urine output
C. Hypoglycemia
D. Diarrhea
E. Abdominal cramping

Nursing Management

Assessment and Analysis

Patients with obesity undergoing bariatric surgery are at risk for complications. Because bariatric surgery is considered a major abdominal surgery, patients can be expected to remain hospitalized for 1 to 2 days. Patients undergoing bariatric surgery should be observed for complications related to both surgery and obesity. Complications specifically related to obesity and bariatric surgery in hospitalized patients include:

- Impaired breathing
- Increased risk of venous thromboembolism
- Increased risk of pressure injury
- Increased risk of skin infections
- Immobility
- Urinary and fecal incontinence
- Infection
- Increased risk of venous thromboembolism
- Anastomosis leak (a leak where dissected bowel is reattached together)
- Peritonitis
- Intestinal obstruction
- Atelectasis and pneumonia
- Dehydration
- Electrolyte imbalance related to vomiting
- Bleeding

Nursing Diagnoses

- **Deficient fluid volume** related to malabsorption secondary to surgical procedure
- **Imbalanced nutrition: less than body requirements** related to poor nutrition prior to surgery and postoperative restriction
- **Impaired physical mobility** related to body habitus and postoperative pain
- **Acute pain** related to surgical incisions
- **Disturbed body image** related to obesity and failed attempts to lose weight
- **Anxiety** related to the surgical procedure

Nursing Interventions

Assessments

- Vital signs, using appropriately sized equipment
  Body temperature, heart rate, respiratory rate, and blood pressure can point to early complications such as infection or bleeding. Elevated heart rate and decreased blood pressure may be secondary to hypovolemia, hemorrhage, or infection. Bariatric-sized blood pressure cuffs are essential to obtain proper readings in patients who are obese.
- Oxygen saturation
  Decreased ventilation due to obesity hypoventilation syndrome (OHS) and opioid analgesics can result in lower oxygen saturation.
- Electrolytes
  The patient is at risk for fluid and electrolyte disturbances, particularly with dumping syndrome.
- Daily weight and intake and output
  Dehydration and fluid overload are common in postoperative patients and can be identified through changes in weight and monitoring of intake and output.
- Skin using a pressure-injury-prevention protocol
  Increased weight and decreased mobility increase the risk of skin breakdown due to pressure as well as increased moisture.
- Skinfolds (breast, groin, neck, abdomen, perianal) for irritation/fungal infections
  Patients with obesity have increased skinfolds, which are prone to skin irritation and infection.
- Incisions and drains
  Signs of bleeding, anastomosis leak, and infection may be observed in incisional drainage and drains.
- Pain
  Postoperative pain not only decreases ventilation and mobility, but it can also be a sign of infection and other complications.

▪ Actions

- Obtain appropriately sized equipment for care (gowns, bed, chair, bedside commode, stretcher, wheelchairs, etc.).
  Properly sized bariatric gowns are needed to provide patient dignity. A bariatric bed should be large enough to ensure the patient can turn and reposition. Skin should not be in contact with bed rails because this can lead to pressure injury. Bariatric chairs, bedside commodes, and wheelchairs/stretchers increase patient mobility, prevent injury, and allow safe patient transport.

- Elevate head of bed 30 to 45 degrees if no contraindications
  Obesity hypoventilation syndrome is worsened when patients are supine or prone. Elevating the head of the bed 30 to 45 degrees optimizes diaphragmatic excursion and minimizes the pressure of abdominal contents on the thoracic cavity.

- Encourage use of incentive spirometer
  Promotes increased lung expansion and decreases risk of atelectasis and pneumonia

- Apply sequential compressive devices as ordered.
  The risk for venous thromboembolism is increased in patients with obesity.

- Encourage self-care and mobility as appropriate.
  Early ambulation and mobility decrease the risk of venous thromboembolism and other complications associated with decreased mobility (atelectasis, pressure injury, constipation, etc.).

- Turn patients with decreased mobility frequently, a minimum of every 2 hours, using additional staff as needed.
  Skin injury is common in hospitalized patients who are obese and have decreased mobility, in part because of the difficulty in achieving rotational pressure relief for all body surfaces.

- Use slide and transfer assistance devices as appropriate.
  Proper equipment is essential for the safety of the patient and nursing staff when repositioning or transferring patients who are obese. Skin shearing and back injuries can be prevented.

- Assist patient with skin care.
  Patients with obesity commonly have difficulty with toileting and bathing, which, along with increased skinfolds, makes patients more prone to skin breakdown and infection.

- Administer pain medication.
  Pain management improves early ambulation and the use of the incentive spirometry. Intravenous patient-controlled analgesia is the suggested method of pain control in the first 24 to 48 hours after surgery or until the patient can transition to oral pain management.

- Do not reposition a nasogastric tube (NGT); monitor the NGT for patency if applicable.
  Repositioning or insertion of an NGT can perforate the new gastric staple or suture lines.

- Introduce clear liquids as ordered.
  Dehydration is common after bariatric surgery, so introducing and encouraging small sips of clear liquids as ordered decreases the risk of a fluid volume deficit.

- Inform transportation and other departments of weight prior to transport.
  Hospital equipment is often not properly sized for patients who are obese or overweight. In addition, some tests may not be able to be performed on certain equipment, and accommodations may need to be made before the patient arrives. Alerting staff early to bring proper equipment or prepare for the patient decreases patient embarrassment and decreases the risk of injury.

- Collaborate with appropriate members of the healthcare team: wound ostomy care nurse for skin assessment and specialty bed recommendation; physical therapy and occupational therapy; respiratory therapy; social services; clinical pharmacist; nutrition services.
  Obesity is a complex disease, and proper care of this patient population requires a collaborative approach with other healthcare experts.

▪ Teaching

- Incentive spirometry, coughing, and deep-breathing exercises
  Decrease risk of pneumonia and atelectasis

- Sequential compression devices
  Decrease risk of venous thromboembolism

- Ambulation
  Decreases risk of pneumonia, atelectasis, and venous thromboembolism

- Postoperative lifting restrictions
  Decrease hernia development or suture disruption

- Postoperative and recovery activity
  Exercise should begin in the immediate postoperative period to decrease the risk of operative complications and to begin lifelong healthy weight-management practices.

- Postoperative dietary restrictions
  Decrease risk of dehydration, suture disruption, and vomiting

- Medication side effects
  Pain medications may cause drowsiness and constipation. Patients should not drive, drink alcohol, or operate machinery while taking opioid pain medications. Patients should be taught about the increased risk of constipation as a side effect of opioid medications.

- Care of wounds/drains
  Wounds should be kept clean, dry, and covered. Jackson-Pratt drains should be emptied when they are half-full to decrease pull on the surgical site and should be kept clean to prevent infection.

- Signs and symptoms to report to the healthcare provider
  Shortness of breath, tachycardia, severe abdominal pain, fever, rigors, purulent discharge or redness at wounds, and hypotension can be indicative of life-threatening complications, such as pulmonary embolism, anastomosis leak, or infection, and need to be immediately reported to the healthcare provider.

- Signs of dumping syndrome
  Symptoms include nausea, vomiting, diarrhea, diaphoresis, tachycardia, salivation, fatigue, and dizziness, and this complication places the patient at risk of fluid and electrolyte disorders.

- Available support groups
  Patients who attend support groups are more likely to have better outcomes.

Connection Check 68.7

In which position does the nurse place the patient to minimize complications in the patient with OHS?

A. Prone with hips elevated
B. Head of bed elevated 30 to 45 degrees
C. Side-lying with head flat
D. Head of bed elevated 90 degrees

> **Safety Alert** Never insert or reposition a nasogastric or orogastric tube on a patient who has had bariatric surgery because it can disrupt the suture line.

Evaluating Care Outcomes

Obesity is a complex, multifactorial condition. Diet; exercise; and behavioral, pharmacological, and surgical interventions are available to treat the condition, and the primary expected outcome is weight loss. Community nursing interventions are crucial to decreasing the prevalence and reoccurrence of obesity. Prevention of complications related to obesity in hospitalized patients is important. The postoperative care of patients undergoing bariatric surgery is similar to that of patients undergoing other abdominal surgeries but has the added risks of pre-existing obesity. Nurses play a critical role in the follow-up of patients who have had postoperative bariatric surgery by monitoring for complications, supporting dietary and lifestyle changes, monitoring for nutritional deficiencies, and advocating for social support.

Connection Check 68.8

Which statement by the patient being discharged after gastric bypass surgery indicates the need for further teaching?

A. "I may need to take a multivitamin every day."
B. "I may develop constipation while I am taking pain medications."
C. "I should not lift anything heavy until cleared by the surgeon."
D. "I should drink at least one cup of fluids with every meal."

Making Connections

CASE STUDY: WRAP-UP

Ms. Wiley undergoes gastric bypass surgery and has an uneventful postoperative course. On postoperative day 2, her bowel sounds return, the NGT is removed, and she is allowed sips of clear liquids. She is discharged to home the following day with instructions to monitor her temperature every 4 hours and to contact the surgeon if she has an elevated temperature, nausea and vomiting, or increased pain. She is to return to the bariatric surgeon for postoperative follow-up in 7 to 10 days.

Case Study Questions

1. Ms. Wiley is 5 ft 6 in. tall and weighs 256 lb. The nurse calculates her BMI to be which value?
   A. 19 kg/m²
   B. 34 kg/m²
   C. 41 kg/m²
   D. 49 kg/m²

2. Ms. Wiley asks if she qualifies for bariatric surgery. What is the best response by the nurse?
   A. "No. You are healthy and therefore do not qualify for bariatric surgery."
   B. "Yes. You meet the BMI criteria, but I would not recommend bariatric surgery for someone so young. I know someone who died from it."
   C. "No. You do not meet the BMI criteria for bariatric surgery."
   D. "Yes. You meet the BMI criteria, but there are several other factors that determine whether someone should have bariatric surgery."

3. Ms. Wiley wants to know the key difference between the Roux-en-Y and adjustable gastric banding. Which explanation by the nurse is most accurate?
   A. "Some surgeons just prefer one over the other."
   B. "Roux-en-Y is a combination of a restrictive surgery and a malabsorptive surgery."
   C. "Adjustable gastric banding is designed to be temporary."
   D. "Roux-en-Y is a type of adjustable gastric banding."

4. The nurse is caring for Ms. Wiley in the presurgical suite. The patient asks, "Will you hold my hand? I am getting nervous. My mom told me this morning that I could die from this surgery." Which action by the nurse is best?
   A. Patting the patient on the shoulder and covering her up
   B. Asking her if she would like some alprazolam (Xanax) to calm her down
   C. Holding her hand and listening to her concerns
   D. Explaining that the percentage of people who die from bariatric surgery is small

5. The nurse is caring for Ms. Wiley in the post-anesthesia recovery unit. The patient is 2 hours post–gastric bypass surgery and has a nasogastric tube (NGT). The orders state that the NGT should be hooked up to low continuous suction. There is scant blood-tinged drainage coming from the tube. What action should the nurse take?
   A. Call the surgeon right away.
   B. Reposition the NGT.
   C. Discontinue the NGT.
   D. Document the findings.

CHAPTER SUMMARY

On the basis of body mass index (BMI), patients are classified as underweight, normal weight, overweight, or obese (class 1, 2, or 3). Obesity occurs when energy expenditure is less than caloric intake. Obesity is a complex phenomenon involving genetic, behavioral, environmental, and biochemical processes. Obesity increases mortality and morbidity, such as diabetes, sleep apnea, hypertension, and gallbladder disease.

Diet, exercise, and behavioral treatment should be implemented in patients with a BMI greater than or equal to 30 kg/m^2 or greater than or equal to 25 kg/m^2 with risk factors. The pharmacological treatment of obesity is limited but should be considered in patients who have not been successful with diet, exercise, and behavioral treatment who have a BMI greater than or equal to 30 kg/m^2 or a BMI greater than or equal to 27 kg/m^2 with other risk factors.

Bariatric surgery is considered in patients who have been unsuccessful with diet, exercise, and behavioral and pharmacological treatments and have a BMI of greater than or equal to 40 kg/m^2 or a BMI of greater than or equal to 35 kg/m^2 with additional comorbidities. There are three main types of bariatric surgery: restrictive, malabsorptive, and combination. Patients with obesity are at increased risk of respiratory, circulatory, and skin-related issues during hospitalizations. Complications vary depending on the type of bariatric surgery. Pulmonary embolism and infection are common complications that nursing interventions can significantly reduce.

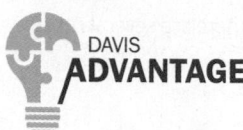

DAVIS
ADVANTAGE

To explore learning resources for this chapter, go to **Davis Advantage** and find:
- Answers to in-text questions
- Chapter Resources and Activities
- NCLEX®-Style Chapter Review Questions
- Bibliography

Chapter 69

Substance Use Disorders in the Adult Population

Wanda Edwards

Finding Connections

CASE STUDY: EPISODE 1

Follow this patient throughout the chapter.

Ms. Mary Litfield is a 64-year-old widowed female who is admitted on Monday to the surgical service of a general hospital for resection of colon cancer. Her operation is very successful, but on Wednesday, when she is about to be transferred from the step-down unit to a regular surgical bed, there is a change in her condition. She becomes confused, anxious, and tremulous. Her pulse and blood pressure are elevated, and she seems to be responding to visual hallucinations. Her surgical team initially suspects pneumonia or a postoperative infection, but her temperature and white blood cell count are both normal, and her abdomen is soft. Radiographic examination of her chest and abdomen demonstrate no new problems, but abdominal ultrasonography reveals a fatty liver. Mary's nurse suspects alcohol withdrawal and calls her family to obtain more information. Mary's daughter tells the nurse that she has been worried about Mary's drinking. The death of her husband 2 years ago was very hard on her, but his life insurance provided enough money for her to take early retirement from her job as a high school English teacher. She has been spending a lot of time alone at home, not going out with her old friends, seems less interested in her two young grandchildren, and is sometimes irritable with them. Mary and her husband used to enjoy one or two cocktails together in the evenings, but her daughter expresses concern that her drinking may have increased...

INTRODUCTION

Substances such as drugs, alcohol, and tobacco are abused for varied and complicated reasons. Substance abuse is the use of a substance in amounts that are harmful to the abuser or others, impacting individuals, families, and society. The individual who abuses substances may neglect important obligations or role responsibilities at home, school, or work. Ongoing interpersonal problems, such as the loss of friends or a marital separation, may occur. There may be family disintegration, loss of employment, failure in school, domestic violence, or child abuse. The individual who is abusing substances may expose him- or herself to dangerous situations, such as driving while intoxicated or having unprotected sex with a stranger. The substance use may continue even when the substance user is aware of actual and potential negative consequences. Society also pays a significant cost. The cost to the U.S. economy is estimated at hundreds of billions of dollars and includes increased healthcare costs, crime-related costs, and costs associated with lost productivity.

DIAGNOSTIC CRITERIA OF SUBSTANCE USE DISORDERS

In the *Diagnostic and Statistical Manual of Mental Disorders* (4th edition, Text Revision; *DSM-IV-TR*), "abuse" and "dependence" were defined as diagnoses. Dependence was considered a more severe form of substance abuse. In the fifth edition (*DSM-5*), the diagnosis of "**substance use disorder (SUD)**" replaces "abuse and dependence." The *DSM-5* describes the essential feature of an SUD as "a cluster of cognitive, behavioral, and physiological symptoms indicating that the individual continues using the substance despite significant substance-related problems." For a diagnosis of an SUD based on the *DSM-5*, the pattern of substance use must be problematic, must be associated with clinically significant manifestations, and at least 2 of 11 possible symptoms or criteria must be present (Table 69.1). The severity of an SUD is determined by the number of symptoms present: mild (two or three symptoms), moderate (four or five symptoms), or severe (six or more symptoms). In the *DSM-5*, the specific substance used is included as part of the diagnosis. If an individual uses alcohol and the use meets the criteria for an SUD, the diagnosis is **alcohol use disorder (AUD)**; an individual who uses marijuana has a diagnosis of cannabis use disorder if the marijuana use meets the criteria for an SUD.

Tolerance, **withdrawal**, and **craving**—three symptoms of **physical dependence**—are also clinical manifestations that may be evident with the diagnosis of an SUD. Dependence occurs because the body naturally adapts to regular exposure to a substance. The adaptation may lead to tolerance, withdrawal, or both. When tolerance develops, more of the substance is required to achieve the same effect. If a person who has an AUD has developed tolerance to alcohol, the person may be able to walk and talk with a **blood alcohol level (BAL)** that would seriously incapacitate the inexperienced drinker. Withdrawal is the occurrence of physical or emotional clinical manifestations if the substance is decreased or abruptly stopped.

Physical dependence may lead to craving (strong desire or persistent thoughts about the substance), which may be triggered by external or internal factors. External triggers include places, people, or things associated with the substance use patterns of the substance user. Internal triggers include emotional or physical symptoms of withdrawal.

Physical dependence is a separate condition from SUD. When medications with addictive properties are prescribed for an individual, it is not uncommon for the individual to develop physical dependence without engaging in the maladaptive behaviors that define an SUD. One example is a patient with cancer who is prescribed an opiate for pain; physical dependence may develop even when opiates are used as prescribed. Careful assessment and interprofessional team collaboration are essential for the accurate identification of clinical manifestations of physical dependence and for

Table 69.1 Diagnosis of a Substance Use Disorder

Impaired Control	Social Impairment	Risky Use	Pharmacological Criteria
Criteria 1–4	*Criteria 5–7*	*Criteria 8–9*	*Criteria 10–11*
1. Substance is often taken in larger amounts or over a longer period than was intended.	5. Recurrent substance use resulting in a failure to fulfill major role obligations at work, school, or home	8. Recurrent substance use in situations in which it is physically hazardous	10. Tolerance: a. A need for markedly increased amounts of substance to achieve intoxication or desired effect b. A markedly diminished effect with continued use of the same amount of substance
2. There is a persistent desire or unsuccessful efforts to cut down or control substance use.	6. Continued substance use despite having persistent or recurrent social or interpersonal problems caused or exacerbated by the effects of alcohol	9. Substance use is continued despite knowledge of having a persistent or recurrent physical or psychological problem that is likely to have been caused or exacerbated by substance.	11. Withdrawal: a. The characteristic withdrawal syndrome for substance (refer to Criteria A and B of the criteria set for substance withdrawal in the *DSM-5*) b. Substance (or a closely related substance) is taken to relieve or avoid withdrawal symptoms.
3. A great deal of time is spent in activities necessary to obtain substance, use substance, or recover from its effects.	7. Important social, occupational, or recreational activities are given up or reduced because of substance use.		
4. Craving, or a strong desire or urge to use substance			

DSM-5, Diagnostic and Statistical Manual of Mental Disorders, 5th edition.
A substance use disorder is a problematic pattern of substance use leading to clinically significant impairment or distress, as manifested by at least 2 of the 11 criteria listed in this chart, occurring within a 12-month time period.
The *DSM-5* criteria for Criterion A diagnosis of a substance use disorder fits into one of four broad categories: impaired control, social impairment, risky use, and pharmacological criteria.
Source: American Psychiatric Association. (2013). *Diagnostic and statistical manual of mental disorders* (5th ed.). Arlington, VA: Author, pp. 483–484.

determining the appropriate plan of action. If an individual on prescription pain medication develops tolerance to the prescribed medication, modification of the medication dose or frequency of dosing to adequately control pain may be required. The same individual may require further assessment to identify and address SUDs if symptoms are present that suggest the presence of an SUD.

Connection Check 69.1

The patient with an SUD diagnosis may demonstrate which symptoms? (*Select all that apply.*)

A. Failure to fulfill major role obligations at work, home, or school

B. Recurrent use in situations in which it is physically hazardous

C. Continued use despite having persistent or recurrent social or interpersonal problems caused or exacerbated by the effects of the substance

D. Withdrawal from the substance when the dose is decreased or stopped

E. Successful attempts to cut down

EPIDEMIOLOGY

Prevalence

The development and manifestation of an SUD are influenced by genetic, psychosocial, and environmental factors. Common substances associated with hazardous or harmful use include alcohol, tobacco, and illicit drugs, including prescribed medications when used for nonmedical purposes (Table 69.2). In the United States, alcohol is the most commonly used drug; tobacco and marijuana are close seconds. Although tobacco and alcohol are legal, the patterns of use by individuals who use one or both of these substances frequently meet the criteria for a tobacco or alcohol use disorder. In 2016, 136.7 million people aged 12 and older in the United States (50% of the population) reported current use of alcohol. Among current alcohol users, 16.3 million (11.9%) met the criteria for heavy use, defined as five or more drinks on the same occasion on each of 5 or more days in the past 30 days. The rate of heavy drinking was highest among young adults aged 18 to 25 (57.1%). In 2016, the prevalence of any drinking; binge drinking, defined as drinking five or more alcoholic drinks on the same occasion on at least 1 day in the past 30 days; and heavy drinking

Table 69.2 Commonly Used Addictive Substances

Substance Category and Generic and Brand or Chemical Name	Examples of Commercial and Street Names	How Used
TOBACCO		
Tobacco Nicotine	Cigarettes	Smoked
	E-cigarettes	Vaped (inhalation of vapors produced by an electronic/battery-operated device)
	Smokeless tobacco (chewing tobacco, snuff)	Chewed, sniffed
CANNABINOIDS		
Cannabis/Hashish Marijuana	Hashish: Hash, hash oil, hemp	Smoked, swallowed, vaped
	Marijuana: Aunt Mary, BC bud, blunt (marijuana cigar), boom, chronic, dope, gangster, ganja, grass, hash, herb, hydro, indo, joint, kif, Mary Jane, mota, pot, reefer, sinsemilla, skunk, smoke, weed, yerba	
DEPRESSANTS		
Alcohol Ethanol/alcohol	Booze, brew, juice, sauce, hooch	Swallowed
Barbiturates *Phenobarbital, Amytal, Nembutal, Seconal*	Barbs, reds, red birds, phennies, yellow jackets	Injected, swallowed, snorted
Benzodiazepines *Ativan, Halcion, Klonopin, Librium, Valium, Xanax*	*Ativan, Halcion, Klonopin, Librium, Valium, Xanax*: Candy, downers, sleeping pills	Swallowed, injected
Flunitrazepam/*Rohypnol*	*Rohypnol*: Forget-me pill, Mexican Valium, R2, Roche, roofies, roofinol, rope, rophies	
Gamma-hydroxybutyric acid (GHB)	*Gamma-hydroxybutyrate*: G, Georgia home boy, liquid ecstasy	
Methaqualone/*Quaalude*	*Quaalude, Sopor, Parest*: Ludes, mandrex, quad, quay	
HALLUCINOGENS		
Phencyclidine (PCP and analogues)	*Phencyclidine (PCP)*: PCP, angel dust, supergrass, boat, peace pill, tic tac, zoom, Shermans, hog	Injected, snorted, smoked, swallowed
Ketamine/Ketalar	*Ketamine:* Cat Valium, K, special K, vitamin K, kit kat	
Other Hallucinogens *Ayahuasca* (Combination of Psychotria viridis plant, which contains DMT, and *Banisteriopsis caapi* vine, which contains an MAO inhibitor)	*Aya, Yagé, Hoasca*	Brewed and ingested as tea
Lysergic acid diethylamide: acid/LSD	*Lysergic acid diethylamide:* Acid, blotter, boomers, cubes, microdot, yellow sunshines	Swallowed, absorbed through mouth tissues, smoked
Mescaline	*Mescaline:* Buttons, cactus, mesc, peyote	
Psilocybin	*Psilocybin:* Magic mushrooms, mushrooms, shrooms	

Table 69.2 Commonly Used Addictive Substances—cont'd

Substance Category and Generic and Brand or Chemical Name	Examples of Commercial and Street Names	How Used
OPIOIDS AND MORPHINE DERIVATIVES		
Codeine	*Empirin with Codeine, Fiorinal with Codeine, Robitussin-AC, Tylenol with Codeine:* Captain Cody, Cody, schoolboy; (with glutethimide) doors and fours, loads, pancakes and syrup	Injected, swallowed, smoked, snorted
Fentanyl and fentanyl analogues Actiq, Duragesic	*Actiq, Duragesic, Sublimaze:* Apache, China girl, dance fever, friend, jackpot, murder 8, TNT	
Heroin Diacetylmorphine	*Diacetylmorphine:* Brown sugar, dope, H, horse, junk, skag, skunk, smack, white horse	
Morphine Roxanol, Duramorph	*Roxanol, Duramorph:* M, Miss Emma, monkey, white stuff	
Opium Laudanum, paregoric	*Laudanum, paregoric:* Big O, black stuff, block, gum, hop	
Oxycodone HCL OxyContin	*OxyContin:* Oxy, OC, killer	
Hydrocodone bitartrate Acetaminophen/Vicodin	*Vicodin:* Vike, Watson-387	
STIMULANTS		
Amphetamine Biphetamine, Dexedrine	*Biphetamine, Dexedrine:* Bennies, black beauties, crosses, hearts, LA turnaround, speed, truck drivers, uppers	Injected, swallowed, smoked, snorted
Cocaine	*Cocaine hydrochloride:* Blow, bump, C, candy, Charlie, coke, crack, flake, rock, snow, toot	
Methamphetamine Desoxyn	*Desoxyn:* Chalk, crank, crystal, crystal meth, fire, glass, go fast, ice, meth, speed	
Methylphenidate	*Ritalin:* JIF, MPH, R-ball, Skippy, the smart drug, vitamin R	
3,4-Methylenedioxymethamphetamine MDMA	*MDMA:* Adam, clarity, ecstasy, Eve, lover's speed, Molly, peace, STP, X, XTC	
	Note: MDMA is a synthetic psychoactive drug with properties similar to those of both stimulant amphetamines and the hallucinogen mescaline.	

among college students (aged 18–22) was higher as compared to others in the same age group. There is wide variation in the prevalence of alcohol use among individual communities within the United States. In 2016, the prevalence of alcohol use was higher in the Northeast (36%) and Midwest (37%) and lower in the South (27%) and West (28%).

Although the legal drinking age is 21 in all states in the United States, there is a high prevalence of alcohol use among individuals between 12 and 20 years of age. In 2016 about 7.3 million young people (19.3%) under age 21 reported using alcohol during the past 30 days. Among current

underage users, approximately 4.5 million (12.1%) were binge drinkers, and 1.1 million (2.8%) were heavy drinkers. The rate of alcohol use among persons 12 to 20 was lower in 2017 compared to 2012. However, underage use of alcohol is still a significant public health issue.

The use of alcohol among women of childbearing age increases the risk of fetal alcohol spectrum disorders and other disorders associated with substance use among pregnant women. In the United States, 9.4% of pregnant women aged 15 to 44 reported current alcohol use, 2.3% reported binge drinking, and 0.4% reported heavy drinking.

Among nonpregnant women in the same age group, 55.4% reported alcohol use, 24.6% reported binge drinking, and 5.3% reported heavy drinking.

Although marijuana is legal now in some areas, it is the most commonly used illegal substance, with an estimated 24 million people (8.9% of the population) reporting use in 2016, up from 19.8 million users in 2013. It is estimated that 1 in 11 people who use marijuana develop a cannabis use disorder and that an estimated 1% of the American population meets the diagnostic criteria for a cannabis use disorder.

An estimated 4.6 million young adults and older were current users of illicit drugs other than marijuana in 2016. Nonmedical use of prescription medications accounted for the next highest number of illegal substances used (5.3 million persons, or 2.3% of the population). Individuals who used prescription psychotherapeutic medications for nonmedical purposes included 3.3 million misusers of pain relievers (1.4%), 2 million misusers of tranquilizers (0.7), 1.7 million misusers of stimulants (0.6%), and 500,000 misusers of sedatives (0.2%). The prevalence of past-month illicit substance use in the United States in 2016 was 10.6% (Box 69.1).

Once on the decline, heroin use has increased over the past decade, and this rise is attributed largely to young people who are smoking or sniffing the drug rather than injecting it. The prevalence of opioid use, including heroin, in the United States in 2016 was 1.4% of the young adult and adult population.

Methamphetamine use has seen a dramatic increase over the last 25 years in the United States. Initially observed primarily in Hawaii and the western United States, methamphetamine abuse quickly spread eastward. In 2016, there were 700,000 users in the United States. Although cocaine use has declined since its popularity soared in the 1980s and 1990s, the appeal of cocaine as a stimulant continues. In 2016, of the young adults and older adults in the U.S. population, 9% reported the use of cocaine during the past month.

Substance use is a factor in many preventable injuries and deaths. In the United States in 2015, 2,333 teens aged 16 to 19 were killed and 235,845 required emergency treatment for injuries suffered in motor vehicle crashes. In 2016, alcohol was a factor in 28% of all traffic deaths (10,497) in the United States; 15% involved a driver aged 15 to 20. There is a significant link between alcohol use and motor vehicle crashes, homicides, alcohol poisoning, falls, burns, drowning, and suicides. One in four patients admitted to medical and surgical services in general hospitals has an AUD.

Compared to 2013, drug-poisoning deaths in the United States increased among all age groups in 2016. There were 63,632 drug-poisoning deaths in 2016 compared to 43,982 in 2013. Natural and synthetic opioids such as oxycodone and hydrocodone were responsible for 14,487 poisoning deaths, and 15,469 drug-poisoning deaths involved heroin. Frequently, when drug poisoning is the cause of death, toxicology tests reveal the presence of more than one drug. In 2016, fentanyl or another synthetic opioid was involved in 50% of all overdose deaths in the United States, with fentanyl responsible for 19,413 deaths in 2016.

Risk Factors

Multiple risk factors are associated with SUDs (Box 69.2). It is evident that no independent factor is sufficient to cause a SUD; rather, a complex interaction of multiple factors is responsible. Not everyone who has an opportunity to use an addictive substance does so, and not everyone who uses an addictive substance develops an SUD. Many individuals with biological, social, or environmental risk factors who use one or more substances do not develop an SUD.

Genetics

Genetics influences the risk for SUDs. Research supports a genetic component for nicotine, alcohol, cocaine, opioid, and cannabis use disorders (see Genetic Connections:

Box 69.1 Prescription Drug Abuse: A National Epidemic

- Prescription medications, such as those used to treat pain, attention deficit disorders, and anxiety, are being abused at a rate second only to marijuana among illicit drug users.
- In 2016, an estimated 11.8 million people reported misusing opioids in the past year. Among people who misused opioids, 11.5 million misused prescription pain relievers, and 948,000 used heroin.
- Among those who reported nonmedical use of a prescription medication, 5.3 million persons, or 2.3% of the U.S. population reported nonmedical use of prescription medication within the past 30 days.
- In 2016, drug-poisoning deaths were higher than in previous years. There were 63,632 drug-poisoning deaths in 2016 compared to 43,982 in 2013. Natural and synthetic opioids such as oxycodone and hydrocodone were responsible for 14,487 poisoning deaths, and 15,469 drug-poisoning deaths involved heroin.

Box 69.2 Risk Factors for Substance Use Disorders

- Biology/genetics
- Ethnicity/gender/age
- Presence of other mental health disorders
- Early drug use
- Peer group pressure
- Childhood adverse advents/history of sexual abuse
- Increased stress/crisis
- Home environment/family beliefs and attitudes
- Academic failure or poor social skills

Alcohol Use Disorders). Of course, an individual with the genetic predisposition for an AUD or another SUD cannot develop a disorder if the person does not drink alcohol or use drugs. The interaction of biology and environment truly determines whether an individual develops an SUD.

Genetic Connections

Alcohol Use Disorders

Rates of alcohol use disorders are substantially higher in the relatives of people with an alcohol use disorder than in relatives of people who do not have an alcohol use disorder, even in cases of people who have been adopted and not raised by their biological parent. It has been postulated that the genes a person is born with, in combination with environmental influences, account for about half of a person's vulnerability to substance use disorders (SUDs). With rapidly increasing access to online databases and data from genomic studies, including the Genome-Wide Association Studies catalog, genomic studies will quickly add to the understanding of the role of genetics in the development of SUDs.

Ethnicity, Gender, Education, and Mental Health Disorders

A person's ethnicity, gender, and level of education and the presence of other mental health disorders are also associated with the risk of developing an SUD. Males are almost twice as likely as females to have an SUD. However, women are almost twice as likely as men to develop a sedative, hypnotic, or anxiolytic use disorder. In the United States, the prevalence of AUDs is significantly higher among men, Caucasians, Native Americans, younger and unmarried adults, and those with lower incomes.

Education is identified as a factor associated with the nonmedical use of prescription stimulants. When compared to individuals in the same age group, nonmedical use of Adderall was higher among college students. Recently reported statistics among college students in the United States demonstrate that the use of illicit drugs was highest for Caucasians (25.1%), followed by Hispanics (21.5%), then African Americans (19.7%) and Asians (9.4%). Looking at ethnicity as a risk factor for the use of illicit substances, the highest use rates were reported among persons of two or more races (17.4%) and Native Hawaiians or Other Pacific Islanders (14.0%), followed by American Indians or Alaska Natives (12.3%), African Americans (10.5%), Caucasians (9.5%), and Hispanics (8.8%). The lowest rate was reported among Asians (3.3%).

Individuals with other mental health disorders are at much higher risk than the general population of developing an SUD by approximately two to one. Associated mental health disorders include mood, anxiety, and personality disorders; eating disorders; attention deficit-hyperactivity disorder (ADHD); and conduct disorders in childhood.

Age

A person's age at the initial use of an addictive substance is a strong risk factor for subsequent substance use problems. Often, initial substance use takes place in adolescence. When adolescent individuals first try an addictive substance, they might not be fully aware of the effect of the drug or the dangers and consequences of drug use. Adolescents' brains (Fig. 69.1) are still developing in the areas that govern decision making, judgment, and self-control, making them especially prone to risk-taking behaviors, including trying addictive substances. The likelihood of developing an AUD has been found to quadruple if drinking begins before the age of 15. The harmful effects of the drugs themselves on the developing brain may further increase the chances of future substance use problems. Once there has been an initial exposure to alcohol and other addictive substances, the likelihood of going on to use other drugs increases. Research has shown that teens who have an AUD and smoke marijuana are more likely to go on to use drugs such as cocaine and heroin. Stress is also strongly associated with the development of SUDs, with adverse events in childhood being a particularly significant risk factor. Adolescents are more likely to develop problems at times of change or increased stress, such as when there is a divorce, change in schools, or death in the family. Women are more likely than

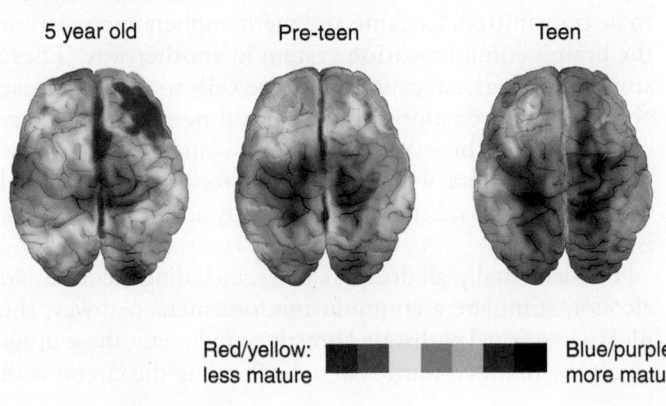

Red/yellow: less mature   Blue/purple: more mature

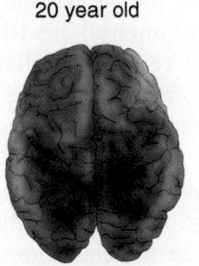

FIGURE 69.1 National Institute of Drug Abuse (NIDA) images of brain development in healthy children and teens (aged 5–20).

men to say their heavy drinking followed a crisis, such as miscarriage, divorce, or unemployment, or a recent departure of a child from the home. The use of alcohol is also increasing among adults aged 65 years or older.

The method of administration of a drug also increases its addictive potential. Smoking a drug or injecting it into a vein allows the drug to enter the brain within seconds. This intense, almost immediate "high" and the fact that the rush can fade in a few minutes may drive some individuals to repeated drug use in an attempt to recapture the initial pleasurable state.

Psychosocial Risk Factors

Although there is no one reason why people decide to use drugs, one of the simplest reasons that people use drugs and alcohol is to *feel good*. Most addictive substances produce intense feelings of pleasure, making them highly desirable. Depending on the substance, the associated feelings can be those of power, increased self-confidence, increased energy, or a sense of creativity. For example, persons who use cocaine and other stimulants (such as methamphetamine) often experience an inflated sense of self and describe feeling energized and ready to take on anything. People who use heroin or marijuana often feel very relaxed and "mellow" after the initial euphoria.

Alcohol and other drugs are often portrayed as enhancing the enjoyment of social interactions. Many find that the shared activity of using drugs or drinking with others makes them feel part of a group, which is socially reinforcing. This can make stopping drinking or drugs all the more difficult. Not only does the substance user have to give up familiar activities, locations, and established socializing patterns on the path to recovery, but friendships with individuals who continue to use may also have to be relinquished.

Another reason people use drugs is to *feel better*. Not uncommonly, people who suffer from social anxiety, stress-related disorders, and depression begin abusing drugs in an attempt to lessen feelings of distress. Stress can play an important role in the initiation and maintenance of drug use and the relapse back to the use of drugs and alcohol. Significant associations are found between SUDs and co-occurring mental health illness, including mood, anxiety, and personality disorders. The term "self-medicating" refers to individuals who take drugs in an attempt to cope with genuinely difficult problems such as stress, trauma, and the symptoms of mental health disorders. It is important, however, to remember that these drugs are not prescribed medications, and they frequently exacerbate the very conditions they are being used to relieve.

Just as some individuals use drugs to *feel good* or *feel better*, others use them in an attempt to *be the best*. With increasing pressure on individuals to achieve more in the classroom, in the boardroom, or on the court, more individuals are using drugs to enhance their cognitive and athletic performance. College campuses across the nation have seen dramatic increases in the numbers of students abusing stimulant drugs such as methylphenidate (Ritalin) and dextroamphetamine (Adderall) in an effort to achieve established goals, such as staying awake and focused during long hours of studying or working.

Connection Check 69.2

The nurse recognizes that which patient(s) are at risk for developing problems with substance abuse? *(Select all that apply.)*

A. The 14-year-old girl whose family has just moved and who is smoking and drinking after school with friends
B. The 17-year-old senior in high school who has untreated ADHD and whose mother has an AUD
C. The 32-year-old mother of two with a past history of binge drinking in college whose husband just left her
D. The 52-year-old executive with severe back pain who typically drinks cocktails in the evenings after work
E. The 64-year-old recently retired man who has an occasional drink in the evening after work

---

HOW PSYCHOACTIVE DRUGS AFFECT THE BRAIN

To understand how an SUD can be considered a disease, the nurse must appreciate the intricate communication system going on inside the brain. To function normally, the brain must maintain a careful balance of neurotransmitters. These small molecules carry messages between nerve cells (neurons) to help regulate the body's function and behavior. **Psychoactive drugs** are chemicals that, in one way or another, tap into this communication system and disrupt the way the neurons normally send, receive, and process information. There are at least two ways that drugs are able to do this: (1) by imitating the brain's natural chemical messengers (neurotransmitters) and/or (2) by overstimulating the "reward circuit" of the brain.

Researchers have found that marijuana and heroin can activate neurons because they have a structure similar to that of a natural neurotransmitter and thus are able to "fool" the brain's receptors, causing abnormal messages to be transmitted. Cocaine and methamphetamine disrupt the brain's communication system in another way. These stimulant drugs can cause the nerve cells to either release abnormally large amounts of natural neurotransmitters or prevent the brain's transporters from recycling these neurotransmitters, which is required to shut off the signal between neurons. Either way, a greatly amplified message is produced.

Fundamentally, all drugs of abuse, including nicotine and alcohol, stimulate a common reinforcement pathway, the **pleasure reward pathway**. Directly or indirectly, these drugs target the brain's reward system by flooding the circuit with dopamine. Dopamine is present in regions of the brain that control movement, emotion, motivation, and feelings of pleasure. The dopaminergic system normally responds to natural behaviors that are linked to survival, such as eating or spending time with loved ones. The overstimulation of the dopaminergic system, which produces euphoric effects, sets in motion a pattern that "teaches" people to repeat the behavior of abusing drugs. As a person continues to abuse drugs and alcohol, the brain starts to adapt to these chemical changes by producing less dopamine or by reducing the number of dopamine receptors in the reward circuit. As a result, dopamine's impact on the reward circuit is lessened, reducing the abuser's ability to enjoy the drugs and the things that previously brought pleasure. This conditioning leads individuals with an SUD to experience uncontrollable cravings when they see a place or person they associate with the drug experience (trigger) even when the drug itself is not available.

With ongoing exposure, the brain may become insensitive to the effects of drugs or alcohol. This, in turn, can cause the individual to require larger amounts of the drug (tolerance) to achieve the euphoria or "dopamine high." Long-term use causes changes in other brain chemical systems and circuits as well. Glutamate is a neurotransmitter that influences the reward circuit and the ability to learn. Alteration of glutaminergic function by an SUD can impair cognitive function. Brain imaging studies of individuals with one or more SUDs show changes in areas of the brain that are critical to judgment, decision making, learning and memory, and behavior control. Together, these changes can cause a person with an SUD to seek out and take drugs compulsively despite adverse consequences.

Connection Check 69.3

Which reaction in the brain results from drugs causing overwhelming surges of dopamine?
A. Production of more of the neurotransmitter
B. Increase in the number of receptors that can receive and transmit signals
C. An increased ability to respond to pleasure
D. A decreased ability to respond to pleasure

SUBSTANCES AND CLINICAL MANIFESTATIONS

In virtually every practice setting, nurses encounter patients struggling with one or more SUDs. There are general physical, behavioral, and psychosocial signs the nurse should be alert to that may indicate a patient is abusing drugs and/or alcohol (Box 69.3). To provide safe and individualized care, it is helpful for the nurse to be aware of categories and names of substances commonly used by persons with SUDs, examples of commercial and street names, and methods and routes of use (see Table 69.2) and their clinical manifestations.

Box 69.3 Physical, Behavioral, and Psychological Signs of Hazardous Substance Use

Physical Signs
- Bloodshot eyes
- Pupils larger or smaller than usual
- Changes in appetite
- Sudden weight loss or gain
- Changes in sleep patterns
- Deterioration of physical appearance and personal grooming habits
- Unusual smells on breath, body, or clothing
- Tremors, slurred speech, or impaired coordination

Behavioral Signs
- Poor performance or missed days at school or work
- Financial troubles; unexplained need for money; may borrow or steal to get money
- Secretive or suspicious behaviors
- Change in peer group, hangouts, favorite activities, or hobbies
- Frequently getting into trouble (fights, accidents, illegal activities)

Psychological Signs
- Unexplained changes in personality or attitude
- Sudden mood swings, irritability, or angry outbursts
- Periods of unusual hyperactivity, agitation, or giddiness
- Lack of motivation; appears lethargic or "spaced out"
- Appears fearful, anxious, or paranoid for no apparent reason

Connection Check 69.4

The nurse working in the pediatric clinic is performing substance abuse screenings on all children aged 12 to 18 as part of a community effort to identify at-risk teens. The nurse should consider which teen at greatest risk?
A. The 13-year-old girl who has recently been irritable and moody
B. The 14-year-old boy being treated for diagnosed ADHD with prescription stimulants
C. The 15-year-old who recently entered high school and appears down, reports trouble sleeping, and has difficulty concentrating
D. The 17-year-old cheerleader who quits the squad, suddenly changes her group of friends, and has been acting very secretive at home

Alcohol

Categories of Alcohol Use

Alcohol use can be defined by the pattern of use and amount consumed (e.g., binge or heavy) or by the number of symptoms and consequences associated with its use (e.g., mild, moderate, or severe). The amount of alcohol consumed and the pattern of use are also indicators of an individual's risk (i.e., low, moderate, or high) of developing an AUD. According to guidelines developed by the National Institute on Alcohol Abuse and Alcoholism, persons at risk for developing an AUD are men who consume more than 4 drinks and women who consume more than 3 drinks on a single occasion or more than 14 drinks in a week for men and more than 7 for women. The guidelines for persons aged 65 and older are the same as the guidelines for women under 65. Heavy alcohol use is defined as five or more drinks on the same occasion on each of 5 or more days in the past 30 days. Binge drinking is defined as drinking five or more alcoholic drinks on the same occasion on at least 1 day in the past 30 days or a pattern of drinking that brings BALs to 80 mg/dL. This typically occurs after four drinks for women and five drinks for men are consumed within about 2 hours.

The category of "moderate" alcohol consumption is used for individuals whose alcohol use falls between abstinence (i.e., no use of alcohol) and heavy use. According to the Dietary Guidelines for Americans, moderate drinking is up to one drink per day for women and up to two drinks per day for men. In the United States, a standard drink is any drink that contains about 14 g of pure alcohol. Among individual alcohol users, the definition of one "standard" drink may vary. In Figure 69.2, examples are given of a "standard" drink based on the choice of alcoholic beverage—beer, malt liquor, table wine, or 80-proof spirits. Table 69.3 quantifies the number of standard drinks in common container sizes sold in the United States. According to Table 69.3, if an individual reports drinking one beer daily, clarification of the meaning of *beer* (beer or malt liquor) and the size of the container (12, 24, or 40 oz) is needed to more accurately estimate the number of "standard" drinks consumed daily.

Effects

Alcohol is a central nervous system depressant that affects several areas of the brain (Fig. 69.3). When alcohol reaches the brain, it interferes with communication between nerve cells by interacting with the receptors on some cells.

Alcohol enhances inhibitory nerve pathway activity at gamma-aminobutyric acid A ($GABA_A$) receptors, which has the effect of making a person sluggish. Additionally, alcohol reduces excitatory neurotransmission at glutamate N-methyl-D-aspartate receptor (NMDA) receptors, serving to further enhance sluggishness. Although the entire brain is affected, the cerebellum, responsible for balance, coordination, and movement, and the frontal lobes, responsible for cognition, memory, thought, and learning, are most heavily affected by alcohol consumption.

The short-term effects of alcohol vary on the basis of a number of factors, such as a person's size, the setting, the amount and time of consumption, hydration levels, and whether a heavy meal is being consumed. In general, though, in low doses, alcohol's effects include euphoria, mild stimulation, relaxation, and lowered inhibitions. In higher doses, alcohol causes drowsiness and symptoms of **intoxication**, such as slurred speech, decreased reaction time, further disinhibition, nausea/vomiting, emotional volatility, loss of coordination, visual distortions, impaired memory, nystagmus, unsteady gait, sexual dysfunction, and loss of consciousness. Both the quantity of alcohol ingested and the rate of the rise of the BAL determine the level of intoxication (Table 69.4). Changes in behavior and functional abilities are usually observable at BALs of 20 mg/dL or higher. Examples of behaviors and functional ability at BALs of 20 to 40 mg/dL are shown in Table 68.4 along with the equivalent blood alcohol concentration (BAC) in grams per deciliter (g/dL) and percentage of alcohol in the blood. The amount of ingested alcohol required to reach a specific BAL varies among individuals. Body weight, gender, and percentage of body fat influence the BAL. **Blackouts** are intervals of time for which the intoxicated person cannot recall key details of events. They are thought to be much more common in social drinkers than previously assumed and occur during a rapid rise in BAL, such as when a person drinks quickly or drinks on an empty stomach.

The long-term effects of alcohol abuse are associated with a wide range of physical and mental health disorders, including liver and heart disease, hypertension, risk for infectious diseases, nutritional deficiencies, depression, certain cancers, infertility, and AUD, to name a few (Box 69.4). Women who consume less alcohol and for a shorter period of time than men are at higher risk of developing alcohol-related health problems. Studies also report that women with an AUD are up to twice as likely as men to die from alcohol-related causes such as suicide, accidents, and illnesses. Alcohol has been implicated in more than 200 types of disease and injury, almost 75% of all rapes, and up to 70% of all incidents of domestic violence. Annually, 696,000 students between the ages of 18 and 24 are assaulted by another student who has been drinking; 97,000 students between the ages of 18 and 24 report experiencing alcohol-related sexual assault or date rape. In the United States, alcohol is the third-leading preventable cause of death. Nearly 88,000 people die annually from alcohol-related causes. In 2013, 10,076 fatalities were related to alcohol-impaired

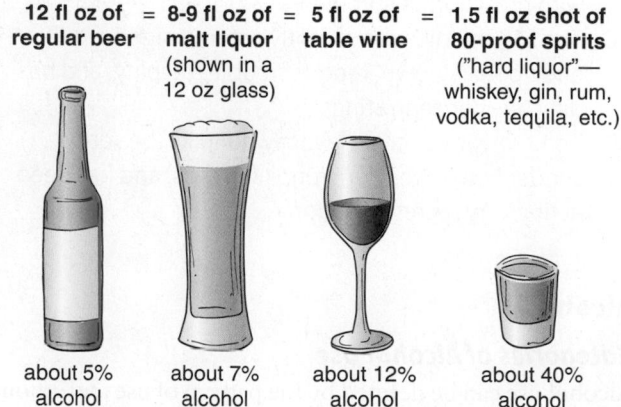

| 12 fl oz of regular beer | = | 8-9 fl oz of malt liquor (shown in a 12 oz glass) | = | 5 fl oz of table wine | = | 1.5 fl oz shot of 80-proof spirits ("hard liquor"— whiskey, gin, rum, vodka, tequila, etc.) |

about 5% alcohol   about 7% alcohol   about 12% alcohol   about 40% alcohol

FIGURE 69.2 Examples of a "standard" drink based on the choice of alcoholic beverage, beer, malt liquor, table wine, or 80-proof spirits.

Table 69.3 Number of Standard Drinks in a Container (Bottle or Can)

Type of Beverage	Sample of Containers/Sizes Sold	Number of "Standard" Drinks in the Container
Regular beer	12 oz	0.8 "standard" drink
		A little less than the equivalent of 1 standard drink
Malt liquor	12 oz	1.4 standard drinks
	24 oz	2.8 standard drinks
	40 oz	4.7 standard drinks
Table wine 750 mL standard: Common bottle size for most distributed wine	750 mL = 25.36 oz	5 standard drinks
80-proof spirits (whiskey, gin, rum, vodka tequila, etc.)	Pint: 12.7 oz = 375 mL	8.5 standard drinks
	Fifth: 25.36 oz = 750 mL	16.9 standard drinks

Adapted from information from U.S. Department of Health and Human Services, National Institutes of Health, & National Institute of Alcohol Abuse and Alcoholism (NIAAA). (n.d.). *Drink size calculator.* Retrieved from http://pubs.niaaa.nih.gov/publications/UnderageDrinking/UnderageFact.htm Retrieved from http://rethinkingdrinking.niaaa.nih.gov/Tools/Calculators/drink-size-calculator.aspx

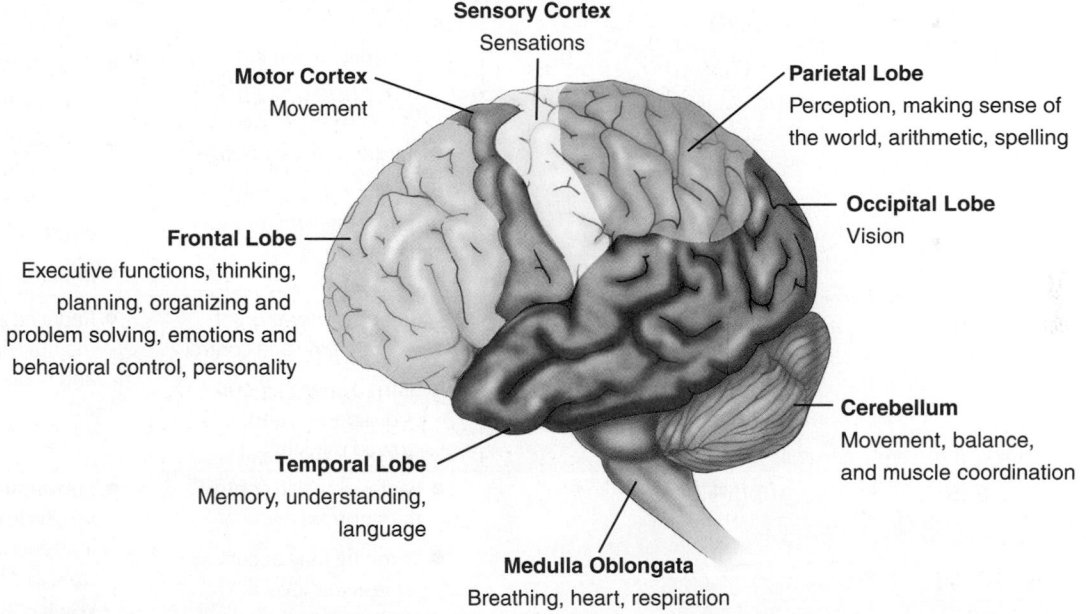

FIGURE 69.3 Schematic drawing of the human brain. Although all areas are affected, the cerebellum, responsible for balance, coordination, and movement, and the frontal lobes, responsible for cognition, memory, thought, and learning, are most heavily affected by alcohol consumption.

driving (30.8% of all driving fatalities). More than 10% of U.S. children live with a parent with issues related to alcohol consumption.

Alcohol and Pregnancy

Alcohol is a known teratogen, a substance that can harm the fetus. Fetal alcohol syndrome is a constellation of birth defects that includes poor growth, developmental delay, heart defects, and craniofacial abnormalities. When a woman drinks during pregnancy, alcohol crosses the placental barrier and enters the bloodstream of the fetus in levels that equal or exceed that of the mother. Newborns have been known to go through alcohol withdrawal and to require benzodiazepines for treatment after delivery. Alcohol can also pass through breast milk to the baby.

Age-Related Considerations

As a person ages, blood flow, metabolism, and excretion all diminish. In the older adult population, where health may already be deteriorating, alcohol serves to cause new health concerns or exacerbate old ones. The change in physical health complicates alcohol absorption and metabolism, can interfere with medications, and can lead to falls and associated complications.

Table 69.4 **Comparison of Equivalent Measures of the Blood Alcohol Level, Blood Alcohol Concentration, and Percentage of Alcohol in Blood**

Blood Alcohol Level (BAL) (mg/dL)	Blood Alcohol Concentration (BAC) (g/dL)	Percentage of Alcohol (Weight/Volume) Parts Alcohol per 1,000 Parts Blood	Typical Effect	Effect on Driving
20	0.02	0.02% Two-tenths of 1% of the person's blood volume is alcohol	• Some loss of judgment • Relaxation • Feels slightly warmer even in cold temperature • Mood euphoric	• Decline in visual functions (rapid tracking of a moving target) • Decline in ability to perform two tasks at the same time (divided attention)
50	0.05	0.05%	• Difficulty focusing eyes on an object • Judgment impaired • Usually good feeling • Less alert • Release of inhibition	• Reduced coordination • Reduced ability to track moving objects • Difficulty steering • Reduced response to emergency driving situations
80	0.08	0.08%	• Poor muscle coordination (e.g., balance, speech, vision, reaction time, and hearing) • Harder to detect danger • Judgment, self-control, reasoning, and memory are impaired	• Impaired concentration • Short-term memory loss • Impaired speed control • Reduced information processing capability (e.g., signal detection, visual search) • Impaired perception
100	0.10	0.10%	• Clear deterioration of reaction time and control • Slurred speech, poor coordination, and slowed thinking	• Reduced ability to maintain lane position and brake appropriately
150	0.15	0.15%	• Far less muscle control than normal • Vomiting may occur (unless this level is reached slowly or a person has developed a tolerance for alcohol) • Major loss of balance	• Substantial impairment in vehicle control, inattention to driving task, and in necessary visual and auditory information processing
180	0.18	0.18%	Dysphonic, anxious, restless, nausea	
250	0.25	0.25%	Confused, needs assistance walking	
300	0.30	0.30%	Loss of consciousness	
Greater than or equal to 400	Greater than or equal to 0.40	Greater than or equal to 0.40%	Respiratory depression, coma, potential death	

Adapted from U.S. Department of Health and Human Services, Centers for Disease Control and Prevention (CDC) & National Center for Injury Prevention and Control, Division of Unintentional Injury Prevention. (2015). *Effects of blood alcohol concentration (BAC)*. Retrieved from http://www.cdc.gov/Motorvehiclesafety/impaired_driving/bac.html

Note: The information on the CDC Web site was gathered from a variety of sources, including the National Highway Traffic Safety Administration, the National Institute on Alcohol Abuse and Alcoholism, the American Medical Association, the National Commission Against Drunk Driving, and http://www.webMD.com.

Box 69.4 Manifestations of Chronic Alcohol Use

- Anxiety
- Bleeding disorders
- Cardiomyopathy
- Certain cancers
- Cirrhosis
- Delirium
- Depression
- Erectile dysfunction
- Gastrointestinal disorders
- Hypertension
- Insomnia
- Korsakoff's syndrome
- Nutritional deficiency
- Osteoporosis
- Recurrent falls
- Self-care deficient
- Spider angiomas
- Weight loss
- Wernicke's encephalopathy

Table 69.5 Common Findings of Alcohol Withdrawal Syndrome

Early to Mild AWS (6–12 Hours)	Moderate AWS (12–48 Hours)	Severe AWS (48–72 Hours)
• Fine tremor	• Increased tremor	• Tremors become uncontrollable shaking
• Mild diaphoresis	• Diaphoresis	• Diaphoresis becomes profuse
• Increased heart rate	• Tachycardia	
• Increased blood pressure	• Blood pressure continues to increase	• Hypertension, tachycardia, and tachypnea worsen, and hyperthermia may occur
• Nausea/Vomiting	• Nausea and vomiting worsen	
• Anorexia		• Seizures may present
• Headache	• Increasingly anxious, distressed, or agitated	• Mental status worsens to extreme agitation, fluctuating disorientation, confusion, and hallucinations—alcohol withdrawal delirium tremens or DTs
• Anxiety		
• Irritability		
• Insomnia	• Marked insomnia	
• May be demanding or aggressive in interactions	• May experience transient confusion or hallucinations	
• Sensitivity to light and sounds		

AWS, Alcohol withdrawal syndrome.

Nutritional Deficiencies

Because very heavy drinkers take in most of their calories through alcohol rather than food, a large percentage of persons with an AUD are found to have a deficiency in thiamine. Thiamine (vitamin B_1) is vital for carbohydrate metabolism and for the proper functioning of neurotransmitters. Thiamine also plays a key role in protecting neurons from injury, and a thiamine deficiency is one of the main mechanisms of alcohol-related brain injury. Long-term thiamine depletion in the brain can lead to serious central nervous system (CNS) disorders, such as **Wernicke–Korsakoff's syndrome.** Wernicke–Korsakoff's syndrome is a neurocognitive disorder that consists of two separate syndromes; an acute, short-lived, severe condition called *Wernicke's encephalopathy* and a long-lasting and debilitating condition known as *Korsakoff's psychosis.* The clinical manifestations of Wernicke's encephalopathy include mental confusion, paralysis of the nerves that move the eyes (i.e., oculomotor disturbances), and difficulty with muscle coordination. Korsakoff's psychosis is a chronic and debilitating syndrome characterized by persistent learning and memory problems.

Withdrawal Symptoms

Almost all people with an AUD who have been chronic heavy drinkers experience some level of withdrawal symptomatology if they suddenly stop drinking or significantly decrease the amount of alcohol consumed. The clinical presentation can range from mild tremors, anxiety, and discomfort to life-threatening seizures and **delirium tremens**—which can include confusion, hallucinations, autonomic instability, and death. When the depressant effect of alcohol is removed, every mechanism overreacts within hours of the last drink, resulting in alcohol withdrawal syndrome (AWS; Table 69.5).

Many factors determine whether a person is considered as having a high risk for complicated withdrawal, including a previous history of significant withdrawal, multiple previous detoxifications, comorbid illnesses, and recent drinking at high levels.

Treatment

Various treatments are available to help people with an AUD, and depending on the circumstances, AUD treatment may involve a brief intervention, an outpatient program or counseling, medications, or a residential inpatient stay. Specific treatment for alcohol withdrawal may be inpatient or outpatient. The majority of people with an AUD with mild to moderate withdrawal symptoms can be treated on an outpatient basis. Some need to be hospitalized in a facility that specializes in detoxification and can provide close monitoring of vital signs and assessment of withdrawal symptoms. Medically managed detoxification generally includes the use of benzodiazepines. Alcoholics Anonymous (AA) plays a major role in the treatment of AUDs nationwide and has been proven to be an extremely effective treatment approach. The AA 12-step program (Box 69.5), essential to so many people with an AUD for the day-by-day

Box 69.5 The 12 Steps of Alcoholics Anonymous

1. We admitted we were powerless over alcohol—that our lives had become unmanageable.
2. Came to believe that a Power greater than ourselves could restore us to sanity.
3. Made a decision to turn our will and our lives over to the care of God *as we understood Him.*
4. Made a searching and fearless moral inventory of ourselves.
5. Admitted to God, to ourselves, and to another human being the exact nature of our wrongs.
6. Were entirely ready to have God remove all these defects of character.
7. Humbly asked Him to remove our shortcomings.
8. Made a list of all persons we had harmed, and became willing to make amends to them all.
9. Made direct amends to such people wherever possible, except when to do so would injure them or others.
10. Continued to take personal inventory and when we were wrong promptly admitted it.
11. Sought through prayer and meditation to improve our conscious contact with God, *as we understood Him*, praying only for knowledge of His will for us and the power to carry that out.
12. Having had a spiritual awakening as the result of these Steps, we tried to carry this message to alcoholics, and to practice these principles in all our affairs.

support they need, works best when combined with other forms of therapy such as psychotherapy and medical care.

Currently, there are only three medications that are approved by the U.S. Food and Drug Administration (FDA) for the treatment of AUD. Disulfiram (Antabuse) was the first medication approved for the treatment of AUD, and it works by causing a severe adverse reaction when someone taking the medication consumes alcohol. Naltrexone (ReVia and Depade) works by blocking in the brain the "high" that people experience when they drink or take drugs such as heroin or cocaine. Acamprosate (Campral) is the most recently approved medication treatment for AUD, and it works by reducing the physical distress and emotional discomfort people experience when they quit drinking.

Connection Check 69.5

The nurse monitors for which clinical manifestations in the patient diagnosed with early alcohol withdrawal?
A. Anxiety, stomach cramping, and aching muscles
B. Restlessness, diaphoresis, and sensitivity to lights and sounds
C. Autonomic hyperactivity, hallucinations, and global confusion
D. Depression, hunger, and fatigue

Sedative-Hypnotics

The sedative-hypnotics, sometimes referred to as *depressants*, are a diverse group of medications that are generally classified on the basis of their medical effects on the body. All reduce the activity of the CNS. Most do so by enhancing the actions of the neurotransmitter GABA and decreasing the activity of the reticular activating system in the brainstem, which in turn causes a reduction in the level of consciousness. Sedatives cause a mild depression of the CNS, decrease excitability and anxiety, and have a muscle-relaxing property sought by many abusers of drugs. Hypnotics, on the other hand, induce sleep. Increasing the dose of a sedative can cause a hypnotic effect, and increasing the dose even further can produce an anesthetic state, a deep depression of the CNS. This group of agents includes the benzodiazepines, barbiturates, and various agents not belonging to either of these categories. The use of alcohol, also a CNS depressant, with any of these medications potentiates the effects of the medication and can lead to an additive and dangerous reaction.

Barbiturates

Barbiturates are defined as any of a group of barbituric acid derivatives used in medicine as sedatives and hypnotics. They have considerable medical value but can easily be misused. Initial use can cause loss of inhibition, euphoria, and behavioral stimulation. Chronic nonmedical use of barbiturates causes a cumulative toxic effect on the CNS. Delirium can develop with increased doses or when used in the presence of other medical or psychiatric conditions.

Barbiturates still enjoy some use as anticonvulsants and anesthetic agents but have been almost entirely replaced by the benzodiazepines as legitimate anxiolytics, medications used in the treatment of anxiety. Because of the potential for barbiturates to cause respiratory depression, they are much more dangerous in cases of overdose.

Benzodiazepines

Benzodiazepines are minor tranquilizers, anxiolytics, or antianxiety agents often prescribed for short-term treatment of medical and mental health conditions, such as anxiety, acute stress reaction, and panic attacks. The primary action of the minor tranquilizers is on the limbic system, which serves as the intermediary between the hypothalamus and the cerebral cortex and appears to control emotion. Specific agents, including diazepam (Valium), lorazepam (Ativan), oxazepam (Serax), and chlordiazepoxide (Librium), are frequently employed to treat acute alcohol withdrawal. The more sedating benzodiazepines with intermediate half-lives, such as triazolam (Halcion), estazolam (ProSom), and temazepam (Restoril), are prescribed for short-term treatment of sleep disorders. Benzodiazepines are also used to treat anxiety disorders in the geriatric population but should be used with caution (see Geriatric/Gerontological Considerations: Benzodiazepines).

Geriatric/Gerontological Considerations

Benzodiazepines

- The biological half-life of benzodiazepines is significantly longer for older adults compared to younger adults.
- Starting doses must be much lower than those given to younger adults and should be adjusted to the individual to prevent oversedation.
- Susceptibility to the side effects of these medications, including dizziness, drowsiness, unsteady gait, and confusion, increases with age, putting older adults at greater risk for falls and accidents.

People of all ages tend to view these medications differently than "street drugs" and may not realize the potential for **addiction**, a complex condition leading to compulsive use of a substance despite its harmful effects. Findings in a previous survey indicated that 40% of teens believed that even if these medications are not prescribed by a provider, they are much safer to use than illegal drugs. Physical and psychological dependence can easily develop with repeated use and resemble dependence on alcohol and the barbiturates. Tolerance is common, and doses must be increased to obtain the desired results. Adverse effects of chronic benzodiazepine use can include a general deterioration in physical and mental health, cognitive impairment, behavioral problems, anxiety, depression, loss of sex drive, agoraphobia (extreme fear of entering open or crowded places, leaving own home, or being in places from which escape is difficult), social phobia, an altered perception of self and environment, and an inability to experience or express feelings. Chronic abusers may experience paradoxical effects such as aggression, violence, impulsivity, irritability, and suicidal behavior.

Miscellaneous Agents

Flunitrazepam

Flunitrazepam (Rohypnol) is a highly potent, intermediate-acting benzodiazepine derivative that is prescribed outside the United States for the treatment of severe cases of insomnia and as a preanesthetic. Although this medication is neither manufactured nor approved for sale in the United States, it is legally prescribed in over 60 countries (including Mexico, Colombia, and some European countries) and is often smuggled into the United States. It is often referred to as the "date rape" drug due to its amnesia-inducing effects. Flunitrazepam's effects include sedation, muscle relaxation, relief from anxiety, and prevention of convulsions. The effects of flunitrazepam are stronger than those of other benzodiazepines, appearing 15 to 20 minutes after administration and lasting approximately 4 to 6 hours. Some residual effects can be found for 12 hours or more. Flunitrazepam causes partial amnesia, and individuals are frequently unable to remember events that they experienced while under the influence of the drug. It can also be used to boost the high of heroin and modulate the effects of cocaine. It also cannot be detected in a urinalysis.

Flunitrazepam is usually consumed orally, often combined with alcohol, or by crushing tablets and snorting the powder. As with the other CNS depressants, chronic use of Rohypnol can lead to psychological and physical dependence and produce a withdrawal syndrome when the medication is discontinued, necessitating a 3- to 5-day inpatient detoxification admission that follows accepted protocols for benzodiazepine withdrawal syndrome.

Methaqualone

Methaqualone (Quaalude) is a popular nonbarbiturate sedative-hypnotic that is commonly abused in the United States. At higher doses, excessive CNS depression results, much like that produced by barbiturates—drowsiness, dizziness, decreased alertness and concentration.

Gamma-Hydroxybutyric Acid

Gamma-hydroxybutyric acid (GHB; Xyrem) is a CNS depressant that was approved in 2002 by the FDA, with severe restrictions, for use in the treatment of the sleep disorder narcolepsy. Gamma-hydroxybutyric acid, often referred to as "liquid ecstasy," is gaining popularity as a club drug and is used for its ability to produce euphoric and hallucinatory states. Some bodybuilders abuse GHB to aid in fat reduction and muscle building because of its anabolic effects. Like flunitrazepam, GHB is available in tasteless, colorless, and odorless forms; is frequently combined with alcohol; and has been used to commit sexual assaults because of its ability to sedate and incapacitate unsuspecting victims.

Gamma-hydroxybutyric acid is found naturally in the CNS. When ingested, GHB acts on at least two receptors, including the $GABA_B$ receptor and a specific GHB-binding site. Gamma-hydroxybutyric acid is rapidly absorbed after ingestion and takes 20 to 60 minutes, depending on the dose, to reach a maximal plasma concentration. Clinical effects become evident approximately 5 to 15 minutes after ingestion and can last up to several hours. Its effects include euphoria, disinhibition, enhanced sensuality, and feelings of kinship with others. Its relaxant properties cause the heart rate and respiration to slow and can interfere with blood circulation, motor coordination, balance, and speech. Other adverse effects may include nausea, vomiting, loss of reflexes, tremors, delusions, seizures, and amnesia. Taken in higher amounts, GHB can cause unconsciousness, seizures, severe respiratory depression, and coma. Gamma-hydroxybutyric acid can be addictive if used for prolonged periods. Chronic abusers who stop using GHB suddenly may experience withdrawal symptoms that include increased heart rate, hallucinations, sweating, insomnia, and seizures.

Withdrawal and Treatment

Discontinuing prolonged use of high doses of CNS depressants can lead to serious clinical manifestations of withdrawal, such as insomnia, nausea, vomiting, tremors, anxiety, restlessness, agitation, muscle spasms or twitching, dizziness, orthostatic hypotension, sweating, irritability, fearfulness, depression, or psychosis. Because the medications work by slowing the brain's activity, when a person stops taking a CNS depressant, this activity can rebound to the point that seizures occur. Abrupt withdrawal from benzodiazepines likely precipitates an acute syndrome resembling alcohol withdrawal and can be quite complicated and prolonged depending on the amount the person was taking. Improved psychomotor and cognitive functioning, particularly in older adults, is usually seen after discontinuation of benzodiazepines.

The treatment for withdrawal is based on the severity of the symptoms and the patient's individual profile, including overall health status, comorbidities, and age. Detoxification requires a cautious and gradual reduction of these medications. After initial detoxification, the treatment for dependence on CNS depressants is much like that of other drugs and includes cognitive-behavioral therapies, psychoeducation, and comprehensive care in a supportive environment.

Marijuana

The hemp plant *Cannabis sativa* is a potent substance that alters mood, perceptions, and sensations. The potency can vary significantly depending on the source and selection of plant materials. The psychoactive properties of marijuana are produced by delta-9-tetrahydrocannabinol (THC), the main active chemical found in cannabis. In 1974, the average THC content of illicit marijuana was less than 1%. The more recent use of hydroponic solution, however, has produced marijuana plants with THC concentrations ranging from 18% to 24% on average.

The THC binds to and overstimulates cannabinoid receptors found in areas of the brain responsible for movement, coordination, learning and memory, judgment, perception, and concentration. Marijuana enhances the senses and brings on feelings of relaxation and well-being. Marijuana is also used medicinally to relieve pain, reduce nausea and vomiting, and stimulate the appetite. Marijuana is usually smoked, and the effects of the drug can be felt within 10 minutes and can last from 1 to 3 hours.

Although marijuana was long thought to be a "benign" recreational drug, its use can have serious consequences. It can result in red eyes with dilated pupils, increased blood pressure and heart rate, impaired balance and coordination, difficulty concentrating and decreased memory, slowed reaction time, anxiety, paranoid thinking, and psychosis. Marijuana abuse has also been linked to low achievement, delinquent behavior, and poor family relationships.

Marijuana also contains known toxins and cancer-causing chemicals that are stored in fat cells for as long as several months. Smoking three to four cannabis cigarettes a day is associated with the same degree of acute and chronic bronchitis and the same degree of damage to the bronchial mucosa as smoking 20 or more tobacco cigarettes a day. The long-term use is implicated in respiratory disease, heart attack, stroke, stomach ulcers, and other health problems.

Withdrawal and Treatment

Although it is not thought to produce physical dependence, marijuana use can produce a strong psychological dependence, and new research is revealing a marijuana withdrawal syndrome. The clinical presentation includes decreased appetite, nausea, weight loss, headaches, irritability, anxiety, anger, aggressive behavior, restlessness, depressed mood, sleep disturbances, strange dreams, and cravings. Generally, only mild and symptomatic pharmacological treatment is needed.

Opiates/Opioids

Opiates are narcotic analgesics derived from the opium poppy plant grown in Asia and Central and South America. The term **opioid** refers to narcotic analgesics that are either semisynthetic or fully synthetic but can also refer to the entire family of both opiates and opioids. Morphine and codeine are both considered natural opiates. Semisynthetic opioids include hydrocodone (Vicodin), hydromorphone (Dilaudid), meperidine (Demerol), oxycodone (Percocet, Percodan, and OxyContin), and the highly addictive drug heroin. Synthetic opioids are fentanyl (Duragesic), propoxyphene (Darvon), pentazocine (Talwin), and methadone.

Opioids act by attaching to specific proteins called *opioid receptors* (mu receptors) that are found in the brain, spinal cord, gastrointestinal tract, and other organs in the body. Opiates can be classified as **full agonists**, **partial agonists**, or **antagonists** depending on their actions at the mu receptor. Full agonists bind to and activate receptors until all opioid receptors are occupied. Partial agonists behave like agonists but do not cause full receptor activation. Opioids such as Demerol and heroin are agonists; buprenorphine is a partial agonist. Antagonists bind to the same receptor but do not cause activity. They prevent the opiate "high" while simultaneously blockading the receptor to other agonists. Naloxone is an antagonist.

Opioids reduce the intensity of pain signals reaching the brain and affect the brain areas controlling emotion, which diminishes the effects of the painful stimulus (Fig. 69.4). They can produce drowsiness, mental confusion, nausea, and constipation, and depending on the amount taken, they can depress respiration. These drugs also produce feelings of euphoria, relaxation, and contentment, making them highly reinforcing psychologically. Consequently, there is a high potential for nonmedical use of opioids and the development of an opioid use disorder.

Prescription Narcotics

These medications are commonly prescribed because they are extremely effective for the treatment of pain. Because of their common use, most abusers can get them from family and friends or directly from providers. In recent years, among young adults and older adults who used prescription opiates, 27% obtained them through a prescription from their healthcare provider. Other sources include from friends or relatives for free (26%), buying from friends or relatives (23%), or buying from a drug dealer (15%).

Limbic System
Opiates can change the limbic system which controls emotions and increases feelings of pleasure

Brainstem
Opiates can depress breathing by changing neurochemical activity in the brainstem where automatic body functions are controlled

Spinal Cord
Opiates can block pain messages transmitted through the spinal cord from the body

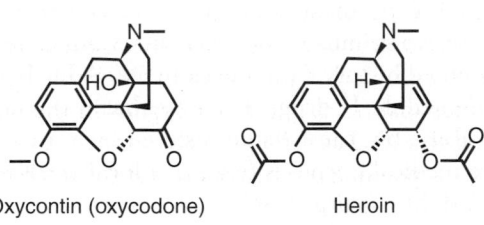

Oxycontin (oxycodone)   Heroin

FIGURE 69.4 Locations in the brain affected by opiates. The chemical structures of OxyContin and heroin are similar and bind to the same receptors in the brain.

In addition to nonmedical use, more people are being exposed to prescription opiates legitimately to treat pain due to an aging population (see Geriatric/Gerontological Considerations: Prescription Narcotics) and more sports-related injuries in the younger population. The consistent use of prescription narcotics can lead to physical dependence with characteristic withdrawal signs (Table 69.6). Tolerance may

Table 69.6 Opioid Withdrawal Symptoms

Initial	Cravings, anxiety, runny nose (rhinorrhea), yawning, excess tears (lacrimation), perspiration, and minor stomach cramps
12–72 hours	Hot and cold flashes, loss of appetite, nausea, vomiting, diarrhea, goose bumps, muscle twitching and aching muscles and bones, insomnia, increased blood pressure, fever, tachycardia
24–48 hours	Significant muscle and bone aches along with powerful muscle spasms that cause violent kicking motions ("kicking the habit")

accompany the physical dependence, resulting in the need to take higher doses of the medication to get the same effect. When this occurs, it can be very difficult for a provider to know if the patient is developing a drug problem or has a real medical need for higher doses to control the symptoms. If the provider believes it to be a drug problem, the medication is discontinued, which can sometimes lead the dependent patient to seek out the opiates someplace else.

Geriatric/Gerontological Considerations

Prescription Narcotics

- Persons 65 or older comprise only 13% of the population yet account for more than one-third of total outpatient spending on prescription medications in the United States.
- Older persons are more likely to be prescribed long-term and multiple prescriptions.
- Some experience cognitive decline, which could lead to improper use of medications.
- Older adults on a fixed income may take another person's remaining medication to save money.
- High rates of comorbid illnesses, age-related changes in medication metabolism, and the potential for medication interactions increase the risk of danger in geriatrics.
- The use of over-the-counter medicines, dietary supplements, and alcohol can compound any adverse health consequences resulting from prescription medication abuse.

Heroin

Heroin is a highly addictive drug that is processed from morphine and usually appears as a white or brown powder or as a black, sticky substance. It is injected, snorted, or smoked and rapidly delivered to the brain. Short-term effects of heroin include a surge of euphoria ("rush"), dry mouth, a feeling of heaviness of the extremities, a warm flushing of the skin, and clouded thinking. This is followed by alternating wakeful and drowsy states.

Like other opioids, heroin depresses breathing, and overdoses can be fatal. Users who inject the drug are at particular risk for infectious diseases such as HIV/AIDS and hepatitis. Pulmonary complications may result from the poor health of the abuser as well as from heroin's depressing effects on respiration. Injecting heroin can also contribute to valvular infections due to the possibility of introducing bacteria into the bloodstream. It can also lead to collapsed veins, cellulitis, and abscesses. Repeated IV injections can cause vascular sclerosis and lead the injectors to inject subcutaneously or intramuscularly. Resulting infections such as necrotizing fasciitis can lead to disfigurement or death.

Treatment

Because of the withdrawal syndrome that develops when doses are significantly reduced or stopped, treatment for an opiate use disorder usually begins with medically assisted detoxification using buprenorphine (Suboxone, Buprenex) in tapered doses. Buprenorphine is also gaining popularity as an effective maintenance medication to prevent relapse. Buprenorphine, a partial agonist, produces less risk for overdose, fewer withdrawal effects when stopped, and a lower level of dependence than the more reinforcing agonist, methadone. Some chronic abusers, however, may not respond to buprenorphine and may require maintenance treatment with methadone. Methadone has been used effectively for more than 30 years to treat opiate use disorders. It is a full agonist; it binds with the opioid receptors but has a controlled-release effect that greatly reduces the addiction risk while reducing withdrawal symptoms and drug cravings. Naltrexone (ReVia, Vivitrol), an antagonist, blocks opioids from binding to their receptors and thus prevents substance users from feeling the effects of the drug.

In 2017, the FDA approved the NSS-2 Bridge device to treat opioid withdrawal. The NSS-2 Bridge is a tiny electrical nerve stimulator placed behind the patient's ear. A battery-powered chip emits electrical pulses to stimulate branches of certain cranial nerves, and these stimulations may provide relief from opioid withdrawal symptoms. The device is used during the acute physical withdrawal phase. In 2018 the FDA approved lofexidine (Lucemyra) for use in reducing symptoms associated with opioid withdrawal in adults. Lofexidine is a central alpha-2 adrenergic agonist indicated for the mitigation of opioid withdrawal symptoms to facilitate abrupt opioid discontinuation in adults.

In cases of life-threatening overdose, naloxone (Narcan), another antagonist, is used to counteract the effects of opiates. It reverses the respiratory depression but also has the effect of triggering immediate withdrawal. The best treatment outcomes for opiate use disorders are achieved when available medications are used in conjunction with behavioral and cognitive therapies.

Stimulants

Stimulants are a class of psychoactive drugs that temporarily elevate mood, increase feelings of well-being, and increase energy and alertness. Some stimulant drugs are legal and widely used for legitimate medical purposes, and others are used as illicit drugs. All can be highly addictive. The therapeutic effect of stimulants is achieved by slow and steady increases of dopamine, which is similar to the natural production of the chemical by the brain. The doses prescribed by providers start low and increase gradually until a therapeutic effect is reached. When taken in doses and routes other than those prescribed, stimulants can increase brain dopamine in a rapid and highly amplified manner. Examples of stimulants include amphetamines, methylphenidate (Ritalin), cocaine, methamphetamine, and MDMA (3,4-methylenedioxymethamphetamine), better known as "ecstasy" (see Table 69.2). Taken repeatedly or in high doses, stimulants can cause anxiety, hostility, paranoia, and even psychosis. Further, taking high doses of a stimulant may result in dangerously high body temperatures, irregular heartbeat, cardiovascular failure, or seizures.

Amphetamines and Methylphenidate

Amphetamines, such as dextroamphetamine (Dexedrine, Adderall) and methylphenidate (Ritalin, Concerta), are stimulants generally prescribed by providers for a small number of medical problems, including ADHD, narcolepsy, and occasionally depression. For those who take these medications to improve properly diagnosed conditions, they can be transforming, greatly enhancing a person's quality of life. The dramatic increase in stimulant prescriptions over the last two decades has led to a greater availability and increased risk for diversion and nonmedical use. Like other addictive prescription medications, stimulants are frequently being used without a legitimate prescription or in doses higher or in ways other than prescribed (crushed or snorted).

Cocaine

Cocaine is one of the most addictive recreational drugs available. Its use as a stimulant goes back thousands of years, with a documented history dating back to 500 A.D. Today, cocaine is a Schedule II drug, meaning that it has high potential for abuse but can be administered by a provider for legitimate medical purposes (e.g., as a local anesthetic for ear, eye, and throat surgeries).

Effects

The mechanism of action of cocaine, like that of other substances of abuse, is related to its ability to modify the action of dopamine in the brain's "pleasure reward pathway." Cocaine promotes dopamine transmission by binding to a protein called the *dopamine transporter*, which in turn inhibits the removal of dopamine and ultimately leads to increased activation of the dopaminergic reward pathway. This increased activation leads to the feelings of euphoria and the "high" associated with cocaine use. Cocaine provides a reward that the user learns to obtain in the most efficient manner possible. Unlike learning to obtain natural rewards, such as food, sex, or social cooperation, cocaine results in a pathological form of reward-seeking and ultimately takes precedence over adaptive social and personal behaviors. Cocaine administration results in an increase in dopamine that is markedly greater in terms of both amplitude and duration than what is physiologically induced by a novel, rewarding stimulus. Cocaine's reinforcing value impels repeated drug use. Studies have demonstrated that animals will work very hard for cocaine, such as pressing a bar 10,000 times after a single injection of the drug. These animals choose cocaine over food and water and take lethal doses if supply is not limited.

The increased energy and mental alertness and the feelings of exhilaration in acute cocaine intoxication can quickly turn to irritability, agitation, and restlessness. The euphoric state is replaced in relatively short order by withdrawal, characterized by anxiety, paranoia, depression, and even suicidality. These contrasting mood states signal the brain to use more in an attempt to regain the "high." Cravings for the drug are a cardinal feature of cocaine use disorders and are significant because of the potential to trigger use and relapse. Strong psychological dependence, tolerance, and varying degrees of physical dependence can ensue.

The complications associated with chronic use of cocaine are varied, and virtually every organ system is affected by chronic cocaine use because of the vasoconstriction and neuronal death that occurs. Cocaine abuse has been associated with cardiovascular, pulmonary, neurological, infectious, gastrointestinal, hematological, and obstetrical complications, as well as homeostatic disturbances. The method of administration strongly influences the pathophysiological processes that develop in persons using cocaine. Respiratory complications, usually associated with smoked cocaine, can range from exacerbation of asthma or wheezing to pulmonary edema, acute respiratory distress syndrome, bacterial pneumonia, pneumothorax, and eosinophilic pneumonitis or "crack lung." Intranasal cocaine is often responsible for atrophy of the nasal mucosa, rhinitis, rhinorrhea, bleeding, loss of the sense of smell, and vasculitis. Necrosis and perforation of the nasal septum have occurred in more severe cases. Patients often present in the emergency department with chest pain or with depression or psychosis during a psychiatric evaluation. Significant morbidity, seizures, coma, and sudden death are all possible during periods of intoxication and withdrawal.

Treatment

The current treatment for cocaine use disorders is primarily focused on the psychosocial models of cognitive-behavioral, motivational, and rewards therapy, typically combined with support groups and counseling. Pharmacological treatment for cocaine use disorders has proven challenging over the years, and to date, no medication with proven efficacy is available for the treatment of cocaine or stimulant use disorders. Dopamine agonists, GABA enhancers, adrenergic blockers, and stimulant medications have all shown some promise. More recently, a cocaine vaccine that would block the effects of cocaine has been studied and shows promise for relapse prevention when used in combination with more traditional psychotherapeutic models.

Methamphetamine

Methamphetamine (MA) is a highly addictive psychostimulant that has proven to be a serious worldwide public health problem. Methamphetamine can be synthesized at home using a straightforward, one-step process of reduction of ephedrine or pseudoephedrine, making it easy and inexpensive to produce. There has been an expansive proliferation of "mom-and-pop" meth laboratories along with larger criminal "super-lab" organizations in Mexico, Canada, and the United States that has led some regions to have near epidemics of MA-use disorders. The most predominant

form of MA currently consumed, d-methamphetamine hydrochloride, commonly referred to by the street name "crystal" or "ice," is also the most potent, with purity levels often above 80%. Methamphetamine's high purity level, combined with the almost immediate onset of effects produced by inhalation or injection, can quickly lead to the development of an MA-use disorder.

Effects

Methamphetamine acts on the brain's reward pathway like no other substance or pleasure-generating activity, with a two-fold mechanism of action that causes an extreme surge in dopamine of almost 3.5 times the amount produced by cocaine and 12 times that produced by sex. In addition to blocking the reuptake of dopamine, like cocaine does, MA stimulates the release of dopamine and other catecholamines in the CNS, resulting in levels of dopamine that are about 1,200% more than the baseline level found in a normal brain. Methamphetamine also has a significantly greater elimination half-life (8–13 hours) than many other psychostimulants, such as cocaine (1–3 hours), leading to behavioral and psychological effects that last substantially longer than those of other drugs. It can take up to 2 days to eliminate a single dose. Additionally, MA also has relatively high lipid solubility, allowing more rapid transfer of the drug across the blood–brain barrier.

The acute effects of MA are like those of the other stimulants; however, methamphetamine has the ability to increase energy to the point that users feel "superhuman," making it particularly appealing. The enhanced sexual experiences that many users report put individuals at increased risk for contracting sexually transmitted infections, including HIV. There is significant morbidity associated with acute and chronic MA abuse, including respiratory, cardiovascular, renal, and infectious complications. Many MA users rapidly lose their teeth, a condition known as "meth mouth" that is caused by a combination of dry mouth, poor oral hygiene, consumption of high-sugar beverages, and bruxism (tooth grinding). Additionally, MA exposure in utero has been associated with low birth weight and cognitive deficits in infants.

Unlike cocaine use, long-term MA exposure has been shown in numerous studies to result in extensive neural damage that is associated with cognitive impairments, including deficits in attention, memory, and executive function. This neurotoxicity may play a critical role in the individual's inability to regulate and control the use of the drug. There is a strong psychological dependence associated with MA use, along with substantial evidence that heavy use can lead to progressive social and occupational deterioration. Mood and psychotic disorders are not uncommon and can persist months or years after use has ceased.

Treatment

Multiple medication trials have been tried over the years to identify pharmacotherapy treatment for MA-use disorders, including experiments with selective serotonin reuptake inhibitors, tricyclic antidepressants medications, monoamine oxidase inhibitors (MAOIs), the GABAergic medications gabapentin (Neurontin) and baclofen (Lioresal), and the anti-nausea medication ondansetron (Zofran), all with inconclusive or negative results. Second-generation atypical antipsychotics and agents that increase dopamine levels are being studied along with other, more diverse approaches. The treatment of MA complications is primarily supportive and needs an interprofessional approach. The effectiveness of psychotherapy and behavioral treatments has reliably demonstrated a clinical benefit with minimal potential for side effects.

 Safety   Methamphetamine and Women Alert

- Methamphetamine can be appealing to women because of the potential for significant weight loss, increased energy, and mood-enhancing properties.
- Women have been found to transition from initiation of drug use to regular use of MA in less time than men who use.
- Women who use MA are often in abusive relationships and engage in antisocial behaviors, including drug trafficking, and report difficulty controlling violent tendencies.
- Depression and anxiety due to chronic use have been found to be more severe in women than in men.
- Women are now entering treatment settings with primary diagnoses of MA-use disorder in higher numbers than men.

MDMA (3,4-methylenedioxymethamphetamine)

MDMA, or ecstasy, is a synthetic psychoactive drug that is similar to the stimulant MA and the hallucinogen mescaline. In 2014, the National Survey on Drug Use and Health reported that more than 17 million people aged 12 and older had used MDMA at least once, which is an increase from the 11 million reported 10 years earlier. In a 2016 annual survey of teen drug use by the National Institute of Drug Abuse (NIDA), 2.7% of 12th graders, 1.8% of 10th graders, and 1% of 8th graders reported using MDMA.

Effects

MDMA, usually taken orally as a capsule or tablet, produces feelings of emotional warmth, euphoria, and increased energy along with distortions in time, perception, and tactile experiences. As opposed to dopamine, serotonin is the neurotransmitter primarily affected by MDMA. The serotonin system plays an important role in regulating mood, aggression, sexual activity, sleep, and sensitivity to pain. MDMA binds to the serotonin transporter and thereby increases and prolongs the serotonin signal. It also causes excessive release of serotonin from the neurons. MDMA has similar effects on the neurotransmitter norepinephrine, which can cause the increases in blood pressure and pulse that are seen in ecstasy use.

Like other drugs of abuse, MDMA can be dangerous to overall health and even lethal at times. The increased blood pressure and pulse caused by MDMA increase the cardiovascular risks. In high doses, MDMA can interfere with the body's ability to regulate temperature, which can lead to sharp increases in hyperthermia and result in liver, kidney, and cardiovascular system failure or death. Ecstasy is often taken in combination with alcohol or other drugs, and ecstasy tablets can also contain other substances, such as ephedrine, dextromethorphan, ketamine, caffeine, and cocaine, making MDMA use potentially more dangerous.

Treatment

Although there are no current pharmacological treatments for MDMA-use disorders, behavioral interventions used in the treatment of other SUDs have been shown to be the most effective. Cognitive-behavioral interventions that help modify the patient's thinking, expectancies, and behaviors related to the drug use and increase coping skills are particularly helpful, especially in combination with drug abuse support groups such as Narcotics Anonymous (NA).

CASE STUDY: EPISODE 2

Mary is given a diagnosis of delirium tremens, an AWS characterized by global confusion, autonomic hyperactivity, and hallucinations. The nurse assesses Mary's AWS using the CIWA-Ar, a tool that assesses the presence and severity of AWS (Fig. 69.5). On the basis of a total score of 20, she contacts the nurse practitioner working with Mary's team. Mary is given lorazepam (Ativan) 2 mg intramuscularly immediately and monitored every hour for 4 hours. After 4 hours, Mary is less confused and less tremulous. Monitoring of Mary's status is ongoing. The CIWA-Ar is repeated every 4 hours. Lorazepam 2 mg PO is ordered every 4 hours for a CIWA-Ar score between 10 and 19. Lorazepam is discontinued when the CIWA-Ar score is less than 10. Her stay in the hospital is prolonged by 3 days, 2 of which are spent in the step-down unit. Her vital signs stabilize, and she becomes more coherent.

On her final day in the hospital, the nurse who first spoke to her family goes to check on her. Mary acknowledges that she has been drinking more since retirement and the death of her husband. She is skeptical of the idea that her hospital complications have been caused by alcohol withdrawal because "nothing like that has ever happened to me before." She denies having a drinking problem and insists that she can abstain for as long as necessary if it is required. Mary's daughter comes to pick her up and asks the nurse to "do something" because she is worried about Mary's ability to recover from the surgery and do the necessary follow-up if her drinking continues. The nurse asks to meet with Mary and her daughter to discuss ongoing treatment, but Mary is packed up and leaves the hospital before the meeting can take place…

Clinical Institute Withdrawal Assessment of Alcohol Scale, Revised (CIWA-AR)

Patient: _____ Date: _____ Time: _____ (24 hour clock, midnight = 00:00)

Pulse or heart rate, taken for one minute: _____ Blood Pressure: _____

Nausea and Vomiting—Ask "Do you feel sick to your stomach? Have you vomited?"
Observation:
0 No nausea and no vomiting
1 Mild nausea with no vomiting
2
3
4 Intermittent nausea with dry heaves
5
6
7 Constant nausea, frequent dry heaves, and vomiting

Tremor—Arms extended and fingers spread apart
Observation:
0 No tremor
1 Not visible, but can be felt fingertip to fingertip
2
3
4 Moderate, with patient's arms extended
5
6
7 Severe, even with arms not extended

Paroxysmal Sweats
Observation:
0 No sweat visible
1 Barely perceptible sweating, palms moist
2
3
4 Beads of sweat obvious on forehead
5
6
7 Drenching sweats

Anxiety—Ask "Do you feel nervous?"
Observation:
0 No anxiety, at ease
1 Mildly anxious
2
3
4 Moderately anxious, or guarded, so anxiety is inferred
5
6
7 Equivalent to acute panic states as seen in severe delirium or acute schizophrenic reactions

Agitation
Observation:
0 Normal activity
1 Somewhat more than normal activity
2
3
4 Moderately fidgety and restless
5
6
7 Paces back and forth during most of the interview, or constantly thrashes about

Tactile Disturbances—Ask "Have you any itching, pins and needles sensations, any burning, any numbness, or do you feel bugs crawling on or under your skin?"
Observation:
0 None
1 Very mild itching, pins and needles, burning, or numbness
2 Mild itching, pins and needles, burning, or numbness
3 Moderate itching, pins and needles, burning, or numbness
4 Moderately severe hallucinations
5 Severe hallucinations
6 Extremely severe hallucinations
7 Continuous hallucinations

Auditory Disturbances—Ask "Are you more aware of sounds around you? Are they harsh? Do they frighten you? Are you hearing anything that is disturbing to you? Are you hearing things you know are not there?"
Observation:
0 Not Present
1 Very mild harshness or ability to frighten
2 Mild harshness or ability to frighten
3 Moderate harshness or ability to frighten
4 Moderately severe hallucinations
5 Severe hallucinations
6 Extremely severe hallucinations
7 Continuous hallucinations

Visual Disturbances—Ask "Does the light appear to be too bright? Is its color different? Does it hurt your eyes? Are you seeing anything that is disturbing to you? Are you seeing things you know are not there?"
Observation:
0 Not Present
1 Very mild sensitivity
2 Mild sensitivity
3 Moderate sensitivity
4 Moderately severe hallucinations
5 Severe hallucinations
6 Extremely severe hallucinations
7 Continuous hallucinations

Headache, fullness in head—Ask "Does your head feel different? Does it feel like there is a band around your head?" Do not rate for dizziness or lightheadedness. Otherwise, rate severity.
Observation:
0 Not Present
1 Very mild
2 Mild
3 Moderate
4 Moderately severe
5 Severe
6 Very severe
7 Extremely severe

Orientation and Clouding of Sensorium—Ask "What day is this? Where are you? Who am I?"
Observation:
0 Oriented and can do serial additions
1 Cannot do serial additions or is uncertain about date
2 Disoriented for date by no more than 2 calendar days
3 Disoriented for date by more than 2 calendar days
4 Disoriented for place/or person

Total CIWA-Ar Score _____
Rater's Initials _____
Maximum Possible Score 67

Patients scoring less than 10 do not usually need additional medication for withdrawal.

The CIWA-Ar is *not* copyrighted and may be reproduced freely.

FIGURE 69.5 Clinical Institute Withdrawal Assessment of Alcohol Scale, Revised (CIWA-Ar).

MEDICAL MANAGEMENT: SCREENING AND INTERVENTIONS

Similar to other chronic, relapsing diseases, such as diabetes, asthma, or heart disease, SUDs can be successfully managed. Effective treatment approaches include screening to identify the problem and interventions that are tailored to each patient's drug use patterns and particular strengths, challenges, resources, and needs.

For those who receive substance abuse treatment, the hospital emergency department (ED) may serve as an initial entry point. Common presenting complaints are chest pain and injuries, whether from falls, violence, spousal and child abuse, or other accidents directly related to the substance abuse. The ED is an appropriate and convenient setting for immediate interventions and represents a unique access point for directing patients with SUDs to appropriate treatment programs. Screening and brief interventions are particularly suited to the ED and the hospital setting. Adults admitted to hospitals and/or EDs may be particularly receptive to an intervention because the adverse event is current. Although the stress and emotion of the crisis situation may interfere with learning, it can also make people more receptive to health advice and recommendations. Nurses are well placed to provide interventions in the clinical setting that capitalize on a "teachable moment" and a "window of opportunity." As with other chronic diseases, it is not uncommon for a person to relapse and begin abusing drugs again. Relapse, however, does not signal failure; rather, it indicates that treatment needs to be reinstated or adjusted or that alternative treatment is needed to help the individual regain control and recover.

Many people with an SUD deny having a problem and do not independently seek help. However, to be effective, treatment does not necessarily need to be voluntary. Sanctions or enticements from family, employers, or the criminal justice system can significantly increase treatment entry, retention rates, and the ultimate success of drug treatment interventions.

Screening

Research has demonstrated that screening for substance use combined with brief interventions in primary care settings can be cost-effective, practical techniques to use with people at risk for and those with actual drinking problems. Screening, brief intervention, and referral to treatment (SBIRT) is an example of an evidence-based approach. Screening followed by 3 to 5 minutes of simple advice from a healthcare professional helps many patients reduce their drinking. The Web site of the Substance Abuse and Mental Health Services Administration (SAMHSA) of the U.S. Department of Health and Human Services has information on SBIRT training and related resources.

Screening tools and approaches include:

- SBIRT
- CAGE questionnaire
- AUDIT-C

Screening, Brief Intervention, and Referral to Treatment

Implementation of the **screening, brief intervention, and referral to treatment (SBIRT)** approach is designed for early identification of individuals with an SUD. The SBIRT approach is suited to identify individuals at risk for substance use disorders and to plan early interventions. The brief intervention focuses on increasing insight and awareness regarding substance use and motivation toward behavioral change. Emergency departments, trauma centers, primary health clinics, and other community healthcare venues provide opportunities for early intervention with at-risk substance users before more serious consequences occur. Screening quickly assesses the severity of substance use and identifies the appropriate level of treatment. Those individuals deemed to be at risk receive a brief intervention that focuses on raising their awareness of substance abuse and motivating them to change their behavior. Patients who need more extensive treatment receive referrals to specialty care. Research has demonstrated that SBIRT is effective and that approaching patients during the "teachable moment" of their hospital or primary care visit helps change drinking behavior (see Evidence-Based Practice).

Evidence-Based Practice

Substance Use Outcomes After SBIRT Implementation

This study used the screening, brief intervention, and referral treatment (SBIRT) to estimate changes in behaviors in patients with substance use disorders before and 6 months after the implementation of SBIRT. Using a pre/post design and previously collected performance-monitoring data, data from a sample of 17,575 patients were used to compare pre-SBIRT substance use and substance use 6 months after receiving SBIRT services. Results demonstrated a large and statistically significant decrease for most measures of substance use, including a 35.6% decrease in the prevalence of alcohol use, a 43.4% decrease in heavy drinking, and 75.8% decrease in illicit drug use. The findings of this study support the continued use of SBIRT to monitor substance use reduction in adults.

Aldridge, A., Linford, R., & Bray, J. (2017). Substance use outcomes of patients served by a large US implementation of screening, brief intervention and referral to treatment (SBIRT). *Addiction, 112*(s2), 43–53.

CAGE Questionnaire

The CAGE questionnaire is a widely used tool for assessing alcohol use. One "yes" answer suggests the patient needs closer assessment; two "yes" answers is highly correlated with AUDs (Box 69.6).

Box 69.6 CAGE Questionnaire

Two "yes" responses indicate that the possibility of alcoholism should be investigated further. The questionnaire asks the following questions:

1. Have you ever felt you needed to **C**ut down on your drinking?
2. Have people **A**nnoyed you by criticizing your drinking?
3. Have you ever felt **G**uilty about drinking?
4. Have you ever felt you needed a drink first thing in the morning (**E**ye-opener) to steady your nerves or to get rid of a hangover?

AUDIT-C

The AUDIT-C is a standardized, three-question tool that focuses on consumption and evaluates the severity of alcohol use. It is a short version of the original 10-question AUDIT questionnaire (Fig. 69.6).

AUDIT-C	
Q1: How often did you have a drink containing alcohol in the past year?	
Answer	Points
Never	0
Monthly or less	1
Two to four times a month	2
Two to three times a week	3
Four or more times a week	4
Q2: How many drinks did you have on a typical day when you were drinking in the past year?	
Answer	Points
None, I do not drink	0
1 or 2	0
3 or 4	1
5 or 6	2
7 to 9	3
10 or more	4
Q3: How often did you have six or more drinks on one occasion in the past year?	
Answer	Points
Never	0
Less than monthly	1
Monthly	2
Weekly	3
Daily or almost daily	4

The AUDIT-C is scored on a scale of 0-12 (scores of 0 reflect no alcohol use). In men, a score of 4 or more is considered positive; in women, a score of 3 or more is considered positive. Generally, the higher the AUDIT-C score, the more likely it is that the patient's drinking is affecting his/her health and safety.

FIGURE 69.6 The Alcohol Use Disorders Identification Test–Consumption (AUDIT-C).

Treatment approaches and individual programs continue to evolve and diversify. Approaches involve pharmacotherapy; detoxification and treatment of acute withdrawal symptoms; maintenance therapy; and relapse prevention that includes 12-step programs, behavioral therapy, motivational interviewing techniques, and counseling. Finally, there needs to be a comprehensive substance abuse treatment approach that treats not only the abuse disorder but also any comorbidities that complicate recovery. Table 69.7 provides an overview of disorders and complications associated with substance use and SUDs.

Pharmacotherapy

Pharmacotherapy is used in conjunction with behavioral and supportive therapy. Medications can be used to help reestablish normal brain function, manage withdrawal symptoms, and prevent relapse and diminish cravings. As discussed earlier, there are medications proven to help treat opioid use disorders (buprenorphine, methadone, naloxone, lofexidine) and AUDs (disulfiram, naltrexone, acamprosate). Others are being developed to treat stimulant (cocaine, MA) and cannabis (marijuana) use disorders.

Detoxification

Detoxification is the process by which the body clears itself of drugs. It is often accompanied by unpleasant and sometimes even fatal side effects caused by withdrawal. Easing withdrawal symptoms is important in the initiation of treatment. The process of detoxification is often managed with medications in an inpatient or outpatient setting that provides medical supervision and is sometimes referred to as "medically managed" or "medically assisted withdrawal." Medically assisted detoxification can safely manage the acute physical symptoms of withdrawal but is only the first stage of SUD treatment. It is rarely sufficient by itself to help individuals with an SUD to achieve long-term recovery. Detoxification needs to be followed by a formal assessment and referral for subsequent SUD treatment.

Maintenance and Relapse Prevention

12-Step Meetings—Alcoholics Anonymous and Other 12-Step Programs

Alcoholics Anonymous and many other 12-step fellowships, such as Narcotics Anonymous, are international, nonprofessional organizations composed of individuals who all share a common problem of an AUD or another SUD. Members share their experiences, strengths, and hopes with each other in order to stay sober and help others to achieve sobriety. The 12-step model of Alcoholics Anonymous (see Box 69.5) promotes the achievement of sobriety and the maintenance of lifetime recovery by encouraging members to take proactive steps on a daily basis to monitor their mental, emotional, physical, and spiritual condition. Balance in life is stressed in order to "protect sobriety" and "prevent relapse." Working with a sponsor and developing a sober network are critical to the success of this approach.

Table 69.7 Common Disorders and Complications Associated With Substance Use or Substance Use Disorder

Condition	Related to
Carcinoma—esophageal	Alcohol and tobacco alone or in combination
Carcinoma—liver, hepatocellular	Heavy alcohol for several years
Carcinoma—pancreas	Smoking associated with pancreatic cancer and delays healing
Cirrhosis—alcohol-induced Laënnec's cirrhosis	Chronic alcoholism + malnutrition
Delirium	Alcohol poisoning
	Overdose of an opiate or another drug
	Drug-related physical syndromes
Depression	May be evident during or after substance use
Gout	Decreased clotting ability associated with alcoholic beverages, especially beer, contributes to increased production of uric acid
Hypertension	Heavy alcohol intake
Hypothermia	Alcohol use
	High risk of hypothermia related to dilation of blood vessels and poor judgment
Nutritional deficiencies, including thiamine deficiency	Alcohol
Wernicke–Korsakoff's syndrome	Chronic alcohol use
Pancreatitis	Alcohol associated with 1 in 3 cases of pancreatitis
Poisoning, accidental or intentional	Alcohol, opioids
Pre- and postoperative complications	Alcohol, smoking
Traumatic injuries	Alcohol and other substances that impair alertness or judgment
Withdrawal	Related to decreasing or stopping alcohol, an opiate, or another substance with a history of a discontinuation syndrome, when there has been a pattern of regular use.

Behavioral Therapy

Behavioral therapy helps patients engage in the treatment process, modify their attitudes and behaviors related to drug abuse, and increase healthy life skills. These treatments also enhance the effectiveness of medications and help people stay in treatment longer. The most commonly used behavioral treatment is **cognitive-behavioral therapy**, which seeks to help patients recognize, avoid, and cope with the situations in which they are most likely to abuse drugs or alcohol.

Contingency management, another form of behavioral therapy, uses motivational incentives (tokens, money, and privileges) to encourage abstinence from drugs. The three key principles of contingency management are identified as follows: (1) frequently monitor the behavior the individual is trying to achieve (abstinence); (2) provide tangible, immediate positive reinforcers each time the behavior occurs; and (3) when the behavior does not occur, withhold the positive reinforcers.

Motivational Interviewing

Motivational interviewing capitalizes on the readiness of individuals to change behavior and enter treatment by combining personal feedback with an empathetic approach. The motivational interviewing approach uses open-ended questions, affirmations, reflective listening, and summaries. This approach attempts to meet the individual where the person is rather than where the person should be, finding out what is important to the individual and using that as motivation for change. A 15- to 20-minute session using the motivational interviewing has been quite effective.

Individualized Counseling

Individualized drug counseling includes the content and structure of the patient's recovery program and focuses on reducing or stopping illicit drug or alcohol use, as well as addressing related areas of impaired functioning, such as employment status, illegal activity, and family/social relations. Through an emphasis on short-term behavioral goals, individualized counseling helps the patient develop coping strategies and tools to abstain from drug use and maintain abstinence. The addiction counselor encourages 12-step participation (at least one or two times per week) and makes referrals for needed supplemental medical, psychiatric, employment, and other services.

Group Counseling

Many therapeutic settings use group therapy to capitalize on the social reinforcement offered by peer discussion and to help promote drug-free lifestyles. Research has demonstrated that when group therapy is offered in conjunction with individualized drug counseling or is formatted to reflect the principles of cognitive-behavioral therapy or contingency management, positive outcomes are achieved. Currently, researchers are testing conditions in which group therapy can be standardized and made more community-friendly.

Internet

The Internet may offer a treatment-delivery alternative for persons who cannot easily access more traditional drug treatment services either because of limited financial resources or the availability of specific services. Many Web sites now exist that offer information and support for individuals, families, teachers, and communities. The National Institutes of Health published preliminary findings on Web-based treatment for rural women with alcohol problems and found that barriers to professional care were greatest in rural areas; these barriers include limited financial resources, a scarcity of gender-focused services, privacy issues, and stigma associated with alcohol abuse among women. Other barriers are the fact that any lay-led support groups in these areas, such as AA, tend to be frequented by men, and there are generally no childcare services offered. The Internet may prove to be a viable option for women who struggle with one or more SUDs.

Comprehensive Substance Abuse Treatment Approach

The high rate of comorbidity between drug use disorders and other mental health disorders demonstrates the need for a comprehensive approach to interventions that identify, evaluate, and treat each disorder concurrently. Programs that utilize a comprehensive treatment approach are designed to help the patient learn to avoid relapse and include extensive substance abuse and psychiatric evaluations, individual and group therapy, behavioral therapy, pharmacotherapy, education, social services, promotion of 12-step programs, and treatment of any comorbid psychiatric illness. Often, these programs involve individual reflection about how problems with substance abuse first developed, the direct and indirect costs of substance abuse, the triggers for substance use, relapse prevention strategies, ways to enhance coping skills, and spiritual issues. They also assist the patient in exploring motivations to change, building skills to resist drug use, replacing drug-using activities with constructive and rewarding activities, improving problem-solving skills, and nurturing better interpersonal relationships.

Programs that use a more comprehensive treatment approach assess patients for the presence of HIV/AIDS, hepatitis B and C, tuberculosis, and other infectious diseases, as well as provide targeted risk-reduction counseling to help patients modify or change behaviors that place them at risk of contracting or spreading infectious diseases. Targeted counseling specifically focused on reducing infectious disease risk can help patients further reduce or avoid substance-related and other high-risk behaviors.

Treatment Settings

Treatment for SUDs is delivered in many different settings. In the United States, there are thousands of specialized drug treatment facilities that provide counseling, behavioral therapy, medication, case management, and other types of services to persons with SUDs. Along with specialized drug treatment facilities, drug abuse and SUDs are treated in jails, providers' offices, and mental health clinics by a variety of professionals, including counselors, physicians, psychiatrists, psychologists, nurses, and social workers. Treatment is delivered in outpatient, inpatient, and residential settings. Although specific treatment approaches often are associated with particular treatment settings, a variety of therapeutic interventions or services can be included in any given setting.

Inpatient Hospital-Based Treatment

Hospital-based treatment takes place on a general hospital unit and serves those persons who, along with their SUD, have concurrent acute medical or psychiatric problems. The length of stay on these units is generally shorter than in free-standing SUD treatment centers. In many cases, individuals are referred to a longer outpatient or residential program from the hospital-based unit to continue with SUD treatment.

Freestanding Residential Substance Use Disorder Treatment Centers

A freestanding residential SUD treatment center is a stand-alone facility that specializes in the treatment of SUDs and dual diagnoses. Patients generally reside within the treatment facility 24 hours a day under the care of a team of addiction professionals. Although these SUD treatment programs may have other components of care, such as day treatment, partial hospitalization, or outpatient therapy, their main focus lies in providing 24-hour residential care for their patients. Freestanding SUD treatment programs are also capable of providing drug and alcohol detoxification, but not all SUD treatment programs offer this service in-house. The average length of stay for private insurance in these SUD treatment centers is approximately 21 days. A residential center that is federally funded may have a length of stay that is approximately 3 to 6 months.

Long-Term Drug Treatment Programs

Long-term SUD treatment programs are designed for people who have completed anywhere from 14 to 30 days of residential SUD treatment and, for a variety of reasons, require additional residential treatment. Reasons that persons may need long-term treatment may be that they are still displaying drug-seeking behavior after completion of a 30-day SUD treatment program, they have experienced a relapse after a short-term stay in a SUD treatment center, or more time is needed in a structured setting to resolve outstanding clinical issues. The average length of stay in a long-term SUD treatment center is approximately 90 days. Originally designed to treat impaired professionals, the additional time in long-term SUD treatment proved so positive that many SUD treatment facilities began referring other patients. Today, it is not uncommon for all types of people to access long-term SUD treatment.

Outpatient Substance Use Disorder Treatment Programs

Patients participating in outpatient SUD treatment programs generally reside at home and attend the program several evenings or days during the week. Outpatient services are provided to individuals at a variety of intensity levels (i.e., education classes, outpatient treatment, and intensive outpatient treatment). This type of treatment costs less than residential or inpatient treatment and often is more suitable for people with jobs or extensive social supports. This is often the first-line treatment for persons who are newer to treatment or who do not have insurance coverage for more intensive residential treatment. Outpatient programs provide therapeutic activities and interventions for patients to assist them in their recovery from substance abuse while they maintain residence and employment in the community. The focus of the programs is on SUD treatment and the provision of ancillary services. It should be noted that low-intensity programs may only offer drug education.

Opioid Treatment Programs

Opioid treatment programs provide medication-assisted therapy with methadone and/or buprenorphine for the treatment of opiate use disorders and SUDs related to the nonmedical use of prescription painkillers. The extent of services offered varies from simple medication dispensing to comprehensive outpatient programs that provide opiate-replacement medication along with treatment for any co-morbid psychiatric or medical issues, individual and group counseling, behavioral therapy, contingency management treatment, and other treatment approaches are also aspects of these opioid treatment programs.

Long-Term Residential Settings (Therapeutic Communities)

Long-term residential treatment provides care 24 hours a day, generally in nonhospital settings. The best-known residential treatment model is the therapeutic community (TC), with planned lengths of stay between 6 and 12 months. Therapeutic communities differ from other treatment approaches principally in their use of the community treatment staff and those in recovery as a key agent of change. Substance use disorders are viewed in the context of an individual's social and psychological deficits, and treatment focuses on developing personal accountability and responsibility as well as learning to live socially productive lives. Treatment is highly structured and can be confrontational at times, with activities designed to help residents examine damaging beliefs, self-concepts, and destructive patterns of behavior and adopt new, more harmonious, and constructive ways to interact with others. These are programs based in the community and may include faith-based programs connected with a church or religious organization. Patients live at these facilities, attend groups and various rehabilitative classes, and are often assigned work duties as part of the treatment. These programs offer "rehab from the ground up," including job skills training, GED® programs, and other forms of assistance to prepare patients to be productive members of society. Research shows that TCs can be modified to treat individuals with special needs, including adolescents, women, homeless individuals, people with severe mental health disorders, and individuals in the criminal justice system.

Halfway Houses, Recovery Houses, and Transitional Houses

Halfway houses, recovery houses, and transitional houses provide clean and sober living environments where groups of people reside together while recovering from SUDs. House managers are often in later stages of recovery and can mentor others to try to stay clean and sober. Patients can be in various stages of recovery. Facilities are shared (bedrooms, bathrooms, and kitchen). Each house varies in the amount of structure and rules, including a possible "blackout period" where the patient may not be able to leave the house unescorted. Recovery houses do not take health insurance, and they each set their own prices. Patients are required to attend AA/NA meetings and can also benefit from being involved with an outpatient treatment program.

Treatment Within the Criminal Justice System

Research has found that combining criminal justice sanctions with drug treatment can be effective in decreasing drug abuse and related crime. It has also demonstrated that individuals under legal coercion tend to stay in treatment longer and do as well or better than those not under legal pressure. Often, drug abusers come into contact with the criminal justice system earlier than other health or social systems, presenting opportunities for intervention and treatment prior to, during, after, or in lieu of incarceration, which may ultimately interrupt and shorten a career of drug use. Unfortunately, only a small percentage of all inmates with SUDs receive any treatment during incarceration. Studies have indicated that if all inmates who needed treatment and aftercare services received such services and just over 10% remained substance- and crime-free and employed, the nation would break even in a year.

NURSING MANAGEMENT

With an understanding of common risk factors associated with SUDs, clinical manifestations of commonly used addictive substances, symptoms of intoxication, and withdrawal issues, nurses are prepared to identify at-risk individuals and use the information to individualize a plan of care. To ensure patient safety when caring for persons with a SUD, it is important to consider the primary diagnosis and any comorbid or co-occurring SUDs and psychiatric or other medical diagnoses.

Substance abuse causes, complicates, or coexists with other illnesses that may require admission to the hospital setting. The clinical manifestations of substance abuse are often subtle, caused by a comorbid condition or the substance abuse itself, and may not be recognized among the more obvious indicators of the admitting diagnoses. This is also complicated by denial on the part of the patient. The cornerstone of assessment for substance abuse problems is establishing rapport and taking a thorough history from the patient and from outside informants, including family, friends, and other providers. The nurse must communicate to the patient that there is no judgment, that information will be kept confidential, and that the nurse is there to help.

Assessment and Analysis

Clinical manifestations observed in the patient with SUDs may be related to intoxication, withdrawal, and longer-term physiological and psychological changes associated with specific SUDs. In some cases, the toxic effect of the substance directly damages body organs. Second, the route or method of administration may cause health problems (e.g., skin infections). Third, lifestyle factors associated with substance abuse cause illnesses (e.g., malnutrition and poor hygiene). Increased risk taking or impairment in judgment while under the influence of drugs or alcohol may result in injuries or life-threatening situations that require hospitalization. Whatever the reason for hospitalization, if a patient has participated in hazardous use of substances, there is a risk for withdrawal once use has ceased or dosages are decreased. Several opioid withdrawal scales are available for identifying and quantifying the severity of opioid withdrawal symptoms. Validated tools include:

- The Objective Opioid Withdrawal Scale (OOWS), which relies on clinical observation
- The Subjective Opioid Withdrawal Scale (SOWS), which records the patient's rating of opioid withdrawal on a 16-item scale
- The Clinical Opioid Withdrawal Scale (COWS), which includes 11 items and contains both objective and subjective signs and symptoms of opioid withdrawal

All nurses should have current, working knowledge of usual intoxication and withdrawal symptoms and other health conditions associated with hazardous use and SUDs (Table 69.8).

Table 69.8 Common Indicators of Intoxication, Withdrawal, or Other Health Concerns Associated With Substance Use Disorders

Intoxication	Withdrawal	Other
• Drowsiness	• Changes in vital signs	• Malnutrition
• Slurred speech	• Tremulousness	• Poor dentition
• Impaired balance and coordination	• Nausea/vomiting	• Track marks
• Difficulty focusing	• Headache	• Abscesses
• Decreased alertness and concentration	• Poor appetite	• Presence of infectious diseases
• Mood lability	• Diarrhea	• Abnormal laboratory values
• Strange, aggressive, or paranoid behavior	• Diaphoresis	• Histories suggesting nonepileptic seizures, liver disease, gastric bleeding, or pancreatitis
• Constricted or dilated pupils	• Complaints of muscle aches	• History of motor vehicle accidents, falls, fires, or suicide attempts
• Changes in vital signs	• Disturbed sleep	• History of noncompliance
	• Sensitivity to light and sounds	• Drug-seeking behavior
	• Hallucinations	• Homelessness
	• Confusion	• Lack of social supports
	• Seizures	• History of legal, social, occupational problems
	• Anxiety	• History of aggression
	• Depression/suicidality	
	• Irritability/hostility	
	• Cravings	
	• Drug-seeking behavior	
	• Manipulative behavior	

Nursing Diagnoses

- **Alteration in comfort:** Physical pain or discomfort related to craving or withdrawal from substances
- **Sensory perception alteration** related to withdrawal from substances
- **Potential for injury** related to withdrawal from substances
- **Alteration in nutrition less than body requirements** related to poor dietary intake secondary to drug or alcohol use and decreased appetite with accompanying N/V secondary to withdrawal
- **Sleep pattern disturbance** related to withdrawal from substances
- **Anxiety** related to the distress of withdrawal and absence of usual coping mechanism
- **Hopelessness** related to chronic nature of the disease and past failed attempts at recovery
- **Knowledge deficit** related to the withdrawal process and treatment, recovery planning, and relapse prevention

Nursing Interventions

Assessments

- Vital signs
  Increased pulse, blood pressure, and temperature may be signs of autonomic hyperactivity and indicate withdrawal. Vital signs are a useful index of the severity of substance withdrawal. Frequent monitoring is required to ensure safety, treat withdrawal symptoms, and promote comfort.
- Mental status examination
  Withdrawal symptoms may be unpredictable. Changes from baseline may indicate increased severity of withdrawal or other physiological or psychiatric problems. Prompt response reduces the risk of worsening clinical manifestations. Comorbid psychiatric problems are common in persons who abuse substances. Diagnosis and treatment may aid in recovery from illicit substances. Patients withdrawing from substances may have impaired reality testing.
- Nutritional status
  Albumin and total protein may be decreased; vitamin deficiencies may be present, reflecting malnutrition/ malabsorption associated with drug and/or alcohol abuse.
- Blood alcohol/drug levels
  Determine the substance used and the risk for substance withdrawal. The alcohol level may or may not be severely elevated depending on the amount consumed and the length of time between consumption and testing. These levels provide an indication of tolerance and the risk for complicated withdrawal. Numerous controlled/illicit substances may be identified in a polydrug screen that could also cause symptoms of withdrawal.
- Complete blood count (CBC)
  Decreased hemoglobin/hematocrit may reflect such problems as iron-deficiency anemia or acute/chronic gastrointestinal bleeding associated with chronic alcohol use. The white blood cell count may be increased with infections associated with drug and alcohol use.
- Glucose
  Hyperglycemia/hypoglycemia may be present related to pancreatitis, malnutrition, or depletion of liver glycogen stores associated with drug and/or alcohol use.
- Serum electrolytes
  Hypokalemia and hypomagnesemia are common with AUD.
- Liver function studies
  Creatine kinase (CK), lactate dehydrogenase (LDH), aspartate aminotransferase (AST), alanine aminotransferase (ALT), and amylase may be elevated, reflecting liver or pancreatic damage associated with drug and/or alcohol abuse.
- Human immunodeficiency virus (HIV), hepatitis C virus (HCV), and tuberculosis (TB) testing as indicated
  Infection with HIV, HCV, and TB is a possibility because of the risky lifestyle behaviors of individuals with an SUD. These disorders require treatment and may complicate or confound withdrawal.
- Electrocardiogram (ECG)
  Dysrhythmias, cardiomyopathies, and/or ischemia may be present because of the direct effect of alcohol on the cardiac muscle and/or conduction system, as well as the effects of electrolyte imbalance.
- Chest x-ray
  May reveal pneumonia or chronic lung disorders associated with tobacco use, which is often associated with drug and/or alcohol abuse
- Comprehensive medical, psychiatric, and substance use/abuse history and physical examination
  Establishing an appropriate diagnosis and determining if acute intoxication/overdose is present are essential in determining the appropriate treatment. An estimated 15% to 20% of hospitalized patients are dependent on alcohol. To prevent AWS in hospitalized patients, nurses need to assess the pattern of alcohol use. Medical and psychiatric problems that may have been masked by substance use may reappear.
- CAGE questionnaire (see Box 69.6)
  The CAGE questionnaire is a widely used tool for assessing alcohol use. One "yes" answer suggests the patient needs closer assessment; two "yes" answers is highly correlated with AUDs.
- AUDIT-C (see Fig. 69.6)
  The AUDIT-C is a standardized, three-question tool that focuses on consumption and evaluates for the severity of alcohol use. The AUDIT-C is a short version of the original 10-question AUDIT questionnaire.
- CIWA-Ar (see Fig. 69.5).
  The CIWA-Ar is a widely used standardized assessment tool that assesses the presence of 10 symptoms of ethyl alcohol (ETOH) withdrawal, such as tremor and hallucinations (visual, tactile, and other types of hallucinations are associated with alcohol withdrawal). The higher the score, the more severe the withdrawal. It allows the nurse to identify and assess the severity of symptoms in order to intervene and medicate appropriately.

- SBIRT
  The SBIRT approach is designed for early identification of individuals with an SUD or risk for SUDs, early determination of the severity of identified SUDs, implementation of an appropriate level of brief intervention, and referral to the appropriate level of treatment.

■ Actions

- Establish and maintain airway.
  Required if the patient is acutely intoxicated or has overdosed. Excessive somnolence increases the risk of airway compromise. Additionally, with vomiting along with a decreased level of consciousness, there is also an increased risk of aspiration.
- Provide adequate fluids and electrolytes.
  Abnormalities in fluid and electrolyte levels should be corrected. Intravenous fluid may be necessary in patients with more severe withdrawal because of excessive fluid loss through hyperthermia, sweating, and vomiting. Intravenous fluid should not be administered routinely in patients with less severe withdrawal because these patients may become overhydrated.
- Administer medications to treat withdrawal symptoms and specific SUD as ordered.
  - Opioid use disorder (OUD) treatment
    - Lofexidine
      A central alpha-2 adrenergic agonist for use in reducing symptoms associated with opioid withdrawal in adults
    - Methadone
      A full agonist that binds with the opioid receptors but has a controlled-release effect that greatly reduces the addiction risk while reducing withdrawal symptoms and drug cravings
    - Buprenorphine
      A partial agonist, it has actions like agonists but does not cause full receptor activation. There is less risk for overdose, fewer withdrawal effects when stopped, and a lower level of dependence than with the more reinforcing agonist, methadone.
    - Naloxone
      An antagonist, it blocks opioids from binding to their receptors and thus prevents substance users from feeling the effects of the drug. It is also used to reverse the respiratory depression seen with acute overdose.
  - AUD treatment
    - Disulfiram
      It works by causing a severe adverse reaction (nausea/vomiting) when someone taking the drug drinks alcohol.
    - Naltrexone
      Blocks the "high" that people experience when they drink or take drugs such as heroin or cocaine
    - Acamprosate
      This medication reduces the physical distress and emotional discomfort people experience when they quit drinking.
    - Multivitamins, folate, and thiamine
      Individuals with an AUD have poor nutrition and may be deficient in thiamine and folate. Thiamine is essential for the metabolism of glucose. A patient who is deficient in thiamine is at risk for acute and chronic mental status changes associated with Wernicke–Korsakoff's syndrome. Folate, crucial for the formation of red blood cells and protein metabolism, helps to treat or prevent anemia.
- Promote adequate nutrition.
  Nutrition is especially important for the individual recovering from an SUD because these patients are likely to be nutritionally depleted because of poor diet or impaired absorption of nutrients.
- Maintain a calm environment with appropriate lighting.
  Patients in withdrawal need a quiet environment with appropriate lighting. Excessive stimulation may exacerbate the effects of withdrawal.
- Establish rapport by using a nonjudgmental, caring, and competent approach.
  Builds trust and minimizes resistance; demonstrates acceptance of patient as worthy human being and one deserving of care
- Provide psychological support and instill hope that successful recovery is possible.
  Hopelessness is often present if the patient has made several attempts at rehabilitation and suffered relapses.
- Consult social work, case management, or psychiatry to plan for longer-term treatment.
  Detoxification alone is insufficient for long-term recovery from substances. Ultimately, the goal is to prepare the person for entry into a rehabilitation program, with the hope of long-term abstinence.

■ Teaching

- Educate the patient on symptoms and treatment of withdrawal.
  Make the patient a partner in care; signs may be subtle and may need to rely on patient report of symptoms.
- Disease process and general health education
  Patients need to have an appreciation of the physical, psychological, cognitive, and behavioral changes and conditions that are associated with drug use and SUDs.
- Recovery planning and relapse prevention education
  Patients need to learn treatment options and ways to develop sober support systems that will facilitate long-term recovery. They need to learn ways to identify, avoid, and cope with triggers.
- Educate the patient on basic concepts of 12 steps and how to locate meetings in his or her area after discharge.
  It is important to understand what the 12 steps are and what they can offer for recovery because they have helped millions achieve and maintain sobriety.
- Stress management
  It is important that the patient increases his or her repertoire of effective coping mechanisms in order to better avoid destructive coping such as drug abuse.
- Post-acute withdrawal syndrome (PAWS)
  The symptoms of PAWS may occur because the brain's ability to react to stress has been weakened by long-term

substance use. Post-acute withdrawal syndrome can last from months to a year to several decades, with the symptoms entering into periods of relative remission between periods of instability. Patients need to be aware of the signs and symptoms of PAWS, understand that it is a normal part of recovery, and learn ways to cope in order to maintain sobriety.

Evaluating Care Outcomes

With prompt recognition and treatment, complications from acute withdrawal may be avoided, physiological status stabilized, and injury prevented, and the patient reports significantly decreased discomfort related to withdrawal. Expected outcomes include stable vital signs, mental status, fluid and electrolyte status, and weight. A well-managed patient with an SUD understands the disorder, actively states personal responsibility for recovery, and is compliant with the treatment program best suited to his or her individual needs.

Making Connections

CASE STUDY: WRAP-UP

At her daughter's urging, Mary abstains from alcohol for several weeks and makes a successful recovery from her surgery, but 2 months later, she is back in the hospital with a broken hip, sustained in a fall down her basement stairs. She spends a day in the ED waiting for a bed, and when she returns to the unit, she is already tremulous and hallucinating. The nurse makes the diagnoses of

- Potential for injury related to alcohol withdrawal
- Alteration in sensory perception (such as visual illusions or hallucinations) related to alcohol withdrawal

Mary is again assessed using the CIWA-Ar and is treated with lorazepam. The nurse monitors her vital signs at frequent intervals and uses the CIWA-Ar to assess withdrawal symptoms and response to the medication. She implements seizure and fall precautions. Mary has IV fluids running and is receiving a multivitamin, folic acid, and thiamine. The nurse is providing a calm, quiet, supportive environment, as well as reality orientation as needed. Mary begins to improve significantly on the second day. Her hip replacement surgery goes well, and she is beginning to bear weight again. The nurse now believes it to be a good time to start educating Mary about alcohol-related disorders and recovery planning. The nurse understands that simply treating the withdrawal is not enough and that Mary needs ongoing treatment to address her AUD. She asks the provider to get a substance use treatment referral from social work. Mary is visited by her daughter, son-in-law, and granddaughter and by an old friend of

hers who has been in recovery for many years. Mary attends an AA group that meets in the hospital and is expressing interest in starting substance abuse treatment after she is discharged.

Case Study Questions

1. During Mary's first admission, prior to transferring her from the step-down unit, the nurse observes symptoms of AWS. On the basis of her length of time in the hospital and Mary's symptoms, the nurse knows Mary's symptoms indicate which stage of AWS?
   A. Severe AWS
   B. Moderate AWS
   C. Mild AWS
   D. Early AWS

2. During her first admission, which factor(s) place Mary at greatest risk of developing severe AWS? *(Select all that apply.)*
   A. Diaphoresis
   B. Age
   C. Drinking history
   D. Recent surgery
   E. Pain

3. The nurse caring for Mary incorporates which nursing diagnosis into the plan of care? *(Select all that apply.)*
   A. Alteration in comfort: discomfort related to withdrawal
   B. Risk for injury related to withdrawal
   C. Anxiety related to the distress of withdrawal
   D. Imbalanced nutrition: less than body requirement
   E. Dysfunctional family processes

4. The nurse includes which assessments for Mary related to the status of AWS? *(Select all that apply.)*
   A. Vital signs
   B. CIWA-Ar score
   C. CAGE score
   D. Mental status
   E. Respiratory status

5. The nurse includes which of the following information in Mary's teaching plan? *(Select all that apply.)*
   A. How to cope with triggers and cravings
   B. Importance of good nutrition
   C. Substance abuse treatment options
   D. How much alcohol is acceptable to drink
   E. Importance of building a support network

CHAPTER SUMMARY

The United States has one of the highest levels of substance use disorders (SUDs) in the world. An SUD is defined as a maladaptive pattern of substance use that results in recurrent and significant adverse consequences. The severity of SUDs is classified as mild, moderate, or severe. A severe SUD is characterized by compulsive drug seeking and use despite harmful consequences. A SUD is a chronic, relapsing brain disease that often results in individuals developing tolerance to drugs or alcohol over time and manifesting a withdrawal syndrome when use stops or decreases after prolonged heavy use.

People in all age groups from any background could be at risk for developing an SUD. As with many other diseases, genetics influences a person's risk of developing an SUD. Additionally, ethnicity, age of first use, gender, stress, and the presence of other mental health disorders are also strongly associated with the risk of developing SUDs.

Psychoactive drugs are chemicals that in one way or another tap into the brain's communication system and disrupt the way the neurons normally send, receive, and process information. As the person continues to abuse drugs or alcohol, the brain starts to adapt to these chemical changes by producing less dopamine or by reducing the number of dopamine receptors in the reward circuit. As a result, dopamine's impact on the reward circuit is lessened, reducing the abuser's ability to enjoy the drugs and the things that previously brought pleasure.

Nurses in virtually every practice setting encounter patients struggling with SUDs and need to be aware of commonly used substances and their clinical manifestations in order to provide optimal care for patients. There are physical, behavioral, and psychosocial signs that all nurses should be alert to that may indicate a patient is abusing drugs and/or alcohol. Any sudden or obvious changes in hygiene, sleep, energy, eating patterns, weight, health, behavior, performance, personality, or attitude can be a sign that a person is abusing substances.

Substance abuse causes, complicates, or coexists with other illnesses that require admission to general hospital units. Millions of ED visits each year are connected to substance use, including the nonmedical use of prescription medications, adverse reactions to drugs, or other drug-related consequences. Nonmedical use of prescription opioids and access to fentanyl has led to a dramatic increase in deaths from unintentional drug overdose. Although alcohol is legal, it is also a frequently abused drug. About 3 in every 10 adults in the United States consume sufficient alcohol to elevate their risk of physical and psychosocial problems, and 1 in 4 patients admitted to medical and surgical services in general hospitals has an alcohol use disorder (AUD). Many of these patients experience withdrawal from drugs or alcohol once they come into the hospital and no longer have access to the substance. Nurses need to be able to recognize symptoms of withdrawal so that treatment can be initiated and progression to more serious withdrawal can be prevented. Almost all people with an AUD who have been chronic heavy drinkers experience some level of withdrawal symptoms when they suddenly stop drinking or significantly decrease the amount of alcohol they drink. Alcohol withdrawal, in particular, can be very serious and can put patients at risk for serious harm if not adequately treated early on in the hospital stay. Early signs of alcohol withdrawal can present as anxiety and restlessness, sensitivity to light and sounds, autonomic hyperactivity, mild tremor, nausea, and headache. If there is not continued monitoring and appropriate pharmacotherapy initiated for moderate withdrawal symptoms, they can progress to life-threatening seizures and delirium tremens, which can include confusion, hallucinations, autonomic instability, and death. Aside from continued assessment of the patient and pharmacological treatment for symptoms of withdrawal, nursing care includes the provision of adequate nutrition and rest in a quiet, safe, and supportive environment.

Detoxification is rarely sufficient by itself to help individuals achieve long-term recovery, so it should be followed by a formal assessment and referral to subsequent SUD treatment. Treatment approaches that are tailored to each patient's substance use patterns and any co-occurring medical, psychiatric, and social problems can help individuals with an SUD stop drug and alcohol use, avoid relapse, and successfully recover their lives. Treatment for an SUD is delivered in many different settings, using a variety of behavioral and pharmacological approaches. Unfortunately, most people who require treatment for an SUD do not get the help they need. Nurses are in a unique position to intervene with these patients and can provide valuable education about relapse prevention and recovery planning, stress management, treatment options, and signs and symptoms of post-acute withdrawal symptoms.

DAVIS ADVANTAGE | To explore learning resources for this chapter, go to **Davis Advantage** and find:
- Answers to in-text questions
- Chapter Resources and Activities
- NCLEX®-Style Chapter Review Questions
- Bibliography

Chapter 70

Emergency, Trauma, and Environmental Injuries

Monica Filburn and Nancy Sullivan

LEARNING OUTCOMES

Content in this chapter is designed to support the learner in:

1. Stating the prevalence of trauma in our society
2. Identifying the roles of healthcare professionals on the emergency care team
3. Discussing the priorities of care in the field
4. Examining hospital emergency/trauma care priorities
5. Describing common mechanisms of injury
6. Defining major complications of trauma
7. Describing the prevalence of environmental emergencies
8. Explaining the pathophysiological processes of environmental emergencies
9. Correlating clinical manifestations with the pathophysiological processes of
   a. Poisoning
   b. Hypothermia
   c. Hyperthermia
   d. Snakebites
   e. Spider bites
   f. Drowning
10. Describing the diagnostic results used to confirm the diagnoses of selected emergencies
11. Discussing the medical management of selected emergencies
12. Developing a comprehensive plan of nursing care for patients with selected emergencies

ESSENTIAL TERMS

Acceleration
Active external rewarming
Antivenin
Blunt trauma
Cavitation
Compression
Conduction
Convection
C-spine stabilization
Deceleration
Decontamination
Envenomation
Evaporation
Exsanguination
Fragmentation
Golden period
Heat cramps
Heat edema
Heat exhaustion
Heat stress
Heat stroke
Heat syncope
Hemotoxic
Hyperthermia
Internal rewarming
Mechanism of injury

Mild hypothermia
Moderate hypothermia
Motor vehicle collision (MVC)
Neurotoxic
Passive external rewarming
Penetrating trauma
Primary survey
Profile
Rapid fluid infuser
Rhabdomyolysis
Secondary survey
Severe hypothermia
Shearing
Systemic loxoscelism
Thermoregulation
Trauma triad of death
Traumatic aneurysm
Triage
Tumble
Venom
Yaw

CONCEPTS

- Assessment
- Fluid and Electrolyte Balance
- Medication
- Nursing Roles
- Oxygenation
- Perfusion
- pH Regulation
- Safety
- Thermoregulation
- Trauma

Finding Connections

CASE STUDY: EPISODE 1

Follow this patient throughout the chapter.

On a hot Saturday summer night, three male teenagers are at a friend's house for a house party. While they are leaving the house at approximately 1 a.m., a vehicle drives by and starts shooting at them and at the house. One male is shot in the head, another male is able to run away and call 911. The third is shot in the torso. On the arrival of emergency medical personnel at the scene, the team finds two victims. The first victim is found to be shot in the head and has no vital signs or signs of life. He is declared dead at the scene. The second victim is found to have two gunshot wounds. The EMS team quickly stabilizes, packages, and starts to transport the patient to the nearest trauma center.

Prehospital EMS consultation to the level I hospital emergency department (ED) and trauma center: 19-year-old male with a gunshot wound to the right shoulder and lower back. Vital signs: heart rate: 120 bpm; blood pressure: 120/60 mm Hg; respiratory rate: 24 breaths/minute; pulse oximetry: 90% on room air, 98% on 100% nonrebreather (NRB) mask; GCS: 15; IV: 18 g left antecubital; ETA: 2 minutes...

EMERGENCY NURSING

Emergency nursing is a specialty practice in the nursing profession that requires the rapid assessment and treatment of patients, particularly during the initial phase of acute illness and trauma. Emergency nurses provide episodic care for individuals of all ages and cultures who may present with real or perceived alterations of health that require a primary evaluation and often a timely intervention. To provide quality patient care for people of all ages, emergency nurses must possess both general and specific knowledge about a wide variety of health topics ranging from sore throat to heart attack. Emergency nurses must tackle diverse tasks with professionalism, efficiency, and caring.

TRAUMA

Epidemiology of Trauma

In the United States, an unintentional injury is the third leading cause of death for all ages but is the leading cause of death for those aged 1 to 44 (Fig. 70.1). Falls are the leading cause of unintentional injury; **motor vehicle collisions (MVCs)** are the leading cause of death. Unintentional injury is also the leading cause for lost work years

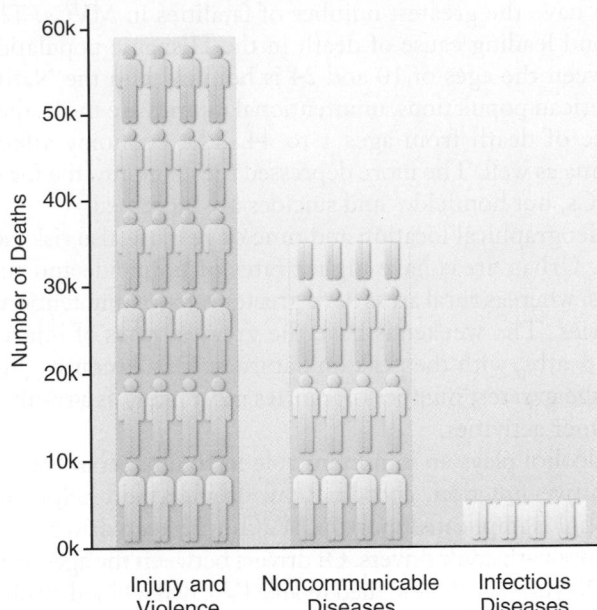

Leading Causes of Death

(y-axis: Number of Deaths, 0k–60k; x-axis categories: Injury and Violence, Noncommunicable Diseases, Infectious Diseases)

FIGURE 70.1 Unintentional injury is the leading cause of death for those aged 1 to 44 years in the United States.

because trauma affects mostly a younger population in its prime. Not only does trauma (fatal or nonfatal) affect the patients, it also affects their family, friends, and employers because they have to adjust to the changes brought about by the injury.

Age is a risk factor. The majority of deaths associated with motor vehicle trauma occur in individuals aged between 15 and 45 years. Patients older than 65 years of age have the greatest risk of dying from unintentional injury because of multiple factors such as comorbidities. Older adults also have a statistically higher occurrence of diaphragm laceration/rupture, heart laceration, hemo/pneumothorax, lung contusion/laceration, and rib and sternum fracture when compared with other age groups.

Gender is also a risk factor of trauma. Females are most likely to fall; however, males are at twice the risk for injury than females in motor vehicle–related collisions. There are a number of factors that affect this statistic such as higher risk-taking behavior, participation in more hazardous activities, occupation, and cultural norms. However, females sustain 80% of hip fractures. Females are also at greater risk for injury and death when the cause of injury is associated with intimate partner abuse. Males are much more likely to sustain and die from a penetrating injury than females.

Race and socioeconomic background are other risk factors of trauma. There are many reasons for this, although they are not completely understood. The higher the income, the lower the death rate, irrespective of the mechanism of injury or race. African Americans have the highest rate of homicide in the population. The pedestrian death rate is almost two times higher in African Americans than Caucasians. African American women have the highest rate of intimate partner violence injuries. The highest rate for suicide is found in the Caucasian population, and Caucasian men have the greatest number of fatalities in MVCs. The second leading cause of death in the Hispanic population between the ages of 10 and 24 is homicide. In the Native American populations, unintentional injuries are the leading cause of death from ages 1 to 44. The economy affects trauma as well. The more depressed the economy, the fewer MVCs, but homicides and suicides are increased.

Geographical location and time of year are also risk factors. Urban areas have higher rates of homicide and suicides, whereas rural areas have greater rates of unintentional injuries. The weekends have the greatest rates of injuries and deaths, with the peak on Saturday. Of all months, July has the greatest number of injuries most likely as a result of summer activities.

Alcohol plays an important role in trauma. It influences cognitive function, coordination, balance, and judgment. Alcohol is implicated more in MVCs with teen drivers than in those with adult drivers. Of drivers between the ages of 15 and 20 years, 25% who died in an MVC had a blood alcohol level (BAL) of 0.08% or greater. Tobacco may not have an important role as a risk factor for trauma; however, it does affect morbidity and mortality. Smoking increases the morbidity and mortality associated with trauma secondary to the smoking-related health issues. Substance abuse is found in all socioeconomic and educational levels. There is no clear evidence that connects drug use and trauma, but it should be considered when thinking about causes and risk factors of trauma.

Connection Check 70.1

As an emergency nurse in an inner-city ED, you are responsible for developing a trauma prevention program for your community. Who will be your priority patient population?
A. 10- to 34-year-old African American males
B. 10- to 34-year-old Caucasian females
C. 75+-year-olds
D. 10- to 34-year-old Hispanic males

Emergency/Trauma Care Centers

Trauma care is ideally provided by professionals working in institutions designated as trauma centers. Trauma centers are hospitals specially equipped to provide comprehensive emergency care to patients suffering from a traumatic injury. They came into existence from the realization that traumatic injury is a disease process requiring specialized multidisciplinary treatment and resources. Trauma centers have been shown to improve outcomes for trauma patients. To be designated as a trauma center, certain criteria must be met. The hospital must maintain a specialty trained workforce that is prepared to provide a range of emergency care 24/7 and must also ensure access to the equipment that is needed to provide immediate lifesaving care to critically injured patients.

In the United States, hospitals are designated as level I, II, III, or IV trauma centers on the basis of the depth of the resources and available personnel (Box 70.1). Some states have five designated levels, in which case level V (level 5) is the lowest. The American College of Surgeons (ACS) outlines the criteria for each designation level and verifies the presence of the resources recommended for optimal care of trauma patients. The general differentiation is that higher level trauma centers have trauma surgeons and other specialists, such as neurosurgeons and orthopedic surgeons, available as well as highly sophisticated medical diagnostic

Box 70.1 Levels of Trauma Centers (TCs)

Level I
- Regional resource hospital that is central to the trauma care system
- Provides total care for every aspect of injury from prevention through rehabilitation
- Maintains resources and personnel for patient care, education, and research; usually in university-based teaching hospital
- Provides leadership in education, research, and system planning to all hospitals caring for injured patients in the region
- Meets minimum requirement for volume of trauma patients

Level II
- Provides comprehensive trauma care, regardless of the severity of injury
- Might be most prevalent facility in a community and manages majority of trauma patients or supplements the activity of a level I trauma center (TC)
- Can be an academic institution or a public or private community facility located in an urban, suburban, or rural area
- Where no level I TC exists, is responsible for education and system leadership

Level III
- Provides prompt assessment, resuscitation, emergency surgery, and stabilization and arranges transfer to a higher-level facility when necessary
- Maintains continuous general surgery coverage
- Has transfer agreements and standardization treatment protocols to plan for care of injured patients
- Provides back-up care for rural and/or community hospitals

Level IV
- Rural facility that supplements care within the larger trauma system
- Provides initial evaluation and assessment of injured patients
- Must have 24-hour emergency coverage by a provider
- Has transfer agreements and a good working relationship with the nearest level I, II, or III TC

Source: Centers for Disease Control and Prevention. (2012, January 13). Guidelines for field triage of injured patients: Recommendations of the National Expert Panel on Field Triage, 2011. Retrieved from http://www.cdc.gov/mmwr/preview/mmwrhtml/rr6101a1.htm

equipment. Lower-level trauma centers may be able to provide only initial care and stabilization and arrange for transfer of the injured patient to a higher level of care.

To maintain trauma center designation, the hospital must ensure that all staff members receive ongoing education in trauma and maintain their competency in trauma care. Life support equipment, blood and blood products, and diagnostic tools need to be maintained in the highest state of readiness so that they are available when the patient arrives.

Prehospital Care

According to R. Adams Cowley, MD, the father of trauma medicine, there is a **"golden hour,"** now known as a **"golden period"** – the critical time between when an injury occurs, and definitive care is initiated. During this period, if bleeding is uncontrolled and there is inadequate tissue perfusion, damage occurs throughout the entire body. If bleeding and tissue oxygenation are not quickly controlled, the patient's chances of survival drop. This critical period may be much less than an hour for some patients, while others have more time. It is the prehospital provider who is responsible for recognizing the urgency of the situation and transporting the patient as quickly as possible to a hospital that can provide definitive care.

Priorities of Prehospital Care
Stabilization

At the scene, emergency medical providers such as emergency medical technicians (EMTs) or paramedics are the primary care providers. They use "field triage" to evaluate the severity of the injury. The initial assessment they perform drives decisions involving the management and transportation of the patient. The patient's respiratory, circulatory, and neurological systems are all quickly assessed to identify life-threatening conditions that require urgent intervention and resuscitation. The goal is to minimize time spent on the scene.

There is a systematic method to rapidly assess patients presenting with traumatic injury. This process is guided by the mnemonic "ABCD": airway (A); breathing (B); circulation (C); and disability (D). This sequence maximizes the ability of the body to oxygenate blood and deliver oxygen (O_2) to the tissues. The first step is A for airway, which must be checked to make sure it is open and clear while maintaining C-spine stabilization. **C-spine stabilization** is when a patient is in a supine position with the spine in neutral alignment (no rotation or bending of the spine); this position protects the patient from spinal cord damage and minimizes further damage. If a patient is able to vocalize, there is likely a stable airway. Gasping, gurgling, or no respirations at all often indicate a compromised airway in need of emergent definitive management. Step B is for breathing: ventilation and oxygenation, which can rapidly be assessed by auscultating for breath sounds in both lung fields and checking O_2 saturation via pulse oximetry. All patients must be placed on O_2. For patients who are found not breathing on their own, the prehospital provider must start assisting ventilation with a bag-valve mask device with supplemental O_2. Step C is for circulation: checking perfusion and assessing for hemorrhage and circulatory system compromise or failure. During this stage of assessment, palpating pulses and measuring blood pressure can determine the adequacy of circulation. Management of circulatory compromise includes hemorrhage control. Direct pressure is the most effective way of stopping external hemorrhage. The patient may also need IV insertion to provide IV fluids while in transport. Step D is for disability: neurological function. The goal is to determine the patient's level of consciousness.

Transport

If life-threatening conditions are identified, the patient should receive necessary emergency care described above, be rapidly "packaged" (the process of preparing a patient for transport) and transported to the nearest appropriate trauma facility. Important factors to be considered in determining appropriate transportation type and destination is the mechanism of injury and transportation time to the medical facility. If the transport time by ground is too long, air transportation may be necessary. If there is no air transportation or close trauma facility, the patient should be taken to the closest facility for stabilization then transported to a trauma center. Other special considerations such as age, pregnancy greater than 20 weeks, and bleeding disorders are also considered when determining the level of care necessary for the patient.

If in doubt, the EMS team may consult the trauma center and the closest facility to obtain guidance on the best initial treatment location of the patient. It is always recommended to notify the receiving hospital in advance so that the trauma team can assemble before the patient's arrival.

Connection Check 70.2

The nurse understands priority prehospital interventions include which of the following?

A. Transporting the patient as quickly as possible to the nearest trauma center

B. Treating all injuries found and then transporting the patient

C. Notifying the local hospital of the transport of a trauma patient and transporting the patient quickly

D. Assessing the patient using ABCs, treating life-threatening conditions, then transport to the hospital

---

Hospital Care

Hospital Personnel

Once the injured patient has been delivered to the trauma center, the aim of the trauma team is to provide safe and efficient evaluation and treatment. The team must identify all injuries and initiate definitive management of such injuries in an expedient matter. The staff at trauma centers are specially trained to function smoothly in the most challenging and chaotic circumstances.

The response of hospital personnel depends on the type of trauma patient presenting. Many trauma centers designate a tiered response based on the severity of the injuries. The more seriously injured a patient, the more hospital resources are activated to respond. The core trauma team is composed of many people working around a single patient. It is vital that everyone on the team knows their role and has the skills, equipment, and support to safely care for the patient. Typical roles of the trauma team include the following: trauma team leader, airway provider, surgical provider, nurses, respiratory therapy, radiologist, clinical technician (a highly trained nursing assistant or EMT), clinical pharmacist, social work and/or pastoral care, and ancillary support staff (Fig. 70.2).

The team leader typically does not physically touch the patient but orchestrates the care of the patient through delegation and supervision of the other providers and staff in the room. The team leader establishes priorities for the patient's care and authorizes interventions based on the assessment of the patient and all diagnostic results. If there are several providers attempting to initiate orders or carry out procedures independently, the care of the patient can be uncoordinated and confusing for team members. The team

leader must be clear and in control of the situation; the captain of the team. The trauma room should be quiet so that all members of the team can hear the voice of the team leader.

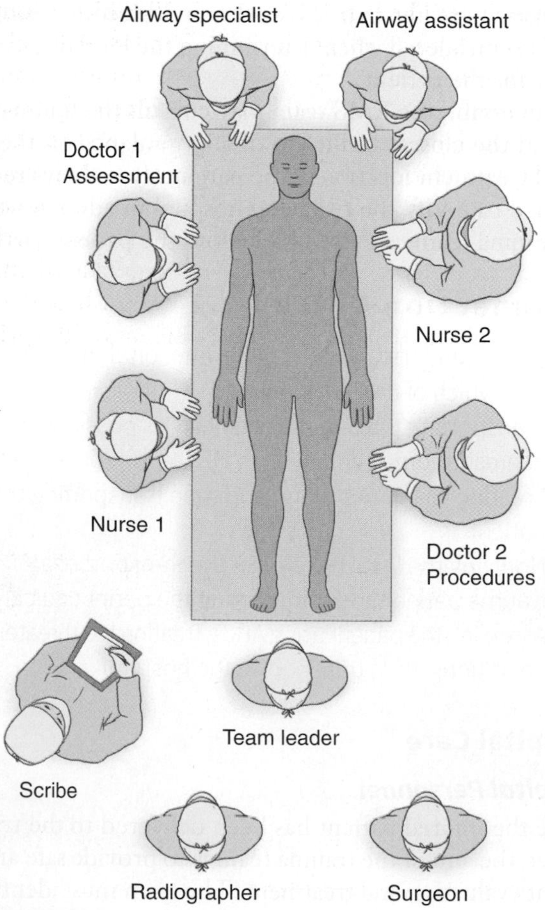

The airway, surgical, and ED providers are responsible for establishing and maintaining an airway, ordering medications, and performing surgical procedures at the direction of the team leader. At least one of the providers is typically assigned to perform the **primary survey** (the first quick assessment and initial management of life-threatening injuries). Some overlap in roles is necessary between the general surgeons and ED providers to ensure that tasks continue simultaneously, and no time is lost.

In the management of a trauma patient, nursing is typically responsible for administration of all medications and IV fluids as well as setup of equipment for wound management and surgical procedures. The **rapid fluid infuser** is sometimes used to administer blood or boluses of fluid to the injured patient who has lost large volumes of blood. When it is in use, a nurse is dedicated to its management, ensuring empty fluid bags are replaced as necessary and fluid intake is closely monitored. During the patient's care, one nurse typically serves in the role of a scribe and is responsible for the full documentation of the trauma assessment and care. Records must include the details of the patient's care, such as time of arrival, personnel present at call, physical findings, and fluids and drugs administered. After the patient has been stabilized, nursing staff are responsible for providing updates to the family (Box 70.2).

Clinical technicians, EMTs, or paramedics may be delegated duties within their scope of practice, such as establishing IV access, performing chest compressions during cardiopulmonary resuscitation, preparing equipment,

FIGURE 70.2 The trauma team.

Box 70.2 Family Presence During Trauma Resuscitation

The concept of family presence during trauma resuscitation (FPTR) remains controversial. Healthcare workers have expressed concern that the witness of the resuscitation of a severely injured trauma patient may be inappropriate for the family, but studies support that family members who were present benefited from the experience. They gained better understanding of the situation. A recent study reported that this is especially true in pediatric trauma: the ability of the parent to support the child is extremely important to both the parent and child. FPTR is a growing trend and should be considered unless family behaviors interfere with resuscitative efforts. A designated nurse case manager, social worker or clergy should be assigned to the family during resuscitation to assure their own psychosocial needs and knowledge deficits are being met and addressed. If the family is not present, nursing staff is responsible for giving frequent updates to the family.

obtaining vital signs, and placing the patient on a cardiac monitor. Clinical pharmacists are excellent resources in the care of the trauma patient as they provide expert support in the pharmacological management of the patient. A radiologist is necessary to evaluate the many x-rays and scans typically performed in the trauma assessment. Social workers and ED nursing case management are helpful in serving as liaisons with the families who are often in need of support as their loved one is cared for by the team. Ancillary staff members in the room retrieve equipment and supplies and run blood samples to the laboratory.

Connection Check 70.3

The nurse caring for a trauma patient understands which team member will establish priorities for the patient's care and authorize the interventions and procedures?

A. Trauma surgeon
B. Trauma team leader
C. Anesthesiologist
D. Radiologist

Triage

Triage is the sorting of patients based on their need for treatment and the resources available to provide that treatment. The triage nurse must quickly identify patients who need to be seen immediately and those who can safely wait for treatment. This is based on a quick assessment often including vital signs, which allows the nurse to assign an acuity level. There are several different triage systems used in hospitals, but priorities are universal. As in the survey for prehospital providers, triage and acuity are based on the ABCD priorities: **A**irway with C-spine precautions, **B**reathing, **C**irculation with hemorrhage control, and **D**isability and resource management. The importance of rapid and accurate triage is necessary for optimal patient outcomes.

Trauma Assessment

Trauma assessments are broken down into a primary survey and secondary survey. They should be performed on all trauma patients even if they do not appear to be seriously injured. In addition to gaining information on the patient's presenting condition, the initial assessment includes obtaining

limited subjective information about major injuries and mechanism of injury from the prehospital providers, patient, or family members. A more detailed report is received during the secondary survey.

Primary Survey

The **primary survey** begins immediately on the patient's arrival to the hospital. The purpose of a rapid primary survey is to identify life-threatening conditions and simultaneously institute management of these conditions. Similar to the prehospital assessment, it follows the ABCDs with the addition of E. "E" stands for "exposure/environment" (Table 70.1). The primary survey starts with an **A**irway assessment. The airway needs to be inspected for injuries that may result in airway obstruction. If the patient is talking, there are likely no airway issues, but the airway requires frequent reassessment later. Once the airway has been quickly assessed, **B**reathing, or ventilation, needs to be quickly assessed because it can be affected by numerous thoracic injuries and can be life threatening. Ineffective breathing patterns may indicate life-threatening injuries.

Key components of the **C**irculatory assessment are pulses, heart rate, skin color, blood pressure, capillary refill, and any obvious signs of bleeding, internal or external. A **D**isability assessment is a brief neurological assessment that measures the patient's level of consciousness. This is done using the Glasgow Coma Scale (GCS) (Box 70.3). The GCS provides a quick assessment of neurological abilities or disabilities. The best GCS score is 15, which is found in a person with no deficits or injuries. The lowest GCS score a patient can receive is 3. This is a person who is nonresponsive or is intubated and heavily sedated. Pupils should also be assessed for size, shape, equality, and reaction to light as well as looking for lateralizing signs that may help locate an area of brain injury. Finally, **exposure** means to completely undress the patient so that obvious and potential injuries, both front and back, can be quickly identified. Exposure also includes measures to prevent hypothermia. With a large trauma team, these assessments of the primary survey can be done simultaneously.

Secondary Survey

The **secondary survey** is performed after the primary survey is complete and lifesaving interventions have been

Table 70.1 ABCDE: The Primary Survey

Letter	Body System	Assessment
A	Airway	Airway with C-spine precautions which is especially important if airway is not patent
B	Breathing	Evaluate ventilation; apply high-flow O$_2$
C	Circulation	Evaluate perfusion and bleeding; includes hemorrhage control
D	Disability	Evaluate neurological status and evaluate resources necessary for the care of the patient
E	Exposure/Environment	Complete assessment of the patient; prevent hypothermia

Box 70.3 Glasgow Coma Scale

Eye Opening Response

4 = Spontaneous
3 = To verbal stimuli
2 = To pain
1 = None

Verbal Response

5 = Oriented
4 = Confused
3 = Inappropriate words
2 = Incoherent
1 = None

Motor Response

6 = Obeys commands
5 = Localizes pain
4 = Withdraws from pain
3 = Flexion to pain; decorticate
2 = Extension to pain; decerebrate
1 = None

Total Scores

15: Best score possible. Patient opens eyes spontaneously (E=4), is oriented (V=5), and obeys commands (M=6)
13–15: Minor brain injury
9–12: Moderate brain injury
8 or less: Severe brain injury
3: Worst score possible (cannot have a score lower then 3). The patient is not opening eyes (E=1), is making no sounds (V=1), and is flaccid/not following any commands (M=1).

A patient who is intubated and heavily sedated may have a Glasgow Coma Scale score of 3 as well.

Adapted from Teasdale, G., & Jennett, B. (1974). Assessment of coma and impaired consciousness: A practical scale. *Lancet, 2*(7872), 81–84.

initiated. This survey identifies the other injuries that the primary survey did not assess along with pertinent information about the patient such as other comorbidities. It is during the secondary survey that pain should be assessed. At the start of the secondary survey, a complete set of vital signs should be obtained again. If they are abnormal, the team may need to return to the primary survey and reassess. If vital signs remain normal, then a head-to-toe assessment should be completed, including the posterior surfaces. Also, it is during this time that the trauma team is gathering critical information about the event from the patient, prehospital providers, witnesses, and family. In an MVC, information about where the patient was in the car, the use or nonuse of safety devices, the speed, location and extent of car damage, and where the patient was found and in what condition helps to create a high index of suspicion for injuries. Additionally, determination of the sequence of events, such as whether the patient was able to get out of the vehicle independently or if the damage was so significant

that the patient had to be extricated by emergency personnel is important. Entrapment can result in greater injury and may prolong the transport time. This delay is important when considering the "golden period." With penetrating trauma, knowing the weapon, type of gun, or length of the knife or other sharp object, how many shots were heard, how close the patient was to the weapon, and size of the assailant help develop a high index of suspicion of injuries.

Intervention

Priority interventions include airway, breathing, circulation, disability, and environment.

Airway

Airway priority interventions include (A) open airway; (B) provide oxygen; and (C) prepare for an advanced airway. If the airway is not patent, open and clear the airway using the jaw thrust (Fig. 70.3) maneuver and suction. The chin-lift (Fig. 70.4) maneuver is another option for opening the airway. If the patient's tongue has fallen backward and obstructed the airway, both maneuvers allow the airway to become unobstructed but the jaw thrust maneuver is always used for trauma patients when spinal cord injury is suspected to prevent primary or further injury to the spinal cord (see Safety Alert). The jaw thrust is also very effective at creating a good seal with the face mask of a bag-mask

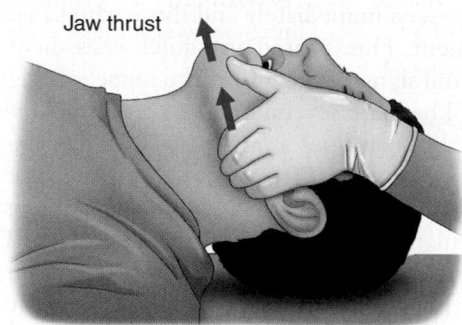

FIGURE 70.3 Jaw-thrust technique of opening airway.

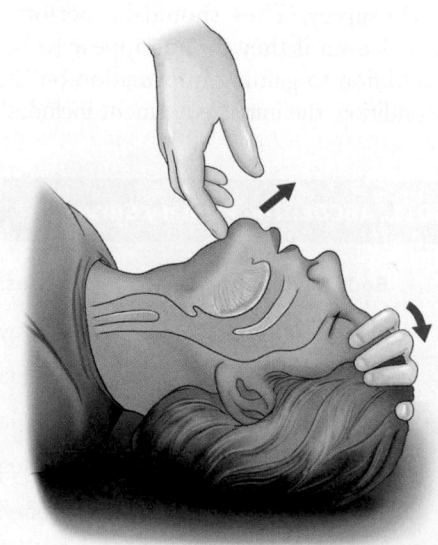

FIGURE 70.4 Chin-lift technique of opening airway.

device. Care must be taken to not hyperextend the neck with either maneuver. If necessary, an oropharyngeal or nasopharyngeal airway can be placed. At this stage, preparations for endotracheal intubation or a surgical airway, cricothyroidotomy, should be implemented if indicated.

 Safety Alert **Assessing airway in a trauma patient:**

There is always a high index of suspicion for C-spine injury after trauma. It is essential to maintain C-spine precautions and use the jaw thrust maneuver when assessing airway and breathing and when placing a definitive airway, if necessary.

Provider Protection:

Always wear full protective gear to guard against splashes with body fluid. While exposing patients, be on the lookout for sharp objects that may be on them or in their clothing.

Breathing

Breathing priority interventions include (A) providing oxygen and (B) diagnosing and treating life-threatening breathing injuries. All trauma patients should receive O_2 via face mask and placed on pulse oximetry to properly measure oxygenation changes. Chest x-rays should be done to check for life-threatening chest injuries along with appropriate laboratory studies, such as arterial blood gases. Any abnormal assessment findings should be acted on. For instance, patient respiratory distress, hemodynamic instability and/or decreased breath sounds on the injured side should raise the suspicion for a pneumothorax that should be confirmed by chest x-ray (CXR) and treated with chest tube placement. A pneumothorax occurs when air enters the pleural space between the visceral and parietal pleurae partially collapsing the lung. If the pneumothorax is evolving quickly or untreated, it may lead to a tension pneumothorax. A tension pneumothorax is caused when the air entering the pleural space cannot escape on expiration, increasing the intrathoracic pressure. This results in a fully collapsed lung and a mediastinal shift that compresses the heart, trachea, great vessels, and uninjured lung. Please refer to Chapter 27 for more in-depth details regarding pneumothorax. If tension pneumothorax occurs, it may be necessary to perform a needle thoracostomy (needle decompression); the insertion of a needle into the pleural space on the side of the pneumothorax. This procedure allows the air that has accumulated in the pleural space to escape (Fig. 70.5). This is followed by tube thoracostomy (chest tube) placement and again, confirmed by CXR.

Circulation

Circulation priority interventions include (A) IV access; and (B) fluid resuscitation. Vascular access is essential. The patient needs one or two large-bore (18-gauge or larger) IV catheters to allow for fluid and medication administration.

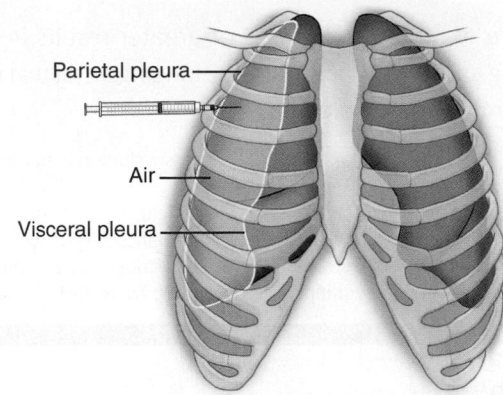

Parietal pleura

Air

Visceral pleura

FIGURE 70.5 Needle thoracostomy: insertion of a needle into the pleural space, allowing the accumulated air to escape and prevent a pneumothorax from becoming a tension pneumothorax.

If venous access is difficult, the patient should be prepared for insertion of a central line. An intraosseous catheter, a catheter placed into the marrow cavity of a bone, is also an option for fluid or medication administration when peripheral blood vessels are inaccessible. As a last resort, a surgical cutdown may be performed. This is an emergency procedure that surgically exposes a vein, typically the saphenous vein, allowing placement of an IV catheter under direct visualization of the vessel.

Fluid resuscitation is dictated by the patient's condition. Typically, this starts with the judicious infusion use of warmed isotonic crystalloid solution. Blood products are indicated if there is excessive bleeding. If the patient is severely hypotensive or has suffered extensive blood loss, fluids may be placed in pressure bags or administered through a rapid infusion device that can infuse about 1,000 mL of warmed fluid per minute but recent evidence suggests a more judicious use of fluids (see Evidence-Based Practice: Fluid Resuscitation).

Evidence-Based Practice

Fluid Resuscitation

Previous fluid replacement strategies in severe trauma began with the rapid infusion of crystalloid solutions, but recent research suggests that a balanced resuscitation strategy for severe hemorrhagic shock may have better outcomes. First, minimization of crystalloids and the use of balanced crystalloids: normal saline and Ringer's lactate rather than just normal saline. Second, a 1:1:1 blood product ratio for infusions and last, permissive hypotension. Based on significant experiential evidence in the military population, an approach using limited resuscitation with crystalloids and a blood product ratio of equal amounts of packed red blood cells with fresh frozen plasma and platelets may have a positive impact on overall survival. Additionally, maintaining a mean arterial pressure of 50 rather than 65 or greater results in less bleeding and reduces the risk of dislodging a clot that may have formed to stop bleeding.

Cantle, P. M., & Cotton, B. A. (2017). Balanced resuscitation in trauma management. *Surgical Clinics, 97*(5), 999–1014.
Self, W. H., Semler, M. W., Wanderer, J. P., Ehrenfeld, J. M., Byrne, D. W., Wang, L.,. . .& Shaw, A. D. (2017). Saline versus balanced crystalloids for intravenous fluid therapy in the emergency department: study protocol for a cluster-randomized, multiple-crossover trial. *Trials, 18*(1), 178.

Disability

Maintaining spinal immobilization is essential in trauma patients with a risk of spinal cord injury. Also, if during the primary survey the patient is found to have a decreased level of consciousness, there should be further investigation in the secondary survey, including a detailed neurological evaluation and imaging of the brain and spinal cord.

Exposure/Environment

An environmental priority intervention is to control the environment to prevent hypothermia. Warming blankets, warmed fluids, and continual temperature monitoring are essential to help prevent the **trauma triad of death** (Box 70.4).

Further Secondary Survey Interventions

During the secondary survey further laboratory, radiographical, ultrasound, and other diagnostic studies should be performed. A valuable diagnostic tool is a focused assessment with sonography for trauma (FAST). This is an ultrasound that looks for free fluid in the abdominal cavity, pericardium, or pelvis. If the FAST examination is positive, it typically indicates the presence of blood. The patient with a positive FAST requires emergency surgery to find the source of the bleeding and repair of the injury. Other

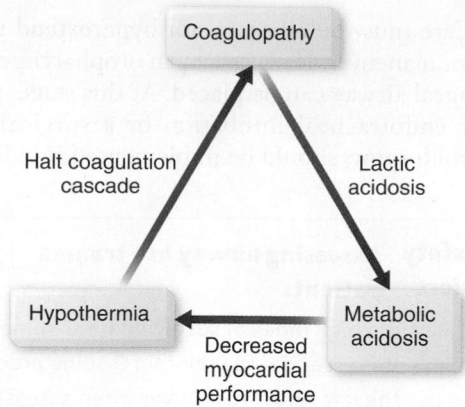

FIGURE 70.6 Trauma triad of death. Hypothermia results in peripheral vasoconstriction, which decreases oxygenation, causing hypoperfusion and lactic acidosis as well as coagulopathy. The acidosis also results in decreased myocardial performance.

interventions include the insertion of a Foley catheter to monitor urine output and renal function. If blood is present at the urinary meatus, further evaluation is required before a Foley catheter is inserted because of the potential of injury to the urinary structures. Additionally, the insertion of a gastric tube to empty the stomach and prevent aspiration is essential especially for a patient where bag-valve mask ventilation has been used. Nasogastric tubes are not recommended in patients with significant facial trauma because of the potential presence of fractures that may result in intracranial insertion of the tube. Once the secondary survey has been completed, definitive interventions are performed, or initial surgical stabilization is performed if the patient is too ill to tolerate definitive procedures (see Evidence-Based Practice: Damage Control Surgery).

Box 70.4 Trauma Triad of Death

The **trauma triad of death** is a term describing the lethal combination of hypothermia, metabolic acidosis, and coagulopathy (Fig. 70.6) in the trauma patient. Hypothermia, a preventable contributory factor, is caused by a number of factors, such as massive hemorrhage, sepsis, exposure, fluid resuscitation without warm fluid, and certain medications (muscle relaxers, sedatives, anesthetics, and/or opioids). Hypothermia causes peripheral vasoconstriction, which decreases oxygenation, causing hypoperfusion and lactic acidosis. This leads to reduced efficiency of the heart muscle, which then further reduces the O_2 delivery. Also, as the body temperature drops, coagulation is inhibited, resulting in bleeding (coagulopathy). Without interruption in the cycle, principally by preventing hypothermia, the consequential sequelae of the "trauma triad of death" may result in serious complications and death.

Evidence-Based Practice

Damage Control Surgery

Damage control surgery is indicated for a select group of trauma patients that present in physiological extremis or at the point of death and require immediate surgical control of hemorrhage and contamination. It is a concept that originated in the military many years ago and has been refined in more recent years due to conflicts in the Middle East and by trauma physicians in the civilian sector. It has demonstrated success in increasing survival rate in patients in severe hemorrhagic shock by 50%. It uses a staged surgical approach after initial resuscitation, avoiding long, complicated procedures on unstable patients and focusing instead on stabilizing potentially fatal problems at the initial operation. The philosophy of this type of management is to abbreviate surgical interventions before the development of irreversible physiological endpoints; avoiding or correcting the lethal triad of hypothermia, acidosis, and coagulopathy before definitive surgical management. The stages are:

1. Stop hemorrhage, control contamination, perform temporary closure of wounds.
2. Correct physiologic abnormalities in the critical care setting through intensive monitoring, ensuring adequate fluid resuscitation, warming, and correcting coagulopathy.
3. Definitive operative management

Weber, D. G., & Bendinelli, C. (2017). Damage control surgery for emergency general surgery. In *Acute Care Surgery Handbook* (pp. 387-401). Springer: Cham.

Connection Check 70.4

The nurse understands the purpose of damage control surgery is which of the following? Select all that apply.
A. Control hemorrhage
B. Prevent renal failure
C. Prevent contamination
D. Avoid further surgery
E. Control hypoxia

Mechanism of Injury

Mechanism of injury is defined as the transference of energy from an external force to the body of the patient. Understanding the type of mechanism of injury: blunt or penetrating, region of the body affected, and how severely the force was applied helps determine the extent of injury.

Blunt Trauma

Blunt trauma is when the energy transference does not cause disruption to the skin, making these injuries more difficult to see. Mechanisms of energy transference that cause blunt trauma injuries are deceleration and acceleration forces, compression, and shearing. **Deceleration** is when the body has been moving and comes to an abrupt stop. **Acceleration**

is a sudden increase in speed. Acceleration is often followed by deceleration. An example of deceleration is a motor vehicle traveling at 50 mph that hits a brick wall, causing the vehicle to come to a sudden stop. All passengers inside the vehicle come to a sudden stop, typically against a hard surface in the car. An example of acceleration is a pedestrian standing on the side of the road who is hit by a moving vehicle, causing the pedestrian to be thrown 20 feet. Deceleration forces are applied when the pedestrian hits the ground. **Compression** injuries are as they sound—organs or tissues compressed between two immovable surfaces such as bones or a steering wheel. **Shearing** occurs when skin or tissue slides in opposite but parallel directions. Although blunt trauma injuries may be more difficult to see on first assessment, they are frequently very severe and widespread. The most common forms of blunt trauma are MVCs, motorcycle crashes, pedestrians struck, bicycle injuries, sports (football) injuries, falls, and assaults.

Blunt Thoracic Trauma

Thoracic injuries can be some of the most life-threatening injuries. Many vital organs are located in the thoracic cavity: heart, lungs, and aorta. These injuries can cause airway disruptions, and/or serious circulatory alterations. Isolated blunt trauma thoracic injuries are not common and should generate a high suspicion for related abdominal injuries.

The primary mechanism of blunt trauma to the thoracic cavity is from compression causing the chest wall to be displaced inward with impact, such as when the chest hits the steering wheel during an MVC. Rapid deceleration is often the force involved with compression injuries. When the body stops moving forward after it hits an object, the internal organs still continue to move forward until they hit something (Fig. 70.7). The heart tends to hit the sternum, the lungs hit the ribs, and the aorta can be pressed up against the spine. It is these types of movements that often also cause shearing injuries.

Blunt Cardiac Injury

Blunt cardiac injury (BCI), one form of thoracic trauma, can be anything from a myocardial contusion to a cardiac rupture. The most common causes of BCIs are high-speed

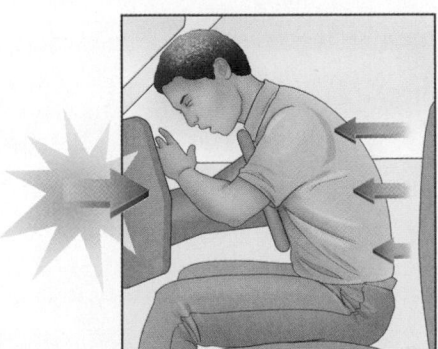
The chest hits the steering wheel and the body stops moving

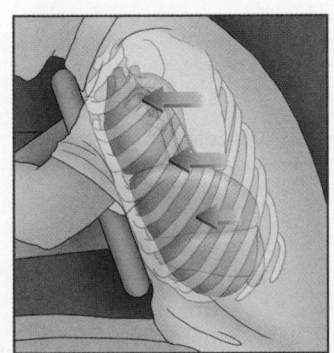
The internal organs continue to move forward until they hit something

FIGURE 70.7 Rapid deceleration and compression injuries in motor vehicle crashes.

MVC impacts and falls from heights where there is a direct impact on the chest. Sternum fractures can result in right ventricular perforation, and fractured ribs can lacerate either the right or left ventricle. Blunt cardiac injuries can also happen due to deceleration and shearing forces. An example is injury to the descending aorta. Unlike the heart, aortic arch, and ascending aorta, the descending aorta is tightly restrained to the posterior thoracic wall and vertebral column. This predisposes the descending aorta to shearing injuries. When the body is rapidly decelerated, the heart and ascending aorta continue to move forward while the descending aorta cannot. This can cause a tear in the aorta at the junction of the aorta that can move freely and the section that is restrained (Fig. 70.8). This tear can be a complete transection of the aorta, causing immediate death due to **exsanguinations** (extreme loss of blood volume), or it can be a partial tear, a **traumatic aneurysm.** A traumatic aneurysm is caused by a partial or incomplete laceration of the layers of the aorta wall (Fig. 70.9). Both can cause ischemia and a hematoma that causes a weakened area in the aorta wall, allowing an aneurysm to form (see Chapter 31 for more information on aneurysms). This traumatic aneurysm can rupture anywhere from minutes to days from the time of injury.

Compression injury to the heart can occur when the heart is compressed between the sternum and spine or when a heavy object is crushing a person on the chest. When the heart becomes compressed, it can result in cardiac contusion and dysrhythmias. The most common dysrhythmia is sinus tachycardia, which may be caused by other reasons such as hypotension as well as cardiac contusion. Other dysrhythmias noted are premature ventricular contractions. Cardiac compression can also happen when a pneumothorax progresses to a tension pneumothorax compressing the heart, trachea, great vessels, and uninjured lung. Worst case, cardiac contusion can result in nonperfusing rhythms such as ventricular fibrillation or ventricular tachycardia and cardiac arrest. (Chapter 29 discusses dysrhythmias in detail.)

Blunt Pulmonary Injuries

Rib Fractures. The most common thoracic traumatic injury is rib fracture. Rib fractures can be seen in many types of blunt trauma to the thorax: the steering wheel hitting the chest in an MVC, a baseball bat to the rib cage, a fall landing on the chest or side. The sternum and ribs resist energy forces better than other bones of the body and provide protection to the vital thoracic organs. If these bones are fractured, significant injuries to the underlying structures must be evaluated because of the force necessary to fracture these bones. Understanding which ribs are fractured can help identify associated intrathoracic injuries (Table 70.2). When a rib fracture produces a free-floating sternum or there is a fracture of two or more ribs in two or more places, a condition called *flail chest* results. Clinically, this condition can be identified by paradoxical motion of the flailed segment of chest wall during spontaneous respiration.

Pneumothorax, Hemothorax, and Pulmonary Contusion.
Rib fractures and flail chests can cause pneumothorax or hemothorax when the sharp edges of the broken ribs perforate the chest wall, causing a loss of the negative intrapleural pressure. This can cause a partial or total lung collapse. Once a pneumothorax has developed, tension pneumothorax, as discussed previously, may occur. Traumatic hemothorax is caused by a laceration in the lung or intercostal vessel.

Pulmonary contusion is another possible injury caused by blunt thoracic trauma. Before impact, whether in an MVC or fall, a person instinctively takes a deep breath and holds it, closing the glottis and sealing off the lungs. As when a paper bag full of air is suddenly compressed, when the chest wall is suddenly compressed, the lungs can rupture; but more typically, they become contused. Pulmonary contusion leads to pulmonary edema with blood collecting in the alveoli, causing poor gas exchange, decreased lung compliance, and increased pulmonary vascular resistance.

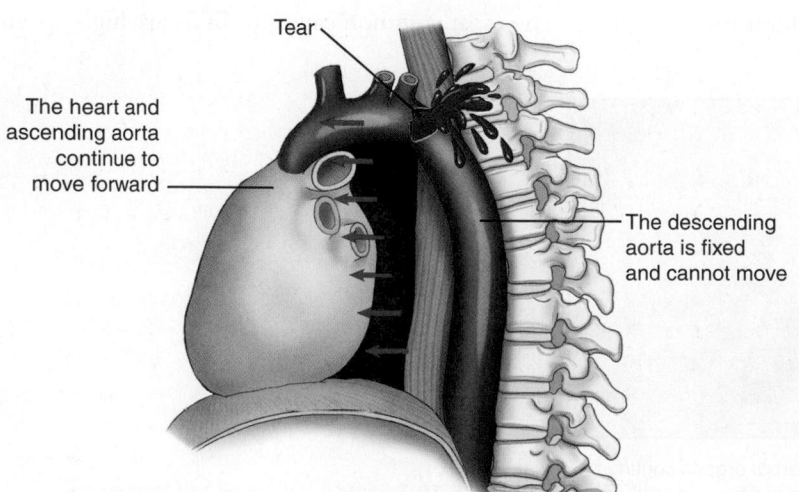

FIGURE 70.8 Sheared descending aorta: when the body rapidly decelerates and the heart and ascending aorta continue to move forward while the descending aorta cannot, causing a tear in the aorta.

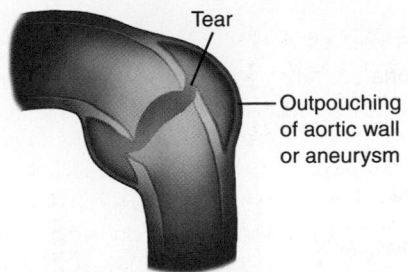

Tear

Outpouching
of aortic wall
or aneurysm

FIGURE 70.9 Traumatic aortic aneurysm caused by a partial or incomplete laceration of the layers of the aorta wall.

Table 70.2 Injuries Associated With Rib Fractures

Rib Fracture	Associated Injuries
Upper ribs (1–3)— protected by scapula, clavicle, humerus; these fractures indicate great energy was necessary to cause damage	• Scapula, clavicle, sternal, humerus fractures • Head, neck, spinal cord injuries • Great vessel injuries • Lung injuries • Blunt cardiac injuries
Middle ribs (4–9) most commonly injured	• Pneumothorax • Hemothorax • Pulmonary contusion • Muscle injuries • Blood vessel injuries
Lower ribs (10–12)	• Liver, spleen, and intra-abdominal injuries

Blunt Abdominal Trauma

Abdominal organs are more vulnerable to injury than those in the thorax because of the lack of protection from the sternum and rib cage. They are separated into two categories by density: solid and hollow (Box 70.5). The solid organs are dense masses of very vascular tissue. The hollow organs are less dense because of the presence of a cavity that is filled with air or digestive matter. This is important to understand and differentiate when looking at potential for traumatic injuries. Like blunt thoracic trauma, blunt abdominal trauma injuries result from compression, shearing, and acceleration/deceleration. Blunt abdominal trauma may be associated with damage to the viscera (internal organs), which can result in massive blood loss or the spilling of intestinal contents into the peritoneal space, and peritonitis. The manifestation of these injuries is often subtle and requires a high index of suspicion during patient evaluation. Motor vehicle crashes are the leading cause of blunt abdominal injuries.

Compression Injuries

Compression injuries in the abdomen are caused by the vertebral column pressing the internal organs into an external structure, causing them to bruise or rupture. This external

Box 70.5 Abdominal Organ Categories by Density

Solid Abdominal Organs

• Liver
• Spleen
• Kidneys
• Pancreas
• Adrenal glands
• Ovaries

Hollow Abdominal Organs

• Bladder
• Large intestines
• Small intestines
• Stomach
• Uterus

structure could be a steering wheel or dashboard in an MVC or the ground after a fall from a height. The sudden increase in pressure caused by compression frequently injures the solid organs. This overpressure within the abdomen can also cause the diaphragm to tear or be ruptured (Fig. 70.10). Diaphragm injuries can affect ventilation by allowing the abdomen organs and blood from an intra-abdominal hemorrhage to enter the thoracic cavity. This can result in compression of the lung or heart, and worst case from cardiac compression, cardiac tamponade.

Shearing Injuries

Rapid deceleration produces shearing forces, causing tears or ruptures in organs. When the body stops moving forward, the internal organs continue to move forward in the abdomen, causing tears at the point of attachment to the abdominal wall. Blood vessels that enter these organs may also be torn. The kidneys, spleen, and large and small intestines (mesenteric attachments) are known for being highly susceptible to shearing injuries.

Liver lacerations often occur during rapid deceleration events secondary to its impact with the ligamentum teres. This ligament divides the left part of the liver into medial and lateral sections. The liver is supported by the diaphragm and not by any fixed structure. When the body experiences a rapid deceleration, the liver keeps moving in a downward fashion onto the ligamentum teres. This movement onto the ligament can cause a tear in the liver.

Safety restraints such as seat belts provide significant protection but when not used correctly can cause injury. If the lap belt of a seat belt is not placed correctly, it can cause shearing injuries to the lower abdomen, such as rupture of the small bowel or colon.

Pelvic Fractures

Also, as a result of blunt abdominal trauma, pelvic fractures can be seen in MVCs, pedestrians struck, and falls.

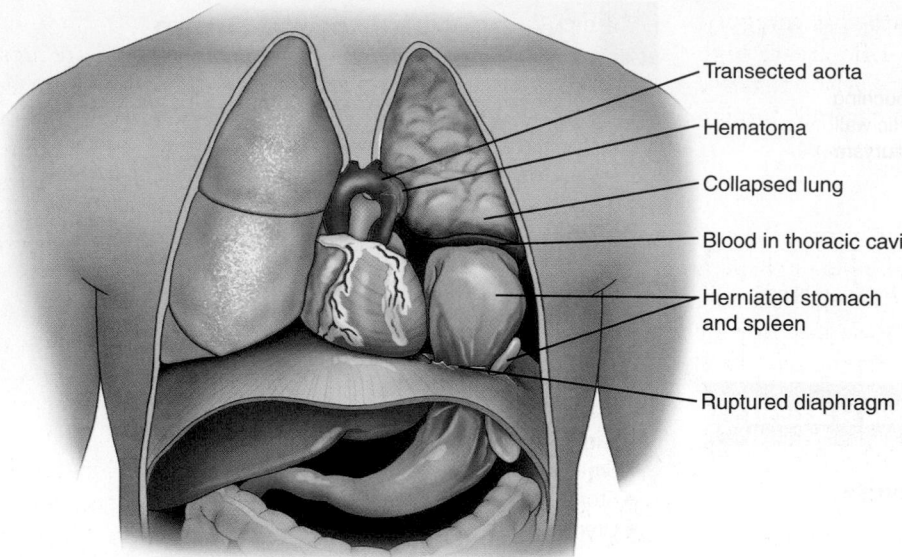

Transected aorta

Hematoma

Collapsed lung

Blood in thoracic cavity

Herniated stomach and spleen

Ruptured diaphragm

FIGURE 70.10 Diaphragmatic rupture allowing abdominal organs and blood from an intra-abdominal hemorrhage to enter the thoracic cavity, resulting in compression of the lung or heart and shearing injuries.

They can be stable or unstable fractures, with unstable being the most dangerous. Genitourinary injuries are noted in approximately 10% of those patients with pelvic fractures. These include bladder ruptures, ureteral transections, and urethral disruptions. In severe, unstable pelvic fractures, there can be circulatory disruption, both venous and arterial.

Penetrating Trauma

Penetrating trauma is defined as injuries produced by a foreign object penetrating the tissue. Knives, guns, or ice picks are the most common cause of penetrating trauma. However, anything that penetrates the skin, such as glass from a broken windshield, can be a cause of trauma. Foreign objects that cause penetrating trauma are often classified according to the amount of energy they or their projectiles produce:

- Low-energy: knife or other sharp objects thrown by hand; also glass from an MVC or another falling object
- Medium-energy: handguns
- High-energy: military or hunting rifles

The energy created by the foreign object dissipates into the surrounding tissues, causing injury. The extent of the damage is affected by three main factors: the character of the wounding object, its velocity, and the characteristics of the tissues that it passes through. Penetrating injuries can be like an iceberg; the injury one sees on the skin may be minor compared to the significant injury beneath the surface.

Gunshot Wound

Many bullets do not travel in a linear fashion once entering the body. Direction can change after contact with different density tissues or by hitting bone. Noting entrance and exit wounds can help determine the anatomical structures in the bullet's pathway. Also, to help estimate the damage that can be done by a bullet it is important to understand the type of bullet and the factors that affect its movement and action: cavitation, velocity, profile, tumble, yaw, and fragmentation.

Cavitation

Cavitation is associated with shock waves that compress the tissues and travel ahead and to the sides of the bullet—the energy exchange between the missile/bullet and the body tissue it is passing through. There can be a permanent cavitation caused by the track of the bullet and a temporary cavitation (Fig. 70.11) in which the wound cavity is temporarily stretched outward as a result of a pressure wave created in the tissue in the wake of the bullet. The elasticity in the tissue struck by the missile determines the size of the permanent cavity created. The permanent cavity in muscle is relatively small because muscle has more elasticity and can expand and return back to shape. An organ such as the liver has very little elasticity, and thus the permanent cavity created is much larger.

Velocity

Velocity is the speed of a traveling object and is the most significant determinant of its wounding capability. The velocity affects the extent of cavitation and tissue deformation. Low-velocity missiles have little disruptive effect on tissues; they have a small radius of distribution around the center tract of injury. These low-velocity missiles push the tissues aside along a path without creating a

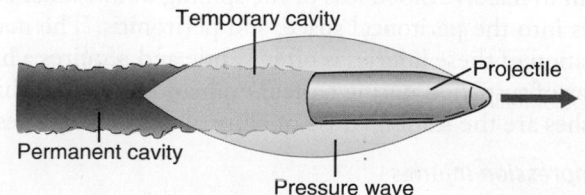

Temporary cavity

Projectile

Permanent cavity

Pressure wave

FIGURE 70.11 Cavitation injury; permanent or temporary cavitation caused by the track of the bullet where the wound cavity is stretched outward as a result of a pressure wave created in the wake of the bullet.

large cavitation. Most sidearms fall into this category. High-velocity missiles such as from a rifle create high cavitation and high-energy transference. Also, negative pressure behind a high-velocity missile can pull foreign matter into the wound, causing contamination.

Profile

Profile describes the initial size of the projectile and changes, if any, at the time of impact. The bullet shape is specifically designed to be aerodynamic, with minimal drag through the air but more drag when it passes through body tissues. If it becomes deformed when it hits the skin, then it impacts a larger area, creates more drag, and has a much greater energy exchange, causing a larger cavitation and more injury. This is why hollow-point bullets (bullets that flatten and spread on impact) cause more damage.

Tumble and Yaw

Tumble is when the bullet assumes a different angle once inside the body. This creates more drag inside the body than air. **Yaw,** also known as the wobble of the bullet, is the deviation of the tip of the bullet from the straight axis of flight as it comes out of the barrel. It should come out going straight but spinning. The higher the velocity, the longer it should take for the bullet to yaw. The longer it takes a bullet to yaw after entering tissue, the deeper the maximum injury.

Fragmentation

Fragmentation is when the missile/bullet breaks up to produce multiple parts which causes more drag and energy exchange. There can be fragmentation upon leaving the weapon, such as shotgun pellets, and there can be fragmentation upon entering the body, which can be passive or active. Active fragmentation is when a bullet has an explosive that detonates inside the body, whereas passive fragmentation is when the bullet has a soft nose that contains small fragments that break off on impact. Fragmentation can happen when the bullet hits bone, creating not only bullet fragments but also bony fragments. Figure 70.12 illustrates tumble, yaw, hollow point, and fragmentation.

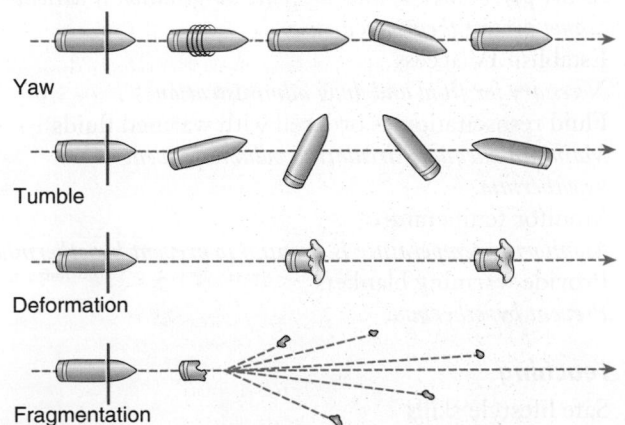

FIGURE 70.12 Yaw, tumble, deformation (hollow-point bullet), fragmentation.

Stabbing

Penetrating injuries caused by low-energy weapons are most often hand-driven such as a knife. Broken glass from a broken window shield in an MVC can cause penetrating trauma if it enters the body. Foreign bodies causing penetrating trauma can produce damage only with their sharp points or edges. Less cavitation occurs with low-energy injuries, and the injury pathway is much easier to determine by tracing the path of the weapon as it entered the body. As with gunshot wounds, stab wounds can have more extensive damage on the inside that is not visible upon external examination. The amount of damage done is based on the potential scope of movement of the inserted object, the length of the object, and the density of the tissue affected. Knowing the position of the patient and the attacker and the type of weapon used can help identify the projected path of injury. A single stab wound can penetrate several body cavities such as thoracic and abdominal cavities.

Connection Check 70.5

A 30-year-old female driver who was in a front-end, high-speed MVC is admitted to the ED. She had a seat belt on, but the car did not have any air bags. There was severe front-end damage with spidering of the windshield in front of the driver's seat and a bent steering wheel. The nurse caring for this patient should anticipate and monitor for which injuries?

A. Sternal/rib, T-spine, pelvic fracture injuries
B. Head, cervical-spine (C-spine), sternal/rib, cardiac contusion, hollow abdominal organ injuries
C. Head, C-spine, solid abdominal organ injuries
D. Sternal/rib, collarbone fracture, pelvic fracture, facial fracture injuries

Complications of Trauma

Hemorrhage

Hemorrhage is a serious and common complication of trauma. It is the leading cause of preventable death after injury if not controlled. Obvious causes of hemorrhage include abdominal or chest trauma injuring organs or vessels. The major sources of abdominal bleeding in blunt trauma are injuries to the spleen or liver. Both organs are very vascular and prone to shearing and lacerations. Chest damage resulting in a massive hemothorax may cause not only blood loss (1,500 mL or one-third or more of the patient's blood in the intrapleural space) but also a tension pneumothorax due to airway compression. Vessel damage, especially damage to arteries, can result in exsanguination if not quickly controlled. Hemorrhage can also occur as a result of fractures (Table 70.3). Pelvic or femur fractures can be a source of major hemorrhage that needs to be controlled by stabilizing the fractures.

Airway Compromise

Airway compromise can occur because of direct damage to the airway, injury to the surrounding tissue, or secondary issues such as a decreased level of consciousness. Direct injury

Table 70.3 Approximate Blood Losses From Fractures	
Bone	**Blood Loss**
Rib fracture	125 mL
Ulna or radius fracture	250–500 mL
Tibia or fibula fracture	500–1,000 mL
Femur fracture	1,500 mL
Pelvic fracture	1–3 L (retroperitoneal hematoma)

due to blunt or penetrating trauma or as a result of smoke inhalation may result in the loss of an effective airway, requiring the insertion of an artificial airway through intubation. Trauma to the surrounding tissue such as facial and neck trauma that results in excessive bleeding or swelling may also result in airway compromise requiring intubation to maintain a patent airway. A decrease in level of consciousness, administration of a sedative or pain medication, hypovolemia, or hypoxemia may result in the patient's inability to protect his or her airway or in an ineffective breathing pattern, again requiring the insertion of an artificial airway.

Additional potential causes of airway compromise are the presence of rib fractures and flat supine patient positioning. Both increase the work of breathing. Patients with rib fractures, especially in the geriatric population, may tire when breathing against rib fractures. Flat supine positioning to ensure C-spine immobilization increases the work of breathing and can also increase the risk of aspiration if vomiting were to occur.

Sepsis

Sepsis is a potential complication in the critically injured trauma patient. The injuries themselves and the invasive interventions necessary to treat the injuries put the patient at risk for infection. The trauma itself is thought to be one cause of the initiation of a systemic inflammatory response. Recognizing the signs and symptoms of sepsis and treating it early can help prevent serious complications and death. See Chapter 14 for more information on shock and sepsis.

Connection Check 70.6

The trauma nurse anticipates which of the following complications when treating an intoxicated homeless patient after he was hit by a car in the snow? The patient is in C-spine immobilization, has an open femur fracture, a pelvic fracture, abdominal tenderness, and a GCS of 12. *(Select all that apply.)*
A. Decreased hemoglobin and hematocrit
B. Decreased SpO$_2$
C. Tension pneumothorax
D. Sepsis
E. Decreased PaCO$_2$

Nursing Management
Assessment and Analysis
The clinical manifestations seen in a trauma patient are dictated by the mechanism of injury and area of the body impacted. Blunt trauma of the chest can result in compression, shearing, deceleration or acceleration injuries. Penetrating trauma to the abdomen can result excessive bleeding especially when a very vascular organ such as the liver is impacted.

Nursing Diagnoses
- **Impaired tissue perfusion**
- **Ineffective breathing patterns**
- **Impaired gas exchange**

Nursing Interventions
■ *Assessment*
- **A**irway
  Assess for possible airway obstruction that would impair ventilation.
- **B**reathing
  Assess for the ineffective breathing patterns that may indicate life-threatening injuries.
- **C**irculation
  Assess pulses, heart rate, skin color, blood pressure, capillary refill, and any obvious signs of bleeding; internal or external that would indicate ineffective perfusion.
- **D**isability
  Assess the GCS to determine the patient's level of consciousness and determine if further evaluation and treatment are necessary.
- **E**xpose
  Completely undress the patient so that obvious and potential injuries, both front and back, can be quickly identified.

■ *Actions*
- Open airway using c-spine precautions
  Assure patent airway
- Provide oxygen
  Optimize oxygenation
- Prepare for an advanced airway
  Assure patent airway and adequate oxygenation if patient cannot protect their own airway.
- Establish IV access
  Necessary for fluid and drug administration
- Fluid resuscitation as ordered with warmed fluids
  Maintain adequate circulating volume/prevent hypothermia.
- Monitor temperature
  Monitoring temperature is essential to prevent hypothermia.
- Provide warming blankets
  Prevent hypothermia.

■ *Teaching*
- Safe lifestyle skills
  Avoid high-risk behaviors and/or potential situations that may result in unintentional injury.

CASE STUDY: EPISODE 2

On arrival to the trauma bay, the patient is sitting up and yelling that he cannot breathe. VSs: HR: 130 bpm; BP: 100/55 mm Hg; RR: 30, SpO$_2$, 98% on 100% NRB. There is a single gunshot wound to the right shoulder and a single gunshot wound to the right upper quadrant of the abdomen, no other wounds. On assessment, there are minimal breath sounds on the right, positive breath sounds on the left. The trachea is midline. The prehospital providers had performed a needle decompression to the right chest to release accumulated air due to a pneumothorax...

POISONING

The definition of a poison is any substance that is harmful to the body when ingested, inhaled, injected, or absorbed through the skin. Too much of any substance can be poisonous. If the person taking or giving a substance did not mean to cause harm, then it is an unintentional poisoning. Unintentional poisonings include the excessive use of drugs or chemicals for recreational purposes. It also includes the accidental exposure to drugs or chemicals for nonrecreational purposes such as a child ingesting cleaning fluid. If the substance is given or taken with the intention of causing harm, then it is an intentional poisoning. Intentional poisoning can be done with the aim to commit a crime or with the goal of committing suicide.

Epidemiology

Poisonings involve people of all ages across all socioeconomic, cultural, and religious boundaries. According to the Centers for Disease Control and Prevention (CDC), a total of 55,403 individuals died of drug-induced causes in the United States in 2015. In 2017, the CDC stated that an estimated 75,000 children (18-years of age and younger) are seen in emergency departments each year because of unintentional medication poisoning. The most common poison exposures are due to analgesics, cleaning substances, cosmetics, foreign bodies, plants, sedative-hypnotics and antipsychotics, and cough and cold preparations. Fatalities most commonly result from the ingestion of analgesics, sedative-hypnotics, antipsychotics, antidepressants, street drugs, cardiovascular medications, or alcohol.

From 2012 through 2014, the number of drug overdose deaths per year increased by 23% (from 38,329 to 47,056 in 2014). According to the 2015 statistics, this number continues to increase substantially. The most commonly used drugs resulting in overdose include ten drugs in three classes: opioids (heroin, oxycodone, methadone, hydrocodone, and fentanyl); benzodiazepines (alprazolam and diazepam); and stimulants (cocaine and methamphetamine). A new public health epidemic emerging in the United States is the number of overdose deaths due to prescription painkillers. The number of overdose deaths from these medications is greater than the deaths from heroin and cocaine combined. This growing trend is resulting in a call to change the way prescribers address patients with pain-related issues. Opium-based prescription pain medication is discussed in detail in Chapter 69.

Pathophysiology and Clinical Manifestations

Common poisoning agents include:

- Salicylates
- Acetaminophen
- Sedatives/hypnotics; barbiturates, benzodiazepines
- Antidepressants
- Cardiovascular medications such as beta blockers
- Alcohol

Salicylates are a class of medications that include aspirin or aspirin-containing compounds such as Pepto-Bismol, Kaopectate, Maalox, and some topical creams. Risk factors for salicylate poisoning include accidental ingestion by young children, chronic exposure seen with adults older than age 70, dehydration, renal disease resulting in decreased renal clearance, and disorders or conditions associated with increased bleeding risk such as alcoholism, ulcers, use of anticoagulants, and concomitant use of other NSAIDs such as ibuprofen.

Acetaminophen toxicity is the result of either intentional or unintentional poisoning. Intentional poisonings are typically suicide attempts. They are seen more often in females 15 to 24 years old or older than 40. If females are older than 40, the effects of acetaminophen toxicity are more likely to be severe. Unintentional poisoning can occur when someone is unfamiliar with the appropriate dosing or unknowingly takes two or more medications that contain acetaminophen at the same time. Also, patients with chronic liver disease are predisposed to acetaminophen toxicity because of the impaired ability of the liver to metabolize the medication. Acetaminophen overdose can result in significant liver damage.

Sedatives-hypnotics: barbiturates and benzodiazepines are central nervous system (CNS) depressants. Most severe sedative-hypnotic poisonings are deliberate or suicidal in nature. Risk factors for toxicity include present or history of alcohol or drug abuse, emphysema, asthma, bronchitis or other chronic lung disease, mental depression, sleep apnea, kidney or liver disease, and elderly age. Antidepressant (tricyclic antidepressant [TCA]) medication toxicity is seen most frequently in the young. Overdose of serotonin reuptake inhibitors (SSRIs) antidepressants is also seen. SSRIs are generally safer than TCAs but in severe cases, serotonin toxicity can be fatal. Toxicity to cardiovascular medications such as beta blockers can be seen in children and adults. With young children, toxicity typically occurs through the accidental exposure to adults' unsecured medications. With adults, toxicity is typically intentional.

Risk factors for alcohol toxicity are many. A small child can get a lethal dose of alcohol by drinking a very small amount. Young people, teenagers, or college students are more likely to binge drink. It occurs more frequently in males, but women are more vulnerable to the effects of alcohol. Small, thin people are also more vulnerable to the effects of alcohol because the body absorbs the alcohol more rapidly. Overall health plays a role. Chronic health conditions make a person more vulnerable to life-threatening symptoms of alcohol toxicity. Conditions such as diabetes may cause a person to experience dangerously low blood sugar levels during and after ingesting alcohol. Finally, the combination of alcohol and medications greatly increases the risk for fatal alcohol overdose. It is important to note that a growing trend in the presentation of alcohol withdrawal in hospitalized patients is occurring. Patients who drink daily, no matter the amount, should be closely monitored for signs and symptoms of acute withdrawal. Table 70.4 outlines the pathophysiology and clinical manifestations of the poisoning agents.

Table 70.4 Pathophysiology and Clinical Manifestations of the Poisoning Agents

Poisoning Agent	Pathophysiology	Clinical Manifestation
Salicylates	Salicylate Toxicity: Acid-base disturbances • Toxicity impairs cellular respiration, stimulating the respiratory centers in the medulla to increase O_2 consumption (hyperventilation) causing respiratory alkalosis. • Salicylate levels greater than 35 mg/dL cause increases in rate and depth of respirations. • Salicylates enter cells and poison mitochondria, causing a metabolic acidosis. Glucose metabolism With the increase in cellular metabolic activity, the patient may develop clinical hypoglycemia; glucose levels may be within normal range, but the intracellular glucose is depleted. Fluid and electrolytes • Dehydration with significant poisoning due to increased gastrointestinal (GI) tract losses (vomiting) and insensible fluid losses (hyperpnea and hyperthermia) • Decreased renal clearance secondary to dehydration Bleeding Impaired blood clotting and platelet dysfunction	• Presentation of toxicity is dependent on dose, acute vs. chronic ingestion, and the patient's age. • Adult patients with acute poisoning usually present with a mixed respiratory alkalosis and metabolic acidosis. Children present with metabolic acidosis. • Early Symptoms (< 30 mg/dL) Nausea, vomiting, diaphoresis and tinnitus, vertigo, hyperventilation, tachycardia, abdominal pain, occasional hematemesis, and hyperactivity • Toxicity Progression (30–70 mg/dL) Agitation, delirium, hallucinations, convulsions, lethargy, and stupor may occur. • Severe Toxicity (> 70 mg/dL) Hyperthermia (especially in young children) Rhabdomyolysis: muscle damage resulting in the release of myoglobin into the bloodstream to be excreted by the kidneys; this eventually causes damage to the kidney, acute renal failure. Respiratory failure may eventually develop.
Acetaminophen	Hepatotoxicity: • *Glutathione* is a naturally occurring antioxidant that is in all the cells of the body, with the highest concentration in the liver. It is critically important in the detoxification and elimination of free radicals. An acute overdose of acetaminophen depletes glutathione (GSH) stores in the liver. Loss of	Acetaminophen poisoning can cause gastroenteritis within hours and hepatotoxicity 1 to 3 days after ingestion. Acute Overdose: • Greater than 150 mg/kg (about 7.5 g in adults) within 24 hours • Phase I: 0–24 Hours: anorexia, nausea, and vomiting, diaphoresis • Phase II: 24–72 Hours: right upper quadrant abdominal pain

Table 70.4 Pathophysiology and Clinical Manifestations of the Poisoning Agents—cont'd

Poisoning Agent	Pathophysiology	Clinical Manifestation
	glutathione causes *N*-acetyl-p-benzoquinone imine (NAPQI), the principal toxic metabolite of acetaminophen, to accumulate and cause hepatocellular necrosis and damage to other organs.	• Phase III: 72–96 Hours: vomiting and symptoms of liver failure, potentially renal failure • Phase IV: 5 Days: resolution of hepatotoxicity or progresses into multisystem organ failure
Sedatives/ hypnotics Benzodiazepines Barbiturates	Sedative-hypnotics are CNS depressants. The main effect is respiratory depression, especially for patients with preexisting pulmonary conditions. which may increase with the ingestion of alcohol or other depressant medications. These medications concentrate in the adipose tissue of the body, taking it longer to be eliminated.	• CNS depression • Slurred speech • Ataxia • Altered (most commonly depressed) mental status • Respiratory depression Severe Overdose – Progression of Symptoms • Stuporous • Comatose • Difficult or slow breathing • Severe nausea or vomiting • Slowed heart rate • Heart failure • Lung failure Skin changes such as ecchymosis or blisters, referred to as barbiturate blisters, are seen with barbiturate, carbon monoxide or benzodiazepines poisoning over pressure areas. The exact mechanism for the development of these blisters is not entirely understood; however, pressure, friction, and local hypoxia have been implicated as causes.

Antidepressants	Tricyclic antidepressants are rapidly absorbed and distributed into tissues. In excessive amounts, they can produce neurotoxicity. Anticholinergic side effects are also seen due to the altered levels of the neurotransmitter acetylcholine at the neuromuscular junction due to inhibition of reuptake or blocking at the receptor sites.
	
	Acetylcholine dilates blood vessels; decreases heart rate; constricts bronchioles; increases the production of mucus in the respiratory tract; produces contractions or cramping of the intestines; stimulates the production of saliva, sweat, and tears; and constricts the pupil of the eye. Anticholinergic side effects therefore are the opposite of acetylcholine.
		Anticholinergic effects:
		
		• "Red as a beet"—Cutaneous vasodilation occurs as a means to dissipate heat (flushed face).
		
		• "Dry as a bone" (anhidrosis)—dry skin
		
		• "Hot as a hare" (anhydrotic hyperthermia)—Interference with normal heat dissipation mechanisms (i.e., sweating) frequently leads to hyperthermia.
		
		• "Blind as a bat" (nonreactive mydriasis)—Anticholinergic medications generally produce pupillary dilation and ineffective accommodation that frequently manifests as blurry vision.
		
		• "Mad as a hatter" (delirium; hallucinations)
		
		• Urinary retention
		
		• Dry mouth and eyes
		
		• Tachycardia
		
		• Delayed gastric empting
		
		• Anti–alpha-adrenergic effects:
		  • Hypotension
		• Cardiac effects:
		  • QTc prolongation
		  • QRS widening
		  • Ventricular tachycardia—torsade des pointes

Continued

Table 70.4   Pathophysiology and Clinical Manifestations of the Poisoning Agents—cont'd

Poisoning Agent	Pathophysiology	Clinical Manifestation

		• Central nervous system:
		  • Restlessness
		  • Delirium and coma
		  • Seizures
		• Noncardiogenic pulmonary edema
		
		SSRI Toxicity: altered mental status, tremors, agitation, fever, diarrhea, coma, hyper or hypotension, or muscle rigidity. Muscle rigidity can lead to rhabdomyolysis which can cause renal failure

Cardiovascular medications Beta blockers	Beta blockers—cardiovascular class of medications that affects the heart by controlling the rate or intensity of cardiac contraction, blood vessel diameter, or blood volume	**Beta Blocker Toxicity:** • Bradycardia • Hypotension (due to decreased cardiac output, which may impair myocardial perfusion) • Arrhythmias • Hypothermia • Hypoglycemia • Seizures • Decreased systemic vascular resistance (SVR) • Cardiogenic shock Symptoms may be seen as early as 20 minutes after ingestion, but it is more common to see them within 1–2 hours.
Alcohol	• Alcohol (ethanol) is absorbed into the blood system and the fluids surrounding various tissues and inside of the cells. The concentration of alcohol in blood and tissue depends on the amount of total body water because alcohol is soluble in water. • The liver metabolizes and eliminates alcohol in the body. • The mean rate of alcohol elimination is 100 mg/kg/hr for a 70-kg person. • Alcohol toxicity occurs when someone drinks so much alcohol that the liver cannot metabolize it fast enough, causing dangerously high blood alcohol levels.	Common symptoms of alcohol intoxication include: • Slurred speech • Euphoria • Impaired balance • Loss of muscle coordination (ataxia) • Flushed face • Vomiting • Red eyes • Reduced inhibition • Erratic behavior

SSRI, Elective serotonin reuptake inhibitor.

Management

Medical Management

Diagnosis and Treatment

Diagnosis and treatment vary depending on the specific medication or substance ingested or exposed to and the levels that remain in the body. Table 70.5 details the diagnostics and treatment for common poisoning agents.

Decontamination

The definition of **decontamination** is the process of removing or neutralizing a substance to decrease absorption. Regardless of the poison, decontamination is the first step in treating the patient. The most common form is gastrointestinal (GI) decontamination (Table 70.6). Other types of decontamination include flushing the exposed body area or eyes with water to remove or neutralize the substance. Once

Table 70.5 Diagnostics and Treatments for Common Poisoning Agents

Agent	Diagnostics	Treatment
Salicylates	<ul><li>Serum salicylate level—greater than 100 mg/dL for acute toxicity or greater than 60 mg/dL with chronic overdose</li><li>Urine pH—excretion of salicylates increases when urine pH increases</li><li>ABGs—to determine acidosis (salicylates more toxic if pH is low)</li><li>Arterial lactate—increases in the face of metabolic acidosis—lactate levels are good prognostic indicators</li><li>Electrolytes—may be abnormal because of excessive vomiting, diarrhea, and insensible fluid losses</li><li>Glucose—increased metabolic activity produces hypoglycemia</li><li>PT/aPTT and CBC—may have alterations because of bleeding and platelet malfunction</li></ul>	**IV Fluids** To correct volume and electrolyte abnormalities **Medications**<ul><li>Activated charcoal (see Table 70.6)—binds residual aspirin in the gastrointestinal tract if bowel sounds present; repeat dose every 4 hours until charcoal appears in the stool</li><li>Sodium bicarbonate to increase urine pH (alkalize urine), causing alkaline diuresis to occur; making the pH of the urine more alkaline increases clearance of an acid-type medication (e.g., salicylates)</li></ul>**Hemodialysis** Indications: coma, renal, hepatic, pulmonary failure, pulmonary edema, severe acid-base disturbances **Evaluation and Ongoing Monitoring**<ul><li>Repeat laboratory tests and salicylate levels until the level peaks</li><li>Monitor urine pH every 2 hours to maintain pH at 7.5–8.5 during alkalization therapy</li><li>Treatment to remove salicylates can result in hypokalemia; therefore potassium must be carefully monitored during treatment.</li></ul>
Acetaminophen	<ul><li>Serum acetaminophen levels to determine severity of toxicity</li><li>Liver function tests (AST—aspartate aminotransferase, *ALT*—alanine aminotransferase, albumin, bilirubin, alkaline phosphatase) to determine extent of injury to the liver</li><li>PT/aPTT—clotting abnormalities may occur as a result of liver damage</li></ul>	**Medications**<ul><li>Activated charcoal (see Table 70.6) to decrease absorption</li><li>*N*-acetylcysteine, an amino acid, is given by mouth or IV to prevent or minimize hepatotoxicity</li></ul>**Evaluation and Ongoing Monitoring**<ul><li>Acetaminophen levels</li><li>Liver function tests</li></ul>
Sedatives/ hypnotics Benzodiazepines Barbiturates	<ul><li>Medication levels</li><li>Serum glucose to rule out hypoglycemia</li><li>Serum and urine drug screen</li><li>ABGs—to assess level of respiratory depression</li></ul>	**Medications**<ul><li>Flumazenil is the antidote for benzodiazepines, but its risk for withdrawal symptoms such as seizures may outweigh its benefits</li><li>Activated charcoal (see Table 70.6)</li></ul>**Hemodialysis** for severe cases **Supportive Care**<ul><li>Rapid airway, breathing, and circulation assessment</li><li>Endotracheal intubation if respiratory depression severe</li><li>Oxygen</li><li>IV access</li><li>Cardiac monitoring</li><li>End tidal CO_2 (i.e., capnography)</li></ul>

Continued

Table 70.5 Diagnostics and Treatments for Common Poisoning Agents—cont'd

Agent	Diagnostics	Treatment
		Evaluation and Ongoing Monitoring • Repeat drug levels • Assess respiratory status, hemodynamic status, and level of consciousness
Antidepressants Tricyclic antidepressant (TCA)	• ECG to assess for cardiac conduction abnormalities (this is particularly important in TCA ingestions) • Serum glucose level to rule out hypoglycemia as the cause of any alteration in mental status • Acetaminophen and salicylate levels to rule out these common co-ingestions	**IV Fluids** Administer IV normal saline fluids for hypotension **Medications** • Activated charcoal (see Table 70.6) should be given continuously for very high drug levels • Administer sodium bicarbonate IV for serum alkalization (goal is pH 7.5) to reduce the cardiotoxic effects (e.g., QRS prolongation 100 milliseconds or greater, myocardial depression) in tricyclic overdoses • Administer benzodiazepines for tricyclic-induced seizures • Administer antiarrhythmic medications for arrhythmias **Supportive Care** • Airway—protect the airway (endotracheal intubation) • Breathing—assist with breathing (supplemental O_2) • Circulation • Continuous cardiac monitoring • IV access **GI Decontamination** Gastric lavage to remove pill fragments regardless of the suspected drug ingestion (TCA delays gastric empting, which allows pill fragments to remain in the stomach for a longer period of time) **Evaluation and Ongoing Monitoring** • Hemodynamic and respiratory status • Continuous monitoring • Foley catheter
Cardiovascular medications Beta blockers	• Serum glucose test—high beta blocker levels may be associated with hypoglycemia • Serum electrolytes—hypokalemia may contribute to cardiac arrhythmias; co-ingestions or concomitant medical conditions may alter other serum electrolytes • Cardiac enzymes to rule out myocardial infarction in any hemodynamically unstable patient • ABGs—managing acid-base balance • CXR to rule out pulmonary edema • ECG—to identify arrhythmias	**Medications** • Activated charcoal (see Table 70.6) to decrease absorption • Glucagon—antidote • D50 if hypoglycemic • Benzodiazepines for seizures if present • Hemodialysis for extremely high levels **Supportive Care** • Initial treatment is primarily supportive and includes fluid resuscitation, which is essential to correct vasodilation and low cardiac filling pressures • Supplemental O_2

Table 70.5 Diagnostics and Treatments for Common Poisoning Agents—cont'd

Agent	Diagnostics	Treatment
		Evaluation and Ongoing Monitoring ● Cardiac monitoring ● Hemodynamic monitoring ● Serum glucose levels
Alcohol	● Alcohol level ● Glucose to test for hypoglycemia	**IV Fluids** ● IV fluids with thiamine to prevent Wernicke-Korsakoff's syndrome—syndrome may cause seizures ● Benzodiazepines for seizures that may occur related to alcohol withdrawal **Evaluation and Ongoing Monitoring** Assess for alcohol withdrawal such as agitation, delirium tremens, confusion, seizures

ABG, Arterial blood gas; *CBC,* complete blood count; *CNS,* central nervous system; *CXR,* chest x-ray; *ECG,* electrocardiogram; *IV,* intravenous; *PT/aPTT,* prothrombin time/activated partial thromboplastin time; *TCA,* tricyclic antidepressant.

Table 70.6 Decontamination

	Practice	Contraindications/Precautions	Comments
Activated charcoal	● Activated charcoal is an emergency decontaminant administered via the gastrointestinal (GI) tract. It works by binding with the ingested/absorbed chemical/drugs to reduce the absorption into the body. ● Patient may drink the charcoal; if vomiting or unconscious, instill charcoal through a NG or OG tube ● Should be initiated as soon as possible (within 60 minutes) after ingestion of the poison	Contraindicated in caustic or corrosive ingestions, decreased or absent bowel sounds, or substances that do not bind with the charcoal, such as heavy metals	May require multiple doses
Cathartic	● Use magnesium sulfate, magnesium citrate, sorbitol ● Mix with charcoal and administer orally, or NG/OG tube	Contraindicated in patients without bowel sounds or patients who have preexisting renal and cardiac failure	● One-time dose ● May be used to enhance elimination of activated charcoal ● May cause vomiting or severe diarrhea
Gastric lavage	● Tap water is instilled and withdrawn from the stomach with an orogastric or nasogastric tube to allow for tablet fragments to be retrieved. ● Lavage until the fluid return appears free of the substance ● After lavage, a second 25-g dose of charcoal can be instilled.	● Potential for aspiration ● Use with caution with ingestion of caustics or corrosives ● Contraindicated in co-ingestion of sharp objects and nontoxic substances **Precautions** Endotracheal intubation should be done before lavage in patients	Consider instilling charcoal 25-g dose through the tube before lavage because lavage sometimes forces substances farther into the GI tract

Continued

Table 70.6 Decontamination—cont'd

	Practice	Contraindications/Precautions	Comments
		with an altered level of consciousness or a weak gag reflex to prevent aspiration.	
Whole bowel irrigation	Nonabsorbable evacuant solution GI tract flushes given at a rate of 1–2 L/hr or 25–40 mL/kg/hr via NG or OG tube for adults in cases of: • Serious poisonings due to sustained-release preparations or substances that are not adsorbed by charcoal (e.g., heavy metals) • Drug packets (e.g., latex-coated packets of heroin or cocaine ingested by body packers) • A suspected bezoar (a mass found trapped in the GI system)	• Precaution in paediatric patients • Contraindicated in patients with known GI disease or at risk for ileus, perforation, or obstruction	May cause nausea, vomiting, abdominal cramping, electrolyte imbalance
Irrigation (ocular)	Irrigation of the eye with copious amounts of water or saline for chemical exposures		• Alkali exposures require longer irrigation of the eye. • Eye pH should return to neutral before discontinuation of irrigation.
Irrigation (dermal exposures)	Remove all contaminated clothing Thoroughly wash the whole body including hair and nails	Wear PPE	

GI, Gastrointestinal; *NG,* nasogastric; *OG,* orogastric; *PPE,* personal protective equipment.

commonly used, syrup of ipecac, is discouraged by poison control centers in out-of-hospital situations.

Nursing Management

Assessment and Analysis

The general appearance and clinical manifestations seen with poisoning are related to the specific substance, type and amount of exposure, and complicating comorbidities. For example, level of consciousness changes manifested as drowsiness, sedation, euphoria, impaired memory and judgment, changes in speech patterns, ataxia, or depression may be present with barbiturates or alcohol poisoning because of CNS depression. Tachypnea, crackles on auscultation, and respiratory distress may be seen with salicylate poisonings because of the body's attempt to compensate for the decrease in cellular respiration and the increased O$_2$ consumption, which causes respiratory alkalosis. Tachycardia and/or hypotension may be present in any type of poisoning that results in excessive vomiting, diarrhea, or blood loss due to bleeding, such as salicylate overdose. It should be evaluated in relation to other presenting symptoms such as a prolonged QTs or cardiac dysrhythmias, which may be seen with overdose of tricyclics and cardiovascular medications.

Nursing Diagnoses

• **Risk for ineffective airway clearance**
• **Ineffective breathing patterns**
• **Impaired gas exchange**
• **Risk for aspiration**

Nursing Interventions

▪ *Assessment*

• Vital signs
  Hypotension and tachycardia may be present in many types of poisonings as a result of volume loss from vomiting and diarrhea; an overdose of beta blockers that affects the heart by controlling the rate or intensity of cardiac contraction, blood vessel diameter, or blood volume may result in hypotension and bradycardia.
• Pulse oximetry
  Many common poisoning agents result in a decreased level of consciousness, potentially resulting in respiratory depression and hypoxia.
• Neurological assessment
  Many types of poisoning cause a decreased level of consciousness, confusion, delirium, or seizures.
• Continuous cardiac monitoring
  Antidepressants and cardiovascular medications such as beta blockers can cause dangerous dysrhythmias and

bradycardia. Alkalization therapy for salicylate poisoning may deplete potassium, increasing the potential for cardiac dysrhythmias.

- Laboratory assessment
  - Toxicology screen - serum and urine
    A tox screen is essential in determining the type and amount of poison in the patient.
  - Arterial blood gases
    Salicylate levels greater than 35 mg/dL cause increases in rate and depth of respirations, resulting in respiratory alkalosis. Salicylates enter cells disrupting mitochondrial function, causing a metabolic acidosis.
  - Potassium
    Alkalization therapy for salicylate poisoning may deplete potassium.
  - Serum glucose
    Hypoglycemia must be ruled out as a cause of decreased level of consciousness; with the increase in cellular metabolic activity with salicylate poisoning, the patient may develop clinical hypoglycemia.
  - Urine pH
    Making the pH of the urine more alkaline increases the clearance of acid-type medications such as salicylates.
  - Complete blood count/Clotting studies
    Salicylate poisoning impairs blood clotting and platelet dysfunction and may result in bleeding.
  - Liver function tests
    Acetaminophen overdoses lead to impaired liver function, resulting in elevated liver enzymes.
  - Repeat urine and serum medication levels
    Necessary to assess level of medication or alcohol in the system and assess adequacy of treatment

■ Actions

- Airway management, including supplemental O$_2$ and preparations for intubation
  Airway compromise may be present because of the decreased level of consciousness.
- Establish IV access
  Necessary to facilitate fluid and medication administration for the treatment of the overdose
- ECG
  To assess for cardiac conduction abnormalities due to poisoning or potassium depletion
- Administer medications as ordered
  - IV fluids with thiamine
    Alcoholics are prone to thiamine depletion, making them susceptible to Wernicke-Korsakoff's syndrome, which may cause seizures.
  - Benzodiazepines
    For tricyclic- or alcohol withdrawal–induced seizures
  - Flumazenil
    Flumazenil is the antidote for benzodiazepine overdose.
  - Sodium bicarbonate
    To increase urine pH (alkalize urine) causing alkaline diuresis, increasing clearance of acid-type medications such as salicylates

- N-acetylcysteine
  An amino acid is given by mouth or IV to prevent or minimize hepatotoxicity with acetaminophen toxicity.
- Activated charcoal
  Decontamination agent that works by binding with the poison, preventing or slowing absorption into the system
- Glucagon
  Administered for beta blocker toxicity; enhances myocardial contractility and heart rate
- Prepare for decontamination through GI, ocular, or dermal irrigation or flushing
  To enhance elimination of the poison, which helps reverse the effects of the overdose

■ *Teaching*

- Careful use of over-the-counter (OTC) medications— read the labels, be aware of maximum daily doses
  Misuse or overuse of OTC medications such as acetaminophen may be dangerous; many OTC products contain aspirin.
- Review early signs of toxicity or overdose with patients/family
  Facilitate early identification and prompt treatment in the event of overdose
- Review dangers of alcohol and/or sedative abuse as well as dangers of abrupt withdrawal
  Alcohol and sedative abuse has serious and long-term consequences. Abrupt withdrawal is life threatening and may result in seizures.
- Precaution in the use of aspirin with children suffering a viral disorder
  Aspirin has been linked with Reye's syndrome in children. Reye's syndrome is a disorder resulting in sometimes fatal neurological and hepatic changes.

Evaluating Care Outcomes

Poisoning may be managed with prompt recognition and treatment. A well-managed patient is discharged with adequate respiratory effort and is hemodynamically stable, understanding the cause and future risk of poisoning. If poisoning was intentional, the patient is discharged to a psychiatric facility for treatment in hopes of preventing further suicide attempts.

Connection Check 70.7

The nurse is caring for a patient coming into the ED unconscious after taking an overdose of an unknown substance approximately 1 hour ago. Which of the following actions should the nurse take first?

A. Initiate gastric lavage

B. Insert two large-bore IVs

C. Assess vital signs with pulse oximetry

D. Insert nasogastric tube

INJURIES RELATED TO THERMOREGULATION

The human body strives to maintain normal body temperature at 98.6°F (37.1°C) regardless of environmental factors. **Thermoregulation** is a physiological response that occurs in the anterior (cooling) and posterior (heating) hypothalamus. The hypothalamus responds to temperature information sent to the brain from peripheral and central thermoreceptors in the skin, limb muscles, and spinal cord.

The body's response to cool environments is to minimize heat loss through cutaneous vasoconstriction, increasing heat production by shivering, mobilization of carbohydrate reserves, and elevation of the basal metabolic rate. Heat is dissipated through **convection** (being exposed to cool air or water), **conduction** (loss of heat to cold object), or **evaporation** (sweating). In response to overheating, the body initiates cutaneous vasodilation to shunt blood to the skin surface, increasing heat loss through convection and conduction. The body also activates the sweat glands causing perspiration, which helps cool the body. Fig. 70.13 illustrates the maintenance of temperature homeostasis. Sweating is the body's primary cooling mechanism, but it may also cause a loss of sodium, potassium, and body fluids. It is important to assess for dehydration and replace fluid and electrolytes.

Hypothermia

Epidemiology

The incidence of hypothermia is increasing in the United States. Between 2003 and 2013, there were greater than 13,400 hypothermia deaths, with annual rates ranging from 0.3 to 0.5 per 100,000 persons. A report from the CDC in 2015, indicated that this statistic may be increasing. The growing trend is a combination of colder more drastic

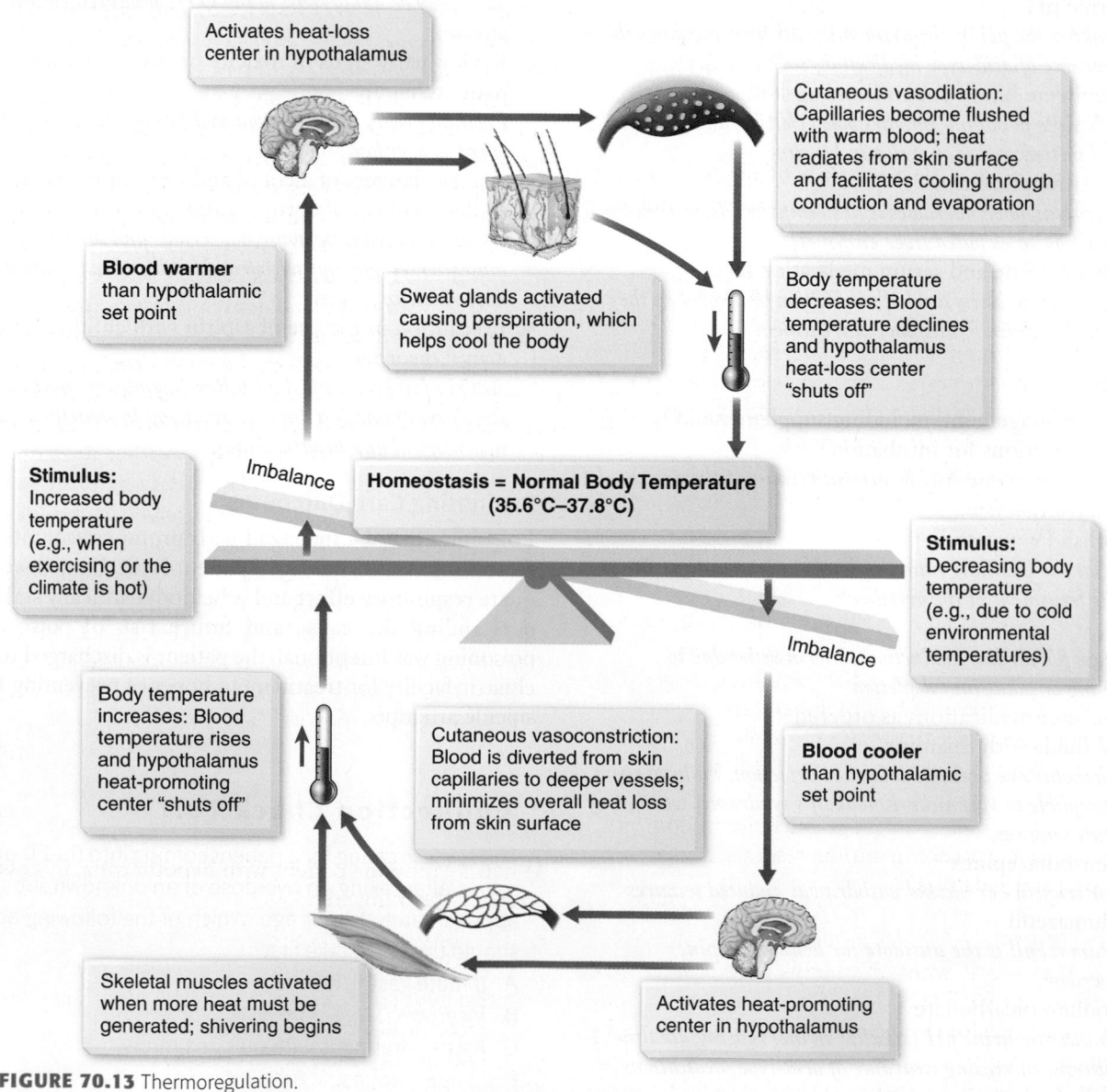

FIGURE 70.13 Thermoregulation.

winters with cold spells and the increasing number of homeless populations. Risk factors for hypothermia include the following:

- In older adults
  - Ability to regulate body temperature and to sense cold may lessen with age.
  - More likely to have medical conditions that will affect temperature regulation
  - May not be able to communicate when they are cold or may not be mobile enough to get to a warm location
- The very young
  - Children lose heat faster than adults because of a larger percentage of body surface area for their weight.
  - Children will lose more heat through the head (largest body surface area in young children).
  - Children may not have the judgment to dress properly in cold weather or to get out of the cold when they should.
  - Infants have less efficient mechanisms for generating heat, putting them at risk for hypothermia.
- Psychiatric problems/Diminished capacity
  - Condition(s) interferes with judgment (i.e., may not dress appropriately for the weather or understand the risk of cold weather)
  - People with dementia may wander from home or get lost easily, making them more likely to be stranded outside in cold or wet weather.
- Alcohol and drug use
  - Alcohol may make your body feel warm inside, but it causes your blood vessels to dilate, or expand, resulting in more rapid heat loss from the surface of your skin.
  - Using alcohol or recreational drugs can affect your judgment about the need to get inside or wear warm clothes in cold weather conditions.
  - If a person is intoxicated and passes out in cold weather, the risk of hypothermia is high.
- Certain medical conditions
  - Some medical conditions affect the body's ability to regulate body temperature such as hypothyroidism, poor nutrition, stroke, severe arthritis, Parkinson's disease, trauma, spinal cord injuries, and burns.
  - Some medical conditions affect sensation in the body's extremities, such as peripheral neuropathy with diabetes, dehydration, or any condition that limits activity or restrains the normal flow of blood.
- Medications
  - Some medications can change the body's ability to regulate, such as certain antidepressants, antipsychotics, and sedatives.

Pathophysiology and Clinical Manifestations

Mild hypothermia is when the body's core temperature drops to 89.6°F to 95°F (32°C to 35°C). The human body tries to compensate for decreases in body temperature by stimulating the sympathetic nervous system to shiver and increase heart rate, blood pressure, respirations, and promote peripheral vasoconstriction. Tachypnea causes a decrease in carbon dioxide (CO_2) levels, resulting in a respiratory alkalosis. Hyperglycemia may be present because of a decrease in glucose use by the cells and a decrease in insulin secretion due to an increase in corticosteroid levels. Cold diuresis develops as a result of peripheral vasoconstriction, hyperglycemia, and decreased renal tubular absorption. Other symptoms, including mild confusion, ataxia, and diminished fine motor movements, may also be present in patients with mild hypothermia because of the shifts in metabolic state.

Moderate hypothermia is when the body's core temperature drops to 82.4°F to 89.6°F (28°C to 32°C). As the body's temperature continues to lower, shivering becomes more violent and eventually stops. There is deterioration in the patient's mental status (agitation, hallucinations) that, if left untreated, progress to coma. Pupils dilate, and movements become less coordinated as a result of CNS depression. Blood shunts away from the skin surface to preserve heat as part of the body's compensatory mechanism. Compensatory mechanisms begin to fail, resulting in bradycardia, hypoventilation, and hypoxemia. Myocardial irritability begins to develop with increasing bradycardia and decrease in spontaneous depolarization of the pacemaker cells. This change in cell excitability increases the risk for dysrhythmias such as atrial fibrillation, ventricular fibrillation, and ventricular tachycardia. The metabolic rate slows and respiratory and lactic acidosis develops. In addition, patients develop hypokalemia because potassium shifts into the cell.

Severe hypothermia is when the body's core temperature is lower than 82.4°F (28°C). At this temperature, the body begins to shut down. When the patient reaches this point, compensatory mechanisms that cause vasoconstriction and shunting of blood away from the skin to vital organs in an effort to retain heat completely fail. There is a massive dilation of vessels moving blood back to the surface of the skin, causing further cooling and also resulting in further deterioration of cardiovascular, respiratory, and neurological functions. Compromised cardiovascular functions include decreased cardiac output, arterial pressure, and basal metabolic rate (20% of basal metabolic rate), resulting in severe cerebral hypoperfusion. Patients become severely hypotensive, myocardial irritability worsens, and muscle rigidity develops. Eventually, the body completely shuts down and the patient dies.

Frostbite is another complication associated with cold weather exposure (see Box 70.6).

Management

Medical Management

Diagnosis

When treating the patient with hypothermia, it is essential to assess the following:

- Mechanism of exposure
  - Ambient temperature
  - Enclosed or open space; was the person in a protected area out in the open
  - Did the exposure include water?
- Time of exposure

Box 70.6 Frostbite

In response to cold temperatures, the vessels in the skin constrict allowing less warm blood to flow to the affected areas causing freezing of the tissues. Hands, feet, and the face are the areas most typically affected. There are four stages or grades of frostbite:

Stage 1: Frostnip
- Superficial skin surface damage
- Initial symptom is numbness with an area of pallor and edema
- Damage is not permanent

Stage 2:
- Clear blisters are evident with hardened skin
- Over time the affected area becomes black, dries, and peels
- There is typically no tissue loss

Stage 3:
- Tissues below the superficial skin layers freeze
- Blood blisters and a blue-grey discoloration appears
- Pain is persistent and blackened eschar develops

Stage 4:
- Tissue damage extends to muscle and bone
- Involves complete tissue necrosis and permanent damage

Treatment
- Prevention is the best treatment
- Move to warm environment, remove wet clothing and place affected tissue in warm water or, if water not available, use body heat for warming—place fingers under the arms. Do not rewarm in the prehospital environment if there is a possibility of refreezing before arriving at the hospital for definitive care. That can exacerbate tissue damage. Avoid walking on frostbitten feet as that can cause more tissue damage.
- Most effective treatment is immersion in warm water. Successful rewarming is evident when the tissue is red and soft to the touch. This process is painful so analgesia may be necessary. More severe frostbite may require thrombolysis due to clot formation in affected tissue. Very severe tissue damage may require amputation.

- Length of time since the incident
- Predisposing factors such as mental status, alcohol, drugs
- Past medical history that may predispose the patient to hypothermia.

Laboratory and diagnostic tests are detailed in Table 70.7.

Treatment

Treatment priorities are the same as for any trauma patient: focus on the ABCs. Ensure an adequate airway and effective ventilation, insert an IV line, and start IV fluids. The specific treatment varies depending on the degree of hypothermia. **Passive external rewarming** can be used for mild hypothermia. **Active external rewarming** is used for mild to moderate hypothermia, and **internal rewarming** is used for moderate to severe hypothermia. See Table 70.8 for a description of rewarming techniques.

Safety Alert Complications in Rewarming the Patient With Hypothermia

- Rewarming the core at a prescribed rate is important to prevent significant complications. Rewarming too rapidly can cause hyperkalemia as potassium shifts out of the cells and a condition known as "afterdrop." Afterdrop is defined as a precipitous reduction in core temperature due to redistribution of body heat to improperly warmed peripheral tissues, with rapid shunting of cold blood from the periphery to the core as the direct result of vasodilation. This causes a bolus of cold, hyperkalemic, acidotic blood to return from the periphery to the heart, which results in a biochemical injury that leads to severe hypotension and dysrhythmias.
- Limit invasive procedures and overall movement of the patient when severely hypothermic because of a greater susceptibility to dysrhythmias.
- If cardiac arrest is suspected:
  - Hypotension and bradycardia are expected when core temperature is low. The patient may appear pulseless and lifeless. A longer than usual attempt should be made to determine pulselessness; 45 to 60 seconds. If there is no pulse, cardiopulmonary resuscitation should be initiated. Resuscitation medications and defibrillation are not effective until the patient's temperature is above 86°F (30°C). Defibrillation should be attempted one time, but if ineffective, further attempts are deferred until temperature reaches higher than 86°F (30°C). Advanced cardiac life-support medications such as antiarrhythmics, vasopressors, and inotropes are ineffective at low body temperatures so are usually not given. Conversely, very mild hypothermia is recommended after cardiac arrest to slow the metabolic rate and decrease cerebral injury (see Evidence-Based Practice: Therapeutic Hypothermia).

Evidence-Based Practice

Therapeutic Hypothermia

In 2015, the American Heart Association recommended therapeutic hypothermia, targeted temperature management between 89.6°F (32°C) and 96.8°F (36°C), for patients who have had a return of spontaneous circulation (ROSC) after cardiac arrest but are still demonstrating a decreased level of consciousness. Reducing body temperature will reduce cerebral metabolic rate, reducing the risk of anoxic brain injury. Hypothermia induction may begin as soon as the patient has ROSC and should continue for at least 24 hours.

Neumar, R. W., Shuster, M., Callaway, C. W., Gent, L. M., Atkins, D. L., Bhanji, F.,. . .Hazinski, M. F. (2015). Part 1: Executive summary 2015 American Heart Association guidelines update for cardiopulmonary resuscitation and emergency cardiovascular care. *Circulation*, *132*(18 Suppl. 2), S315–S367.

Table 70.7 Laboratory and Diagnostic Tests

Laboratory Test	Rationale
Arterial blood gas	Assess for metabolic acidosis, respiratory alkalosis, or both
Electrolytes	Abnormalities in blood chemistries may indicate the degree of hypothermia and necessary treatment
Glucose	Depending on the level of hypothermia, may see an increase or decrease in blood glucose
CBC Hemoglobin, hematocrit	Cold diuresis and subsequent loss of fluid causes hemoconcentration of the blood
Coagulation studies (PT/aPTT)	Hypothermia inhibits the coagulation cascade
Other diagnostics	
ECG	Hypothermia causes heart to become irritable, resulting in changes to ECG, changes to electrical conduction
Chest radiograph	Assess for aspiration pneumonia, vascular congestion, pulmonary edema
Head CT	Rule out significant injury causing changes in LOC different from hypothermia
Serum and urine toxicology	Rule out drugs or alcohol involvement
Pregnancy test	Should be completed on women of childbearing years to determine pregnancy status

CBC, Complete blood cell count; *CT,* computed tomography; *ECG,* electrocardiogram; *LOC,* level of consciousness; *PT/aPTT,* partial thromboplastin time/activated partial thromboplastin time.

Table 70.8 Rewarming Strategies

Category	Strategies
Passive external rewarming	Used for mild hypothermia and focuses on preventing further heat loss: Move to a warmer environment Remove all wet clothing and dry the patient Cover the patient with warmed blankets and wrap the head to prevent heat loss
Active external rewarming	Used for mild to moderate hypothermia: External heat sources such as heat lamps and forced warm air blankets
Active internal rewarming	Used for moderate to severe hypothermia: <u>Least invasive</u> Warmed humidified O_2—increases core temperature and reduces heat loss due to evaporation Warmed IV fluids O_2 and fluids should be warmed to 40°C–42°C <u>More invasive rewarming methods</u> Peritoneal, bladder, and thoracic lavage with warmed fluids Open thoracotomy (surgical opening into thorax) followed by thoracic lavage and cardiac massage in cardiopulmonary arrest. Cardiopulmonary bypass or extracorporeal membrane oxygenation (ECMO)—blood is circulated extracorporeally (outside of the body), oxygenated, warmed and returned to the body; allows the heart to warm and provides adequate cardiac output. This is the preferred method of rewarming for the cardiac arrest patient because it reduces the risk of intractable cardiorespiratory failure while providing adequate circulation and oxygenation

Nursing Management

Assessment and Analysis

The clinical manifestations are directly related to the severity of the hypothermia. Shivering is the body's first compensatory mechanism in an attempt to raise the body's temperature. Muscle groups around the vital organs begin to shake in small movements in an attempt to create warmth by expending energy. Other compensatory mechanisms are activated as core body temperature decreases, such as vasoconstriction to shunt blood away from the skin to vital organs. As compensatory mechanisms fail, massive vasodilation occurs, resulting in profound changes in neurological, respiratory, and cardiovascular status.

Nursing Diagnoses

- **Ineffective airway clearance**
- **Impaired gas exchange**
- **Deficient fluid volume**
- **Hypothermia**
- **Impaired skin integrity**

Nursing Interventions

■ Assessment

- Vital signs including temperature (rectal temperature or automatic continuous temperature probe should be used) and pulse oximetry
  Initial temperature to determine degree of hypothermia, then ongoing vital sign monitoring to assess effectiveness of treatment. Initial vital signs reflect tachycardia and hypertension resulting from stimulation of the sympathetic nervous system in an attempt to compensate for the hypothermia. Hypotension and bradycardia may eventually occur because of massive dilation.
- Neurological status
  Profound hypothermia produces a deterioration in neurological status.
- Laboratory values
  - Arterial blood gases
    Blood gases may reflect a metabolic acidosis secondary to decreased flow and shunting and/or respiratory alkalosis due to tachypnea.
  - Potassium
    Hypokalemia occurs initially because of cellular shifts. Later during rewarming, hyperkalemia may occur.
  - Glucose
    Monitor glucose because of the risk for hyperglycemia and hypoglycemia.

■ Actions

- Administer O_2; prepare to intubate with severe respiratory depression
  Airway compromise may be present because of a decreased level of consciousness.
- Continuous cardiac monitoring
  Myocardial irritability develops with a decrease in spontaneous depolarization of the pacemaker cells. This change in cell excitability increases the risk for dysrhythmias such as atrial fibrillation, ventricular fibrillation, and ventricular tachycardia.

- Establish IV access
  Necessary for administration of warm fluids and medications
- Prepare for appropriate rewarming technique
  - Remove from cold environment
  - Remove wet clothing
  - Dry patient
  - Warm blankets
  - Heat lamp
  - Warmed IV fluids
  - Peritoneal, bladder, and thoracic lavage with warmed fluids
  - Cardiopulmonary bypass/extracorporeal membrane oxygenation (ECMO)
    Warming techniques increase in complexity and invasiveness as hypothermia worsens.

■ Teaching

- Signs and symptoms of early hypothermia
  With knowledge, the patient may be able to avoid more severe or profound hypothermia.
- The risk of overindulgence in alcohol or recreational drugs and hypothermia
  Alcohol may make a person's body feel warm inside, but it causes blood vessels to dilate, resulting in more rapid heat loss from the surface of the skin. Using alcohol or recreational drugs can affect judgment about the need to get inside or wear warm clothes in cold weather conditions. If a person is intoxicated and passes out in cold weather, the risk of hypothermia is high.

Evaluating Care Outcomes

Managing a patient with hypothermia varies according to the degree of hypothermia. Successful treatment requires prompt assessment, continuous monitoring, and careful rewarming. A well-managed patient is discharged with a normal temperature, dysrhythmia free, and an understanding of how to avoid future occurrences.

Connection Check 70.8

The nurse should monitor for which clinical manifestations in the patient diagnosed with mild hypothermia? *(Select all that apply.)*

A. Ataxia
B. Shivering
C. Cardiac dysrhythmias
D. Oliguria
E. Hypoglycemia

Hyperthermia

Epidemiology

Hyperthermia is considered a body temperature of more than 103°F (39.4°C) and occurs when the body produces or absorbs more heat than it can dissipate. Hyperthermia is a medical emergency and requires immediate treatment to prevent disability or death. Data from a 2009/2010 Nationwide

Emergency Department sample demonstrated there were approximately 4,100 ED visits each year associated with heat stroke and heat-related illnesses. Heatstroke and deaths from excessive heat exposure are more common during summers with prolonged heat waves. Morbidity and mortality from heatstroke are associated with the duration of the temperature elevation. Delayed therapy is associated with a higher mortality rate of 80% from heatstroke. Mortality is highest among the elderly population, patients with preexisting disease, those confined to a bed, and those who are socially isolated.

Risk factors for hyperthermia include:

- Very young, less than 5 years of age
  - Produce proportionally more metabolic heat
  - Core body temperature rises faster in response to dehydration
  - Smaller organ system that is not as efficient in dissipating heat
- Older adults, older than 65 years of age
  - More commonly have a chronic illness that interferes with normal thermoregulation such as chronic lung or heart disease
  - More likely to be taking medication that alters the body's response to heat:
    - Phenothiazines, which depress the hypothalamus (temperature regulation center in the body)
    - Anticholinergic medications, which inhibit sweating
    - Diuretics, which cause or exacerbate dehydration
    - TCAs and amphetamines, which stimulate the hypothalamus and increase muscle activity
    - Beta blockers or calcium channel blockers, which decrease the body's cardiovascular response to heat
- Patients with an illness that causes a fever
- Patients that have diabetes, peripheral vascular disease, or uncontrolled hypertension
- Patients who have taken drugs or alcohol
- Athletes exercising strenuously in hot climates
- Obese people who generate more heat during activity and dissipate heat more slowly

Pathophysiology and Clinical Manifestations

The hypothalamus in the brain helps the body maintain a normal temperature by balancing heat production and heat loss. During hot weather or in a hot environment, the body works to regulate its internal temperature by producing sweat, which cools the body as it evaporates. A humid environment reduces evaporation of sweat and decreases cooling. When the sweat does not evaporate effectively, or the person is not sweating at all, there is likelihood for a heat-related illness. **Heat cramps** are painful, involuntary muscle spasms of the arms, legs, or abdomen that occur because of sweating profusely during strenuous activity. It is postulated that the loss of sodium, magnesium, or calcium is responsible for the muscle cramps. The cramps generally last 1 to 3 minutes. The muscles are tender and hard, and the patient may have some involuntary twitching. The skin is moist and cool. Generally, the patient's vital signs are within normal limits, and the temperature is either normal

or slightly elevated. **Heat edema** occurs when exposure to a hot environment causes swelling of the feet, ankles, and hands. **Heat stress** occurs when your body can no longer regulate your temperature and you become too hot.

Heat syncope occurs when standing still for an extended period or when moving too quickly from sitting to standing while in the heat. This occurs in response to a sudden drop in perfusion to the brain as the body tries to cool itself by diverting blood flow to the skin through peripheral dilation. As a result of peripheral dilation and gravity, blood pools in the legs and the blood pressure drops. As a response to the pooling in the lower extremities, the patient experiences dizziness, vertigo, tunnel vision, weakness, and nausea before finally losing consciousness.

Heat exhaustion occurs when a person performs strenuous activity in a hot environment for an extended time without drinking enough fluid to replace sodium and water lost from profuse sweating. Symptoms include fatigue, weakness, dizziness, headache, nausea, vomiting, and muscle cramps. A patient with heat exhaustion may have some confusion but does not have significant neurological impairment. Patients may also be tachycardic, hypotensive, and tachypneic. The patient's temperature is usually higher than 100.4°F (38°C) and lower than 104°F (40°C).

Heat stroke is a medical emergency. The body's thermoregulatory mechanism has failed, and the body temperature rises uncontrollably. Immediate intervention is necessary to prevent organ damage and death. Classic heatstroke develops over several days during a heat wave and typically affects elderly, sedentary people with preexisting conditions. Patients usually present with red, dry skin; the patient has stopped sweating altogether. However, moist skin does not rule out the presence of heatstroke. Exertional heatstroke generally occurs in younger healthy people who are participating in strenuous physical activity. They have signs and symptoms of heat exhaustion but also have CNS dysfunction, which may appear as confusion, irrational behavior, delirium, seizures, or coma. Core temperature is greater than 104°F (40°C) in heatstroke. Without immediate intervention, pulmonary edema, dysrhythmias, and **rhabdomyolysis**, a condition in which skeletal muscle cells break down, releasing oxygen-carrying myoglobin potentially precipitating renal failure, may occur. Eventually, hypovolemic and cardiogenic shock and multiorgan failure occur.

Management
Medical Management

Treatment is dependent upon the category of heat-related illness. It is vital to reduce the patient's core temperature as quickly as possible to decrease the probability of serious complications. All interventions start with removal to a cooler environment and hydration. Heat stress or heat edema may require nothing more than removing to a cooler environment. The patient with heat syncope requires safety maneuvers to help prevent injury from falling. After being gently helped to the floor, the patient should be placed in the recovery position until full recovery of consciousness.

Heat cramping requires rehydration with oral fluids containing electrolytes to correct the fluid and electrolyte loss.

Cooling interventions for the patient with heat exhaustion include moving the patient to a cool environment, having the patient lie down and elevate his or her feet, removal of extra clothing, and encouraging the patient to drink cool, nonalcoholic beverages. For this purpose, sports drinks, water, and fruit juices are best. Additional cooling interventions include the application of a cool cloth or towel to the skin or encouraging the individual to shower, bathe, or sponge off with cool water. In the hospital, cooling blankets, ice packs, or fans are interventions utilized to cool the patients. Fluid replacement with IV 0.9% normal saline solutions may be necessary if vital signs are abnormal or the patient is unable to tolerate oral fluid replacement. Patients should rest for at least 24 hours before resuming normal activity.

Immediate emergency intervention is required if the victim is exhibiting signs of heatstroke. Reducing the patient's temperature (to approximately 102.2°F [39°C]) is the number one priority because the duration of elevated temperature is the primary determinant of outcome. Particular attention to airway, breathing, and circulation is essential in resuscitating the patient adequately. The heatstroke patient requires intensive hemodynamic monitoring as well as monitoring a continuous core temperature. This patient also requires administration of IV fluids. Avoid aggressive fluid resuscitation in these patients because it puts the patient at risk for pulmonary edema due to fluid overload. A Foley catheter is essential for accurate measurement of intake and output. Cooling methods include ice packs to the axilla and groin, cooling blankets or fans, and submersion in tepid water if the patient's condition allows. Along with immediate active cooling, take the necessary steps to stop excessive heat production. Treat agitation and shivering with benzodiazepines.

Nursing Management
Assessment and Analysis
The clinical manifestations of hyperthermia are consistent with the degree of increased temperature. Patients with early stage or mild hyperthermia such as heat stress or heat syncope sweat profusely. Patients with heat exhaustion manifest some mild symptoms of CNS dysfunction such as confusion, but patients with heat stroke manifest severe symptoms of CNS dysfunction such as delirium and seizures. Severe heatstroke results in dysrhythmias and cardiac and/or respiratory failure.

Nursing Diagnoses
- **Ineffective airway clearance**
- **Impaired gas exchange**
- **Deficient fluid volume**

Nursing Interventions
Assessment
- Vital signs with temperature
  Continual monitoring of temperature is essential to determine the severity of hyperthermia and effectiveness of the

  intervention. Hypotension and tachycardia may be present because of fluid loss.
- Neurological status
  Signs of CNS dysfunction such as confusion occur with heatstroke.
- Skin assessment
  Patients sweat profusely during early stages of hyperthermia; the skin becomes flushed and dry in later stages.

Actions
- Move the patient into a cool environment
  Removing the patient from the heat source reduces the impact of radiant heat.
- Encourage intake of oral fluids such as cool nonalcoholic beverages, fruit juices, or sports drinks
  Replaces circulating volume
- Administer IV fluids as necessary
  Replace circulating volume when fluid by mouth is not adequate or possible because of CNS dysfunction
- Active cooling methods
  - Sponge bath
  - Ice packs in the axilla/groin
  - Cooling blanket/fans
  - Submerge in tepid water if condition allows
    Reduce body temperature through convection and conduction

Teaching
- Avoid hyperthermia
  - Avoid excessive activity in high-heat environments
  - Drink plenty of fluids in the heat and while exercising
  - Know the signs and symptoms of hyperthermia
    Prevention of hyperthermia is safer than treating hyperthermia.

Evaluating Care Outcomes
The best treatment of hyperthermia is prevention. Evaluating heat risk in the environment, modulating activity as necessary in a hot environment, and drinking plenty of fluids are first steps at prevention. A well-managed patient is discharged alert and oriented, safe from injury or falls, and hemodynamically stable with a normal temperature and an understanding of how to avoid future occurrences of hyperthermia.

Connection Check 70.9

The nurse is caring for patient who came into the ED with a temperature of 105°F (40.6°C). This patient was found at home in an apartment without air conditioning; the current heat wave has temperatures higher than 100°F (37.8°C) for the last 3 days. Which of the following actions should the nurse plan to take first?

A. Apply cooling blankets
B. Obtain laboratory specimens
C. Establish IV access
D. Administer Tylenol

SNAKEBITES

Epidemiology

Snakebites are a significant problem worldwide. They account for approximately 125,000 deaths per year worldwide, although they are less common in the United States than in other parts of the world. In the United States, approximately 5,000 snakebites per year are reported to the American Association of Poison Control Centers, with a fatality rate of reported cases of 0.06%. These deaths are often in the age extremes—children and elderly—and in those who do not receive **antivenin** or its administration is delayed. Reporting snakebites is not mandatory, so many snakebites may go unreported, and not everyone seeks treatment for snakebites. About 25% of bites are believed to be dry bites, bites in which there is no envenomation, the injection of venom into the victim.

The largest group of venomous snakes in North America is the Viperid subfamily Crotalinae, also known as pit vipers. This has three genera with more than 30 species of rattlesnakes, water moccasins/cottonmouths, and copperheads. This group of snakes causes 95% of the snakebites in the United States, followed by coral snakes and a small number of imported exotic snakes.

Snakebites tend to occur during the warmer months (April through October) when snakes are more active. The peak months are July and August, when more people are outside and active as well. Warmer, more southern states such as Georgia, Louisiana, North Carolina, Florida, Texas, California, and Arizona have the largest number of reported snakebites.

Snakes are often found in tall grass and leaf piles, lying under logs or rocks, in rock/log piles, or basking on warm rocks. When snakes are surprised, they may bite. The majority (98%) of snakebites are on the extremities. Of the extremities bitten, most bites occur on the hands or arms. These are bites associated with attempting to handle or kill the snake. Even a dead snake is dangerous. The bite reflex in a recently killed snake remains intact even if the snake has been decapitated. Of those who have been bitten by a snake in the United States, about 77% are male and 70% are adults older than 20 years old.

Pathophysiology and Clinical Manifestations

When a venomous snake bites and injects venom through its fangs, the process is called **envenomation**. **Venom** differs from species to species but is typically a complex mixture of enzymes and proteins designed to immobilize and digest prey. Immobilization occurs because of the **neurotoxic** properties of venom, blocking the transmission of acetylcholine at the neuromuscular junction, causing weakness or paralysis. Venom can also be **hemotoxic**, causing the destruction of red blood cells. The venom of Crotalinae results in increased capillary permeability allowing the shift of fluid, red blood cells, and albumin into the site of envenomation. These are local effects that are seen at the site of injury. Clinical manifestations include local swelling and ecchymosis. At the site of the bite, fang marks, teeth marks, and/or scratches are visible (Fig. 70.14). With envenomation, there is edema and erythema at the site and the surrounding tissues, which occurs usually within 30 to 60 minutes. Ecchymosis may appear around the bite site within 3 to 6 hours in moderate or severe envenomation. Within 8 hours, serous and/or hemorrhagic bullae usually appear at the bite site. The edema is usually limited to dermal and subcutaneous tissues. Rarely, severe envenomation may cause compartment syndrome, substantial amounts of serous fluid within the subcutaneous tissue causing compression of the muscle, nerves, and blood vessels. With rattlesnake bites, necrosis (or cell/tissue death) around the bite site is common. The necrosis is caused by the enzymes/toxins within the rattlesnake venom that cause hemolysis and the decreased perfusion to the involved tissue due to the increase in capillary membrane permeability. Most soft tissue venom effects peak within 2 to 4 days.

There are systemic effects that occur while the venom is circulated through the vascular system. Systemic effects include damage at the cellular level, weakening vascular walls, causing muscle breakdown, and initiating the coagulation cascade. This results in excessive clotting abnormalities similar to disseminated intravascular coagulation (DIC) discussed in Chapter 14. The toxic systemic effects can be seen in the lungs, kidneys, myocardium, peritoneum, and CNS. In severe Crotalinae bites, specifically rattlesnake, it is common to see significant thrombocytopenia (greatly decreased platelet count). The thrombocytopenia may be asymptomatic

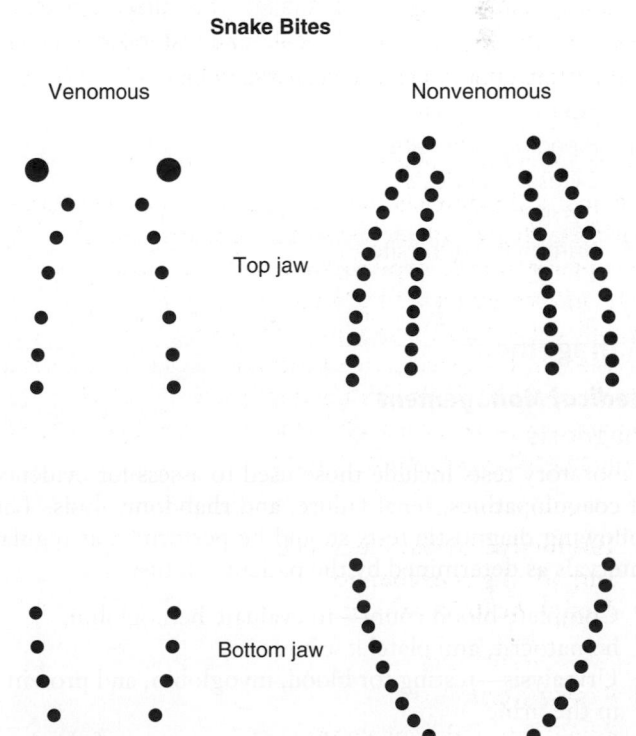

FIGURE 70.14 Bite mark differences between venomous and nonvenomous snakes.

or symptomatic with spontaneous bleeding. Other coagulopathies may occur leading to a DIC-like syndrome causing more bleeding. Most often, patients hemorrhage from the bite site, mucous membranes, and venipuncture sites. They may develop epistaxis (bloody nose), hematemesis (bloody emesis), hematuria (blood in urine), gingival bleeding, or hematochezia (blood in stool). Later, hypovolemia occurs while blood loss continues, and fluids pool in the microcirculation as a result of the increased capillary permeability. Severe hypotension, rhabdomyolysis, hemolysis, nephrotoxic venom effects, or DIC-like syndrome may cause renal failure in severe envenomation snakebites. Decreasing circulating blood volume contributes to cardiac failure. The end result is shock, lactic acidosis and, in severe cases, multisystem organ failure.

Clinical manifestations from coral snake bites differ in several significant ways. Coral snakes leave smaller wounds due to having shorter fangs and smaller mouths. Coral snake envenomation may resemble dry bites as a result of minimal swelling and pain. Neurological manifestations of the neurotoxic effects may be delayed for 12 hours. These symptoms are often cranial-nerve palsies that cause ptosis, dysphagia, diplopia, dyspnea, dysarthria, blurred vision, and respiratory paralysis. Other symptoms may include increased salivation, weakness, lethargy, drowsiness, euphoria, and tremors. These bites may eventually result in respiratory failure secondary to systemic neuromuscular blockade.

Connection Check 70.10

The nurse is caring for a patient bitten by a rattlesnake 3 hours before admission to the ED. The nurse correlates which of the following clinical manifestations with a venomous snakebite? *(Select all that apply.)*

A. Edema at the site
B. Bleeding at the site
C. Excessive diuresis
D. Dysrhythmias
E. Numbness at the site

Management

Medical Management

Diagnosis

Laboratory tests include those used to assess for evidence of coagulopathies, renal failure, and rhabdomyolysis. The following diagnostic tests should be performed at regular intervals as determined by the patient's status:

- Complete blood count—to evaluate hemoglobin, hematocrit, and platelet values
- Urinalysis—testing for blood, myoglobin, and protein in the urine
- Coagulation studies—evaluate the presence of clotting abnormalities and DIC

- Renal studies—elevated blood urea nitrogen (BUN) and creatinine indicate renal failure
- Electrolytes—potassium may be elevated in renal failure
- Serum creatine kinase (CK)—increases because of muscle breakdown; will be elevated in rhabdomyolysis

Diagnostic studies for a coral snake envenomation are aimed toward detection of respiratory failure and may include blood gas measurement, capnography, pulmonary function testing, and continuous pulse oximetry.

Treatment

Medical treatment is dependent on the type of snake involved. Medical treatment for a Crotalinae bite is based on the symptoms and the severity of envenomation. Patients who do not show immediate signs of envenomation should be observed for 12 hours. If the patient does not develop any local or systemic signs after 12 hours, discharge home is indicated.

For severe envenomation, antivenin administration is the recommended treatment. Prior to administration, consultation with a medical toxicologist through the poison control center should be performed. The antivenin provided to patients with severe Crotalinae envenomation is called Crotalidae Polyvalent Immune Fab (Ovine) (FabAV). When FabAV is infused to a patient with a Crotalinae bite, the Fab fragments bind the venom in the intravascular space to allow excretion through the kidneys. Antivenin is most effective when given within 4 to 6 hours after envenomation. The tissue swelling and ecchymosis around the bite site should be evaluated to determine the appropriate dose. The adequacy of the dose is based on improvement of vital signs—a decrease in tachycardia and tachypnea and an increase in blood pressure, partial or complete reversal of the coagulopathies, and improvement of systemic findings such as diarrhea, vomiting, pain, altered mental status, or oral paresthesias.

The patient should be closely monitored while receiving antivenin because reactions may occur. If the patient experiences signs of acute hypersensitivity, the antivenin infusion should be stopped immediately. Epinephrine (1:1,000 [1 mg/mL] 0.3 to 0.5 mg intramuscularly), diphenhydramine, inhaled albuterol, and IV corticosteroids should be available to treat the anaphylactic reaction. The antivenin may be restarted at a lower infusion rate after the acute hypersensitivity has been treated. This patient should be continually monitored in an intensive care setting over 24 hours after the antivenin administration to observe for signs of immediate or recurrent toxicity. For coagulopathies, do not transfuse platelets or fresh frozen plasma (FFP) because the Crotalinae venom inactivates them. The only time a patient with a Crotalinae bite should receive platelets or FFP is when there is significant bleeding uncontrolled by high-dose antivenin administration.

A bite from a coral snake involves serial detailed neurological examinations for at least 12 hours. If the patient has clinical evidence for ventilatory failure, then prompt endotracheal intubation is warranted. Antivenin specific for coral snake is again the recommended treatment. This antivenin is not as readily available, so consultation with a medical toxicologist or poison control center may be necessary to locate available antivenin or for advice regarding alternative clinical treatment. The poison control number should be readily available.

Do not apply a tourniquet, ice, or alcohol to the affected extremity. Previously, these treatments were recommended, but they have been found to have minimal effect. Additionally, the tourniquet can damage tissue, blood vessels, nerves, and tendons. The wound care is the same for all snakes. The wound should be cleansed, and the patient should receive tetanus prophylaxis if the immunization is outdated or unknown. It is not recommended to provide antibiotics for snakebites unless the wound is heavily contaminated.

Nursing Management

Assessment and Analysis

A Crotalinae bite with envenomation produces swelling, pain, blistering, and ecchymosis due to proteins in venom breaking down muscle and blood vessels and triggering the clotting cascade. Later clinical manifestations include signs of ventilatory decompensation, rhabdomyolysis, compartment syndrome, and signs of coagulopathies such as bleeding from the wound, IV sites, and mucous membranes. The clinical manifestations associated with a coral snake bite are due to the neurotoxic effects of the venom. Muscular weakness, ptosis, and dysphagia are common signs. Later manifestations include respiratory failure.

Nursing Diagnoses
- **Impaired gas exchange**
- **Deficient fluid volume**
- **Impaired mobility**

Nursing Interventions

▪ Assessments
- Vital signs
  Tachycardia, hypotension, and tachypnea may be present because of fluid volume loss due to bleeding and increased capillary permeability causing leakage into the tissues. Worsening vital signs indicate either worsening of systemic reaction (before antivenin), anaphylaxis reaction to antivenin, or needing a higher dose of antivenin. The adequacy of the antivenin dose is also based on improvement of vital signs.
- Pulse oximetry
  Decreased O_2 saturation and increases in respiratory distress may indicate a venomous coral snake bite.
- Skin assessment
  A venomous bite produces edema, bleeding, ecchymosis, and pain at the site; a venomous coral snake does not produce significant inflammation in the localized tissue.
- Laboratory assessment
  - Renal studies
    Blood urea nitrogen and creatinine are elevated in renal failure which is a risk with rhabdomyolysis.
  - Coagulation studies
    Coagulation studies will be prolonged.
- Urinalysis
  Urinalysis reveals myoglobin, indicating the presence of rhabdomyolysis.
- Electrolytes, specifically potassium
  Potassium may become elevated with decreased renal function.

▪ Actions
- Continuous cardiac monitoring
  Dysrhythmias may be present with elevated potassium in renal failure.
- Administer IV fluids as ordered
  IV fluids help maintain intravascular volume, preventing hypotension. The treatment of rhabdomyolysis involves administration of large volumes of IV fluids to flush the kidneys and maintain urine output.
- Administer antivenin as ordered
  Antivenin is the recommended treatment to counteract the neurotoxic and hemotoxic effects of venom.
- Keep affected extremity immobilized in a functional position below the level of the heart
  Reduces blood flow to the heart and the spread of the venom
- Remove tight clothing and jewelry from affected extremity
  These objects could act as a tourniquet if swelling is present
- Keep patient calm
  Enables identification of symptoms as related to the snakebite and not the autonomic manifestations of nausea, vomiting, tachycardia, diaphoresis, and diarrhea caused by the terror of a snake bite

▪ Teaching
- Discharge instructions: return to the ED immediately if they develop swelling, redness, increase in pain, epistaxis, fever, dark or bloody urine, shortness of breath, vomiting, diaphoresis, any change in mental status, or any other symptoms besides mild pain at the site.
  These signs may indicate inadequate treatment with antivenin, requiring repeated dosing.
- Avoid handling snakes, including dead snakes. When possible, avoid tall grass, piles of wood, piles of rock, and other snake hiding places. While outdoors in the warmer months when snakes are most active, people should wear long pants and thick or leather boots and be aware of where they are placing their feet and hands at all times.
  Snakebite prevention: snakes have bite reflex even after death.

Evaluating Care Outcomes

Careful, ongoing assessment, prompt treatment with antivenin, and IV fluids as dictated by patient presentation are necessary for successful management of a snakebite. A well-managed patient remains calm and is discharged with stable vital signs and the knowledge of when to return to the hospital if conditions change.

SPIDER BITES

Epidemiology

There are no national or international registries for spider bites, nor is there mandatory reporting; therefore, global epidemiological information is somewhat difficult to obtain. However, according to the data collected by the American Association of Poison Control Centers, almost half of all spider bites within the United States are reportedly caused by black widow or brown recluse spiders, each causing nearly 2,500 envenomations each year. These data are based mostly on self-report and are not 100% reliable because these bites are often misdiagnosed. Ulcerating or necrotic wounds, which are assumed to be a result of a spider bite, can be caused by a myriad of other insect-induced, infectious, or physical sources.

Pathophysiology and Clinical Manifestations

Most spider bites are not dangerous to humans and produce only mild, local erythema. However, there are a few species of spiders in the United States that are known to produce more serious reactions, namely the brown recluse (*Loxosceles*), the black widow (*Latrodectus*), and the hobo spider (*Tegenaria agrestis*). These spiders have been associated with significant disease and have been known to cause death, though rarely and more commonly in small children or the elderly.

The brown recluse spider (*Loxosceles*) is found mostly in the southwestern United States and is known for its characteristic violin pattern on its back. Brown recluse spider venom contains multiple enzymes that make it hemotoxic. Its bite sometimes progresses to extensive local necrosis but rarely to hemolytic reactions. The exact mechanism of this reaction has not been conclusively determined. The typical course progresses from an initially painless bite to painful blistering that occurs within 2 to 8 hours of the bite and then progresses to more serious ulceration within 72 hours. Approximately 20% of the time, necrosis eventually forms. The bite then slowly heals over the course of several weeks to months. **Systemic loxoscelism**; arthralgias, fever, rash, and vomiting followed by hemolytic anemia, thrombocytopenia, DIC, acute renal failure, and very rarely coma, is uncommon. If it does occur, it presents within 72 hours of the bite.

The black widow spider (*Latrodectus*) is found throughout North America but is more common in the southwestern United States. The spider, identified by a red color on the underside of its abdomen, releases a neurotoxic venom with its bite. This neurotoxin causes massive presynaptic release of neurotransmitters, thereby causing diffuse muscle pains, spasms and rigidity, and extreme stomach pain. Associated symptoms also include arthralgias, fever, hypertension, vomiting, and hyperreflexia. This resulting condition, latrodectism, usually resolves in 3 to 7 days. It rarely results in death.

The hobo spider, most commonly found in the Pacific Northwest, is large and brown with distinct yellow markings on its abdomen. A bite from the hobo spider can result in extensive dermal necrosis and permanent scarring. It is characterized by a completely painless initial bite, progressing to painful induration and erythema within 30 minutes, then multiple small blisters within 15 to 35 hours, and then finally progressing to serous exudate encrusting a cratered wound within 72 hours. These lesions generally heal spontaneously. Systemic symptoms include severe headache, vomiting, weakness, fatigue, and vision impairment within 10 hours of the bite.

Management

Medical Management

Once a person has been bitten, serious sequelae can usually be prevented if the spider species is identified early and the person receives the appropriate medical treatment quickly, especially if a venomous spider bite is suspected. In general, bites can be treated with oral or IV analgesics and antihistamines and antibiotic treatment for secondary wound infections. A tetanus vaccine is suggested for prophylaxis because spider bites can become infected with tetanus spores. Occasionally, systemic symptoms result, and further monitoring in the hospital setting is warranted.

Treatment for a Brown Recluse Bite

Recommended laboratory tests include complete blood count, serum glucose, platelet count, BUN and creatinine levels, partial thromboplastin time/activated partial thromboplastin time (PT/aPTT), fibrinogen, renal function tests, and urinalysis. These studies are aimed at identifying signs of hemolysis and intravascular coagulation. Treatment may include oral corticosteroids, dapsone, colchicine, or hyperbaric oxygenation, all of which work to reduce the effects of the dermonecrosis—necrosis of the skin caused by the venom. Antibiotics may be indicated if signs of infection exist. Some recommend early excision of the bite site. An antivenin is under investigation but is not universally available.

Treatment for a Black Widow Bite

Laboratory tests may include complete blood count, blood glucose, CK, and urinalysis and often identify leukocytosis, elevated CK levels, and proteinuria. Treatment includes opioids or muscle relaxants. Calcium gluconate 10% IV may relieve muscle rigidity. Antivenin is available but is often only used to treat those who do not respond promptly to the other treatments first. If warranted, the antivenin has high therapeutic efficacy and has little risks.

Treatment for a Hobo Bite

Treatment is symptomatic and includes excision of the necrotic tissue as indicated.

Nursing Management

Assessment and Analysis

The clinical manifestations of spider bites are unique to the type of spider. The venom of the brown recluse and hobo spiders contains enzymes that are hemotoxic and result in local tissue necrosis. The black widow venom is neurotoxic and causes diffuse pain as a result.

Nursing Diagnoses

- **Impaired skin integrity**
- **Pain**
- **Ineffective airway clearance**

Nursing Interventions

▣ *Assessments*

- Vital signs
  The black widow spider bite may result in hypertension.
- Pain assessment
  Spider bites can result in severe pain at the site.
- Skin assessment; color, size, and drainage
  These characteristics may help identify the type of spider involved.

▣ *Actions*

- Cleanse wound thoroughly
  Minimizes risk of infection
- Apply cold compresses and elevate the affected extremity
  Minimizes swelling
- Administer medications as ordered
  - Antivenin if available
    Antivenin counteracts the neurotoxic and hemotoxic effects of venom spider bites.
  - Pain medication
    Spider bites can be very painful.
  - Antibiotics
    To treat infection if necessary
  - Tetanus
    For prophylaxis because spider bites can become infected with tetanus spores

▣ *Teaching*

- Wound care
  Keeping the wound clean and reporting any changes or worsening immediately to the provider

Evaluating Care Outcomes

Successful treatment of a spider bite requires prompt intervention, administration of antivenin if available, and symptom management. A well-managed patient is discharged home hemodynamically stable with pain under control and clear wound care instructions.

Connection Check 70.11

The nurse is caring for a patient who presents 4 hours after a spider bite to the hand. The hand is slightly swollen, and there are areas of redness and painful blistering. The nurse correlates these symptoms with what type of spider bite?

A. Brown recluse
B. Black widow
C. Hobo spider
D. Tarantula

DROWNING

Epidemiology

Drowning accounts for more than one-half million deaths worldwide. It is difficult to get an accurate number of drowning and near-drowning victims because of differences in terminology and reporting requirements. The outcome of drowning is either death or survival. The term "drowned" typically means that the victim died as a result of drowning. A victim survives drowning if he or she is successfully resuscitated from cardiac or respiratory arrest and is discharged from the hospital. It is also termed *survival from drowning* if the victim dies from other causes in which the death is not directly due to the drowning. Drowning is classified as witnessed when the episode is observed or unwitnessed when the victim is found in the water.

Risk factors for drowning include but are not limited to:

- Alcohol use
- Assault
- Drug abuse
- Head trauma
- Hypothermia
- Severe weather
- Water sport accidents
- Younger age (0–5 years)
- Inability to swim
- Open water swimming in severe currents, riptides, waves, and cold water temperatures

Pathophysiology and Clinical Manifestations

The pathophysiology of drowning starts with submersion in water and the victim's automatic or voluntary response of holding his/her breath. There is a depletion of oxygen and a buildup of CO_2. As the victim remains under water, he or she starts to breathe in water without any gas exchange occurring, further decreasing oxygenation. The respiratory and circulatory systems collapse. Neurologically, the victim ultimately suffers seizures, coma, and death. Fig. 70.15 illustrates the pathophysiology associated with the drowning process.

Cardiovascular System

Initially, the victim is hypertensive and tachycardic with activation of the sympathetic nervous system. While hypoxia, acidosis, and hypothermia worsen, the victim becomes bradycardic, pulmonary hypertension develops, and there is a decreased cardiac output. Atrial fibrillation and other arrhythmias may occur, ultimately progressing to asystole.

Respiratory System

Because of impaired or nonexistent ventilation, hypoxia, hypercarbia, and acidemia occur.

Neurological System

Development of hypoxia from drowning causes CNS dysfunction. It begins within 5 minutes of inadequate

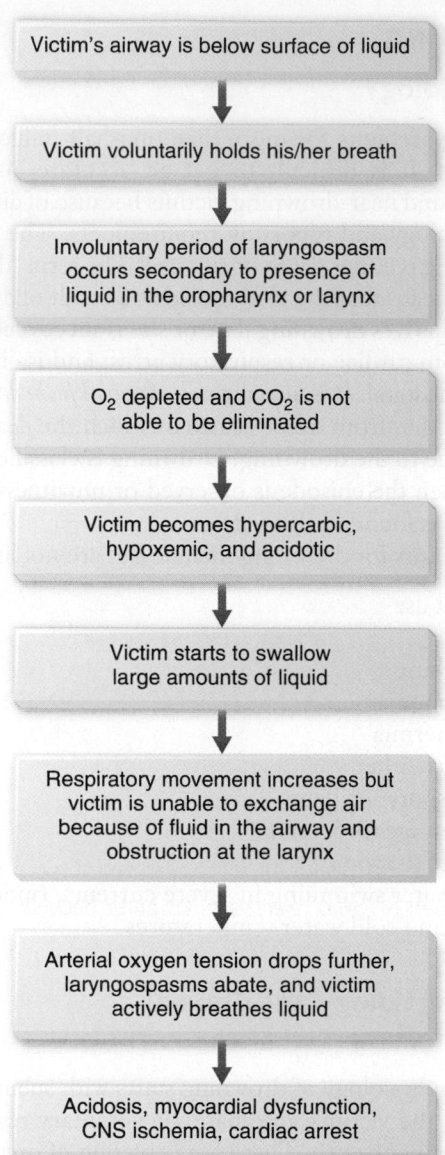

Victim's airway is below surface of liquid

↓

Victim voluntarily holds his/her breath

↓

Involuntary period of laryngospasm occurs secondary to presence of liquid in the oropharynx or larynx

↓

O_2 depleted and CO_2 is not able to be eliminated

↓

Victim becomes hypercarbic, hypoxemic, and acidotic

↓

Victim starts to swallow large amounts of liquid

↓

Respiratory movement increases but victim is unable to exchange air because of fluid in the airway and obstruction at the larynx

↓

Arterial oxygen tension drops further, laryngospasms abate, and victim actively breathes liquid

↓

Acidosis, myocardial dysfunction, CNS ischemia, cardiac arrest

FIGURE 70.15 Drowning process.

oxygenation. This is the leading cause of morbidity and mortality in drowning victims. The clinical manifestation ranges from confusion and disorientation to coma, seizures, and death.

Complications

If the victim survives, approximately 70% will develop acute respiratory failure. This develops due to aspirated fluid, increased capillary permeability, and neurogenic pulmonary edema. Decrease in lung compliance is the result of surfactant washout and dysfunction resulting in atelectasis, ventilation-perfusion mismatch, and intrapulmonary shunting.

Management

Medical Management

Diagnostic and Laboratory Tests

- Arterial blood gases are done to assess respiratory status.

- Chest x-ray may reveal the presence of infiltrates or aspiration.

Examination should focus on the respiratory, cardiovascular, and neurological systems. Dyspnea, wheeze, and crackles suggest aspiration, while the level of consciousness may have prognostic relevance. Examine for signs of trauma or other medical conditions.

Treatment

The initial priorities in a drowning victim are to restore oxygenation, ventilation, and perfusion. Ventilatory support with supplemental O_2 is required. Further support with noninvasive ventilation or intubation may be required depending on the severity of the respiratory failure and the patient's level of consciousness. Intensive care management is directed at treating hypoxia, maintaining cardiovascular stability, neuroprotection, and prevention and/or management of infection likely present due to aspirated fluid. Hypothermia is common in drowning victims. Medications and defibrillation are not likely to be successful if the patient's core temperature is lower than 86°F (30°C). Slow, active rewarming should be instituted as soon as possible to facilitate resuscitation priorities. Ultimately, prevention and/or treatment of multiorgan failure may be necessary.

Nursing Management

Assessment and Analysis

The clinical manifestations of drowning are directly related to the amount of time the victim has been submerged underwater. Respiratory effects range from respiratory distress to respiratory failure and apnea. Cardiovascular effects range from hypertension and tachycardia secondary to the initiation of the sympathetic nervous system to cardiovascular collapse secondary to lack of oxygen. Neurovascular effects may be as minimal as slight confusion to no response, again secondary to lack of oxygen.

Nursing Diagnoses

- **Impaired gas exchange**
- **Hypothermia**
- **Decreased level of consciousness**

Nursing Interventions

- **Assessment**
- Vital signs
  Initial vital signs indicate hypertension and tachycardia; later, because of hypoxia, acidosis, and hypothermia, bradycardia and hypotension result.
- Arterial blood gases
  Blood gases indicate respiratory and metabolic acidosis due to the inability to clear CO_2 and inadequate oxygenation.
- Neurological assessment
  Neurological assessment varies depending upon the amount of time the patient was submerged and hypoxic; the more hypoxia, the more profound the neurological deterioration.

Actions

- Administer 100% nonrebreather mask
  Administer O₂ to maintain adequate saturation to support vital bodily functions.
- Prepare for intubation
  Intubation may be necessary if the patient's respiratory and/or neurological status has deteriorated to the point the victim cannot protect the airway.
- Continuous cardiac monitoring
  Continuous monitoring allows for early detection of bradycardia or dysrhythmias.
- Insert IV
  An IV is necessary for the administration of IV fluids to support cardiovascular status and administration of medications.
- Anticipate cardiopulmonary resuscitation (CPR)
  In severe and prolonged drowning, cardiopulmonary arrest is likely, necessitating CPR.

Teaching

- Water safety—careful observation of children, use of life preservers, limit alcohol, learn to swim
  The best treatment of drowning is prevention.

Evaluating Care Outcomes

Successful intervention is possible if submersion time is minimal. The longer underwater, the more dire the outcome. A well-managed patient is one who is discharged with minimal to no respiratory, circulatory, or neurological sequelae. This patient understands the hazards of water and takes the necessary safety precautions for himself/herself and family. The best cure is prevention.

Making Connections

CASE STUDY: WRAP-UP

The 19-year-old gunshot patient is still complaining of shortness of breath. A needle decompression was done in the field to release air because of the pneumothorax, preventing a tension pneumothorax. Initial assessment confirms minimal breath sounds on the right, requiring a right-sided chest tube with positive air and blood return in the chest tube. The patient's breathing becomes less shallow and labored. A second IV is placed, laboratory tests are drawn, and warm fluids are hung. On further assessment, patient has a wound to the right lower back, which is tender to palpation. Current VSs HR: 135 bpm; BP: 90/50 mm Hg; RR: 22 breaths/minute; O₂ 99% with 100% NRB mask in place, temperature 97.7°F (36.5°C). A FAST examination is performed and is positive. The operating room (OR) is alerted and the patient is prepared to go to the OR STAT. In the OR, the bleeding is controlled. The patient is moved to the ICU, where he begins to stabilize.

Case Study Questions

1. After receiving the report from the field provider about the patient, the trauma nurse anticipates and prepares for which initial interventions? *(Select all that apply.)*
   A. Chest tube placement
   B. Rapid fluid infuser
   C. Open chest massage
   D. Intubation
   E. Magnetic resonance imaging

2. The nurse recognizes this patient is at risk for developing which complications? *(Select all that apply.)*
   A. Infection
   B. Airway compromise
   C. Hypovolemia
   D. Rhabdomyolysis
   E. Seizures

3. What symptom should prompt a quick intervention from the nurse in this case?
   A. Hypertensive
   B. Hypothermic
   C. Anxious
   D. Tachycardic

4. In addition to the trauma surgeon and nurse, what other members of the team are essential at the bedside in this patient's care? *(Select all that apply.)*
   A. Airway provider
   B. Radiology
   C. Clinical technician
   D. Laboratory technician
   E. Pharmacist

5. The nurse is responsible for which of the following functions as part of the trauma team? *(Select all that apply.)*
   A. Documentation
   B. Medication administration
   C. Airway management
   D. Management of rapid fluid infuser
   E. Central line insertion

CHAPTER SUMMARY

In the United States, unintentional injury is the fifth leading cause of death for all ages. Trauma centers are hospitals specially equipped to provide comprehensive emergency care to patients suffering from a traumatic injury. A designated trauma center must maintain a specialty-trained workforce that is prepared to provide a range of emergency care 24/7 and must also ensure access to the equipment that is needed to provide immediate life-saving care. Roles in a trauma team include a trauma team leader, nurses, airway provider, surgical provider, respiratory therapy, radiologist, and clinical technician, pharmacist, social work and/or pastoral care, and support staff.

The prehospital provider is responsible for recognizing the urgency of the trauma situation, providing initial care based on the ABCs, and transporting the patient as quickly as possible to a hospital. Once at the hospital, the patient undergoes a primary survey based on the ABCDEs, emergency treatment is provided as necessary, and then a more thorough secondary assessment is performed.

It is important to understand the mechanism of injury because that may help determine the scope and extent of injuries. Mechanisms of injury may be characterized as blunt or penetrating injuries. In blunt trauma, there is no penetration of the skin. Mechanisms of energy transference that often cause blunt trauma injuries are deceleration and acceleration forces, compression, and shearing. Penetrating trauma is defined as injuries produced by a foreign object penetrating the tissue. The energy created by the foreign object dissipates into the surrounding tissues, causing injury.

A poison is any substance that is harmful to your body when ingested, inhaled, injected, or absorbed through the skin. Prompt recognition and treatment are essential. Common clinical manifestations include respiratory depression, excessive vomiting, diarrhea, bradycardia, hypotension, and arrhythmias, depending on the poison. Definitive treatment is specific for each poison, but decontamination—removing or neutralizing a substance to decrease absorption—is an important component of care for all.

Thermoregulation is a physiological response the body uses to maintain normal body temperature. If body temperature is not maintained, hypothermia or hyperthermia may result. Hypothermia may result in symptoms such as shivering and increased heart rate and blood pressure to myocardial irritability and bradycardia when hypothermia worsens. Depending on the level of hypothermia, treatment involves passive external rewarming, active external rewarming, or active internal rewarming. Depending on the level, hyperthermia results in symptoms such as swelling of the feet, ankles, and hands to fatigue, weakness, dizziness, headache, nausea, vomiting, and muscle cramps. Cooling interventions include moving the patient to a cool environment, removal of extra clothing, applying cool cloths, applying ice packs, and encouraging the patient to drink cool, nonalcoholic beverages.

When a venomous snake bites and injects venom through its fangs, the process is called *envenomation*. Venom immobilizes prey and can be neurotoxic, hemotoxic, and can disrupt fluid balance. Treatment with antivenin is important if available; otherwise, treatment is based on patient symptoms.

Most spider bites are not dangerous to humans, but serious reactions are produced by the bite of the brown recluse, the black widow, and the hobo spider. The effects can be treated if identified early. Spider bites can be treated with antivenin if available, analgesics and antihistamines, and antibiotic treatment for secondary wound infections.

Drowning is a process resulting in primary respiratory impairment from submersion/immersion in water. Oxygenation and removal of CO_2 is impaired, resulting in acidosis, neurological impairment, and myocardial dysfunction. The initial priorities in a drowning victim are to restore oxygenation, ventilation, and perfusion.

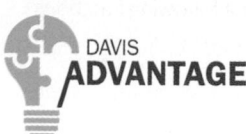

DAVIS
ADVANTAGE

To explore learning resources for this chapter, go to **Davis Advantage** and find:
- Answers to in-text questions
- Chapter Resources and Activities
- NCLEX®-Style Chapter Review Questions
- Bibliography

Chapter 71

Disasters, Mass Casualty Incidents, and Complex Emergencies

Dianne Whyne

Finding Connections

CASE STUDY: EPISODE 1

Follow the scenario throughout the chapter.

The spring of 2011 saw three record-breaking and deadly tornado outbreaks in the United States. In mid-April, a severe storm produced 179 confirmed tornadoes across 16 southern states. Two weeks later, an even larger outbreak spawned at least 336 tornadoes across 21 states. In all, more than 300 people died from tornadoes during the month of April 2011.

Late Sunday afternoon, May 22, 2011, a supercell thunderstorm tracked from extreme southeast Kansas into far southwest Missouri. The National Weather Service issued a tornado warning (Box 71.1) at 5:17 p.m. Central Time Zone that included the city of Joplin, Missouri. Joplin is a city of more than 50,000 with a population density near 1,500 people per square mile. The area's major industries include agriculture, education, health and social services, manufacturing, and retail trade. Two hospitals, Mercy/St. John's Regional Medical Center and the Freeman Health System, provide medical care to the region and serve as the city's emergency medical service (EMS) providers. Joplin is home to Missouri Southern State University, Ozark Christian College, and Messenger College. The Joplin area is located within "Tornado Alley," a part of the central United States that experiences a high frequency of tornadoes each year. Meteorically, this region is ideally situated for the formation of supercell thunderstorms that produce tornadoes rated Enhanced Fujita (EF) scale-2 or higher.

Joplin city residents were given a 24-minute notice of the impending tornado. Twenty-five tornado sirens sounded, and weather alert boxes appeared in the corners of local TV stations. As the EF scale-5 tornado touched down in Joplin, it had maximum winds in excess of 200 mph and was three-fourths to 1-mile wide with a damage path 6-miles long (the entire tornado path was 22.1-miles long and up to 1-mile wide). The tornado's eye was 300-yards wide. This tornado resulted in 161 fatalities and approximately 1,371 injuries. Of the fatalities, 54% died in their homes, 32% died in nonresidential areas, and 14% died in vehicles or out-of-doors. The tornado destroyed 4,380 homes and damaged an additional 3,884 homes, not including 400 businesses and 8 schools. Eighteen thousand vehicles were destroyed, and 4,500 jobs were displaced.

At St. John's Regional Medical Center, a 9-story building, there were 183 patients—patients watching television, visiting with friends, or eating their dinner. There were also 25 patients in the emergency department (ED) and approximately 100 staff members on duty. The announcement over the hospital speakers warned of a potential tornado, and "Plan Gray" was activated.

Plan Gray is the Tornado Emergency Operations Plan. No one panicked, as such calls are routine in Joplin; "Condition Gray" is practiced several times per year. On the inpatient units, patients who were able to walk were placed in hardback chairs or wheelchairs and lined up in the halls; others were rolled into the hallways on their beds, and for those too sick to move, blankets and pillows were placed over them. Staff also pulled shades over windows to shield patients from flying debris. Because the storm was not expected to hit them, hospital visitors watched the storm on TV while they continued their visits. The storm came up quickly and passed over St. John's Hospital in 45 seconds. The hospital sustained a direct hit at approximately 5:41 p.m. At the hospital, just prior to the hit, an employee ran down a corridor shouting, "Take cover! We're gonna get hit!" Seconds later, the air turned cold, the lights flickered and died, and glass exploded from the hospital's windows.

Within seconds, this community of 50,000 was devastated and broken. The tornado flattened whole neighborhoods, splintered homes, debarked trees, and flipped over cars and trucks. Some homes were completely swept away. Immediately following the tornado, emergency responders were deployed to the city to undertake search and rescue efforts. The governor declared a "state of emergency" for the Joplin area shortly after the tornado hit and ordered Missouri National Guard troops into the city…

OVERVIEW OF DISASTERS

Throughout recorded history, disasters have been an integral part of our existence, causing immeasurable amounts of pain and suffering. The term **"disaster"** is used commonly to describe many different events. The 2013 Boston Marathon bombing that killed three people and injured more than 260 others, including 16 who lost limbs, was called a disaster. The 2014 Ebola outbreak that caused more than 28,000 cases worldwide and more than 11,000 deaths was called a public health disaster. The October 2017 mass shooting at an outdoor concert in Las Vegas where a gunman sprayed gunfire on a crowd of 22,000 concert goers,

Box 71.1 Tornado Warning vs Tornado Watch

- A **Tornado Watch** is issued when, although a tornado has not been seen, conditions are very favorable for one to occur at any moment
- A **Tornado Warning** is issued when a tornado has actually been sighted or picked up on radar

killing 58 people and injuring almost 500 was called the worst U.S. mass shooting and a disaster. In September of 2017 a major earthquake that registered a magnitude of 7.1 struck the area around Mexico City, killing 370 people and collapsing more than 40 buildings. That event was called a disaster.

There is no one definition of a disaster. The definition adopted by the World Health Organization (WHO) terms a disaster as "a serious disruption of the functioning of a community or a society causing widespread human, material, economic or environmental losses which exceed the ability of the affected community or society to cope using its own resources." The U.S. **Federal Emergency Management Agency (FEMA)** describes a disaster as "an occurrence of a natural catastrophe, technological accident, or human event that has resulted in severe property damage, deaths, and/or multiple injuries." The U.S. Stafford Act defines a major disaster as "any natural catastrophe (including any hurricane, tornado, storm, high water, wind driven water, tidal wave, tsunami, earthquake, volcanic eruption, landslide, mudslide, snowstorm, or drought), regardless of cause, or any fire, flood, or explosion, in any part of the United States, which in the determination of the President, causes damage of sufficient severity and magnitude to warrant major disaster assistance to supplement the efforts and available resources of states or local governments, and disaster relief organizations to alleviate the damage, loss, hardship, or suffering caused." When the President declares that a major disaster or emergency exists, an array of federal programs are activated to assist in response and recovery efforts. The United Nations defines disasters as "a serious disruption of the functioning of society, causing widespread human, material, or environmental losses which exceed the ability of affected society to cope using only its own resources." Dr. Kathleen J. Tierney, sociologist and internationally known expert on disasters, puts the matter in a different perspective. She defines disasters as "many people trying to do quickly what they do not ordinarily do, in an environment with which they are not familiar." A simpler definition yet is that "a disaster occurs when needs exceed resources following an event."

In general, most disaster events are defined by three main characteristics: (1) an event of destructive magnitude; (2) that kills, injures, or causes human suffering to a significant number of people or the environment; and (3) that requires the need for external assistance. A disaster is a large-scale destructive event that disrupts the infrastructure and normal functioning of a community or society. Disasters can be natural or man-made. This chapter will define and describe types of disasters, complex emergencies, and mass casualty events as well as disaster response.

Complex Emergency

The WHO defines a **complex emergency (CE)** as "situations of disrupted livelihoods and threats to life produced by warfare, civil disturbance and large-scale movements of people, in which any emergency response has to be conducted in a difficult political and security environment." Such "complex emergencies" are characterized by the WHO as involving:

- extensive violence and loss of life
- displacements of populations
- widespread damage to societies and economies
- the need for large-scale, multifaceted humanitarian assistance
- the hindrance or prevention of humanitarian assistance by political and military constraints
- significant security risks for humanitarian relief workers in some areas

According to the United Nations, those suffering the consequences of complex emergencies are primarily civilians (50%-90%) and especially vulnerable populations that include children, women, the elderly, and the disabled. Over the last few decades, complex emergencies have generally become more complex and longer-lasting.

Mass Casualty Incident

A **mass casualty incident (MCI)** refers to any large-scale event in which emergency medical resources such as supplies, medical/rescue personnel, or equipment are overwhelmed by the number and severity of casualties, thus requiring prioritization of medical care by triage. All MCIs are disasters, but not all disasters are MCIs. The term *casualty* includes all persons who are ill, injured, missing, or dead as the result of the incident. The term *incident* is defined as an event that requires scene or casualty management. This may look different in different locales. In a large city with multiple hospitals, hundreds of casualties may be handled locally without any outside assistance. In a rural setting, 10 casualties may overwhelm the single local hospital. A simple definition of an MCI is "when the healthcare needs exceed the healthcare resources." The goal of the response to any MCI is to "do the greatest good for the greatest number of people." Regardless of whether a situation is classified as a disaster, a mass casualty incident, or a complex emergency, an effective triage method is needed to optimize overall patient outcomes. This is done through the process called *disaster triage*.

Disaster Triage

Triage is the process of placing the right patient in the right place at the right time to receive the right level of care. On a daily basis, most EDs in the United States use some form of daily triage to identify those patients who are more critically ill or injured and cannot tolerate a delay in receiving care. The goal of daily triage is to identify and treat the most seriously ill or injured first.

In a disaster situation, there is a paradigm shift in the triage philosophy. Simply stated, the goal of disaster triage is to ensure "doing the most good for the greatest number of people rather than doing everything possible to save every life." This may mean delaying care to selected patients who have little hope of survival or would consume too many resources. In most instances, disaster triage is used only in the most catastrophic situations.

During a disaster event, prehospital personnel arriving at the scene usually establish a casualty collection area. Patients brought to this area are triaged and maybe tagged with a corresponding colored triage tag, provided with basic field care for stabilization, and transported to the most appropriate facility for care. At the hospital, secondary triage is typically performed by Emergency Department (ED) personnel, and then patients are assigned to a treatment area for care.

There are different triage models that can be used to sort patients. At present, no one model is universally accepted as the standard. Two commonly used models are **Simple Triage and Rapid Treatment (START)** and Sort, Assess, Lifesaving Interventions, Treatment, and/or Transport (SALT).

Simple Triage and Rapid Treatment

Simple Triage and Rapid Treatment (START) is one of the most popular triage systems in use in the United States. It uses physiological parameters and is designed to be completed in 60 seconds or less. It is based on three observations: (1) respirations; (2) perfusion (or pulse); and (3) mental status. The mnemonic "RPM" is used as a memory aid. Simple Triage and Rapid Treatment begins by directing all patients who are ambulatory to move to a safe area. These patients are tagged "green," or "minor." These patients are capable of ambulating and understanding directions and have adequate perfusion to follow commands and stay upright. Triage then continues for the remainder of the patients. Patients with no spontaneous respirations receive airway repositioning. If they remain apneic, they are tagged "deceased" by using a black label and receive no further care or interventions. If repositioning the airway initiates respirations, that patient is tagged red or "immediate." Patients with respirations greater than 30 breaths per minute or capillary refill longer than 2 seconds (or who lack a radial pulse) or who are unable to follow simple directions are also tagged "immediate" by using a red triage tag. The remaining patients are tagged "delayed" and are given a yellow tag. The START triage model allows for only two interventions during the triage process: (1) direct pressure to control bleeding and (2) basic airway-opening maneuvers. Disaster triage is not a static activity; the patient's condition may change or there may be a change in available resources. Patients not moved or transferred to a definitive area for care are retriaged on a constant basis.

JumpSTART is a Pediatric Mass Casualty Incident Triage tool. It is an objective triage model designed for triaging infants and young children. It takes into consideration the developmental and physiological differences of children by using breathing as the cornerstone for triage decisions (Fig. 71.1).

Sort, Assess, Lifesaving Interventions, Treatment, and/or Transport Triage

In response to the lack of scientific data regarding the efficacy of mass casualty triage systems, the Centers for Disease Control and Prevention (CDC) formed an interdisciplinary advisory committee to review existing disaster triage models. The advisory committee developed the **Sort, Assess, Lifesaving Interventions, Treatment, and/or Transport (SALT)** model by combining the best features of the existing systems (Fig 71.2). The SALT model can be used to triage both adults and children and is endorsed by several national organizations, including the American College of Emergency Physicians, the American College of Surgeons Committee on Trauma, the American Trauma Society, and the National Association of EMS Physicians.

The first step in the SALT model is to address the "walking wounded." Those who are able to walk are prioritized last; those who cannot follow a command or have an obvious life threat are prioritized first; and those who can follow a command but are unable to walk are prioritized second. The next step is to make lifesaving interventions before assigning a patient to a triage category. Lifesaving interventions include control of major hemorrhage, opening the airway and providing two breaths for child casualties, decompression of a tension pneumothorax, and the use of auto injector antidotes. Finally, triage categories are assigned (delayed, immediate, or expectant) based on breathing, peripheral pulses, respiratory distress, and hemorrhage control. The SALT system of triage is different from the other systems in that there is a grey or "Expectant" category. This category means that the patient may have a life-threatening injury, but current resources are not available to meet the need. As resources become available, this "Expectant" category of patients should be re-evaluated frequently. It is a different method of triage in that there are two phases; a global sorting based on the ability to follow commands and walk, and a triage category assignment based on response to lifesaving interventions. Regardless of the system used, the primary goal of disaster triage is to maximize the number of survivors.

Many casualties will present to the hospital within the first 2 hours of the event. Patients usually arrive at the hospital in two waves. Wave 1 arrives in approximately 15 to 30 minutes. These patients are the walking wounded who were able to self-extricate themselves from the scene and make it to the hospital on their own. Past disasters have shown that 80% to 85% of all disaster casualties will bypass the EMS system and arrive at the hospital on their own. Wave 2 will follow in 30 to 45 minutes. This second group needed assistance for extrication from the scene and were transported by EMS. They are usually more seriously injured than the patients in the first wave.

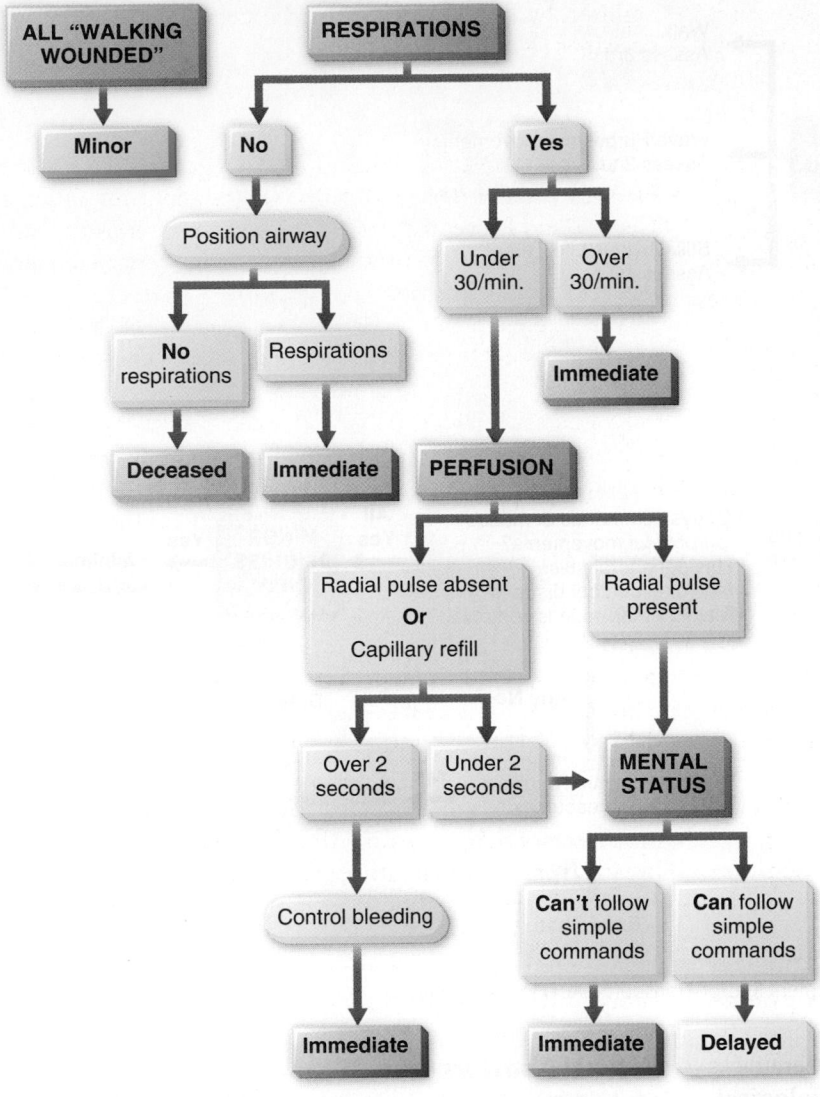

FIGURE 71.1 Adult Simple Triage and Rapid Treatment (START) triage algorithm.

Connection Check 71.1

Which of the following statements best explains the relationship between an MCI and a disaster?

A. All disasters are mass casualty events.
B. All mass casualty events are disasters.
C. Mass casualty events are natural disasters.
D. Mass casualty events are man-made disasters.

Types of Disasters

Disasters are commonly categorized by their origin: natural events, nuclear/radiological events, bioterrorism/emerging infectious diseases, chemical incidents, and explosive/blast incidents. All disasters are unique because of the nature of the affected community in terms of preparedness, affluence, political structure, and baseline health system preparedness.

Terrorism

Terrorism is a particular type of disaster that may or may not produce an MCI. No one definition of terrorism has gained universal acceptance. Title 22 of the United States Code defines terrorism as "premeditated, politically motivated violence perpetrated against noncombatant targets by subnational groups or clandestine agents, usually intended to influence an audience." FEMA defines terrorism as "the use of force or violence against persons or property in violation of the criminal laws of the United States for the purpose of intimidation, coercion, or ransom."

Terrorism is often motivated by religious, political, or other ideological beliefs. Terrorists use threats to (1) create fear among the public; (2) try to convince citizens that their government is powerless to prevent terrorism; and (3) get immediate publicity for their causes. Terrorism differs from other forms of military action in that noncombatants are usually deliberately targeted by the terrorists. Acts of terrorism can include threats of terrorism, assassinations,

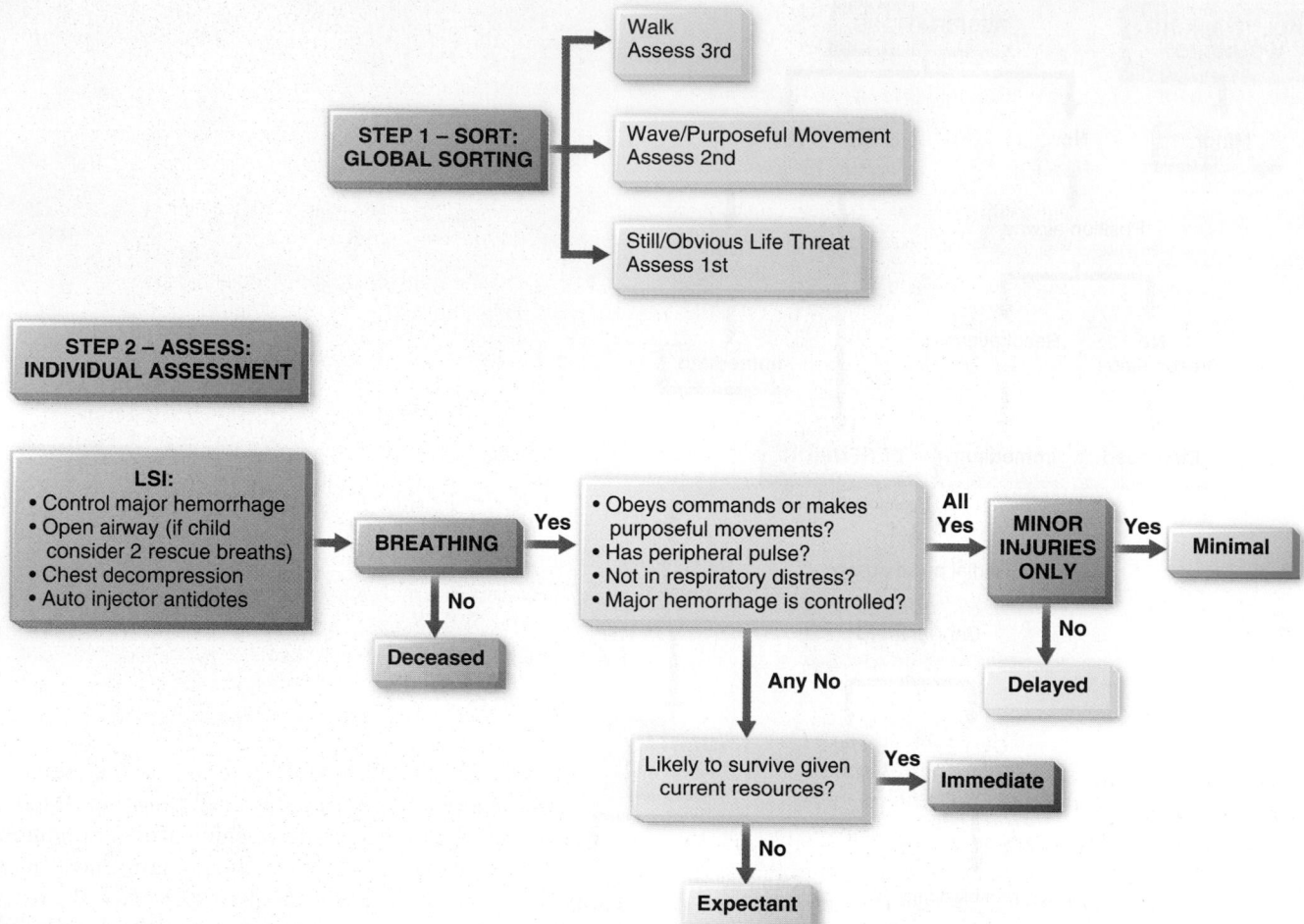

FIGURE 71.2 Sort, Assess, Lifesaving interventions, Treatment and/or Transport (SALT) triage algorithm.

kidnappings, hijackings, bomb scares, bombings, cyberattacks (computer-based), and the use of **chemical, biological, radiological, nuclear, and explosive (CBRNE)** weapons also known as weapons of mass destruction.

A **weapon of mass destruction (WMD)** is defined as "any weapon or device that is intended, or has the capability, to cause death or serious bodily injury to a significant number of people through the release, dissemination, or impact of (1) a toxin or poisonous chemical or their precursors; (2) a disease organism; (3) radiation or radioactivity; or (4) an explosive device." The term "weapon of mass effect" has recently appeared in the literature, and many consider it to be a more appropriate description, considering the large numbers of injuries and deaths that can occur. A WMD may be used by a terrorist(s) to produce an MCI.

Connection Check 71.2

Which of the following factors contributes the most to positive patient outcomes in a mass casualty disaster?

A. On-site patient treatment
B. Disaster triage
C. Transport of all victims to the closest hospital
D. Availability of patient air transportation

Natural Disasters

Natural disasters are numerous and widespread and are part of the human experience. They often result in significant losses, including physical destruction of dwellings, social and economic disruption, human pain, suffering, and injury including loss of life. Some natural disasters are predictable, but most are unpredictable, unpreventable, and uncontrollable. They can be classified as acute or slow in their onset. Natural disasters with a slow onset include blizzards, drought, famine, and pest infestations. Those with an acute onset include floods, earthquakes, tsunamis, tornadoes, volcanic eruptions, and hurricanes. The severity of damage caused by natural disasters is directly associated with the population density in the disaster area, local building codes, community preparedness, and the public communication system. Recovery following a natural disaster is largely dependent on the public's access to information, the speed of disaster relief services, and the political and economic climate of the area. Table 71.1 lists common natural disasters and the resultant possible injuries and medical issues.

Earthquakes

Earthquakes are defined as a sudden rapid shaking of the ground caused by the shifting of the tectonic plates that

Table 71.1 Natural Disasters, Human Impacts, and Medical Issues

Natural Disaster	Potential Injuries and Medical Issues
Earthquake	Skull fractures, spinal cord injuries, hypothermia, wound infections, exacerbation of pulmonary diseases such as asthma, and crush injuries
Tsunami	Drowning, blunt force trauma, crush injuries, impalements, penetrating trauma, closed head injury, eye injuries, pulmonary injury from aspiration of contaminated water, orthopedic injuries
Tornado	Blunt injuries (rapid movement of victims through the air who then strike a stationary object); penetrating ballistics (wind-driven projectiles striking people); crush injuries (from collapse of structures); traumatic injuries to the head, thorax, and abdomen; eye injuries; closed and open brain injuries
Cyclone/Hurricane/ Typhoon	Drowning, electrocution, lacerations, punctures from flying debris, blunt trauma or bone fractures from falling trees and other debris, heart attacks and other stress-related disorders, disrupted wildlife (bites from animals, insects, and snakes), injuries from improper use of chain saws or other power equipment when responding to the event
Blizzard	Orthopedic injuries; acute myocardial infarction; carbon monoxide poisoning; cold exposure; hypothermia; frostbite; frostnip; motor vehicle accidents; head, chest, and abdominal injuries from snowmobile accidents; injuries from the use of power equipment for clearing debris, fallen trees, and snow
Heat wave	Heatstroke, sunstroke, heat cramps, heat exhaustion, fatigue

form the Earth's crust. Where the edges of these tectonic plates meet is referred to as a major **fault line**. The San Andreas Fault in California is an example of a fault line. In the United States, the greatest seismic activity is along the Pacific Coast from Alaska to California. Miles underground, as the Earth's plates move, stressed areas develop and rupture, resulting in the release of tremendous amounts of energy and ground motion. The point of rupture is known as the **epicenter**. The Richter Scale (Table 71.2) is a logarithmic scale that estimates the total energy released by an earthquake. A change of 1 unit on the scale corresponds to a 10-fold change in ground motion and a 32-fold change in radiated energy. Measurements on the scale below a magnitude of 2.0 are not usually felt, and measurements above a magnitude of 5.0 usually cause damage (Box 71.2). Earthquakes can cause buildings and bridges to collapse, disruption of gas service, communication failures, and electric line failures.

A major earthquake can be preceded by less severe preliminary tremors called **foreshocks**. Smaller tremors after the main earthquake are called **aftershocks**. Earthquakes can sometimes trigger landslides, avalanches, flash floods, fires, and huge destructive ocean waves called tsunami. Table 71.3 lists the world's earthquakes with greater than 1,000 dead since 2001.

Tsunami

A **tsunami** is a Japanese word meaning "harbor wave." A tsunami is a tremendously powerful ocean wave that is the result of an underwater earthquake, landslide, or volcano. Tsunami are not a single wave but rather a series of waves spaced minutes to more than 1 hour apart. These waves can travel across the ocean at speeds up to 500 miles per hour depending on the location and the source of the event. A tsunami is relatively unnoticeable until the wave reaches shallow water; then it can come crashing ashore at heights up to 50 feet or more. Historically, tsunami have been reported in all the oceans, but the Pacific Ocean is the most common location. Tsunami can cause buildings to collapse, disruption of utilities, loss of coastal marine systems, and injuries/deaths to coastal populations.

Table 71.2 Richter Scale

Description	Magnitude (Richter Scale)	Number per Year
Great earthquake	Over 8.0	1–2
Major earthquake	7.0–7.9	18
Destructive earthquake	6.0–6.9	120
Damaging earthquake	5.0–5.9	800
Minor earthquake	4.0–4.9	6,200
Smaller usually felt	3.0–3.9	49,000
Detected but not felt	2.0–2.9	300,000

Box 71.2 Earthquake in Nepal (2015)

On April 25, 2015, a magnitude 7.8 earthquake struck Nepal. It was the worst to strike the region in more than 80 years. The area suffered a second 7.3 magnitude quake just 17 days later, on May 12, causing further damage and hardship for those who had survived the initial disaster. Nepal, well known for its rich cultural heritage and extreme tourism, is one of the poorest countries in southeast Asia. The damage done by the quake put a strain on the country's citizens that has lasted many years. Approximately 8 million people were affected. The death toll was around 8,900 with 22,000 suffering injuries. Deaths were also reported in neighboring Tibet and India. Approximately 1.1 million children needed urgent assistance, and 2.8 million people needed humanitarian assistance. Homes and historic temples crumbled, roads damaged and communications made sporadic. The quake triggered an avalanche that killed 19 climbers on Mt. Everest and stranded hundreds at base camp. Entire villages were destroyed without a single home left standing. Water systems in hillside villages were wrecked. Terraced farms and cattle were wiped out by the quake or subsequent landslides, destroying people's entire livelihoods. More than 800,000 homes were destroyed, and 298,000 homes were damaged. The quakes' strongest impact was in remote rural areas that made the response extremely challenging.

Table 71.3 World's Earthquakes With 1,000 or More Dead Since 2001

Date	Region	Magnitude	Fatalities
2015	Nepal	7.3	8,9000
2011	Japan	9.0	28,000
2010	Haiti	7.0	222,570
2009	Indonesia	7.5	1,117
2008	China	7.9	87,587
2006	Indonesia	6.3	5,749
2005	Pakistan	7.6	86,000
2005	Indonesia	8.6	1,313
2004	Sumatra	9.1	227,898
2003	Iran	6.6	31,000
2003	Algeria	6.8	2,286
2002	Afghanistan	6.1	1,000
2001	India	7.7	20,023

Source: U.S. Geological Survey. https://earthquake.usgs.gov/earthquakes/browse/stats.php

Tornadoes

Tornadoes are spawned by severe thunderstorms. There are approximately 1,000 tornadoes each year in the United States. Although most tornadoes remain aloft, those that touch the ground can cause significant damage. The United States has the most severe tornadoes on Earth because of our weather patterns and terrain. Although a tornado is inherently dangerous, it becomes a serious risk only when it threatens a populated area (Fig. 71.3).

Tornadoes can occur in all regions of the United States, but the majority occurs in what has been termed "**Tornado Alley.**" Tornado Alley is a colloquial and popular media term that refers to the area between the Rocky and Appalachian Mountains. Although no U.S. state is entirely free of tornadoes, they are most frequent in the "Plains States." In this area, the cold, dry air from Canada and the Rocky Mountains meets the warm, moist air from the Gulf of Mexico and the hot, dry air from the Sonoran Desert. These combine and produce atmospheric instability and intense thunderstorms. Tornadoes can have a wind velocity of more than 250 miles per hour, and the winds can generate sufficient force to destroy even massive buildings. Tornado severity is rated using the Fujita Scale seen in Table 71.4.

CASE STUDY: EPISODE 2

In 45 seconds, the tornado all but destroyed St. John's Hospital. Patients and visitors were screaming. Everyone in the hospital thought they were going to die. The wind roared with such force that it twisted the top floors of the hospital by several inches. Water pipes burst, the ceiling tiles caved in, and wires were hanging in the air. There were no lights; both power generators were gone from their foundations. Intravenous lines were ripped from patients' arms, and the IV poles became projectiles. All emergency lights and exit signs were ripped from their mounts and were useless, and the exit stairwells were blocked by debris. X-ray machines, respirators, and computer monitors crashed through the air. Doors were ripped off their hinges. The winds were so powerful that items from the hospital such as medications, medical records, and radiographs were found in neighboring counties. Fortunately, most people inside the hospital and the ED were uninjured.

In the town, survivors told harrowing stories of riding out the 200-mph winds in walk-in coolers in restaurants and convenience stores. Some hid in bathtubs and closets, others ran for their lives as the tornado bore down on them. Heavy objects including concrete bumpers and large trucks were tossed up to one-eighth mile.

It was a storm more ferocious than the citizens of Joplin had ever seen. At its height, it plowed a path of destruction three-quarters of a mile wide and kicked debris more than 20,000 feet into the air...

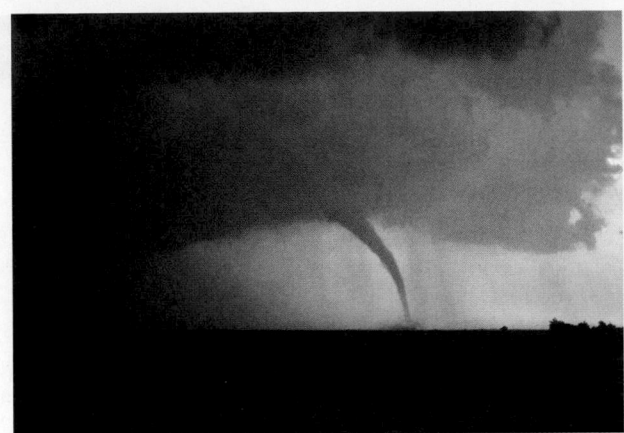

FIGURE 71.3 Tornado.

Table 71.4 Fujita Tornado Scale

Scale Value	Wind Speed Range and Description of Damage
F0	**40–72 mph:** Light damage. Some damage to chimneys; tree branches broken off, shallow-rooted trees pushed over, sign boards damaged.
F1	**73–112 mph:** Moderate damage. The lower limit is the beginning of hurricane wind speed. Roof surfaces peeled off, mobile homes pushed off foundations or overturned, moving autos pushed off roads.
F2	**113–157 mph:** Considerable damage. Roofs torn off houses, mobile homes demolished, boxcars pushed over, large trees snapped off or uprooted, light object missiles generated.
F3	**158–206 mph:** Severe damage. Roofs and some walls torn off well-constructed houses, trains overturned, most trees in a forest uprooted, heavy cars lifted off ground and thrown.
F4	**207–260 mph:** Devastating damage. Well-constructed houses leveled, structures with weak foundations blown off some distance, cars thrown, large missiles generated.
F5	**261–318 mph:** Incredible damage. Strong frame houses lifted off foundations and carried considerable distances, car-sized missiles fly through the air in excess of 100 yards, and trees debarked.

Hurricanes, Cyclones, and Typhoons

Hurricanes, cyclones, and **typhoons** are all the same weather phenomena. The only difference is the location where the storm occurs. All are storm systems that can produce extremely powerful winds, torrential rain, high waves, and damaging storm surges, as well as spawn tornadoes. These storm systems develop over large bodies of warm water and eventually may move over land. They are among the most devastating naturally occurring hazards and are capable of producing large-scale devastation in human populations. Hurricanes are classified according to their intensity using the Saffir-Simpson Scale (Table 71.5 and Box 71.3).

Winter Storms and Blizzards

Winter storms and blizzards are severe, dangerous weather events. Winter storms consisting of extreme cold and heavy snowfall and ice can affect every state except Hawaii. States where cold weather is rare are more severely disrupted by winter storms than states that experience severe winter weather more frequently. Severe winter storms can isolate and disrupt families; shut down schools, businesses, and transportation; and destroy large components of agriculture. Heavily populated areas are particularly impacted when severe storms disrupt communication and electricity as a result of downed power and phone lines. In a severe storm, snow and ice removal from roads can be difficult when the snow and ice accumulate faster than equipment can clear it.

Heat Waves

Heat waves are characterized as extreme summer temperatures with a combination of very high temperatures and very high humidity levels. When these persist over several days and nighttime temperatures do not drop significantly, it is called a *heat wave*. As a result of the heat wave, mortality and morbidity rise. There have been more than 20 serious heat emergencies in the world since 1901, including the deadly 2003 heat wave in Europe that killed more than 35,000, with 15,000 dead in France alone.

Connection Check 71.3

Which of the following is an example of a natural disaster?
A. The 1984 Bhopal, India, methyl isocyanate release
B. The March 20, 1995, sarin incident in Japan
C. The 2007 Virginia Tech campus shootings
D. The 2011 earthquake in Japan

Nuclear/Radiological Events

Exposures to radiation may be accidental or deliberate in origin. An accidental exposure occurred in March 2011 following the Japan earthquake and tsunami. The earthquake and tsunami damaged the Fukushima nuclear power plant, resulting in accidental radiation exposure to hundreds of civilians.

Radiation

Radiation is a form of energy that is present all around us. People are exposed to small amounts of radiation every day. The exposure can be from naturally occurring sources such

Table 71.5 Saffir-Simpson Hurricane Scale

Intensity	Winds (mph)	Storm Surge	Damage Caused
Category 1 *Minimal*	74–95	4–5 ft above normal	Minimal damage to building structures. Damage primarily to unanchored mobile homes, shrubbery, and trees; some coastal road flooding and minor pier damage
Category 2 *Extensive*	96–110	6–8 ft above normal	Some roofing material, door, and window damage; considerable damage to vegetation, mobile homes, and piers; small craft in unprotected anchorages break moorings
Category 3 *Extensive*	111–130	9–12 ft above normal	Structural damage to small residences and utility buildings with a minor amount of curtain wall failure; mobile homes are destroyed; flooding near the coast destroys smaller structures with larger structures damaged by floating debris
Category 4 *Extreme*	131–155	13–18 ft above normal.	More extensive curtain wall failures with some complete roof structure failures on small residences; major beach erosion; major damage to lower floors of structures near the shore
Category 5 *Catastrophic*	Greater than 155	More than 18 ft above normal	Complete roof failure on many residences and industrial buildings; some complete building failures with small utility buildings blown over or away; major damage to lower floors of structures located more than 15 ft above sea level and within 500 yd of the shoreline

Curtain wall, Nonstructural outer covering of buildings designed to keep weather out and occupants in

Box 71.3 Hurricane Maria

Hurricane Maria made its first landfall on the Caribbean island nation of Dominica on September 18, 2017 as a Category 5 storm with winds topping 160 mph - the strongest hurricane on record to make landfall there. With devastating force and 155mph winds the storm hit the U.S. territory of Puerto Rico as a Category 4 hurricane on September 20, 2017. Puerto Rico had not yet fully recovered from Hurricane Irma, which pummeled the island with high winds just two weeks earlier. On Puerto Rico widespread property destruction took place with many structures leveled. The hurricane completely destroyed the island's power grid, leaving all 3.4 million residents without electricity. All communication networks were crippled across the island. Ninety-five percent of cell networks were down. Approximately 80 percent of the territory's agriculture was lost due to the hurricane, with agricultural losses estimated at $780 million. Seven months after the hurricane, the island's healthcare system was still slowly recovering and facing many challenges. Maria caused an estimated $90 billion in damage in Puerto Rico, Florida, and the U.S. Virgin Islands.

as cosmic rays from the sun or from man-made sources such as televisions, microwave ovens, or certain diagnostic tests such as x-ray examinations. Exposures such as these present no health risk to humans. In contrast, **ionizing radiation** can damage our DNA and cause health effects when humans are exposed to sufficiently high doses. There are three basic types of ionizing radiation: alpha, beta, and gamma (Fig. 71.4).

Alpha radiation is a stream of positively charged particles that travel only about an inch in the air. They have no penetration power past the keratinized layer of the skin and can be stopped by thin clothing or a sheet of notebook paper. However, if ingested, inhaled, or introduced into an open wound, alpha radiation can be very damaging because of the energy transfer to the "delicate" cells of the lungs or internal organs.

Beta radiation is a stream of electrons that can be stopped by a few millimeters of aluminum but can penetrate up to a centimeter into human tissue. Large quantities of beta particles impinging on the skin can damage the basal layer of the skin and cause what are commonly referred to as *radiation burns*. As with alpha particles, if the radioactive atoms that emit beta particles are ingested or inhaled, they can cause biological damage.

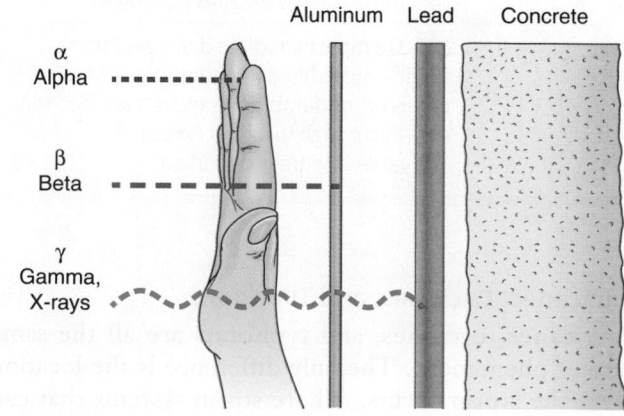

FIGURE 71.4 Radiation penetration.

Gamma radiation is similar to x-rays as it can penetrate the whole body, but unlike x-rays they are more radioactive and can kill cells. Because of its high penetrability, gamma radiation can deliver radiation doses to the internal organs as well as the skin, resulting in damage.

Means of Exposure

Irradiation is the act of "exposing" something or someone to radiation. A person is irradiated when he or she is "exposed" to ionizing radiation from a source outside the body (Fig. 71.5). There is no transfer of radioactive material from the environment to the body, and the person poses no radiological hazard to anyone else. Being exposed to external radiation does not make a person radioactive.

Contamination occurs when people have radioactive material on or in them. A person is externally contaminated when material that contains radioactive atoms is deposited on the skin, clothing, or anywhere it is not desired. A person externally contaminated with radioactive materials will be irradiated until the source of radiation (the radioactive material) is removed from the body, clothing, or wound. Decontamination is typically performed to remove external contamination.

A person is **internally contaminated** if radioactive material is breathed, swallowed, or absorbed through wounds. Treatment for internal contamination includes gastric lavage, cathartics, blocking the uptake to the thyroid by administering potassium iodide, excision of the wound to minimize absorption, dilution, altering the chemistry of the substance, chelation (binding of ions and molecules to render a harmful agent inactive or facilitate excretion), or bronchoalveolar lavage.

Radiation Effects. Radiation can affect the body in a number of ways. The adverse health effects of exposure may not be apparent for many years and can range from mild to serious. Mild effects include skin reddening, and serious effects include cancer and death, depending on the amount of radiation absorbed by the body, the type of radiation, the route of exposure, and the length of time a person was exposed. Exposure to very large doses of radiation may cause death within a few hours or days. Exposure to lower doses of radiation may lead to an increased risk of developing cancer or to other adverse health effects later in life.

If there is a radiation emergency in the United States, local authorities monitor the levels of radiation and determine what protective actions people should take. The appropriate action will depend on the situation. If the radiation emergency involves the release of large amounts of radioactive materials, officials may advise people to "shelter in place," which means to stay in their home or office, or they may be advised to move to another more safe location. It is often less risky to stay inside than to try to evacuate.

There are two types of radiation injury: local radiation injury and acute radiation syndrome. Most radiation injuries are "local" injuries frequently involving only the hands. An acute local injury may occur separately or may coexist with acute radiation syndrome. Local radiation injury patients present with a skin lesion without a history of chemical or thermal burn, an insect bite, or a history of skin disease or allergy. The patient may give a history of possible radiation exposure (such as from a radiography source, x-ray device, or accelerator) or a history of finding and handling an unknown metallic object. Local injuries to the skin, especially the hands, evolve very slowly over time, and symptoms may not manifest for days to weeks after the exposure. The nurse may note the presence of any of the following: erythema, blistering, dry or wet desquamation, epilation, or ulceration.

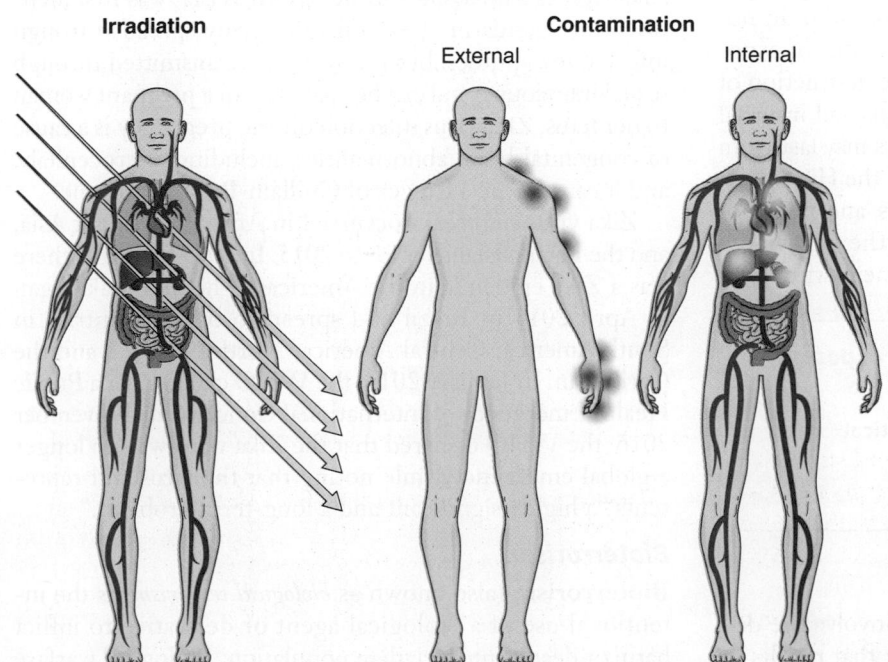

Irradiation

Contamination
External   Internal

FIGURE 71.5 Illustration of radiation exposure. Irradiation: There is no transfer of radioactive material from the environment to the body. External contamination: Radioactive material is deposited on clothing or skin Internal contamination: Radioactive material is breathed, swallowed, or ingested internally.

Conventional wound management is usually ineffective in these cases.

Acute radiation syndrome (ARS) is an acute illness caused by irradiation of the whole body (or a significant portion of it). It follows a somewhat predictable course and is characterized by signs and symptoms that are manifestations of cellular deficiencies and the reactions of various cells, tissues, and organ systems to ionizing radiation. The initial clinical manifestations are nonspecific and may be indistinguishable from those of other illnesses. They include nausea, vomiting, anorexia, diarrhea, fever, and possible mild skin erythema. These symptoms will start within minutes to days after the exposure, will last for minutes to several days, and may come and go. The person usually looks and feels healthy for a short time, after which he or she will become sick again with loss of appetite, fatigue, fever, nausea, vomiting, diarrhea, and possibly even seizures and coma. This seriously ill stage may last from a few hours to several months followed by recovery or death. Each phase of the illness varies in length relative to the radiation dose received. Early onset of anorexia, nausea, vomiting, and malaise is an indication of a high dose of exposure.

People with ARS also typically have some skin damage. This damage may become evident within a few hours after exposure and includes swelling, itching, and redness of the skin (like a bad sunburn). There also can be hair loss. As with other symptoms, the skin may heal for a short time, but this is followed by the return of swelling, itching, and redness days or weeks later. Complete healing of the skin may take from several weeks to a few years depending on the radiation dose the person's skin received. The medical management of ARS is focused mainly on support and recovery of the hematological system. Two major aims are to prevent neutropenia and sepsis.

The chance of survival for people with ARS decreases with increasing radiation doses. Most people who do not recover from ARS will die within several months of exposure. The cause of death in most cases is the destruction of the bone marrow, which results in infections and internal bleeding. For survivors, the recovery process may last from several weeks to 2 years. Many survivors of the Hiroshima and Nagasaki atomic bombs in the 1940s and many of the firefighters who first responded after the Chernobyl Nuclear Power Plant accident in 1986 became ill with ARS.

> ⚠️ **Safety Alert** **Principles for minimizing exposure to radiation**
> - Stay as far away from the source as is practical
> - Use appropriate shielding
> - Limit exposure time

Infectious Disease Disaster

Infectious disease disasters are events that involve the dissemination of a biological agent or disease that results in mass causalities. The occurrence of **emerging infectious diseases (EID)** or remerging infectious diseases in human history is not new. The great plague and the influenza pandemics are well-known historical examples. Humans are in a delicate balance with the microbial coinhabitants of the earth. There will always be emerging pathogens that may cause the next big infectious disease disaster. Emerging infections can be considered an MCI if large numbers of people are affected. Recent examples include Ebola and the Zika virus.

Ebola Virus Disease

Ebola virus disease (EVD) is a rare and deadly disease caused by the Ebola virus. It was first discovered in 1976 near the Ebola River in what is now the Democratic Republic of Congo. Since then, the virus has been infecting people from time to time, leading to outbreaks in several African countries. The Ebola virus spreads to people through direct contact with the body fluids of a person who is sick with or has died from EVD. The virus can also spread to people through direct contact with the blood, body fluids, and tissues of infected fruit bats or primates. Symptoms may appear anywhere from 2 to 21 days after contact with the virus, with an average of 8 to 10 days.

The 2014-2016 Ebola outbreak in West Africa began in a rural setting of southeastern Guinea, spread to urban areas and across borders within weeks to become a global **epidemic**. From 2014 through 2016 there were 28,652 cases of Ebola and 11,325 Ebola deaths. The 2014-2016 Ebola outbreak is a dramatic illustration of the threat of EID. It is also an example of an evolving public health crisis of international concern. The U.S. government took a number of steps to address the 2014-2016 EVD outbreak. One of them resulted in the construction of several **biocontainment units (BCUs)** or Ebola treatment centers across the US.

Zika Virus

Zika virus is a mosquito-borne flavivirus that was first identified in Uganda in 1947. Zika primarily spreads through infected mosquitoes, but it can also be transmitted through sexual intercourse and can be passed from a pregnant woman to her fetus. Zika virus infection during pregnancy is a cause of congenital brain abnormalities, including microcephaly, and it can also be a trigger of Guillain-Barré syndrome.

Zika virus outbreaks occurred in Africa, Southeast Asia, and the Pacific Islands prior to 2015. In 2015 and 2016 there was a Zika epidemic in the Americas. The outbreak began in April 2015 in Brazil and spread to other countries in South America, Central America, North America, and the Caribbean. In January 2016, the WHO called Zika a Public Health Emergency of International Concern. By November 2016, the WHO declared that the Zika virus was no longer a global emergency while noting that the virus still represents "a highly significant and a long-term problem."

Bioterrorism

Bioterrorism (also known as *biological terrorism*) is the intentional use of a biological agent or derivative to inflict harm or death onto a civilian population. Biological warfare differs from bioterrorism in that the target of the attack is military personnel.

Bioterrorism and biological warfare are ancient in its origins, dating back to at least 1346 when Tartar invaders laid siege to the city of Kaffa on the Black Sea. Plague broke out among the invaders. Using catapults designed to throw boulders and fireballs over the walls, the Tartar invaders launched the plague-infected corpses of their dead men into the city. The bodies were quickly dumped into the sea, but the damage was done. Hoping to escape the quickly spreading disease, four ships departed from Kaffa and sailed to Italy. When the ships reached Italy, many sailors onboard were sick, causing the plague to quickly spread throughout Europe. By the time the **pandemic** played itself out 3 years later, between 25% and 35% of Europe's population had fallen victim to the disease.

Bioterrorism has the potential to result in high morbidity and mortality. Organisms and toxins that can be used as biological weapons have been categorized by the CDC into three categories. Agents classified as Category A are easily disseminated or transmitted. They can result in high mortality rates, have the potential for a major public health impact, may cause public panic and social disruption, and may require special action by public health officials. Category B and C agents, although still concerning, are less easily disseminated and result in lower morbidity and mortality rates. A renewed sense of appreciation of the potential of biological weapons came following the anthrax-contaminated letters sent in the United States in late 2001.

Chemical Incidents

Today there are nearly 100,000 known commercial chemicals, and worldwide chemical production is estimated at 400 million tons per year. The CDC divides chemicals into categories by the effects they can have on people exposed to them. Some of these chemicals can cause death by interfering with the nervous system; some inhibit breathing and lead to asphyxiation. Others have caustic effects on contact. Chemical injuries also may accompany and complicate the treatment of conventional injuries in trauma patients. Additionally, exposure can complicate or trigger existing illnesses such as asthma. As a result, treatment of exposure can be complicated. Also, depending on what chemical is encountered, healthcare providers may need to wear different **personal protective equipment (PPE)**, for example, a simple mask and gloves versus a special chemical protection suit and breathing apparatus.

A chemical incident usually involves the release of a vapor or liquid. The type and volume of the agent released is important in determining the type and volume of injuries. An outdoor vapor cloud release is quickly dissipated by the wind and may result in a small number of casualties at the release site. An agent dispersed indoors does not dissipate as easily and can lead to a greater number of casualties. Temperature, humidity, and the type of terrain can also affect the dispersal and the number of casualties. Incidents involving chemicals can be nonintentional/accidental or

intentional. Nonintentional chemical incidents leading to an MCI can occur during the manufacture, storage, or transport of chemical agents (Box 71.4). An intentional chemical disaster is defined as the intentional release or spill of toxic chemicals to harm people and/or the environment (Box 71.5). Some of these compounds can be potential WMDs if used by terrorists.

The early detection of a chemical event is critical, but not all chemical events are immediately apparent. Clues to the detection of a chemical event are (1) a rapid onset of symptoms in patients; (2) large numbers of patients presenting with common symptoms; (3) low-lying clouds or vapors; (4) dying animals or insects; (5) unexplained odors; and (6) concentrations of dead, dying, or sick people at the scene.

Explosions and Blast Events

Explosions occur when a solid or liquid material is rapidly transformed into a gas, and energy is released. The gas expands outward in a high-pressure blast wave that exceeds the speed of sound. Air is highly compressed on the leading edge of the wave, creating a shock or **blast front**. The body of the wave and the associated mass outward movement of ambient air, the **blast wind**, follows the front. Explosive events can occur as a result of an intentional or unintentional incident. Blast trauma from explosives varies greatly depending on the environment (indoors or outdoors), the structural characteristics of the building or vehicle, the presence of reflecting surfaces, and the distance from the blast. **Primary blast injury** is a result of barotrauma, unique to explosions, which causes damage to air-filled organs—the lungs (hemothorax, pneumothorax), gastrointestinal tract (bowel perforation), and auditory system (tympanic membrane rupture). **Secondary blast injuries** refer to trauma caused by projectiles carried by the blast pressure wave

---

Box 71.4 Nonintentional Release in Bhopal, India

A nonintentional chemical event occurred on the evening of December 2–3, 1984, at the Union Carbide plant in Bhopal, India (population 900,000). Approximately 27 tons of methyl isocyanate were accidentally released into the atmosphere. The atmospheric conditions resulted in a gas cloud that moved slowly and relatively close to the ground. The cloud quickly covered the homes of a large number of residents. The release is estimated to have killed at least 3,500 people immediately, and thousands more are said to have since died or been injured as a result of the toxic cloud. An Indian government affidavit in 2006 stated the leak caused 558,125 injuries. They included 38,478 temporary partial injuries and approximately 3,900 severely and permanently disabling injuries. Many pets, farm animals, and livestock near the scene were also killed. This release has been called the world's single most catastrophic chemical event to date.

Box 71.5 Intentional Release in Matsumoto, Japan

An intentional chemical release occurred on March 20, 1995, in Matsumoto, Japan, a city of 200,000 situated at the foot of the Japanese Alps in the heart of Japan. At the peak of the morning rush hour, the chemical agent sarin was released on five different subway trains scheduled to arrive within 4 minutes of each other at the Kasumigaseki Train Station. Entering the trains carrying packets of sarin and umbrellas with sharpened tips, the perpetrators placed the plastic containers of sarin on the floor and then punctured them several times with the sharpened tip of an umbrella. The men then quickly exited the trains and the stations.

Sarin is a volatile nerve agent, which means that it can easily and quickly evaporate from a liquid into a vapor and spread into the environment. People can be exposed to the vapor even if they do not come in contact with the liquid form of sarin. With the punctured packets left on the floor, the sarin was allowed to leak out into the train cars and evaporate. The sarin affected passengers, subway workers, and anyone in the immediate vicinity. Those affected by the sarin experienced a variety of symptoms including bleeding from the nose and mouth, seizures, difficulty breathing, loss of consciousness, nausea and vomiting, and vision problems. Witnesses said that "the subway entrances resembled battlefields." In many cases, the injured simply lay on the ground, many with breathing difficulties. Several of those affected were exposed to sarin only by helping those who had been directly exposed.

Following the event, 4,930 people were seen at Tokyo's hospitals, and of that number, 1,100 were admitted to the hospitals. There were 12 deaths as a result of the attack. The initial report to the hospitals was that there had been a "gas explosion," and hospitals prepared to receive patients with burns and carbon monoxide poisoning. St. Luke's Hospital, closest to the scene, received more than 600 patients within the first 24 hours; of these, 5 patients were in critical condition, 3 were in cardiac arrest, and 2 were unconscious. Because it was not identified initially as a chemical event, no personal protective equipment was worn by the rescuers or the hospital personnel, and no decontamination occurred. This resulted in 10% of the prehospital workers and 23% of the hospital staff experiencing some symptoms (cross-contamination) of sarin exposure.

common weapon is the **dirty bomb**. A dirty bomb is any explosive device that intentionally releases a secondary agent. The secondary agent can be any hazardous (chemical, radiological) or infectious (biological) agent. **Improvised explosive devices (IEDs)** are conventional explosive devices deployed in an unconventional fashion such as a suicide bombing.

Mass Shooting Events/Active Shooters

Mass shootings are man-made disasters. The agreed-upon definition of an active shooter by U.S. government agencies—including the White House, U.S. Department of Justice/FBI, U.S. Department of Education, and U.S. Department of Homeland Security/Federal Emergency Management Agency—is "an individual actively engaged in killing or attempting to kill people in a confined and populated area." In most cases, active shooters use firearms, and there is no pattern or method to their selection of victims.

Active shooter situations are unpredictable and evolve quickly. Typically, the immediate deployment of law enforcement is required to stop the shooting and mitigate harm to victims. Active shooters usually will continue to move throughout buildings or areas until stopped by law enforcement, suicide, or other intervention.

The definition above does not include shootings tied to gang disputes or robberies that went awry, and it does not include shootings that took place in private homes. In an active shooter event, the people who are killed come from every race, religion and socioeconomic background. Their ages range from the unborn to the elderly. Shootings occur without warning in the most mundane places. Most of the victims are chosen not for what they have done but simply for where they happen to be. Mass shootings in America appear to be getting deadlier and happening more frequently (Box 71.6). Some have said "it feels like they've taken hold like a virus."

Connection Check 71.4

Several patients present to the triage nurse in an ED. They are complaining of skin redness, itching, vomiting, and diarrhea. What does the nurse suspect the patients have been exposed to?
A. Radiation
B. Chemical agents
C. Influenza
D. Biotoxin agent

CURRENT CONCEPTS IN DISASTER PREPAREDNESS AND RESPONSE

penetrating any body part. **Tertiary blast injuries** are caused by the individual being propelled by the blast wave and thrown into an object or when a structure collapses and causes injury. Other injuries, quaternary injuries, include exacerbations or complications of preexisting illnesses or injuries as a result of the blast such as burns.

Today's terrorists and insurgents are deploying unique devices and using various delivery tactics for explosives. One

The first response to a disaster is the responsibility of the local government's emergency services, supplemented by neighboring communities and volunteer agencies. If

Box 71.6 Mass Shooting Events

Recent Deadly Shootings

February 14, 2018 – Parkland, Florida – gunfire at a High School – 17 people killed, 12 injured

November 5, 2017 – Sutherland Springs, Texas – gunfire at a small church – 26 people killed, 20 wounded.

October 1, 2017 – Las Vegas, Nevada – gunfire into a crowd of 22,000 at a concert – 58 people killed and 546 injured.

June 12, 2016 – Orlando, Florida – gunfire inside a nightclub, – 49 people killed and 58 injured.

December 2, 2015 – San Bernardino, California – gunfire at an employee gathering – 14 killed, 22 injured.

December 14, 2012 – Newtown, Connecticut – gunfire at an Elementary School – 26 killed (20 children, ages six and seven), 2 injured.

overwhelmed, the local government can turn to the state for assistance. The state responds with state resources such as the National Guard and other state agencies. The state's governor, not the U.S. president, is primarily responsible for the health and welfare of the respective citizens. The governor possesses broad police powers that include the legal authority to order evacuations, commandeer private property, require quarantine, and take other actions to protect public safety. If needed, a state can request outside assistance from other states through the **Emergency Management Assistance Compact (EMAC)**. If they are available, the assisting states can provide resources such as National Guard or medical personnel.

If the disaster event is clearly more than the state and local governments can handle alone, the governor of the affected state may request federal assistance. Federal resources can be mobilized through FEMA. The agency can assist with search and rescue, electrical power, food, water, shelter, and other basic human needs. If FEMA assistance is needed, the agency will evaluate the request and recommend an action to the White House based on the disaster, the local community, and the state's ability to recover. The president can either approve or deny the request. This decision process can take a few hours or several weeks, depending on the nature of the disaster. A governor's request for a major disaster declaration could mean an infusion of federal funds into the state, but the governor of the state must also commit significant state funds and resources to the recovery efforts. If a Presidential Major Disaster Declaration is declared, funding comes from the president's Disaster Relief Fund, which is managed by FEMA, and from disaster aid programs of other participating federal agencies. A Presidential Major Disaster Declaration puts into motion long-term federal recovery programs, some of which are matched by state programs, and is designed to help disaster victims, businesses, and public entities.

National Response Framework

In recent years, the United States has faced an unprecedented series of disasters and emergencies. In October 2011, the first-ever National Preparedness Goal was released. The national goal is "to have a secure and resilient Nation with the capabilities required across the whole community to prevent, protect against, mitigate, respond to, and recover from the threats and hazards that pose the greatest risk to the nation." This goal recognizes the reality that the entire community including the public and private sectors, faith-based and nonprofit organizations, and the general public must continue to work together to build a more prepared and resilient nation. Our national response structures have evolved and improved to meet this goal. The National Response Framework, written in 2008 and revised in 2016, is the disaster plan for the nation. This document establishes a comprehensive, national, all-hazards approach to domestic incident response, from the smallest incident to the largest catastrophe. The framework identifies the key response principles as well as the roles and structures that support the plan. Additionally, it describes special circumstances in which the federal government exercises a larger role in a disaster response, including incidents in which federal interests are involved and catastrophic incidents in which a state requires significant support. The response plan lays the groundwork for first responders, decision makers, and supporting entities to provide a unified national response.

Assessing Risk and Vulnerability

The first step in disaster planning is the development of a **hazard vulnerability analysis (HVA)** and risk assessment. The HVA is an assessment of the risks and consequences of a disaster or critical event occurring in the community. A list of all potential hazards and threats in the region is compiled. The list may be quite lengthy and will vary depending on the location. Factors that should be considered when developing the list include historical records, input from local emergency managers and healthcare providers, and the presence of high-risk local industries, rail lines, stadiums, and airports. Communities should pay special attention to targets of high value to terrorists, including historical monuments. Each hazard is then given a ranking of low, medium, or high probability of occurrence.

Next, the potential consequences of the event are evaluated and rated as high, medium, or low consequence. Things to consider include potential injuries, loss of life, disruption of services, loss of community trust, and business continuity issues. The data can then be put into a matrix that defines the probable events and consequences as high, medium, or low. Disaster planners will then use this grid for planning purposes.

Disaster Phases

Disasters do not just appear one day and go away the next. Rather, they have an occurrence cycle. This cycle entails a series of management phases that include strategies to mitigate hazards and prepare for, respond to, and recover from disasters and their effects (Fig. 71.6).

Mitigation

Mitigation includes activities that eliminate or reduce the chance of occurrence or the effects of an event if it occurs. Disaster mitigation programs have shown that communities can do a lot to prevent major emergencies or disasters from affecting them negatively. If communities cannot prevent disasters, they can at least reduce the damaging impact, for example, requiring roof reinforcements to reduce damage from hurricane winds or passing legislation that prevents new construction in floodplains.

Preparedness

Preparedness, the next phase, is planning how to respond when an emergency or disaster occurs. This step builds an organization's capacity to manage the effects of an event should it occur. These activities help to save lives and minimize damage by preparing people to respond appropriately. Examples include disaster drills, evacuation plans, and fire drills.

Response

Response covers the period during and immediately following a disaster. During this phase, emergency responders and public officials provide emergency assistance to victims of the event and try to reduce the likelihood of further damage.

Recovery

Recovery begins almost concurrently with response activities and is directed at restoring essential services and resuming normal operations. This phase may require a large amount of time, money, and resources.

Incident Command System

The initial challenges met by those responding to a disaster are "how to rapidly gain control of the chaos at the scene," be it in the field or in the hospital ED. The second challenge is how to rapidly organize the personnel resources into a hierarchy of command. This process is referred to as establishing command and control. The **incident command system (ICS)** is an organizational tool that is used to provide the management infrastructure to support any disaster response. The structure is the same regardless of the nature of the disaster. Fig. 71.7 illustrates the hierarchical structure of the ICS.

The ICS is modular and can be expanded or contracted according to the changing needs of the disaster response. The structure is built around five major management activities/functions required in a disaster setting regardless of size or type. The functions are command, operations, planning, logistics, and finance/administration. For some terrorist incidents, a sixth role, intelligence gathering, may be added. Each function is headed by a section chief, and the overall response is led by an incident commander. The ideal span of control is three people, and the maximum is seven persons. Additional functions that aid in the response include liaison, public information, and safety/security. Table 71.6 explains the ICS's roles and responsibilities.

Connection Check 71.5

An ICS is set up at the scene of a disaster. Who has the responsibility for keeping ahead of the disaster by evaluating the status of the resources and determining future resource needs?
A. Incident commander
B. Planning chief
C. Operations chief
D. Logistics chief

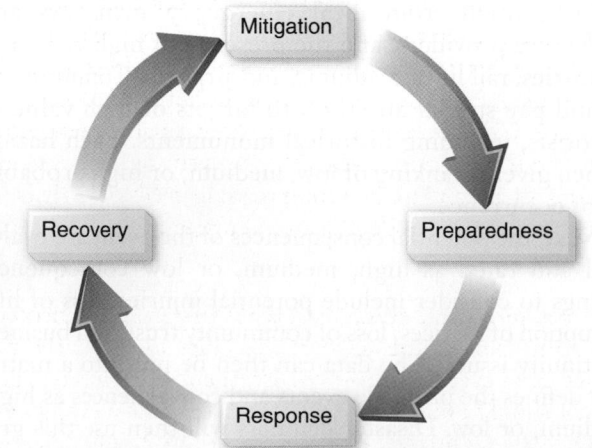

FIGURE 71.6 Disaster cycle. Mitigation: activities that eliminate or reduce the chance of occurrence or the effects of an event if it occurs. Preparedness: planning how to respond when an emergency or disaster occurs. Response: emergency assistance to victims of the event. Recovery: activities directed at restoring essential services and resuming normal operations.

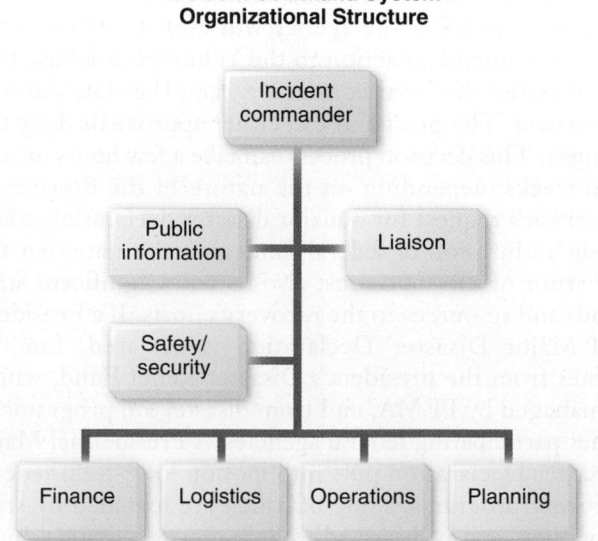

FIGURE 71.7 Disaster incident command organization.

Table 71.6 The Incident Command System

Role	Responsibilities
Incident commander	Responsible for all aspects of the response. This person has the overall authority and responsibility for the entire operation; develops the incident objectives and manages all incident operations. Four section chiefs report to the incident commander. Each section chief is part of the general staff and supervises a team of responders.
Operations chief	Responsible for all tactical operations, including decontamination, rescue/extrication, triage, treatment, transportation, communication, and medical control.
Planning chief	Responsible for continuously evaluating the response and "keeping ahead of the disaster"; maintains resource status, evaluates future resource needs and personnel, maintains all incident records, develops the strategy and action plans with the incident commander for the other section chiefs to implement.
Logistics section chief	Responsible for obtaining and providing services and resources, obtaining equipment needed, and staff support.
Finance/Administration chief	Responsible for documenting all financial costs of the incident including the cost of recovery for services and supplies.
Public information officer	A member of the command staff who is responsible for advising the incident commander on all public information matters relating to the management of the incident. This person also manages the media, public inquiries, warnings, rumor monitoring, and other functions required to gather, verify, coordinate, and disseminate accurate, accessible, and timely information related to the incident.
Safety/Security officer	A member of the command staff who is responsible for monitoring and assessing personnel hazards and unsafe situations.
Liaison officer	A command staff position who acts as the on-scene contact point for assisting agencies.

HOSPITAL RESPONSE TO A DISASTER

Disasters come in all shapes and sizes, and hospitals need to be prepared to respond to virtually any type of event. Some disasters impact a small number of people, produce a few critically injured patients, and put intense demands on the hospital for a short period of time. Others may involve a large number of casualties over the course of several weeks. For disasters such as hurricanes and floods, hospitals are likely to receive advanced warning and are able to activate their disaster plan before the event. For disasters such as earthquakes, tsunamis, chemical plant explosions, industrial accidents, building collapses, and acts of terrorism, there is no advanced warning system. Regardless of the warning, all disaster scenarios carry with them the possibility of many injured patients.

The overall response to a disaster used to focus just on rescuing victims at the scene of the disaster and delivering these victims to the hospital. It was assumed hospitals would always be there, ready to receive all victims. However, the events of September 11, 2001, the anthrax incidents in 2001, and the 2002/2003 SARS cases changed the rules that defined hospital disaster preparedness and response. Following Hurricane Katrina in 2005 and the 2009 H1N1 pandemic, the rules changed again. Currently, disaster preparedness in hospitals is shifting yet again to include internal workplace violence concerns, active shooters, and strategies surrounding Emerging Infectious Diseases. Hospitals need to be accessible, prepared, and functioning at maximum capacity so that they are ready to respond to both external and internal events.

Hospital Preparedness

Hospital preparedness for an MCI is a daunting task. Unique issues must be considered with each type of event. For example, a hospital response to a new highly infectious influenza virus is entirely different from the response to a chemical explosion. It is these differences that hold challenging implications for hospitals. Effectively planning an emergency response requires hospitals to address many details such as staff safety and availability of PPE, decontamination equipment and processes, surge capacity, evacuation plans, addressing mental health or psychosocial issues, debriefing plans, and maintaining readiness. Box 71.7 lists the many important details in hospital preparedness.

Personal Protective Equipment

Personal protective equipment (PPE) is a means of protecting staff from hazardous materials (Fig. 71.8). At the first notice of an event, the hospital emergency planner or safety officer should evaluate the potential hazardous exposure of employees and provide the appropriate PPE. The selection of the appropriate PPE is a complex process and is based on a hazard assessment that (1) identifies the hazards or suspected hazards; (2) identifies the routes of entry of the potential hazard (inhalation, skin absorption, ingestion, and eye or skin contact); and (3) defines the performance of the

Box 71.7 Hospital Preparedness

Disaster plans should address the following:

- Staff safety/personal protective equipment
- Decontamination equipment and processes
- Surge capacity
- Mental health
- Lockdown procedures
- Mass fatality management
- Evacuation
- Altered standards of care
- Allocation of scarce resources
- Mass employee medication prophylaxis
- Internal utility failure
- Workplace violence including active shooters
- Bomb threats
- Civil unrest

PPE materials in providing a barrier to these hazards. The potential exposure of hospital staff is usually a result of proximity to or contact with a patient whose skin and/or clothing may be contaminated with a hazardous substance.

Level A PPE

Level A is the highest level of respiratory, eye, mucous membrane, and skin protection. This level provides protection against gas, vapor, liquid, and oxygen-deficient atmospheres. It includes a totally encapsulating chemical protective suit, often called a "moon suit," with a self-contained breathing apparatus (SCBA), gloves, and boots. This level should be selected when the hazards are unknown or unquantifiable or when the greatest level of protection is required. It provides full protection against liquids and vapors. Generally, this level is not appropriate for hospital staff.

Level B PPE

Level B provides the greatest level of respiratory protection but a lower level of skin protection than Level A. It differs from Level A in that the suit is not fully encapsulated and airtight, but it provides splash protection against liquids.

This level should be selected when the highest level of respiratory protection is necessary, but a lesser level of skin protection is needed. Level B consists of an SCBA, nonencapsulated chemical-resistant garments, gloves, and boots.

Level C PPE

Level C provides the same skin protection as Level B but a lesser level of respiratory protection than Levels A and B. Level C consists of a nonencapsulated chemical-resistant suit (splash protection), air-purifying respirator (APR), gloves, and boots. Level C is used when the type of airborne exposure is known to be guarded against adequately by an APR.

Level D PPE

Level D PPE consists of a surgical gown, mask, and gloves. It provides no additional protection for respiratory or splash hazards, only minimal protection for nuisance contamination.

Decontamination

Decontamination is the reduction or removal of contaminating material from a person or equipment by water and mechanical processes. All hospitals must have the capability to provide some form of patient decontamination. Eliminating contaminants from a patient's skin and clothing is important because it reduces the risk for further absorption or inhalation and helps to prevent others from becoming secondarily exposed or contaminated. During the decontamination procedure, the patient must be monitored for signs of decomposition. Antidotes or other medications may need to be given.

There are three goals for patient decontamination. First, hospitals must not allow contaminated patients to enter the facility. Hospital security staff needs to lock down the entrances and exits in order to protect patients and staff. Ideally, when medically appropriate, patients should be decontaminated at the incident scene. However, complete on-incident scene decontamination may not be possible because of the medical condition of the patient as well as weather conditions and equipment availability. This may

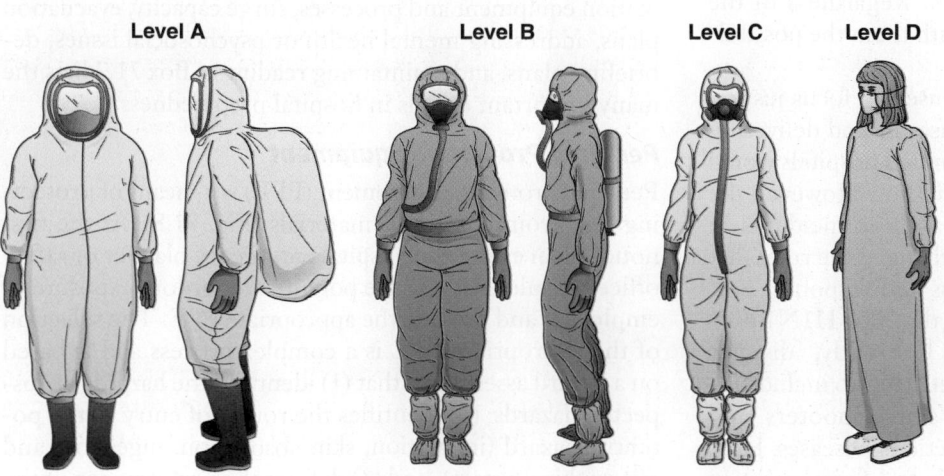

FIGURE 71.8 Levels of personal protective equipment. Level A provides the highest level of respiratory, eye, mucous membrane, and skin protection. Level B provides the highest level of respiratory protection but a lower level of skin protection. Level C provides the same skin protection as Level B but a lower level of respiratory protection. Level D protects from nuisance exposure with mask, gown, and gloves.

require that decontamination sites and triage station be set up immediately outside the hospital ED. If needed, decontamination is carried out prior to triage. This arrangement is essential for security and safety reasons. Second, hospitals should decontaminate patients as rapidly as possible. This means the decontamination equipment must be easily deployable and the staff trained to set it up. Third, hospitals must plan to protect the decontamination team from secondary exposure and injury. This includes having enough decontamination suits, respirators, boots, and gloves on hand to sustain the facility for at least 24 hours with a cadre of staff rotating through the process.

Patient decontamination includes the following procedures:

- Remove the patient's clothing. In general, removing and bagging a patient's clothing eliminates 60% to 90% of the contaminants.
- Wet the patient's skin and wash with soap and water for 5 to 10 minutes. Gentle cleaning of the skin with soap and a soft cloth removes any remaining contaminants.
- Pay special attention to hair, face, hands, and other areas that were exposed but were not covered by clothing.
- Follow washing by a copious rinsing of the patient with tepid water.

Additional elements of decontamination include:

- Determining the level of PPE required for staff to wear.
- Controlling access to the decontamination site as well as the hospital.
- Having a container ready to receive contaminated clothing, valuables, and contaminated supplies.
- Ensuring screens are available for patient privacy.
- Ensuring a collection system for water runoff is available if needed.

The degree of decontamination performed depends on the situation. Anyone suspected of being acutely exposed to or contaminated by a toxic material—whether it is chemical, biological, or radiological—should be provided adequate decontamination.

Surge Capacity

Surge capacity has been defined as the ability of a healthcare system to "expand rapidly and to obtain adequate staff, beds, supplies, and equipment to provide sufficient care to meet the immediate needs of an influx of patients following a large-scale incident or disaster. Hospitals should have surge capacity plans in order to diffuse this imbalance of supply and demand.

Hospital Evacuations

In the traditional approach to disasters, hospitals are viewed as sources of medical care for victims. However, it is important to remember that hospitals also are vulnerable to disasters and may need to close or evacuate depending on the circumstances. Evacuations may be necessary due to fire or damage from a natural disaster such as a hurricane, earthquake or flood. The decision to evacuate a hospital should

be based on the ability of the hospital to meet the medical needs of the patients. Hospitals should have in place plans for either a full or partial evacuation and those plans should be consistent with regulatory requirements. A full evacuation of a hospital should generally be considered a last resort. There are two types of hospital evacuations: "advanced warning events" and "no advanced warning events."

Advanced Warning Events

Hurricanes are the most common example of an advanced warning event. For example, several New Orleans hospitals evacuated their patients prior to Hurricane Katrina in 2005, and in September of 2017 at least 35 hospitals in Florida, Georgia, and South Carolina either closed entirely or ordered partial or complete evacuations ahead of Hurricane Irma.

With advanced warning events, the hospital incident commander has time prior to the event to make a decision but must remember there is a limited opportunity to evacuate. As the event draws nearer, the opportunity for a safe evacuation diminishes. Evacuation requires consideration of two factors: (1) the nature of the event, including its expected arrival time, magnitude, area of impact, and duration; and (2) the anticipated effects on both the hospital and the community. Once notified of an impending disaster, the hospital incident commander may decide to (1) preemptively evacuate the hospital while the hospital structure and surrounding environment are not yet compromised or (2) **shelter in place (SIP).** Sheltering in place is defined as "the need to take immediate shelter in a current location. Shelter in place (SIP) is a rapid and effective way to protect the hospital occupants from an external or internal threat. External threats include: civil unrest or a chemical release. Internal threats include infrastructure damage from an earthquake, flood, or tornado. Since SIP plans will differ depending on the type of event it is important to have plans that are flexible and scalable. Plans should also define what happens to those persons "locked out" when the hospital is "locked down." If the decision is made to shelter in place, as soon as possible after the event, the building's integrity, including the availability of critical utilities (water, sewer, electricity, and heating systems) requires assessment. The utilities must be assessed to determine whether the hospital can continue to provide safe, appropriate medical care or if a postevent evacuation may still be necessary. For example, following Hurricane Katrina, some New Orleans hospitals that did not evacuate prior to the event lost city water, lost all power, or were unable to ensure the safety of patients and staff in the midst of civil unrest. In this case, it was not the hurricane or the subsequent flood that caused the incident commander to order the evacuation, rather it was the damage to city infrastructures and the conditions in the surrounding community.

No Advanced Warning Events

No advanced warning events include earthquakes, building fires, tornadoes, and explosions. Decisions must often be made very quickly in the midst of the disaster or immediately afterward.

Evacuation

Regardless of the warning, successful hospital evacuation requires the symphonic coordination of personnel, transportation, communication and the tracking of patients and materials. Additional considerations during an evacuation include:

- *Sequences of the evacuation*: The most medically fragile and resource-intensive patients are usually evacuated first, as soon as appropriate transportation and staff are available. However, in cases in which all patients are in immediate danger and evacuation must be conducted as quickly as possible, some suggest that the most mobile patients should be evacuated first.
- *Urgency of the evacuation:* It is important to distinguish between an orderly and planned evacuation, in which there is time to move patients in a manner that maximizes safety for all, and a "drop-everything-and-go" evacuation, in which patients and staff are in immediate danger and must exit the unit and/or hospital as quickly as possible. Optimal procedures for safely moving patients may be abandoned in favor of the fastest possible egress.
- *Extent of the evacuation:* A hospital evacuation will be planned differently depending on whether the entire area/community is being evacuated or just one hospital. If just one hospital is being evacuated (e.g., because of a fire), patients can be more easily dispersed among nearby hospitals. In most metro areas, the transport would be for a distance of less than 10 miles, and ambulances could cycle back and forth moving patients.
- *Condition of hospital infrastructure:* Although unlikely to be a problem during an "orderly and planned" evacuation, egress from a hospital may be severely constrained during a "drop-everything-and-go" evacuation. Stairwells or exits may be obscured by smoke or unavailable because of fire. Stairwells may be dark if backup power has failed. Elevators can also be out of service, lengthening the time required to move all patients out of the hospital.
- *Types of patients:* Highly complex patients—especially intensive care unit and other specialty-care patients—may be difficult to place in the surrounding community.
- *Road conditions:* In a disaster where a community and more than one hospital are affected, evacuating transport destinations may be far away. Traffic-choked highways and the lack of refueling stations preventing ambulances from quickly cycling back for repeated evacuation trips could slow the evacuation process.
- *Transportation resources:* Transportation resources include not only the vehicles but also the staff, equipment, and supplies that must accompany the patient in the vehicle.

If a hospital is either fully or partially evacuated, plans should be in place for repopulation of the facility. These plans should identify safety and operational considerations as well as regulatory agency requirements.

Mental Health Considerations

For every person physically injured in a disaster, there are an estimated 4 to 20 psychological victims. The psychological casualties following a disaster may include those who cared for the victims of the disaster, including prehospital workers, ED staff, social workers, and pastoral care staff. In the aftermath of the September 11, 2001, attacks, the Psychiatric Department at St. Vincent's Medical Center, just one of many healthcare facilities in the area, provided counseling to more than 7,000 patients and received more than 10,000 calls to its help line during the first 2 weeks. Hospitals need to make provisions to accommodate and manage these acute mental health needs.

Debriefing

A postevent disaster debriefing should be held within 24 hours of the disaster response. This debriefing should include all participants in the disaster response. The purpose of the debriefing is to critically analyze all aspects of the response and to identify strengths and areas that need to be improved. Additionally, this debriefing allows hospital leadership to begin to identify staff who may need assistance recovering from the disaster response.

Maintaining Readiness

Hospitals and other healthcare organizations must be prepared to handle a large influx of patients with any level of acuity from any disaster event. Disaster drills or disaster exercises are an integral element of preparedness and should be conducted twice yearly. A *disaster drill* or exercise is a controlled, scenario-driven experience designed to demonstrate and evaluate an organization's capability to execute its Emergency Operations Plan (EOP). The goal during an exercise is to assess disaster processes and staff performance when systems are stressed during a simulated emergency. During the exercise, performance should be critiqued to identify deficiencies and opportunities for improvement facilitating modifications/improvements of the EOP. Disaster drills and exercises should test every aspect of the EOP including:

- Setting up the incident command center
- Receiving casualties
- Triage
- Testing communications systems, both internal and external, with response to agencies, including other healthcare organizations
- Evacuating and transporting patients
- Requesting and receiving emergency supplies
- Staff roles and responsibilities
- Utility management
- Safety and security
- Resources and assets, including the following equipment: decontamination, PPE, transportation, communication, and emergency supplies

> **Safety Alert** To maximize the effectiveness of the drill, inject as much "reality" into the exercise as possible such as volunteer moulaged patients (using makeup to simulate injuries), donning PPE, and testing communication devices and messaging. It is also essential to ensure safety for all participants during the drill. To do this, two key elements must be in place:
> 1. All communications during the drill should start and end with "This is a drill."
> 2. A safety officer with the sole responsibility to monitor and respond to any unsafe situations should be identified.

Connection Check 71.6

Which of the following contributes to a successful hospital disaster response?
A. Aggressive resuscitation efforts for patients without a pulse
B. Immediate response for patients as soon as they arrive at the ED
C. Appropriate PPE to protect staff from contamination
D. Decontamination area located within the ED

NURSE'S ROLE DURING A DISASTER

In the United States, nurses constitute the largest sector of the healthcare workforce and are on the front lines of any disaster response. When a disaster strikes, nurses must be ready and able to respond quickly and competently to the array of sudden new demands for care.

Nursing plays a role in all aspects of disaster preparedness, response, and recovery. Nursing plays a major role in mass casualty triage, helping to ensure patients get the most appropriate level of care. This includes differentiating as quickly and as accurately as possible between physiological victims of the event and the "worried well" and manage each appropriately. Nursing also plays a role in putting disaster response plans into action, evacuation, and decontamination when necessary. Obviously, nursing plays a major role in treatment: patient stabilization, medication administration including antidotes or prophylaxis where necessary, and routine or emergency care as part of the healthcare team, as dictated by the patient's condition. Nursing also provides supportive care and mental health support to victims of the disaster.

A great distracter to a nurse's participation in a disaster response is worrying about family and significant others. Staff members whose roles are considered essential must feel comfortable that their family members know what to do in the event of a disaster. Box 71.8 lists some essential elements to be considered in developing a personal/family disaster plan. Comprehensive family disaster planning information is available from the American Red Cross and FEMA.

Connection Check 71.7

Which of the following items is an essential component of your personal disaster plan?
A. Water
B. Fresh fruit
C. Reading material
D. Hazard flares

Box 71.8 Personal/Family Disaster Planning

Disaster Supply Kit

1. Water for 3 to 5 days (remember water for pets also); a normal person needs 2 quarts of water per day
2. Cans of food
3. Food items such as nuts, dried fruit, and other packaged snacks
4. Blanket, small pillow
5. Inflatable bed (may be used as a float if needed)
6. Closable waterproof plastic bags
7. Backpack for carrying items
8. Battery-operated radio (change the batteries every 6 months)
9. Medications to sustain 14 days
10. Personal hygiene items
11. Extra eyeglasses
12. Manual can opener
13. Flashlight with extra batteries
14. Face masks to protect from dust
15. Traffic flares
16. Duct tape and scissors
17. Whistle
18. Plastic sheeting
19. Work gloves
20. One complete change of cloths
21. Heavy duty plastic garbage bags and ties—for personal sanitation uses—and toilet paper
22. Compass
23. Waterproof matches
24. Waterproof markers (used to write a young child's name, address, phone number, and next of kin number on children's feet)
25. Over-the-counter medications for diarrhea, headache, nausea, and vomiting
26. Basic first aid kit
27. Cell phone charger
28. Water purifier kit
29. Sunscreen and insect repellent
30. Cash

Continued

Box 71.8 Personal/Family Disaster Planning—cont'd

Home

1. Draw a floor plan of your home. Mark two escape routes from each room.
2. Make sure everyone in the household knows how to shut off water, gas, and electricity at the main switches.
3. Post emergency phone numbers by the telephones. Teach children how and when to call 911.
4. Identify two meeting places: The first should be near your home in case of fire; the second should be away from your neighborhood in case you cannot return home
5. Keep car gas tank filled.

Documents*

1. Birth certificates
2. Immunization records

3. Homeowners insurance policy with contact information
4. Health records
5. Driver license copy
6. Complete list of medications
7. Copies of health insurance cards
8. All emergency phone numbers for family
9. List of all credit card numbers

Other

1. Consider ways to help neighbors who may need special assistance, such as the elderly or the disabled
2. Make arrangements for pets. Most pets are not allowed in public shelters
3. Identify an out-of-state family member or friend so all your family members have a single point of contact.

* Consider laminating all documents so they are waterproof

Making Connections

CASE STUDY: WRAP-UP

The response within St. John's Hospital went well. When the tornado warning was issued for Joplin, the hospital activated "Code Gray," its tornado response plan. Staff members simply did what they had to do. Patients were moved into safe areas if possible, and the staff braced for the impact. Very shortly after the tornado passed over the hospital, officials decided that the hospital was unsafe and they needed to quickly evacuate their 183 patients. Because elevators were not operating, patients were carried down up to 10 flights of stairs without overhead lighting or air-conditioning. Staff and visitors carried fragile patients down blackened hallways guided by the dim lights of their cell phones. Patients were carried on backboards, canvas slings, doors, wheelchairs, wooden chairs, sheets, and even sagging mattresses. The hospital did attempt to discharge as many patients as possible, but there was nowhere for these patients to go because of the destruction in the surrounding community and the road conditions.

In moving the patients out of the hospital, the first challenge was knowing where and how to start. The patients needed to get to facilities that could handle their medical conditions.

The roads surrounding the hospital were mostly covered with debris, and the heliport was unusable. Plus, landlines and cell phone towers were destroyed, making communication difficult. Fortunately, the city's other hospital was close and had suffered little damage from the tornado, so it was able to accept patients. Ten hospitals in Missouri also accepted patients from St. John's, as did hospitals in nearby Arkansas, Kansas, and Oklahoma.

The hospital staff loaded patients on pickup trucks and did whatever they could to get them to safety. Dozens of ambulances from towns as far as 100 miles away came to offer assistance. Strangers rushed to the hospital in convoys of pickup trucks to help evacuate patients. Within 90 minutes, all the patients were evacuated, and by 2 a.m., the situation at the hospital was largely under control.

Tragically, in Joplin, despite a 24-minute advanced tornado warning, 160 people died and more than 1,000 were injured. There were a number of people who did all the right things, took shelter in the best available place, but still found themselves in situations that weren't survivable; however, given the scale of destruction in Joplin, it is a wonder that more people were not killed or injured. The tornado offers many important lessons about disaster preparedness. The National Weather Service final report had several observations and recommendations.

First, tornado warning communications should be improved to convey a sense of urgency for extreme events. This will compel people to take immediate lifesaving action. Since the first tornado forecast was made in 1948, tornado warning lead times have been increasing and now average 13 minutes; however, societal response to a tornado warning is highly complex and involves a number of factors, such as risk perception and overall credibility of the warning. There is a 70% false tornado alarm rate. Because of this "tornado warning fatigue," the vast majority of Joplin's residents either ignored or were slow to react to the first warning sirens and did not immediately take protective action. To help improve communication, partnerships should be established with technology to develop global positioning system-based warning communications, including the use of text messaging, smart phone applications, and social media. For instance, the City of Joplin used both traditional mechanisms and social media (e.g., Facebook, Twitter, and YouTube) to communicate emergency information to the public.

Second, preparedness is key. Participation in the National Level Exercise 2011 helped to prepare federal, state, regional, local, and private sector personnel to respond effectively. Finally, volunteer effort is essential. It was key in the rapid evacuation of Mercy/St. John's Hospital. Also, on the lighter side, volunteer organizations established a mass shelter for thousands (1,308) of animals made homeless by the tornado.

Case Study Questions

1. What aids communication of a potential tornado?
   A. Frequent tornado warnings
   B. Communication only when the tornado is visible
   C. Social media, text messaging, phone apps
   D. Loud sirens

2. What is the average number of minutes of warning time forecasters can give before a tornado strikes?
   A. 90 minutes
   B. 60 minutes
   C. No advanced warning is possible.
   D. 13 minutes

3. What is the difference between a tornado watch and a tornado warning?
   A. A tornado watch means that a tornado has been spotted. A tornado warning means conditions are good for a tornado to form.
   B. A tornado watch defines an area where tornadoes are possible in the next several hours. A tornado warning means that a tornado has been spotted or that Doppler radar shows a thunderstorm circulation that can spawn a tornado.
   C. A tornado watch defines an area where tornadoes are possible in the next 48 hours. A tornado warning means a tornado has been spotted.
   D. A tornado watch and a tornado warning mean the same thing. They mean conditions are good for a tornado to form.

4. What is the average number of tornadoes in the United States each year?
   A. 500
   B. 5,000
   C. 10,000
   D. 1,000

5. Which of the following actions at St. John's Hospital helped the most in the smooth response to the Tornado?
   A. Preparedness due to frequent practice
   B. Quickly moving patients in darkened hallways
   C. Quickly moving patients in available transportation
   D. Volunteerism from the community

CHAPTER SUMMARY

No country or community is immune to disasters. The last part of the 20th century and the first few years of the 21st century have witnessed an increase in both natural and man-made disasters. A disaster is defined as "a serious disruption of the functioning of a community or a society causing widespread human, material, economic or environmental losses which exceed the ability of the affected community or society to cope using its own resources." A mass casualty incident is any large-scale event in which emergency medical resources such as supplies, medical/rescue personnel, or equipment are overwhelmed by the number and severity of casualties, thus requiring prioritization of medical care by triage. All disasters are not mass casualty events, but all mass casualty events are disasters.

Disasters are commonly categorized by their origin: natural events, nuclear and radiological events, bioterrorism/emerging infection incidents, chemical incidents, and explosive/blast event incidents. Natural disasters can be classified as acute or slow in their onset. Natural disasters with a slow onset include blizzards, drought, famine, and pest infestation. Those with an acute onset include floods, earthquakes, tsunamis, tornadoes, volcanic eruptions, and hurricanes. Exposure to radiation, infection, and chemicals produce different clinical manifestations. Patients with radiation exposure, for example, present with loss of appetite, fatigue, fever, nausea, vomiting, diarrhea, and possibly even seizures and coma. They also have some skin damage that includes swelling, itching, redness of the skin (like a bad sunburn), and hair loss.

The National Response Framework is the disaster plan for the nation. This document establishes a comprehensive, national, all-hazards approach to domestic incident response, from the smallest incident to the largest catastrophe. The framework identifies the key response principles as well as the roles and structures to support the plan.

The incident command system (ICS) is an organizational tool that is used to provide the management infrastructure to support the disaster response. The ICS's roles include:

- Incident commander responsible for all aspects of the response
- Chief of operations responsible for all tactical operations
- Planning chief responsible for continuously evaluating the response and "keeping ahead of the disaster"
- Logistics section chief responsible for obtaining and providing services and resources, obtaining equipment needed, and staff support
- Finance/administration chief responsible for documenting all financial costs of the incident

During the last three decades, the field of disaster management has evolved into a respected profession, and nursing personnel working in these emergencies have proven to be key agents in both the response and recovery phases of disasters. When a disaster strikes, nurses must be ready and able to respond quickly and competently to an array of sudden, new demands such as triaging casualties, assisting with lifesaving care, administering medications, participating or coordinating decontamination or evacuation, and helping ensure positive patient outcomes across a wide range of injuries and conditions. Staff members whose roles are considered essential must also develop a personal/family disaster plan to be certain that their family members know what to do in the event of a disaster.

Since September 11, 2001, much has changed in our world and the nation. We have become more aware of the devastation that can be caused by disasters, no matter the cause. Each individual, family, and community needs to take steps to prepare for a possible disaster. In every community there are several organizations that lead the way to prepare for and recover from a disaster should one strike. An important part of personal disaster preparedness is becoming involved your community disaster organizations.

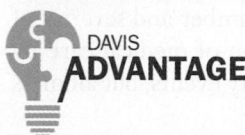

DAVIS ADVANTAGE   To explore learning resources for this chapter, go to **Davis Advantage** and find:
- Answers to in-text questions
- Chapter Resources and Activities
- NCLEX®-Style Chapter Review Questions
- Bibliography

Connection Checks Answer Key

CHAPTER 1

1.1	A, C, and D
1.2	C
1.3	D
1.4	B
1.5	B

CHAPTER 2

2.1	C
2.2	B
2.3	A, B, and C
2.4	B, C, and E
2.5	A, C, and E
2.6	C
2.7	A, B, C, and D
2.8	A, B, C, and D

CHAPTER 3

3.1	B
3.2	D
3.3	B
3.4	A
3.5	C

CHAPTER 4

4.1	B
4.2	D
4.3	B
4.4	C
4.5	A, C, and D

CHAPTER 5

5.1	C
5.2	A, B, and C
5.3	B
5.4	D
5.5	A, B, C, D, and E
5.6	D

CHAPTER 6

6.1	C
6.2	C
6.3	C
6.4	C
6.5	C

CHAPTER 7

7.1	A
7.2	C
7.3	A, B, C, and E
7.4	A and D
7.5	A
7.6	D
7.7	B
7.8	B

CHAPTER 8

8.1	C
8.2	A
8.3	A, B, and C
8.4	D
8.5	B
8.6	D
8.7	B

CHAPTER 9

9.1	B
9.2	C
9.3	B
9.4	B
9.5	C
9.6	D
9.7	D

CHAPTER 10

10.1	A, B, and D
10.2	C
10.3	C
10.4	B
10.5	C
10.6	C
10.7	B
10.8	A, B, and D

CHAPTER 11

11.1	B
11.2	D
11.3	C
11.4	D
11.5	B
11.6	C

CHAPTER 12

12.1	B, C, and D
12.2	B, D, and E
12.3	C

CHAPTER 13

13.1	B
13.2	C
13.3	B
13.4	D
13.5	C
13.6	B

CHAPTER 14

14.1	A and B
14.2	C
14.3	A
14.4	A, B, and C
14.5	B
14.6	D
14.7	D and E
14.8	C
14.9	B

CHAPTER 15

15.1	D
15.2	A, C, and D
15.3	C
15.4	A
15.5	B
15.6	A, B, C, and D

CHAPTER 16

16.1	D
16.2	A, B, C, D, E, and F
16.3	B
16.4	C and D
16.5	D
16.6	A, B, and C

CHAPTER 17

17.1	C
17.2	D
17.3	C, D, and E
17.4	B
17.5	C

CHAPTER 18

18.1 D
18.2 A, C, and D
18.3 C
18.4 C and D
18.5 A, B, D, and E

CHAPTER 19

19.1 C
19.2 B
19.3 C
19.4 B
19.5 C
19.6 A
19.7 A
19.8 C

CHAPTER 20

20.1 C
20.2 B, C, and D
20.3 A, C, and D
20.4 B, C, and D
20.5 C
20.6 A, B, and C
20.7 C
20.8 D
20.9 D
20.10 D

CHAPTER 21

21.1 A, B, C, and E
21.2 B
21.3 D
21.4 A, B, and D
21.5 A

CHAPTER 22

22.1 A
22.2 B
22.3 C
22.4 C
22.5 A
22.6 B

CHAPTER 23

23.1 D
23.2 C
23.3 B
23.4 A
23.5 C
23.6 D

CHAPTER 24

24.1 C
24.2 C
24.3 B

CHAPTER 25

25.1 C
25.2 A, B, and D
25.3 A, B, C, and E
25.4 A
25.5 B, C, and D
25.6 C
25.7 B

CHAPTER 26

26.1 C
26.2 C
26.3 B
26.4 A
26.5 A, B, and D

CHAPTER 27

27.1 B
27.2 B and C
27.3 A
27.4 A
27.5 B
27.6 B
27.7 D

CHAPTER 28

28.1 A
28.2 C
28.3 B
28.4 A, C, and E
28.5 A
28.6 C
28.7 C

CHAPTER 29

29.1 B, C, and D
29.2 A, B, C, and D
29.3 A, B, C, and D
29.4 D
29.5 A and C
29.6 D
29.7 D
29.8 C
29.9 A, B, and D

CHAPTER 30

30.1 B
30.2 C
30.3 C
30.4 B
30.5 C

CHAPTER 31

31.1 A, B, and C
31.2 A, C, and E
31.3 C
31.4 C
31.5 B
31.6 C
31.7 A, C, and E
31.8 A, B, and D
31.9 C
31.10 D

CHAPTER 32

32.1 B
32.2 A
32.3 C
32.4 A
32.5 A
32.6 B, C, and E
32.7 A, B, and D
32.8 D
32.9 B
32.10 A

CHAPTER 33

33.1 A
33.2 D
33.3 C
33.4 A and B
33.5 C
33.6 B
33.7 B
33.8 A and C

CHAPTER 34

34.1 B
34.2 D
34.3 A
34.4 C
34.5 C
34.6 A
34.7 B
34.8 D

CHAPTER 35

35.1	A
35.2	A and D
35.3	A, B, and D
35.4	A
35.5	C
35.6	A, C, and E

CHAPTER 36

36.1	A
36.2	A, B, and C
36.3	C
36.4	A
36.5	A, B, and C
36.6	B
36.7	A
36.8	B, C, and D
36.9	C
36.10	C and D
36.11	B, C, and E
36.12	C
36.13	D

CHAPTER 37

37.1	D
37.2	B
37.3	A
37.4	D
37.5	A, D, and E
37.6	C
37.7	A

CHAPTER 38

38.1	B
38.2	B
38.3	A, B, and D
38.4	C
38.5	D
38.6	A
38.7	C
38.8	D
38.9	D
38.10	C

CHAPTER 39

39.1	A
39.2	C
39.3	C
39.4	B
39.5	C
39.6	C

CHAPTER 40

40.1	C
40.2	B and E
40.3	A
40.4	D
40.5	C
40.6	B, D, and E

CHAPTER 41

41.1	A
41.2	B
41.3	A
41.4	B
41.5	C
41.6	C

CHAPTER 42

42.1	B
42.2	D
42.3	A
42.4	A
42.5	D

CHAPTER 43

43.1	B
43.2	A
43.3	A
43.4	C
43.5	C
43.6	B
43.7	A
43.8	D

CHAPTER 44

44.1	B and D
44.2	A, B, C, and D
44.3	A
44.4	A
44.5	A, C, and D
44.6	D
44.7	A, B, and C
44.8	A, D, and E
44.9	A and B
44.10	A
44.11	B
44.12	A

CHAPTER 45

45.1	C
45.2	B
45.3	A
45.4	D
45.5	C
45.6	A
45.7	A

CHAPTER 46

46.1	A
46.2	A, B, and D
46.3	A, C, and D
46.4	B
46.5	C
46.6	A and D
46.7	C
46.8	D
46.9	C

CHAPTER 47

47.1	C
47.2	A, B, D, and E
47.3	A
47.4	C
47.5	A
47.6	C
47.7	D
47.8	B, C, and D

CHAPTER 48

48.1	A
48.2	C
48.3	A
48.4	C and D
48.5	A
48.6	D
48.7	A
48.8	D

CHAPTER 49

49.1	A, C, D, and E
49.2	C
49.3	B
49.4	A, B, and D
49.5	C
49.6	D

CHAPTER 50

50.1	C
50.2	A
50.3	C
50.4	D
50.5	C
50.6	B
50.7	B
50.8	D
50.9	A, D, and E
50.10	C
50.11	B
50.12	A

CHAPTER 51

51.1	B
51.2	C
51.3	A
51.4	B, C, D, and E
51.5	A, B, C, and D
51.6	B
51.7	A
51.8	B
51.9	B
51.10	A, B, D, and E

CHAPTER 52

52.1	C
52.2	A, B, D, and E
52.3	A
52.4	C
52.5	D
52.6	A

CHAPTER 53

53.1	B
53.2	A, B, and C
53.3	D
53.4	A, B, C, and D
53.5	B
53.6	B
53.7	A
53.8	B

CHAPTER 54

54.1	A
54.2	B
54.3	A
54.4	A
54.5	A
54.6	B
54.7	A
54.8	A

CHAPTER 55

55.1	B
55.2	C
55.3	D
55.4	B
55.5	D
55.6	C

CHAPTER 56

56.1	B, D, and E
56.2	A
56.3	B
56.4	A
56.5	A, C, and D
56.6	B
56.7	D

CHAPTER 57

57.1	B
57.2	A and C
57.3	A
57.4	C
57.5	C
57.6	B
57.7	A, C, and D
57.8	B

CHAPTER 58

58.1	A
58.2	A, B, and C
58.3	A
58.4	B
58.5	B
58.6	B
58.7	B

CHAPTER 59

59.1	C
59.2	C
59.3	C
59.4	B
59.5	B, D, and E
59.6	B

CHAPTER 60

60.1	A, C, and E
60.2	D
60.3	B
60.4	D
60.5	A
60.6	D

CHAPTER 61

61.1	A
61.2	D
61.3	A and C
61.4	B
61.5	A, B, and E
61.6	A

CHAPTER 62

62.1	C
62.2	D
62.3	A, B, C, and D
62.4	B
62.5	D
62.6	D
62.7	B
62.8	C
62.9	D
62.10	C
62.11	A and B
62.12	B
62.13	B

CHAPTER 63

63.1	B
63.2	B
63.3	B
63.4	D
63.5	B

CHAPTER 64

64.1	A
64.2	C
64.3	D
64.4	A, D, and E

CHAPTER 65

65.1	C
65.2	C
65.3	B
65.4	A
65.5	B
65.6	C
65.7	D
65.8	A

CHAPTER 66

66.1   B
66.2   C
66.3   C and D
66.4   D
66.5   D
66.6   A
66.7   D
66.8   B
66.9   A
66.10   A

CHAPTER 67

67.1   D
67.2   B, C, and E
67.3   D
67.4   A
67.5   B, D, and E
67.6   B and E

CHAPTER 68

68.1   B
68.2   A
68.3   A, C, and D
68.4   C
68.5   A
68.6   A, D, and E
68.7   B
68.8   D

CHAPTER 69

69.1   A, B, C, and D
69.2   A, B, C, and D
69.3   D
69.4   D
69.5   B

CHAPTER 70

70.1   A
70.2   D
70.3   B
70.4   A and C
70.5   B
70.6   A, B, and D
70.7   C
70.8   A and B
70.9   A
70.10   A and B
70.11   A

CHAPTER 71

71.1   B
71.2   B
71.3   D
71.4   A
71.5   B
71.6   C
71.7   A

Chapter 3

Fig. 3.1: From Office of Disease Prevention and Health Promotion. (2018b). *Determinants of health*. Retrieved from https://www.healthypeople.gov/2020/topics-objectives/topic/social-determinants-of-health

Fig. 3.2: From Leininger, M. M. (2002). Culture care theory: A major contribution to advance transcultural nursing knowledge and practices. *Journal of Transcultural Nursing, 13*(2), 189–192. doi: 10.1177/10459602013003005. Retrieved from http://www.madeleine-leininger.com/cc/sunrise.pdf

Chapter 6

Fig. 6.1: Copyright © Fancy Images/Fotosearch

Fig. 6.2: Copyright © Corbis Photos/Fotosearch

Fig. 6.4: Copyright © Rauluminate/Thinkstock

Chapter 7

Fig. 7.11: Copyright © 2014 Covidien. All rights reserved. Used with the permission of Covidien.

Fig. 7.12: Copyright © GameFace/Thinkstock

Fig. 7.15: Copyright © Fuse/Getty Images

Chapter 10

Fig. 10.3: Insyte Autoguard, Courtesy and © Becton, Dickinson and Company. Reprinted with permission.

Fig. 10.4: BD SAF-T E-Z set, Courtesy and © Becton, Dickinson and Company. Reprinted with permission.

Fig. 10.12: BD Q-Syte Luer Access Split Septum, Courtesy of BD Medical, Sandy, UT.

Fig. 10.13: Courtesy of Baxter Healthcare Corp., Round Lake, IL.

Chapter 11

Fig. 11.8: Copyright © 2015 Medline Industries, Inc.

Chapter 12

Fig. 12.1: Copyright © Ryan McVay/Thinkstock

Chapter 14

Fig. 14.6: From Goldsmith, L. A., Lazarus, G. S., & Tharp, M. D. (1997). *Adult and pediatric dermatology*. Philadelphia, PA: F. A. Davis Company.

Fig. 14.7: Adapted from Seymour, C. W., Liu, V. X., Iwashyna, T. J., Brunkhorst, F. M., Rea, T. D., Scherag, A., ... Deutschman, C. S. (2016). Assessment of clinical criteria for sepsis: For the Third International Consensus Definitions for Sepsis and Septic Shock (Sepsis-3). *JAMA, 315*(8), 762–774.

Fig. 14.8: From Harmening, D. M. (1997). *Clinical hematology and fundamentals of hemostasis* (3rd ed.). Philadelphia, PA: F. A. Davis Company.

Chapter 15

Fig. 15.4: From World Health Organization. (2009). Surgical safety checklist. Retrieved from http://www.who.int/patientsafety/safesurgery/checklist/en/ © World Health Organization, 2009.

Chapter 16

Fig. 16.2: Copyright © Tyler Olson/Shutterstock

Chapter 18

Fig. 18.1: Adapted from Cowan, M. K. (2012). *Microbiology: A systems approach* (3rd ed.). New York, NY: McGraw-Hill, p. 399.

Chapter 20

Fig. 20.2B: Courtesy of MCP Hahnemann University, Department of Dermatology, Philadelphia, PA.

Chapter 22

Fig. 22.1: Adapted from National Institute of Allergy and Infectious Diseases. (2012). *Replication cycle of HIV*. Retrieved from http://www.niaid.nih.gov/topics/HIVAIDS/Understanding/howHIVCausesAIDS/Pages/howhiv.aspx

Fig. 22.2: From Reeves, J. R. T., & Maibach, H. (1991). *Clinical dermatology illustrated: A regional approach*. Philadelphia, PA: F. A. Davis Company.

Chapter 25

Fig. 25.10: Copyright © AG Industries

Fig. 25.12: Copyright © 2014 Covidien. All rights reserved. Used with the permission of Covidien.

Chapter 26

Fig. 26.1: Adapted from Global Initiative for Asthma. (2018). *Pocket guide for asthma management and prevention for adults and children older than 5 years: A pocket guide for health professionals*. Retrieved from http://www.ginasthma.org

Fig. 26.3: From National Heart, Lung, and Blood Institute, National Institutes of Health, U.S. Department of Health and Human Services. (2007 April). *Asthma action plan* (NIH Publication No. 07-5251). Retrieved from https://www.nhlbi.nih.gov/files/docs/public/lung/asthma_actplan.pdf

Chapter 28

Figs. 28.15, 28.16: From McKinnis, L. N. (2014). *Fundamentals of musculoskeletal imaging* (4th ed.). Philadelphia, PA: F. A. Davis Company.

Fig. 28.17: Image courtesy of Greg Starke, MD.

Chapter 31

Figs. 31.2, 31.5B, 31.5C, 31.5D, 31.7: From McCulloch, J. M., & Kloth, L. C. (2010). *Wound healing: Evidence-based management* (4th ed.). Philadelphia, PA: F. A. Davis Company.

Chapter 33

Fig. 33.13: From Dillon, P. M. (2007). *Nursing health assessment* (2nd ed.). Philadelphia, PA: F. A. Davis Company.

UNFigs. 33.1, 33.2, 33.3, 33.4, 33.5: From Harmening, D. M. (2009). *Clinical hematology and fundamentals of hemostasis* (5th ed.). Philadelphia, PA: F. A. Davis Company.

Chapter 34

Figs. 34.1, 34.4: From Harmening, D. M. (2009). *Clinical hematology and fundamentals of hemostasis* (5th ed.). Philadelphia, PA: F. A. Davis Company.

Fig. 34.2: From Ciesla, B. (2012). *Hematology in practice* (2nd ed.). Philadelphia, PA: F. A. Davis Company.

Chapter 36

Fig. 36.4: Adapted from Fisher, R., Cross, J. H., French, J. A., Higurashi, N., Hirsch, E., Jansen, F. E., ... Zuberi, S. M. (2017). Operational classification of seizure types by the International League Against Epilepsy: Position Paper of the ILAE Commission for Classification and Terminology. *Epilepsia, 58*(4), 522–530.

Chapter 39

Fig. 39.6: Modified from National Institutes of Health, National Institute of Neurological Disorders and Stroke. (n.d.). *Stroke scale*. Retrieved from http://www.ninds.nih.gov/doctors/NIH_Stroke_Scale.pdf

Chapter 40

Figs. 40.10A, 40.10B: From Dillon, P. M. (2007). *Nursing health assessment* (2nd ed.). Philadelphia, PA: F. A. Davis Company.

Chapter 42

Fig. 42.1: From Goldsmith, L. A., Lazarus, G. S., & Tharp, M. D. (1997). *Adult and pediatric dermatology*. Philadelphia, PA: F. A. Davis Company.

Chapter 44

Fig. 44.5: Copyright © Robert Byron/Thinkstock

Fig. 44.6: MiniMed 530G® with Enlite® Insulin Pump and Continuous Glucose Monitoring System. Manufactured by the diabetes division of Medtronic plc.

Chapter 45

Figs. 45.4, 45.8: Courtesy of Wills Eye Hospital, Philadelphia, PA.

Chapter 46

Fig. 46.2C: Copyright © David Kevitch/Thinkstock

Figs. 46.3, 46.4, 46.10, 46.11, 46.18: Courtesy of Wills Eye Hospital, Philadelphia, PA.

Chapter 47

Figs. 47.3, 47.4: Courtesy of Welch Allyn, Inc., Skaneateles Falls, NY.

INDEX

Page numbers followed by "f" denote figures, "t" denote tables, and "b" denote boxes